2 0 0 3

ICD•9•CM

Professional for Hospitals
Volumes 1, 2, and 3

International Classification of Diseases
9th Revision
Clinical Modification

Sixth Edition

Effective October 1, 2002–September 30, 2003

Edited by:
Anita C. Hart, RHIA, CCS, CCS-P
Catherine A. Hopkins, CPC

St. Anthony Publishing/Medicode

Additional copies may be ordered from:

Your local bookstore
or
1-800-INGENIX (464-3649)

IHP ISBN 1-56329-876-7

DISCLAIMER

All the codes, indexes and other material in the ICD-9-CM are compiled from official ICD-9-CM codes and instructions as well as the Medicare regulations and manuals issued or authorized by the Centers for Medicare and Medicaid Services. The code book is designed to provide accurate and authoritative information in regard to the subject covered, and every reasonable effort has been made to ensure the accuracy of the information within these pages. However, the ultimate responsibility for correct coding lies with the provider of services.

Ingenix, Inc., its employees, agents and staff make no representation, warranty or guarantee that this compilation of codes and narratives is error-free or that the use of this code book will prevent differences of opinion or disputes with Medicare or other third-party payers as to the codes that are accepted or the amounts that will be paid to providers of services, and will bear no responsibility or liability for the results or consequences of the use of this code book.

American Academy of Professional Coders (AAPC)
Continuing Education Units Credits: 5 CEUs
Contact AAPC directly for credits: 1.800.626.CODE

St. Anthony Publishing/Medicode

2525 Lake Park Boulevard • Salt Lake City, UT 84120
11410 Isaac Newton Square • Reston, VA 20190

2003 Publications

St.Anthony Publishing/Medicode

The ICD-9-CM System is Changing!

ICD-9-CM Professional for Hospitals, Vols. 1, 2 & 3

Softbound
ISBN: 1-56329-876-7   Item No. 3654 **$74.95**
Available: September 2002

Compact
ISBN: 1-56329-877-5   Item No. 3662 **$74.95**
Available: September 2002

ICD-9-CM Expert for Hospitals, Vols. 1, 2 & 3

Spiral
ISBN: 1-56329-878-3   Item No. 3656 **$94.95**
Available: September 2002

Updateable Binder
ISBN: 1-56329-879-1   Item No. 3539 **$154.95**

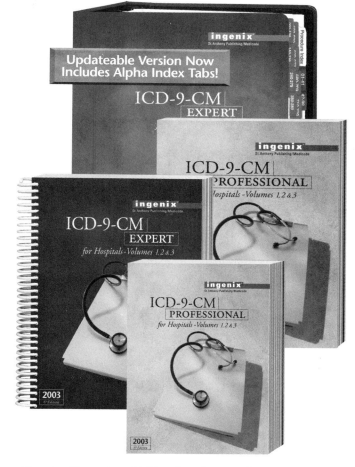

This year, a chapter on New Technologies and Medical Services has been added to the ICD-9-CM code books for Hospitals, and code changes that affect nearly every chapter! Last year, our newly designed pages, featuring intuitive symbols, exclusive color-coding, and additional resources, demonstrated why our customers consider these codes books the BEST!

Professional and Expert editions of ICD-9-CM for Hospitals Feature:

- New and Revised Code Symbols
- Fourth-and Fifth-digit Requirement Alerts
- Complete Official Coding Guidelines
- AHA's *Coding Clinic for ICD-9-CM* References
- Illustrations and Definitions
- Age and Sex Edits
- Nonspecific and Unacceptable Primary Diagnosis Alerts
- Medicare as Secondary Payer Indicators
- Manifestation Code Alerts

- Complex Diagnosis and Major Complication Alerts
- HIV Major Related Diagnosis Alerts
- CC Principal Diagnosis Exclusion List
- CC Diagnosis Symbol
- Crucial Medicare Procedure Code Edits

Expert Editions Also Include These Enhancements:

- Special Reports Via E-mail.
- Complete Principal Diagnosis/MDC/DRG Listing
- Pharmacological List
- CC Code List
- Valid Three-digit Code List

The Expert Updateable Binder Subscriptions Feature:

- Money Saving Update Service
- Three Updates per Year [October (full text), January and July]

Call Toll-Free 1.877.INGENIX (464.3649) or Shop Online at www.IngenixOnline.com

Also Available from your Medical Bookstore or Distributor

060102

ingenix
St. Anthony Publishing/Medicode

2003 ICD-9-CM Code Books for Physicians Volumes 1 & 2

ICD-9-CM Professional for Physicians, Vols. 1 & 2

Softbound
ISBN: 1-56329-872-4   Item No. 3650 **$64.95**
Available: September 2002

Compact
ISBN: 1-56329-873-2   Item No. 3661 **$64.95**
Available: September 2002

ICD-9-CM Expert for Physicians, Vols. 1 & 2

Spiral
ISBN: 1-56329-874-0   Item No. 3652 **$84.95**
Available: September 2002

Updateable Binder
ISBN: 1-56329-875-9   Item No. 3534 **$144.95**

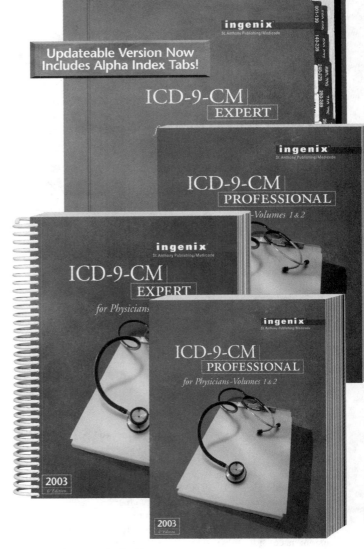

Our page design, featuring intuitive symbols, exclusive color-coding, and additional resources provides a new approach to pertinent coding and reimbursement information. New codes and changes to the ICD-9-CM make our 2003 code books a must buy! Order today and keep currenton all changes!

Professional and Expert Editions of ICD-9-CM for Physicians Feature:

- New and Revised Code Symbols

- Fourth-and Fifth-digit Requirement Alerts

- Complete Official Coding Guidelines

- Age and Sex Edits

- Clinically Oriented Definitions and Illustrations

- Medicare as Secondary Payer Indicators

- Manifestation Code Alerts

- "Other" and "Unspecified" Diagnosis Alerts

- Symbols Identifying V Codes Designated for only Primary or only Secondary Diagnosis Use

Expert Editions Also Include These Enhancements:

- Special Reports Via E-mail.

- Code Tables--Complex coding issues are simplified in coding tables, as developed for I-9 Express

- Valid Three-digit Category List

The _Expert_ Updateable Binder Subscriptions Feature:

- Money Saving Update Service

- Three Updates per Year [October (full text), January and July]

An Exceptional Code Book! An Exceptional Year for ICD-9-CM!

2003 ICD-9-CM Expert for Home Health Services, Nursing Facilities & Hospices, Volumes 1, 2 & 3

Softbound

ISBN: 1-56329-880-5   Item No. 3658 **$129.95**

Available: September 2002

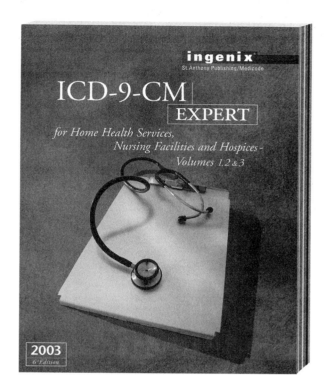

In the healthcare marketplace, this is the only ICD-9-CM code book designed specifically for the needs of the home health, nursing home, and hospice coder. This enhanced code book now includes features that will take the coder to the next level of coding. Code quickly and accurately using this resource filled with important alerts and references specific to each facility type. No other code book exists that explains each prospective payment system in detail or that can serve as a reference for specific coding guidelines.

Inside You Will Find:

- **New Chapter in Volume 3 for New Technologies and Medical Services**

- Illustrations and Definitions

- **Exclusive**—E-mail delivered Special Reports

- Additional Digit Requirement Alerts in the Index and the Tabular Sections

- "10 Steps to Correct Coding" Tutorial

- Excerpts from the Home Health Agency Prospective Payment System (HHA PPS) and Symbols Identifying Clinical Dimension Diagnoses

- Medicare Home Health Manual Section on Coverage Qualifications

- Explanation of the SNF Prospective Payment System (SNF PPS) and Color-coding Indicating ICD-9-CM Codes Associated with Specific RUG-III Categories

- Color-coding and Criteria for Acceptable Non-cancer Diagnoses for Hospice Coverage

- Complete Official Coding Guidelines, Including LTC Guidelines

- Symbols Identifying V Codes Designated for only Primary or only Secondary Diagnosis Use

2003 Publications

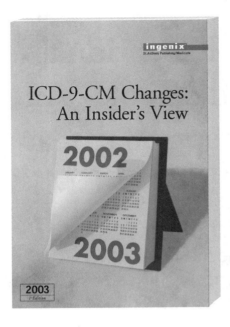

NEW!
CPT® Changes 2003: An Insider's View

7" x 10" Perfect Bound

The American Medical Association and Ingenix Publishing present *CPT® Changes 2003: An Insider's View*, a must-have resource for Physicians' Current Procedural Terminology (CPT®) Professional users! This book serves as a reference tool to understanding each of the CPT® code changes found in CPT® 2003.

In both books you'll find:

- **Every new, revised and deleted code change**—Listed along with a detailed rationale for the change. Index changes, convention changes and instructional note changes are also explained.

- **Organized by ICD-9-CM and CPT® code section and code number**—Includes a separate section that discusses index changes.

- **Illustrated**—Helps orient you to change in code.

- **Clinical Examples/Diagnostic or Procedural Descriptions**— Helps you understand the practical application of the code.

CPT is a registered trademark of the American Medical Association

NEW!
ICD-9-CM Changes 2003: An Insider's View

7" x 10" Perfect Bound
Item No. 4951 **$54.95**
Available: November 2002

A must have resource for ICD-9-CM users! *ICD-9-CM Changes 2003: An Insider's View* serves as a reference tool to understanding each of the ICD-9-CM code changes found in ICD-9-CM 2003.

CPT® Changes for 2003:
- 204 New Codes
- 23 Deleted Codes
- 203 Revised Codes
- Place of Service section added to appendices

ICD-9-CM Changes for 2003:
- 163 New Diagnosis Codes
- 23 Revised Diagnosis Codes
- 25 New Procedure Codes
- 3 Revised Procedure Codes
- New chapter on New Technology and Medical Services in Volume 3
- Changes to conventions and to the index

Call Toll-Free 1.877.INGENIX (1.877.464.3649) or Shop Online at www.IngenixOnLine.com
Also Available from your Medical Bookstore or Distributor   020606

DRG System Changes Impact 12 of the Top 25 DRGs!

2003 DRG Expert
(formerly called the DRG Guidebook)

Compact, Spiral
ISBN: 1-56329-891-0   Item No. 3575 **$99.95**
Available: September 2002

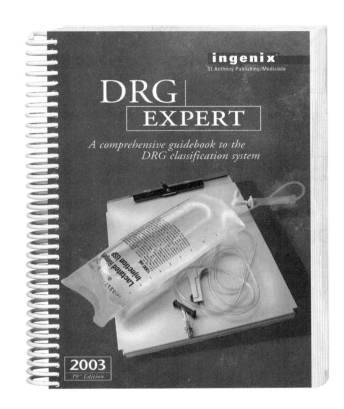

Trust the nation's DRG experts to bring you the DRG guidebook designed specifically for those who need a comprehensive resource for accurate assignment of DRGs, concurrently and retrospectively. The most trusted and comprehensive guidebook to the DRG classification system for 19 years should be your guide to navigate the changes in the DRG system!

NEW—Exclusive Color Coding Helps Hospitals to:

- See at a glance surgical/medical partitioning
- Know if CCs must be assigned and when age limits apply
- Know when certain qualifications for principal or secondary diagnosis must be met
- Identify DRGs targeted for audits

Other Features Include:

- **Organized by Major Diagnositic Category (MDC)**

- **Transfer DRG Alert**—Indicates a DRG selected as a qualified discharge that may be paid by per diem rate

- **Main Term Code Search**—Customized code descriptions that list main conditions or operative terms first

- **Average National Payment**—Listed with every DRG for quick benchmark comparisons

- **Surgical Hierarchy Table**—Quickly shows DRG hierarch for multiple procedure cases

- **Invalid DRG Conversion Table**—Easily track the reassignment of codes to the new DRG

- **Full Listing of All Dx Within a MDC**

- **Numeric and Alphabetic ICD-9-CM Inde**

- **Current CMS Rate Structure** (RW, AMI

- **QuickFlip Color Tabs**—Find the right c of traditional thumb tabs

2003 Publications

St. Anthony Publishing/Medicode

New! DRG Desk Reference—The Book You've Been Requesting!

DRG Desk Reference

Compact, Softbound
ISBN: 1-56329-929-1   Item No. 4282 **$199.95**
Available: September 2002

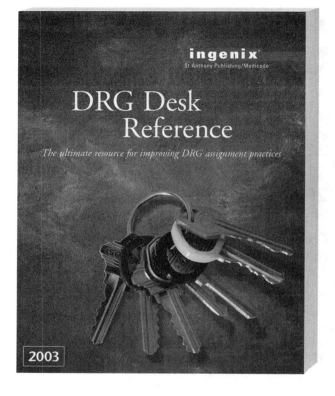

ingenix
St. Anthony Publishing/Medicode

DRG Desk Reference

The ultimate resource for improving DRG assignment practices

2003

A truly comprehensive resource that creates an inpatient coding resource that functions to work efficiently and effectively with either *DRG Expert* or *DRG Guidebook*.

A must-have resource for anyone who assigns DRGs or audits claims for inpatient cases!

DRG Desk Reference **will bring you:**

- **Optimal Reimbursement Indicators**—Quickly identify the top ICD-9-CM diagnosis or procedure codes and key indicators for each DRG to ensure optimal payment while ensuring compliance.

- **Tips for the Encoder Use**r—Many decisions faced by coders using grouper software, or encoder, have significant impact on final DRG assignment. Tips are provided on how to avoid making the wrong decisions.

- **New Technology and Medical Services**—Descriptions of the new technology and medical services and which services will receive add-on payment under the Medicare inpatient prospective payment system.

- **Key Abstracting Field Items**—An in-depth look at the significance of key abstracting fields for DRG assignment and the impact on reimbursement.

- **DRG Assignment Tutorial**—This tutorial will explain the DRG assignment process in clear and understandable language.

- **Coding and Documentation Guidelines for DRG Validation**—Uncover potential coding problems and ensure the accuracy and validity of DRG assignment.

- **Key Complication and Comorbidity Condition (CC) Indicators:**
  Drug Usage and Treatment
  Durable Medical Equipment
  Noninvasive Diagnostic Test Outcomes
  Abnormal EKG Findings
  Abnormal Laboratory Values
  Major Cardiovascular Complications
  Complex Diagnoses
  Organisms

- **DRG Decision Trees**

- **Complete CC List**

- **CC Principal Diagnosis Exclusion List**

- **Relative Weights of Valid DRG**

2003 Publications

ingenix
St. Anthony Publishing/Medicode

Take Charge of Your Chargemaster

Hospital Chargemaster Guide—2003

ISBN: 1-56329-870-8   Item No. 4302 **$199.95**

Available: December 2002

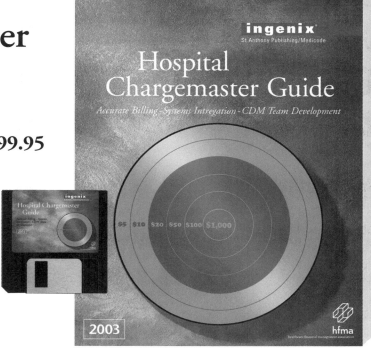

This "consultant in a book" provides step-by-step guidance for implementing and maintaining an accurate hospital chargemaster from a coding, billing, and reimbursement perspective. The *Hospital Chargemaster* provides the HCPCS/Physicians' Current Procedural Terminology (CPT®) codes, applicable revenue codes, Medicare compliance and fraud issues, payment guidelines, and claim submission procedures by clinical department for all chargemaster-driven hospital-based procedures.

- **Step-by-step Guidance to Setting Up and Maintaining an Accurate Charge Description Master.** Helps improve billing accuracy and compliance throughout your facility. Also helps establish a process for reviewing and maintaining the CDM on an annual basis, and makes educating and training clinical department heads and your CDM team easier.

- **Provides Relevant CPT®/HCPCS Code and Revenue Code Combinations for Each Clinical Department.** Takes the guesswork out of assigning revenue codes to each line item on your chargemaster.

- **APC Payment Status Indicators.** Identify how each line item charge should be billed and how it will be reimbursed under APCs or other payment methodology.

- **Easy-to-use Diskette.** Provides templates with recommendations on procedure codes, and descriptions for radiology, laboratory, and other clinical areas to eliminate confusion over code selection.

- **Easy-to-use Tables within each Clinical Department Section.**

- **Recommendations as to How Each HCPCS Code Should Be Described in the CDM.**

- **Department-specific Billing Information and Tips.**

- **Expanded Modifier Section.**

- **Regulations and Reimbursement Information.** Provides new regulatory and reimbursement information for pharmacy, supplies, observation services, and more.

- **Co-published with HFMA.**

CPT is a registered trademark of the American Medical Association

Look to the Source Most People Trust for UB-92 Billing Perfection

UB-92 Editor

Item No. 4787 **$269.95**
*Call for CD multi-user pricing

Available: Now

This one-of-a-kind book, published by "the experts" in UB-92 billing for Medicare, enables you to minimize billing and payment delays. The *UB-92 Editor* walks you through the UB-92 claim form for billing Medicare inpatient and outpatient services. It helps you understand the requirements of each form locator (FL) and revenue code, and provides detailed billing and coding tips for accurate claim submission.

- **EXCLUSIVE — Links HCPCS and Physicians' Current Procedural Terminology (CPT®) Codes to Applicable Revenue Codes.** Helps prevent the most common reasons for rejections(mismatched revenue codes and CPT® or HCPCS codes. Updated to include the latest billing and coding rules for OPPS.

- **EXCLUSIVE — Step-by-step Instructions for Completing the UB-92 Claim Form.** Gives you the most current Medicare billing and coding information for each data element on the UB-92 claim form and ensures accurate submission of inpatient and outpatient claims.

- **Addresses Home Health and SNF Issues, Consolidated Billing, Use of HIPPS Rate Codes and Modifiers.** Increases efficiency and accuracy, ensuring timely payment.

- **CD-ROM with Hypertext and Jump Links.** Provides all of the information available in the hard-copy book with jump links to revenue codes, other form locators, condition codes, occurrence codes, and value codes. Use it to ensure that your claims are submitted accurately to Medicare the first time.

- **Quarterly Updates — Fully Indexed and Tabbed.** New coding and billing tips are highlighted with an arrow, so you know what changed from update to update. Eliminates billing with outdated information. It's easy to find and use the information necessary to bill Medicare.

- **Earn 5 CEUS from AAPC.**

CPT is a registered trademark of the American Medical Association

St. Anthony Publishing/Medicode

Solutions for PFS operational and compliance challenges with proven policies and procedures!

Hospital Toolkit for Patient Financial Services

ISBN: 1-56329-812-0   Item No. 3017 **$249.95**

Available: Now

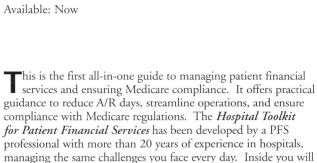

This is the first all-in-one guide to managing patient financial services and ensuring Medicare compliance. It offers practical guidance to reduce A/R days, streamline operations, and ensure compliance with Medicare regulations. The *Hospital Toolkit for Patient Financial Services* has been developed by a PFS professional with more than 20 years of experience in hospitals, managing the same challenges you face every day. Inside you will find strategies you can trust!

- **Expert Management Strategies and Compliance Guidance—Specifically for Your PFS Team.** Combines leading-edge strategies with best practices to reduce AR and increase efficiency. Will help you prevent mistakes that can lead to accounts receivable problems, trigger a compliance audit, or put you under a corporate integrity agreement.

- **Solutions to Patient Accounting and Compliance Problems.** Use proven strategies to establish an effective compliance program, streamline billing, and ensure low levels of accounts receivable.

- **Organized by Function within Patient Financial Services/Patient Accounts.** Presents billing and compliance problems by functional area. Allows you to tackle compliance issues at each stage of the billing process.

- **Templates, Checklists, Procedures, and Worksheets on CD.** Develop procedures for your department, analyze errors, identify risk areas, record results, document actions, and more.

- **Addresses Interdepartmental Issues Central to Patient Accounts Management.** Helps to improve billing accuracy and compliance throughout your facility.

- **Deals with Fraud and Abuse Issues Specific to Patient Accounts.** Calls attention to the compliance issues pertinent to each function within PFS. Incorporates the OIG's compliance guidance for hospitals and the latest high-risk issues identified in the annual OIG work plan.

- **Co-published with HFMA.**

St. Anthony Publishing/Medicode

You Can Depend on Us for Answers to All Your Inpatient and Outpatient Billing Compliance Questions

Medicare Billing Compliance Guide

Item No. 2446 **$279.95**
*Call for CD multi-user pricing

Available: Now

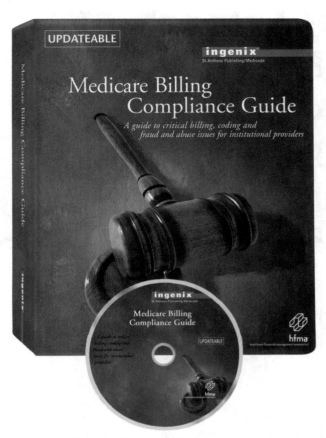

Since 1996 the *Medicare Billing Compliance Guide* has been providing guidance and interpretation of Medicare inpatient and outpatient billing and coding rules for hospitals and institutional providers in a language that your entire staff can understand.

This reliable guide will take you step by step through the Medicare maze of inpatient and outpatient billing and coding issues. Only the *Medicare Billing Compliance Guide* interprets Medicare requirements and translates them into easy-to-understand language, ensuring that you and your staff understand what you must to do stay in compliance.

- **Interpret Medicare Billing Rules and Fraud Issues.** Get easy-to-understand explanations, examples, and interpretations of Medicare billing rules, fraud issues, and OIG compliance program guidance. Plus, get answers to high-risk and complex billing questions affecting your hospital or facility.

- **Complete Coverage of Hospital Billing Rules and Targeted Fraud and Abuse Issues.** Includes complete information on Medicare fraud and abuse, corporate integrity agreements, fraud alerts, compliance program guidance, and OIG hot issues affecting hospitals. Ensures that your billing and coding practices are in compliance with Medicare program requirements. Helps you stay up to date on all of the OIG fraud and abuse initiatives and investigations.

- **A to Z Billing, Coding, and Coverage Rules— Fully Indexed.** Provides a quick, easy-to-use format to find important billing, coding, and coverage issues. Helps you easily find answers to your most pressing billing and coding questions, such as modifiers, medical coverage, observation services, emergency room, medical necessity and local medical review policies.

- **Updates for One Full Year.** Keeps you current with the regulatory changes that affect the accuracy of claim submission and billing operations at your facility.

- **Full Text of Product on CD-ROM in PDF Format.** Electronic solution for researching billing and fraud and abuse issues or problems. The jump links and search capabilities allow you to get the information you need quickly.

- **Co-published with HFMA.**

- **Earn 5 CEUS from AAPC.**

St. Anthony Publishing/Medicode

Take the Mystery Out of Medicare Coverage and Issuing ABNs

Complete Guide to Medicare Coverage Issues

Item No. 3036 **$279.95**
*Call for CD multi-user pricing

Available: Now

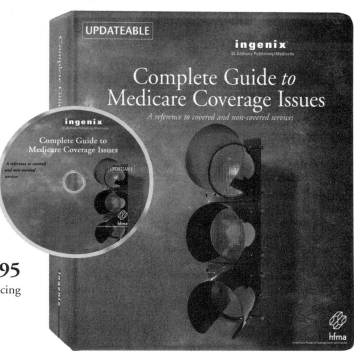

Know exactly which services and items Medicare will pay for, and which it won't, before you submit a claim.

This one-of-a-kind, updateable guide details Medicare's national coverage policies using CMS's official source documents. For any site of service, know what Medicare will and will not cover before submitting claims. Your subscription includes a CD-ROM with the full text of the manual and a newsletter with information about new and existing Medicare coverage for both Part A and Part B services.

- **New — Now Includes Pending National Decisions.**
  You'll have pending decisions available in one resource to help you and your staff manage all national coverage issues affecting Part A and Part B services.

- **Exclusive — Color-coded Coverage Prompts.**
  Know at a glance whether an item or procedure has restricted coverage, enabling you to make accurate coverage decisions promptly and submit bills correctly the first time. Helps prevent costly denials and claim resubmissions. Provides guidance regarding proper documentation for medical necessity, and helps you know when to issue an advance beneficiary notice for noncovered services. Also helps health plans understand Medicare coverage policies.

- **Fully Indexed.** Easily locate a specific item or service.

- **Updates and Coverage Alert Newsletter.** Keep you up to date on all new national Medicare coverage policies and revisions to existing policies.

- **Full Text of Manual on CD-ROM in PDF Format.**
  Electronic solution for researching national coverage decisions and medical necessity issues. Allows you to find key coverage issues and/or specific items and services with the click of a mouse. Other easy-to-use features include hypertext links and electronic bookmarks to take you quickly to the sections of the manual that you use the most.

- **Physicians' Current Procedural Terminology (CPT®) Codes and HCPCS Codes Assigned to National Issues.**
  Helps you identify coverage issues by CPT® or HCPCS code. Includes coverage issues pertaining to medical equipment, devices, procedures, clinical trials, and more!

- **Co-published with HFMA.**

- **Earn 5 CEUS from AAPC.**

CPT is a registered trademark of the American Medical Association

4 Easy Ways to Order

CALL toll-free
1.800.INGENIX
(464.3649)
and mention the
Source Code: FOBA3

SHOP on line at
www.IngenixOnline.com

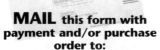

MAIL this form with
payment and/or purchase
order to:
PO Box 27116
Salt Lake City, UT 84127-0116

FAX this order form with
credit card information and /or
purchase order to 801.982.4033

100% Money Back Guarantee

If our merchandise* ever fails to meet your expectations, please contact our Customer Service Department toll-free at 1.800.INGENIX (464.3649) for an immediate response. We will resolve any concern without hesitation.

*Software: Credit will be granted for unopened packages only.

Shipping and Handling	
No. of Items	**Fee**
1	$9.95
2-4	$11.95
5-7	$14.95
8-10	$19.95
11+	Call

PUBLICATION ORDER AND FAX FORM *FOBA3*

Customer No._____   Contact No._____

Purchase Order No._____   Source Code_____
(Attach copy of Purchase Order)

Contact Name _____   Title_____

Company_____

Address _____
(no P.O. Boxes, please)

City_____ State_____ Zip_____

Phone (_____)_____ Fax (_____)_____
(in case we have questions about your order)

IMPORTANT: E-MAIL REQUIRED FOR ORDER CONFIRMATION AND SELECT PRODUCT DELIVERY.

E-mail _____

❏ YES, I WANT TO RECEIVE SPECIAL REPORTS AND INFORMATION VIA E-MAIL.
❏ YES, I WANT TO RECEIVE NEW PRODUCT ANNOUNCEMENTS VIA E-MAIL.

Item #	Qty	Item Description	Price	Total
~~4025~~	~~1~~	~~(SAMPLE) DRG Guidebook~~	~~$89.95~~	~~$89.95~~

Sub Total _____
TX, UT, OH, and VA residents please add applicable sales tax _____
Shipping & handling (see chart) _____
(11 plus items, foreign and Canadian orders, please call for shipping costs)
Total enclosed _____

Payment Options

❏ Check enclosed. (Make payable to Ingenix, Inc.)

❏ Charge my: ❏ MasterCard   ❏ VISA   ❏ AMEX   ❏ Discover

Card # | | | | | | | | | | | | | | | | | | Exp. Date: | | | |
                                                                              MM   YR

❏ Bill Me P.O.#_____

Signature _____

©2002 Ingenix, Inc. All prices subject to change without notice.   *FOBA3*

020601

Preface

Since the federal government implemented diagnosis-related groups (DRGs) on October 1, 1983, medical record professionals and others have had to refer to many sources for ICD-9-CM codes and coding and reimbursement principles.

ICD-9-CM for Hospitals, Volumes 1, 2, and 3, has been designed with the hospital coder in mind. All three volumes of the most recent official government version of ICD-9-CM have been combined into one book.

Our technical experts have drawn upon their extensive hands-on experience to enhance the government's book with valuable features essential to correct coding and reimbursement. Without these enhancements, health information management departments would spend hours locating the information required to code each record accurately. Because of the thoroughness, accuracy, timeliness and ease of use of *ICD-9-CM for Hospitals,* health information departments nationwide have turned to them for their coding needs.

ICD-9-CM for Hospitals includes many of the enhancements described below in direct response to requests from our subscribers. As you review the content, you'll find the following:

- the complete ICD-9-CM official guidelines for coding and reporting, published by the U.S. Department of Health and Human Services and approved by the cooperating parties (American Hospital Association, American Health Information Management Association, Health Care Financing Administration and National Center for Health Statistics)
- all the official ICD-9-CM codes, indexes, notes, footnotes and symbols
- color-highlighted illustrations and clearly worded definitions integrated in the tabular, provide important clinical information
- exclusive color coding, symbols, and footnotes that alert coders to coding and reimbursement issues, including the majority of the Medicare code edits and identification of conditions that significantly affect DRG assignment of cardiovascular and HIV cases.
- the complication and comorbidity (CC) exclusion list, integrated beneath the applicable codes makes it easier to determine complications and comorbidities excluded with a particular principal diagnosis
- the American Hospital Association (AHA's) *Coding Clinic for ICD-9-CM references,* integrated beneath the applicable codes to provide easy reference to official coding advice as designated by the four cooperating parties (AHA, AHIMA, CMS, and NCHS)
- compliance symbol identifying diagnosis codes associated with DRGs targeted by the government for audit

- check fourth- and fifth-digit symbols identify codes that require the addition of a fourth or fifth digit for code specificity and validity
- symbols identify new codes and text revisions and pages are dated to indicate when the changes were made
- synopsis of the code changes for the current year
- color coding and symbol legend at the bottom of each page
- exclusive QuickFlip Color Tabs for quick, easy location of terms and codes in the index and tabular list

Please review "How to Use *ICD-9-CM for Hospital's (Volumes 1, 2, and 3)*" in this section to learn about the features that will help you assign and report correct codes, ensuring appropriate reimbursement.

USE OF OFFICIAL SOURCES

The *ICD-9-CM for Hospitals* contains the official U.S. Department of Health and Human Services, Ninth Revision, Sixth Edition ICD-9-CM codes, effective for the current year.

The color-coding, footnotes and symbols, which identify coding and reimbursement issues, are derived from official federal government sources, including the Medicare code edit (MCE), Version 20.0.

The American Hospital Association (AHA) Coding Clinic for ICD-9-CM references are used with permission of the AHA.

In addition to the editors, the following people have contributed to this book:

Stacy Perry, Desktop Publishing Manager
Kerrie Hornsby, Desktop Publishing Manger
Tracy Betzler, Desktop Publishing Specialist
Irene Day, Desktop Publishing Specialist
Paul Driscoll, Illustrator
Sheri Bernard, Director of Essential Regulatory Products
Lynn Speirs, Managing Editor

IMPORTANT INFORMATION ABOUT YOUR SUBSCRIPTION SERVICE

If you have purchased the updateable *ICD-9-CM Expert for Hospitals,* your subscription includes an updating service throughout the year to keep the code book current and accurate. The January update includes new illustrations and definitions, *AHA Coding Clinic* references for third and fourth quarter, the latest MCEs, and official errata changes. In July you will receive a list of all new, revised, and invalid codes for the upcoming year.

TECHNICAL EDITORS

Anita C. Hart, RHIA, CCS, CCS-P
Product Manager
Ingenix, Inc
Reston, VA

Ms. Hart's experience includes fifteen years conducting and publishing research in clinical medicine and human genetics for Yale University, Massachusetts General Hospital, and Massachusetts Institute of Technology. In addition, Ms. Hart has supervised medical records management, health information management, coding and reimbursement, and worker's compensation issues as the office manager for a physical therapy rehabilitation clinic. Ms. Hart is an expert in physician and facility coding, reimbursement systems, and compliance issues. Ms. Hart developed the *Complete Coding Tutor*, an advanced self-study guide for ICD-9-CM, CPT, and HCPCS Level II coding and served as technical consultant for numerous other publications for hospital and physician practices. Currrently, Ms. Hart is the Product Manager for the ICD-9-CM and DRG product lines.

Catherine A. Hopkins, CPC
Technical Consultant
Ingenix, Inc.
Reston, VA

Ms. Hopkins has 17 years of experience in the healthcare field. Her experience includes six years as office manager and senior coding specialist for a large multi-specialty practice. Ms. Hopkins has written several coding manuals and newsletters and has taught seminars on CPT, HCPCS, and ICD-9-CM coding. She also serves as technical support for various software products.

PRODUCT REVIEW PANEL

DeAnne Bloomquist, RHIT, CCS, Consultant and President, Mid-Continent Coding, Inc

Lori J. Date Daun, RHIT, Coder/Abstractor-OPDQ, Allina-Mercy Hospital

Nan-Jean Dobrowski, RHIT, CCs, Director, Medical Records, Delnor-Community Hospital

Corella Marie Fenwick, CCP, Compliance Auditor/Fiscal Coordinator, GWU, Dept. of Medicine

Gwen Kalor, RHIT, HIM Specialist, Coding, North Memorial Medical Center

Jo Ann Steigerwald, RHIT, Senior Healthcare Consultant, The Wellington Group

Denise Von Dohren, Manager, Reimbursement Planning, Merck & Co.

Carol Wojcik, MS, RHIA, CCS, CCS-P, Coding Supervisor, Central DuPage Hospital

Laura C. Zeranski, RHIA, Consultant, Laura Zeranski and Associates

WHAT TO DO IF YOU HAVE QUESTIONS

If you have any questions about your subscription, call our customer service department toll free at (800) INGENIX (464-3649).

If you have comments on the content of this book, please address them in writing to:
Product Manager, Ingenix, Inc.
11410 Isaac Newton Square,
Reston, VA 20190
Tel no.:(800) 464-3649;
Fax no.: (801) 982-4033

ADDITIONAL COPIES

Contact the customer service order department toll free at (800) INGENIX (464-3649).

Introduction

HISTORY AND FUTURE OF ICD•9

The International Classification of Diseases, Ninth Revision, Clinical Modification (ICD-9-CM) is based on the official version of the World Health Organization's Ninth Revision, International Classification of Diseases (ICD-9). ICD-9 classifies morbidity and mortality information for statistical purposes, and for the indexing of hospital records by disease and operations, for data storage and retrieval.

This modification of ICD-9 supplants the Eighth Revision International Classification of Diseases, Adapted for Use in the United States (ICDA-8) and the Hospital Adaptation of ICDA (H-ICDA).

The concept of extending the International Classification of Diseases for use in hospital indexing was originally developed in response to a need for a more efficient basis for storage and retrieval of diagnostic data. In 1950, the U.S. Public Health Service and the Veterans Administration began independent tests of the International Classification of Diseases for hospital indexing purposes. The following year, the Columbia Presbyterian Medical Center in New York City adopted the International Classification of Diseases, Sixth Revision, with some modifications for use in its medical record department. A few years later, the Commission on Professional and Hospital Activities (CPHA) in Ann Arbor, Mich., adopted the International Classification of Diseases with similar modifications for use in hospitals participating in the Professional Activity Study.

The problem of adapting ICD for indexing hospital records was taken up by the U.S. National Committee on Vital and Health Statistics through its subcommittee on hospital statistics. The subcommittee reviewed the modifications made by the various users of ICD and proposed that uniform changes be made. This was done by a small working party.

In view of the growing interest in the use of the International Classification of Diseases for hospital indexing, a study was undertaken in 1956 by the American Hospital Association and the American Medical Record Association (then the American Association of Medical Record Librarians) of the relative efficiencies of coding systems for diagnostic indexing. This study indicated the International Classification of Diseases provided a suitable and efficient framework for indexing hospital records. The major users of the International Classification of Diseases for hospital indexing purposes then consolidated their experiences, and an adaptation was first published in December 1959. A revision was issued in 1962 and the first "Classification of Operations and Treatments" was included.

In 1966, the international conference for revising the International Classification of Diseases noted the eighth revision of ICD had been constructed with hospital indexing in mind and considered the revised classification suitable, in itself, for hospital use in some countries. However, it was recognized that the basic classification might provide inadequate detail for diagnostic indexing in other countries.

A group of consultants was asked to study the eighth revision of ICD (ICD-8) for applicability to various users in the United States. This group recommended that further detail be provided for coding of hospital and morbidity data. The American Hospital Association was requested to develop the needed adaptation proposals. This was done by an advisory committee (the Advisory Committee to the Central Office on ICDA). In 1968 the United States Public Health Service published the product, Eighth Revision International Classification of Diseases, Adapted for Use in the United States. This became commonly known as ICDA-8, and beginning in 1968 it served as the basis for coding diagnostic data for both official morbidity and mortality statistics in the United States.

In 1968, the CPHA published the Hospital Adaptation of ICDA (H-ICDA) based on both the original ICD-8 and ICDA-8. In 1973, CPHA published a revision of H-ICDA, referred to as H-ICDA-2. Hospitals throughout the United States were divided in their use of these classifications until January 1979, when ICD-9-CM was made the single classification intended primarily for use in the United States, replacing these earlier related, but somewhat dissimilar, classifications.

Physicians have been required by law to submit diagnosis codes for Medicare reimbursement since the passage of the Medicare Catastrophic Coverage Act of 1988. This act requires physician offices to include the appropriate diagnosis codes when billing for services provided to Medicare beneficiaries on or after April 1, 1989. The Health Care Financing Administration designated ICD-9-CM as the coding system physicians must use.

In 1993 the World Health Organization published the newest version of International Classification of Diseases, Tenth Revision, ICD-10. This version contains the greatest number of changes in the history of ICD. There are more codes (5,500 more than ICD-9) to allow more specific reporting of diseases and newly recognized conditions. ICD-10 consists of three volumes; tabular list (volume I), instructions (volume 2) and the alphabetic index (volume 3). It contains 21 chapters including two supplementary ones. The codes are alphanumeric (A00–T98, V01–Y98 and Z00–Z99). Currently ICD-10 is being used in some European countries with implementation expected after the year 2000 in the United States.

ICD-9-CM BACKGROUND

In February 1977, a steering committee was convened by the National Center for Health Statistics to provide advice and counsel in developing a clinical modification of ICD-9. The organizations represented on the steering committee included the following:

• American Association of Health Data Systems
• American Hospital Association
• American Medical Record Association
• Association for Health Records

- Council on Clinical Classifications
- Centers for Medicare and Medicaid Services (formerly known as Health Care Financing Administration,) Department of Health and Human Services
- WHO Center for Classification of Diseases for North America, sponsored by the National Center for Health Statistics, Department of Health and Human Services

The Council on Clinical Classifications was sponsored by the following:

- American Academy of Pediatrics
- American College of Obstetricians and Gynecologists
- American College of Physicians
- American College of Surgeons
- American Psychiatric Association
- Commission on Professional and Hospital Activities

The steering committee met periodically in 1977. Clinical guidance and technical input were provided by task forces on classification from the Council on Clinical Classification's sponsoring organizations.

ICD-9-CM is a clinical modification of the World Health Organization's ICD-9. The term "clinical" is used to emphasize the modification's intent: to serve as a useful tool to classify morbidity data for indexing medical records, medical care review, and ambulatory and other medical care programs, as well as for basic health statistics. To describe the clinical picture of the patient, the codes must be more precise than those needed only for statistical groupings and trend analysis.

CHARACTERISTICS OF ICD-9-CM

ICD-9-CM far exceeds its predecessors in the number of codes provided. The disease classification has been expanded to include health-related conditions and to provide greater specificity at the fifth-digit level of detail. These fifth digits are not optional; they are intended for use in recording the information substantiated in the clinical record.

Volume I (tabular list) of ICD-9-CM contains five appendices:

Appendix A:	Morphology of Neoplasms
Appendix B:	Glossary of Mental Disorders
Appendix C:	Classification of Drugs by American Hospital Formulary Service List Number and Their ICD-9-CM Equivalents
Appendix D:	Classification of Industrial Accidents According to Agency
Appendix E:	List of Three-Digit Categories

These appendices are included as a reference to provide further information about the patient's clinical picture, to further define a diagnostic statement, to aid in classifying new drugs or to reference three-digit categories.

Volume 2 (alphabetic index) of ICD-9-CM contains many diagnostic terms that do not appear in Volume I since the index includes most diagnostic terms currently in use.

Volume 3 (procedure index and procedure tabular) of ICD-9-CM contains codes for operations and procedures. The format for the tabular is the same as Volume 1 disease tabular,

except the codes consist of two digits with one or two digits following the decimal point. Conventions in the index follow Volume 2 conventions except some subterms appear immediately below the main term rather than following alphabetizing rules

THE DISEASE CLASSIFICATION

ICD-9-CM is totally compatible with its parent system, ICD-9, thus meeting the need for comparability of morbidity and mortality statistics at the international level. A few fourth-digit codes were created in existing three-digit rubrics only when the necessary detail could not be accommodated by the use of a fifth-digit subclassification. To ensure that each rubric of ICD-9-CM collapses back to its ICD-9 counterpart the following specifications governed the ICD-9-CM disease classification:

Specifications for the tabular list:

1. Three-digit rubrics and their contents are unchanged from ICD-9.
2. The sequence of three-digit rubrics is unchanged from ICD-9.
3. Three-digit rubrics are not added to the main body of the classification.
4. Unsubdivided three-digit rubrics are subdivided where necessary to
   - add clinical detail
   - isolate terms for clinical accuracy
5. The modification in ICD-9-CM is accomplished by adding a fifth digit to existing ICD-9 rubrics, except as noted under #7 below.
6. The optional dual classification in ICD-9 is modified.
   - Duplicate rubrics are deleted:
     - four-digit manifestation categories duplicating etiology entries
     - manifestation inclusion terms duplicating etiology entries
   - Manifestations of disease are identified, to the extent possible, by creating five-digit codes in the etiology rubrics.
   - When the manifestation of a disease cannot be included in the etiology rubrics, provision for its identification is made by retaining the ICD-9 rubrics used for classifying manifestations of disease.
7. The format of ICD-9-CM is revised from that used in ICD-9.
   - American spelling of medical terms is used.
   - Inclusion terms are indented beneath the titles of codes.
   - Codes not to be used for primary tabulation of disease are printed in italics with the notation, "code first underlying disease."

Specifications for the alphabetic index:

1. The format of the alphabetic index follows that of ICD-9.
2. When two codes are required to indicate etiology and manifestation, the manifestation code appears in brackets (e.g., diabetic cataract 250.5 [366.41]).

How to Use the ICD•9•CM for Hospitals (Volumes 1, 2, & 3)

This *ICD-9-CM for Hospitals* is based on the official version of the International Classification of Diseases, Ninth Revision, Clinical Modification, Sixth Edition, issued by the U.S. Department of Health and Human Services. Annual code changes are implemented by the government and are effective Oct. 1 and valid through Sept. 30 of the following year.

The code book is totally compatible with its parent system, ICD-9, thus meeting the need for comparability of morbidity and mortality statistics at the international level.

This book is consistent with the content of the government's version of ICD-9-CM. However, to accommodate the coder's approach to coding, the alphabetic index has been placed before the tabular list in both the disease and procedure classifications. This allows the user to locate the correct codes in a logical, natural manner by locating the term in the index, then confirming the accuracy of the code in the tabular list.

STEPS TO CORRECT CODING

1. Look up the main term in the alphabetic index and scan the subterm entries as appropriate. Follow any cross-references such as "*see*" and "*see also*." Do not code from the alphabetic index without verifying the accuracy of the code in the tabular list.

2. Locate the code in the numerically arranged tabular list.

3. Observe the punctuation, footnotes, cross-references, color-coded prompts and other conventions described in the 'Conventions' section.

4. To determine the appropriateness of the code selection, read all instructional material:

   - "includes" and "*excludes*" notes
   - "*see*," "*see also*" and "*see category*" cross-references
   - "use additional code" and "*code first underlying disease*" instructions
   - "code also" and "*omit code*" notes
   - fourth- and fifth-digit requirements
   - CC exclusions

5. Consult definitions, relevant illustrations, CC exclusions, color coding and reimbursement prompts, the check fourth- and fifth-digit, age and sex symbols. Refer to the color/symbol legend at the bottom of each page for symbols. Refer to the list of footnotes that is included in the "Additional Conventions" section of this book for a full explanation of a footnote associated with a code.

6. Consult the official ICD-9-CM guidelines for coding and reporting, and refer to the AHA's *Coding Clinic for ICD-9-CM* for coding guidelines governing the use of specific codes.

7. Confirm and transcribe the correct code.

ORGANIZATION

Introduction
The introductory material in this book includes the history and future of ICD-9-CM as well as an overview of the classification system

Official ICD-9-CM Conventions
This section provides a full explanation of all the official footnotes, symbols, instructional notes, and conventions found in the official government version

Additional Conventions
Exclusive color-coding, symbols, and notations have been included in the *ICD-9-CM for Hospitals, Volumes 1, 2 & 3*, to alert coders to important coding and reimbursement issues. This section provides a full explanation of the additional conventions used throughout this book.

Coding Guidelines
Included in this book are the official ICD-9-CM coding guidelines as approved by the four cooperating parties of the ICD-9-CM Coordination and Maintenance Committee. Failure to comply with the official coding guidelines may result in denied or delayed claims.

Synopsis of Code Changes
This section includes a complete listing of all new code changes for the current year.

Disease Classification: Alphabetic Index to Diseases
The Alphabetic Index to Diseases is separated by tabs labeled with the letters of the alphabet, contains diagnostic terms for illnesses, injuries and reasons for encounters with health care professionals. The Table of Drugs and Chemicals is easily located with the tab in this section.

Disease Classification: Tabular List of Diseases
The Tabular List of Diseases arranges the ICD-9-CM codes and descriptors numerically. Tabs divide this section into chapters, identified by the code range on the tab.

The tabular list includes two supplementary classifications:

- V Codes—Supplementary Classification of Factors Influencing Health Status and Contact with Health Services (V01–V83)
- E Codes—Supplementary Classification of External Causes of Injury and Poisoning (E800–E999)

ICD-9-CM includes five official appendixes.

- Appendix A   Morphology of Neoplasms
- Appendix B   Glossary of Mental Disorders
- Appendix C   Classification of Drugs by AHFS List
- Appendix D   Classification of Industrial Accidents
                According to Agency
- Appendix E   List of Three-digit Categories

These appendices are included as a reference to provide further information about the patient's circumstances, help further define a diagnostic statement, maintain a tumor registry and aid in classifying new drugs.

Procedure Classification: Alphabetic Index to Procedures
The Alphabetic Index to Procedures lists common surgical and procedural terminology.

Procedure Classification: Tabular List of Procedures
The Tabular List of Procedures numerically arranges the procedure codes and their descriptors.

RESOURCES
Listed below are the exclusive resources found ONLY in the *ICD-9-CM Expert for Hospitals, Volumes 1, 2 & 3* books.

Dx/MDC/DRG List
Provides the complete list of diagnosis codes and the MDC and DRG to which they group, except when a secondary diagnosis affects DRG assignment for a quick audit.

CC Condition List
A complete list of all codes considered CC (Complications and Comorbidities) that will affect DRG assignment. This an essential auditing tool for assigning the most appropriate DRG.

Pharmacological Listings
The most common generic and brand names of drugs are linked with the disease processes to assist in the identification of CC, thereby improving DRG assignment practices.

Valid Three-digit Code Table
ICD-9-CM is composed of codes with either 3, 4, or 5 digits. A code is invalid if it has not been coded to the full number of digits required for that code. There are a certain number codes that are valid for reporting as three digit codes. A list of the valid three-digit code is included as a convenient reference when auditing claims.

2002 Ingenix, Inc.

ICD-9-CM Official Conventions

ICD-9-CM FOOTNOTES, SYMBOLS, INSTRUCTIONAL NOTES AND CONVENTIONS

This *ICD-9-CM for Hospitals* preserves all the footnotes, symbols, instructional notes and conventions found in the government's official version. Accurate coding depends upon understanding the meaning of these elements.

The following appear in the disease tabular list, unless otherwise noted.

OFFICIAL GOVERNMENT SYMBOLS

§   The section mark preceding a code denotes a footnote on the page. This symbol is used in the Tabular List of Diseases and in the Tabular List of Procedures.

ICD-9-CM CONVENTIONS USED IN THE TABULAR LIST

In addition to the symbols and footnotes above, the ICD-9-CM disease tabular has certain abbreviations, punctuation, symbols and other conventions. Our *ICD-9-CM for Hospitals* preserves these conventions. Proper use of the conventions will lead to efficient and accurate coding.

Abbreviations

NEC   Not elsewhere classifiable

    This abbreviation is used when the ICD-9-CM system does not provide a code specific for the patient's condition.

NOS   Not otherwise specified

    This abbreviation is the equivalent of 'unspecified' and is used only when the coder lacks the information necessary to code to a more specific four-digit subcategory.

[ ]   Brackets enclose synonyms, alternative terminology or explanatory phrases:

    482.2 Pneumonia due to Hemophilus influenzae [H. influenzae]

    Brackets that appear beneath a code indicate the fifth digits that are considered valid fifth digits for the code. This convention is applied for those instances in ICD-9-CM where not all common fifth digits are considered valid for each subcategory within a category.

    715.0 Osteoarthrosis, generalized
    [0,4,9]

    Generalized arthrosis can only be assigned in cases for which the degenerative joint disease involves multiple joints. Therefore, this code is considered for arthrosis in the sites described as unspecified, hand (which consists of multiple joints), or multiple sites. Therefore, only fifth digits 0, 4, and 9 are valid with subcategory 715.0.

( )   Parentheses enclose supplementary words, called nonessential modifiers, that may be present in the narrative description of a disease without affecting the code assignment:

    198.4 Other parts of nervous system
       Meninges (cerebral) (spinal)

:   Colons are used in the tabular list after an incomplete term that needs one or more of the modifiers that follow in order to make it assignable to a given category:

    021.1 Enteric tularemia
       Tularemia:
          cryptogenic
          intestinal
          typhoidal

}   Braces enclose a series of terms, each of which is modified by the statement appearing to the right of the brace:

    560.2 Volvulus

       Knotting
       Strangulation   } of intestine, bowel, or
       Torsion   colon
       Twist

OTHER CONVENTIONS

Boldface   Boldface type is used for all codes and titles in the tabular list.

Italicized   Italicized type is used for all exclusion notes and to identify codes that should not be used for describing the primary diagnosis.

INSTRUCTIONAL NOTES

These notes appear only in the Tabular List of Diseases

Includes An includes note further defines or clarifies the content of the chapter, subchapter, category, sub-category or subclassification. The includes note in the example below applies only to category 461.

Excludes Terms following the word "*Excludes*" are not classified to the chapter, subchapter, category, subcategory or specific subclassification code under which it is found. The note also may provide the location of the excluded diagnosis. Excludes notes are italicized.

461 Acute sinusitis

    INCLUDES abscess
                empyema
                infection   acute, of sinus
                inflammation   (accessory)
                suppuration   (nasal)

    EXCLUDES *chronic or unspecified sinusitis (473.0-473.9)*

Use additional code:

This instruction signals the coder that an additional code should be used if the information is available to provide a more complete picture of that diagnosis.

330 Cerebral degenerations usually manifest in childhood

Use additional code to identify associated mental retardation

Code first underlying disease:

This instruction is used in those categories not intended for primary tabulation of disease. These codes, called manifestation codes, may never be used alone or indicated as the primary diagnosis (i.e., sequenced first). They must always be preceded by another code.

The code and its descriptor appear in italics in the tabular list. The instruction "*Code first underlying disease*" is usually followed by the code or codes for the most common underlying disease (etiology). Record the code for the etiology or origin of the disease, and then record the italicized manifestation code in the next position.

590.81 Pyelitis or pyelonephritis in diseases classified elsewhere

Code first underlying disease as:
tuberculosis (016.0)

Code, if applicable, any causal condition first:

A code with this note may be principal if no causal condition is applicable or known.

590.0 Chronic pyelonephritis

Chronic pyelitis
Chronic pyonephrosis
Code, if applicable, any causal condition first

Omit code

"*Omit code*" is used to instruct the coder that no code is to be assigned. When this instruction is found in the Alphabetic Index to Diseases the medical term should not be coded as a diagnosis.

Metaplasia

cervix—*omit code*

When used in Volume 3, 'omit code' is meant to indicate procedures that do not merit separate code assignments, such as minor procedures preformed in conjunction with more extensive procedures or procedures that represent an operative approach.

Arthrotomy 80.10

as operative approach—*omit code*

2002 Ingenix, Inc.

Additional Conventions

NEW AND REVISED TEXT SYMBOLS

●   A bullet at a code or line of text indicates that that the entry is new.

▲   A triangle in the Tabular List indicates that the code title is revised. In the Alphabetic Index the triangle indicates that a code has changed.

►◄   These symbols appear at the beginning and at the end of a section of new or revised text.

When these symbols appear on a page there will be a date on the lower outside corner of the page indicating the date of the change, (e.g., October 2002).

ADDITIONAL DIGITS REQUIRED

√3ʳᵈ This symbol indicates that the code requires a third digit.

√4ᵗʰ This symbol indicates that the code requires a fourth digit.

√5ᵗʰ This symbol indicates that a code requires a fifth digit.

DEFINITIONS

DEF: This symbol indicates a definition of disease or procedure term. The definition will appear in blue type in the Disease and Procedure Tabular Lists.

AHA *CODING CLINIC FOR ICD-9-CM* REFERENCES

The four cooperating parties have designated the AHA's *Coding Clinic for ICD-9-CM* as the official publication for coding guidelines. The references are identified by the notation AHA: followed by the issue, year and page number.

In the example below, AHA *Coding Clinic for ICD-9-CM*, third quarter 1991, page 15, contains a discussion on code assignment for vitreous hemorrhage:

> **379.23 Vitreous hemorrhage**
> **AHA: 3Q, '91, 15**

The table below explains the abbreviations in the *Coding Clinic* references:

J-F	January/February
M-A	March/April
M-J	May/June
J-A	July/August
S-O	September/October
N-D	November/December
1Q	First quarter
2Q	Second quarter
3Q	Third quarter
4Q	Fourth quarter

MEDICARE CODE EDITS

Fiscal intermediaries use the Medicare Code Editor (MCE) to check the coding accuracy on claims. The Medicare code edits are listed below:

1.   Invalid diagnosis or procedure code
2.   E-code as principal diagnosis
3.   Duplicate of principal diagnosis (PDx) (as applied to a secondary diagnosis)
* 4. Age conflict
* 5. Sex conflict
* 6. Manifestation code as principal diagnosis
* 7. Nonspecific principal diagnosis
* 8. Questionable admission
*9. Unacceptable principal diagnosis
*10. Nonspecific OR procedure
*11. Noncovered procedure
12. Open biopsy check
*13. Bilateral procedure
14. Invalid age
15. Invalid sex
16. Invalid discharge status

Starred edits are identified by colors, symbols or footnotes as described on the next page.

Age and Sex Edit Symbols

The age edits below address MCE edits and are used to detect inconsistencies between the patient's age and diagnosis. They appear in the Tabular List of Diseases to the right of the code description.

Newborn Age: 0

> These diagnoses are intended for newborns and neonates and the patient's age must be 0 years

Pediatric Age: 0-17

> These diagnoses are intended for children and the patient's age must between 0 and 17 years

Maternity Age: 12-55

> These diagnoses are intended for the patients between the age of 12 and 55 years

Adult Age: 15-124

> These diagnoses are intended for the patients between the age of 15 and 124 years.

The sex symbols below address MCE edits and are used to detect inconsistencies between the patient's sex and diagnosis. They appear in the Tabular Lists to the right of the code description:

♂ **Male diagnosis only**

This symbol appears to the right of the code description. This reference appears in the disease tabular list.

♀ **Female diagnosis only**

This symbol appears to the right of the code description. This reference appears in the disease tabular list.

Color Coding

For a quick reference to the color codes and their meaning, refer to the color/symbol legend located at the bottom of each page.

To alert the coder to important reimbursement issues affected by the code assignment, color bars have been added. The colors represent Medicare code edits as well as other reimbursement issues.

Color coding appears in both tabular lists. Some codes carry more than one color. Please note that the same color may appear in the disease and procedure tabular lists, but with different meanings.

Disease Tabular List
Manifestation Code

These codes will appear in italic type as well as with a blue color bar over the code title. A manifestation code is not allowed to be reported as a primary diagnosis because each describes a manifestation of some other underlying disease, not the disease itself. This is also referred to as mandatory multiple coding. Code the underlying disease first. A *'Code first underlying disease'* instructional note will appear with underlying disease codes identified. In the Alphabetic Index these codes are listed as the secondary code in slanted bracket with the code for the underlying disease listed first. Medicare code edit (MCE) 6

Unacceptable PDx

These codes will appear with a gray color bar over the code title. These codes do not describe a current illness or injury, but a circumstance which influences a patient's health status. These are considered an unacceptable principal diagnosis for inpatient admission. Medicare code edit (MCE) 9

Questionable Admission

These codes will also appear with a gray color bar over the code title. These codes identify a condition that usually is insufficient justification for hospital admission. Since these codes are considered an unacceptable principal diagnoses for inpatient admission, they are color coded in the same manner as the "unacceptable PDx codes". Medicare code edit (MCE) 8

Nonspecific PDx

These codes will have a yellow color bar over the code title. While these codes are considered valid ICD-9-CM codes, for inpatients discharged alive, a more specific principal diagnosis should be assigned. These codes are used when the neither the diagnostic statement nor the documentation provides enough information to assign a more specified diagnosis code. These codes may be stated as "Unspecified" or "Not otherwise specified (NOS)." Medicare code edit (MCE) 7

Procedure Tabular List
Non-specific OR Procedure

While this code is a valid unspecific or not otherwise specified (NOS) procedure code, a more precise code should be used. The code is recognized as a nonspecific operating room procedure ONLY if ALL OR procedures performed are coded NOS. Medicare Code Edit (MCE 10)

Valid OR

A procedure that triggers a change in DRG assignment.

Non-OR Procedure

A non-operating room procedure that affects DRG assignment.

Footnotes

All footnotes are identified by a numerical superscript that appears to the upper left of the code:

[1]718.5 Ankylosis of joint

The footnote 1 indicates "Nonspecific PDx = 0". This means that when code 718.50, Ankylosis of the joint, site unspecified, the diagnosis is considered a nonspecific principal diagnosis. While this code may be valid according to ICD-9-CM, a more precise diagnosis should be used for the principal diagnosis for inpatient admission.

The following list identifies the meaning of each footnote number and the classification in which the footnote appears:

Disease Tabular

1   Nonspecific PDx = 0

2   Nonspecific PDx = 9

3   These V codes may be used as principal diagnosis on Medicare patients.

4   This V code, with the fourth digit of 1 or 2, is unacceptable as a principal diagnosis.

5   These codes, with the fourth digit of 0 or 1, may be used as a principal diagnosis for Medicare patients.

6   Rehabilitation codes acceptable as a principal diagnosis when accompanied by a secondary diagnosis reflecting the condition treated.

7   These V codes are acceptable as principal diagnosis when accompanied by a diagnosis of personal history of malignancy. These codes group to DRG 465.

8   Questionable admission = 0

9   The codes with fifth-digit of 1 are considered a major complication condition that causes DRG assignment from DRG 121 to DRG 122.

Procedure Tabular

10   Valid OR procedure code if accompanied by one of the following codes: 37.80, 37.81, 37.82, 37.85, 37.86, 37.87.

11   Valid OR procedure code if accompanied by one of the following codes: 37.80, 37.83.

12   Valid OR procedure code if accompanied by one of the following codes: 37.80, 37.85, 37.86, 37.87.

13   Valid OR procedure code if accompanied by any one of the following codes: 37.80, 37.81, 37.82, 37.83, 37.85, 37.86, 37.87.

2002 Ingenix, Inc.

14 Valid OR procedure code if accompanied by any other pacemaker procedure except 37.72, 37.76.

15 Valid OR procedure code if accompanied by any other pacemaker procedure except 37.70, 37.71, 37.73, 37.76.

16 Nonspecific OR procedure = 0.

17 Noncovered procedure only if none of the following codes are present as either a principal or secondary diagnosis: 200.00-202.08, 202.80-202.98, 204.01, 205.01, 206.01, 207.01, 208.01.

18 Noncovered procedure only if none of the following codes are present as either a principal or secondary diagnosis: 204.00-208.91, 279.12, 279.2, 284.0-284.9

19 Noncovered procedure unless diagnosis code is present from 250.00–250.93 and 585, V42.0 or V43.89

Other Notations

Disease Tabular
CC Exclusion List

A exclusive feature of *ICD-9-CM for Hospitals* is the integration of the government's CC exclusion list with each affected code.

The CC exclusion list indicates secondary diagnosis codes that are excluded as CC conditions with certain principal diagnoses. This exclusion occurs because the cited conditions are inherent to the disease process of the principal diagnosis.

Listed below each code that is considered a complication or comorbidity (CC) diagnosis, are the codes or code ranges of principal diagnosis with which the CC code cannot be used.

In the example below, code 254.1 is normally a CC condition. However, the CC exclusion (CC Excl:) notation indicates that if a code from the listed code ranges is assigned as the principal diagnosis, the secondary diagnosis of 254.0 will not be recognized as a CC condition in DRG assignment.

254.1 Abscess of thymus
CC Excl: 254.0-254.1, 254.8-254.9, 259.8-259.9

CC Condition

A complication or comorbidity diagnosis that may change DRG assignment. A complication is defined as a condition that arises during the hospital stay that extends the length of stay by at least one day in 75 percent of the cases. A comorbidity is a pre-existing condition that will, because of its presence with a specific principal diagnosis, that extends the length of stay by at least one day in 75 percent of the cases.

CC listed with a digit or range of digits indicates the fifth-digit assignments for that code that are considered CC conditions. Example: code 250.1 has a symbol CC 1-3 which means that only 250.11, 250.12, and 250.13 are considered CC conditions. Code 251.0 is not a CC condition.

Major Cardiovascular Complication

A complication that causes the DRG to change from DRG 122 to DRG 121.

Complex Diagnosis

A diagnosis that causes the DRG assignment of a case to change from DRG 125 to DRG 124.

Medicare as Secondary Payer

Specific trauma diagnoses are identified that alert fiscal intermediaries (FIs) that another carrier should be billed first and Medicare billed second if payment from the first payer does not equal or exceed the amount Medicare would pay.

DRG

This symbol indicates the diagnosis is assigned to a diagnosis related group (DRG) that has been targeted for audit. The condition must be thoroughly documented in the medical record to prevent inappropriate coding or "upcoding."

HIV

This symbol indicates that the condition is considered a major HIV related diagnosis. When the condition is coded in combination with a diagnosis of human immunodeficiency virus (HIV), code 042, the case will move from DRG 490 to DRG 489.

Procedure Tabular
Noncovered procedure

A procedure not covered by Medicare. In some instances this procedure may also be identified as a valid operating room (OR) procedure that may trigger a DRG assignment. Even if a DRG assignment is made, Medicare may not reimburse for the noncovered procedure. (MCE 11)

Bilateral Edit

Due to the lack of laterality in ICD-9-CM, there are certain lower extremity joint procedure codes that do not accurately reflect procedures that are performed in one admission on two or more different bilateral joints. To group to DRG 471, Bilateral or Multiple Joint Procedures of Lower Extremity, a case must be coded with a combination of two or more different major lower extremity joint procedures. The bilateral procedure symbol identifies those procedure codes that when coded twice represent the same procedure performed on both of the same bilateral joints of the lower extremity. Otherwise, a code edit will instruct the fiscal intermediary to verify that the two different procedures were performed on two different bilateral joints. (MCE 13)

Summary of Code Changes

DISEASE TABULAR LIST (VOLUME 1)

038	Excludes term added
● 040.82	Toxic shock syndrome Use additional code note added
062.8	Excludes note added
066.3	Includes term deleted
● 066.4	West Nile fever Includes notes added
256.2	Use additional code note added Excludes term deleted
256.3	Use additional code note revised
277.00	Includes note added
● 277.02	Cystic fibrosis with pulmonary manifestations Includes note added Use additional code note added
● 277.03	Cystic fibrosis with gastrointestinal manifestations Excludes note added
● 277.09	Cystic fibrosis with other manifestations
277.7	Use additional code note revised
337.3	Use additional code note revised
357.8	Includes note deleted
● 357.81	Chronic inflammatory demyelinating polyneuritis
● 357.82	Critical illness polyneuropathy Includes note added
● 357.89	Other inflammatory and toxic neuropathy
● 359.81	Critical illness myopathy Includes note added
● 359.89	Other myopathies
● 365.83	Aqueous misdirection Includes note added
368.6	Includes term deleted
402	Use additional code note added
▲ 402.00	Hypertensive heart disease, malignant, without congestive heart failure
▲ 402.01	Hypertensive heart disease, malignant, with ~~congestive~~ heart failure
▲ 402.10	Hypertensive heart disease, benign, without ~~congestive~~ heart failure
▲ 402.11	Hypertensive heart disease, benign, with ~~congestive~~ heart failure
▲ 402.90	Hypertensive heart disease, unspecified, without ~~congestive~~ heart failure
▲ 402.91	Hypertensive heart disease, unspecified, with ~~congestive~~ heart failure
404	Use additional code note added Fifth-digit code definitions revised 0 without mention of ~~congestive~~

	heart failure or renal failure 1 with ~~congestive~~ heart failure 2 with ~~congestive~~ heart failure and renal failure
▲ 404.00	Hypertensive heart and renal disease, malignant, without mention of ~~congestive~~ heart failure or renal failure
▲ 404.01	Hypertensive heart and renal disease, malignant, with ~~congestive~~ heart failure
▲ 404.03	Hypertensive heart and renal disease, malignant, with ~~congestive~~ heart failure and renal failure
▲ 404.10	Hypertensive heart and renal disease, benign, without mention of ~~congestive~~ heart failure or renal failure
▲ 404.11	Hypertensive heart and renal disease, benign, with ~~congestive~~ heart failure
▲ 404.13	Hypertensive heart and renal disease, benign, with ~~congestive~~ heart failure and renal failure
▲ 404.90	Hypertensive heart and renal disease, unspecified, without mention of ~~congestive~~ heart failure or renal failure
▲ 404.91	Hypertensive heart and renal disease, unspecified, with ~~congestive~~ heart failure
▲ 404.93	Hypertensive heart and renal disease, unspecified, with ~~congestive~~ heart failure and renal failure
411.81	Excludes terms revised
● 414.06	Coronary atherosclerosis of coronary artery of transplanted heart
▲ 414.1	Aneurysm ►and dissection◄ of heart
▲ 414.10	►Aneurysm◄ of heart (wall)
▲ 414.11	►Aneurysm◄ of coronary vessels
● 414.12	Dissection of coronary artery
▲ 414.19	Other ►aneurysm of heart◄
427.89	Excludes terms added
428	Excludes term deleted Code, if applicable, note added
▲ 428.0	Congestive heart failure, ►unspecified◄ Excludes note added
● 428.2	Systolic heart failure Excludes note added
● 428.20	Systolic heart failure, unspecified
● 428.21	Systolic heart failure, acute
● 428.22	Systolic heart failure, chronic
● 428.23	Systolic heart failure, acute on chronic

● 428.3	Diastolic heart failure Excludes note added
● 428.30	Diastolic heart failure, unspecified
● 428.31	Diastolic heart failure, acute
● 428.32	Diastolic heart failure, chronic
● 428.33	Diastolic heart failure, acute on chronic
● 428.4	Combined systolic and diastolic heart failure
● 428.40	Combined systolic and diastolic heart failure, unspecified
● 428.41	Combined systolic and diastolic heart failure, acute
● 428.42	Combined systolic and diastolic heart failure, chronic
● 428.43	Combined systolic and diastolic heart failure, acute on chronic
(430-438)	Cerebrovascular Disease section Excludes term added
436	Excludes term added
● 438.6	Late effects of cerebrovascular disease, alterations of sensations Use additional code note added
● 438.7	Late effects of cerebrovascular disease, disturbances of vision Use additional code note added
● 438.83	Other late effects of cerebrovascular disease, facial weakness Includes term added
● 438.84	Other late effects of cerebrovascular disease, ataxia
● 438.85	Other late effects of cerebrovascular disease, vertigo
440	Excludes term added
440.8	Excludes term revised
441.0	Includes note deleted
● 443.2	Other arterial dissection Excludes note added
● 443.21	Dissection of carotid artery
● 443.22	Dissection of iliac artery
● 443.23	Dissection of renal artery
● 443.24	Dissection of vertebral artery
● 443.29	Dissection of other artery
444	Excludes term added
● 445	Atheroembolism Includes note added
● 445.0	Atheroembolism, of extermities
● 445.01	Atheroembolism, upper extermity
● 445.02	Atheroembolism, lower extremity
● 445.8	Atheroembolism, of other sites
● 445.81	Atheroembolism, kidney Use additional code note added
● 445.89	Atheroembolism, other site
447.6	Excludes term revised
● 454.8	Varicose veins of the lower extremities, with other complications Includes note added

►◄ Revised Text   ● New Code   ▲ Revised Code Title

2002 Ingenix, Inc.   **xiii**

▲ 454.9   Varicose veins of lower extremities, ~~without mention of ulcer or inflammation~~ ►asmyptomatic varicose veins◄ Includes term added

459.1   Includes note added
Excludes note added

● 459.10   Postphlebetic syndrome without complications
Includes note added

● 459.11   Postphlebetic syndrome with ulcer

● 459.12   Postphlebetic syndrome with inflammation

● 459.13   Postphlebetic syndrome with ulcer and inflammation

● 459.19   Postphlebetic syndrome with other complication

● 459.3   Chronic venous hypertension (idiopathic)
Includes note added
Excludes note added

● 459.30   Chronic venous hypertension without complications
Includes note added

● 459.31   Chronic venous hypertension with ulcer

● 459.32   Chronic venous hypertension with inflammation

● 459.33   Chronic venous hypertension with ulcer and inflammation

● 459.39   Chronic venous hypertension with other complication

491.2   Includes term deleted

491.20   Includes term deleted

491.21   Includes term deleted

493.2   Includes term added
Excludes term deleted

518.81   Excludes term revised

518.82   Excludes term revised

● 537.84   Dieulafoy lesion (hemorrhagic) of stomach and duodenum

● 569.86   Dieulafoy lesion (hemorrhagic) of intestine

577.8   Excludes term revised

590.0   Code first note deleted
Code, if applicable, note added

593.7   Use additional code note deleted

599.0   Excludes term added

602.3   Includes terms revised
Excludes terms revised

622.1   Includes terms added

▲ 627.2   ►Symptomatic◄ menopausal or female climacteric states

▲ 627.4   ►Symptomatic◄ states associated with artificial menopause

629.0   Excludes term revised

● 633.00   Abdominal pregnancy without intrauterine pregnancy

● 633.01   Abdominal pregnancy with intrauterine pregnancy

● 633.10   Tubal pregnancy without intrauterine pregnancy

● 633.11   Tubal pregnancy with intrauterine pregnancy

● 633.20   Ovarian pregnancy without intrauterine pregnancy

● 633.21   Ovarian pregnancy with intrauterine pregnancy

● 633.80   Other ectopic pregnancy without intrauterine pregnancy

● 633.81   Other ectopic pregnancy with intrauterine pregnancy

● 633.90   Unspecified ectopic pregnancy without intrauterine pregnancy

● 633.91   Unspecified ectopic pregnancy with intrauterine pregnancy

646.6   Includes term revised

647.1   Excludes note added

707.1   Code first note revised
Code, if applicable, terms added

710   Use additional code note deleted

710.1   Use additional code note added

718.7   Excludes terms deleted
Excludes terms added

723.5   Excludes term added

730.1   Includes term deleted

733.4   Excludes term deleted

● 747.83   Persistent fetal circulation
Includes note added

751.7   Excludes term revised

753.0   Code first note deleted

753.15   Code first note deleted

(764-779)   Other conditions originating in the perinatal period section
Fifth-digit subclassification instructions revised

▲ 765   Disorders relating to short gestation and low birthweight

765.0   Instructional note revised
Use additional code note added

765.1   Instrucitonal note revised
Use additional code note added

● 765.2   Disorders relating to short gestation and low birthweight, weeks of gestation

● 765.20   Unspecified weeks of gestation

● 765.21   Less than 24 completed weeks of gestation

● 765.22   24 completed weeks of gestation

● 765.23   25-26 completed weeks of gestation

● 765.24   27-28 completed weeks of gestation

● 765.25   29-30 completed weeks of gestation

● 765.26   31-32 completed weeks of gestation

● 765.27   33-34 completed weeks of gestation

● 765.28   35-36 completed weeks of gestation

● 765.29   37 or more completed weeks of gestation

770.8   Includes note deleted

● 770.81   Primary apnea of newborn
Includes note added

● 770.82   Other apnea of newborn
Includes note added

● 770.83   Cyanotic attacks of newborn

● 770.84   Respiratory failure of newborn
Excludes note added

● 770.89   Other respiratory problems after birth

771.8   Includes note deleted
Use additional code note added

● 771.81   Septicemia [sepsis] of newborn

● 771.82   Urinary tract infection of newborn

● 771.83   Bacteremia of newborn

● 771.89   Other infections specific to the perinatal period
Includes note added

774.5   Code first term revised

● 779.81   Neonatal bradycardia
Excludes note added

● 779.82   Neonatal tachycardia
Excludes note added

● 779.89   Other specified conditions originating in the perinatal period

780.9   Includes note deleted

● 780.91   Fussy infant (baby)

● 780.92   Excessive crying of infant (baby)

● 780.99   Other general symptoms
Includes note added

● 781.93   Ocular torticollis

782.5   Excludes note revised

785.0   Excludes note added

786.03   Excludes term added

786.09   Excludes terms revised

788.3   Code first note deleted
Code, if applicable, note added

790.7   Excludes term added

795.0   Includes note deleted
Excludes note added

● 795.00   Nonspecific abnormal Papanicolaou smear of cervix, unspecified

● 795.01   Atypical squamous cell changes of undetermined significance favor benign (ASCUS favor benign)
Includes note added

● 795.02   Atypical squamous cell changes of undetermined significance favor dysplasia (ASCUS favor dysplasia)
Includes note added

● 795.09   Other nonspecific abnormal Papanicolaou smear of cervix
Includes note added

● 795.31   Nonspecific positive findings for anthrax
Includes term added

● 795.39   Other nonspecific positive culture findings

799.1   Excludes terms revised

(800-829)   Fractures section
Instructional note revised

● 813.45   Torus fracture of radius

● 823.4   Fracture of tibia and fibula, torus fracture

959.01   Excludes term added

991.6   Excludes term revised

995.0   Code first note deleted

● 995.9   Systemic inflammatory response syndrome (SIRS)

● 995.90   Systemic inflammatory response syndrome, unspecified
Includes note added

- 995.91 Systemic inflammatory response syndrome due to infectious process without organ dysfunction
- 995.92 Systemic inflammatory response syndrome due to infectious process with organ dysfunction
  Includes note added
  Use additional code note added
- 995.93 Systemic inflammatory response syndrome due to non-infectious process without organ dysfunction
- 995.94 Systemic inflammatory response syndrome due to non-infectious process with organ dysfunction
  Use additional code note added
- 996.72 Excludes note revised
- 998.31 Disruption of internal operation wound
- 998.32 Disruption of external operation wound
  Includes note added
- V01.81 Contact with or exposure to anthrax
- V01.89 Contact with or exposure to other communicable diseases
- V13.21 Personal history of pre-term labor
  Excludes note added
- V13.29 Personal history of other genital system and obstetric disorders
- V23.41 Pregnancy with history of pre-term labor
- V23.49 Pregnancy with other poor obstetric history
- V46.2 Other dependence on machines, supplemental oxygen
  Includes note added
- ▲ V49.81 ▶Asymptomatic◀ postmenopausal status (age-related) (natural)
- V54.0 Excludes term revised
- V54.1 Aftercare for healing traumatic fracture
- V54.10 Aftercare for healing traumatic fracture of arm, unspecified
- V54.11 Aftercare for healing traumatic fracture of upper arm
- V54.12 Aftercare for healing traumatic fracture of lower arm
- V54.13 Aftercare for healing traumatic fracture of hip
- V54.14 Aftercare for healing traumatic fracture of leg, unspecified
- V54.15 Aftercare for healing traumatic fracture of upper leg
  Excludes note added
- V54.16 Aftercare for healing traumatic fracture of lower leg
- V54.17 Aftercare for healing traumatic fracture of vertebrae
- V54.19 Aftercare for healing traumatic fracture of other bone
- V54.2 Aftercare for healing pathologic fracture
- V54.20 Aftercare for healing pathologic fracture of arm, unspecified
- V54.21 Aftercare for healing pathologic fracture of upper arm

- V54.22 Aftercare for healing pathologic fracture of lower arm
- V54.23 Aftercare for healing pathologic fracture of hip
- V54.24 Aftercare for healing pathologic fracture of leg, unspecified
- V54.25 Aftercare for healing pathologic fracture of upper leg
  Excludes note added
- V54.26 Aftercare for healing pathologic fracture of lower leg
- V54.27 Aftercare for healing pathologic fracture of vertebrae
- V54.29 Aftercare for healing pathologic fracture of other bone
- V54.8 Includes note deleted
- V54.81 Aftercare following joint replacement
  Use additional code note added
- V54.89 Other orthopedic aftercare
  Includes note added
- V58.4 Instructional note added
- V58.42 Aftercare following surgery for neoplasm
  Includes note added
- V58.43 Aftercare following surgery for injury and trauma
  Includes note added
  Excludes note added
- V58.7 Aftercare following surgery to specified body systems, not elsewhere classified
  Instructional note added
- V58.71 Aftercare following surgery of the sense organs, NEC
  Includes note added
- V58.72 Aftercare following surgery of the nervous system, NEC
  Includes note added
  Excludes note added
- V58.73 Aftercare following surgery of the circulatory system, NEC
  Includes note added
- V58.74 Aftercare following surgery of the respiratory system, NEC
  Includes note added
- V58.75 Aftercare following surgery of the teeth, oral cavity and digestive system, NEC
  Includes note added
- V58.76 Aftercare following surgery of the genitourinary system, NEC
  Includes note added
  Excludes note added
- V58.77 Aftercare following surgery of the skin and subcutaneous tissue, NEC
  Includes note added
- V58.78 Aftercare following surgery of the musculoskeletal system, NEC
  Includes note added
- V58.83 Use additional code note added
- ▲ V71.8 Observation ▶and evaluation◀ for other specified suspected conditions
- V71.82 Observation and evaluation for suspected exposure to anthrax

- V71.83 Observation and evaluation for suspected exposure to other biological agent
- V83.8 Other genetic carrier status
- V83.81 Cystic fibrosis gene carrier
- V83.89 Other genetic carrier status
- E885.0 Fall from (nonmotorized) scooter
- E922.5 Accident caused by firearm, and air gun missle, paintball gun
- E955.7 Suicide and self-inflicted injury by firearms, air guns and explosives, paintball gun
- E960-E969 Homicide and injury purposely inflicted by other persons section
  Excludes term added
- (E979) Terrorism (E979) new section
- E979 Terrorism
  Instructional note added
- E979.0 Terrorism involving explosion of marine weapons
  Includes note added
- E979.1 Terrorism involving destruction of aircraft
  Includes note added
- E979.2 Terrorism involving other explosions and fragments
  Includes note added
- E979.3 Terrorism involving fires, conflagration and hot substances
  Includes note added
- E979.4 Terrorism involving firearms
  Includes note added
- E979.5 Terrorism involving nuclear weapons
  Includes note added
- E979.6 Terrorism involving biological weapons
  Includes note added
- E979.7 Terrorism involving chemical weapons
  Includes note added
- E979.8 Terrorism involving other means
  Includes note added
- E979.9 Terrorism, secondary effects
  Instructional note added
  Excludes note added
- E985.7 Injury by paintball gun, undetermined whether accidentally or purposely inflicted
- ▲ E999 Late effect of injury due to war operations wand terrorismx
  Instructional note revised
- E999.0 Late effect of injury due to war operations
- E999.1 Late effect of injury due to terrorism

PROCEDURE TABULAR LIST (VOLUME 3)
- 00 Procedures and interventions, not elsewhere classified
- 00.0 Therapeutic ultrasound
- 00.01 Therapeutic ultrasound of vessels of head and neck
  Includes note added
  Excludes note added

▶◀ Revised Text   ● New Code   ▲ Revised Code Title

▶◀ Revised Text   ● New Code   ▲ Revised Code Title

Coding Guidelines

OFFICIAL ICD-9-CM GUIDELINES FOR CODING AND REPORTING

The Public Health Service and the Centers for Medicare and Medicaid (formerly know as Health Care Financing Administration) of the U.S. Department of Health and Human Services present the following guidelines for coding and reporting using the International Classification of Diseases, 9th Revision, Clinical Modification (ICD-9-CM). These guidelines should be used as a companion document to the official versions of the ICD-9-CM.

These guidelines for coding and reporting have been developed and approved by the cooperating parties for ICD-9-CM: American Hospital Association, American Health Information Management Association, Center for Medicare and Medicaid Services and the National Center for Health Statistics. These guidelines previously appeared in the Coding Clinic for ICD-9-CM, published by the American Hospital Association.

These guidelines have been developed to assist the user in coding and reporting in situations where the ICD-9-CM manual does not provide direction. Coding and sequencing instructions in the three ICD-9-CM manuals take precedence over any guidelines.

These guidelines are not exhaustive. The cooperating parties are continuing to conduct review of these guidelines and develop new guidelines as needed. Users of the ICD-9-CM should be aware that only guidelines approved by the cooperating parties are official. Revision of these guidelines and new guidelines will be published by the U.S. Department of Health and Human Services when they are approved by the cooperating parties.

OUTPATIENT SERVICES

(Hospital-Based and Physician Office)

INPATIENT SERVICES

OFFICIAL GUIDELINES FOR CODING AND REPORTING OUTPATIENT SERVICES (HOSPITAL-BASED AND PHYSICIAN OFFICE)

Introduction

These revised coding guidelines for outpatient diagnoses have been approved for use by hospitals/physicians in coding and reporting hospital-based outpatient services and physician office visits.

The terms encounter and visit are often used interchangeably in describing outpatient service contacts and, therefore, appear together in these guidelines without distinguishing one from the other.

Coding guidelines for outpatient and physician reporting of diagnoses will vary in a number of instances from those for inpatient diagnoses, recognizing that:

The Uniform Hospital Discharge Data Set (UHDDS) definition of principal diagnosis applies only to inpatients in acute, short-term, general hospitals.

Coding guidelines for inconclusive diagnoses (probable, suspected, rule out, etc.) were developed for inpatient reporting and do not apply to outpatients.

Diagnoses often are not established at the time of the initial encounter/visit. It may take two or more visits before the diagnosis is confirmed.

The most critical rule involves beginning the search for the correct code assignment through the Alphabetic Index. Never begin searching initially in the Tabular List as this will lead to coding errors.

Basic Coding Guidelines for Outpatient Services

A. Code Range

   The appropriate code or codes from 001.0 through V82.9 must be used to identify diagnoses, symptoms, conditions, problems, complaints, or other reason(s) for the encounter/visit.

B. Accurate Reporting

   For accurate reporting of ICD-9-CM diagnosis codes, the documentation should describe the patient's condition, using terminology which includes specific diagnoses as well as symptoms, problems, or reasons for the encounter. There are ICD-9-CM codes to describe all of these.

C. Code Selection

   The selection of codes 001.0 through 999.9 will frequently be used to describe the reason for the encounter. These codes are from the section of ICD-9-CM for the classification of diseases and injuries (e.g. infectious and parasitic diseases; neoplasms; symptoms, signs, and ill-defined conditions, etc.).

D. Symptoms, Signs and Ill-defined Conditions

Codes that describe symptoms and signs, as opposed to diagnoses, are acceptable for reporting purposes when an established diagnosis has not been diagnosed (confirmed) by the physician. Chapter 16 of ICD-9-CM, Symptoms, Signs, and Ill-defined conditions (codes 780.0 - 799.9) contain many, but not all codes for symptoms.

E. Circumstances other than Disease or Injury

ICD-9-CM provides codes to deal with encounters for circumstances other than a disease or injury. The Supplementary Classification of factors Influencing Health Status and Contact with Health Services (V01.0- V82.9) is provided to deal with occasions when circumstances other than a disease or injury are recorded as diagnosis or problems. The V codes should be used for encounters of this type. For example, the correct code for a cancer patient who is seen solely for radiotherapy is V58.0, radiotherapy session.

Example:

Discharge diagnosis: Open-angle glaucoma

Reason for visit code: 365.10

Discharge diagnosis: Follow-up examination after surgery

Reason for visit code: V67.0

F. Code Specificity

ICD-9-CM is composed of codes with either 3, 4, or 5 digits. Codes with 3 digits are included in ICD-9-CM as the heading of a category of codes that may be further subdivided by the use of fourth and/or fifth digits which provide greater specificity. A code is invalid if it has not been coded to the full number of digits required for that code.

- Assign three-digit codes only if there are no four-digit codes within that code category.
- Assign four-digit codes only if there is no fifth-digit subclassification for that subcategory.
- Assign the fifth-digit subclassification code for those subcategories where it exists.

Example:

Diagnosis: Acute tonsillitis

Correct code: 463

Diagnosis: Benign neoplasm of colon

Incorrect code: 211

Correct code: 211.3

G. Code Sequence

List first the ICD-9-CM code for the diagnosis, condition, problem, or other reason for encounter/visit shown in the medical record to be chiefly responsible for the services provided. List additional codes that describe any coexisting conditions.

H. Uncertain Diagnosis

Do not code diagnoses documented as "probable", "suspected," "questionable," "rule out," or working diagnosis. Rather, code the condition(s) to the highest degree of certainty for that encounter/visit, such as symptoms, signs, abnormal test results, or other reason for the visit.

Coders should be aware that this is contrary to the coding practices used by health information management departments for coding the diagnoses of hospital inpatients. For inpatient coding, all discharge diagnoses listed as "probable," "suspected," "questionable" or "rule out" would be coded as if the condition existed. Further, coding symptoms for inpatients is generally unacceptable, particularly when there is an established diagnosis. A requirement that conditions listed as "probable," "suspected," "questionable" or "rule out" be coded in the outpatient setting as if the condition existed would lead to significant over-reporting of conditions. Therefore codes for symptoms and signs are appropriate and acceptable for hospital outpatient reporting.

Example:

Reason for visit: Chest pain, code 786.50

Discharge diagnosis: Rule out angina, code 413.9

Correct code: 786.50

Comment: Do not code angina as if it were established; code the reason for the visit.

I. Chronic Disease

Chronic diseases treated on an ongoing basis may be coded and reported as many times as the patient receives treatment and care for the condition(s).

Example:

History of illness: Patient is seen for monthly lumbar epidural block with steroid injection.

Discharge diagnosis: Chronic low back pain, code 724.2

Comment: Report code 724.2, low back pain, for each visit during which the patient receives lumbar-block treatment, regardless of the number or frequency of visits.

J. Coexisting Conditions

Code all documented conditions that coexist at the time of the encounter/visit, and require or affect patient care treatment or management. Do not code conditions that were previously treated and no longer exist. However, history codes (V10- V19) may be used as secondary codes if the historical condition or family history has an impact on current care or influences treatment.

Coders are advised to exercise care in identifying (a) conditions presently existing, (b) conditions no longer existing, (c) residuals (late effects) of conditions no longer existing, and (d) certain postoperative status conditions that require consideration in managing patient care and that warrant coding. Some physicians add to the list of conditions currently being treated any previous surgery or conditions that no longer exist to provide easy reference of the patient's history for recapitulation in the ongoing care of the patient. These conditions should not be coded unless they require or affect patient care treatment or management.

Example:

Chief complaint: Uncontrolled diabetes mellitus, 250.02

Review of systems: Patient has congestive heart failure (428.0) and is curently on Lasix.

Medical history: Patient is status three months post right inguinal herniorrherapy for incarcerated inguinal hernia.

Comment: First code "uncontrolled diabetes mellitus" as the reason for the visit, followed by "congestive heart failure" as a coexisting condition. Do not code the incarcerated inguinal hernia; it was treated successfully.

Code sequence: 250.02, 428.0

K.   Ancillary Diagnostic Services

For patients receiving diagnostic services only during an encounter/visit, sequence first the diagnosis, condition, problem, or other reason for encounter/visit shown in the medical record to be chiefly responsible for the outpatient services provided during the encounter/visit. Codes for other diagnoses (e.g., chronic conditions) may be sequenced as additional diagnoses.

Example:

Chief complaint: Hematuria, code 599.7

Laboratory studies: Intravenous pyelogram, code V72.5

History of illness: Patient was referred to hospital outpatient clinic for intravenous pyelogram only. Will provide patient's physician with the results.

Code sequence: 599.7

L.   Ancillary Therapeutic Services

For patients receiving therapeutic services only during an encounter/visit, sequence first the diagnosis, condition, problem, or other reason for encounter/visit shown in the medical record to be chiefly responsible for the outpatient services provided during the encounter/visit. Codes for other diagnoses (e.g., chronic conditions) may be sequenced as additional diagnoses.

Example:

Chief complaint: Chronic renal failure, code 585

Procedure performed: Hemodialysis, code V56.0

History of illness: Patient is being seen for hemodialysis treatment.

Code sequence: 585

NOTE: The appropriate V code can be listed first for patients receiving the following (the diagnosis or problem for which the service is being performed should be listed second):

- chemotherapy
- radiation therapy
- rehabilitation.

Example:

Chief complaint: Trigone bladder cancer, code 188.0

Procedure performed: Chemotherapy infusion, code V58.1

History of illness: Patient is being seen for second course of five chemotherapy infusions.

Code sequence: V58.1, 188.0

M.   [Guideline M-deleted in the official guidelines]

N.   Preoperative Evaluations

For patient's receiving preoperative evaluations only, sequence a code from category V72.8, Other specified examinations, to describe the pre-op consultations. Assign a code for the condition to describe the reason for the surgery as an additional diagnosis. Code also any findings related to the pre-op evaluation.

Example:

Chief complaint: Rhegmatogenous retinal detachment in left eye, code 361.00

Procedure performed: Preoperative cardiovascular examination, V72.81

History of illness: Patient is being seen for preoperative cardiovascular examination, due to history of myocardial infarction 1 year ago. Patient is scheduled for a repair of his retinal detachment next week.

Code sequence: V72.81, 361.00

O.   Ambulatory Surgery

For ambulatory surgery, code the diagnosis for which the surgery was performed. If the postoperative diagnosis is known to be different from the preoperative diagnosis at the time the diagnosis is confirmed, select the postoperative diagnosis for coding, since it is the most definitive.

Example:

Preoperative diagnosis: Breast mass, code 611.72

Postoperative diagnosis: Fibrocystic breast disease, code 610.3

Comment: Code 610.3 as the reason for the visit because it is the postoperative diagnosis.

OFFICIAL GUIDELINES FOR CODING AND REPORTING INPATIENT SERVICES

1. GENERAL INPATIENT CODING GUIDELINES

  1.1. Use of Both Alphabetic Index and Tabular List

    A. Use both the Alphabetic Index and the Tabular List when locating and assigning a code. Reliance on only the Alphabetic Index or the Tabular List leads to errors in code assignments and less specificity in code selection.

    B. Locate each term in the Alphabetic Index and verify the code selected in the Tabular List. Read and be guided by instructional notations that appear in both the Alphabetic Index and the Tabular List.

  1.2. Level of Specificity in Coding

    Diagnostic and procedure codes are to be used at their highest level of specificity:

- Assign three-digit codes only if there are no four-digit codes within that code category.
- Assign four-digit codes only if there is no fifth-digit subclassification for that category.
- Assign the fifth-digit subclassification code for those categories where it exists.

  1.3. Other (NEC) and Unspecified (NOS) Code Titles

    Codes labeled "other specified" (NEC—not elsewhere classified) or "unspecified" (NOS—not otherwise specified) are used only when neither the diagnostic statement nor a thorough review of the medical record provides adequate information to permit assignment of a more specific code.

- Use the code assignment for "other" or NEC when the information at hand specifies a condition but no separate code for that condition is provided.
- Use "unspecified" (NOS) when the information at hand does not permit either a more specific or "other" code assignment.
- When the Alphabetic Index assigns a code to a category labeled "other (NEC)" or to a category labeled "unspecified (NOS)", refer to the Tabular List and review the titles and inclusion terms in the subdivisions under that particular three-digit category (or subdivision under the four-digit code) to determine if the information at hand can be appropriately assigned to a more specific code.

  1.4. Acute and Chronic Conditions

    If the same condition is described as both acute (subacute) and chronic and separate subentries exist in the Alphabetic Index at the same indentation level, code both and sequence the acute (subacute) code first.

  1.5. Combination Code

    A single code used to classify two diagnoses or a diagnosis with an associated secondary process (manifestation) or an associated complication is called a combination code. Combination codes are identified by referring to subterm entries in the Alphabetic Index and by reading the inclusion and exclusion notes in the Tabular List.

    Assign only the combination code when that code fully identifies the diagnostic conditions involved or when the Alphabetic Index so directs. Multiple coding should not be used when the classification provides a combination code that clearly identifies all of the elements documented in the diagnosis. When the combination code lacks necessary specificity in describing the manifestation or complication, an additional code may be used as a secondary code.

  1.6. Multiple Coding of Diagnoses

    Multiple coding is required for certain conditions not subject to the rules for combination codes.

    Instruction for conditions that require multiple coding appear in the Alphabetic Index and the Tabular List.

    A. Alphabetic Index: Codes for both etiology and manifestation of a disease appear following the subentry term, with the second code in brackets. Assign both codes in the same sequence in which they appear in the Alphabetic Index.

    B. Tabular List: Instructional terms, such as "Code first...," "Use additional code for any...," and "Note...," indicate when to use more than one code.

- "Code first underlying disease" - Assign the codes for both the manifestation and underlying cause. The codes for manifestations cannot be used (designated) as principal diagnosis.
- "Use additional code, to identify manifestation, as ..." - Assign also the code that identifies the manifestation, such as, but not limited to, the examples listed. The codes for manifestations cannot be used (designated) as principal diagnosis.

    C. Apply multiple coding instructions throughout the classification where appropriate, whether or not multiple coding directions appear in the Alphabetic Index or the Tabular List. Avoid indiscriminate multiple coding or irrelevant information, such as symptoms or signs characteristic of the diagnosis.

1.7. Late Effect

A late effect is the residual effect (condition produced) after the acute phase of an illness or injury has terminated. There is no time limit on when a late effect code can be used. The residual may be apparent early, such as in cerebrovascular accident cases, or it may occur months or years later, such as that due to a previous injury.

Coding of late effects requires two codes:

- The residual condition or nature of the late effect
- The cause of the late effect

The residual condition or nature of the late effect is sequenced first, followed by the cause of the late effect, except in those few instances where the code for late effect is followed by a manifestation code identified in the Tabular List and title or the late effect code has been expanded (at the fourth and fifth-digit levels) to include the manifestation(s).

The code for the acute phase of an illness or injury that led to the late effect is never used with a code for the cause of the late effect.

A. Late Effects of Cerebrovascular Disease

Category 438 is used to indicate conditions classifiable to categories 430-437 as the causes of late effects (neurologic deficits), themselves classified elsewhere. These "late effects" include neurologic deficits that persist after initial onset of conditions classifiable to 430-437. The neurologic deficits caused by cerebrovascular disease may be present from the onset or may arise at any time after the onset of the condition classifiable to 430–437.

- Codes from category 438 may be assigned on a health care record with codes from 430–437, if the patient has a current CVA and deficits from an old CVA.
- Assign code V12.59 (and not a code from category 438) as an additional code for history of cerebrovascular disease when no neurologic deficits are present.

1.8. Uncertain Diagnosis

If the diagnosis documented at the time of discharge is qualified as "probable", "suspected", "likely", "questionable", "possible", or "still to be ruled out", code the condition as if it existed or was established. The bases for this guidelines are the diagnostic workup, arrangements for further workup or observation, and initial therapeutic approach that correspond most closely with the established diagnosis.

1.9. Impending or Threatened Condition

Code any condition described at the time of discharge as "impending" or "threatened" as follows:

If it did occur, code as confirmed diagnosis.

If it did not occur, reference the Alphabetic Index to determine if the condition has a subentry term for "impending" or "threatened" and also reference main term entries for Impending and for Threatened.

- If the subterms are listed, assign the given code.
- If the subterms are not listed, code the existing forerunner condition(s) and not the condition described as impending or threatened.

2. SELECTION OF PRINCIPAL DIAGNOSIS

The circumstances of inpatient admission always govern the selection of principal diagnosis. The principal diagnosis is defined in the Uniform Hospital Discharge Data Set (UHDDS) as "that condition established after study to be chiefly responsible for occasioning the admission of the patient to the hospital for care".

In determining principal diagnosis the coding directives in the ICD-9-CM manuals, Volumes I, II, and III, take precedence over all other guidelines.

The importance of consistent, complete documentation in the medical record cannot be overemphasized. Without such documentation the application of all coding guidelines is a difficult, if not impossible, task.

2.1. Codes for symptoms, signs, and ill-defined conditions

Codes for symptoms, signs, and ill-defined conditions from Chapter 16 are not to be used as principal diagnosis when a related definitive diagnosis has been established.

2.2. Codes in brackets

Codes in brackets in the Alphabetic Index can never be sequenced as principal diagnosis. Coding directives require that the codes in brackets be sequenced in the order as they appear in the Alphabetic Index.

2.3. Acute and chronic conditions

If the same condition is described as both acute (subacute) and chronic and separate subentries exist in the Alphabetic Index at the same indentation level, code both and sequence the acute (subacute) code first.

2.4. Two or more interrelated conditions, each potentially meeting the definition for principal diagnosis

When there are two or more interrelated conditions (such as diseases in the same ICD-9-CM chapter or manifestations characteristically associated with a certain disease) potentially meeting the definition of principal diagnosis, either condition may be sequenced first, unless the circumstances of the admission, the therapy provided, the Tabular List, or the Alphabetic Index indicate otherwise.

2.5.   Two or more diagnoses that equally meet the definition for principal diagnosis

In the unusual instance when two or more diagnoses equally meet the criteria for principal diagnosis as determined by the circumstances of admission, diagnostic workup and/or therapy provided, and the Alphabetic Index, Tabular List, or another coding guidelines does not provide sequencing direction, any one of the diagnoses may be sequenced first.

2.6.   Two or more comparative or contrasting conditions

In those rare instances when two or more contrasting or comparative diagnoses are documented as "either/or" (or similar terminology), they are coded as if the diagnoses were confirmed and the diagnoses are sequenced according to the circumstances of the admission. If no further determination can be made as to which diagnosis should be principal, either diagnosis may be sequenced first.

2.7.   A symptom(s) followed by contrasting/comparative diagnoses

When a symptom(s) is followed by contrasting/comparative diagnoses, the symptom code is sequenced first. All the contrasting/comparative diagnoses should be coded as suspected conditions.

2.8.   Codes from the V71.0-V71.9 series, Observation and evaluation for suspected conditions

Codes from the V71.0-V71.9 series are assigned as principal diagnoses for encounters or admissions to evaluate the patient's condition when there is some evidence to suggest the existence of an abnormal condition or following an accident or other incident that ordinarily results in a health problem, and where no supporting evidence for the suspected condition is found and no treatment is currently required. The fact that the patient may be scheduled for continuing observation in the office/clinic setting following discharge does not limit the use of this category.

2.9.   Original treatment plan not carried out

Sequence as the principal diagnosis the condition which after study occasioned the admission to the hospital, even though treatment may not have been carried out due to unforeseen circumstances.

2.10.   Residual condition or nature of late effect

The residual condition or nature of the late effect is sequenced first, followed by the late

effect code for the cause of the residual condition, except in a few instances where the Alphabetic Index or Tabular List directs otherwise.

2.11.   Multiple burns

Sequence first the code that reflects the highest degree of burn when more than one burn is present. (See also Burns guideline 8.3)

2.12.   Multiple injuries

When multiple injuries exist, the code for the most severe injury as determined by the attending physician is sequenced first.

2.13.   Neoplasms

A.   If the treatment is directed at the malignancy, designate the malignancy as the principal diagnosis, except when the purpose of the encounter or hospital admission is for radiotherapy session(s), V58.0, or for chemotherapy session(s), V58.1, in which instance the malignancy is coded and sequenced second.

B.   When a patient is admitted for the purpose of radiotherapy or chemotherapy and develops complications such as uncontrolled nausea and vomiting or dehydration, the principal diagnosis is Encounter for radiotherapy, V58.0, or Encounter for chemotherapy, V58.1.

C.   When an episode of inpatient care involves surgical removal of a primary site or secondary site malignancy followed by adjunct chemotherapy or radiotherapy, code the malignancy as the principal diagnosis, using codes in the 140-198 series or where appropriate in the 200-203 series.

D.   When the reason for admission is to determine the extent of the malignancy, or for a procedure such as paracentesis or thoracentesis, the primary malignancy or appropriate metastatic site is designated as the principal diagnosis, even though chemotherapy or radiotherapy is administered.

E.   When the primary malignancy has been previously excised or eradicated from its site and there is not adjunct treatment directed to that site and no evidence of any remaining malignancy at the primary site, use the appropriate code from the V10 series to indicate the former site of primary malignancy. Any mention of extension, invasion, or metastasis to a nearby structure or organ or to a distant site is coded as a secondary malignant neoplasm to that site and may be the principal diagnosis in the absence of the primary site.

Coding Guidelines—Inpatient

F. When a patient is admitted because of a primary neoplasm with metastasis and treatment is directed toward the secondary site only, the secondary neoplasm is designated as the principal diagnosis even though the primary malignancy is still present.

G. Symptoms, signs, and ill-defined conditions listed in Chapter 16 characteristic of, or associated with, an existing primary or secondary site malignancy cannot be used to replace the malignancy as principal diagnosis, regardless of the number of admissions or encounters for treatment and care of the neoplasm.

H. Coding and sequencing of complications associated with the malignant neoplasm or with the therapy thereof are subject to the following guidelines:

- When admission is for management of an anemia associated with the malignancy, and the treatment is only for anemia, the anemia is designated at the principal diagnosis and is followed by the appropriate code(s) for the malignancy.

- When the admission is for management of an anemia associated with chemotherapy or radiotherapy and the only treatment is for the anemia, the anemia is designated as the principal diagnosis followed by the appropriate code(s) for the malignancy.

- When the admission is for management of dehydration due to the malignancy or the therapy, or a combination of both, and only the dehydration is being treated (intravenous rehydration), the dehydration is designated as the principal diagnosis, followed by the code(s) for the malignancy.

- When the admission is for treatment of a complication resulting from a surgical procedure performed for the treatment of an intestinal malignancy, designate the complication as the principal diagnosis if treatment is directed at resolving the complication.

2.14. Poisoning

When coding a poisoning or reaction to the improper use of a medication (e.g., wrong dose, wrong substance, wrong route of administration) the poisoning code is sequenced first, followed by a code for the manifestation. If there is also a diagnosis of drug abuse or dependence to the substance, the abuse or dependence is coded as an additional code.

2.15. Complications of surgery and other medical care

When the admission is for treatment of a complication resulting from surgery or other medical care, the complication code is sequenced as the principal diagnosis. If the complication is classified to the 996-999 series, an additional code for the specific complication may be assigned.

2.16. Complication of pregnancy

When a patient is admitted because of a condition that is either a complication pregnancy or that is complicating the pregnancy, the code for the obstetric complication is the principal diagnosis. An additional code may be assigned as needed to provide specificity.

3. REPORTING OTHER (ADDITIONAL) DIAGNOSES

A joint effort between the attending physician and coder is essential to achieve complete and accurate documentation, code assignment, and reporting of diagnoses and procedures.

These guidelines have been developed and approved by the Cooperating Parties to assure both the physician and the coder in identifying those diagnoses that are to be reported in addition to the principal diagnosis. Hospitals may record other diagnoses as needed for internal data use.

The UHDDS definitions are used by acute care short-term hospitals to report inpatient data elements in a standardized manner. These data elements and their definitions can be found in the July 31, 1985, Federal Register (Vol. 50, No, 147), pp. 31038-40.

The UHDDS item #11-b defines Other Diagnoses as "all conditions that coexist at the time of admission, that develop subsequently, or that affect the treatment received and/or the length of stay. Diagnoses that relate to an earlier episode which have no bearing on the current hospital stay are to be excluded".

General Rule

For reporting purposes the definition for "other diagnoses" is interpreted as additional conditions that affect patient care in terms of requiring:

- clinical evaluation; or
- therapeutic treatment; or
- diagnostic procedures; or
- extended length of hospital stay; or
- increased nursing care and/or monitoring.

The following guidelines are to be applied in designating "other diagnoses" when neither the Alphabetic Index nor the Tabular List in ICD-9-CM provide direction.

The listing of the diagnoses on the attestation statement is the responsibility of the attending physician.

3.1. Previous conditions

If the physician has included a diagnosis in the final diagnostic statement, such as the discharge summary or the face sheet, it should ordinarily be coded. Some physicians include in the diagnostic statement resolved conditions or diagnoses and status-post procedures from previous admission that have no bearing on the current stay. Such conditions are not to be reported and are coded only if required by hospital policy.

However, history codes (V10-V19) may be used as secondary codes if the historical condition or family history has an impact on current care or influences treatment.

3.2. Diagnoses not listed in the final diagnostic statement

When the physician has documented what appears to be a current diagnosis in the body of the record, but has not included the diagnosis in the final diagnostic statement, the physician should be asked whether the diagnosis should be added.

3.3. Conditions that are an integral part of a disease process

Conditions that are integral to the disease process should not be assigned as additional codes.

3.4. Conditions that are not an integral part of a disease process

Additional conditions that may not be associated routinely with a disease process should be coded when present.

3.5. Abnormal findings

Abnormal findings (laboratory, x-ray, pathologic, and other diagnostic results) are not coded and reported unless the physician indicates their clinical significance. If the findings are outside the normal range and the physician has ordered other tests to evaluate the condition or prescribed treatment, it is appropriate to ask the physician whether the diagnosis should be added.

4. HYPERTENSION

4.1. Hypertension, Essential, or NOS

Assign hypertension (arterial) (essential) (primary) (systemic) (NOS) to category code 401 with the appropriate fourth digit to indicate malignant (.0), benign (.1), or unspecified (.9). Do not use either .0 malignant or .1 benign unless medical record documentation supports such a designation.

4.2. Hypertension with Heart Disease

Certain heart conditions (425.8, 428, 429.0-429.3, 429.8, 429.9) are assigned to a code

from category 402 when a causal relationship is stated (due to hypertension) or implied (hypertensive). Use only the code from category 402.

The same heart conditions (425.8, 428, 429.0-429.3, 429.8, 429.9) with hypertension, but without a stated casual relationship, are coded separately. Sequence according to the circumstances of the admission.

4.3. Hypertensive Renal Disease with Chronic Renal Failure

Assign codes from category 403, Hypertensive renal disease, when conditions classified to categories 585-587 are present. Unlike hypertension with heart disease, ICD-9-CM presumes a cause-and-effect relationship and classifies renal failure with hypertension as hypertensive renal disease.

4.4. Hypertensive Heart and Renal Disease

Assign codes from combination category 404, Hypertensive heart and renal disease, when both hypertensive renal disease and hypertensive heart disease are stated in the diagnosis. Assume a relationship between the hypertension and the renal disease, whether or not the condition is so designated.

4.5. Hypertensive Cerebrovascular Disease.

First assign codes from 430-438, Cerebrovascular disease, then the appropriate hypertension code from categories 401-405.

4.6. Hypertensive Retinopathy

Two codes are necessary to identify the condition. First assign the code from subcategory 362.11, Hypertensive retinopathy, then the appropriate code from categories 401-405 to indicate the type of hypertension.

4.7. Hypertension, Secondary

Two codes are required: one to identify the underlying condition and one from category 405 to identify the hypertension. Sequencing of codes is determined by the reason for admission to the hospital.

4.8. Hypertension, Transient

Assign code 796.2, Elevated blood pressure reading without diagnosis of hypertension, unless patient has an established diagnosis of hypertension. Assign code 642.3x for transient hypertension of pregnancy.

4.9. Hypertension, Controlled

Assign appropriate code from categories 401-405. This diagnostic statement usually refers to an existing state of hypertension under control by therapy.

4.10. Hypertension, Uncontrolled

Uncontrolled hypertension may refer to untreated hypertension or hypertension not responding to current therapeutic regimen. In either case. assign the appropriate code from categories 401-405 to designate the stage and type of hypertension. Code to the type of hypertension.

4.11. Elevated Blood Pressure

For a statement of elevated blood pressure without further specificity, assign code 796.2, Elevated blood pressure reading without diagnosis of hypertension, rather than a code from category 401.

5. OBSTETRICS

Introduction

These guidelines have been developed and approved by the Cooperating Parties in conjunction with the Editorial Advisory Board of Coding Clinic and the American College of Obstetricians and Gynecologists, to assist the coder in coding and reporting obstetric cases. Where feasible, previously published advice has been incorporated. Some advice in these new guidelines may supersede previous advice. The guidelines are provided for reporting purposes. Health care facilities may record additional diagnoses as needed for internal data needs.

5.1. General Rules

A. Obstetric cases require codes from chapter 11, codes in the range 630-677, Complications of Pregnancy, Childbirth, and the Puerperium. Should the physician document that the pregnancy is incidental to the encounter then code V22.2 should be used in place of any chapter 11 codes. It is the physician's responsibility to state that the condition being treated is not affecting the pregnancy.

B. Chapter 11 codes have sequencing priority over codes from other chapters. Additional codes from other chapters may be used in conjunction with chapter 11 codes to further specify conditions.

C. Chapter 11 codes are to be used only on the maternal record, never on the record of the newborn.

D. An outcome of delivery code, V27.0-V27.9, should be included on every maternal record when a delivery has occurred. These codes are not to be used on subsequent records or on the newborn record.

5.2. Selection of Principal Diagnosis

A. The circumstances of the encounter govern the selection of the principal diagnosis.

B. In episodes when no delivery occurs the principal diagnosis should correspond to the principal complication of the pregnancy which necessitated the encounter. Should more than one complication exist, all of which are treated or monitored, any of the complications codes may be sequenced first.

C. When a delivery occurs the principal diagnosis should correspond to the main circumstances or complication of the delivery. In cases of cesarean deliveries, the principal diagnosis should correspond to the reason the cesarean was performed, unless the reason for admission was unrelated to the condition resulting in the cesarean delivery.

D. For routine prenatal visits when no complications are present codes V22.0, Supervision of normal first pregnancy, and V22.1, Supervision of other normal pregnancy, should be used as principal diagnoses. These codes should not be used in conjunction with chapter 11 codes.

E. For prenatal outpatient visits for patients with high-risk pregnancies, a code from category V23, Supervision of high-risk pregnancy, should be used as the principal diagnosis. Secondary chapter 11 codes may be used in conjunction with these codes if appropriate. A thorough review of any pertinent excludes note is necessary to be certain that these V codes are being used properly.

5.3. Chapter 11 Fifth-digits

A. Categories 640-648, 651-676 have required fifth-digits which indicate whether the encounter is antepartum, postpartum and whether a delivery has also occurred.

B. The fifth-digits which are appropriate for each code number are listed in brackets under each code. The fifth-digits on each code should all be consistent with each other. That is, should a delivery occur all of the fifth-digits should indicate the delivery.

5.4. Fetal Conditions Affecting the Management of the Mother.

Codes from category 655, Known or suspected fetal abnormality affecting management of the mother, and category 656, Other fetal and placental problems affecting the management of the mother, are assigned only when the fetal condition is actually responsible for modifying the management of the mother, i.e., by requiring diagnostic studies, additional observation, special care, or termination of pregnancy. The fact that the fetal condition exists does not justify assigning a code from this series to the mother's record.

5.5. Normal Delivery, 650

A. Code 650 is for use in cases when a woman is admitted for a full-term normal delivery and delivers a single, healthy infant without any complications antepartum, during the delivery, or postpartum during the delivery episode.

B. 650 may be used if the patient had a complications at some point during her pregnancy but the complication is not present at the time of the admission for delivery.

C. Code 650 is always a principal diagnosis. It is not to be used if any other code from chapter 11 is needed to describe a current complication of the antenatal, delivery, or perinatal period. Additional codes from other chapters may be used with code 650 if they are not related to or are in any way complicating the pregnancy.

D. V27.0, Single liveborn, is the only outcome of delivery code appropriate for use with 650.

5.6. Procedure Codes

A. In cases of cesarean delivery, the selection of the principal diagnosis should correspond to the reason the cesarean delivery was performed unless the reason for admission was unrelated to the condition resulting in the cesarean delivery.

B. A delivery procedure code should not be used for a woman who has delivered prior to admission to the hospital. Any postpartum repairs should be coded.

5.7. The Postpartum Period

A. The postpartum period begins immediately after delivery and continues for 6 weeks following delivery.

B. A postpartum complication is any complication occurring within the 6 week period.

C. Chapter 11 codes may also be used to describe pregnancy-related complications after the 6 week period should the physician document that a condition is pregnancy related.

D. Postpartum complications that occur during the same admission as the delivery are identified with a fifth digit of "2". Subsequent admissions for postpartum complications should identified with a fifth digit of "4".

E. When the mother delivers outside the hospital prior to admission and is admitted for routine postpartum care and no complications are noted, code V24.0, Postpartum care and examination immediately after delivery, should be assigned as the principal diagnosis.

5.8. Abortions

A. Fifth-digits are required for abortion categories 634-637. Fifth-digit 1, incomplete, indicates that all of the products of conception have not been expelled from the uterus. Fifth-digit 2, complete, indicates that all products of conception have been expelled from the uterus prior to the episode of care.

B. A code from categories 640-648 and 651-657 may be used as additional codes with an abortion code to indicate the complication leading to the abortion.

Fifth digit 3 is assigned with codes from these categories when used with an abortion code because the other fifth digits will not apply. Codes from the 660-669 series are not to be used for complications of abortion.

C. Code 639 is to be used for all complications following abortion. Code 639 cannot be assigned with codes from categories 634-638.

D. Abortion with Liveborn Fetus. When an attempted termination of pregnancy results in a liveborn fetus assign code 644.21, Early onset of delivery, with an appropriate code from category V27, Outcome of Delivery. The procedure code for the attempted termination of pregnancy should also be assigned.

E. Retained Products of Conception following an abortion. Subsequent admissions for retained products of conception following a spontaneous or legally induced abortion are assigned the appropriate code from category 634, Spontaneous abortion, or legally induced abortion, with a fifth digit of "1" (incomplete). This advice is appropriate even when the patient was discharged previously with a discharge diagnosis of complete abortion.

5.9. Code 677, Late effect of complication of pregnancy, childbirth, and the puerperium

A. Code 677, Late effect of complication of pregnancy, childbirth, and the puerperium is for use in those cases when an initial complication of a pregnancy develops a sequelae requiring care or treatment at a future date.

B. This code may be used at any time after the initial postpartum period.

C. This code, like all late effect codes, is to be sequenced following the code describing the sequelae of the complication.

6. NEWBORN GUIDELINES

Definition

The newborn period is defined as beginning at birth and lasting through the 28th day following birth.

The following guidelines are provided for reporting purposes. Hospitals may record other diagnoses as needed for internal data use.

General Rule

All clinically significant conditions noted on routine newborn examination should be coded. A condition is clinically significant if it requires:

- clinical evaluation; or
- therapeutic treatment; or
- diagnostic procedures; or
- extended length of hospital stay; or
- increased nursing care and/or monitoring; or
- has implications for future health care needs.

Note: The newborn guidelines listed above are the same as the general coding guidelines for "other diagnoses," except for the final bullet regarding implications for future health care needs. Whether or not a condition is clinically significant can only be determined by the physician.

6.1. Use of Codes V30-V39

When coding the birth of an infant, assign a code from categories V30-V39, according to the type of birth. A code from this series is assigned as a principal diagnosis, and assigned only once to a newborn at the time of birth.

6.2. Newborn Transfers

If the newborn is transferred to another institution, the V30 series is not used.

6.3. Use of Category V29

A. Assign a code from category V29, Observation and evaluation of newborns and infants for suspected conditions not found, to identify those instances when a healthy newborn is evaluated for a suspected condition that is determined after study not to be present. Do not use a code from category V29 when the patient has identified signs or symptoms of a suspected problem; in such cases, code the sign or symptom.

B. A V29 code is to be used as a secondary code after the V30, Outcome of delivery, code. It may also be assigned as a principal code for readmissions or encounters when the V30 code no longer applies. It is for use only for healthy newborns and infants for which no condition after study is found to be present.

6.4. Maternal Causes of Perinatal Morbidity

Codes from categories 760-763, Maternal causes of perinatal morbidity and mortality, are assigned only when the maternal condition has actually affected the fetus or newborn. The fact that the mother has an associated medical condition or experiences some complication of pregnancy, labor or delivery does not justify the routine assignment of codes from these categories to the newborn record.

6.5. Congenital Anomalies

Assign an appropriate code from categories 740-759, Congenital Anomalies, when a specific abnormality is diagnosed for an infant. Such abnormalities may occur as a set of symptoms or multiple malformations. A code should be assigned for each presenting manifestation of the syndrome if the syndrome is not specifically indexed in ICD-9-CM.

6.6. Coding of Other (Additional) Diagnoses

A. Assign codes for conditions that require treatment or further investigation, prolong the length of stay, or require resource utilization.

B. Assign codes for conditions that have been specified by the physician as having implications for future health care needs.

NOTE: This guideline should not be used for adult patients.

C. Assign a code for Newborn conditions originating in the perinatal period (categories 760-779), as well as complications arising during the current episode of care classified in other chapters, only if the diagnoses have been documented by the responsible physician at the time of transfer or discharge as having affected the fetus or newborn.

D. Insignificant conditions or signs or symptoms that resolve without treatment are not coded.

6.7. Prematurity and Fetal Growth Retardation

Codes from categories 764 and 765 should not be assigned based solely on recorded birthweight or estimated gestational age, but upon the attending physician's clinical assessment of maturity of the infant.

NOTE: Since physicians may utilize different criteria in determining prematurity, do not code the diagnosis of prematurity unless the physician documents this condition.

7. SEPTICEMIA AND SEPTIC SHOCK

When the diagnosis of septicemia with shock or the diagnosis of general sepsis with septic shock is documented, code and list the septicemia first and report the septic shock code as a secondary condition. The septicemia code assignment should identify the type of bacteria if it is known.

Sepsis and septic shock associated with abortion, ectopic pregnancy, and molar pregnancy are classified to category codes in Chapter 11 (630-639).

Negative or inconclusive blood cultures do not preclude a diagnosis of septicemia in patients with clinical evidence of the condition.

8. TRAUMA

8.1. Coding for Multiple Injuries

When coding multiple injuries such as fracture of tibia and fibula, assign separate codes for each injury unless a combination code is provided, in which case the combination code is assigned. Multiple injury codes are provided in ICD-9-CM, but should not be assigned unless information for a more specific code is not available.

A. The code for the most serious injury, as determined by the physician, is sequenced first.

B. Superficial injuries such as abrasions or contusions are not coded when associated with more severe injuries of the same site.

C. When a primary injury results in minor damage to peripheral nerves or blood vessels, the primary injury is sequenced first with additional code(s) from categories 950-957, Injury to nerves and spinal cord, and/or 900-904, Injury to blood vessels. When the primary injury is to the blood vessels or nerves, that injury should be sequenced first.

8.2. Coding for Multiple Fractures

The principle of multiple coding of injuries should be followed in coding multiple fractures. Multiple fractures of specified sites are coded individually by site in accordance with both the provisions within categories 800-829 and the level of detail furnished by medical record content. Combination categories for multiple fractures are provided for use when there is insufficient detail in the medical record (such as trauma cases transferred to another hospital), when the reporting form limits the number of codes that can be used in reporting pertinent clinical data, or when there is insufficient specificity at the fourth-digit or fifth-digit level. More specific guidelines are as follows:

A. Multiple fractures of same limb classifiable to the same three-digit or four-digit category are coded to that category.

B. Multiple unilateral or bilateral fractures of same bone(s) but classified to different fourth-digit subdivisions (bone part) within the same three-digit category are coded individually by site.

C. Multiple fracture categories 819 and 828 classify bilateral fractures of both upper limbs (819) and both lower limbs (828), but without any detail at the fourth-digit level other than open and closed type of fractures.

D. Multiple fractures are sequenced in accordance with the severity of the fracture and the physician should be asked to list the fracture diagnoses in the order of severity.

8.3. Current Burns and Encounters for Late Effects of Burns

Current burns (940-948) are classified by depth, extent and, if desired, by agent (E code). By depth burns are classified as first degree (erythema), second degree (blistering), and third degree (full-thickness involvement).

A. All burns are coded with the highest degree of burn sequenced first.

B. Classify burns of the same local site (three-digit category level, (940-947) but of different degrees to the subcategory identifying the highest degree recorded in the diagnosis.

C. Non-healing burns are coded as acute burns. Necrosis of burned skin should be coded as a non-healed burn.

D. Assign code 958.3, Posttraumatic wound infection, not elsewhere classified, as an additional code for any documented infected burn site.

E. When coding multiple burns, assign separate codes for each burn site. Category 946 Burns of Multiple specified sites, should only be used if the location of the burns are not documented. Category 949, Burn, unspecified, is extremely vague and should rarely be used.

F. Assign codes from category 948, Burns classified according to extent of body surface involved, when the site of the burn is not specified or when there is a need for additional data. It is advisable to use category 948 as additional coding when needed to provide data for evaluating burn mortality, such as that needed by burn units. It is also advisable to use category 948 as an additional code for reporting purposes when there is mention of a third-degree burn involving 20 percent or more of the body surface. In assigning a code from category 948:

- Four-digit codes are used to identify the percentage of total body surface involved in a burn (all degree).

- Fifth-digits are assigned to identify the percentage of body surface involved in third-degree burn.

- Fifth-digit zero (0) is assigned when less than 10 percent or when no body surface is involved in a third-degree burn.

Category 948 is based on the classic "rule of nines" in estimating body surface involved: head and neck are assigned nine percent, each arm nine percent, each leg 18 percent, the anterior trunk 18 percent, posterior trunk 18 percent, and genitalia one percent. Physicians may change these percentage assignments where necessary to accommodate infants and children who have proportionately larger heads than adults and patients who have large buttocks, thighs, or abdomen that involve burns.

G. Encounters for the treatment of the late effects of burns (i.e., scars or joint contractures) should be coded to the residual condition (sequelae) followed by the appropriate late effect code (906.5-906.9). A late effect E code may also be used, if desired.

H. When appropriate, both a sequelae with a late effect code, and a current burn code may be assigned on the same record.

8.4. Debridement of Wound, Infection, or Burn

A. For coding purposes, excisional debridement, 86.22, is assigned only when the procedure is performed by a physician.

B. For coding purposes, nonexcisional debridement performed by the physician or nonphysician health care professional is assigned to 86.28. Any "excisional" type procedure performed by a nonphysician is assigned to 86. 28.

9. ADVERSE EFFECTS AND POISONING

The properties of certain drugs, medicinal and biological substances or combinations of such substances, may cause toxic reactions. The occurrence of drug toxicity is classified in ICD-9-CM as follows:

9.1. Adverse Effect

When the drug was correctly prescribed and properly administered, code the reaction plus the appropriate code from the E930-E949 series.

Adverse effects of therapeutic substances correctly prescribed and properly administered (toxicity, synergistic reaction, side effect, and idiosyncratic reaction) may be due to (1) differences among patients, such as age, sex, disease, and genetic factors, and (2) drug-related factors, such as type of drug, route of administration, duration of therapy, dosage, and bioavailability.

Codes from the E930-E949 series must be used to identify the causative substance for an adverse effect of drug, medicinal and biological substances, correctly prescribed and properly administered. The effect, such as tachycardia, delirium, gastrointestinal hemorrhaging, vomiting, hypokalemia, hepatitis, renal failure, or respiratory failure, is coded and followed by the appropriate code from the E930-E949 series.

9.2. Poisoning

Poisoning when an error was made in drug prescription or in the administration of the drug by physician, nurse, patient, or other person, use the appropriate code from the 960-979 series. If an overdose of a drug was intentionally taken or administered and resulted in drug toxicity, it would be coded as a poisoning (960-979 series). If a nonprescribed drug or medicinal agent was taken in combination with a correctly prescribed and properly administered drug, any drug toxicity or other reaction resulting from the interaction of the two drugs would be classified as a poisoning.

10. HUMAN IMMUNODEFICIENCY VIRUS (HIV) INFECTIONS

10.1. Code only confirmed cases of HIV infection/illness.

This is an exception to guideline 1.8 which states "If the diagnosis documented at the time of discharge is qualified as 'probable,' 'suspected,' 'likely,' 'questionable,' 'possible,' or 'still to be ruled out,' code the condition as if it existed or was established..."

In this context, "confirmation" does not require documentation of positive serology or culture for HIV; the physician's diagnostic statement that the patient is HIV positive, or has an HIV-related illness is sufficient.

10.2. Selection of HIV code

042 Human Immunodeficiency Virus [HIV] Disease

Patients with an HIV-related illness should be coded to 042, Human Immunodeficiency Virus [HIV] Disease.

V08 Asymptomatic Human Immunodeficiency Virus [HIV] Infection

Patients with physician-documented asymptomatic HIV infections who have never had an HIV-related illness should be coded to V08, Asymptomatic Human Immunodeficiency Virus [HIV] Infection.

795.71 Nonspecific Serologic Evidence of Human Immunodeficiency Virus [HIV]

Code 795.71, Nonspecific serologic evidence of human immunodeficiency virus [HIV], should be used for patients (including infants) with inconclusive HIV test results.

10.3. Previously diagnosed HIV-related illness

Patients with any known prior diagnosis of an HIV-related illness should be coded to 042. Once a patient had developed an HIV-related illness, the patient should always be assigned code 042 on every subsequent admission. Patients previously diagnosed with any HIV illness (042) should never be assigned to 795.71 or V 08.

10.4. Sequencing

The sequencing of diagnoses for patients with HIV-related illnesses follows guideline 2 for selection of principal diagnosis. That is, the circumstances of admission govern the selection of principal diagnosis, "that condition established after study to be chiefly responsible for occasioning the admission of the patient to the hospital for care."

Patients who are admitted for an HIV-related illness should be assigned a minimum of two codes: first assign code 042 to identify the HIV disease and then sequence additional codes to identify the other diagnoses. If a patient is admitted for an HIV-related condition, the principal diagnosis should be 042, followed by additional diagnosis codes for all reported HIV-related conditions.

If a patient with HIV disease is admitted for an unrelated condition (such as a traumatic injury), the code for the unrelated condition (e.g., the nature of injury code) should be the principal diagnosis. Other diagnoses would be 042 followed by additional diagnosis codes for all reported HIV-related conditions.

Whether the patient is newly diagnosed or has had previous admissions for HIV conditions (or has expired) is irrelevant to the sequencing decision.

10.5. HIV Infection in Pregnancy, Childbirth and the Puerperium

During pregnancy, childbirth or the puerperium, a patient admitted because of an HIV-related illness should receive a principal diagnosis of 647.6X, Other specified infectious and parasitic diseases in the mother classifiable elsewhere, but complicating the pregnancy, childbirth or the puerperium, followed by 042 and the code(s) for the HIV-related illness(es). This is an exception to the sequencing rule found in 10.4 above.

Patients with asymptomatic HIV infection status admitted during pregnancy, childbirth, or the puerperium should receive codes of 647.6X and V08.

10.6. Asymptomatic HIV Infection

V08 Asymptomatic human immunodeficiency virus [HIV] infection, is to be applied when the patient without any documentation of symptoms is listed as being "HIV positive," "known HIV," "HIV test positive," or similar terminology. Do not use this code if the term "AIDS" is used or if the patient is treated for any HIV-related illness or is described as having any condition(s) resulting from his/her HIV positive status; use 042 in these cases.

10.7. Inconclusive Laboratory Test for HIV

Patients with inconclusive HIV serology, but no definitive diagnosis or manifestations of the illness may be assigned code 795.71.Inconclusive serologic test for Human Immunodeficiency Virus [HIV]

10.8. Testing for HIV

If the patient is asymptomatic but wishes to know his/her HIV status, use code V73.89, Screening for other specified viral disease. Use code V69.8, Other problems related to lifestyle, as a secondary code if an asymptomatic patient is in a known high-risk group for HIV. Should a patient with signs or symptoms or illness, or a confirmed HIV related diagnosis be tested for HIV code the signs and symptoms or the diagnosis. An additional counseling code V65.44 may be used if counseling is provided during the encounter for the test.

When the patient returns to be informed of his/her HIV test results use code V65.44, HIV counseling, if the results of the test are negative. If the results are positive but the patient is asymptomatic use code V08, Asymptomatic HIV infection. If the results are positive and the patient is symptomatic use code 042, HIV infection, with codes for the HIV related symptoms or diagnosis. The HIV counseling code may also be used if counseling is provided for patients with positive test results.

11. GUIDELINES FOR CODING EXTERNAL CAUSES OF INJURIES, POISONINGS AND ADVERSE EFFECTS OF DRUGS (E Codes)

Introduction

These guidelines are provided for those who are currently collecting E codes in order that there will be standardization in the process. If your institution plans to begin collecting E codes, these guidelines are to be applied. The use of E codes are supplemental to the application of basic ICD-9-CM codes. E codes are never to be recorded as principal diagnosis (first listed in the outpatient setting) and are not required for reporting to the Health Care Financing Administration.

Injuries are a major cause of mortality, morbidity and disability. In the United States, the care of patients who suffer intentional and unintentional injuries and poisonings contributes significantly to the increase in medical care costs. External causes of injury and poisoning codes (E codes) are intended to provide data for injury research and evaluation of injury prevention strategies. E codes capture how the injury or poisoning happened (cause), the intent (unintentional or accidental; or intentional, such as suicide or assault), and the place where the event occurred. Some major categories of E codes include:

- transport accidents
- poisoning and adverse effects of drugs, medicinal substances and biologicals
- accidental falls
- accidents caused by fire and flames
- accidents due to natural and environmental factors
- late effects of accidents, assaults or self injury
- assaults or purposely inflicted injury
- suicide or self inflicted injury

These guidelines apply for the coding and collection of E code from records in hospitals, outpatient clinics, emergency departments, other ambulatory care settings and physician offices except when other specific guidelines apply. (See Reporting Diagnostic Guidelines for Hospital-based Outpatient Services/Reporting Requirements for Physician Billing.)

11.1. General E Code Coding Guidelines

A. An E code may be used with any code in the range of 001-V83.89 which indicates an injury, poisoning, or adverse effect due to an external cause.

B. Assign the appropriate E-code for all initial treatments of an injury, poisoning, or adverse effect of drugs.

C. Use a late effect E code for subsequent visits when a late effect of the initial injury or poisoning is being treated. There is no late effect E code for adverse effects of drugs.

D. Use the full range of E codes to completely describe the cause, the intent and the place of occurrence, if applicable, for all injuries, poisonings, and adverse effects of drugs.

E. Assign as many E codes as necessary to fully explain each cause. If only one E code can be recorded, assign the E code most related to the principal diagnosis.

F. The selection of the appropriate E code is guided by the Index to External Causes which is located after the alphabetical index to diseases and by Inclusion and Exclusion notes in the Tabular List.

G. An E code can never be a principal (first listed) diagnosis.

11.2. Place of Occurrence Guideline

Use an additional code from category E849 to indicate the Place of Occurrence for injuries and poisonings. The Place of Occurrence describes the place where the event occurred and not the patient's activity at the time of the event.

Do not use E849.9 if the place of occurrence is not stated.

11.3. Poisonings and Adverse Effects of Drugs, Medicinal and Biological Substances Guidelines

A. Do not code directly from the Table of Drugs and Chemicals. Always refer back to the Tabular List.

B. Use as many codes as necessary to describe completely all drugs, medicinal or biological substances.

C. If the same E code would describe the causative agent for more than one adverse reaction, assign the code only once.

D. If two or more drugs, medicinal or biological substances are reported, code each individually unless the combination code is listed in the Table of Drugs and Chemicals. In that case, assign the E code for the combination.

E. When a reaction results from the interaction of a drug(s) and alcohol, use poisoning codes and E codes for both.

F. If the reporting format limits the number of E codes that can be used in reporting clinical data, code the one most related to the principal diagnosis. Include at least one from each category (cause, intent, place) if possible.

- If there are different fourth digit codes in the same three digit category, use the code for "Other specified" of that category. If there is no "Other specified" code in that category, use the appropriate "Unspecified" code in that category.

- If the codes are in different three digit categories, assign the appropriate E code for other multiple drugs and medicinal substances.

11.4. Multiple Cause E Code Coding Guidelines

If two or more events cause separate injuries, an E code should be assigned for each cause. The first listed E code will be selected in the following order:

- E codes for child and adult abuse take priority over all other E code—see Child and Adult abuse guidelines
- E codes for cataclysmic events take priority over all other E codes except child and adult abuse
- E codes for transport accidents take priority over all other E codes except cataclysmic events and child and adult abuse

The first listed E code should correspond to the cause of the most serious diagnosis due to an assault, accident, or self-harm, following the order of hierarchy listed above.

11.5. Child and Adult Abuse Guideline

    A.   When the cause of an injury or neglect is intentional child or adult abuse, the first listed E code should be assigned from categories E960-E968, Homicide and injury purposely inflicted by other persons, (except category E967). An E code from category E967, Child and adult battering and other maltreatment, should be added as an additional code to identify the perpetrator, if known.

    B.   In cases of neglect when the intent is determined to be accidental E code E904.0, Abandonment or neglect of infant and helpless person, should be the first listed E code.

11.6. Unknown or Suspected Intent Guideline

    A.   If the intent (accident, self-harm, assault) of the cause of an injury or poisoning is unknown or unspecified, code the intent as undetermined E980-E989.

    B.   If the intent (accident, self-harm, assault) of the cause of an injury or poisoning is questionable, probable or suspected, code the intent as undetermined E980-E989.

11.7. Undetermined Cause

When the intent of an injury or poisoning is known, but the cause is unknown, use codes: E928.9, Unspecified accident, E958.9, Suicide and self-inflicted injury by unspecified means, and E968.9, Assault by unspecified means.

These E codes should rarely be used as the documentation in the medical record, in both the inpatient and outpatient settings, should normally provide sufficient detail to determine the cause of the injury.

11.8. Late Effects of External Cause Guidelines

    A.   Late effect E codes exist for injuries and poisonings but not for adverse effects of drugs, misadventures and surgical complications.

    B.   A late effect E code (E929, E959, E969, E977, E989, or E999) should be used with any report of a late effect or sequela resulting from a previous injury or poisoning (905-909).

    C.   A late effect E code should nev er be used with a related current nature of injury code.

11.9. Misadventures and Complications of Care Guidelines

    A.   Assign a code in the range of E870-E876 if misadventures are stated by the physician.

    B.   Assign a code in the range of E878-E879 if the physician attributes an abnormal reaction or later complication to a surgical or medical procedure, but does not mention misadventure at the time of the procedure as the cause of the reaction.

A

AAV (disease) (illness) (infection) — *see* Human immunodeficiency virus (disease) (illness) (infection)

Abactio — *see* Abortion, induced

Abactus venter — *see* Abortion, induced

Abarognosis 781.99

Abasia (-astasia) 307.9
  atactica 781.3
  choreic 781.3
  hysterical 300.11
  paroxysmal trepidant 781.3
  spastic 781.3
  trembling 781.3
  trepidans 781.3

Abderhalden-Kaufmann-Lignac syndrome (cystinosis) 270.0

Abdomen, abdominal — *see also* condition
  accordion 306.4
  acute 789.0 ✔5ᵗʰ
  angina 557.1
  burst 868.00
  convulsive equivalent (*see also* Epilepsy) 345.5 ✔5ᵗʰ
  heart 746.87
  muscle deficiency syndrome 756.79
  obstipum 756.79

Abdominalgia 789.0 ✔5ᵗʰ
  periodic 277.3

Abduction contracture, hip or other joint — *see* Contraction, joint

Abercrombie's syndrome (amyloid degeneration) 277.3

Aberrant (congenital) — *see also* Malposition, congenital
  adrenal gland 759.1
  blood vessel NEC 747.60
    arteriovenous NEC 747.60
    cerebrovascular 747.81
    gastrointestinal 747.61
    lower limb 747.64
    renal 747.62
    spinal 747.82
    upper limb 747.63
  breast 757.6
  endocrine gland NEC 759.2
  gastrointestinal vessel (peripheral) 747.61
  hepatic duct 751.69
  lower limb vessel (peripheral) 747.64
  pancreas 751.7
  parathyroid gland 759.2
  peripheral vascular vessel NEC 747.60
  pituitary gland (pharyngeal) 759.2
  renal blood vessel 747.62
  sebaceous glands, mucous membrane, mouth 750.26
  spinal vessel 747.82
  spleen 759.0
  testis (descent) 752.51
  thymus gland 759.2
  thyroid gland 759.2
  upper limb vessel (peripheral) 747.63

Aberratio
  lactis 757.6
  testis 752.51

Aberration — *see also* Anomaly
  chromosome — *see* Anomaly, chromosome(s)
  distantial 368.9
  mental (*see also* Disorder, mental, nonpsychotic) 300.9

Abetalipoproteinemia 272.5

Abionarce 780.79

Abiotrophy 799.8

Ablatio
  placentae — *see* Placenta, ablatio
  retinae (*see also* Detachment, retina) 361.9

Ablation
  pituitary (gland) (with hypofunction) 253.7
  placenta — *see* Placenta, ablatio
  uterus 621.8

Ablepharia, ablepharon, ablephary 743.62

Ablepsia — *see* Blindness

Ablepsy — *see* Blindness

Ablutomania 300.3

Abnormal, abnormality, abnormalities — *see also* Anomaly
  acid-base balance 276.4
    fetus or newborn — *see* Distress, fetal
  adaptation curve, dark 368.63
  alveolar ridge 525.9
  amnion 658.9 ✔5ᵗʰ
    affecting fetus or newborn 762.9
  anatomical relationship NEC 759.9
  apertures, congenital, diaphragm 756.6
  auditory perception NEC 388.40
  autosomes NEC 758.5
    13 758.1
    18 758.2
    21 or 22 758.0
    D₁ 758.1
    E₃ 758.2
    G 758.0
  ballistocardiogram 794.39
  basal metabolic rate (BMR) 794.7
  biosynthesis, testicular androgen 257.2
  blood level (of)
    cobalt 790.6
    copper 790.6
    iron 790.6
    lithium 790.6
    magnesium 790.6
    mineral 790.6
    zinc 790.6
  blood pressure
    elevated (without diagnosis of hypertension) 796.2
    low (*see also* Hypotension) 458.9
      reading (incidental) (isolated) (nonspecific) 796.3
  bowel sounds 787.5
  breathing behavior — *see* Respiration
  caloric test 794.19
  cervix (acquired) NEC 622.9
    congenital 752.40
    in pregnancy or childbirth 654.6 ✔5ᵗʰ
      causing obstructed labor 660.2 ✔5ᵗʰ
        affecting fetus or newborn 763.1
  chemistry, blood NEC 790.6
  chest sounds 786.7
  chorion 658.9 ✔5ᵗʰ
    affecting fetus or newborn 762.9
  chromosomal NEC 758.89
    analysis, nonspecific result 795.2
    autosomes (*see also* Abnormal, autosomes NEC) 758.5
    fetal, (suspected) affecting management of pregnancy 655.1 ✔5ᵗʰ
    sex 758.81
  clinical findings NEC 796.4
  communication — *see* Fistula
  configuration of pupils 379.49
  coronary
    artery 746.85
    vein 746.9
  cortisol-binding globulin 255.8
  course, Eustachian tube 744.24
  dentofacial NEC 524.9
    functional 524.5
    specified type NEC 524.8
  development, developmental NEC 759.9
    bone 756.9
    central nervous system 742.9
  direction, teeth 524.3
  Dynia (*see also* Defect, coagulation) 286.9
  Ebstein 746.2
  echocardiogram 793.2
  echoencephalogram 794.01
  echogram NEC — *see* Findings, abnormal, structure
  electrocardiogram (ECG) (EKG) 794.31
  electroencephalogram (EEG) 794.02
  electromyogram (EMG) 794.17
    ocular 794.14
  electro-oculogram (EOG) 794.12
  electroretinogram (ERG) 794.11
  erythrocytes 289.9
    congenital, with perinatal jaundice 282.9 [774.0]
  Eustachian valve 746.9
  excitability under minor stress 301.9

Abnormal, abnormality, abnormalities — *see also* Anomaly — *continued*
  fat distribution 782.9
  feces 787.7
  fetal heart rate — *see* Distress, fetal
  fetus NEC
    affecting management of pregnancy — *see* Pregnancy, management affected by, fetal
    causing disproportion 653.7 ✔5ᵗʰ
      affecting fetus or newborn 763.1
      causing obstructed labor 660.1 ✔5ᵗʰ
        affecting fetus or newborn 763.1
  findings without manifest disease — *see* Findings, abnormal
  fluid
    amniotic 792.3
    cerebrospinal 792.0
    peritoneal 792.9
    pleural 792.9
    synovial 792.9
    vaginal 792.9
  forces of labor NEC 661.9 ✔5ᵗʰ
    affecting fetus or newborn 763.7
  form, teeth 520.2
  function studies
    auditory 794.15
    bladder 794.9
    brain 794.00
    cardiovascular 794.30
    endocrine NEC 794.6
    kidney 794.4
    liver 794.8
    nervous system
      central 794.00
      peripheral 794.19
    oculomotor 794.14
    pancreas 794.9
    placenta 794.9
    pulmonary 794.2
    retina 794.11
    special senses 794.19
    spleen 794.9
    thyroid 794.5
    vestibular 794.16
  gait 781.2
    hysterical 300.11
  gastrin secretion 251.5
  globulin
    cortisol-binding 255.8
    thyroid-binding 246.8
  glucagon secretion 251.4
  glucose tolerance test 790.2
    in pregnancy, childbirth, or puerperium 648.8 ✔5ᵗʰ
    fetus or newborn 775.0
  gravitational (G) forces or states 994.9
  hair NEC 704.2
  hard tissue formation in pulp 522.3
  head movement 781.0
  heart
    rate
      fetus, affecting liveborn infant
        before the onset of labor 763.81
        during labor 763.82
        unspecified as to time of onset 763.83
      intrauterine
        before the onset of labor 763.81
        during labor 763.82
        unspecified as to time of onset 763.83
      newborn
        before the onset of labor 763.81
        during labor 763.82
        unspecified as to time of onset 763.83
    shadow 793.2
    sounds NEC 785.3
  hemoglobin (*see also* Disease, hemoglobin) 282.7
    trait — *see* Trait, hemoglobin, abnormal
  hemorrhage, uterus — *see* Hemorrhage, uterus
  histology NEC 795.4
  increase
    in
      appetite 783.6
      development 783.9
  involuntary movement 781.0
  jaw closure 524.5

✔4ᵗʰ Fourth-digit Required   ✔5ᵗʰ Fifth-digit Required   ▶◀ Revised Text   ● New Line   ▲ Revised Code

Abnormal, abnormality, abnormalities — *see also* Anomaly — *continued*
- karyotype 795.2
- knee jerk 796.1
- labor NEC 661.9 ✓5ᵗʰ
  - affecting fetus or newborn 763.7
- laboratory findings — *see* Findings, abnormal
- length, organ or site, congenital — *see* Distortion
- loss of height 781.91
- loss of weight 783.21
- lung shadow 793.1
- mammogram 793.80
  - microcalcification 793.81
- Mantoux test 795.5
- membranes (fetal)
  - affecting fetus or newborn 762.9
  - complicating pregnancy 658.8 ✓5ᵗʰ
- menstruation — *see* Menstruation
- metabolism (*see also* condition) 783.9
- movement 781.0
  - disorder NEC 333.90
    - specified NEC 333.99
  - head 781.0
  - involuntary 781.0
  - specified type NEC 333.99
- muscle contraction, localized 728.85
- myoglobin (Aberdeen) (Annapolis) 289.9
- narrowness, eyelid 743.62
- optokinetic response 379.57
- organs or tissues of pelvis NEC
  - in pregnancy or childbirth 654.9 ✓5ᵗʰ
    - affecting fetus or newborn 763.89
    - causing obstructed labor 660.2 ✓5ᵗʰ
      - affecting fetus or newborn 763.1
- origin — *see* Malposition, congenital
- palmar creases 757.2
- Papanicolaou (smear)
  - cervix 795.00 ▲
    - atypical squamous cell changes of undetermined significance ●
    - favor benign (ASCUS favor benign) 795.01 ●
    - favor dysplasia (ASCUS favor dysplasia) 795.02 ●
    - nonspecific finding NEC 795.09 ●
  - other site 795.1
- parturition
  - affecting fetus or newborn 763.9
  - mother — *see* Delivery, complicated
- pelvis (bony) — *see* Deformity, pelvis
- percussion, chest 786.7
- periods (grossly) (*see also* Menstruation) 626.9
- phonocardiogram 794.39
- placenta — *see* Placenta, abnormal
- plantar reflex 796.1
- plasma protein — *see* Deficiency, plasma, protein
- pleural folds 748.8
- position — *see also* Malposition
  - gravid uterus 654.4 ✓5ᵗʰ
    - causing obstructed labor 660.2 ✓5ᵗʰ
      - affecting fetus or newborn 763.1
- posture NEC 781.92
- presentation (fetus) — *see* Presentation, fetus, abnormal
- product of conception NEC 631
- puberty — *see* Puberty
- pulmonary
  - artery 747.3
  - function, newborn 770.89 ▲
  - test results 794.2
  - ventilation, newborn 770.89 ▲
    - hyperventilation 786.01
- pulsations in neck 785.1
- pupil reflexes 379.40
- quality of milk 676.8 ✓5ᵗʰ
- radiological examination 793.9
  - abdomen NEC 793.6
  - biliary tract 793.3
  - breast 793.89
    - mammogram NOS 793.80
    - mammographic microcalcification 793.81
  - gastrointestinal tract 793.4
  - genitourinary organs 793.5
  - head 793.0
  - intrathoracic organ NEC 793.2

Abnormal, abnormality, abnormalities — *see also* Anomaly — *continued*
- radiological examination — *continued*
  - lung (field) 793.1
  - musculoskeletal system 793.7
  - retroperitoneum 793.6
  - skin and subcutaneous tissue 793.9
  - skull 793.0
- red blood cells 790.09
  - morphology 790.09
  - volume 790.09
- reflex NEC 796.1
- renal function test 794.4
- respiration signs — *see* Respiration
- response to nerve stimulation 794.10
- retinal correspondence 368.34
- rhythm, heart — *see also* Arrhythmia
  - fetus — *see* Distress, fetal
- saliva 792.4
- scan
  - brain 794.09
  - kidney 794.4
  - liver 794.8
  - lung 794.2
  - thyroid 794.5
- secretion
  - gastrin 251.5
  - glucagon 251.4
- semen 792.2
- serum level (of)
  - acid phosphatase 790.5
  - alkaline phosphatase 790.5
  - amylase 790.5
  - enzymes NEC 790.5
  - lipase 790.5
- shape
  - cornea 743.41
  - gallbladder 751.69
  - gravid uterus 654.4 ✓5ᵗʰ
    - affecting fetus or newborn 763.89
    - causing obstructed labor 660.2 ✓5ᵗʰ
      - affecting fetus or newborn 763.1
  - head (*see also* Anomaly, skull) 756.0
  - organ or site, congenital NEC — *see* Distortion
- sinus venosus 747.40
- size
  - fetus, complicating delivery 653.5 ✓5ᵗʰ
    - causing obstructed labor 660.1 ✓5ᵗʰ
  - gallbladder 751.69
  - head (*see also* Anomaly, skull) 756.0
  - organ or site, congenital NEC — *see* Distortion
  - teeth 520.2
- skin and appendages, congenital NEC 757.9
- soft parts of pelvis — *see* Abnormal, organs or tissues of pelvis
- spermatozoa 792.2
- sputum (amount) (color) (excessive) (odor) (purulent) 786.4
- stool NEC 787.7
  - bloody 578.1
    - occult 792.1
  - bulky 787.7
  - color (dark) (light) 792.1
  - content (fat) (mucus) (pus) 792.1
  - occult blood 792.1
- synchondrosis 756.9
- test results without manifest disease — *see* Findings, abnormal
- thebesian valve 746.9
- thermography — *see* Findings, abnormal, structure
- threshold, cones or rods (eye) 368.63
- thyroid-binding globulin 246.8
- thyroid product 246.8
- toxicology (findings) NEC 796.0
- tracheal cartilage (congenital) 748.3
- transport protein 273.8
- ultrasound results — *see* Findings, abnormal, structure
- umbilical cord
  - affecting fetus or newborn 762.6
  - complicating delivery 663.9 ✓5ᵗʰ
  - specified NEC 663.8 ✓5ᵗʰ
- union
  - cricoid cartilage and thyroid cartilage 748.3
  - larynx and trachea 748.3

Abnormal, abnormality, abnormalities — *see also* Anomaly — *continued*
- union — *continued*
  - thyroid cartilage and hyoid bone 748.3
- urination NEC 788.69
  - psychogenic 306.53
  - stream
    - intermittent 788.61
    - slowing 788.62
    - splitting 788.61
    - weak 788.62
- urine (constituents) NEC 791.9
- uterine hemorrhage (*see also* Hemorrhage, uterus) 626.9
  - climacteric 627.0
  - postmenopausal 627.1
- vagina (acquired) (congenital)
  - in pregnancy or childbirth 654.7 ✓5ᵗʰ
    - affecting fetus or newborn 763.89
    - causing obstructed labor 660.2 ✓5ᵗʰ
      - affecting fetus or newborn 763.1
- vascular sounds 785.9
- vectorcardiogram 794.39
- visually evoked potential (VEP) 794.13
- vulva (acquired) (congenital)
  - in pregnancy or childbirth 654.8 ✓5ᵗʰ
    - affecting fetus or newborn 763.89
    - causing obstructed labor 660.2 ✓5ᵗʰ
      - affecting fetus or newborn 763.1
- weight
  - gain 783.1
    - of pregnancy 646.1 ✓5ᵗʰ
      - with hypertension — *see* Toxemia, of pregnancy
  - loss 783.21
- x-ray examination — *see* Abnormal, radiological examination

Abnormally formed uterus — *see* Anomaly, uterus

Abnormity (any organ or part) — *see* Anomaly

ABO
- hemolytic disease 773.1
- incompatibility reaction 999.6

Abocclusion 524.2

Abolition, language 784.69

Aborter, habitual or recurrent NEC
- without current pregnancy 629.9
- current abortion (*see also* Abortion, spontaneous) 634.9 ✓5ᵗʰ
  - affecting fetus or newborn 761.8
- observation in current pregnancy 646.3 ✓5ᵗʰ

Abortion (complete) (incomplete) (inevitable) (with retained products of conception) 637.9 ✓5ᵗʰ

> *Note — Use the following fifth-digit subclassification with categories 634–637:*
>
> 0   *unspecified*
> 1   *incomplete*
> 2   *complete*

- with
  - complication(s) (any) following previous abortion — *see* category 639 ✓4ᵗʰ
  - damage to pelvic organ (laceration) (rupture) (tear) 637.2 ✓5ᵗʰ
  - embolism (air) (amniotic fluid) (blood clot) (pulmonary) (pyemic) (septic) (soap) 637.6 ✓5ᵗʰ
  - genital tract and pelvic infection 637.0 ✓5ᵗʰ
  - hemorrhage, delayed or excessive 637.1 ✓5ᵗʰ
  - metabolic disorder 637.4 ✓5ᵗʰ
  - renal failure (acute) 637.3 ✓5ᵗʰ
  - sepsis (genital tract) (pelvic organ) 637.0 ✓5ᵗʰ
    - urinary tract 637.7 ✓5ᵗʰ
  - shock (postoperative) (septic) 637.5 ✓5ᵗʰ
  - specified complication NEC 637.7 ✓5ᵗʰ
  - toxemia 637.3 ✓5ᵗʰ
  - unspecified complication(s) 637.8 ✓5ᵗʰ
  - urinary tract infection 637.7 ✓5ᵗʰ
- accidental — *see* Abortion, spontaneous
- artificial — *see* Abortion, induced
- attempted (failed) — *see* Abortion, failed
- criminal — *see* Abortion, illegal
- early — *see* Abortion, spontaneous
- elective — *see* Abortion, legal

Abortion — *continued*
  failed (legal) 638.9
    with
      damage to pelvic organ (laceration)
        (rupture) (tear) 638.2
      embolism (air) (amniotic fluid) (blood clot)
        (pulmonary) (pyemic) (septic) (soap)
        638.6
      genital tract and pelvic infection 638.0
      hemorrhage, delayed or excessive 638.1
      metabolic disorder 638.4
      renal failure (acute) 638.3
      sepsis (genital tract) (pelvic organ) 638.0
        urinary tract 638.7
      shock (postoperative) (septic) 638.5
      specified complication NEC 638.7
      toxemia 638.3
      unspecified complication(s) 638.8
      urinary tract infection 638.7
  fetal indication — *see* Abortion, legal
  fetus 779.6
  following threatened abortion — *see* Abortion,
    by type
  habitual or recurrent (care during pregnancy)
    646.3 ✓5ᵗʰ
    with current abortion (*see also* Abortion,
      spontaneous) 634.9 ✓5ᵗʰ
      affecting fetus or newborn 761.8
    without current pregnancy 629.9
  homicidal — *see* Abortion, illegal
  illegal 636.9 ✓5ᵗʰ
    with
      damage to pelvic organ (laceration)
        (rupture) (tear) 636.2 ✓5ᵗʰ
      embolism (air) (amniotic fluid) (blood clot)
        (pulmonary) (pyemic) (septic) (soap)
        636.6 ✓5ᵗʰ
      genital tract and pelvic infection
        636.0 ✓5ᵗʰ
      hemorrhage, delayed or excessive
        636.1 ✓5ᵗʰ
      metabolic disorder 636.4 ✓5ᵗʰ
      renal failure 636.3 ✓5ᵗʰ
      sepsis (genital tract) (pelvic organ)
        636.0 ✓5ᵗʰ
        urinary tract 636.7 ✓5ᵗʰ
      shock (postoperative) (septic) 636.5 ✓5ᵗʰ
      specified complication NEC 636.7 ✓5ᵗʰ
      toxemia 636.3 ✓5ᵗʰ
      unspecified complication(s) 636.8 ✓5ᵗʰ
      urinary tract infection 636.7 ✓5ᵗʰ
    fetus 779.6
  induced 637.9 ✓5ᵗʰ
    illegal — *see* Abortion, illegal
    legal indications — *see* Abortion, legal
    medical indications — *see* Abortion, legal
    therapeutic — *see* Abortion, legal
  late — *see* Abortion, spontaneous
  legal (legal indication) (medical indication)
    (under medical supervision) 635.9 ✓5ᵗʰ
    with
      damage to pelvic organ (laceration)
        (rupture) (tear) 635.2 ✓5ᵗʰ
      embolism (air) (amniotic fluid) (blood clot)
        (pulmonary) (pyemic) (septic) (soap)
        635.6 ✓5ᵗʰ
      genital tract and pelvic infection
        635.0 ✓5ᵗʰ
      hemorrhage, delayed or excessive
        635.1 ✓5ᵗʰ
      metabolic disorder 635.4 ✓5ᵗʰ
      renal failure (acute) 635.3 ✓5ᵗʰ
      sepsis (genital tract) (pelvic organ)
        635.0 ✓5ᵗʰ
        urinary tract 635.7 ✓5ᵗʰ
      shock (postoperative) (septic) 635.5 ✓5ᵗʰ
      specified complication NEC 635.7 ✓5ᵗʰ
      toxemia 635.3 ✓5ᵗʰ
      unspecified complication(s) 635.8 ✓5ᵗʰ
      urinary tract infection 635.7 ✓5ᵗʰ
    fetus 779.6
  medical indication — *see* Abortion, legal
  mental hygiene problem — *see* Abortion, legal
  missed 632
  operative — *see* Abortion, legal
  psychiatric indication — *see* Abortion, legal

Abortion — *continued*
  recurrent — *see* Abortion, spontaneous
  self-induced — *see* Abortion, illegal
  septic — *see* Abortion, by type, with sepsis
  spontaneous 634.9 ✓5ᵗʰ
    with
      damage to pelvic organ (laceration)
        (rupture) (tear) 634.2 ✓5ᵗʰ
      embolism (air) (amniotic fluid) (blood clot)
        (pulmonary) (pyemic) (septic) (soap)
        634.6 ✓5ᵗʰ
      genital tract and pelvic infection
        634.0 ✓5ᵗʰ
      hemorrhage, delayed or excessive
        634.1 ✓5ᵗʰ
      metabolic disorder 634.4 ✓5ᵗʰ
      renal failure 634.3 ✓5ᵗʰ
      sepsis (genital tract) (pelvic organ)
        634.0 ✓5ᵗʰ
        urinary tract 634.7 ✓5ᵗʰ
      shock (postoperative) (septic) 634.5 ✓5ᵗʰ
      specified complication NEC 634.7 ✓5ᵗʰ
      toxemia 634.3 ✓5ᵗʰ
      unspecified complication(s) 634.8 ✓5ᵗʰ
      urinary tract infection 634.7 ✓5ᵗʰ
    fetus 761.8
    threatened 640.0 ✓5ᵗʰ
      affecting fetus or newborn 762.1
  surgical — *see* Abortion, legal
  therapeutic — *see* Abortion, legal
  threatened 640.0 ✓5ᵗʰ
    affecting fetus or newborn 762.1
  tubal — *see* Pregnancy, tubal
  voluntary — *see* Abortion, legal

Abortus fever 023.9

Aboulomania 301.6

Abrachia 755.20

Abrachiatism 755.20

Abrachiocephalia 759.89

Abrachiocephalus 759.89

Abrami's disease (acquired hemolytic jaundice)
  283.9

Abramov-Fiedler myocarditis (acute isolated
  myocarditis) 422.91

Abrasion — *see also* Injury, superficial, by site
  cornea 918.1
  dental 521.2
  teeth, tooth (dentifrice) (habitual) (hard tissues)
    (occupational) (ritual) (traditional) (wedge
    defect) 521.2

Abrikossov's tumor (M9580/0) — *see also*
  Neoplasm, connective tissue, benign
  malignant (M9580/3) — *see* Neoplasm,
    connective tissue, malignant

Abrism 988.8

Abruption, placenta — *see* Placenta, abruptio

Abruptio placentae — *see* Placenta, abruptio

Abscess (acute) (chronic) (infectional)
  (lymphangitic) (metastatic) (multiple)
  (pyogenic) (septic) (with lymphangitis) (*see
  also* Cellulitis) 682.9
  abdomen, abdominal
    cavity — *see* Abscess, peritoneum
    wall 682.2
  abdominopelvic — *see* Abscess, peritoneum
  accessory sinus (chronic) (*see also* Sinusitis)
    473.9
  adrenal (capsule) (gland) 255.8
  alveolar 522.5
    with sinus 522.7
  amebic 006.3
    bladder 006.8
    brain (with liver or lung abscess) 006.5
    liver (without mention of brain or lung
      abscess) 006.3
      with
        brain abscess (and lung abscess)
        006.5
        lung abscess 006.4
    lung (with liver abscess) 006.4
      with brain abscess 006.5
    seminal vesicle 006.8
    specified site NEC 006.8
    spleen 006.8

Abscess (*see also* Cellulitis) — *continued*
  anaerobic 040.0
  ankle 682.6
  anorectal 566
  antecubital space 682.3
  antrum (chronic) (Highmore) (*see also* Sinusitis,
    maxillary) 473.0
  anus 566
  apical (tooth) 522.5
    with sinus (alveolar) 522.7
  appendix 540.1
  areola (acute) (chronic) (nonpuerperal) 611.0
    puerperal, postpartum 675.1 ✓5ᵗʰ
  arm (any part, above wrist) 682.3
  artery (wall) 447.2
  atheromatous 447.2
  auditory canal (external) 380.10
  auricle (ear) (staphylococcal) (streptococcal)
    380.10
  axilla, axillary (region) 682.3
    lymph gland or node 683
  back (any part) 682.2
  Bartholin's gland 616.3
    with
      abortion — *see* Abortion, by type, with
        sepsis
      ectopic pregnancy (*see also* categories
        633.0-633.9) 639.0
      molar pregnancy (*see also* categories 630-
        632) 639.0
    complicating pregnancy or puerperium
      646.6 ✓5ᵗʰ
    following
      abortion 639.0
      ectopic or molar pregnancy 639.0
  bartholinian 616.3
  Bezold's 383.01
  bile, biliary, duct or tract (*see also*
    Cholecystitis) 576.8
  bilharziasis 120.1
  bladder (wall) 595.89
    amebic 006.8
  bone (subperiosteal) (*see also* Osteomyelitis)
    730.0 ✓5ᵗʰ
    accessory sinus (chronic) (*see also* Sinusitis)
      473.9
    acute 730.0 ✓5ᵗʰ
    chronic or old 730.1 ✓5ᵗʰ
    jaw (lower) (upper) 526.4
    mastoid — *see* Mastoiditis, acute
    petrous (*see also* Petrositis) 383.20
    spinal (tuberculous) (*see also* Tuberculosis)
      015.0 ✓5ᵗʰ *[730.88]*
      nontuberculous 730.08
  bowel 569.5
  brain (any part) 324.0
    amebic (with liver or lung abscess) 006.5
    cystic 324.0
    late effect — *see* category 326
    otogenic 324.0
    tuberculous (*see also* Tuberculosis)
      013.3 ✓5ᵗʰ
  breast (acute) (chronic) (nonpuerperal) 611.0
    newborn 771.5
    puerperal, postpartum 675.1 ✓5ᵗʰ
    tuberculous (*see also* Tuberculosis)
      017.9 ✓5ᵗʰ
  broad ligament (chronic) (*see also* Disease,
    pelvis, inflammatory) 614.4
    acute 614.3
  Brodie's (chronic) (localized) (*see also*
    Osteomyelitis) 730.1 ✓5ᵗʰ
  bronchus 519.1
  buccal cavity 528.3
  bulbourethral gland 597.0
  bursa 727.89
    pharyngeal 478.29
  buttock 682.5
  canaliculus, breast 611.0
  canthus 372.20
  cartilage 733.99
  cecum 569.5   ▲
    with appendicitis 540.1   ●
  cerebellum, cerebellar 324.0
    late effect — *see* category 326
  cerebral (embolic) 324.0
    late effect — *see* category 326

Abscess (*see also* Cellulitis) — *continued*
 cervical (neck region) 682.1
  lymph gland or node 683
   stump (*see also* Cervicitis) 616.0
 cervix (stump) (uteri) (*see also* Cervicitis) 616.0
 cheek, external 682.0
  inner 528.3
 chest 510.9
  with fistula 510.0
  wall 682.2
 chin 682.0
 choroid 363.00
 ciliary body 364.3
 circumtonsillar 475
 cold (tuberculous) — *see also* Tuberculosis, abscess
  articular — *see* Tuberculosis, joint
 colon (wall) 569.5
 colostomy or enterostomy 569.61
 conjunctiva 372.00
 connective tissue NEC 682.9
 cornea 370.55
  with ulcer 370.00
 corpus
  cavernosum 607.2
  luteum (*see also* Salpingo-oophoritis) 614.2
 Cowper's gland 597.0
 cranium 324.0
 cul-de-sac (Douglas') (posterior) (*see also* Disease, pelvis, inflammatory) 614.4
  acute 614.3
 dental 522.5
  with sinus (alveolar) 522.7
 dentoalveolar 522.5
  with sinus (alveolar) 522.7
 diaphragm, diaphragmatic — *see* Abscess, peritoneum
 digit NEC 681.9
 Douglas' cul-de-sac or pouch (*see also* Disease, pelvis, inflammatory) 614.4
  acute 614.3
 Dubois' 090.5
 ductless gland 259.8
 ear
  acute 382.00
  external 380.10
  inner 386.30
  middle — *see* Otitis media
 elbow 682.3
 endamebic — *see* Abscess, amebic
 entamebic — *see* Abscess, amebic
 enterostomy 569.61
 epididymis 604.0
 epidural 324.9
  brain 324.0
   late effect — *see* category 326
  spinal cord 324.1
 epiglottis 478.79
 epiploon, epiploic — *see* Abscess, peritoneum
 erysipelatous (*see also* Erysipelas) 035
 esophagus 530.19
 ethmoid (bone) (chronic) (sinus) (*see also* Sinusitis, ethmoidal) 473.2
 external auditory canal 380.10
 extradural 324.9
  brain 324.0
   late effect — *see* category 326
  spinal cord 324.1
 extraperitoneal — *see* Abscess, peritoneum
 eye 360.00
 eyelid 373.13
 face (any part, except eye) 682.0
 fallopian tube (*see also* Salpingo-oophoritis) 614.2
 fascia 728.89
 fauces 478.29
 fecal 569.5
 femoral (region) 682.6
 filaria, filarial (*see also* Infestation, filarial) 125.9
 finger (any) (intrathecal) (periosteal) (subcutaneous) (subcuticular) 681.00
 fistulous NEC 682.9
 flank 682.2
 foot (except toe) 682.7
 forearm 682.3
 forehead 682.0

Abscess (*see also* Cellulitis) — *continued*
 frontal (sinus) (chronic) (*see also* Sinusitis, frontal) 473.1
 gallbladder (*see also* Cholecystitis, acute) 575.0
 gastric 535.0 ✓5ᵗʰ
 genital organ or tract NEC
  female 616.9
   with
    abortion — *see* Abortion, by type, with sepsis
    ectopic pregnancy (*see also* categories 633.0-633.9) 639.0
    molar pregnancy (*see also* categories 630-632) 639.0
   following
    abortion 639.0
    ectopic or molar pregnancy 639.0
   puerperal, postpartum, childbirth 670 ✓5ᵗʰ
  male 608.4
 genitourinary system, tuberculous (*see also* Tuberculosis) 016.9 ✓5ᵗʰ
 gingival 523.3
 gland, glandular (lymph) (acute) NEC 683
 glottis 478.79
 gluteal (region) 682.5
 gonorrheal NEC (*see also* Gonococcus) 098.0
 groin 682.2
 gum 523.3
 hand (except finger or thumb) 682.4
 head (except face) 682.8
 heart 429.89
 heel 682.7
 helminthic (*see also* Infestation, by specific parasite) 128.9
 hepatic 572.0
  amebic (*see also* Abscess, liver, amebic) 006.3
  duct 576.8
 hip 682.6
  tuberculous (active) (*see also* Tuberculosis) 015.1 ✓5ᵗʰ
 ileocecal 540.1
 ileostomy (bud) 569.61
 iliac (region) 682.2
  fossa 540.1
 iliopsoas (tuberculous) (*see also* Tuberculosis) 015.0 ✓5ᵗʰ [730.88]
  nontuberculous 728.89
 infraclavicular (fossa) 682.3
 inguinal (region) 682.2
  lymph gland or node 683
 intersphincteric (anus) 566
 intestine, intestinal 569.5
  rectal 566
 intra-abdominal (*see also* Abscess, peritoneum) 567.2
  postoperative 998.59
 intracranial 324.0
  late effect — *see* category 326
 intramammary — *see* Abscess, breast
 intramastoid (*see also* Mastoiditis, acute) 383.00
 intraorbital 376.01
 intraperitoneal — *see* Abscess, peritoneum
 intraspinal 324.1
  late effect — *see* category 326
 intratonsillar 475
 iris 364.3
 ischiorectal 566
 jaw (bone) (lower) (upper) 526.4
  skin 682.0
 joint (*see also* Arthritis, pyogenic) 711.0 ✓5ᵗʰ
  vertebral (tuberculous) (*see also* Tuberculosis) 015.0 ✓5ᵗʰ [730.88]
  nontuberculous 724.8
 kidney 590.2
  with
   abortion — *see* Abortion, by type, with urinary tract infection
   calculus 592.0
   ectopic pregnancy (*see also* categories 633.0-633.9) 639.8
   molar pregnancy (*see also* categories 630-632) 639.8

Abscess (*see also* Cellulitis) — *continued*
 kidney — *continued*
  complicating pregnancy or puerperium 646.6 ✓5ᵗʰ
   affecting fetus or newborn 760.1
  following
   abortion 639.8
   ectopic or molar pregnancy 639.8
 knee 682.6
  joint 711.06
  tuberculous (active) (*see also* Tuberculosis) 015.2 ✓5ᵗʰ
 labium (majus) (minus) 616.4
  complicating pregnancy, childbirth, or puerperium 646.6 ✓5ᵗʰ
 lacrimal (passages) (sac) (*see also* Dacryocystitis) 375.30
  caruncle 375.30
  gland (*see also* Dacryoadenitis) 375.00
 lacunar 597.0
 larynx 478.79
 lateral (alveolar) 522.5
  with sinus 522.7
 leg, except foot 682.6
 lens 360.00
 lid 373.13
 lingual 529.0
  tonsil 475
 lip 528.5
 Littre's gland 597.0
 liver 572.0
  amebic 006.3
   with
    brain abscess (and lung abscess) 006.5
    lung abscess 006.4
   due to Entamoeba histolytica 006.3
  dysenteric (*see also* Abscess, liver, amebic) 006.3
  pyogenic 572.0
  tropical (*see also* Abscess, liver, amebic) 006.3
 loin (region) 682.2
 lumbar (tuberculous) (*see also* Tuberculosis) 015.0 ✓5ᵗʰ [730.88]
  nontuberculous 682.2
 lung (miliary) (putrid) 513.0
  amebic (with liver abscess) 006.4
   with brain abscess 006.5
 lymph, lymphatic, gland or node (acute) 683
  any site, except mesenteric 683
  mesentery 289.2
 lymphangitic, acute — *see* Cellulitis
 malar 526.4
 mammary gland — *see* Abscess, breast
 marginal (anus) 566
 mastoid (process) (*see also* Mastoiditis, acute) 383.00
  subperiosteal 383.01
 maxilla, maxillary 526.4
  molar (tooth) 522.5
   with sinus 522.7
  premolar 522.5
  sinus (chronic) (*see also* Sinusitis, maxillary) 473.0
 mediastinum 513.1
 meibomian gland 373.12
 meninges (*see also* Meningitis) 320.9
 mesentery, mesenteric — *see* Abscess, peritoneum
 mesosalpinx (*see also* Salpingo-oophoritis) 614.2
 milk 675.1 ✓5ᵗʰ
 Monro's (psoriasis) 696.1
 mons pubis 682.2
 mouth (floor) 528.3
 multiple sites NEC 682.9
 mural 682.2
 muscle 728.89
 myocardium 422.92
 nabothian (follicle) (*see also* Cervicitis) 616.0
 nail (chronic) (with lymphangitis) 681.9
  finger 681.02
  toe 681.11
 nasal (fossa) (septum) 478.1
  sinus (chronic) (*see also* Sinusitis) 473.9
 nasopharyngeal 478.29

✓4ᵗʰ Fourth-digit Required   ✓5ᵗʰ Fifth-digit Required   ▶◀ Revised Text   ● New Line   ▲ Revised Code

Abscess (*see also* Cellulitis) — *continued*
  nates 682.5
  navel 682.2
    newborn NEC 771.4
  neck (region) 682.1
    lymph gland or node 683
  nephritic (*see also* Abscess, kidney) 590.2
  nipple 611.0
    puerperal, postpartum 675.0 ✔5ᵗʰ
  nose (septum) 478.1
    external 682.0
  omentum — *see* Abscess, peritoneum
  operative wound 998.59
  orbit, orbital 376.01
  ossifluent — *see* Abscess, bone
  ovary, ovarian (corpus luteum) (*see also* Salpingo-oophoritis) 614.2
  oviduct (*see also* Salpingo-oophoritis) 614.2
  palate (soft) 528.3
    hard 526.4
  palmar (space) 682.4
  pancreas (duct) 577.0
  paradontal 523.3
  parafrenal 607.2
  parametric, parametrium (chronic) (*see also* Disease, pelvis, inflammatory) 614.4
    acute 614.3
  paranephric 590.2
  parapancreatic 577.0
  parapharyngeal 478.22
  pararectal 566
  parasinus (*see also* Sinusitis) 473.9
  parauterine (*see also* Disease, pelvis, inflammatory) 614.4
    acute 614.3
  paravaginal (*see also* Vaginitis) 616.10
  parietal region 682.8
  parodontal 523.3
  parotid (duct) (gland) 527.3
    region 528.3
  parumbilical 682.2
    newborn 771.4
  pectoral (region) 682.2
  pelvirectal — *see* Abscess, peritoneum
  pelvis, pelvic
    female (chronic) (*see also* Disease, pelvis, inflammatory) 614.4
      acute 614.3
    male, peritoneal (cellular tissue) — *see* Abscess, peritoneum
    tuberculous (*see also* Tuberculosis) 016.9 ✔5ᵗʰ
  penis 607.2
    gonococcal (acute) 098.0
      chronic or duration of 2 months or over 098.2
  perianal 566
  periapical 522.5
    with sinus (alveolar) 522.7
  periappendiceal 540.1
  pericardial 420.99
  pericecal 540.1
  pericemental 523.3
  pericholecystic (*see also* Cholecystitis, acute) 575.0
  pericoronal 523.3
  peridental 523.3
  perigastric 535.0 ✔5ᵗʰ
  perimetric (*see also* Disease, pelvis, inflammatory) 614.4
    acute 614.3
  perinephric, perinephritic (*see also* Abscess, kidney) 590.2
  perineum, perineal (superficial) 682.2
    deep (with urethral involvement) 597.0
    urethra 597.0
  periodontal (parietal) 523.3
    apical 522.5
  periosteum, periosteal (*see also* Periostitis) 730.3 ✔5ᵗʰ
    with osteomyelitis (*see also* Osteomyelitis) 730.2 ✔5ᵗʰ
      acute or subacute 730.0 ✔5ᵗʰ
      chronic or old 730.1 ✔5ᵗʰ
  peripleuritic 510.9
    with fistula 510.0
  periproctic 566
  periprostatic 601.2

Abscess (*see also* Cellulitis) — *continued*
  perirectal (staphylococcal) 566
  perirenal (tissue) (*see also* Abscess, kidney) 590.2
  perisinuous (nose) (*see also* Sinusitis) 473.9
  peritoneum, peritoneal (perforated) (ruptured) 567.2
    with
      abortion — *see* Abortion, by type, with sepsis
      appendicitis 540.1
      ectopic pregnancy (*see also* categories 633.0-633.9) 639.0
      molar pregnancy (*see also* categories 630-632) 639.0
    following
      abortion 639.0
      ectopic or molar pregnancy 639.0
    pelvic, female (*see also* Disease, pelvis, inflammatory) 614.4
      acute 614.3
    postoperative 998.59
    puerperal, postpartum, childbirth 670 ✔4ᵗʰ
    tuberculous (*see also* Tuberculosis) 014.0 ✔5ᵗʰ
  peritonsillar 475
  perityphlic 540.1
  periureteral 593.89
  periurethral 597.0
    gonococcal (acute) 098.0
      chronic or duration of 2 months or over 098.2
  periuterine (*see also* Disease, pelvis, inflammatory) 614.4
    acute 614.3
  perivesical 595.89
  pernicious NEC 682.9
  petrous bone — *see* Petrositis
  phagedenic NEC 682.9
    chancroid 099.0
  pharynx, pharyngeal (lateral) 478.29
  phlegmonous NEC 682.9
  pilonidal 685.0
  pituitary (gland) 253.8
  pleura 510.9
    with fistula 510.0
  popliteal 682.6
  postanal 566
  postcecal 540.1
  postlaryngeal 478.79
  postnasal 478.1
  postpharyngeal 478.24
  posttonsillar 475
  posttyphoid 002.0
  Pott's (*see also* Tuberculosis) 015.0 ✔5ᵗʰ [730.88]
  pouch of Douglas (chronic) (*see also* Disease, pelvis, inflammatory) 614.4
  premammary — *see* Abscess, breast
  prepatellar 682.6
  prostate (*see also* Prostatitis) 601.2
    gonococcal (acute) 098.12
      chronic or duration of 2 months or over 098.32
  psoas (tuberculous) (*see also* Tuberculosis) 015.0 ✔5ᵗʰ [730.88]
    nontuberculous 728.89
  pterygopalatine fossa 682.8
  pubis 682.2
  puerperal — Puerperal, abscess, by site
  pulmonary — *see* Abscess, lung
  pulp, pulpal (dental) 522.0
    finger 681.01
    toe 681.10
  pyemic — *see* Septicemia
  pyloric valve 535.0 ✔5ᵗʰ
  rectovaginal septum 569.5
  rectovesical 595.89
  rectum 566
  regional NEC 682.9
  renal (*see also* Abscess, kidney) 590.2
  retina 363.00
  retrobulbar 376.01
  retrocecal — *see* Abscess, peritoneum
  retrolaryngeal 478.79
  retromammary — *see* Abscess, breast
  retroperineal 682.2

Abscess (*see also* Cellulitis) — *continued*
  retroperitoneal — *see* Abscess, peritoneum
  retropharyngeal 478.24
    tuberculous (*see also* Tuberculosis) 012.8 ✔5ᵗʰ
  retrorectal 566
  retrouterine (*see also* Disease, pelvis, inflammatory) 614.4
    acute 614.3
  retrovesical 595.89
  root, tooth 522.5
    with sinus (alveolar) 522.7
  round ligament (*see also* Disease, pelvis, inflammatory) 614.4
    acute 614.3
  rupture (spontaneous) NEC 682.9
  sacrum (tuberculous) (*see also* Tuberculosis) 015.0 ✔5ᵗʰ [730.88]
    nontuberculous 730.08
  salivary duct or gland 527.3
  scalp (any part) 682.8
  scapular 730.01
  sclera 379.09
  scrofulous (*see also* Tuberculosis) 017.2 ✔5ᵗʰ
  scrotum 608.4
  seminal vesicle 608.0
    amebic 006.8
  septal, dental 522.5
    with sinus (alveolar) 522.7
  septum (nasal) 478.1
  serous (*see also* Periostitis) 730.3 ✔5ᵗʰ
  shoulder 682.3
  side 682.2
  sigmoid 569.5
  sinus (accessory) (chronic) (nasal) (*see also* Sinusitis) 473.9
    intracranial venous (any) 324.0
    late effect — *see* category 326
  Skene's duct or gland 597.0
  skin NEC 682.9
    tuberculous (primary) (*see also* Tuberculosis) 017.0 ✔5ᵗʰ
  sloughing NEC 682.9
  specified site NEC 682.8
    amebic 006.8
  spermatic cord 608.4
  sphenoidal (sinus) (*see also* Sinusitis, sphenoidal) 473.3
  spinal
    cord (any part) (staphylococcal) 324.1
      tuberculous (*see also* Tuberculosis) 013.5 ✔5ᵗʰ
    epidural 324.1
  spine (column) (tuberculous) (*see also* Tuberculosis) 015.0 ✔5ᵗʰ [730.88]
    nontuberculous 730.08
  spleen 289.59
    amebic 006.8
  staphylococcal NEC 682.9
  stitch 998.59
  stomach (wall) 535.0 ✔5ᵗʰ
  strumous (tuberculous) (*see also* Tuberculosis) 017.2 ✔5ᵗʰ
  subarachnoid 324.9
    brain 324.0
    cerebral 324.0
    late effect — *see* category 326
    spinal cord 324.1
  subareolar — *see also* Abscess, breast
    puerperal, postpartum 675.1 ✔5ᵗʰ
  subcecal 540.1
  subcutaneous NEC 682.9
  subdiaphragmatic — *see* Abscess, peritoneum
  subdorsal 682.2
  subdural 324.9
    brain 324.0
    late effect — *see* category 326
    spinal cord 324.1
  subgaleal 682.8
  subhepatic — *see* Abscess, peritoneum
  sublingual 528.3
    gland 527.3
  submammary — *see* Abscess, breast
  submandibular (region) (space) (triangle) 682.0
    gland 527.3
  submaxillary (region) 682.0
    gland 527.3

Abscess (*see also* Cellulitis) — *continued*
  submental (pyogenic) 682.0
    gland 527.3
  subpectoral 682.2
  subperiosteal — *see* Abscess, bone
  subperitoneal — *see* Abscess, peritoneum
  subphrenic — *see also* Abscess, peritoneum
    postoperative 998.59
  subscapular 682.2
  subungual 681.9
  suburethral 597.0
  sudoriparous 705.89
  suppurative NEC 682.9
  supraclavicular (fossa) 682.3
  suprahepatic — *see* Abscess, peritoneum
  suprapelvic (*see also* Disease, pelvis,
      inflammatory) 614.4
    acute 614.3
  suprapubic 682.2
  suprarenal (capsule) (gland) 255.8
  sweat gland 705.89
  syphilitic 095.8
  teeth, tooth (root) 522.5
    with sinus (alveolar) 522.7
    supporting structures NEC 523.3
  temple 682.0
  temporal region 682.0
  temporosphenoidal 324.0
    late effect — *see* category 326
  tendon (sheath) 727.89
  testicle — *see* Orchitis
  thecal 728.89
  thigh (acquired) 682.6
  thorax 510.9
    with fistula 510.0
  throat 478.29
  thumb (intrathecal) (periosteal) (subcutaneous)
      (subcuticular) 681.00
  thymus (gland) 254.1
  thyroid (gland) 245.0
  toe (any) (intrathecal) (periosteal)
      (subcutaneous) (subcuticular) 681.10
  tongue (staphylococcal) 529.0
  tonsil(s) (lingual) 475
  tonsillopharyngeal 475
  tooth, teeth (root) 522.5
    with sinus (alveolar) 522.7
    supporting structure NEC 523.3
  trachea 478.9
  trunk 682.2
  tubal (*see also* Salpingo-oophoritis) 614.2
  tuberculous — *see* Tuberculosis, abscess
  tubo-ovarian (*see also* Salpingo-oophoritis)
      614.2
  tunica vaginalis 608.4
  umbilicus NEC 682.2
    newborn 771.4
  upper arm 682.3
  upper respiratory 478.9
  urachus 682.2
  urethra (gland) 597.0
  urinary 597.0
  uterus, uterine (wall) (*see also* Endometritis)
      615.9
    ligament (*see also* Disease, pelvis,
        inflammatory) 614.4
      acute 614.3
    neck (*see also* Cervicitis) 616.0
  uvula 528.3
  vagina (wall) (*see also* Vaginitis) 616.10
  vaginorectal (*see also* Vaginitis) 616.10
  vas deferens 608.4
  vermiform appendix 540.1
  vertebra (column) (tuberculous) (*see also*
      Tuberculosis) 015.0 ✓5ᵗʰ *[730.88]*
    nontuberculous 730.0 ✓5ᵗʰ
  vesical 595.89
  vesicouterine pouch (*see also* Disease, pelvis,
      inflammatory) 614.4
  vitreous (humor) (pneumococcal) 360.04
  vocal cord 478.5
  von Bezold's 383.01
  vulva 616.4
    complicating pregnancy, childbirth, or
        puerperium 646.6 ✓5ᵗʰ
  vulvovaginal gland (*see also* Vaginitis) 616.3
  web-space 682.4
  wrist 682.4

Absence (organ or part) (complete or partial)
  acoustic nerve 742.8
  adrenal (gland) (congenital) 759.1
    acquired V45.79
  albumin (blood) 273.8
  alimentary tract (complete) (congenital) (partial)
      751.8
    lower 751.5
    upper 750.8
  alpha-fucosidase 271.8
  alveolar process (acquired) 525.8
    congenital 750.26
  anus, anal (canal) (congenital) 751.2
  aorta (congenital) 747.22
  aortic valve (congenital) 746.89
  appendix, congenital 751.2
  arm (acquired) V49.60
    above elbow V49.66
    below elbow V49.65
    congenital (*see also* Deformity, reduction,
        upper limb) 755.20
      lower — *see* Absence, forearm, congenital
      upper (complete) (partial) (with absence of
          distal elements, incomplete) 755.24
        with
          complete absence of distal elements
              755.21
          forearm (incomplete) 755.23
  artery (congenital) (peripheral) NEC (*see also*
      Anomaly, peripheral vascular system)
      747.60
    brain 747.81
    cerebral 747.81
    coronary 746.85
    pulmonary 747.3
    umbilical 747.5
  atrial septum 745.69
  auditory canal (congenital) (external) 744.01
  auricle (ear) (with stenosis or atresia of
      auditory canal), congenital 744.01
  bile, biliary duct (common) or passage
      (congenital) 751.61
  bladder (acquired) V45.74
    congenital 753.8
  bone (congenital) NEC 756.9
    marrow 284.9
      acquired (secondary) 284.8
      congenital 284.0
      hereditary 284.0
      idiopathic 284.9
    skull 756.0
  bowel sounds 787.5
  brain 740.0
    specified part 742.2
  breast(s) (acquired) V45.71
    congenital 757.6
  broad ligament (congenital) 752.19
  bronchus (congenital) 748.3
  calvarium, calvaria (skull) 756.0
  canaliculus lacrimalis, congenital 743.65
  carpal(s) (congenital) (complete) (partial) (with
      absence of distal elements, incomplete)
      (*see also* Deformity, reduction, upper
      limb) 755.28
    with complete absence of distal elements
        755.21
  cartilage 756.9
  caudal spine 756.13
  cecum (acquired) (postoperative)
      (posttraumatic) V45.72
    congenital 751.2
  cementum 520.4
  cerebellum (congenital) (vermis) 742.2
  cervix (acquired) (uteri) V45.77
    congenital 752.49
  chin, congenital 744.89
  cilia (congenital) 743.63
    acquired 374.89
  circulatory system, part NEC 747.89
  clavicle 755.51
  clitoris (congenital) 752.49
  coccyx, congenital 756.13
  cold sense (*see also* Disturbance, sensation)
      782.0
  colon (acquired) (postoperative) V45.72
    congenital 751.2

Absence — *continued*
  congenital
    lumen — *see* Atresia
    organ or site NEC — *see* Agenesis
    septum — *see* Imperfect, closure
  corpus callosum (congenital) 742.2
  cricoid cartilage 748.3
  diaphragm (congenital) (with hernia) 756.6
    with obstruction 756.6
  digestive organ(s) or tract, congenital (complete)
      (partial) 751.8
    acquired V45.79
    lower 751.5
    upper 750.8
  ductus arteriosus 747.89
  duodenum (acquired) (postoperative) V45.72
    congenital 751.1
  ear, congenital 744.09
    acquired V45.79
    auricle 744.01
    external 744.01
    inner 744.05
    lobe, lobule 744.21
    middle, except ossicles 744.03
      ossicles 744.04
    ossicles 744.04
  ejaculatory duct (congenital) 752.8
  endocrine gland NEC (congenital) 759.2
  epididymis (congenital) 752.8
    acquired V45.77
  epiglottis, congenital 748.3
  epileptic (atonic) (typical) (*see also* Epilepsy)
      345.0 ✓5ᵗʰ
  erythrocyte 284.9
  erythropoiesis 284.9
    congenital 284.0
  esophagus (congenital) 750.3
  Eustachian tube (congenital) 744.24
  extremity (acquired)
    congenital (*see also* Deformity, reduction)
        755.4
    lower V49.70
    upper V49.60
  extrinsic muscle, eye 743.69
  eye (acquired) V45.78
    adnexa (congenital) 743.69
    congenital 743.00
    muscle (congenital) 743.69
  eyelid (fold), congenital 743.62
    acquired 374.89
  face
    bones NEC 756.0
    specified part NEC 744.89
  fallopian tube(s) (acquired) V45.77
    congenital 752.19
  femur, congenital (complete) (partial) (with
      absence of distal elements, incomplete)
      (*see also* Deformity, reduction, lower
      limb) 755.34
    with
      complete absence of distal elements
          755.31
      tibia and fibula (incomplete) 755.33
  fibrin 790.92
  fibrinogen (congenital) 286.3
    acquired 286.6
  fibula, congenital (complete) (partial) (with
      absence of distal elements, incomplete)
      (*see also* Deformity, reduction, lower
      limb) 755.37
    with
      complete absence of distal elements
          755.31
      tibia 755.35
        with
          complete absence of distal elements
              755.31
          femur (incomplete) 755.33
            with complete absence of distal
                elements 755.31
  finger (acquired) V49.62
    congenital (complete) (partial) (*see also*
        Deformity, reduction, upper limb)
        755.29
      meaning all fingers (complete) (partial)
          755.21
      transverse 755.21

Absence — *continued*
  fissures of lungs (congenital) 748.5
  foot (acquired) V49.73
    congenital (complete) 755.31
  forearm (acquired) V49.65
    congenital (complete) (partial) (with absence
        of distal elements, incomplete) (*see
        also* Deformity, reduction, upper limb)
        755.25
      with
        complete absence of distal elements
            (hand and fingers) 755.21
        humerus (incomplete) 755.23
  fovea centralis 743.55
  fucosidase 271.8
  gallbladder (acquired) V45.79
    congenital 751.69
  gamma globulin (blood) 279.00
  genital organs
    acquired V45.77
    congenital
      female 752.8
        external 752.49
        internal NEC 752.8
      male 752.8
        penis 752.69
  genitourinary organs, congenital NEC 752.8
  glottis 748.3
  gonadal, congenital NEC 758.6
  hair (congenital) 757.4
    acquired — *see* Alopecia
  hand (acquired) V49.63
    congenital (complete) (*see also* Deformity,
        reduction, upper limb) 755.21
  heart (congenital) 759.89
    acquired — *see* Status, organ replacement
  heat sense (*see also* Disturbance, sensation)
      782.0
  humerus, congenital (complete) (partial) (with
      absence of distal elements, incomplete)
      (*see also* Deformity, reduction, upper
      limb) 755.24
    with
      complete absence of distal elements
          755.21
      radius and ulna (incomplete) 755.23
  hymen (congenital) 752.49
  ileum (acquired) (postoperative) (posttraumatic)
      V45.72
    congenital 751.1
  immunoglobulin, isolated NEC 279.03
    IgA 279.01
    IgG 279.03
    IgM 279.02
  incus (acquired) 385.24
    congenital 744.04
  internal ear (congenital) 744.05
  intestine (acquired) (small) V45.72
    congenital 751.1
      large 751.2
    large V45.72
      congenital 751.2
  iris (congenital) 743.45
  jaw — *see* Absence, mandible
  jejunum (acquired) V45.72
    congenital 751.1
  joint, congenital NEC 755.8
  kidney(s) (acquired) V45.73
    congenital 753.0
  labium (congenital) (majus) (minus) 752.49
  labyrinth, membranous 744.05
  lacrimal apparatus (congenital) 743.65
  larynx (congenital) 748.3
  leg (acquired) V49.70
    above knee V49.76
    below knee V49.75
    congenital (partial) (unilateral) (*see also*
        Deformity, reduction, lower limb)
        755.31
      lower (complete) (partial) (with absence of
          distal elements, incomplete) 755.35
        with
          complete absence of distal elements
              (foot and toes) 755.31
          thigh (incomplete) 755.33
            with complete absence of distal
                elements 755.31

Absence — *continued*
  leg — *continued*
    congenital — *continued*
      upper — *see* Absence, femur
  lens (congenital) 743.35
    acquired 379.31
  ligament, broad (congenital) 752.19
  limb (acquired)
    congenital (complete) (partial) (*see also*
        Deformity, reduction) 755.4
      lower 755.30
        complete 755.31
        incomplete 755.32
        longitudinal — *see* Deficiency, lower
            limb, longitudinal
        transverse 755.31
      upper 755.20
        complete 755.21
        incomplete 755.22
        longitudinal — *see* Deficiency, upper
            limb, longitudinal
        transverse 755.21
    lower NEC V49.70
    upper NEC V49.60
  lip 750.26
  liver (congenital) (lobe) 751.69
  lumbar (congenital) (vertebra) 756.13
    isthmus 756.11
    pars articularis 756.11
  lumen — *see* Atresia
  lung (bilateral) (congenital) (fissure) (lobe)
      (unilateral) 748.5
    acquired (any part) V45.76
  mandible (congenital) 524.09
  maxilla (congenital) 524.09
  menstruation 626.0
  metacarpal(s), congenital (complete) (partial)
      (with absence of distal elements,
      incomplete) (*see also* Deformity,
      reduction, upper limb) 755.28
    with all fingers, complete 755.21
  metatarsal(s), congenital (complete) (partial)
      (with absence of distal elements,
      incomplete) (*see also* Deformity,
      reduction, lower limb) 755.38
    with complete absence of distal elements
        755.31
  muscle (congenital) (pectoral) 756.81
    ocular 743.69
  musculoskeletal system (congenital) NEC 756.9
  nail(s) (congenital) 757.5
  neck, part 744.89
  nerve 742.8
  nervous system, part NEC 742.8
  neutrophil 288.0
  nipple (congenital) 757.6
  nose (congenital) 748.1
    acquired 738.0
  nuclear 742.8
  ocular muscle (congenital) 743.69
  organ
    of Corti (congenital) 744.05
    or site
      acquired V45.79
      congenital NEC 759.89
  osseous meatus (ear) 744.03
  ovary (acquired) V45.77
    congenital 752.0
  oviduct (acquired) V45.77
    congenital 752.19
  pancreas (congenital) 751.7
    acquired (postoperative) (posttraumatic)
        V45.79
  parathyroid gland (congenital) 759.2
  parotid gland(s) (congenital) 750.21
  patella, congenital 755.64
  pelvic girdle (congenital) 755.69
  penis (congenital) 752.69
    acquired V45.77
  pericardium (congenital) 746.89
  perineal body (congenital) 756.81
  phalange(s), congenital 755.4
    lower limb (complete) (intercalary) (partial)
        (terminal) (*see also* Deformity,
        reduction, lower limb) 755.39
      meaning all toes (complete) (partial)
          755.31

Absence — *continued*
  phalange(s), congenital — *continued*
    lower limb (*see also* Deformity, reduction,
        lower limb) — *continued*
      transverse 755.31
    upper limb (complete) (intercalary) (partial)
        (terminal) (*see also* Deformity,
        reduction, upper limb) 755.29
      meaning all digits (complete) (partial)
          755.21
      transverse 755.21
  pituitary gland (congenital) 759.2
  postoperative — *see* Absence, by site, acquired
  prostate (congenital) 752.8
    acquired V45.77
  pulmonary
    artery 747.3
    trunk 747.3
    valve (congenital) 746.01
    vein 747.49
  punctum lacrimale (congenital) 743.65
  radius, congenital (complete) (partial) (with
      absence of distal elements, incomplete)
      755.26
    with
      complete absence of distal elements
          755.21
      ulna 755.25
        with
          complete absence of distal elements
              755.21
          humerus (incomplete) 755.23
  ray, congenital 755.4
    lower limb (complete) (partial) (*see also*
        Deformity, reduction, lower limb)
        755.38
      meaning all rays 755.31
      transverse 755.31
    upper limb (complete) (partial) (*see also*
        Deformity, reduction, upper limb)
        755.28
      meaning all rays 755.21
      transverse 755.21
  rectum (congenital) 751.2
    acquired V45.79
  red cell 284.9
    acquired (secondary) 284.8
    congenital 284.0
    hereditary 284.0
    idiopathic 284.9
  respiratory organ (congenital) NEC 748.9
  rib (acquired) 738.3
    congenital 756.3
  roof of orbit (congenital) 742.0
  round ligament (congenital) 752.8
  sacrum, congenital 756.13
  salivary gland(s) (congenital) 750.21
  scapula 755.59
  scrotum, congenital 752.8
  seminal tract or duct (congenital) 752.8
    acquired V45.77
  septum (congenital) — *see also* Imperfect,
      closure, septum
    atrial 745.69
      and ventricular 745.7
    between aorta and pulmonary artery 745.0
    ventricular 745.3
      and atrial 745.7
  sex chromosomes 758.81
  shoulder girdle, congenital (complete) (partial)
      755.59
  skin (congenital) 757.39
  skull bone 756.0
    with
      anencephalus 740.0
      encephalocele 742.0
      hydrocephalus 742.3
        with spina bifida (*see also* Spina
            bifida) 741.0 ✔5ᵗʰ
      microcephalus 742.1
  spermatic cord (congenital) 752.8
  spinal cord 742.59
  spine, congenital 756.13
  spleen (congenital) 759.0
    acquired V45.79
  sternum, congenital 756.3

Absence — *continued*
- stomach (acquired) (partial) (postoperative) V45.75
  - with postgastric surgery syndrome 564.2
  - congenital 750.7
- submaxillary gland(s) (congenital) 750.21
- superior vena cava (congenital) 747.49
- tarsal(s), congenital (complete) (partial) (with absence of distal elements, incomplete) (*see also* Deformity, reduction, lower limb) 755.38
- teeth, tooth (congenital) 520.0
  - with abnormal spacing 524.3
  - acquired 525.10
    - with malocclusion 524.3
    - due to
      - caries 525.13
      - extraction 525.10
      - periodontal disease 525.12
      - trauma 525.11
- tendon (congenital) 756.81
- testis (congenital) 752.8
  - acquired V45.77
- thigh (acquired) 736.89
- thumb (acquired) V49.61
  - congenital 755.29
- thymus gland (congenital) 759.2
- thyroid (gland) (surgical) 246.8
  - with hypothyroidism 244.0
  - cartilage, congenital 748.3
  - congenital 243
- tibia, congenital (complete) (partial) (with absence of distal elements, incomplete) (*see also* Deformity, reduction, lower limb) 755.36
  - with
    - complete absence of distal elements 755.31
    - fibula 755.35
      - with
        - complete absence of distal elements 755.31
        - femur (incomplete) 755.33
          - with complete absence of distal elements 755.31
- toe (acquired) V49.72
  - congenital (complete) (partial) 755.39
    - meaning all toes 755.31
    - transverse 755.31
  - great V49.71
- tongue (congenital) 750.11
- tooth, teeth, (congenital) 520.0
  - with abnormal spacing 524.3
  - acquired 525.10
    - with malocclusion 524.3
    - due to
      - caries 525.13
      - extraction 525.10
      - periodontal disease 525.12
      - trauma 525.11
- trachea (cartilage) (congenital) (rings) 748.3
- transverse aortic arch (congenital) 747.21
- tricuspid valve 746.1
- ulna, congenital (complete) (partial) (with absence of distal elements, incomplete) (*see also* Deformity, reduction, upper limb) 755.27
  - with
    - complete absence of distal elements 755.21
    - radius 755.25
      - with
        - complete absence of distal elements 755.21
        - humerus (incomplete) 755.23
- umbilical artery (congenital) 747.5
- ureter (congenital) 753.4
  - acquired V45.74
- urethra, congenital 753.8
  - acquired V45.74
- urinary system, part NEC, congenital 753.8
  - acquired V45.74
- uterus (acquired) V45.77
  - congenital 752.3
- uvula (congenital) 750.26
- vagina, congenital 752.49
  - acquired V45.77

Absence — *continued*
- vas deferens (congenital) 752.8
  - acquired V45.77
- vein (congenital) (peripheral) NEC (*see also* Anomaly, peripheral vascular system) 747.60
  - brain 747.81
  - great 747.49
  - portal 747.49
  - pulmonary 747.49
- vena cava (congenital) (inferior) (superior) 747.49
- ventral horn cell 742.59
- ventricular septum 745.3
- vermis of cerebellum 742.2
- vertebra, congenital 756.13
- vulva, congenital 752.49

Absentia epileptica (*see also* Epilepsy) 345.0 ✓5ᵗʰ
Absinthemia (*see also* Dependence) 304.6 ✓5ᵗʰ
Absinthism (*see also* Dependence) 304.6 ✓5ᵗʰ
Absorbent system disease 459.89
Absorption
- alcohol, through placenta or breast milk 760.71
- antibiotics, through placenta or breast milk 760.74
- anti-infective, through placenta or breast milk 760.74
- chemical NEC 989.9
  - specified chemical or substance — *see* Table of Drugs and Chemicals
  - through placenta or breast milk (fetus or newborn) 760.70
    - alcohol 760.71
    - anti-infective agents 760.74
    - cocaine 760.75
    - "crack" 760.75
    - diethylstilbestrol [DES] 760.76
    - hallucinogenic agents 760.73
    - medicinal agents NEC 760.79
    - narcotics 760.72
    - obstetric anesthetic or analgesic drug 763.5
    - specified agent NEC 760.79
    - suspected, affecting management of pregnancy 655.5 ✓5ᵗʰ
- cocaine, through placenta or breast milk 760.75
- drug NEC (*see also* Reaction, drug)
  - through placenta or breast milk (fetus or newborn) 760.70
    - alcohol 760.71
  - through placenta or breast milk (fetus or newborn) — *continued*
    - anti-infective agents 760.74
    - cocaine 760.75
    - "crack" 760.75
    - diethylstilbestrol [DES] 760.76
    - hallucinogenic agents 760.73
    - medicinal agents NEC 760.79
    - narcotics 760.72
    - obstetric anesthetic or analgesic drug 763.5
    - specified agent NEC 760.79
    - suspected, affecting management of pregnancy 655.5 ✓5ᵗʰ
- fat, disturbance 579.8
- hallucinogenic agents, through placenta or breast milk 760.73
- immune sera, through placenta or breast milk 760.79
- lactose defect 271.3
- medicinal agents NEC, through placenta or breast milk 760.79
- narcotics, through placenta or breast milk 760.72
- noxious substance, — *see* Absorption, chemical
- protein, disturbance 579.8
- pus or septic, general — *see* Septicemia
- quinine, through placenta or breast milk 760.74
- toxic substance, — *see* Absorption, chemical
- uremic — *see* Uremia

Abstinence symptoms or syndrome
- alcohol 291.81
- drug 292.0

Abt-Letterer-Siwe syndrome (acute histiocytosis X) (M9722/3) 202.5 ✓5ᵗʰ
Abulia 799.8
Abulomania 301.6
Abuse
- adult 995.80
  - emotional 995.82
  - multiple forms 995.85
  - neglect (nutritional) 995.84
  - physical 995.81
  - psychological 995.82
  - sexual 995.83
- alcohol (*see also* Alcoholism) 305.0 ✓5ᵗʰ
  - dependent 303.9 ✓5ᵗʰ
  - non-dependent 305.0 ✓5ᵗʰ
- child 995.50
  - counseling
    - perpetrator
      - non-parent V62.83
      - parent V61.22
    - victim V61.21
  - emotional 995.51
  - multiple forms 995.59
  - neglect (nutritional) 995.52
  - psychological 995.51
  - physical 995.54
    - shaken infant syndrome 995.55
  - sexual 995.53
- drugs, nondependent 305.9 ✓5ᵗʰ

> Note — Use the following fifth-digit subclassification with the following codes: 305.0, 305.2-305.9:
>
> | 0 | unspecified | 2 | episodic |
> |---|---|---|---|
> | 1 | continuous | 3 | in remission |

- amphetamine type 305.7 ✓5ᵗʰ
- antidepressants 305.8 ✓5ᵗʰ
- barbiturates 305.4 ✓5ᵗʰ
- caffeine 305.9 ✓5ᵗʰ
- cannabis 305.2 ✓5ᵗʰ
- cocaine type 305.6 ✓5ᵗʰ
- hallucinogens 305.3 ✓5ᵗʰ
- hashish 305.2 ✓5ᵗʰ
- LSD 305.3 ✓5ᵗʰ
- marijuana 305.2 ✓5ᵗʰ
- mixed 305.9 ✓5ᵗʰ
- morphine type 305.5 ✓5ᵗʰ
- opioid type 305.5 ✓5ᵗʰ
- phencyclidine (PCP) 305.9 ✓5ᵗʰ
- specified NEC 305.9 ✓5ᵗʰ
- tranquilizers 305.4 ✓5ᵗʰ
- spouse 995.80
- tobacco 305.1

Acalcerosis 275.40
Acalcicosis 275.40
Acalculia 784.69
- developmental 315.1
Acanthocheilonemiasis 125.4
Acanthocytosis 272.5
Acanthokeratodermia 701.1
Acantholysis 701.8
- bullosa 757.39
Acanthoma (benign) (M8070/0) — *see also* Neoplasm, by site, benign
- malignant (M8070/3) — *see* Neoplasm, by site, malignant
Acanthosis (acquired) (nigricans) 701.2
- adult 701.2
- benign (congenital) 757.39
- congenital 757.39
- glycogenic
  - esophagus 530.89
- juvenile 701.2
- tongue 529.8
Acanthrocytosis 272.5
Acapnia 276.3
Acarbia 276.2
Acardia 759.89
Acardiacus amorphus 759.89
Acardiotrophia 429.1
Acardius 759.89

Acariasis 133.9
  sarcoptic 133.0
Acaridiasis 133.9
Acarinosis 133.9
Acariosis 133.9
Acarodermatitis 133.9
  urticarioides 133.9
Acarophobia 300.29
Acatalasemia 277.8
Acatalasia 277.8
Acatamathesia 784.69
Acataphasia 784.5
Acathisia 781.0
  due to drugs 333.99
Acceleration, accelerated
  atrioventricular conduction 426.7
  idioventricular rhythm 427.89
Accessory (congenital)
  adrenal gland 759.1
  anus 751.5
  appendix 751.5
  atrioventricular conduction 426.7
  auditory ossicles 744.04
  auricle (ear) 744.1
  autosome(s) NEC 758.5
    21 or 22 758.0
  biliary duct or passage 751.69
  bladder 753.8
  blood vessels (peripheral) (congenital) NEC (*see also* Anomaly, peripheral vascular system) 747.60
    cerebral 747.81
    coronary 746.85
  bone NEC 756.9
    foot 755.67
  breast tissue, axilla 757.6
  carpal bones 755.56
  cecum 751.5
  cervix 752.49
  chromosome(s) NEC 758.5
    13-15 758.1
    16-18 758.2
    21 or 22 758.0
    autosome(s) NEC 758.5
    D_1 758.1
    E_3 758.2
    G 758.0
    sex 758.81
  coronary artery 746.85
  cusp(s), heart valve NEC 746.89
    pulmonary 746.09
  cystic duct 751.69
  digits 755.00
  ear (auricle) (lobe) 744.1
  endocrine gland NEC 759.2
  external os 752.49
  eyelid 743.62
  eye muscle 743.69
  face bone(s) 756.0
  fallopian tube (fimbria) (ostium) 752.19
  fingers 755.01
  foreskin 605
  frontonasal process 756.0
  gallbladder 751.69
  genital organ(s)
    female 752.8
      external 752.49
      internal NEC 752.8
    male NEC 752.8
      penis 752.69
  genitourinary organs NEC 752.8
  heart 746.89
    valve NEC 746.89
      pulmonary 746.09
  hepatic ducts 751.69
  hymen 752.49
  intestine (large) (small) 751.5
  kidney 753.3
  lacrimal canal 743.65
  leaflet, heart valve NEC 746.89
    pulmonary 746.09
  ligament, broad 752.19
  liver (duct) 751.69
  lobule (ear) 744.1
  lung (lobe) 748.69

Accessory — *continued*
  muscle 756.82
  navicular of carpus 755.56
  nervous system, part NEC 742.8
  nipple 757.6
  nose 748.1
  organ or site NEC — *see* Anomaly, specified type NEC
  ovary 752.0
  oviduct 752.19
  pancreas 751.7
  parathyroid gland 759.2
  parotid gland (and duct) 750.22
  pituitary gland 759.2
  placental lobe — *see* Placenta, abnormal
  preauricular appendage 744.1
  prepuce 605
  renal arteries (multiple) 747.62
  rib 756.3
    cervical 756.2
  roots (teeth) 520.2
  salivary gland 750.22
  sesamoids 755.8
  sinus — *see* condition
  skin tags 757.39
  spleen 759.0
  sternum 756.3
  submaxillary gland 750.22
  tarsal bones 755.67
  teeth, tooth 520.1
    causing crowding 524.3
  tendon 756.89
  thumb 755.01
  thymus gland 759.2
  thyroid gland 759.2
  toes 755.02
  tongue 750.13
  tragus 744.1
  ureter 753.4
  urethra 753.8
  urinary organ or tract NEC 753.8
  uterus 752.2
  vagina 752.49
  valve, heart NEC 746.89
    pulmonary 746.09
  vertebra 756.19
  vocal cords 748.3
  vulva 752.49
Accident, accidental — *see also* condition
  birth NEC 767.9
  cardiovascular (*see also* Disease, cardiovascular) 429.2
  cerebral (*see also* Disease, cerebrovascular, acute) 436
  cerebrovascular (current) (CVA) (*see also* Disease, cerebrovascular, acute) 436
    healed or old V12.59
    impending 435.9
    late effect — *see* Late effect(s) (of) cerebrovascular disease
    postoperative 997.02   ●
  coronary (*see also* Infarct, myocardium) 410.9 ✔5ᵗʰ
  craniovascular (*see also* Disease, cerebrovascular, acute) 436
  during pregnancy, to mother
    affecting fetus or newborn 760.5
  heart, cardiac (*see also* Infarct, myocardium) 410.9 ✔5ᵗʰ
  intrauterine 779.89   ▲
  vascular — *see* Disease, cerebrovascular, acute
Accommodation
  disorder of 367.51
    drug-induced 367.89
    toxic 367.89
  insufficiency of 367.4
  paralysis of 367.51
    hysterical 300.11
  spasm of 367.53
Accouchement — *see* Delivery
Accreta placenta (without hemorrhage) 667.0 ✔5ᵗʰ
  with hemorrhage 666.0 ✔5ᵗʰ
Accretio cordis (nonrheumatic) 423.1
Accretions on teeth 523.6
Accumulation secretion, prostate 602.8
Acephalia, acephalism, acephaly 740.0

Acephalic 740.0
Acephalobrachia 759.89
Acephalocardia 759.89
Acephalocardius 759.89
Acephalochiria 759.89
Acephalochirus 759.89
Acephalogaster 759.89
Acephalostomus 759.89
Acephalothorax 759.89
Acephalus 740.0
Acetonemia 790.6
  diabetic 250.1 ✔5ᵗʰ
Acetonglycosuria 982.8
Acetonuria 791.6
Achalasia 530.0
  cardia 530.0
  digestive organs congenital NEC 751.8
  esophagus 530.0
  pelvirectal 751.3
  psychogenic 306.4
  pylorus 750.5
  sphincteral NEC 564.89
Achard-Thiers syndrome (adrenogenital) 255.2
Ache(s) — *see* Pain
Acheilia 750.26
Acheiria 755.21
Achillobursitis 726.71
Achillodynia 726.71
Achlorhydria, achlorhydric 536.0
  anemia 280.9
  diarrhea 536.0
  neurogenic 536.0
  postvagotomy 564.2
  psychogenic 306.4
  secondary to vagotomy 564.2
Achloroblepsia 368.52
Achloropsia 368.52
Acholia 575.8
Acholuric jaundice (familial) (splenomegalic) (*see also* Spherocytosis) 282.0
  acquired 283.9
Achondroplasia 756.4
Achrestic anemia 281.8
Achroacytosis, lacrimal gland 375.00
  tuberculous (*see also* Tuberculosis) 017.3 ✔5ᵗʰ
Achroma, cutis 709.00
Achromate (congenital) 368.54
Achromatopia 368.54
Achromatopsia (congenital) 368.54
Achromia
  congenital 270.2
  parasitica 111.0
  unguium 703.8
Achylia
  gastrica 536.8
    neurogenic 536.3
    psychogenic 306.4
  pancreatica 577.1
Achylosis 536.8
Acid
  burn — *see also* Burn, by site
    from swallowing acid — *see* Burn, internal organs
  deficiency
    amide nicotinic 265.2
    amino 270.9
    ascorbic 267
    folic 266.2
    nicotinic (amide) 265.2
    pantothenic 266.2
  intoxication 276.2
  peptic disease 536.8
  stomach 536.8
    psychogenic 306.4
Acidemia 276.2
  arginosuccinic 270.6
  fetal
    affecting management of pregnancy 656.3 ✔5ᵗʰ
    before onset of labor, in liveborn infant 768.2

Acidemia — *continued*
> fetal — *continued*
>> during labor, in liveborn infant 768.3
>> intrauterine — *see* Distress, fetal 656.3 ✓5ᵗʰ
>> unspecified as to time of onset, in liveborn infant 768.4
> pipecolic 270.7

Acidity, gastric (high) (low) 536.8
> psychogenic 306.4

Acidocytopenia 288.0

Acidocytosis 288.3

Acidopenia 288.0

Acidosis 276.2
> diabetic 250.1 ✓5ᵗʰ
> fetal, affecting management of pregnancy 756.8 ✓5ᵗʰ
> fetal, affecting newborn 768.9   ▲
> kidney tubular 588.8
> lactic 276.2
> metabolic NEC 276.2
>> with respiratory acidosis 276.4
>> late, of newborn 775.7
> renal
>> hyperchloremic 588.8
>> tubular (distal) (proximal) 588.8
> respiratory 276.2
>> complicated by
>>> metabolic acidosis 276.4
>>> metabolic alkalosis 276.4

Aciduria 791.9
> arginosuccinic 270.6
> beta-aminoisobutyric (BAIB) 277.2
> glycolic 271.8
> methylmalonic 270.3
>> with glycinemia 270.7
> organic 270.9
> orotic (congenital) (hereditary) (pyrimidine deficiency) 281.4

Acladiosis 111.8
> skin 111.8

Aclasis
> diaphyseal 756.4
> tarsoepiphyseal 756.59

Acleistocardia 745.5

Aclusion 524.4

Acmesthesia 782.0

Acne (pustular) (vulgaris) 706.1
> agminata (*see also* Tuberculosis) 017.0 ✓5ᵗʰ
> artificialis 706.1
> atrophica 706.0
> cachecticorum (Hebra) 706.1
> conglobata 706.1
> conjunctiva 706.1
> cystic 706.1
> decalvans 704.09
> erythematosa 695.3
> eyelid 706.1
> frontalis 706.0
> indurata 706.1
> keloid 706.1
> lupoid 706.0
> necrotic, necrotica 706.0
>> miliaris 704.8
> nodular 706.1
> occupational 706.1
> papulosa 706.1
> rodens 706.0
> rosacea 695.3
> scorbutica 267
> scrofulosorum (Bazin) (*see also* Tuberculosis) 017.0 ✓5ᵗʰ
> summer 692.72
> tropical 706.1
> varioliformis 706.0

Acneiform drug eruptions 692.3

Acnitis (primary) (*see also* Tuberculosis) 017.0 ✓5ᵗʰ

Acomia 704.00

Acontractile bladder 344.61

Aconuresis (*see also* Incontinence) 788.30

Acosta's disease 993.2

Acousma 780.1

Acoustic — *see* condition

Acousticophobia 300.29

Acquired — *see* condition

Acquired immune deficiency syndrome — *see* Human immunodeficiency virus (disease) (illness) (infection)

Acquired immunodeficiency syndrome — *see* Human immunodeficiency virus (disease) (illness) (infection)

Acragnosis 781.99

Acrania 740.0

Acroagnosis 781.99

Acroasphyxia, chronic 443.89

Acrobrachycephaly 756.0

Acrobystiolith 608.89

Acrobystitis 607.2

Acrocephalopolysyndactyly 755.55

Acrocephalosyndactyly 755.55

Acrocephaly 756.0

Acrochondrohyperplasia 759.82

Acrocyanosis 443.89
> newborn 770.83   ▲

Acrodermatitis 686.8
> atrophicans (chronica) 701.8
> continua (Hallopeau) 696.1
> enteropathica 686.8
> Hallopeau's 696.1
> perstans 696.1
> pustulosa continua 696.1
> recalcitrant pustular 696.1

Acrodynia 985.0

Acrodysplasia 755.55

Acrohyperhidrosis 780.8

Acrokeratosis verruciformis 757.39

Acromastitis 611.0

Acromegaly, acromegalia (skin) 253.0

Acromelalgia 443.89

Acromicria acromikria 756.59

Acronyx 703.0

Acropachy, thyroid (*see also* Thyrotoxicosis) 242.9 ✓5ᵗʰ

Acropachyderma 757.39

Acroparesthesia 443.89
> simple (Schultz's type) 443.89
> vasomotor (Nothnagel's type) 443.89

Acropathy thyroid (*see also* Thyrotoxicosis) 242.9 ✓5ᵗʰ

Acrophobia 300.29

Acroposthitis 607.2

Acroscleriasis (*see also* Scleroderma) 710.1

Acroscleroderma (*see also* Scleroderma) 710.1

Acrosclerosis (*see also* Scleroderma) 710.1

Acrosphacelus 785.4

Acrosphenosyndactylia 755.55

Acrospiroma, eccrine (M8402/0) — *see* Neoplasm, skin, benign

Acrostealgia 732.9

Acrosyndactyly (*see also* Syndactylism) 755.10

Acrotrophodynia 991.4

Actinic — *see also* condition
> cheilitis (due to sun) 692.72
>> chronic NEC 692.74
>> due to radiation, except from sun 692.82
> conjunctivitis 370.24
> dermatitis (due to sun) (*see also* Dermatitis, actinic 692.70
>> due to
>>> roentgen rays or radioactive substance 692.82
>>> ultraviolet radiation, except from sun 692.82
>>> sun NEC 692.70
> elastosis solare 692.74
> granuloma 692.73
> keratitis 370.24
> ophthalmia 370.24
> reticuloid 692.73

Actinobacillosis, general 027.8

Actinobacillus
> lignieresii 027.8
> mallei 024
> muris 026.1

Actinocutitis NEC (*see also* Dermatitis, actinic) 692.70

Actinodermatitis NEC (*see also* Dermatitis, actinic) 692.70

Actinomyces
> israelii (infection) — *see* Actinomycosis
> muris-ratti (infection) 026.1

Actinomycosis, actinomycotic 039.9
> with
>> pneumonia 039.1
> abdominal 039.2
> cervicofacial 039.3
> cutaneous 039.0
> pulmonary 039.1
> specified site NEC 039.8
> thoracic 039.1

Actinoneuritis 357.89   ▲

Action, heart
> disorder 427.9
>> postoperative 997.1
> irregular 427.9
>> postoperative 997.1
>> psychogenic 306.2

Active — *see* condition

Activity decrease, functional 780.99   ▲

Acute — *see also* condition
> abdomen NEC 789.0 ✓5ᵗʰ
> gallbladder (*see also* Cholecystitis, acute) 575.0

Acyanoblepsia 368.53

Acyanopsia 368.53

Acystia 753.8

Acystinervia — *see* Neurogenic, bladder

Acystineuria — *see* Neurogenic, bladder

Adactylia, adactyly (congenital) 755.4
> lower limb (complete) (intercalary) (partial) (terminal) (*see also* Deformity, reduction, lower limb) 755.39
>> meaning all digits (complete) (partial) 755.31
>> transverse (complete) (partial) 755.31
> upper limb (complete) (intercalary) (partial) (terminal) (*see also* Deformity, reduction, upper limb) 755.29
>> meaning all digits (complete) (partial) 755.21
>> transverse (complete) (partial) 755.21

Adair-Dighton syndrome (brittle bones and blue sclera, deafness) 756.51

Adamantinoblastoma (M9310/0) — *see* Ameloblastoma

Adamantinoma (M9310/0) — *see* Ameloblastoma

Adamantoblastoma (M9310/0) — *see* Ameloblastoma

Adams-Stokes (-Morgagni) disease or syndrome (syncope with heart block) 426.9

Adaptation reaction (*see also* Reaction, adjustment) 309.9

Addiction — *see also* Dependence
> absinthe 304.6 ✓5ᵗʰ
> alcoholic (ethyl) (methyl) (wood) 303.9 ✓5ᵗʰ
>> complicating pregnancy, childbirth, or puerperium 648.4 ✓5ᵗʰ
>>> affecting fetus or newborn 760.71
>> suspected damage to fetus affecting management of pregnancy 655.4 ✓5ᵗʰ
> drug (*see also* Dependence) 304.9 ✓5ᵗʰ
> ethyl alcohol 303.9 ✓5ᵗʰ
> heroin 304.0 ✓5ᵗʰ
> hospital 301.51
> methyl alcohol 303.9 ✓5ᵗʰ
> methylated spirit 303.9 ✓5ᵗʰ
> morphine (-like substances) 304.0 ✓5ᵗʰ
> nicotine 305.1
> opium 304.0 ✓5ᵗʰ
> tobacco 305.1
> wine 303.9 ✓5ᵗʰ

Addison's
> anemia (pernicious) 281.0
> disease (bronze) (primary adrenal insufficiency) 255.4
>> tuberculous (*see also* Tuberculosis) 017.6 ✓5ᵗʰ
> keloid (morphea) 701.0
> melanoderma (adrenal cortical hypofunction) 255.4

✓4ᵗʰ Fourth-digit Required   ✓5ᵗʰ Fifth-digit Required   ▶◀ Revised Text   ● New Line   ▲ Revised Code

Addison-Biermer anemia (pernicious) 281.0

Addison-Gull disease — *see* Xanthoma

Addisonian crisis or melanosis (acute
  adrenocortical insufficiency) 255.4

Additional — *see also* Accessory
  chromosome(s) 758.5
    13-15 758.1
    16-18 758.2
    21 758.0
    autosome(s) NEC 758.5
    sex 758.81

Adduction contracture, hip or other joint — *see*
  Contraction, joint

Adenasthenia gastrica 536.0

Aden fever 061

Adenitis (*see also* Lymphadenitis) 289.3
  acute, unspecified site 683
    epidemic infectious 075
  axillary 289.3
    acute 683
    chronic or subacute 289.1
  Bartholin's gland 616.8
  bulbourethral gland (*see also* Urethritis) 597.89
  cervical 289.3
    acute 683
    chronic or subacute 289.1
  chancroid (Ducrey's bacillus) 099.0
  chronic (any lymph node, except mesenteric)
      289.1
    mesenteric 289.2
  Cowper's gland (*see also* Urethritis) 597.89
  epidemic, acute 075
  gangrenous 683
  gonorrheal NEC 098.89
  groin 289.3
    acute 683
    chronic or subacute 289.1
  infectious 075
  inguinal (region) 289.3
    acute 683
    chronic or subacute 289.1
  lymph gland or node, except mesenteric 289.3
    acute 683
    chronic or subacute 289.1
    mesenteric (acute) (chronic) (nonspecific)
        (subacute) 289.2
  mesenteric (acute) (chronic) (nonspecific)
      (subacute) 289.2
    due to Pasteurella multocida (P. septica)
        027.2
  parotid gland (suppurative) 527.2
  phlegmonous 683
  salivary duct or gland (any) (recurring)
      (suppurative) 527.2
  scrofulous (*see also* Tuberculosis) 017.2 ☑5ᵗʰ
  septic 289.3
  Skene's duct or gland (*see also* Urethritis)
      597.89
  strumous, tuberculous (*see also* Tuberculosis)
      017.2 ☑5ᵗʰ
  subacute, unspecified site 289.1
  sublingual gland (suppurative) 527.2
  submandibular gland (suppurative) 527.2
  submaxillary gland (suppurative) 527.2
  suppurative 683
  tuberculous — *see* Tuberculosis, lymph gland
  urethral gland (*see also* Urethritis) 597.89
  venereal NEC 099.8
  Wharton's duct (suppurative) 527.2

Adenoacanthoma (M8570/3) — *see* Neoplasm, by
  site, malignant

Adenoameloblastoma (M9300/0) 213.1
  upper jaw (bone) 213.0

Adenocarcinoma (M8140/3) — *see also*
  Neoplasm, by site, malignant

> *Note* — *The following list of adjectival
> modifiers is not exhaustive. A description of
> adenocarcinoma that does not appear in this
> list should be coded in the same manner as
> carcinoma with that description. Thus,
> "mixed acidophil-basophil adenocarcinoma,"
> should be coded in the same manner as
> "mixed acidophil-basophil carcinoma," which
> appears in the list under "Carcinoma."*
>
> *Except where otherwise indicated, the
> morphological varieties of adenocarcinoma in
> the list should be coded by site as for
> "Neoplasm, malignant."*

  with
    apocrine metaplasia (M8573/3)
    cartilaginous (and osseous) metaplasia
        (M8571/3)
    osseous (and cartilaginous) metaplasia
        (M8571/3)
    spindle cell metaplasia (M8572/3)
    squamous metaplasia (M8570/3)
  acidophil (M8280/3)
    specified site — *see* Neoplasm, by site,
        malignant
    unspecified site 194.3
  acinar (M8550/3)
  acinic cell (M8550/3)
  adrenal cortical (M8370/3) 194.0
  alveolar (M8251/3)
    and
      epidermoid carcinoma, mixed (M8560/3)
      squamous cell carcinoma, mixed
          (M8560/3)
  apocrine (M8401/3)
    breast — *see* Neoplasm, breast, malignant
    specified site NEC — *see* Neoplasm, skin,
        malignant
    unspecified site 173.9
  basophil (M8300/3)
    specified site — *see* Neoplasm, by site,
        malignant
    unspecified site 194.3
  bile duct type (M8160/3)
    liver 155.1
    specified site NEC — *see* Neoplasm, by site,
        malignant
    unspecified site 155.1
  bronchiolar (M8250/3) — *see* Neoplasm, lung,
      malignant
  ceruminous (M8420/3) 173.2
  chromophobe (M8270/3)
    specified site — *see* Neoplasm, by site,
        malignant
    unspecified site 194.3
  clear cell (mesonephroid type) (M8310/3)
  colloid (M8480/3)
  cylindroid type (M8200/3)
  diffuse type (M8145/3)
    specified site — *see* Neoplasm, by site,
        malignant
    unspecified site 151.9
  duct (infiltrating) (M8500/3)
    with Paget's disease (M8541/3) — *see*
        Neoplasm, breast, malignant
    specified site — *see* Neoplasm, by site,
        malignant
    unspecified site 174.9
  embryonal (M9070/3)
  endometrioid (M8380/3) — *see* Neoplasm, by
      site, malignant
  eosinophil (M8280/3)
    specified site — *see* Neoplasm, by site
        malignant
    unspecified site 194.3
  follicular (M8330/3)
    and papillary (M8340/3) 193
    moderately differentiated type (M8332/3) 193
    pure follicle type (M8331/3) 193
    specified site — *see* Neoplasm, by site,
        malignant
    trabecular type (M8332/3) 193
    unspecified type 193
    well differentiated type (M8331/3) 193
  gelatinous (M8480/3)

Adenocarcinoma — *see also* Neoplasm, by site,
  malignant — *continued*
  granular cell (M8320/3)
  Hürthle cell (M8290/3) 193
  in
    adenomatous
      polyp (M8210/3)
      polyposis coli (M8220/3) 153.9
    polypoid adenoma (M8210/3)
    tubular adenoma (M8210/3)
    villous adenoma (M8261/3)
  infiltrating duct (M8500/3)
    with Paget's disease (M8541/3) — *see*
        Neoplasm, breast, malignant
    specified site — *see* Neoplasm, by site,
        malignant
    unspecified site 174.9
  inflammatory (M8530/3)
    specified site — *see* Neoplasm, by site,
        malignant
    unspecified site 174.9
  in situ (M8140/2) — *see* Neoplasm, by site, in
      situ
  intestinal type (M8144/3)
    specified site — *see* Neoplasm, by site,
        malignant
    unspecified site 151.9
  intraductal (noninfiltrating) (M8500/2)
    papillary (M8503/2)
      specified site — *see* Neoplasm, by site, in
          situ
      unspecified site 233.0
    specified site — *see* Neoplasm, by site, in
        situ
    unspecified site 233.0
  islet cell (M8150/3)
    and exocrine, mixed (M8154/3)
      specified site — *see* Neoplasm, by site,
          malignant
      unspecified site 157.9
    pancreas 157.4
    specified site NEC — *see* Neoplasm, by site,
        malignant
    unspecified site 157.4
  lobular (M8520/3)
    specified site — *see* Neoplasm, by site,
        malignant
    unspecified site 174.9
  medullary (M8510/3)
  mesonephric (M9110/3)
  mixed cell (M8323/3)
  mucinous (M8480/3)
  mucin-producing (M8481/3)
  mucoid (M8480/3) — *see also* Neoplasm, by
      site, malignant
    cell (M8300/3)
      specified site — *see* Neoplasm, by site,
          malignant
      unspecified site 194.3
  nonencapsulated sclerosing (M8350/3) 193
  oncocytic (M8290/3)
  oxyphilic (M8290/3)
  papillary (M8260/3)
    and follicular (M8340/3) 193
    intraductal (noninfiltrating) (M8503/2)
      specified site — *see* Neoplasm, by site, in
          situ
      unspecified site 233.0
    serous (M8460/3)
      specified site — *see* Neoplasm, by site,
          malignant
      unspecified site 183.0
  papillocystic (M8450/3)
    specified site — *see* Neoplasm, by site,
        malignant
    unspecified site 183.0
  pseudomucinous (M8470/3)
    specified site — *see* Neoplasm, by site,
        malignant
    unspecified site 183.0
  renal cell (M8312/3) 189.0
  sebaceous (M8410/3)
  serous (M8441/3) — *see also* Neoplasm, by
      site, malignant
    papillary
      specified site — *see* Neoplasm, by site
          malignant

Addison-Biermer anemia — Adenocarcinoma

Adenocarcinoma — *see also* Neoplasm, by site,
   malignant — *continued*
   serous — *see also* Neoplasm, by site, malignant
      — *continued*
      papillary — *continued*
         unspecified site 183.0
   signet ring cell (M8490/3)
   superficial spreading (M8143/3)
   sweat gland (M8400/3) — *see* Neoplasm, skin,
      malignant
   trabecular (M8190/3)
   tubular (M8211/3)
   villous (M8262/3)
   water-clear cell (M8322/3) 194.1
Adenofibroma (M9013/0)
   clear cell (M8313/0) — *see* Neoplasm, by site,
      benign
   endometrioid (M8381/0) 220
      borderline malignancy (M8381/1) 236.2
      malignant (M8381/3) 183.0
   mucinous (M9015/0)
      specified site — *see* Neoplasm, by site,
         benign
      unspecified site 220
   prostate 600.2
   serous (M9014/0)
      specified site — *see* Neoplasm, by site,
         benign
      unspecified site 220
   specified site — *see* Neoplasm, by site, benign
   unspecified site 220
Adenofibrosis
   breast 610.2
   endometrioid 617.0
Adenoiditis 474.01
   acute 463
   chronic 474.01
      with chronic tonsillitis 474.02
Adenoids (congenital) (of nasal fossa) 474.9
   hypertrophy 474.12
   vegetations 474.2
Adenolipomatosis (symmetrical) 272.8
Adenolymphoma (M8561/0)
   specified site — *see* Neoplasm, by site, benign
   unspecified 210.2
Adenoma (sessile) (M8140/0) — *see also*
   Neoplasm, by site, benign

> *Note* — Except where otherwise indicated,
> the morphological varieties of adenoma in the
> list below should be coded by site as for
> "Neoplasm, benign."

   acidophil (M8280/0)
      specified site — *see* Neoplasm, by site,
         benign
      unspecified site 227.3
   acinar (cell) (M8550/0)
   acinic cell (M8550/0)
   adrenal (cortex) (cortical) (functioning)
      (M8370/0) 227.0
      clear cell type (M8373/0) 227.0
      compact cell type (M8371/0) 227.0
      glomerulosa cell type (M8374/0) 227.0
      heavily pigmented variant (M8372/0) 227.0
      mixed cell type (M8375/0) 227.0
   alpha cell (M8152/0)
      pancreas 211.7
      specified site NEC — *see* Neoplasm, by site,
         benign
      unspecified site 211.7
   alveolar (M8251/0)
   apocrine (M8401/0)
      breast 217
      specified site NEC — *see* Neoplasm, skin,
         benign
      unspecified site 216.9
   basal cell (M8147/0)
   basophil (M8300/0)
      specified site — *see* Neoplasm, by site,
         benign
      unspecified site 227.3
   beta cell (M8151/0)
      pancreas 211.7

Adenoma — *see also* Neoplasm, by site, benign —
   continued
   beta cell — *continued*
      specified site NEC — *see* Neoplasm, by site,
         benign
      unspecified site 211.7
   bile duct (M8160/0) 211.5
   black (M8372/0) 227.0
   bronchial (M8140/1) 235.7
      carcinoid type (M8240/3) — *see* Neoplasm,
         lung, malignant
      cylindroid type (M8200/3) — *see* Neoplasm,
         lung, malignant
   ceruminous (M8420/0) 216.2
   chief cell (M8321/0) 227.1
   chromophobe (M8270/0)
      specified site — *see* Neoplasm, by site,
         benign
      unspecified site 227.3
   clear cell (M8310/0)
   colloid (M8334/0)
      specified site — *see* Neoplasm, by site,
         benign
      unspecifted site 226
   cylindroid type, bronchus (M8200/3) — *see*
      Neoplasm, lung, malignant
   duct (M8503/0)
   embryonal (M8191/0)
   endocrine, multiple (M8360/1)
      single specified site — *see* Neoplasm, by site,
         uncertain behavior
      two or more specified sites 237.4
      unspecified site 237.4
   endometrioid (M8380/0) — *see also* Neoplasm,
      by site, benign
      borderline malignancy (M8380/1) — *see*
         Neoplasm, by site, uncertain behavior
   eosinophil (M8280/0)
      specified site — *see* Neoplasm, by site,
         benign
      unspecified site 227.3
   fetal (M8333/0)
      specified site — *see* Neoplasm, by site,
         benign
      unspecified site 226
   follicular (M8330/0)
      specified site — *see* Neoplasm, by site,
         benign
      unspecified site 226
   hepatocellular (M8170/0) 211.5
   Hürthle cell (M8290/0) 226
   intracystic papillary (M8504/0)
   islet cell (functioning) (M8150/0)
      pancreas 211.7
      specified site NEC — *see* Neoplasm, by site,
         benign
      unspecified site 211.7
   liver cell (M8170/0) 211.5
   macrofollicular (M8334/0)
      specified site NEC — *see* Neoplasm, by site,
         benign
      unspecified site 226
   malignant, malignum (M8140/3) — *see*
      Neoplasm, by site, malignant
   mesonephric (M9110/0)
   microfollicular (M8333/0)
      specified site — *see* Neoplasm, by site,
         benign
      unspecified site 226
   mixed cell (M8323/0)
   monomorphic (M8146/0)
   mucinous (M8480/0)
   mucoid cell (M8300/0)
      specified site — *see* Neoplasm, by site,
         benign
      unspecified site 227.3
   multiple endocrine (M8360/1)
      single specified site — *see* Neoplasm, by site,
         uncertain behavior
      two or more specified sites 237.4
      unspecified site 237.4
   nipple (M8506/0) 217
   oncocytic (M8290/0)
   oxyphilic (M8290/0)
   papillary (M8260/0) — *see also* Neoplasm, by
      site, benign
      intracystic (M8504/0)
   papillotubular (M8263/0)

Adenoma — *see also* Neoplasm, by site, benign —
   continued
   Pick's tubular (M8640/0)
      specified site — *see* Neoplasm, by site,
         benign
      unspecified site
         female 220
         male 222.0
   pleomorphic (M8940/0)
   polypoid (M8210/0)
   prostate (benign) 600.2
   rete cell 222.0
   sebaceous, sebaceum (gland) (senile) (M8410/0)
      — *see also* Neoplasm, skin, benign
      disseminata 759.5
   Sertoli cell (M8640/0)
      specified site — *see* Neoplasm, by site,
         benign
      unspecified site
         female 220
         male 222.0
   skin appendage (M8390/0) — *see* Neoplasm,
      skin, benign
   sudoriferous gland (M8400/0) — *see* Neoplasm,
      skin, benign
   sweat gland or duct (M8400/0) — *see*
      Neoplasm, skin, benign
   testicular (M8640/0)
      specified site — *see* Neoplasm, by site,
         benign
      unspecified site
         female 220
         male 222.0
   thyroid 226
   trabecular (M8190/0)
   tubular (M8211/0) — *see also* Neoplasm, by
      site, benign
      papillary (M8460/3)
      Pick's (M8640/0)
         specified site — *see* Neoplasm, by site,
            benign
         unspecified site
            female 220
            male 222.0
   tubulovillous (M8263/0)
   villoglandular (M8263/0)
   villous (M8261/1) — *see* Neoplasm, by site,
      uncertain behavior
   water-clear cell (M8322/0) 227.1
   wolffian duct (M9110/0)
Adenomatosis (M8220/0)
   endocrine (multiple) (M8360/1)
      single specified site — *see* Neoplasm, by site,
         uncertain behavior
      two or more specified sites 237.4
      unspecified site 237.4
   erosive of nipple (M8506/0) 217
   pluriendocrine — *see* Adenomatosis, endocrine
   pulmonary (M8250/1) 235.7
      malignant (M8250/3) — *see* Neoplasm, lung,
         malignant
   specified site — *see* Neoplasm, by site, benign
   unspecified site 211.3
Adenomatous
   cyst, thyroid (gland) — *see* Goiter, nodular
   goiter (nontoxic) (*see also* Goiter, nodular)
      241.9
      toxic or with hyperthyroidism 242.3 ✓5ᵗʰ
Adenomyoma (M8932/0) — *see also* Neoplasm,
   by site, benign
   prostate 600.2
Adenomyometritis 617.0
Adenomyosis (uterus) (internal) 617.0
Adenopathy (lymph gland) 785.6
   inguinal 785.6
   mediastinal 785.6
   mesentery 785.6
   syphilitic (secondary) 091.4
   tracheobronchial 785.6
      tuberculous (*see also* Tuberculosis)
         012.1 ✓5ᵗʰ
         primary, progressive 010.8 ✓5ᵗʰ
   tuberculous (*see also* Tuberculosis, lymph
      gland) 017.2 ✓5ᵗʰ
      tracheobronchial 012.1 ✓5ᵗʰ
         primary, progressive 010.8 ✓5ᵗʰ

Adenopharyngitis 462
Adenophlegmon 683
Adenosalpingitis 614.1
Adenosarcoma (M8960/3) 189.0
Adenosclerosis 289.3
Adenosis
  breast (sclerosing) 610.2
  vagina, congenital 752.49
Adentia (complete) (partial) (*see also* Absence, teeth) 520.0
Adherent
  labium (minus) 624.4
  pericardium (nonrheumatic) 423.1
    rheumatic 393
  placenta 667.0 ✓5th
    with hemorrhage 666.0 ✓5th
  prepuce 605
  scar (skin) NEC 709.2
  tendon in scar 709.2
Adhesion(s), adhesive (postinfectional) (postoperative)
  abdominal (wall) (*see also* Adhesions, peritoneum) 568.0
  amnion to fetus 658.8 ✓5th
    affecting fetus or newborn 762.8
  appendix 543.9
  arachnoiditis — *see* Meningitis
  auditory tube (Eustachian) 381.89
  bands — *see also* Adhesions, peritoneum
    cervix 622.3
    uterus 621.5
  bile duct (any) 576.8
  bladder (sphincter) 596.8
  bowel (*see also* Adhesions, peritoneum) 568.0
  cardiac 423.1
    rheumatic 398.99
  cecum (*see also* Adhesions, peritoneum) 568.0
  cervicovaginal 622.3
    congenital 752.49
    postpartal 674.8 ✓5th
    old 622.3
  cervix 622.3
  clitoris 624.4
  colon (*see also* Adhesions, peritoneum) 568.0
  common duct 576.8
  congenital — *see also* Anomaly, specified type NEC
    fingers (*see also* Syndactylism, fingers) 755.11
    labium (majus) (minus) 752.49
    omental, anomalous 751.4
    ovary 752.0
    peritoneal 751.4
    toes (*see also* Syndactylism, toes) 755.13
    tongue (to gum or roof of mouth) 750.12
  conjunctiva (acquired) (localized) 372.62
    congenital 743.63
    extensive 372.63
  cornea — *see* Opacity, cornea
  cystic duct 575.8
  diaphragm (*see also* Adhesions, peritoneum) 568.0
  due to foreign body — *see* Foreign body
  duodenum (*see also* Adhesions, peritoneum) 568.0
    with obstruction 537.3
  ear, middle — *see* Adhesions, middle ear
  epididymis 608.89
  epidural — *see* Adhesions, meninges
  epiglottis 478.79
  Eustachian tube 381.89
  eyelid 374.46
    postoperative 997.99
      surgically created V45.69
  gallbladder (*see also* Disease, gallbladder) 575.8
  globe 360.89
  heart 423.1
    rheumatic 398.99
  ileocecal (coil) (*see also* Adhesions, peritoneum) 568.0
  ileum (*see also* Adhesions, peritoneum) 568.0
  intestine (postoperative) (*see also* Adhesions, peritoneum) 568.0

Adhesion(s), adhesive — *continued*
  intestine (*see also* Adhesions, peritoneum) — *continued*
    with obstruction 560.81
      with hernia — *see also* Hernia, by site, with obstruction
        gangrenous — *see* Hernia, by site, with gangrene
  intra-abdominal (*see also* Adhesions, peritoneum) 568.0
  iris 364.70
    to corneal graft 996.79
  joint (*see also* Ankylosis) 718.5 ✓5th
  kidney 593.89
  labium (majus) (minus), congenital 752.49
  liver 572.8
  lung 511.0
  mediastinum 519.3
  meninges 349.2
    cerebral (any) 349.2
      congenital 742.4
    congenital 742.8
    spinal (any) 349.2
      congenital 742.59
    tuberculous (cerebral) (spinal) (*see also* Tuberculosis, meninges) 013.0 ✓5th
  mesenteric (*see also* Adhesions, peritoneum) 568.0
  middle ear (fibrous) 385.10
    drum head 385.19
      to
        incus 385.11
        promontorium 385.13
        stapes 385.12
    specified NEC 385.19
  nasal (septum) (to turbinates) 478.1
  nerve NEC 355.9
    spinal 355.9
      root 724.9
        cervical NEC 723.4
        lumbar NEC 724.4
        lumbosacral 724.4
        thoracic 724.4
  ocular muscle 378.60
  omentum (*see also* Adhesions, peritoneum) 568.0
  organ or site, congenital NEC — *see* Anomaly, specified type NEC
  ovary 614.6
    congenital (to cecum, kidney, or omentum) 752.0
  parauterine 614.6
  parovarian 614.6
  pelvic (peritoneal)
    female (postoperative) (postinfection) 614.6
    male (postoperative) (postinfection) (*see also* Adhesions, peritoneum) 568.0
    postpartal (old) 614.6
    tuberculous (*see also* Tuberculosis) 016.9 ✓5th
  penis to scrotum (congenital) 752.69
  periappendiceal (*see also* Adhesions, peritoneum) 568.0
  pericardium (nonrheumatic) 423.1
    rheumatic 393
    tuberculous (*see also* Tuberculosis) 017.9 ✓5th [420.0]
  pericholecystic 575.8
  perigastric (*see also* Adhesions, peritoneum) 568.0
  periovarian 614.6
  periprostatic 602.8
  perirectal (*see also* Adhesions, peritoneum) 568.0
  perirenal 593.89
  peritoneum, peritoneal (fibrous) (postoperative) 568.0
    with obstruction (intestinal) 560.81
      with hernia — *see also* Hernia, by site, with obstruction
        gangrenous — *see* Hernia, by site, with gangrene
    duodenum 537.3
    congenital 751.4
    female (postoperative) (postinfective) 614.6
    pelvic, female 614.6
    pelvic, male 568.0
    postpartal, pelvic 614.6

Adhesion(s), adhesive — *continued*
  peritoneum, peritoneal — *continued*
    to uterus 614.6
  peritubal 614.6
  periureteral 593.89
  periuterine 621.5
  perivesical 596.8
  perivesicular (seminal vesicle) 608.89
  pleura, pleuritic 511.0
    tuberculous (*see also* Tuberculosis, pleura) 012.0 ✓5th
  pleuropericardial 511.0
  postoperative (gastrointestinal tract) (*see also* Adhesions, peritoneum) 568.0
    eyelid 997.99
      surgically created V45.69
    pelvic female 614.9
    pelvic male 568.0
    urethra 598.2
  postpartal, old 624.4
  preputial, prepuce 605
  pulmonary 511.0
  pylorus (*see also* Adhesions, peritoneum) 568.0
  Rosenmüller's fossa 478.29
  sciatic nerve 355.0
  seminal vesicle 608.89
  shoulder (joint) 726.0
  sigmoid flexure (*see also* Adhesions, peritoneum) 568.0
  spermatic cord (acquired) 608.89
    congenital 752.8
  spinal canal 349.2
    nerve 355.9
      root 724.9
        cervical NEC 723.4
        lumbar NEC 724.4
        lumbosacral 724.4
        thoracic 724.4
  stomach (*see also* Adhesions, peritoneum) 568.0
  subscapular 726.2
  tendonitis 726.90
    shoulder 726.0
  testicle 608.89
  tongue (congenital) (to gum or roof of mouth) 750.12
    acquired 529.8
  trachea 519.1
  tubo-ovarian 614.6
  tunica vaginalis 608.89
  ureter 593.89
  uterus 621.5
    to abdominal wall 614.6
    in pregnancy or childbirth 654.4 ✓5th
      affecting fetus or newborn 763.89
  vagina (chronic) (postoperative) (postradiation) 623.2
  vaginitis (congenital) 752.49
  vesical 596.8
  vitreous 379.29
Adie (-Holmes) syndrome (tonic pupillary reaction) 379.46
Adiponecrosis neonatorum 778.1
Adiposa dolorosa 272.8
Adiposalgia 272.8
Adiposis
  cerebralis 253.8
  dolorosa 272.8
  tuberosa simplex 272.8
Adiposity 278.00
  heart (*see also* Degeneration, myocardial) 429.1
  localized 278.1
Adiposogenital dystrophy 253.8
Adjustment
  prosthesis or other device — *see* Fitting of
  reaction — *see* Reaction, adjustment
Administration, prophylactic
  antibiotics V07.39
  antitoxin, any V07.2
  antivenin V07.2
  chemotherapeutic agent NEC V07.39
  chemotherapy V07.39
  diphtheria antitoxin V07.2
  fluoride V07.31
  gamma globulin V07.2
  immune sera (gamma globulin) V07.2

Administration, prophylactic — *continued*
  passive immunization agent V07.2
  RhoGAM V07.2
Admission (encounter)
  as organ donor — *see* Donor
  by mistake V68.9
  for
    adequacy testing (for)
      hemodialysis V56.31
      peritoneal dialysis V56.32
    adjustment (of)
      artificial
        arm (complete) (partial) V52.0
        eye V52.2
        leg (complete) (partial) V52.1
      brain neuropacemaker V53.02
      breast
        implant V52.4
        prosthesis V52.4
      cardiac device V53.39
        defibrillator, automatic implantable
          V53.32
        pacemaker V53.31
          carotid sinus V53.39
      catheter
        non-vascular V58.82
        vascular V58.81
      cerebral ventricle (communicating) shunt
        V53.01
      colostomy belt V55.3
      contact lenses V53.1
      cystostomy device V53.6
      dental prosthesis V52.3
      device NEC V53.9
        abdominal V53.5
        cardiac V53.39
          defibrillator, automatic implantable
            V53.32
          pacemaker V53.31
        carotid sinus V53.39
        cerebral ventricle (communicating)
          shunt V53.01
        intrauterine contraceptive V25.1
        nervous system V53.09
        orthodontic V53.4
        prosthetic V52.9
          breast V52.4
          dental V52.3
          eye V52.2
          specified type NEC V52.8
        special senses V53.09
        substitution
          auditory V53.09
          nervous system V53.09
          visual V53.09
        urinary V53.6
      dialysis catheter
        extracorporeal V56.1
        peritoneal V56.2
      diaphragm (contraceptive) V25.02
      hearing aid V53.2
      ileostomy device V55.2
      intestinal appliance or device NEC V53.5
      intrauterine contraceptive device V25.1
      neuropacemaker (brain) (peripheral nerve)
        (spinal cord) V53.02
      orthodontic device V53.4
      orthopedic (device) V53.7
        brace V53.7
        cast V53.7
        shoes V53.7
      pacemaker
        brain V53.02
        cardiac V53.31
        carotid sinus V53.39
        peripheral nerve V53.02
        spinal cord V53.02
      prosthesis V52.9
        arm (complete) (partial) V52.0
        breast V52.4
        dental V52.3
        eye V52.2
        leg (complete) (partial) V52.1
        specified type NEC V52.8
      spectacles V53.1
      wheelchair V53.8

Admission — *continued*
  for — *continued*
    adoption referral or proceedings V68.89
    aftercare (*see also* Aftercare) V58.9
      cardiac pacemaker V53.31
      chemotherapy V58.1
      dialysis
        extracorporeal (renal) V56.0
        peritoneal V56.8
        renal V56.0
      fracture (*see also* Aftercare, fracture)
        V54.9
      medical NEC V58.89
      orthopedic V54.9
        specified care NEC V54.89   ▲
      pacemaker device
        brain V53.02
        cardiac V53.31
        carotid sinus V53.39
        nervous system V53.02
        spinal cord V53.02
      postoperative NEC V58.49
        wound closure, planned V58.41
      postpartum
        immediately after delivery V24.0
        routine follow-up V24.2
      postradiation V58.0
      radiation therapy V58.0
      removal of
        non-vascular catheter V58.82
        vascular catheter V58.81
      specified NEC V58.89
      surgical NEC V58.49
        wound closure, planned V58.41
    artificial insemination V26.1
    attention to artificial opening (of) V55.9
      artificial vagina V55.7
      colostomy V55.3
      cystostomy V55.5
      enterostomy V55.4
      gastrostomy V55.1
      ileostomy V55.2
      jejunostomy V55.4
      nephrostomy V55.6
      specified site NEC V55.8
        intestinal tract V55.4
        urinary tract V55.6
      tracheostomy V55.0
      ureterostomy V55.6
      urethrostomy V55.6
    battery replacement
      cardiac pacemaker V53.31
    boarding V65.0
    breast
      augmentation or reduction V50.1
      removal, prophylactic V50.41
    change of
      cardiac pacemaker (battery) V53.31
      carotid sinus pacemaker V53.39
      catheter in artificial opening — *see*
        Attention to, artificial, opening
      dressing V58.3
      fixation device
        external V54.89   ▲
        internal V54.0
      Kirschner wire V54.89   ▲
      neuropacemaker device (brain)
        (peripheral nerve) (spinal cord)
        V53.02
      pacemaker device
        brain V53.02
        cardiac V53.31
        carotid sinus V53.39
        nervous system V53.02
      plaster cast V54.89   ▲
      splint, external V54.89   ▲
      Steinmann pin V54.89   ▲
      surgical dressing V58.3
      traction device V54.89   ▲
    checkup only V70.0
    chemotherapy V58.1
    circumcision, ritual or routine (in absence of
      medical indication) V50.2
    clinical research investigation (control)
      (normal comparison) (participant)
      V70.7

Admission — *continued*
  for — *continued*
    closure of artificial opening — *see* Attention
      to, artificial, opening
    contraceptive
      counseling V25.09
      management V25.9
        specified type NEC V25.8
    convalescence following V66.9
      chemotherapy V66.2
      psychotherapy V66.3
      radiotherapy V66.1
      surgery V66.0
      treatment (for) V66.5
        combined V66.6
        fracture V66.4
        mental disorder NEC V66.3
        specified condition NEC V66.5
    cosmetic surgery NEC V50.1
      following healed injury or operation V51
    counseling (*see also* Counseling) V65.40
      without complaint or sickness V65.49
      contraceptive management V25.09
      dietary V65.3
      exercise V65.41
      for
        nonattending third party V65.1
        victim of abuse
          child V61.21
          partner or spouse V61.11
      genetic V26.3
      gonorrhea V65.45
      HIV V65.44
      human immunodeficiency virus V65.44
      injury prevention V65.43
      procreative management V26.4
      sexually transmitted disease NEC V65.45
        HIV V65.44
      specified reason NEC V65.49
      substance use and abuse V65.42
      syphilis V65.45
      victim of abuse
        child V61.21
        partner or spouse V61.11
    desensitization to allergens V07.1
    dialysis V56.0
      catheter
        fitting and adjustment
          extracorporeal V56.1
          peritoneal V56.2
        removal or replacement
          extracorporeal V56.1
          peritoneal V56.2
      extracorporeal (renal) V56.0
      peritoneal V56.8
      renal V56.0
    dietary surveillance and counseling V65.3
    drug monitoring, therapeutic V58.83
    ear piercing V50.3
    elective surgery V50.9
      breast
        augmentation or reduction V50.1
        removal, prophylactic V50.41
      circumcision, ritual or routine (in
        absence of medical indication)
        V50.2
      cosmetic NEC V50.1
        following healed injury or operation
          V51
      ear piercing V50.3
      face-lift V50.1
      hair transplant V50.0
      plastic
        cosmetic NEC V50.1
        following healed injury or operation
          V51
      prophylactic organ removal V50.49
        breast V50.41
        ovary V50.42
      repair of scarred tissue (following healed
        injury or operation) V51
      specified type NEC V50.8
    end-of-life care V66.7
    examination (*see also* Examination) V70.9
      administrative purpose NEC V70.3
      adoption V70.3

| ✔4ᵗʰ Fourth-digit Required | ✔5ᵗʰ Fifth-digit Required | ►◄ Revised Text | ● New Line | ▲ Revised Code |

Admission — *continued*
  for — *continued*
    examination (*see also* Examination) —
      continued
      allergy V72.7
      at health care facility V70.0
      athletic team V70.3
      camp V70.3
      cardiovascular, preoperative V72.81
      clinical research investigation (control)
        (participant) V70.7
      dental V72.2
      developmental testing (child) (infant)
        V20.2
      donor (potential) V70.8
      driver's license V70.3
      ear V72.1
      employment V70.5
      eye V72.0
      follow-up (routine) — *see* Examination,
        follow-up
      for admission to
        old age home V70.3
        school V70.3
      general V70.9
        specified reason NEC V70.8
      gynecological V72.3
      health supervision (child) (infant) V20.2
      hearing V72.1
      immigration V70.3
      insurance certification V70.3
      laboratory V72.6
      marriage license V70.3
      medical (general) (*see also* Examination,
        medical) V70.9
      medicolegal reasons V70.4
      naturalization V70.3
      pelvic (annual) (periodic) V72.3
      postpartum checkup V24.2
      pregnancy (possible) (unconfirmed) V72.4
      preoperative V72.84
        cardiovascular V72.81
        respiratory V72.82
        specified NEC V72.83
      prison V70.3
      psychiatric (general) V70.2
        requested by authority V70.1
      radiological NEC V72.5
      respiratory, preoperative V72.82
      school V70.3
      screening — *see* Screening
      skin hypersensitivity V72.7
      specified type NEC V72.85
      sport competition V70.3
      vision V72.0
      well baby and child care V20.2
    exercise therapy V57.1
    face-lift, cosmetic reason V50.1
    fitting (of)
      artificial
        arm (complete) (partial) V52.0
        eye V52.2
        leg (complete) (partial) V52.1
      biliary drainage tube V58.82
      brain neuropacemaker V53.02
      breast V52.4
        implant V52.4
        prosthesis V52.4
      cardiac pacemaker V53.31
      catheter
        non-vascular V58.82
        vascular V58.81
      cerebral ventricle (communicating) shunt
        V53.01
      chest tube V58.82
      colostomy belt V55.2
      contact lenses V53.1
      cystostomy device V53.6
      dental prosthesis V52.3
      device NEC V53.9
        abdominal V53.5
        cerebral ventricle (communicating)
          shunt V53.01
        intrauterine contraceptive V25.1
        nervous system V53.09
        orthodontic V53.4

Admission — *continued*
  for — *continued*
    fitting — *continued*
      device NEC — *continued*
        prosthetic V52.9
          breast V52.4
          dental V52.3
          eye V52.2
          special senses V53.09
        substitution
          auditory V53.09
          nervous system V53.09
          visual V53.09
      diaphragm (contraceptive) V25.02
      fistula (sinus tract) drainage tube V58.82
      hearing aid V53.2
      ileostomy device V55.2
      intestinal appliance or device NEC V53.5
      intrauterine contraceptive device V25.1
      neuropacemaker (brain) (peripheral nerve)
        (spinal cord) V53.02
      orthodontic device V53.4
      orthopedic (device) V53.7
        brace V53.7
        cast V53.7
        shoes V53.7
      pacemaker
        brain V53.02
        cardiac V53.31
        carotid sinus V53.39
        spinal cord V53.02
      pleural drainage tube V58.82
      prosthesis V52.9
        arm (complete) (partial) V52.0
        breast V52.4
        dental V52.3
        eye V52.2
        leg (complete) (partial) V52.1
        specified type NEC V52.8
      spectacles V53.1
      wheelchair V53.8
    follow-up examination (routine) (following)
      V67.9
      cancer chemotherapy V67.2
      chemotherapy V67.2
      high-risk medication NEC V67.51
      injury NEC V67.59
      psychiatric V67.3
      psychotherapy V67.3
      radiotherapy V67.1
      specified surgery NEC V67.09
      surgery V67.00
        vaginal pap smear V67.01
      treatment (for) V67.9
        combined V67.6
        fracture V67.4
        involving high-risk medication NEC
          V67.51
        mental disorder V67.3
        specified NEC V67.59
    hair transplant, for cosmetic reason V50.0
    health advice, education, or instruction
      V65.4
    hospice care V66.7
    insertion (of)
      subdermal implantable contraceptive
        V25.5
    intrauterine device
      insertion V25.1
      management V25.42
    investigation to determine further
      disposition V63.8
    isolation V07.0
    issue of
      medical certificate NEC V68.0
      repeat prescription NEC V68.1
        contraceptive device NEC V25.49
    kidney dialysis V56.0
    mental health evaluation V70.2
      requested by authority V70.1
    nonmedical reason NEC V68.89
    nursing care evaluation V63.8
    observation (without need for further
      medical care) (*see also* Observation)
      V71.9
      accident V71.4

Admission — *continued*
  for — *continued*
    observation (*see also* Observation) —
      continued
      alleged rape or seduction V71.5
      criminal assault V71.6
      following accident V71.4
        at work V71.3
      foreign body ingestion V71.89
      growth and development variations,
        childhood V21.0
      inflicted injury NEC V71.6
      ingestion of deleterious agent or foreign
        body V71.89
      injury V71.6
      malignant neoplasm V71.1
      mental disorder V71.09
      newborn — *see* Observation, suspected,
        condition, newborn
      rape V71.5
      specified NEC V71.89
      suspected disorder V71.9
        abuse V71.81
        accident V71.4
          at work V71.3
        benign neoplasm V71.89
        cardiovascular V71.7
        exposure   ●
          anthrax V71.82   ●
          biological agent NEC V71.83 ●
        heart V71.7
        inflicted injury NEC V71.6
        malignant neoplasm V71.1
        mental NEC V71.09
        neglect V71.81
        specified condition NEC V71.89
        tuberculosis V71.2
      tuberculosis V71.2
    occupational therapy V57.21
    organ transplant, donor — *see* Donor
    ovary, ovarian removal, prophylactic V50.42
    palliative care V66.7
    Papanicolaou smear
      cervix V76.2
        for suspected malignant neoplasm
          V76.2
          no disease found V71.1
        routine, as part of gynecological
          examination V72.3
      vaginal V76.47
        following hysterectomy for malignant
          condition V67.01
    passage of sounds or bougie in artificial
      opening — *see* Attention to, artificial,
      opening
    paternity testing V70.4
    peritoneal dialysis V56.32
    physical therapy NEC V57.1
    plastic surgery
      cosmetic NEC V50.1
      following healed injury or operation V51
    postmenopausal hormone replacement
      therapy V07.4
    postpartum observation
      immediately after delivery V24.0
      routine follow-up V24.2
    poststerilization (for restoration) V26.0
    procreative management V26.9
      specified type NEC V26.8
    prophylactic
      administration of
        antibiotics V07.39
        antitoxin, any V07.2
        antivenin V07.2
        chemotherapeutic agent NEC V07.39
        chemotherapy NEC V07.39
        diphtheria antitoxin V07.2
        fluoride V07.31
        gamma globulin V07.2
        immune sera (gamma globulin) V07.2
        RhoGAM V07.2
        tetanus antitoxin V07.2
      breathing exercises V57.0
      chemotherapy NEC V07.39
        fluoride V07.31
      measure V07.9
        specified type NEC V07.8

Admission — *continued*
  for — *continued*
    prophylactic — *continued*
      organ removal V50.49
        breast V50.41
        ovary V50.42
      psychiatric examination (general) V70.2
        requested by authority V70.1
      radiation management V58.0
      radiotherapy V58.0
      reforming of artificial opening — *see*
          Attention to, artificial, opening
      rehabilitation V57.9
        multiple types V57.89
        occupational V57.21
        orthoptic V57.4
        orthotic V57.81
        physical NEC V57.1
        specified type NEC V57.89
        speech V57.3
        vocational V57.22
      removal of
        cardiac pacemaker V53.31
        cast (plaster) V54.89 ▲
        catheter from artificial opening — *see*
            Attention to, artificial, opening
        cerebral ventricle (communicating) shunt
            V53.01
        cystostomy catheter V55.5
        device
          cerebral ventricle (communicating)
              shunt V53.01
          fixation
            external V54.89 ▲
            internal V54.0
          intrauterine contraceptive V25.42
          traction, external V54.89 ▲
        dressing V58.3
        fixation device
          external V54.89 ▲
          internal V54.0
        intrauterine contraceptive device V25.42
        Kirschner wire V54.89 ▲
        neuropacemaker (brain) (peripheral nerve)
            (spinal cord) V53.02
        orthopedic fixation device
          external V54.89 ▲
          internal V54.0
        pacemaker device
          brain V53.02
          cardiac V53.31
          carotid sinus V53.39
          nervous system V53.02
        plaster cast V54.89 ▲
        plate (fracture) V54.0
        rod V54.0
        screw (fracture) V54.0
        splint, traction V54.89 ▲
        Steinmann pin V54.89 ▲
        subdermal implantable contraceptive
            V25.43
        surgical dressing V58.3
        sutures V58.3
        traction device, external V54.89 ▲
        ureteral stent V53.6
      repair of scarred tissue (following healed
          injury or operation) V51
      reprogramming of cardiac pacemaker
          V53.31
      restoration of organ continuity
          (poststerilization) (tuboplasty)
          (vasoplasty) V26.0
      sensitivity test — *see also* Test, skin
        allergy NEC V72.7
        bacterial disease NEC V74.9
        Dick V74.8
        Kveim V82.89
        Mantoux V74.1
        mycotic infection NEC V75.4
        parasitic disease NEC V75.8
        Schick V74.3
        Schultz-Charlton V74.8
      social service (agency) referral or evaluation
          V63.8
      speech therapy V57.3
      sterilization V25.2

Admission — *continued*
  for — *continued*
    suspected disorder (ruled out) (without need
        for further care) — *see* Observation
    terminal care V66.7
    tests only — *see* Test
    therapeutic drug monitoring V58.83
    therapy
      blood transfusion, without reported
          diagnosis V58.2
      breathing exercises V57.0
      chemotherapy V58.1
        prophylactic NEC V07.39
          fluoride V07.31
      dialysis (intermittent) (treatment)
        extracorporeal V56.0
        peritoneal V56.8
        renal V56.0
        specified type NEC V56.8
      exercise (remedial) NEC V57.1
        breathing V57.0
      long-term (current) drug use NEC V58.69
        antibiotics V58.62
        anticoagulant V58.61
      occupational V57.21
      orthoptic V57.4
      physical NEC V57.1
      radiation V58.0
      speech V57.3
      vocational V57.22
    toilet or cleaning
      of artificial opening — *see* Attention to,
          artificial, opening
      of non-vascular catheter V58.82
      of vascular catheter V58.81
    tubal ligation V25.2
    tuboplasty for previous sterilization V26.0
    vaccination, prophylactic (against)
      arthropod-borne virus, viral NEC V05.1
        disease NEC V05.1
        encephalitis V05.0
      Bacille Calmette Guérin (BCG) V03.2
      BCG V03.2
      chickenpox V05.4
      cholera alone V03.0
        with typhoid-paratyphoid (cholera +
            TAB) V06.0
      common cold V04.7
      dengue V05.1
      diphtheria alone V03.5
      diphtheria-tetanus [Td] without pertussis
          V06.5
      diphtheria-tetanus-pertussis (DTP) V06.1
        with
          poliomyelitis (DTP + polio) V06.3
          typhoid-paratyphoid (DTP + TAB)
              V06.2
      disease (single) NEC V05.9
        bacterial NEC V03.9
          specified type NEC V03.89
        combinations NEC V06.9
          specified type NEC V06.8
        specified type NEC V05.8
      encephalitis, viral, arthropod-borne V05.0
      Hemophilus infuenzae, type B [Hib]
          V03.81
      hepatitis, viral V05.3
      immune sera (gamma globulin) V07.2
      influenza V04.8
        with
          Streptococcus pneumoniae
              [pneumococcus] V06.6
      Leishmaniasis V05.2
      measles alone V04.2
      measles-mumps-rubella (MMR) V06.4
      mumps alone V04.6
        with measles and rubella (MMR) V06.4
      not done because of contraindication
          V64.0
      pertussis alone V03.6
      plague V03.3
      pneumonia V03.82
      poliomyelitis V04.0
        with diphtheria-tetanus-pertussis
            (DTP+ polio) V06.3
      rabies V04.5

Admission — *continued*
  for — *continued*
    vaccination, prophylactic — *continued*
      rubella alone V04.3
        with measles and mumps (MMR)
            V06.4
      smallpox V04.1
      specified type NEC V05.8
      Streptococcus pneumoniae
          [pneumococcus] V03.82
        with
          influenza V06.6
      tetanus toxoid alone V03.7
        with diphtheria [Td] V06.5
          and pertussis (DTP) V06.1
      tuberculosis (BCG) V03.2
      tularemia V03.4
      typhoid alone V03.1
        with diphtheria-tetanus-pertussis (TAB
            + DTP) V06.2
      typhoid-paratyphoid alone (TAB) V03.1
      typhus V05.8
      varicella (chicken pox) V05.4
      viral encephalitis, arthropod-borne V05.0
      viral hepatitis V05.3
      yellow fever V04.4
    vasectomy V25.2
    vasoplasty for previous sterilization V26.0
    vision examination V72.0
    vocational therapy V57.22
    waiting period for admission to other facility
        V63.2
      undergoing social agency investigation
          V63.8
    well baby and child care V20.2
    x-ray of chest
      for suspected tuberculosis V71.2
      routine V72.5
Adnexitis (suppurative) (*see also* Salpingo-
    oophoritis) 614.2
Adolescence NEC V21.2
Adoption
  agency referral V68.89
  examination V70.3
  held for V68.89
Adrenal gland — *see* condition
Adrenalism 255.9
  tuberculous (*see also* Tuberculosis) 017.6 ✓5ᵗʰ
Adrenalitis, adrenitis 255.8
  meningococcal hemorrhagic 036.3
Adrenarche, precocious 259.1
Adrenocortical syndrome 255.2
Adrenogenital syndrome (acquired) (congenital)
    255.2
  iatrogenic, fetus or newborn 760.79
Adventitious bursa — *see* Bursitis
Adynamia (episodica) (hereditary) (periodic) 359.3
Adynamic
  ileus or intestine (*see also* Ileus) 560.1
  ureter 753.22
Aeration lung, imperfect, newborn 770.5
Aerobullosis 993.3
Aerocele — *see* Embolism, air
Aerodermectasia
  subcutaneous (traumatic) 958.7
    surgical 998.81
  surgical 998.81
Aerodontalgia 993.2
Aeroembolism 993.3
Aerogenes capsulatus infection (*see also*
    Gangrene, gas) 040.0
Aero-otitis media 993.0
Aerophagy, aerophagia 306.4
  psychogenic 306.4
Aerosinusitis 993.1
Aerotitis 993.0
Affection, affections — *see also* Disease
  sacroiliac (joint), old 724.6
  shoulder region NEC 726.2
Afibrinogenemia 286.3
  acquired 286.6
  congenital 286.3

✓4ᵗʰ Fourth-digit Required   ✓5ᵗʰ Fifth-digit Required   ▶◀ Revised Text   ● New Line   ▲ Revised Code

Afibrinogenemia — *continued*
  postpartum 666.3 ☑5ᵗʰ
African
  sleeping sickness 086.5
  tick fever 087.1
  trypanosomiasis 086.5
    Gambian 086.3
    Rhodesian 086.4
Aftercare V58.9
  artificial openings — *see* Attention to, artificial,
    opening
  blood transfusion without reported diagnosis
    V58.2
  breathing exercise V57.0
  cardiac device V53.39
    defibrillator, automatic implantable V53.32
    pacemaker V53.31
      carotid sinus V53.39
  carotid sinus pacemaker V53.39
  cerebral ventricle (communicating) shunt
    V53.01
  chemotherapy session (adjunctive)
    (maintenance) V58.1
  defibrillator, automatic implantable cardiac
    V53.32
  exercise (remedial) (therapeutic) V57.1
    breathing V57.0
  extracorporeal dialysis (intermittent)
    (treatment) V56.0
  following surgery NEC V58.49
    for
      injury V58.43   ●
      neoplasm V58.42   ●
      trauma V58.43   ●
    joint replacement V58.81   ●
    of
      circulatory system V58.73   ●
      digestive system V58.75   ●
      genital organs V58.76   ●
      genitourinary system V58.76   ●
      musculoskeletal system V58.78   ●
      nervous system V58.72   ●
      oral cavity V58.75   ●
      respiratory system V58.74   ●
      sense organs V58.71   ●
      skin V58.77   ●
      subcutaneous tissue V58.77   ●
      teeth V58.75   ●
      urinary system V58.76   ●
    wound closure, planned V58.41
  fracture V54.9
    healing V54.89   ●
      pathologic   ●
        arm V54.20   ●
          lower V54.22   ●
          upper V54.21   ●
        hip V54.23   ●
        leg V54.24   ●
          lower V54.26   ●
          upper V54.25   ●
        specified site NEC V54.29   ●
        vertebrae V54.27   ●
      traumatic   ●
        arm V54.10   ●
          lower V54.12   ●
          upper V54.11   ●
        hip V54.13   ●
        leg V54.14   ●
          lower V54.16   ●
          upper V54.15   ●
        specified site NEC V54.19   ●
        vertebrae V54.17   ●
    removal of
      external fixation device V54.89   ▲
      internal fixation device V54.0
    specified care NEC V54.89   ▲
  gait training V57.1
    for use of artificial limb(s) V57.81
  involving
    dialysis (intermittent) (treatment)
      extracorporeal V56.0
      peritoneal V56.8
      renal V56.0
    gait training V57.1
      for use of artificial limb(s) V57.81
    orthoptic training V57.4

Aftercare — *continued*
  involving — *continued*
    orthotic training V57.81
    radiotherapy session V58.0
    removal of
      dressings V58.3
      fixation device
        external V54.89   ▲
        internal V54.0
      fracture plate V54.0
      pins V54.0
      plaster cast V54.89   ▲
      rods V54.0
      screws V54.0
      surgical dressings V58.3
      sutures V58.3
      traction device, external V54.89   ▲
    neuropacemaker (brain) (peripheral nerve)
      (spinal cord) V53.02
    occupational therapy V57.21
    orthodontic V58.5
    orthopedic V54.9
      change of external fixation or traction device
        V54.89   ▲
      following joint replacement V54.81   ●
      removal of fixation device
        external V54.89   ▲
        internal V54.0
      specified care NEC V54.89   ▲
    orthoptic training V57.4
    orthotic training V57.81
    pacemaker
      brain V53.02
      cardiac V53.31
      carotid sinus V53.39
      peripheral nerve V53.02
      spinal cord V53.02
    peritoneal dialysis (intermittent) (treatment)
      V56.8
    physical therapy NEC V57.1
      breathing exercises V57.0
    radiotherapy session V58.0
    rehabilitation procedure V57.9
      breathing exercises V57.0
      multiple types V57.89
      occupational V57.21
      orthoptic V57.4
      orthotic V57.81
      physical therapy NEC V57.1
      remedial exercises V57.1
      specified type NEC V57.89
      speech V57.3
      therapeutic exercises V57.1
      vocational V57.22
    renal dialysis (intermittent) (treatment) V56.0
    specified type NEC V58.89
      removal of non-vascular catheter V58.82
      removal of vascular catheter V58.81
    speech therapy V57.3
    vocational rehabilitation V57.22
After-cataract 366.50
  obscuring vision 366.53
  specified type, not obscuring vision 366.52
Agalactia 676.4 ☑5ᵗʰ
Agammaglobulinemia 279.00
  with lymphopenia 279.2
  acquired (primary) (secondary) 279.06
  Bruton's X-linked 279.04
  infantile sex-linked (Bruton's) (congenital)
    279.04
  Swiss-type 279.2
Aganglionosis (bowel) (colon) 751.3
AGCUS (atypical glandular cell changes of   ●
    undetermined significance)
  favor benign 795.01   ●
  favor dysplasia 795.02   ●
Age (old) (*see also* Senile) 797
Agenesis — *see also* Absence, by site, congenital
  acoustic nerve 742.8
  adrenal (gland) 759.1
  alimentary tract (complete) (partial) NEC 751.8
    lower 751.2
    upper 750.8
  anus, anal (canal) 751.2
  aorta 747.22
  appendix 751.2

Agenesis — *see also* Absence, by site, congenital
  — *continued*
  arm (complete) (partial) (*see also* Deformity,
    reduction, upper limb) 755.20
  artery (peripheral) NEC (*see also* Anomaly,
    peripheral vascular system) 747.60
    brain 747.81
    coronary 746.85
    pulmonary 747.3
    umbilical 747.5
  auditory (canal) (external) 744.01
  auricle (ear) 744.01
  bile, biliary duct or passage 751.61
  bone NEC 756.9
  brain 740.0
    specified part 742.2
  breast 757.6
  bronchus 748.3
  canaliculus lacrimalis 743.65
  carpus NEC (*see also* Deformity, reduction,
    upper limb) 755.28
  cartilage 756.9
  cecum 751.2
  cerebellum 742.2
  cervix 752.49
  chin 744.89
  cilia 743.63
  circulatory system, part NEC 747.89
  clavicle 755.51
  clitoris 752.49
  coccyx 756.13
  colon 751.2
  corpus callosum 742.2
  cricoid cartilage 748.3
  diaphragm (with hernia) 756.6
  digestive organ(s), or tract (complete) (partial)
      NEC 751.8
    lower 751.2
    upper 750.8
  ductus arteriosus 747.89
  duodenum 751.1
  ear NEC 744.09
    auricle 744.01
    lobe 744.21
  ejaculatory duct 752.8
  endocrine (gland) NEC 759.2
  epiglottis 748.3
  esophagus 750.3
  Eustachian tube 744.24
  extrinsic muscle, eye 743.69
  eye 743.00
    adnexa 743.69
  eyelid (fold) 743.62
  face
    bones NEC 756.0
    specified part NEC 744.89
  fallopian tube 752.19
  femur NEC (*see also* Absence, femur,
      congenital) 755.34
  fibula NEC (*see also* Absence, fibula,
      congenital) 755.37
  finger NEC (*see also* Absence, finger,
      congenital) 755.29
  foot (complete) (*see also* Deformity, reduction,
      lower limb) 755.31
  gallbladder 751.69
  gastric 750.8
  genitalia, genital (organ)
    female 752.8
      external 752.49
      internal NEC 752.8
    male 752.8
      penis 752.69
  glottis 748.3
  gonadal 758.6
  hair 757.4
  hand (complete) (*see also* Deformity, reduction,
      upper limb) 755.21
  heart 746.89
    valve NEC 746.89
      aortic 746.89
      mitral 746.89
      pulmonary 746.01
  hepatic 751.69
  humerus NEC (*see also* Absence, humerus,
      congenital) 755.24
  hymen 752.49
  ileum 751.1

☑4ᵗʰ Fourth-digit Required   ☑5ᵗʰ Fifth-digit Required   ►◄ Revised Text   ● New Line   ▲ Revised Code

Agenesis — *see also* Absence, by site, congenital
— *continued*
 incus 744.04
 intestine (small) 751.1
  large 751.2
 iris (dilator fibers) 743.45
 jaw 524.09
 jejunum 751.1
 kidney(s) (partial) (unilateral) 753.0
 labium (majus) (minus) 752.49
 labyrinth, membranous 744.05
 lacrimal apparatus (congenital) 743.65
 larynx 748.3
 leg NEC (*see also* Deformity, reduction, lower
  limb) 755.30
 lens 743.35
 limb (complete) (partial) (*see also* Deformity,
  reduction) 755.4
  lower NEC 755.30
  upper 755.20
 lip 750.26
 liver 751.69
 lung (bilateral) (fissures) (lobe) (unilateral)
  748.5
 mandible 524.09
 maxilla 524.09
 metacarpus NEC 755.28
 metatarsus NEC 755.38
 muscle (any) 756.81
 musculoskeletal system NEC 756.9
 nail(s) 757.5
 neck, part 744.89
 nerve 742.8
 nervous system, part NEC 742.8
 nipple 757.6
 nose 748.1
 nuclear 742.8
 organ
  of Corti 744.05
  or site not listed — *see* Anomaly, specified
   type NEC
 osseous meatus (ear) 744.03
 ovary 752.0
 oviduct 752.19
 pancreas 751.7
 parathyroid (gland) 759.2
 patella 755.64
 pelvic girdle (complete) (partial) 755.69
 penis 752.69
 pericardium 746.89
 perineal body 756.81
 pituitary (gland) 759.2
 prostate 752.8
 pulmonary
  artery 747.3
  trunk 747.3
  vein 747.49
 punctum lacrimale 743.65
 radioulnar NEC (*see also* Absence, forearm,
  congenital) 755.25
 radius NEC (*see also* Absence, radius,
  congenital) 755.26
 rectum 751.2
 renal 753.0
 respiratory organ NEC 748.9
 rib 756.3
 roof of orbit 742.0
 round ligament 752.8
 sacrum 756.13
 salivary gland 750.21
 scapula 755.59
 scrotum 752.8
 seminal duct or tract 752.8
 septum
  atrial 745.69
  between aorta and pulmonary artery 745.0
  ventricular 745.3
 shoulder girdle (complete) (partial) 755.59
 skull (bone) 756.0
  with
   anencephalus 740.0
   encephalocele 742.0
   hydrocephalus 742.3
    with spina bifida (*see also* Spina
     bifida) 741.0 ✓5ᵗʰ
   microcephalus 742.1
 spermatic cord 752.8
 spinal cord 742.59

Agenesis — *see also* Absence, by site, congenital
— *continued*
 spine 756.13
  lumbar 756.13
   isthmus 756.11
   pars articularis 756.11
 spleen 759.0
 sternum 756.3
 stomach 750.7
 tarsus NEC 755.38
 tendon 756.81
 testicular 752.8
 testis 752.8
 thymus (gland) 759.2
 thyroid (gland) 243
  cartilage 748.3
 tibia NEC (*see also* Absence, tibia, congenital)
  755.36
 tibiofibular NEC 755.35
 toe (complete) (partial) (*see also* Absence, toe,
  congenital) 755.39
 tongue 750.11
 trachea (cartilage) 748.3
 ulna NEC (*see also* Absence, ulna, congenital)
  755.27
 ureter 753.4
 urethra 753.8
 urinary tract NEC 753.8
 uterus 752.3
 uvula 750.26
 vagina 752.49
 vas deferens 752.8
 vein(s) (peripheral) NEC (*see also* Anomaly,
  peripheral vascular system) 747.60
  brain 747.81
  great 747.49
  portal 747.49
  pulmonary 747.49
 vena cava (inferior) (superior) 747.49
 vermis of cerebellum 742.2
 vertebra 756.13
  lumbar 756.13
   isthmus 756.11
   pars articularis 756.11
 vulva 752.49
Ageusia (*see also* Disturbance, sensation) 781.1
Aggressiveness 301.3
Aggressive outburst (*see also* Disturbance,
 conduct) 312.0 ✓5ᵗʰ
 in children and adolescents 313.9
Aging skin 701.8
Agitated — *see* condition
Agitation 307.9
 catatonic (*see also* Schizophrenia) 295.2 ✓5ᵗʰ
Aglossia (congenital) 750.11
Aglycogenosis 271.0
Agnail (finger) (with lymphangitis) 681.02
Agnosia (body image) (tactile) 784.69
 verbal 784.69
  auditory 784.69
   secondary to organic lesion 784.69
  developmental 315.8
  secondary to organic lesion 784.69
  visual 784.69
   developmental 315.8
   secondary to organic lesion 784.69
 visual 368.16
  developmental 315.31
Agoraphobia 300.22
 with panic attacks 300.21
Agrammatism 784.69
Agranulocytopenia 288.0
Agranulocytosis (angina) (chronic) (cyclical)
 (genetic) (infantile) (periodic) (pernicious)
 288.0
Agraphia (absolute) 784.69
 with alexia 784.61
 developmental 315.39
Agrypnia (*see also* Insomnia) 780.52
Ague (*see also* Malaria) 084.6
 brass-founders' 985.8
 dumb 084.6
 tertian 084.1
Agyria 742.2

Ahumada-del Castillo syndrome (nonpuerperal
 galactorrhea and amenorrhea) 253.1
AIDS 042
AIDS-associated retrovirus (disease) (illness) 042
 infection — *see* Human immunodeficiency
  virus, infection
AIDS-associated virus (disease) (illness) 042
 infection — *see* Human immunodeficiency
  virus, infection
AIDS-like disease (illness) (syndrome) 042
AIDS-related complex 042
AIDS-related conditions 042
AIDS-related virus (disease) (illness) 042
 infection — *see* Human immunodeficiency
  virus, infection
AIDS virus (disease) (illness) 042
 infection — *see* Human immunodeficiency
  virus, infection
Ailment, heart — *see* Disease, heart
Ailurophobia 300.29
Ainhum (disease) 136.0
Air
 anterior mediastinum 518.1
 compressed, disease 993.3
 embolism (any site) (artery) (cerebral) 958.0
  with
   abortion — *see* Abortion, by type, with
    embolism
   ectopic pregnancy (*see also* categories
    633.0-633.9) 639.6
   molar pregnancy (*see also* categories 630-
    632) 639.6
  due to implanted device — *see*
   Complications, due to (presence of)
   any device, implant, or graft classified
   to 996.0-996.5 NEC
  following
   abortion 639.6
   ectopic or molar pregnancy 639.6
  infusion, perfusion, or transfusion 999.1
  in pregnancy, childbirth, or puerperium
   673.0 ✓5ᵗʰ
  traumatic 958.0
 hunger 786.09
  psychogenic 306.1
 leak (lung) (pulmonary) (thorax) 512.8
  iatrogenic 512.1
  postoperative 512.1
 rarefied, effects of — *see* Effect, adverse, high
  altitude
 sickness 994.6
Airplane sickness 994.6
Akathisia, acathisia 781.0
 due to drugs 333.99
Akinesia algeria 352.6
Akiyami 100.89
Akureyri disease (epidemic neuromyasthenia)
 049.8
Alacrima (congenital) 743.65
Alactasia (hereditary) 271.3
Alalia 784.3
 developmental 315.31
  receptive-expressive 315.32
 secondary to organic lesion 784.3
Alaninemia 270.8
Alastrim 050.1
Albarrán's disease (colibacilluria) 791.9
Albers-Schönberg's disease (marble bones)
 756.52
Albert's disease 726.71
Albinism, albino (choroid) (cutaneous) (eye)
 (generalized) (isolated) (ocular)
 (oculocutaneous) (partial) 270.2
Albinismus 270.2
Albright (-Martin) (-Bantam) disease
 (pseudohypoparathyroidism) 275.49
Albright (-McCune) (-Sternberg) syndrome
 (osteitis fibrosa disseminata) 756.59
Albuminous — *see* condition
Albuminuria, albuminuric (acute) (chronic)
 (subacute) 791.0

Agenesis — Albuminuria

Albuminuria, albuminuric — *continued*
Bence-Jones 791.0
cardiac 785.9
complicating pregnancy, childbirth, or
puerperium 646.2 ✓5ᵗʰ
with hypertension — *see* Toxemia, of
pregnancy
affecting fetus or newborn 760.1
cyclic 593.6
gestational 646.2 ✓5ᵗʰ
gravidarum 646.2 ✓5ᵗʰ
with hypertension — *see* Toxemia, of
pregnancy
affecting fetus or newborn 760.1
heart 785.9
idiopathic 593.6
orthostatic 593.6
postural 593.6
pre-eclamptic (mild) 642.4 ✓5ᵗʰ
affecting fetus or newborn 760.0
severe 642.5 ✓5ᵗʰ
affecting fetus or newborn 760.0
recurrent physiologic 593.6
scarlatinal 034.1
Albumosuria 791.0
Bence-Jones 791.0
myelopathic (M9730/3) 203.0 ✓5ᵗʰ
Alcaptonuria 270.2
Alcohol, alcoholic
abstinence 291.81
acute intoxication 305.0 ✓5ᵗʰ
with dependence 303.0 ✓5ᵗʰ
addiction (*see also* Alcoholism) 303.9 ✓5ᵗʰ
maternal
with suspected fetal damage affecting
management of pregnancy
655.4 ✓5ᵗʰ
affecting fetus or newborn 760.71
amnestic disorder, persisting 291.1
anxiety 291.89
brain syndrome, chronic 291.2
cardiopathy 425.5
chronic (*see also* Alcoholism) 303.9 ✓5ᵗʰ
cirrhosis (liver) 571.2
delirium 291.0
acute 291.0
chronic 291.1
tremens 291.0
withdrawal 291.0
dementia NEC 291.2
deterioration 291.2
drunkenness (simple) 305.0 ✓5ᵗʰ
hallucinosis (acute) 291.3
insanity 291.9
intoxication (acute) 305.0 ✓5ᵗʰ
with dependence 303.0 ✓5ᵗʰ
pathological 291.4
jealousy 291.5
Korsakoff's, Korsakov's, Korsakow's 291.1
liver NEC 571.3
acute 571.1
chronic 571.2
mania (acute) (chronic) 291.9
mood 291.89
paranoia 291.5
paranoid (type) psychosis 291.5
pellagra 265.2
poisoning, accidental (acute) NEC 980.9
specified type of alcohol — *see* Table of
Drugs and Chemicals
psychosis (*see also* Psychosis, alcoholic) 291.9
Korsakoff's, Korsakov's, Korsakow's 291.1
polyneuritic 291.1
with
delusions 291.5
hallucinations 291.3
withdrawal symptoms, syndrome NEC 291.81
delirium 291.0
hallucinosis 291.3

Alcoholism 303.9 ✓5ᵗʰ

Note — *Use the following fifth-digit
subclassification with category 303:*

0	*unspecified*
1	*continuous*
2	*episodic*
3	*in remission*

with psychosis (*see also* Psychosis, alcoholic)
291.9
acute 303.0 ✓5ᵗʰ
chronic 303.9 ✓5ᵗʰ
with psychosis 291.9
complicating pregnancy, childbirth, or
puerperium 648.4 ✓5ᵗʰ
affecting fetus or newborn 760.71
history V11.3
Korsakoff's, Korsakov's, Korsakow's 291.1
suspected damage to fetus affecting
management of pregnancy 655.4 ✓5ᵗʰ
Alder's anomaly or syndrome (leukocyte
granulation anomaly) 288.2
Alder-Reilly anomaly (leukocyte granulation)
288.2
Aldosteronism (primary) (secondary) 255.1
congenital 255.1
Aldosteronoma (M8370/1) 237.2
Aldrich (-Wiskott) syndrome (eczema-
thrombocytopenia) 279.12
Aleppo boil 085.1
Aleukemic — *see* condition
Aleukia
congenital 288.0
hemorrhagica 284.9
acquired (secondary) 284.8
congenital 284.0
idiopathic 284.9
splenica 289.4
Alexia (congenital) (developmental) 315.01
secondary to organic lesion 784.61
Algoneurodystrophy 733.7
Algophobia 300.29
Alibert's disease (mycosis fungoides) (M9700/3)
202.1 ✓5ᵗʰ
Alibert-Bazin disease (M9700/3) 202.1 ✓5ᵗʰ
Alice in Wonderland syndrome 293.89
Alienation, mental (*see also* Psychosis) 298.9
Alkalemia 276.3
Alkalosis 276.3
metabolic 276.3
with respiratory acidosis 276.4
respiratory 276.3
Alkaptonuria 270.2
Allen-Masters syndrome 620.6
Allergic bronchopulmonary aspergillosis 518.6
Allergy, allergic (reaction) 995.3
air-borne substance (*see also* Fever, hay) 477.9
specified allergen NEC 477.8
alveolitis (extrinsic) 495.9
due to
Aspergillus clavatus 495.4
cryptostroma corticale 495.6
organisms (fungal, thermophilic
actinomycete, other) growing in
ventilation (air conditioning
systems) 495.7
specified type NEC 495.8
anaphylactic shock 999.4
due to food — *see* Anaphylactic shock, due
to, food
angioneurotic edema 995.1
animal (dander) (epidermal) (hair) 477.8
arthritis (*see also* Arthritis, allergic) 716.2 ✓5ᵗʰ
asthma — *see* Asthma
bee sting (anaphylactic shock) 989.5
biological — *see* Allergy, drug
bronchial asthma — *see* Asthma
conjunctivitis (eczematous) 372.14
dander (animal) 477.8
dandruff 477.8
dermatitis (venenata) — *see* Dermatitis

Allergy, allergic — *continued*
diathesis V15.09
drug, medicinal substance, and biological (any)
(correct medicinal substance properly
administered) (external) (internal) 995.2
wrong substance given or taken NEC 977.9
specified drug or substance — *see* Table
of Drugs and Chemicals
dust (house) (stock) 477.8
eczema — *see* Eczema
endophthalmitis 360.19
epidermal (animal) 477.8
feathers 477.8
food (any) (ingested) 693.1
atopic 691.8
in contact with skin 692.5
gastritis 535.4 ✓5ᵗʰ
gastroenteritis 558.3
gastrointestinal 558.3
grain 477.0
grass (pollen) 477.0
asthma (*see also* Asthma) 493.0 ✓5ᵗʰ
hay fever 477.0
hair (animal) 477.8
hay fever (grass) (pollen) (ragweed) (tree) (*see
also* Fever, hay) 477.9
history (of) V15.09
to
eggs V15.03
food additives V15.05
insect bite V15.06
latex V15.07
milk products V15.02
nuts V15.05
peanuts V15.01
radiographic dye V15.08
seafood V15.04
specified food NEC V15.05
spider bite V15.06
horse serum — *see* Allergy, serum
inhalant 477.9
dust 477.8
pollen 477.0
specified allergen other than pollen 477.8
kapok 477.8
medicine — *see* Allergy, drug
migraine 346.2 ✓5ᵗʰ
pannus 370.62
pneumonia 518.3
pollen (any) (hay fever) 477.0
asthma (*see also* Asthma) 493.0 ✓5ᵗʰ
primrose 477.0
primula 477.0
purpura 287.0
ragweed (pollen) (Senecio jacobae) 477.0
asthma (*see also* Asthma) 493.0 ✓5ᵗʰ
hay fever 477.0
respiratory (*see also* Allergy, inhalant) 477.9
due to
drug — *see* Allergy, drug
food — *see* Allergy, food
rhinitis (*see also* Fever, hay) 477.9
due to food 477.1
rose 477.0
Senecio jacobae 477.0
serum (prophylactic) (therapeutic) 999.5
anaphylactic shock 999.4
shock (anaphylactic) (due to adverse effect of
correct medicinal substance properly
administered) 995.0
food — *see* Anaphylactic shock, due to, food
from serum or immunization 999.5
anaphylactic 999.4
sinusitis (*see also* Fever, hay) 477.9
skin reaction 692.9
specified substance — *see* Dermatitis, due
to
tree (any) (hay fever) (pollen) 477.0
asthma (*see also* Asthma) 493.0 ✓5ᵗʰ
upper respiratory (*see also* Fever, hay) 477.9
urethritis 597.89
urticaria 708.0
vaccine — *see* Allergy, serum
Allescheriosis 117.6
Alligator skin disease (ichthyosis congenita)
757.1
acquired 701.1

✓4ᵗʰ Fourth-digit Required   ✓5ᵗʰ Fifth-digit Required   ▶◀ Revised Text   ● New Line   ▲ Revised Code

Allocheiria, allochiria (*see also* Disturbance, sensation) 782.0
Almeida's disease (Brazilian blastomycosis) 116.1
Alopecia (atrophicans) (pregnancy) (premature) (senile) 704.00
  adnata 757.4
  areata 704.01
  celsi 704.01
  cicatrisata 704.09
  circumscripta 704.01
  congenital, congenitalis 757.4
  disseminata 704.01
  effluvium (telogen) 704.02
  febrile 704.09
  generalisata 704.09
  hereditaria 704.09
  marginalis 704.01
  mucinosa 704.09
  postinfectional 704.09
  seborrheica 704.09
  specific 091.82
  syphilitic (secondary) 091.82
  telogen effluvium 704.02
  totalis 704.09
  toxica 704.09
  universalis 704.09
  x-ray 704.09
Alpers' disease 330.8
Alpha-lipoproteinemia 272.4
Alpha thalassemia 282.4
Alphos 696.1
Alpine sickness 993.2
Alport's syndrome (hereditary hematurianephropathy-deafness) 759.89
Alteration (of), altered
  awareness 780.09
    transient 780.02
  consciousness 780.09
    persistent vegetative state 780.03
    transient 780.02
  mental status 780.99   ▲
Alternaria (infection) 118
Alternating — *see* condition
Altitude, high (effects) — *see* Effect, adverse, high altitude
Aluminosis (of lung) 503
Alvarez syndrome (transient cerebral ischemia) 435.9
Alveolar capillary block syndrome 516.3
Alveolitis
  allergic (extrinsic) 495.9
    due to organisms (fungal, thermophilic actinomycete, other) growing in ventilation (air conditioning systems) 495.7
    specified type NEC 495.8
  due to
    Aspergillus clavatus 495.4
    Cryptostroma corticale 495.6
  fibrosing (chronic) (cryptogenic) (lung) 516.3
    idiopathic 516.3
    rheumatoid 714.81
  jaw 526.5
  sicca dolorosa 526.5
Alveolus, alveolar — *see* condition
Alymphocytosis (pure) 279.2
Alymphoplasia, thymic 279.2
Alzheimer's
  dementia (senile)
    with behavioral disturbance 331.0 *[294.11]*
    without behavioral disturbance 331.0 *[294.10]*
  disease or sclerosis 331.0
    with dementia — *see* Alzheimer's, dementia
Amastia (*see also* Absence, breast) 611.8
Amaurosis (acquired) (congenital) (*see also* Blindness) 369.00
  fugax 362.34
  hysterical 300.11
  Leber's (congenital) 362.76
  tobacco 377.34
  uremic — *see* Uremia

Amaurotic familial idiocy (infantile) (juvenile) (late) 330.1
Ambisexual 752.7
Amblyopia (acquired) (congenital) (partial) 368.00
  color 368.59
    acquired 368.55
  deprivation 368.02
  ex anopsia 368.00
  hysterical 300.11
  nocturnal 368.60
    vitamin A deficiency 264.5
  refractive 368.03
  strabismic 368.01
  suppression 368.01
  tobacco 377.34
  toxic NEC 377.34
  uremic — *see* Uremia
Ameba, amebic (histolytica) — *see also* Amebiasis
  abscess 006.3
    bladder 006.8
    brain (with liver and lung abscess) 006.5
    liver 006.3
      with
        brain abscess (and lung abscess) 006.5
        lung abscess 006.4
    lung (with liver abscess) 006.4
      with brain abscess 006.5
    seminal vesicle 006.8
    spleen 006.8
  carrier (suspected of) V02.2
  meningoencephalitis
    due to Naegleria (gruberi) 136.2
    primary 136.2
Amebiasis NEC 006.9
  with
    brain abscess (with liver or lung abscess) 006.5
    liver abscess (without mention of brain or lung abscess) 006.3
    lung abscess (with liver abscess) 006.4
      with brain abscess 006.5
  acute 006.0
  bladder 006.8
  chronic 006.1
  cutaneous 006.6
  cutis 006.6
  due to organism other than Entamoeba histolytica 007.8
  hepatic (*see also* Abscess, liver, amebic) 006.3
  nondysenteric 006.2
  seminal vesicle 006.8
  specified
    organism NEC 007.8
    site NEC 006.8
Ameboma 006.8
Amelia 755.4
  lower limb 755.31
  upper limb 755.21
Ameloblastoma (M9310/0) 213.1
  jaw (bone) (lower) 213.1
    upper 213.0
  long bones (M9261/3) — *see* Neoplasm, bone, malignant
  malignant (M9310/3) 170.1
    jaw (bone) (lower) 170.1
      upper 170.0
  mandible 213.1
  tibial (M9261/3) 170.7
Amelogenesis imperfecta 520.5
  nonhereditaria (segmentalis) 520.4
Amenorrhea (primary) (secondary) 626.0
  due to ovarian dysfunction 256.8
  hyperhormonal 256.8
Amentia (*see also* Retardation, mental) 319
  Meynert's (nonalcoholic) 294.0
    alcoholic 291.1
  nevoid 759.6
American
  leishmaniasis 085.5
  mountain tick fever 066.1
  trypanosomiasis — *see* Trypanosomiasis, American
Ametropia (*see also* Disorder, accommodation) 367.9

Amianthosis 501
Amimia 784.69
Amino acid
  deficiency 270.9
    anemia 281.4
  metabolic disorder (*see also* Disorder, amino acid) 270.9
Aminoaciduria 270.9
  imidazole 270.5
Amnesia (retrograde) 780.99   ▲
  auditory 784.69
    developmental 315.31
    secondary to organic lesion 784.69
  hysterical or dissociative type 300.12
  psychogenic 300.12
  transient global 437.7
Amnestic (confabulatory) syndrome 294.0
  alcohol induced 291.1
  drug-induced 292.83
  posttraumatic 294.0
Amniocentesis screening (for) V28.2
  alphafetoprotein level, raised V28.1
  chromosomal anomalies V28.0
Amnion, amniotic — *see also* condition
  nodosum 658.8 ✔5ᵗʰ
Amnionitis (complicating pregnancy) 658.4 ✔5ᵗʰ
  affecting fetus or newborn 762.7
Amoral trends 301.7
Amotio retinae (*see also* Detachment, retina) 361.9
Ampulla
  lower esophagus 530.89
  phrenic 530.89
Amputation
  any part of fetus, to facilitate delivery 763.89
  cervix (supravaginal) (uteri) 622.8
    in pregnancy or childbirth 654.6 ✔5ᵗʰ
      affecting fetus or newborn 763.89
  clitoris — *see* Wound, open, clitoris
  congenital
    lower limb 755.31
    upper limb 755.21
  neuroma (traumatic) — *see also* Injury, nerve, by site
    surgical complication (late) 997.61
  penis — *see* Amputation, traumatic, penis
  status (without complication) — *see* Absence, by site, acquired
  stump (surgical) (posttraumatic)
    abnormal, painful, or with complication (late) 997.60
    healed or old NEC — *see also* Absence, by site, acquired
      lower V49.70
      upper V49.60
  traumatic (complete) (partial)

> *Note* — "Complicated" includes traumatic amputation with delayed healing, delayed treatment, foreign body, or infection.

  arm 887.4
    at or above elbow 887.2
      complicated 887.3
    below elbow 887.0
      complicated 887.1
    both (bilateral) (any level(s)) 887.6
      complicated 887.7
    complicated 887.5
  finger(s) (one or both hands) 886.0
    with thumb(s) 885.0
      complicated 885.1
    complicated 886.1
  foot (except toe(s) only) 896.0
    and other leg 897.6
      complicated 897.7
    both (bilateral) 896.2
      complicated 896.3
    complicated 896.1
  toe(s) only (one or both feet) 895.0
    complicated 895.1
  genital organ(s) (external) NEC 878.8
    complicated 878.9
  hand (except finger(s) only) 887.0
    and other arm 887.6

Amputation — *continued*
  traumatic — *continued*
    hand — *continued*
      and other arm — *continued*
        complicated 887.7
        both (bilateral) 887.6
          complicated 887.7
        complicated 887.1
        finger(s) (one or both hands) 886.0
          with thumb(s) 885.0
            complicated 885.1
          complicated 886.1
        thumb(s) (with fingers of either hand) 885.0
          complicated 885.1
    head 874.9
    late effect — *see* Late, effects (of), amputation
    leg 897.4
      and other foot 897.6
        complicated 897.7
      at or above knee 897.2
        complicated 897.3
      below knee 897.0
        complicated 897.1
      both (bilateral) 897.6
        complicated 897.7
      complicated 897.5
    lower limb(s) except toe(s) — *see* Amputation, traumatic, leg
    nose — *see* Wound, open, nose
    penis 878.0
      complicated 878.1
    sites other than limbs — *see* Wound, open, by site
    thumb(s) (with finger(s) of either hand) 885.0
      complicated 885.1
    toe(s) (one or both feet) 895.0
      complicated 895.1
    upper limb(s) — *see* Amputation, traumatic, arm

Amputee (bilateral) (old) — *see also* Absence, by site, acquired V49.70

Amusia 784.69
  developmental 315.39
  secondary to organic lesion 784.69

Amyelencephalus 740.0

Amyelia 742.59

Amygdalitis — *see* Tonsillitis

Amygdalolith 474.8

Amyloid disease or degeneration 277.3
  heart 277.3 *[425.7]*

Amyloidosis (familial) (general) (generalized) (genetic) (primary) (secondary) 277.3
  with lung involvement 277.3 *[517.8]*
  heart 277.3 *[425.7]*
  nephropathic 277.3 *[583.81]*
  neuropathic (Portuguese) (Swiss) 277.3 *[357.4]*
  pulmonary 277.3 *[517.8]*
  systemic, inherited 277.3

Amylopectinosis (brancher enzyme deficiency) 271.0

Amylophagia 307.52

Amyoplasia, congenita 756.89

Amyotonia 728.2
  congenita 358.8

Amyotrophia, amyotrophy, amyotrophic 728.2
  congenita 756.89
  diabetic 250.6 ☑5ᵗʰ *[358.1]*
  lateral sclerosis (syndrome) 335.20
  neuralgic 353.5
  sclerosis (lateral) 335.20
  spinal progressive 335.21

Anacidity, gastric 536.0
  psychogenic 306.4

Anaerosis of newborn 768.9 ▲

Analbuminemia 273.8

Analgesia (*see also* Anesthesia) 782.0

Analphalipoproteinemia 272.5

Anaphylactic shock or reaction (correct substance properly administered) 995.0
  due to
    food 995.60
      additives 995.66
      crustaceans 995.62
      eggs 995.68
      fish 995.65
      fruits 995.63
      milk products 995.67
      nuts (tree) 995.64
      peanuts 995.61
      seeds 995.64
      specified NEC 995.69
      tree nuts 995.64
      vegetables 995.63
    immunization 999.4
    overdose or wrong substance given or taken 977.9
      specified drug — *see* Table of Drugs and Chemicals
    serum 999.4
  following sting(s) 989.5
  purpura 287.0
  serum 999.4

Anaphylactoid shock or reaction — *see* Anaphylactic shock

Anaphylaxis — *see* Anaphylactic shock

Anaplasia, cervix 622.1

Anarthria 784.5

Anarthritic rheumatoid disease 446.5

Anasarca 782.3
  cardiac (*see also* Failure, heart) 428.0
  fetus or newborn 778.0
  lung 514
  nutritional 262
  pulmonary 514
  renal (*see also* Nephrosis) 581.9

Anaspadias 752.62

Anastomosis
  aneurysmal — *see* Aneurysm
  arteriovenous, congenital NEC (*see also* Anomaly, arteriovenous) 747.60
    ruptured, of brain (*see also* Hemorrhage, subarachnoid) 430
  intestinal 569.89
    complicated NEC 997.4
      involving urinary tract 997.5
  retinal and choroidal vessels 743.58
    acquired 362.17

Anatomical narrow angle (glaucoma) 365.02

Ancylostoma (infection) (infestation) 126.9
  americanus 126.1
  braziliense 126.2
  caninum 126.8
  ceylanicum 126.3
  duodenale 126.0
  Necator americanus 126.1

Ancylostomiasis (intestinal) 126.9
  Ancylostoma
    americanus 126.1
    caninum 126.8
    ceylanicum 126.3
    duodenale 126.0
    braziliense 126.2
    Necator americanus 126.1

Anders' disease or syndrome (adiposis tuberosa simplex) 272.8

Andersen's glycogen storage disease 271.0

Anderson's disease 272.7

Andes disease 993.2

Andrews' disease (bacterid) 686.8

Androblastoma (M8630/1)
  benign (M8630/0)
    specified site — *see* Neoplasm, by site, benign
    unspecified site
      female 220
      male 222.0
  malignant (M8630/3)
    specified site — *see* Neoplasm, by site, malignant
    unspecified site
      female 183.0

Androblastoma — *continued*
  malignant — *continued*
    unspecified site — *continued*
      male 186.9
  specified site — *see* Neoplasm, by site, uncertain behavior
  tubular (M8640/0)
    with lipid storage (M8641/0)
      specified site — *see* Neoplasm, by site, benign
      unspecified site
        female 220
        male 222.0
    specified site — *see* Neoplasm, by site, benign
    unspecified site
      female 220
      male 222.0
  unspecified site
    female 236.2
    male 236.4

Android pelvis 755.69
  with disproportion (fetopelvic) 653.3 ☑5ᵗʰ
    affecting fetus or newborn 763.1
    causing obstructed labor 660.1 ☑5ᵗʰ
      affecting fetus or newborn 763.1

Anectasis, pulmonary (newborn or fetus) 770.5

Anemia 285.9
  with
    disorder of
      anaerobic glycolysis 282.3
      pentose phosphate pathway 282.2
    koilonychia 280.9
    6-phosphogluconic dehydrogenase deficiency 282.2
  achlorhydric 280.9
  achrestic 281.8
  Addison's (pernicious) 281.0
  Addison-Biermer (pernicious) 281.0
  agranulocytic 288.0
  amino acid deficiency 281.4
  aplastic 284.9
    acquired (secondary) 284.8
    congenital 284.0
    constitutional 284.0
    due to
      chronic systemic disease 284.8
      drugs 284.8
      infection 284.8
      radiation 284.8
    idiopathic 284.9
    myxedema 244.9
    of or complicating pregnancy 648.2 ☑5ᵗʰ
    red cell (acquired) (pure) (with thymoma) 284.8
      congenital 284.0
    specified type NEC 284.8
    toxic (paralytic) 284.8
  aregenerative 284.9
    congenital 284.0
  asiderotic 280.9
  atypical (primary) 285.9
  autohemolysis of Selwyn and Dacie (type I) 282.2
  autoimmune hemolytic 283.0
  Baghdad Spring 282.2
  Balantidium coli 007.0
  Biermer's (pernicious) 281.0
  blood loss (chronic) 280.0
    acute 285.1
  bothriocephalus 123.4
  brickmakers' (*see also* Ancylostomiasis) 126.9
  cerebral 437.8
  childhood 285.9
  chlorotic 280.9
  chronica congenita aregenerativa 284.0
  chronic simple 281.9
  combined system disease NEC 281.0 *[336.2]*
    due to dietary deficiency 281.1 *[336.2]*
  complicating pregnancy or childbirth 648.2 ☑5ᵗʰ
  congenital (following fetal blood loss) 776.5
    aplastic 284.0
    due to isoimmunization NEC 773.2
    Heinz-body 282.7
    hereditary hemolytic NEC 282.9
    nonspherocytic
      Type I 282.2

Anemia — Anemia

Anemia — *continued*
  congenital — *continued*
    nonspherocytic — *continued*
      Type II 282.3
    pernicious 281.0
    spherocytic (*see also* Spherocytosis) 282.0
  Cooley's (erythroblastic) 282.4
  crescent — *see* Disease, sickle-cell
  cytogenic 281.0
  Dacie's (nonspherocytic)
    type I 282.2
    type II 282.3
  Davidson's (refractory) 284.9
  deficiency 281.9
    2, 3 diphosphoglycurate mutase 282.3
    2, 3 PG 282.3
    6-PGD 282.2
    6-phosphogluronic dehydrogenase 282.2
    amino acid 281.4
    combined B$_{12}$ and folate 281.3
    enzyme, drug-induced (hemolytic) 282.2
    erythrocytic glutathione 282.2
    folate 281.2
      dietary 281.2
      drug-induced 281.2
    folic acid 281.2
      dietary 281.2
      drug-induced 281.2
    G-6-PD 282.2
    GGS-R 282.2
    glucose-6-phosphate dehydrogenase (G-6-PD) 282.2
    glucose-phosphate isomerase 282.3
    glutathione peroxidase 282.2
    glutathione reductase 282.2
    glyceraldehyde phosphate dehydrogenase 282.3
    GPI 282.3
    G SH 282.2
    hexokinase 282.3
    iron (Fe) 280.9
      specified NEC 280.8
    nutritional 281.9
      with
        poor iron absorption 280.9
        specified deficiency NEC 281.8
      due to inadequate dietary iron intake 280.1
      specified type NEC 281.8
    of or complicating pregnancy 648.2 ✓5ᵗʰ
    pentose phosphate pathway 282.2
    PFK 282.3
    phosphofructo-aldolase 282.3
    phosphofructokinase 282.3
    phosphoglycerate kinase 282.3
    PK 282.3
    protein 281.4
    pyruvate kinase (PK) 282.3
    TPI 282.3
    triosephosphate isomerase 282.3
    vitamin B$_{12}$ NEC 281.1
      dietary 281.1
      pernicious 281.0
  Diamond-Blackfan (congenital hypoplastic) 284.0
  dibothriocephalus 123.4
  dimorphic 281.9
  diphasic 281.8
  diphtheritic 032.89
  Diphyllobothrium 123.4
  drepanocytic (*see also* Disease, sickle-cell) 282.60
  due to
    blood loss (chronic) 280.0
      acute 285.1
    defect of Embden-Meyerhof pathway glycolysis 282.3
    disorder of glutathione metabolism 282.2
    fetal blood loss 776.5
    fish tapeworm (D. latum) infestation 123.4
    glutathione metabolism disorder 282.2
    hemorrhage (chronic) 280.0
      acute 285.1
    hexose monophosphate (HMP) shunt deficiency 282.2
    impaired absorption 280.9

Anemia — *continued*
  due to — *continued*
    loss of blood (chronic) 280.0
      acute 285.1
    myxedema 244.9
    Necator americanus 126.1
    prematurity 776.6
    selective vitamin B$_{12}$ malabsorption with proteinuria 281.1
  Dyke-Young type (secondary) (symptomatic) 283.9
  dyserythropoietic (congenital) (types I, II, III) 285.8
  dyshemopoietic (congenital) 285.8
  Egypt (*see also* Ancylostomiasis) 126.9
  elliptocytosis (*see also* Elliptocytosis) 282.1
  enzyme deficiency, drug-induced 282.2
  epidemic (*see also* Ancylostomiasis) 126.9
  erythroblastic
    familial 282.4
    fetus or newborn (*see also* Disease, hemolytic) 773.2
    late 773.5
  erythrocytic glutathione deficiency 282.2
  essential 285.9
  Faber's (achlorhydric anemia) 280.9
  factitious (self-induced blood letting) 280.0
  familial erythroblastic (microcytic) 282.4
  Fanconi's (congenital pancytopenia) 284.0
  favism 282.2
  fetal, following blood loss 776.5
  fetus or newborn
    due to
      ABO
        antibodies 773.1
        incompatibility, maternal/fetal 773.1
        isoimmunization 773.1
      Rh
        antibodies 773.0
        incompatibility, maternal/fetal 773.0
        isoimmunization 773.0
    following fetal blood loss 776.5
  fish tapeworm (D. latum) infestation 123.4
  folate (folic acid) deficiency 281.2
    dietary 281.2
    drug-induced 281.2
  folate malabsorption, congenital 281.2
  folic acid deficiency 281.2
    dietary 281.2
    drug-induced 281.2
  G-6-PD 282.2
  general 285.9
  glucose-6-phosphate dehydrogenase deficiency 282.2
  glutathione-reductase deficiency 282.2
  goat's milk 281.2
  granulocytic 288.0
  Heinz-body, congenital 282.7
  hemoglobin deficiency 285.9
  hemolytic 283.9
    acquired 283.9
      with hemoglobinuria NEC 283.2
      autoimmune (cold type) (idiopathic) (primary) (secondary) (symptomatic) (warm type) 283.0
      due to
        cold reactive antibodies 283.0
        drug exposure 283.0
        warm reactive antibodies 283.0
      fragmentation 283.19
      idiopathic (chronic) 283.9
      infectious 283.19
        autoimmune 283.0
      non-autoimmune NEC 283.10
      toxic 283.19
      traumatic cardiac 283.19
    acute 283.9
      due to enzyme deficiency NEC 282.3
      fetus or newborn (*see also* Disease, hemolytic) 773.2
      late 773.5
      Lederer's (acquired infectious hemolytic anemia) 283.19
    autoimmune (acquired) 283.0
    chronic 282.9
      idiopathic 283.9
    cold type (secondary) (symptomatic) 283.0

Anemia — *continued*
  hemolytic — *continued*
    congenital (spherocytic) (*see also* Spherocytosis) 282.0
      nonspherocytic — *see* Anemia, hemolytic, nonspherocytic, congenital
    drug-induced 283.0
      enzyme deficiency 282.2
    due to
      cardiac conditions 283.19
      drugs 283.0
      enzyme deficiency NEC 282.3
        drug-induced 282.2
      presence of shunt or other internal prosthetic device 283.19
      thrombotic thrombocytopenic purpura 446.6
    elliptocytic (*see also* Elliptocytosis) 282.1
    familial 282.9
    hereditary 282.9
      due to enzyme deficiency NEC 282.3
      specified NEC 282.8
    idiopathic (chronic) 283.9
    infectious (acquired) 283.19
    mechanical 283.19
    microangiopathic 283.19
    non-autoimmune NEC 283.10
    nonspherocytic
      congenital or hereditary NEC 282.3
        glucose-6-phosphate dehydrogenase deficiency 282.2
        pyruvate kinase (PK) deficiency 282.3
        type I 282.2
        type II 282.3
      type I 282.2
      type II 282.3
    of or complicating pregnancy 648.2 ✓5ᵗʰ
    resulting from presence of shunt or other internal prosthetic device 283.19
    secondary 283.19
      autoimmune 283.0
    sickle-cell — *see* Disease, sickle-cell
    Stransky-Regala type (Hb-E) (*see also* Disease, hemoglobin) 282.7
    symptomatic 283.19
      autoimmune 283.0
    toxic (acquired) 283.19
    uremic (adult) (child) 283.11
    warm type (secondary) (symptomatic) 283.0
  hemorrhagic (chronic) 280.0
    acute 285.1
  HEMPAS 285.8
  hereditary erythroblast multinuclearity-positive acidified serum test 285.8
  Herrick's (hemoglobin S disease) 282.61
  hexokinase deficiency 282.3
  high A$_2$ 282.4
  hookworm (*see also* Ancylostomiasis) 126.9
  hypochromic (idiopathic) (microcytic) (normoblastic) 280.9
    with iron loading 285.0
    due to blood loss (chronic) 280.0
      acute 285.1
    familial sex linked 285.0
    pyridoxine-responsive 285.0
  hypoplasia, red blood cells 284.8
    congenital or familial 284.0
  hypoplastic (idiopathic) 284.9
    congenital 284.0
    familial 284.0
    of childhood 284.0
  idiopathic 285.9
    hemolytic, chronic 283.9
  in
    chronic illness NEC 285.29
    end-stage renal disease 285.21
    neoplastic disease 285.22
  infantile 285.9
  infective, infectional 285.9
  intertropical (*see also* Ancylostomiasis) 126.9
  iron (Fe) deficiency 280.9
    due to blood loss (chronic) 280.0
      acute 285.1
    of or complicating pregnancy 648.2 ✓5ᵗʰ
    specified NEC 280.8
  Jaksch's (pseudoleukemia infantum) 285.8

Anemia — *continued*
- Joseph-Diamond-Blackfan (congenital hypoplastic) 284.0
- labyrinth 386.50
- Lederer's (acquired infectious hemolytic anemia) 283.19
- leptocytosis (hereditary) 282.4
- leukoerythroblastic 285.8
- macrocytic 281.9
  - nutritional 281.2
  - of or complicating pregnancy 648.2 ✓5ᵗʰ
  - tropical 281.2
- malabsorption (familial), selective B₁₂ with proteinuria 281.1
- malarial (*see also* Malaria) 084.6
- malignant (progressive) 281.0
- malnutrition 281.9
- marsh (*see also* Malaria) 084.6
- Mediterranean (with hemoglobinopathy) 282.4
- megaloblastic 281.9
  - combined B₁₂ and folate deficiency 281.3
  - nutritional (of infancy) 281.2
  - of infancy 281.2
  - of or complicating pregnancy 648.2 ✓5ᵗʰ
  - refractory 281.3
  - specified NEC 281.3
- megalocytic 281.9
- microangiopathic hemolytic 283.19
- microcytic (hypochromic) 280.9
  - due to blood loss (chronic) 280.0
    - acute 285.1
  - familial 282.4
  - hypochromic 280.9
- microdrepanocytosis 282.4
- miners' (*see also* Ancylostomiasis) 126.9
- myelopathic 285.8
- myelophthisic (normocytic) 285.8
- newborn (*see also* Disease, hemolytic) 773.2
  - due to isoimmunization (*see also* Disease, hemolytic) 773.2
  - late, due to isoimmunization 773.5
  - posthemorrhagic 776.5
- nonregenerative 284.9
- nonspherocytic hemolytic — *see* Anemia, hemolytic, nonspherocytic
- normocytic (infectional) (not due to blood loss) 285.9
  - due to blood loss (chronic) 280.0
    - acute 285.1
  - myelophthisic 284.8
- nutritional (deficiency) 281.9
  - with
    - poor iron absorption 280.9
    - specified deficiency NEC 281.8
  - due to inadequate dietary iron intake 280.1
  - megaloblastic (of infancy) 281.2
- of childhood (*see also* Thalassemia) 282.4
- of chronic illness NEC 285.29
- of or complicating pregnancy 648.2 ✓5ᵗʰ
  - affecting fetus or newborn 760.8
- of prematurity 776.6
- orotic aciduric (congenital) (hereditary) 281.4
- osteosclerotic 289.8
- ovalocytosis (hereditary) (*see also* Elliptocytosis) 282.1
- paludal (*see also* Malaria) 084.6
- pentose phosphate pathway deficiency 282.2
- pernicious (combined system disease) (congenital) (dorsolateral spinal degeneration) (juvenile) (myelopathy) (neuropathy) (posterior sclerosis) (primary) (progressive) (spleen) 281.0
  - of or complicating pregnancy 648.2 ✓5ᵗʰ
- pleochromic 285.9
  - of sprue 281.8
- portal 285.8
- posthemorrhagic (chronic) 280.0
  - acute 285.1
  - newborn 776.5
- pressure 285.9
- primary 285.9
- profound 285.9
- progressive 285.9
  - malignant 281.0
  - pernicious 281.0
- protein-deficiency 281.4
- pseudoleukemica infantum 285.8
- puerperal 648.2 ✓5ᵗʰ

Anemia — *continued*
- pure red cell 284.8
  - congenital 284.0
- pyridoxine-responsive (hypochromic) 285.0
- pyruvate kinase (PK) deficiency 282.3
- refractoria sideroblastica 285.0
- refractory (primary) 284.9
  - with hemochromatosis 285.0
  - megaloblastic 281.3
  - sideroblastic 285.0
  - sideropenic 280.9
- Rietti-Greppi-Micheli (thalassemia minor) 282.4
- scorbutic 281.8
- secondary (to) 285.9
  - blood loss (chronic) 280.0
    - acute 285.1
  - hemorrhage 280.0
    - acute 285.1
  - inadequate dietary iron intake 280.1
- semiplastic 284.9
- septic 285.9
- sickle-cell (*see also* Disease, sickle-cell) 282.60
- sideroachrestic 285.0
- sideroblastic (acquired) (any type) (congenital) (drug-induced) (due to disease) (hereditary) (primary) (refractory) (secondary) (sex-linked hypochromic) (vitamin B₆ responsive) 285.0
- sideropenic (refractory) 280.9
  - due to blood loss (chronic) 280.0
    - acute 285.1
- simple chronic 281.9
- specified type NEC 285.8
- spherocytic (hereditary) (*see also* Spherocytosis) 282.0
- splenic 285.8
  - familial (Gaucher's) 272.7
- splenomegalic 285.8
- stomatocytosis 282.8
- syphilitic 095.8
- target cell (oval) 282.4
- thalassemia 282.4
- thrombocytopenic (*see also* Thrombocytopenia) 287.5
- toxic 284.8
- triosephosphate isomerase deficiency 282.3
- tropical, macrocytic 281.2
- tuberculous (*see also* Tuberculosis) 017.9 ✓5ᵗʰ
- vegan's 281.1
- vitamin
  - B₆-responsive 285.0
  - B₁₂ deficiency (dietary) 281.1
    - pernicious 281.0
- von Jaksch's (pseudoleukemia infantum) 285.8
- Witts' (achlorhydric anemia) 280.9
- Zuelzer (-Ogden) (nutritional megaloblastic anemia) 281.2

Anencephalus, anencephaly 740.0
- fetal, affecting management of pregnancy 655.0 ✓5ᵗʰ

Anergasia (*see also* Psychosis, organic) 294.9
- senile 290.0

Anesthesia, anesthetic 782.0
- complication or reaction NEC 995.2
  - due to
    - correct substance properly administered 995.2
    - overdose or wrong substance given 968.4
    - specified anesthetic — *see* Table of Drugs and Chemicals
- cornea 371.81
- death from
  - correct substance properly administered 995.4
  - during delivery 668.9 ✓5ᵗʰ
  - overdose or wrong substance given 968.4
  - specified anesthetic — *see* Table of Drugs and Chemicals
- eye 371.81
- functional 300.11
- hyperesthetic, thalamic 348.8
- hysterical 300.11
- local skin lesion 782.0
- olfactory 781.1
- sexual (psychogenic) 302.72

Anesthesia, anesthetic — *continued*
- shock
  - due to
    - correct substance properly administered 995.4
    - overdose or wrong substance given 968.4
    - specified anesthetic — *see* Table of Drugs and Chemicals
- skin 782.0
- tactile 782.0
- testicular 608.9
- thermal 782.0

Anetoderma (maculosum) 701.3

Aneuploidy NEC 758.5

Aneurin deficiency 265.1

Aneurysm (anastomotic) (artery) (cirsoid) (diffuse) (false) (fusiform) (multiple) (ruptured) (saccular) (varicose) 442.9
- abdominal (aorta) 441.4
  - ruptured 441.3
  - syphilitic 093.0
- aorta, aortic (nonsyphilitic) 441.9
  - abdominal 441.4
    - dissecting 441.02
    - ruptured 441.3
    - syphilitic 093.0
  - arch 441.2
    - ruptured 441.1
  - arteriosclerotic NEC 441.9
    - ruptured 441.5
  - ascending 441.2
    - ruptured 441.1
  - congenital 747.29
  - descending 441.9
    - abdominal 441.4
      - ruptured 441.3
    - ruptured 441.5
    - thoracic 441.2
      - ruptured 441.1
  - dissecting 441.00
    - abdominal 441.02
    - thoracic 441.01
    - thoracoabdominal 441.03
  - due to coarctation (aorta) 747.10
  - ruptured 441.5
  - sinus, right 747.29
  - syphilitic 093.0
  - thoracoabdominal 441.7
    - ruptured 441.6
  - thorax, thoracic (arch) (nonsyphilitic) 441.2
    - dissecting 441.01
    - ruptured 441.1
    - syphilitic 093.0
  - transverse 441.2
    - ruptured 441.1
  - valve (heart) (*see also* Endocarditis, aortic) 424.1
- arteriosclerotic NEC 442.9
  - cerebral 437.3
    - ruptured (*see also* Hemorrhage, subarachnoid) 430
- arteriovenous (congenital) (peripheral) NEC (*see also* Anomaly, arteriovenous) 747.60
  - acquired NEC 447.0
    - brain 437.3
      - ruptured (*see also* Hemorrhage subarachnoid) 430
    - coronary 414.11
    - pulmonary 417.0
  - brain (cerebral) 747.81
    - ruptured (*see also* Hemorrhage, subarachnoid) 430
  - coronary 746.85
  - pulmonary 747.3
  - retina 743.58
  - specified site NEC 747.89
    - acquired 447.0
  - traumatic (*see also* Injury, blood vessel, by site) 904.9
- basal — *see* Aneurysm, brain
- berry (congenital) (ruptured) (*see also* Hemorrhage, subarachnoid) 430
- brain 437.3
  - arteriosclerotic 437.3
    - ruptured (*see also* Hemorrhage, subarachnoid) 430

Aneurysm — *continued*
  brain — *continued*
    arteriovenous 747.81
      acquired 437.3
        ruptured (*see also* Hemorrhage,
          subarachnoid) 430
      ruptured (*see also* Hemorrhage,
        subarachnoid) 430
    berry (congenital) (ruptured) (*see also*
      Hemorrhage, subarachnoid) 430
    congenital 747.81
      ruptured (*see also* Hemorrhage,
        subarachnoid) 430
    meninges 437.3
      ruptured (*see also* Hemorrhage,
        subarachnoid) 430
    miliary (congenital) (ruptured) (*see also*
      Hemorrhage, subarachnoid) 430
    mycotic 421.0
      ruptured (*see also* Hemorrhage,
        subarachnoid) 430
    nonruptured 437.3
    ruptured (*See also* Hemorrhage,
      subarachnoid) 430
    syphilitic 094.87
    syphilitic (hemorrhage) 094.87
    traumatic — *see* Injury, intracranial
  cardiac (false) (*see also* Aneurysm, heart)
    414.10
  carotid artery (common) (external) 442.81
    internal (intracranial portion) 437.3
      extracranial portion 442.81
      ruptured into brain (*see also*
        Hemorrhage, subarachnoid) 430
    syphilitic 093.89
      intracranial 094.87
  cavernous sinus (*see also* Aneurysm, brain)
    437.3
    arteriovenous 747.81
      ruptured (*see also* Hemorrhage,
        subarachnoid) 430
    congenital 747.81
      ruptured (*see also* Hemorrhage,
        subarachnoid) 430
  celiac 442.84
  central nervous system, syphilitic 094.89
  cerebral — *see* Aneurysm, brain
  chest — *see* Aneurysm, thorax
  circle of Willis (*see also* Aneurysm, brain) 437.3
    congenital 747.81
      ruptured (*see also* Hemorrhage,
        subarachnoid) 430
    ruptured (*see also* Hemorrhage,
      subarachnoid) 430
  common iliac artery 442.2
  congenital (peripheral) NEC 747.60
    brain 747.81
      ruptured (*see also* Hemorrhage,
        subarachnoid) 430
    cerebral — *see* Aneurysm, brain, congenital
    coronary 746.85
    gastrointestinal 747.61
    lower limb 747.64
    pulmonary 747.3
    renal 747.62
    retina 743.58
    specified site NEC 747.89
    spinal 747.82
    upper limb 747.63
  conjunctiva 372.74
  conus arteriosus (*see also* Aneurysm, heart)
    414.10
  coronary (arteriosclerotic) (artery) (vein) (*see
    also* Aneurysm, heart) 414.11
    arteriovenous 746.85
    congenital 746.85
    syphilitic 093.89
  cylindrical 441.9
    ruptured 441.5
    syphilitic 093.9
  dissecting 442.9
    aorta (any part) 441.00
      abdominal 441.02
      thoracic 441.01
      thoracoabdominal 441.03
    syphilitic 093.9

Aneurysm — *continued*
  ductus arteriosus 747.0
  embolic — *see* Embolism, artery
  endocardial, infective (any valve) 421.0
  femoral 442.3
  gastroduodenal 442.84
  gastroepiploic 442.84
  heart (chronic or with a stated duration of over
    8 weeks) (infectional) (wall) 414.10
    acute or with a stated duration of 8 weeks
      or less (*see also* Infarct, myocardium)
      410.9 ✓5ᵗʰ
    congenital 746.89
    valve — *see* Endocarditis
  hepatic 442.84
  iliac (common) 442.2
  infective (any valve) 421.0
  innominate (nonsyphilitic) 442.89
    syphilitic 093.89
  interauricular septum (*see also* Aneurysm,
    heart) 414.10
  interventricular septum (*see also* Aneurysm,
    heart) 414.10
  intracranial — *see* Aneurysm, brain
  intrathoracic (nonsyphilitic) 441.2
    ruptured 441.1
    syphilitic 093.0
  jugular vein 453.8
  lower extremity 442.3
  lung (pulmonary artery) 417.1
  malignant 093.9
  mediastinal (nonsyphilitic) 442.89
    syphilitic 093.89
  miliary (congenital) (ruptured) (*see also*
    Hemorrhage, subarachnoid) 430
  mitral (heart) (valve) 424.0
  mural (arteriovenous) (heart) (*see also*
    Aneurysm, heart) 414.10
  mycotic, any site 421.0
    ruptured, brain (*see also* Hemorrhage,
      subarachnoid) 430
  myocardium (*see also* Aneurysm, heart) 414.10
  neck 442.81
  pancreaticoduodenal 442.84
  patent ductus arteriosus 747.0
  peripheral NEC 442.89
    congenital NEC (*see also* Aneurysm,
      congenital) 747.60
  popliteal 442.3
  pulmonary 417.1
    arteriovenous 747.3
      acquired 417.0
    syphilitic 093.89
    valve (heart) (*see also* Endocarditis,
      pulmonary) 424.3
  racemose 442.9
    congenital (peripheral) NEC 747.60
  radial 442.0
  Rasmussen's (*see also* Tuberculosis) 011.2 ✓5ᵗʰ
  renal 442.1
  retinal (acquired) 362.17
    congenital 743.58
    diabetic 250.5 ✓5ᵗʰ [362.01]
  sinus, aortic (of Valsalva) 747.29
  specified site NEC 442.89
  spinal (cord) 442.89
    congenital 747.82
    syphilitic (hemorrhage) 094.89
  spleen, splenic 442.83
  subclavian 442.82
    syphilitic 093.89
  superior mesenteric 442.84
  syphilitic 093.9
    aorta 093.0
    central nervous system 094.89
    congenital 090.5
    spine, spinal 094.89
  thoracoabdominal 441.7
    ruptured 441.6
  thorax, thoracic (arch) (nonsyphilitic) 441.2
    dissecting 441.0 ✓5ᵗʰ
    ruptured 441.1
    syphilitic 093.0
  traumatic (complication) (early) — *see* Injury,
    blood vessel, by site
  tricuspid (heart) (valve) — *see* Endocarditis,
    tricuspid
  ulnar 442.0

Aneurysm — *continued*
  upper extremity 442.0
  valve, valvular — *see* Endocarditis
  venous 456.8
    congenital NEC (*see also* Aneurysm,
      congenital) 747.60
  ventricle (arteriovenous) (*see also* Aneurysm,
    heart) 414.10
  visceral artery NEC 442.84
Angiectasis 459.89
Angiectopia 459.9
Angiitis 447.6
  allergic granulomatous 446.4
  hypersensitivity 446.20
    Goodpasture's syndrome 446.21
    specified NEC 446.29
  necrotizing 446.0
  Wegener's (necrotizing respiratory
    granulomatosis) 446.4
Angina (attack) (cardiac) (chest) (effort) (heart)
  (pectoris) (syndrome) (vasomotor) 413.9
  abdominal 557.1
  agranulocytic 288.0
  aphthous 074.0
  catarrhal 462
  crescendo 411.1
  croupous 464.4
  cruris 443.9
    due to atherosclerosis NEC (*see also*
      Arteriosclerosis, extremities) 440.20
  decubitus 413.0
  diphtheritic (membranous) 032.0
  erysipelatous 034.0
  erythematous 462
  exudative, chronic 476.0
  faucium 478.29
  gangrenous 462
    diphtheritic 032.0
  infectious 462
  initial 411.1
  intestinal 557.1
  ludovici 528.3
  Ludwig's 528.3
  malignant 462
    diphtheritic 032.0
  membranous 464.4
    diphtheritic 032.0
  mesenteric 557.1
  monocytic 075
  nocturnal 413.0
  phlegmonous 475
    diphtheritic 032.0
  preinfarctional 411.1
  Prinzmetal's 413.1
  progressive 411.1
  pseudomembranous 101
  psychogenic 306.2
  pultaceous, diphtheritic 032.0
  scarlatinal 034.1
  septic 034.0
  simple 462
  stable NEC 413.9
  staphylococcal 462
  streptococcal 034.0
  stridulous, diphtheritic 032.3
  syphilitic 093.9
    congenital 090.5
  tonsil 475
  trachealis 464.4
  unstable 411.1
  variant 413.1
  Vincent's 101
Angioblastoma (M9161/1) — *see* Neoplasm,
  connective tissue, uncertain behavior
Angiocholecystitis (*see also* Cholecystitis, acute)
  575.0
Angiocholitis (*see also* Cholecystitis, acute) 576.1
Angiodysgensis spinalis 336.1
Angiodysplasia (intestinalis) (intestine) 569.84
  with hemorrhage 569.85
  duodenum 537.82
    with hemorrhage 537.83
  stomach 537.82
    with hemorrhage 537.83

Aneurysm — Angiodysplasia

Angioedema (allergic) (any site) (with urticaria) 995.1
  hereditary 277.6
Angioendothelioma (M9130/1) — *see also* Neoplasm, by site, uncertain behavior
  benign (M9130/0) (*see also* Hemangioma, by site) 228.00
  bone (M9260/3) — *see* Neoplasm, bone, malignant
  Ewing's (M9260/3) — *see* Neoplasm, bone, malignant
  nervous system (M9130/0) 228.09
Angiofibroma (M9160/0) — *see also* Neoplasm, by site, benign
  juvenile (M9160/0) 210.7
    specified site — *see* Neoplasm, by site, benign
    unspecified site 210.7
Angiohemophilia (A) (B) 286.4
Angioid streaks (choroid) (retina) 363.43
Angiokeratoma (M9141/0) — *see also* Neoplasm, skin, benign
  corporis diffusum 272.7
Angiokeratosis
  diffuse 272.7
Angioleiomyoma (M8894/0) — *see* Neoplasm, connective tissue, benign
Angioleucitis 683
Angiolipoma (M8861/0) (*see also* Lipoma, by site) 214.9
  infiltrating (M8861/1) — *see* Neoplasm, connective tissue, uncertain behavior
Angioma (M9120/0) (*see also* Hemangioma, by site) 228.00
  capillary 448.1
  hemorrhagicum hereditaria 448.0
  malignant (M9120/3) — *see* Neoplasm, connective tissue, malignant
  pigmentosum et atrophicum 757.33
  placenta — *see* Placenta, abnormal
  plexiform (M9131/0) — *see* Hemangioma, by site
  senile 448.1
  serpiginosum 709.1
  spider 448.1
  stellate 448.1
Angiomatosis 757.32
  bacillary 083.8
  corporis diffusum universale 272.7
  cutaneocerebral 759.6
  encephalocutaneous 759.6
  encephalofacial 759.6
  encephalotrigeminal 759.6
  hemorrhagic familial 448.0
  hereditary familial 448.0
  heredofamilial 448.0
  meningo-oculofacial 759.6
  multiple sites 228.09
  neuro-oculocutaneous 759.6
  retina (Hippel's disease) 759.6
  retinocerebellosa 759.6
  retinocerebral 759.6
  systemic 228.09
Angiomyolipoma (M8860/0)
  specified site — *see* Neoplasm, connective tissue, benign
  unspecified site 223.0
Angiomyoliposarcoma (M8860/3) — *see* Neoplasm, connective tissue, malignant
Angiomyoma (M8894/0) — *see* Neoplasm, connective tissue, benign
Angiomyosarcoma (M8894/3) — *see* Neoplasm, connective tissue, malignant
Angioneurosis 306.2
Angioneurotic edema (allergic) (any site) (with urticaria) 995.1
  hereditary 277.6
Angiopathia, angiopathy 459.9
  diabetic (peripheral) 250.7 ✓5ᵗʰ [443.81]
  peripheral 443.9
    diabetic 250.7 ✓5ᵗʰ [443.81]
    specified type NEC 443.89
  retinae syphilitica 093.89

Angiopathia, angiopathy — *continued*
  retinalis (juvenilis) 362.18
    background 362.10
    diabetic 250.5 ✓5ᵗʰ [362.01]
    proliferative 362.29
    tuberculous (*see also* Tuberculosis) 017.3 ✓5ᵗʰ [362.18]
Angiosarcoma (M9120/3) — *see* Neoplasm, connective tissue, malignant
Angiosclerosis — *see* Arteriosclerosis
Angioscotoma, enlarged 368.42
Angiospasm 443.9
  brachial plexus 353.0
  cerebral 435.9
  cervical plexus 353.2
  nerve
    arm 354.9
      axillary 353.0
      median 354.1
      ulnar 354.2
    autonomic (*see also* Neuropathy, peripheral, autonomic) 337.9
    axillary 353.0
    leg 355.8
      plantar 355.6
    lower extremity — *see* Angiospasm, nerve, leg
    median 354.1
    peripheral NEC 355.9
    spinal NEC 355.9
    sympathetic (*see also* Neuropathy, peripheral, autonomic) 337.9
    ulnar 354.2
    upper extremity — *see* Angiospasm, nerve, arm
  peripheral NEC 443.9
  traumatic 443.9
    foot 443.9
    leg 443.9
  vessel 443.9
Angiospastic disease or edema 443.9
Anguillulosis 127.2
Angulation
  cecum (*see also* Obstruction, intestine) 560.9
  coccyx (acquired) 738.6
    congenital 756.19
  femur (acquired) 736.39
    congenital 755.69
  intestine (large) (small) (*see also* Obstruction, intestine) 560.9
  sacrum (acquired) 738.5
    congenital 756.19
  sigmoid (flexure) (*see also* Obstruction, intestine) 560.9
  spine (*see also* Curvature, spine) 737.9
  tibia (acquired) 736.89
    congenital 755.69
  ureter 593.3
  wrist (acquired) 736.09
    congenital 755.59
Angulus infectiosus 686.8
Anhedonia 302.72
Anhidrosis (lid) (neurogenic) (thermogenic) 705.0
Anhydration 276.5
  with
    hypernatremia 276.0
    hyponatremia 276.1
Anhydremia 276.5
  with
    hypernatremia 276.0
    hyponatremia 276.1
Anidrosis 705.0
Aniridia (congenital) 743.45
Anisakiasis (infection) (infestation) 127.1
Anisakis larva infestation 127.1
Aniseikonia 367.32
Anisocoria (pupil) 379.41
  congenital 743.46
Anisocytosis 790.09
Anisometropia (congenital) 367.31
Ankle — *see* condition
Ankyloblepharon (acquired) (eyelid) 374.46
  filiforme (adnatum) (congenital) 743.62

Ankyloblepharon — *continued*
  total 743.62
Ankylodactly (*see also* Syndactylism) 755.10
Ankyloglossia 750.0
Ankylosis (fibrous) (osseous) 718.50
  ankle 718.57
  any joint, produced by surgical fusion V45.4
  cricoarytenoid (cartilage) (joint) (larynx) 478.79
  dental 521.6
  ear ossicle NEC 385.22
    malleus 385.21
  elbow 718.52
  finger 718.54
  hip 718.55
  incostapedial joint (infectional) 385.22
  joint, produced by surgical fusion NEC V45.4
  knee 718.56
  lumbosacral (joint) 724.6
  malleus 385.21
  multiple sites 718.59
  postoperative (status) V45.4
  sacroiliac (joint) 724.6
  shoulder 718.51
  specified site NEC 718.58
  spine NEC 724.9
  surgical V45.4
  teeth, tooth (hard tissues) 521.6
  temporomandibular joint 524.61
  wrist 718.53
Ankylostoma — *see* Ancylostoma
Ankylostomiasis (intestinal) — *see* Ancylostomiasis
Ankylurethria (*see also* Stricture, urethra) 598.9
Annular — *see also* condition
  detachment, cervix 622.8
  organ or site, congenital NEC — *see* Distortion
  pancreas (congenital) 751.7
Anodontia (complete) (partial) (vera) 520.0
  with abnormal spacing 524.3
  acquired 525.10
    causing malocclusion 524.3
    due to
      caries 525.13
      extraction 525.10
      periodontal disease 525.12
      trauma 525.11
Anomaly, anomalous (congenital) (unspecified type) 759.9
  abdomen 759.9
  abdominal wall 756.70
  acoustic nerve 742.9
  adrenal (gland) 759.1
  Alder (-Reilly) (leukocyte granulation) 288.2
  alimentary tract 751.9
    lower 751.5
    specified type NEC 751.8
    upper (any part, except tongue) 750.9
      tongue 750.10
        specified type NEC 750.19
  alveolar ridge (process) 525.8
  ankle (joint) 755.69
  anus, anal (canal) 751.5
  aorta, aortic 747.20
    arch 747.21
    coarctation (postductal) (preductal) 747.10
    cusp or valve NEC 746.9
    septum 745.0
    specified type NEC 747.29
  aorticopulmonary septum 745.0
  apertures, diaphragm 756.6
  appendix 751.5
  aqueduct of Sylvius 742.3
    with spina bifida (*see also* Spina bifida) 741.0 ✓5ᵗʰ
  arm 755.50
    reduction (*see also* Deformity, reduction, upper limb) 755.20
  arteriovenous (congenital) (peripheral) NEC 747.60
    brain 747.81
    cerebral 747.81
    coronary 746.85
    gastrointestinal 747.61
    lower limb 747.64
    renal 747.62
    specified site NEC 747.69

Anomaly, anomalous — *continued*
  arteriovenous — *continued*
    spinal 747.82
    upper limb 747.63
  artery (*see also* Anomaly, peripheral vascular
      system) NEC 747.60
    brain 747.81
    cerebral 747.81
    coronary 746.85
    eye 743.9
    pulmonary 747.3
    renal 747.62
    retina 743.9
    umbilical 747.5
  arytenoepiglottic folds 748.3
  atrial
    bands 746.9
    folds 746.9
    septa 745.5
  atrioventricular
    canal 745.69
    common 745.69
    conduction 426.7
    excitation 426.7
    septum 745.4
  atrium — *see* Anomaly, atrial
  auditory canal 744.3
    specified type NEC 744.29
      with hearing impairment 744.02
  auricle
    ear 744.3
      causing impairment of hearing 744.02
    heart 746.9
      septum 745.5
  autosomes, autosomal NEC 758.5
  Axenfeld's 743.44
  back 759.9
  band
    atrial 746.9
    heart 746.9
    ventricular 746.9
  Bartholin's duct 750.9
  biliary duct or passage 751.60
    atresia 751.61
  bladder (neck) (sphincter) (trigone) 753.9
    specified type NEC 753.8
  blood vessel 747.9
    artery — *see* Anomaly, artery
    peripheral vascular — *see* Anomaly,
      peripheral vascular system
    vein — *see* Anomaly, vein
  bone NEC 756.9
    ankle 755.69
    arm 755.50
    chest 756.3
    cranium 756.0
    face 756.0
    finger 755.50
    foot 755.67
    forearm 755.50
    frontal 756.0
    head 756.0
    hip 755.63
    leg 755.60
    lumbosacral 756.10
    nose 748.1
    pelvic girdle 755.60
    rachitic 756.4
    rib 756.3
    shoulder girdle 755.50
    skull 756.0
      with
        anencephalus 740.0
        encephalocele 742.0
        hydrocephalus 742.3
          with spina bifida (*see also* Spina
            bifida) 741.0 ✔5ᵗʰ
        microcephalus 742.1
    toe 755.66
  brain 742.9
    multiple 742.4
    reduction 742.2
    specified type NEC 742.4
    vessel 747.81
  branchial cleft NEC 744.49
    cyst 744.42
    fistula 744.41

Anomaly, anomalous — *continued*
  branchial cleft NEC — *continued*
    persistent 744.41
    sinus (external) (internal) 744.41
  breast 757.9
  broad ligament 752.10
    specified type NEC 752.19
  bronchus 748.3
  bulbar septum 745.0
  bulbus cordis 745.9
    persistent (in left ventricle) 745.8
  bursa 756.9
  canal of Nuck 752.9
  canthus 743.9
  capillary NEC (*see also* Anomaly, peripheral
      vascular system) 747.60
  cardiac 746.9
    septal closure 745.9
      acquired 429.71
    valve NEC 746.9
      pulmonary 746.00
      specified type NEC 746.89
  cardiovascular system 746.9
    complicating pregnancy, childbirth, or
      puerperium 648.5 ✔5ᵗʰ
  carpus 755.50
  cartilage, trachea 748.3
  cartilaginous 756.9
  caruncle, lacrimal, lachrymal 743.9
  cascade stomach 750.7
  cauda equina 742.59
  cecum 751.5
  cerebral — *see also* Anomaly, brain vessels
    747.81
  cerebrovascular system 747.81
  cervix (uterus) 752.40
    with doubling of vagina and uterus 752.2
    in pregnancy or childbirth 654.6 ✔5ᵗʰ
      affecting fetus or newborn 763.89
      causing obstructed labor 660.2 ✔5ᵗʰ
        affecting fetus or newborn 763.1
  Chédiak-Higashi (-Steinbrinck) (congenital
      gigantism of peroxidase granules) 288.2
  cheek 744.9
  chest (wall) 756.3
  chin 744.9
    specified type NEC 744.89
  chordae tendineae 746.9
  choroid 743.9
    plexus 742.9
  chromosomes, chromosomal 758.9
    13 (13-15) 758.1
    18 (16-18) 758.2
    21 or 22 758.0
    autosomes NEC (*see also* Abnormality,
      autosomes) 758.5
      deletion 758.3
    Christchurch 758.3
    D₁ 758.1
    E₃ 758.2
    G 758.0
    mitochondrial 758.9
    mosaics 758.89
    sex 758.81
      complement, XO 758.6
      complement, XXX 758.81
      complement, XXY 758.7
      complement, XYY 758.81
      gonadal dysgenesis 758.6
      Klinefelter's 758.7
      Turner's 758.6
    trisomy 21 758.0
  cilia 743.9
  circulatory system 747.9
    specified type NEC 747.89
  clavicle 755.51
  clitoris 752.40
  coccyx 756.10
  colon 751.5
  common duct 751.60
  communication
    coronary artery 746.85
    left ventricle with right atrium 745.4
  concha (ear) 744.3
  connection
    renal vessels with kidney 747.62
    total pulmonary venous 747.41

Anomaly, anomalous — *continued*
  connective tissue 756.9
    specified type NEC 756.89
  cornea 743.9
    shape 743.41
    size 743.41
    specified type NEC 743.49
  coronary
    artery 746.85
    vein 746.89
  cranium — *see* Anomaly, skull
  cricoid cartilage 748.3
  cushion, endocardial 745.60
    specified type NEC 745.69
  cystic duct 751.60
  dental arch relationship 524.2
  dentition 520.6
  dentofacial NEC 524.9
    functional 524.5
    specified type NEC 524.8
  dermatoglyphic 757.2
  Descemet's membrane 743.9
    specified type NEC 743.49
  development
    cervix 752.40
    vagina 752.40
    vulva 752.40
  diaphragm, diaphragmatic (apertures) NEC
    756.6
  digestive organ(s) or system 751.9
    lower 751.5
    specified type NEC 751.8
    upper 750.9
  distribution, coronary artery 746.85
  ductus
    arteriosus 747.0
    Botalli 747.0
  duodenum 751.5
  dura 742.9
    brain 742.4
    spinal cord 742.59
  ear 744.3
    causing impairment of hearing 744.00
      specified type NEC 744.09
    external 744.3
      causing impairment of hearing 744.02
      specified type NEC 744.29
    inner (causing impairment of hearing)
      744.05
    middle, except ossicles (causing impairment
      of hearing) 744.03
      ossicles 744.04
    ossicles 744.04
    prominent auricle 744.29
    specified type NEC 744.29
      with hearing impairment 744.09
  Ebstein's (heart) 746.2
    tricuspid valve 746.2
  ectodermal 757.9
  Eisenmenger's (ventricular septal defect) 745.4
  ejaculatory duct 752.9
    specified type NEC 752.8
  elbow (joint) 755.50
  endocardial cushion 745.60
    specified type NEC 745.69
  endocrine gland NEC 759.2
  epididymis 752.9
  epiglottis 748.3
  esophagus 750.9
    specified type NEC 750.4
  Eustachian tube 744.3
    specified type NEC 744.24
  eye (any part) 743.9
    adnexa 743.9
      specified type NEC 743.69
    anophthalmos 743.00
    anterior
      chamber and related structures 743.9
        angle 743.9
          specified type NEC 743.44
        specified type NEC 743.44
      segment 743.9
        combined 743.48
        multiple 743.48
        specified type NEC 743.49
    cataract (*see also* Cataract) 743.30
    glaucoma (*see also* Buphthalmia) 743.20

Anomaly, anomalous — *continued*
- eye — *continued*
  - lid 743.9
    - specified type NEC 743.63
  - microphthalmos (*see also* Microphthalmos) 743.10
  - posterior segment 743.9
    - specified type NEC 743.59
    - vascular 743.58
    - vitreous 743.9
      - specified type NEC 743.51
  - ptosis (eyelid) 743.61
  - retina 743.9
    - specified type NEC 743.59
  - sclera 743.9
    - specified type NEC 743.47
  - specified type NEC 743.8
- eyebrow 744.89
- eyelid 743.9
  - specified type NEC 743.63
- face (any part) 744.9
  - bone(s) 756.0
  - specified type NEC 744.89
- fallopian tube 752.10
  - specified type NEC 752.19
- fascia 756.9
  - specified type NEC 756.89
- femur 755.60
- fibula 755.60
- finger 755.50
  - supernumerary 755.01
  - webbed (*see also* Syndactylism, fingers) 755.11
- fixation, intestine 751.4
- flexion (joint) 755.9
  - hip or thigh (*see also* Dislocation, hip, congenital) 754.30
- folds, heart 746.9
- foot 755.67
- foramen
  - Botalli 745.5
  - ovale 745.5
- forearm 755.50
- forehead (*see also* Anomaly, skull) 756.0
- form, teeth 520.2
- fovea centralis 743.9
- frontal bone (*see also* Anomaly, skull) 756.0
- gallbladder 751.60
- Gartner's duct 752.11
- gastrointestinal tract 751.9
  - specified type NEC 751.8
  - vessel 747.61
- genitalia, genital organ(s) or system
  - female 752.9
    - external 752.40
      - specified type NEC 752.49
    - internal NEC 752.9
  - male (external and internal) 752.9
    - epispadias 752.62
    - hidden penis 752.65
    - hydrocele, congenital 778.6
    - hypospadias 752.61
    - micropenis 752.64
    - testis, undescended 752.51
      - retractile 752.52
  - specified type NEC 752.8
- genitourinary NEC 752.9
- Gerbode 745.4
- globe (eye) 743.9
- glottis 748.3
- granulation or granulocyte, genetic 288.2
  - constitutional 288.2
  - leukocyte 288.2
- gum 750.9
- gyri 742.9
- hair 757.9
  - specified type NEC 757.4
- hand 755.50
- hard tissue formation in pulp 522.3
- head (*see also* Anomaly, skull) 756.0
- heart 746.9
  - auricle 746.9
  - bands 746.9
  - fibroelastosis cordis 425.3
  - folds 746.9
  - malposition 746.87
  - maternal, affecting fetus or newborn 760.3

Anomaly, anomalous — *continued*
- heart — *continued*
  - obstructive NEC 746.84
  - patent ductus arteriosus (Botalli) 747.0
  - septum 745.9
    - acquired 429.71
    - aortic 745.0
    - aorticopulmonary 745.0
    - atrial 745.5
    - auricular 745.5
    - between aorta and pulmonary artery 745.0
    - endocardial cushion type 745.60
      - specified type NEC 745.69
    - interatrial 745.5
    - interventricular 745.4
      - with pulmonary stenosis or atresia, dextraposition of aorta, and hypertrophy of right ventricle 745.2
      - acquired 429.71
    - specified type NEC 745.8
    - ventricular 745.4
      - with pulmonary stenosis or atresia, dextraposition of aorta, and hypertrophy of right ventricle 745.2
      - acquired 429.71
  - specified type NEC 746.89
  - tetralogy of Fallot 745.2
  - valve NEC 746.9
    - aortic 746.9
      - atresia 746.89
      - bicuspid valve 746.4
      - insufficiency 746.4
      - specified type NEC 746.89
      - stenosis 746.3
        - subaortic 746.81
        - supravalvular 747.22
    - mitral 746.9
      - atresia 746.89
      - insufficiency 746.6
      - specified type NEC 746.89
      - stenosis 746.5
    - pulmonary 746.00
      - atresia 746.01
      - insufficiency 746.09
      - stenosis 746.02
        - infundibular 746.83
        - subvalvular 746.83
    - tricuspid 746.9
      - atresia 746.1
      - stenosis 746.1
  - ventricle 746.9
- heel 755.67
- Hegglin's 288.2
- hemianencephaly 740.0
- hemicephaly 740.0
- hemicrania 740.0
- hepatic duct 751.60
- hip (joint) 755.63
- hourglass
  - bladder 753.8
  - gallbladder 751.69
  - stomach 750.7
- humerus 755.50
- hymen 752.40
- hypersegmentation of neutrophils, hereditary 288.2
- hypophyseal 759.2
- ileocecal (coil) (valve) 751.5
- ileum (intestine) 751.5
- ilium 755.60
- integument 757.9
  - specified type NEC 757.8
- intervertebral cartilage or disc 756.10
- intestine (large) (small) 751.5
  - fixational type 751.4
- iris 743.9
  - specified type NEC 743.46
- ischium 755.60
- jaw NEC 524.9
  - closure 524.5
  - size (major) NEC 524.00
  - specified type NEC 524.8
- jaw-cranial base relationship 524.10
  - specified NEC 524.19

Anomaly, anomalous — *continued*
- jejunum 751.5
- joint 755.9
  - hip
    - dislocation (*see also* Dislocation, hip, congenital) 754.30
    - predislocation (*see also* Subluxation, congenital, hip) 754.32
    - preluxation (*see also* Subluxation, congenital, hip) 754.32
    - subluxation (*see also* Subluxation, congenital, hip) 754.32
  - lumbosacral 756.10
    - spondylolisthesis 756.12
    - spondylosis 756.11
  - multiple arthrogryposis 754.89
  - sacroiliac 755.69
- Jordan's 288.2
- kidney(s) (calyx) (pelvis) 753.9
  - vessel 747.62
- Klippel-Feil (brevicollis) 756.16
- knee (joint) 755.64
- labium (majus) (minus) 752.40
- labyrinth, membranous (causing impairment of hearing) 744.05
- lacrimal
  - apparatus, duct or passage 743.9
    - specified type NEC 743.65
  - gland 743.9
    - specified type NEC 743.64
- Langdon Down (mongolism) 758.0
- larynx, laryngeal (muscle) 748.3
  - web, webbed 748.2
- leg (lower) (upper) 755.60
  - reduction NEC (*see also* Deformity, reduction, lower limb) 755.30
- lens 743.9
  - shape 743.36
  - specified type NEC 743.39
- leukocytes, genetic 288.2
  - granulation (constitutional) 288.2
- lid (fold) 743.9
- ligament 756.9
  - broad 752.10
  - round 752.9
- limb, except reduction deformity 755.9
  - lower 755.60
    - reduction deformity (*see also* Deformity, reduction, lower limb) 755.30
    - specified type NEC 755.69
  - upper 755.50
    - reduction deformity (*see also* Deformity, reduction, upper limb) 755.20
    - specified type NEC 755.59
- lip 750.9
  - harelip (*see also* Cleft, lip) 749.10
  - specified type NEC 750.26
- liver (duct) 751.60
  - atresia 751.69
- lower extremity 755.60
  - vessel 747.64
- lumbosacral (joint) (region) 756.10
- lung (fissure) (lobe) NEC 748.60
  - agenesis 748.5
  - specified type NEC 748.69
- lymphatic system 759.9
- Madelung's (radius) 755.54
- mandible 524.9
  - size NEC 524.00
- maxilla 524.9
  - size NEC 524.00
- May (-Hegglin) 288.2
- meatus urinarius 753.9
  - specified type NEC 753.8
- meningeal bands or folds, constriction of 742.8
- meninges 742.9
  - brain 742.4
  - spinal 742.59
- meningocele (*see also* Spina bifida) 741.9 ✓5ᵗʰ
- mesentery 751.9
- metacarpus 755.50
- metatarsus 755.67
- middle ear, except ossicles (causing impairment of hearing) 744.03
  - ossicles 744.04
- mitral (leaflets) (valve) 746.9
  - atresia 746.89

Anomaly — Anomaly

Anomaly, anomalous — *continued*
mitral — *continued*
  insufficiency 746.6
  specified type NEC 746.89
  stenosis 746.5
mouth 750.9
  specified type NEC 750.26
multiple NEC 759.7
  specified type NEC 759.89
muscle 756.9
  eye 743.9
    specified type NEC 743.69
  specified type NEC 756.89
musculoskeletal system, except limbs 756.9
  specified type NEC 756.9
nail 757.9
  specified type NEC 757.5
narrowness, eyelid 743.62
nasal sinus or septum 748.1
neck (any part) 744.9
  specified type NEC 744.89
nerve 742.9
  acoustic 742.9
    specified type NEC 742.8
  optic 742.9
    specified type NEC 742.8
  specified type NEC 742.8
nervous system NEC 742.9
  brain 742.9
    specified type NEC 742.4
  specified type NEC 742.8
neurological 742.9
nipple 757.9
nonteratogenic NEC 754.89
nose, nasal (bone) (cartilage) (septum) (sinus) 748.1
ocular muscle 743.9
omphalomesenteric duct 751.0
opening, pulmonary veins 747.49
optic
  disc 743.9
    specified type NEC 743.57
  nerve 742.9
opticociliary vessels 743.9
orbit (eye) 743.9
  specified type NEC 743.66
organ
  of Corti (causing impairment of hearing) 744.05
  or site 759.9
    specified type NEC 759.89
origin
  both great arteries from same ventricle 745.11
  coronary artery 746.85
  innominate artery 747.69
  left coronary artery from pulmonary artery 746.85
  pulmonary artery 747.3
  renal vessels 747.62
  subclavian artery (left) (right) 747.21
osseous meatus (ear) 744.03
ovary 752.0
oviduct 752.10
palate (hard) (soft) 750.9
  cleft (*see also* Cleft, palate) 749.00
pancreas (duct) 751.7
papillary muscles 746.9
parathyroid gland 759.2
paraurethral ducts 753.9
parotid (gland) 750.9
patella 755.64
Pelger-Huët (hereditary hyposegmentation) 288.2
pelvic girdle 755.60
  specified type NEC 755.69
pelvis (bony) 755.60
  complicating delivery 653.0 ☑5ᵗʰ
  rachitic 268.1
    fetal 756.4
penis (glans) 752.69
pericardium 746.89
peripheral vascular system NEC 747.60
  gastrointestinal 747.61
  lower limb 747.64
  renal 747.62
  specified site NEC 747.69

Anomaly, anomalous — *continued*
peripheral vascular system NEC — *continued*
  spinal 747.82
  upper limb 747.63
Peter's 743.44
pharynx 750.9
  branchial cleft 744.41
  specified type NEC 750.29
Pierre Robin 756.0
pigmentation NEC 709.00
  congenital 757.33
pituitary (gland) 759.2
pleural folds 748.8
portal vein 747.40
position tooth, teeth 524.3
preauricular sinus 744.46
prepuce 752.9
prostate 752.9
pulmonary 748.60
  artery 747.3
  circulation 747.3
  specified type NEC 748.69
  valve 746.00
    atresia 746.01
    insufficiency 746.09
    specified type NEC 746.09
    stenosis 746.02
      infundibular 746.83
      subvalvular 746.83
  vein 747.40
  venous
    connection 747.49
      partial 747.42
      total 747.41
    return 747.49
      partial 747.42
      total (TAPVR) (complete) (subdiaphragmatic) (supradiaphrag-matic) 747.41
pupil 743.9
pylorus 750.9
  hypertrophy 750.5
  stenosis 750.5
rachitic, fetal 756.4
radius 755.50
rectovaginal (septum) 752.40
rectum 751.5
refraction 367.9
renal 753.9
  vessel 747.62
respiratory system 748.9
  specified type NEC 748.8
rib 756.3
  cervical 756.2
Rieger's 743.44
rings, trachea 748.3
rotation — *see also* Malrotation
  hip or thigh (*see also* Subluxation, congenital, hip) 754.32
round ligament 752.9
sacroiliac (joint) 755.69
sacrum 756.10
saddle
  back 754.2
  nose 754.0
    syphilitic 090.5
salivary gland or duct 750.9
  specified type NEC 750.26
scapula 755.50
sclera 743.9
  specified type NEC 743.47
scrotum 752.9
sebaceous gland 757.9
seminal duct or tract 752.9
sense organs 742.9
  specified type NEC 742.8
septum
  heart — *see* Anomaly, heart, septum
  nasal 748.1
sex chromosomes NEC (*see also* Anomaly, chromosomes) 758.81
shoulder (girdle) (joint) 755.50
  specified type NEC 755.59
sigmoid (flexure) 751.5
sinus of Valsalva 747.29
site NEC 759.9
skeleton generalized NEC 756.50

Anomaly, anomalous — *continued*
skin (appendage) 757.9
  specified type NEC 757.39
skull (bone) 756.0
  with
    anencephalus 740.0
    encephalocele 742.0
    hydrocephalus 742.3
      with spina bifida (*see also* Spina bifida) 741.0 ☑5ᵗʰ
    microcephalus 742.1
specified type NEC
  adrenal (gland) 759.1
  alimentary tract (complete) (partial) 751.8
    lower 751.5
    upper 750.8
  ankle 755.69
  anus, anal (canal) 751.5
  aorta, aortic 747.29
    arch 747.21
  appendix 751.5
  arm 755.59
  artery (peripheral) NEC (*see also* Anomaly, peripheral vascular system) 747.60
    brain 747.81
    coronary 746.85
    eye 743.58
    pulmonary 747.3
    retinal 743.58
    umbilical 747.5
  auditory canal 744.29
    causing impairment of hearing 744.02
  bile duct or passage 751.69
  bladder 753.8
    neck 753.8
  bone(s) 756.9
    arm 755.59
    face 756.0
    leg 755.69
    pelvic girdle 755.69
    shoulder girdle 755.59
    skull 756.0
      with
        anencephalus 740.0
        encephalocele 742.0
        hydrocephalus 742.3
          with spina bifida (*see also* Spina bifida) 741.0 ☑5ᵗʰ
        microcephalus 742.1
  brain 742.4
  breast 757.6
  broad ligament 752.19
  bronchus 748.3
  canal of Nuck 752.8
  cardiac septal closure 745.8
  carpus 755.59
  cartilaginous 756.9
  cecum 751.5
  cervix 752.49
  chest (wall) 756.3
  chin 744.89
  ciliary body 743.46
  circulatory system 747.89
  clavicle 755.51
  clitoris 752.49
  coccyx 756.19
  colon 751.5
  common duct 751.69
  connective tissue 756.89
  cricoid cartilage 748.3
  cystic duct 751.69
  diaphragm 756.6
  digestive organ(s) or tract 751.8
    lower 751.5
    upper 750.8
  duodenum 751.5
  ear 744.29
    auricle 744.29
      causing impairment of hearing 744.02
    causing impairment of hearing 744.09
    inner (causing impairment of hearing) 744.05
    middle, except ossicles 744.03
      ossicles 744.04
  ejaculatory duct 752.8
  endocrine 759.2
  epiglottis 748.3

☑4ᵗʰ Fourth-digit Required   ☑5ᵗʰ Fifth-digit Required   ▶◀ Revised Text   ● New Line   ▲ Revised Code

Anomaly, anomalous — *continued*
specified type NEC — *continued*
esophagus 750.4
Eustachian tube 744.24
eye 743.8
lid 743.63
muscle 743.69
face 744.89
bone(s) 756.0
fallopian tube 752.19
fascia 756.89
femur 755.69
fibula 755.69
finger 755.59
foot 755.67
fovea centralis 743.55
gallbladder 751.69
Gartner's duct 752.8
gastrointestinal tract 751.8
genitalia, genital organ(s)
female 752.8
external 752.49
internal NEC 752.8
male 752.8
penis 752.69
genitourinary tract NEC 752.8
glottis 748.3
hair 757.4
hand 755.59
heart 746.89
valve NEC 746.89
pulmonary 746.09
hepatic duct 751.69
hydatid of Morgagni 752.8
hymen 752.49
integument 757.8
intestine (large) (small) 751.5
fixational type 751.4
iris 743.46
jejunum 751.5
joint 755.8
kidney 753.3
knee 755.64
labium (majus) (minus) 752.49
labyrinth, membranous 744.05
larynx 748.3
leg 755.69
lens 743.39
limb, except reduction deformity 755.8
lower 755.69
reduction deformity (*see also*
Deformity, reduction, lower limb)
755.30
upper 755.59
reduction deformity (*see also*
Deformity, reduction, upper
limb) 755.20
lip 750.26
liver 751.69
lung (fissure) (lobe) 748.69
meatus urinarius 753.8
metacarpus 755.59
mouth 750.26
muscle 756.89
eye 743.69
musculoskeletal system, except limbs 756.9
nail 757.5
neck 744.89
nerve 742.8
acoustic 742.8
optic 742.8
nervous system 742.8
nipple 757.6
nose 748.1
organ NEC 759.89
of Corti 744.05
osseous meatus (ear) 744.03
ovary 752.0
oviduct 752.19
pancreas 751.7
parathyroid 759.2
patella 755.64
pelvic girdle 755.69
penis 752.69
pericardium 746.89

Anomaly, anomalous — *continued*
specified type NEC — *continued*
peripheral vascular system NEC (*see also*
Anomaly, peripheral vascular system)
747.60
pharynx 750.29
pituitary 759.2
prostate 752.8
radius 755.59
rectum 751.5
respiratory system 748.8
rib 756.3
round ligament 752.8
sacrum 756.19
salivary duct or gland 750.26
scapula 755.59
sclera 743.47
scrotum 752.8
seminal duct or tract 752.8
shoulder girdle 755.59
site NEC 759.89
skin 757.39
skull (bone(s)) 756.0
with
anencephalus 740.0
encephalocele 742.0
hydrocephalus 742.3
with spina bifida (*see also* Spina
bifida) 741.0 ✓5th
microcephalus 742.1
specified organ or site NEC 759.89
spermatic cord 752.8
spinal cord 742.59
spine 756.19
spleen 759.0
sternum 756.3
stomach 750.7
tarsus 755.67
tendon 756.89
testis 752.8
thorax (wall) 756.3
thymus 759.2
thyroid (gland) 759.2
cartilage 748.3
tibia 755.69
toe 755.66
tongue 750.19
trachea (cartilage) 748.3
ulna 755.59
urachus 753.7
ureter 753.4
obstructive 753.29
urethra 753.8
obstructive 753.6
urinary tract 753.8
uterus 752.3
uvula 750.26
vagina 752.49
vascular NEC (*see also* Anomaly, peripheral
vascular system) 747.60
brain 747.81
vas deferens 752.8
vein(s) (peripheral) NEC (*see also* Anomaly,
peripheral vascular system) 747.60
brain 747.81
great 747.49
portal 747.49
pulmonary 747.49
vena cava (inferior) (superior) 747.49
vertebra 756.19
vulva 752.49
spermatic cord 752.9
spine, spinal 756.10
column 756.10
cord 742.9
meningocele (*see also* Spina bifida)
741.9 ✓5th
specified type NEC 742.59
spina bifida (*see also* Spina bifida)
741.9 ✓5th
vessel 747.82
meninges 742.59
nerve root 742.9
spleen 759.0
Sprengel's 755.52
sternum 756.3

Anomaly, anomalous — *continued*
stomach 750.9
specified type NEC 750.7
submaxillary gland 750.9
superior vena cava 747.40
talipes — *see* Talipes
tarsus 755.67
with complete absence of distal elements
755.31
teeth, tooth NEC 520.9
position 524.3
spacing 524.3
tendon 756.9
specified type NEC 756.89
termination
coronary artery 746.85
testis 752.9
thebesian valve 746.9
thigh 755.60
flexion (*see also* Subluxation, congenital,
hip) 754.32
thorax (wall) 756.3
throat 750.9
thumb 755.50
supernumerary 755.01
thymus gland 759.2
thyroid (gland) 759.2
cartilage 748.3
tibia 755.60
saber 090.5
toe 755.66
supernumerary 755.02
webbed (*see also* Syndactylism, toes) 755.13
tongue 750.10
specified type NEC 750.19
trachea, tracheal 748.3
cartilage 748.3
rings 748.3
tragus 744.3
transverse aortic arch 747.21
trichromata 368.59
trichromatopsia 368.59
tricuspid (leaflet) (valve) 746.9
atresia 746.1
Ebstein's 746.2
specified type NEC 746.89
stenosis 746.1
trunk 759.9
Uhl's (hypoplasia of myocardium, right
ventricle) 746.84
ulna 755.50
umbilicus 759.9
artery 747.5
union, trachea with larynx 748.3
unspecified site 759.9
upper extremity 755.50
vessel 747.63
urachus 753.7
specified type NEC 753.7
ureter 753.9
obstructive 753.20
specified type NEC 753.4
obstructive 753.29
urethra (valve) 753.9
obstructive 753.6
specified type NEC 753.8
urinary tract or system (any part, except
urachus) 753.9
specified type NEC 753.8
urachus 753.7
uterus 752.3
with only one functioning horn 752.3
in pregnancy or childbirth 654.0 ✓5th
affecting fetus or newborn 763.89
causing obstructed labor 660.2 ✓5th
affecting fetus or newborn 763.1
uvula 750.9
vagina 752.40
valleculae 748.3
valve (heart) NEC 746.9
formation, ureter 753.29
pulmonary 746.00
specified type NEC 746.89
vascular NEC (*see also* Anomaly, peripheral
vascular system) 747.60
ring 747.21
vas deferens 752.9

Anomaly, anomalous — *continued*
vein(s) (peripheral) NEC (*see also* Anomaly, peripheral vascular system) 747.60
  brain 747.81
  cerebral 747.81
  coronary 746.89
  great 747.40
    specified type NEC 747.49
  portal 747.40
  pulmonary 747.40
  retina 743.9
  vena cava (inferior) (superior) 747.40
  venous return (pulmonary) 747.49
    partial 747.42
    total 747.41
  ventricle, ventricular (heart) 746.9
    bands 746.9
    folds 746.9
    septa 745.4
  vertebra 756.10
  vesicourethral orifice 753.9
  vessels NEC (*see also* Anomaly, peripheral vascular system) 747.60
    optic papilla 743.9
  vitelline duct 751.0
  vitreous humor 743.9
    specified type NEC 743.51
  vulva 752.40
  wrist (joint) 755.50
Anomia 784.69
Anonychia 757.5
  acquired 703.8
Anophthalmos, anophthalmus (clinical) (congenital) (globe) 743.00
  acquired V45.78
Anopsia (altitudinal) (quadrant) 368.46
Anorchia 752.8
Anorchism, anorchidism 752.8
Anorexia 783.0
  hysterical 300.11
  nervosa 307.1
Anosmia (*see also* Disturbance, sensation) 781.1
  hysterical 300.11
  postinfectional 478.9
  psychogenic 306.7
  traumatic 951.8
Anosognosia 780.99 ▲
Anosphrasia 781.1
Anosteoplasia 756.50
Anotia 744.09
Anovulatory cycle 628.0
Anoxemia 799.0
  newborn 768.9 ▲
Anoxia 799.0
  altitude 993.2
  cerebral 348.1
    with
      abortion — *see* Abortion, by type, with specified complication NEC
      ectopic pregnancy (*see also* categories 633.0-633.9) 639.8
      molar pregnancy (*see also* categories 630-632) 639.8
    complicating
      delivery (cesarean) (instrumental) 669.4 ✓5ᵗʰ
      ectopic or molar pregnancy 639.8
      obstetric anesthesia or sedation 668.2 ✓5ᵗʰ
    during or resulting from a procedure 997.01
    following
      abortion 639.8
      ectopic or molar pregnancy 639.8
    newborn (*see also* Distress, fetal, liveborn infant) 768.9
  due to drowning 994.1
  fetal, affecting newborn 768.9 ▲
  heart — *see* Insufficiency, coronary
  high altitude 993.2
  intrauterine
    fetal death (before onset of labor) 768.0
      during labor 768.1
    liveborn infant — *see* Distress, fetal, liveborn infant

Anoxia — *continued*
  myocardial — *see* Insufficiency, coronary
  newborn 768.9
    mild or moderate 768.6
    severe 768.5
  pathological 799.0
Anteflexion — *see* Anteversion
Antenatal
  care, normal pregnancy V22.1
    first V22.0
  screening (for) V28.9
    based on amniocentesis NEC V28.2
      chromosomal anomalies V28.0
      raised alphafetoprotein levels V28.1
    chromosomal anomalies V28.0
    fetal growth retardation using ultrasonics V28.4
    isoimmunization V28.5
    malformations using ultrasonics V28.3
    raised alphafetoprotein levels in amniotic fluid V28.1
    specified condition NEC V28.8
    Streptococcus B V28.6
Antepartum — *see* condition
Anterior — *see also* condition
  spinal artery compression syndrome 721.1
Antero-occlusion 524.2
Anteversion
  cervix (*see also* Anteversion, uterus) 621.6
  femur (neck), congenital 755.63
  uterus, uterine (cervix) (postinfectional) (postpartal, old) 621.6
    congenital 752.3
    in pregnancy or childbirth 654.4 ✓5ᵗʰ
      affecting fetus or newborn 763.89
      causing obstructed labor 660.2 ✓5ᵗʰ
        affecting fetus or newborn 763.1
Anthracosilicosis (occupational) 500
Anthracosis (lung) (occupational) 500
  lingua 529.3
Anthrax 022.9
  with pneumonia 022.1 [484.5]
  colitis 022.2
  cutaneous 022.0
  gastrointestinal 022.2
  intestinal 022.2
  pulmonary 022.1
  respiratory 022.1
  septicemia 022.3
  specified manifestation NEC 022.8
Anthropoid pelvis 755.69
  with disproportion (fetopelvic) 653.2 ✓5ᵗʰ
    affecting fetus or newborn 763.1
    causing obstructed labor 660.1 ✓5ᵗʰ
      affecting fetus or newborn 763.1
Anthropophobia 300.29
Antibioma, breast 611.0
Antibodies
  maternal (blood group) (*see also* Incompatibility) 656.2 ✓5ᵗʰ
    anti-D, cord blood 656.1 ✓5ᵗʰ
      fetus or newborn 773.0
Antibody deficiency syndrome
  agammaglobulinemic 279.00
  congenital 279.04
  hypogammaglobulinemic 279.00
Anticoagulant, circulating (*see also* Circulating anticoagulants) 286.5
Antimongolism syndrome 758.3
Antimonial cholera 985.4
Antisocial personality 301.7
Antithrombinemia (*see also* Circulating anticoagulants) 286.5
Antithromboplastinemia (*see also* Circulating anticoagulants) 286.5
Antithromboplastinogenemia (*see also* Circulating anticoagulants) 286.5
Antitoxin complication or reaction — *see* Complications, vaccination
Anton (-Babinski) syndrome (hemiasomatognosia) 307.9
Antritis (chronic) 473.0
  acute 461.0

Antrum, antral — *see* condition
Anuria 788.5
  with
    abortion — *see* Abortion, by type, with renal failure
    ectopic pregnancy (*see also* categories 633.0-633.9) 639.3
    molar pregnancy (*see also* categories 630-632) 639.3
  calculus (impacted) (recurrent) 592.9
    kidney 592.0
    ureter 592.1
  congenital 753.3
  due to a procedure 997.5
  following
    abortion 639.3
    ectopic or molar pregnancy 639.3
  newborn 753.3
  postrenal 593.4
  puerperal, postpartum, childbirth 669.3 ✓5ᵗʰ
  specified as due to a procedure 997.5
  sulfonamide
    correct substance properly administered 788.5
    overdose or wrong substance given or taken 961.0
  traumatic (following crushing) 958.5
Anus, anal — *see* condition
Anusitis 569.49
Anxiety (neurosis) (reaction) (state) 300.00
  alcohol-induced 291.89
  depression 300.4
  drug-induced 292.89
  due to or associated with physical condition 293.84
  generalized 300.02
  hysteria 300.20
  in
    acute stress reaction 308.0
    transient adjustment reaction 309.24
  panic type 300.01
  separation, abnormal 309.21
  syndrome (organic) (transient) 293.84
Aorta, aortic — *see* condition
Aortectasia 441.9
Aortitis (nonsyphilitic) 447.6
  arteriosclerotic 440.0
  calcific 447.6
  Döhle-Heller 093.1
  luetic 093.1
  rheumatic (*see also* Endocarditis, acute, rheumatic) 391.1
  rheumatoid — *see* Arthritis, rheumatoid
  specific 093.1
  syphilitic 093.1
    congenital 090.5
Apethetic thyroid storm (*see also* Thyrotoxicosis) 242.9 ✓5ᵗʰ
Apepsia 536.8
  achlorhydric 536.0
  psychogenic 306.4
Aperistalsis, esophagus 530.0
Apert's syndrome (acrocephalosyndactyly) 755.55
Apert-Gallais syndrome (adrenogenital) 255.2
Apertognathia 524.2
Aphagia 787.2
  psychogenic 307.1
Aphakia (acquired) (bilateral) (postoperative) (unilateral) 379.31
  congenital 743.35
Aphalangia (congenital) 755.4
  lower limb (complete) (intercalary) (partial) (terminal) 755.39
    meaning all digits (complete) (partial) 755.31
    transverse 755.31
  upper limb (complete) (intercalary) (partial) (terminal) 755.29
    meaning all digits (complete) (partial) 755.21
    transverse 755.21

Aphasia (amnestic) (ataxic) (auditory) (Broca's)
(choreatic) (classic) (expressive) (global)
(ideational) (ideokinetic) (ideomotor) (jargon)
(motor) (nominal) (receptive) (semantic)
(sensory) (syntactic) (verbal) (visual)
(Wernicke's) 784.3
  developmental 315.31
  syphilis, tertiary 094.89
  uremic — *see* Uremia

Aphemia 784.3
  uremic — *see* Uremia

Aphonia 784.41
  clericorum 784.49
  hysterical 300.11
  organic 784.41
  psychogenic 306.1

Aphthae, aphthous — *see also* condition
  Bednar's 528.2
  cachectic 529.0
  epizootic 078.4
  fever 078.4
  oral 528.2
  stomatitis 528.2
  thrush 112.0
  ulcer (oral) (recurrent) 528.2
    genital organ(s) NEC
      female 629.8
      male 608.89
    larynx 478.79

Apical — *see* condition

Aplasia — *see also* Agenesis
  alveolar process (acquired) 525.8
    congenital 750.26
  aorta (congenital) 747.22
  aortic valve (congenital) 746.89
  axialis extracorticalis (congenital) 330.0
  bone marrow (myeloid) 284.9
    acquired (secondary) 284.8
    congenital 284.0
    idiopathic 284.9
  brain 740.0
    specified part 742.2
  breast 757.6
  bronchus 748.3
  cementum 520.4
  cerebellar 742.2
  congenital pure red cell 284.0
  corpus callosum 742.2
  erythrocyte 284.8
    congenital 284.0
  extracortical axial 330.0
  eye (congenital) 743.00
  fovea centralis (congenital) 743.55
  germinal (cell) 606.0
  iris 743.45
  labyrinth, membranous 744.05
  limb (congenital) 755.4
    lower NEC 755.30
    upper NEC 755.20
  lung (bilateral) (congenital) (unilateral) 748.5
  nervous system NEC 742.8
  nuclear 742.8
  ovary 752.0
  Pelizaeus-Merzbacher 330.0
  prostate (congenital) 752.8
  red cell (pure) (with thymoma) 284.8
    acquired (secondary) 284.8
    congenital 284.0
    hereditary 284.0
    of infants 284.0
    primary 284.0
  round ligament (congenital) 752.8
  salivary gland 750.21
  skin (congenital) 757.39
  spinal cord 742.59
  spleen 759.0
  testis (congenital) 752.8
  thymic, with immunodeficiency 279.2
  thyroid 243
  uterus 752.3
  ventral horn cell 742.59

Apleuria 756.3

Apnea, apneic (spells) 786.03
  newborn, neonatorum 770.81 ▲
    essential 770.81 ●

Apnea, apneic — *continued*
  newborn, neonatorum — *continued*
    obstructive 770.82 ●
    primary 770.81 ●
    sleep 770.81 ●
    specified NEC 770.82 ●
  psychogenic 306.1
  sleep NEC 780.57
    with
      hypersomnia 780.53
      hyposomnia 780.51
      insomnia 780.51
      sleep disturbance NEC 780.57

Apneumatosis newborn 770.4

Apodia 755.31

Apophysitis (bone) (*see also* Osteochondrosis)
732.9
  calcaneus 732.5
  juvenile 732.6

Apoplectiform convulsions (*see also* Disease,
cerebrovascular, acute) 436

Apoplexia, apoplexy, apoplectic (*see also*
Disease, cerebrovascular, acute) 436
  abdominal 569.89
  adrenal 036.3
  attack 436
  basilar (*see also* Disease, cerebrovascular,
acute) 436
  brain (*see also* Disease, cerebrovascular, acute)
436
  bulbar (*see also* Disease, cerebrovascular,
acute) 436
  capillary (*see also* Disease, cerebrovascular,
acute) 436
  cardiac (*see also* Infarct, myocardium)
410.9 ✓5ᵗʰ
  cerebral (*see also* Disease, cerebrovascular
acute) 436
  chorea (*see also* Disease, cerebrovascular,
acute) 436
  congestive (*see also* Disease, cerebrovascular,
acute) 436
    newborn 767.4
  embolic (*see also* Embolism, brain) 434.1 ✓5ᵗʰ
  fetus 767.0
  fit (*see also* Disease, cerebrovascular, acute)
436
  healed or old V12.59
  heart (auricle) (ventricle) (*see also* Infarct,
myocardium) 410.9 ✓5ᵗʰ
  heat 992.0
  hemiplegia (*see also* Disease, cerebrovascular,
acute) 436
  hemorrhagic (stroke) (*see also* Hemorrhage,
brain) 432.9
  ingravescent (*see also* Disease, cerebrovascular,
acute) 436
  late effect — *see* Late effect(s) (of)
cerebrovascular disease
  lung — *see* Embolism, pulmonary
  meninges, hemorrhagic (*see also* Hemorrhage,
subarachnoid) 430
  neonatorum 767.0
  newborn 767.0
  pancreatitis 577.0
  placenta 641.2 ✓5ᵗʰ
  progressive (*see also* Disease, cerebrovascular,
acute) 436
  pulmonary (artery) (vein) — *see* Embolism,
pulmonary
  sanguineous (*see also* Disease,
cerebrovascular, acute) 436
  seizure (*see also* Disease, cerebrovascular,
acute) 436
  serous (*see also* Disease, cerebrovascular,
acute) 436
  spleen 289.59
  stroke (*see also* Disease, cerebrovascular,
acute) 436
  thrombotic (*see also* Thrombosis, brain)
434.0 ✓5ᵗʰ
  uremic — *see* Uremia
  uteroplacental 641.2 ✓5ᵗʰ

Appendage
  fallopian tube (cyst of Morgagni) 752.11
  intestine (epiploic) 751.5

Appendage — *continued*
  preauricular 744.1
  testicular (organ of Morgagni) 752.8

Appendicitis 541
  with
    perforation, peritonitis (generalized), or
rupture 540.0
      with peritoneal abscess 540.1
    peritoneal abscess 540.1
  acute (catarrhal) (fulminating) (gangrenous)
(inflammatory) (obstructive) (retrocecal)
(suppurative) 540.9
    with
      perforation, peritonitis, or rupture 540.0
        with peritoneal abscess 540.1
      peritoneal abscess 540.1
  amebic 006.8
  chronic (recurrent) 542
  exacerbation — *see* Appendicitis, acute
  fulminating — *see* Appendicitis, acute
  gangrenous — *see* Appendicitis, acute
  healed (obliterative) 542
  interval 542
  neurogenic 542
  obstructive 542
  pneumococcal 541
  recurrent 542
  relapsing 542
  retrocecal 541
  subacute (adhesive) 542
  subsiding 542
  suppurative — *see* Appendicitis, acute
  tuberculous (*see also* Tuberculosis) 014.8 ✓5ᵗʰ

Appendiclausis 543.9

Appendicolithiasis 543.9

Appendicopathia oxyurica 127.4

Appendix, appendicular — *see also* condition
  Morgagni (male) 752.8
    fallopian tube 752.11

Appetite
  depraved 307.52
  excessive 783.6
    psychogenic 307.51
  lack or loss (*see also* Anorexia) 783.0
    nonorganic origin 307.59
  perverted 307.52
    hysterical 300.11

Apprehension, apprehensiveness (abnormal)
(state) 300.00
  specified type NEC 300.09

Approximal wear 521.1

Apraxia (classic) (ideational) (ideokinetic)
(ideomotor) (motor) 784.69
  oculomotor, congenital 379.51
  verbal 784.69

Aptyalism 527.7

Aqueous misdirection 365.83 ●

Arabicum elephantiasis (*see also* Infestation,
filarial) 125.9

Arachnidism 989.5

Arachnitis — *see* Meningitis

Arachnodactyly 759.82

Arachnoidism 989.5

Arachnoiditis (acute) (adhesive) (basic) (brain)
(cerebrospinal) (chiasmal) (chronic) (spinal)
(*see also* Meningitis) 322.9
  meningococcal (chronic) 036.0
  syphilitic 094.2
  tuberculous (*see also* Tuberculosis meninges)
013.0 ✓5ᵗʰ

Araneism 989.5

Arboencephalitis, Australian 062.4

Arborization block (heart) 426.6

Arbor virus, arbovirus (infection) NEC 066.9

ARC 042

Arches — *see* condition

Arcuatus uterus 752.3

Arcus (cornea)
  juvenilis 743.43
    interfering with vision 743.42
  senilis 371.41

Arc-welders' lung 503

✓4ᵗʰ Fourth-digit Required   ✓5ᵗʰ Fifth-digit Required   ▶◀ Revised Text   ● New Line   ▲ Revised Code

Arc-welders' syndrome (photokeratitis) 370.24
Areflexia 796.1
Areola — *see* condition
Argentaffinoma (M8241/1) — *see also* Neoplasm, by site, uncertain behavior
  benign (M8241/0) — *see* Neoplasm, by site, benign
  malignant (M8241/3) — *see* Neoplasm, by site, malignant
  syndrome 259.2
Argentinian hemorrhagic fever 078.7
Arginosuccinicaciduria 270.6
Argonz-Del Castillo syndrome (nonpuerperal galactorrhea and amenorrhea) 253.1
Argyll-Robertson phenomenon, pupil, or syndrome (syphilitic) 094.89
  atypical 379.45
  nonluetic 379.45
  nonsyphilitic 379.45
  reversed 379.45
Argyria, argyriasis NEC 985.8
  conjunctiva 372.55
  cornea 371.16
  from drug or medicinal agent
    correct substance properly administered 709.09
    overdose or wrong substance given or taken 961.2
Arhinencephaly 742.2
Arias-Stella phenomenon 621.3
Ariboflavinosis 266.0
Arizona enteritis 008.1
Arm — *see* condition
Armenian disease 277.3
Arnold-Chiari obstruction or syndrome (*see also* Spina bifida) 741.0 ☑5ᵗʰ
  type I 348.4
  type II (*see also* Spina bifida) 741.0 ☑5ᵗʰ
  type III 742.0
  type IV 742.2
Arrest, arrested
  active phase of labor 661.1 ☑5ᵗʰ
    affecting fetus or newborn 763.7
  any plane in pelvis
    complicating delivery 660.1 ☑5ᵗʰ
      affecting fetus or newborn 763.1
  bone marrow (*see also* Anemia, aplastic) 284.9
  cardiac 427.5
    with
      abortion — *see* Abortion, by type, with specified complication NEC
      ectopic pregnancy (*see also* categories 633.0-633.9) 639.8
      molar pregnancy (*see also* categories 630-632) 639.8
    complicating
      anesthesia
        correct substance properly administered 427.5
        obstetric 668.1 ☑5ᵗʰ
        overdose or wrong substance given 968.4
          specified anesthetic — *see* Table of Drugs and Chemicals
      delivery (cesarean) (instrumental) 669.4 ☑5ᵗʰ
      ectopic or molar pregnancy 639.8
      surgery (nontherapeutic) (therapeutic) 997.1
    fetus or newborn 779.89 ▲
    following
      abortion 639.8
      ectopic or molar pregnancy 639.8
    postoperative (immediate) 997.1
      long-term effect of cardiac surgery 429.4
  cardiorespiratory (*see also* Arrest, cardiac) 427.5
  deep transverse 660.3 ☑5ᵗʰ
    affecting fetus or newborn 763.1
  development or growth
    bone 733.91
    child 783.40

Arrest, arrested — *continued*
  development or growth — *continued*
    fetus 764.9 ☑5ᵗʰ
      affecting management of pregnancy 656.5 ☑5ᵗʰ
    tracheal rings 748.3
    epiphyseal 733.91
    granulopoiesis 288.0
    heart — *see* Arrest, cardiac
    respiratory 799.1
      newborn 770.89 ▲
    sinus 426.6
    transverse (deep) 660.3 ☑5ᵗʰ
      affecting fetus or newborn 763.1
Arrhenoblastoma (M8630/1)
  benign (M8630/0)
    specified site — *see* Neoplasm, by site, benign
    unspecified site
      female 220
      male 222.0
  malignant (M8630/3)
    specified site — *see* Neoplasm, by site, malignant
    unspecified site
      female 183.0
      male 186.9
  specified site — *see* Neoplasm, by site, uncertain behavior
  unspecified site
    female 236.2
    male 236.4
Arrhinencephaly 742.2
  due to
    trisomy 13 (13-15) 758.1
    trisomy 18 (16-18) 758.2
Arrhythmia (auricle) (cardiac) (cordis) (gallop rhythm) (juvenile) (nodal) (reflex) (sinus) (supraventricular) (transitory) (ventricle) 427.9
  bigeminal rhythm 427.89
  block 426.9
  bradycardia 427.89
  contractions, premature 427.60
  coronary sinus 427.89
  ectopic 427.89
  extrasystolic 427.60
  postoperative 997.1
  psychogenic 306.2
  vagal 780.2
Arrillaga-Ayerza syndrome (pulmonary artery sclerosis with pulmonary hypertension) 416.0
Arsenical
  dermatitis 692.4
  keratosis 692.4
  pigmentation 985.1
    from drug or medicinal agent
      correct substance properly administered 709.09
      overdose or wrong substance given or taken 961.1
Arsenism 985.1
  from drug or medicinal agent
    correct substance properly administered 692.4
    overdose or wrong substance given or taken 961.1
Arterial — *see* condition
Arteriectasis 447.8
Arteriofibrosis — *see* Arteriosclerosis
Arteriolar sclerosis — *see* Arteriosclerosis
Arteriolith — *see* Arteriosclerosis
Arteriolitis 447.6
  necrotizing, kidney 447.5
  renal — *see* Hypertension, kidney
Arteriolosclerosis — *see* Arteriosclerosis
Arterionephrosclerosis (*see also* Hypertension, kidney) 403.90
Arteriopathy 447.9
Arteriosclerosis, arteriosclerotic (artery) (deformans) (diffuse) (disease) (endarteritis) (general) (obliterans) (obliterative) (occlusive) (senile) (with calcification) 440.9

Arteriosclerosis, arteriosclerotic — *continued*
  with
    gangrene 440.24
    psychosis (*see also* Psychosis, arteriosclerotic) 290.40
    ulceration 440.23
  aorta 440.0
  arteries of extremities — *see* Arteriosclerosis, extremities
  basilar (artery) (*see also* Occlusion, artery, basilar) 433.0 ☑5ᵗʰ
  brain 437.0
  bypass graft
    coronary artery 414.05
      autologous artery (gastroepiploic) (internal mammary) 414.04
      autologous vein 414.02
      nonautologous biological 414.03
    extremity 440.30
      autologous vein 440.31
      nonautologous biological 440.32
  cardiac — *see* Arteriosclerosis, coronary
  cardiopathy — *see* Arteriosclerosis, coronary
  cardiorenal (*see also* Hypertension, cardiorenal) 404.90
  cardiovascular (*see also* Disease, cardiovascular) 429.2
  carotid (artery) (common) (internal) (*see also* Occlusion, artery, carotid) 433.1 ☑5ᵗʰ
  central nervous system 437.0
  cerebral 437.0
    late effect — *see* Late effect(s) (of) cerebrovascular disease
  cerebrospinal 437.0
  cerebrovascular 437.0
  coronary (artery) 414.00
    graft — *see* Arteriosclerosis, bypass graft
    native artery 414.01
    of transplanted heart 414.06 ●
  extremities (native artery) NEC 440.20
    bypass graft 440.30
      autologous vein 440.31
      nonautologous biological 440.32
    claudication (intermittent) 440.21
      and
        gangrene 440.24
        rest pain 440.22
          and
            gangrene 440.24
            ulceration 440.23
              and gangrene 440.24
          ulceration 440.23
            and gangrene 440.24
      gangrene 440.24
      rest pain 440.22
        and
          gangrene 440.24
          ulceration 440.23
            and gangrene 440.24
    specified site NEC 440.29
    ulceration 440.23
      and gangrene 440.24
  heart (disease) — *see also* Arteriosclerosis, coronary
    valve 424.99
      aortic 424.1
      mitral 424.0
      pulmonary 424.3
      tricuspid 424.2
  kidney (*see also* Hypertension, kidney) 403.90
  labyrinth, labyrinthine 388.00
  medial NEC 440.20
  mesentery (artery) 557.1
  Mönckeberg's 440.20
  myocarditis 429.0
  nephrosclerosis (*see also* Hypertension, kidney) 403.90
  peripheral (of extremities) — *see* Arteriosclerosis, extremities
  precerebral 433.9 ☑5ᵗʰ
    specified artery NEC 433.8 ☑5ᵗʰ
  pulmonary (idiopathic) 416.0
  renal (*see also* Hypertension, kidney) 403.90
    arterioles (*see also* Hypertension, kidney) 403.90
    artery 440.1
  retinal (vascular) 440.8 *[362.13]*

Arteriosclerosis, arteriosclerotic — *continued*
  specified artery NEC 440.8
    with gangrene 440.8 *[785.4]*
  spinal (cord) 437.0
  vertebral (artery) (*see also* Occlusion, artery,
      vertebral) 433.2 ✓5ᵗʰ

Arteriospasm 443.9

Arteriovenous — *see* condition

Arteritis 447.6
  allergic (*see also* Angiitis, hypersensitivity)
      446.20
  aorta (nonsyphilitic) 447.6
    syphilitic 093.1
  aortic arch 446.7
  brachiocephalica 446.7
  brain 437.4
    syphilitic 094.89
  branchial 446.7
  cerebral 437.4
    late effect — *see* Late effect(s) (of)
        cerebrovascular disease
    syphilitic 094.89
  coronary (artery) — *see also* Arteriosclerosis,
      coronary
    rheumatic 391.9
      chronic 398.99
    syphilitic 093.89
  cranial (left) (right) 446.5
  deformans — *see* Arteriosclerosis
  giant cell 446.5
  necrosing or necrotizing 446.0
  nodosa 446.0
  obliterans — *see also* Arteriosclerosis
    subclaviocarotica 446.7
  pulmonary 417.8
  retina 362.18
  rheumatic — *see* Fever, rheumatic
  senile — *see* Arteriosclerosis
  suppurative 447.2
  syphilitic (general) 093.89
    brain 094.89
    coronary 093.89
    spinal 094.89
  temporal 446.5
  young female, syndrome 446.7

Artery, arterial — *see* condition

Arthralgia (*see also* Pain, joint) 719.4 ✓5ᵗʰ
  allergic (*see also* Pain, joint) 719.4 ✓5ᵗʰ
  in caisson disease 993.3
  psychogenic 307.89
  rubella 056.71
  Salmonella 003.23
  temporomandibular joint 524.62

Arthritis, arthritic (acute) (chronic) (subacute)
    716.9 ✓5ᵗʰ
  meaning Osteoarthritis — *see* Osteoarthrosis

> *Note* — *Use the following fifth-digit*
> *subclassification with categories 711-712,*
> *715-716:*
>
> | | |
> |---|---|
> | *0* | *site unspecified* |
> | *1* | *shoulder region* |
> | *2* | *upper arm* |
> | *3* | *forearm* |
> | *4* | *hand* |
> | *5* | *pelvic region and thigh* |
> | *6* | *lower leg* |
> | *7* | *ankle and foot* |
> | *8* | *other specified sites* |
> | *9* | *multiple sites* |

  allergic 716.2 ✓5ᵗʰ
  ankylosing (crippling) (spine) 720.0
    sites other than spine 716.9 ✓5ᵗʰ
  atrophic 714.0
    spine 720.9
  back (*see also* Arthritis, spine) 721.90
  Bechterew's (ankylosing spondylitis) 720.0
  blennorrhagic 098.50
  cervical, cervicodorsal (*see also* Spondylosis,
      cervical) 721.0
  Charcôt's 094.0 *[713.5]*
    diabetic 250.6 ✓5ᵗʰ *[713.5]*
    syringomyelic 336.0 *[713.5]*

Arthritis, arthritic — *continued*
  Charcôt's — *continued*
    tabetic 094.0 *[713.5]*
  chylous (*see also* Filariasis) 125.9 *[711.7]* ✓5ᵗʰ
  climacteric NEC 716.3 ✓5ᵗʰ
  coccyx 721.8
  cricoarytenoid 478.79
  crystal (-induced) — *see* Arthritis, due to
      crystals
  deformans (*see also* Osteoarthrosis) 715.9 ✓5ᵗʰ
    spine 721.90
      with myelopathy 721.91
  degenerative (*see also* Osteoarthrosis)
      715.9 ✓5ᵗʰ
    idiopathic 715.09
    polyarticular 715.09
    spine 721.90
      with myelopathy 721.91
  dermatoarthritis, lipoid 272.8 *[713.0]*
  due to or associated with
    acromegaly 253.0 *[713.0]*
    actinomycosis 039.8 *[711.4]* ✓5ᵗʰ
    amyloidosis 277.3 *[713.7]*
    bacterial disease NEC 040.89 *[711.4]* ✓5ᵗʰ
    Behçet's syndrome 136.1 *[711.2]* ✓5ᵗʰ
    blastomycosis 116.0 *[711.6]* ✓5ᵗʰ
    brucellosis (*see also* Brucellosis)
        023.9 *[711.4]* ✓5ᵗʰ
    caisson disease 993.3
    coccidioidomycosis 114.3 *[711.6]* ✓5ᵗʰ
    coliform (Escherichia coli) 711.0 ✓5ᵗʰ
    colitis, ulcerative (*see also* Colitis, ulcerative)
        556.9 *[713.1]*
    cowpox 051.0 *[711.5]* ✓5ᵗʰ
    crystals — *see also* Gout
      dicalcium phosphate 275.49 *[712.1]*
      pyrophosphate 275.49 *[712.2]*
      specified NEC 275.49 *[712.8]*
    dermatoarthritis, lipoid 272.8 *[713.0]*
    dermatological disorder NEC 709.9 *[713.3]*
    diabetes 250.6 ✓5ᵗʰ *[713.5]*
    diphtheria 032.89 *[711.4]* ✓5ᵗʰ
    dracontiasis 125.7 *[711.7]* ✓5ᵗʰ
    dysentery 009.0 *[711.3]* ✓5ᵗʰ
    endocrine disorder NEC 259.9 *[713.0]*
    enteritis NEC 009.1 *[711.3]* ✓5ᵗʰ
      infectious (*see also* Enteritis, infectious)
          009.0 *[711.3]* ✓5ᵗʰ
        specified organism NEC 008.8
            [711.3] ✓5ᵗʰ
      regional (*see also* Enteritis, regional)
          555.9 *[713.1]*
      specified organism NEC 008.8 *[711.3]* ✓5ᵗʰ
    epiphyseal slip, nontraumatic (old)
        716.8 ✓5ᵗʰ
    erysipelas 035 *[711.4]* ✓5ᵗʰ
    erythema
      epidemic 026.1
      multiforme 695.1 *[713.3]*
      nodosum 695.2 *[713.3]*
    Escherichia coli 711.0 ✓5ᵗʰ
    filariasis NEC 125.9 *[711.7]* ✓5ᵗʰ
    gastrointestinal condition NEC 569.9 *[713.1]*
    glanders 024 *[711.4]* ✓5ᵗʰ
    Gonococcus 098.50
    gout 274.0
    H. influenzae 711.0 ✓5ᵗʰ
    helminthiasis NEC 128.9 *[711.7]* ✓5ᵗʰ
    hematological disorder NEC 289.9 *[713.2]*
    hemochromatosis 275.0 *[713.0]*
    hemoglobinopathy NEC (*see also* Disease,
        hemoglobin) 282.7 *[713.2]*
    hemophilia (*see also* Hemophilia) 286.0
        [713.2]
    Hemophilus influenzae (H. influenzae)
        711.0 ✓5ᵗʰ
    Henoch (-Schönlein) purpura 287.0 *[713.6]*
    histoplasmosis NEC (*see also*
        Histoplasmosis) 115.99 *[711.6]* ✓5ᵗʰ
    hyperparathyroidism 252.0 *[713.0]*
    hypersensitivity reaction NEC 995.3 *[713.6]*
    hypogammaglobulinemia (*see also*
        Hypogamma-globulinemia) 279.00
        [713.0]
    hypothyroidism NEC 244.9 *[713.0]*
    infection (*see also* Arthritis, infectious)
        711.9 ✓5ᵗʰ

Arthritis, arthritic — *continued*
  due to or associated with — *continued*
    infectious disease NEC 136.9 *[711.8]* ✓5ᵗʰ
    leprosy (*see also* Leprosy) 030.9 *[711.4]* ✓5ᵗʰ
    leukemia NEC (M9800/3) 208.9 ✓5ᵗʰ *[713.2]*
    lipoid dermatoarthritis 272.8 *[713.0]*
    Lyme disease 088.81 *[711.8]* ✓5ᵗʰ
    Mediterranean fever, familial 277.3 *[713.7]*
    meningococcal infection 036.82
    metabolic disorder NEC 277.9 *[713.0]*
    multiple myelomatosis (M9730/3) 203.0 ✓5ᵗʰ
        [713.2]
    mumps 072.79 *[711.5]* ✓5ᵗʰ
    mycobacteria 031.8 *[711.4]* ✓5ᵗʰ
    mycosis NEC 117.9 *[711.6]* ✓5ᵗʰ
    neurological disorder NEC 349.9 *[713.5]*
    ochronosis 270.2 *[713.0]*
    O'Nyong Nyong 066.3 *[711.5]* ✓5ᵗʰ
    parasitic disease NEC 136.9 *[711.8]* ✓5ᵗʰ
    paratyphoid fever (*see also* Fever,
        paratyphoid) 002.9 *[711.3]* ✓5ᵗʰ
    Pneumococcus 711.0 ✓5ᵗʰ
    poliomyelitis (*see also* Poliomyelitis)
        045.9 ✓5ᵗʰ *[711.5]* ✓5ᵗʰ
    Pseudomonas 711.0 ✓5ᵗʰ
    psoriasis 696.0
    pyogenic organism (E. coli) (H. influenzae)
        (Pseudomonas) (Streptococcus)
        711.0 ✓5ᵗʰ
    rat-bite fever 026.1 *[711.4]* ✓5ᵗʰ
    regional enteritis (*see also* Enteritis,
        regional) 555.9 *[713.1]*
    Reiter's disease 099.3 *[711.1]* ✓5ᵗʰ
    respiratory disorder NEC 519.9 *[713.4]*
    reticulosis, malignant (M9720/3) 202.3 ✓5ᵗʰ
        [713.2]
    rubella 056.71
    salmonellosis 003.23
    sarcoidosis 135 *[713.7]*
    serum sickness 999.5 *[713.6]*
    Staphylococcus 711.0 ✓5ᵗʰ
    Streptococcus 711.0 ✓5ᵗʰ
    syphilis (*see also* Syphilis) 094.0 *[711.4]* ✓5ᵗʰ
    syringomyelia 336.0 *[713.5]*
    thalassemia 282.4 *[713.2]*
    tuberculosis (*see also* Tuberculosis,
        arthritis) 015.9 ✓5ᵗʰ *[711.4]* ✓5ᵗʰ
    typhoid fever 002.0 *[711.3]* ✓5ᵗʰ
    ulcerative colitis (*see also* Colitis, ulcerative)
        556.9 *[713.1]*
    urethritis
      nongonococcal (*see also* Urethritis,
          nongonococcal) 099.40 *[711.1]* ✓5ᵗʰ
      nonspecific (*see also* Urethritis,
          nongonococcal) 099.40 *[711.1]* ✓5ᵗʰ
      Reiter's 099.3 *[711.1]* ✓5ᵗʰ
    viral disease NEC 079.99 *[711.5]* ✓5ᵗʰ
  erythema epidemic 026.1
  gonococcal 098.50
  gouty (acute) 274.0
  hypertrophic (*see also* Osteoarthrosis)
      715.9 ✓5ᵗʰ
    spine 721.90
      with myelopathy 721.91
  idiopathic, blennorrheal 099.3
  in caisson disease 993.3 *[713.8]*
  infectious or infective (acute) (chronic)
      (subacute) NEC 711.9 ✓5ᵗʰ
    nonpyogenic 711.9 ✓5ᵗʰ
    spine 720.9
  inflammatory NEC 714.9
  juvenile rheumatoid (chronic) (polyarticular)
      714.30
    acute 714.31
    monoarticular 714.33
    pauciarticular 714.32
  lumbar (*see also* Spondylosis, lumbar) 721.3
  meningococcal 036.82
  menopausal NEC 716.3 ✓5ᵗʰ
  migratory — *see* Fever, rheumatic
  neuropathic (Charcôt's) 094.0 *[713.5]*
    diabetic 250.6 ✓5ᵗʰ *[713.5]*
    nonsyphilitic NEC 349.9 *[713.5]*
    syringomyelic 336.0 *[713.5]*
    tabetic 094.0 *[713.5]*
  nodosa (*see also* Osteoarthrosis) 715.9 ✓5ᵗʰ
    spine 721.90
      with myelopathy 721.91

Arthritis, arthritic — *continued*
  nonpyogenic NEC 716.9 ✓5ᵗʰ
    spine 721.90
      with myelopathy 721.91
  ochronotic 270.2 *[713.0]*
  palindromic (see also Rheumatism,
      palindromic) 719.3 ✓5ᵗʰ
  pneumococcal 711.0 ✓5ᵗʰ
  postdysenteric 009.0 *[711.3]* ✓5ᵗʰ
  postrheumatic, chronic (Jaccoud's) 714.4
  primary progressive 714.0
    spine 720.9
  proliferative 714.0
    spine 720.0
  psoriatic 696.0
  purulent 711.0 ✓5ᵗʰ
  pyogenic or pyemic 711.0 ✓5ᵗʰ
  rheumatic 714.0
    acute or subacute — see Fever, rheumatic
    chronic 714.0
    spine 720.9
  rheumatoid (nodular) 714.0
    with
      splenoadenomegaly and leukopenia 714.1
      visceral or systemic involvement 714.2
    aortitis 714.89
    carditis 714.2
    heart disease 714.2
    juvenile (chronic) (polyarticular) 714.30
      acute 714.31
      monoarticular 714.33
      pauciarticular 714.32
    spine 720.0
  rubella 056.71
  sacral, sacroiliac, sacrococcygeal (see also
      Spondylosis, sacral) 721.3
  scorbutic 267
  senile or senescent (see also Osteoarthrosis)
      715.9 ✓5ᵗʰ
    spine 721.90
      with myelopathy 721.91
  septic 711.0 ✓5ᵗʰ
  serum (nontherapeutic) (therapeutic) 999.5
      [713.6]
  specified form NEC 716.8 ✓5ᵗʰ
  spine 721.90
    with myelopathy 721.91
    atrophic 720.9
    degenerative 721.90
      with myelopathy 721.91
    hypertrophic (with deformity) 721.90
      with myelopathy 721.91
    infectious or infective NEC 720.9
    Marie-Strümpell 720.0
    nonpyogenic 721.90
      with myelopathy 721.91
    pyogenic 720.9
    rheumatoid 720.0
    traumatic (old) 721.7
    tuberculous (see also Tuberculosis)
        015.0 ✓5ᵗʰ *[720.81]*
  staphylococcal 711.0 ✓5ᵗʰ
  streptococcal 711.0 ✓5ᵗʰ
  suppurative 711.0 ✓5ᵗʰ
  syphilitic 094.0 *[713.5]*
    congenital 090.49 *[713.5]*
  syphilitica deformans (Charcôt) 094.0 *[713.5]*
  temporomandibular joint 524.69
  thoracic (see also Spondylosis, thoracic) 721.2
  toxic of menopause 716.3 ✓5ᵗʰ
  transient 716.4 ✓5ᵗʰ
  traumatic (chronic) (old) (post) 716.1 ✓5ᵗʰ
    current injury — see nature of injury
  tuberculous (see also Tuberculosis, arthritis)
      015.9 ✓5ᵗʰ *[711.4]* ✓5ᵗʰ
  urethritica 099.3 *[711.1]* ✓5ᵗʰ
  urica, uratic 274.0
  venereal 099.3 *[711.1]* ✓5ᵗʰ
  vertebral (see also Arthritis, spine) 721.90
  villous 716.8 ✓5ᵗʰ
  von Bechterew's 720.0
Arthrocele (see also Effusion, joint) 719.0 ✓5ᵗʰ
Arthrochondritis — see Arthritis
Arthrodesis status V45.4
Arthrodynia (see also Pain, joint) 719.4 ✓5ᵗʰ
  psychogenic 307.89

Arthrodysplasia 755.9
Arthrofibrosis, joint (see also Ankylosis)
    718.5 ✓5ᵗʰ
Arthrogryposis 728.3
  multiplex, congenita 754.89
Arthrokatadysis 715.35
Arthrolithiasis 274.0
Arthro-onychodysplasia 756.89
Arthro-osteo-onychodysplasia 756.89
Arthropathy (see also Arthritis) 716.9 ✓5ᵗʰ

Note — Use the following fifth-digit
subclassification with categories 711-712,
716:

    0   site unspecified
    1   shoulder region
    2   upper arm
    3   forearm
    4   hand
    5   pelvic region and thigh
    6   lower leg
    7   ankle and foot
    8   other specified sites
    9   multiple sites

  Behçets 136.1 *[711.2]* ✓5ᵗʰ
  Charcôt's 094.0 *[713.5]*
    diabetic 250.6 ✓5ᵗʰ *[713.5]*
    syringomyelic 336.0 *[713.5]*
    tabetic 094.0 *[713.5]*
  crystal (-induced) — see Arthritis, due to
      crystals
  gouty 274.0
  neurogenic, neuropathic (Charcôt's) (tabetic)
      094.0 *[713.5]*
    diabetic 250.6 ✓5ᵗʰ *[713.5]*
    nonsyphilitic NEC 349.9 *[713.5]*
    syringomyelic 336.0 *[713.5]*
  postdysenteric NEC 009.0 *[711.3]* ✓5ᵗʰ
  postrheumatic, chronic (Jaccoud's) 714.4
  psoriatic 696.0
  pulmonary 731.2
  specified NEC 716.8 ✓5ᵗʰ
  syringomyelia 336.0 *[713.5]*
  tabes dorsalis 094.0 *[713.5]*
  tabetic 094.0 *[713.5]*
  transient 716.4 ✓5ᵗʰ
  traumatic 716.1 ✓5ᵗʰ
  uric acid 274.0
Arthophyte (see also Loose, body, joint) 718.1 ✓5ᵗʰ
Arthrophytis 719.80
  ankle 719.87
  elbow 719.82
  foot 719.87
  hand 719.84
  hip 719.85
  knee 719.86
  multiple sites 719.89
  pelvic region 719.85
  shoulder (region) 719.81
  specified site NEC 719.88
  wrist 719.83
Arthropyosis (see also Arthritis, pyogenic)
    711.0 ✓5ᵗʰ
Arthrosis (deformans) (degenerative) (see also
    Osteoarthrosis) 715.9 ✓5ᵗʰ
  Charcôt's 094.0 *[713.5]*
  polyarticular 715.09
  spine (see also Spondylosis) 721.90
Arthus' phenomenon 995.2
  due to
    correct substance properly administered
        995.2
    overdose or wrong substance given or taken
        977.9
      specified drug — see Table of Drugs and
          Chemicals
    serum 999.5
Articular — see also condition
  disc disorder (reducing or non-reducing)
      524.63
  spondylolisthesis 756.12

Artificial
  device (prosthetic) — see Fitting, device
  insemination V26.1
  menopause (states) (symptoms) (syndrome)
      627.4
  opening status (functioning) (without
      complication) V44.9
    anus (colostomy) V44.3
    colostomy V44.3
    cystostomy V44.50
      appendico-vesicostomy V44.52
      cutaneous-vesicostomy V44.51
      specified type NEC V44.59
    enterostomy V44.4
    gastrostomy V44.1
    ileostomy V44.2
    intestinal tract NEC V44.4
    jejunostomy V44.4
    nephrostomy V44.6
    specified site NEC V44.8
    tracheostomy V44.0
    ureterostomy V44.6
    urethrostomy V44.6
    urinary tract NEC V44.6
    vagina V44.7
    vagina status V44.7
ARV (disease) (illness) (infection) — see Human
    immunodeficiency virus (disease) (illness)
    (infection)
Arytenoid — see condition
Asbestosis (occupational) 501
Asboe-Hansen's disease (incontinentia
    pigmenti) 757.33
Ascariasis (intestinal) (lung) 127.0
Ascaridiasis 127.0
Ascaris 127.0
  lumbricoides (infestation) 127.0
  pneumonia 127.0
Ascending — see condition
Aschoff's bodies (see also Myocarditis,
    rheumatic) 398.0
Ascites 789.5
  abdominal NEC 789.5
  cancerous (M80000/6) 197.6
  cardiac 428.0
  chylous (nonfilarial) 457.8
    filarial (see also Infestation, filarial) 125.9
  congenital 778.0
  due to S. japonicum 120.2
  fetal, causing fetopelvic disproportion 653.7 ✓5ᵗʰ
  heart 428.0
  joint (see also Effusion, joint) 719.0 ✓5ᵗʰ
  malignant (M8000/6) 197.6
  pseudochylous 789.5
  syphilitic 095.2
  tuberculous (see also Tuberculosis) 014.0 ✓5ᵗʰ
Ascorbic acid (vitamin C) **deficiency** (scurvy) 267
ASCUS (atypical squamous cell changes of ●
    undetermined significance) ●
  favor benign 795.01 ●
  favor dysplasia 795.02 ●
ASCVD (arteriosclerotic cardiovascular disease)
    429.2
Aseptic — see condition
Asherman's syndrome 621.5
Asialia 527.7
Asiatic cholera (see also Cholera) 001.9
Asocial personality or trends 301.7
Asomatognosia 781.8
Aspergillosis 117.3
  with pneumonia 117.3 *[484.6]*
  allergic bronchopulmonary 518.6
  nonsyphilitic NEC 117.3
Aspergillus (flavus) (fumigatus) (infection)
    (terreus) 117.3
Aspermatogenesis 606.0
Aspermia (testis) 606.0
Asphyxia, asphyxiation (by) 799.0
  antenatal — see Distress, fetal
  bedclothes 994.7
  birth (see also Ashpyxia, newborn) 768.9
  bunny bag 994.7
  carbon monoxide 986

Asphyxia, asphyxiation — *continued*
caul (*see also* Asphyxia, newborn)
cave-in 994.7
 crushing — *see* Injury, internal, intrathoracic organs
constriction 994.7
crushing — *see* Injury, internal, intrathoracic organs
drowning 994.1
fetal, affecting newborn 768.9 ▲
food or foreign body (in larynx) 933.1
 bronchioles 934.8
 bronchus (main) 934.1
 lung 934.8
 nasopharynx 933.0
 nose, nasal passages 932
 pharynx 933.0
 respiratory tract 934.9
  specified part NEC 934.8
 throat 933.0
 trachea 934.0
gas, fumes, or vapor NEC 987.9
 specified — *see* Table of Drugs and Chemicals
gravitational changes 994.7
hanging 994.7
inhalation — *see* Inhalation
intrauterine
 fetal death (before onset of labor) 768.0
  during labor 768.1
 liveborn infant — *see* Distress, fetal, liveborn infant
local 443.0
mechanical 994.7
 during birth (*see also* Distress, fetal) 768.9 ▲
mucus 933.1
 bronchus (main) 934.1
 larynx 933.1
 lung 934.8
 nasal passages 932
 newborn 770.1
 pharynx 933.0
 respiratory tract 934.9
  specfied part NEC 934.8
 throat 933.0
 trachea 934.0
 vaginal (fetus or newborn) 770.1
newborn 768.9
 blue 768.6
 livida 768.6
 mild or moderate 768.6
 pallida 768.5
 severe 768.5
 white 768.5
pathological 799.0
plastic bag 994.7
postnatal (*see also* Asphyxia, newborn) 768.9
 mechanical 994.7
pressure 994.7
reticularis 782.61
strangulation 994.7
submersion 994.1
traumatic NEC — *see* Injury, internal, intrathoracic organs
vomiting, vomitus — *see* Asphyxia, food or foreign body

Aspiration
acid pulmonary (syndrome) 997.3
 obstetric 668.0 ✓5ᵗʰ
amniotic fluid 770.1
bronchitis 507.0
contents of birth canal 770.1
fetal pneumonitis 770.1
food, foreign body, or gasoline (with asphyxiation) — *see* Asphyxia, food or foreign body
meconium 770.1
mucus 933.1
 into
  bronchus (main) 934.1
  lung 934.8
  respiratory tract 934.9
   specified part NEC 934.8
  trachea 934.0
 newborn 770.1
 vaginal (fetus or newborn) 770.1

Aspiration — *continued*
newborn 770.1
pneumonia 507.0
pneumonitis 507.0
 fetus or newborn 770.1
 obstetric 668.0 ✓5ᵗʰ
syndrome of newborn (massive) (meconium) 770.1
vernix caseosa 770.1

Asplenia 759.0
with mesocardia 746.87

Assam fever 085.0

Assimilation, pelvis
with disproportion 653.2 ✓5ᵗʰ
 affecting fetus or newborn 763.1
 causing obstructed labor 660.1 ✓5ᵗʰ
  affecting fetus or newborn 763.1

Assmann's focus (*see also* Tuberculosis) 011.0 ✓5ᵗʰ

Astasia (-asbasia) 307.9
hysterical 300.11

Asteatosis 706.8
cutis 706.8

Astereognosis 780.99 ▲

Asterixis 781.3
in liver disease 572.8

Asteroid hyalitis 379.22

Asthenia, asthenic 780.79
cardiac (*see also* Failure, heart) 428.9
 psychogenic 306.2
cardiovascular (*see also* Failure, heart) 428.9
 psychogenic 306.2
heart (*see also* Failure, heart) 428.9
 psychogenic 306.2
hysterical 300.11
myocardial (*see also* Failure, heart) 428.9
 psychogenic 306.2
nervous 300.5
neurocirculatory 306.2
neurotic 300.5
psychogenic 300.5
psychoneurotic 300.5
psychophysiologic 300.5
reaction, psychoneurotic 300.5
senile 797
Stiller's 780.79
tropical anhidrotic 705.1

Asthenopia 368.13
accommodative 367.4
hysterical (muscular) 300.11
psychogenic 306.7

Asthenospermia 792.2

Asthma, asthmatic (bronchial) (catarrh) (spasmodic) 493.9 ✓5ᵗʰ

> *Note* — *Use the following fifth-digit subclassification with category 493:*
>
> 0   *without mention of status asthmaticus or acute exacerbation or unspecified*
> 1   *with status asthmaticus*
> 2   *with acute exacerbation*

with
 chronic obstructive pulmonary disease (COPD) 493.2 ✓5ᵗʰ
 hay fever 493.0 ✓5ᵗʰ
 rhinitis, allergic 493.0 ✓5ᵗʰ
allergic 493.9 ✓5ᵗʰ
 stated cause (external allergen) 493.0 ✓5ᵗʰ
atopic 493.0 ✓5ᵗʰ
cardiac (*see also* Failure, ventricular, left) 428.1
cardiobronchial (*see also* Failure, ventricular, left) 428.1
cardiorenal (*see also* Hypertension, cardiorenal) 404.90
childhood 493.0 ✓5ᵗʰ
colliers' 500
croup 493.9 ✓5ᵗʰ
detergent 507.8
due to
 detergent 507.8
 inhalation of fumes 506.3
 internal immunological process 493.0 ✓5ᵗʰ
endogenous (intrinsic) 493.1 ✓5ᵗʰ

Asthma, asthmatic — *continued*
eosinophilic 518.3
exogenous (cosmetics) (dander or dust) (drugs) (dust) (feathers) (food) (hay) (platinum) (pollen) 493.0 ✓5ᵗʰ
extrinsic 493.0 ✓5ᵗʰ
grinders' 502
hay 493.0 ✓5ᵗʰ
heart (*see also* Failure, ventricular, left) 428.1
IgE 493.0 ✓5ᵗʰ
infective 493.1 ✓5ᵗʰ
intrinsic 493.1 ✓5ᵗʰ
Kopp's 254.8
late-onset 493.1 ✓5ᵗʰ
meat-wrappers' 506.9
Millar's (laryngismus stridulus) 478.75
millstone makers' 502
miners' 500
Monday morning 504
New Orleans (epidemic) 493.0 ✓5ᵗʰ
platinum 493.0 ✓5ᵗʰ
pneumoconiotic (occupational) NEC 505
potters' 502
psychogenic 316 [493.9] ✓5ᵗʰ
pulmonary eosinophilic 518.3
red cedar 495.8
Rostan's (*see also* Failure, ventricular, left) 428.1
sandblasters' 502
sequoiosis 495.8
stonemasons' 502
thymic 254.8
tuberculous (*see also* Tuberculosis, pulmonary) 011.9 ✓5ᵗʰ
Wichmann's (laryngismus stridulus) 478.75
wood 495.8

Astigmatism (compound) (congenital) 367.20
irregular 367.22
regular 367.21

Astroblastoma (M9430/3)
nose 748.1
specified site — *see* Neoplasm, by site, malignant
unspecified site 191.9

Astrocytoma (cystic) (M9400/3)
anaplastic type (M9401/3)
 specified site — *see* Neoplasm, by site, malignant
 unspecified site 191.9
fibrillary (M9420/3)
 specified site — *see* Neoplasm, by site, malignant
 unspecified site 191.9
fibrous (M9420/3)
 specified site — *see* Neoplasm, by site, malignant
 unspecified site 191.9
gemistocytic (M9411/3)
 specified site — *see* Neoplasm, by site, malignant
 unspecified site 191.9
juvenile (M9421/3)
 specified site — *see* Neoplasm, by site, malignant
 unspecified site 191.9
nose 748.1
pilocytic (M9421/3)
 specified site — *see* Neoplasm, by site, malignant
 unspecified site 191.9
piloid (M9421/3)
 specified site — *see* Neoplasm, by site, malignant
 unspecified site 191.9
protoplasmic (M9410/3)
 specified site — *see* Neoplasm, by site, malignant
 unspecified site 191.9
specified site — *see* Neoplasm, by site, malignant
subependymal (M9383/1) 237.5
 giant cell (M9384/1) 237.5
unspecified site 191.9

Astroglioma (M9400/3)
nose 748.1
specified site — *see* Neoplasm, by site, malignant
unspecified site 191.9

Asymbolia — Atresia

Asymbolia 784.60
Asymmetrical breathing 786.09
Asymmetry — *see also* Distortion
   chest 786.9
   face 754.0
   jaw NEC 524.12
      maxillary 524.11
   pelvis with disproportion 653.0 ✓5ᵗʰ
      affecting fetus or newborn 763.1
      causing obstructed labor 660.1 ✓5ᵗʰ
         affecting fetus or newborn 763.1
Asynergia 781.3
Asynergy 781.3
   ventricular 429.89
Asystole (heart) (*see also* Arrest, cardiac) 427.5
Ataxia, ataxy, ataxic 781.3
   acute 781.3
   brain 331.89
   cerebellar 334.3
      hereditary (Marie's) 334.2
      in
         alcoholism 303.9 ✓5ᵗʰ [334.4]
         myxedema (*see also* Myxedema) 244.9
            [334.4]
         neoplastic disease NEC 239.9 [334.4]
   cerebral 331.89
   family, familial 334.2
      cerebral (Marie's) 334.2
      spinal (Friedreich's) 334.0
   Friedreich's (heredofamilial) (spinal) 334.0
   frontal lobe 781.3
   gait 781.2
      hysterical 300.11
   general 781.3
   hereditary NEC 334.2
      cerebellar 334.2
      spastic 334.1
      spinal 334.0
   heredofamilial (Marie's) 334.2
   hysterical 300.11
   locomotor (progressive) 094.0
      diabetic 250.6 ✓5ᵗʰ [337.1]
   Marie's (cerebellar) (heredofamilial) 334.2
   nonorganic origin 307.9
   partial 094.0
   postchickenpox 052.7
   progressive locomotor 094.0
   psychogenic 307.9
   Sanger-Brown's 334.2
   spastic 094.0
      hereditary 334.1
      syphilitic 094.0
   spinal
      hereditary 334.0
      progressive locomotor 094.0
   telangiectasia 334.8
Ataxia-telangiectasia 334.8
Atelectasis (absorption collapse) (complete)
      (compression) (massive) (partial)
      (postinfective) (pressure collapse)
      (pulmonary) (relaxation) 518.0
   newborn (congenital) (partial) 770.5
      primary 770.4
   primary 770.4
   tuberculous (*see also* Tuberculosis, pulmonary)
      011.9 ✓5ᵗʰ
Ateleiosis, ateliosis 253.3
Atelia — *see* Distortion
Ateliosis 253.3
Atelocardia 746.9
Atelomyelia 742.59
Athelia 757.6
Atheroembolism
   extremity
      lower 445.02   ●
      upper 445.01   ●
   kidney 445.81   ●
   specified site NEC 445.89   ●
Atheroma, atheromatous (*see also*
      Arteriosclerosis) 440.9
   aorta, aortic 440.0
      valve (*see also* Endocarditis, aortic) 424.1
   artery — *see* Arteriosclerosis

Atheroma, atheromatous (*see also*
      Arteriosclerosis) — *continued*
   basilar (artery) (*see also* Occlusion, artery,
      basilar) 433.0 ✓5ᵗʰ
   carotid (artery) (common) (internal) (*see also*
      Occlusion, artery, carotid) 433.1 ✓5ᵗʰ
   cerebral (arteries) 437.0
   coronary (artery) — *see* Arteriosclerosis,
      coronary
   degeneration — *see* Arteriosclerosis
   heart, cardiac — *see* Arteriosclerosis, coronary
   mitral (valve) 424.0
   myocardium, myocardial — *see*
      Arteriosclerosis, coronary
   pulmonary valve (heart) (*see also* Endocarditis,
      pulmonary) 424.3
   skin 706.2
   tricuspid (heart) (valve) 424.2
   valve, valvular — *see* Endocarditis
   vertebral (artery) (*see also* Occlusion, artery,
      vertebral) 433.2 ✓5ᵗʰ
Atheromatosis — *see also* Arteriosclerosis
   arterial, congenital 272.8
Atherosclerosis — *see also* Arteriosclerosis
Athetosis (acquired) 781.0
   bilateral 333.7
   congenital (bilateral) 333.7
   double 333.7
   unilateral 781.0
Athlete's
   foot 110.4
   heart 429.3
Athletic team examination V70.3
Athrepsia 261
Athyrea (acquired) (*see also* Hypothyroidism)
      244.9
   congenital 243
Athyreosis (congenital) 243
   acquired — *see* Hypothyroidism
Athyroidism (acquired) (*see also* Hypothyroidism)
      244.9
   congenital 243
Atmospheric pyrexia 992.0
Atonia, atony, atonic
   abdominal wall 728.2
   bladder (sphincter) 596.4
      neurogenic NEC 596.54
         with cauda equina syndrome 344.61
   capillary 448.9
   cecum 564.89
      psychogenic 306.4
   colon 564.89
      psychogenic 306.4
   congenital 779.89
   dyspepsia 536.3
      psychogenic 306.4
   intestine 564.89
      psychogenic 306.4
   stomach 536.3
      neurotic or psychogenic 306.4
      psychogenic 306.4
   uterus 666.1 ✓5ᵗʰ
      affecting fetus or newborn 763.7
   vesical 596.4
Atopy NEC V15.09
Atransferrinemia, congenital 273.8
Atresia, atretic (congenital) 759.89
   alimentary organ or tract NEC 751.8
      lower 751.2
      upper 750.8
   ani, anus, anal (canal) 751.2
   aorta 747.22
      with hypoplasia of ascending aorta and
         defective development of left ventricle
         (with mitral valve atresia) 746.7
      arch 747.11
      ring 747.21
   aortic (orifice) (valve) 746.89
      arch 747.11
   aqueduct of Sylvius 742.3
      with spina bifida (*see also* Spina bifida)
         741.0 ✓5ᵗʰ
   artery NEC (*see also* Atresia, blood vessel)
      747.60
      cerebral 747.81

Atresia, atretic — *continued*
   artery NEC (*see also* Atresia, blood vessel) —
         continued
      coronary 746.85
      eye 743.58
      pulmonary 747.3
      umbilical 747.5
   auditory canal (external) 744.02
   bile, biliary duct (common) or passage 751.61
      acquired (*see also* Obstruction, biliary)
         576.2
   bladder (neck) 753.6
   blood vessel (peripheral) NEC 747.60
      cerebral 747.81
      gastrointestinal 747.61
      lower limb 747.64
      pulmonary artery 747.3
      renal 747.62
      spinal 747.82
      upper limb 747.63
   bronchus 748.3
   canal, ear 744.02
   cardiac
      valve 746.89
         aortic 746.89
         mitral 746.89
         pulmonary 746.01
         tricuspid 746.1
   cecum 751.2
   cervix (acquired) 622.4
      congenital 752.49
      in pregnancy or childbirth 654.6 ✓5ᵗʰ
         affecting fetus or newborn 763.89
         causing obstructed labor 660.2 ✓5ᵗʰ
            affecting fetus or newborn 763.1
   choana 748.0
   colon 751.2
   cystic duct 751.61
      acquired 575.8
         with obstruction (*see also* Obstruction,
            gallbladder) 575.2
   digestive organs NEC 751.8
   duodenum 751.1
   ear canal 744.02
   ejaculatory duct 752.8
   epiglottis 748.3
   esophagus 750.3
   Eustachian tube 744.24
   fallopian tube (acquired) 628.2
      congenital 752.19
   follicular cyst 620.0
   foramen of
      Luschka 742.3
         with spina bifida (*see also* Spina bifida)
            741.0 ✓5ᵗʰ
      Magendie 742.3
         with spina bifida (*see also* Spina bifida)
            741.0 ✓5ᵗʰ
   gallbladder 751.69
   genital organ
      external
         female 752.49
         male NEC 752.8
            penis 752.69
      internal
         female 752.8
         male 752.8
   glottis 748.3
   gullet 750.3
   heart
      valve NEC 746.89
         aortic 746.89
         mitral 746.89
         pulmonary 746.01
         tricuspid 746.1
   hymen 752.42
      acquired 623.3
      postinfective 623.3
   ileum 751.1
   intestine (small) 751.1
      large 751.2
   iris, filtration angle (*see also* Buphthalmia)
      743.20
   jejunum 751.1
   kidney 753.3
   lacrimal, apparatus 743.65
      acquired — *see* Stenosis, lacrimal

Atresia, atretic — *continued*
  larynx 748.3
  ligament, broad 752.19
  lung 748.5
  meatus urinarius 753.6
  mitral valve 746.89
    with atresia or hypoplasia of aortic orifice or
      valve, with hypoplasia of ascending
      aorta and defective development of left
      ventricle 746.7
  nares (anterior) (posterior) 748.0
  nasolacrimal duct 743.65
  nasopharynx 748.8
  nose, nostril 748.0
    acquired 738.0
  organ or site NEC — *see* Anomaly, specified
    type NEC
  osseous meatus (ear) 744.03
  oviduct (acquired) 628.2
    congenital 752.19
  parotid duct 750.23
    acquired 527.8
  pulmonary (artery) 747.3
    valve 746.01
    vein 747.49
  pulmonic 746.01
  pupil 743.46
  rectum 751.2
  salivary duct or gland 750.23
    acquired 527.8
  sublingual duct 750.23
    acquired 527.8
  submaxillary duct or gland 750.23
    acquired 527.8
  trachea 748.3
  tricuspid valve 746.1
  ureter 753.29
  ureteropelvic junction 753.21
  ureterovesical orifice 753.22
  urethra (valvular) 753.6
  urinary tract NEC 753.29
  uterus 752.3
    acquired 621.8
  vagina (acquired) 623.2
    congenital 752.49
    postgonococcal (old) 098.2
    postinfectional 623.2
    senile 623.2
  vascular NEC (*see also* Atresia, blood vessel)
    747.60
    cerebral 747.81
  vas deferens 752.8
  vein NEC (*see also* Atresia, blood vessel) 747.60
    cardiac 746.89
    great 747.49
    portal 747.49
    pulmonary 747.49
  vena cava (inferior) (superior) 747.49
  vesicourethral orifice 753.6
  vulva 752.49
    acquired 624.8
Atrichia, atrichosis 704.00
  congenital (universal) 757.4
Atrioventricularis commune 745.69
Atrophia — *see also* Atrophy
  alba 709.09
  cutis 701.8
    idiopathica progressiva 701.8
    senilis 701.8
  dermatological, diffuse (idiopathic) 701.8
  flava hepatis (acuta) (subacuta) (*see also*
    Necrosis, liver) 570
  gyrata of choroid and retina (central) 363.54
    generalized 363.57
  senilis 797
    dermatological 701.8
  unguium 703.8
    congenita 757.5
Atrophoderma, atrophodermia 701.9
  diffusum (idiopathic) 701.8
  maculatum 701.3
    et striatum 701.3
      due to syphilis 095.8
    syphilitic 091.3
  neuriticum 701.8
  pigmentosum 757.33
  reticulatum symmetricum faciei 701.8

Atrophoderma, atrophodermia — *continued*
  senile 701.8
  symmetrical 701.8
  vermiculata 701.8
Atrophy, atrophic
  adrenal (autoimmune) (capsule) (cortex) (gland)
    255.4
    with hypofunction 255.4
  alveolar process or ridge (edentulous) 525.2
  appendix 543.9
  Aran-Duchenne muscular 335.21
  arm 728.2
  arteriosclerotic — *see* Arteriosclerosis
  arthritis 714.0
    spine 720.9
  bile duct (any) 576.8
  bladder 596.8
  blanche (of Milian) 701.3
  bone (senile) 733.99
    due to
      disuse 733.7
      infection 733.99
      tabes dorsalis (neurogenic) 094.0
    posttraumatic 733.99
  brain (cortex) (progressive) 331.9
    with dementia 290.10
    Alzheimer's 331.0
      with dementia — *see* Alzheimer's,
        dementia
    circumscribed (Pick's) 331.1
      with dementia
        with behavioral disturbance 331.1
          [294.11]
        without behavioral disturbance 331.1
          [294.10]
    congenital 742.4
    hereditary 331.9
    senile 331.2
  breast 611.4
    puerperal, postpartum 676.3 ✓5ᵗʰ
  buccal cavity 528.9
  cardiac (brown) (senile) (*see also* Degeneration,
    myocardial) 429.1
  cartilage (infectional) (joint) 733.99
  cast, plaster of Paris 728.2
  cerebellar — *see* Atrophy, brain
  cerebral — *see* Atrophy, brain
  cervix (endometrium) (mucosa) (myometrium)
    (senile) (uteri) 622.8
    menopausal 627.8
  Charcôt-Marie-Tooth 356.1
  choroid 363.40
    diffuse secondary 363.42
    hereditary (*see also* Dystrophy, choroid)
      363.50
      gyrate
        central 363.54
        diffuse 363.57
        generalized 363.57
    senile 363.41
  ciliary body 364.57
  colloid, degenerative 701.3
  conjunctiva (senile) 372.89
  corpus cavernosum 607.89
  cortical (*see also* Atrophy, brain) 331.9
  Cruveilhier's 335.21
  cystic duct 576.8
  dacryosialadenopathy 710.2
  degenerative
    colloid 701.3
    senile 701.3
  Déjérine-Thomas 333.0
  diffuse idiopathic, dermatological 701.8
  disuse
    bone 733.7
    muscle 728.2
  Duchenne-Aran 335.21
  ear 388.9
  edentulous alveolar ridge 525.2
  emphysema, lung 492.8
  endometrium (senile) 621.8
    cervix 622.8
  enteric 569.89
  epididymis 608.3
  eyeball, cause unknown 360.41
  eyelid (senile) 374.50
  facial (skin) 701.9

Atrophy, atrophic — *continued*
  facioscapulohumeral (Landouzy-Déjérine) 359.1
  fallopian tube (senile), acquired 620.3
  fatty, thymus (gland) 254.8
  gallbladder 575.8
  gastric 537.89
  gastritis (chronic) 535.1 ✓5ᵗʰ
  gastrointestinal 569.89
  genital organ, male 608.89
  glandular 289.3
  globe (phthisis bulbi) 360.41
  gum 523.2
  hair 704.2
  heart (brown) (senile) (*see also* Degeneration,
    myocardial) 429.1
  hemifacial 754.0
    Romberg 349.89
  hydronephrosis 591
  infantile 261
    paralysis, acute (*see also* Poliomyelits, with
      paralysis) 045.1 ✓5ᵗʰ
  intestine 569.89
  iris (generalized) (postinfectional) (sector
    shaped) 364.59
    essential 364.51
    progressive 364.51
    sphincter 364.54
  kidney (senile) (*see also* Sclerosis, renal) 587
    with hypertension (*see also* Hypertension,
      kidney) 403.90
    congenital 753.0
    hydronephrotic 591
    infantile 753.0
  lacrimal apparatus (primary) 375.13
    secondary 375.14
  Landouzy-Déjérine 359.1
  laryngitis, infection 476.0
  larynx 478.79
  Leber's optic 377.16
  lip 528.5
  liver (acute) (subacute) (*see also* Necrosis, liver)
    570
    chronic (yellow) 571.8
    yellow (congenital) 570
      with
        abortion — *see* Abortion, by type, with
          specified complication NEC
        ectopic pregnancy (*see also* categories
          633.0-633.9) 639.8
        molar pregnancy (*see also* categories
          630-632) 639.8
      chronic 571.8
      complicating pregnancy 646.7 ✓5ᵗʰ
      following
        abortion 639.8
        ectopic or molar pregnancy 639.8
      from injection, inoculation or transfusion
        (onset within 8 months after
        administration) — *see* Hepatitis,
        viral
      healed 571.5
      obstetric 646.7 ✓5ᵗʰ
      postabortal 639.8
      postimmunization — *see* Hepatitis, viral
      posttransfusion — *see* Hepatitis, viral
      puerperal, postpartum 674.8 ✓5ᵗʰ
  lung (senile) 518.89
    congenital 748.69
  macular (dermatological) 701.3
    syphilitic, skin 091.3
      striated 095.8
  muscle, muscular 728.2
    disuse 728.2
    Duchenne-Aran 335.21
    extremity (lower) (upper) 728.2
    familial spinal 335.11
    general 728.2
    idiopathic 728.2
    infantile spinal 335.0
    myelopathic (progressive) 335.10
    myotonic 359.2
    neuritic 356.1
    neuropathic (peroneal) (progressive) 356.1
    peroneal 356.1
    primary (idiopathic) 728.2
    progressive (familial) (hereditary) (pure)
      335.21

Atrophy — Audible tinnitus

Atrophy, atrophic — *continued*
  muscle, muscular — *continued*
    progressive — *continued*
      adult (spinal) 335.19
      infantile (spinal) 335.0
      juvenile (spinal) 335.11
      spinal 335.10
        adult 335.19
        Aran-Duchenne 335.10
        hereditary or familial 335.11
        infantile 335.0
      pseudohypertrophic 359.1
      spinal (progressive) 335.10
        adult 335.19
        Aran-Duchenne 335.21
        familial 335.11
        hereditary 335.11
        infantile 335.0
        juvenile 335.11
      syphilitic 095.6
  myocardium (*see also* Degeneration, myocardial) 429.1
  myometrium (senile) 621.8
    cervix 622.8
  myotatic 728.2
  myotonia 359.2
  nail 703.8
    congenital 757.5·
  nasopharynx 472.2
  nerve — *see also* Disorder, nerve
    abducens 378.54
    accessory 352.4
    acoustic or auditory 388.5
    cranial 352.9
      first (olfactory) 352.0
      second (optic) (*see also* Atrophy, optic nerve) 377.10
      third (oculomotor)(partial) 378.51
        total 378.52
      fourth (trochlear) 378.53
      fifth (trigeminal) 350.8
      sixth (abducens) 378.54
      seventh (facial) 351.8
      eighth (auditory) 388.5
      ninth (glossopharyngeal) 352.2
      tenth (pneumogastric) (vagus) 352.3
      eleventh (accessory) 352.4
      twelfth (hypoglossal) 352.5
    facial 351.8
    glossopharyngeal 352.2
    hypoglossal 352.5
    oculomotor (partial) 378.51
    total 378.52
    olfactory 352.0
    peripheral 355.9
    pneumogastric 352.3
    trigeminal 350.8
    trochlear 378.53
    vagus (pneumogastric) 352.3
  nervous system, congenital 742.8
  neuritic (*see also* Disorder, nerve) 355.9
  neurogenic NEC 355.9
    bone
      tabetic 094.0
  nutritional 261
  old age 797
  olivopontocerebellar 333.0
  optic nerve (ascending) (descending) (infectional) (nonfamilial) (papillomacular bundle) (postretinal) (secondary NEC) (simple) 377.10
    associated with retinal dystrophy 377.13
    dominant hereditary 377.16
    glaucomatous 377.14
    hereditary (dominant) (Leber's) 377.16
    Leber's (hereditary) 377.16
    partial 377.15
    postinflammatory 377.12
    primary 377.11
    syphilitic 094.84
      congenital 090.49
      tabes dorsalis 094.0
  orbit 376.45
  ovary (senile), acquired 620.3
  oviduct (senile), acquired 620.3
  palsy, diffuse 335.20
  pancreas (duct) (senile) 577.8

Atrophy, atrophic — *continued*
  papillary muscle 429.81
  paralysis 355.9
  parotid gland 527.0
  patches skin 701.3
    senile 701.8
  penis 607.89
  pharyngitis 472.1
  pharynx 478.29
  pluriglandular 258.8
  polyarthritis 714.0
  prostate 602.2
  pseudohypertrophic 359.1
  renal (*see also* Sclerosis, renal) 587
  reticulata 701.8
  retina (*see also* Degeneration, retina) 362.60
    hereditary (*see also* Dystrophy, retina) 362.70
  rhinitis 472.0
  salivary duct or gland 527.0
  scar NEC 709.2
  sclerosis, lobar (of brain) 331.0
    with dementia
      with behavioral disturbance 331.1
        [294.11]
      without behavioral disturbance 331.1
        [294.10]
  scrotum 608.89
  seminal vesicle 608.89
  senile 797
    degenerative, of skin 701.3
  skin (patches) (senile) 701.8
  spermatic cord 608.89
  spinal (cord) 336.8
    acute 336.8
    muscular (chronic) 335.10
      adult 335.19
      familial 335.11
      juvenile 335.10
    paralysis 335.10
      acute (*see also* Poliomyelitis, with paralysis) 045.1
  spine (column) 733.99
  spleen (senile) 289.59
  spots (skin) 701.3
    senile 701.8
  stomach 537.89
  striate and macular 701.3
    syphilitic 095.8
  subcutaneous 701.9
    due to injection 999.9
  sublingual gland 527.0
  submaxillary gland 527.0
  Sudeck's 733.7
  suprarenal (autoimmune) (capsule) (gland) 255.4
    with hypofunction 255.4
  tarso-orbital fascia, congenital 743.66
  testis 608.3
  thenar, partial 354.0
  throat 478.29
  thymus (fat) 254.8
  thyroid (gland) 246.8
    with
      cretinism 243
      myxedema 244.9
    congenital 243
  tongue (senile) 529.8
    papillae 529.4
    smooth 529.4
  trachea 519.1
  tunica vaginalis 608.89
  turbinate 733.99
  tympanic membrane (nonflaccid) 384.82
    flaccid 384.81
  ulcer (*see also* Ulcer, skin) 707.9
  upper respiratory tract 478.9
  uterus, uterine (acquired) (senile) 621.8
    cervix 622.8
    due to radiation (intended effect) 621.8
  vagina (senile) 627.3
  vascular 459.89
  vas deferens 608.89
  vertebra (senile) 733.99
  vulva (primary) (senile) 624.1
  Werdnig-Hoffmann 335.0

Atrophy, atrophic — *continued*
  yellow (acute) (congenital) (liver) (subacute) (*see also* Necrosis, liver) 570
    chronic 571.8
    resulting from administration of blood, plasma, serum, or other biological substance (within 8 months of administration) — *see* Hepatitis, viral

Attack
  akinetic (*see also* Epilepsy) 345.0 ✓5ᵗʰ
  angina — *see* Angina
  apoplectic (*see also* Disease, cerebrovascular, acute) 436
  benign shuddering 333.93
  bilious — *see* Vomiting
  cataleptic 300.11
  cerebral (*see also* Disease, cerebrovascular, acute) 436
  coronary (*see also* Infarct, myocardium) 410.9 ✓5ᵗʰ
  cyanotic, newborn 770.83 ▲
  epileptic (*see also* Epilepsy) 345.9 ✓5ᵗʰ
  epileptiform 780.39
  heart (*see also* Infarct, myocardium) 410.9 ✓5ᵗʰ
  hemiplegia (*see also* Disease, cerebrovascular, acute) 436
  hysterical 300.11
  jacksonian (*see also* Epilepsy) 345.5 ✓5ᵗʰ
  myocardium, myocardial (*see also* Infarct, myocardium) 410.9 ✓5ᵗʰ
  myoclonic (*see also* Epilepsy) 345.1 ✓5ᵗʰ
  panic 300.01
  paralysis (*see also* Disease, cerebrovascular, acute) 436
  paroxysmal 780.39
  psychomotor (*see also* Epilepsy) 345.4 ✓5ᵗʰ
  salaam (*see also* Epilepsy) 345.6 ✓5ᵗʰ
  schizophreniform (*see also* Schizophrenia) 295.4 ✓5ᵗʰ
  sensory and motor 780.39
  syncope 780.2
  toxic, cerebral 780.39
  transient ischemic (TIA) 435.9
  unconsciousness 780.2
    hysterical 300.11
  vasomotor 780.2
  vasovagal (idiopathic) (paroxysmal) 780.2

Attention to
  artificial opening (of) V55.9
    digestive tract NEC V55.4
    specified site NEC V55.8
    urinary tract NEC V55.6
    vagina V55.7
  colostomy V55.3
  cystostomy V55.5
  gastrostomy V55.1
  ileostomy V55.2
  jejunostomy V55.4
  nephrostomy V55.6
  surgical dressings V58.3
  sutures V58.3
  tracheostomy V55.0
  ureterostomy V55.6
  urethrostomy V55.6

Attrition
  gum 523.2
  teeth (excessive) (hard tissues) 521.1

Atypical — *see also* condition
  distribution, vessel (congenital) (peripheral) NEC 747.60
  endometrium 621.9
  glandular cell changes of undetermined significance ●
    favor benign (AGCUS favor benign) 795.01 ●
    favor dysplasia (AGCUS favor dysplasia) 795.02 ●
  kidney 593.89
  squamous cell changes of undetermined significance ●
    favor benign (ASCUS favor benign) 795.01 ●
    favor dysplasia (ASCUS favor dysplasia) 795.02 ●

Atypism, cervix 622.1

Audible tinnitus (*see also* Tinnitus) 388.30

✓4ᵗʰ Fourth-digit Required   ✓5ᵗʰ Fifth-digit Required   ▶◀ Revised Text   ● New Line   ▲ Revised Code

Auditory — *see* condition

Audry's syndrome (acropachyderma) 757.39

Aujeszky's disease 078.89

Aura, jacksonian (*see also* Epilepsy) 345.5 ✓5ᵗʰ

Aurantiasis, cutis 278.3

Auricle, auricular — *see* condition

Auriculotemporal syndrome 350.8

Australian
Q fever 083.0
X disease 062.4

Autism, autistic (child) (infantile) 299.0 ✓5ᵗʰ

Autodigestion 799.8

Autoerythrocyte sensitization 287.2

Autographism 708.3

Autoimmune
cold sensitivity 283.0
disease NEC 279.4
hemolytic anemia 283.0
thyroiditis 245.2

Autoinfection, septic — *see* Septicemia

Autointoxication 799.8

Automatism 348.8
epileptic (*see also* Epilepsy) 345.4 ✓5ᵗʰ
paroxysmal, idiopathic (*see also* Epilepsy)
345.4 ✓5ᵗʰ

Autonomic, autonomous
bladder 596.54
neurogenic NEC 596.54
with cauda equina 344.61
dysreflexia 337.3
faciocephalalgia (*see also* Neuropathy,
peripheral, autonomic) 337.9
hysterical seizure 300.11
imbalance (*see also* Neuropathy, peripheral,
autonomic) 337.9

Autophony 388.40

Autosensitivity, erythrocyte 287.2

Autotopagnosia 780.99

Autotoxemia 799.8

Autumn — *see* condition

Avellis' syndrome 344.89

Aviators
disease or sickness (*see also* Effect, adverse,
high altitude) 993.2
ear 993.0
effort syndrome 306.2

Avitaminosis (multiple NEC) (*see also* Deficiency,
vitamin) 269.2
A 264.9
B 266.9
with
beriberi 265.0
pellagra 265.2
B₁ 265.1
B₂ 266.0
B₆ 266.1
B₁₂ 266.2
C (with scurvy) 267
D 268.9
with
osteomalacia 268.2
rickets 268.0
E 269.1
G 266.0
H 269.1
K 269.0
multiple 269.2
nicotinic acid 265.2
P 269.1

Avulsion (traumatic) 879.8
blood vessel — *see* Injury, blood vessel, by site
cartilage — *see also* Dislocation, by site
knee, current (*see also* Tear, meniscus)
836.2
symphyseal (inner), complicating delivery
665.6 ✓5ᵗʰ
complicated 879.9
diaphragm — *see* Injury, internal, diaphragm
ear — *see* Wound, open, ear
epiphysis of bone — *see* Fracture, by site
external site other than limb — *see* Wound,
open, by site
eye 871.3

Avulsion — *continued*
fingernail — *see* Wound, open, finger
fracture — *see* Fracture, by site
genital organs, external — *see* Wound, open,
genital organs
head (intracranial) NEC — *see also* Injury,
intracranial, with open intracranial
wound
complete 874.9
external site NEC 873.8
complicated 873.9
internal organ or site — *see* Injury, internal, by
site
joint — *see also* Dislocation, by site
capsule — *see* Sprain, by site
ligament — *see* Sprain, by site
limb — *see also* Amputation, traumatic, by site
skin and subcutaneous tissue — *see*
Wound, open, by site
muscle — *see* Sprain, by site
nerve (root) — *see* Injury, nerve, by site
scalp — *see* Wound, open, scalp
skin and subcutaneous tissue — *see* Wound,
open, by site
symphyseal cartilage (inner), complicating
delivery 665.6 ✓5ᵗʰ
tendon — *see also* Sprain, by site
with open wound — *see* Wound, open, by
site
toenail — *see* Wound, open, toe(s)
tooth 873.63
complicated 873.73

Awareness of heart beat 785.1

Axe grinders' disease 502

Axenfeld's anomaly or syndrome 743.44

Axilla, axillary — *see also* condition
breast 757.6

Axonotmesis — *see* Injury, nerve, by site

Ayala's disease 756.89

Ayerza's disease or syndrome (pulmonary artery
sclerosis with pulmonary hypertension)
416.0

Azoospermia 606.0

Azotemia 790.6
meaning uremia (*see also* Uremia) 586

Aztec ear 744.29

Azorean disease (of the nervous system) 334.8

Azygos lobe, lung (fissure) 748.69

B

Baader's syndrome (erythema multiforme
exudativum) 695.1

Baastrup's syndrome 721.5

Babesiasis 088.82

Babesiosis 088.82

Babington's disease (familial hemorrhagic
telangiectasia) 448.0

Babinski's syndrome (cardiovascular syphilis)
093.89

Babinski-Fröhlich syndrome (adiposogenital
dystrophy) 253.8

Babinski-Nageotte syndrome 344.89

Bacillary — *see* condition

Bacilluria 791.9
asymptomatic, in pregnancy or puerperium
646.5 ✓5ᵗʰ
tuberculous (*see also* Tuberculosis) 016.9 ✓5ᵗʰ

Bacillus — *see also* Infection, bacillus
abortus infection 023.1
anthracis infection 022.9
coli
infection 041.4
generalized 038.42
intestinal 008.00
pyemia 038.42
septicemia 038.42
Flexner's 004.1
fusiformis infestation 101
mallei infection 024
Shiga's 004.0
suipestifer infection (*see also* Infection,
Salmonella) 003.9

Back — *see* condition

Backache (postural) 724.5
psychogenic 307.89
sacroiliac 724.6

Backflow (pyelovenous) (*see also* Disease, renal)
593.9

Backknee (*see also* Genu, recurvatum) 736.5

Bacteremia 790.7
with
sepsis — *see* Septicemia
during
labor 659.3 ✓5ᵗʰ
pregnancy 647.8 ✓5ᵗʰ
newborn 771.83 ▲

Bacteria
in blood (*see also* Bacteremia) 790.7
in urine (*see also* Bacteriuria) 599.0

Bacterial — *see* condition

Bactericholia (*see also* Cholecystitis, acute) 575.0

Bacterid, bacteride (Andrews' pustular) 686.8

Bacteriuria, bacteruria 791.9
with
urinary tract infection 599.0
asymptomatic 791.9
in pregnancy or puerperium 646.5 ✓5ᵗʰ
affecting fetus or newborn 760.1

Bad
breath 784.9
heart — *see* Disease, heart
trip (*see also* Abuse, drugs, nondependent)
305.3 ✓5ᵗʰ

Baehr-Schiffrin disease (thrombotic
thrombocytopenic purpura) 446.6

Baelz's disease (cheilitis glandularis
apostematosa) 528.5

Baerensprung's disease (eczema marginatum)
110.3

Bagassosis (occupational) 495.1

Baghdad boil 085.1

Bagratuni's syndrome (temporal arteritis) 446.5

Baker's
cyst (knee) 727.51
tuberculous (*see also* Tuberculosis)
015.2 ✓5ᵗʰ
itch 692.82

Bakwin-Krida syndrome (craniometaphyseal
dysplasia) 756.89

Balanitis (circinata) (gangraenosa) (infectious)
(vulgaris) 607.1
amebic 006.8
candidal 112.2
chlamydial 099.53
due to Ducrey's bacillus 099.0
erosiva circinata et gangraenosa 607.1
gangrenous 607.1
gonococcal (acute) 098.0
chronic or duration of 2 months or over
098.2
nongonococcal 607.1
phagedenic 607.1
venereal NEC 099.8
xerotica obliterans 607.81

Balanoposthitis 607.1
chlamydial 099.53
gonococcal (acute) 098.0
chronic or duration of 2 months or over
098.2
ulcerative NEC 099.8

Balanorrhagia — *see* Balanitis

Balantidiasis 007.0

Balantidiosis 007.0

Balbuties, balbutio 307.0

Bald
patches on scalp 704.00
tongue 529.4

Baldness (*see also* Alopecia) 704.00

Balfour's disease (chloroma) 205.3 ✓5ᵗʰ

Balint's syndrome (psychic paralysis of visual
fixation) 368.16

Balkan grippe 083.0

Auditory — Balkan grippe

Ball
food 938
hair 938
Ballantyne (-Runge) syndrome (postmaturity)
766.2
Balloon disease (*see also* Effect, adverse, high
altitude) 993.2
Ballooning posterior leaflet syndrome 424.0
Baló's disease or concentric sclerosis 341.1
Bamberger's disease (hypertrophic pulmonary
osteoarthropathy) 731.2
Bamberger-Marie disease (hypertrophic
pulmonary osteoarthropathy) 731.2
Bamboo spine 720.0
Bancroft's filariasis 125.0
Band(s)
adhesive (*see also* Adhesions, peritoneum)
568.0
amniotic 658.8 ✓5ᵗʰ
affecting fetus or newborn 762.8
anomalous or congenital — *see also* Anomaly,
specified type NEC
atrial 746.9
heart 746.9
intestine 751.4
omentum 751.4
ventricular 746.9
cervix 622.3
gallbladder (congenital) 751.69
intestinal (adhesive) (*see also* Adhesions,
peritoneum) 568.0
congenital 751.4
obstructive (*see also* Obstruction, intestine)
560.81
periappendiceal (congenital) 751.4
peritoneal (adhesive) (*see also* Adhesions,
peritoneum) 568.0
with intestinal obstruction 560.81
congenital 751.4
uterus 621.5
vagina 623.2
Bandl's ring (contraction)
complicating delivery 661.4 ✓5ᵗʰ
affecting fetus or newborn 763.7
Bang's disease (Brucella abortus) 023.1
Bangkok hemorrhagic fever 065.4
Bannister's disease 995.1
Bantam-Albright-Martin disease
(pseudohypoparathyroidism) 275.49
Banti's disease or syndrome (with cirrhosis)
(with portal hypertension) — *see* Cirrhosis,
liver
Bar
calcaneocuboid 755.67
calcaneonavicular 755.67
cubonavicular 755.67
prostate 600.9
talocalcaneal 755.67
Baragnosis 780.99   ▲
Barasheh, barashek 266.2
Barcoo disease or rot (*see also* Ulcer, skin) 707.9
Bard-Pic syndrome (carcinoma, head of pancreas)
157.0
Bärensprung's disease (eczema marginatum)
110.3
Baritosis 503
Barium lung disease 503
Barlow's syndrome (meaning mitral valve
prolapse) 424.0
Barlow (-Möller) disease or syndrome (meaning
infantile scurvy) 267
Barodontalgia 993.2
Baron Münchausen syndrome 301.51
Barosinusitis 993.1
Barotitis 993.0
Barotrauma 993.2
odontalgia 993.2
otitic 993.0
sinus 993.1
Barraquer's disease or syndrome (progressive
lipodystrophy) 272.6

Barré-Guillain syndrome 357.0
Barré-Liéou syndrome (posterior cervical
sympathetic) 723.2
Barrel chest 738.3
Barrett's syndrome or ulcer (chronic peptic ulcer
of esophagus) 530.2
Bársony-Polgár syndrome (corkscrew esophagus)
530.5
Bársony-Teschendorf syndrome (corkscrew
esophagus) 530.5
Bartholin's
adenitis (*see also* Bartholinitis) 616.8
gland — *see* condition
Bartholinitis (suppurating) 616.8
gonococcal (acute) 098.0
chronic or duration of 2 months or over
098.2
Bartonellosis 088.0
Bartter's syndrome (secondary
hyperaldosteronism with juxtaglomerular
hyperplasia) 255.1
Basal — *see* condition
Basan's (hidrotic) ectodermal dysplasia 757.31
Baseball finger 842.13
Basedow's disease or syndrome (exophthalmic
goiter) 242.0 ✓5ᵗʰ
Basic — *see* condition
Basilar — *see* condition
Bason's (hidrotic) ectodermal dysplasia 757.31
Basopenia 288.0
Basophilia 288.8
Basophilism (corticoadrenal) (Cushing's)
(pituitary) (thymic) 255.0
Bassen-Kornzweig syndrome
(abetalipoproteinemia) 272.5
Bat ear 744.29
Bateman's
disease 078.0
purpura (senile) 287.2
Bathing cramp 994.1
Bathophobia 300.23
Batten's disease, retina 330.1 *[362.71]*
Batten-Mayou disease 330.1 *[362.71]*
Batten-Steinert syndrome 359.2
Battered
adult (syndrome) 995.81
baby or child (syndrome) 995.54
spouse (syndrome) 995.81
Battey mycobacterium infection 031.0
Battledore placenta — *see* Placenta, abnormal
Battle exhaustion (*see also* Reaction, stress,
acute) 308.9
**Baumgarten-Cruveilhier (cirrhosis) disease, or
syndrome** 571.5
Bauxite
fibrosis (of lung) 503
workers' disease 503
Bayle's disease (dementia paralytica) 094.1
Bazin's disease (primary) (*see also* Tuberculosis)
017.1 ✓5ᵗʰ
Beach ear 380.12
Beaded hair (congenital) 757.4
Beard's disease (neurasthenia) 300.5
Bearn-Kunkel (-Slater) syndrome (lupoid
hepatitis) 571.49
Beat
elbow 727.2
hand 727.2
knee 727.2
Beats
ectopic 427.60
escaped, heart 427.60
postoperative 997.1
premature (nodal) 427.60
atrial 427.61
auricular 427.61
postoperative 997.1
specified type NEC 427.69

Beats — *continued*
premature (nodal) — *continued*
supraventricular 427.61
ventricular 427.69
Beau's
disease or syndrome (*see also* Degeneration,
myocardial) 429.1
lines (transverse furrows on fingernails) 703.8
Bechterew's disease (ankylosing spondylitis)
720.0
Bechterew-Strümpell-Marie syndrome
(ankylosing spondylitis) 720.0
Beck's syndrome (anterior spinal artery
occlusion) 433.8 ✓5ᵗʰ
Becker's
disease (idiopathic mural endomyocardial
disease) 425.2
dystrophy 359.1
Beckwith (-Wiedemann) syndrome 759.89
Bedclothes, asphyxiation or suffocation by
994.7
Bednar's aphthae 528.2
Bedsore 707.0
with gangrene 707.0 *[785.4]*
Bedwetting (*see also* Enuresis) 788.36
Beer-drinkers' heart (disease) 425.5
Bee sting (with allergic or anaphylactic shock)
989.5
Begbie's disease (exophthalmic goiter) 242.0 ✓5ᵗʰ
Behavior disorder, disturbance — *see also*
Disturbance, conduct
antisocial, without manifest psychiatric
disorder
adolescent V71.02
adult V71.01
child V71.02
dyssocial, without manifest psychiatric disorder
adolescent V71.02
adult V71.01
child V71.02
high risk — *see* Problem
Behçet's syndrome 136.1
Behr's disease 362.50
Beigel's disease or morbus (white piedra) 111.2
Bejel 104.0
Bekhterev's disease (ankylosing spondylitis)
720.0
Bekhterev-Strümpell-Marie syndrome
(ankylosing spondylitis) 720.0
Belching (*see also* Eructation) 787.3
Bell's
disease (*see also* Psychosis, affective) 296.0 ✓5ᵗʰ
mania (*see also* Psychosis, affective) 296.0 ✓5ᵗʰ
palsy, paralysis 351.0
infant 767.5
newborn 767.5
syphilitic 094.89
spasm 351.0
**Bence-Jones albuminuria, albuminosuria, or
proteinuria** 791.0
Bends 993.3
Benedikt's syndrome (paralysis) 344.89
Benign — *see also* condition
cellular changes, cervix 795.09   ●
prostate
hyperplasia 600.0
neoplasm 222.2
Bennett's
disease (leukemia) 208.9 ✓5ᵗʰ
fracture (closed) 815.01
open 815.11
Benson's disease 379.22
Bent
back (hysterical) 300.11
nose 738.0
congenital 754.0
Bereavement V62.82
as adjustment reaction 309.0
Berger's paresthesia (lower limb) 782.0
Bergeron's disease (hysteroepilepsy) 300.11

✓4ᵗʰ Fourth-digit Required   ✓5ᵗʰ Fifth-digit Required   ▶◀ Revised Text   ● New Line   ▲ Revised Code

Beriberi (acute) (atrophic) (chronic) (dry) (subacute) (wet) 265.0
  with polyneuropathy 265.0 *[357.4]*
    heart (disease) 265.0 *[425.7]*
    leprosy 030.1
    neuritis 265.0 *[357.4]*
Berlin's disease or edema (traumatic) 921.3
Berloque dermatitis 692.72
Bernard-Horner syndrome (*see also* Neuropathy, peripheral, autonomic) 337.9
Bernard-Sergent syndrome (acute adrenocortical insufficiency) 255.4
Bernard-Soulier disease or thrombopathy 287.1
Bernhardt's disease or paresthesia 355.1
Bernhardt-Roth disease or syndrome (paresthesia) 355.1
Bernheim's syndrome (*see also* Failure, heart) 428.0
Bertielliasis 123.8
Bertolotti's syndrome (sacralization of fifth lumbar vertebra) 756.15
Berylliosis (acute) (chronic) (lung) (occupational) 503
Besnier's
  lupus pernio 135
  prurigo (atopic dermatitis) (infantile eczema) 691.8
Besnier-Boeck disease or sarcoid 135
Besnier-Boeck-Schaumann disease (sarcoidosis) 135
Best's disease 362.76
Bestiality 302.1
Beta-adrenergic hyperdynamic circulatory state 429.82
Beta-aminoisobutyric aciduria 277.2
Beta-mercaptolactate-cysteine disulfiduria 270.0
Beta thalassemia (major) (minor) (mixed) 282.4
Beurmann's disease (sporotrichosis) 117.1
Bezoar 938
  intestine 936
  stomach 935.2
Bezold's abscess (*see also* Mastoiditis) 383.01
Bianchi's syndrome (aphasia-apraxia-alexia) 784.69
Bicornuate or bicornis uterus 752.3
  in pregnancy or childbirth 654.0 ✓5th
    with obstructed labor 660.2 ✓5th
      affecting fetus or newborn 763.1
    affecting fetus or newborn 763.89
Bicuspid aortic valve 746.4
Biedl-Bardet syndrome 759.89
Bielschowsky's disease 330.1
Bielschowsky-Jansky
  amaurotic familial idiocy 330.1
  disease 330.1
Biemond's syndrome (obesity, polydactyly, and mental retardation) 759.89
Biermer's anemia or disease (pernicious anemia) 281.0
Biett's disease 695.4
Bifid (congenital) — *see also* Imperfect, closure
  apex, heart 746.89
  clitoris 752.49
  epiglottis 748.3
  kidney 753.3
  nose 748.1
  patella 755.64
  scrotum 752.8
  toe 755.66
  tongue 750.13
  ureter 753.4
  uterus 752.3
  uvula 749.02
    with cleft lip (*see also* Cleft, palate, with cleft lip) 749.20
Biforis uterus (suprasimplex) 752.3
Bifurcation (congenital) — *see also* Imperfect, closure
  gallbladder 751.69
  kidney pelvis 753.3

Bifurcation — *see also* Imperfect, closure — *continued*
  renal pelvis 753.3
  rib 756.3
  tongue 750.13
  trachea 748.3
  ureter 753.4
  urethra 753.8
  uvula 749.02
    with cleft lip (*see also* Cleft, palate, with cleft lip) 749.20
  vertebra 756.19
Bigeminal pulse 427.89
Bigeminy 427.89
Big spleen syndrome 289.4
Bilateral — *see* condition
Bile duct — *see* condition
Bile pigments in urine 791.4
Bilharziasis (*see also* Schistosomiasis) 120.9
  chyluria 120.0
  cutaneous 120.3
  galacturia 120.0
  hematochyluria 120.0
  intestinal 120.1
  lipemia 120.9
  lipuria 120.0
  Oriental 120.2
  piarhemia 120.9
  pulmonary 120.2
  tropical hematuria 120.0
  vesical 120.0
Biliary — *see* condition
Bilious (attack) — *see also* Vomiting
  fever, hemoglobinuric 084.8
Bilirubinuria 791.4
Biliuria 791.4
Billroth's disease
  meningocele (*see also* Spina bifida) 741.9 ✓5th
Bilobate placenta — *see* Placenta, abnormal
Bilocular
  heart 745.7
  stomach 536.8
Bing-Horton syndrome (histamine cephalgia) 346.2 ✓5th
Binswanger's disease or dementia 290.12
Biörck (-Thorson) syndrome (malignant carcinoid) 259.2
Biparta, bipartite — *see also* Imperfect, closure
  carpal scaphoid 755.59
  patella 755.64
  placenta — *see* Placenta, abnormal
  vagina 752.49
Bird
  face 756.0
  fanciers' lung or disease 495.2
Bird's disease (oxaluria) 271.8
Birth
  abnormal fetus or newborn 763.9
  accident, fetus or newborn — *see* Birth, injury
  complications in mother — *see* Delivery, complicated
  compression during NEC 767.9
  defect — *see* Anomaly
  delayed, fetus 763.9
  difficult NEC, affecting fetus or newborn 763.9
  dry, affecting fetus or newborn 761.1
  forced, NEC, affecting fetus or newborn 763.89
  forceps, affecting fetus or newborn 763.2
  hematoma of sternomastoid 767.8
  immature 765.1 ✓5th
    extremely 765.0 ✓5th
  inattention, after or at 995.52
  induced, affecting fetus or newborn 763.89
  infant — *see* Newborn
  injury NEC 767.9
    adrenal gland 767.8
    basal ganglia 767.0
    brachial plexus (paralysis) 767.6
    brain (compression) (pressure) 767.0
    cerebellum 767.0
    cerebral hemorrhage 767.0
    conjunctiva 767.8
    eye 767.8

Birth — *continued*
  injury NEC — *continued*
    fracture
      bone, any except clavicle or spine 767.3
      clavicle 767.2
      femur 767.3
      humerus 767.3
      long bone 767.3
      radius and ulna 767.3
      skeleton NEC 767.3
      skull 767.3
      spine 767.4
      tibia and fibula 767.3
    hematoma 767.8
      liver (subcapsular) 767.8
      mastoid 767.8
      skull 767.1
      sternomastoid 767.8
      testes 767.8
      vulva 767.8
    intracranial (edema) 767.0
    laceration
      brain 767.0
      by scalpel 767.8
      peripheral nerve 767.7
    liver 767.8
    meninges
      brain 767.0
      spinal cord 767.4
    nerves (cranial, peripheral) 767.7
      brachial plexus 767.6
      facial 767.5
    paralysis 767.7
      brachial plexus 767.6
      Erb (-Duchenne) 767.6
      facial nerve 767.5
      Klumpke (-Déjérine) 767.6
      radial nerve 767.6
      spinal (cord) (hemorrhage) (laceration) (rupture) 767.4
    rupture
      intracranial 767.0
      liver 767.8
      spinal cord 767.4
      spleen 767.8
      viscera 767.8
    scalp 767.1
    scalpel wound 767.8
    skeleton NEC 767.3
    specified NEC 767.8
    spinal cord 767.4
    spleen 767.8
    subdural hemorrhage 767.0
    tentorial, tear 767.0
    testes 767.8
    vulva 767.8
  instrumental, NEC, affecting fetus or newborn 763.2
  lack of care, after or at 995.52
  multiple
    affected by maternal complications of pregnancy 761.5
    healthy liveborn — *see* Newborn, multiple
  neglect, after or at 995.52
  newborn — *see* Newborn
  palsy or paralysis NEC 767.7
  precipitate, fetus or newborn 763.6
  premature (infant) 765.1 ✓5th
  prolonged, affecting fetus or newborn 763.9
  retarded, fetus or newborn 763.9
  shock, newborn 779.89   ▲
  strangulation or suffocation
    due to aspiration of amniotic fluid 770.1
    mechanical 767.8
  trauma NEC 767.9
  triplet
    affected by maternal complications of pregnancy 761.5
    healthy liveborn — *see* Newborn, multiple
  twin
    affected by maternal complications of pregnancy 761.5
    healthy liveborn — *see* Newborn, twin
  ventouse, affecting fetus or newborn 763.3
Birthmark 757.32
Bisalbuminemia 273.8

Beriberi — Bisalbuminemia

Biskra button 085.1

Bite(s)
  with intact skin surface — *see* Contusion
  animal — *see* Wound, open, by site
    intact skin surface — *see* Contusion
  centipede 989.5
  chigger 133.8
  fire ant 989.5
  flea — *see* Injury, superficial, by site
  human (open wound) — *see also* Wound, open,
    by site
    intact skin surface — *see* Contusion
  insect
    nonvenomous — *see* Injury, superficial, by
      site
    venomous 989.5
  mad dog (death from) 071
  poisonous 989.5
  red bug 133.8
  reptile 989.5
    nonvenomous — *see* Wound, open, by site
  snake 989.5
    nonvenomous — *see* Wound, open, by site
  spider (venomous) 989.5
    nonvenomous — *see* Injury, superficial, by
      site
  venomous 989.5

Biting
  cheek or lip 528.9
  nail 307.9

Black
  death 020.9
  eye NEC 921.0
  hairy tongue 529.3
  lung disease 500

Blackfan-Diamond anemia or syndrome
  (congenital hypoplastic anemia) 284.0

Blackhead 706.1

Blackout 780.2

Blackwater fever 084.8

Bladder — *see* condition

Blast
  blindness 921.3
  concussion — *see* Blast, injury
  injury 869.0
    with open wound into cavity 869.1
    abdomen or thorax — *see* Injury, internal,
      by site
    brain (*see also* Concussion, brain) 850.9
      with skull fracture — *see* Fracture, skull
    ear (acoustic nerve trauma) 951.5
      with perforation, tympanic membrane —
        see Wound, open, ear, drum
    lung (*see also* Injury, internal, lung) 861.20
    otitic (explosive) 388.11

Blastomycosis, blastomycotic (chronic)
  (cutaneous) (disseminated) (lung)
  (pulmonary) (systemic) 116.0
  Brazilian 116.1
  European 117.5
  keloidal 116.2
  North American 116.0
  primary pulmonary 116.0
  South American 116.1

Bleb(s) 709.8
  emphysematous (bullous) (diffuse) (lung)
    (ruptured) (solitary) 492.0
  filtering, eye (postglaucoma) (status) V45.69
    with complication 997.99
      postcataract extraction (complication)
        997.99
  lung (ruptured) 492.0
    congenital 770.5
  subpleural (emphysematous) 492.0

Bleeder (familial) (hereditary) (*see also* Defect,
  coagulation) 286.9
  nonfamilial 286.9

Bleeding (*see also* Hemorrhage) 459.0
  anal 569.3
  anovulatory 628.0
  atonic, following delivery 666.1 √5ᵗʰ
  capillary 448.9
  due to subinvolution 621.1
    puerperal 666.2 √5ᵗʰ
  ear 388.69

Bleeding (*see also* Hemorrhage) — *continued*
  excessive, associated with menopausal onset
    627.0
  familial (*see also* Defect, coagulation) 286.9
  following intercourse 626.7
  gastrointestinal 578.9
  gums 523.8
  hemorrhoids — *see* Hemorrhoids, bleeding
  intermenstrual
    irregular 626.6
    regular 626.5
  intraoperative 998.11
  irregular NEC 626.4
  menopausal 627.0
  mouth 528.9
  nipple 611.79
  nose 784.7
  ovulation 626.5
  postclimacteric 627.1
  postcoital 626.7
  postmenopausal 627.1
    following induced menopause 627.4
  postoperative 998.11
  preclimacteric 627.0
  puberty 626.3
    excessive, with onset of menstrual periods
      626.3
  rectum, rectal 569.3
  tendencies (*see also* Defect, coagulation) 286.9
  throat 784.8
  umbilical stump 772.3
  umbilicus 789.9
  unrelated to menstrual cycle 626.6
  uterus, uterine 626.9
    climacteric 627.0
    dysfunctional 626.8
    functional 626.8
    unrelated to menstrual cycle 626.6
  vagina, vaginal 623.8
    functional 626.8
  vicarious 625.8

Blennorrhagia, blennorrhagic — *see* Blennorrhea

Blennorrhea (acute) 098.0
  adultorum 098.40
  alveolaris 523.4
  chronic or duration of 2 months or over 098.2
  gonococcal (neonatorum) 098.40
  inclusion (neonatal) (newborn) 771.6
  neonatorum 098.40

Blepharelosis (*see also* Entropion) 374.00

Blepharitis (eyelid) 373.00
  angularis 373.01
  ciliaris 373.00
    with ulcer 373.01
  marginal 373.00
    with ulcer 373.01
  scrofulous (*see also* Tuberculosis) 017.3 √5ᵗʰ
    [373.00]
  squamous 373.02
  ulcerative 373.01

Blepharochalasis 374.34
  congenital 743.62

Blepharoclonus 333.81

Blepharoconjunctivitis (*see also* Conjunctivitis)
  372.20
  angular 372.21
  contact 372.22

Blepharophimosis (eyelid) 374.46
  congenital 743.62

Blepharoplegia 374.89

Blepharoptosis 374.30
  congenital 743.61

Blepharopyorrhea 098.49

Blepharospasm 333.81

Blessig's cyst 362.62

Blighted ovum 631

Blind
  bronchus (congenital) 748.3
  eye — *see also* Blindness
    hypertensive 360.42
    hypotensive 360.41
  loop syndrome (postoperative) 579.2
  sac, fallopian tube (congenital) 752.19
  spot, enlarged 368.42
  tract or tube (congenital) NEC — *see* Atresia

Blindness (acquired) (congenital) (both eyes)
  369.00
  blast 921.3
    with nerve injury — *see* Injury, nerve, optic
  Bright's — *see* Uremia
  color (congenital) 368.59
    acquired 368.55
    blue 368.53
    green 368.52
    red 368.51
    total 368.54
  concussion 950.9
  cortical 377.75
  day 368.10 ▲
    acquired 368.10 ▲
    congenital 368.10 ▲
    hereditary 368.10 ▲
    specified type NEC 368.10 ▲
  due to
    injury NEC 950.9
    refractive error — *see* Error, refractive
  eclipse (total) 363.31
  emotional 300.11
  hysterical 300.11
  legal (both eyes) (USA definition) 369.4
    with impairment of better (less impaired) eye
      near-total 369.02
      with
        lesser eye impairment 369.02
          near-total 369.04
          total 369.03
      profound 369.05
      with
        lesser eye impairment 369.05
          near-total 369.07
          profound 369.08
          total 369.06
      severe 369.21
      with
        lesser eye impairment 369.21
          blind 369.11
          near-total 369.13
          profound 369.14
          severe 369.22
          total 369.12
    total
      with lesser eye impairment
        total 369.01
  mind 784.69
  moderate
    both eyes 369.25
      with impairment of lesser eye (specified
        as)
        blind, not further specified 369.15
        low vision, not further specified 369.23
        near-total 369.17
        profound 369.18
        severe 369.24
        total 369.16
    one eye 369.74
      with vision of other eye (specified as)
        near-normal 369.75
        normal 369.76
  near-total
    both eyes 369.04
      with impairment of lesser eye (specified
        as)
        blind, not further specified 369.02
        total 369.03
    one eye 369.64
      with vision of other eye (specified as)
        near-normal 369.65
        normal 369.66
  night 368.60
    acquired 368.62
    congenital (Japanese) 368.61
    hereditary 368.61
    specified type NEC 368.69
    vitamin A deficiency 264.5
  nocturnal — *see* Blindness, night
  one eye 369.60
    with low vision of other eye 369.10
  profound
    both eyes 369.08
      with impairment of lesser eye (specified
        as)
      blind, not further specified 369.05

Blindness — *continued*
  profound — *continued*
    both eyes — *continued*
      with impairment of lesser eye (specified as) — *continued*
        near-total 369.07
        total 369.06
    one eye 369.67
      with vision of other eye (specified as)
        near-normal 369.68
        normal 369.69
  psychic 784.69
  severe
    both eyes 369.22
      with impairment of lesser eye (specified as)
        blind, not further specified 369.11
        low vision, not further specified 369.21
        near-total 369.13
        profound 369.14
        total 369.12
    one eye 369.71
      with vision of other eye (specified as)
        near-normal 369.72
        normal 369.73
  snow 370.24
  sun 363.31
  temporary 368.12
  total
    both eyes 369.01
    one eye 369.61
      with vision of other eye (specified as)
        near-normal 369.62
        normal 369.63
  transient 368.12
  traumatic NEC 950.9
  word (developmental) 315.01
    acquired 784.61
    secondary to organic lesion 784.61
Blister — *see also* Injury, superficial, by site
  beetle dermatitis 692.89
  due to burn — *see* Burn, by site, second degree
  fever 054.9
  multiple, skin, nontraumatic 709.8
Bloating 787.3
Bloch-Siemens syndrome (incontinentia pigmenti) 757.33
Bloch-Stauffer dyshormonal dermatosis 757.33
Bloch-Sulzberger disease or syndrome (incontinentia pigmenti) (melanoblastosis) 757.33
Block
  alveolar capillary 516.3
  arborization (heart) 426.6
  arrhythmic 426.9
  atrioventricular (AV) (incomplete) (partial) 426.10
    with
      2:1 atrioventricular response block 426.13
      atrioventricular dissociation 426.0
      first degree (incomplete) 426.11
      second degree (Mobitz type I) 426.13
        Mobitz (type) II 426.12
      third degree 426.0
    complete 426.0
      congenital 746.86
    congenital 746.86
    Mobitz (incomplete)
      type I (Wenckebach's) 426.13
      type II 426.12
    partial 426.13
  auriculoventricular (*see also* Block, atrioventricular) 426.10
    complete 426.0
      congenital 746.86
    congenital 746.86
  bifascicular (cardiac) 426.53
  bundle branch (complete) (false) (incomplete) 426.50
    bilateral 426.53
    left (complete) (main stem) 426.3
      with right bundle branch block 426.53

Block — *continued*
  bundle branch — *continued*
    left — *continued*
      anterior fascicular 426.2
        with
          posterior fascicular block 426.3
          right bundle branch block 426.52
        hemiblock 426.2
        incomplete 426.2
          with right bundle branch block 426.53
        posterior fascicular 426.2
          with
            anterior fascicular block 426.3
            right bundle branch block 426.51
    right 426.4
      with
        left bundle branch block (incomplete) (main stem) 426.53
        left fascicular block 426.53
          anterior 426.52
          posterior 426.51
        Wilson's type 426.4
  cardiac 426.9
  conduction 426.9
    complete 426.0
  Eustachian tube (*see also* Obstruction, Eustachian tube) 381.60
  fascicular (left anterior) (left posterior) 426.2
  foramen Magendie (acquired) 331.3
    congenital 742.3
      with spina bifida (*see also* Spina bifida) 741.0 ✓5ᵗʰ
  heart 426.9
    first degree (atrioventricular) 426.11
    second degree (atrioventricular) 426.13
    third degree (atrioventricular) 426.0
    bundle branch (complete) (false) (incomplete) 426.50
      bilateral 426.53
      left (*see also* Block, bundle branch, left) 426.3
      right (*see also* Block, bundle branch, right) 426.4
    complete (atrioventricular) 426.0
    congenital 746.86
    incomplete 426.13
    intra-atrial 426.6
    intraventricular NEC 426.6
    sinoatrial 426.6
    specified type NEC 426.6
  hepatic vein 453.0
  intraventricular (diffuse) (myofibrillar) 426.6
    bundle branch (complete) (false) (incomplete) 426.50
      bilateral 426.53
      left (*see also* Block, bundle branch, left) 426.3
      right (*see also* Block, bundle branch, right) 426.4
  kidney (*see also* Disease, renal) 593.9
    postcystoscopic 997.5
  myocardial (*see also* Block, heart) 426.9
  nodal 426.10
  optic nerve 377.49
  organ or site (congenital) NEC — *see* Atresia
  parietal 426.6
  peri-infarction 426.6
  portal (vein) 452
  sinoatrial 426.6
  sinoauricular 426.6
  spinal cord 336.9
  trifascicular 426.54
  tubal 628.2
  vein NEC 453.9
Blocq's disease or syndrome (astasia-abasia) 307.9
Blood
  constituents, abnormal NEC 790.6
  disease 289.9
    specified NEC 289.8
  donor V59.01
    other blood components V59.09
    stem cells V59.02
    whole blood V59.01

Blood — *continued*
  dyscrasia 289.9
    with
      abortion — *see* Abortion, by type, with hemorrhage, delayed or excessive
      ectopic pregnancy (*see also* categories 633.0-633.9) 639.1
      molar pregnancy (*see also* categories 630-632) 639.1
    fetus or newborn NEC 776.9
    following
      abortion 639.1
      ectopic or molar pregnancy 639.1
    puerperal, postpartum 666.3 ✓5ᵗʰ
  flukes NEC (*see also* Infestation, Schistosoma) 120.9
  in
    feces (*see also* Melena) 578.1
      occult 792.1
    urine (*see also* Hematuria) 599.7
  mole 631
  occult 792.1
  poisoning (*see also* Septicemia) 038.9
  pressure
    decreased, due to shock following injury 958.4
    fluctuating 796.4
    high (*see also* Hypertension) 401.9
      incidental reading (isolated) (nonspecific), without diagnosis of hypertension 796.2
    low (*see also* Hypotension) 458.9
      incidental reading (isolated) (nonspecific), without diagnosis of hypotension 796.3
  spitting (*see also* Hemoptysis) 786.3
  staining cornea 371.12
  transfusion
    without reported diagnosis V58.2
      donor V59.01
        stem cells V59.02
    reaction or complication — *see* Complications, transfusion
  tumor — *see* Hematoma
  vessel rupture — *see* Hemorrhage
  vomiting (*see also* Hematemesis) 578.0
Blood-forming organ disease 289.9
Bloodgood's disease 610.1
Bloodshot eye 379.93
Bloom (-Machacek) (-Torre) syndrome 757.39
Blotch, palpebral 372.55
Blount's disease (tibia vara) 732.4
Blount-Barber syndrome (tibia vara) 732.4
Blue
  baby 746.9
  bloater 491.20
    with acute bronchitis or exacerbation 491.21
  diaper syndrome 270.0
  disease 746.9
  dome cyst 610.0
  drum syndrome 381.02
  sclera 743.47
    with fragility of bone and deafness 756.51
  toe syndrome — *see* Atherosclerosis
Blueness (*see also* Cyanosis) 782.5
Blurring, visual 368.8
Blushing (abnormal) (excessive) 782.62
Boarder, hospital V65.0
  infant V65.0
Bockhart's impetigo (superficial folliculitis) 704.8
Bodechtel-Guttmann disease (subacute sclerosing panencephalitis) 046.2
Boder-Sedgwick syndrome (ataxia-telangiectasia) 334.8
Body, bodies
  Aschoff (*see also* Myocarditis, rheumatic) 398.0
  asteroid, vitreous 379.22
  choroid, colloid (degenerative) 362.57
    hereditary 362.77
  cytoid (retina) 362.82
  drusen (retina) (*see also* Drusen) 362.57
    optic disc 377.21
  fibrin, pleura 511.0

Body, bodies — *continued*
foreign — *see* Foreign body
Hassall-Henle 371.41
loose
  joint (*see also* Loose, body, joint) 718.1 ✓5ᵗʰ
    knee 717.6
  knee 717.6
  sheath, tendon 727.82
Mallory's 034.1
Mooser 081.0
Negri 071
rice (joint) (*see also* Loose, body, joint) 718.1 ✓5ᵗʰ
  knee 717.6
rocking 307.3

Boeck's
disease (sarcoidosis) 135
lupoid (miliary) 135
sarcoid 135

Boerhaave's syndrome (spontaneous esophageal rupture) 530.4

Boggy
cervix 622.8
uterus 621.8

Boil (*see also* Carbuncle) 680.9
abdominal wall 680.2
Aleppo 085.1
ankle 680.6
anus 680.5
arm (any part, above wrist) 680.3
auditory canal, external 680.0
axilla 680.3
back (any part) 680.2
Baghdad 085.1
breast 680.2
buttock 680.5
chest wall 680.2
corpus cavernosum 607.2
Delhi 085.1
ear (any part) 680.0
eyelid 373.13
face (any part, except eye) 680.0
finger (any) 680.4
flank 680.2
foot (any part) 680.7
forearm 680.3
Gafsa 085.1
genital organ, male 608.4
gluteal (region) 680.5
groin 680.2
hand (any part) 680.4
head (any part, except face) 680.8
heel 680.7
hip 680.6
knee 680.6
labia 616.4
lacrimal (*see also* Dacryocystitis) 375.30
  gland (*see also* Dacryoadenitis) 375.00
  passages (duct) (sac) (*see also* Dacryocystitis) 375.30
leg, any part except foot 680.6
multiple sites 680.9
natal 085.1
neck 680.1
nose (external) (septum) 680.0
orbit, orbital 376.01
partes posteriores 680.5
pectoral region 680.2
penis 607.2
perineum 680.2
pinna 680.0
scalp (any part) 680.8
scrotum 608.4
seminal vesicle 608.0
shoulder 680.3
skin NEC 680.9
specified site NEC 680.8
spermatic cord 608.4
temple (region) 680.0
testis 608.4
thigh 680.6
thumb 680.4
toe (any) 680.7
tropical 085.1
trunk 680.2
tunica vaginalis 608.4
umbilicus 680.2

Boil (*see also* Carbuncle) — *continued*
upper arm 680.3
vas deferens 608.4
vulva 616.4
wrist 680.4

Bold hives (*see also* Urticaria) 708.9

Bolivian hemorrhagic fever 078.7

Bombé, iris 364.74

Bomford-Rhoads anemia (refractory) 284.9

Bone — *see* condition

Bonnevie-Ullrich syndrome 758.6

Bonnier's syndrome 386.19

Bonvale Dam fever 780.79

Bony block of joint 718.80
ankle 718.87
elbow 718.82
foot 718.87
hand 718.84
hip 718.85
knee 718.86
multiple sites 718.89
pelvic region 718.85
shoulder (region) 718.81
specified site NEC 718.88
wrist 718.83

Borderline
intellectual functioning V62.89
pelvis 653.1 ✓5ᵗʰ
  with obstruction during labor 660.1 ✓5ᵗʰ
    affecting fetus or newborn 763.1
psychosis (*see also* Schizophrenia) 295.5 ✓5ᵗʰ
  of childhood (*see also* Psychosis, childhood) 299.8 ✓5ᵗʰ
schizophrenia (*see also* Schizophrenia) 295.5 ✓5ᵗʰ

Borna disease 062.9

Bornholm disease (epidemic pleurodynia) 074.1

Borrelia vincentii (mouth) (pharynx) (tonsils) 101

Bostock's catarrh (*see also* Fever, hay) 477.9

Boston exanthem 048

Botalli, ductus (patent) (persistent) 747.0

Bothriocephalus latus infestation 123.4

Botulism 005.1

Bouba (*see also* Yaws) 102.9

Bouffée délirante 298.3

Bouillaud's disease or syndrome (rheumatic heart disease) 391.9

Bourneville's disease (tuberous sclerosis) 759.5

Boutonneuse fever 082.1

Boutonniere
deformity (finger) 736.21
hand (intrinsic) 736.21

Bouveret (-Hoffmann) disease or syndrome (paroxysmal tachycardia) 427.2

Bovine heart — *see* Hypertrophy, cardiac

Bowel — *see* condition

Bowen's
dermatosis (precancerous) (M8081/2) — *see* Neoplasm, skin, in situ
disease (M8081/2) — *see* Neoplasm, skin, in situ
epithelioma (M8081/2) — *see* Neoplasm, skin, in situ
type
  epidermoid carcinoma in situ (M8081/2) — *see* Neoplasm, skin, in situ
  intraepidermal squamous cell carcinoma (M8081/2) — *see* Neoplasm, skin, in situ

Bowing
femur 736.89
  congenital 754.42
fibula 736.89
  congenital 754.43
forearm 736.09
  away from midline (cubitus valgus) 736.01
  toward midline (cubitus varus) 736.02
leg(s), long bones, congenital 754.44
radius 736.09
  away from midline (cubitus valgus) 736.01
  toward midline (cubitus varus) 736.02

Bowing — *continued*
tibia 736.89
  congenital 754.43

Bowleg(s) 736.42
congenital 754.44
rachitic 268.1

Boyd's dysentery 004.2

Brachial — *see* condition

Brachman-de Lange syndrome (Amsterdam dwarf, mental retardation, and brachycephaly) 759.89

Brachycardia 427.89

Brachycephaly 756.0

Brachymorphism and ectopia lentis 759.89

Bradley's disease (epidemic vomiting) 078.82

Bradycardia 427.89
chronic (sinus) 427.81
newborn 779.81   ▲
nodal 427.89
postoperative 997.1
reflex 337.0
sinoatrial 427.89
  with paroxysmal tachyarrhythmia or tachycardia 427.81
    chronic 427.81
sinus 427.89
  with paroxysmal tachyarrhythmia or tachycardia 427.81
    chronic 427.81
  persistent 427.81
  severe 427.81
tachycardia syndrome 427.81
vagal 427.89

Bradypnea 786.09

Brailsford's disease 732.3
radial head 732.3
tarsal scaphoid 732.5

Brailsford-Morquio disease or syndrome (mucopolysac-charidosis IV) 277.5

Brain — *see also* condition
death 348.8
syndrome (acute) (chronic) (nonpsychotic) (organic) (with neurotic reaction) (with behavioral reaction) (*see also* Syndrome, brain) 310.9
  with
    presenile brain disease 290.10
    psychosis, psychotic reaction (*see also* Psychosis, organic) 294.9
  congenital (*see also* Retardation, mental) 319

Branched-chain amino-acid disease 270.3

Branchial — *see* condition

Branchopulmonitis — *see* Pneumonia, broncho-

Brandt's syndrome (acrodermatitis enteropathica) 686.8

Brash (water) 787.1

Brass-founders', ague 985.8

Bravais-Jacksonian epilepsy (*see also* Epilepsy) 345.5 ✓5ᵗʰ

Braxton Hicks contractions 644.1 ✓5ᵗʰ

Braziers' disease 985.8

Brazilian
blastomycosis 116.1
leishmaniasis 085.5

Break
cardiorenal — *see* Hypertension, cardiorenal
retina (*see also* Defect, retina) 361.30

Breakbone fever 061

Breakdown
device, implant, or graft — *see* Complications, mechanical
nervous (*see also* Disorder, mental, nonpsychotic) 300.9
perineum 674.2 ✓5ᵗʰ

Breast — *see* condition

Breast feeding difficulties 676.8 ✓5ᵗʰ

Breath
foul 784.9
holder, child 312.81
holding spells 786.9
shortness 786.05

Breathing
- asymmetrical 786.09
- bronchial 786.09
- exercises V57.0
- labored 786.09
- mouth 784.9
- periodic 786.09
- tic 307.20

Breathlessness 786.09

Breda's disease (*see also* Yaws) 102.9

Breech
- delivery, affecting fetus or newborn 763.0
- extraction, affecting fetus or newborn 763.0
- presentation (buttocks) (complete) (frank) 652.2 ✓5ᵗʰ
  - with successful version 652.1 ✓5ᵗʰ
  - before labor, affecting fetus or newborn 761.7
  - during labor, affecting fetus or newborn 763.0

Breisky's disease (kraurosis vulvae) 624.0

Brennemann's syndrome (acute mesenteric lymphadenitis) 289.2

Brenner's
- tumor (benign) (M9000/0) 220
  - borderline malignancy (M9000/1) 236.2
  - malignant (M9000/3) 183.0
  - proliferating (M9000/1) 236.2

Bretonneau's disease (diphtheritic malignant angina) 032.0

Breus' mole 631

Brevicollis 756.16

Bricklayers' itch 692.89

Brickmakers' anemia 126.9

Bridge
- myocardial 746.85

Bright's
- blindness — *see* Uremia
- disease (*see also* Nephritis) 583.9
  - arteriosclerotic (*see also* Hypertension, kidney) 403.90

Brill's disease (recrudescent typhus) 081.1
- flea-borne 081.0
- louse-borne 081.1

Brill-Symmers disease (follicular lymphoma) (M9690/3) 202.0 ✓5ᵗʰ

Brill-Zinsser disease (recrudescent typhus) 081.1

Brinton's disease (linitis plastica) (M8142/3) 151.9

Brion-Kayser disease (*see also* Fever, paratyphoid) 002.9

Briquet's disorder or syndrome 300.81

Brissaud's
- infantilism (infantile myxedema) 244.9
- motor-verbal tic 307.23

Brissaud-Meige syndrome (infantile myxedema) 244.9

Brittle
- bones (congenital) 756.51
- nails 703.8
  - congenital 757.5

Broad — *see also* condition
- beta disease 272.2
- ligament laceration syndrome 620.6

Brock's syndrome (atelectasis due to enlarged lymph nodes) 518.0

Brocq's disease 691.8
- atopic (diffuse) neurodermatitis 691.8
- lichen simplex chronicus 698.3
- parakeratosis psoriasiformis 696.2
- parapsoriasis 696.2

Brocq-Duhring disease (dermatitis herpetiformis) 694.0

Brodie's
- abscess (localized) (chronic) (*see also* Osteomyelitis) 730.1 ✓5ᵗʰ
- disease (joint) (*see also* Osteomyelitis) 730.1 ✓5ᵗʰ

Broken
- arches 734
  - congenital 755.67

Broken — *continued*
- back — *see* Fracture, vertebra, by site
- bone — *see* Fracture, by site
- compensation — *see* Disease, heart
- implant or internal device — *see* listing under Complications, mechanical
- neck — *see* Fracture, vertebra, cervical
- nose 802.0
  - open 802.1
- tooth, teeth 873.63
  - complicated 873.73

Bromhidrosis 705.89

Bromidism, bromism
- acute 967.3
  - correct substance properly administered 349.82
  - overdose or wrong substance given or taken 967.3
- chronic (*see also* Dependence) 304.1 ✓5ᵗʰ

Bromidrosiphobia 300.23

Bromidrosis 705.89

Bronchi, bronchial — *see* condition

Bronchiectasis (cylindrical) (diffuse) (fusiform) (localized) (moniliform) (postinfectious) (recurrent) (saccular) 494.0
- with acute exacerbation 494.1
- congenital 748.61
- tuberculosis (*see also* Tuberculosis) 011.5 ✓5ᵗʰ

Bronchiolectasis — *see* Bronchiectasis

Bronchiolitis (acute) (infectious) (subacute) 466.19
- with
  - bronchospasm or obstruction 466.19
  - influenza, flu, or grippe 487.1
- catarrhal (acute) (subacute) 466.19
- chemical 506.0
  - chronic 506.4
- chronic (obliterative) 491.8
- due to external agent — *see* Bronchitis, acute, due to
- fibrosa obliterans 491.8
- influenzal 487.1
- obliterans 491.8
  - with organizing pneumonia (B.O.O.P.) 516.8
  - status post lung transplant 996.84
- obliterative (chronic) (diffuse) (subacute) 491.8
  - due to fumes or vapors 506.4
- respiratory syncytial virus 466.11
- vesicular — *see* Pneumonia, broncho-

Bronchitis (diffuse) (hypostatic) (infectious) (inflammatory) (simple) 490
- with
  - emphysema — *see* Emphysema
  - influenza, flu, or grippe 487.1
  - obstruction airway, chronic 491.20
    - with acute exacerbation 491.21
  - tracheitis 490
    - acute or subacute 466.0
      - with bronchospasm or obstruction 466.0
    - chronic 491.8
- acute or subacute 466.0
  - with
    - bronchospasm 466.0
    - chronic
      - bronchitis (obstructive) 491.21
      - obstructive pulmonary disease (COPD) 491.21
    - obstruction 466.0
    - tracheitis 466.0
  - chemical (due to fumes or vapors) 506.0
  - due to
    - fumes or vapors 506.0
    - radiation 508.8
- allergic (acute) (*see also* Asthma) 493.9 ✓5ᵗʰ
- arachidic 934.1
- aspiration 507.0
  - due to fumes or vapors 506.0
- asthmatic (acute) 493.90
  - with
    - acute exacerbation 493.92
    - status asthmaticus 493.91
  - chronic 493.2 ✓5ᵗʰ   ▲
- capillary 466.19
  - with bronchospasm or obstruction 466.19

Bronchitis — *continued*
- capillary — *continued*
  - chronic 491.8
- caseous (*see also* Tuberculosis) 011.3 ✓5ᵗʰ
- Castellani's 104.8
- catarrhal 490
  - acute — *see* Bronchitis, acute
  - chronic 491.0
- chemical (acute) (subacute) 506.0
  - chronic 506.4
  - due to fumes or vapors (acute) (subacute) 506.0
    - chronic 506.4
- chronic 491.9
  - with
    - tracheitis (chronic) 491.8
    - asthmatic 493.2 ✓5ᵗʰ   ▲
  - catarrhal 491.0
  - chemical (due to fumes and vapors) 506.4
  - due to
    - fumes or vapors (chemical) (inhalation) 506.4
    - radiation 508.8
    - tobacco smoking 491.0
  - mucopurulent 491.1
  - obstructive 491.20
    - with acute bronchitis or acute exacerbation 491.21
  - purulent 491.1
  - simple 491.0
  - specified type NEC 491.8
- croupous 466.0
  - with bronchospasm or obstruction 466.0
  - due to fumes or vapors 506.0
- emphysematous 491.20
  - with acute bronchitis or acute exacerbation 491.21
- exudative 466.0
- fetid (chronic) (recurrent) 491.1
- fibrinous, acute or subacute 466.0
  - with bronchospasm or obstruction 466.0
- grippal 487.1
- influenzal 487.1
- membranous, acute or subacute 466.0
  - with bronchospasm or obstruction 466.0
- moulders' 502
- mucopurulent (chronic) (recurrent) 491.1
  - acute or subacute 466.0
- non-obstructive 491.0
- obliterans 491.8
- obstructive (chronic) 491.20
  - with acute bronchitis or acute exacerbation 491.21
- pituitous 491.1
- plastic (inflammatory) 466.0
- pneumococcal, acute or subacute 466.0
  - with bronchospasm or obstruction 466.0
- pseudomembranous 466.0
- purulent (chronic) (recurrent) 491.1
  - acute or subacute 466.0
    - with bronchospasm or obstruction 466.0
- putrid 491.1
- scrofulous (*see also* Tuberculosis) 011.3 ✓5ᵗʰ
- senile 491.9
- septic, acute or subacute 466.0
  - with bronchospasm or obstruction 466.0
- smokers' 491.0
- spirochetal 104.8
- suffocative, acute or subacute 466.0
- summer (*see also* Asthma) 493.9 ✓5ᵗʰ
- suppurative (chronic) 491.1
  - acute or subacute 466.0
- tuberculous (*see also* Tuberculosis) 011.3 ✓5ᵗʰ
- ulcerative 491.8
  - Vincent's 101
- Vincent's 101
- viral, acute or subacute 466.0

Bronchoalveolitis 485

Bronchoaspergillosis 117.3

Bronchocele
- meaning
  - dilatation of bronchus 519.1
  - goiter 240.9

Bronchogenic carcinoma 162.9

Bronchohemisporosis 117.9

Broncholithiasis 518.89
  tuberculous (*see also* Tuberculosis) 011.3 ✓5ᵗʰ
Bronchomalacia 748.3
Bronchomoniliasis 112.89
Bronchomycosis 112.89
Bronchonocardiosis 039.1
Bronchopleuropneumonia — *see* Pneumonia, broncho-
Bronchopneumonia — *see* Pneumonia, broncho-
Bronchopneumonitis — *see* Pneumonia, broncho-
Bronchopulmonary — *see* condition
Bronchorrhagia 786.3
  newborn 770.3
  tuberculous (*see also* Tuberculosis) 011.3 ✓5ᵗʰ
Bronchorrhea (chronic) (purulent) 491.0
  acute 466.0
Bronchospasm 519.1
  with
    asthma — *see* Asthma
    bronchiolitis
      due to respiratory syncytial virus 466.11
    bronchitis — *see* Bronchitis
    chronic obstructive pulmonary disease (COPD) 496
    emphysema — *see* Emphysema
      due to external agent — *see* Condition, respiratory, acute, due to
Bronchospirochetosis 104.8
Bronchostenosis 519.1
Bronchus — *see* condition
Bronze, bronzed
  diabetes 275.0
  disease (Addison's) (skin) 255.4
    tuberculous (*see also* Tuberculosis) 017.6 ✓5ᵗʰ
Brooke's disease or tumor (M8100/0) — *see* Neoplasm, skin, benign
Brown's tendon sheath syndrome 378.61
Brown enamel of teeth (hereditary) 520.5
Brown-Séquard's paralysis (syndrome) 344.89
Brow presentation complicating delivery 652.4 ✓5ᵗʰ
Brucella, brucellosis (infection) 023.9
  abortus 023.1
  canis 023.3
  dermatitis, skin 023.9
  melitensis 023.0
  mixed 023.8
  suis 023.2
Bruck's disease 733.99
Bruck-de Lange disease or syndrome (Amsterdam dwarf, mental retardation, and brachycephaly) 759.89
Brugada syndrome 746.89
Brugsch's syndrome (acropachyderma) 757.39
Brug's filariasis 125.1
Bruhl's disease (splenic anemia with fever) 285.8
Bruise (skin surface intact) — *see also* Contusion
  with
    fracture — *see* Fracture, by site
    open wound — *see* Wound, open, by site
    internal organ (abdomen, chest, or pelvis) — *see* Injury, internal, by site
  umbilical cord 663.6 ✓5ᵗʰ
    affecting fetus or newborn 762.6
Bruit 785.9
  arterial (abdominal) (carotid) 785.9
  supraclavicular 785.9
Brushburn — *see* Injury, superficial, by site
Bruton's X-linked agammaglobulinemia 279.04
Bruxism 306.8
Bubbly lung syndrome 770.7
Bubo 289.3
  blennorrhagic 098.89
  chancroidal 099.0
  climatic 099.1
  due to Hemophilus ducreyi 099.0
  gonococcal 098.89
  indolent NEC 099.8
  inguinal NEC 099.8

Bubo — *continued*
  inguinal NEC — *continued*
    chancroidal 099.0
    climatic 099.1
    due to H. ducreyi 099.0
  scrofulous (*see also* Tuberculosis) 017.2 ✓5ᵗʰ
  soft chancre 099.0
  suppurating 683
  syphilitic 091.0
    congenital 090.0
  tropical 099.1
  venereal NEC 099.8
  virulent 099.0
Bubonic plague 020.0
Bubonocele — *see* Hernia, inguinal
Buccal — *see* condition
Buchanan's disease (juvenile osteochondrosis of iliac crest) 732.1
Buchem's syndrome (hyperostosis corticalis) 733.3
Buchman's disease (osteochondrosis, juvenile) 732.1
Bucket handle fracture (semilunar cartilage) (*see also* Tear, meniscus) 836.2
Budd-Chiari syndrome (hepatic vein thrombosis) 453.0
Budgerigar-fanciers' disease or lung 495.2
Büdinger-Ludloff-Läwen disease 717.89
Buerger's disease (thromboangiitis obliterans) 443.1
Bulbar — *see* condition
Bulbus cordis 745.9
  persistent (in left ventricle) 745.8
Bulging fontanels (congenital) 756.0
Bulimia 783.6
  nonorganic origin 307.51
Bulky uterus 621.2
Bulla(e) 709.8
  lung (emphysematous) (solitary) 492.0
Bullet wound — *see also* Wound, open, by site
  fracture — *see* Fracture, by site, open
  internal organ (abdomen, chest, or pelvis) — *see* Injury, internal, by site, with open wound
  intracranial — *see* Laceration, brain, with open wound
Bullis fever 082.8
Bullying (*see also* Disturbance, conduct) 312.0 ✓5ᵗʰ
Bundle
  branch block (complete) (false) (incomplete) 426.50
    bilateral 426.53
    left (*see also* Block, bundle branch, left) 426.3
      hemiblock 426.2
    right (*see also* Block, bundle branch, right) 426.4
  of His — *see* condition
  of Kent syndrome (anomalous atrioventricular excitation) 426.7
Bungpagga 040.81
Bunion 727.1
Bunionette 727.1
Bunyamwera fever 066.3
Buphthalmia, buphthalmos (congenital) 743.20
  associated with
    keratoglobus, congenital 743.22
    megalocornea 743.22
    ocular anomalies NEC 743.22
  isolated 743.21
  simple 743.21
Bürger-Grütz disease or syndrome (essential familial hyperlipemia) 272.3
Buried roots 525.3
Burke's syndrome 577.8
Burkitt's
  tumor (M9750/3) 200.2 ✓5ᵗʰ
  type malignant, lymphoma, lymphoblastic, or undifferentiated (M9750/3) 200.2 ✓5ᵗʰ

Burn (acid) (cathode ray) (caustic) (chemical) (electric heating appliance) (electricity) (fire) (flame) (hot liquid or object) (irradiation) (lime) (radiation) (steam) (thermal) (x-ray) 949.0

> *Note — Use the following fifth-digit subclassification with category 948 to indicate the percent of body surface with third degree burn:*
>
> 0   *Less than 10% or unspecified*
> 1   *10–19%*
> 2   *20–29%*
> 3   *30–39%*
> 4   *40–49%*
> 5   *50–59%*
> 6   *60–69%*
> 7   *70–79%*
> 8   *80–89%*
> 9   *90% or more of body surface*

  with
    blisters — *see* Burn, by site, second degree
    erythema — *see* Burn, by site, first degree
    skin loss (epidermal) — *see also* Burn, by site, second degree
      full thickness — *see also* Burn, by site, third degree
        with necrosis of underlying tissues — *see* Burn, by site, third degree, deep
  first degree — *see* Burn, by site, first degree
  second degree — *see* Burn, by site, second degree
  third degree — *see* Burn, by site, third degree
    deep — *see* Burn, by site, third degree, deep
  abdomen, abdominal (muscle) (wall) 942.03
    with
      trunk — *see* Burn, trunk, multiple sites
    first degree 942.13
    second degree 942.23
    third degree 942.33
      deep 942.43
        with loss of body part 942.53
  ankle 945.03
    with
      lower limb(s) — *see* Burn, leg, multiple sites
    first degree 945.13
    second degree 945.23
    third degree 945.33
      deep 945.43
        with loss of body part 945.53
  anus — *see* Burn, trunk, specified site NEC
  arm(s) 943.00
    first degree 943.10
    second degree 943.20
    third degree 943.30
      deep 943.40
        with loss of body part 943.50
    lower — *see* Burn, forearm(s)
    multiple sites, except hand(s) or wrist(s) 943.09
      first degree 943.19
      second degree 943.29
      third degree 943.39
        deep 943.49
          with loss of body part 943.59
    upper 943.03
      first degree 943.13
      second degree 943.23
      third degree 943.33
        deep 943.43
          with loss of body part 943.53
  auditory canal (external) — *see* Burn, ear
  auricle (ear) — *see* Burn, ear
  axilla 943.04
    with
      upper limb(s) except hand(s) or wrist(s) — *see* Burn, arm(s), multiple sites
    first degree 943.14
    second degree 943.24
    third degree 943.34
      deep 943.44
        with loss of body part 943.54

Burn — *continued*
　back 942.04
　　with
　　　trunk — *see* Burn, trunk, multiple sites
　　first degree 942.14
　　second degree 942.24
　　third degree 942.34
　　　deep 942.44
　　　　with loss of body part 942.54
　biceps
　　brachii — *see* Burn, arm(s), upper
　　femoris — *see* Burn, thigh
　breast(s) 942.01
　　with
　　　trunk — *see* Burn, trunk, multiple sites
　　first degree 942.11
　　second degree 942.21
　　third degree 942.31
　　　deep 942.41
　　　　with loss of body part 942.51
　brow — *see* Burn, forehead
　buttock(s) — *see* Burn, back
　canthus (eye) 940.1
　　chemical 940.0
　cervix (uteri) 947.4
　cheek (cutaneous) 941.07
　　with
　　　face or head — *see* Burn, head, multiple sites
　　first degree 941.17
　　second degree 941.27
　　third degree 941.37
　　　deep 941.47
　　　　with loss of body part 941.57
　chest wall (anterior) 942.02
　　with
　　　trunk — *see* Burn, trunk, multiple sites
　　first degree 942.12
　　second degree 942.22
　　third degree 942.32
　　　deep 942.42
　　　　with loss of body part 942.52
　chin 941.04
　　with
　　　face or head — *see* Burn, head, multiple sites
　　first degree 941.14
　　second degree 941.24
　　third degree 941.34
　　　deep 941.44
　　　　with loss of body part 941.54
　clitoris — *see* Burn, genitourinary organs, external
　colon 947.3
　conjunctiva (and cornea) 940.4
　　chemical
　　　acid 940.3
　　　alkaline 940.2
　cornea (and conjunctiva) 940.4
　　chemical
　　　acid 940.3
　　　alkaline 940.2
　costal region — *see* Burn, chest wall
　due to ingested chemical agent — *see* Burn, internal organs
　ear (auricle) (canal) (drum) (external) 941.01
　　with
　　　face or head — *see* Burn, head, multiple sites
　　first degree 941.11
　　second degree 941.21
　　third degree 941.31
　　　deep 941.41
　　　　with loss of a body part 941.51
　elbow 943.02
　　with
　　　hand(s) and wrist(s) — *see* Burn, multiple specified sites
　　　upper limb(s) except hand(s) or wrist(s) — *see also* Burn, arm(s), multiple sites
　　first degree 943.12
　　second degree 943.22
　　third degree 943.32
　　　deep 943.42
　　　　with loss of body part 943.52

Burn — *continued*
　electricity, electric current — *See* Burn, by site
　entire body — *see* Burn, multiple, specified sites
　epididymis — *see* Burn, genitourinary organs, external
　epigastric region — *see* Burn, abdomen
　epiglottis 947.1
　esophagus 947.2
　extent (percent of body surface)
　　less than 10 percent 948.0 ✓5ᵗʰ
　　10-19 percent 948.1 ✓5ᵗʰ
　　20-29 percent 948.2 ✓5ᵗʰ
　　30-39 percent 948.3 ✓5ᵗʰ
　　40-49 percent 948.4 ✓5ᵗʰ
　　50-59 percent 948.5 ✓5ᵗʰ
　　60-69 percent 948.6 ✓5ᵗʰ
　　70-79 percent 948.7 ✓5ᵗʰ
　　80-89 percent 948.8 ✓5ᵗʰ
　　90 percent or more 948.9 ✓5ᵗʰ
　extremity
　　lower — *see* Burn, leg
　　upper — *see* Burn, arm(s)
　eye(s) (and adnexa) (only) 940.9
　　with
　　　face, head, or neck 941.02
　　　　first degree 941.12
　　　　second degree 941.22
　　　　third degree 941.32
　　　　　deep 941.42
　　　　　　with loss of body part 941.52
　　　other sites (classifiable to more than one category in 940-945) — *see* Burn, multiple, specified sites
　　　resulting rupture and destruction of eyeball 940.5
　　specified part — *see* Burn, by site
　eyeball — *see also* Burn, eye with resulting rupture and destruction of eyeball 940.5
　eyelid(s) 940.1
　　chemical 940.0
　face — *see* Burn, head
　finger (nail) (subungual) 944.01
　　with
　　　hand(s) — *see* Burn, hand(s), multiple sites
　　　other sites — *see* Burn, multiple, specified sites
　　　thumb 944.04
　　　　first degree 944.14
　　　　second degree 944.24
　　　　third degree 944.34
　　　　　deep 944.44
　　　　　　with loss of body part 944.54
　　first degree 944.11
　　second degree 944.21
　　third degree 944.31
　　　deep 944.41
　　　　with loss of body part 944.51
　　multiple (digits) 944.03
　　　with thumb — *see* Burn, finger, with thumb
　　　first degree 944.13
　　　second degree 944.23
　　　third degree 944.33
　　　　deep 944.43
　　　　　with loss of body part 944.53
　flank — *see* Burn, abdomen
　foot 945.02
　　with
　　　lower limb(s) — *see* Burn, leg, multiple sites
　　first degree 945.12
　　second degree 945.22
　　third degree 945.32
　　　deep 945.42
　　　　with loss of body part 945.52
　forearm(s) 943.01
　　with
　　　upper limb(s) except hand(s) or wrist(s) — *see* Burn, arm(s), multiple sites
　　first degree 943.11
　　second degree 943.21
　　third degree 943.31
　　　deep 943.41
　　　　with loss of body part 943.51

Burn — *continued*
　forehead 941.07
　　with
　　　face or head — *see* Burn, head, multiple sites
　　first degree 941.17
　　second degree 941.27
　　third degree 941.37
　　　deep 941.47
　　　　with loss of body part 941.57
　fourth degree — *see* Burn, by site, third degree, deep
　friction — *see* Injury, superficial, by site
　from swallowing caustic or corrosive substance NEC — *see* Burn, internal organs
　full thickness — *see* Burn, by site, third degree
　gastrointestinal tract 947.3
　genitourinary organs
　　external 942.05
　　　with
　　　　trunk — *see* Burn, trunk, multiple sites
　　　first degree 942.15
　　　second degree 942.25
　　　third degree 942.35
　　　　deep 942.45
　　　　　with loss of body part 942.55
　　internal 947.8
　globe (eye) — *see* Burn, eyeball
　groin — *see* Burn, abdomen
　gum 947.0
　hand(s) (phalanges) (and wrist) 944.00
　　first degree 944.10
　　second degree 944.20
　　third degree 944.30
　　　deep 944.40
　　　　with loss of body part 944.50
　　back (dorsal surface) 944.06
　　　first degree 944.16
　　　second degree 944.26
　　　third degree 944.36
　　　　deep 944.46
　　　　　with loss of body part 944.56
　　multiple sites 944.08
　　　first degree 944.18
　　　second degree 944.28
　　　third degree 944.38
　　　　deep 944.48
　　　　　with loss of body part 944.58
　head (and face) 941.00
　　eye(s) only 940.9
　　　specified part — *see* Burn, by site
　　first degree 941.10
　　second degree 941.20
　　third degree 941.30
　　　deep 941.40
　　　　with loss of body part 941.50
　　multiple sites 941.09
　　　with eyes — *see* Burn, eyes, with face, head, or neck
　　　first degree 941.19
　　　second degree 941.29
　　　third degree 941.39
　　　　deep 941.49
　　　　　with loss of body part 941.59
　heel — *see* Burn, foot
　hip — *see* Burn, trunk, specified site NEC
　iliac region — *see* Burn, trunk, specified site NEC
　infected 958.3
　inhalation (*see also* Burn, internal organs) 947.9
　internal organs 947.9
　　from caustic or corrosive substance (swallowing) NEC 947.9
　　specified NEC (*see also* Burn, by site) 947.8
　interscapular region — *see* Burn, back
　intestine (large) (small) 947.3
　iris — *see* Burn, eyeball
　knee 945.05
　　with
　　　lower limb(s) — *see* Burn, leg, multiple sites
　　first degree 945.15
　　second degree 945.25

Burn — *continued*
  knee — *continued*
    third degree 945.35
      deep 945.45
        with loss of body part 945.55
  labium (majorus) (minus) — *see* Burn, genitourinary organs, external
  lacrimal apparatus, duct, gland, or sac 940.1
    chemical 940.0
  larynx 947.1
  late effect — *see* Late, effects (of), burn
  leg 945.00
    first degree 945.10
    second degree 945.20
    third degree 945.30
      deep 945.40
        with loss of body part 945.50
    lower 945.04
      with other part(s) of lower limb(s) — *see* Burn, leg, multiple sites
      first degree 945.14
      second degree 945.24
      third degree 945.34
        deep 945.44
          with loss of body part 945.54
    multiple sites 945.09
      first degree 945.19
      second degree 945.29
      third degree 945.39
        deep 945.49
          with loss of body part 945.59
    upper — *see* Burn, thigh
  lightning — *see* Burn, by site
  limb(s)
    lower (including foot or toe(s)) — *see* Burn, leg
    upper (except wrist and hand) — *see* Burn, arm(s)
  lip(s) 941.03
    with
      face or head — *see* Burn, head, multiple sites
    first degree 941.13
    second degree 941.23
    third degree 941.33
      deep 941.43
        with loss of body part 941.53
  lumbar region — *see* Burn, back
  lung 947.1
  malar region — *see* Burn, cheek
  mastoid region — *see* Burn, scalp
  membrane, tympanic — *see* Burn, ear
  midthoracic region — *see* Burn, chest wall
  mouth 947.0
  multiple (*see also* Burn, unspecified) 949.0
    specified sites classifiable to more than one category in 940-945 946.0
      first degree 946.1
      second degree 946.2
      third degree 946.3
        deep 946.4
          with loss of body part 946.5
  muscle, abdominal — *see* Burn, abdomen
  nasal (septum) — *see* Burn, nose
  neck 941.08
    with
      face or head — *see* Burn, head, multiple sites
    first degree 941.18
    second degree 941.28
    third degree 941.38
      deep 941.48
        with loss of body part 941.58
  nose (septum) 941.05
    with
      face or head — *see* Burn, head, multiple sites
    first degree 941.15
    second degree 941.25
    third degree 941.35
      deep 941.45
        with loss of body part 941.55
  occipital region — *see* Burn, scalp
  orbit region 940.1
    chemical 940.0
  oronasopharynx 947.0
  palate 947.0

Burn — *continued*
  palm(s) 944.05
    with
      hand(s) and wrist(s) — *see* Burn, hand(s), multiple sites
    first degree 944.15
    second degree 944.25
    third degree 944.35
      deep 944.45
        with loss of a body part 944.55
  parietal region — *see* Burn, scalp
  penis — *see* Burn, genitourinary organs, external
  perineum — *see* Burn, genitourinary organs, external
  periocular area 940.1
    chemical 940.0
  pharynx 947.0
  pleura 947.1
  popliteal space — *see* Burn, knee
  prepuce — *see* Burn, genitourinary organs, external
  pubic region — *see* Burn, genitourinary organs, external
  pudenda — *see* Burn, genitourinary organs, external
  rectum 947.3
  sac, lacrimal 940.1
    chemical 940.0
  sacral region — *see* Burn, back
  salivary (ducts) (glands) 947.0
  scalp 941.06
    with
      face or neck — *see* Burn, head, multiple sites
    first degree 941.16
    second degree 941.26
    third degree 941.36
      deep 941.46
        with loss of body part 941.56
  scapular region 943.06
    with
      upper limb(s), except hand(s) or wrist(s) — *see* Burn, arm(s), multiple sites
    first degree 943.16
    second degree 943.26
    third degree 943.36
      deep 943.46
        with loss of body part 943.56
  sclera — *see* Burn, eyeball
  scrotum — *see* Burn, genitourinary organs, external
  septum, nasal — *see* Burn, nose
  shoulder(s) 943.05
    with
      hand(s) and wrist(s) — *see* Burn, multiple, specified sites
      upper limb(s), except hand(s) or wrist(s) — *see* Burn, arm(s), multiple sites
    first degree 943.15
    second degree 943.25
    third degree 943.35
      deep 943.45
        with loss of body part 943.55
  skin NEC (*see also* Burn, unspecified) 949.0
  skull — *see* Burn, head
  small intestine 947.3
  sternal region — *see* Burn, chest wall
  stomach 947.3
  subconjunctival — *see* Burn, conjunctiva
  subcutaneous — *see* Burn, by site, third degree
  submaxillary region — *see* Burn, head
  submental region — *see* Burn, chin
  sun — *see* Sunburn
  supraclavicular fossa — *see* Burn, neck
  supraorbital — *see* Burn, forehead
  temple — *see* Burn, scalp
  temporal region — *see* Burn, scalp
  testicle — *see* Burn, genitourinary organs, external
  testis — *see* Burn, genitourinary organs, external
  thigh 945.06
    with
      lower limb(s) — *see* Burn, leg, multiple sites

Burn — *continued*
  thigh — *continued*
    first degree 945.16
    second degree 945.26
    third degree 945.36
      deep 945.46
        with loss of body part 945.56
  thorax (external) — *see* Burn, chest wall
  throat 947.0
  thumb(s) (nail) (subungual) 944.02
    with
      finger(s) — *see* Burn, finger, with other sites, thumb
      hand(s) and wrist(s) — *see* Burn, hand(s), multiple sites
    first degree 944.12
    second degree 944.22
    third degree 944.32
      deep 944.42
        with loss of body part 944.52
  toe (nail) (subungual) 945.01
    with
      lower limb(s) — *see* Burn, leg, multiple sites
    first degree 945.11
    second degree 945.21
    third degree 945.31
      deep 945.41
        with loss of body part 945.51
  tongue 947.0
  tonsil 947.0
  trachea 947.1
  trunk 942.00
    first degree 942.10
    second degree 942.20
    third degree 942.30
      deep 942.40
        with loss of body part 942.50
    multiple sites 942.09
      first degree 942.19
      second degree 942.29
      third degree 942.39
        deep 942.49
          with loss of body part 942.59
    specified site NEC 942.09
      first degree 942.19
      second degree 942.29
      third degree 942.39
        deep 942.49
          with loss of body part 942.59
  tunica vaginalis — *see* Burn, genitourinary organs, external
  tympanic membrane — *see* Burn, ear
  tympanum — *see* Burn, ear
  ultraviolet 692.82
  unspecified site (multiple) 949.0
    with extent of body surface involved specified
      less than 10 percent 948.0 ✓5ᵗʰ
      10-19 percent 948.1 ✓5ᵗʰ
      20-29 percent 948.2 ✓5ᵗʰ
      30-39 percent 948.3 ✓5ᵗʰ
      40-49 percent 948.4 ✓5ᵗʰ
      50-59 percent 948.5 ✓5ᵗʰ
      60-69 percent 948.6 ✓5ᵗʰ
      70-79 percent 948.7 ✓5ᵗʰ
      80-89 percent 948.8 ✓5ᵗʰ
      90 percent or more 948.9 ✓5ᵗʰ
    first degree 949.1
    second degree 949.2
    third degree 949.3
      deep 949.4
        with loss of body part 949.5
  uterus 947.4
  uvula 947.0
  vagina 947.4
  vulva — *see* Burn, genitourinary organs, external
  wrist(s) 944.07
    with
      hand(s) — *see* Burn, hand(s), multiple sites
    first degree 944.17
    second degree 944.27
    third degree 944.37
      deep 944.47
        with loss of body part 944.57

Burnett's syndrome (milk-alkali) 999.9

Burnier's syndrome (hypophyseal dwarfism) 253.3

Burning
  feet syndrome 266.2
  sensation (*see also* Disturbance, sensation) 782.0
    tongue 529.6

Burns' disease (osteochondrosis, lower ulna) 732.3

Bursa — *see also* condition
  pharynx 478.29

Bursitis NEC 727.3
  Achilles tendon 726.71
  adhesive 726.90
    shoulder 726.0
  ankle 726.79
  buttock 726.5
  calcaneal 726.79
  collateral ligament
    fibular 726.63
    tibial 726.62
  Duplay's 726.2
  elbow 726.33
  finger 726.8
  foot 726.79
  gonococcal 098.52
  hand 726.4
  hip 726.5
  infrapatellar 726.69
  ischiogluteal 726.5
  knee 726.60
  occupational NEC 727.2
  olecranon 726.33
  pes anserinus 726.61
  pharyngeal 478.29
  popliteal 727.51
  prepatellar 726.65
  radiohumeral 727.3
  scapulohumeral 726.19
    adhesive 726.0
  shoulder 726.10
    adhesive 726.0
  subacromial 726.19
    adhesive 726.0
  subcoracoid 726.19
  subdeltoid 726.19
    adhesive 726.0
  subpatellar 726.69
  syphilitic 095.7
  Thornwaldt's, Tornwaldt's (pharyngeal) 478.29
  toe 726.79
  trochanteric area 726.5
  wrist 726.4

Burst stitches or sutures (complication of surgery) ▶(external)◀ 998.32 ▲
  internal 998.31 ●

Buruli ulcer 031.1

Bury's disease (erythema elevatum diutinum) 695.89

Buschke's disease or scleredema (adultorum) 710.1

Busquet's disease (osteoperiostitis) (*see also* Osteomyelitis) 730.1 ✓5ᵗʰ

Busse-Buschke disease (cryptococcosis) 117.5

Buttock — *see* condition

Button
  Biskra 085.1
  Delhi 085.1
  oriental 085.1

Buttonhole hand (intrinsic) 736.21

Bwamba fever (encephalitis) 066.3

Byssinosis (occupational) 504

Bywaters' syndrome 958.5

C

Cacergasia 300.9

Cachexia 799.4
  cancerous (M8000/3) 199.1
  cardiac — *see* Disease, heart

Cachexia — *continued*
  dehydration 276.5
    with
      hypernatremia 276.0
      hyponatremia 276.1
  due to malnutrition 261
  exophthalmic 242.0 ✓5ᵗʰ
  heart — *see* Disease, heart
  hypophyseal 253.2
  hypopituitary 253.2
  lead 984.9
    specified type of lead — *see* Table of Drugs and Chemicals
  malaria 084.9
  malignant (M8000/3) 199.1
  marsh 084.9
  nervous 300.5
  old age 797
  pachydermic — *see* Hypothyroidism
  paludal 084.9
  pituitary (postpartum) 253.2
  renal (*see also* Disease, renal) 593.9
  saturnine 984.9
    specified type of lead — *see* Table of Drugs and Chemicals
  senile 797
  Simmonds' (pituitary cachexia) 253.2
  splenica 289.59
  strumipriva (*see also* Hypothyroidism) 244.9
  tuberculous NEC (*see also* Tuberculosis) 011.9 ✓5ᵗʰ

Café au lait spots 709.09

Caffey's disease or syndrome (infantile cortical hyperostosis) 756.59

Caisson disease 993.3

Caked breast (puerperal, postpartum) 676.2 ✓5ᵗʰ

Cake kidney 753.3

Calabar swelling 125.2

Calcaneal spur 726.73

Calcaneoapophysitis 732.5

Calcaneonavicular bar 755.67

Calcareous — *see* condition

Calcicosis (occupational) 502

Calciferol (vitamin D) deficiency 268.9
  with
    osteomalacia 268.2
    rickets (*see also* Rickets) 268.0

Calcification
  adrenal (capsule) (gland) 255.4
    tuberculous (*see also* Tuberculosis) 017.6 ✓5ᵗʰ
  aorta 440.0
  artery (annular) — *see* Arteriosclerosis
  auricle (ear) 380.89
  bladder 596.8
    due to S. hematobium 120.0
  brain (cortex) — *see* Calcification, cerebral
  bronchus 519.1
  bursa 727.82
  cardiac (*see also* Degeneration, myocardial) 429.1
  cartilage (postinfectional) 733.99
  cerebral (cortex) 348.8
    artery 437.0
  cervix (uteri) 622.8
  choroid plexus 349.2
  conjunctiva 372.54
  corpora cavernosa (penis) 607.89
  cortex (brain) — *see* Calcification, cerebral
  dental pulp (nodular) 522.2
  dentinal papilla 520.4
  disc, intervertebral 722.90
    cervical, cervicothoracic 722.91
    lumbar, lumbosacral 722.93
    thoracic, thoracolumbar 722.92
  fallopian tube 620.8
  falx cerebri — *see* Calcification, cerebral
  fascia 728.89
  gallbladder 575.8
  general 275.40
  heart (*see also* Degeneration, myocardial) 429.1
    valve — *see* Endocarditis
  intervertebral cartilage or disc (postinfectional) 722.90
    cervical, cervicothoracic 722.91

Calcification — *continued*
  intervertebral cartilage or disc — *continued*
    lumbar, lumbosacral 722.93
    thoracic, thoracolumbar 722.92
  intracranial — *see* Calcification, cerebral
  intraspinal ligament 728.89
  joint 719.80
    ankle 719.87
    elbow 719.82
    foot 719.87
    hand 719.84
    hip 719.85
    knee 719.86
    multiple sites 719.89
    pelvic region 719.85
    shoulder (region) 719.81
    specified site NEC 719.88
    wrist 719.83
  kidney 593.89
    tuberculous (*see also* Tuberculosis) 016.0 ✓5ᵗʰ
  larynx (senile) 478.79
  lens 366.8
  ligament 728.89
    intraspinal 728.89
    knee (medial collateral) 717.89
  lung 518.89
    active 518.89
    postinfectional 518.89
    tuberculous (*see also* Tuberculosis, pulmonary) 011.9 ✓5ᵗʰ
  lymph gland or node (postinfectional) 289.3
    tuberculous (*see also* Tuberculosis, lymph gland) 017.2 ✓5ᵗʰ
  massive (paraplegic) 728.10
  medial NEC (*see also* Arteriosclerosis, extremities) 440.20
  meninges (cerebral) 349.2
  metastatic 275.40
  Mönckeberg's — *see* Arteriosclerosis
  muscle 728.10
    heterotopic, postoperative 728.13
  myocardium, myocardial (*see also* Degeneration, myocardial) 429.1
  ovary 620.8
  pancreas 577.8
  penis 607.89
  periarticular 728.89
  pericardium (*see also* Pericarditis) 423.8
  pineal gland 259.8
  pleura 511.0
    postinfectional 518.89
    tuberculous (*see also* Tuberculosis, pleura) 012.0 ✓5ᵗʰ
  pulp (dental) (nodular) 522.2
  renal 593.89
  Rider's bone 733.99
  sclera 379.16
  semilunar cartilage 717.89
  spleen 289.59
  subcutaneous 709.3
  suprarenal (capsule) (gland) 255.4
  tendon (sheath) 727.82
    with bursitis, synovitis or tenosynovitis 727.82
  trachea 519.1
  ureter 593.89
  uterus 621.8
  vitreous 379.29

Calcified — *see also* Calcification
  hematoma NEC 959.9

Calcinosis (generalized) (interstitial) (tumoral) (universalis) 275.49
  circumscripta 709.3
  cutis 709.3
  intervertebralis 275.49 [722.90]
  Raynaud's
    phenomenonsclerodactylytelangiectasis (CRST) 710.1

Calcium
  blood
    high (*see also* Hypercalcemia) 275.42
    low (*see also* Hypocalcemia) 275.41
  deposits — *see also* Calcification, by site
    in bursa 727.82

Calcium — *continued*
  deposits — *see also* Calcification, by site —
      continued
    in tendon (sheath) 727.82
      with bursitis, synovitis or tenosynovitis
          727.82
  salts or soaps in vitreous 379.22
Calciuria 791.9
Calculi — *see* Calculus
Calculosis, intrahepatic — *see*
    Choledocholithiasis
Calculus, calculi, calculous 592.9
  ampulla of Vater — *see* Choledocholithiasis
  anuria (impacted) (recurrent) 592.0
  appendix 543.9
  bile duct (any) — *see* Choledocholithiasis
  biliary — *see* Cholelithiasis
  bilirubin, multiple — *see* Cholelithiasis
  bladder (encysted) (impacted) (urinary) 594.1
    diverticulum 594.0
  bronchus 518.89
  calyx (kidney) (renal) 592.0
    congenital 753.3
  cholesterol (pure) (solitary) — *see* Cholelithiasis
  common duct (bile) — *see* Choledocholithiasis
  conjunctiva 372.54
  cystic 594.1
    duct — *see* Cholelithiasis
  dental 523.6
    subgingival 523.6
    supragingival 523.6
  epididymis 608.89
  gallbladder — *see also* Cholelithiasis
    congenital 751.69
  hepatic (duct) — *see* Choledocholithiasis
  intestine (impaction) (obstruction) 560.39
  kidney (impacted) (multiple) (pelvis) (recurrent)
        (staghorn) 592.0
    congenital 753.3
  lacrimal (passages) 375.57
  liver (impacted) — *see* Choledocholithiasis
  lung 518.89
  nephritic (impacted) (recurrent) 592.0
  nose 478.1
  pancreas (duct) 577.8
  parotid gland 527.5
  pelvis, encysted 592.0
  prostate 602.0
  pulmonary 518.89
  renal (impacted) (recurrent) 592.0
    congenital 753.3
  salivary (duct) (gland) 527.5
  seminal vesicle 608.89
  staghorn 592.0
  Stensen's duct 527.5
  sublingual duct or gland 527.5
    congenital 750.26
  submaxillary duct, gland, or region 527.5
  suburethral 594.8
  tonsil 474.8
  tooth, teeth 523.6
  tunica vaginalis 608.89
  ureter (impacted) (recurrent) 592.1
  urethra (impacted) 594.2
  urinary (duct) (impacted) (passage) (tract) 592.9
    lower tract NEC 594.9
      specified site 594.8
  vagina 623.8
  vesical (impacted) 594.1
  Wharton's duct 527.5
Caliectasis 593.89
California
  disease 114.0
  encephalitis 062.5
Caligo cornea 371.03
Callositas, callosity (infected) 700
Callus (infected) 700
  bone 726.91
  excessive, following fracture — *see also* Late,
      effect (of), fracture
Calvé (-Perthes) disease (osteochondrosis,
    femoral capital) 732.1
Calvities (*see also* Alopecia) 704.00
Cameroon fever (*see also* Malaria) 084.6
Camptocormia 300.11

Camptodactyly (congenital) 755.59
Camurati-Engelmann disease (diaphyseal
    sclerosis) 756.59
Canal — *see* condition
Canaliculitis (lacrimal) (acute) 375.31
  Actinomyces 039.8
  chronic 375.41
Canavan's disease 330.0
Cancer (M8000/3) — *see also* Neoplasm, by site,
    malignant

> Note — The term "cancer" when modified by
> an adjective or adjectival phrase indicating a
> morphological type should be coded in the
> same manner as "carcinoma" with that
> adjective or phrase. Thus, "squamous-cell
> cancer" should be coded in the same manner
> as "squamous-cell carcinoma," which
> appears in the list under "Carcinoma."

  bile duct type (M8160/3), liver 155.1
  hepatocellular (M8170/3) 155.0
Cancerous (M8000/3) — *see* Neoplasm, by site,
    malignant
Cancerphobia 300.29
Cancrum oris 528.1
Candidiasis, candidal 112.9
  with pneumonia 112.4
  balanitis 112.2
  congenital 771.7
  disseminated 112.5
  endocarditis 112.81
  esophagus 112.84
  intertrigo 112.3
  intestine 112.85
  lung 112.4
  meningitis 112.83
  mouth 112.0
  nails 112.3
  neonatal 771.7
  onychia 112.3
  otitis externa 112.82
  otomycosis 112.82
  paronychia 112.3
  perionyxis 112.3
  pneumonia 112.4
  pneumonitis 112.4
  skin 112.3
  specified site NEC 112.89
  systemic 112.5
  urogenital site NEC 112.2
  vagina 112.1
  vulva 112.1
  vulvovaginitis 112.1
Candidiosis — *see* Candidiasis
Candiru infection or infestation 136.8
Canities (premature) 704.3
  congenital 757.4
Canker (mouth) (sore) 528.2
  rash 034.1
Cannabinosis 504
Canton fever 081.9
Cap
  cradle 690.11
Capillariasis 127.5
Capillary — *see* condition
Caplan's syndrome 714.81
Caplan-Colinet syndrome 714.81
Capsule — *see* condition
Capsulitis (joint) 726.90
  adhesive (shoulder) 726.0
  hip 726.5
  knee 726.60
  labyrinthine 387.8
  thyroid 245.9
  wrist 726.4
Caput
  crepitus 756.0
  medusae 456.8
  succedaneum 767.1
Carapata disease 087.1
Carate — *see* Pinta

Carboxyhemoglobinemia 986
Carbuncle 680.9
  abdominal wall 680.2
  ankle 680.6
  anus 680.5
  arm (any part, above wrist) 680.3
  auditory canal, external 680.0
  axilla 680.3
  back (any part) 680.2
  breast 680.2
  buttock 680.5
  chest wall 680.2
  corpus cavernosum 607.2
  ear (any part) (external) 680.0
  eyelid 373.13
  face (any part except eye) 680.0
  finger (any) 680.4
  flank 680.2
  foot (any part) 680.7
  forearm 680.3
  genital organ (male) 608.4
  gluteal (region) 680.5
  groin 680.2
  hand (any part) 680.4
  head (any part except face) 680.8
  heel 680.7
  hip 680.6
  kidney (*see also* Abscess, kidney) 590.2
  knee 680.6
  labia 616.4
  lacrimal
    gland (*see also* Dacryoadenitis) 375.00
    passages (duct) (sac) (*see also*
        Dacryocystitis) 375.30
  leg, any part except foot 680.6
  lower extremity, any part except foot 680.6
  malignant 022.0
  multiple sites 680.9
  neck 680.1
  nose (external) (septum) 680.0
  orbit, orbital 376.01
  partes posteriores 680.5
  pectoral region 680.2
  penis 607.2
  perineum 680.2
  pinna 680.0
  scalp (any part) 680.8
  scrotum 608.4
  seminal vesicle 608.0
  shoulder 680.3
  skin NEC 680.9
  specified site NEC 680.8
  spermatic cord 608.4
  temple (region) 680.0
  testis 608.4
  thigh 680.6
  thumb 680.4
  toe (any) 680.7
  trunk 680.2
  tunica vaginalis 608.4
  umbilicus 680.2
  upper arm 680.3
  urethra 597.0
  vas deferens 608.4
  vulva 616.4
  wrist 680.4
Carbunculus (*see also* Carbuncle) 680.9
Carcinoid (tumor) (M8240/1) — *see also*
    Neoplasm, by site, uncertain behavior
  and struma ovarii (M9091/1) 236.2
  argentaffin (M8241/1) — *see* Neoplasm, by site,
      uncertain behavior
    malignant (M8241/3) — *see* Neoplasm, by
        site, malignant
  benign (M9091/0) 220
  composite (M8244/3) — *see* Neoplasm, by site,
      malignant
  goblet cell (M8243/3) — *see* Neoplasm, by site,
      malignant
  malignant (M8240/3) — *see* Neoplasm, by site,
      malignant
  nonargentaffin (M8242/1) — *see also*
      Neoplasm, by site, uncertain behavior
    malignant (M8242/3) — *see* Neoplasm, by
        site, malignant
  strumal (M9091/1) 236.2
  syndrome (intestinal) (metastatic) 259.2

✔4ᵗʰ Fourth-digit Required   ✔5ᵗʰ Fifth-digit Required   ►◄ Revised Text   ● New Line   ▲ Revised Code

Carcinoid — *see also* Neoplasm, by site,
      uncertain behavior — *continued*
   type bronchial adenoma (M8240/3) — *see*
      Neoplasm, lung, malignant
Carcinoidosis 259.2
Carcinoma (M8010/3) — *see also* Neoplasm, by
      site, malignant

> *Note — Except where otherwise indicated,*
> *the morphological varieties of carcinoma in*
> *the list below should be coded by site as for*
> *"Neoplasm, malignant."*

   with
      apocrine metaplasia (M8573/3)
      cartilaginous (and osseous) metaplasia
         (M8571/3)
      osseous (and cartilaginous) metaplasia
         (M8571/3)
      productive fibrosis (M8141/3)
      spindle cell metaplasia (M8572/3)
      squamous metaplasia (M8570/3)
   acidophil (M8280/3)
      specified site — *see* Neoplasm, by site,
         malignant
      unspecified site 194.3
   acidophil-basophil, mixed (M8281/3)
      specified site — *see* Neoplasm, by site,
         malignant
      unspecified site 194.3
   acinar (cell) (M8550/3)
   acinic cell (M8550/3)
   adenocystic (M8200/3)
   adenoid
      cystic (M8200/3)
      squamous cell (M8075/3)
   adenosquamous (M8560/3)
   adnexal (skin) (M8390/3) — *see* Neoplasm,
      skin, malignant
   adrenal cortical (M8370/3) 194.0
   alveolar (M8251/3)
      cell (M8250/3) — *see* Neoplasm, lung,
         malignant
   anaplastic type (M8021/3)
   apocrine (M8401/3)
      breast — *see* Neoplasm, breast, malignant
      specified site NEC — *see* Neoplasm, skin,
         malignant
      unspecified site 173.9
   basal cell (pigmented) (M8090/3) — *see also*
      Neoplasm, skin, malignant
      fibro-epithelial type (M8093/3) — *see*
         Neoplasm, skin, malignant
      morphea type (M8092/3) — *see* Neoplasm,
         skin, malignant
      multicentric (M8091/3) — *see* Neoplasm,
         skin, malignant
   basaloid (M8123/3)
   basal-squamous cell, mixed (M8094/3) — *see*
      Neoplasm, skin, malignant
   basophil (M8300/3)
      specified site — *see* Neoplasm, by site,
         malignant
      unspecified site 194.3
   basophil-acidophil, mixed (M8281/3)
      specified site — *see* Neoplasm, by site,
         malignant
      unspecified site 194.3
   basosquamous (M8094/3) — *see* Neoplasm,
      skin, malignant
   bile duct type (M8160/3)
      and hepatocellular, mixed (M8180/3) 155.0
         liver 155.1
      specified site NEC — *see* Neoplasm, by site,
         malignant
      unspecified site 155.1
   branchial or branchiogenic 146.8
   bronchial or bronchogenic — *see* Neoplasm,
      lung, malignant
   bronchiolar (terminal) (M8250/3) — *see*
      Neoplasm, lung, malignant
   bronchiolo-alveolar (M8250/3) — *see*
      Neoplasm, lung, malignant
   bronchogenic (epidermoid) 162.9
   C cell (M8510/3)
      specified site — *see* Neoplasm, by site,
         mailignant
      unspecified site 193

Carcinoma — *see also* Neoplasm, by site,
      malignant — *continued*
   ceruminous (M8420/3) 173.2
   chorionic (M9100/3)
      specified site — *see* Neoplasm, by site,
         malignant
      unspecified site
         female 181
         male 186.9
   chromophobe (M8270/3)
      specified site — *see* Neoplasm, by site,
         malignant
      unspecified site 194.3
   clear cell (mesonephroid type) (M8310/3)
   cloacogenic (M8124/3)
      specified site — *see* Neoplasm, by site,
         malignant
      unspecified site 154.8
   colloid (M8480/3)
   cribriform (M8201/3)
   cylindroid type (M8200/3)
   diffuse type (M8145/3)
      specified site — *see* Neoplasm, by site,
         malignant
      unspecified site 151.9
   duct (cell) (M8500/3)
      with Paget's disease (M8541/3) — *see*
         Neoplasm, breast, malignant
      infiltrating (M8500/3)
         specified site — *see* Neoplasm, by site,
            malignant
         unspecified site 174.9
   ductal (M8500/3)
   ductular, infiltrating (M8521/3)
   embryonal (M9070/3)
      and teratoma, mixed (M9081/3)
      combined with choriocarcinoma (M9101/3)
         — *see* Neoplasm, by site, malignant
      infantile type (M9071/3)
      liver 155.0
      polyembryonal type (M9072/3)
   endometrioid (M8380/3)
   eosinophil (M8280/3)
      specified site — *see* Neoplasm, by site,
         malignant
      unspecified site 194.3
   epidermoid (M8070/3) — *see also* Carcinoma,
      squamous cell
      and adenocarcinoma, mixed (M8560/3)
      in situ, Bowen's type (M8081/2) — *see*
         Neoplasm, skin, malignant
      intradermal — *see* Neoplasm, skin, in situ
   fibroepithelial type basal cell (M8093/3) — *see*
      Neoplasm, skin, malignant
   follicular (M8330/3)
      and papillary (mixed) (M8340/3) 193
      moderately differentiated type (M8332/3)
         193
      pure follicle type (M8331/3) 193
      specified site — *see* Neoplasm, by site,
         malignant
      trabecular type (M8332/3) 193
      unspecified site 193
      well differentiated type (M8331/3) 193
   gelatinous (M8480/3)
   giant cell (M8031/3)
      and spindle cell (M8030/3)
   granular cell (M8320/3)
   granulosa cell (M8620/3) 183.0
   hepatic cell (M8170/3) 155.0
   hepatocellular (M8170/3) 155.0
      and bile duct, mixed (M8180/3) 155.0
   hepatocholangiolitic (M8180/3) 155.0
   Hürthle cell (thyroid) 193
   hypernephroid (M8311/3)
   in
      adenomatous
         polyp (M8210/3)
         polyposis coli (M8220/3) 153.9
      pleomorphic adenoma (M8940/3)
      polypoid adenoma (M8210/3)
      situ (M8010/3) — *see* Carcinoma, in situ
      tubular adenoma (M8210/3)
      villous adenoma (M8261/3)
   infiltrating duct (M8500/3)
      with Paget's disease (M8541/3) — *see*
         Neoplasm, breast, malignant

Carcinoma — *see also* Neoplasm, by site,
      malignant — *continued*
   infiltrating duct — *continued*
      specified site — *see* Neoplasm, by site,
         malignant
      unspecified site 174.9
   inflammatory (M8530/3)
      specified site — *see* Neoplasm, by site,
         malignant
      unspecified site 174.9
   in situ (M8010/2) — *see also* Neoplasm, by
      site, in situ
      epidermoid (M8070/2) — *see also* Neoplasm,
         by site, in situ
         with questionable stromal invasion
            (M8076/2)
            specified site — *see* Neoplasm, by site,
               in situ
            unspecified site 233.1
         Bowen's type (M8081/2) — *see*
            Neoplasm, skin, in situ
      intraductal (M8500/2)
         specified site — *see* Neoplasm, by site, in
            situ
         unspecified site 233.0
      lobular (M8520/2)
         specified site — *see* Neoplasm, by site, in
            situ
         unspecified site 233.0
      papillary (M8050/2) — *see* Neoplasm, by
         site, in situ
      squamous cell (M8070/2) — *see also*
         Neoplasm, by site, in situ
         with questionable stromal invasion
            (M8076/2)
            specified site — *see* Neoplasm, by site,
               in situ
            unspecified site 233.1
      transitional cell (M8120/2) — *see* Neoplasm,
         by site, in situ
   intestinal type (M8144/3)
      specified site — *see* Neoplasm, by site,
         malignant
      unspecified site 151.9
   intraductal (noninfiltrating) (M8500/2)
      papillary (M8503/2)
         specified site — *see* Neoplasm, by site, in
            situ
         unspecified site 233.0
      specified site — *see* Neoplasm, by site, in
         situ
      unspecified site 233.0
   intraepidermal (M8070/2) — *see also*
      Neoplasm, skin, in situ
      squamous cell, Bowen's type (M8081/2) —
         see Neoplasm, skin, in situ
   intraepithelial (M8010/2) — *see also* Neoplasm,
      by site, in situ
      squamous cell (M8072/2) — *see* Neoplasm,
         by site, in situ
   intraosseous (M9270/3) 170.1
      upper jaw (bone) 170.0
   islet cell (M8150/3)
      and exocrine, mixed (M8154/3)
         specified site — *see* Neoplasm, by site,
            malignant
         unspecified site 157.9
      pancreas 157.4
      specified site NEC — *see* Neoplasm, by site,
         malignant
      unspecified site 157.4
   juvenile, breast (M8502/3) — *see* Neoplasm,
      breast, malignant
   Kulchitsky's cell (carcinoid tumor of intestine)
      259.2
   large cell (M8012/3)
      squamous cell, nonkeratinizing type
         (M8072/3)
   Leydig cell (testis) (M8650/3)
      specified site — *see* Neoplasm, by site,
         malignant
      unspecified site 186.9
         female 183.0
         male 186.9
   liver cell (M8170/3) 155.0

Carcinoma — see also Neoplasm, by site, malignant — continued
lobular (infiltrating) (M8520/3)
  non-infiltrating (M8520/3)
    specified site — see Neoplasm, by site, in situ
    unspecified site 233.0
  specified site — see Neoplasm, by site, malignant
  unspecified site 174.9
lymphoepithelial (M8082/3)
medullary (M8510/3)
  with
    amyloid stroma (M8511/3)
      specified site — see Neoplasm, by site, malignant
      unspecified site 193
    lymphoid stroma (M8512/3)
      specified site — see Neoplasm, by site, malignant
      unspecified site 174.9
mesometanephric (M9110/3)
mesonephric (M9110/3)
metastatic (M8010/6) — see Metastasis, cancer
metatypical (M8095/3) — see Neoplasm, skin, malignant
morphea type basal cell (M8092/3) — see Neoplasm, skin, malignant
mucinous (M8480/3)
mucin-producing (M8481/3)
mucin-secreting (M8481/3)
mucoepidermoid (M8430/3)
mucoid (M8480/3)
  cell (M8300/3)
    specified site — see Neoplasm, by site, malignant
    unspecified site 194.3
mucous (M8480/3)
nonencapsulated sclerosing (M8350/3) 193
noninfiltrating
  intracystic (M8504/2) — see Neoplasm, by site, in situ
  intraductal (M8500/2)
    papillary (M8503/2)
      specified site — see Neoplasm, by site, in situ
      unspecified site 233.0
    specified site — see Neoplasm, by site, in situ
    unspecified site 233.0
  lobular (M8520/2)
    specified site — see Neoplasm, by site, in situ
    unspecified site 233.0
oat cell (M8042/3)
  specified site — see Neoplasm, by site, malignant
  unspecified site 162.9
odontogenic (M9270/3) 170.1
  upper jaw (bone) 170.0
onocytic (M8290/3)
oxyphilic (M8290/3)
papillary (M8050/3)
  and follicular (mixed) (M8340/3) 193
  epidermoid (M8052/3)
  intraductal (noninfiltrating) (M8503/2)
    specified site — see Neoplasm, by site, in situ
    unspecified site 233.0
  serous (M8460/3)
    specified site — see Neoplasm, by site, malignant
    surface (M8461/3)
      specified site — see Neoplasm, by site, malignant
      unspecified site 183.0
    unspecified site 183.0
  squamous cell (M8052/3)
  transitional cell (M8130/3)
papillocystic (M8450/3)
  specified site — see Neoplasm, by site, malignant
  unspecified site 183.0
parafollicular cell (M8510/3)
  specified site — see Neoplasm, by site, malignant
  unspecified site 193

Carcinoma — see also Neoplasm, by site, malignant — continued
pleomorphic (M8022/3)
polygonal cell (M8034/3)
prickle cell (M8070/3)
pseudoglandular, squamous cell (M8075/3)
pseudomucinous (M8470/3)
  specified site — see Neoplasm, by site, malignant
  unspecified site 183.0
pseudosarcomatous (M8033/3)
regaud type (M8082/3) — see Neoplasm, nasopharynx, malignant
renal cell (M8312/3) 189.0
reserve cell (M8041/3)
round cell (M8041/3)
Schmincke (M8082/3) — see Neoplasm, nasopharynx, malignant
Schneiderian (M8121/3)
  specified site — see Neoplasm, by site, malignant
  unspecified site 160.0
scirrhous (M8141/3)
sebaceous (M8410/3) — see Neoplasm, skin, malignant
secondary (M8010/6) — see Neoplasm, by site, malignant, secondary
secretory, breast (M8502/3) — see Neoplasm, breast, malignant
serous (M8441/3)
  papillary (M8460/3)
    specified site — see Neoplasm, by site, malignant
    unspecified site 183.0
  surface, papillary (M8461/3)
    specified site — see Neoplasm, by site, malignant
    unspecified site 183.0
Sertoli cell (M8640/3)
  specified site — see Neoplasm, by site, malignant
  unspecified site 186.9
signet ring cell (M8490/3)
  metastatic (M8490/6) — see Neoplasm, by site, secondary
simplex (M8231/3)
skin appendage (M8390/3) — see Neoplasm, skin, malignant
small cell (M8041/3)
  fusiform cell type (M8043/3)
  squamous cell, non-keratinizing type (M8073/3)
solid (M8230/3)
  with amyloid stroma (M8511/3)
    specified site — see Neoplasm, by site, malignant
    unspecified site 193
spheroidal cell (M8035/3)
spindle cell (M8032/3)
  and giant cell (M8030/3)
spinous cell (M8070/3)
squamous (cell) (M8070/3)
  adenoid type (M8075/3)
  and adenocarcinoma, mixed (M8560/3)
  intraepidermal, Bowen's type — see Neoplasm, skin, in situ
  keratinizing type (large cell) (M8071/3)
  large cell, non-keratinizing type (M8072/3)
  microinvasive (M8076/3)
    specified site — see Neoplasm, by site, malignant
    unspecified site 180.9
  non-keratinizing type (M8072/3)
  papillary (M8052/3)
  pseudoglandular (M8075/3)
  small cell, non-keratinizing type (M8073/3)
  spindle cell type (M8074/3)
  verrucous (M805l/3)
superficial spreading (M8143/3)
sweat gland (M8400/3) — see Neoplasm, skin, malignant
theca cell (M8600/3) 183.0
thymic (M8580/3) 164.0
trabecular (M8190/3)
transitional (cell) (M8120/3)
  papillary (M8130/3)
  spindle cell type (M8122/3)

Carcinoma — see also Neoplasm, by site, malignant — continued
tubular (M8211/3)
undifferentiated type (M8020/3)
urothelial (M8120/3)
ventriculi 151.9
verrucous (epidermoid) (squamous cell) (M8051/3)
villous (M8262/3)
water-clear cell (M8322/3) 194.1
wolffian duct (M9110/3)

Carcinomaphobia 300.29

Carcinomatosis
peritonei (M8010/6) 197.6
specified site NEC (M8010/3) — see Neoplasm, by site, malignant
unspecified site (M8010/6) 199.0

Carcinosarcoma (M8980/3) — see also Neoplasm, by site, malignant
embryonal type (M8981/3) — see Neoplasm, by site, malignant

Cardia, cardial — see condition

Cardiac — see also condition
death — see Disease, heart
device
  defibrillator, automatic implantable V45.02
  in situ NEC V45.00
  pacemaker
    cardiac
      fitting or adjustment V53.31
      in situ V45.01
    carotid sinus
      fitting or adjustment V53.39
      in situ V45.09
pacemaker — see Cardiac, device, pacemaker
tamponade 423.9

Cardialgia (see also Pain, precordial) 786.51

Cardiectasis — see Hypertrophy, cardiac

Cardiochalasia 530.81

Cardiomalacia (see also Degeneration, myocardial) 429.1

Cardiomegalia glycogenica diffusa 271.0

Cardiomegaly (see also Hypertrophy, cardiac) 429.3
congenital 746.89
glycogen 271.0
hypertensive (see also Hypertension, heart) 402.90
idiopathic 429.3

Cardiomyoliposis (see also Degeneration, myocardial) 429.1

Cardiomyopathy (congestive) (constrictive) (familial) (infiltrative) (obstructive) (restrictive) (sporadic) 425.4
alcoholic 425.5
amyloid 277.3 [425.7]
beriberi 265.0 [425.7]
cobalt-beer 425.5
congenital 425.3
due to
  amyloidosis 277.3 [425.7]
  beriberi 265.0 [425.7]
  cardiac glycogenosis 271.0 [425.7]
  Chagas' disease 086.0
  Friedreich's ataxia 334.0 [425.8]
  hypertension —see Hypertension, with, heart involvement
  mucopolysaccharidosis 277.5 [425.7]
  myotonia atrophica 359.2 [425.8]
  progressive muscular dystrophy 359.1 [425.8]
  sarcoidosis 135 [425.8]
glycogen storage 271.0 [425.7]
hypertensive — see Hypertension, with, heart involvement
hypertrophic
  nonobstructive 425.4
  obstructive 425.1
    congenital 746.84
idiopathic (concentric) 425.4
in
  Chagas' disease 086.0
  sarcoidosis 135 [425.8]
ischemic 414.8

Cardiomyopathy — *continued*
metabolic NEC 277.9 *[425.7]*
  amyloid 277.3 *[425.7]*
  thyrotoxic (*see also* Thyrotoxicosis)
    242.9 ✓5ᵗʰ *[425.7]*
  thyrotoxicosis (*see also* Thyrotoxicosis)
    242.9 ✓5ᵗʰ *[425.7]*
  nutritional 269.9 *[425.7]*
    beriberi 265.0 *[425.7]*
obscure of Africa 425.2
postpartum 674.8 ✓5ᵗʰ
primary 425.4
secondary 425.9
thyrotoxic (*see also* Thyrotoxicosis) 242.9 ✓5ᵗʰ
    [425.7]
toxic NEC 425.9
tuberculous (*see also* Tuberculosis) 017.9 ✓5ᵗʰ
    [425.8]
Cardionephritis — *see* Hypertension, cardiorenal
Cardionephropathy — *see* Hypertension,
  cardiorenal
Cardionephrosis — *see* Hypertension, cardiorenal
Cardioneurosis 306.2
Cardiopathia nigra 416.0
Cardiopathy (*see also* Disease, heart) 429.9
hypertensive (*see also* Hypertension, heart)
    402.90
idiopathic 425.4
mucopolysaccharidosis 277.5 *[425.7]*
Cardiopericarditis (*see also* Pericarditis) 423.9
Cardiophobia 300.29
Cardioptosis 746.87
Cardiorenal — *see* condition
Cardiorrhexis (*see also* Infarct, myocardium)
    410.9 ✓5ᵗʰ
Cardiosclerosis — *see* Arteriosclerosis, coronary
Cardiosis — *see* Disease, heart
Cardiospasm (esophagus) (reflex) (stomach) 530.0
congenital 750.7
Cardiostenosis — *see* Disease, heart
Cardiosymphysis 423.1
Cardiothyrotoxicosis — *see* Hyperthyroidism
Cardiovascular — *see* condition
Carditis (acute) (bacterial) (chronic) (subacute)
    429.89
Coxsackie 074.20
hypertensive (*see also* Hypertension, heart)
    402.90
meningococcal 036.40
rheumatic — *see* Disease, heart, rheumatic
rheumatoid 714.2
Care (of)
child (routine) V20.1
convalescent following V66.9
  chemotherapy V66.2
  medical NEC V66.5
  psychotherapy V66.3
  radiotherapy V66.1
  surgery V66.0
  surgical NEC V66.0
  treatment (for) V66.5
    combined V66.6
    fracture V66.4
    mental disorder NEC V66.3
    specified type NEC V66.5
end-of-life V66.7
family member (handicapped) (sick)
  creating problem for family V61.49
  provided away from home for holiday relief
    V60.5
  unavailable, due to
    absence (person rendering care) (sufferer)
      V60.4
    inability (any reason) of person rendering
      care V60.4
holiday relief V60.5
hospice V66.7
lack of (at or after birth) (infant) (child) 995.52
  adult 995.84
lactation of mother V24.1
palliative V66.7
postpartum
  immediately after delivery V24.0
  routine follow-up V24.2

Care (of) — *continued*
prenatal V22.1
  first pregnancy V22.0
  high risk pregnancy V23.9
    specified problem NEC V23.89
terminal V66.7
unavailable, due to
  absence of person rendering care V60.4
  inability (any reason) of person rendering
    care V60.4
well baby V20.1
Caries (bone) (*see also* Tuberculosis, bone)
    015.9 ✓5ᵗʰ *[730.8]* ✓5ᵗʰ
arrested 521.04
cementum 521.03
cerebrospinal (tuberculous) 015.0 ✓5ᵗʰ *[730.88]*
dental (acute) (chronic) (incipient) (infected)
    521.09
  with pulp exposure 521.03
  extending to
    dentine 521.02
    pulp 521.03
  other specified NEC 521.09
dentin (acute) (chronic) 521.02
enamel (acute) (chronic) (incipient) 521.01
external meatus 380.89
hip (*see also* Tuberculosis) 015.1 ✓5ᵗʰ *[730.85]*
knee 015.2 ✓5ᵗʰ *[730.86]*
labyrinth 386.8
limb NEC 015.7 ✓5ᵗʰ *[730.88]*
mastoid (chronic) (process) 383.1
middle ear 385.89
nose 015.7 ✓5ᵗʰ *[730.88]*
orbit 015.7 ✓5ᵗʰ *[730.88]*
ossicle 385.24
petrous bone 383.20
sacrum (tuberculous) 015.0 ✓5ᵗʰ *[730.88]*
spine, spinal (column) (tuberculous) 015.0 ✓5ᵗʰ
    [730.88]
syphilitic 095.5
  congenital 090.0 *[730.8]* ✓5ᵗʰ
teeth (internal) 521.00
  initial 521.01
vertebra (column) (tuberculous) 015.0 ✓5ᵗʰ
    [730.88]
Carini's syndrome (ichthyosis congenita) 757.1
Carious teeth 521.00
Carneous mole 631
Carnosinemia 270.5
Carotid body or sinus syndrome 337.0
Carotidynia 337.0
Carotinemia (dietary) 278.3
Carotinosis (cutis) (skin) 278.3
Carpal tunnel syndrome 354.0
Carpenter's syndrome 759.89
Carpopedal spasm (*see also* Tetany) 781.7
Carpoptosis 736.05
Carrier (suspected) **of**
amebiasis V02.2
bacterial disease (meningococcal,
    staphylococcal, streptococcal) NEC
    V02.59
cholera V02.0
cystic fibrosis gene V83.81   ●
defective gene V83.89   ▲
diphtheria V02.4
dysentery (bacillary) V02.3
  amebic V02.2
Endamoeba histolytica V02.2
gastrointestinal pathogens NEC V02.3
genetic defect V83.89   ▲
gonorrhea V02.7
group B streptococcus V02.51
HAA (hepatitis Australian-antigen) V02.61
hemophilia A (asymptomatic) V83.01
  symptomatic V83.02
hepatitis V02.60
  Australian-antigen (HAA) V02.61
  B V02.61
  C V02.62
  serum V02.61
  specified type NEC V02.69
  viral V02.60
infective organism NEC V02.9
malaria V02.9

Carrier (suspected) **of** — *continued*
paratyphoid V02.3
Salmonella V02.3
  typhosa V02.1
serum hepatitis V02.61
Shigella V02.3
Staphylococcus NEC V02.59
Streptococcus NEC V02.52
  group B V02.51
typhoid V02.1
venereal disease NEC V02.8
Carrión's disease (Bartonellosis) 088.0
Car sickness 994.6
Carter's
relapsing fever (Asiatic) 087.0
Cartilage — *see* condition
Caruncle (inflamed)
abscess, lacrimal (*see also* Dacryocystitis)
    375.30
conjunctiva 372.00
  acute 372.00
eyelid 373.00
labium (majus) (minus) 616.8
lacrimal 375.30
urethra (benign) 599.3
vagina (wall) 616.8
Cascade stomach 537.6
Caseation lymphatic gland (*see also*
    Tuberculosis) 017.2 ✓5ᵗʰ
Caseous
bronchitis — *see* Tuberculosis, pulmonary
meningitis 013.0 ✓5ᵗʰ
pneumonia — *see* Tuberculosis, pulmonary
Cassidy (-Scholte) syndrome (malignant
    carcinoid) 259.2
Castellani's bronchitis 104.8
Castleman's tumor or lymphoma (mediastinal
    lymph node hyperplasia) 785.6
Castration, traumatic 878.2
complicated 878.3
Casts in urine 791.7
Cat's ear 744.29
Catalepsy 300.11
catatonic (acute) (*see also* Schizophrenia)
    295.2 ✓5ᵗʰ
hysterical 300.11
schizophrenic (*see also* Schizophrenia)
    295.2 ✓5ᵗʰ
Cataphasia 307.0
Cataplexy (idiopathic) 347
Cataract (anterior cortical) (anterior polar) (black)
    (capsular) (central) (cortical) (hypermature)
    (immature) (incipient) (mature) 366.9
anterior
  and posterior axial embryonal 743.33
  pyramidal 743.31
  subcapsular polar
    infantile, juvenile, or presenile 366.01
    senile 366.13
associated with
  calcinosis 275.40 *[366.42]*
  craniofacial dysostosis 756.0 *[366.44]*
  galactosemia 271.1 *[366.44]*
  hypoparathyroidism 252.1 *[366.42]*
  myotonic disorders 359.2 *[366.43]*
  neovascularization 366.33
blue dot 743.39
cerulean 743.39
complicated NEC 366.30
congenital 743.30
  capsular or subcapsular 743.31
  cortical 743.32
  nuclear 743.33
  specified type NEC 743.39
  total or subtotal 743.34
  zonular 743.32
coronary (congenital) 743.39
  acquired 366.12
cupuliform 366.14
diabetic 250.5 ✓5ᵗʰ *[366.41]*
drug-induced 366.45
due to
  chalcosis 360.24 *[366.34]*

Cardiomyopathy — Cataract

Cataract — *continued*
  due to — *continued*
    chronic choroiditis (*see also* Choroiditis)
      363.20 *[366.32]*
    degenerative myopia 360.21 *[366.34]*
    glaucoma (*see also* Glaucoma) 365.9
      [366.31]
    infection, intraocular NEC 366.32
    inflammatory ocular disorder NEC 366.32
    iridocyclitis, chronic 364.10 *[366.33]*
    pigmentary retinal dystrophy 362.74
      [366.34]
    radiation 366.46
  electric 366.46
  glassblowers' 366.46
  heat ray 366.46
  heterochromic 366.33
  in eye disease NEC 366.30
  infantile (*see also* Cataract, juvenile) 366.00
  intumescent 366.12
  irradiational 366.46
  juvenile 366.00
    anterior subcapsular polar 366.01
    combined forms 366.09
    cortical 366.03
    lamellar 366.03
    nuclear 366.04
    posterior subcapsular polar 366.02
    specified NEC 366.09
    zonular 366.03
  lamellar 743.32
    infantile, juvenile, or presenile 366.03
  morgagnian 366.18
  myotonic 359.2 *[366.43]*
  myxedema 244.9 *[366.44]*
  nuclear 366.16
  posterior, polar (capsular) 743.31
    infantile, juvenile, or presenile 366.02
    senile 366.14
  presenile (*see also* Cataract, juvenile) 366.00
  punctate
    acquired 366.12
    congenital 743.39
  secondary (membrane) 366.50
    obscuring vision 366.53
    specified type, not obscuring vision 366.52
  senile 366.10
    anterior subcapsular polar 366.13
    combined forms 366.19
    cortical 366.15
    hypermature 366.18
    immature 366.12
    incipient 366.12
    mature 366.17
    nuclear 366.16
    posterior subcapsular polar 366.14
    specified NEC 366.19
    total or subtotal 366.17
  snowflake 250.5 ✓5ᵗʰ *[366.41]*
  specified NEC 366.8
  subtotal (senile) 366.17
    congenital 743.34
  sunflower 360.24 *[366.34]*
  tetanic NEC 252.1 *[366.42]*
  total (mature) (senile) 366.17
    congenital 743.34
    localized 366.21
    traumatic 366.22
  toxic 366.45
  traumatic 366.20
    partially resolved 366.23
    total 366.22
  zonular (perinuclear) 743.32
    infantile, juvenile, or presenile 366.03

Cataracta 366.10
  brunescens 366.16
  cerulea 743.39
  complicata 366.30
  congenita 743.30
  coralliformis 743.39
  coronaria (congenital) 743.39
    acquired 366.12
  diabetic 250.5 ✓5ᵗʰ *[366.41]*
  floriformis 360.24 *[366.34]*
  membranacea
    accreta 366.50
    congenita 743.39
  nigra 366.16

Catarrh, catarrhal (inflammation) (*see also*
  condition) 460
  acute 460
  asthma, asthmatic (*see also* Asthma) 493.9 ✓5ᵗʰ
  Bostock's (*see also* Fever, hay) 477.9
  bowel — *see* Enteritis
  bronchial 490
    acute 466.0
    chronic 491.0
    subacute 466.0
  cervix, cervical (canal) (uteri) — *see* Cervicitis
  chest (*see also* Bronchitis) 490
  chronic 472.0
  congestion 472.0
  conjunctivitis 372.03
  due to syphilis 095.9
    congenital 090.0
  enteric — *see* Enteritis
  epidemic 487.1
  Eustachian 381.50
  eye (acute) (vernal) 372.03
  fauces (*see also* Pharyngitis) 462
  febrile 460
  fibrinous acute 466.0
  gastroenteric — *see* Enteritis
  gastrointestinal — *see* Enteritis
  gingivitis 523.0
  hay (*see also* Fever, hay) 477.9
  infectious 460
  intestinal — *see* Enteritis
  larynx (*see also* Laryngitis, chronic) 476.0
  liver 070.1
    with hepatic coma 070.0
  lung (*see also* Bronchitis) 490
    acute 466.0
    chronic 491.0
  middle ear (chronic) — *see* Otitis media,
    chronic
  mouth 528.0
  nasal (chronic) (*see also* Rhinitis) 472.0
    acute 460
  nasobronchial 472.2
  nasopharyngeal (chronic) 472.2
    acute 460
  nose — *see* Catarrh, nasal
  ophthalmia 372.03
  pneumococcal, acute 466.0
  pulmonary (*see also* Bronchitis) 490
    acute 466.0
    chronic 491.0
  spring (eye) 372.13
  suffocating (*see also* Asthma) 493.9 ✓5ᵗʰ
  summer (hay) (*see also* Fever, hay) 477.9
  throat 472.1
  tracheitis 464.10
    with obstruction 464.11
  tubotympanal 381.4
    acute (*see also* Otitis media, acute,
      nonsuppurative) 381.00
    chronic 381.10
  vasomotor (*see also* Fever, hay) 477.9
  vesical (bladder) — *see* Cystitis

Catarrhus aestivus (*see also* Fever, hay) 477.9

Catastrophe, cerebral (*see also* Disease,
  cerebrovascular, acute) 436

Catatonia, catatonic (acute) 781.99
  with
    affective psychosis — *see* Psychosis,
      affective
  agitation 295.2 ✓5ᵗʰ
  Churg-Strauss syndrome 446.4
  dementia (praecox) 295.2 ✓5ᵗʰ
  due to or associated with physical condition
    293.89
  excitation 295.2 ✓5ᵗʰ
  excited type 295.2 ✓5ᵗʰ
  schizophrenia 295.2 ✓5ᵗʰ
  stupor 295.2 ✓5ᵗʰ

Cat-scratch — *see also* Injury, superficial disease
  or fever 078.3

Cauda equina — *see also* condition
  syndrome 344.60

Cauliflower ear 738.7

Caul over face 768.9

Causalgia 355.9
  lower limb 355.71
  upper limb 354.4

Cause
  external, general effects NEC 994.9
  not stated 799.9
  unknown 799.9

Caustic burn — *see also* Burn, by site
  from swallowing caustic or corrosive substance
    — *see* Burn, internal organs

Cavare's disease (familial periodic paralysis)
  359.3

Cave-in, injury
  crushing (severe) (*see also* Crush, by site)
    869.1
  suffocation 994.7

Cavernitis (penis) 607.2
  lymph vessel — *see* Lymphangioma

Cavernositis 607.2

Cavernous — *see* condition

Cavitation of lung (*see also* Tuberculosis)
  011.2 ✓5ᵗʰ
  nontuberculous 518.89
  primary, progressive 010.8 ✓5ᵗʰ

Cavity
  lung — *see* Cavitation of lung
  optic papilla 743.57
  pulmonary — *see* Cavitation of lung
  teeth 521.00
  vitreous (humor) 379.21

Cavovarus foot, congenital 754.59

Cavus foot (congenital) 754.71
  acquired 736.73

Cazenave's
  disease (pemphigus) NEC 694.4
  lupus (erythematosus) 695.4

Cecitis — *see* Appendicitis

Cecocele — *see* Hernia

Cecum — *see* condition

Celiac
  artery compression syndrome 447.4
  disease 579.0
  infantilism 579.0

Cell, cellular — *see also* condition
  anterior chamber (eye) (positive aqueous ray)
    364.04

Cellulitis (diffuse) (with lymphangitis) (*see also*
  Abscess) 682.9
  abdominal wall 682.2
  anaerobic (*see also* Gas gangrene) 040.0
  ankle 682.6
  anus 566
  areola 611.0
  arm (any part, above wrist) 682.3
  auditory canal (external) 380.10
  axilla 682.3
  back (any part) 682.2
  breast 611.0
    postpartum 675.1 ✓5ᵗʰ
  broad ligament (*see also* Disease, pelvis,
    inflammatory) 614.4
    acute 614.3
  buttock 682.5
  cervical (neck region) 682.1
  cervix (uteri) (*see also* Cervicitis) 616.0
  cheek, external 682.0
    internal 528.3
  chest wall 682.2
  chronic NEC 682.9
  corpus cavernosum 607.2
  digit 681.9
  Douglas' cul-de-sac or pouch (chronic) (*see also*
    Disease, pelvis, inflammatory) 614.4
    acute 614.3
  drainage site (following operation) 998.59
  ear, external 380.10
  enterostomy 569.61
  erysipelar (*see also* Erysipelas) 035
  eyelid 373.13
  face (any part, except eye) 682.0
  finger (intrathecal) (periosteal) (subcutaneous)
    (subcuticular) 681.00
  flank 682.2
  foot (except toe) 682.7

Cellulitis (*see also* Abscess) — *continued*
  forearm 682.3
  gangrenous (*see also* Gangrene) 785.4
  genital organ NEC
    female — *see* Abscess, genital organ, female
    male 608.4
  glottis 478.71
  gluteal (region) 682.5
  gonococcal NEC 098.0
  groin 682.2
  hand (except finger or thumb) 682.4
  head (except face) NEC 682.8
  heel 682.7
  hip 682.6
  jaw (region) 682.0
  knee 682.6
  labium (majus) (minus) (*see also* Vulvitis)
    616.10
  larynx 478.71
  leg, except foot 682.6
  lip 528.5
  mammary gland 611.0
  mouth (floor) 528.3
  multiple sites NEC 682.9
  nasopharynx 478.21
  navel 682.2
    newborn NEC 771.4
  neck (region) 682.1
  nipple 611.0
  nose 478.1
    external 682.0
  orbit, orbital 376.01
  palate (soft) 528.3
  pectoral (region) 682.2
  pelvis, pelvic
    with
      abortion — *see* Abortion, by type, with
        sepsis
      ectopic pregnancy (*see also* categories
        633.0— 633.9) 639.0
      molar pregnancy (*see also* categories
        630— 632) 639.0
    female (*see also* Disease, pelvis,
      inflammatory) 614.4
      acute 614.3
    following
      abortion 639.0
      ectopic or molar pregnancy 639.0
    male (*see also* Abscess, peritoneum) 567.2
    puerperal, postpartum, childbirth 670 ✓4ᵗʰ
  penis 607.2
  perineal, perineum 682.2
  perirectal 566
  peritonsillar 475
  periurethral 597.0
  periuterine (*see also* Disease, pelvis,
    inflammatory) 614.4
    acute 614.3
  pharynx 478.21
  phlegmonous NEC 682.9
  rectum 566
  retromammary 611.0
  retroperitoneal (*see also* Peritonitis) 567.2
  round ligament (*see also* Disease, pelvis,
    inflammatory) 614.4
    acute 614.3
  scalp (any part) 682.8
    dissecting 704.8
  scrotum 608.4
  seminal vesicle 608.0
  septic NEC 682.9
  shoulder 682.3
  specified sites NEC 682.8
  spermatic cord 608.4
  submandibular (region) (space) (triangle) 682.0
    gland 527.3
  submaxillary 528.3
    gland 527.3
  submental (pyogenic) 682.0
    gland 527.3
  suppurative NEC 682.9
  testis 608.4
  thigh 682.6
  thumb (intrathecal) (periosteal) (subcutaneous)
    (subcuticular) 681.00
  toe (intrathecal) (periosteal) (subcutaneous)
    (subcuticular) 681.10

Cellulitis (*see also* Abscess) — *continued*
  tonsil 475
  trunk 682.2
  tuberculous (primary) (*see also* Tuberculosis)
    017.0 ✓5ᵗʰ
  tunica vaginalis 608.4
  umbilical 682.2
    newborn NEC 771.4
  vaccinal 999.3
  vagina — *see* Vaginitis
  vas deferens 608.4
  vocal cords 478.5
  vulva (*see also* Vulvitis) 616.10
  wrist 682.4

Cementoblastoma, benign (M9273/0) 213.1
  upper jaw (bone) 213.0

Cementoma (M9273/0) 213.1
  gigantiform (M9276/0) 213.1
    upper jaw (bone) 213.0
  upper jaw (bone) 213.0

Cementoperiostitis 523.4

Cephalgia, cephalagia (*see also* Headache) 784.0
  histamine 346.2 ✓5ᵗʰ
  nonorganic origin 307.81
  psychogenic 307.81
  tension 307.81

Cephalhematocele, cephalematocele
  due to birth injury 767.1
  fetus or newborn 767.1
  traumatic (*see also* Contusion, head) 920

Cephalhematoma, cephalematoma (calcified)
  due to birth injury 767.1
  fetus or newborn 767.1
  traumatic (*see also* Contusion, head) 920

Cephalic — *see* condition

Cephalitis — *see* Encephalitis

Cephalocele 742.0

Cephaloma — *see* Neoplasm, by site, malignant

Cephalomenia 625.8

Cephalopelvic — *see* condition

Cercomoniasis 007.3

Cerebellitis — *see* Encephalitis

Cerebellum (cerebellar) — *see* condition

Cerebral — *see* condition

Cerebritis — *see* Encephalitis

Cerebrohepatorenal syndrome 759.89

Cerebromacular degeneration 330.1

Cerebromalacia (*see also* Softening, brain)
    434.9 ✓5ᵗʰ

Cerebrosidosis 272.7

Cerebrospasticity — *see* Palsy, cerebral

Cerebrospinal — *see* condition

Cerebrum — *see* condition

Ceroid storage disease 272.7

Cerumen (accumulation) (impacted) 380.4

Cervical — *see also* condition
  auricle 744.43
  rib 756.2

Cervicalgia 723.1

Cervicitis (acute) (chronic) (nonvenereal)
    (subacute) (with erosion or ectropion) 616.0
  with
    abortion — *see* Abortion, by type, with
      sepsis
    ectopic pregnancy (*see also* categories
      633.0-633.9) 639.0
    molar pregnancy (*see also* categories 630-
      632) 639.0
    ulceration 616.0
  chlamydial 099.53
  complicating pregnancy or puerperium
    646.6 ✓5ᵗʰ
    affecting fetus or newborn 760.8
  following
    abortion 639.0
    ectopic or molar pregnancy 639.0
  gonococcal (acute) 098.15
    chronic or duration of 2 months or more
      098.35
  senile (atrophic) 616.0
  syphilitic 095.8
  trichomonal 131.09

Cervicitis — *continued*
  tuberculous (*see also* Tuberculosis) 016.7 ✓5ᵗʰ

Cervicoaural fistula 744.49

Cervicocolpitis (emphysematosa) (*see also*
    Cervicitis) 616.0

Cervix — *see* condition

Cesarean delivery, operation or section NEC
    669.7 ✓5ᵗʰ
  affecting fetus or newborn 763.4
  post mortem, affecting fetus or newborn 761.6
  previous, affecting management of pregnancy
    654.2 ✓5ᵗʰ

Céstan's syndrome 344.89

Céstan-Chenais paralysis 344.89

Céstan-Raymond syndrome 433.8 ✓5ᵗʰ

Cestode infestation NEC 123.9
  specified type NEC 123.8

Cestodiasis 123.9

Chabert's disease 022.9

Chacaleh 266.2

Chafing 709.8

Chagas' disease (*see also* Trypanosomiasis,
    American) 086.2
  with heart involvement 086.0

Chagres fever 084.0

Chalasia (cardiac sphincter) 530.81

Chalazion 373.2

Chalazoderma 757.39

Chalcosis 360.24
  cornea 371.15
  crystalline lens 360.24 *[366.34]*
  retina 360.24

Chalicosis (occupational) (pulmonum) 502

Chancre (any genital site) (hard) (indurated)
    (infecting) (primary) (recurrent) 091.0
  congenital 090.0
  conjunctiva 091.2
  Ducrey's 099.0
  extragenital 091.2
  eyelid 091.2
  Hunterian 091.0
  lip (syphilis) 091.2
  mixed 099.8
  nipple 091.2
  Nisbet's 099.0
  of
    carate 103.0
    pinta 103.0
    yaws 102.0
  palate, soft 091.2
  phagedenic 099.0
  Ricord's 091.0
  Rollet's (syphilitic) 091.0
  seronegative 091.0
  seropositive 091.0
  simple 099.0
  soft 099.0
    bubo 099.0
  urethra 091.0
  yaws 102.0

Chancriform syndrome 114.1

Chancroid 099.0
  anus 099.0
  penis (Ducrey's bacillus) 099.0
  perineum 099.0
  rectum 099.0
  scrotum 099.0
  urethra 099.0
  vulva 099.0

Chandipura fever 066.8

Chandler's disease (osteochondritis dissecans,
    hip) 732.7

Change(s) (of) — *see also* Removal of
  arteriosclerotic — *see* Arteriosclerosis
  battery
    cardiac pacemaker V53.31
  bone 733.90
    diabetic 250.8 ✓5ᵗʰ *[731.8]*
    in disease, unknown cause 733.90
  bowel habits 787.99

Change(s) (of) — *see also* Removal of — *continued*
  cardiorenal (vascular) (*see also* Hypertension, cardiorenal) 404.90
  cardiovascular — *see* Disease, cardiovascular
  circulatory 459.9
  cognitive or personality change of other type, nonpsychotic 310.1
  color, teeth, tooth
    during formation 520.8
    posteruptive 521.7
  contraceptive device V25.42
  cornea, corneal
    degenerative NEC 371.40
    membrane NEC 371.30
    senile 371.41
  coronary (*see also* Ischemia, heart) 414.9
  degenerative
    chamber angle (anterior) (iris) 364.56
    ciliary body 364.57
    spine or vertebra (*see also* Spondylosis) 721.90
  dental pulp, regressive 522.2
  dressing V58.3
  fixation device V54.89 ▲
    external V54.89 ▲
    internal V54.0
  heart — *see also* Disease, heart
  hip joint 718.95
  hyperplastic larynx 478.79
  hypertrophic
    nasal sinus (*see also* Sinusitis) 473.9
    turbinate, nasal 478.0
    upper respiratory tract 478.9
  inflammatory — *see* Inflammation
  joint (*see also* Derangement, joint) 718.90
    sacroiliac 724.6
  Kirschner wire V54.89 ▲
  knee 717.9
  macular, congenital 743.55
  malignant (M—— /3) — *see also* Neoplasm, by site, malignant

> *Note* — for malignant change occurring in a neoplasm, use the appropriate M code with behavior digit /3 e.g., malignant change in uterine fibroid — M8890/3. For malignant change occurring in a nonneoplastic condition (e.g., gastric ulcer) use the M code M8000/3.

  mental (status) NEC 780.99 ▲
    due to or associated with physical condition — *see* Syndrome, brain
  myocardium, myocardial — *see* Degeneration, myocardial
  of life (*see also* Menopause) 627.2
  pacemaker battery (cardiac) V53.31
  peripheral nerve 355.9
  personality (nonpsychotic) NEC 310.1
  plaster cast V54.89 ▲
  refractive, transient 367.81
  regressive, dental pulp 522.2
  retina 362.9
    myopic (degenerative) (malignant) 360.21
    vascular appearance 362.13
  sacroiliac joint 724.6
  scleral 379.19
    degenerative 379.16
  senile (*see also* Senility) 797
  sensory (*see also* Disturbance, sensation) 782.0
  skin texture 782.8
  spinal cord 336.9
  splint, external V54.89 ▲
  subdermal implantable contraceptive V25.5
  suture V58.3
  traction device V54.89 ▲
  trophic 355.9
    arm NEC 354.9
    leg NEC 355.8
    lower extremity NEC 355.8
    upper extremity NEC 354.9
  vascular 459.9
  vasomotor 443.9
  voice 784.49
    psychogenic 306.1
Changing sleep-work schedule, affecting sleep 307.45
Changuinola fever 066.0

Chapping skin 709.8
Character
  depressive 301.12
Charcôt's
  arthropathy 094.0 [713.5]
  cirrhosis — *see* Cirrhosis, biliary
  disease 094.0
    spinal cord 094.0
  fever (biliary) (hepatic) (intermittent) — *see* Choledocholithiasis
  joint (disease) 094.0 [713.5]
    diabetic 250.6 ✓5ᵗʰ [713.5]
    syringomyelic 336.0 [713.5]
  syndrome (intermittent claudication) 443.9
    due to atherosclerosis 440.21
Charcôt-Marie-Tooth disease, paralysis, or syndrome 356.1
Charleyhorse (quadriceps) 843.8
  muscle, except quadriceps — *see* Sprain, by site
Charlouis' disease (*see also* Yaws) 102.9
Chauffeur's fracture — *see* Fracture, ulna, lower end
Cheadle (-Möller) (-Barlow) disease or syndrome (infantile scurvy) 267
Checking (of)
  contraceptive device (intrauterine) V25.42
  device
    fixation V54.89 ▲
      external V54.89 ▲
      internal V54.0
    traction V54.89 ▲
  Kirschner wire V54.89 ▲
  plaster cast V54.89 ▲
  splint, external V54.89 ▲
Checkup
  following treatment — *see* Examination
  health V70.0
  infant (not sick) V20.2
  pregnancy (normal) V22.1
    first V22.0
    high risk pregnancy V23.9
      specified problem NEC V23.89
Chédiak-Higashi (-Steinbrinck) anomaly, disease, or syndrome (congenital gigantism of peroxidase granules) 288.2
Cheek — *see also* condition
  biting 528.9
Cheese itch 133.8
Cheese washers' lung 495.8
Cheilitis 528.5
  actinic (due to sun) 692.72
    chronic NEC 692.72
      due to radiation, except from sun 692.82
    due to radiation, except from sun 692.82
  acute 528.5
  angular 528.5
  catarrhal 528.5
  chronic 528.5
  exfoliative 528.5
  gangrenous 528.5
  glandularis apostematosa 528.5
  granulomatosa 351.8
  infectional 528.5
  membranous 528.5
  Miescher's 351.8
  suppurative 528.5
  ulcerative 528.5
  vesicular 528.5
Cheilodynia 528.5
Cheilopalatoschisis (*see also* Cleft, palate, with cleft lip) 749.20
Cheilophagia 528.9
Cheiloschisis (*see also* Cleft, lip) 749.10
Cheilosis 528.5
  with pellagra 265.2
  angular 528.5
  due to
    dietary deficiency 266.0
    vitamin deficiency 266.0
Cheiromegaly 729.89
Cheiropompholyx 705.81
Cheloid (*see also* Keloid) 701.4

Chemical burn — *see also* Burn, by site
  from swallowing chemical — *see* Burn, internal organs
Chemodectoma (M8693/1) — *see* Paraganglioma, nonchromaffin
Chemoprophylaxis NEC V07.39
Chemosis, conjunctiva 372.73
Chemotherapy
  convalescence V66.2
  encounter (for) V58.1
  maintenance V58.1
  prophylactic NEC V07.39
    fluoride V07.31
Cherubism 526.89
Chest — *see* condition
Cheyne-Stokes respiration (periodic) 786.04
Chiari's
  disease or syndrome (hepatic vein thrombosis) 453.0
  malformation
    type I 348.4
    type II (*see also* Spina bifida) 741.0 ✓5ᵗʰ
    type III 742.0
    type IV 742.2
  network 746.89
Chiari-Frommel syndrome 676.6 ✓5ᵗʰ
Chicago disease (North American blastomycosis) 116.0
Chickenpox (*see also* Varicella) 052.9
  vaccination and inoculation (prophylactic) V05.4
Chiclero ulcer 085.4
Chiggers 133.8
Chignon 111.2
  fetus or newborn (from vacuum extraction) 767.1
Chigoe disease 134.1
Chikungunya fever 066.3
Chilaiditi's syndrome (subphrenic displacement, colon) 751.4
Chilblains 991.5
  lupus 991.5
Child
  behavior causing concern V61.20
Childbed fever 670 ✓4ᵗʰ
Childbirth — *see also* Delivery
  puerperal complications — *see* Puerperal
Childhood, period of rapid growth V21.0
Chill(s) 780.99 ▲
  with fever 780.6
  congestive 780.99 ▲
    in malarial regions 084.6
  septic — *see* Septicemia
  urethral 599.84
Chilomastigiasis 007.8
Chin — *see* condition
Chinese dysentery 004.9
Chiropractic dislocation (*see also* Lesion, nonallopathic, by site) 739.9
Chitral fever 066.0
Chlamydia, chlamydial — *see* condition
Chloasma 709.09
  cachecticorum 709.09
  eyelid 374.52
    congenital 757.33
    hyperthyroid 242.0 ✓5ᵗʰ
  gravidarum 646.8 ✓5ᵗʰ
  idiopathic 709.09
  skin 709.09
  symptomatic 709.09
Chloroma (M9930/3) 205.3 ✓5ᵗʰ
Chlorosis 280.9
  Egyptian (*see also* Ancylostomiasis) 126.9
  miners' (*see also* Ancylostomiasis) 126.9
Chlorotic anemia 280.9
Chocolate cyst (ovary) 617.1
Choked
  disk or disc — *see* Papilledema
  on food, phlegm, or vomitus NEC (*see also* Asphyxia, food) 933.1
  phlegm 933.1

Choked — *continued*
  while vomiting NEC (*see also* Asphyxia, food) 933.1
Chokes (resulting from bends) 993.3
Choking sensation 784.9
Cholangiectasis (*see also* Disease, gallbladder) 575.8
Cholangiocarcinoma (M8160/3)
  and hepatocellular carcinoma, combined (M8180/3) 155.0
  liver 155.1
  specified site NEC — *see* Neoplasm, by site, malignant
  unspecified site 155.1
Cholangiohepatitis 575.8
  due to fluke infestation 121.1
Cholangiohepatoma (M8180/3) 155.0
Cholangiolitis (acute) (chronic) (extrahepatic) (gangrenous) 576.1
  intrahepatic 575.8
  paratyphoidal (*see also* Fever, paratyphoid) 002.9
  typhoidal 002.0
Cholangioma (M8160/0) 211.5
  malignant — *see* Cholangiocarcinoma
Cholangitis (acute) (ascending) (catarrhal) (chronic) (infective) (malignant) (primary) (recurrent) (sclerosing) (secondary) (stenosing) (suppurative) 576.1
  chronic nonsuppurative destructive 571.6
  nonsuppurative destructive (chronic) 571.6
Cholecystdocholithiasis — *see* Choledocholithiasis
Cholecystitis 575.10
  with
    calculus, stones in
      bile duct (common) (hepatic) — *see* Choledocholithiasis
      gallbladder — *see* Cholelithiasis
  acute 575.0
  acute and chronic 575.12
  chronic 575.11
  emphysematous (acute) (*see also* Cholecystitis, acute) 575.0
  gangrenous (*see also* Cholecystitis, acute) 575.0
  paratyphoidal, current (*see also* Fever, paratyphoid) 002.9
  suppurative (*see also* Cholecystitis, acute) 575.0
  typhoidal 002.0
Choledochitis (suppurative) 576.1
Choledocholith — *see* Choledocholithiasis
Choledocholithiasis 574.5 ✓5ᵗʰ

> *Note* — *Use the following fifth-digit subclassification with category 574:*
>
> 0   *without mention of obstruction*
> 1   *with obstruction*

  with
    cholecystitis 574.4 ✓5ᵗʰ
      acute 574.3 ✓5ᵗʰ
      chronic 574.4 ✓5ᵗʰ
    cholelithiasis 574.9 ✓5ᵗʰ
      with
        cholecystitis 574.7 ✓5ᵗʰ
          acute 574.6 ✓5ᵗʰ
            and chronic 574.8 ✓5ᵗʰ
          chronic 574.7 ✓5ᵗʰ
Cholelithiasis (impacted) (multiple) 574.2 ✓5ᵗʰ

> *Note* — *Use the following fifth-digit subclassification with category 574:*
>
> 0   *without mention of obstruction*
> 1   *with obstruction*

  with
    cholecystitis 574.1 ✓5ᵗʰ
      acute 574.0 ✓5ᵗʰ
      chronic 574.1 ✓5ᵗʰ

Cholelithiasis — *continued*
  with — *continued*
    choledocholithiasis 574.9 ✓5ᵗʰ
      with
        cholecystitis 574.7 ✓5ᵗʰ
          acute 574.6 ✓5ᵗʰ
            and chronic 574.8 ✓5ᵗʰ
          chronic cholecystitis 574.7 ✓5ᵗʰ
Cholemia (*see also* Jaundice) 782.4
  familial 277.4
  Gilbert's (familial nonhemolytic) 277.4
Cholemic gallstone — *see* Cholelithiasis
Choleperitoneum, choleperitonitis (*see also* Disease, gallbladder) 567.8
Cholera (algid) (Asiatic) (asphyctic) (epidemic) (gravis) (Indian) (malignant) (morbus) (pestilential) (spasmodic) 001.9
  antimonial 985.4
  carrier (suspected) of V02.0
  classical 001.0
  contact V01.0
  due to
    Vibrio
      cholerae (Inaba, Ogawa, Hikojima serotypes) 001.0
      El Tor 001.1
  El Tor 001.1
  exposure to V01.0
  vaccination, prophylactic (against) V03.0
Cholerine (*see also* Cholera) 001.9
Cholestasis 576.8
Cholesteatoma (ear) 385.30
  attic (primary) 385.31
  diffuse 385.35
  external ear (canal) 380.21
  marginal (middle ear) 385.32
    with involvement of mastoid cavity 385.33
    secondary (with middle ear involvement) 385.33
  mastoid cavity 385.30
  middle ear (secondary) 385.32
    with involvement of mastoid cavity 385.33
  postmastoidectomy cavity (recurrent) 383.32
  primary 385.31
  recurrent, postmastoidectomy cavity 383.32
  secondary (middle ear) 385.32
    with involvement of mastoid cavity 385.33
Cholesteatosis (middle ear) (*see also* Cholesteatoma) 385.30
  diffuse 385.35
Cholesteremia 272.0
Cholesterin
  granuloma, middle ear 385.82
  in vitreous 379.22
Cholesterol
  deposit
    retina 362.82
    vitreous 379.22
  imbibition of gallbladder (*see also* Disease, gallbladder) 575.6
Cholesterolemia 272.0
  essential 272.0
  familial 272.0
  hereditary 272.0
Cholesterosis, cholesterolosis (gallbladder) 575.6
  with
    cholecystitis — *see* Cholecystitis
    cholelithiasis — *see* Cholelithiasis
  middle ear (*see also* Cholesteatoma) 385.30
Cholocolic fistula (*see also* Fistula, gallbladder) 575.5
Choluria 791.4
Chondritis (purulent) 733.99
  costal 733.6
    Tietze's 733.6
  patella, posttraumatic 717.7
  posttraumatica patellae 717.7
  tuberculous (active) (*see also* Tuberculosis) 015.9 ✓5ᵗʰ
    intervertebral 015.0 ✓5ᵗʰ [730.88]
Chondroangiopathia calcarea seu punctate 756.59

Chondroblastoma (M9230/0) — *see also* Neoplasm, bone, benign
  malignant (M9230/3) — *see* Neoplasm, bone, malignant
Chondrocalcinosis (articular) (crystal deposition) (dihydrate) (*see also* Arthritis, due to, crystals) 275.49 [712.3] ✓5ᵗʰ
  due to
    calcium pyrophosphate 275.49 [712.2] ✓5ᵗʰ
    dicalcium phosphate crystals 275.49 [712.1] ✓5ᵗʰ
    pyrophosphate crystals 275.49 [712.2] ✓5ᵗʰ
Chondrodermatitis nodularis helicis 380.00
Chondrodysplasia 756.4
  angiomatose 756.4
  calcificans congenita 756.59
  epiphysialis punctata 756.59
  hereditary deforming 756.4
Chondrodystrophia (fetalis) 756.4
  calcarea 756.4
  calcificans congenita 756.59
  fetalis hypoplastica 756.59
  hypoplastica calcinosa 756.59
  punctata 756.59
  tarda 277.5
Chondrodystrophy (familial) (hypoplastic) 756.4
Chondroectodermal dysplasia 756.55
Chondrolysis 733.99
Chondroma (M9220/0) — *see also* Neoplasm cartilage, benign
  juxtacortical (M9221/0) — *see* Neoplasm, bone, benign
  periosteal (M9221/0) — *see* Neoplasm, bone, benign
Chondromalacia 733.92
  epiglottis (congenital) 748.3
  generalized 733.92
  knee 717.7
  larynx (congenital) 748.3
  localized, except patella 733.92
  patella, patellae 717.7
  systemic 733.92
  tibial plateau 733.92
  trachea (congenital) 748.3
Chondromatosis (M9220/1) — *see* Neoplasm, cartilage, uncertain behavior
Chondromyxosarcoma (M9220/3) — *see* Neoplasm, cartilage, malignant
Chondro-osteodysplasia (Morquio- Brailsford type) 277.5
Chondro-osteodystrophy 277.5
Chondro-osteoma (M9210/0) — *see* Neoplasm, bone, benign
Chondropathia tuberosa 733.6
Chondrosarcoma (M9220/3) — *see also* Neoplasm, cartilage, malignant
  juxtacortical (M9221/3) — *see* Neoplasm, bone, malignant
  mesenchymal (M9240/3) — *see* Neoplasm, connective tissue, malignant
Chordae tendineae rupture (chronic) 429.5
Chordee (nonvenereal) 607.89
  congenital 752.63
  gonococcal 098.2
Chorditis (fibrinous) (nodosa) (tuberosa) 478.5
Chordoma (M9370/3) — *see* Neoplasm, by site, malignant
Chorea (gravis) (minor) (spasmodic) 333.5
  with
    heart involvement — *see* Chorea with rheumatic heart disease
    rheumatic heart disease (chronic, inactive, or quiescent) (conditions classifiable to 393-398) — *see also* Rheumatic heart condition involved
      active or acute (conditions classifiable to 391) 392.0
  acute — *see* Chorea, Sydenham's
  apoplectic (*see also* Disease, cerebrovascular, acute) 436
  chronic 333.4
  electric 049.8
  gravidarum — *see* Eclampsia, pregnancy

Chorea — *continued*
  habit 307.22
  hereditary 333.4
  Huntington's 333.4
  posthemiplegic 344.89
  pregnancy — *see* Eclampsia, pregnancy
  progressive 333.4
    chronic 333.4
    hereditary 333.4
  rheumatic (chronic) 392.9
    with heart disease or involvement — *see*
      Chorea, with rheumatic heart disease
  senile 333.5
  Sydenham's 392.9
    with heart involvement — *see* Chorea, with
      rheumatic heart disease
    nonrheumatic 333.5
  variabilis 307.23
Choreoathetosis (paroxysmal) 333.5
Chorioadenoma (destruens) (M9100/1) 236.1
Chorioamnionitis 658.4 ✓5ᵗʰ
  affecting fetus or newborn 762.7
Chorioangioma (M9120/0) 219.8
Choriocarcinoma (M9100/3)
  combined with
    embryonal carcinoma (M9101/3) — *see*
      Neoplasm, by site, malignant
    teratoma (M9101/3) — *see* Neoplasm, by
      site, malignant
  specified site — *see* Neoplasm, by site,
    malignant
  unspecified site
    female 181
    male 186.9
Chorioencephalitis, lymphocytic (acute) (serous)
  049.0
Chorioepithelioma (M9100/3) — *see*
  Choriocarcinoma
Choriomeningitis (acute) (benign) (lymphocytic)
  (serous) 049.0
Chorionepithelioma (M9100/3) — *see*
  Choriocarcinoma
Chorionitis (*see also* Scleroderma) 710.1
Chorioretinitis 363.20
  disseminated 363.10
    generalized 363.13
    in
      neurosyphilis 094.83
      secondary syphilis 091.51
    peripheral 363.12
    posterior pole 363.11
    tuberculous (*see also* Tuberculosis)
      017.3 ✓5ᵗʰ [363.13]
  due to
    histoplasmosis (*see also* Histoplasmosis)
      115.92
    toxoplasmosis (acquired) 130.2
      congenital (active) 771.2
  focal 363.00
    juxtapapillary 363.01
    peripheral 363.04
    posterior pole NEC 363.03
  juxtapapillaris, juxtapapillary 363.01
  progressive myopia (degeneration) 360.21
  syphilitic (secondary) 091.51
    congenital (early) 090.0 [363.13]
      late 090.5 [363.13]
    late 095.8 [363.13]
  tuberculous (*see also* Tuberculosis) 017.3 ✓5ᵗʰ
    [363.13]
Choristoma — *see* Neoplasm, by site, benign
Choroid — *see* condition
Choroideremia, choroidermia (initial stage) (late
  stage) (partial or total atrophy) 363.55
Choroiditis (*see also* Chorioretinitis) 363.20
  leprous 030.9 [363.13]
  senile guttate 363.41
  sympathetic 360.11
  syphilitic (secondary) 091.51
    congenital (early) 090.0 [363.13]
      late 090.5 [363.13]
    late 095.8 [363.13]
  Tay's 363.41
  tuberculous (*see also* Tuberculosis) 017.3 ✓5ᵗʰ
    [363.13]

Choroidopathy NEC 363.9
  degenerative (*see also* Degeneration, choroid)
    363.40
  hereditary (*see also* Dystrophy, choroid) 363.50
  specified type NEC 363.8
Choroidoretinitis — *see* Chorioretinitis
Choroidosis, central serous 362.41
Choroidretinopathy, serous 362.41
Christian's syndrome (chronic histiocytosis X)
  277.8
Christian-Weber disease (nodular nonsuppurative
  panniculitis) 729.30
Christmas disease 286.1
Chromaffinoma (M8700/0) — *see also* Neoplasm,
  by site, benign
  malignant (M8700/3) — *see* Neoplasm, by site,
    malignant
Chromatopsia 368.59
Chromhidrosis, chromidrosis 705.89
Chromoblastomycosis 117.2
Chromomycosis 117.2
Chromophytosis 111.0
Chromotrichomycosis 111.8
Chronic — *see* condition
Churg-Strauss syndrome 446.4
Chyle cyst, mesentery 457.8
Chylocele (nonfilarial) 457.8
  filarial (*see also* Infestation, filarial) 125.9
  tunica vaginalis (nonfilarial) 608.84
    filarial (*see also* Infestation, filarial) 125.9
Chylomicronemia (fasting) (with
  hyperprebetalipoproteinemia) 272.3
Chylopericardium (acute) 420.90
Chylothorax (nonfilarial) 457.8
  filarial (*see also* Infestation, filarial) 125.9
Chylous
  ascites 457.8
  cyst of peritoneum 457.8
  hydrocele 603.9
  hydrothorax (nonfilarial) 457.8
    filarial (*see also* Infestation, filarial) 125.9
Chyluria 791.1
  bilharziasis 120.0
  due to
    Brugia (malayi) 125.1
    Wuchereria (bancrofti) 125.0
      malayi 125.1
  filarial (*see also* Infestation, filarial) 125.9
  filariasis (*see also* Infestation, filarial) 125.9
  nonfilarial 791.1
Cicatricial (deformity) — *see* Cicatrix
Cicatrix (adherent) (contracted) (painful) (vicious)
  709.2
  adenoid 474.8
  alveolar process 525.8
  anus 569.49
  auricle 380.89
  bile duct (*see also* Disease, biliary) 576.8
  bladder 596.8
  bone 733.99
  brain 348.8
  cervix (postoperative) (postpartal) 622.3
    in pregnancy or childbirth 654.6 ✓5ᵗʰ
      causing obstructed labor 660.2 ✓5ᵗʰ
  chorioretinal 363.30
    disseminated 363.35
    macular 363.32
    peripheral 363.34
    posterior pole NEC 363.33
  choroid — *see* Cicatrix, chorioretinal
  common duct (*see also* Disease, biliary) 576.8
  congenital 757.39
  conjunctiva 372.64
  cornea 371.00
    tuberculous (*see also* Tuberculosis)
      017.3 ✓5ᵗʰ [371.05]
  duodenum (bulb) 537.3
  esophagus 530.3
  eyelid 374.46
    with
      ectropion — *see* Ectropion
      entropion — *see* Entropion
  hypopharynx 478.29

Cicatrix — *continued*
  knee, semilunar cartilage 717.5
  lacrimal
    canaliculi 375.53
    duct
      acquired 375.56
      neonatal 375.55
    punctum 375.52
    sac 375.54
  larynx 478.79
  limbus (cystoid) 372.64
  lung 518.89
  macular 363.32
    disseminated 363.35
    peripheral 363.34
  middle ear 385.89
  mouth 528.9
  muscle 728.89
  nasolacrimal duct
    acquired 375.56
    neonatal 375.55
  nasopharynx 478.29
  palate (soft) 528.9
  penis 607.89
  prostate 602.8
  rectum 569.49
  retina 363.30
    disseminated 363.35
    macular 363.32
    peripheral 363.34
    posterior pole NEC 363.33
  semilunar cartilage — *see* Derangement,
    meniscus
  seminal vesicle 608.89
  skin 709.2
    infected 686.8
    postinfectional 709.2
    tuberculous (*see also* Tuberculosis)
      017.0 ✓5ᵗʰ
  specified site NEC 709.2
  throat 478.29
  tongue 529.8
  tonsil (and adenoid) 474.8
  trachea 478.9
  tuberculous NEC (*see also* Tuberculosis)
    011.9 ✓5ᵗʰ
  ureter 593.89
  urethra 599.84
  uterus 621.8
  vagina 623.4
    in pregnancy or childbirth 654.7 ✓5ᵗʰ
      causing obstructed labor 660.2 ✓5ᵗʰ
  vocal cord 478.5
  wrist, constricting (annular) 709.2
CIN I [cervical intraepithelial neoplasia I] 622.1
CIN II [cervical intraepithelial neoplasia II] 622.1
CIN III [cervical intraepithelial neoplasia III] 233.1
Cinchonism
  correct substance properly administered 386.9
  overdose or wrong substance given or taken
    961.4
Circine herpes 110.5
Circle of Willis — *see* condition
Circular — *see also* condition
  hymen 752.49
Circulating anticoagulants 286.5
  following childbirth 666.3 ✓5ᵗʰ
  postpartum 666.3 ✓5ᵗʰ
Circulation
  collateral (venous), any site 459.89
  defective 459.9
    congenital 747.9
    lower extremity 459.89
  embryonic 747.9
  failure 799.8
    fetus or newborn 779.89   ▲
    peripheral 785.59
  fetal, persistent 747.83   ▲
  heart, incomplete 747.9
Circulatory system — *see* condition
Circulus senilis 371.41
Circumcision
  in absence of medical indication V50.2
  ritual V50.2
  routine V50.2

Circumscribed — *see* condition
Circumvallata placenta — *see* Placenta, abnormal
Cirrhosis, cirrhotic 571.5
  with alcoholism 571.2
  alcoholic (liver) 571.2
  atrophic (of liver) — *see* Cirrhosis, portal
  Baumgarten-Cruveilhier 571.5
  biliary (cholangiolitic) (cholangitic) (cholestatic) (extrahepatic) (hypertrophic) (intrahepatic) (nonobstructive) (obstructive) (pericholangiolitic) (posthepatic) (primary) (secondary) (xanthomatous) 571.6
    due to
      clonorchiasis 121.1
      flukes 121.3
  brain 331.9
  capsular — *see* Cirrhosis, portal
  cardiac 571.5
    alcoholic 571.2
  central (liver) — *see* Cirrhosis, liver
  Charcôt's 571.6
  cholangiolitic — *see* Cirrhosis, biliary
  cholangitic — *see* Cirrhosis, biliary
  cholestatic — *see* Cirrhosis, biliary
  clitoris (hypertrophic) 624.2
  coarsely nodular 571.5
  congestive (liver) — *see* Cirrhosis, cardiac
  Cruveilhier-Baumgarten 571.5
  cryptogenic (of liver) 571.5
    alcoholic 571.2
  dietary (*see also* Cirrhosis, portal) 571.5
  due to
    bronzed diabetes 275.0
    congestive hepatomegaly — *see* Cirrhosis, cardiac
    cystic fibrosis 277.00
    hemochromatosis 275.0
    hepatolenticular degeneration 275.1
    passive congestion (chronic) — *see* Cirrhosis, cardiac
    Wilson's disease 275.1
    xanthomatosis 272.2
  extrahepatic (obstructive) — *see* Cirrhosis, biliary
  fatty 571.8
    alcoholic 571.0
  florid 571.2
  Glisson's — *see* Cirrhosis, portal
  Hanot's (hypertrophic) — *see* Cirrhosis, biliary
  hepatic — *see* Cirrhosis, liver
  hepatolienal — *see* Cirrhosis, liver
  hobnail — *see* Cirrhosis, portal
  hypertrophic — *see also* Cirrhosis, liver
    biliary — *see* Cirrhosis, biliary
    Hanot's — *see* Cirrhosis, biliary
  infectious NEC — *see* Cirrhosis, portal
  insular — *see* Cirrhosis, portal
  intrahepatic (obstructive) (primary) (secondary) — *see* Cirrhosis, biliary
  juvenile (*see also* Cirrhosis, portal) 571.5
  kidney (*see also* Sclerosis, renal) 587
  Laennec's (of liver) 571.2
    nonalcoholic 571.5
  liver (chronic) (hepatolienal) (hypertrophic) (nodular) (splenomegalic) (unilobar) 571.5
    with alcoholism 571.2
    alcoholic 571.2
    congenital (due to failure of obliteration of umbilical vein) 777.8
    cryptogenic 571.5
      alcoholic 571.2
    fatty 571.8
      alcoholic 571.0
    macronodular 571.5
      alcoholic 571.2
    micronodular 571.5
      alcoholic 571.2
    nodular, diffuse 571.5
      alcoholic 571.2
    pigmentary 275.0
    portal 571.5
      alcoholic 571.2
    postnecrotic 571.5
      alcoholic 571.2
    syphilitic 095.3

Cirrhosis, cirrhotic — *continued*
  lung (chronic) (*see also* Fibrosis, lung) 515
  macronodular (of liver) 571.5
    alcoholic 571.2
  malarial 084.9
  metabolic NEC 571.5
  micronodular (of liver) 571.5
    alcoholic 571.2
  monolobular — *see* Cirrhosis, portal
  multilobular — *see* Cirrhosis, portal
  nephritis (*see also* Sclerosis, renal) 587
  nodular — *see* Cirrhosis, liver
  nutritional (fatty) 571.5
  obstructive (biliary) (extrahepatic) (intrahepatic) — *see* Cirrhosis, biliary
  ovarian 620.8
  paludal 084.9
  pancreas (duct) 577.8
  pericholangiolitic — *see* Cirrhosis, biliary
  periportal — *see* Cirrhosis, portal
  pigment, pigmentary (of liver) 275.0
  portal (of liver) 571.5
    alcoholic 571.2
  posthepatitic (*see also* Cirrhosis, postnecrotic) 571.5
  postnecrotic (of liver) 571.5
    alcoholic 571.2
  primary (intrahepatic) — *see* Cirrhosis, biliary
  pulmonary (*see also* Fibrosis, lung) 515
  renal (*see also* Sclerosis, renal) 587
  septal (*see also* Cirrhosis, postnecrotic) 571.5
  spleen 289.51
  splenomegalic (of liver) — *see* Cirrhosis, liver
  stasis (liver) — *see* Cirrhosis, liver
  stomach 535.4 ✔5ᵗʰ
  Todd's (*see also* Cirrhosis, biliary) 571.6
  toxic (nodular) — *see* Cirrhosis, postnecrotic
  trabecular — *see* Cirrhosis, postnecrotic
  unilobar — *see* Cirrhosis, liver
  vascular (of liver) — *see* Cirrhosis, liver
  xanthomatous (biliary) (*see also* Cirrhosis, biliary) 571.6
    due to xanthomatosis (familial) (metabolic) (primary) 272.2
Cistern, subarachnoid 793.0
Citrullinemia 270.6
Citrullinuria 270.6
Ciuffini-Pancoast tumor (M8010/3) (carcinoma, pulmonary apex) 162.3
Civatte's disease or poikiloderma 709.09
Clam diggers' itch 120.3
Clap — *see* Gonorrhea
Clark's paralysis 343.9
Clarke-Hadfield syndrome (pancreatic infantilism) 577.8
Clastothrix 704.2
Claude's syndrome 352.6
Claude Bernard-Horner syndrome (*see also* Neuropathy, peripheral, autonomic) 337.9
Claudication, intermittent 443.9
  cerebral (artery) (*see also* Ischemia, cerebral, transient) 435.9
  due to atherosclerosis 440.21
  spinal cord (arteriosclerotic) 435.1
    syphilitic 094.89
  spinalis 435.1
  venous (axillary) 453.8
Claudicatio venosa intermittens 453.8
Claustrophobia 300.29
Clavus (infected) 700
Clawfoot (congenital) 754.71
  acquired 736.74
Clawhand (acquired) 736.06
  congenital 755.59
Clawtoe (congenital) 754.71
  acquired 735.5
Clay eating 307.52
Clay shovelers' fracture — *see* Fracture, vertebra, cervical
Cleansing of artificial opening (*see also* Attention to artificial opening) V55.9
Cleft (congenital) — *see also* Imperfect, closure
  alveolar process 525.8

Cleft — *see also* Imperfect, closure — *continued*
  branchial (persistent) 744.41
    cyst 744.42
  clitoris 752.49
  cricoid cartilage, posterior 748.3
  facial (*see also* Cleft, lip) 749.10
  lip 749.10
    with cleft palate 749.20
      bilateral (lip and palate) 749.24
        with unilateral lip or palate 749.25
        complete 749.23
        incomplete 749.24
      unilateral (lip and palate) 749.22
        with bilateral lip or palate 749.25
        complete 749.21
        incomplete 749.22
    bilateral 749.14
      with cleft palate, unilateral 749.25
      complete 749.13
      incomplete 749.14
    unilateral 749.12
      with cleft palate, bilateral 749.25
      complete 749.11
      incomplete 749.12
  nose 748.1
  palate 749.00
    with cleft lip 749.20
      bilateral (lip and palate) 749.24
        with unilateral lip or palate 749.25
        complete 749.23
        incomplete 749.24
      unilateral (lip and palate) 749.22
        with bilateral lip or palate 749.25
        complete 749.21
        incomplete 749.22
    bilateral 749.04
      with cleft lip, unilateral 749.25
      complete 749.03
      incomplete 749.04
    unilateral 749.02
      with cleft lip, bilateral 749.25
      complete 749.01
      incomplete 749.02
  penis 752.69
  posterior, cricoid cartilage 748.3
  scrotum 752.8
  sternum (congenital) 756.3
  thyroid cartilage (congenital) 748.3
  tongue 750.13
  uvula 749.02
    with cleft lip (*see also* Cleft, lip, with cleft palate) 749.20
  water 366.12
Cleft hand (congenital) 755.58
Cleidocranial dysostosis 755.59
Cleidotomy, fetal 763.89
Cleptomania 312.32
Clérambault's syndrome 297.8
  erotomania 302.89
Clergyman's sore throat 784.49
Click, clicking
  systolic syndrome 785.2
Clifford's syndrome (postmaturity) 766.2
Climacteric (*see also* Menopause) 627.2
  arthritis NEC (*see also* Arthritis, climacteric) 716.3 ✔5ᵗʰ
  depression (*see also* Psychosis, affective) 296.2 ✔5ᵗʰ
  disease 627.2
    recurrent episode 296.3 ✔5ᵗʰ
    single episode 296.2 ✔5ᵗʰ
  female (symptoms) 627.2
  male (symptoms) (syndrome) 608.89
  melancholia (*see also* Psychosis, affective) 296.2 ✔5ᵗʰ
    recurrent episode 296.3 ✔5ᵗʰ
    single episode 296.2 ✔5ᵗʰ
  paranoid state 297.2
  paraphrenia 297.2
  polyarthritis NEC 716.39
    male 608.89
  symptoms (female) 627.2
Clinical research investigation (control) (participant) V70.7
Clinodactyly 755.59

Clitoris — *see* condition
Cloaca, persistent 751.5
Clonorchiasis 121.1
Clonorchiosis 121.1
Clonorchis infection, liver 121.1
Clonus 781.0
Closed bite 524.2
Closure
　artificial opening (*see also* Attention to artificial
　　opening) V55.9
　congenital, nose 748.0
　cranial sutures, premature 756.0
　defective or imperfect NEC — *see* Imperfect,
　　closure
　fistula, delayed — *see* Fistula
　fontanelle, delayed 756.0
　foramen ovale, imperfect 745.5
　hymen 623.3
　interauricular septum, defective 745.5
　interventricular septum, defective 745.4
　lacrimal duct 375.56
　　congenital 743.65
　　neonatal 375.55
　nose (congenital) 748.0
　　acquired 738.0
　vagina 623.2
　valve — *see* Endocarditis
　vulva 624.8
Clot (blood)
　artery (obstruction) (occlusion) (*see also*
　　Embolism) 444.9
　bladder 596.7
　brain (extradural or intradural) (*see also*
　　Thrombosis, brain) 434.0 ✓5ᵗʰ
　　late effects — *see* Late effect(s) (of)
　　　cerebrovascular disease
　circulation 444.9
　heart (*see also* Infarct, myocardium) 410.9 ✓5ᵗʰ
　vein (*see also* Thrombosis) 453.9
Clotting defect NEC (*see also* Defect, coagulation)
　286.9
Clouded state 780.09
　epileptic (*see also* Epilepsy) 345.9 ✓5ᵗʰ
　paroxysmal (idiopathic) (*see also* Epilepsy)
　　345.9 ✓5ᵗʰ
Clouding
　corneal graft 996.51
Cloudy
　antrum, antra 473.0
　dialysis effluent 792.5
Clouston's (hidrotic) ectodermal dysplasia
　757.31
Clubbing of fingers 781.5
Clubfinger 736.29
　acquired 736.29
　congenital 754.89
Clubfoot (congenital) 754.70
　acquired 736.71
　equinovarus 754.51
　paralytic 736.71
Club hand (congenital) 754.89
　acquired 736.07
Clubnail (acquired) 703.8
　congenital 757.5
Clump kidney 753.3
Clumsiness 781.3
　syndrome 315.4
Cluttering 307.0
Clutton's joints 090.5
Coagulation, intravascular (diffuse)
　(disseminated) (*see also* Fibrinolysis) 286.6
　newborn 776.2
Coagulopathy (*see also* Defect, coagulation) 286.9
　consumption 286.6
　intravascular (disseminated) NEC 286.6
　　newborn 776.2
Coalition
　calcaneoscaphoid 755.67
　calcaneus 755.67
　tarsal 755.67
Coal miners'
　elbow 727.2
　lung 500

Coal workers' lung or pneumoconiosis 500
Coarctation
　aorta (postductal) (preductal) 747.10
　pulmonary artery 747.3
Coated tongue 529.3
Coats' disease 362.12
Cocainism (*see also* Dependence) 304.2 ✓5ᵗʰ
Coccidioidal granuloma 114.3
Coccidioidomycosis 114.9
　with pneumonia 114.0
　cutaneous (primary) 114.1
　disseminated 114.3
　extrapulmonary (primary) 114.1
　lung 114.5
　　acute 114.0
　　chronic 114.4
　　primary 114.0
　meninges 114.2
　primary (pulmonary) 114.0
　　acute 114.0
　prostate 114.3
　pulmonary 114.5
　　acute 114.0
　　chronic 114.4
　　primary 114.0
　specified site NEC 114.3
Coccidioidosis 114.9
　lung 114.5
　　acute 114.0
　　chronic 114.4
　　primary 114.0
　meninges 114.2
Coccidiosis (colitis) (diarrhea) (dysentery) 007.2
Cocciuria 791.9
Coccus in urine 791.9
Coccydynia 724.79
Coccygodynia 724.79
Coccyx — *see* condition
Cochin-China
　diarrhea 579.1
　　anguilluliasis 127.2
　ulcer 085.1
Cock's peculiar tumor 706.2
Cockayne's disease or syndrome (microcephaly
　and dwarfism) 759.89
Cockayne-Weber syndrome (epidermolysis
　bullosa) 757.39
Cocked-up toe 735.2
Codman's tumor (benign chondroblastoma)
　(M9230/0) — *see* Neoplasm, bone, benign
Coenurosis 123.8
Coffee workers' lung 495.8
Cogan's syndrome 370.52
　congenital oculomotor apraxia 379.51
　nonsyphilitic interstitial keratitis 370.52
Coiling, umbilical cord — *see* Complications,
　umbilical cord
Coitus, painful (female) 625.0
　male 608.89
　psychogenic 302.76
Cold 460
　with influenza, flu, or grippe 487.1
　abscess — *see also* Tuberculosis, abscess
　　articular — *see* Tuberculosis, joint
　agglutinin
　　disease (chronic) or syndrome 283.0
　　hemoglobinuria 283.0
　　　paroxysmal (cold) (nocturnal) 283.2
　allergic (*see also* Fever, hay) 477.9
　bronchus or chest — *see* Bronchitis
　　with grippe or influenza 487.1
　common (head) 460
　　vaccination, prophylactic (against) V04.7
　deep 464.10
　effects of 991.9
　　specified effect NEC 991.8
　excessive 991.9
　　specified effect NEC 991.8
　exhaustion from 991.8
　exposure to 991.9
　　specified effect NEC 991.8
　grippy 487.1
　head 460

Cold — *continued*
　injury syndrome (newborn) 778.2
　intolerance 780.99　　　　　　　　　　　　　　▲
　on lung — *see* Bronchitis
　rose 477.0
　sensitivity, autoimmune 283.0
　virus 460
Coldsore (*see also* Herpes, simplex) 054.9
Colibacillosis 041.4
　generalized 038.42
Colibacilluria 791.9
Colic (recurrent) 789.0 ✓5ᵗʰ
　abdomen 789.0 ✓5ᵗʰ
　　psychogenic 307.89
　appendicular 543.9
　appendix 543.9
　bile duct — *see* Choledocholithiasis
　biliary — *see* Cholelithiasis
　bilious — *see* Cholelithiasis
　common duct — *see* Choledocholithiasis
　Devonshire NEC 984.9
　　specified type of lead — *see* Table of Drugs
　　　and Chemicals
　flatulent 787.3
　gallbladder or gallstone — *see* Cholelithiasis
　gastric 536.8
　hepatic (duct) — *see* Choledocholithiasis
　hysterical 300.11
　infantile 789.0 ✓5ᵗʰ
　intestinal 789.0 ✓5ᵗʰ
　kidney 788.0
　lead NEC 984.9
　　specified type of lead — *see* Table of Drugs
　　　and Chemicals
　liver (duct) — *see* Choledocholithiasis
　mucous 564.9
　　psychogenic 316 *[564.9]*
　nephritic 788.0
　painter's NEC 984.9
　pancreas 577.8
　psychogenic 306.4
　renal 788.0
　saturnine NEC 984.9
　　specified type of lead — *see* Table of Drugs
　　　and Chemicals
　spasmodic 789.0 ✓5ᵗʰ
　ureter 788.0
　urethral 599.84
　　due to calculus 594.2
　uterus 625.8
　　menstrual 625.3
　vermicular 543.9
　virus 460
　worm NEC 128.9
Colicystitis (*see also* Cystitis) 595.9
Colitis (acute) (catarrhal) (croupous) (cystica
　superficialis) (exudative) (hemorrhagic)
　(noninfectious) (phlegmonous) (presumed
　noninfectious) 558.9
　adaptive 564.9
　allergic 558.3
　amebic (*see also* Amebiasis) 006.9
　　nondysenteric 006.2
　anthrax 022.2
　bacillary (*see also* Infection, Shigella) 004.9
　balantidial 007.0
　chronic 558.9
　　ulcerative (*see also* Colitis, ulcerative) 556.9
　coccidial 007.2
　dietetic 558.9
　due to radiation 558.1
　functional 558.9
　gangrenous 009.0
　giardial 007.1
　granulomatous 555.1
　gravis (*see also* Colitis, ulcerative) 556.9
　infectious (*see also* Enteritis, due to, specific
　　organism) 009.0
　　presumed 009.1
　ischemic 557.9
　　acute 557.0
　　chronic 557.1
　　due to mesenteric artery insufficiency 557.1
　membranous 564.9
　　psychogenic 316 *[564.9]*

Colitis — *continued*
  mucous 564.9
    psychogenic 316 [564.9]
  necrotic 009.0
  polyposa (*see also* Colitis, ulcerative) 556.9
  protozoal NEC 007.9
  pseudomembranous 008.45
  pseudomucinous 564.9
  regional 555.1
  segmental 555.1
  septic (*see also* Enteritis, due to, specific organism) 009.0
  spastic 564.9
    psychogenic 316 [564.9]
  staphylococcus 008.41
    food 005.0
  thromboulcerative 557.0
  toxic 558.2
  transmural 555.1
  trichomonal 007.3
  tuberculous (ulcerative) 014.8 ✓5ᵗʰ
  ulcerative (chronic) (idiopathic) (nonspecific) 556.9
    entero- 556.0
    fulminant 557.0
    ileo- 556.1
    left-sided 556.5
    procto- 556.2
    proctosigmoid 556.3
    psychogenic 316 [556] ✓4ᵗʰ
    specified NEC 556.8
    universal 556.6
Collagen disease NEC 710.9
  nonvascular 710.9
  vascular (allergic) (*see also* Angiitis, hypersensitivity) 446.20
Collagenosis (*see also* Collagen disease) 710.9
  cardiovascular 425.4
  mediastinal 519.3
Collapse 780.2
  adrenal 255.8
  cardiorenal (*see also* Hypertension, cardiorenal) 404.90
  cardiorespiratory 785.51
    fetus or newborn 779.89   ▲
  cardiovascular (*see also* Disease, heart) 785.51
    fetus or newborn 779.89   ▲
  circulatory (peripheral) 785.59
    with
      abortion — *see* Abortion, by type, with shock
      ectopic pregnancy (*see also* categories 633.0-633.9) 639.5
      molar pregnancy (*see also* categories 630-632) 639.5
    during or after labor and delivery 669.1 ✓5ᵗʰ
    fetus or newborn 779.89   ▲
    following
      abortion 639.5
      ectopic or molar pregnancy 639.5
  during or after labor and delivery 669.1 ✓5ᵗʰ
    fetus or newborn 779.89   ▲
  external ear canal 380.50
    secondary to
      inflammation 380.53
      surgery 380.52
      trauma 380.51
  general 780.2
  heart — *see* Disease, heart
  heat 992.1
  hysterical 300.11
  labyrinth, membranous (congenital) 744.05
  lung (massive) (*see also* Atelectasis) 518.0
    pressure, during labor 668.0 ✓5ᵗʰ
  myocardial — *see* Disease, heart
  nervous (*see also* Disorder, mental, nonpsychotic) 300.9
  neurocirculatory 306.2
  nose 738.0
  postoperative (cardiovascular) 998.0
  pulmonary (*see also* Atelectasis) 518.0
    fetus or newborn 770.5
      partial 770.5
      primary 770.4
  thorax 512.8
    iatrogenic 512.1
    postoperative 512.1

Collapse — *continued*
  trachea 519.1
  valvular — *see* Endocarditis
  vascular (peripheral) 785.59
    with
      abortion — *see* Abortion, by type, with shock
      ectopic pregnancy (*see also* categories 633.0-633.9) 639.5
      molar pregnancy (*see also* categories 630-632) 639.5
    cerebral (*see also* Disease, cerebrovascular, acute) 436
    during or after labor and delivery 669.1 ✓5ᵗʰ
    fetus or newborn 779.89   ▲
    following
      abortion 639.5
      ectopic or molar pregnancy 639.5
  vasomotor 785.59
  vertebra 733.13
Collateral — *see also* condition
  circulation (venous) 459.89
  dilation, veins 459.89
Colles' fracture (closed) (reversed) (separation) 813.41
  open 813.51
Collet's syndrome 352.6
Collet-Sicard syndrome 352.6
Colliculitis urethralis (*see also* Urethritis) 597.89
Colliers'
  asthma 500
  lung 500
  phthisis (*see also* Tuberculosis) 011.4 ✓5ᵗʰ
Collodion baby (ichthyosis congenita) 757.1
Colloid milium 709.3
Coloboma NEC 743.49
  choroid 743.59
  fundus 743.52
  iris 743.46
  lens 743.36
  lids 743.62
  optic disc (congenital) 743.57
    acquired 377.23
  retina 743.56
  sclera 743.47
Coloenteritis — *see* Enteritis
Colon — *see* condition
Coloptosis 569.89
Color
  amblyopia NEC 368.59
    acquired 368.55
  blindness NEC (congenital) 368.59
    acquired 368.55
Colostomy
  attention to V55.3
  fitting or adjustment V53.5
  malfunctioning 569.62
  status V44.3
Colpitis (*see also* Vaginitis) 616.10
Colpocele 618.6
Colpocystitis (*see also* Vaginitis) 616.10
Colporrhexis 665.4 ✓5ᵗʰ
Colpospasm 625.1
Column, spinal, vertebral — *see* condition
Coma 780.01
  apoplectic (*see also* Disease, cerebrovascular, acute) 436
  diabetic (with ketoacidosis) 250.3 ✓5ᵗʰ
    hyperosmolar 250.2 ✓5ᵗʰ
  eclamptic (*see also* Eclampsia) 780.39
  epileptic 345.3
  hepatic 572.2
  hyperglycemic 250.2 ✓5ᵗʰ
  hyperosmolar (diabetic) (nonketotic) 250.2 ✓5ᵗʰ
  hypoglycemic 251.0
    diabetic 250.3 ✓5ᵗʰ
  insulin 250.3 ✓5ᵗʰ
    hypersmolar 250.2 ✓5ᵗʰ
    non-diabetic 251.0
    organic hyperinsulinism 251.0
  Kussmaul's (diabetic) 250.3 ✓5ᵗʰ
  liver 572.2
  newborn 779.2

Coma — *continued*
  prediabetic 250.2 ✓5ᵗʰ
  uremic — *see* Uremia
Combat fatigue (*see also* Reaction, stress, acute) 308.9
Combined — *see* condition
Comedo 706.1
Comedocarcinoma (M8501/3) — *see also* Neoplasm, breast, malignant
  noninfiltrating (M8501/2)
    specified site — *see* Neoplasm, by site, in situ
    unspecified site 233.0
Comedomastitis 610.4
Comedones 706.1
  lanugo 757.4
Comma bacillus, carrier (suspected) of V02.3
Comminuted fracture — *see* Fracture, by site
Common
  aortopulmonary trunk 745.0
  atrioventricular canal (defect) 745.69
  atrium 745.69
  cold (head) 460
    vaccination, prophylactic (against) V04.7
  truncus (arteriosus) 745.0
  ventricle 745.3
Commotio (current)
  cerebri (*see also* Concussion, brain) 850.9
    with skull fracture — *see* Fracture, skull, by site
  retinae 921.3
  spinalis — *see* Injury, spinal, by site
Commotion (current)
  brain (without skull fracture) (*see also* Concussion, brain) 850.9
    with skull fracture — *see* Fracture, skull, by site
  spinal cord — *see* Injury, spinal, by site
Communication
  abnormal — *see also* Fistula
    between
      base of aorta and pulmonary artery 745.0
      left ventricle and right atrium 745.4
      pericardial sac and pleural sac 748.8
      pulmonary artery and pulmonary vein 747.3
    congenital, between uterus and anterior abdominal wall 752.3
      bladder 752.3
      intestine 752.3
      rectum 752.3
    left ventricular— right atrial 745.4
    pulmonary artery— pulmonary vein 747.3
Compensation
  broken — *see* Failure, heart
  failure — *see* Failure, heart
  neurosis, psychoneurosis 300.11
Complaint — *see also* Disease
  bowel, functional 564.9
    psychogenic 306.4
  intestine, functional 564.9
    psychogenic 306.4
  kidney (*see also* Disease, renal) 593.9
  liver 573.9
  miners' 500
Complete — *see* condition
Complex
  cardiorenal (*see also* Hypertension, cardiorenal) 404.90
  castration 300.9
  Costen's 524.60
  ego-dystonic homosexuality 302.0
  Eisenmenger's (ventricular septal defect) 745.4
  homosexual, ego-dystonic 302.0
  hypersexual 302.89
  inferiority 301.9
  jumped process
    spine — *see* Dislocation, vertebra
  primary, tuberculosis (*see also* Tuberculosis) 010.0 ✓5ᵗʰ
  Taussig-Bing (transposition, aorta and overriding pulmonary artery) 745.11

✓4ᵗʰ Fourth-digit Required   ✓5ᵗʰ Fifth-digit Required   ▶◀ Revised Text   ● New Line   ▲ Revised Code

Complications

abortion NEC — *see* categories 634-639
accidental puncture or laceration during a
  procedure 998.2
amputation stump (late) (surgical) 997.60
  traumatic — *see* Amputation, traumatic
anastomosis (and bypass) NEC — *see also*
  Complications, due to (presence of) any
  device, implant, or graft classified to
  996.0-996.5 NEC
  hemorrhage NEC 998.11
  intestinal (internal) NEC 997.4
    involving urinary tract 997.5
  mechanical — *see* Complications,
    mechanical, graft
  urinary tract (involving intestinal tract)
    997.5
anesthesia, anesthetic NEC (*see also*
  Anesthesia, complication) 995.2
  in labor and delivery 668.9 ✓5th
    affecting fetus or newborn 763.5
    cardiac 668.1 ✓5th
    central nervous system 668.2 ✓5th
    pulmonary 668.0 ✓5th
    specified type NEC 668.8 ✓5th
aortocoronary (bypass) graft 996.03
  atherosclerosis — *see* Arteriosclerosis,
    coronary
  embolism 996.72
  occlusion NEC 996.72
  thrombus 996.72
arthroplasty 996.4
artificial opening
  cecostomy 569.60
  colostomy 569.60
  cystostomy 997.5
  enterostomy 569.60
  gastrostomy 536.40
  ileostomy 569.60
  jejunostomy 569.60
  nephrostomy 997.5
  tracheostomy 519.00
  ureterostomy 997.5
  urethrostomy 997.5
bile duct implant (prosthetic) NEC 996.79
  infection or inflammation 996.69
  mechanical 996.59
bleeding (intraoperative) (postoperative) 998.11
blood vessel graft 996.1
  aortocoronary 996.03
    atherosclerosis — *see* Arteriosclerosis,
      coronary
    embolism 996.72
    occlusion NEC 996.72
    thrombus 996.72
  atherosclerosis — *see* Arteriosclerosis,
    extremities
  embolism 996.74
  occlusion NEC 996.74
  thrombus 996.74
bone growth stimulator 996.78
  infection or inflammation 996.67
bone marrow transplant 996.85
breast implant (prosthetic) NEC 996.79
  infection or inflammation 996.69
  mechanical 996.54
bypass — *see also* Complications, anastomosis
  aortocoronary 996.03
    atherosclerosis — *see* Arteriosclerosis,
      coronary
    embolism 996.72
    occlusion NEC 996.72
    thrombus 996.72
  carotid artery 996.1
    atherosclerosis — *see* Arteriosclerosis,
      extremities
    embolism 996.74
    occulsion NEC 996.74
    thrombus 996.74
cardiac (*see also* Disease, heart) 429.9
  device, implant, or graft NEC 996.72
    infection or inflammation 996.61
    long-term effect 429.4
    mechanical (*see also* Complications,
      mechanical, by type) 996.00
    valve prosthesis 996.71
      infection or inflammation 996.61

Complications — *continued*
 cardiac (*see also* Disease, heart) — *continued*
  postoperative NEC 997.1
    long-term effect 429.4
 cardiorenal (*see also* Hypertension, cardiorenal)
  404.90
 carotid artery bypass graft 996.1
  atherosclerosis — *see* Arteriosclerosis,
    extremities
  embolism 996.74
  occlusion NEC 996.74
  thrombus 996.74
 cataract fragments in eye 998.82
 catheter device NEC — *see also* Complications,
  due to (presence of) any device, implant,
  or graft classified to 996.0-996.5 NEC
  mechanical — *see* Complications,
    mechanical, catheter
 cecostomy 569.60
 cesarean section wound 674.3 ✓5th
 chin implant (prosthetic) NEC 996.79
  infection or inflammation 996.69
  mechanical 996.59
 colostomy (enterostomy) 569.60
  specified type NEC 569.69
 contraceptive device, intrauterine NEC 996.76
  infection 996.65
  inflammation 996.65
  mechanical 996.32
 cord (umbilical) — *see* Complications, umbilical
  cord
 cornea
  due to
    contact lens 371.82
 coronary (artery) bypass (graft) NEC 996.03
  atherosclerosis — *see* Arterio-sclerosis,
    coronary
  embolism 996.72
  infection or inflammation 996.61
  mechanical 996.03
  occlusion NEC 996.72
  specified type NEC 996.72
  thrombus 996.72
 cystostomy 997.5
 delivery 669.9 ✓5th
  procedure (instrumental) (manual) (surgical)
    669.4 ✓5th
  specified type NEC 669.8 ✓5th
 dialysis (hemodialysis) (peritoneal) (renal) NEC
  999.9
  catheter NEC — *see also* Complications, due
    to (presence of) any device, implant or
    graft classified to 996.0-996.5 NEC
    infection or inflammation 996.62
      peritoneal 996.68
    mechanical 996.1
      peritoneal 996.56
 due to (presence of) any device, implant, or
  graft classified to 996.0-996.5 NEC
  996.70
  with infection or inflammation — *see*
    Complications, infection or
    inflammation, due to (presence of) any
    device, implant, or graft classified to
    996.0-996.5 NEC
  arterial NEC 996.74
    coronary NEC 996.03
      atherosclerosis — *see* Arteriosclerosis,
        coronary
      embolism 996.72
      occlusion NEC 996.72
      specified type NEC 996.72
      thrombus 996.72
    renal dialysis 996.73
  arteriovenous fistula or shunt NEC 996.74
  bone growth stimulator 996.78
  breast NEC 996.70
  cardiac NEC 996.72
    defibrillator 996.72
    pacemaker 996.72
    valve prosthesis 996.71
  catheter NEC 996.79
    spinal 996.75
    urinary, indwelling 996.76
    vascular NEC 996.74
      renal dialysis 996.73
    ventricular shunt 996.75

Complications — *continued*
 due to (presence of) any device, implant, or
  graft classified to 996.0-996.5 NEC —
  continued
  coronary (artery) bypass (graft) NEC 996.03
    atherosclerosis — *see* Arteriosclerosis,
      coronary
    embolism 996.72
    occlusion NEC 996.72
    thrombus 996.72
  electrodes
    brain 996.75
    heart 996.72
  gastrointestinal NEC 996.79
  genitourinary NEC 996.76
  heart valve prosthesis NEC 996.71
  infusion pump 996.74
  internal
    joint prosthesis 996.77
    orthopedic NEC 996.78
    specified type NEC 996.79
  intrauterine contraceptive device NEC
    996.76
  joint prosthesis, internal NEC 996.77
  mechanical — *see* Complications,
    mechanical
  nervous system NEC 996.75
  ocular lens NEC 996.79
  orbital NEC 996.79
  orthopedic NEC 996.78
    joint, internal 996.77
  renal dialysis 996.73
  specified type NEC 996.79
  urinary catheter, indwelling 996.76
  vascular NEC 996.74
  ventricular shunt 996.75
 during dialysis NEC 999.9
 ectopic or molar pregnancy NEC 639.9
 electroshock therapy NEC 999.9
 enterostomy 569.60
  specified type NEC 569.69
 external (fixation) device with internal
  component(s) NEC 996.78
  infection or inflammation 996.67
  mechanical 996.4
 extracorporeal circulation NEC 999.9
 eye implant (prosthetic) NEC 996.79
  infection or inflammation 996.69
  mechanical
    ocular lens 996.53
    orbital globe 996.59
 gastrointestinal, postoperative NEC (*see also*
  Complications, surgical procedures)
  997.4
 gastrostomy 536.40
  specified type NEC 536.49
 genitourinary device, implant or graft NEC
  996.76
  infection or inflammation 996.65
    urinary catheter, indwelling 996.64
  mechanical (*see also* Complications,
    mechanical, by type) 996.30
  specified NEC 996.39
 graft (bypass) (patch) NEC — *see also*
  Complications, due to (presence of) any
  device, implant, or graft classified to
  996.0-996.5 NEC
  bone marrow 996.85
  corneal NEC 996.79
    infection or inflammation 996.69
    rejection or reaction 996.51
  mechanical — *see* Complications,
    mechanical, graft
  organ (immune or nonimmune cause)
    (partial) (total) 996.80
    bone marrow 996.85
    heart 996.83
    intestines 996.87
    kidney 996.81
    liver 996.82
    lung 996.84
    pancreas 996.86
    specified NEC 996.89
  skin NEC 996.79
    infection or inflammation 996.69

Complications — *continued*
  graft (bypass) (patch) NEC — *see also*
    Complications, due to (presence of) any
    device, implant, or graft classified to
    996.0-996.5 NEC — *continued*
    skin NEC — *continued*
      rejection 996.52
        artificial 996.55
        decellularized allodermis 996.55
  heart — *see also* Disease, heart transplant
    (immune or nonimmune cause) 996.83
  hematoma (intraoperative) (postoperative)
    998.12
  hemorrhage (intraoperative) (postoperative)
    998.11
  hyperalimentation therapy NEC 999.9
  immunization (procedure) — *see*
    Complications, vaccination
  implant — *see also* Complications, due to
    (presence of) any device, implant, or graft
    classified to 996.0-996.5 NEC
    mechanical — *see* Complications,
      mechanical, implant
  infection and inflammation
    due to (presence of) any device, implant or
      graft classified to 996.0-996.5 NEC
      996.60
      arterial NEC 996.62
        coronary 996.61
        renal dialysis 996.62
      arteriovenous fistula or shunt 996.62
      bone growth stimulator 996.67
      breast 996.69
      cardiac 996.61
      catheter NEC 996.69
        peritoneal 996.68
        spinal 996.63
        urinary, indwelling 996.64
        vascular NEC 996.62
        ventricular shunt 996.63
      coronary artery bypass 996.61
      electrodes
        brain 996.63
        heart 996.61
      gastrointestinal NEC 996.69
      genitourinary NEC 996.65
        indwelling urinary catheter 996.64
      heart valve 996.61
      infusion pump 996.62
      intrauterine contraceptive device 996.65
      joint prosthesis, internal 996.66
      ocular lens 996.69
      orbital (implant) 996.69
      orthopedic NEC 996.67
        joint, internal 996.66
      specified type NEC 996.69
      urinary catheter, indwelling 996.64
      ventricular shunt 996.63
  infusion (procedure) 999.9
    blood — *see* Complications, transfusion
    infection NEC 999.3
    sepsis NEC 999.3
  inhalation therapy NEC 999.9
  injection (procedure) 999.9
    drug reaction (*see also* Reaction, drug) 995.2
    infection NEC 999.3
    sepsis NEC 999.3
    serum (prophylactic) (therapeutic) — *see*
      Complications, vaccination
    vaccine (any) — *see* Complications,
      vaccination
  inoculation (any) — *see* Complications,
    vaccination
  internal device (catheter) (electronic) (fixation)
    (prosthetic) NEC — *see also*
    Complications, due to (presence of) any
    device, implant, or graft classified to
    996.0-996.5 NEC
    mechanical — *see* Complications,
      mechanical
  intestinal transplant (immune or nonimmune
    cause) 996.87
  intraoperative bleeding or hemorrhage 998.11
  intrauterine contraceptive device 996.76 — *see*
    also Complications, contraceptive device
    with fetal damage affecting management of
      pregnancy 655.8 ✓5ᵗʰ

Complications — *continued*
  intrauterine contraceptive device 996.76 — *see*
    also Complications, contraceptive device
    — *continued*
    infection or inflammation 996.65
  jejunostomy 569.60
  kidney transplant (immune or nonimmune
    cause) 996.81
  labor 669.9 ✓5ᵗʰ
    specified condition NEC 669.8 ✓5ᵗʰ
  liver transplant (immune or nonimmune cause)
    996.82
  lumbar puncture 349.0
  mechanical
    anastomosis — *see* Complications,
      mechanical, graft
    bypass — *see* Complications, mechanical,
      graft
    catheter NEC 996.59
      cardiac 996.09
      cystostomy 996.39
      dialysis (hemodialysis) 996.1
        peritoneal 996.56
      during a procedure 998.2
      urethral, indwelling 996.31
    colostomy 569.62
    device NEC 996.59
      balloon (counterpulsation), intra-aortic
        996.1
      cardiac 996.00
        automatic implantable defibrillator
          996.04
        long-term effect 429.4
        specified NEC 996.09
      contraceptive, intrauterine 996.32
      counterpulsation, intra-aortic 996.1
      fixation, external, with internal
        components 996.4
      fixation, internal (nail, rod, plate) 996.4
      genitourinary 996.30
        specified NEC 996.39
      nervous system 996.2
      orthopedic, internal 996.4
      prosthetic NEC 996.59
      umbrella, vena cava 996.1
      vascular 996.1
    dorsal column stimulator 996.2
    electrode NEC 996.59
      brain 996.2
      cardiac 996.01
      spinal column 996.2
    enterostomy 569.62
    fistula, arteriovenous, surgically created
      996.1
    gastrostomy 536.42
    graft NEC 996.52
      aortic (bifurcation) 996.1
      aortocoronary bypass 996.03
      blood vessel NEC 996.1
      bone 996.4
      cardiac 996.00
      carotid artery bypass 996.1
      cartilage 996.4
      corneal 996.51
      coronary bypass 996.03
      decellularized allodermis 996.55
      genitourinary 996.30
        specified NEC 996.39
      muscle 996.4
      nervous system 996.2
      organ (immune or nonimmune cause)
        996.80
        heart 996.83
        intestines 996.87
        kidney 996.81
        liver 996.82
        lung 996.84
        pancreas 996.86
        specified NEC 996.89
      orthopedic, internal 996.4
      peripheral nerve 996.2
      prosthetic NEC 996.59
      skin 996.52
        artificial 996.55
      specified NEC 996.59
      tendon 996.4

Complications — *continued*
  mechanical — *continued*
    graft NEC — *continued*
      tissue NEC 996.52
      tooth 996.59
      ureter, without mention of resection
        996.39
      vascular 996.1
    heart valve prosthesis 996.02
      long-term effect 429.4
    implant NEC 996.59
      cardiac 996.00
        automatic implantable defibrillator
          996.04
        long-term effect 429.4
        specified NEC 996.09
      electrode NEC 996.59
        brain 996.2
        cardiac 996.01
        spinal column 996.2
      genitourinary 996.30
      nervous system 996.2
      orthopedic, internal 996.4
      prosthetic NEC 996.59
        in
          bile duct 996.59
          breast 996.54
          chin 996.59
          eye
            ocular lens 996.53
            orbital globe 996.59
      vascular 996.1
    nonabsorbable surgical material 996.59
    pacemaker NEC 996.59
      brain 996.2
      cardiac 996.01
      nerve (phrenic) 996.2
    patch — *see* Complications, mechanical,
      graft
    prosthesis NEC 996.59
      bile duct 996.59
      breast 996.54
      chin 996.59
      ocular lens 996.53
      reconstruction, vas deferens 996.39
    reimplant NEC 996.59
      extremity (*see also* Complications,
        reattached, extremity) 996.90
      organ (*see also* Complications,
        transplant, organ, by site) 996.80
    repair — *see* Complications, mechanical,
      graft
    shunt NEC 996.59
      arteriovenous, surgically created 996.1
      ventricular (communicating) 996.2
    stent NEC 996.59
    tracheostomy 519.02
    vas deferens reconstruction 996.39
  medical care NEC 999.9
    cardiac NEC 997.1
    gastrointestinal NEC 997.4
    nervous system NEC 997.00
    peripheral vascular NEC 997.2
    respiratory NEC 997.3
    urinary NEC 997.5
    vascular
      mesenteric artery 997.71
      other vessels 997.79
      peripheral vessels 997.2
      renal artery 997.72
  nephrostomy 997.5
  nervous system
    device, implant, or graft NEC 349.1
      mechanical 996.2
    postoperative NEC 997.00
  obstetric 669.9 ✓5ᵗʰ
    procedure (instrumental) (manual) (surgical)
      669.4 ✓5ᵗʰ
    specified NEC 669.8 ✓5ᵗʰ
    surgical wound 674.3 ✓5ᵗʰ
  ocular lens implant NEC 996.79
    infection or inflammation 996.69
    mechanical 996.53
  organ transplant — *see* Complications,
    transplant, organ, by site

Complications — *continued*
  orthopedic device, implant, or graft
    internal (fixation) (nail) (plate) (rod) NEC
        996.78
      infection or inflammation 996.67
      joint prosthesis 996.77
        infection or inflammation 996.66
      mechanical 996.4
    pacemaker (cardiac) 996.72
      infection or inflammation 996.61
      mechanical 996.01
    pancreas transplant (immune or nonimmune
        cause) 996.86
  perfusion NEC 999.9
  perineal repair (obstetrical) 674.3 ✓5ᵗʰ
    disruption 674.2 ✓5ᵗʰ
  pessary (uterus) (vagina) — *see* Complications,
      contraceptive device
  phototherapy 990
  postcystoscopic 997.5
  postmastoidectomy NEC 383.30
  postoperative — *see* Complications, surgical
      procedures
  pregnancy NEC 646.9 ✓5ᵗʰ
    affecting fetus or newborn 761.9
  prosthetic device, internal NEC — *see also*
      Complications, due to (presence of) any
      device, implant or graft classified to
      996.0-996.5 NEC
    mechanical NEC (*see also* Complications,
        mechanical) 996.59
  puerperium NEC (*see also* Puerperal) 674.9 ✓5ᵗʰ
  puncture, spinal 349.0
  pyelogram 997.5
  radiation 990
  radiotherapy 990
  reattached
    body part, except extremity 996.99
    extremity (infection) (rejection) 996.90
      arm(s) 996.94
      digit(s) (hand) 996.93
        foot 996.95
      finger(s) 996.93
      foot 996.95
      forearm 996.91
      hand 996.92
      leg 996.96
      lower NEC 996.96
      toe(s) 996.95
      upper NEC 996.94
  reimplant NEC — *see also* Complications, to
      (presence of) any device, implant, or graft
      classified to 996.0-996.5 NEC
    bone marrow 996.85
    extremity (*see also* Complications,
        reattached, extremity) 996.90
      due to infection 996.90
    mechanical — *see* Complications,
        mechanical, reimplant
    organ (immune or nonimmune cause)
        (partial) (total) (*see also* Complications,
        transplant, organ, by site) 996.80
  renal allograft 996.81
  renal dialysis — *see* Complications, dialysis
  respiratory 519.9
    device, implant or graft NEC 996.79
      infection or inflammation 996.69
      mechanical 996.59
    distress syndrome, adult, following trauma
        or surgery 518.5
    insufficiency, acute, postoperative 518.5
    postoperative NEC 997.3
    therapy NEC 999.9
  sedation during labor and delivery 668.9 ✓5ᵗʰ
    affecting fetus or newborn 763.5
    cardiac 668.1 ✓5ᵗʰ
    central nervous system 668.2 ✓5ᵗʰ
    pulmonary 668.0 ✓5ᵗʰ
    specified type NEC 668.8 ✓5ᵗʰ
  seroma (intraoperative) (postoperative)
      (noninfected) 998.13
    infected 998.51
  shunt NEC — *see also* Complications, due to
      (presence of) any device, implant, or graft
      classified to 996.0-996.5 NEC
    mechanical — *see* Complications,
        mechanical, shunt

Complications — *continued*
  specified body system NEC
    device, implant, or graft NEC — *see*
        Complications, due to (presence of)
        any device, implant, or graft classified
        to 996.0-996.5 NEC
    postoperative NEC 997.99
  spinal puncture or tap 349.0
  stoma, external
    gastrointestinal tract
      colostomy 569.60
      enterostomy 569.60
      gastrostomy 536.40
    urinary tract 997.5
  surgical procedures 998.9
    accidental puncture or laceration 998.2
    amputation stump (late) 997.60
    anastomosis — *see* Complications,
        anastomosis
    burst stitches or sutures ▶(external)◀
        998.32   ▲
      internal 998.31   ●
    cardiac 997.1
      long-term effect following cardiac surgery
          429.4
    cataract fragments in eye 998.82
    catheter device — *see* Complications,
        catheter device
    cecostomy malfunction 569.62
    colostomy malfunction 569.62
    cystostomy malfunction 997.5
    dehiscence (of incision) ▶(external)◀
        998.32   ▲
      internal 998.31   ●
    dialysis NEC (*see also* Complications,
        dialysis) 999.9
    disruption
      anastomosis (internal) — *see*
          Complications, mechanical, graft
      internal suture (line) 998.31   ▲
      wound ▶(external)◀ 998.32   ▲
        internal 998.31   ●
    dumping syndrome (postgastrectomy) 564.2
    elephantiasis or lymphedema 997.99
      postmastectomy 457.0
    emphysema (surgical) 998.81
    enterostomy malfunction 569.62
    evisceration 998.32   ▲
    fistula (persistent postoperative) 998.6
    foreign body inadvertently left in wound
        (sponge) (suture) (swab) 998.4
    from nonabsorbable surgical material
        (Dacron) (mesh) (permanent suture)
        (reinforcing) (Teflon) — *see*
        Complications, due to (presence of)
        any device, implant, or graft classified
        to 996.0-996.5 NEC
    gastrointestinal NEC 997.4
    gastrostomy malfunction 536.42
    hematoma 998.12
    hemorrhage 998.11
    ileostomy malfunction 569.62
    internal prosthetic device NEC (*see also*
        Complications, internal device) 996.70
      hemolytic anemia 283.19
      infection or inflammation 996.60
      malfunction — *see* Complications,
          mechanical
      mechanical complication — *see*
          Complications, mechanical
      thrombus 996.70
    jejunostomy malfunction 569.62
    nervous system NEC 997.00
    obstruction, internal anastomosis — *see*
        Complications, mechanical, graft
    other body system NEC 997.99
    peripheral vascular NEC 997.2
    postcardiotomy syndrome 429.4
    postcholecystectomy syndrome 576.0
    postcommissurotomy syndrome 429.4
    postgastrectomy dumping syndrome 564.2
    postmastectomy lymphedema syndrome
        457.0
    postmastoidectomy 383.30
      cholesteatoma, recurrent 383.32
      cyst, mucosal 383.31
      granulation 383.33

Complications — *continued*
  surgical procedures — *continued*
    postmastoidectomy — *continued*
      inflammation, chronic 383.33
    postvagotomy syndrome 564.2
    postvalvulotomy syndrome 429.4
    reattached extremity (infection) (rejection)
        (*see also* Complications, reattached,
        extremity) 996.90
    respiratory NEC 997.3
    seroma 998.13
    shock (endotoxic) (hypovolemic) (septic)
        998.0
    shunt, prosthetic (thrombus) — *see also*
        Complications, due to (presence of)
        any device, implant, or graft classified
        to 996.0-996.5 NEC
      hemolytic anemia 283.19
    specified complication NEC 998.89
    stitch abscess 998.59
    transplant — *see* Complications, graft
    ureterostomy malfunction 997.5
    urethrostomy malfunction 997.5
    urinary NEC 997.5
    vascular
      mesenteric artery 997.71
      other vessels 997.79
      peripheral vessels 997.2
      renal artery 997.72
    wound infection 998.59
  therapeutic misadventure NEC 999.9
    surgical treatment 998.9
  tracheostomy 519.00
  transfusion (blood) (lymphocytes) (plasma) NEC
      999.8
    atrophy, liver, yellow, subacute (within 8
        months of administration) — *see*
        Hepatitis, viral
    bone marrow 996.85
    embolism
      air 999.1
      thrombus 999.2
    hemolysis NEC 999.8
      bone marrow 996.85
    hepatitis (serum) (type B) (within 8 months
        after administration) — *see* Hepatitis,
        viral
    incompatibility reaction (ABO) (blood group)
        999.6
      Rh (factor) 999.7
    infection 999.3
    jaundice (serum) (within 8 months after
        administration) — *see* Hepatitis, viral
    sepsis 999.3
    shock or reaction NEC 999.8
      bone marrow 996.85
    subacute yellow atrophy of liver (within 8
        months after administration) — *see*
        Hepatitis, viral
    thromboembolism 999.2
  transplant NEC — *see also* Complications, due
      to (presence of) any device, implant, or
      graft classified to 996.0-996.5 NEC
    bone marrow 996.85
    organ (immune or nonimmune cause)
        (partial) (total) 996.80
      bone marrow 996.85
      heart 996.83
      intestines 996.87
      kidney 996.81
      liver 996.82
      lung 996.84
      pancreas 996.86
      specified NEC 996.89
  trauma NEC (early) 958.8
  ultrasound therapy NEC 999.9
  umbilical cord
    affecting fetus or newborn 762.6
    complicating delivery 663.9 ✓5ᵗʰ
      affecting fetus or newborn 762.6
      specified type NEC 663.8 ✓5ᵗʰ
  urethral catheter NEC 996.76
    infection or inflammation 996.64
    mechanical 996.31
  urinary, postoperative NEC 997.5
  vaccination 999.9
    anaphylaxis NEC 999.4

Complications — *continued*
vaccination — *continued*
cellulitis 999.3
encephalitis or encephalomyelitis 323.5
hepatitis (serum) (type B) (within 8 months after administration) — *see* Hepatitis, viral
infection (general) (local) NEC 999.3
jaundice (serum) (within 8 months after administration) — *see* Hepatitis, viral
meningitis 997.09 *[321.8]*
myelitis 323.5
protein sickness 999.5
reaction (allergic) 999.5
Herxheimer's 995.0
serum 999.5
sepsis 999.3
serum intoxication, sickness, rash, or other serum reaction NEC 999.5
shock (allergic) (anaphylactic) 999.4
subacute yellow atrophy of liver (within 8 months after administration) — *see* Hepatitis, viral
vaccinia (generalized) 999.0
localized 999.3
vascular
device, implant, or graft NEC 996.74
infection or inflammation 996.62
mechanical NEC 996.1
cardiac (*see also* Complications, mechanical, by type) 996.00
following infusion, perfusion, or transfusion 999.2
postoperative NEC 997.2
mesenteric artery 997.71
other vessels 997.79
peripheral vessels 997.2
renal artery 997.72
ventilation therapy NEC 999.9
Compound presentation, complicating delivery 652.8 ✓5ᵗʰ
causing obstructed labor 660.0 ✓5ᵗʰ
Compressed air disease 993.3
Compression
with injury — *see* specific injury
arm NEC 354.9
artery 447.1
celiac, syndrome 447.4
brachial plexus 353.0
brain (stem) 348.4
due to
contusion, brain — *see* Contusion, brain
injury NEC — *see also* Hemorrhage, brain, traumatic
birth — *see* Birth, injury, brain
laceration, brain — *see* Laceration, brain
osteopathic 739.0
bronchus 519.1
by cicatrix — *see* Cicatrix
cardiac 423.9
cauda equina 344.60
with neurogenic bladder 344.61
celiac (artery) (axis) 447.4
cerebral — *see* Compression, brain
cervical plexus 353.2
cord (umbilical) — *see* Compression, umbilical cord
cranial nerve 352.9
second 377.49
third (partial) 378.51
total 378.52
fourth 378.53
fifth 350.8
sixth 378.54
seventh 351.8
divers' squeeze 993.3
duodenum (external) (*see also* Obstruction, duodenum) 537.3
during birth 767.9
esophagus 530.3
congenital, external 750.3
Eustachian tube 381.63
facies (congenital) 754.0
fracture — *see* Fracture, by site
heart — *see* Disease, heart

Compression — *continued*
intestine (*see also* Obstruction, intestine) 560.9
with hernia — *see* Hernia, by site, with obstruction
laryngeal nerve, recurrent 478.79
leg NEC 355.8
lower extremity NEC 355.8
lumbosacral plexus 353.1
lung 518.89
lymphatic vessel 457.1
medulla — *see* Compression, brain
nerve NEC — *see also* Disorder, nerve
arm NEC 354.9
autonomic nervous system (*see also* Neuropathy, peripheral, autonomic) 337.9
axillary 353.0
cranial NEC 352.9
due to displacement of intervertebral disc 722.2
with myelopathy 722.70
cervical 722.0
with myelopathy 722.71
lumbar, lumbosacral 722.10
with myelopathy 722.73
thoracic, thoracolumbar 722.11
with myelopathy 722.72
iliohypogastric 355.79
ilioinguinal 355.79
leg NEC 355.8
lower extremity NEC 355.8
median (in carpal tunnel) 354.0
obturator 355.79
optic 377.49
plantar 355.6
posterior tibial (in tarsal tunnel) 355.5
root (by scar tissue) NEC 724.9
cervical NEC 723.4
lumbar NEC 724.4
lumbosacral 724.4
thoracic 724.4
saphenous 355.79
sciatic (acute) 355.0
sympathetic 337.9
traumatic — *see* Injury, nerve
ulnar 354.2
upper extremity NEC 354.9
peripheral — *see* Compression, nerve
spinal (cord) (old or nontraumatic) 336.9
by displacement of intervertebral disc — *see* Displacement, intervertebral disc
nerve
root NEC 724.9
postoperative 722.80
cervical region 722.81
lumbar region 722.83
thoracic region 722.82
traumatic — *see* Injury, nerve, spinal
traumatic — *see* Injury, nerve, spinal
spondylogenic 721.91
cervical 721.1
lumbar, lumbosacral 721.42
thoracic 721.41
traumatic — *see also* Injury, spinal, by site
with fracture, vertebra — *see* Fracture, vertebra, by site, with spinal cord injury
spondylogenic — *see* Compression, spinal cord, spondylogenic
subcostal nerve (syndrome) 354.8
sympathetic nerve NEC 337.9
syndrome 958.5
thorax 512.8
iatrogenic 512.1
postoperative 512.1
trachea 519.1
congenital 748.3
ulnar nerve (by scar tissue) 354.2
umbilical cord
affecting fetus or newborn 762.5
cord prolapsed 762.4
complicating delivery 663.2 ✓5ᵗʰ
cord around neck 663.1 ✓5ᵗʰ
cord prolapsed 663.0 ✓5ᵗʰ
upper extremity NEC 354.9
ureter 593.3
urethra — *see* Stricture, urethra

Compression — *continued*
vein 459.2
vena cava (inferior) (superior) 459.2
vertebral NEC — *see* Compression, spinal (cord)
Compulsion, compulsive
eating 307.51
neurosis (obsessive) 300.3
personality 301.4
states (mixed) 300.3
swearing 300.3
in Gilles de la Tourette's syndrome 307.23
tics and spasms 307.22
water drinking NEC (syndrome) 307.9
Concato's disease (pericardial polyserositis) 423.2
peritoneal 568.82
pleural — *see* Pleurisy
Concavity, chest wall 738.3
Concealed
hemorrhage NEC 459.0
penis 752.65
Concentric fading 368.12
Concern (normal) about sick person in family V61.49
Concrescence (teeth) 520.2
Concretio cordis 423.1
rheumatic 393
Concretion — *see also* Calculus
appendicular 543.9
canaliculus 375.57
clitoris 624.8
conjunctiva 372.54
eyelid 374.56
intestine (impaction) (obstruction) 560.39
lacrimal (passages) 375.57
prepuce (male) 605
female (clitoris) 624.8
salivary gland (any) 527.5
seminal vesicle 608.89
stomach 537.89
tonsil 474.8
Concussion (current) 850.9
with
loss of consciousness 850.5
brief (less than one hour) 850.1
moderate (1-24 hours) 850.2
prolonged (more than 24 hours) (with complete recovery) (with return to pre-existing conscious level) 850.3
without return to pre-existing conscious level 850.4
mental confusion or disorientation (without loss of consciousness) 850.0
with loss of consciousness — *see* Concussion, with, loss of consciousness
without loss of consciousness 850.0
blast (air) (hydraulic) (immersion) (underwater) 869.0
with open wound into cavity 869.1
abdomen or thorax — *see* Injury, internal, by site
brain — *see* Concussion, brain
ear (acoustic nerve trauma) 951.5
with perforation, tympanic membrane — *see* Wound, open, ear drum
thorax — *see* Injury, internal, intrathoracic organs NEC
brain or cerebral (without skull fracture) 850.9
with
loss of consciousness 850.5
brief (less than one hour) 850.1
moderate (1-24 hours) 850.2
prolonged (more than 24 hours) (with complete recovery) (with return to pre-existing conscious level) 850.3
without return to pre-existing conscious level 850.4
mental confusion or disorientation (without loss of consciousness) 850.0
with loss of consciousness — *see* Concussion, brain, with, loss of consciousness

✓4ᵗʰ Fourth-digit Required   ✓5ᵗʰ Fifth-digit Required   ▶◀ Revised Text   ● New Line   ▲ Revised Code

Concussion — *continued*
  brain or cerebral — *continued*
    with — *continued*
      skull fracture — *see* Fracture, skull, by
          site
      without loss of consciousness 850.0
  cauda equina 952.4
  cerebral — *see* Concussion, brain
  conus medullaris (spine) 952.4
  hydraulic — *see* Concussion, blast
  internal organs — *see* Injury, internal, by site
  labyrinth — *see* Injury, intracranial
  ocular 921.3
  osseous labyrinth — *see* Injury, intracranial
  spinal (cord) — *see also* Injury, spinal, by site
    due to
      broken
        back — *see* Fracture, vertebra, by site,
            with spinal cord injury
        neck — *see* Fracture, vertebra,
            cervical, with spinal cord injury
      fracture, fracture dislocation, or
          compression fracture of spine or
          vertebra — *see* Fracture, vertebra,
          by site, with spinal cord injury
  syndrome 310.2
  underwater blast — *see* Concussion, blast
Condition — *see also* Disease
  psychiatric 298.9
  respiratory NEC 519.9
    acute or subacute NEC 519.9
      due to
        external agent 508.9
          specified type NEC 508.8
        fumes or vapors (chemical) (inhalation)
            506.3
        radiation 508.0
    chronic NEC 519.9
      due to
        external agent 508.9
          specified type NEC 508.8
        fumes or vapors (chemical) (inhalation)
            506.4
        radiation 508.1
    due to
      external agent 508.9
        specified type NEC 508.8
      fumes or vapors (chemical) (inhalation)
          506.9
Conduct disturbance (*see also* Disturbance,
    conduct) 312.9
  adjustment reaction 309.3
  hyperkinetic 314.2
Condyloma NEC 078.10
  acuminatum 078.11
  gonorrheal 098.0
  latum 091.3
  syphilitic 091.3
    congenital 090.0
  venereal, syphilitic 091.3
Confinement — *see* Delivery
Conflagration — *see also* Burn, by site
  asphyxia (by inhalation of smoke, gases, fumes,
      or vapors) 987.9
  specified agent — *see* Table of Drugs and
      Chemicals
Conflict
  family V61.9
    specified circumstance NEC V61.8
  interpersonal NEC V62.81
  marital V61.10
    involving divorce or estrangement V61.0
  parent-child V61.20
  partner V61.10
Confluent — *see* condition
Confusion, confused (mental) (state) (*see also*
    State, confusional) 298.9
  acute 293.0
  epileptic 293.0
  postoperative 293.9
  psychogenic 298.2
  reactive (from emotional stress, psychological
      trauma) 298.2
  subacute 293.1
Congelation 991.9

Congenital — *see also* condition
  aortic septum 747.29
  intrinsic factor deficiency 281.0
  malformation — *see* Anomaly
Congestion, congestive (chronic) (passive)
  asphyxia, newborn 768.9
  bladder 596.8
  bowel 569.89
  brain (*see also* Disease, cerebrovascular NEC)
      437.8
    malarial 084.9
  breast 611.79
  bronchi 519.1
  bronchial tube 519.1
  catarrhal 472.0
  cerebral — *see* Congestion, brain
  cerebrospinal — *see* Congestion, brain
  chest 514
  chill 780.99   ▲
    malarial (*see also* Malaria) 084.6
  circulatory NEC 459.9
  conjunctiva 372.71
  due to disturbance of circulation 459.9
  duodenum 537.3
  enteritis — *see* Enteritis
  eye 372.71
  fibrosis syndrome (pelvic) 625.5
  gastroenteritis — *see* Enteritis
  general 799.8
  glottis 476.0
  heart (*see also* Failure, heart) 428.0
  hepatic 573.0
  hypostatic (lung) 514
  intestine 569.89
  intracranial — *see* Congestion, brain
  kidney 593.89
  labyrinth 386.50
  larynx 476.0
  liver 573.0
  lung 514
    active or acute (*see also* Pneumonia) 486
      congenital 770.0
    chronic 514
    hypostatic 514
    idiopathic, acute 518.5
    passive 514
  malaria, malarial (brain) (fever) (*see also*
      Malaria) 084.6
  medulla — *see* Congestion, brain
  nasal 478.1
  orbit, orbital 376.33
    inflammatory (chronic) 376.10
      acute 376.00
  ovary 620.8
  pancreas 577.8
  pelvic, female 625.5
  pleural 511.0
  prostate (active) 602.1
  pulmonary — *see* Congestion, lung
  renal 593.89
  retina 362.89
  seminal vesicle 608.89
  spinal cord 336.1
  spleen 289.51
    chronic 289.51
  stomach 537.89
  trachea 464.11
  urethra 599.84
  uterus 625.5
    with subinvolution 621.1
  viscera 799.8
Congestive — *see* Congestion
Conical
  cervix 622.6
  cornea 371.60
  teeth 520.2
Conjoined twins 759.4
  causing disproportion (fetopelvic) 653.7 ✔5ᵗʰ
Conjugal maladjustment V61.10
  involving divorce or estrangement V61.0
Conjunctiva — *see* condition
Conjunctivitis (exposure) (infectious)
    (nondiphtheritic) (pneumococcal) (pustular)
    (staphylococcal) (streptococcal) NEC 372.30
  actinic 370.24
  acute 372.00

Conjunctivitis NEC — *continued*
  acute — *continued*
    atopic 372.05
    contagious 372.03
    follicular 372.02
    hemorrhagic (viral) 077.4
  adenoviral (acute) 077.3
  allergic (chronic) 372.14
    with hay fever 372.05
  anaphylactic 372.05
  angular 372.03
  Apollo (viral) 077.4
  atopic 372.05
  blennorrhagic (neonatorum) 098.40
  catarrhal 372.03
  chemical 372.05
  chlamydial 077.98
    due to
      Chlamydia trachomatis — *see* Trachoma
        paratrachoma 077.0
  chronic 372.10
    allergic 372.14
    follicular 372.12
    simple 372.11
    specified type NEC 372.14
    vernal 372.13
  diphtheritic 032.81
  due to
    dust 372.05
    enterovirus type 70 077.4
    erythema multiforme 695.1 *[372.33]*
    filariasis (*see also* Filariasis) 125.9 *[372.15]*
    mucocutaneous
      disease NEC 372.33
      leishmaniasis 085.5 *[372.15]*
    Reiter's disease 099.3 *[372.33]*
    syphilis 095.8 *[372.10]*
    toxoplasmosis (acquired) 130.1
      congenital (active) 771.2
    trachoma — *see* Trachoma
  dust 372.05
  eczematous 370.31
  epidemic 077.1
    hemorrhagic 077.4
  follicular (acute) 372.02
    adenoviral (acute) 077.3
    chronic 372.12
  glare 370.24
  gonococcal (neonatorum) 098.40
  granular (trachomatous) 076.1
    late effect 139.1
  hemorrhagic (acute) (epidemic) 077.4
  herpetic (simplex) 054.43
    zoster 053.21
  inclusion 077.0
  infantile 771.6
  influenzal 372.03
  Koch-Weeks 372.03
  light 372.05
  medicamentosa 372.05
  membranous 372.04
  meningococcic 036.89
  Morax-Axenfeld 372.02
  mucopurulent NEC 372.03
  neonatal 771.6
    gonococcal 098.40
  Newcastle's 077.8
  nodosa 360.14
  of Beal 077.3
  parasitic 372.15
    filariasis (*see also* Filariasis) 125.9 *[372.15]*
    mucocutaneous leishmaniasis 085.5
        [372.15]
  Parinaud's 372.02
  petrificans 372.39
  phlyctenular 370.31
  pseudomembranous 372.04
    diphtheritic 032.81
  purulent 372.03
  Reiter's 099.3 *[372.33]*
  rosacea 695.3 *[372.31]*
  serous 372.01
    viral 077.99
  simple chronic 372.11
  specified NEC 372.39
  sunlamp 372.04
  swimming pool 077.0

Contraction — Contusion

Contraction, contracture, contracted — *continued*
muscle NEC — *continued*
  congenital 756.89
    sternocleidomastoid 754.1
  extraocular 378.60
  eye (extrinsic) (*see also* Strabismus) 378.9
    paralytic (*see also* Strabismus, paralytic) 378.50
  flaccid 728.85
  hysterical 300.11
  ischemic (Volkmann's) 958.6
  paralytic 728.85
  posttraumatic 958.6
  psychogenic 306.0
    specified as conversion reaction 300.11
myotonic 728.85
neck (*see also* Torticollis) 723.5
  congenital 754.1
  psychogenic 306.0
ocular muscle (*see also* Strabismus) 378.9
  paralytic (*see also* Strabismus, paralytic) 378.50
organ or site, congenital NEC — *see* Atresia
outlet (pelvis) — *see* Contraction, pelvis
palmar fascia 728.6
paralytic
  joint (*see also* Contraction, joint) 718.4 ✓5ᵗʰ
  muscle 728.85
    ocular (*see also* Strabismus, paralytic) 378.50
pelvis (acquired) (general) 738.6
  affecting fetus or newborn 763.1
  complicating delivery 653.1 ✓5ᵗʰ
    causing obstructed labor 660.1 ✓5ᵗʰ
    generally contracted 653.1 ✓5ᵗʰ
      causing obstructed labor 660.1 ✓5ᵗʰ
    inlet 653.2 ✓5ᵗʰ
      causing obstructed labor 660.1 ✓5ᵗʰ
    midpelvic 653.8 ✓5ᵗʰ
      causing obstructed labor 660.1 ✓5ᵗʰ
    midplane 653.8 ✓5ᵗʰ
      causing obstructed labor 660.1 ✓5ᵗʰ
    outlet 653.3 ✓5ᵗʰ
      causing obstructed labor 660.1 ✓5ᵗʰ
plantar fascia 728.71
premature
  atrial 427.61
  auricular 427.61
  auriculoventricular 427.61
  heart (junctional) (nodal) 427.60
  supraventricular 427.61
  ventricular 427.69
prostate 602.8
pylorus (*see also* Pylorospasm) 537.81
rectosigmoid (*see also* Obstruction, intestine) 560.9
rectum, rectal (sphincter) 564.89
  psychogenic 306.4
ring (Bandl's) 661.4 ✓5ᵗʰ
  affecting fetus or newborn 763.7
scar — *see* Cicatrix
sigmoid (*see also* Obstruction, intestine) 560.9
socket, eye 372.64
spine (*see also* Curvature, spine) 737.9
stomach 536.8
  hourglass 536.8
    congenital 750.7
    psychogenic 306.4
  psychogenic 306.4
tendon (sheath) (*see also* Short, tendon) 727.81
toe 735.8
ureterovesical orifice (postinfectional) 593.3
urethra 599.84
uterus 621.8
  abnormal 661.9 ✓5ᵗʰ
    affecting fetus or newborn 763.7
  clonic, hourglass or tetanic 661.4 ✓5ᵗʰ
    affecting fetus or newborn 763.7
  dyscoordinate 661.4 ✓5ᵗʰ
    affecting fetus or newborn 763.7
  hourglass 661.4 ✓5ᵗʰ
    affecting fetus or newborn 763.7
  hypotonic NEC 661.2 ✓5ᵗʰ
    affecting fetus or newborn 763.7
  incoordinate 661.4 ✓5ᵗʰ
    affecting fetus or newborn 763.7

Contraction, contracture, contracted — *continued*
uterus — *continued*
  inefficient or poor 661.2 ✓5ᵗʰ
    affecting fetus or newborn 763.7
  irregular 661.2 ✓5ᵗʰ
    affecting fetus or newborn 763.7
  tetanic 661.4 ✓5ᵗʰ
    affecting fetus or newborn 763.7
vagina (outlet) 623.2
vesical 596.8
  neck or urethral orifice 596.0
visual field, generalized 368.45
Volkmann's (ischemic) 958.6
Contusion (skin surface intact) 924.9
with
  crush injury — *see* Crush
  dislocation — *see* Dislocation, by site
  fracture — *see* Fracture, by site
  internal injury — *see also* Injury, internal, by site
    heart — *see* Contusion, cardiac
    kidney — *see* Contusion, kidney
    liver — *see* Contusion, liver
    lung — *see* Contusion, lung
    spleen — *see* Contusion, spleen
  intracranial injury — *see* Injury, intracranial
  nerve injury — *see* Injury, nerve
  open wound — *see* Wound, open, by site
abdomen, abdominal (muscle) (wall) 922.2
  organ(s) NEC 868.00
adnexa, eye NEC 921.9
ankle 924.21
  with other parts of foot 924.20
arm 923.9
  lower (with elbow) 923.10
  upper 923.03
    with shoulder or axillary region 923.09
auditory canal (external) (meatus) (and other part(s) of neck, scalp, or face, except eye) 920
auricle, ear (and other part(s) of neck, scalp, or face except eye) 920
axilla 923.02
  with shoulder or upper am 923.09
back 922.31
bone NEC 924.9
brain (cerebral) (membrane) (with hemorrhage) 851.8 ✓5ᵗʰ

Note — Use the following fifth-digit subclassification with categories 851-854:

  0   unspecified state of consciousness

  1   with no loss of consciousness

  2   with brief [less than one hour] loss of consciousness

  3   with moderate [1-24 hours] loss of consciousness

  4   with prolonged [more than 24 hours] loss of consciousness and return to pre-existing conscious level

  5   with prolonged [more than 24 hours] loss of consciousness, without return to pre-existing conscious level

  Use fifth-digit to designate when a patient is unconscious and dies before regaining consciousness, regardless of the duration of the loss of consciousness

  6   with loss of consciousness of unspecified duration

  9   with concussion, unspecified

---

  with
    open intracranial wound 851.9 ✓5ᵗʰ
    skull fracture — *see* Fracture, skull, by site
  cerebellum 851.4 ✓5ᵗʰ
    with open intracranial wound 851.5 ✓5ᵗʰ
  cortex 851.0 ✓5ᵗʰ
    with open intracranial wound 851.1 ✓5ᵗʰ
  occipital lobe 851.4 ✓5ᵗʰ
    with open intracranial wound 851.5 ✓5ᵗʰ

Contusion — *continued*
brain — *continued*
  stem 851.4 ✓5ᵗʰ
    with open intracranial wound 851.5 ✓5ᵗʰ
breast 922.0
brow (and other part(s) of neck, scalp, or face, except eye) 920
buttock 922.32
canthus 921.1
cardiac 861.01
  with open wound into thorax 861.11
cauda equina (spine) 952.4
cerebellum — *see* Contusion, brain, cerebellum
cerebral — *see* Contusion, brain
cheek(s) (and other part(s) of neck, scalp, or face, except eye) 920
chest (wall) 922.1
chin (and other part(s) of neck, scalp, or face, except eye) 920
clitoris 922.4
conjunctiva 921.1
conus medullaris (spine) 952.4
cornea 921.3
corpus cavernosum 922.4
cortex (brain) (cerebral) — *see* Contusion, brain, cortex
costal region 922.1
ear (and other part(s) of neck, scalp, or face except eye) 920
elbow 923.11
  with forearm 923.10
epididymis 922.4
epigastric region 922.2
eye NEC 921.9
eyeball 921.3
eyelid(s) (and periocular area) 921.1
face (and neck, or scalp, any part except eye) 920
femoral triangle 922.2
fetus or newborn 772.6
finger(s) (nail) (subungual) 923.3
flank 922.2
foot (with ankle) (excluding toe(s)) 924.20
forearm (and elbow) 923.10
forehead (and other part(s) of neck, scalp, or face, except eye) 920
genital organs, external 922.4
globe (eye) 921.3
groin 922.2
gum(s) (and other part(s) of neck, scalp, or face, except eye) 920
hand(s) (except fingers alone) 923.20
head (any part, except eye) (and face) (and neck) 920
heart — *see* Contusion, cardiac
heel 924.20
hip 924.01
  with thigh 924.00
iliac region 922.2
inguinal region 922.2
internal organs (abdomen, chest, or pelvis) NEC — *see* Injury, internal, by site
interscapular region 922.33
iris (eye) 921.3
kidney 866.01
  with open wound into cavity 866.11
knee 924.11
  with lower leg 924.10
labium (majus) (minus) 922.4
lacrimal apparatus, gland, or sac 921.1
larynx (and other part(s) of neck, scalp, or face, except eye) 920
late effect — *see* Late, effects (of), contusion
leg 924.5
  lower (with knee) 924.10
lens 921.3
lingual (and other part(s) of neck, scalp, or face, except eye) 920
lip(s) (and other part(s) of neck, scalp, or face, except eye) 920
liver 864.01
  with
    laceration — *see* Laceration, liver
    open wound into cavity 864.11
lower extremity 924.5
  multiple sites 924.4
lumbar region 922.31

Contusion — *continued*
lung 861.21
  with open wound into thorax 861.31
malar region (and other part(s) of neck, scalp, or face, except eye) 920
mandibular joint (and other part(s) of neck, scalp, or face, except eye) 920
mastoid region (and other part(s) of neck, scalp. or face, except eye) 920
membrane, brain — *see* Contusion, brain
midthoracic region 922.1
mouth (and other part(s) of neck, scalp, or face, except eye) 920
multiple sites (not classifiable to same three-digit category) 924.8
  lower limb 924.4
  trunk 922.8
  upper limb 923.8
muscle NEC 924.9
myocardium — *see* Contusion, cardiac
nasal (septum) (and other part(s) of neck, scalp, or face, except eye) 920
neck (and scalp, or face any part, except eye) 920
nerve — *see* Injury, nerve, by site
nose (and other part(s) of neck, scalp, or face, except eye) 920
occipital region (scalp) (and neck or face, except eye) 920
  lobe — *see* Contusion, brain, occipital lobe
orbit (region) (tissues) 921.2
palate (soft) (and other part(s) of neck, scalp, or face, except eye) 920
parietal region (scalp) (and neck, or face, except eye) 920
  lobe — *see* Contusion, brain
penis 922.4
pericardium — *see* Contusion, cardiac
perineum 922.4
periocular area 921.1
pharynx (and other part(s) of neck, scalp, or face, except eye) 920
popliteal space (*see also* Contusion, knee) 924.11
prepuce 922.4
pubic region 922.4
pudenda 922.4
pulmonary — *see* Contusion, lung
quadriceps femoralis 924.00
rib cage 922.1
sacral region 922.32
salivary ducts or glands (and other part(s) of neck, scalp, or face, except eye) 920
scalp (and neck, or face any part, except eye) 920
scapular region 923.01
  with shoulder or upper arm 923.09
sclera (eye) 921.3
scrotum 922.4
shoulder 923.00
  with upper arm or axillar regions 923.09
skin NEC 924.9
skull 920
spermatic cord 922.4
spinal cord — *see also* Injury, spinal, by site
  cauda equina 952.4
  conus medullaris 952.4
spleen 865.01
  with open wound into cavity 865.11
sternal region 922.1
stomach — *see* Injury, internal, stomach
subconjunctival 921.1
subcutaneous NEC 924.9
submaxillary region (and other part(s) of neck, scalp, or face, except eye) 920
submental region (and other part(s) of neck, scalp, or face, except eye) 920
subperiosteal NEC 924.9
supraclavicular fossa (and other part(s) of neck, scalp, or face, except eye) 920
supraorbital (and other part(s) of neck, scalp, or face, except eye) 920
temple (region) (and other part(s) of neck, scalp, or face, except eye) 920
testis 922.4
thigh (and hip) 924.00

Contusion — *continued*
thorax 922.1
  organ — *see* Injury, internal, intrathoracic
throat (and other part(s) of neck, scalp, or face, except eye) 920
thumb(s) (nail) (subungual) 923.3
toe(s) (nail) (subungual) 924.3
tongue (and other part(s) of neck, scalp, or face, except eye) 920
trunk 922.9
  multiple sites 922.8
  specified site — *see* Contusion, by site
tunica vaginalis 922.4
tympanum (membrane) (and other part(s) of neck, scalp, or face, except eye) 920
upper extremity 923.9
  multiple sites 923.8
uvula (and other part(s) of neck, scalp, or face, except eye) 920
vagina 922.4
vocal cord(s) (and other part(s) of neck, scalp, or face, except eye) 920
vulva 922.4
wrist 923.21
  with hand(s), except finger(s) alone 923.20
Conus (any type) (congenital) 743.57
acquired 371.60
medullaris syndrome 336.8
Convalescence (following) V66.9
chemotherapy V66.2
medical NEC V66.5
psychotherapy V66.3
radiotherapy V66.1
surgery NEC V66.0
treatment (for) NEC V66.5
  combined V66.6
  fracture V66.4
  mental disorder NEC V66.3
  specified disorder NEC V66.5
Conversion
hysteria, hysterical, any type 300.11
laparoscopic surgical procedure to open procedure V64.4
neurosis, any 300.11
reaction, any 300.11
Converter, tuberculosis (test reaction) 795.5
Convulsions (idiopathic) 780.39
apoplectiform (*see also* Disease, cerebrovascular, acute) 436
brain 780.39
cerebral 780.39
cerebrospinal 780.39
due to trauma NEC — *see* Injury, intracranial
eclamptic (*see also* Eclampsia) 780.39
epileptic (*see also* Epilepsy) 345.9 ✓5ᵗʰ
epileptiform (*see also* Seizure, epileptiform) 780.39
epileptoid (*see also* Seizure, epileptiform) 780.39
ether
  anesthetic
    correct substance properly administered 780.39
    overdose or wrong substance given 968.2
  other specified type — *see* Table of Drugs and Chemicals
febrile 780.31
generalized 780.39
hysterical 300.11
infantile 780.39
  epilepsy — *see* Epilepsy
internal 780.39
jacksonian (*see also* Epilepsy) 345.5 ✓5ᵗʰ
myoclonic 333.2
newborn 779.0
paretic 094.1
pregnancy (nephritic) (uremic) — *see* Eclampsia, pregnancy
psychomotor (*see also* Epilepsy) 345.4 ✓5ᵗʰ
puerperal, postpartum — *see* Eclampsia, pregnancy
recurrent 780.39
  epileptic — *see* Epilepsy
reflex 781.0
repetitive 780.39
  epileptic — *see* Epilepsy

Convulsions — *continued*
salaam (*see also* Epilepsy) 345.6 ✓5ᵗʰ
scarlatinal 034.1
spasmodic 780.39
tetanus, tetanic (*see also* Tetanus) 037
thymic 254.8
uncinate 780.39
uremic 586
Convulsive — *see also* Convulsions
disorder or state 780.39
  epileptic — *see* Epilepsy
equivalent, abdominal (*see also* Epilepsy) 345.5 ✓5ᵗʰ
Cooke-Apert-Gallais syndrome (adrenogenital) 255.2
Cooley's anemia (erythroblastic) 282.4
Coolie itch 126.9
Cooper's
disease 610.1
hernia — *see* Hernia, Cooper's
Coordination disturbance 781.3
Copper wire arteries, retina 362.13
Copra itch 133.8
Coprolith 560.39
Coprophilia 302.89
Coproporphyria, hereditary 277.1
Coprostasis 560.39
with hernia — *see also* Hernia, by site, with obstruction
  gangrenous — *see* Hernia, by site, with gangrene
Cor
biloculare 745.7
bovinum — *see* Hypertrophy, cardiac
bovis — *see also* Hypertrophy, cardiac
pulmonale (chronic) 416.9
  acute 415.0
triatriatum, triatrium 746.82
triloculare 745.8
  biatriatum 745.3
  biventriculare 745.69
Corbus' disease 607.1
Cord — *see also* condition
around neck (tightly) (with compression)
  affecting fetus or newborn 762.5
  complicating delivery 663.1 ✓5ᵗʰ
    without compression 663.3 ✓5ᵗʰ
      affecting fetus or newborn 762.6
bladder NEC 344.61
  tabetic 094.0
prolapse
  affecting fetus or newborn 762.4
  complicating delivery 663.0 ✓5ᵗʰ
Cord's angiopathy (*see also* Tuberculosis) 017.3 ✓5ᵗʰ *[362.18]*
Cordis ectopia 746.87
Corditis (spermatic) 608.4
Corectopia 743.46
Cori type glycogen storage disease — *see* Disease, glycogen storage
Cork-handlers' disease or lung 495.3
Corkscrew esophagus 530.5
Corlett's pyosis (impetigo) 684
Corn (infected) 700
Cornea — *see also* condition
donor V59.5
guttata (dystrophy) 371.57
plana 743.41
Cornelia de Lange's syndrome (Amsterdam dwarf, mental retardation, and brachycephaly) 759.89
Cornual gestation or pregnancy — *see* Pregnancy, cornual
Cornu cutaneum 702.8
Coronary (artery) — *see also* condition
arising from aorta or pulmonary trunk 746.85
Corpora — *see also* condition
amylacea (prostate) 602.8
cavernosa — *see* condition
Corpulence (*see also* Obesity) 278.0 ✓5ᵗʰ
Corpus — *see* condition

✓4ᵗʰ Fourth-digit Required   ✓5ᵗʰ Fifth-digit Required   ►◄ Revised Text   ● New Line   ▲ Revised Code

Corrigan's disease — Creutzfeldt-Jakob disease

Corrigan's disease — see Insufficiency, aortic
Corrosive burn — see Burn, by site
Corsican fever (see also Malaria) 084.6
Cortical — see also condition
  blindness 377.75
  necrosis, kidney (bilateral) 583.6
Corticoadrenal — see condition
Corticosexual syndrome 255.2
Coryza (acute) 460
  with grippe or influenza 487.1
  syphilitic 095.8
    congenital (chronic) 090.0
Costen's syndrome or complex 524.60
Costiveness (see also Constipation) 564.00
Costochondritis 733.6
Cotard's syndrome (paranoia) 297.1
Cot death 798.0
Cotungo's disease 724.3
Cough 786.2
  with hemorrhage (see also Hemoptysis) 786.3
  affected 786.2
  bronchial 786.2
    with grippe or influenza 487.1
  chronic 786.2
  epidemic 786.2
  functional 306.1
  hemorrhagic 786.3
  hysterical 300.11
  laryngeal, spasmodic 786.2
  nervous 786.2
  psychogenic 306.1
  smokers' 491.0
  tea tasters' 112.89
Counseling NEC V65.40
  without complaint or sickness V65.49
  abuse victim NEC V62.89
      child V61.21
      partner V61.11
      spouse V61.11
  child abuse, maltreatment, or neglect V61.21
  contraceptive NEC V25.09
      device (intrauterine) V25.02
      maintenance V25.40
        intrauterine contraceptive device V25.42
        oral contraceptive (pill) V25.41
        specified type NEC V25.49
        subdermal implantable V25.43
      management NEC V25.9
      oral contraceptive (pill) V25.01
      prescription NEC V25.02
        oral contraceptive (pill) V25.01
          repeat prescription V25.41
        repeat prescription V25.40
      subdermal implantable V25.43
      surveillance NEC V25.40
  dietary V65.3
  excercise V65.41
  explanation of
      investigation finding NEC V65.49
      medication NEC V65.49
  family planning V25.09
  for nonattending third party V65.1
  genetic V26.3
  gonorrhea V65.45
  health (advice) (education) (instruction) NEC
      V65.49
  HIV V65.44
  human immunodeficiency virus V65.44
  injury prevention V65.43
  marital V61.10
  medical (for) V65.9
      boarding school resident V60.6
      condition not demonstrated V65.5
      feared complaint and no disease found
        V65.5
      institutional resident V60.6
      on behalf of another V65.1
      person living alone V60.3
  parent-child conflict V61.20
      specified problem NEC V61.29
  partner abuse
      perpetrator V61.12
      victim V61.11

Counseling NEC — continued
  perpetrator of
      child abuse V62.83
        parental V61.22
      partner abuse V61.12
      spouse abuse V61.12
  procreative V65.49
  sex NEC V65.49
      transmitted disease NEC V65.45
        HIV V65.44
  specified reason NEC V65.49
  spousal abuse
      perpetrator V61.12
      victim V61.11
  substance use and abuse V65.42
  syphilis V65.45
  victim (of)
      abuse NEC V62.89
      child abuse V61.21
      partner abuse V61.11
      spousal abuse V61.11
Coupled rhythm 427.89
Couvelaire uterus (complicating delivery) — see
      Placenta, separation
Cowper's gland — see condition
Cowperitis (see also Urethritis) 597.89
  gonorrheal (acute) 098.0
      chronic or duration of 2 months or over
        098.2
Cowpox (abortive) 051.0
  due to vaccination 999.0
  eyelid 051.0 [373.5]
      postvaccination 999.0 [373.5]
Coxa
  plana 732.1
  valga (acquired) 736.31
      congenital 755.61
      late effect of rickets 268.1
  vara (acquired) 736.32
      congenital 755.62
      late effect of rickets 268.1
Coxae malum senilis 715.25
Coxalgia (nontuberculous) 719.45
  tuberculous (see also Tuberculosis) 015.1 ✓5ᵗʰ
      [730.85]
Coxalgic pelvis 736.30
Coxitis 716.65
Coxsackie (infection) (virus) 079.2
  central nervous system NEC 048
  endocarditis 074.22
  enteritis 008.67
  meningitis (aseptic) 047.0
  myocarditis 074.23
  pericarditis 074.21
  pharyngitis 074.0
  pleurodynia 074.1
  specific disease NEC 074.8
Crabs, meaning pubic lice 132.2
Crack baby 760.75
Cracked nipple 611.2
  puerperal, postpartum 676.1 ✓5ᵗʰ
Cradle cap 690.11
Craft neurosis 300.89
Craigiasis 007.8
Cramp(s) 729.82
  abdominal 789.0 ✓5ᵗʰ
  bathing 994.1
  colic 789.0 ✓5ᵗʰ
      psychogenic 306.4
  due to immersion 994.1
  extremity (lower) (upper) NEC 729.82
  fireman 992.2
  heat 992.2
  hysterical 300.11
  immersion 994.1
  intestinal 789.0 ✓5ᵗʰ
      psychogenic 306.4
  linotypist's 300.89
      organic 333.84
  muscle (extremity) (general) 729.82
      due to immersion 994.1
      hysterical 300.11
  occupational (hand) 300.89
      organic 333.84

Cramp(s) — continued
  psychogenic 307.89
  salt depletion 276.1
  stoker 992.2
  stomach 789.0 ✓5ᵗʰ
  telegraphers' 300.89
      organic 333.84
  typists' 300.89
      organic 333.84
  uterus 625.8
      menstrual 625.3
  writers' 333.84
      organic 333.84
      psychogenic 300.89
Cranial — see condition
Cranioclasis, fetal 763.89
Craniocleidodysostosis 755.59
Craniofenestria (skull) 756.0
Craniolacunia (skull) 756.0
Craniopagus 759.4
Craniopathy, metabolic 733.3
Craniopharyngeal — see condition
Craniopharyngioma (M9350/1) 237.0
Craniorachischisis (totalis) 740.1
Cranioschisis 756.0
Craniostenosis 756.0
Craniosynostosis 756.0
Craniotabes (cause unknown) 733.3
  rachitic 268.1
  syphilitic 090.5
Craniotomy, fetal 763.89
Cranium — see condition
Craw-craw 125.3
Creaking joint 719.60
  ankle 719.67
  elbow 719.62
  foot 719.67
  hand 719.64
  hip 719.65
  knee 719.66
  multiple sites 719.69
  pelvic region 719.65
  shoulder (region) 719.61
  specified site NEC 719.68
  wrist 719.63
Creeping
  eruption 126.9
  palsy 335.21
  paralysis 335.21
Crenated tongue 529.8
Creotoxism 005.9
Crepitus
  caput 756.0
  joint 719.60
      ankle 719.67
      elbow 719.62
      foot 719.67
      hand 719.64
      hip 719.65
      knee 719.66
      multiple sites 719.69
      pelvic region 719.65
      shoulder (region) 719.61
      specified site NEC 719.68
      wrist 719.63
Crescent or conus choroid, congenital 743.57
Cretin, cretinism (athyrotic) (congenital)
      (endemic) (metabolic) (nongoitrous)
      (sporadic) 243
  goitrous (sporadic) 246.1
  pelvis (dwarf type) (male type) 243
      with disproportion (fetopelvic) 653.1 ✓5ᵗʰ
        affecting fetus or newborn 763.1
        causing obstructed labor 660.1 ✓5ᵗʰ
          affecting fetus or newborn 763.1
  pituitary 253.3
Cretinoid degeneration 243
Creutzfeldt-Jakob disease (syndrome) 046.1
  with dementia
      with behavioral disturbance 046.1 [294.11]
      without behavioral disturbance 046.1
        [294.10]

▲

Crib death 798.0
Cribriform hymen 752.49
Cri-du-chat syndrome 758.3
Crigler-Najjar disease or syndrome (congenital hyperbilirubinemia) 277.4
Crimean hemorrhagic fever 065.0
Criminalism 301.7
Crisis
  abdomen 789.0 ☑5ᵗʰ
  addisonian (acute adrenocortical insufficiency) 255.4
  adrenal (cortical) 255.4
  asthmatic — see Asthma
  brain, cerebral (see also Disease, cerebrovascular, acute) 436
  celiac 579.0
  Dietl's 593.4
  emotional NEC 309.29
    acute reaction to stress 308.0
    adjustment reaction 309.9
    specific to childhood and adolescence 313.9
  gastric (tabetic) 094.0
  glaucomatocyclitic 364.22
  heart (see also Failure, heart) 428.9
  hypertensive — see Hypertension
  nitritoid
    correct substance properly administered 458.2
    overdose or wrong substance given or taken 961.1
  oculogyric 378.87
    psychogenic 306.7
  Pel's 094.0
  psychosexual identity 302.6
  rectum 094.0
  renal 593.81
  sickle cell 282.62
  stomach (tabetic) 094.0
  tabetic 094.0
  thyroid (see also Thyrotoxicosis) 242.9 ☑5ᵗʰ
  thyrotoxic (see also Thyrotoxicosis) 242.9 ☑5ᵗʰ
  vascular — see Disease, cerebrovascular, acute
Crocq's disease (acrocyanosis) 443.89
Crohn's disease (see also Enteritis, regional) 555.9
Cronkhite-Canada syndrome 211.3
Crooked septum, nasal 470
Cross
  birth (of fetus) complicating delivery 652.3 ☑5ᵗʰ
    with successful version 652.1 ☑5ᵗʰ
    causing obstructed labor 660.0 ☑5ᵗʰ
  bite, anterior or posterior 524.2
  eye (see also Esotropia) 378.00
Crossed ectopia of kidney 753.3
Crossfoot 754.50
Croup, croupous (acute) (angina) (catarrhal) (infective) (inflammatory) (laryngeal) (membranous) (nondiphtheritic) (pseudomembranous) 464.4
  asthmatic (see also Asthma) 493.9 ☑5ᵗʰ
  bronchial 466.0
  diphtheritic (membranous) 032.3
  false 478.75
  spasmodic 478.75
    diphtheritic 032.3
  stridulous 478.75
    diphtheritic 032.3
Crouzon's disease (craniofacial dysostosis) 756.0
Crowding, teeth 524.3
CRST syndrome (cutaneous systemic sclerosis) 710.1
Cruchet's disease (encephalitis lethargica) 049.8
Cruelty in children (see also Disturbance, conduct) 312.9
Crural ulcer (see also Ulcer, lower extremity) 707.10
Crush, crushed, crushing (injury) 929.9
  with
    fracture — see Fracture, by site
  abdomen 926.19
    internal — see Injury, internal, abdomen
  ankle 928.21
    with other parts of foot 928.20

Crush, crushed, crushing — continued
  arm 927.9
    lower (and elbow) 927.10
    upper 927.03
      with shoulder or axillary region 927.09
  axilla 927.02
    with shoulder or upper arm 927.09
  back 926.11
  breast 926.19
  buttock 926.12
  cheek 925.1
  chest — see Injury, internal, chest
  ear 925.1
  elbow 927.11
    with forearm 927.10
  face 925.1
  finger(s) 927.3
    with hand(s) 927.20
      and wrist(s) 927.21
  flank 926.19
  foot, excluding toe(s) alone (with ankle) 928.20
  forearm (and elbow) 927.10
  genitalia, external (female) (male) 926.0
    internal — see Injury, internal, genital organ NEC
  hand, except finger(s) alone (and wrist) 927.20
  head — see Fracture, skull, by site
  heel 928.20
  hip 928.01
    with thigh 928.00
  internal organ (abdomen, chest, or pelvis) — see Injury, internal, by site
  knee 928.11
    with leg, lower 928.10
  labium (majus) (minus) 926.0
  larynx 925.2
  late effect — see Late, effects (of), crushing
  leg 928.9
    lower 928.10
      and knee 928.11
    upper 928.00
  limb
    lower 928.9
      multiple sites 928.8
    upper 927.9
      multiple sites 927.8
  multiple sites NEC 929.0
  neck 925.2
  nerve — see Injury, nerve, by site
  nose 802.0
    open 802.1
  penis 926.0
  pharynx 925.2
  scalp 925.1
  scapular region 927.01
    with shoulder or upper arm 927.09
  scrotum 926.0
  shoulder 927.00
    with upper arm or axillary region 927.09
  skull or cranium — see Fracture, skull, by site
  spinal cord — see Injury, spinal, by site
  syndrome (complication of trauma) 958.5
  testis 926.0
  thigh (with hip) 928.00
  throat 925.2
  thumb(s) (and fingers) 927.3
  toe(s) 928.3
    with foot 928.20
      and ankle 928.21
  tonsil 925.2
  trunk 926.9
    chest — see Injury, internal, intrathoracic organs NEC
    internal organ — see Injury, internal, by site
    multiple sites 926.8
    specified site NEC 926.19
  vulva 926.0
  wrist 927.21
    with hand(s), except fingers alone 927.20
Crusta lactea 690.11
Crusts 782.8
Crutch paralysis 953.4
Cruveilhier's disease 335.21
Cruveilhier-Baumgarten cirrhosis, disease, or syndrome 571.5

Cruz-Chagas disease (see also Trypanosomiasis) 086.2
Cryoglobulinemia (mixed) 273.2
Crypt (anal) (rectal) 569.49
Cryptitis (anal) (rectal) 569.49
Cryptococcosis (European) (pulmonary) (systemic) 117.5
Cryptococcus 117.5
  epidermicus 117.5
  neoformans, infection by 117.5
Cryptopapillitis (anus) 569.49
Cryptophthalmos (eyelid) 743.06
Cryptorchid, cryptorchism, cryptorchidism 752.51
Cryptosporidiosis 007.4
Cryptotia 744.29
Crystallopathy
  calcium pyrophosphate (see also Arthritis) 275.49 [712.2]
  dicalcium phosphate (see also Arthritis) 275.49 [712.1]
  gouty 274.0
  pyrophosphate NEC (see also Arthritis) 275.49 [712.2]
  uric acid 274.0
Crystalluria 791.9
Csillag's disease (lichen sclerosus or atrophicus) 701.0
Cuban itch 050.1
Cubitus
  valgus (acquired) 736.01
    congenital 755.59
    late effect of rickets 268.1
  varus (acquired) 736.02
    congenital 755.59
    late effect of rickets 268.1
Cultural deprivation V62.4
Cupping of optic disc 377.14
Curling's ulcer — see Ulcer, duodenum
Curling esophagus 530.5
Curschmann (-Batten) (-Steinert) disease or syndrome 359.2
Curvature
  organ or site, congenital NEC — see Distortion
  penis (lateral) 752.69
  Pott's (spinal) (see also Tuberculosis) 015.0 ☑5ᵗʰ [737.43]
  radius, idiopathic, progressive (congenital) 755.54
  spine (acquired) (angular) (idiopathic) (incorrect) (postural) 737.9
    congenital 754.2
    due to or associated with
      Charcôt-Marie-Tooth disease 356.1 [737.40]
      mucopolysaccharidosis 277.5 [737.40]
      neurofibromatosis 237.71 [737.40]
      osteitis
        deformans 731.0 [737.40]
        fibrosa cystica 252.0 [737.40]
      osteoporosis (see also Osteoporosis) 733.00 [737.40]
      poliomyelitis (see also Poliomyelitis) 138 [737.40]
      tuberculosis (Pott's curvature) (see also Tuberculosis) 015.0 ☑5ᵗʰ [737.43]
    kyphoscoliotic (see also Kyphoscoliosis) 737.30
    kyphotic (see also Kyphosis) 737.10
    late effect of rickets 268.1 [737.40]
    Pott's 015.0 ☑5ᵗʰ [737.40]
    scoliotic (see also Scoliosis) 737.30
    specified NEC 737.8
    tuberculous 015.0 ☑5ᵗʰ [737.40]
Cushing's
  basophilism, disease, or syndrome (iatrogenic) (idiopathic) (pituitary basophilism) (pituitary dependent) 255.0
  ulcer — see Ulcer, peptic
Cushingoid due to steroid therapy
  correct substance properly administered 255.0
  overdose or wrong substance given or taken 962.0

Cut (external) — *see* Wound, open, by site
Cutaneous — *see also* condition
  hemorrhage 782.7
  horn (cheek) (eyelid) (mouth) 702.8
  larva migrans 126.9
Cutis — *see also* condition
  hyperelastic 756.83
    acquired 701.8
  laxa 756.83
    senilis 701.8
  marmorata 782.61
  osteosis 709.3
  pendula 756.83
    acquired 701.8
  rhomboidalis nuchae 701.8
  verticis gyrata 757.39
    acquired 701.8
Cyanopathy, newborn 770.83 ▲
Cyanosis 782.5
  autotoxic 289.7
  common atrioventricular canal 745.69
  congenital 770.83 ▲
  conjunctiva 372.71
  due to
    endocardial cushion defect 745.60
    nonclosure, foramen botalli 745.5
    patent foramen botalli 745.5
    persistent foramen ovale 745.5
  enterogenous 289.7
  fetus or newborn 770.83 ▲
  ostium primum defect 745.61
  paroxysmal digital 443.0
  retina, retinal 362.10
Cycle
  anovulatory 628.0
  menstrual, irregular 626.4
Cyclencephaly 759.89
Cyclical vomiting 536.2
  psychogenic 306.4
Cyclitic membrane 364.74
Cyclitis (*see also* Iridocyclitis) 364.3
  acute 364.00
    primary 364.01
    recurrent 364.02
  chronic 364.10
    in
      sarcoidosis 135 *[364.11]*
      tuberculosis (*see also* Tuberculosis)
        017.3 ✓5ᵗʰ *[364.11]*
  Fuchs' heterochromic 364.21
  granulomatous 364.10
  lens induced 364.23
  nongranulomatous 364.00
  posterior 363.21
  primary 364.01
  recurrent 364.02
  secondary (noninfectious) 364.04
    infectious 364.03
  subacute 364.00
    primary 364.01
    recurrent 364.02
Cyclokeratitis — *see* Keratitis
Cyclophoria 378.44
Cyclopia, cyclops 759.89
Cycloplegia 367.51
Cyclospasm 367.53
Cyclosporiasis 007.5
Cyclothymia 301.13
Cyclothymic personality 301.13
Cyclotropia 378.33
Cyesis — *see* Pregnancy
Cylindroma (M8200/3) — *see also* Neoplasm, by
    site, malignant
  eccrine dermal (M8200/0) — *see* Neoplasm,
    skin, benign
  skin (M8200/0) — *see* Neoplasm, skin, benign
Cylindruria 791.7
Cyllosoma 759.89
Cynanche
  diphtheritic 032.3
  tonsillaris 475
Cynorexia 783.6
Cyphosis — *see* Kyphosis

Cyprus fever (*see also* Brucellosis) 023.9
Cyriax's syndrome (slipping rib) 733.99
Cyst (mucus) (retention) (serous) (simple)

Note — In general, cysts are not neoplastic
and are classified to the appropriate category
for disease of the specified anatomical site.
This generalization does not apply to certain
types of cysts which are neoplastic in nature,
for example, dermoid, nor does it apply to
cysts of certain structures, for example,
branchial cleft, which are classified as
developmental anomalies.

The following listing includes some of the
most frequently reported sites of cysts as
well as qualifiers which indicate the type of
cyst. The latter qualifiers usually are not
repeated under the anatomical sites. Since
the code assignment for a given site may
vary depending upon the type of cyst, the
coder should refer to the listings under the
specified type of cyst before consideration is
given to the site.

  accessory, fallopian tube 752.11
  adenoid (infected) 474.8
  adrenal gland 255.8
    congenital 759.1
  air, lung 518.89
  allantoic 753.7
  alveolar process (jaw bone) 526.2
  amnion, amniotic 658.8 ✓5ᵗʰ
  anterior chamber (eye) 364.60
    exudative 364.62
    implantation (surgical) (traumatic) 364.61
    parasitic 360.13
  anterior nasopalatine 526.1
  antrum 478.1
  anus 569.49
  apical (periodontal) (tooth) 522.8
  appendix 543.9
  arachnoid, brain 348.0
  arytenoid 478.79
  auricle 706.2
  Baker's (knee) 727.51
    tuberculous (*see also* Tuberculosis)
      015.2 ✓5ᵗʰ
  Bartholin's gland or duct 616.2
  bile duct (*see also* Disease, biliary) 576.8
  bladder (multiple) (trigone) 596.8
  Blessig's 362.62
  blood, endocardial (*see also* Endocarditis)
    424.90
  blue dome 610.0
  bone (local) 733.20
    aneurysmal 733.22
    jaw 526.2
      developmental (odontogenic) 526.0
      fissural 526.1
      latent 526.89
    solitary 733.21
    unicameral 733.21
  brain 348.0
    congenital 742.4
    hydatid (*see also* Echinococcus) 122.9
    third ventricle (colloid) 742.4
  branchial (cleft) 744.42
  branchiogenic 744.42
  breast (benign) (blue dome) (pedunculated)
      (solitary) (traumatic) 610.0
    involution 610.4
    sebaceous 610.8
  broad ligament (benign) 620.8
    embryonic 752.11
  bronchogenic (mediastinal) (sequestration)
    518.89
    congenital 748.4
  buccal 528.4
  bulbourethral gland (Cowper's) 599.89
  bursa, bursal 727.49
    pharyngeal 478.26
  calcifying odontogenic (M9301/0) 213.1
    upper jaw (bone) 213.0
  canal of Nuck (acquired) (serous) 629.1
    congenital 752.41
  canthus 372.75

Cyst — *continued*
  carcinomatous (M8010/3) — *see* Neoplasm, by
      site, malignant
  cartilage (joint) — *see* Derangement, joint
  cauda equina 336.8
  cavum septi pellucidi NEC 348.0
  celomic (pericardium) 746.89
  cerebellopontine (angle) — *see* Cyst, brain
  cerebellum — *see* Cyst, brain
  cerebral — *see* Cyst, brain
  cervical lateral 744.42
  cervix 622.8
    embryonal 752.41
    nabothian (gland) 616.0
  chamber, anterior (eye) 364.60
    exudative 364.62
    implantation (surgical) (traumatic) 364.61
    parasitic 360.13
  chiasmal, optic NEC (*see also* Lesion, chiasmal)
    377.54
  chocolate (ovary) 617.1
  choledochal (congenital) 751.69
    acquired 576.8
  choledochus 751.69
  chorion 658.8 ✓5ᵗʰ
  choroid plexus 348.0
  chyle, mesentery 457.8
  ciliary body 364.60
    exudative 364.64
    implantation 364.61
    primary 364.63
  clitoris 624.8
  coccyx (*see also* Cyst, bone) 733.20
  colloid
    third ventricle (brain) 742.4
    thyroid gland — *see* Goiter
  colon 569.89
  common (bile) duct (*see also* Disease, biliary)
    576.8
  congenital NEC 759.89
    adrenal glands 759.1
    epiglottis 748.3
    esophagus 750.4
    fallopian tube 752.11
    kidney 753.10
      multiple 753.19
      single 753.11
    larynx 748.3
    liver 751.62
    lung 748.4
    mediastinum 748.8
    ovary 752.0
    oviduct 752.11
    pancreas 751.7
    periurethral (tissue) 753.8
    prepuce NEC 752.69
      penis 752.69
    sublingual 750.26
    submaxillary gland 750.26
    thymus (gland) 759.2
    tongue 750.19
    ureterovesical orifice 753.4
    vulva 752.41
  conjunctiva 372.75
  cornea 371.23
  corpora quadrigemina 348.0
  corpus
    albicans (ovary) 620.2
    luteum (ruptured) 620.1
  Cowper's gland (benign) (infected) 599.89
  cranial meninges 348.0
  craniobuccal pouch 253.8
  craniopharyngeal pouch 253.8
  cystic duct (*see also* Disease, gallbladder) 575.8
  Cysticercus (any site) 123.1
  Dandy-Walker 742.3
    with spina bifida (*see also* Spina bifida)
      741.0 ✓5ᵗʰ
  dental 522.8
    developmental 526.0
    eruption 526.0
    lateral periodontal 526.0
    primordial (keratocyst) 526.0
    root 522.8
  dentigerous 526.0
    mandible 526.0
    maxilla 526.0

Cyst — *continued*
dermoid (M9084/0) — *see also* Neoplasm, by
    site, benign
    with malignant transformation (M9084/3)
        183.0
    implantation
        external area or site (skin) NEC 709.8
        iris 364.61
        skin 709.8
        vagina 623.8
        vulva 624.8
    mouth 528.4
    oral soft tissue 528.4
    sacrococcygeal 685.1
        with abscess 685.0
developmental of ovary, ovarian 752.0
dura (cerebral) 348.0
    spinal 349.2
ear (external) 706.2
echinococcal (*see also* Echinococcus) 122.9
embryonal
    cervix uteri 752.41
    genitalia, female external 752.41
    uterus 752.3
    vagina 752.41
endometrial 621.8
    ectopic 617.9
endometrium (uterus) 621.8
    ectopic — *see* Endometriosis
enteric 751.5
enterogenous 751.5
epidermal (inclusion) (*see also* Cyst, skin)
    706.2
epidermoid (inclusion) (*see also* Cyst, skin)
    706.2
    mouth 528.4
    not of skin — *see* Cyst, by site
    oral soft tissue 528.4
epididymis 608.89
epiglottis 478.79
epiphysis cerebri 259.8
epithelial (inclusion) (*see also* Cyst, skin) 706.2
epoophoron 752.11
eruption 526.0
esophagus 530.89
ethmoid sinus 478.1
eye (retention) 379.8
    congenital 743.03
    posterior segment, congenital 743.54
eyebrow 706.2
eyelid (sebaceous) 374.84
    infected 373.13
    sweat glands or ducts 374.84
falciform ligament (inflammatory) 573.8
fallopian tube 620.8
female genital organs NEC 629.8
fimbrial (congenital) 752.11
fissural (oral region) 526.1
follicle (atretic) (graafian) (ovarian) 620.0
    nabothian (gland) 616.0
follicular (atretic) (ovarian) 620.0
    dentigerous 526.0
frontal sinus 478.1
gallbladder or duct 575.8
ganglion 727.43
Gartner's duct 752.11
gas, of mesentery 568.89
gingiva 523.8
gland of moll 374.84
globulomaxillary 526.1
graafian follicle 620.0
granulosal lutein 620.2
hemangiomatous (M9121/0) (*see also*
    Hemangioma) 228.00
hydatid (*see also* Echinococcus) 122.9
    fallopian tube (Morgagni) 752.11
    liver NEC 122.8
    lung NEC 122.9
    Morgagni 752.8
        fallopian tube 752.11
    specified site NEC 122.9
hymen 623.8
    embryonal 752.41
hypopharynx 478.26
hypophysis, hypophyseal (duct) (recurrent)
    253.8
    cerebri 253.8

Cyst — *continued*
implantation (dermoid)
    anterior chamber (eye) 364.61
    external area or site (skin) NEC 709.8
    iris 364.61
    vagina 623.8
    vulva 624.8
incisor, incisive canal 526.1
inclusion (epidermal) (epithelial) (epidermoid)
    (mucous) (squamous) (*see also* Cyst, skin)
    706.2
    not of skin — *see* Neoplasm, by site, benign
intestine (large) (small) 569.89
intracranial — *see* Cyst, brain
intraligamentous 728.89
    knee 717.89
intrasellar 253.8
iris (idiopathic) 364.60
    exudative 364.62
    implantation (surgical) (traumatic) 364.61
    miotic pupillary 364.55
    parasitic 360.13
Iwanoff's 362.62
jaw (bone) (aneurysmal) (extravasation)
    (hemorrhagic) (traumatic) 526.2
    developmental (odontogenic) 526.0
    fissural 526.1
keratin 706.2
kidney (congenital) 753.10
    acquired 593.2
    calyceal (*see also* Hydronephrosis) 591
    multiple 753.19
    pyelogenic (*see also* Hydronephrosis) 591
    simple 593.2
    single 753.11
    solitary (not congenital) 593.2
labium (majus) (minus) 624.8
    sebaceous 624.8
lacrimal
    apparatus 375.43
    gland or sac 375.12
larynx 478.79
lens 379.39
    congenital 743.39
lip (gland) 528.5
liver 573.8
    congenital 751.62
    hydatid (*see also* Echinococcus) 122.8
        granulosis 122.0
        multilocularis 122.5
lung 518.89
    congenital 748.4
    giant bullous 492.0
lutein 620.1
lymphangiomatous (M9173/0) 228.1
lymphoepithelial
    mouth 528.4
    oral soft tissue 528.4
macula 362.54
malignant (M8000/3) — *see* Neoplasm, by site,
    malignant
mammary gland (sweat gland) (*see also* Cyst,
    breast) 610.0
mandible 526.2
    dentigerous 526.0
    radicular 522.8
maxilla 526.2
    dentigerous 526.0
    radicular 522.8
median
    anterior maxillary 526.1
    palatal 526.1
mediastinum (congenital) 748.8
meibomian (gland) (retention) 373.2
    infected 373.12
membrane, brain 348.0
meninges (cerebral) 348.0
    spinal 349.2
meniscus knee 717.5
mesentery, mesenteric (gas) 568.89
    chyle 457.8
    gas 568.89
mesonephric duct 752.8
mesothelial
    peritoneum 568.89
    pleura (peritoneal) 569.89
milk 611.5

Cyst — *continued*
miotic pupillary (iris) 364.55
Morgagni (hydatid) 752.8
    fallopian tube 752.11
mouth 528.4
mullerian duct 752.8
multilocular (ovary) (M8000/1) 239.5
myometrium 621.8
nabothian (follicle) (ruptured) 616.0
nasal sinus 478.1
nasoalveolar 528.4
nasolabial 528.4
nasopalatine (duct) 526.1
    anterior 526.1
nasopharynx 478.26
neoplastic (M8000/1) — *see also* Neoplasm, by
    site, unspecified nature
    benign (M8000/0) — *see* Neoplasm, by site,
        benign
    uterus 621.8
nervous system — *see* Cyst, brain
neuroenteric 742.59
neuroepithelial ventricle 348.0
nipple 610.0
nose 478.1
    skin of 706.2
odontogenic, developmental 526.0
omentum (lesser) 568.89
    congenital 751.8
oral soft tissue (dermoid) (epidermoid)
    (lymphoepithelial) 528.4
ora serrata 361.19
orbit 376.81
ovary, ovarian (twisted) 620.2
    adherent 620.2
    chocolate 617.1
    corpus
        albicans 620.2
        luteum 620.1
    dermoid (M9084/0) 220
    developmental 752.0
    due to failure of involution NEC 620.2
    endometrial 617.1
    follicular (atretic) (graafian) (hemorrhagic)
        620.0
    hemorrhagic 620.2
    in pregnancy or childbirth 654.4 ☑5ᵗʰ
        affecting fetus or newborn 763.89
        causing obstructed labor 660.2 ☑5ᵗʰ
            affecting fetus or newborn 763.1
    multilocular (M8000/1) 239.5
    pseudomucinous (M8470/0) 220
    retention 620.2
    serous 620.2
    theca lutein 620.2
    tuberculous (*see also* Tuberculosis)
        016.6 ☑5ᵗʰ
    unspecified 620.2
oviduct 620.8
palatal papilla (jaw) 526.1
palate 526.1
    fissural 526.1
    median (fissural) 526.1
palatine, of papilla 526.1
pancreas, pancreatic 577.2
    congenital 751.7
    false 577.2
    hemorrhagic 577.2
    true 577.2
paranephric 593.2
para ovarian 752.11
paraphysis, cerebri 742.4
parasitic NEC 136.9
parathyroid (gland) 252.8
paratubal (fallopian) 620.8
paraurethral duct 599.89
paroophoron 752.11
parotid gland 527.6
    mucous extravasation or retention 527.6
parovarian 752.11
pars planus 364.60
    exudative 364.64
    primary 364.63

Cyst — *continued*
  pelvis, female
    in pregnancy or childbirth 654.4 ✔5ᵗʰ
      affecting fetus or newborn 763.89
      causing obstructed labor 660.2 ✔5ᵗʰ
        affecting fetus or newborn 763.1
  penis (sebaceous) 607.89
  periapical 522.8
  pericardial (congenital) 746.89
    acquired (secondary) 423.8
  pericoronal 526.0
  perineural (Tarlov's) 355.9
  periodontal 522.8
    lateral 526.0
  peripancreatic 577.2
  peripelvic (lymphatic) 593.2
  peritoneum 568.89
    chylous 457.8
  pharynx (wall) 478.26
  pilonidal (infected) (rectum) 685.1
    with abscess 685.0
    malignant (M9084/3) 173.5
  pituitary (duct) (gland) 253.8
  placenta (amniotic) — *see* Placenta, abnormal
  pleura 519.8
  popliteal 727.51
  porencephalic 742.4
    acquired 348.0
  postanal (infected) 685.1
    with abscess 685.0
  posterior segment of eye, congenital 743.54
  postmastoidectomy cavity 383.31
  preauricular 744.47
  prepuce 607.89
    congenital 752.69
  primordial (jaw) 526.0
  prostate 600.3
  pseudomucinous (ovary) (M8470/0) 220
  pudenda (sweat glands) 624.8
  pupillary, miotic 364.55
    sebaceous 624.8
  radicular (residual) 522.8
  radiculodental 522.8
  ranular 527.6
  Rathke's pouch 253.8
  rectum (epithelium) (mucous) 569.49
  renal — *see* Cyst, kidney
  residual (radicular) 522.8
  retention (ovary) 620.2
  retina 361.19
    macular 362.54
    parasitic 360.13
    primary 361.13
    secondary 361.14
  retroperitoneal 568.89
  sacrococcygeal (dermoid) 685.1
    with abscess 685.0
  salivary gland or duct 527.6
    mucous extravasation or retention 527.6
  Sampson's 617.1
  sclera 379.19
  scrotum (sebaceous) 706.2
    sweat glands 706.2
  sebaceous (duct) (gland) 706.2
    breast 610.8
    eyelid 374.84
    genital organ NEC
      female 629.8
      male 608.89
    scrotum 706.2
  semilunar cartilage (knee) (multiple) 717.5
  seminal vesicle 608.89
  serous (ovary) 620.2
  sinus (antral) (ethmoidal) (frontal) (maxillary) (nasal) (sphenoidal) 478.1
  Skene's gland 599.89
  skin (epidermal) (epidermoid, inclusion) (epithelial) (inclusion) (retention) (sebaceous) 706.2
    breast 610.8
    eyelid 374.84
    genital organ NEC
      female 629.8
      male 608.89
    neoplastic 216.3
    scrotum 706.2
  sweat gland or duct 705.89

Cyst — *continued*
  solitary
    bone 733.21
    kidney 593.2
  spermatic cord 608.89
  sphenoid sinus 478.1
  spinal meninges 349.2
  spine (*see also* Cyst, bone) 733.20
  spleen NEC 289.59
    congenital 759.0
    hydatid (*see also* Echinococcus) 122.9
  spring water (pericardium) 746.89
  subarachnoid 348.0
    intrasellar 793.0
  subdural (cerebral) 348.0
    spinal cord 349.2
  sublingual gland 527.6
    mucous extravasation or retention 527.6
  submaxillary gland 527.6
    mucous extravasation or retention 527.6
  suburethral 599.89
  suprarenal gland 255.8
  suprasellar — *see* Cyst, brain
  sweat gland or duct 705.89
  sympathetic nervous system 337.9
  synovial 727.40
    popliteal space 727.51
  Tarlov's 355.9
  tarsal 373.2
  tendon (sheath) 727.42
  testis 608.89
  theca-lutein (ovary) 620.2
  Thornwaldt's, Tornwaldt's 478.26
  thymus (gland) 254.8
  thyroglossal (duct) (infected) (persistent) 759.2
  thyroid (gland) 246.2
    adenomatous — *see* Goiter, nodular
    colloid (*see also* Goiter) 240.9
  thyrolingual duct (infected) (persistent) 759.2
  tongue (mucous) 529.8
  tonsil 474.8
  tooth (dental root) 522.8
  tubo-ovarian 620.8
    inflammatory 614.1
  tunica vaginalis 608.89
  turbinate (nose) (*see also* Cyst, bone) 733.20
  Tyson's gland (benign) (infected) 607.89
  umbilicus 759.89
  urachus 753.7
  ureter 593.89
  ureterovesical orifice 593.89
    congenital 753.4
  urethra 599.84
  urethral gland (Cowper's) 599.89
  uterine
    ligament 620.8
      embryonic 752.11
    tube 620.8
  uterus (body) (corpus) (recurrent) 621.8
    embryonal 752.3
  utricle (ear) 386.8
    prostatic 599.89
  utriculus masculinus 599.89
  vagina, vaginal (squamous cell) (wall) 623.8
    embryonal 752.41
    implantation 623.8
    inclusion 623.8
  vallecula, vallecular 478.79
  ventricle, neuroepithelial 348.0
  verumontanum 599.89
  vesical (orifice) 596.8
  vitreous humor 379.29
  vulva (sweat glands) 624.8
    congenital 752.41
    implantation 624.8
    inclusion 624.8
    sebaceous gland 624.8
  vulvovaginal gland 624.8
  wolffian 752.8

Cystadenocarcinoma (M8440/3) — *see also* Neoplasm, by site, malignant
  bile duct type (M8161/3) 155.1
  endometrioid (M8380/3) — *see* Neoplasm, by site, malignant

Cystadenocarcinoma — *see also* Neoplasm, by site, malignant — *continued*
  mucinous (M8470/3)
    papillary (M8471/3)
      specified site — *see* Neoplasm, by site, malignant
      unspecified site 183.0
    specified site — *see* Neoplasm, by site, malignant
    unspecified site 183.0
  papillary (M8450/3)
    mucinous (M8471/3)
      specified site — *see* Neoplasm, by site, malignant
      unspecified site 183.0
    pseudomucinous (M8471/3)
      specified site — *see* Neoplasm, by site, malignant
      unspecified site 183.0
    serous (M8460/3)
      specified site — *see* Neoplasm, by site, malignant
      unspecified site 183.0
    specified site — *see* Neoplasm, by site, malignant
    unspecified 183.0
  pseudomucinous (M8470/3)
    papillary (M8471/3)
      specified site — *see* Neoplasm, by site, malignant
      unspecified site 183.0
    specified site — *see* Neoplasm, by site, malignant
    unspecified site 183.0
  serous (M8441/3)
    papillary (M8460/3)
      specified site — *see* Neoplasm, by site, malignant
      unspecified site 183.0
    specified site — *see* Neoplasm, by site, malignant
    unspecified site 183.0

Cystadenofibroma (M9013/0)
  clear cell (M8313/0) — *see* Neoplasm, by site, benign
  endometrioid (M8381/0) 220
    borderline malignancy (M8381/1) 236.2
    malignant (M8381/3) 183.0
  mucinous (M9015/0)
    specified site — *see* Neoplasm, by site, benign
    unspecified site 220
  serous (M9014/0)
    specified site — *see* Neoplasm, by site, benign
    unspecified site 220
  specified site — *see* Neoplasm, by site, benign
  unspecified site 220

Cystadenoma (M8440/0) — *see also* Neoplasm, by site, benign
  bile duct (M8161/0) 211.5
  endometrioid (M8380/0) — *see also* Neoplasm, by site, benign
    borderline malignancy (M8380/1) — *see* Neoplasm, by site, uncertain behavior
  malignant (M8440/3) — *see* Neoplasm, by site, malignant
  mucinous (M8470/0)
    borderline malignancy (M8470/1)
      specified site — *see* Neoplasm, uncertain behavior
      unspecified site 236.2
    papillary (M8471/0)
      borderline malignancy (M8471/1)
        specified site — *see* Neoplasm, by site, uncertain behavior
        unspecified site 236.2
      specified site — *see* Neoplasm, by site, benign
      unspecified site 220
    specified site — *see* Neoplasm, by site, benign
    unspecified site 220
  papillary (M8450/0)
    borderline malignancy (M8450/1)
      specified site — *see* Neoplasm, by site, uncertain behavior

Cystadenoma — *see also* Neoplasm, by site,
    benign — *continued*
  papillary — *continued*
    borderline malignancy — *continued*
      unspecified site 236.2
    lymphomatosum (M8561/0) 210.2
    mucinous (M8471/0)
      borderline malignancy (M8471/1)
        specified site — *see* Neoplasm, by site,
          uncertain behavior
        unspecified site 236.2
      specified site — *see* Neoplasm, by site,
        benign
      unspecified site 220
    pseudomucinous (M8471/0)
      borderline malignancy (M8471/1)
        specified site — *see* Neoplasm, by site,
          uncertain behavior
        unspecified site 236.2
      specified site — *see* Neoplasm, by site,
        benign
      unspecified site 220
    serous (M8460/0)
      borderline malignancy (M8460/1)
        specified site — *see* Neoplasm, by site,
          uncertain behavior
        unspecified site 236.2
      specified site — *see* Neoplasm, by site,
        benign
      unspecified site 220
    specified site — *see* Neoplasm, by site,
      benign
    unspecified site 220
  pseudomucinous (M8470/0)
    borderline malignancy (M8470/1)
      specified site — *see* Neoplasm, by site,
        uncertain behavior
      unspecified site 236.2
    papillary (M8471/0)
      borderline malignancy (M8471/1)
        specified site — *see* Neoplasm, by site,
          uncertain behavior
        unspecified site 236.2
      specified site — *see* Neoplasm, by site,
        benign
      unspecified site 220
    specified site — *see* Neoplasm, by site,
      benign
    unspecified site 220
  serous (M8441/0)
    borderline malignancy (M8441/1)
      specified site — *see* Neoplasm, by site,
        uncertain behavior
      unspecified site 236.2
    papillary (M8460/0)
      borderline malignancy (M8460/1)
        specified site — *see* Neoplasm, by site,
          uncertain behavior
        unspecified site 236.2
      specified site — *see* Neoplasm, by site,
        benign
      unspecified site 220
    specified site — *see* Neoplasm, by site,
      benign
    unspecified site 220
  thyroid 226
Cystathioninemia 270.4
Cystathioninuria 270.4
Cystic — *see also* condition
  breast, chronic 610.1
  corpora lutea 620.1
  degeneration, congenital
    brain 742.4
    kidney 753.10
  disease
    breast, chronic 610.1
    kidney, congenital 753.10
      medullary 753.16
      multiple 753.19
      polycystic — *see* Polycystic, kidney
      single 753.11
      specified NEC 753.19
    liver, congenital 751.62
    lung 518.89
      congenital 748.4

Cystic — *see also* condition — *continued*
  disease — *continued*
    pancreas, congenital 751.7
    semilunar cartilage 717.5
  duct — *see* condition
  eyeball, congenital 743.03
  fibrosis (pancreas) 277.00
    with ●
      manifestations ●
        gastrointestinal 277.03 ●
        pulmonary 277.02 ●
        specified NEC 277.09 ●
      meconium ileus 277.01 ●
      pulmonary exacerbation 277.02 ●
  hygroma (M9173/0) 228.1
  kidney, congenital 753.10
    medullary 753.16
    multiple 753.19
    polycystic — *see* Polycystic, kidney
    single 753.11
    specified NEC 753.19
  liver, congenital 751.62
  lung 518.89
    congenital 748.4
  mass — *see* Cyst
  mastitis, chronic 610.1
  ovary 620.2
  pancreas, congenital 751.7
Cysticerciasis 123.1
Cysticercosis (mammary) (subretinal) 123.1
Cysticercus 123.1
  cellulosae infestation 123.1
Cystinosis (malignant) 270.0
Cystinuria 270.0
Cystitis (bacillary) (colli) (diffuse) (exudative)
  (hemorrhagic) (purulent) (recurrent) (septic)
  (suppurative) (ulcerative) 595.9
  with
    abortion — *see* Abortion, by type, with
      urinary tract infection
    ectopic pregnancy (*see also* categories
      633.0-633.9) 639.8
    fibrosis 595.1
    leukoplakia 595.1
    malakoplakia 595.1
    metaplasia 595.1
    molar pregnancy (*see also* categories 630-
      632) 639.8
  actinomycotic 039.8 *[595.4]*
  acute 595.0
    of trigone 595.3
  allergic 595.89
  amebic 006.8 *[595.4]*
  bilharzial 120.9 *[595.4]*
  blennorrhagic (acute) 098.11
    chronic or duration of 2 months or more
      098.31
  bullous 595.89
  calculous 594.1
    chlamydial 099.53
  chronic 595.2
    interstitial 595.1
    of trigone 595.3
  complicating pregnancy, childbirth, or
    puerperium 646.6 ✔5ᵗʰ
    affecting fetus or newborn 760.1
  cystic(a) 595.81
  diphtheritic 032.84
  echinococcal
    granulosus 122.3 *[595.4]*
    multilocularis 122.6 *[595.4]*
  emphysematous 595.89
  encysted 595.81
  follicular 595.3
  following
    abortion 639.8
    ectopic or molar pregnancy 639.8
  gangrenous 595.89
  glandularis 595.89
  gonococcal (acute) 098.11
    chronic or duration of 2 months or more
      098.31
  incrusted 595.89
  interstitial 595.1
  irradiation 595.82
  irritation 595.89

Cystitis — *continued*
  malignant 595.89
  monilial 112.2
  of trigone 595.3
  panmural 595.1
  polyposa 595.89
  prostatic 601.3
  radiation 595.82
  Reiter's (abacterial) 099.3
  specified NEC 595.89
  subacute 595.2
  submucous 595.1
  syphilitic 095.8
  trichomoniasis 131.09
  tuberculous (*see also* Tuberculosis) 016.1 ✔5ᵗʰ
  ulcerative 595.1
Cystocele (-rectocele)
  female (without uterine prolapse) 618.0
    with uterine prolapse 618.4
      complete 618.3
      incomplete 618.2
  in pregnancy or childbirth 654.4 ✔5ᵗʰ
    affecting fetus or newborn 763.89
    causing obstructed labor 660.2 ✔5ᵗʰ
      affecting fetus or newborn 763.1
  male 596.8
Cystoid
  cicatrix limbus 372.64
  degeneration macula 362.53
Cystolithiasis 594.1
Cystoma (M8440/0) — *see also* Neoplasm, by
  site, benign
  endometrial, ovary 617.1
  mucinous (M8470/0)
    specified site — *see* Neoplasm, by site,
      benign
    unspecified site 220
  serous (M8441/0)
    specified site — *see* Neoplasm, by site,
      benign
    unspecified site 220
  simple (ovary) 620.2
Cystoplegia 596.53
Cystoptosis 596.8
Cystopyelitis (*see also* Pyelitis) 590.80
Cystorrhagia 596.8
Cystosarcoma phyllodes (M9020/1) 238.3
  benign (M9020/0) 217
  malignant (M9020/3) — *see* Neoplasm, breast,
    malignant
Cystostomy status V44.50
  appendico-vesicostomy V44.52
  cutaneous-vesicostomy V44.51
  specified type NEC V44.59
  with complication 997.5
Cystourethritis (*see also* Urethritis) 597.89
Cystourethrocele (*see also* Cystocele)
  female (without uterine prolapse) 618.0
    with uterine prolapse 618.4
      complete 618.3
      incomplete 618.2
  male 596.8
Cytomegalic inclusion disease 078.5
  congenital 771.1
Cytomycosis, reticuloendothelial (*see also*
  Histoplasmosis, American) 115.00

✔4ᵗʰ Fourth-digit Required   ✔5ᵗʰ Fifth-digit Required   ►◄ Revised Text   ● New Line   ▲ Revised Code

D

Daae (-Finsen) disease (epidemic pleurodynia) 074.1

Dabney's grip 074.1

Da Costa's syndrome (neurocirculatory asthenia) 306.2

Dacryoadenitis, dacryadenitis 375.00
  acute 375.01
  chronic 375.02

Dacryocystitis 375.30
  acute 375.32
  chronic 375.42
  neonatal 771.6
  phlegmonous 375.33
  syphilitic 095.8
    congenital 090.0
  trachomatous, active 076.1
    late effect 139.1
  tuberculous (*see also* Tuberculosis) 017.3 ✓5ᵗʰ

Dacryocystoblenorrhea 375.42

Dacryocystocele 375.43

Dacryolith, dacryolithiasis 375.57

Dacryoma 375.43

Dacryopericystitis (acute) (subacute) 375.32
  chronic 375.42

Dacryops 375.11

Dacryosialadenopathy, atrophic 710.2

Dacryostenosis 375.56
  congenital 743.65

Dactylitis 686.9
  bone (*see also* Osteomyelitis) 730.2 ✓5ᵗʰ
  sickle cell 282.61
  syphilitic 095.5
  tuberculous (*see also* Tuberculosis) 015.5 ✓5ᵗʰ

Dactylolysis opontaned 136.0

Dactylosymphysis (*see also* Syndactylism) 755.10

Damage
  arteriosclerotic — *see* Arteriosclerosis
  brain 348.9
    anoxic, hypoxic 348.1
      during or resulting from a procedure 997.01
    child NEC 343.9
    due to birth injury 767.0
    minimal (child) (*see also* Hyperkinesia) 314.9
    newborn 767.0
  cardiac — *see also* Disease, heart
  cardiorenal (vascular) (*see also* Hypertension, cardiorenal) 404.90
  central nervous system — *see* Damage, brain
  cerebral NEC — *see* Damage, brain
  coccyx, complicating delivery 665.6 ✓5ᵗʰ
  coronary (*see also* Ischemia, heart) 414.9
  eye, birth injury 767.8
  heart — *see also* Disease, heart
    valve — *see* Endocarditis
  hypothalamus NEC 348.9
  liver 571.9
    alcoholic 571.3
  myocardium (*see also* Degeneration, myocardial) 429.1
  pelvic
    joint or ligament, during delivery 665.6 ✓5ᵗʰ
    organ NEC
      with
        abortion — *see* Abortion, by type, with damage to pelvic organs
        ectopic pregnancy (*see also* categories 633.0-633.9) 639.2
        molar pregnancy (*see also* categories 630-632) 639.2
      during delivery 665.5 ✓5ᵗʰ
      following
        abortion 639.2
        ectopic or molar pregnancy 639.2
  renal (*see also* Disease, renal) 593.9
  skin, solar 692.79
    acute 692.72
    chronic 692.74
  subendocardium, subendocardial (*see also* Degeneration, myocardial) 429.1
  vascular 459.9

Dameshek's syndrome (erythroblastic anemia) 282.4

Dana-Putnam syndrome (subacute combined sclerosis with pernicious anemia) 281.0 [336.2]

Danbolt (-Closs) syndrome (acrodermatitis enteropathica) 686.8

Dandruff 690.18

Dandy fever 061

Dandy-Walker deformity or syndrome (atresia, foramen of Magendie) 742.3
  with spina bifida (*see also* Spina bifida) 741.0 ✓5ᵗʰ

Dangle foot 736.79

Danielssen's disease (anesthetic leprosy) 030.1

Danlos' syndrome 756.83

Darier's disease (congenital) (keratosis follicularis) 757.39
  due to vitamin A deficiency 264.8
  meaning erythema annulare centrifugum 695.0

Darier-Roussy sarcoid 135

Darling's
  disease (*see also* Histoplasmosis, American) 115.00
  histoplasmosis (*see also* Histoplasmosis, American) 115.00

Dartre 054.9

Darwin's tubercle 744.29

Davidson's anemia (refractory) 284.9

Davies' disease 425.0

Davies-Colley syndrome (slipping rib) 733.99

Dawson's encephalitis 046.2

Day blindness (*see also* Blindness, day) 368.60

Dead
  fetus
    retained (in utero) 656.4 ✓5ᵗʰ
      early pregnancy (death before 22 completed weeks gestation) 632
      late (death after 22 completed weeks gestation) 656.4 ✓5ᵗʰ
    syndrome 641.3 ✓5ᵗʰ
  labyrinth 386.50
  ovum, retained 631

Deaf and dumb NEC 389.7

Deaf mutism (acquired) (congenital) NEC 389.7
  endemic 243
  hysterical 300.11
  syphilitic, congenital 090.0

Deafness (acquired) (bilateral) (both ears) (complete) (congenital) (hereditary) (middle ear) (partial) (unilateral) 389.9
  with blue sclera and fragility of bone 756.51
  auditory fatigue 389.9
  aviation 993.0
    nerve injury 951.5
  boilermakers' 951.5
  central 389.14
    with conductive hearing loss 389.2
  conductive (air) 389.00
    with sensorineural hearing loss 389.2
    combined types 389.08
    external ear 389.01
    inner ear 389.04
    middle ear 389.03
    multiple types 389.08
    tympanic membrane 389.02
  emotional (complete) 300.11
  functional (complete) 300.11
  high frequency 389.8
  hysterical (complete) 300.11
  injury 951.5
  low frequency 389.8
  mental 784.69
  mixed conductive and sensorineural 389.2
  nerve 389.12
    with conductive hearing loss 389.2
  neural 389.12
    with conductive hearing loss 389.2
  noise-induced 388.12
    nerve injury 951.5
  nonspeaking 389.7

Deafness — *continued*
  perceptive 389.10
    with conductive hearing loss 389.2
    central 389.14
    combined types 389.18
    multiple types 389.18
    neural 389.12
    sensory 389.11
  psychogenic (complete) 306.7
  sensorineural (*see also* Deafness, perceptive) 389.10
  sensory 389.11
    with conductive hearing loss 389.2
  specified type NEC 389.8
  sudden NEC 388.2
  syphilitic 094.89
  transient ischemic 388.02
  transmission — *see* Deafness, conductive
  traumatic 951.5
  word (secondary to organic lesion) 784.69
    developmental 315.31

Death
  after delivery (cause not stated) (sudden) 674.9 ✓5ᵗʰ
  anesthetic
    due to
      correct substance properly administered 995.4
      overdose or wrong substance given 968.4
        specified anesthetic — *see* Table of Drugs and Chemicals
    during delivery 668.9 ✓5ᵗʰ
  brain 348.8
  cardiac — *see* Disease, heart
  cause unknown 798.2
  cot (infant) 798.0
  crib (infant) 798.0
  fetus, fetal (cause not stated) (intrauterine) 779.9
    early, with retention (before 22 completed weeks gestation) 632
    from asphyxia or anoxia (before labor) 768.0
      during labor 768.1
    late, affecting management of pregnancy (after 22 completed weeks gestation) 656.4 ✓5ᵗʰ
  from pregnancy NEC 646.9 ✓5ᵗʰ
  instantaneous 798.1
  intrauterine (*see also* Death, fetus) 779.9
    complicating pregnancy 656.4 ✓5ᵗʰ
  maternal, affecting fetus or newborn 761.6
  neonatal NEC 779.9
  sudden (cause unknown) 798.1
    during delivery 669.9 ✓5ᵗʰ
      under anesthesia NEC 668.9 ✓5ᵗʰ
    infant, syndrome (SIDS) 798.0
    puerperal, during puerperium 674.9 ✓5ᵗʰ
  unattended (cause unknown) 798.9
  under anesthesia NEC
    due to
      correct substance properly administered 995.4
      overdose or wrong substance given 968.4
        specified anesthetic — *see* Table of Drugs and Chemicals
    during delivery 668.9 ✓5ᵗʰ
  violent 798.1

de Beurmann-Gougerot disease (sporotrichosis) 117.1

Debility (general) (infantile) (postinfectional) 799.3
  with nutritional difficulty 269.9
  congenital or neonatal NEC 779.9
  nervous 300.5
  old age 797
  senile 797

Débove's disease (splenomegaly) 789.2

Decalcification
  bone (*see also* Osteoporosis) 733.00
  teeth 521.8

Decapitation 874.9
  fetal (to facilitate delivery) 763.89

Decapsulation, kidney 593.89

Decay
  dental 521.00
  senile 797
  tooth, teeth 521.00

Decensus, uterus — *see* Prolapse, uterus
Deciduitis (acute)
    with
        abortion — *see* Abortion, by type, with
            sepsis
        ectopic pregnancy (*see also* categories
            633.0-633.9) 639.0
        molar pregnancy (*see also* categories 630-
            632) 639.0
    affecting fetus or newborn 760.8
    following
        abortion 639.0
        ectopic or molar pregnancy 639.0
    in pregnancy 646.6 ✔5ᵗʰ
    puerperal, postpartum 670 ✔4ᵗʰ
Deciduoma malignum (M9100/3) 181
Deciduous tooth (retained) 520.6
Decline (general) (*see also* Debility) 799.3
Decompensation
    cardiac (acute) (chronic) (*see also* Disease,
        heart) 429.9
        failure — *see* Failure, heart
    cardiorenal (*see also* Hypertension, cardiorenal)
        404.90
    cardiovascular (*see also* Disease,
        cardiovascular) 429.2
    heart (*see also* Disease, heart) 429.9
        failure — *see* Failure, heart
    hepatic 572.2
    myocardial (acute) (chronic) (*see also* Disease,
        heart) 429.9
        failure — *see* Failure, heart
    respiratory 519.9
Decompression sickness 993.3
Decrease, decreased
    blood
        platelets (*see also* Thrombocytopenia) 287.5
        pressure 796.3
            due to shock following
                injury 958.4
                operation 998.0
    cardiac reserve — *see* Disease, heart
    estrogen 256.39
        postablative 256.2
    fetal movements 655.7 ✔5ᵗʰ
    fragility of erythrocytes 289.8
    function
        adrenal (cortex) 255.4
            medulla 255.5
        ovary in hypopituitarism 253.4
        parenchyma of pancreas 577.8
        pituitary (gland) (lobe) (anterior) 253.2
            posterior (lobe) 253.8
    functional activity 780.99   ▲
    glucose 790.2
    haptoglobin (serum) NEC 273.8
    platelets (*see also* Thrombocytopenia) 287.5
    pulse pressure 785.9
    respiration due to shock following injury 958.4
    tear secretion NEC 375.15
    tolerance
        fat 579.8
        glucose 790.2
        salt and water 276.9
    vision NEC 369.9
Decubital gangrene 707.0 *[785.4]*
Decubiti (*see also* Decubitus) 707.0
Decubitus (ulcer) 707.0
    with gangrene 707.0 *[785.4]*
Deepening acetabulum 718.85
Defect, defective 759.9
    3-beta-hydroxysteroid dehydrogenase 255.2
    11-hydroxylase 255.2
    21-hydroxylase 255.2
    abdominal wall, congenital 756.70
    aorticopulmonary septum 745.0
    aortic septal 745.0
    atrial septal (ostium secundum type) 745.5
        acquired 429.71
        ostium primum type 745.61
        sinus venosus 745.8
    atrioventricular
        canal 745.69
        septum 745.4
            acquired 429.71

Defect, defective — *continued*
    atrium secundum 745.5
        acquired 429.71
    auricular septal 745.5
        acquired 429.71
    bilirubin excretion 277.4
    biosynthesis, testicular androgen 257.2
    bulbar septum 745.0
    butanol-insoluble iodide 246.1
    chromosome — *see* Anomaly, chromosome
    circulation (acquired) 459.9
        congenital 747.9
        newborn 747.9
    clotting NEC (*see also* Defect, coagulation)
        286.9
    coagulation (factor) (*see also* Deficiency,
        coagulation factor) 286.9
        with
            abortion — *see* Abortion, by type, with
                hemorrhage
            ectopic pregnancy (*see also* categories
                634-638) 639.1
            molar pregnancy (*see also* categories
                630-632) 639.1
        acquired (any) 286.7
        antepartum or intrapartum 641.3 ✔5ᵗʰ
            affecting fetus or newborn 762.1
        causing hemorrhage of pregnancy or delivery
            641.3 ✔5ᵗʰ
        due to
            liver disease 286.7
            vitamin K deficiency 286.7
        newborn, transient 776.3
        postpartum 666.3 ✔5ᵗʰ
        specified type NEC 286.3
    conduction (heart) 426.9
        bone (*see also* Deafness, conductive) 389.00
    congenital, organ or site NEC — *see also*
        Anomaly
        circulation 747.9
        Descemet's membrane 743.9
            specified type NEC 743.49
        diaphragm 756.6
        ectodermal 757.9
        esophagus 750.9
        pulmonic cusps — *see* Anomaly, heart valve
        respiratory system 748.9
            specified type NEC 748.8
    cushion endocardial 745.60
    dentin (hereditary) 520.5
    Descemet's membrane (congenital) 743.9
        acquired 371.30
        specific type NEC 743.49
    deutan 368.52
    developmental — *see also* Anomaly, by site
        cauda equina 742.59
        left ventricle 746.9
            with atresia or hypoplasia of aortic orifice
                or valve, with hypoplasia of
                ascending aorta 746.7
            in hypoplastic left heart syndrome 746.7
        testis 752.9
        vessel 747.9
    diaphragm
        with elevation, eventration, or hernia — *see*
            Hernia, diaphragm
        congenital 756.6
            with elevation, eventration, or hernia
                756.6
            gross (with elevation, eventration, or
                hernia) 756.6
    ectodermal, congenital 757.9
    Eisenmenger's (ventricular septal defect) 745.4
    endocardial cushion 745.60
        specified type NEC 745.69
    esophagus, congenital 750.9
    extensor retinaculum 728.9
    fibrin polymerization (*see also* Defect,
        coagulation) 286.3
    filling
        biliary tract 793.3
        bladder 793.5
        gallbladder 793.3
        kidney 793.5
        stomach 793.4
        ureter 793.5
    fossa ovalis 745.5

Defect, defective — *continued*
    gene, carrier (suspected) of V83.89   ▲
    Gerbode 745.4
    glaucomatous, without elevated tension 365.89
    Hageman (factor) (*see also* Defect, coagulation)
        286.3
    hearing (*see also* Deafness) 389.9
    high grade 317
    homogentisic acid 270.2
    interatrial septal 745.5
        acquired 429.71
    interauricular septal 745.5
        acquired 429.71
    interventricular septal 745.4
        with pulmonary stenosis or atresia,
            dextraposition of aorta, and
            hypertrophy of right ventricle 745.2
        acquired 429.71
        in tetralogy of Fallot 745.2
    iodide trapping 246.1
    iodotyrosine dehalogenase 246.1
    kynureninase 270.2
    learning, specific 315.2
    mental (*see also* Retardation, mental) 319
    osteochondral NEC 738.8
    ostium
        primum 745.61
        secundum 745.5
    pericardium 746.89
    peroxidase-binding 246.1
    placental blood supply — *see* Placenta,
        insufficiency
    platelet (qualitative) 287.1
        constitutional 286.4
    postural, spine 737.9
    protan 368.51
    pulmonic cusps, congenital 746.00
    renal pelvis 753.9
        obstructive 753.29
        specified type NEC 753.3
    respiratory system, congenital 748.9
        specified type NEC 748.8
    retina, retinal 361.30
        with detachment (*see also* Detachment,
            retina, with retinal defect) 361.00
        multiple 361.33
            with detachment 361.02
        nerve fiber bundle 362.85
        single 361.30
            with detachment 361.01
    septal (closure) (heart) NEC 745.9
        acquired 429.71
        atrial 745.5
        specified type NEC 745.8
    speech NEC 784.5
        developmental 315.39
        secondary to organic lesion 784.5
    Taussig-Bing (transposition, aorta and
        overriding pulmonary artery) 745.11
    teeth, wedge 521.2
    thyroid hormone synthesis 246.1
    tritan 368.53
    ureter 753.9
        obstructive 753.29
    vascular (acquired) (local) 459.9
        congenital (peripheral) NEC 747.60
            gastrointestinal 747.61
            lower limb 747.64
            renal 747.62
            specified NEC 747.69
            spinal 747.82
            upper limb 747.63
    ventricular septal 745.4
        with pulmonary stenosis or atresia,
            dextraposition of aorta, and
            hypertrophy of right ventricle 745.2
        acquired 429.71
        atrioventricular canal type 745.69
        between infundibulum and anterior portion
            745.4
        in tetralogy of Fallot 745.2
        isolated anterior 745.4
    vision NEC 369.9
    visual field 368.40
        arcuate 368.43
        heteronymous, bilateral 368.47
        homonymous, bilateral 368.46

Defect, defective — *continued*
  visual field — *continued*
    localized NEC 368.44
    nasal step 368.44
    peripheral 368.44
    sector 368.43
  voice 784.40
  wedge, teeth (abrasion) 521.2
Defeminization syndrome 255.2
Deferentitis 608.4
  gonorrheal (acute) 098.14
    chronic or duration of 2 months or over 098.34
Defibrination syndrome (*see also* Fibrinolysis) 286.6
Deficiency, deficient
  3-beta-hydroxysteroid dehydrogenase 255.2
  6-phosphogluconic dehydrogenase (anemia) 282.2
  11-beta-hydroxylase 255.2
  17-alpha-hydroxylase 255.2
  18-hydroxysteroid dehydrogenase 255.2
  20-alpha-hydroxylase 255.2
  21-hydroxylase 255.2
  abdominal muscle syndrome 756.79
  accelerator globulin (Ac G) (blood) (*see also* Defect, coagulation) 286.3
  AC globulin (congenital) (*see also* Defect, coagulation) 286.3
    acquired 286.7
  activating factor (blood) (*see also,* Defect, coagulation) 286.3
  adenohypophyseal 253.2
  adenosine deaminase 277.2
  aldolase (hereditary) 271.2
  alpha-1-antitrypsin 277.6
  alpha-1-trypsin inhibitor 277.6
  alpha-fucosidase 271.8
  alpha-lipoprotein 272.5
  alpha-mannosidase 271.8
  amino acid 270.9
  anemia — *see* Anemia, deficiency
  aneurin 265.1
    with beriberi 265.0
  antibody NEC 279.00
  antidiuretic hormone 253.5
  antihemophilic
    factor (A) 286.0
      B 286.1
      C 286.2
    globulin (AHG) NEC 286.0
  antitrypsin 277.6
  argininosuccinate synthetase or lyase 270.6
  ascorbic acid (with scurvy) 267
  autoprothrombin
    I (*see also* Defect, coagulation) 286.3
    II 286.1
    C (*see also* Defect, coagulation) 286.3
  bile salt 579.8
  biotin 266.2
  biotinidase 277.6
  bradykinase-1 277.6
  brancher enzyme (amylopectinosis) 271.0
  calciferol 268.9
    with
      osteomalacia 268.2
      rickets (*see also* Rickets) 268.0
  calcium 275.40
    dietary 269.3
  calorie, severe 261
  carbamyl phosphate synthetase 270.6
  cardiac (*see also* Insufficiency, myocardial) 428.0
  carnitine palmityl transferase 791.3
  carotene 264.9
  Carr factor (*see also* Defect, coagulation) 286.9
  central nervous system 349.9
  ceruloplasmin 275.1
  cevitamic acid (with scurvy) 267
  choline 266.2
  Christmas factor 286.1
  chromium 269.3
  citrin 269.1
  clotting (blood) (*see also* Defect, coagulation) 286.9

Deficiency, deficient — *continued*
  coagulation factor NEC 286.9
    with
      abortion — *see* Abortion, by type, with hemorrhage
      ectopic pregnancy (*see also* categories 634-638) 639.1
      molar pregnancy (*see also* categories 630-632) 639.1
    acquired (any) 286.7
    antepartum or intrapartum 641.3 ✓5ᵗʰ
      affecting fetus or newborn 762.1
    due to
      liver disease 286.7
      vitamin K deficiency 286.7
    newborn, transient 776.3
    postpartum 666.3 ✓5ᵗʰ
    specified type NEC 286.3
  color vision (congenital) 368.59
    acquired 368.55
  combined, two or more coagulation factors (*see also* Defect, coagulation) 286.9
  complement factor NEC 279.8
  contact factor (*see also* Defect, coagulation) 286.3
  copper NEC 275.1
  corticoadrenal 255.4
  craniofacial axis 756.0
  cyanocobalamin (vitamin B_{12}) 266.2
  debrancher enzyme (limit dextrinosis) 271.0
  desmolase 255.2
  diet 269.9
  dihydrofolate reductase 281.2
  dihydropteridine reductase 270.1
  disaccharidase (intestinal) 271.3
  disease NEC 269.9
  ear(s) V48.8
  edema 262
  endocrine 259.9
  enzymes, circulating NEC (*see also* Deficiency, by specific enzyme) 277.6
  ergosterol 268.9
    with
      osteomalacia 268.2
      rickets (*see also* Rickets) 268.0
  erythrocytic glutathione (anemia) 282.2
  eyelid(s) V48.8
  factor (*See also* Defect, coagulation) 286.9
    I (congenital) (fibrinogen) 286.3
      antepartum or intrapartum 641.3 ✓5ᵗʰ
        affecting fetus or newborn 762.1
      newborn, transient 776.3
      postpartum 666.3 ✓5ᵗʰ
    II (congenital) (prothrombin) 286.3
    V (congenital) (labile) 286.3
    VII (congenital) (stable) 286.3
    VIII (congenital) (functional) 286.0
      with
        functional defect 286.0
        vascular defect 286.4
    IX (Christmas) (congenital) (functional) 286.1
    X (congenital) (Stuart-Prower) 286.3
    XI (congenital) (plasma thromboplastin antecedent) 286.2
    XII (congenital) (Hageman) 286.3
    XIII (congenital) (fibrin stabilizing) 286.3
    Hageman 286.3
    multiple (congenital) 286.9
      acquired 286.7
  fibrinase (*see also* Defect, coagulation) 286.3
  fibrinogen (congenital) (*see also* Defect, coagulation) 286.3
    acquired 286.6
  fibrin-stabilizing factor (congenital) (*see also* Defect, coagulation) 286.3
  finger — *see* Absence, finger
  fletcher factor (*see also* Defect, coagulation) 286.9
  fluorine 269.3
  folate, anemia 281.2
  folic acid (vitamin B_6) 266.2
    anemia 281.2
  fructokinase 271.2
  fructose-1, 6-diphosphate 271.2
  fructose-1-phosphate aldolase 271.2
  FSH (follicle-stimulating hormone) 253.4
  fucosidase 271.8

Deficiency, deficient — *continued*
  galactokinase 271.1
  galactose-1-phosphate uridyl transferase 271.1
  gamma globulin in blood 279.00
  glass factor (*see also* Defect, coagulation) 286.3
  glucocorticoid 255.4
  glucose-6-phosphatase 271.0
  glucose-6-phosphate dehydrogenase anemia 282.2
  glucuronyl transferase 277.4
  glutathione-reductase (anemia) 282.2
  glycogen synthetase 271.0
  growth hormone 253.3
  Hageman factor (congenital) (*see also* Defect, coagulation) 286.3
  head V48.0
  hemoglobin (*see also* Anemia) 285.9
  hepatophosphorylase 271.0
  hexose monophosphate (HMP) shunt 282.2
  HGH (human growth hormone) 253.3
  HG-PRT 277.2
  homogentisic acid oxidase 270.2
  hormone — *see also* Deficiency, by specific hormone
    anterior pituitary (isolated) (partial) NEC 253.4
      growth (human) 253.3
    follicle-stimulating 253.4
    growth (human) (isolated) 253.3
    human growth 253.3
    interstitial cell-stimulating 253.4
    luteinizing 253.4
    melanocyte-stimulating 253.4
    testicular 257.2
  human growth hormone 253.3
  humoral 279.00
    with
      hyper-IgM 279.05
        autosomal recessive 279.05
        X-linked 279.05
      increased IgM 279.05
    congenital hypogammaglobulinemia 279.04
    non-sex-linked 279.06
    selective immunoglobulin NEC 279.03
      IgA 279.01
      IgG 279.03
      IgM 279.02
        increased 279.05
    specified NEC 279.09
  hydroxylase 255.2
  hypoxanthine-guanine phosphoribosyltransferase (HG-PRT) 277.2
  ICSH (interstitial cell-stimulating hormone) 253.4
  immunity NEC 279.3
    cell-mediated 279.10
      with
        hyperimmunoglob-ulinemia 279.2
        thrombocytopenia and eczema 279.12
      specified NEC 279.19
    combined (severe) 279.2
      syndrome 279.2
    common variable 279.06
    humoral NEC 279.00
    IgA (secretory) 279.01
    IgG 279.03
    IgM 279.02
  immunoglobulin, selective NEC 279.03
    IgA 279.01
    IgG 279.03
    IgM 279.02
  inositol (B complex) 266.2
  interferon 279.4
  internal organ V47.0
  interstitial cell-stimulating hormone (ICSH) 253.4
  intrinsic factor (Castle's) (congenital) 281.0
  intrinsic (urethral) sphincter (ISD) 599.82
  invertase 271.3
  iodine 269.3
  iron, anemia 280.9
  labile factor (congenital) (*see also* Defect, coagulation) 286.3
    acquired 286.7
  lacrimal fluid (acquired) 375.15
    congenital 743.64
  lactase 271.3

Deficiency, deficient — *continued*
 Laki-Lorand factor (*see also* Defect,
  coagulation) 286.3
 lecithin-cholesterol acyltranferase 272.5
 LH (luteinizing hormone) 253.4
 limb V49.0
  lower V49.0
   congenital (*see also* Deficiency, lower
    limb, congenital) 755.30
  upper V49.0
   congenital (*see also* Deficiency, upper
    limb, congenital) 755.20
 lipocaic 577.8
 lipoid (high-density) 272.5
 lipoprotein (familial) (high density) 272.5
 liver phosphorylase 271.0
 lower limb V49.0
  congenital 755.30
   with complete absence of distal elements
    755.31
   longitudinal (complete) (partial) (with
    distal deficiencies, incomplete)
    755.32
    with complete absence of distal
     elements 755.31
    combined femoral, tibial, fibular
     (incomplete) 755.33
    femoral 755.34
    fibular 755.37
    metatarsal(s) 755.38
    phalange(s) 755.39
     meaning all digits 755.31
    tarsal(s) 755.38
    tibia 755.36
    tibiofibular 755.35
   transverse 755.31
 luteinizing hormone (LH) 253.4
 lysosomal alpha-1, 4 glucosidase 271.0
 magnesium 275.2
 mannosidase 271.8
 melanocyte-stimulating hormone (MSH) 253.4
 menadione (vitamin K) 269.0
  newborn 776.0
 mental (familial) (hereditary) (*see also*
  Retardation, mental) 319
 mineral NEC 269.3
 molybdenum 269.3
 moral 301.7
 multiple, syndrome 260
 myocardial (*see also* Insufficiency myocardial)
  428.0
 myophosphorylase 271.0
 NADH (DPNH)-methemoglobin-reductase
  (congenital) 289.7
 NADH-diaphorase or reductase (congenital)
  289.7
 neck V48.1
 niacin (amide) (-tryptophan) 265.2
 nicotinamide 265.2
 nicotinic acid (amide) 265.2
 nose V48.8
 number of teeth (*see also* Anodontia) 520.0
 nutrition, nutritional 269.9
  specified NEC 269.8
 ornithine transcarbamylase 270.6
 ovarian 256.39
 oxygen (*see also* Anoxia) 799.0
 pantothenic acid 266.2
 parathyroid (gland) 252.1
 phenylalanine hydroxylase 270.1
 phosphofructokinase 271.2
 phosphoglucomutase 271.0
 phosphohexosisomerase 271.0
 phosphorylase kinase, liver 271.0
 pituitary (anterior) 253.2
  posterior 253.5
 placenta — *see* Placenta, insufficiency
 plasma
  cell 279.00
  protein (paraproteinemia) (pyroglobulinemia)
   273.8
   gamma globulin 279.00
  thromboplastin
   antecedent (PTA) 286.2
   component (PTC) 286.1
 platelet NEC 287.1
  constitutional 286.4

Deficiency, deficient — *continued*
 polyglandular 258.9
 potassium (K) 276.8
 proaccelerin (congenital) (*see also* Defect,
  congenital) 286.3
  acquired 286.7
 proconvertin factor (congenital) (*see also*
  Defect, coagulation) 286.3
  acquired 286.7
 prolactin 253.4
 protein 260
  anemia 281.4
  plasma — *see* Deficiency, plasma protein
 prothrombin (congenital) (*see also* Defect
  coagulation) 286.3
  acquired 286.7
 Prower factor (*see also* Defect, coagulation)
  286.3
 PRT 277.2
 pseudocholinesterase 289.8
 psychobiological 301.6
 PTA 286.2
 PTC 286.1
 purine nucleoside phosphorylase 277.2
 pyracin (alpha) (Beta) 266.1
 pyridoxal 266.1
 pyridoxamine 266.1
 pyridoxine (derivatives) 266.1
 pyruvate kinase (PK) 282.3
 riboflavin (vitamin B_2) 266.0
 saccadic eye movements 379.57
 salivation 527.7
 salt 276.1
 secretion
  ovary 256.39
  salivary gland (any) 527.7
  urine 788.5
 selenium 269.3
 serum
  antitrypsin, familial 277.6
  protein (congenital) 273.8
 smooth pursuit movements (eye) 379.58
 sodium (Na) 276.1
 SPCA (*see also* Defect, coagulation) 286.3
 specified NEC 269.8
 stable factor (congenital) (*see also* Defect,
  coagulation) 286.3
  acquired 286.7
 Stuart (-Prower) factor (*see also* Defect,
  coagulation) 286.3
 sucrase 271.3
 sucrase-isomaltase 271.3
 sulfite oxidase 270.0
 syndrome, multiple 260
 thiamine, thiaminic (chloride) 265.1
 thrombokinase (*see also* Defect, coagulation)
  286.3
  newborn 776.0
 thrombopoieten 287.3
 thymolymphatic 279.2
 thyroid (gland) 244.9
 tocopherol 269.1
 toe — *see* Absence, toe
 tooth bud (*see also* Anodontia) 520.0
 trunk V48.1
 UDPG-glycogen transferase 271.0
 upper limb V49.0
  congenital 755.20
   with complete absence of distal elements
    755.21
   longitudinal (complete) (partial) (with
    distal deficiencies, incomplete)
    755.22
    carpal(s) 755.28
    combined humeral, radial, ulnar
     (incomplete) 755.23
    humeral 755.24
    metacarpal(s) 755.28
    phalange(s) 755.29
     meaning all digits 755.21
    radial 755.26
    radioulnar 755.25
    ulnar 755.27
   transverse (complete) (partial) 755.21
 vascular 459.9
 vasopressin 253.5
 viosterol (*see also* Deficiency, calciferol) 268.9

Deficiency, deficient — *continued*
 vitamin (multiple) NEC 269.2
  A 264.9
   with
    Bitôt's spot 264.1
     corneal 264.2
      with corneal ulceration 264.3
    keratomalacia 264.4
    keratosis, follicular 264.8
    night blindness 264.5
    scar of cornea, xerophthalmic 264.6
    specified manifestation NEC 264.8
     ocular 264.7
    xeroderma 264.8
    xerophthalmia 264.7
    xerosis
     conjunctival 264.0
      with Bitôt's spot 264.1
     corneal 264.2
      with corneal ulceraton 264.3
  B (complex) NEC 266.9
   with
    beriberi 265.0
    pellagra 265.2
   specified type NEC 266.2
  B_1 NEC 265.1
   beriberi 265.0
  B_2 266.0
  B_6 266.1
  B_{12} 266.2
  B_9 (folic acid) 266.2
  C (ascorbic acid) (with scurvy) 267
  D (calciferol) (ergosterol) 268.9
   with
    osteomalacia 268.2
    rickets (*see also* Rickets) 268.0
  E 269.1
  folic acid 266.2
  G 266.0
  H 266.2
  K 269.0
   of newborn 776.0
  nicotinic acid 265.2
  P 269.1
  PP 265.2
  specified NEC 269.1
  zinc 269.3
Deficient — *see also* Deficiency
 blink reflex 374.45
 craniofacial axis 756.0
 number of teeth (*see also* Anodontia) 520.0
 secretion of urine 788.5
Deficit
 neurologic NEC 781.99
  due to
   cerebrovascular lesion (*see also* Disease,
    cerebrovascular, acute) 436
   late effect — *see* Late effect(s) (of)
    cerebrovascular disease
   transient ischemic attack 435.9
 oxygen 799.0
Deflection
 radius 736.09
 septum (acquired) (nasal) (nose) 470
 spine — *see* Curvature, spine
 turbinate (nose) 470
Defluvium
 capillorum (*see also* Alopecia) 704.00
 ciliorum 374.55
 unguium 703.8
Deformity 738.9
 abdomen, congenital 759.9
 abdominal wall
  acquired 738.8
  congenital 756.70
  muscle deficiency syndrome 756.79
 acquired (unspecified site) 738.9
  specified site NEC 738.8
 adrenal gland (congenital) 759.1
 alimentary tract, congenital 751.9
  lower 751.5
  specified type NEC 751.8
  upper (any part, except tongue) 750.9
   specified type NEC 750.8
   tongue 750.10
    specified type NEC 750.19

Deficiency — Deformity

Deformity — *continued*
  ankle (joint) (acquired) 736.70
    abduction 718.47
    congenital 755.69
    contraction 718.47
    specified NEC 736.79   ●
  anus (congenital) 751.5
    acquired 569.49
  aorta (congenital) 747.20
    acquired 447.8
    arch 747.21
      acquired 447.8
    coarctation 747.10
  aortic
    arch 747.21
      acquired 447.8
    cusp or valve (congenital) 746.9
        acquired (*see also* Endocarditis, aortic) 424.1
    ring 747.21
  appendix 751.5
  arm (acquired) 736.89
    congenital 755.50
  arteriovenous (congenital) (peripheral) NEC 747.60
    gastrointestinal 747.61
    lower limb 747.64
    renal 747.62
    specified NEC 747.69
    spinal 747.82
    upper limb 747.63
  artery (congenital) (peripheral) NEC (*see also* Deformity, vascular) 747.60
    acquired 447.8
    cerebral 747.81
    coronary (congenital) 746.85
      acquired (*see also* Ischemia, heart) 414.9
    retinal 743.9
    umbilical 747.5
  atrial septal (congenital) (heart) 745.5
  auditory canal (congenital) (external) (*see also* Deformity, ear) 744.3
    acquired 380.50
  auricle
    ear (congenital) (*see also* Deformity, ear) 744.3
      acquired 380.32
    heart (congenital) 746.9
  back (acquired) — *see* Deformity, spine
  Bartholin's duct (congenital) 750.9
  bile duct (congenital) 751.60
    acquired 576.8
      with calculus, choledocholithiasis, or stones — *see* Choledocholithiasis
  biliary duct or passage (congenital) 751.60
    acquired 576.8
      with calculus, choledocholithiasis, or stones — *see* Choledocholithiasis
  bladder (neck) (spincter) (trigone) (acquired) 596.8
    congenital 753.9
  bone (acquired) NEC 738.9
    congenital 756.9
    turbinate 738.0
  boutonniere (finger) 736.21
  brain (congenital) 742.9
    acquired 348.8
    multiple 742.4
    reduction 742.2
    vessel (congenital) 747.81
  breast (acquired) 611.8
    congenital 757.9
  bronchus (congenital) 748.3
    acquired 519.1
  bursa, congenital 756.9
  canal of Nuck 752.9
  canthus (congenital) 743.9
    acquired 374.89
  capillary (acquired) 448.9
    congenital NEC (*see also* Deformity, vascular) 747.60
  cardiac — *see* Deformity, heart
  cardiovascular system (congenital) 746.9
  caruncle, lacrimal (congenital) 743.9
    acquired 375.69
  cascade, stomach 537.6
  cecum (congenital) 751.5
    acquired 569.89

Deformity — *continued*
  cerebral (congenital) 742.9
    acquired 348.8
  cervix (acquired) (uterus) 622.8
    congenital 752.40
  cheek (acquired) 738.19
    congenital 744.9
  chest (wall) (acquired) 738.3
    congenital 754.89
    late effect of rickets 268.1
  chin (acquired) 738.19
    congenital 744.9
  choroid (congenital) 743.9
    acquired 363.8
    plexus (congenital) 742.9
      acquired 349.2
  cicatricial — *see* Cicatrix
  cilia (congenital) 743.9
    acquired 374.89
  circulatory system (congenital) 747.9
  clavicle (acquired) 738.8
    congenital 755.51
  clitoris (congenital) 752.40
    acquired 624.8
  clubfoot — *see* Clubfoot
  coccyx (acquired) 738.6
    congenital 756.10
  colon (congenital) 751.5
    acquired 569.89
  concha (ear) (congenital) (*see also* Deformity, ear) 744.3
    acquired 380.32
  congenital, organ or site not listed (*see also* Anomaly) 759.9
  cornea (congenital) 743.9
    acquired 371.70
  coronary artery (congenital) 746.85
    acquired (*see also* Ischemia, heart) 414.9
  cranium (acquired) 738.19
    congenital (*see also* Deformity, skull, congenital) 756.0
  cricoid cartilage (congenital) 748.3
    acquired 478.79
  cystic duct (congenital) 751.60
    acquired 575.8
  Dandy-Walker 742.3
    with spina bifida (*see also* Spina bifida) 741.0 ✓5ᵗʰ
  diaphragm (congenital) 756.6
    acquired 738.8
  digestive organ(s) or system (congenital) NEC 751.9
    specified type NEC 751.8
  ductus arteriosus 747.0
  duodenal bulb 537.89
  duodenum (congenital) 751.5
    acquired 537.89
  dura (congenital) 742.9
    brain 742.4
      acquired 349.2
    spinal 742.59
      acquired 349.2
  ear (congenital) 744.3
    acquired 380.32
    auricle 744.3
      causing impairment of hearing 744.02
    causing impairment of hearing 744.00
    external 744.3
      causing impairment of hearing 744.02
    internal 744.05
    lobule 744.3
    middle 744.03
      ossicles 744.04
    ossicles 744.04
  ectodermal (congenital) NEC 757.9
    specified type NEC 757.8
  ejaculatory duct (congenital) 752.9
    acquired 608.89
  elbow (joint) (acquired) 736.00
    congenital 755.50
    contraction 718.42
  endocrine gland NEC 759.2
  epididymis (congenital) 752.9
    acquired 608.89
    torsion 608.2
  epiglottis (congenital) 748.3
    acquired 478.79

Deformity — *continued*
  esophagus (congenital) 750.9
    acquired 530.89
  Eustachian tube (congenital) NEC 744.3
    specified type NEC 744.24
  extremity (acquired) 736.9
    congenital, except reduction deformity 755.9
      lower 755.60
      upper 755.50
    reduction — *see* Deformity, reduction
  eye (congenital) 743.9
    acquired 379.8
    muscle 743.9
  eyebrow (congenital) 744.89
  eyelid (congenital) 743.9
    acquired 374.89
    specified type NEC 743.62
  face (acquired) 738.19
    congenital (any part) 744.9
      due to intrauterine malposition and pressure 754.0
  fallopian tube (congenital) 752.10
    acquired 620.8
  femur (acquired) 736.89
    congenital 755.60
  fetal
    with fetopelvic disproportion 653.7 ✓5ᵗʰ
      affecting fetus or newborn 763.1
    causing obstructed labor 660.1 ✓5ᵗʰ
      affecting fetus or newborn 763.1
    known or suspected, affecting management of pregnancy 655.9 ✓5ᵗʰ
  finger (acquired) 736.20
    boutonniere type 736.21
    congenital 755.50
    flexion contracture 718.44
    swan neck 736.22
  flexion (joint) (acquired) 736.9
    congenital NEC 755.9
    hip or thigh (acquired) 736.39
      congenital (*see also* Subluxation, congenital, hip) 754.32
  foot (acquired) 736.70
    cavovarus 736.75
      congenital 754.59
    congenital NEC 754.70
      specified type NEC 754.79
    valgus (acquired) 736.79
      congenital 754.60
        specified type NEC 754.69
    varus (acquired) 736.79
      congenital 754.50
        specified type NEC 754.59
  forearm (acquired) 736.00
    congenital 755.50
  forehead (acquired) 738.19
    congenital (*see also* Deformity, skull, congenital) 756.0
  frontal bone (acquired) 738.19
    congenital (*see also* Deformity, skull, congenital) 756.0
  gallbladder (congenital) 751.60
    acquired 575.8
  gastrointestinal tract (congenital) NEC 751.9
    acquired 569.89
    specified type NEC 751.8
  genitalia, genital organ(s) or system NEC
    congenital 752.9
    female (congenital) 752.9
      acquired 629.8
      external 752.40
      internal 752.9
    male (congenital) 752.9
      acquired 608.89
  globe (eye) (congenital) 743.9
    acquired 360.89
  gum (congenital) 750.9
    acquired 523.9
  gunstock 736.02
  hand (acquired) 736.00
    claw 736.06
    congenital 755.50
    minus (and plus) (intrinsic) 736.09
    pill roller (intrinsic) 736.09
    plus (and minus) (intrinsic) 736.09
    swan neck (intrinsic) 736.09

✓4ᵗʰ Fourth-digit Required   ✓5ᵗʰ Fifth-digit Required   ▶◀ Revised Text   ● New Line   ▲ Revised Code

Deformity — *continued*
head (acquired) 738.10
  congenital (*see also* Deformity, skull
    congenital) 756.0
  specified NEC 738.19
heart (congenital) 746.9
  auricle (congenital) 746.9
  septum 745.9
    auricular 745.5
    specified type NEC 745.8
    ventricular 745.4
  valve (congenital) NEC 746.9
    acquired — *see* Endocarditis
    pulmonary (congenital) 746.00
    specified type NEC 746.89
  ventricle (congenital) 746.9
heel (acquired) 736.76
  congenital 755.67
hepatic duct (congenital) 751.60
  acquired 576.8
    with calculus, choledocholithiasis, or
      stones — *see* Choledocholithiasis
hip (joint) (acquired) 736.30
  congenital NEC 755.63
  flexion 718.45
    congenital (*see also* Subluxation,
      congenital, hip) 754.32
hourglass — *see* Contraction, hourglass
humerus (acquired) 736.89
  congenital 755.50
hymen (congenital) 752.40
hypophyseal (congenital) 759.2
ileocecal (coil) (valve) (congenital) 751.5
  acquired 569.89
ileum (intestine) (congenital) 751.5
  acquired 569.89
ilium (acquired) 738.6
  congenital 755.60
integument (congenital) 757.9
intervertebral cartilage or disc (acquired) — *see*
  also Displacement, intervertebral disc
  congenital 756.10
intestine (large) (small) (congenital) 751.5
  acquired 569.89
iris (acquired) 364.75
  congenital 743.9
  prolapse 364.8
ischium (acquired) 738.6
  congenital 755.60
jaw (acquired) (congenital) NEC 524.9
  due to intrauterine malposition and
    pressure 754.0
joint (acquired) NEC 738.8
  congenital 755.9
  contraction (abduction) (adduction)
    (extension) (flexion) — *see* Contraction,
    joint
kidney(s) (calyx) (pelvis) (congenital) 753.9
  acquired 593.89
  vessel 747.62
    acquired 459.9
Klippel-Feil (brevicollis) 756.16
knee (acquired) NEC 736.6
  congenital 755.64
labium (majus) (minus) (congenital) 752.40
  acquired 624.8
lacrimal apparatus or duct (congenital) 743.9
  acquired 375.69
larynx (muscle) (congenital) 748.3
  acquired 478.79
  web (glottic) (subglottic) 748.2
leg (lower) (upper) (acquired) NEC 736.89
  congenital 755.60
    reduction — *see* Deformity, reduction,
      lower limb
lens (congenital) 743.9
  acquired 379.39
lid (fold) (congenital) 743.9
  acquired 374.89
ligament (acquired) 728.9
  congenital 756.9
limb (acquired) 736.9
  congenital, except reduction deformity 755.9
    lower 755.60
      reduction (*see also* Deformity,
       reduction, lower limb) 755.30

Deformity — *continued*
limb — *continued*
  congenital, except reduction deformity —
    continued
    upper 755.50
      reduction (*see also* Deformity,
       reduction, upper limb) 755.20
  specified NEC 736.89
lip (congenital) NEC 750.9
  acquired 528.5
  specified type NEC 750.26
liver (congenital) 751.60
  acquired 573.8
  duct (congenital) 751.60
    acquired 576.8
      with calculus, choledocholithiasis, or
       stones — *see* Choledocholithi-
       asis
lower extremity — *see* Deformity, leg
lumbosacral (joint) (region) (congenital) 756.10
  acquired 738.5
lung (congenital) 748.60
  acquired 518.89
  specified type NEC 748.69
lymphatic system, congenital 759.9
Madelung's (radius) 755.54
maxilla (acquired) (congenital) 524.9
meninges or membrane (congenital) 742.9
  brain 742.4
    acquired 349.2
  spinal (cord) 742.59
    acquired 349.2
mesentery (congenital) 751.9
  acquired 568.89
metacarpus (acquired) 736.00
  congenital 755.50
metatarsus (acquired) 736.70
  congenital 754.70
middle ear, except ossicles (congenital) 744.03
  ossicles 744.04
mitral (leaflets) (valve) (congenital) 746.9
  acquired — *see* Endocarditis, mitral
  Ebstein's 746.89
  parachute 746.5
  specified type NEC 746.89
  stenosis, congenital 746.5
mouth (acquired) 528.9
  congenital NEC 750.9
    specified type NEC 750.26
multiple, congenital NEC 759.7
  specified type NEC 759.89
muscle (acquired) 728.9
  congenital 756.9
    specified type NEC 756.89
    sternocleidomastoid (due to intrauterine
      malposition and pressure) 754.1
musculoskeletal system, congenital NEC 756.9
  specified type NEC 756.9
nail (acquired) 703.9
  congenital 757.9
nasal — *see* Deformity, nose
neck (acquired) NEC 738.2
  congenital (any part) 744.9
    sternocleidomastoid 754.1
nervous system (congenital) 742.9
nipple (congenital) 757.9
  acquired 611.8
nose, nasal (cartilage) (acquired) 738.0
  bone (turbinate) 738.0
  congenital 748.1
    bent 754.0
    squashed 754.0
  saddle 738.0
    syphilitic 090.5
  septum 470
    congenital 748.1
  sinus (wall) (congenital) 748.1
    acquired 738.0
  syphilitic (congenital) 090.5
    late 095.8
ocular muscle (congenital) 743.9
  acquired 378.60
opticociliary vessels (congenital) 743.9
orbit (congenital) (eye) 743.9
  acquired NEC 376.40
    associated with craniofacial deformities
      376.44

Deformity — *continued*
orbit — *continued*
  acquired NEC — *continued*
    due to
      bone disease 376.43
      surgery 376.47
      trauma 376.47
organ of Corti (congenital) 744.05
ovary (congenital) 752.0
  acquired 620.8
oviduct (congenital) 752.10
  acquired 620.8
palate (congenital) 750.9
  acquired 526.89
  cleft (congenital) (*see also* Cleft, palate)
    749.00
  hard, acquired 526.89
  soft, acquired 528.9
pancreas (congenital) 751.7
  acquired 577.8
parachute, mitral valve 746.5
parathyroid (gland) 759.2
parotid (gland) (congenital) 750.9
  acquired 527.8
patella (acquired) 736.6
  congenital 755.64
pelvis, pelvic (acquired) (bony) 738.6
  with disproportion (fetopelvic) 653.0 ✓5ᵗʰ
    affecting fetus or newborn 763.1
    causing obstructed labor 660.1 ✓5ᵗʰ
      affecting fetus or newborn 763.1
  congenital 755.60
  rachitic (late effect) 268.1
penis (glans) (congenital) 752.9
  acquired 607.89
pericardium (congenital) 746.9
  acquired — *see* Pericarditis
pharynx (congenital) 750.9
  acquired 478.29
Pierre Robin (congenital) 756.0
pinna (acquired) 380.32
  congenital 744.3
pituitary (congenital) 759.2
pleural folds (congenital) 748.8
portal vein (congenital) 747.40
posture *see* Curvature, spine
prepuce (congenital) 752.9
  acquired 607.89
prostate (congenital) 752.9
  acquired 602.8
pulmonary valve — *see* Endocarditis,
  pulmonary
pupil (congenital) 743.9
  acquired 364.75
pylorus (congenital) 750.9
  acquired 537.89
rachitic (acquired), healed or old 268.1
radius (acquired) 736.00
  congenital 755.50
    reduction — *see* Deformity, reduction,
      upper limb
rectovaginal septum (congenital) 752.40
  acquired 623.8
rectum (congenital) 751.5
  acquired 569.49
reduction (extremity) (limb) 755.4
  brain 742.2
  lower limb 755.30
    with complete absence of distal elements
      755.31
    longitudinal (complete) (partial) (with
      distal deficiencies, incomplete)
      755.32
      with complete absence of distal
       elements 755.31
      combined femoral, tibial, fibular
       (incomplete) 755.33
      femoral 755.34
      fibular 755.37
      metatarsal(s) 755.38
      phalange(s) 755.39
       meaning all digits 755.31
      tarsal(s) 755.38
      tibia 755.36
      tibiofibular 755.35
    transverse 755.31

✓4ᵗʰ Fourth-digit Required ✓5ᵗʰ Fifth-digit Required ▶◀ Revised Text ● New Line ▲ Revised Code

Deformity — *continued*
  reduction — *continued*
    upper limb 755.20
      with complete absence of distal elements 755.21
      longitudinal (complete) (partial) (with distal deficiencies, incomplete) 755.22
        with complete absence of distal elements 755.21
        carpal(s) 755.28
        combined humeral, radial, ulnar (incomplete) 755.23
        humeral 755.24
        metacarpal(s) 755.28
        phalange(s) 755.29
          meaning all digits 755.21
        radial 755.26
        radioulnar 755.25
        ulnar 755.27
        transverse (complete) (partial) 755.21
  renal — *see* Deformity, kidney
  respiratory system (congenital) 748.9
    specified type NEC 748.8
  rib (acquired) 738.3
    congenital 756.3
      cervical 756.2
  rotation (joint) (acquired) 736.9
    congenital 755.9
    hip or thigh 736.39
      congenital (*see also* Subluxation, congenital, hip) 754.32
  sacroiliac joint (congenital) 755.69
    acquired 738.5
  sacrum (acquired) 738.5
    congenital 756.10
  saddle
    back 737.8
    nose 738.0
      syphilitic 090.5
  salivary gland or duct (congenital) 750.9
    acquired 527.8
  scapula (acquired) 736.89
    congenital 755.50
  scrotum (congenital) 752.9
    acquired 608.89
  sebaceous gland, acquired 706.8
  seminal tract or duct (congenital) 752.9
    acquired 608.89
  septum (nasal) (acquired) 470
    congenital 748.1
  shoulder (joint) (acquired) 736.89
    congenital 755.50
      specified type NEC 755.59
    contraction 718.41
  sigmoid (flexure) (congenital) 751.5
    acquired 569.89
  sinus of Valsalva 747.29
  skin (congenital) 757.9
    acquired NEC 709.8
  skull (acquired) 738.19
    congenital 756.0
      with
        anencephalus 740.0
        encephalocele 742.0
        hydrocephalus 742.3
          with spina bifida (*see also* Spina bifida) 741.0 ✓5ᵗʰ
        microcephalus 742.1
      due to intrauterine malposition and pressure 754.0
  soft parts, organs or tissues (of pelvis)
    in pregnancy or childbirth NEC 654.9 ✓5ᵗʰ
      affecting fetus or newborn 763.89
      causing obstructed labor 660.2 ✓5ᵗʰ
        affecting fetus or newborn 763.1
  spermatic cord (congenital) 752.9
    acquired 608.89
      torsion 608.2
  spinal
    column — *see* Deformity, spine
    cord (congenital) 742.9
      acquired 336.8
      vessel (congenital) 747.82
    nerve root (congenital) 742.9
      acquired 724.9

Deformity — *continued*
  spine (acquired) NEC 738.5
    congenital 756.10
      due to intrauterine malposition and pressure 754.2
    kyphoscoliotic (*see also* Kyphoscoliosis) 737.30
    kyphotic (*see also* Kyphosis) 737.10
    lordotic (*see also* Lordosis) 737.20
    rachitic 268.1
    scoliotic (*see also* Scoliosis) 737.30
  spleen
    acquired 289.59
    congenital 759.0
  Sprengel's (congenital) 755.52
  sternum (acquired) 738.3
    congenital 756.3
  stomach (congenital) 750.9
    acquired 537.89
  submaxillary gland (congenital) 750.9
    acquired 527.8
  swan neck (acquired)
    finger 736.22
    hand 736.09
  talipes — *see* Talipes
  teeth, tooth NEC 520.9
  testis (congenital) 752.9
    acquired 608.89
      torsion 608.2
  thigh (acquired) 736.89
    congenital 755.60
  thorax (acquired) (wall) 738.3
    congenital 754.89
    late effect of rickets 268.1
  thumb (acquired) 736.20
    congenital 755.50
  thymus (tissue) (congenital) 759.2
  thyroid (gland) (congenital) 759.2
    cartilage 748.3
      acquired 478.79
  tibia (acquired) 736.89
    congenital 755.60
    saber 090.5
  toe (acquired) 735.9
    congenital 755.66
    specified NEC 735.8
  tongue (congenital) 750.10
    acquired 529.8
  tooth, teeth NEC 520.9
  trachea (rings) (congenital) 748.3
    acquired 519.1
  transverse aortic arch (congenital) 747.21
  tricuspid (leaflets) (valve) (congenital) 746.9
    acquired — *see* Endocarditis, tricuspid
    atresia or stenosis 746.1
    specified type NEC 746.89
  trunk (acquired) 738.3
    congenital 759.9
  ulna (acquired) 736.00
    congenital 755.50
  upper extremity — *see* Deformity, arm
  urachus (congenital) 753.7
  ureter (opening) (congenital) 753.9
    acquired 593.89
  urethra (valve) (congenital) 753.9
    acquired 599.84
  urinary tract or system (congenital) 753.9
    urachus 753.7
  uterus (congenital) 752.3
    acquired 621.8
  uvula (congenital) 750.9
    acquired 528.9
  vagina (congenital) 752.40
    acquired 623.8
  valve, valvular (heart) (congenital) 746.9
    acquired — *see* Endocarditis
    pulmonary 746.00
    specified type NEC 746.89
  vascular (congenital) (peripheral) NEC 747.60
    acquired 459.9
  vas deferens (congenital) 752.9
    acquired 608.89
  vein (congenital) NEC (*see also* Deformity, vascular) 747.60
    brain 747.81
    coronary 746.9
    great 747.40

Deformity — *continued*
  vena cava (inferior) (superior) (congenital) 747.40
  vertebra — *see* Deformity, spine
  vesicourethral orifice (acquired) 596.8
    congenital NEC 753.9
      specified type NEC 753.8
  vessels of optic papilla (congenital) 743.9
  visual field (contraction) 368.45
  vitreous humor (congenital) 743.9
    acquired 379.29
  vulva (congenital) 752.40
    acquired 624.8
  wrist (joint) (acquired) 736.00
    congenital 755.50
    contraction 718.43
    valgus 736.03
      congenital 755.59
    varus 736.04
      congenital 755.59

Degeneration, degenerative
  adrenal (capsule) (gland) 255.8
    with hypofunction 255.4
    fatty 255.8
    hyaline 255.8
    infectional 255.8
    lardaceous 277.3
  amyloid (any site) (general) 277.3
  anterior cornua, spinal cord 336.8
  aorta, aortic 440.0
    fatty 447.8
    valve (heart) (*see also* Endocarditis, aortic) 424.1
  arteriovascular — *see* Arteriosclerosis
  artery, arterial (atheromatous) (calcareous) — *see also* Arteriosclerosis
    amyloid 277.3
    lardaceous 277.3
    medial NEC (*see also* Arteriosclerosis, extremities) 440.20
  articular cartilage NEC (*see also* Disorder, cartilage, articular) 718.0 ✓5ᵗʰ
    elbow 718.02
    knee 717.5
    patella 717.7
    shoulder 718.01
    spine (*see also* Spondylosis) 721.90
  atheromatous — *see* Arteriosclerosis
  bacony (any site) 277.3
  basal nuclei or ganglia NEC 333.0
  bone 733.90
  brachial plexus 353.0
  brain (cortical) (progressive) 331.9
    arteriosclerotic 437.0
    childhood 330.9
      specified type NEC 330.8
    congenital 742.4
    cystic 348.0
      congenital 742.4
    familial NEC 331.89
    grey matter 330.8
    heredofamilial NEC 331.89
    in
      alcoholism 303.9 ✓5ᵗʰ [331.7]
      beriberi 265.0 [331.7]
      cerebrovascular disease 437.9 [331.7]
      congenital hydrocephalus 742.3 [331.7]
        with spina bifida (*see also* Spina bifida) 741.0 ✓5ᵗʰ [331.7]
      Fabry's disease 272.7 [330.2]
      Gaucher's disease 272.7 [330.2]
      Hunter's disease or syndrome 277.5 [330.3]
      lipidosis
        cerebral 330.1
        generalized 272.7 [330.2]
      mucopolysaccharidosis 277.5 [330.3]
      myxedema (*see also* Myxedema) 244.9 [331.7]
      neoplastic disease NEC (M8000/1) 239.9 [331.7]
      Niemann-Pick disease 272.7 [330.2]
      sphingolipidosis 272.7 [330.2]
      vitamin B_{12} deficiency 266.2 [331.7]
    motor centers 331.89
    senile 331.2
    specified type NEC 331.89

Deformity — Degeneration

Degeneration — Degeneration

Degeneration, degenerative — *continued*
breast — *see* Disease, breast
Bruch's membrane 363.40
bundle of His 426.50
   left 426.3
   right 426.4
calcareous NEC 275.49
capillaries 448.9
   amyloid 277.3
   fatty 448.9
   lardaceous 277.3
cardiac (brown) (calcareous) (fatty) (fibrous)
   (hyaline) (mural) (muscular) (pigmentary)
   (senile) (with arteriosclerosis) (*see also*
   Degeneration, myocardial) 429.1
   valve, valvular — *see* Endocarditis
cardiorenal (*see also* Hypertension, cardiorenal)
   404.90
cardiovascular (*see also* Disease,
   cardiovascular) 429.2
   renal (*see also* Hypertension, cardiorenal)
     404.90
cartilage (joint) — *see* Derangement, joint
cerebellar NEC 334.9
   primary (hereditary) (sporadic) 334.2
cerebral — *see* Degeneration, brain
cerebromacular 330.1
cerebrovascular 437.1
   due to hypertension 437.2
   late effect — *see* Late effect(s) (of)
     cerbrovascular disease
cervical plexus 353.2
cervix 622.8
   due to radiation (intended effect) 622.8
     adverse effect or misadventure 622.8
changes, spine or vertebra (*see also*
   Spondylosis) 721.90
chitinous 277.3
chorioretinal 363.40
   congenital 743.53
   hereditary 363.50
choroid (colloid) (drusen) 363.40
   hereditary 363.50
   senile 363.41
     diffuse secondary 363.42
cochlear 386.8
collateral ligament (knee) (medial) 717.82
   lateral 717.81
combined (spinal cord) (subacute) 266.2 *[336.2]*
   with anemia (pernicious) 281.0 *[336.2]*
     due to dietary deficiency 281.1 *[336.2]*
   due to vitamin B$_{12}$ deficiency anemia
     (dietary) 281.1 *[336.2]*
conjunctiva 372.50
   amyloid 277.3 *[372.50]*
cornea 371.40
   calcerous 371.44
   familial (hereditary) (*see also* Dystrophy,
     cornea) 371.50
     macular 371.55
     reticular 371.54
   hyaline (of old scars) 371.41
   marginal (Terrien's) 371.48
   mosaic (shagreen) 371.41
   nodular 371.46
   peripheral 371.48
   senile 371.41
cortical (cerebellar) (parenchymatous) 334.2
   alcoholic 303.9 ✓5ᵗʰ *[334.4]*
   diffuse, due to arteriopathy 437.0
corticostriatal-spinal 334.8
cretinoid 243
cruciate ligament (knee) (posterior) 717.84
   anterior 717.83
cutis 709.3
   amyloid 277.3
dental pulp 522.2
disc disease — *see* Degeneration, intervertebral
   disc
dorsolateral (spinal cord) — *see* Degeration,
   combined
endocardial 424.90
extrapyramidal NEC 333.90
eye NEC 360.40
   macular (*see also* Degeneration, macula)
     362.50
     congenital 362.75
     hereditary 362.76

Degeneration, degenerative — *continued*
fatty (diffuse) (general) 272.8
   liver 571.8
     alcoholic 571.0
   localized site — *see* Degeneration, by site,
     fatty
   placenta — *see* Placenta, abnormal
globe (eye) NEC 360.40
   macular — *see* Degeneration, macula
grey matter 330.8
heart (brown) (calcareous) (fatty) (fibrous)
   (hyaline) (mural) (muscular) (pigmentary)
   (senile) (with arteriosclerosis) (*see also*
   Degeneration, myocardial) 429.1
   amyloid 277.3 *[425.7]*
   atheromatous —*see* Arteriosclerosis,
     coronary
   gouty 274.82
   hypertensive (*see also* Hypertension, heart)
     402.90
   ischemic 414.9
   valve, valvular — *see* Endocarditis
hepatolenticular (Wilson's) 275.1
hepatorenal 572.4
heredofamilial
   brain NEC 331.89
   spinal cord NEC 336.8
hyaline (diffuse) (generalized) 728.9
   localized — *see also* Degeneration, by site
     cornea 371.41
     keratitis 371.41
hypertensive vascular — *see* Hypertension
infrapatellar fat pad 729.31
internal semilunar cartilage 717.3
intervertebral disc 722.6
   with myelopathy 722.70
   cervical, cervicothoracic 722.4
     with myelopathy 722.71
   lumbar, lumbosacral 722.52
     with myelopathy 722.73
   thoracic, thoracolumbar 722.51
     with myelopathy 722.72
intestine 569.89
   amyloid 277.3
   lardaceous 277.3
iris (generalized) (*see also* Atrophy, iris) 364.59
   pigmentary 364.53
   pupillary margin 364.54
ischemic — *see* Ischemia
joint disease (*see also* Osteoarthrosis)
   715.9 ✓5ᵗʰ
   multiple sites 715.09
   spine (*see also* Spondylosis) 721.90
kidney (*see also* Sclerosis, renal 587
   amyloid 277.3 *[583.81]*
   cyst, cystic (multiple) (solitary) 593.2
     congenital (*see also* Cystic, disease,
      kidney) 753.10
   fatty 593.89
   fibrocystic (congenital) 753.19
   lardaceous 277.3 *[583.81]*
   polycystic (congenital) 753.12
     adult type (APKD) 753.13
     autosomal dominant 753.13
     autosomal recessive 753.14
     childhood type (CPKD) 753.14
     infantile type 753.14
   waxy 277.3 *[583.81]*
Kuhnt-Junius (retina) 362.52
labyrinth, osseous 386.8
lacrimal passages, cystic 375.12
lardaceous (any site) 277.3
lateral column (posterior), spinal cord (*see also*
   Degeneration, combined) 266.2 *[336.2]*
lattice 362.63
lens 366.9
   infantile, juvenile, or presenile 366.00
   senile 366.10
lenticular (familial) (progressive) (Wilson's) (with
   cirrhosis of liver) 275.1
   striate artery 437.0
lethal ball, prosthetic heart valve 996.02
ligament
   collateral (knee) (medial) 717.82
     lateral 717.81
   cruciate (knee) (posterior) 717.84
     anterior 717.83

Degeneration, degenerative — *continued*
liver (diffuse) 572.8
   amyloid 277.3
   congenital (cystic) 751.62
   cystic 572.8
     congenital 751.62
   fatty 571.8
     alcoholic 571.0
   hypertrophic 572.8
   lardaceous 277.3
   parenchymatous, acute or subacute (*see
     also* Necrosis, liver) 570
   pigmentary 572.8
   toxic (acute) 573.8
   waxy 277.3
lung 518.89
lymph gland 289.3
   hyaline 289.3
   lardaceous 277.3
macula (acquired) (senile) 362.50
   atrophic 362.51
   Best's 362.76
   congenital 362.75
   cystic 362.54
   cystoid 362.53
   disciform 362.52
   dry 362.51
   exudative 362.52
   familial pseudoinflammatory 362.77
   hereditary 362.76
   hole 362.54
   juvenile (Stargardt's) 362.75
   nonexudative 362.51
   pseudohole 362.54
   wet 362.52
medullary — *see* Degeneration, brain
membranous labyrinth, congenital (causing
   impairment of hearing) 744.05
meniscus — *see* Derangement, joint
microcystoid 362.62
mitral — *see* Insufficiency, mitral
Mönckeberg's (*see also* Arteriosclerosis,
   extremities) 440.20
moral 301.7
motor centers, senile 331.2
mural (*see also* Degeneration, myocardial)
   429.1
   heart, cardiac (*see also* Degeneration,
     myocardial) 429.1
   myocardium, myocardial (*see also*
     Degeneration, myocardial) 429.1
muscle 728.9
   fatty 728.9
   fibrous 728.9
   heart (*see also* Degeneration, myocardial)
     429.1
   hyaline 728.9
muscular progressive 728.2
myelin, central nervous system NEC 341.9
myocardium, myocardial (brown) (calcareous)
   (fatty) (fibrous) (hyaline) (mural)
   (muscular) (pigmentary) (senile) (with
   arteriosclerosis) 429.1
   with rheumatic fever (conditions classifiable
     to 390) 398.0
     active, acute, or subacute 391.2
       with chorea 392.0
     inactive or quiescent (with chorea) 398.0
   amyloid 277.3 *[425.7]*
   congenital 746.89
   fetus or newborn 779.89   ▲
   gouty 274.82
   hypertensive (*see also* Hypertension, heart)
     402.90
   ischemic 414.8
   rheumatic (*see also* Degeneration,
     myocardium, with rheumatic fever)
     398.0
   syphilitic 093.82
nasal sinus (mucosa) (*see also* Sinusitis) 473.9
   frontal 473.1
   maxillary 473.0
nerve — *see* Disorder, nerve
nervous system 349.89
   amyloid 277.3 *[357.4]*
   autonomic (*see also* Neuropathy, peripheral,
     autonomic) 337.9
   fatty 349.89

Degeneration, degenerative — *continued*
  nervous system — *continued*
    peripheral autonomic NEC (*see also*
        Neuropathy, peripheral, autonomic)
        337.9
  nipple 611.9
  nose 478.1
  oculoacousticocerebral, congenital (progressive)
      743.8
  olivopontocerebellar (familial) (hereditary) 333.0
  osseous labyrinth 386.8
  ovary 620.8
    cystic 620.2
    microcystic 620.2
  pallidal, pigmentary (progressive) 333.0
  pancreas 577.8
    tuberculous (*see also* Tuberculosis)
        017.9 ✓5ᵗ
  papillary muscle 429.81
  paving stone 362.61
  penis 607.89
  peritoneum 568.89
  pigmentary (diffuse) (general)
    localized — *see* Degeneration, by site
    pallidal (progressive) 333.0
    secondary 362.65
  pineal gland 259.8
  pituitary (gland) 253.8
  placenta (fatty) (fibrinoid) (fibroid) — *see*
      Placenta, abnormal
  popliteal fat pad 729.31
  posterolateral (spinal cord) (*see also*
      Degeneration, combined) 266.2 *[336.2]*
  pulmonary valve (heart) (*see also* Endocarditis,
      pulmonary) 424.3
  pulp (tooth) 522.2
  pupillary margin 364.54
  renal (*see also* Sclerosis, renal) 587
    fibrocystic 753.19
    polycystic 753.12
      adult type (APKD) 753.13
      autosomal dominant 753.13
      autosomal recessive 753.14
      childhood type (CPKD) 753.14
      infantile type 753.14
  reticuloendothelial system 289.8
  retina (peripheral) 362.60
    with retinal defect (*see also* Detachment,
        retina, with retinal defect) 361.00
    cystic (senile) 362.50
    cystoid 362.53
    hereditary (*see also* Dystrophy, retina)
        362.70
      cerebroretinal 362.71
      congenital 362.75
      juvenile (Stargardt's) 362.75
      macula 362.76
    Kuhnt-Junius 362.52
    lattice 362.63
    macular (*see also* Degeneration, macula)
        362.50
    microcystoid 362.62
    palisade 362.63
    paving stone 362.61
    pigmentary (primary) 362.74
      secondary 362.65
    posterior pole (*see also* Degeneration,
        macula) 362.50
    secondary 362.66
    senile 362.60
      cystic 362.53
      reticular 362.64
  saccule, congenital (causing impairment of
      hearing) 744.05
  sacculocochlear 386.8
  senile 797
    brain 331.2
    cardiac, heart, or myocardium (*see also*
        Degeneration, myocardial) 429.1
    motor centers 331.2
    reticle 362.64
    retina, cystic 362.50
    vascular — *see* Arteriosclerosis
  silicone rubber poppet (prosthetic valve) 996.02
  sinus (cystic) (*see also* Sinusitis) 473.9
    polypoid 471.1

Degeneration, degenerative — *continued*
  skin 709.3
    amyloid 277.3
    colloid 709.3
  spinal (cord) 336.8
    amyloid 277.3
    column 733.90
    combined (subacute) (*see also* Degeneration,
        combined) 266.2 *[336.2]*
      with anemia (pernicious) 281.0 *[336.2]*
    dorsolateral (*see also* Degeneration,
        combined) 266.2 *[336.2]*
    familial NEC 336.8
    fatty 336.8
    funicular (*see also* Degeneration, combined)
        266.2 *[336.2]*
    heredofamilial NEC 336.8
    posterolateral (*see also* Degeneration,
        combined) 266.2 *[336.2]*
    subacute combined — *see* Degeneration,
        combined
    tuberculous (*see also* Tuberculosis)
        013.8 ✓5ᵗ
  spine 733.90
  spleen 289.59
    amyloid 277.3
    lardaceous 277.3
  stomach 537.89
    lardaceous 277.3
  strionigral 333.0
  sudoriparous (cystic) 705.89
  suprarenal (capsule) (gland) 255.8
    with hypofunction 255.4
  sweat gland 705.89
  synovial membrane (pulpy) 727.9
  tapetoretinal 362.74
    adult or presenile form 362.50
  testis (postinfectional) 608.89
  thymus (gland) 254.8
    fatty 254.8
    lardaceous 277.3
  thyroid (gland) 246.8
  tricuspid (heart) (valve) *see* Endocarditis,
      tricuspid
  tuberculous NEC (*see also* Tuberculosis)
      011.9 ✓5ᵗ
  turbinate 733.90
  uterus 621.8
    cystic 621.8
  vascular (senile) — *see also* Arteriosclerosis
    hypertensive — *see* Hypertension
  vitreoretinal (primary) 362.73
    secondary 362.66
  vitreous humor (with infiltration) 379.21
  wallerian NEC — *see* Disorder, nerve
  waxy (any site) 277.3
  Wilson's hepatolenticular 275.1

Deglutition
  paralysis 784.9
    hysterical 300.11
  pneumonia 507.0

Degos' disease or syndrome 447.8

**Degradation disorder, branched-chain amino
    acid** 270.3

Dehiscence
  anastomosis — *see* Complications, anastomosis
  cesarean wound 674.1 ✓5ᵗ
  episiotomy 674.2 ✓5ᵗ
  operation wound 998.32 ▲
    internal 998.31 ●
  perineal wound (postpartum) 674.2 ✓5ᵗ
  postoperative 998.32 ▲
    abdomen 998.32 ▲
      internal 998.31 ●
    internal 998.31 ●
  uterine wound 674.1 ✓5ᵗ

Dehydration (cachexia) 276.5
  with
    hypernatremia 276.0 ●
    hyponatremia 276.1 ●
  newborn 775.5

Deiters' nucleus syndrome 386.19

Déjérine's disease 356.0

Déjérine-Klumpke paralysis 767.6

Déjérine-Roussy syndrome 348.8

Déjérine-Sottas disease or neuropathy
    (hypertrophic) 356.0

Déjérine-Thomas atrophy or syndrome 333.0

de Lange's syndrome (Amsterdam dwarf, mental
    retardation, and brachycephaly) 759.89

Delay, delayed
  adaptation, cones or rods 368.63
  any plane in pelvis
    affecting fetus or newborn 763.1
    complicating delivery 660.1 ✓5ᵗ
  birth or delivery NEC 662.1 ✓5ᵗ
    affecting fetus or newborn 763.89
    second twin, triplet, or multiple mate
        662.3 ✓5ᵗ
  closure — *see also* Fistula
    cranial suture 756.0
    fontanel 756.0
  coagulation NEC 790.92
  conduction (cardiac) (ventricular) 426.9
  delivery NEC 662.1 ✓5ᵗ
    second twin, triplet, etc. 662.3 ✓5ᵗ
      affecting fetus or newborn 763.89
  development
    in childhood 783.40
      physiological 783.40
    intellectual NEC 315.9
    learning NEC 315.2
    reading 315.00
    sexual 259.0
    speech 315.39
      associated with hyperkinesis 314.1
    spelling 315.09
  gastric emptying 536.8
  menarche 256.39
    due to pituitary hypofunction 253.4
  menstruation (cause unknown) 626.8
  milestone in childhood 783.42
  motility — *see* Hypomotility
  passage of meconium (newborn) 777.1
  primary respiration 768.9
  puberty 259.0
  sexual maturation, female 259.0

Del Castillo's syndrome (germinal aplasia) 606.0

Déleage's disease 359.89 ▲

Delhi (boil) (button) (sore) 085.1

Delinquency (juvenile) 312.9
  group (*see also* Disturbance, conduct)
      312.2 ✓5ᵗ
  neurotic 312.4

Delirium, delirious 780.09
  acute (psychotic) 293.0
  alcoholic 291.0
    acute 291.0
    chronic 291.1
  alcoholicum 291.0
  chronic (*see also* Psychosis) 293.89
    due to or associated with physical condition
        — *see* Psychosis, organic
  drug-induced 292.81
  eclamptic (*see also* Eclampsia) 780.39
  exhaustion (*see also* Reaction, stress, acute)
      308.9
  hysterical 300.11
  in
    presenile dementia 290.11
    senile dementia 290.3
  induced by drug 292.81
  manic, maniacal (acute) (*see also* Psychosis,
      affective) 296.0 ✓5ᵗ
    recurrent episode 296.1 ✓5ᵗ
    single episode 296.0 ✓5ᵗ
  puerperal 293.9
  senile 290.3
  subacute (psychotic) 293.1
  thyroid (*see also* Thyrotoxicosis) 242.9 ✓5ᵗ
  traumatic — *see also* Injury, intracranial
    with
      lesion, spinal cord — *see* Injury, spinal,
          by site
      shock, spinal — *see* Injury, spinal, by site
    tremens (impending) 291.0
  uremic — *see* Uremia
  withdrawal
    alcoholic (acute) 291.0
      chronic 291.1
    drug 292.0

Degeneration — Delirium (vertical right margin)

Delivery

Note — Use the following fifth-digit subclassification with categories 640-648, 651-676:

0	unspecified as to episode of care
1	delivered, with or without mention of antepartum condition
2	delivered, with mention of postpartum complication
3	antepartum condition or complication
4	postpartum condition or complication

breech (assisted) (spontaneous) 652.2 ✓5th
   affecting fetus or newborn 763.0
   extraction NEC 669.6 ✓5th
cesarean (for) 669.7 ✓5th
   abnormal
      cervix 654.6 ✓5th
      pelvic organs or tissues 654.9 ✓5th
      pelvis (bony) (major) NEC 653.0 ✓5th
      presentation or position 652.9 ✓5th
         in multiple gestation 652.6 ✓5th
      size, fetus 653.5 ✓5th
      soft parts (of pelvis) 654.9 ✓5th
      uterus, congenital 654.0 ✓5th
      vagina 654.7 ✓5th
      vulva 654.8 ✓5th
   abruptio placentae 641.2 ✓5th
   acromion presentation 652.8 ✓5th
      affecting fetus or newborn 763.4
   anteversion, cervix or uterus 654.4 ✓5th
   atony, uterus 666.1 ✓5th
   bicornis or bicornuate uterus 654.0 ✓5th
   breech presentation 652.2 ✓5th
   brow presentation 652.4 ✓5th
   cephalopelvic disproportion (normally formed fetus) 653.4 ✓5th
   chin presentation 652.4 ✓5th
   cicatrix of cervix 654.6 ✓5th
   contracted pelvis (general) 653.1 ✓5th
      inlet 653.2 ✓5th
      outlet 653.3 ✓5th
   cord presentation or prolapse 663.0 ✓5th
   cystocele 654.4 ✓5th
   deformity (acquired) (congenital)
      pelvic organs or tissues NEC 654.9 ✓5th
      pelvis (bony) NEC 653.0 ✓5th
   displacement, uterus NEC 654.4 ✓5th
   disproportion NEC 653.9 ✓5th
   distress
      fetal 656.8 ✓5th
      maternal 669.0 ✓5th
   eclampsia 642.6 ✓5th
   face presentation 652.4 ✓5th
   failed
      forceps 660.7 ✓5th
      trial of labor NEC 660.6 ✓5th
      vacuum extraction 660.7 ✓5th
      ventouse 660.7 ✓5th
   fetal deformity 653.7 ✓5th
   fetal-maternal hemorrhage 656.0 ✓5th
   fetus, fetal
      distress 656.8 ✓5th
      prematurity 656.8 ✓5th
   fibroid (tumor) (uterus) 654.1 ✓5th
   footling 652.8 ✓5th
      with successful version 652.1 ✓5th
   hemorrhage (antepartum) (intrapartum) NEC 641.9 ✓5th
   hydrocephalic fetus 653.6 ✓5th
   incarceration of uterus 654.3 ✓5th
   incoordinate uterine action 661.4 ✓5th
   inertia, uterus 661.2 ✓5th
      primary 661.0 ✓5th
      secondary 661.1 ✓5th
   lateroversion, uterus or cervix 654.4 ✓5th
   mal lie 652.9 ✓5th
   malposition
      fetus 652.9 ✓5th
         in multiple gestation 652.6 ✓5th
      pelvic organs or tissues NEC 654.9 ✓5th
      uterus NEC or cervix 654.4 ✓5th
   malpresentation NEC 652.9 ✓5th
      in multiple gestation 652.6 ✓5th

Delivery — continued
cesarean — continued
   maternal
      diabetes mellitus 648.0 ✓5th
      heart disease NEC 648.6 ✓5th
   meconium in liquor 656.8 ✓5th
      staining only 792.3
   oblique presentation 652.3 ✓5th
   oversize fetus 653.5 ✓5th
   pelvic tumor NEC 654.9 ✓5th
   placental insufficiency 656.5 ✓5th
   placenta previa 641.0 ✓5th
      with hemorrhage 641.1 ✓5th
   poor dilation, cervix 661.0 ✓5th
   preeclampsia 642.4 ✓5th
      severe 642.5 ✓5th
   previous
      cesarean delivery 654.2 ✓5th
      surgery (to)
         cervix 654.6 ✓5th
         gynecological NEC 654.9 ✓5th
         uterus NEC 654.9 ✓5th
            previous cesarean delivery 654.2 ✓5th
         vagina 654.7 ✓5th
   prolapse
      arm or hand 652.7 ✓5th
      uterus 654.4 ✓5th
   prolonged labor 662.1 ✓5th
   rectocele 654.4 ✓5th
   retroversion, uterus or cervix 654.3 ✓5th
   rigid
      cervix 654.6 ✓5th
      pelvic floor 654.4 ✓5th
      perineum 654.8 ✓5th
      vagina 654.7 ✓5th
      vulva 654.8 ✓5th
   sacculation, pregnant uterus 654.4 ✓5th
   scar(s)
      cervix 654.6 ✓5th
      cesarean delivery 654.2 ✓5th
      uterus NEC 654.9 ✓5th
         due to previous cesarean delivery 654.2 ✓5th
   Shirodkar suture in situ 654.5 ✓5th
   shoulder presentation 652.8 ✓5th
   stenosis or stricture, cervix 654.6 ✓5th
   transverse presentation or lie 652.3 ✓5th
   tumor, pelvic organs or tissues NEC 654.4 ✓5th
   umbilical cord presentation or prolapse 663.0 ✓5th
completely normal case — see category 650
complicated (by) NEC 669.9 ✓5th
   abdominal tumor, fetal 653.7 ✓5th
      causing obstructed labor 660.1 ✓5th
   abnormal, abnormality of
      cervix 654.6 ✓5th
         causing obstructed labor 660.2 ✓5th
      forces of labor 661.9 ✓5th
      formation of uterus 654.0 ✓5th
      pelvic organs or tissues 654.9 ✓5th
         causing obstructed labor 660.2 ✓5th
      pelvis (bony) (major) NEC 653.0 ✓5th
         causing obstructed labor 660.1 ✓5th
      presentation or position NEC 652.9 ✓5th
         causing obstructed labor 660.0 ✓5th
      size, fetus 653.5 ✓5th
         causing obstructed labor 660.1 ✓5th
      soft parts (of pelvis) 654.9 ✓5th
         causing obstructed labor 660.2 ✓5th
      uterine contractions NEC 661.9 ✓5th
      uterus (formation) 654.0 ✓5th
         causing obstructed labor 660.2 ✓5th
      vagina 654.7 ✓5th
         causing obstructed labor 660.2 ✓5th
   abnormally formed uterus (any type) (congenital) 654.0 ✓5th
      causing obstructed labor 660.2 ✓5th
   acromion presentation 652.8 ✓5th
      causing obstructed labor 660.0 ✓5th
   adherent placenta 667.0 ✓5th
      with hemorrhage 666.0 ✓5th
   adhesions, uterus (to abdominal wall) 654.4 ✓5th

Delivery — continued
complicated (by) NEC — continued
   advanced maternal age NEC 659.6 ✓5th
      multigravida 659.6 ✓5th
      primigravida 659.5 ✓5th
   air embolism 673.0 ✓5th
   amnionitis 658.4 ✓5th
   amniotic fluid embolism 673.1 ✓5th
   anesthetic death 668.9 ✓5th
   annular detachment, cervix 665.3 ✓5th
   antepartum hemorrhage — see Delivery, complicated, hemorrhage
   anteversion, cervix or uterus 654.4 ✓5th
      causing obstructed labor 660.2 ✓5th
   apoplexy 674.0 ✓5th
      placenta 641.2 ✓5th
   arrested active phase 661.1 ✓5th
   asymmetrical pelvis bone 653.0 ✓5th
      causing obstructed labor 660.1 ✓5th
   atony, uterus (hypotonic) (inertia) 666.1 ✓5th
      hypertonic 661.4 ✓5th
   Bandl's ring 661.4 ✓5th
   battledore placenta — see Placenta, abnormal
   bicornis or bicornuate uterus 654.0 ✓5th
      causing obstructed labor 660.2 ✓5th
   birth injury to mother NEC 665.9 ✓5th
   bleeding (see also Delivery, complicated, hemorrhage) 641.9 ✓5th
   breech presentation (assisted) (buttocks) (complete) (frank) (spontaneous) 652.2 ✓5th
      with successful version 652.1 ✓5th
   brow presentation 652.4 ✓5th
   cephalopelvic disproportion (normally formed fetus) 653.4 ✓5th
      causing obstructed labor 660.1 ✓5th
   cerebral hemorrhage 674.0 ✓5th
   cervical dystocia 661.0 ✓5th
   chin presentation 652.4 ✓5th
      causing obstructed labor 660.0 ✓5th
   cicatrix
      cervix 654.6 ✓5th
         causing obstructed labor 660.2 ✓5th
      vagina 654.7 ✓5th
         causing obstructed labor 660.2 ✓5th
   colporrhexis 665.4 ✓5th
      with perineal laceration 664.0 ✓5th
   compound presentation 652.8 ✓5th
      causing obstructed labor 660.0 ✓5th
   compression of cord (umbilical) 663.2 ✓5th
      around neck 663.1 ✓5th
      cord prolapsed 663.0 ✓5th
   contraction, contracted pelvis 653.1 ✓5th
      causing obstructed labor 660.1 ✓5th
      general 653.1 ✓5th
         causing obstructed labor 660.1 ✓5th
      inlet 653.2 ✓5th
         causing obstructed labor 660.1 ✓5th
      midpelvic 653.8 ✓5th
         causing obstructed labor 660.1 ✓5th
      midplane 653.8 ✓5th
         causing obstructed labor 660.1 ✓5th
      outlet 653.3 ✓5th
         causing obstructed labor 660.1 ✓5th
   contraction ring 661.4 ✓5th
   cord (umbilical) 663.9 ✓5th
      around neck, tightly or with compression 663.1 ✓5th
         without compression 663.3 ✓5th
      bruising 663.6 ✓5th
      complication NEC 663.9 ✓5th
         specified type NEC 663.8 ✓5th
      compression NEC 663.2 ✓5th
      entanglement NEC 663.3 ✓5th
         with compression 663.2 ✓5th
      forelying 663.0 ✓5th
      hematoma 663.6 ✓5th
      marginal attachment 663.8 ✓5th
      presentation 663.0 ✓5th
      prolapse (complete) (occult) (partial) 663.0 ✓5th
      short 663.4 ✓5th
      specified complication NEC 663.8 ✓5th
      thrombosis (vessels) 663.6 ✓5th
      vascular lesion 663.6 ✓5th

Delivery — Delivery

Delivery — *continued*
complicated (by) NEC — *continued*
  cord — *continued*
    velamentous insertion 663.8 ✓5ᵗʰ
    Couvelaire uterus 641.2 ✓5ᵗʰ
    cretin pelvis (dwarf type) (male type) 653.1 ✓5ᵗʰ
      causing obstructed labor 660.1 ✓5ᵗʰ
    crossbirth 652.3 ✓5ᵗʰ
      with successful version 652.1 ✓5ᵗʰ
      causing obstructed labor 660.0 ✓5ᵗʰ
    cyst (Gartner's duct) 654.7 ✓5ᵗʰ
    cystocele 654.4 ✓5ᵗʰ
      causing obstructed labor 660.2 ✓5ᵗʰ
    death of fetus (near term) 656.4 ✓5ᵗʰ
      early (before 22 completed weeks gestation) 632
    deformity (acquired) (congenital)
      fetus 653.7 ✓5ᵗʰ
        causing obstructed labor 660.1 ✓5ᵗʰ
      pelvic organs or tissues NEC 654.9 ✓5ᵗʰ
        causing obstructed labor 660.2 ✓5ᵗʰ
      pelvis (bony) NEC 653.0 ✓5ᵗʰ
        causing obstructed labor 660.1 ✓5ᵗʰ
    delay, delayed
      delivery in multiple pregnancy 662.3 ✓5ᵗʰ
      due to locked mates 660.5 ✓5ᵗʰ
      following rupture of membranes (spontaneous) 658.2 ✓5ᵗʰ
        artificial 658.3 ✓5ᵗʰ
    depressed fetal heart tones 659.7 ✓5ᵗʰ
    diastasis recti 665.8 ✓5ᵗʰ
    dilation
      bladder 654.4 ✓5ᵗʰ
        causing obstructed labor 660.2 ✓5ᵗʰ
      cervix, incomplete, poor or slow 661.0 ✓5ᵗʰ
    diseased placenta 656.7 ✓5ᵗʰ
    displacement uterus NEC 654.4 ✓5ᵗʰ
      causing obstructed labor 660.2 ✓5ᵗʰ
    disproportion NEC 653.9 ✓5ᵗʰ
      causing obstructed labor 660.1 ✓5ᵗʰ
    disruptio uteri — *see* Delivery, complicated, rupture, uterus
    distress
      fetal 656.8 ✓5ᵗʰ
      maternal 669.0 ✓5ᵗʰ
    double uterus (congenital) 654.0 ✓5ᵗʰ
      causing obstructed labor 660.2 ✓5ᵗʰ
    dropsy amnion 657 ✓4ᵗʰ
    dysfunction, uterus 661.9 ✓5ᵗʰ
      hypertonic 661.4 ✓5ᵗʰ
      hypotonic 661.2 ✓5ᵗʰ
        primary 661.0 ✓5ᵗʰ
        secondary 661.1 ✓5ᵗʰ
      incoordinate 661.4 ✓5ᵗʰ
    dystocia
      cervical 661.0 ✓5ᵗʰ
      fetal — *see* Delivery, complicated, abnormal presentation
      maternal — *see* Delivery, complicated, prolonged labor
      pelvic — *see* Delivery, complicated, contraction pelvis
      positional 652.8 ✓5ᵗʰ
      shoulder girdle 660.4 ✓5ᵗʰ
    eclampsia 642.6 ✓5ᵗʰ
    ectopic kidney 654.4 ✓5ᵗʰ
      causing obstructed labor 660.2 ✓5ᵗʰ
    edema, cervix 654.6 ✓5ᵗʰ
      causing obstructed labor 660.2 ✓5ᵗʰ
    effusion, amniotic fluid 658.1 ✓5ᵗʰ
    elderly multigravida 659.6 ✓5ᵗʰ
    elderly primigravida 659.5 ✓5ᵗʰ
    embolism (pulmonary) 673.2 ✓5ᵗʰ
      air 673.0 ✓5ᵗʰ
      amniotic fluid 673.1 ✓5ᵗʰ
      blood clot 673.2 ✓5ᵗʰ
      cerebral 674.0 ✓5ᵗʰ
      fat 673.8 ✓5ᵗʰ
      pyemic 673.3 ✓5ᵗʰ
      septic 673.3 ✓5ᵗʰ
    entanglement, umbilical cord 663.3 ✓5ᵗʰ
      with compression 663.2 ✓5ᵗʰ
        around neck (with compression) 663.1 ✓5ᵗʰ
    eversion, cervix or uterus 665.2 ✓5ᵗʰ

Delivery — *continued*
complicated (by) NEC — *continued*
  excessive
    fetal growth 653.5 ✓5ᵗʰ
      causing obstructed labor 660.1 ✓5ᵗʰ
    size of fetus 653.5 ✓5ᵗʰ
      causing obstructed labor 660.1 ✓5ᵗʰ
  face presentation 652.4 ✓5ᵗʰ
    causing obstructed labor 660.0 ✓5ᵗʰ
    to pubes 660.3 ✓5ᵗʰ
  failure, fetal head to enter pelvic brim 652.5 ✓5ᵗʰ
    causing obstructed labor 660.0 ✓5ᵗʰ
  fetal
    acid-base balance 656.8 ✓5ᵗʰ
    death (near term) NEC 656.4 ✓5ᵗʰ
      early (before 22 completed weeks gestation) 632
    deformity 653.7 ✓5ᵗʰ
      causing obstructed labor 660.1 ✓5ᵗʰ
    distress 656.8 ✓5ᵗʰ
    heart rate or rhythm 659.7 ✓5ᵗʰ
  fetopelvic disproportion 653.4 ✓5ᵗʰ
    causing obstructed labor 660.1 ✓5ᵗʰ
  fever during labor 659.2 ✓5ᵗʰ
  fibroid (tumor) (uterus) 654.1 ✓5ᵗʰ
    causing obstructed labor 660.2 ✓5ᵗʰ
  fibromyomata 654.1 ✓5ᵗʰ
    causing obstructed labor 660.2 ✓5ᵗʰ
  forelying umbilical cord 663.0 ✓5ᵗʰ
  fracture of coccyx 665.6 ✓5ᵗʰ
  hematoma 664.5 ✓5ᵗʰ
    broad ligament 665.7 ✓5ᵗʰ
    ischial spine 665.7 ✓5ᵗʰ
    pelvic 665.7 ✓5ᵗʰ
    perineum 664.5 ✓5ᵗʰ
    soft tissues 665.7 ✓5ᵗʰ
    subdural 674.0 ✓5ᵗʰ
    umbilical cord 663.6 ✓5ᵗʰ
    vagina 665.7 ✓5ᵗʰ
    vulva or perineum 664.5 ✓5ᵗʰ
  hemorrhage (uterine) (antepartum) (intrapartum) (pregnancy) 641.9 ✓5ᵗʰ
    accidental 641.2 ✓5ᵗʰ
    associated with
      afibrinogenemia 641.3 ✓5ᵗʰ
      coagulation defect 641.3 ✓5ᵗʰ
        hyperfibrinolysis 641.3 ✓5ᵗʰ
        hypofibrinogenemia 641.3 ✓5ᵗʰ
    cerebral 674.0 ✓5ᵗʰ
    due to
      low-lying placenta 641.1 ✓5ᵗʰ
      placenta previa 641.1 ✓5ᵗʰ
      premature separation of placenta (normally implanted) 641.2 ✓5ᵗʰ
      retained placenta 666.0 ✓5ᵗʰ
      trauma 641.8 ✓5ᵗʰ
      uterine leiomyoma 641.8 ✓5ᵗʰ
    marginal sinus rupture 641.2 ✓5ᵗʰ
    placenta NEC 641.9 ✓5ᵗʰ
    postpartum (atonic) (immediate) (within 24 hours) 666.1 ✓5ᵗʰ
      with retained or trapped placenta 666.0 ✓5ᵗʰ
      delayed 666.2 ✓5ᵗʰ
      secondary 666.2 ✓5ᵗʰ
      third stage 666.0 ✓5ᵗʰ
  hourglass contraction, uterus 661.4 ✓5ᵗʰ
  hydramnios 657 ✓5ᵗʰ
  hydrocephalic fetus 653.6 ✓5ᵗʰ
    causing obstructed labor 660.1 ✓5ᵗʰ
  hydrops fetalis 653.7 ✓5ᵗʰ
    causing obstructed labor 660.1 ✓5ᵗʰ
  hypertension — *see* Hypertension, complicating pregnancy
  hypertonic uterine dysfunction 661.4 ✓5ᵗʰ
  hypotonic uterine dysfunction 661.2 ✓5ᵗʰ
  impacted shoulders 660.4 ✓5ᵗʰ
  incarceration, uterus 654.3 ✓5ᵗʰ
    causing obstructed labor 660.2 ✓5ᵗʰ
  incomplete dilation (cervix) 661.0 ✓5ᵗʰ
  incoordinate uterus 661.4 ✓5ᵗʰ
  indication NEC 659.9 ✓5ᵗʰ
    specified type 659.8 ✓5ᵗʰ
  inertia, uterus 661.2 ✓5ᵗʰ
    hypertonic 661.4 ✓5ᵗʰ

Delivery — *continued*
complicated (by) NEC — *continued*
  inertia, uterus — *continued*
    hypotonic 661.2 ✓5ᵗʰ
    primary 661.0 ✓5ᵗʰ
    secondary 661.1 ✓5ᵗʰ
  infantile
    genitalia 654.4 ✓5ᵗʰ
      causing obstructed labor 660.2 ✓5ᵗʰ
    uterus (os) 654.4 ✓5ᵗʰ
      causing obstructed labor 660.2 ✓5ᵗʰ
  injury (to mother) NEC 665.9 ✓5ᵗʰ
  intrauterine fetal death (near term) NEC 656.4 ✓5ᵗʰ
    early (before 22 completed weeks gestation) 632
  inversion, uterus 665.2 ✓5ᵗʰ
  kidney, ectopic 654.4 ✓5ᵗʰ
    causing obstructed labor 660.2 ✓5ᵗʰ
  knot (true), umbilical cord 663.2 ✓5ᵗʰ
  labor, premature (before 37 completed weeks gestation) 644.2 ✓5ᵗʰ
  laceration 664.9 ✓5ᵗʰ
    anus (spincter) 664.2 ✓5ᵗʰ
      with mucosa 664.3 ✓5ᵗʰ
    bladder (urinary) 665.5 ✓5ᵗʰ
    bowel 665.5 ✓5ᵗʰ
    central 664.4 ✓5ᵗʰ
    cervix (uteri) 665.3 ✓5ᵗʰ
    fourchette 664.0 ✓5ᵗʰ
    hymen 664.0 ✓5ᵗʰ
    labia (majora) (minora) 664.0 ✓5ᵗʰ
    pelvic
      floor 664.1 ✓5ᵗʰ
      organ NEC 665.5 ✓5ᵗʰ
    perineum, perineal 664.4 ✓5ᵗʰ
      first degree 664.0 ✓5ᵗʰ
      second degree 664.1 ✓5ᵗʰ
      third degree 664.2 ✓5ᵗʰ
      fourth degree 664.3 ✓5ᵗʰ
      central 664.4 ✓5ᵗʰ
      extensive NEC 664.4 ✓5ᵗʰ
      muscles 664.1 ✓5ᵗʰ
      skin 664.0 ✓5ᵗʰ
      slight 664.0 ✓5ᵗʰ
    peritoneum 665.5 ✓5ᵗʰ
    periurethral tissue 665.5 ✓5ᵗʰ
    rectovaginal (septum) (without perineal laceration) 665.4 ✓5ᵗʰ
      with perineum 664.2 ✓5ᵗʰ
        with anal rectal mucosa 664.3 ✓5ᵗʰ
    skin (perineum) 664.0 ✓5ᵗʰ
    specified site or type NEC 664.8 ✓5ᵗʰ
    sphincter ani 664.2 ✓5ᵗʰ
      with mucosa 664.3 ✓5ᵗʰ
    urethra 665.5 ✓5ᵗʰ
    uterus 665.1 ✓5ᵗʰ
      before labor 665.0 ✓5ᵗʰ
    vagina, vaginal (deep) (high) (sulcus) (wall) (without perineal laceration) 665.4 ✓5ᵗʰ
      with perineum 664.0 ✓5ᵗʰ
      muscles, with perineum 664.1 ✓5ᵗʰ
    vulva 664.0 ✓5ᵗʰ
  lateroversion, uterus or cervix 654.4 ✓5ᵗʰ
    causing obstructed labor 660.2 ✓5ᵗʰ
  locked mates 660.5 ✓5ᵗʰ
  low implantation of placenta — *see* Delivery, complicated, placenta, previa
  mal lie 652.9 ✓5ᵗʰ
  malposition
    fetus NEC 652.9 ✓5ᵗʰ
      causing obstructed labor 660.0 ✓5ᵗʰ
    pelvic organs or tissues NEC 654.9 ✓5ᵗʰ
      causing obstructed labor 660.2 ✓5ᵗʰ
    placenta 641.1 ✓5ᵗʰ
      without hemorrhage 641.0 ✓5ᵗʰ
    uterus NEC or cervix 654.4 ✓5ᵗʰ
      causing obstructed labor 660.2 ✓5ᵗʰ
  malpresentation 652.9 ✓5ᵗʰ
    causing obstructed labor 660.0 ✓5ᵗʰ
  marginal sinus (bleeding) (rupture) 641.2 ✓5ᵗʰ
  maternal hypotension syndrome 669.2 ✓5ᵗʰ
  meconium in liquor 656.8 ✓5ᵗʰ

Delivery — *continued*
  complicated (by) NEC — *continued*
    membranes, retained — *see* Delivery,
      complicated, placenta, retained
    mentum presentation 652.4 ✓5ᵗʰ
      causing obstructed labor 660.0 ✓5ᵗʰ
    metrorrhagia (myopathia) — *see* Delivery,
      complicated, hemorrhage
    metrorrhexis — *see* Delivery, complicated,
      rupture, uterus
    multiparity (grand) 659.4 ✓5ᵗʰ
    myelomeningocele, fetus 653.7 ✓5ᵗʰ
      causing obstructed labor 660.1 ✓5ᵗʰ
    Nägele's pelvis 653.0 ✓5ᵗʰ
      causing obstructed labor 660.1 ✓5ᵗʰ
    nonengagement, fetal head 652.5 ✓5ᵗʰ
      causing obstructed labor 660.0 ✓5ᵗʰ
    oblique presentation 652.3 ✓5ᵗʰ
      causing obstructed labor 660.0 ✓5ᵗʰ
    obstetric
      shock 669.1 ✓5ᵗʰ
      trauma NEC 665.9 ✓5ᵗʰ
    obstructed labor 660.9 ✓5ᵗʰ
      due to
        abnormality pelvic organs or tissues
          (conditions classifiable to 654.0-
          654.9) 660.2 ✓5ᵗʰ
        deep transverse arrest 660.3 ✓5ᵗʰ
        impacted shoulders 660.4 ✓5ᵗʰ
        locked twins 660.5 ✓5ᵗʰ
        malposition and malpresentation of
          fetus (conditions classifiable to
          652.0-652.9) 660.0 ✓5ᵗʰ
        persistent occipitoposterior 660.3 ✓5ᵗʰ
        shoulder dystocia 660.4 ✓5ᵗʰ
    occult prolapse of umbilical cord 663.0 ✓5ᵗʰ
    oversize fetus 653.5 ✓5ᵗʰ
      causing obstructed labor 660.1 ✓5ᵗʰ
    pathological retraction ring, uterus
      661.4 ✓5ᵗʰ
    pelvic
      arrest (deep) (high) (of fetal head)
        (transverse) 660.3 ✓5ᵗʰ
      deformity (bone) — *see also* Deformity,
        pelvis, with disproportion
        soft tissue 654.9 ✓5ᵗʰ
          causing obstructed labor 660.2 ✓5ᵗʰ
      tumor NEC 654.9 ✓5ᵗʰ
        causing obstructed labor 660.2 ✓5ᵗʰ
    penetration, pregnant uterus by instrument
      665.1 ✓5ᵗʰ
    perforation — *see* Delivery, complicated,
      laceration
    persistent
      hymen 654.8 ✓5ᵗʰ
        causing obstructed labor 660.2 ✓5ᵗʰ
      occipitoposterior 660.3 ✓5ᵗʰ
    placenta, placental
      ablatio 641.2 ✓5ᵗʰ
      abnormality 656.7 ✓5ᵗʰ
        with hemorrhage 641.2 ✓5ᵗʰ
      abruptio 641.2 ✓5ᵗʰ
      accreta 667.0 ✓5ᵗʰ
        with hemorrhage 666.0 ✓5ᵗʰ
      adherent (without hemorrhage) 667.0 ✓5ᵗʰ
        with hemorrhage 666.0 ✓5ᵗʰ
      apoplexy 641.2 ✓5ᵗʰ
      battledore placenta — *see* Placenta,
        abnormal 663.8 ✓5ᵗʰ
      detachment (premature) 641.2 ✓5ᵗʰ
      disease 656.7 ✓5ᵗʰ
      hemorrhage NEC 641.9 ✓5ᵗʰ
      increta (without hemorrhage) 667.0 ✓5ᵗʰ
        with hemorrhage 666.0 ✓5ᵗʰ
      low (implantation) 641.0 ✓5ᵗʰ
        without hemorrhage 641.0 ✓5ᵗʰ
      malformation 656.7 ✓5ᵗʰ
        with hemorrhage 641.2 ✓5ᵗʰ
      malposition 641.1 ✓5ᵗʰ
        without hemorrhage 641.0 ✓5ᵗʰ
      marginal sinus rupture 641.2 ✓5ᵗʰ
      percreta 667.0 ✓5ᵗʰ
        with hemorrhage 666.0 ✓5ᵗʰ
      premature separation 641.2 ✓5ᵗʰ
      previa (central) (lateral) (marginal) partial)
        641.1 ✓5ᵗʰ

Delivery — *continued*
  complicated (by) NEC — *continued*
    placenta, placental — *continued*
      previa — *continued*
        without hemorrhage 641.0 ✓5ᵗʰ
        retained (with hemorrhage) 666.0 ✓5ᵗʰ
          without hemorrhage 667.0 ✓5ᵗʰ
      rupture of marginal sinus 641.2 ✓5ᵗʰ
      separation (premature) 641.2 ✓5ᵗʰ
      trapped 666.0 ✓5ᵗʰ
        without hemorrhage 667.0 ✓5ᵗʰ
      vicious insertion 641.1 ✓5ᵗʰ
    polyhydramnios 657 ✓4ᵗʰ
    polyp, cervix 654.6 ✓5ᵗʰ
      causing obstructed labor 660.2 ✓5ᵗʰ
    precipitate labor 661.3 ✓5ᵗʰ
    premature
      labor (before 37 completed weeks
        gestation) 644.2 ✓5ᵗʰ
      rupture, membranes 658.1 ✓5ᵗʰ
        delayed delivery following 658.2 ✓5ᵗʰ
    presenting umbilical cord 663.0 ✓5ᵗʰ
    previous
      cesarean delivery 654.2 ✓5ᵗʰ
      surgery
        cervix 654.6 ✓5ᵗʰ
          causing obstructed labor 660.2 ✓5ᵗʰ
        gynecological NEC 654.9 ✓5ᵗʰ
          causing obstructed labor 660.2 ✓5ᵗʰ
        perineum 654.8 ✓5ᵗʰ
        uterus NEC 654.9 ✓5ᵗʰ
          due to previous cesarean delivery
            654.2 ✓5ᵗʰ
        vagina 654.7 ✓5ᵗʰ
          causing obstructed labor 660.2 ✓5ᵗʰ
        vulva 654.8 ✓5ᵗʰ
    primary uterine inertia 661.0 ✓5ᵗʰ
    primipara, elderly or old 659.5 ✓5ᵗʰ
    prolapse
      arm or hand 652.7 ✓5ᵗʰ
        causing obstructed labor 660.0 ✓5ᵗʰ
      cord (umbilical) 663.0 ✓5ᵗʰ
      fetal extremity 652.8 ✓5ᵗʰ
      foot or leg 652.8 ✓5ᵗʰ
        causing obstructed labor 660.0 ✓5ᵗʰ
      umbilical cord (complete) (occult) (partial)
        663.0 ✓5ᵗʰ
      uterus 654.4 ✓5ᵗʰ
        causing obstructed labor 660.2 ✓5ᵗʰ
    prolonged labor 662.1 ✓5ᵗʰ
      first stage 662.0 ✓5ᵗʰ
      second stage 662.2 ✓5ᵗʰ
      active phase 661.2 ✓5ᵗʰ
      due to
        cervical dystocia 661.0 ✓5ᵗʰ
        contraction ring 661.4 ✓5ᵗʰ
        tetanic uterus 661.4 ✓5ᵗʰ
        uterine inertia 661.2 ✓5ᵗʰ
          primary 661.0 ✓5ᵗʰ
          secondary 661.1 ✓5ᵗʰ
      latent phase 661.0 ✓5ᵗʰ
    pyrexia during labor 659.2 ✓5ᵗʰ
    rachitic pelvis 653.2 ✓5ᵗʰ
      causing obstructed labor 660.1 ✓5ᵗʰ
    rectocele 654.4 ✓5ᵗʰ
      causing obstructed labor 660.2 ✓5ᵗʰ
    retained membranes or portions of placenta
      666.2 ✓5ᵗʰ
      without hemorrhage 667.1 ✓5ᵗʰ
    retarded (prolonged) birth 662.1 ✓5ᵗʰ
    retention secundines (with hemorrhage)
      666.2 ✓5ᵗʰ
      without hemorrhage 667.1 ✓5ᵗʰ
    retroversion, uterus or cervix 654.3 ✓5ᵗʰ
      causing obstructed labor 660.2 ✓5ᵗʰ
    rigid
      cervix 654.6 ✓5ᵗʰ
        causing obstructed labor 660.2 ✓5ᵗʰ
      pelvic floor 654.4 ✓5ᵗʰ
        causing obstructed labor 660.2 ✓5ᵗʰ
      perineum or vulva 654.8 ✓5ᵗʰ
        causing obstructed labor 660.2 ✓5ᵗʰ
      vagina 654.7 ✓5ᵗʰ
        causing obstructed labor 660.2 ✓5ᵗʰ
    Robert's pelvis 653.0 ✓5ᵗʰ
      causing obstructed labor 660.1 ✓5ᵗʰ

Delivery — *continued*
  complicated (by) NEC — *continued*
    rupture — *see also* Delivery, complicated,
      laceration
      bladder (urinary) 665.5 ✓5ᵗʰ
      cervix 665.3 ✓5ᵗʰ
      marginal sinus 641.2 ✓5ᵗʰ
      membranes, premature 658.1 ✓5ᵗʰ
      pelvic organ NEC 665.5 ✓5ᵗʰ
      perineum (without mention of other
        laceration) — *see* Delivery,
        complicated, laceration, perineum
      peritoneum 665.5 ✓5ᵗʰ
      urethra 665.5 ✓5ᵗʰ
      uterus (during labor) 665.1 ✓5ᵗʰ
        before labor 665.0 ✓5ᵗʰ
    sacculation, pregnant uterus 654.4 ✓5ᵗʰ
    sacral teratomas, fetal 653.7 ✓5ᵗʰ
      causing obstructed labor 660.1 ✓5ᵗʰ
    scar(s)
      cervix 654.6 ✓5ᵗʰ
        causing obstructed labor 660.2 ✓5ᵗʰ
      cesarean delivery 654.2 ✓5ᵗʰ
        causing obstructed labor 660.2 ✓5ᵗʰ
      perineum 654.8 ✓5ᵗʰ
        causing obstructed labor 660.2 ✓5ᵗʰ
      uterus NEC 654.9 ✓5ᵗʰ
        causing obstructed labor 660.2 ✓5ᵗʰ
        due to previous cesarean delivery
          654.2 ✓5ᵗʰ
      vagina 654.7 ✓5ᵗʰ
        causing obstructed labor 660.2 ✓5ᵗʰ
      vulva 654.8 ✓5ᵗʰ
        causing obstructed labor 660.2 ✓5ᵗʰ
    scoliotic pelvis 653.0 ✓5ᵗʰ
      causing obstructed labor 660.1 ✓5ᵗʰ
    secondary uterine inertia 661.1 ✓5ᵗʰ
    secundines, retained — *see* Delivery,
      complicated, placenta, retained
    separation
      placenta (premature) 641.2 ✓5ᵗʰ
      pubic bone 665.6 ✓5ᵗʰ
      symphysis pubis 665.6 ✓5ᵗʰ
    septate vagina 654.7 ✓5ᵗʰ
      causing obstructed labor 660.2 ✓5ᵗʰ
    shock (birth) (obstetric) (puerperal)
      669.1 ✓5ᵗʰ
    short cord syndrome 663.4 ✓5ᵗʰ
    shoulder
      girdle dystocia 660.4 ✓5ᵗʰ
      presentation 652.8 ✓5ᵗʰ
        causing obstructed labor 660.0 ✓5ᵗʰ
    Siamese twins 653.7 ✓5ᵗʰ
      causing obstructed labor 660.1 ✓5ᵗʰ
    slow slope active phase 661.2 ✓5ᵗʰ
    spasm
      cervix 661.4 ✓5ᵗʰ
      uterus 661.4 ✓5ᵗʰ
    spondylolisthesis, pelvis 653.3 ✓5ᵗʰ
      causing obstructed labor 660.1 ✓5ᵗʰ
    spondylolysis (lumbosacral) 653.3 ✓5ᵗʰ
      causing obstructed labor 660.1 ✓5ᵗʰ
    spondylosis 653.0 ✓5ᵗʰ
      causing obstructed labor 660.1 ✓5ᵗʰ
    stenosis or stricture
      cervix 654.6 ✓5ᵗʰ
        causing obstructed labor 660.2 ✓5ᵗʰ
      vagina 654.7 ✓5ᵗʰ
        causing obstructed labor 660.2 ✓5ᵗʰ
    sudden death, unknown cause 669.9 ✓5ᵗʰ
    tear (pelvic organ) (*see also* Delivery,
      complicated, laceration) 664.9 ✓5ᵗʰ
    teratomas, sacral, fetal 653.7 ✓5ᵗʰ
      causing obstructed labor 660.1 ✓5ᵗʰ
    tetanic uterus 661.4 ✓5ᵗʰ
    tipping pelvis 653.0 ✓5ᵗʰ
      causing obstructed labor 660.1 ✓5ᵗʰ
    transverse
      arrest (deep) 660.3 ✓5ᵗʰ
      presentation or lie 652.3 ✓5ᵗʰ
        with successful version 652.1 ✓5ᵗʰ
        causing obstructed labor 660.0 ✓5ᵗʰ
    trauma (obstetrical) NEC 665.9 ✓5ᵗʰ
    tumor
      abdominal, fetal 653.7 ✓5ᵗʰ
        causing obstructed labor 660.1 ✓5ᵗʰ

Delivery — *continued*
  complicated (by) NEC — *continued*
    tumor — *continued*
      pelvic organs or tissues NEC 654.9 √5th
        causing obstructed labor 660.2 √5th
    umbilical cord (*see also* Delivery, complicated, cord) 663.9 √5th
      around neck tightly, or with compression 663.1 √5th
      entanglement NEC 663.3 √5th
        with compression 663.2 √5th
      prolapse (complete) (occult) (partial) 663.0 √5th
    unstable lie 652.0 √5th
      causing obstructed labor 660.0 √5th
    uterine
      inertia (*see also* Delivery, complicated, inertia, uterus) 661.2 √5th
      spasm 661.4 √5th
    vasa previa 663.5 √5th
    velamentous insertion of cord 663.8 √5th
    young maternal age 659.8 √5th
  delayed NEC 662.1 √5th
    following rupture of membranes (spontaneous) 658.2 √5th
      artificial 658.3 √5th
    second twin, triplet, etc. 662.3 √5th
  difficult NEC 669.9 √5th
    previous, affecting management of pregnancy or childbirth V23.49 ▲
    specified type NEC 669.8 √5th
  early onset (spontaneous) 644.2 √5th
  footling 652.8 √5th
    with successful version 652.1 √5th
  forceps NEC 669.5 √5th
    affecting fetus or newborn 763.2
  missed (at or near term) 656.4 √5th
  multiple gestation NEC 651.9 √5th
    with fetal loss and retention of one or more fetus(es) 651.6 √5th
    specified type NEC 651.8 √5th
      with fetal loss and retention of one or more fetus(es) 651.6 √5th
  nonviable infant 656.4 √5th
  normal — *see* category 650
  precipitate 661.3 √5th
    affecting fetus or newborn 763.6
  premature NEC (before 37 completed weeks gestation) 644.2 √5th
    previous, affecting management of pregnancy V23.41 ▲
  quadruplet NEC 651.2 √5th
    with fetal loss and retention of one or more fetus(es) 651.5 √5th
  quintuplet NEC 651.8 √5th
    with fetal loss and retention of one or more fetus(es) 651.6 √5th
  sextuplet NEC 651.8 √5th
    with fetal loss and retention of one or more fetus(es) 651.6 √5th
  specified complication NEC 669.8 √5th
  stillbirth (near term) NEC 656.4 √5th
    early (before 22 completed weeks gestation) 632
  term pregnancy (live birth) NEC — *see* category 650
    stillbirth NEC 656.4 √5th
  threatened premature 644.2 √5th
  triplets NEC 651.1 √5th
    with fetal loss and retention of one or more fetus(es) 651.4 √5th
    delayed delivery (one or more mates) 662.3 √5th
    locked mates 660.5 √5th
  twins NEC 651.0 √5th
    with fetal loss and retention of one fetus 651.3 √5th
    delayed delivery (one or more mates) 662.3 √5th
    locked mates 660.5 √5th
  uncomplicated — *see* category 650
  vacuum extractor NEC 669.5 √5th
    affecting fetus or newborn 763.3
  ventouse NEC 669.5 √5th
    affecting fetus or newborn 763.3
Dellen, cornea 371.41

Delusions (paranoid) 297.9
  grandiose 297.1
  parasitosis 300.29
  systematized 297.1
Dementia 294.8
  alcoholic (*see also* Psychosis, alcoholic) 291.2
  Alzheimer's — *see* Alzheimer's dementia
  arteriosclerotic (simple type) (uncomplicated) 290.40
    with
      acute confusional state 290.41
      delirium 290.41
      delusional features 290.42
      depressive features 290.43
    depressed type 290.43
    paranoid type 290.42
  Binswanger's 290.12
  catatonic (acute) (*see also* Schizophrenia) 295.2 √5th
  congenital (*see also* Retardation, mental) 319
  degenerative 290.9
    presenile-onset — *see* Dementia, presenile
    senile-onset — *see* Dementia, senile
  developmental (*see also* Schizophrenia) 295.9 √5th
  dialysis 294.8
    transient 293.9
  due to or associated with condition(s) classified elsewhere
    Alzheimer's
      with behavioral disturbance 331.0 *[294.11]*
      without behavioral disturbance 331.0 *[294.10]*
    cerebral lipidoses
      with behavioral disturbance 330.1 *[294.11]*
      without behavioral disturbance 330.1 *[294.10]*
    epilepsy
      with behavioral disturbance 345.9 √5th *[294.11]*
      without behavioral disturbance 345.9 √5th *[294.10]*
    hepatolenticular degeneration
      with behavioral disturbance 275.1 *[294.11]*
      without behavioral disturbance 275.1 *[294.10]*
    HIV
      with behavioral disturbance 042 *[294.11]*
      without behavioral disturbance 042 *[294.10]*
    Huntington's chorea
      with behavioral disturbance 333.4 *[294.11]*
      without behavioral disturbance 333.4 *[294.10]*
    Jakob-Creutzfeldt disease
      with behavioral disturbance 046.1 *[294.11]*
      without behavioral disturbance 046.1 *[294.10]*
    multiple sclerosis
      with behavioral disturbance 340 *[294.11]*
      without behavioral disturbance 340 *[294.10]*
    neurosyphilis
      with behavioral disturbance 094.9 *[294.11]*
      without behavioral disturbance 094.9 *[294.10]*
    Pelizaeus-Merzbacher disease
      with behavioral disturbance 333.0 *[294.11]*
      without behavioral disturbance 333.0 *[294.10]*
    Pick's disease
      with behavioral disturbance 331.1 *[294.11]*
      without behavioral disturbance 331.1 *[294.10]*
    polyarteritis nodosa
      with behavioral disturbance 446.0 *[294.11]*

Dementia — *continued*
  due to or associated with condition(s) classified elsewhere — *continued*
    polyarteritis nodosa — *continued*
      without behavioral disturbance 446.0 *[294.10]*
    syphilis
      with behavioral disturbance 094.1 *[294.11]*
      without behavioral disturbance 094.1 *[294.10]*
    Wilson's disease
      with behavioral disturbance 275.1 *[294.11]*
      without behavioral disturbance 275.1 *[294.10]*
  hebephrenic (acute) 295.1 √5th
  Heller's (infantile psychosis) (*see also* Psychosis, childhood) 299.1 √5th
  idiopathic 290.9
    presenile-onset — *see* Dementia, presenile
    senile-onset — *see* Dementia, senile
  in
    arteriosclerotic brain disease 290.40
    senility 290.0
  induced by drug 292.82
  infantile, infantilia (*see also* Psychosis, childhood) 299.0 √5th
  multi-infarct (cerebrovascular) (*see also* Dementia, arteriosclerotic) 290.40
  old age 290.0
  paralytica, paralytic 094.1
    juvenilis 090.40
    syphilitic 094.1
      congenital 090.40
    tabetic form 094.1
  paranoid (*see also* Schizophrenia) 295.3 √5th
  paraphrenic (*see also* Schizophrenia) 295.3 √5th
  paretic 094.1
  praecox (*see also* Schizophrenia) 295.9 √5th
  presenile 290.10
    with
      acute confusional state 290.11
      delirium 290.11
      delusional features 290.12
      depressive features 290.13
    depressed type 290.13
    paranoid type 290.12
    simple type 290.10
    uncomplicated 290.10
  primary (acute) (*see also* Schizophrenia) 295.0 √5th
  progressive, syphilitic 094.1
  puerperal — *see* Psychosis, puerperal
  schizophrenic (*see also* Schizophrenia) 295.9 √5th
  senile 290.0
    with
      acute confusional state 290.3
      delirium 290.3
      delusional features 290.20
      depressive features 290.21
    depressed type 290.21
    exhaustion 290.0
    paranoid type 290.20
  simple type (acute) (*see also* Schizophrenia) 295.0 √5th
  simplex (acute) (*see also* Schizophrenia) 295.0 √5th
  syphilitic 094.1
  uremic — *see* Uremia
  vascular 290.40
Demerol dependence (*see also* Dependence) 304.0 √5th
Demineralization, ankle (*see also* Osteoporosis) 733.00
Demodex folliculorum (infestation) 133.8
de Morgan's spots (senile angiomas) 448.1
Demyelinating
  polyneuritis, chronic inflammatory 357.81 ▲
Demyelination, demyelinization
  central nervous system 341.9
    specified NEC 341.8
  corpus callosum (central) 341.8
  global 340

Dengue — Dependence

Dengue (fever) 061
    sandfly 061
    vaccination, prophylactic (against) V05.1
    virus hemorrhagic fever 065.4

Dens
    evaginatus 520.2
    in dente 520.2
    invaginatus 520.2

Density
    increased, bone (disseminated) (generalized)
        (spotted) 733.99
    lung (nodular) 518.89

Dental — *see also* condition
    examination only V72.2

Dentia praecox 520.6

Denticles (in pulp) 522.2

Dentigerous cyst 526.0

Dentin
    irregular (in pulp) 522.3
    opalescent 520.5
    secondary (in pulp) 522.3
    sensitive 521.8

Dentinogenesis imperfecta 520.5

Dentinoma (M9271/0) 213.1
    upper jaw (bone) 213.0

Dentition 520.7
    abnormal 520.6
    anomaly 520.6
    delayed 520.6
    difficult 520.7
    disorder of 520.6
    precocious 520.6
    retarded 520.6

Denture sore (mouth) 528.9

Dependence

> *Note — Use the following fifth-digit*
> *subclassification with category 304:*
>
>   0   unspecified
>   1   continuous
>   2   episodic
>   3   in remission

    with
        withdrawal symptoms
            alcohol 291.81
            drug 292.0
    14-hydroxy-dihydromorphinone 304.0 ✓5th
    absinthe 304.6 ✓5th
    acemorphan 304.0 ✓5th
    acetanilid(e) 304.6 ✓5th
    acetorphine 304.0 ✓5th
    acetyldihydrocodeine 304.0 ✓5th
    acetyldihydrocodeinone 304.0 ✓5th
    Adalin 304.1 ✓5th
    Afghanistan black 304.3 ✓5th
    agrypnal 304.1 ✓5th
    alcohol, alcoholic (ethyl) (methyl) (wood)
        303.9 ✓5th
        maternal, with suspected fetal damage
            affecting management of pregnancy
            655.4 ✓5th
    allobarbitone 304.1 ✓5th
    allonal 304.1 ✓5th
    allylisopropylacetylurea 304.1 ✓5th
    alphaprodine (hydrochloride) 304.0 ✓5th
    Alurate 304.1 ✓5th
    Alvodine 304.0 ✓5th
    amethocaine 304.6 ✓5th
    amidone 304.0 ✓5th
    amidopyrine 304.6 ✓5th
    aminopyrine 304.6 ✓5th
    amobarbital 304.1 ✓5th
    amphetamine(s) (type) (drugs classifiable to
        969.7) 304.4 ✓5th
    amylene hydrate 304.6 ✓5th
    amylobarbitone 304.1 ✓5th
    amylocaine 304.6 ✓5th
    Amytal (sodium) 304.1 ✓5th
    analgesic (drug) NEC 304.6 ✓5th
        synthetic with morphine-like effect
            304.0 ✓5th

Dependence — *continued*
    anesthetic (agent) (drug) (gas) (general) (local)
        NEC 304.6 ✓5th
    Angel dust 304.6 ✓5th
    anileridine 304.0 ✓5th
    antipyrine 304.6 ✓5th
    aprobarbital 304.1 ✓5th
    aprobarbitone 304.1 ✓5th
    atropine 304.6 ✓5th
    Avertin (bromide) 304.6 ✓5th
    barbenyl 304.1 ✓5th
    barbital(s) 304.1 ✓5th
    barbitone 304.1 ✓5th
    barbiturate(s) (compounds) (drugs classifiable
        to 967.0) 304.1 ✓5th
    barbituric acid (and compounds) 304.1 ✓5th
    benzedrine 304.4 ✓5th
    benzylmorphine 304.0 ✓5th
    Beta-chlor 304.1 ✓5th
    bhang 304.3 ✓5th
    blue velvet 304.0 ✓5th
    Brevital 304.1 ✓5th
    bromal (hydrate) 304.1 ✓5th
    bromide(s) NEC 304.1 ✓5th
    bromine compounds NEC 304.1 ✓5th
    bromisovalum 304.1 ✓5th
    bromoform 304.1 ✓5th
    Bromo-seltzer 304.1 ✓5th
    bromural 304.1 ✓5th
    butabarbital (sodium) 304.1 ✓5th
    butabarpal 304.1 ✓5th
    butallylonal 304.1 ✓5th
    butethal 304.1 ✓5th
    buthalitone (sodium) 304.1 ✓5th
    Butisol 304.1 ✓5th
    butobarbitone 304.1 ✓5th
    butyl chloral (hydrate) 304.1 ✓5th
    caffeine 304.4 ✓5th
    cannabis (indica) (sativa) (resin) (derivatives)
        (type) 304.3 ✓5th
    carbamazepine 304.6 ✓5th
    Carbrital 304.1 ✓5th
    carbromal 304.1 ✓5th
    carisoprodol 304.6 ✓5th
    Catha (edulis) 304.4 ✓5th
    chloral (betaine) (hydrate) 304.1 ✓5th
    chloralamide 304.1 ✓5th
    chloralformamide 304.1 ✓5th
    chloralose 304.1 ✓5th
    chlordiazepoxide 304.1 ✓5th
    Chloretone 304.1 ✓5th
    chlorobutanol 304.1 ✓5th
    chlorodyne 304.1 ✓5th
    chloroform 304.6 ✓5th
    Cliradon 304.0 ✓5th
    coca (leaf) and derivatives 304.2 ✓5th
    cocaine 304.2 ✓5th
        hydrochloride 304.2 ✓5th
        salt (any) 304.2 ✓5th
    codeine 304.0 ✓5th
    combination of drugs (excluding morphine or
        opioid type drug) NEC 304.8 ✓5th
        morphine or opioid type drug with any other
            drug 304.7 ✓5th
    croton-chloral 304.1 ✓5th
    cyclobarbital 304.1 ✓5th
    cyclobarbitone 304.1 ✓5th
    dagga 304.3 ✓5th
    Delvinal 304.1 ✓5th
    Demerol 304.0 ✓5th
    desocodeine 304.0 ✓5th
    desomorphine 304.0 ✓5th
    desoxyephedrine 304.4 ✓5th
    DET 304.5 ✓5th
    dexamphetamine 304.4 ✓5th
    dexedrine 304.4 ✓5th
    dextromethorphan 304.0 ✓5th
    dextromoramide 304.0 ✓5th
    dextronorpseudoephedrine 304.4 ✓5th
    dextrorphan 304.0 ✓5th
    diacetylmorphine 304.0 ✓5th
    Dial 304.1 ✓5th
    diallylbarbituric acid 304.1 ✓5th
    diamorphine 304.0 ✓5th
    diazepam 304.1 ✓5th
    dibucaine 304.6 ✓5th
    dichloroethane 304.6 ✓5th
    diethyl barbituric acid 304.1 ✓5th

Dependence — *continued*
    diethylsulfone-diethylmethane 304.1 ✓5th
    difencloxazine 304.0 ✓5th
    dihydrocodeine 304.0 ✓5th
    dihydrocodeinone 304.0 ✓5th
    dihydrohydroxycodeinone 304.0 ✓5th
    dihydroisocodeine 304.0 ✓5th
    dihydromorphine 304.0 ✓5th
    dihydromorphinone 304.0 ✓5th
    dihydroxcodeinone 304.0 ✓5th
    Dilaudid 304.0 ✓5th
    dimenhydrinate 304.6 ✓5th
    dimethylmeperidine 304.0 ✓5th
    dimethyltriptamine 304.5 ✓5th
    Dionin 304.0 ✓5th
    diphenoxylate 304.6 ✓5th
    dipipanone 304.0 ✓5th
    d-lysergic acid diethylamide 304.5 ✓5th
    DMT 304.5 ✓5th
    Dolophine 304.0 ✓5th
    DOM 304.2 ✓5th
    Doriden 304.1 ✓5th
    dormiral 304.1 ✓5th
    Dormison 304.1 ✓5th
    Dromoran 304.0 ✓5th
    drug NEC 304.9 ✓5th
        analgesic NEC 304.6 ✓5th
        combination (excluding morphine or opioid
            type drug) NEC 304.8 ✓5th
            morphine or opioid type drug with any
                other drug 304.7 ✓5th
        complicating pregnancy, childbirth, or
            puerperium 648.3 ✓5th
            affecting fetus or newborn 779.5
        hallucinogenic 304.5 ✓5th
        hypnotic NEC 304.1 ✓5th
        narcotic NEC 304.9 ✓5th
        psychostimulant NEC 304.4 ✓5th
        sedative 304.1 ✓5th
        soporific NEC 304.1 ✓5th
        specified type NEC 304.6 ✓5th
        suspected damage to fetus affecting
            management of pregnancy 655.5 ✓5th
        synthetic, with morphine-like effect
            304.0 ✓5th
        tranquilizing 304.1 ✓5th
    duboisine 304.6 ✓5th
    ectylurea 304.1 ✓5th
    Endocaine 304.6 ✓5th
    Equanil 304.1 ✓5th
    Eskabarb 304.1 ✓5th
    ethchlorvynol 304.1 ✓5th
    ether (ethyl) (liquid) (vapor) (vinyl) 304.6 ✓5th
    ethidene 304.6 ✓5th
    ethinamate 304.1 ✓5th
    ethoheptazine 304.6 ✓5th
    ethyl
        alcohol 303.9 ✓5th
        bromide 304.6 ✓5th
        carbamate 304.6 ✓5th
        chloride 304.6 ✓5th
        morphine 304.0 ✓5th
    ethylene (gas) 304.6 ✓5th
        dichloride 304.6 ✓5th
    ethylidene chloride 304.6 ✓5th
    etilfen 304.1 ✓5th
    etorphine 304.0 ✓5th
    etoval 304.1 ✓5th
    eucodal 304.0 ✓5th
    euneryl 304.1 ✓5th
    Evipal 304.1 ✓5th
    Evipan 304.1 ✓5th
    fentanyl 304.0 ✓5th
    ganja 304.3 ✓5th
    gardenal 304.1 ✓5th
    gardenpanyl 304.1 ✓5th
    gelsemine 304.6 ✓5th
    Gelsemium 304.6 ✓5th
    Gemonil 304.1 ✓5th
    glucochloral 304.1 ✓5th
    glue (airplane) (sniffing) 304.6 ✓5th
    glutethimide 304.1 ✓5th
    hallucinogenics 304.5 ✓5th
    hashish 304.3 ✓5th
    headache powder NEC 304.6 ✓5th
    Heavenly Blue 304.5 ✓5th
    hedonal 304.1 ✓5th
    hemp 304.3 ✓5th

Dependence — *continued*
heptabarbital 304.1 ✓5ᵗʰ
Heptalgin 304.0 ✓5ᵗʰ
heptobarbitone 304.1 ✓5ᵗʰ
heroin 304.0 ✓5ᵗʰ
   salt (any) 304.0 ✓5ᵗʰ
hexethal (sodium) 304.1 ✓5ᵗʰ
hexobarbital 304.1 ✓5ᵗʰ
Hycodan 304.0 ✓5ᵗʰ
hydrocodone 304.0 ✓5ᵗʰ
hydromorphinol 304.0 ✓5ᵗʰ
hydromorphinone 304.0 ✓5ᵗʰ
hydromorphone 304.0 ✓5ᵗʰ
hydroxycodeine 304.0 ✓5ᵗʰ
hypnotic NEC 304.1 ✓5ᵗʰ
Indian hemp 304.3 ✓5ᵗʰ
intranarcon 304.1 ✓5ᵗʰ
Kemithal 304.1 ✓5ᵗʰ
ketobemidone 304.0 ✓5ᵗʰ
khat 304.4 ✓5ᵗʰ
kif 304.3 ✓5ᵗʰ
Lactuca (virosa) extract 304.1 ✓5ᵗʰ
lactucarium 304.1 ✓5ᵗʰ
laudanum 304.0 ✓5ᵗʰ
Lebanese red 304.3 ✓5ᵗʰ
Leritine 304.0 ✓5ᵗʰ
lettuce opium 304.1 ✓5ᵗʰ
Levanil 304.1 ✓5ᵗʰ
Levo-Dromoran 304.0 ✓5ᵗʰ
levo-iso-methadone 304.0 ✓5ᵗʰ
levorphanol 304.0 ✓5ᵗʰ
Librium 304.1 ✓5ᵗʰ
Lomotil 304.6 ✓5ᵗʰ
Lotusate 304.1 ✓5ᵗʰ
LSD (-25) (and derivatives) 304.5 ✓5ᵗʰ
Luminal 304.1 ✓5ᵗʰ
lysergic acid 304.5 ✓5ᵗʰ
   amide 304.5 ✓5ᵗʰ
maconha 304.3 ✓5ᵗʰ
magic mushroom 304.5 ✓5ᵗʰ
marihuana 304.3 ✓5ᵗʰ
MDA (methylene dioxyamphetamine) 304.4 ✓5ᵗʰ
Mebaral 304.1 ✓5ᵗʰ
Medinal 304.1 ✓5ᵗʰ
Medomin 304.1 ✓5ᵗʰ
megahallucinogenics 304.5 ✓5ᵗʰ
meperidine 304.0 ✓5ᵗʰ
mephobarbital 304.1 ✓5ᵗʰ
meprobamate 304.1 ✓5ᵗʰ
mescaline 304.5 ✓5ᵗʰ
methadone 304.0 ✓5ᵗʰ
methamphetamine(s) 304.4 ✓5ᵗʰ
methaqualone 304.1 ✓5ᵗʰ
metharbital 304.1 ✓5ᵗʰ
methitural 304.1 ✓5ᵗʰ
methobarbitone 304.1 ✓5ᵗʰ
methohexital 304.1 ✓5ᵗʰ
methopholine 304.6 ✓5ᵗʰ
methyl
   alcohol 303.9 ✓5ᵗʰ
   bromide 304.6 ✓5ᵗʰ
   morphine 304.0 ✓5ᵗʰ
   sulfonal 304.1 ✓5ᵗʰ
methylated spirit 303.9 ✓5ᵗʰ
methylbutinol 304.6 ✓5ᵗʰ
methyldihydromorphinone 304.0 ✓5ᵗʰ
methylene
   chloride 304.6 ✓5ᵗʰ
   dichloride 304.6 ✓5ᵗʰ
   dioxyamphetamine (MDA) 304.4 ✓5ᵗʰ
methylaparafynol 304.1 ✓5ᵗʰ
methylphenidate 304.4 ✓5ᵗʰ
methyprylone 304.1 ✓5ᵗʰ
metopon 304.0 ✓5ᵗʰ
Miltown 304.1 ✓5ᵗʰ
morning glory *seeds* 304.5 ✓5ᵗʰ
morphinan(s) 304.0 ✓5ᵗʰ
morphine (sulfate) (sulfite) (type) (drugs classifiable to 965.00-965.09) 304.0 ✓5ᵗʰ
morphine or opioid type drug (drugs classifiable to 965.00-965.09) with any other drug 304.7 ✓5ᵗʰ
morphinol(s) 304.0 ✓5ᵗʰ
morphinon 304.0 ✓5ᵗʰ
morpholinylethylmorphine 304.0 ✓5ᵗʰ
mylomid 304.1 ✓5ᵗʰ
myristicin 304.5 ✓5ᵗʰ
narcotic (drug) NEC 304.9 ✓5ᵗʰ

Dependence — *continued*
nealbarbital 304.1 ✓5ᵗʰ
nealbarbitone 304.1 ✓5ᵗʰ
Nembutal 304.1 ✓5ᵗʰ
Neonal 304.1 ✓5ᵗʰ
Neraval 304.1 ✓5ᵗʰ
Neravan 304.1 ✓5ᵗʰ
neurobarb 304.1 ✓5ᵗʰ
nicotine 305.1
Nisentil 304.0 ✓5ᵗʰ
nitrous oxide 304.6 ✓5ᵗʰ
Noctec 304.1 ✓5ᵗʰ
Noludar 304.1 ✓5ᵗʰ
nonbarbiturate sedatives and tranquilizers with similar effect 304.1 ✓5ᵗʰ
noptil 304.1 ✓5ᵗʰ
normorphine 304.0 ✓5ᵗʰ
noscapine 304.0 ✓5ᵗʰ
Novocaine 304.6 ✓5ᵗʰ
Numorphan 304.0 ✓5ᵗʰ
nunol 304.1 ✓5ᵗʰ
Nupercaine 304.6 ✓5ᵗʰ
Oblivon 304.1 ✓5ᵗʰ
on
   aspirator V46.0
   hyperbaric chamber V46.8
   iron lung V46.1
   machine (enabling) V46.9
      specified type NEC V46.8
   Possum (Patient-Operated-Selector-Mechanism) V46.8
   renal dialysis machine V45.1
   respirator V46.1
   supplemental oxygen V46.2   ●
opiate 304.0 ✓5ᵗʰ
opioids 304.0 ✓5ᵗʰ
opioid type drug 304.0 ✓5ᵗʰ
   with any other drug 304.7 ✓5ᵗʰ
opium (alkaloids) (derivatives) (tincture) 304.0 ✓5ᵗʰ
ortal 304.1 ✓5ᵗʰ
Oxazepam 304.1 ✓5ᵗʰ
oxycodone 304.0 ✓5ᵗʰ
oxymorphone 304.0 ✓5ᵗʰ
Palfium 304.0 ✓5ᵗʰ
Panadol 304.6 ✓5ᵗʰ
pantopium 304.0 ✓5ᵗʰ
pantopon 304.0 ✓5ᵗʰ
papaverine 304.0 ✓5ᵗʰ
paracetamol 304.6 ✓5ᵗʰ
paracodin 304.0 ✓5ᵗʰ
paraldehyde 304.1 ✓5ᵗʰ
paregoric 304.0 ✓5ᵗʰ
Parzone 304.0 ✓5ᵗʰ
PCP (phencyclidine) 304.6 ✓5ᵗʰ
Pearly Gates 304.5 ✓5ᵗʰ
pentazocine 304.0 ✓5ᵗʰ
pentobarbital 304.1 ✓5ᵗʰ
pentobarbitone (sodium) 304.1 ✓5ᵗʰ
Pentothal 304.1 ✓5ᵗʰ
Percaine 304.6 ✓5ᵗʰ
Percodan 304.0 ✓5ᵗʰ
Perichlor 304.1 ✓5ᵗʰ
Pernocton 304.1 ✓5ᵗʰ
Pernoston 304.1 ✓5ᵗʰ
peronine 304.0 ✓5ᵗʰ
pethidine (hydrochloride) 304.0 ✓5ᵗʰ
petrichloral 304.1 ✓5ᵗʰ
peyote 304.5 ✓5ᵗʰ
Phanodron 304.1 ✓5ᵗʰ
phenacetin 304.6 ✓5ᵗʰ
phenadoxone 304.0 ✓5ᵗʰ
phenaglycodol 304.1 ✓5ᵗʰ
phenazocine 304.0 ✓5ᵗʰ
phencyclidine 304.6 ✓5ᵗʰ
phenmetrazine 304.4 ✓5ᵗʰ
phenobal 304.1 ✓5ᵗʰ
phenobarbital 304.1 ✓5ᵗʰ
phenobarbitone 304.1 ✓5ᵗʰ
phenomorphan 304.0 ✓5ᵗʰ
phenonyl 304.1 ✓5ᵗʰ
phenoperidine 304.0 ✓5ᵗʰ
pholcodine 304.0 ✓5ᵗʰ
piminodine 304.0 ✓5ᵗʰ
Pipadone 304.0 ✓5ᵗʰ
Pitkin's solution 304.6 ✓5ᵗʰ
Placidyl 304.1 ✓5ᵗʰ
polysubstance 304.8 ✓5ᵗʰ

Dependence — *continued*
Pontocaine 304.6 ✓5ᵗʰ
pot 304.3 ✓5ᵗʰ
potassium bromide 304.1 ✓5ᵗʰ
Preludin 304.4 ✓5ᵗʰ
Prinadol 304.0 ✓5ᵗʰ
probarbital 304.1 ✓5ᵗʰ
procaine 304.6 ✓5ᵗʰ
propanal 304.1 ✓5ᵗʰ
propoxyphene 304.6 ✓5ᵗʰ
psilocibin 304.5 ✓5ᵗʰ
psilocin 304.5 ✓5ᵗʰ
psilocybin 304.5 ✓5ᵗʰ
psilocyline 304.5 ✓5ᵗʰ
psilocyn 304.5 ✓5ᵗʰ
psychedelic agents 304.5 ✓5ᵗʰ
psychostimulant NEC 304.4 ✓5ᵗʰ
psychotomimetic agents 304.5 ✓5ᵗʰ
pyrahexyl 304.3 ✓5ᵗʰ
Pyramidon 304.6 ✓5ᵗʰ
quinalbarbitone 304.1 ✓5ᵗʰ
racemoramide 304.0 ✓5ᵗʰ
racemorphan 304.0 ✓5ᵗʰ
Rela 304.6 ✓5ᵗʰ
scopolamine 304.6 ✓5ᵗʰ
secobarbital 304.1 ✓5ᵗʰ
Seconal 304.1 ✓5ᵗʰ
sedative NEC 304.1 ✓5ᵗʰ
   nonbarbiturate with barbiturate effect 304.1 ✓5ᵗʰ
Sedormid 304.1 ✓5ᵗʰ
sernyl 304.1 ✓5ᵗʰ
sodium bromide 304.1 ✓5ᵗʰ
Soma 304.6 ✓5ᵗʰ
Somnal 304.1 ✓5ᵗʰ
Somnos 304.1 ✓5ᵗʰ
Soneryl 304.1 ✓5ᵗʰ
soporific (drug) NEC 304.1 ✓5ᵗʰ
specified drug NEC 304.6 ✓5ᵗʰ
speed 304.4 ✓5ᵗʰ
spinocaine 304.6 ✓5ᵗʰ
Stovaine 304.6 ✓5ᵗʰ
STP 304.5 ✓5ᵗʰ
stramonium 304.6 ✓5ᵗʰ
Sulfonal 304.1 ✓5ᵗʰ
sulfonethylmethane 304.1 ✓5ᵗʰ
sulfonmethane 304.1 ✓5ᵗʰ
Surital 304.1 ✓5ᵗʰ
synthetic drug with morphine-like effect 304.0 ✓5ᵗʰ
talbutal 304.1 ✓5ᵗʰ
tetracaine 304.6 ✓5ᵗʰ
tetrahydrocannabinol 304.3 ✓5ᵗʰ
tetronal 304.1 ✓5ᵗʰ
THC 304.3 ✓5ᵗʰ
thebacon 304.0 ✓5ᵗʰ
thebaine 304.0 ✓5ᵗʰ
thiamil 304.1 ✓5ᵗʰ
thiamylal 304.1 ✓5ᵗʰ
thiopental 304.1 ✓5ᵗʰ
tobacco 305.1
toluene, toluol 304.6 ✓5ᵗʰ
tranquilizer NEC 304.1 ✓5ᵗʰ
   nonbarbiturate with barbiturate effect 304.1 ✓5ᵗʰ
tribromacetaldehyde 304.6 ✓5ᵗʰ
tribromethanol 304.6 ✓5ᵗʰ
tribromomethane 304.6 ✓5ᵗʰ
trichloroethanol 304.6 ✓5ᵗʰ
trichoroethyl phosphate 304.1 ✓5ᵗʰ
triclofos 304.1 ✓5ᵗʰ
Trional 304.1 ✓5ᵗʰ
Tuinal 304.1 ✓5ᵗʰ
Turkish Green 304.3 ✓5ᵗʰ
urethan(e) 304.6 ✓5ᵗʰ
Valium 304.1 ✓5ᵗʰ
Valmid 304.1 ✓5ᵗʰ
veganin 304.0 ✓5ᵗʰ
veramon 304.1 ✓5ᵗʰ
Veronal 304.1 ✓5ᵗʰ
versidyne 304.6 ✓5ᵗʰ
vinbarbital 304.1 ✓5ᵗʰ
vinbarbitone 304.1 ✓5ᵗʰ
vinyl bitone 304.1 ✓5ᵗʰ
vitamin B₆ 266.1
wine 303.9 ✓5ᵗʰ
Zactane 304.6 ✓5ᵗʰ

✓4ᵗʰ Fourth-digit Required   ✓5ᵗʰ Fifth-digit Required   ▶◀ Revised Text   ● New Line   ▲ Revised Code

Dependency
  passive 301.6
  reactions 301.6

Depersonalization (episode, in neurotic state)
    (neurotic) (syndrome) 300.6

Depletion
  carbohydrates 271.9
  complement factor 279.8
  extracellular fluid 276.5
    plasma 276.5
  potassium 276.8
    nephropathy 588.8
  salt or sodium 276.1
    causing heat exhaustion or prostration
        992.4
    nephropathy 593.9
  volume 276.5
    extracellular fluid 276.5
    plasma 276.5

Deposit
  argentous, cornea 371.16
  bone, in Boeck's sarcoid 135
  calcareous, calcium — see Calcification
  cholesterol
    retina 362.82
    skin 709.3
    vitreous (humor) 379.22
  conjunctival 372.56
  cornea, corneal NEC 371.10
    argentous 371.16
    in
        cystinosis 270.0 [371.15]
        mucopolysaccharidosis 277.5 [371.15]
  crystalline, vitreous (humor) 379.22
  hemosiderin, in old scars of cornea 371.11
  metallic, in lens 366.45
  skin 709.3
  teeth, tooth (betel) (black) (green) (materia alba)
        (orange) (soft) (tobacco) 523.6
  urate, in kidney (see also Disease, renal) 593.9

Depraved appetite 307.52

Depression 311
  acute (see also Psychosis, affective) 296.2 ✓5ᵗʰ
    recurrent episode 296.3 ✓5ᵗʰ
    single episode 296.2 ✓5ᵗʰ
  agitated (see also Psychosis, affective)
        296.2 ✓5ᵗʰ
    recurrent episode 296.3 ✓5ᵗʰ
    single episode 296.2 ✓5ᵗʰ
  anaclitic 309.21
  anxiety 300.4
  arches 734
    congenital 754.61
  autogenous (see also Psychosis, affective)
        296.2 ✓5ᵗʰ
    recurrent episode 296.3 ✓5ᵗʰ
    single episode 296.2 ✓5ᵗʰ
  basal metabolic rate (BMR) 794.7
  bone marrow 289.9
  central nervous system 799.1
    newborn 779.2
  cerebral 331.9
    newborn 779.2
  cerebrovascular 437.8
    newborn 779.2
  chest wall 738.3
  endogenous (see also Psychosis, affective)
        296.2 ✓5ᵗʰ
    recurrent episode 296.3 ✓5ᵗʰ
    single episode 296.2 ✓5ᵗʰ
  functional activity 780.99   ▲
  hysterical 300.11
  involutional, climacteric, or menopausal (see
        also Psychosis, affective) 296.2 ✓5ᵗʰ
    recurrent episode 296.3 ✓5ᵗʰ
    single episode 296.2 ✓5ᵗʰ
  manic (see also Psychosis, affective) 296.80
  medullary 348.8
    newborn 779.2
  mental 300.4
  metatarsal heads — see Depression, arches
  metatarsus — see Depression, arches
  monopolar (see also Psychosis, affective)
        296.2 ✓5ᵗʰ
    recurrent episode 296.3 ✓5ᵗʰ
    single episode 296.2 ✓5ᵗʰ
  nervous 300.4

Depression — continued
  neurotic 300.4
  nose 738.0
  postpartum 648.4 ✓5ᵗʰ
  psychogenic 300.4
    reactive 298.0
  psychoneurotic 300.4
  psychotic (see also Psychosis, affective)
        296.2 ✓5ᵗʰ
    reactive 298.0
    recurrent episode 296.3 ✓5ᵗʰ
    single episode 296.2 ✓5ᵗʰ
  reactive 300.4
    neurotic 300.4
    psychogenic 298.0
    psychoneurotic 300.4
    psychotic 298.0
  recurrent 296.3 ✓5ᵗʰ
  respiratory center 348.8   ▲
    newborn 770.89
  scapula 736.89
  senile 290.21
  situational (acute) (brief) 309.0
    prolonged 309.1
  skull 754.0
  sternum 738.3
  visual field 368.40

Depressive reaction — see also Reaction,
      depressive
  acute (transient) 309.0
    with anxiety 309.28
  prolonged 309.1
  situational (acute) 309.0
    prolonged 309.1

Deprivation
  cultural V62.4
  emotional V62.89
    affecting
        adult 995.82
        infant or child 995.51
  food 994.2
    specific substance NEC 269.8
  protein (familial) (kwashiorkor) 260
  social V62.4
    affecting
        adult 995.82
        infant or child 995.51
  symptoms, syndrome
    alcohol 291.81
    drug 292.0
  vitamins (see also Deficiency, vitamin) 269.2
  water 994.3

de Quervain's
  disease (tendon sheath) 727.04
  thyroiditis (subacute granulomatous thyroiditis)
        245.1

Derangement
  ankle (internal) 718.97
    current injury (see also Dislocation, ankle)
        837.0
    recurrent 718.37
  cartilage (articular) NEC (see also Disorder,
      cartilage, articular) 718.0 ✓5ᵗʰ
    knee 717.9
      recurrent 718.36
    recurrent 718.3 ✓5ᵗʰ
  collateral ligament (knee) (medial) (tibial)
        717.82
    current injury 844.1
      lateral (fibular) 844.0
    lateral (fibular) 717.81
      current injury 844.0
  cruciate ligament (knee) (posterior) 717.84
    anterior 717.83
      current injury 844.2
    current injury 844.2
  elbow (internal) 718.92
    current injury (see also Dislocation, elbow)
        832.00
    recurrent 718.32
  gastrointestinal 536.9
  heart — see Disease, heart
  hip (joint) (internal) (old) 718.95
    current injury (see also Dislocation, hip)
        835.00
    recurrent 718.35

Derangement — continued
  intervertebral disc — see Displacement,
      intervertebral disc
  joint (internal) 718.90
    ankle 718.97
      current injury — see also Dislocation, by
          site
        knee, meniscus or cartilage (see also
            Tear, meniscus) 836.2
    elbow 718.92
    foot 718.97
    hand 718.94
    hip 718.95
    knee 717.9
    multiple sites 718.99
    pelvic region 718.95
    recurrent 718.30
      ankle 718.37
      elbow 718.32
      foot 718.37
      hand 718.34
      hip 718.35
      knee 718.36
      multiple sites 718.39
      pelvic region 718.35
      shoulder (region) 718.31
      specified site NEC 718.38
      temporomandibular (old) 524.69
      wrist 718.33
    shoulder (region) 718.91
    specified site NEC 718.98
    spine NEC 724.9
    temporomandibular 524.69
    wrist 718.93
  knee (cartilage) (internal) 717.9
    current injury (see also Tear, meniscus)
        836.2
    ligament 717.89
      capsular 717.85
      collateral — see Derangement, collateral
          ligament
      cruciate — see Derangement, cruciate
          ligament
      specified NEC 717.85
    recurrent 718.36
  low back NEC 724.9
  meniscus NEC (knee) 717.5
    current injury (see also Tear, meniscus)
        836.2
    lateral 717.40
      anterior horn 717.42
      posterior horn 717.43
      specified NEC 717.49
    medial 717.3
      anterior horn 717.1
      posterior horn 717.2
    recurrent 718.3 ✓5ᵗʰ
    site other than knee — see Disorder,
        cartilage, articular
  mental (see also Psychosis) 298.9
  rotator cuff (recurrent) (tear) 726.10
    current 840.4
  sacroiliac (old) 724.6
    current — see Dislocation, sacroiliac
  semilunar cartilage (knee) 717.5
    current injury 836.2
      lateral 836.1
      medial 836.0
    recurrent 718.3 ✓5ᵗʰ
  shoulder (internal) 718.91
    current injury (see also Dislocation,
        shoulder) 831.00
    recurrent 718.31
  spine (recurrent) NEC 724.9
    current — see Dislocation, spine
  temporomandibular (internal) (joint) (old)
        524.69
    current — see Dislocation, jaw

Dercum's disease or syndrome (adiposis
      dolorosa) 272.8

Derealization (neurotic) 300.6

Dermal — see condition

Dermaphytid — see Dermatophytosis

Dermatergosis — see Dermatitis

Dependency — Dermatergosis

Dermatitis (allergic) (contact) (occupational)
(venenata) 692.9
ab igne 692.82
acneiform 692.9
actinic (due to sun) 692.70
   acute 692.72
   chronic NEC 692.74
   other than from sun NEC 692.82
ambustionis
   due to
      burn or scald — *see* Burn, by site
      sunburn (*see also* Sunburn) 692.71
amebic 006.6
ammonia 691.0
anaphylactoid NEC 692.9
arsenical 692.4
artefacta 698.4
   psychogenic 316 *[698.4]*
asthmatic 691.8
atopic (allergic) (intrinsic) 691.8
   psychogenic 316 *[691.8]*
atrophicans 701.8
   diffusa 701.8
   maculosa 701.3
berlock, berloque 692.72
blastomycetic 116.0
blister beetle 692.89
Brucella NEC 023.9
bullosa 694.9
   striata pratensis 692.6
bullous 694.9
   mucosynechial, atrophic 694.60
      with ocular involvement 694.61
   seasonal 694.8
calorica
   due to
      burn or scald — *see* Burn, by site
      cold 692.89
      sunburn (*see also* Sunburn) 692.71
caterpillar 692.89
cercarial 120.3
combustionis
   due to
      burn or scald — *see* Burn, by site
      sunburn (*see also* Sunburn) 692.71
congelationis 991.5
contusiformis 695.2
diabetic 250.8 ☑5ᵗʰ
diaper 691.0
diphtheritica 032.85
due to
   acetone 692.2
   acids 692.4
   adhesive plaster 692.4
   alcohol (skin contact) (substances
      classifiable to 980.0-980.9) 692.4
      taken internally 693.8
   alkalis 692.4
   allergy NEC 692.9
   ammonia (household) (liquid) 692.4
   arnica 692.3
   arsenic 692.4
      taken internally 693.8
   blister beetle 692.89
   cantharides 692.3
   carbon disulphide 692.2
   caterpillar 692.89
   caustics 692.4
   cereal (ingested) 693.1
      contact with skin 692.5
   chemical(s) NEC 692.4
      internal 693.8
      irritant NEC 692.4
      taken internally 693.8
   chlorocompounds 692.2
   coffee (ingested) 693.1
      contact with skin 692.5
   cold weather 692.89
   cosmetics 692.81
   cyclohexanes 692.2
   deodorant 692.81
   detergents 692.0
   dichromate 692.4

Dermatitis — *continued*
due to — *continued*
   drugs and medicinals (correct substance
      properly administered) (internal use)
      693.0
      external (in contact with skin) 692.3
         wrong substance given or taken 976.9
            specified substance — *see* Table of
               Drugs and Chemicals
      wrong substance given or taken 977.9
         specified substance — *see* Table of
            Drugs and Chemicals
   dyes 692.89
      hair 692.89
   epidermophytosis — *see* Dermatophytosis
   esters 692.2
   external irritant NEC 692.9
      specified agent NEC 692.89
   eye shadow 692.81
   fish (ingested) 693.1
      contact with skin 692.5
   flour (ingested) 693.1
      contact with skin 692.5
   food (ingested) 693.1
      in contact with skin 692.5
   fruit (ingested) 693.1
      contact with skin 692.5
   fungicides 692.3
   furs 692.89
   glycols 692.2
   greases NEC 692.1
   hair dyes 692.89
   hot
      objects and materials — *see* Burn, by
         site
      weather or places 692.89
   hydrocarbons 692.2
   infrared rays, except from sun 692.82
      solar NEC (*see also* Dermatitis, due to,
         sun) 692.70
   ingested substance 693.9
      drugs and medicinals (*see also*
         Dermatitis, due to, drugs and
         medicinals) 693.0
      food 693.1
      specified substance NEC 693.8
   ingestion or injection of chemical 693.8
      drug (correct substance properly
         administered) 693.0
      wrong substance given or taken 977.9
         specified substance — *see* Table of
            Drugs and Chemicals
   insecticides 692.4
   internal agent 693.9
      drugs and medicinals (*see also*
         Dermatitis, due to, drugs and
         medicinals) 693.0
      food (ingested) 693.1
      in contact with skin 692.5
      specified agent NEC 693.8
   iodine 692.3
   iodoform 692.3
   irradiation 692.82
   jewelry 692.83
   keratolytics 692.3
   ketones 692.2
   lacquer tree (Rhus verniciflua) 692.6
   light NEC (*see also* Dermatitis, due to, sun)
      692.70
      other 692.82
   low temperature 692.89
   mascara 692.81
   meat (ingested) 693.1
      contact with skin 692.5
   mercury, mercurials 692.3
   metals 692.83
   milk (ingested) 693.1
      contact with skin 692.5
   Neomycin 692.3
   nylon 692.4
   oils NEC 692.1
   paint solvent 692.2
   pediculocides 692.3
   petroleum products (substances classifiable
      to 981) 692.4
   phenol 692.3

Dermatitis — *continued*
due to — *continued*
   photosensitiveness, photosensitivity (sun)
      692.72
      other light 692.82
   plants NEC 692.6
   plasters, medicated (any) 692.3
   plastic 692.4
   poison
      ivy (Rhus toxicodendron) 692.6
      oak (Rhus diversiloba) 692.6
      plant or vine 692.6
      sumac (Rhus venenata) 692.6
      vine (Rhus radicans) 692.6
   preservatives 692.89
   primrose (primula) 692.6
   primula 692.6
   radiation 692.82
      sun NEC (*see also* Dermatitis, due to,
         sun) 692.70
      tanning bed 692.82
   radioactive substance 692.82
   radium 692.82
   ragweed (Senecio jacobae) 692.6
   Rhus (diversiloba) (radicans) (toxicodendron)
      (venenata) (verniciflua) 692.6
   rubber 692.4
   scabicides 692.3
   Senecio jacobae 692.6
   solar radiation — *see* Dermatitis, due to,
      sun
   solvents (any) (substances classifiable to
      982.0-982.8) 692.2
      chlorocompound group 692.2
      cyclohexane group 692.2
      ester group 692.2
      glycol group 692.2
      hydrocarbon group 692.2
      ketone group 692.2
      paint 692.2
   specified agent NEC 692.89
   sun 692.70
      acute 692.72
      chronic NEC 692.74
      specified NEC 692.79
   sunburn (*see also* Sunburn) 692.71
   sunshine NEC (*see also* Dermatitis, due to,
      sun) 692.70
   tanning bed 692.82
   tetrachlorethylene 692.2
   toluene 692.2
   topical medications 692.3
   turpentine 692.2
   ultraviolet rays, except from sun 692.82
      sun NEC (*see also* Dermatitis, due to,
         sun) 692.82
   vaccine or vaccination (correct substance
      properly administered) 693.0
      wrong substance given or taken
         bacterial vaccine 978.8
            specified — *see* Table of Drugs and
               Chemicals
         other vaccines NEC 979.9
            specified — *see* Table of Drugs and
               Chemicals
   varicose veins (*see also* Varicose, vein,
      inflamed or infected) 454.1
   x-rays 692.82
dyshydrotic 705.81
dysmenorrheica 625.8
eczematoid NEC 692.9
   infectious 690.8
eczematous NEC 692.9
epidemica 695.89
erysipelatosa 695.81
escharotica — *see* Burn, by site
exfoliativa, exfoliative 695.89
   generalized 695.89
   infantum 695.81
   neonatorum 695.81
eyelid 373.31
   allergic 373.32
   contact 373.32
   eczematous 373.31
   herpes (zoster) 053.20
      simplex 054.41

Dermatitis — *continued*
  eyelid — *continued*
    infective 373.5
      due to
        actinomycosis 039.3 *[373.5]*
        herpes
          simplex 054.41
          zoster 053.20
        impetigo 684 *[373.5]*
        leprosy (*see also* Leprosy)
          030.0 *[373.4]*
        lupus vulgaris (tuberculous) (*see also*
          Tuberculosis) 017.0 ✓5ᵗʰ *[373.4]*
        mycotic dermatitis (*see also*
          Dermatomycosis) 111.9 *[373.5]*
        vaccinia 051.0 *[373.5]*
          postvaccination 999.0 *[373.5]*
        yaws (*see also* Yaws) 102.9 *[373.4]*
  facta, factitia 698.4
    psychogenic 316 *[698.4]*
  ficta 698.4
    psychogenic 316 *[698.4]*
  flexural 691.8
  follicularis 704.8
  friction 709.8
  fungus 111.9
    specified type NEC 111.8
  gangrenosa, gangrenous (infantum) (*see also*
    Gangrene) 785.4
  gestationis 646.8 ✓5ᵗʰ
  gonococcal 098.89
  gouty 274.89
  harvest mite 133.8
  heat 692.89
  herpetiformis (bullous) (erythematous)
    (pustular) (vesicular) 694.0
    juvenile 694.2
    senile 694.5
  hiemalis 692.89
  hypostatic, hypostatica 454.1
    with ulcer 454.2
  impetiginous 684
  infantile (acute) (chronic) (intertriginous)
    (intrinsic) (seborrheic) 690.12
  infectiosa eczematoides 690.8
  infectious (staphylococcal) (streptococcal) 686.9
    eczematoid 690.8
  infective eczematoid 690.8
  Jacquet's (diaper dermatitis) 691.0
  leptus 133.8
  lichenified NEC 692.9
  lichenoid, chronic 701.0
  lichenoides purpurica pigmentosa 709.1
  meadow 692.6
  medicamentosa (correct substance properly
    administered) (internal use) (*see also*
    Dermatitis, due to, drugs, or medicinals)
    693.0
    due to contact with skin 692.3
  mite 133.8
  multiformis 694.0
    juvenile 694.2
    senile 694.5
  napkin 691.0
  neuro 698.3
  neurotica 694.0
  nummular NEC 692.9
  osteatosis, osteatotic 706.8
  papillaris capillitii 706.1
  pellagrous 265.2
  perioral 695.3
  perstans 696.1
  photosensitivity (sun) 692.72
    other light 692.82
  pigmented purpuric lichenoid 709.1
  polymorpha dolorosa 694.0
  primary irritant 692.9
  pruriginosa 694.0
  pruritic NEC 692.9
  psoriasiform nodularis 696.2
  psychogenic 316
  purulent 686.00
  pustular contagious 051.2
  pyococcal 686.00
  pyocyaneus 686.09
  pyogenica 686.00
  radiation 692.82

Dermatitis — *continued*
  repens 696.1
  Ritter's (exfoliativa) 695.81
  Schamberg's (progressive pigmentary
    dermatosis) 709.09
  schistosome 120.3
  seasonal bullous 694.8
  seborrheic 690.10
    infantile 690.12
  sensitization NEC 692.9
  septic (*see also* Septicemia) 686.00
    gonococcal 098.89
  solar, solare NEC (*see also* Dermatitis, due to,
    sun) 692.70
  stasis 459.81
    due to
      postphlebitic syndrome 459.12 ▲
        with ulcer 459.13 ●
      varicose veins — *see* Varicose
    ulcerated or with ulcer (varicose) 454.2
  sunburn (*see also* Sunburn) 692.71
  suppurative 686.00
  traumatic NEC 709.8
  trophoneurotica 694.0
  ultraviolet, except from sun 692.82
    due to sun NEC (*see also* Dermatitis, due to,
      sun) 692.70
  varicose 454.1
    with ulcer 454.2
  vegetans 686.8
  verrucosa 117.2
  xerotic 706.8

Dermatoarthritis, lipoid 272.8 *[713.0]*

Dermatochalasia, dermatochalasis 374.87

Dermatofibroma (lenticulare) (M8832/0) — *see*
  also Neoplasm, skin, benign
  protuberans (M8832/1) — *see* Neoplasm, skin,
    uncertain behavior

Dermatofibrosarcoma (protuberans) (M8832/3)
  — *see* Neoplasm, skin, malignant

Dermatographia 708.3

Dermatolysis (congenital) (exfoliativa) 757.39
  acquired 701.8
  eyelids 374.34
  palpebrarum 374.34
  senile 701.8

Dermatomegaly NEC 701.8

Dermatomucomyositis 710.3

Dermatomycosis 111.9
  furfuracea 111.0
  specified type NEC 111.8

Dermatomyositis (acute) (chronic) 710.3

Dermatoneuritis of children 985.0

Dermatophiliasis 134.1

Dermatophytide — *see* Dermatophytosis

Dermatophytosis (Epidermophyton) (infection)
  (microsporum) (tinea) (Trichophyton) 110.9
  beard 110.0
  body 110.5
  deep seated 110.6
  fingernails 110.1
  foot 110.4
  groin 110.3
  hand 110.2
  nail 110.1
  perianal (area) 110.3
  scalp 110.0
  scrotal 110.8
  specified site NEC 110.8
  toenails 110.1
  vulva 110.8

Dermatopolyneuritis 985.0

Dermatorrhexis 756.83
  acquired 701.8

Dermatosclerosis (*see also* Scleroderma) 710.1
  localized 701.0

Dermatosis 709.9
  Andrews' 686.8
  atopic 691.8
  Bowen's (M8081/2) — *see* Neoplasm, skin, in
    situ
  bullous 694.9
    specified type NEC 694.8
  erythematosquamous 690.8

Dermatosis — *continued*
  exfoliativa 695.89
  factitial 698.4
  gonococcal 098.89
  herpetiformis 694.0
    juvenile 694.2
    senile 694.5
  hysterical 300.11
  Linear IgA 694.8   ●
  menstrual NEC 709.8
  neutrophilic, acute febrile 695.89
  occupational (*see also* Dermatitis) 692.9
  papulosa nigra 709.8
  pigmentary NEC 709.00
    progressive 709.09
    Schamberg's 709.09
    Siemens-Bloch 757.33
  progressive pigmentary 709.09
  psychogenic 316
  pustular subcorneal 694.1
  Schamberg's (progressive pigmentary) 709.09
  senile NEC 709.3
  Unna's (seborrheic dermatitis) 690.10

Dermographia 708.3

Dermographism 708.3

Dermoid (cyst) (M9084/0) — *see also* Neoplasm,
  by site, benign
  with malignant transformation (M9084/3)
    183.0

Dermopathy
  infiltrative, with throtoxicosis 242.0 ✓5ᵗʰ
  senile NEC 709.3

Dermophytosis — *see* Dermatophytosis

Descemet's membrane — *see* condition

Descemetocele 371.72

Descending — *see* condition

Descensus uteri (complete) (incomplete) (partial)
  (without vaginal wall prolapse) 618.1
  with mention of vaginal wall proplapse — *see*
    Prolapse, uterovaginal

Desensitization to allergens V07.1

Desert
  rheumatism 114.0
  sore (*see also* Ulcer, skin) 707.9

Desertion (child) (newborn) 995.52
  adult 995.84

Desmoid (extra-abdominal) (tumor) (M8821/1) —
  see also Neoplasm, connective tissue,
  uncertain behavior
  abdominal (M8822/1) — *see* Neoplasm,
    connective tissue, uncertain behavior

Despondency 300.4

Desquamative dermatitis NEC 695.89

Destruction
  articular facet (*see also* Derangement, joint)
    718.9 ✓5ᵗʰ
    vertebra 724.9
  bone 733.90
    syphilitic 095.5
  joint (*see also* Derangement, joint) 718.9 ✓5ᵗʰ
    sacroiliac 724.6
  kidney 593.89
  live fetus to facilitate birth NEC 763.89
  ossicles (ear) 385.24
  rectal sphincter 569.49
  septum (nasal) 478.1
  tuberculous NEC (*see also* Tuberculosis)
    011.9 ✓5ᵗʰ
  tympanic membrane 384.82
  tympanum 385.89
  vertebral disc — *see* Degeneration,
    intervertebral disc

Destructiveness (*see also* Disturbance, conduct)
  312.9
  adjustment reaction 309.3

Detachment
  cartilage — *see also* Sprain, by site
    knee — *see* Tear, meniscus
  cervix, annular 622.8
    complicating delivery 665.3 ✓5ᵗʰ
  choroid (old) (postinfectional) (simple)
    (spontaneous) 363.70
    hemorrhagic 363.72

Side tab: **Dermatitis — Detachment**

✓4ᵗʰ Fourth-digit Required   ✓5ᵗʰ Fifth-digit Required   ▶◀ Revised Text   ● New Line   ▲ Revised Code

Detachment — *continued*
  choroid — *continued*
    serous 363.71
  knee, medial meniscus (old) 717.3
    current injury 836.0
  ligament — *see* Sprain, by site
  placenta (premature) — *see* Placenta,
      separation
  retina (recent) 361.9
    with retinal defect (rhegmatogenous) 361.00
      giant tear 361.03
      multiple 361.02
      partial
        with
          giant tear 361.03
          multiple defects 361.02
          retinal dialysis (juvenile) 361.04
          single defect 361.01
        retinal dialysis (juvenile) 361.04
        single 361.01
      subtotal 361.05
      total 361.05
    delimited (old) (partial) 361.06
    old
      delimited 361.06
      partial 361.06
      total or subtotal 361.07
    pigment epithelium (RPE) (serous) 362.42
      exudative 362.42
      hemorrhagic 362.43
    rhegmatogenous (*see also* Detachment,
        retina, with retinal defect) 361.00
    serous (without retinal defect) 361.2
    specified type NEC 361.89
    traction (with vitreoretinal organization)
        361.81
  vitreous humor 379.21
Detergent asthma 507.8
Deterioration
  epileptic
    with behavioral disturbance 345.9 [294.11]
    without behavioral disturbance
        345.9 [294.10]
  heart, cardiac (*see also* Degeneration,
      myocardial) 429.1
  mental (*see also* Psychosis) 298.9
  myocardium, myocardial (*see also*
      Degeneration, myocardial) 429.1
  senile (simple) 797
  transplanted organ — *see* Complications,
      transplant, organ, by site
de Toni-Fanconi syndrome (cystinosis) 270.0
Deuteranomaly 368.52
Deuteranopia (anomalous trichromat) (complete)
    (incomplete) 368.52
Deutschländer's disease — *see* Fracture, foot
Development
  abnormal, bone 756.9
  arrested 783.40
    bone 733.91
    child 783.40
    due to malnutrition (protein-calorie) 263.2
    fetus or newborn 764.9 ✓5ᵗʰ
    tracheal rings (congenital) 748.3
  defective, congenital — *see also* Anomaly
    cauda equina 742.59
    left ventricle 746.9
      with atresia or hypoplasia of aortic orifice
          or valve with hypoplasia of
          ascending aorta 746.7
      in hypoplastic left heart syndrome 746.7
  delayed (*see also* Delay, development) 783.40
    arithmetical skills 315.1
    language (skills) 315.31
      expressive 315.31
      mixed receptive-expressive 315.32
    learning skill, specified NEC 315.2
    mixed skills 315.5
    motor coordination 315.4
    reading 315.00
    specified
      learning skill NEC 315.2
      type NEC, except learning 315.8
    speech 315.39
      associated with hyperkinesia 314.1
      phonological 315.39

Development — *continued*
  delayed (*see also* Delay, development) —
      continued
    spelling 315.09
  imperfect, congenital — *see also* Anomaly
    heart 746.9
    lungs 748.60
  improper (fetus or newborn) 764.9 ✓5ᵗʰ
  incomplete (fetus or newborn) 764.9 ✓5ᵗʰ
    affecting management of pregnancy
        656.5 ✓5ᵗʰ
    bronchial tree 748.3
    organ or site not listed — *see* Hypoplasia
    respiratory system 748.9
  sexual, precocious NEC 259.1
  tardy, mental (*see also* Retardation, mental)
      319
  written expression 315.2
Developmental — *see* condition
Devergie's disease (pityriasis rubra pilaris) 696.4
Deviation
  conjugate (eye) 378.87
    palsy 378.81
    spasm, spastic 378.82
  esophagus 530.89
  eye, skew 378.87
  midline (jaw) (teeth) 524.2
    specified site NEC — *see* Malposition
  organ or site, congenital NEC — *see*
      Malposition, congenital
  septum (acquired) (nasal) 470
    congenital 754.0
  sexual 302.9
    bestiality 302.9
    coprophilia 302.89
    ego-dystonic
      homosexuality 302.0
      lesbianism 302.0
    erotomania 302.89
      Clérambault's 297.8
    exhibitionism (sexual) 302.4
    fetishism 302.81
      transvestic 302.3
    frotteurism 302.89
    homosexuality, ego-dystonic 302.0
      pedophilic 302.2
    lesbianism, ego-dystonic 302.0
    masochism 302.83
    narcissism 302.89
    necrophilia 302.89
    nymphomania 302.89
    pederosis 302.2
    pedophilia 302.2
    sadism 302.84
    sadomasochism 302.84
    satyriasis 302.89
    specified type NEC 302.89
    transvestic fetishism 302.3
    transvestism 302.3
    voyeurism 302.82
    zoophilia (erotica) 302.1
  teeth, midline 524.2
  trachea 519.1
  ureter (congenital) 753.4
Devic's disease 341.0
Device
  cerebral ventricle (communicating) in situ
      V45.2
  contraceptive — *see* Contraceptive, device
  drainage, cerebrospinal fluid V45.2
Devil's
  grip 074.1
  pinches (purpura simplex) 287.2
Devitalized tooth 522.9
Devonshire colic 984.9
  specified type of lead — *see* Table of Drugs and
      Chemicals
Dextraposition, aorta 747.21
  with ventricular septal defect, pulmonary
      stenosis or atresia, and hypertrophy of
      right ventricle 745.2
  in tetralogy of Fallot 745.2
Dextratransposition, aorta 745.11
Dextrinosis, limit (debrancher enzyme deficiency)
    271.0

Dextrocardia (corrected) (false) (isolated)
    (secondary) (true) 746.87
  with
    complete transposition of viscera 759.3
    situs inversus 759.3
Dextroversion, kidney (left) 753.3
Dhobie itch 110.3
Diabetes, diabetic (brittle) (congenital) (familial)
    (mellitus) (severe) (slight) (without
    complication) 250.0 ✓5ᵗʰ

> *Note* — *Use the following fifth-digit*
> *subclassification with category 250:*
>
> 0   *type II [non-insulin dependent type]*
>   *[NIDDM type] [adult-onset type] or*
>   *unspecified type, not stated as*
>   *uncontrolled*
>
> 1   *type I [insulin dependent type]*
>   *[IDDM type] [juvenile type], not*
>   *stated as uncontrolled*
>
> 2   *type II [non-insulin dependent type]*
>   *[NIDDM type] [adult-onset type] or*
>   *unspecified type, uncontrolled*
>
> 3   *type I [insulin dependent type]*
>   *[IDDM] [juvenile type], uncontrolled*

  with
    coma (with ketoacidosis) 250.3 ✓5ᵗʰ
      hyperosmolar (nonketotic) 250.2 ✓5ᵗʰ
    complication NEC 250.9 ✓5ᵗʰ
      specified NEC 250.8 ✓5ᵗʰ
    gangrene 250.7 ✓5ᵗʰ [785.4]
    hyperosmolarity 250.2 ✓5ᵗʰ
    ketosis, ketoacidosis 250.1 ✓5ᵗʰ
    osteomyelitis 250.8 ✓5ᵗʰ [731.8]
    specified manisfestations NEC 250.8 ✓5ᵗʰ
  acetonemia 250.1 ✓5ᵗʰ
  acidosis 250.1 ✓5ᵗʰ
  amyotrophy 250.6 ✓5ᵗʰ [358.1]
  angiopathy, peripheral 250.7 ✓5ᵗʰ [443.81]
  asymptomatic 790.2
  autonomic neuropathy (peripheral)
      250.6 ✓5ᵗʰ [337.1]
  bone change 250.8 ✓5ᵗʰ [731.8]
  bronze, bronzed 275.0
  cataract 250.5 ✓5ᵗʰ [366.41]
  chemical 790.2
    complicating pregnancy, childbirth, or
        puerperium 648.8 ✓5ᵗʰ
  coma (with ketoacidosis) 250.3 ✓5ᵗʰ
    hyperglycemic 250.3 ✓5ᵗʰ
    hyperosmolar (nonketotic) 250.2 ✓5ᵗʰ
    hypoglycemic 250.3 ✓5ᵗʰ
    insulin 250.3 ✓5ᵗʰ
  complicating pregnancy, childbirth, or
      puerperium (maternal) 648.0 ✓5ᵗʰ
    affecting fetus or newborn 775.0
  complication NEC 250.9 ✓5ᵗʰ
    specified NEC 250.8 ✓5ᵗʰ
  dorsal sclerosis 250.6 ✓5ᵗʰ [340] ✓5ᵗʰ
  dwarfism-obesity syndrome 258.1
  gangrene 250.7 ✓5ᵗʰ [785.4]
  gastroparesis 250.6 ✓5ᵗʰ [536.3]
  gestational 648.8 ✓5ᵗʰ
    complicating pregnancy, childbirth, or
        puerperium 648.8 ✓5ᵗʰ
  glaucoma 250.5 ✓5ᵗʰ [365.44]
  glomerulosclerosis (intercapillary)
      250.4 ✓5ᵗʰ [581.81]
  glycogenosis, secondary 250.8 ✓5ᵗʰ [259.8]
  hemochromatosis 275.0
  hyperosmolar coma 250.2 ✓5ᵗʰ
  hyperosmolarity 250.2 ✓5ᵗʰ
  hypertension-nephrosis syndrome
      250.4 ✓5ᵗʰ [581.81]
  hypoglycemia 250.8 ✓5ᵗʰ
  hypoglycemic shock 250.8 ✓5ᵗʰ
  insipidus 253.5
    nephrogenic 588.1
    pituitary 253.5
    vasopressin-resistant 588.1
  intercapillary glomerulosclerosis
      250.4 ✓5ᵗʰ [581.81]
  iritis 250.5 ✓5ᵗʰ [364.42]
  ketosis, ketoacidosis 250.1 ✓5ᵗʰ

Detachment — Diabetes

Diabetes — Difficulty (side tab)

Diabetes, diabetic — *continued*
    Kimmelstiel (-Wilson) disease or syndrome
        (intercapillary glomerulosclerosis)
        250.4 ✓5ᵗʰ [581.81]
    Lancereaux's (diabetes mellitus with marked
        emaciation) 250.8 ✓5ᵗʰ [261]
    latent (chemical) 790.2
        complicating pregnancy, childbirth, or
            puerperium 648. ✓5ᵗʰ
    lipoidosis 250.8 ✓5ᵗʰ [272.7]
    macular edema 250.5 ✓5ᵗʰ [362.01]
    maternal
        with manifest disease in the infant 775.1
        affecting fetus or newborn 775.0
    microaneurysms, retinal 250.5 ✓5ᵗʰ [362.01]
    mononeuropathy 250.6 ✓5ᵗʰ [355.9]
    neonatal, transient 775.1
    nephropathy 250.4 ✓5ᵗʰ [583.81]
    nephrosis (syndrome) 250.4 ✓5ᵗʰ [581.81]
    neuralgia 250.6 ✓5ᵗʰ [357.2]
    neuritis 250.6 ✓5ᵗʰ [357.2]
    neurogenic arthropathy 250.6 ✓5ᵗʰ [713.5]
    neuropathy 250.6 ✓5ᵗʰ [357.2]
    nonclinical 790.2
    osteomyelitis 250.8 ✓5ᵗʰ [731.8]
    peripheral autonomic neuropathy
        250.6 ✓5ᵗʰ [337.1]
    phosphate 275.3
    polyneuropathy 250.6 ✓5ᵗʰ [357.2]
    renal (true) 271.4
    retinal
        edema 250.5 ✓5ᵗʰ [362.01]
        hemorrhage 250.5 ✓5ᵗʰ [362.01]
        microaneurysms 250.5 ✓5ᵗʰ [362.01]
    retinitis 250.5 ✓5ᵗʰ [362.01]
    retinopathy 250.5 ✓5ᵗʰ [362.01]
        background 250.5 ✓5ᵗʰ [362.01]
        proliferative 250.5 ✓5ᵗʰ [362.02]
    steroid induced
        correct substance properly administered
            251.8
        overdose or wrong substance given or taken
            962.0
    stress 790.2
    subclinical 790.2
    subliminal 790.2
    sugar 250.0 ✓5ᵗʰ
    ulcer (skin) 250.8 ✓5ᵗʰ [707.9]
        lower extremity 250.8 ✓5ᵗʰ [707.10]
            ankle 250.8 [707.13]
            calf 250.8 [707.12]
            foot 250.8 [707.15]
            heel 250.8 [707.14]
            knee 250.8 [707.19]
            specified site NEC 250.8 [707.19]
            thigh 250.8 [707.11]
            toes 250.8 [707.15]
        specified site NEC 250.8 ✓5ᵗʰ [707.8]
    xanthoma 250.8 ✓5ᵗʰ [272.2]
Diacyclothrombopathia 287.1
Diagnosis deferred 799.9
Dialysis (intermittent) (treatment)
    anterior retinal (juvenile) (with detachment)
        361.04
    extracorporeal V56.0
    peritoneal V56.8
    renal V56.0
        status only V45.1
    specified type NEC V56.8
Diamond-Blackfan anemia or syndrome
    (congenital hypoplastic anemia) 284.0
Diamond-Gardener syndrome (autoerythrocyte
    sensitization) 287.2
Diaper rash 691.0
Diaphoresis (excessive) NEC 780.8
Diaphragm — *see* condition
Diaphragmalgia 786.52
Diaphragmitis 519.4
Diaphyseal aclasis 756.4
Diaphysitis 733.99

Diarrhea, diarrheal (acute) (autumn) (bilious)
    (bloody) (catarrhal) (choleraic) (chronic)
    (gravis) (green) (infantile) (lienteric)
    (noninfectious) (presumed noninfectious)
    (putrefactive) (secondary) (sporadic)
    (summer) (symptomatic) (thermic) 787.91
    achlorhydric 536.0
    allergic 558.3
    amebic (*see also* Amebiasis) 006.9
        with abscess — *see* Abscess, amebic
        acute 006.0
        chronic 006.1
        nondysenteric 006.2
    bacillary — *see* Dysentery, bacillary
    bacterial NEC 008.5
    balantidial — 007.0
    bile salt-induced 579.8
    cachectic NEC 787.91
    chilomastix 007.8
    choleriformis 001.1
    coccidial 007.2
    Cochin-China 579.1
        anguilluliasis 127.2
        psilosis 579.1
    Dientamoeba 007.8
    dietetic 787.91
    due to
        achylia gastrica 536.8
        Aerobacter aerogenes 008.2 ✓5ᵗʰ
        Bacillus coli — *see* Enteritis, E. coli
        bacteria NEC 008.5
        bile salts 579.8
        Capillaria
            hepatica 128.8
            philippinensis 127.5
        Clostridium perfringens (C) (F) 008.46
        Enterobacter aerogenes 008.2 ✓5ᵗʰ
        enterococci 008.49
        Escherichia coli — *see* Enteritis, E. coli
        Giardia lamblia 007.1
        Heterophyes heterophyes 121.6
        irritating foods 787.91
        Metagonimus yokogawai 121.5
        Necator americanus 126.1
        Paracolobactrum arizonae 008.1
        Paracolon bacillus NEC 008.47
            Arizona 008.1
        Proteus (bacillus) (mirabilis) (Morganii) 008.3
        Pseudomonas aeruginosa 008.42
        S. japonicum 120.2
        specified organism NEC 008.8
            bacterial 008.49
            viral NEC 008.69
        Staphylococcus 008.41
        Streptococcus 008.49
            anaerobic 008.46
        Strongyloides stercoralis 127.2
        Trichuris trichiuria 127.3
        virus NEC (*see also* Enteritis, viral) 008.69
    dysenteric 009.2
        due to specified organism NEC 008.8
    dyspeptic 787.91
    endemic 009.3
        due to specified organism NEC 008.8
    epidemic 009.2
        due to specified organism NEC 008.8
    fermentative 787.91
    flagellate 007.9
    Flexner's (ulcerative) 004.1
    functional 564.5
        following gastrointestinal surgery 564.4
        psychogenic 306.4
    giardial 007.1
    Giardia lamblia 007.1
    hill 579.1
    hyperperistalsis (nervous) 306.4
    infectious 009.2
        due to specified organism NEC 008.8
        presumed 009.3
    inflammatory 787.91
        due to specified organism NEC 008.8
    malarial (*see also* Malaria) 084.6
    mite 133.8
    mycotic 117.9
    nervous 306.4
    neurogenic 564.5
    parenteral NEC 009.2

Diarrhea, diarrheal — *continued*
    postgastrectomy 564.4
    postvagotomy 564.4
    prostaglandin induced 579.8
    protozoal NEC 007.9
    psychogenic 306.4
    septic 009.2
        due to specified organism NEC 008.8
        specified organism NEC 008.8
            bacterial 008.49
            viral NEC 008.69
        Staphylococcus 008.41
        Streptococcus 008.49
            anaerobic 008.46
    toxic 558.2
    travelers' 009.2
        due to specified organism NEC 008.8
    trichomonal 007.3
    tropical 579.1
    tuberculous 014.8 ✓5ᵗʰ
    ulcerative (chronic) (*see also* Colitis, ulcerative)
        556.9
    viral (*see also* Enteritis, viral) 008.8
    zymotic NEC 009.2
Diastasis
    cranial bones 733.99
        congenital 756.0
    joint (traumatic) — *see* Dislocation, by site
    muscle 728.84
        congenital 756.89
    recti (abdomen) 728.84
        complicating delivery 665.8 ✓5ᵗʰ
        congenital 756.79
Diastema, teeth, tooth 524.3
Diastematomyelia 742.51
Diataxia, cerebral, infantile 343.0
Diathesis
    allergic V15.09
    bleeding (familial) 287.9
    cystine (familial) 270.0
    gouty 274.9
    hemorrhagic (familial) 287.9
        newborn NEC 776.0
    oxalic 271.8
    scrofulous (*see also* Tuberculosis) 017.2 ✓5ᵗʰ
    spasmophilic (*see also* Tetany) 781.7
    ulcer 536.9
    uric acid 274.9
Diaz's disease or osteochondrosis 732.5
Dibothriocephaliasis 123.4
    larval 123.5
Dibothriocephalus (infection) (infestation) (latus)
    123.4
    larval 123.5
Dicephalus 759.4
Dichotomy, teeth 520.2
Dichromat, dichromata (congenital) 368.59
Dichromatopsia (congenital) 368.59
Dichuchwa 104.0
Dicroceliasis 121.8
Didelphys, didelphic (*see also* Double uterus)
    752.2
Didymitis (*see also* Epididymitis) 604.90
Died — *see also* Death
    without
        medical attention (cause unknown) 798.9
        sign of disease 798.2
Dientamoeba diarrhea 007.8
Dietary
    inadequacy or deficiency 269.9
    surveillance and counseling V65.3
Dietl's crisis 593.4
Dieulafoy ►lesion (hemorrhagic)◄
    of   ●
        duodenum 537.84   ●
        intestine 569.86   ●
        stomach 537.84   ●
Difficult
    birth, affecting fetus or newborn 763.9
    delivery NEC 669.9 ✓5ᵗʰ
Difficulty
    feeding 783.3
        breast 676.8 ✓5ᵗʰ

Difficulty — *continued*
  feeding — *continued*
    newborn 779.3
    nonorganic (infant) NEC 307.59
  mechanical, gastroduodenal stoma 537.89
  reading 315.00
  specific, spelling 315.09
  swallowing (*see also* Dysphagia) 787.2
  walking 719.7 ✔5ᵗʰ
Diffuse — *see* condition
Diffused ganglion 727.42
DiGeorge's syndrome (thymic hypoplasia) 279.11
Digestive — *see* condition
Di Guglielmo's disease or syndrome (M9841/3) 207.0 ✔5ᵗʰ
Diktyoma (M9051/3) — *see* Neoplasm, by site, malignant
Dilaceration, tooth 520.4
Dilatation
  anus 564.89
    venule — *see* Hemorrhoids
  aorta (focal) (general) (*see also* Aneurysm, aorta) 441.9
    congenital 747.29
    infectional 093.0
    ruptured 441.5
    syphilitic 093.0
  appendix (cystic) 543.9
  artery 447.8
  bile duct (common) (cystic) (congenital) 751.69
    acquired 576.8
  bladder (sphincter) 596.8
    congenital 753.8
    in pregnancy or childbirth 654.4 ✔5ᵗʰ
      causing obstructed labor 660.2 ✔5ᵗʰ
        affecting fetus or newborn 763.1
  blood vessel 459.89
  bronchus, bronchi 494.0
    with acute exacerbation 494.1
  calyx (due to obstruction) 593.89
  capillaries 448.9
  cardiac (acute) (chronic) (*see also* Hypertrophy, cardiac) 429.3
    congenital 746.89
    valve NEC 746.89
      pulmonary 746.09
    hypertensive (*see also* Hypertension, heart) 402.90
  cavum septi pellucidi 742.4
  cecum 564.89
    psychogenic 306.4
  cervix (uteri) — *see also* Incompetency, cervix
    incomplete, poor, slow
      affecting fetus or newborn 763.7
      complicating delivery 661.0 ✔5ᵗʰ
        affecting fetus or newborn 763.7
  colon 564.7
    congenital 751.3
    due to mechanical obstruction 560.89
    psychogenic 306.4
  common bile duct (congenital) 751.69
    acquired 576.8
      with calculus, choledocholithiasis, or stones — *see* Choledocholithiasis
  cystic duct 751.69
    acquired (any bile duct) 575.8
  duct, mammary 610.4
  duodenum 564.89
  esophagus 530.89
    congenital 750.4
    due to
      achalasia 530.0
      cardiospasm 530.0
  Eustachian tube, congenital 744.24
  fontanel 756.0
  gallbladder 575.8
    congenital 751.69
  gastric 536.8
    acute 536.1
    psychogenic 306.4
  heart (acute) (chronic) (*see also* Hypertrophy, cardiac) 429.3
    congenital 746.89
    hypertensive (*see also* Hypertension, heart) 402.90

Dilatation — *continued*
  heart (*see also* Hypertrophy, cardiac) — *continued*
    valve — *see also* Endocarditis
      congenital 746.89
  ileum 564.89
    psychogenic 306.4
  inguinal rings — *see* Hernia, inguinal
  jejunum 564.89
    psychogenic 306.4
  kidney (calyx) (collecting structures) (cystic) (parenchyma) (pelvis) 593.89
  lacrimal passages 375.69
  lymphatic vessel 457.1
  mammary duct 610.4
  Meckel's diverticulum (congenital) 751.0
  meningeal vessels, congenital 742.8
  myocardium (acute) (chronic) (*see also* Hypertrophy, cardiac) 429.3
  organ or site, congenital NEC — *see* Distortion
  pancreatic duct 577.8
  pelvis, kidney 593.89
  pericardium — *see* Pericarditis
  pharynx 478.29
  prostate 602.8
  pulmonary
    artery (idiopathic) 417.8
      congenital 747.3
    valve, congenital 746.09
  pupil 379.43
  rectum 564.89
  renal 593.89
  saccule vestibularis, congenital 744.05
  salivary gland (duct) 527.8
  sphincter ani 564.89
  stomach 536.8
    acute 536.1
    psychogenic 306.4
  submaxillary duct 527.8
  trachea, congenital 748.3
  ureter (idiopathic) 593.89
    congenital 753.20
    due to obstruction 593.5
  urethra (acquired) 599.84
  vasomotor 443.9
  vein 459.89
  ventricular, ventricle (acute) (chronic) (*see also* Hypertrophy, cardiac) 429.3
    cerebral, congenital 742.4
    hypertensive (*see also* Hypertension, heart) 402.90
  venule 459.89
    anus — *see* Hemorrhoids
  vesical orifice 596.8
Dilated, dilation — *see* Dilatation
Diminished
  hearing (acuity) (*see also* Deafness) 389.9
  pulse pressure 785.9
  vision NEC 369.9
  vital capacity 794.2
Diminuta taenia 123.6
Diminution, sense or sensation (cold) (heat) (tactile) (vibratory) (*see also* Disturbance, sensation) 782.0
Dimitri-Sturge-Weber disease (encephalocutaneous angiomatosis) 759.6
Dimple
  parasacral 685.1
    with abscess 685.0
  pilonidal 685.1
    with abscess 685.0
  postanal 685.1
    with abscess 685.0
Dioctophyma renale (infection) (infestation) 128.8
Dipetalonemiasis 125.4
Diphallus 752.69
Diphtheria, diphtheritic (gangrenous) (hemorrhagic) 032.9
  carrier (suspected) of V02.4
  cutaneous 032.85
  cystitis 032.84
  faucial 032.0
  infection of wound 032.85
  inoculation (anti) (not sick) V03.5
  laryngeal 032.3
  myocarditis 032.82

Diphtheria, diphtheritic — *continued*
  nasal anterior 032.2
  nasopharyngeal 032.1
  neurological complication 032.89
  peritonitis 032.83
  specified site NEC 032.89
Diphyllobothriasis (intestine) 123.4
  larval 123.5
Diplacusis 388.41
Diplegia (upper limbs) 344.2
  brain or cerebral 437.8
  congenital 343.0
  facial 351.0
    congenital 352.6
  infantile or congenital (cerebral) (spastic) (spinal) 343.0
  lower limbs 344.1
  syphilitic, congenital 090.49
Diplococcus, diplococcal — *see* condition
Diplomyelia 742.59
Diplopia 368.2
  refractive 368.15
Dipsomania (*see also* Alcoholism) 303.9 ✔5ᵗʰ
  with psychosis (*see also* Psychosis, alcoholic) 291.9
Dipylidiasis 123.8
  intestine 123.8
Direction, teeth, abnormal 524.3
Dirt-eating child 307.52
Disability
  heart — *see* Disease, heart
  learning NEC 315.2
  special spelling 315.09
Disarticulation (*see also* Derangement, joint) 718.9 ✔5ᵗʰ
  meaning
    amputation
      status — *see* Absence, by site
      traumatic — *see* Amputation, traumatic
    dislocation, traumatic or congenital — *see* Dislocation
Disaster, cerebrovascular (*see also* Disease, cerebrovascular, acute) 436
Discharge
  anal NEC 787.99
  breast (female) (male) 611.79
  conjunctiva 372.89
  continued locomotor idiopathic (*see also* Epilepsy) 345.5 ✔5ᵗʰ
  diencephalic autonomic idiopathic (*see also* Epilepsy) 345.5 ✔5ᵗʰ
  ear 388.60
    blood 388.69
    cerebrospinal fluid 388.61
  excessive urine 788.42
  eye 379.93
  nasal 478.1
  nipple 611.79
  patterned motor idiopathic (*see also* Epilepsy) 345.5 ✔5ᵗʰ
  penile 788.7
  postnasal — *see* Sinusitis
  sinus, from mediastinum 510.0
  umbilicus 789.9
  urethral 788.7
    bloody 599.84
  vaginal 623.5
Discitis 722.90
  cervical, cervicothoracic 722.91
  lumbar, lumbosacral 722.93
  thoracic, thoracolumbar 722.92
Discogenic syndrome — *see* Displacement, intervertebral disc
Discoid
  kidney 753.3
  meniscus, congenital 717.5
  semilunar cartilage 717.5
Discoloration
  mouth 528.9
  nails 703.8
  teeth 521.7
    due to
      drugs 521.7

Discoloration — *continued*
teeth — *continued*
  due to — *continued*
    metals (copper) (silver) 521.7
    pulpal bleeding 521.7
  during formation 520.8
  posteruptive 521.7

Discomfort
chest 786.59
visual 368.13

Discomycosis — *see* Actinomycosis

Discontinuity, ossicles, ossicular chain 385.23

Discrepancy
leg length (acquired) 736.81
  congenital 755.30
uterine size-date 646.8 ✓5ᵗʰ

Discrimination
political V62.4
racial V62.4
religious V62.4
sex V62.4

Disease, diseased — *see also* Syndrome
Abrami's (acquired hemolytic jaundice) 283.9
absorbent system 459.89
accumulation — *see* Thesaurismosis
acid-peptic 536.8
Acosta's 993.2
Adams-Stokes (-Morgagni) (syncope with heart
  block) 426.9
Addison's (bronze) (primary adrenal
  insufficiency) 255.4
  anemia (pernicious) 281.0
  tuberculous (*see also* Tuberculosis)
    017.6 ✓5ᵗʰ
Addison-Gull — *see* Xanthoma
adenoids (and tonsils) (chronic) 474.9
adrenal (gland) (capsule) (cortex) 255.9
  hyperfunction 255.3
  hypofunction 255.4
  specified type NEC 255.8
ainhum (dactylolysis spontanea) 136.0
akamushi (scrub typhus) 081.2
Akureyri (epidemic neuromyasthenia) 049.8
Albarrán's (colibacilluria) 791.9
Albers-Schönberg's (marble bones) 756.52
Albert's 726.71
Albright (-Martin) (-Bantam) 275.49
Alibert's (mycosis fungoides) (M9700/3)
  202.1 ✓5ᵗʰ
Alibert-Bazin (M9700/3) 202.1 ✓5ᵗʰ
alimentary canal 569.9
alligator skin (ichthyosis congenita) 757.1
  acquired 701.1
Almeida's (Brazilian blastomycosis) 116.1
Alpers' 330.8
alpine 993.2
altitude 993.2
alveoli, teeth 525.9
Alzheimer's — *see* Alzheimer's
amyloid (any site) 277.3
anarthritic rheumatoid 446.5
Anders' (adiposis tuberosa simplex) 272.8
Andersen's (glycogenosis IV) 271.0
Anderson's (angiokeratoma corporis diffusum)
  272.7
Andes 993.2
Andrews' (bacterid) 686.8
angiospastic, angiospasmodic 443.9
  cerebral 435.9
    with transient neurologic deficit 435.9
  vein 459.89
anterior
  chamber 364.9
  horn cell 335.9
    specified type NEC 335.8
antral (chronic) 473.0
  acute 461.0
anus NEC 569.49
aorta (nonsyphilitic) 447.9
  syphilitic NEC 093.89
aortic (heart) (valve) (*see also* Endocarditis,
  aortic) 424.1
apollo 077.4
aponeurosis 726.90
appendix 543.9
aqueous (chamber) 364.9

Disease, diseased — *see also* Syndrome —
continued
arc-welders' lung 503
Armenian 277.3
Arnold-Chiari (*see also* Spina bifida) 741.0 ✓5ᵗʰ
arterial 447.9
  occlusive (*see also* Occlusion, by site)
    444.22
    with embolus or thrombus — *see*
      Occlusion, by site
    due to stricture or stenosis 447.1
  specified type NEC 447.8
arteriocardiorenal (*see also* Hypertension,
  cardiorenal) 404.90
arteriolar (generalized) (obliterative) 447.9
  specified type NEC 447.8
arteriorenal — *see* Hypertension, kidney
arteriosclerotic — *see also* Arteriosclerosis
  cardiovascular 429.2
  coronary — *see* Arteriosclerosis, coronary
  heart — *see* Arteriosclerosis, coronary
  vascular — *see* Arteriosclerosis
artery 447.9
  cerebral 437.9
  coronary — *see* Arteriosclerosis, coronary
  specified type NEC 447.8
arthropod-borne NEC 088.9
  specified type NEC 088.89
Asboe-Hansen's (incontinentia pigmenti) 757.33
atticoantral, chronic (with posterior or superior
  marginal perforation of ear drum) 382.2
auditory canal, ear 380.9
Aujeszky's 078.89
auricle, ear NEC 380.30
Australian X 062.4
autoimmune NEC 279.4
  hemolytic (cold type) (warm type) 283.0
  parathyroid 252.1
  thyroid 245.2
aviators' (*see also* Effect, adverse, high altitude)
  993.2
ax(e)-grinders' 502
Ayala's 756.89
Ayerza's (pulmonary artery sclerosis with
  pulmonary hypertension) 416.0
Azorean (of the nervous system) 334.8
Babington's (familial hemorrhagic
  telangiectasia) 448.0
back bone NEC 733.90
bacterial NEC 040.89
  zoonotic NEC 027.9
    specified type NEC 027.8
Baehr-Schiffrin (thrombotic thrombocytopenic
  purpura) 446.6
Baelz's (cheilitis glandularis apostematosa)
  528.5
Baerensprung's (eczema marginatum) 110.3
Balfour's (chloroma) 205.3 ✓5ᵗʰ
balloon (*see also* Effect, adverse, high altitude)
  993.2
Baló's 341.1
Bamberger (-Marie) (hypertrophic pulmonary
  osteoarthropathy) 731.2
Bang's (Brucella abortus) 023.1
Bannister's 995.1
Banti's (with cirrhosis) (with portal
  hypertension) — *see* Cirrhosis, liver
Barcoo (*see also* Ulcer, skin) 707.9
barium lung 503
Barlow (-Möller) (infantile scurvy) 267
barometer makers' 985.0
Barraquer (-Simons) (progressive lipodystrophy)
  272.6
basal ganglia 333.90
  degenerative NEC 333.0
  specified NEC 333.89
Basedow's (exophthalmic goiter) 242.0 ✓5ᵗʰ
basement membrane NEC 583.89
  with
    pulmonary hemorrhage (Goodpasture's
      syndrome) 446.21 [583.81]
Bateman's 078.0
  purpura (senile) 287.2
Batten's 330.1 [362.71]
Batten-Mayou (retina) 330.1 [362.71]
Batten-Steinert 359.2
Battey 031.0

Disease, diseased — *see also* Syndrome —
continued
Baumgarten-Cruveilhier (cirrhosis of liver)
  571.5
bauxite-workers' 503
Bayle's (dementia paralytica) 094.1
Bazin's (primary) (*see also* Tuberculosis)
  017.1 ✓5ᵗʰ
Beard's (neurasthenia) 300.5
Beau's (*see also* Degeneration, myocardial)
  429.1
Bechterew's (ankylosing spondylitis) 720.0
Becker's (idiopathic mural endomyocardial
  disease) 425.2
Begbie's (exophthalmic goiter) 242.0 ✓5ᵗʰ
Behr's 362.50
Beigel's (white piedra) 111.2
Bekhterev's (ankylosing spondylitis) 720.0
Bell's (*see also* Psychosis, affective) 296.0 ✓5ᵗʰ
Bennett's (leukemia) 208.9 ✓5ᵗʰ
Benson's 379.22
Bergeron's (hysteroepilepsy) 300.11
Berlin's 921.3
Bernard-Soulier (thrombopathy) 287.1
Bernhardt (-Roth) 355.1
beryllium 503
Besnier-Boeck (-Schaumann) (sarcoidosis) 135
Best's 362.76
Beurmann's (sporotrichosis) 117.1
Bielschowsky (-Jansky) 330.1
Biermer's (pernicious anemia) 281.0
Biett's (discoid lupus erythematosus) 695.4
bile duct (*see also* Disease, biliary) 576.9
biliary (duct) (tract) 576.9
  with calculus, choledocholithiasis, or stones
    — *see* Choledocholithiasis
Billroth's (meningocele) (*see also* Spina bifida)
  741.9 ✓5ᵗʰ
Binswanger's 290.12
Bird's (oxaluria) 271.8
bird fanciers' 495.2
black lung 500
bladder 596.9
  specified NEC 596.8
bleeder's 286.0
Bloch-Sulzberger (incontinentia pigmenti)
  757.33
Blocq's (astasia-abasia) 307.9
blood (-forming organs) 289.9
  specified NEC 289.8
  vessel 459.9
Bloodgood's 610.1
Blount's (tibia vara) 732.4
blue 746.9
Bodechtel-Guttmann (subacute sclerosing
  panencephalitis) 046.2
Boeck's (sarcoidosis) 135
bone 733.90
  fibrocystic NEC 733.29
    jaw 526.2
  marrow 289.9
  Paget's (osteitis deformans) 731.0
  specified type NEC 733.99
  von Rechlinghausen's (osteitis fibrosa
    cystica) 252.0
Bonfils' — *see* Disease, Hodgkin's
Borna 062.9
Bornholm (epidemic pleurodynia) 074.1
Bostock's (*see also* Fever, hay) 477.9
Bouchard's (myopathic dilatation of the
  stomach) 536.1
Bouillaud's (rheumatic heart disease) 391.9
Bourneville (-Brissaud) (tuberous sclerosis)
  759.5
Bouveret (-Hoffmann) (paroxysmal tachycardia)
  427.2
bowel 569.9
  functional 564.9
    psychogenic 306.4
Bowen's (M8081/2) — *see* Neoplasm, skin, in
  situ
Bozzolo's (multiple myeloma) (M973/3)
  203.0 ✓5ᵗʰ
Bradley's (epidemic vomiting) 078.82
Brailsford's 732.3
  radius, head 732.3
  tarsal, scaphoid 732.5

Disease, diseased — *see also* Syndrome — *continued*
  Brailsford-Morquio (mucopolysaccharidosis IV) 277.5
  brain 348.9
    Alzheimer's 331.0
      with dementia — *see* Alzheimer's, dementia
    arterial, artery 437.9
    arteriosclerotic 437.0
    congenital 742.9
    degenerative — *see* Degeneration, brain
    inflammatory — *see also* Encephalitis
      late effect — *see* category 326
    organic 348.9
      arteriosclerotic 437.0
    parasitic NEC 123.9
    Pick's 331.1
      with dementia
        with behavioral disturbance 331.1 *[294.11]*
        without behavioral disturbance 331.1 *[294.10]*
    senile 331.2
  brazier's 985.8
  breast 611.9
    cystic (chronic) 610.1
    fibrocystic 610.1
    inflammatory 611.0
    Paget's (M8540/3) 174.0
    puerperal, postpartum NEC 676.3 ✓5ᵗʰ
    specified NEC 611.8
  Breda's (*see also* Yaws) 102.9
  Breisky's (kraurosis vulvae) 624.0
  Bretonneau's (diphtheritic malignant angina) 032.0
  Bright's (*see also* Nephritis) 583.9
    arteriosclerotic (*see also* Hypertension, kidney) 403.90
  Brill's (recrudescent typhus) 081.1
    flea-borne 081.0
    louse-borne 081.1
  Brill-Symmers (follicular lymphoma) (M9690/3) 202.0 ✓5ᵗʰ
  Brill-Zinsser (recrudescent typhus) 081.1
  Brinton's (leather bottle stomach) (M8142/3) 151.9
  Brion-Kayser (*see also* Fever, paratyphoid) 002.9
  broad
    beta 272.2
    ligament, noninflammatory 620.9
      specified NEC 620.8
  Brocq's 691.8
    meaning
      atopic (diffuse) neurodermatitis 691.8
      dermatitis herpetiformis 694.0
      lichen simplex chronicus 698.3
      parapsoriasis 696.2
      prurigo 698.2
  Brocq-Duhring (dermatitis herpetiformis) 694.0
  Brodie's (joint) (*see also* Osteomyelitis) 730.1 ✓5ᵗʰ
  bronchi 519.1
  bronchopulmonary 519.1
  bronze (Addison's) 255.4
    tuberculous (*see also* Tuberculosis) 017.6 ✓5ᵗʰ
  Brown-Séquard 344.89
  Bruck's 733.99
  Bruck-de Lange (Amsterdam dwarf, mental retardation and brachycephaly) 759.89
  Bruhl's (splenic anemia with fever) 285.8
  Bruton's (X-linked agammaglobulinemia) 279.04
  buccal cavity 528.9
  Buchanan's (juvenile osteochondrosis, iliac crest) 732.1
  Buchman's (osteochondrosis juvenile) 732.1
  Budgerigar-fanciers' 495.2
  Büdinger-Ludloff-Läwen 717.89
  Buerger's (thromboangiitis obliterans) 443.1
  Bürger-Grütz (essential familial hyperlipemia) 272.3
  Burns' (lower ulna) 732.3
  bursa 727.9
  Bury's (erythema elevatum diutinum) 695.89

Disease, diseased — *see also* Syndrome — *continued*
  Buschke's 710.1
  Busquet's (*see also* Osteomyelitis) 730.1 ✓5ᵗʰ
  Busse-Buschke (cryptococcosis) 117.5
  C_2 (*see also* Alcoholism) 303.9 ✓5ᵗʰ
  Caffey's (infantile cortical hyperostosis) 756.59
  caisson 993.3
  calculous 592.9
  California 114.0
  Calvé (-Perthes) (osteochondrosis, femoral capital) 732.1
  Camurati-Engelmann (diaphyseal sclerosis) 756.59
  Canavan's 330.0
  capillaries 448.9
  Carapata 087.1
  cardiac — *see* Disease, heart
  cardiopulmonary, chronic 416.9
  cardiorenal (arteriosclerotic) (hepatic) (hypertensive) (vascular) (*see also* Hypertension, cardiorenal) 404.90
  cardiovascular (arteriosclerotic) 429.2
    congenital 746.9
    hypertensive (*see also* Hypertension, heart) 402.90
      benign 402.10
      malignant 402.00
    renal (*see also* Hypertension, cardiorenal) 404.90
    syphilitic (asymptomatic) 093.9
  carotid gland 259.8
  Carrión's (Bartonellosis) 088.0
  cartilage NEC 733.90
    specified NEC 733.99
  Castellani's 104.8
  cat-scratch 078.3
  Cavare's (familial periodic paralysis) 359.3
  Cazenave's (pemphigus) 694.4
  cecum 569.9
  celiac (adult) 579.0
    infantile 579.0
  cellular tissue NEC 709.9
  central core 359.0
  cerebellar, cerebellum — *see* Disease, brain
  cerebral (*see also* Disease, brain) 348.9
    arterial, artery 437.9
    degenerative — *see* Degeneration, brain
  cerebrospinal 349.9
  cerebrovascular NEC 437.9
    acute 436
      embolic — *see* Embolism, brain
      late effect — *see* Late effect(s) (of) cerebrovascular disease
      puerperal, postpartum, childbirth 674.0 ✓5ᵗʰ
      thrombotic — *see* Thrombosis, brain
    arteriosclerotic 437.0
    embolic — *see* Embolism, brain
    ischemic, generalized NEC 437.1
    late effect — *see* Late effect(s) (of) cerebrovascular disease
    occlusive 437.1
    puerperal, postpartum, childbirth 674.0 ✓5ᵗʰ
    specified type NEC 437.8
    thrombotic — *see* Thrombosis, brain
  ceroid storage 272.7
  cervix (uteri)
    inflammatory 616.9
      specified NEC 616.8
    noninflammatory 622.9
      specified NEC 622.8
  Chabert's 022.9
  Chagas' (*see also* Trypanosomiasis, American) 086.2
  Chandler's (osteochondritis dissecans, hip) 732.7
  Charcots' (joint) 094.0 *[713.5]*
    spinal cord 094.0
  Charcôt-Marie-Tooth 356.1
  Charlouis' (*see also* Yaws) 102.9
  Cheadle (-Möller) (-Barlow) (infantile scurvy) 267
  Chédiak-Steinbrinck (-Higashi) (congenital gigantism of peroxidase granules) 288.2
  cheek, inner 528.9
  chest 519.9

Disease, diseased — *see also* Syndrome — *continued*
  Chiari's (hepatic vein thrombosis) 453.0
  Chicago (North American blastomycosis) 116.0
  chignon (white piedra) 111.2
  chigoe, chigo (jigger) 134.1
  childhood granulomatous 288.1
  Chinese liver fluke 121.1
  chlamydial NEC 078.88
  cholecystic (*see also* Disease, gallbladder) 575.9
  choroid 363.9
    degenerative (*see also* Degeneration, choroid) 363.40
    hereditary (*see also* Dystrophy, choroid) 363.50
    specified type NEC 363.8
  Christian's (chronic histiocytosis X) 277.8
  Christian-Weber (nodular nonsuppurative panniculitis) 729.30
  Christmas 286.1
  ciliary body 364.9
  circulatory (system) NEC 459.9
    chronic, maternal, affecting fetus or newborn 760.3
    specified NEC 459.89
    syphilitic 093.9
      congenital 090.5
  Civatte's (poikiloderma) 709.09
  climacteric 627.2
    male 608.89
  coagulation factor deficiency (congenital) (*see also* Defect, coagulation) 286.9
  Coats' 362.12
  coccidiodal pulmonary 114.5
    acute 114.0
    chronic 114.4
    primary 114.0
    residual 114.4
  Cockayne's (microcephaly and dwarfism) 759.89
  Cogan's 370.52
  cold
    agglutinin 283.0
      or hemoglobinuria 283.0
        paroxysmal (cold) (nocturnal) 283.2
    hemagglutinin (chronic) 283.0
  collagen NEC 710.9
    nonvascular 710.9
    specified NEC 710.8
    vascular (allergic) (*see also* Angiitis, hypersensitivity) 446.20
  colon 569.9
    functional 564.9
      congenital 751.3
    ischemic 557.0
  combined system (of spinal cord) 266.2 *[336.2]*
    with anemia (pernicious) 281.0 *[336.2]*
  compressed air 993.3
  Concato's (pericardial polyserositis) 423.2
    peritoneal 568.82
    pleural — *see* Pleurisy
  congenital NEC 799.8
  conjunctiva 372.9
    chlamydial 077.98
      specified NEC 077.8
    specified type NEC 372.89
    viral 077.99
      specified NEC 077.8
  connective tissue, diffuse (*see also* Disease, collagen) 710.9
  Conor and Bruch's (boutonneuse fever) 082.1
  Conradi (-Hünermann) 756.59
  Cooley's (erythroblastic anemia) 282.4
  Cooper's 610.1
  Corbus' 607.1
  cork-handlers' 495.3
  cornea (*see also* Keratopathy) 371.9
  coronary (*see also* Ischemia, heart) 414.9
    congenital 746.85
    ostial, syphilitic 093.20
      aortic 093.22
      mitral 093.21
      pulmonary 093.24
      tricuspid 093.23
  Corrigan's — *see* Insufficiency, aortic
  Cotugno's 724.3
  Coxsackie (virus) NEC 074.8

Disease, diseased — *see also* Syndrome —
continued
cranial nerve NEC 352.9
Creutzfeldt-Jakob 046.1
    with dementia
        with behavioral disturbance
            046.1 *[294.11]*
        without behavioral disturbance
            046.1 *[294.10]*
Crigler-Najjar (congenital hyperbilirubinemia)
    277.4
Crocq's (acrocyanosis) 443.89
Crohn's (intestine) (*see also* Enteritis, regional)
    555.9
Crouzon's (craniofacial dysostosis) 756.0
Cruchet's (encephalitis lethargica) 049.8
Cruveilhier's 335.21
Cruz-Chagas (*see also* Trypanosomiasis,
    American) 086.2
crystal deposition (*see also* Arthritis, due to,
    crystals) 712.9 ✓5ᵗʰ
Csillag's (lichen sclerosus et atrophicus) 701.0
Curschmann's 359.2
Cushing's (pituitary basophilism) 255.0
cystic
    breast (chronic) 610.1
    kidney, congenital (*see also* Cystic, disease,
        kidney) 753.10
    liver, congenital 751.62
    lung 518.89
        congenital 748.4
    pancreas 577.2
        congenital 751.7
    renal, congenital (*see also* Cystic, disease,
        kidney) 753.10
    semilunar cartilage 717.5
cysticercus 123.1
cystine storage (with renal sclerosis) 270.0
cytomegalic inclusion (generalized) 078.5
    with
        pneumonia 078.5 *[484.1]*
    congenital 771.1
Daae (-Finsen) (epidemic pleurodynia) 074.1
dancing 297.8
Danielssen's (anesthetic leprosy) 030.1
Darier's (congenital) (keratosis follicularis)
    757.39
    erythema annulare centrifugum 695.0
    vitamin A deficiency 264.8
Darling's (histoplasmosis) (*see also*
    Histoplasmosis, American) 115.00
Davies' 425.0
de Beurmann-Gougerot (sporotrichosis) 117.1
Débove's (splenomegaly) 789.2
deer fly (*see also* Tularemia) 021.9
deficiency 269.9
degenerative — *see also* Degeneration
    disc — *see* Degeneration, intervertebral disc
Degos' 447.8
Déjérine (-Sottas) 356.0
Déléage's 359.89 ▲
demyelinating, demyelinizating (brain stem)
    (central nervous system) 341.9
    multiple sclerosis 340
    specified NEC 341.8
de Quervain's (tendon sheath) 727.04
    thyroid (subacute granulomatous thyroiditis)
        245.1
Dercum's (adiposis dolorosa) 272.8
Deutschländer's — *see* Fracture, foot
Devergie's (pityriasis rubra pilaris) 696.4
Devic's 341.0
diaphorase deficiency 289.7
diaphragm 519.4
diarrheal, infectious 009.2
diatomaceous earth 502
Diaz's (osteochondrosis astragalus) 732.5
digestive system 569.9
Di Guglielmo's (erythemic myelosis) (M9841/3)
    207.0 ✓5ᵗʰ
Dimitri-Sturge-Weber (encephalocutaneous
    angiomatosis) 759.6
disc, degenerative — *see* Degeneration,
    intervertebral disc
discogenic (*see also* Disease, intervertebral
    disc) 722.90
diverticular — *see* Diverticula
Down's (mongolism) 758.0

Disease, diseased — *see also* Syndrome —
continued
Dubini's (electric chorea) 049.8
Dubois' (thymus gland) 090.5
Duchenne's 094.0
    locomotor ataxia 094.0
    muscular dystrophy 359.1
    paralysis 335.22
    pseudohypertrophy, muscles 359.1
Duchenne-Griesinger 359.1
ductless glands 259.9
Duhring's (dermatitis herpetiformis) 694.0
Dukes (-Filatov) 057.8
duodenum NEC 537.9
    specified NEC 537.89
Duplay's 726.2
Dupré's (meningism) 781.6
Dupuytren's (muscle contracture) 728.6
Durand-Nicolas-Favre (climatic bubo) 099.1
Duroziez's (congenital mitral stenosis) 746.5
Dutton's (trypanosomiasis) 086.9
Eales' 362.18
ear (chronic) (inner) NEC 388.9
    middle 385.9
        adhesive (*see also* Adhesions, middle ear)
            385.10
        specified NEC 385.89
Eberth's (typhoid fever) 002.0
Ebstein's
    heart 746.2
    meaning diabetes 250.4 ✓5ᵗʰ *[581.81]*
Echinococcus (*see also* Echinococcus) 122.9
ECHO virus NEC 078.89
Economo's (encephalitis lethargica) 049.8
Eddowes' (brittle bones and blue sclera) 756.51
Edsall's 992.2
Eichstedt's (pityriasis versicolor) 111.0
Ellis-van Creveld (chondroectodermal
    dysplasia) 756.55
endocardium — *see* Endocarditis
endocrine glands or system NEC 259.9
    specified NEC 259.8
endomyocardial, idiopathic mural 425.2
Engel-von Recklinghausen (osteitis fibrosa
    cystica) 252.0
Engelmann's (diaphyseal sclerosis) 756.59
English (rickets) 268.0
Engman's (infectious eczematoid dermatitis)
    690.8
enteroviral, enterovirus NEC 078.89
    central nervous system NEC 048
epidemic NEC 136.9
epididymis 608.9
epigastric, functional 536.9
    psychogenic 306.4
Erb (-Landouzy) 359.1
Erb-Goldflam 358.0
Erichsen's (railway spine) 300.16
esophagus 530.9
    functional 530.5
    psychogenic 306.4
Eulenburg's (congenital paramyotonia) 359.2
Eustachian tube 381.9
Evans' (thrombocytopenic purpura) 287.3
external auditory canal 380.9
extrapyramidal NEC 333.90
eye 379.90
    anterior chamber 364.9
    inflammatory NEC 364.3
    muscle 378.9
eyeball 360.9
eyelid 374.9
eyeworm of Africa 125.2
Fabry's (angiokeratoma corporis diffusum)
    272.7
facial nerve (seventh) 351.9
    newborn 767.5
Fahr-Volhard (malignant nephrosclerosis)
    403.00
fallopian tube, noninflammatory 620.9
    specified NEC 620.8
familial periodic 277.3
    paralysis 359.3
Fanconi's (congenital pancytopenia) 284.0
Farber's (disseminated lipogranulomatosis)
    272.8
fascia 728.9
    inflammatory 728.9

Disease, diseased — *see also* Syndrome —
continued
Fauchard's (periodontitis) 523.4
Favre-Durand-Nicolas (climatic bubo) 099.1
Favre-Racouchot (elastoidosis cutanea
    nodularis) 701.8
Fede's 529.0
Feer's 985.0
Felix's (juvenile osteochondrosis, hip) 732.1
Fenwick's (gastric atrophy) 537.89
Fernels' (aortic aneurysm) 441.9
fibrocaseous, of lung (*see also* Tuberculosis,
    pulmonary) 011.9 ✓5ᵗʰ
fibrocystic — *see also* Fibrocystic, disease
    newborn 277.01
Fiedler's (leptospiral jaundice) 100.0
fifth 057.0
Filatoff's (infectious mononucleosis) 075
Filatov's (infectious mononucleosis) 075
file-cutters' 984.9
    specified type of lead — *see* Table of Drugs
        and Chemicals
filterable virus NEC 078.89
fish skin 757.1
    acquired 701.1
Flajani (-Basedow) (exophthalmic goiter)
    242.0 ✓5ᵗʰ
Flatau-Schilder 341.1
flax-dressers' 504
Fleischner's 732.3
flint 502
fluke — *see* Infestation, fluke
Følling's (phenylketonuria) 270.1
foot and mouth 078.4
foot process 581.3
Forbes' (glycogenosis III) 271.0
Fordyce's (ectopic sebaceous glands) (mouth)
    750.26
Fordyce-Fox (apocrine miliaria) 705.82
Fothergill's
    meaning scarlatina anginosa 034.1
    neuralgia (*see also* Neuralgia, trigeminal)
        350.1
Fournier's 608.83
fourth 057.8
Fox (-Fordyce) (apocrine miliaria) 705.82
Francis' (*see also* Tularemia) 021.9
Franklin's (heavy chain) 273.2
Frei's (climatic bubo) 099.1
Freiberg's (flattening metarsal) 732.5
Friedländer's (endarteritis obliterans) — *see*
    Arteriosclerosis
Friedreich's
    combined systemic or ataxia 334.0
    facial hemihypertrophy 756.0
    myoclonia 333.2
Fröhlich's (adiposogenital dystrophy) 253.8
Frommel's 676.6 ✓5ᵗʰ
frontal sinus (chronic) 473.1
    acute 461.1
Fuller's earth 502
fungus, fungous NEC 117.9
Gaisböck's (polycythemia hypertonica) 289.0
gallbladder 575.9
    congenital 751.60
Gamna's (siderotic splenomegaly) 289.51
Gamstorp's (adynamia episodica hereditaria)
    359.3
Gandy-Nanta (siderotic splenomegaly) 289.51
gannister (occupational) 502
Garré's (*see also* Osteomyelitis) 730.1 ✓5ᵗʰ
gastric (*see also* Disease, stomach) 537.9
gastrointestinal (tract) 569.9
    amyloid 277.3
    functional 536.9
        psychogenic 306.4
Gaucher's (adult) (cerebroside lipidosis)
    (infantile) 272.7
Gayet's (superior hemorrhagic
    polioencephalitis) 265.1
Gee (-Herter) (-Heubner) (-Thaysen) (nontropical
    sprue) 579.0
generalized neoplastic (M8000/6) 199.0
genital organs NEC
    female 629.9
        specified NEC 629.8
    male 608.9
Gerhardt's (erythromelalgia) 443.89

Disease — Disease

Disease, diseased — *see also* Syndrome — *continued*
Gerlier's (epidemic vertigo) 078.81
Gibert's (pityriasis rosea) 696.3
Gibney's (perispondylitis) 720.9
Gierke's (glycogenosis I) 271.0
Gilbert's (familial nonhemolytic jaundice) 277.4
Gilchrist's (North American blastomycosis) 116.0
Gilford (-Hutchinson) (progeria) 259.8
Gilles de la Tourette's (motor-verbal tic) 307.23
Giovannini's 117.9
gland (lymph) 289.9
Glanzmann's (hereditary hemorrhagic thrombasthenia) 287.1
glassblowers' 527.1
Glénard's (enteroptosis) 569.89
Glisson's (*see also* Rickets) 268.0
glomerular
    membranous, idiopathic 581.1
    minimal change 581.3
glycogen storage (Andersen's) (Cori types 1-7) (Forbes') (McArdle-Schmid-Pearson) (Pompe's) (types I-VII) 271.0
    cardiac 271.0 [425.7]
    generalized 271.0
    glucose-6-phosphatase deficiency 271.0
    heart 271.0 [425.7]
    hepatorenal 271.0
    liver and kidneys 271.0
    myocardium 271.0 [425.7]
    von Gierke's (glycogenosis I) 271.0
Goldflam-Erb 358.0
Goldscheider's (epidermolysis bullosa) 757.39
Goldstein's (familial hemorrhagic telangiectasia) 448.0
gonococcal NEC 098.0
Goodall's (epidemic vomiting) 078.82
Gordon's (exudative enteropathy) 579.8
Gougerot's (trisymptomatic) 709.1
Gougerot-Carteaud (confluent reticulate papillomatosis) 701.8
Gougerot-Hailey-Hailey (benign familial chronic pemphigus) 757.39
graft-versus-host (bone marrow) 996.85
    due to organ transplant NEC — *see* Complications, transplant, organ
grain-handlers' 495.8
Grancher's (splenopneumonia) — *see* Pneumonia
granulomatous (childhood) (chronic) 288.1
graphite lung 503
Graves' (exophthalmic goiter) 242.0 ✓5ᵗʰ
Greenfield's 330.0
green monkey 078.89
Griesinger's (*see also* Ancylostomiasis) 126.9
grinders' 502
Grisel's 723.5
Gruby's (tinea tonsurans) 110.0
Guertin's (electric chorea) 049.8
Guillain-Barré 357.0
Guinon's (motor-verbal tic) 307.23
Gull's (thyroid atrophy with myxedema) 244.8
Gull and Sutton's — *see* Hypertension, kidney
gum NEC 523.9
Günther's (congenital erythropoietic porphyria) 277.1
gynecological 629.9
    specified NEC 629.8
H 270.0
Haas' 732.3
Habermann's (acute parapsoriasis varioliformis) 696.2
Haff 985.1
Hageman (congenital factor XII deficiency) (*see also* Defect, congenital) 286.3
Haglund's (osteochondrosis os tibiale externum) 732.5
Hagner's (hypertrophic pulmonary osteoarthropathy) 731.2
Hailey-Hailey (benign familial chronic pemphigus) 757.39
hair (follicles) NEC 704.9
    specified type NEC 704.8
Hallervorden-Spatz 333.0
Hallopeau's (lichen sclerosus et atrophicus) 701.0

Disease, diseased — *see also* Syndrome — *continued*
Hamman's (spontaneous mediastinal emphysema) 518.1
hand, foot, and mouth 074.3
Hand-Schüller-Christian (chronic histiocytosis X) 277.8
Hanot's — *see* Cirrhosis, biliary
Hansen's (leprosy) 030.9
    benign form 030.1
    malignant form 030.0
Harada's 363.22
Harley's (intermittent hemoglobinuria) 283.2
Hart's (pellagra-cerebellar ataxia renal aminoaciduria) 270.0
Hartnup (pellagra-cerebellar ataxia renal aminoaciduria) 270.0
Hashimoto's (struma lymphomatosa) 245.2
Hb — *see* Disease, hemoglobin
heart (organic) 429.9
    with
        acute pulmonary edema (*see also* Failure, ventricular, left) 428.1
            hypertensive 402.91
                with renal failure 404.91
                benign 402.11
                    with renal failure 404.11
                malignant 402.01
                    with renal failure 404.01
        kidney disease — *see* Hypertension, cardiorenal
        rheumatic fever (conditions classifiable to 390)
            active 391.9
                with chorea 392.0
            inactive or quiescent (with chorea) 398.90
    amyloid 277.3 [425.7]
    aortic (valve) (*see also* Endocarditis, aortic) 424.1
    arteriosclerotic or sclerotic (minimal) (senile) — *see* Arteriosclerosis, coronary
    artery — *see* Arteriosclerosis, coronary
    atherosclerotic — *see* Arteriosclerosis, coronary
    beer drinkers' 425.5
    beriberi 265.0 [425.7]
    black 416.0
    congenital NEC 746.9
        cyanotic 746.9
        maternal, affecting fetus or newborn 760.3
        specified type NEC 746.89
    congestive (*see also* Failure, heart) 428.0
    coronary 414.9
    cryptogenic 429.9
    due to
        amyloidosis 277.3 [425.7]
        beriberi 265.0 [425.7]
        cardiac glycogenosis 271.0 [425.7]
        Friedreich's ataxia 334.0 [425.8]
        gout 274.82
        mucopolysaccharidosis 277.5 [425.7]
        myotonia atrophica 359.2 [425.8]
        progressive muscular dystrophy 359.1 [425.8]
        sarcoidosis 135 [425.8]
    fetal 746.9
        inflammatory 746.89
    fibroid (*see also* Myocarditis) 429.0
    functional 427.9
        postoperative 997.1
        psychogenic 306.2
    glycogen storage 271.0 [425.7]
    gonococcal NEC 098.85
    gouty 274.82
    hypertensive (*see also* Hypertension, heart) 402.90
        benign 402.10
        malignant 402.00
    hyperthyroid (*see also* Hyperthyroidism) 242.9 ✓5ᵗʰ [425.7]
    incompletely diagnosed — *see* Disease, heart
    ischemic (chronic) (*see also* Ischemia, heart) 414.9

Disease, diseased — *see also* Syndrome — *continued*
heart — *continued*
    ischemic (*see also* Ischemia, heart) — *continued*
        acute (*see also* Infarct, myocardium)
            without myocardial infarction 411.89
                with coronary (artery) occlusion 411.81
            asymptomatic 412
            diagnosed on ECG or other special investigation but currently presenting no symptoms 412
    kyphoscoliotic 416.1
    mitral (*see also* Endocarditis, mitral) 394.9
    muscular (*see also* Degeneration, myocardial) 429.1
    postpartum 674.8 ✓5ᵗʰ
    psychogenic (functional) 306.2
    pulmonary (chronic) 416.9
        acute 415.0
        specified NEC 416.8
    rheumatic (chronic) (inactive) (old) (quiescent) (with chorea) 398.90
        active or acute 391.9
            with chorea (active) (rheumatic) (Sydenham's) 392.0
            specified type NEC 391.8
        maternal, affecting fetus or newborn 760.3
    rheumatoid — *see* Arthritis, rheumatoid
    sclerotic — *see* Arteriosclersis, coronary
    senile (*see also* Myocarditis) 429.0
    specified type NEC 429.89
    syphilitic 093.89
        aortic 093.1
            aneurysm 093.0
            asymptomatic 093.89
        congenital 090.5
    thyroid (gland) (*see also* Hyper-thyroidism) 242.9 ✓5ᵗʰ [425.7]
    thyrotoxic (*see also* Thyrotoxicosis) 242.9 ✓5ᵗʰ [425.7]
    tuberculous (*see also* Tuberculosis) 017.9 ✓5ᵗʰ [425.8]
    valve, valvular (obstructive) (regurgitant) — *see also* Endocarditis
        congenital NEC (*see also* Anomaly, heart, valve) 746.9
            pulmonary 746.00
            specified type NEC 746.89
    vascular — *see* Disease, cardiovascular
heavy-chain (gamma G) 273.2
Heberden's 715.04
Hebra's
    dermatitis exfoliativa 695.89
    erythema multiforme exudativum 695.1
    pityriasis
        maculata et circinata 696.3
        rubra 695.89
            pilaris 696.4
    prurigo 698.2
Heerfordt's (uveoparotitis) 135
Heidenhain's 290.10
    with dementia 290.10
Heilmeyer-Schöner (M9842/3) 207.1 ✓5ᵗʰ
Heine-Medin (*see also* Poliomyelitis) 045.9 ✓5ᵗʰ
Heller's (*see also* Psychosis, childhood) 299.1 ✓5ᵗʰ
Heller-Döhle (syphilitic aortitis) 093.1
hematopoietic organs 289.9
hemoglobin (Hb) 282.7
    with thalassemia 282.4
    abnormal (mixed) NEC 282.7
        with thalassemia 282.4
    AS genotype 282.5
    Bart's 282.7
    C (Hb-C) 282.7
        with other abnormal hemoglobin NEC 282.7
        elliptocytosis 282.7
        Hb-S 282.63
        sickle-cell 282.63
        thalassemia 282.4
    constant spring 282.7

Disease, diseased — *see also* Syndrome — continued

hemoglobin — *continued*
  D (Hb-D) 282.7
    with other abnormal hemoglobin NEC 282.7
    Hb-S 282.69
    sickle-cell 282.69
    thalassemia 282.4
  E (Hb-E) 282.7
    with other abnormal hemoglobin NEC 282.7
    Hb-S 282.69
    sickle-cell 282.69
    thalassemia 282.4
  elliptocytosis 282.7
  F (Hb-F) 282.7
  G (Hb-G) 282.7
  H (Hb-H) 282.4
  hereditary persistence, fetal (HPFH) ("Swiss variety") 282.7
  high fetal gene 282.7
  I thalassemia 282.4
  M 289.7
  S — *see* Disease, sickle-cell, Hb-S
  spherocytosis 282.7
  unstable, hemolytic 282.7
  Zurich (Hb-Zurich) 282.7
hemolytic (fetus) (newborn) 773.2
  autoimmune (cold type) (warm type) 283.0
  due to or with
    incompatibility
      ABO (blood group) 773.1
      blood (group) (Duffy) (Kell) (Kidd) (Lewis) (M) (S) NEC 773.2
      Rh (blood group) (factor) 773.0
      Rh negative mother 773.0
  unstable hemoglobin 282.7
hemorrhagic 287.9
  newborn 776.0
Henoch (-Schönlein) (purpura nervosa) 287.0
hepatic — *see* Disease, liver
hepatolenticular 275.1
heredodegenerative NEC
  brain 331.89
  spinal cord 336.8
Hers' (glycogenosis VI) 271.0
Herter (-Gee) (-Heubner) (nontropical sprue) 579.0
Herxheimer's (diffuse idiopathic cutaneous atrophy) 701.8
Heubner's 094.89
Heubner-Herter (nontropical sprue) 579.0
high fetal gene or hemoglobin thalassemia 282.4
Hildenbrand's (typhus) 081.9
hip (joint) NEC 719.95
  congenital 755.63
  suppurative 711.05
  tuberculous (*see also* Tuberculosis) 015.1 ✓5ᵗʰ [730.85]
Hippel's (retinocerebral angiomatosis) 759.6
Hirschfeld's (acute diabetes mellitus) (*see also* Diabetes) 250.0 ✓5ᵗʰ
Hirschsprung's (congenital megacolon) 751.3
His (-Werner) (trench fever) 083.1
HIV 042
Hodgkin's (M9650/3) 201.9 ✓5ᵗʰ

> Note — Use the following fifth-digit subclassification with category 201:
>
> 0   *unspecifed site*
> 1   *lymph nodes of head, face, and neck*
> 2   *intrathoracic lymp nodes*
> 3   *intra-abdominal lymph nodes*
> 4   *lymph nodes of axilla and upper limb*
> 5   *lymph nodes of inguinal region and lower limb*
> 6   *intrapelvic lymph nodes*
> 7   *spleen*
> 8   *lymph nodes of multiple sites*

Disease, diseased — *see also* Syndrome — continued

Hodgkin's — *continued*
  lymphocytic
    depletion (M9653/3) 201.7 ✓5ᵗʰ
      diffuse fibrosis (M9654/3) 201.7 ✓5ᵗʰ
      reticular type (M9655/3) 201.7 ✓5ᵗʰ
    predominance (M9651/3) 201.4 ✓5ᵗʰ
  lymphocytic-histiocytic predominance (M9651/3) 201.4 ✓5ᵗʰ
  mixed cellularity (M9652/3) 201.6 ✓5ᵗʰ
  nodular sclerosis (M9656/3) 201.5 ✓5ᵗʰ
    cellular phase (M9657/3) 201.5 ✓5ᵗʰ
Hodgson's 441.9
  ruptured 441.5
Hoffa (-Kastert) (liposynovitis prepatellaris) 272.8
Holla (*see also* Spherocytosis) 282.0
homozygous-Hb-S 282.61
hoof and mouth 078.4
hookworm (*see also* Ancylostomiasis) 126.9
Horton's (temporal arteritis) 446.5
host-versus-graft (immune or nonimmune cause) 996.80
  bone marrow 996.85
  heart 996.83
  intestines 996.87
  kidney 996.81
  liver 996.82
  lung 996.84
  pancreas 996.86
  specified NEC 996.89
HPFH (hereditary persistence of fetal hemoglobin) ("Swiss variety") 282.7
Huchard's (continued arterial hypertension) 401.9
Huguier's (uterine fibroma) 218.9
human immunodeficiency (virus) 042
hunger 251.1
Hunt's
  dyssynergia cerebellaris myoclonica 334.2
  herpetic geniculate ganglionitis 053.11
Huntington's 333.4
Huppert's (multiple myeloma) (M9730/3) 203.0 ✓5ᵗʰ
Hurler's (mucopolysaccharidosis I) 277.5
Hutchinson's, meaning
  angioma serpiginosum 709.1
  cheiropompholyx 705.81
  prurigo estivalis 692.72
Hutchinson-Boeck (sarcoidosis) 135
Hutchinson-Gilford (progeria) 259.8
hyaline (diffuse) (generalized) 728.9
  membrane (lung) (newborn) 769
hydatid (*see also* Echinococcus) 122.9
Hyde's (prurigo nodularis) 698.3
hyperkinetic (*see also* Hyperkinesia) 314.9
  heart 429.82
hypertensive (*see also* Hypertension) 401.9
hypophysis 253.9
  hyperfunction 253.1
  hypofunction 253.2
Iceland (epidemic neuromyasthenia) 049.8
I cell 272.7
ill-defined 799.8
immunologic NEC 279.9
immunoproliferative 203.8 ✓5ᵗʰ
inclusion 078.5
  salivary gland 078.5
infancy, early NEC 779.9
infective NEC 136.9
inguinal gland 289.9
internal semilunar cartilage, cystic 717.5
intervertebral disc 722.90
  with myelopathy 722.70
  cervical, cervicothoracic 722.91
    with myelopathy 722.71
  lumbar, lumbosacral 722.93
    with myelopathy 722.73
  thoracic, thoracolumbar 722.92
    with myelopathy 722.72
intestine 569.9
  functional 564.9
    congenital 751.3
    psychogenic 306.4
  lardaceous 277.3

Disease, diseased — *see also* Syndrome — continued

intestine — *continued*
  organic 569.9
  protozoal NEC 007.9
iris 364.9
iron
  metabolism 275.0
  storage 275.0
Isambert's (*see also* Tuberculosis, larynx) 012.3 ✓5ᵗʰ
Iselin's (osteochondrosis, fifth metatarsal) 732.5
Island (scrub typhus) 081.2
itai-itai 985.5
Jadassohn's (maculopapular erythroderma) 696.2
Jadassohn-Pellizari's (anetoderma) 701.3
Jakob-Creutzfeldt 046.1
  with dementia
    with behavioral disturbance 046.1 [294.11]
    without behavioral disturbance 046.1 [294.10]
Jaksch (-Luzet) (pseudoleukemia infantum) 285.8
Janet's 300.89
Jansky-Bielschowsky 330.1
jaw NEC 526.9
  fibrocystic 526.2
Jensen's 363.05
Jeune's (asphyxiating thoracic dystrophy) 756.4
jigger 134.1
Johnson-Stevens (erythema multiforme exudativum) 695.1
joint NEC 719.9 ✓5ᵗʰ
  ankle 719.97
  Charcôt 094.0 [713.5]
  degenerative (*see also* Osteoarthrosis) 715.9 ✓5ᵗʰ
    multiple 715.09
    spine (*see also* Spondylosis) 721.90
  elbow 719.92
  foot 719.97
  hand 719.94
  hip 719.95
  hypertrophic (chronic) (degenerative) (*see also* Osteoarthrosis) 715.9 ✓5ᵗʰ
    spine (*see also* Spondylosis) 721.90
  knee 719.96
  Luschka 721.90
  multiple sites 719.99
  pelvic region 719.95
  sacroiliac 724.6
  shoulder (region) 719.91
  specified site NEC 719.98
  spine NEC 724.9
    pseudarthrosis following fusion 733.82
    sacroiliac 724.6
  wrist 719.93
Jourdain's (acute gingivitis) 523.0
Jüngling's (sarcoidosis) 135
Kahler (-Bozzolo) (multiple myeloma) (M9730/3) 203.0 ✓5ᵗʰ
Kalischer's 759.6
Kaposi's 757.33
  lichen ruber 697.8
    acuminatus 696.4
    moniliformis 697.8
  xeroderma pigmentosum 757.33
Kaschin-Beck (endemic polyarthritis) 716.00
  ankle 716.07
  arm 716.02
    lower (and wrist) 716.03
    upper (and elbow) 716.02
  foot (and ankle) 716.07
  forearm (and wrist) 716.03
  hand 716.04
  leg 716.06
    lower 716.06
    upper 716.05
  multiple sites 716.09
  pelvic region (hip) (thigh) 716.05
  shoulder region 716.01
  specified site NEC 716.08
Katayama 120.2
Kawasaki 446.1
Kedani (scrub typhus) 081.2

Disease, diseased — *see also* Syndrome — *continued*
  kidney (functional) (pelvis) (*see also* Disease, renal) 593.9
    cystic (congenital) 753.10
      multiple 753.19
      single 753.11
      specified NEC 753.19
    fibrocystic (congenital) 753.19
    in gout 274.10
    polycystic (congenital) 753.12
      adult type (APKD) 753.13
      autosomal dominant 753.13
      autosomal recessive 753.14
      childhood type (CPKD) 753.14
      infantile type 753.14
  Kienböck's (carpal lunate) (wrist) 732.3
  Kimmelstiel (-Wilson) (intercapillary glomerulosclerosis) 250.4 ✓5ᵗʰ [581.81]
  Kinnier Wilson's (hepatolenticular degeneration) 275.1
  kissing 075
  Kleb's (*see also* Nephritis) 583.9
  Klinger's 446.4
  Klippel's 723.8
  Klippel-Feil (brevicollis) 756.16
  knight's 911.1
  Köbner's (epidermolysis bullosa) 757.39
  Koenig-Wichmann (pemphigus) 694.4
  Köhler's
    first (osteoarthrosis juvenilis) 732.5
    second (Freiberg's infraction, metatarsal head) 732.5
    patellar 732.4
    tarsal navicular (bone) (osteoarthrosis juvenilis) 732.5
  Köhler-Freiberg (infraction, metatarsal head) 732.5
  Köhler-Mouchet (osteoarthrosis juvenilis) 732.5
  Köhler-Pellegrini-Stieda (calcification, knee joint) 726.62
  König's (osteochondritis dissecans) 732.7
  Korsakoff's (nonalcoholic) 294.0
    alcoholic 291.1
  Kostmann's (infantile genetic agranulocytosis) 288.0
  Krabbe's 330.0
  Kraepelin-Morel (*see also* Schizophrenia) 295.9 ✓5ᵗʰ
  Kraft-Weber-Dimitri 759.6
  Kufs' 330.1
  Kugelberg-Welander 335.11
  Kuhnt-Junius 362.52
  Kümmell's (-Verneuil) (spondylitis) 721.7
  Kundrat's (lymphosarcoma) 200.1 ✓5ᵗʰ
  kuru 046.0
  Kussmaul (-Meier) (polyarteritis nodosa) 446.0
  Kyasanur Forest 065.2
  Kyrle's (hyperkeratosis follicularis in cutem penetrans) 701.1
  labia
    inflammatory 616.9
      specified NEC 616.8
    noninflammatory 624.9
      specified NEC 624.8
  labyrinth, ear 386.8
  lacrimal system (apparatus) (passages) 375.9
    gland 375.00
    specified NEC 375.89
  Lafora's 333.2
  Lagleyze-von Hippel (retinocerebral angiomatosis) 759.6
  Lancereaux-Mathieu (leptospiral jaundice) 100.0
  Landry's 357.0
  Lane's 569.89
  lardaceous (any site) 277.3
  Larrey-Weil (leptospiral jaundice) 100.0
  Larsen (-Johansson) (juvenile osteopathia patellae) 732.4
  larynx 478.70
  Lasègue's (persecution mania) 297.9
  Leber's 377.16
  Lederer's (acquired infectious hemolytic anemia) 283.19
  Legg's (capital femoral osteochondrosis) 732.1

Disease, diseased — *see also* Syndrome — *continued*
  Legg-Calvé-Perthes (capital femoral osteochondrosis) 732.1
  Legg-Calvé-Waldenström (femoral capital osteochondrosis) 732.1
  Legg-Perthes (femoral capital osteochrondosis) 732.1
  Legionnaires' 482.84
  Leigh's 330.8
  Leiner's (exfoliative dermatitis) 695.89
  Leloir's (lupus erythematosus) 695.4
  Lenegre's 426.0
  lens (eye) 379.39
  Leriche's (osteoporosis, post-traumatic) 733.7
  Letterer-Siwe (acute histiocytosis X) (M9722/3) 202.5 ✓5ᵗʰ
  Lev's (acquired complete heart block) 426.0
  Lewandowski's (*see also* Tuberculosis) 017.0 ✓5ᵗʰ
  Lewandowski-Lutz (epidermodysplasia verruciformis) 078.19
  Leyden's (periodic vomiting) 536.2
  Libman-Sacks (verrucous endocarditis) 710.0 [424.91]
  Lichtheim's (subacute combined sclerosis with pernicious anemia) 281.0 [336.2]
  ligament 728.9
  light chain 203.0 ✓5ᵗʰ
  Lightwood's (renal tubular acidosis) 588.8
  Lignac's (cystinosis) 270.0
  Lindau's (retinocerebral angiomatosis) 759.6
  Lindau-von Hippel (angiomatosis retinocerebellosa) 759.6
  lip NEC 528.5
  lipidosis 272.7
  lipoid storage NEC 272.7
  Lipschütz's 616.50
  Little's — *see* Palsy, cerebral
  liver 573.9
    alcoholic 571.3
      acute 571.1
      chronic 571.3
    chronic 571.9
      alcoholic 571.3
    cystic, congenital 751.62
    drug-induced 573.3
    due to
      chemicals 573.3
        fluorinated agents 573.3
        hypersensitivity drugs 573.3
        isoniazids 573.3
    fibrocystic (congenital) 751.62
    glycogen storage 271.0
    organic 573.9
    polycystic (congenital) 751.62
  Lobo's (keloid blastomycosis) 116.2
  Lobstein's (brittle bones and blue sclera) 756.51
  locomotor system 334.9
  Lorain's (pituitary dwarfism) 253.3
  Lou Gehrig's 335.20
  Lucas-Championnière (fibrinous bronchitis) 466.0
  Ludwig's (submaxillary cellulitis) 528.3
  luetic — *see* Syphilis
  lumbosacral region 724.6
  lung NEC 518.89
    black 500
    congenital 748.60
    cystic 518.89
      congenital 748.4
    fibroid (chronic) (*see also* Fibrosis, lung) 515
    fluke 121.2
      Oriental 121.2
    in
      amyloidosis 277.3 [517.8]
      polymyositis 710.4 [517.8]
      sarcoidosis 135 [517.8]
      Sjögren's syndrome 710.2 [517.8]
      syphilis 095.1
      systemic lupus erythematosus 710.0 [517.8]
      systemic sclerosis 710.1 [517.2]
    interstitial (chronic) 515
      acute 136.3
    nonspecific, chronic 496

Disease, diseased — *see also* Syndrome — *continued*
  lung NEC — *continued*
    obstructive (chronic) (COPD) 496
      with
        acute exacerbation NEC 491.21
        alveolitis, allergic (*see also* Alveolitis, allergic) 495.9
        asthma (chronic) (obstructive) 493.2 ✓5ᵗʰ
        bronchiectasis 494.0
          with acute exacerbation 494.1
        bronchitis (chronic) 491.20
          with acute exacerbation 491.21
        emphysema NEC 492.8
      diffuse (with fibrosis) 496
    polycystic 518.89
      asthma (chronic) (obstructive) 493.2 ✓5ᵗʰ
      congenital 748.4
    purulent (cavitary) 513.0
    restrictive 518.89
    rheumatoid 714.81
      diffuse interstitial 714.81
    specified NEC 518.89
  Lutembacher's (atrial septal defect with mitral stenosis) 745.5
  Lutz-Miescher (elastosis perforans serpiginosa) 701.1
  Lutz-Splendore-de Almeida (Brazilian blastomycosis) 116.1
  Lyell's (toxic epidermal necrolysis) 695.1
    due to drug
      correct substance properly administered 695.1
      overdose or wrong substance given or taken 977.9
        specific drug — *see* Table of Drugs and Chemicals
  Lyme 088.81
  lymphatic (gland) (system) 289.9
    channel (noninfective) 457.9
    vessel (noninfective) 457.9
      specified NEC 457.8
  lymphoproliferative (chronic) (M9970/1) 238.7
  Machado-Joseph 334.8
  Madelung's (lipomatosis) 272.8
  Madura (actinomycotic) 039.9
    mycotic 117.4
  Magitot's 526.4
  Majocchi's (purpura annularis telangiectodes) 709.1
  malarial (*see also* Malaria) 084.6
  Malassez's (cystic) 608.89
  Malibu 919.8
    infected 919.9
  malignant (M8000/3) — *see also* Neoplasm, by site, malignant
    previous, affecting management of pregnancy V23.8 ✓5ᵗʰ
  Manson's 120.1
  maple bark 495.6
  maple syrup (urine) 270.3
  Marburg (virus) 078.89
  Marchiafava (-Bignami) 341.8
  Marfan's 090.49
    congenital syphilis 090.49
    meaning Marfan's syndrome 759.82
  Marie-Bamberger (hypertrophic pulmonary osteoarthropathy) (secondary) 731.2
    primary or idiopathic (acropachyderma) 757.39
    pulmonary (hypertrophic osteoarthropathy) 731.2
  Marie-Strümpell (ankylosing spondylitis) 720.0
  Marion's (bladder neck obstruction) 596.0
  Marsh's (exophthalmic goiter) 242.0 ✓5ᵗʰ
  Martin's 715.27
  mast cell 757.33
    systemic (M9741/3) 202.6 ✓5ᵗʰ
  mastoid (*see also* Mastoiditis) 383.9
    process 385.9
  maternal, unrelated to pregnancy NEC, affecting fetus or newborn 760.9
  Mathieu's (leptospiral jaundice) 100.0
  Mauclaire's 732.3
  Mauriac's (erythema nodosum syphiliticum) 091.3 ✓5ᵗʰ

Disease — Disease

Disease, diseased — *see also* Syndrome —
  continued
Maxcy's 081.0
McArdle (-Schmid-Pearson) (glycogenosis V)
  271.0
mediastinum NEC 519.3
Medin's (*see also* Poliomyelitis) 045.9 ✔5ᵗʰ
Mediterranean (with hemoglobinopathy) 282.4
medullary center (idiopathic) (respiratory) 348.8
Meige's (chronic hereditary edema) 757.0
Meleda 757.39
Ménétrier's (hypertrophic gastritis) 535.2 ✔5ᵗʰ
Ménière's (active) 386.00
  cochlear 386.02
  cochleovestibular 386.01
  inactive 386.04
  in remission 386.04
  vestibular 386.03
meningeal — *see* Meningitis
mental (*see also* Psychosis) 298.9
Merzbacher-Pelizaeus 330.0
mesenchymal 710.9
mesenteric embolic 557.0
metabolic NEC 277.9
metal polishers' 502
metastatic — *see* Metastasis
Mibelli's 757.39
microdrepanocytic 282.4
Miescher's 709.3
Mikulicz's (dryness of mouth, absent or
  decreased lacrimation) 527.1
Milkman (-Looser) (osteomalacia with
  pseudofractures) 268.2
Miller's (osteomalacia) 268.2
Mills' 335.29
Milroy's (chronic hereditary edema) 757.0
Minamata 985.0
Minor's 336.1
Minot's (hemorrhagic disease, newborn) 776.0
Minot-von Willebrand-Jürgens
  (angiohemophilia) 286.4
Mitchell's (erythromelalgia) 443.89
mitral — *see* Endocarditis, mitral
Mljet (mal de Meleda) 757.39
Möbius', Moebius' 346.8 ✔5ᵗʰ
Moeller's 267
Möller (-Barlow) (infantile scurvy) 267
Mönckeberg's (*see also* Arteriosclerosis,
  extremities) 440.20
Mondor's (thrombophlebitis of breast) 451.89
Monge's 993.2
Morel-Kraepelin (*see also* Schizophrenia)
  295.9 ✔5ᵗʰ
Morgagni's (syndrome) (hyperostosis frontalis
  interna) 733.3
Morgagni-Adams-Stokes (syncope with heart
  block) 426.9
Morquio (-Brailsford) (-Ullrich)
  (mucopolysaccharidosis IV) 277.5
Morton's (with metatarsalgia) 355.6
Morvan's 336.0
motor neuron (bulbar) (mixed type) 335.20
Mouchet's (juvenile osteochondrosis, foot)
  732.5
mouth 528.9
Moyamoya 437.5
Mucha's (acute parapsoriasis varioliformis)
  696.2
mu-chain 273.2
mucolipidosis (I) (II) (III) 272.7
Münchmeyer's (exostosis luxurians) 728.11
Murri's (intermittent hemoglobinuria) 283.2
muscle 359.9
  inflammatory 728.9
  ocular 378.9
musculoskeletal system 729.9
mushroom workers' 495.5
Myà's (congenital dilation, colon) 751.3
mycotic 117.9
myeloproliferative (chronic) (M9960/1) 238.7
myocardium, myocardial (*see also*
  Degeneration, myocardial) 429.1
  hypertensive (*see also* Hypertension, heart)
    402.90
  primary (idiopathic) 425.4
myoneural 358.9
Naegeli's 287.1

Disease, diseased — *see also* Syndrome —
  continued
nail 703.9
  specified type NEC 703.8
Nairobi sheep 066.1
nasal 478.1
  cavity NEC 478.1
  sinus (chronic) — *see* Sinusitis
navel (newborn) NEC 779.89 ▲
nemaline body 359.0
neoplastic, generalized (M8000/6) 199.0
nerve — *see* Disorder, nerve
nervous system (central) 349.9
  autonomic, peripheral (*see also* Neuropathy,
    peripheral, autonomic) 337.9
  congenital 742.9
  inflammatory — *see* Encephalitis
  parasympathetic (*see also* Neuropathy,
    peripheral, autonomic) 337.9
  peripheral NEC 355.9
  specified NEC 349.89
  sympathetic (*see also* Neuropathy,
    peripheral, autonomic) 337.9
  vegetative (*see also* Neuropathy, peripheral,
    autonomic) 337.9
Nettleship's (urticaria pigmentosa) 757.33
Neumann's (pemphigus vegetans) 694.4
neurologic (central) NEC (*see also* Disease,
  nervous system) 349.9
  peripheral NEC 355.9
neuromuscular system NEC 358.9
Newcastle 077.8
Nicolas (-Durand) — Favre (climatic bubo)
  099.1
Niemann-Pick (lipid histiocytosis) 272.7
nipple 611.9
  Paget's (M8540/3) 174.0
Nishimoto (-Takeuchi) 437.5
nonarthropod-borne NEC 078.89
  central nervous system NEC 049.9
  enterovirus NEC 078.89
non-autoimmune hemolytic NEC 283.10
Nonne-Milroy-Meige (chronic hereditary edema)
  757.0
Norrie's (congenital progressive
  oculoacousticocerebral degeneration)
  743.8
nose 478.1
nucleus pulposus — *see* Disease, intervertebral
  disc
nutritional 269.9
  maternal, affecting fetus or newborn 760.4
oasthouse, urine 270.2
obliterative vascular 447.1
Odelberg's (juvenile osteochondrosis) 732.1
Oguchi's (retina) 368.61
Ohara's (*see also* Tularemia) 021.9
Ollier's (chondrodysplasia) 756.4
Opitz's (congestive splenomegaly) 289.51
Oppenheim's 358.8
Oppenheim-Urbach (necrobiosis lipoidica
  diabeticorum) 250.8 ✔5ᵗʰ *[709.3]*
optic nerve NEC 377.49
orbit 376.9
  specified NEC 376.89
Oriental liver fluke 121.1
Oriental lung fluke 121.2
Ormond's 593.4
Osgood's tibia (tubercle) 732.4
Osgood-Schlatter 732.4
Osler (-Vaquez) (polycythemia vera) (M9950/1)
  238.4
Osler-Rendu (familial hemorrhagic
  telangiectasia) 448.0
osteofibrocystic 252.0
Otto's 715.35
outer ear 380.9
ovary (noninflammatory) NEC 620.9
  cystic 620.2
  polycystic 256.4
  specified NEC 620.8
Owren's (congenital) (*see also* Defect,
  coagulation) 286.3
Paas' 756.59
Paget's (osteitis deformans) 731.0
  with infiltrating duct carcinoma of the
    breast (M8541/3) — *see* Neoplasm,
    breast, malignant

Disease, diseased — *see also* Syndrome —
  continued
Paget's — *continued*
  bone 731.0
    osteosarcoma in (M9184/3) — *see*
      Neoplasm, bone, malignant
  breast (M8540/3) 174.0
  extramammary (M8542/3) — *see also*
    Neoplasm, skin, malignant
    anus 154.3
      skin 173.5
  malignant (M8540/3)
    breast 174.0
    specified site NEC (M8542/3) — *see*
      Neoplasm, skin, malignant
    unspecified site 174.0
  mammary (M8540/3) 174.0
  nipple (M8540/3) 174.0
palate (soft) 528.9
Paltauf-Sternberg 201.9 ✔5ᵗʰ
pancreas 577.9
  cystic 577.2
    congenital 751.7
  fibrocystic 277.00
Panner's 732.3
  capitellum humeri 732.3
  head of humerus 732.3
  tarsal navicular (bone) (osteochondrosis)
    732.5
panvalvular — *see* Endocarditis, mitral
parametrium 629.9
parasitic NEC 136.9
  cerebral NEC 123.9
  intestinal NEC 129
  mouth 112.0
  skin NEC 134.9
  specified type — *see* Infestation
  tongue 112.0
parathyroid (gland) 252.9
  specified NEC 252.8
Parkinson's 332.0
parodontal 523.9
Parrot's (syphilitic osteochondritis) 090.0
Parry's (exophthalmic goiter) 242.0 ✔5ᵗʰ
Parson's (exophthalmic goiter) 242.0 ✔5ᵗʰ
Pavy's 593.6
Paxton's (white piedra) 111.2
Payr's (splenic flexure syndrome) 569.89
pearl-workers' (chronic osteomyelitis) (*see also*
  Osteomyelitis) 730.1 ✔5ᵗʰ
Pel-Ebstein — *see* Disease, Hodgkin's
Pelizaeus-Merzbacher 330.0
  with dementia
    with behavioral disturbance
      330.0 *[294.11]*
    without behavioral disturbance
      330.0 *[294.10]*
Pellegrini-Stieda (calcification, knee joint)
  726.62
pelvis, pelvic
  female NEC 629.9
    specified NEC 629.8
  gonococcal (acute) 098.19
    chronic or duration of 2 months or over
      098.39
  infection (*see also* Disease, pelvis,
    inflammatory) 614.9
  inflammatory (female) (PID) 614.9
    with
      abortion — *see* Abortion, by type, with
        sepsis
      ectopic pregnancy (*see also* categories
        (633.0-633.9) 639.0
      molar pregnancy (*see also* categories
        630-632) 639.0
    acute 614.3
    chronic 614.4
    complicating pregnancy 646.6 ✔5ᵗʰ
      affecting fetus or newborn 760.8
    following
      abortion 639.0
      ectopic or molar pregnancy 639.0
    peritonitis (acute) 614.5
      chronic NEC 614.7
    puerperal, postpartum, childbirth
      670 ✔4ᵗʰ
    specified NEC 614.8

Disease, diseased — *see also* Syndrome — *continued*

pelvis, pelvic — *continued*
  organ, female NEC 629.9
    specified NEC 629.8
    peritoneum, female NEC 629.9
      specified NEC 629.8
penis 607.9
  inflammatory 607.2
peptic NEC 536.9
  acid 536.8
periapical tissues NEC 522.9
pericardium 423.9
  specified type NEC 423.8
perineum
  female
    inflammatory 616.9
      specified NEC 616.8
    noninflammatory 624.9
      specified NEC 624.8
  male (inflammatory) 682.2
periodic (familial) (Reimann's) NEC 277.3
  paralysis 359.3
periodontal NEC 523.9
  specified NEC 523.8
periosteum 733.90
peripheral
  arterial 443.9
  autonomic nervous system (*see also* Neuropathy, autonomic) 337.9
  nerve NEC (*see also* Neuropathy) 356.9
    multiple — *see* Polyneuropathy
  vascular 443.9
    specified type NEC 443.89
peritoneum 568.9
  pelvic, female 629.9
    specified NEC 629.8
Perrin-Ferraton (snapping hip) 719.65
persistent mucosal (middle ear) (with posterior or superior marginal perforation of ear drum) 382.2
Perthes' (capital femoral osteochondrosis) 732.1
Petit's (*see also* Hernia, lumbar) 553.8
Peutz-Jeghers 759.6
Peyronie's 607.89
Pfeiffer's (infectious mononucleosis) 075
pharynx 478.20
Phocas' 610.1
photochromogenic (acid-fast bacilli) (pulmonary) 031.0
  nonpulmonary 031.9
Pick's
  brain 331.1
    with dementia
      with behavioral disturbance 331.1 *[294.11]*
      without behavioral disturbance 331.1 *[294.10]*
  cerebral atrophy 331.1
    with dementia
      with behavioral disturbance 331.1 *[294.11]*
      without behavioral disturbance 331.1 *[294.10]*
  lipid histiocytosis 272.7
  liver (pericardial pseudocirrhosis of liver) 423.2
  pericardium (pericardial pseudocirrhosis of liver) 423.2
  polyserositis (pericardial pseudocirrhosis of liver) 423.2
Pierson's (osteochondrosis) 732.1
pigeon fanciers' or breeders' 495.2
pineal gland 259.8
pink 985.0
Pinkus' (lichen nitidus) 697.1
pinworm 127.4
pituitary (gland) 253.9
  hyperfunction 253.1
  hypofunction 253.2
pituitary snuff-takers' 495.8
placenta
  affecting fetus or newborn 762.2
  complicating pregnancy or childbirth 656.7 ✔5ᵗʰ
pleura (cavity) (*see also* Pleurisy) 511.0
Plummer's (toxic nodular goiter) 242.3 ✔5ᵗʰ

Disease, diseased — *see also* Syndrome — *continued*

pneumatic
  drill 994.9
  hammer 994.9
policeman's 729.2
Pollitzer's (hidradenitis suppurativa) 705.83
polycystic (congenital) 759.89
  kidney or renal 753.12
    adult type (APKD) 753.13
    autosomal dominant 753.13
    autosomal recessive 753.14
    childhood type (CPKD) 753.14
    infantile type 753.14
  liver or hepatic 751.62
  lung or pulmonary 518.89
    congenital 748.4
  ovary, ovaries 256.4
  spleen 759.0
Pompe's (glycogenosis II) 271.0
Poncet's (tuberculous rheumatism) (*see also* Tuberculosis) 015.9 ✔5ᵗʰ
Posada-Wernicke 114.9
Potain's (pulmonary edema) 514
Pott's (*see also* Tuberculosis) 015.0 ✔5ᵗʰ *[730.88]*
  osteomyelitis 015.0 ✔5ᵗʰ *[730.88]*
  paraplegia 015.0 ✔5ᵗʰ *[730.88]*
  spinal curvature 015.0 ✔5ᵗʰ *[737.43]*
  spondylitis 015.0 ✔5ᵗʰ *[720.81]*
Potter's 753.0
Poulet's 714.2
pregnancy NEC (*see also* Pregnancy) 646.9 ✔5ᵗʰ
Preiser's (osteoporosis) 733.09
Pringle's (tuberous sclerosis) 759.5
Profichet's 729.9
prostate 602.9
  specified type NEC 602.8
protozoal NEC 136.8
  intestine, intestinal NEC 007.9
pseudo-Hurler's (mucolipidosis III) 272.7
psychiatric (*see also* Psychosis) 298.9
psychotic (*see also* Psychosis) 298.9
Puente's (simple glandular cheilitis) 528.5
puerperal NEC (*see also* Puerperal) 674.9 ✔5ᵗʰ
pulmonary — *see also* Disease, lung
  amyloid 277.3 *[517.8]*
  artery 417.9
  circulation, circulatory 417.9
    specified NEC 417.8
  diffuse obstructive (chronic) 496
    with
      acute exacerbation NEC 491.21
      asthma (chronic) (obstructive) 493.2 ✔5ᵗʰ
  heart (chronic) 416.9
    specified NEC 416.8
  hypertensive (vascular) 416.0
    cardiovascular 416.0
  obstructive diffuse (chronic) 496
    with
      acute exacerbation NEC 491.21
      asthma (chronic) (obstructive) 493.2 ✔5ᵗʰ
      bronchitis (chronic) 491.20
        with acute exacerbation 491.21
  valve (*see also* Endocarditis, pulmonary) 424.3
pulp (dental) NEC 522.9
pulseless 446.7
Putnam's (subacute combined sclerosis with pernicious anemia) 281.0 *[336.2]*
Pyle (-Cohn) (craniometaphyseal dysplasia) 756.89
pyramidal tract 333.90
Quervain's
  tendon sheath 727.04
  thyroid (subacute granulomatous thyroiditis) 245.1
Quincke's — *see* Edema, angioneurotic
Quinquaud (acne decalvans) 704.09
rag sorters' 022.1
Raynaud's (paroxysmal digital cyanosis) 443.0
reactive airway — *see* Asthma
Recklinghausen's (M9540/1) 237.71
  bone (osteitis fibrosa cystica) 252.0
Recklinghausen-Applebaum (hemochromatosis) 275.0

Disease, diseased — *see also* Syndrome — *continued*

Reclus' (cystic) 610.1
rectum NEC 569.49
Refsum's (heredopathia atactica polyneuritiformis) 356.3
Reichmann's (gastrosuccorrhea) 536.8
Reimann's (periodic) 277.3
Reiter's 099.3
renal (functional) (pelvis) 593.9
  with
    edema (*see also* Nephrosis) 581.9
    exudative nephritis 583.89
    lesion of interstitial nephritis 583.89
    stated generalized cause — *see* Nephritis
  acute — *see* Nephritis, acute
  basement membrane NEC 583.89
    with
      pulmonary hemorrhage (Goodpasture's syndrome) 446.21 *[583.81]*
  chronic — *see* Nephritis, chronic
  complicating pregnancy or puerperium NEC 646.2 ✔5ᵗʰ
    with hypertension — *see* Toxemia, of pregnancy
    affecting fetus or newborn 760.1
  cystic, congenital (*see also* Cystic, disease, kidney) 753.10
  diabetic 250.4 ✔5ᵗʰ *[583.81]*
  due to
    amyloidosis 277.3 *[583.81]*
    diabetes mellitus 250.4 ✔5ᵗʰ *[583.81]*
    systemic lupus erythematosis 710.0 *[583.81]*
  end-stage 585
  exudative 583.89
  fibrocystic (congenital) 753.19
  gonococcal 098.19 *[583.81]*
  gouty 274.10
  hypertensive (*see also* Hypertension, kidney) 403.90
  immune complex NEC 583.89
  interstitial (diffuse) (focal) 583.89
  lupus 710.0 *[583.81]*
  maternal, affecting fetus or newborn 760.1
    hypertensive 760.0
  phosphate-losing (tubular) 588.0
  polycystic (congenital) 753.12
    adult type (APKD) 753.13
    autosomal dominant 753.13
    autosomal recessive 753.14
    childhood type (CPKD) 753.14
    infantile type 753.14
  specified lesion or cause NEC (*see also* Glomerulonephritis) 583.89
  subacute 581.9
  syphilitic 095.4
  tuberculous (*see also* Tuberculosis) 016.0 ✔5ᵗʰ *[583.81]*
  tubular (*see also* Nephrosis, tubular) 584.5
Rendu-Osler-Weber (familial hemorrhagic telangiectasia) 448.0
renovascular (arteriosclerotic) (*see also* Hypertension, kidney) 403.90
respiratory (tract) 519.9
  acute or subacute (upper) NEC 465.9
    due to fumes or vapors 506.3
    multiple sites NEC 465.8
    noninfectious 478.9
    streptococcal 034.0
  chronic 519.9
    arising in the perinatal period 770.7
    due to fumes or vapors 506.4
  due to
    aspiration of liquids or solids 508.9
    external agents NEC 508.9
      specified NEC 508.8
    fumes or vapors 506.9
      acute or subacute NEC 506.3
      chronic 506.4
  fetus or newborn NEC 770.9
  obstructive 496
  specified type NEC 519.8
  upper (acute) (infectious) NEC 465.9
    multiple sites NEC 465.8
    noninfectious NEC 478.9
    streptococcal 034.0

Disease — Disease

Disease, diseased — *see also* Syndrome — *continued*

retina, retinal NEC 362.9
    Batten's or Batten-Mayou 330.1 *[362.71]*
    degeneration 362.89
    vascular lesion 362.17
rheumatic (*see also* Arthritis) 716.8 ✓5ᵗʰ
    heart — *see* Disease, heart, rheumatic
rheumatoid (heart) — *see* Arthritis, rheumatoid
rickettsial NEC 083.9
    specified type NEC 083.8
Riedel's (ligneous thyroiditis) 245.3
Riga (-Fede) (cachectic aphthae) 529.0
Riggs' (compound periodontitis) 523.4
Ritter's 695.81
Rivalta's (cervicofacial actinomycosis) 039.3
Robles' (onchocerciasis) 125.3 *[360.13]*
Roger's (congenital interventricular septal defect) 745.4
Rokitansky's (*see also* Necrosis, liver) 570
Romberg's 349.89
Rosenthal's (factor XI deficiency) 286.2
Rossbach's (hyperchlorhydria) 536.8
    psychogenic 306.4
Roth (-Bernhardt) 355.1
Runeberg's (progressive pernicious anemia) 281.0
Rust's (tuberculous spondylitis) (*see also* Tuberculosis) 015.0 ✓5ᵗʰ *[720.81]*
Rustitskii's (multiple myeloma) (M9730/3) 203.0 ✓5ᵗʰ
Ruysch's (Hirschsprung's disease) 751.3
Sachs (-Tay) 330.1
sacroiliac NEC 724.6
salivary gland or duct NEC 527.9
    inclusion 078.5
        streptococcal 034.0
    virus 078.5
Sander's (paranoia) 297.1
Sandhoff's 330.1
sandworm 126.9
Savill's (epidemic exfoliative dermatitis) 695.89
Schamberg's (progressive pigmentary dermatosis) 709.09
Schaumann's (sarcoidosis) 135
Schenck's (sporotrichosis) 117.1
Scheuermann's (osteochondrosis) 732.0
Schilder (-Flatau) 341.1
Schimmelbusch's 610.1
Schlatter's tibia (tubercle) 732.4
Schlatter-Osgood 732.4
Schmorl's 722.30
    cervical 722.39
    lumbar, lumbosacral 722.32
    specified region NEC 722.39
    thoracic, thoracolumbar 722.31
Scholz's 330.0
Schönlein (-Henoch) (purpura rheumatica) 287.0
Schottmüller's (*see also* Fever, paratyphoid) 002.9
Schüller-Christian (chronic histiocytosis X) 277.8
Schultz's (agranulocytosis) 288.0
Schwalbe-Ziehen-Oppenheimer 333.6
Schweninger-Buzzi (macular atrophy) 701.3
sclera 379.19
scrofulous (*see also* Tuberculosis) 017.2 ✓5ᵗʰ
scrotum 608.9
sebaceous glands NEC 706.9
Secretan's (posttraumatic edema) 782.3
semilunar cartilage, cystic 717.5
seminal vesicle 608.9
Senear-Usher (pemphigus erythematosus) 694.4
serum NEC 999.5
Sever's (osteochondrosis calcaneum) 732.5
Sézary's (reticulosis) (M9701/3) 202.2 ✓5ᵗʰ
Shaver's (bauxite pneumoconiosis) 503
Sheehan's (postpartum pituitary necrosis) 253.2
shimamushi (scrub typus) 081.2
shipyard 077.1
sickle cell 282.60
    with
        crisis 282.62
        Hb-S disease 282.61

Disease, diseased — *see also* Syndrome — *continued*

sickle cell — *continued*
    with — *continued*
        other abnormal hemoglobin (Hb-D) (Hb-E) (Hb-G) (Hb-J) (Hb-K) (Hb-O) (Hb-P) (high fetal gene) 282.69
    elliptocytosis 282.60
    Hb-C 282.63
    Hb-S 282.61
        with
            crisis 282.62
            Hb-C 282.63
            other abnormal hemoglobin (Hb-D) (Hb-E) (Hb-G) (Hb-J) (Hb-K) (Hb-O) (Hb-P) (high fetal gene) 282.69
    spherocytosis 282.60
    thalassemia 282.4
Siegal-Cattan-Mamou (periodic) 277.3
silo fillers' 506.9
Simian B 054.3
Simmonds' (pituitary cachexia) 253.2
Simons' (progressive lipodystrophy) 272.6
Sinding-Larsen (juvenile osteopathia patellae) 732.4
sinus — *see also* Sinusitis
    brain 437.9
    specified NEC 478.1
Sirkari's 085.0
sixth 057.8
Sjögren (-Gougerot) 710.2
    with lung involvement 710.2 *[517.8]*
Skevas-Zerfus 989.5
skin NEC 709.9
    due to metabolic disorder 277.9
    specified type NEC 709.8
sleeping 347
    meaning sleeping sickness (*see also* Trypanosomiasis) 086.5
small vessel 443.9
Smith-Strang (oasthouse urine) 270.2
Sneddon-Wilkinson (subcorneal pustular dermatosis) 694.1
South African creeping 133.8
Spencer's (epidemic vomiting) 078.82
Spielmeyer-Stock 330.1
Spielmeyer-Vogt 330.1
spine, spinal 733.90
    combined system (*see also* Degeneration, combined) 266.2 *[336.2]*
        with pernicious anemia 281.0 *[336.2]*
    cord NEC 336.9
        congenital 742.9
    demyelinating NEC 341.8
    joint (*see also* Disease, joint, spine) 724.9
        tuberculous 015.0 ✓5ᵗʰ *[730.8]* ✓5ᵗʰ
spinocerebellar 334.9
    specified NEC 334.8
spleen (organic) (postinfectional) 289.50
    amyloid 277.3
    lardaceous 277.3
    polycystic 759.0
    specified NEC 289.59
sponge divers' 989.5
Stanton's (melioidosis) 025
Stargardt's 362.75
Steinert's 359.2
Sternberg's — *see* Disease, Hodgkin's
Stevens-Johnson (erythema multiforme exudativum) 695.1
Sticker's (erythema infectiosum) 057.0
Stieda's (calcification, knee joint) 726.62
Still's (juvenile rheumatoid arthritis) 714.30
Stiller's (asthenia) 780.79
Stokes' (exophthalmic goiter) 242.0 ✓5ᵗʰ
Stokes-Adams (syncope with heart block) 426.9
Stokvis (-Talma) (enterogenous cyanosis) 289.7
stomach NEC (organic) 537.9
    functional 536.9
        psychogenic 306.4
    lardaceous 277.3
stonemasons' 502
storage
    glycogen (*see also* Disease, glycogen storage) 271.0
    lipid 272.7
    mucopolysaccharide 277.5

Disease, diseased — *see also* Syndrome — *continued*

striatopallidal system 333.90
    specified NEC 333.89
Strümpell-Marie (ankylosing spondylitis) 720.0
Stuart's (congenital factor X deficiency) (*see also* Defect, coagulation) 286.3
Stuart-Prower (congenital factor X deficiency) (*see also* Defect, coagulation) 286.3
Sturge (-Weber) (-Dimitri) (encephalocutaneous angiomatosis) 759.6
Stuttgart 100.89
Sudeck's 733.7
supporting structures of teeth NEC 525.9
suprarenal (gland) (capsule) 255.9
    hyperfunction 255.3
    hypofunction 255.4
Sutton's 709.09
Sutton and Gull's — *see* Hypertension, kidney
sweat glands NEC 705.9
    specified type NEC 705.89
sweating 078.2
Sweeley-Klionsky 272.4
Swift (-Feer) 985.0
swimming pool (bacillus) 031.1
swineherd's 100.89
Sylvest's (epidemic pleurodynia) 074.1
Symmers (follicular lymphoma) (M9690/3) 202.0 ✓5ᵗʰ
sympathetic nervous system (*see also* Neuropathy, peripheral, autonomic) 337.9
synovium 727.9
syphilitic — *see* Syphilis
systemic tissue mast cell (M9741/3) 202.6 ✓5ᵗʰ
Taenzer's 757.4
Takayasu's (pulseless) 446.7
Talma's 728.85
Tangier (familial high-density lipoprotein deficiency) 272.5
Tarral-Besnier (pityriasis rubra pilaris) 696.4
Tay-Sachs 330.1
Taylor's 701.8
tear duct 375.69
teeth, tooth 525.9
    hard tissues NEC 521.9
    pulp NEC 522.9
tendon 727.9
    inflammatory NEC 727.9
terminal vessel 443.9
testis 608.9
Thaysen-Gee (nontropical sprue) 579.0
Thomsen's 359.2
Thomson's (congenital poikiloderma) 757.33
Thornwaldt's, Tornwaldt's (pharyngeal bursitis) 478.29
throat 478.20
    septic 034.0
thromboembolic (*see also* Embolism) 444.9
thymus (gland) 254.9
    specified NEC 254.8
thyroid (gland) NEC 246.9
    heart (*see also* Hyperthyroidism) 242.9 ✓5ᵗʰ *[425.7]*
    lardaceous 277.3
    specified NEC 246.8
Tietze's 733.6
Tommaselli's
    correct substance properly administered 599.7
    overdose or wrong substance given or taken 961.4
tongue 529.9
tonsils, tonsillar (and adenoids) (chronic) 474.9
    specified NEC 474.8
tooth, teeth 525.9
    hard tissues NEC 521.9
    pulp NEC 522.9
Tornwaldt's (pharyngeal bursitis) 478.29
Tourette's 307.23
trachea 519.1
tricuspid — *see* Endocarditis, tricuspid
triglyceride-storage, type I, II, III 272.7
triple vessel (coronary arteries) — *see* Arteriosclerosis, coronary
trisymptomatic, Gourgerot's 709.1
trophoblastic (*see also* Hydatidiform mole) 630
    previous, affecting management of pregnancy V23.1

✓4ᵗʰ Fourth-digit Required   ✓5ᵗʰ Fifth-digit Required   ▶◀ Revised Text   ● New Line   ▲ Revised Code

Disease, diseased — *see also* Syndrome — *continued*
 tsutsugamushi (scrub typhus) 081.2
 tube (fallopian), noninflammatory 620.9
  specified NEC 620.8
 tuberculous NEC (*see also* Tuberculosis) 011.9 ✔5ᵗʰ
 tubo-ovarian
  inflammatory (*see also* Salpingo-oophoritis) 614.2
  noninflammatory 620.9
   specified NEC 620.8
 tubotympanic, chronic (with anterior perforation of ear drum) 382.1
 tympanum 385.9
 Uhl's 746.84
 umbilicus (newborn) NEC 779.89   ▲
 Underwood's (sclerema neonatorum) 778.1
 undiagnosed 799.9
 Unna's (seborrheic dermatitis) 690.18
 unstable hemoglobin hemolytic 282.7
 Unverricht (-Lundborg) 333.2
 Urbach-Oppenheim (necrobiosis lipoidica diabeticorum) 250.8 ✔5ᵗʰ [709.3]
 Urbach-Wiethe (lipoid proteinosis) 272.8
 ureter 593.9
 urethra 599.9
  specified type NEC 599.84
 urinary (tract) 599.9
  bladder 596.9
   specified NEC 596.8
  maternal, affecting fetus or newborn 760.1
 Usher-Senear (pemphigus erythematosus) 694.4
 uterus (organic) 621.9
  infective (*see also* Endometritis) 615.9
  inflammatory (*see also* Endometritis) 615.9
  noninflammatory 621.9
   specified type NEC 621.8
 uveal tract
  anterior 364.9
  posterior 363.9
 vagabonds' 132.1
 vagina, vaginal
  inflammatory 616.9
   specified NEC 616.8
  noninflammatory 623.9
   specified NEC 623.8
 Valsuani's (progressive pernicious anemia, puerperal) 648.2 ✔5ᵗʰ
  complicating pregnancy or puerperium 648.2 ✔5ᵗʰ
 valve, valvular — *see* Endocarditis
 van Bogaert-Nijssen (-Peiffer) 330.0
 van Creveld-von Gierke (glycogenosis I) 271.0
 van den Bergh's (enterogenous cyanosis) 289.7
 van Neck's (juvenile osteochondrosis) 732.1
 Vaquez (-Osler) (polycythemia vera) (M9950/1) 238.4
 vascular 459.9
  arteriosclerotic — *see* Arteriosclerosis
  hypertensive — *see* Hypertension
  obliterative 447.1
   peripheral 443.9
  occlusive 459.9
  peripheral (occlusive) 443.9
   in diabetes mellitus 250.7 ✔5ᵗʰ [443.81]
   specified type NEC 443.89
 vas deferens 608.9
 vasomotor 443.9
 vasopastic 443.9
 vein 459.9
 venereal 099.9
  chlamydial NEC 099.50
   anus 099.52
   bladder 099.53
   cervix 099.53
   epididymis 099.54
   genitourinary NEC 099.55
    lower 099.53
     specified NEC 099.54
   pelvic inflammatory disease 099.54
   perihepatic 099.56
   peritoneum 099.56
   pharynx 099.51
   rectum 099.52
   specified site NEC 099.54

Disease, diseased — *see also* Syndrome — *continued*
 venereal — *continued*
  chlamydial NEC — *continued*
   testis 099.54
   vagina 099.53
   vulva 099.53
  fifth 099.1
  sixth 099.1
  complicating pregnancy, childbirth, or puerperium 647.2 ✔5ᵗʰ
  specified nature or type NEC 099.8
   chlamydial — *see* Disease, venereal, chlamydial
 Verneuil's (syphilitic bursitis) 095.7
 Verse's (calcinosis intervertebralis) 275.49 [722.90]
 vertebra, vertebral NEC 733.90
  disc — *see* Disease, Intervertebral disc
 vibration NEC 994.9
 Vidal's (lichen simplex chronicus) 698.3
 Vincent's (trench mouth) 101
 Virchow's 733.99
 virus (filterable) NEC 078.89
  arbovirus NEC 066.9
  arthropod-borne NEC 066.9
  central nervous system NEC 049.9
   specified type NEC 049.8
  complicating pregnancy, childbirth, or puerperium 647.6 ✔5ᵗʰ
  contact (with) V01.7
  exposure to V01.7
  Marburg 078.89
  maternal
   with fetal damage affecting management of pregnancy 655.3 ✔5ᵗʰ
  nonarthropod-borne NEC 078.89
   central nervous sytem NEC 049.9
    specified NEC 049.8
 vitreous 379.29
 vocal cords NEC 478.5
 Vogt's (Cecile) 333.7
 Vogt-Spielmeyer 330.1
 Volhard-Fahr (malignant nephrosclerosis) 403.00
 Volkmann's
  acquired 958.6
 von Bechterew's (ankylosing spondylitis) 720.0
 von Economo's (encephalitis lethargica) 049.8
 von Eulenburg's (congenital paramyotonia) 359.2
 von Gierke's (glycogenosis I) 271.0
 von Graefe's 378.72
 von Hippel's (retinocerebral angiomatosis) 759.6
 von Hippel-Lindau (angiomatosis retinocerebellosa) 759.6
 von Jaksch's (pseudoleukemia infantum) 285.8
 von Recklinghausen's (M9540/1) 237.71
  bone (osteitis fibrosa cystica) 252.0
 von Recklinghausen-Applebaum (hemochromatosis) 275.0
 von Willebrand (-Jürgens) (angiohemophilia) 286.4
 von Zambusch's (lichen sclerosus et atrophicus) 701.0
 Voorhoeve's (dyschondroplasia) 756.4
 Vrolik's (osteogenesis imperfecta) 756.51
 vulva
  noninflammatory 624.9
   specified NEC 624.8
 Wagner's (colloid milium) 709.3
 Waldenström's (osteochondrosis capital femoral) 732.1
 Wallgren's (obstruction of splenic vein with collateral circulation) 459.89
 Wardrop's (with lymphangitis) 681.9
  finger 681.02
  toe 681.11
 Wassilieff's (leptospiral jaundice) 100.0
 wasting NEC 799.4
  due to malnutrition 261
  paralysis 335.21
 Waterhouse-Friderichsen 036.3
 waxy (any site) 277.3
 Weber-Christian (nodular nonsuppurative panniculitis) 729.30

Disease, diseased — *see also* Syndrome — *continued*
 Wegner's (syphilitic osteochondritis) 090.0
 Weil's (leptospral jaundice) 100.0
  of lung 100.0
 Weir Mitchell's (erythromelalgia) 443.89
 Werdnig-Hoffmann 335.0
 Werlhof's (*see also* Purpura, thrombocytopenic) 287.3
 Wermer's 258.0
 Werner's (progeria adultorum) 259.8
 Werner-His (trench fever) 083.1
 Werner-Schultz (agranulocytosis) 288.0
 Wernicke's (superior hemorrhagic polioencephalitis) 265.1
 Wernicke-Posadas 114.9
 Whipple's (intestinal lipodystrophy) 040.2
 whipworm 127.3
 white
  blood cell 288.9
   specified NEC 288.8
  spot 701.0
 White's (congenital) (keratosis follicularis) 757.39
 Whitmore's (melioidosis) 025
 Widal-Abrami (acquired hemolytic jaundice) 283.9
 Wilkie's 557.1
 Wilkinson-Sneddon (subcorneal pustular dermatosis) 694.1
 Willis' (diabetes mellitus) (*see also* Diabetes) 250.0 ✔5ᵗʰ
 Wilson's (hepatolenticular degeneration) 275.1
 Wilson-Brocq (dermatitis exfoliativa) 695.89
 winter vomiting 078.82
 Wise's 696.2
 Wohlfart-Kugelberg-Welander 335.11
 Woillez's (acute idiopathic pulmonary congestion) 518.5
 Wolman's (primary familial xanthomatosis) 272.7
 wool-sorters' 022.1
 Zagari's (xerostomia) 527.7
 Zahorsky's (exanthem subitum) 057.8
 Ziehen-Oppenheim 333.6
 zoonotic, bacterial NEC 027.9
  specified type NEC 027.8
Disfigurement (due to scar) 709.2
 head V48.6
 limb V49.4
 neck V48.7
 trunk V48.7

Disgerminoma — *see* Dysgerminoma

Disinsertion, retina 361.04

Disintegration, complete, of the body 799.8
 traumatic 869.1

Disk kidney 753.3

Dislocatable hip, congenital (*see also* Dislocation, hip, congenital) 754.30

Dislocation (articulation) (closed) (displacement) (simple) (subluxation) 839.8

Note — "Closed" includes simple, complete, partial, uncomplicated, and unspecified dislocation.

"Open" includes dislocation specified as infected or compound and dislocation with foreign body.

"Chronic," "habitual," "old," or "recurrent" dislocations should be coded as indicated under the entry "Dislocation, recurrent," and "pathological" as indicated under the entry "Dislocation, pathological."

For late effect of dislocation see Late, effect, dislocation.

 with fracture — *see* Fracture, by site
 acromioclavicular (joint) (closed) 831.04
  open 831.14
 anatomical site (closed)
  specified NEC 839.69
   open 839.79
  unspecified or ill-defined 839.8
   open 839.9

Disease — Dislocation

Dislocation — continued

ankle (scaphoid bone) (closed) 837.0
  open 837.1
arm (closed) 839.8
  open 839.9
astragalus (closed) 837.0
  open 837.1
atlanto-axial (closed) 839.01
  open 839.11
atlas (closed) 839.01
  open 839.11
axis (closed) 839.02
  open 839.12
back (closed) 839.8
  open 839.9
Bell-Daly 723.8
breast bone (closed) 839.61
  open 839.71
capsule, joint — see Dislocation, by site
carpal (bone) — see Dislocation, wrist
carpometacarpal (joint) (closed) 833.04
  open 833.14
cartilage (joint) — see also Dislocation, by site
  knee — see Tear, meniscus
cervical, cervicodorsal, or cervicothoracic
  (spine) (vertebra) — see Dislocation,
  vertebra, cervical
chiropractic (see also Lesion, nonallopathic)
  739.9
chondrocostal — see Dislocation, costochondral
chronic — see Dislocation, recurrent
clavicle (closed) 831.04
  open 831.14
coccyx (closed) 839.41
  open 839.51
collar bone (closed) 831.04
  open 831.14
compound (open) NEC 839.9
congenital NEC 755.8
  hip (see also Dislocation, hip, congenital)
    754.30
  lens 743.37
  rib 756.3
  sacroiliac 755.69
  spine NEC 756.19
  vertebra 756.19
coracoid (closed) 831.09
  open 831.19
costal cartilage (closed) 839.69
  open 839.79
costochondral (closed) 839.69
  open 839.79
cricoarytenoid articulation (closed) 839.69
  open 839.79
cricothyroid (cartilage) articulation (closed)
  839.69
  open 839.79
dorsal vertebrae (closed) 839.21
  open 839.31
ear ossicle 385.23
elbow (closed) 832.00
  anterior (closed) 832.01
    open 832.11
  congenital 754.89
  divergent (closed) 832.09
    open 832.19
  lateral (closed) 832.04
    open 832.14
  medial (closed) 832.03
    open 832.13
  open 832.10
  posterior (closed) 832.02
    open 832.12
  recurrent 718.32
  specified type NEC 832.09
    open 832.19
eye 360.81
  lateral 376.36
eyeball 360.81
  lateral 376.36
femur
  distal end (closed) 836.50
    anterior 836.52
      open 836.62
    lateral 836.53
      open 836.63

Dislocation — continued

femur — continued
  distal end — continued
    medial 836.54
      open 836.64
    open 836.60
    posterior 836.51
      open 836.61
  proximal end (closed) 835.00
    anterior (pubic) 835.03
      open 835.13
    obturator 835.02
      open 835.12
    open 835.10
    posterior 835.01
      open 835.11
fibula
  distal end (closed) 837.0
    open 837.1
  proximal end (closed) 836.59
    open 836.69
finger(s) (phalanx) (thumb) (closed) 834.00
  interphalangeal (joint) 834.02
    open 834.12
  metacarpal (bone), distal end 834.01
    open 834.11
  metacarpophalangeal (joint) 834.01
    open 834.11
  open 834.10
  recurrent 718.34
foot (closed) 838.00
  open 838.10
  recurrent 718.37
forearm (closed) 839.8
  open 839.9
fracture — see Fracture, by site
glenoid (closed) 831.09
  open 831.19
habitual — see Dislocation, recurrent
hand (closed) 839.8
  open 839.9
hip (closed) 835.00
  anterior 835.03
    obturator 835.02
      open 835.12
    open 835.13
  congenital (unilateral) 754.30
    with subluxation of other hip 754.35
    bilateral 754.31
  developmental 718.75
  open 835.10
  posterior 835.01
    open 835.11
  recurrent 718.35
humerus (closed) 831.00
  distal end (see also Dislocation, elbow)
    832.00
  open 831.10
  proximal end (closed) 831.00
    anterior (subclavicular) (subcoracoid)
      (subglenoid) (closed) 831.01
      open 831.11
    inferior (closed) 831.03
      open 831.13
    open 831.10
    posterior (closed) 831.02
      open 831.12
implant — see Complications, mechanical
incus 385.23
infracoracoid (closed) 831.01
  open 831.11
innominate (pubic juntion) (sacral junction)
  (closed) 839.69
  acetabulum (see also Dislocation, hip)
    835.00
  open 839.79
interphalangeal (joint)
  finger or hand (closed) 834.02
    open 834.12
  foot or toe (closed) 838.06
    open 838.16
jaw (cartilage) (meniscus) (closed) 830.0
  open 830.1
  recurrent 524.69
joint NEC (closed) 839.8
  developmental 718.7 [5th]
  open 839.9

Dislocation — continued

joint NEC — continued
  pathological — see Dislocation, pathological
  recurrent — see Dislocation, recurrent
knee (closed) 836.50
  anterior 836.51
    open 836.61
  congenital (with genu recurvatum) 754.41
  habitual 718.36
  lateral 836.54
    open 836.64
  medial 836.53
    open 836.63
  old 718.36
  open 836.60
  posterior 836.52
    open 836.62
  recurrent 718.36
  rotatory 836.59
    open 836.69
lacrimal gland 375.16
leg (closed) 839.8
  open 839.9
lens (crystalline) (complete) (partial) 379.32
  anterior 379.33
  congenital 743.37
  ocular implant 996.53
  posterior 379.34
  traumatic 921.3
ligament — see Dislocation, by site
lumbar (vertebrae) (closed) 839.20
  open 839.30
lumbosacral (vertebrae) (closed) 839.20
  congenital 756.19
  open 839.30
mandible (closed) 830.0
  open 830.1
maxilla (inferior) (closed) 830.0
  open 830.1
meniscus (knee) — see also Tear, meniscus
  other sites — see Dislocation, by site
metacarpal (bone)
  distal end (closed) 834.01
    open 834.11
  proximal end (closed) 833.05
    open 833.15
metacarpophalangeal (joint) (closed) 834.01
  open 834.11
metatarsal (bone) (closed) 838.04
  open 838.14
metatarsophalangeal (joint) (closed) 838.05
  open 838.15
midcarpal (joint) (closed) 833.03
  open 833.13
midtarsal (joint) (closed) 838.02
  open 838.12
Monteggia's — see Dislocation, hip
multiple locations (except fingers only or toes
  only) (closed) 839.8
  open 839.9
navicular (bone) foot (closed) 837.0
  open 837.1
neck (see also Dislocation, vertebra, cervical)
  839.00
Nélaton's — see Dislocation, ankle
nontraumatic (joint) — see Dislocation,
  pathological
nose (closed) 839.69
  open 839.79
not recurrent, not current injury — see
  Dislocation, pathological
occiput from atlas (closed) 839.01
  open 839.11
old — see Dislocation, recurrent
open (compound) NEC 839.9
ossicle, ear 385.23
paralytic (flaccid) (spastic) — see Dislocation,
  pathological
patella (closed) 836.3
  congenital 755.64
  open 836.4
pathological NEC 718.20
  ankle 718.27
  elbow 718.22
  foot 718.27
  hand 718.24
  hip 718.25
  knee 718.26

Dislocation — *continued*
pathological NEC — *continued*
lumbosacral joint 724.6
multiple sites 718.29
pelvic region 718.25
sacroiliac 724.6
shoulder (region) 718.21
specified site NEC 718.28
spine 724.8
sacroiliac 724.6
wrist 718.23
pelvis (closed) 839.69
acetabulum (*see also* Dislocation, hip) 835.00
open 839.79
phalanx
foot or toe (closed) 838.09
open 838.19
hand or finger (*see also* Dislocation, finger) 834.00
postpoliomyelitic — *see* Dislocation, pathological
prosthesis, internal — *see* Complications, mechanical
radiocarpal (joint) (closed) 833.02
open 833.12
radioulnar (joint)
distal end (closed) 833.01
open 833.11
proximal end (*see also* Dislocation, elbow) 832.00
radius
distal end (closed) 833.00
open 833.10
proximal end (closed) 832.01
open 832.11
recurrent (*see also* Derangement, joint, recurrent) 718.3 ✓5ᵗʰ
elbow 718.32
hip 718.35
joint NEC 718.38
knee 718.36
lumbosacral (joint) 724.6
patella 718.36
sacroiliac 724.6
shoulder 718.31
temporomandibular 524.69
rib (cartilage) (closed) 839.69
congenital 756.3
open 839.79
sacrococcygeal (closed) 839.42
open 839.52
sacroiliac (joint) (ligament) (closed) 839.42
congenital 755.69
open 839.52
recurrent 724.6
sacrum (closed) 839.42
open 839.52
scaphoid (bone)
ankle or foot (closed) 837.0
open 837.1
wrist (closed) (*see also* Dislocation, wrist) 833.00
open 833.10
scapula (closed) 831.09
open 831.19
semilunar cartilage, knee — *see* Tear, meniscus
septal cartilage (nose) (closed) 839.69
open 839.79
septum (nasal) (old) 470
sesamoid bone — *see* Dislocation, by site
shoulder (blade) (ligament) (closed) 831.00
anterior (subclavicular) (subcoracoid) (subglenoid) (closed) 831.01
open 831.11
chronic 718.31
inferior 831.03
open 831.13
open 831.10
posterior (closed) 831.02
open 831.12
recurrent 718.31
skull — *see* Injury, intracranial
Smith's — *see* Dislocation, foot
spine (articular process) (*see also* Dislocation, vertebra) (closed) 839.40
atlanto-axial (closed) 839.01

Dislocation — *continued*
spine (*see also* Dislocation, vertebra) — *continued*
atlanto-axial — *continued*
open 839.11
recurrent 723.8
cervical, cervicodorsal, cervicothoracic (closed) (*see also* Dislocation, vertebrae, cervical) 839.00
open 839.10
recurrent 723.8
coccyx 839.41
open 839.51
congenital 756.19
due to birth trauma 767.4
open 839.50
recurrent 724.9
sacroiliac 839.42
recurrent 724.6
sacrum (sacrococcygeal) (sacroiliac) 839.42
open 839.52
spontaneous — *see* Dislocation, pathological
sternoclavicular (joint) (closed) 839.61
open 839.71
sternum (closed) 839.61
open 839.71
subastragalar — *see* Dislocation, foot
subglenoid (closed) 831.01
open 831.11
symphysis
jaw (closed) 830.0
open 830.1
mandibular (closed) 830.0
open 830.1
pubis (closed) 839.69
open 839.79
tarsal (bone) (joint) 838.01
open 838.11
tarsometatarsal (joint) 838.03
open 838.13
temporomandibular (joint) (closed) 830.0
open 830.1
recurrent 524.69
thigh
distal end (*see also* Dislocation, femur, distal end) 836.50
proximal end (*see also* Dislocation, hip) 835.00
thoracic (vertebrae) (closed) 839.21
open 839.31
thumb(s) (*see also* Dislocation, finger) 834.00
thyroid cartilage (closed) 839.69
open 839.79
tibia
distal end (closed) 837.0
open 837.1
proximal end (closed) 836.50
anterior 836.51
open 836.61
lateral 836.54
open 836.64
medial 836.53
open 836.63
open 836.60
posterior 836.52
open 836.62
rotatory 836.59
open 836.69
tibiofibular
distal (closed) 837.0
open 837.1
superior (closed) 836.59
open 836.69
toe(s) (closed) 838.09
open 838.19
trachea (closed) 839.69
open 839.79
ulna
distal end (closed) 833.09
open 833.19
proximal end — *see* Dislocation, elbow
vertebra (articular process) (body) (closed) 839.40
cervical, cervicodorsal or cervicothoracic (closed) 839.00
first (atlas) 839.01
open 839.11

Dislocation — *continued*
vertebra — *continued*
cervical, cervicodorsal or cervicothoracic — *continued*
second (axis) 839.02
open 839.12
third 839.03
open 839.13
fourth 839.04
open 839.14
fifth 839.05
open 839.15
sixth 839.06
open 839.16
seventh 839.07
open 839.17
congential 756.19
multiple sites 839.08
open 839.18
open 839.10
congenital 756.19
dorsal 839.21
open 839.31
recurrent 724.9
lumbar, lumbosacral 839.20
open 839.30
open NEC 839.50
recurrent 724.9
specified region NEC 839.49
open 839.59
thoracic 839.21
open 839.31
wrist (carpal bone) (scaphoid) (semilunar) (closed) 833.00
carpometacarpal (joint) 833.04
open 833.14
metacarpal bone, proximal end 833.05
open 833.15
midcarpal (joint) 833.03
open 833.13
open 833.10
radiocarpal (joint) 833.02
open 833.12
radioulnar (joint) 833.01
open 833.11
recurrent 718.33
specified site NEC 833.09
open 833.19
xiphoid cartilage (closed) 839.61
open 839.71

Dislodgement
artificial skin graft 996.55
decellularized allodermis graft 996.55

Disobedience, hostile (covert) (overt) (*see also* Disturbance, conduct) 312.0 ✓5ᵗʰ

Disorder — *see also* Disease
academic underachievement, childhood and adolescence 313.83
accommodation 367.51
drug-induced 367.89
toxic 367.89
adjustment (*see also* Reaction, adjustment) 309.9
adrenal (capsule) (cortex) (gland) 255.9
specified type NEC 255.8
adrenogenital 255.2
affective (*see also* Psychosis, affective) 296.90
atypical 296.81
aggressive, unsocialized (*see also* Disturbance, conduct) 312.0 ✓5ᵗʰ
alcohol, alcoholic (*see also* Alcohol) 291.9
allergic — *see* Allergy
amnestic (*see also* Amnestic syndrome) 294.0
amino acid (metabolic) (*see also* Disturbance, metabolism, amino acid) 270.9
albinism 270.2
alkaptonuria 270.2
argininosuccinicaciduria 270.6
beta-amino-isobutyricaciduria 277.2
cystathioninuria 270.4
cystinosis 270.0
cystinuria 270.0
glycinuria 270.0
homocystinuria 270.4
imidazole 270.5
maple syrup (urine) disease 270.3

Dislocation — Disorder

Disorder — *see also* Disease — *continued*
  amino acid (*see also* Disturbance, metabolism, amino acid) — *continued*
    neonatal, transitory 775.8
    oasthouse urine disease 270.2
    ochronosis 270.2
    phenylketonuria 270.1
    phenylpyruvic oligophrenia 270.1
    purine NEC 277.2
    pyrimidine NEC 277.2
    renal transport NEC 270.0
    specified type NEC 270.8
    transport NEC 270.0
      renal 270.0
    xanthinuria 277.2
  anaerobic glycolysis with anemia 282.3
  anxiety (*see also* Anxiety) 300.00
    due to or associated with physical condition 293.84
  arteriole 447.9
    specified type NEC 447.8
  artery 447.9
    specified type NEC 447.8
  articulation — *see* Disorder, joint
  Asperger's 299.8 ✓5ᵗʰ
  attachment of infancy 313.89
  attention deficit 314.00
    with hyperactivity 314.01
    predominantly
      combined hyperactive/inattentive 314.01
      hyperactive/impulsive 314.01
      inattentive 314.00
    residual type 314.8
  autoimmune NEC 279.4
    hemolytic (cold type) (warm type) 283.0
    parathyroid 252.1
    thyroid 245.2
  autistic 299.0 ✓5ᵗʰ
  avoidant, childhood or adolescence 313.21
  balance
    acid-base 276.9
      mixed (with hypercapnia) 276.4
    electrolyte 276.9
    fluid 276.9
  behavior NEC (*see also* Disturbance, conduct) 312.9
  bilirubin excretion 277.4
  bipolar (affective) (alternating) (type I) (*see also* Psychosis, affective) 296.7
    atypical 296.7
    currently
      depressed 296.5 ✓5ᵗʰ
      hypomanic 296.4 ✓5ᵗʰ
      manic 296.4 ✓5ᵗʰ
    mixed 296.6 ✓5ᵗʰ
    type II (recurrent major depressive episodes with hypomania) 296.89
  bladder 596.9
    functional NEC 596.59
    specified NEC 596.8
  bone NEC 733.90
    specified NEC 733.99
  brachial plexus 353.0
  branched-chain amino-acid degradation 270.3
  breast 611.9
    puerperal, postpartum 676.3 ✓5ᵗʰ
    specified NEC 611.8
  Briquet's 300.81
  bursa 727.9
    shoulder region 726.10
  carbohydrate metabolism, congenital 271.9
  cardiac, functional 427.9
    postoperative 997.1
    psychogenic 306.2
  cardiovascular, psychogenic 306.2
  cartilage NEC 733.90
    articular 718.00
      ankle 718.07
      elbow 718.02
      foot 718.07
      hand 718.04
      hip 718.05
      knee 717.9
      multiple sites 718.09
      pelvic region 718.05
      shoulder region 718.01

Disorder — *see also* Disease — *continued*
  cartilage NEC — *continued*
    articular — *continued*
      specified
        site NEC 718.08
        type NEC 733.99
      wrist 718.03
  catatonic — *see* Catatonia
  cervical region NEC 723.9
  cervical root (nerve) NEC 353.2
  character NEC (*see also* Disorder, personality) 301.9
  coagulation (factor) (*see also* Defect, coagulation) 286.9
    factor VIII (congenital) (functional) 286.0
    factor IX (congenital) (functional) 286.1
    neonatal, transitory 776.3
  coccyx 724.70
    specified NEC 724.79
  colon 569.9
    functional 564.9
      congenital 751.3
  cognitive 294.9
  conduct (*see also* Disturbance, conduct) 312.9
    adjustment reaction 309.3
    adolescent onset type 312.82
    childhood onset type 312.81
    compulsive 312.30
      specified type NEC 312.39
    hyperkinetic 314.2
    socialized (type) 312.20
      aggressive 312.23
      unaggressive 312.21
    specified NEC 312.89
  conduction, heart 426.9
    specified NEC 426.89
  convulsive (secondary) (*see also* Convulsions) 780.39
    due to injury at birth 767.0
    idiopathic 780.39
  coordination 781.3
  cornea NEC 371.89
    due to contact lens 371.82
  corticosteroid metabolism NEC 255.2
  cranial nerve — *see* Disorder, nerve, cranial
  cyclothymic 301.13
  degradation, branched-chain amino acid 270.3
  delusional 297.9
  dentition 520.6
  depressive NEC 311
    atypical 296.82
    major (*see also* Psychosis, affective) 296.2 ✓5ᵗʰ
      recurrent episode 296.3 ✓5ᵗʰ
      single episode 296.2 ✓5ᵗʰ
  development, specific 315.9
    associated with hyperkinesia 314.1
    language 315.31
    learning 315.2
      arithmetical 315.1
      reading 315.00
    mixed 315.5
    motor coordination 315.4
    specified type NEC 315.8
    speech 315.39
  diaphragm 519.4
  digestive 536.9
    fetus or newborn 777.9
      specified NEC 777.8
    psychogenic 306.4
  disintegrative (childhood) 299.1 ✓5ᵗʰ
  dissociative 300.14
    identity 300.14
  dysmorphic body 300.7
  dysthymic 300.4
  ear 388.9
    degenerative NEC 388.00
    external 380.9
      specified 380.89
    pinna 380.30
    specified type NEC 388.8
    vascular NEC 388.00
  eating NEC 307.50
  electrolyte NEC 276.9
    with
      abortion — *see* Abortion, by type, with metabolic disorder

Disorder — *see also* Disease — *continued*
  electrolyte NEC — *continued*
    with — *continued*
      ectopic pregnancy (*see also* categories 633.0-633.9) 639.4
      molar pregnancy (*see also* categories 630-632) 639.4
    acidosis 276.2
      metabolic 276.2
      respiratory 276.2
    alkalosis 276.3
      metabolic 276.3
      respiratory 276.3
    following
      abortion 639.4
      ectopic or molar pregnancy 639.4
    neonatal, transitory NEC 775.5
  emancipation as adjustment reaction 309.22
  emotional (*see also* Disorder, mental, nonpsychotic) V40.9
  endocrine 259.9
    specified type NEC 259.8
  esophagus 530.9
    functional 530.5
    psychogenic 306.4
  explosive
    intermittent 312.34
    isolated 312.35
  expressive language 315.31
  eye 379.90
    globe — *see* Disorder, globe
    ill-defined NEC 379.99
    limited duction NEC 378.63
    specified NEC 379.8
  eyelid 374.9
    degenerative 374.50
    sensory 374.44
    specified type NEC 374.89
    vascular 374.85
  factitious — *see* Illness, factitious
  factor, coagulation (*see also* Defect, coagulation) 286.9
    VIII (congenital) (functional) 286.0
    IX (congenital) (funcitonal) 286.1
  fascia 728.9
  feeding — *see* Feeding
  female sexual arousal 302.72
  fluid NEC 276.9
  gastric (functional) 536.9
    motility 536.8
    psychogenic 306.4
    secretion 536.8
  gastrointestinal (functional) NEC 536.9
    newborn (neonatal) 777.9
      specified NEC 777.8
    psychogenic 306.4
  gender (child) 302.6
    adult 302.85
  gender identity (childhood) 302.6
    adult-life 302.85
  genitourinary system, psychogenic 306.50
  globe 360.9
    degenerative 360.20
      specified NEC 360.29
    specified type NEC 360.89
  hearing — *see also* Deafness
    conductive type (air) (*see also* Deafness, conductive) 389.00
    mixed conductive and sensorineural 389.2
    nerve 389.12
    perceptive (*see also* Deafness, perceptive) 389.10
    sensorineural type NEC (*see also* Deafness, perceptive) 389.10
  heart action 427.9
    postoperative 997.1
  hematological, transient neonatal 776.9
    specified type NEC 776.8
  hematopoietic organs 289.9
  hemorrhagic NEC 287.9
    due to circulating anticoagulants 286.5
    specified type NEC 287.8
  hemostasis (*see also* Defect, coagulation) 286.9
  homosexual conflict 302.0
  hypomanic (chronic) 301.11

✓4ᵗʰ Fourth-digit Required   ✓5ᵗʰ Fifth-digit Required   ▶◀ Revised Text   ● New Line   ▲ Revised Code

Disorder — *see also* Disease — *continued*
  identity
    childhood and adolescence 313.82
      gender 302.6
    gender 302.6
  immune mechanism (immunity) 279.9
    single complement (C-C) 279.8
    specified type NEC 279.8
  impulse control (*see also* Disturbance, conduct, compulsive) 312.30
  infant sialic acid storage 271.8
  integument, fetus or newborn 778.9
    specified type NEC 778.8
  interactional psychotic (childhood) (*see also* Psychosis, childhood) 299.1 ✓5ᵗʰ
  intermittent explosive 312.34
  intervertebral disc 722.90
    cervical, cervicothoracic 722.91
    lumbar, lumbosacral 722.93
    thoracic, thoracolumbar 722.92
  intestinal 569.9
    functional NEC 564.9
      congenital 751.3
      postoperative 564.4
    psychogenic 306.4
  introverted, of childhood and adolescence 313.22
  iron, metabolism 275.0
  isolated explosive 312.35
  joint NEC 719.90
    ankle 719.97
    elbow 719.92
    foot 719.97
    hand 719.94
    hip 719.95
    knee 719.96
    multiple sites 719.99
    pelvic region 719.95
    psychogenic 306.0
    shoulder (region) 719.91
    specified site NEC 719.98
    temporomandibular 524.60
      specified NEC 524.69
    wrist 719.93
  kidney 593.9
    functional 588.9
      specified NEC 588.8
  labyrinth, labyrinthine 386.9
    specified type NEC 386.8
  lactation 676.9 ✓5ᵗʰ
  language (developmental) (expressive) 315.31
    mixed (receptive) (receptive-expressive) 315.32
  ligament 728.9
  ligamentous attachments, peripheral — *see also* Enthesopathy
    spine 720.1
  limb NEC 729.9
    psychogenic 306.0
  lipid
    metabolism, congenital 272.9
    storage 272.7
  lipoprotein deficiency (familial) 272.5
  low back NEC 724.9
    psychogenic 306.0
  lumbosacral
    plexus 353.1
    root (nerve) NEC 353.4
  lymphoproliferative (chronic) NEC (M9970/1) 238.7
  male erectile 302.72
    organic origin 607.84
  major depressive (*see also* Psychosis, affective) 296.2 ✓5ᵗʰ
    recurrent episode 296.3 ✓5ᵗʰ
    single episode 296.2 ✓5ᵗʰ
  manic (*see also* Psychosis, affective) 296.0 ✓5ᵗʰ
    atypical 296.81
  meniscus NEC (*see also* Disorder, cartilage, articular) 718.0 ✓5ᵗʰ
  menopausal 627.9
    specified NEC 627.8
  menstrual 626.9
    psychogenic 306.52
    specified NEC 626.8
  mental (nonpsychotic) 300.9
    affecting management of pregnancy, childbirth, or puerperium 648.4 ✓5ᵗʰ

Disorder — *see also* Disease — *continued*
  mental — *continued*
    drug-induced 292.9
      hallucinogen persisting perception 292.89
      specified type NEC 292.89
    due to or associated with
      alcoholism 291.9
      drug consumption NEC 292.9
        specified type NEC 292.89
      physical condition NEC 293.9
    induced by drug 292.9
      specified type NEC 292.89
    neurotic (*see also* Neurosis) 300.9
    presenile 310.1
      psychotic NEC 290.10
    previous, affecting management of pregnancy V23.8 ✓5ᵗʰ
    psychoneurotic (*see also* Neurosis) 300.9
    psychotic (*see also* Psychosis) 298.9
      senile 290.20
    specific, following organic brain damage 310.9
      cognitive or personality change of other type 310.1
      frontal lobe syndrome 310.0
      postconcussional syndrome 310.2
      specified type NEC 310.8
  metabolism NEC 277.9
    with
      abortion — *see* Abortion, by type with metabolic disorder
      ectopic pregnancy (*see also* categories 633.0-633.9) 639.4
      molar pregnancy (*see also* categories 630-632) 639.4
    alkaptonuria 270.2
    amino acid (*see also* Disorder, amino acid) 270.9
      specified type NEC 270.8
    ammonia 270.6
    arginine 270.6
    argininosuccinic acid 270.6
    basal 794.7
    bilirubin 277.4
    calcium 275.40
    carbohydrate 271.9
      specified type NEC 271.8
    cholesterol 272.9
    citrulline 270.6
    copper 275.1
    corticosteroid 255.2
    cystine storage 270.0
    cystinuria 270.0
    fat 272.9
    following
      abortion 639.4
      ectopic or molar pregnancy 639.4
    fructosemia 271.2
    fructosuria 271.2
    fucosidosis 271.8
    galactose-1-phosphate uridyl transferase 271.1
    glutamine 270.7
    glycine 270.7
    glycogen storage NEC 271.0
      hepatorenal 271.0
    hemochromatosis 275.0
    in labor and delivery 669.0 ✓5ᵗʰ
    iron 275.0
    lactose 271.3
    lipid 272.9
      specified type NEC 272.8
      storage 272.7
    lipoprotein — *see also* Hyperlipemia
      deficiency (familial) 272.5
    lysine 270.7
    magnesium 275.2
    mannosidosis 271.8
    mineral 275.9
      specified type NEC 275.8
    mucopolysaccharide 277.5
    nitrogen 270.9
    ornithine 270.6
    oxalosis 271.8
    pentosuria 271.8
    phenylketonuria 270.1
    phosphate 275.3

Disorder — *see also* Disease — *continued*
  metabolism NEC — *continued*
    phosphorous 275.3
    plasma protein 273.9
      specified type NEC 273.8
    porphyrin 277.1
    purine 277.2
    pyrimidine 277.2
    serine 270.7
    sodium 276.9
    specified type NEC 277.8
    steroid 255.2
    threonine 270.7
    urea cycle 270.6
    xylose 271.8
  micturition NEC 788.69
    psychogenic 306.53
  misery and unhappiness, of childhood and adolescence 313.1
  mitral valve 424.0
  mood — *see* Psychosis, affective
  motor tic 307.20
    chronic 307.22
    transient, childhood 307.21
  movement NEC 333.90
    hysterical 300.11
    specified type NEC 333.99
    stereotypic 307.3
  mucopolysaccharide 277.5
  muscle 728.9
    psychogenic 306.0
    specified type NEC 728.3
  muscular attachments, peripheral — *see also* Enthesopathy
    spine 720.1
  musculoskeletal system NEC 729.9
    psychogenic 306.0
  myeloproliferative (chronic) NEC (M9960/1) 238.7
  myoneural 358.9
    due to lead 358.2
    specified type NEC 358.8
    toxic 358.2
  myotonic 359.2
  neck region NEC 723.9
  nerve 349.9
    abducens NEC 378.54
    accessory 352.4
    acoustic 388.5
    auditory 388.5
    auriculotemporal 350.8
    axillary 353.0
    cerebral — *see* Disorder, nerve, cranial
    cranial 352.9
      first 352.0
      second 377.49
      third
        partial 378.51
        total 378.52
      fourth 378.53
      fifth 350.9
      sixth 378.54
      seventh NEC 351.9
      eighth 388.5
      ninth 352.2
      tenth 352.3
      eleventh 352.4
      twelfth 352.5
      multiple 352.6
    entrapment — *see* Neuropathy, entrapment
    facial 351.9
      specified NEC 351.8
    femoral 355.2
    glossopharyngeal NEC 352.2
    hypoglossal 352.5
    iliohypogastric 355.79
    ilioinguinal 355.79
    intercostal 353.8
    lateral
      cutaneous of thigh 355.1
      popliteal 355.3
    lower limb NEC 355.8
    medial, popliteal 355.4
    median NEC 354.1
    obturator 355.79

Disorder — *see also* Disease — *continued*
  nerve — *continued*
    oculomotor
      partial 378.51
      total 378.52
    olfactory 352.0
    optic 377.49
      ischemic 377.41
      nutritional 377.33
      toxic 377.34
    peroneal 355.3
    phrenic 354.8
    plantar 355.6
    pneumogastric 352.3
    posterior tibial 355.5
    radial 354.3
    recurrent laryngeal 352.3
    root 353.9
      specified NEC 353.8
    saphenous 355.79
    sciatic NEC 355.0
    specified NEC 355.9
      lower limb 355.79
      upper limb 354.8
    spinal 355.9
    sympathetic NEC 337.9
    trigeminal 350.9
      specified NEC 350.8
    trochlear 378.53
    ulnar 354.2
    upper limb NEC 354.9
    vagus 352.3
  nervous system NEC 349.9
    autonomic (peripheral) (*see also* Neuropathy,
      peripheral, autonomic) 337.9
    cranial 352.9
    parasympathetic (*see also* Neuropathy,
      peripheral, autonomic) 337.9
    specified type NEC 349.89
    sympathetic (*see also* Neuropathy,
      peripheral, autonomic) 337.9
    vegetative (*see also* Neuropathy, peripheral,
      autonomic) 337.9
  neurohypophysis NEC 253.6
  neurological NEC 781.99
    peripheral NEC 355.9
  neuromuscular NEC 358.9
    hereditary NEC 359.1
    specified NEC 358.8
    toxic 358.2
  neurotic 300.9
    specified type NEC 300.89
  neutrophil, polymorphonuclear (functional)
    288.1
  obsessive-compulsive 300.3
  oppositional, childhood and adolescence 313.81
  optic
    chiasm 377.54
      associated with
        inflammatory disorders 377.54
        neoplasm NEC 377.52
          pituitary 377.51
        pituitary disorders 377.51
        vascular disorders 377.53
    nerve 377.49
    radiations 377.63
    tracts 377.63
  orbit 376.9
    specified NEC 376.89
  overanxious, of childhood and adolescence
    313.0
  pancreas, internal secretion (other than
    diabetes mellitus) 251.9
    specified type NEC 251.8
  panic 300.01
    with agoraphobia 300.21
  papillary muscle NEC 429.81
  paranoid 297.9
    induced 297.3
    shared 297.3
  parathyroid 252.9
    specified type NEC 252.8
  paroxysmal, mixed 780.39
  pentose phosphate pathway with anemia 282.2
  personality 301.9
    affective 301.10
    aggressive 301.3

Disorder — *see also* Disease — *continued*
  personality — *continued*
    amoral 301.7
    anancastic, anankastic 301.4
    antisocial 301.7
    asocial 301.7
    asthenic 301.6
    boderline 301.83
    compulsive 301.4
    cyclothymic 301.13
    dependent-passive 301.6
    dyssocial 301.7
    emotional instability 301.59
    epileptoid 301.3
    explosive 301.3
    following organic brain damage 310.1
    histrionic 301.50
    hyperthymic 301.11
    hypomanic (chronic) 301.11
    hypothymic 301.12
    hysterical 301.50
    immature 301.89
    inadequate 301.6
    introverted 301.21
    labile 301.59
    moral deficiency 301.7
    obsessional 301.4
    obsessive (-compulsive) 301.4
    overconscientious 301.4
    paranoid 301.0
    passive (-dependent) 301.6
    passive-aggressive 301.84
    pathological NEC 301.9
    pseudosocial 301.7
    psychopathic 301.9
    schizoid 301.20
      introverted 301.21
      schizotypal 301.22
    schizotypal 301.22
    seductive 301.59
    type A 301.4
    unstable 301.59
  pervasive developmental, childhood-onset
    299.8 ☑5ᵗʰ
  pigmentation, choroid (congenital) 743.53 ☑4ᵗʰ
  pinna 380.30
    specified type NEC 380.39
  pituitary, thalamic 253.9
    anterior NEC 253.4
    iatrogenic 253.7
    postablative 253.7
    specified NEC 253.8
  pityriasis-like NEC 696.8
  platelets (blood) 287.1
  polymorphonuclear neutrophils (functional)
    288.1
  porphyrin metabolism 277.1
  postmenopausal 627.9
    specified type NEC 627.8
  posttraumatic stress 309.81
    acute 308.3
    brief 308.3
    chronic 309.81
  premenstrual dysphoric 625.4   ●
  psoriatic-like NEC 696.8
  psychic, with diseases classified elsewhere 316
  psychogenic NEC (*see also* condition) 300.9
    allergic NEC
      respiratory 306.1
    anxiety 300.00
      atypical 300.00
      generalized 300.02
    appetite 307.50
    articulation, joint 306.0
    asthenic 300.5
    blood 306.8
    cardiovascular (system) 306.2
    compulsive 300.3
    cutaneous 306.3
    depressive 300.4
    digestive (system) 306.4
    dysmenorrheic 306.52
    dyspneic 306.1
    eczematous 306.3
    endocrine (system) 306.6
    eye 306.7
    feeding 307.59
    functional NEC 306.9

Disorder — *see also* Disease — *continued*
  psychogenic NEC (*see also* condition) —
      continued
    gastric 306.4
    gastrointestinal (system) 306.4
    genitourinary (system) 306.50
    heart (function) (rhythm) 306.2
    hemic 306.8
    hyperventilatory 306.1
    hypochondriacal 300.7
    hysterical 300.10
    intestinal 306.4
    joint 306.0
    learning 315.2
    limb 306.0
    lymphatic (system) 306.8
    menstrual 306.52
    micturition 306.53
    monoplegic NEC 306.0
    motor 307.9
    muscle 306.0
    musculoskeletal 306.0
    neurocirculatory 306.2
    obsessive 300.3
    occupational 300.89
    organ or part of body NEC 306.9
    organs of special sense 306.7
    paralytic NEC 306.0
    phobic 300.20
    physical NEC 306.9
    pruritic 306.3
    rectal 306.4
    respiratory (system) 306.1
    rheumatic 306.0
    sexual (function) 302.70
      specified type NEC 302.79
    skin (allergic) (eczematous) (pruritic) 306.3
    sleep 307.40
      initiation or maintenance 307.41
        persistent 307.42
        transient 307.41
      specified type NEC 307.49
    specified part of body NEC 306.8
    stomach 306.4
  psychomotor NEC 307.9
    hysterical 300.11
  psychoneurotic (*see also* Neurosis) 300.9
    mixed NEC 300.89
  psychophysiologic (*see also* Disorder,
      psychosomatic) 306.9
  psychosexual identity (childhood) 302.6
    adult-life 302.85
  psychosomatic NEC 306.9
    allergic NEC
      respiratory 306.1
    articulation, joint 306.0
    cardiovascular (system) 306.2
    cutaneous 306.3
    digestive (system) 306.4
    dysmenorrheic 306.52
    dyspneic 306.1
    endocrine (system) 306.6
    eye 306.7
    gastric 306.4
    gastrointestinal (system) 306.4
    genitourinary (system) 306.50
    heart (functional) (rhythm) 306.2
    hyperventilatory 306.1
    intestinal 306.4
    joint 306.0
    limb 306.0
    lymphatic (system) 306.8
    menstrual 306.52
    micturition 306.53
    monoplegic NEC 306.0
    muscle 306.0
    musculoskeletal 306.0
    neurocirculatory 306.2
    organs of special sense 306.7
    paralytic NEC 306.0
    pruritic 306.3
    rectal 306.4
    respiratory (system) 306.1
    rheumatic 306.0
    sexual (function) 302.70
    specified type NEC 302.79
    skin 306.3
    specified part of body NEC 306.8

Disorder — Disorder

Disorder — *see also* Disease — *continued*
  psychosomatic NEC — *continued*
    stomach 306.4
  psychotic — *see* Psychosis
  purine metabolism NEC 277.2
  pyrimidine metabolism NEC 277.2
  reactive attachment (of infancy or early
      childhood) 313.89
  reading, developmental 315.00
  reflex 796.1
  renal function, impaired 588.9
    specified type NEC 588.8
  renal transport NEC 588.8
  respiration, respiratory NEC 519.9
    due to
      aspiration of liquids or solids 508.9
      inhalation of fumes or vapors 506.9
    psychogenic 306.1
  retina 362.9
    specified type NEC 362.89
  sacroiliac joint NEC 724.6
  sacrum 724.6
  schizo-affective (*see also* Schizophrenia)
      295.7 ✓5ᵗʰ
  schizoid, childhood or adolescence 313.22
  schizophreniform 295.4 ✓5ᵗʰ
  schizotypal personality 301.22
  secretion, thyrocalcitonin 246.0
  seizure 780.39
    recurrent 780.39
    epileptic — *see* Epilepsy
  sense of smell 781.1
    psychogenic 306.7
  separation anxiety 309.21
  sexual (*see also* Deviation, sexual) 302.9
    function, psychogenic 302.70
  shyness, of childhood and adolescence 313.21
  single complement (C-C) 279.8
  skin NEC 709.9
    fetus or newborn 778.9
      specified type 778.8
    psychogenic (allergic) (eczematous) (pruritic)
        306.3
    specified type NEC 709.8
    vascular 709.1
  sleep 780.50
    with apnea — *see* Apnea, sleep
    circadian rhythm 307.45
    initiation or maintenance (*see also*
        Insomnia) 780.52
      nonorganic origin (transient) 307.41
        persistent 307.42
    nonorganic origin 307.40
      specified type NEC 307.49
    specified NEC 780.59
  social, of childhood and adolescence 313.22
    specified NEC 780.59
  soft tissue 729.9
  somatization 300.81
  somatoform (atypical) (undifferentiated) 300.82
    severe 300.81
  speech NEC 784.5
    nonorganic origin 307.9
  spine NEC 724.9
    ligamentous or muscular attachments,
        peripheral 720.1
  steroid metabolism NEC 255.2
  stomach (functional) (*see also* Disorder, gastric)
      536.9
    psychogenic 306.4
  storage, iron 275.0
  stress (*see also* Reaction, stress, acute) 308.9
    posttraumatic
      acute 308.3
      brief 308.3
      chronic 309.81
  substitution 300.11
  suspected — *see* Observation
  synovium 727.9
  temperature regulation, fetus or newborn 778.4
  temporomandibular joint NEC 524.60
    specified NEC 524.69
  tendon 727.9
    shoulder region 726.10
  thoracic root (nerve) NEC 353.3
  thyrocalcitonin secretion 246.0

Disorder — *see also* Disease — *continued*
  thyroid (gland) NEC 246.9
    specified type NEC 246.8
  tic 307.20
    chronic (motor or vocal) 307.22
    motor-verbal 307.23
    organic origin 333.1
    transient of childhood 307.21
  tooth NEC 525.9
    development NEC 520.9
      specified type NEC 520.8
    eruption 520.6
      with abnormal position 524.3
    specified type NEC 525.8
  transport, carbohydrate 271.9
    specified type NEC 271.8
  tubular, phosphate-losing 588.0
  tympanic membrane 384.9
  unaggressive, unsocialized (*see also*
      Disturbance, conduct) 312.1 ✓5ᵗʰ
  undersocialized, unsocialized (*see also*
      Disturbance, conduct)
    aggressive (type) 312.0 ✓5ᵗʰ
    unaggressive (type) 312.1 ✓5ᵗʰ
  vision, visual NEC 368.9
    binocular NEC 368.30
    cortex 377.73
      associated with
        inflammatory disorders 377.73
        neoplasms 377.71
        vascular disorders 377.72
    pathway NEC 377.63
      associated with
        inflammatory disorders 377.63
        neoplasms 377.61
        vascular disorders 377.62
  wakefulness (*see also* Hypersomnia) 780.54
    nonorganic origin (transient) 307.43
      persistent 307.44

Disorganized globe 360.29
Displacement, displaced

> Note — For acquired displacement of bones,
> cartilage, joints, tendons, due to injury, see
> also Dislocation.
>
> Displacements at ages under one year
> should be considered congenital, provided
> there is no indication the condition was
> acquired after birth.

  acquired traumatic of bone, cartilage, joint,
      tendon NEC (without fracture) (*see also*
      Dislocation) 839.8
    with fracture — *see* Fracture, by site
  adrenal gland (congenital) 759.1
  appendix, retrocecal (congenital) 751.5
  auricle (congenital) 744.29
  bladder (acquired) 596.8
    congenital 753.8
  brachial plexus (congenital) 742.8
  brain stem, caudal 742.4
  canaliculus lacrimalis 743.65
  cardia, through esophageal hiatus 750.6
  cerebellum, caudal 742.4
  cervix (*see also* Malposition, uterus) 621.6
  colon (congenital) 751.4
  device, implant, or graft — *see* Complications,
      mechanical
  epithelium
    columnar of cervix 622.1
    cuboidal, beyond limits of external os
        (uterus) 752.49
  esophageal mucosa into cardia of stomach,
      congenital 750.4
  esophagus (acquired) 530.89
    congenital 750.4
  eyeball (acquired) (old) 376.36
    congenital 743.8
    current injury 871.3
    lateral 376.36
  fallopian tube (acquired) 620.4
    congenital 752.19
    opening (congenital) 752.19
  gallbladder (congenital) 751.69

Displacement, displaced — *continued*
  gastric mucosa 750.7
    into
      duodenum 750.7
      esophagus 750.7
      Meckel's diverticulum, congenital 750.7
  globe (acquired) (lateral) (old) 376.36
    current injury 871.3
  graft
    artificial skin graft 996.55
    decellularized allodermis graft 996.55
  heart (congenital) 746.87
    acquired 429.89
  hymen (congenital) (upward) 752.49
  internal prothesis NEC — *see* Complications,
      mechanical
  intervertebral disc (with neuritis, radiculutis,
      sciatica, or other pain) 722.2
    with myelopathy 722.70
    cervical, cervicodorsal, cervicothoracic 722.0
      with myelopathy 722.71
      due to major trauma — *see* Dislocation,
          vertebra, cervical
    due to major trauma — *see* Dislocation,
        vertebra
  intervertebral disc
    lumbar, lumbosacral 722.10
      with myelopathy 722.73
      due to major trauma — *see* Dislocation,
          vertebra, lumbar
    thoracic, thoracolumbar 722.11
      with myelopathy 722.72
      due to major trauma — *see* Dislocation,
          vertebra, thoracic
  intrauterine device 996.32
  kidney (acquired) 593.0
    congenital 753.3
  lacrimal apparatus or duct (congenital) 743.65
  macula (congenital) 743.55
  Meckel's diverticulum (congenital) 751.0
  nail (congenital) 757.5
    acquired 703.8
  opening of Wharton's duct in mouth 750.26
  organ or site, congenital NEC — *see*
      Malposition, congenital
  ovary (acquired) 620.4
    congenital 752.0
    free in peritoneal cavity (congenital) 752.0
    into hernial sac 620.4
  oviduct (acquired) 620.4
    congenital 752.19
  parathyroid (gland) 252.8
  parotid gland (congenital) 750.26
  punctum lacrimale (congenital) 743.65
  sacroiliac (congenital) (joint) 755.69
    current injury — *see* Dislocation, sacroiliac
    old 724.6
  spine (congenital) 756.19
  spleen, congenital 759.0
  stomach (congenital) 750.7
    acquired 537.89
  subglenoid (closed) 831.01
  sublingual duct (congenital) 750.26
  teeth, tooth 524.3
  tongue (congenital) (downward) 750.19
  trachea (congenital) 748.3
  ureter or ureteric opening or orifice (congenital)
      753.4
  uterine opening of oviducts or fallopian tubes
      752.19
  uterus, uterine (*see also* Malposition, uterus)
      621.6
    congenital 752.3
  ventricular septum 746.89
    with rudimentary ventricle 746.89
  xyphoid bone (process) 738.3
Disproportion 653.9 ✓5ᵗʰ
  affecting fetus or newborn 763.1
  caused by
    conjoined twins 653.7 ✓5ᵗʰ
    contraction, pelvis (general) 653.1 ✓5ᵗʰ
      inlet 653.2 ✓5ᵗʰ
      midpelvic 653.8 ✓5ᵗʰ
      midplane 653.8 ✓5ᵗʰ
      outlet 653.3 ✓5ᵗʰ
    fetal
      ascites 653.7 ✓5ᵗʰ
      hydrocephalus 653.6 ✓5ᵗʰ

Disproportion — *continued*
 caused by — *continued*
  fetal — *continued*
   hydrops 653.7 ✓5ᵗʰ
   meningomyelocele 653.7 ✓5ᵗʰ
   sacral teratoma 653.7 ✓5ᵗʰ
   tumor 653.7 ✓5ᵗʰ
   hydrocephalic fetus 653.6 ✓5ᵗʰ
   pelvis, pelvic, abnormality (bony) NEC 653.0 ✓5ᵗʰ
   unusually large fetus 653.5 ✓5ᵗʰ
  causing obstructed labor 660.1 ✓5ᵗʰ
  cephalopelvic, normally formed fetus 653.4 ✓5ᵗʰ
   causing obstructed labor 660.1 ✓5ᵗʰ
  fetal NEC 653.5 ✓5ᵗʰ
   causing obstructed labor 660.1 ✓5ᵗʰ
  fetopelvic, normally formed fetus 653.4 ✓5ᵗʰ
   causing obstructed labor 660.1 ✓5ᵗʰ
  mixed maternal and fetal origin, normally formed fetus 653.4 ✓5ᵗʰ
  pelvis, pelvic (bony) NEC 653.1 ✓5ᵗʰ
   causing obstructed labor 660.1 ✓5ᵗʰ
  specified type NEC 653.8 ✓5ᵗʰ

Disruption
 cesarean wound 674.1 ✓5ᵗʰ
 family V61.0
 gastrointestinal anastomosis 997.4
 ligament(s) — *see also* Sprain
  knee
   current injury — *see* Dislocation knee
   old 717.89
    capsular 717.85
    collateral (medial) 717.82
     lateral 717.81
    cruciate (posterior) 717.84
     anterior 717.83
    specified site NEC 717.85
 marital V61.10
  involving divorce or estrangement V61.0
 operation wound ▶(external)◀ 998.32 ▲
  internal 998.31 ●
 organ transplant, anastomosis site — *see* Complications, transplant, organ, by site
 ossicles, ossicular chain 385.23
  traumatic — *see* Fracture, skull, base
 parenchyma
  liver (hepatic) — *see* Laceration, liver, major
  spleen — *see* Laceration, spleen, parenchyma, massive
 phase-shift, of 24-hour sleep-wake cycle 780.55
  nonorganic origin 307.45
 sleep-wake cycle (24-hour) 780.55
  circadian rhythm 307.45
  nonorganic origin 307.45
 suture line (external) 998.32 ▲
  internal 998.31 ▲
 wound
  cesarean operation 674.1 ✓5ᵗʰ
  episiotomy 674.2 ✓5ᵗʰ
  operation 998.32 ▲
   cesarean 674.1 ✓5ᵗʰ
   internal 998.31 ●
  perineal (obstetric) 674.2 ✓5ᵗʰ
  uterine 674.1 ✓5ᵗʰ

Disruptio uteri — *see also* Rupture, uterus
 complicating delivery — *see* Delivery, complicated, rupture, uterus

Dissatisfaction with
 employment V62.2
 school environment V62.3

Dissecting — *see* condition

Dissection
 aorta 441.00
  abdominal 441.02
  thoracic 441.01
  thoracoabdominal 441.03
 artery, arterial ●
  carotid 443.21 ●
  coronary 414.12 ●
  iliac 443.22 ●
  renal 443.23 ●
  specified NEC 443.29 ●
  vertebral 443.24 ●
 vascular 459.9
 wound — *see* Wound, open, by site

Disseminated — *see* condition

Dissociated personality NEC 300.15

Dissociation
 auriculoventricular or atrioventricular (any degree) (AV) 426.89
  with heart block 426.0
 interference 426.89
 isorhythmic 426.89
 rhythm
  atrioventricular (AV) 426.89
  interference 426.89

Dissociative
 identity disorder 300.14
 reaction NEC 300.15

Dissolution, vertebra (*see also* Osteoporosis) 733.00

Distention
 abdomen (gaseous) 787.3
 bladder 596.8
 cecum 569.89
 colon 569.89
 gallbladder 575.8
 gaseous (abdomen) 787.3
 intestine 569.89
 kidney 593.89
 liver 573.9
 seminal vesicle 608.89
 stomach 536.8
  acute 536.1
  psychogenic 306.4
 ureter 593.5
 uterus 621.8

Distichia, distichiasis (eyelid) 743.63

Distoma hepaticum infestation 121.3

Distomiasis 121.9
 bile passages 121.3
  due to Clonorchis sinensis 121.1
 hemic 120.9
 hepatic (liver) 121.3
  due to Clonorchis sinensis (clonorchiasis) 121.1
 intestinal 121.4
 liver 121.3
  due to Clonorchis sinensis 121.1
 lung 121.2
 pulmonary 121.2

Distomolar (fourth molar) 520.1
 causing crowding 524.3

Disto-occlusion 524.2

Distortion (congenital)
 adrenal (gland) 759.1
 ankle (joint) 755.69
 anus 751.5
 aorta 747.29
 appendix 751.5
 arm 755.59
 artery (peripheral) NEC (*see also* Distortion, peripheral vascular system) 747.60
  cerebral 747.81
  coronary 746.85
  pulmonary 747.3
  retinal 743.58
  umbilical 747.5
 auditory canal 744.29
  causing impairment of hearing 744.02
 bile duct or passage 751.69
 bladder 753.8
 brain 742.4
 bronchus 748.3
 cecum 751.5
 cervix (uteri) 752.49
 chest (wall) 756.3
 clavicle 755.51
 clitoris 752.49
 coccyx 756.19
 colon 751.5
 common duct 751.69
 cornea 743.41
 cricoid cartilage 748.3
 cystic duct 751.69
 duodenum 751.5
 ear 744.29
  auricle 744.29
   causing impairment of hearing 744.02
  causing impairment of hearing 744.09
  external 744.29
   causing impairment of hearing 744.02

Distortion — *continued*
 ear — *continued*
  inner 744.05
  middle, except ossicles 744.03
   ossicles 744.04
  ossicles 744.04
 endocrine (gland) NEC 759.2
 epiglottis 748.3
 Eustachian tube 744.24
 eye 743.8
  adnexa 743.69
 face bone(s) 756.0
 fallopian tube 752.19
 femur 755.69
 fibula 755.69
 finger(s) 755.59
 foot 755.67
 gallbladder 751.69
 genitalia, genital organ(s)
  female 752.8
   external 752.49
   internal NEC 752.8
  male 752.8
   penis 752.69
 glottis 748.3
 gyri 742.4
 hand bone(s) 755.59
 heart (auricle) (ventricle) 746.89
  valve (cusp) 746.89
 hepatic duct 751.69
 humerus 755.59
 hymen 752.49
 ileum 751.5
 intestine (large) (small) 751.5
  with anomalous adhesions, fixation or malrotation 751.4
 jaw NEC 524.8
 jejunum 751.5
 kidney 753.3
 knee (joint) 755.64
 labium (majus) (minus) 752.49
 larynx 748.3
 leg 755.69
 lens 743.36
 liver 751.69
 lumbar spine 756.19
  with disproportion (fetopelvic) 653.0 ✓5ᵗʰ
   affecting fetus or newborn 763.1
   causing obstructed labor 660.1 ✓5ᵗʰ
 lumbosacral (joint) (region) 756.19
 lung (fissures) (lobe) 748.69
 nerve 742.8
 nose 748.1
 organ
  of Corti 744.05
  or site not listed — *see* Anomaly, specified type NEC
 ossicles, ear 744.04
 ovary 752.0
 oviduct 752.19
 pancreas 751.7
 parathyroid (gland) 759.2
 patella 755.64
 peripheral vascular system NEC 747.60
  gastrointestinal 747.61
  lower limb 747.64
  renal 747.62
  spinal 747.82
  upper limb 747.63
 pituitary (gland) 759.2
 radius 755.59
 rectum 751.5
 rib 756.3
 sacroiliac joint 755.69
 sacrum 756.19
 scapula 755.59
 shoulder girdle 755.59
 site not listed — *see* Anomaly, specified type NEC
 skull bone(s) 756.0
  with
   anencephalus 740.0
   encephalocele 742.0
   hydrocephalus 742.3
    with spina bifida (*see also* Spina bifida) 741.0 ✓5ᵗʰ
   microcephalus 742.1

✓4ᵗʰ Fourth-digit Required ✓5ᵗʰ Fifth-digit Required ▶◀ Revised Text ● New Line ▲ Revised Code

114 — Volume 2 • October 2002   *2003 ICD•9•CM*

Distortion — *continued*
spinal cord 742.59
spine 756.19
spleen 759.0
sternum 756.3
thorax (wall) 756.3
thymus (gland) 759.2
thyroid (gland) 759.2
cartilage 748.3
tibia 755.69
toe(s) 755.66
tongue 750.19
trachea (cartilage) 748.3
ulna 755.59
ureter 753.4
causing obstruction 753.20
urethra 753.8
causing obstruction 753.6
uterus 752.3
vagina 752.49
vein (peripheral) NEC (*see also* Distortion,
peripheral vascular system) 747.60
great 747.49
portal 747.49
pulmonary 747.49
vena cava (inferior) (superior) 747.49
vertebra 756.19
visual NEC 368.15
shape or size 368.14
vulva 752.49
wrist (bones) (joint) 755.59

Distress
abdomen 789.0 ☑5ᵗʰ
colon 789.0 ☑5ᵗʰ
emotional V40.9
epigastric 789.0 ☑5ᵗʰ
fetal (syndrome) 768.4
affecting management of pregnancy or
childbirth 656.8 ☑5ᵗʰ   ▲
liveborn infant 768.4
first noted
before onset of labor 768.2
during labor or delivery 768.3
stillborn infant (death before onset of labor)
768.0
death during labor 768.1
gastrointestinal (functional) 536.9
psychogenic 306.4
intestinal (functional) NEC 564.9
psychogenic 306.4
intrauterine — *see* Distress, fetal
leg 729.5
maternal 669.0 ☑5ᵗʰ
mental V40.9
respiratory 786.09
acute (adult) 518.82
adult syndrome (following shock, surgery,
or trauma) 518.5
specified NEC 518.82
fetus or newborn 770.89   ▲
syndrome (idiopathic) (newborn) 769
stomach 536.9
psychogenic 306.4

Distribution vessel, atypical NEC 747.60
coronary artery 746.85
spinal 747.82

Districhiasis 704.2

Disturbance — *see also* Disease
absorption NEC 579.9
calcium 269.3
carbohydrate 579.8
fat 579.8
protein 579.8
specified type NEC 579.8
vitamin (*see also* Deficiency, vitamin) 269.2
acid-base equilibrium 276.9
activity and attention, simple, with
hyperkinesis 314.01
amino acid (metabolic) (*see also* Disorder,
amino acid) 270.9
imidazole 270.5
maple syrup (urine) disease 270.3
transport 270.0
assimilation, food 579.9
attention, simple 314.00
with hyperactivity 314.01

Disturbance — *see also* Disease — *continued*
auditory, nerve, except deafness 388.5
behavior (*see also* Disturbance, conduct) 312.9
blood clotting (hypoproteinemia) (mechanism)
(*see also* Defect, coagulation) 286.9
central nervous system NEC 349.9
cerebral nerve NEC 352.9
circulatory 459.9
conduct 312.9
adjustment reaction 309.3
adolescent onset type 312.82
childhood onset type 312.81

Note — *Use the following fifth-digit
subclassification with categories
312.0–312.2:*

0	*unspecified*
1	*mild*
2	*moderate*
3	*severe*

compulsive 312.30
intermittent explosive disorder 312.34
isolated explosive disorder 312.35
kleptomania 312.32
pathological gambling 312.31
pyromania 312.33
hyperkinetic 314.2
intermittent explosive 312.34
isolated explosive 312.35
mixed with emotions 312.4
socialized (type) 312.20
aggressive 312.23
unaggressive 312.21
specified type NEC 312.89
undersocialized, unsocialized
aggressive (type) 312.0 ☑5ᵗʰ
unaggressive (type) 312.1 ☑5ᵗʰ
coordination 781.3
cranial nerve NEC 352.9
deep sensibility — *see* Disturbance, sensation
digestive 536.9
psychogenic 306.4
electrolyte — *see* Imbalance, electrolyte
emotions specific to childhood and adolescence
313.9
with
academic underachievement 313.83
anxiety and fearfulness 313.0
elective mutism 313.23
identity disorder 313.82
jealousy 313.3
misery and unhappiness 313.1
oppositional disorder 313.81
overanxiousness 313.0
sensitivity 313.21
shyness 313.21
social withdrawal 313.22
withdrawal reaction 313.22
involving relationship problems 313.3
mixed 313.89
specified type NEC 313.89
endocrine (gland) 259.9
neonatal, transitory 775.9
specified NEC 775.8
equilibrium 780.4
feeding (elderly) (infant) 783.3
newborn 779.3
nonorganic origin NEC 307.59
psychogenic NEC 307.59
fructose metabolism 271.2
gait 781.2
hysterical 300.11
gastric (functional) 536.9
motility 536.8
psychogenic 306.4
secretion 536.8
gastrointestinal (functional) 536.9
psychogenic 306.4
habit, child 307.9
hearing, except deafness 388.40
heart, functional (conditions classifiable to 426,
427, 428)
due to presence of (cardiac) prosthesis 429.4
postoperative (immediate) 997.1
long-term effect of cardiac surgery 429.4

Disturbance — *see also* Disease — *continued*
heart, functional — *continued*
psychogenic 306.2
hormone 259.9
innervation uterus, sympathetic,
parasympathetic 621.8
keratinization NEC
gingiva 523.1
lip 528.5
oral (mucosa) (soft tissue) 528.7
tongue 528.7
labyrinth, labyrinthine (vestibule) 386.9
learning, specific NEC 315.2
memory (*see also* Amnesia) 780.99   ▲
mild, following organic brain
damage 310.1
mental (*see also* Disorder, mental) 300.9
associated with diseases classified elsewhere
316
metabolism (acquired) (congenital) (*see also*
Disorder, metabolism) 277.9
with
abortion — *see* Abortion, by type, with
metabolic disorder
ectopic pregnancy (*see also* categories
633.0-633.9) 639.4
molar pregnancy (*see also* categories 630-
632) 639.4
amino acid (*see also* Disorder, amino acid)
270.9
aromatic NEC 270.2
branched-chain 270.3
specified type NEC 270.8
straight-chain NEC 270.7
sulfur-bearing 270.4
transport 270.0
ammonia 270.6
arginine 270.6
argininosuccinic acid 270.6
carbohydrate NEC 271.9
cholesterol 272.9
citrulline 270.6
cystathionine 270.4
fat 272.9
following
abortion 639.4
ectopic or molar pregnancy 639.4
general 277.9
carbohydrate 271.9
iron 275.0
phosphate 275.3
sodium 276.9
glutamine 270.7
glycine 270.7
histidine 270.5
homocystine 270.4
in labor or delivery 669.0 ☑5ᵗʰ
iron 275.0
isoleucine 270.3
leucine 270.3
lipoid 272.9
specified type NEC 272.8
lysine 270.7
methionine 270.4
neonatal, transitory 775.9
specified type NEC 775.8
nitrogen 788.9
ornithine 270.6
phosphate 275.3
phosphatides 272.7
serine 270.7
sodium NEC 276.9
threonine 270.7
tryptophan 270.2
tyrosine 270.2
urea cycle 270.6
valine 270.3
motor 796.1
nervous functional 799.2
neuromuscular mechanism (eye) due to
syphilis 094.84
nutritional 269.9
nail 703.8
ocular motion 378.87
psychogenic 306.7
oculogyric 378.87
psychogenic 306.7

Distortion — Disturbance

Disturbance — Dizziness

Disturbance — *see also* Disease — *continued*
oculomotor NEC 378.87
  psychogenic 306.7
olfactory nerve 781.1
optic nerve NEC 377.49
oral epithelium, including tongue 528.7
personality (pattern) (trait) (*see also* Disorder, personality) 301.9
  following organic brain damage 310.1
polyglandular 258.9
psychomotor 307.9
pupillary 379.49
reflex 796.1
rhythm, heart 427.9
  postoperative (immediate) 997.1
    long-term effect of cardiac surgery 429.4
  psychogenic 306.2
salivary secretion 527.7
sensation (cold) (heat) (localization) (tactile discrimination localization) (texture) (vibratory) NEC 782.0
  hysterical 300.11
  skin 782.0
  smell 781.1
  taste 781.1
sensory (*see also* Disturbance, sensation) 782.0
  innervation 782.0
situational (transient) (*see also* Reaction, adjustment) 309.9
  acute 308.3
sleep 780.50
  with apnea — *see* Apnea, sleep
  initiation or maintenance (*see also* Insomnia) 780.52
    nonorganic origin 307.41
  nonorganic origin 307.40
    specified type NEC 307.49
  specified NEC 780.59
    nonorganic origin 307.49
  wakefulness (*see also* Hypersomnia) 780.54
    nonorganic origin 307.43
sociopathic 301.7
speech NEC 784.5
  developmental 315.39
    associated with hyperkinesis 314.1
  secondary to organic lesion 784.5
stomach (functional) (*see also* Disturbance, gastric) 536.9
sympathetic (nerve) (*see also* Neuropathy, peripheral, autonomic) 337.9
temperature sense 782.0
  hysterical 300.11
tooth
  eruption 520.6
  formation 520.4
  structure, hereditary NEC 520.5
touch (*see also* Disturbance, sensation) 782.0
vascular 459.9
  arteriosclerotic — *see* Arteriosclerosis
vasomotor 443.9
vasospastic 443.9
vestibular labyrinth 386.9
vision, visual NEC 368.9
  psychophysical 368.16
  specified NEC 368.8
  subjective 368.10
voice 784.40
wakefulness (initiation or maintenance) (*see also* Hypersomnia) 780.54
  nonorganic origin 307.43

Disulfiduria, beta-mercaptolactate-cysteine 270.0

Disuse atrophy, bone 733.7

Ditthomska syndrome 307.81

Diuresis 788.42

Divers'
  palsy or paralysis 993.3
  squeeze 993.3

Diverticula, diverticulosis, diverticulum (acute) (multiple) (perforated) (ruptured) 562.10
  with diverticulitis 562.11
  aorta (Kommerell's) 747.21
  appendix (noninflammatory) 543.9
  bladder (acquired) (sphincter) 596.3
    congenital 753.8
  broad ligament 620.8

Diverticula, diverticulosis, diverticulum — *continued*
bronchus (congenital) 748.3
  acquired 494.0
    with acute exacerbation 494.1
calyx, calyceal (kidney) 593.89
cardia (stomach) 537.1
cecum 562.10
  with
    diverticulitis 562.11
      with hemorrhage 562.13
    hemorrhage 562.12
  congenital 751.5
colon (acquired) 562.10
  with
    diverticulitis 562.11
      with hemorrhage 562.13
    hemorrhage 562.12
  congenital 751.5
duodenum 562.00
  with
    diverticulitis 562.01
      with hemorrhage 562.03
    hemorrhage 562.02
  congenital 751.5
epiphrenic (esophagus) 530.6
esophagus (congenital) 750.4
  acquired 530.6
  epiphrenic 530.6
  pulsion 530.6
  traction 530.6
  Zenker's 530.6
Eustachian tube 381.89
fallopian tube 620.8
gallbladder (congenital) 751.69
gastric 537.1
heart (congenital) 746.89
ileum 562.00
  with
    diverticulitis 562.01
      with hemorrhage 562.03
    hemorrhage 562.02
intestine (large) 562.10
  with
    diverticulitis 562.11
      with hemorrhage 562.13
    hemorrhage 562.12
  congenital 751.5
  small 562.00
    with
      diverticulitis 562.01
        with hemorrhage 562.03
      hemorrhage 562.02
    congenital 751.5
jejunum 562.00
  with
    diverticulitis 562.01
      with hemorrhage 562.03
    hemorrhage 562.02
kidney (calyx) (pelvis) 593.89
  with calculus 592.0
Kommerell's 747.21
laryngeal ventricle (congenital) 748.3
Meckel's (displaced) (hypertrophic) 751.0
midthoracic 530.6
organ or site, congenital NEC — *see* Distortion
pericardium (conginital) (cyst) 746.89
  acquired (true) 423.8
pharyngoesophageal (pulsion) 530.6
pharynx (congenital) 750.27
pulsion (esophagus) 530.6
rectosigmoid 562.10
  with
    diverticulitis 562.11
      with hemorrhage 562.13
    hemorrhage 562.12
  congenital 751.5
rectum 562.10
  with
    diverticulitis 562.11
      with hemorrhage 562.13
    hemorrhage 562.12
renal (calyces) (pelvis) 593.89
  with calculus 592.0
Rokitansky's 530.6
seminal vesicle 608.0

Diverticula, diverticulosis, diverticulum — *continued*
sigmoid 562.10
  with
    diverticulitis 562.11
      with hemorrhage 562.13
    hemorrhage 562.12
  congenital 751.5
small intestine 562.00
  with
    diverticulitis 562.01
      with hemorrhage 562.03
    hemorrhage 562.02
stomach (cardia) (juxtacardia) (juxtapyloric) (acquired) 537.1
  congenital 750.7
subdiaphragmatic 530.6
trachea (congenital) 748.3
  acquired 519.1
traction (esophagus) 530.6
ureter (acquired) 593.89
  congenital 753.4
ureterovesical orifice 593.89
urethra (acquired) 599.2
  congenital 753.8
ventricle, left (congenital) 746.89
vesical (urinary) 596.3
  congenital 753.8
Zenker's (esophagus) 530.6

Diverticulitis (acute) (*see also* Diverticula) 562.11
with hemorrhage 562.13
bladder (urinary) 596.3
cecum (perforated) 562.11
  with hemorrhage 562.13
colon (perforated) 562.11
  with hemorrhage 562.13
duodenum 562.01
  with hemorrhage 562.03
esophagus 530.6
ileum (perforated) 562.01
  with hemorrhage 562.03
intestine (large) (perforated) 562.11
  with hemorrhage 562.13
  small 562.01
    with hemorrhage 562.03
jejunum (perforated) 562.01
  with hemorrhage 562.03
Meckel's (perforated) 751.0
pharyngoesophageal 530.6
rectosigmoid (perforated) 562.11
  with hemorrhage 562.13
rectum 562.11
  with hemorrhage 562.13
sigmoid (old) (perforated) 562.11
  with hemorrhage 562.13
small intestine (perforated) 562.01
  with hemorrhage 562.03
vesical (urinary) 596.3

Diverticulosis — *see* Diverticula

Division
cervix uteri 622.8
  external os into two openings by frenum 752.49
external (cervical) into two openings by frenum 752.49
glans penis 752.69
hymen 752.49
labia minora (congenital) 752.49
ligament (partial or complete) (current) — *see also* Sprain, by site
  with open wound — *see* Wound, open, by site
muscle (partial or complete) (current) — *see also* Sprain, by site
  with open wound — *see* Wound, open, by site
nerve — *see* Injury, nerve, by site
penis glans 752.69
spinal cord — *see* Injury, spinal, by site
vein 459.9
  traumatic — *see* Injury, vascular, by site

Divorce V61.0

Dix-Hallpike neurolabyrinthitis 386.12

Dizziness 780.4
hysterical 300.11
psychogenic 306.9

Doan-Wiseman syndrome (primary splenic neutropenia) 288.0
Dog bite — *see* Wound, open, by site
Döhle-Heller aortitis 093.1
Döhle body-panmyelopathic syndrome 288.2
Dolichocephaly, dolichocephalus 754.0
Dolichocolon 751.5
Dolichostenomelia 759.82
Donohue's syndrome (leprechaunism) 259.8
Donor
  blood V59.01
    other blood components V59.09
    stem cells V59.02
    whole blood V59.01
  bone V59.2
    marrow V59.3
  cornea V59.5
  heart V59.8
  kidney V59.4
  liver V59.6
  lung V59.8
  lymphocyte V59.8
  organ V59.9
    specified NEC V59.8
  potential, examination of V70.8
  skin V59.1
  specified organ or tissue NEC V59.8
  stem cells V59.02
  tissue V59.9
    specified type NEC V59.8
Donovanosis (granuloma venereum) 099.2
DOPS (diffuse obstructive pulmonary syndrome) 496
Double
  albumin 273.8
  aortic arch 747.21
  auditory canal 744.29
  auricle (heart) 746.82
  bladder 753.8
  external (cervical) os 752.49
  kidney with double pelvis (renal) 753.3
  larynx 748.3
  meatus urinarius 753.8
  organ or site NEC — *see* Accessory
  orifice
    heart valve NEC 746.89
    pulmonary 746.09
  outlet, right ventricle 745.11
  pelvis (renal) with double ureter 753.4
  penis 752.69
  tongue 750.13
  ureter (one or both sides) 753.4
    with double pelvis (renal) 753.4
  urethra 753.8
  urinary meatus 753.8
  uterus (any degree) 752.2
    with doubling of cervix and vagina 752.2
    in pregnancy or childbirth 654.0 ✓5th
      affecting fetus or newborn 763.89
  vagina 752.49
    with doubling of cervix and uterus 752.2
  vision 368.2
  vocal cords 748.3
  vulva 752.49
  whammy (syndrome) 360.81
Douglas' pouch, cul-de-sac — *see* condition
Down's disease or syndrome (mongolism) 758.0
Down-growth, epithelial (anterior chamber) 364.61
Dracontiasis 125.7
Dracunculiasis 125.7
Drancunculosis 125.7
Drainage
  abscess (spontaneous) — *see* Abscess
  anomalous pulmonary veins to hepatic veins or right atrium 747.41
  stump (amputation) (surgical) 997.62
  suprapubic, bladder 596.8
Dream state, hysterical 300.13
Drepanocytic anemia (*see also* Disease, sickle cell) 282.60
Dresbach's syndrome (elliptocytosis) 282.1

Dreschlera (infection) 118
  hawaiiensis 117.8
Dressler's syndrome (postmyocardial infarction) 411.0
Dribbling (post-void) 788.35
Drift, ulnar 736.09
Drinking (alcohol) — *see also* Alcoholism
  excessive, to excess NEC (*see also* Abuse, drugs, nondependent) 305.0 ✓5th
    bouts, periodic 305.0 ✓5th
    continual 303.9 ✓5th
    episodic 305.0 ✓5th
    habitual 303.9 ✓5th
    periodic 305.0 ✓5th
Drip, postnasal (chronic) — *see* Sinusitis
Drivers' license examination V70.3
Droop
  Cooper's 611.8
  facial 781.99
Drop
  finger 736.29
  foot 736.79
  hematocrit (precipitous) 790.01
  toe 735.8
  wrist 736.05
Dropped
  dead 798.1
  heart beats 426.6
Dropsy, dropsical (*see also* Edema) 782.3
  abdomen 789.5
  amnion (*see also* Hydramnios) 657 ✓5th
  brain — *see* Hydrocephalus
  cardiac (*see also* Failure, heart) 428.0
  cardiorenal (*see also* Hypertension, cardiorenal) 404.90
  chest 511.9
  fetus or newborn 778.0
    due to isoimmunization 773.3
  gangrenous (*see also* Gangrene) 785.4
  heart (*see also* Failure, heart) 428.0
  hepatic — *see* Cirrhosis, liver
  infantile — *see* Hydrops, fetalis
  kidney (*see also* Nephrosis) 581.9
  liver — *see* Cirrhosis, liver
  lung 514
  malarial (*see also* Malaria) 084.9
  neonatorum — *see* Hydrops, fetalis
  nephritic 581.9
  newborn — *see* Hydrops, fetalis
  nutritional 269.9
  ovary 620.8
  pericardium (*see also* Pericarditis) 423.9
  renal (*see also* Nephrosis) 581.9
  uremic — *see* Uremia
Drowned, drowning 994.1
  lung 518.5
Drowsiness 780.09
Drug — *see also* condition
  addiction (*see also* listing under Dependence) 304.9 ✓5th
  adverse effect NEC, correct substance properly administered 995.2
  dependence (*see also* listing under Dependence) 304.9 ✓5th
  habit (*see also* listing under Dependence) 304.9 ✓5th
  overdose — *see* Table of Drugs and Chemicals
  poisoning — *see* Table of Drugs and Chemicals
  therapy (maintenance) status NEC V58.1
    anticoagulant V58.61
    long-term (current) use V58.69
      antibiotics V58.62
  wrong substance given or taken in error — *see* Table of Drugs and Chemicals
Drunkenness (*see also* Abuse, drugs, nondependent) 305.0 ✓5th
  acute in alcoholism (*see also* Alcoholism) 303.0 ✓5th
  chronic (*see also* Alcoholism) 303.9 ✓5th
  pathologic 291.4
  simple (acute) 305.0 ✓5th
    in alcoholism 303.0 ✓5th
  sleep 307.47

Drusen
  optic disc or papilla 377.21
  retina (colloid) (hyaloid degeneration) 362.57
    hereditary 362.77
Drusenfieber 075
Dry, dryness — *see also* condition
  eye 375.15
    syndrome 375.15
  larynx 478.79
  mouth 527.7
  nose 478.1
  skin syndrome 701.1
  socket (teeth) 526.5
  throat 478.29
DSAP (disseminated superficial actinic porokeratosis) 692.75
Duane's retraction syndrome 378.71
Duane-Stilling-Türk syndrome (ocular retraction syndrome) 378.71
Dubin-Johnson disease or syndrome 277.4
Dubini's disease (electric chorea) 049.8
Dubois' abscess or disease 090.5
Duchenne's
  disease 094.0
    locomotor ataxia 094.0
    muscular dystrophy 359.1
    pseudohypertrophy, muscles 359.1
  paralysis 335.22
  syndrome 335.22
Duchenne-Aran myelopathic, muscular atrophy (nonprogressive) (progressive) 335.21
Duchenne-Griesinger disease 359.1
Ducrey's
  bacillus 099.0
  chancre 099.0
  disease (chancroid) 099.0
Duct, ductus — *see* condition
Duengero 061
Duhring's disease (dermatitis herpetiformis) 694.0
Dukes (-Filatov) disease 057.8
Dullness
  cardiac (decreased) (increased) 785.3
Dumb ague (*see also* Malaria) 084.6
Dumbness (*see also* Aphasia) 784.3
Dumdum fever 085.0
Dumping syndrome (postgastrectomy) 564.2
  nonsurgical 536.8
Duodenitis (nonspecific) (peptic) 535.60
  with hemorrhage 535.61
  due to
    Strongyloides stercoralis 127.2
Duodenocholangitis 575.8
Duodenum, duodenal — *see* condition
Duplay's disease, periarthritis, or syndrome 726.2
Duplex — *see also* Accessory
  kidney 753.3
  placenta — *see* Placenta, abnormal
  uterus 752.2
Duplication — *see also* Accessory
  anus 751.5
  aortic arch 747.21
  appendix 751.5
  biliary duct (any) 751.69
  bladder 753.8
  cecum 751.5
    and appendix 751.5
  clitoris 752.49
  cystic duct 751.69
  digestive organs 751.8
  duodenum 751.5
  esophagus 750.4
  fallopian tube 752.19
  frontonasal process 756.0
  gallbladder 751.69
  ileum 751.5
  intestine (large) (small) 751.5
  jejunum 751.5
  kidney 753.3
  liver 751.69
  nose 748.1

Duplication — *see also* Accessory — *continued*
  pancreas 751.7
  penis 752.69
  respiratory organs NEC 748.9
  salivary duct 750.22
  spinal cord (incomplete) 742.51
  stomach 750.7
  ureter 753.4
  vagina 752.49
  vas deferens 752.8
  vocal cords 748.3
Dupré's disease or syndrome (meningism) 781.6
Dupuytren's
  contraction 728.6
  disease (muscle contracture) 728.6
  fracture (closed) 824.4
    ankle (closed) 824.4
      open 824.5
    fibula (closed) 824.4
      open 824.5
    open 824.5
    radius (closed) 813.42
      open 813.52
  muscle contracture 728.6
Durand-Nicolas-Favre disease (climatic bubo) 099.1
Duroziez's disease (congenital mitral stenosis) 746.5
Dust
  conjunctivitis 372.05
  reticulation (occupational) 504
Dutton's
  disease (trypanosomiasis) 086.9
  relapsing fever (West African) 087.1
Dwarf, dwarfism 259.4
  with infantilism (hypophyseal) 253.3
  achondroplastic 756.4
  Amsterdam 759.89
  bird-headed 759.89
  congenital 259.4
  constitutional 259.4
  hypophyseal 253.3
  infantile 259.4
  Levi type 253.3
  Lorain-Levi (pituitary) 253.3
  Lorain type (pituitary) 253.3
  metatropic 756.4
  nephrotic-glycosuric, with hypophosphatemic rickets 270.0
  nutritional 263.2
  ovarian 758.6
  pancreatic 577.8
  pituitary 253.3
  polydystrophic 277.5
  primordial 253.3
  psychosocial 259.4
  renal 588.0
    with hypertension — *see* Hypertension, kidney
  Russell's (uterine dwarfism and craniofacial dysostosis) 759.89
Dyke-Young anemia or syndrome (acquired macrocytic hemolytic anemia) (secondary) (symptomatic) 283.9
Dynia abnormality (*see also* Defect, coagulation) 286.9
Dysacousis 388.40
Dysadrenocortism 255.9
  hyperfunction 255.3
  hypofunction 255.4
Dysarthria 784.5
Dysautonomia (*see also* Neuropathy, peripheral, autonomic) 337.9
  familial 742.8
Dysbarism 993.3
Dysbasia 719.7 ✓5ᵗʰ
  angiosclerotica intermittens 443.9
    due to atherosclerosis 440.21
  hysterical 300.11
  lordotica (progressiva) 333.6
  nonorganic origin 307.9
  psychogenic 307.9
Dysbetalipoproteinemia (familial) 272.2
Dyscalculia 315.1

Dyschezia (*see also* Constipation) 564.00
Dyschondroplasia (with hemangiomata) 756.4
  Voorhoeve's 756.4
Dyschondrosteosis 756.59
Dyschromia 709.00
Dyscollagenosis 710.9
Dyscoria 743.41
Dyscraniopyophalangy 759.89
Dyscrasia
  blood 289.9
    with antepartum hemorrhage 641.3 ✓5ᵗʰ
    fetus or newborn NEC 776.9
    hemorrhage, subungual 287.8
    puerperal, postpartum 666.3 ✓5ᵗʰ
  ovary 256.8
  plasma cell 273.9
  pluriglandular 258.9
  polyglandular 258.9
Dysdiadochokinesia 781.3
Dysectasia, vesical neck 596.8
Dysendocrinism 259.9
Dysentery, dysenteric (bilious) (catarrhal) (diarrhea) (epidemic) (gangrenous) (hemorrhagic) (infectious) (sporadic) (tropical) (ulcerative) 009.0
  abscess, liver (*see also* Abscess, amebic) 006.3
  amebic (*see also* Amebiasis) 006.9
    with abscess — *see* Abscess, amebic
    acute 006.0
    carrier (suspected) of V02.2
    chronic 006.1
  arthritis (*see also* Arthritis, due to, dysentery) 009.0 [711.3] ✓5ᵗʰ
    bacillary 004.9 [711.3] ✓5ᵗʰ
  asylum 004.9
  bacillary 004.9
    arthritis 004.9 [711.3] ✓5ᵗʰ
    Boyd 004.2
    Flexner 004.1
    Schmitz (-Stutzer) 004.0
    Shiga 004.0
    Shigella 004.9
      group A 004.0
      group B 004.1
      group C 004.2
      group D 004.3
      specified type NEC 004.8
    Sonne 004.3
    specified type NEC 004.8
  bacterium 004.9
  balantidial 007.0
  Balantidium coli 007.0
  Boyd's 004.2
  Chilomastix 007.8
  Chinese 004.9
  choleriform 001.1
  coccidial 007.2
  Dientamoeba fragilis 007.8
  due to specified organism NEC — *see* Enteritis, due to, by organism
  Embadomonas 007.8
  Endolimax nana — *see* Dysentery, amebic
  Entamoba, entamebic — *see* Dysentery, amebic
  Flexner's 004.1
  Flexner-Boyd 004.2
  giardial 007.1
  Giardia lamblia 007.1
  Hiss-Russell 004.1
  lamblia 007.1
  leishmanial 085.0
  malarial (*see also* Malaria) 084.6
  metazoal 127.9
  Monilia 112.89
  protozoal NEC 007.9
  Russell's 004.8
  salmonella 003.0
  schistosomal 120.1
  Schmitz (-Stutzer) 004.0
  Shiga 004.0
  Shigella NEC (*see also* Dysentery, bacillary) 004.9
    boydii 004.2
    dysenteriae 004.0
      Schmitz 004.0
      Shiga 004.0

Dysentery, dysenteric — *continued*
  Shigella NEC (*see also* Dysentery, bacillary) — *continued*
    flexneri 004.1
    Group A 004.0
    Group B 004.1
    Group C 004.2
    Group D 004.3
    Schmitz 004.0
    Shiga 004.0
    Sonnei 004.3
  Sonne 004.3
  strongyloidiasis 127.2
  trichomonal 007.3
  tuberculous (*see also* Tuberculosis) 014.8 ✓5ᵗʰ
  viral (*see also* Enteritis, viral) 008.8
Dysequilibrium 780.4
Dysesthesia 782.0
  hysterical 300.11
Dysfibrinogenemia (congenital) (*see also* Defect, coagulation) 286.3
Dysfunction
  adrenal (cortical) 255.9
    hyperfunction 255.3
    hypofunction 255.4
  associated with sleep stages or arousal from sleep 780.56
    nonorganic origin 307.47
  bladder NEC 596.59
  bleeding, uterus 626.8
  brain, minimal (*see also* Hyperkinesia) 314.9
  cerebral 348.3
  colon 564.9
    psychogenic 306.4
  colostomy or enterostomy 569.62
  cystic duct 575.8
  diastolic 429.9
    with heart failure — *see* Failure, heart
    due to
      cardiomyopathy — *see* Cardiomyopathy
      hypertension — *see* Hypertension, heart
  endocrine NEC 259.9
  endometrium 621.8
  enteric stoma 569.62
  enterostomy 569.62
  Eustachian tube 381.81
  gallbladder 575.9
  gastrointestinal 536.9
  gland, glandular NEC 259.9
  heart 427.9
    postoperative (immediate) 997.1
      long-term effect of cardiac surgery 429.4
  hemoglobin 288.8
  hepatic 573.9
  hepatocellular NEC 573.9
  hypophysis 253.9
    hyperfunction 253.1
    hypofunction 253.2
    posterior lobe 253.6
      hypofunction 253.5
  kidney (*see also* Disease, renal) 593.9
  labyrinthine 386.50
    specified NEC 386.58
  liver 573.9
    constitutional 277.4
  minimal brain (child) (*see also* Hyperkinesia) 314.9
  ovary, ovarian 256.9
    hyperfunction 256.1
      estrogen 256.0
    hypofunction 256.39
      postablative 256.2
    postablative 256.2
    specified NEC 256.8
  papillary muscle 429.81
    with myocardial infarction 410.8 ✓5ᵗʰ
  parathyroid 252.8
    hyperfunction 252.0
    hypofunction 252.1
  pineal gland 259.8
  pituitary (gland) 253.9
    hyperfunction 253.1
    hypofunction 253.2
    posterior 253.6
      hypofunction 253.5
  placental — *see* Placenta, insufficiency
  platelets (blood) 287.1

Dysfunction — *continued*
polyglandular 258.9
  specified NEC 258.8
psychosexual 302.70
  with
    dyspareunia (functional) (psychogenic)
      302.76
    frigidity 302.72
    impotence 302.72
    inhibition
      orgasm
        female 302.73
        male 302.74
      sexual
        desire 302.71
        excitement 302.72
    premature ejaculation 302.75
    sexual aversion 302.79
    specified disorder NEC 302.79
    vaginismus 306.51
pylorus 537.9
rectum 564.9
  psychogenic 306.4
segmental (*see also* Dysfunction, somatic)
    739.9
senile 797
sinoatrial node 427.81
somatic 739.9
  abdomen 739.9
  acromioclavicular 739.7
  cervical 739.1
  cervicothoracic 739.1
  costochondral 739.8
  costovertebral 739.8
  extremities
    lower 739.6
    upper 739.7
  head 739.0
  hip 739.5
  lumbar, lumbosacral 739.3
  occipitocervical 739.0
  pelvic 739.5
  pubic 739.5
  rib cage 739.8
  sacral 739.4
  sacrococcygeal 739.4
  sacroiliac 739.4
  specified site NEC 739.9
  sternochondral 739.8
  sternoclavicular 739.7
  temporomandibular 739.0
  thoracic, thoracolumbar 739.2
stomach 536.9
  psychogenic 306.4
suprarenal 255.9
  hyperfunction 255.3
  hypofunction 255.4
symbolic NEC 784.60
  specified type NEC 784.69
temporomandibular (joint) (joint-pain-
    syndrome) NEC 524.60
  specified NEC 524.69
testicular 257.9
  hyperfunction 257.0
  hypofunction 257.2
  specified type NEC 257.8
thymus 254.9
thyroid 246.9
  complicating pregnancy, childbirth or
    puerperium 648.1 ✓5ᵗʰ
  hyperfunction — *see* Hyperthyroidism
  hypofunction — *see* Hypothyroidism
uterus, complicating delivery 661.9 ✓5ᵗʰ
  affecting fetus or newborn 763.7
  hypertonic 661.4 ✓5ᵗʰ
  hypotonic 661.2 ✓5ᵗʰ
    primary 661.0 ✓5ᵗʰ
    secondary 661.1 ✓5ᵗʰ
velopharyngeal (acquired) 528.9
  congenital 750.29
ventricular 429.9
  with congestive heart failure (*see also*
    Failure, heart) 428.0
  due to
    cardiomyopathy — *see* Cardiomyopathy
    hypertension — *see* Hypertension, heart
vesicourethral NEC 596.59

Dysfunction — *continued*
vestibular 386.50
  specified type NEC 386.58
Dysgammaglobulinemia 279.06
Dysgenesis
gonadal (due to chromosomal anomaly) 758.6
  pure 752.7
kidney(s) 753.0
ovarian 758.6
renal 753.0
reticular 279.2
seminiferous tubules 758.6
tidal platelet 287.3
Dysgerminoma (M9060/3)
specified site — *see* Neoplasm, by site,
    malignant
unspecified site
  female 183.0
  male 186.9
Dysgeusia 781.1
Dysgraphia 781.3
Dyshidrosis 705.81
Dysidrosis 705.81
Dysinsulinism 251.8
Dyskaryotic cervical smear 795.09 ▲
Dyskeratosis (*see also* Keratosis) 701.1
bullosa hereditaria 757.39
cervix 622.1
congenital 757.39
follicularis 757.39
  vitamin A deficiency 264.8
gingiva 523.8
oral soft tissue NEC 528.7
tongue 528.7
uterus NEC 621.8
Dyskinesia 781.3
biliary 575.8
esophagus 530.5
hysterical 300.11
intestinal 564.89
nonorganic origin 307.9
orofacial 333.82
psychogenic 307.9
tardive (oral) 333.82
Dyslalia 784.5
developmental 315.39
Dyslexia 784.61
developmental 315.02
secondary to organic lesion 784.61
Dysmaturity (*see also* Immaturity) 765.1 ✓5ᵗʰ
lung 770.4
pulmonary 770.4
Dysmenorrhea (essential) (exfoliative) (functional)
    (intrinsic) (membranous) (primary)
    (secondary) 625.3
  psychogenic 306.52
Dysmetabolic syndrome X 277.7
Dysmetria 781.3
Dysmorodystrophia mesodermalis congenita
    759.82
Dysnomia 784.3
Dysorexia 783.0
hysterical 300.11
Dysostosis
cleidocranial, cleidocranialis 755.59
craniofacial 756.0
Fairbank's (idiopathic familial generalized
    osteophytosis) 756.50
mandibularis 756.0
mandibulofacial, incomplete 756.0
multiplex 277.5
orodigitofacial 759.89
Dyspareunia (female) 625.0
male 608.89
psychogenic 302.76
Dyspepsia (allergic) (congenital) (fermentative)
    (flatulent) (functional) (gastric)
    (gastrointestinal) (neurogenic) (occupational)
    (reflex) 536.8
acid 536.8
atonic 536.3
  psychogenic 306.4

Dyspepsia — *continued*
diarrhea 787.91
  psychogenic 306.4
intestinal 564.89
  psychogenic 306.4
nervous 306.4
neurotic 306.4
psychogenic 306.4
Dysphagia 787.2
functional 300.11
hysterical 300.11
nervous 300.11
psychogenic 306.4
sideropenic 280.8
spastica 530.5
Dysphagocytosis, congenital 288.1
Dysphasia 784.5
Dysphonia 784.49
clericorum 784.49
functional 300.11
hysterical 300.11
psychogenic 306.1
spastica 478.79
Dyspigmentation — *see also* Pigmentation
eyelid (acquired) 374.52
Dyspituitarism 253.9
hyperfunction 253.1
hypofunction 253.2
posterior lobe 253.6
Dysplasia — *see also* Anomaly
artery
  fibromuscular NEC 447.8
    carotid 447.8
    renal 447.3
bladder 596.8
bone (fibrous) NEC 733.29
  diaphyseal, progressive 756.59
  jaw 526.89
  monostotic 733.29
  polyostotic 756.54
  solitary 733.29
brain 742.9
bronchopulmonary, fetus or newborn 770.7
cervix (uteri) 622.1
  cervical intraepithelial neoplasia I [CIN I]
    622.1
  cervical intraepithelial neoplasia II [CIN II]
    622.1
  cervical intraepithelial neoplasia III [CIN III]
    233.1
  CIN I 622.1
  CIN II 622.1
  CIN III 233.1
chondroectodermal 756.55
chondromatose 756.4
craniocarpotarsal 759.89
craniometaphyseal 756.89
dentinal 520.5
diaphyseal, progressive 756.59
ectodermal (anhidrotic) (Bason) (Clouston's)
    (congenital) (Feinmesser) (hereditary)
    (hidrotic) (Marshall) (Robinson's) 757.31
epiphysealis 756.9
  multiplex 756.56
  punctata 756.59
epiphysis 756.9
  multiple 756.56
epithelial
  epiglottis 478.79
  uterine cervix 622.1
erythroid NEC 289.8
eye (*see also* Microphthalmos) 743.10
familial metaphyseal 756.89
fibromuscular, artery NEC 447.8
  carotid 447.8
  renal 447.3
fibrous
  bone NEC 733.29
  diaphyseal, progressive 756.59
  jaw 526.89
  monostotic 733.29
  polyostotic 756.54
  solitary 733.29
high grade squamous intraepithelial
    (HGSIL) 622.1

Dysplasia — Dystrophy

Dysplasia — *see also* Anomaly — *continued*
  hip (congenital) 755.63
    with dislocation (*see also* Dislocation, hip, congenital) 754.30
  hypohidrotic ectodermal 757.31
  joint 755.8
  kidney 753.15
  leg 755.69
  linguofacialis 759.89
  low grade squamous intraepithelial (LGSIL) 622.1   ●
  lung 748.5
  macular 743.55
  mammary (benign) (gland) 610.9
    cystic 610.1
    specified type NEC 610.8
  metaphyseal 756.9
    familial 756.89
  monostotic fibrous 733.29
  muscle 756.89
  myeloid NEC 289.8
  nervous system (general) 742.9
  neuroectodermal 759.6
  oculoauriculovertebral 756.0
  oculodentodigital 759.89
  olfactogenital 253.4
  osteo-onycho-arthro (hereditary) 756.89
  periosteum 733.99
  polyostotic fibrous 756.54
  progressive diaphyseal 756.59
  prostate 602.3
    intraepithelial neoplasia I [PIN I] 602.3
    intraepithelial neoplasia II [PIN II] 602.3
    intraepithelial neoplasia III [PIN III] 233.4
  renal 753.15
  renofacialis 753.0
  retinal NEC 743.56
  retrolental 362.21
  spinal cord 742.9
  thymic, with immunodeficiency 279.2
  vagina 623.0
  vocal cord 478.5
  vulva 624.8
    intraepithelial neoplasia I [VIN I] 624.8
    intraepithelial neoplasia II [VIN II] 624.8
    intraepithelial neoplasia III [VIN III] 233.3
    VIN I 624.8
    VIN II 624.8
    VIN III 233.3

Dyspnea (nocturnal) (paroxysmal) 786.09
  asthmatic (bronchial) (*see also* Asthma) 493.9 ✓5ᵗʰ
    with bronchitis (*see also* Asthma) 493.9 ✓5ᵗʰ
      chronic 493.2 ✓5ᵗʰ   ▲
    cardiac (*see also* Failure, ventricular, left) 428.1
  cardiac (*see also* Failure, ventricular, left) 428.1
  functional 300.11
  hyperventilation 786.01
  hysterical 300.11
  Monday morning 504
  newborn 770.89   ▲
  psychogenic 306.1
  uremic — *see* Uremia

Dyspraxia 781.3
  syndrome 315.4

Dysproteinemia 273.8
  transient with copper deficiency 281.4

Dysprothrombinemia (constitutional) (*see also* Defect, coagulation) 286.3

Dysreflexia, autonomic 337.3

Dysrhythmia
  cardiac 427.9
    postoperative (immediate) 997.1
      long-term effect of cardiac surgery 429.4
    specified type NEC 427.89
  cerebral or cortical 348.3

Dyssecretosis, mucoserous 710.2

Dyssocial reaction, without manifest psychiatric disorder
  adolescent V71.02
  adult V71.01
  child V71.02

Dyssomnia NEC 780.56
  nonorganic origin 307.47

Dyssplenism 289.4

Dyssynergia
  biliary (*see also* Disease, biliary) 576.8
  cerebellaris myoclonica 334.2
  detrusor sphincter (bladder) 596.55
  ventricular 429.89

Dystasia, hereditary areflexic 334.3

Dysthymia 300.4

Dysthymic disorder 300.4

Dysthyroidism 246.9

Dystocia 660.9 ✓5ᵗʰ
  affecting fetus or newborn 763.1
  cervical 661.0 ✓5ᵗʰ
    affecting fetus or newborn 763.7
  contraction ring 661.4 ✓5ᵗʰ
    affecting fetus or newborn 763.7
  fetal 660.9 ✓5ᵗʰ
    abnormal size 653.5 ✓5ᵗʰ
      affecting fetus or newborn 763.1
    deformity 653.7 ✓5ᵗʰ
  maternal 660.9 ✓5ᵗʰ
    affecting fetus or newborn 763.1
  positional 660.0 ✓5ᵗʰ
    affecting fetus or newborn 763.1
  shoulder (girdle) 660.4 ✓5ᵗʰ
    affecting fetus or newborn 763.1
  uterine NEC 661.4 ✓5ᵗʰ
    affecting fetus or newborn 763.7

Dystonia
  deformans progressiva 333.6
  due to drugs 333.7
  lenticularis 333.6
  musculorum deformans 333.6
  torsion (idiopathic) 333.6
    fragments (of) 333.89
    symptomatic 333.7

Dystonic
  movements 781.0

Dystopia kidney 753.3

Dystrophy, dystrophia 783.9
  adiposogenital 253.8
  asphyxiating thoracic 756.4
  Becker's type 359.1
  brevicollis 756.16
  Bruch's membrane 362.77
  cervical (sympathetic) NEC 337.0
  chondro-osseus with punctate epiphyseal dysplasia 756.59
  choroid (hereditary) 363.50
    central (areolar) (partial) 363.53
      total (gyrate) 363.54
    circinate 363.53
    circumpapillary (partial) 363.51
      total 363.52
    diffuse
      partial 363.56
      total 363.57
    generalized
      partial 363.56
      total 363.57
    gyrate
      central 363.54
      generalized 363.57
    helicoid 363.52
    peripapillary — *see* Dystrophy, choroid, circumpapillary
    serpiginous 363.54
  cornea (hereditary) 371.50
    anterior NEC 371.52
    Cogan's 371.52
    combined 371.57
    crystalline 371.56
    endothelial (Fuchs') 371.57
    epithelial 371.50
      juvenile 371.51
      microscopic cystic 371.52
    granular 371.53
    lattice 371.54
    macular 371.55
    marginal (Terrien's) 371.48
    Meesman's 371.51
    microscopic cystic (epithelial) 371.52
    nodular, Salzmann's 371.46
    polymorphous 371.58
    posterior NEC 371.58
    ring-like 371.52
    Salzmann's nodular 371.46

Dystrophy, dystrophia — *continued*
  cornea — *continued*
    stromal NEC 371.56
  dermatochondrocorneal 371.50
  Duchenne's 359.1
  due to malnutrition 263.9
  Erb's 359.1
  familial
    hyperplastic periosteal 756.59
    osseous 277.5
  foveal 362.77
  Fuchs', cornea 371.57
  Gowers' muscular 359.1
  hair 704.2
  hereditary, progressive muscular 359.1
  hypogenital, with diabetic tendency 759.81
  Landouzy-Déjérine 359.1
  Leyden-Möbius 359.1
  mesodermalis congenita 759.82
  muscular 359.1
    congenital (hereditary) 359.0
      myotonic 359.2
    distal 359.1
    Duchenne's 359.1
    Erb's 359.1
    fascioscapulohumeral 359.1
    Gowers' 359.1
    hereditary (progressive) 359.1
    Landouzy-Déjérine 359.1
    limb-girdle 359.1
    myotonic 359.2
    progressive (hereditary) 359.1
      Charcôt-Marie-Tooth 356.1
    pseudohypertrophic (infantile) 359.1
  myocardium, myocardial (*see also* Degeneration, myocardial) 429.1
  myotonic 359.2
  myotonica 359.2
  nail 703.8
    congenital 757.5
  neurovascular (traumatic) (*see also* Neuropathy, peripheral, autonomic) 337.9
  nutritional 263.9
  ocular 359.1
  oculocerebrorenal 270.8
  oculopharyngeal 359.1
  ovarian 620.8
  papillary (and pigmentary) 701.1
  pelvicrural atrophic 359.1
  pigmentary (*see also* Acanthosis) 701.2
  pituitary (gland) 253.8
  polyglandular 258.8
  posttraumatic sympathetic — *see* Dystrophy, sympathetic
  progressive ophthalmoplegic 359.1
  retina, retinal (hereditary) 362.70
    albipunctate 362.74
    Bruch's membrane 362.77
    cone, progressive 362.75
    hyaline 362.77
    in
      Bassen-Kornzweig syndrome 272.5 [362.72]
      cerebroretinal lipidosis 330.1 [362.71]
      Refsum's disease 356.3 [362.72]
      systemic lipidosis 272.7 [362.71]
    juvenile (Stargardt's) 362.75
    pigmentary 362.74
    pigment epithelium 362.76
    progressive cone (-rod) 362.75
    pseudoinflammatory foveal 362.77
    rod, progressive 362.75
    sensory 362.75
    vitelliform 362.76
  Salzmann's nodular 371.46
  scapuloperoneal 359.1
  skin NEC 709.9
  sympathetic (posttraumatic) (reflex) 337.20
    lower limb 337.22
    specified NEC 337.29
    upper limb 337.21
  tapetoretinal NEC 362.74
  thoracic asphyxiating 756.4
  unguium 703.8
    congenital 757.5
  vitreoretinal (primary) 362.73
    secondary 362.66
  vulva 624.0

Dysuria 788.1
 psychogenic 306.53

E

Eagle-Barrett syndrome 756.71
Eales' disease (syndrome) 362.18
Ear — *see also* condition
 ache 388.70
  otogenic 388.71
  referred 388.72
 lop 744.29
 piercing V50.3
 swimmers' acute 380.12
 tank 380.12
 tropical 111.8 *[380.15]*
 wax 380.4
Earache 388.70
 otogenic 388.71
 referred 388.72
Eaton-Lambert syndrome (*see also* Neoplasm, by site, malignant) 199.1 *[358.1]*
Eberth's disease (typhoid fever) 002.0
Ebstein's
 anomaly or syndrome (downward displacement, tricuspid valve into right ventricle) 746.2
 disease (diabetes) 250.4 ✓5ᵗʰ *[581.81]*
Eccentro-osteochondrodysplasia 277.5
Ecchondroma (M9210/0) — *see* Neoplasm, bone, benign
Ecchondrosis (M9210/1) 238.0
Ecchordosis physaliphora 756.0
Ecchymosis (multiple) 459.89
 conjunctiva 372.72
 eye (traumatic) 921.0
 eyelids (traumatic) 921.1
 newborn 772.6
 spontaneous 782.7
 traumatic — *see* Contusion
Echinococciasis — *see* Echinococcus
Echinococcosis — *see* Echinococcus
Echinococcus (infection) 122.9
 granulosus 122.4
  liver 122.0
  lung 122.1
  orbit 122.3 *[376.13]*
  specified site NEC 122.3
  thyroid 122.2
 liver NEC 122.8
  granulosus 122.0
  multilocularis 122.5
 lung NEC 122.9
  granulosus 122.1
  multilocularis 122.6
 multilocularis 122.7
  liver 122.5
  specified site NEC 122.6
 orbit 122.9 *[376.13]*
  granulosus 122.3 *[376.13]*
  multilocularis 122.6 *[376.13]*
 specified site NEC 122.9
  granulosus 122.3
  multilocularis 122.6 *[376.13]*
 thyroid NEC 122.9
  granulosus 122.2
  multilocularis 122.6
Echinorhynchiasis 127.7
Echinostomiasis 121.8
Echolalia 784.69
ECHO virus infection NEC 079.1
Eclampsia, eclamptic (coma) (convulsions) (delirium) 780.39
 female, child-bearing age NEC — *see* Eclampsia, pregnancy
 gravidarum — *see* Eclampsia, pregnancy
 male 780.39
 not associated with pregnancy or childbirth 780.39
 pregnancy, childbirth, or puerperium 642.6 ✓5ᵗʰ
  with pre-existing hypertension 642.7 ✓5ᵗʰ
  affecting fetus or newborn 760.0
 uremic 586
Eclipse blindness (total) 363.31

Economic circumstance affecting care V60.9
 specified type NEC V60.8
Economo's disease (encephalitis lethargica) 049.8
Ectasia, ectasis
 aorta (*see also* Aneurysm, aorta) 441.9
  ruptured 441.5
 breast 610.4
 capillary 448.9
 cornea (marginal) (postinfectional) 371.71
 duct (mammary) 610.4
 kidney 593.89
 mammary duct (gland) 610.4
 papillary 448.9
 renal 593.89
 salivary gland (duct) 527.8
 scar, cornea 371.71
 sclera 379.11
Ecthyma 686.8
 contagiosum 051.2
 gangrenosum 686.09
 infectiosum 051.2
Ectocardia 746.87
Ectodermal dysplasia, congenital 757.31
Ectodermosis erosiva pluriorificialis 695.1
Ectopic, ectopia (congenital) 759.89
 abdominal viscera 751.8
  due to defect in anterior abdominal wall 756.79
 ACTH syndrome 255.0
 adrenal gland 759.1
 anus 751.5
 auricular beats 427.61
 beats 427.60
 bladder 753.5
 bone and cartilage in lung 748.69
 brain 742.4
 breast tissue 757.6
 cardiac 746.87
 cerebral 742.4
 cordis 746.87
 endometrium 617.9
 gallbladder 751.69
 gastric mucosa 750.7
 gestation — *see* Pregnancy, ectopic
 heart 746.87
 hormone secretion NEC 259.3
 hyperparathyroidism 259.3
 kidney (crossed) (intrathoracic) (pelvis) 753.3
  in pregnancy or childbirth 654.4 ✓5ᵗʰ
   causing obstructed labor 660.2 ✓5ᵗʰ
 lens 743.37
 lentis 743.37
 mole — *see* Pregnancy, ectopic
 organ or site NEC — *see* Malposition, congenital
 ovary 752.0
 pancreas, pancreatic tissue 751.7
 pregnancy — *see* Pregnancy, ectopic
 pupil 364.75
 renal 753.3
 sebaceous glands of mouth 750.26
 secretion
  ACTH 255.0
  adrenal hormone 259.3
  adrenalin 259.3
  adrenocorticotropin 255.0
  antidiuretic hormone (ADH) 259.3
  epinephrine 259.3
  hormone NEC 259.3
  norepinephrine 259.3
  pituitary (posterior) 259.3
 spleen 759.0
 testis 752.51
 thyroid 759.2
 ureter 753.4
 ventricular beats 427.69
 vesicae 753.5
Ectrodactyly 755.4
 finger (*see also* Absence, finger, congenital) 755.29
 toe (*see also* Absence, toe, congenital) 755.39
Ectromelia 755.4
 lower limb 755.30
 upper limb 755.20
Ectropion 374.10
 anus 569.49

Ectropion — *continued*
 cervix 622.0
  with mention of cervicitis 616.0
 cicatricial 374.14
 congenital 743.62
 eyelid 374.10
  cicatricial 374.14
  congenital 743.62
  mechanical 374.12
  paralytic 374.12
  senile 374.11
  spastic 374.13
 iris (pigment epithelium) 364.54
 lip (congenital) 750.26
  acquired 528.5
 mechanical 374.12
 paralytic 374.12
 rectum 569.49
 senile 374.11
 spastic 374.13
 urethra 599.84
 uvea 364.54
Eczema (acute) (allergic) (chronic) (erythematous) (fissum) (occupational) (rubrum) (squamous) 692.9
 asteatotic 706.8
 atopic 691.8
 contact NEC 692.9
 dermatitis NEC 692.9
 due to specified cause — *see* Dermatitis, due to
 dyshidrotic 705.81
 external ear 380.22
 flexural 691.8
 gouty 274.89
 herpeticum 054.0
 hypertrophicum 701.8
 hypostatic — *see* Varicose, vein
 impetiginous 684
 infantile (acute) (chronic) (due to any substance) (intertriginous) (seborrheic) 690.12
 intertriginous NEC 692.9
  infantile 690.12
 intrinsic 691.8
 lichenified NEC 692.9
 marginatum 110.3
 nummular 692.9
 pustular 686.8
 seborrheic 690.18
  infantile 690.12
 solare 692.72
 stasis (lower extremity) 454.1
  ulcerated 454.2
 vaccination, vaccinatum 999.0
 varicose (lower extremity) — *see* Varicose, vein
 verrucosum callosum 698.3
Eczematoid, exudative 691.8
Eddowes' syndrome (brittle bone and blue sclera) 756.51
Edema, edematous 782.3
 with nephritis (*see also* Nephrosis) 581.9
 allergic 995.1
 angioneurotic (allergic) (any site) (with urticaria) 995.1
  hereditary 277.6
 angiospastic 443.9
 Berlin's (traumatic) 921.3
 brain 348.5
  due to birth injury 767.8
  fetus or newborn 767.8
 cardiac (*see also* Failure, heart) 428.0
 cardiovascular (*see also* Failure, heart) 428.0
 cerebral — *see* Edema, brain
 cerebrospinal vessel — *see* Edema, brain
 cervix (acute) (uteri) 622.8
  puerperal, postpartum 674.8 ✓5ᵗʰ
 chronic hereditary 757.0
 circumscribed, acute 995.1
  hereditary 277.6
 complicating pregnancy (gestational) 646.1 ✓5ᵗʰ
  with hypertension — *see* Toxemia, of pregnancy
 conjunctiva 372.73
 connective tissue 782.3
 cornea 371.20
  due to contact lenses 371.24
  idiopathic 371.21

Edema — Effect

Edema, edematous — *continued*
cornea — *continued*
  secondary 371.22
 due to
  lymphatic obstruction — *see* Edema,
    lymphatic
  salt retention 276.0
epiglottis — *see* Edema, glottis
essential, acute 995.1
 hereditary 277.6
extremities, lower — *see* Edema, legs
eyelid NEC 374.82
familial, hereditary (legs) 757.0
famine 262
fetus or newborn 778.5
genital organs
 female 629.8
 male 608.86
gestational 646.1 ✓5ᵗʰ
 with hypertension — *see* Toxemia, of
  pregnancy
glottis, glottic, glottides (obstructive) (passive)
  478.6
 allergic 995.1
  hereditary 277.6
 due to external agent — *see* Condition,
  respiratory, acute, due to specified
  agent
heart (*see also* Failure, heart) 428.0
 newborn 779.89 ▲
heat 992.7
hereditary (legs) 757.0
inanition 262
infectious 782.3
intracranial 348.5
 due to injury at birth 767.8
iris 364.8
joint (*see also* Effusion, joint) 719.0 ✓5ᵗʰ
larynx (*see also* Edema, glottis) 478.6
legs 782.3
 due to venous obstruction 459.2
 hereditary 757.0
localized 782.3
 due to venous obstruction 459.2
  lower extremity 459.2
lower extremities — *see* Edema, legs
lung 514
 acute 518.4
  with heart disease or failure (*see also*
    Failure, ventricular, left) 428.1
   congestive 428.0
  chemical (due to fumes or vapors) 506.1
  due to
   external agent(s) NEC 508.9
    specified NEC 508.8
   fumes and vapors (chemical)
    (inhalation) 506.1
   radiation 508.0
 chemical (acute) 506.1
  chronic 506.4
 chronic 514
  chemical (due to fumes or vapors) 506.4
  due to
   external agent(s) NEC 508.9
    specified NEC 508.8
   fumes or vapors (chemical) (inhalation)
    506.4
   radiation 508.1
 due to
  external agent 508.9
   specified NEC 508.8
  high altitude 993.2
  near drowning 994.1
 postoperative 518.4
 terminal 514
lymphatic 457.1
 due to mastectomy operation 457.0
macula 362.83
 cystoid 362.53
 diabetic 250.5 ✓5ᵗʰ *[362.01]*
malignant (*see also* Gangrene, gas) 040.0
Milroy's 757.0
nasopharynx 478.25
neonatorum 778.5
nutritional (newborn) 262
 with dyspigmentation, skin and hair 260
optic disc or nerve — *see* Papilledema

Edema, edematous — *continued*
orbit 376.33
 circulatory 459.89
palate (soft) (hard) 528.9
pancrease 577.8
penis 607.83
periodic 995.1
 hereditary 277.6
pharynx 478.25
pitting 782.3
pulmonary — *see* Edema, lung
Quincke's 995.1
 hereditary 277.6
renal (*see also* Nephrosis) 581.9
retina (localized) (macular) (peripheral) 362.83
 cystoid 362.53
 diabetic 250.5 ✓5ᵗʰ *[362.01]*
salt 276.0
scrotum 608.86
seminal vesicle 608.86
spermatic cord 608.86
spinal cord 336.1
starvation 262
stasis (*see also* Hypertension, venous) ●
 459.30 ●
subconjunctival 372.73
subglottic (*see also* Edema, glottis) 478.6
supraglottic (*see also* Edema, glottis) 478.6
testis 608.86
toxic NEC 782.3
traumatic NEC 782.3
tunica vaginalis 608.86
vas deferens 608.86
vocal cord — *see* Edema, glottis
vulva (acute) 624.8

Edentia (complete) (partial) (*see also* Absence,
  tooth) 520.0
acquired 525.10
 due to
  caries 525.13
  extraction 525.10
  periodontal disease 525.12
  specified NEC 525.19
  trauma 525.11
causing malocclusion 524.3
congenital (deficiency of tooth buds) 520.0

Edentulism 525.10

Edsall's disease 992.2

Educational handicap V62.3

Edwards' syndrome 758.2

Effect, adverse NEC
abnormal gravitation (G) forces or states 994.9
air pressure — *see* Effect, adverse, atmospheric
  pressure
altitude (high) — *see* Effect, adverse, high
  altitude
anesthetic
 in labor and delivery NEC 668.9 ✓5ᵗʰ
  affecting fetus or newborn 763.5
antitoxin — *see* Complications, vaccination
atmospheric pressure 993.9
 due to explosion 993.4
 high 993.3
 low — *see* Effect, adverse, high altitude
 specified effect NEC 993.8
biological, correct substance properly
  administered (*see also* Effect, adverse,
  drug) 995.2
blood (derivatives) (serum) (transfusion) — *see*
  Complications, transfusion
chemical substance NEC 989.9
 specified — *see* Table of Drugs and
  Chemicals
cobalt, radioactive (*see also* Effect, adverse,
  radioactive substance) 990
cold (temperature) (weather) 991.9
 chilblains 991.5
 frostbite — *see* Frostbite
 specified effect NEC 991.8
drugs and medicinals NEC 995.2
 correct substance properly administered
  995.2
 overdose or wrong substance given or taken
  977.9
  specified drug — *see* Table of Drugs and
    Chemicals

Effect, adverse NEC — *continued*
electric current (shock) 994.8
 burn — *see* Burn, by site
electricity (electrocution) (shock) 994.8
 burn — *see* Burn, by site
exertion (excessive) 994.5
exposure 994.9
 exhaustion 994.4
external cause NEC 994.9
fallout (radioactive) NEC 990
fluoroscopy NEC 990
foodstuffs
 allergic reaction (*see also* Allergy, food)
  693.1
  anaphylactic shock due to food NEC
    995.60
 noxious 988.9
  specified type NEC (*see also* Poisoning, by
    name of noxious foodstuff) 988.8
gases, fumes, or vapors — *see* Table of Drugs
  and Chemicals
glue (airplane) sniffing 304.6 ✓5ᵗʰ
heat — *see* Heat
high altitude NEC 993.2
 anoxia 993.2
 on
  ears 993.0
  sinuses 993.1
 polycythemia 289.0
hot weather — *see* Heat
hunger 994.2
immersion, foot 991.4
immunization — *see* Complications,
  vaccination
immunological agents — *see* Complications,
  vaccination
implantation (removable) of isotope or radium
  NEC 990
infrared (radiation) (rays) NEC 990
 burn — *see* Burn, by site
 dermatitis or eczema 692.82
infusion — *see* Complications, infusion
ingestion or injection of isotope (therapeutic)
  NEC 990
irradiation NEC (*see also* Effect, adverse,
  radiation) 990
isotope (radioactive) NEC 990
lack of care (child) (infant) (newborn) 995.52
 adult 995.84
lightning 994.0
 burn — *see* Burn, by site
Lirugin — *see* Complications, vaccination
medicinal substance, correct, properly
  administered (*see also* Effect, adverse,
  drugs) 995.2
mesothorium NEC 990
motion 994.6
noise, inner ear 388.10
overheated places — *see* Heat
polonium NEC 990
psychosocial, of work environment V62.1
radiation (diagnostic) (fallout) (infrared) (natural
  source) (therapeutic) (tracer) (ultraviolet)
  (x-ray) NEC 990
 with pulmonary manifestations
  acute 508.0
  chronic 508.1
 dermatitis or eczema 692.82
  due to sun NEC (*see also* Dermatitis, due
    to, sun) 692.70
 fibrosis of lungs 508.1
 maternal with suspected damage to fetus
  affecting management of pregnancy
  655.6 ✓5ᵗʰ
 pneumonitis 508.0
radioactive substance NEC 990
 dermatitis or eczema 692.82
radioactivity NEC 990
radiotherapy NEC 990
 dermatitis or eczema 692.82
radium NEC 990
reduced temperature 991.9
 frostbite — *see* Frostbite
 immersion, foot (hand) 991.4
 specified effect NEC 991.8
roentgenography NEC 990
roentgenoscopy NEC 990

✓4ᵗʰ Fourth-digit Required   ✓5ᵗʰ Fifth-digit Required   ▶◀ Revised Text   ● New Line   ▲ Revised Code

Effect, adverse NEC — *continued*
　roentgen rays NEC 990
　serum (prophylactic) (therapeutic) NEC 999.5
　specified NEC 995.89
　　external cause NEC 994.9
　strangulation 994.7
　submersion 994.1
　teletherapy NEC 990
　thirst 994.3
　transfusion — *see* Complications, transfusion
　ultraviolet (radiation) (rays) NEC 990
　　burn — *see also* Burn, by site
　　　from sun (*see also* Sunburn) 692.71
　　dermatitis or eczema 692.82
　　　due to sun NEC (*see also* Dermatitis, due
　　　　to, sun) 692.70
　uranium NEC 990
　vaccine (any) — *see* Complications, vaccination
　weightlessness 994.9
　whole blood — *see also* Complications,
　　transfusion
　　overdose or wrong substance given (*see also*
　　　Table of Drugs and Chemicals) 964.7
　working environment V62.1
　x-rays NEC 990
　　dermatitis or eczema 692.82
Effects, late — *see* Late, effect (of)
Effect, remote
　of cancer — *see* condition
Effluvium, telogen 704.02
Effort
　intolerance 306.2
　syndrome (aviators) (psychogenic) 306.2
Effusion
　amniotic fluid (*see also* Rupture, membranes,
　　premature) 658.1 ✔5ᵗʰ
　brain (serous) 348.5
　bronchial (*see also* Bronchitis) 490
　cerebral 348.5
　cerebrospinal (*see also* Meningitis) 322.9
　　vessel 348.5
　chest — *see* Effusion, pleura
　intracranial 348.5
　joint 719.00
　　ankle 719.07
　　elbow 719.02
　　foot 719.07
　　hand 719.04
　　hip 719.05
　　knee 719.06
　　multiple sites 719.09
　　pelvic region 719.05
　　shoulder (region) 719.01
　　specified site NEC 719.08
　　wrist 719.03
　meninges (*see also* Meningitis) 322.9
　pericardium, pericardial (*see also* Pericarditis)
　　423.9
　　acute 420.90
　peritoneal (chronic) 568.82
　pleura, pleurisy, pleuritic, pleuropericardial
　　511.9
　　bacterial, nontuberculous 511.1
　　fetus or newborn 511.9
　　malignant 197.2
　　nontuberculous 511.9
　　　bacterial 511.1
　　pneumococcal 511.1
　　staphylococcal 511.1
　　streptococcal 511.1
　　traumatic 862.29
　　　with open wound 862.39
　　tuberculous (*see also* Tuberculosis, pleura)
　　　012.0 ✔5ᵗʰ
　　　primary progressive 010.1 ✔5ᵗʰ
　pulmonary — *see* Effusion, pleura
　spinal (*see also* Meningitis) 322.9
　thorax, thoracic — *see* Effusion, pleura
Eggshell nails 703.8
　congenital 757.5
Ego-dystonic
　homosexuality 302.0
　lesbianism 302.0
Egyptian splenomegaly 120.1
Ehlers-Danlos syndrome 756.83

Ehrlichiosis 082.40
　chaffeensis 082.41
　specified type NEC 082.49
Eichstedt's disease (pityriasis versicolor) 111.0
Eisenmenger's complex or syndrome
　(ventricular septal defect) 745.4
Ejaculation, semen
　painful 608.89
　　psychogenic 306.59
　premature 302.75
　retrograde 608.87
Ekbom syndrome (restless legs) 333.99
Ekman's syndrome (brittle bones and blue sclera)
　756.51
Elastic skin 756.83
　acquired 701.8
Elastofibroma (M8820/0) — *see* Neoplasm,
　connective tissue, benign
Elastoidosis
　cutanea nodularis 701.8
　cutis cystica et comedonica 701.8
Elastoma 757.39
　juvenile 757.39
　Miescher's (elastosis perforans serpiginosa)
　　701.1
Elastomyofibrosis 425.3
Elastosis 701.8
　atrophicans 701.8
　perforans serpiginosa 701.1
　reactive perforating 701.1
　senilis 701.8
　solar (actinic) 692.74
Elbow — *see* condition
Electric
　current, electricity, effects (concussion) (fatal)
　　(nonfatal) (shock) 994.8
　　burn — *see* Burn, by site
　feet (foot) syndrome 266.2
Electrocution 994.8
Electrolyte imbalance 276.9
　with
　　abortion — *see* Abortion, by type with
　　　metabolic disorder
　　ectopic pregnancy (*see also* categories
　　　633.0-633.9) 639.4
　　hyperemesis gravidarum (before 22
　　　completed weeks gestation) 643.1 ✔5ᵗʰ
　　molar pregnancy (*see also* categories 630-
　　　632) 639.4
　following
　　abortion 639.4
　　ectopic or molar pregnancy 639.4
Elephant man syndrome 237.71
Elephantiasis (nonfilarial) 457.1
　arabicum (*see also* Infestation, filarial) 125.9
　congenita hereditaria 757.0
　congenital (any site) 757.0
　due to
　　Brugia (malayi) 125.1
　　mastectomy operation 457.0
　　Wuchereria (bancrofti) 125.0
　　　malayi 125.1
　eyelid 374.83
　filarial (*see also* Infestation, filarial) 125.9
　filariensis (*see also* Infestation, filarial) 125.9
　gingival 523.8
　glandular 457.1
　graecorum 030.9
　lymphangiectatic 457.1
　lymphatic vessel 457.1
　　due to mastectomy operation 457.0
　neuromatosa 237.71
　postmastectomy 457.0
　scrotum 457.1
　streptococcal 457.1
　surgical 997.99
　　postmastectomy 457.0
　telangiectodes 457.1
　vulva (nonfilarial) 624.8
Elevated — *see* Elevation
Elevation
　17-ketosteroids 791.9
　acid phosphatase 790.5
　alkaline phosphatase 790.5

Elevation — *continued*
　amylase 790.5
　antibody titers 795.79
　basal metabolic rate (BMR) 794.7
　blood pressure (*see also* Hypertension) 401.9
　　reading (incidental) (isolated) (nonspecific),
　　　no diagnosis or hypertension 796.2
　body temperature (of unknown origin) (*see also*
　　Pyrexia) 780.6
　conjugate, eye 378.81
　diaphragm, congenital 756.6
　immunoglobulin level 795.79
　indolacetic acid 791.9
　lactic acid dehydrogenase (LDH) level 790.4
　lipase 790.5
　prostate specific antigen (PSA) 790.93
　renin 790.99
　　in hypertension (*see also* Hypertension,
　　　renovascular) 405.91
　Rh titer 999.7
　scapula, congenital 755.52
　sedimentation rate 790.1
　SGOT 790.4
　SGPT 790.4
　transaminase 790.4
　vanillylmandelic acid 791.9
　venous pressure 459.89
　VMA 791.9
Elliptocytosis (congenital) (hereditary) 282.1
　Hb-C (disease) 282.7
　hemoglobin disease 282.7
　sickle-cell (disease) 282.60
　　trait 282.5
Ellis-van Creveld disease or syndrome
　(chondroectodermal dysplasia) 756.55
Ellison-Zollinger syndrome (gastric
　hypersecretion with pancreatic islet cell
　tumor) 251.5
Elongation, elongated (congenital) — *see also*
　Distortion
　bone 756.9
　cervix (uteri) 752.49
　　acquired 622.6
　　hypertrophic 622.6
　colon 751.5
　common bile duct 751.69
　cystic duct 751.69
　frenulum, penis 752.69
　labia minora, acquired 624.8
　ligamentum patellae 756.89
　petiolus (epiglottidis) 748.3
　styloid bone (process) 733.99
　tooth, teeth 520.2
　uvula 750.26
　　acquired 528.9
Elschnig bodies or pearls 366.51
El Tor cholera 001.1
Emaciation (due to malnutrition) 261
Emancipation disorder 309.22
Embadomoniasis 007.8
Embarrassment heart, cardiac — *see* Disease,
　heart
Embedded tooth, teeth 520.6
　with abnormal position (same or adjacent
　　tooth) 524.3
　root only 525.3
Embolic — *see* condition
Embolism 444.9
　with
　　abortion — *see* Abortion, by type, with
　　　embolism
　　ectopic pregnancy (*see also* categories
　　　633.0-633.9) 639.6
　　molar pregnancy (*see also* categories 630-
　　　632) 639.6
　air (any site) 958.0
　　with
　　　abortion — *see* Abortion, by type, with
　　　　embolism
　　　ectopic pregnancy (*see also* categories
　　　　633.0-633.9) 639.6
　　　molar pregnancy (*see also* categories 630-
　　　　632) 639.6

Embolism — *continued*
  air — *continued*
    due to implanted device — *see*
      Complications, due to (presence of)
      any device, implant, or graft classified
      to 996.0-996.5 NEC
    following
      abortion 639.6
      ectopic or molar pregnancy 639.6
      infusion, perfusion, or transfusion 999.1
    in pregnancy, childbirth, or puerperium
      673.0 ✓5ᵗʰ
    traumatic 958.0
  amniotic fluid (pulmonary) 673.1 ✓5ᵗʰ
    with
      abortion — *see* Abortion, by type, with
        embolism
      ectopic pregnancy (*see also* categories
        633.0-633.9) 639.6
      molar pregnancy (*see also* categories 630-
        632) 639.6
    following
      abortion 639.6
      ectopic or molar pregnancy 639.6
  aorta, aortic 444.1
    abdominal 444.0
    bifurcation 444.0
    saddle 444.0
    thoracic 444.1
  artery 444.9
    auditory, internal 433.8 ✓5ᵗʰ
    basilar (*see also* Occlusion, artery, basilar)
      433.0 ✓5ᵗʰ
    bladder 444.89
    carotid (common) (internal) (*see also*
      Occlusion, artery, carotid) 433.1 ✓5ᵗʰ
    cerebellar (anterior inferior) (posterior
      inferior) (superior) 433.8 ✓5ᵗʰ
    cerebral (*see also* Embolism, brain)
      434.1 ✓5ᵗʰ
    choroidal (anterior) 433.8 ✓5ᵗʰ
    communicating posterior 433.8 ✓5ᵗʰ
    coronary (*see also* Infarct, myocardium)
      410.9 ✓5ᵗʰ
      without myocardial infarction 411.81
    extremity 444.22
      lower 444.22
      upper 444.21
    hypophyseal 433.8 ✓5ᵗʰ
    mesenteric (with gangrene) 557.0
    ophthalmic (*see also* Occlusion, retina)
      362.30
    peripheral 444.22
    pontine 433.8 ✓5ᵗʰ
    precerebral NEC — *see* Occlusion, artery,
      precerebral
    pulmonary — *see* Embolism, pulmonary
    renal 593.81
    retinal (*see also* Occlusion, retina) 362.30
    specified site NEC 444.89
    vertebral (*see also* Occlusion, artery,
      vertebral) 433.2 ✓5ᵗʰ
  auditory, internal 433.8 ✓5ᵗʰ
  basilar (artery) (*see also* Occlusion, artery,
    basilar) 433.0 ✓5ᵗʰ
  birth, mother — *see* Embolism, obstetrical
  blood-clot
    with
      abortion — *see* Abortion, by type, with
        embolism
      ectopic pregnancy (*see also* categories
        633.0-633.9) 639.6
      molar pregnancy (*see also* categories 630-
        632) 639.6
    following
      abortion 639.6
      ectopic or molar pregnancy 639.6
    in pregnancy, childbirth, or puerperium
      673.2 ✓5ᵗʰ
  brain 434.1 ✓5ᵗʰ
    with
      abortion — *see* Abortion, by type, with
        embolism
      ectopic pregnancy (*see also* categories
        633.0-633.9) 639.6
      molar pregnancy (*see also* categories 630-
        632) 639.6

Embolism — *continued*
  brain — *continued*
    following
      abortion 639.6
      ectopic or molar pregnancy 639.6
    late effect — *see* Late effect(s) (of)
      cerebrovascular disease
    puerperal, postpartum, childbirth 674.0 ✓5ᵗʰ
  capillary 448.9
  cardiac (*see also* Infarct, myocardium)
    410.9 ✓5ᵗʰ
  carotid (artery) (common) (internal) (*see also*
    Occlusion, artery, carotid) 433.1 ✓5ᵗʰ
  cavernous sinus (venous) — *see* Embolism,
    intracranial venous sinus
  cerebral (*see also* Embolism, brain) 434.1 ✓5ᵗʰ
  cholesterol — *see* Atheroembolism   ●
  choroidal (anterior) (artery) 433.8 ✓5ᵗʰ
  coronary (artery or vein) (systemic) (*see also*
    Infarct, myocardium) 410.9 ✓5ᵗʰ
    without myocardial infarction 411.81
  due to (presence of) any device, implant, or
    graft classifiable to 996.0-996.5 — *see*
    Complications, due to (presence of) any
    device, implant, or graft classified to
    996.0-996.5 NEC
  encephalomalacia (*see also* Embolism, brain)
    434.1 ✓5ᵗʰ
  extremities 444.22
    lower 444.22
    upper 444.21
  eye 362.30
  fat (cerebral) (pulmonary) (systemic) 958.1
    with
      abortion — *see* Abortion, by type, with
        embolism
      ectopic pregnancy (*see also* categories
        633.0-633.9) 639.6
      molar pregnancy (*see also* categories 630-
        632) 639.6
    complicating delivery or puerperium
      673.8 ✓5ᵗʰ
    following
      abortion 639.6
      ectopic or molar pregnancy 639.6
    in pregnancy, childbirth, or the puerperium
      673.8 ✓5ᵗʰ
  femoral (artery) 444.22
    vein 453.8
  following
    abortion 639.6
    ectopic or molar pregnancy 639.6
    infusion, perfusion, or transfusion
      air 999.1
      thrombus 999.2
  heart (fatty) (*see also* Infarct, myocardium)
    410.9 ✓5ᵗʰ
  hepatic (vein) 453.0
  iliac (artery) 444.81
  iliofemoral 444.81
  in pregnancy, childbirth, or puerperium
    (pulmonary) — *see* Embolism, obstetrical
  intestine (artery) (vein) (with gangrene) 557.0
  intracranial (*see also* Embolism, brain)
    434.1 ✓5ᵗʰ
    venous sinus (any) 325
      late effect — *see* category 326
      nonpyogenic 437.6
        in pregnancy or puerperium 671.5 ✓5ᵗʰ
  kidney (artery) 593.81
  lateral sinus (venous) — *see* Embolism,
    intracranial venous sinus
  longitudinal sinus (venous) — *see* Embolism,
    intracranial venous sinus
  lower extremity 444.22
  lung (massive) — *see* Embolism, pulmonary
  meninges (*see also* Embolism, brain) 434.1 ✓5ᵗʰ
  mesenteric (artery) (with gangrene) 557.0
  multiple NEC 444.9
  obstetrical (pulmonary) 673.2 ✓5ᵗʰ
    air 673.0 ✓5ᵗʰ
    amniotic fluid (pulmonary) 673.1 ✓5ᵗʰ
    blood-clot 673.2 ✓5ᵗʰ
    cardiac 674.8 ✓5ᵗʰ
    fat 673.8 ✓5ᵗʰ
    heart 674.8 ✓5ᵗʰ
    pyemic 673.3 ✓5ᵗʰ

Embolism — *continued*
  obstetrical — *continued*
    septic 673.3 ✓5ᵗʰ
    specified NEC 674.8 ✓5ᵗʰ
  ophthalmic (*see also* Occlusion, retina) 362.30
  paradoxical NEC 444.9
  penis 607.82
  peripheral arteries NEC 444.22
    lower 444.22
    upper 444.21
  pituitary 253.8
  popliteal (artery) 444.22
  portal (vein) 452
  postoperative NEC 997.2
    cerebral 997.02
    mesenteric artery 997.71
    other vessels 997.79
    peripheral vascular 997.2
    pulmonary 415.11
    renal artery 997.72
  precerebral artery (*see also* Occlusion, artery,
    precerebral) 433.9 ✓5ᵗʰ
  puerperal — *see* Embolism, obstetrical
  pulmonary (artery) (vein) 415.1 ✓5ᵗʰ
    with
      abortion — *see* Abortion, by type, with
        embolism
      ectopic pregnancy (*see also* categories
        633.0-633.9) 639.6
      molar pregnancy (*see also* categories 630-
        632) 639.6
    following
      abortion 639.6
      ectopic or molar pregnancy 639.6
    iatrogenic 415.11
    in pregnancy, childbirth, or puerperium —
      see Embolism, obstetrical
    postoperative 415.11
  pyemic (multiple) 038.9
    with
      abortion — *see* Abortion, by type, with
        embolism
      ectopic pregnancy (*see also* categories
        633.0-633.9) 639.6
      molar pregnancy (*see also* categories 630-
        632) 639.6
    Aerobacter aerogenes 038.49
    enteric gram-negative bacilli 038.40
    Enterobacter aerogenes 038.49
    Escherichia coli 038.42
    following
      abortion 639.6
      ectopic or molar pregnancy 639.6
    Hemophilus influenzae 038.41
    pneumococcal 038.2
    Proteus vulgaris 038.49
    Pseudomonas (aeruginosa) 038.43
    puerperal, postparztum, childbirth (any
      organism) 673.3 ✓5ᵗʰ
    Serratia 038.44
    specified organism NEC 038.8
    staphylococcal 038.10
      aureus 038.11
      specified organism NEC 038.19
    streptococcal 038.0
  renal (artery) 593.81
    vein 453.3
  retina, retinal (*see also* Occlusion, retina)
    362.30
  saddle (aorta) 444.0
  septicemic — *see* Embolism, pyemic
  sinus — *see* Embolism, intracranial venous
    sinus
  soap
    with
      abortion — *see* Abortion, by type, with
        embolism
      ectopic pregnancy (*see also* categories
        633.0-633.9) 639.6
      molar pregnancy (*see also* categories 630-
        632) 639.6
    following
      abortion 639.6
      ectopic or molar pregnancy 639.6
  spinal cord (nonpyogenic) 336.1
    in pregnancy or puerperium 671.5 ✓5ᵗʰ

Embolism — *continued*
  spinal cord — *continued*
    pyogenic origin 324.1
      late effect — *see* category 326
  spleen, splenic (artery) 444.89
  thrombus (thromboembolism) following
      infusion, perfusion, or transfusion 999.2
  upper extremity 444.21
  vein 453.9
    with inflammation or phlebitis — *see*
        Thrombophlebitis
    cerebral (*see also* Embolism, brain)
        434.1 ✔5ᵗʰ
    coronary (*see also* Infarct, myocardium)
        410.9 ✔5ᵗʰ
      without myocardial infarction 411.81
    hepatic 453.0
    mesenteric (with gangrene) 557.0
    portal 452
    pulmonary — *see* Embolism, pulmonary
    renal 453.3
    specified NEC 453.8
      with inflammation or phlebitis — *see*
          Thrombophlebitis
  vena cava (inferior) (superior) 453.2
  vessels of brain (*see also* Embolism, brain)
      434.1 ✔5ᵗʰ

Embolization — *see* Embolism

Embolus — *see* Embolism

Embryoma (M9080/1) — *see also* Neoplasm, by
    site, uncertain behavior
  benign (M9080/0 — *see* Neoplasm, by site,
      benign
  kidney (M8960/3) 189.0
  liver (M8970/3) 155.0
  malignant (M9080/3) — *see also* Neoplasm, by
      site, malignant
    kidney (M8960/3) 189.0
    liver (M8970/3) 155.0
    testis (M9070/3) 186.9
      undescended 186.0
  testis (M9070/3) 186.9
    undescended 186.0

Embryonic
  circulation 747.9
  heart 747.9
  vas deferens 752.8

Embryopathia NEC 759.9

Embryotomy, fetal 763.89

Embryotoxon 743.43
  interfering with vision 743.42

Emesis — *see also* Vomiting
  gravidarum — *see* Hyperemesis, gravidarum

Emissions, nocturnal (semen) 608.89

Emotional
  crisis — *see* Crisis, emotional
  disorder (*see also* Disorder, mental) 300.9
  instability (excessive) 301.3
  overlay — *see* Reaction, adjustment
  upset 300.9

Emotionality, pathological 301.3

Emotogenic disease (*see also* Disorder,
    psychogenic) 306.9

Emphysema (atrophic) (centriacinar)
    (centrilobular) (chronic) (diffuse) (essential)
    (hypertrophic) (interlobular) (lung)
    (obstructive) (panlobular) (paracicatricial)
    (paracinar) (postural) (pulmonary) (senile)
    (subpleural) (traction) (unilateral)
    (unilobular) (vesicular) 492.8
  with
    bronchitis
      acute and chronic 491.21
      chronic 491.20
        with acute bronchitis or acute
            exacerbation 491.21
  bullous (giant) 492.0
  cellular tissue 958.7
    surgical 998.81
  compensatory 518.2
  congenital 770.2
  conjunctiva 372.89
  connective tissue 958.7
    surgical 998.81

Emphysema — *continued*
  due to fumes or vapors 506.4
  eye 376.89
  eyelid 374.85
    surgical 998.81
    traumatic 958.7
  fetus or newborn (interstitial) (mediastinal)
      (unilobular) 770.2
  heart 416.9
  interstitial 518.1
    congenital 770.2
    fetus or newborn 770.2
  laminated tissue 958.7
    surgical 998.81
  mediastinal 518.1
    fetus or newborn 770.2
  newborn (interstitial) (mediastinal) (unilobular)
      770.2
  obstructive diffuse with fibrosis 492.8
  orbit 376.89
  subcutaneous 958.7
    due to trauma 958.7
    nontraumatic 518.1
    surgical 998.81
  surgical 998.81
  thymus (gland) (congenital) 254.8
  traumatic 958.7
  tuberculous (*see also* Tuberculosis, pulmonary)
      011.9 ✔5ᵗʰ

Employment examination (certification) V70.5

Empty sella (turcica) syndrome 253.8

Empyema (chest) (diaphragmatic) (double)
    (encapsulated) (general) (interlobar) (lung)
    (medial) (necessitatis) (perforating chest wall)
    (pleura) (pneumococcal) (residual)
    (sacculated) (streptococcal)
    (supradiaphragmatic) 510.9
  with fistula 510.0
  accessory sinus (chronic) (*see also* Sinusitis)
      473.9
  acute 510.9
    with fistula 510.0
  antrum (chronic) (*see also* Sinusitis, maxillary)
      473.0
  brain (any part) (*see also* Abcess, brain) 324.0
  ethmoidal (sinus) (chronic) (*see also* Sinusitis,
      ethmoidal) 473.2
  extradural (*see also* Abscess, extradural) 324.9
  frontal (sinus) (chronic) (*see also* Sinusitis,
      frontal) 473.1
  gallbladder (*see also* Cholecystitis, acute) 575.0
  mastoid (process) (acute) (*see also* Mastoiditis,
      acute) 383.00
  maxilla, maxillary 526.4
    sinus (chronic) (*see also* Sinusitis, maxillary)
        473.0
  nasal sinus (chronic) (*see also* Sinusitis) 473.9
  sinus (accessory) (nasal) (*see also* Sinusitis)
      473.9
  sphenoidal (chronic) (sinus) (*see also* Sinusitis,
      sphenoidal) 473.3
  subarachnoid (*see also* Abscess, extradural)
      324.9
  subdural (*see also* Abscess, extradural) 324.9
  tuberculous (*see also* Tuberculosis, pleura)
      012.0 ✔5ᵗʰ
  ureter (*see also* Ureteritis) 593.89
  ventricular (*see also* Abscess, brain) 324.0

Enameloma 520.2

Encephalitis (bacterial) (chronic) (hemorrhagic)
    (idiopathic) (nonepidemic) (spurious)
    (subacute) 323.9
  acute — *see also* Encephalitis, viral
    disseminated (postinfectious) NEC
        136.9 [323.6]
      postimmunization or postvaccination
          323.5
    inclusional 049.8
    inclusion body 049.8
    necrotizing 049.8
  arboviral, arbovirus NEC 064
  arthropod-borne (*see also* Encephalitis, viral,
      arthropod-borne) 064
  Australian X 062.4
  Bwamba fever 066.3
  California (virus) 062.5
  Central European 063.2

Encephalitis — *continued*
  Czechoslovakian 063.2
  Dawson's (inclusion body) 046.2
  diffuse sclerosing 046.2
  due to
    actinomycosis 039.8 [323.4]
    cat-scratch disease 078.3 [323.0]
    infectious mononucleosis 075 [323.0]
    malaria (*see also* Malaria) 084.6 [323.2]
    Negishi virus 064
    ornithosis 073.7 [323.0]
    prophylactic inoculation against smallpox
        323.5
    rickettsiosis (*see also* Rickettsiosis)
        083.9 [323.1]
    rubella 056.01
    toxoplasmosis (acquired) 130.0
      congenital (active) 771.2 [323.4]
    typhus (fever) (*see also* Typhus)
        081.9 [323.1]
    vaccination (smallpox) 323.5
  Eastern equine 062.2
  endemic 049.8
  epidemic 049.8
  equine (acute) (infectious) (viral) 062.9
    Eastern 062.2
    Venezuelan 066.2
    Western 062.1
  Far Eastern 063.0
  following vaccination or other immunization
      procedure 323.5
  herpes 054.3
  Ilheus (virus) 062.8
  inclusion body 046.2
  infectious (acute) (virus) NEC 049.8
  influenzal 487.8 [323.4]
    lethargic 049.8
  Japanese (B type) 062.0
  La Crosse 062.5
  Langat 063.8
  late effect — *see* Late, effect, encephalitis
  lead 984.9 [323.7]
  lethargic (acute) (infectious) (influenzal) 049.8
  lethargica 049.8
  louping ill 063.1
  lupus 710.0 [323.8]
  lymphatica 049.0
  Mengo 049.8
  meningococcal 036.1
  mumps 072.2
  Murray Valley 062.4
  myoclonic 049.8
  Negishi virus 064
  otitic NEC 382.4 [323.4]
  parasitic NEC 123.9 [323.4]
  periaxialis (concentrica) (diffusa) 341.1
  postchickenpox 052.0
  postexanthematous NEC 057.9 [323.6]
  postimmunization 323.5
  postinfectious NEC 136.9 [323.6]
  postmeasles 055.0
  posttraumatic 323.8
  postvaccinal (smallpox) 323.5
  postvaricella 052.0
  postviral NEC 079.99 [323.6]
    postexanthematous 057.9 [323.6]
      specified NEC 057.8 [323.6]
  Powassan 063.8
  progressive subcortical (Binswanger's) 290.12
  Rio Bravo 049.8
  rubella 056.01
  Russian
    autumnal 062.0
    spring-summer type (taiga) 063.0
  saturnine 984.9 [323.7]
  Semliki Forest 062.8
  serous 048
  slow-acting virus NEC 046.8
  specified cause NEC 323.8
  St. Louis type 062.3
  subacute sclerosing 046.2
  subcorticalis chronica 290.12
  summer 062.0
  suppurative 324.0
  syphilitic 094.81
    congenital 090.41
  tick-borne 063.9
  torula, torular 117.5 [323.4]

Encephalitis — *continued*
toxic NEC 989.9 *[323.7]*
toxoplasmic (acquired) 130.0
congenital (active) 771.2 *[323.4]*
trichinosis 124 *[323.4]*
Trypanosomiasis (*see also* Trypanosomiasis) 086.9 *[323.2]*
tuberculous (*see also* Tuberculosis) 013.6 ✓5ᵗʰ
type B (Japanese) 062.0
type C 062.3
van Bogaert's 046.2
Venezuelan 066.2
Vienna type 049.8
viral, virus 049.9
arthropod-borne NEC 064
mosquito-borne 062.9
Australian X disease 062.4
California virus 062.5
Eastern equine 062.2
Ilheus virus 062.8
Japanese (B type) 062.0
Murray Valley 062.4
specified type NEC 062.8
St. Louis 062.3
type B 062.0
type C 062.3
Western equine 062.1
tick-borne 063.9
biundulant 063.2
Central European 063.2
Czechoslovakian 063.2
diphasic meningoencephalitis 063.2
Far Eastern 063.0
Langat 063.8
louping ill 063.1
Powassan 063.8
Russian spring-summer (taiga) 063.0
specified type NEC 063.8
vector unknown 064
slow acting NEC 046.8
specified type NEC 049.8
vaccination, prophylactic (against) V05.0
von Economo's 049.8
Western equine 062.1
West Nile type 066.4 ▲
Encephalocele 742.0
orbit 376.81
Encephalocystocele 742.0
Encephalomalacia (brain) (cerebellar) (cerebral) (cerebrospinal) (*see also* Softening, brain) 434.9 ✓5ᵗʰ
due to
hemorrhage (*see also* Hemorrhage, brain) 431
recurrent spasm of artery 435.9
embolic (cerebral) (*see also* Embolism, brain) 434.1 ✓5ᵗʰ
subcorticalis chronicus arteriosclerotica 290.12
thrombotic (*see also* thrombosis, brain) 434.0 ✓5ᵗʰ
Encephalomeningitis — *see* Meningoencephalitis
Encephalomeningocele 742.0
Encephalomeningomyelitis — *see* Meningoencephalitis
Encephalomeningopathy (*see also* Meningoencephalitis) 349.9
Encephalomyelitis (chronic) (granulomatous) (hemorrhagic necrotizing, acute) (myalgic, benign) (*see also* Encephalitis) 323.9
abortive disseminated 049.8
acute disseminated (postinfectious) 136.9 *[323.6]*
postimmunization 323.5
due to or resulting from vaccination (any) 323.5
equine (acute) (infectious) 062.9
Eastern 062.2
Venezuelan 066.2
Western 062.1
funicularis infectiosa 049.8
late effect — *see* Late, effect, encephalitis
Munch-Peterson's 049.8
postchickenpox 052.0
postimmunization 323.5
postmeasles 055.0
postvaccinal (smallpox) 323.5

Encephalomyelitis (*see also* Encephalitis) — *continued*
rubella 056.01
specified cause NEC 323.8
syphilitic 094.81
Encephalomyelocele 742.0
Encephalomyelomeningitis — *see* Meningoencephalitis
Encephalomyeloneuropathy 349.9
Encephalomyelopathy 349.9
subacute necrotizing (infantile) 330.8
Encephalomyeloradiculitis (acute) 357.0
Encephalomyeloradiculoneuritis (acute) 357.0
Encephalomyeloradiculopathy 349.9
Encephalomyocarditis 074.23
Encephalopathia hyperbilirubinemica, newborn 774.7
due to isoimmunization (conditions classifiable to 773.0-773.2) 773.4
Encephalopathy (acute) 348.3
alcoholic 291.2
anoxic — *see* Damage, brain, anoxic
arteriosclerotic 437.0
late effect — *see* Late effect(s) (of) cerebrovascular disease
bilirubin, newborn 774.7
due to isoimmunization 773.4
congenital 742.9
demyelinating (callosal) 341.8
due to
birth injury (intracranial) 767.8
dialysis 294.8
transient 293.9
hyperinsulinism — *see* Hyperinsulinism
influenza (virus) 487.8
lack of vitamin (*see also* Deficiency, vitamin) 269.2
nicotinic acid deficiency 291.2
serum (nontherapeutic) (therapeutic) 999.5
syphilis 094.81
trauma (postconcussional) 310.2
current (*see also* Concussion, brain) 850.9
with skull fracture — *see* Fracture, skull, by site, with intracranial injury
vaccination 323.5
hepatic 572.2
hyperbilirubinemic, newborn 774.7
due to isoimmunization (conditions classifiable to 773.0-773.2) 773.4
hypertensive 437.2
hypoglycemic 251.2
hypoxic — *see* Damage, brain, anoxic
infantile cystic necrotizing (congenital) 341.8
lead 984.9 *[323.7]*
leukopolio 330.0
metabolic (toxic) — *see* Delirium
necrotizing, subacute 330.8
pellagrous 265.2
portal-systemic 572.2
postcontusional 310.2
posttraumatic 310.2
saturnine 984.9 *[323.7]*
spongiform, subacute (viral) 046.1
subacute
necrotizing 330.8
spongiform 046.1
viral, spongiform 046.1
subcortical progressive (Schilder) 341.1
chronic (Binswanger's) 290.12
toxic 349.82
metabolic — *see* Delirium
traumatic (postconcussional) 310.2
current (*see also* Concussion, brain) 850.9
with skull fracture — *see* Fracture, skull, by site, with intracranial injury
vitamin B deficiency NEC 266.9
Wernicke's (superior hemorrhagic polioencephalitis) 265.1
Encephalorrhagia (*see also* Hemorrhage, brain) 432.9
healed or old V12.59
late effect — *see* Late effect(s) (of) cerebrovascular disease

Encephalosis, posttraumatic 310.2
Enchondroma (M9220/0) — *see also* Neoplasm, bone, benign
multiple, congenital 756.4
Enchondromatosis (cartilaginous) (congenital) (multiple) 756.4
Enchondroses, multiple (cartilaginous) (congenital) 756.4
Encopresis (*see also* Incontinence, feces) 787.6
nonorganic origin 307.7
Encounter for — *see also* Admission for
administrative purpose only V68.9
referral of patient without examination or treatment V68.81
specified purpose NEC V68.89
chemotherapy V58.1
end-of-life care V66.7
hospice care V66.7
palliative care V66.7
paternity testing V70.4
radiotherapy V58.0
screening mammogram NEC V76.12
for high-risk patient V76.11
terminal care V66.7
Encystment — *see* Cyst
End-of-life care V66.7
Endamebiasis — *see* Amebiasis
Endamoeba — *see* Amebiasis
Endarteritis (bacterial, subacute) (infective) (septic) 447.6
brain, cerebral or cerebrospinal 437.4
late effect — *see* Late effect(s) (of) cerebrovascular disease
coronary (artery) — *see* Arteriosclerosis, coronary
deformans — *see* Arteriosclerosis
embolic (*see also* Embolism) 444.9
obliterans — *see* Arteriosclerosis
pulmonary 417.8
pulmonary 417.8
retina 362.18
senile — *see* Arteriosclerosis
syphilitic 093.89
brain or cerebral 094.89
congenital 090.5
spinal 094.89
tuberculous (*see also* Tuberculosis) 017.9 ✓5ᵗʰ
Endemic — *see* condition
Endocarditis (chronic) (indeterminate) (interstitial) (marantic) (nonbacterial thrombotic) (residual) (sclerotic) (sclerous) (senile) (valvular) 424.90
with
rheumatic fever (conditions classifiable to 390)
active — *see* Endocarditis, acute, rheumatic
inactive or quiescent (with chorea) 397.9
acute or subacute 421.9
rheumatic (aortic) (mitral) (pulmonary) (tricuspid) 391.1
with chorea (acute) (rheumatic) (Sydenham's) 392.0
aortic (heart) (nonrheumatic) (valve) 424.1
with
mitral (valve) disease 396.9
active or acute 391.1
with chorea (acute) (rheumatic) (Sydenham's) 392.0
rheumatic fever (conditions classifiable to 390)
active — *see* Endocarditis, acute, rheumatic
inactive or quiescent (with chorea) 395.9
with mitral disease 396.9
acute or subacute 421.9
arteriosclerotic 424.1
congenital 746.89
hypertensive 424.1
rheumatic (chronic) (inactive) 395.9
with mitral (valve) disease 396.9
active or acute 391.1
with chorea (acute) (rheumatic) (Sydenham's) 392.0

Endocarditis — *continued*
   aortic — *continued*
      rheumatic — *continued*
         active or acute 391.1
            with chorea (acute) (rheumatic)
               (Sydenham's) 392.0
         specified cause, except rheumatic 424.1
      syphilitic 093.22
   arteriosclerotic or due to arteriosclerosis
      424.99
   atypical verrucous (Libman-Sacks)
      710.0 *[424.91]*
   bacterial (acute) (any valve) (chronic) (subacute)
      421.0
   blastomycotic 116.0 *[421.1]*
   candidal 112.81
   congenital 425.3
   constrictive 421.0
   Coxsackie 074.22
   due to
      blastomycosis 116.0 *[421.1]*
      candidiasis 112.81
      Coxsackie (virus) 074.22
      disseminated lupus erythematosus
         710.0 *[424.91]*
      histoplasmosis (*see also* Histoplasmosis)
         115.94
      hypertension (benign) 424.99
      moniliasis 112.81
      prosthetic cardiac valve 996.61
      Q fever 083.0 *[421.1]*
      serratia marcescens 421.0
      typhoid (fever) 002.0 *[421.1]*
   fetal 425.3
   gonococcal 098.84
   hypertensive 424.99
   infectious or infective (acute) (any valve)
      (chronic) (subacute) 421.0
   lenta (acute) (any valve) (chronic) (subacute)
      421.0
   Libman-Sacks 710.0 *[424.91]*
   Loeffler's (parietal fibroplastic) 421.0
   malignant (acute) (any valve) (chronic)
      (subacute) 421.0
   meningococcal 036.42
   mitral (chronic) (double) (fibroid) (heart)
      (inactive) (valve) (with chorea) 394.9
      with
         aortic (valve) disease 396.9
            active or acute 391.1
               with chorea (acute) (rheumatic)
                  (Sydenham's) 392.0
         rheumatic fever (conditions classifiable to
            390)
            active — *see* Endocarditis, acute,
               rheumatic
            inactive or quiescent (with chorea)
               394.9
               with aortic valve disease 396.9
      active or acute 391.1
         with chorea (acute) (rheumatic)
            (Sydenham's) 392.0
            bacterial 421.0
      arteriosclerotic 424.0
      congenital 746.89
      hypertensive 424.0
      nonrheumatic 424.0
         acute or subacute 421.9
      syphilitic 093.21
   monilial 112.81
   mycotic (acute) (any valve) (chronic) (subacute)
      421.0
   pneumococcic (acute) (any valve) (chronic)
      (subacute) 421.0
   pulmonary (chronic) (heart) (valve) 424.3
      with
         rheumatic fever (conditions classifiable to
            390)
            active — *see* Endocarditis, acute,
               rheumatic
            inactive or quiescent (with chorea)
               397.1
      acute or subacute 421.9
         rheumatic 391.1
            with chorea (acute) (rheumatic)
               (Sydenham's) 392.0

Endocarditis — *continued*
   pulmonary — *continued*
      arteriosclerotic or due to arteriosclerosis
         424.3
      congenital 746.09
      hypertensive or due to hypertension (benign)
         424.3
      rheumatic (chronic) (inactive) (with chorea)
         397.1
         active or acute 391.1
            with chorea (acute) (rheumatic)
               (Sydenham's) 392.0
      syphilitic 093.24
   purulent (acute) (any valve) (chronic) (subacute)
      421.0
   rheumatic (chronic) (inactive) (with chorea)
      397.9
      active or acute (aortic) (mitral) (pulmonary)
         (tricuspid) 391.1
         with chorea (acute) (rheumatic)
            (Sydenham's) 392.0
   septic (acute) (any valve) (chronic) (subacute)
      421.0
   specified cause, except rheumatic 424.99
   streptococcal (acute) (any valve) (chronic)
      (subacute) 421.0
   subacute — *see* Endocarditis, acute
   suppurative (any valve) (acute) (chronic)
      (subacute) 421.0
   syphilitic NEC 093.20
   toxic (*see also* Endocarditis, acute) 421.9
   tricuspid (chronic) (heart) (inactive) (rheumatic)
      (valve) (with chorea) 397.0
      with
         rheumatic fever (conditions classifiable to
            390)
            active — *see* Endocarditis, acute,
               rheumatic
            inactive or quiescent (with chorea)
               397.0
      active or acute 391.1
         with chorea (acute) (rheumatic)
            (Sydenham's) 392.0
      arteriosclerotic 424.2
      congenital 746.89
      hypertensive 424.2
      nonrheumatic 424.2
         acute or subacute 421.9
      specified cause, except rheumatic 424.2
      syphilitic 093.23
   tuberculous (*see also* Tuberculosis)
      017.9 ✓5ᵗʰ *[424.91]*
   typhoid 002.0 *[421.1]*
   ulcerative (acute) (any valve) (chronic)
      (subacute) 421.0
   vegetative (acute) (any valve) (chronic)
      (subacute) 421.0
   verrucous (acute) (any valve) (chronic)
      (subacute) NEC 710.0 *[424.91]*
      nonbacterial 710.0 *[424.91]*
      nonrheumatic 710.0 *[424.91]*

Endocardium, endocardial — *see also* condition
   cushion defect 745.60
      specified type NEC 745.69

Endocervicitis (*see also* Cervicitis) 616.0
   due to
      intrauterine (contraceptive) device 996.65
   gonorrheal (acute) 098.15
      chronic or duration of 2 months or over
         098.35
   hyperplastic 616.0
   syphilitic 095.8
   trichomonal 131.09
   tuberculous (*see also* Tuberculosis) 016.7 ✓5ᵗʰ

Endocrine — *see* condition

Endocrinopathy, pluriglandular 258.9

Endodontitis 522.0

Endomastoiditis (*see also* Mastoiditis) 383.9

Endometrioma 617.9

Endometriosis 617.9
   appendix 617.5
   bladder 617.8
   bowel 617.5
   broad ligament 617.3
   cervix 617.0
   colon 617.5

Endometriosis — *continued*
   cul-de-sac (Douglas') 617.3
   exocervix 617.0
   fallopian tube 617.2
   female genital organ NEC 617.8
   gallbladder 617.8
   in scar of skin 617.6
   internal 617.0
   intestine 617.5
   lung 617.8
   myometrium 617.0
   ovary 617.1
   parametrium 617.3
   pelvic peritoneum 617.3
   peritoneal (pelvic) 617.3
   rectovaginal septum 617.4
   rectum 617.5
   round ligament 617.3
   skin 617.6
   specified site NEC 617.8
   stromal (M8931/1) 236.0
   umbilicus 617.8
   uterus 617.0
      internal 617.0
   vagina 617.4
   vulva 617.8

Endometritis (nonspecific) (purulent) (septic)
      (suppurative) 615.9
   with
      abortion — *see* Abortion, by type, with
         sepsis
      ectopic pregnancy (*see also* categories
         633.0-633.9) 639.0
      molar pregancy (*see also* categories 630-632)
         639.0
   acute 615.0
   blennorrhagic 098.16
      acute 098.16
      chronic or duration of 2 months or over
         098.36
   cervix, cervical (*see also* Cervicitis) 616.0
      hyperplastic 616.0
   chronic 615.1
   complicating pregnancy 646.6 ✓5ᵗʰ
      affecting fetus or newborn 760.8
   decidual 615.9
   following
      abortion 639.0
      ectopic or molar pregnancy 639.0
   gonorrheal (acute) 098.16
      chronic or duration of 2 months or over
         098.36
   hyperplastic 621.3
      cervix 616.0
   polypoid — *see* Endometritis, hyperplastic
   puerperal, postpartum, childbirth 670 ✓4ᵗʰ
   senile (atrophic) 615.9
   subacute 615.0
   tuberculous (*see also* Tuberculosis) 016.7 ✓5ᵗʰ

Endometrium — *see* condition

Endomyocardiopathy, South African 425.2

Endomyocarditis — *see* Endocarditis

Endomyofibrosis 425.0

Endomyometritis (*see also* Endometritis) 615.9

Endopericarditis — *see* Endocarditis

Endoperineuritis — *see* Disorder, nerve

Endophlebitis (*see also* Phlebitis) 451.9
   leg 451.2
      deep (vessels) 451.19
      superficial (vessels) 451.0
   portal (vein) 572.1
   retina 362.18
   specified site NEC 451.89
   syphilitic 093.89

Endophthalmia (*see also* Endophthalmitis)
      360.00
   gonorrheal 098.42

Endophthalmitis (globe) (infective) (metastatic)
      (purulent) (subacute) 360.00
   acute 360.01
   chronic 360.03
   parasitis 360.13
   phacoanaphylactic 360.19
   specified type NEC 360.19
   sympathetic 360.11

Endosalpingioma — Enteritis

Endosalpingioma (M9111/1) 236.2
Endosteitis — *see* Osteomyelitis
Endothelioma, bone (M9260/3) — *see* Neoplasm, bone, malignant
Endotheliosis 287.8
   hemorrhagic infectional 287.8
Endotoxic shock 785.59
Endotrachelitis (*see also* Cervicitis) 616.0
Enema rash 692.89
Engel-von Recklinghausen disease or syndrome (osteitis fibrosa cystica) 252.0
Engelmann's disease (diaphyseal sclerosis) 756.9
English disease (*see also* Rickets) 268.0
Engman's disease (infectious eczematoid dermatitis) 690.8
Engorgement
   breast 611.79
     newborn 778.7
     puerperal, postpartum 676.2 ✓5ᵗʰ
   liver 573.9
   lung 514
   pulmonary 514
   retina, venous 362.37
   stomach 536.8
   venous, retina 362.37
Enlargement, enlarged — *see also* Hypertrophy
   abdomen 789.3 ✓5ᵗʰ
   adenoids 474.12
     and tonsils 474.10
   alveolar process or ridge 525.8
   apertures of diaphragm (congenital) 756.6
   blind spot, visual field 368.42
   gingival 523.8
   heart, cardiac (*see also* Hypertrophy, cardiac) 429.3
   lacrimal gland, chronic 375.03
   liver (*see also* Hypertrophy, liver) 789.1
   lymph gland or node 785.6
   orbit 376.46
   organ or site, congenital NEC — *see* Anomaly, specified type NEC
   parathyroid (gland) 252.0
   pituitary fossa 793.0
   prostate ►(simple) (soft)◄ 600.0
   sella turcica 793.0
   spleen (*see also* Splenomegaly) 789.2
     congenital 759.0
   thymus (congenital) (gland) 254.0
   thyroid (gland) (*see also* Goiter) 240.9
   tongue 529.8
   tonsils 474.11
     and adenoids 474.10
   uterus 621.2
Enophthalmos 376.50
   due to
     atrophy of orbital tissue 376.51
     surgery 376.52
     trauma 376.52
Enostosis 526.89
Entamebiasis — *see* Amebiasis
Entamebic — *see* Amebiasis
Entanglement, umbilical cord(s) 663.3 ✓5ᵗʰ
   with compression 663.2 ✓5ᵗʰ
   affecting fetus or newborn 762.5
   around neck with compression 663.1 ✓5ᵗʰ
   twins in monoamniotic sac 663.2 ✓5ᵗʰ
Enteralgia 789.0 ✓5ᵗʰ
Enteric — *see* condition
Enteritis (acute) (catarrhal) (choleraic) (chronic) (congestive) (diarrheal) (exudative) (follicular) (hemorrhagic) (infantile) (lienteric) (noninfectious) (perforative) (phlegmonous) (presumed noninfectious) (pseudomembranous) 558.9
   adaptive 564.9
   aertrycke infection 003.0
   allergic 558.3
   amebic (*see also* Amebiasis) 006.9
     with abscess — *see* Abscess, amebic
     acute 006.0
       with abscess — *see* Abscess, amebic
       nondysenteric 006.2

Enteritis — *continued*
   amebic (*see also* Amebiasis) — *continued*
     chronic 006.1
       with abscess — *see* Abscess, amebic
       nondysenteric 006.2
     nondysenteric 006.2
   anaerobic (cocci) (gram-negative) (gram-positive) (mixed) NEC 008.46
   bacillary NEC 004.9
   bacterial NEC 008.5
     specified NEC 008.49
   Bacteroides (fragilis) (melaninogeniscus) (oralis) 008.46
   Butyrivibrio (fibriosolvens) 008.46
   Campylobacter 008.43
   Candida 112.85
   Chilomastix 007.8
   choleriformis 001.1
   chronic 558.9
     ulcerative (*see also* Colitis, ulcerative) 556.9
   cicatrizing (chronic) 555.0
   Clostridium
     botulinum 005.1
     difficile 008.45
     haemolyticum 008.46
     novyi 008.46
     perfringens (C) (F) 008.46
     specified type NEC 008.46
   coccidial 007.2
   dietetic 558.9
   due to
     achylia gastrica 536.8
     adenovirus 008.62
     Aerobacter aerogenes 008.2 ✓5ᵗʰ
     anaerobes — *see* Enteritis, anaerobic
     Arizona (bacillus) 008.1
     astrovirus 008.66
     Bacillus coli — *see* Enteritis, E. coli 008.0 ✓5ᵗʰ
     bacteria NEC 008.5
       specified NEC 008.49
     Bacteroides 008.46
     Butyrivibrio (fibriosolvens)
     Calcivirus 008.65
     Camplyobacter 008.43
     Clostridium — *see* Enteritis, Clostridium
     Cockle agent 008.64
     Coxsackie (virus) 008.67
     Ditchling agent 008.64
     ECHO virus 008.67
     Enterobacter aerogenes 008.2 ✓5ᵗʰ
     enterococci 008.49
     enterovirus NEC 008.67
     Escherichia coli — *see* Enteritis, E. coli 008.0 ✓5ᵗʰ
     Eubacterium 008.46
     Fusobacterium (nucleatum) 008.46
     gram-negative bacteria NEC 008.47
       anaerobic NEC 008.46
     Hawaii agent 008.63
     irritating foods 558.9
     Klebsiella aerogenes 008.47
     Marin County agent 008.66
     Montgomery County agent 008.63
     Norwalk-like agent 008.63
     Norwalk virus 008.63
     Otofuke agent 008.63
     Paracolobactrum arizonae 008.1
     paracolon bacillus NEC 008.47
       Arizona 008.1
     Paramatta agent 008.64
     Peptococcus 008.46
     Peptostreptococcus 008.46
     Proprionibacterium 008.46
     Proteus (bacillus) (mirabilis) (morganii) 008.3
     Pseudomonas aeruginosa 008.42
     Rotavirus 008.61
     Sapporo agent 008.63
     small round virus (SRV) NEC 008.64
       featureless NEC 008.63
       structured NEC 008.63
     Snow Mountain (SM) agent 008.63
     specified
       bacteria NEC 008.49
       organism, nonbacterial NEC 008.8
       virus (NEC) 008.69
     Staphylococcus 008.41

Enteritis — *continued*
   due to — *continued*
     Streptococcus 008.49
       anaerobic 008.46
     Taunton agent 008.63
     Torovirus 008.69
     Treponema 008.46
     Veillonella 008.46
     virus 008.8
       specified type NEC 008.69
     Wollan (W) agent 008.64
     Yersinia enterocolitica 008.44
   dysentery — *see* Dysentery
   E. coli 008.00
     enterohemorrhagic 008.04
     enteroinvasive 008.03
     enteropathogenic 008.01
     enterotoxigenic 008.02
     specified type NEC 008.09
   el tor 001.1
   embadomonial 007.8
   epidemic 009.0
   Eubacterium 008.46
   fermentative 558.9
   fulminant 557.0
   Fusobacterium (nucleatum) 008.46
   gangrenous (*see also* Enteritis, due to, by organism) 009.0
   giardial 007.1
   gram-negative bacteria NEC 008.47
     anaerobic NEC 008.46
   infectious NEC (*see also* Enteritis, due to, by organism) 009.0
     presumed 009.1
   influenzal 487.8
   ischemic 557.9
     acute 557.0
     chronic 557.1
     due to mesenteric artery insufficiency 557.1
   membranous 564.9
   mucous 564.9
   myxomembranous 564.9
   necrotic (*see also* Enteritis, due to, by organism) 009.0
   necroticans 005.2
   necrotizing of fetus or newborn 777.5
   neurogenic 564.9
   newborn 777.8
     necrotizing 777.5
   parasitic NEC 129
   paratyphoid (fever) (*see also* Fever, paratyphoid) 002.9
   Peptococcus 008.46
   Peptostreptococcus 008.46
   Proprionibacterium 008.46
   protozoal NEC 007.9
   radiation 558.1
   regional (of) 555.9
     intestine
       large (bowel, colon, or rectum) 555.1
         with small intestine 555.2
       small (duodenum, ileum, or jejunum) 555.0
         with large intestine 555.2
   Salmonella infection 003.0
   salmonellosis 003.0
   segmental (*see also* Enteritis, regional) 555.9
   septic (*see also* Enteritis, due to, by organism) 009.0
   Shigella 004.9
   simple 558.9
   spasmodic 564.9
   spastic 564.9
   staphylococcal 008.41
     due to food 005.0
   streptococcal 008.49
     anaerobic 008.46
   toxic 558.2
   Treponema (denticola) (macrodentium) 008.46
   trichomonal 007.3
   tuberculous (*see also* Tuberculosis) 014.8 ✓5ᵗʰ
   typhosa 002.0
   ulcerative (chronic) (*see also* Colitis, ulcerative) 556.9
   Veillonella 008.46
   viral 008.8
     adenovirus 008.62

Enteritis — *continued*
  viral — *continued*
    enterovirus 008.67
    specified virus NEC 008.69
    Yersinia enterocolitica 008.44
    zymotic 009.0

Enteroarticular syndrome 099.3

Enterobiasis 127.4

Enterobius vermicularis 127.4

Enterocele (*see also* Hernia) 553.9
  pelvis, pelvic (acquired) (congenital) 618.6
  vagina, vaginal (acquired) (congenital) 618.6

Enterocolitis — *see also* Enteritis
  fetus or newborn 777.8
    necrotizing 777.5
  fulminant 557.0
  granulomatous 555.2
  hemorrhagic (acute) 557.0
    chronic 557.1
  necrotizing (acute) membranous 557.0
  primary necrotizing 777.5
  pseudomembranous 008.45
  radiation 558.1
    newborn 777.5
  ulcerative 556.0

Enterocystoma 751.5

Enterogastritis — *see* Enteritis

Enterogenous cyanosis 289.7

Enterolith, enterolithiasis (impaction) 560.39
  with hernia — *see also* Hernia, by site, with obstruction
    gangrenous — *see* Hernia, by site, with gangrene

Enteropathy 569.9
  exudative (of Gordon) 579.8
  gluten 579.0
  hemorrhagic, terminal 557.0
  protein-losing 579.8

Enteroperitonitis (*see also* Peritonitis) 567.9

Enteroptosis 569.89

Enterorrhagia 578.9

Enterospasm 564.9
  psychogenic 306.4

Enterostenosis (*see also* Obstruction, intestine) 560.9

Enterostomy status V44.4
  with complication 569.60

Enthesopathy 726.39
  ankle and tarsus 726.70
  elbow region 726.30
    specified NEC 726.39
  hip 726.5
  knee 726.60
  peripheral NEC 726.8
  shoulder region 726.10
    adhesive 726.0
  spinal 720.1
  wrist and carpus 726.4

Entrance, air into vein — *see* Embolism, air

Entrapment, nerve — *see* Neuropathy, entrapment

Entropion (eyelid) 374.00
  cicatricial 374.04
  congenital 743.62
  late effect of trachoma (healed) 139.1
  mechanical 374.02
  paralytic 374.02
  senile 374.01
  spastic 374.03

Enucleation of eye (current) (traumatic) 871.3

Enuresis 788.30
  habit disturbance 307.6
  nocturnal 788.36
    psychogenic 307.6
  nonorganic origin 307.6
  psychogenic 307.6

Enzymopathy 277.9

Eosinopenia 288.0

Eosinophilia 288.3
  allergic 288.3
  hereditary 288.3
  idiopathic 288.3

Eosinophilia — *continued*
  infiltrative 518.3
  Loeffler's 518.3
  myalgia syndrome 710.5
  pulmonary (tropical) 518.3
  secondary 288.3
  tropical 518.3

Eosinophilic — *see also* condition
  fasciitis 728.89
  granuloma (bone) 277.8
  infiltration lung 518.3

Ependymitis (acute) (cerebral) (chronic) (granular) (*see also* Meningitis) 322.9

Ependymoblastoma (M9392/3)
  specified site — *see* Neoplasm, by site, malignant
  unspecified site 191.9

Ependymoma (epithelial) (malignant) (M9391/3)
  anaplastic type (M9392/3)
    specified site — *see* Neoplasm, by site, malignant
    unspecified site 191.9
  benign (M9391/0)
    specified site — *see* Neoplasm, by site, benign
    unspecified site 225.0
  myxopapillary (M9394/1) 237.5
  papillary (M9393/1) 237.5
  specified site — *see* Neoplasm, by site, malignant
  unspecified site 191.9

Ependymopathy 349.2
  spinal cord 349.2

Ephelides, ephelis 709.09

Ephemeral fever (*see also* Pyrexia) 780.6

Epiblepharon (congenital) 743.62

Epicanthus, epicanthic fold (congenital) (eyelid) 743.63

Epicondylitis (elbow) (lateral) 726.32
  medial 726.31

Epicystitis (*see also* Cystitis) 595.9

Epidemic — *see* condition

Epidermidalization, cervix — *see* condition

Epidermidization, cervix — *see* condition

Epidermis, epidermal — *see* condition

Epidermization, cervix — *see* condition

Epidermodysplasia verruciformis 078.19

Epidermoid
  cholesteatoma — *see* Cholesteatoma
  inclusion (*see also* Cyst, skin) 706.2

Epidermolysis
  acuta (combustiformis) (toxica) 695.1
  bullosa 757.39
  necroticans combustiformis 695.1
    due to drug
      correct substance properly administered 695.1
      overdose or wrong substance given or taken 977.9
      specified drug — *see* Table of Drugs and Chemicals

Epidermophytid — *see* Dermatophytosis

Epidermophytosis (infected) — *see* Dermatophytosis

Epidermosis, ear (middle) (*see also* Cholesteatoma) 385.30

Epididymis — *see* condition

Epididymitis (nonvenereal) 604.90
  with abscess 604.0
  acute 604.99
  blennorrhagic (acute) 098.0
    chronic or duration of 2 months or over 098.2
  caseous (*see also* Tuberculosis) 016.4 ✓5ᵗʰ
  chlamydial 099.54
  diphtheritic 032.89 [604.91]
  filarial 125.9 [604.91]
  gonococcal (acute) 098.0
    chronic or duration of 2 months or over 098.2
  recurrent 604.99
  residual 604.99
  syphilitic 095.8 [604.91]

Epididymitis — *continued*
  tuberculous (*see also* Tuberculosis) 016.4 ✓5ᵗʰ

Epididymo-orchitis (*see also* Epididymitis) 604.90
  with abscess 604.0
  chlamydial 099.54
  gonococcal (acute) 098.13
    chronic or duration of 2 months or over 098.33

Epidural — *see* condition

Epigastritis (*see also* Gastritis) 535.5 ✓5ᵗʰ

Epigastrium, epigastric — *see* condition

Epigastrocele (*see also* Hernia, epigastric) 553.29

Epiglottiditis (acute) 464.30
  with obstruction 464.31
  chronic 476.1
  viral 464.30
    with obstruction 464.31

Epiglottis — *see* condition

Epiglottitis (acute) 464.30
  with obstruction 464.31
  chronic 476.1
  viral 464.30
    with obstruction 464.31

Epignathus 759.4

Epilepsia
  partialis continua (*see also* Epilepsy) 345.7 ✓5ᵗʰ
  procursiva (*see also* Epilepsy) 345.8 ✓5ᵗʰ

Epilepsy, epileptic (idiopathic) 345.9 ✓5ᵗʰ

> *Note* — use the following fifth-digit subclassification with categories 345.0, 345.1, 345.4–345.9:
> 0 *without mention of intractable epilepsy*
> 1 *with intractable epilepsy*

  abdominal 345.5 ✓5ᵗʰ
  absence (attack) 345.0 ✓5ᵗʰ
  akinetic 345.0 ✓5ᵗʰ
    psychomotor 345.4 ✓5ᵗʰ
  automatism 345.4 ✓5ᵗʰ
  autonomic diencephalic 345.5 ✓5ᵗʰ
  brain 345.9 ✓5ᵗʰ
  Bravais-Jacksonian 345.5 ✓5ᵗʰ
  cerebral 345.9 ✓5ᵗʰ
  climacteric 345.9 ✓5ᵗʰ
  clonic 345.1 ✓5ᵗʰ
  clouded state 345.9 ✓5ᵗʰ
  coma 345.3
  communicating 345.4 ✓5ᵗʰ
  congenital 345.9 ✓5ᵗʰ
  convulsions 345.9 ✓5ᵗʰ
  cortical (focal) (motor) 345.5 ✓5ᵗʰ
  cursive (running) 345.8 ✓5ᵗʰ
  cysticercosis 123.1
  deterioration
    with behavioral disturbance 345.9 ✓5ᵗʰ [294.11]
    without behavioral disturbance 345.9 ✓5ᵗʰ [294.10]
  due to syphilis 094.89
  equivalent 345.5 ✓5ᵗʰ
  fit 345.9 ✓5ᵗʰ
  focal (motor) 345.5 ✓5ᵗʰ
  gelastic 345.8 ✓5ᵗʰ
  generalized 345.9 ✓5ᵗʰ
    convulsive 345.1 ✓5ᵗʰ
    flexion 345.1 ✓5ᵗʰ
    nonconvulsive 345.0 ✓5ᵗʰ
  grand mal (idiopathic) 345.1 ✓5ᵗʰ
  Jacksonian (motor) (sensory) 345.5 ✓5ᵗʰ
  Kojevnikoff's, Kojevnikov's, Kojewnikoff's 345.7 ✓5ᵗʰ
  laryngeal 786.2
  limbic system 345.4 ✓5ᵗʰ
  major (motor) 345.1 ✓5ᵗʰ
  minor 345.0 ✓5ᵗʰ
  mixed (type) 345.9 ✓5ᵗʰ
  motor partial 345.5 ✓5ᵗʰ
  musicogenic 345.1 ✓5ᵗʰ
  myoclonus, myoclonic 345.1 ✓5ᵗʰ
    progressive (familial) 333.2
  nonconvulsive, generalized 345.0 ✓5ᵗʰ
  parasitic NEC 123.9

Epilepsy — Eruption

Epilepsy, epileptic — *continued*
  partial (focalized) 345.5 ✔5th
    with
      impairment of consciousness 345.4 ✔5th
      memory and ideational disturbances
        345.4 ✔5th
    abdominal type 345.5 ✔5th
    motor type 345.5 ✔5th
    psychomotor type 345.4 ✔5th
    psychosensory type 345.4 ✔5th
    secondarily generalized 345.4 ✔5th
    sensory type 345.5 ✔5th
    somatomotor type 345.5 ✔5th
    somatosensory type 345.5 ✔5th
    temporal lobe type 345.4 ✔5th
    visceral type 345.5 ✔5th
    visual type 345.5 ✔5th
  peripheral 345.9 ✔5th
  petit mal 345.0 ✔5th
  photokinetic 345.8 ✔5th
  progressive myoclonic (familial) 333.2
  psychic equivalent 345.5 ✔5th
  psychomotor 345.4 ✔5th
  psychosensory 345.4 ✔5th
  reflex 345.1 ✔5th
  seizure 345.9 ✔5th
  senile 345.9 ✔5th
  sensory-induced 345.5 ✔5th
  sleep 347
  somatomotor type 345.5 ✔5th
  somatosensory 345.5 ✔5th
  specified type NEC 345.8 ✔5th
  status (grand mal) 345.3
    focal motor 345.7 ✔5th
    petit mal 345.2
    psychomotor 345.7 ✔5th
    temporal lobe 345.7 ✔5th
  symptomatic 345.9 ✔5th
  temporal lobe 345.4 ✔5th
  tonic (-clonic) 345.1 ✔5th
  traumatic (injury unspecified) 907.0
    injury specified — *see* Late, effect (of)
      specified injury
  twilight 293.0
  uncinate (gyrus) 345.4 ✔5th
  Unverricht (-Lundborg) (familial myoclonic)
    333.2
  visceral 345.5 ✔5th
  visual 345.5 ✔5th
Epileptiform
  convulsions 780.39
  seizure 780.39
Epiloia 759.5
Epimenorrhea 626.2
Epipharyngitis (*see also* Nasopharyngitis) 460
Epiphora 375.20
  due to
    excess lacrimation 375.21
    insufficient drainage 375.22
Epiphyseal arrest 733.91
  femoral head 732.2
Epiphyseolysis, epiphysiolysis (*see also*
  Osteochondrosis) 732.9
Epiphysitis (*see also* Osteochondrosis) 732.9
  juvenile 732.6
  marginal (Scheuermann's) 732.0
  os calcis 732.5
  syphilitic (congenital) 090.0
  vertebral (Scheuermann's) 732.0
Epiplocele (*see also* Hernia) 553.9
Epiploitis (*see also* Peritonitis) 567.9
Epiplosarcomphalocele (*see also* Hernia,
  umbilicus) 553.1
Episcleritis 379.00
  gouty 274.89 [379.09]
  nodular 379.02
  periodica fugax 379.01
    angioneurotic — *see* Edema, angioneurotic
  specified NEC 379.09
  staphylococcal 379.00
  suppurative 379.00
  syphilitic 095.0
  tuberculous (*see also* Tuberculosis)
    017.3 ✔5th [379.09]

Episode
  brain (*see also* Disease, cerebrovascular, acute)
    436
  cerebral (*see also* Disease, cerebrovascular,
    acute) 436
  depersonalization (in neurotic state) 300.6
  hyporesponsive 780.09
  psychotic (*see also* Psychosis) 298.9
    organic, transient 293.9
  schizophrenic (acute) NEC (*see also*
    Schizophrenia) 295.4 ✔5th
Epispadias
  female 753.8
  male 752.62
Episplenitis 289.59
Epistaxis (multiple) 784.7
  hereditary 448.0
  vicarious menstruation 625.8
Epithelioma (malignant) (M8011/3) — *see also*
  Neoplasm, by site, malignant
  adenoides cysticum (M8100/0) — *see*
    Neoplasm, skin, benign
  basal cell (M8090/3) — *see* Neoplasm, skin,
    malignant
  benign (M8011/0) — *see* Neoplasm, by site,
    benign
  Bowen's (M8081/2) — *see* Neoplasm, skin, in
    situ
  calcifying (benign) (Malherbe's) (M8110/0) —
    see Neoplasm, skin, benign
  external site — *see* Neoplasm, skin, malignant
  intraepidermal, Jadassohn (M8096/0) — *see*
    Neoplasm, skin, benign
  squamous cell (M8070/3) — *see* Neoplasm, by
    site, malignant
Epitheliopathy
  pigment, retina 363.15
  posterior multifocal placoid (acute) 363.15
Epithelium, epithelial — *see* condition
Epituberculosis (allergic) (with atelectasis) (*see
  also* Tuberculosis) 010.8 ✔5th
Eponychia 757.5
Epstein's
  nephrosis or syndrome (*see also* Nephrosis)
    581.9
  pearl (mouth) 528.4
Epstein-Barr infection (viral) 075
  chronic 780.79 [139.8]
Epulis (giant cell) (gingiva) 523.8
Equinia 024
Equinovarus (congenital) 754.51
  acquired 736.71
Equivalent
  convulsive (abdominal) (*see also* Epilepsy)
    345.5 ✔5th
  epileptic (psychic) (*see also* Epilepsy) 345.5 ✔5th
Erb's
  disease 359.1
  palsy, paralysis (birth) (brachial) (newborn)
    767.6
    spinal (spastic) syphilitic 094.89
  pseudohypertrophic muscular dystrophy 359.1
Erb (-Duchenne) paralysis (birth injury)
  (newborn) 767.6
Erb-Goldflam disease or syndrome 358.0
Erdheim's syndrome (acromegalic
  macrospondylitis) 253.0
Erection, painful (persistent) 607.3
Ergosterol deficiency (vitamin D) 268.9
  with
    osteomalacia 268.2
    rickets (*see also* Rickets) 268.0
Ergotism (ergotized grain) 988.2
  from ergot used as drug (migraine therapy)
    correct substance properly administered
      349.82
    overdose or wrong substance given or taken
      975.0
Erichsen's disease (railway spine) 300.16
Erlacher-Blount syndrome (tibia vara) 732.4
Erosio interdigitalis blastomycetica 112.3

Erosion
  artery NEC 447.2
    without rupture 447.8
  arteriosclerotic plaque — *see* Arteriosclerosis,
    by site
  bone 733.99
  bronchus 519.1
  cartilage (joint) 733.99
  cervix (uteri) (acquired) (chronic) (congenital)
    622.0
    with mention of cervicitis 616.0
  cornea (recurrent) (*see also* Keratitis) 371.42
    traumatic 918.1
  dental (idiopathic) (occupational) 521.3
  duodenum, postpyloric — *see* Ulcer, duodenum
  esophagus 530.89
  gastric 535.4 ✔5th
  intestine 569.89
  lymphatic vessel 457.8
  pylorus, pyloric (ulcer) 535.4 ✔5th
  sclera 379.16
  spine, aneurysmal 094.89
  spleen 289.59
  stomach 535.4 ✔5th
  teeth (idiopathic) (occupational) 521.3
    due to
      medicine 521.3
      persistent vomiting 521.3
  urethra 599.84
  uterus 621.8
  vertebra 733.99
Erotomania 302.89
  Clérambault's 297.8
Error
  in diet 269.9
  refractive 367.9
    astigmatism (*see also* Astigmatism) 367.20
    drug-induced 367.89
    hypermetropia 367.0
    hyperopia 367.0
    myopia 367.1
    presbyopia 367.4
    toxic 367.89
Eructation 787.3
  nervous 306.4
  psychogenic 306.4
Eruption
  creeping 126.9
  drug — *see* Dermatitis, due to, drug
  Hutchinson, summer 692.72
  Kaposi's varicelliform 054.0
  napkin (psoriasiform) 691.0
  polymorphous
    light (sun) 692.72
      other source 692.82
  psoriasiform, napkin 691.0
  recalcitrant pustular 694.8
  ringed 695.89
  skin (*see also* Dermatitis) 782.1
    creeping (meaning hookworm) 126.9
    due to
      chemical(s) NEC 692.4
        internal use 693.8
      drug — *see* Dermatitis, due to, drug
      prophylactic inoculation or vaccination
        against disease — *see* Dermatitis,
        due to, vaccine
      smallpox vaccination NEC — *see*
        Dermatitis, due to, vaccine
  erysipeloid 027.1
  feigned 698.4
  Hutchinson, summer 692.72
  Kaposi's, varicelliform 054.0
    vaccinia 999.0
  lichenoid, axilla 698.3
  polymorphous, due to light 692.72
  toxic NEC 695.0
  vesicular 709.8
  teeth, tooth
    accelerated 520.6
    delayed 520.6
    difficult 520.6
    disturbance of 520.6
    in abnormal sequence 520.6
    incomplete 520.6
    late 520.6

Eruption — *continued*
  teeth, tooth — *continued*
    natal 520.6
    neonatal 520.6
    obstructed 520.6
    partial 520.6
    persistent primary 520.6
    premature 520.6
  vesicular 709.8
Erysipelas (gangrenous) (infantile) (newborn) (phlegmonous) (suppurative) 035
  external ear 035 *[380.13]*
  puerperal, postpartum, childbirth 670 ✓5ᵗʰ
Erysipelatoid (Rosenbach's) 027.1
Erysipeloid (Rosenbach's) 027.1
Erythema, erythematous (generalized) 695.9
  ab igne — *see* Burn, by site, first degree
  annulare (centrifugum) (rheumaticum) 695.0
  arthriticum epidemicum 026.1
  brucellum (*see also* Brucellosis) 023.9
  bullosum 695.1
  caloricum — *see* Burn, by site, first degree
  chronicum migrans 088.81
    chronicum 088.81
  circinatum 695.1
  diaper 691.0
  due to
    chemical (contact) NEC 692.4
      internal 693.8
    drug (internal use) 693.0
      contact 692.3
  elevatum diutinum 695.89
  endemic 265.2
  epidemic, arthritic 026.1
  figuratum perstans 695.0
  gluteal 691.0
  gyratum (perstans) (repens) 695.1
  heat — *see* Burn, by site, first degree
  ichthyosiforme congenitum 757.1
  induratum (primary) (scrofulosorum) (*see also* Tuberculosis) 017.1 ✓5ᵗʰ
    nontuberculous 695.2
  infantum febrile 057.8
  infectional NEC 695.9
  infectiosum 057.0
  inflammation NEC 695.9
  intertrigo 695.89
  iris 695.1
  lupus (discoid) (localized) (*see also* Lupus erythematosus) 695.4
  marginatum 695.0
    rheumaticum — *see* Fever, rheumatic
  medicamentosum — *see* Dermatitis, due to, drug
  migrans 529.1
    chronicum 088.81
  multiforme 695.1
    bullosum 695.1
    conjunctiva 695.1
    exudativum (Hebra) 695.1
    pemphigoides 694.5
  napkin 691.0
  neonatorum 778.8
  nodosum 695.2
    tuberculous (*see also* Tuberculosis) 017.1 ✓5ᵗʰ
  nummular, nummulare 695.1
  palmar 695.0
  palmaris hereditarium 695.0
  pernio 991.5
  perstans solare 692.72
  rash, newborn 778.8
  scarlatiniform (exfoliative) (recurrent) 695.0
  simplex marginatum 057.8
  solare (*see also* Sunburn) 692.71
  streptogenes 696.5
  toxic, toxicum NEC 695.0
    newborn 778.8
  tuberculous (primary) (*see also* Tuberculosis) 017.0 ✓5ᵗʰ
  venenatum 695.0
Erythematosus — *see* condition
Erythematous — *see* condition
Erythermalgia (primary) 443.89
Erythralgia 443.89
Erythrasma 039.0

Erythredema 985.0
  polyneuritica 985.0
  polyneuropathy 985.0
Erythremia (acute) (M9841/3) 207.0 ✓5ᵗʰ
  chronic (M9842/3) 207.1 ✓5ᵗʰ
  secondary 289.0
Erythroblastopenia (acquired) 284.8
  congenital 284.0
Erythroblastophthisis 284.0
Erythroblastosis (fetalis) (newborn) 773.2
  due to
    ABO
      antibodies 773.1
      incompatibility, maternal/fetal 773.1
      isoimmunization 773.1
    Rh
      antibodies 773.0
      incompatibility, maternal/fetal 773.0
      isoimmunization 773.0
Erythrocyanosis (crurum) 443.89
Erythrocythemia — *see* Erythremia
Erythrocytopenia 285.9
Erythrocytosis (megalosplenic)
  familial 289.6
  oval, hereditary (*see also* Elliptocytosis) 282.1
  secondary 289.0
  stress 289.0
Erythroderma (*see also* Erythema) 695.9
  desquamativa (in infants) 695.89
  exfoliative 695.89
  ichthyosiform, congenital 757.1
  infantum 695.89
  maculopapular 696.2
  neonatorum 778.8
  psoriaticum 696.1
  secondary 695.9
Erythrogenesis imperfecta 284.0
Erythroleukemia (M9840/3) 207.0 ✓5ᵗʰ
Erythromelalgia 443.89
Erythromelia 701.8
Erythropenia 285.9
Erythrophagocytosis 289.9
Erythrophobia 300.23
Erythroplakia
  oral mucosa 528.7
  tongue 528.7
Erythroplasia (Queyrat) (M8080/2)
  specified site — *see* Neoplasm, skin, in situ
  unspecified site 233.5
Erythropoiesis, idiopathic ineffective 285.0
Escaped beats, heart 427.60
  postoperative 997.1
Esoenteritis — *see* Enteritis
Esophagalgia 530.89
Esophagectasis 530.89
  due to cardiospasm 530.0
Esophagismus 530.5
Esophagitis (alkaline) (chemical) (chronic) (infectional) (necrotic) (peptic) (postoperative) (regurgitant) 530.10
  acute 530.12
  candidal 112.84
  reflux 530.11
  specified NEC 530.19
  tuberculous (*see also* Tuberculosis) 017.8 ✓5ᵗʰ
  ulcerative 530.19
Esophagocele 530.6
Esophagodynia 530.89
Esophagomalacia 530.89
Esophagoptosis 530.89
Esophagospasm 530.5
Esophagostenosis 530.3
Esophagostomiasis 127.7
Esophagotracheal — *see* condition
Esophagus — *see* condition
Esophoria 378.41
  convergence, excess 378.84
  divergence, insufficiency 378.85
Esotropia (nonaccommodative) 378.00
  accommodative 378.35

Esotropia — *continued*
  alternating 378.05
    with
      A pattern 378.06
      specified noncomitancy NEC 378.08
      V pattern 378.07
      X pattern 378.08
      Y pattern 378.08
    intermittent 378.22
  intermittent 378.20
    alternating 378.22
    monocular 378.21
  monocular 378.01
    with
      A pattern 378.02
      specified noncomitancy NEC 378.04
      V pattern 378.03
      X pattern 378.04
      Y pattern 378.04
    intermittent 378.21
Espundia 085.5
Essential — *see* condition
Esterapenia 289.8
Esthesioneuroblastoma (M9522/3) 160.0
Esthesioneurocytoma (M9521/3) 160.0
Esthesioneuroepithelioma (M9523/3) 160.0
Esthiomene 099.1
Estivo-autumnal
  fever 084.0
  malaria 084.0
Estrangement V61.0
Estriasis 134.0
Ethanolaminuria 270.8
Ethanolism (*see also* Alcoholism) 303.9 ✓5ᵗʰ
Ether dependence, dependency (*see also* Dependence) 304.6 ✓5ᵗʰ
Etherism (*see also* Dependence) 304.6 ✓5ᵗʰ
Ethmoid, ethmoidal — *see* condition
Ethmoiditis (chronic) (nonpurulent) (purulent) (*see also* Sinusitis, ethmoidal) 473.2
  influenzal 487.1
  Woakes' 471.1
Ethylism (*see also* Alcoholism) 303.9 ✓5ᵗʰ
Eulenburg's disease (congenital paramyotonia) 359.2
Eunuchism 257.2
Eunuchoidism 257.2
  hypogonadotropic 257.2
European blastomycosis 117.5
Eustachian — *see* condition
Euthyroid sick syndrome 790.94
Euthyroidism 244.9
Evaluation
  fetal lung maturity 659.8
  for suspected condition (*see also* Observation) V71.9
    abuse V71.81
    exposure
      anthrax V71.82 ●
      biologic agent NEC V71.83 ●
    neglect V71.81
    newborn — *see* Observation, suspected, condition, newborn
    specified condition NEC V71.89
  mental health V70.2
    requested by authority V70.1
  nursing care V63.8
  social service V63.8
Evan's syndrome (thrombocytopenic purpura) 287.3
Eventration
  colon into chest — *see* Hernia, diaphragm
  diaphragm (congenital) 756.6
Eversion
  bladder 596.8
  cervix (uteri) 622.0
    with mention of cervicitis 616.0
  foot NEC 736.79
    congenital 755.67
  lacrimal punctum 375.51
  punctum lacrimale (postinfectional) (senile) 375.51

Eversion — continued
- ureter (meatus) 593.89
- urethra (meatus) 599.84
- uterus 618.1
  - complicating delivery 665.2 ☑5ᵗʰ
    - affecting fetus or newborn 763.89
  - puerperal, postpartum 674.8 ☑5ᵗʰ

Evisceration
- birth injury 767.8
- bowel (congenital) — see Hernia, ventral
- congenital (see also Hernia, ventral) 553.29
- operative wound 998.32 ▲
- traumatic NEC 869.1
  - eye 871.3

Evulsion — see Avulsion

Ewing's
- angioendothelioma (M9260/3) — see Neoplasm, bone, malignant
- sarcoma (M9260/3) — see Neoplasm, bone, malignant
- tumor (M9260/3) — see Neoplasm, bone, malignant

Exaggerated lumbosacral angle (with impinging spine) 756.12

Examination (general) (routine) (of) (for) V70.9
- allergy V72.7
- annual V70.0
- cardiovascular preoperative V72.81
- cervical Papanicolaou smear V76.2
  - as a part of routine gynecological examination V72.3
- child care (routine) V20.2
- clinical research investigation (normal control patient) (participant) V70.7
- dental V72.2
- developmental testing (child) (infant) V20.2
- donor (potential) V70.8
- ear V72.1
- eye V72.0
- following
  - accident (motor vehicle) V71.4
  - alleged rape or seduction (victim or culprit) V71.5
  - inflicted injury (victim or culprit) NEC V71.6
  - rape or seduction, alleged (victim or culprit) V71.5
  - treatment (for) V67.9
    - combined V67.6
    - fracture V67.4
    - involving high-risk medication NEC V67.51
    - mental disorder V67.3
    - specified condition NEC V67.59
- follow-up (routine) (following) V67.9
  - cancer chemotherapy V67.2
  - chemotherapy V67.2
  - disease NEC V67.59
  - high-risk medication NEC V67.51
  - injury NEC V67.59
  - population survey V70.6
  - postpartum V24.2
  - psychiatric V67.3
  - psychotherapy V67.3
  - radiotherapy V67.1
  - specified surgery NEC V67.09
  - surgery V67.00
    - vaginal pap smear V67.01
- gynecological V72.3
  - for contraceptive maintenance V25.40
    - intrauterine device V25.42
    - pill V25.41
    - specified method NEC V25.49
- health (of)
  - armed forces personnel V70.5
  - checkup V70.0
  - child, routine V20.2
  - defined subpopulation NEC V70.5
  - inhabitants of institutions V70.5
  - occupational V70.5
  - pre-employment screening V70.5
  - preschool children V70.5
    - for admission to school V70.3
  - prisoners V70.5
    - for entrance into prison V70.3
  - prostitutes V70.5
  - refugees V70.5

Examination — continued
- health — continued
  - school children V70.5
  - students V70.5
- hearing V72.1
- infant V20.2
- laboratory V72.6
- lactating mother V24.1
- medical (for) (of) V70.9
  - administrative purpose NEC V70.3
  - admission to
    - old age home V70.3
    - prison V70.3
    - school V70.3
  - adoption V70.3
  - armed forces personnel V70.5
  - at health care facility V70.0
  - camp V70.3
  - child, routine V20.2
  - clinical research investigation (control) (normal comparison) (participant) V70.7
  - defined subpopulation NEC V70.5
  - donor (potential) V70.8
  - driving license V70.3
  - general V70.9
    - routine V70.0
    - specified reason NEC V70.8
  - immigration V70.3
  - inhabitants of institutions V70.5
  - insurance certification V70.3
  - marriage V70.3
  - medicolegal reasons V70.4
  - naturalization V70.3
  - occupational V70.5
  - population survey V70.6
  - pre-employment V70.5
  - preschool children V70.5
    - for admission to school V70.3
  - prison V70.3
  - prisoners V70.5
    - for entrance into prison V70.3
  - prostitutes V70.5
  - refugees V70.5
  - school children V70.5
  - specified reason NEC V70.8
  - sport competition V70.3
  - students V70.5
- medicolegal reason V70.4
- pelvic (annual) (periodic) V72.3
- periodic (annual) (routine) V70.0
- postpartum
  - immediately after delivery V24.0
  - routine follow-up V24.2
- pregnancy (unconfirmed) (possible) V72.4
- prenatal V22.1
  - first pregnancy V22.0
  - high-risk pregnancy V23.9
    - specified problem NEC V23.8 ☑5ᵗʰ
- preoperative V72.84
  - cardiovascular V72.81
  - respiratory V72.82
  - specified NEC V72.83
- psychiatric V70.2
  - follow-up not needing further care V67.3
  - requested by authority V70.1
- radiological NEC V72.5
- respiratory preoperative V72.82
- screening — see Screening
- sensitization V72.7
- skin V72.7
  - hypersensitivity V72.7
- special V72.9
- specified type or reason NEC V72.85
  - preoperative V72.83
  - specified NEC V72.83
- teeth V72.2
- victim or culprit following
  - alleged rape or seduction V71.5
  - inflicted injury NEC V71.6
- vaginal Papanicolaou smear V76.47
  - following hysterectomy for malignant condition V67.01
- vision V72.0
- well baby V20.2

Exanthem, exanthema (see also Rash) 782.1
- Boston 048
- epidemic, with meningitis 048
- lichenoid psoriasiform 696.2
- subitum 057.8
- viral, virus NEC 057.9
  - specified type NEC 057.8

Excess, excessive, excessively
- alcohol level in blood 790.3
- carbohydrate tissue, localized 278.1
- carotene (dietary) 278.3
- cold 991.9
  - specified effect NEC 991.8
- convergence 378.84
- crying of infant (baby) 780.92 ●
- development, breast 611.1
- diaphoresis 780.8
- divergence 378.85
- drinking (alcohol) NEC (see also Abuse, drugs, nondependent) 305.0 ☑5ᵗʰ
  - continual (see also Alcoholism) 303.9 ☑5ᵗʰ
  - habitual (see also Alcoholism) 303.9 ☑5ᵗʰ
- eating 783.6
- eyelid fold (congenital) 743.62
- fat 278.00
  - in heart (see also Degeneration, myocardial) 429.1
  - tissue, localized 278.1
- foreskin 605
- gas 787.3
- gastrin 251.5
- glucagon 251.4
- heat (see also Heat) 992.9
- large
  - colon 564.7
    - congenital 751.3
  - fetus or infant 766.0
    - with obstructed labor 660.1 ☑5ᵗʰ
      - affecting management of pregnancy 656.6 ☑5ᵗʰ
    - causing disproportion 653.5 ☑5ᵗʰ
  - newborn (weight of 4500 grams or more) 766.0
  - organ or site, congenital NEC — see Anomaly, specified type NEC
- lid fold (congenital) 743.62
- long
  - colon 751.5
  - organ or site, congenital NEC — see Anomaly, specified type NEC
  - umbilical cord (entangled)
    - affecting fetus or newborn 762.5
    - in pregnancy or childbirth 663.3 ☑5ᵗʰ
      - with compression 663.2 ☑5ᵗʰ
- menstruation 626.2
- number of teeth 520.1
  - causing crowding 524.3
- nutrients (dietary) NEC 783.6
- potassium (K) 276.7
- salivation (see also Ptyalism) 527.7
- secretion — see also Hypersecretion
  - milk 676.6 ☑5ᵗʰ
  - sputum 786.4
  - sweat 780.8
- short
  - organ or site, congenital NEC — see Anomaly, specified type NEC
  - umbilical cord
    - affecting fetus or newborn 762.6
    - in pregnancy or childbirth 663.4 ☑5ᵗʰ
- skin NEC 701.9
  - eyelid 743.62
    - acquired 374.30
- sodium (Na) 276.0
- sputum 786.4
- sweating 780.8
- tearing (ducts) (eye) (see also Epiphora) 375.20
- thirst 783.5
  - due to deprivation of water 994.3
- vitamin
  - A (dietary) 278.2
    - administered as drug (chronic) (prolonged excessive intake) 278.2
      - reaction to sudden overdose 963.5

Excess, excessive, excessively — *continued*
  vitamin — *continued*
    D (dietary) 278.4
      administered as drug (chronic) (prolonged excessive intake) 278.4
        reaction to sudden overdose 963.5
  weight 278.00
    gain 783.1
      of pregnancy 646.1 ✓5ᵗʰ
    loss 783.21

Excitability, abnormal, under minor stress 309.29

Excitation
  catatonic (*see also* Schizophrenia) 295.2 ✓5ᵗʰ
  psychogenic 298.1
  reactive (from emotional stress, psychological trauma) 298.1

Excitement
  manic (*see also* Psychosis, affective) 296.0 ✓5ᵗʰ
    recurrent episode 296.1 ✓5ᵗʰ
    single episode 296.0 ✓5ᵗʰ
  mental, reactive (from emotional stress, psychological trauma) 298.1
  state, reactive (from emotional stress, psychological trauma) 298.1

Excluded pupils 364.76

Excoriation (traumatic) (*see also* Injury, superficial, by site) 919.8
  neurotic 698.4

Excyclophoria 378.44

Excyclotropia 378.33

Exencephalus, exencephaly 742.0

Exercise
  breathing V57.0
  remedial NEC V57.1
  therapeutic NEC V57.1

Exfoliation, teeth due to systemic causes 525.0

Exfoliative — *see also* condition dermatitis 695.89

Exhaustion, exhaustive (physical NEC) 780.79
  battle (*see also* Reaction, stress, acute) 308.9
  cardiac (*see also* Failure, heart) 428.9
  delirium (*see also* Reaction, stress, acute) 308.9
  due to
    cold 991.8
    excessive exertion 994.5
    exposure 994.4
  fetus or newborn 779.89 ▲
  heart (*see also* Failure, heart) 428.9
  heat 992.5
    due to
      salt depletion 992.4
      water depletion 992.3
  manic (*see also* Psychosis, affective) 296.0 ✓5ᵗʰ
    recurrent episode 296.1 ✓5ᵗʰ
    single episode 296.0 ✓5ᵗʰ
  maternal, complicating delivery 669.8 ✓5ᵗʰ
    affecting fetus or newborn 763.89
  mental 300.5
  myocardium, myocardial (*see also* Failure, heart) 428.9
  nervous 300.5
  old age 797
  postinfectional NEC 780.79
  psychogenic 300.5
  psychosis (*see also* Reaction, stress, acute) 308.9
  senile 797
    dementia 290.0

Exhibitionism (sexual) 302.4

Exomphalos 756.79

Exophoria 378.42
  convergence, insufficiency 378.83
  divergence, excess 378.85

Exophthalmic
  cachexia 242.0 ✓5ᵗʰ
  goiter 242.0 ✓5ᵗʰ
  ophthalmoplegia 242.0 ✓5ᵗʰ [376.22]

Exophthalmos 376.30
  congenital 743.66
  constant 376.31
  endocrine NEC 259.9 [376.22]
  hyperthyroidism 242.0 ✓5ᵗʰ [376.21]

Exophthalmos — *continued*
  intermittent NEC 376.34
  malignant 242.0 ✓5ᵗʰ [376.21]
  pulsating 376.35
    endocrine NEC 259.9 [376.22]
  thyrotoxic 242.0 ✓5ᵗʰ [376.21]

Exostosis 726.91
  cartilaginous (M9210/0) — *see* Neoplasm, bone, benign
  congenital 756.4
  ear canal, external 380.81
  gonococcal 098.89
  hip 726.5
  intracranial 733.3
  jaw (bone) 526.81
  luxurians 728.11
  multiple (cancellous) (congenital) (hereditary) 756.4
  nasal bones 726.91
  orbit, orbital 376.42
  osteocartilaginous (M9210/0) — *see* Neoplasm, bone, benign
  spine 721.8
    with spondylosis — *see* Spondylosis
  syphilitic 095.5
  wrist 726.4

Exotropia 378.10
  alternating 378.15
    with
      A pattern 378.16
      specified noncomitancy NEC 378.18
      V pattern 378.17
      X pattern 378.18
      Y pattern 378.18
    intermittent 378.24
  intermittent 378.20
    alternating 378.24
    monocular 378.23
  monocular 378.11
    with
      A pattern 378.12
      specified noncomitancy NEC 378.14
      V pattern 378.13
      X pattern 378.14
      Y pattern 378.14
    intermittent 378.23

Explanation of
  investigation finding V65.4
  medication V65.4

Exposure 994.9
  cold 991.9
    specified effect NEC 991.8
  effects of 994.9
  exhaustion due to 994.4
  to
    AIDS virus V01.7
    anthrax V01.81 ●
    asbestos V15.84
    body fluids (hazardous) V15.85
    cholera V01.0
    communicable disease V01.9
      specified type NEC V01.89 ▲
    German measles V01.4
    gonorrhea V01.6
    hazardous body fluids V15.85
    HIV V01.7
    human immunodeficiency virus V01.7
    lead V15.86
    parasitic disease V01.89 ▲
    poliomyelitis V01.2
    potentially hazardous body fluids V15.85
    rabies V01.5
    rubella V01.4
    smallpox V01.3
    syphilis V01.6
    tuberculosis V01.1
    venereal disease V01.6
    viral disease NEC V01.7

Exsanguination, fetal 772.0

Exstrophy
  abdominal content 751.8
  bladder (urinary) 753.5

Extensive — *see* condition

Extra — *see also* Accessory
  rib 756.3
    cervical 756.2

Extraction
  with hook 763.89
  breech NEC 669.6 ✓5ᵗʰ
    affecting fetus or newborn 763.0
  cataract postsurgical V45.61
  manual NEC 669.8 ✓5ᵗʰ
    affecting fetus or newborn 763.89

Extrasystole 427.60
  atrial 427.61
  postoperative 997.1
  ventricular 427.69

Extrauterine gestation or pregnancy — *see* Pregnancy, ectopic

Extravasation
  blood 459.0
    lower extremity 459.0
  chyle into mesentery 457.8
  pelvicalyceal 593.4
  pyelosinus 593.4
  urine 788.8
    from ureter 788.8

Extremity — *see* condition

Extrophy — *see* Exstrophy

Extroversion
  bladder 753.5
  uterus 618.1
    complicating delivery 665.2 ✓5ᵗʰ
      affecting fetus or newborn 763.89
    postpartal (old) 618.1

Extrusion
  breast implant (prosthetic) 996.54
  device, implant, or graft — *see* Complications, mechanical
  eye implant (ball) (globe) 996.59
  intervertebral disc — *see* Displacement, intervertebral disc
  lacrimal gland 375.43
  mesh (reinforcing) 996.59
  ocular lens implant 996.53
  prosthetic device NEC — *see* Complications, mechanical
  vitreous 379.26

Exudate, pleura — *see* Effusion, pleura

Exudates, retina 362.82

Exudative — *see* condition

Eye, eyeball, eyelid — *see* condition

Eyestrain 368.13

Eyeworm disease of Africa 125.2

F

Faber's anemia or syndrome (achlorhydric anemia) 280.9

Fabry's disease (angiokeratoma corporis diffusum) 272.7

Face, facial — *see* condition

Facet of cornea 371.44

Faciocephalalgia, autonomic (*see also* Neuropathy, peripheral, autonomic) 337.9

Facioscapulohumeral myopathy 359.1

Factitious disorder, illness — *see* Illness, factitious

Factor
  deficiency — *see* Deficiency, factor
  psychic, associated with diseases classified elsewhere 316
  risk — *see* Problem

Fahr-Volhard disease (malignant nephrosclerosis) 403.00

Failure, failed
  adenohypophyseal 253.2
  attempted abortion (legal) (*see also* Abortion, failed) 638.9
  bone marrow (anemia) 284.9
    acquired (secondary) 284.8
    congenital 284.0
    idiopathic 284.9
  cardiac (*see also* Failure, heart) 428.9
    newborn 779.89 ▲
  cardiorenal (chronic) 428.9
    hypertensive (*see also* Hypertension, cardiorenal) 404.93

Failure — Failure

Failure, failed — *continued*
  cardiorespiratory 799.1
    specified during or due to a procedure 997.1
      long-term effect of cardiac surgery 429.4
  cardiovascular (chronic) 428.9
  cerebrovascular 437.8
  cervical dilatation in labor 661.0 ✓5ᵗʰ
    affecting fetus or newborn 763.7
  circulation, circulatory 799.8
    fetus or newborn 779.89 ▲
    peripheral 785.50
  compensation — *see* Disease, heart
  congestive (*see also* Failure, heart) 428.0
  coronary (*see also* Insufficiency, coronary) 411.89
  descent of head (at term) 652.5 ✓5ᵗʰ
    affecting fetus or newborn 763.1
    in labor 660.0 ✓5ᵗʰ
      affecting fetus or newborn 763.1
  device, implant, or graft — *see* Complications, mechanical
  engagement of head NEC 652.5 ✓5ᵗʰ
    in labor 660.0 ✓5ᵗʰ
  extrarenal 788.9
  fetal head to enter pelvic brim 652.5 ✓5ᵗʰ
    affecting fetus or newborn 763.1
    in labor 660.0 ✓5ᵗʰ
      affecting fetus or newborn 763.1
  forceps NEC 660.7 ✓5ᵗʰ
    affecting fetus or newborn 763.1
  fusion (joint) (spinal) 996.4
  growth in childhood 783.43
  heart (acute) (sudden) 428.9
    with
      abortion — *see* Abortion, by type, with specified complication NEC
      acute pulmonary edema (*see also* Failure, ventricular, left) 428.1
        with congestion ▶(*see also* Failure, heart)◀ 428.0
      decompensation (*see also* Failure, heart) 428.0
      dilation — *see* Disease, heart
      ectopic pregnancy (*see also* categories 633.0-633.9) 639.8
      molar pregnancy (*see also* categories 630-632) 639.8
    arteriosclerotic 440.9
    combined left-right sided 428.0
    combined systolic and diastolic 428.40 ●
      acute 428.41 ●
      acute on chronic 428.43 ●
      chronic 428.42 ●
    compensated (*see also* Failure, heart) 428.0
    complicating
      abortion — *see* Abortion, by type, with specified complication NEC
      delivery (cesarean) (instrumental) 669.4 ✓5ᵗʰ
      ectopic pregnancy (*see also* categories 633.0-633.9) 639.8
      molar pregnancy (*see also* categories 630-632) 639.8
      obstetric anesthesia or sedation 668.1 ✓5ᵗʰ
      surgery 997.1
    congestive (compensated) (decompensated) ▶(*see also* Failure, heart)◀ 428.0
      with rheumatic fever (conditions classifiable to 390)
        active 391.8
        inactive or quiescent (with chorea) 398.91
      fetus or newborn 779.89 ▲
      hypertensive (*see also* Hypertension, heart) 402.90
        with renal disease (*see also* Hypertension, cardiorenal) 404.91
          with renal failure 404.93
        benign 402.11
        malignant 402.01
      rheumatic (chronic) (inactive) (with chorea) 398.91
        active or acute 391.8
          with chorea (Sydenham's) 392.0

Failure, failed — *continued*
  heart — *continued*
    decompensated (*see also* Failure, heart) 428.0
    degenerative (*see also* Degeneration, myocardial) 429.1
    diastolic 428.30 ●
      acute 428.31 ●
      acute on chronic 428.33 ●
      chronic 428.32 ●
    due to presence of (cardiac) prosthesis 429.4
    fetus or newborn 779.89 ▲
    following
      abortion 639.8
      cardiac surgery 429.4
      ectopic or molar pregnancy 639.8
    high output NEC 428.9
    hypertensive (*see also* Hypertension, heart) 402.91
      with renal disease (*see also* Hypertension, cardiorenal) 404.91
        with renal failure 404.93
      benign 402.11
      malignant 402.01
    left (ventricular) (*see also* Failure, ventricular, left) 428.1
      with right-sided failure ▶(*see also* Failure, heart)◀ 428.0
    low output (syndrome) NEC 428.9
    organic — *see* Disease, heart
    postoperative (immediate) 997.1
      long term effect of cardiac surgery 429.4
    rheumatic (chronic) (congestive) (inactive) 398.91
    right (secondary to left heart failure, conditions classifiable to 428.1) (ventricular) (*see also* Failure, heart) 428.0
    senile 797
    specified during or due to a procedure 997.1
      long-term effect of cardiac surgery 429.4
    systolic 428.20 ●
      acute 428.21 ●
      acute on chronic 428.23 ●
      chronic 428.22 ●
    thyrotoxic (*see also* Thyrotoxicosis) 242.9 ✓5ᵗʰ [425.7]
    valvular — *see* Endocarditis
  hepatic 572.8
    acute 570
    due to a procedure 997.4
  hepatorenal 572.4
  hypertensive heart (*see also* Hypertension, heart) 402.91
    benign 402.11
    malignant 402.01
  induction (of labor) 659.1 ✓5ᵗʰ
    abortion (legal) (*see also* Abortion, failed) 638.9
    affecting fetus or newborn 763.89
    by oxytocic drugs 659.1 ✓5ᵗʰ
    instrumental 659.0 ✓5ᵗʰ
    mechanical 659.0 ✓5ᵗʰ
    medical 659.1 ✓5ᵗʰ
    surgical 659.0 ✓5ᵗʰ
  initial alveolar expansion, newborn 770.4
  involution, thymus (gland) 254.8
  kidney — *see* Failure, renal
  lactation 676.4 ✓5ᵗʰ
  Leydig's cell, adult 257.2
  liver 572.8
    acute 570
  medullary 799.8
  mitral — *see* Endocarditis, mitral
  myocardium, myocardial (*see also* Failure, heart) 428.9
    chronic (*see also* Failure, heart) 428.0
    congestive (*see also* Failure, heart) 428.0
  ovarian (primary) 256.39
    iatrogenic 256.2
    postablative 256.2
    postirradiation 256.2
    postsurgical 256.2
  ovulation 628.0
  prerenal 788.9

Failure, failed — *continued*
  renal 586
    with
      abortion — *see* Abortion, by type, with renal failure
      ectopic pregnancy (*see also* categories 633.0-633.9) 639.3
      edema (*see also* Nephrosis) 581.9
      hypertension (*see also* Hypertension, kidney) 403.91
      hypertensive heart disease (conditions classifiable to 402) 404.92
        with heart failure 404.93
        benign 404.12
          with heart failure 404.13
        malignant 404.02
          with heart failure 404.03
      molar pregnancy (*see also* categories 630-632) 639.3
      tubular necrosis (acute) 584.5
    acute 584.9
      with lesion of
        necrosis
          cortical (renal) 584.6
          medullary (renal) (papillary) 584.7
          tubular 584.5
        specified pathology NEC 584.8
    chronic 585
      hypertensive or with hypertension (*see also* Hypertension, kidney) 403.91
    due to a procedure 997.5
    following
      abortion 639.3
      crushing 958.5
      ectopic or molar pregnancy 639.3
      labor and delivery (acute) 669.3 ✓5ᵗʰ
    hypertensive (*see also* Hypertension, kidney) 403.91
    puerperal, postpartum 669.3 ✓5ᵗʰ
  respiration, respiratory 518.81
    acute 518.81
    acute and chronic 518.84
    center 348.8
      newborn 770.84 ▲
    chronic 518.83
    due to trauma, surgery or shock 518.5
    newborn 770.84 ▲
  rotation
    cecum 751.4
    colon 751.4
    intestine 751.4
    kidney 753.3
  segmentation — *see also* Fusion
    fingers (*see also* Syndactylism, fingers) 755.11
    toes (*see also* Syndactylism, toes) 755.13
  seminiferous tubule, adult 257.2
  senile (general) 797
    with psychosis 290.20
  testis, primary (seminal) 257.2
  to progress 661.2 ✓5ᵗʰ
  to thrive
    adult 783.7
    child 783.41
  transplant 996.80
    bone marrow 996.85
    organ (immune or nonimmune cause) 996.80
      bone marrow 996.85
      heart 996.83
      intestines 996.87
      kidney 996.81
      liver 996.82
      lung 996.84
      pancreas 996.86
      specified NEC 996.89
    skin 996.52
      artificial 996.55
      decellularized allodermis 996.55
      temporary allograft or pigskin graft — *omit code*
  trial of labor NEC 660.6 ✓5ᵗʰ
    affecting fetus or newborn 763.1
  urinary 586
  vacuum extraction
    abortion — *see* Abortion, failed
    delivery NEC 660.7 ✓5ᵗʰ

◼4ᵗʰ Fourth-digit Required   ✓5ᵗʰ Fifth-digit Required   ▶◀ Revised Text   ● New Line   ▲ Revised Code

Failure, failed — *continued*
  vacuum extraction — *continued*
    delivery NEC — *continued*
      affecting fetus or newborn 763.1
    ventouse NEC 660.7 ✓5ᵗʰ
      affecting fetus or newborn 763.1
  ventricular (*see also* Failure, heart) 428.9
    left 428.1
      with rheumatic fever (conditions
        classifiable to 390)
        active 391.8
          with chorea 392.0
        inactive or quiescent (with chorea)
          398.91
      hypertensive (*see also* Hypertension,
        heart) 402.91
        benign 402.11
        malignant 402.01
      rheumatic (chronic) (inactive) (with
        chorea) 398.91
        active or acute 391.8
          with chorea 392.0
    right (*see also* Failure, heart) 428.0
  vital centers, fetus or newborn 779.8
  weight gain in childhood 783.41
Fainting (fit) (spell) 780.2
Falciform hymen 752.49
Fall, maternal, affecting fetus or newborn
  760.5
Fallen arches 734
Falling, any organ or part — *see* Prolapse
Fallopian
  insufflation
    fertility testing V26.21
    following sterilization reversal V26.22
  tube — *see* condition
Fallot's
  pentalogy 745.2
  tetrad or tetralogy 745.2
  triad or trilogy 746.09
Fallout, radioactive (adverse effect) NEC 990
False — *see also* condition
  bundle branch block 426.50
  bursa 727.89
  croup 478.75
  joint 733.82
  labor (pains) 644.1 ✓5ᵗʰ
  opening, urinary, male 752.69
  passage, urethra (prostatic) 599.4
  positive
    serological test for syphilis 795.6
    Wassermann reaction 795.6
  pregnancy 300.11
Family, familial — *see also* condition
  disruption V61.0
  planning advice V25.09
  problem V61.9
    specified circumstance NEC V61.8
Famine 994.2
  edema 262
Fanconi's anemia (congenital pancytopenia)
  284.0
Fanconi (-de Toni) (-Debré) syndrome
  (cystinosis) 270.0
Farber (-Uzman) syndrome or disease
  (disseminated lipogranulomatosis) 272.8
Farcin 024
Farcy 024
Farmers'
  lung 495.0
  skin 692.74
Farsightedness 367.0
Fascia — *see* condition
Fasciculation 781.0
Fasciculitis optica 377.32
Fasciitis 729.4
  eosinophilic 728.89
  necrotizing 728.86
  nodular 728.79
  perirenal 593.4
  plantar 728.71
  pseudosarcomatous 728.79

Fasciitis — *continued*
  traumatic (old) NEC 728.79
    current — *see* Sprain, by site
Fasciola hepatica infestation 121.3
Fascioliasis 121.3
Fasciolopsiasis (small intestine) 121.4
Fasciolopsis (small intestine) 121.4
Fast pulse 785.0
Fat
  embolism (cerebral) (pulmonary) (systemic)
    958.1
    with
      abortion — *see* Abortion, by type, with
        embolism
      ectopic pregnancy (*see also* categories
        633.0-633.9) 639.6
      molar pregnancy (*see also* categories 630-
        632) 639.6
    complicating delivery or puerperium
      673.8 ✓5ᵗʰ
    following
      abortion 639.6
      ectopic or molar pregnancy 639.6
    in pregnancy, childbirth, or the puerperium
      673.8 ✓5ᵗʰ
  excessive 278.00
    in heart (*see also* Degeneration, myocardial)
      429.1
  general 278.00
  hernia, herniation 729.30
    eyelid 374.34
    knee 729.31
    orbit 374.34
    retro-orbital 374.34
    retropatellar 729.31
    specified site NEC 729.39
  indigestion 579.8
  in stool 792.1
  localized (pad) 278.1
    heart (*see also* Degeneration, myocardial)
      429.1
    knee 729.31
    retropatellar 729.31
  necrosis — *see also* Fatty, degeneration breast
    (aseptic)
    (segmental) 611.3
    mesentery 567.8
    omentum 567.8
  pad 278.1
Fatal syncope 798.1
Fatigue 780.79
  auditory deafness (*see also* Deafness) 389.9
  chronic 780.7 ✓5ᵗʰ
  chronic, syndrome 780.71
  combat (*see also* Reaction, stress, acute) 308.9
  during pregnancy 646.8 ✓5ᵗʰ
  general 780.79
    psychogenic 300.5
  heat (transient) 992.6
  muscle 729.89
  myocardium (*see also* Failure, heart) 428.9
  nervous 300.5
  neurosis 300.5
  operational 300.89
  postural 729.89
  posture 729.89
  psychogenic (general) 300.5
  senile 797
  syndrome NEC 300.5
    chronic 780.71
  undue 780.79
  voice 784.49
Fatness 278.00
Fatty — *see also* condition
  apron 278.1
  degeneration (diffuse) (general) NEC 272.8
    localized — *see* Degeneration, by site, fatty
    placenta — *see* Placenta, abnormal
  heart (enlarged) (*see also* Degeneration,
    myocardial) 429.1
  infiltration (diffuse) (general) (*see also*
    Degeneration, by site, fatty) 272.8
    heart (enlarged) (*see also* Degeneration,
      myocardial) 429.1
  liver 571.8
    alcoholic 571.0

Fatty — *see also* condition — *continued*
  necrosis — *see* Degeneration, fatty
  phanerosis 272.8
Fauces — *see* condition
Fauchard's disease (periodontitis) 523.4
Faucitis 478.29
Faulty — *see also* condition
  position of teeth 524.3
Favism (anemia) 282.2
Favre-Racouchot disease (elastoidosis cutanea
  nodularis) 701.8
Favus 110.9
  beard 110.0
  capitis 110.0
  corporis 110.5
  eyelid 110.8
  foot 110.4
  hand 110.2
  scalp 110.0
  specified site NEC 110.8
Fear, fearfullness (complex) (reaction) 300.20
  child 313.0
  of
    animals 300.29
    closed spaces 300.29
    crowds 300.29
    eating in public 300.23
    heights 300.29
    open spaces 300.22
      with panic attacks 300.21
    public speaking 300.23
    streets 300.22
      with panic attacks 300.21
    travel 300.22
      with panic attacks 300.21
    washing in public 300.23
  transient 308.0
Feared complaint unfounded V65.5
Febricula (continued) (simple) (*see also* Pyrexia)
  780.6
Febrile (*see also* Pyrexia) 780.6
  convulsion 780.31
  seizure 780.31
Febris (*see also* Fever) 780.6
  aestiva (*see also* Fever, hay) 477.9
  flava (*see also* Fever, yellow) 060.9
  melitensis 023.0
  pestis (*see also* Plague) 020.9
  puerperalis 672 ✓5ᵗʰ
  recurrens (*see also* Fever, relapsing) 087.9
    pediculo vestimenti 087.0
  rubra 034.1
  typhoidea 002.0
  typhosa 002.0
Fecal — *see* condition
Fecalith (impaction) 560.39
  with hernia — *see also* Hernia, by site, with
    obstruction
    gangrenous — *see* Hernia, by site, with
      gangrene
  appendix 543.9
  congenital 777.1
Fede's disease 529.0
Feeble-minded 317
Feeble rapid pulse due to shock following
  injury 958.4
Feeding
  faulty (elderly) (infant) 783.3
    newborn 779.3
  formula check V20.2
  improper (elderly) (infant) 783.3
    newborn 779.3
  problem (elderly) (infant) 783.3
    newborn 779.3
    nonorganic origin 307.59
Feer's disease 985.0
Feet — *see* condition
Feigned illness V65.2
Feil-Klippel syndrome (brevicollis) 756.16
Feinmesser's (hidrotic) **ectodermal dysplasia**
  757.31

✓4ᵗʰ Fourth-digit Required   ✓5ᵗʰ Fifth-digit Required   ▶◀ Revised Text   ● New Line   ▲ Revised Code

Felix's disease (juvenile osteochondrosis, hip) 732.1
Felon (any digit) (with lymphangitis) 681.01
  herpetic 054.6
Felty's syndrome (rheumatoid arthritis with splenomegaly and leukopenia) 714.1
Feminism in boys 302.6
Feminization, testicular 257.8
  with pseudohermaphroditism, male 257.8
Femoral hernia — see Hernia, femoral
Femora vara 736.32
Femur, femoral — see condition
Fenestrata placenta — see Placenta, abnormal
Fenestration, fenestrated — see also Imperfect, closure
  aorta-pulmonary 745.0
  aorticopulmonary 745.0
  aortopulmonary 745.0
  cusps, heart valve NEC 746.89
    pulmonary 746.09
  hymen 752.49
  pulmonic cusps 746.09
Fenwick's disease 537.89
Fermentation (gastric) (gastrointestinal) (stomach) 536.8
  intestine 564.89
    psychogenic 306.4
  psychogenic 306.4
Fernell's disease (aortic aneurysm) 441.9
Fertile eunuch syndrome 257.2
Fertility, meaning multiparity — see Multiparity
Fetal alcohol syndrome 760.71
Fetalis uterus 752.3
Fetid
  breath 784.9
  sweat 705.89
Fetishism 302.81
  transvestic 302.3
Fetomaternal hemorrhage
  affecting management of pregnancy 656.0 ✔5th
  fetus or newborn 772.0
Fetus, fetal — see also condition
  papyraceous 779.89
  type lung tissue 770.4 ▲
Fever 780.6
  with chills 780.6
    in malarial regions (see also Malaria) 084.6
  abortus NEC 023.9
  Aden 061
  African tick-borne 087.1
  American
    mountain tick 066.1
    spotted 082.0
  and ague (see also Malaria) 084.6
  aphthous 078.4
  arbovirus hemorrhagic 065.9
  Assam 085.0
  Australian A or Q 083.0
  Bangkok hemorrhagic 065.4
  biliary, Charcôt's intermittent — see Choledocholithiasis
  bilious, hemoglobinuric 084.8
  blackwater 084.8
  blister 054.9
  Bonvale Dam 780.79
  boutonneuse 082.1
  brain 323.9
    late effect — see category 326
  breakbone 061
  Bullis 082.8
  Bunyamwera 066.3
  Burdwan 085.0
  Bwamba (encephalitis) 066.3
  Cameroon (see also Malaria) 084.6
  Canton 081.9
  catarrhal (acute) 460
    chronic 472.0
  cat-scratch 078.3
  cerebral 323.9
    late effect — see category 326
  cerebrospinal (meningococcal) (see also Meningitis, cerebrospinal) 036.0
  Chagres 084.0

Fever — continued
  Chandipura 066.8
  changuinola 066.0
  Charcôt's (biliary) (hepatic) (intermittent) see Choledocholithiasis
  Chikungunya (viral) 066.3
    hemorrhagic 065.4
  childbed 670 ✔4th
  Chitral 066.0
  Colombo (see also Fever, paratyphoid) 002.9
  Colorado tick (virus) 066.1
  congestive
    malarial (see also Malaria) 084.6
    remittent (see also Malaria) 084.6
  Congo virus 065.0
  continued 780.6
    malarial 084.0
  Corsican (see also Malaria) 084.6
  Crimean hemorrhagic 065.0
  Cyprus (see also Brucellosis) 023.9
  dandy 061
  deer fly (see also Tularemia) 021.9
  dehydration, newborn 778.4
  dengue (virus) 061
    hemorrhagic 065.4
  desert 114.0
  due to heat 992.0
  Dumdum 085.0
  enteric 002.0
  ephemeral (of unknown origin) (see also Pyrexia) 780.6
  epidemic, hemorrhagic of the Far East 065.0
  erysipelatous (see also Erysipelas) 035
  estivo-autumnal (malarial) 084.0
  etiocholanolone 277.3
  famine — see also Fever, relapsing
    meaning typhus — see Typhus
  Far Eastern hemorrhagic 065.0
  five day 083.1
  Fort Bragg 100.89
  gastroenteric 002.0
  gastromalarial (see also Malaria) 084.6
  Gibraltar (see also Brucellosis) 023.9
  glandular 075
  Guama (viral) 066.3
  Haverhill 026.1
  hay (allergic) (with rhinitis) 477.9
    with
      asthma (bronchial) (see also Asthma) 493.0 ✔5th
    due to
      dander 477.8
      dust 477.8
      fowl 477.8
      pollen, any plant or tree 477.0
      specified allergen other than pollen 477.8
  heat (effects) 992.0
  hematuric, bilious 084.8
  hemoglobinuric (malarial) 084.8
    bilious 084.8
  hemorrhagic (arthropod-borne) NEC 065.9
    with renal syndrome 078.6
    arenaviral 078.7
    Argentine 078.7
    Bangkok 065.4
    Bolivian 078.7
    Central Asian 065.0
    chikungunya 065.4
    Crimean 065.0
    dengue (virus) 065.4
    Ebola 065.8
    epidemic 078.6
      of Far East 065.0
    Far Eastern 065.0
    Junin virus 078.7
    Korean 078.6
    Kyasanur forest 065.2
    Machupo virus 078.7
    mite-borne NEC 065.8
    mosquito-borne 065.4
    Omsk 065.1
    Philippine 065.4
    Russian (Yaroslav) 078.6
    Singapore 065.4
    Southeast Asia 065.4
    Thailand 065.4
    tick-borne NEC 065.3

Fever — continued
  hepatic (see also Cholecystitis) 575.8
    intermittent (Charcôt's) — see Choledocholithiasis
  herpetic (see also Herpes) 054.9
  Hyalomma tick 065.0
  icterohemorrhagic 100.0
  inanition 780.6
    newborn 778.4
  infective NEC 136.9
  intermittent (bilious) (see also Malaria) 084.6
    hepatic (Charcôt) — see Choledocholithiasis
    of unknown origin (see also Pyrexia) 780.6
    pernicious 084.0
  iodide
    correct substance properly administered 780.6
    overdose or wrong substance given or taken 975.5
  Japanese river 081.2
  jungle yellow 060.0
  Junin virus, hemorrhagic 078.7
  Katayama 120.2
  Kedani 081.2
  Kenya 082.1
  Korean hemorrhagic 078.6
  Lassa 078.89
  Lone Star 082.8
  lung — see Pneumonia
  Machupo virus, hemorrhagic 078.7
  malaria, malarial (see also Malaria) 084.6
  Malta (see also Brucellosis) 023.9
  Marseilles 082.1
  marsh (see also Malaria) 084.6
  Mayaro (viral) 066.3
  Mediterranean (see also Brucellosis) 023.9
    familial 277.3
    tick 082.1
  meningeal — see Meningitis
  metal fumes NEC 985.8
  Meuse 083.1
  Mexican — see Typhus, Mexican
  Mianeh 087.1
  miasmatic (see also Malaria) 084.6
  miliary 078.2
  milk, female 672 ✔4th
  mill 504
  mite-borne hemorrhagic 065.8
  Monday 504
  mosquito-borne NEC 066.3
    hemorrhagic NEC 065.4
  mountain 066.1
    meaning
      Rocky Mountain spotted 082.0
      undulant fever (see also Brucellosis) 023.9
    tick (American) 066.1
  Mucambo (viral) 066.3
  mud 100.89
  Neapolitan (see also Brucellosis) 023.9
  neutropenic 288.0
  nine-mile 083.0
  nonexanthematous tick 066.1
  North Asian tick-borne typhus 082.2
  Omsk hemorrhagic 065.1
  O'nyong-nyong (viral) 066.3
  Oropouche (viral) 066.3
  Oroya 088.0
  paludal (see also Malaria) 084.6
  Panama 084.0
  pappataci 066.0
  paratyphoid 002.9
    A 002.1
    B (Schöttmüller's) 002.2
    C (Hirschfeld) 002.3
  parrot 073.9
  periodic 277.3
  pernicious, acute 084.0
  persistent (of unknown origin) (see also Pyrexia) 780.6
  petechial 036.0
  pharyngoconjunctival 077.2
    adenoviral type 3 077.2
  Philippine hemorrhagic 065.4
  phlebotomus 066.0
  Piry 066.8
  Pixuna (viral) 066.3
  Plasmodium ovale 084.3

Fever — *continued*

pleural (*see also* Pleurisy) 511.0
pneumonic — *see* Pneumonia
polymer fume 987.8
postoperative 998.89
due to infection 998.59
pretibial 100.89
puerperal, postpartum 672 ✓4th
putrid — *see* Septicemia
pyemic — *see* Septicemia
Q 083.0
with pneumonia 083.0 [484.8]
quadrilateral 083.0
quartan (malaria) 084.2
Queensland (coastal) 083.0
seven-day 100.89
Quintan (A) 083.1
quotidian 084.0
rabbit (*see also* Tularemia) 021.9
rat-bite 026.9
due to
Spirillum minor or minus 026.0
Spirochaeta morsus muris 026.0
Streptobacillus moniliformis 026.1
recurrent — *see* Fever, relapsing
relapsing 087.9
Carter's (Asiatic) 087.0
Dutton's (West African) 087.1
Koch's 087.9
louse-borne (epidemic) 087.0
Novy's (American) 087.1
Obermeyer's (European) 087.0
spirillum NEC 087.9
tick-borne (endemic) 087.1
remittent (bilious) (congestive) (gastric) (*see also* Malaria) 084.6
rheumatic (active) (acute) (chronic) (subacute) 390
with heart involvement 391.9
carditis 391.9
endocarditis (aortic) (mitral) (pulmonary) (tricuspid) 391.1
multiple sites 391.8
myocarditis 391.2
pancarditis, acute 391.8
pericarditis 391.0
specified type NEC 391.8
valvulitis 391.1
inactive or quiescent with cardiac hypertrophy 398.99
carditis 398.90
endocarditis 397.9
aortic (valve) 395.9
with mitral (valve) disease 396.9
mitral (valve) 394.9
with aortic (valve) disease 396.9
pulmonary (valve) 397.1
tricuspid (valve) 397.0
heart conditions (classifiable to 429.3, 429.6, 429.9) 398.99
failure (congestive) (conditions classifiable to 428.0, 428.9) 398.91
left ventricular failure (conditions classifiable to 428.1) 398.91
myocardial degeneration (conditions classifiable to 429.1) 398.0
myocarditis (conditions classifiable to 429.0) 398.0
pancarditis 398.99
pericarditis 393
Rift Valley (viral) 066.3
Rocky Mountain spotted 082.0
rose 477.0
Ross river (viral) 066.3
Russian hemorrhagic 078.6
sandfly 066.0
San Joaquin (valley) 114.0
São Paulo 082.0
scarlet 034.1
septic — *see* Septicemia
seven-day 061
Japan 100.89
Queensland 100.89
shin bone 083.1
Singapore hemorrhagic 065.4
solar 061

Fever — *continued*

sore 054.9
South African tick-bite 087.1
Southeast Asia hemorrhagic 065.4
spinal — *see* Meningitis
spirillary 026.0
splenic (*see also* Anthrax) 022.9
spotted (Rocky Mountain) 082.0
American 082.0
Brazilian 082.0
Colombian 082.0
meaning
cerebrospinal meningitis 036.0
typhus 082.9
spring 309.23
steroid
correct substance properly administered 780.6
overdose or wrong substance given or taken 962.0
streptobacillary 026.1
subtertian 084.0
Sumatran mite 081.2
sun 061
swamp 100.89
sweating 078.2
swine 003.8
sylvatic yellow 060.0
Tahyna 062.5
tertian — *see* Malaria, tertian
Thailand hemorrhagic 065.4
thermic 992.0
three day 066.0
with Coxsackie exanthem 074.8
tick
American mountain 066.1
Colorado 066.1
Kemerovo 066.1
Mediterranean 082.1
mountain 066.1
nonexanthematous 066.1
Quaranfil 066.1
tick-bite NEC 066.1
tick-borne NEC 066.1
hemorrhagic NEC 065.3
transitory of newborn 778.4
trench 083.1
tsutsugamushi 081.2
typhogastric 002.0
typhoid (abortive) (ambulant) (any site) (hemorrhagic) (infection) (intermittent) (malignant) (rheumatic) 002.0
typhomalarial (*see also* Malaria) 084.6
typhus — *see* Typhus
undulant (*see also* Brucellosis) 023.9
unknown origin (*see also* Pyrexia) 780.6
uremic — *see* Uremia
uveoparotid 135
valley (Coccidioidomycosis) 114.0
Venezuelan equine 066.2
Volhynian 083.1
Wesselsbron (viral) 066.3
West
African 084.8
Nile (viral) 066.4 ▲
Whitmore's 025
Wolhynian 083.1
worm 128.9
Yaroslav hemorrhagic 078.6
yellow 060.9
jungle 060.0
sylvatic 060.0
urban 060.1
vaccination, prophylactic (against) V04.4
Zika (viral) 066.3

Fibrillation

atrial (established) (paroxysmal) 427.31
auricular (atrial) (established) 427.31
cardiac (ventricular) 427.41
coronary (*see also* Infarct, myocardium) 410.9 ✓5th
heart (ventricular) 427.41
muscular 728.9
postoperative 997.1
ventricular 427.41

Fibrin

ball or bodies, pleural (sac) 511.0
chamber, anterior (eye) (gelatinous exudate) 364.04
Fibrinogenolysis (hemorrhagic) — *see* Fibrinolysis
Fibrinogenopenia (congenital) (hereditary) (*see also* Defect, coagulation) 286.3
acquired 286.6
Fibrinolysis (acquired) (hemorrhagic) (pathologic) 286.6
with
abortion — *see* Abortion, by type, with hemorrhage, delayed or excessive
ectopic pregnancy (*see also* categories 633.0-633.9) 639.1
molar pregnancy (*see also* categories 630-632) 639.1
antepartum or intrapartum 641.3 ✓5th
affecting fetus or newborn 762.1
following
abortion 639.1
ectopic or molar pregnancy 639.1
newborn, transient 776.2
postpartum 666.3 ✓5th
Fibrinopenia (hereditary) (*see also* Defect, coagulation) 286.3
acquired 286.6
Fibrinopurulent — *see* condition
Fibrinous — *see* condition
Fibroadenoma (M9010/0)
cellular intracanalicular (M9020/0) 217
giant (intracanalicular) (M9020/0) 217
intracanalicular (M9011/0)
cellular (M9020/0) 217
giant (M9020/0) 217
specified site — *see* Neoplasm, by site, benign
unspecified site 217
juvenile (M9030/0) 217
pericanicular (M9012/0)
specified site — *see* Neoplasm, by site, benign
unspecified site 217
phyllodes (M9020/0) 217
prostate 600.2
specified site — *see* Neoplasm, by site, benign
unspecified site 217
Fibroadenosis, breast (chronic) (cystic) (diffuse) (periodic) (segmental) 610.2
Fibroangioma (M9160/0) — *see also* Neoplasm, by site, benign
juvenile (M9160/0)
specified site — *see* Neoplasm, by site, benign
unspecified site 210.7
Fibrocellulitis progressiva ossificans 728.11
Fibrochondrosarcoma (M9220/3) — *see* Neoplasm, cartilage, malignant
Fibrocystic
disease 277.00
bone NEC 733.29
breast 610.1
jaw 526.2
kidney (congenital) 753.19
liver 751.62
lung 518.89
congenital 748.4
pancreas 277.00
kidney (congenital) 753.19
Fibrodysplasia ossificans multiplex (progressiva) 728.11
Fibroelastosis (cordis) (endocardial) (endomyocardial) 425.3
Fibroid (tumor) (M8890/0) — *see also* Neoplasm, connective tissue, benign
disease, lung (chronic) (*see also* Fibrosis, lung) 515
heart (disease) (*see also* Myocarditis) 429.0
induration, lung (chronic) (*see also* Fibrosis, lung) 515
in pregnancy or childbirth 654.1 ✓5th
affecting fetus or newborn 763.89
causing obstructed labor 660.2 ✓5th
affecting fetus or newborn 763.1

✓4th Fourth-digit Required   ✓5th Fifth-digit Required   ▶◀ Revised Text   ● New Line   ▲ Revised Code

Fibroid — *see also* Neoplasm, connective tissue, benign — *continued*
liver — *see* Cirrhosis, liver
lung (*see also* Fibrosis, lung) 515
pneumonia (chronic) (*see also* Fibrosis, lung) 515
uterus (M8890/0) (*see also* Leiomyoma, uterus) 218.9

Fibrolipoma (M8851/0) (*see also* Lipoma, by site) 214.9

Fibroliposarcoma (M8850/3) — *see* Neoplasm, connective tissue, malignant

Fibroma (M8810/0) — *see also* Neoplasm, connective tissue, benign
ameloblastic (M9330/0) 213.1
upper jaw (bone) 213.0
bone (nonossifying) 733.99
ossifying (M9262/0) — *see* Neoplasm, bone, benign
cementifying (M9274/0) — *see* Neoplasm, bone, benign
chondromyxoid (M9241/0) — *see* Neoplasm, bone, benign
desmoplastic (M8823/1) — *see* Neoplasm, connective tissue, uncertain behavior
facial (M8813/0) — *see* Neoplasm, connective tissue, benign
invasive (M8821/1) — *see* Neoplasm, connective tissue, uncertain behavior
molle (M8851/0) (*see also* Lipoma, by site) 214.9
myxoid (M8811/0) — *see* Neoplasm, connective tissue, benign
nasopharynx, nasopharyngeal (juvenile) (M9160/0) 210.7
nonosteogenic (nonossifying) — *see* Dysplasia, fibrous
odontogenic (M9321/0) 213.1
upper jaw (bone) 213.0
ossifying (M9262/0) — *see* Neoplasm, bone, benign
periosteal (M8812/0 — *see* Neoplasm, bone, benign
prostate 600.2
soft (M8851/0) (*see also* Lipoma, by site) 214.9

Fibromatosis
abdominal (M8822/1) — *see* Neoplasm, connective tissue, uncertain behavior
aggressive (M8821/1) — *see* Neoplasm, connective tissue, uncertain behavior
Dupuytren's 728.6
gingival 523.8
plantar fascia 728.71
proliferative 728.79
pseudosarcomatous (proliferative) (subcutaneous) 728.79
subcutaneous pseudosarcomatous (proliferative) 728.79

Fibromyalgia 729.1

Fibromyoma (M8890/0) — *see also* Neoplasm, connective tissue, benign
uterus (corpus) (*see also* Leiomyoma, uterus) 218.9
in pregnancy or childbirth 654.1 ✓5ᵗʰ
affecting fetus or newborn 763.89
causing obstructed labor 660.2 ✓5ᵗʰ
affecting fetus or newborn 763.1

Fibromyositis (*see also* Myositis) 729.1
scapulohumeral 726.2

Fibromyxolipoma (M8852/0) (*see also* Lipoma, by site) 214.9

Fibromyxoma (M8811/0) — *see* Neoplasm, connective tissue, benign

Fibromyxosarcoma (M8811/3) — *see* Neoplasm, connective tissue, malignant

Fibro-odontoma, ameloblastic (M9290/0) 213.1
upper jaw (bone) 213.0

Fibro-osteoma (M9262/0) — *see* Neoplasm, bone, benign

Fibroplasia, retrolental 362.21

Fibropurulent — *see* condition

Fibrosarcoma (M8810/3) — *see also* Neoplasm, connective tissue, malignant
ameloblastic (M9330/3) 170.1
upper jaw (bone) 170.0

Fibrosarcoma — *see also* Neoplasm, connective tissue, malignant — *continued*
congenital (M8814/3) — *see* Neoplasm, connective tissue, malignant
fascial (M8813/3) — *see* Neoplasm, connective tissue, malignant
infantile (M8814/3) — *see* Neoplasm, connective tissue, malignant
odontogenic (M9330/3) 170.1
upper jaw (bone) 170.0
periosteal (M8812/3) — *see* Neoplasm, bone, malignant

Fibrosclerosis
breast 610.3
corpora cavernosa (penis) 607.89
familial multifocal NEC 710.8
multifocal (idiopathic) NEC 710.8
penis (corpora cavernosa) 607.89

Fibrosis, fibrotic
adrenal (gland) 255.8
alveolar (diffuse) 516.3
amnion 658.8 ✓5ᵗʰ
anal papillae 569.49
anus 569.49
appendix, appendiceal, noninflammatory 543.9
arteriocapillary — *see* Arteriosclerosis
bauxite (of lung) 503
biliary 576.8
due to Clonorchis sinensis 121.1
bladder 596.8
interstitial 595.1
localized submucosal 595.1
panmural 595.1
bone, diffuse 756.59
breast 610.3
capillary — *see also* Arteriosclerosis
lung (chronic) (*see also* Fibrosis, lung) 515
cardiac (*see also* Myocarditis) 429.0
cervix 622.8
chorion 658.8 ✓5ᵗʰ
corpus cavernosum 607.89
cystic (of pancreas) 277.00
with ●
manifestations ●
gastrointestinal 277.03 ●
pulmonary 277.02 ●
specified NEC 277.09 ●
meconium ileus 277.01 ●
pulmonary exacerbation 277.02 ●
due to (presence of) any device, implant, or graft — *see* Complications, due to (presence of) any device, implant, or graft classified to 996.0-996.5 NEC
ejaculatory duct 608.89
endocardium (*see also* Endocarditis) 424.90
endomyocardial (African) 425.0
epididymis 608.89
eye muscle 378.62
graphite (of lung) 503
heart (*see also* Myocarditis) 429.0
hepatic — *see* Cirrhosis, liver due to Clonorchis sinensis 121.1
hepatolienal — *see* Cirrhosis, liver
hepatosplenic — *see* Cirrhosis, liver
infrapatellar fat pad 729.31
interstitial pulmonary, newborn 770.7
intrascrotal 608.89
kidney (*see also* Sclerosis, renal) 587
liver — *see* Cirrhosis, liver
lung (atrophic) (capillary) (chronic) (confluent) (massive) (perialveolar) (peribronchial) 515
with
anthracosilicosis (occupational) 500
anthracosis (occupational) 500
asbestosis (occupational) 501
bagassosis (occupational) 495.1
bauxite 503
berylliosis (occupational) 503
byssinosis (occupational) 504
calcicosis (occupational) 502
chalicosis (occupational) 502
dust reticulation (occupational) 504
farmers' lung 495.0
gannister disease (occupational) 502
graphite 503
pneumonoconiosis (occupational) 505

Fibrosis, fibrotic — *continued*
lung — *continued*
with — *continued*
pneumosiderosis (occupational) 503
siderosis (occupational) 503
silicosis (occupational) 502
tuberculosis (*see also* Tuberculosis) 011.4 ✓5ᵗʰ
diffuse (idiopathic) (interstitial) 516.3
due to
bauxite 503
fumes or vapors (chemical) inhalation 506.4
graphite 503
following radiation 508.1
postinflammatory 515
silicotic (massive) (occupational) 502
tuberculous (*see also* Tuberculosis) 011.4 ✓5ᵗʰ
lymphatic gland 289.3
median bar 600.9
mediastinum (idiopathic) 519.3
meninges 349.2
muscle NEC 728.2
iatrogenic (from injection) 999.9
myocardium, myocardial (*see also* Myocarditis) 429.0
oral submucous 528.8
ovary 620.8
oviduct 620.8
pancreas 577.8
cystic 277.00
with ●
manifestations ●
gastrintestinal 277.03 ●
pulmonary 277.02 ●
specified NEC 277.09 ●
meconium ileus 277.01 ●
pulmonary exacerbation 277.02 ●
penis 607.89
periappendiceal 543.9
periarticular (*see also* Ankylosis) 718.5 ✓5ᵗʰ
pericardium 423.1
perineum, in pregnancy or childbirth 654.8 ✓5ᵗʰ
affecting fetus or newborn 763.89
causing obstructed labor 660.2 ✓5ᵗʰ
affecting fetus or newborn 763.1
perineural NEC 355.9
foot 355.6
periureteral 593.89
placenta — *see* Placenta, abnormal
pleura 511.0
popliteal fat pad 729.31
preretinal 362.56
prostate (chronic) 600.9
pulmonary (chronic) (*see also* Fibrosis, lung) 515
alveolar capillary block 516.3
interstitial
diffuse (idiopathic) 516.3
newborn 770.7
radiation — *see* Effect, adverse, radiation
rectal sphincter 569.49
retroperitoneal, idiopathic 593.4
scrotum 608.89
seminal vesicle 608.89
senile 797
skin NEC 709.2
spermatic cord 608.89
spleen 289.59
bilharzial (*see also* Schistosomiasis) 120.9
subepidermal nodular (M8832/0) — *see* Neoplasm, skin, benign
submucous NEC 709.2
oral 528.8
tongue 528.8
syncytium — *see* Placenta, abnormal
testis 608.89
chronic, due to syphilis 095.8
thymus (gland) 254.8
tunica vaginalis 608.89
ureter 593.89
urethra 599.84
uterus (nonneoplastic) 621.8
bilharzial (*see also* Schistosomiasis) 120.9
neoplastic (*see also* Leiomyoma, uterus) 218.9

Fibrosis, fibrotic — *continued*
  vagina 623.8
  valve, heart (*see also* Endocarditis) 424.90
  vas deferens 608.89
  vein 459.89
    lower extremities 459.89
  vesical 595.1
Fibrositis (periarticular) (rheumatoid) 729.0
  humeroscapular region 726.2
  nodular, chronic
    Jaccoud's 714.4
    rheumatoid 714.4
  ossificans 728.11
  scapulohumeral 726.2
Fibrothorax 511.0
Fibrotic — *see* Fibrosis
Fibrous — *see* condition
Fibroxanthoma (M8831/0) — *see also* Neoplasm,
    connective tissue, benign
  atypical (M8831/1) — *see* Neoplasm,
    connective tissue, uncertain behavior
  malignant (M8831/3) — *see* Neoplasm,
    connective tissue, malignant
Fibroxanthosarcoma (M8831/3) — *see* Neoplasm,
    connective tissue, malignant
Fiedler's
  disease (leptospiral jaundice) 100.0
  myocarditis or syndrome (acute isolated
    myocarditis) 422.91
Fiessinger-Leroy (-Reiter) syndrome 099.3
Fiessinger-Rendu syndrome (erythema
    muliforme exudativum) 695.1
Fifth disease (eruptive) 057.0
  venereal 099.1
Filaria, filarial — *see* Infestation, filarial
Filariasis (*see also* Infestation, filarial) 125.9
  bancroftian 125.0
  Brug's 125.1
  due to
    bancrofti 125.0
    Brugia (Wuchereria) (malayi) 125.1
    Loa loa 125.2
    malayi 125.1
    organism NEC 125.6
    Wuchereria (bancrofti) 125.0
      malayi 125.1
  Malayan 125.1
  ozzardi 125.1
  specified type NEC 125.6
Filatoff's, Filatov's, Filatow's disease (infectious
    mononucleosis) 075
File-cutters' disease 984.9
  specified type of lead — *see* Table of Drugs and
    Chemicals
Filling defect
  biliary tract 793.3
  bladder 793.5
  duodenum 793.4
  gallbladder 793.3
  gastrointestinal tract 793.4
  intestine 793.4
  kidney 793.5
  stomach 793.4
  ureter 793.5
Filtering bleb, eye (postglaucoma) (status)
    V45.69
  with complication or rupture 997.99
  postcataract extraction (complication) 997.99
Fimbrial cyst (congenital) 752.11
Fimbriated hymen 752.49
Financial problem affecting care V60.2
Findings, abnormal, without diagnosis
    (examination) (laboratory test) 796.4
  17-ketosteroids, elevated 791.9
  acetonuria 791.6
  acid phosphatase 790.5
  albumin-globulin ratio 790.99
  albuminuria 791.0
  alcohol in blood 790.3
  alkaline phosphatase 790.5
  amniotic fluid 792.3
  amylase 790.5
  anisocytosis 790.09
  antenatal screening 796.5

Findings, abnormal, without diagnosis —
    continued
  anthrax, positive 795.31   ●
  antibody titers, elevated 795.79
  anticardiolipin antibody 795.79
  antigen-antibody reaction 795.79
  antiphospholipid antibody 795.79
  bacteriuria 791.9
  ballistocardiogram 794.39
  bicarbonate 276.9
  bile in urine 791.4
  bilirubin 277.4
  bleeding time (prolonged) 790.92
  blood culture, positive 790.7
  blood gas level 790.91
  blood sugar level 790.2
    high 790.2
    low 251.2
  calcium 275.40
  carbonate 276.9
  casts, urine 791.7
  catecholamines 791.9
  cells, urine 791.7
  cerebrospinal fluid (color) (content) (pressure)
    792.0
  chloride 276.9
  cholesterol 272.9
  chromosome analysis 795.2
  chyluria 791.1
  circulation time 794.39
  cloudy dialysis effluent 792.5
  cloudy urine 791.9
  coagulation study 790.92
  cobalt, blood 790.6
  color of urine (unusual) NEC 791.9
  copper, blood 790.6
  crystals, urine 791.9
  culture, positive NEC 795.39   ▲
    blood 790.7
    HIV V08
    human immunodeficiency virus V08
    nose 795.39   ▲
    skin lesion NEC 795.39   ▲
    spinal fluid 792.0
    sputum 795.39   ▲
    stool 792.1
    throat 795.39   ▲
    urine 791.9
    viral
      human immunodeficiency V08
    wound 795.39   ▲
  echocardiogram 793.2
  echoencephalogram 794.01
  echogram NEC — *see* Findings, abnormal,
    structure
  electrocardiogram (ECG) (EKG) 794.31
  electroencephalogram (EEG) 794.02
  electrolyte level, urinary 791.9
  electromyogram (EMG) 794.17
    ocular 794.14
  electro-oculogram (EOG) 794.12
  electroretinogram (ERG) 794.11
  enzymes, serum NEC 790.5
  fibrinogen titer coagulation study 790.92
  filling defect — *see* Filling defect
  function study NEC 794.9
    auditory 794.15
    bladder 794.9
    brain 794.00
    cardiac 794.30
    endocrine NEC 794.6
      thyroid 794.5
    kidney 794.4
    liver 794.8
    nervous system
      central 794.00
      peripheral 794.19
    oculomotor 794.14
    pancreas 794.9
    placenta 794.9
    pulmonary 794.2
    retina 794.11
    special senses 794.19
    spleen 794.9
    vestibular 794.16
  gallbladder, nonvisualization 793.3
  glucose 790.2
    tolerance test 790.2

Findings, abnormal, without diagnosis —
    continued
  glycosuria 791.5
  heart
    shadow 793.2
    sounds 785.3
  hematinuria 791.2
  hematocrit
    drop (precipitous) 790.01
    elevated 282.7
    low 285.9
  hematologic NEC 790.99
  hematuria 599.7
  hemoglobin
    elevated 282.7
    low 285.9
  hemoglobinuria 791.2
  histological NEC 795.4
  hormones 259.9
  immunoglobulins, elevated 795.79
  indolacetic acid, elevated 791.9
  iron 790.6
  karyotype 795.2
  ketonuria 791.6
  lactic acid dehydrogenase (LDH) 790.4
  lipase 790.5
  lipids NEC 272.9
  lithium, blood 790.6
  lung field (coin lesion) (shadow) 793.1
  magnesium, blood 790.6
  mammogram 793.80
    microcalcification 793.81
  mediastinal shift 793.2
  melanin, urine 791.9
  microbiologic NEC 795.39   ▲
  mineral, blood NEC 790.6
  myoglobinuria 791.3
  nasal swab, anthrax 795.31   ●
  nitrogen derivatives, blood 790.6
  nonvisualization of gallbladder 793.3
  nose culture, positive 795.39   ▲
  odor of urine (unusual) NEC 791.9
  oxygen saturation 790.91
  Papanicolaou (smear) 795.1
    cervix 795.00   ▲
      atypical squamous cell changes of   ●
        undetermined significance   ●
        favor benign (ASCUS favor benign) ●
          795.01
        favor dysplasia (ASCUS favor ●
          dysplasia) 795.02
      dyskaryotic 795.09   ●
      nonspecific finding NEC 795.09   ●
    other site 795.1
  peritoneal fluid 792.9
  phonocardiogram 794.39
  phosphorus 275.3
  pleural fluid 792.9
  pneumoencephalogram 793.0
  PO$_2$-oxygen ratio 790.91
  poikilocytosis 790.09
  potassium
    deficiency 276.8
    excess 276.7
  PPD 795.5
  prostate specific antigen (PSA) 790.93
  protein, serum NEC 790.99
  proteinuria 791.0
  prothrombin time (partial) (prolonged) (PT)
    (PTT) 790.92
  pyuria 791.9
  radiologic (x-ray) 793.9
    abdomen 793.6
    biliary tract 793.3
    breast 793.89
      abnormal mammogram NOS 793.80
      mammographic microcalcification 793.81
    gastrointestinal tract 793.4
    genitourinary organs 793.5
    head 793.0
    intrathoracic organs NEC 793.2
    lung 793.1
    musculoskeletal 793.7
    placenta 793.9
    retroperitoneum 793.6
    skin 793.9
    skull 793.0

Fibrosis — Findings

✔4ᵗʰ Fourth-digit Required   ✔5ᵗʰ Fifth-digit Required   ►◄ Revised Text   ● New Line   ▲ Revised Code

Findings, abnormal, without diagnosis — *continued*
radiologic — *continued*
subcutaneous tissue 793.9
red blood cell 790.09
count 790.09
morphology 790.09
sickling 790.09
volume 790.09
saliva 792.4
scan NEC 794.9
bladder 794.9
bone 794.9
brain 794.09
kidney 794.4
liver 794.8
lung 794.2
pancreas 794.9
placental 794.9
spleen 794.9
thyroid 794.5
sedimentation rate, elevated 790.1
semen 792.2
serological (for)
human immunodeficiency virus (HIV)
inconclusive 795.71
positive V08
syphilis — *see* Findings, serology for syphilis
serology for syphilis
false positive 795.6
positive 097.1
false 795.6
follow-up of latent syphilis — *see* Syphilis, latent
only finding — *see* Syphilis, latent
serum 790.99
blood NEC 790.99
enzymes NEC 790.5
proteins 790.99
SGOT 790.4
SGPT 790.4
sickling of red blood cells 790.09
skin test, positive 795.79
tuberculin (without active tuberculosis) 795.5
sodium 790.6
deficiency 276.1
excess 276.0
spermatozoa 792.2
spinal fluid 792.0
culture, positive 792.0
sputum culture, positive 795.39 ▲
for acid-fast bacilli 795.39 ▲
stool NEC 792.1
bloody 578.1
occult 792.1
color 792.1
culture, positive 792.1
occult blood 792.1
structure, body (echogram) (thermogram) (ultrasound) (x-ray) NEC 793.9
abdomen 793.6
breast 793.89
abnormal mammogram 793.80
mammographic microcalcification 793.81
gastrointestinal tract 793.4
genitourinary organs 793.5
head 793.0
echogram (ultrasound) 794.01
intrathoracic organs NEC 793.2
lung 793.1
musculoskeletal 793.7
placenta 793.9
retroperitoneum 793.6
skin 793.9
subcutaneous tissue NEC 793.9
synovial fluid 792.9
thermogram — *see* Finding, abnormal, structure
throat culture, positive 795.39 ▲
thyroid (function) 794.5
metabolism (rate) 794.5
scan 794.5
uptake 794.5
total proteins 790.99
toxicology (drugs) (heavy metals) 796.0
transaminase (level) 790.4

Findings, abnormal, without diagnosis — *continued*
triglycerides 272.9
tuberculin skin test (without active tuberculosis) 795.5
ultrasound — *see also* Finding, abnormal, structure
cardiogram 793.2
uric acid, blood 790.6
urine, urinary constituents 791.9
acetone 791.6
albumin 791.0
bacteria 791.9
bile 791.4
blood 599.7
casts or cells 791.7
chyle 791.1
culture, positive 791.9
glucose 791.5
hemoglobin 791.2
ketone 791.6
protein 791.0
pus 791.9
sugar 791.5
vaginal fluid 792.9
vanillylmandelic acid, elevated 791.9
vectorcardiogram (VCG) 794.39
ventriculogram (cerebral) 793.0
VMA, elevated 791.9
Wassermann reaction
false positive 795.6
positive 097.1
follow-up of latent syphilis — *see* Syphilis, latent
only finding — *see* Syphilis, latent
white blood cell 288.9
count 288.9
elevated 288.8
low 288.0
differential 288.9
morphology 288.9
wound culture 795.39 ▲
xerography 793.89
zinc, blood 790.6

Finger — *see* condition
Fire, St. Anthony's (*see also* Erysipelas) 035
Fish
hook stomach 537.89
meal workers' lung 495.8

Fisher's syndrome 357.0
Fissure, fissured
abdominal wall (congenital) 756.79
anus, anal 565.0
congenital 751.5
buccal cavity 528.9
clitoris (congenital) 752.49
ear, lobule (congenital) 744.29
epiglottis (congenital) 748.3
larynx 478.79
congenital 748.3
lip 528.5
congenital (*see also* Cleft, lip) 749.10
nipple 611.2
puerperal, postpartum 676.1 ✓5ᵗʰ
palate (congenital) (*see also* Cleft, palate) 749.00
postanal 565.0
rectum 565.0
skin 709.8
streptococcal 686.9
spine (congenital) (*see also* Spina bifida) 741.9 ✓5ᵗʰ
sternum (congenital) 756.3
tongue (acquired) 529.5
congenital 750.13
Fistula (sinus) 686.9
abdomen (wall) 569.81
bladder 596.2
intestine 569.81
ureter 593.82
uterus 619.2
abdominorectal 569.81
abdominosigmoidal 569.81
abdominothoracic 510.0
abdominouterine 619.2
congenital 752.3

Fistula — *continued*
abdominovesical 596.2
accessory sinuses (*see also* Sinusitis) 473.9
actinomycotic — *see* Actinomycosis
alveolar
antrum (*see also* Sinusitis, maxillary) 473.0
process 522.7
anorectal 565.1
antrobuccal (*see also* Sinusitis, maxillary) 473.0
antrum (*see also* Sinusitis, maxillary) 473.0
anus, anal (infectional) (recurrent) 565.1
congenital 751.5
tuberculous (*see also* Tuberculosis) 014.8 ✓5ᵗʰ
aortic sinus 747.29
aortoduodenal 447.2
appendix, appendicular 543.9
arteriovenous (acquired) 447.0
brain 437.3
congenital 747.81
ruptured (*see also* Hemorrhage, subarachnoid) 430
ruptured (*see also* Hemorrhage, subarachnoid) 430
cerebral 437.3
congenital 747.81
congenital (peripheral) 747.60
brain — *see* Fistula, arteriovenous, brain, congenital
coronary 746.85
gastrointestinal 747.61
lower limb 747.64
pulmonary 747.3
renal 747.62
specified NEC 747.69
upper limb 747.63
coronary 414.19
congenital 746.85
heart 414.19
pulmonary (vessels) 417.0
congenital 747.3
surgically created (for dialysis) V45.1
complication NEC 996.73
atherosclerosis — *see* Arteriosclerosis, extremities
embolism 996.74
infection or inflammation 996.62
mechanical 996.1
occlusion NEC 996.74
thrombus 996.74
traumatic — *see* Injury, blood vessel, by site
artery 447.2
aural 383.81
congenital 744.49
auricle 383.81
congenital 744.49
Bartholin's gland 619.8
bile duct (*see also* Fistula, biliary) 576.4
biliary (duct) (tract) 576.4
congenital 751.69
bladder (neck) (sphincter) 596.2
into seminal vesicle 596.2
bone 733.99
brain 348.8
arteriovenous — *see* Fistula, arteriovenous, brain
branchial (cleft) 744.41
branchiogenous 744.41
breast 611.0
puerperal, postpartum 675.1 ✓5ᵗʰ
bronchial 510.0
bronchocutaneous, bronchomediastinal, bronchopleural, bronchopleuromediastinal (infective) 510.0
tuberculous (*see also* Tuberculosis) 011.3 ✓5ᵗʰ
bronchoesophageal 530.89
congenital 750.3
buccal cavity (infective) 528.3
canal, ear 380.89
carotid-cavernous
congenital 747.81
with hemorrhage 430

Fistula — *continued*
  carotid-cavernous — *continued*
    traumatic 900.82
      with hemorrhage (*see also* Hemorrhage,
        brain, traumatic) 853.0 ✓5ᵗʰ
      late effect 908.3
  cecosigmoidal 569.81
  cecum 569.81
  cerebrospinal (fluid) 349.81
  cervical, lateral (congenital) 744.41
  cervicoaural (congenital) 744.49
  cervicosigmoidal 619.1
  cervicovesical 619.0
  cervix 619.8
  chest (wall) 510.0
  cholecystocolic (*see also* Fistula, gallbladder)
    575.5
  cholecystocolonic (*see also* Fistula, gallbladder)
    575.5
  cholecystoduodenal (*see also* Fistula,
    gallbladder) 575.5
  cholecystoenteric (*see also* Fistula, gallbladder)
    575.5
  cholecystogastric (*see also* Fistula, gallbladder)
    575.5
  cholecystointestinal (*see also* Fistula,
    gallbladder) 575.5
  choledochoduodenal 576.4
  cholocolic (*see also* Fistula, gallbladder) 575.5
  coccyx 685.1
    with abscess 685.0
  colon 569.81
  colostomy 569.69
  colovaginal (acquired) 619.1
  common duct (bile duct) 576.4
  congenital, NEC — *see* Anomaly, specified type
    NEC
  cornea, causing hypotony 360.32
  coronary, arteriovenous 414.19
    congenital 746.85
  costal region 510.0
  cul-de-sac, Douglas' 619.8
  cutaneous 686.9
  cystic duct (*see also* Fistula, gallbladder) 575.5
    congenital 751.69
  dental 522.7
  diaphragm 510.0
    bronchovisceral 510.0
    pleuroperitoneal 510.0
    pulmonoperitoneal 510.0
  duodenum 537.4
  ear (canal) (external) 380.89
  enterocolic 569.81
  enterocutaneous 569.81
  enteroenteric 569.81
  entero-uterine 619.1
    congenital 752.3
  enterovaginal 619.1
    congenital 752.49
  enterovesical 596.1
  epididymis 608.89
    tuberculous (*see also* Tuberculosis)
      016.4 ✓5ᵗʰ
  esophagobronchial 530.89
    congenital 750.3
  esophagocutaneous 530.89
  esophagopleurocutaneous 530.89
  esophagotracheal 530.84
    congenital 750.3
  esophagus 530.89
    congenital 750.4
  ethmoid (*see also* Sinusitis, ethmoidal) 473.2
  eyeball (cornea) (sclera) 360.32
  eyelid 373.11
  fallopian tube (external) 619.2
  fecal 569.81
    congenital 751.5
  from periapical lesion 522.7
  frontal sinus (*see also* Sinusitis, frontal) 473.1
  gallbladder 575.5
    with calculus, cholelithiasis, stones (*see also*
      Cholelithiasis) 574.2 ✓5ᵗʰ
    congenital 751.69
  gastric 537.4
  gastrocolic 537.4
    congenital 750.7
    tuberculous (*see also* Tuberculosis)
      014.8 ✓5ᵗʰ

Fistula — *continued*
  gastroenterocolic 537.4
  gastroesophageal 537.4
  gastrojejunal 537.4
  gastrojejunocolic 537.4
  genital
    organs
      female 619.9
        specified site NEC 619.8
      male 608.89
    tract-skin (female) 619.2
  hepatopleural 510.0
  hepatopulmonary 510.0
  horseshoe 565.1
  ileorectal 569.81
  ileosigmoidal 569.81
  ileostomy 569.69
  ileovesical 596.1
  ileum 569.81
  in ano 565.1
    tuberculous (*see also* Tuberculosis)
      014.8 ✓5ᵗʰ
  inner ear (*see also* Fistula, labyrinth) 386.40
  intestine 569.81
  intestinocolonic (abdominal) 569.81
  intestinoureteral 593.82
  intestinouterine 619.1
  intestinovaginal 619.1
    congenital 752.49
  intestinovesical 596.1
  involving female genital tract 619.9
    digestive-genital 619.1
    genital tract-skin 619.2
    specified site NEC 619.8
    urinary-genital 619.0
  ischiorectal (fossa) 566
  jejunostomy 569.69
  jejunum 569.81
  joint 719.89
    ankle 719.87
    elbow 719.82
    foot 719.87
    hand 719.84
    hip 719.85
    knee 719.86
    multiple sites 719.89
    pelvic region 719.85
    shoulder (region) 719.81
    specified site NEC 719.88
    tuberculous — *see* Tuberculosis, joint
    wrist 719.83
  kidney 593.89
  labium (majus) (minus) 619.8
  labyrinth, labyrinthine NEC 386.40
    combined sites 386.48
    multiple sites 386.48
    oval window 386.42
    round window 386.41
    semicircular canal 386.43
  lacrimal, lachrymal (duct) (gland) (sac) 375.61
  lacrimonasal duct 375.61
  laryngotracheal 748.3
  larynx 478.79
  lip 528.5
    congenital 750.25
  lumbar, tuberculous (*see also* Tuberculosis)
    015.0 ✓5ᵗʰ [730.8] ✓5ᵗʰ
  lung 510.0
  lymphatic (node) (vessel) 457.8
  mamillary 611.0
  mammary (gland) 611.0
    puerperal, postpartum 675.1 ✓5ᵗʰ
  mastoid (process) (region) 383.1
  maxillary (*see also* Sinusitis, maxillary) 473.0
  mediastinal 510.0
  mediastinobronchial 510.0
  mediastinocutaneous 510.0
  middle ear 385.89
  mouth 528.3
  nasal 478.1
    sinus (*see also* Sinusitis) 473.9
  nasopharynx 478.29
  nipple — *see* Fistula, breast
  nose 478.1
  oral (cutaneous) 528.3
    maxillary (*see also* Sinusitis, maxillary)
      473.0

Fistula — *continued*
  oral — *continued*
    nasal (with cleft palate) (*see also* Cleft,
      palate) 749.00
  orbit, orbital 376.10
  oro-antral (*see also* Sinusitis, maxillary) 473.0
  oval window (internal ear) 386.42
  oviduct (external) 619.2
  palate (hard) 526.89
    soft 528.9
  pancreatic 577.8
  pancreaticoduodenal 577.8
  parotid (gland) 527.4
    region 528.3
  pelvoabdominointestinal 569.81
  penis 607.89
  perianal 565.1
  pericardium (pleura) (sac) (*see also* Pericarditis)
    423.8
  pericecal 569.81
  perineal — *see* Fistula, perineum
  perineorectal 569.81
  perineosigmoidal 569.81
  perineo-urethroscrotal 608.89
  perineum, perineal (with urethral involvement)
    NEC 599.1
    tuberculous (*see also* Tuberculosis)
      017.9 ✓5ᵗʰ
    ureter 593.82
  perirectal 565.1
    tuberculous (*see also* Tuberculosis)
      014.8 ✓5ᵗʰ
  peritoneum (*see also* Peritonitis) 567.2
  periurethral 599.1
  pharyngo-esophageal 478.29
  pharynx 478.29
    branchial cleft (congenital) 744.41
  pilonidal (infected) (rectum) 685.1
    with abscess 685.0
  pleura, pleural, pleurocutaneous,
    pleuroperitoneal 510.0
    stomach 510.0
    tuberculous (*see also* Tuberculosis)
      012.0 ✓5ᵗʰ
  pleuropericardial 423.8
  postauricular 383.81
  postoperative, persistent 998.6
  preauricular (congenital) 744.46
  prostate 602.8
  pulmonary 510.0
    arteriovenous 417.0
      congenital 747.3
    tuberculous (*see also* Tuberculosis,
      pulmonary) 011.9 ✓5ᵗʰ
  pulmonoperitoneal 510.0
  rectolabial 619.1
  rectosigmoid (intercommunicating) 569.81
  rectoureteral 593.82
  rectourethral 599.1
    congenital 753.8
  rectouterine 619.1
    congenital 752.3
  rectovaginal 619.1
    congenital 752.49
    old, postpartal 619.1
    tuberculous (*see also* Tuberculosis)
      014.8 ✓5ᵗʰ
  rectovesical 596.1
    congenital 753.8
  rectovesicovaginal 619.1
  rectovulvar 619.1
    congenital 752.49
  rectum (to skin) 565.1
    tuberculous (*see also* Tuberculosis)
      014.8 ✓5ᵗʰ
  renal 593.89
  retroauricular 383.81
  round window (internal ear) 386.41
  salivary duct or gland 527.4
    congenital 750.24
  sclera 360.32
  scrotum (urinary) 608.89
    tuberculous (*see also* Tuberculosis)
      016.5 ✓5ᵗʰ
  semicircular canals (internal ear) 386.43
  sigmoid 569.81
    vesicoabdominal 596.1

Fistula — *continued*
  sigmoidovaginal 619.1
    congenital 752.49
  skin 686.9
    ureter 593.82
    vagina 619.2
  sphenoidal sinus (*see also* Sinusitis,
      sphenoidal) 473.3
  splenocolic 289.59
  stercoral 569.81
  stomach 537.4
  sublingual gland 527.4
    congenital 750.24
  submaxillary
    gland 527.4
      congenital 750.24
    region 528.3
  thoracic 510.0
    duct 457.8
  thoracicoabdominal 510.0
  thoracicogastric 510.0
  thoracicointestinal 510.0
  thoracoabdominal 510.0
  thoracogastric 510.0
  thorax 510.0
  thyroglossal duct 759.2
  thyroid 246.8
  trachea (congenital) (external) (internal) 748.3
  tracheoesophageal 530.84
    congenital 750.3
    following tracheostomy 519.09
  traumatic
    arteriovenous (*see also* Injury, blood vessel,
        by site) 904.9
    brain — *see* Injury, intracranial
  tuberculous — *see* Tuberculosis, by site
  typhoid 002.0
  umbilical 759.89
  umbilico-urinary 753.8
  urachal, urachus 753.7
  ureter (persistent) 593.82
  ureteroabdominal 593.82
  ureterocervical 593.82
  ureterorectal 593.82
  ureterosigmoido-abdominal 593.82
  ureterovaginal 619.0
  ureterovesical 596.2
  urethra 599.1
    congenital 753.8
    tuberculous (*see also* Tuberculosis)
        016.3 ✓5ᵗʰ
  urethroperineal 599.1
  urethroperineovesical 596.2
  urethrorectal 599.1
    congenital 753.8
  urethroscrotal 608.89
  urethrovaginal 619.0
  urethrovesical 596.2
  urethrovesicovaginal 619.0
  urinary (persistent) (recurrent) 599.1
  uteroabdominal (anterior wall) 619.2
    congenital 752.3
  uteroenteric 619.1
  uterofecal 619.1
  uterointestinal 619.1
    congenital 752.3
  uterorectal 619.1
    congenital 752.3
  uteroureteric 619.0
  uterovaginal 619.8
  uterovesical 619.0
    congenital 752.3
  uterus 619.8
  vagina (wall) 619.8
    postpartal, old 619.8
  vaginocutaneous (postpartal) 619.2
  vaginoileal (acquired) 619.1
  vaginoperineal 619.2
  vesical NEC 596.2
  vesicoabdominal 596.2
  vesicocervicovaginal 619.0
  vesicocolic 596.1
  vesicocutaneous 596.2
  vesicoenteric 596.1
  vesicointestinal 596.1
  vesicometrorectal 619.1
  vesicoperineal 596.2

Fistula — *continued*
  vesicorectal 596.1
    congenital 753.8
  vesicosigmoidal 596.1
  vesicosigmoidovaginal 619.1
  vesicoureteral 596.2
  vesicoureterovaginal 619.0
  vesicourethral 596.2
  vesicourethrorectal 596.1
  vesicouterine 619.0
    congenital 752.3
  vesicovaginal 619.0
  vulvorectal 619.1
    congenital 752.49

Fit 780.39
  apoplectic (*see also* Disease, cerebrovascular,
      acute) 436
    late effect — *see* Late effect(s) (of)
        cerebrovascular disease
  epileptic (*see also* Epilepsy) 345.9 ✓5ᵗʰ
  fainting 780.2
  hysterical 300.11
  newborn 779.0

Fitting (of)
  artificial
    arm (complete) (partial) V52.0
    breast V52.4
    eye(s) V52.2
    leg(s) (complete) (partial) V52.1
  brain neuropacemaker V53.02
  cardiac pacemaker V53.31
  carotid sinus pacemaker V53.39
  cerebral ventricle (communicating) shunt
      V53.01
  colostomy belt V53.5
  contact lenses V53.1
  cystostomy device V53.6
  defibrillator, automatic implantable cardiac
      V53.32
  dentures V52.3
  device NEC V53.9
    abdominal V53.5
    cardiac
      defibrillator, automatic implantable
          V53.32
      pacemaker V53.31
      specified NEC V53.39
    cerebral ventricle (communicating) shunt
        V53.01
    intrauterine contraceptive V25.1
    nervous system V53.09
    orthodontic V53.4
    orthoptic V53.1
    prosthetic V52.9
      breast V52.4
      dental V52.3
      eye V52.2
      specified type NEC V52.8
    special senses V53.09
    substitution
      auditory V53.09
      nervous system V53.09
      visual V53.09
    urinary V53.6
  diaphragm (contraceptive) V25.02
  glasses (reading) V53.1
  hearing aid V53.2
  ileostomy device V53.5
  intestinal appliance or device NEC V53.5
  intrauterine contraceptive device V25.1
  neuropacemaker (brain) (peripheral nerve)
      (spinal cord) V53.02
  orthodontic device V53.4
  orthopedic (device) V53.7
    brace V53.7
    cast V53.7
    corset V53.7
    shoes V53.7
  pacemaker (cardiac) V53.31
    brain V53.02
    carotid sinus V53.39
    peripheral nerve V53.02
    spinal cord V53.02
  prosthesis V52.9
    arm (complete) (partial) V52.0
    breast V52.4
    dental V52.3

Fitting — *continued*
  prosthesis — *continued*
    eye V52.2
    leg (complete) (partial) V52.1
    specified type NEC V52.8
  spectacles V53.1
  wheelchair V53.8

Fitz's syndrome (acute hemorrhagic pancreatitis)
577.0

Fitz-Hugh and Curtis syndrome (gonococcal
peritonitis) 098.86

Fixation
  joint — *see* Ankylosis
  larynx 478.79
  pupil 364.76
  stapes 385.22
    deafness (*see also* Deafness, conductive)
        389.04
  uterus (acquired) — *see* Malposition, uterus
  vocal cord 478.5

Flaccid — *see also* condition
  foot 736.79
  forearm 736.09
  palate, congenital 750.26

Flail
  chest 807.4
    newborn 767.3
  joint (paralytic) 718.80
    ankle 718.87
    elbow 718.82
    foot 718.87
    hand 718.84
    hip 718.85
    knee 718.86
    multiple sites 718.89
    pelvic region 718.85
    shoulder (region) 718.81
    specified site NEC 718.88
    wrist 718.83

Flajani (-Basedow) syndrome or disease
(exophthalmic goiter) 242.0 ✓5ᵗʰ

Flap, liver 572.8

Flare, anterior chamber (aqueous) (eye) 364.04

Flashback phenomena (drug) (hallucinogenic)
292.89

Flat
  chamber (anterior) (eye) 360.34
  chest, congenital 754.89
  electroencephalogram (EEG) 348.8
  foot (acquired) (fixed type) (painful) (postural)
      (spastic) 734
    congenital 754.61
      rocker bottom 754.61
      vertical talus 754.61
    rachitic 268.1
    rocker bottom (congenital) 754.61
    vertical talus, congenital 754.61
  organ or site, congenital NEC — *see* Anomaly,
      specified type NEC
  pelvis 738.6
    with disproportion (fetopelvic) 653.2 ✓5ᵗʰ
      affecting fetus or newborn 763.1
      causing obstructed labor 660.1 ✓5ᵗʰ
        affecting fetus or newborn 763.1
    congenital 755.69

Flatau-Schilder disease 341.1

Flattening
  head, femur 736.39
  hip 736.39
  lip (congenital) 744.89
  nose (congenital) 754.0
    acquired 738.0

Flatulence 787.3

Flatus 787.3
  vaginalis 629.8

Flax dressers' disease 504

Flea bite — *see* Injury, superficial, by site

Fleischer (-Kayser) ring (corneal pigmentation)
275.1 [371.14]

Fleischner's disease 732.3

Fleshy mole 631

Flexibilitas cerea (*see also* Catalepsy) 300.11

Flexion
  cervix (*see also* Malposition, uterus) 621.6
  contracture, joint (*see also* Contraction, joint)
    718.4 ✔5ᵗʰ
  deformity, joint (*see also* Contraction, joint)
    718.4 ✔5ᵗʰ
    hip, congenital (*see also* Subluxation,
      congenital, hip) 754.32
  uterus (*see also* Malposition, uterus) 621.6
Flexner's
  bacillus 004.1
  diarrhea (ulcerative) 004.1
  dysentery 004.1
Flexner-Boyd dysentery 004.2
Flexure — *see* condition
Floater, vitreous 379.24
Floating
  cartilage (joint) (*see also* Disorder, cartilage,
    articular) 718.0 ✔5ᵗʰ
    knee 717.6
  gallbladder (congenital) 751.69
  kidney 593.0
    congenital 753.3
  liver (congenital) 751.69
  rib 756.3
  spleen 289.59
Flooding 626.2
Floor — *see* condition
Floppy
  infant NEC 781.99
  valve syndrome (mitral) 424.0
Flu — *see also* Influenza
  gastric NEC 008.8
Fluctuating blood pressure 796.4
Fluid
  abdomen 789.5
  chest (*see also* Pleurisy, with effusion) 511.9
  heart (*see also* Failure, heart) 428.0
  joint (*see also* Effusion, joint) 719.0 ✔5ᵗʰ
  loss (acute) 276.5
    with
      hypernatremia 276.0
      hyponatremia 276.1
  lung — *see also* Edema, lung encysted 511.8
  peritoneal cavity 789.5
  pleural cavity (*see also* Pleurisy, with effusion)
    511.9
  retention 276.6
Flukes NEC (*see also* Infestation, fluke) 121.9
  blood NEC (*see also* Infestation, Schistosoma)
    120.9
  liver 121.3
Fluor (albus) (vaginalis) 623.5
  trichomonal (Trichomonas vaginalis) 131.00
Fluorosis (dental) (chronic) 520.3
Flushing 782.62
  menopausal 627.2
Flush syndrome 259.2
Flutter
  atrial or auricular 427.32
  heart (ventricular) 427.42
    atrial 427.32
  impure 427.32
  postoperative 997.1
  ventricular 427.42
Flux (bloody) (serosanguineous) 009.0
Focal — *see* condition
Fochier's abscess — *see* Abscess, by site
Focus, Assmann's (*see also* Tuberculosis)
  011.0 ✔5ᵗʰ
Fogo selvagem 694.4
Foix-Alajouanine syndrome 336.1
Folds, anomalous — *see also* Anomaly, specified
    type NEC
  Bowman's membrane 371.31
  Descemet's membrane 371.32
  epicanthic 743.63
  heart 746.89
  posterior segment of eye, congenital 743.54
Folie à deux 297.3
Follicle
  cervix (nabothian) (ruptured) 616.0
  graafian, ruptured, with hemorrhage 620.0

Follicle — *continued*
  nabothian 616.0
Folliclis (primary) (*see also* Tuberculosis)
  017.0 ✔5ᵗʰ
Follicular — *see also* condition
  cyst (atretic) 620.0
Folliculitis 704.8
  abscedens et suffodiens 704.8
  decalvans 704.09
  gonorrheal (acute) 098.0
    chronic or duration of 2 months or more
      098.2
  keloid, keloidalis 706.1
  pustular 704.8
  ulerythematosa reticulata 701.8
Folliculosis, conjunctival 372.02
Følling's disease (phenylketonuria) 270.1
Follow-up (examination) (routine) (following)
    V67.9
  cancer chemotherapy V67.2
  chemotherapy V67.2
  fracture V67.4
  high-risk medication V67.51
  injury NEC V67.59
  postpartum
    immediately after delivery V24.0
    routine V24.2
  psychiatric V67.3
  psychotherapy V67.3
  radiotherapy V67.1
  specified condition NEC V67.59
  specified surgery NEC V67.09
  surgery V67.00
    vaginal pap smear V67.01
  treatment V67.9
    combined NEC V67.6
    fracture V67.4
    involving high-risk medication NEC V67.51
    mental disorder V67.3
    specified NEC V67.59
Fong's syndrome (hereditary
    osteoonychodysplasia) 756.89
Food
  allergy 693.1
  anaphylactic shock — *see* Anaphylactic shock,
    due to, food
  asphyxia (from aspiration or inhalation) (*see
    also* Asphyxia, food) 933.1
  choked on (*see also* Asphyxia, food) 933.1
  deprivation 994.2
    specified kind of food NEC 269.8
  intoxication (*see also* Poisoning, food) 005.9
  lack of 994.2
  poisoning (*see also* Poisoning, food) 005.9
  refusal or rejection NEC 307.59
  strangulation or suffocation (*see also* Asphyxia,
    food) 933.1
  toxemia (*see also* Poisoning, food) 005.9
Foot — *see also* condition
  and mouth disease 078.4
  process disease 581.3
Foramen ovale (nonclosure) (patent) (persistent)
    745.5
Forbes' (glycogen storage) disease 271.0
Forbes-Albright syndrome (nonpuerperal
    amenorrhea and lactation associated with
    pituitary tumor) 253.1
Forced birth or delivery NEC 669.8 ✔5ᵗʰ
  affecting fetus or newborn NEC 763.89
Forceps
  delivery NEC 669.6 ✔5ᵗʰ
    affecting fetus or newborn 763.2
Fordyce's disease (ectopic sebaceous glands)
    (mouth) 750.26
Fordyce-Fox disease (apocrine miliaria) 705.82
Forearm — *see* condition
Foreign body

> Note — For foreign body with open wound or
> other injury, see Wound, open, or the type of
> injury specified.

  accidentally left during a procedure 998.4

Foreign body — *continued*
  anterior chamber (eye) 871.6
    magnetic 871.5
      retained or old 360.51
    retained or old 360.61
  ciliary body (eye) 871.6
    magnetic 871.5
      retained or old 360.52
    retained or old 360.62
  entering through orifice (current) (old)
    accessory sinus 932
    air passage (upper) 933.0
      lower 934.8
    alimentary canal 938
    alveolar process 935.0
    antrum (Highmore) 932
    anus 937
    appendix 936
    asphyxia due to (*see also* Asphyxia, food)
      933.1
    auditory canal 931
    auricle 931
    bladder 939.0
    bronchioles 934.8
    bronchus (main) 934.1
    buccal cavity 935.0
    canthus (inner) 930.1
    cecum 936
    cervix (canal) uterine 939.1
    coil, ileocecal 936
    colon 936
    conjunctiva 930.1
    conjunctival sac 930.1
    cornea 930.0
    digestive organ or tract NEC 938
    duodenum 936
    ear (external) 931
    esophagus 935.1
    eye (external) 930.9
      combined sites 930.8
      intraocular — *see* Foreign body, by site
      specified site NEC 930.8
    eyeball 930.8
      intraocular — *see* Foreign body,
        intraocular
    eyelid 930.1
      retained or old 374.86
    frontal sinus 932
    gastrointestinal tract 938
    genitourinary tract 939.9
    globe 930.8
      penetrating 871.6
        magnetic 871.5
          retained or old 360.50
        retained or old 360.60
    gum 935.0
    Highmore's antrum 932
    hypopharynx 933.0
    ileocecal coil 936
    ileum 936
    inspiration (of) 933.1
    intestine (large) (small) 936
    lacrimal apparatus, duct, gland, or sac
      930.2
    larynx 933.1
    lung 934.8
    maxillary sinus 932
    mouth 935.0
    nasal sinus 932
    nasopharynx 933.0
    nose (passage) 932
    nostril 932
    oral cavity 935.0
    palate 935.0
    penis 939.3
    pharynx 933.0
    pyriform sinus 933.0
    rectosigmoid 937
      junction 937
    rectum 937
    respiratory tract 934.9
      specified part NEC 934.8
    sclera 930.1
    sinus 932
      accessory 932
      frontal 932
      maxillary 932

Foreign body — *continued*
  entering through orifice — *continued*
    sinus — *continued*
      nasal 932
      pyriform 933.0
    small intestine 936
    stomach (hairball) 935.2
    suffocation by (*see also* Asphyxia, food)
      933.1
    swallowed 938
      tongue 933.0
    tear ducts or glands 930.2
    throat 933.0
    tongue 935.0
      swallowed 933.0
    tonsil, tonsillar 933.0
      fossa 933.0
    trachea 934.0
    ureter 939.0
    urethra 939.0
    uterus (any part) 939.1
    vagina 939.2
    vulva 939.2
    wind pipe 934.0
  granuloma (old) 728.82
    bone 733.99
    in operative wound (inadvertently left) 998.4
      due to surgical material intentionally left
        — *see* Complications, due to
        (presence of) any device, implant, or
        graft classified to 996.0-996.5 NEC
    muscle 728.82
    skin 709.4
    soft tissue 709.4
    subcutaneous tissue 709.4
  in
    bone (residual) 733.99
    open wound — *see* Wound, open, by site
      complicated
    soft tissue (residual) 729.6
  inadvertently left in operation wound (causing
    adhesions, obstruction, or perforation)
    998.4
  ingestion, ingested NEC 938
  inhalation or inspiration (*see also* Asphyxia,
    food) 933.1
  internal organ, not entering through an orifice
    — *see* Injury, internal, by site, with open
    wound
  intraocular (nonmagnetic 871.6
    combined sites 871.6
      magnetic 871.5
        retained or old 360.59
      retained or old 360.69
    magnetic 871.5
      retained or old 360.50
    retained or old 360.60
    specified site NEC 871.6
      magnetic 871.5
        retained or old 360.59
      retained or old 360.69
    iris (nonmagnetic) 871.6
      magnetic 871.5
        retained or old 360.52
      retained or old 360.62
    lens (nonmagnetic) 871.6
      magnetic 871.5
        retained or old 360.53
      retained or old 360.63
  lid, eye 930.1
  ocular muscle 870.4
    retained or old 376.6
  old or residual
    bone 733.99
    eyelid 374.86
    middle ear 385.83
    muscle 729.6
      ocular 376.6
    retrobulbar 376.6
    skin 729.6
      with granuloma 709.4
    soft tissue 729.6
      with granuloma 709.4
    subcutaneous tissue 729.6
      with granuloma 709.4
  operation wound, left accidentally 998.4

Foreign body — *continued*
  orbit 870.4
    retained or old 376.6
  posterior wall, eye 871.6
    magnetic 871.5
      retained or old 360.55
    retained or old 360.65
  respiratory tree 934.9
    specified site NEC 934.8
  retained (old) (nonmagnetic) (in)
    anterior chamber (eye) 360.61
      magnetic 360.51
    ciliary body 360.62
      magnetic 360.52
    eyelid 374.86
    globe 360.60
      magnetic 360.50
    intraocular 360.60
      magnetic 360.50
      specified site NEC 360.69
        magnetic 360.59
    iris 360.62
      magnetic 360.52
    lens 360.63
      magnetic 360.53
    muscle 729.6
    orbit 376.6
    posterior wall of globe 360.65
      magnetic 360.55
    retina 360.65
      magnetic 360.55
      retrobulbar 376.6
      soft tissue 729.6
      vitreous 360.64
        magnetic 360.54
    skin 729.6
      with granuloma 709.4
    soft tissue 729.6
      with granuloma 709.4
    subcutaneous tissue 729.6
      with granuloma 709.4
  retina 871.6
    magnetic 871.5
      retained or old 360.55
    retained or old 360.65
  superficial, without major open wound (*see*
    also Injury, superficial, by site) 919.6
  swallowed NEC 938
  vitreous (humor) 871.6
    magnetic 871.5
      retained or old 360.54
    retained or old 360.64

Forking, aqueduct of Sylvius 742.3
  with spina bifida (*see also* Spina bifida)
    741.0 ✓5ᵗʰ

Formation
  bone in scar tissue (skin) 709.3
  connective tissue in vitreous 379.25
  Elschnig pearls (postcataract extraction) 366.51
  hyaline in cornea 371.49
  sequestrum in bone (due to infection) (*see also*
    Osteomyelitis) 730.1 ✓5ᵗʰ
  valve
    colon, congenital 751.5
    ureter (congenital) 753.29

Formication 782.0

Fort Bragg fever 100.89

Fossa — *see also* condition
  pyriform — *see* condition

Foster-Kennedy syndrome 377.04

Fothergill's
  disease, meaning scarlatina anginosa 034.1
  neuralgia (*see also* Neuralgia, trigeminal) 350.1

Foul breath 784.9

Found dead (cause unknown) 798.9

Foundling V20.0

Fournier's disease (idiopathic gangrene) 608.83

Fourth
  cranial nerve — *see* condition
  disease 057.8
  molar 520.1

Foville's syndrome 344.89

Fox's
  disease (apocrine miliaria) 705.82
  impetigo (contagiosa) 684

Fox-Fordyce disease (apocrine miliaria) 705.82

Fracture (abduction) (adduction) (avulsion)
  (compression) (crush) (dislocation) (oblique)
  (separation) (closed) 829.0

> *Note — For fracture of any of the following*
> *sites with fracture of other bones — see*
> *Fracture, multiple.*
> *"Closed" includes the following descriptions*
> *of fractures, with or without delayed healing,*
> *unless they are specified as open or*
> *compound:*
>
> | | |
> |---|---|
> | comminuted | linear |
> | depressed | simple |
> | elevated | slipped epiphysis |
> | fissured | spiral |
> | greenstick | unspecified |
> | impacted | |
>
> *"Open" includes the following descriptions of*
> *fractures, with or without delayed healing:*
>
> | | |
> |---|---|
> | compound | puncture |
> | infected | with foreign body |
> | missile | |
>
> *For late effect of fracture, see Late, effect,*
> *fracture, by site.*

  with
    internal injuries in same region (conditions
      classifiable to 860-869) — *see also*
      Injury, internal, by site pelvic region —
      see Fracture, pelvis
  acetabulum (with visceral injury) (closed) 808.0
    open 808.1
  acromion (process) (closed) 811.01
    open 811.11
  alveolus (closed) 802.8
    open 802.9
  ankle (malleolus) (closed) 824.8
    bimalleolar (Dupuytren's) (Pott's) 824.4
      open 824.5
    bone 825.21
      open 825.31
    lateral malleolus only (fibular) 824.2
      open 824.3
    medial malleolus only (tibial) 824.0
      open 824.1
      open 824.9
    pathologic 733.16
    talus 825.21
      open 825.31
    trimalleolar 824.6
      open 824.7
  antrum — *see* Fracture, skull, base
  arm (closed) 818.0
    and leg(s) (any bones) 828.0
      open 828.1
    both (any bones) (with rib(s)) (with sternum)
      819.0
      open 819.1
    lower 813.80
      open 813.90
    open 818.1
    upper — *see* Fracture, humerus
  astragalus (closed) 825.21
    open 825.31
  atlas — *see* Fracture, vertebra, cervical, first
  axis — *see* Fracture, vertebra, cervical, second
  back — *see* Fracture, vertebra, by site
  Barton's — *see* Fracture, radius, lower end
  basal (skull) — *see* Fracture, skull, base
  Bennett's (closed) 815.01
    open 815.11
  bimalleolar (closed) 824.4
    open 824.5
  bone (closed) NEC 829.0
    birth injury NEC 767.3
    open 829.1
    pathologic NEC (*see also* Fracture,
      pathologic) 733.10
    stress NEC (*see also* Fracture, stress)
      733.95
  boot top — *see* Fracture, fibula
  boxers' — *see* Fracture, metacarpal bone(s)
  breast bone — *see* Fracture, sternum

✓4ᵗʰ Fourth-digit Required   ✓5ᵗʰ Fifth-digit Required   ▶◀ Revised Text   ● New Line   ▲ Revised Code

Fracture — *continued*
  bucket handle (semilunar cartilage) — *see* Tear, meniscus
  bursting — *see* Fracture, phalanx, hand, distal
  calcaneus (closed) 825.0
    open 825.1
  capitate (bone) (closed) 814.07
    open 814.17
  capitellum (humerus) (closed) 812.49
    open 812.59
  carpal bone(s) (wrist NEC) (closed) 814.00
    open 814.10
    specified site NEC 814.09
      open 814.19
  cartilage, knee (semilunar) — *see* Tear, meniscus
  cervical — *see* Fracture, vertebra, cervical
  chauffeur's — *see* Fracture, ulna, lower end
  chisel — *see* Fracture, radius, upper end
  clavicle (interligamentous part) (closed) 810.00
    acromial end 810.03
      open 810.13
    due to birth trauma 767.2
    open 810.10
    shaft (middle third) 810.02
      open 810.12
    sternal end 810.01
      open 810.11
  clayshovelers' — *see* Fracture, vertebra, cervical
  coccyx — *see also* Fracture, vertebra, coccyx
    complicating delivery 665.6 ☑5ᵗʰ
  collar bone — *see* Fracture, clavicle
  Colles' (reversed) (closed) 813.41
    open 813.51
  comminuted — *see* Fracture, by site
  compression — *see also* Fracture, by site
    nontraumatic — *see* Fracture, pathologic
  congenital 756.9
  coracoid process (closed) 811.02
    open 811.12
  coronoid process (ulna) (closed) 813.02
    mandible (closed) 802.23
      open 802.33
    open 813.12
  costochondral junction — *see* Fracture, rib
  costosternal junction — *see* Fracture, rib
  cranium — *see* Fracture, skull, by site
  cricoid cartilage (closed) 807.5
    open 807.6
  cuboid (ankle) (closed) 825.23
    open 825.33
  cuneiform
    foot (closed) 825.24
      open 825.34
    wrist (closed) 814.03
      open 814.13
  due to
    birth injury — *see* Birth injury, fracture
    gunshot — *see* Fracture, by site, open
    neoplasm — *see* Fracture, pathologic
    osteoporosis — *see* Fracture, pathologic
  Dupuytren's (ankle) (fibula) (closed) 824.4
    open 824.5
    radius 813.42
      open 813.52
  Duverney's — *see* Fracture, ilium
  elbow — *see also* Fracture, humerus, lower end
    olecranon (process) (closed) 813.01
      open 813.11
    supracondylar (closed) 812.41
      open 812.51
  ethmoid (bone) (sinus) — *see* Fracture, skull, base
  face bone(s) (closed) NEC 802.8
    with
      other bone(s) — *see* Fracture, multiple, skull
      skull — *see also* Fracture, skull
        involving other bones — *see* Fracture, multiple, skull
    open 802.9
  fatigue — *see* Fracture, march
  femur, femoral (closed) 821.00
    cervicotrochanteric 820.03
      open 820.13
    condyles, epicondyles 821.21
      open 821.31

Fracture — *continued*
  femur, femoral — *continued*
    distal end — *see* Fracture, femur, lower end
    epiphysis (separation)
      capital 820.01
        open 820.11
      head 820.01
        open 820.11
      lower 821.22
        open 821.32
      trochanteric 820.01
        open 820.11
      upper 820.01
        open 820.11
    head 820.09
      open 820.19
    lower end or extremity (distal end) (closed) 821.20
      condyles, epicondyles 821.21
        open 821.31
      epiphysis (separation) 821.22
        open 821.32
      multiple sites 821.29
        open 821.39
      open 821.30
      specified site NEC 821.29
        open 821.39
      supracondylar 821.23
        open 821.33
      T-shaped 821.21
        open 821.31
    neck (closed) 820.8
      base (cervicotrochanteric) 820.03
        open 820.13
      extracapsular 820.20
        open 820.30
      intertrochanteric (section) 820.21
        open 820.31
      intracapsular 820.00
        open 820.10
      intratrochanteric 820.21
        open 820.31
      midcervical 820.02
        open 820.12
      open 820.9
      pathologic 733.14
        specified part NEC 733.15
      specified site NEC 820.09
        open 820.19
      transcervical 820.02
        open 820.12
      transtrochanteric 820.20
        open 820.30
    open 821.10
    pathologic 733.14
      specified part NEC 733.15
    peritrochanteric (section) 820.20
      open 820.30
    shaft (lower third) (middle third) (upper third) 821.01
      open 821.11
    subcapital 820.09
      open 820.19
    subtrochanteric (region) (section) 820.22
      open 820.32
    supracondylar 821.23
      open 821.33
    transepiphyseal 820.01
      open 820.11
    trochanter (greater) (lesser) (*see also* Fracture, femur, neck, by site) 820.20
      open 820.30
    T-shaped, into knee joint 821.21
      open 821.31
    upper end 820.8
      open 820.9
  fibula (closed) 823.81
    with tibia 823.82
      open 823.92
    distal end 824.8
      open 824.9
    epiphysis
      lower 824.8
        open 824.9
      upper — *see* Fracture, fibula, upper end

Fracture — *continued*
  fibula — *continued*
    head — *see* Fracture, fibula, upper end
    involving ankle 824.2
      open 824.3
    lower end or extremity 824.8
      open 824.9
    malleolus (external) (lateral) 824.2
      open 824.3
    open NEC 823.91
    pathologic 733.16
    proximal end — *see* Fracture, fibula, upper end
    shaft 823.21
      with tibia 823.22
        open 823.32
      open 823.31
    stress 733.93
    torus 823.41 ●
      with tibia 823.42 ●
    upper end or extremity (epiphysis) (head) (proximal end) (styloid) 823.01
      with tibia 823.02
        open 823.12
      open 823.11
  finger(s), of one hand (closed) (*see also* Fracture, phalanx, hand) 816.00
    with
      metacarpal bone(s), of same hand 817.0
        open 817.1
      thumb of same hand 816.03
        open 816.13
    open 816.10
  foot, except toe(s) alone (closed) 825.20
    open 825.30
  forearm (closed) NEC 813.80
    lower end (distal end) (lower epiphysis) 813.40
      open 813.50
    open 813.90
    shaft 813.20
      open 813.30
    upper end (proximal end) (upper epiphysis) 813.00
      open 813.10
  fossa, anterior, middle, or posterior — *see* Fracture, skull, base
  frontal (bone) — *see also* Fracture, skull, vault
    sinus — *see* Fracture, skull, base
  Galeazzi's — *see* Fracture, radius, lower end
  glenoid (cavity) (fossa) (scapula) (closed) 811.03
    open 811.13
  Gosselin's — *see* Fracture, ankle
  greenstick — *see* Fracture, by site
  grenade-throwers' — *see* Fracture, humerus, shaft
  gutter — *see* Fracture, skull, vault
  hamate (closed) 814.08
    open 814.18
  hand, one (closed) 815.00
    carpals 814.00
      open 814.10
      specified site NEC 814.09
        open 814.19
    metacarpals 815.00
      open 815.10
    multiple, bones of one hand 817.0
      open 817.1
    open 815.10
    phalanges (*see also* Fracture, phalanx, hand) 816.00
      open 816.10
  healing
    aftercare ▶(*see also* Aftercare, fracture)◀ V54.89 ▲
    change of cast V54.89 ▲
    complications — *see* condition
    convalescence V66.4 ●
    removal of
      cast V54.89 ▲
      fixation device
        external V54.89 ▲
        internal V54.0
  heel bone (closed) 825.0
    open 825.1
  hip (closed) (*see also* Fracture, femur, neck) 820.8

Fracture — *continued*
  hip (*see also* Fracture, femur, neck) — *continued*
    open 820.9
    pathologic 733.14
  humerus (closed) 812.20
    anatomical neck 812.02
      open 812.12
    articular process (*see also* Fracture humerus, condyle(s)) 812.44
      open 812.54
    capitellum 812.49
      open 812.59
    condyle(s) 812.44
      lateral (external) 812.42
        open 812.52
      medial (internal epicondyle) 812.43
        open 812.53
        open 812.54
    distal end — *see* Fracture, humerus, lower end
    epiphysis
      lower (*see also* Fracture, humerus, condyle(s)) 812.44
        open 812.54
      upper 812.09
        open 812.19
    external condyle 812.42
      open 812.52
    great tuberosity 812.03
      open 812.13
    head 812.09
      open 812.19
    internal epicondyle 812.43
      open 812.53
    lesser tuberosity 812.09
      open 812.19
    lower end or extremity (distal end) (*see also* Fracture, humerus, by site) 812.40
      multiple sites NEC 812.49
        open 812.59
      open 812.50
      specified site NEC 812.49
        open 812.59
    neck 812.01
      open 812.11
    open 812.30
    pathologic 733.11
    proximal end — *see* Fracture, humerus, upper end
    shaft 812.21
      open 812.31
    supracondylar 812.41
      open 812.51
    surgical neck 812.01
      open 812.11
    trochlea 812.49
      open 812.59
    T-shaped 812.44
      open 812.54
    tuberosity — *see* Fracture, humerus, upper end
    upper end or extremity (proximal end) (*see also* Fracture, humerus, by site) 812.00
      open 812.10
      specified site NEC 812.09
        open 812.19
  hyoid bone (closed) 807.5
    open 807.6
  hyperextension — *see* Fracture, radius, lower end
  ilium (with visceral injury) (closed) 808.41
    open 808.51
  impaction, impacted — *see* Fracture, by site
  incus — *see* Fracture, skull, base
  innominate bone (with visceral injury) (closed) 808.49
    open 808.59
  instep, of one foot (closed) 825.20
    with toe(s) of same foot 827.0
      open 827.1
    open 825.30
  internal
    ear — *see* Fracture, skull, base
    semilunar cartilage, knee — *see* Tear, meniscus, medial

Fracture — *continued*
  intertrochanteric — *see* Fracture, femur, neck, intertrochanteric
  ischium (with visceral injury) (closed) 808.42
    open 808.52
  jaw (bone) (lower) (closed) (*see also* Fracture, mandible) 802.20
    angle 802.25
      open 802.35
    open 802.30
    upper — *see* Fracture, maxilla
  knee
    cap (closed) 822.0
      open 822.1
    cartilage (semilunar) — *see* Tear, meniscus
  labyrinth (osseous) — *see* Fracture, skull, base
  larynx (closed) 807.5
    open 807.6
  late effect — *see* Late, effects (of), fracture
  Le Fort's — *see* Fracture, maxilla
  leg (closed) 827.0
    with rib(s) or sternum 828.0
      open 828.1
    both (any bones) 828.0
      open 828.1
    lower — *see* Fracture, tibia
    open 827.1
    upper — *see* Fracture, femur
  limb
    lower (multiple) (closed) NEC 827.0
      open 827.1
    upper (multiple) (closed) NEC 818.0
      open 818.1
  long bones, due to birth trauma — *see* Birth injury, fracture
  lumbar — *see* Fracture, vertebra, lumbar
  lunate bone (closed) 814.02
    open 814.12
  malar bone (closed) 802.4
    open 802.5
  Malgaigne's (closed) 808.43
    open 808.53
  malleolus (closed) 824.8
    bimalleolar 824.4
      open 824.5
    lateral 824.2
      and medial — *see also* Fracture, malleolus, bimalleolar
        with lip of tibia — *see* Fracture, malleolus, trimalleolar
      open 824.3
    medial (closed) 824.0
      and lateral — *see also* Fracture, malleolus, bimalleolar
        with lip of tibia — *see* Fracture, malleolus, trimalleolar
      open 824.1
    open 824.9
    trimalleolar (closed) 824.6
      open 824.7
  malleus — *see* Fracture, skull, base
  malunion 733.81
  mandible (closed) 802.20
    angle 802.25
      open 802.35
    body 802.28
      alveolar border 802.27
        open 802.37
      open 802.38
      symphysis 802.26
        open 802.36
    condylar process 802.21
      open 802.31
    coronoid process 802.23
      open 802.33
    multiple sites 802.29
      open 802.39
    open 802.30
    ramus NEC 802.24
      open 802.34
    subcondylar 802.22
      open 802.32
  manubrium — *see* Fracture, sternum
  march 733.95   ▲
    fibula 733.94   ●
    metatarsals 733.94   ●
    tibia 733.94   ●

Fracture — *continued*
  maxilla, maxillary (superior) (upper jaw) (closed) 802.4
    inferior — *see* Fracture, mandible
    open 802.5
  meniscus, knee — *see* Tear, meniscus
  metacarpus, metacarpal (bone(s)), of one hand (closed) 815.00
    with phalanx, phalanges, hand (finger(s)) (thumb) of same hand 817.0
      open 817.1
    base 815.02
      first metacarpal 815.01
        open 815.11
      open 815.12
      thumb 815.01
        open 815.11
    multiple sites 815.09
      open 815.19
    neck 815.04
      open 815.14
    open 815.10
    shaft 815.03
      open 815.13
  metatarsus, metatarsal (bone(s)), of one foot (closed) 825.25
    with tarsal bone(s) 825.29
      open 825.39
    open 825.35
  Monteggia's (closed) 813.03
    open 813.13
  Moore's — *see* Fracture, radius, lower end
    multangular bone (closed)
      larger 814.05
        open 814.15
      smaller 814.06
        open 814.16
    multiple (closed) 829.0

> Note — *Multiple fractures of sites classifiable to the same three- or four-digit category are coded to that category, except for sites classifiable to 810-818 or 820-827 in different limbs.*
> *Multiple fractures of sites classifiable to different fourth-digit subdivisions within the same three-digit category should be dealt with according to coding rules.*
> *Multiple fractures of sites classifiable to different three-digit categories (identifiable from the listing under "Fracture"), and of sites classifiable to 810-818 or 820-827 in different limbs should be coded according to the following list, which should be referred to in the following priority order: skull or face bones, pelvis or vertebral column, legs, arms.*

      arm (multiple bones in same arm except in hand alone) (sites classifiable to 810-817 with sites classifiable to a different three-digit category in 810-817 in same arm) (closed) 818.0
        open 818.1
      arms, both or arm(s) with rib(s) or sternum (sites classifiable to 810-818 with sites classifiable to same range of categories in other limb or to 807) (closed) 819.0
        open 819.1
      bones of trunk NEC (closed) 809.0
        open 809.1
      hand, metacarpal bone(s) with phalanx or phalanges of same hand (sites classifiable to 815 with sites classifiable to 816 in same hand) (closed) 817.0
        open 817.1
      leg (multiple bones in same leg) (sites classifiable to 820-826 with sites classifiable to a different three-digit category in that range in same leg) (closed) 827.0
        open 827.1
      legs, both or leg(s) with arm(s), rib(s), or sternum (sites classifiable to 820-827 with sites classifiable to same range of categories in other leg or to 807 or 810-819) (closed) 828.0
        open 828.1

Fracture — *continued*
 Moore's — *see* Fracture, radius, lower end
 multangular bone — *continued*
  open 829.1
 pelvis with other bones except skull or face
   bones (sites classifiable to 808 with
   sites classifiable to 805-807 or 810-
   829) (closed) 809.0
  open 809.1
 skull, specified or unspecified bones, or face
   bone(s) with any other bone(s) (sites
   classifiable to 800-803 with sites
   classifiable to 805-829) (closed)
   804.0 ✓5ᵗʰ

> Note — Use the following fifth-digit
> subclassification with categories 800, 801,
> 803, and 804:
>
> 0   unspecified state of consciousness
> 1   with no loss of consciousness
> 2   with brief [less than one hour] loss
>   of consciousness
> 3   with moderate [1-24 hours] loss of
>   consciousness
> 4   with prolonged [more than 24 hours]
>   loss of consciousness and return to
>   pre-existing conscious level
> 5   with prolonged [more than 24 hours]
>   loss of consciousness, without
>   return to pre-existing conscious level
> Use fifth-digit 5 to designate when a
>   patient is unconscious and dies
>   before regaining consciousness,
>   regardless of the duration of the
>   loss of consciousness
> 6   with loss of consciousness of
>   unspecified duration
> 9   with concussion, unspecified

  with
    contusion, cerebral 804.1 ✓5ᵗʰ
    epidural hemorrhage 804.2 ✓5ᵗʰ
    extradural hemorrhage 804.2 ✓5ᵗʰ
    hemorrhage (intracranial) NEC
      804.3 ✓5ᵗʰ
    intracranial injury NEC 804.4 ✓5ᵗʰ
    laceration, cerebral 804.1 ✓5ᵗʰ
    subarachnoid hemorrhage 804.2 ✓5ᵗʰ
    subdural hemorrhage 804.2 ✓5ᵗʰ
  open 804.5 ✓5ᵗʰ
    with
      contusion, cerebral 804.6 ✓5ᵗʰ
      epidural hemorrhage 804.7 ✓5ᵗʰ
      extradural hemorrhage 804.7 ✓5ᵗʰ
      hemorrhage (intracranial) NEC
        804.8 ✓5ᵗʰ
      intracranial injury NEC 804.9 ✓5ᵗʰ
      laceration, cerebral 804.6 ✓5ᵗʰ
      subarachnoid hemorrhage
        804.7 ✓5ᵗʰ
      subdural hemorrhage 804.7 ✓5ᵗʰ
 vertebral column with other bones, except
   skull or face bones (sites classifiable to
   805 or 806 with sites classifiable to
   807-808 or 810-829) (closed) 809.0
  open 809.1
 nasal (bone(s)) (closed) 802.0
  open 802.1
  sinus — *see* Fracture, skull, base
 navicular
  carpal (wrist) (closed) 814.01
   open 814.11
  tarsal (ankle) (closed) 825.22
   open 825.32
 neck — *see* Fracture, vertebra, cervical
 neural arch — *see* Fracture, vertebra, by site
 nonunion 733.82
 nose, nasal, (bone) (septum) (closed) 802.0
  open 802.1
 occiput — *see* Fracture, skull, base
 odontoid process — *see* Fracture, vertebra,
   cervical
 olecranon (process) (ulna) (closed) 813.01
  open 813.11
 open 829.1

Fracture — *continued*
 orbit, orbital (bone) (region) (closed) 802.8
  floor (blow-out) 802.6
   open 802.7
  open 802.9
  roof — *see* Fracture, skull, base
  specified part NEC 802.8
   open 802.9
 os
  calcis (closed) 825.0
   open 825.1
  magnum (closed) 814.07
   open 814.17
  pubis (with visceral injury) (closed) 808.2
   open 808.3
  triquetrum (closed) 814.03
   open 814.13
 osseous
  auditory meatus — *see* Fracture, skull, base
  labyrinth — *see* Fracture, skull, base
    ossicles, auditory (incus) (malleus)
    (stapes) — *see* Fracture, skull, base
 osteoporotic — *see* Fracture, pathologic
 palate (closed) 802.8
  open 802.9
 paratrooper — *see* Fracture, tibia, lower end
 parietal bone — *see* Fracture, skull, vault
 parry — *see* Fracture, Monteggia's
 patella (closed) 822.0
  open 822.1
 pathologic (cause unknown) 733.10
  ankle 733.16
  femur (neck) 733.14
   specified NEC 733.15
  fibula 733.16
  hip 733.14
  humerus 733.11
  radius 733.12
  specified site NEC 733.19
  tibia 733.16
  ulna 733.12
  vertebrae (collapse) 733.13
  wrist 733.12
 pedicle (of vertebral arch) — *see* Fracture,
   vertebra, by site
 pelvis, pelvic (bone(s)) (with visceral injury)
   (closed) 808.8
  multiple (with disruption of pelvic circle)
    808.43
   open 808.53
  open 808.9
  rim (closed) 808.49
   open 808.59
 peritrochanteric (closed) 820.20
  open 820.30
 phalanx, phalanges, of one
  foot (closed) 826.0
   with bone(s) of same lower limb 827.0
    open 827.1
   open 826.1
  hand (closed) 816.00
   with metacarpal bone(s) of same hand
     817.0
    open 817.1
   distal 816.02
    open 816.12
   middle 816.01
    open 816.11
   multiple sites NEC 816.03
    open 816.13
   open 816.10
   proximal 816.01
    open 816.11
 pisiform (closed) 814.04
  open 814.14
 pond — *see* Fracture, skull, vault
 Pott's (closed) 824.4
  open 824.5
 prosthetic device, internal — *see*
   Complications, mechanical
 pubis (with visceral injury) (closed) 808.2
  open 808.3
 Quervain's (closed) 814.01
  open 814.11
 radius (alone) (closed) 813.81
  with ulna NEC 813.83
   open 813.93

Fracture — *continued*
 radius — *continued*
  distal end — *see* Fracture, radius, lower end
  epiphysis
   lower — *see* Fracture, radius, lower end
   upper — *see* Fracture, radius, upper end
  head — *see* Fracture, radius, upper end
  lower end or extremity (distal end) (lower
    epiphysis) 813.42
   with ulna (lower end) 813.44
    open 813.54
   torus 813.45   ●
    open 813.52
  neck — *see* Fracture, radius, upper end
  open NEC 813.91
  pathologic 733.12
  proximal end — *see* Fracture, radius, upper
    end
  shaft (closed) 813.21
   with ulna (shaft) 813.23
    open 813.33
   open 813.31
  upper end 813.07
   with ulna (upper end) 813.08
    open 813.18
   epiphysis 813.05
    open 813.15
   head 813.05
    open 813.15
   multiple sites 813.07
    open 813.17
   neck 813.06
    open 813.16
   open 813.17
   specified site NEC 813.07
    open 813.17
 ramus
  inferior or superior (with visceral injury)
    (closed) 808.2
   open 808.3
  ischium — *see* Fracture, ischium
  mandible 802.24
   open 802.34
 rib(s) (closed) 807.0

> Note — Use the following fifth-digit
> subclassification with categories 807.0-
> 807.1:
>
> 0   rib(s), unspecified
> 1   one rib
> 2   two ribs
> 3   three ribs
> 4   four ribs
> 5   five ribs
> 6   six ribs
> 7   seven ribs
> 8   eight or more ribs
> 9   multiple ribs, unspecified

  with flail chest (open) 807.4
  open 807.1 ✓5ᵗʰ
 root, tooth 873.63
  complicated 873.73
 sacrum — *see* Fracture, vertebra, sacrum
 scaphoid
  ankle (closed) 825.22
   open 825.32
  wrist (closed) 814.01
   open 814.11
 scapula (closed) 811.00
  acromial, acromion (process) 811.01
   open 811.11
  body 811.09
   open 811.19
  coracoid process 811.02
   open 811.12
  glenoid (cavity) (fossa) 811.03
   open 811.13
  neck 811.03
   open 811.13
  open 811.10
 semilunar
  bone, wrist (closed) 814.02
   open 814.12

Fracture — *continued*
 semilunar — *continued*
  cartilage (interior) (knee) — *see* Tear,
    meniscus
 sesamoid bone — *see* Fracture, by site
 Shepherd's (closed) 825.21
  open 825.31
 shoulder — *see also* Fracture, humerus, upper
   end
  blade — *see* Fracture, scapula
 silverfork — *see* Fracture, radius, lower end
 sinus (ethmoid) (frontal) (maxillary) (nasal)
   (sphenoidal) — *see* Fracture, skull, base
 Skillern's — *see* Fracture, radius, shaft
 skull (multiple NEC) (with face bones) (closed)
   803.0 ✓5ᵗʰ

Note — *Use the following fifth digit
subclassification with categories 800, 801,
803, and 804:*

 0 *unspecified state of consciousness*
 1 *with no loss of consciousness*
 2 *with brief [less than one hour] loss
    of consciousness*
 3 *with moderate [1-24 hours] loss of
    consciousness*
 4 *with prolonged [more than 24 hours]
    loss of consciousness and return to
    pre-existing conscious level*
 5 *with prolonged [more than 24 hours]
    loss of consciousness, without
    return to pre-existing conscious level*

 *Use fifth-digit 5 to designate when a
 patient is unconscious and dies
 before regaining consciousness,
 regardles of the duration of loss of
 consciousness*

 6 *with loss of consciousness of
    unspecified duration*
 9 *with concussion, unspecified*

---

  with
   contusion, cerebral 803.1 ✓5ᵗʰ
   epidural hemorrhage 803.2 ✓5ᵗʰ
   extradural hemorrhage 803.2 ✓5ᵗʰ
   hemorrhage (intracranial) NEC 803.3 ✓5ᵗʰ
   intracranial injury NEC 803.4 ✓5ᵗʰ
   laceration, cerebral 803.1 ✓5ᵗʰ
   other bones — *see* Fracture, multiple,
     skull
   subarachnoid hemorrhage 803.2 ✓5ᵗʰ
   subdural hemorrhage 803.2 ✓5ᵗʰ
  base (antrum) (ethmoid bone) (fossa)
    (internal ear) (nasal sinus) (occiput)
    (sphenoid) (temporal bone) (closed)
    801.0 ✓5ᵗʰ
   with
    contusion, cerebral 801.1 ✓5ᵗʰ
    epidural hemorrhage 801.2 ✓5ᵗʰ
    extradural hemorrhage 801.2 ✓5ᵗʰ
    hemorrhage (intracranial) NEC
      801.3 ✓5ᵗʰ
    intracranial injury NEC 801.4 ✓5ᵗʰ
    laceration, cerebral 801.1 ✓5ᵗʰ
    subarachnoid hemorrhage 801.2 ✓5ᵗʰ
    subdural hemorrhage 801.2 ✓5ᵗʰ
   open 801.5 ✓5ᵗʰ
    with
     contusion, cerebral 801.6 ✓5ᵗʰ
     epidural hemorrhage 801.7 ✓5ᵗʰ
     extradural hemorrhage 801.7 ✓5ᵗʰ
     hemorrhage (intracranial) NEC
       801.8 ✓5ᵗʰ
     intracranial injury NEC 801.9 ✓5ᵗʰ
     laceration, cerebral 801.6 ✓5ᵗʰ
     subarachnoid hemorrhage
       801.7 ✓5ᵗʰ
     subdural hemorrhage 801.7 ✓5ᵗʰ
  birth injury 767.3
  face bones — *see* Fracture, face bones
  open 803.5 ✓5ᵗʰ
   with
    contusion, cerebral 803.6 ✓5ᵗʰ
    epidural hemorrhage 803.7 ✓5ᵗʰ
    extradural hemorrhage 803.7 ✓5ᵗʰ

Fracture — *continued*
 skull — *continued*
  open — *continued*
   with — *continued*
    hemorrhage (intracranial) NEC
      803.8 ✓5ᵗʰ
    intracranial injury NEC 803.9 ✓5ᵗʰ
    laceration, cerebral 803.6 ✓5ᵗʰ
    subarachnoid hemorrhage 803.7 ✓5ᵗʰ
    subdural hemorrhage 803.7 ✓5ᵗʰ
  vault (frontal bone) (parietal bone) (vertex)
    (closed) 800.0 ✓5ᵗʰ
   with
    contusion, cerebral 800.1 ✓5ᵗʰ
    epidural hemorrhage 800.2 ✓5ᵗʰ
    extradural hemorrhage 800.2 ✓5ᵗʰ
    hemorrhage (intracranial) NEC
      800.3 ✓5ᵗʰ
    intracranial injury NEC 800.4 ✓5ᵗʰ
    laceration, cerebral 800.1 ✓5ᵗʰ
    subarachnoid hemorrhage 800.2 ✓5ᵗʰ
    subdural hemorrhage 800.2 ✓5ᵗʰ
   open 800.5 ✓5ᵗʰ
    with
     contusion, cerebral 800.6 ✓5ᵗʰ
     epidural hemorrhage 800.7 ✓5ᵗʰ
     extradural hemorrhage 800.7 ✓5ᵗʰ
     hemorrhage (intracranial) NEC
       800.8 ✓5ᵗʰ
     intracranial injury NEC 800.9 ✓5ᵗʰ
     laceration, cerebral 800.6 ✓5ᵗʰ
     subarachnoid hemorrhage
       800.7 ✓5ᵗʰ
     subdural hemorrhage 800.7 ✓5ᵗʰ
 Smith's 813.41
  open 813.51
 sphenoid (bone) (sinus) — *see* Fracture, skull,
   base
 spine — *see also* Fracture, vertebra, by site due
   to birth trauma 767.4
 spinous process — *see* Fracture, vertebra, by
   site
 spontaneous — *see* Fracture, pathologic
 sprinters' — *see* Fracture, ilium
 stapes — *see* Fracture, skull, base
 stave — *see also* Fracture, metacarpus,
   metacarpal bone(s)
  spine — *see* Fracture, tibia, upper end
 sternum (closed) 807.2
  with flail chest (open) 807.4
  open 807.3
 Stieda's — *see* Fracture, femur, lower end
 stress 733.95
  fibula 733.93
  metatarsals 733.94
  specified site NEC 733.95
  tibia 733.93
 styloid process
  metacarpal (closed) 815.02
   open 815.12
  radius — *see* Fracture, radius, lower end
  temporal bone — *see* Fracture, skull, base
  ulna — *see* Fracture, ulna, lower end
 supracondylar, elbow 812.41
  open 812.51
 symphysis pubis (with visceral injury) (closed)
   808.2
  open 808.3
 talus (ankle bone) (closed) 825.21
  open 825.31
 tarsus, tarsal bone(s) (with metatarsus) of one
   foot (closed) NEC 825.29
  open 825.39
 temporal bone (styloid) — *see* Fracture, skull,
   base
 tendon — *see* Sprain, by site
 thigh — *see* Fracture, femur, shaft
 thumb (and finger(s)) of one hand (closed) (*see
   also* Fracture, phalanx, hand) 816.00
  with metacarpal bone(s) of same hand 817.0
  open 817.1
  metacarpal(s) — *see* Fracture, metacarpus
  open 816.10
 thyroid cartilage (closed) 807.5
  open 807.6

Fracture — *continued*
 tibia (closed) 823.80
  with fibula 823.82
   open 823.92
  condyles — *see* Fracture, tibia, upper end
  distal end 824.8
   open 824.9
  epiphysis
   lower 824.8
    open 824.9
   upper — *see* Fracture, tibia, upper end
  head (involving knee joint) — *see* Fracture,
    tibia, upper end
  intercondyloid eminence — *see* Fracture,
    tibia, upper end
  involving ankle 824.0
   open 824.0
  malleolus (internal) (medial) 824.0
   open 824.1
  open NEC 823.90
  pathologic 733.16
  proximal end — *see* Fracture, tibia, upper
    end
  shaft 823.20
   with fibula 823.22
    open 823.32
   open 823.30
  spine — *see* Fracture, tibia, upper end
  stress 733.93
  torus 823.40   ●
   with tibia 823.42
  tuberosity — *see* Fracture, tibia, upper end
  upper end or extremity (condyle) (epiphysis)
    (head) (spine) (proximal end)
    (tuberosity) 823.00
   with fibula 823.02
    open 823.12
   open 823.10
 toe(s), of one foot (closed) 826.0
  with bone(s) of same lower limb 827.0
   open 827.1
  open 826.1
 tooth (root) 873.63
  complicated 873.73   ●
 torus   ●
  fibula 823.41   ●
   with tibia 823.42   ●
  radius 813.45   ●
  tibia 823.40   ●
   with fibula 823.42   ●
 trachea (closed) 807.5
  open 807.6
 transverse process — *see* Fracture, vertebra, by
   site
 trapezium (closed) 814.05
  open 814.15
 trapezoid bone (closed) 814.06
  open 814.16
 trimalleolar (closed) 824.6
  open 824.7
 triquetral (bone) (closed) 814.03
  open 814.13
 trochanter (greater) (lesser) (closed) (*see also*
   Fracture, femur, neck, by site) 820.20
  open 820.30
 trunk (bones) (closed) 809.0
  open 809.1
 tuberosity (external) — *see* Fracture, by site
 ulna (alone) (closed) 813.82
  with radius NEC 813.83
   open 813.93
  coronoid process (closed) 813.02
   open 813.12
  distal end — *see* Fracture, ulna, lower end
  epiphysis
   lower — *see* Fracture, ulna, lower end
   upper — *see* Fracture, ulna, upper end
  head — *see* Fracture, ulna, lower end
  lower end (distal end) (head) (lower
    epiphysis) (styloid process) 813.43
   with radius (lower end) 813.44
    open 813.54
   open 813.53
  olecranon process (closed) 813.01
   open 813.11
  open NEC 813.92

Fracture — *continued*
  ulna — *continued*
    pathologic 733.12
    proximal end — *see* Fracture, ulna, upper
      end
    shaft 813.22
      with radius (shaft) 813.23
        open 813.33
      open 813.32
    styloid process — *see* Fracture, ulna, lower
      end
    transverse — *see* Fracture, ulna, by site
    upper end (epiphysis) 813.04
      with radius (upper end) 813.08
        open 813.18
      multiple sites 813.04
        open 813.14
      open 813.14
      specified site NEC 813.04
        open 813.14
  unciform (closed) 814.08
    open 814.18
  vertebra, vertebral (back) (body) (column)
    (neural arch) (pedicle) (spine) (spinous
    process) (transverse process) (closed)
    805.8
    with
      hematomyelia — *see* Fracture, vertebra,
        by site, with spinal cord injury
      injury to
        cauda equina — *see* Fracture,
          vertebra, sacrum, with spinal
          cord injury
        nerve — *see* Fracture, vertebra, by
          site, with spinal cord injury
      paralysis — *see* Fracture, vertebra, by
        site, with spinal cord injury
      paraplegia — *see* Fracture, vertebra, by
        site, with spinal cord injury
      quadriplegia — *see* Fracture, vertebra, by
        site, with spinal cord injury
      spinal concussion — *see* Fracture,
        vertebra, by site, with spinal cord
        injury
      spinal cord injury (closed) NEC 806.8

> *Note — Use the following fifth-digit
> subclassification with categories 806.0-
> 806.3:*
>
> C_1-C_4 *or unspecified level and* D_1-D_6 (T_1-T_6)
> *or unspecified level with*
>
> 0   *unspecified spinal cord injury*
> 1   *complete lesion of cord*
> 2   *anterior cord syndrome*
> 3   *central cord syndrome*
> 4   *specified injury NEC*
>
> C_5-C_7 *level and* D_7-D_{12} *level with:*
>
> 5   *unspecified spinal cord injury*
> 6   *complete lesion of cord*
> 7   *anterior cord syndrome*
> 8   *central cord syndrome*
> 9   *specified injury NEC*

    cervical 806.0 ✓5ᵗʰ
      open 806.1 ✓5ᵗʰ
    dorsal, dorsolumbar 806.2 ✓5ᵗʰ
      open 806.3 ✓5ᵗʰ
      open 806.9
    thoracic, thoracolumbar 806.2 ✓5ᵗʰ
      open 806.3 ✓5ᵗʰ
  atlanto-axial — *see* Fracture, vertebra,
    cervical
  cervical (hangman) (teardrop) (closed) 805.00
    with spinal cord injury — *see* Fracture,
      vertebra, with spinal cord injury,
      cervical
    first (atlas) 805.01
      open 805.11
    second (axis) 805.02
      open 805.12
    third 805.03
      open 805.13
    fourth 805.04
      open 805.14

Fracture — *continued*
  vertebra, vertebral — *continued*
    cervical — *continued*
      fifth 805.05
        open 805.15
      sixth 805.06
        open 805.16
      seventh 805.07
        open 805.17
      multiple sites 805.08
        open 805.18
      open 805.10
  coccyx (closed) 805.6
    with spinal cord injury (closed) 806.60
      cauda equina injury 806.62
        complete lesion 806.61
          open 806.71
        open 806.72
      open 806.70
      specified type NEC 806.69
        open 806.79
    open 805.7
  collapsed 733.13
  compression, not due to trauma 733.13
  dorsal (closed) 805.2
    with spinal cord injury — *see* Fracture,
      vertebra, with spinal cord injury,
      dorsal
    open 805.3
  dorsolumbar (closed) 805.2
    with spinal cord injury — *see* Fracture,
      vertebra, with spinal cord injury,
      dorsal
    open 805.3
  due to osteoporosis 733.13
  fetus or newborn 767.4
  lumbar (closed) 805.4
    with spinal cord injury (closed) 806.4
      open 806.5
    open 805.5
  nontraumatic 733.13
  open NEC 805.9
  pathologic (any site) 733.13
  sacrum (closed) 805.6
    with spinal cord injury 806.60
      cauda equina injury 806.62
        complete lesion 806.61
          open 806.71
        open 806.72
      open 806.70
      specified type NEC 806.69
        open 806.79
    open 805.7
  site unspecified (closed) 805.8
    with spinal cord injury (closed) 806.8
      open 806.9
    open 805.9
  stress (any site) 733.95
  thoracic (closed) 805.2
    with spinal cord injury — *see* Fracture,
      vertebra, with spinal cord injury,
      thoracic
    open 805.3
  vertex — *see* Fracture, skull, vault
  vomer (bone) 802.0
    open 802.1
  Wagstaffe's — *see* Fracture, ankle
  wrist (closed) 814.00
    open 814.10
    pathologic 733.12
  xiphoid (process) — *see* Fracture, sternum
  zygoma (zygomatic arch) (closed) 802.4
    open 802.5
Fragile X syndrome 759.83
Fragilitas
  crinium 704.2
  hair 704.2
  ossium 756.51
    with blue sclera 756.51
  unguium 703.8
    congenital 757.5
Fragility
  bone 756.51
    with deafness and blue sclera 756.51
  capillary (hereditary) 287.8

Fragility — *continued*
  hair 704.2
  nails 703.8
Fragmentation — *see* Fracture, by site
Frambesia, frambesial (tropica) (*see also* Yaws)
  102.9
  initial lesion or ulcer 102.0
  primary 102.0
Frambeside
  gummatous 102.4
  of early yaws 102.2
Frambesioma 102.1
Franceschetti's syndrome (mandibulofacial
  dysotosis) 756.0
Francis' disease (*see also* Tularemia) 021.9
Frank's essential thrombocytopenia (*see also*
  Purpura, thrombocytopenic) 287.3
Franklin's disease (heavy chain) 273.2
Fraser's syndrome 759.89
Freckle 709.09
  malignant melanoma in (M8742/3) — *see*
    Melanoma
  melanotic (of Hutchinson) (M8742/2) — *see*
    Neoplasm, skin, in situ
Freeman-Sheldon syndrome 759.89
Freezing 991.9
  specified effect NEC 991.8
Frei's disease (climatic bubo) 099.1
Freiberg's
  disease (osteochondrosis, second metatarsal)
    732.5
  infraction of metatarsal head 732.5
  osteochondrosis 732.5
Fremitus, friction, cardiac 785.3
Frenulum linguae 750.0
Frenum
  external os 752.49
  tongue 750.0
Frequency (urinary) NEC 788.41
  micturition 788.41
  nocturnal 788.43
  psychogenic 306.53
Frey's syndrome (auriculotemporal syndrome)
  350.8
Friction
  burn (*see also* Injury, superficial, by site) 919.0
  fremitus, cardiac 785.3
  precordial 785.3
  sounds, chest 786.7
Friderichsen-Waterhouse syndrome or disease
  036.3
Friedländer's
  B (bacillus) NEC (*see also* condition) 041.3
    sepsis or septicemia 038.49
  disease (endarteritis obliterans) — *see*
    Arteriosclerosis
Friedreich's
  ataxia 334.0
  combined systemic disease 334.0
  disease 333.2
    combined systemic 334.0
  myoclonia 333.2
  sclerosis (spinal cord) 334.0
Friedrich-Erb-Arnold syndrome
  (acropachyderma) 757.39
Frigidity 302.72
  psychic or psychogenic 302.72
Fröhlich's disease or syndrome (adiposogenital
  dystrophy) 253.8
Froin's syndrome 336.8
Frommel's disease 676.6 ✓5ᵗʰ
Frommel-Chiari syndrome 676.6 ✓5ᵗʰ
Frontal — *see also* condition
  lobe syndrome 310.0
Frostbite 991.3
  face 991.0
  foot 991.2
  hand 991.1
  specified site NEC 991.3
Frotteurism 302.89

✓4ᵗʰ Fourth-digit Required   ✓5ᵗʰ Fifth-digit Required   ▶◀ Revised Text   ● New Line   ▲ Revised Code

Frozen 991.9
  pelvis 620.8
  shoulder 726.0
Fructosemia 271.2
Fructosuria (benign) (essential) 271.2
Fuchs'
  black spot (myopic) 360.21
  corneal dystrophy (endothelial) 371.57
  heterochromic cyclitis 364.21
Fucosidosis 271.8
Fugue 780.99   ▲
  hysterical (dissociative) 300.13
  reaction to exceptional stress (transient) 308.1
Fuller Albright's syndrome (osteitis fibrosa
    disseminata) 756.59
Fuller's earth disease 502
Fulminant, fulminating — *see* condition
Functional — see condition
Fundus — *see also* condition
  flavimaculatus 362.76
Fungemia 117.9
Fungus, fungous
  cerebral 348.8
  disease NEC 117.9
  infection — *see* Infection, fungus
  testis (*see also* Tuberculosis) 016.5 ✓5ᵗʰ *[608.81]*
Funiculitis (acute) 608.4
  chronic 608.4
  endemic 608.4
  gonococcal (acute) 098.14
    chronic or duration of 2 months or over
      098.34
  tuberculous (*see also* Tuberculosis) 016.5 ✓5ᵗʰ
Funnel
  breast (acquired) 738.3
    congenital 754.81
    late effect of rickets 268.1
  chest (acquired) 738.3
    congenital 754.81
    late effect of rickets 268.1
  pelvis (acquired) 738.6
    with disproportion (fetopelvic) 653.3 ✓5ᵗʰ
      affecting fetus or newborn 763.1
      causing obstructed labor 660.1 ✓5ᵗʰ
        affecting fetus or newborn 763.1
    congenital 755.69
    tuberculous (*see also* Tuberculosis)
      016.9 ✓5ᵗʰ
F.U.O. (*see also* Pyrexia) 780.6
Furfur 690.18
  microsporon 111.0
Furor, paroxysmal (idiopathic) (*see also* Epilepsy)
  345.8 ✓5ᵗʰ
Furriers' lung 495.8
Furrowed tongue 529.5
  congenital 750.13
Furrowing nail(s) (transverse) 703.8
  congenital 757.5
Furuncle 680.9
  abdominal wall 680.2
  ankle 680.6
  anus 680.5
  arm (any part, above wrist) 680.3
  auditory canal, external 680.0
  axilla 680.3
  back (any part) 680.2
  breast 680.2
  buttock 680.5
  chest wall 680.2
  corpus cavernosum 607.2
  ear (any part) 680.0
  eyelid 373.13
  face (any part, except eye) 680.0
  finger (any) 680.4
  flank 680.2
  foot (any part) 680.7
  forearm 680.3
  gluteal (region) 680.5
  groin 680.2
  hand (any part) 680.4
  head (any part, except face) 680.8
  heel 680.7

Furuncle — *continued*
  hip 680.6
  kidney (*see also* Abscess, kidney) 590.2
  knee 680.6
  labium (majus) (minus) 616.4
  lacrimal
    gland (*see also* Dacryoadenitis) 375.00
    passages (duct) (sac) (*see also*
      Dacryocystitis) 375.30
  leg, any part except foot 680.6
  malignant 022.0
  multiple sites 680.9
  neck 680.1
  nose (external) (septum) 680.0
  orbit 376.01
  partes posteriores 680.5
  pectoral region 680.2
  penis 607.2
  perineum 680.2
  pinna 680.0
  scalp (any part) 680.8
  scrotum 608.4
  seminal vesicle 608.0
  shoulder 680.3
  skin NEC 680.9
  specified site NEC 680.8
  spermatic cord 608.4
  temple (region) 680.0
  testis 604.90
  thigh 680.6
  thumb 680.4
  toe (any) 680.7
  trunk 680.2
  tunica vaginalis 608.4
  umbilicus 680.2
  upper arm 680.3
  vas deferens 608.4
  vulva 616.4
  wrist 680.4
Furunculosis (*see also* Furuncle) 680.9
  external auditory meatus 680.0 *[380.13]*
Fusarium (infection) 118
Fusion, fused (congenital)
  anal (with urogenital canal) 751.5
  aorta and pulmonary artery 745.0
  astragaloscaphoid 755.67
  atria 745.5
  atrium and ventricle 745.69
  auditory canal 744.02
  auricles, heart 745.5
  binocular, with defective stereopsis 368.33
  bone 756.9
  cervical spine — *see* Fusion, spine
  choanal 748.0
  commissure, mitral valve 746.5
  cranial sutures, premature 756.0
  cusps, heart valve NEC 746.89
    mitral 746.5
    tricuspid 746.89
  ear ossicles 744.04
  fingers (*see also* Syndactylism, fingers) 755.11
  hymen 752.42
  hymeno-urethral 599.89
    causing obstructed labor 660.1 ✓5ᵗʰ
      affecting fetus or newborn 763.1
  joint (acquired) — *see also* Ankylosis
    congenital 755.8
  kidneys (incomplete) 753.3
  labium (majus) (minus) 752.49
  larynx and trachea 748.3
  limb 755.8
    lower 755.69
    upper 755.59
  lobe, lung 748.5
  lumbosacral (acquired) 724.6
    congenital 756.15
    surgical V45.4
  nares (anterior) (posterior) 748.0
  nose, nasal 748.0
  nostril(s) 748.0
  organ or site NEC — *see* Anomaly, specified
    type NEC
  ossicles 756.9
    auditory 744.04
  pulmonary valve segment 746.02

Fusion, fused — *continued*
  pulmonic cusps 746.02
  ribs 756.3
  sacroiliac (acquired) (joint) 724.6
    congenital 755.69
    surgical V45.4
  skull, imperfect 756.0
  spine (acquired) 724.9
    arthrodesis status V45.4
    congenital (vertebra) 756.15
    postoperative status V45.4
  sublingual duct with submaxillary duct at
    opening in mouth 750.26
  talonavicular (bar) 755.67
  teeth, tooth 520.2
  testes 752.8
  toes (*see also* Syndactylism, toes) 755.13
  trachea and esophagus 750.3
  twins 759.4
  urethral-hymenal 599.89
  vagina 752.49
  valve cusps — *see* Fusion, cusps, heart valve
  ventricles, heart 745.4
  vertebra (arch) — *see* Fusion, spine
  vulva 752.49
Fusospirillosis (mouth) (tongue) (tonsil) 101
Fussy infant (baby) 780.91   ●

G

Gafsa boil 085.1
Gain, weight (abnormal) (excessive) (*see also*
  Weight, gain) 783.1
Gaisböck's disease or syndrome
  (polycythemia hypertonica) 289.0
Gait
  abnormality 781.2
    hysterical 300.11
  ataxic 781.2
    hysterical 300.11
  disturbance 781.2
    hysterical 300.11
  paralytic 781.2
  scissor 781.2
  spastic 781.2
  staggering 781.2
    hysterical 300.11
Galactocele (breast) (infected) 611.5
  puerperal, postpartum 676.8 ✓5ᵗʰ
Galactophoritis 611.0
  puerperal, postpartum 675.2 ✓5ᵗʰ
Galactorrhea 676.6 ✓5ᵗʰ
  not associated with childbirth 611.6
Galactosemia (classic) (congenital) 271.1
Galactosuria 271.1
Galacturia 791.1
  bilharziasis 120.0
Galen's vein — *see* condition
Gallbladder — *see also* condition
  acute (*see also* Disease, gallbladder) 575.0
Gall duct — *see* condition
Gallop rhythm 427.89
Gallstone (cholemic) (colic) (impacted) — *see also*
  Cholelithiasis
  causing intestinal obstruction 560.31
Gambling, pathological 312.31
Gammaloidosis 277.3
Gammopathy 273.9
  macroglobulinemia 273.3
  monoclonal (benign) (essential) (idiopathic)
    (with lymphoplasmacytic dyscrasia) 273.1
Gamna's disease (siderotic splenomegaly) 289.51
Gampsodactylia (congenital) 754.71
Gamstorp's disease (adynamia episodica
  hereditaria) 359.3
Gandy-Nanta disease (siderotic splenomegaly)
  289.51
**Gang activity, without manifest psychiatric
  disorder** V71.09
  adolescent V71.02
  adult V71.01
  child V71.02
Gangliocytoma (M9490/0) — *see* Neoplasm,
  connective tissue, benign
Ganglioglioma (M9505/1) — *see* Neoplasm, by
  site, uncertain behavior
Ganglion 727.43
  joint 727.41
  of yaws (early) (late) 102.6
  periosteal (*see also* Periostitis) 730.3 ✓5ᵗʰ
  tendon sheath (compound) (diffuse) 727.42
  tuberculous (*see also* Tuberculosis) 015.9 ✓5ᵗʰ
Ganglioneuroblastoma (M9490/3) — *see*
  Neoplasm, connective tissue, malignant
Ganglioneuroma (M9490/0) — *see also*
  Neoplasm, connective tissue, benign
  malignant (M9490/3) — *see* Neoplasm,
    connective tissue, malignant
Ganglioneuromatosis (M9491/0) — *see*
  Neoplasm, connective tissue, benign
Ganglionitis
  fifth nerve (*see also* Neuralgia, trigeminal)
    350.1
  gasserian 350.1
  geniculate 351.1
    herpetic 053.11
    newborn 767.5
  herpes zoster 053.11
  herpetic geniculate (Hunt's syndrome) 053.11
Gangliosidosis 330.1

Gangosa 102.5
Gangrene, gangrenous (anemia) (artery) (cellulitis)
  (dermatitis) (dry) (infective) (moist)
  (pemphigus) (septic) (skin) (stasis) (ulcer)
  785.4
  with
    arteriosclerosis (native artery) 440.24
      bypass graft 440.30
        autologous vein 440.31
        nonautologous biological 440.32
    diabetes (mellitus) 250.7 ✓5ᵗʰ [785.4]
  abdomen (wall) 785.4
    arteriosclerosis 440.29 [785.4]
  adenitis 683
  alveolar 526.5
  angina 462
    diphtheritic 032.0
  anus 569.49
  appendices epiploicae — *see* Gangrene,
    mesentery
  appendix — *see* Appendicitis, acute
  arteriosclerotic — *see* Arteriosclerosis, with,
    gangrene
  auricle 785.4
  Bacillus welchii (*see also* Gangrene, gas) 040.0
  bile duct (*see also* Cholangitis) 576.8
  bladder 595.89
  bowel — *see* Gangrene, intestine
  cecum — *see* Gangrene, intestine
  Clostridium perfringens or welchii (*see also*
    Gangrene, gas) 040.0
  colon — *see* Gangrene, intestine
  connective tissue 785.4
  cornea 371.40
  corpora cavernosa (infective) 607.2
    noninfective 607.89
  cutaneous, spreading 785.4
  decubital 707.0 [785.4]
  diabetic (any site) 250.7 ✓5ᵗʰ [785.4]
  dropsical 785.4
  emphysematous (*see also* Gangrene, gas) 040.0
  epidemic (ergotized grain) 988.2
  epididymis (infectional) (*see also* Epididymitis)
    604.99
  erysipelas (*see also* Erysipelas) 035
  extremity (lower) (upper) 785.4
  gallbladder or duct (*see also* Cholecystitis,
    acute) 575.0
  gas (bacillus) 040.0
    with
      abortion — *see* Abortion, by type, with
        sepsis
      ectopic pregnancy (*see also* categories
        633.0-633.9) 639.0
      molar pregnancy (*see also* categories 630-
        632) 639.0
    following
      abortion 639.0
      ectopic or molar pregnancy 639.0
    puerperal, postpartum, childbirth 670 ✓4ᵗʰ
  glossitis 529.0
  gum 523.8
  hernia — *see* Hernia, by site, with gangrene
  hospital noma 528.1
  intestine, intestinal (acute) (hemorrhagic)
    (massive) 557.0
    with
      hernia — *see* Hernia, by site, with
        gangrene
      mesenteric embolism or infarction 557.0
      obstruction (*see also* Obstruction,
        intestine) 560.9
  laryngitis 464.00
    with obstruction 464.01
  liver 573.8
  lung 513.0
    spirochetal 104.8
  lymphangitis 457.2
  Meleney's (cutaneous) 686.09
  mesentery 557.0
    with
      embolism or infarction 557.0
      intestinal obstruction (*see also*
        Obstruction, intestine) 560.9
  mouth 528.1
  noma 528.1
  orchitis 604.90

Gangrene, gangrenous — *continued*
  ovary (*see also* Salpingo-oophoritis) 614.2
  pancreas 577.0
  penis (infectional) 607.2
    noninfective 607.89
  perineum 785.4
  pharynx 462
  septic 034.0
  pneumonia 513.0
  Pott's 440.24
  presenile 443.1
  pulmonary 513.0
  pulp, tooth 522.1
  quinsy 475
  Raynaud's (symmetric gangrene) 443.0 [785.4]
  rectum 569.49
  retropharyngeal 478.24
  rupture — *see* Hernia, by site, with gangrene
  scrotum 608.4
    noninfective 608.83
  senile 440.24
  sore throat 462
  spermatic cord 608.4
    noninfective 608.89
  spine 785.4
  spirochetal NEC 104.8
  spreading cutaneous 785.4
  stomach 537.89
  stomatitis 528.1
  symmetrical 443.0 [785.4]
  testis (infectional) (*see also* Orchitis) 604.99
    noninfective 608.89
  throat 462
    diphtheritic 032.0
  thyroid (gland) 246.8
  tonsillitis (acute) 463
  tooth (pulp) 522.1
  tuberculous NEC (*see also* Tuberculosis)
    011.9 ✓5ᵗʰ
  tunica vaginalis 608.4
    noninfective 608.89
  umbilicus 785.4
  uterus (*see also* Endometritis) 615.9
  uvulitis 528.3
  vas deferens 608.4
    noninfective 608.89
  vulva (*see also* Vulvitis) 616.10
Gannister disease (occupational) 502
  with tuberculosis — *see* Tuberculosis,
    pulmonary
Ganser's syndrome, hysterical 300.16
Gardner-Diamond syndrome (autoerythrocyte
  sensitization) 287.2
Gargoylism 277.5
Garré's
  disease (*see also* Osteomyelitis) 730.1 ✓5ᵗʰ
  osteitis (sclerosing) (*see also* Osteomyelitis)
    730.1 ✓5ᵗʰ
  osteomyelitis (*see also* Osteomyelitis) 730.1 ✓5ᵗʰ
Garrod's pads, knuckle 728.79
Gartner's duct
  cyst 752.11
  persistent 752.11
Gas
  asphyxia, asphyxiation, inhalation, poisoning,
    suffocation NEC 987.9
    specified gas — *see* Table of Drugs and
      Chemicals
  bacillus gangrene or infection — *see* Gas,
    gangrene
  cyst, mesentery 568.89
  excessive 787.3
  gangrene 040.0
    with
      abortion — *see* Abortion, by type, with
        sepsis
      ectopic pregnancy (*see also* categories
        633.0-633.9) 639.0
      molar pregnancy (*see also* categories 630-
        632) 639.0
    following
      abortion 639.0
      ectopic or molar pregnancy 639.0
    puerperal, postpartum, childbirth 670 ✓4ᵗʰ
  on stomach 787.3
  pains 787.3

✓4ᵗʰ Fourth-digit Required   ✓5ᵗʰ Fifth-digit Required   ►◄ Revised Text   ● New Line   ▲ Revised Code

Gastradenitis 535.0 E
Gastralgia 536.8
  psychogenic 307.89
Gastrectasis, gastrectasia 536.1
  psychogenic 306.4
Gastric — *see* condition
Gastrinoma (M8153/1)
  malignant (M8153/3)
    pancreas 157.4
    specified site NEC — *see* Neoplasm, by site,
      malignant
    unspecified site 157.4
  specified site — *see* Neoplasm, by site,
    uncertain behavior
  unspecified site 235.5
Gastritis 535.5 ✓5ᵗʰ

> *Note* — *Use the following fifth-digit
> subclassification for category 535:*
>
>   0   *without mention of hemorrhage*
>   1   *with hemorrhage*

  acute 535.0 ✓5ᵗʰ
  alcoholic 535.3 ✓5ᵗʰ
  allergic 535.4 ✓5ᵗʰ
  antral 535.4 ✓5ᵗʰ
  atrophic 535.1 ✓5ᵗʰ
  atrophic-hyperplastic 535.1 ✓5ᵗʰ
  bile-induced 535.4 ✓5ᵗʰ
  catarrhal 535.0 ✓5ᵗʰ
  chronic (atrophic) 535.1 ✓5ᵗʰ
  cirrhotic 535.4 ✓5ᵗʰ
  corrosive (acute) 535.4 ✓5ᵗʰ
  dietetic 535.4 ✓5ᵗʰ
  due to diet deficiency 269.9 [535.4]
  eosinophilic 535.4 ✓5ᵗʰ
  erosive 535.4 ✓5ᵗʰ
  follicular 535.4 ✓5ᵗʰ
    chronic 535.1 ✓5ᵗʰ
  giant hypertrophic 535.2 ✓5ᵗʰ
  glandular 535.4 ✓5ᵗʰ
    chronic 535.1 ✓5ᵗʰ
  hypertrophic (mucosa) 535.2 ✓5ᵗʰ
    chronic giant 211.1
  irritant 535.4 ✓5ᵗʰ
  nervous 306.4
  phlegmonous 535.0 ✓5ᵗʰ
  psychogenic 306.4
  sclerotic 535.4 ✓5ᵗʰ
  spastic 536.8
  subacute 535.0 ✓5ᵗʰ
  superficial 535.4 ✓5ᵗʰ
  suppurative 535.0 ✓5ᵗʰ
  toxic 535.4 ✓5ᵗʰ
  tuberculous (*see also* Tuberculosis) 017.9 ✓5ᵗʰ
Gastrocarcinoma (M8010/3) 151.9
Gastrocolic — *see* condition
Gastrocolitis — *see* Enteritis
Gastrodisciasis 121.8
Gastroduodenitis (*see also* Gastritis) 535.5 ✓5ᵗʰ
  catarrhal 535.0 ✓5ᵗʰ
  infectional 535.0 ✓5ᵗʰ
  virus, viral 008.8
    specified type NEC 008.69
Gastrodynia 536.8
Gastroenteritis (acute) (catarrhal) (congestive)
  (hemorrhagic) (noninfectious) (*see also*
  Enteritis) 558.9
  aertrycke infection 003.0
  allergic 558.3
  chronic 558.9
    ulcerative (*see also* Colitis, ulcerative) 556.9
  dietetic 558.9
  due to
    food poisoning (*see also* Poisoning, food)
      005.9
    radiation 558.1
  epidemic 009.0
  functional 558.9
  infectious (*see also* Enteritis, due to, by
    organism) 009.0
    presumed 009.1
  salmonella 003.0
  septic (*see also* Enteritis, due to, by organism)
    009.0

Gastroenteritis — *continued*
  toxic 558.2
  tuberculous (*see also* Tuberculosis) 014.8 ✓5ᵗʰ
  ulcerative (*see also* Colitis, ulcerative) 556.9
  viral NEC 008.8
    specified type NEC 008.69
  zymotic 009.0
Gastroenterocolitis — *see* Enteritis
Gastroenteropathy, protein-losing 579.8
Gastroenteroptosis 569.89
**Gastroesophageal laceration-hemorrhage
syndrome** 530.7
Gastroesophagitis 530.19
Gastrohepatitis (*see also* Gastritis) 535.5 ✓5ᵗʰ
Gastrointestinal — *see* condition
Gastrojejunal — *see* condition
Gastrojejunitis (*see also* Gastritis) 535.5 ✓5ᵗʰ
Gastrojejunocolic — *see* condition
Gastroliths 537.89
Gastromalacia 537.89
Gastroparalysis 536.8
  diabetic 250.6 ✓5ᵗʰ [536.3]
Gastroparesis 536.3
  diabetic 250.6 ✓5ᵗʰ [536.3]
Gastropathy, exudative 579.8
Gastroptosis 537.5
Gastrorrhagia 578.0
Gastorrhea 536.8
  psychogenic 306.4
Gastroschisis (congenital) 756.79
  acquired 569.89
Gastrospasm (neurogenic) (reflex) 536.8
  neurotic 306.4
  psychogenic 306.4
Gastrostaxis 578.0
Gastrostenosis 537.89
Gastrostomy
  attention to V55.1
  complication 536.40
    specified type 536.49
  infection 536.41
  malfunctioning 536.42
  status V44.1
Gastrosuccorrhea (continous) (intermittent) 536.8
  neurotic 306.4
  psychogenic 306.4
Gaucher's
  disease (adult) (cerebroside lipidosis) (infantile)
    272.7
  hepatomegaly 272.7
  splenomegaly (cerebroside lipidosis) 272.7
Gayet's disease (superior hemorrhagic
  polioencephalitis) 265.1
Gayet-Wernicke's syndrome (superior
  hemorrhagic polioencephalitis) 265.1
**Gee (-Herter) (-Heubner) (-Thaysen) disease or
syndrome** (nontropical sprue) 579.0
Gélineau's syndrome 347
Gemination, teeth 520.2
Gemistocytoma (M9411/3)
  specified site — *see* Neoplasm, by site,
    malignant
  unspecified site 191.9
General, generalized — *see* condtion
Genital — *see* condition
Genito-anorectal syndrome 099.1
Genitourinary system — *see* condition
Genu
  congenital 755.64
  extrorsum (acquired) 736.42
    congenital 755.64
    late effects of rickets 268.1
  introrsum (acquired) 736.41
    congenital 755.64
    late effects of rickets 268.1
  rachitic (old) 268.1
  recurvatum (acquired) 736.5
    congenital 754.40
      with dislocation of knee 754.41
    late effects or rickets 268.1

Genu — *continued*
  valgum (acquired) (knock-knee) 736.41
    congenital 755.64
    late effects of rickets 268.1
  varum (acquired) (bowleg) 736.42
    congenital 755.64
    late effect of rickets 268.1
Geographic tongue 529.1
Geophagia 307.52
Geotrichosis 117.9
  intestine 117.9
  lung 117.9
  mouth 117.9
Gephyrophobia 300.29
Gerbode defect 745.4
Gerhardt's
  disease (erythromelalgia) 443.89
  syndrome (vocal cord paralysis) 478.30
Gerlier's disease (epidemic vertigo) 078.81
German measles 056.9
  exposure to V01.4
Germinoblastoma (diffuse) (M9614/3) 202.8 ✓5ᵗʰ
  follicular (M9692/3) 202.0 ✓5ᵗʰ
Germinoma (M9064/3) — *see* Neoplasm, by site,
  malignant
Gerontoxon 371.41
Gerstmann's syndrome (finger agnosia) 784.69
Gestation (period) — *see also* Pregnancy
  ectopic NEC (*see also* Pregnancy, ectopic)
    633.90 ▲
      with intrauterine pregnancy 633.91 ●
Gestational proteinuria 646.2 ✓5ᵗʰ
  with hypertension — *see* Toxemia, of pregnancy
Ghon tubercle primary infection (*see also*
  Tuberculosis) 010.0 ✓5ᵗʰ
Ghost
  teeth 520.4
  vessels, cornea 370.64
Ghoul hand 102.3
Giant
  cell
    epulis 523.8
    peripheral (gingiva) 523.8
    tumor, tendon sheath 727.02
  colon (congenital) 751.3
  esophagus (congenital) 750.4
  kidney 753.3
  urticaria 995.1
    hereditary 277.6
Giardia lamblia infestation 007.1
Giardiasis 007.1
Gibert's disease (pityriasis rosea) 696.3
Gibraltar fever — *see* Brucellosis
Giddiness 780.4
  hysterical 300.11
  psychogenic 306.9
Gierke's disease (glycogenosis I) 271.0
Gigantism (cerebral) (hypophyseal) (pituitary)
  253.0
Gilbert's disease or cholemia (familial
  nonhemolytic jaundice) 277.4
Gilchrist's disease (North American
  blastomycosis) 116.0
Gilford (-Hutchinson) disease or syndrome
  (progeria) 259.8
Gilles de la Tourette's disease (motor-verbal tic)
  307.23
Gillespie's syndrome (dysplasia
  oculodentodigitalis) 759.89
Gingivitis 523.1
  acute 523.0
    necrotizing 101
  catarrhal 523.0
  chronic 523.1
  desquamative 523.1
  expulsiva 523.4
  hyperplastic 523.1
  marginal, simple 523.1
  necrotizing, acute 101
  pellagrous 265.2
  ulcerative 523.1
    acute necrotizing 101

Gastradenitis — Gingivitis

Gingivitis — *continued*
Vincent's 101
Gingivoglossitis 529.0
Gingivopericementitis 523.4
Gingivosis 523.1
Gingivostomatitis 523.1
herpetic 054.2
Giovannini's disease 117.9
Gland, glandular — *see* condition
Glanders 024
Glanzmann (-Naegeli) disease or thrombasthenia 287.1
Glassblowers' disease 527.1
Glaucoma (capsular) (inflammatory) (noninflammatory) (primary) 365.9
with increased episcleral venous pressure 365.82
absolute 360.42
acute 365.22
narrow angle 365.22
secondary 365.60
angle closure 365.20
acute 365.22
chronic 365.23
intermittent 365.21
interval 365.21
residual stage 365.24
subacute 365.21
borderline 365.00
chronic 365.11
noncongestive 365.11
open angle 365.11
simple 365.11
closed angle — *see* Glaucoma, angle closure
congenital 743.20
associated with other eye anomalies 743.22
simple 743.21
congestive — *see* Glaucoma, narrow angle
corticosteroid-induced (glaucomatous stage) 365.31
residual stage 365.32
hemorrhagic 365.60
hypersecretion 365.81
in or with
aniridia 743.45 *[365.42]*
Axenfeld's anomaly 743.44 *[365.41]*
concussion of globe 921.3 *[365.65]*
congenital syndromes NEC 759.89 *[365.44]*
dislocation of lens
anterior 379.33 *[365.59]*
posterior 379.34 *[365.59]*
disorder of lens NEC 365.59
epithelial down-growth 364.61 *[365.64]*
glaucomatocyclitic crisis 364.22 *[365.62]*
hypermature cataract 366.18 *[365.51]*
hyphema 364.41 *[365.63]*
inflammation, ocular 365.62
iridocyclitis 364.3 *[365.62]*
iris
anomalies NEC 743.46 *[365.42]*
atrophy, essential 364.51 *[365.42]*
bombé 364.74 *[365.61]*
rubeosis 364.42 *[365.63]*
microcornea 743.41 *[365.43]*
neurofibromatosis 237.71 *[365.44]*
ocular
cysts NEC 365.64
disorders NEC 365.60
trauma 365.65
tumors NEC 365.64
postdislocation of lens
anterior 379.33 *[365.59]*
posterior 379.34 *[365.59]*
pseudoexfoliation of capsule 366.11 *[365.52]*
pupillary block or seclusion 364.74 *[365.61]*
recession of chamber angle 364.77 *[365.65]*
retinal vein occlusion 362.35 *[365.63]*
Rieger's anomaly or syndrome 743.44 *[365.41]*
rubeosis of iris 364.42 *[365.63]*
seclusion of pupil 364.74 *[365.61]*
spherophakia 743.36 *[365.59]*
Sturge-Weber (-Dimitri) syndrome 759.6 *[365.44]*
systemic syndrome NEC 365.44

Glaucoma — *continued*
in or with — *continued*
tumor of globe 365.64
vascular disorders NEC 365.63
infantile 365.14
congenital 743.20
associated with other eye anomalies 743.22
simple 743.21
juvenile 365.14
low tension 365.12
malignant 365.83 ▲
narrow angle (primary) 365.20
acute 365.22
chronic 365.23
intermittent 365.21
interval 365.21
residual stage 365.24
subacute 365.21
newborn 743.20
associated with other eye anomalies 743.22
simple 743.21
noncongestive (chronic) 365.11
nonobstructive (chronic) 365.11
obstructive 365.60
due to lens changes 365.59
open angle 365.10
with
borderline intraocular pressure 365.01
cupping of optic discs 365.01
primary 365.11
residual stage 365.15
phacolytic 365.51
with hypermature cataract 366.18 *[365.51]*
pigmentary 365.13
postinfectious 365.60
pseudoexfoliation 365.52
with pseudoexfoliation of capsule 366.11 *[365.52]*
secondary NEC 365.60
simple (chronic) 365.11
simplex 365.11
steroid responders 365.03
suspect 365.00
syphilitic 095.8
traumatic NEC 365.65
newborn 767.8
tuberculous (*see also* Tuberculosis) 017.3 ☑5ᵗʰ *[365.62]*
wide angle (*see also* Glaucoma, open angle) 365.10
Glaucomatous flecks (subcapsular) 366.31
Glazed tongue 529.4
Gleet 098.2
Glénard's disease or syndrome (enteroptosis) 569.89
Glinski-Simmonds syndrome (pituitary cachexia) 253.2
Glioblastoma (multiforme) (M9440/3)
with sarcomatous component (M9442/3)
specified site — *see* Neoplasm, by site, malignant
unspecified site 191.9
giant cell (M9441/3)
specified site — *see* Neoplasm, by site, malignant
unspecified site 191.9
specified site — *see* Neoplasm, by site, malignant
unspecified site 191.9
Glioma (malignant) (M9380/3)
astrocytic (M9400/3)
specified site — *see* Neoplasm, by site, malignant
unspecified site 191.9
mixed (M9382/3)
specified site — *see* Neoplasm, by site, malignant
unspecified site 191.9
nose 748.1
specified site NEC — *see* Neoplasm, by site, malignant
subependymal (M9383/1) 237.5
unspecified site 191.9
Gliomatosis cerebri (M9381/3) 191.0

Glioneuroma (M9505/1) — *see* Neoplasm, by site, uncertain behavior
Gliosarcoma (M9380/3)
specified site — *see* Neoplasm, by site, malignant
unspecified site 191.9
Gliosis (cerebral) 349.89
spinal 336.0
Glisson's
cirrhosis — *see* Cirrhosis, portal
disease (*see also* Rickets) 268.0
Glissonitis 573.3
Globinuria 791.2
Globus 306.4
hystericus 300.11
Glomangioma (M8712/0) (*see also* Hemangioma) 228.00
Glomangiosarcoma (M8710/3) — *see* Neoplasm, connective tissue, malignant
Glomerular nephritis (*see also* Nephritis) 583.9
Glomerulitis (*see also* Nephritis) 583.9
Glomerulonephritis (*see also* Nephritis) 583.9
with
edema (*see also* Nephrosis) 581.9
lesion of
exudative nephritis 583.89
interstitial nephritis (diffuse) (focal) 583.89
necrotizing glomerulitis 583.4
acute 580.4
chronic 582.4
renal necrosis 583.9
cortical 583.6
medullary 583.7
specified pathology NEC 583.89
acute 580.89
chronic 582.89
necrosis, renal 583.9
cortical 583.6
medullary (papillary) 583.7
specified pathology or lesion NEC 583.89
acute 580.9
with
exudative nephritis 580.89
interstitial nephritis (diffuse) (focal) 580.89
necrotizing glomerulitis 580.4
extracapillary with epithelial crescents 580.4
poststreptococcal 580.0
proliferative (diffuse) 580.0
rapidly progressive 580.4
specified pathology NEC 580.89
arteriolar (*see also* Hypertension, kidney) 403.90
arteriosclerotic (*see also* Hypertension, kidney) 403.90
ascending (*see also* Pyelitis) 590.80
basement membrane NEC 583.89
with
pulmonary hemorrhage (Goodpasture's syndrome) 446.21 *[583.81]*
chronic 582.9
with
exudative nephritis 582.89
interstitial nephritis (diffuse) (focal) 582.89
necrotizing glomerulitis 582.4
specified pathology or lesion NEC 582.89
endothelial 582.2
extracapillary with epithelial crescents 582.4
hypocomplementemic persistent 582.2
lobular 582.2
membranoproliferative 582.2
membranous 582.1
and proliferative (mixed) 582.2
sclerosing 582.1
mesangiocapillary 582.2
mixed membranous and proliferative 582.2
proliferative (diffuse) 582.0
rapidly progressive 582.4
sclerosing 582.1
cirrhotic — *see* Sclerosis, renal
desquamative — *see* Nephrosis

Glomerulonephritis (*see also* Nephritis) —
continued
  due to or associated with
    amyloidosis 277.3 *[583.81]*
      with nephrotic syndrome 277.3 *[581.81]*
      chronic 277.3 *[582.81]*
    diabetes mellitus 250.4 √5ᵗʰ *[583.81]*
      with nephrotic syndrome
        250.4 √5ᵗʰ *[581.81]*
    diphtheria 032.89 *[580.81]*
    gonococcal infection (acute) 098.19 *[583.81]*
      chronic or duration of 2 months or over
        098.39 *[583.81]*
    infectious hepatitis 070.9 *[580.81]*
    malaria (with nephrotic syndrome)
      084.9 *[581.81]*
    mumps 072.79 *[580.81]*
    polyarteritis (nodosa) (with nephrotic
      syndrome) 446.0 *[581.81]*
    specified pathology NEC 583.89
      acute 580.89
      chronic 582.89
    streptotrichosis 039.8 *[583.81]*
    subacute bacterial endocarditis
      421.0 *[580.81]*
    syphilis (late) 095.4
      congenital 090.5 *[583.81]*
      early 091.69 *[583.81]*
    systemic lupus erythematosus 710.0 *[583.81]*
      with nephrotic syndrome 710.0 *[581.81]*
      chronic 710.0 *[582.81]*
    tuberculosis (*see also* Tuberculosis)
      016.0 √5ᵗʰ *[583.81]*
    typhoid fever 002.0 *[580.81]*
  extracapillary with epithelial crescents 583.4
    acute 580.4
    chronic 582.4
  exudative 583.89
    acute 580.89
    chronic 582.89
  focal (*see also* Nephritis) 583.9
    embolic 580.4
  granular 582.89
  granulomatous 582.89
  hydremic (*see also* Nephrosis) 581.9
  hypocomplementemic persistent 583.2
    with nephrotic syndrome 581.2
    chronic 582.2
  immune complex NEC 583.89
  infective (*see also* Pyelitis) 590.80
  interstitial (diffuse) (focal) 583.89
    with nephrotic syndrome 581.89
    acute 580.89
    chronic 582.89
  latent or quiescent 582.9
  lobular 583.2
    with nephrotic syndrome 581.2
    chronic 582.2
  membranoproliferative 583.2
    with nephrotic syndrome 581.2
    chronic 582.2
  membranous 583.1
    with nephrotic syndrome 581.1
    and proliferative (mixed) 583.2
      with nephrotic syndrome 581.2
      chronic 582.2
    chronic 582.1
    sclerosing 582.1
      with nephrotic syndrome 581.1
  mesangiocapillary 583.2
    with nephrotic syndrome 581.2
    chronic 582.2
  minimal change 581.3
  mixed membranous and proliferative 583.2
    with nephrotic syndrome 581.2
    chronic 582.2
  necrotizing 583.4
    acute 580.4
    chronic 582.4
  nephrotic (*see also* Nephrosis) 581.9
  old — *see* Glomerulonephritis, chronic
  parenchymatous 581.89
  poststreptococcal 580.0
  proliferative (diffuse) 583.0
    with nephrotic syndrome 581.0
    acute 580.0
    chronic 582.0

Glomerulonephritis (*see also* Nephritis) —
continued
  purulent (*see also* Pyelitis) 590.80
  quiescent — *see* Nephritis, chronic
  rapidly progressive 583.4
    acute 580.4
    chronic 582.4
  sclerosing membranous (chronic) 582.1
    with nephrotic syndrome 581.1
  septic (*see also* Pyelitis) 590.80
  specified pathology or lesion NEC 583.89
    with nephrotic syndrome 581.89
    acute 580.89
    chronic 582.89
  suppurative (acute) (disseminated) (*see also*
    Pyelitis) 590.80
  toxic — *see* Nephritis, acute
  tubal, tubular — *see* Nephrosis, tubular
  type II (Ellis) — *see* Nephrosis
  vascular — *see* Hypertension, kidney
Glomerulosclerosis (*see also* Sclerosis, renal) 587
  focal 582.1
    with nephrotic syndrome 581.1
  intercapillary (nodular) (with diabetes)
    250.4 √5ᵗʰ *[581.81]*
Glossagra 529.6
Glossalgia 529.6
Glossitis 529.0
  areata exfoliativa 529.1
  atrophic 529.4
  benign migratory 529.1
  gangrenous 529.0
  Hunter's 529.4
  median rhomboid 529.2
  Moeller's 529.4
  pellagrous 265.2
Glossocele 529.8
Glossodynia 529.6
  exfoliativa 529.4
Glossoncus 529.8
Glossophytia 529.3
Glossoplegia 529.8
Glossoptosis 529.8
Glossopyrosis 529.6
Glossotrichia 529.3
Glossy skin 710.9
Glottis — *see* condition
Glottitis — *see* Glossitis
Glucagonoma (M8152/0)
  malignant (M8152/3)
    pancreas 157.4
    specified site NEC — *see* Neoplasm, by site,
      malignant
    unspecified site 157.4
  pancreas 211.7
  specified site NEC — *see* Neoplasm, by site,
    benign
  unspecified site 211.7
Glucoglycinuria 270.7
Glue ear syndrome 381.20
Glue sniffing (airplane glue) (*see also*
  Dependence) 304.6 √5ᵗʰ
Glycinemia (with methylmalonic acidemia) 270.7
Glycinuria (renal) (with ketosis) 270.0
Glycogen
  infiltration (*see also* Disease, glycogen storage)
    271.0
  storage disease (*see also* Disease, glycogen
    storage) 271.0
Glycogenosis (*see also* Disease, glycogen storage)
  271.0
  cardiac 271.0 *[425.7]*
  Cori, types I-VII 271.0
  diabetic, secondary 250.8 √5ᵗʰ *[259.8]*
  diffuse (with hepatic cirrhosis) 271.0
  generalized 271.0
  glucose-6-phosphatase deficiency 271.0
  hepatophosphorylase deficiency 271.0
  hepatorenal 271.0
  myophosphorylase deficiency 271.0
Glycopenia 251.2
Glycoprolinuria 270.8

Glycosuria 791.5
  renal 271.4
Gnathostoma (spinigerum) (infection) (infestation)
  128.1
  wandering swellings from 128.1
Gnathostomiasis 128.1
Goiter (adolescent) (colloid) (diffuse) (dipping) (due
  to iodine deficiency) (endemic) (euthyroid)
  (heart) (hyperplastic) (internal)
  (intrathoracic) (juvenile) (mixed type)
  (nonendemic) (parenchymatous) (plunging)
  (sporadic) (subclavicular) (substernal) 240.9
  with
    hyperthyroidism (recurrent) (*see also* Goiter,
      toxic) 242.0 √5ᵗʰ
    thyrotoxicosis (*see also* Goiter, toxic)
      242.0 √5ᵗʰ
  adenomatous (*see also* Goiter, nodular) 241.9
  cancerous (M8000/3) 193
  complicating pregnancy, childbirth, or
    puerperium 648.1 √5ᵗʰ
  congenital 246.1
  cystic (*see also* Goiter, nodular) 241.9
  due to enzyme defect in synthesis of thyroid
    hormone (butane-insoluble iodine)
    (coupling) (deiodinase) (iodide trapping or
    organificaiton) (iodotyrosine
    dehalogenase) (peroxidase) 246.1
  dyshormonogenic 246.1
  exophthalmic (*see also* Goiter, toxic) 242.0 √5ᵗʰ
  familial (with deaf-mutism) 243
  fibrous 245.3
  lingual 759.2
  lymphadenoid 245.2
  malignant (M8000/3) 193
  multinodular (nontoxic) 241.1
    toxic or with hyperthyroidism (*see also*
      Goiter, toxic) 242.2 √5ᵗʰ
  nodular (nontoxic) 241.9
    with
      hyperthyroidism (*see also* Goiter, toxic)
        242.3 √5ᵗʰ
      thyrotoxicosis (*see also* Goiter, toxic)
        242.3 √5ᵗʰ
    endemic 241.9
    exophthalmic (diffuse) (*see also* Goiter, toxic)
      242.0 √5ᵗʰ
    multinodular (nontoxic) 241.1
    sporadic 241.9
    toxic (*see also* Goiter, toxic) 242.3 √5ᵗʰ
    uninodular (nontoxic) 241.0
  nontoxic (nodular) 241.9
    multinodular 241.1
    uninodular 241.0
  pulsating (*see also* Goiter, toxic) 242.0 √5ᵗʰ
  simple 240.0
  toxic 242.0 √5ᵗʰ

---

*Note — Use the following fifth-digit
subclassification with category 242:*

  *0   without mention of thyrotoxic crisis or
        storm*
  *1   with mention of thyrotoxic crisis or
        storm*

---

    adenomatous 242.3 √5ᵗʰ
      multinodular 242.2 √5ᵗʰ
      uninodular 242.1 √5ᵗʰ
    multinodular 242.2 √5ᵗʰ
    nodular 242.3 √5ᵗʰ
      multinodular 242.2 √5ᵗʰ
      uninodular 242.1 √5ᵗʰ
    uninodular 242.1 √5ᵗʰ
  uninodular (nontoxic) 241.0
    toxic or with hyperthyroidism (*see also*
      Goiter, toxic) 242.1 √5ᵗʰ
Goldberg (-Maxwell) (-Morris) **syndrome**
  (testicular feminization) 257.8
Goldblatt's
  hypertension 440.1
  kidney 440.1
Goldenhar's syndrome (oculoauriculovertebral
  dysplasia) 756.0
Goldflam-Erb disease or syndrome 358.0
Goldscheider's disease (epidermolysis bullosa)
  757.39

Goldstein's disease (familial hemorrhagic telangiectasia) 448.0

Golfer's elbow 726.32

Goltz-Gorlin syndrome (dermal hypoplasia) 757.39

Gonadoblastoma (M9073/1)
  specified site — *see* Neoplasm, by site uncertain behavior
  unspecified site
    female 236.2
    male 236.4

Gonecystitis (*see also* Vesiculitis) 608.0

Gongylonemiasis 125.6
  mouth 125.6

Goniosynechiae 364.73

Gonococcemia 098.89

Gonococcus, gonococcal (disease) (infection) (*see also* condition) 098.0
  anus 098.7
  bursa 098.52
  chronic NEC 098.2
  complicating pregnancy, childbirth, or puerperium 647.1 ☑5ᵗʰ
    affecting fetus or newborn 760.2
  conjunctiva, conjunctivitis (neonatorum) 098.40
  dermatosis 098.89
  endocardium 098.84
  epididymo-orchitis 098.13
    chronic or duration of 2 months or over 098.33
  eye (newborn) 098.40
  fallopian tube (chronic) 098.37
    acute 098.17
  genitourinary (acute) (organ) (system) (tract) (*see also* Gonnorrhea) 098.0
    lower 098.0
      chronic 098.2
    upper 098.10
      chronic 098.30
  heart NEC 098.85
  joint 098.50
  keratoderma 098.81
  keratosis (blennorrhagica) 098.81
  lymphatic (gland) (node) 098.89
  meninges 098.82
  orchitis (acute) 098.13
    chronic or duration of 2 months or over 098.33
  pelvis (acute) 098.19
    chronic or duration of 2 months or over 098.39
  pericarditis 098.83
  peritonitis 098.86
  pharyngitis 098.6
  pharynx 098.6
  proctitis 098.7
  pyosalpinx (chronic) 098.37
    acute 098.17
  rectum 098.7
  septicemia 098.89
  skin 098.89
  specified site NEC 098.89
  synovitis 098.51
  tendon sheath 098.51
  throat 098.6
  urethra (acute) 098.0
    chronic or duration of 2 months or over 098.2
  vulva (acute) 098.0
    chronic or duration of 2 months or over 098.2

Gonocytoma (M9073/1)
  specified site — *see* Neoplasm, by site, uncertain behavior
  unspecified site
    female 236.2
    male 236.4

Gonorrhea 098.0
  acute 098.0
  Bartholin's gland (acute) 098.0
    chronic or duration of 2 months or over 098.2
  bladder (acute) 098.11
    chronic or duration of 2 months or over 098.31

Gonorrhea — *continued*
  carrier (suspected of) V02.7
  cervix (acute) 098.15
    chronic or duration of 2 months or over 098.35
  chronic 098.2
  complicating pregnancy, childbirth, or puerperium 647.1 ☑5ᵗʰ
    affecting fetus or newborn 760.2
  conjunctiva, conjunctivitis (neonatorum) 098.40
  contact V01.6
  Cowper's gland (acute) 098.0
    chronic or duration of 2 months or over 098.2
  duration of two months or over 098.2
  exposure to V01.6
  fallopian tube (chronic) 098.37
    acute 098.17
  genitourinary (acute) (organ) (system) (tract) 098.0
    chronic 098.2
    duration of two months or over 098.2
  kidney (acute) 098.19
    chronic or duration of 2 months or over 098.39
  ovary (acute) 098.19
    chronic or duration of 2 months or over 098.39
  pelvis (acute) 098.19
    chronic or duration of 2 months or over 098.39
  penis (acute) 098.0
    chronic or duration of 2 months or over 098.2
  prostate (acute) 098.12
    chronic or duration of 2 months or over 098.32
  seminal vesicle (acute) 098.14
    chronic or duration of 2 months or over 098.34
  specified site NEC — *see* Gonococcus
  spermatic cord (acute) 098.14
    chronic or duration of 2 months or over 098.34
  urethra (acute) 098.0
    chronic or duration of 2 months or over 098.2
  vagina (acute) 098.0
    chronic or duration of 2 months or over 098.2
  vas deferens (acute) 098.14
    chronic or duration of 2 months or over 098.34
  vulva (acute) 098.0
    chronic or duration of 2 months or over 098.2

Goodpasture's syndrome (pneumorenal) 446.21

Gopalan's syndrome (burning feet) 266.2

Gordon's disease (exudative enteropathy) 579.8

Gorlin-Chaudhry-Moss syndrome 759.89

Gougerot's syndrome (trisymptomatic) 709.1

Gougerot-Blum syndrome (pigmented purpuric lichenoid dermatitis) 709.1

Gougerot-Carteaud disease or syndrome (confluent reticulate papillomatosis) 701.8

Gougerot-Hailey-Hailey disease (benign familial chronic pemphigus) 757.39

Gougerot (-Houwer) - Sjögren syndrome (keratoconjunctivitis sicca) 710.2

Gouley's syndrome (constrictive pericarditis) 423.2

Goundou 102.6

Gout, gouty 274.9
  with specified manifestations NEC 274.89
  arthritis (acute) 274.0
  arthropathy 274.0
  degeneration, heart 274.82
  diathesis 274.9
  eczema 274.89
  episcleritis 274.89 [379.09]
  external ear (tophus) 274.81
  glomerulonephritis 274.10
  iritis 274.89 [364.11]
  joint 274.0

Gout, gouty — *continued*
  kidney 274.10
  lead 984.9
    specified type of lead — *see* Table of Drugs and Chemicals
  nephritis 274.10
  neuritis 274.89 [357.4]
  phlebitis 274.89 [451.9]
  rheumatic 714.0
  saturnine 984.9
    specified type of lead — *see* Table of Drugs and Chemicals
  spondylitis 274.0
  synovitis 274.0
  syphilitic 095.8
  tophi 274.0
    ear 274.81
    heart 274.82
    specified site NEC 274.82

Gowers'
  muscular dystrophy 359.1
  syndrome (vasovagal attack) 780.2

Gowers-Paton-Kennedy syndrome 377.04

Gradenigo's syndrome 383.02

Graft-versus-host disease (bone marrow) 996.85
  due to organ transplant NEC — *see* Complications, transplant, organ

Graham Steell's murmur (pulmonic regurgitation) (*see also* Endocarditis, pulmonary) 424.3

Grain-handlers' disease or lung 495.8

Grain mite (itch) 133.8

Grand
  mal (idiopathic) (*see also* Epilepsy) 345.1 ☑5ᵗʰ
    hysteria of Charcôt 300.11
    nonrecurrent or isolated 780.39
  multipara
    affecting management of labor and delivery 659.4 ☑5ᵗʰ
    status only (not pregnant) V61.5

Granite workers' lung 502

Granular — *see also* condition
  inflammation, pharynx 472.1
  kidney (contracting) (*see also* Sclerosis, renal) 587
  liver — *see* Cirrhosis, liver
  nephritis — *see* Nephritis

Granulation tissue, abnormal — *see also* Granuloma
  abnormal or excessive 701.5
  postmastoidectomy cavity 383.33
  postoperative 701.5
  skin 701.5

Granulocytopenia, granulocytopenic (primary) 288.0
  malignant 288.0

Granuloma NEC 686.1
  abdomen (wall) 568.89
    skin (pyogenicum) 686.1
      from residual foreign body 709.4
  annulare 695.89
  anus 569.49
  apical 522.6
  appendix 543.9
  aural 380.23
  beryllium (skin) 709.4
    lung 503
  bone (*see also* Osteomyelitis) 730.1 ☑5ᵗʰ
    eosinophilic 277.8
    from residual foreign body 733.99
  canaliculus lacrimalis 375.81
  cerebral 348.8
  cholesterin, middle ear 385.82
  coccidioidal (progressive) 114.3
    lung 114.4
    meninges 114.2
    primary (lung) 114.0
  colon 569.89
  conjunctiva 372.61
  dental 522.6
  ear, middle (cholesterin) 385.82
    with otitis media — *see* Otitis media
  eosinophilic 277.8
    bone 277.8
    lung 277.8

Granuloma NEC — *continued*
  eosinophilic — *continued*
    oral mucosa 528.9
  exuberant 701.5
  eyelid 374.89
  facial
    lethal midline 446.3
    malignant 446.3
  faciale 701.8
  fissuratum (gum) 523.8
  foot NEC 686.1
  foreign body (in soft tissue) NEC 728.82
    bone 733.99
    in operative wound 998.4
    muscle 728.82
    skin 709.4
    subcutaneous tissue 709.4
  fungoides 202.1 ☑5ᵗʰ
  gangraenescens 446.3
  giant cell (central) (jaw) (reparative) 526.3
    gingiva 523.8
    peripheral (gingiva) 523.8
  gland (lymph) 289.3
  Hodgkin's (M9661/3) 201.1 ☑5ᵗʰ
  ileum 569.89
  infectious NEC 136.9
  inguinale (Donovan) 099.2
    venereal 099.2
  intestine 569.89
  iridocyclitis 364.10
  jaw (bone) 526.3
    reparative giant cell 526.3
  kidney (*see also* Infection, kidney) 590.9
  lacrimal sac 375.81
  larynx 478.79
  lethal midline 446.3
  lipid 277.8
  lipoid 277.8
  liver 572.8
  lung (infectious) (*see also* Fibrosis, lung) 515
    coccidioidal 114.4
    eosinophilic 277.8
  lymph gland 289.3
  Majocchi's 110.6
  malignant, face 446.3
  mandible 526.3
  mediastinum 519.3
  midline 446.3
  monilial 112.3
  muscle 728.82
    from residual foreign body 728.82
  nasal sinus (*see also* Sinusitis) 473.9
  operation wound 998.59
    foreign body 998.4
    stitch (external) 998.89
      internal organ 996.7 ☑5ᵗʰ
      internal wound 998.89
    talc 998.7
  oral mucosa, eosinophilic or pyogenic 528.9
  orbit, orbital 376.11
  paracoccidioidal 116.1
  penis, venereal 099.2
  periapical 522.6
  peritoneum 568.89
    due to ova of helminths NEC (*see also*
      Helminthiasis) 128.9
  postmastoidectomy cavity 383.33
  postoperative — *see* Granuloma, operation
    wound
  prostate 601.8
  pudendi (ulcerating) 099.2
  pudendorum (ulcerative) 099.2
  pulp, internal (tooth) 521.4
  pyogenic, pyogenicum (skin) 686.1
    maxillary alveolar ridge 522.6
    oral mucosa 528.9
  rectum 569.49
  reticulohistiocytic 277.8
  rubrum nasi 705.89
  sarcoid 135
  Schistosoma 120.9
  septic (skin) 686.1
  silica (skin) 709.4
  sinus (accessory) (infectional) (nasal) (*see also*
    Sinusitis) 473.9
  skin (pyogenicum) 686.1
    from foreign body or material 709.4
  sperm 608.89

Granuloma NEC — *continued*
  spine
    syphilitic (epidural) 094.89
    tuberculous (*see also* Tuberculosis)
      015.0 ☑5ᵗʰ *[730.88]*
  stitch (postoperative) 998.89
    internal wound 998.89
  suppurative (skin) 686.1
  suture (postoperative) 998.89
    internal wound 998.89
  swimming pool 031.1
  talc 728.82
    in operation wound 998.7
  telangiectaticum (skin) 686.1
  trichophyticum 110.6
  tropicum 102.4
  umbilicus 686.1
    newborn 771.4
  urethra 599.84
  uveitis 364.10
  vagina 099.2
  venereum 099.2
  vocal cords 478.5
  Wegener's (necrotizing respiratory
    granulomatosis) 446.4
Granulomatosis NEC 686.1
  disciformis chronica et progressiva 709.3
  infantiseptica 771.2
  lipoid 277.8
  lipohagic, intestinal 040.2
  miliary 027.0
  necrotizing, respiratory 446.4
  progressive, septic 288.1
  Wegener's (necrotizing respiratory) 446.4
Granulomatous tissue — *see* Granuloma
Granulosis rubra nasi 705.89
Graphite fibrosis (of lung) 503
Graphospasm 300.89
  organic 333.84
Grating scapula 733.99
Gravel (urinary) (*see also* Calculus) 592.9
Graves' disease (exophthalmic goiter) (*see also*
  Goiter, toxic) 242.0 ☑5ᵗʰ
Gravis — *see* condition
Grawitz's tumor (hypernephroma) (M8312/3)
  189.0
Grayness, hair (premature) 704.3
  congenital 757.4
Gray or grey syndrome (chloramphenicol)
  (newborn) 779.4
Greenfield's disease 330.0
Green sickness 280.9
Greenstick fracture — *see* Fracture, by site
Greig's syndrome (hypertelorism) 756.0
Griesinger's disease (*see also* Ancylostomiasis)
  126.9
Grinders'
  asthma 502
  lung 502
  phthisis (*see also* Tuberculosis) 011.4 ☑5ᵗʰ
Grinding, teeth 306.8
Grip
  Dabney's 074.1
  devil's 074.1
Grippe, grippal — *see also* Influenza
  Balkan 083.0
  intestinal 487.8
  summer 074.8
Grippy cold 487.1
Grisel's disease 723.5
Groin — *see* condition
Grooved
  nails (transverse) 703.8
  tongue 529.5
    congenital 750.13
Ground itch 126.9
Growing pains, children 781.99
Growth (fungoid) (neoplastic) (new) (M8000/1) —
  see also Neoplasm, by site, unspecified
  nature
  adenoid (vegetative) 474.12

Growth — *see also* Neoplasm, by site, unspecified
  nature — *continued*
  benign (M8000/0) — *see* Neoplasm, by site,
    benign
  fetal, poor 764.9 ☑5ᵗʰ
    affecting management of pregnancy
      656.5 ☑5ᵗʰ
  malignant (M8000/3) — *see* Neoplasm, by site,
    malignant
  rapid, childhood V21.0
  secondary (M8000/6) — *see* Neoplasm, by site,
    malignant, secondary
Gruber's hernia — *see* Hernia, Gruber's
Gruby's disease (tinea tonsurans) 110.0
G-trisomy 758.0
Guama fever 066.3
Gubler (-Millard) paralysis or syndrome 344.89
Guérin-Stern syndrome (arthorgryposis multiplex
  congenita) 754.89
Guertin's disease (electric chorea) 049.8
Guillain-Barré disease or syndrome 357.0
Guinea worms (infection) (infestation) 125.7
Guinon's disease (motor-verbal tic) 307.23
Gull's disease (thyroid atrophy with myxedema)
  244.8
Gull and Sutton's disease — *see* Hypertension,
  kidney
Gum — *see* condition
Gumboil 522.7
Gumma (syphilitic) 095.9
  artery 093.89
    cerebral or spinal 094.89
  bone 095.5
    of yaws (late) 102.6
  brain 094.89
  cauda equina 094.89
  central nervous system NEC 094.9
  ciliary body 095.8 *[364.11]*
  congenital 090.5
    testis 090.5
  eyelid 095.8 *[373.5]*
  heart 093.89
  intracranial 094.89
  iris 095.8 *[364.11]*
  kidney 095.4
  larynx 095.8
  leptomeninges 094.2
  liver 095.3
  meninges 094.2
  myocardium 093.82
  nasopharynx 095.8
  neurosyphilitic 094.9
  nose 095.8
  orbit 095.8
  palate (soft) 095.8
  penis 095.8
  pericardium 093.81
  pharynx 095.8
  pituitary 095.8
  scrofulous (see also Tuberculosis) 017.0 ☑5ᵗʰ
  skin 095.8
  specified site NEC 095.8
  spinal cord 094.89
  tongue 095.8
  tonsil 095.8
  trachea 095.8
  tuberculous (*see also* Tuberculosis) 017.0 ☑5ᵗʰ
  ulcerative due to yaws 102.4
  ureter 095.8
  yaws 102.4
    bone 102.6
Gunn's syndrome (jaw-winking syndrome) 742.8
Gunshot wound — *see also* Wound, open, by site
  fracture — *see* Fracture, by site, open
  internal organs (abdomen, chest, or pelvis) —
    see Injury, internal, by site, with open
    wound
  intracranial — *see* Laceration, brain, with open
    intracranial wound
Günther's disease or syndrome (congenital
  erythropoietic porphyria) 277.1
Gustatory hallucination 780.1
Gynandrism 752.7

Gynanadroblastoma (M8632/1)
  specified site — *see* Neoplasm, by site,
    uncertain behavior
  unspecified site
    female 236.2
    male 236.4
Gynandromorphism 752.7
Gynatresia (congenital) 752.49
Gynecoid pelvis, male 738.6
Gynecological examination V72.3
  for contraceptive maintenance V25.40
Gynecomastia 611.1
Gynephobia 300.29
Gyrate scalp 757.39

H

Haas' disease (osteochondrosis head of humerus)
  732.3
Habermann's disease (acute parapsoriasis
  varioliformis) 696.2
Habit, habituation
  chorea 307.22
  disturbance, child 307.9
  drug (*see also* Dependence) 304.9 ✓5ᵗʰ
  laxative (*see also* Abuse, drugs, nondependent)
    305.9 ✓5ᵗʰ
  spasm 307.20
    chronic 307.22
    transient of childhood 307.21
  tic 307.20
    chronic 307.22
    transient of childhood 307.21
  use of
    nonprescribed drugs (*see also* Abuse, drugs,
      nondependent) 305.9 ✓5ᵗʰ
    patent medicines (*see also* Abuse, drugs,
      nondependent) 305.9 ✓5ᵗʰ
  vomiting 536.2
Hadfield-Clarke syndrome (pancreatic
  infantilism) 577.8
Haff disease 985.1
Hageman factor defect, deficiency, or disease
  (*see also* Defect, coagulation) 286.3
Haglund's disease (osteochondrosis os tibiale
  externum) 732.5
Haglund-Läwen-Fründ syndrome 717.89
Hagner's disease (hypertrophic pulmonary
  osteoarthropathy) 731.2
Hag teeth, tooth 524.3
Hailey-Hailey disease (benign familial chronic
  pemphigus) 757.39
Hair — *see also* condition
  plucking 307.9
Hairball in stomach 935.2
Hairy black tongue 529.3
Half vertebra 756.14
Halitosis 784.9
Hallermann-Streiff syndrome 756.0
Hallervorden-Spatz disease or syndrome 333.0
Hallopeau's
  acrodermatitis (continua) 696.1
  disease (lichen sclerosis et atrophicus) 701.0
Hallucination (auditory) (gustatory) (olfactory)
  (tactile) 780.1
  alcoholic 291.3
  drug-induced 292.12
  visual 368.16
Hallucinosis 298.9
  alcoholic (acute) 291.3
  drug-induced 292.12
Hallus — *see* Hallux
Hallux 735.9
  malleus (acquired) 735.3
  rigidus (acquired) 735.2
    congenital 755.66
    late effects of rickets 268.1
  valgus (acquired) 735.0
    congenital 755.66
  varus (acquired) 735.1
    congenital 755.66

Halo, visual 368.15
Hamartoblastoma 759.6
Hamartoma 759.6
  epithelial (gingival), odontogenic, central, or
    peripheral (M9321/0) 213.1
    upper jaw (bone) 213.0
  vascular 757.32
Hamartosis, hamartoses NEC 759.6
Hamman's disease or syndrome (spontaneous
  mediastinal emphysema) 518.1
Hamman-Rich syndrome (diffuse interstitial
  pulmonary fibrosis) 516.3
Hammer toe (acquired) 735.4
  congenital 755.66
  late effects of rickets 268.1
Hand — *see* condition
Hand-Schüller-Christian disease or syndrome
  (chronic histiocytosis x) 277.8
Hand-foot syndrome 282.61
Hanging (asphyxia) (strangulation) (suffocation)
  994.7
Hangnail (finger) (with lymphangitis) 681.02
Hangover (alcohol) (*see also* Abuse, drugs,
  nondependent) 305.0 ✓5ᵗʰ
Hanot's cirrhosis or disease — *see* Cirrhosis,
  biliary
Hanot-Chauffard (-Troisier) syndrome (bronze
  diabetes) 275.0
Hansen's disease (leprosy) 030.9
  benign form 030.1
  malignant form 030.0
Harada's disease or syndrome 363.22
Hard chancre 091.0
Hard firm prostate 600.1
Hardening
  artery — *see* Arteriosclerosis
  brain 348.8
  liver 571.8
Hare's syndrome (M8010/3) (carcinoma,
  pulmonary apex) 162.3
Harelip (*see also* Cleft, lip) 749.10
Harkavy's syndrome 446.0
Harlequin (fetus) 757.1
  color change syndrome 779.89 ▲
Harley's disease (intermittent hemoglobinuria)
  283.2
Harris'
  lines 733.91
  syndrome (organic hyperinsulinism) 251.1
Hart's disease or syndrome (pellagra-cerebellar
  ataxia-renal aminoaciduria) 270.0
Hartmann's pouch (abnormal sacculation of
  gallbladder neck) 575.8
  of intestine V44.3
    attention to V55.3
Hartnup disease (pellagra-cerebellar ataxia-renal
  aminoaciduria) 270.0
Harvester lung 495.0
Hashimoto's disease or struma (struma
  lymphomatosa) 245.2
Hassell-Henle bodies (corneal warts) 371.41
Haut mal (*see also* Epilepsy) 345.1 ✓5ᵗʰ
Haverhill fever 026.1
Hawaiian wood rose dependence 304.5 ✓5ᵗʰ
Hawkins' keloid 701.4
Hay
  asthma (*see also* Asthma) 493.0 ✓5ᵗʰ
  fever (allergic) (with rhinitis) 477.9
    with asthma (bronchial) (*see also* Asthma)
      493.0 ✓5ᵗʰ
    allergic, due to grass, pollen, ragweed, or
      tree 477.0
    conjunctivitis 372.05
    due to
      dander 477.8
      dust 477.8
      fowl 477.8
      pollen 477.0
      specified allergen other than pollen 477.8

Hayem-Faber syndrome (achlorhydric anemia)
  280.9
Hayem-Widal syndrome (acquired hemolytic
  jaundice) 283.9
Haygarth's nodosities 715.04
Hazard-Crile tumor (M8350/3) 193
Hb (abnormal)
  disease — *see* Disease, hemoglobin
  trait — *see* Trait
H disease 270.0
Head — *see also* condition
  banging 307.3
Headache 784.0
  allergic 346.2 ✓5ᵗʰ
  cluster 346.2 ✓5ᵗʰ
  due to
    loss, spinal fluid 349.0
    lumbar puncture 349.0
    saddle block 349.0
  emotional 307.81
  histamine 346.2 ✓5ᵗʰ
  lumbar puncture 349.0
  menopausal 627.2
  migraine 346.9 ✓5ᵗʰ
  nonorganic origin 307.81
  postspinal 349.0
  psychogenic 307.81
  psychophysiologic 307.81
  sick 346.1 ✓5ᵗʰ
  spinal 349.0
    complicating labor and   ●
      delivery 668.8 ✓5ᵗʰ   ●
    postpartum 668.8 ✓5ᵗʰ   ●
  spinal fluid loss 349.0
  tension 307.81
  vascular 784.0
    migraine type 346.9 ✓5ᵗʰ
  vasomotor 346.9 ✓5ᵗʰ
Health
  advice V65.4
  audit V70.0
  checkup V70.0
  education V65.4
  hazard (*see also* History of) V15.9
    specified cause NEC V15.89
  instruction V65.4
  services provided because (of)
    boarding school residence V60.6
    holiday relief for person providing home care
      V60.5
    inadequate
      housing V60.1
      resources V60.2
    lack of housing V60.0
    no care available in home V60.4
    person living alone V60.3
    poverty V60.3
    residence in institution V60.6
    specified cause NEC V60.8
    vacation relief for person providing home
      care V60.5
Healthy
  donor (*see also* Donor) V59.9
  infant or child
    accompanying sick mother V65.0
    receiving care V20.1
  person
    accompanying sick relative V65.0
    admitted for sterilization V25.2
    receiving prophylactic inoculation or
      vaccination (*see also* Vaccination,
      prophylactic) V05.9
Hearing examination V72.1
Heart — *see* condition
Heartburn 787.1
  psychogenic 306.4
Heat (effects) 992.9
  apoplexy 992.0
  burn — *see also* Burn, by site
    from sun (*see also* Sunburn) 692.71
  collapse 992.1
  cramps 992.2
  dermatitis or eczema 692.89
  edema 992.7
  erythema — *see* Burn, by site

Gynanadroblastoma — Heat

✓4ᵗʰ Fourth-digit Required   ✓5ᵗʰ Fifth-digit Required   ►◄ Revised Text   ● New Line   ▲ Revised Code

Heat — continued
excessive 992.9
  specified effect NEC 992.8
exhaustion 992.5
  anhydrotic 992.3
  due to
    salt (and water) depletion 992.4
    water depletion 992.3
fatigue (transient) 992.6
fever 992.0
hyperpyrexia 992.0
prickly 705.1
prostration — see Heat, exhaustion
pyrexia 992.0
rash 705.1
specified effect NEC 992.8
stroke 992.0
sunburn (see also Sunburn) 692.71
syncope 992.1
Heavy-chain disease 273.2
Heavy-for-dates (fetus or infant) 766.1
4500 grams or more 766.0
exceptionally 766.0
Hebephrenia, hebephrenic (acute) (see also
Schizophrenia) 295.1 ✓5ᵗʰ
dementia (praecox) (see also Schizophrenia)
295.1 ✓5ᵗʰ
schizophrenia (see also Schizophrenia)
295.1 ✓5ᵗʰ
Heberden's
disease or nodes 715.04
syndrome (angina pectoris) 413.9
Hebra's disease
dermatitis exfoliativa 695.89
erythema multiforme exudativum 695.1
pityriasis 695.89
  maculata et circinata 696.3
  rubra 695.89
    pilaris 696.4
prurigo 698.2
Hebra, nose 040.1
Hedinger's syndrome (malignant carcinoid) 259.2
Heel — see condition
Heerfordt's disease or syndrome (uveoparotitis)
135
Hegglin's anomaly or syndrome 288.2
Heidenhain's disease 290.10
with dementia 290.10
Heilmeyer-Schöner disease (M9842/3) 207.1 ✓5ᵗʰ
Heine-Medin disease (see also Poliomyelitis)
045.9 ✓5ᵗʰ
Heinz-body anemia, congenital 282.7
Heller's disease or syndrome (infantile
psychosis) (see also Psychosis, childhood)
299.1 ✓5ᵗʰ
H.E.L.L.P 642.5 ✓5ᵗʰ
Helminthiasis (see also Infestation, by specific
parasite) 128.9
Ancylostoma (see also Ancylostoma) 126.9
intestinal 127.9
  mixed types (types classifiable to more than
    one of the titles 120.0-127.7) 127.8
  specified type 127.7
mixed types (intestinal) (types classifiable to
  more than one of the titles 120.0-127.7)
  127.8
Necator americanus 126.1
specified type NEC 128.8
Trichinella 124
Heloma 700
Hemangioblastoma (M9161/1) — see also
Neoplasm, connective tissue, uncertain
behavior
malignant (M9161/3) — see Neoplasm,
connective tissue, malignant
Hemangioblastomatosis, cerebelloretinal 759.6
Hemangioendothelioma (M9130/1) — see also
Neoplasm, by site, uncertain behavior
benign (M9130/0) 228.00
bone (diffuse) (M9130/3) — see Neoplasm,
bone, malignant
malignant (M9130/3) — see Neoplasm,
connective tissue, malignant

Hemangioendothelioma — see also Neoplasm, by
site, uncertain behavior — continued
nervous system (M9130/0) 228.09
Hemangioendotheliosarcoma (M9130/3) — see
Neoplasm, connective tissue, malignant
Hemangiofibroma (M9160/0) — see Neoplasm,
by site, benign
Hemangiolipoma (M8861/0) — see Lipoma
Hemangioma (M9120/0) 228.00
arteriovenous (M9123/0) — see Hemangioma,
by site
brain 228.02
capillary (M9131/0) — see Hemangioma, by
site
cavernous (M9121/0) — see Hemangioma, by
site
central nervous system NEC 228.09
choroid 228.09
heart 228.09
infantile (M9131/0) — see Hemangioma, by site
intra-abdominal structures 228.04
intracranial structures 228.02
intramuscular (M9132/0) — see Hemangioma,
by site
iris 228.09
juvenile (M9131/0) — see Hemangioma, by site
malignant (M9120/3) — see Neoplasm,
connective tissue, malignant
meninges 228.09
  brain 228.02
  spinal cord 228.09
peritoneum 228.04
placenta — see Placenta, abnormal
plexiform (M9131/0) — see Hemangioma, by
site
racemose (M9123/0) — see Hemangioma, by
site
retina 228.03
retroperitoneal tissue 228.04
sclerosing (M8832/0) — see Neoplasm, skin,
benign
simplex (M9131/0) — see Hemangioma, by site
skin and subcutaneous tissue 228.01
specified site NEC 228.09
spinal cord 228.09
venous (M9122/0) — see Hemangioma, by site
verrucous keratotic (M9142/0) — see
Hemangioma, by site
Hemangiomatosis (systemic) 757.32
involving single site — see Hemangioma
Hemangiopericytoma (M9150/1) — see also
Neoplasm, connective tissue, uncertain
behavior
benign (M9150/0) — see Neoplasm, connective
tissue, benign
malignant (M9150/3) — see Neoplasm,
connective tissue, malignant
Hemangiosarcoma (M9120/3) — see Neoplasm,
connective tissue, malignant
Hemarthrosis (nontraumatic) 719.10
ankle 719.17
elbow 719.12
foot 719.17
hand 719.14
hip 719.15
knee 719.16
multiple sites 719.19
pelvic region 719.15
shoulder (region) 719.11
specified site NEC 719.18
traumatic — see Sprain, by site
wrist 719.13
Hematemesis 578.0
with ulcer — see Ulcer, by site, with
hemorrhage
due to S. japonicum 120.2
Goldstein's (familial hemorrhagic telangiectasia)
448.0
newborn 772.4
  due to swallowed maternal blood 777.3
Hematidrosis 705.89
Hematinuria (see also Hemoglobinuria) 791.2
malarial 084.8
paroxysmal 283.2
Hematite miners' lung 503

Hematobilia 576.8
Hematocele (congenital) (diffuse) (idiopathic)
608.83
broad ligament 620.7
canal of Nuck 629.0
cord male 608.83
fallopian tube 620.8
female NEC 629.0
ischiorectal 569.89
male NEC 608.83
ovary 629.0
pelvis, pelvic
  female 629.0
    with ectopic pregnancy (see also
      Pregnancy, ectopic) 633.90   ▲
    with intrauterine pregnancy 633.91●
  male 608.83
periuterine 629.0
retrouterine 629.0
scrotum 608.83
spermatic cord (diffuse) 608.83
testis 608.84
traumatic — see Injury, internal, pelvis
tunica vaginalis 608.83
uterine ligament 629.0
uterus 621.4
vagina 623.6
vulva 624.5
Hematocephalus 742.4
Hematochezia (see also Melena) 578.1
Hematochyluria (see also Infestation, filarial)
125.9
Hematocolpos 626.8
Hematocornea 371.12
Hematogenous — see condition
Hematoma (skin surface intact) (traumatic) — see
also Contusion

> Note — Hematomas are coded according to
> origin and the nature and site of the
> hematoma or the accompanying injury.
> Hematomas of unspecified origin are coded
> as injuries of the sites involved, except:
>
> (a) hematomas of genital organs which
>   are coded as diseases of the organ
>   involved unless they complicate
>   pregnancy or delivery
>
> (b) hematomas of the eye which are
>   coded as diseases of the eye.
>   For late effect of hematoma
>   classifiable to 920-924 see Late,
>   effect, contusion

with
  crush injury — see Crush
  fracture — see Fracture, by site
  injury of internal organs — see also Injury,
    internal, by site
    kidney — see Hematoma, kidney
      traumatic
    liver — see Hematoma, liver, traumatic
    spleen — see Hematoma, spleen
  nerve injury — see Injury, nerve
  open wound — see Wound, open, by site
  skin surface intact — see Contusion
abdomen (wall) — see Contusion, abdomen
amnion 658.8 ✓5ᵗʰ
aorta, dissecting 441.00
  abdominal 441.02
  thoracic 441.01
  thoracoabdominal 441.03
arterial (complicating trauma) 904.9
  specified site — see Injury, blood vessel, by
    site
auricle (ear) 380.31
birth injury 767.8
  skull 767.1

Hematoma — *see also* Contusion — *continued*
　brain (traumatic) 853.0 ☑5ᵗʰ

> Note — Use the following fifth-digit subclassification with categories 851-854:
>
> 0　unspecified state of consciousness
> 1　with no loss of consciousness
> 2　with brief [less than one hour] loss of consciousness
> 3　with moderate [1-24 hours] loss of consciousness
> 4　with prolonged [more than 24 hours] loss of consciousness and return to pre-existing conscious level
> 5　with prolonged [more than 24 hours] loss of consciousness, without return to pre-existing conscious level
>
> Use fifth-digit 5 to designate when a patient is unconscious and dies before regaining consciousness, regardless of the duration of the loss of consciousness
>
> 6　with loss of consciousness of unspecified duration
> 9　with concussion, unspecified

　　with
　　　cerebral
　　　　contusion — *see* Contusion, brain
　　　　laceration — *see* Laceration, brain
　　　open intracranial wound 853.1 ☑5ᵗʰ
　　　skull fracture — *see* Fracture, skull, by site
　　extradural or epidural 852.4 ☑5ᵗʰ
　　　with open intracranial wound 852.5 ☑5ᵗʰ
　　　fetus or newborn 767.0
　　　nontraumatic 432.0
　　fetus or newborn NEC 767.0
　　nontraumatic (*see also* Hemorrhage, brain) 431
　　　epidural or extradural 432.0
　　　newborn NEC 772.8
　　　subarachnoid, arachnoid, or meningeal (*see also* Hemorrhage, subarachnoid) 430
　　　subdural (*see also* Hemorrhage, subdural) 432.1
　　subarachnoid, arachnoid, or meningeal 852.0 ☑5ᵗʰ
　　　with open intracranial wound 852.1 ☑5ᵗʰ
　　　fetus or newborn 772.2
　　　nontraumatic (*see also* Hemorrhage, subarachnoid) 430
　　subdural 852.2 ☑5ᵗʰ
　　　with open intracranial wound 852.3 ☑5ᵗʰ
　　　fetus or newborn (localized) 767.0
　　　nontraumatic (*see also* Hemorrhage, subdural) 432.1
　breast (nontraumatic) 611.8
　broad ligament (nontraumatic) 620.7
　　complicating delivery 665.7 ☑5ᵗʰ
　　traumatic — *see* Injury, internal, broad ligament
　calcified NEC 959.9
　capitis 920
　　due to birth injury 767.1
　　newborn 767.1
　cerebral — *see* Hematoma, brain
　cesarean section wound 674.3 ☑5ᵗʰ
　chorion — *see* Placenta, abnormal
　complicating delivery (perineum) (vulva) 664.5 ☑5ᵗʰ
　　pelvic 665.7 ☑5ᵗʰ
　　vagina 665.7 ☑5ᵗʰ
　corpus
　　cavernosum (nontraumatic) 607.82
　　luteum (nontraumatic) (ruptured) 620.1
　dura (mater) — *see* Hematoma, brain, subdural
　epididymis (nontraumatic) 608.83
　epidural (traumatic) — *see also* Hematoma, brain, extradural
　　spinal — *see* Injury, spinal, by site
　episiotomy 674.3 ☑5ᵗʰ
　external ear 380.31

Hematoma — *see also* Contusion — *continued*
　extradural — *see also* Hematoma, brain, extradural
　　fetus or newborn 767.0
　　nontraumatic 432.0
　　　fetus or newborn 767.0
　fallopian tube 620.8
　genital organ (nontraumatic)
　　female NEC 629.8
　　male NEC 608.83
　　traumatic (external site) 922.4
　　　internal — *see* Injury, internal, genital organ
　graafian follicle (ruptured) 620.0
　internal organs (abdomen, chest, or pelvis) — *see also* Injury, internal, by site
　　kidney — *see* Hematoma, kidney, traumatic
　　liver — *see* Hematoma, liver, traumatic
　　spleen — *see* Hematoma, brain
　intracrainal — *see* Hematoma, brain
　kidney, cystic 593.81
　　traumatic 866.01
　　　with open wound into cavity 866.11
　labia (nontraumatic) 624.5
　lingual (and other parts of neck, scalp, or face, except eye) 920
　liver (subcapsular) 573.8
　　birth injury 767.8
　　fetus or newborn 767.8
　　traumatic NEC 864.01
　　　with
　　　　laceration — *see* Laceration, liver
　　　　open wound into cavity 864.11
　mediastinum — *see* Injury, internal, mediastinum
　menges, meningeal (brain) — *see also* Hematoma, brain, subarachnoid
　　spinal — *see* Injury, spinal, by site
　mesosalpinx (nontraumatic) 620.8
　　traumatic — *see* Injury, internal, pelvis
　muscle (traumatic — *see* Contusion, by site
　nasal (septum) (and other part(s) of neck, scalp, or face, except eye) 920
　obstetrical surgical wound 674.3 ☑5ᵗʰ
　orbit, orbital (nontraumatic) 376.32
　　traumatic 921.2
　ovary (corpus luteum) (nontraumatic) 620.1
　　traumatic — *see* Injury, internal, ovary
　pelvis (female) (nontraumatic) 629.8
　　complicating delivery 665.7 ☑5ᵗʰ
　　male 608.83
　　traumatic — *see also* Injury, internal, pelvis
　　　specified organ NEC (*see also* Injury, internal, pelvis) 867.6
　penis (nontraumatic) 607.82
　pericranial (and neck, or face any part, except eye) 920
　　due to injury at birth 767.1
　perineal wound (obstetrical) 674.3 ☑5ᵗʰ
　　complicating delivery 664.5 ☑5ᵗʰ
　perirenal, cystic 593.81
　pinna 380.31
　placenta — *see* Placenta, abnormal
　postoperative 998.12
　retroperitoneal (nontraumatic) 568.81
　　traumatic — *see* Injury, internal, retroperitoneum
　retropubic, male 568.81
　scalp (and neck, or face any part, except eye) 920
　　fetus or newborn 767.1
　scrotum (nontraumatic) 608.83
　　traumatic 922.4
　seminal vesicle (nontraumatic) 608.83
　　traumatic — *see* Injury, internal, seminal, vesicle
　spermatic cord — *see also* Injury, internal, spermatic cord
　　nontraumatic 608.83
　spinal (cord) (meninges) — *see also* Injury, spinal, by site
　　fetus or newborn 767.4
　　nontraumatic 336.1
　spleen 865.01
　　with
　　　laceration — *see* Laceration, spleen
　　　open wound into cavity 865.11

Hematoma — *see also* Contusion — *continued*
　sternocleidomastoid, birth injury 767.8
　sternomastoid, birth injury 767.8
　subarachnoid — *see also* Hematoma, brain, subarachnoid
　　fetus or newborn 772.2
　　nontraumatic (*see also* Hemorrhage, subarachnoid) 430
　　newborn 772.2
　subdural — *see also* Hematoma, brain, subdural
　　fetus or newborn (localized) 767.0
　　nontraumatic (*see also* Hemorrhage, subdural) 432.1
　subperiosteal (syndrome) 267
　　traumatic — *see* Hematoma, by site
　superficial, fetus or newborn 772.6
　syncytium — *see* Placenta, abnormal
　testis (nontraumatic) 608.83
　　birth injury 767.8
　　traumatic 922.4
　tunica vaginalis (nontraumatic) 608.83
　umbilical cord 663.6 ☑5ᵗʰ
　　affecting fetus or newborn 762.6
　uterine ligament (nontraumatic) 620.7
　　traumatic — *see* Injury, internal, pelvis
　uterus 621.4
　　traumatic — *see* Injury, internal, pelvis
　vagina (nontraumatic) (ruptured) 623.6
　　complicating delivery 665.7 ☑5ᵗʰ
　　traumatic 922.4
　vas deferens (nontraumatic) 608.83
　　traumatic — *see* Injury, internal, vas deferens
　vitreous 379.23
　vocal cord 920
　vulva (nontraumatic) 624.5
　　complicating delivery 664.5 ☑5ᵗʰ
　　fetus or newborn 767.8
　　traumatic 922.4

Hematometra 621.4

Hematomyelia 336.1
　with fracture of vertebra (*see also* Fracture, vertebra, by site, with spinal cord injury) 806.8
　fetus or newborn 767.4

Hematomyelitis 323.9
　late effect — *see* category 326

Hematoperitoneum (*see also* Hemoperitoneum) 568.81

Hematopneumothorax (*see also* Hemothorax) 511.8

Hematoporphyria (acquired) (congenital) 277.1

Hematoporphyrinuria (acquired) (congenital) 277.1

Hematorachis, hematorrhachis 336.1
　fetus or newborn 767.4

Hematosalpinx 620.8
　with
　　ectopic pregnancy (*see also* categories 633.0-633.9) 639.2
　　molar pregnancy (*see also* categories 630-632) 639.2
　　infectional (*see also* Salpingo-oophoritis) 614.2

Hematospermia 608.82

Hematothorax (*see also* Hemothorax) 511.8

Hematotympanum 381.03

Hematuria (benign) (essential) (idiopathic) 599.7
　due to S. hematobium 120.0
　endemic 120.0
　intermittent 599.7
　malarial 084.8
　paroxysmal 599.7
　sulfonamide
　　correct substance properly administered 599.7
　　overdose or wrong substance given or taken 961.0
　tropical (bilharziasis) 120.0
　tuberculous (*see also* Tuberculosis) 016.9 ☑5ᵗʰ

Hematuric bilious fever 084.8

Hemeralopia 368.10　　　　　　　　　　　▲

☑4ᵗʰ Fourth-digit Required　　☑5ᵗʰ Fifth-digit Required　　►◄ Revised Text　　● New Line　　▲ Revised Code

Hemiabiotrophy 799.8
Hemi-akinesia 781.8
Hemianalgesia (see also Disturbance, sensation) 782.0
Hemianencephaly 740.0
Hemianesthesia (see also Disturbance, sensation) 782.0
Hemianopia, hemianopsia (altitudinal) (homonymous) 368.46
  binasal 368.47
  bitemporal 368.47
  heteronymous 368.47
  syphilitic 095.8
Hemiasomatognosia 307.9
Hemiathetosis 781.0
Hemiatrophy 799.8
  cerebellar 334.8
  face 349.89
    progressive 349.89
  fascia 728.9
  leg 728.2
  tongue 529.8
Hemiballism(us) 333.5
Hemiblock (cardiac) (heart) (left) 426.2
Hemicardia 746.89
Hemicephalus, hemicephaly 740.0
Hemichorea 333.5
Hemicrania 346.9 ✓5ᵗʰ
  congenital malformation 740.0
Hemidystrophy — see Hemiatrophy
Hemiectromelia 755.4
Hemihypalgesia (see also Disturbance, sensation) 782.0
Hemihypertrophy (congenital) 759.89
  cranial 756.0
Hemihypesthesia (see also Disturbance, sensation) 782.0
Hemi-inattention 781.8
Hemimelia 755.4
  lower limb 755.30
    paraxial (complete) (incomplete) (intercalary) (terminal) 755.32
      fibula 755.37
      tibia 755.36
    transverse (complete) (partial) 755.31
  upper limb 755.20
    paraxial (complete) (incomplete) (intercalary) (terminal) 755.22
      radial 755.26
      ulnar 755.27
    transverse (complete) (partial) 755.21
Hemiparalysis (see also Hemiplegia) 342.9 ✓5ᵗʰ
Hemiparesis (see also Hemiplegia) 342.9 ✓5ᵗʰ
Hemiparesthesia (see also Disturbance, sensation) 782.0
Hemiplegia 342.9 ✓5ᵗʰ
  acute (see also Disease, cerebrovascular, acute) 436
  alternans facialis 344.89
  apoplectic (see also Disease, cerebrovascular, acute) 436
    late effect or residual
      affecting
        dominant side 438.21
        nondominant side 438.22
        unspecified side 438.20
  arteriosclerotic 437.0
    late effect or residual
      affecting
        dominant side 438.21
        nondominant side 438.22
        unspecified side 438.20
  ascending (spinal) NEC 344.89
  attack (see also Disease, cerebrovascular, acute) 436
  brain, cerebral (current episode) 437.8
    congenital 343.1
  cerebral — see Hemiplegia, brain
  congenital (cerebral) (spastic) (spinal) 343.1
  conversion neurosis (hysterical) 300.11

Hemiplegia — continued
  cortical — see Hemiplegia, brain
  due to
    arteriosclerosis 437.0
      late effect or residual
        affecting
          dominant side 438.21
          nondominant side 438.22
          unspecified side 438.20
    cerebrovascular lesion (see also Disease, cerebrovascular, acute) 436
      late effect
        affecting
          dominant side 438.21
          nondominant side 438.22
          unspecified side 438.20
  embolic (current) (see also Embolism, brain) 434.1 ✓5ᵗʰ
    late effect
      affecting
        dominant side 438.21
        nondominant side 438.22
        unspecified side 438.20
  flaccid 342.0
  hypertensive (current episode) 437.8
  infantile (postnatal) 343.4
  late effect
    birth injury, intracranial or spinal 343.4
    cerebrovascular lesion — see Late effect(s) (of) cerebrovascular disease
    viral encephalitis 139.0
  middle alternating NEC 344.89
  newborn NEC 767.0
  seizure (current episode) (see also Disease, cerebrovascular, acute) 436
  spastic 342.1
    congenital or infantile 343.1
  specified NEC 342.8
  thrombotic (current) (see also Thrombosis, brain) 434.0 ✓5ᵗʰ
    late effect — see Late effect(s) (of) cerebrovascular disease
Hemisection, spinal cord — see Fracture, vertebra, by site, with spinal cord injury
Hemispasm 781.0
  facial 781.0
Hemispatial neglect 781.8
Hemisporosis 117.9
Hemitremor 781.0
Hemivertebra 756.14
Hemobilia 576.8
Hemocholecyst 575.8
Hemochromatosis (acquired) (diabetic) (hereditary) (liver) (myocardium) (primary idiopathic) (secondary) 275.0
  with refractory anemia 285.0
Hemodialysis V56.0
Hemoglobin — see also condition
  abnormal (disease) — see Disease, hemoglobin
  AS genotype 282.5
  fetal, hereditary persistence 282.7
  high-oxygen-affinity 289.0
  low NEC 285.9
  S (Hb-S), heterozygous 282.5
Hemoglobinemia 283.2
  due to blood transfusion NEC 999.8
    bone marrow 996.85
  paroxysmal 283.2
Hemoglobinopathy (mixed) (see also Disease, hemoblobin) 282.7
  with thalassemia 282.4
  sickle-cell 282.60
    with thalassemia 282.4
Hemoglobinuria, hemoglobinuric 791.2
  with anemia, hemolytic, acquired (chronic) NEC 283.2
  cold (agglutinin) (paroxysmal) (with Raynaud's syndrome) 283.2
  due to
    exertion 283.2
    hemolysis (from external causes) NEC 283.2
  exercise 283.2
  fever (malaria) 084.8
  infantile 791.2

Hemoglobinuria, hemoglobinuric — continued
  intermittent 283.2
  malarial 084.8
  march 283.2
  nocturnal (paroxysmal) 283.2
  paroxysmal (cold) (nocturnal) 283.2
Hemolymphangioma (M9175/0) 228.1
Hemolysis
  fetal — see Jaundice, fetus or newborn
  intravascular (disseminated) NEC 286.6
    with
      abortion — see Abortion, by type, with hemorrhage, delayed or excessive
      ectopic pregnancy (see also categories 633.0-633.9) 639.1
      hemorrhage of pregnancy 641.3 ✓5ᵗʰ
        affecting fetus or newborn 762.1
      molar pregnancy (see also categories 630-632) 639.1
    acute 283.2
    following
      abortion 639.1
      ectopic or molar pregnancy 639.1
  neonatal — see Jaundice, fetus or newborn
  transfusion NEC 999.8
    bone marrow 996.85
Hemolytic — see also condition
  anemia — see Anemia, hemolytic
  uremic syndrome 283.11
Hemometra 621.4
Hemopericardium (with effusion) 423.0
  newborn 772.8
  traumatic (see also Hemothorax, traumatic) 860.2
    with open wound into thorax 860.3
Hemoperitoneum 568.81
  infectional (see also Peritonitis) 567.2
  traumatic — see Injury, internal, peritoneum
Hemophilia (familial) (hereditary) 286.0
  A 286.0
    carrier (asymptomatic) V83.01
      symptomatic V83.02
  acquired 286.5 ●
  B (Leyden) 286.1
  C 286.2
  calcipriva (see also Fibrinolysis) 286.7
  classical 286.0
  nonfamilial 286.7
  vascular 286.4
Hemophilus influenzae NEC 041.5
  arachnoiditis (basic) (brain) (spinal) 320.0
    late effect — see category 326
  bronchopneumonia 482.2
  cerebral ventriculitis 320.0
    late effect — see category 326
  cerebrospinal inflammation 320.0
    late effect — see category 326
  infection NEC 041.5
  leptomeningitis 320.0
    late effect — see category 326
  meningitis (cerebral) (cerebrospinal) (spinal) 320.0
    late effect — see category 326
  meningomyelitis 320.0
    late effect — see category 326
  pachymeningitis (adhesive) (fibrous) (hemorrhagic) (hypertrophic) (spinal) 320.0
    late effect — see category 326
  pneumonia (broncho-) 482.2
Hemophthalmos 360.43
Hemopneumothorax (see also Hemothorax) 511.8
  traumatic 860.4
    with open wound into thorax 860.5
Hemoptysis 786.3
  due to Paragonimus (westermani) 121.2
  newborn 770.3
  tuberculous (see also Tuberculosis, pulmonary) 011.9 ✓5ᵗʰ
Hemorrhage, hemorrhagic (nontraumatic) 459.0
  abdomen 459.0
  accidental (antepartum) 641.2 ✓5ᵗʰ
    affecting fetus or newborn 762.1
  adenoid 474.8

Hemorrhage, hemorrhagic — *continued*
 adrenal (capsule) (gland) (medulla) 255.4
  newborn 772.5
 after labor — *see* Hemorrhage, postpartum
 alveolar
  lung, newborn 770.3
  process 525.8
 alveolus 525.8
 amputation stump (surgical) 998.11
  secondary, delayed 997.69
 anemia (chronic) 280.0
  acute 285.1
 antepartum — *see* Hemorrhage, pregnancy
 anus (sphincter) 569.3
 apoplexy (stroke) 432.9
 arachnoid — *see* Hemorrhage, subarachnoid
 artery NEC 459.0
  brain (*see also* Hemorrhage, brain) 431
  middle meningeal — *see* Hemorrhage,
   subarachnoid
 basilar (ganglion) (*see also* Hemorrhage, brain)
  431
 bladder 596.8
 blood dyscrasia 289.9
 bowel 578.9
  newborn 772.4
 brain (miliary) (nontraumatic) 431
  with
   birth injury 767.0
   arachnoid — *see* Hemorrhage, subarachnoid
   due to
    birth injury 767.0
    rupture of aneurysm (congenital) (*see
     also* Hemorrhage, subarachnoid)
     430
     mycotic 431
    syphilis 094.89
   epidural or extradural — *see* Hemorrhage,
    extradural
   fetus or newborn (anoxic) (hypoxic) (due to
    birth trauma) (nontraumatic) 767.0
    intraventricular 772.10
     grade I 772.11
     grade II 772.12
     grade III 772.13
     grade IV 772.14
   iatrogenic 997.02
   postoperative 997.02
   puerperal, postpartum, childbirth 674.0 ✓5ᵗʰ
   stem 431
   subarachnoid, arachnoid, or meningeal —
    see Hemorrhage, subarachnoid
   subdural — *see* Hemorrhage, subdural
   traumatic NEC 853.0 ✓5ᵗʰ

Note — *Use the following fifth-digit
subclassification with categories 851-854:*

 0   unspecified state of consciousness

 1   with no loss of consciousness

 *2   with brief [less than one hour] loss of
      consciousness*

 *3   with moderate [1-24 hours] loss of
      consciousness*

 *4   with prolonged [more than 24 hours]
      loss of consciousness and return to
      pre-existing conscious level*

 *5   with prolonged [more than 24 hours]
      loss of consciousness, without return
      to pre-existing conscious level*

 *Use fifth-digit 5 to designate when a patient
 is unconscious and dies before
 regaining consciousness, regardless
 of the duration of the loss of
 consciousness*

 *6   with loss of consciousness of
      unspecified duration*

 9   with concussion, unspecified

---

   with
    cerebral
     contusion — *see* Contusion, brain
     laceration — *see* Laceration, brain
    open intracranial wound 853.1 ✓5ᵗʰ
    skull fracture — *see* Fracture, skull,
     by site

Hemorrhage, hemorrhagic — *continued*
 brain — *continued*
  traumatic NEC — *continued*
   extradural or epidural 852.4 ✓5ᵗʰ
    with open intracranial wound
     852.5 ✓5ᵗʰ
   subarachnoid 852.0 ✓5ᵗʰ
    with open intracranial wound
     852.1 ✓5ᵗʰ
   subdural 852.2 ✓5ᵗʰ
    with open intracranial wound
     852.3 ✓5ᵗʰ
 breast 611.79
 bronchial tube — *see* Hemorrhage, lung
 bronchopulmonary — *see* Hemorrhage, lung
 bronchus (cause unknown) (*see also*
  Hemorrhage, lung) 786.3
 bulbar (*see also* Hemorrhage, brain) 431
 bursa 727.89
 capillary 448.9
  primary 287.8
 capsular — *see* Hemorrhage, brain
 cardiovascular 429.89
 cecum 578.9
 cephalic (*see also* Hemorrhage, brain) 431
 cerebellar (*see also* Hemorrhage, brain) 431
 cerebellum (*see also* Hemorrhage, brain) 431
 cerebral (*see also* Hemorrhage, brain) 431
  fetus or newborn (anoxic) (traumatic) 767.0
 cerebromeningeal (*see also* Hemorrhage, brain)
  431
 cerebrospinal (*see also* Hemorrhage, brain) 431
 cerebrum (*see also* Hemorrhage, brain) 431
 cervix (stump) (uteri) 622.8
 cesarean section wound 674.3 ✓5ᵗʰ
 chamber, anterior (eye) 364.41
 childbirth — *see* Hemorrhage, complicating,
  delivery
 choroid 363.61
  expulsive 363.62
 ciliary body 364.41
 cochlea 386.8
 colon — *see* Hemorrhage, intestine
 complicating
  delivery 641.9 ✓5ᵗʰ
   affecting fetus or newborn 762.1
   associated with
    afibrinogenemia 641.3 ✓5ᵗʰ
     affecting fetus or newborn 763.89
    coagulation defect 641.3 ✓5ᵗʰ
     affecting fetus or newborn 763.89
    hyperfibrinolysis 641.3 ✓5ᵗʰ
     affecting fetus or newborn 763.89
    hypofibrinogenemia 641.3 ✓5ᵗʰ
     affecting fetus or newborn 763.89
   due to
    low-lying placenta 641.1 ✓5ᵗʰ
     affecting fetus or newborn 762.0
    placenta previa 641.1 ✓5ᵗʰ
     affecting fetus or newborn 762.0
    premature separation of placenta
     641.2 ✓5ᵗʰ
     affecting fetus or newborn 762.1
    retained
     placenta 666.0 ✓5ᵗʰ
     secundines 666.2 ✓5ᵗʰ
    trauma 641.8 ✓5ᵗʰ
     affecting fetus or newborn 763.89
    uterine leiomyoma 641.8 ✓5ᵗʰ
     affecting fetus or newborn 763.89
  surgical procedure 998.11
 concealed NEC 459.0
 congenital 772.9
 conjunctiva 372.72
  newborn 772.8
 cord, newborn 772.0
  slipped ligature 772.3
  stump 772.3
 corpus luteum (ruptured) 620.1
 cortical (*see also* Hemorrhage, brain) 431
 cranial 432.9
 cutaneous 782.7
  newborn 772.6
 cyst, pancreas 577.2
 cystitis — *see* Cystitis

Hemorrhage, hemorrhagic — *continued*
 delayed
  with
   abortion — *see* Abortion, by type, with
    hemorrhage, delayed or excessive
   ectopic pregnancy (*see also* categories
    633.0-633.9) 639.1
   molar pregnancy (*see also* categories 630-
    632) 639.1
  following
   abortion 639.1
   ectopic or molar pregnancy 639.1
  postpartum 666.2 ✓5ᵗʰ
 diathesis (familial) 287.9
  newborn 776.0
 disease 287.9
  newborn 776.0
  specified type NEC 287.8
 disorder 287.9
  due to circulating anticoagulants 286.5
  specified type NEC 287.8
 due to
  any device, implant or graft (presence of)
   classifiable to 996.0-996.5 — *see*
   Complications, due to (presence of)
   any device, implant, or graft classified
   to 996.0-996.5 NEC
  circulating anticoagulant 286.5
 duodenum, duodenal 537.89
  ulcer — *see* Ulcer, duodenum, with
   hemorrhage
 dura mater — *see* Hemorrhage, subdural
 endotracheal — *see* Hemorrhage, lung
 epidural — *see* Hemorrhage, extradural
 episiotomy 674.3 ✓5ᵗʰ
 esophagus 530.82
  varix (*see also* Varix, esophagus, bleeding)
   456.0
 excessive
  with
   abortion — *see* Abortion, by type, with
    hemorrhage, delayed or excessive
   ectopic pregnancy (*see also* categories
    633.0-633.9) 639.1
   molar pregnancy (*see also* categories 630-
    632) 639.1
  following
   abortion 639.1
   ectopic or molar pregnancy 639.1
 external 459.0
 extradural (traumatic) — *see also* Hemorrhage,
  brain, traumatic, extradural
  birth injury 767.0
  fetus or newborn (anoxic) (traumatic) 767.0
  nontraumatic 432.0
 eye 360.43
  chamber (anterior) (aqueous) 364.41
  fundus 362.81
 eyelid 374.81
 fallopian tube 620.8
 fetomaternal 772.0
  affecting management of pregnancy or
   puerperium 656.0 ✓5ᵗʰ
 fetus, fetal 772.0
  from
   cut end of co-twin's cord 772.0
   placenta 772.0
   ruptured cord 772.0
   vasa previa 772.0
  into
   co-twin 772.0
   mother's circulation 772.0
    affecting management of pregnancy or
     puerperium 656.0 ✓5ᵗʰ
 fever (*see also* Fever, hemorrhagic) 065.9
  with renal syndrome 078.6
  arthropod-borne NEC 065.9
  Bangkok 065.4
  Crimean 065.0
  dengue virus 065.4
  epidemic 078.6
  Junin virus 078.7
  Korean 078.6
  Machupo virus 078.7
  mite-borne 065.8
  mosquito-borne 065.4
  Philippine 065.4

Hemorrhage, hemorrhagic — *continued*
  fever (*see also* Fever, hemorrhagic) — *continued*
    Russian (Yaroslav) 078.6
    Singapore 065.4
    southeast Asia 065.4
    Thailand 065.4
    tick-borne NEC 065.3
  fibrinogenolysis (*see also* Fibrinolysis) 286.6
  fibrinolytic (acquired) (*see also* Fibrinolysis)
    286.6
  fontanel 767.1
  from tracheostomy stoma 519.09
  fundus, eye 362.81
  funis
    affecting fetus or newborn 772.0
    complicating delivery 663.8 ✓5ᵗʰ
  gastric (*see also* Hemorrhage, stomach) 578.9
  gastroenteric 578.9
    newborn 772.4
  gastrointestinal (tract) 578.9
    newborn 772.4
  genitourinary (tract) NEC 599.89
  gingiva 523.8
  globe 360.43
  gravidarum — *see* Hemorrhage, pregnancy
  gum 523.8
  heart 429.89
  hypopharyngeal (throat) 784.8
  intermenstrual 626.6
    irregular 626.6
    regular 626.5
  internal (organs) 459.0
    capsule (*see also* Hemorrhage, brain) 431
    ear 386.8
    newborn 772.8
  intestine 578.9
    congenital 772.4
    newborn 772.4
  into
    bladder wall 596.7
    bursa 727.89
    corpus luysii (*see also* Hemorrhage, brain)
      431
  intra-abdominal 459.0
    during or following surgery 998.11
  intra-alveolar, newborn (lung) 770.3
  intracerebral (*see also* Hemorrhage, brain) 431
  intracranial NEC 432.9
    puerperal, postpartum, childbirth 674.0 ✓5ᵗʰ
    traumatic — *see* Hemorrhage, brain,
      traumatic
  intramedullary NEC 336.1
  intraocular 360.43
  intraoperative 998.11
  intrapartum — *see* Hemorrhage, complicating,
      delivery
  intrapelvic
    female 629.8
    male 459.0
  intraperitoneal 459.0
  intrapontine (*see also* Hemorrhage, brain) 431
  intrauterine 621.4
    complicating delivery — *see* Hemorrhage,
      complicating, delivery
    in pregnancy or childbirth — *see*
      Hemorrhage, pregnancy
    postpartum (*see also* Hemorrhage,
      postpartum) 666.1 ✓5ᵗʰ
  intraventricular (*see also* Hemorrhage, brain)
      431
    fetus or newborn (anoxic) (traumatic) 772.10
      grade I 772.11
      grade II 772.12
      grade III 772.13
      grade IV 772.14
  intravesical 596.7
  iris (postinfectional) (postinflammatory) (toxic)
      364.41
  joint (nontraumatic) 719.10
    ankle 719.17
    elbow 719.12
    foot 719.17
    forearm 719.13
    hand 719.14
    hip 719.15
    knee 719.16
    lower leg 719.16
    multiple sites 719.19

Hemorrhage, hemorrhagic — *continued*
  joint — *continued*
    pelvic region 719.15
    shoulder (region) 719.11
    specified site NEC 719.18
    thigh 719.15
    upper arm 719.12
    wrist 719.13
  kidney 593.81
  knee (joint) 719.16
  labyrinth 386.8
  leg NEC 459.0
  lenticular striate artery (*see also* Hemorrhage,
      brain) 431
  ligature, vessel 998.11
  liver 573.8
  lower extremity NEC 459.0
  lung 786.3
    newborn 770.3
    tuberculous (*see also* Tuberculosis,
      pulmonary) 011.9 ✓5ᵗʰ
  malaria 084.8
  marginal sinus 641.2 ✓5ᵗʰ
  massive subaponeurotic, birth injury 767.1
  maternal, affecting fetus or newborn 762.1
  mediastinum 786.3
  medulla (*see also* Hemorrhage, brain) 431
  membrane (brain) (*see also* Hemorrhage,
      subarachnoid) 430
    spinal cord — *see* Hemorrhage, spinal cord
  meninges, meningeal (brain) (middle) (*see also*
      Hemorrhage, subarachnoid) 430
    spinal cord — *see* Hemorrhage, spinal cord
  mesentery 568.81
  metritis 626.8
  midbrain (*see also* Hemorrhage, brain) 431
  mole 631
  mouth 528.9
  mucous membrane NEC 459.0
    newborn 728.8 ✓5ᵗʰ
  muscle 728.89
  nail (subungual) 703.8
  nasal turbinate 784.7
    newborn 772.8
  nasopharynx 478.29
  navel, newborn 772.3
  newborn 772.9
    adrenal 772.5
    alveolar (lung) 770.3
    brain (anoxic) (hypoxic) (due to birth
      trauma) 767.0
    cerebral (anoxic) (hypoxic) (due to birth
      trauma) 767.0
    conjunctiva 772.8
    cutaneous 772.6
    diathesis 776.0
    due to vitamin K deficiency 776.0
    gastrointestinal 772.4
    internal (organs) 772.8
    intestines 772.4
    intra-alveolar (lung) 770.3
    intracranial (from any perinatal cause) 767.0
    intraventricular (from any perinatal cause)
      772.10
      grade I 772.11
      grade II 772.12
      grade III 772.13
      grade IV 772.14
    lung 770.3
    pulmonary (massive) 770.3
    spinal cord, traumatic 767.4
    stomach 772.4
    subaponeurotic (massive) 767.1
    subarachnoid (from any perinatal cause)
      772.2
    subconjunctival 772.8
    umbilicus 772.0
      slipped ligature 772.3
      vasa previa 772.0
  nipple 611.79
  nose 784.7
    newborn 772.8
  obstetrical surgical wound 674.3 ✓5ᵗʰ
  omentum 568.89
    newborn 772.4
  optic nerve (sheath) 377.42
  orbit 376.32
  ovary 620.1

Hemorrhage, hemorrhagic — *continued*
  oviduct 620.8
  pancreas 577.8
  parathyroid (gland) (spontaneous) 252.8
  parturition — *see* Hemorrhage, complicating,
      delivery
  penis 607.82
  pericardium, paricarditis 423.0
  perineal wound (obstetrical) 674.3 ✓5ᵗʰ
  peritoneum, peritoneal 459.0
  peritonsillar tissue 474.8
    after operation on tonsils 998.11
    due to infection 475
  petechial 782.7
  pituitary (gland) 253.8
  placenta NEC 641.9 ✓5ᵗʰ
    affecting fetus or newborn 762.1
    from surgical or instrumental damage
      641.8 ✓5ᵗʰ
      affecting fetus or newborn 762.1
    previa 641.8 ✓5ᵗʰ
      affecting fetus or newborn 762.0
  pleura — *see* Hemorrhage, lung
  polioencephalitis, superior 265.1
  polymyositis — *see* Polymyositis
  pons (*see also* Hemorrhage, brain) 431
  pontine (*see also* Hemorrhage, brain) 431
  popliteal 459.0
  postcoital 626.7
  postextraction (dental) 998.11
  postmenopausal 627.1
  postnasal 784.7
  postoperative 998.11
  postpartum (atonic) (following delivery of
      placenta) 666. ✓5ᵗʰ
    delayed or secondary (after 24 hours)
      666.2 ✓5ᵗʰ
    retained placenta 666.0 ✓5ᵗʰ
    third stage 666.0 ✓5ᵗʰ
  pregnancy (concealed) 641.9 ✓5ᵗʰ
    accidental 641.2 ✓5ᵗʰ
      affecting fetus or newborn 762.1
    affecting fetus or newborn 762.1
    before 22 completed weeks gestation
      640.9 ✓5ᵗʰ
      affecting fetus or newborn 762.1
    due to
      abruptio placenta 641.2 ✓5ᵗʰ
        affecting fetus or newborn 762.1
      afibrinogenemia or other coagulation
        defect (conditions classifiable to
        286.0-286.9) 641.3 ✓5ᵗʰ
        affecting fetus or newborn 762.1
      coagulation defect 641.3 ✓5ᵗʰ
        affecting fetus or newborn 762.1
      hyperfibrinolysis 641.3 ✓5ᵗʰ
        affecting fetus or newborn 762.1
      hypofibrinogenemia 641.3 ✓5ᵗʰ
        affecting fetus or newborn 762.1
      leiomyoma, uterus 641.8 ✓5ᵗʰ
        affecting fetus or newborn 762.1
      low-lying placenta 641.1 ✓5ᵗʰ
        affecting fetus or newborn 762.1
      marginal sinus (rupture) 641.2 ✓5ᵗʰ
        affecting fetus or newborn 762.1
      placenta previa 641.1 ✓5ᵗʰ
        affecting fetus or newborn 762.0
      premature separation of placenta
        (normally implanted) 641.2 ✓5ᵗʰ
        affecting fetus or newborn 762.1
      threatend abortion 640.0 ✓5ᵗʰ
        affecting fetus or newborn 762.1
      trauma 641.8 ✓5ᵗʰ
        affecting fetus or newborn 762.1
    early (before 22 completed weeks gestation)
      640.9 ✓5ᵗʰ
      affecting fetus or newborn 762.1
    previous, affecting management of
      pregnancy or childbirth V23.49   ▲
    unavoidable — *see* Hemorrhage, pregnancy,
      due to placenta previa
  prepartum (mother) — *see* Hemorrhage,
      pregnancy
  preretinal, cause unspecified 362.81
  prostate 602.1
  puerperal (*see also* Hemorrhage, postpartum)
      666.1 ✓5ᵗʰ

✓4ᵗʰ Fourth-digit Required   ✓5ᵗʰ Fifth-digit Required   ▶◀ Revised Text   ● New Line   ▲ Revised Code

Hepatitis — continued
  infectious, infective (acute) (chronic) (subacute)
      070.1
    with hepatic coma 070.0
  inoculation — see Hepatitis, viral
  interstitial (chronic) 571.49
    acute 570
  lupoid 571.49
  malarial 084.9 [573.2]
  malignant (see also Necrosis, liver) 570
  neonatal (toxic) 774.4
  newborn 774.4
  parenchymatous (acute) (see also Necrosis,
      liver) 570
  peliosis 573.3
  persistent, chronic 571.41
  plasma cell 571.49
  postimmunization — see Hepatitis, viral
  postnecrotic 571.49
  posttransfusion — see Hepatitis, viral
  recurrent 571.49
  septic 573.3
  serum — see Hepatitis, viral
    carrier (suspected of) V02.61
  subacute (see also Necrosis, liver) 570
  suppurative (diffuse) 572.0
  syphilitic (late) 095.3
    congenital (early) 090.0 [573.2]
      late 090.5 [573.2]
    secondary 091.62
  toxic (noninfectious) 573.3
    fetus or newborn 774.4
  tuberculous (see also Tuberculosis) 017.9 ✓5ᵗʰ
  viral (acute) (anicteric) (cholangiolitic)
      (cholestatic) (chronic) (subacute) 070.9
    with hepatic coma 070.6
    AU-SH type virus — see Hepatitis, viral, type
        B
    Australian antigen — see Hepatitis, viral,
        type B
    B-antigen — see Hepatitis, viral, type B
    Coxsackie 074.8 [573.1]
    cytomegalic inclusion 078.5 [573.1]
    IH (virus) — see Hepatitis, viral, type A
    infectious hepatitis, viral, type A
    serum hepatitis virus — see Hepatitis, viral,
        type B
    SH — see Hepatitis, viral, type B
    specified type NEC 070.59
      with hepatic coma 070.49
    type A 070.1
      with hepatic coma 070.0
    type B (acute) 070.30
      with
        hepatic coma 070.20
          with hepatitis delta 070.21
        hepatitis delta 070.31
          with hepatic coma 070.21
      carrier status V02.61
      chronic 070.32
        with
          hepatic coma 070.22
            with hepatitis delta 070.23
          hepatitis delta 070.33
            with hepatic coma 070.23
    type C (acute) 070.51
      with hepatic coma 070.41
      carrier status V02.62
      chronic 070.54
        with hepatic coma 070.44
    type delta (with hepatitis B carrier state)
        070.52
      with
        active hepatitis B disease — see
            Hepatitis, viral, type B
        hepatic coma 070.42
    type E 070.53
      with hepatic coma 070.43
    vaccination and inoculation (prophylactic)
        V05.3
    Waldenstrom's (lupoid hepatitis) 571.49
Hepatization, lung (acute) — see also
      Pneumonia, lobar
    chronic (see also Fibrosis, lung) 515
Hepatoblastoma (M8970/3) 155.0
Hepatocarcinoma (M8170/3) 155.0
Hepatocholangiocarcinoma (M8180/3) 155.0

Hepatocholangioma, benign (M8180/0) 211.5
Hepatocholangitis 573.8
Hepatocystitis (see also Cholecystitis) 575.10
Hepatodystrophy 570
Hepatolenticular degeneration 275.1
Hepatolithiasis — see Choledocholithiasis
Hepatoma (malignant) (M8170/3) 155.0
    benign (M8170/0) 211.5
    congenital (M8970/3) 155.0
    embryonal (M8970/3) 155.0
Hepatomegalia glycogenica diffusa 271.0
Hepatomegaly (see also Hypertrophy, liver) 789.1
    congenital 751.69
      syphilitic 090.0
    due to Clonorchis sinensis 121.1
    Gaucher's 272.7
    syphilitic (congenital) 090.0
Hepatoptosis 573.8
Hepatorrhexis 573.8
Hepatosis, toxic 573.8
Hepatosplenomegaly 571.8
    due to S. japonicum 120.2
    hyperlipemic (Burger-Grutz type) 272.3
Herald patch 696.3
Hereditary — see condition
Heredodegeneration 330.9
    macular 362.70
Heredopathia atactica polyneuritiformis 356.3
Heredosyphilis (see also Syphilis, congenital)
      090.9 ✓5ᵗʰ
Hermaphroditism (true) 752.7
    with specified chromosomal anomaly — see
        Anomaly, chromosomes, sex
Hernia, hernial (acquired) (recurrent) 553.9
    with
      gangrene (obstructed) NEC 551.9
      obstruction NEC 552.9
        and gangrene 551.9
    abdomen (wall) — see Hernia, ventral
    abdominal, specified site NEC 553.8
      with
        gangrene (obstructed) 551.8
        obstruction 552.8
          and gangrene 551.8
    appendix 553.8
      with
        gangrene (obstructed) 551.8
        obstruction 552.8
          and gangrene 551.8
    bilateral (inguinal) — see Hernia, inguinal
    bladder (sphincter)
      congenital (female) (male) 756.71
      female 618.0
      male 596.8
    brain 348.4
      congenital 742.0
    broad ligament 553.8
    cartilage, vertebral — see Displacement,
        intervertebral disc
    cerebral 348.4
      congenital 742.0
      endaural 742.0
    ciliary body 364.8
      traumatic 871.1
    colic 553.9
      with
        gangrene (obstructed) 551.9
        obstruction 552.9
          and gangrene 551.9
    colon 553.9
      with
        gangrene (obstructed) 551.9
        obstruction 552.9
          and gangrene 551.9
    colostomy (stoma) 569.69
    Cooper's (retroperitoneal) 553.8
      with
        gangrene (obstructed) 551.8
        obstruction 552.8
          and gangrene 551.8
    crural — see Hernia, femoral

Hernia, hernial — continued
  diaphragm, diaphragmatic 553.3
    with
      gangrene (obstructed) 551.3
      obstruction 552.3
        and gangrene 551.3
    congenital 756.6
    due to gross defect of diaphragm 756.6
    traumatic 862.0
      with open wound into cavity 862.1
  direct (inguinal) — see Hernia, inguinal
  disc, intervertebral — see Displacement,
      intervertebral disc
  diverticulum, intestine 553.9
    with
      gangrene (obstructed) 551.9
      obstruction 552.9
        and gangrene 551.9
  double (inguinal) — see Hernia, inguinal
  duodenojejunal 553.8
    with
      gangrene (obstructed) 551.8
      obstruction 552.8
        and gangrene 551.8
  en glissade — see Hernia, inguinal
  enterostomy (stoma) 569.69
  epigastric 553.29
    with
      gangrene (obstruction) 551.29
      obstruction 552.29
        and gangrene 551.29
    recurrent 553.21
      with
        gangrene (obstructed) 551.21
        obstruction 552.21
          and gangrene 551.21
  esophageal hiatus (sliding) 553.3
    with
      gangrene (obstructed) 551.3
      obstruction 552.3
        and gangrene 551.3
    congenital 750.6
  external (inguinal) — see Hernia, inguinal
  fallopian tube 620.4
  fascia 728.89
  fat 729.30
    eyelid 374.34
    orbital 374.34
    pad 729.30
      eye, eyelid 374.34
      knee 729.31
      orbit 374.34
      popliteal (space) 729.31
      specified site NEC 729.39
  femoral (unilateral) 553.00
    with
      gangrene (obstructed) 551.00
      obstruction 552.00
        with gangrene 551.0 ✓5ᵗʰ
    bilateral 553.02
      gangrenous (obstructed) 551.02
      obstructed 552.02
        with gangrene 551.02
      recurrent 553.03
        gangrenous (obstructed) 551.03
        obstructed 552.03
          with gangrene 551.03
    recurrent (unilateral) 553.01
      bilateral 553.03
        gangrenous (obstructed) 551.03
        obstructed 552.03
          with gangrene 551.03
      gangrenous (obstructed) 551.01
      obstructed 552.01
        with gangrene
  foramen
    Bochdalek 553.3
      with
        gangrene (obstructed) 551.3
        obstruction 552.3
          and gangrene 551.3
      congenital 756.6
    magnum 348.4
    Morgagni, Morgagnian 553.3
      with
        gangrene 551.3

Hernia, hernial — *continued*
  foramen — *continued*
    Morgagni, Morgagnian — *continued*
      with — *continued*
        obstruction 552.3
          and gangrene 551.3
      congenital 756.6
  funicular (umbilical) 553.1
    with
      gangrene (obstructed) 551.1
      obstruction 552.1
        and gangrene 551.1
    spermatic cord — *see* Hernia, inguinal
  gangrenous — *see* Hernia, by site, with
    gangrene
  gastrointestinal tract 553.9
    with
      gangrene (obstructed) 551.9
      obstruction 552.9
        and gangrene 551.9
  gluteal — *see* Hernia, femoral
  Gruber's (internal mesogastric) 553.8
    with
      gangrene (obstructed) 551.8
      obstruction 552.8
        and gangrene 551.8
  Hesselbach's 553.8
    with
      gangrene (obstructed) 551.8
      obstruction 552.8
        and gangrene 551.8
  hiatal (esophageal) (sliding) 553.3
    with
      gangrene (obstructed) 551.3
      obstruction 552.3
        and gangrene 551.3
    congenital 750.6
  incarcerated (*see also* Hernia, by site, with
    obstruction) 552.9
    gangrenous (*see also* Hernia, by site, with
      gangrene) 551.9
  incisional 553.21
    with
      gangrene (obstructed) 551.21
      obstruction 552.21
        and gangrene 551.21
    lumbar — *see* Hernia, lumbar
    recurrent 553.21
      with
        gangrene (obstructed) 551.21
        obstruction 552.21
          and gangrene 551.21
  indirect (inguinal) — *see* Hernia, inguinal
  infantile — *see* Hernia, inguinal
  infrapatellar fat pad 729.31
  inguinal (direct) (double) (encysted) (external)
    (funicular) (indirect) (infantile) (internal)
    (interstitial) (oblique) (scrotal) (sliding)
    550.9 ✓5ᵗʰ

> *Note* — *Use the following fifth-digit subclassification with category 550:*
>
> 0   *unilateral or unspecified (not specified as recurrent)*
> 1   *unilateral or unspecified, recurrent*
> 2   *bilateral (not specified as recurrent)*
> 3   *bilateral, recurrent*

    with
      gangrene (obstructed) 550.0 ✓5ᵗʰ
      obstruction 550.1 ✓5ᵗʰ
        and gangrene 550.0 ✓5ᵗʰ
  internal 553.8
    with
      gangrene (obstructed) 551.8
      obstruction 552.8
        and gangrene 551.8
    inguinal — *see* Hernia, inguinal
  interstitial 553.9
    with
      gangrene (obstructed) 551.9
      obstruction 552.9
        and gangrene 551.9
    inguinal — *see* Hernia, inguinal
  intervertebral cartilage or disc — *see*
    Displacement, intervertebral disc

Hernia, hernial — *continued*
  intestine, intestinal 553.9
    with
      gangrene (obstructed) 551.9
      obstruction 552.9
        and gangrene 551.9
  intra-abdominal 553.9
    with
      gangrene (obstructed) 551.9
      obstruction 552.9
        and gangrene 551.9
  intraparietal 553.9
    with
      gangrene (obstructed) 551.9
      obstruction 552.9
        and gangrene 551.9
  iris 364.8
    traumatic 871.1
  irreducible (*see also* Hernia, by site, with
    obstruction) 552.9
    gangrenous (with obstruction) (*see also*
      Hernia, by site, with gangrene) 551.9
  ischiatic 553.8
    with
      gangrene (obstructed) 551.8
      obstruction 552.8
        and gangrene 551.8
  ischiorectal 553.8
    with
      gangrene (obstructed) 551.8
      obstruction 552.8
        and gangrene 551.8
  lens 379.32
    traumatic 871.1
  linea
    alba — *see* Hernia, epigastric
    semilunaris — *see* Hernia, spigelian
  Littre's (diverticular) 553.9
    with
      gangrene (obstructed) 551.9
      obstruction 552.9
        and gangrene 551.9
  lumbar 553.8
    with
      gangrene (obstructed) 551.8
      obstruction 552.8
        and gangrene 551.8
    intervertebral disc 722.10
  lung (subcutaneous) 518.89
    congenital 748.69
  mediastinum 519.3
  mesenteric (internal) 553.8
    with
      gangrene (obstructed) 551.8
      obstruction 552.8
        and gangrene 551.8
  mesocolon 553.8
    with
      gangrene (obstructed) 551.8
      obstruction 552.8
        and gangrene 551.8
  muscle (sheath) 728.89
  nucleus pulposus — *see* Displacement,
    intervertebral disc
  oblique (inguinal) — *see* Hernia, inguinal
  obstructive (*see also* Hernia, by site, with
    obstruction) 552.9
    gangrenous (with obstruction) (*see also*
      Hernia, by site, with gangrene) 551.9
  obturator 553.8
    with
      gangrene (obstructed) 551.8
      obstruction 552.8
        and gangrene 551.8
  omental 553.8
    with
      gangrene (obstructed) 551.8
      obstruction 552.8
        and gangrene 551.8
  orbital fat (pad) 374.34
  ovary 620.4
  oviduct 620.4
  paracolostomy (stoma) 569.69
  paraduodenal 553.8
    with
      gangrene (obstructed) 551.8
      obstruction 552.8
        and gangrene 551.8

Hernia, hernial — *continued*
  paraesophageal 553.3
    with
      gangrene (obstructed) 551.3
      obstruction 552.3
        and gangrene 551.3
    congenital 750.6
  parahiatal 553.3
    with
      gangrene (obstructed) 551.3
      obstruction 552.3
        and gangrene 551.3
  paraumbilical 553.1
    with
      gangrene (obstructed) 551.1
      obstruction 552.1
        and gangrene 551.1
  parietal 553.9
    with
      gangrene (obstructed) 551.9
      obstruction 552.9
        and gangrene 551.9
  perineal 553.8
    with
      gangrene (obstructed) 551.8
      obstruction 552.8
        and gangrene 551.8
  peritoneal sac, lesser 553.8
    with
      gangrene (obstructed) 551.8
      obstruction 552.8
        and gangrene 551.8
  popliteal fat pad 729.31
  postoperative 553.21
    with
      gangrene (obstructed) 551.21
      obstruction 552.21
        and gangrene 551.21
  pregnant uterus 654.4 ✓5ᵗʰ
  prevesical 596.8
  properitoneal 553.8
    with
      gangrene (obstructed) 551.8
      obstruction 552.8
        and gangrene 551.8
  pudendal 553.8
    with
      gangrene (obstructed) 551.8
      obstruction 552.8
        and gangrene 551.8
  rectovaginal 618.6
  retroperitoneal 553.8
    with
      gangrene (obstructed) 551.8
      obstruction 552.8
        and gangrene 551.8
  Richter's (parietal) 553.9
    with
      gangrene (obstructed) 551.9
      obstruction 552.9
        and gangrene 551.9
  Rieux's, Riex's (retrocecal) 553.8
    with
      gangrene (obstructed) 551.8
      obstruction 552.8
        and gangrene 551.8
  sciatic 553.8
    with
      gangrene (obstructed) 551.8
      obstruction 552.8
        and gangrene 551.8
  scrotum, scrotal — *see* Hernia, inguinal
  sliding (inguinal) — *see also* Hernia, inguinal
    hiatus — *see* Hernia, hiatal
  spigelian 553.29
    with
      gangrene (obstructed) 551.29
      obstruction 552.29
        and gangrene 551.29
  spinal (*see also* Spina bifida) 741.9 ✓5ᵗʰ
    with hydrocephalus 741.0 ✓5ᵗʰ
  strangulated (*see also* Hernia, by site, with
    obstruction) 552.9
    gangrenous (with obstruction) (*see also*
      Hernia, by site, with gangrene) 551.9
  supraumbilicus (linea alba) — *see* Hernia,
    epigastric

Hernia, hernial — *continued*
  tendon 727.9
  testis (nontraumatic) 550.9
    meaning
      scrotal hernia 550.9
      symptomatic late syphilis 095.8
  Treitz's (fossa) 553.8
    with
      gangrene (obstructed) 551.8
      obstruction 552.8
        and gangrene 551.8
  tunica
    albuginea 608.89
    vaginalis 752.8
  umbilicus, umbilical 553.1
    with
      gangrene (obstructed) 551.1
      obstruction 552.1
        and gangrene 551.1
  ureter 593.89
    with obstruction 593.4
  uterus 621.8
    pregnant 654.4 ✓5ᵗʰ
  vaginal (posterior) 618.6
  Velpeau's (femoral) (*see also* Hernia, femoral)
      553.00
  ventral 553.20
    with
      gangrene (obstructed) 551.20
      obstruction 552.20
        and gangrene 551.20
    recurrent 553.21
      with
        gangrene (obstructed) 551.21
        obstruction 552.21
          and gangrene 551.21
  vesical
    congenital (female) (male) 756.71
    female 618.0
    male 596.8
  vitreous (into anterior chamber) 379.21
    traumatic 871.1
Herniation — *see also* Hernia
  brain (stem) 348.4
  cerebral 348.4
  gastric mucosa (into duodenal bulb) 537.89
  mediastinum 519.3
  nucleus pulposus — *see* Displacement,
      intervertebral disc
Herpangina 074.0
Herpes, herpetic 054.9
  auricularis (zoster) 053.71
    simplex 054.73
  blepharitis (zoster) 053.20
    simplex 054.41
  circinate 110.5
  circinatus 110.5
    bullous 694.5
  conjunctiva (simplex) 054.43
    zoster 053.21
  cornea (simplex) 054.43
    disciform (simplex) 054.43
    zoster 053.21
  encephalitis 054.3
  eye (zoster) 053.29
    simplex 054.40
  eyelid (zoster) 053.20
    simplex 054.41
  febrilis 054.9
  fever 054.9
  geniculate ganglionitis 053.11
  genital, genitalis 054.10
    specified site NEC 054.19
  gestationis 646.8 ✓5ᵗʰ
  gingivostomatitis 054.2
  iridocyclitis (simplex) 054.44
    zoster 053.22
  iris (any site) 695.1
  iritis (simplex) 054.44
  keratitis (simplex) 054.43
    dendritic 054.42
    disciform 054.43
    interstitial 054.43
      zoster 053.21
  keratoconjunctivitis (simplex) 054.43
    zoster 053.21

Herpes, herpetic — *continued*
  labialis 054.9
    meningococcal 036.89
  lip 054.9
  meningitis (simplex) 054.72
    zoster 053.0
  ophthalmicus (zoster) 053.20
    simplex 054.40
  otitis externa (zoster) 053.71
    simplex 054.73
  penis 054.13
  perianal 054.10
  pharyngitis 054.79
  progenitalis 054.10
  scrotum 054.19
  septicemia 054.4 ✓5ᵗʰ
  simplex 054.9
    complicated 054.8
      ophthalmic 054.40
        specified NEC 054.49
      specified NEC 054.79
    congenital 771.2
    external ear 054.73
    keratitis 054.43
      dendritic 054.42
    meningitis 054.72
    neuritis 054.79
    specified complication NEC 054.79
      ophthalmic 054.49
    visceral 054.71
  stomatitis 054.2
  tonsurans 110.0
    maculosus (of Hebra) 696.3
  visceral 054.71
  vulva 054.12
  vulvovaginitis 054.11
  whitlow 054.6
  zoster 053.9
    auricularis 053.71
    complicated 053.8
      specified NEC 053.79
    conjunctiva 053.21
    cornea 053.21
    ear 053.71
    eye 053.29
    geniculate 053.11
    keratitis 053.21
      interstitial 053.21
    neuritis 053.10
    ophthalmicus(a) 053.20
    oticus 053.71
    otitis externa 053.71
    specified complication NEC 053.79
    specified site NEC 053.9
  zosteriform, intermediate type 053.9
Herrick's
  anemia (hemoglobin S disease) 282.61
  syndrome (hemoglobin S disease) 282.61
Hers' disease (glycogenosis VI) 271.0
Herter's infantilism (nontropical sprue) 579.0
Herter (-Gee) disease or syndrome (nontropical
    sprue) 579.0
Herxheimer's disease (diffuse idiopathic
    cutaneous atrophy) 701.8
Herxheimer's reaction 995.0
Hesselbach's hernia — *see* Hernia, Hesselbach's
Heterochromia (congenital) 743.46
  acquired 364.53
  cataract 366.33
  cyclitis 364.21
  hair 704.3
  iritis 364.21
  retained metallic foreign body 360.62
    magnetic 360.52
  uveitis 364.21
Heterophoria 378.40
  alternating 378.45
  vertical 378.43
Heterophyes, small intestine 121.6
Heterophyiasis 121.6
Heteropsia 368.8
Heterotopia, heterotopic — *see also* Malposition,
    congenital
  cerebralis 742.4
  pancreas, pancreatic 751.7

Heterotopia, heterotopic — *see also* Malposition,
    congenital — *continued*
  spinalis 742.59
Heterotropia 378.30
  intermittent 378.20
    vertical 378.31
  vertical (constant) (intermittent) 378.31
Heubner's disease 094.89
Heubner-Herter disease or syndrome
    (nontropical sprue) 579.0
Hexadactylism 755.0 ✓5ᵗʰ
Heyd's syndrome (hepatorenal) 572.4
HGSIL (high grade squamous intraepithelial ●
    dysplasia) 622.1 ●
Hibernoma (M8880/0) — *see* Lipoma
Hiccough 786.8
  epidemic 078.89
  psychogenic 306.1
Hiccup (*see also* Hiccough) 786.8
Hicks (-Braxton) contractures 644.1 ✓5ᵗʰ
Hidden penis 752.65
Hidradenitis (axillaris) (suppurative) 705.83
Hidradenoma (nodular) (M8400/0) — *see also*
    Neoplasm, skin, benign
  clear cell (M8402/0) — *see* Neoplasm, skin,
    benign
  papillary (M8405/0) — *see* Neoplasm, skin,
    benign
Hidrocystoma (M8404/0) — *see* Neoplasm, skin,
    benign
High
  A₂ anemia 282.4
  altitude effects 993.2
    anoxia 993.2
    on
      ears 993.0
      sinuses 993.1
    polycythemia 289.0
  arch
    foot 755.67
    palate 750.26
  artery (arterial) tension (*see also* Hypertension)
      401.9
    without diagnosis of hypertension 796.2
  basal metabolic rate (BMR) 794.7
  blood pressure (*see also* Hypertension) 401.9
    incidental reading (isolated) (nonspecific), no
      diagnosis of hypertension 796.2
  compliance bladder 596.4
  diaphragm (congenital) 756.6
  frequency deafness (congenital) (regional) 389.8
  head at term 652.5 ✓5ᵗʰ
    affecting fetus or newborn 763.1
  output failure (cardiac) (*see also* Failure, heart)
      428.9
  oxygen-affinity hemoglobin 289.0
  palate 750.26
  risk
    behavior — *see* Problem
    family situation V61.9
      specified circumstance NEC V61.8
    individual NEC V62.89
    infant NEC V20.1
    patient taking drugs (prescribed) V67.51
      nonprescribed (*see also* Abuse, drugs,
        nondependent) 305.9 ✓5ᵗʰ
    pregnancy V23.9
      inadequate prenatal care V23.7
      specified problem NEC V23.8 ✓5ᵗʰ
  temperature (of unknown origin) (*see also*
      Pyrexia) 780.6
  thoracic rib 756.3
Hildenbrand's disease (typhus) 081.9
Hilger's syndrome 337.0
Hill diarrhea 579.1
Hilliard's lupus (*see also* Tuberculosis) 017.0 ✓5ᵗʰ
Hilum — *see* condition
Hip — *see* condition
Hippel's disease (retinocerebral angiomatosis)
    759.6
Hippus 379.49
Hirschfeld's disease (acute diabetes mellitus) (*see
    also* Diabetes) 250.0 ✓5ᵗʰ

Hirschsprung's disease or megacolon
(congenital) 751.3
Hirsuties (*see also* Hypertrichosis) 704.1
Hirsutism (*see also* Hypertrichosis) 704.1
Hirudiniasis (external) (internal) 134.2
His-Werner disease (trench fever) 083.1
Hiss-Russell dysentery 004.1
Histamine cephalgia 346.2 ✓5ᵗʰ
Histidinemia 270.5
Histidinuria 270.5
Histiocytoma (M8832/0) — *see also* Neoplasm,
skin, benign
fibrous (M8830/0) — *see also* Neoplasm, skin,
benign
atypical (M8830/1) — *see* Neoplasm,
connective tissue, uncertain behavior
malignant (M8830/3) — *see* Neoplasm,
connective tissue, malignant
Histiocytosis (acute) (chronic) (subacute) 277.8
acute differentiated progressive (M9722/3)
202.5 ✓5ᵗʰ
cholesterol 277.8
essential 277.8
lipid, lipoid (essential) 272.7
lipochrome (familial) 288.1
malignant (M9720/3) 202.3 ✓5ᵗʰ
X (chronic) 277.8
acute (progressive) (M9722/3) 202.5 ✓5ᵗʰ
Histoplasmosis 115.90
with
endocarditis 115.94
meningitis 115.91
pericarditis 115.93
pneumonia 115.95
retinitis 115.92
specified manifestation NEC 115.99
African (due to Histoplasma duboisii) 115.10
with
endocarditis 115.14
meningitis 115.11
pericarditis 115.13
pneumonia 115.15
retinitis 115.12
specified manifestation NEC 115.19
American (due to Histoplasma capsulatum)
115.00
with
endocarditis 115.04
meningitis 115.01
pericarditis 115.03
pneumonia 115.05
retinitis 115.02
specified manifestation NEC 115.09
Darling's — *see* Histoplasmosis, American
large form (*see also* Histoplasmosis, African)
115.10
lung 115.05
small form (*see also* Histoplasmosis, American)
115.00
History (personal) of
abuse
emotional V15.42
neglect V15.42
physical V15.41
sexual V15.41
affective psychosis V11.1
alcoholism V11.3
specified as drinking problem (*see also*
Abuse, drugs, nondependent)
305.0 ✓5ᵗʰ
allergy to
analgesic agent NEC V14.6
anesthetic NEC V14.4
antibiotic agent NEC V14.1
penicillin V14.0
anti-infective agent NEC V14.3
diathesis V15.09
drug V14.9
specified type NEC V14.8
eggs V15.03
food additives V15.05
insect bite V15.06
latex V15.07
medicinal agents V14.9
specified type NEC V14.8

History (personal) of — *continued*
allergy to — *continued*
milk products V15.02
narcotic agent NEC V14.5
nuts V15.05
peanuts V15.01
penicillin V14.0
radiographic dye V15.08
seafood V15.04
serum V14.7
specified food NEC V15.05
specified nonmedicinal agents NEC V15.09
spider bite V15.06
sulfa V14.2
sulfonamides V14.2
therapeutic agent NEC V15.09
vaccine V14.7
anemia V12.3
arthritis V13.4
benign neoplasm of brain V12.41
blood disease V12.3
calculi, urinary V13.01
cardiovascular disease V12.50
myocardial infarction 412
child abuse V15.41
cigarette smoking V15.82
circulatory system disease V12.50
myocardial infarction 412
congenital malformation V13.69
contraception V15.7
diathesis, allergic V15.09
digestive system disease V12.70
peptic ulcer V12.71
polyps, colonic V12.72
specified NEC V12.79
disease (of) V13.9
blood V12.3
blood-forming organs V12.3
cardiovascular system V12.50
circulatory system V12.50
digestive system V12.70
peptic ulcer V12.71
polyps, colonic V12.72
specified NEC V12.79
infectious V12.00
malaria V12.03
poliomyelitis V12.02
specified NEC V12.09
tuberculosis V12.01
parasitic V12.00
specified NEC V12.09
respiratory system V12.6
skin V13.3
specified site NEC V13.8
subcutaneous tissue V13.3
trophoblastic V13.1
affecting management of pregnant V23.1
disorder (of) V13.9
endocrine V12.2
genital system V13.29   ▲
hematological V12.3
immunity V12.2
mental V11.9
affective type V11.1
manic-depressive V11.1
neurosis V11.2
schizophrenia V11.0
specified type NEC V11.8
metabolic V12.2
musculoskeletal NEC V13.5
nervous system V12.40
specified type NEC V12.49
obstetric V13.29   ▲
affecting management of current
pregnancy V23.49   ▲
pre-term labor V23.41   ●
pre-term labor V13.21   ●
sense organs V12.40
specified type NEC V12.49
specified site NEC V13.8
urinary system V13.00
calculi V13.01
specified NEC V13.09
drug use
nonprescribed (*see also* Abuse, drugs,
nondependent) 305.9 ✓5ᵗʰ

History (personal) of — *continued*
drug use — *continued*
patent (*see also* Abuse, drugs,
nondependent) 305.9 ✓5ᵗʰ
effect NEC of external cause V15.89
embolism (pulmonary) V12.51
emotional abuse V15.42
endocrine disorder V12.2
family
allergy V19.6
anemia V18.2
arteriosclerosis V17.4
arthritis V17.7
asthma V17.5
blindness V19.0
blood disorder NEC V18.3
cardiovascular disease V17.4
cerebrovascular disease V17.1
chronic respiratory condition NEC V17.6
congenital anomalies V19.5
consanguinity V19.7
coronary artery disease V17.3
cystic fibrosis V18.1
deafness V19.2
diabetes mellitus V18.0
digestive disorders V18.5
disease or disorder (of)
allergic V19.6
blood NEC V18.3
cardiovascular NEC V17.4
cerebrovascular V17.1
coronary artery V17.3
digestive V18.5
ear NEC V19.3
endocrine V18.1
eye NEC V19.1
genitourinary NEC V18.7
hypertensive V17.4
infectious V18.8
ischemic heart V17.3
kidney V18.69
polycystic V18.61
mental V17.0
metabolic V18.1
musculoskeletal NEC V17.8
neurological NEC V17.2
parasitic V18.8
psychiatric condition V17.0
skin condition V19.4
ear disorder NEC V19.3
endocrine disease V18.1
epilepsy V17.2
eye disorder NEC V19.1
genitourinary disease NEC V18.7
glomerulonephritis V18.69
gout V18.1
hay fever V17.6
hearing loss V19.2
hematopoietic neoplasia V16.7
Hodgkin's disease V16.7
Huntington's chorea V17.2
hydrocephalus V19.5
hypertension V17.4
hypospadias V13.61
infectious disease V18.8
ischemia heart disease V17.3
kidney disease V18.69
polycystic V18.61
leukemia V16.6
lymphatic malignant neoplasia NEC V16.7
malignant neoplasm (of) NEC V16.9
anorectal V16.0
anus V16.0
appendix V16.0
bladder V16.59
bone V16.8
brain V16.8
breast V16.3
male V16.8
bronchus V16.1
cecum V16.0
cervix V16.49
colon V16.0
duodenum V16.0
esophagus V16.0
eye V16.8
gallbladder V16.0

✓4ᵗʰ Fourth-digit Required   ✓5ᵗʰ Fifth-digit Required   ►◄ Revised Text   ● New Line   ▲ Revised Code

History (personal) of — *continued*
  family — *continued*
    malignant neoplasm (of) NEC — *continued*
      gastrointestinal tract V16.0
      genital organs V16.40
      hemopoietic NEC V16.7
      ileum V16.0
      ilium V16.8
      intestine V16.0
      intrathoracic organs NEC V16.2
      kidney V16.51
      larynx V16.2
      liver V16.0
      lung V16.1
      lymphatic NEC V16.7
      ovary V16.41
      oviduct V16.41
      pancreas V16.0
      penis V16.49
      prostate V16.42
      rectum V16.0
      respiratory organs NEC V16.2
      skin V16.8
      specified site NEC V16.8
      stomach V16.0
      testis V16.43
      trachea V16.1
      ureter V16.59
      urethra V16.59
      urinary organs V16.59
      uterus V16.49
      vagina V16.49
      vulva V16.49
    mental retardation V18.4
    metabolic disease NEC V18.1
    mongolism V19.5
    multiple myeloma V16.7
    musculoskeletal disease NEC V17.8
    nephritis V18.69
    nephrosis V18.69
    parasitic disease V18.8
    polycystic kidney disease V18.61
    psychiatric disorder V17.0
    psychosis V17.0
    retardation, mental V18.4
    retinitis pigmentosa V19.1
    schizophrenia V17.0
    skin conditions V19.4
    specified condition NEC V19.8
    stroke (cerebrovascular) V17.1
    visual loss V19.0
  genital system disorder V13.29   ▲
    pre-term labor V13.21   ●
  health hazard V15.9
    specified cause NEC V15.89
  Hodgkin's disease V10.72
  immunity disorder V12.2
  infectious disease V12.00
    malaria V12.03
    poliomyelitis V12.02
    specified NEC V12.09
    tuberculosis V12.01
  injury NEC V15.5
  insufficient prenatal care V23.7
  irradiation V15.3
  leukemia V10.60
    lymphoid V10.61
    monocytic V10.63
    myeloid V10.62
    specified type NEC V10.69
  little or no prenatal care V23.7
  low birth weight (*see also* Status, low birth
    weight) V21.30
  lymphosarcoma V10.71
  malaria V12.03
  malignant neoplasm (of) V10.9
    accessory sinus V10.22
    adrenal V10.88
    anus V10.06
    bile duct V10.09
    bladder V10.51
    bone V10.81
    brain V10.85
    breast V10.3
    bronchus V10.11
    cervix uteri V10.41
    colon V10.05

History (personal) of — *continued*
  malignant neoplasm (of) — *continued*
    connective tissue NEC V10.89
    corpus uteri V10.42
    digestive system V10.00
      specified part NEC V10.09
    duodenum V10.09
    endocrine gland NEC V10.88
    epididymis V10.48
    esophagus V10.03
    eye V10.84
    fallopian tube V10.44
    female genital organ V10.40
      specified site NEC V10.44
    gallbladder V10.09
    gastrointestinal tract V10.00
    gum V10.02
    hematopoietic NEC V10.79
    hypopharynx V10.02
    ileum V10.09
    intrathoracic organs NEC V10.20
    jejunum V10.09
    kidney V10.52
    large intestine V10.05
    larynx V10.21
    lip V10.02
    liver V10.07
    lung V10.11
    lymphatic NEC V10.79
    lymph glands or nodes NEC V10.79
    male genital organ V10.45
      specified site NEC V10.49
    mediastinum V10.29
    melanoma (of skin) V10.82
    middle ear V10.22
    mouth V10.02
      specified part NEC V10.02
    nasal cavities V10.22
    nasopharynx V10.02
    nervous system NEC V10.86
    nose V10.22
    oropharynx V10.02
    ovary V10.43
    pancreas V10.09
    parathyroid V10.88
    penis V10.49
    pharynx V10.02
    pineal V10.88
    pituitary V10.88
    placenta V10.44
    pleura V10.29
    prostate V10.46
    rectosigmoid junction V10.06
    rectum V10.06
    renal pelvis V10.53
    respiratory organs NEC V10.20
    salivary gland V10.02
    skin V10.83
      melanoma V10.82
    small intestine NEC V10.09
    soft tissue NEC V10.89
    specified site NEC V10.89
    stomach V10.04
    testis V10.47
    thymus V10.29
    thyroid V10.87
    tongue V10.01
    trachea V10.12
    ureter V10.59
    urethra V10.59
    urinary organ V10.50
    uterine adnexa V10.44
    uterus V10.42
    vagina V10.44
    vulva V10.44
  manic-depressive psychosis V11.1
  mental disorder V11.9
    affective type V11.1
    manic-depressive V11.1
    neurosis V11.2
    schizophrenia V11.0
    specified type NEC V11.8
  metabolic disorder V12.2
  musculoskeletal disorder NEC V13.5
  myocardial infarction 412
  neglect (emotional) V15.42
  nervous system disorder V12.40
    specified type NEC V12.49

History (personal) of — *continued*
  neurosis V11.2
  noncompliance with medical treatment V15.81
  nutritional deficiency V12.1
  obstetric disorder V13.29   ●
    affecting management of current
      pregnancy V23.49   ▲
      pre-term labor V23.41   ●
    pre-term labor V13.41   ●
  parasitic disease V12.00
    specified NEC V12.09
  perinatal problems V13.7
    low birth weight (*see also* Status, low birth
      weight) V21.30
  physical abuse V15.41
  poisoning V15.6
  poliomyelitis V12.02
  polyps, colonic V12.72
  poor obstetric V13.49   ▲
    affecting management of current   ●
      pregnancy V23.49   ●
      pre-term labor V23.41   ●
    pre-term labor V13.41   ●
  psychiatric disorder V11.9
    affective type V11.1
    manic-depressive V11.1
    neurosis V11.2
    schizophrenia V11.0
    specified type NEC V11.8
  psychological trauma V15.49
    emotional abuse V15.42
    neglect V15.42
    physical abuse V15.41
    rape V15.41
  psychoneurosis V11.2
  radiation therapy V15.3
  rape V15.41
  respiratory system disease V12.6
  reticulosarcoma V10.71
  schizophrenia V11.0
  skin disease V13.3
  smoking (tobacco) V15.82
  subcutaneous tissue disease V13.3
  surgery (major) to
    great vessels V15.1
    heart V15.1
    major organs NEC V15.2
  thrombophlebitis V12.52
  thrombosis V12.51
  tobacco use V15.82
  trophoblastic disease V13.1
    affecting management of pregnancy V23.1
  tuberculosis V12.01
  ulcer, peptic V12.71
  urinary system disorder V13.00
    calculi V13.01
    specified NEC V13.09

HIV infection (disease) (illness) — *see* Human
  immunodeficiency virus (disease) (illness)
  (infection)

Hives (bold) (*see also* Urticaria) 708.9

Hoarseness 784.49

Hobnail liver — *see* Cirrhosis, portal

Hobo, hoboism V60.0

Hodgkins
  disease (M9650/3) 201.9 ✔5ᵗʰ
    lymphocytic
      depletion (M9653/3) 201.7 ✔5ᵗʰ
        diffuse fibrosis (M9654/3) 201.7 ✔5ᵗʰ
        reticular type (M9655/3) 201.7 ✔5ᵗʰ
      predominance (M9651/3) 201.4 ✔5ᵗʰ
    lymphocytic-histiocytic predominance
      (M9651/3) 201.4 ✔5ᵗʰ
    mixed cellularity (M9652/3) 201.6 ✔5ᵗʰ
    nodular sclerosis (M9656/3) 201.5 ✔5ᵗʰ
      cellular phase (M9657/3) 201.5 ✔5ᵗʰ
  granuloma (M9661/3) 201.1 ✔5ᵗʰ
  lymphogranulomatosis (M9650/3) 201.9 ✔5ᵗʰ
  lymphoma (M9650/3) 201.9 ✔5ᵗʰ
  lymphosarcoma (M9650/3) 201.9 ✔5ᵗʰ
  paragranuloma (M9660/3) 201.0 ✔5ᵗʰ
  sarcoma (M9662/3) 201.2 ✔5ᵗʰ

Hodgson's disease (aneurysmal dilatation of
  aorta) 441.9
  ruptured 441.5

Hodi-potsy 111.0

Hoffa (-Kastert) disease or syndrome
(liposynovitis prepatellaris) 272.8
Hoffman's syndrome 244.9 *[359.5]*
Hoffmann-Bouveret syndrome (paroxysmal
tachycardia) 427.2
Hole
macula 362.54
optic disc, crater-like 377.22
retina (macula) 362.54
round 361.31
with detachment 361.01
Holla disease (*see also* Spherocytosis) 282.0
Holländer-Simons syndrome (progressive
lipodystrophy) 272.6
Hollow foot (congenital) 754.71
acquired 736.73
Holmes' syndrome (visual disorientation) 368.16
Holoprosencephaly 742.2
due to
trisomy 13 758.1
trisomy 18 758.2
Holthouse's hernia — *see* Hernia, inguinal
Homesickness 309.89
Homocystinemia 270.4
Homocystinuria 270.4
Homologous serum jaundice (prophylactic)
(therapeutic) — *see* Hepatitis, viral
Homosexuality — *omit code*
ego-dystonic 302.0
pedophilic 302.2
problems with 302.0
Homozygous Hb-S disease 282.61
Honeycomb lung 518.89
congenital 748.4
Hong Kong ear 117.3
HOOD (hereditary osteo-onychodysplasia) 756.89
Hooded
clitoris 752.49
penis 752.69
Hookworm (anemia) (disease) (infestation) — *see*
Ancylostomiasis
Hoppe-Goldflam syndrome 358.0
Hordeolum (external) (eyelid) 373.11
internal 373.12
Horn
cutaneous 702.8
cheek 702.8
eyelid 702.8
penis 702.8
iliac 756.89
nail 703.8
congenital 757.5
papillary 700
Horner's
syndrome (*see also* Neuropathy, peripheral,
autonomic) 337.9
traumatic 954.0
teeth 520.4
Horseshoe kidney (congenital) 753.3
Horton's
disease (temporal arteritis) 446.5
headache or neuralgia 346.2 ☑5ᵗʰ
Hospice care V66.7
Hospitalism (in children) NEC 309.83
Hourglass contraction, contracture
bladder 596.8
gallbladder 575.2
congenital 751.69
stomach 536.8
congenital 750.7
psychogenic 306.4
uterus 661.4 ☑5ᵗʰ
affecting fetus or newborn 763.7
Household circumstance affecting care V60.9
specified type NEC V60.8
Housemaid's knee 727.2
Housing circumstance affecting care V60.9
specified type NEC V60.8
Huchard's disease (continued arterial
hypertension) 401.9

Hudson-Stähli lines 371.11
Huguier's disease (uterine fibroma) 218.9
Hum, venous — *omit code*
Human bite (open wound) — *see also* Wound,
open, by site
intact skin surface — *see* Contusion
Human immunodeficiency virus (disease)
(illness) 042
infection V08
with symptoms, symptomatic 042
Human immunodeficiency virus-2 infection
079.53
Human immunovirus (disease) (illness) (infection)
— *see* Human immunodeficiency virus
(disease) (illness) (infection)
Human papillomavirus 079.4
Human T-cell lymphotrophic virus-I infection
079.51
Human T-cell lymphotrophic virus-II infection
079.52
Human T-cell lymphotrophic virus-III (disease)
(illness) (infection) — *see* Human
immunodeficiency virus (disease) (illness)
(infection)
HTLV-I infection 079.51
HTLV-II infection 079.52
HTLV-III (disease) (illness) (infection) — *see*
Human immunodeficiency virus (disease)
(illness) (infection)
HTLV-III/LAV (disease) (illness) (infection) — *see*
Human immunodeficiency virus (disease)
(illness) (infection)
Humpback (acquired) 737.9
congenital 756.19
Hunchback (acquired) 737.9
congenital 756.19
Hunger 994.2
air, psychogenic 306.1
disease 251.1
Hunner's ulcer (*see also* Cystitis) 595.1
Hunt's
neuralgia 053.11
syndrome (herpetic geniculate ganglionitis)
053.11
dyssynergia cerebellaris myoclonica 334.2
Hunter's glossitis 529.4
Hunter (-Hurler) syndrome
(mucopolysaccharidosis II) 277.5
Hunterian chancre 091.0
Huntington's
chorea 333.4
disease 333.4
Huppert's disease (multiple myeloma) (M9730/3)
203.0 ☑5ᵗʰ
Hurier (-Hunter) disease or syndrome
(mucopolysaccharidosis II) 277.5
Hürthle cell
adenocarcinoma (M8290/3) 193
adenoma (M8290/0) 226
carcinoma (M8290/3) 193
tumor (M8290/0) 226
Hutchinson's
disease meaning
angioma serpiginosum 709.1
cheiropompholyx 705.81
prurigo estivalis 692.72
summer eruption, or summer prurigo
692.72
incisors 090.5
melanotic freckle (M8742/2) — *see also*
Neoplasm, skin, in situ
malignant melanoma in (M8742/3) — *see*
Melanoma
teeth or incisors (congenital syphilis) 090.5
Hutchinson-Boeck disease or syndrome
(sarcoidosis) 135
Hutchinson-Gilford disease or syndrome
(progeria) 259.8
Hyaline
degeneration (diffuse) (generalized) 728.9
localized — *see* Degeneration, by site

Hyaline — *continued*
membrane (disease) (lung) (newborn) 769
Hyalinosis cutis et mucosae 272.8
Hyalin plaque, sclera, senile 379.16
Hyalitis (asteroid) 379.22
syphilitic 095.8
Hydatid
cyst or tumor — *see also* Echinococcus
fallopian tube 752.11
mole — *see* Hydatidiform mole
Morgagni (congenital) 752.8
fallopian tube 752.11
Hydatidiform mole (benign) (complicating
pregnancy) (delivered) (undelivered) 630
invasive (M9100/1) 236.1
malignant (M9100/1) 236.1
previous, affecting management of pregnancy
V23.1
Hydatidosis — *see* Echinococcus
Hyde's disease (prurigo nodularis) 698.3
Hydradenitis 705.83
Hydradenoma (M8400/0) — *see* Hidradenoma
Hydralazine lupus or syndrome
correct substance properly administered 695.4
overdose or wrong substance given or taken
972.6
Hydramnios 657 ☑4ᵗʰ
affecting fetus or newborn 761.3
Hydrancephaly 742.3
with spina bifida (*see also* Spina bifida)
741.0 ☑5ᵗʰ
Hydranencephaly 742.3
with spina bifida (*see also* Spina bifida)
741.0 ☑5ᵗʰ
Hydrargyrism NEC 985.0
Hydrarthrosis (*see also* Effusion, joint) 719.0 ☑5ᵗʰ
gonococcal 098.50
intermittent (*see also* Rheumatism,
palindromic) 719.3 ☑5ᵗʰ
of yaws (early) (late) 102.6
syphilitic 095.8
congenital 090.5
Hydremia 285.9
Hydrencephalocele (congenital) 742.0
Hydrencephalomeningocele (congenital) 742.0
Hydroa 694.0
aestivale 692.72
gestationis 646.8 ☑5ᵗʰ
herpetiformis 694.0
pruriginosa 694.0
vacciniforme 692.72
Hydroadenitis 705.83
Hydrocalycosis (*see also* Hydronephrosis) 591
congenital 753.29
Hydrocalyx (*see also* Hydronephrosis) 591
Hydrocele (calcified) (chylous) (idiopathic)
(infantile) (inguinal canal) (recurrent) (senile)
(spermatic cord) (testis) (tunica vaginalis)
603.9
canal of Nuck (female) 629.1
male 603.9
congenital 778.6
encysted 603.0
congenital 778.6
female NEC 629.8
infected 603.1
round ligament 629.8
specified type NEC 603.8
congenital 778.6
spinalis (*see also* Spina bifida) 741.9 ☑5ᵗʰ
vulva 624.8
Hydrocephalic fetus
affecting management or pregnancy 655.0 ☑5ᵗʰ
causing disproportion 653.6 ☑5ᵗʰ
with obstructed labor 660.1 ☑5ᵗʰ
affecting fetus or newborn 763.1
Hydrocephalus (acquired) (external) (internal)
(malignant) (noncommunicating)
(obstructive) (recurrent) 331.4
aqueduct of Sylvius structure 742.3
with spina bifida (*see also* Spina bifida)
741.0 ☑5ᵗʰ

☑4ᵗʰ Fourth-digit Required   ☑5ᵗʰ Fifth-digit Required   ▶◀ Revised Text   ● New Line   ▲ Revised Code

Sidebar: Hydrocephalus — Hyperelectrolytemia

Hydrocephalus — continued
  chronic 742.3
    with spina bifida (*see also* Spina bifida) 741.0 ✓5ᵗ
  communicating 331.3
  congenital (external) (internal) 742.3
    with spina bifida (*see also* Spina bifida) 741.0 ✓5ᵗ
  due to
    structure of aqueduct of Sylvius 742.3
      with spina bifida (*see also* Spina bifida) 741.0 ✓5ᵗ
    toxoplasmosis (congenital) 771.2
  fetal affecting management of pregnancy 655.0 ✓5ᵗ
  foramen Magendie block (acquired) 331.3
    congenital 742.3
      with spina bifida (*see also* Spina bifida) 741.0 ✓5ᵗ
  newborn 742.3
    with spina bifida (*see also* Spina bifida) 741.0 ✓5ᵗ
  otitic 331.4
  syphilitic, congenital 090.49
  tuberculous (*see also* Tuberculosis) 013.8 ✓5ᵗ
Hydrocolpos (congenital) 623.8
Hydrocystoma (M8404/0) — *see* Neoplasm, skin, benign
Hydroencephalocele (congenital) 742.0
Hydroencephalomeningocele (congenital) 742.0
Hydrohematopneumothorax (*see also* Hemothorax) 511.8
Hydromeningitis — *see* Meningitis
Hydromeningocele (spinal) (*see also* Spina bifida) 741.9 ✓5ᵗ
  cranial 742.0
Hydrometra 621.8
Hydrometrocolpos 623.8
Hydromicrocephaly 742.1
Hydromphalus (congenital) (since birth) 757.39
Hydromyelia 742.53
Hydromyelocele (*see also* Spina bifida) 741.9 ✓5ᵗ
Hydronephrosis 591
  atrophic 591
  congenital 753.29
  due to S. hematobium 120.0
  early 591
  functionless (infected) 591
  infected 591
  intermittent 591
  primary 591
  secondary 591
  tuberculous (*see also* Tuberculosis) 016.0 ✓5ᵗ
Hydropericarditis (*see also* Pericarditis) 423.9
Hydropericardium (*see also* Pericarditis) 423.9
Hydroperitoneum 789.5
Hydrophobia 071
Hydrophthalmos (*see also* Buphthalmia) 743.20
Hydropneumohemothorax (*see also* Hemothorax) 511.8
Hydropneumopericarditis (*see also* Pericarditis) 423.9
Hydropneumopericardium (*see also* Pericarditis) 423.9
Hydropneumothorax 511.8
  nontuberculous 511.8
    bacterial 511.1
  pneumococcal 511.1
  staphylococcal 511.1
  streptococcal 511.1
  traumatic 860.0
    with open wound into thorax 860.1
  tuberculous (*see also* Tuberculosis, pleura) 012.0 ✓5ᵗ
Hydrops 782.3
  abdominis 789.5
  amnii (complicating pregnancy) (*see also* Hydramnios) 657 ✓4ᵗ
  articulorum intermittens (*see also* Rheumatism, palindromic) 719.3 ✓5ᵗ
  cardiac (*see also* Failure, heart) 428.0
  congenital — *see* Hydrops, fetalis

Hydrops — continued
  endolymphatic (*see also* Disease, Ménière's) 386.00
  fetal(is) or newborn 778.0
    due to isoimmunization 773.3
    not due to isoimmunization 778.0
  gallbladder 575.3
  idiopathic (fetus or newborn) 778.0
  joint (see also Effusion, joint) 719.0 ✓5ᵗ
  labyrinth (*see also* Disease, Ménière's) 386.00
  meningeal NEC 331.4
  nutritional 262
  pericardium — *see* Pericarditis
  pleura (*see also* Hydrothorax) 511.8
  renal (*see also* Nephrosis) 581.9
  spermatic cord (*see also* Hydrocele) 603.9
Hydropyonephrosis (*see also* Pyelitis) 590.80
  chronic 590.00
Hydrorachis 742.53
Hydrorrhea (nasal) 478.1
  gravidarum 658.1 ✓5ᵗ
  pregnancy 658.1 ✓5ᵗ
Hydrosadenitis 705.83
Hydrosalpinx (fallopian tube) (follicularis) 614.1
Hydrothorax (double) (pleural) 511.8
  chylous (nonfilarial) 457.8
    filaria (*see also* Infestation, filarial) 125.9
  nontuberculous 511.8
    bacterial 511.1
  pneumococcal 511.1
  staphylococcal 511.1
  streptococcal 511.1
  traumatic 862.29
    with open wound into thorax 862.39
  tuberculous (*see also* Tuberculosis, pleura) 012.0 ✓5ᵗ
Hydroureter 593.5
  congenital 753.22
Hydroureteronephrosis (*see also* Hydronephrosis) 591
Hydrourethra 599.84
Hydroxykynureninuria 270.2
Hydroxyprolinemia 270.8
Hydroxyprolinuria 270.8
Hygroma (congenital) (cystic) (M9173/0) 228.1
  prepatellar 727.3
  subdural — *see* Hematoma, subdural
Hymen — *see* condition
Hymenolepiasis (diminuta) (infection) (infestation) (nana) 123.6
Hymenolepis (diminuta) (infection) (infestation) (nana) 123.6
Hypalgesia (*see also* Disturbance, sensation) 782.0
Hyperabduction syndrome 447.8
Hyperacidity, gastric 536.8
  psychogenic 306.4
Hyperactive, hyperactivity
  basal cell, uterine cervix 622.1
  bladder 596.51
  bowel (syndrome) 564.9
    sounds 787.5
  cervix epithelial (basal) 622.1
  child 314.01
  colon 564.9
  gastrointestinal 536.8
    psychogenic 306.4
  intestine 564.9
  labyrinth (unilateral) 386.51
    with loss of labyrinthine reactivity 386.58
    bilateral 386.52
  nasal mucous membrane 478.1
  stomach 536.8
  thyroid (gland) (*see also* Thyrotoxicosis) 242.9 ✓5ᵗ
Hyperacusis 388.42
Hyperadrenalism (cortical) 255.3
  medullary 255.6
Hyperadrenocorticism 255.3
  congenital 255.2
  iatrogenic
    correct substance properly administered 255.3

Hyperadrenocorticism — continued
  iatrogenic — continued
    overdose or wrong substance given or taken 962.0
Hyperaffectivity 301.11
Hyperaldosteronism (atypical) (hyperplastic) (normoaldosteronal) (normotensive) (primary) (secondary) 255.1
Hyperalgesia (*see also* Disturbance, sensation) 782.0
Hyperalimentation 783.6
  carotene 278.3
  specified NEC 278.8
  vitamin A 278.2
  vitamin D 278.4
Hyperaminoaciduria 270.9
  arginine 270.6
  citrulline 270.6
  cystine 270.0
  glycine 270.0
  lysine 270.7
  ornithine 270.6
  renal (types I, II, III) 270.0
Hyperammonemia (congenital) 270.6
Hyperamnesia 780.99 ▲
Hyperamylasemia 790.5
Hyperaphia 782.0
Hyperazotemia 791.9
Hyperbetalipoproteinemia (acquired) (essential) (familial) (hereditary) (primary) (secondary) 272.0
  with prebetalipoproteinemia 272.2
Hyperbilirubinemia 782.4
  congenital 277.4
  constitutional 277.4
  neonatal (transient) (*see also* Jaundice, fetus or newborn) 774.6
  of prematurity 774.2
Hyperbilirubinemica encephalopathia, newborn 774.7
  due to isoimmunization 773.4
Hypercalcemia, hypercalcemic (idiopathic) 275.42
  nephropathy 588.8
Hypercalcinuria 275.40
Hypercapnia 786.09
  with mixed acid-base disorder 276.4
  fetal, affecting newborn 770.89 ▲
Hypercarotinemia 278.3
Hypercementosis 521.5
Hyperchloremia 276.9
Hyperchlorhydria 536.8
  neurotic 306.4
  psychogenic 306.4
Hypercholesterinemia — *see* Hypercholesterolemia
Hypercholesterolemia 272.0
  with hyperglyceridemia, endogenous 272.2
  essential 272.0
  familial 272.0
  hereditary 272.0
  primary 272.0
  pure 272.0
Hypercholesterolosis 272.0
Hyperchylia gastrica 536.8
  psychogenic 306.4
Hyperchylomicronemia (familial) (with hyperbetalipoproteinemia) 272.3
Hypercoagulation syndrome 289.8
Hypercorticosteronism
  correct substance properly administered 255.3
  overdose or wrong substance given or taken 962.0
Hypercortisonism
  correct substance properly administered 255.3
  overdose or wrong substance given or taken 962.0
Hyperdynamic beta-adrenergic state or syndrome (circulatory) 429.82
Hyperelectrolytemia 276.9

Hyperemesis 536.2
  arising during pregnancy — *see* Hyperemesis, gravidarum
  gravidarum (mild) (before 22 completed weeks gestation) 643.0 ☑5ᵗʰ
    with
      carbohydrate depletion 643.1 ☑5ᵗʰ
      dehydration 643.1 ☑5ᵗʰ
      electrolyte imbalance 643.1 ☑5ᵗʰ
      metabolic disturbance 643.1 ☑5ᵗʰ
      affecting fetus or newborn 761.8
      severe (with metabolic disturbance) 643.1 ☑5ᵗʰ
  psychogenic 306.4
Hyperemia (acute) 780.99   ▲
  anal mucosa 569.49
  bladder 596.7
  cerebral 437.8
  conjunctiva 372.71
  ear, internal, acute 386.30
  enteric 564.89
  eye 372.71
  eyelid (active) (passive) 374.82
  intestine 564.89
  iris 364.41
  kidney 593.81
  labyrinth 386.30
  liver (active) (passive) 573.8
  lung 514
  ovary 620.8
  passive 780.99   ▲
  pulmonary 514
  renal 593.81
  retina 362.89
  spleen 289.59
  stomach 537.89
Hyperesthesia (body surface) (*see also* Disturbance, sensation) 782.0
  larynx (reflex) 478.79
    hysterical 300.11
  pharynx (reflex) 478.29
Hyperestrinism 256.0
Hyperestrogenism 256.0
Hyperestrogenosis 256.0
Hyperextension, joint 718.80
  ankle 718.87
  elbow 718.82
  foot 718.87
  hand 718.84
  hip 718.85
  knee 718.86
  multiple sites 718.89
  pelvic region 718.85
  shoulder (region) 718.81
  specified site NEC 718.88
  wrist 718.83
Hyperfibrinolysis — *see* Fibrinolysis
Hyperfolliculinism 256.0
Hyperfructosemia 271.2
Hyperfunction
  adrenal (cortex) 255.3
    androgenic, acquired benign 255.3
    medulla 255.6
    virilism 255.2
  corticoadrenal NEC 255.3
  labyrinth — *see* Hyperactive, labyrinth
  medulloadrenal 255.6
  ovary 256.1
    estrogen 256.0
  pancreas 577.8
  parathyroid (gland) 252.0
  pituitary (anterior) (gland) (lobe) 253.1
  testicular 257.0
Hypergammaglobulinemia 289.8
  monoclonal, benign (BMH) 273.1
  polyclonal 273.0
  Waldenström's 273.0
Hyperglobulinemia 273.8
Hyperglycemia 790.6
  maternal
    affecting fetus or newborn 775.0
    manifest diabetes in infant 775.1
  postpancreatectomy (complete) (partial) 251.3

Hyperglyceridemia 272.1
  endogenous 272.1
  essential 272.1
  familial 272.1
  hereditary 272.1
  mixed 272.3
  pure 272.1
Hyperglycinemia 270.7
Hypergonadism
  ovarian 256.1
  testicular (infantile) (primary) 257.0
Hyperheparinemia (*see also* Circulating anticoagulants) 286.5
Hyperhidrosis, hyperidrosis 780.8
  psychogenic 306.3
Hyperhistidinemia 270.5
Hyperinsulinism (ectopic) (functional) (organic) NEC 251.1
  iatrogenic 251.0
  reactive 251.2
  spontaneous 251.2
  therapeutic misadventure (from administration of insulin) 962.3
Hyperiodemia 276.9
Hyperirritability (cerebral), in newborn 779.1
Hyperkalemia 276.7
Hyperkeratosis (*see also* Keratosis) 701.1
  cervix 622.1
  congenital 757.39
  cornea 371.89
  due to yaws (early) (late) (palmar or plantar) 102.3
  eccentrica 757.39
  figurata centrifuga atrophica 757.39
  follicularis 757.39
    in cutem penetrans 701.1
  limbic (cornea) 371.89
  palmoplantaris climacterica 701.1
  pinta (carate) 103.1
  senile (with pruritus) 702.0
  tongue 528.7
  universalis congenita 757.1
  vagina 623.1
  vocal cord 478.5
  vulva 624.0
Hyperkinesia, hyperkinetic (disease) (reaction) (syndrome) 314.9
  with
    attention deficit — *see* Disorder, attention deficit
    conduct disorder 314.2
    developmental delay 314.1
    simple disturbance of activity and attention 314.01
    specified manifestation NEC 314.8
  heart (disease) 429.82
  of childhood or adolescence NEC 314.9
Hyperlacrimation (*see also* Epiphora) 375.20
Hyperlipemia (*see also* Hyperlipidemia) 272.4
Hyperlipidemia 272.4
  carbohydrate-induced 272.1'
  combined 272.4
  endogenous 272.1
  exogenous 272.3
  fat-induced 272.3
  group
    A 272.0
    B 272.1
    C 272.2
    D 272.3
  mixed 272.2
  specified type NEC 272.4
Hyperlipidosis 272.7
  hereditary 272.7
Hyperlipoproteinemia (acquired) (essential) (familial) (hereditary) (primary) (secondary) 272.4
  Fredrickson type
    I 272.3
    IIa 272.0
    IIb 272.2
    III 272.2
    IV 272.1
    V 272.3

Hyperlipoproteinemia — *continued*
  low-density-lipoid-type (LDL) 272.0
  very-low-density-lipoid-type (VLDL) 272.1
Hyperlucent lung, unilateral 492.8
Hyperluteinization 256.1
Hyperlysinemia 270.7
Hypermagnesemia 275.2
  neonatal 775.5
Hypermaturity (fetus or newborn) 766.2
Hypermenorrhea 626.2
Hypermetabolism 794.7
Hypermethioninemia 270.4
Hypermetropia (congenital) 367.0
Hypermobility
  cecum 564.9
  coccyx 724.71
  colon 564.9
    psychogenic 306.4
  ileum 564.89
  joint (acquired) 718.80
    ankle 718.87
    elbow 718.82
    foot 718.87
    hand 718.84
    hip 718.85
    knee 718.86
    multiple sites 718.89
    pelvic region 718.85
    shoulder (region) 718.81
    specified site NEC 718.88
    wrist 718.83
  kidney, congenital 753.3
  meniscus (knee) 717.5
  scapula 718.81
  stomach 536.8
    psychogenic 306.4
  syndrome 728.5
  testis, congenital 752.52
  urethral 599.81
Hypermotility
  gastrointestinal 536.8
  intestine 564.9
    psychogenic 306.4
  stomach 536.8
Hypernasality 784.49
Hypernatremia 276.0
  with water depletion 276.0
Hypernephroma (M8312/3) 189.0
Hyperopia 367.0
Hyperorexia 783.6
Hyperornithinemia 270.6
Hyperosmia (*see also* Disturbance, sensation) 781.1
Hyperosmolality 276.0
Hyperosteogenesis 733.99
Hyperostosis 733.99
  calvarial 733.3
  cortical 733.3
    infantile 756.59
  frontal, internal of skull 733.3
  interna frontalis 733.3
  monomelic 733.99
  skull 733.3
    congenital 756.0
  vertebral 721.8
    with spondylosis — *see* Spondylosis
    ankylosing 721.6
Hyperovarianism 256.1
Hyperovarism, hyperovaria 256.1
Hyperoxaluria (primary) 271.8
Hyperoxia 987.8
Hyperparathyroidism 252.0
  ectopic 259.3
  secondary, of renal origin 588.8
Hyperpathia (*see also* Disturbance, sensation) 782.0
  psychogenic 307.80
Hyperperistalsis 787.4
  psychogenic 306.4
Hyperpermeability, capillary 448.9
Hyperphagia 783.6

Hyperphenylalaninemia 270.1
Hyperphoria 378.40
 alternating 378.45
Hyperphosphatemia 275.3
Hyperpiesia (see also Hypertension) 401.9
Hyperpiesis (see also Hypertension) 401.9
Hyperpigmentation — see Pigmentation
Hyperpinealism 259.8
Hyperpipecolatemia 270.7
Hyperpituitarism 253.1
Hyperplasia, hyperplastic
 adenoids (lymphoid tissue) 474.12
  and tonsils 474.10
 adrenal (capsule) (cortex) (gland) 255.8
  with
   sexual precocity (male) 255.2
   virilism, adrenal 255.2
   virilization (female) 255.2
  congenital 255.2
  due to excess ACTH (ectopic) (pituitary)
   255.0
  medulla 255.8
 alpha cells (pancreatic)
  with
   gastrin excess 251.5
   glucagon excess 251.4
 appendix (lymphoid) 543.0
 artery, fibromuscular NEC 447.8
  carotid 447.8
  renal 447.3
 bone 733.99
  marrow 289.9
 breast (see also Hypertrophy, breast) 611.1
 carotid artery 447.8
 cementation, cementum (teeth) (tooth) 521.5
 cervical gland 785.6
 cervix (uteri) 622.1
  basal cell 622.1
  congenital 752.49
  endometrium 622.1
  polypoid 622.1
 chin 524.05
 clitoris, congenital 752.49
 dentin 521.5
 endocervicitis 616.0
 endometrium, endometrial (adenomatous)
   (atypical) (cystic) (glandular) (polypoid)
   (uterus) 621.3
  cervix 622.1
 epithelial 709.8
  focal, oral, including tongue 528.7
  mouth (focal) 528.7
  nipple 611.8
  skin 709.8
  tongue (focal) 528.7
  vaginal wall 623.0
 erythroid 289.9
 fascialis ossificans (progressiva) 728.11
 fibromuscular, artery NEC 447.8
  carotid 447.8
  renal 447.3
 genital
  female 629.8
  male 608.89
 gingiva 523.8
 glandularis
  cystica uteri 621.3
  endometrium (uterus) 621.3
  interstitialis uteri 621.3
 granulocytic 288.8
 gum 523.8
 hymen, congenital 752.49
 islands of Langerhans 251.1
 islet cell (pancreatic) 251.9
  alpha cells
   with excess
    gastrin 251.5
    glucagon 251.4
  beta cells 251.1
 juxtaglomerular (complex) (kidney) 593.89
 kidney (congenital) 753.3
 liver (congenital) 751.69
 lymph node (gland) 785.6
 lymphoid (diffuse) (nodular) 785.6
  appendix 543.0

Hyperplasia, hyperplastic — continued
 lymphoid — continued
  intestine 569.89
 mandibular 524.02
  alveolar 524.72
  unilateral condylar 526.89
 Marchand multiple nodular (liver) — see
   Cirrhosis, postnecrotic
 maxillary 524.01
  alveolar 524.71
 medulla, adrenal 255.8
 myometrium, myometrial 621.2
 nose (lymphoid) (polypoid) 478.1
 oral soft tissue (inflammatory) (irritative)
   (mucosa) NEC 528.9
  gingiva 523.8
  tongue 529.8
 organ or site, congenital NEC — see Anomaly,
   specified type NEC
 ovary 620.8
 palate, papillary 528.9
 pancreatic islet cells 251.9
  alpha
   with excess
    gastrin 251.5
    glucagon 251.4
  beta 251.1
 parathyroid (gland) 252.0
 persistent, vitreous (primary) 743.51
 pharynx (lymphoid) 478.29
 prostate 600.9 ▲
  adenofibromatous 600.2
  nodular 600.1
 renal artery (fibromuscular) 447.3
 reticuloendothelial (cell) 289.9
 salivary gland (any) 527.1
 Schimmelbusch's 610.1
 suprarenal (capsule) (gland) 255.8
 thymus (gland) (persistent) 254.0
 thyroid (see also Goiter) 240.9
  primary 242.0 ✓5ᵗʰ
  secondary 242.2 ✓5ᵗʰ
 tonsil (lymphoid tissue) 474.11
  and adenoids 474.10
 urethrovaginal 599.89
 uterus, uterine (myometrium) 621.2
  endometrium 621.3
 vitreous (humor), primary persistent 743.51
 vulva 624.3
 zygoma 738.11
Hyperpnea (see also Hyperventilation) 786.01
Hyperpotassemia 276.7
Hyperprebetalipoproteinemia 272.1
 with chylomicronemia 272.3
 familial 272.1
Hyperprolactinemia 253.1
Hyperprolinemia 270.8
Hyperproteinemia 273.8
Hyperprothrombinemia 289.8
Hyperpselaphesia 782.0
Hyperpyrexia 780.6
 heat (effects of) 992.0
 malarial (see also Malaria) 084.6
 malignant, due to anesthetic 995.86
 rheumatic — see Fever, rheumatic
 unknown origin (see also Pyrexia) 780.6
Hyperreactor, vascular 780.2
Hyperreflexia 796.1
 bladder, autonomic 596.54
  with cauda equina 344.61
 detrusor 344.61
Hypersalivation (see also Ptyalism) 527.7
Hypersarcosinemia 270.8
Hypersecretion
 ACTH 255.3
 androgens (ovarian) 256.1
 calcitonin 246.0
 corticoadrenal 255.3
 cortisol 255.0
 estrogen 256.0
 gastric 536.8
  psychogenic 306.4
 gastrin 251.5
 glucagon 251.4

Hypersecretion — continued
 hormone
  ACTH 255.3
  anterior pituitary 253.1
  growth NEC 253.0
  ovarian androgen 256.1
  testicular 257.0
  thyroid stimulating 242.8 ✓5ᵗʰ
 insulin — see Hyperinsulinism
 lacrimal glands (see also Epiphora) 375.20
 medulloadrenal 255.6
 milk 676.6 ✓5ᵗʰ
 ovarian androgens 256.1
 pituitary (anterior) 253.1
 salivary gland (any) 527.7
 testicular hormones 257.0
 thyrocalcitonin 246.0
 upper respiratory 478.9
Hypersegmentation, hereditary 288.2
 eosinophils 288.2
 neutrophil nuclei 288.2
Hypersensitive, hypersensitiveness,
  hypersensitivity — see also Allergy
 angiitis 446.20
  specified NEC 446.29
 carotid sinus 337.0
 colon 564.9
  psychogenic 306.4
 DNA (deoxyribonucleic acid) NEC 287.2
 drug (see also Allergy, drug) 995.2
 esophagus 530.89
 insect bites — see Injury, superficial, by site
 labyrinth 386.58
 pain (see also Disturbance, sensation) 782.0
 pneumonitis NEC 495.9
 reaction (see also Allergy) 995.3
  upper respiratory tract NEC 478.8
 stomach (allergic) (nonallergic) 536.8
  psychogenic 306.4
Hypersomatotropism (classic) 253.0
Hypersomnia 780.54
 with sleep apnea 780.53
 nonorganic origin 307.43
  persistent (primary) 307.44
  transient 307.43
Hypersplenia 289.4
Hypersplenism 289.4
Hypersteatosis 706.3
Hyperstimulation, ovarian 256.1
Hypersuprarenalism 255.3
Hypersusceptibility — see Allergy
Hyper-TBG-nemia 246.8
Hypertelorism 756.0
 orbit, orbital 376.41

	Malignant	Benign	Unspecified
Hypertension, hypertensive (arterial) (arteriolar) (crisis) (degeneration) (disease) (essential) (fluctuating) (idiopathic) (intermittent) (labile) (low renin) (orthostatic) (paroxysmal) (primary) (systemic) (uncontrolled) (vascular)	401.0	401.1	401.9
with			
heart involvement (conditions classifiable to 425.8, 428, 429.0-429.3, 429.8, 429.9 due to hypertension) (*see also* Hypertension, heart)	402.00	402.10	402.90
with kidney involvement — *see* Hypertension, cardiorenal			
renal involvement (only conditions classifiable to 585, 586, 587) (excludes conditions classifiable to 584) (*see also* Hypertension, kidney)	403.00	403.10	403.90
renal sclerosis or failure	403.00	403.10	403.90
with heart involvement — *see* Hypertension, cardiorenal			
failure (and sclerosis) (*see also* Hypertension, kidney)	403.01	403.11	403.91
sclerosis without failure (*see also* Hypertension, kidney)	403.00	403.10	403.90
accelerated — (*see also* Hypertension, by type, malignant)	401.0	—	—
antepartum — *see* Hypertension, complicating pregnancy, childbirth, or the puerperium			
cardiorenal (disease)	404.00	404.10	404.90
with			
heart failure	404.01	404.11	404.91
and renal failure	404.03	404.13	404.93
renal failure	404.02	404.12	404.92
and heart failure	404.03	404.13	404.93
cardiovascular disease (arteriosclerotic) (sclerotic)	402.00	402.10	402.90
with			
heart failure	402.01	402.11	402.91
renal involvement (conditions classifiable to 403) (*see also* Hypertension, cardiorenal)	404.00	404.10	404.90
cardiovascular renal (disease) (sclerosis) (*see also* Hypertension, cardiorenal)	404.00	404.10	404.90
cerebrovascular disease NEC	437.2	437.2	437.2
complicating pregnancy, childbirth, or the puerperium	642.2 ✓5ᵗʰ	642.0	642.9 ✓5ᵗʰ
with			
albuminuria (and edema) (mild)	—	—	642.4 ✓5ᵗʰ
severe	—	—	642.5 ✓5ᵗʰ
edema (mild)	—	—	642.4 ✓5ᵗʰ
severe	—	—	642.5 ✓5ᵗʰ
heart disease	642.2 ✓5ᵗʰ	642.2 ✓5ᵗʰ	642.2 ✓5ᵗʰ
and renal disease	642.2 ✓5ᵗʰ	642.2 ✓5ᵗʰ	642.2 ✓5ᵗʰ
renal disease	642.2 ✓5ᵗʰ	642.2 ✓5ᵗʰ	642.2 ✓5ᵗʰ
and heart disease	642.2 ✓5ᵗʰ	642.2 ✓5ᵗʰ	642.2 ✓5ᵗʰ
chronic	642.2 ✓5ᵗʰ	642.0 ✓5ᵗʰ	642.0 ✓5ᵗʰ
with pre-eclampsia or eclampsia	642.7 ✓5ᵗʰ	642.7 ✓5ᵗʰ	642.7 ✓5ᵗʰ
fetus or newborn	760.0	760.0	760.0
essential	—	642.0	642.0 ✓5ᵗʰ
with pre-eclampsia or eclampsia	—	642.7 ✓5ᵗʰ	642.7 ✓5ᵗʰ
fetus or newborn	760.0	760.0	760.0
fetus or newborn	760.0	760.0	760.0
gestational	—	—	642.3 ✓5ᵗʰ
pre-existing	642.2 ✓5ᵗʰ	642.0	642.0 ✓5ᵗʰ
with pre-eclampsia or eclampsia	642.7 ✓5ᵗʰ	642.7 ✓5ᵗʰ	642.7 ✓5ᵗʰ
fetus or newborn	760.0	760.0	760.0
secondary to renal disease	642.1 ✓5ᵗʰ	642.1 ✓5ᵗʰ	642.1 ✓5ᵗʰ
with pre-eclampsia or eclampsia	642.7 ✓5ᵗʰ	642.7 ✓5ᵗʰ	642.7 ✓5ᵗʰ
fetus or newborn	760.0	760.0	760.0
transient	—	—	642.3 ✓5ᵗʰ
due to			
aldosteronism, primary	405.09	405.19	405.99
brain tumor	405.09	405.19	405.99
bulbar poliomyelitis	405.09	405.19	405.99
calculus			
kidney	405.09	405.19	405.99
ureter	405.09	405.19	405.99
coarctation, aorta	405.09	405.19	405.99
Cushing's disease	405.09	405.19	405.99
glomerulosclerosis (*see also* Hypertension, kidney)	403.00	403.10	403.90
periarteritis nodosa	405.09	405.19	405.99
pheochromocytoma	405.09	405.19	405.99
polycystic kidney(s)	405.09	405.19	405.99

✓4ᵗʰ Fourth-digit Required   ✓5ᵗʰ Fifth-digit Required   ▶◀ Revised Text   ● New Line   ▲ Revised Code

Hypertension — Hypertension

Hypertension — Hypertension

	Malignant	Benign	Unspecified
Hypertension, hypertensive — *continued*			
due to — *continued*			
polycythemia	405.09	405.19	405.99
porphyria	405.09	405.19	405.99
pyelonephritis	405.09	405.19	405.99
renal (artery)			
aneurysm	405.01	405.11	405.91
anomaly	405.01	405.11	405.91
embolism	405.01	405.11	405.91
fibromuscular hyperplasia	405.01	405.11	405.91
occlusion	405.01	405.11	405.91
stenosis	405.01	405.11	405.91
thrombosis	405.01	405.11	405.91
encephalopathy	437.2	437.2	437.2
gestational (transient) NEC	—	—	642.3 ✓5ᵗʰ
Goldblatt's	440.1	440.1	440.1
heart (disease) (conditions classifiable to 425.8, 428, 429.0-429.3, 429.8, 429.9 due to hypertension)	402.00	402.10	402.90
with heart failure	402.01	402.11	402.91
hypertensive kidney disease (conditions classifiable to 403) (*see also* Hypertension, cardiorenal)	404.00	404.10	404.90
renal sclerosis (*see also* Hypertension, cardiorenal)	404.00	404.10	404.90
intracranial, benign	—	348.2	—
intraocular	—	—	365.04
kidney	403.00	403.10	403.90
with			
heart involvement (conditions classifiable to 425.8, 428, 429.0-429.3, 429.8, 429.9 due to hypertension) (*see also* Hypertension, cardiorenal)	404.00	404.10	404.90
hypertensive heart (disease) (conditions classifiable to 402) (*see also* Hypertension, cardiorenal)	404.00	404.10	404.90
lesser circulation	—	—	416.0
necrotizing	401.0	—	—
ocular	—	—	365.04
portal (due to chronic liver disease)	—	—	572.3
postoperative	—	—	997.91
psychogenic	—	—	306.2
puerperal, postpartum — *see* Hypertension, complicating pregnancy, childbirth, or the puerperium			
pulmonary (artery)	—	—	416.8
with cor pulmonale (chronic)	—	—	416.8
acute	—	—	415.0
idiopathic	—	—	416.0
primary	—	—	416.0
of newborn	—	—	747.83 ●
secondary	—	—	416.8
renal (disease) (*see also* Hypertension, kidney)	403.00	403.10	403.90
renovascular NEC	405.01	405.11	405.91
secondary NEC	405.09	405.19	405.99
due to			
aldosteronism, primary	405.09	405.19	405.99
brain tumor	405.09	405.19	405.99
bulbar poliomyelitis	405.09	405.19	405.99
calculus			
kidney	405.09	405.19	405.99
ureter	405.09	405.19	405.99
coarctation, aorta	405.09	405.19	405.99
Cushing's disease	405.09	405.19	405.99
glomerulosclerosis (*see also* Hypertension, kidney)	403.00	403.10	403.90
periarteritis nodosa	405.09	405.19	405.99
pheochromocytoma	405.09	405.19	405.99
polycystic kidney(s)	405.09	405.19	405.99
polycythemia	405.09	405.19	405.99
porphyria	405.09	405.19	405.99
pyelonephritis	405.09	405.19	405.99
renal (artery)			
aneurysm	405.01	405.11	405.91
anomaly	405.01	405.11	405.91
embolism	405.01	405.11	405.91
fibromuscular hyperplasia	405.01	405.11	405.91
occlusion	405.01	405.11	405.91
stenosis	405.01	405.11	405.91
thrombosis	405.01	405.11	405.91
transient	—	—	796.2
of pregnancy	—	—	642.3 ✓5ᵗʰ

	Malignant	Benign	Unspecified
Hypertension, hypertensive — *continued*			
venous, chronic (asymptomatic) (idiopathic)	—	—	459.30 ●
due to			●
deep vein thrombosis (see also Syndrome, postphlebetic)	—	—	459.10 ●
with			●
complication, NEC	—	—	459.39 ●
inflammation	—	—	459.32 ●
with ulcer	—	—	459.33 ●
ulcer	—	—	459.31 ●
with inflammation	—	—	459.33 ●

Hyperthecosis, ovary 256.8

Hyperthermia (of unknown origin) (*see also* Pyrexia) 780.6
  malignant (due to anesthesia) 995.86
  newborn 778.4

Hyperthymergasia (*see also* Psychosis, affective) 296.0 ✓5th
  reactive (from emotional stress, psychological trauma) 298.1
  recurrent episode 296.1 ✓5th
  single episode 296.0 ✓5th

Hyperthymism 254.8

Hyperthyroid (recurrent) — *see* Hyperthyroidism

Hyperthyroidism (latent) (preadult) (recurrent) (without goiter) 242.9 ✓5th

> *Note* — *Use the following fifth-digit subclassification with category 242:*
>
> 0   *without mention of thyrotoxic crisis or storm*
>
> 1   *with mention of thyrotoxic crisis or storm*

  with
    goiter (diffuse) 242.0 ✓5th
      adenomatous 242.3 ✓5th
        multinodular 242.2 ✓5th
        uninodular 242.1 ✓5th
      nodular 242.3 ✓5th
        multinodular 242.2 ✓5th
        uninodular 242.1 ✓5th
    thyroid nodule 242.1 ✓5th
  complicating pregnancy, childbirth, or puerperium 648.1 ✓5th
  neonatal (transient) 775.3

Hypertonia — *see* Hypertonicity

Hypertonicity
  bladder 596.51
  fetus or newborn 779.89 ▲
  gastrointestinal (tract) 536.8
  infancy 779.89 ▲
    due to electrolyte imbalance 779.89 ▲
  muscle 728.85
  stomach 536.8
    psychogenic 306.4
  uterus, uterine (contractions) 661.4 ✓5th
    affecting fetus or newborn 763.7

Hypertony — *see* Hypertonicity

Hypertransaminemia 790.4

Hypertrichosis 704.1
  congenital 757.4
  eyelid 374.54
  lanuginosa 757.4
    acquired 704.1

Hypertriglyceridemia, essential 272.1

Hypertrophy, hypertrophic
  adenoids (infectional) 474.12
    and tonsils (faucial) (infective) (lingual) (lymphoid) 474.10
  adrenal 255.8
  alveolar process or ridge 525.8
  anal papillae 569.49
  apocrine gland 705.82
  artery NEC 447.8
    carotid 447.8
    congenital (peripheral) NEC 747.60
      gastrointestinal 747.61
      lower limb 747.64
      renal 747.62
      specified NEC 747.69
      spinal 747.82
      upper limb 747.63
  arthritis (chronic) (*see also* Osteoarthrosis) 715.9 ✓5th
    spine (*see also* Spondylosis) 721.90
  arytenoid 478.79
  asymmetrical (heart) 429.9
  auricular — *see* Hypertrophy, cardiac
  Bartholin's gland 624.8
  bile duct 576.8
  bladder (sphincter) (trigone) 596.8
  blind spot, visual field 368.42
  bone 733.99

2003 ICD•9•CM

October 2002 • Volume 2 — 175

Hypertension — Hypertrophy

Hypertrophy, hypertrophic — *continued*
  brain 348.8
  breast 611.1
    cystic 610.1
    fetus or newborn 778.7
    fibrocystic 610.1
    massive pubertal 611.1
    puerperal, postpartum 676.3 ✓5ᵗʰ
    senile (parenchymatous) 611.1
  cardiac (chronic) (idiopathic) 429.3
    with
        rheumatic fever (conditions classifiable to
            390)
          active 391.8
            with chorea 392.0
          inactive or quiescent (with chorea)
            398.99
    congenital NEC 746.89
    fatty (*see also* Degeneration, myocardial)
        429.1
    hypertensive (*see also* Hypertension, heart)
        402.90
    rheumatic (with chorea) 398.99
        active or acute 391.8
          with chorea 392.0
    valve (*see also* Endocarditis) 424.90
        congenital NEC 746.89
  cartilage 733.99
  cecum 569.89
  cervix (uteri) 622.6
    congenital 752.49
    elongation 622.6
  clitoris (cirrhotic) 624.2
    congenital 752.49
  colon 569.89
    congenital 751.3
  conjunctiva, lymphoid 372.73
  cornea 371.89
  corpora cavernosa 607.89
  duodenum 537.89
  endometrium (uterus) 621.3
    cervix 622.6
  epididymis 608.89
  esophageal hiatus (congenital) 756.6
    with hernia — *see* Hernia, diaphragm
  eyelid 374.30
  falx, skull 733.99
  fat pad 729.30
    infrapatellar 729.31
    knee 729.31
    orbital 374.34
    popliteal 729.31
    prepatellar 729.31
    retropatellar 729.31
    specified site NEC 729.39
  foot (congenital) 755.67
  frenum, frenulum (tongue) 529.8
    linguae 529.8
    lip 528.5
  gallbladder or cystic duct 575.8
  gastric mucosa 535.2 ✓5ᵗʰ
  gingiva 523.8
  gland, glandular (general) NEC 785.6
  gum (mucous membrane) 523.8
  heart (idiopathic) — *see also* Hypertrophy,
      cardiac
    valve — *see also* Endocarditis
      congenital NEC 746.89
  hemifacial 754.0
  hepatic — *see* Hypertrophy, liver
  hiatus (esophageal) 756.6
  hilus gland 785.6
  hymen, congenital 752.49
  ileum 569.89
  infrapatellar fat pad 729.31
  intestine 569.89
  jejunum 569.89
  kidney (compensatory) 593.1
    congenital 753.3
  labial frenulum 528.5
  labium (majus) (minus) 624.3
  lacrimal gland, chronic 375.03
  ligament 728.9
    spinal 724.8
  linguae frenulum 529.8
  lingual tonsil (infectional) 474.11

Hypertrophy, hypertrophic — *continued*
  lip (frenum) 528.5
    congenital 744.81
  liver 789.1
    acute 573.8
    cirrhotic — *see* Cirrhosis, liver
    congenital 751.69
    fatty — *see* Fatty, liver
  lymph gland 785.6
    tuberculous — *see* Tuberculosis, lymph
        gland
  mammary gland — *see* Hypertrophy, breast
  maxillary frenuium 528.5
  Meckel's diverticulum (congenital) 751.0
  medial meniscus, acquired 717.3
  median bar 600.9
  mediastinum 519.3
  meibomian gland 373.2
  meniscus, knee, congenital 755.64
  metatarsal head 733.99
  metatarsus 733.99
  mouth 528.9
  mucous membrane
    alveolar process 523.8
    nose 478.1
    turbinate (nasal) 478.0
  muscle 728.9
  muscular coat, artery NEC 447.8
    carotid 447.8
    renal 447.3
  myocardium (*see also* Hypertrophy, cardiac)
      429.3
    idiopathic 425.4
  myometrium 621.2
  nail 703.8
    congenital 757.5
  nasal 478.1
    alae 478.1
    bone 738.0
    cartilage 478.1
    mucous membrane (septum) 478.1
    sinus (*see also* Sinusitis) 473.9
    turbinate 478.0
  nasopharynx, lymphoid (infectional) (tissue)
      (wall) 478.29
  neck, uterus 622.6
  nipple 611.1
  normal aperture diaphragm (congenital) 756.6
  nose (*see also* Hypertrophy, nasal) 478.1
  orbit 376.46
  organ or site, congenital NEC — *see* Anomaly,
      specified type NEC
  osteoarthropathy (pulmonary) 731.2
  ovary 620.8
  palate (hard) 526.89
    soft 528.9
  pancreas (congenital) 751.7
  papillae
    anal 569.49
    tongue 529.3
  parathyroid (gland) 252.0
  parotid gland 527.1
  penis 607.89
  phallus 607.89
    female (clitoris) 624.2
  pharyngeal tonsil 474.12
  pharyngitis 472.1
  pharynx 478.29
    lymphoid (infectional) (tissue) (wall) 478.29
  pituitary (fossa) (gland) 253.8
  popliteal fat pad 729.31
  preauricular (lymph) gland (Hampstead) 785.6
  prepuce (congenital) 605
    female 624.2
  prostate (asymptomatic) (early) (recurrent)
      600.9
    adenofibromatous 600.2
    benign 600.0
    congenital 752.8
  pseudoedematous hypodermal 757.0
  pseudomuscular 359.1
  pylorus (muscle) (sphincter) 537.0
    congenital 750.5
    infantile 750.5
  rectal sphincter 569.49
  rectum 569.49
  renal 593.1
  rhinitis (turbinate) 472.0

Hypertrophy, hypertrophic — *continued*
  salivary duct or gland 527.1
    congenital 750.26
  scaphoid (tarsal) 733.99
  scar 701.4
  scrotum 608.89
  sella turcica 253.8
  seminal vesicle 608.89
  sigmoid 569.89
  skin condition NEC 701.9
  spermatic cord 608.89
  spinal ligament 728.9
  spleen — *see* Splenomegaly
  spondylitis (spine) (*see also* Spondylosis)
      721.90
  stomach 537.89
  subaortic stenosis (idiopathic) 425.1
  sublingual gland 527.1
    congenital 750.26
  submaxillary gland 527.1
  suprarenal (gland) 255.8
  tendon 727.9
  testis 608.89
    congenital 752.8
  thymic, thymus (congenital) (gland) 254.0
  thyroid (gland) (*see also* Goiter) 240.9
    primary 242.0 ✓5ᵗʰ
    secondary 242.2 ✓5ᵗʰ
  toe (congenital) 755.65
    acquired 735.8
  tongue 529.8
    congenital 750.15
    frenum 529.8
    papillae (foliate) 529.3
  tonsil (faucial) (infective) (lingual) (lymphoid)
      474.11
    with
        adenoiditis 474.01
        tonsillitis 474.00
          and adenoiditis 474.02
        and adenoids 474.10
  tunica vaginalis 608.89
  turbinate (mucous membrane) 478.0
  ureter 593.89
  urethra 599.84
  uterus 621.2
    puerperal, postpartum 674.8 ✓5ᵗʰ
  uvula 528.9
  vagina 623.8
  vas deferens 608.89
  vein 459.89
  ventricle, ventricular (heart) (left) (right) — *see
      also* Hypertrophy, cardiac
    congenital 746.89
    due to hypertension (left) (right) (*see also*
        Hypertension, heart) 402.90
      benign 402.10
      malignant 402.00
    right with ventricular septal defect,
        pulmonary stenosis or atresia, and
        dextraposition of aorta 745.2
  verumontanum 599.89
  vesical 596.8
  vocal cord 478.5
  vulva 624.3
    stasis (nonfilarial) 624.3
Hypertropia (intermittent) (periodic) 378.31
Hypertyrosinemia 270.2
Hyperuricemia 790.6
Hypervalinemia 270.3
Hyperventilation (tetany) 786.01
  hysterical 300.11
  psychogenic 306.1
  syndrome 306.1
Hyperviscidosis 277.00
Hyperviscosity (of serum) (syndrome) NEC 273.3
  polycythemic 289.0
  sclerocythemic 282.8
Hypervitaminosis (dietary) NEC 278.8
  A (dietary) 278.2
  D (dietary) 278.4
  from excessive administration or use of vitamin
      preparations (chronic) 278.8
    reaction to sudden overdose 963.5

Hypertrophy — Hypervitaminosis

Hypervitaminosis (dietary) NEC
  from excessive administration or use of vitamin
    preparations — *continued*
    vitamin A 278.2
      reaction to sudden overdose 963.5
    vitamin D 278.4
      reaction to sudden overdose 963.5
    vitamin K
      correct substance properly administered
        278.8
      overdose or wrong substance given or
        taken 964.3
Hypervolemia 276.6
Hypesthesia (*see also* Disturbance, sensation)
    782.0
    cornea 371.81
Hyphema (anterior chamber) (ciliary body) (iris)
    364.41
    traumatic 921.3
Hyphemia — *see* Hyphema
Hypoacidity, gastric 536.8
    psychogenic 306.4
Hypoactive labyrinth (function) — *see*
    Hypofunction, labyrinth
Hypoadrenalism 255.4
    tuberculous (*see also* Tuberculosis) 017.6 ☑5ᵗʰ
Hypoadrenocorticism 255.4
    pituitary 253.4
Hypoalbuminemia 273.8
Hypoalphalipoproteinemia 272.5
Hypobarism 993.2
Hypobaropathy 993.2
Hypobetalipoproteinemia (familial) 272.5
Hypocalcemia 275.41
    cow's milk 775.4
    dietary 269.3
    neonatal 775.4
    phosphate-loading 775.4
Hypocalcification, teeth 520.4
Hypochloremia 276.9
Hypochlorhydria 536.8
    neurotic 306.4
    psychogenic 306.4
Hypocholesteremia 272.5
Hypochondria (reaction) 300.7
Hypochondriac 300.7
Hyponchondriasis 300.7
Hypochromasia blood cells 280.9
Hypochromic anemia 280.9
    due to blood loss (chronic) 280.0
      acute 285.1
    microcytic 280.9
Hypocoagulability (*see also* Defect, coagulation)
    286.9
Hypocomplementemia 279.8
Hypocythemia (progressive) 284.9
Hypodontia (*see also* Anodontia) 520.0
Hypoeosinophilia 288.8
Hypoesthesia (*see also* Disturbance, sensation)
    782.0
    cornea 371.81
    tactile 782.0
Hypoestrinism 256.39
Hypoestrogenism 256.39
Hypoferremia 280.9
    due to blood loss (chronic) 280.0
Hypofertility
    female 628.9
    male 606.1
Hypofibrinogenemia 286.3
    acquired 286.6
    congenital 286.3
Hypofunction
    adrenal (gland) 255.4
      cortex 255.4
      medulla 255.5
      specified NEC 255.5
    cerebral 331.9
    corticoadrenal NEC 255.4
    intestinal 564.89

Hypofunction — *continued*
    labyrinth (unilateral) 386.53
      with loss of labyrinthine reactivity 386.55
      bilateral 386.54
        with loss of labyrinthine reactivity 386.56
    Leydig cell 257.2
    ovary 256.39
      postablative 256.2
    pituitary (anterior) (gland) (lobe) 253.2
      posterior 253.5
    testicular 257.2
      iatrogenic 257.1
      postablative 257.1
      postirradiation 257.1
      postsurgical 257.1
Hypogammaglobulinemia 279.00
    acquired primary 279.06
    non-sex-linked, congenital 279.06
    sporadic 279.06
    transient of infancy 279.09
Hypogenitalism (congenital) (female) (male) 752.8
    penis 752.69
Hypoglycemia (spontaneous) 251.2
    coma 251.0
      diabetic 250.3 ☑5ᵗʰ
    diabetic 250.8 ☑5ᵗʰ
    due to insulin 251.0
      therapeutic misadventure 962.3
    familial (idiopathic) 251.2
    following gastrointestinal surgery 579.3
    infantile (idiopathic) 251.2
    in infant of diabetic mother 775.0
    leucine-induced 270.3
    neonatal 775.6
    reactive 251.2
    specified NEC 251.1
Hypoglycemic shock 251.0
    diabetic 250.8 ☑5ᵗʰ
    due to insulin 251.0
    functional (syndrome) 251.1
Hypogonadism
    female 256.39
    gonadotrophic (isolated) 253.4
    hypogonadotropic (isolated) (with anosmia)
      253.4
    isolated 253.4
    male 257.2
    ovarian (primary) 256.39
    pituitary (secondary) 253.4
    testicular (primary) (secondary) 257.2
Hypohidrosis 705.0
Hypohidrotic ectodermal dysplasia 757.31
Hypoidrosis 705.0
Hypoinsulinemia, postsurgical 251.3
    postpancreatectomy (complete) (partial) 251.3
Hypokalemia 276.8
Hypokinesia 780.99   ▲
Hypoleukia splenica 289.4
Hypoleukocytosis 288.8
Hypolipidemia 272.5
Hypolipoproteinemia 272.5
Hypomagnesemia 275.2
    neonatal 775.4
Hypomania, hypomanic reaction (*see also*
    Psychosis, affective) 296.0 ☑5ᵗʰ
    recurrent episode 296.1 ☑5ᵗʰ
    single episode 296.0 ☑5ᵗʰ
Hypomastia (congenital) 757.6
Hypomenorrhea 626.1
Hypometabolism 783.9
Hypomotility
    gastrointestinal tract 536.8
      psychogenic 306.4
    intestine 564.89
      psychogenic 306.4
    stomach 536.8
      psychogenic 306.4
Hyponasality 784.49
Hyponatremia 276.1
Hypo-ovarianism 256.39
Hypo-ovarism 256.39

Hypoparathyroidism (idiopathic) (surgically
    induced) 252.1
    neonatal 775.4
Hypopharyngitis 462
Hypophoria 378.40
Hypophosphatasia 275.3
Hypophosphatemia (acquired) (congenital)
    (familial) 275.3
    renal 275.3
Hypophyseal, hypophysis — *see also* condition
    dwarfism 253.3
    gigantism 253.0
    syndrome 253.8
Hypophyseothalamic syndrome 253.8
Hypopiesis — *see* Hypotension
Hypopigmentation 709.00
    eyelid 374.53
Hypopinealism 259.8
Hypopituitarism (juvenile) (syndrome) 253.2
    due to
      hormone therapy 253.7
      hypophysectomy 253.7
      radiotherapy 253.7
    postablative 253.7
    postpartum hemorrhage 253.2
Hypoplasia, hypoplasis 759.89
    adrenal (gland) 759.1
    alimentary tract 751.8
      lower 751.2
      upper 750.8
    anus, anal (canal) 751.2
    aorta 747.22
    aortic
      arch (tubular) 747.10
      orifice or valve with hypoplasia of ascending
        aorta and defective development of left
        ventricle (with mitral valve atresia)
        746.7
    appendix 751.2
    areola 757.6
    arm (*see also* Absence, arm, congenital) 755.20
    artery (congenital) (peripheral) NEC 747.60
      brain 747.81
      cerebral 747.81
      coronary 746.85
      gastrointestinal 747.61
      lower limb 747.64
      pulmonary 747.3
      renal 747.62
      retinal 743.58
      specified NEC 747.69
      spinal 747.82
      umbilical 747.5
      upper limb 747.63
    auditory canal 744.29
      causing impairment of hearing 744.02
    biliary duct (common) or passage 751.61
    bladder 753.8
    bone NEC 756.9
      face 756.0
      malar 756.0
      mandible 524.04
        alveolar 524.74
      marrow 284.9
        acquired (secondary) 284.8
        congenital 284.0
        idiopathic 284.9
      maxilla 524.03
        alveolar 524.73
      skull (*see also* Hypoplasia, skull) 756.0
    brain 742.1
      gyri 742.2
      specified part 742.2
    breast (areola) 757.6
    bronchus (tree) 748.3
    cardiac 746.89
      valve — *see* Hypoplasia, heart, valve
      vein 746.89
    carpus (*see also* Absence, carpal, congenital)
      755.28
    cartilaginous 756.9
    cecum 751.2
    cementum 520.4
      hereditary 520.5
    cephalic 742.1

Hypoplasia — Hypothyroidism

Hypoplasia, hypoplasis — *continued*
  cerebellum 742.2
  cervix (uteri) 752.49
  chin 524.06
  clavicle 755.51
  coccyx 756.19
  colon 751.2
  corpus callosum 742.2
  cricoid cartilage 748.3
  dermal, focal (Goltz) 757.39
  digestive organ(s) or tract NEC 751.8
      lower 751.2
      upper 750.8
  ear 744.29
      auricle 744.23
      lobe 744.29
      middle, except ossicles 744.03
          ossicles 744.04
      ossicles 744.04
  enamel of teeth (neonatal) (postnatal) (prenatal) 520.4
      hereditary 520.5
  endocrine (gland) NEC 759.2
  endometrium 621.8
  epididymis 752.8
  epiglottis 748.3
  erythroid, congenital 284.0
  erythropoietic, chronic acquired 284.8
  esophagus 750.3
  Eustachian tube 744.24
  eye (*see also* Microphthalmos) 743.10
      lid 743.62
  face 744.89
      bone(s) 756.0
  fallopian tube 752.19
  femur (*see also* Absence, femur, congenital) 755.34
  fibula (*see also* Absence, fibula, congenital) 755.37
  finger (*see also* Absence, finger, congenital) 755.29
  focal dermal 757.39
  foot 755.31
  gallbladder 751.69
  genitalia, genital organ(s)
      female 752.8
          external 752.49
          internal NEC 752.8
      in adiposogenital dystrophy 253.8
      male 752.8
          penis 752.69
  glottis 748.3
  hair 757.4
  hand 755.21
  heart 746.89
      left (complex) (syndrome) 746.7
      valve NEC 746.89
          pulmonary 746.01
  humerus (*see also* Absence, humerus, congenital) 755.24
  hymen 752.49
  intestine (small) 751.1
      large 751.2
  iris 743.46
  jaw 524.09
  kidney(s) 753.0
  labium (majus) (minus) 752.49
  labyrinth, membranous 744.05
  lacrimal duct (apparatus) 743.65
  larynx 748.3
  leg (*see also* Absence, limb, congenital, lower) 755.30
  limb 755.4
      lower (*see also* Absence, limb, congenital, lower) 755.30
      upper (*see also* Absence, limb, congenital, upper) 755.20
  liver 751.69
  lung (lobe) 748.5
  mammary (areolar) 757.6
  mandibular 524.04
      alveolar 524.74
      unilateral condylar 526.89
  maxillary 524.03
      alveolar 524.73
  medullary 284.9
  megakaryocytic 287.3

Hypoplasia, hypoplasis — *continued*
  metacarpus (*see also* Absence, metacarpal, congenital) 755.28
  metatarsus (*see also* Absence, metatarsal, congenital) 755.38
  muscle 756.89
      eye 743.69
  myocardium (congenital) (Uhl's anomaly) 746.84
  nail(s) 757.5
  nasolacrimal duct 743.65
  nervous system NEC 742.8
  neural 742.8
  nose, nasal 748.1
  ophthalmic (*see also* Microphthalmos) 743.10
  organ
      of Corti 744.05
      or site NEC — *see* Anomaly, by site
  osseous meatus (ear) 744.03
  ovary 752.0
  oviduct 752.19
  pancreas 751.7
  parathyroid (gland) 759.2
  parotid gland 750.26
  patella 755.64
  pelvis, pelvic girdle 755.69
  penis 752.69
  peripheral vascular system (congenital) NEC 747.60
      gastrointestinal 747.61
      lower limb 747.64
      renal 747.62
      specified NEC 747.69
      spinal 747.82
      upper limb 747.63
  pituitary (gland) 759.2
  pulmonary 748.5
      arteriovenous 747.3
      artery 747.3
      valve 746.01
  punctum lacrimale 743.65
  radioulnar (*see also* Absence, radius, congenital, with ulna) 755.25
  radius (*see also* Absence, radius, congenital) 755.26
  rectum 751.2
  respiratory system NEC 748.9
  rib 756.3
  sacrum 756.19
  scapula 755.59
  shoulder girdle 755.59
  skin 757.39
  skull (bone) 756.0
      with
          anencephalus 740.0
          encephalocele 742.0
          hydrocephalus 742.3
              with spina bifida (*see also* Spina bifida) 741.0 ✓5ᵗʰ
          microcephalus 742.1
  spinal (cord) (ventral horn cell) 742.59
      vessel 747.82
  spine 756.19
  spleen 759.0
  sternum 756.3
  tarsus (*see also* Absence, tarsal, congenital) 755.38
  testis, testicle 752.8
  thymus (gland) 279.11
  thyroid (gland) 243
      cartilage 748.3
  tibiofibular (*see also* Absence, tibia, congenital, with fibula) 755.35
  toe (*see also* Absence, toe, congenital) 755.39
  tongue 750.16
  trachea (cartilage) (rings) 748.3
  Turner's (tooth) 520.4
  ulna (*see also* Absence, ulna, congenital) 755.27
  umbilical artery 747.5
  ureter 753.29
  uterus 752.3
  vagina 752.49
  vascular (peripheral) NEC (*see also* Hypoplasia, peripheral vascular system) 747.60
      brain 747.81

Hypoplasia, hypoplasis — *continued*
  vein(s) (peripheral) NEC (*see also* Hypoplasia, peripheral vascular system) 747.60
      brain 747.81
      cardiac 746.89
      great 747.49
      portal 747.49
      pulmonary 747.49
  vena cava (inferior) (superior) 747.49
  vertebra 756.19
  vulva 752.49
  zonule (ciliary) 743.39
  zygoma 738.12

Hypopotassemia 276.8

Hypoproaccelerinemia (*see also* Defect, coagulation) 286.3

Hypoproconvertinemia (congenital) (*see also* Defect, coagulation) 286.3

Hypoproteinemia (essential) (hypermetabolic) (idiopathic) 273.8

Hypoproteinosis 260

Hypoprothrombinemia (congenital) (hereditary) (idiopathic) (*see also* Defect, coagulation) 286.3
  acquired 286.7
  newborn 776.3

Hypopselaphesia 782.0

Hypopyon (anterior chamber) (eye) 364.05
  iritis 364.05
  ulcer (cornea) 370.04

Hypopyrexia 780.99   ▲

Hyporeflex 796.1

Hyporeninemia, extreme 790.99
  in primary aldosteronism 255.1

Hyporesponsive episode 780.09

Hyposecretion
  ACTH 253.4
  ovary 256.39
      postblative 256.2
  salivary gland (any) 527.7

Hyposegmentation of neutrophils, hereditary 288.2

Hyposiderinemia 280.9

Hyposmolality 276.1
  syndrome 276.1

Hyposomatotropism 253.3

Hyposomnia (*see also* Insomnia) 780.52

Hypospadias (male) 752.61
  female 753.8

Hypospermatogenesis 606.1

Hyposphagma 372.72

Hyposplenism 289.59

Hypostasis, pulmonary 514

Hypostatic — *see* condition

Hyposthenuria 593.89

Hyposuprarenalism 255.4

Hypo-TBG-nemia 246.8

Hypotension (arterial) (constitutional) 458.9
  chronic 458.1
  iatrogenic 458.2
  maternal, syndrome (following labor and delivery) 669.2 ✓5ᵗʰ
  orthostatic (chronic) 458.0
      dysautonomic-dyskinetic syndrome 333.0
  permanent idiopathic 458.1
  postoperative 458.2
  postural 458.0
  specified type NEC 458.8
  transient 796.3

Hypothermia (accidental) 991.6
  anesthetic 995.89
  newborn NEC 778.3
  not associated with low environmental temperature 780.99   ▲

Hypothymergasia (*see also* Psychosis, affective) 296.2 ✓5ᵗʰ
  recurrent episode 296.3 ✓5ᵗʰ
  single episode 296.2 ✓5ᵗʰ

Hypothyroidism (acquired) 244.9
  complicating pregnancy, childbirth, or puerperium 648.1 ✓5ᵗʰ
  congenital 243

Hypothyroidism — *continued*
  due to
    ablation 244.1
      radioactive iodine 244.1
      surgical 244.0
    iodine (administration) (ingestion) 244.2
      radioactive 244.1
    irradiation therapy 244.1
    p-aminosalicylic acid (PAS) 244.3
    phenylbutazone 244.3
    resorcinol 244.3
    specified cause NEC 244.8
    surgery 244.0
  goitrous (sporadic) 246.1
  iatrogenic NEC 244.3
  iodine 244.2
  pituitary 244.8
  postablative NEC 244.1
  postsurgical 244.0
  primary 244.9
  secondary NEC 244.8
  specified cause NEC 244.8
  sporadic goitrous 246.1

Hypotonia, hypotonicity, hypotony 781.3
  benign congenital 358.8
  bladder 596.4
  congenital 779.89
    benign 358.8
  eye 360.30 ▲
    due to
      fistula 360.32
      ocular disorder NEC 360.33
    following loss of aqueous or vitreous 360.33
    primary 360.31
  infantile muscular (benign) 359.0
  muscle 728.9
  uterus, uterine (contractions) — *see* Inertia, uterus

Hypotrichosis 704.09
  congenital 757.4
  lid (congenital) 757.4
    acquired 374.55
  postinfectional NEC 704.09

Hypotropia 378.32

Hypoventilation 786.09

Hypovitaminosis (*see also* Deficiency, vitamin) 269.2

Hypovolemia 276.5
  surgical shock 998.0
  traumatic (shock) 958.4

Hypoxemia (*see also* Anoxia) 799.0

Hypoxia (*see also* Anoxia) 799.0
  cerebral 348.1
    during or resulting from a procedure 997.01
    newborn 768.9
      mild or moderate 768.6
      severe 768.5
  fetal, affecting newborn 768.9 ▲
  intrauterine — *see* Distress, fetal
  myocardial (*see also* Insufficiency, coronary) 411.89
    arteriosclerotic — *see* Arteriosclerosis, coronary
  newborn 768.9 ▲

Hypsarrhythmia (*see also* Epilepsy) 345.6 ✓5ᵗʰ

Hysteralgia, pregnant uterus 646.8 ✓5ᵗʰ

Hysteria, hysterical 300.10
  anxiety 300.20
  Charcôt's gland 300.11
  conversion (any manifestation) 300.11
  dissociative type NEC 300.15
  psychosis, acute 298.1

Hysteroepilepsy 300.11

Hysterotomy, affecting fetus or newborn 763.89

I

Iatrogenic syndrome of excess cortisol 255.0

Iceland disease (epidemic neuromyasthenia) 049.8

Ichthyosis (congenita) 757.1
  acquired 701.1
  fetalis gravior 757.1

Ichthyosis — *continued*
  follicularis 757.1
  hystrix 757.39
  lamellar 757.1
  lingual 528.6
  palmaris and plantaris 757.39
  simplex 757.1
  vera 757.1
  vulgaris 757.1

Ichthyotoxism 988.0
  bacterial (*see also* Poisoning, food) 005.9

Icteroanemia, hemolytic (acquired) 283.9
  congenital (*see also* Spherocytosis) 282.0

Icterus (*see also* Jaundice) 782.4
  catarrhal — *see* Icterus, infectious
  conjunctiva 782.4
    newborn 774.6
  epidemic — *see* Icterus, infectious
  febrilis — *see* Icterus, infectious
  fetus or newborn — *see* Jaundice, fetus or newborn
  gravis (*see also* Necrosis, liver) 570
    complicating pregnancy 646.7 ✓5ᵗʰ
      affecting fetus or newborn 760.8
    fetus or newborn NEC 773.0
    obstetrical 646.7 ✓5ᵗʰ
      affecting fetus or newborn 760.8
  hematogenous (acquired) 283.9
  hemolytic (acquired) 283.9
    congenital (*see also* Spherocytosis) 282.0
  hemorrhagic (acute) 100.0
    leptospiral 100.0
    newborn 776.0
    spirochetal 100.0
  infectious 070.1
    with hepatic coma 070.0
    leptospiral 100.0
    spirochetal 100.0
  intermittens juvenilis 277.4
  malignant (*see also* Necrosis, liver) 570
  neonatorum (*see also* Jaundice, fetus or newborn) 774.6
  pernicious (*see also* Necrosis, liver) 570
  spirochetal 100.0

Ictus solaris, solis 992.0

Identity disorder 313.82
  dissociative 300.14
  gender role (child) 302.6
    adult 302.85
  psychosexual (child) 302.6
    adult 302.85

Idioglossia 307.9

Idiopathic — *see* condition

Idiosyncrasy (*see also* Allergy) 995.3
  drug, medicinal substance, and biological — *see* Allergy, drug

Idiot, idiocy (congenital) 318.2
  amaurotic (Bielschowsky) (-Jansky) (family) (infantile (late)) (juvenile (late)) (Vogt-Spielmeyer) 330.1
  microcephalic 742.1
  Mongolian 758.0
  oxycephalic 756.0

Id reaction (due to bacteria) 692.89

IgE asthma 493.0 ✓5ᵗʰ

Ileitis (chronic) (*see also* Enteritis) 558.9
  infectious 009.0
  noninfectious 558.9
  regional (ulcerative) 555.0
    with large intestine 555.2
  segmental 555.0
    with large intestine 555.2
  terminal (ulcerative) 555.0
    with large intestine 555.2

Ileocolitis (*see also* Enteritis) 558.9
  infectious 009.0
  regional 555.2
  ulcerative 556.1

Ileostomy status V44.2
  with complication 569.60

Ileotyphus 002.0

Ileum — *see* condition

Ileus (adynamic) (bowel) (colon) (inhibitory) (intestine) (neurogenic) (paralytic) 560.1
  arteriomesenteric duodenal 537.2
  due to gallstone (in intestine) 560.31
  duodenal, chronic 537.2
  following gastrointestinal surgery 997.4
  gallstone 560.31
  mechanical (*see also* Obstruction, intestine) 560.9
  meconium 777.1
    due to cystic fibrosis 277.01
  myxedema 564.89
  postoperative 997.4
  transitory, newborn 777.4

Iliac — *see* condition

Iliotibial band friction syndrome 728.89

Ill, louping 063.1

Illegitimacy V61.6

Illness — *see also* Disease
  factitious 300.19
    with
      combined physical and psychological symptoms 300.19
      physical symptoms 300.19
      psychological symptoms 300.16
    chronic (with physical symptoms) 301.51
  heart — *see* Disease, heart
  manic-depressive (*see also* Psychosis, affective) 296.80
  mental (*see also* Disorder, mental) 300.9

Imbalance 781.2
  autonomic (*see also* Neuropathy, peripheral, autonomic) 337.9
  electrolyte 276.9
    with
      abortion — *see* Abortion, by type, with metabolic disorder
      ectopic pregnancy (*see also* categories 633.0-633.9) 639.4
      hyperemesis gravidarum (before 22 completed weeks gestation) 643.1 ✓5ᵗʰ
      molar pregnancy (*see also* categories 630-632) 639.4
    following
      abortion 639.4
      ectopic or molar pregnancy 639.4
    neonatal, transitory NEC 775.5
  endocrine 259.9
  eye muscle NEC 378.9
    heterophoria — *see* Heterophoria
  glomerulotubular NEC 593.89
  hormone 259.9
  hysterical (*see also* Hysteria) 300.10
  labyrinth NEC 386.50
  posture 729.9
  sympathetic (*see also* Neuropathy, peripheral, autonomic) 337.9

Imbecile, imbecility 318.0
  moral 301.7
  old age 290.9
  senile 290.9
  specified IQ — *see* IQ
  unspecified IQ 318.0

Imbedding, intrauterine device 996.32

Imbibition, cholesterol (gallbladder) 575.6

Imerslund (-Gräsbeck) syndrome (anemia due to familial selective vitamin B₁₂ malabsorption) 281.1

Iminoacidopathy 270.8

Iminoglycinuria, familial 270.8

Immature — *see also* Immaturity
  personality 301.89

Immaturity 765.1 ✓5ᵗʰ
  extreme 765.0 ✓5ᵗʰ
  fetus or infant light-for-dates — *see* Light-for-dates
  lung, fetus or newborn 770.4
  organ or site NEC — *see* Hypoplasia
  pulmonary, fetus or newborn 770.4
  reaction 301.89
  sexual (female) (male) 259.0

Immersion 994.1
- foot 991.4
- hand 991.4

Immobile, immobility
- intestine 564.89
- joint — see Ankylosis
- syndrome (paraplegic) 728.3

Immunization
- ABO
  - affecting management of pregnancy 656.2 ✓5ᵗʰ
    - fetus or newborn 773.1
  - complication — see Complications, vaccination
- Rh factor
  - affecting management of pregnancy 656.1 ✓5ᵗʰ
    - fetus or newborn 773.0
  - from transfusion 999.7

Immunodeficiency 279.3
- with
  - adenosine-deaminase deficiency 279.2
  - defect, predominant
    - B-cell 279.00
    - T-cell 279.10
  - hyperimmunoglobulinemia 279.2
  - lymphopenia, hereditary 279.2
  - thrombocytopenia and eczema 279.12
  - thymic
    - aplasia 279.2
    - dysplasia 279.2
- autosomal recessive, Swiss-type 279.2
- common variable 279.06
- severe combined (SCID) 279.2
- to Rh factor
  - affecting management of pregnancy 656.1 ✓5ᵗʰ
    - fetus or newborn 773.0
- X-linked, with increased IgM 279.05

Immunotherapy, prophylactic V07.2

Impaction, impacted
- bowel, colon, rectum 560.30
  - with hernia — see also Hernia, by site, with obstruction
    - gangrenous — see Hernia, by site, with gangrene
  - by
    - calculus 560.39
    - gallstone 560.31
  - fecal 560.39
  - specified type NEC 560.39
- calculus — see Calculus
- cerumen (ear) (external) 380.4
- cuspid 520.6
  - with abnormal position (same or adjacent tooth) 524.3
- dental 520.6
  - with abnormal position (same or adjacent tooth) 524.3
- fecal, feces 560.39
  - with hernia — see also Hernia, by site, with obstruction
    - gangrenous — see Hernia, by site, with gangrene
- fracture — see Fracture, by site
- gallbladder — see Cholelithiasis
- gallstone(s) — see Cholelithiasis
  - in intestine (any part) 560.31
- intestine(s) 560.30
  - with hernia — see also Hernia, by site, with obstruction
    - grangrenous — see Hernia, by site, with gangrene
  - by
    - calculus 560.39
    - gallstone 560.31
  - fecal 560.39
  - specified type NEC 560.39
- intrauterine device (IUD) 996.32
- molar 520.6
  - with abnormal position (same or adjacent tooth) 524.3
- shoulder 660.4 ✓5ᵗʰ
  - affecting fetus or newborn 763.1
- tooth, teeth 520.6
  - with abnormal position (same or adjacent tooth) 524.3

Impaction, impacted — continued
- turbinate 733.99

Impaired, impairment (function)
- arm V49.1
  - movement, involving
    - musculoskeletal system V49.1
    - nervous system V49.2
- auditory discrimination 388.43
- back V48.3
- body (entire) V49.89
- hearing (see also Deafness) 389.9
- heart — see Disease, heart
- kidney (see also Disease, renal) 593.9
  - disorder resulting from 588.9
    - specified NEC 588.8
- leg V49.1
  - movement, involving
    - musculoskeletal system V49.1
    - nervous system V49.2
- limb V49.1
  - movement, involving
    - musculoskeletal system V49.1
    - nervous system V49.2
- liver 573.8
- mastication 524.9
- mobility
  - ear ossicles NEC 385.22
  - incostapedial joint 385.22
  - malleus 385.21
- myocardium, myocardial (see also Insufficiency, myocardial) 428.0
- neuromusculoskeletal NEC V49.89
  - back V48.3
  - head V48.2
  - limb V49.2
  - neck V48.3
  - spine V48.3
  - trunk V48.3
- rectal sphincter 787.99
- renal (see also Disease, renal) 593.9
  - disorder resulting from 588.9
    - specified NEC 588.8
- spine V48.3
- vision NEC 369.9
  - both eyes NEC 369.3
  - moderate 369.74
    - both eyes 369.25
      - with impairment of lesser eye (specified as)
        - blind, not further specified 369.15
        - low vision, not further specified 369.23
        - near-total 369.17
        - profound 369.18
        - severe 369.24
        - total 369.16
    - one eye 369.74
      - with vision of other eye (specified as)
        - near-normal 369.75
        - normal 369.76
  - near-total 369.64
    - both eyes 369.04
      - with impairment of lesser eye (specified as)
        - blind, not further specified 369.02
        - total 369.03
    - one eye 369.64
      - with vision of other eye (specified as)
        - near normal 369.65
        - normal 369.66
  - one eye 369.60
    - with low vision of other eye 369.10
  - profound 369.67
    - both eyes 369.08
      - with impairment of lesser eye (specified as)
        - blind, not further specified 369.05
        - near-total 369.07
        - total 369.06
    - one eye 369.67
      - with vision of other eye (specified as)
        - near-normal 369.68
        - normal 369.69

Impaired, impairment — continued
- vision NEC — continued
  - severe 369.71
    - both eyes 369.22
      - with impairment of lesser eye (specified as)
        - blind, not further specified 369.11
        - low vision, not further specified 369.21
        - near-total 369.13
        - profound 369.14
        - total 369.12
    - one eye 369.71
      - with vision of other eye (specified as)
        - near-normal 369.72
        - normal 369.73
  - total
    - both eyes 369.01
    - one eye 369.61
      - with vision of other eye (specified as)
        - near-normal 369.62
        - normal 369.63

Impaludism — see Malaria

Impediment, speech NEC 784.5
- psychogenic 307.9
- secondary to organic lesion 784.5

Impending
- cerebrovascular accident or attack 435.9
- coronary syndrome 411.1
- delirium tremens 291.0
- myocardial infarction 411.1

Imperception, auditory (acquired) (congenital) 389.9

Imperfect
- aeration, lung (newborn) 770.5
- closure (congenital)
  - alimentary tract NEC 751.8
    - lower 751.5
    - upper 750.8
  - atrioventricular ostium 745.69
  - atrium (secundum) 745.5
    - primum 745.61
  - branchial cleft or sinus 744.41
  - choroid 743.59
  - cricoid cartilage 748.3
  - cusps, heart valve NEC 746.89
    - pulmonary 746.09
  - ductus
    - arteriosus 747.0
    - Botalli 747.0
  - ear drum 744.29
    - causing impairment of hearing 744.03
  - endocardial cushion 745.60
  - epiglottis 748.3
  - esophagus with communication to bronchus or trachea 750.3
  - Eustachian valve 746.89
  - eyelid 743.62
  - face, facial (see also Cleft, lip) 749.10
  - foramen
    - Botalli 745.5
    - ovale 745.5
  - genitalia, genital organ(s) or system
    - female 752.8
      - external 752.49
      - internal NEC 752.8
      - uterus 752.3
    - male 752.8
      - penis 752.69
  - glottis 748.3
  - heart valve (cusps) NEC 746.89
  - interatrial ostium or septum 745.5
  - interauricular ostium or septum 745.5
  - interventricular ostium or septum 745.4
  - iris 743.46
  - kidney 753.3
  - larynx 748.3
  - lens 743.36
  - lip (see also Cleft, lip) 749.10
  - nasal septum or sinus 748.1
  - nose 748.1
  - omphalomesenteric duct 751.0
  - optic nerve entry 743.57
  - organ or site NEC — see Anomaly, specified type, by site

Imperfect — *continued*
closure — *continued*
    ostium
        interatrial 745.5
        interauricular 745.5
        interventricular 745.4
    palate (*see also* Cleft, palate) 749.00
    preauricular sinus 744.46
    retina 743.56
    roof of orbit 742.0
    sclera 743.47
    septum
        aortic 745.0
        aorticopulmonary 745.0
        atrial (secundum) 745.5
            primum 745.61
        between aorta and pulmonary artery
            745.0
        heart 745.9
        interatrial (secundum) 745.5
            primum 745.61
        interauricular (secundum) 745.5
            primum 745.61
        interventricular 745.4
            with pulmonary stenosis or atresia,
                dextraposition of aorta, and
                hypertrophy of right ventricle
                745.2
            in tetralogy of Fallot 745.2
        nasal 748.1
        ventricular 745.4
            with pulmonary stenosis or atresia,
                dextraposition of aorta, and
                hypertrophy of right ventricle
                745.2
            in tetralogy of Fallot 745.2
    skull 756.0
        with
            anencephalus 740.0
            encephalocele 742.0
            hydrocephalus 742.3
                with spina bifida (*see also* Spina
                    bifida) 741.0 ✓5ᵗʰ
            microcephalus 742.1
    spine (with meningocele) (*see also* Spina
        bifida) 741.90
    thyroid cartilage 748.3
    trachea 748.3
    tympanic membrane 744.29
        causing impairment of hearing 744.03
    uterus (with communication to bladder,
        intestine, or rectum) 752.3
    uvula 749.02
        with cleft lip (*see also* Cleft, palate, with
            cleft lip) 749.20
    vitelline duct 751.0
development — *see* Anomaly, by site
erection 607.84
fusion — *see* Imperfect, closure
inflation lung (newborn) 770.5
intestinal canal 751.5
poise 729.9
rotation — *see* Malrotation
septum, ventricular 745.4
Imperfectly descended testis 752.51
Imperforate (congenital) — *see also* Atresia
anus 751.2
bile duct 751.61
cervix (uteri) 752.49
esophagus 750.3
hymen 752.42
intestine (small) 751.1
    large 751.2
jejunum 751.1
pharynx 750.29
rectum 751.2
salivary duct 750.23
urethra 753.6
urinary meatus 753.6
vagina 752.49
Impervious (congenital) — *see also* Atresia
anus 751.2
bile duct 751.61
esophagus 750.3
intestine (small) 751.1
    large 751.5
rectum 751.2
urethra 753.6

Impetiginization of other dermatoses 684
Impetigo (any organism) (any site) (bullous)
    (circinate) (contagiosa) (neonatorum)
    (simplex) 684
Bockhart's (superficial folliculitis) 704.8
external ear 684 *[380.13]*
eyelid 684 *[373.5]*
Fox's (contagiosa) 684
furfuracea 696.5
herpetiformis 694.3
    nonobstetrical 694.3
staphylococcal infection 684
ulcerative 686.8
vulgaris 684
Impingement, soft tissue between teeth 524.2
Implant, endometrial 617.9
Implantation
anomalous — *see also* Anomaly, specified type,
    by site
    ureter 753.4
cyst
    external area or site (skin) NEC 709.8
    iris 364.61
    vagina 623.8
    vulva 624.8
dermoid (cyst)
    external area or site (skin) NEC 709.8
    iris 364.61
    vagina 623.8
    vulva 624.8
placenta, low or marginal — *see* Placenta
    previa
Impotence (sexual) (psychogenic) 302.72
organic origin NEC 607.84
Impoverished blood 285.9
Impression, basilar 756.0
Imprisonment V62.5
Improper
development, infant 764.9 ✓5ᵗʰ
Improperly tied umbilical cord (causing
    hemorrhage) 772.3
Impulses, obsessional 300.3
Impulsive neurosis 300.3
Inaction, kidney (*see also* Disease, renal) 593.9
Inactive — *see* condition
Inadequate, inadequacy
biologic 301.6
cardiac and renal — *see* Hypertension,
    cardiorenal
constitutional 301.6
development
    child 783.40
    fetus 764.9 ✓5ᵗʰ
        affecting management of pregnancy
            656.5 ✓5ᵗʰ
    genitalia
        after puberty NEC 259.0
        congenital — *see* Hypoplasia, genitalia
    lungs 748.5
    organ or site NEC — *see* Hypoplasia, by site
dietary 269.9
education V62.3
environment
    economic problem V60.2
    household condition NEC V60.1
    poverty V60.2
    unemployment V62.0
functional 301.6
household care, due to
    family member
        handicapped or ill V60.4
        temporarily away from home V60.4
            on vacation V60.5
    technical defects in home V60.1
    temporary absence from home of person
        rendering care V60.4
housing (heating) (space) V60.1
material resources V60.2
mental (*see also* Retardation, mental) 319
nervous system 799.2
personality 301.6
prenatal care in current pregnancy V23.7
pulmonary
    function 786.09
        newborn 770.89   ▲
    ventilation, newborn 770.89   ▲

Inadequate, inadequacy — *continued*
respiration 786.09
    newborn 770.89   ▲
social 301.6
Inanition 263.9
with edema 262
due to
    deprivation of food 994.2
    malnutrition 263.9
fever 780.6
Inappropriate secretion
ACTH 255.0
antidiuretic hormone (ADH) (excessive) 253.6
    deficiency 253.5
ectopic hormone NEC 259.3
pituitary (posterior) 253.6
Inattention after or at birth 995.52
Inborn errors of metabolism — *see* Disorder,
    metabolism
Incarceration, incarcerated
bubonocele — *see also* Hernia, inguinal, with
    obstruction
    gangrenous — *see* Hernia, inguinal, with
        gangrene
colon (by hernia) — *see also* Hernia, by site
    with obstruction
    gangrenous — *see* Hernia, by site, with
        gangrene
enterocele 552.9
    gangrenous 551.9
epigastrocele 552.29
    gangrenous 551.29
epiplocele 552.9
    gangrenous 551.9
exomphalos 552.1
    gangrenous 551.1
fallopian tube 620.8
hernia — *see also* Hernia, by site, with
    obstruction
    gangrenous — *see* Hernia, by site, with
        gangrene
iris, in wound 871.1
lens, in wound 871.1
merocele (*see also* Hernia, femoral, with
    obstruction) 552.00
omentum (by hernia) — *see also* Hernia, by
    site, with obstruction
    gangrenous — *see* Hernia, by site, with
        gangrene
omphalocele 756.79
rupture (meaning hernia) (*see also* Hernia, by
    site, with obstruction) 552.9
    gangrenous (*see also* Hernia, by site, with
        gangrene) 551.9
sarcoepiplocele 552.9
    gangrenous 551.9
sarcoepiplomphalocele 552.1
    with gangrene 551.1
uterus 621.8
    gravid 654.3 ✓5ᵗʰ
        causing obstructed labor 660.2 ✓5ᵗʰ
            affecting fetus or newborn 763.1
Incident, cerebrovascular (*see also* Disease,
    cerebrovascular, acute) 436
Incineration (entire body) (from fire,
    conflagration, electricity, or lightning) — *see*
    Burn, multiple, specified sites
Incised wound
external — *see* Wound, open, by site
internal organs (abdomen, chest, or pelvis) —
    see Injury, internal, by site, with open
    wound
Incision, incisional
hernia — *see* Hernia, incisional
surgical, complication — *see* Complications,
    surgical procedures
traumatic
    external — *see* Wound, open, by site
    internal organs (abdomen, chest, or pelvis)
        — *see* Injury, internal, by site, with
        open wound
Inclusion
azurophilic leukocytic 288.2
blennorrhea (neonatal) (newborn) 771.6
cyst — *see* Cyst, skin
gallbladder in liver (congenital) 751.69

✓4ᵗʰ Fourth-digit Required   ✓5ᵗʰ Fifth-digit Required   ▶◀ Revised Text   ● New Line   ▲ Revised Code

Incompatibility
 ABO
  affecting management of pregnancy
   656.2 ☑5ᵗʰ
  fetus or newborn 773.1
  infusion or transfusion reaction 999.6
 blood (group) (Duffy) (E) (K(ell)) (Kidd) (Lewis)
  (M) (N) (P) (S) NEC
  affecting management of pregnancy
   656.2 ☑5ᵗʰ
  fetus or newborn 773.2
  infusion or transfusion reaction 999.6
 marital V61.10
  involving divorce or estrangement V61.0
 Rh (blood group) (factor)
  affecting management of pregnancy
   656.1 ☑5ᵗʰ
  fetus or newborn 773.0
  infusion or transfusion reaction 999.7
 Rhesus — see Incompatibility, Rh
Incompetency, incompetence, incompetent
 annular
  aortic (valve) (see also Insufficiency, aortic)
   424.1
  mitral (valve) — (see also Insufficiency,
   mitral) 424.0
  pulmonary valve (heart) (see also
   Endocarditis, pulmonary) 424.3
 aortic (valve) (see also Insufficiency, aortic)
  424.1
  syphilitic 093.22
 cardiac (orifice) 530.0
  valve — see Endocarditis
 cervix, cervical (os) 622.5
  in pregnancy 654.5 ☑5ᵗʰ
   affecting fetus or newborn 761.0
 esophagogastric (junction) (sphincter) 530.0
 heart valve, congenital 746.89
 mitral (valve) — see Insufficiency, mitral
 papillary muscle (heart) 429.81
 pelvic fundus 618.8
 pulmonary valve (heart) (see also Endocarditis,
  pulmonary) 424.3
  congenital 746.09
 tricuspid (annular) (rheumatic) (valve) (see also
  Endocarditis, tricuspid) 397.0
 valvular — see Endocarditis
 vein, venous (saphenous) (varicose) (see also
  Varicose, vein) 454.9
 velopharyngeal (closure)
  acquired 528.9
  congenital 750.29
Incomplete — see also condition
 bladder emptying 788.21
 expansion lungs (newborn) 770.5
 gestation (liveborn) — see Immaturity
 rotation — see Malrotation
Incontinence 788.30
 without sensory awareness 788.34
 anal sphincter 787.6
 continuous leakage 788.37
 feces 787.6
  due to hysteria 300.11
  nonorganic origin 307.7
 hysterical 300.11
 mixed (male) (female) (urge and stress) 788.33
 overflow 788.39
 paradoxical 788.39
 rectal 787.6
 specified NEC 788.39
 stress (female) 625.6
  male NEC 788.32
 urethral sphincter 599.84
 urge 788.31
  and stress (male) (female) 788.33
 urine 788.30
  active 788.30
  male 788.30
   stress 788.32
    and urge 788.33
  neurogenic 788.39
  nonorganic origin 307.6
  stress (female) 625.6
   male NEC 788.32
  urge 788.31
   and stress 788.33
Incontinentia pigmenti 757.33

Incoordinate
 uterus (action) (contractions) 661.4 ☑5ᵗʰ
  affecting fetus or newborn 763.7
Incoordination
 esophageal-pharyngeal (newborn) 787.2
 muscular 781.3
 papillary muscle 429.81
Increase, increased
 abnormal, in development 783.9
 androgens (ovarian) 256.1
 anticoagulants (antithrombin) (anti-VIIIa) (anti-
  IXa) (anti-Xa) (anti-XIa) 286.5
  postpartum 666.3 ☑5ᵗʰ
 cold sense (see also Disturbance, sensation)
  782.0
 estrogen 256.0
 function
  adrenal (cortex) 255.3
   medulla 255.6
  pituitary (anterior) (gland) (lobe) 253.1
   posterior 253.6
 heat sense (see also Disturbance, sensation)
  782.0
 intracranial pressure 781.99
  injury at birth 767.8
 light reflex of retina 362.13
 permeability, capillary 448.9
 pressure
  intracranial 781.99
   injury at birth 767.8
  intraocular 365.00
 pulsations 785.9
 pulse pressure 785.9
 sphericity, lens 743.36
 splenic activity 289.4
 venous pressure 459.89
  portal 572.3
Incrustation, cornea, lead or zinc 930.0
Incyclophoria 378.44
Incyclotropia 378.33
Indeterminate sex 752.7
India rubber skin 756.83
Indicanuria 270.2
Indigestion (bilious) (functional) 536.8
 acid 536.8
 catarrhal 536.8
 due to decomposed food NEC 005.9
 fat 579.8
 nervous 306.4
 psychogenic 306.4
Indirect — see condition
Indolent bubo NEC 099.8
Induced
 abortion — see Abortion, induced
 birth, affecting fetus or newborn 763.89
 delivery — see Delivery
 labor — see Delivery
Induration, indurated
 brain 348.8
 breast (fibrous) 611.79
  puerperal, postpartum 676.3 ☑5ᵗʰ
 broad ligament 620.8
 chancre 091.0
  anus 091.1
  congenital 090.0
  extragenital NEC 091.2
 corpora cavernosa (penis) (plastic) 607.89
 liver (chronic) 573.8
  acute 573.8
 lung (black) (brown) (chronic) (fibroid) (see also
  Fibrosis, lung) 515
  essential brown 275.0 [516.1]
 penile 607.89
 phlebitic — see Phlebitis
 skin 782.8
 stomach 537.89
Induratio penis plastica 607.89
Industrial — see condition
Inebriety (see also Abuse, drugs, nondependent)
 305.0 ☑5ᵗʰ
Inefficiency
 kidney (see also Disease, renal) 593.9
 thyroid (acquired) (gland) 244.9
Inelasticity, skin 782.8

Inequality, leg (acquired) (length) 736.81
 congenital 755.30
Inertia
 bladder 596.4
  neurogenic 596.54
   with cauda equina syndrome 344.61
 stomach 536.8
  psychogenic 306.4
 uterus, uterine 661.2 ☑5ᵗʰ
  affecting fetus or newborn 763.7
  primary 661.0 ☑5ᵗʰ
  secondary 661.1 ☑5ᵗʰ
 vesical 596.4
  neurogenic 596.54
   with cauda equina 344.61
Infant — see also condition
 excessive crying of 780.92 ●
 fussy (baby) 780.91 ●
 held for adoption V68.89
 newborn — see Newborn
 syndrome of diabetic mother 775.0
"Infant Hercules" syndrome 255.2
Infantile — see also condition
 genitalia, genitals 259.0
  in pregnancy or childbirth NEC 654.4 ☑5ᵗʰ
   affecting fetus or newborn 763.89
   causing obstructed labor 660.2 ☑5ᵗʰ
    affecting fetus or newborn 763.1
 heart 746.9
 kidney 753.3
 lack of care 995.52
 macula degeneration 362.75
 melanodontia 521.05
 os, uterus (see also Infantile, genitalia) 259.0
 pelvis 738.6
  with disproportion (fetopelvic) 653.1 ☑5ᵗʰ
   affecting fetus or newborn 763.1
   causing obstructed labor 660.1 ☑5ᵗʰ
    affecting fetus or newborn 763.1
 penis 259.0
 testis 257.2
 uterus (see also Infantile, genitalia) 259.0
 vulva 752.49
Infantilism 259.9
 with dwarfism (hypophyseal) 253.3
 Brissaud's (infantile myxedema) 244.9
 celiac 579.0
 Herter's (nontropical sprue) 579.0
 hypophyseal 253.3
 hypothalamic (with obesity) 253.8
 idiopathic 259.9
 intestinal 579.0
 pancreatic 577.8
 pituitary 253.3
 renal 588.0
 sexual (with obesity) 259.0
Infants, healthy liveborn — see Newborn
Infarct, infarction
 adrenal (capsule) (gland) 255.4
 amnion 658.8 ☑5ᵗʰ
 anterior (with contiguous portion of
  intraventricular septum) NEC (see also
  Infarct, myocardium) 410.1 ☑5ᵗʰ
 appendices epiploicae 557.0
 bowel 557.0
 brain (stem) 434.91
  embolic (see also Embolism, brain) 434.11
  healed or old without residuals V12.59
  iatrogenic 997.02
  postoperative 997.02
  puerperal, postpartum, childbirth 674.0 ☑5ᵗʰ
  thrombotic (see also Thrombosis, brain)
   434.01
 breast 611.8
 Brewer's (kidney) 593.81
 cardiac (see also Infarct, myocardium)
  410.9 ☑5ᵗʰ
 cerebellar (see also Infarct, brain) 434.91
  embolic (see also Embolism, brain) 434.11
 cerebral (see also Infarct, brain) 434.91
  embolic (see also Embolism, brain) 434.11
 chorion 658.8 ☑5ᵗʰ
 colon (acute) (agnogenic) (embolic)
  (hemorrhagic) (nonocclusive)
  (nonthrombotic) (occlusive) (segmental)
  (thrombotic) (with gangrene) 557.0

☑4ᵗʰ Fourth-digit Required   ☑5ᵗʰ Fifth-digit Required   ▶◀ Revised Text   ● New Line   ▲ Revised Code

Infarct, infarction — *continued*

coronary artery (*see also* Infarct, myocardium) 410.9 ☑5ᵗʰ
embolic (*see also* Embolism) 444.9
fallopian tube 620.8
gallbladder 575.8
heart (*see also* Infarct, myocardium) 410.9 ☑5ᵗʰ
hepatic 573.4
hypophysis (anterior lobe) 253.8
impending (myocardium) 411.1
intestine (acute) (agnogenic) (embolic) (hemorrhagic) (nonocclusive) (nonthrombotic) (occlusive) (thrombotic) (with gangrene) 557.0
kidney 593.81
liver 573.4
lung (embolic) (thrombotic) 415.1 ☑5ᵗʰ
  with
    abortion — *see* Abortion, by type, with embolism
    ectopic pregnancy (*see also* categories 633.0-633.9) 639.6
    molar pregnancy (*see also* categories 630-632) 639.6
  following
    abortion 639.6
    ectopic or molar pregnancy 639.6
  iatrogenic 415.11
  in pregnancy, childbirth, or puerperium — *see* Embolism, obstetrical
  postoperative 415.11
lymph node or vessel 457.8
medullary (brain) — *see* Infarct, brain
meibomian gland (eyelid) 374.85
mesentery, mesenteric (embolic) (thrombotic) (with gangrene) 557.0
midbrain — *see* Infarct, brain
myocardium, myocardial (acute or with a stated duration of 8 weeks or less) (with hypertension) 410.9 ☑5ᵗʰ

> *Note* — *Use the following fifth-digit subclassification with category 410:*
>
> 0   *episode unspecified*
> 1   *initial episode*
> 2   *subsequent episode without recurrence*

  with symptoms after 8 weeks from date of infarction 414.8
  anterior (wall) (with contiguous portion of intraventricular septum) NEC 410.1 ☑5ᵗʰ
  anteroapical (with contiguous portion of intraventricular septum) 410.1 ☑5ᵗʰ
  anterolateral (wall) 410.0 ☑5ᵗʰ
  anteroseptal (with contiguous portion of intraventricular septum) 410.1 ☑5ᵗʰ
  apical-lateral 410.5 ☑5ᵗʰ
  atrial 410.8 ☑5ᵗʰ
  basal-lateral 410.5 ☑5ᵗʰ
  chronic (with symptoms after 8 weeks from date of infarction) 414.8
  diagnosed on ECG, but presenting no symptoms 412
  diaphragmatic wall (with contiguous portion of intraventricular septum) 410.4 ☑5ᵗʰ
  healed or old, currently presenting no symptoms 412
  high lateral 410.5 ☑5ᵗʰ
  impending 411.1
  inferior (wall) (with contiguous portion of intraventricular septum) 410.4 ☑5ᵗʰ
  inferolateral (wall) 410.2 ☑5ᵗʰ
  inferoposterior wall 410.3 ☑5ᵗʰ
  lateral wall 410.5 ☑5ᵗʰ
  nontransmural 410.7 ☑5ᵗʰ
  papillary muscle 410.8 ☑5ᵗʰ
  past (diagnosed on ECG or other special investigation, but currently presenting no symptoms) 412
    with symptoms NEC 414.8
  posterior (strictly) (true) (wall) 410.6 ☑5ᵗʰ
  posterobasal 410.6 ☑5ᵗʰ
  posteroinferior 410.3 ☑5ᵗʰ
  posterolateral 410.5 ☑5ᵗʰ

Infarct, infarction — *continued*

myocardium, myocardial — *continued*
  previous, currently presenting no symptoms 412
  septal 410.8 ☑5ᵗʰ
  specified site NEC 410.8 ☑5ᵗʰ
  subendocardial 410.7 ☑5ᵗʰ
  syphilitic 093.82
nontransmural 410.7 ☑5ᵗʰ
omentum 557.0
ovary 620.8
pancreas 577.8
papillary muscle (*see also* Infarct, myocardium) 410.8 ☑5ᵗʰ
parathyroid gland 252.8
pituitary (gland) 253.8
placenta (complicating pregnancy) 656.7 ☑5ᵗʰ
  affecting fetus or newborn 762.2
pontine — *see* Infarct, brain
posterior NEC (*see also* Infarct, myocardium) 410.6 ☑5ᵗʰ
prostate 602.8
pulmonary (artery) (hemorrhagic) (vein) 415.1 ☑5ᵗʰ
  with
    abortion — *see* Abortion, by type, with embolism
    ectopic pregnancy (*see also* categories 633.0-633.9) 639.6
    molar pregnancy (*see also* categories 630-632) 639.6
  following
    abortion 639.6
    ectopic or molar pregnancy 639.6
  iatrogenic 415.11
  in pregnancy, childbirth, or puerperium — *see* Embolism, obstetrical
  postoperative 415.11
renal 593.81
  embolic or thrombotic 593.81
retina, retinal 362.84
  with occlusion — *see* Occlusion, retina
spinal (acute) (cord) (embolic) (nonembolic) 336.1
spleen 289.59
  embolic or thrombotic 444.89
subchorionic — *see* Infarct, placenta
subendocardial (*see also* Infarct, myocardium) 410.7 ☑5ᵗʰ
suprarenal (capsule) (gland) 255.4
syncytium — *see* Infarct, placenta
testis 608.83
thrombotic (*see also* Thrombosis) 453.9
  artery, arterial — *see* Embolism
thyroid (gland) 246.3
ventricle (heart) (*see also* Infarct, myocardium) 410.9 ☑5ᵗʰ

Infecting — *see* condition

Infection, infected, infective (opportunistic) 136.9
with lymphangitis — *see* Lymphangitis
abortion — *see* Abortion, by type, with sepsis
abscess (skin) — *see* Abscess, by site
Absidia 117.7
Acanthocheilonema (perstans) 125.4
  streptocerca 125.6
accessory sinus (chronic) (*see also* Sinusitis) 473.9
Achorion — *see* Dermatophytosis
Acremonium falciforme 117.4
acromioclavicular (joint) 711.91
actinobacillus
  lignieresii 027.8
  mallei 024
  muris 026.1
actinomadura — *see* Actinomycosis
Actinomyces (israelii) — *see also* Actinomycosis
  muris-ratti 026.1
Actinomycetales (actinomadura) (Actinomyces) (Nocardia) (Streptomyces) — *see* Actinomycosis
actinomycotic NEC (*see also* Actinomycosis) 039.9
adenoid (chronic) 474.01
  acute 463
  and tonsil (chronic) 474.02
    acute or subacute 463

Infection, infected, infective — *continued*

adenovirus NEC 079.0
  in diseases classified elsewhere — *see* category 079 ☑4ᵗʰ
  unspecified nature or site 079.0
Aerobacter aerogenes NEC 041.85
  enteritis 008.2
aerogenes capsulatus (*see also* Gangrene, gas) 040.0
aertrycke (*see also* Infection, Salmonella) 003.9
ajellomyces dermatitidis 116.0
alimentary canal NEC (*see also* Enteritis, due to, by organism) 009.0
Allescheria boydii 117.6
Alternaria 118
alveolus, alveolar (process) (pulpal origin) 522.4
ameba, amebic (histolytica) (*see also* Amebiasis) 006.9
  acute 006.0
  chronic 006.1
  free-living 136.2
  hartmanni 007.8
  specified
    site NEC 006.8
    type NEC 007.8
amniotic fluid or cavity 658.4 ☑5ᵗʰ
  affecting fetus or newborn 762.7
anaerobes (cocci) (gram-negative) (gram-positive) (mixed) NEC 041.84
anal canal 569.49
Ancylostoma braziliense 126.2
Angiostrongylus cantonensis 128.8
anisakiasis 127.1
Anisakis larva 127.1
anthrax (*see also* Anthrax) 022.9
antrum (chronic) (*see also* Sinusitis, maxillary) 473.0
anus (papillae) (sphincter) 569.49
arbor virus NEC 066.9
arbovirus NEC 066.9
argentophil-rod 027.0
Ascaris lumbricoides 127.0
ascomycetes 117.4
Aspergillus (flavus) (fumigatus) (terreus) 117.3
atypical
  acid-fast (bacilli) (*see also* Mycobacterium, atypical) 031.9
  mycobacteria (*see also* Mycobacterium, atypical) 031.9
auditory meatus (circumscribed) (diffuse) (external) (*see also* Otitis, externa) 380.10
auricle (ear) (*see also* Otitis, externa) 380.10
axillary gland 683
Babesiasis 088.82
Babesiosis 088.82
Bacillus NEC 041.89
  abortus 023.1
  anthracis (*see also* Anthrax) 022.9
  cereus (food poisoning) 005.89
  coli — *see* Infection, Escherichia coli
  coliform NEC 041.85
  Ducrey's (any location) 099.0
  Flexner's 004.1
  fragilis NEC 041.82
  Friedländer's NEC 041.3
  fusiformis 101
  gas (gangrene) (*see also* Gangrene, gas) 040.0
  mallei 024
  melitensis 023.0
  paratyphoid, paratyphosus 002.9
    A 002.1
    B 002.2
    C 002.3
  Schmorl's 040.3
  Shiga 004.0
  suipestifer (*see also* Infection, Salmonella) 003.9
  swimming pool 031.1
  typhosa 002.0
  welchii (*see also* Gangrene, gas) 040.0
  Whitmore's 025
bacterial NEC 041.9
  specified NEC 041.89
    anaerobic NEC 041.84
    gram-negative NEC 041.85
      anaerobic NEC 041.84

☑4ᵗʰ Fourth-digit Required   ☑5ᵗʰ Fifth-digit Required   ▶◀ Revised Text   ● New Line   ▲ Revised Code

Infection, infected, infective — *continued*

Bacterium
  paratyphosum 002.9
    A 002.1
    B 002.2
    C 002.3
  typhosum 002.0
Bacteroides (fragilis) (melaninogenicus) (oralis) NEC 041.84
balantidium coli 007.0
Bartholin's gland 616.8
Basidiobolus 117.7
Bedsonia 079.98
  specified NEC 079.88
bile duct 576.1
bladder (*see also* Cystitis) 595.9
Blastomyces, blastomycotic 116.0
  brasiliensis 116.1
  dermatitidis 116.0
  European 117.5
  Loboi 116.2
  North American 116.0
  South American 116.1
blood stream — *see* Septicemia
bone 730.9 ✓5ᵗʰ
  specified — *see* Osteomyelitis
Bordetella 033.9
  bronchiseptica 033.8
  parapertussis 033.1
  pertussis 033.0
Borrelia
  bergdorfi 088.81
  vincentii (mouth) (pharynx) (tonsil) 101
brain (*see also* Encephalitis) 323.9
  late effect — *see* category 326
  membranes — (*see also* Meningitis) 322.9
  septic 324.0
    late effect — *see* category 326
    meninges (*see also* Meningitis) 320.9
branchial cyst 744.42
breast 611.0
  puerperal, postpartum 675.2 ✓5ᵗʰ
    with nipple 675.9 ✓5ᵗʰ
      specified type NEC 675.8 ✓5ᵗʰ
    nonpurulent 675.2 ✓5ᵗʰ
    purulent 675.1 ✓5ᵗʰ
bronchus (*see also* Bronchitis) 490
  fungus NEC 117.9
Brucella 023.9
  abortus 023.1
  canis 023.3
  melitensis 023.0
  mixed 023.8
  suis 023.2
Brugia (Wuchereria) malayi 125.1
bursa — *see* Bursitis
buttocks (skin) 686.9
Candida (albicans) (tropicalis) (*see also* Candidiasis) 112.9
  congenital 771.7
Candiru 136.8
Capillaria
  hepatica 128.8
  philippinensis 127.5
cartilage 733.99
cat liver fluke 121.0
cellulitis — *see* Cellulitis, by site
Cephalosporum falciforme 117.4
Cercomonas hominis (intestinal) 007.3
cerebrospinal (*see also* Meningitis) 322.9
  late effect — *see* category 326
cervical gland 683
cervix (*see also* Cervicitis) 616.0
cesarean section wound 674.3 ✓5ᵗʰ
Chilomastix (intestinal) 007.8
Chlamydia 079.98
  specified NEC 079.88
cholera (*see also* Cholera) 001.9
chorionic plate 658.8 ✓5ᵗʰ
Cladosporium
  bantianum 117.8
  carrionii 117.2
  mansoni 111.1
  trichoides 117.8
  wernecki 111.1
Clonorchis (sinensis) (liver) 121.1

Infection, infected, infective — *continued*

Clostridium (haemolyticum) (novyi) NEC 041.84
  botulinum 005.1
  congenital 771.89 ▲
  histolyticum (*see also* Gangrene, gas) 040.0
  oedematiens (*see also* Gangrene, gas) 040.0
  perfringens 041.83
    due to food 005.2
  septicum (*see also* Gangrene, gas) 040.0
  sordellii (*see also* Gangrene, gas) 040.0
  welchii (*see also* Gangrene, gas) 040.0
    due to food 005.2
Coccidioides (immitis) (*see also* Coccidioidomycosis) 114.9
coccus NEC 041.89
colon (*see also* Enteritis, due to, by organism) 009.0
  bacillus — *see* Infection, Escherichia coli
colostomy or enterostomy 569.61
common duct 576.1
complicating pregnancy, childbirth, or puerperium NEC 647.9 ✓5ᵗʰ
  affecting fetus or newborn 760.2
Condiobolus 117.7
congenital NEC 771.89 ▲
  Candida albicans 771.7
  chronic 771.2
  clostridial 771.89 ▲
  cytomegalovirus 771.1
  Escherichia coli 771.89 ▲
  hepatitis, viral 771.2
  herpes simplex 771.2
  listeriosis 771.2
  malaria 771.2
  poliomyelitis 771.2
  rubella 771.0
  Salmonella 771.89 ▲
  streptococcal 771.89 ▲
  toxoplasmosis 771.2
  tuberculosis 771.2
  urinary (tract) 771.82 ▲
  vaccinia 771.2
corpus luteum (*see also* Salpingo-oophoritis) 614.2
Corynebacterium diphtheriae — *see* Diphtheria
Coxsackie (*see also* Coxsackie) 079.2
  endocardium 074.22
  heart NEC 074.20
  in diseases classified elsewhere — *see* category 079 ✓5ᵗʰ
  meninges 047.0
  myocardium 074.23
  pericardium 074.21
  pharynx 074.0
  specified disease NEC 074.8
  unspecified nature or site 079.2
Cryptococcus neoformans 117.5
Cryptosporidia 007.4
Cunninghamella 117.7
cyst — *see* Cyst
Cysticercus cellulosae 123.1
cytomegalovirus 078.5
  congenital 771.1
dental (pulpal origin) 522.4
deuteromycetes 117.4
Dicrocoelium dendriticum 121.8
Dipetalonema (perstans) 125.4
  streptocerca 125.6
diphtherial — *see* Diphtheria
Diphyllobothrium (adult) (latum) (pacificum) 123.4
  larval 123.5
Diplogonoporus (grandis) 123.8
Dipylidium (caninum) 123.8
Dirofilaria 125.6
dog tapeworm 123.8
Dracunculus medinensis 125.7
Dreschlera 118
  hawaiiensis 117.8
Ducrey's bacillus (any site) 099.0
due to or resulting from
  device, implant, or graft (any) (presence of) — *see* Complications, infection and inflammation, due to (presence of) any device, implant, or graft classified to 996.0-996.5 NEC

Infection, infected, infective — *continued*

due to or resulting from — *continued*
  injection, inoculation, infusion, transfusion, or vaccination (prophylactic) (therapeutic) 999.3
  injury NEC — *see* Wound, open, by site, complicated
  surgery 998.59
duodenum 535.6 ✓5ᵗʰ
ear — *see also* Otitis
  external (*see also* Otitis, externa) 380.10
  inner (*see also* Labyrinthitis) 386.30
  middle — *see* Otitis, media
Eaton's agent NEC 041.81
Eberthella typhosa 002.0
Ebola 065.8
echinococcosis 122.9
Echinococcus (*see also* Echinococcus) 122.9
Echinostoma 121.8
ECHO virus 079.1
  in diseases classified elsewhere — *see* category 079 ✓4ᵗʰ
  unspecified nature or site 079.1
Ehrlichiosis 082.40
  chaffeensis 082.41
  specified type NEC 082.49
Endamoeba — *see* Infection, ameba
endocardium (*see also* Endocarditis) 421.0
endocervix (*see also* Cervicitis) 616.0
Entamoeba — *see* Infection, ameba
enteric (*see also* Enteritis, due to, by organism) 009.0
Enterobacter aerogenes NEC 041.85
Enterobius vermicularis 127.4
enterococcus NEC 041.04
enterovirus NEC 079.89
  central nervous system NEC 048
  enteritis 008.67
  meningitis 047.9
Entomophthora 117.7
Epidermophyton — *see* Dermatophytosis
epidermophytosis — *see* Dermatophytosis
episiotomy 674.3 ✓5ᵗʰ
Epstein-Barr virus 075
  chronic 780.79 [139.8]
erysipeloid 027.1
Erysipelothrix (insidiosa) (rhusiopathiae) 027.1
erythema infectiosum 057.0
Escherichia coli NEC 041.4
  congenital 771.89 ▲
  enteritis — *see* Enteritis, E. coli
  generalized 038.42
  intestinal — *see* Enteritis, E. coli
ethmoidal (chronic) (sinus) (*see also* Sinusitis, ethmoidal) 473.2
Eubacterium 041.84
Eustachian tube (ear) 381.50
  acute 381.51
  chronic 381.52
exanthema subitum 057.8
external auditory canal (meatus) (*see also* Otitis, externa) 380.10
eye NEC 360.00
eyelid 373.9
  specified NEC 373.8
fallopian tube (*see also* Salpingo-oophoritis) 614.2
fascia 728.89
Fasciola
  gigantica 121.3
  hepatica 121.3
Fasciolopsis (buski) 121.4
fetus (intra-amniotic) — *see* Infection, congenital
filarial — *see* Infestation, filarial
finger (skin) 686.9
  abscess (with lymphangitis) 681.00
    pulp 681.01
  cellulitis (with lymphangitis) 681.00
  distal closed space (with lymphangitis) 681.00
  nail 681.02
    fungus 110.1
fish tapeworm 123.4
  larval 123.5
flagellate, intestinal 007.9
fluke — *see* Infestation, fluke

Infection, infected, infective — *continued*
 focal
  teeth (pulpal origin) 522.4
  tonsils 474.00
   and adenoids 474.02
 Fonsecaea
  compactum 117.2
  pedrosoi 117.2
 food (*see also* Poisoning, food) 005.9
 foot (skin) 686.9
  fungus 110.4
 Francisella tularensis (*see also* Tularemia)
   021.9
 frontal sinus (chronic) (*see also* Sinusitis,
   frontal) 473.1
 fungus NEC 117.9
  beard 110.0
  body 110.5
  dermatiacious NEC 117.8
  foot 110.4
  groin 110.3
  hand 110.2
  nail 110.1
  pathogenic to compromised host only 118
  perianal (area) 110.3
  scalp 110.0
  scrotum 110.8
  skin 111.9
   foot 110.4
   hand 110.2
  toenails 110.1
  trachea 117.9
 Fusarium 118
 Fusobacterium 041.84
 gallbladder (*see also* Cholecystitis, acute) 575.0
 Gardnerella vaginalis 041.89   ●
 gas bacillus (*see also* Gas, gangrene) 040.0
 gastric (*see also* Gastritis) 535.5 ☑5ᵗʰ
 Gastrodiscoides hominis 121.8
 gastroenteric (*see also* Enteritis, due to, by
   organism) 009.0
 gastrointestinal (*see also* Enteritis, due to, by
   organism) 009.0
 gastrostomy 536.41
 generalized NEC (*see also* Septicemia) 038.9
 genital organ or tract NEC
  female 614.9
   with
    abortion — *see* Abortion, by type, with
      sepsis
    ectopic pregnancy (*see also* categories
      633.0-633.9) 639.0
    molar pregnancy (*see also* categories
      630-632) 639.0
   complicating pregnancy 646.6 ☑5ᵗʰ
    affecting fetus or newborn 760.8
   following
    abortion 639.0
    ectopic or molar pregnancy 639.0
   puerperal, postpartum, childbirth
     670 ☑4ᵗʰ
    minor or localized 646.6 ☑5ᵗʰ
     affecting fetus or newborn 760.8
  male 608.4
 genitourinary tract NEC 599.0
 Ghon tubercle, primary (*see also* Tuberculosis)
   010.0 ☑5ᵗʰ
 Giardia lamblia 007.1
 gingival (chronic) 523.1
  acute 523.0
  Vincent's 101
 glanders 024
 Glenosporopsis amazonica 116.2
 Gnathostoma spinigerum 128.1
 Gongylonema 125.6
 gonococcal NEC (*see also* Gonococcus) 098.0
 gram-negative bacilli NEC 041.85
  anaerobic 041.84
 guinea worm 125.7
 gum (*see also* Infection, gingival) 523.1
 Hantavirus 079.81
 heart 429.89
 Helicobacter pylori (H. pylori) 041.86
 helminths NEC 128.9
  intestinal 127.9
   mixed (types classifiable to more than one
     category in 120.0-127.7) 127.8

Infection, infected, infective — *continued*
 helminths NEC — *continued*
  intestinal — *continued*
   specified type NEC 127.7
   specified type NEC 128.8
 Hemophilus influenzae NEC 041.5
  generalized 038.41
 herpes (simplex) (*see also* Herpes, simplex)
   054.9
  congenital 771.2
  zoster (*see also* Herpes, zoster) 053.9
   eye NEC 053.29
 Heterophyes heterophyes 121.6
 Histoplasma (*see also* Histoplasmosis) 115.90
  capsulatum (*see also* Histoplasmosis,
    American) 115.00
  duboisii (*see also* Histoplasmosis, African)
    115.10
 HIV V08
  with symptoms, symptomatic 042
 hookworm (*see also* Ancylostomiasis) 126.9
 human immunodeficiency virus V08
  with symptoms, symptomatic 042
 human papillomavirus 079.4
 hydrocele 603.1
 hydronephrosis 591
 Hymenolepis 123.6
 hypopharynx 478.29
 inguinal glands 683
  due to soft chancre 099.0
 intestine, intestinal (*see also* Enteritis, due to,
   by organism) 009.0
 intrauterine (*see also* Endometritis) 615.9
  complicating delivery 646.6 ☑5ᵗʰ
 isospora belli or hominis 007.2
 Japanese B encephalitis 062.0
 jaw (bone) (acute) (chronic) (lower) (subacute)
   (upper) 526.4
 joint — *see* Arthritis, infectious or infective
 kidney (cortex) (hematogenous) 590.9
  with
   abortion — *see* Abortion, by type, with
     urinary tract infection
   calculus 592.0
   ectopic pregnancy (*see also* categories
     633.0-633.9) 639.8
   molar pregnancy (*see also* categories 630-
     632) 639.8
  complicating pregnancy or puerperium
    646.6 ☑5ᵗʰ
   affecting fetus or newborn 760.1
  following
   abortion 639.8
   ectopic or molar pregnancy 639.8
  pelvis and ureter 590.3
 Klebsiella pneumoniae NEC 041.3
 knee (skin) NEC 686.9
  joint — *see* Arthritis, infectious
 Koch's (*see also* Tuberculosis, pulmonary)
   011.9 ☑5ᵗʰ
 labia (majora) (minora) (*see also* Vulvitis)
   616.10
 lacrimal
  gland (*see also* Dacryoadenitis) 375.00
  passages (duct) (sac) (*see also*
    Dacryocystitis) 375.30
 larynx NEC 478.79
 leg (skin) NEC 686.9
 Leishmania (*see also* Leishmaniasis) 085.9
  braziliensis 085.5
  donovani 085.0
  Ethiopica 085.3
  furunculosa 085.1
  infantum 085.0
  mexicana 085.4
  tropica (minor) 085.1
   major 085.2
 Leptosphaeria senegalensis 117.4
 leptospira (*see also* Leptospirosis) 100.9
  Australis 100.89
  Bataviae 100.89
  pyrogenes 100.89
  specified type NEC 100.89
 leptospirochetal NEC (*see also* Leptospirosis)
   100.9
 Leptothrix — *see* Actinomycosis

Infection, infected, infective — *continued*
 Listeria monocytogenes (listeriosis) 027.0
  congenital 771.2
 liver fluke — *see* Infestation, fluke, liver
 Loa loa 125.2
  eyelid 125.2 *[373.6]*
 Loboa loboi 116.2
 local, skin (staphylococcal) (streptococcal)
   NEC 686.9
  abscess — *see* Abscess, by site
  cellulitis — *see* Cellulitis, by site
  ulcer (*see also* Ulcer, skin) 707.9
 Loefflerella
  mallei 024
  whitmori 025
 lung 518.89
  atypical Mycobacterium 031.0
   tuberculous (*see also* Tuberculosis,
     pulmonary) 011.9 ☑5ᵗʰ
  basilar 518.89
  chronic 518.89
  fungus NEC 117.9
  spirochetal 104.8
  virus — *see* Pneumonia, virus
 lymph gland (axillary) (cervical) (inguinal) 683
  mesenteric 289.2
 lymphoid tissue, base of tongue or posterior
   pharynx, NEC 474.00
 madurella
  grisea 117.4
  mycetomii 117.4
 major
  with
   abortion — *see* Abortion, by type, with
     sepsis
   ectopic pregnancy (*see also* categories
     633.0-633.9) 639.0
   molar pregnancy (*see also* categories 630-
     632) 639.0
  following
   abortion 639.0
   ectopic or molar pregnancy 639.0
  puerperal, postpartum, childbirth 670 ☑4ᵗʰ
 Malassezia furfur 111.0
 Malleomyces
  mallei 024
  pseudomallei 025
 mammary gland 611.0
  puerperal, postpartum 675.2 ☑5ᵗʰ
 Mansonella (ozzardi) 125.5
 mastoid (suppurative) — *see* Mastoiditis
 maxilla, maxillary 526.4
  sinus (chronic) (*see also* Sinusitis, maxillary)
    473.0
 mediastinum 519.2
 medina 125.7
 meibomian
  cyst 373.12
  gland 373.12
 melioidosis 025
 meninges (*see also* Meningitis) 320.9
 meningococcal (*see also* condition) 036.9
  brain 036.1
  cerebrospinal 036.0
  endocardium 036.42
  generalized 036.2
  meninges 036.0
  meningococcemia 036.2
  specified site NEC 036.89
 mesenteric lymph nodes or glands NEC 289.2
 Metagonimus 121.5
 metatarsophalangeal 711.97
 microorganism resistant to drugs — *see*
   Resistance (to), drugs by microorganisms
 Microsporidia 136.8
 microsporum, microsporic — *see*
   Dermatophytosis
 Mima polymorpha NEC 041.85
 mixed flora NEC 041.89
 Monilia (*see also* Candidiasis) 112.9
  neonatal 771.7
 Monosporium apiospermum 117.6
 mouth (focus) NEC 528.9
  parasitic 112.0
 Mucor 117.7
 muscle NEC 728.89

Infection, infected, infective — *continued*
  mycelium NEC 117.9
  mycetoma
    actinomycotic NEC (*see also* Actinomycosis)
      039.9
    mycotic NEC 117.4
  Mycobacterium, mycobacterial (*see also*
      Mycobacterium) 031.9
  mycoplasma NEC 041.81
  mycotic NEC 117.9
    pathogenic to compromised host only 118
    skin NEC 111.9
    systemic 117.9
  myocardium NEC 422.90
  nail (chronic) (with lymphangitis) 681.9
    finger 681.02
      fungus 110.1
    ingrowing 703.0
    toe 681.11
      fungus 110.1
  nasal sinus (chronic) (*see also* Sinusitis) 473.9
  nasopharynx (chronic) 478.29
    acute 460
  navel 686.9
    newborn 771.4
  Neisserian — *see* Gonococcus
  Neotestudina rosatii 117.4
  newborn, generalized 771.89   ▲
  nipple 611.0
    puerperal, postpartum 675.0 ✓5ᵗʰ
      with breast 675.9 ✓5ᵗʰ
        specified type NEC 675.8 ✓5ᵗʰ
  Nocardia — *see* Actinomycosis
  nose 478.1
  nostril 478.1
  obstetrical surgical wound 674.3 ✓5ᵗʰ
  Oesophagostomum (apiostomum) 127.7
  Oestrus ovis 134.0
  Oidium albicans (*see also* Candidiasis) 112.9
  Onchocerca (volvulus) 125.3
    eye 125.3 [360.13]
    eyelid 125.3 [373.6]
  operation wound 998.59
  Opisthorchis (felineus) (tenuicollis) (viverrini)
      121.0
  orbit 376.00
    chronic 376.10
  ovary (*see also* Salpingo-oophoritis) 614.2
  Oxyuris vermicularis 127.4
  pancreas 577.0
  Paracoccidioides brasiliensis 116.1
  Paragonimus (westermani) 121.2
  parainfluenza virus 079.89
  parameningococcus NEC 036.9
    with meningitis 036.0
  parasitic NEC 136.9
  paratyphoid 002.9
    Type A 002.1
    Type B 002.2
    Type C 002.3
  paraurethral ducts 597.89
  parotid gland 527.2
  Pasteurella NEC 027.2
    multocida (cat-bite) (dog-bite) 027.2
    pestis (*see also* Plague) 020.9
    pseudotuberculosis 027.2
    septica (cat-bite) (dog-bite) 027.2
    tularensis (*see also* Tularemia) 021.9
  pelvic, female (*see also* Disease, pelvis,
      inflammatory) 614.9
  penis (glans) (retention) NEC 607.2
    herpetic 054.13
  Peptococcus 041.84
  Peptostreptococcus 041.84
  periapical (pulpal origin) 522.4
  peridental 523.3
  perineal wound (obstetrical) 674.3 ✓5ᵗʰ
  periodontal 523.3
  periorbital 376.00
    chronic 376.10
  perirectal 569.49
  perirenal (*see also* Infection, kidney) 590.9
  peritoneal (*see also* Peritonitis) 567.9
  periureteral 593.89
  periurethral 597.89
  Petriellidium boydii 117.6

Infection, infected, infective — *continued*
  pharynx 478.29
    Coxsackievirus 074.0
    phlegmonous 462
    posterior, lymphoid 474.00
  Phialophora
    gougerotii 117.8
    jeanselmei 117.8
    verrucosa 117.2
  Piedraia hortai 111.3
  pinna, acute 380.11
  pinta 103.9
    intermediate 103.1
    late 103.2
    mixed 103.3
    primary 103.0
  pinworm 127.4
  pityrosporum furfur 111.0
  pleuropneumonia-like organisms NEC (PPLO)
      041.81
  pneumococcal NEC 041.2
    generalized (purulent) 038.2
  Pneumococcus NEC 041.2
  postoperative wound 998.59
  posttraumatic NEC 958.3
  postvaccinal 999.3
  prepuce NEC 607.1
  Proprionibacterium 041.84
  prostate (capsule) (*see also* Prostatitis) 601.9
  Proteus (mirabilis) (morganii) (vulgaris)
      NEC 041.6
    enteritis 008.3
  protozoal NEC 136.8
    intestinal NEC 007.9
  Pseudomonas NEC 041.7
    mallei 024
    pneumonia 482.1
    pseudomallei 025
  psittacosis 073.9
  puerperal, postpartum (major) 670 ✓4ᵗʰ
    minor 646.6 ✓5ᵗʰ
  pulmonary — *see* Infection, lung
  purulent — *see* Abscess
  putrid, generalized — *see* Septicemia
  pyemic — *see* Septicemia
  Pyrenochaeta romeroi 117.4
  Q fever 083.0
  rabies 071
  rectum (sphincter) 569.49
  renal (*see also* Infection, kidney) 590.9
    pelvis and ureter 590.3
  resistant to drugs — *see* Resistance (to), drugs
      by microorganisms
  respiratory 519.8
    chronic 519.8
    influenzal (acute) (upper) 487.1
    lung 518.89
    rhinovirus 460
    syncytial virus 079.6
    upper (acute) (infectious) NEC 465.9
      with flu, grippe, or influenza 487.1
      influenzal 487.1
      multiple sites NEC 465.8
      streptococcal 034.0
      viral NEC 465.9
  respiratory syncytial virus (RSV) 079.6
  resulting from presence of shunt or other
      internal prosthetic device — *see*
      Complications, infection and
      inflammation, due to (presence of) any
      device, implant, or graft classified to
      996.0-996.5 NEC
  retrovirus 079.50
    human immunodeficiency virus type 2 [HIV
      2] 079.53
    human T-cell lymphotrophic virus type I
      [HTLV-I] 079.51
    human T-cell lymphotrophic virus type II
      [HTLV-II] 079.52
    specified NEC 079.59
  Rhinocladium 117.1
  Rhinosporidium (*seeberi*) 117.0
  rhinovirus
    in diseases classified elsewhere — *see*
      category 079 ✓4ᵗʰ
    unspecified nature or site 079.3
  Rhizopus 117.7
  rickettsial 083.9

Infection, infected, infective — *continued*
  rickettsialpox 083.2
  rubella (*see also* Rubella) 056.9
    congenital 771.0
  Saccharomyces (*see also* Candidiasis) 112.9
  Saksenaea 117.7
  salivary duct or gland (any) 527.2
  Salmonella (aertrycke) (callinarum)
      (choleraesuis) (enteritidis) (suipestifer)
      (typhimurium) 003.9
    with
      arthritis 003.23
      gastroenteritis 003.0
      localized infection 003.20
        specified type NEC 003.29
      meningitis 003.21
      osteomyelitis 003.24
      pneumonia 003.22
      septicemia 003.1
      specified manifestation NEC 003.8
    congenital 771.89   ▲
    due to food (poisoning) (any serotype) (*see*
      also Poisoning, food, due to,
      Salmonella)
    hirschfeldii 002.3
    localized 003.20
      specified type NEC 003.29
    paratyphi 002.9
      A 002.1
      B 002.2
      C 002.3
    schottmuelleri 002.2
    specified type NEC 003.8
    typhi 002.0
    typhosa 002.0
  saprophytic 136.8
  Sarcocystis, lindemanni 136.5
  scabies 133.0
  Schistosoma — *see* Infestation, Schistosoma
  Schmorl's bacillus 040.3
  scratch or other superficial injury — *see* Injury,
      superficial, by site
  scrotum (acute) NEC 608.4
  secondary, burn or open wound (dislocation)
      (fracture) 958.3
  seminal vesicle (*see also* Vesiculitis) 608.0
  septic
    generalized — *see* Septicemia
    localized, skin (*see also* Abscess) 682.9
  septicemic — *see* Septicemia
  seroma 998.51
  Serratia (marcescens) 041.85
    generalized 038.44
  sheep liver fluke 121.3
  Shigella 004.9
    boydii 004.2
    dysenteriae 004.0
    flexneri 004.1
    group
      A 004.0
      B 004.1
      C 004.2
      D 004.3
    Schmitz (-Stutzer) 004.0
    schmitzii 004.0
    shiga 004.0
    sonnei 004.3
    specified type NEC 004.8
  Sin Nombre virus 079.81
  sinus (*see also* Sinusitis) 473.9
    pilonidal 685.1
      with abscess 685.0
    skin NEC 686.9
  Skene's duct or gland (*see also* Urethritis)
      597.89
  skin (local) (staphylococcal) (streptococcal)
      NEC 686.9
    abscess — *see* Abscess, by site
    cellulitis — *see* Cellulitis, by site
    due to fungus 111.9
      specified type NEC 111.8
    mycotic 111.9
      specified type NEC 111.8
    ulcer (*see also* Ulcer, skin) 707.9
  slow virus 046.9
    specified condition NEC 046.8
  Sparganum (mansoni) (proliferum) 123.5

✓4ᵗʰ Fourth-digit Required   ✓5ᵗʰ Fifth-digit Required   ▶◀ Revised Text   ● New Line   ▲ Revised Code

Infection, infected, infective — *continued*
  spermatic cord NEC 608.4
  sphenoidal (chronic) (sinus) (*see also* Sinusitis,
    sphenoidal 473.3)
  Spherophorus necrophorus 040.3
  spinal cord NEC (*see also* Encephalitis) 323.9
    abscess 324.1
      late effect — *see* category 326
    late effect — *see* category 326
    meninges — *see* Meningitis
    streptococcal 320.2
  Spirillum
    minus or minor 026.0
    morsus muris 026.0
    obermeieri 087.0
  spirochetal NEC 104.9
    lung 104.8
    specified nature or site NEC 104.8
  spleen 289.59
  Sporothrix schenckii 117.1
  Sporotrichum (schenckii) 117.1
  Sporozoa 136.8
  staphylococcal NEC 041.10
    aureus 041.11
    food poisoning 005.0
    generalized (purulent) 038.10
      aureus 038.11
      specified organism NEC 038.19
    pneumonia 482.40
      aureus 482.41
      specified type NEC 482.49
    septicemia 038.10
      aureus 038.11
      specified organism NEC 038.19
    specified NEC 041.19
  steatoma 706.2
  Stellantchasmus falcatus 121.6
  Streptobacillus moniliformis 026.1
  streptococcal NEC 041.00
    congenital 771.89   ▲
    generalized (purulent) 038.0
    Group
      A 041.01
      B 041.02
      C 041.03
      D [enterococcus] 041.04
      G 041.05
    pneumonia — *see* Pneumonia, streptococcal
      482.3 ✓5ᵗʰ
    septicemia 038.0
    sore throat 034.0
    specified NEC 041.09
  Streptomyces — *see* Actinomycosis
  streptotrichosis — *see* Actinomycosis
  Strongyloides (stercoralis) 127.2
  stump (amputation) (posttraumatic) (surgical)
    997.62
    traumatic — *see* Amputation, traumatic, by
      site, complicated
  subcutaneous tissue, local NEC 686.9
  submaxillary region 528.9
  suipestifer (*see also* Infection, Salmonella)
    003.9
  swimming pool bacillus 031.1
  syphilitic — *see* Syphilis
  systemic — *see* Septicemia
  Taenia — *see* Infestation, Taenia
  Taeniarhynchus saginatus 123.2
  tapeworm — *see* Infestation, tapeworm
  tendon (sheath) 727.89
  Ternidens diminutus 127.7
  testis (*see also* Orchitis) 604.90
  thigh (skin) 686.9
  threadworm 127.4
  throat 478.29
    pneumococcal 462
    staphylococcal 462
    streptococcal 034.0
    viral NEC (*see also* Pharyngitis) 462
  thumb (skin) 686.9
    abscess (with lymphangitis) 681.00
      pulp 681.01
    cellulitis (with lymphangitis) 681.00
    nail 681.02
  thyroglossal duct 529.8
  toe (skin) 686.9
    abscess (with lymphangitis) 681.10

Infection, infected, infective — *continued*
  toe — *continued*
    cellulitis (with lymphangitis) 681.10
    nail 681.11
      fungus 110.1
  tongue NEC 529.0
    parasitic 112.0
  tonsil (faucial) (lingual) (pharyngeal) 474.00
    acute or subacute 463
    and adenoid 474.02
    tag 474.00
  tooth, teeth 522.4
    periapical (pulpal origin) 522.4
    peridental 523.3
    periodontal 523.3
    pulp 522.0
    socket 526.5
  Torula histolytica 117.5
  Toxocara (cani) (cati) (felis) 128.0
  Toxoplasma gondii (*see also* Toxoplasmosis)
    130.9
  trachea, chronic 491.8
    fungus 117.9
  traumatic NEC 958.3
  trematode NEC 121.9
  trench fever 083.1
  Treponema
    denticola 041.84
    macrodenticum 041.84
    pallidum (*see also* Syphillis) 097.9
  Trichinella (spiralis) 124
  Trichomonas 131.9
    bladder 131.09
    cervix 131.09
    hominis 007.3
    intestine 007.3
    prostate 131.03
    specified site NEC 131.8
    urethra 131.02
    urogenitalis 131.00
    vagina 131.01
    vulva 131.01
  Trichophyton, trichophytid — *see*
    Dermatophytosis
  Trichosporon (beigelii) cutaneum 111.2
  Trichostrongylus 127.6
  Trichuris (trichiuria) 127.3
  Trombicula (irritans) 133.8
  Trypanosoma (*see also* Trypanosomiasis) 086.9
    cruzi 086.2
  tubal (*see also* Salpingo-oophoritis) 614.2
  tuberculous NEC (*see also* Tuberculosis)
    011.9 ✓5ᵗʰ
  tubo-ovarian (*see also* Salpingo-oophoritis)
    614.2
  tunica vaginalis 608.4
  tympanic membrane — *see* Myringitis
  typhoid (abortive) (ambulant) (bacillus) 002.0
  typhus 081.9
    flea-borne (endemic) 081.0
    louse-borne (epidemic) 080
    mite-borne 081.2
    recrudescent 081.1
    tick-borne 082.9
      African 082.1
      North Asian 082.2
  umbilicus (septic) 686.9
    newborn NEC 771.4
  ureter 593.89
  urethra (*see also* Urethritis) 597.80
  urinary (tract) NEC 599.0
    with
      abortion — *see* Abortion, by type, with
        urinary tract infection
      ectopic pregnancy (*see also* categories
        633.0-633.9) 639.8
      molar pregnancy (*see also* categories 630-
        632) 639.8
    candidal 112.2
    complicating pregnancy, childbirth, or
      puerperium 646.6 ✓5ᵗʰ
      affecting fetus or newborn 760.1
      asymptomatic 646.5 ✓5ᵗʰ
        affecting fetus or newborn 760.1
    diplococcal (acute) 098.0
      chronic 098.2

Infection, infected, infective — *continued*
  urinary (tract) NEC — *continued*
    due to Trichomonas (vaginalis) 131.00
      following
        abortion 639.8
        ectopic or molar pregnancy 639.8
      gonococcal (acute) 098.0
        chronic or duration of 2 months or
          over 098.2
      newborn 771.82   ▲
    trichomonal 131.00
    tuberculous (*see also* Tuberculosis)
      016.3 ✓5ᵗʰ
  uterus, uterine (*see also* Endometritis) 615.9
  utriculus masculinus NEC 597.89
  vaccination 999.3
  vagina (granulation tissue) (wall) (*see also*
    Vaginitis) 616.10
  varicella 052.9
  varicose veins — *see* Varicose, veins
  variola 050.9
    major 050.0
    minor 050.1
  vas deferens NEC 608.4
  Veillonella 041.84
  verumontanum 597.89
  vesical (*see also* Cystitis) 595.9
  Vibrio
    cholerae 001.0
      El Tor 001.1
    parahaemolyticus (food poisoning) 005.4
    vulnificus 041.85
  Vincent's (gums) (mouth) (tonsil) 101
  virus, viral 079.99
    adenovirus
      in diseases classified elsewhere — *see*
        category 079 ✓4ᵗʰ
      unspecified nature or site 079.0
    central nervous system NEC 049.9
      enterovirus 048
        meningitis 047.9
          specified type NEC 047.8
        slow virus 046.9
          specified condition NEC 046.8
    chest 519.8
    conjunctivitis 077.99
      specified type NEC 077.8
    Coxsackie (*see also* Infection, Coxsackie)
      079.2
    Ebola 065.8
    ECHO
      in diseases classified elsewhere — *see*
        category 079 ✓4ᵗʰ
      unspecified nature or site 079.1
    encephalitis 049.9
      arthropod-borne NEC 064
      tick-borne 063.9
        specified type NEC 063.8
    enteritis NEC (*see also* Enteritis, viral) 008.8
    exanthem NEC 057.9
    Hantavirus 079.81
    human papilloma 079.4
    in diseases classified elsewhere — *see*
      category 079 ✓4ᵗʰ
    intestine (*see also* Enteritis, viral) 008.8
    lung — *see* Pneumonia, viral
    respiratory syncytial (RSV) 079.6
    retrovirus 079.50
    rhinovirus
      in diseases classified elsewhere — *see*
        category 079 ✓4ᵗʰ
      unspecified nature or site 079.3
    salivary gland disease 078.5
    slow 046.9
      specified condition NEC 046.8
    specified type NEC 079.89
      in diseases classified elsewhere — *see*
        category 079 ✓4ᵗʰ
    unspecified nature or site 079.99
    warts NEC 078.10
  vulva (*see also* Vulvitis) 616.10
  whipworm 127.3
  Whitmore's bacillus 025
  wound (local) (posttraumatic) NEC 958.3
    with
      dislocation — *see* Dislocation, by site,
        open

Infection — Infection

Infection, infected, infective — *continued*
wound` — *continued*
with — *continued*
fracture — *see* Fracture, by site, open
open wound — *see* Wound, open, by site,
complicated
postoperative 998.59
surgical 998.59
Wuchereria 125.0
bancrofti 125.0
malayi 125.1
yaws — *see* Yaws
yeast (*see also* Candidiasis) 112.9
yellow fever (*see also* Fever, yellow) 060.9
Yersinia pestis (*see also* Plague) 020.9
Zeis' gland 373.12
zoonotic bacterial NEC 027.9
Zopfia senegalensis 117.4
Infective, infectious — *see* condition
Inferiority complex 301.9
constitutional psychopathic 301.9
Infertility
female 628.9
associated with
adhesions, peritubal 614.6 *[628.2]*
anomaly
cervical mucus 628.4
congenital
cervix 628.4
fallopian tube 628.2
uterus 628.3
vagina 628.4
anovulation 628.0
dysmucorrhea 628.4
endometritis, tuberculous (*see also*
Tuberculosis) 016.7 ✓5ᵗʰ *[628.3]*
Stein-Leventhal syndrome 256.4 *[628.0]*
due to
adiposogenital dystrophy 253.8 *[628.1]*
anterior pituitary disorder NEC
253.4 *[628.1]*
hyperfunction 253.1 *[628.1]*
cervical anomaly 628.4
fallopian tube anomaly 628.2
ovarian failure 256.39 *[628.0]*
Stein-Leventhal syndrome 256.4 *[628.0]*
uterine anomaly 628.3
vaginal anomaly 628.4
nonimplantation 628.3
origin
cervical 628.4
pituitary-hypothalamus NEC
253.8 *[628.1]*
anterior pituitary NEC 253.4 *[628.1]*
hyperfunction NEC 253.1 *[628.1]*
dwarfism 253.3 *[628.1]*
panhypopituitarism 253.2 *[628.1]*
specified NEC 628.8
tubal (block) (occlusion) (stenosis) 628.2
adhesions 614.6 *[628.2]*
uterine 628.3
vaginal 628.4
previous, requiring supervision of pregnancy
V23.0
male 606.9
absolute 606.0
due to
azoospermia 606.0
drug therapy 606.8
extratesticular cause NEC 606.8
germinal cell
aplasia 606.0
desquamation 606.1
hypospermatogenesis 606.1
infection 606.8
obstruction, afferent ducts 606.8
oligospermia 606.1
radiation 606.8
spermatogenic arrest (complete) 606.0
incomplete 606.1
systemic disease 606.8
Infestation 134.9
Acanthocheilonema (perstans) 125.4
streptocerca 125.6
Acariasis 133.9
demodex folliculorum 133.8

Infestation — *continued*
Acariasis — *continued*
Sarcoptes scabiei 133.0
trombiculae 133.8
Agamofilaria streptocerca 125.6
Ancylostoma, Ankylostoma 126.9
americanum 126.1
braziliense 126.2
canium 126.8
ceylanicum 126.3
duodenale 126.0
new world 126.1
old world 126.0
Angiostrongylus cantonensis 128.8
anisakiasis 127.1
Anisakis larva 127.1
arthropod NEC 134.1
Ascaris lumbricoides 127.0
Bacillus fusiformis 101
Balantidium coli 007.0
beef tapeworm 123.2
Bothriocephalus (latus) 123.4
larval 123.5
broad tapeworm 123.4
larval 123.5
Brugia malayi 125.1
Candiru 136.8
Capillaria
hepatica 128.8
philippinensis 127.5
cat liver fluke 121.0
Cercomonas hominis (intestinal) 007.3
cestodes 123.9
specified type NEC 123.8
chigger 133.8
chigoe 134.1
Chilomastix 007.8
Clonorchis (sinensis) (liver) 121.1
coccidia 007.2
complicating pregnancy, childbirth, or
puerperium 647.9 ✓5ᵗʰ
affecting fetus or newborn 760.8
Cysticercus cellulosae 123.1
Demodex folliculorum 133.8
Dermatobia (hominis) 134.0
Dibothriocephalus (latus) 123.4
larval 123.5
Dicrocoelium dendriticum 121.8
Diphyllobothrium (adult) (intestinal) (latum)
(pacificum) 123.4
larval 123.5
Diplogonoporus (grandis) 123.8
Dipylidium (caninum) 123.8
Distoma hepaticum 121.3
dog tapeworm 123.8
Dracunculus medinensis 125.7
dragon worm 125.7
dwarf tapeworm 123.6
Echinococcus (*see also* Echinococcus) 122.9
Echinostoma ilocanum 121.8
Embadomonas 007.8
Endamoeba (histolytica) — *see* Infection,
ameba
Entamoeba (histolytica) — *see* Infection, ameba
Enterobius vermicularis 127.4
Epidermophyton — *see* Dermatophytosis
eyeworm 125.2
Fasciola
gigantica 121.3
hepatica 121.3
Fasciolopsis (buski) (small intestine) 121.4
filarial 125.9
due to
Acanthocheilonema (perstans) 125.4
streptocerca 125.6
Brugia (Wuchereria) malayi 125.1
Dracunculus medinensis 125.7
guinea worms 125.7
Mansonella (ozzardi) 125.5
Onchocerca volvulus 125.3
eye 125.3 *[360.13]*
eyelid 125.3 *[373.6]*
Wuchereria (bancrofti) 125.0
malayi 125.1
specified type NEC 125.6
fish tapeworm 123.4
larval 123.5

Infestation — *continued*
Fasciolopsis — *continued*
fluke 121.9
blood NEC (*see also* Schistosomiasis) 120.9
cat liver 121.0
intestinal (giant) 121.4
liver (sheep) 121.3
cat 121.0
Chinese 121.1
clonorchiasis 121.1
fascioliasis 121.3
Oriental 121.1
lung (oriental) 121.2
sheep liver 121.3
fly larva 134.0
Gasterophilus (intestinalis) 134.0
Gastrodiscoides hominis 121.8
Giardia lamblia 007.1
Gnathostoma (spinigerum) 128.1
Gongylonema 125.6
guinea worm 125.7
helminth NEC 128.9
intestinal 127.9
mixed (types classifiable to more than one
category in 120.0-127.7) 127.8
specified type NEC 127.7
specified type NEC 128.8
Heterophyes heterophyes (small intestine)
121.6
hookworm (*see also* Infestation, ancylostoma)
126.9
Hymenolepis (diminuta) (nana) 123.6
intestinal NEC 129
leeches (aquatic) (land) 134.2
Leishmania — *see* Leishmaniasis
lice (*see also* Infestation, pediculus) 132.9
Linguatulidae, linguatula (pentastoma) (serrata)
134.1
Loa loa 125.2
eyelid 125.2 *[373.6]*
louse (*see also* Infestation, pediculus) 132.9
body 132.1
head 132.0
pubic 132.2
maggots 134.0
Mansonella (ozzardi) 125.5
medina 125.7
Metagonimus yokogawai (small intestine) 121.5
Microfilaria streptocerca 125.3
eye 125.3 *[360.13]*
eyelid 125.3 *[373.6]*
Microsporon furfur 111.0
microsporum — *see* Dermatophytosis
mites 133.9
scabic 133.0
specified type NEC 133.8
Monilia (albicans) (*see also* Candidiasis) 112.9
vagina 112.1
vulva 112.1
mouth 112.0
Necator americanus 126.1
nematode (intestinal) 127.9
Ancylostoma (*see also* Ancylostoma) 126.9
Ascaris lumbricoides 127.0
conjunctiva NEC 128.9
Dioctophyma 128.8
Enterobius vermicularis 127.4
Gnathostoma spinigerum 128.1
Oesophagostomum (apiostomum) 127.7
Physaloptera 127.4
specified type NEC 127.7
Strongyloides stercoralis 127.2
Ternidens diminutus 127.7
Trichinella spiralis 124
Trichostrongylus 127.6
Trichuris (trichiuria) 127.3
Oesophagostomum (apiostomum) 127.7
Oestrus ovis 134.0
Onchocerca (volvulus) 125.3
eye 125.3 *[360.13]*
eyelid 125.3 *[373.6]*
Opisthorchis (felineus) (tenuicollis) (viverrini)
121.0
Oxyuris vermicularis 127.4
Paragonimus (westermani) 121.2
parasite, parasitic NEC 136.9
eyelid 134.9 *[373.6]*

✓4ᵗʰ Fourth-digit Required   ✓5ᵗʰ Fifth-digit Required   ►◄ Revised Text   ● New Line   ▲ Revised Code

Infestation — *continued*
  parasite, parasitic NEC — *continued*
    intestinal 129
    mouth 112.0
    orbit 376.13
    skin 134.9
    tongue 112.0
  pediculus 132.9
    capitis (humanus) (any site) 132.0
    corporis (humanus) (any site) 132.1
    eyelid 132.0 *[373.6]*
    mixed (classifiable to more than one
        category in 132.0-132.2) 132.3
    pubis (any site) 132.2
  phthirus (pubis) (any site) 132.2
    with any infestation classifiable to 132.0,
        132.1 and 132.3
  pinworm 127.4
  pork tapeworm (adult) 123.0
  protozoal NEC 136.8
  pubic louse 132.2
  rat tapeworm 123.6
  red bug 133.8
  roundworm (large) NEC 127.0
  sand flea 134.1
  saprophytic NEC 136.8
  Sarcoptes scabiei 133.0
  scabies 133.0
  Schistosoma 120.9
    bovis 120.8
    cercariae 120.3
    hematobium 120.0
    intercalatum 120.8
    japonicum 120.2
    mansoni 120.1
    mattheii 120.8
    specified
      site — *see* Schistosomiasis
      type NEC 120.8
    spindale 120.8
  screw worms 134.0
  skin NEC 134.9
  Sparganum (mansoni) (proliferum) 123.5
    larval 123.5
  specified type NEC 134.8
  Spirometra larvae 123.5
  Sporozoa NEC 136.8
  Stellantchasmus falcatus 121.6
  Strongyloides 127.2
  Strongylus (gibsoni) 127.7
  Taenia 123.3
    diminuta 123.6
    Echinococcus (*see also* Echinococcus) 122.9
    mediocanellata 123.2
    nana 123.6
    saginata (mediocanellata) 123.2
    solium (intestinal form) 123.0
      larval form 123.1
  Taeniarhynchus saginatus 123.2
  tapeworm 123.9
    beef 123.2
    broad 123.4
      larval 123.5
    dog 123.8
    dwarf 123.6
    fish 123.4
      larval 123.5
    pork 123.0
    rat 123.6
  Ternidens diminutus 127.7
  Tetranychus molestissimus 133.8
  threadworm 127.4
  tongue 112.0
  Toxocara (cani) (cati) (felis) 128.0
  trematode(s) NEC 121.9
  Trichina spiralis 124
  Trichinella spiralis 124
  Trichocephalus 127.3
  Trichomonas 131.9
    bladder 131.09
    cervix 131.09
    intestine 007.3
    prostate 131.03
    specified site NEC 131.8
    urethra (female) (male) 131.02
    urogenital 131.00

Infestation — *continued*
  Trichomonas — *continued*
    vagina 131.01
    vulva 131.01
  Trichophyton — *see* Dermatophytosis
  Trichostrongylus instabilis 127.6
  Trichuris (trichiuria) 127.3
  Trombicula (irritans) 133.8
  Trypanosoma — *see* Trypanosomiasis
  Tunga penetrans 134.1
  Uncinaria americana 126.1
  whipworm 127.3
  worms NEC 128.9
    intestinal 127.9
  Wuchereria 125.0
    bancrofti 125.0
    malayi 125.1

Infiltrate, infiltration
  with an iron compound 275.0
  amyloid (any site) (generalized) 277.3
  calcareous (muscle) NEC 275.49
    localized — *see* Degeneration, by site
  calcium salt (muscle) 275.49
  corneal (*see also* Edema, cornea) 371.20
  eyelid 373.9
  fatty (diffuse) (generalized) 272.8
    localized — *see* Degeneration, by site, fatty
  glycogen, glycogenic (*see also* Disease, glycogen
    storage) 271.0
  heart, cardiac
    fatty (*see also* Degeneration, myocardial)
      429.1
    glycogenic 271.0 *[425.7]*
  inflammatory in vitreous 379.29
  kidney (*see also* Disease, renal) 593.9
  leukemic (M9800/3) — *see* Leukemia
  liver 573.8
    fatty — *see* Fatty, liver
    glycogen (*see also* Disease, glycogen storage)
      271.0
  lung (*see also* Infiltrate, pulmonary) 518.3
    eosinophilic 518.3
    x-ray finding only 793.1
  lymphatic (*see also* Leukemia, lymphatic)
    204.9 ✔5ᵗʰ
    gland, pigmentary 289.3
  muscle, fatty 728.9
  myelogenous (*see also* Leukemia, myeloid)
    205.9 ✔5ᵗʰ
  myocardium, myocardial
    fatty (*see also* Degeneration, myocardial)
      429.1
    glycogenic 271.0 *[425.7]*
  pulmonary 518.3
    with
      eosinophilia 518.3
      pneumonia — *see* Pneumonia, by type
    x-ray finding only 793.1
  Ranke's primary (*see also* Tuberculosis)
    010.0 ✔5ᵗʰ
  skin, lymphocytic (benign) 709.8
  thymus (gland) (fatty) 254.8
  urine 788.8
  vitreous humor 379.29

Infirmity 799.8
  senile 797

Inflammation, inflamed, inflammatory (with
  exudation)
  abducens (nerve) 378.54
  accessory sinus (chronic) (*see also* Sinusitis)
    473.9
  adrenal (gland) 255.8
  alimentary canal — *see* Enteritis
  alveoli (teeth) 526.5
    scorbutic 267
  amnion — *see* Amnionitis
  anal canal 569.49
  antrum (chronic) (*see also* Sinusitis, maxillary)
    473.0
  anus 569.49
  appendix (*see also* Appendicitis) 541
  arachnoid — *see* Meningitis
  areola 611.0
    puerperal, postpartum 675.0 ✔5ᵗʰ
  areolar tissue NEC 686.9
  artery — *see* Arteritis

Inflammation, inflamed, inflammatory —
  continued
  auditory meatus (external) (*see also* Otitis,
    externa) 380.10
  Bartholin's gland 616.8
  bile duct or passage 576.1
  bladder (*see also* Cystitis) 595.9
  bone — *see* Osteomyelitis
  bowel (*see also* Enteritis) 558.9
  brain (*see also* Encephalitis) 323.9
    late effect — *see* category 326
    membrane — *see* Meningitis
  breast 611.0
    puerperal, postpartum 675.2 ✔5ᵗʰ
  broad ligament (*see also* Disease, pelvis,
    inflammatory) 614.4
    acute 614.3
  bronchus — *see* Bronchitis
  bursa — *see* Bursitis
  capsule
    liver 573.3
    spleen 289.59
  catarrhal (*see also* Catarrh) 460
    vagina 616.10
  cecum (*see also* Appendicitis) 541
  cerebral (*see also* Encephalitis) 323.9
    late effect — *see* category 326
    membrane — *see* Meningitis
  cerebrospinal (*see also* Meningitis) 322.9
    late effect — *see* category 326
    meningococcal 036.0
    tuberculous (*see also* Tuberculosis)
      013.6 ✔5ᵗʰ
  cervix (uteri) (*see also* Cervicitis) 616.0
  chest 519.9
  choroid NEC (*see also* Choroiditis) 363.20
  cicatrix (tissue) — *see* Cicatrix
  colon (*see also* Enteritis) 558.9
    granulomatous 555.1
    newborn 558.9
  connective tissue (diffuse) NEC 728.9
  cornea (*see also* Keratitis) 370.9
    with ulcer (*see also* Ulcer, cornea) 370.00
  corpora cavernosa (penis) 607.2
  cranial nerve — *see* Disorder, nerve, cranial
  diarrhea — *see* Diarrhea
  disc (intervertebral) (space) 722.90
    cervical, cervicothoracic 722.91
    lumbar, lumbosacral 722.93
    thoracic, thoracolumbar 722.92
  Douglas' cul-de-sac or pouch (chronic) (*see also*
    Disease, pelvis, inflammatory) 614.4
    acute 614.3
  due to (presence of) any device, implant, or
    graft classifiable to 996.0-996.5 — *see*
    Complications, infection and
    inflammation, due to (presence of) any
    device, implant, or graft classified to
    996.0-996.5 NEC
  duodenum 535.6 ✔5ᵗʰ
  dura mater — *see* Meningitis
  ear — *see also* Otitis
    external (*see also* Otitis, externa) 380.10
    inner (*see also* Labyrinthitis) 386.30
    middle — *see* Otitis media
  esophagus 530.10
  ethmoidal (chronic) (sinus) (*see also* Sinusitis,
    ethmoidal) 473.2
  Eustachian tube (catarrhal) 381.50
    acute 381.51
    chronic 381.52
  extrarectal 569.49
  eye 379.99
  eyelid 373.9
    specified NEC 373.8
  fallopian tube (*see also* Salpingo-oophoritis)
    614.2
  fascia 728.9
  fetal membranes (acute) 658.4 ✔5ᵗʰ
    affecting fetus or newborn 762.7
  follicular, pharynx 472.1
  frontal (chronic) (sinus) (*see also* Sinusitis,
    frontal) 473.1
  gallbladder (*see also* Cholecystitis, acute) 575.0
  gall duct (*see also* Cholecystitis) 575.10
  gastrointestinal (*see also* Enteritis) 558.9

Infestation — Inflammation

Inflammation — Inhalation

Inflammation, inflamed, inflammatory —
continued
genital organ (diffuse) (internal)
female 614.9
with
abortion — *see* Abortion, by type, with
sepsis
ectopic pregnancy (*see also* categories
633.0-633.9) 639.0
molar pregnancy (*see also* categories
630-632) 639.0
complicating pregnancy, childbirth, or
puerperium 646.6 ✓5ᵗʰ
affecting fetus or newborn 760.8
following
abortion 639.0
ectopic or molar pregnancy 639.0
male 608.4
gland (lymph) (*see also* Lymphadenitis) 289.3
glottis (*see also* Laryngitis) 464.00
with obstruction 464.01
granular, pharynx 472.1
gum 523.1
heart (*see also* Carditis) 429.89
hepatic duct 576.8
hernial sac — *see* Hernia, by site
ileum (*see also* Enteritis) 558.9
terminal or regional 555.0
with large intestine 555.2
intestine (*see also* Enteritis) 558.9
intervertebral disc 722.90
cervical, cervicothoracic 722.91
lumbar, lumbosacral 722.93
thoracic, thoracolumbar 722.92
jaw (acute) (bone) (chronic) (lower) (suppurative)
(upper) 526.4
jejunum — *see* Enteritis
joint NEC (*see also* Arthritis) 716.9 ✓5ᵗʰ
sacroiliac 720.2
kidney (*see also* Nephritis) 583.9
knee (joint) 716.66
tuberculous (active) (*see also* Tuberculosis)
015.2 ✓5ᵗʰ
labium (majus) (minus) (*see also* Vulvitis)
616.10
lacrimal
gland (*see also* Dacryoadenitis) 375.00
passages (duct) (sac) (*see also*
Dacryocystitis) 375.30
larynx (*see also* Laryngitis) 464.00
with obstruction 464.01
diphtheritic 032.3
leg NEC 686.9
lip 528.5
liver (capsule) (*see also* Hepatitis) 573.3
acute 570
chronic 571.40
suppurative 572.0
lung (acute) (*see also* Pneumonia) 486
chronic (interstitial) 518.89
lymphatic vessel (*see also* Lymphangitis) 457.2
lymph node or gland (*see also* Lymphadenitis)
289.3
mammary gland 611.0
puerperal, postpartum 675.2 ✓5ᵗʰ
maxilla, maxillary 526.4
sinus (chronic) (*see also* Sinusitis, maxillary)
473.0
membranes of brain or spinal cord — *see*
Meningitis
meninges — *see* Meningitis
mouth 528.0
muscle 728.9
myocardium (*see also* Myocarditis) 429.0
nasal sinus (chronic) (*see also* Sinusitis) 473.9
nasopharynx — *see* Nasopharyngitis
navel 686.9
newborn NEC 771.4
nerve NEC 729.2
nipple 611.0
puerperal, postpartum 675.0 ✓5ᵗʰ
nose 478.1
suppurative 472.0
oculomotor nerve 378.51
optic nerve 377.30
orbit (chronic) 376.10
acute 376.00

Inflammation, inflamed, inflammatory —
continued
orbit — *continued*
chronic 376.10
ovary (*see also* Salpingo-oophoritis) 614.2
oviduct (*see also* Salpingo-oophoritis) 614.2
pancreas — *see* Pancreatitis
parametrium (chronic) (*see also* Disease, pelvis,
inflammatory) 614.4
acute 614.3
parotid region 686.9
gland 527.2
pelvis, female (*see also* Disease, pelvis,
inflammatory) 614.9
penis (corpora cavernosa) 607.2
perianal 569.49
pericardium (*see also* Pericarditis) 423.9
perineum (female) (male) 686.9
perirectal 569.49
peritoneum (*see also* Peritonitis) 567.9
periuterine (*see also* Disease, pelvis,
inflammatory) 614.9
perivesical (*see also* Cystitis) 595.9
petrous bone (*see also* Petrositis) 383.20
pharynx (*see also* Pharyngitis) 462
follicular 472.1
granular 472.1
pia mater — *see* Meningitis
pleura — *see* Pleurisy
postmastoidectomy cavity 383.30
chronic 383.33
prostate (*see also* Prostatitis) 601.9
rectosigmoid — *see* Rectosigmoiditis
rectum (*see also* Proctitis) 569.49
respiratory, upper (*see also* Infection,
respiratory, upper) 465.9
chronic, due to external agent — *see*
Condition, respiratory, chronic, due to,
external agent
due to
fumes or vapors (chemical) (inhalation)
506.2
radiation 508.1
retina (*see also* Retinitis) 363.20
retrocecal (*see also* Appendicitis) 541
retroperitoneal (*see also* Peritonitis) 567.9
salivary duct or gland (any) (suppurative) 527.2
scorbutic, alveoli, teeth 267
scrotum 608.4
sigmoid — *see* Enteritis
sinus (*see also* Sinusitis) 473.9
Skene's duct or gland (*see also* Urethritis)
597.89
skin 686.9
spermatic cord 608.4
sphenoidal (sinus) (*see also* Sinusitis,
sphenoidal) 473.3
spinal
cord (*see also* Encephalitis) 323.9
late effect — *see* category 326
membrane — *see* Meningitis
nerve — *see* Disorder, nerve
spine (*see also* Spondylitis) 720.9
spleen (capsule) 289.59
stomach — *see* Gastritis
stricture, rectum 569.49
subcutaneous tissue NEC 686.9
suprarenal (gland) 255.8
synovial (fringe) (membrane) — *see* Bursitis
tendon (sheath) NEC 726.90
testis (*see also* Orchitis) 604.90
thigh 686.9
throat (*see also* Sore throat) 462
thymus (gland) 254.8
thyroid (gland) (*see also* Thyroiditis) 245.9
tongue 529.0
tonsil — *see* Tonsillitis
trachea — *see* Tracheitis
trochlear nerve 378.53
tubal (*see also* Salpingo-oophoritis) 614.2
tuberculous NEC (*see also* Tuberculosis)
011.9 ✓5ᵗʰ
tubo-ovarian (*see also* Salpingo-oophoritis)
614.2
tunica vaginalis 608.4
tympanic membrane — *see* Myringitis
umbilicus, umbilical 686.9
newborn NEC 771.4

Inflammation, inflamed, inflammatory —
continued
uterine ligament (*see also* Disease, pelvis,
inflammatory) 614.4
acute 614.3
uterus (catarrhal) (*see also* Endometritis) 615.9
uveal tract (anterior) (*see also* Iridocyclitis)
364.3
posterior — *see* Chorioretinitis
sympathetic 360.11
vagina (*see also* Vaginitis) 616.10
vas deferens 608.4
vein (*see also* Phlebitis) 451.9
thrombotic 451.9
cerebral (*see also* Thrombosis, brain)
434.0 ✓5ᵗʰ
leg 451.2
deep (vessels) NEC 451.19
superficial (vessels) 451.0
lower extremity 451.2
deep (vessels) NEC 451.19
superficial (vessels) 451.0
vocal cord 478.5
vulva (*see also* Vulvitis) 616.10
Inflation, lung imperfect (newborn) 770.5
Influenza, influenzal 487.1
with
bronchitis 487.1
bronchopneumonia 487.0
cold (any type) 487.1
digestive manifestations 487.8
hemoptysis 487.1
involvement of
gastrointestinal tract 487.8
nervous system 487.8
laryngitis 487.1
manifestations NEC 487.8
respiratory 487.1
pneumonia 487.0
pharyngitis 487.1
pneumonia (any form classifiable to 480-
483, 485-486) 487.0
respiratory manifestations NEC 487.1
sinusitis 487.1
sore throat 487.1
tonsillitis 487.1
tracheitis 487.1
upper respiratory infection (acute) 487.1
abdominal 487.8
Asian 487.1
bronchial 487.1
bronchopneumonia 487.0
catarrhal 487.1
epidemic 487.1
gastric 487.8
intestinal 487.8
laryngitis 487.1
maternal affecting fetus or newborn 760.2
manifest influenza in infant 771.2
pharyngitis 487.1
pneumonia (any form) 487.0
respiratory (upper) 487.1
stomach 487.8
vaccination, prophylactic (against) V04.8
Influenza-like disease 487.1
Infraction, Freiberg's (metatarsal head) 732.5
**Infusion complication, misadventure, or
reaction** — *see* Complication, infusion
Ingestion
chemical — *see* Table of Drugs and Chemicals
drug or medicinal substance
overdose or wrong substance given or taken
977.9
specified drug — *see* Table of Drugs and
Chemicals
foreign body NEC (*see also* Foreign body) 938
Ingrowing
hair 704.8
nail (finger) (toe) (infected) 703.0
Inguinal — *see also* condition
testis 752.51
Inhalation
carbon monoxide 986
flame
mouth 947.0

✓4ᵗʰ Fourth-digit Required   ✓5ᵗʰ Fifth-digit Required   ▶◀ Revised Text   ● New Line   ▲ Revised Code

Inhalation — *continued*
  flame — *continued*
    lung 947.1
  food or foreign body (*see also* Asphyxia, food or foreign body) 933.1
  gas, fumes, or vapor (noxious) 987.9
    specified agent — *see* Table of Drugs and Chemicals
  liquid or vomitus (*see also* Asphyxia, food or foreign body) 933.1
    lower respiratory tract NEC 934.9
  meconium (fetus or newborn) 770.1
  mucus (*see also* Asphyxia, mucus) 933.1
  oil (causing suffocation) (*see also* Asphyxia, food or foreign body) 933.1
  pneumonia — *see* Pneumonia, aspiration
  smoke 987.9
  steam 987.9
  stomach contents or secretions (*see also* Asphyxia, food or foreign body) 933.1
    in labor and delivery 668.0 ✓5ᵗʰ

Inhibition, inhibited
  academic as adjustment reaction 309.23
  orgasm
    female 302.73
    male 302.74
  sexual
    desire 302.71
    excitement 302.72
  work as adjustment reaction 309.23

Inhibitor, systemic lupus erythematosus (presence of) 286.5

Iniencephalus, iniencephaly 740.2

Injected eye 372.74

Injury 959.9

> *Note* — *For abrasion, insect bite (nonvenomous), blister, or scratch, see Injury, superficial.*
>
> *For laceration, traumatic rupture, tear, or penetrating wound of internal organs, such as heart, lung, liver, kidney, pelvic organs, whether or not accompanied by open wound in the same region, see Injury, internal.*
>
> *For nerve injury, see Injury, nerve.*
>
> *For late effect of injuries classifiable to 850-854, 860-869, 900-919, 950-959, see Late, effect, injury, by type.*

  abdomen, abdominal (viscera) — *see also* Injury, internal, abdomen
    muscle or wall 959.1
  acoustic, resulting in deafness 951.5
  adenoid 959.09
  adrenal (gland) — *see* Injury, internal, adrenal
  alveolar (process) 959.09
  ankle (and foot) (and knee) (and leg, except thigh) 959.7
  anterior chamber, eye 921.3
  anus 959.1
  aorta (thoracic) 901.0
    abdominal 902.0
  appendix — *see* Injury, internal, appendix
  arm, upper (and shoulder) 959.2
  artery (complicating trauma) (*see also* Injury, blood vessel, by site) 904.9
    cerebral or meningeal (*see also* Hemorrhage, brain, traumatic, subarachnoid) 852.0 ✓5ᵗʰ
  auditory canal (external) (meatus) 959.09
  auricle, auris, ear 959.09
  axilla 959.2
  back 959.1
  bile duct — *see* Injury, internal, bile duct
  birth — *see also* Birth, injury
    canal NEC, complicating delivery 665.9 ✓5ᵗʰ
  bladder (sphincter) — *see* Injury, internal, bladder
  blast (air) (hydraulic) (immersion) (underwater) NEC 869.0
    with open wound into cavity NEC 869.1
    abdomen or thorax — *see* Injury, internal, by site
    brain — *see* Concussion, brain

Injury — *continued*
  blast — *continued*
    ear (acoustic nerve trauma) 951.5
      with perforation of tympanic membrane — *see* Wound, open, ear, drum
  blood vessel NEC 904.9
    abdomen 902.9
      multiple 902.87
      specified NEC 902.89
    aorta (thoracic) 901.0
      abdominal 902.0
    arm NEC 903.9
    axillary 903.00
      artery 903.01
      vein 903.02
    azygos vein 901.89
    basilic vein 903.1
    brachial (artery) (vein) 903.1
    bronchial 901.89
    carotid artery 900.00
      common 900.01
      external 900.02
      internal 900.03
    celiac artery 902.20
      specified branch NEC 902.24
    cephalic vein (arm) 903.1
    colica dextra 902.26
    cystic
      artery 902.24
      vein 902.39
    deep plantar 904.6
    digital (artery) (vein) 903.5
    due to accidental puncture or laceration during procedure 998.2
    extremity
      lower 904.8
        multiple 904.7
        specified NEC 904.7
      upper 903.9
        multiple 903.8
        specified NEC 903.8
    femoral
      artery (superficial) 904.1
        above profunda origin 904.0
        common 904.0
      vein 904.2
    gastric
      artery 902.21
      vein 902.39
    head 900.9
      intracranial — *see* Injury, intracranial
      multiple 900.82
      specified NEC 900.89
    hemiazygos vein 901.89
    hepatic
      artery 902.22
      vein 902.11
    hypogastric 902.59
      artery 902.51
      vein 902.52
    ileocolic
      artery 902.26
      vein 902.31
    iliac 902.50
      artery 902.53
      specified branch NEC 902.59
      vein 902.54
    innominate
      artery 901.1
      vein 901.3
    intercostal (artery) (vein) 901.81
    jugular vein (external) 900.81
      internal 900.1
    leg NEC 904.8
    mammary (artery) (vein) 901.82
    mesenteric
      artery 902.20
        inferior 902.27
        specified branch NEC 902.29
        superior (trunk) 902.25
          branches, primary 902.26
      vein 902.39
        inferior 902.32
        superior (and primary subdivisions) 902.31

Injury — *continued*
  blood vessel NEC — *continued*
    neck 900.9
      multiple 900.82
      specified NEC 900.89
    ovarian 902.89
      artery 902.81
      vein 902.82
    palmar artery 903.4
    pelvis 902.9
      multiple 902.87
      specified NEC 902.89
    plantar (deep) (artery) (vein) 904.6
    popliteal 904.40
      artery 904.41
      vein 904.42
    portal 902.33
    pulmonary 901.40
      artery 901.41
      vein 901.42
    radial (artery) (vein) 903.2
    renal 902.40
      artery 902.41
      specified NEC 902.49
      vein 902.42
    saphenous
      artery 904.7
      vein (greater) (lesser) 904.3
    splenic
      artery 902.23
      vein 902.34
    subclavian
      artery 901.1
      vein 901.3
    suprarenal 902.49
    thoracic 901.9
      multiple 901.83
      specified NEC 901.89
    tibial 904.50
      artery 904.50
        anterior 904.51
        posterior 904.53
      vein 904.50
        anterior 904.52
        posterior 904.54
    ulnar (artery) (vein) 903.3
    uterine 902.59
      artery 902.55
      vein 902.56
    vena cava
      inferior 902.10
        specified branches NEC 902.19
      superior 901.2
  brachial plexus 953.4
    newborn 767.6
  brain NEC (*see also* Injury, intracranial) 854.0 ✓5ᵗʰ
  breast 959.1
  broad ligament — *see* Injury, internal, broad ligament
  bronchus, bronchi — *see* Injury, internal, bronchus
  brow 959.09
  buttock 959.1
  canthus, eye 921.1
  cathode ray 990
  cauda equina 952.4
    with fracture, vertebra — *see* Fracture, vertebra, sacrum
  cavernous sinus (*see also* Injury, intracranial) 854.0 ✓5ᵗʰ
  cecum — *see* Injury, internal, cecum
  celiac ganglion or plexus 954.1
  cerebellum (*see also* Injury, intracranial) 854.0 ✓5ᵗʰ
  cervix (uteri) — *see* Injury, internal, cervix
  cheek 959.09
  chest — *see also* Injury, internal, chest
    wall 959.1
  childbirth — *see also* Birth, injury
    maternal NEC 665.9 ✓5ᵗʰ
  chin 959.09
  choroid (eye) 921.3
  clitoris 959.1
  coccyx 959.1
    complicating delivery 665.6 ✓5ᵗʰ
  colon — *see* Injury, internal, colon

Injury — *continued*
  common duct — *see* Injury, internal, common duct
  conjunctiva 921.1
    superficial 918.2
  cord
    spermatic — *see* Injury, internal, spermatic cord
    spinal — *see* Injury, spinal, by site
  cornea 921.3
    abrasion 918.1
      due to contact lens 371.82
    penetrating — *see* Injury, eyeball, penetrating
    superficial 918.1
      due to contact lens 371.82
  cortex (cerebral) (*see also* Injury, intracranial) 854.0 ✓5ᵗʰ
    visual 950.3
  costal region 959.1
  costochondral 959.1
  cranial
    bones — *see* Fracture, skull, by site
    cavity (*see also* Injury, intracranial) 854.0 ✓5ᵗʰ
    nerve — *see* Injury, nerve, cranial
  crushing — *see* Crush
  cutaneous sensory nerve
    lower limb 956.4
    upper limb 955.5 ✓5ᵗʰ
  delivery — *see also* Birth, injury
    maternal NEC 665.9 ✓5ᵗʰ
  Descemet's membrane — *see* Injury, eyeball, penetrating
  diaphragm — *see* Injury, internal, diaphragm
  duodenum — *see* Injury, internal, duodenum
  ear (auricle) (canal) (drum) (external) 959.09
  elbow (and forearm) (and wrist) 959.3
  epididymis 959.1
  epigastric region 959.1
  epiglottis 959.09
  epiphyseal, current — *see* Fracture, by site
  esophagus — *see* Injury, internal, esophagus
  Eustachian tube 959.09
  extremity (lower) (upper) NEC 959.8
  eye 921.9
    penetrating eyeball — *see* Injury, eyeball, penetrating
    superficial 918.9
  eyeball 921.3
    penetrating 871.7
      with
        partial loss (of intraocular tissue) 871.2
        prolapse or exposure (of intraocular tissue) 871.1
      without prolapse 871.0
      foreign body (nonmagnetic) 871.6
        magnetic 871.5
    superficial 918.9
  eyebrow 959.09
  eyelid(s) 921.1
    laceration — *see* Laceration, eyelid
    superficial 918.0
  face (and neck) 959.09
  fallopian tube — *see* Injury, internal, fallopian tube
  finger(s) (nail) 959.5
  flank 959.1
  foot (and ankle) (and knee) (and leg except thigh) 959.7
  forceps NEC 767.9
    scalp 767.1
  forearm (and elbow) (and wrist) 959.3
  forehead 959.09
  gallbladder — *see* Injury, internal, gallbladder
  gasserian ganglion 951.2
  gastrointestinal tract — *see* Injury, internal, gastrointestinal tract
  genital organ(s)
    with
      abortion — *see* Abortion, by type, with, damage to pelvic organs
      ectopic pregnancy (*see also* categories 633.0-633.9) 639.2
      molar pregnancy (*see also* categories 630-632) 639.2

Injury — *continued*
  genital organ(s) — *continued*
    external 959.1
    following
      abortion 639.2
      ectopic or molar pregnancy 639.2
    internal — *see* Injury, internal, genital organs
    obstetrical trauma NEC 665. ✓5ᵗʰ
      affecting fetus or newborn 763.89
  gland
    lacrimal 921.1
      laceration 870.8
    parathyroid 959.09
    salivary 959.09
    thyroid 959.09
  globe (eye) (*see also* Injury, eyeball) 921.3
  grease gun — *see* Wound, open, by site, complicated
  groin 959.1
  gum 959.09
  hand(s) (except fingers) 959.4
  head NEC 959.01
    with
      loss of consciousness 850.5 ●
      skull fracture — *see* Fracture, skull, by site
  heart — *see* Injury, internal, heart
  heel 959.7
  hip (and thigh) 959.6
  hymen 959.1
  hyperextension (cervical) (vertebra) 847.0
  ileum — *see* Injury, internal, ileum
  iliac region 959.1
  infrared rays NEC 990
  instrumental (during surgery) 998.2
    birth injury — *see* Birth, injury
    nonsurgical (*see also* Injury, by site) 959.9
    obstetrical 665.9 ✓5ᵗʰ
      affecting fetus or newborn 763.89
      bladder 665.5 ✓5ᵗʰ
      cervix 665.3 ✓5ᵗʰ
      high vaginal 665.4 ✓5ᵗʰ
      perineal NEC 664.9 ✓5ᵗʰ
      urethra 665.5 ✓5ᵗʰ
      uterus 665.5 ✓5ᵗʰ
  internal 869.0

> *Note* — For injury of internal organ(s) by foreign body entering through a natural orifice (e.g., inhaled, ingested, or swallowed) — *see* Foreign body, entering through orifice.
>
> For internal injury of any of the following sites with internal injury of any other of the sites — *see* Injury, internal, multiple.

    with
      fracture
        open wound into cavity 869.1
        pelvis — *see* Fracture, pelvis
        specified site, except pelvis — *see* Injury, internal, by site
    abdomen, abdominal (viscera) NEC 868.00
      with
        fracture, pelvis — *see* Fracture, pelvis
        open wound into cavity 868.10
      specified site NEC 868.09
        with open wound into cavity 868.19
    adrenal (gland) 868.01
      with open wound into cavity 868.11
    aorta (thoracic) 901.0
      abdominal 902.0
    appendix 863.85
      with open wound into cavity 863.95
    bile duct 868.02
      with open wound into cavity 868.12
    bladder (sphincter) 867.0
      with
        abortion — *see* Abortion, by type, with damage to pelvic organs
        ectopic pregnancy (*see also* categories 633.0-633.9) 639.2
        molar pregnancy (*see also* categories 630-632) 639.2
        open wound into cavity 867.1

Injury — *continued*
  internal — *continued*
    bladder — *continued*
      following
        abortion 639.2
        ectopic or molar pregnancy 639.2
      obstetrical trauma 665.5 ✓5ᵗʰ
        affecting fetus or newborn 763.89
    blood vessel — *see* Injury, blood vessel, by site
    broad ligament 867.6
      with open wound into cavity 867.7
    bronchus, bronchi 862.21
      with open wound into cavity 862.31
    cecum 863.89
      with open wound into cavity 863.99
    cervix (uteri) 867.4
      with
        abortion — *see* Abortion, by type, with damage to pelvic organs
        ectopic pregnancy (*see also* categories 633.0-633.9) 639.2
        molar pregnancy (*see also* categories 630-632) 639.2
        open wound into cavity 867.5
      following
        abortion 639.2
        ectopic or molar pregnancy 639.2
      obstetrical trauma 665.3 ✓5ᵗʰ
        affecting fetus or newborn 763.89
    chest (*see also* Injury, internal, intrathoracic organs) 862.8
      with open wound into cavity 862.9
    colon 863.40
      with
        open wound into cavity 863.50
        rectum 863.46
          with open wound into cavity 863.56
      ascending (right) 863.41
        with open wound into cavity 863.51
      descending (left) 863.43
        with open wound into cavity 863.53
      multiple sites 863.46
        with open wound into cavity 863.56
      sigmoid 863.44
        with open wound into cavity 863.54
      specified site NEC 863.49
        with open wound into cavity 863.59
      transverse 863.42
        with open wound into cavity 863.52
    common duct 868.02
      with open wound into cavity 868.12
    complicating delivery 665.9 ✓5ᵗʰ
      affecting fetus or newborn 763.89
    diaphragm 862.0
      with open wound into cavity 862.1
    duodenum 863.21
      with open wound into cavity 863.31
    esophagus (intrathoracic) 862.22
      with open wound into cavity 862.32
      cervical region 874.4
        complicated 874.5
    fallopian tube 867.6
      with open wound into cavity 867.7
    gallbladder 868.02
      with open wound into cavity 868.12
    gastrointestinal tract NEC 863.80
      with open wound into cavity 863.90
    genital organ NEC 867.6
      with open wound into cavity 867.7
    heart 861.00
      with open wound into thorax 861.10
    ileum 863.29
      with open wound into cavity 863.39
    intestine NEC 863.89
      with open wound into cavity 863.99
      large NEC 863.40
        with open wound into cavity 863.50
      small NEC 863.20
        with open wound into cavity 863.30
    intra-abdominal (organ) 868.00
      with open wound into cavity 868.10
      multiple sites 868.09
        with open wound into cavity 868.19
      specified site NEC 868.09
        with open wound into cavity 868.19

Injury — *continued*
  internal — *continued*
    intrathoracic organs (multiple) 862.8
      with open wound into cavity 862.9
      diaphragm (only) — *see* Injury, internal,
        diaphragm
      heart (only) — *see* Injury, internal, heart
      lung (only) — *see* Injury, internal, lung
      specified site NEC 862.29
        with open wound into cavity 862.39
    intrauterine (*see also* Injury, internal,
      uterus) 867.4
      with open wound into cavity 867.5
    jejunum 863.29
      with open wound into cavity 863.39
    kidney (subcapsular) 866.00
      with
        disruption of parenchyma (complete)
          866.03
          with open wound into cavity 866.13
        hematoma (without rupture of capsule)
          866.01
          with open wound into cavity 866.11
        laceration 866.02
          with open wound into cavity 866.12
        open wound into cavity 866.10
    liver 864.00
      with
        contusion 864.01
          with open wound into cavity 864.11
        hematoma 864.01
          with open wound into cavity 864.11
        laceration 864.05
          with open wound into cavity 864.15
          major (disruption of hepatic
            parenchyma) 864.04
            with open wound into cavity
              864.14
          minor (capsule only) 864.02
            with open wound into cavity
              864.12
          moderate (involving parenchyma)
            864.03
            with open wound into cavity
              864.13
          multiple 864.04
        stellate 864.04
          with open wound into cavity
            864.14
        open wound into cavity 864.10
    lung 861.20
      with open wound into thorax 861.30
      hemopneumothorax — *see*
        Hemopneumothorax, traumatic
      hemothorax — *see* Hemothorax,
        traumatic
      pneumohemothorax — *see*
        Pneumohemothorax, traumatic
      pneumothorax — *see* Pneumothorax,
        traumatic
    mediastinum 862.29
      with open wound into cavity 862.39
    mesentery 863.89
      with open wound into cavity 863.99
    mesosalpinx 867.6
      with open wound into cavity 867.7
    multiple 869.0

> *Note* — Multiple internal injuries of sites
> classifiable to the same three- or four-digit
> category should be classified to that
> category.
>
> Multiple injuries classifiable to different
> fourth-digit subdivisions of 861 (heart and
> lung injuries) should be dealt with according
> to coding rules.

      internal
        with open wound into cavity 869.1
      intra-abdominal organ (sites classifiable
        to 863-868)
        with
          intrathoracic organ(s) (sites
            classifiable to 861-862) 869.0
            with open wound into cavity
              869.1

Injury — *continued*
  internal — *continued*
    multiple — *continued*
      intra-abdominal organ — *continued*
        with — *continued*
          other intra-abdominal organ(s)
            (sites classifiable to 863-868,
            except where classifiable to
            the same three-digit category)
            868.09
            with open wound into cavity
              868.19
      intrathoracic organ (sites classifiable to
        861-862)
        with
          intra-abdominal organ(s) (sites
            classifiable to 863-868) 869.0
            with open wound into cavity
              869.1
          other intrathoracic organ(s) (sites
            classifiable to 861-862, except
            where classifiable to the same
            three-digit category) 862.8
            with open wound into cavity
             862.9
      myocardium — *see* Injury, internal, heart
    ovary 867.6
      with open wound into cavity 867.7
    pancreas (multiple sites) 863.84
      with open wound into cavity 863.94
      body 863.82
        with open wound into cavity 863.92
      head 863.81
        with open wound into cavity 863.91
      tail 863.83
        with open wound into cavity 863.93
    pelvis, pelvic (organs) (viscera) 867.8
      with
        fracture, pelvis — *see* Fracture, pelvis
        open wound into cavity 867.9
      specified site NEC 867.6
        with open wound into cavity 867.7
    peritoneum 868.03
      with open wound into cavity 868.13
    pleura 862.29
      with open wound into cavity 862.39
    prostate 867.6
      with open wound into cavity 867.7
    rectum 863.45
      with
        colon 863.46
          with open wound into cavity 863.56
        open wound into cavity 863.55
    retroperitoneum 868.04
      with open wound into cavity 868.14
    round ligament 867.6
      with open wound into cavity 867.7
    seminal vesicle 867.6
      with open wound into cavity 867.7
    spermatic cord 867.6
      with open wound into cavity 867.7
      scrotal — *see* Wound, open, spermatic
        cord
    spleen 865.00
      with
        disruption of parenchyma (massive)
          865.04
          with open wound into cavity 865.14
        hematoma (without rupture of capsule)
          865.01
          with open wound into cavity 865.11
        open wound into cavity 865.10
        tear, capsular 865.02
          with open wound into cavity 865.12
          extending into parenchyma 865.03
            with open wound into cavity
              865.13
    stomach 863.0
      with open wound into cavity 863.1
    suprarenal gland (multiple) 868.01
      with open wound into cavity 868.11
    thorax, thoracic (cavity) (organs) (multiple)
      (*see also* Injury, internal, intrathoracic
      organs) 862.8
      with open wound into cavity 862.9
    thymus (gland) 862.29
      with open wound into cavity 862.39

Injury — *continued*
  internal — *continued*
    trachea (intrathoracic) 862.29
      with open wound into cavity 862.39
      cervical region (*see also* Wound, open,
        trachea) 874.02
    ureter 867.2
      with open wound into cavity 867.3
    urethra (sphincter) 867.0
      with
        abortion — *see* Abortion, by type, with
          damage to pelvic organs
        ectopic pregnancy (*see also* categories
          633.0-633.9) 639.2
        molar pregnancy (*see also* categories
          630-632) 639.2
        open wound into cavity 867.1
      following
        abortion 639.2
        ectopic or molar pregnancy 639.2
      obstetrical trauma 665.5 ✓5ᵗʰ
        affecting fetus or newborn 763.89
    uterus 867.4
      with
        abortion — *see* Abortion, by type, with
          damage to pelvic organs
        ectopic pregnancy (*see also* categories
          633.0-633.9) 639.2
        molar pregnancy (*see also* categories
          630-632) 639.2
        open wound into cavity 867.5
      following
        abortion 639.2
        ectopic or molar pregnancy 639.2
      obstetrical trauma NEC 665.5 ✓5ᵗʰ
        affecting fetus or newborn 763.89
    vas deferens 867.6
      with open wound into cavity 867.7
    vesical (sphincter) 867.0
      with open wound into cavity 867.1
    viscera (abdominal) (*see also* Injury,
      internal, multiple) 868.00
      with
        fracture, pelvis — *see* Fracture, pelvis
        open wound into cavity 868.10
      thoracic NEC (*see also* Injury, internal,
        intrathoracic organs) 862.8
        with open wound into cavity 862.9
  interscapular region 959.1
  intervertebral disc 959.1
  intestine — *see* Injury, internal, intestine
  intra-abdominal (organs) NEC — *see* Injury,
    internal, intra-abdominal
  intracranial 854.0 ✓5ᵗʰ

> *Note* — Use the following fifth-digit
> subclassification with categories 851-854:
>
> 0   unspecified state of consciousness
> 1   with no loss of consciousness
> 2   with brief [less than one hour] loss
>   of consciousness
> 3   with moderate [1-24 hours] loss of
>   consciousness
> 4   with prolonged [more than 24 hours]
>   loss of consciousness and return to
>   pre-existing conscious level
> 5   with prolonged [more than 24 hours]
>   loss of consciousness, without
>   return to pre-existing conscious level
>   Use fifth-digit 5 to designate when a
>   patient is unconscious and dies
>   before regaining consciousness,
>   regardless of the duration of the
>   loss of consciousness
> 6   with loss of consciousness of
>   unspecified duration
> 9   with concussion, unspecified

    with
      open intracranial wound 854.1 ✓5ᵗʰ
      skull fracture — *see* Fracture, skull, by
        site
    contusion 851.8 ✓5ᵗʰ
      with open intracranial wound 851.9 ✓5ᵗʰ

Injury — *continued*
  intracranial — *continued*
    contusion — *continued*
      brain stem 851.4 ✓5ᵗʰ
        with open intracranial wound
          851.5 ✓5ᵗʰ
      cerebellum 851.4 ✓5ᵗʰ
        with open intracranial wound
          851.5 ✓5ᵗʰ
      cortex (cerebral) 851.0 ✓5ᵗʰ
        with open intracranial wound
          851.2 ✓5ᵗʰ
    hematoma — *see* Injury, intracranial,
      hemorrhage
    hemorrhage 853.0 ✓5ᵗʰ
      with
        laceration — *see* Injury, intracranial,
          laceration
        open intracranial wound 853.1 ✓5ᵗʰ
      extradural 852.4 ✓5ᵗʰ
        with open intracranial wound
          852.5 ✓5ᵗʰ
      subarachnoid 852.0 ✓5ᵗʰ
        with open intracranial wound
          852.1 ✓5ᵗʰ
      subdural 852.2 ✓5ᵗʰ
        with open intracranial wound
          852.3 ✓5ᵗʰ
    laceration 851.8 ✓5ᵗʰ
      with open intracranial wound 851.9 ✓5ᵗʰ
      brain stem 851.6 ✓5ᵗʰ
        with open intracranial wound
          851.7 ✓5ᵗʰ
      cerebellum 851.6 ✓5ᵗʰ
        with open intracranial wound
          851.7 ✓5ᵗʰ
      cortex (cerebral) 851.2 ✓5ᵗʰ
        with open intracranial wound
          851.3 ✓5ᵗʰ
  intraocular — *see* Injury, eyeball, penetrating
  intrathoracic organs (multiple) — *see* Injury,
    internal, intrathoracic organs
  intrauterine — *see* Injury, internal, intrauterine
  iris 921.3
    penetrating — *see* Injury, eyeball,
      penetrating
  jaw 959.09
  jejunum — *see* Injury, internal, jejunum
  joint NEC 959.9
    old or residual 718.80
      ankle 718.87
      elbow 718.82
      foot 718.87
      hand 718.84
      hip 718.85
      knee 718.86
      multiple sites 718.89
      pelvic region 718.85
      shoulder (region) 718.81
      specified site NEC 718.88
      wrist 718.83
  kidney — *see* Injury, internal, kidney
  knee (and ankle) (and foot) (and leg, except
    thigh) 959.7
  labium (majus) (minus) 959.1
  labyrinth, ear 959.09
  lacrimal apparatus, gland, or sac 921.1
    laceration 870.8
  larynx 959.09
  late effect — *see* Late, effects (of), injury
  leg except thigh (and ankle) (and foot) (and
    knee) 959.7
    upper or thigh 959.6
  lens, eye 921.3
    penetrating — *see* Injury, eyeball,
      penetrating
  lid, eye — *see* Injury, eyelid
  lip 959.09
  liver — *see* Injury, internal, liver
  lobe, parietal — *see* Injury, intracranial
  lumbar (region) 959.1
    plexus 953.5
  lumbosacral (region) 959.1
    plexus 953.5
  lung — *see* Injury, internal, lung
  malar region 959.09
  mastoid region 959.09

Injury — *continued*
  maternal, during pregnancy, affecting fetus or
    newborn 760.5
  maxilla 959.09
  mediastinum — *see* Injury, internal,
    mediastinum
  membrane
    brain (*see also* Injury, intracranial)
      854.0 ✓5ᵗʰ
    tympanic 959.09
  meningeal artery — *see* Hemorrhage, brain,
    traumatic, subarachnoid
  meninges (cerebral) — *see* Injury, intracranial
  mesenteric
    artery — *see* Injury, blood vessel,
      mesenteric, artery
    plexus, inferior 954.1
    vein — *see* Injury, blood vessel, mesenteric,
      vein
  mesentery — *see* Injury, internal, mesentery
  mesosalpinx — *see* Injury, internal,
    mesosalpinx
  middle ear 959.09
  midthoracic region 959.1
  mouth 959.09
  multiple (sites not classifiable to the same four-
    digit category in 959.0-959.7) 959.8
    internal 869.0
      with open wound into cavity 869.1
  musculocutaneous nerve 955.4
  nail
    finger 959.5
    toe 959.7
  nasal (septum) (sinus) 959.09
  nasopharynx 959.09
  neck (and face) 959.09
  nerve 957.9
    abducens 951.3
    abducent 951.3
    accessory 951.6
    acoustic 951.5
    ankle and foot 956.9
    anterior crural, femoral 956.1
    arm (*see also* Injury, nerve, upper limb)
      955.9
    auditory 951.5
    axillary 955.0
    brachial plexus 953.4
    cervical sympathetic 954.0
    cranial 951.9
      first or olfactory 951.8
      second or optic 950.0
      third or oculomotor 951.0
      fourth or trochlear 951.1
      fifth or trigeminal 951.2
      sixth or abducens 951.3
      seventh or facial 951.4
      eighth, acoustic, or auditory 951.5
      ninth or glossopharyngeal 951.8
      tenth, pneumogastric, or vagus 951.8
      eleventh or accessory 951.6
      twelfth or hypoglossal 951.7
      newborn 767.7
    cutaneous sensory
      lower limb 956.4
      upper limb 955.5 ✓5ᵗʰ
    digital (finger) 955.6
      toe 956.5
    facial 951.4
      newborn 767.5
    femoral 956.1
    finger 955.9
    foot and ankle 956.9
    forearm 955.9
    glossopharyngeal 951.8
    hand and wrist 955.9
    head and neck, superficial 957.0
    hypoglossal 951.7
    involving several parts of body 957.8
    leg (*see also* Injury, nerve, lower limb) 956.9
    lower limb 956.9
      multiple 956.8
      specified site NEC 956.5
    lumbar plexus 953.5
    lumbosacral plexus 953.5
    median 955.1
      forearm 955.1

Injury — *continued*
  nerve — *continued*
    median — *continued*
      wrist and hand 955.1
    multiple (in several parts of body) (sites not
      classifiable to the same three-digit
      category) 957.8
    musculocutaneous 955.4
    musculospiral 955.3
      upper arm 955.3
    oculomotor 951.0
    olfactory 951.8
    optic 950.0
    pelvic girdle 956.9
      multiple sites 956.8
      specified site NEC 956.5
    peripheral 957.9
      multiple (in several regions) (sites not
        classifiable to the same three-digit
        category) 957.8
      specified site NEC 957.1
    peroneal 956.3
      ankle and foot 956.3
      lower leg 956.3
    plantar 956.5
    plexus 957.9
      celiac 954.1
      mesenteric, inferior 954.1
      spinal 953.9
        brachial 953.4
        lumbosacral 953.5
        multiple sites 953.8
      sympathetic NEC 954.1
    pneumogastric 951.8
    radial 955.3
      wrist and hand 955.3
    sacral plexus 953.5
    sciatic 956.0
      thigh 956.0
    shoulder girdle 955.9
      multiple sites 955.8
      specified site NEC 955.7
    specified site NEC 957.1
    spinal 953.9
      plexus — *see* Injury, nerve, plexus, spinal
      root 953.9
        cervical 953.0
        dorsal 953.1
        lumbar 953.2
        multiple sites 953.8
        sacral 953.3
    splanchnic 954.1
    sympathetic NEC 954.1
      cervical 954.0
    thigh 956.9
    tibial 956.5
      ankle and foot 956.2
      lower leg 956.5
      posterior 956.2
    toe 956.9
    trigeminal 951.2
    trochlear 951.1
    trunk, excluding shoulder and pelvic girdles
      954.9
      specified site NEC 954.8
      sympathetic NEC 954.1
    ulnar 955.2
      forearm 955.2
      wrist (and hand) 955.2
    upper limb 955.9
      multiple 955.8
      specified site NEC 955.7
    vagus 951.8
    wrist and hand 955.9
  nervous system, diffuse 957.8
  nose (septum) 959.09
  obstetrical NEC 665.9 ✓5ᵗʰ
    affecting fetus or newborn 763.89
  occipital (region) (scalp) 959.09
    lobe (*see also* Injury, intracranial) 854.0 ✓5ᵗʰ
  optic 950.9
    chiasm 950.1
    cortex 950.3
    nerve 950.0
    pathways 950.2

Injury — *continued*
  orbit, orbital (region) 921.2
    penetrating 870.3
      with foreign body 870.4
  ovary — *see* Injury, internal, ovary
  paint-gun — *see* Wound, open, by site,
    complicated
  palate (soft) 959.09
  pancreas — *see* Injury, internal, pancreas
  parathyroid (gland) 959.09
  parietal (region) (scalp) 959.09
    lobe — *see* Injury, intracranial
  pelvic
    floor 959.1
      complicating delivery 664.1 ✓5th
        affecting fetus or newborn 763.89
      joint or ligament, complicating delivery
        665.6 ✓5th
      affecting fetus or newborn 763.89
    organs — *see also* Injury, internal, pelvis
      with
        abortion — *see* Abortion, by type, with
          damage to pelvic organs
        ectopic pregnancy (*see also* categories
          633.0-633.9) 639.2
        molar pregnancy (*see also* categories
          633.0-633.9) 639.2
      following
        abortion 639.2
        ectopic or molar pregnancy 639.2
      obstetrical trauma 665.5 ✓5th
        affecting fetus or newborn 763.89
  pelvis 959.1
  penis 959.1
  perineum 959.1
  peritoneum — *see* Injury, internal, peritoneum
  periurethral tissue
    with
      abortion — *see* Abortion, by type, with
        damage to pelvic organs
      ectopic pregnancy (*see also* categories
        633.0-633.9) 639.2
      molar pregnancy (*see also* categories 630-
        632) 639.2
    complicating delivery 665.5 ✓5th
      affecting fetus or newborn 763.89
    following
      abortion 639.2
      ectopic or molar pregnancy 639.2
  phalanges
    foot 959.7
    hand 959.5
  pharynx 959.09
  pleura — *see* Injury, internal, pleura
  popliteal space 959.7
  prepuce 959.1
  prostate — *see* Injury, internal, prostate
  pubic region 959.1
  pudenda 959.1
  radiation NEC 990
  radioactive substance or radium NEC 990
  rectovaginal septum 959.1
  rectum — *see* Injury, internal, rectum
  retina 921.3
    penetrating — *see* Injury, eyeball,
      penetrating
  retroperitoneal — *see* Injury, internal,
    retroperitoneum
  roentgen rays NEC 990
  round ligament — *see* Injury, internal, round
    ligament
  sacral (region) 959.1
    plexus 953.5
  sacroiliac ligament NEC 959.1
  sacrum 959.1
  salivary ducts or glands 959.09
  scalp 959.09
    due to birth trauma 767.1
    fetus or newborn 767.1
  scapular region 959.2
  sclera 921.3
    penetrating — *see* Injury, eyeball,
      penetrating
    superficial 918.2
  scrotum 959.1
  seminal vesicle — *see* Injury, internal, seminal
    vesicle
  shoulder (and upper arm) 959.2

Injury — *continued*
  sinus
    cavernous (*see also* Injury, intracranial)
      854.0 ✓5th
    nasal 959.09
  skeleton NEC, birth injury 767.3
  skin NEC 959.9
  skull — *see* Fracture, skull, by site
  soft tissue (of external sites) (severe) — *see*
    Wound, open, by site
  specified site NEC 959.8
  spermatic cord — *see* Injury, internal,
    spermatic cord
  spinal (cord) 952.9
    with fracture, vertebra — *see* Fracture,
      vertebra, by site, with spinal cord
      injury
    cervical (C₁-C₄) 952.00
      with
        anterior cord syndrome 952.02
        central cord syndrome 952.03
        complete lesion of cord 952.01
        incomplete lesion NEC 952.04
        posterior cord syndrome 952.04
      C₅-C₇ level 952.05
        with
          anterior cord syndrome 952.07
          central cord syndrome 952.08
          complete lesion of cord 952.06
          incomplete lesion NEC 952.09
          posterior cord syndrome 952.09
        specified type NEC 952.09
      specified type NEC 952.04
    dorsal (D₁-D₆) (T₁-T₆) (thoracic) 952.10
      with
        anterior cord syndrome 952.12
        central cord syndrome 952.13
        complete lesion of cord 952.11
        incomplete lesion NEC 952.14
        posterior cord syndrome 952.14
      D₇-D₁₂ level (T₇-T₁₂) 952.15
        with
          anterior cord syndrome 952.17
          central cord syndrome 952.18
          complete lesion of cord 952.16
          incomplete lesion NEC 952.19
          posterior cord syndrome 952.19
        specified type NEC 952.19
      specified type NEC 952.14
    lumbar 952.2
    multiple sites 952.8
    nerve (root) NEC — *see* Injury, nerve, spinal,
      root
    plexus 953.9
      brachial 953.4
      lumbosacral 953.5
      multiple sites 953.8
    sacral 952.3
    thoracic (*see also* Injury, spinal, dorsal)
      952.10
  spleen — *see* Injury, internal, spleen
  stellate ganglion 954.1
  sternal region 959.1
  stomach — *see* Injury, internal, stomach
  subconjunctival 921.1
  subcutaneous 959.9
  subdural — *see* Injury, intracranial
  submaxillary region 959.09
  submental region 959.09
  subungual
    fingers 959.5
    toes 959.7
  superficial 919 ✓4th

Injury — *continued*
  superficial — *continued*

> **Note** — Use the following fourth-digit
> subdivisions with categories 910-919:
>
>   0 *Abrasion or friction burn without
>   mention of infection*
>   1 *Abrasion or friction burn, infected*
>   2 *Blister without mention of infection*
>   3 *Blister, infected*
>   4 *Insect bite, nonvenomous, without
>   mention of infection*
>   5 *Insect bite, nonvenomous, infected*
>   6 *Superficial foreign body (splinter)
>   without major open wound and
>   without mention of infection*
>   7 *Superficial foreign body (splinter)
>   without major open wound, infected*
>   8 *Other and unspecified superficial
>   injury without mention of infection*
>   9 *Other and unspecified superficial
>   injury, infected*
>
> *For late effects of superficial injury, see
> category 906.2.*

  abdomen, abdominal (muscle) (wall) (and
    other part(s) of trunk) 911 ✓4th
  ankle (and hip, knee, leg, or thigh) 916 ✓4th
  anus (and other part(s) of trunk) 911 ✓4th
  arm 913 ✓4th
    upper (and shoulder) 912 ✓4th
  auditory canal (external) (meatus) (and other
    part(s) of face, neck, or scalp, except
    eye) 910 ✓4th
  axilla (and upper arm) 912 ✓4th
  back (and other part(s) of trunk) 911 ✓4th
  breast (and other part(s) of trunk) 911 ✓4th
  brow (and other part(s) of face, neck, or
    scalp, except eye) 910 ✓4th
  buttock (and other part(s) of trunk) 911 ✓4th
  canthus, eye 918.0
  cheek(s) (and other part(s) of face, neck, or
    scalp, except eye) 910 ✓4th
  chest wall (and other part(s) of trunk)
    911 ✓4th
  chin (and other part(s) of face, neck, or
    scalp, except eye) 910 ✓4th
  clitoris (and other part(s) of trunk) 911 ✓4th
  conjunctiva 918.2
  cornea 918.1
    due to contact lens 371.82
  costal region (and other part(s) of trunk)
    911 ✓4th
  ear(s) (auricle) (canal) (drum) (external) (and
    other part(s) of face, neck, or scalp,
    except eye) 910 ✓4th
  elbow (and forearm) (and wrist) 913 ✓4th
  epididymis (and other part(s) of trunk)
    911 ✓4th
  epigastric region (and other part(s) of trunk)
    911 ✓4th
  epiglottis (and other part(s) of face, neck, or
    scalp, except eye) 910 ✓4th
  eye(s) (and adnexa) NEC 918.9
  eyelid(s) (and periocular area) 918.0
  face (any part(s), except eye) (and neck or
    scalp) 910 ✓4th
  finger(s) (nail) (any) 915 ✓4th
  flank (and other part(s) of trunk) 911 ✓4th
  foot (phalanges) (and toe(s)) 917 ✓4th
  forearm (and elbow) (and wrist) 913 ✓4th
  forehead (and other part(s) of face, neck, or
    scalp, except eye) 910 ✓4th
  globe (eye) 918.9
  groin (and other part(s) of trunk) 911 ✓4th
  gum(s) (and other part(s) of face, neck, or
    scalp, except eye) 910 ✓4th
  hand(s) (except fingers alone) 914 ✓4th
  head (and other part(s) of face, neck, or
    scalp, except eye) 910 ✓4th
  heel (and foot or toe) 917 ✓4th
  hip (and ankle, knee, leg, or thigh) 916 ✓4th
  iliac region (and other part(s) of trunk)
    911 ✓4th

✓4th Fourth-digit Required   ✓5th Fifth-digit Required   ▶◀ Revised Text   ● New Line   ▲ Revised Code

Injury — *continued*
  superficial — *continued*
    interscapular region (and other part(s) of trunk) 911 ✔4ᵗʰ
    iris 918.9
    knee (and ankle, hip, leg, or thigh) 916 ✔4ᵗʰ
    labium (majus) (minus) (and other part(s) of trunk) 911 ✔4ᵗʰ
    lacrimal (apparatus) (gland) (sac) 918.0
    leg (lower) (upper) (and ankle, hip, knee, or thigh) 916 ✔4ᵗʰ
    lip(s) (and other part(s) of face, neck, or scalp, except eye) 910 ✔4ᵗʰ
    lower extremity (except foot) 916 ✔4ᵗʰ
    lumbar region (and other part(s) of trunk) 911 ✔4ᵗʰ
    malar region (and other part(s) of face, neck, or scalp, except eye) 910 ✔4ᵗʰ
    mastoid region (and other part(s) of face, neck, or scalp, except eye) 910 ✔4ᵗʰ
    midthoracic region (and other part(s) of trunk) 911 ✔4ᵗʰ
    mouth (and other part(s) of face, neck, or scalp, except eye) 910 ✔4ᵗʰ
    multiple sites (not classifiable to the same three-digit category) 919 ✔4ᵗʰ
    nasal (septum) (and other part(s) of face, neck, or scalp, except eye) 910 ✔4ᵗʰ
    neck (and face or scalp, any part(s), except eye) 910 ✔4ᵗʰ
    nose (septum) (and other part(s) of face, neck, or scalp, except eye) 910 ✔4ᵗʰ
    occipital region (and other part(s) of face, neck, or scalp, except eye) 910 ✔4ᵗʰ
    orbital region 918.0
    palate (soft) (and other part(s) of face, neck, or scalp, except eye) 910 ✔4ᵗʰ
    parietal region (and other part(s) of face, neck, or scalp, except eye) 910 ✔4ᵗʰ
    penis (and other part(s) of trunk) 911 ✔4ᵗʰ
    perineum (and other part(s) of trunk) 911 ✔4ᵗʰ
    periocular area 918.0
    pharynx (and other part(s) of face, neck, or scalp, except eye) 910 ✔4ᵗʰ
    popliteal space (and ankle, hip, leg, or thigh) 916 ✔4ᵗʰ
    prepuce (and other part(s) of trunk) 911 ✔4ᵗʰ
    pubic region (and other part(s) of trunk) 911 ✔4ᵗʰ
    pudenda (and other part(s) of trunk) 911 ✔4ᵗʰ
    sacral region (and other part(s) of trunk) 911 ✔4ᵗʰ
    salivary (ducts) (glands) (and other part(s) of face, neck, or scalp, except eye) 910 ✔4ᵗʰ
    scalp (and other part(s) of face or neck, except eye) 910 ✔4ᵗʰ
    scapular region (and upper arm) 912 ✔4ᵗʰ
    sclera 918.2
    scrotum (and other part(s) of trunk) 911 ✔4ᵗʰ
    shoulder (and upper arm) 912 ✔4ᵗʰ
    skin NEC 919 ✔4ᵗʰ
    specified site(s) NEC 919 ✔4ᵗʰ
    sternal region (and other part(s) of trunk) 911 ✔4ᵗʰ
    subconjunctival 918.2
    subcutaneous NEC 919 ✔4ᵗʰ
    submaxillary region (and other part(s) of face, neck, or scalp, except eye) 910 ✔4ᵗʰ
    submental region (and other part(s) of face, neck, or scalp, except eye) 910 ✔4ᵗʰ
    supraclavicular fossa (and other part(s) of face, neck or scalp, except eye) 910 ✔4ᵗʰ
    supraorbital 918.0
    temple (and other part(s) of face, neck, or scalp, except eye) 910 ✔4ᵗʰ
    temporal region (and other part(s) of face, neck, or scalp, except eye) 910 ✔4ᵗʰ
    testis (and other part(s) of trunk) 911 ✔4ᵗʰ
    thigh (and ankle, hip, knee, or leg) 916 ✔4ᵗʰ
    thorax, thoracic (external) (and other part(s) of trunk) 911 ✔4ᵗʰ
    throat (and other part(s) of face, neck, or scalp, except eye) 910 ✔4ᵗʰ
    thumb(s) (nail) 915 ✔4ᵗʰ

Injury — *continued*
  superficial — *continued*
    toe(s) (nail) (subungual) (and foot) 917 ✔4ᵗʰ
    tongue (and other part(s) of face, neck, or scalp, except eye) 910 ✔4ᵗʰ
    tooth, teeth 521.2
    trunk (any part(s)) 911 ✔4ᵗʰ
    tunica vaginalis (and other part(s) of trunk) 911 ✔4ᵗʰ
    tympanum, tympanic membrane (and other part(s) of face, neck, or scalp, except eye) 910 ✔4ᵗʰ
    upper extremity NEC 913 ✔4ᵗʰ
    uvula (and other part(s) of face, neck, or scalp, except eye) 910 ✔4ᵗʰ
    vagina (and other part(s) of trunk) 911 ✔4ᵗʰ
    vulva (and other part(s) of trunk) 911 ✔4ᵗʰ
    wrist (and elbow) (and forearm) 913 ✔4ᵗʰ
  supraclavicular fossa 959.1
  supraorbital 959.09
  surgical complication (external or internal site) 998.2
  symphysis pubis 959.1
    complicating delivery 665.6 ✔5ᵗʰ
      affecting fetus or newborn 763.89
  temple 959.09
  temporal region 959.09
  testis 959.1
  thigh (and hip) 959.6
  thorax, thoracic (external) 959.1
    cavity — *see* Injury, internal, thorax
    internal — *see* Injury, internal, intrathoracic organs
  throat 959.09
  thumb(s) (nail) 959.5
  thymus — *see* Injury, internal, thymus
  thyroid (gland) 959.09
  toe (nail) (any) 959.7
  tongue 959.09
  tonsil 959.09
  tooth NEC 873.63
    complicated 873.73
  trachea — *see* Injury, internal, trachea
  trunk 959.1
  tunica vaginalis 959.1
  tympanum, tympanic membrane 959.09
  ultraviolet rays NEC 990
  ureter — *see* Injury, internal, ureter
  urethra (sphincter) — *see* Injury, internal, urethra
  uterus — *see* Injury, internal, uterus
  uvula 959.09
  vagina 959.1
  vascular — *see* Injury, blood vessel
  vas deferens — *see* Injury, internal, vas deferens
  vein (*see also* Injury, blood vessel, by site) 904.9
  vena cava
    inferior 902.10
    superior 901.2
  vesical (sphincter) — *see* Injury, internal, vesical
  viscera (abdominal) — *see also* Injury, internal, viscera
    with fracture, pelvis — *see* Fracture, pelvis
  visual 950.9
    cortex 950.3
  vitreous (humor) 871.2
  vulva 959.1
  whiplash (cervical spine) 847.0
  wringer — *see* Crush, by site
  wrist (and elbow) (and forearm) 959.3
  x-ray NEC 990

Inoculation — *see also* Vaccination
  complication or reaction — *see* Complication, vaccination

Insanity, insane (*see also* Psychosis) 298.9
  adolescent (*see also* Schizophrenia) 295.9 ✔5ᵗʰ
  alternating (*see also* Psychosis, affective, circular) 296.7
  confusional 298.9
    acute 293.0
    subacute 293.1
  delusional 298.9

Insanity, insane (*see also* Psychosis) — *continued*
  paralysis, general 094.1
    progressive 094.1
  paresis, general 094.1
  senile 290.20

Insect
  bite — *see* Injury, superficial, by site
  venomous, poisoning by 989.5

Insemination, artificial V26.1

Insertion
  cord (umbilical) lateral or velamentous 663.8 ✔5ᵗʰ
    affecting fetus or newborn 762.6
  intrauterine contraceptive device V25.1
  placenta, vicious — *see* Placenta, previa
  subdermal implantable contraceptive V25.5
  velamentous, umbilical cord 663.8 ✔5ᵗʰ
    affecting fetus or newborn 762.6

Insolation 992.0
  meaning sunstroke 992.0

Insomnia 780.52
  with sleep apnea 780.51
  nonorganic origin 307.41
    persistent (primary) 307.42
    transient 307.41
  subjective complaint 307.49

Inspiration
  food or foreign body (*see also* Asphyxia, food or foreign body) 933.1
  mucus (*see also* Asphyxia, mucus) 933.1

Inspissated bile syndrome, newborn 774.4

Instability
  detrusor 596.59
  emotional (excessive) 301.3
  joint (posttraumatic) 718.80
    ankle 718.87
    elbow 718.82
    foot 718.87
    hand 718.84
    hip 718.85
    knee 718.86
    lumbosacral 724.6
    multiple sites 718.89
    pelvic region 718.85
    sacroiliac 724.6
    shoulder (region) 718.81
    specified site NEC 718.88
    wrist 718.83
  lumbosacral 724.6
  nervous 301.89
  personality (emotional) 301.59
  thyroid, paroxysmal 242.9 ✔5ᵗʰ
  urethral 599.83
  vasomotor 780.2

Insufficiency, insufficient
  accommodation 367.4
  adrenal (gland) (acute) (chronic) 255.4
    medulla 255.5
    primary 255.4
    specified NEC 255.5
  adrenocortical 255.4
  anus 569.49
  aortic (valve) 424.1
    with
      mitral (valve) disease 396.1
        insufficiency, incompetence, or regurgitation 396.3
        stenosis or obstruction 396.1
      stenosis or obstruction 424.1
        with mitral (valve) disease 396.8
    congenital 746.4
    rheumatic 395.1
      with
        mitral (valve) disease 396.1
          insufficiency, incompetence, or regurgitation 396.3
          stenosis or obstruction 396.1
        stenosis or obstruction 395.2
          with mitral (valve) disease 396.8
    specified cause NEC 424.1
    syphilitic 093.22
  arterial 447.1
    basilar artery 435.0
    carotid artery 435.8
    cerebral 437.1
    coronary (acute or subacute) 411.89

Insufficiency, insufficient — *continued*
  arterial — *continued*
    mesenteric 557.1
    peripheral 443.9
    precerebral 435.9
    vertebral artery 435.1
    vertebrobasilar 435.3
  arteriovenous 459.9
  basilar artery 435.0
  biliary 575.8
  cardiac (*see also* Insufficiency, myocardial) 428.0
    complicating surgery 997.1
    due to presence of (cardiac) prosthesis 429.4
    postoperative 997.1
      long-term effect of cardiac surgery 429.4
    specified during or due to a procedure 997.1
      long-term effect of cardiac surgery 429.4
  cardiorenal (*see also* Hypertension, cardiorenal) 404.90
  cardiovascular (*see also* Disease, cardiovascular) 429.2
    renal (*see also* Hypertension, cardiorenal) 404.90
  carotid artery 435.8
  cerebral (vascular) 437.9
  cerebrovascular 437.9
    with transient focal neurological signs and symptoms 435.9
    acute 437.1
      with transient focal neurological signs and symptoms 435.9
  circulatory NEC 459.9
    fetus or newborn 779.89 ▲
  convergence 378.83
  coronary (acute or subacute) 411.89
    chronic or with a stated duration of over 8 weeks 414.8
  corticoadrenal 255.4
  dietary 269.9
  divergence 378.85
  food 994.2
  gastroesophageal 530.89
  gonadal
    ovary 256.39
    testis 257.2
  gonadotropic hormone secretion 253.4
  heart — *see also* Insufficiency, myocardial
    fetus or newborn 779.89 ▲
    valve (*see also* Endocarditis) 424.90
      congenital NEC 746.89
  hepatic 573.8
  idiopathic autonomic 333.0
  kidney ▶(acute) (chronic)◀ 593.9
  labyrinth, labyrinthine (function) 386.53
    bilateral 386.54
    unilateral 386.53
  lacrimal 375.15
  liver 573.8
  lung (acute) (*see also* Insufficiency, pulmonary) 518.82
    following trauma, surgery, or shock 518.5
    newborn 770.89 ▲
  mental (congenital) (*see also* Retardation, mental) 319
  mesenteric 557.1
  mitral (valve) 424.0
    with
      aortic (valve) disease 396.3
        insufficiency, incompetence, or regurgitation 396.3
        stenosis or obstruction 396.2
      obstruction or stenosis 394.2
        with aortic valve disease 396.8
    congenital 746.6
    rheumatic 394.1
      with
        aortic (valve) disease 396.3
          insufficiency, incompetence, or regurgitation 396.3
          stenosis or obstruction 396.2
        obstruction or stenosis 394.2
          with aortic valve disease 396.8
        active or acute 391.1
          with chorea, rheumatic (Sydenham's) 392.0
    specified cause, except rheumatic 424.0

Insufficiency, insufficient — *continued*
  muscle
    heart — *see* Insufficiency, myocardial
    ocular (*see also* Strabismus) 378.9
  myocardial, myocardium (with arteriosclerosis) 428.0
    with rheumatic fever (conditions classifiable to 390)
      active, acute, or subacute 391.2
        with chorea 392.0
      inactive or quiescent (with chorea) 398.0
    congenital 746.89
    due to presence of (cardiac) prosthesis 429.4
    fetus or newborn 779.89 ▲
    following cardiac surgery 429.4
    hypertensive (*see also* Hypertension, heart) 402.91
      benign 402.11
      malignant 402.01
    postoperative 997.1
      long-term effect of cardiac surgery 429.4
    rheumatic 398.0
      active, acute, or subacute 391.2
        with chorea (Sydenham's) 392.0
    syphilitic 093.82
  nourishment 994.2
  organic 799.8
  ovary 256.39
    postablative 256.2
  pancreatic 577.8
  parathyroid (gland) 252.1
  peripheral vascular (arterial) 443.9
  pituitary (anterior) 253.2
    posterior 253.5
  placental — *see* Placenta, insufficiency
  platelets 287.5
  prenatal care in current pregnancy V23.7
  progressive pluriglandular 258.9
  pseudocholinesterase 289.8
  pulmonary (acute) 518.82
    following
      shock 518.5
      surgery 518.5
      trauma 518.5
    newborn 770.89 ▲
    valve (*see also* Endocarditis, pulmonary) 424.3
      congenital 746.09
  pyloric 537.0
  renal ▶(acute) (chronic)◀ 593.9
    due to a procedure 997.5
  respiratory 786.09
    acute 518.82
      following shock, surgery, or trauma 518.5
    newborn 770.89 ▲
  rotation — *see* Malrotation
  suprarenal 255.4
    medulla 255.5
  tarso-orbital fascia, congenital 743.66
  tear film 375.15
  testis 257.2
  thyroid (gland) (acquired) — *see also* Hypothyroidism
    congenital 243
  tricuspid (*see also* Endocarditis, tricuspid) 397.0
    congenital 746.89
    syphilitic 093.23
  urethral sphincter 599.84
  valve, valvular (heart) (*see also* Endocarditis) 424.90
  vascular 459.9
    intestine NEC 557.9
    mesenteric 557.1
    peripheral 443.9
    renal (*see also* Hypertension, kidney) 403.90
  velopharyngeal
    acquired 528.9
    congenital 750.29
  venous (peripheral) 459.81
  ventricular — *see* Insufficiency, myocardial
  vertebral artery 435.1
  vertebrobasilar artery 435.3
  weight gain during pregnancy 646.8 ✓5ᵗʰ
  zinc 269.3

Insufflation
  fallopian
    fertility testing V26.21
    following sterilization reversal V26.22
  meconium 770.1
Insular — *see* condition
Insulinoma (M8151/0)
  malignant (M8151/3)
    pancreas 157.4
    specified site — *see* Neoplasm, by site, malignant
    unspecified site 157.4
  pancreas 211.7
  specified site — *see* Neoplasm, by site, benign
  unspecified site 211.7
Insuloma — *see* Insulinoma
Insult
  brain 437.9
    acute 436
  cerebral 437.9
    acute 436
  cerebrovascular 437.9
    acute 436
  vascular NEC 437.9
    acute 436
Insurance examination (certification) V70.3
Intemperance (*see also* Alcoholism) 303.9 ✓5ᵗʰ
Interception of pregnancy (menstrual extraction) V25.3
Intermenstrual
  bleeding 626.6
    irregular 626.6
    regular 626.5
  hemorrhage 626.6
    irregular 626.6
    regular 626.5
  pain(s) 625.2
Intermittent — *see* condition
Internal — *see* condition
Interproximal wear 521.1
Interruption
  aortic arch 747.11
  bundle of His 426.50
  fallopian tube (for sterilization) V25.2
  phase-shift, sleep cycle 307.45
  repeated REM-sleep 307.48
  sleep
    due to perceived environmental disturbances 307.48
    phase-shift, of 24-hour sleep-wake cycle 307.45
    repeated REM-sleep type 307.48
  vas deferens (for sterilization) V25.2
Intersexuality 752.7
Interstitial — *see* condition
Intertrigo 695.89
  labialis 528.5
Intervertebral disc — *see* condition
Intestine, intestinal — *see also* condition
  flu 487.8
Intolerance
  carbohydrate NEC 579.8
  cardiovascular exercise, with pain (at rest) (with less than ordinary activity) (with ordinary activity) V47.2
  cold 780.99 ▲
  dissacharide (hereditary) 271.3
  drug
    correct substance properly administered 995.2
    wrong substance given or taken in error 977.9
      specified drug — *see* Table of Drugs and Chemicals
  effort 306.2
  fat NEC 579.8
  foods NEC 579.8
  fructose (hereditary) 271.2
  glucose (-galactose) (congenital) 271.3
  gluten 579.0
  lactose (hereditary) (infantile) 271.3
  lysine 270.7
  milk NEC 579.8
  protein (familial) 270.7
  starch NEC 579.8

Intolerance — *continued*
  sucrose (-isomaltose) (congenital) 271.3
Intoxicated NEC (*see also* Alcoholism) 305.0 ☑5ᵗʰ
Intoxication
  acid 276.2
  acute
    alcoholic 305.0 ☑5ᵗʰ
      with alcoholism 303.0 ☑5ᵗʰ
      hangover effects 305.0 ☑5ᵗʰ
    caffeine 305.9 ☑5ᵗʰ
    hallucinogenic (*see also* Abuse, drugs, nondependent) 305.3 ☑5ᵗʰ
  alcohol (acute) 305.0 ☑5ᵗʰ
    with alcoholism 303.0 ☑5ᵗʰ
    hangover effects 305.0 ☑5ᵗʰ
    idiosyncratic 291.4
    pathological 291.4
  alimentary canal 558.2
  ammonia (hepatic) 572.2
  chemical — *see also* Table of Drugs and Chemicals
    via placenta or breast milk 760.70
      alcohol 760.71
      anti-infective agents 760.74
      cocaine 760.75
      "crack" 760.75
      hallucinogenic agents NEC 760.73
      medicinal agents NEC 760.79
  chemical — *see also* Table of Drugs and Chemicals — *continued*
    via placenta or breast milk — *continued*
      narcotics 760.72
      obstetric anesthetic or analgesic drug 763.5
      specified agent NEC 760.79
      suspected, affecting management of pregnancy 655.5 ☑5ᵗʰ
  cocaine, through placenta or breast milk 760.75
  delirium
    alcohol 291.0
    drug 292.81
  drug
    with delirium 292.81
    correct substance properly administered (*see also* Allergy, drug) 995.2
    newborn 779.4
    obstetric anesthetic or sedation 668.9 ☑5ᵗʰ
      affecting fetus or newborn 763.5
    overdose or wrong substance given or taken — *see* Table of Drugs and Chemicals
    pathologic 292.2
    specific to newborn 779.4
    via placenta or breast milk 760.70
      alcohol 760.71
      anti-infective agents 760.74
      cocaine 760.75
      "crack" 760.75
      hallucinogenic agents 760.73
      medicinal agents NEC 760.79
      narcotics 760.72
      obstetric anesthetic or analgesic drug 763.5
      specified agent NEC 760.79
      suspected, affecting management of pregnancy 655.5 ☑5ᵗʰ
  enteric — *see* Intoxication, intestinal
  fetus or newborn, via placenta or breast milk 760.70
    alcohol 760.71
    anti-infective agents 760.74
    cocaine 760.75
    "crack" 760.75
    hallucinogenic agents 760.73
    medicinal agents NEC 760.79
    narcotics 760.72
    obstetric anesthetic or analgesic drug 763.5
    specified agent NEC 760.79
    suspected, affecting management of pregnancy 655.5 ☑5ᵗʰ
  food — *see* Poisoning, food
  gastrointestinal 558.2
  hallucinogenic (acute) 305.3 ☑5ᵗʰ
  hepatocerebral 572.2
  idiosyncratic alcohol 291.4
  intestinal 569.89
    due to putrefaction of food 005.9

Intoxication — *continued*
  methyl alcohol (*see also* Alcoholism) 305.0 ☑5ᵗʰ
    with alcoholism 303.0 ☑5ᵗʰ
  pathologic 291.4
    drug 292.2
  potassium (K) 276.7
  septic
    with
      abortion — *see* Abortion, by type, with sepsis
      ectopic pregnancy (*see also* categories 633.0-633.9) 639.0
      molar pregnancy (*see also* categories 630-632) 639.0
    during labor 659.3 ☑5ᵗʰ
    following
      abortion 639.0
      ectopic or molar pregnancy 639.0
    generalized — *see* Septicemia
    puerperal, postpartum, childbirth 670 ☑4ᵗʰ
  serum (prophylactic) (therapeutic) 999.5
  uremic — *see* Uremia
  water 276.6
Intracranial — *see* condition
Intrahepatic gallbladder 751.69
Intraligamentous — *see also* condition
  pregnancy — *see* Pregnancy, cornual
Intraocular — *see also* condition
  sepsis 360.00
Intrathoracic — *see also* condition
  kidney 753.3
  stomach — *see* Hernia, diaphragm
Intrauterine contraceptive device
  checking V25.42
  insertion V25.1
  in situ V45.51
  management V25.42
  prescription V25.02
    repeat V25.42
  reinsertion V25.42
  removal V25.42
Intraventricular — *see* condition
Intrinsic deformity — *see* Deformity
Intrusion, repetitive, of sleep (due to environmental disturbances) (with atypical polysomnographic features) 307.48
Intumescent, lens (eye) NEC 366.9
  senile 366.12
Intussusception (colon) (enteric) (intestine) (rectum) 560.0
  appendix 543.9
  congenital 751.5
  fallopian tube 620.8
  ileocecal 560.0
  ileocolic 560.0
  ureter (with obstruction) 593.4
Invagination
  basilar 756.0
  colon or intestine 560.0
Invalid (since birth) 799.8
Invalidism (chronic) 799.8
Inversion
  albumin-globulin (A-G) ratio 273.8
  bladder 596.8
  cecum (*see also* Intussusception) 560.0
  cervix 622.8
  nipple 611.79
    congenital 757.6
    puerperal, postpartum 676.3 ☑5ᵗʰ
  optic papilla 743.57
  organ or site, congenital NEC — *see* Anomaly, specified type NEC
  sleep rhythm 780.55
    nonorganic origin 307.45
  testis (congenital) 752.51
  uterus (postinfectional) (postpartal, old) 621.7
    chronic 621.7
    complicating delivery 665.2 ☑5ᵗʰ
      affecting fetus or newborn 763.89
  vagina — *see* Prolapse, vagina
Investigation
  allergens V72.7
  clinical research (control) (normal comparison) (participant) V70.7

Inviability — *see* Immaturity
Involuntary movement, abnormal 781.0
Involution, involutional — *see also* condition
  breast, cystic or fibrocystic 610.1
  depression (*see also* Psychosis, affective) 296.2 ☑5ᵗʰ
    recurrent episode 296.3 ☑5ᵗʰ
    single episode 296.2 ☑5ᵗʰ
  melancholia (*see also* Psychosis, affective) 296.2 ☑5ᵗʰ
    recurrent episode 296.3 ☑5ᵗʰ
    single episode 296.2 ☑5ᵗʰ
  ovary, senile 620.3
  paranoid state (reaction) 297.2
  paraphrenia (climacteric) (menopause) 297.2
  psychosis 298.8
  thymus failure 254.8
IQ
  under 20 318.2
  20-34 318.1
  35-49 318.0
  50-70 317
IRDS 769
Irideremia 743.45
Iridis rubeosis 364.42
  diabetic 250.5 ☑5ᵗʰ *[364.42]*
Iridochoroiditis (panuveitis) 360.12
Iridocyclitis NEC 364.3
  acute 364.00
    primary 364.01
    recurrent 364.02
  chronic 364.10
    in
      lepromatous leprosy 030.0 *[364.11]*
      sarcoidosis 135 *[364.11]*
      tuberculosis (*see also* Tuberculosis) 017.3 ☑5ᵗʰ *[364.11]*
  due to allergy 364.04
  endogenous 364.01
  gonococcal 098.41
  granulomatous 364.10
  herpetic (simplex) 054.44
    zoster 053.22
  hypopyon 364.05
  lens induced 364.23
  nongranulomatous 364.00
  primary 364.01
  recurrent 364.02
  rheumatic 364.10
  secondary 364.04
    infectious 364.03
    noninfectious 364.04
  subacute 364.00
    primary 364.01
    recurrent 364.02
  sympathetic 360.11
  syphilitic (secondary) 091.52
  tuberculous (chronic) (*see also* Tuberculosis) 017.3 ☑5ᵗʰ *[364.11]*
Iridocyclochoroiditis (panuveitis) 360.12
Iridodialysis 364.76
Iridodonesis 364.8
Iridoplegia (complete) (partial) (reflex) 379.49
Iridoschisis 364.52
Iris — *see* condition
Iritis 364.3
  acute 364.00
    primary 364.01
    recurrent 364.02
  chronic 364.10
    in
      sarcoidosis 135 *[364.11]*
      tuberculosis (*see also* Tuberculosis) 017.3 ☑5ᵗʰ *[364.11]*
  diabetic 250.5 ☑5ᵗʰ *[364.42]*
  due to
    allergy 364.04
    herpes simplex 054.44
    leprosy 030.0 *[364.11]*
  endogenous 364.01
  gonococcal 098.41
  gouty 274.89 *[364.11]*
  granulomatous 364.10
  hypopyon 364.05
  lens induced 364.23

Iritis — *continued*
  nongranulomatous 364.00
  papulosa 095.8 *[364.11]*
  primary 364.01
  recurrent 364.02
  rheumatic 364.10
  secondary 364.04
    infectious 364.03
    noninfectious 364.04
  subacute 364.00
    primary 364.01
    recurrent 364.02
  sympathetic 360.11
  syphilitic (secondary) 091.52
    congenital 090.0 *[364.11]*
    late 095.8 *[364.11]*
  tuberculous (*see also* Tuberculosis)
    017.3 ✓5ᵗʰ *[364.11]*
  uratic 274.89 *[364.11]*
Iron
  deficiency anemia 280.9
  metabolism disease 275.0
  storage disease 275.0
Iron-miners' lung 503
Irradiated enamel (tooth, teeth) 521.8
Irradiation
  burn — *see* Burn, by site
  effects, adverse 990
Irreducible, irreducibility — *see* condition
Irregular, irregularity
  action, heart 427.9
  alveolar process 525.8
  bleeding NEC 626.4
  breathing 786.09
  colon 569.89
  contour of cornea 743.41
    acquired 371.70
  dentin in pulp 522.3
  eye movements NEC 379.59
  menstruation (cause unknown) 626.4
  periods 626.4
  prostate 602.9
  pupil 364.75
  respiratory 786.09
  septum (nasal) 470
  shape, organ or site, congenital NEC — *see*
    Distortion
  sleep-wake rhythm (non-24-hour) 780.55
    nonorganic origin 307.45
  vertebra 733.99
Irritability (nervous) 799.2
  bladder 596.8
    neurogenic 596.54
      with cauda equina syndrome 344.61
  bowel (syndrome) 564.1
  bronchial (*see also* Bronchitis) 490
  cerebral, newborn 779.1
  colon 564.1
    psychogenic 306.4
  duodenum 564.89
  heart (psychogenic) 306.2
  ileum 564.89
  jejunum 564.89
  myocardium 306.2
  rectum 564.89
  stomach 536.9
    psychogenic 306.4
  sympathetic (nervous system) (*see also*
    Neuropathy, peripheral, autonomic) 337.9
  urethra 599.84
  ventricular (heart) (psychogenic) 306.2
Irritable — *see* Irritability
Irritation
  anus 569.49
  axillary nerve 353.0
  bladder 596.8
  brachial plexus 353.0
  brain (traumatic) (*see also* Injury, intracranial)
    854.0 ✓5ᵗʰ
    nontraumatic — *see* Encephalitis
  bronchial (*see also* Bronchitis) 490
  cerebral (traumatic) (*see also* Injury,
    intracranial) 854.0 ✓5ᵗʰ
    nontraumatic — *see* Encephalitis
  cervical plexus 353.2
  cervix (*see also* Cervicitis) 616.0

Irritation — *continued*
  choroid, sympathetic 360.11
  cranial nerve — *see* Disorder, nerve, cranial
  digestive tract 536.9
    psychogenic 306.4
  gastric 536.9
    psychogenic 306.4
  gastrointestinal (tract) 536.9
    functional 536.9
    psychogenic 306.4
  globe, sympathetic 360.11
  intestinal (bowel) 564.9
  labyrinth 386.50
  lumbosacral plexus 353.1
  meninges (traumatic) (*see also* Injury,
    intracranial) 854.0 ✓5ᵗʰ
    nontraumatic — *see* Meningitis
  myocardium 306.2
  nerve — *see* Disorder, nerve
  nervous 799.2
  nose 478.1
  penis 607.89
  perineum 709.9
  peripheral
    autonomic nervous system (*see also*
      Neuropathy, peripheral, autonomic)
      337.9
    nerve — *see* Disorder, nerve
  peritoneum (*see also* Peritonitis) 567.9
  pharynx 478.29
  plantar nerve 355.6
  spinal (cord) (traumatic) — *see also* Injury,
    spinal, by site
    nerve — *see also* Disorder, nerve
      root NEC 724.9
      traumatic — *see* Injury, nerve, spinal
    nontraumatic — *see* Myelitis
  stomach 536.9
    psychogenic 306.4
  sympathetic nerve NEC (*see also* Neuropathy,
    peripheral, autonomic) 337.9
  ulnar nerve 354.2
  vagina 623.9
Isambert's disease 012.3 ✓5ᵗʰ
Ischemia, ischemic 459.9
  basilar artery (with transient neurologic deficit)
    435.0
  bone NEC 733.40
  bowel (transient) 557.9
    acute 557.0
    chronic 557.1
    due to mesenteric artery insufficiency 557.1
  brain — *see also* Ischemia, cerebral
    recurrent focal 435.9
  cardiac (*see also* Ischemia, heart) 414.9
  cardiomyopathy 414.8
  carotid artery (with transient neurologic deficit)
    435.8
  cerebral (chronic) (generalized) 437.1
    arteriosclerotic 437.0
    intermittent (with transient neurologic
      deficit) 435.9
    puerperal, postpartum, childbirth 674.0 ✓5ᵗʰ
    recurrent focal (with transient neurologic
      deficit) 435.9
    transient (with transient neurologic deficit)
      435.9
  colon 557.9
    acute 557.0
    chronic 557.1
    due to mesenteric artery insufficiency 557.1
  coronary (chronic) (*see also* Ischemia, heart)
    414.9
  heart (chronic or with a stated duration of over
    8 weeks) 414.9
    acute or with a stated duration of 8 weeks
      or less (*see also* Infarct, myocardium)
      410.9 ✓5ᵗʰ
      without myocardial infarction 411.89
        with coronary (artery) occlusion
          411.81
    subacute 411.89
  intestine (transient) 557.9
    acute 557.0
    chronic 557.1
    due to mesenteric artery insufficiency 557.1
  kidney 593.81

Ischemia, ischemic — *continued*
  labyrinth 386.50
  muscles, leg 728.89
  myocardium, myocardial (chronic or with a
    stated duration of over 8 weeks) 414.8
    acute (*see also* Infarct, myocardium)
      410.9 ✓5ᵗʰ
      without myocardial infarction 411.89
        with coronary (artery) occlusion
          411.81
  renal 593.81
  retina, retinal 362.84
  small bowel 557.9
    acute 557.0
    chronic 557.1
    due to mesenteric artery insufficiency 557.1
  spinal cord 336.1
  subendocardial (*see also* Insufficiency,
    coronary) 411.89
  vertebral artery (with transient neurologic
    deficit) 435.1
Ischialgia (*see also* Sciatica) 724.3
Ischiopagus 759.4
Ischium, ischial — *see* condition
Ischomenia 626.8
Ischuria 788.5
Iselin's disease or osteochondrosis 732.5
Islands of
  parotid tissue in
    lymph nodes 750.26
    neck structures 750.26
  submaxillary glands in
    fascia 750.26
    lymph nodes 750.26
    neck muscles 750.26
Islet cell tumor, pancreas (M8150/0) 211.7
Isoimmunization NEC (*see also* Incompatibility)
    656.2 ✓5ᵗʰ
  fetus or newborn 773.2
    ABO blood groups 773.1
    Rhesus (Rh) factor 773.0
Isolation V07.0
  social V62.4
Isosporosis 007.2
Issue
  medical certificate NEC V68.0
    cause of death V68.0
    fitness V68.0
    incapacity V68.0
  repeat prescription NEC V68.1
    appliance V68.1
    contraceptive V25.40
      device NEC V25.49
        intrauterine V25.42
        specified type NEC V25.49
      pill V25.41
    glasses V68.1
    medicinal substance V68.1
Itch (*see also* Pruritus) 698.9
  bakers' 692.89
  barbers' 110.0
  bricklayers' 692.89
  cheese 133.8
  clam diggers' 120.3
  coolie 126.9
  copra 133.8
  Cuban 050.1
  dew 126.9
  dhobie 110.3
  eye 379.99
  filarial (*see also* Infestation, filarial) 125.9
  grain 133.8
  grocers' 133.8
  ground 126.9
  harvest 133.8
  jock 110.3
  Malabar 110.9
    beard 110.0
    foot 110.4
    scalp 110.0
  meaning scabies 133.0
  Norwegian 133.0
  perianal 698.0
  poultrymen's 133.8

Itch — Ixodiasis

Itch (*see also* Pruritus) — *continued*
   sarcoptic 133.0
   scrub 134.1
   seven year V61.10
      meaning scabies 133.0
   straw 133.8
   swimmers' 120.3
   washerwoman's 692.4
   water 120.3
   winter 698.8
Itsenko-Cushing syndrome (pituitary
   basophilism) 255.0
Ivemark's syndrome (asplenia with congenital
   heart disease) 759.0
Ivory bones 756.52
Ixodes 134.8
Ixodiasis 134.8

J

Jaccoud's nodular fibrositis, chronic (Jaccoud's syndrome) 714.4
Jackson's
  membrane 751.4
  paralysis or syndrome 344.89
  veil 751.4
Jacksonian
  epilepsy (*see also* Epilepsy) 345.5 ✓5ᵗʰ
  seizures (focal) (*see also* Epilepsy) 345.5 ✓5ᵗʰ
Jacob's ulcer (M8090/3) — *see* Neoplasm, skin, malignant, by site
Jacquet's dermatitis (diaper dermatitis) 691.0
Jadassohn's
  blue nevus (M8780/0) — *see* Neoplasm, skin, benign
  disease (maculopapular erythroderma) 696.2
  intraepidermal epithelioma (M8096/0) — *see* Neoplasm, skin, benign
Jadassohn-Lewandowski syndrome (pachyonychia congenita) 757.5
Jadassohn-Pellizari's disease (anetoderma) 701.3
Jadassohn-Tièche nevus (M8780/0) — *see* Neoplasm, skin, benign
Jaffe-Lichtenstein (-Uehlinger) syndrome 252.0
Jahnke's syndrome (encephalocutaneous angiomatosis) 759.6
Jakob-Creutzfeldt disease or syndrome 046.1
  with dementia
    with behavioral disturbance 046.1 [294.11]
    without behavioral disturbance 046.1 [294.10]
Jaksch (-Luzet) disease or syndrome (pseudoleukemia infantum) 285.8
Jamaican
  neuropathy 349.82
  paraplegic tropical ataxic-spastic syndrome 349.82
Janet's disease (psychasthenia) 300.89
Janiceps 759.4
Jansky-Bielschowsky amaurotic familial idiocy 330.1
Japanese
  B type encephalitis 062.0
  river fever 081.2
  seven-day fever 100.89
Jaundice (yellow) 782.4
  acholuric (familial) (splenomegalic) (*see also* Spherocytosis) 282.0
    acquired 283.9
  breast milk 774.39
  catarrhal (acute) 070.1
    with hepatic coma 070.0
    chronic 571.9
    epidemic — *see* Jaundice, epidemic
  cholestatic (benign) 782.4
  chronic idiopathic 277.4
  epidemic (catarrhal) 070.1
    with hepatic coma 070.0
    leptospiral 100.0
    spirochetal 100.0
  febrile (acute) 070.1
    with hepatic coma 070.0
    leptospiral 100.0
    spirochetal 100.0
  fetus or newborn 774.6
    due to or associated with
      ABO
        antibodies 773.1
        incompatibility, maternal/fetal 773.1
        isoimmunization 773.1
      absence or deficiency of enzyme system for bilirubin conjugation (congenital) 774.39
      blood group incompatibility NEC 773.2
      breast milk inhibitors to conjugation 774.39
        associated with preterm delivery 774.2
      bruising 774.1
      Crigler-Najjar syndrome 277.4 [774.31]
      delayed conjugation 774.30
        associated with preterm delivery 774.2
        development 774.39

Jaundice — *continued*
  fetus or newborn — *continued*
    due to or associated with — *continued*
      drugs or toxins transmitted from mother 774.1
      G-6-PD deficiency 282.2 [774.0]
      galactosemia 271.1 [774.5]
      Gilbert's syndrome 277.4 [774.31]
      hepatocellular damage 774.4
      hereditary hemolytic anemia (*see also* Anemia, hemolytic) 282.9 [774.0]
      hypothyroidism, congenital 243 [774.31]
      incompatibility, maternal/fetal NEC 773.2
      infection 774.1
      inspissated bile syndrome 774.4
      isoimmunization NEC 773.2
      mucoviscidosis 277.01 [774.5]
      obliteration of bile duct, congenital 751.61 [774.5]
      polycythemia 774.1
      preterm delivery 774.2
      red cell defect 282.9 [774.0]
      Rh
        antibodies 773.0
        incompatibility, maternal/fetal 773.0
        isoimmunization 773.0
      spherocytosis (congenital) 282.0 [774.0]
      swallowed maternal blood 774.1
    physiological NEC 774.6
  from injection, inoculation, infusion, or transfusion (blood) (plasma) (serum) (other substance) (onset within 8 months after administration) — *see* Hepatitis, viral
  Gilbert's (familial nonhemolytic) 277.4
  hematogenous 283.9
  hemolytic (acquired) 283.9
    congenital (*see also* Spherocytosis) 282.0
  hemorrhagic (acute) 100.0
    leptospiral 100.0
    newborn 776.0
  hemorrhagic
    spirochetal 100.0
  hepatocellular 573.8
  homologous (serum) — *see* Hepatitis, viral
  idiopathic, chronic 277.4
  infectious (acute) (subacute) 070.1
    with hepatic coma 070.0
    leptospiral 100.0
    spirochetal 100.0
  leptospiral 100.0
  malignant (*see also* Necrosis, liver) 570
  newborn (physiological) (*see also* Jaundice, fetus or newborn) 774.6
  nonhemolytic, congenital familial (Gilbert's) 277.4
  nuclear, newborn (*see also* Kernicterus of newborn) 774.7
  obstructive NEC (*see also* Obstruction, biliary) 576.8
  postimmunization — *see* Hepatitis, viral
  posttransfusion — *see* Hepatitis, viral
  regurgitation (*see also* Obstruction, biliary) 576.8
  serum (homologous) (prophylactic) (therapeutic) — *see* Hepatitis, viral
  spirochetal (hemorrhagic) 100.0
  symptomatic 782.4
    newborn 774.6
Jaw — *see* condition
Jaw-blinking 374.43
  congenital 742.8
Jaw-winking phenomenon or syndrome 742.8
Jealousy
  alcoholic 291.5
  childhood 313.3
  sibling 313.3
Jejunitis (*see also* Enteritis) 558.9
Jejunostomy status V44.4
Jejunum, jejunal — *see* condition
Jensen's disease 363.05
Jericho boil 085.1
Jerks, myoclonic 333.2

Jeune's disease or syndrome (asphyxiating thoracic dystrophy) 756.4
Jigger disease 134.1
Job's syndrome (chronic granulomatous disease) 288.1
Jod-Basedow phenomenon 242.8 ✓5ᵗʰ
Johnson-Stevens disease (erythema multiforme exudativum) 695.1
Joint — *see also* condition
  Charcôt's 094.0 [713.5]
  false 733.82
  flail — *see* Flail, joint
  mice — *see* Loose, body, joint, by site
  sinus to bone 730.9 ✓5ᵗʰ
  von Gies' 095.8
Jordan's anomaly or syndrome 288.2
Josephs-Diamond-Blackfan anemia (congenital hypoplastic) 284.0
Joubert syndrome 759.89
Jumpers' knee 727.2
Jungle yellow fever 060.0
Jüngling's disease (sarcoidosis) 135
Junin virus hemorrhagic fever 078.7
Juvenile — *see also* condition
  delinquent 312.9
    group (*see also* Disturbance, conduct) 312.2 ✓5ᵗʰ
  neurotic 312.4

K

Kahler (-Bozzolo) disease (multiple myeloma) (M9730/3) 203.0 ✓5ᵗʰ
Kakergasia 300.9
Kakke 265.0
Kala-azar (Indian) (infantile) (Mediterranean) (Sudanese) 085.0
Kalischer's syndrome (encephalocutaneous angiomatosis) 759.6
Kallmann's syndrome (hypogonadotropic hypogonadism with anosmia) 253.4
Kanner's syndrome (autism) (*see also* Psychosis, childhood) 299.0 ✓5ᵗʰ
Kaolinosis 502
Kaposi's
  disease 757.33
    lichen ruber 696.4
      acuminatus 696.4
      moniliformis 697.8
    xeroderma pigmentosum 757.33
  sarcoma (M9140/3) 176.9
    adipose tissue 176.1
    aponeurosis 176.1
    artery 176.1
    blood vessel 176.1
    bursa 176.1
    connective tissue 176.1
    external genitalia 176.8
    fascia 176.1
    fatty tissue 176.1
    fibrous tissue 176.1
    gastrointestinal tract NEC 176.3
    ligament 176.1
    lung 176.4
    lymph
      gland(s) 176.5
      node(s) 176.5
    lymphatic(s) NEC 176.1
    muscle (skeletal) 176.1
    oral cavity NEC 176.8
    palate 176.2
    scrotum 176.8
    skin 176.0
    soft tissue 176.1
    specified site NEC 176.8
    subcutaneous tissue 176.1
    synovia 176.1
    tendon (sheath) 176.1
    vein 176.1
    vessel 176.1
    viscera NEC 176.9
    vulva 176.8

Kaposi's — *continued*
  varicelliform eruption 054.0
    vaccinia 999.0
Kartagener's syndrome or triad (sinusitis, bronchiectasis, situs inversus) 759.3
Kasabach-Merritt syndrome (capillary hemangioma associated with thrombocytopenic purpura) 287.3
Kaschin-Beck disease (endemic polyarthritis) — *see* Disease, Kaschin-Beck
Kast's syndrome (dyschondroplasia with hemangiomas) 756.4
Katatonia (*see also* Schizophrenia) 295.2 ✓5ᵗʰ
Katayama disease or fever 120.2
Kathisophobia 781.0
Kawasaki disease 446.1
Kayser-Fleischer ring (cornea) (pseudosclerosis) 275.1 *[371.14]*
Kaznelson's syndrome (congenital hypoplastic anemia) 284.0
Kedani fever 081.2
Kelis 701.4
Kelly (-Patterson) syndrome (sideropenic dysphagia) 280.8
Keloid, cheloid 701.4
  Addison's (morphea) 701.0
  cornea 371.00
  Hawkins' 701.4
  scar 701.4
Keloma 701.4
Kenya fever 082.1
Keratectasia 371.71
  congenital 743.41
Keratitis (nodular) (nonulcerative) (simple) (zonular) NEC 370.9
  with ulceration (*see also* Ulcer, cornea) 370.00
  actinic 370.24
  arborescens 054.42
  areolar 370.22
  bullosa 370.8
  deep — *see* Keratitis, interstitial
  dendritic(a) 054.42
  desiccation 370.34
  diffuse interstitial 370.52
  disciform(is) 054.43
    varicella 052.7 *[370.44]*
  epithelialis vernalis 372.13 *[370.32]*
  exposure 370.34
  filamentary 370.23
  gonococcal (congenital) (prenatal) 098.43
  herpes, herpetic (simplex) NEC 054.43
    zoster 053.21
  hypopyon 370.04
  in
    chickenpox 052.7 *[370.44]*
    exanthema (*see also* Exanthem) 057.9 *[370.44]*
    paravaccinia (*see also* Paravaccinia) 051.9 *[370.44]*
    smallpox (*see also* Smallpox) 050.9 *[370.44]*
    vernal conjunctivitis 372.13 *[370.32]*
  interstitial (nonsyphilitic) 370.50
    with ulcer (*see also* Ulcer, cornea) 370.00
    diffuse 370.52
    herpes, herpetic (simplex) 054.43
      zoster 053.21
    syphilitic (congenital) (hereditary) 090.3
    tuberculous (*see also* Tuberculosis) 017.3 ✓5ᵗʰ *[370.59]*
  lagophthalmic 370.34
  macular 370.22
  neuroparalytic 370.35
  neurotrophic 370.35
  nummular 370.22
  oyster-shuckers' 370.8
  parenchymatous — *see* Keratitis, interstitial
  petrificans 370.8
  phlyctenular 370.31
  postmeasles 055.71
  punctata, punctate 370.21
    leprosa 030.0 *[370.21]*
    profunda 090.3
    superficial (Thygeson's) 370.21
  purulent 370.8

Keratitis — *continued*
  pustuliformis profunda 090.3
  rosacea 695.3 *[370.49]*
  sclerosing 370.54
  specified type NEC 370.8
  stellate 370.22
  striate 370.22
  superficial 370.20
    with conjunctivitis (*see also* Keratoconjunctivitis) 370.40
    punctate (Thygeson's) 370.21
  suppurative 370.8
  syphilitic (congenital) (prenatal) 090.3
  trachomatous 076.1
    late effect 139.1
  tuberculous (phlyctenular) (*see also* Tuberculosis) 017.3 ✓5ᵗʰ *[370.31]*
  ulcerated (*see also* Ulcer, cornea) 370.00
  vesicular 370.8
  welders' 370.24
  xerotic (*see also* Keratomalacia) 371.45
    vitamin A deficiency 264.4
Keratoacanthoma 238.2
Keratocele 371.72
Keratoconjunctivitis (*see also* Keratitis) 370.40
  adenovirus type 8 077.1
  epidemic 077.1
  exposure 370.34
  gonococcal 098.43
  herpetic (simplex) 054.43
    zoster 053.21
  in
    chickenpox 052.7 *[370.44]*
    exanthema (*see also* Exanthem) 057.9 *[370.44]*
    paravaccinia (*see also* Paravaccinia) 051.9 *[370.44]*
    smallpox (*see also* Smallpox) 050.9 *[370.44]*
  infectious 077.1
  neurotrophic 370.35
  phlyctenular 370.31
  postmeasles 055.71
  shipyard 077.1
  sicca (Sjögren's syndrome) 710.2
    not in Sjögren's syndrome 370.33
  specified type NEC 370.49
  tuberculous (phlyctenular) (*see also* Tuberculosis) 017.3 ✓5ᵗʰ *[370.31]*
Keratoconus 371.60
  acute hydrops 371.62
  congenital 743.41
  stable 371.61
Keratocyst (dental) 526.0
Keratoderma, keratodermia (congenital) (palmaris et plantaris) (symmetrical) 757.39
  acquired 701.1
  blennorrhagica 701.1
    gonococcal 098.81
  climacterium 701.1
  eccentrica 757.39
  gonorrheal 098.81
  punctata 701.1
  tylodes, progressive 701.1
Keratodermatocele 371.72
Keratoglobus 371.70
  congenital 743.41
    associated with buphthalmos 743.22
Keratohemia 371.12
Keratoiritis (*see also* Iridocyclitis) 364.3
  syphilitic 090.3
  tuberculous (*see also* Tuberculosis) 017.3 ✓5ᵗʰ *[364.11]*
Keratolysis exfoliativa (congenital) 757.39
  acquired 695.89
  neonatorum 757.39
Keratoma 701.1
  congenital 757.39
  malignum congenitale 757.1
  palmaris et plantaris hereditarium 757.39
  senile 702.0
Keratomalacia 371.45
  vitamin A deficiency 264.4
Keratomegaly 743.41
Keratomycosis 111.1
  nigricans (palmaris) 111.1

Keratopathy 371.40
  band (*see also* Keratitis) 371.43
  bullous (*see also* Keratitis) 371.23
  degenerative (*see also* Degeneration, cornea) 371.40
    hereditary (*see also* Dystrophy, cornea) 371.50
  discrete colliquative 371.49
Keratoscleritis, tuberculous (*see also* Tuberculosis) 017.3 ✓5ᵗʰ *[370.31]*
Keratosis 701.1
  actinic 702.0
  arsenical 692.4
  blennorrhagica 701.1
    gonococcal 098.81
  congenital (any type) 757.39
  ear (middle) (*see also* Cholesteatoma) 385.30
  female genital (external) 629.8
  follicular, vitamin A deficiency 264.8
  follicularis 757.39
    acquired 701.1
    congenital (acneiformis) (Siemens') 757.39
    spinulosa (decalvans) 757.39
    vitamin A deficiency 264.8
  gonococcal 098.81
  larynx, laryngeal 478.79
  male genital (external) 608.89
  middle ear (*see also* Cholesteatoma) 385.30
  nigricans 701.2
    congenital 757.39
  obturans 380.21
  palmaris et plantaris (symmetrical) 757.39
  penile 607.89
  pharyngeus 478.29
  pilaris 757.39
    acquired 701.1
  punctata (palmaris et plantaris) 701.1
  scrotal 608.89
  seborrheic 702.19
    inflamed 702.11
  senilis 702.0
  solar 702.0
  suprafollicularis 757.39
  tonsillaris 478.29
  vagina 623.1
  vegetans 757.39
  vitamin A deficiency 264.8
Kerato-uveitis (*see also* Iridocyclitis) 364.3
Keraunoparalysis 994.0
Kerion (celsi) 110.0
Kernicterus of newborn (not due to isoimmunization) 774.7
  due to isoimmunization (conditions classifiable to 773.0-773.2) 773.4
Ketoacidosis 276.2
  diabetic 250.1 ✓5ᵗʰ
Ketonuria 791.6
  branched-chain, intermittent 270.3
Ketosis 276.2
  diabetic 250.1 ✓5ᵗʰ
Kidney — *see* condition
Kienböck's
  disease 732.3
    adult 732.8
  osteochondrosis 732.3
Kimmelstiel (-Wilson) disease or syndrome (intercapillary glomerulosclerosis) 250.4 ✓5ᵗʰ *[581.81]*
Kink, kinking
  appendix 543.9
  artery 447.1
  cystic duct, congenital 751.61
  hair (acquired) 704.2
  ileum or intestine (*see also* Obstruction, intestine) 560.9
  Lane's (*see also* Obstruction, intestine) 560.9
  organ or site, congenital NEC — *see* Anomaly, specified type NEC, by site
  ureter (pelvic junction) 593.3
    congenital 753.20
  vein(s) 459.2
    caval 459.2
    peripheral 459.2
Kinnier Wilson's disease (hepatolenticular degeneration) 275.1

Kissing
  osteophytes 721.5
  spine 721.5
  vertebra 721.5
Klauder's syndrome (erythema multiforme, exudativum) 695.1
Klebs' disease (*see also* Nephritis) 583.9
Klein-Waardenburg syndrome (ptosisepicanthus) 270.2
Kleine-Levin syndrome 349.89
Kleptomania 312.32
Klinefelter's syndrome 758.7
Klinger's disease 446.4
Klippel's disease 723.8
Klippel-Feil disease or syndrome (brevicollis) 756.16
Klippel-Trenaunay syndrome 759.89
Klumpke (-Déjérine) palsy, paralysis (birth) (newborn) 767.6
Klüver-Bucy (-Terzian) syndrome 310.0
Knee — *see* condition
Knifegrinders' rot (*see also* Tuberculosis) 011.4 ✓5ᵗʰ
Knock-knee (acquired) 736.41
  congenital 755.64
Knot
  intestinal, syndrome (volvulus) 560.2
  umbilical cord (true) 663.2 ✓5ᵗʰ
    affecting fetus or newborn 762.5
Knots, surfer 919.8
  infected 919.9
Knotting (of)
  hair 704.2
  intestine 560.2
Knuckle pads (Garrod's) 728.79
Köbner's disease (epidermolysis bullosa) 757.39
Koch's
  infection (*see also* Tuberculosis, pulmonary) 011.9 ✓5ᵗʰ
  relapsing fever 087.9
Koch-Weeks conjunctivitis 372.03
Koenig-Wichman disease (pemphigus) 694.4
Köhler's disease (osteochondrosis) 732.5
  first (osteochondrosis juvenilis) 732.5
    second (Freiburg's infarction, metatarsal head) 732.5
  patellar 732.4
  tarsal navicular (bone) (osteoarthrosis juvenilis) 732.5
Köhler-Mouchet disease (osteoarthrosis juvenilis) 732.5
Köhler-Pellegrini-Stieda disease or syndrome (calcification, knee joint) 726.62
Koilonychia 703.8
  congenital 757.5
Kojevnikov's, Kojewnikoff's epilepsy (*see also* Epilepsy) 345.7 ✓5ᵗʰ
König's
  disease (osteochondritis dissecans) 732.7
  syndrome 564.89
Koniophthisis (*see also* Tuberculosis) 011.4 ✓5ᵗʰ
Koplik's spots 055.9
Kopp's asthma 254.8
Korean hemorrhagic fever 078.6
Korsakoff (-Wernicke) disease, psychosis, or syndrome (nonalcoholic) 294.0
  alcoholic 291.1
Korsakov's disease — *see* Korsakoff's disease
Korsakow's disease — *see* Korsakoff's disease
Kostmann's disease or syndrome (infantile genetic agranulocytosis) 288.0
Krabbe's
  disease (leukodystrophy) 330.0
  syndrome
    congenital muscle hypoplasia 756.89
    cutaneocerebral angioma 759.6
Kraepelin-Morel disease (*see also* Schizophrenia) 295.9 ✓5ᵗʰ
Kraft-Weber-Dimitri disease 759.6

Kraurosis
  ani 569.49
  penis 607.0
  vagina 623.8
  vulva 624.0
Kreotoxism 005.9
Krukenberg's
  spindle 371.13
  tumor (M8490/6) 198.6
Kufs' disease 330.1
Kugelberg-Welander disease 335.11
Kuhnt-Junius degeneration or disease 362.52
Kulchitsky's cell carcinoma (carcinoid tumor of intestine) 259.2
Kümmell's disease or spondylitis 721.7
Kundrat's disease (lymphosarcoma) 200.1 ✓5ᵗʰ
Kunekune — *see* Dermatophytosis
Kunkel syndrome (lupoid hepatitis) 571.49
Kupffer cell sarcoma (M9124/3) 155.0
Kuru 046.0
Kussmaul's
  coma (diabetic) 250.3 ✓5ᵗʰ
  disease (polyarteritis nodosa) 446.0
  respiration (air hunger) 786.09
Kwashiorkor (marasmus type) 260
Kyasanur Forest disease 065.2
Kyphoscoliosis, kyphoscoliotic (acquired) (*see also* Scoliosis) 737.30
  congenital 756.19
  due to radiation 737.33
  heart (disease) 416.1
  idiopathic 737.30
    infantile
      progressive 737.32
      resolving 737.31
  late effect of rickets 268.1 *[737.43]*
  specified NEC 737.39
  thoracogenic 737.34
  tuberculous (*see also* Tuberculosis) 015.0 ✓5ᵗʰ *[737.43]*
Kyphosis, kyphotic (acquired) (postural) 737.10
  adolescent postural 737.0
  congenital 756.19
  dorsalis juvenilis 732.0
  due to or associated with
    Charcôt-Marie-Tooth disease 356.1 *[737.41]*
    mucopolysaccharidosis 277.5 *[737.41]*
    neurofibromatosis 237.71 *[737.41]*
    osteitis
      deformans 731.0 *[737.41]*
      fibrosa cystica 252.0 *[737.41]*
    osteoporosis (*see also* Osteoporosis) 733.0 ✓5ᵗʰ *[737.41]*
    poliomyelitis (*see also* Poliomyelitis) 138 *[737.41]*
    radiation 737.11
    tuberculosis (*see also* Tuberculosis) 015.0 ✓5ᵗʰ *[737.41]*
  Kümmell's 721.7
  late effect of rickets 268.1 *[737.41]*
  Morquio-Brailsford type (spinal) 277.5 *[737.41]*
  pelvis 738.6
  postlaminectomy 737.12
  specified cause NEC 737.19
  syphilitic, congenital 090.5 *[737.41]*
  tuberculous (*see also* Tuberculosis) 015.0 ✓5ᵗʰ *[737.41]*
Kyrle's disease (hyperkeratosis follicularis in cutem penetrans) 701.1

L

Labia, labium — *see* condition
Labiated hymen 752.49
Labile
  blood pressure 796.2
  emotions, emotionality 301.3
  vasomotor system 443.9
Labioglossal paralysis 335.22
Labium leporinum (*see also* Cleft, lip) 749.10
Labor (*see also* Delivery)
  with complications — *see* Delivery, complicated

Labor (*see also* Delivery) — *continued*
  abnormal NEC 661.9 ✓5ᵗʰ
    affecting fetus or newborn 763.7
  arrested active phase 661.1 ✓5ᵗʰ
    affecting fetus or newborn 763.7
  desultory 661.2 ✓5ᵗʰ
    affecting fetus or newborn 763.7
  dyscoordinate 661.4 ✓5ᵗʰ
    affecting fetus or newborn 763.7
  early onset (22-36 weeks gestation) 644.2 ✓5ᵗʰ
  failed
    induction 659.1 ✓5ᵗʰ
      mechanical 659.0 ✓5ᵗʰ
      medical 659.1 ✓5ᵗʰ
      surgical 659.0 ✓5ᵗʰ
    trial (vaginal delivery) 660.6 ✓5ᵗʰ
  false 644.1 ✓5ᵗʰ
  forced or induced, affecting fetus or newborn 763.89
  hypertonic 661.4 ✓5ᵗʰ
    affecting fetus or newborn 763.7
  hypotonic 661.2 ✓5ᵗʰ
    primary 661.0 ✓5ᵗʰ
      affecting fetus or newborn 763.7
    secondary 661.1 ✓5ᵗʰ
      affecting fetus or newborn 763.7
  incoordinate 661.4 ✓5ᵗʰ
    affecting fetus or newborn 763.7
  irregular 661.2 ✓5ᵗʰ
    affecting fetus or newborn 763.7
  long — *see* Labor, prolonged
  missed (at or near term) 656.4 ✓5ᵗʰ
  obstructed NEC 660.9 ✓5ᵗʰ
    affecting fetus or newborn 763.1
    specified cause NEC 660.8 ✓5ᵗʰ
      affecting fetus or newborn 763.1
  pains, spurious 644.1 ✓5ᵗʰ
  precipitate 661.3 ✓5ᵗʰ
    affecting fetus or newborn 763.6
  premature 644.2 ✓5ᵗʰ
    threatened 644.0 ✓5ᵗʰ
  prolonged or protracted 662.1 ✓5ᵗʰ
    affecting fetus or newborn 763.89
    first stage 662.0 ✓5ᵗʰ
      affecting fetus or newborn 763.89
    second stage 662.2 ✓5ᵗʰ
      affecting fetus or newborn 763.89
  threatened NEC 644.1 ✓5ᵗʰ
  undelivered 644.1 ✓5ᵗʰ
Labored breathing (*see also* Hyperventilation) 786.09
Labyrinthitis (inner ear) (destructive) (latent) 386.30
  circumscribed 386.32
  diffuse 386.31
  focal 386.32
  purulent 386.33
  serous 386.31
  suppurative 386.33
  syphilitic 095.8
  toxic 386.34
  viral 386.35
Laceration — *see also* Wound, open, by site
  accidental, complicating surgery 998.2
  Achilles tendon 845.09
    with open wound 892.2
  anus (sphincter) 863.89
    with
      abortion — *see* Abortion, by type, with damage to pelvic organs
      ectopic pregnancy (*see also* categories 633.0-633.9) 639.2
      molar pregnancy (*see also* categories 630-632) 639.2
    complicating delivery 664.2 ✓5ᵗʰ
      with laceration of anal or rectal mucosa 664.3 ✓5ᵗʰ
    following
      abortion 639.2
      ectopic or molar pregnancy 639.2
    nontraumatic, nonpuerperal 565.0
  bladder (urinary)
    with
      abortion — *see* Abortion, by type, with damage to pelvic organs

Laceration — Laceration

Laceration — *see also* Wound, open, by site — *continued*
 bladder (urinary) — *continued*
  with — *continued*
   ectopic pregancy (*see also* categories 633.0-633.9) 639.2
   molar pregnancy (*see also* categories 630-632) 639.2
  following
   abortion 639.2
   ectopic or molar pregnancy 639.2
  obstetrical trauma 665.5 ✓5ᵗʰ
 blood vessel — *see* Injury, blood vessel, by site
 bowel
  with
   abortion — *see* Abortion, by type, with damage to pelvic organs
   ectopic pregnancy (*see also* categories 633.0-633.9) 639.2
   molar pregnancy (*see also* categories 630-632) 639.2
  following
   abortion 639.2
   ectopic or molar pregnancy 639.2
  obstetrical trauma 665.5 ✓5ᵗʰ
 brain (with hemorrhage) (cerebral) (membrane) 851.8 ✓5ᵗʰ
 brain (cerebral) (membrane) 851.8 ✓5ᵗʰ

> *Note* — *Use the following fifth-digit subclassification with categories 851–854:*
>
> *0   unspecified state of consciousness*
> *1   with no loss of consciousness*
> *2   with brief [less than one hour] loss of consciousness*
> *3   with moderate [1-24 hours] loss of consciousness*
> *4   with prolonged [more than 24 hours] loss of consciousness and return to pre-existing conscious level*
> *5   with prolonged [more than 24 hours] loss of consciousness, without return to pre-existing conscious level*
>
> *Use fifth-digit 5 to designate when a patient is unconscious and dies before regaining consciousness, regardless of the duration of the loss of consciousness*
>
> *6   with loss of consciousness of unspecified duration*
> *9   with concussion, unspecified*

  with
   open intracranial wound 851.9 ✓5ᵗʰ
   skull fracture — *see* Fracture, skull, by site
  cerebellum 851.6 ✓5ᵗʰ
   with open intracranial wound 851.7 ✓5ᵗʰ
  cortex 851.2 ✓5ᵗʰ
   with open intracranial wound 851.3 ✓5ᵗʰ
  during birth 767.0
  stem 851.6 ✓5ᵗʰ
   with open intracranial wound 851.7 ✓5ᵗʰ
 broad ligament
  with
   abortion — *see* Abortion, by type, with damage to pelvic organs
   ectopic pregnancy (*see also* categories 633.0-633.9) 639.2
   molar pregnancy (*see also* categories 630-632) 639.2
  following
   abortion 639.2
   ectopic or molar pregnancy 639.2
  nontraumatic 620.6
  obstetrical trauma 665.6 ✓5ᵗʰ
  syndrome (nontraumatic) 620.6
 capsule, joint — *see* Sprain, by site
 cardiac — *see* Laceration, heart
 causing eversion of cervix uteri (old) 622.0
 central, complicating delivery 664.4 ✓5ᵗʰ
 cerebellum — *see* Laceration, brain, cerebellum
 cerebral — *see also* Laceration, brain during birth 767.0

Laceration — *see also* Wound, open, by site — *continued*
 cervix (uteri)
  with
   abortion — *see* Abortion, by type, with damage to pelvic organs
   ectopic pregnancy (*see also* categories 633.0-633.9) 639.2
   molar pregnancy (*see also* categories 630-632) 639.2
  following
   abortion 639.2
   ectopic or molar pregnancy 639.2
  nonpuerperal, nontraumatic 622.3
  obstetrical trauma (current) 665.3 ✓5ᵗʰ
  old (postpartal) 622.3
  traumatic — *see* Injury, internal, cervix
 chordae heart 429.5
 complicated 879.9
 cornea — *see* Laceration, eyeball
  superficial 918.1
 cortex (cerebral) — *see* Laceration, brain, cortex
 esophagus 530.89
 eye(s) — *see* Laceration, ocular
 eyeball NEC 871.4
  with prolapse or exposure of intraocular tissue 871.1
  penetrating — *see* Penetrating wound, eyeball
  specified as without prolapse of intraocular tissue 871.0
 eyelid NEC 870.8
  full thickness 870.1
   involving lacrimal passages 870.2
  skin (and periocular area) 870.0
   penetrating — *see* Penetrating wound, orbit
 fourchette
  with
   abortion — *see* Abortion, by type, with damage to pelvic organs
   ectopic pregnancy (*see also* categories 633.0-633.9) 639.2
   molar pregnancy (*see also* categories 630-632) 639.2
  complicating delivery 664.0 ✓5ᵗʰ
  following
   abortion 639.2
   ectopic or molar pregnancy 639.2
 heart (without penetration of heart chambers) 861.02
  with
   open wound into thorax 861.12
   penetration of heart chambers 861.03
    with open wound into thorax 861.13
 hernial sac — *see* Hernia, by site
 internal organ (abdomen) (chest) (pelvis) NEC — *see* Injury, internal, by site
 kidney (parenchyma) 866.02
  with
   complete disruption of parenchyma (rupture) 866.03
    with open wound into cavity 866.13
   open wound into cavity 866.12
 labia
  complicating delivery 664.0 ✓5ᵗʰ
 ligament — *see also* Sprain, by site
  with open wound — *see* Wound, open, by site
 liver 864.05
  with open wound into cavity 864.15
  major (disruption of hepatic parenchyma) 864.04
   with open wound into cavity 864.14
  minor (capsule only) 864.02
   with open wound into cavity 864.12
  moderate (involving parenchyma without major disruption) 864.03
   with open wound into cavity 864.13
  multiple 864.04
   with open wound into cavity 864.14
  stellate 864.04
   with open wound into cavity 864.14
 lung 861.22
  with open wound into thorax 861.32
 meninges — *see* Laceration, brain

Laceration — *see also* Wound, open, by site — *continued*
 meniscus (knee) (*see also* Tear, meniscus) 836.2
  old 717.5
  site other than knee — *see also* Sprain, by site
   old NEC (*see also* Disorder, cartilage, articular) 718.0 ✓5ᵗʰ
 muscle — *see also* Sprain, by site
  with open wound — *see* Wound, open, by site
 myocardium — *see* Laceration, heart
 nerve — *see* Injury, nerve, by site
 ocular NEC (*see also* Laceration, eyeball) 871.4
  adnexa NEC 870.8
   penetrating 870.3
    with foreign body 870.4
  orbit (eye) 870.8
   penetrating 870.3
    with foreign body 870.4
 pelvic
  floor (muscles)
   with
    abortion — *see* Abortion, by type, with damage to pelvic organs
    ectopic pregnancy (*see also* categories 633.0-633.9) 639.2
    molar pregnancy (*see also* categories 630-632) 639.2
   complicating delivery 664.1 ✓5ᵗʰ
   following
    abortion 639.2
    ectopic or molar pregnancy 639.2
   nonpuerperal 618.7
   old (postpartal) 618.7
  organ NEC
   with
    abortion — *see* Abortion, by type, with damage to pelvic organs
    ectopic pregnancy (*see also* categories 633.0-633.9) 639.2
    molar pregnancy (*see also* categories 630-632) 639.2
   complicating delivery 665.5 ✓5ᵗʰ
    affecting fetus or newborn 763.89
   following
    abortion 639.2
    ectopic or molar pregnancy 639.2
   obstetrical trauma 665.5 ✓5ᵗʰ
 perineum, perineal (old) (postpartal) 618.7
  with
   abortion — *see* Abortion, by type, with damage to pelvic floor
   ectopic pregnancy (*see also* categories 633.0-633.9) 639.2
   molar pregnancy (*see also* categories 630-632) 639.2
  complicating delivery 664.4 ✓5ᵗʰ
   first degree 664.0 ✓5ᵗʰ
   second degree 664.1 ✓5ᵗʰ
   third degree 664.2 ✓5ᵗʰ
   fourth degree 664.3 ✓5ᵗʰ
   central 664.4 ✓5ᵗʰ
   involving
    anal sphincter 664.2 ✓5ᵗʰ
    fourchette 664.0 ✓5ᵗʰ
    hymen 664.0 ✓5ᵗʰ
    labia 664.0 ✓5ᵗʰ
    pelvic floor 664.1 ✓5ᵗʰ
    perineal muscles 664.1 ✓5ᵗʰ
    rectovaginal septum 664.2 ✓5ᵗʰ
     with anal mucosa 664.3 ✓5ᵗʰ
    skin 664.0 ✓5ᵗʰ
    sphincter (anal) 664.2 ✓5ᵗʰ
     with anal mucosa 664.3 ✓5ᵗʰ
    vagina 664.0 ✓5ᵗʰ
    vaginal muscles 664.1 ✓5ᵗʰ
    vulva 664.0 ✓5ᵗʰ
   secondary 674.2 ✓5ᵗʰ
  following
   abortion 639.2
   ectopic or molar pregnancy 639.2
 male 879.6
  complicated 879.7
 muscles, complicating delivery 664.1 ✓5ᵗʰ

Laceration — *see also* Wound, open, by site — *continued*
  perineum, perineal — *continued*
    nonpuerperal, current injury 879.6
      complicated 879.7
    secondary (postpartal) 674.2 ✓5ᵗʰ
  peritoneum
    with
      abortion — *see* Abortion, by type, with damage to pelvic organs
      ectopic pregnancy (*see also* categories 633.0-633.9) 639.2
      molar pregnancy (*see also* categories 630-632) 639.2
    following
      abortion 639.2
      ectopic or molar pregnancy 639.2
    obstetrical trauma 665.5 ✓5ᵗʰ
  periurethral tissue
    with
      abortion — *see* Abortion, by type, with damage to pelvic organs
      ectopic pregnancy (*see also* categories 633.0-633.9) 639.2
      molar pregnancy (*see also* categories 630-632) 639.2
    following
      abortion 639.2
      ectopic or molar pregnancy 639.2
    obstetrical trauma 665.5 ✓5ᵗʰ
  rectovaginal (septum)
    with
      abortion — *see* Abortion, by type, with damage to pelvic organs
      ectopic pregnancy (*see also* categories 633.0-633.9) 639.2
      molar pregnancy (*see also* categories 630-632) 639.2
    complicating delivery 665.4 ✓5ᵗʰ
      with perineum 664.2 ✓5ᵗʰ
        involving anal or rectal mucosa 664.3 ✓5ᵗʰ
    following
      abortion 639.2
      ectopic or molar pregnancy 639.2
    nonpuerperal 623.4
    old (postpartal) 623.4
  spinal cord (meninges) — *see also* Injury, spinal, by site
    due to injury at birth 767.4
    fetus or newborn 767.4
  spleen 865.09
    with
      disruption of parenchyma (massive) 865.04
        with open wound into cavity 865.14
      open wound into cavity 865.19
    capsule (without disruption of parenchyma) 865.02
      with open wound into cavity 865.12
    parenchyma 865.03
      with open wound into cavity 865.13
      massive disruption (rupture) 865.04
        with open wound into cavity 865.14
  tendon 848.9
    with open wound — *see* Wound, open, by site
    Achilles 845.09
      with open wound 892.2
    lower limb NEC 844.9
      with open wound NEC 894.2
    upper limb NEC 840.9
      with open wound NEC 884.2
  tentorium cerebelli — *see* Laceration, brain, cerebellum
  tongue 873.64
    complicated 873.74
  urethra
    with
      abortion — *see* Abortion, by type, with damage to pelvic organs
      ectopic pregnancy (*see also* categories 633.0-633.9) 639.2
      molar pregnancy (*see also* categories 630-632) 639.2

Laceration — *see also* Wound, open, by site — *continued*
  urethra — *continued*
    following
      abortion 639.2
      ectopic or molar pregnancy 639.2
    nonpuerperal, nontraumatic 599.84
    obstetrical trauma 665.5 ✓5ᵗʰ
  uterus
    with
      abortion — *see* Abortion, by type, with damage to pelvic organs
      ectopic pregnancy (*see also* categories 633.0-633.9) 639.2
      molar pregnancy (*see also* categories 630-632) 639.2
    following
      abortion 639.2
      ectopic or molar pregnancy 639.2
    nonpuerperal, nontraumatic 621.8
    obstetrical trauma NEC 665.8 ✓5ᵗʰ ▲
    old (postpartal) 621.8
  vagina
    with
      abortion — *see* Abortion, by type, with damage to pelvic organs
      ectopic pregnancy (*see also* categories 633.0-633.9) 639.2
      molar pregnancy (*see also* categories 630-632) 639.2
      perineal involvement, complicating delivery 664.0 ✓5ᵗʰ
    complicating delivery 665.4 ✓5ᵗʰ
      first degree 664.0 ✓5ᵗʰ
      second degree 664.1 ✓5ᵗʰ
      third degree 664.2 ✓5ᵗʰ
      fourth degree 664.3 ✓5ᵗʰ
      high 665.4 ✓5ᵗʰ
      muscles 664.1 ✓5ᵗʰ
      sulcus 665.4 ✓5ᵗʰ
      wall 665.4 ✓5ᵗʰ
    following
      abortion 639.2
      ectopic or molar pregnancy 639.2
    nonpuerperal, nontraumatic 623.4
    old (postpartal) 623.4
  valve, heart — *see* Endocarditis
  vulva
    with
      abortion — *see* Abortion, by type, with damage to pelvic organs,
      ectopic pregnancy (*see also* categories 633.0-633.9) 639.2
      molar pregnancy (*see also* categories 630-632) 639.2
    complicating delivery 664.0 ✓5ᵗʰ
    following
      abortion 639.2
      ectopic or molar pregnancy 639.2
    nonpuerperal, nontraumatic 624.4
    old (postpartal) 624.4

Lachrymal — *see* condition

Lachrymonasal duct — *see* condition

Lack of
  appetite (*see also* Anorexia) 783.0
  care
    in home V60.4
    of adult 995.84
    of infant (at or after birth) 995.52
  coordination 781.3
  development — *see also* Hypoplasia
    physiological in childhood 783.40
  education V62.3
  energy 780.79
  financial resources V60.2
  food 994.2
    in environment V60.8
  growth in childhood 783.43
  heating V60.1
  housing (permanent) (temporary) V60.0
    adequate V60.1
  material resources V60.2
  medical attention 799.8
  memory (*see also* Amnesia) 780.99 ▲
    mild, following organic brain damage 310.1
  ovulation 628.0

Lack of — *continued*
  person able to render necessary care V60.4
  physical exercise V69.0
  physiologic development in childhood 783.40
  prenatal care in current pregnancy V23.7
  shelter V60.0
  water 994.3

Lacrimal — *see* condition

Lacrimation, abnormal (*see also* Epiphora) 375.20

Lacrimonasal duct — *see* condition

Lactation, lactating (breast) (puerperal) (postpartum)
  defective 676.4 ✓5ᵗʰ
  disorder 676.9 ✓5ᵗʰ
    specified type NEC 676.8 ✓5ᵗʰ
  excessive 676.6 ✓5ᵗʰ
  failed 676.4 ✓5ᵗʰ
  mastitis NEC 675.2 ✓5ᵗʰ
  mother (care and/or examination) V24.1
  nonpuerperal 611.6
  suppressed 676.5 ✓5ᵗʰ

Lacticemia 271.3
  excessive 276.2

Lactosuria 271.3

Lacunar skull 756.0

Laennec's cirrhosis (alcoholic) 571.2
  nonalcoholic 571.5

Lafora's disease 333.2

Lag, lid (nervous) 374.41

Lagleyze-von Hippel disease (retinocerebral angiomatosis) 759.6

Lagophthalmos (eyelid) (nervous) 374.20
  cicatricial 374.23
  keratitis (*see also* Keratitis) 370.34
  mechanical 374.22
  paralytic 374.21

La grippe — *see* Influenza

Lahore sore 085.1

Lakes, venous (cerebral) 437.8

Laki-Lorand factor deficiency (*see also* Defect, coagulation) 286.3

Lalling 307.9

Lambliasis 007.1

Lame back 724.5

Lancereaux's diabetes (diabetes mellitus with marked emaciation) 250.8 ✓5ᵗʰ *[261]*

Landouzy-Déjérine dystrophy (fascioscapulohumeral atrophy) 359.1

Landry's disease or paralysis 357.0

Landry-Guillain-Barré syndrome 357.0

Lane's
  band 751.4
  disease 569.89
  kink (*see also* Obstruction, intestine) 560.9

Langdon Down's syndrome (mongolism) 758.0

Language abolition 784.69

Lanugo (persistent) 757.4

Laparoscopic surgical procedure converted to open procedure V64.4

Lardaceous
  degeneration (any site) 277.3
  disease 277.3
  kidney 277.3 *[583.81]*
  liver 277.3

Large
  baby (regardless of gestational age) 766.1
    exceptionally (weight of 4500 grams or more) 766.0
    of diabetic mother 775.0
  ear 744.22
  fetus — *see also* Oversize, fetus
    causing disproportion 653.5 ✓5ᵗʰ
      with obstructed labor 660.1 ✓5ᵗʰ
  for dates
    fetus or newborn (regardless of gestational age) 766.1
      affecting management of pregnancy 656.6 ✓5ᵗʰ
      exceptionally (weight of 4500 grams or more) 766.0

Large — *continued*
  physiological cup 743.57
  waxy liver 277.3
  white kidney — *see* Nephrosis

Larsen's syndrome (flattened facies and multiple
    congenital dislocations) 755.8

Larsen-Johansson disease (juvenile osteopathia
    patellae) 732.4

Larva migrans
  cutaneous NEC 126.9
    ancylostoma 126.9
  of Diptera in vitreous 128.0
  visceral NEC 128.0

Laryngeal — *see also* condition syncope 786.2

Laryngismus (acute) (infectious) (stridulous)
    478.75
  congenital 748.3
  diphtheritic 032.3

Laryngitis (acute) (edematous) (fibrinous)
    (gangrenous) (infective) (infiltrative)
    (malignant) (membranous) (phlegmonous)
    (pneumococcal) (pseudomembranous)
    (septic) (subglottic) (suppurative) (ulcerative)
    (viral) 464.00
  with
    influenza, flu, or grippe 487.1
    obstruction 464.01
    tracheitis (*see also* Laryngotracheitis) 464.20
      with obstruction 464.21
      acute 464.20
        with obstruction 464.21
      chronic 476.1
  atrophic 476.0
  Borrelia vincentii 101
  catarrhal 476.0
  chronic 476.0
    with tracheitis (chronic) 476.1
    due to external agent — *see* Condition,
      respiratory, chronic, due to
  diphtheritic (membranous) 032.3
  due to external agent — *see* Inflammation,
    respiratory, upper, due to
  H. influenzae 464.00
    with obstruction 464.01
  Hemophilus influenzae 464.00
    with obstruction 464.01
  hypertrophic 476.0
  influenzal 487.1
  pachydermic 478.79
  sicca 476.0
  spasmodic 478.75
    acute 464.00
      with obstruction 464.01
  streptococcal 034.0
  stridulous 478.75
  syphilitic 095.8
    congenital 090.5
  tuberculous (*see also* Tuberculosis, larynx)
    012.3 ☑5ᵗʰ
  Vincent's 101

Laryngocele (congenital) (ventricular) 748.3

Laryngofissure 478.79
  congenital 748.3

Laryngomalacia (congenital) 748.3

Laryngopharyngitis (acute) 465.0
  chronic 478.9
    due to external agent — *see* Condition,
      respiratory, chronic, due to
    due to external agent — *see* Inflammation,
      respiratory, upper, due to
  septic 034.0

Laryngoplegia (*see also* Paralysis, vocal cord)
    478.30

Laryngoptosis 478.79

Laryngospasm 478.75
  due to external agent — *see* Condition,
    respiratory, acute, due to

Laryngostenosis 478.74
  congenital 748.3

Laryngotracheitis (acute) (infectional) (viral) (*see*
    also Laryngitis) 464.20
  with obstruction 464.21
  atrophic 476.1
  Borrelia vincenti 101

Laryngotracheitis (*see also* Laryngitis) —
    continued
  catarrhal 476.1
  chronic 476.1
    due to external agent — *see* Condition,
      respiratory, chronic, due to
  diphtheritic (membranous) 032.3
  due to external agent — *see* Inflammation,
    respiratory, upper, due to
  H. influenzae 464.20
    with obstruction 464.21
  hypertrophic 476.1
  influenzal 487.1
  pachydermic 478.75
  sicca 476.1
  spasmodic 478.75
    acute 464.20
      with obstruction 464.21
  streptococcal 034.0
  stridulous 478.75
  syphilitic 095.8
    congenital 090.5
  tuberculous (*see also* Tuberculosis, larynx)
    012.3 ☑5ᵗʰ
  Vincent's 101

Laryngotracheobronchitis (*see also* Bronchitis)
    490
  acute 466.0
  chronic 491.8
  viral 466.0

Laryngotracheobronchopneumonitis — *see*
    Pneumonia, broncho-

Larynx, laryngeal — *see* condition

Lasègue's disease (persecution mania) 297.9

Lassa fever 078.89

Lassitude (*see also* Weakness) 780.79

Late — *see also* condition
  effect(s) (of) — *see also* condition
    abscess
      intracranial or intraspinal (conditions
        classifiable to 324) — *see* category
        326
    adverse effect of drug, medicinal or
      biological substance 909.5
    amputation
      postoperative (late) 997.60
      traumatic (injury classifiable to 885-887
        and 895-897) 905.9
    burn (injury classifiable to 948-949) 906.9
      extremities NEC (injury classifiable to 943
        or 945) 906.7

      hand or wrist (injury classifiable to
        944) 906.6
      eye (injury classifiable to 940) 906.5
      face, head, and neck (injury classifiable
        to 941) 906.5
      specified site NEC (injury classifiable to
        942 and 946-947) 906.8
    cerebrovascular disease (conditions
      classifiable to 430-437) 438.9
      with
        alterations of sensations 438.6 ●
        aphasia 438.11
        apraxia 438.81
        ataxia 438.84 ●
        cognitive deficits 438.0 ●
        disturbances of vision 438.7 ●
        dysphagia 438.82
        dysphasia 438.12
        facial droop 438.83 ●
        facial weakness 438.83 ●
        hemiplegia/hemiparesis
          affecting
            dominant side 438.21
            nondominant side 438.22
            unspecified side 438.20
        monoplegia of lower limb
          affecting
            dominant side 438.41
            nondominant side 438.42
            unspecified side 438.40
        monoplegia of upper limb
          affecting
            dominant side 438.31

Late — *see also* condition — *continued*
  effect(s) (of) — *see also* condition — *continued*
    cerebrovascular disease — *continued*
      with — *continued*
        monoplegia of upper limb — *continued*
          affecting — *continued*
            nondominant side 438.32
            unspecified side 438.30
        paralytic syndrome NEC
          affecting
            bilateral 438.53
            dominant side 438.51
            nondominant side 438.52
            unspecified side 438.50
        speech and language deficit 438.10
        vertigo 438.85 ●
      specified type NEC 438.89
    childbirth complication(s) 677
    complication(s) of
      childbirth 677
      delivery 677
      pregnancy 677
      puerperium 677
      surgical and medical care (conditions
        classifiable to 996-999) 909.3
    complication(s) of — *continued*
      trauma (conditions classifiable to 958)
        908.6
    contusion (injury classifiable to 920-924)
      906.3
    crushing (injury classifiable to 925-929)
      906.4
    delivery complication(s) 677
    dislocation (injury classifiable to 830-839)
      905.6
    encephalitis or encephalomyelitis (conditions
      classifiable to 323) — *see* category 326
      in infectious diseases 139.8
      viral (conditions classifiable to 049.8,
        049.9, 062-064) 139.0
    external cause NEC (conditions classifiable
      to 995) 909.9
    certain conditions classifiable to
      categories 991-994 909.4
    foreign body in orifice (injury classifiable to
      930-939) 908.5
    fracture (multiple) (injury classifiable to 828-
      829) 905.5
      extremity
        lower (injury classifiable to 821-827)
          905.4
          neck of femur (injury classifiable to
            820) 905.3
        upper (injury classifiable to 810-819)
          905.2
      face and skull (injury classifiable to 800-
        804) 905.0
      skull and face (injury classifiable to 800-
        804) 905.0
      spine and trunk (injury classifiable to
        805 and 807-809) 905.1
        with spinal cord lesion (injury
          classifiable to 806) 907.2
    infection
      pyogenic, intracranial — *see* category 326
    infectious diseases (conditions classifiable to
      001-136) NEC 139.8
    injury (injury classifiable to 959) 908.9
      blood vessel 908.3
        abdomen and pelvis (injury classifiable
          to 902) 908.4
        extremity (injury classifiable to 903-
          904) 908.3
        head and neck (injury classifiable to
          900) 908.3
        intracranial (injury classifiable to
          850-854) 907.0
          with skull fracture 905.0
        thorax (injury classifiable to 901)
          908.4
      internal organ NEC (injury classifiable to
        867 and 869) 908.2
        abdomen (injury classifiable to 863-
          866 and 868) 908.1
        thorax (injury classifiable to 860-862)
          908.0

Large — Late

Late — *see also* condition — *continued*
  effect(s) (of) — *see also* condition — *continued*
    injury — *continued*
      intracranial (injury classifiable to 850-854) 907.0
        with skull fracture (injury classifiable to 800-801 and 803-804) 905.0
      nerve NEC (injury classifiable to 957) 907.9
        cranial (injury classifiable to 950-951) 907.1
        peripheral NEC (injury classifiable to 957) 907.9
          lower limb and pelvic girdle (injury classifiable to 956) 907.5
          upper limb and shoulder girdle (injury classifiable to 955) 907.4
      roots and plexus(es), spinal (injury classifiable to 953) 907.3
      trunk (injury classifiable to 954) 907.3
      spinal
        cord (injury classifiable to 806 and 952) 907.2
        nerve root(s) and plexus(es) (injury classifiable to 953) 907.3
      superficial (injury classifiable to 910-919) 906.2
      tendon (tendon injury classifiable to 840-848, 880-884 with .2, and 890-894 with .2) 905.8
    meningitis
      bacterial (conditions classifiable to 320) — *see* category 326
      unspecified cause (conditions classifiable to 322) — *see* category 326
    myelitis (*see also* Late, effect(s) (of), encephalitis) — *see* category 326
    parasitic diseases (conditions classifiable to 001-136 NEC) 139.8
    phlebitis or thrombophlebitis of intracranial venous sinuses (conditions classifiable to 325) — *see* category 326
    poisoning due to drug, medicinal or biological substance (conditions classifiable to 960-979) 909.0
    poliomyelitis, acute (conditions classifiable to 045) 138
    pregnancy complication(s) 677
    puerperal complication(s) 677
    radiation (conditions classifiable to 990) 909.2
    rickets 268.1
    sprain and strain without mention of tendon injury (injury classifiable to 840-848, except tendon injury) 905.7
      tendon involvement 905.8
    toxic effect of
      drug, medicinal or biological substance (conditions classifiable to 960-979) 909.0
      nonmedical substance (conditions classifiable to 980-989) 909.1
    trachoma (conditions classifiable to 076) 139.1
    tuberculosis 137.0
      bones and joints (conditions classifiable to 015) 137.3
      central nervous system (conditions classifiable to 013) 137.1
      genitourinary (conditions classifiable to 016) 137.2
      pulmonary (conditions classifiable to 010-012) 137.0
      specified organs NEC (conditions classifiable to 014, 017-018) 137.4
    viral encephalitis (conditions classifiable to 049.8, 049.9, 062-064) 139.0
    wound, open
      extremity (injury classifiable to 880-884 and 890-894, except .2) 906.1
      tendon (injury classifiable to 880-884 with .2 and 890-894 with.2) 905.8
      head, neck, and trunk (injury classifiable to 870-879) 906.0

Latent — *see* condition
Lateral — *see* condition
Laterocession — *see* Lateroversion
Lateroflexion — *see* Lateroversion
Lateroversion
  cervix — *see* Lateroversion, uterus
  uterus, uterine (cervix) (postinfectional) (postpartal, old) 621.6
    congenital 752.3
    in pregnancy or childbirth 654.4 ✓5ᵗʰ
      affecting fetus or newborn 763.89
Lathyrism 988.2
Launois' syndrome (pituitary gigantism) 253.0
Launois-Bensaude's lipomatosis 272.8
Launois-Cléret syndrome (adiposogenital dystrophy) 253.8
Laurence-Moon-Biedl syndrome (obesity, polydactyly, and mental retardation) 759.89
LAV (disease) (illness) (infection) — *see* Human immunodeficiency virus (disease) (illness) (infection)
LAV/HTLV-III (disease) (illness) (infection) — *see* Human immunodeficiency virus (disease) (illness) (infection)
Lawford's syndrome (encephalocutaneous angiomatosis) 759.6
Lax, laxity — *see also* Relaxation
  ligament 728.4
  skin (acquired) 701.8
    congenital 756.83
Laxative habit (*see also* Abuse, drugs, nondependent) 305.9 ✓5ᵗʰ
Lazy leukocyte syndrome 288.0
Lead — *see also* condition
  exposure to V15.86
  incrustation of cornea 371.15
  poisoning 984.9
    specified type of lead — *see* Table of Drugs and Chemicals
Lead miners' lung 503
Leakage
  amniotic fluid 658.1 ✓5ᵗʰ
    with delayed delivery 658.2 ✓5ᵗʰ
    affecting fetus or newborn 761.1
  bile from drainage tube (T tube) 997.4
  blood (microscopic), fetal, into maternal circulation 656.0 ✓5ᵗʰ
    affecting management of pregnancy or puerperium 656.0 ✓5ᵗʰ
  device, implant, or graft — *see* Complications, mechanical
  spinal fluid at lumbar puncture site 997.09
  urine, continuous 788.37
Leaky heart — *see* Endocarditis
Learning defect, specific NEC (strephosymbolia) 315.2
Leather bottle stomach (M8142/3) 151.9
Leber's
  congenital amaurosis 362.76
  optic atrophy (hereditary) 377.16
Lederer's anemia or disease (acquired infectious hemolytic anemia) 283.19
Lederer-Brill syndrome (acquired infectious hemolytic anemia) 283.19
Leeches (aquatic) (land) 134.2
Left-sided neglect 781.8
Leg — *see* condition
Legal investigation V62.5
Legg (-Calvé) -Perthes disease or syndrome (osteochondrosis, femoral capital) 732.1
Legionnaires' disease 482.84
Leigh's disease 330.8
Leiner's disease (exfoliative dermatitis) 695.89
Leiofibromyoma (M8890/0) — *see also* Leiomyoma
  uterus (cervix) (corpus) (*see also* Leiomyoma, uterus) 218.9
Leiomyoblastoma (M8891/1) — *see* Neoplasm, connective tissue, uncertain behavior

Leiomyofibroma (M8890/0) — *see also* Neoplasm, connective tissue, benign
  uterus (cervix) (corpus) (*see also* Leiomyoma, uterus) 218.9
Leiomyoma (M8890/0) — *see also* Neoplasm, connective tissue, benign
  bizarre (M8893/0) — *see* Neoplasm, connective tissue, benign
  cellular (M8892/1) — *see* Neoplasm, connective tissue, uncertain behavior
  epithelioid (M8891/1) — *see* Neoplasm, connective tissue, uncertain behavior
  prostate (polypoid) 600.2
  uterus (cervix) (corpus) 218.9
    interstitial 218.1
    intramural 218.1
    submucous 218.0
    subperitoneal 218.2
    subserous 218.2
  vascular (M8894/0) — *see* Neoplasm, connective tissue, benign
Leiomyomatosis (intravascular) (M8890/1) — *see* Neoplasm, connective tissue, uncertain behavior
Leiomyosarcoma (M8890/3) — *see also* Neoplasm, connective tissue, malignant
  epithelioid (M8891/3) — *see* Neoplasm, connective tissue, malignant
Leishmaniasis 085.9
  American 085.5
    cutaneous 085.4
    mucocutaneous 085.5
  Asian desert 085.2
  Brazilian 085.5
  cutaneous 085.9
    acute necrotizing 085.2
    American 085.4
    Asian desert 085.2
    diffuse 085.3
    dry form 085.1
    Ethiopian 085.3
    eyelid 085.5 *[373.6]*
    late 085.1
    lepromatous 085.3
    recurrent 085.1
    rural 085.2
    ulcerating 085.1
    urban 085.1
    wet form 085.2
    zoonotic form 085.2
  dermal — *see also* Leishmaniasis, cutaneous
    post kala-azar 085.0
  eyelid 085.5 *[373.6]*
  infantile 085.0
  Mediterranean 085.0
  mucocutaneous (American) 085.5
  naso-oral 085.5
  nasopharyngeal 085.5
  Old World 085.1
  tegumentaria diffusa 085.4
  vaccination, prophylactic (against) V05.2
  visceral (Indian) 085.0
Leishmanoid, dermal — *see also* Leishmaniasis, cutaneous
  post kala-azar 085.0
Leloir's disease 695.4
Lenegre's disease 426.0
Lengthening, leg 736.81
Lennox's syndrome (*see also* Epilepsy) 345.0 ✓5ᵗʰ
Lens — *see* condition
Lenticonus (anterior) (posterior) (congenital) 743.36
Lenticular degeneration, progressive 275.1
Lentiglobus (posterior) (congenital) 743.36
Lentigo (congenital) 709.09
  juvenile 709.09
  Maligna (M8742/2) — *see also* Neoplasm, skin, in situ
    melanoma (M8742/3) — *see* Melanoma
  senile 709.09
Leonine leprosy 030.0
Leontiasis
  ossium 733.3
  syphilitic 095.8
    congenital 090.5

Léopold-Lévi's syndrome (paroxysmal thyroid instability) 242.9 ✔5th
Lepore hemoglobin syndrome 282.4
Lepothrix 039.0
Lepra 030.9
  Willan's 696.1
Leprechaunism 259.8
Lepromatous leprosy 030.0
Leprosy 030.9
  anesthetic 030.1
  beriberi 030.1
  borderline (group B) (infiltrated) (neuritic) 030.3
  cornea (see also Leprosy, by type) 030.9 [371.89]
  dimorphous (group B) (infiltrated) (lepromatous) (neuritic) (tuberculoid) 030.3
  eyelid 030.0 [373.4]
  indeterminate (group I) (macular) (neuritic) (uncharacteristic) 030.2
  leonine 030.0
  lepromatous (diffuse) (infiltrated) (macular) (neuritic) (nodular) (type L) 030.0
  macular (early) (neuritic) (simple) 030.2
  maculoanesthetic 030.1
  mixed 030.0
  neuro 030.1
  nodular 030.0
  primary neuritic 030.3
  specified type or group NEC 030.8
  tubercular 030.1
  tuberculoid (macular) (maculoanesthetic) (major) (minor) (neuritic) (type T) 030.1
Leptocytosis, hereditary 282.4
Leptomeningitis (chronic) (circumscribed) (hemorrhagic) (nonsuppurative) (see also Meningitis) 322.9
  aseptic 047.9
    adenovirus 049.1
    Coxsackie virus 047.0
    ECHO virus 047.1
    enterovirus 047.9
    lymphocytic choriomeningitis 049.0
  epidemic 036.0
  late effect — see category 326
  meningococcal 036.0
  pneumococcal 320.1
  syphilitic 094.2
  tuberculous (see also Tuberculosis, meninges) 013.0 ✔5th
Leptomeningopathy (see also Meningitis) 322.9
Leptospiral — see condition
Leptospirochetal — see condition
Leptospirosis 100.9
  autumnalis 100.89
  canicula 100.89
  grippotyphosa 100.89
  hebdomidis 100.89
  icterohemorrhagica 100.0
  nanukayami 100.89
  pomona 100.89
  Weil's disease 100.0
Leptothricosis — see Actinomycosis
Leptothrix infestation — see Actinomycosis
Leptotricosis — see Actinomycosis
Leptus dermatitis 133.8
Léris pleonosteosis 756.89
Léri-Weill syndrome 756.59
Leriche's syndrome (aortic bifurcation occlusion) 444.0
Lermoyez's syndrome (see also Disease, Ménière's) 386.00
Lesbianism — omit code
  ego-dystonic 302.0
  problems with 302.0
Lesch-Nyhan syndrome (hypoxanthineguanine-phosphoribosyltransferase deficiency) 277.2
Lesion
  abducens nerve 378.54
  alveolar process 525.8
  anorectal 569.49
  aortic (valve) — see Endocarditis, aortic
  auditory nerve 388.5
  basal ganglion 333.90

Lesion — continued
  bile duct (see also Disease, biliary) 576.8
  bladder 596.9
  bone 733.90
  brachial plexus 353.0
  brain 348.8
    congenital 742.9
    vascular (see also Lesion, cerebrovascular) 437.9
      degenerative 437.1
      healed or old without residuals V12.59
      hypertensive 437.2
      late effect — see Late effect(s) (of) cerebrovascular disease
  buccal 528.9
  calcified — see Calcification
  canthus 373.9
  carate — see Pinta, lesions
  cardia 537.89
  cardiac — see also Disease, heart
    congenital 746.9
    valvular — see Endocarditis
  cauda equina 344.60
    with neurogenic bladder 344.61
  cecum 569.89
  cerebral — see Lesion, brain
  cerebrovascular (see also Disease, cerebrovascular NEC) 437.9
    degenerative 437.1
      healed or old without residuals V12.59
    hypertensive 437.2
    specified type NEC 437.8
  cervical root (nerve) NEC 353.2
  chiasmal 377.54
    associated with
      inflammatory disorders 377.54
      neoplasm NEC 377.52
        pituitary 377.51
      pituitary disorders 377.51
      vascular disorders 377.53
  chorda tympani 351.8
  coin, lung 793.1
  colon 569.89
  congenital — see Anomaly
  conjunctiva 372.9
  coronary artery (see also Ischemia, heart) 414.9
  cranial nerve 352.9
    first 352.0
    second 377.49
    third
      partial 378.51
      total 378.52
    fourth 378.53
    fifth 350.9
    sixth 378.54
    seventh 351.9
    eighth 388.5
    ninth 352.2
    tenth 352.3
    eleventh 352.4
    twelfth 352.5
  cystic — see Cyst
  degenerative — see Degeneration
  dermal (skin) 709.9
  Dieulafoy (hemorrhagic) ●
    of ●
      duodenum 537.84 ●
      intestine 569.86 ●
      stomach 537.84 ●
  duodenum 537.89
    with obstruction 537.3
  eyelid 373.9
  gasserian ganglion 350.8
  gastric 537.89
  gastroduodenal 537.89
  gastrointestinal 569.89
  glossopharyngeal nerve 352.2
  heart (organic) — see also Disease, heart
    vascular — see Disease, cardiovascular
  helix (ear) 709.9
  hyperchromic, due to pinta (carate) 103.1
  hyperkeratotic (see also Hyperkeratosis) 701.1
  hypoglossal nerve 352.5
  hypopharynx 478.29
  hypothalamic 253.9
  ileocecal coil 569.89
  ileum 569.89

Lesion — continued
  iliohypogastric nerve 355.79
  ilioinguinal nerve 355.79
  in continuity — see Injury, nerve, by site
  inflammatory — see Inflammation
  intestine 569.89
  intracerebral — see Lesion, brain
  intrachiasmal (optic) (see also Lesion, chiasmal) 377.54
  intracranial, space-occupying NEC 784.2
  joint 719.90
    ankle 719.97
    elbow 719.92
    foot 719.97
    hand 719.94
    hip 719.95
    knee 719.96
    multiple sites 719.99
    pelvic region 719.95
    sacroiliac (old) 724.6
    shoulder (region) 719.91
    specified site NEC 719.98
    wrist 719.93
  keratotic (see also Keratosis) 701.1
  kidney (see also Disease, renal) 593.9
  laryngeal nerve (recurrent) 352.3
  leonine 030.0
  lip 528.5
  liver 573.8
  lumbosacral
    plexus 353.1
    root (nerve) NEC 353.4
  lung 518.89
    coin 793.1
  maxillary sinus 473.0
  mitral — see Endocarditis, mitral
  motor cortex 348.8
  nerve (see also Disorder, nerve) 355.9
  nervous system 349.9
    congenital 742.9
  nonallopathic NEC 739.9
    in region (of)
      abdomen 739.9
      acromioclavicular 739.7
      cervical, cervicothoracic 739.1
      costochondral 739.8
      costovertebral 739.8
      extremity
        lower 739.6
        upper 739.7
      head 739.0
      hip 739.5
      lower extremity 739.6
      lumbar, lumbosacral 739.3
      occipitocervical 739.0
      pelvic 739.5
      pubic 739.5
      rib cage 739.8
      sacral, sacrococcygeal, sacroiliac 739.4
      sternochondral 739.8
      sternoclavicular 739.7
      thoracic, thoracolumbar 739.2
      upper extremity 739.7
  nose (internal) 478.1
  obstructive — see Obstruction
  obturator nerve 355.79
  occlusive
    artery — see Embolism, artery
  organ or site NEC — see Disease, by site
  osteolytic 733.90
  paramacular, of retina 363.32
  peptic 537.89
  periodontal, due to traumatic occlusion 523.8
  perirectal 569.49
  peritoneum (granulomatous) 568.89
  pigmented (skin) 709.00
  pinta — see Pinta, lesions
  polypoid — see Polyp
  prechiasmal (optic) (see also Lesion, chiasmal) 377.54
  primary — see also Syphilis, primary
    carate 103.0
    pinta 103.0
    yaws 102.0
  pulmonary 518.89
    valve (see also Endocarditis, pulmonary) 424.3

Lesion — *continued*
  pylorus 537.89
  radiation NEC 990
  radium NEC 990
  rectosigmoid 569.89
  retina, retinal — *see also* Retinopathy
    vascular 362.17
  retroperitoneal 568.89
  romanus 720.1
  sacroiliac (joint) 724.6
  salivary gland 527.8
    benign lymphoepithelial 527.8
  saphenous nerve 355.79
  secondary — *see* Syphilis, secondary
  sigmoid 569.89
  sinus (accessory) (nasal) (*see also* Sinusitis)
    473.9
  skin 709.9
    suppurative 686.00
  SLAP (superior glenoid labrum) 840.7
  space-occupying, intracranial NEC 784.2
  spinal cord 336.9
    congenital 742.9
    traumatic (complete) (incomplete)
        (transverse) — *see also* Injury, spinal,
        by site
      with
        broken
          back — *see* Fracture, vertebra, by
            site, with spinal cord injury
          neck — *see* Fracture, vertebra,
            cervical, with spinal cord
            injury
        fracture, vertebra — *see* Fracture,
          vertebra, by site, with spinal
          cord injury
  spleen 289.50
  stomach 537.89
  superior glenoid labrum (SLAP) 840.7
  syphilitic — *see* Syphilis
  tertiary — *see* Syphilis, tertiary
  thoracic root (nerve) 353.3
  tonsillar fossa 474.9
  tooth, teeth 525.8
    white spot 521.01
  traumatic NEC (*see also* nature and site of
    injury) 959.9
  tricuspid (valve) — *see* Endocarditis, tricuspid
  trigeminal nerve 350.9
  ulcerated or ulcerative — *see* Ulcer
  uterus NEC 621.9
  vagina 623.8
  vagus nerve 352.3
  valvular — *see* Endocarditis
  vascular 459.9
    affecting central nervous system (*see also*
      Lesion, cerebrovascular) 437.9
    following trauma (*see also* Injury, blood
      vessel, by site) 904.9
    retina 362.17
    traumatic — *see* Injury, blood vessel, by site
    umbilical cord 663.6 ✓4ᵗʰ
      affecting fetus or newborn 762.6
  visual
    cortex NEC (*see also* Disorder, visual, cortex)
      377.73
    pathway NEC (*see also* Disorder, visual,
      pathway) 377.63
  warty — *see* Verruca
  white spot, on teeth 521.01
  x-ray NEC 990
Lethargic — *see* condition
Lethargy 780.79
Letterer-Siwe disease (acute histiocytosis X)
  (M9722/3) 202.5 ✓5ᵗʰ
Leucinosis 270.3
Leucocoria 360.44
Leucosarcoma (M9850/3) 207.8 ✓5ᵗʰ
Leukasmus 270.2

Leukemia, leukemic (congenital) (M9800/3)
  208.9 ✓5ᵗʰ

> Note — Use the following fifth-digit
> subclassification for categories 203–208:
>
> 0   without mention of remission
> 1   with remission

  acute NEC (M9801/3) 208.0 ✓5ᵗʰ
  aleukemic NEC (M9804/3) 208.8 ✓5ᵗʰ
    granulocytic (M9864/3) 205.8 ✓5ᵗʰ
  basophilic (M9870/3) 205.1 ✓5ᵗʰ
  blast (cell) (M9801/3) 208.0 ✓5ᵗʰ
  blastic (M9801/3) 208.0 ✓5ᵗʰ
    granulocytic (M9861/3) 205.0 ✓5ᵗʰ
  chronic NEC (M9803/3) 208.1 ✓5ᵗʰ
  compound (M9810/3) 207.8 ✓5ᵗʰ
  eosinophilic (M9880/3) 205.1 ✓5ᵗʰ
  giant cell (M9910/3) 207.2 ✓5ᵗʰ
  granulocytic (M9860/3) 205.9 ✓5ᵗʰ
    acute (M9861/3) 205.0 ✓5ᵗʰ
    aleukemic (M9864/3) 205.8 ✓5ᵗʰ
    blastic (M9861/3) 205.0 ✓5ᵗʰ
    chronic (M9863/3) 205.1 ✓5ᵗʰ
    subacute (M9862/3) 205.2 ✓5ᵗʰ
    subleukemic (M9864/3) 205.8 ✓5ᵗʰ
  hairy cell (M9940/3) 202.4 ✓5ᵗʰ
  hemoblastic (M9801/3) 208.0 ✓5ᵗʰ
  histiocytic (M9890/3) 206.9 ✓5ᵗʰ
  lymphatic (M9820/3) 204.9 ✓5ᵗʰ
    acute (M9821/3) 204.0 ✓5ᵗʰ
    aleukemic (M9824/3) 204.8 ✓5ᵗʰ
    chronic (M9823/3) 204.1 ✓5ᵗʰ
    subacute (M9822/3) 204.2 ✓5ᵗʰ
    subleukemic (M9824/3) 204.8 ✓5ᵗʰ
  lymphoblastic (M9821/3) 204.0 ✓5ᵗʰ
  lymphocytic (M9820/3) 204.9 ✓5ᵗʰ
    acute (M9821/3) 204.0 ✓5ᵗʰ
    aleukemic (M9824/3) 204.8 ✓5ᵗʰ
    chronic (M9823/3) 204.1 ✓5ᵗʰ
    subacute (M9822/3) 204.2 ✓5ᵗʰ
    subleukemic (M9824/3) 204.8 ✓5ᵗʰ
  lymphogenous (M9820/3) — *see* Leukemia,
    lymphoid
  lymphoid (M9820/3) 204.9 ✓5ᵗʰ
    acute (M9821/3) 204.0 ✓5ᵗʰ
    aleukemic (M9824/3) 204.8 ✓5ᵗʰ
    blastic (M9821/3) 204.0 ✓5ᵗʰ
    chronic (M9823/3) 204.1 ✓5ᵗʰ
    subacute (M9822/3) 204.2 ✓5ᵗʰ
    subleukemic (M9824/3) 204.8 ✓5ᵗʰ
  lymphosarcoma cell (M9850/3) 207.8 ✓5ᵗʰ
  mast cell (M9900/3) 207.8 ✓5ᵗʰ
  megakaryocytic (M9910/3) 207.2 ✓5ᵗʰ
  megakaryocytoid (M9910/3) 207.2 ✓5ᵗʰ
  mixed (cell) (M9810/3) 207.8 ✓5ᵗʰ
  monoblastic (M9891/3) 206.0 ✓5ᵗʰ
  monocytic (Schilling-type) (M9890/3) 206.9 ✓5ᵗʰ
    acute (M9891/3) 206.0 ✓5ᵗʰ
    aleukemic (M9894/3) 206.8 ✓5ᵗʰ
    chronic (M9893/3) 206.1 ✓5ᵗʰ
    Naegeli-type (M9863/3) 205.1 ✓5ᵗʰ
    subacute (M9892/3) 206.2 ✓5ᵗʰ
    subleukemic (M9894/3) 206.8 ✓5ᵗʰ
  monocytoid (M9890/3) 206.9 ✓5ᵗʰ
    acute (M9891/3) 206.0 ✓5ᵗʰ
    aleukemic (M9894/3) 206.8 ✓5ᵗʰ
    chronic (M9893/3) 206.1 ✓5ᵗʰ
    myelogenous (M9863/3) 205.1 ✓5ᵗʰ
    subacute (M9892/3) 206.2 ✓5ᵗʰ
    subleukemic (M9894/3) 206.8 ✓5ᵗʰ
  monomyelocytic (M9860/3) — *see* Leukemia,
    myelomonocytic
  myeloblastic (M9861/3) 205.0 ✓5ᵗʰ
  myelocytic (M9863/3) 205.1 ✓5ᵗʰ
    acute (M9861/3) 205.0 ✓5ᵗʰ
  myelogenous (M9860/3) 205.9 ✓5ᵗʰ
    acute (M9861/3) 205.0 ✓5ᵗʰ
    aleukemic (M9864/3) 205.8 ✓5ᵗʰ
    chronic (M9863/3) 205.1 ✓5ᵗʰ
    monocytoid (M9863/3) 205.1 ✓5ᵗʰ
    subacute (M9862/3) 205.2 ✓5ᵗʰ
    subleukemic (M9864) 205.8 ✓5ᵗʰ
  myeloid (M9860/3) 205.9 ✓5ᵗʰ
    acute (M9861/3) 205.0 ✓5ᵗʰ
    aleukemic (M9864/3) 205.8 ✓5ᵗʰ
    chronic (M9863/3) 205.1 ✓5ᵗʰ

Leukemia, leukemic — *continued*
  myeloid — *continued*
    subacute (M9862/3) 205.2 ✓5ᵗʰ
    subleukemic (M9864/3) 205.8 ✓5ᵗʰ
  myelomonocytic (M9860/3) 205.9 ✓5ᵗʰ
    acute (M9861/3) 205.0 ✓5ᵗʰ
    chronic (M9863/3) 205.1 ✓5ᵗʰ
  Naegeli-type monocytic (M9863/3) 205.1 ✓5ᵗʰ
  neutrophilic (M9865/3) 205.1 ✓5ᵗʰ
  plasma cell (M9830/3) 203.1 ✓5ᵗʰ
  plasmacytic (M9830/3) 203.1 ✓5ᵗʰ
  prolymphocytic (M9825/3) — *see* Leukemia,
    lymphoid
  promyelocytic, acute (M9866/3) 205.0 ✓5ᵗʰ
  Schilling-type monocytic (M9890/3) — *see*
    Leukemia, monocytic
  stem cell (M9801/3) 208.0 ✓5ᵗʰ
  subacute NEC (M9802/3) 208.2 ✓5ᵗʰ
  subleukemic NEC (M9804/3) 208.8 ✓5ᵗʰ
  thrombocytic (M9910/3) 207.2 ✓5ᵗʰ
  undifferentiated (M9801/3) 208.0 ✓5ᵗʰ
Leukemoid reaction (lymphocytic) (monocytic)
  (myelocytic) 288.8
Leukoclastic vasculitis 446.29
Leukocoria 360.44
Leukocythemia — *see* Leukemia
Leukocytosis 288.8
  basophilic 288.8
  eosinophilic 288.3
  lymphocytic 288.8
  monocytic 288.8
  neutrophilic 288.8
Leukoderma 709.09
  syphilitic 091.3
    late 095.8
Leukodermia (*see also* Leukoderma) 709.09
Leukodystrophy (cerebral) (globoid cell)
  (metachromatic) (progressive) (sudanophilic)
  330.0
Leukoedema, mouth or tongue 528.7
Leukoencephalitis
  acute hemorrhagic (postinfectious) NEC
    136.9 [323.6]
    postimmunization or postvaccinal 323.5
  subacute sclerosing 046.2
    van Bogaert's 046.2
  van Bogaert's (sclerosing) 046.2
Leukoencephalopathy (*see also* Encephalitis)
  323.9
  acute necrotizing hemorrhagic (postinfectious)
    136.9 [323.6]
    postimmunization or postvaccinal 323.5
  metachromatic 330.0
  multifocal (progressive) 046.3
  progressive multifocal 046.3
Leukoerythroblastosis 289.0
Leukoerythrosis 289.0
Leukokeratosis (*see also* Leukoplakia) 702.8
  mouth 528.6
  nicotina palati 528.7
  tongue 528.6
Leukokoria 360.44
Leukokraurosis vulva, vulvae 624.0
Leukolymphosarcoma (M9850/3) 207.8 ✓5ᵗʰ
Leukoma (cornea) (interfering with central vision)
  371.03
  adherent 371.04
Leukomalacia, periventricular 779.7
Leukomelanopathy, hereditary 288.2
Leukonychia (punctata) (striata) 703.8
  congenital 757.5
Leukopathia
  unguium 703.8
    congenital 757.5
Leukopenia 288.0
  cyclic 288.0
  familial 288.0
  malignant 288.0
  periodic 288.0
  transitory neonatal 776.7
Leukopenic — *see* condition
Leukoplakia 702.8
  anus 569.49

Leukoplakia — *continued*
　　bladder (postinfectional) 596.8
　　buccal 528.6
　　cervix (uteri) 622.2
　　esophagus 530.83
　　gingiva 528.6
　　kidney (pelvis) 593.89
　　larynx 478.79
　　lip 528.6
　　mouth 528.6
　　oral soft tissue (including tongue) (mucosa)
　　　　528.6
　　palate 528.6
　　pelvis (kidney) 593.89
　　penis (infectional) 607.0
　　rectum 569.49
　　syphilitic 095.8
　　tongue 528.6
　　tonsil 478.29
　　ureter (postinfectional) 593.89
　　urethra (postinfectional) 599.84
　　uterus 621.8
　　vagina 623.1
　　vesical 596.8
　　vocal cords 478.5
　　vulva 624.0
Leukopolioencephalopathy 330.0
Leukorrhea (vagina) 623.5
　　due to trichomonas (vaginalis) 131.00
　　trichomonal (Trichomonas vaginalis) 131.00
Leukosarcoma (M9850/3) 207.8 ✓5ᵗʰ
Leukosis (M9800/3) — *see* Leukemia
Lev's disease or syndrome (acquired complete
　　heart block) 426.0
Levi's syndrome (pituitary dwarfism) 253.3
Levocardia (isolated) 746.87
　　with situs inversus 759.3
Levulosuria 271.2
Lewandowski's disease (primary) (*see also*
　　Tuberculosis) 017.0 ✓5ᵗʰ
Lewandowski-Lutz disease (epidermodysplasia
　　verruciformis) 078.19
Leyden's disease (periodic vomiting) 536.2
Leyden-Möbius dystrophy 359.1
Leydig cell
　　carcinoma (M8650/3)
　　　specified site — *see* Neoplasm, by site,
　　　　malignant
　　　unspecified site
　　　　female 183.0
　　　　male 186.9
　　tumor (M8650/1)
　　　benign (M8650/0)
　　　　specified site — *see* Neoplasm, by site,
　　　　　benign
　　　　unspecified site
　　　　　female 220
　　　　　male 222.0
　　　malignant (M8650/3)
　　　　specified site — *see* Neoplasm, by site,
　　　　　malignant
　　　　unspecified site
　　　　　female 183.0
　　　　　male 186.9
　　　specified site — *see* Neoplasm, by site,
　　　　uncertain behavior
　　　unspecified site
　　　　female 236.2
　　　　male 236.4
Leydig-Sertoli cell tumor (M8631/0)
　　specified site — *see* Neoplasm, by site, benign
　　unspecified site
　　　female 220
　　　male 222.0
LGSIL (low grade squamous intraepithelial ●
　　dysplasia) 622.1 ●
Liar, pathologic 301.7
Libman-Sacks disease or syndrome
　　710.0 *[424.91]*
Lice (infestation) 132.9
　　body (pediculus corporis) 132.1
　　crab 132.2
　　head (pediculus capitis) 132.0

Lice — *continued*
　　mixed (classifiable to more than one of the
　　　categories 132.0-132.2) 132.3
　　pubic (pediculus pubis) 132.2
Lichen 697.9
　　albus 701.0
　　annularis 695.89
　　atrophicus 701.0
　　corneus obtusus 698.3
　　myxedematous 701.8
　　nitidus 697.1
　　pilaris 757.39
　　　acquired 701.1
　　planopilaris 697.0
　　planus (acute) (chronicus) (hypertrophic)
　　　(verrucous) 697.0
　　　morphoeicus 701.0
　　　sclerosus (et atrophicus) 701.0
　　ruber 696.4
　　　acuminatus 696.4
　　　moniliformis 697.8
　　　obtusus corneus 698.3
　　　of Wilson 697.0
　　　planus 697.0
　　selerosus (et atrophicus) 701.0
　　scrofulosus (primary) (*see also* Tuberculosis)
　　　017.0 ✓5ᵗʰ
　　simplex (Vidal's) 698.3
　　　chronicus 698.3
　　　circumscriptus 698.3
　　spinulosus 757.39
　　　mycotic 117.9
　　striata 697.8
　　urticatus 698.2
Lichenification 698.3
　　nodular 698.3
Lichenoides tuberculosis (primary) (*see also*
　　Tuberculosis) 017.0 ✓5ᵗʰ
Lichtheim's disease or syndrome (subacute
　　combined sclerosis with pernicious anemia)
　　281.0 *[336.2]*
Lien migrans 289.59
Lientery (*see also* Diarrhea) 787.91
　　infectious 009.2
Life circumstance problem NEC V62.89
Li-Fraumeni cancer syndrome 758.3
Ligament — *see* condition
Light-for-dates (infant) 764.0 ✓5ᵗʰ
　　with signs of fetal malnutrition 764.1 ✓5ᵗʰ
　　affecting management of pregnancy 656.5 ✓5ᵗʰ
Light-headedness 780.4
Lightning (effects) (shock) (stroke) (struck by)
　　994.0
　　burn — *see* Burn, by site
　　foot 266.2
Lightwood's disease or syndrome (renal tubular
　　acidosis) 588.8
Lignac's disease (cystinosis) 270.0
Lignac (-de Toni) (-Fanconi) (-Debré) syndrome
　　(cystinosis) 270.0
Lignac (-Fanconi) syndrome (cystinosis) 270.0
Ligneous thyroiditis 245.3
Likoff's syndrome (angina in menopausal
　　women) 413.9
Limb — *see* condition
Limitation of joint motion (*see also* Stiffness,
　　joint) 719.5 ✓5ᵗʰ
　　sacroiliac 724.6
Limit dextrinosis 271.0
Limited
　　cardiac reserve — *see* Disease, heart
　　duction, eye NEC 378.63
Lindau's disease (retinocerebral angiomatosis)
　　759.6
Lindau (-von Hippel) disease (angiomatosis
　　retinocerebellosa) 759.6
Linea corneae senilis 371.41
Lines
　　Beau's (transverse furrows on fingernails)
　　　703.8
　　Harris' 733.91
　　Hudson-Stähli 371.11
　　Stähli's 371.11

Lingua
　　geographical 529.1
　　nigra (villosa) 529.3
　　plicata 529.5
　　　congenital 750.13
　　tylosis 528.6
Lingual (tongue) — *see also* condition
　　thyroid 759.2
Linitis (gastric) 535.4 ✓5ᵗʰ
　　plastica (M8142/3) 151.9
Lioderma essentialis (cum melanosis et
　　telangiectasia) 757.33
Lip — *see also* condition
　　biting 528.9
Lipalgia 272.8
Lipedema — *see* Edema
Lipemia (*see also* Hyperlipidemia) 272.4
　　retina, retinalis 272.3
Lipidosis 272.7
　　cephalin 272.7
　　cerebral (infantile) (juvenile) (late) 330.1
　　cerebroretinal 330.1 *[362.71]*
　　cerebroside 272.7
　　cerebrospinal 272.7
　　chemically-induced 272.7
　　cholesterol 272.7
　　diabetic 250.8 ✓5ᵗʰ *[272.7]*
　　dystopic (hereditary) 272.7
　　glycolipid 272.7
　　hepatosplenomegalic 272.3
　　hereditary, dystopic 272.7
　　sulfatide 330.0
Lipoadenoma (M8324/0) — *see* Neoplasm, by
　　site, benign
Lipoblastoma (M8881/0) — *see* Lipoma, by site
Lipoblastomatosis (M8881/0) — *see* Lipoma, by
　　site
Lipochondrodystrophy 277.5
Lipochrome histiocytosis (familial) 288.1
Lipodystrophia progressiva 272.6
Lipodystrophy (progressive) 272.6
　　insulin 272.6
　　intestinal 040.2
Lipofibroma (M8851/0) — *see* Lipoma, by site
Lipoglycoproteinosis 272.8
Lipogranuloma, sclerosing 709.8
Lipogranulomatosis (disseminated) 272.8
　　kidney 272.8
Lipoid — *see also* condition
　　histiocytosis 272.7
　　　essential 272.7
　　nephrosis (*see also* Nephrosis) 581.3
　　proteinosis of Urbach 272.8
Lipoidemia (*see also* Hyperlipidemia) 272.4
Lipoidosis (*see also* Lipidosis) 272.7
Lipoma (M8850/0) 214.9
　　breast (skin) 214.1
　　face 214.0
　　fetal (M8881/0) — *see also* Lipoma, by site
　　　fat cell (M8880/0) — *see* Lipoma, by site
　　infiltrating (M8856/0) — *see* Lipoma, by site
　　intra-abdominal 214.3
　　intramuscular (M8856/0) — *see* Lipoma, by
　　　site
　　intrathoracic 214.2
　　kidney 214.3
　　mediastinum 214.2
　　muscle 214.8
　　peritoneum 214.3
　　retroperitoneum 214.3
　　skin 214.1
　　　face 214.0
　　spermatic cord 214.4
　　spindle cell (M8857/0) — *see* Lipoma, by site
　　stomach 214.3
　　subcutaneous tissue 214.1
　　　face 214.0
　　thymus 214.2
　　thyroid gland 214.2
Lipomatosis (dolorosa) 272.8
　　epidural 214.8
　　fetal (M8881/0) — *see* Lipoma, by site

Lipomatosis — *continued*
  Launois-Bensaude's 272.8
Lipomyohemangioma (M8860/0)
  specified site — *see* Neoplasm, connective
      tissue, benign
  unspecified site 223.0
Lipomyoma (M8860/0)
  specified site — *see* Neoplasm, connective
      tissue, benign
  unspecified site 223.0
Lipomyxoma (M8852/0) — *see* Lipoma, by site
Lipomyxosarcoma (M8852/3) — *see* Neoplasm,
      connective tissue, malignant
Lipophagocytosis 289.8
Lipoproteinemia (alpha) 272.4
  broad-beta 272.2
  floating-beta 272.2
  hyper-pre-beta 272.1
Lipoproteinosis (Rössle-Urbach-Wiethe) 272.8
Liposarcoma (M8850/3) — *see also* Neoplasm,
      connective tissue, malignant
  differentiated type (M8851/3) — *see* Neoplasm,
      connective tissue, malignant
  embryonal (M8852/3) — *see* Neoplasm,
      connective tissue, malignant
  mixed type (M8855/3) — *see* Neoplasm,
      connective tissue, malignant
  myxoid (M8852/3) — *see* Neoplasm, connective
      tissue, malignant
  pleomorphic (M8854/3) — *see* Neoplasm,
      connective tissue, malignant
  round cell (M8853/3) — *see* Neoplasm,
      connective tissue, malignant
  well differentiated type (M8851/3) — *see*
      Neoplasm, connective tissue, malignant
Lipsynovitis prepatellaris 272.8
Lipping
  cervix 622.0
  spine (*see also* Spondylosis) 721.90
  vertebra (*see also* Spondylosis) 721.90
Lip pits (mucus), congenital 750.25
Lipschütz disease or ulcer 616.50
Lipuria 791.1
  bilharziasis 120.0
Liquefaction, vitreous humor 379.21
Lisping 307.9
Lissauer's paralysis 094.1
Lissencephalia, lissencephaly 742.2
Listerellose 027.0
Listeriose 027.0
Listeriosis 027.0
  congenital 771.2
  fetal 771.2
  suspected fetal damage affecting management
      of pregnancy 655.4 ✓5ᵗʰ
Listlessness 780.79
Lithemia 790.6
Lithiasis — *see also* Calculus
  hepatic (duct) — *see* Choledocholithiasis
  urinary 592.9
Lithopedion 779.9
  affecting management of pregnancy 656.8 ✓5ᵗʰ
Lithosis (occupational) 502
  with tuberculosis — *see* Tuberculosis,
      pulmonary
Lithuria 791.9
Litigation V62.5
Little
  league elbow 718.82
  stroke syndrome 435.9
Little's disease — *see* Palsy, cerebral
Littre's
  gland — *see* condition
  hernia — *see* Hernia, Littre's
Littritis (*see also* Urethritis) 597.89
Livedo 782.61
  annularis 782.61
  racemose 782.61
  reticularis 782.61
Live flesh 781.0

Liver — *see also* condition
  donor V59.6
Livida, asphyxia
  newborn 768.6
Living
  alone V60.3
      with handicapped person V60.4
Lloyd's syndrome 258.1
Loa loa 125.2
Loasis 125.2
Lobe, lobar — *see* condition
Lobo's disease or blastomycosis 116.2
Lobomycosis 116.2
Lobotomy syndrome 310.0
Lobstein's disease (brittle bones and blue sclera)
      756.51
Lobster-claw hand 755.58
Lobulation (congenital) — *see also* Anomaly,
      specified type NEC, by site
  kidney, fetal 753.3
  liver, abnormal 751.69
  spleen 759.0
Lobule, lobular — *see* condition
Local, localized — *see* condition
Locked bowel or intestine (*see also* Obstruction,
      intestine) 560.9
Locked-in state 344.81
Locked twins 660.5 ✓5ᵗʰ
  affecting fetus or newborn 763.1
Locking
  joint (*see also* Derangement, joint) 718.90
  knee 717.9
Lockjaw (*see also* Tetanus) 037
Locomotor ataxia (progressive) 094.0
Löffler's
  endocarditis 421.0
  eosinophilia or syndrome 518.3
  pneumonia 518.3
  syndrome (eosinophilic pneumonitis) 518.3
Löfgren's syndrome (sarcoidosis) 135
Loiasis 125.2
  eyelid 125.2 [373.6]
Loneliness V62.89
Lone star fever 082.8
Long labor 662.1 ✓5ᵗʰ
  affecting fetus or newborn 763.89
  first stage 662.0 ✓5ᵗʰ
  second stage 662.2 ✓5ᵗʰ
Longitudinal stripes or grooves, nails 703.8
  congenital 757.5
Long-term (current) drug use V58.69
  antibiotics V58.62
  anticoagulants V58.61
Loop
  intestine (*see also* Volvulus) 560.2
  intrascleral nerve 379.29
  vascular on papilla (optic) 743.57
Loose — *see also* condition
  body
      in tendon sheath 727.82
      joint 718.10
          ankle 718.17
          elbow 718.12
          foot 718.17
          hand 718.14
          hip 718.15
          knee 717.6
          multiple sites 718.19
          pelvic region 718.15
          prosthetic implant — *see* Complications,
              mechanical
          shoulder (region) 718.11
          specified site NEC 718.18
          wrist 718.13
  cartilage (joint) (*see also* Loose, body, joint)
      718.1 ✓5ᵗʰ
      knee 717.6
  facet (vertebral) 724.9
  prosthetic implant — *see* Complications,
      mechanical

Loose — *see also* condition — *continued*
  sesamoid, joint (*see also* Loose, body, joint)
      718.1 ✓5ᵗʰ
  tooth, teeth 525.8
Loosening epiphysis 732.9
Looser (-Debray) -Milkman syndrome
  (osteomalacia with pseudofractures) 268.2
Lop ear (deformity) 744.29
Lorain's disease or syndrome (pituitary
      dwarfism) 253.3
Lorain-Levi syndrome (pituitary dwarfism) 253.3
Lordosis (acquired) (postural) 737.20
  congenital 754.2
  due to or associated with
      Charcôt-Marie-Tooth disease 356.1 [737.42]
      mucopolysaccharidosis 277.5 [737.42]
      neurofibromatosis 237.71 [737.42]
      osteitis
          deformans 731.0 [737.42]
          fibrosa cystica 252.0 [737.42]
      osteoporosis (*see also* Osteoporosis)
          733.00 [737.42]
      poliomyelitis (*see also* Poliomyelitis)
          138 [737.42]
      tuberculosis (*see also* Tuberculosis)
          015.0 ✓5ᵗʰ [737.42]
  late effect of rickets 268.1 [737.42]
  postlaminectomy 737.21
  postsurgical NEC 737.22
  rachitic 268.1 [737.42]
  specified NEC 737.29
  tuberculous (*see also* Tuberculosis)
      015.0 ✓5ᵗʰ [737.42]
Loss
  appetite 783.0
      hysterical 300.11
      nonorganic origin 307.59
      psychogenic 307.59
  blood — *see* Hemorrhage
  central vision 368.41
  consciousness 780.09
      transient 780.2
  control, sphincter, rectum 787.6
      nonorganic origin 307.7
  ear ossicle, partial 385.24
  elasticity, skin 782.8
  extremity or member, traumatic, current — *see*
      Amputation, traumatic
  fluid (acute) 276.5
      with
          hypernatremia 276.0
          hyponatremia 276.1
      fetus or newborn 775.5
  hair 704.00
  hearing — *see also* Deafness
      central 389.14
      conductive (air) 389.00
          with sensorineural hearing loss 389.2
          combined types 389.08
          external ear 389.01
          inner ear 389.04
          middle ear 389.03
          multiple types 389.08
          tympanic membrane 389.02
      mixed type 389.2
      nerve 389.12
      neural 389.12
      noise-induced 388.12
      perceptive NEC (*see also* Loss, hearing,
          sensorineural) 389.10
      sensorineural 389.10
          with conductive hearing loss 389.2
          central 389.14
          combined types 389.18
          multiple types 389.18
          neural 389.12
          sensory 389.11
      sensory 389.11
      specified type NEC 389.8
      sudden NEC 388.2
  height 781.91
  labyrinthine reactivity (unilateral) 386.55
      bilateral 386.56
  memory (*see also* Amnesia) 780.99 ▲
      mild, following organic brain damage 310.1

Loss — Lymphadenitis (left margin vertical text)

Loss — *continued*
  mind (*see also* Psychosis) 298.9
  organ or part — *see* Absence, by site, acquired
  sensation 782.0
  sense of
    smell (*see also* Disturbance, sensation) 781.1
    taste (*see also* Disturbance, sensation) 781.1
    touch (*see also* Disturbance, sensation) 781.1
  sight (acquired) (complete) (congenital) *see* Blindness
  spinal fluid
    headache 349.0
  substance of
    bone (*see also* Osteoporosis) 733.00
    cartilage 733.99
      ear 380.32
    vitreous (humor) 379.26
  tooth, teeth
    acquired 525.10
      due to
        caries 525.13
        extraction 525.10
        periodontal disease 525.12
        specified NEC 525.19
        trauma 525.11
  vision, visual (*see also* Blindness) 369.9
    both eyes (*see also* Blindness, both eyes) 369.3
    complete (*see also* Blindness, both eyes) 369.00
    one eye 369.8
    sudden 368.11
    transient 368.12
  vitreous 379.26
  voice (*see also* Aphonia) 784.41
  weight (cause unknown) 783.21
Lou Gehrig's disease 335.20
Louis-Bar syndrome (ataxia-telangiectasia) 334.8
Louping ill 063.1
Lousiness — *see* Lice
Low
  back syndrome 724.2
  basal metabolic rate (BMR) 794.7
  birthweight 765.1 ✓5ᵗʰ
    extreme (less than 1000 grams) 765.0 ✓5ᵗʰ
    for gestational age 764.0 ✓5ᵗʰ
    status (*see also* Status, low birth weight) V21.30
  bladder compliance 596.52
  blood pressure (*see also* Hypotension) 458.9
    reading (incidental) (isolated) (nonspecific) 796.3
  cardiac reserve — *see* Disease, heart
  compliance bladder 596.52
  frequency deafness — *see* Disorder, hearing
  function — *see also* Hypofunction
    kidney (*see also* Disease, renal) 593.9
    liver 573.9
  hemoglobin 285.9
  implantation, placenta — *see* Placenta, previa
  insertion, placenta — *see* placenta, previa
  lying
    kidney 593.0
    organ or site, congenital — *see* Malposition, congenital
    placenta — *see* Placenta, previa
  output syndrome (cardiac) (*see also* Failure, heart) 428.9
  platelets (blood) (*see also* Thrombocytopenia) 287.5
  reserve, kidney (*see also* Disease, renal) 593.9
  salt syndrome 593.9
  tension glaucoma 365.12
  vision 369.9
    both eyes 369.20
    one eye 369.70
Lowe (-Terrey-MacLachlan) syndrome (oculocerebrorenal dystrophy) 270.8
Lower extremity — *see* condition
Lown (-Ganong) -Levine syndrome (short P-R interval, normal QRS complex, and paroxysmal supraventricular tachycardia) 426.81

LSD reaction (*see also* Abuse, drugs, nondependent) 305.3 ✓5ᵗʰ
L-shaped kidney 753.3
Lucas-Championnière disease (fibrinous bronchitis) 466.0
Lucey-Driscoll syndrome (jaundice due to delayed conjugation) 774.30
Ludwig's
  angina 528.3
  disease (submaxillary cellulitis) 528.3
Lues (venerea), luetic — *see* Syphilis
Luetscher's syndrome (dehydration) 276.5
Lumbago 724.2
  due to displacement, intervertebral disc 722.10
Lumbalgia 724.2
  due to displacement, intervertebral disc 722.10
Lumbar — *see* condition
Lumbarization, vertebra 756.15
Lumbermen's itch 133.8
Lump — *see also* Mass
  abdominal 789.3 ✓5ᵗʰ
  breast 611.72
  chest 786.6
  epigastric 789.3 ✓5ᵗʰ
  head 784.2
  kidney 753.3
  liver 789.1
  lung 786.6
  mediastinal 786.6
  neck 784.2
  nose or sinus 784.2
  pelvic 789.3 ✓5ᵗʰ
  skin 782.2
  substernal 786.6
  throat 784.2
  umbilicus 789.3 ✓5ᵗʰ
Lunacy (*see also* Psychosis) 298.9
Lunatomalacia 732.3
Lung — *see also* condition
  donor V59.8
  drug addict's 417.8
  mainliners' 417.8
  vanishing 492.0
Lupoid (miliary) **of Boeck** 135
Lupus 710.0
  Cazenave's (erythematosus) 695.4
  discoid (local) 695.4
  disseminated 710.0
  erythematosus (discoid) (local) 695.4
    disseminated 710.0
    eyelid 373.34
    systemic 710.0
      with
        encephalitis 710.0 [323.8]
        lung involvement 710.0 [517.8]
      inhibitor (presence of) 286.5
  exedens 017.0 ✓5ᵗʰ
  eyelid (*see also* Tuberculosis) 017.0 ✓5ᵗʰ [373.4]
  Hilliard's 017.0 ✓5ᵗʰ
  hydralazine
    correct substance properly administered 695.4
    overdose or wrong substance given or taken 972.6
  miliaris disseminatus faciei 017.0 ✓5ᵗʰ
  nephritis 710.0 [583.81]
    acute 710.0 [580.81]
    chronic 710.0 [582.81]
  nontuberculous, not disseminated 695.4
  pernio (Besnier) 135
  tuberculous (*see also* Tuberculosis) 017.0 ✓5ᵗʰ
    eyelid (*see also* Tuberculosis) 017.0 ✓5ᵗʰ [373.4]
  vulgaris 017.0 ✓5ᵗʰ
Luschka's joint disease 721.90
Luteinoma (M8610/0) 220
Lutembacher's disease or syndrome (atrial septal defect with mitral stenosis) 745.5
Luteoma (M8610/0) 220
Lutz-Miescher disease (elastosis perforans serpiginosa) 701.1
Lutz-Splendore-de Almeida disease (Brazilian blastomycosis) 116.1

Luxatio
  bulbi due to birth injury 767.8
  coxae congenita (*see also* Dislocation, hip, congenital) 754.30
  erecta — *see* Dislocation, shoulder
  imperfecta — *see* Sprain, by site
  perinealis — *see* Dislocation, hip
Luxation — *see also* Dislocation, by site
  eyeball 360.81
    due to birth injury 767.8
    lateral 376.36
  genital organs (external) NEC — *see* Wound, open, genital organs
  globe (eye) 360.81
    lateral 376.36
  lacrimal gland (postinfectional) 375.16
  lens (old) (partial) 379.32
    congenital 743.37
      syphilitic 090.49 [379.32]
    Marfan's disease 090.49
    spontaneous 379.32
  penis — *see* Wound, open, penis
  scrotum — *see* Wound, open, scrotum
  testis — *see* Wound, open, testis
L-xyloketosuria 271.8
Lycanthropy (*see also* Psychosis) 298.9
Lyell's disease or syndrome (toxic epidermal necrolysis) 695.1
  due to drug
    correct substance properly administered 695.1
    overdose or wrong substance given or taken 977.9
      specified drug — *see* Table of Drugs and Chemicals
Lyme disease 088.81
Lymph
  gland or node — *see* condition
  scrotum (*see also* Infestation, filarial) 125.9
Lymphadenitis 289.3
  with
    abortion — *see* Abortion, by type, with sepsis
    ectopic pregnancy (*see also* categories 633.0-633.9) 639.0
    molar pregnancy (*see also* categories 630-632) 639.0
  acute 683
    mesenteric 289.2
  any site, except mesenteric 289.3
    acute 683
    chronic 289.1
    mesenteric (acute) (chronic) (nonspecific) (subacute) 289.2
    subacute 289.1
      mesenteric 289.2
  breast, puerperal, postpartum 675.2 ✓5ᵗʰ
  chancroidal (congenital) 099.0
  chronic 289.1
    mesenteric 289.2
  dermatopathic 695.89
  due to
    anthracosis (occupational) 500
    Brugia (Wuchereria) malayi 125.1
    diphtheria (toxin) 032.89
    lymphogranuloma venereum 099.1
    Wuchereria bancrofti 125.0
  following
    abortion 639.0
    ectopic or molar pregnancy 639.0
  generalized 289.3
  gonorrheal 098.89
  granulomatous 289.1
  infectional 683
  mesenteric (acute) (chronic) (nonspecific) (subacute) 289.2
    due to Bacillus typhi 002.0
    tuberculous (*see also* Tuberculosis) 014.8 ✓5ᵗʰ
  mycobacterial 031.8
  purulent 683
  pyogenic 683
  regional 078.3
  septic 683
  streptococcal 683
  subacute, unspecified site 289.1

Lymphadenitis — *continued*
 suppurative 683
 syphilitic (early) (secondary) 091.4
  late 095.8
 tuberculous — *see* Tuberculosis, lymph gland
 venereal 099.1
Lymphadenoid goiter 245.2
Lymphadenopathy (general) 785.6
 due to toxoplasmosis (acquired) 130.7
  congenital (active) 771.2
Lymphadenopathy-associated virus (disease)
  (illness) (infection) — *see* Human
  immunodeficiency virus (disease) (illness)
  (infection)
Lymphadenosis 785.6
 acute 075
Lymphangiectasis 457.1
 conjunctiva 372.89
 postinfectional 457.1
 scrotum 457.1
Lymphangiectatic elephantiasis, nonfilarial
 457.1
Lymphangioendothelioma (M9170/0) 228.1
 malignant (M9170/3) — *see* Neoplasm,
  connective tissue, malignant
Lymphangioma (M9170/0) 228.1
 capillary (M9171/0) 228.1
 cavernous (M9172/0) 228.1
 cystic (M9173/0) 228.1
 malignant (M9170/3) — *see* Neoplasm,
  connective tissue, malignant
Lymphangiomyoma (M9174/0) 228.1
Lymphangiomyomatosis (M9174/1) — *see*
 Neoplasm, connective tissue, uncertain
 behavior
Lymphangiosarcoma (M9170/3) — *see*
 Neoplasm, connective tissue, malignant
Lymphangitis 457.2
 with
  abortion — *see* Abortion, by type, with
   sepsis
  abscess — *see* Abscess, by site
  cellulitis — *see* Abscess, by site
  ectopic pregnancy (*see also* categories
   633.0-633.9) 639.0
  molar pregnancy (*see also* categories 630-
   632) 639.0
 acute (with abscess or cellulitis) 682.9
  specified site — *see* Abscess, by site
 breast, puerperal, postpartum 675.2 ✓5th
 chancroidal 099.0
 chronic (any site) 457.2
 due to
  Brugia (Wuchereria) malayi 125.1
  Wuchereria bancrofti 125.0
 following
  abortion 639.0
  ectopic or molar pregnancy 639.0
 gangrenous 457.2
 penis
  acute 607.2
  gonococcal (acute) 098.0
   chronic or duration of 2 months or more
    098.2
 puerperal, postpartum, childbirth 670 ✓4th
 strumous, tuberculous (*see also* Tuberculosis)
  017.2 ✓5th
 subacute (any site) 457.2
 tuberculous — *see* Tuberculosis, lymph gland
Lymphatic (vessel) — *see* condition
Lymphatism 254.8
 scrofulous (*see also* Tuberculosis) 017.2 ✓5th
Lymphectasia 457.1
Lymphedema (*see also* Elephantiasis) 457.1
 acquired (chronic) 457.1
 chronic hereditary 757.0
 congenital 757.0
 idiopathic hereditary 757.0
 praecox 457.1
 secondary 457.1
 surgical NEC 997.99
  postmastectomy (syndrome) 457.0
Lymph-hemangioma (M9120/0) — *see*
 Hemangioma, by site

Lymphoblastic — *see* condition
Lymphoblastoma (diffuse) (M9630/3) 200.1 ✓5th
 giant follicular (M9690/3) 202.0 ✓5th
 macrofollicular (M9690/3) 202.0 ✓5th
Lymphoblastosis, acute benign 075
Lymphocele 457.8
Lymphocythemia 288.8
Lymphocytic — *see also* condition
 chorioencephalitis (acute) (serous) 049.0
 choriomeningitis (acute) (serous) 049.0
Lymphocytoma (diffuse) (malignant) (M9620/3)
 200.1 ✓5th
Lymphocytomatosis (M9620/3) 200.1 ✓5th
Lymphocytopenia 288.8
Lymphocytosis (symptomatic) 288.8
 infectious (acute) 078.89
Lymphoepithelioma (M8082/3) — *see* Neoplasm,
 by site, malignant
Lymphogranuloma (malignant) (M9650/3)
 201.9 ✓5th
 inguinale 099.1
 venereal (any site) 099.1
  with stricture of rectum 099.1
 venereum 099.1
Lymphogranulomatosis (malignant) (M9650/3)
 201.9 ✓5th
 benign (Boeck's sarcoid) (Schaumann's) 135
 Hodgkin's (M9650/3) 201.9 ✓5th
Lymphoid — *see* condition
Lympholeukoblastoma (M9850/3) 207.8 ✓5th
Lympholeukosarcoma (M9850/3) 207.8 ✓5th
Lymphoma (malignant) (M9590/3) 202.8 ✓5th

> *Note* — *Use the following fifth-digit*
> *subclassification with categories 200–202:*
>
> 0 *unspecified site*
> 1 *lymph nodes of head, face, and*
>   *neck*
> 2 *intrathoracic lymph nodes*
> 3 *intra-abdominal lymph nodes*
> 4 *lymph nodes of axilla and upper*
>   *limb*
> 5 *lymph nodes of inguinal region and*
>   *lower limb*
> 6 *intrapelvic lymph nodes*
> 7 *spleen*
> 8 *lymph nodes of multiple sites*

 benign (M9590/0) — *see* Neoplasm, by site,
  benign
 Burkitt's type (lymphoblastic) (undifferentiated)
  (M9750/3) 200.2 ✓5th
 Castleman's (mediastinal lymph node
  hyperplasia) 785.6
 centroblastic-centrocytic
  diffuse (M9614/3) 202.8 ✓5th
  follicular (M9692/3) 202.0 ✓5th
 centroblastic type (diffuse) (M9632/3)
  202.8 ✓5th
  follicular (M9697/3) 202.0 ✓5th
 centrocytic (M9622/3) 202.8 ✓5th
 compound (M9613/3) 200.8 ✓5th
 convoluted cell type (lymphoblastic) (M9602/3)
  202.8 ✓5th
 diffuse NEC (M9590/3) 202.8 ✓5th
 follicular (giant) (M9690/3) 202.0 ✓5th
  center cell (diffuse) (M9615/3) 202.8 ✓5th
  cleaved (diffuse) (M9623/3) 202.8 ✓5th
   follicular (M9695/3) 202.0 ✓5th
  non-cleaved (diffuse) (M9633/3)
   202.8 ✓5th
   follicular (M9698/3) 202.0 ✓5th
  centroblastic-centrocytic (M9692/3)
   202.0 ✓5th
  centroblastic type (M9697/3) 202.0 ✓5th
  lymphocytic
   intermediate differentiation (M9694/3)
    202.0 ✓5th
   poorly differentiated (M9696/3) 202.0 ✓5th
  mixed (cell type) (lymphocytic-histiocytic)
   (small cell and large cell) (M9691/3)
    202.0 ✓5th

Lymphoma — *continued*
 germinocytic (M9622/3) 202.8 ✓5th
 giant, follicular or follicle (M9690/3) 202.0 ✓5th
 histiocytic (diffuse) (M9640/3) 200.0 ✓5th
  nodular (M9642/3) 200.0 ✓5th
  pleomorphic cell type (M9641/3) 200.0 ✓5th
 Hodgkin's (M9650/3) (*see also* Disease,
  Hodgkin's) 201.9 ✓5th
 immunoblastic (type) (M9612/3) 200.8 ✓5th
 large cell (M9640/3) 200.0 ✓5th
  nodular (M9642/3) 200.0 ✓5th
  pleomorphic cell type (M9641/3) 200.0 ✓5th
 lymphoblastic (diffuse) (M9630/3) 200.1 ✓5th
  Burkitt's type (M9750/3) 200.2 ✓5th
  convoluted cell type (M9602/3) 202.8 ✓5th
 lymphocytic (cell type) (diffuse) (M9620/3)
  200.1 ✓5th
  with plasmacytoid differentiation, diffuse
   (M9611/3) 200.8 ✓5th
  intermediate differentiation (diffuse)
   (M9621/3) 200.1 ✓5th
   follicular (M9694/3) 202.0 ✓5th
   nodular (M9694/3) 202.0 ✓5th
  nodular (M9690/3) 202.0 ✓5th
  poorly differentiated (diffuse) (M9630/3)
   200.1 ✓5th
   follicular (M9696/3) 202.0 ✓5th
   nodular (M9696/3) 202.0 ✓5th
  well differentiated (diffuse) (M9620/3)
   200.1 ✓5th
   follicular (M9693/3) 202.0 ✓5th
   nodular (M9693/3) 202.0 ✓5th
 lymphocytic-histiocytic, mixed (diffuse)
  (M9613/3) 200.8 ✓5th
  follicular (M9691/3) 202.0 ✓5th
  nodular (M9691/3) 202.0 ✓5th
 lymphoplasmacytoid type (M9611/3) 200.8 ✓5th
 lymphosarcoma type (M9610/3) 200.1 ✓5th
 macrofollicular (M9690/3) 202.0 ✓5th
 mixed cell type (diffuse) (M9613/3) 200.8 ✓5th
  follicular (M9691/3) 202.0 ✓5th
  nodular (M9691/3) 202.0 ✓5th
 nodular (M9690/3) 202.0 ✓5th
  histiocytic (M9642/3) 200.0 ✓5th
  lymphocytic (M9690/3) 202.0 ✓5th
   intermediate differentiation (M9694/3)
    202.0 ✓5th
   poorly differentiated (M9696/3) 202.0 ✓5th
  mixed (cell type) (lymphocytic-histiocytic)
   (small cell and large cell) (M9691/3)
    202.0 ✓5th
 non-Hodgkin's type NEC (M9591/3) 202.8 ✓5th
 reticulum cell (type) (M9640/3) 200.0 ✓5th
 small cell and large cell, mixed (diffuse)
  (M9613/3) 200.8 ✓5th
  follicular (M9691/3) 202.0 ✓5th
  nodular (9691/3) 202.0 ✓5th
 stem cell (type) (M9601/3) 202.8 ✓5th
 T-cell 202.1 ✓5th
 undifferentiated (cell type) (non-Burkitt's)
  (M9600/3) 202.8 ✓5th
  Burkitt's type (M9750/3) 200.2 ✓5th
Lymphomatosis (M9590/3) — *see also*
 Lymphoma
 granulomatous 099.1
Lymphopathia
 venereum 099.1
 veneris 099.1
Lymphopenia 288.8
 familial 279.2
Lymphoreticulosis, benign (of inoculation) 078.3
Lymphorrhea 457.8
Lymphosarcoma (M9610/3) 200.1 ✓5th
 diffuse (M9610/3) 200.1 ✓5th
  with plasmacytoid differentiation (M9611/3)
   200.8 ✓5th
  lymphoplasmacytic (M9611/3) 200.8 ✓5th
 follicular (giant) (M9690/3) 202.0 ✓5th
  lymphoblastic (M9696/3) 202.0 ✓5th
  lymphocytic, intermediate differentiation
   (M9694/3) 202.0 ✓5th
  mixed cell type (M9691/3) 202.0 ✓5th
 giant follicular (M9690/3) 202.0 ✓5th
 Hodgkin's (M9650/3) 201.9 ✓5th
 immunoblastic (M9612/3) 200.8 ✓5th

✓4th Fourth-digit Required ✓5th Fifth-digit Required ▶◀ Revised Text ● New Line ▲ Revised Code

Lymphosarcoma — *continued*
  lymphoblastic (diffuse) (M9630/3) 200.1 ✓5ᵗʰ
    follicular (M9696/3) 202.0 ✓5ᵗʰ
    nodular (M9696/3) 202.0 ✓5ᵗʰ
  lymphocytic (diffuse) (M9620/3) 200.1 ✓5ᵗʰ
    intermediate differentiation (diffuse)
      (M9621/3) 200.1 ✓5ᵗʰ
      follicular (M9694/3) 202.0 ✓5ᵗʰ
      nodular (M9694/3) 202.0 ✓5ᵗʰ
  mixed cell type (diffuse) (M9613/3) 200.8 ✓5ᵗʰ
    follicular (M9691/3) 202.0 ✓5ᵗʰ
    nodular (M9691/3) 202.0 ✓5ᵗʰ
  nodular (M9690/3) 202.0 ✓5ᵗʰ
    lymphoblastic (M9696/3) 202.0 ✓5ᵗʰ
    lymphocytic, intermediate differentiation
      (M9694/3) 202.0 ✓5ᵗʰ
    mixed cell type (M9691/3) 202.0 ✓5ᵗʰ
  prolymphocytic (M9631/3) 200.1 ✓5ᵗʰ
  reticulum cell (M9640/3) 200.0 ✓5ᵗʰ
Lymphostasis 457.8
Lypemania (*see also* Melancholia) 296.2 ✓5ᵗʰ
Lyssa 071

M

Macacus ear 744.29
Maceration
  fetus (cause not stated) 779.9
  wet feet, tropical (syndrome) 991.4
Machado-Joseph disease 334.8
Machupo virus hemorrhagic fever 078.7
Macleod's syndrome (abnormal transradiancy, one lung) 492.8
Macrocephalia, macrocephaly 756.0
Macrocheilia (congenital) 744.81
Macrochilia (congenital) 744.81
Macrocolon (congenital) 751.3
Macrocornea 743.41
  associated with buphthalmos 743.22
Macrocytic — *see* condition
Macrocytosis 289.8
Macrodactylia, macrodactylism (fingers)
  (thumbs) 755.57
  toes 755.65
Macrodontia 520.2
Macroencephaly 742.4
Macrogenia 524.05
Macrogenitosomia (female) (male) (praecox) 255.2
Macrogingivae 523.8
Macroglobulinemia (essential) (idiopathic)
  (monoclonal) (primary) (syndrome)
  (Waldenström's) 273.3
Macroglossia (congenital) 750.15
  acquired 529.8
Macrognathia, macrognathism (congenital)
  524.00
  mandibular 524.02
    alveolar 524.72
  maxillary 524.01
    alveolar 524.71
Macrogyria (congenital) 742.4
Macrohydrocephalus (*see also* Hydrocephalus)
  331.4
Macromastia (*see also* Hypertrophy, breast) 611.1
Macropsia 368.14
Macrosigmoid 564.7
  congenital 751.3
Macrospondylitis, acromegalic 253.0
Macrostomia (congenital) 744.83
Macrotia (external ear) (congenital) 744.22
Macula
  cornea, corneal
    congenital 743.43
      interfering with vision 743.42
    interfering with central vision 371.03
    not interfering with central vision 371.02
  degeneration (*see also* Degeneration, macula)
    362.50
    hereditary (*see also* Dystrophy, retina)
      362.70

Macula — *continued*
  edema, cystoid 362.53
Maculae ceruleae 132.1
Macules and papules 709.8
Maculopathy, toxic 362.55
Madarosis 374.55
Madelung's
  deformity (radius) 755.54
  disease (lipomatosis) 272.8
  lipomatosis 272.8
Madness (*see also* Psychosis) 298.9
  myxedema (acute) 293.0
    subacute 293.1
Madura
  disease (actinomycotic) 039.9
    mycotic 117.4
  foot (actinomycotic) 039.4
    mycotic 117.4
Maduromycosis (actinomycotic) 039.9
  mycotic 117.4
Maffucci's syndrome (dyschondroplasia with hemangiomas) 756.4
Magenblase syndrome 306.4
Main en griffe (acquired) 736.06
  congenital 755.59
Maintenance
  chemotherapy regimen or treatment V58.1
  dialysis regimen or treatment
    extracorporeal (renal) V56.0
    peritoneal V56.8
    renal V56.0
  drug therapy or regimen V58.1
  external fixation NEC V54.89 ▲
  radiotherapy V58.0
  traction NEC V54.89 ▲
Majocchi's
  disease (purpura annularis telangiectodes)
    709.1
  granuloma 110.6
Major — *see* condition
Mal
  cerebral (idiopathic) (*see also* Epilepsy)
    345.9 ✓5ᵗʰ
  comital (*see also* Epilepsy) 345.9 ✓5ᵗʰ
  de los pintos (*see also* Pinta) 103.9
  de Meleda 757.39
  de mer 994.6
  lie — *see* Presentation, fetal
  perforant (*see also* Ulcer, lower extremity)
    707.15
Malabar itch 110.9
  beard 110.0
  foot 110.4
  scalp 110.0
Malabsorption 579.9
  calcium 579.8
  carbohydrate 579.8
  disaccharide 271.3
  drug-induced 579.8
  due to bacterial overgrowth 579.8
  fat 579.8
  folate, congenital 281.2
  galactose 271.1
  glucose-galactose (congenital) 271.3
  intestinal 579.9
  isomaltose 271.3
  lactose (hereditary) 271.3
  methionine 270.4
  monosaccharide 271.8
  postgastrectomy 579.3
  postsurgical 579.3
  protein 579.8
  sucrose (-isomaltose) (congenital) 271.3
  syndrome 579.9
    postgastrectomy 579.3
    postsurgical 579.3
Malacia, bone 268.2
  juvenile (*see also* Rickets) 268.0
  Kienböck's (juvenile) (lunate) (wrist) 732.3
    adult 732.8
Malacoplakia
  bladder 596.8
  colon 569.89
  pelvis (kidney) 593.89

Malacoplakia — *continued*
  ureter 593.89
  urethra 599.84
Malacosteon 268.2
  juvenile (*see also* Rickets) 268.0
Maladaptation — *see* Maladjustment
Maladie de Roger 745.4
Maladjustment
  conjugal V61.10
    involving divorce or estrangement V61.0
  educational V62.3
  family V61.9
    specified circumstance NEC V61.8
  marital V61.10
    involving divorce or estrangement V61.0
  occupational V62.2
  simple, adult (*see also* Reaction, adjustment)
    309.9
  situational acute (*see also* Reaction,
    adjustment) 309.9
  social V62.4
Malaise 780.79
Malakoplakia — *see* Malacoplakia
Malaria, malarial (fever) 084.6
  algid 084.9
  any type, with
    algid malaria 084.9
    blackwater fever 084.8
    fever
      blackwater 084.8
      hemoglobinuric (bilious) 084.8
    hemoglobinuria, malarial 084.8
    hepatitis 084.9 [573.2]
    nephrosis 084.9 [581.81]
    pernicious complication NEC 084.9
      cardiac 084.9
      cerebral 084.9
  cardiac 084.9
  carrier (suspected) of V02.9
  cerebral 084.9
  complicating pregnancy, childbirth, or
    puerperium 647.4 ✓5ᵗʰ
  congenital 771.2
  congestion, congestive 084.6
    brain 084.9
  continued 084.0
  estivo-autumnal 084.0
  falciparum (malignant tertian) 084.0
  hematinuria 084.8
  hematuria 084.8
  hemoglobinuria 084.8
  hemorrhagic 084.6
  induced (therapeutically) 084.7
    accidental — *see* Malaria, by type
  liver 084.9 [573.2]
  malariae (quartan) 084.2
  malignant (tertian) 084.0
  mixed infections 084.5
  monkey 084.4
  ovale 084.3
  pernicious, acute 084.0
  Plasmodium, P.
    falciparum 084.0
    malariae 084.2
    ovale 084.3
    vivax 084.1
  quartan 084.2
  quotidian 084.0
  recurrent 084.6
    induced (therapeutically) 084.7
      accidental — *see* Malaria, by type
  remittent 084.6
  specified types NEC 084.4
  spleen 084.6
  subtertian 084.0
  tertian (benign) 084.1
    malignant 084.0
  tropical 084.0
  typhoid 084.6
  vivax (benign tertian) 084.1
Malassez's disease (testicular cyst) 608.89
Malassimilation 579.9
Maldescent, testis 752.51

✓4ᵗʰ Fourth-digit Required   ✓5ᵗʰ Fifth-digit Required   ▶◀ Revised Text   ● New Line   ▲ Revised Code

Maldevelopment — see also Anomaly, by site
brain 742.9
colon 751.5
hip (joint) 755.63
congenital dislocation (see also Dislocation, hip, congenital) 754.30
mastoid process 756.0
middle ear, except ossicles 744.03
ossicles 744.04
newborn (not malformation) 764.9
ossicles, ear 744.04
spine 756.10
toe 755.66

Male type pelvis 755.69
with disproportion (fetopelvic) 653.2
affecting fetus or newborn 763.1
causing obstructed labor 660.1
affecting fetus or newborn 763.1

Malformation (congenital) — see also Anomaly
bone 756.9
bursa 756.9
circulatory system NEC 747.9
specified type NEC 747.89
Chiari
type I 348.4
type II (see also Spina bifida) 741.0
type III 742.0
type IV 742.2
cochlea 744.05
digestive system NEC 751.9
lower 751.5
specified type NEC 751.8
upper 750.9
eye 743.9
gum 750.9
heart NEC 746.9
specified type NEC 746.89
valve 746.9
internal ear 744.05
joint NEC 755.9
specified type NEC 755.8
Mondini's (congenital) (malformation, cochlea) 744.05
muscle 756.9
nervous system (central) 742.9
pelvic organs or tissues
in pregnancy or childbirth 654.9
affecting fetus or newborn 763.89
causing obstructed labor 660.2
affecting fetus or newborn 763.1
placenta (see also Placenta, abnormal) 656.7
respiratory organs 748.9
specified type NEC 748.8
Rieger's 743.44
sense organs NEC 742.9
specified type NEC 742.8
skin 757.9
specified type NEC 757.8
spinal cord 742.9
teeth, tooth NEC 520.9
tendon 756.9
throat 750.9
umbilical cord (complicating delivery) 663.9
affecting fetus or newborn 762.6
umbilicus 759.9
urinary system NEC 753.9
specified type NEC 753.8

Malfunction — see also Dysfunction
arterial graft 996.1
cardiac pacemaker 996.01
catheter device — see Complications, mechanical, catheter
colostomy 569.62
cystostomy 997.5
device, implant, or graft NEC — see Complications, mechanical
enteric stoma 569.62
enterostomy 569.62
gastroenteric 536.8
gastrostomy 536.42
nephrostomy 997.5
pacemaker — see Complications, mechanical, pacemaker
prosthetic device, internal — see Complications, mechanical
tracheostomy 519.02

Malfunction — see also Dysfunction — continued
vascular graft or shunt 996.1

Malgaigne's fracture (closed) 808.43
open 808.53

Malherbe's
calcifying epithelioma (M8110/0) — see Neoplasm, skin, benign
tumor (M8110/0) — see Neoplasm, skin, benign

Malibu disease 919.8
infected 919.9

Malignancy (M8000/3) — see Neoplasm, by site, malignant

Malignant — see condition

Malingerer, malingering V65.2

Mallet, finger (acquired) 736.1
congenital 755.59
late effect of rickets 268.1

Malleus 024

Mallory's bodies 034.1

Mallory-Weiss syndrome 530.7

Malnutrition (calorie) 263.9
complicating pregnancy 648.9
degree
first 263.1
second 263.0
third 262
mild 263.1
moderate 263.0
severe 261
protein-calorie 262
fetus 764.2
"light-for-dates" 764.1
following gastrointestinal surgery 579.3
intrauterine or fetal 764.2
fetus or infant "light-for-dates" 764.1
lack of care, or neglect (child) (infant) 995.52
adult 995.84
malignant 260
mild 263.1
moderate 263.0
protein 260
protein-calorie 263.9
severe 262
specified type NEC 263.8
severe 261
protein-calorie NEC 262

Malocclusion (teeth) 524.4
due to
abnormal swallowing 524.5
accessory teeth (causing crowding) 524.3
dentofacial abnormality NEC 524.8
impacted teeth (causing crowding) 524.3
missing teeth 524.3
mouth breathing 524.5
supernumerary teeth (causing crowding) 524.3
thumb sucking 524.5
tongue, lip, or finger habits 524.5
temporomandibular (joint) 524.69

Malposition
cardiac apex (congenital) 746.87
cervix — see Malposition, uterus
congenital
adrenal (gland) 759.1
alimentary tract 751.8
lower 751.5
upper 750.8
aorta 747.21
appendix 751.5
arterial trunk 747.29
artery (peripheral) NEC (see also Malposition, congenital, peripheral vascular system) 747.60
coronary 746.85
pulmonary 747.3
auditory canal 744.29
causing impairment of hearing 744.02
auricle (ear) 744.29
causing impairment of hearing 744.02
cervical 744.43
biliary duct or passage 751.69
bladder (mucosa) 753.8
exteriorized or extroverted 753.5
brachial plexus 742.8

Malposition — continued
congenital — continued
brain tissue 742.4
breast 757.6
bronchus 748.3
cardiac apex 746.87
cecum 751.5
clavicle 755.51
colon 751.5
digestive organ or tract NEC 751.8
lower 751.5
upper 750.8
ear (auricle) (external) 744.29
ossicles 744.04
endocrine (gland) NEC 759.2
epiglottis 748.3
Eustachian tube 744.24
eye 743.8
facial features 744.89
fallopian tube 752.19
finger(s) 755.59
supernumerary 755.01
foot 755.67
gallbladder 751.69
gastrointestinal tract 751.8
genitalia, genital organ(s) or tract
female 752.8
external 752.49
internal NEC 752.8
male 752.8
penis 752.69
glottis 748.3
hand 755.59
heart 746.87
dextrocardia 746.87
with complete transposition of viscera 759.3
hepatic duct 751.69
hip (joint) (see also Dislocation, hip, congenital) 754.30
intestine (large) (small) 751.5
with anomalous adhesions, fixation, or malrotation 751.4
joint NEC 755.8
kidney 753.3
larynx 748.3
limb 755.8
lower 755.69
upper 755.59
liver 751.69
lung (lobe) 748.69
nail(s) 757.5
nerve 742.8
nervous system NEC 742.8
nose, nasal (septum) 748.1
organ or site NEC — see Anomaly, specified type NEC, by site
ovary 752.0
pancreas 751.7
parathyroid (gland) 759.2
patella 755.64
peripheral vascular system 747.60
gastrointestinal 747.61
lower limb 747.64
renal 747.62
specified NEC 747.69
spinal 747.82
upper limb 747.63
pituitary (gland) 759.2
respiratory organ or system NEC 748.9
rib (cage) 756.3
supernumerary in cervical region 756.2
scapula 755.59
shoulder 755.59
spinal cord 742.59
spine 756.19
spleen 759.0
sternum 756.3
stomach 750.7
symphysis pubis 755.69
testis (undescended) 752.51
thymus (gland) 759.2
thyroid (gland) (tissue) 759.2
cartilage 748.3
toe(s) 755.66
supernumerary 755.02
tongue 750.19

Malposition — Martin's disease

Malposition — *continued*
  congenital — *continued*
    trachea 748.3
    uterus 752.3
    vein(s) (peripheral) NEC (*see also*
        Malposition, congenital, peripheral
        vascular system) 747.60
      great 747.49
      portal 747.49
      pulmonary 747.49
    vena cava (inferior) (superior) 747.49
  device, implant, or graft — *see* Complications,
      mechanical
  fetus NEC — (*see also* Presentation, fetal)
      652.9 ✓5ᵗʰ
    with successful version 652.1 ✓5ᵗʰ
      affecting fetus or newborn 763.1
    before labor, affecting fetus or newborn
        761.7
    causing obstructed labor 660.0 ✓5ᵗʰ
    in multiple gestation (one fetus or more)
        652.6 ✓5ᵗʰ
      with locking 660.5 ✓5ᵗʰ
      causing obstructed labor 660.0 ✓5ᵗʰ
  gallbladder — (*see also* Disease, gallbladder)
      575.8
  gastrointestinal tract 569.89
    congenital 751.8
  heart (*see also* Malposition, congenital, heart)
      746.87
  intestine 569.89
    congenital 751.5
  pelvic organs or tissues
    in pregnancy or childbirth 654.4 ✓5ᵗʰ
      affecting fetus or newborn 763.89
      causing obstructed labor 660.2 ✓5ᵗʰ
        affecting fetus or newborn 763.1
  placenta — *see* Placenta, previa
  stomach 537.89
    congenital 750.7
  tooth, teeth (with impaction) 524.3
  uterus or cervix (acquired) (acute) (adherent)
      (any degree) (asymptomatic)
      (postinfectional) (postpartal, old) 621.6
    anteflexion or anteversion (*see also*
        Anteversion, uterus) 621.6
    congenital 752.3
    flexion 621.6
      lateral (*see also* Lateroversion, uterus)
          621.6
    in pregnancy or childbirth 654.4 ✓5ᵗʰ
      affecting fetus or newborn 763.89
      causing obstructed labor 660.2 ✓5ᵗʰ
        affecting fetus or newborn 763.1
    inversion 621.6
    lateral (flexion) (version) (*see also*
        Lateroversion, uterus) 621.6
    lateroflexion (*see also* Lateroversion, uterus)
        621.6
    lateroversion (*see also* Lateroversion, uterus)
        621.6
    retroflexion or retroversion (*see also*
        Retroversion, uterus) 621.6

Malposture 729.9

Malpresentation, fetus — (*see also* Presentation,
    fetal) 652.9 ✓5ᵗʰ

Malrotation
  cecum 751.4
  colon 751.4
  intestine 751.4
  kidney 753.3

Malta fever (*see also* Brucellosis) 023.9

Maltosuria 271.3

Maltreatment (of)
  adult 995.80
    emotional 995.82
    multiple forms 995.85
    neglect (nutritional) 995.84
    physical 995.81
    psychological 995.82
    sexual 995.83
  child 995.50
    emotional 995.51
    multiple forms 995.59
    neglect (nutritional) 995.52

Maltreatment — *continued*
  child — *continued*
    physical 995.54
      shaken infant syndrome 995.55
    psychological 995.51
    sexual 995.53
  spouse 995.80 — (*see also* Maltreatment,
      adult)

Malt workers' lung 495.4

Malum coxae senilis 715.25

Malunion, fracture 733.81

Mammillitis (*see also* Mastitis) 611.0
  puerperal, postpartum 675.2 ✓5ᵗʰ

Mammitis (*see also* Mastitis) 611.0
  puerperal, postpartum 675.2 ✓5ᵗʰ

Mammographic microcalcification 793.81

Mammoplasia 611.1

Management
  contraceptive V25.9
    specified type NEC V25.8
  procreative V26.9
    specified type NEC V26.8

Mangled NEC (*see also* nature and site of injury)
    959.9

Mania (monopolar) — (*see also* Psychosis,
    affective) 296.0 ✓5ᵗʰ
  alcoholic (acute) (chronic) 291.9
  Bell's — *see* Mania, chronic
  chronic 296.0 ✓5ᵗʰ
    recurrent episode 296.1 ✓5ᵗʰ
    single episode 296.0 ✓5ᵗʰ
  compulsive 300.3
  delirious (acute) 296.0 ✓5ᵗʰ
    recurrent episode 296.1 ✓5ᵗʰ
    single episode 296.0 ✓5ᵗʰ
  epileptic (*see also* Epilepsy) 345.4 ✓5ᵗʰ
  hysterical 300.10
  inhibited 296.89
  puerperal (after delivery) 296.0 ✓5ᵗʰ
    recurrent episode 296.1 ✓5ᵗʰ
    single episode 296.0 ✓5ᵗʰ
  recurrent episode 296.1 ✓5ᵗʰ
  senile 290.8
  single episode 296.0 ✓5ᵗʰ
  stupor 296.89
  stuporous 296.89
  unproductive 296.89

**Manic-depressive insanity, psychosis, reaction,
  or syndrome** (*see also* Psychosis, affective)
    296.80
  circular (alternating) 296.7
    currently
      depressed 296.5 ✓5ᵗʰ
      episode unspecified 296.7
      hypomanic, previously depressed
          296.4 ✓5ᵗʰ
      manic 296.4 ✓5ᵗʰ
    mixed 296.6 ✓5ᵗʰ
  depressed (type), depressive 296.2 ✓5ᵗʰ
    atypical 296.82
    recurrent episode 296.3 ✓5ᵗʰ
    single episode 296.2 ✓5ᵗʰ
  hypomanic 296.0 ✓5ᵗʰ
    recurrent episode 296.1 ✓5ᵗʰ
    single episode 296.0 ✓5ᵗʰ
  manic 296.0 ✓5ᵗʰ
    atypical 296.81
    recurrent episode 296.1 ✓5ᵗʰ
    single episode 296.0 ✓5ᵗʰ
  mixed NEC 296.89
  perplexed 296.89
  stuporous 296.89

Manifestations, rheumatoid
  lungs 714.81
  pannus — *see* Arthritis, rheumatoid
  subcutaneous nodules — *see* Arthritis,
      rheumatoid

Mankowsky's syndrome (familial dysplastic
    osteopathy) 731.2

Mannoheptulosuria 271.8

Mannosidosis 271.8

Manson's
  disease (schistosomiasis) 120.1
  pyosis (pemphigus contagiosus) 684
  schistosomiasis 120.1

Mansonellosis 125.5

Manual — *see* condition

Maple bark disease 495.6

Maple bark-strippers' lung 495.6

Maple syrup (urine) disease or syndrome 270.3

Marable's syndrome (celiac artery compression)
    447.4

Marasmus 261
  brain 331.9
  due to malnutrition 261
  intestinal 569.89
  nutritional 261
  senile 797
  tuberculous NEC (*see also* Tuberculosis)
      011.9 ✓5ᵗʰ

Marble
  bones 756.52
  skin 782.61

Marburg disease (virus) 078.89

March
  foot 733.94 ▲
  hemoglobinuria 283.2

Marchand multiple nodular hyperplasia (liver)
    571.5

Marchesani (-Weill) syndrome (brachymorphism
    and ectopia lentis) 759.89

Marchiafava (-Bignami) disease or syndrome
    341.8

Marchiafava-Micheli syndrome (paroxysmal
    nocturnal hemoglobinuria) 283.2

Marcus Gunn's syndrome (jaw-winking
    syndrome) 742.8

Marfan's
  congenital syphilis 090.49
  disease 090.49
  syndrome (arachnodactyly) 759.82
    meaning congenital syphilis 090.49
      with luxation of lens 090.49 [379.32]

Marginal
  implantation, placenta — *see* Placenta, previa
  placenta — *see* Placenta, previa
  sinus (hemorrhage) (rupture) 641.2 ✓5ᵗʰ
    affecting fetus or newborn 762.1

Marie's
  cerebellar ataxia 334.2
  syndrome (acromegaly) 253.0

Marie-Bamberger disease or syndrome
    (hypertrophic) (pulmonary) (secondary)
    731.2
  idiopathic (acropachyderma) 757.39
  primary (acropachyderma) 757.39

Marie-Charcôt-Tooth neuropathic atrophy,
    muscle 356.1

Marie-Strümpell arthritis or disease (ankylosing
    spondylitis) 720.0

Marihuana, marijuana
  abuse (*see also* Abuse, drugs, nondependent)
      305.2 ✓5ᵗʰ
  dependence (*see also* Dependence) 304.3 ✓5ᵗʰ

Marion's disease (bladder neck obstruction)
    596.0

Marital conflict V61.10

Mark
  port wine 757.32
  raspberry 757.32
  strawberry 757.32
  stretch 701.3
  tattoo 709.09

Maroteaux-Lamy syndrome
    (mucopolysaccharidosis VI) 277.5

Marriage license examination V70.3

Marrow (bone)
  arrest 284.9
  megakaryocytic 287.3
  poor function 289.9

Marseilles fever 082.1

Marsh's disease (exophthalmic goiter) 242.0 ✓5ᵗʰ

Marshall's (hidrotic) **ectodermal dysplasia**
    757.31

Marsh fever (*see also* Malaria) 084.6

Martin's disease 715.27

Martin-Albright syndrome
(pseudohypoparathyroidism) 275.49

Martorell-Fabre syndrome (pulseless disease) 446.7

Masculinization, female, with adrenal hyperplasia 255.2

Masculinovoblastoma (M8670/0) 220

Masochism 302.83

Masons' lung 502

Mass
  abdominal 789.3 ✓5th
  anus 787.99
  bone 733.90
  breast 611.72
  cheek 784.2
  chest 786.6
  cystic — see Cyst
  ear 388.8
  epigastric 789.3 ✓5th
  eye 379.92
  female genital organ 625.8
  gum 784.2
  head 784.2
  intracranial 784.2
  joint 719.60
    ankle 719.67
    elbow 719.62
    foot 719.67
    hand 719.64
    hip 719.65
    knee 719.66
    multiple sites 719.69
    pelvic region 719.65
    shoulder (region) 719.61
    specified site NEC 719.68
    wrist 719.63
  kidney (see also Disease, kidney) 593.9
  lung 786.6
  lymph node 785.6
  malignant (M8000/3) — see Neoplasm, by site, malignant
  mediastinal 786.6
  mouth 784.2
  muscle (limb) 729.89
  neck 784.2
  nose or sinus 784.2
  palate 784.2
  pelvis, pelvic 789.3 ✓5th
  penis 607.89
  perineum 625.8
  rectum 787.99
  scrotum 608.89
  skin 782.2
  specified organ NEC — see Disease of specified organ or site
  splenic 789.2
  substernal 786.6
    thyroid (see also Goiter) 240.9
  superficial (localized) 782.2
  testes 608.89
  throat 784.2
  tongue 784.2
  umbilicus 789.3 ✓5th
  uterus 625.8
  vagina 625.8
  vulva 625.8

Massive — see condition

Mastalgia 611.71
  psychogenic 307.89

Mast cell
  disease 757.33
    systemic (M9741/3) 202.6 ✓5th
  leukemia (M9900/3) 207.8 ✓5th
  sarcoma (M9742/3) 202.6 ✓5th
  tumor (M9740/1) 238.5
    malignant (M9740/3) 202.6 ✓5th

Masters-Allen syndrome 620.6

Mastitis (acute) (adolescent) (diffuse) (interstitial) (lobular) (nonpuerperal) (nonsuppurative) (parenchymatous) (phlegmonous) (simple) (subacute) (suppurative) 611.0
  chronic (cystic) (fibrocystic) 610.1
  cystic 610.1
    Schimmelbusch's type 610.1
  fibrocystic 610.1

Mastitis — continued
  infective 611.0
  lactational 675.2 ✓5th
  lymphangitis 611.0
  neonatal (noninfective) 778.7
    infective 771.5
  periductal 610.4
  plasma cell 610.4
  puerperal, postpartum, (interstitial) (nonpurulent) (parenchymatous) 675.2 ✓5th
    purulent 675.1 ✓5th
    stagnation 676.2 ✓5th
  puerperalis 675.2 ✓5th
  retromammary 611.0
    puerperal, postpartum 675.1 ✓5th
  submammary 611.0
    puerperal, postpartum 675.1 ✓5th

Mastocytoma (M9740/1) 238.5
  malignant (M9740/3) 202.6 ✓5th

Mastocytosis 757.33
  malignant (M9741/3) 202.6 ✓5th
  systemic (M9741/3) 202.6 ✓5th

Mastodynia 611.71
  psychogenic 307.89

Mastoid — see condition

Mastoidalgia (see also Otalgia) 388.70

Mastoiditis (coalescent) (hemorrhagic) (pneumococcal) (streptococcal) (suppurative) 383.9
  acute or subacute 383.00
    with
      Gradenigo's syndrome 383.02
      petrositis 383.02
      specified complication NEC 383.02
      subperiosteal abscess 383.01
  chronic (necrotic) (recurrent) 383.1
  tuberculous (see also Tuberculosis) 015.6 ✓5th

Mastopathy, mastopathia 611.9
  chronica cystica 610.1
  diffuse cystic 610.1
  estrogenic 611.8
  ovarian origin 611.8

Mastoplasia 611.1

Masturbation 307.9

Maternal condition, affecting fetus or newborn
  acute yellow atrophy of liver 760.8
  albuminuria 760.1
  anesthesia or analgesia 763.5
  blood loss 762.1
  chorioamnionitis 762.7
  circulatory disease, chronic (conditions classifiable to 390-459, 745-747) 760.3
  congenital heart disease (conditions classifiable to 745-746) 760.3
  cortical necrosis of kidney 760.1
  death 761.6
  diabetes mellitus 775.0
    manifest diabetes in the infant 775.1
  disease NEC 760.9
    circulatory system, chronic (conditions classifiable to 390-459, 745-747) 760.3
    genitourinary system (conditions classifiable to 580-599) 760.1
    respiratory (conditions classifiable to 490-519, 748) 760.3
  eclampsia 760.0
  hemorrhage NEC 762.1
  hepatitis acute, malignant, or subacute 760.8
  hyperemesis (gravidarum) 761.8
  hypertension (arising during pregnancy) (conditions classifiable to 642) 760.0
  infection
    disease classifiable to 001-136 760.2
    genital tract NEC 760.8
    urinary tract 760.1
  influenza 760.2
    manifest influenza in the infant 771.2
  injury (conditions classifiable to 800-996) 760.5
  malaria 760.2
    manifest malaria in infant or fetus 771.2
  malnutrition 760.4
  necrosis of liver 760.8
  nephritis (conditions classifiable to 580-583) 760.1

Maternal condition, affecting fetus or newborn — continued
  nephrosis (conditions classifiable to 581) 760.1
  noxious substance transmitted via breast milk or placenta 760.70
    alcohol 760.71
    anti-infective agents 760.74
    cocaine 760.75
    "crack" 760.75
    diethylstilbestrol [DES] 760.76
    hallucinogenic agents 760.73
    medicinal agents NEC 760.79
    narcotics 760.72
    obstetric anesthetic or analgesic drug 760.72
    specified agent NEC 760.79
  nutritional disorder (conditions classifiable to 260-269) 760.4
  operation unrelated to current delivery 760.6
  preeclampsia 760.0
  pyelitis or pyelonephritis, arising during pregnancy (conditions classifiable to 590) 760.1
  renal disease or failure 760.1
  respiratory disease, chronic (conditions classifiable to 490-519, 748) 760.3
  rheumatic heart disease (chronic) (conditions classifiable to 393-398) 760.3
  rubella (conditions classifiable to 056) 760.2
    manifest rubella in the infant or fetus 771.0
  surgery unrelated to current delivery 760.6
    to uterus or pelvic organs 763.89
  syphilis (conditions classifiable to 090-097) 760.2
    manifest syphilis in the infant or fetus 090.0
  thrombophlebitis 760.3
  toxemia (of pregnancy) 760.0
    preeclamptic 760.0
  toxoplasmosis (conditions classifiable to 130) 760.2
    manifest toxoplasmosis in the infant or fetus 771.2
  transmission of chemical substance through the placenta 760.70
    alcohol 760.71
    anti-infective 760.74
    cocaine 760.75
    "crack" 760.75
    diethylstilbestrol [DES] 760.76
    hallucinogenic agents 760.73
    narcotics 760.72
    specified substance NEC 760.79
  uremia 760.1
  urinary tract conditions (conditions classifiable to 580-599) 760.1
  vomiting (pernicious) (persistent) (vicious) 761.8

Maternity — see Delivery

Matheiu's disease (leptospiral jaundice) 100.0

Mauclaire's disease or osteochondrosis 732.3

Maxcy's disease 081.0

Maxilla, maxillary — see condition

May (-Hegglin) anomaly or syndrome 288.2

Mayaro fever 066.3

Mazoplasia 610.8

MBD (minimal brain dysfunction), child (see also Hyperkinesia) 314.9

McArdle (-Schmid-Pearson) disease or syndrome (glycogenosis V) 271.0

McCune-Albright syndrome (osteitis fibrosa disseminata) 756.59

MCLS (mucocutaneous lymph node syndrome) 446.1

McQuarrie's syndrome (idiopathic familial hypoglycemia) 251.2

Measles (black) (hemorrhagic) (suppressed) 055.9
  with
    encephalitis 055.0
    keratitis 055.71
    keratoconjunctivitis 055.71
    otitis media 055.2
    pneumonia 055.1
  complication 055.8
    specified type NEC 055.79
  encephalitis 055.0

Measles — *continued*
　French 056.9
　German 056.9
　keratitis 055.71
　keratoconjunctivitis 055.71
　liberty 056.9
　otitis media 055.2
　pneumonia 055.1
　specified complications NEC 055.79
　vaccination, prophylactic (against) V04.2
Meatitis, urethral (*see also* Urethritis) 597.89
Meat poisoning — *see* Poisoning, food
Meatus, meatal — *see* condition
Meat-wrappers' asthma 506.9
Meckel's
　diverticulitis 751.0
　diverticulum (displaced) (hypertrophic) 751.0
Meconium
　aspiration 770.1
　delayed passage in newborn 777.1
　ileus 777.1
　　due to cystic fibrosis 277.01
　in liquor 792.3
　　noted during delivery 656.8 ✔5ᵗʰ
　insufflation 770.1
　obstruction
　　fetus or newborn 777.1
　　　in mucoviscidosis 277.01
　passage of 792.3
　　noted during delivery — *omit code*
　peritonitis 777.6
　plug syndrome (newborn) NEC 777.1
Median — *see also* condition
　arcuate ligament syndrome 447.4
　bar (prostate) 600.9
　　vesical orifice 600.9
　rhomboid glossitis 529.2
Mediastinal shift 793.2
Mediastinitis (acute) (chronic) 519.2
　actinomycotic 039.8
　syphilitic 095.8
　tuberculous (*see also* Tuberculosis) 012.8 ✔5ᵗʰ
Mediastinopericarditis (*see also* Pericarditis) 423.9
　acute 420.90
　chronic 423.8
　　rheumatic 393
　rheumatic, chronic 393
Mediastinum, mediastinal — *see* condition
Medical services provided for — *see* Health, services provided because (of)
Medicine poisoning (by overdose) (wrong substance given or taken in error) 977.9
　specified drug or substance — *see* Table of Drugs and Chemicals
Medin's disease (poliomyelitis) 045.9 ✔5ᵗʰ
Mediterranean
　anemia (with other hemoglobinopathy) 282.4
　disease or syndrome (hemipathic) 282.4
　fever (*see also* Brucellosis) 023.9
　　familial 277.3
　kala-azar 085.0
　leishmaniasis 085.0
　tick fever 082.1
Medulla — *see* condition
Medullary
　cystic kidney 753.16
　sponge kidney 753.17
Medullated fibers
　optic (nerve) 743.57
　retina 362.85
Medulloblastoma (M9470/3)
　desmoplastic (M9471/3) 191.6
　specified site — *see* Neoplasm, by site, malignant
　unspecified site 191.6
Medulloepithelioma (M9501/3) — *see also* Neoplasm, by site, malignant
　teratoid (M9502/3) — *see* Neoplasm, by site, malignant
Medullomyoblastoma (M9472/3)
　specified site — *see* Neoplasm, by site, malignant

Medullomyoblastoma — *continued*
　unspecified site 191.6
Meekeren-Ehlers-Danlos syndrome 756.83
Megacaryocytic — *see* condition
Megacolon (acquired) (functional) (not Hirschsprung's disease) 564.7
　aganglionic 751.3
　congenital, congenitum 751.3
　Hirschsprung's (disease) 751.3
　psychogenic 306.4
　toxic (*see also* Colitis, ulcerative) 556.9
Megaduodenum 537.3
Megaesophagus (functional) 530.0
　congenital 750.4
Megakaryocytic — *see* condition
Megalencephaly 742.4
Megalerythema (epidermicum) (infectiosum) 057.0
Megalia, cutis et ossium 757.39
Megaloappendix 751.5
Megalocephalus, megalocephaly NEC 756.0
Megalocornea 743.41
　associated with buphthalmos 743.22
Megalocytic anemia 281.9
Megalodactylia (fingers) (thumbs) 755.57
　toes 755.65
Megaloduodenum 751.5
Megaloesophagus (functional) 530.0
　congenital 750.4
Megalogastria (congenital) 750.7
Megalomania 307.9
Megalophthalmos 743.8
Megalopsia 368.14
Megalosplenia (*see also* Splenomegaly) 789.2
Megaloureter 593.89
　congenital 753.22
Megarectum 569.49
Megasigmoid 564.7
　congenital 751.3
Megaureter 593.89
　congenital 753.22
Megrim 346.9 ✔5ᵗʰ
Meibomian
　cyst 373.2
　　infected 373.12
　gland — *see* condition
　infarct (eyelid) 374.85
　stye 373.11
Meibomitis 373.12
Meige
　-Milroy disease (chronic hereditary edema) 757.0
　syndrome (blepharospasm-oromandibular dystonia) 333.82
Melalgia, nutritional 266.2
Melancholia (*see also* Psychosis, affective) 296.90
　climacteric 296.2 ✔5ᵗʰ
　　recurrent episode 296.3 ✔5ᵗʰ
　　single episode 296.2 ✔5ᵗʰ
　hypochondriac 300.7
　intermittent 296.2 ✔5ᵗʰ
　　recurrent episode 296.3 ✔5ᵗʰ
　　single episode 296.2 ✔5ᵗʰ
　involutional 296.2 ✔5ᵗʰ
　　recurrent episode 296.3 ✔5ᵗʰ
　　single episode 296.2 ✔5ᵗʰ
　menopausal 296.2 ✔5ᵗʰ
　　recurrent episode 296.3 ✔5ᵗʰ
　　single episode 296.2 ✔5ᵗʰ
　puerperal 296.2 ✔5ᵗʰ
　reactive (from emotional stress, psychological trauma) 298.0
　recurrent 296.3 ✔5ᵗʰ
　senile 290.21
　stuporous 296.2 ✔5ᵗʰ
　　recurrent episode 296.3 ✔5ᵗʰ
　　single episode 296.2 ✔5ᵗʰ
Melanemia 275.0
Melanoameloblastoma (M9363/0) — *see* Neoplasm, bone, benign
Melanoblastoma (M8720/3) — *see* Melanoma

Melanoblastosis
　Block-Sulzberger 757.33
　cutis linearis sive systematisata 757.33
Melanocarcinoma (M8720/3) — *see* Melanoma
Melanocytoma, eyeball (M8726/0) 224.0
Melanoderma, melanodermia 709.09
　Addison's (primary adrenal insufficiency) 255.4
Melanodontia, infantile 521.05
Melanodontoclasia 521.05
Melanoepithelioma (M8720/3) — *see* Melanoma
Melanoma (malignant) (M8720/3) 172.9

> *Note — Except where otherwise indicated, the morphological varieties of melanoma in the list below should be coded by site as for "Melanoma (malignant)". Internal sites should be coded to malignant neoplasm of those sites.*

　abdominal wall 172.5
　ala nasi 172.3
　amelanotic (M8730/3) — *see* Melanoma, by site
　ankle 172.7
　anus, anal 154.3
　　canal 154.2
　arm 172.6
　auditory canal (external) 172.2
　auricle (ear) 172.2
　auricular canal (external) 172.2
　axilla 172.5
　axillary fold 172.5
　back 172.5
　balloon cell (M8722/3) — *see* Melanoma, by site
　benign (M8720/0) — *see* Neoplasm, skin, benign
　breast (female) (male) 172.5
　brow 172.3
　buttock 172.5
　canthus (eye) 172.1
　cheek (external) 172.3
　chest wall 172.5
　chin 172.3
　choroid 190.6
　conjunctiva 190.3
　ear (external) 172.2
　epithelioid cell (M8771/3) — *see also* Melanoma, by site
　　and spindle cell, mixed (M8775/3) — *see* Melanoma, by site
　external meatus (ear) 172.2
　eye 190.9
　eyebrow 172.3
　eyelid (lower) (upper) 172.1
　face NEC 172.3
　female genital organ (external) NEC 184.4
　finger 172.6
　flank 172.5
　foot 172.7
　forearm 172.6
　forehead 172.3
　foreskin 187.1
　gluteal region 172.5
　groin 172.5
　hand 172.6
　heel 172.7
　helix 172.2
　hip 172.7
　in
　　giant pigmented nevus (M8761/3) — *see* Melanoma, by site
　　Hutchinson's melanotic freckle (M8742/3) — *see* Melanoma, by site
　　junctional nevus (M8740/3) — *see* Melanoma, by site
　　precancerous melanosis (M8741/3) — *see* Melanoma, by site
　interscapular region 172.5
　iris 190.0
　jaw 172.3
　juvenile (M8770/0) — *see* Neoplasm, skin, benign
　knee 172.7
　labium
　　majus 184.1
　　minus 184.2

Melanoma — *continued*
  lacrimal gland 190.2
  leg 172.7
  lip (lower) (upper) 172.0
  liver 197.7
  lower limb NEC 172.7
  male genital organ (external) NEC 187.9
  meatus, acoustic (external) 172.2
  meibomian gland 172.1
  metastatic
    of or from specified site — *see* Melanoma, by site
    site not of skin — *see* Neoplasm, by site, malignant, secondary
    to specified site — *see* Neoplasm, by site, malignant, secondary
    unspecified site 172.9
  nail 172.9
    finger 172.6
    toe 172.7
  neck 172.4
  nodular (M8721/3) — *see* Melanoma, by site
  nose, external 172.3
  orbit 190.1
  penis 187.4
  perianal skin 172.5
  perineum 172.5
  pinna 172.2
  popliteal (fossa) (space) 172.7
  prepuce 187.1
  pubes 172.5
  pudendum 184.4
  retina 190.5
  scalp 172.4
  scrotum 187.7
  septum nasal (skin) 172.3
  shoulder 172.6
  skin NEC 172.8
  spindle cell (M8772/3) — *see also* Melanoma, by site
    type A (M8773/3) 190.0
    type B (M8774/3) 190.0
  submammary fold 172.5
  superficial spreading (M8743/3) — *see* Melanoma, by site
  temple 172.3
  thigh 172.7
  toe 172.7
  trunk NEC 172.5
  umbilicus 172.5
  upper limb NEC 172.6
  vagina vault 184.0
  vulva 184.4
Melanoplakia 528.9
Melanosarcoma (M8720/3) — *see also* Melanoma
  epithelioid cell (M8771/3) — *see* Melanoma
Melanosis 709.09
  addisonian (primary adrenal insufficiency) 255.4
    tuberculous (*see also* Tuberculosis) 017.6 ✔5ᵗʰ
  adrenal 255.4
  colon 569.89
  conjunctiva 372.55
    congenital 743.49
  corii degenerativa 757.33
  cornea (presenile) (senile) 371.12
    congenital 743.43
      interfering with vision 743.42
    prenatal 743.43
      interfering with vision 743.42
  eye 372.55
    congenital 743.49
  jute spinners' 709.09
  lenticularis progressiva 757.33
  liver 573.8
  precancerous (M8741/2) — *see also* Neoplasm, skin, in situ
    malignant melanoma in (M8741/3) — *see* Melanoma
  Riehl's 709.09
  sclera 379.19
    congenital 743.47
  suprarenal 255.4
  tar 709.09
  toxic 709.09
Melanuria 791.9

MELAS 758.89
Melasma 709.09
  adrenal (gland) 255.4
  suprarenal (gland) 255.4
Melena 578.1
  due to
    swallowed maternal blood 777.3
    ulcer — *see* Ulcer, by site, with hemorrhage
  newborn 772.4
    due to swallowed maternal blood 777.3
Meleney's
  gangrene (cutaneous) 686.09
  ulcer (chronic undermining) 686.09
Melioidosis 025
Melitensis, febris 023.0
Melitococcosis 023.0
Melkersson (-Rosenthal) syndrome 351.8
Mellitus, diabetes — *see* Diabetes
Melorheostosis (bone) (leri) 733.99
Meloschisis 744.83
Melotia 744.29
Membrana
  capsularis lentis posterior 743.39
  epipapillaris 743.57
Membranacea placenta — *see* Placenta, abnormal
Membranaceous uterus 621.8
Membrane, membranous — *see also* condition
  folds, congenital — *see* Web
    Jackson's 751.4
  over face (causing asphyxia), fetus or newborn 768.9
  premature rupture — *see* Rupture, membranes, premature
  pupillary 364.74
    persistent 743.46
  retained (complicating delivery) (with hemorrhage) 666.2 ✔5ᵗʰ
    without hemorrhage 667.1 ✔5ᵗʰ
  secondary (eye) 366.50
  unruptured (causing asphyxia) 768.9
  vitreous humor 379.25
Membranitis, fetal 658.4 ✔5ᵗʰ
  affecting fetus or newborn 762.7
Memory disturbance, loss or lack (*see also* Amnesia) 780.99 ▲
  mild, following organic brain damage 310.1
Menadione (vitamin K) deficiency 269.0
Menarche, precocious 259.1
Mendacity, pathologic 301.7
Mende's syndrome (ptosis-epicanthus) 270.2
Mendelson's syndrome (resulting from a procedure) 997.3
  obstetric 668.0 ✔5ᵗʰ
Ménétrier's disease or syndrome (hypertrophic gastritis) 535.2 ✔5ᵗʰ
Ménière's disease, syndrome, or vertigo 386.00
  cochlear 386.02
  cochleovestibular 386.01
  inactive 386.04
  in remission 386.04
  vestibular 386.03
Meninges, meningeal — *see* condition
Meningioma (M9530/0) — *see also* Neoplasm, meninges, benign
  angioblastic (M9535/0) — *see* Neoplasm, meninges, benign
  angiomatous (M9534/0) — *see* Neoplasm, meninges, benign
  endotheliomatous (M9531/0) — *see* Neoplasm, meninges, benign
  fibroblastic (M9532/0) — *see* Neoplasm, meninges, benign
  fibrous (M9532/0) — *see* Neoplasm, meninges, benign
  hemangioblastic (M9535/0) — *see* Neoplasm, meninges, benign
  hemangiopericytic (M9536/0) — *see* Neoplasm, meninges, benign
  malignant (M9530/3) — *see* Neoplasm, meninges, malignant
  meningiothelial (M9531/0) — *see* Neoplasm, meninges, benign

Meningioma — *see also* Neoplasm, meninges, benign — *continued*
  meningotheliomatous (M9531/0) — *see* Neoplasm, meninges, benign
  mixed (M9537/0) — *see* Neoplasm, meninges, benign
  multiple (M9530/1) 237.6
  papillary (M9538/1) 237.6
  psammomatous (M9533/0) — *see* Neoplasm, meninges, benign
  syncytial (M9531/0) — *see* Neoplasm, meninges, benign
  transitional (M9537/0) — *see* Neoplasm, meninges, benign
Meningiomatosis (diffuse) (M9530/1) 237.6
Meningism (*see also* Meningismus) 781.6
Meningismus (infectional) (pneumococcal) 781.6
  due to serum or vaccine 997.09 [321.8]
  influenzal NEC 487.8
Meningitis (basal) (basic) (basilar) (brain) (cerebral) (cervical) (congestive) (diffuse) (hemorrhagic) (infantile) (membranous) (metastatic) (nonspecific) (pontine) (progressive) (simple) (spinal) (subacute) (sympathetica) (toxic) 322.9
  abacterial NEC (*see also* Meningitis, aseptic) 047.9
  actinomycotic 039.8 [320.7]
  adenoviral 049.1
  Aerobacter aerogenes 320.82
    anaerobes (cocci) (gram-negative) (gram-positive) (mixed) (NEC) 320.81
  arbovirus NEC 066.9 [321.2]
    specified type NEC 066.8 [321.2]
  aseptic (acute) NEC 047.9
    adenovirus 049.1
    Coxsackievirus 047.0
    due to
      adenovirus 049.1
      Coxsackievirus 047.0
      ECHO virus 047.1
      enterovirus 047.9
      mumps 072.1
      poliovirus (*see also* Poliomyelitis) 045.2 ✔5ᵗʰ [321.2]
    ECHO virus 047.1
    herpes (simplex) virus 054.72
      zoster 053.0
    leptospiral 100.81
    lymphocytic choriomeningitis 049.0
    noninfective 322.0
  Bacillus pyocyaneus 320.89
  bacterial NEC 320.9
    anaerobic 320.81
    gram-negative 320.82
      anaerobic 320.81
  Bacteroides (fragilis) (oralis) (melaninogenicus) 320.81
  cancerous (M8000/6) 198.4
  candidal 112.83
  carcinomatous (M8010/6) 198.4
  caseous (*see also* Tuberculosis, meninges) 013.0 ✔5ᵗʰ
  cerebrospinal (acute) (chronic) (diplococcal) (endemic) (epidemic) (fulminant) (infectious) (malignant) (meningococcal) (sporadic) 036.0
    carrier (suspected) of V02.59
  chronic NEC 322.2
  clear cerebrospinal fluid NEC 322.0
  Clostridium (haemolyticum) (novyi) NEC 320.81
  coccidioidomycosis 114.2
  Coxsackievirus 047.0
  cryptococcal 117.5 [321.0]
  diplococcal 036.0
    gram-negative 036.0
    gram-positive 320.1
  Diplococcus pneumoniae 320.1
  due to
    actinomycosis 039.8 [320.7]
    adenovirus 049.1
    coccidiomycosis 114.2
    enterovirus 047.9
      specified NEC 047.8
    histoplasmosis (*see also* Histoplasmosis) 115.91
    Listerosis 027.0 [320.7]

Meningitis — *continued*
  due to — *continued*
    Lyme disease 088.81 *[320.7]*
    moniliasis 112.83
    mumps 072.1
    neurosyphilis 094.2
    nonbacterial organisms NEC 321.8
    oidiomycosis 112.83
    poliovirus (*see also* Poliomyelitis)
      045.2 ☑5ᵗʰ *[321.2]*
    preventive immunization, inoculation, or
      vaccination 997.09 *[321.8]*
    sarcoidosis 135 *[321.4]*
    sporotrichosis 117.1 *[321.1]*
    syphilis 094.2
      acute 091.81
      congenital 090.42
      secondary 091.81
    trypanosomiasis (*see also* Trypanosomiasis)
      086.9 *[321.3]*
    whooping cough 033.9 *[320.7]*
  E. coli 320.82
  ECHO virus 047.1
  endothelial-leukocytic, benign, recurrent 047.9
  Enterobacter aerogenes 320.82
  enteroviral 047.9
    specified type NEC 047.8
  enterovirus 047.9
    specified NEC 047.8
  eosinophilic 322.1
  epidemic NEC 036.0
  Escherichia coli (E. coli) 320.82
  Eubacterium 320.81
  fibrinopurulent NEC 320.9
    specified type NEC 320.89
  Friedländer (bacillus) 320.82
  fungal NEC 117.9 *[321.1]*
  Fusobacterium 320.81
  gonococcal 098.82
  gram-negative bacteria NEC 320.82
    anaerobic 320.81
    cocci 036.0
      specified NEC 320.82
  gram-negative cocci NEC 036.0
    specified NEC 320.82
  gram-positive cocci NEC 320.9
  H. influenzae 320.0
  herpes (simplex) virus 054.72
    zoster 053.0
  infectious NEC 320.9
  influenzal 320.0
  Klebsiella pneumoniae 320.82
  late effect — *see* Late, effect, meningitis
  leptospiral (aseptic) 100.81
  Listerella (monocytogenes) 027.0 *[320.7]*
  Listeria monocytogenes 027.0 *[320.7]*
  lymphocytic (acute) (benign) (serous) 049.0
    choriomeningitis virus 049.0
  meningococcal (chronic) 036.0
  Mima polymorpha 320.82
  Mollaret's 047.9
  monilial 112.83
  mumps (virus) 072.1
  mycotic NEC 117.9 *[321.1]*
  Neisseria 036.0
  neurosyphilis 094.2
  nonbacterial NEC (*see also* Meningitis, aseptic)
    047.9
  nonpyogenic NEC 322.0
  oidiomycosis 112.83
  ossificans 349.2
  Peptococcus 320.81
  Peptostreptococcus 320.81
  pneumococcal 320.1
  poliovirus (*see also* Poliomyelitis)
    045.2 ☑5ᵗʰ *[321.2]*
  Proprionibacterium 320.81
  Proteus morganii 320.82
  Pseudomonas (aeruginosa) (pyocyaneus) 320.82
  purulent NEC 320.9
    specified organism NEC 320.89
  pyogenic NEC 320.9
    specified organism NEC 320.89
  Salmonella 003.21
  septic NEC 320.9
    specified organism NEC 320.89
  serosa circumscripta NEC 322.0

Meningitis — *continued*
  serous NEC (*see also* Meningitis, aseptic) 047.9
    lymphocytic 049.0
    syndrome 348.2
  Serratia (marcescens) 320.82
  specified organism NEC 320.89
  sporadic cerebrospinal 036.0
  sporotrichosis 117.1 *[321.1]*
  staphylococcal 320.3
  sterile 997.09
  streptococcal (acute) 320.2
  suppurative 320.9
    specified organism NEC 320.89
  syphilitic 094.2
    acute 091.81
    congenital 090.42
    secondary 091.81
  torula 117.5 *[321.0]*
  traumatic (complication of injury) 958.8
  Treponema (denticola) (Macrodenticum) 320.81
  trypanosomiasis 086.1 *[321.3]*
  tuberculous (*see also* Tuberculosis, meninges)
    013.0 ☑5ᵗʰ
  typhoid 002.0 *[320.7]*
  Veillonella 320.81
  Vibrio vulnificus 320.82
  viral, virus NEC (*see also* Meningitis, aseptic)
    047.9
  Wallgren's (*see also* Meningitis, aseptic) 047.9
Meningocele (congenital) (spinal) (*see also* Spina
    bifida) 741.9 ☑5ᵗʰ
  acquired (traumatic) 349.2
  cerebral 742.0
  cranial 742.0
Meningocerebritis — *see* Meningoencephalitis
Meningococcemia (acute) (chronic) 036.2
Meningococcus, meningococcal (*see also*
    condition) 036.9
  adrenalitis, hemorrhagic 036.3
  carditis 036.40
  carrier (suspected) of V02.59
  cerebrospinal fever 036.0
  encephalitis 036.1
  endocarditis 036.42
  infection NEC 036.9
  meningitis (cerebrospinal) 036.0
  myocarditis 036.43
  optic neuritis 036.81
  pericarditis 036.41
  septicemia (chronic) 036.2
Meningoencephalitis (*see also* Encephalitis)
    323.9
  acute NEC 048
  bacterial, purulent, pyogenic, or septic — *see*
    Meningitis
  chronic NEC 094.1
  diffuse NEC 094.1
  diphasic 063.2
  due to
    actinomycosis 039.8 *[320.7]*
    blastomycosis NEC (*see also* Blastomycosis)
      116.0 *[323.4]*
    free-living amebae 136.2
    Listeria monocytogenes 027.0 *[320.7]*
    Lyme disease 088.81 *[320.7]*
    mumps 072.2
    Naegleria (amebae) (gruberi) (organisms)
      136.2
    rubella 056.01
    sporotrichosis 117.1 *[321.1]*
    toxoplasmosis (acquired) 130.0
      congenital (active) 771.2 *[323.4]*
    Trypanosoma 086.1 *[323.2]*
  epidemic 036.0
  herpes 054.3
  herpetic 054.3
  H. influenzae 320.0
  infectious (acute) 048
  influenzal 320.0
  late effect — *see* category 326
  Listeria monocytogenes 027.0 *[320.7]*
  lymphocytic (serous) 049.0
  mumps 072.2
  parasitic NEC 123.9 *[323.4]*
  pneumococcal 320.1
  primary amebic 136.2
  rubella 056.01

Meningoencephalitis (*see also* Encephalitis) —
    continued
  serous 048
    lymphocytic 049.0
  specific 094.2
  staphylococcal 320.3
  streptococcal 320.2
  syphilitic 094.2
  toxic NEC 989.9 *[323.7]*
    due to
      carbon tetrachloride 987.8 *[323.7]*
      hydroxyquinoline derivatives poisoning
        961.3 *[323.7]*
      lead 984.9 *[323.7]*
      mercury 985.0 *[323.7]*
      thallium 985.8 *[323.7]*
  toxoplasmosis (acquired) 130.0
  trypanosomic 086.1 *[323.2]*
  tuberculous (*see also* Tuberculosis, meninges)
    013.0 ☑5ᵗʰ
  virus NEC 048
Meningoencephalocele 742.0
  syphilitic 094.89
  congenital 090.49
Meningoencephalomyelitis (*see also*
    Meningoencephalitis) 323.9
  acute NEC 048
    disseminated (postinfectious) 136.9 *[323.6]*
      postimmunization or postvaccination
        323.5
    due to
      actinomycosis 039.8 *[320.7]*
      torula 117.5 *[323.4]*
      toxoplasma or toxoplasmosis (acquired)
        130.0
        congenital (active) 771.2 *[323.4]*
    late effect — *see* category 326
Meningoencephalomyelopathy (*see also*
    Meningoencephalomyelitis) 349.9
Meningoencephalopathy (*see also*
    Meningoencephalitis) 348.3
Meningoencephalopoliomyelitis (*see also*
    Poliomyelitis, bulbar) 045.0 ☑5ᵗʰ
  late effect 138
Meningomyelitis (*see also* Meningoencephalitis)
    323.9
  blastomycotic NEC (*see also* Blastomycosis)
    116.0 *[323.4]*
  due to
    actinomycosis 039.8 *[320.7]*
    blastomycosis (*see also* Blastomycosis)
      116.0 *[323.4]*
    Meningococcus 036.0
    sporotrichosis 117.1 *[323.4]*
    torula 117.5 *[323.4]*
  late effect — *see* category 326
  lethargic 049.8
  meningococcal 036.0
  syphilitic 094.2
  tuberculous (*see also* Tuberculosis, meninges)
    013.0 ☑5ᵗʰ
Meningomyelocele (*see also* Spina bifida)
    741.9 ☑5ᵗʰ
  syphilitic 094.89
Meningomyeloneuritis — *see*
    Meningoencephalitis
Meningoradiculitis — *see* Meningitis
Meningovascular — *see* condition
Meniscocytosis 282.60
Menkes' syndrome — *see* Syndrome, Menkes'
Menolipsis 626.0
Menometrorrhagia 626.2
Menopause, menopausal (symptoms) (syndrome)
    627.2
  arthritis (any site) NEC 716.3 ☑5ᵗʰ
  artificial 627.4
  bleeding 627.0
  crisis 627.2
  depression (*see also* Psychosis, affective)
    296.2 ☑5ᵗʰ
    agitated 296.2 ☑5ᵗʰ
      recurrent episode 296.3 ☑5ᵗʰ
      single episode 296.2 ☑5ᵗʰ

Menopause, menopausal — *continued*
depression (*see also* Psychosis, affective) — *continued*
  psychotic 296.2 ☑5ᵗʰ
    recurrent episode 296.3 ☑5ᵗʰ
    single episode 296.2 ☑5ᵗʰ
  recurrent episode 296.3 ☑5ᵗʰ
  single episode 296.2 ☑5ᵗʰ
  melancholia (*see also* Psychosis, affective) 296.2 ☑5ᵗʰ
    recurrent episode 296.3 ☑5ᵗʰ
    single episode 296.2 ☑5ᵗʰ
  paranoid state 297.2
  paraphrenia 297.2
  postsurgical 627.4
  premature 256.31
    postirradiation 256.2
    postsurgical 256.2
  psychoneurosis 627.2
  psychosis NEC 298.8
  surgical 627.4
  toxic polyarthritis NEC 716.39
Menorrhagia (primary) 626.2
  climacteric 627.0
  menopausal 627.0
  postclimacteric 627.1
  postmenopausal 627.1
  preclimacteric 627.0
  premenopausal 627.0
  puberty (menses retained) 626.3
Menorrhalgia 625.3
Menoschesis 626.8
Menostaxis 626.2
Menses, retention 626.8
Menstrual — *see also* Menstruation
  cycle, irregular 626.4
  disorders NEC 626.9
  extraction V25.3
  fluid, retained 626.8
  molimen 625.4
  period, normal V65.5
  regulation V25.3
Menstruation
  absent 626.0
  anovulatory 628.0
  delayed 626.8
  difficult 625.3
  disorder 626.9
    psychogenic 306.52
    specified NEC 626.8
  during pregnancy 640.8 ☑5ᵗʰ
  excessive 626.2
  frequent 626.2
  infrequent 626.1
  irregular 626.4
  latent 626.8
  membranous 626.8
  painful (primary) (secondary) 625.3
    psychogenic 306.52
  passage of clots 626.2
  precocious 626.8
  protracted 626.8
  retained 626.8
  retrograde 626.8
  scanty 626.1
  suppression 626.8
  vicarious (nasal) 625.8
Mentagra (*see also* Sycosis) 704.8
Mental — *see also* condition
  deficiency (*see also* Retardation, mental) 319
  deterioration (*see also* Psychosis) 298.9
  disorder (*see also* Disorder, mental) 300.9
  exhaustion 300.5
  insufficiency (congenital) (*see also* Retardation, mental) 319
  observation without need for further medical care NEC V71.09
  retardation (*see also* Retardation, mental) 319
  subnormality (*see also* Retardation, mental) 319
    mild 317
    moderate 318.0
    profound 318.2
    severe 318.1
  upset (*see also* Disorder, mental) 300.9

Meralgia paresthetica 355.1
Mercurial — *see* condition
Mercurialism NEC 985.0
Merergasia 300.9
MERFF 758.89
Merkel cell tumor — *see* Neoplasm, by site, malignant
Merocele (*see also* Hernia, femoral) 553.00
Meromelia 755.4
  lower limb 755.30
    intercalary 755.32
      femur 755.34
        tibiofibular (complete) (incomplete) 755.33
      fibula 755.37
      metatarsal(s) 755.38
      tarsal(s) 755.38
      tibia 755.36
      tibiofibular 755.35
    terminal (complete) (partial) (transverse) 755.31
    longitudinal 755.32
      metatarsal(s) 755.38
      phalange(s) 755.39
      tarsal(s) 755.38
    transverse 755.31
  upper limb 755.20
    intercalary 755.22
      carpal(s) 755.28
      humeral 755.24
        radioulnar (complete) (incomplete) 755.23
      metacarpal(s) 755.28
      phalange(s) 755.29
      radial 755.26
      radioulnar 755.25
      ulnar 755.27
    terminal (complete) (partial) (transverse) 755.21
    longitudinal 755.22
      carpal(s) 755.28
      metacarpal(s) 755.28
      phalange(s) 755.29
    transverse 755.21
Merosmia 781.1
Merycism — *see also* Vomiting
  psychogenic 307.53
Merzbacher-Pelizaeus disease 330.0
Mesaortitis — *see* Aortitis
Mesarteritis — *see* Arteritis
Mesencephalitis (*see also* Encephalitis) 323.9
  late effect — *see* category 326
Mesenchymoma (M8990/1) — *see also* Neoplasm, connective tissue, uncertain behavior
  benign (M8990/0) — *see* Neoplasm, connective tissue, benign
  malignant (M8990/3) — *see* Neoplasm, connective tissue, malignant
Mesentery, mesenteric — *see* condition
Mesiodens, mesiodentes 520.1
  causing crowding 524.3
Mesio-occlusion 524.2
Mesocardia (with asplenia) 746.87
Mesocolon — *see* condition
Mesonephroma (malignant) (M9110/3) — *see also* Neoplasm, by site, malignant
  benign (M9110/0) — *see* Neoplasm, by site, benign
Mesophlebitis — *see* Phlebitis
Mesostromal dysgenesis 743.51
Mesothelioma (malignant) (M9050/3) — *see also* Neoplasm, by site, malignant
  benign (M9050/0) — *see* Neoplasm, by site, benign
  biphasic type (M9053/3) — *see also* Neoplasm, by site, malignant
    benign (M9053/0) — *see* Neoplasm, by site, benign
  epithelioid (M9052/3) — *see also* Neoplasm, by site, malignant
    benign (M9052/0) — *see* Neoplasm, by site, benign

Mesothelioma — *see also* Neoplasm, by site, malignant — *continued*
  fibrous (M9051/3) — *see also* Neoplasm, by site, malignant
    benign (M9051/0) — *see* Neoplasm, by site, benign
Metabolism disorder 277.9
  specified type NEC 277.8
Metagonimiasis 121.5
Metagonimus infestation (small intestine) 121.5
Metal
  pigmentation (skin) 709.00
  polishers' disease 502
Metalliferous miners' lung 503
Metamorphopsia 368.14
Metaplasia
  bone, in skin 709.3
  breast 611.8
  cervix — *omit code*
  endometrium (squamous) 621.8
  intestinal, of gastric mucosa 537.89
  kidney (pelvis) (squamous) (*see also* Disease, renal) 593.89
  myelogenous 289.8
  myeloid (agnogenic) (megakaryocytic) 289.8
  spleen 289.59
  squamous cell
    amnion 658.8 ☑5ᵗʰ
    bladder 596.8
    cervix — *see* condition
    trachea 519.1
    tracheobronchial tree 519.1
    uterus 621.8
      cervix — *see* condition
Metastasis, metastatic
  abscess — *see* Abscess
  calcification 275.40
  cancer, neoplasm, or disease
    from specified site (M8000/3) — *see* Neoplasm, by site, malignant
    to specified site (M8000/6) — *see* Neoplasm, by site, secondary
  deposits (in) (M8000/6) — *see* Neoplasm, by site, secondary
  pneumonia 038.8 [484.8]
  spread (to) (M8000/6) — *see* Neoplasm, by site, secondary
Metatarsalgia 726.70
  anterior 355.6
  due to Freiberg's disease 732.5
  Morton's 355.6
Metatarsus, metatarsal — *see also* condition
  abductus valgus (congenital) 754.60
  adductus varus (congenital) 754.53
  primus varus 754.52
  valgus (adductus) (congenital) 754.60
  varus (abductus) (congenital) 754.53
  primus 754.52
Methemoglobinemia 289.7
  acquired (with sulfhemoglobinemia) 289.7
  congenital 289.7
  enzymatic 289.7
  Hb-M disease 289.7
  hereditary 289.7
  toxic 289.7
Methemoglobinuria (*see also* Hemoglobinuria) 791.2
Methioninemia 270.4
Metritis (catarrhal) (septic) (suppurative) (*see also* Endometritis) 615.9
  blennorrhagic 098.16
    chronic or duration of 2 months or over 098.36
  cervical (*see also* Cervicitis) 616.0
  gonococcal 098.16
    chronic or duration of 2 months or over 098.36
  hemorrhagic 626.8
  puerperal, postpartum, childbirth 670 ☑5ᵗʰ
  tuberculous (*see also* Tuberculosis) 016.7 ☑5ᵗʰ
Metropathia hemorrhagica 626.8
Metroperitonitis (*see also* Peritonitis, pelvic, female) 614.5

Metrorrhagia 626.6
arising during pregnancy — *see* Hemorrhage, pregnancy
postpartum NEC 666.2 ✓5ᵗʰ
primary 626.6
psychogenic 306.59
puerperal 666.2 ✓5ᵗʰ
Metrorrhexis — *see* Rupture, uterus
Metrosalpingitis (*see also* Salpingo-oophoritis) 614.2
Metrostaxis 626.6
Metrovaginitis (*see also* Endometritis) 615.9
gonococcal (acute) 098.16
chronic or duration of 2 months or over 098.36
Mexican fever — *see* Typhus, Mexican
Meyenburg-Altherr-Uehlinger syndrome 733.99
Meyer-Schwickerath and Weyers syndrome (dysplasia oculodentodigitalis) 759.89
Meynert's amentia (nonalcoholic) 294.0
alcoholic 291.1
Mibelli's disease 757.39
Mice, joint (*see also* Loose, body, joint) 718.1 ✓5ᵗʰ
knee 717.6
Micheli-Rietti syndrome (thalassemia minor) 282.4
Michotte's syndrome 721.5
Micrencephalon, micrencephaly 742.1
Microaneurysm, retina 362.14
diabetic 250.5 ✓5ᵗʰ [362.01]
Microangiopathy 443.9
diabetic (peripheral) 250.7 ✓5ᵗʰ [443.81]
retinal 250.5 ✓5ᵗʰ [362.01]
peripheral 443.9
diabetic 250.7 ✓5ᵗʰ [443.81]
retinal 362.18
diabetic 250.5 ✓5ᵗʰ [362.01]
thrombotic 446.6
Moschcowitz's (thrombotic thrombocytopenic purpura) 446.6
Microcalcification, mammographic 793.81
Microcephalus, microcephalic, microcephaly 742.1
due to toxoplasmosis (congenital) 771.2
Microcheilia 744.82
Microcolon (congenital) 751.5
Microcornea (congenital) 743.41
Microcytic — *see* condition
Microdontia 520.2
Microdrepanocytosis (thalassemia-Hb-S disease) 282.4
Microembolism
atherothrombotic — *see* Atheroembolism ●
retina 362.33
Microencephalon 742.1
Microfilaria streptocerca infestation 125.3
Microgastria (congenital) 750.7
Microgenia 524.0 ✓5ᵗʰ
Microgenitalia (congenital) 752.8
penis 752.64
Microglioma (M9710/3)
specified site — *see* Neoplasm, by site, malignant
unspecified site 191.9
Microglossia (congenital) 750.16
Micrognathia, micrognathism (congenital) 524.00
mandibular 524.04
alveolar 524.74
maxillary 524.03
alveolar 524.73
Microgyria (congenital) 742.2
Microinfarct, heart (*see also* Insufficiency, coronary) 411.89
Microlithiasis, alveolar, pulmonary 516.2
Micromyelia (congenital) 742.59
Micropenis 752.64
Microphakia (congenital) 743.36
Microphthalmia (congenital) (*see also* Microphthalmos) 743.10

Microphthalmos (congenital) 743.10
associated with eye and adnexal anomalies NEC 743.12
due to toxoplasmosis (congenital) 771.2
isolated 743.11
simple 743.11
syndrome 759.89
Micropsia 368.14
Microsporidiosis 136.8
Microsporon furfur infestation 111.0
Microsporosis (*see also* Dermatophytosis) 110.9
nigra 111.1
Microstomia (congenital) 744.84
Microthelia 757.6
Microthromboembolism — *see* Embolism
Microtia (congenital) (external ear) 744.23
Microtropia 378.34
Micturition
disorder NEC 788.69
psychogenic 306.53
frequency 788.41
psychogenic 306.53
nocturnal 788.43
painful 788.1
psychogenic 306.53
Middle
ear — *see* condition
lobe (right) syndrome 518.0
Midplane — *see* condition
Miescher's disease 709.3
cheilitis 351.8
granulomatosis disciformis 709.3
Miescher-Leder syndrome or granulomatosis 709.3
Mieten's syndrome 759.89
Migraine (idiopathic) 346.9 ✓5ᵗʰ
with aura 346.0 ✓5ᵗʰ
abdominal (syndrome) 346.2 ✓5ᵗʰ
allergic (histamine) 346.2 ✓5ᵗʰ
atypical 346.1 ✓5ᵗʰ
basilar 346.2 ✓5ᵗʰ
classical 346.0 ✓5ᵗʰ
common 346.1 ✓5ᵗʰ
hemiplegic 346.8 ✓5ᵗʰ
lower-half 346.2 ✓5ᵗʰ
menstrual 625.4
ophthalmic 346.8 ✓5ᵗʰ
ophthalmoplegic 346.8 ✓5ᵗʰ
retinal 346.2 ✓5ᵗʰ
variant 346.2 ✓5ᵗʰ
Migrant, social V60.0
Migratory, migrating — *see also* condition
person V60.0
testis, congenital 752.52
Mikulicz's disease or syndrome (dryness of mouth, absent or decreased lacrimation) 527.1
Milian atrophia blanche 701.3
Miliaria (crystallina) (rubra) (tropicalis) 705.1
apocrine 705.82
Miliary — *see* condition
Milium (*see also* Cyst, sebaceous) 706.2
colloid 709.3
eyelid 374.84
Milk
crust 690.11
excess secretion 676.6 ✓5ᵗʰ
fever, female 672 ✓5ᵗʰ
poisoning 988.8
retention 676.2 ✓5ᵗʰ
sickness 988.8
spots 423.1
Milkers' nodes 051.1
Milk-leg (deep vessels) 671.4 ✓5ᵗʰ
complicating pregnancy 671.3 ✓5ᵗʰ
nonpuerperal 451.19
puerperal, postpartum, childbirth 671.4 ✓5ᵗʰ
Milkman (-Looser) disease or syndrome (osteomalacia with pseudofractures) 268.2
Milky urine (*see also* Chyluria) 791.1
Millar's asthma (laryngismus stridulus) 478.75
Millard-Gubler paralysis or syndrome 344.89

Millard-Gubler-Foville paralysis 344.89
Miller's disease (osteomalacia) 268.2
Miller Fisher's syndrome 357.0
Milles' syndrome (encephalocutaneous angiomatosis) 759.6
Mills' disease 335.29
Millstone makers' asthma or lung 502
Milroy's disease (chronic hereditary edema) 757.0
Miners' — *see also* condition
asthma 500
elbow 727.2
knee 727.2
lung 500
nystagmus 300.89
phthisis (*see also* Tuberculosis) 011.4 ✓5ᵗʰ
tuberculosis (see also Tuberculosis) 011.4 ✓5ᵗʰ
Minkowski-Chauffard syndrome (*see also* Spherocytosis) 282.0
Minor — *see* condition
Minor's disease 336.1
Minot's disease (hemorrhagic disease, newborn) 776.0
Minot-von Willebrand (-Jürgens) disease or syndrome (angiohemophilia) 286.4
Minus (and plus) hand (intrinsic) 736.09
Miosis (persistent) (pupil) 379.42
Mirizzi's syndrome (hepatic duct stenosis) (*see also* Obstruction, biliary) 576.2
with calculus, cholelithiasis, or stones — *see* Choledocholithiasis
Mirror writing 315.09
secondary to organic lesion 784.69
Misadventure (prophylactic) (therapeutic) (*see also* Complications) 999.9
administration of insulin 962.3
infusion — *see* Complications, infusion
local applications (of fomentations, plasters, etc.) 999.9
burn or scald — *see* Burn, by site
medical care (early) (late) NEC 999.9
adverse effect of drugs or chemicals — *see* Table of Drugs and Chemicals
burn or scald — *see* Burn, by site
radiation NEC 990
radiotherapy NEC 990
surgical procedure (early) (late) — *see* Complications, surgical procedure
transfusion — *see* Complications, transfusion
vaccination or other immunological procedure — *see* Complications, vaccination
Misanthropy 301.7
Miscarriage — *see* Abortion, spontaneous
Mischief, malicious, child (*see also* Disturbance, conduct) 312.0 ✓5ᵗʰ
Misdirection ●
aqueous 365.83 ●
Mismanagement, feeding 783.3
Misplaced, misplacement
kidney (*see also* Disease, renal) 593.0
congenital 753.3
organ or site, congenital NEC — *see* Malposition, congenital
Missed
abortion 632
delivery (at or near term) 656.4 ✓5ᵗʰ
labor (at or near term) 656.4 ✓5ᵗʰ
Missing — *see also* Absence
teeth (acquired) 525.10
congenital (see also Anodontia) 520.0
due to
caries 525.13
extraction 525.10
periodontal disease 525.12
specified NEC 525.19 ●
trauma 525.11
vertebrae (congenital) 756.13
Misuse of drugs NEC (*see also* Abuse, drug, nondependent) 305.9 ✓5ᵗʰ
Mitchell's disease (erythromelalgia) 443.89
Mite(s)
diarrhea 133.8
grain (itch) 133.8

Mite(s) — *continued*
  hair follicle (itch) 133.8
  in sputum 133.8
Mitral — *see* condition
Mittelschmerz 625.2
Mixed — *see* condition
Mljet disease (mal de Meleda) 757.39
Mobile, mobility
  cecum 751.4
  coccyx 733.99
  excessive — *see* Hypermobility
  gallbladder 751.69
  kidney 593.0
    congenital 753.3
  organ or site, congenital NEC — *see*
    Malposition, congenital
  spleen 289.59
Mobitz heart block (atrioventricular) 426.10
  type I (Wenckebach's) 426.13
  type II 426.12
Möbius'
  disease 346.8 ✔5ᵗʰ
  syndrome
    congenital oculofacial paralysis 352.6
    ophthalmoplegic migraine 346.8 ✔5ᵗʰ
Moeller (-Barlow) disease (infantile scurvy) 267
  glossitis 529.4
Mohr's syndrome (types I and II) 759.89
Mola destruens (M9100/1) 236.1
Molarization, premolars 520.2
Molar pregnancy 631
  hydatidiform (delivered) (undelivered) 630
Mold(s)
  in vitreous 117.9
Molding, head (during birth) 767.3
Mole (pigmented) (M8720/0) — *see also*
    Neoplasm, skin, benign
  blood 631
  Breus' 631
  cancerous (M8720/3) — *see* Melanoma
  carneous 631
  destructive (M9100/1) 236.1
  ectopic — *see* Pregnancy, ectopic
  fleshy 631
  hemorrhagic 631
  hydatid, hydatidiform (benign) (complicating
    pregnancy) (delivered) (undelivered) (*see
    also* Hydatidiform mole) 630
    invasive (M9100/1) 236.1
    malignant (M9100/1) 236.1
    previous, affecting management of
      pregnancy V23.1
  invasive (hydatidiform) (M9100/1) 236.1
  malignant
    meaning
      malignant hydatidiform mole (9100/1)
        236.1
      melanoma (M8720/3) — *see* Melanoma
  nonpigmented (M8730/0) — *see* Neoplasm,
    skin, benign
  pregnancy NEC 631
  skin (M8720/0) — *see* Neoplasm, skin, benign
  tubal — *see* Pregnancy, tubal
  vesicular (*see also* Hydatidiform mole) 630
Molimen, molimina (menstrual) 625.4
Mollaret's meningitis 047.9
Mollities (cerebellar) (cerebral) 437.8
  ossium 268.2
Molluscum
  contagiosum 078.0
  epitheliale 078.0
  fibrosum (M8851/0) — *see* Lipoma, by site
  pendulum (M8851/0) — *see* Lipoma, by site
**Mönckeberg's arteriosclerosis, degeneration,
  disease, or sclerosis** (*see also*
    Arteriosclerosis, extremities) 440.20
Monday fever 504
Monday morning dyspnea or asthma 504
Mondini's malformation (cochlea) 744.05
Mondor's disease (thrombophlebitis of breast)
    451.89

**Mongolian, mongolianism, mongolism,
  mongoloid** 758.0
  spot 757.33
Monilethrix (congenital) 757.4
Monilia infestation — *see* Candidiasis
Moniliasis — *see also* Candidiasis
  neonatal 771.7
  vulvovaginitis 112.1
Monoarthritis 716.60
  ankle 716.67
  arm 716.62
    lower (and wrist) 716.63
    upper (and elbow) 716.62
  foot (and ankle) 716.67
  forearm (and wrist) 716.63
  hand 716.64
  leg 716.66
    lower 716.66
    upper 716.65
  pelvic region (hip) (thigh) 716.65
  shoulder (region) 716.61
  specified site NEC 716.68
Monoblastic — *see* condition
Monochromatism (cone) (rod) 368.54
Monocytic — *see* condition
Monocytosis (symptomatic) 288.8
Monofixation syndrome 378.34
Monomania (*see also* Psychosis) 298.9
Mononeuritis 355.9
  cranial nerve — *see* Disorder, nerve, cranial
  femoral nerve 355.2
  lateral
    cutaneous nerve of thigh 355.1
    popliteal nerve 355.3
  lower limb 355.8
    specified nerve NEC 355.79
  medial popliteal nerve 355.4
  median nerve 354.1
  multiplex 354.5
  plantar nerve 355.6
  posterior tibial nerve 355.5
  radial nerve 354.3
  sciatic nerve 355.0
  ulnar nerve 354.2
  upper limb 354.9
    specified nerve NEC 354.8
  vestibular 388.5
Mononeuropathy (*see also* Mononeuritis) 355.9
  diabetic NEC 250.6 ✔5ᵗʰ [355.9]
    lower limb 250.6 ✔5ᵗʰ [355.8]
    upper limb 250.6 ✔5ᵗʰ [354.9]
  iliohypogastric 355.79
  ilioinguinal 355.79
  obturator 355.79
  saphenous 355.79
Mononucleosis, infectious 075
  with hepatitis 075 [573.1]
Monoplegia 344.5
  brain (current episode) (*see also* Paralysis,
    brain) 437.8
    fetus or newborn 767.8
  cerebral (current episode) (*see also* Paralysis,
    brain) 437.8
  congenital or infantile (cerebral) (spastic)
    (spinal) 343.3
  embolic (current) (*see also* Embolism, brain)
    434.1 ✔5ᵗʰ
    late effect — *see* Late effect(s) (of)
      cerebrovascular disease
  infantile (cerebral) (spastic) (spinal) 343.3
  lower limb 344.30
    affecting
      dominant side 344.31
      nondominant side 344.32
    due to late effect of cerebrovascular accident
      — *see* Late effect(s) (of)
        cerebrovascular accident
  newborn 767.8
  psychogenic 306.0
    specified as conversion reaction 300.11
  thrombotic (current) (*see also* Thrombosis,
    brain) 434.0 ✔5ᵗʰ
    late effect — *see* Late effect(s) (of)
      cerebrovascular disease
  transient 781.4

Monoplegia — *continued*
  upper limb 344.40
    affecting
      dominant side 344.41
      nondominant side 344.42
    due to late effect of cerebrovascular accident
      — *see* Late effect(s) (of)
        cerebrovascular accident
Monorchism, monorchidism 752.8
Monster, monstrosity — *see* Anomaly
Monteggia's fracture (closed) 813.03
  open 813.13
Mood swings
  brief compensatory 296.99
  rebound 296.99
Moore's syndrome (*see also* Epilepsy) 345.5 ✔5ᵗʰ
Mooren's ulcer (cornea) 370.07
Mooser-Neill reaction 081.0
Mooser bodies 081.0
Moral
  deficiency 301.7
  imbecility 301.7
Morax-Axenfeld conjunctivitis 372.03
Morbilli (*see also* Measles) 055.9
Morbus
  anglicus, anglorum 268.0
  Beigel 111.2
  caducus (*see also* Epilepsy) 345.9 ✔5ᵗʰ
  caeruleus 746.89
  celiacus 579.0
  comitialis (see also Epilepsy) 345.9 ✔5ᵗʰ
  cordis — *see also* Disease, heart
    valvulorum — *see* Endocarditis
  coxae 719.95
    tuberculous (*see also* Tuberculosis)
      015.1 ✔5ᵗʰ
  hemorrhagicus neonatorum 776.0
  maculosus neonatorum 772.6
  renum 593.0
  senilis (*see also* Osteoarthrosis) 715.9 ✔5ᵗʰ
Morel-Kraepelin disease (*see also* Schizophrenia)
    295.9 ✔5ᵗʰ
Morel-Moore syndrome (hyperostosis frontalis
    interna) 733.3
Morel-Morgagni syndrome (hyperostosis
    interna) 733.3
Morgagni
  cyst, organ, hydatid, or appendage 752.8
    fallopian tube 752.11
  disease or syndrome (hyperostosis frontalis
    interna) 733.3
Morgagni-Adams-Stokes syndrome (syncope with
    heart block) 426.9
Morgagni-Stewart-Morel syndrome (hyperostosis
    frontalis interna) 733.3
Moria (*see also* Psychosis) 298.9
Morning sickness 643.0 ✔5ᵗʰ
Moron 317
Morphea (guttate) (linear) 701.0
Morphine dependence (*see also* Dependence)
    304.0 ✔5ᵗʰ
Morphinism (*see also* Dependence) 304.0 ✔5ᵗʰ
Morphinomania (*see also* Dependence) 304.0 ✔5ᵗʰ
Morphoea 701.0
**Morquio (-Brailsford) (-Ullrich) disease or
  syndrome** (mucopolysaccharidosis IV) 277.5
  kyphosis 277.5
Morris syndrome (testicular feminization) 257.8
Morsus humanus (open wound) — *see also*
    Wound, open, by site
  skin surface intact — *see* Contusion
Mortification (dry) (moist) (*see also* Gangrene)
    785.4
Morton's
  disease 355.6
  foot 355.6
  metatarsalgia (syndrome) 355.6
  neuralgia 355.6
  neuroma 355.6
  syndrome (metatarsalgia) (neuralgia) 355.6
  toe 355.6

Morvan's disease — Mycosis

Morvan's disease 336.0
Mosaicism, mosaic (chromosomal) 758.9
  autosomal 758.5
  sex 758.81
Moschcowitz's syndrome (thrombotic thrombocytopenic purpura) 446.6
Mother yaw 102.0
Motion sickness (from travel, any vehicle) (from roundabouts or swings) 994.6
Mottled teeth (enamel) (endemic) (nonendemic) 520.3
Mottling enamel (endemic) (nonendemic) (teeth) 520.3
Mouchet's disease 732.5
Mould(s) (in vitreous) 117.9
Moulders'
  bronchitis 502
  tuberculosis (see also Tuberculosis) 011.4 ✓5ᵗʰ
Mounier-Kuhn syndrome 494.0
  with acute exacerbation 494.1
Mountain
  fever — see Fever, mountain
  sickness 993.2
    with polycythemia, acquired 289.0
    acute 289.0
  tick fever 066.1
Mouse, joint (see also Loose, body, joint) 718.1 ✓5ᵗʰ
  knee 717.6
Mouth — see condition
Movable
  coccyx 724.71
  kidney (see also Disease, renal) 593.0
    congenital 753.3
  organ or site, congenital NEC — see Malposition, congenital
  spleen 289.59
Movement
  abnormal (dystonic) (involuntary) 781.0
  decreased fetal 655.7 ✓5ᵗʰ
  paradoxical facial 374.43
Moya Moya disease 437.5
Mozart's ear 744.29
Mucha's disease (acute parapsoriasis varioliformis) 696.2
Mucha-Haberman syndrome (acute parapsoriasis varioliformis) 696.2
Mu-chain disease 273.2
Mucinosis (cutaneous) (papular) 701.8
Mucocele
  appendix 543.9
  buccal cavity 528.9
  gallbladder (see also Disease, gallbladder) 575.3
  lacrimal sac 375.43
  orbit (eye) 376.81
  salivary gland (any) 527.6
  sinus (accessory) (nasal) 478.1
  turbinate (bone) (middle) (nasal) 478.1
  uterus 621.8
Mucocutaneous lymph node syndrome (acute) (febrile) (infantile) 446.1
Mucoenteritis 564.9
Mucolipidosis I, II, III 272.7
Mucopolysaccharidosis (types 1-6) 277.5
  cardiopathy 277.5 [425.7]
Mucormycosis (lung) 117.7
Mucositis — see also Inflammation by site
  necroticans agranulocytica 288.0
Mucous — see also condition
  patches (syphilitic) 091.3
    congenital 090.0
Mucoviscidosis 277.00
  with meconium obstruction 277.01
Mucus
  asphyxia or suffocation (see also Asphyxia, mucus) 933.1
    newborn 770.1
  in stool 792.1
  plug (see also Asphyxia, mucus) 933.1
    aspiration, of newborn 770.1

Mucus — continued
  plug (see also Asphyxia, mucus) — continued
    tracheobronchial 519.1
      newborn 770.1
Muguet 112.0
Mulberry molars 090.5
Mullerian mixed tumor (M8950/3) — see Neoplasm, by site, malignant
Multicystic kidney 753.19
Multilobed placenta — see Placenta, abnormal
Multinodular prostate 600.1
Multiparity V61.5
  affecting
    fetus or newborn 763.89
    management of
      labor and delivery 659.4 ✓5ᵗʰ
      pregnancy V23.3
  requiring contraceptive management (see also Contraception) V25.9
Multipartita placenta — see Placenta, abnormal
Multiple, multiplex — see also condition
  birth
    affecting fetus or newborn 761.5
    healthy liveborn — see Newborn, multiple
  digits (congenital) 755.00
    fingers 755.01
    toes 755.02
  organ or site NEC — see Accessory
  personality 300.14
  renal arteries 747.62
Mumps 072.9
  with complication 072.8
    specified type NEC 072.79
  encephalitis 072.2
  hepatitis 072.71
  meningitis (aseptic) 072.1
  meningoencephalitis 072.2
  oophoritis 072.79
  orchitis 072.0
  pancreatitis 072.3
  polyneuropathy 072.72
  vaccination, prophylactic (against) V04.6
Mumu (see also Infestation, filarial) 125.9
Münchausen syndrome 301.51
Münchmeyer's disease or syndrome (exostosis luxurians) 728.11
Mural — see condition
Murmur (cardiac) (heart) (nonorganic) (organic) 785.2
  abdominal 787.5
  aortic (valve) (see also Endocarditis, aortic) 424.1
  benign — omit code
  cardiorespiratory 785.2
  diastolic — see condition
  Flint (see also Endocarditis, aortic) 424.1
  functional — omit code
  Graham Steell (pulmonic regurgitation) (see also Endocarditis, pulmonary) 424.3
  innocent — omit code
  insignificant — omit code
  midsystolic 785.2
  mitral (valve) — see Stenosis, mitral
  physiologic — see condition
  presystolic, mitral — see Insufficiency, mitral
  pulmonic (valve) (see also Endocarditis, pulmonary) 424.3
  Still's (vibratory) — omit code
  systolic (valvular) — see condition
  tricuspid (valve) — see Endocarditis, tricuspid
  undiagnosed 785.2
  valvular — see condition
  vibratory — omit code
Murri's disease (intermittent hemoglobinuria) 283.2
Muscae volitantes 379.24
Muscle, muscular — see condition
Musculoneuralgia 729.1
Mushrooming hip 718.95
Mushroom workers' (pickers') lung 495.5
Mutism (see also Aphasia) 784.3
  akinetic 784.3
  deaf (acquired) (congenital) 389.7

Mutism (see also Aphasia) — continued
  elective (selective) 313.23
    adjustment reaction 309.83
  hysterical 300.11
Myà's disease (congenital dilation, colon) 751.3
Myalgia (intercostal) 729.1
  eosinophilia syndrome 710.5
  epidemic 074.1
    cervical 078.89
  psychogenic 307.89
  traumatic NEC 959.9
Myasthenia, myasthenic 358.0
  cordis — see Failure, heart
  gravis 358.0
    neonatal 775.2
    pseudoparalytica 358.0
  stomach 536.8
    psychogenic 306.4
  syndrome
    in
      botulism 005.1 [358.1]
      diabetes mellitus 250.6 ✓5ᵗʰ [358.1]
      hypothyroidism (see also Hypothyroidism) 244.9 [358.1]
      malignant neoplasm NEC 199.1 [358.1]
      pernicious anemia 281.0 [358.1]
      thyrotoxicosis (see also Thyrotoxicosis) 242.9 ✓5ᵗʰ [358.1]
Mycelium infection NEC 117.9
Mycetismus 988.1
Mycetoma (actinomycotic) 039.9
  bone 039.8
    mycotic 117.4
  foot 039.4
    mycotic 117.4
  madurae 039.9
    mycotic 117.4
  maduromycotic 039.9
    mycotic 117.4
  mycotic 117.4
  nocardial 039.9
Mycobacteriosis — see Mycobacterium
Mycobacterium, mycobacterial (infection) 031.9
  acid-fast (bacilli) 031.9
  anonymous (see also Mycobacterium, atypical) 031.9
  atypical (acid-fast bacilli) 031.9
    cutaneous 031.1
    pulmonary 031.0
      tuberculous (see also Tuberculosis, pulmonary) 011.9 ✓5ᵗʰ
    specified site NEC 031.8
  avium 031.0
    intracellulare complex bacteremia (MAC) 031.2
  balnei 031.1
  Battey 031.0
  cutaneous 031.1
  disseminated 031.2
    avium-intracellulare complex (DMAC) 031.2
  fortuitum 031.0
  intracellulare (battey bacillus) 031.0
  kakerifu 031.8
  kansasii 031.0
  kasongo 031.8
  leprae — see Leprosy
  luciflavum 031.0
  marinum 031.1
  pulmonary 031.0
    tuberculous (see also Tuberculosis, pulmonary) 011.9 ✓5ᵗʰ
  scrofulaceum 031.1
  tuberculosis (human, bovine) — see also Tuberculosis
    avian type 031.0
  ulcerans 031.1
  xenopi 031.0
Mycosis, mycotic 117.9
  cutaneous NEC 111.9
  ear 111.8 [380.15]
  fungoides (M9700/3) 202.1 ✓5ᵗʰ
  mouth 112.0
  pharynx 117.9
  skin NEC 111.9
  stomatitis 112.0
  systemic NEC 117.9

Mycosis, mycotic — *continued*
tonsil 117.9
vagina, vaginitis 112.1
Mydriasis (persistent) (pupil) 379.43
Myelatelia 742.59
Myelinoclasis, perivascular, acute
(postinfectious) NEC 136.9 *[323.6]*
postimmunization or postvaccinal 323.5
Myelinosis, central pontine 341.8
Myelitis (acute) (ascending) (cerebellar)
(childhood) (chronic) (descending) (diffuse)
(disseminated) (pressure) (progressive)
(spinal cord) (subacute) (transverse) (*see also*
Encephalitis) 323.9
late effect — *see* category 326
optic neuritis in 341.0
postchickenpox 052.7
postvaccinal 323.5
syphilitic (transverse) 094.89
tuberculous (*see also* Tuberculosis) 013.6 ✓5ᵗʰ
virus 049.9
Myeloblastic — *see* condition
Myelocele (*see also* Spina bifida) 741.9 ✓5ᵗʰ
with hydrocephalus 741.0 ✓5ᵗʰ
Myelocystocele (*see also* Spina bifida) 741.9 ✓5ᵗʰ
Myelocytic — *see* condition
Myelocytoma 205.1 ✓5ᵗʰ
Myelodysplasia (spinal cord) 742.59
meaning myelodysplastic syndrome — *see*
Syndrome, myelodysplastic
Myeloencephalitis — *see* Encephalitis
Myelofibrosis (osteosclerosis) 289.8
Myelogenous — *see* condition
Myeloid — *see* condition
Myelokathexis 288.0
Myeloleukodystrophy 330.0
Myelolipoma (M8870/0) — *see* Neoplasm, by site,
benign
Myeloma (multiple) (plasma cell) (plasmacytic)
(M9730/3) 203.0 ✓5ᵗʰ
monostotic (M9731/1) 238.6
solitary (M9731/1) 238.6
Myelomalacia 336.8
Myelomata, multiple (M9730/3) 203.0 ✓5ᵗʰ
Myelomatosis (M9730/3) 203.0 ✓5ᵗʰ
Myelomeningitis — *see* Meningoencephalitis
Myelomeningocele (spinal cord) (*see also* Spina
bifida) 741.9 ✓5ᵗʰ
fetal, causing fetopelvic disproportion 653.7 ✓5ᵗʰ
Myelo-osteo-musculodysplasia hereditaria
756.89
Myelopathic — *see* condition
Myelopathy (spinal cord) 336.9
cervical 721.1
diabetic 250.6 ✓5ᵗʰ *[336.3]*
drug-induced 336.8
due to or with
carbon tetrachloride 987.8 *[323.7]*
degeneration or displacement, intervertebral
disc 722.70
cervical, cervicothoracic 722.71
lumbar, lumbosacral 722.73
thoracic, thoracolumbar 722.72
hydroxyquinoline derivatives 961.3 *[323.7]*
infection — *see* Encephalitis
intervertebral disc disorder 722.70
cervical, cervicothoracic 722.71
lumbar, lumbosacral 722.73
thoracic, thoracolumbar 722.72
lead 984.9 *[323.7]*
mercury 985.0 *[323.7]*
neoplastic disease (*see also* Neoplasm, by
site) 239.9 *[336.3]*
pernicious anemia 281.0 *[336.3]*
spondylosis 721.91
cervical 721.1
lumbar, lumbosacral 721.42
thoracic 721.41
thallium 985.8 *[323.7]*
lumbar, lumbosacral 721.42
necrotic (subacute) 336.1
radiation-induced 336.8

Myelopathy — *continued*
spondylogenic NEC 721.91
cervical 721.1
lumbar, lumbosacral 721.42
thoracic 721.41
thoracic 721.41
toxic NEC 989.9 *[323.7]*
transverse (*see also* Encephalitis) 323.9
vascular 336.1
Myeloproliferative disease (M9960/1) 238.7
Myeloradiculitis (*see also* Polyneuropathy) 357.0
Myeloradiculodysplasia (spinal) 742.59
Myelosarcoma (M9930/3) 205.3 ✓5ᵗʰ
Myelosclerosis 289.8
with myeloid metaplasia (M9961/1) 238.7
disseminated, of nervous system 340
megakaryocytic (M9961/1) 238.7
Myelosis (M9860/3) (*see also* Leukemia, myeloid)
205.9 ✓5ᵗʰ
acute (M9861/3) 205.0 ✓5ᵗʰ
aleukemic (M9864/3) 205.8 ✓5ᵗʰ
chronic (M9863/3) 205.1 ✓5ᵗʰ
erythremic (M9840/3) 207.0 ✓5ᵗʰ
acute (M9841/3) 207.0 ✓5ᵗʰ
megakaryocytic (M9920/3) 207.2 ✓5ᵗʰ
nonleukemic (chronic) 288.8
subacute (M9862/3) 205.2 ✓5ᵗʰ
Myesthenia — *see* Myasthenia
Myiasis (cavernous) 134.0
orbit 134.0 *[376.13]*
Myoadenoma, prostate 600.2
Myoblastoma
granular cell (M9580/0) — *see also* Neoplasm,
connective tissue, benign
malignant (M9580/3) — *see* Neoplasm,
connective tissue, malignant
tongue (M9580/0) 210.1
Myocardial — *see* condition
Myocardiopathy (congestive) (constrictive)
(familial) (hypertrophic nonobstructive)
(idiopathic) (infiltrative) (obstructive)
(primary) (restrictive) (sporadic) 425.4
alcoholic 425.5
amyloid 277.3 *[425.7]*
beriberi 265.0 *[425.7]*
cobalt-beer 425.5
due to
amyloidosis 277.3 *[425.7]*
beriberi 265.0 *[425.7]*
cardiac glycogenosis 271.0 *[425.7]*
Chagas' disease 086.0
Friedreich's ataxia 334.0 *[425.8]*
influenza 487.8 *[425.8]*
mucopolysaccharidosis 277.5 *[425.7]*
myotonia atrophica 359.2 *[425.8]*
progressive muscular dystrophy 359.1
[425.8]
sarcoidosis 135 *[425.8]*
glycogen storage 271.0 *[425.7]*
hypertrophic obstructive 425.1
metabolic NEC 277.9 *[425.7]*
nutritional 269.9 *[425.7]*
obscure (African) 425.2
postpartum 674.8 ✓5ᵗʰ
secondary 425.9
thyrotoxic (*see also* Thyrotoxicosis)
242.9 ✓5ᵗʰ *[425.7]*
toxic NEC 425.9
Myocarditis (fibroid) (interstitial) (old)
(progressive) (senile) (with arteriosclerosis)
429.0
with
rheumatic fever (conditions classifiable to
390) 398.0
active (*see also* Myocarditis, acute,
rheumatic) 391.2
inactive or quiescent (with chorea) 398.0
active (nonrheumatic) 422.90
rheumatic 391.2
with chorea (acute) (rheumatic)
(Sydenham's) 392.0
acute or subacute (interstitial) 422.90
due to Streptococcus (beta-hemolytic) 391.2
idiopathic 422.91

Myocarditis — *continued*
acute or subacute — *continued*
rheumatic 391.2
with chorea (acute) (rheumatic)
(Sydenham's) 392.0
specified type NEC 422.99
aseptic of newborn 074.23
bacterial (acute) 422.92
chagasic 086.0
chronic (interstitial) 429.0
congenital 746.89
constrictive 425.4
Coxsackie (virus) 074.23
diphtheritic 032.82
due to or in
Coxsackie (virus) 074.23
diphtheria 032.82
epidemic louse-borne typhus 080 *[422.0]*
influenza 487.8 *[422.0]*
Lyme disease 088.81 *[422.0]*
scarlet fever 034.1 *[422.0]*
toxoplasmosis (acquired) 130.3
tuberculosis (*see also* Tuberculosis)
017.9 ✓5ᵗʰ *[422.0]*
typhoid 002.0 *[422.0]*
typhus NEC 081.9 *[422.0]*
eosinophilic 422.91
epidemic of newborn 074.23
Fiedler's (acute) (isolated) (subacute) 422.91
giant cell (acute) (subacute) 422.91
gonococcal 098.85
granulomatous (idiopathic) (isolated)
(nonspecific) 422.91
hypertensive (*see also* Hypertension, heart)
402.90
idiopathic 422.91
granulomatous 422.91
infective 422.92
influenzal 487.8 *[422.0]*
isolated (diffuse) (granulomatous) 422.91
malignant 422.99
meningococcal 036.43
nonrheumatic, active 422.90
parenchymatous 422.90
pneumococcal (acute) (subacute) 422.92
rheumatic (chronic) (inactive) (with chorea)
398.0
active or acute 391.2
with chorea (acute) (rheumatic)
(Sydenham's) 392.0
septic 422.92
specific (giant cell) (productive) 422.91
staphylococcal (acute) (subacute) 422.92
suppurative 422.92
syphilitic (chronic) 093.82
toxic 422.93
rheumatic (*see also* Myocarditis, acute
rheumatic) 391.2
tuberculous (*see also* Tuberculosis)
017.9 ✓5ᵗʰ *[422.0]*
typhoid 002.0 *[422.0]*
valvular — *see* Endocarditis
viral, except Coxsackie 422.91
Coxsackie 074.23
of newborn (Coxsackie) 074.23
Myocardium, myocardial — *see* condition
Myocardosis (*see also* Cardiomyopathy) 425.4
Myoclonia (essential) 333.2
epileptica 333.2
Friedrich's 333.2
massive 333.2
Myoclonic
epilepsy, familial (progressive) 333.2
jerks 333.2
Myoclonus (familial essential) (multifocal)
(simplex) 333.2
facial 351.8
massive (infantile) 333.2
pharyngeal 478.29
Myodiastasis 728.84
Myoendocarditis — *see also* Endocarditis
acute or subacute 421.9
Myoepithelioma (M8982/0) — *see* Neoplasm, by
site, benign
Myofascitis (acute) 729.1
low back 724.2

Myofibroma — **Narrowing**

Myofibroma (M8890/0) — *see also* Neoplasm, connective tissue, benign
 uterus (cervix) (corpus) (*see also* Leiomyoma) 218.9
Myofibrosis 728.2
 heart (*see also* Myocarditis) 429.0
 humeroscapular region 726.2
 scapulohumeral 726.2
Myofibrositis (*see also* Myositis) 729.1
 scapulohumeral 726.2
Myogelosis (occupational) 728.89
Myoglobinuria 791.3
Myoglobulinuria, primary 791.3
Myokymia — *see also* Myoclonus
 facial 351.8
Myolipoma (M8860/0)
 specified site — *see* Neoplasm, connective tissue, benign
 unspecified site 223.0
Myoma (M8895/0) — *see also* Neoplasm, connective tissue, benign
 cervix (stump) (uterus) (*see also* Leiomyoma) 218.9
 malignant (M8895/3) — *see* Neoplasm, connective tissue, malignant
 prostate 600.2
 uterus (cervix) (corpus) (*see also* Leiomyoma) 218.9
  in pregnancy or childbirth 654.1 ✓5ᵗʰ
   affecting fetus or newborn 763.89
   causing obstructed labor 660.2 ✓5ᵗʰ
    affecting fetus or newborn 763.1
Myomalacia 728.9
 cordis, heart (*see also* Degeneration, myocardial) 429.1
Myometritis (*see also* Endometritis) 615.9
Myometrium — *see* condition
Myonecrosis, clostridial 040.0
Myopathy 359.9
 alcoholic 359.4
 amyloid 277.3 [359.6]
 benign congenital 359.0
 central core 359.0
 centronuclear 359.0
 congenital (benign) 359.0
 critical illness 359.81 ●
 distal 359.1
 due to drugs 359.4
 endocrine 259.9 [359.5]
  specified type NEC 259.8 [359.5]
 extraocular muscles 376.82
 facioscapulohumeral 359.1
 in
  Addison's disease 255.4 [359.5]
  amyloidosis 277.3 [359.6]
  cretinism 243 [359.5]
  Cushing's syndrome 255.0 [359.5]
  disseminated lupus erythematosus 710.0 [359.6]
  giant cell arteritis 446.5 [359.6]
  hyperadrenocorticism NEC 255.3 [359.5]
  hyperparathyroidism 252.0 [359.5]
  hypopituitarism 253.2 [359.5]
  hypothyroidism (*see also* Hypothyroidism) 244.9 [359.5]
  malignant neoplasm NEC (M8000/3) 199.1 [359.6]
  myxedema (*see also* Myxedema) 244.9 [359.5]
  polyarteritis nodosa 446.0 [359.6]
  rheumatoid arthritis 714.0 [359.6]
  sarcoidosis 135 [359.6]
  scleroderma 710.1 [359.6]
  Sjögren's disease 710.2 [359.6]
  thyrotoxicosis (*see also* Thyrotoxicosis) 242.9 ✓5ᵗʰ [359.5]
 inflammatory 359.89 ▲
 intensive care (ICU) 359.81 ▲
 limb-girdle 359.1
 myotubular 359.0
 necrotizing, acute 359.81 ●
 nemaline 359.0
 ocular 359.1
 oculopharyngeal 359.1
 of critical illness 359.81 ●

Myopathy — *continued*
 primary 359.89 ▲
 progressive NEC 359.89 ▲
 quadriplegic, acute 359.81 ●
 rod body 359.0
 scapulohumeral 359.1
 specified type NEC 359.89 ▲
 toxic 359.4
Myopericarditis (*see also* Pericarditis) 423.9
Myopia (axial) (congenital) (increased curvature or refraction, nucleus of lens) 367.1
 degenerative, malignant 360.21
 malignant 360.21
 progressive high (degenerative) 360.21
Myosarcoma (M8895/3) — *see* Neoplasm, connective tissue, malignant
Myosis (persistent) 379.42
 stromal (endolymphatic) (M8931/1) 236.0
Myositis 729.1
 clostridial 040.0
 due to posture 729.1
 epidemic 074.1
 fibrosa or fibrous (chronic) 728.2
  Volkmann's (complicating trauma) 958.6
 infective 728.0
 interstitial 728.81
 multiple — *see* Polymyositis
 occupational 729.1
 orbital, chronic 376.12
 ossificans 728.12
  circumscribed 728.12
  progressive 728.11
  traumatic 728.12
 progressive fibrosing 728.11
 purulent 728.0
 rheumatic 729.1
 rheumatoid 729.1
 suppurative 728.0
 syphilitic 095.6
 traumatic (old) 729.1
Myospasia impulsiva 307.23
Myotonia (acquisita) (intermittens) 728.85
 atrophica 359.2
 congenita 359.2
 dystrophica 359.2
Myotonic pupil 379.46
Myriapodiasis 134.1
Myringitis
 with otitis media — *see* Otitis media
 acute 384.00
  specified type NEC 384.09
 bullosa hemorrhagica 384.01
 bullous 384.01
 chronic 384.1
Mysophobia 300.29
Mytilotoxism 988.0
Myxadenitis labialis 528.5
Myxedema (adult) (idiocy) (infantile) (juvenile) (thyroid gland) (*see also* Hypothyroidism) 244.9
 circumscribed 242.9 ✓5ᵗʰ
 congenital 243
 cutis 701.8
 localized (pretibial) 242.9 ✓5ᵗʰ
 madness (acute) 293.0
  subacute 293.1
 papular 701.8
 pituitary 244.8
 postpartum 674.8 ✓5ᵗʰ
 pretibial 242.9 ✓5ᵗʰ
 primary 244.9
Myxochondrosarcoma (M9220/3) — *see* Neoplasm, cartilage, malignant
Myxofibroma (M8811/0) — *see also* Neoplasm, connective tissue, benign
 odontogenic (M9320/0) 213.1
  upper jaw (bone) 213.0
Myxofibrosarcoma (M8811/3) — *see* Neoplasm, connective tissue, malignant
Myxolipoma (M8852/0) (*see also* Lipoma, by site) 214.9
Myxoliposarcoma (M8852/3) — *see* Neoplasm, connective tissue, malignant

Myxoma (M8840/0) — *see also* Neoplasm, connective tissue, benign
 odontogenic (M9320/0) 213.1
  upper jaw (bone) 213.0
Myxosarcoma (M8840/3) — *see* Neoplasm, connective tissue, malignant

N

Naegeli's
 disease (hereditary hemorrhagic thrombasthenia) 287.1
 leukemia, monocytic (M9863/3) 205.1 ✓5ᵗʰ
 syndrome (incontinentia pigmenti) 757.33
Naffziger's syndrome 353.0
Naga sore (*see also* Ulcer, skin) 707.9
Nägele's pelvis 738.6
 with disproportion (fetopelvic) 653.0 ✓5ᵗʰ
  affecting fetus or newborn 763.1
  causing obstructed labor 660.1 ✓5ᵗʰ
   affecting fetus or newborn 763.1
Nager-de Reynier syndrome (dysostosis mandibularis) 756.0
Nail — *see also* condition
 biting 307.9
 patella syndrome (hereditary osteoonychodysplasia) 756.89
Nanism, nonosomia (*see also* Dwarfism) 259.4
 hypophyseal 253.3
 pituitary 253.3
 renis, renalis 588.0
Nanukayami 100.89
Napkin rash 691.0
Narcissism 301.81
Narcolepsy 347
Narcosis
 carbon dioxide (respiratory) 786.09
 due to drug
  correct substance properly administered 780.09
  overdose or wrong substance given or taken 977.9
   specified drug — *see* Table of Drugs and Chemicals
Narcotism (chronic) (*see also* listing under Dependence) 304.9 ✓5ᵗʰ
 acute
  correct substance properly administered 349.82
  overdose or wrong substance given or taken 967.8
   specified drug — *see* Table of Drugs and Chemicals
Narrow
 anterior chamber angle 365.02
 pelvis (inlet) (outlet) — *see* Contraction, pelvis
Narrowing
 artery NEC 447.1
  auditory, internal 433.8 ✓5ᵗʰ
  basilar 433.0 ✓5ᵗʰ
   with other precerebral artery 433.3 ✓5ᵗʰ
    bilateral 433.3 ✓5ᵗʰ
  carotid 433.1 ✓5ᵗʰ
   with other precerebral artery 433.3 ✓5ᵗʰ
    bilateral 433.3 ✓5ᵗʰ
  cerebellar 433.8 ✓5ᵗʰ
  choroidal 433.8 ✓5ᵗʰ
  communicating posterior 433.8 ✓5ᵗʰ
  coronary — *see also* Arteriosclerosis, coronary
   congenital 746.85
    due to syphilis 090.5
  hypophyseal 433.8 ✓5ᵗʰ
  pontine 433.8 ✓5ᵗʰ
  precerebral NEC 433.9 ✓5ᵗʰ
   multiple or bilateral 433.3 ✓5ᵗʰ
   specified NEC 433.8 ✓5ᵗʰ
  vertebral 433.2 ✓5ᵗʰ
   with other precerebral artery 433.3 ✓5ᵗʰ
    bilateral 433.3 ✓5ᵗʰ
  auditory canal (external) (*see also* Stricture, ear canal, acquired) 380.50
  cerebral arteries 437.0
  cicatricial — *see* Cicatrix

Narrowing — *continued*
congenital — *see* Anomaly, congenital
coronary artery — *see* Narrowing, artery, coronary
ear, middle 385.22
Eustachian tube (*see also* Obstruction, Eustachian tube) 381.60
eyelid 374.46
congenital 743.62
intervertebral disc or space NEC — *see* Degeneration, intervertebral disc
joint space, hip 719.85
larynx 478.74
lids 374.46
congenital 743.62
mesenteric artery (with gangrene) 557.0
palate 524.8
palpebral fissure 374.46
retinal artery 362.13
ureter 593.3
urethra (*see also* Stricture, urethra) 598.9

Narrowness, abnormal, eyelid 743.62
Nasal — *see* condition
Nasolacrimal — *see* condition
Nasopharyngeal — *see also* condition
bursa 478.29
pituitary gland 759.2
torticollis 723.5
Nasopharyngitis (acute) (infective) (subacute) 460
chronic 472.2
due to external agent — *see* Condition, respiratory, chronic, due to
due to external agent — *see* Condition, respiratory, due to
septic 034.0
streptococcal 034.0
suppurative (chronic) 472.2
ulcerative (chronic) 472.2
Nasopharynx, nasopharyngeal — *see* condition
Natal tooth, teeth 520.6
Nausea (*see also* Vomiting) 787.02
with vomiting 787.01
epidemic 078.82
gravidarum — *see* Hyperemesis, gravidarum
marina 994.6
Navel — *see* condition
Neapolitan fever (*see also* Brucellosis) 023.9
Nearsightedness 367.1
Near-syncope 780.2
Nebécourt's syndrome 253.3
Nebula, cornea (eye) 371.01
congenital 743.43
interfering with vision 743.42
Necator americanus infestation 126.1
Necatoriasis 126.1
Neck — *see* condition
Necrencephalus (*see also* Softening, brain) 437.8
Necrobacillosis 040.3
Necrobiosis 799.8
brain or cerebral (*see also* Softening, brain) 437.8
lipoidica 709.3
diabeticorum 250.8 ✓5ᵗʰ [709.3]
Necrodermolysis 695.1
Necrolysis, toxic epidermal 695.1
due to drug
correct substance properly administered 695.1
overdose or wrong substance given or taken 977.9
specified drug — *see* Table of Drugs and Chemicals
Necrophilia 302.89
Necrosis, necrotic
adrenal (capsule) (gland) 255.8
antrum, nasal sinus 478.1
aorta (hyaline) (*see also* Aneurysm, aorta) 441.9
cystic medial 441.00
abdominal 441.02
thoracic 441.01
thoracoabdominal 441.03
ruptured 441.5

Necrosis, necrotic — *continued*
arteritis 446.0
artery 447.5
aseptic, bone 733.40
femur (head) (neck) 733.42
medial condyle 733.43
humoral head 733.41
medial femoral condyle 733.43
specific site NEC 733.49
talus 733.44
avascular, bone NEC (*see also* Necrosis, aseptic, bone) 733.40
bladder (aseptic) (sphincter) 596.8
bone (*see also* Osteomyelitis) 730.1 ✓5ᵗʰ
acute 730.0 ✓5ᵗʰ
aseptic or avascular 733.40
femur (head) (neck) 733.42
medial condyle 733.43
humoral head 733.41
medial femoral condyle 733.43
specified site NEC 733.49
talus 733.44
ethmoid 478.1
ischemic 733.40
jaw 526.4
marrow 289.8
Paget's (osteitis deformans) 731.0
tuberculous — *see* Tuberculosis, bone
brain (softening) (*see also* Softening, brain) 437.8
breast (aseptic) (fat) (segmental) 611.3
bronchus, bronchi 519.1
central nervous system NEC (*see also* Softening, brain) 437.8
cerebellar (*see also* Softening, brain) 437.8
cerebral (softening) (*see also* Softening, brain) 437.8
cerebrospinal (softening) (*see also* Softening, brain) 437.8
cornea (*see also* Keratitis) 371.40
cortical, kidney 583.6
cystic medial (aorta) 441.00
abdominal 441.02
thoracic 441.01
thoracoabdominal 441.03
dental 521.09
pulp 522.1
due to swallowing corrosive substance — *see* Burn, by site
ear (ossicle) 385.24
esophagus 530.89
ethmoid (bone) 478.1
eyelid 374.50
fat, fatty (generalized) (*see also* Degeneration, fatty) 272.8
breast (aseptic) (segmental) 611.3
intestine 569.89
localized — *see* Degeneration, by site, fatty
mesentery 567.8
omentum 567.8
pancreas 577.8
peritoneum 567.8
skin (subcutaneous) 709.3
newborn 778.1
femur (aseptic) (avascular) 733.42
head 733.42
medial condyle 733.43
neck 733.42
gallbladder (*see also* Cholecystitis, acute) 575.0
gangrenous 785.4
gastric 537.89
glottis 478.79
heart (myocardium) — *see* Infarct, myocardium
hepatic (*see also* Necrosis, liver) 570
hip (aseptic) (avascular) 733.42
intestine (acute) (hemorrhagic) (massive) 557.0
ischemic 785.4
jaw 526.4
kidney (bilateral) 583.9
acute 584.9
cortical 583.6
acute 584.6
with
abortion — *see* Abortion, by type, with renal failure
ectopic pregnancy (*see also* categories 633.0-633.9) 639.3

Necrosis, necrotic — *continued*
kidney — *continued*
cortical — *continued*
acute — *continued*
with — *continued*
molar pregnancy (*see also* categories 630-632) 639.3
complicating pregnancy 646.2 ✓5ᵗʰ
affecting fetus or newborn 760.1
following labor and delivery 669.3 ✓5ᵗʰ
medullary (papillary) (*see also* Pyelitis) 590.80
in
acute renal failure 584.7
nephritis, nephropathy 583.7
papillary (*see also* Pyelitis) 590.80
in
acute renal failure 584.7
nephritis, nephropathy 583.7
tubular 584.5
with
abortion — *see* Abortion, by type, with renal failure
ectopic pregnancy (*see also* categories 633.0-633.9) 639.3
molar pregnancy (*see also* categories 630-632) 639.3
complicating
abortion 639.3
ectopic or molar pregnancy 639.3
pregnancy 646.2 ✓5ᵗʰ
affecting fetus or newborn 760.1
following labor and delivery 669.3 ✓5ᵗʰ
traumatic 958.5
larynx 478.79
liver (acute) (congenital) (diffuse) (massive) (subacute) 570
with
abortion — *see* Abortion, by type, with specified complication NEC
ectopic pregnancy (*see also* categories 633.0-633.9) 639.8
molar pregnancy (*see also* categories 630-632) 639.8
complicating pregnancy 646.7 ✓5ᵗʰ
affecting fetus or newborn 760.8
following
abortion 639.8
ectopic or molar pregnancy 639.8
obstetrical 646.7 ✓5ᵗʰ
postabortal 639.8
puerperal, postpartum 674.8 ✓5ᵗʰ
toxic 573.3
lung 513.0
lymphatic gland 683
mammary gland 611.3
mastoid (chronic) 383.1
mesentery 557.0
fat 567.8
mitral valve — *see* Insufficiency, mitral
myocardium, myocardial — *see* Infarct, myocardium
nose (septum) 478.1
omentum 557.0
with mesenteric infarction 557.0
fat 567.8
orbit, orbital 376.10
ossicles, ear (aseptic) 385.24
ovary (*see also* Salpingo-oophoritis) 614.2
pancreas (aseptic) (duct) (fat) 577.8
acute 577.0
infective 577.0
papillary, kidney (*see also* Pyelitis) 590.80
peritoneum 557.0
with mesenteric infarction 557.0
fat 567.8
pharynx 462
in granulocytopenia 288.0
phosphorus 983.9
pituitary (gland) (postpartum) (Sheehan) 253.2
placenta (*see also* Placenta, abnormal) 656.7 ✓5ᵗʰ
pneumonia 513.0
pulmonary 513.0
pulp (dental) 522.1
pylorus 537.89
radiation — *see* Necrosis, by site

Narrowing — Necrosis

Necrosis, necrotic — *continued*
  radium — *see* Necrosis, by site
  renal — *see* Necrosis, kidney
  sclera 379.19
  scrotum 608.89
  skin or subcutaneous tissue 709.8
    due to burn — see Burn, by site
    gangrenous 785.4
  spine, spinal (column) 730.18
    acute 730.18
    cord 336.1
  spleen 289.59
  stomach 537.89
  stomatitis 528.1
  subcutaneous fat 709.3
    fetus or newborn 778.1
  subendocardial — *see* Infarct, myocardium
  suprarenal (capsule) (gland) 255.8
  teeth, tooth 521.09
  testis 608.89
  thymus (gland) 254.8
  tonsil 474.8
  trachea 519.1
  tuberculous NEC — *see* Tuberculosis
  tubular (acute) (anoxic) (toxic) 584.5
    due to a procedure 997.5
  umbilical cord, affecting fetus or newborn
    762.6
  vagina 623.8
  vertebra (lumbar) 730.18
    acute 730.18
    tuberculous (*see also* Tuberculosis)
      015.0 ✓5ᵗʰ *[730.8]* ✓5ᵗʰ
  vesical (aseptic) (bladder) 596.8
  x-ray — *see* Necrosis, by site
Necrospermia 606.0
Necrotizing angiitis 446.0
Negativism 301.7
Neglect (child) (newborn) NEC 995.52
  adult 995.84
  after or at birth 995.52
  hemispatial 781.8
  left-sided 781.8
  sensory 781.8
  visuospatial 781.8
Negri bodies 071
Neill-Dingwall syndrome (microcephaly and
  dwarfism) 759.89
Neisserian infection NEC — *see* Gonococcus
Nematodiasis NEC (*see also* Infestation,
  Nematode) 127.9
  ancylostoma (*see also* Ancylostomiasis) 126.9
Neoformans cryptococcus infection 117.5
Neonatal — *see also* condition
  teeth, tooth 520.6
Neonatorum — *see* condition

Neoplasm, neoplastic	Malignant			Benign	Uncertain Behavior	Unspecified
	Primary	Secondary	Ca in situ			
	199.1	199.1	234.9	229.9	238.9	239.9

Notes — 1. The list below gives the code numbers for neoplasms by anatomical site. For each site there are six possible code numbers according to whether the neoplasm in question is malignant, benign, in situ, of uncertain behavior, or of unspecified nature. The description of the neoplasm will often indicate which of the six columns is appropriate; e.g., malignant melanoma of skin, benign fibroadenoma of breast, carcinoma in situ of cervix uteri.

Where such descriptors are not present, the remainder of the Index should be consulted where guidance is given to the appropriate column for each morphological (histological) variety listed; e.g., Mesonephroma — see Neoplasm, malignant; Embryoma — see also Neoplasm, uncertain behavior; Disease, Bowen's — see Neoplasm, skin, in situ. However, the guidance in the Index can be overridden if one of the descriptors mentioned above is present; e.g., malignant adenoma of colon is coded to 153.9 and not to 211.3 as the adjective "malignant" overrides the Index entry "Adenoma — see also Neoplasm, benign."

2. Sites marked with the sign * (e.g., face NEC*) should be classified to malignant neoplasm of skin of these sites if the variety of neoplasm is a squamous cell carcinoma or an epidermoid carcinoma, and to benign neoplasm of skin of these sites if the variety of neoplasm is a papilloma (any type).

	Primary	Secondary	Ca in situ	Benign	Uncertain Behavior	Unspecified
abdomen, abdominal	195.2	198.89	234.8	229.8	238.8	239.8
cavity	195.2	198.89	234.8	229.8	238.8	239.8
organ	195.2	198.89	234.8	229.8	238.8	239.8
viscera	195.2	198.89	234.8	229.8	238.8	239.8
wall	173.5	198.2	232.5	216.5	238.2	239.2
connective tissue	171.5	198.89	—	215.5	238.1	239.2
abdominopelvic	195.8	198.89	234.8	229.8	238.8	239.8
accessory sinus — see Neoplasm, sinus						
acoustic nerve	192.0	198.4	—	225.1	237.9	239.7
acromion (process)	170.4	198.5	—	213.4	238.0	239.2
adenoid (pharynx) (tissue)	147.1	198.89	230.0	210.7	235.1	239.0
adipose tissue (see also Neoplasm, connective tissue)	171.9	198.89	—	215.9	238.1	239.2
adnexa (uterine)	183.9	198.82	233.3	221.8	236.3	239.5
adrenal (cortex) (gland) (medulla)	194.0	198.7	234.8	227.0	237.2	239.7
ala nasi (external)	173.3	198.2	232.3	216.3	238.2	239.2
alimentary canal or tract NEC	159.9	197.8	230.9	211.9	235.5	239.0
alveolar	143.9	198.89	230.0	210.4	235.1	239.0
mucosa	143.9	198.89	230.0	210.4	235.1	239.0
lower	143.1	198.89	230.0	210.4	235.1	239.0
upper	143.0	198.89	230.0	210.4	235.1	239.0
ridge or process	170.1	198.5	—	213.1	238.0	239.2
carcinoma	143.9	—	—	—	—	—
lower	143.1	—	—	—	—	—
upper	143.0	—	—	—	—	—
lower	170.1	198.5	—	213.1	238.0	239.2
mucosa	143.9	198.89	230.0	210.4	235.1	239.0
lower	143.1	198.89	230.0	210.4	235.1	239.0
upper	143.0	198.89	230.0	210.4	235.1	239.0
upper	170.0	198.5	—	213.0	238.0	239.2
sulcus	145.1	198.89	230.0	210.4	235.1	239.0
alveolus	143.9	198.89	230.0	210.4	235.1	239.0
lower	143.1	198.89	230.0	210.4	235.1	239.0
upper	143.0	198.89	230.0	210.4	235.1	239.0
ampulla of Vater	156.2	197.8	230.8	211.5	235.3	239.0
ankle NEC*	195.5	198.89	232.7	229.8	238.8	239.8
anorectum, anorectal (junction)	154.8	197.5	230.7	211.4	235.2	239.0
antecubital fossa or space*	195.4	198.89	232.6	229.8	238.8	239.8
antrum (Highmore) (maxillary)	160.2	197.3	231.8	212.0	235.9	239.1
pyloric	151.2	197.8	230.2	211.1	235.2	239.0
tympanicum	160.1	197.3	231.8	212.0	235.9	239.1
anus, anal	154.3	197.5	230.6	211.4	235.5	239.0
canal	154.2	197.5	230.5	211.4	233.5	239.0
contiguous sites with rectosigmoid junction or rectum	154.8	—	—	—	—	—
margin	173.5	198.2	232.5	216.5	238.2	239.2
skin	173.5	198.2	232.5	216.5	238.2	239.2
sphincter	154.2	197.5	230.5	211.4	235.5	239.0
aorta (thoracic)	171.4	198.89	—	215.4	238.1	239.2
abdominal	171.5	198.89	—	215.5	238.1	239.2
aortic body	194.6	198.89	—	227.6	237.3	239.7
aponeurosis	171.9	198.89	—	215.9	238.1	239.2
palmar	171.2	198.89	—	215.2	238.1	239.2
plantar	171.3	198.89	—	215.3	238.1	239.2
appendix	153.5	197.5	230.3	211.3	235.2	239.0
arachnoid (cerebral)	192.1	198.4	—	225.2	237.6	239.7
spinal	192.3	198.4	—	225.4	237.6	239.7

✔4ᵗʰ Fourth-digit Required   ✔5ᵗʰ Fifth-digit Required   ▶◀ Revised Text   ● New Line   ▲ Revised Code

	Malignant					
	Primary	**Secondary**	**Ca in situ**	**Benign**	**Uncertain Behavior**	**Unspecified**
Neoplasm, neoplastic — *continued*						
areola (female)	174.0	198.81	233.0	217	238.3	239.3
male	175.0	198.81	233.0	217	238.3	239.3
arm NEC*	195.4	198.89	232.6	229.8	238.8	239.8
artery — *see* Neoplasm, connective tissue						
aryepiglottic fold	148.2	198.89	230.0	210.8	235.1	239.0
hypopharyngeal aspect	148.2	198.89	230.0	210.8	235.1	239.0
laryngeal aspect	161.1	197.3	231.0	212.1	235.6	239.1
marginal zone	148.2	198.89	230.0	210.8	235.1	239.0
arytenoid (cartilage)	161.3	197.3	231.0	212.1	235.6	239.1
fold — *see* Neoplasm, aryepiglottic						
atlas	170.2	198.5	—	213.2	238.0	239.2
atrium, cardiac	164.1	198.89	—	212.7	238.8	239.8
auditory						
canal (external) (skin)	173.2	198.2	232.2	216.2	238.2	239.2
internal	160.1	197.3	231.8	212.0	235.9	239.1
nerve	192.0	198.4	—	225.1	237.9	239.7
tube	160.1	197.3	231.8	212.0	235.9	239.1
opening	147.2	198.89	230.0	210.7	235.1	239.0
auricle, ear	173.2	198.2	232.2	216.2	238.2	239.2
cartilage	171.0	198.89	—	215.0	238.1	239.2
auricular canal (external)	173.2	198.2	232.2	216.2	238.2	239.2
internal	160.1	197.3	231.8	212.0	235.9	239.1
autonomic nerve or nervous system NEC	171.9	198.89	—	215.9	238.1	239.2
axilla, axillary	195.1	198.89	234.8	229.8	238.8	239.8
fold	173.5	198.2	232.5	216.5	238.2	239.2
back NEC*	195.8	198.89	232.5	229.8	238.8	239.8
Bartholin's gland	184.1	198.82	233.3	221.2	236.3	239.5
basal ganglia	191.0	198.3	—	225.0	237.5	239.6
basis pedunculi	191.7	198.3	—	225.0	237.5	239.6
bile or biliary (tract)	156.9	197.8	230.8	211.5	235.3	239.0
canaliculi (biliferi) (intrahepatic)	155.1	197.8	230.8	211.5	235.3	239.0
canals, interlobular	155.1	197.8	230.8	211.5	235.3	239.0
contiguous sites	156.8	—	—	—	—	—
duct or passage (common) (cystic) (extrahepatic)	156.1	197.8	230.8	211.5	235.3	239.0
contiguous sites with gallbladder	156.8	—	—	—	—	—
interlobular	155.1	197.8	230.8	211.5	235.3	239.0
intrahepatic	155.1	197.8	230.8	211.5	235.3	239.0
and extrahepatic	156.9	197.8	230.8	211.5	235.3	239.0
bladder (urinary)	188.9	198.1	233.7	223.3	236.7	239.4
contiguous sites	188.8	—	—	—	—	—
dome	188.1	198.1	233.7	223.3	236.7	239.4
neck	188.5	198.1	233.7	223.3	236.7	239.4
orifice	188.9	198.1	233.7	223.3	236.7	239.4
ureteric	188.6	198.1	233.7	223.3	236.7	239.4
urethral	188.5	198.1	233.7	223.3	236.7	239.4
sphincter	188.8	198.1	233.7	223.3	236.7	239.4
trigone	188.0	198.1	233.7	223.3	236.7	239.4
urachus	188.7	—	233.7	223.3	236.7	239.4
wall	188.9	198.1	233.7	223.3	236.7	239.4
anterior	188.3	198.1	233.7	223.3	236.7	239.4
lateral	188.2	198.1	233.7	223.3	236.7	239.4
posterior	188.4	198.1	233.7	223.3	236.7	239.4
blood vessel — *see* Neoplasm, connective tissue						
bone (periosteum)	170.9	198.5	—	213.9	238.0	239.2

Note — Carcinomas and adenocarcinomas, of any type other than intraosseous or odontogenic, of the sites listed under "Neoplasm, bone" should be considered as constituting metastatic spread from an unspecified primary site and coded to 198.5 for morbidity coding and to 199.1 for underlying cause of death coding.

acetabulum	170.6	198.5	—	213.6	238.0	239.2
acromion (process)	170.4	198.5	—	213.4	238.0	239.2
ankle	170.8	198.5	—	213.8	238.0	239.2
arm NEC	170.4	198.5	—	213.4	238.0	239.2
astragalus	170.8	198.5	—	213.8	238.0	239.2
atlas	170.2	198.5	—	213.2	238.0	239.2
axis	170.2	198.5	—	213.2	238.0	239.2
back NEC	170.2	198.5	—	213.2	238.0	239.2
calcaneus	170.8	198.5	—	213.8	238.0	239.2

	Malignant					
	Primary	Secondary	Ca in situ	Benign	Uncertain Behavior	Unspecified
Neoplasm, neoplastic — *continued*						
bone — *continued*						
calvarium	170.0	198.5	—	213.0	238.0	239.2
carpus (any)	170.5	198.5	—	213.5	238.0	239.2
cartilage NEC	170.9	198.5	—	213.9	238.0	239.2
clavicle	170.3	198.5	—	213.3	238.0	239.2
clivus	170.0	198.5	—	213.0	238.0	239.2
coccygeal vertebra	170.6	198.5	—	213.6	238.0	239.2
coccyx	170.6	198.5	—	213.6	238.0	239.2
costal cartilage	170.3	198.5	—	213.3	238.0	239.2
costovertebral joint	170.3	198.5	—	213.3	238.0	239.2
cranial	170.0	198.5	—	213.0	238.0	239.2
cuboid	170.8	198.5	—	213.8	238.0	239.2
cuneiform	170.9	198.5	—	213.9	238.0	239.2
ankle	170.8	198.5	—	213.8	238.0	239.2
wrist	170.5	198.5	—	213.5	238.0	239.2
digital	170.9	198.5	—	213.9	238.0	239.2
finger	170.5	198.5	—	213.5	238.0	239.2
toe	170.8	198.5	—	213.8	238.0	239.2
elbow	170.4	198.5	—	213.4	238.0	239.2
ethmoid (labyrinth)	170.0	198.5	—	213.0	238.0	239.2
face	170.0	198.5	—	213.0	238.0	239.2
lower jaw	170.1	198.5	—	213.1	238.0	239.2
femur (any part)	170.7	198.5	—	213.7	238.0	239.2
fibula (any part)	170.7	198.5	—	213.7	238.0	239.2
finger (any)	170.5	198.5	—	213.5	238.0	239.2
foot	170.8	198.5	—	213.8	238.0	239.2
forearm	170.4	198.5	—	213.4	238.0	239.2
frontal	170.0	198.5	—	213.0	238.0	239.2
hand	170.5	198.5	—	213.5	238.0	239.2
heel	170.8	198.5	—	213.8	238.0	239.2
hip	170.6	198.5	—	213.6	238.0	239.2
humerus (any part)	170.4	198.5	—	213.4	238.0	239.2
hyoid	170.0	198.5	—	213.0	238.0	239.2
ilium	170.6	198.5	—	213.6	238.0	239.2
innominate	170.6	198.5	—	213.6	238.0	239.2
intervertebral cartilage or disc	170.2	198.5	—	213.2	238.0	239.2
ischium	170.6	198.5	—	213.6	238.0	239.2
jaw (lower)	170.1	198.5	—	213.1	238.0	239.2
upper	170.0	198.5	—	213.0	238.0	239.2
knee	170.7	198.5	—	213.7	238.0	239.2
leg NEC	170.7	198.5	—	213.7	238.0	239.2
limb NEC	170.9	198.5	—	213.9	238.0	239.2
lower (long bones)	170.7	198.5	—	213.7	238.0	239.2
short bones	170.8	198.5	—	213.8	238.0	239.2
upper (long bones)	170.4	198.5	—	213.4	238.0	239.2
short bones	170.5	198.5	—	213.5	238.0	239.2
long	170.9	198.5	—	213.9	238.0	239.2
lower limbs NEC	170.7	198.5	—	213.7	238.0	239.2
upper limbs NEC	170.4	198.5	—	213.4	238.0	239.2
malar	170.0	198.5	—	213.0	238.0	239.2
mandible	170.1	198.5	—	213.1	238.0	239.2
marrow NEC	202.9 ✓5ᵗʰ	198.5	—	—	—	238.7
mastoid	170.0	198.5	—	213.0	238.0	239.2
maxilla, maxillary (superior)	170.0	198.5	—	213.0	238.0	239.2
inferior	170.1	198.5	—	213.1	238.0	239.2
metacarpus (any)	170.5	198.5	—	213.5	238.0	239.2
metatarsus (any)	170.8	198.5	—	213.8	238.0	239.2
navicular (ankle)	170.8	198.5	—	213.8	238.0	239.2
hand	170.5	198.5	—	213.5	238.0	239.2
nose, nasal	170.0	198.5	—	213.0	238.0	239.2
occipital	170.0	198.5	—	213.0	238.0	239.2
orbit	170.0	198.5	—	213.0	238.0	239.2
parietal	170.0	198.5	—	213.0	238.0	239.2
patella	170.8	198.5	—	213.8	238.0	239.2
pelvic	170.6	198.5	—	213.6	238.0	239.2

	Malignant			Benign	Uncertain Behavior	Unspecified
	Primary	Secondary	Ca in situ	Benign	Uncertain Behavior	Unspecified
Neoplasm, neoplastic — *continued*						
bone — *continued*						
phalanges	170.9	198.5	—	213.9	238.0	239.2
foot	170.8	198.5	—	213.8	238.0	239.2
hand	170.5	198.5	—	213.5	238.0	239.2
pubic	170.6	198.5	—	213.6	238.0	239.2
radius (any part)	170.4	198.5	—	213.4	238.0	239.2
rib	170.3	198.5	—	213.3	238.0	239.2
sacral vertebra	170.6	198.5	—	213.6	238.0	239.2
sacrum	170.6	198.5	—	213.6	238.0	239.2
scaphoid (of hand)	170.5	198.5	—	213.5	238.0	239.2
of ankle	170.8	198.5	—	213.8	238.0	239.2
scapula (any part)	170.4	198.5	—	213.4	238.0	239.2
sella turcica	170.0	198.5	—	213.0	238.0	239.2
short	170.9	198.5	—	213.9	238.0	239.2
lower limb	170.8	198.5	—	213.8	238.0	239.2
upper limb	170.5	198.5	—	213.5	238.0	239.2
shoulder	170.4	198.5	—	213.4	238.0	239.2
skeleton, skeletal NEC	170.9	198.5	—	213.9	238.0	239.2
skull	170.0	198.5	—	213.0	238.0	239.2
sphenoid	170.0	198.5	—	213.0	238.0	239.2
spine, spinal (column)	170.2	198.5	—	213.2	238.0	239.2
coccyx	170.6	198.5	—	213.6	238.0	239.2
sacrum	170.6	198.5	—	213.6	238.0	239.2
sternum	170.3	198.5	—	213.3	238.0	239.2
tarsus (any)	170.8	198.5	—	213.8	238.0	239.2
temporal	170.0	198.5	—	213.0	238.0	239.2
thumb	170.5	198.5	—	213.5	238.0	239.2
tibia (any part)	170.7	198.5	—	213.7	238.0	239.2
toe (any)	170.8	198.5	—	213.8	238.0	239.2
trapezium	170.5	198.5	—	213.5	238.0	239.2
trapezoid	170.5	198.5	—	213.5	238.0	239.2
turbinate	170.0	198.5	—	213.0	238.0	239.2
ulna (any part)	170.4	198.5	—	213.4	238.0	239.2
unciform	170.5	198.5	—	213.5	238.0	239.2
vertebra (column)	170.2	198.5	—	213.2	238.0	239.2
coccyx	170.6	198.5	—	213.6	238.0	239.2
sacrum	170.6	198.5	—	213.6	238.0	239.2
vomer	170.0	198.5	—	213.0	238.0	239.2
wrist	170.5	198.5	—	213.5	238.0	239.2
xiphoid process	170.3	198.5	—	213.3	238.0	239.2
zygomatic	170.0	198.5	—	213.0	238.0	239.2
book-leaf (mouth)	145.8	198.89	230.0	210.4	235.1	239.0
bowel — *see* Neoplasm, intestine						
brachial plexus	171.2	198.89	—	215.2	238.1	239.2
brain NEC	191.9	198.3	—	225.0	237.5	239.6
basal ganglia	191.0	198.3	—	225.0	237.5	239.6
cerebellopontine angle	191.6	198.3	—	225.0	237.5	239.6
cerebellum NOS	191.6	198.3	—	225.0	237.5	239.6
cerebrum	191.0	198.3	—	225.0	237.5	239.6
choroid plexus	191.5	198.3	—	225.0	237.5	239.6
contiguous sites	191.8	—	—	—	—	—
corpus callosum	191.8	198.3	—	225.0	237.5	239.6
corpus striatum	191.0	198.3	—	225.0	237.5	239.6
cortex (cerebral)	191.0	198.3	—	225.0	237.5	239.6
frontal lobe	191.1	198.3	—	225.0	237.5	239.6
globus pallidus	191.0	198.3	—	225.0	237.5	239.6
hippocampus	191.2	198.3	—	225.0	237.5	239.6
hypothalamus	191.0	198.3	—	225.0	237.5	239.6
internal capsule	191.0	198.3	—	225.0	237.5	239.6
medulla oblongata	191.7	198.3	—	225.0	237.5	239.6
meninges	192.1	198.4	—	225.2	237.6	239.7
midbrain	191.7	198.3	—	225.0	237.5	239.6
occipital lobe	191.4	198.3	—	225.0	237.5	239.6
parietal lobe	191.3	198.3	—	225.0	237.5	239.6
peduncle	191.7	198.3	—	225.0	237.5	239.6
pons	191.7	198.3	—	225.0	237.5	239.6

	Malignant				Uncertain Behavior	Unspecified
	Primary	Secondary	Ca in situ	Benign		
Neoplasm, neoplastic — *continued*						
brain NEC — *continued*						
stem	191.7	198.3	—	225.0	237.5	239.6
tapetum	191.8	198.3	—	225.0	237.5	239.6
temporal lobe	191.2	198.3	—	225.0	237.5	239.6
thalamus	191.0	198.3	—	225.0	237.5	239.6
uncus	191.2	198.3	—	225.0	237.5	239.6
ventricle (floor)	191.5	198.3	—	225.0	237.5	239.6
branchial (cleft) (vestiges)	146.8	198.89	230.0	210.6	235.1	239.0
breast (connective tissue) (female) (glandular tissue) (soft parts)	174.9	198.81	233.0	217	238.3	239.3
areola	174.0	198.81	233.0	217	238.3	239.3
male	175.0	198.81	233.0	217	238.3	239.3
axillary tail	174.6	198.81	233.0	217	238.3	239.3
central portion	174.1	198.81	233.0	217	238.3	239.3
contiguous sites	174.8	—	—	—	—	—
ectopic sites	174.8	198.81	233.0	217	238.3	239.3
inner	174.8	198.81	233.0	217	238.3	239.3
lower	174.8	198.81	233.0	217	238.3	239.3
lower-inner quadrant	174.3	198.81	233.0	217	238.3	239.3
lower-outer quadrant	174.5	198.81	233.0	217	238.3	239.3
male	175.9	198.81	233.0	217	238.3	239.3
areola	175.0	198.81	233.0	217	238.3	239.3
ectopic tissue	175.9	198.81	233.0	217	238.3	239.3
nipple	175.0	198.81	233.0	217	238.3	239.3
mastectomy site (skin)	173.5	198.2	—	—	—	—
specified as breast tissue	174.8	198.81	—	—	—	—
midline	174.8	198.81	233.0	217	238.3	239.3
nipple	174.0	198.81	233.0	217	238.3	239.3
male	175.0	198.81	233.0	217	238.3	239.3
outer	174.8	198.81	233.0	217	238.3	239.3
skin	173.5	198.2	232.5	216.5	238.2	239.2
tail (axillary)	174.6	198.81	233.0	217	238.3	239.3
upper	174.8	198.81	233.0	217	238.3	239.3
upper-inner quadrant	174.2	198.81	233.0	217	238.3	239.3
upper-outer quadrant	174.4	198.81	233.0	217	238.3	239.3
broad ligament	183.3	198.82	233.3	221.0	236.3	239.5
bronchiogenic, bronchogenic (lung)	162.9	197.0	231.2	212.3	235.7	239.1
bronchiole	162.9	197.0	231.2	212.3	235.7	239.1
bronchus	162.9	197.0	231.2	212.3	235.7	239.1
carina	162.2	197.0	231.2	212.3	235.7	239.1
contiguous sites with lung or trachea	162.8	—	—	—	—	—
lower lobe of lung	162.5	197.0	231.2	212.3	235.7	239.1
main	162.2	197.0	231.2	212.3	235.7	239.1
middle lobe of lung	162.4	197.0	231.2	212.3	235.7	239.1
upper lobe of lung	162.3	197.0	231.2	212.3	235.7	239.1
brow	173.3	198.2	232.3	216.3	238.2	239.2
buccal (cavity)	145.9	198.89	230.0	210.4	235.1	239.0
commissure	145.0	198.89	230.0	210.4	235.1	239.0
groove (lower) (upper)	145.1	198.89	230.0	210.4	235.1	239.0
mucosa	145.0	198.89	230.0	210.4	235.1	239.0
sulcus (lower) (upper)	145.1	198.89	230.0	210.4	235.1	239.0
bulbourethral gland	189.3	198.1	233.9	223.81	236.99	239.5
bursa — *see* Neoplasm, connective tissue						
buttock NEC*	195.3	198.89	232.5	229.8	238.8	239.8
calf*	195.5	198.89	232.7	229.8	238.8	239.8
calvarium	170.0	198.5	—	213.0	238.0	239.2
calyx, renal	189.1	198.0	233.9	223.1	236.91	239.5
canal						
anal	154.2	197.5	230.5	211.4	235.5	239.0
auditory (external)	173.2	198.2	232.2	216.2	238.2	239.2
auricular (external)	173.2	198.2	232.2	216.2	238.2	239.2
canaliculi, biliary (biliferi) (intrahepatic)	155.1	197.8	230.8	211.5	235.3	239.0
canthus (eye) (inner) (outer)	173.1	198.2	232.1	216.1	238.2	239.2
capillary — *see* Neoplasm, connective tissue						
caput coli	153.4	197.5	230.3	211.3	235.2	239.0
cardia (gastric)	151.0	197.8	230.2	211.1	235.2	239.0
cardiac orifice (stomach)	151.0	197.8	230.2	211.1	235.2	239.0

	Malignant					
	Primary	**Secondary**	**Ca in situ**	**Benign**	**Uncertain Behavior**	**Unspecified**
Neoplasm, neoplastic — *continued*						
cardio-esophageal junction	151.0	197.8	230.2	211.1	235.2	239.0
cardio-esophagus	151.0	197.8	230.2	211.1	235.2	239.0
carina (trachea) (bronchus)	162.2	197.0	231.2	212.3	235.7	239.1
carotid (artery)	171.0	198.89	—	215.0	238.1	239.2
body	194.5	198.89	—	227.5	237.3	239.7
carpus (any bone)	170.5	198.5	—	213.5	238.0	239.2
cartilage (articular) (joint) NEC — *see also* Neoplasm, bone	170.9	198.5	—	213.9	238.0	239.2
arytenoid	161.3	197.3	231.0	212.1	235.6	239.1
auricular	171.0	198.89	—	215.0	238.1	239.2
bronchi	162.2	197.3	—	212.3	235.7	239.1
connective tissue — *see* Neoplasm, connective tissue						
costal	170.3	198.5	—	213.3	238.0	239.2
cricoid	161.3	197.3	231.0	212.1	235.6	239.1
cuneiform	161.3	197.3	231.0	212.1	235.6	239.1
ear (external)	171.0	198.89	—	215.0	238.1	239.2
ensiform	170.3	198.5	—	213.3	238.0	239.2
epiglottis	161.1	197.3	231.0	212.1	235.6	239.1
anterior surface	146.4	198.89	230.0	210.6	235.1	239.0
eyelid	171.0	198.89	—	215.0	238.1	239.2
intervertebral	170.2	198.5	—	213.2	238.0	239.2
larynx, laryngeal	161.3	197.3	231.0	212.1	235.6	239.1
nose, nasal	160.0	197.3	231.8	212.0	235.9	239.1
pinna	171.0	198.89	—	215.0	238.1	239.2
rib	170.3	198.5	—	213.3	238.0	239.2
semilunar (knee)	170.7	198.5	—	213.7	238.0	239.2
thyroid	161.3	197.3	231.0	212.1	235.6	239.1
trachea	162.0	197.3	231.1	212.2	235.7	239.1
cauda equina	192.2	198.3	—	225.3	237.5	239.7
cavity						
buccal	145.9	198.89	230.0	210.4	235.1	239.0
nasal	160.0	197.3	231.8	212.0	235.9	239.1
oral	145.9	198.89	230.0	210.4	235.1	239.0
peritoneal	158.9	197.6	—	211.8	235.4	239.0
tympanic	160.1	197.3	231.8	212.0	235.9	239.1
cecum	153.4	197.5	230.3	211.3	235.2	239.0
central						
nervous system — *see* Neoplasm, nervous system						
white matter	191.0	198.3	—	225.0	237.5	239.6
cerebellopontine (angle)	191.6	198.3	—	225.0	237.5	239.6
cerebellum, cerebellar	191.6	198.3	—	225.0	237.5	239.6
cerebrum, cerebral (cortex) (hemisphere) (white matter)	191.0	198.3	—	225.0	237.5	239.6
meninges	192.1	198.4	—	225.2	237.6	239.7
peduncle	191.7	198.3	—	225.0	237.5	239.6
ventricle (any)	191.5	198.3	—	225.0	237.5	239.6
cervical region	195.0	198.89	234.8	229.8	238.8	239.8
cervix (cervical) (uteri) (uterus)	180.9	198.82	233.1	219.0	236.0	239.5
canal	180.0	198.82	233.1	219.0	236.0	239.5
contiguous sites	180.8	—	—	—	—	—
endocervix (canal) (gland)	180.0	198.82	233.1	219.0	236.0	239.5
exocervix	180.1	198.82	233.1	219.0	236.0	239.5
external os	180.1	198.82	233.1	219.0	236.0	239.5
internal os	180.0	198.82	233.1	219.0	236.0	239.5
nabothian gland	180.0	198.82	233.1	219.0	236.0	239.5
squamocolumnar junction	180.8	198.82	233.1	219.0	236.0	239.5
stump	180.8	198.82	233.1	219.0	236.0	239.5
cheek	195.0	198.89	234.8	229.8	238.8	239.8
external	173.3	198.2	232.3	216.3	238.2	239.2
inner aspect	145.0	198.89	230.0	210.4	235.1	239.0
internal	145.0	198.89	230.0	210.4	235.1	239.0
mucosa	145.0	198.89	230.0	210.4	235.1	239.0
chest (wall) NEC	195.1	198.89	234.8	229.8	238.8	239.8
chiasma opticum	192.0	198.4	—	225.1	237.9	239.7
chin	173.3	198.2	232.3	216.3	238.2	239.2
choana	147.3	198.89	230.0	210.7	235.1	239.0
cholangiole	155.1	197.8	230.8	211.5	235.3	239.0
choledochal duct	156.1	197.8	230.8	211.5	235.3	239.0

	Malignant					
	Primary	Secondary	Ca in situ	Benign	Uncertain Behavior	Unspecified
Neoplasm, neoplastic — *continued*						
choroid	190.6	198.4	234.0	224.6	238.8	239.8
plexus	191.5	198.3	—	225.0	237.5	239.6
ciliary body	190.0	198.4	234.0	224.0	238.8	239.8
clavicle	170.3	198.5	—	213.3	238.0	239.2
clitoris	184.3	198.82	233.3	221.2	236.3	239.5
clivus	170.0	198.5	—	213.0	238.0	239.2
cloacogenic zone	154.8	197.5	230.7	211.4	235.5	239.0
coccygeal						
body or glomus	194.6	198.89	—	227.6	237.3	239.7
vertebra	170.6	198.5	—	213.6	238.0	239.2
coccyx	170.6	198.5	—	213.6	238.0	239.2
colon — *see also* Neoplasm, intestine, large and rectum	154.0	197.5	230.4	211.4	235.2	239.0
column, spinal — *see* Neoplasm, spine						
columnella	173.3	198.2	232.3	216.3	238.2	239.2
commissure						
labial, lip	140.6	198.89	230.0	210.4	235.1	239.0
laryngeal	161.0	197.3	231.0	212.1	235.6	239.1
common (bile) duct	156.1	197.8	230.8	211.5	235.3	239.0
concha	173.2	198.2	232.2	216.2	238.2	239.2
nose	160.0	197.3	231.8	212.0	235.9	239.1
conjunctiva	190.3	198.4	234.0	224.3	238.8	239.8
connective tissue NEC	171.9	198.89	—	215.9	238.1	239.2

Note — *For neoplasms of connective tissue (blood vessel, bursa, fascia, ligament, muscle, peripheral nerves, sympathetic and parasympathetic nerves and ganglia, synovia, tendon, etc.) or of morphological types that indicate connective tissue, code according to the list under "Neoplasm, connective tissue"; for sites that do not appear in this list, code to neoplasm of that site; e.g.,*

> *liposarcoma, shoulder 171.2*
> *leiomyosarcoma, stomach 151.9*
> *neurofibroma, chest wall 215.4*

Morphological types that indicate connective tissue appear in the proper place in the alphabetic index with the instruction "see Neoplasm, connective tissue..."

	Primary	Secondary	Ca in situ	Benign	Uncertain Behavior	Unspecified
abdomen	171.5	198.89	—	215.5	238.1	239.2
abdominal wall	171.5	198.89	—	215.5	238.1	239.2
ankle	171.3	198.89	—	215.3	238.1	239.2
antecubital fossa or space	171.2	198.89	—	215.2	238.1	239.2
arm	171.2	198.89	—	215.2	238.1	239.2
auricle (ear)	171.0	198.89	—	215.0	238.1	239.2
axilla	171.4	198.89	—	215.4	238.1	239.2
back	171.7	198.89	—	215.7	238.1	239.2
breast (female) (*see also* Neoplasm, breast)	174.9	198.81	233.0	217	238.3	239.3
male	175.9	198.81	233.0	217	238.3	239.3
buttock	171.6	198.89	—	215.6	238.1	239.2
calf	171.3	198.89	—	215.3	238.1	239.2
cervical region	171.0	198.89	—	215.0	238.1	239.2
cheek	171.0	198.89	—	215.0	238.1	239.2
chest (wall)	171.4	198.89	—	215.4	238.1	239.2
chin	171.0	198.89	—	215.0	238.1	239.2
contiguous sites	171.8	—	—	—	—	—
diaphragm	171.4	198.89	—	215.4	238.1	239.2
ear (external)	171.0	198.89	—	215.0	238.1	239.2
elbow	171.2	198.89	—	215.2	238.1	239.2
extrarectal	171.6	198.89	—	215.6	238.1	239.2
extremity	171.8	198.89	—	215.8	238.1	239.2
lower	171.3	198.89	—	215.3	238.1	239.2
upper	171.2	198.89	—	215.2	238.1	239.2
eyelid	171.0	198.89	—	215.0	238.1	239.2
face	171.0	198.89	—	215.0	238.1	239.2
finger	171.2	198.89	—	215.2	238.1	239.2
flank	171.7	198.89	—	215.7	238.1	239.2
foot	171.3	198.89	—	215.3	238.1	239.2
forearm	171.2	198.89	—	215.2	238.1	239.2
forehead	171.0	198.89	—	215.0	238.1	239.2
gluteal region	171.6	198.89	—	215.6	238.1	239.2
great vessels NEC	171.4	198.89	—	215.4	238.1	239.2
groin	171.6	198.89	—	215.6	238.1	239.2
hand	171.2	198.89	—	215.2	238.1	239.2
head	171.0	198.89	—	215.0	238.1	239.2

	Malignant					
	Primary	Secondary	Ca in situ	Benign	Uncertain Behavior	Unspecified
Neoplasm, neoplastic — *continued*						
connective tissue NEC — *continued*						
heel	171.3	198.89	—	215.3	238.1	239.2
hip	171.3	198.89	—	215.3	238.1	239.2
hypochondrium	171.5	198.89	—	215.5	238.1	239.2
iliopsoas muscle	171.6	198.89	—	215.5	238.1	239.2
infraclavicular region	171.4	198.89	—	215.4	238.1	239.2
inguinal (canal) (region)	171.6	198.89	—	215.6	238.1	239.2
intrathoracic	171.4	198.89	—	215.4	238.1	239.2
ischorectal fossa	171.6	198.89	—	215.6	238.1	239.2
jaw	143.9	198.89	230.0	210.4	235.1	239.0
knee	171.3	198.89	—	215.3	238.1	239.2
leg	171.3	198.89	—	215.3	238.1	239.2
limb NEC	171.9	198.89	—	215.8	238.1	239.2
lower	171.3	198.89	—	215.3	238.1	239.2
upper	171.2	198.89	—	215.2	238.1	239.2
nates	171.6	198.89	—	215.6	238.1	239.2
neck	171.0	198.89	—	215.0	238.1	239.2
orbit	190.1	198.4	234.0	224.1	238.8	239.8
pararectal	171.6	198.89	—	215.6	238.1	239.2
para-urethral	171.6	198.89	—	215.6	238.1	239.2
paravaginal	171.6	198.89	—	215.6	238.1	239.2
pelvis (floor)	171.6	198.89	—	215.6	238.1	239.2
pelvo-abdominal	171.8	198.89	—	215.8	238.1	239.2
perineum	171.6	198.89	—	215.6	238.1	239.2
perirectal (tissue)	171.6	198.89	—	215.6	238.1	239.2
periurethral (tissue)	171.6	198.89	—	215.6	238.1	239.2
popliteal fossa or space	171.3	198.89	—	215.3	238.1	239.2
presacral	171.6	198.89	—	215.6	238.1	239.2
psoas muscle	171.5	198.89	—	215.5	238.1	239.2
pterygoid fossa	171.0	198.89	—	215.0	238.1	239.2
rectovaginal septum or wall	171.6	198.89	—	215.6	238.1	239.2
rectovesical	171.6	198.89	—	215.6	238.1	239.2
retroperitoneum	158.0	197.6	—	211.8	235.4	239.0
sacrococcygeal region	171.6	198.89	—	215.6	238.1	239.2
scalp	171.0	198.89	—	215.0	238.1	239.2
scapular region	171.4	198.89	—	215.4	238.1	239.2
shoulder	171.2	198.89	—	215.2	238.1	239.2
skin (dermis) NEC	173.9	198.2	232.9	216.9	238.2	239.2
submental	171.0	198.89	—	215.0	238.1	239.2
supraclavicular region	171.0	198.89	—	215.0	238.1	239.2
temple	171.0	198.89	—	215.0	238.1	239.2
temporal region	171.0	198.89	—	215.0	238.1	239.2
thigh	171.3	198.89	—	215.3	238.1	239.2
thoracic (duct) (wall)	171.4	198.89	—	215.4	238.1	239.2
thorax	171.4	198.89	—	215.4	238.1	239.2
thumb	171.2	198.89	—	215.2	238.1	239.2
toe	171.3	198.89	—	215.3	238.1	239.2
trunk	171.7	198.89	—	215.7	238.1	239.2
umbilicus	171.5	198.89	—	215.5	238.1	239.2
vesicorectal	171.6	198.89	—	215.6	238.1	239.2
wrist	171.2	198.89	—	215.2	238.1	239.2
conus medullaris	192.2	198.3	—	225.3	237.5	239.7
cord (true) (vocal)	161.0	197.3	231.0	212.1	235.6	239.1
false	161.1	197.3	231.0	212.1	235.6	239.1
spermatic	187.6	198.82	233.6	222.8	236.6	239.5
spinal (cervical) (lumbar) (thoracic)	192.2	198.3	—	225.3	237.5	239.7
cornea (limbus)	190.4	198.4	234.0	224.4	238.8	239.8
corpus						
albicans	183.0	198.6	233.3	220	236.2	239.5
callosum, brain	191.8	198.3	—	225.0	237.5	239.6
cavernosum	187.3	198.82	233.5	222.1	236.6	239.5
gastric	151.4	197.8	230.2	211.1	235.2	239.0
penis	187.3	198.82	233.5	222.1	236.6	239.5
striatum, cerebrum	191.0	198.3	—	225.0	237.5	239.6
uteri	182.0	198.82	233.2	219.1	236.0	239.5
isthmus	182.1	198.82	233.2	219.1	236.0	239.5

	Malignant					
	Primary	**Secondary**	**Ca in situ**	**Benign**	**Uncertain Behavior**	**Unspecified**
Neoplasm, neoplastic — *continued*						
cortex						
adrenal	194.0	198.7	234.8	227.0	237.2	239.7
cerebral	191.0	198.3	—	225.0	237.5	239.6
costal cartilage	170.3	198.5	—	213.3	238.0	239.2
costovertebral joint	170.3	198.5	—	213.3	238.0	239.2
Cowper's gland	189.3	198.1	233.9	223.81	236.99	239.5
cranial (fossa, any)	191.9	198.3	—	225.0	237.5	239.6
meninges	192.1	198.4	—	225.2	237.6	239.7
nerve (any)	192.0	198.4	—	225.1	237.9	239.7
craniobuccal pouch	194.3	198.89	234.8	227.3	237.0	239.7
craniopharyngeal (duct) (pouch)	194.3	198.89	234.8	227.3	237.0	239.7
cricoid	148.0	198.89	230.0	210.8	235.1	239.0
cartilage	161.3	197.3	231.0	212.1	235.6	239.1
cricopharynx	148.0	198.89	230.0	210.8	235.1	239.0
crypt of Morgagni	154.8	197.5	230.7	211.4	235.2	239.0
crystalline lens	190.0	198.4	234.0	224.0	238.8	239.8
cul-de-sac (Douglas')	158.8	197.6	—	211.8	235.4	239.0
cuneiform cartilage	161.3	197.3	231.0	212.1	235.6	239.1
cutaneous — *see* Neoplasm, skin						
cutis — *see* Neoplasm, skin						
cystic (bile) duct (common)	156.1	197.8	230.8	211.5	235.3	239.0
dermis — *see* Neoplasm, skin						
diaphragm	171.4	198.89	—	215.4	238.1	239.2
digestive organs, system, tube, or tract NEC	159.9	197.8	230.9	211.9	235.5	239.0
contiguous sites with peritoneum	159.8	—	—	—	—	—
disc, intervertebral	170.2	198.5	—	213.2	238.0	239.2
disease, generalized	199.0	199.0	234.9	229.9	238.9	199.0
disseminated	199.0	199.0	234.9	229.9	238.9	199.0
Douglas' cul-de-sac or pouch	158.8	197.6	—	211.8	235.4	239.0
duodenojejunal junction	152.8	197.4	230.7	211.2	235.2	239.0
duodenum	152.0	197.4	230.7	211.2	235.2	239.0
dura (cranial) (mater)	192.1	198.4	—	225.2	237.6	239.7
cerebral	192.1	198.4	—	225.2	237.6	239.7
spinal	192.3	198.4	—	225.4	237.6	239.7
ear (external)	173.2	198.2	232.2	216.2	238.2	239.2
auricle or auris	173.2	198.2	232.2	216.2	238.2	239.2
canal, external	173.2	198.2	232.2	216.2	238.2	239.2
cartilage	171.0	198.89	—	215.0	238.1	239.2
external meatus	173.2	198.2	232.2	216.2	238.2	239.2
inner	160.1	197.3	231.8	212.0	235.9	239.8 ▲
lobule	173.2	198.2	232.2	216.2	238.2	239.2
middle	160.1	197.3	231.8	212.0	235.9	239.8 ▲
contiguous sites with accessory sinuses or nasal cavities	160.8	—	—	—	—	—
skin	173.2	198.2	232.2	216.2	238.2	239.2
earlobe	173.2	198.2	232.2	216.2	238.2	239.2
ejaculatory duct	187.8	198.82	233.6	222.8	236.6	239.5
elbow NEC*	195.4	198.89	232.6	229.8	238.8	239.8
endocardium	164.1	198.89	—	212.7	238.8	239.8
endocervix (canal) (gland)	180.0	198.82	233.1	219.0	236.0	239.5
endocrine gland NEC	194.9	198.89	—	227.9	237.4	239.7
pluriglandular NEC	194.8	198.89	234.8	227.8	237.4	239.7
endometrium (gland) (stroma)	182.0	198.82	233.2	219.1	236.0	239.5
ensiform cartilage	170.3	198.5	—	213.3	238.0	239.2
enteric — *see* Neoplasm, intestine						
ependyma (brain)	191.5	198.3	—	225.0	237.5	239.6
epicardium	164.1	198.89	—	212.7	238.8	239.8
epididymis	187.5	198.82	233.6	222.3	236.6	239.5
epidural	192.9	198.4	—	225.9	237.9	239.7
epiglottis	161.1	197.3	231.0	212.1	235.6	239.1
anterior aspect or surface	146.4	198.89	230.0	210.6	235.1	239.0
cartilage	161.3	197.3	231.0	212.1	235.6	239.1
free border (margin)	146.4	198.89	230.0	210.6	235.1	239.0
junctional region	146.5	198.89	230.0	210.6	235.1	239.0
posterior (laryngeal) surface	161.1	197.3	231.0	212.1	235.6	239.1
suprahyoid portion	161.1	197.3	231.0	212.1	235.6	239.1
esophagogastric junction	151.0	197.8	230.2	211.1	235.2	239.0

	Malignant					
	Primary	Secondary	Ca in situ	Benign	Uncertain Behavior	Unspecified
Neoplasm, neoplastic — *continued*						
esophagus	150.9	197.8	230.1	211.0	235.5	239.0
abdominal	150.2	197.8	230.1	211.0	235.5	239.0
cervical	150.0	197.8	230.1	211.0	235.5	239.0
contiguous sites	150.8	—	—	—	—	—
distal (third)	150.5	197.8	230.1	211.0	235.5	239.0
lower (third)	150.5	197.8	230.1	211.0	235.5	239.0
middle (third)	150.4	197.8	230.1	211.0	235.5	239.0
proximal (third)	150.3	197.8	230.1	211.0	235.5	239.0
specified part NEC	150.8	197.8	230.1	211.0	235.5	239.0
thoracic	150.1	197.8	230.1	211.0	235.5	239.0
upper (third)	150.3	197.8	230.1	211.0	235.5	239.0
ethmoid (sinus)	160.3	197.3	231.8	212.0	235.9	239.1
bone or labyrinth	170.0	198.5	—	213.0	238.0	239.2
Eustachian tube	160.1	197.3	231.8	212.0	235.9	239.1
exocervix	180.1	198.82	233.1	219.0	236.0	239.5
external						
meatus (ear)	173.2	198.2	232.2	216.2	238.2	239.2
os, cervix uteri	180.1	198.82	233.1	219.0	236.0	239.5
extradural	192.9	198.4	—	225.9	237.9	239.7
extrahepatic (bile) duct	156.1	197.8	230.8	211.5	235.3	239.0
contiguous sites with gallbladder	156.8	—	—	—	—	—
extraocular muscle	190.1	198.4	234.0	224.1	238.8	239.8
extrarectal	195.3	198.89	234.8	229.8	238.8	239.8
extremity*	195.8	198.89	232.8	229.8	238.8	239.8
lower*	195.5	198.89	232.7	229.8	238.8	239.8
upper*	195.4	198.89	232.6	229.8	238.8	239.8
eye NEC	190.9	198.4	234.0	224.9	238.8	239.8
contiguous sites	190.8	—	—	—	—	—
specified sites NEC	190.8	198.4	234.0	224.8	238.8	239.8
eyeball	190.0	198.4	234.0	224.0	238.8	239.8
eyebrow	173.3	198.2	232.3	216.3	238.2	239.2
eyelid (lower) (skin) (upper)	173.1	198.2	232.1	216.1	238.2	239.2
cartilage	171.0	198.89	—	215.0	238.1	239.2
face NEC*	195.0	198.89	232.3	229.8	238.8	239.8
fallopian tube (accessory)	183.2	198.82	233.3	221.0	236.3	239.5
falx (cerebelli) (cerebri)	192.1	198.4	—	225.2	237.6	239.7
fascia — *see also* Neoplasm, connective tissue						
palmar	171.2	198.89	—	215.2	238.1	239.2
plantar	171.3	198.89	—	215.3	238.1	239.2
fatty tissue — *see* Neoplasm, connective tissue						
fauces, faucial NEC	146.9	198.89	230.0	210.6	235.1	239.0
pillars	146.2	198.89	230.0	210.6	235.1	239.0
tonsil	146.0	198.89	230.0	210.5	235.1	239.0
femur (any part)	170.7	198.5	—	213.7	238.0	239.2
fetal membrane	181	198.82	233.2	219.8	236.1	239.5
fibrous tissue — *see* Neoplasm, connective tissue						
fibula (any part)	170.7	198.5	—	213.7	238.0	239.2
filum terminale	192.2	198.3	—	225.3	237.5	239.7
finger NEC*	195.4	198.89	232.6	229.8	238.8	239.8
flank NEC*	195.8	198.89	232.5	229.8	238.8	239.8
follicle, nabothian	180.0	198.82	233.1	219.0	236.0	239.5
foot NEC*	195.5	198.89	232.7	229.8	238.8	239.8
forearm NEC*	195.4	198.89	232.6	229.8	238.8	239.8
forehead (skin)	173.3	198.2	232.3	216.3	238.2	239.2
foreskin	187.1	198.82	233.5	222.1	236.6	239.5
fornix						
pharyngeal	147.3	198.89	230.0	210.7	235.1	239.0
vagina	184.0	198.82	233.3	221.1	236.3	239.5
fossa (of)						
anterior (cranial)	191.9	198.3	—	225.0	237.5	239.6
cranial	191.9	198.3	—	225.0	237.5	239.6
ischiorectal	195.3	198.89	234.8	229.8	238.8	239.8
middle (cranial)	191.9	198.3	—	225.0	237.5	239.6
pituitary	194.3	198.89	234.8	227.3	237.0	239.7
posterior (cranial)	191.9	198.3	—	225.0	237.5	239.6
pterygoid	171.0	198.89	—	215.0	238.1	239.2

	Malignant			Benign	Uncertain Behavior	Unspecified
	Primary	Secondary	Ca in situ			
Neoplasm, neoplastic — *continued*						
fossa (of) — *continued*						
pyriform	148.1	198.89	230.0	210.8	235.1	239.0
Rosenmüller	147.2	198.89	230.0	210.7	235.1	239.0
tonsillar	146.1	198.89	230.0	210.6	235.1	239.0
fourchette	184.4	198.82	233.3	221.2	236.3	239.5
frenulum						
labii — *see* Neoplasm, lip, internal						
linguae	141.3	198.89	230.0	210.1	235.1	239.0
frontal						
bone	170.0	198.5	—	213.0	238.0	239.2
lobe, brain	191.1	198.3	—	225.0	237.5	239.6
meninges	192.1	198.4	—	225.2	237.6	239.7
pole	191.1	198.3	—	225.0	237.5	239.6
sinus	160.4	197.3	231.8	212.0	235.9	239.1
fundus						
stomach	151.3	197.8	230.2	211.1	235.2	239.0
uterus	182.0	198.82	233.2	219.1	236.0	239.5
gall duct (extrahepatic)	156.1	197.8	230.8	211.5	235.3	239.0
intrahepatic	155.1	197.8	230.8	211.5	235.3	239.0
gallbladder	156.0	197.8	230.8	211.5	235.3	239.0
contiguous sites with extrahepatic bile ducts	156.8	—	—	—	—	—
ganglia (*see also* Neoplasm, connective tissue)	171.9	198.89	—	215.9	238.1	239.2
basal	191.0	198.3	—	225.0	237.5	239.6
ganglion (*see also* Neoplasm, connective tissue)	171.9	198.89	—	215.9	238.1	239.2
cranial nerve	192.0	198.4	—	225.1	237.9	239.7
Gartner's duct	184.0	198.82	233.3	221.1	236.3	239.5
gastric — *see* Neoplasm, stomach						
gastrocolic	159.8	197.8	230.9	211.9	235.5	239.0
gastroesophageal junction	151.0	197.8	230.2	211.1	235.2	239.0
gastrointestinal (tract) NEC	159.9	197.8	230.9	211.9	235.5	239.0
generalized	199.0	199.0	234.9	229.9	238.9	199.0
genital organ or tract						
female NEC	184.9	198.82	233.3	221.9	236.3	239.5
contiguous sites	184.8	—	—	—	—	—
specified site NEC	184.8	198.82	233.3	221.8	236.3	239.5
male NEC	187.9	198.82	233.6	222.9	236.6	239.5
contiguous sites	187.8	—	—	—	—	—
specified site NEC	187.8	198.82	233.6	222.8	236.6	239.5
genitourinary tract						
female	184.9	198.82	233.3	221.9	236.3	239.5
male	187.9	198.82	233.6	222.9	236.6	239.5
gingiva (alveolar) (marginal)	143.9	198.89	230.0	210.4	235.1	239.0
lower	143.1	198.89	230.0	210.4	235.1	239.0
mandibular	143.1	198.89	230.0	210.4	235.1	239.0
maxillary	143.0	198.89	230.0	210.4	235.1	239.0
upper	143.0	198.89	230.0	210.4	235.1	239.0
gland, glandular (lymphatic) (system) — *see also* Neoplasm, lymph gland						
endocrine NEC	194.9	198.89	—	227.9	237.4	239.7
salivary — *see* Neoplasm, salivary, gland						
glans penis	187.2	198.82	233.5	222.1	236.6	239.5
globus pallidus	191.0	198.3	—	225.0	237.5	239.6
glomus						
coccygeal	194.6	198.89	—	227.6	237.3	239.7
jugularis	194.6	198.89	—	227.6	237.3	239.7
glosso-epiglottic fold(s)	146.4	198.89	230.0	210.6	235.1	239.0
glossopalatine fold	146.2	198.89	230.0	210.6	235.1	239.0
glossopharyngeal sulcus	146.1	198.89	230.0	210.6	235.1	239.0
glottis	161.0	197.3	231.0	212.1	235.6	239.1
gluteal region*	195.3	198.89	232.5	229.8	238.8	239.8
great vessels NEC	171.4	198.89	—	215.4	238.1	239.2
groin NEC*	195.3	198.89	232.5	229.8	238.8	239.8
gum	143.9	198.89	230.0	210.4	235.1	239.0
contiguous sites	143.8	—	—	—	—	—
lower	143.1	198.89	230.0	210.4	235.1	239.0
upper	143.0	198.89	230.0	210.4	235.1	239.0
hand NEC*	195.4	198.89	232.6	229.8	238.8	239.8

☑4ᵗʰ Fourth-digit Required   ☑5ᵗʰ Fifth-digit Required   ►◄ Revised Text   ● New Line   ▲ Revised Code

	Malignant					
	Primary	Secondary	Ca in situ	Benign	Uncertain Behavior	Unspecified
Neoplasm, neoplastic — *continued*						
head NEC*	195.0	198.89	232.4	229.8	238.8	239.8
heart	164.1	198.89	—	212.7	238.8	239.8
contiguous sites with mediastinum or thymus	164.8	—	—	—	—	—
heel NEC*	195.5	198.89	232.7	229.8	238.8	239.8
helix	173.2	198.2	232.2	216.2	238.2	239.2
hematopoietic, hemopoietic tissue NEC	202.8 ✓5ᵗʰ	198.89	—	—	—	238.7
hemisphere, cerebral	191.0	198.3	—	225.0	237.5	239.6
hemorrhoidal zone	154.2	197.5	230.5	211.4	235.5	239.0
hepatic	155.2	197.7	230.8	211.5	235.3	239.0
duct (bile)	156.1	197.8	230.8	211.5	235.3	239.0
flexure (colon)	153.0	197.5	230.3	211.3	235.2	239.0
primary	155.0	—	—	—	—	—
hilus of lung	162.2	197.0	231.2	212.3	235.7	239.1
hip NEC*	195.5	198.89	232.7	229.8	238.8	239.8
hippocampus, brain	191.2	198.3	—	225.0	237.5	239.6
humerus (any part)	170.4	198.5	—	213.4	238.0	239.2
hymen	184.0	198.82	233.3	221.1	236.3	239.5
hypopharynx, hypopharyngeal NEC	148.9	198.89	230.0	210.8	235.1	239.0
contiguous sites	148.8	—	—	—	—	—
postcricoid region	148.0	198.89	230.0	210.8	235.1	239.0
posterior wall	148.3	198.89	230.0	210.8	235.1	239.0
pyriform fossa (sinus)	148.1	198.89	230.0	210.8	235.1	239.0
specified site NEC	148.8	198.89	230.0	210.8	235.1	239.0
wall	148.9	198.89	230.0	210.8	235.1	239.0
posterior	148.3	198.89	230.0	210.8	235.1	239.0
hypophysis	194.3	198.89	234.8	227.3	237.0	239.7
hypothalamus	191.0	198.3	—	225.0	237.5	239.6
ileocecum, ileocecal (coil) (junction) (valve)	153.4	197.5	230.3	211.3	235.2	239.0
ileum	152.2	197.4	230.7	211.2	235.2	239.0
ilium	170.6	198.5	—	213.6	238.0	239.2
immunoproliferative NEC	203.8 ✓5ᵗʰ	—	—	—	—	—
infraclavicular (region)*	195.1	198.89	232.5	229.8	238.8	239.8
inguinal (region)*	195.3	198.89	232.5	229.8	238.8	239.8
insula	191.0	198.3	—	225.0	237.5	239.6
insular tissue (pancreas)	157.4	197.8	230.9	211.7	235.5	239.0
brain	191.0	198.3	—	225.0	237.5	239.6
interarytenoid fold	148.2	198.89	230.0	210.8	235.1	239.0
hypopharyngeal aspect	148.2	198.89	230.0	210.8	235.1	239.0
laryngeal aspect	161.1	197.3	231.0	212.1	235.6	239.1
marginal zone	148.2	198.89	230.0	210.8	235.1	239.0
interdental papillae	143.9	198.89	230.0	210.4	235.1	239.0
lower	143.1	198.89	230.0	210.4	235.1	239.0
upper	143.0	198.89	230.0	210.4	235.1	239.0
internal						
capsule	191.0	198.3	—	225.0	237.5	239.6
os (cervix)	180.0	198.82	233.1	219.0	236.0	239.5
intervertebral cartilage or disc	170.2	198.5	—	213.2	238.0	239.2
intestine, intestinal	159.0	197.8	230.7	211.9	235.2	239.0
large	153.9	197.5	230.3	211.3	235.2	239.0
appendix	153.5	197.5	230.3	211.3	235.2	239.0
caput coli	153.4	197.5	230.3	211.3	235.2	239.0
cecum	153.4	197.5	230.3	211.3	235.2	239.0
colon	153.9	197.5	230.3	211.3	235.2	239.0
and rectum	154.0	197.5	230.4	211.4	235.2	239.0
ascending	153.6	197.5	230.3	211.3	235.2	239.0
caput	153.4	197.5	230.3	211.3	235.2	239.0
contiguous sites	153.8	—	—	—	—	—
descending	153.2	197.5	230.3	211.3	235.2	239.0
distal	153.2	197.5	230.3	211.3	235.2	239.0
left	153.2	197.5	230.3	211.3	235.2	239.0
pelvic	153.3	197.5	230.3	211.3	235.2	239.0
right	153.6	197.5	230.3	211.3	235.2	239.0
sigmoid (flexure)	153.3	197.5	230.3	211.3	235.2	239.0
transverse	153.1	197.5	230.3	211.3	235.2	239.0
contiguous sites	153.8	—	—	—	—	—

	Malignant					
	Primary	**Secondary**	**Ca in situ**	**Benign**	**Uncertain Behavior**	**Unspecified**
Neoplasm, neoplastic — *continued*						
intestine, intestinal — *continued*						
large — *continued*						
hepatic flexure	153.0	197.5	230.3	211.3	235.2	239.0
ileocecum, ileocecal (coil) (valve)	153.4	197.5	230.3	211.3	235.2	239.0
sigmoid flexure (lower) (upper)	153.3	197.5	230.3	211.3	235.2	239.0
splenic flexure	153.7	197.5	230.3	211.3	235.2	239.0
small	152.9	197.4	230.7	211.2	235.2	239.0
contiguous sites	152.8	—	—	—	—	—
duodenum	152.0	197.4	230.7	211.2	235.2	239.0
ileum	152.2	197.4	230.7	211.2	235.2	239.0
jejunum	152.1	197.4	230.7	211.2	235.2	239.0
tract NEC	159.0	197.8	230.7	211.9	235.2	239.0
intra-abdominal	195.2	198.89	234.8	229.8	238.8	239.8
intracranial NEC	191.9	198.3	—	225.0	237.5	239.6
intrahepatic (bile) duct	155.1	197.8	230.8	211.5	235.3	239.0
intraocular	190.0	198.4	234.0	224.0	238.8	239.8
intraorbital	190.1	198.4	234.0	224.1	238.8	239.8
intrasellar	194.3	198.89	234.8	227.3	237.0	239.7
intrathoracic (cavity) (organs NEC)	195.1	198.89	234.8	229.8	238.8	239.8
contiguous sites with respiratory organs	165.8	—	—	—	—	—
iris	190.0	198.4	234.0	224.0	238.8	239.8
ischiorectal (fossa)	195.3	198.89	234.8	229.8	238.8	239.8
ischium	170.6	198.5	—	213.6	238.0	239.2
island of Reil	191.0	198.3	—	225.0	237.5	239.6
islands or islets of Langerhans	157.4	197.8	230.9	211.7	235.5	239.0
isthmus uteri	182.1	198.82	233.2	219.1	236.0	239.5
jaw	195.0	198.89	234.8	229.8	238.8	239.8
bone	170.1	198.5	—	213.1	238.0	239.2
carcinoma	143.9	—	—	—	—	—
lower	143.1	—	—	—	—	—
upper	143.0	—	—	—	—	—
lower	170.1	198.5	—	213.1	238.0	239.2
upper	170.0	198.5	—	213.0	238.0	239.2
carcinoma (any type) (lower) (upper)	195.0	—	—	—	—	—
skin	173.3	198.2	232.3	216.3	238.2	239.2
soft tissues	143.9	198.89	230.0	210.4	235.1	239.0
lower	143.1	198.89	230.0	210.4	235.1	239.0
upper	143.0	198.89	230.0	210.4	235.1	239.0
jejunum	152.1	197.4	230.7	211.2	235.2	239.0
joint NEC (*see also* Neoplasm, bone)	170.9	198.5	—	213.9	238.0	239.2
acromioclavicular	170.4	198.5	—	213.4	238.0	239.2
bursa or synovial membrane — *see* Neoplasm, connective tissue						
costovertebral	170.3	198.5	—	213.3	238.0	239.2
sternocostal	170.3	198.5	—	213.3	238.0	239.2
temporomandibular	170.1	198.5	—	213.1	238.0	239.2
junction						
anorectal	154.8	197.5	230.7	211.4	235.5	239.0
cardioesophageal	151.0	197.8	230.2	211.1	235.2	239.0
esophagogastric	151.0	197.8	230.2	211.1	235.2	239.0
gastroesophageal	151.0	197.8	230.2	211.1	235.2	239.0
hard and soft palate	145.5	198.89	230.0	210.4	235.1	239.0
ileocecal	153.4	197.5	230.3	211.3	235.2	239.0
pelvirectal	154.0	197.5	230.4	211.4	235.2	239.0
pelviureteric	189.1	198.0	233.9	223.1	236.91	239.5
rectosigmoid	154.0	197.5	230.4	211.4	235.2	239.0
squamocolumnar, of cervix	180.8	198.82	233.1	219.0	236.0	239.5
kidney (parenchyma)	189.0	198.0	233.9	223.0	236.91	239.5
calyx	189.1	198.0	233.9	223.1	236.91	239.5
hilus	189.1	198.0	233.9	223.1	236.91	239.5
pelvis	189.1	198.0	233.9	223.1	236.91	239.5
knee NEC*	195.5	198.89	232.7	229.8	238.8	239.8
labia (skin)	184.4	198.82	233.3	221.2	236.3	239.5
majora	184.1	198.82	233.3	221.2	236.3	239.5
minora	184.2	198.82	233.3	221.2	236.3	239.5
labial — *see also* Neoplasm, lip						
sulcus (lower) (upper)	145.1	198.89	230.0	210.4	235.1	239.0

| | \multicolumn{3}{Malignant} | | | | |
	Primary	Secondary	Ca in situ	Benign	Uncertain Behavior	Unspecified
Neoplasm, neoplastic — *continued*						
labium (skin)	184.4	198.82	233.3	221.2	236.3	239.5
majus	184.1	198.82	233.3	221.2	236.3	239.5
minus	184.2	198.82	233.3	221.2	236.3	239.5
lacrimal						
canaliculi	190.7	198.4	234.0	224.7	238.8	239.8
duct (nasal)	190.7	198.4	234.0	224.7	238.8	239.8
gland	190.2	198.4	234.0	224.2	238.8	239.8
punctum	190.7	198.4	234.0	224.7	238.8	239.8
sac	190.7	198.4	234.0	224.7	238.8	239.8
Langerhans, islands or islets	157.4	197.8	230.9	211.7	235.5	239.0
laryngopharynx	148.9	198.89	230.0	210.8	235.1	239.0
larynx, laryngeal NEC	161.9	197.3	231.0	212.1	235.6	239.1
aryepiglottic fold	161.1	197.3	231.0	212.1	235.6	239.1
cartilage (arytenoid) (cricoid) (cuneiform) (thyroid)	161.3	197.3	231.0	212.1	235.6	239.1
commissure (anterior) (posterior)	161.0	197.3	231.0	212.1	235.6	239.1
contiguous sites	161.8	—	—	—	—	—
extrinsic NEC	161.1	197.3	231.0	212.1	235.6	239.1
meaning hypopharynx	148.9	198.89	230.0	210.8	235.1	239.0
interarytenoid fold	161.1	197.3	231.0	212.1	235.6	239.1
intrinsic	161.0	197.3	231.0	212.1	235.6	239.1
ventricular band	161.1	197.3	231.0	212.1	235.6	239.1
leg NEC*	195.5	198.89	232.7	229.8	238.8	239.8
lens, crystalline	190.0	198.4	234.0	224.0	238.8	239.8
lid (lower) (upper)	173.1	198.2	232.1	216.1	238.2	239.2
ligament — *see also* Neoplasm, connective tissue						
broad	183.3	198.82	233.3	221.0	236.3	239.5
Mackenrodt's	183.8	198.82	233.3	221.8	236.3	239.5
non-uterine — *see* Neoplasm, connective tissue						
round	183.5	198.82	—	221.0	236.3	239.5
sacro-uterine	183.4	198.82	—	221.0	236.3	239.5
uterine	183.4	198.82	—	221.0	236.3	239.5
utero-ovarian	183.8	198.82	233.3	221.8	236.3	239.5
uterosacral	183.4	198.82	—	221.0	236.3	239.5
limb*	195.8	198.89	232.8	229.8	238.8	239.8
lower*	195.5	198.89	232.7	229.8	238.8	239.8
upper*	195.4	198.89	232.6	229.8	238.8	239.8
limbus of cornea	190.4	198.4	234.0	224.4	238.8	239.8
lingual NEC (*see also* Neoplasm, tongue)	141.9	198.89	230.0	210.1	235.1	239.0
lingula, lung	162.3	197.0	231.2	212.3	235.7	239.1
lip (external) (lipstick area) (vermillion border)	140.9	198.89	230.0	210.0	235.1	239.0
buccal aspect — *see* Neoplasm, lip, internal						
commissure	140.6	198.89	230.0	210.4	235.1	239.0
contiguous sites	140.8	—	—	—	—	—
with oral cavity or pharynx	149.8	—	—	—	—	—
frenulum — *see* Neoplasm, lip, internal						
inner aspect — *see* Neoplasm, lip, internal						
internal (buccal) (frenulum) (mucosa) (oral)	140.5	198.89	230.0	210.0	235.1	239.0
lower	140.4	198.89	230.0	210.0	235.1	239.0
upper	140.3	198.89	230.0	210.0	235.1	239.0
lower	140.1	198.89	230.0	210.0	235.1	239.0
internal (buccal) (frenulum) (mucosa) (oral)	140.4	198.89	230.0	210.0	235.1	239.0
mucosa — *see* Neoplasm, lip, internal						
oral aspect — *see* Neoplasm, lip, internal						
skin (commissure) (lower) (upper)	173.0	198.2	232.0	216.0	238.2	239.2
upper	140.0	198.89	230.0	210.0	235.1	239.0
internal (buccal) (frenulum) (mucosa) (oral)	140.3	198.89	230.0	210.0	235.1	239.0
liver	155.2	197.7	230.8	211.5	235.3	239.0
primary	155.0	—	—	—	—	—
lobe						
azygos	162.3	197.0	231.2	212.3	235.7	239.1
frontal	191.1	198.3	—	225.0	237.5	239.6
lower	162.5	197.0	231.2	212.3	235.7	239.1
middle	162.4	197.0	231.2	212.3	235.7	239.1
occipital	191.4	198.3	—	225.0	237.5	239.6
parietal	191.3	198.3	—	225.0	237.5	239.6

	Malignant					
	Primary	Secondary	Ca in situ	Benign	Uncertain Behavior	Unspecified
Neoplasm, neoplastic — *continued*						
lobe — *continued*						
temporal	191.2	198.3	—	225.0	237.5	239.6
upper	162.3	197.0	231.2	212.3	235.7	239.1
lumbosacral plexus	171.6	198.4	—	215.6	238.1	239.2
lung	162.9	197.0	231.2	212.3	235.7	239.1
azgos lobe	162.3	197.0	231.2	212.3	235.7	239.1
carina	162.2	197.0	231.2	212.3	235.7	239.1
contiguous sites with bronchus or trachea	162.8	—	—	—	—	—
hilus	162.2	197.0	231.2	212.3	235.7	239.1
lingula	162.3	197.0	231.2	212.3	235.7	239.1
lobe NEC	162.9	197.0	231.2	212.3	235.7	239.1
lower lobe	162.5	197.0	231.2	212.3	235.7	239.1
main bronchus	162.2	197.0	231.2	212.3	235.7	239.1
middle lobe	162.4	197.0	231.2	212.3	235.7	239.1
upper lobe	162.3	197.0	231.2	212.3	235.7	239.1
lymph, lymphatic						
channel NEC (*see also* Neoplasm, connective tissue)	171.9	198.89	—	215.9	238.1	239.2
gland (secondary)	—	196.9	—	229.0	238.8	239.8
abdominal	—	196.2	—	229.0	238.8	239.
aortic	—	196.2	—	229.0	238.8	239.8
arm	—	196.3	—	229.0	238.8	239.8
auricular (anterior) (posterior)	—	196.0	—	229.0	238.8	239.8
axilla, axillary	—	196.3	—	229.0	238.8	239.8
brachial	—	196.3	—	229.0	238.8	239.8
bronchial	—	196.1	—	229.0	238.8	239.8
bronchopulmonary	—	196.1	—	229.0	238.8	239.8
celiac	—	196.2	—	229.0	238.8	239.8
cervical	—	196.0	—	229.0	238.8	239.8
cervicofacial	—	196.0	—	229.0	238.8	239.8
Cloquet	—	196.5	—	229.0	238.8	239.8
colic	—	196.2	—	229.0	238.8	239.8
common duct	—	196.2	—	229.0	238.8	239.8
cubital	—	196.3	—	229.0	238.8	239.8
diaphragmatic	—	196.1	—	229.0	238.8	239.8
epigastric, inferior	—	196.6	—	229.0	238.8	239.8
epitrochlear	—	196.3	—	229.0	238.8	239.8
esophageal	—	196.1	—	229.0	238.8	239.8
face	—	196.0	—	229.0	238.8	239.8
femoral	—	196.5	—	229.0	238.8	239.8
gastric	—	196.2	—	229.0	238.8	239.8
groin	—	196.5	—	229.0	238.8	239.8
head	—	196.0	—	229.0	238.8	239.8
hepatic	—	196.2	—	229.0	238.8	239.8
hilar (pulmonary)	—	196.1	—	229.0	238.8	239.8
splenic	—	196.2	—	229.0	238.8	239.8
hypogastric	—	196.6	—	229.0	238.8	239.8
ileocolic	—	196.2	—	229.0	238.8	239.8
iliac	—	196.6	—	229.0	238.8	239.8
infraclavicular	—	196.3	—	229.0	238.8	239.8
inguina, inguinal	—	196.5	—	229.0	238.8	239.8
innominate	—	196.1	—	229.0	238.8	239.8
intercostal	—	196.1	—	229.0	238.8	239.8
intestinal	—	196.2	—	229.0	238.8	239.8
intra-abdominal	—	196.2	—	229.0	238.8	239.8
intrapelvic	—	196.6	—	229.0	238.8	239.8
intrathoracic	—	196.1	—	229.0	238.8	239.9
jugular	—	196.0	—	229.0	238.8	239.8
leg	—	196.5	—	229.0	238.8	239.8
limb						
lower	—	196.5	—	229.0	238.8	239.8
upper	—	196.3	—	229.0	238.8	239.8
lower limb	—	196.5	—	229.0	238.8	238.9
lumbar	—	196.2	—	229.0	238.8	239.8
mandibular	—	196.0	—	229.0	238.8	239.8
mediastinal	—	196.1	—	229.0	238.8	239.8
mesenteric (inferior) (superior)	—	196.2	—	229.0	238.8	239.8

	Malignant					
	Primary	**Secondary**	**Ca in situ**	**Benign**	**Uncertain Behavior**	**Unspecified**
Neoplasm, neoplastic — *continued*						
lymph, lymphatic — *continued*						
gland — *continued*						
midcolic	—	196.2	—	229.0	238.8	239.8
multiple sites in categories 196.0-196.6	—	196.8	—	229.0	238.8	239.8
neck	—	196.0	—	229.0	238.8	239.8
obturator	—	196.6	—	229.0	238.8	239.8
occipital	—	196.0	—	229.0	238.8	239.8
pancreatic	—	196.2	—	229.0	238.8	239.8
para-aortic	—	196.2	—	229.0	238.8	239.8
paracervical	—	196.6	—	229.0	238.8	239.8
parametrial	—	196.6	—	229.0	238.8	239.8
parasternal	—	196.1	—	229.0	238.8	239.8
parotid	—	196.0	—	229.0	238.8	239.8
pectoral	—	196.3	—	229.0	238.8	239.8
pelvic	—	196.6	—	229.0	238.8	239.8
peri-aortic	—	196.2	—	229.0	238.8	239.8
peripancreatic	—	196.2	—	229.0	238.8	239.8
popliteal	—	196.5	—	229.0	238.8	239.8
porta hepatis	—	196.2	—	229.0	238.8	239.8
portal	—	196.2	—	229.0	238.8	239.8
preauricular	—	196.0	—	229.0	238.8	239.8
prelaryngeal	—	196.0	—	229.0	238.8	239.8
presymphysial	—	196.6	—	229.0	238.8	239.8
pretracheal	—	196.0	—	229.0	238.8	239.8
primary (any site) NEC	202.9 ✓5ᵗʰ	—	—	—	—	—
pulmonary (hiler)	—	196.1	—	229.0	238.8	239.8
pyloric	—	196.2	—	229.0	238.8	239.8
retroperitoneal	—	196.2	—	229.0	238.8	239.8
retropharyngeal	—	196.0	—	229.0	238.8	239.8
Rosenmüller's	—	196.5	—	229.0	238.8	239.8
sacral	—	196.6	—	229.0	238.8	239.8
scalene	—	196.0	—	229.0	238.8	239.8
site NEC	—	196.9	—	229.0	238.8	239.8
splenic (hilar)	—	196.2	—	229.0	238.8	239.8
subclavicular	—	196.3	—	229.0	238.8	239.8
subinguinal	—	196.5	—	229.0	238.8	239.8
sublingual	—	196.0	—	229.0	238.8	239.8
submandibular	—	196.0	—	229.0	238.8	239.8
submaxillary	—	196.0	—	229.0	238.8	239.8
submental	—	196.0	—	229.0	238.8	239.8
subscapular	—	196.3	—	229.0	238.8	239.8
supraclavicular	—	196.0	—	229.0	238.8	239.8
thoracic	—	196.1	—	229.0	238.8	239.8
tibial	—	196.5	—	229.0	238.8	239.8
tracheal	—	196.1	—	229.0	238.8	239.8
tracheobronchial	—	196.1	—	229.0	238.8	239.8
upper limb	—	196.3	—	229.0	238.8	239.8
Virchow's	—	196.0	—	229.0	238.8	239.8
node — *see also* Neoplasm, lymph gland						
primary NEC	202.9 ✓5ᵗʰ	—	—	—	—	—
vessel (*see also* Neoplasm, connective tissue)	171.9	198.89	—	215.9	238.1	239.2
Nackenrodt's ligament	183.8	198.82	233.3	221.8	236.3	239.5
malar	170.0	198.5	—	213.0	238.0	239.2
region — *see* Neoplasm, cheek						
mammary gland — *see* Neoplasm, breast						
mandible	170.1	198.5	—	213.1	238.0	239.2
alveolar						
mucose	143.1	198.89	230.0	210.4	235.1	239.0
ridge or process	170.1	198.5	—	213.1	238.0	239.2
carcinoma	143.1	—	—	—	—	—
carcinoma	143.1	—	—	—	—	—
marrow (bone) NEC	202.9 ✓5ᵗʰ	198.5	—	—	—	238.7
mastectomy site (skin)	173.5	198.2	—	—	—	—
specified as breast tissue	174.8	198.81	—	—	—	—
mastoid (air cells) (antrum) (cavity)	160.1	197.3	231.8	212.0	235.9	239.1
bone or process	170.0	198.5	—	213.0	238.0	239.2

■4ᵗʰ Fourth-digit Required   ✓5ᵗʰ Fifth-digit Required   ▶◀ Revised Text   ● New Line   ▲ Revised Code

Neoplasm, neoplastic — continued	Malignant			Benign	Uncertain Behavior	Unspecified
	Primary	Secondary	Ca in situ	Benign	Uncertain Behavior	Unspecified
maxilla, maxillary (superior)	170.0	198.5	—	213.0	238.0	239.2
alveolar						
mucosa	143.0	198.89	230.0	210.4	235.1	239.0
ridge or process	170.0	198.5	—	213.0	238.0	239.2
carcinoma	143.0	—	—	—	—	—
antrum	160.2	197.3	231.8	212.0	235.9	239.1
carcinoma	143.0	—	—	—	—	—
inferior — see Neoplasm, mandible						
sinus	160.2	197.3	231.8	212.0	235.9	239.1
meatus						
external (ear)	173.2	198.2	232.2	216.2	238.2	239.2
Meckel's diverticulum	152.3	197.4	230.7	211.2	235.2	239.0
mediastinum, mediastinal	164.9	197.1	—	212.5	235.8	239.8
anterior	164.2	197.1	—	212.5	235.8	239.8
contiguous sites with heart and thymus	164.8	—	—	—	—	—
posterior	164.3	197.1	—	212.5	235.8	239.8
medulla						
adrenal	194.0	198.7	234.8	227.0	237.2	239.7
oblongata	191.7	198.3	—	225.0	237.5	239.6
meibomian gland	173.1	198.2	232.1	216.1	238.2	239.2
melanoma — see Melanoma						
meninges (brain) (cerebral) (cranial) (intracranial)	192.1	198.4	—	225.2	237.6	239.7
spinal (cord)	192.3	198.4	—	225.4	237.6	239.7
meniscus, knee joint (lateral) (medial)	170.7	198.5	—	213.7	238.0	239.2
mesentery, mesenteric	158.8	197.6	—	211.8	235.4	239.0
mesoappendix	158.8	197.6	—	211.8	235.4	239.0
mesocolon	158.8	197.6	—	211.8	235.4	239.0
mesopharynx — see Neoplasm, oropharynx						
mesosalpinx	183.3	198.82	233.3	221.0	236.3	239.5
mesovarium	183.3	198.82	233.3	221.0	236.3	239.5
metacarpus (any bone)	170.5	198.5	—	213.5	238.0	239.2
metastatic NEC — see also Neoplasm, by site, secondary	—	199.1	—	—	—	—
metatarsus (any bone)	170.8	198.5	—	213.8	238.0	239.2
midbrain	191.7	198.3	—	225.0	237.5	239.6
milk duct — see Neoplasm, breast						
mons						
pubis	184.4	198.82	233.3	221.2	236.3	239.5
veneris	184.4	198.82	233.3	221.2	236.3	239.5
motor tract	192.9	198.4	—	225.9	237.9	239.7
brain	191.9	198.3	—	225.0	237.5	239.6
spinal	192.2	198.3	—	225.3	237.5	239.7
mouth	145.9	198.89	230.0	210.4	235.1	239.0
contiguous sites	145.8	—	—	—	—	—
floor	144.9	198.89	230.0	210.3	235.1	239.0
anterior portion	144.0	198.89	230.0	210.3	235.1	239.0
contiguous sites	144.8	—	—	—	—	—
lateral portion	144.1	198.89	230.0	210.3	235.1	239.0
roof	145.5	198.89	230.0	210.4	235.1	239.0
specified part NEC	145.8	198.89	230.0	210.4	235.1	239.0
vestibule	145.1	198.89	230.0	210.4	235.1	239.0
mucosa						
alveolar (ridge or process)	143.9	198.89	230.0	210.4	235.1	239.0
lower	143.1	198.89	230.0	210.4	235.1	239.0
upper	143.0	198.89	230.0	210.4	235.1	239.0
buccal	145.0	198.89	230.0	210.4	235.1	239.0
cheek	145.0	198.89	230.0	210.4	235.1	239.0
lip — see Neoplasm, lip, internal						
nasal	160.0	197.3	231.8	212.0	235.9	239.1
oral	145.0	198.89	230.0	210.4	235.1	239.0
Müllerian duct						
female	184.8	198.82	233.3	221.8	236.3	239.5
male	187.8	198.82	233.6	222.8	236.6	239.5
multiple sites NEC	199.0	199.0	234.9	229.9	238.9	199.0
muscle — see also Neoplasm, connective tissue						
extraocular	190.1	198.4	234.0	224.1	238.8	239.8
myocardium	164.1	198.89	—	212.7	238.8	239.8

	Malignant					
	Primary	**Secondary**	**Ca in situ**	**Benign**	**Uncertain Behavior**	**Unspecified**
Neoplasm, neoplastic — *continued*						
myometrium	182.0	198.82	233.2	219.1	236.0	239.5
myopericardium	164.1	198.89	—	212.7	238.8	239.8
nabothian gland (follicle)	180.0	198.82	233.1	219.0	236.0	239.5
nail	173.9	198.2	232.9	216.9	238.2	239.2
finger	173.6	198.2	232.6	216.6	238.2	239.2
toe	173.7	198.2	232.7	216.7	238.2	239.2
nares, naris (anterior) (posterior)	160.0	197.3	231.8	212.0	235.9	239.1
nasal — *see* Neoplasm, nose						
nasolabial groove	173.3	198.2	232.3	216.3	238.2	239.2
nasolacrimal duct	190.7	198.4	234.0	224.7	238.8	239.8
nasopharynx, nasopharyngeal	147.9	198.89	230.0	210.7	235.1	239.0
contiguous sites	147.8	—	230.0	—	—	—
floor	147.3	198.89	230.0	210.7	235.1	239.0
roof	147.0	198.89	230.0	210.7	235.1	239.0
specified site NEC	147.8	198.89	230.0	210.7	235.1	239.0
wall	147.9	198.89	230.0	210.7	235.1	239.0
anterior	147.3	198.89	230.0	210.7	235.1	239.0
lateral	147.2	198.89	230.0	210.7	235.1	239.0
posterior	147.1	198.89	230.0	210.7	235.1	239.0
superior	147.0	198.89	230.0	210.7	235.1	239.0
nates	173.5	198.2	232.5	216.5	238.2	239.2
neck NEC*	195.0	198.89	234.8	229.8	238.8	239.8
nerve (autonomic) (ganglion) (parasympathetic) (peripheral) (sympathetic) — *see also* Neoplasm, connective tissue						
abducens	192.0	198.4	—	225.1	237.9	239.7
accessory (spinal)	192.0	198.4	—	225.1	237.9	239.7
acoustic	192.0	198.4	—	225.1	237.9	239.7
auditory	192.0	198.4	—	225.1	237.9	239.7
brachial	171.2	198.89	—	215.2	238.1	239.2
cranial (any)	192.0	198.4	—	225.1	237.9	239.7
facial	192.0	198.4	—	225.1	237.9	239.7
femoral	171.3	198.89	—	215.3	238.1	239.2
glossopharyngeal	192.0	198.4	—	225.1	237.9	239.7
hypoglossal	192.0	198.4	—	225.1	237.9	239.7
intercostal	171.4	198.89	—	215.4	238.1	239.2
lumbar	171.7	198.89	—	215.7	238.1	239.2
median	171.2	198.89	—	215.2	238.1	239.2
obturator	171.3	198.89	—	215.3	238.1	239.2
oculomotor	192.0	198.4	—	225.1	237.9	239.7
olfactory	192.0	198.4	—	225.1	237.9	239.7
optic	192.0	198.4	—	225.1	237.9	239.7
peripheral NEC	171.9	198.89	—	215.9	238.1	239.2
radial	171.2	198.89	—	215.2	238.1	239.2
sacral	171.6	198.89	—	215.6	238.1	239.2
sciatic	171.3	198.89	—	215.3	238.1	239.2
spinal NEC	171.9	198.89	—	215.9	238.1	239.2
trigeminal	192.0	198.4	—	225.1	237.9	239.7
trochlear	192.0	198.4	—	225.1	237.9	239.7
ulnar	171.2	198.89	—	215.2	238.1	239.2
vagus	192.0	198.4	—	225.1	237.9	239.7
nervous system (central) NEC	192.9	198.4	—	225.9	237.9	239.7
autonomic NEC	171.9	198.89	—	215.9	238.1	239.2
brain — *see also* Neoplasm, brain						
membrane or meninges	192.1	198.4	—	225.2	237.6	239.7
contiguous sites	192.8	—	—	—	—	—
parasympathetic NEC	171.9	198.89	—	215.9	238.1	239.2
sympathetic NEC	171.9	198.89	—	215.9	238.1	239.2
nipple (female)	174.0	198.81	233.0	217	238.3	239.3
male	175.0	198.81	233.0	217	238.3	239.3
nose, nasal	195.0	198.89	234.8	229.8	238.8	239.8
ala (external)	173.3	198.2	232.3	216.3	238.2	239.2
bone	170.0	198.5	—	213.0	238.0	239.2
cartilage	160.0	197.3	231.8	212.0	235.9	239.1
cavity	160.0	197.3	231.8	212.0	235.9	239.1
contiguous sites with accessory sinuses or middle ear	160.8	—	—	—	—	—
choana	147.3	198.89	230.0	210.7	235.1	239.0

	Malignant					
	Primary	Secondary	Ca in situ	Benign	Uncertain Behavior	Unspecified
Neoplasm, neoplastic — *continued*						
nose, nasal — *continued*						
external (skin)	173.3	198.2	232.3	216.3	238.2	239.2
fossa	160.0	197.3	231.8	212.0	235.9	239.1
internal	160.0	197.3	231.8	212.0	235.9	239.1
mucosa	160.0	197.3	231.8	212.0	235.9	239.1
septum	160.0	197.3	231.8	212.0	235.9	239.1
posterior margin	147.3	198.89	230.0	210.7	235.1	239.0
sinus — *see* Neoplasm, sinus						
skin	173.3	198.2	232.3	216.3	238.2	239.2
turbinate (mucosa)	160.0	197.3	231.8	212.0	235.9	239.1
bone	170.0	198.5	—	213.0	238.0	239.2
vestibule	160.0	197.3	231.8	212.0	235.9	239.1
nostril	160.0	197.3	231.8	212.0	235.9	239.1
nucleus pulposus	170.2	198.5	—	213.2	238.0	239.2
occipital						
bone	170.0	198.5	—	213.0	238.0	239.2
lobe or pole, brain	191.4	198.3	—	225.0	237.5	239.6
odontogenic — *see* Neoplasm, jaw bone						
oesophagus — *see* Neoplasm, esophagus						
olfactory nerve or bulb	192.0	198.4	—	225.1	237.9	239.7
olive (brain)	191.7	198.3	—	225.0	237.5	239.6
omentum	158.8	197.6	—	211.8	235.4	239.0
operculum (brain)	191.0	198.3	—	225.0	237.5	239.6
optic nerve, chiasm, or tract	192.0	198.4	—	225.1	237.9	239.7
oral (cavity)	145.9	198.89	230.0	210.4	235.1	239.0
contiguous sites with lip or pharynx	149.8	—	—	—	—	—
ill-defined	149.9	198.89	230.0	210.4	235.1	239.0
mucosa	145.9	198.89	230.0	210.4	235.1	239.0
orbit	190.1	198.4	234.0	224.1	238.8	239.8
bone	170.0	198.5	—	213.0	238.0	239.2
eye	190.1	198.4	234.0	224.1	238.8	239.8
soft parts	190.1	198.4	234.0	224.1	238.8	239.8
organ of Zuckerkandl	194.6	198.89	—	227.6	237.3	239.7
oropharynx	146.9	198.89	230.0	210.6	235.1	239.0
branchial cleft (vestige)	146.8	198.89	230.0	210.6	235.1	239.0
contiguous sites	146.8	—	—	—	—	—
junctional region	146.5	198.89	230.0	210.6	235.1	239.0
lateral wall	146.6	198.89	230.0	210.6	235.1	239.0
pillars of fauces	146.2	198.89	230.0	210.6	235.1	239.0
posterior wall	146.7	198.89	230.0	210.6	235.1	239.0
specified part NEC	146.8	198.89	230.0	210.6	235.1	239.0
vallecula	146.3	198.89	230.0	210.6	235.1	239.0
os						
external	180.1	198.82	233.1	219.0	236.0	239.5
internal	180.0	198.82	233.1	219.0	236.0	239.5
ovary	183.0	198.6	233.3	220	236.2	239.5
oviduct	183.2	198.82	233.3	221.0	236.3	239.5
palate	145.5	198.89	230.0	210.4	235.1	239.0
hard	145.2	198.89	230.0	210.4	235.1	239.0
junction of hard and soft palate	145.5	198.89	230.0	210.4	235.1	239.0
soft	145.3	198.89	230.0	210.4	235.1	239.0
nasopharyngeal surface	147.3	198.89	230.0	210.7	235.1	239.0
posterior surface	147.3	198.89	230.0	210.7	235.1	239.0
superior surface	147.3	198.89	230.0	210.7	235.1	239.0
palatoglossal arch	146.2	198.89	230.0	210.6	235.1	239.0
palatopharyngeal arch	146.2	198.89	230.0	210.6	235.1	239.0
pallium	191.0	198.3	—	225.0	237.5	239.6
palpebra	173.1	198.2	232.1	216.1	238.2	239.2
pancreas	157.9	197.8	230.9	211.6	235.5	239.0
body	157.1	197.8	230.9	211.6	235.5	239.0
contiguous sites	157.8	—	—	—	—	—
duct (of Santorini) (of Wirsung)	157.3	197.8	230.9	211.6	235.5	239.0
ectopic tissue	157.8	197.8	230.9	211.6	235.5	239.0
head	157.0	197.8	230.9	211.6	235.5	239.0
islet cells	157.4	197.8	230.9	211.7	235.5	239.0

	Malignant			Benign	Uncertain Behavior	Unspecified
	Primary	Secondary	Ca in situ			
Neoplasm, neoplastic — *continued*						
pancreas — *continued*						
neck	157.8	197.8	230.9	211.6	235.5	239.0
tail	157.2	197.8	230.9	211.6	235.5	239.0
para-aortic body	194.6	198.89	—	227.6	237.3	239.7
paraganglion NEC	194.6	198.89	—	227.6	237.3	239.7
parametrium	183.4	198.82	—	221.0	236.3	239.5
paranephric	158.0	197.6	—	211.8	235.4	239.0
pararectal	195.3	198.89	—	229.8	238.8	239.8
parasagittal (region)	195.0	198.89	234.8	229.8	238.8	239.8
parasellar	192.9	198.4	—	225.9	237.9	239.7
parathyroid (gland)	194.1	198.89	234.8	227.1	237.4	239.7
paraurethral	195.3	198.89	—	229.8	238.8	239.8
gland	189.4	198.1	233.9	223.89	236.99	239.5
paravaginal	195.3	198.89	—	229.8	238.8	239.8
parenchyma, kidney	189.0	198.0	233.9	223.0	236.91	239.5
parietal						
bone	170.0	198.5	—	213.0	238.0	239.2
lobe, brain	191.3	198.3	—	225.0	237.5	239.6
paroophoron	183.3	198.82	233.3	221.0	236.3	239.5
parotid (duct) (gland)	142.0	198.89	230.0	210.2	235.0	239.0
parovarium	183.3	198.82	233.3	221.0	236.3	239.5
patella	170.8	198.5	—	213.8	238.0	239.2
peduncle, cerebral	191.7	198.3	—	225.0	237.5	239.6
pelvirectal junction	154.0	197.5	230.4	211.4	235.2	239.0
pelvis, pelvic	195.3	198.89	234.8	229.8	238.8	239.8
bone	170.6	198.5	—	213.6	238.0	239.2
floor	195.3	198.89	234.8	229.8	238.8	239.8
renal	189.1	198.0	233.9	223.1	236.91	239.5
viscera	195.3	198.89	234.8	229.8	238.8	239.8
wall	195.3	198.89	234.8	229.8	238.8	239.8
pelvo-abdominal	195.8	198.89	234.8	229.8	238.8	239.8
penis	187.4	198.82	233.5	222.1	236.6	239.5
body	187.3	198.82	233.5	222.1	236.6	239.5
corpus (cavernosum)	187.3	198.82	233.5	222.1	236.6	239.5
glans	187.2	198.82	233.5	222.1	236.6	239.5
skin NEC	187.4	198.82	233.5	222.1	236.6	239.5
periadrenal (tissue)	158.0	197.6	—	211.8	235.4	239.0
perianal (skin)	173.5	198.2	232.5	216.5	238.2	239.2
pericardium	164.1	198.89	—	212.7	238.8	239.8
perinephric	158.0	197.6	—	211.8	235.4	239.0
perineum	195.3	198.89	234.8	229.8	238.8	239.8
periodontal tissue NEC	143.9	198.89	230.0	210.4	235.1	239.0
periosteum — *see* Neoplasm, bone						
peripancreatic	158.0	197.6	—	211.8	235.4	239.0
peripheral nerve NEC	171.9	198.89	—	215.9	238.1	239.2
perirectal (tissue)	195.3	198.89	—	229.8	238.8	239.8
perirenal (tissue)	158.0	197.6	—	211.8	235.4	239.0
peritoneum, peritoneal (cavity)	158.9	197.6	—	211.8	235.4	239.0
contiguous sites	158.8	—	—	—	—	—
with digestive organs	159.8	—	—	—	—	—
parietal	158.8	197.6	—	211.8	235.4	239.0
pelvic	158.8	197.6	—	211.8	235.4	239.0
specified part NEC	158.8	197.6	—	211.8	235.4	239.0
peritonsillar (tissue)	195.0	198.89	234.8	229.8	238.8	239.8
periurethral tissue	195.3	198.89	—	229.8	238.8	239.8
phalanges	170.9	198.5	—	213.9	238.0	239.2
foot	170.8	198.5	—	213.8	238.0	239.2
hand	170.5	198.5	—	213.5	238.0	239.2
pharynx, pharyngeal	149.0	198.89	230.0	210.9	235.1	239.0
bursa	147.1	198.89	230.0	210.7	235.1	239.0
fornix	147.3	198.89	230.0	210.7	235.1	239.0
recess	147.2	198.89	230.0	210.7	235.1	239.0
region	149.0	198.89	230.0	210.9	235.1	239.0
tonsil	147.1	198.89	230.0	210.7	235.1	239.0
wall (lateral) (posterior)	149.0	198.89	230.0	210.9	235.1	239.0

✓4ᵗʰ Fourth-digit Required   ✓5ᵗʰ Fifth-digit Required   ▶◀ Revised Text   ● New Line   ▲ Revised Code

	Malignant					
	Primary	Secondary	Ca in situ	Benign	Uncertain Behavior	Unspecified
Neoplasm, neoplastic — *continued*						
pia mater (cerebral) (cranial)	192.1	198.4	—	225.2	237.6	239.7
spinal	192.3	198.4	—	225.4	237.6	239.7
pillars of fauces	146.2	198.89	230.0	210.6	235.1	239.0
pineal (body) (gland)	194.4	198.89	234.8	227.4	237.1	239.7
pinna (ear) NEC	173.2	198.2	232.2	216.2	238.2	239.2
cartilage	171.0	198.89	—	215.0	238.1	239.2
piriform fossa or sinus	148.1	198.89	230.0	210.8	235.1	239.0
pituitary (body) (fossa) (gland) (lobe)	194.3	198.89	234.8	227.3	237.0	239.7
placenta	181	198.82	233.2	219.8	236.1	239.5
pleura, pleural (cavity)	163.9	197.2	—	212.4	235.8	239.1
contiguous sites	163.8	—	—	—	—	—
parietal	163.0	197.2	—	212.4	235.8	239.1
visceral	163.1	197.2	—	212.4	235.8	239.1
plexus						
brachial	171.2	198.89	—	215.2	238.1	239.2
cervical	171.0	198.89	—	215.0	238.1	239.2
choroid	191.5	198.3	—	225.0	237.5	239.6
lumbosacral	171.6	198.89	—	215.6	238.1	239.2
sacral	171.6	198.89	—	215.6	238.1	239.2
pluri-endocrine	194.8	198.89	234.8	227.8	237.4	239.7
pole						
frontal	191.1	198.3	—	225.0	237.5	239.6
occipital	191.4	198.3	—	225.0	237.5	239.6
pons (varolii)	191.7	198.3	—	225.0	237.5	239.6
popliteal fossa or space*	195.5	198.89	234.8	229.8	238.8	239.8
postcricoid (region)	148.0	198.89	230.0	210.8	235.1	239.0
posterior fossa (cranial)	191.6	198.3	—	225.0	237.5	239.6
postnasal space	147.9	198.89	230.0	210.7	235.1	239.0
prepuce	187.1	198.82	233.5	222.1	236.6	239.5
prepylorus	151.1	197.8	230.2	211.1	235.2	239.0
presacral (region)	195.3	198.89	—	229.8	238.8	239.8
prostate (gland)	185	198.82	233.4	222.2	236.5	239.5
utricle	189.3	198.1	233.9	223.81	236.99	239.5
pterygoid fossa	171.0	198.89	—	215.0	238.1	239.2
pubic bone	170.6	198.5	—	213.6	238.0	239.2
pudenda, pudendum (female)	184.4	198.82	233.3	221.2	236.3	239.5
pulmonary	162.9	197.0	231.2	212.3	235.7	239.1
putamen	191.0	198.3	—	225.0	237.5	239.6
pyloric						
antrum	151.2	197.8	230.2	211.1	235.2	239.0
canal	151.1	197.8	230.2	211.1	235.2	239.0
pylorus	151.1	197.8	230.2	211.1	235.2	239.0
pyramid (brain)	191.7	198.3	—	225.0	237.5	239.6
pyriform fossa or sinus	148.1	198.89	230.0	210.8	235.1	239.0
radius (any part)	170.4	198.5	—	213.4	238.0	239.2
Rathke's pouch	194.3	198.89	234.8	227.3	237.0	239.7
rectosigmoid (colon) (junction)	154.0	197.5	230.4	211.4	235.2	239.0
contiguous sites with anus or rectum	154.8	—	—	—	—	—
rectouterine pouch	158.8	197.6	—	211.8	235.4	239.0
rectovaginal septum or wall	195.3	198.89	234.8	229.8	238.8	239.8
rectovesical septum	195.3	198.89	234.8	229.8	238.8	239.8
rectum (ampulla)	154.1	197.5	230.4	211.4	235.2	239.0
and colon	154.0	197.5	230.4	211.4	235.2	239.0
contiguous sites with anus or rectosigmoid junction	154.8	—	—	—	—	—
renal	189.0	198.0	233.9	223.0	236.91	239.5
calyx	189.1	198.0	233.9	223.1	236.91	239.5
hilus	189.1	198.0	233.9	223.1	236.91	239.5
parenchyma	189.0	198.0	233.9	223.0	236.91	239.5
pelvis	189.1	198.0	233.9	223.1	236.91	239.5
respiratory						
organs or system NEC	165.9	197.3	231.9	212.9	235.9	239.1
contiguous sites with intrathoracic organs	165.8	—	—	—	—	—
specified sites NEC	165.8	197.3	231.8	212.8	235.9	239.1
tract NEC	165.9	197.3	231.9	212.9	235.9	239.1
upper	165.0	197.3	231.9	212.9	235.9	239.1
retina	190.5	198.4	234.0	224.5	238.8	239.8

✓4ᵗʰ Fourth-digit Required   ✓5ᵗʰ Fifth-digit Required   ▶◀ Revised Text   ● New Line   ▲ Revised Code

	Malignant					
	Primary	Secondary	Ca in situ	Benign	Uncertain Behavior	Unspecified
Neoplasm, neoplastic — *continued*						
retrobulbar	190.1	198.4	—	224.1	238.8	239.8
retrocecal	158.0	197.6	—	211.8	235.4	239.0
retromolar (area) (triangle) (trigone)	145.6	198.89	230.0	210.4	235.1	239.0
retro-orbital	195.0	198.89	234.8	229.8	238.8	239.8
retroperitoneal (space) (tissue)	158.0	197.6	—	211.8	235.4	239.0
contiguous sites	158.8	—	—	—	—	—
retroperitoneum	158.0	197.6	—	211.8	235.4	239.0
contiguous sites	158.8	—	—	—	—	—
retropharyngeal	149.0	198.89	230.0	210.9	235.1	239.0
retrovesical (septum)	195.3	198.89	234.8	229.8	238.8	239.8
rhinencephalon	191.0	198.3	—	225.0	237.5	239.6
rib	170.3	198.5	—	213.3	238.0	239.2
Rosenmüller's fossa	147.2	198.89	230.0	210.7	235.1	239.0
round ligament	183.5	198.82	—	221.0	236.3	239.5
sacrococcyx, sacrococcygeal	170.6	198.5	—	213.6	238.0	239.2
region	195.3	198.89	234.8	229.8	238.8	239.8
sacrouterine ligament	183.4	198.82	—	221.0	236.3	239.5
sacrum, sacral (vertebra)	170.6	198.5	—	213.6	238.0	239.2
salivary gland or duct (major)	142.9	198.89	230.0	210.2	235.0	239.0
contiguous sites	142.8	—	—	—	—	—
minor NEC	145.9	198.89	230.0	210.4	235.1	239.0
parotid	142.0	198.89	230.0	210.2	235.0	239.0
pluriglandular	142.8	198.89	230.0	210.2	235.0	239.0
sublingual	142.2	198.89	230.0	210.2	235.0	239.0
submandibular	142.1	198.89	230.0	210.2	235.0	239.0
submaxillary	142.1	198.89	230.0	210.2	235.0	239.0
salpinx (uterine)	183.2	198.82	233.3	221.0	236.3	239.5
Santorini's duct	157.3	197.8	230.9	211.6	235.5	239.0
scalp	173.4	198.2	232.4	216.4	238.2	239.2
scapula (any part)	170.4	198.5	—	213.4	238.0	239.2
scapular region	195.1	198.89	234.8	229.8	238.8	239.8
scar NEC (*see also* Neoplasm, skin)	173.9	198.2	232.9	216.9	238.2	239.2
sciatic nerve	171.3	198.89	—	215.3	238.1	239.2
sclera	190.0	198.4	234.0	224.0	238.8	239.8
scrotum (skin)	187.7	198.82	233.6	222.4	236.6	239.5
sebaceous gland — *see* Neoplasm, skin						
sella turcica	194.3	198.89	234.8	227.3	237.0	239.7
bone	170.0	198.5	—	213.0	238.0	239.2
semilunar cartilage (knee)	170.7	198.5	—	213.7	238.0	239.2
seminal vesicle	187.8	198.82	233.6	222.8	236.6	239.5
septum						
nasal	160.0	197.3	231.8	212.0	235.9	239.1
posterior margin	147.3	198.89	230.0	210.7	235.1	239.0
rectovaginal	195.3	198.89	234.8	229.8	238.8	239.8
rectovesical	195.3	198.89	234.8	229.8	238.8	239.8
urethrovaginal	184.9	198.82	233.3	221.9	236.3	239.5
vesicovaginal	184.9	198.82	233.3	221.9	236.3	239.5
shoulder NEC*	195.4	198.89	232.6	229.8	238.8	239.8
sigmoid flexure (lower) (upper)	153.3	197.5	230.3	211.3	235.2	239.0
sinus (accessory)	160.9	197.3	231.8	212.0	235.9	239.1
bone (any)	170.0	198.5	—	213.0	238.0	239.2
contiguous sites with middle ear or nasal cavities	160.8	—	—	—	—	—
ethmoidal	160.3	197.3	231.8	212.0	235.9	239.1
frontal	160.4	197.3	231.8	212.0	235.9	239.1
maxillary	160.2	197.3	231.8	212.0	235.9	239.1
nasal, paranasal NEC	160.9	197.3	231.8	212.0	235.9	239.1
pyriform	148.1	198.89	230.0	210.8	235.1	239.0
sphenoidal	160.5	197.3	231.8	212.0	235.9	239.1
skeleton, skeletal NEC	170.9	198.5	—	213.9	238.0	239.2
Skene's gland	189.4	198.1	233.9	223.89	236.99	239.5
skin NEC	173.9	198.2	232.9	216.9	238.2	239.2
abdominal wall	173.5	198.2	232.5	216.5	238.2	239.2
ala nasi	173.3	198.2	232.3	216.3	238.2	239.2
ankle	173.7	198.2	232.7	216.7	238.2	239.2
antecubital space	173.6	198.2	232.6	216.6	238.2	239.2
anus	173.5	198.2	232.5	216.5	238.2	239.2

| | Malignant | | | | | |
	Primary	Secondary	Ca in situ	Benign	Uncertain Behavior	Unspecified
Neoplasm, neoplastic — *continued*						
skin NEC — *continued*						
arm	173.6	198.2	232.6	216.6	238.2	239.2
auditory canal (external)	173.2	198.2	232.2	216.2	238.2	239.2
auricle (ear)	173.2	198.2	232.2	216.2	238.2	239.2
auricular canal (external)	173.2	198.2	232.2	216.2	238.2	239.2
axilla, axillary fold	173.5	198.2	232.5	216.5	238.2	239.2
back	173.5	198.2	232.5	216.5	238.2	239.2
breast	173.5	198.2	232.5	216.5	238.2	239.2
brow	173.3	198.2	232.3	216.3	238.2	239.2
buttock	173.5	198.2	232.5	216.5	238.2	239.2
calf	173.7	198.2	232.7	216.7	238.2	239.2
canthus (eye) (inner) (outer)	173.1	198.2	232.1	216.1	238.2	239.2
cervical region	173.4	198.2	232.4	216.4	238.2	239.2
cheek (external)	173.3	198.2	232.3	216.3	238.2	239.2
chest (wall)	173.5	198.2	232.5	216.5	238.2	239.2
chin	173.3	198.2	232.3	216.3	238.2	239.2
clavicular area	173.5	198.2	232.5	216.5	238.2	239.2
clitoris	184.3	198.82	233.3	221.2	236.3	239.5
columnella	173.3	198.2	232.3	216.3	238.2	239.2
concha	173.2	198.2	232.2	216.2	238.2	239.2
contiguous sites	173.8	—	—	—	—	—
ear (external)	173.2	198.2	232.2	216.2	238.2	239.2
elbow	173.6	198.2	232.6	216.6	238.2	239.2
eyebrow	173.3	198.2	232.3	216.3	238.2	239.2
eyelid	173.1	198.2	232.1	216.1	238.2	239.2
face NEC	173.3	198.2	232.3	216.3	238.2	239.2
female genital organs (external)	184.4	198.82	233.3	221.2	236.3	239.5
clitoris	184.3	198.82	233.3	221.2	236.3	239.5
labium NEC	184.4	198.82	233.3	221.2	236.3	239.5
majus	184.1	198.82	233.3	221.2	236.3	239.5
minus	184.2	198.82	233.3	221.2	236.3	239.5
pudendum	184.4	198.82	233.3	221.2	236.3	239.5
vulva	184.4	198.82	233.3	221.2	236.3	239.5
finger	173.6	198.2	232.6	216.6	238.2	239.2
flank	173.5	198.2	232.5	216.5	238.2	239.2
foot	173.7	198.2	232.7	216.7	238.2	239.2
forearm	173.6	198.2	232.6	216.6	238.2	239.2
forehead	173.3	198.2	232.3	216.3	238.2	239.2
glabella	173.3	198.2	232.3	216.3	238.2	239.2
gluteal region	173.5	198.2	232.5	216.5	238.2	239.2
groin	173.5	198.2	232.5	216.5	238.2	239.2
hand	173.6	198.2	232.6	216.6	238.2	239.2
head NEC	173.4	198.2	232.4	216.4	238.2	239.2
heel	173.7	198.2	232.7	216.7	238.2	239.2
helix	173.2	198.2	232.2	216.2	238.2	239.2
hip	173.7	198.2	232.7	216.7	238.2	239.2
infraclavicular region	173.5	198.2	232.5	216.5	238.2	239.2
inguinal region	173.5	198.2	232.5	216.5	238.2	239.2
jaw	173.3	198.2	232.3	216.3	238.2	239.2
knee	173.7	198.2	232.7	216.7	238.2	239.2
labia						
majora	184.1	198.82	233.3	221.2	236.3	239.5
minora	184.2	198.82	233.3	221.2	236.3	239.5
leg	173.7	198.2	232.7	216.7	238.2	239.2
lid (lower) (upper)	173.1	198.2	232.1	216.1	238.2	239.2
limb NEC	173.9	198.2	232.9	216.9	238.2	239.5
lower	173.7	198.2	232.7	216.7	238.2	239.2
upper	173.6	198.2	232.6	216.6	238.2	239.2
lip (lower) (upper)	173.0	198.2	232.0	216.0	238.2	239.2
male genital organs	187.9	198.82	233.6	222.9	236.6	239.5
penis	187.4	198.82	233.5	222.1	236.6	239.5
prepuce	187.1	198.82	233.5	222.1	236.6	239.5
scrotum	187.7	198.82	233.6	222.4	236.6	239.5
mastectomy site	173.5	198.2	—	—	—	—
specified as breast tissue	174.8	198.81	—	—	—	—
meatus, acoustic (external)	173.2	198.2	232.2	216.2	238.2	239.2

✓4ᵀ Fourth-digit Required   ✓5ᵀ Fifth-digit Required   ▶◀ Revised Text   ● New Line   ▲ Revised Code

	Malignant					
	Primary	Secondary	Ca in situ	Benign	Uncertain Behavior	Unspecified
Neoplasm, neoplastic — *continued*						
skin NEC — *continued*						
melanoma — *see* Melanoma						
nates	173.5	198.2	232.5	216.5	238.2	239.0
neck	173.4	198.2	232.4	216.4	238.2	239.2
nose (external)	173.3	198.2	232.3	216.3	238.2	239.2
palm	173.6	198.2	232.6	216.6	238.2	239.2
palpebra	173.1	198.2	232.1	216.1	238.2	239.2
penis NEC	187.4	198.82	233.5	222.1	236.6	239.5
perianal	173.5	198.2	232.5	216.5	238.2	239.2
perineum	173.5	198.2	232.5	216.5	238.2	239.2
pinna	173.2	198.2	232.2	216.2	238.2	239.2
plantar	173.7	198.2	232.7	216.7	238.2	239.2
popliteal fossa or space	173.7	198.2	232.7	216.7	238.2	239.2
prepuce	187.1	198.82	233.5	222.1	236.6	239.5
pubes	173.5	198.2	232.5	216.5	238.2	239.2
sacrococcygeal region	173.5	198.2	232.5	216.5	238.2	239.2
scalp	173.4	198.2	232.4	216.4	238.2	239.2
scapular region	173.5	198.2	232.5	216.5	238.2	239.2
scrotum	187.7	198.82	233.6	222.4	236.6	239.5
shoulder	173.6	198.2	232.6	216.6	238.2	239.2
sole (foot)	173.7	198.2	232.7	216.7	238.2	239.2
specified sites NEC	173.8	198.2	232.8	216.8	232.8	239.2
submammary fold	173.5	198.2	232.5	216.5	238.2	239.2
supraclavicular region	173.4	198.2	232.4	216.4	238.2	239.2
temple	173.3	198.2	232.3	216.3	238.2	239.2
thigh	173.7	198.2	232.7	216.7	238.2	239.2
thoracic wall	173.5	198.2	232.5	216.5	238.2	239.2
thumb	173.6	198.2	232.6	216.6	238.2	239.2
toe	173.7	198.2	232.7	216.7	238.2	239.2
tragus	173.2	198.2	232.2	216.2	238.2	239.2
trunk	173.5	198.2	232.5	216.5	238.2	239.2
umbilicus	173.5	198.2	232.5	216.5	238.2	239.2
vulva	184.4	198.82	233.3	221.2	236.3	239.5
wrist	173.6	198.2	232.6	216.6	238.2	239.2
skull	170.0	198.5	—	213.0	238.0	239.2
soft parts or tissues — *see* Neoplasm, connective tissue						
specified site NEC	195.8	198.89	234.8	229.8	238.8	239.8
spermatic cord	187.6	198.82	233.6	222.8	236.6	239.5
sphenoid	160.5	197.3	231.8	212.0	235.9	239.1
bone	170.0	198.5	—	213.0	238.0	239.2
sinus	160.5	197.3	231.8	212.0	235.9	239.1
sphincter						
anal	154.2	197.5	230.5	211.4	235.5	239.0
of Oddi	156.1	197.8	230.8	211.5	235.3	239.0
spine, spinal (column)	170.2	198.5	—	213.2	238.0	239.2
bulb	191.7	198.3	—	225.0	237.5	239.6
coccyx	170.6	198.5	—	213.6	238.0	239.2
cord (cervical) (lumbar) (sacral) (thoracic)	192.2	198.3	—	225.3	237.5	239.7
dura mater	192.3	198.4	—	225.4	237.6	239.7
lumbosacral	170.2	198.5	—	213.2	238.0	239.2
membrane	192.3	198.4	—	225.4	237.6	239.7
meninges	192.3	198.4	—	225.4	237.6	239.7
nerve (root)	171.9	198.89	—	215.9	238.1	239.2
pia mater	192.3	198.4	—	225.4	237.6	239.7
root	171.9	198.89	—	215.9	238.1	239.2
sacrum	170.6	198.5	—	213.6	238.0	239.2
spleen, splenic NEC	159.1	197.8	230.9	211.9	235.5	239.0
flexure (colon)	153.7	197.5	230.3	211.3	235.2	239.0
stem, brain	191.7	198.3	—	225.0	237.5	239.6
Stensen's duct	142.0	198.89	230.0	210.2	235.0	239.0
sternum	170.3	198.5	—	213.3	238.0	239.2
stomach	151.9	197.8	230.2	211.1	235.2	239.0
antrum (pyloric)	151.2	197.8	230.2	211.1	235.2	239.0
body	151.4	197.8	230.2	211.1	235.2	239.0
cardia	151.0	197.8	230.2	211.1	235.2	239.0
cardiac orifice	151.0	197.8	230.2	211.1	235.2	239.0

☑4ᵗʰ Fourth-digit Required   ☑5ᵗʰ Fifth-digit Required   ▶◀ Revised Text   ● New Line   ▲ Revised Code

	Malignant					
	Primary	Secondary	Ca in situ	Benign	Uncertain Behavior	Unspecified
Neoplasm, neoplastic — *continued*						
stomach — *continued*						
contiguous sites	151.8	—	—	—	—	—
corpus	151.4	197.8	230.2	211.1	235.2	239.0
fundus	151.3	197.8	230.2	211.1	235.2	239.0
greater curvature NEC	151.6	197.8	230.2	211.1	235.2	239.0
lesser curvature NEC	151.5	197.8	230.2	211.1	235.2	239.0
prepylorus	151.1	197.8	230.2	211.1	235.2	239.0
pylorus	151.1	197.8	230.2	211.1	235.2	239.0
wall NEC	151.9	197.8	230.2	211.1	235.2	239.0
anterior NEC	151.8	197.8	230.2	211.1	235.2	239.0
posterior NEC	151.8	197.8	230.2	211.1	235.2	239.0
stroma, endometrial	182.0	198.82	233.2	219.1	236.0	239.5
stump, cervical	180.8	198.82	233.1	219.0	236.0	239.5
subcutaneous (nodule) (tissue) NEC — *see* Neoplasm, connective tissue						
subdural	192.1	198.4	—	225.2	237.6	239.7
subglottis, subglottic	161.2	197.3	231.0	212.1	235.6	239.1
sublingual	144.9	198.89	230.0	210.3	235.1	239.0
gland or duct	142.2	198.89	230.0	210.2	235.0	239.0
submandibular gland	142.1	198.89	230.0	210.2	235.0	239.0
submaxillary gland or duct	142.1	198.89	230.0	210.2	235.0	239.0
submental	195.0	198.89	234.8	229.8	238.8	239.8
subpleural	162.9	197.0	—	212.3	235.7	239.1
substernal	164.2	197.1	—	212.5	235.8	239.8
sudoriferous, sudoriparous gland, site unspecified	173.9	198.2	232.9	216.9	238.2	239.2
specified site — *see* Neoplasm, skin						
supraclavicular region	195.0	198.89	234.8	229.8	238.8	239.8
supraglottis	161.1	197.3	231.0	212.1	235.6	239.1
suprarenal (capsule) (cortex) (gland) (medulla)	194.0	198.7	234.8	227.0	237.2	239.7
suprasellar (region)	191.9	198.3	—	225.0	237.5	239.6
sweat gland (apocrine) (eccrine), site unspecified	173.9	198.2	232.9	216.9	238.2	239.2
specified site — *see* Neoplasm, skin						
sympathetic nerve or nervous system NEC	171.9	198.89	—	215.9	238.1	239.2
symphysis pubis	170.6	198.5	—	213.6	238.0	239.2
synovial membrane — *see* Neoplasm, connective tissue						
tapetum, brain	191.8	198.3	—	225.0	237.5	239.6
tarsus (any bone)	170.8	198.5	—	213.8	238.0	239.2
temple (skin)	173.3	198.2	232.3	216.3	238.2	239.2
temporal						
bone	170.0	198.5	—	213.0	238.0	239.2
lobe or pole	191.2	198.3	—	225.0	237.5	239.6
region	195.0	198.89	234.8	229.8	238.8	239.8
skin	173.3	198.2	232.3	216.3	238.2	239.2
tendon (sheath) — *see* Neoplasm, connective tissue						
tentorium (cerebelli)	192.1	198.4	—	225.2	237.6	239.7
testis, testes (descended) (scrotal)	186.9	198.82	233.6	222.0	236.4	239.5
ectopic	186.0	198.82	233.6	222.0	236.4	239.5
retained	186.0	198.82	233.6	222.0	236.4	239.5
undescended	186.0	198.82	233.6	222.0	236.4	239.5
thalamus	191.0	198.3	—	225.0	237.5	239.6
thigh NEC*	195.5	198.89	234.8	229.8	238.8	239.8
thorax, thoracic (cavity) (organs NEC)	195.1	198.89	234.8	229.8	238.8	239.8
duct	171.4	198.89	—	215.4	238.1	239.2
wall NEC	195.1	198.89	234.8	229.8	238.8	239.8
throat	149.0	198.89	230.0	210.9	235.1	239.0
thumb NEC*	195.4	198.89	232.6	229.8	238.8	239.8
thymus (gland)	164.0	198.89	—	212.6	235.8	239.8
contiguous sites with heart and mediastinum	164.8	—	—	—	—	—
thyroglossal duct	193	198.89	234.8	226	237.4	239.7
thyroid (gland)	193	198.89	234.8	226	237.4	239.7
cartilage	161.3	197.3	231.0	212.1	235.6	239.1
tibia (any part)	170.7	198.5	—	213.7	238.0	239.2
toe NEC*	195.5	198.89	232.7	229.8	238.8	239.8
tongue	141.9	198.89	230.0	210.1	235.1	239.0
anterior (two-thirds) NEC	141.4	198.89	230.0	210.1	235.1	239.0
dorsal surface	141.1	198.89	230.0	210.1	235.1	239.0
ventral surface	141.3	198.89	230.0	210.1	235.1	239.0

✓4ᵗʰ Fourth-digit Required   ✓5ᵗʰ Fifth-digit Required   ▶◀ Revised Text   ● New Line   ▲ Revised Code

	Malignant					
	Primary	**Secondary**	**Ca in situ**	**Benign**	**Uncertain Behavior**	**Unspecified**
Neoplasm, neoplastic — *continued*						
tongue — *continued*						
base (dorsal surface)	141.0	198.89	230.0	210.1	235.1	239.0
border (lateral)	141.2	198.89	230.0	210.1	235.1	239.0
contiguous sites	141.8	—	—	—	—	—
dorsal surface NEC	141.1	198.89	230.0	210.1	235.1	239.0
fixed part NEC	141.0	198.89	230.0	210.1	235.1	239.0
foreamen cecum	141.1	198.89	230.0	210.1	235.1	239.0
frenulum linguae	141.3	198.89	230.0	210.1	235.1	239.0
junctional zone	141.5	198.89	230.0	210.1	235.1	239.0
margin (lateral)	141.2	198.89	230.0	210.1	235.1	239.0
midline NEC	141.1	198.89	230.0	210.1	235.1	239.0
mobile part NEC	141.4	198.89	230.0	210.1	235.1	239.0
posterior (third)	141.0	198.89	230.0	210.1	235.1	239.0
root	141.0	198.89	230.0	210.1	235.1	239.0
surface (dorsal)	141.1	198.89	230.0	210.1	235.1	239.0
base	141.0	198.89	230.0	210.1	235.1	239.0
ventral	141.3	198.89	230.0	210.1	235.1	239.0
tip	141.2	198.89	230.0	210.1	235.1	239.0
tonsil	141.6	198.89	230.0	210.1	235.1	239.0
tonsil	146.0	198.89	230.0	210.5	235.1	239.0
fauces, faucial	146.0	198.89	230.0	210.5	235.1	239.0
lingual	141.6	198.89	230.0	210.1	235.1	239.0
palatine	146.0	198.89	230.0	210.5	235.1	239.0
pharyngeal	147.1	198.89	230.0	210.7	235.1	239.0
pillar (anterior) (posterior)	146.2	198.89	230.0	210.6	235.1	239.0
tonsillar fossa	146.1	198.89	230.0	210.6	235.1	239.0
tooth socket NEC	143.9	198.89	230.0	210.4	235.1	239.0
trachea (cartilage) (mucosa)	162.0	197.3	231.1	212.2	235.7	239.1
contiguous sites with bronchus or lung	162.8	—	—	—	—	—
tracheobronchial	162.8	197.3	231.1	212.2	235.7	239.1
contiguous sites with lung	162.8	—	—	—	—	—
tragus	173.2	198.2	232.2	216.2	238.2	239.2
trunk NEC*	195.8	198.89	232.5	229.8	238.8	239.8
tubo-ovarian	183.8	198.82	233.3	221.8	236.3	239.5
tunica vaginalis	187.8	198.82	233.6	222.8	236.6	239.5
turbinate (bone)	170.0	198.5	—	213.0	238.0	239.2
nasal	160.0	197.3	231.8	212.0	235.9	239.1
tympanic cavity	160.1	197.3	231.8	212.0	235.9	239.1
ulna (any part)	170.4	198.5	—	213.4	238.0	239.2
umbilicus, umbilical	173.5	198.2	232.5	216.5	238.2	239.2
uncus, brain	191.2	198.3	—	225.0	237.5	239.6
unknown site or unspecified	199.1	199.1	234.9	229.9	238.9	239.9
urachus	188.7	198.1	233.7	223.3	236.7	239.4
ureter, ureteral	189.2	198.1	233.9	223.2	236.91	239.5
orifice (bladder)	188.6	198.1	233.7	223.3	236.7	239.4
ureter-bladder junction)	188.6	198.1	233.7	223.3	236.7	239.4
urethra, urethral (gland)	189.3	198.1	233.9	223.81	236.99	239.5
orifice, internal	188.5	198.1	233.7	223.3	236.7	239.4
urethrovaginal (septum)	184.9	198.82	233.3	221.9	236.3	239.5
urinary organ or system NEC	189.9	198.1	233.9	223.9	236.99	239.5
bladder — *see* Neoplasm, bladder						
contiguous sites	189.8	—	—	—	—	—
specified sites NEC	189.8	198.1	233.9	223.89	236.99	239.5
utero-ovarian	183.8	198.82	233.3	221.8	236.3	239.5
ligament	183.3	198.82	—	221.0	236.3	239.5
uterosacral ligament	183.4	198.82	—	221.0	236.3	239.5
uterus, uteri, uterine	179	198.82	233.2	219.9	236.0	239.5
adnexa NEC	183.9	198.82	233.3	221.8	236.3	239.5
contiguous sites	183.8	—	—	—	—	—
body	182.0	198.82	233.2	219.1	236.0	239.5
contiguous sites	182.8	—	—	—	—	—
cervix	180.9	198.82	233.1	219.0	236.0	239.5
tornu	182.0	198.82	233.2	219.1	236.0	239.5
corpus	182.0	198.82	233.2	219.1	236.0	239.5
endocervix (canal) (gland)	180.0	198.82	233.1	219.0	236.0	239.5
endometrium	182.0	198.82	233.2	219.1	236.0	239.5

Neoplasm, neoplastic — continued	Malignant			Benign	Uncertain Behavior	Unspecified
	Primary	Secondary	Ca in situ	Benign	Uncertain Behavior	Unspecified
uterus, uteri, uterine — continued						
exocervix	180.1	198.82	233.1	219.0	236.0	239.5
external os	180.1	198.82	233.1	219.0	236.0	239.5
fundus	182.0	198.82	233.2	219.1	236.0	239.5
internal os	180.0	198.82	233.1	219.0	236.0	239.5
isthmus	182.1	198.82	233.2	219.1	236.0	239.5
ligament	183.4	198.82	—	221.0	236.3	239.5
broad	183.3	198.82	233.3	221.0	236.3	239.5
round	183.5	198.82	—	221.0	236.3	239.5
lower segment	182.1	198.82	233.2	219.1	236.0	239.5
myometrium	182.0	198.82	233.2	219.1	236.0	239.5
squamocolumnar junction	180.8	198.82	233.1	219.0	236.0	239.5
tube	183.2	198.82	233.3	221.0	236.3	239.5
utricle, prostatic	189.3	198.1	233.9	223.81	236.99	239.5
uveal tract	190.0	198.4	234.0	224.0	238.8	239.8
uvula	145.4	198.89	230.0	210.4	235.1	239.0
vagina, vaginal (fornix) (vault) (wall)	184.0	198.82	233.3	221.1	236.3	239.5
vaginovesical	184.9	198.82	233.3	221.9	236.3	239.5
septum	194.9	198.82	233.3	221.9	236.3	239.5
vallecula (epiglottis)	146.3	198.89	230.0	210.6	235.1	239.0
vascular — see Neoplasm, connective tissue						
vas deferens	187.6	198.82	233.6	222.8	236.6	239.5
Vater's ampulla	156.2	197.8	230.8	211.5	235.3	239.0
vein, venous — see Neoplasm, connective tissue						
vena cava (abdominal) (inferior)	171.5	198.89	—	215.5	238.1	239.2
superior	171.4	198.89	—	215.4	238.1	239.2
ventricle (cerebral) (floor) (fourth) (lateral) (third)	191.5	198.3	—	225.0	237.5	239.6
cardiac (left) (right)	164.1	198.89	—	212.7	238.8	239.8
ventricular band of larynx	161.1	197.3	231.0	212.1	235.6	239.1
ventriculus — see Neoplasm, stomach						
vermillion border — see Neoplasm, lip						
vermis, cerebellum	191.6	198.3	—	225.0	237.5	239.6
vertebra (column)	170.2	198.5	—	213.2	238.0	239.2
coccyx	170.6	198.5	—	213.6	238.0	239.2
sacrum	170.6	198.5	—	213.6	238.0	239.2
vesical — see Neoplasm, bladder						
vesicle, seminal	187.8	198.82	233.6	222.8	236.6	239.5
vesicocervical tissue	184.9	198.82	233.3	221.9	236.3	239.5
vesicorectal	195.3	198.89	234.8	229.8	238.8	239.8
vesicovaginal	184.9	198.82	233.3	221.9	236.3	239.5
septum	184.9	198.82	233.3	221.9	236.3	239.5
vessel (blood) — see Neoplasm, connective tissue						
vestibular gland, greater	184.1	198.82	233.3	221.2	236.3	239.5
vestibule						
mouth	145.1	198.89	230.0	210.4	235.1	239.0
nose	160.0	197.3	231.8	212.0	235.9	239.1
Virchow's gland	—	196.0	—	229.0	238.8	239.8
viscera NEC	195.8	198.89	234.8	229.8	238.8	239.8
vocal cords (true)	161.0	197.3	231.0	212.1	235.6	239.1
false	161.1	197.3	231.0	212.1	235.6	239.1
vomer	170.0	198.5	—	213.0	238.0	239.2
vulva	184.4	198.82	233.3	221.2	236.3	239.5
vulvovaginal gland	184.4	198.82	233.3	221.2	236.3	239.5
Waldeyer's ring	149.1	198.89	230.0	210.9	235.1	239.0
Wharton's duct	142.1	198.89	230.0	210.2	235.0	239.0
white matter (central) (cerebral)	191.0	198.3	—	225.0	237.5	239.6
windpipe	162.0	197.3	231.1	212.2	235.7	239.1
Wirsung's duct	157.3	197.8	230.9	211.6	235.5	239.0
wolffian (body) (duct)						
female	184.8	198.82	233.3	221.8	236.3	239.5
male	187.8	198.82	233.6	222.8	236.6	239.5
womb — see Neoplasm, uterus						
wrist NEC*	195.4	198.89	232.6	229.8	238.8	239.8
xiphoid process	170.3	198.5	—	213.3	238.0	239.2
Zuckerkandl's organ	194.6	198.89	—	227.6	237.3	239.7

Neoplasm, uterus — Neoplasm, Zuckerkandl's organ

✓4ᵗʰ Fourth-digit Required   ✓5ᵗʰ Fifth-digit Required   ▶◀ Revised Text   ● New Line   ▲ Revised Code

Neovascularization
  choroid 362.16
  ciliary body 364.42
  cornea 370.60
    deep 370.63
    localized 370.61
  iris 364.42
  retina 362.16
  subretinal 362.16
Nephralgia 788.0
Nephritis, nephritic (albuminuric) (azotemic)
    (congenital) (degenerative) (diffuse)
    (disseminated) (epithelial) (familial) (focal)
    (granulomatous) (hemorrhagic) (infantile)
    (nonsuppurative, excretory) (uremic) 583.9
  with
    edema — see Nephrosis
    lesion of
      glomerulonephritis
        hypocomplementemic persistent 583.2
          with nephrotic syndrome 581.2
          chronic 582.2
        lobular 583.2
          with nephrotic syndrome 581.2
          chronic 582.2
        membranoproliferative 583.2
          with nephrotic syndrome 581.2
          chronic 582.2
        membranous 583.1
          with nephrotic syndrome 581.1
          chronic 582.1
        mesangiocapillary 583.2
          with nephrotic syndrome 581.2
          chronic 582.2
        mixed membranous and proliferative
            583.2
          with nephrotic syndrome 581.2
          chronic 582.2
        proliferative (diffuse) 583.0
          with nephrotic syndrome 581.0
          acute 580.0
          chronic 582.0
        rapidly progressive 583.4
          acute 580.4
          chronic 582.4
      interstitial nephritis (diffuse) (focal)
          583.89
        with nephrotic syndrome 581.89
        acute 580.89
        chronic 582.89
      necrotizing glomerulitis 583.4
        acute 580.4
        chronic 582.4
      renal necrosis 583.9
        cortical 583.6
        medullary 583.7
      specified pathology NEC 583.89
        with nephrotic syndrome 581.89
        acute 580.89
        chronic 582.89
    necrosis, renal 583.9
      cortical 583.6
      medullary (papillary) 583.7
    nephrotic syndrome (see also Nephrosis)
        581.9
    papillary necrosis 583.7
    specified pathology NEC 583.89
  acute 580.9
    extracapillary with epithelial crescents 580.4
    hypertensive (see also Hypertension, kidney)
        403.90
    necrotizing 580.4
    poststreptococcal 580.0
    proliferative (diffuse) 580.0
    rapidly progressive 580.4
    specified pathology NEC 580.89
  amyloid 277.3 [583.81]
    chronic 277.3 [582.81]
  arteriolar (see also Hypertension, kidney)
      403.90
  arteriosclerotic (see also Hypertension, kidney)
      403.90
  ascending (see also Pyelitis) 590.80
  atrophic 582.9

Nephritis, nephritic — continued
  basement membrane NEC 583.89
    with
      pulmonary hemorrhage (Goodpasture's
          syndrome) 446.21 [583.81]
  calculous, calculus 592.0
  cardiac (see also Hypertension, kidney) 403.90
  cardiovascular (see also Hypertension, kidney)
      403.90
  chronic 582.9
    arteriosclerotic (see also Hypertension,
        kidney) 403.90
    hypertensive (see also Hypertension, kidney)
        403.90
  cirrhotic (see also Sclerosis, renal) 587
  complicating pregnancy, childbirth, or
      puerperium 646.2 ✔5ᵗʰ
    with hypertension 642.1 ✔5ᵗʰ
      affecting fetus or newborn 760.0
      affecting fetus or newborn 760.1
  croupous 580.9
  desquamative — see Nephrosis
  due to
    amyloidosis 277.3 [583.81]
      chronic 277.3 [582.81]
    arteriosclerosis (see also Hypertension,
        kidney) 403.90
    diabetes mellitus 250.4 ✔5ᵗʰ [583.81]
      with nephrotic syndrome
          250.4 ✔5ᵗʰ [581.81]
    diphtheria 032.89 [580.81]
    gonococcal infection (acute) 098.19 [583.81]
      chronic or duration of 2 months or over
          098.39 [583.81]
    gout 274.10
    infectious hepatitis 070.9 [580.81]
    mumps 072.79 [580.81]
    specified kidney pathology NEC 583.89
      acute 580.89
      chronic 582.89
    streptotrichosis 039.8 [583.81]
    subacute bacterial endocarditis 421.0
    systemic lupus erythematosus
        710.0 [583.81]
      chronic 710.0 [582.81]
    typhoid fever 002.0 [580.81]
  endothelial 582.2
  end stage (chronic) (terminal) NEC 585
  epimembranous 581.1
  exudative 583.89
    with nephrotic syndrome 581.89
    acute 580.89
    chronic 582.89
  gonococcal (acute) 098.19 [583.81]
    chronic or duration of 2 months or over
        098.39 [583.81]
  gouty 274.10
  hereditary (Alport's syndrome) 759.89
  hydremic — see Nephrosis
  hypertensive (see also Hypertension, kidney)
      403.90
  hypocomplementemic persistent 583.2
    with nephrotic syndrome 581.2
    chronic 582.2
  immune complex NEC 583.89
  infective (see also Pyelitis) 590.80
  interstitial (diffuse) (focal) 583.89
    with nephrotic syndrome 581.89
    acute 580.89
    chronic 582.89
  latent or quiescent — see Nephritis, chronic
  lead 984.9
    specified type of lead — see Table of Drugs
        and Chemicals
  lobular 583.2
    with nephrotic syndrome 581.2
    chronic 582.2
  lupus 710.0 [583.81]
    acute 710.0 [580.81]
    chronic 710.0 [582.81]
  membranoproliferative 583.2
    with nephrotic syndrome 581.2
    chronic 582.2
  membranous 583.1
    with nephrotic syndrome 581.1
    chronic 582.1

Nephritis, nephritic — continued
  mesangiocapillary 583.2
    with nephrotic syndrome 581.2
    chronic 582.2
  minimal change 581.3
  mixed membranous and proliferative 583.2
    with nephrotic syndrome 581.2
    chronic 582.2
  necrotic, necrotizing 583.4
    acute 580.4
    chronic 582.4
  nephrotic — see Nephrosis
  old — see Nephritis, chronic
  parenchymatous 581.89
  polycystic 753.12
    adult type (APKD) 753.13
    autosomal dominant 753.13
    autosomal recessive 753.14
    childhood type (CPKD) 753.14
    infantile type 753.14
  poststreptococcal 580.0
  pregnancy — see Nephritis, complicating
      pregnancy
  proliferative (diffuse) 583.0
    with nephrotic syndrome 581.0
    acute 580.0
    chronic 582.0
  purulent (see also Pyelitis) 590.80
  rapidly progressive 583.4
    acute 580.4
    chronic 582.4
  salt-losing or salt-wasting (see also Disease,
      renal) 593.9
  saturnine 984.9
    specified type of lead — see Table of Drugs
        and Chemicals
  septic (see also Pyelitis) 590.80
  specified pathology NEC 583.89
    acute 580.89
    chronic 582.89
  staphylococcal (see also Pyelitis) 590.80
  streptotrichosis 039.8 [583.81]
  subacute (see also Nephrosis) 581.9
  suppurative (see also Pyelitis) 590.80
  syphilitic (late) 095.4
    congenital 090.5 [583.81]
    early 091.69 [583.81]
  terminal (chronic) (end-stage) NEC 585
  toxic — see Nephritis, acute
  tubal, tubular — see Nephrosis, tubular
  tuberculous (see also Tuberculosis)
      016.0 ✔5ᵗʰ [583.81]
  type II (Ellis) — see Nephrosis
  vascular — see Hypertension, kidney
  war 580.9
Nephroblastoma (M8960/3) 189.0
  epithelial (M8961/3) 189.0
  mesenchymal (M8962/3) 189.0
Nephrocalcinosis 275.49
Nephrocystitis, pustular (see also Pyelitis)
    590.80
Nephrolithiasis (congenital) (pelvis) (recurrent)
    592.0
  uric acid 274.11
Nephroma (M8960/3) 189.0
  mesoblastic (M8960/1) 236.9 ✔5ᵗʰ
Nephronephritis (see also Nephrosis) 581.9
Nephronopthisis 753.16
Nephropathy (see also Nephritis) 583.9
  with
    exudative nephritis 583.89
    interstitial nephritis (diffuse) (focal) 583.89
    medullary necrosis 583.7
    necrosis 583.9
      cortical 583.6
      medullary or papillary 583.7
    papillary necrosis 583.7
    specified lesion or cause NEC 583.89
  analgesic 583.89
    with medullary necrosis, acute 584.7
  arteriolar (see also Hypertension, kidney)
      403.90
  arteriosclerotic (see also Hypertension, kidney)
      403.90
  complicating pregnancy 646.2 ✔5ᵗʰ
  diabetic 250.4 ✔5ᵗʰ [583.81]

(vertical left margin) **Neovascularization — Nephropathy**

■4ᵗʰ Fourth-digit Required   ✔5ᵗʰ Fifth-digit Required   ►◄ Revised Text   ● New Line   ▲ Revised Code

Nephropathy (*see also* Nephritis) — *continued*
   gouty 274.10
      specified type NEC 274.19
   hypercalcemic 588.8
   hypertensive (*see also* Hypertension, kidney)
      403.90
   hypokalemic (vacuolar) 588.8
   obstructive 593.89
      congenital 753.20
   phenacetin 584.7
   phosphate-losing 588.0
   potassium depletion 588.8
   proliferative (*see also* Nephritis, proliferative)
      583.0
   protein-losing 588.8
   salt-losing or salt-wasting (*see also* Disease,
      renal) 593.9
   sickle-cell (*see also* Disease, sickle-cell)
      282.60 [583.81]
   toxic 584.5
   vasomotor 584.5
   water-losing 588.8
Nephroptosis (*see also* Disease, renal) 593.0
   congenital (displaced) 753.3
Nephropyosis (*see also* Abscess, kidney) 590.2
Nephrorrhagia 593.81
Nephrosclerosis (arteriolar) (arteriosclerotic)
   (chronic) (hyaline) (*see also* Hypertension,
   kidney) 403.90
   gouty 274.10
   hyperplastic (arteriolar) (*see also* Hypertension,
      kidney) 403.90
   senile (*see also* Sclerosis, renal) 587
Nephrosis, nephrotic (Epstein's) (syndrome)
   581.9
   with
      lesion of
         focal glomerulosclerosis 581.1
         glomerulonephritis
            endothelial 581.2
            hypocomplementemic persistent 581.2
            lobular 581.2
            membranoproliferative 581.2
            membranous 581.1
            mesangiocapillary 581.2
            minimal change 581.3
            mixed membranous and proliferative
               581.2
            proliferative 581.0
         segmental hyalinosis 581.1
         specified pathology NEC 581.89
   acute — *see* Nephrosis, tubular
   anoxic — *see* Nephrosis, tubular
   arteriosclerotic (*see also* Hypertension, kidney)
      403.90
   chemical — *see* Nephrosis, tubular
   cholemic 572.4
   complicating pregnancy, childbirth, or
      puerperium — *see* Nephritis,
      complicating pregnancy
   diabetic 250.4 ✓5ᵗʰ [581.81]
   hemoglobinuric — *see* Nephrosis, tubular
   in
      amyloidosis 277.3 [581.81]
      diabetes mellitus 250.4 ✓5ᵗʰ [581.81]
      epidemic hemorrhagic fever 078.6
      malaria 084.9 [581.81]
      polyarteritis 446.0 [581.81]
      systemic lupus erythematosus
         710.0 [581.81]
   ischemic — *see* Nephrosis, tubular
   lipoid 581.3
   lower nephron — *see* Nephrosis, tubular
   lupoid 710.0 [581.81]
   lupus 710.0 [581.81]
   malarial 084.9 [581.81]
   minimal change 581.3
   necrotizing — *see* Nephrosis, tubular
   osmotic (sucrose) 588.8
   polyarteritic 446.0 [581.81]
   radiation 581.9
   specified lesion or cause NEC 581.89
   syphilitic 095.4
   toxic — *see* Nephrosis, tubular

Nephrosis, nephrotic — *continued*
   tubular (acute) 584.5
      due to a procedure 997.5
      radiation 581.9
Nephrosonephritis hemorrhagic (endemic) 078.6
Nephrostomy status V44.6
   with complication 997.5
Nerve — *see* condition
Nerves 799.2
Nervous (*see also* condition) 799.2
   breakdown 300.9
   heart 306.2
   stomach 306.4
   tension 799.2
Nervousness 799.2
Nesidioblastoma (M8150/0)
   pancreas 211.7
   specified site NEC — *see* Neoplasm, by site,
      benign
   unspecified site 211.7
Netherton's syndrome (ichthyosiform
   erythroderma) 757.1
Nettle rash 708.8
Nettleship's disease (urticaria pigmentosa)
   757.33
Neumann's disease (pemphigus vegetans) 694.4
Neuralgia, neuralgic (acute) (*see also* Neuritis)
   729.2
   accessory (nerve) 352.4
   acoustic (nerve) 388.5
   ankle 355.8
   anterior crural 355.8
   anus 787.99
   arm 723.4
   auditory (nerve) 388.5
   axilla 353.0
   bladder 788.1
   brachial 723.4
   brain — *see* Disorder, nerve, cranial
   broad ligament 625.9
   cerebral — *see* Disorder, nerve, cranial
   ciliary 346.2 ✓5ᵗʰ
   cranial nerve — *see also* Disorder, nerve,
      cranial
      fifth or trigeminal (*see also* Neuralgia,
         trigeminal) 350.1
   ear 388.71
      middle 352.1
   facial 351.8
   finger 354.9
   flank 355.8
   foot 355.8
   forearm 354.9
   Fothergill's (*see also* Neuralgia, trigeminal)
      350.1
      postherpetic 053.12
   glossopharyngeal (nerve) 352.1
   groin 355.8
   hand 354.9
   heel 355.8
   Horton's 346.2 ✓5ᵗʰ
   Hunt's 053.11
   hypoglossal (nerve) 352.5
   iliac region 355.8
   infraorbital (*see also* Neuralgia, trigeminal)
      350.1
   inguinal 355.8
   intercostal (nerve) 353.8
      postherpetic 053.19
   jaw 352.1
   kidney 788.0
   knee 355.8
   loin 355.8
   malarial (*see also* Malaria) 084.6
   mastoid 385.89
   maxilla 352.1
   median thenar 354.1
   metatarsal 355.6
   middle ear 352.1
   migrainous 346.2 ✓5ᵗʰ
   Morton's 355.6
   nerve, cranial — *see* Disorder, nerve, cranial
   nose 352.0
   occipital 723.8

Neuralgia, neuralgic (*see also* Neuritis) —
      continued
   ophthalmic 377.30
      postherpetic 053.19
   optic (nerve) 377.30
   penis 607.9
   perineum 355.8
   pleura 511.0
   postherpetic NEC 053.19
      geniculate ganglion 053.11
      ophthalmic 053.19
      trifacial 053.12
      trigeminal 053.12
   pubic region 355.8
   radial (nerve) 723.4
   rectum 787.99
   sacroiliac joint 724.3
   sciatic (nerve) 724.3
   scrotum 608.9
   seminal vesicle 608.9
   shoulder 354.9
   Sluder's 337.0
   specified nerve NEC — *see* Disorder, nerve
   spermatic cord 608.9
   sphenopalatine (ganglion) 337.0
   subscapular (nerve) 723.4
   suprascapular (nerve) 723.4
   testis 608.89
   thenar (median) 354.1
   thigh 355.8
   tongue 352.5
   trifacial (nerve) (*see also* Neuralgia, trigeminal)
      350.1
   trigeminal (nerve) 350.1
      postherpetic 053.12
   tympanic plexus 388.71
   ulnar (nerve) 723.4
   vagus (nerve) 352.3
   wrist 354.9
   writers' 300.89
      organic 333.84
Neurapraxia — *see* Injury, nerve, by site
Neurasthenia 300.5
   cardiac 306.2
   gastric 306.4
   heart 306.2
   postfebrile 780.79
   postviral 780.79
Neurilemmoma (M9560/0) — *see also* Neoplasm,
      connective tissue, benign
   acoustic (nerve) 225.1
   malignant (M9560/3) — *see also* Neoplasm,
      connective tissue, malignant
   acoustic (nerve) 192.0
Neurilemmosarcoma (M9560/3) — *see* Neoplasm,
      connective tissue, malignant
Neurilemoma — *see* Neurilemmoma
Neurinoma (M9560/0) — *see* Neurilemmoma
Neurinomatosis (M9560/1) — *see also* Neoplasm,
      connective tissue, uncertain behavior
   centralis 759.5
Neuritis (*see also* Neuralgia) 729.2
   abducens (nerve) 378.54
   accessory (nerve) 352.4
   acoustic (nerve) 388.5
      syphilitic 094.86
   alcoholic 357.5
      with psychosis 291.1
   amyloid, any site 277.3 [357.4]
   anterior crural 355.8
   arising during pregnancy 646.4 ✓5ᵗʰ
   arm 723.4
   ascending 355.2
   auditory (nerve) 388.5
   brachial (nerve) NEC 723.4
      due to displacement, intervertebral disc
         722.0
   cervical 723.4
   chest (wall) 353.8
   costal region 353.8
   cranial nerve — *see also* Disorder, nerve,
      cranial
      first or olfactory 352.0
      second or optic 377.30
      third or oculomotor 378.52
      fourth or trochlear 378.53

Neuritis (*see also* Neuralgia) — *continued*
  cranial nerve — *see also* Disorder, nerve,
      cranial — *continued*
    fifth or trigeminal (*see also* Neuralgia,
        trigeminal) 350.1
    sixth or abducens 378.54
    seventh or facial 351.8
      newborn 767.5
    eighth or acoustic 388.5
    ninth or glossopharyngeal 352.1
    tenth or vagus 352.3
    eleventh or accessory 352.4
    twelfth or hypoglossal 352.5
  Déjérine-Sottas 356.0
  diabetic 250.6 ✓5ᵗʰ *[357.2]*
  diphtheritic 032.89 *[357.4]*
  due to
    beriberi 265.0 *[357.4]*
    displacement, prolapse, protrusion, or
        rupture of intervertebral disc 722.2
      cervical 722.0
      lumbar, lumbosacral 722.10
      thoracic, thoracolumbar 722.11
    herniation, nucleus pulposus 722.2
      cervical 722.0
      lumbar, lumbosacral 722.10
      thoracic, thoracolumbar 722.11
  endemic 265.0 *[357.4]*
  facial (nerve) 351.8
    newborn 767.5
  general — *see* Polyneuropathy
  geniculate ganglion 351.1
    due to herpes 053.11
  glossopharyngeal (nerve) 352.1
  gouty 274.89 *[357.4]*
  hypoglossal (nerve) 352.5
  ilioinguinal (nerve) 355.8
  in diseases classified elsewhere — *see*
      Polyneuropathy, in
  infectious (multiple) 357.0
  intercostal (nerve) 353.8
  interstitial hypertrophic progressive NEC 356.9
  leg 355.8
  lumbosacral NEC 724.4
  median (nerve) 354.1
    thenar 354.1
  multiple (acute) (infective) 356.9
    endemic 265.0 *[357.4]*
  multiplex endemica 265.0 *[357.4]*
  nerve root (*see also* Radiculitis) 729.2
  oculomotor (nerve) 378.52
  olfactory (nerve) 352.0
  optic (nerve) 377.30
    in myelitis 341.0
    meningococcal 036.81
  pelvic 355.8
  peripheral (nerve) — *see also* Neuropathy,
      peripheral
    complicating pregnancy or puerperium
        646.4 ✓5ᵗʰ
    specified nerve NEC — *see* Mononeuritis
  pneumogastric (nerve) 352.3
  postchickenpox 052.7
  postherpetic 053.19
  progressive hypertrophic interstitial NEC 356.9
  puerperal, postpartum 646.4 ✓5ᵗʰ
  radial (nerve) 723.4
  retrobulbar 377.32
    syphilitic 094.85
  rheumatic (chronic) 729.2
  sacral region 355.8
  sciatic (nerve) 724.3
    due to displacement of intervertebral disc
        722.10
  serum 999.5
  specified nerve NEC — *see* Disorder, nerve
  spinal (nerve) 355.9
    root (*see also* Radiculitis) 729.2
  subscapular (nerve) 723.4
  suprascapular (nerve) 723.4
  syphilitic 095.8
  thenar (median) 354.1
  thoracic NEC 724.4
  toxic NEC 357.7
  trochlear (nerve) 378.53
  ulnar (nerve) 723.4
  vagus (nerve) 352.3

Neuroangiomatosis, encephalofacial 759.6
Neuroastrocytoma (M9505/1) — *see* Neoplasm,
    by site, uncertain behavior
Neuro-avitaminosis 269.2
Neuroblastoma (M9500/3)
  olfactory (M9522/3) 160.0
  specified site — *see* Neoplasm, by site,
      malignant
  unspecified site 194.0
Neurochorioretinitis (*see also* Chorioretinitis)
    363.20
Neurocirculatory asthenia 306.2
Neurocytoma (M9506/0) — *see* Neoplasm, by
    site, benign
Neurodermatitis (circumscribed) (circumscripta)
    (local) 698.3
  atopic 691.8
  diffuse (Brocq) 691.8
  disseminated 691.8
  nodulosa 698.3
Neuroencephalomyelopathy, optic 341.0
Neuroepithelioma (M9503/3) — *see also*
    Neoplasm, by site, malignant
  olfactory (M9521/3) 160.0
Neurofibroma (M9540/0) — *see also* Neoplasm,
    connective tissue, benign
  melanotic (M9541/0) — *see* Neoplasm,
      connective tissue, benign
  multiple (M9540/1) 237.70
    type 1 237.71
    type 2 237.72
  plexiform (M9550/0) — *see* Neoplasm,
      connective tissue, benign
Neurofibromatosis (multiple) (M9540/1) 237.70
  acoustic 237.72
  malignant (M9540/3) — *see* Neoplasm,
      connective tissue, malignant
  type 1 237.71
  type 2 237.72
  von Recklinghausen's 237.71
Neurofibrosarcoma (M9540/3) — *see* Neoplasm,
    connective tissue, malignant
Neurogenic — *see also* condition
  bladder (atonic) (automatic) (autonomic)
      (flaccid) (hypertonic) (hypotonic) (inertia)
      (infranuclear) (irritable) (motor)
      (nonreflex) (nuclear) (paralysis) (reflex)
      (sensory) (spastic) (supranuclear)
      (uninhibited) 596.54
    with cauda equina syndrome 344.61
  bowel 564.81
  heart 306.2
Neuroglioma (M9505/1) — *see* Neoplasm, by site,
    uncertain behavior
Neurolabyrinthitis (of Dix and Hallpike) 386.12
Neurolathyrism 988.2
Neuroleprosy 030.1
Neuroleptic malignant syndrome 333.92
Neurolipomatosis 272.8
Neuroma (M9570/0) — *see also* Neoplasm,
    connective tissue, benign
  acoustic (nerve) (M9560/0) 225.1
  amputation (traumatic) — *see also* Injury,
      nerve, by site
    surgical complication (late) 997.61
  appendix 211.3
  auditory nerve 225.1
  digital 355.6
    toe 355.6
  interdigital (toe) 355.6
  intermetatarsal 355.6
  Morton's 355.6
  multiple 237.70
    type 1 237.71
    type 2 237.72
  nonneoplastic 355.9
    arm NEC 354.9
    leg NEC 355.8
    lower extremity NEC 355.8
    specified site NEC — *see* Mononeuritis, by
        site
    upper extremity NEC 354.9
  optic (nerve) 225.1
  plantar 355.6

Neuroma — *see also* Neoplasm, connective tissue,
    benign — *continued*
  plexiform (M9550/0) — *see* Neoplasm,
      connective tissue, benign
  surgical (nonneoplastic) 355.9
    arm NEC 354.9
    leg NEC 355.8
    lower extremity NEC 355.8
    upper extremity NEC 354.9
  traumatic — *see also* Injury, nerve, by site
  old — *see* Neuroma, nonneoplastic
Neuromyalgia 729.1
Neuromyasthenia (epidemic) 049.8
Neuromyelitis 341.8
  ascending 357.0
  optica 341.0
Neuromyopathy NEC 358.9
Neuromyositis 729.1
Neuronevus (M8725/0) — *see* Neoplasm, skin,
    benign
Neuronitis 357.0
  ascending (acute) 355.2
  vestibular 386.12
Neuroparalytic — *see* condition
Neuropathy, neuropathic (*see also* Disorder,
    nerve) 355.9
  acute motor 357.82 ●
  alcoholic 357.5
    with psychosis 291.1
  arm NEC 354.9
  autonomic (peripheral) — *see* Neuropathy,
      peripheral, autonomic
  axillary nerve 353.0
  brachial plexus 353.0
  cervical plexus 353.2
  chronic
    progressive segmentally demyelinating
        357.89 ▲
    relapsing demyelinating 357.89 ▲
  congenital sensory 356.2
  Déjérine-Sottas 356.0
  diabetic 250.6 ✓5ᵗʰ *[357.2]*
  entrapment 355.9
    iliohypogastric nerve 355.79
    ilioinguinal nerve 355.79
    lateral cutaneous nerve of thigh 355.1
    median nerve 354.0
    obturator nerve 355.79
    peroneal nerve 355.3
    posterior tibial nerve 355.5
    saphenous nerve 355.79
    ulnar nerve 354.2
  facial nerve 351.9
  hereditary 356.9
    peripheral 356.0
    sensory (radicular) 356.2
  hypertrophic
    Charcôt-Marie-Tooth 356.1
    Déjérine-Sottas 356.0
    interstitial 356.9
    Refsum 356.3
  intercostal nerve 354.8
  ischemic — *see* Disorder, nerve
  Jamaican (ginger) 357.7
  leg NEC 355.8
  lower extremity NEC 355.8
  lumbar plexus 353.1
  median nerve 354.1
  motor ●
    acute 357.82 ●
  multiple (acute) (chronic) (*see also*
      Polyneuropathy) 356.9
  optic 377.39
    ischemic 377.41
    nutritional 377.33
    toxic 377.34
  peripheral (nerve) (*see also* Polyneuropathy)
      356.9
    arm NEC 354.9
    autonomic 337.9
      amyloid 277.3 *[337.1]*
      idiopathic 337.0
      in
        amyloidosis 277.3 *[337.1]*
        diabetes (mellitus) 250.6 ✓5ᵗʰ *[337.1]*
        diseases classified elsewhere 337.1

Neuropathy, neuropathic (see also Disorder, nerve) — continued
  nerve) — continued
  peripheral (see also Polyneuropathy) —
      continued
    autonomic — continued
      in — continued
        gout 274.89 [337.1]
        hyperthyroidism 242.9 ✔5ᵗʰ [337.1]
    due to
      antitetanus scrum 357.6
      arsenic 357.7
      drugs 357.6
      lead 357.7
      organophosphate compounds 357.7
      toxic agent NEC 357.7
    hereditary 356.0
    idiopathic 356.9
      progresive 356.4
      specified type NEC 356.8
    in diseases classified elsewhere — see
        Polyneuropathy, in
    leg NEC 355.8
    lower extremity NEC 355.8
    upper extremity NEC 354.9
  plantar nerves 355.6
  progressive hypertrophic interstitial 356.9
  radicular NEC 729.2
    brachial 723.4
    cervical NEC 723.4
    hereditary sensory 356.2
    lumbar 724.4
    lumbosacral 724.4
    thoracic NEC 724.4
  sacral plexus 353.1
  sciatic 355.0
  spinal nerve NEC 355.9
    root (see also Radiculitis) 729.2
  toxic 357.7
  trigeminal sensory 350.8
  ulnar nerve 354.2
  upper extremity NEC 354.9
  uremic 585 [357.4]
  vitamin B₁₂ 266.2 [357.4]
    with anemia (pernicious) 281.0 [357.4]
      due to dietary deficiency 281.1 [357.4]

Neurophthisis — (see also Disorder, nerve
    peripheral) 356.9
  diabetic 250.6 ✔5ᵗʰ [357.2]

Neuropraxia — see Injury, nerve

Neuroretinitis 363.05
  syphilitic 094.85

Neurosarcoma (M9540/3) — see Neoplasm,
    connective tissue, malignant

Neurosclerosis — see Disorder, nerve

Neurosis, neurotic 300.9
  accident 300.16
  anancastic, anankastic 300.3
  anxiety (state) 300.00
    generalized 300.02
    panic type 300.01
  asthenic 300.5
  bladder 306.53
  cardiac (reflex) 306.2
  cardiovascular 306.2
  climacteric, unspecified type 627.2
  colon 306.4
  compensation 300.16
  compulsive, compulsion 300.3
  conversion 300.11
  craft 300.89
  cutaneous 306.3
  depersonalization 300.6
  depressive (reaction) (type) 300.4
  endocrine 306.6
  environmental 300.89
  fatigue 300.5
  functional (see also Disorder, psychosomatic)
      306.9
  gastric 306.4
  gastrointestinal 306.4
  genitourinary 306.50
  heart 306.2
  hypochondriacal 300.7
  hysterical 300.10
    conversion type 300.11
    dissociative type 300.15

Neurosis, neurotic — continued
  impulsive 300.3
  incoordination 306.0
    larynx 306.1
    vocal cord 306.1
  intestine 306.4
  larynx 306.1
    hysterical 300.11
    sensory 306.1
  menopause, unspecified type 627.2
  mixed NEC 300.89
  musculoskeletal 306.0
  obsessional 300.3
    phobia 300.3
  obsessive-compulsive 300.3
  occupational 300.89
  ocular 306.7
  oral 307.0
  organ (see also Disorder, psychosomatic) 306.9
  pharynx 306.1
  phobic 300.20
  posttraumatic (acute) (situational) 308.3
    chronic 309.81
  psychasthenic (type) 300.89
  railroad 300.16
  rectum 306.4
  respiratory 306.1
  rumination 306.4
  senile 300.89
  sexual 302.70
  situational 300.89
  specified type NEC 300.89
  state 300.9
    with depersonalization episode 300.6
  stomach 306.4
  vasomotor 306.2
  visceral 306.4
  war 300.16

Neurospongioblastosis diffusa 759.5

Neurosyphilis (arrested) (early) (inactive) (late)
    (latent) (recurrent) 094.9
  with ataxia (cerebellar) (locomotor) (spastic)
      (spinal) 094.0
  acute meningitis 094.2
  aneurysm 094.89
  arachnoid (adhesive) 094.2
  arteritis (any artery) 094.89
  asymptomatic 094.3
  congenital 090.40
  dura (mater) 094.89
  general paresis 094.1
  gumma 094.9
  hemorrhagic 094.9
  juvenile (asymptomatic) (meningeal) 090.40
  leptomeninges (aseptic) 094.2
  meningeal 094.2
  meninges (adhesive) 094.2
  meningovascular (diffuse) 094.2
  optic atrophy 094.84
  parenchymatous (degenerative) 094.1
  paresis (see also Paresis, general) 094.1
  paretic (see also Paresis, general) 094.1
  relapse 094.9
  remission in (sustained) 094.9
  serological 094.3
  specified nature or site NEC 094.89
  tabes (dorsalis) 094.0
    juvenile 090.40
  tabetic 094.0
    juvenile 090.40
  taboparesis 094.1
    juvenile 090.40
  thrombosis 094.89
  vascular 094.89

Neurotic (see also Neurosis) 300.9
  excoriation 698.4
    psychogenic 306.3

Neurotmesis — see Injury, nerve, by site

Neurotoxemia — see Toxemia

Neutroclusion 524.2

Neutropenia, neutropenic (chronic) (cyclic) (drug-
    induced) (genetic) (idiopathic) (immune)
    (infantile) (malignant) (periodic) (pernicious)
    (primary) (splenic) (splenomegaly) (toxic)
    288.0
  chronic hypoplastic 288.0

Neutropenia, neutropenic — continued
  congenital (nontransient) 288.0
  fever 288.0
  neonatal, transitory (isoimmune) (maternal
      transfer) 776.7

Neutrophilia, hereditary giant 288.2

Nevocarcinoma (M8720/3) — see Melanoma

Nevus (M8720/0) — see also Neoplasm, skin,
    benign

> Note — Except where otherwise indicated,
> varieties of nevus in the list below that are
> followed by a morphology code number (M----
> /0) should be coded by site as for
> "Neoplasm, skin, benign."

  acanthotic 702.8
  achromic (M8730/0)
  amelanotic (M8730/0)
  anemic, anemicus 709.09
  angiomatous (M9120/0) (see also Hemangioma)
      228.00
  araneus 448.1
  avasculosus 709.09
  balloon cell (M8722/0)
  bathing trunk (M8761/1) 238.2
  blue (M8780/0)
    cellular (M8790/0)
    giant (M8790/0)
    Jadassohn's (M8780/0)
    malignant (M8780/3) — see Melanoma
  capillary (M9131/0) (see also Hemangioma)
      228.00
  cavernous (M9121/0) (see also Hemangioma)
      228.00
  cellular (M8720/0)
    blue (M8790/0)
  comedonicus 757.33
  compound (M8760/0)
  conjunctiva (M8720/0) 224.3
  dermal (M8750/0)
    and epidermal (M8760/0)
  epithelioid cell (and spindle cell) (M8770/0)
  flammeus 757.32
    osteohypertrophic 759.89
  hairy (M8720/0)
  halo (M8723/0)
  hemangiomatous (M9120/0) (see also
      Hemangioma) 228.00
  intradermal (M8750/0)
  intraepidermal (M8740/0)
  involuting (M8724/0)
  Jadassohn's (blue) (M8780/0)
  junction, junctional (M8740/0)
    malignant melanoma in (M8740/3) — see
        Melanoma
  juvenile (M8770/0)
  lymphatic (M9170/0) 228.1
  magnocellular (M8726/0)
    specified site — see Neoplasm, by site,
        benign
    unspecified site 224.0
  malignant (M8720/3) — see Melanoma
  meaning hemangioma (M9120/0) (see also
      Hemangioma) 228.00
  melanotic (pigmented) (M8720/0)
  multiplex 759.5
  nonneoplastic 448.1
  nonpigmented (M8730/0)
  nonvascular (M8720/0)
  oral mucosa, white sponge 750.26
  osteohypertrophic, flammeus 759.89
  papillaris (M8720/0)
  papillomatosus (M8720/0)
  pigmented (M8720/0)
    giant (M8761/1) — see also Neoplasm, skin,
        uncertain behavior
    malignant melanoma in (M8761/3) — see
        Melanoma
    systematicus 757.33
  pilosus (M8720/0)
  port wine 757.32
  sanguineous 757.32
  sebaceous (senile) 702.8
  senile 448.1
  spider 448.1
  spindle cell (and epithelioid cell) (M8770/0)

Neuropathy — Nevus

Nevus — Normoblastosis

Normocytic anemia (infectional) 285.9
  due to blood loss (chronic) 280.0
    acute 285.1
Norrie's disease (congenital) (progressive
  oculoacousticocerebral degeneration) 743.8
North American blastomycosis 116.0
Norwegian itch 133.0
Nose, nasal — *see* condition
Nosebleed 784.7
Nosomania 298.9
Nosophobia 300.29
Nostalgia 309.89
Notch of iris 743.46
Notched lip, congenital (*see also* Cleft, lip)
  749.10
Notching nose, congenital (tip) 748.1
Nothnagel's
  syndrome 378.52
  vasomotor acroparesthesia 443.89
Novy's relapsing fever (American) 087.1
Noxious
  foodstuffs, poisoning by
    fish 988.0
    fungi 988.1
    mushrooms 988.1
    plants (food) 988.2
    shellfish 988.0
    specified type NEC 988.8
    toadstool 988.1
  substances transmitted through placenta or
    breast milk 760.70
    alcohol 760.71
    anti-infective agents 760.74
    cocaine 760.75
    "crack" 760.75
    diethylstilbestrol (DES) 760.76
    hallucinogenic agents NEC 760.73
    medicinal agents NEC 760.79
    narcotics 760.72
    obstetric anesthetic or analgesic 763.5
    specified agent NEC 760.79
    suspected, affecting management of
      pregnancy 655.5 ✓5ᵗʰ
Nuchal hitch (arm) 652.8 ✓5ᵗʰ
Nucleus pulposus — *see* condition
Numbness 782.0
Nuns' knee 727.2
Nursemaid's
  elbow 832.0 ✓5ᵗʰ
  shoulder 831.0 ✓5ᵗʰ
Nutmeg liver 573.8
Nutrition, deficient or insufficient (particular
  kind of food) 269.9
  due to
    insufficient food 994.2
    lack of
      care (child) (infant) 995.52
        adult 995.84
      food 994.2
Nyctalopia (*see also* Blindness, night) 368.60
  vitamin A deficiency 264.5
Nycturia 788.43
  psychogenic 306.53
Nymphomania 302.89
Nystagmus 379.50
  associated with vestibular system disorders
    379.54
  benign paroxysmal positional 386.11
  central positional 386.2
  congenital 379.51
  deprivation 379.53
  dissociated 379.55
  latent 379.52
  miners' 300.89
  positional
    benign paroxysmal 386.11
    central 386.2
  specified NEC 379.56
  vestibular 379.54
  visual deprivation 379.53

✓4ᵗʰ Fourth-digit Required   ✓5ᵗʰ Fifth-digit Required   ▶◀ Revised Text   ● New Line   ▲ Revised Code

O

Oasthouse urine disease 270.2
Obermeyer's relapsing fever (European) 087.0
Obesity (constitutional) (exogenous) (familial)
  (nutritional) (simple) 278.00
  adrenal 255.8
  due to hyperalimentation 278.00
  endocrine NEC 259.9
  endogenous 259.9
  Fröhlich's (adiposogenital dystrophy) 253.8
  glandular NEC 259.9
  hypothyroid (see also Hypothyroidism) 244.9
  morbid 278.01
  of pregnancy 646.1
  pituitary 253.8
  thyroid (see also Hypothyroidism) 244.9
Oblique — see also condition
  lie before labor, affecting fetus or newborn
    761.7
Obliquity, pelvis 738.6
Obliteration
  abdominal aorta 446.7
  appendix (lumen) 543.9
  artery 447.1
  ascending aorta 446.7
  bile ducts 576.8
    with calculus, choledocholithiasis, or stones
      — see Choledocholithiasis
    congenital 751.61
      jaundice from 751.61 [774.5]
  common duct 576.8
    with calculus, choledocholithiasis, or stones
      — see Choledocholithiasis
    congenital 751.61
  cystic duct 575.8
    with calculus, choledocholithiasis, or stones
      — see Choledocholithiasis
  disease, arteriolar 447.1
  endometrium 621.8
  eye, anterior chamber 360.34
  fallopian tube 628.2
  lymphatic vessel 457.1
    postmastectomy 457.0
  organ or site, congenital NEC — see Atresia
  placental blood vessels — see Placenta,
    abnormal
  supra-aortic branches 446.7
  ureter 593.89
  urethra 599.84
  vein 459.9
  vestibule (oral) 525.8
Observation (for) V71.9
  without need for further medical care V71.9
  accident NEC V71.4
    at work V71.3
  criminal V71.6
  deleterious agent ingestion V71.89
  disease V71.9
    cardiovascular V71.7
    heart V71.7
    mental V71.09
    specified condition NEC V71.89
  foreign body ingestion V71.89
  growth and development variations V21.8
  injuries (accidental) V71.4
    inflicted NEC V71.6
      during alleged rape or seduction V71.5
  malignant neoplasm, suspected V71.1
  postpartum
    immediately after delivery V24.0
    routine follow-up V24.2
  pregnancy
    high-risk V23.9
      specified problem NEC V23.8
    normal (without complication) V22.1
      with nonobstetric complication V22.2
      first V22.0
  rape or seduction, alleged V71.5
    injury during V71.5
  suicide attempt, alleged V71.89
  suspected (undiagnosed) (unproven)
    abuse V71.81
    cardiovascular disease V71.7
    child or wife battering victim V71.6
    concussion (cerebral) V71.6

Observation — continued
  suspected — continued
    condition NEC V71.89
      infant — see Observation, suspected,
        condition, newborn
      newborn V29.9
        cardiovascular disease V29.8
        congenital anomaly V29.8
        genetic V29.3
        infectious V29.0
        ingestion foreign object V29.8
        injury V29.8
        metabolic V29.3
        neoplasm V29.8
        neurological V29.1
        poison, poisoning V29.8
        respiratory V29.2
        specified NEC V29.8
    exposure ●
      anthrax V71.82 ●
      biologic agent NEC V71.83 ●
    infectious disease not requiring isolation
      V71.89
    malignant neoplasm V71.1
    mental disorder V71.09
    neglect V71.81
    neoplasm
      benign V71.89
      malignant V71.1
    specified condition NEC V71.89
    tuberculosis V71.2
  tuberculosis, suspected V71.2
Obsession, obsessional 300.3
  ideas and mental images 300.3
  impulses 300.3
  neurosis 300.3
  phobia 300.3
  psychasthenia 300.3
  ruminations 300.3
  state 300.3
  syndrome 300.3
Obsessive-compulsive 300.3
  neurosis 300.3
  reaction 300.3
Obstetrical trauma NEC (complicating delivery)
  665.9
  with
    abortion — see Abortion, by type, with
      damage to pelvic organs
    ectopic pregnancy (see also categories
      633.0-633.9) 639.2
    molar pregnancy (see also categories 630-
      632) 639.2
  affecting fetus or newborn 763.89
  following
    abortion 639.2
    ectopic or molar pregnancy 639.2
Obstipation (see also Constipation) 564.00
  psychogenic 306.4
Obstruction, obstructed, obstructive
  airway NEC 519.8
    with
      allergic alveolitis NEC 495.9
      asthma NEC (see also Asthma) 493.9
      bronchiectasis 494.0
        with acute exacerbation 494.1
      bronchitis (chronic) (see also Bronchitis,
        with, obstruction) 491.20
      emphysema NEC 492.8
    chronic 496
      with
        allergic alveolitis NEC 495.5
        asthma NEC (see also Asthma)
          493.2
        bronchiectasis 494.0
          with acute exacerbation 494.1
        bronchitis (chronic) (see also
          Bronchitis, with, obstruction)
          491.20
        emphysema NEC 492.8
    due to
      bronchospasm 519.1
      foreign body 934.9
      inhalation of fumes or vapors 506.9
      laryngospasm 478.75

Obstruction, obstructed, obstructive —
  continued
  alimentary canal (see also Obstruction,
    intestine) 560.9
  ampulla of Vater 576.2
    with calculus, cholelithiasis, or stones — see
      Choledocholithiasis
  aortic (heart) (valve) (see also Stenosis, aortic)
    424.1
    rheumatic (see also Stenosis, aortic,
      rheumatic) 395.0
  aortoiliac 444.0
  aqueduct of Sylvius 331.4
    congenital 742.3
      with spina bifida (see also Spina bifida)
        741.0
  Arnold-Chiari (see also Spina bifida) 741.0
  artery (see also Embolism, artery) 444.9
    basilar (complete) (partial) (see also
      Occlusion, artery, basilar) 433.0
    carotid (complete) (partial) (see also
      Occlusion, artery, carotid) 433.1
    precerebral — see Occlusion, artery,
      precerebral NEC
    retinal (central) (see also Occlusion, retina)
      362.30
    vertebral (complete) (partial) (see also
      Occlusion, artery, vertebral) 433.2
  asthma (chronic) (with obstructive pulmonary
    disease) 493.2
  band (intestinal) 560.81
  bile duct or passage (see also Obstruction,
    biliary) 576.2
    congenital 751.61
      jaundice from 751.61 [774.5]
  biliary (duct) (tract) 576.2
    with calculus 574.51
      with cholecystitis (chronic) 574.41
        acute 574.31
    congenital 751.61
      jaundice from 751.61 [774.5]
    gallbladder 575.2
      with calculus 574.21
        with cholecystitis (chronic) 574.11
          acute 574.01
  bladder neck (acquired) 596.0
    congenital 753.6
  bowel (see also Obstruction, intestine) 560.9
  bronchus 519.1
  canal, ear (see also Stricture, ear canal,
    acquired) 380.50
  cardia 537.89
  caval veins (inferior) (superior) 459.2
  cecum (see also Obstruction, intestine) 560.9
  circulatory 459.9
  colon (see also Obstruction, intestine) 560.9
    sympathicotonic 560.89
  common duct (see also Obstruction, biliary)
    576.2
    congenital 751.61
  coronary (artery) (heart) — see also
    Arteriosclerosis, coronary
    acute (see also Infarct, myocardium)
      410.9
      without myocardial infarction 411.81
  cystic duct (see also Obstruction, gallbladder)
    575.2
    congenital 751.61
  device, implant, or graft — see Complications,
    due to (presence of) any device, implant,
    or graft classified to 996.0-996.5 NEC
  due to foreign body accidentally left in
    operation wound 998.4
  duodenum 537.3
    congenital 751.1
    due to
      compression NEC 537.3
      cyst 537.3
      intrinsic lesion or disease NEC 537.3
      scarring 537.3
      torsion 537.3
      ulcer 532.91
      volvulus 537.3
  ejaculatory duct 608.89
  endocardium 424.90
    arteriosclerotic 424.99
      specified cause, except rheumatic 424.99

Obstruction, obstructed, obstructive —
continued
  esophagus 530.3
  eustachian tube (complete) (partial) 381.60
    cartilaginous
      extrinsic 381.63
      intrinsic 381.62
    due to
      cholesteatoma 381.61
      osseous lesion NEC 381.61
      polyp 381.61
    osseous 381.61
  fallopian tube (bilateral) 628.2
  fecal 560.39
    with hernia — *see also* Hernia, by site, with
      obstruction
      gangrenous — *see* Hernia, by site, with
        gangrene
  foramen of Monro (congenital) 742.3
    with spina bifida (*see also* Spina bifida)
      741.0 ✓5ᵗʰ
  foreign body — *see* Foreign body
  gallbladder 575.2
    with calculus, cholelithiasis, or stones
      574.21
      with cholecystitis (chronic) 574.11
        acute 574.01
    congenital 751.69
      jaundice from 751.69 [774.5]
  gastric outlet 537.0
  gastrointestinal (*see also* Obstruction,
    intestine) 560.9
  glottis 478.79
  hepatic 573.8
    duct (*see also* Obstruction, biliary) 576.2
      congenital 751.61
  icterus (*see also* Obstruction, biliary) 576.8
    congenital 751.61
  ileocecal coil (*see also* Obstruction, intestine)
    560.9
  ileum (*see also* Obstruction, intestine) 560.9
  iliofemoral (artery) 444.81
  internal anastomosis — *see* Complications,
    mechanical, graft
  intestine (mechanical) (neurogenic)
    (paroxysmal) (postinfectional) (reflex)
    560.9
    with
      adhesions (intestinal) (peritoneal) 560.81
      hernia — *see also* Hernia, by site, with
        obstruction
        gangrenous — *see* Hernia, by site,
          with gangrene
    adynamic (*see also* Ileus) 560.1
    by gallstone 560.31
    congenital or infantile (small) 751.1
      large 751.2
    due to
      Ascaris lumbricoides 127.0
      mural thickening 560.89
      procedure 997.4
        involving urinary tract 997.5
    impaction 560.39
    infantile — *see* Obstruction, intestine,
      congenital
    newborn
      due to
        fecaliths 777.1
        inspissated milk 777.2
        meconium (plug) 777.1
          in mucoviscidosis 277.01
      transitory 777.4
    specified cause NEC 560.89
    transitory, newborn 777.4
    volvulus 560.2
  intracardiac ball valve prosthesis 996.02
  jaundice (*see also* Obstruction, biliary) 576.8
    congenital 751.61
  jejunum (*see also* Obstruction, intestine) 560.9
  kidney 593.89
  labor 660.9 ✓5ᵗʰ
    affecting fetus or newborn 763.1
    by
      bony pelvis (conditions classifiable to
        653.0-653.9) 660.1 ✓5ᵗʰ
      deep transverse arrest 660.3 ✓5ᵗʰ
      impacted shoulder 660.4 ✓5ᵗʰ

Obstruction, obstructed, obstructive —
continued
  labor — *continued*
    by — *continued*
      locked twins 660.5 ✓5ᵗʰ
      malposition (fetus) (conditions classifiable
        to 652.0-652.9) 660.0 ✓5ᵗʰ
        head during labor 660.3 ✓5ᵗʰ
      persistent occipitoposterior position
        660.3 ✓5ᵗʰ
      soft tissue, pelvic (conditions classifiable
        to 654.0-654.9) 660.2 ✓5ᵗʰ
  lacrimal
    canaliculi 375.53
    congenital 743.65
    punctum 375.52
    sac 375.54
  lacrimonasal duct 375.56
    congenital 743.65
    neonatal 375.55
  lacteal, with steatorrhea 579.2
  laryngitis (*see also* Laryngitis) 464.01
  larynx 478.79
    congenital 748.3
  liver 573.8
    cirrhotic (*see also* Cirrhosis, liver) 571.5
  lung 518.89
    with
      asthma — *see* Asthma
      bronchitis (chronic) 491.2 ✓5ᵗʰ
      emphysema NEC 492.8
    airway, chronic 496
    chronic NEC 496
      with
        asthma (chronic) (obstructive)
          493.2 ✓5ᵗʰ
    disease, chronic 496
      with
        asthma (chronic) (obstructive)
          493.2 ✓5ᵗʰ
    emphysematous 492.8
  lymphatic 457.1
  meconium
    fetus or newborn 777.1
      in mucoviscidosis 277.01
    newborn due to fecaliths 777.1
  mediastinum 519.3
  mitral (rheumatic) — *see* Stenosis, mitral
  nasal 478.1
    duct 375.56
      neonatal 375.55
    sinus — *see* Sinusitis
  nasolacrimal duct 375.56
    congenital 743.65
    neonatal 375.55
  nasopharynx 478.29
  nose 478.1
  organ or site, congenital NEC — *see* Atresia
  pancreatic duct 577.8
  parotid gland 527.8
  pelviureteral junction (*see also* Obstruction,
    ureter) 593.4
  pharynx 478.29
  portal (circulation) (vein) 452
  prostate 600.9
    valve (urinary) 596.0
  pulmonary
    valve (heart) (*see also* Endocarditis,
      pulmonary) 424.3
    vein, isolated 747.49
  pyemic — *see* Septicemia
  pylorus (acquired) 537.0
    congenital 750.5
    infantile 750.5
  rectosigmoid (*see also* Obstruction, intestine)
    560.9
  rectum 569.49
  renal 593.89
  respiratory 519.8
    chronic 496
  retinal (artery) (vein) (central) (*see also*
    Occlusion, retina) 362.30
  salivary duct (any) 527.8
    with calculus 527.5
  sigmoid (*see also* Obstruction, intestine) 560.9
  sinus (accessory) (nasal) (*see also* Sinusitis)
    473.9

Obstruction, obstructed, obstructive —
continued
  Stensen's duct 527.8
  stomach 537.89
    acute 536.1
    congenital 750.7
  submaxillary gland 527.8
    with calculus 527.5
  thoracic duct 457.1
  thrombotic — *see* Thrombosis
  tooth eruption 520.6
  trachea 519.1
  tracheostomy airway 519.09
  tricuspid — *see* Endocarditis, tricuspid
  upper respiratory, congenital 748.8
  ureter (functional) 593.4
    congenital 753.20
    due to calculus 592.1
  ureteropelvic junction, congenital 753.21
  ureterovesical junction, congenital 753.22
  urethra 599.6
    congenital 753.6
  urinary (moderate) 599.6
    organ or tract (lower) 599.6
    prostatic valve 596.0
  uropathy 599.6
  uterus 621.8
  vagina 623.2
  valvular — *see* Endocarditis
  vascular graft or shunt 996.1
    atherosclerosis — *see* Arteriosclerosis,
      coronary
    embolism 996.74
    occlusion NEC 996.74
    thrombus 996.74
  vein, venous 459.2
    caval (inferior) (superior) 459.2
    thrombotic — *see* Thrombosis
  vena cava (inferior) (superior) 459.2
  ventricular shunt 996.2
  vesical 596.0
  vesicourethral orifice 596.0
  vessel NEC 459.9

Obturator — *see* condition

Occlusal wear, teeth 521.1

Occlusion
  anus 569.49
    congenital 751.2
    infantile 751.2
  aortoiliac (chronic) 444.0
  aqueduct of Sylvius 331.4
    congenital 742.3
      with spina bifida (*see also* Spina bifida)
        741.0 ✓5ᵗʰ
  arteries of extremities, lower 444.22
    without thrombus or embolus (*see also*
      Arteriosclerosis, extremities) 440.20
    due to stricture or stenosis 447.1
    upper 444.21
      without thrombus or embolus (*see also*
        Arteriosclerosis, extremities) 440.20
      due to stricture or stenosis 447.1
  artery NEC (*see also* Embolism, artery) 444.9
    auditory, internal 433.8 ✓5ᵗʰ
    basilar 433.0 ✓5ᵗʰ
      with other precerebral artery 433.3 ✓5ᵗʰ
      bilateral 433.3 ✓5ᵗʰ
    brain or cerebral (*see also* Infarct, brain)
      434.9 ✓5ᵗʰ
    carotid 433.1 ✓5ᵗʰ
      with other precerebral artery 433.3 ✓5ᵗʰ
      bilateral 433.3 ✓5ᵗʰ
    cerebellar (anterior inferior) (posterior
      inferior) (superior) 433.8 ✓5ᵗʰ
    cerebral (*see also* Infarct, brain) 434.9 ✓5ᵗʰ
    choroidal (anterior) 433.8 ✓5ᵗʰ
    communicating posterior 433.8 ✓5ᵗʰ
    coronary (thrombotic) (*see also* Infarct,
      myocardium) 410.9 ✓5ᵗʰ
      acute 410.9 ✓5ᵗʰ
        without myocardial infarction
          411.81
      healed or old 412
    hypophyseal 433.8 ✓5ᵗʰ
    iliac 444.81

Occlusion — *continued*
  artery NEC (*see also* Embolism, artery) — *continued*
    mesenteric (embolic) (thrombotic) (with gangrene) 557.0
    pontine 433.8 ✔5ᵗʰ
    precerebral NEC 433.9 ✔5ᵗʰ
      late effect — *see* Late effect(s) (of) cerebrovascular disease
      multiple or bilateral 433.3 ✔5ᵗʰ
      puerperal, postpartum, childbirth 674.0 ✔5ᵗʰ
      specified NEC 433.8 ✔5ᵗʰ
    renal 593.81
    retinal — *see* Occlusion, retina, artery
    spinal 433.8 ✔5ᵗʰ
    vertebral 433.2 ✔5ᵗʰ
      with other precerebral artery 433.3 ✔5ᵗʰ
      bilateral 433.3 ✔5ᵗʰ
  basilar (artery) — *see also* Occlusion, artery, basilar
  bile duct (any) (*see also* Obstruction, biliary) 576.2
  bowel (*see also* Obstruction, intestine) 560.9
  brain (artery) (vascular) (*see also* Infarct, brain) 434.9 ✔5ᵗʰ
  breast (duct) 611.8
  carotid (artery) (common) (internal) — *see* Occlusion, artery, carotid
  cerebellar (anterior inferior) (artery) (posterior inferior) (superior) 433.8 ✔5ᵗʰ
  cerebral (artery) (*see also* Infarct, brain) 434.9 ✔5ᵗʰ
  cerebrovascular (*see also* Infarct, brain) 434.9 ✔5ᵗʰ
    diffuse 437.0
  cervical canal (*see also* Stricture, cervix) 622.4
    by falciparum malaria 084.0
  cervix (uteri) (*see also* Stricture, cervix) 622.4
  choanal 748.0
  choroidal (artery) 433.8 ✔5ᵗʰ
  colon (*see also* Obstruction, intestine) 560.9
  communicating posterior artery 433.8 ✔5ᵗʰ
  coronary (artery) (thrombotic) (*see also* Infarct, myocardium) 410.9 ✔5ᵗʰ
    acute 410.9 ✔5ᵗʰ
      without myocardial infarction 411.81
    healed or old 412
    without myocardial infarction 411.81
  cystic duct (*see also* Obstruction, gallbladder) 575.2
    congenital 751.69
  embolic — *see* Embolism
  fallopian tube 628.2
    congenital 752.19
  gallbladder (*see also* Obstruction, gallbladder) 575.2
    congenital 751.69
      jaundice from 751.69 [774.5]
  gingiva, traumatic 523.8
  hymen 623.3
    congenital 752.42
  hypophyseal (artery) 433.8 ✔5ᵗʰ
  iliac artery 444.81
  intestine (*see also* Obstruction, intestine) 560.9
  kidney 593.89
  lacrimal apparatus — *see* Stenosis, lacrimal
  lung 518.89
  lymph or lymphatic channel 457.1
  mammary duct 611.8
  mesenteric artery (embolic) (thrombotic) (with gangrene) 557.0
  nose 478.1
    congenital 748.0
  organ or site, congenital NEC — *see* Atresia
  oviduct 628.2
    congenital 752.19
  periodontal, traumatic 523.8
  peripheral arteries (lower extremity) 444.22
    without thrombus or embolus (*see also* Arteriosclerosis, extremities) 440.20
    due to stricture or stenosis 447.1
    upper extremity 444.21
      without thrombus or embolus (*see also* Arteriosclerosis, extremities) 440.20
      due to stricture or stenosis 447.1
  pontine (artery) 433.8 ✔5ᵗʰ
  posterior lingual, of mandibular teeth 524.2

Occlusion — *continued*
  precerebral artery — *see* Occlusion, artery, precerebral NEC
  puncta lacrimalia 375.52
  pupil 364.74
  pylorus (*see also* Stricture, pylorus) 537.0
  renal artery 593.81
  retina, retinal (vascular) 362.30
    artery, arterial 362.30
      branch 362.32
      central (total) 362.31
      partial 362.33
      transient 362.34
      tributary 362.32
    vein 362.30
      branch 362.36
      central (total) 362.35
      incipient 362.37
      partial 362.37
      tributary 362.36
  spinal artery 433.8 ✔5ᵗʰ
  stent
    coronary 996.72
  teeth (mandibular) (posterior lingual) 524.2
  thoracic duct 457.1
  tubal 628.2
  ureter (complete) (partial) 593.4
    congenital 753.29
  urethra (*see also* Stricture, urethra) 598.9
    congenital 753.6
  uterus 621.8
  vagina 623.2
  vascular NEC 459.9
  vein — *see* Thrombosis
  vena cava (inferior) (superior) 453.2
  ventricle (brain) NEC 331.4
  vertebral (artery) — *see* Occlusion, artery, vertebral
  vessel (blood) NEC 459.9
  vulva 624.8
Occlusio pupillae 364.74
Occupational
  problems NEC V62.2
  therapy V57.21
Ochlophobia 300.29
Ochronosis (alkaptonuric) (congenital) (endogenous) 270.2
  with chloasma of eyelid 270.2
Ocular muscle — *see also* condition
  myopathy 359.1
  torticollis 781.93
Oculoauriculovertebral dysplasia 756.0
Oculogyric
  crisis or disturbance 378.87
    psychogenic 306.7
Oculomotor syndrome 378.81
Oddi's sphincter spasm 576.5
Odelberg's disease (juvenile osteochondrosis) 732.1
Odontalgia 525.9
Odontoameloblastoma (M9311/0) 213.1
  upper jaw (bone) 213.0
Odontoclasia 521.05
Odontoclasis 873.63
  complicated 873.73
Odontodysplasia, regional 520.4
Odontogenesis imperfecta 520.5
Odontoma (M9280/0) 213.1
  ameloblastic (M9311/0) 213.1
    upper jaw (bone) 213.0
  calcified (M9280/0) 213.1
    upper jaw (bone) 213.0
  complex (M9282/0) 213.1
    upper jaw (bone) 213.0
  compound (M9281/0) 213.1
    upper jaw (bone) 213.0
  fibroameloblastic (M9290/0) 213.1
    upper jaw (bone) 213.0
  follicular 526.0
  upper jaw (bone) 213.0
Odontomyelitis (closed) (open) 522.0
Odontonecrosis 521.09
Odontorrhagia 525.8

Odontosarcoma, ameloblastic (M9290/3) 170.1
  upper jaw (bone) 170.0
Odynophagia 787.2
Oesophagostomiasis 127.7
Oesophagostomum infestation 127.7
Oestriasis 134.0
Ogilvie's syndrome (sympathicotonic colon obstruction) 560.89
Oguchi's disease (retina) 368.61
Ohara's disease (*see also* Tularemia) 021.9
Oidiomycosis (*see also* Candidiasis) 112.9
Oidiomycotic meningitis 112.83
Oidium albicans infection (*see also* Candidiasis) 112.9
Old age 797
  dementia (of) 290.0
Olfactory — *see* condition
Oligemia 285.9
Oligergasia (*see also* Retardation, mental) 319
Oligoamnios 658.0 ✔5ᵗʰ
  affecting fetus or newborn 761.2
Oligoastrocytoma, mixed (M9382/3)
  specified site — *see* Neoplasm, by site, malignant
  unspecified site 191.9
Oligocythemia 285.9
Oligodendroblastoma (M9460/3)
  specified site — *see* Neoplasm, by site, malignant
  unspecified site 191.9
Oligodendroglioma (M9450/3)
  anaplastic type (M9451/3)
    specified site — *see* Neoplasm, by site, malignant
    unspecified site 191.9
  specified site — *see* Neoplasm, by site, malignant
  unspecified site 191.9
Oligodendroma — *see* Oligodendroglioma
Oligodontia (*see also* Anodontia) 520.0
Oligoencephalon 742.1
Oligohydramnios 658.0 ✔5ᵗʰ
  affecting fetus or newborn 761.2
  due to premature rupture of membranes 658.1 ✔5ᵗʰ
    affecting fetus or newborn 761.2
Oligohydrosis 705.0
Oligomenorrhea 626.1
Oligophrenia (*see also* Retardation, mental) 319
  phenylpyruvic 270.1
Oligospermia 606.1
Oligotrichia 704.09
  congenita 757.4
Oliguria 788.5
  with
    abortion — *see* Abortion, by type, with renal failure
    ectopic pregnancy (*see also* categories 633.0-633.9) 639.3
    molar pregnancy (*see also* categories 630-632) 639.3
  complicating
    abortion 639.3
    ectopic or molar pregnancy 639.3
    pregnancy 646.2 ✔5ᵗʰ
      with hypertension — *see* Toxemia, of pregnancy
  due to a procedure 997.5
  following labor and delivery 669.3 ✔5ᵗʰ
  heart or cardiac — *see* Failure, heart
  puerperal, postpartum 669.3 ✔5ᵗʰ
  specified due to a procedure 997.5
Ollier's disease (chondrodysplasia) 756.4
Omentitis (*see also* Peritonitis) 567.9
Omentocele (*see also* Hernia, omental) 553.8
Omentum, omental — *see* condition
Omphalitis (congenital) (newborn) 771.4
  not of newborn 686.9
  tetanus 771.3
Omphalocele 756.79
Omphalomesenteric duct, persistent 751.0

Omphalorrhagia, newborn 772.3
Omsk hemorrhagic fever 065.1
Onanism 307.9
Onchocerciasis 125.3
   eye 125.3 [360.13]
Onchocercosis 125.3
Oncocytoma (M8290/0) — see Neoplasm, by site, benign
Ondine's curse 348.8
Oneirophrenia (see also Schizophrenia) 295.4 ☑5ᵗʰ
Onychauxis 703.8
   congenital 757.5
Onychia (with lymphangitis) 681.9
   dermatophytic 110.1
   finger 681.02
   toe 681.11
Onychitis (with lymphangitis) 681.9
   finger 681.02
   toe 681.11
Onychocryptosis 703.0
Onychodystrophy 703.8
   congenital 757.5
Onychogryphosis 703.8
Onychogryposis 703.8
Onycholysis 703.8
Onychomadesis 703.8
Onychomalacia 703.8
Onychomycosis 110.1
   finger 110.1
   toe 110.1
Onycho-osteodysplasia 756.89
Onychophagy 307.9
Onychoptosis 703.8
Onychorrhexis 703.8
   congenital 757.5
Onychoschizia 703.8
Onychotrophia (see also Atrophy, nail) 703.8
O'nyong-nyong fever 066.3
Onyxis (finger) (toe) 703.0
Onyxitis (with lymphangitis) 681.9
   finger 681.02
   toe 681.11
Oophoritis (cystic) (infectional) (interstitial) (see also Salpingo-oophoritis) 614.2
   complicating pregnancy 646.6 ☑5ᵗʰ
   fetal (acute) 752.0
   gonococcal (acute) 098.19
     chronic or duration of 2 months or over 098.39
   tuberculous (see also Tuberculosis) 016.6 ☑5ᵗʰ
Opacity, opacities
   cornea 371.00
     central 371.03
     congenital 743.43
       interfering with vision 743.42
     degenerative (see also Degeneration, cornea) 371.40
     hereditary (see also Dystrophy, cornea) 371.50
     inflammatory (see also Keratitis) 370.9
     late effect of trachoma (healed) 139.1
     minor 371.01
     peripheral 371.02
   enamel (fluoride) (nonfluoride) (teeth) 520.3
   lens (see also Cataract) 366.9
   snowball 379.22
   vitreous (humor) 379.24
     congenital 743.51
Opalescent dentin (hereditary) 520.5
Open, opening
   abnormal, organ or site, congenital — see Imperfect, closure
   angle with
     borderline intraocular pressure 365.01
     cupping of discs 365.01
   bite (anterior) (posterior) 524.2
   false — see Imperfect, closure
   wound — see Wound, open, by site

Operation
   causing mutilation of fetus 763.89
   destructive, on live fetus, to facilitate birth 763.89
   for delivery, fetus or newborn 763.89
   maternal, unrelated to current delivery, affecting fetus or newborn 760.6
Operational fatigue 300.89
Operative — see condition
Operculitis (chronic) 523.4
   acute 523.3
Operculum, retina 361.32
   with detachment 361.01
Ophiasis 704.01
Ophthalmia (see also Conjunctivitis) 372.30
   actinic rays 370.24
   allergic (acute) 372.05
     chronic 372.14
   blennorrhagic (neonatorum) 098.40
   catarrhal 372.03
   diphtheritic 032.81
   Egyptian 076.1
   electric, electrica 370.24
   gonococcal (neonatorum) 098.40
   metastatic 360.11
   migraine 346.8 ☑5ᵗʰ
   neonatorum, newborn 771.6
     gonococcal 098.40
   nodosa 360.14
   phlyctenular 370.31
     with ulcer (see also Ulcer, cornea) 370.00
   sympathetic 360.11
Ophthalmitis — see Ophthalmia
Ophthalmocele (congenital) 743.66
Ophthalmoneuromyelitis 341.0
Ophthalmopathy, infiltrative with thyrotoxicosis 242.0 ☑5ᵗʰ
Ophthalmoplegia (see also Strabismus) 378.9
   anterior internuclear 378.86
   ataxia-areflexia syndrome 357.0
   bilateral 378.9
   diabetic 250.5 ☑5ᵗʰ [378.86]
   exophthalmic 242.0 ☑5ᵗʰ [376.22]
   external 378.55
     progressive 378.72
     total 378.56
   interna(l) (complete) (total) 367.52
   internuclear 378.86
   migraine 346.8 ☑5ᵗʰ
   painful 378.55
   Parinaud's 378.81
   progressive external 378.72
   supranuclear, progressive 333.0
   total (external) 378.56
     internal 367.52
   unilateral 378.9
Opisthognathism 524.00
Opisthorchiasis (felineus) (tenuicollis) (viverrini) 121.0
Opisthotonos, opisthotonus 781.0
Opitz's disease (congestive splenomegaly) 289.51
Opiumism (see also Dependence) 304.0 ☑5ᵗʰ
Oppenheim's disease 358.8
Oppenheim-Urbach disease or syndrome (necrobiosis lipoidica diabeticorum) 250.8 ☑5ᵗʰ [709.3]
Opsoclonia 379.59
Optic nerve — see condition
Orbit — see condition
Orchioblastoma (M9071/3) 186.9
Orchitis (nonspecific) (septic) 604.90
   with abscess 604.0
   blennorrhagic (acute) 098.13
     chronic or duration of 2 months or over 098.33
   diphtheritic 032.89 [604.91]
   filarial 125.9 [604.91]
   gangrenous 604.99
   gonococcal (acute) 098.13
     chronic or duration of 2 months or over 098.33
   mumps 072.0
   parotidea 072.0

Orchitis — continued
   suppurative 604.99
   syphilitic 095.8 [604.91]
   tuberculous (see also Tuberculosis) 016.5 ☑5ᵗʰ [608.81]
Orf 051.2
Organic — see also condition
   heart — see Disease, heart
   insufficiency 799.8
Oriental
   bilharziasis 120.2
   schistosomiasis 120.2
   sore 085.1
Orifice — see condition
Origin, both great vessels from right ventricle 745.11
Ormond's disease or syndrome 593.4
Ornithosis 073.9
   with
     complication 073.8
       specified NEC 073.7
     pneumonia 073.0
     pneumonitis (lobular) 073.0
Orodigitofacial dysostosis 759.89
Oropouche fever 066.3
Orotaciduria, oroticaciduria (congenital) (hereditary) (pyrimidine deficiency) 281.4
Oroya fever 088.0
Orthodontics V58.5
   adjustment V53.4
   aftercare V58.5
   fitting V53.4
Orthopnea 786.02
Orthoptic training V57.4
Os, uterus — see condition
Osgood-Schlatter
   disease 732.4
   osteochondrosis 732.4
Osler's
   disease (M9950/1) (polycythemia vera) 238.4
   nodes 421.0
Osler-Rendu disease (familial hemorrhagic telangiectasia) 448.0
Osler-Vaquez disease (M9950/1) (polycythemia vera) 238.4
Osler-Weber-Rendu syndrome (familial hemorrhagic telangiectasia) 448.0
Osmidrosis 705.89
Osseous — see condition
Ossification
   artery — see Arteriosclerosis
   auricle (ear) 380.39
   bronchus 519.1
   cardiac (see also Degeneration, myocardial) 429.1
   cartilage (senile) 733.99
   coronary (artery) — see Arteriosclerosis, coronary
   diaphragm 728.10
   ear 380.39
     middle (see also Otosclerosis) 387.9
   falx cerebri 349.2
   fascia 728.10
   fontanel
     defective or delayed 756.0
     premature 756.0
   heart (see also Degeneration, myocardial) 429.1
     valve — see Endocarditis
   larynx 478.79
   ligament
     posterior longitudinal 724.8
       cervical 723.7
   meninges (cerebral) 349.2
     spinal 336.8
   multiple, eccentric centers 733.99
   muscle 728.10
     heterotopic, postoperative 728.13
   myocardium, myocardial (see also Degeneration, myocardial) 429.1
   penis 607.81
   periarticular 728.89
   sclera 379.16
   tendon 727.82

Ossification — *continued*
trachea 519.1
tympanic membrane (*see also* Tympanosclerosis) 385.00
vitreous (humor) 360.44

Osteitis (*see also* Osteomyelitis) 730.2 ✓5ᵗʰ
acute 730.0 ✓5ᵗʰ
alveolar 526.5
chronic 730.1 ✓5ᵗʰ
condensans (ilii) 733.5
deformans (Paget's) 731.0
due to or associated with malignant neoplasm (*see also* Neoplasm, bone, malignant) 170.9 *[731.1]*
due to yaws 102.6
fibrosa NEC 733.29
cystica (generalisata) 252.0
disseminata 756.59
osteoplastica 252.0
fragilitans 756.51
Garré's (sclerosing) 730.1 ✓5ᵗʰ
infectious (acute) (subacute) 730.0 ✓5ᵗʰ
chronic or old 730.1 ✓5ᵗʰ
jaw (acute) (chronic) (lower) (neonatal) (suppurative) (upper) 526.4
parathyroid 252.0
petrous bone (*see also* Petrositis) 383.20
pubis 733.5
sclerotic, nonsuppurative 730.1 ✓5ᵗʰ
syphilitic 095.5
tuberculosa
cystica (of Jüngling) 135
multiplex cystoides 135

Osteoarthritica spondylitis (spine) (*see also* Spondylosis) 721.90

Osteoarthritis (*see also* Osteoarthrosis) 715.9 ✓5ᵗʰ
distal interphalangeal 715.9 ✓5ᵗʰ
hyperplastic 731.2
interspinalis (*see also* Spondylosis) 721.90
spine, spinal NEC (*see also* Spondylosis) 721.90

Osteoarthropathy (*see also* Osteoarthrosis) 715.9 ✓5ᵗʰ
chronic idiopathic hypertrophic 757.39
familial idiopathic 757.39
hypertrophic pulmonary 731.2
secondary 731.2
idiopathic hypertrophic 757.39
primary hypertrophic 731.2
pulmonary hypertrophic 731.2
secondary hypertrophic 731.2

Osteoarthrosis (degenerative) (hypertrophic) (rheumatoid) 715.9 ✓5ᵗʰ

Note — Use the following fifth-digit subclassification with category 715:

0   site unspecified
1   shoulder region
2   upper arm
3   forearm
4   hand
5   pelvic region and thigh
6   lower leg
7   ankle and foot
8   other specified sites except spine
9   multiple sites

Deformans alkaptonurica 270.2
generalized 715.09
juvenilis (Köhler's) 732.5
localized 715.3 ✓5ᵗʰ
idiopathic 715.1 ✓5ᵗʰ
primary 715.1 ✓5ᵗʰ
secondary 715.2 ✓5ᵗʰ
multiple sites, not specified as generalized 715.89
polyarticular 715.09
spine (*see also* Spondylosis) 721.90
temporomandibular joint 524.69

Osteoblastoma (M9200/0) — *see* Neoplasm, bone, benign

Osteochondritis (*see also* Osteochondrosis) 732.9
dissecans 732.7
hip 732.7

Osteochondritis (*see also* Osteochondrosis) — *continued*
ischiopubica 732.1
multiple 756.59
syphilitic (congenital) 090.0

Osteochondrodermodysplasia 756.59

Osteochondrodystrophy 277.5
deformans 277.5
familial 277.5
fetalis 756.4

Osteochondrolysis 732.7

Osteochondroma (M9210/0) — *see also* Neoplasm, bone, benign
multiple, congenital 756.4

Osteochondromatosis (M9210/1) 238.0
synovial 727.82

Osteochondromyxosarcoma (M9180/3) — *see* Neoplasm, bone, malignant

Osteochondropathy NEC 732.9

Osteochondrosarcoma (M9180/3) — *see* Neoplasm, bone, malignant

Osteochondrosis 732.9
acetabulum 732.1
adult spine 732.8
astragalus 732.5
Blount's 732.4
Buchanan's (juvenile osteochondrosis of iliac crest) 732.1
Buchman's (juvenile osteochondrosis) 732.1
Burns' 732.3
calcaneus 732.5
capitular epiphysis (femur) 732.1
carpal
lunate (wrist) 732.3
scaphoid 732.3
coxae juvenilis 732.1
deformans juvenilis (coxae) (hip) 732.1
Scheuermann's 732.0
spine 732.0
tibia 732.4
vertebra 732.0
Diaz's (astragalus) 732.5
dissecans (knee) (shoulder) 732.7
femoral capital epiphysis 732.1
femur (head) (juvenile) 732.1
foot (juvenile) 732.5
Freiberg's (disease) (second metatarsal) 732.5
Haas' 732.3
Haglund's (os tibiale externum) 732.5
hand (juvenile) 732.3
head of
femur 732.1
humerus (juvenile) 732.3
hip (juvenile) 732.1
humerus (juvenile) 732.3
iliac crest (juvenile) 732.1
ilium (juvenile) 732.1
ischiopubic synchondrosis 732.1
Iselin's (osteochondrosis fifth metatarsal) 732.5
juvenile, juvenilis 732.6
arm 732.3
capital femoral epiphysis 732.1
capitellum humeri 732.3
capitular epiphysis 732.1
carpal scaphoid 732.3
clavicle, sternal epiphysis 732.6
coxae 732.1
deformans 732.1
foot 732.5
hand 732.3
hip and pelvis 732.1
lower extremity, except foot 732.4
lunate, wrist 732.3
medial cuneiform bone 732.5
metatarsal (head) 732.5
metatarsophalangeal 732.5
navicular, ankle 732.5
patella 732.4
primary patellar center (of Köhler) 732.4
specified site NEC 732.6
spine 732.0
tarsal scaphoid 732.5
tibia (epiphysis) (tuberosity) 732.4
upper extremity 732.3
vertebra (body) (Calvé) 732.0
epiphyseal plates (of Scheuermann) 732.0

Osteochondrosis — *continued*
Kienböck's (disease) 732.3
Köhler's (disease) (navicular, ankle) 732.5
patellar 732.4
tarsal navicular 732.5
Legg-Calvé-Perthes (disease) 732.1
lower extremity (juvenile) 732.4
lunate bone 732.3
Mauclaire's 732.3
metacarpal heads (of Mauclaire) 732.3
metatarsal (fifth) (head) (second) 732.5
navicular, ankle 732.5
os calcis 732.5
Osgood-Schlatter 732.4
os tibiale externum 732.5
Panner's 732.3
patella (juvenile) 732.4
patellar center
primary (of Köhler) 732.4
secondary (of Sinding-Larsen) 732.4
pelvis (juvenile) 732.1
Pierson's 732.1
radial head (juvenile) 732.3
Scheuermann's 732.0
Sever's (calcaneum) 732.5
Sinding-Larsen (secondary patellar center) 732.4
spine (juvenile) 732.0
adult 732.8
symphysis pubis (of Pierson) (juvenile) 732.1
syphilitic (congenital) 090.0
tarsal (navicular) (scaphoid) 732.5
tibia (proximal) (tubercle) 732.4
tuberculous — *see* Tuberculosis, bone
ulna 732.3
upper extremity (juvenile) 732.3
van Neck's (juvenile osteochondrosis) 732.1
vertebral (juvenile) 732.0
adult 732.8

Osteoclastoma (M9250/1) 238.0
malignant (M9250/3) — *see* Neoplasm, bone, malignant

Osteocopic pain 733.90

Osteodynia 733.90

Osteodystrophy
azotemic 588.0
chronica deformans hypertrophica 731.0
congenital 756.50
specified type NEC 756.59
deformans 731.0
fibrosa localisata 731.0
parathyroid 252.0
renal 588.0

Osteofibroma (M9262/0) — *see* Neoplasm, bone, benign

Osteofibrosarcoma (M9182/3) — *see* Neoplasm, bone, malignant

Osteogenesis imperfecta 756.51

Osteogenic — *see* condition

Osteoma (M9180/0) — *see also* Neoplasm, bone, benign
osteoid (M9191/0) — *see also* Neoplasm, bone, benign
giant (M9200/0) — *see* Neoplasm, bone, benign

Osteomalacia 268.2
chronica deformans hypertrophica 731.0
due to vitamin D deficiency 268.2
infantile (*see also* Rickets) 268.0
juvenile (*see also* Rickets) 268.0
pelvis 268.2
vitamin D-resistant 275.3

Osteomalacic bone 268.2

Osteomalacosis 268.2

Osteomyelitis (general) (infective) (localized) (neonatal) (purulent) (pyogenic) (septic) (staphylococcal) (streptococcal) (suppurative) (with periostitis) 730.2 ✓5ᵗʰ

> Note — Use the following fifth-digit subclassification with category 730:
>
> 0   site unspecified
> 1   shoulder region
> 2   upper arm
> 3   forearm
> 4   hand
> 5   pelvic region and thigh
> 6   lower leg
> 7   ankle and foot
> 8   other specified sites
> 9   multiple sites

  acute or subacute 730.0 ✓5ᵗʰ
  chronic or old 730.1 ✓5ᵗʰ
  due to or associated with
    diabetes mellitus 250.8 ✓5ᵗʰ [731.8]
    tuberculosis (see also Tuberculosis, bone)
      015.9 ✓5ᵗʰ [730.8] ✓5ᵗʰ
      limb bones 015.5 ✓5ᵗʰ [730.8] ✓5ᵗʰ
      specified bones NEC
        015.7 ✓5ᵗʰ [730.8] ✓5ᵗʰ
      spine 015.0 ✓5ᵗʰ [730.8] ✓5ᵗʰ
      typhoid 002.0 [730.8] ✓5ᵗʰ
  Garré's 730.1 ✓5ᵗʰ
  jaw (acute) (chronic) (lower) (neonatal) (suppurative) (upper) 526.4
  nonsuppurating 730.1 ✓5ᵗʰ
  orbital 376.03
  petrous bone (see also Petrositis) 383.20
  Salmonella 003.24
  sclerosing, nonsuppurative 730.1 ✓5ᵗʰ
  sicca 730.1 ✓5ᵗʰ
  syphilitic 095.5
    congenital 090.0 [730.8] ✓5ᵗʰ
  tuberculous — see Tuberculosis, bone
  typhoid 002.0 [730.8] ✓5ᵗʰ
Osteomyelofibrosis 289.8
Osteomyelosclerosis 289.8
Osteonecrosis 733.40 ▲
  meaning osteomyelitis 730.1 ✓5ᵗʰ ●
Osteo-onycho-arthro dysplasia 756.89
Osteo-onychodysplasia, hereditary 756.89
Osteopathia
  condensans disseminata 756.53
  hyperostotica multiplex infantilis 756.59
  hypertrophica toxica 731.2
  striata 756.4
Osteopathy resulting from poliomyelitis (see also Poliomyelitis) 045.9 ✓5ᵗʰ [730.7]
  familial dysplastic 731.2
Osteopecilia 756.53
Osteopenia 733.90
Osteoperiostitis (see also Osteomyelitis) 730.2 ✓5ᵗʰ
  ossificans toxica 731.2
  toxica ossificans 731.2
Osteopetrosis (familial) 756.52
Osteophyte — see Exostosis
Osteophytosis — see Exostosis
Osteopoikilosis 756.53
Osteoporosis (generalized) 733.00
  circumscripta 731.0
  disuse 733.03
  drug-induced 733.09
  idiopathic 733.02
  postmenopausal 733.01
  posttraumatic 733.7
  screening V82.81
  senile 733.01
  specified type NEC 733.09
Osteoporosis-osteomalacia syndrome 268.2
Osteopsathyrosis 756.51
Osteoradionecrosis, jaw 526.89
Osteosarcoma (M9180/3) — see also Neoplasm, bone, malignant
  chondroblastic (M9181/3) — see Neoplasm, bone, malignant

Osteosarcoma (M9180/3) — see also Neoplasm, bone, malignant — continued
  fibroblastic (M9182/3) — see Neoplasm, bone, malignant
  in Paget's disease of bone (M9184/3) — see Neoplasm, bone, malignant
  juxtacortical (M9190/3) — see Neoplasm, bone, malignant
  parosteal (M9190/3) — see Neoplasm, bone, malignant
  telangiectatic (M9183/3) — see Neoplasm, bone, malignant
Osteosclerosis 756.52
  fragilis (generalisata) 756.52
  myelofibrosis 289.8
Osteosclerotic anemia 289.8
Osteosis
  acromegaloid 757.39
  cutis 709.3
  parathyroid 252.0
  renal fibrocystic 588.0
Österreicher-Turner syndrome 756.89
Ostium
  atrioventriculare commune 745.69
  primum (arteriosum) (defect) (persistent) 745.61
  secundum (arteriosum) (defect) (patent) (persistent) 745.5
Ostrum-Furst syndrome 756.59
Otalgia 388.70
  otogenic 388.71
  referred 388.72
Othematoma 380.31
Otitic hydrocephalus 348.2
Otitis 382.9
  with effusion 381.4
    purulent 382.4
    secretory 381.4
    serous 381.4
    suppurative 382.4
  acute 382.9
  adhesive (see also Adhesions, middle ear) 385.10
  chronic 382.9
    with effusion 381.3
    mucoid, mucous (simple) 381.20
    purulent 382.3
    secretory 381.3
    serous 381.10
    suppurative 382.3
  diffuse parasitic 136.8
  externa (acute) (diffuse) (hemorrhagica) 380.10
    actinic 380.22
    candidal 112.82
    chemical 380.22
    chronic 380.23
      mycotic — see Otitis, externa, mycotic
      specified type NEC 380.23
    circumscribed 380.10
    contact 380.22
    due to
      erysipelas 035 [380.13]
      impetigo 684 [380.13]
      seborrheic dermatitis 690.10 [380.13]
    eczematoid 380.22
    furuncular 680.0 [380.13]
    infective 380.10
      chronic 380.16
    malignant 380.14
    mycotic (chronic) 380.15
      due to
        aspergillosis 117.3 [380.15]
        moniliasis 112.82
        otomycosis 111.8 [380.15]
    reactive 380.22
    specified type NEC 380.22
    tropical 111.8 [380.15]
  insidiosa (see also Otosclerosis) 387.9
  interna (see also Labyrinthitis) 386.30
  media (hemorrhagic) (staphylococcal) (streptococcal) 382.9
    acute 382.9
      with effusion 381.00
      allergic 381.04
        mucoid 381.05
        sanguineous 381.06

Otitis — continued
  media — continued
    acute — continued
      allergic — continued
        serous 381.04
      catarrhal 381.00
      exudative 381.00
      mucoid 381.02
        allergic 381.05
      necrotizing 382.00
        with spontaneous rupture of ear drum 382.01
        in
          influenza 487.8 [382.02]
          measles 055.2
          scarlet fever 034.1 [382.02]
      nonsuppurative 381.00
      purulent 382.00
        with spontaneous rupture of ear drum 382.01
      sanguineous 381.03
        allergic 381.06
      secretory 381.01
      seromucinous 381.02
      serous 381.01
        allergic 381.04
      suppurative 382.00
        with spontaneous rupture of ear drum 382.01
        due to
          influenza 487.8 [382.02]
          scarlet fever 034.1 [382.02]
      transudative 381.00
    adhesive (see also Adhesions, middle ear) 385.10
    allergic 381.4
      acute 381.04
        mucoid 381.05
        sanguineous 381.06
        serous 381.04
      chronic 381.3
    catarrhal 381.4
      acute 381.00
      chronic (simple) 381.10
    chronic 382.9
      with effusion 381.3
      adhesive (see also Adhesions, middle ear) 385.10
      allergic 381.3
      atticoantral, suppurative (with posterior or superior marginal perforation of ear drum) 382.2
      benign suppurative (with anterior perforation of ear drum) 382.1
      catarrhal 381.10
      exudative 381.3
      mucinous 381.20
      mucoid, mucous (simple) 381.20
      mucosanguineous 381.29
      nonsuppurative 381.3
      purulent 382.3
      secretory 381.3
      seromucinous 381.3
      serosanguineous 381.19
      serous (simple) 381.10
      suppurative 382.3
        atticoantral (with posterior or superior marginal perforation of ear drum) 382.2
        benign (with anterior perforation of ear drum) 382.1
        tuberculous (see also Tuberculosis) 017.4 ✓5ᵗʰ
        tubotympanic 382.1
      transudative 381.3
    exudative 381.4
      acute 381.00
      chronic 381.3
    fibrotic (see also Adhesions, middle ear) 385.10
    mucoid, mucous 381.4
      acute 381.02
      chronic (simple) 381.20
    mucosanguineous, chronic 381.29
    nonsuppurative 381.4
      acute 381.00
      chronic 381.3
    postmeasles 055.2

Otitis — *continued*
  media — *continued*
    purulent 382.4
      acute 382.00
        with spontaneous rupture of ear drum 382.01
      chronic 382.3
    sanguineous, acute 381.03
      allergic 381.06
    secretory 381.4
      acute or subacute 381.01
      chronic 381.3
    seromucinous 381.4
      acute or subacute 381.02
      chronic 381.3
    serosanguineous, chronic 381.19
    serous 381.4
      acute or subacute 381.01
      chronic (simple) 381.10
    subacute — *see* Otitis, media, acute
    suppurative 382.4
      acute 382.00
        with spontaneous rupture of ear drum 382.01
      chronic 382.3
        atticoantral 382.2
        benign 382.1
        tuberculous (*see also* Tuberculosis) 017.4 ✓5ᵗʰ
        tubotympanic 382.1
    transudative 381.4
      acute 381.00
      chronic 381.3
    tuberculous (*see also* Tuberculosis) 017.4 ✓5ᵗʰ
  postmeasles 055.2
Otoconia 386.8
Otolith syndrome 386.19
Otomycosis 111.8 *[380.15]*
  in
    aspergillosis 117.3 *[380.15]*
    moniliasis 112.82
Otopathy 388.9
Otoporosis (*see also* Otosclerosis) 387.9
Otorrhagia 388.69
  traumatic — *see* nature of injury
Otorrhea 388.60
  blood 388.69
  cerebrospinal (fluid) 388.61
Otosclerosis (general) 387.9
  cochlear (endosteal) 387.2
  involving
    otic capsule 387.2
    oval window
      nonobliterative 387.0
      obliterative 387.1
    round window 387.2
  nonobliterative 387.0
  obliterative 387.1
  specified type NEC 387.8
Otospongiosis (*see also* Otosclerosis) 387.9
Otto's disease or pelvis 715.35
Outburst, aggressive (*see also* Disturbance, conduct) 312.0 ✓5ᵗʰ
  in children and adolescents 313.9
Outcome of delivery
  multiple birth NEC V27.9
    all liveborn V27.5
    all stillborn V27.7
    some liveborn V27.6
    unspecified V27.9
  single V27.9
    liveborn V27.0
    stillborn V27.1
  twins V27.9
    both liveborn V27.2
    both stillborn V27.4
    one liveborn, one stillborn V27.3
Outlet — *see also* condition
  syndrome (thoracic) 353.0
Outstanding ears (bilateral) 744.29
Ovalocytosis (congenital) (hereditary) (*see also* Elliptocytosis) 282.1

Ovarian — *see also* condition
  pregnancy — *see* Pregnancy, ovarian
  remnant syndrome 620.8
  vein syndrome 593.4
Ovaritis (cystic) (*see also* Salpingo-oophoritis) 614.2
Ovary, ovarian — *see* condition
Overactive — *see also* Hyperfunction
  bladder 596.51
  eye muscle (*see also* Strabismus) 378.9
  hypothalamus 253.8
  thyroid (*see also* Thyrotoxicosis) 242.9 ✓5ᵗʰ
Overactivity, child 314.01
Overbite (deep) (excessive) (horizontal) (vertical) 524.2
Overbreathing (*see also* Hyperventilation) 786.01
Overconscientious personality 301.4
Overdevelopment — *see also* Hypertrophy
  breast (female) (male) 611.1
  nasal bones 738.0
  prostate, congenital 752.8
Overdistention — *see* Distention
Overdose, overdosage (drug) 977.9
  specified drug or substance — *see* Table of Drugs and Chemicals
Overeating 783.6
  with obesity 278.0 ✓5ᵗʰ
  nonorganic origin 307.51
Overexertion (effects) (exhaustion) 994.5
Overexposure (effects) 994.9
  exhaustion 994.4
Overfeeding (*see also* Overeating) 783.6
Overgrowth, bone NEC 733.99
Overheated (effects) (places) — *see* Heat
Overinhibited child 313.0
Overjet 524.2
Overlaid, overlying (suffocation) 994.7
Overlapping toe (acquired) 735.8
  congenital (fifth toe) 755.66
Overload
  fluid 276.6
  potassium (K) 276.7
  sodium (Na) 276.0
Overnutrition (*see also* Hyperalimentation) 783.6
Overproduction — *see also* Hypersecretion
  ACTH 255.3
  cortisol 255.0
  growth hormone 253.0
  thyroid-stimulating hormone (TSH) 242.8 ✓5ᵗʰ
Overriding
  aorta 747.21
  finger (acquired) 736.29
    congenital 755.59
  toe (acquired) 735.8
    congenital 755.66
Oversize
  fetus (weight of 4500 grams or more) 766.0
    affecting management of pregnancy 656.6 ✓5ᵗʰ
    causing disproportion 653.5 ✓5ᵗʰ
      with obstructed labor 660.1 ✓5ᵗʰ
        affecting fetus or newborn 763.1
Overstimulation, ovarian 256.1
Overstrained 780.79
  heart — *see* Hypertrophy, cardiac
Overweight (*see also* Obesity) 278.00
Overwork 780.79
Oviduct — *see* condition
Ovotestis 752.7
Ovulation (cycle)
  failure or lack of 628.0
  pain 625.2
Ovum
  blighted 631
  dropsical 631
  pathologic 631
Owren's disease or syndrome (parahemophilia) (*see also* Defect, coagulation) 286.3
Oxalosis 271.8
Oxaluria 271.8

Ox heart — *see* Hypertrophy, cardiac
OX syndrome 758.6
Oxycephaly, oxycephalic 756.0
  syphilitic, congenital 090.0
Oxyuriasis 127.4
Oxyuris vermicularis (infestation) 127.4
Ozena 472.0

Pacemaker syndrome 429.4
Pachyderma, pachydermia 701.8
  laryngis 478.5
  laryngitis 478.79
  larynx (verrucosa) 478.79
Pachydermatitis 701.8
Pachydermatocele (congenital) 757.39
  acquired 701.8
Pachydermatosis 701.8
Pachydermoperiostitis
  secondary 731.2
Pachydermoperiostosis
  primary idiopathic 757.39
  secondary 731.2
Pachymeningitis (adhesive) (basal) (brain) (cerebral) (cervical) (chronic) (circumscribed) (external) (fibrous) (hemorrhagic) (hypertrophic) (internal) (purulent) (spinal) (suppurative) (*see also* Meningitis) 322.9
  gonococcal 098.82
Pachyonychia (congenital) 757.5
  acquired 703.8
Pachyperiosteodermia
  primary or idiopathic 757.39
  secondary 731.2
Pachyperiostosis
  primary or idiopathic 757.39
  secondary 731.2
Pacinian tumor (M9507/0) — *see* Neoplasm, skin, benign
Pads, knuckle or Garrod's 728.79
Paget's disease (osteitis deformans) 731.0
  with infiltrating duct carcinoma of the breast (M8541/3) — *see* Neoplasm, breast, malignant
  bone 731.0
    osteosarcoma in (M9184/3) — *see* Neoplasm, bone, malignant
  breast (M8540/3) 174.0
  extramammary (M8542/3) — *see also* Neoplasm, skin, malignant
    anus 154.3
    skin 173.5
  malignant (M8540/3)
    breast 174.0
    specified site NEC (M8542/3) — *see* Neoplasm, skin, malignant
    unspecified site 174.0
  mammary (M8540/3) 174.0
  necrosis of bone 731.0
  nipple (M8540/3) 174.0
  osteitis deformans 731.0
Paget-Schroetter syndrome (intermittent venous claudication) 453.8
Pain(s)
  abdominal 789.0 ✓5ᵗʰ
  adnexa (uteri) 625.9
  alimentary, due to vascular insufficiency 557.9
  anginoid (*see also* Pain, precordial) 786.51 anus 569.42
  arch 729.5
  arm 729.5
  back (postural) 724.5
    low 724.2
    psychogenic 307.89
  bile duct 576.9
  bladder 788.9
  bone 733.90
  breast 611.71
    psychogenic 307.89
  broad ligament 625.9
  cartilage NEC 733.90
  cecum 789.0 ✓5ᵗʰ

Pain(s) — *continued*
- cervicobrachial 723.3
- chest (central) 786.50
  - atypical 786.59
  - midsternal 786.51
  - musculoskeletal 786.59
  - noncardiac 786.59
  - substernal 786.51
  - wall (anterior) 786.52
- coccyx 724.79
- colon 789.0 ✓5ᵗʰ
- common duct 576.9
- coronary — *see* Angina
- costochondral 786.52
- diaphragm 786.52
- due to (presence of) any device, implant, or graft classifiable to 996.0-996.5 — *see* Complications, due to (presence of) any device, implant, or graft classified to 996.0-996.5 NEC
- ear (*see also* Otalgia) 388.70
- epigastric, epigastrium 789.0 ✓5ᵗʰ
- extremity (lower) (upper) 729.5
- eye 379.91
- face, facial 784.0
  - atypical 350.2
  - nerve 351.8
- false (labor) 644.1 ✓5ᵗʰ
- female genital organ NEC 625.9
  - psychogenic 307.89
- finger 729.5
- flank 789.0 ✓5ᵗʰ
- foot 729.5
- gallbladder 575.9
- gas (intestinal) 787.3
- gastric 536.8
- generalized 780.99 ▲
- genital organ
  - female 625.9
  - male 608.9
  - psychogenic 307.89
- groin 789.0 ✓5ᵗʰ
- growing 781.99
- hand 729.5
- head (*see also* Headache) 784.0
- heart (see also Pain, precordial) 786.51
- infraorbital (*see also* Neuralgia, trigeminal) 350.1
- intermenstrual 625.2
- jaw 526.9
- joint 719.40
  - ankle 719.47
  - elbow 719.42
  - foot 719.47
  - hand 719.44
  - hip 719.45
  - knee 719.46
  - multiple sites 719.49
  - pelvic region 719.45
  - psychogenic 307.89
  - shoulder (region) 719.41
  - specified site NEC 719.48
  - wrist 719.43
- kidney 788.0
- labor, false or spurious 644.1 ✓5ᵗʰ
- laryngeal 784.1
- leg 729.5
- limb 729.5
- low back 724.2
- lumbar region 724.2
- mastoid (*see also* Otalgia) 388.70
- maxilla 526.9
- metacarpophalangeal (joint) 719.44
- metatarsophalangeal (joint) 719.47
- mouth 528.9
- muscle 729.1
  - intercostal 786.59
- nasal 478.1
- nasopharynx 478.29
- neck NEC 723.1
  - psychogenic 307.89
- nerve NEC 729.2
- neuromuscular 729.1
- nose 478.1
- ocular 379.91
- ophthalmic 379.91
- orbital region 379.91
- osteocopic 733.90

Pain(s) — *continued*
- ovary 625.9
  - psychogenic 307.89
- over heart (*see also* Pain, precordial) 786.51
- ovulation 625.2
- pelvic (female) 625.9
  - male NEC 789.0 ✓5ᵗʰ
    - psychogenic 307.89
  - psychogenic 307.89
- penis 607.9
  - psychogenic 307.89
- pericardial (*see also* Pain, precordial) 786.51
- perineum
  - female 625.9
  - male 608.9
- pharynx 478.29
- pleura, pleural, pleuritic 786.52
- post-operative — *see* Pain, by site
- preauricular 388.70
- precordial (region) 786.51
  - psychogenic 307.89
- psychogenic 307.80
  - cardiovascular system 307.89
  - gastrointestinal system 307.89
  - genitourinary system 307.89
  - heart 307.89
  - musculoskeletal system 307.89
  - respiratory system 307.89
  - skin 306.3
- radicular (spinal) (*see also* Radiculitis) 729.2
- rectum 569.42
- respiration 786.52
- retrosternal 786.51
- rheumatic NEC 729.0
  - muscular 729.1
- rib 786.50
- root (spinal) (*see also* Radiculitis) 729.2
- round ligament (stretch) 625.9
- sacroiliac 724.6
- sciatic 724.3
- scrotum 608.9
  - psychogenic 307.89
- seminal vesicle 608.9
- sinus 478.1
- skin 782.0
- spermatic cord 608.9
- spinal root (*see also* Radiculitis) 729.2
- stomach 536.8
  - psychogenic 307.89
- substernal 786.51
- temporomandibular (joint) 524.62
- temporomaxillary joint 524.62
- testis 608.9
  - psychogenic 307.89
- thoracic spine 724.1
  - with radicular and visceral pain 724.4
- throat 784.1
- tibia 733.90
- toe 729.5
- tongue 529.6
- tooth 525.9
- trigeminal (*see also* Neuralgia, trigeminal) 350.1
- umbilicus 789.0 ✓5ᵗʰ
- ureter 788.0
- urinary (organ) (system) 788.0
- uterus 625.9
  - psychogenic 307.89
- vagina 625.9
- vertebrogenic (syndrome) 724.5
- vesical 788.9
- vulva 625.9
- xiphoid 733.90

Painful — *see also* Pain
- arc syndrome 726.19
- coitus
  - female 625.0
  - male 608.89
  - psychogenic 302.76
- ejaculation (semen) 608.89
  - psychogenic 302.79
- erection 607.3
- feet syndrome 266.2
- menstruation 625.3
  - psychogenic 306.52
- micturition 788.1
- ophthalmoplegia 378.55

Painful — *see also* Pain — *continued*
- respiration 786.52
- scar NEC 709.2
- urination 788.1
- wire sutures 998.89

Painters' colic 984.9
- specified type of lead — *see* Table of Drugs and Chemicals

Palate — *see* condition

Palatoplegia 528.9

Palatoschisis (*see also* Cleft, palate) 749.00

Palilalia 784.69

Palindromic arthritis (*see also* Rheumatism, palindromic) 719.3 ✓5ᵗʰ

Palliative care V66.7

Pallor 782.61
- temporal, optic disc 377.15

Palmar — *see also* condition
- fascia — *see* condition

Palpable
- cecum 569.89
- kidney 593.89
- liver 573.9
- lymph nodes 785.6
- ovary 620.8
- prostate 602.9
- spleen (*see also* Splenomegaly) 789.2
- uterus 625.8

Palpitation (heart) 785.1
- psychogenic 306.2

Palsy (*see also* Paralysis) 344.9
- atrophic diffuse 335.20
- Bell's 351.0
  - newborn 767.5
- birth 767.7
- brachial plexus 353.0
  - fetus or newborn 767.6
- brain — *see also* Palsy, cerebral
  - noncongenital or noninfantile 344.89
    - due to vascular lesion — *see* category 438 ✓4ᵗʰ
    - late effect — *see* Late effect(s) (of) cerebrovascular disease
  - syphilitic 094.89
    - congenital 090.49
- bulbar (chronic) (progressive) 335.22
  - pseudo NEC 335.23
  - supranuclear NEC 344.8 ✓5ᵗʰ
- cerebral (congenital) (infantile) (spastic) 343.9
  - athetoid 333.7
  - diplegic 343.0
    - due to previous vascular lesion — *see* category 438 ✓4ᵗʰ
    - late effect — *see* Late effect(s) (of) cerebrovascular disease
  - hemiplegic 343.1
  - monoplegic 343.3
  - noncongenital or noninfantile 437.8
    - due to previous vascular lesion — *see* category 438 ✓4ᵗʰ
    - late effect — *see* Late effect(s) (of) cerebrovascular disease
  - paraplegic 343.0
  - quadriplegic 343.2
  - spastic, not congenital or infantile 344.8 ✓5ᵗʰ
  - syphilitic 094.89
    - congenital 090.49
  - tetraplegic 343.2
- cranial nerve — *see also* Disorder, nerve, cranial
  - multiple 352.6
- creeping 335.21
- divers' 993.3
- Erb's (birth injury) 767.6
- facial 351.0
  - newborn 767.5
- glossopharyngeal 352.2
- Klumpke (-Déjérine) 767.6
- lead 984.9
  - specified type of lead — *see* Table of Drugs and Chemicals
- median nerve (tardy) 354.0
- peroneal nerve (acute) (tardy) 355.3
- progressive supranuclear 333.0
- pseudobulbar NEC 335.23

Pain(s) — Palsy

Palsy (see also Paralysis) — continued
  radial nerve (acute) 354.3
  seventh nerve 351.0
    newborn 767.5
  shaking (see also Parkinsonism) 332.0
  spastic (cerebral) (spinal) 343.9
    hemiplegic 343.1
  specified nerve NEC — see Disorder, nerve
  supranuclear NEC 356.8
    progressive 333.0
  ulnar nerve (tardy) 354.2
  wasting 335.21

Paltauf-Sternberg disease 201.9 ✓5ᵗʰ

Paludism — see Malaria

Panama fever 084.0

Panaris (with lymphangitis) 681.9
  finger 681.02
  toe 681.11

Panaritium (with lymphangitis) 681.9
  finger 681.02
  toe 681.11

Panarteritis (nodosa) 446.0
  brain or cerebral 437.4

Pancake heart 793.2
  with cor pulmonale (chronic) 416.9

Pancarditis (acute) (chronic) 429.89
  with
    rheumatic
      fever (active) (acute) (chronic) (subacute)
        391.8
        inactive or quiescent 398.99
  rheumatic, acute 391.8
    chronic or inactive 398.99

Pancoast's syndrome or tumor (carcinoma,
  pulmonary apex) (M8010/3) 162.3

Pancoast-Tobias syndrome (M8010/3)
  (carcinoma, pulmonary apex) 162.3

Pancolitis 556.6

Pancreas, pancreatic — see condition

Pancreatitis 577.0
  acute (edematous) (hemorrhagic) (recurrent)
    577.0
  annular 577.0
  apoplectic 577.0
  calcercous 577.0
  chronic (infectious) 577.1
    recurrent 577.1
  cystic 577.2
  fibrous 577.8
  gangrenous 577.0
  hemorrhagic (acute) 577.0
  interstitial (chronic) 577.1
    acute 577.0
  malignant 577.0
  mumps 072.3
  painless 577.1
  recurrent 577.1
  relapsing 577.1
  subacute 577.0
  suppurative 577.0
  syphilitic 095.8

Pancreatolithiasis 577.8

Pancytolysis 289.9

Pancytopenia (acquired) 284.8
  with malformations 284.0
  congenital 284.0

Panencephalitis — see also Encephalitis
  subacute, sclerosing 046.2

Panhematopenia 284.8
  congenital 284.0
  constitutional 284.0
  splenic, primary 289.4

Panhemocytopenia 284.8
  congenital 284.0
  constitutional 284.0

Panhypogonadism 257.2

Panhypopituitarism 253.2
  prepubertal 253.3

Panic (attack) (state) 300.01
  reaction to exceptional stress (transient) 308.0

Panmyelopathy, familial constitutional 284.0

Panmyelophthisis 284.9
  acquired (secondary) 284.8

Panmyelophthisis — continued
  congenital 284.0
  idiopathic 284.9

Panmyelosis (acute) (M9951/1) 238.7

Panner's disease 732.3
  capitellum humeri 732.3
  head of humerus 732.3
  tarsal navicular (bone) (osteochondrosis) 732.5

Panneuritis endemica 265.0 [357.4]

Panniculitis 729.30
  back 724.8
  knee 729.31
  neck 723.6
  nodular, nonsuppurative 729.30
  sacral 724.8
  specified site NEC 729.39

Panniculus adiposus (abdominal) 278.1

Pannus 370.62
  allergic eczematous 370.62
  degenerativus 370.62
  keratic 370.62
  rheumatoid — see Arthritis, rheumatoid
  trachomatosus, trachomatous (active) 076.1
    [370.62]
    late effect 139.1

Panophthalmitis 360.02

Panotitis — see Otitis media

Pansinusitis (chronic) (hyperplastic) (nonpurulent)
  (purulent) 473.8
  acute 461.8
  due to fungus NEC 117.9
  tuberculous (see also Tuberculosis) 012.8 ✓5ᵗʰ

Panuveitis 360.12
  sympathetic 360.11

Panvalvular disease — see Endocarditis, mitral

Papageienkrankheit 073.9

Papanicolaou smear
  cervix (screening test) V76.2
    as part of gynecological examination V72.3
    for suspected malignant neoplasm V76.2
      no disease found V71.1
    nonspecific abnormal finding 795.00 ▲
      atypical squamous cell changes of ●
        undetermined significance ●
      favor benign (ASCUS favor benign) ●
        795.01
      favor dysplasia (ASCUS favor ●
        dysplasia) 795.02
      nonspecific finding NEC 795.09 ●
      unsatisfactory 795.09 ●
  other specified site — see also Screening,
    malignant neoplasm
    for suspected malignant neoplasm — see
      also Screening, malignant neoplasm
      no disease found V71.1
    nonspecific abnormal finding 795.1
  vagina V76.47
    following hysterectomy for malignant
      condition V67.01

Papilledema 377.00
  associated with
    decreased ocular pressure 377.02
    increased intracranial pressure 377.01
    retinal disorder 377.03
  choked disc 377.00
  infectional 377.00

Papillitis 377.31
  anus 569.49
  chronic lingual 529.4
  necrotizing, kidney 584.7
  optic 377.31
  rectum 569.49
  renal, necrotizing 584.7
  tongue 529.0

Papilloma (M8050/0) — see also Neoplasm, by
  site, benign

Note — Except where otherwise indicated,
the morphological varieties of papilloma in
the list below should be coded by site as for
"Neoplasm, benign."

  acuminatum (female) (male) 078.1 ✓5ᵗʰ

Papilloma (M8050/0) — see also Neoplasm, by
  site, benign — continued
  bladder (urinary) (transitional cell) (M8120/1)
    236.7
    benign (M8120/0) 223.3
  choroid plexus (M9390/0) 225.0
    anaplastic type (M9390/3) 191.5
    malignant (M9390/3) 191.5
  ductal (M8503/0)
  dyskeratotic (M8052/0)
  epidermoid (M8052/0)
  hyperkeratotic (M8052/0)
  intracystic (M8504/0)
  intraductal (M8503/0)
  inverted (M8053/0)
  keratotic (M8052/0)
  parakeratotic (M8052/0)
  pinta (primary) 103.0
  renal pelvis (transitional cell) (M8120/1) 236.99
    benign (M8120/0) 223.1
  Schneiderian (M8121/0)
    specified site — see Neoplasm, by site,
      benign
    unspecified site 212.0
  serous surface (M8461/0)
    borderline malignancy (M8461/1)
      specified site — see Neoplasm, by site,
        uncertain behavior
      unspecified site 236.2
    specified site — see Neoplasm, by site,
      benign
    unspecified site 220
  squamous (cell) (M8052/0)
  transitional (cell) (M8120/0)
    bladder (urinary) (M8120/1) 236.7
    inverted type (M8121/1) — see Neoplasm,
      by site, uncertain behavior
    renal pelvis (M8120/1) 236.91
    ureter (M8120/1) 236.91
  ureter (transitional cell) (M8120/1) 236.91
    benign (M8120/0) 223.2
  urothelial (M8120/1) — see Neoplasm, by site,
    uncertain behavior
  verrucous (M8051/0)
  villous (M8261/1) — see Neoplasm, by site,
    uncertain behavior
  yaws, plantar or palmar 102.1

Papillomata, multiple, of yaws 102.1

Papillomatosis (M8060/0) — see also Neoplasm,
  by site, benign
  confluent and reticulate 701.8
  cutaneous 701.8
  ductal, breast 610.1
  Gougerot-Carteaud (confluent reticulate) 701.8
  intraductal (diffuse) (M8505/0) — see
    Neoplasm, by site, benign
  subareolar duct (M8506/0) 217

Papillon-Léage and Psaume syndrome
  (orodigitofacial dysostosis) 759.89

Papule 709.8
  carate (primary) 103.0
  fibrous, of nose (M8724/0) 216.3
  pinta (primary) 103.0

Papulosis, malignant 447.8

Papyraceous fetus 779.89   ▲
  complicating pregnancy 646.0 ✓5ᵗʰ

Paracephalus 759.7

Parachute mitral valve 746.5

Paracoccidioidomycosis 116.1
  mucocutaneous-lymphangitic 116.1
  pulmonary 116.1
  visceral 116.1

Paracoccidiomycosis — see
  Paracoccidioidomycosis

Paracusis 388.40

Paradentosis 523.5

Paradoxical facial movements 374.43

Paraffinoma 999.9

Paraganglioma (M8680/1)
  adrenal (M8700/0) 227.0
    malignant (M8700/3) 194.0
  aortic body (M8691/1) 237.3
    malignant (M8691/3) 194.6
  carotid body (M8692/1) 237.3
    malignant (M8692/3) 194.5

Paraganglioma — *continued*
  chromaffin (M8700/0) — *see also* Neoplasm, by site, benign
    malignant (M8700/3) — *see* Neoplasm, by site, malignant
  extra-adrenal (M8693/1)
    malignant (M8693/3)
      specified site — *see* Neoplasm, by site, malignant
      unspecified site 194.6
    specified site — *see* Neoplasm, by site, uncertain behavior
    unspecified site 237.3
  glomus jugulare (M8690/1) 237.3
    malignant (M8690/3) 194.6
  jugular (M8690/1) 237.3
    malignant (M8680/3)
      specified site — *see* Neoplasm, by site, malignant
      unspecified site 194.6
  nonchromaffin (M8693/1)
    malignant (M8693/3)
      specified site — *see* Neoplasm, by site, malignant
      unspecified site 194.6
    specified site — *see* Neoplasm, by site, uncertain behavior
    unspecified site 237.3
  parasympathetic (M8682/1)
    specified site — *see* Neoplasm, by site, uncertain behavior
    unspecified site 237.3
  specified site — *see* Neoplasm, by site, uncertain behavior
  sympathetic (M8681/1)
    specified site — *see* Neoplasm, by site, uncertain behavior
    unspecified site 237.3
  unspecified site 237.3

Parageusia 781.1
  psychogenic 306.7

Paragonimiasis 121.2

Paragranuloma, Hodgkin's (M9660/3) 201.0 ✓5ᵗʰ

Parahemophilia (*see also* Defect, coagulation) 286.3

Parakeratosis 690.8
  psoriasiformis 696.2
  variegata 696.2

Paralysis, paralytic (complete) (incomplete) 344.9
  with
    broken
      back — *see* Fracture, vertebra, by site, with spinal cord injury
      neck — *see* Fracture, vertebra, cervical, with spinal cord injury
    fracture, vertebra — *see* Fracture, vertebra, by site, with spinal cord injury
    syphilis 094.89
  abdomen and back muscles 355.9
  abdominal muscles 355.9
  abducens (nerve) 378.54
  abductor 355.9
    lower extremity 355.8
    upper extremity 354.9
  accessory nerve 352.4
  accommodation 367.51
    hysterical 300.11
  acoustic nerve 388.5
  agitans 332.0
    arteriosclerotic 332.0
  alternating 344.89
    oculomotor 344.89
  amyotrophic 335.20
  ankle 355.8
  anterior serratus 355.9
  anus (sphincter) 569.49
  apoplectic (current episode) (*see also* Disease, cerebrovascular, acute) 436
    late effect — *see* Late effect(s) (of) cerebrovascular disease
  arm 344.40
    affecting
      dominant side 344.41
      nondominant side 344.42
    both 344.2
    due to old CVA — *see* category 438 ✓4ᵗʰ

Paralysis, paralytic — *continued*
  arm — *continued*
    hysterical 300.11
    late effect — *see* Late effect(s) (of) cerebrovascular disease
    psychogenic 306.0transient 781.4
      traumatic NEC (*see also* Injury, nerve, upper limb) 955.9
  arteriosclerotic (current episode) 437.0
    late effect — *see* Late effect(s) (of) cerebrovascular disease
  ascending (spinal), acute 357.0
  associated, nuclear 344.89
  asthenic bulbar 358.0
  ataxic NEC 334.9
    general 094.1
  athetoid 333.7
  atrophic 356.9
    infantile, acute (*see also* Poliomyelitis, with paralysis) 045.1 ✓5ᵗʰ
    muscle NEC 355.9
    progressive 335.21
    spinal (acute) (*see also* Poliomyelitis, with paralysis) 045.1 ✓5ᵗʰ
  attack (*see also* Disease, cerebrovascular, acute) 436
  axillary 353.0
  Babinski-Nageotte's 344.89
  Bell's 351.0
    newborn 767.5
  Benedikt's 344.89
  birth (injury) 767.7
    brain 767.0
    intracranial 767.0
    spinal cord 767.4
  bladder (sphincter) 596.53
    neurogenic 596.54
      with cauda equina syndrome 344.61
    puerperal, postpartum, childbirth 665.5 ✓5ᵗʰ
    sensory 344.61
      with cauda equina 344.61
    spastic 344.61
      with cauda equina 344.61
  bowel, colon, or intestine (*see also* Ileus) 560.1
  brachial plexus 353.0
    due to birth injury 767.6
    newborn 767.6
  brain
    congenital — *see* Palsy, cerebral
    current episode 437.8
    diplegia 344.2
    due to previous vascular lesion — *see* category 438 ✓4ᵗʰ
    hemiplegia 342.9
      due to previous vascular lesion — *see* category 438 ✓4ᵗʰ
      late effect — *see* Late effect(s) (of) cerebrovascular disease
    infantile — *see* Palsy, cerebral
    late effect — *see* Late effect(s) (of) cerebrovascular disease
    monoplegia — *see also* Monoplegia
      due to previous vascular lesion — *see* category 438 ✓4ᵗʰ
      late effect — *see* Late effect(s) (of) cerebrovascular disease
    paraplegia 344.1
    quadriplegia — *see* Quadriplegia
    syphilitic, congenital 090.49
    triplegia 344.89
  bronchi 519.1
  Brown-Séquard's 344.89
  bulbar (chronic) (progressive) 335.22
    infantile (*see also* Poliomyelitis, bulbar) 045.0 ✓5ᵗʰ
    poliomyelitic (*see also* Poliomyelitis, bulbar) 045.0 ✓5ᵗʰ
    pseudo 335.23
    supranuclear 344.89
  bulbospinal 358.0
  cardiac (*see also* Failure, heart) 428.9
  cerebral
    current episode 437.8
    spastic, infantile — *see* Palsy, cerebral
  cerebrocerebellar 437.8
    diplegic infantile 343.0

Paralysis, paralytic — *continued*
  cervical
    plexus 353.2
    sympathetic NEC 337.0
  Céstan-Chenais 344.89
  Charcôt-Marie-Tooth type 356.1
  childhood — *see* Palsy, cerebral
  Clark's 343.9
  colon (*see also* Ileus) 560.1
  compressed air 993.3
  compression
    arm NEC 354.9
    cerebral — *see* Paralysis, brain
    leg NEC 355.8
    lower extremity NEC 355.8
    upper extremity NEC 354.9
  congenital (cerebral) (spastic) (spinal) — *see* Palsy, cerebral
  conjugate movement (of eye) 378.81
    cortical (nuclear) (supranuclear) 378.81
  convergence 378.83
  cordis (*see also* Failure, heart) 428.9
  cortical (*see also* Paralysis, brain) 437.8
  cranial or cerebral nerve (*see also* Disorder, nerve, cranial) 352.9
  creeping 335.21
  crossed leg 344.89
  crutch 953.4
  deglutition 784.9
    hysterical 300.11
  dementia 094.1
  descending (spinal) NEC 335.9
  diaphragm (flaccid) 519.4
    due to accidental section of phrenic nerve during procedure 998.2
  digestive organs NEC 564.89
  diplegic — *see* Diplegia
  divergence (nuclear) 378.85
  divers' 993.3
  Duchenne's 335.22
  due to intracranial or spinal birth injury — *see* Palsy, cerebral
  embolic (current episode) (*see also* Embolism, brain) 434.1 ✓5ᵗʰ
    late effect — *see* Late effect(s) (of) cerebrovascular disease
  enteric (*see also* Ileus) 560.1
    with hernia — *see* Hernia, by site, with obstruction
  Erb's syphilitic spastic spinal 094.89
  Erb (-Duchenne) (birth) (newborn) 767.6
  esophagus 530.8 ✓5ᵗʰ
  essential, infancy (*see also* Poliomyelitis) 045.9 ✓5ᵗʰ
  extremity
    lower — *see* Paralysis, leg
    spastic (hereditary) 343.3
      noncongenital or noninfantile 344.1
    transient (cause unknown) 781.4
    upper — *see* Paralysis, arm
  eye muscle (extrinsic) 378.55
    intrinsic 367.51
  facial (nerve) 351.0
    birth injury 767.5
    congenital 767.5
    following operation NEC 998.2
    newborn 767.5
  familial 359.3
    periodic 359.3
    spastic 334.1
  fauces 478.29
  finger NEC 354.9
  foot NEC 355.8
  gait 781.2
  gastric nerve 352.3
  gaze 378.81
  general 094.1
    ataxic 094.1
    insane 094.1
    juvenile 090.40
    progressive 094.1
    tabetic 094.1
  glossopharyngeal (nerve) 352.2
  glottis (*see also* Paralysis, vocal cord) 478.30
  gluteal 353.4
  Gubler (-Millard) 344.89
  hand 354.9
    hysterical 300.11

Paralysis, paralytic — *continued*
  hand — *continued*
    psychogenic 306.0
  heart (*see also* Failure, heart) 428.9
  hemifacial, progressive 349.89
  hemiplegic — *see* Hemiplegia
  hyperkalemic periodic (familial) 359.3
  hypertensive (current episode) 437.8
  hypoglossal (nerve) 352.5
  hypokalemic periodic 359.3
  Hyrtl's sphincter (rectum) 569.49
  hysterical 300.11
  ileus (*see also* Ileus) 560.1
  infantile (*see also* Poliomyelitis) 045.9 ☑5ᵗʰ
    atrophic acute 045.1 ☑5ᵗʰ
    bulbar 045.0 ☑5ᵗʰ
    cerebral — *see* Palsy, cerebral
    paralytic 045.1 ☑5ᵗʰ
    progressive acute 045.9 ☑5ᵗʰ
    spastic — *see* Palsy, cerebral
    spinal 045.9 ☑5ᵗʰ
  infective (*see also* Poliomyelitis) 045.9 ☑5ᵗʰ
  inferior nuclear 344.9
  insane, general or progressive 094.1
  internuclear 378.86
  interosseous 355.9
  intestine (*see also* Ileus) 560.1
  intracranial (current episode) (*see also* Paralysis, brain) 437.8
    due to birth injury 767.0
  iris 379.49
    due to diphtheria (toxin) 032.81 *[379.49]*
  ischemic, Volkmann's (complicating trauma) 958.6
  Jackson's 344.8 ☑5ᵗʰ
  jake 357.7
  Jamaica ginger (jake) 357.7
  juvenile general 090.40
  Klumpke (-Déjérine) (birth) (newborn) 767.6
  labioglossal (laryngeal) (pharyngeal) 335.22
  Landry's 357.0
  laryngeal nerve (recurrent) (superior) (*see also* Paralysis, vocal cord) 478.30
  larynx (*see also* Paralysis, vocal cord) 478.30
    due to diphtheria (toxin) 032.3
  late effect
    due to
      birth injury, brain or spinal (cord) — *see* Palsy, cerebral
      edema, brain or cerebral — *see* Paralysis, brain
    lesion
      cerebrovascular — *see* category 438 ☑4ᵗʰ
        late effect — *see* Late effect(s) (of) cerebrovascular disease
      spinal (cord) — *see* Paralysis, spinal
  lateral 335.24
  lead 984.9
    specified type of lead — *see* Table of Drugs and Chemicals
  left side — *see* Hemiplegia
  leg 344.30
    affecting
      dominant side 344.31
      nondominant side 344.32
    both (*see also* Paraplegia) 344.1
    crossed 344.89
    hysterical 300.11
    psychogenic 306.0
    transient or transitory 781.4
      traumatic NEC (*see also* Injury, nerve, lower limb) 956.9
  levator palpebrae superioris 374.31
  limb NEC 344.5
    all four — *see* Quadriplegia
    quadriplegia — *see* Quadriplegia
  lip 528.5
  Lissauer's 094.1
  local 355.9
  lower limb — *see also* Paralysis, leg
    both (*see also* Paraplegia) 344.1
  lung 518.89
    newborn 770.89   ▲
  median nerve 354.1
  medullary (tegmental) 344.89

Paralysis, paralytic — *continued*
  mesencephalic NEC 344.89
    tegmental 344.89
  middle alternating 344.89
  Millard-Gubler-Foville 344.89
  monoplegic — *see* Monoplegia
  motor NEC 344.9
    cerebral — *see* Paralysis, brain
    spinal — *see* Paralysis, spinal
  multiple
    cerebral — *see* Paralysis, brain
    spinal — *see* Paralysis, spinal
  muscle (flaccid) 359.9
    due to nerve lesion NEC 355.9
    eye (extrinsic) 378.55
      intrinsic 367.51
      oblique 378.51
    iris sphincter 364.8
    ischemic (complicating trauma) (Volkmann's) 958.6
    pseudohypertrophic 359.1
  muscular (atrophic) 359.9
    progressive 335.21
  musculocutaneous nerve 354.9
  musculospiral 354.9
  nerve — *see also* Disorder, nerve
    third or oculomotor (partial) 378.51
      total 378.52
    fourth or trochlear 378.53
    sixth or abducens 378.54
    seventh or facial 351.0
      birth injury 767.5
      due to
        injection NEC 999.9
        operation NEC 997.09
      newborn 767.5
    accessory 352.4
    auditory 388.5
    birth injury 767.7
    cranial or cerebral (*see also* Disorder, nerve, cranial) 352.9
    facial 351.0
      birth injury 767.5
      newborn 767.5
    laryngeal (*see also* Paralysis, vocal cord) 478.30
    newborn 767.7
    phrenic 354.8
      newborn 767.7
    radial 354.3
      birth injury 767.6
      newborn 767.6
    syphilitic 094.89
    traumatic NEC (*see also* Injury, nerve, by site) 957.9
    trigeminal 350.9
    ulnar 354.2
  newborn NEC 767.0
  normokalemic periodic 359.3
  obstetrical, newborn 767.7
  ocular 378.9
  oculofacial, congenital 352.6
  oculomotor (nerve) (partial) 378.51
    alternating 344.89
    external bilateral 378.55
    total 378.52
  olfactory nerve 352.0
  palate 528.9
  palatopharyngolaryngeal 352.6
  paratrigeminal 350.9
  periodic (familial) (hyperkalemic) (hypokalemic) (normokalemic) (secondary) 359.3
  peripheral
    autonomic nervous system — *see* Neuropathy, peripheral, autonomic
    nerve NEC 355.9
  peroneal (nerve) 355.3
  pharynx 478.29
  phrenic nerve 354.8
  plantar nerves 355.6
  pneumogastric nerve 352.3
  poliomyelitis (current) (*see also* Poliomyelitis, with paralysis) 045.1 ☑5ᵗʰ
    bulbar 045.0 ☑5ᵗʰ
  popliteal nerve 355.3
  pressure (*see also* Neuropathy, entrapment) 355.9

Paralysis, paralytic — *continued*
  progressive 335.21
    atrophic 335.21
    bulbar 335.22
    general 094.1
    hemifacial 349.89
    infantile, acute (*see also* Poliomyelitis) 045.9 ☑5ᵗʰ
    multiple 335.20
  pseudobulbar 335.23
  pseudohypertrophic 359.1
    muscle 359.1
  psychogenic 306.0
  pupil, pupillary 379.49
  quadriceps 355.8
  quadriplegic (*see also* Quadriplegia) 344.0
  radial nerve 354.3
    birth injury 767.6
  rectum (sphincter) 569.49
  rectus muscle (eye) 378.55
  recurrent laryngeal nerve (*see also* Paralysis, vocal cord) 478.30
  respiratory (muscle) (system) (tract) 786.09
    center NEC 344.89
      fetus or newborn 770.89   ▲
    congenital 768.9
    newborn 768.9
  right side — *see* Hemiplegia
  Saturday night 354.3
  saturnine 984.9
    specified type of lead — *see* Table of Drugs and Chemicals
  sciatic nerve 355.0
  secondary — *see* Paralysis, late effect
  seizure (cerebral) (current episode) (*see also* Disease, cerebrovascular, acute) 436
    late effect — *see* Late effect(s) (of) cerebrovascular disease
  senile NEC 344.9
  serratus magnus 355.9
  shaking (*see also* Parkinsonism) 332.0
  shock (*see also* Disease, cerebrovascular, acute) 436
    late effect — *see* Late effect(s) (of) cerebrovascular disease
  shoulder 354.9
  soft palate 528.9
  spasmodic — *see* Paralysis, spastic
  spastic 344.9
    cerebral infantile — *see* Palsy, cerebral
    congenital (cerebral) — *see* Palsy, cerebral
    familial 334.1
    hereditary 334.1
    infantile 343.9
    noncongenital or noninfantile, cerebral 344.9
    syphilitic 094.0
      spinal 094.89
  sphincter, bladder (*see also* Paralysis, bladder) 596.53
  spinal (cord) NEC 344.1
    accessory nerve 352.4
    acute (*see also* Poliomyelitis) 045.9 ☑5ᵗʰ
    ascending acute 357.0
    atrophic (acute) (*see also* Poliomyelitis, with paralysis) 045.1 ☑5ᵗʰ
      spastic, syphilitic 094.89
    congenital NEC 343.9
    hemiplegic — *see* Hemiplegia
    hereditary 336.8
    infantile (*see also* Poliomyelitis) 045.9 ☑5ᵗʰ
    late effect NEC 344.89
    monoplegic — *see* Monoplegia
    nerve 355.9
    progressive 335.10
    quadriplegic — *see* Quadriplegia
    spastic NEC 343.9
    traumatic — *see* Injury, spinal, by site
  sternomastoid 352.4
  stomach 536.3
    nerve 352.3
  stroke (current episode) (*see also* Disease, cerebrovascular, acute) 436
    late effect — *see* Late effect(s) (of) cerebrovascular disease
  subscapularis 354.8
  superior nuclear NEC 334.9

Paralysis, paralytic — *continued*
  supranuclear 356.8
  sympathetic
    cervical NEC 337.0
      nerve NEC (*see also* Neuropathy, peripheral,
        autonomic) 337.9
      nervous system — *see* Neuropathy,
        peripheral, autonomic
  syndrome 344.9
    specified NEC 344.89
  syphilitic spastic spinal (Erb's) 094.89
  tabetic general 094.1
  thigh 355.8
  throat 478.29
    diphtheritic 032.0
    muscle 478.29
  thrombotic (current episode) (*see also*
      Thrombosis, brain) 434.0 ✓5ᵗʰ
    late effect — *see* Late effect(s) (of)
      cerebrovascular disease
    old — *see* category 438 ✓4ᵗʰ
  thumb NEC 354.9
  tick (-bite) 989.5
  Todd's (postepileptic transitory paralysis) 344.89
  toe 355.6
  tongue 529.8
  transient
    arm or leg NEC 781.4
    traumatic NEC (*see also* Injury, nerve, by
      site) 957.9
  trapezius 352.4
  traumatic, transient NEC (*see also* Injury,
    nerve, by site) 957.9
  trembling (*see also* Parkinsonism) 332.0
  triceps brachii 354.9
  trigeminal nerve 350.9
  trochlear nerve 378.53
  ulnar nerve 354.2
  upper limb — *see also* Paralysis, arm
    both (*see also* Diplegia) 344.2
  uremic — *see* Uremia
  uveoparotitic 135
  uvula 528.9
    hysterical 300.11
    postdiphtheritic 032.0
  vagus nerve 352.3
  vasomotor NEC 337.9
  velum palati 528.9
  vesical (*see also* Paralysis, bladder) 596.53
  vestibular nerve 388.5
  visual field, psychic 368.16
  vocal cord 478.30
    bilateral (partial) 478.33
      complete 478.34
    complete (bilateral) 478.34
    unilateral (partial) 478.31
      complete 478.32
  Volkmann's (complicating trauma) 958.6
  wasting 335.21
  Weber's 344.89
  wrist NEC 354.9
Paramedial orifice, urethrovesical 753.8
Paramenia 626.9
Parametritis (chronic) (*see also* Disease, pelvis,
    inflammatory) 614.4
  acute 614.3
  puerperal, postpartum, childbirth 670 ✓4ᵗʰ
Parametrium, parametric — *see* condition
Paramnesia (*see also* Amnesia) 780.99 ▲
Paramolar 520.1
  causing crowding 524.3
Paramyloidosis 277.3
Paramyoclonus multiplex 333.2
Paramyotonia 359.2
  congenita 359.2
Paraneoplastic syndrome — *see* condition
Parangi (*see also* Yaws) 102.9
Paranoia 297.1
  alcoholic 291.5
  querulans 297.8
  senile 290.20
Paranoid
  dementia (*see also* Schizophrenia) 295.3 ✓5ᵗʰ
    praecox (acute) 295.3 ✓5ᵗʰ
    senile 290.20

Paranoid — *continued*
  personality 301.0
  psychosis 297.9
    alcoholic 291.5
    climacteric 297.2
    drug-induced 292.11
    involutional 297.2
    menopausal 297.2
    protracted reactive 298.4
    psychogenic 298.4
      acute 298.3
    senile 290.20
  reaction (chronic) 297.9
    acute 298.3
  schizophrenia (acute) (*see also* Schizophrenia)
    295.3 ✓5ᵗʰ
  state 297.9
    alcohol-induced 291.5
    climacteric 297.2
    drug-induced 292.11
    due to or associated with
      arteriosclerosis (cerebrovascular) 290.42
      presenile brain disease 290.12
      senile brain disease 290.20
    involutional 297.2
    menopausal 297.2
    senile 290.20
    simple 297.0
    specified type NEC 297.8
  tendencies 301.0
  traits 301.0
  trends 301.0
  type, psychopathic personality 301.0
Paraparesis (*see also* Paralysis) 344.9
Paraphasia 784.3
Paraphilia (*see also* Deviation, sexual) 302.9
Paraphimosis (congenital) 605
  chancroidal 099.0
Paraphrenia, paraphrenic (late) 297.2
  climacteric 297.2
  dementia (*see also* Schizophrenia) 295.3 ✓5ᵗʰ
  involutional 297.2
  menopausal 297.2
  schizophrenia (acute) (*see also* Schizophrenia)
    295.3 ✓5ᵗʰ
Paraplegia 344.1
  with
    broken back — *see* Fracture, vertebra, by
      site, with spinal cord injury
    fracture, vertebra — *see* Fracture, vertebra,
      by site, with spinal cord injury
  ataxic — *see* Degeneration, combined, spinal
    cord
  brain (current episode) (*see also* Paralysis,
    brain) 437.8
  cerebral (current episode) (*see also* Paralysis,
    brain) 437.8
  congenital or infantile (cerebral) (spastic)
    (spinal) 343.0
  cortical — *see* Paralysis, brain
  familial spastic 334.1
  functional (hysterical) 300.11
  hysterical 300.11
  infantile 343.0
  late effect 344.1
  Pott's (*see also* Tuberculosis)
    015.0 ✓5ᵗʰ [730.88]
  psychogenic 306.0
  spastic
    Erb's spinal 094.89
    hereditary 334.1
    not infantile or congenital 344.1
  spinal (cord)
    traumatic NEC — *see* Injury, spinal, by site
    syphilitic (spastic) 094.89
  traumatic NEC — *see* Injury, spinal, by site
Paraproteinemia 273.2
  benign (familial) 273.1
  monoclonal 273.1
  secondary to malignant or inflammatory
    disease 273.1
Parapsoriasis 696.2
  en plaques 696.2
  guttata 696.2

Parapsoriasis — *continued*
  lichenoides chronica 696.2
  retiformis 696.2
  varioliformis (acuta) 696.2
Parascarlatina 057.8
Parasitic — *see also* condition
  disease NEC (*see also* Infestation, parasitic)
    136.9
    contact V01.89 ▲
    exposure to V01.89 ▲
    intestinal NEC 129
    skin NEC 134.9
  stomatitis 112.0
  sycosis 110.0
    beard 110.0
    scalp 110.0
  twin 759.4
Parasitism NEC 136.9
  intestinal NEC 129
  skin NEC 134.9
  specified — *see* Infestation
Parasitophobia 300.29
Parasomnia 780.59
  nonorganic origin 307.47
Paraspadias 752.69
Paraspasm facialis 351.8
Parathyroid gland — *see* condition
Parathyroiditis (autoimmune) 252.1
Parathyroprival tetany 252.1
Paratrachoma 077.0
Paratyphilitis (*see also* Appendicitis) 541
Paratyphoid (fever) — *see* Fever, paratyphoid
Paratyphus — *see* Fever, paratyphoid
Paraurethral duct 753.8
Para-urethritis 597.89
  gonococcal (acute) 098.0
    chronic or duration of 2 months or over
      098.2
Paravaccinia NEC 051.9
  milkers' node 051.1
Paravaginitis (*see also* Vaginitis) 616.10
Parencephalitis (*see also* Encephalitis) 323.9
  late effect — *see* category 326
Parergasia 298.9
Paresis (*see also* Paralysis) 344.9
  accommodation 367.51
  bladder (spastic) (sphincter) (*see also* Paralysis,
    bladder) 596.53
    tabetic 094.0
  bowel, colon, or intestine (*see also* Ileus) 560.1
  brain or cerebral — *see* Paralysis, brain
  extrinsic muscle, eye 378.55
  general 094.1
    arrested 094.1
    brain 094.1
    cerebral 094.1
    insane 094.1
    juvenile 090.40
      remission 090.49
    progressive 094.1
    remission (sustained) 094.1
    tabetic 094.1
  heart (*see also* Failure, heart) 428.9
  infantile (*see also* Poliomyelitis) 045.9 ✓5ᵗʰ
  insane 094.1
  juvenile 090.40
  late effect — *see* Paralysis, late effect
  luetic (general) 094.1
  peripheral progressive 356.9
  pseudohypertrophic 359.1
  senile NEC 344.9
  stomach 536.3
  syphilitic (general) 094.1
    congenital 090.40
  transient, limb 781.4
  vesical (sphincter) NEC 596.53
Paresthesia (*see also* Disturbance, sensation)
    782.0
  Berger's (paresthesia of lower limb) 782.0
  Bernhardt 355.1
  Magnan's 782.0
Paretic — *see* condition

Parinaud's
    conjunctivitis 372.02
    oculoglandular syndrome 372.02
    ophthalmoplegia 378.81
    syndrome (paralysis of conjugate upward gaze) 378.81
Parkes Weber and Dimitri syndrome
    (encephalocutaneous angiomatosis) 759.6
Parkinson's disease, syndrome, or tremor — see Parkinsonism
Parkinsonism (arteriosclerotic) (idiopathic) (primary) 332.0
    associated with orthostatic hypotension (idiopathic) (symptomatic) 333.0
    due to drugs 332.1
    secondary 332.1
    syphilitic 094.82
Parodontitis 523.4
Parodontosis 523.5
Paronychia (with lymphangitis) 681.9
    candidal (chronic) 112.3
    chronic 681.9
        candidal 112.3
        finger 681.02
        toe 681.11
    finger 681.02
    toe 681.11
    tuberculous (primary) (see also Tuberculosis) 017.0 ✓5ᵗʰ
Parorexia NEC 307.52
    hysterical 300.11
Parosmia 781.1
    psychogenic 306.7
Parotid gland — see condition
Parotiditis (see also Parotitis) 527.2
    epidemic 072.9
    infectious 072.9
Parotitis 527.2
    allergic 527.2
    chronic 527.2
    epidemic (see also Mumps) 072.9
    infectious (see also Mumps) 072.9
    noninfectious 527.2
    nonspecific toxic 527.2
    not mumps 527.2
    postoperative 527.2
    purulent 527.2
    septic 527.2
    suppurative (acute) 527.2
    surgical 527.2
    toxic 527.2
Paroxysmal — see also condition
    dyspnea (nocturnal) 786.09
Parrot's disease (syphilitic osteochondritis) 090.0
Parrot fever 073.9
Parry's disease or syndrome (exophthalmic goiter) 242.0 ✓5ᵗʰ
Parry-Romberg syndrome 349.89
Parson's disease (exophthalmic goiter) 242.0 ✓5ᵗʰ
Parsonage-Aldren-Turner syndrome 353.5
Parsonage-Turner syndrome 353.5
Pars planitis 363.21
Particolored infant 757.39
Parturition — see Delivery
Passage
    false, urethra 599.4
    of sounds or bougies (see also Attention to artificial opening) V55.9
Passive — see condition
Pasteurella septica 027.2
Pasteurellosis (see also Infection, Pasteurella) 027.2
PAT (paroxysmal atrial tachycardia) 427.0
Patau's syndrome (trisomy D) 758.1
Patch
    herald 696.3
Patches
    mucous (syphilitic) 091.3
        congenital 090.0
    smokers' (mouth) 528.6
Patellar — see condition

Patellofemoral syndrome 719.46
Patent — see also Imperfect closure
    atrioventricular ostium 745.69
    canal of Nuck 752.41
    cervix 622.5
        complicating pregnancy 654.5 ✓5ᵗʰ
            affecting fetus or newborn 761.0
    ductus arteriosus or Botalli 747.0
    Eustachian
        tube 381.7
        valve 746.89
    foramen
        Botalli 745.5
        ovale 745.5
    interauricular septum 745.5
    interventricular septum 745.4
    omphalomesenteric duct 751.0
    os (uteri) — see Patent, cervix
    ostium secundum 745.5
    urachus 753.7
    vitelline duct 751.0
Paternity testing V70.4
Paterson's syndrome (sideropenic dysphagia) 280.8
Paterson (-Brown) (-Kelly) syndrome (sideropenic dysphagia) 280.8
Paterson-Kelly syndrome or web (sideropenic dysphagia) 280.8
Pathologic, pathological — see also condition
    asphyxia 799.0
    drunkenness 291.4
    emotionality 301.3
    liar 301.7
    personality 301.9
    resorption, tooth 521.4
    sexuality (see also Deviation, sexual) 302.9
Pathology (of) — see Disease
Patterned motor discharge, idiopathic (see also Epilepsy) 345.5 ✓5ᵗʰ
Patulous — see also Patent
    anus 569.49
    Eustachian tube 381.7
Pause, sinoatrial 427.81
Pavor nocturnus 307.46
Pavy's disease 593.6
Paxton's disease (white piedra) 111.2
Payr's disease or syndrome (splenic flexure syndrome) 569.89
Pearls
    Elschnig 366.51
    enamel 520.2
Pearl-workers' disease (chronic osteomyelitis) (see also Osteomyelitis) 730.1 ✓5ᵗʰ
Pectenitis 569.49
Pectenosis 569.49
Pectoral — see condition
Pectus
    carinatum (congenital) 754.82
        acquired 738.3
        rachitic (see also Rickets) 268.0
    excavatum (congenital) 754.81
        acquired 738.3
        rachitic (see also Rickets) 268.0
    recurvatum (congenital) 754.81
        acquired 738.3
Pedatrophia 261
Pederosis 302.2
Pediculosis (infestation) 132.9
    capitis (head louse) (any site) 132.0
    corporis (body louse) (any site) 132.1
    eyelid 132.0 [373.6]
    mixed (classifiable to more than one category in 132.0-132.2) 132.3
    pubis (pubic louse) (any site) 132.2
    vestimenti 132.1
    vulvae 132.2
Pediculus (infestation) — see Pediculosis
Pedophilia 302.2
Peg-shaped teeth 520.2
Pel's crisis 094.0
Pel-Ebstein disease — see Disease, Hodgkin's
Pelade 704.01

Pelger-Huët anomaly or syndrome (hereditary hyposegmentation) 288.2
Peliosis (rheumatica) 287.0
Pelizaeus-Merzbacher
    disease 330.0
    sclerosis, diffuse cerebral 330.0
Pellagra (alcoholic or with alcoholism) 265.2
    with polyneuropathy 265.2 [357.4]
Pellagra-cerebellar-ataxia-renal aminoaciduria syndrome 270.0
Pellegrini's disease (calcification, knee joint) 726.62
Pellegrini (-Stieda) disease or syndrome (calcification, knee joint) 726.62
Pellizzi's syndrome (pineal) 259.8
Pelvic — see also condition
    congestion-fibrosis syndrome 625.5
    kidney 753.3
Pelvioectasis 591
Pelviolithiasis 592.0
Pelviperitonitis
    female (see also Peritonitis, pelvic, female) 614.5
    male (see also Peritonitis) 567.2
Pelvis, pelvic — see also condition or type
    infantile 738.6
    Nägele's 738.6
    obliquity 738.6
    Robert's 755.69
Pemphigoid 694.5
    benign, mucous membrane 694.60
        with ocular involvement 694.61
    bullous 694.5
    cicatricial 694.60
        with ocular involvement 694.61
    juvenile 694.2
Pemphigus 694.4
    benign 694.5
        chronic familial 757.39
    Brazilian 694.4
    circinatus 694.0
    congenital, traumatic 757.39
    conjunctiva 694.61
    contagiosus 684
    erythematodes 694.4
    erythematosus 694.4
    foliaceus 694.4
    frambesiodes 694.4
    gangrenous (see also Gangrene) 785.4
    malignant 694.4
    neonatorum, newborn 684
    ocular 694.61
    papillaris 694.4
    seborrheic 694.4
    South American 694.4
    syphilitic (congenital) 090.0
    vegetans 694.4
    vulgaris 694.4
    wildfire 694.4
Pendred's syndrome (familial goiter with deafmutism) 243
Pendulous
    abdomen 701.9
        in pregnancy or childbirth 654.4 ✓5ᵗʰ
            affecting fetus or newborn 763.89
    breast 611.8
Penetrating wound — see also Wound, open, by site
    with internal injury — see Injury, internal, by site, with open wound
    eyeball 871.7
        with foreign body (nonmagnetic) 871.6
            magnetic 871.5
    ocular (see also Penetrating wound, eyeball) 871.7
        adnexa 870.3
            with foreign body 870.4
        orbit 870.3
            with foreign body 870.4
Penetration, pregnant uterus by instrument
    with
        abortion — see Abortion, by type, with damage to pelvic organs

---

▟4ᵗʰ Fourth-digit Required   ▟5ᵗʰ Fifth-digit Required   ▶◀ Revised Text   ● New Line   ▲ Revised Code

Penetration, pregnant uterus by instrument — *continued*
  with — *continued*
    ectopic pregnancy (*see also* categories 633.0-633.9) 639.2
    molar pregnancy (*see also* categories 630-632) 639.2
  complication of delivery 665.1 ☑5ᵗʰ
    affecting fetus or newborn 763.89
  following
    abortion 639.2
    ectopic or molar pregnancy 639.2
Penfield's syndrome (*see also* Epilepsy) 345.5 ☑5ᵗʰ
Penicilliosis of lung 117.3
Penis — *see* condition
Penitis 607.2
Penta X syndrome 758.81
Pentalogy (of Fallot) 745.2
Pentosuria (benign) (essential) 271.8
Peptic acid disease 536.8
Peregrinating patient V65.2
Perforated — *see* Perforation
Perforation, perforative (nontraumatic)
  antrum (*see also* Sinusitis, maxillary) 473.0
  appendix 540.0
    with peritoneal abscess 540.1
  atrial septum, multiple 745.5
  attic, ear 384.22
    healed 384.81
  bile duct, except cystic (*see also* Disease, biliary) 576.3
    cystic 575.4
  bladder (urinary) 596.6
    with
      abortion — *see* Abortion, by type, with damage to pelvic organs
      ectopic pregnancy (*see also* categories 633.0-633.9) 639.2
      molar pregnancy (*see also* categories 630-632) 639.2
    following
      abortion 639.2
      ectopic or molar pregnancy 639.2
    obstetrical trauma 665.5 ☑5ᵗʰ
  bowel 569.83
    with
      abortion — *see* Abortion, by type, with damage to pelvic organs
      ectopic pregnancy (*see also* categories 633.0-633.9) 639.2
      molar pregnancy (*see also* categories 630-632) 639.2
    fetus or newborn 777.6
    following
      abortion 639.2
      ectopic or molar pregnancy 639.2
    obstetrical trauma 665.5 ☑5ᵗʰ
  broad ligament
    with
      abortion — *see* Abortion, by type, with damage to pelvic organs
      ectopic pregnancy (*see also* categories 633.0-633.9) 639.2
      molar pregnancy (*see also* categories 630-632) 639.2
    following
      abortion 639.2
      ectopic or molar pregnancy 639.2
    obstetrical trauma 665.6 ☑5ᵗʰ
  by
    device, implant, or graft — *see* Complications, mechanical
    foreign body left accidentally in operation wound 998.4
    instrument (any) during a procedure, accidental 998.2
  cecum 540.0
    with peritoneal abcess 540.1
  cervix (uteri) — *see also* Injury, internal, cervix
    with
      abortion — *see* Abortion, by type, with damage to pelvic organs
      ectopic pregnancy (*see also* categories 633.0-633.9) 639.2

Perforation, perforative — *continued*
  cervix (uteri) — *see also* Injury, internal, cervix — *continued*
    with — *continued*
      molar pregnancy (*see also* categories 630-632) 639.2
    following
      abortion 639.2
      ectopic or molar pregnancy 639.2
    obstetrical trauma 665.3 ☑5ᵗʰ
  colon 569.83
  common duct (bile) 576.3
  cornea (*see also* Ulcer, cornea) 370.00
    due to ulceration 370.06
  cystic duct 575.4
  diverticulum (*see also* Diverticula) 562.10
    small intestine 562.00
  duodenum, duodenal (ulcer) — *see* Ulcer, duodenum, with perforation
  ear drum — *see* Perforation, tympanum
  enteritis — *see* Enteritis
  esophagus 530.4
  ethmoidal sinus (*see also* Sinusitis, ethmoidal) 473.2
  foreign body (external site) — *see also* Wound, open, by site, complicated
    internal site, by ingested object — *see* Foreign body
  frontal sinus (*see also* Sinusitis, frontal) 473.1
  gallbladder or duct (*see also* Disease, gallbladder) 575.4
  gastric (ulcer) — *see* Ulcer, stomach, with perforation
  heart valve — *see* Endocarditis
  ileum (*see also* Perforation, intestine) 569.83
  instrumental
    external — *see* Wound, open, by site
    pregnant uterus, complicating delivery 665.9 ☑5ᵗʰ
    surgical (accidental) (blood vessel) (nerve) (organ) 998.2
  intestine 569.83
    with
      abortion — *see* Abortion, by type, with damage to pelvic organs
      ectopic pregnancy (*see also* categories 633.0-633.9) 639.2
      molar pregnancy (*see also* categories 630-632) 639.2
    fetus or newborn 777.6
    obstetrical trauma 665.5 ☑5ᵗʰ
    ulcerative NEC 569.83
  jejunum, jejunal 569.83
    ulcer — *see* Ulcer, gastrojejunal, with perforation
  mastoid (antrum) (cell) 383.89
  maxillary sinus (*see also* Sinusitis, maxillary) 473.0
  membrana tympani — *see* Perforation, tympanum
  nasal
    septum 478.1
      congenital 748.1
      syphilitic 095.8
    sinus (*see also* Sinusitis) 473.9
      congenital 748.1
  palate (hard) 526.89
    soft 528.9
      syphilitic 095.8
        syphilitic 095.8
  palatine vault 526.89
    syphilitic 095.8
      congenital 090.5
  pelvic
    floor
      with
        abortion — *see* Abortion, by type, with damage to pelvic organs
        ectopic pregnancy (*see also* categories 633.0-633.9) 639.2
        molar pregnancy (*see also* categories 630-632) 639.2
      obstetrical trauma 664.1 ☑5ᵗʰ
    organ
      with
        abortion — *see* Abortion, by type, with damage to pelvic organs

Perforation, perforative — *continued*
  pelvic — *continued*
    organ — *continued*
      with — *continued*
        ectopic pregnancy (*see also* categories 633.0-633.9) 639.2
        molar pregnancy (*see also* categories 630-632) 639.2
      following
        abortion 639.2
        ectopic or molar pregnancy 639.2
      obstetrical trauma 665.5 ☑5ᵗʰ
  perineum — *see* Laceration, perineum
  periurethral tissue
    with
      abortion — *see* Abortion, by type, with damage to pelvic organs
      ectopic pregnancy (*see also* categories 630-632) 639.2
      molar pregnancy (*see also* categories 630-632) 639.2
  pharynx 478.29
  pylorus, pyloric (ulcer) — *see* Ulcer, stomach, with perforation
  rectum 569.49
  sigmoid 569.83
  sinus (accessory) (chronic) (nasal) (*see also* Sinusitis) 473.9
  sphenoidal sinus (*see also* Sinusitis, sphenoidal) 473.3
  stomach (due to ulcer) — *see* Ulcer, stomach, with perforation
  surgical (accidental) (by instrument) (blood vessel) (nerve) (organ) 998.2
  traumatic
    external — *see* Wound, open, by site
    eye (*see also* Penetrating wound, ocular) 871.7
    internal organ — *see* Injury, internal, by site
  tympanum (membrane) (persistent posttraumatic) (postinflammatory) 384.20
    with
      otitis media — *see* Otitis media
    attic 384.22
    central 384.21
    healed 384.81
    marginal NEC 384.23
    multiple 384.24
    pars flaccida 384.22
    total 384.25
    traumatic — *see* Wound, open, ear, drum
  typhoid, gastrointestinal 002.0
  ulcer — *see* Ulcer, by site, with perforation
  ureter 593.89
  urethra
    with
      abortion — *see* Abortion, by type, with damage to pelvic organs
      ectopic pregnancy (*see also* categories 633.0-633.9) 639.2
      molar pregnancy (*see also* categories 630-632) 639.2
    following
      abortion 639.2
      ectopic or molar pregnancy 639.2
    obstetrical trauma 665.5 ☑5ᵗʰ
  uterus — *see also* Injury, internal, uterus
    with
      abortion — *see* Abortion, by type, with damage to pelvic organs
      ectopic pregnancy (*see also* categories 633.0-633.9) 639.2
      molar pregnancy (*see also* categories 630-632) 639.2
    by intrauterine contraceptive device 996.32
    following
      abortion 639.2
      ectopic or molar pregnancy 639.2
    obstetrical trauma — *see* Injury, internal, uterus, obstetrical trauma
  uvula 528.9
    syphilitic 095.8
  vagina — *see* Laceration, vagina
  viscus NEC 799.8
    traumatic 868.00
      with open wound into cavity 868.10
Periadenitis mucosa necrotica recurrens 528.2

Periangiitis 446.0
Periantritis 535.4 ✓5ᵗʰ
Periappendicitis (acute) (*see also* Appendicitis) 541
Periarteritis (disseminated) (infectious) (necrotizing) (nodosa) 446.0
Periarthritis (joint) 726.90
  Duplay's 726.2
  gonococcal 098.50
  humeroscapularis 726.2
  scapulohumeral 726.2
  shoulder 726.2
  wrist 726.4
Periarthrosis (angioneural) — *see* Periarthritis
Peribronchitis 491.9
  tuberculous (*see also* Tuberculosis) 011.3 ✓5ᵗʰ
Pericapsulitis, adhesive (shoulder) 726.0
Pericarditis (granular) (with decompensation) (with effusion) 423.9
  with
    rheumatic fever (conditions classifiable to 390)
      active (*see also* Pericarditis, rheumatic) 391.0
      inactive or quiescent 393
  actinomycotic 039.8 *[420.0]*
  acute (nonrheumatic) 420.90
    with chorea (acute) (rheumatic) (Sydenham's) 392.0
    bacterial 420.99
    benign 420.91
    hemorrhagic 420.90
    idiopathic 420.91
    infective 420.90
    nonspecific 420.91
    rheumatic 391.0
      with chorea (acute) (rheumatic) (Sydenham's) 392.0
    sicca 420.90
    viral 420.91
  adhesive or adherent (external) (internal) 423.1
    acute — *see* Pericarditis, acute
    rheumatic (external) (internal) 393
  amebic 006.8 *[420.0]*
  bacterial (acute) (subacute) (with serous or seropurulent effusion) 420.99
  calcareous 423.2
  cholesterol (chronic) 423.8
    acute 420.90
  chronic (nonrheumatic) 423.8
    rheumatic 393
  constrictive 423.2
  Coxsackie 074.21
  due to
    actinomycosis 039.8 *[420.0]*
    amebiasis 006.8 *[420.0]*
    Coxsackie (virus) 074.21
    histoplasmosis (*see also* Histoplasmosis) 115.93
    nocardiosis 039.8 *[420.0]*
    tuberculosis (*see also* Tuberculosis) 017.9 ✓5ᵗʰ *[420.0]*
  fibrinocaseous (*see also* Tuberculosis) 017.9 ✓5ᵗʰ *[420.0]*
  fibrinopurulent 420.99
  fibrinous — *see* Pericarditis, rheumatic
  fibropurulent 420.99
  fibrous 423.1
  gonococcal 098.83
  hemorrhagic 423.0
  idiopathic (acute) 420.91
  infective (acute) 420.90
  meningococcal 036.41
  neoplastic (chronic) 423.8
    acute 420.90
  nonspecific 420.91
  obliterans, obliterating 423.1
  plastic 423.1
  pneumococcal (acute) 420.99
  postinfarction 411.0
  purulent (acute) 420.99
  rheumatic (active) (acute) (with effusion) (with pneumonia) 391.0
    with chorea (acute) (rheumatic) (Sydenham's) 392.0
  chronic or inactive (with chorea) 393

Pericarditis — *continued*
  septic (acute) 420.99
  serofibrinous — *see* Pericarditis, rheumatic
  staphylococcal (acute) 420.99
  streptococcal (acute) 420.99
  suppurative (acute) 420.99
  syphilitic 093.81
  tuberculous (acute) (chronic) (*see also* Tuberculosis) 017.9 ✓5ᵗʰ *[420.0]*
  uremic 585 *[420.0]*
  viral (acute) 420.91
Pericardium, pericardial — *see* condition
Pericellulitis (*see also* Cellulitis) 682.9
Pericementitis 523.4
  acute 523.3
  chronic (suppurative) 523.4
Pericholecystitis (*see also* Cholecystitis) 575.10
Perichondritis
  auricle 380.00
    acute 380.01
    chronic 380.02
  bronchus 491.9
  ear (external) 380.00
    acute 380.01
    chronic 380.02
  larynx 478.71
    syphilitic 095.8
    typhoid 002.0 *[478.71]*
  nose 478.1
  pinna 380.00
    acute 380.01
    chronic 380.02
  trachea 478.9
Periclasia 523.5
Pericolitis 569.89
Pericoronitis (chronic) 523.4
  acute 523.3
Pericystitis (*see also* Cystitis) 595.9
Pericytoma (M9150/1) — *see also* Neoplasm, connective tissue, uncertain behavior
  benign (M9150/0) — *see* Neoplasm, connective tissue, benign
  malignant (M9150/3) — *see* Neoplasm, connective tissue, malignant
Peridacryocystitis, acute 375.32
Peridiverticulitis (*see also* Diverticulitis) 562.11
Periduodenitis 535.6 ✓5ᵗʰ
Periendocarditis (*see also* Endocarditis) 424.90
  acute or subacute 421.9
Periepididymitis (*see also* Epididymitis) 604.90
Perifolliculitis (abscedens) 704.8
  capitis, abscedens et suffodiens 704.8
  dissecting, scalp 704.8
  scalp 704.8
  superficial pustular 704.8
Perigastritis (acute) 535.0 ✓5ᵗʰ
Perigastrojejunitis (acute) 535.0 ✓5ᵗʰ
Perihepatitis (acute) 573.3
  chlamydial 099.56
  gonococcal 098.86
Peri-ileitis (subacute) 569.89
Perilabyrinthitis (acute) — *see* Labyrinthitis
Perimeningitis — *see* Meningitis
Perimetritis (*see also* Endometritis) 615.9
Perimetrosalpingitis (*see also* Salpingo-oophoritis) 614.2
Perinephric — *see* condition
Perinephritic — *see* condition
Perinephritis (*see also* Infection, kidney) 590.9
  purulent (*see also* Abscess, kidney) 590.2
Perineum, perineal — *see* condition
Perineuritis NEC 729.2
Periodic — *see also* condition
  disease (familial) 277.3
  edema 995.1
    hereditary 277.6
  fever 277.3
  paralysis (familial) 359.3
  peritonitis 277.3
  polyserositis 277.3
  somnolence 347

Periodontal
  cyst 522.8
  pocket 523.8
Periodontitis (chronic) (complex) (compound) (local) (simplex) 523.4
  acute 523.3
  apical 522.6
    acute (pulpal origin) 522.4
Periodontoclasia 523.5
Periodontosis 523.5
Periods — *see also* Menstruation
  heavy 626.2
  irregular 626.4
Perionychia (with lymphangitis) 681.9
  finger 681.02
  toe 681.11
Perioophoritis (*see also* Salpingo-oophoritis) 614.2
Periorchitis (*see also* Orchitis) 604.90
Periosteum, periosteal — *see* condition
Periostitis (circumscribed) (diffuse) (infective) 730.3 ✓5ᵗʰ

> *Note — Use the following fifth-digit subclassification with category 730:*
>
> 0   *site unspecified*
> 1   *shoulder region*
> 2   *upper arm*
> 3   *forearm*
> 4   *hand*
> 5   *pelvic region and thigh*
> 6   *lower leg*
> 7   *ankle and foot*
> 8   *other specified sites*
> 9   *multiple sites*

  with osteomyelitis (*see also* Osteomyelitis) 730.2 ✓5ᵗʰ
    acute or subacute 730.0 ✓5ᵗʰ
    chronic or old 730.1 ✓5ᵗʰ
  albuminosa, albuminosus 730.3 ✓5ᵗʰ
  alveolar 526.5
  alveolodental 526.5
  dental 526.5
  gonorrheal 098.89
  hyperplastica, generalized 731.2
  jaw (lower) (upper) 526.4
  monomelic 733.99
  orbital 376.02
  syphilitic 095.5
    congenital 090.0 *[730.8]* ✓5ᵗʰ
    secondary 091.61
  tuberculous (*see also* Tuberculosis, bone) 015.9 ✓5ᵗʰ *[730.8]* ✓5ᵗʰ
  yaws (early) (hypertrophic) (late) 102.6
Periostosis (*see also* Periostitis) 730.3 ✓5ᵗʰ
  with osteomyelitis (*see also* Osteomyelitis) 730.2 ✓5ᵗʰ
    acute or subacute 730.0 ✓5ᵗʰ
    chronic or old 730.1 ✓5ᵗʰ
  hyperplastic 756.59
Periphlebitis (*see also* Phlebitis) 451.9
  lower extremity 451.2
    deep (vessels) 451.19
    superficial (vessels) 451.0
  portal 572.1
  retina 362.18
  superficial (vessels) 451.0
  tuberculous (*see also* Tuberculosis) 017.9 ✓5ᵗʰ
    retina 017.3 ✓5ᵗʰ *[362.18]*
Peripneumonia — *see* Pneumonia
Periproctitis 569.49
Periprostatitis (*see also* Prostatitis) 601.9
Perirectal — *see* condition
Perirenal — *see* condition
Perisalpingitis (*see also* Salpingo-oophoritis) 614.2
Perisigmoiditis 569.89
Perisplenitis (infectional) 289.59
Perispondylitis — *see* Spondylitis
Peristalsis reversed or visible 787.4

Peritendinitis (see also Tenosynovitis) 726.90
  adhesive (shoulder) 726.0
Perithelioma (M9150/1) — see Pericytoma
Peritoneum, peritoneal — see also condition
  equilibration test V56.32
Peritonitis (acute) (adhesive) (fibrinous)
  (hemorrhagic) (idiopathic) (localized)
  (perforative) (primary) (with adhesions) (with
  effusion) 567.9
  with or following
    abortion — see Abortion, by type, with
      sepsis
    abscess 567.2
    appendicitis 540.0
      with peritoneal abcess 540.1
    ectopic pregnancy (see also categories
      633.0-633.9) 639.0
    molar pregnancy (see also categories 630-
      632) 639.0
  aseptic 998.7
  bacterial 567.2
  bile, biliary 567.8
  chemical 998.7
  chlamydial 099.56
  chronic proliferative 567.8
  congenital NEC 777.6
  diaphragmatic 567.2
  diffuse NEC 567.2
  diphtheritic 032.83
  disseminated NEC 567.2
  due to
    bile 567.8
    foreign
      body or object accidentally left during a
        procedure (instrument) (sponge)
        (swab) 998.4
      substance accidentally left during a
        procedure (chemical) (powder) (talc)
        998.7
    talc 998.7
    urine 567.8
  fibrinopurulent 567.2
  fibrinous 567.2
  fibrocaseous (see also Tuberculosis) 014.0 ✓5ᵗʰ
  fibropurulent 567.2
  general, generalized (acute) 567.2
  gonococcal 098.86
  in infective disease NEC 136.9 [567.0]
  meconium (newborn) 777.6
  pancreatic 577.8
  paroxysmal, benign 277.3
  pelvic
    female (acute) 614.5
      chronic NEC 614.7
        with adhesions 614.6
      puerperal, postpartum, childbirth
        670 ✓4ᵗʰ
    male (acute) 567.2
  periodic (familial) 277.3
  phlegmonous 567.2
  pneumococcal 567.1
  postabortal 639.0
  proliferative, chronic 567.8
  puerperal, postpartum, childbirth 670 ✓4ᵗʰ
  purulent 567.2
  septic 567.2
  staphylococcal 567.2
  streptococcal 567.2
  subdiaphragmatic 567.2
  subphrenic 567.2
  suppurative 567.2
  syphilitic 095.2
    congenital 090.0 [567.0]
  talc 998.7
  tuberculous (see also Tuberculosis) 014.0 ✓5ᵗʰ
  urine 567.8
Peritonsillar — see condition
Peritonsillitis 475
Perityphlitis (see also Appendicitis) 541
Periureteritis 593.89
Periurethral — see condition
Periurethritis (gangrenous) 597.89
Periuterine — see condition
Perivaginitis (see also Vaginitis) 616.10
Perivasculitis, retinal 362.18

Perivasitis (chronic) 608.4
Periventricular leukomalacia 779.7
Perivesiculitis (seminal) (see also Vesiculitis)
  608.0
Perlèche 686.8
  due to
    moniliasis 112.0
    riboflavin deficiency 266.0
Pernicious — see condition
Pernio, perniosis 991.5
Persecution
  delusion 297.9
  social V62.4
Perseveration (tonic) 784.69
Persistence, persistent (congenital) 759.89
  anal membrane 751.2
  arteria stapedia 744.04
  atrioventricular canal 745.69
  bloody ejaculate 792.2
  branchial cleft 744.41
  bulbus cordis in left ventricle 745.8
  canal of Cloquet 743.51
  capsule (opaque) 743.51
  cilioretinal artery or vein 743.51
  cloaca 751.5
  communication — see Fistula, congenital
  convolutions
    aortic arch 747.21
    fallopian tube 752.19
    oviduct 752.19
    uterine tube 752.19
  double aortic arch 747.21
  ductus
    arteriosus 747.0
    Botalli 747.0
  fetal
    circulation 747.83   ▲
    form of cervix (uteri) 752.49
    hemoglobin (hereditary) ("Swiss variety")
      282.7
    pulmonary hypertension 747.83 ▲
  foramen
    Botalli 745.5
    ovale 745.5
  Gartner's duct 752.11
  hemoglobin, fetal (hereditary) (HPFH) 282.7
  hyaloid
    artery (generally incomplete) 743.51
    system 743.51
  hymen (tag)
    in pregnancy or childbirth 654.8 ✓5ᵗʰ
      causing obstructed labor 660.2 ✓5ᵗʰ
  lanugo 757.4
  left
    posterior cardinal vein 747.49
    root with right arch of aorta 747.21
    superior vena cava 747.49
  Meckel's diverticulum 751.0
  mesonephric duct 752.8
    fallopian tube 752.11
  mucosal disease (middle ear) (with posterior or
    superior marginal perforation of ear
    drum) 382.2
  nail(s), anomalous 757.5
  occiput, anterior or posterior 660.3 ✓5ᵗʰ
    fetus or newborn 763.1
  omphalomesenteric duct 751.0
  organ or site NEC — see Anomaly, specified
    type NEC
  ostium
    atrioventriculare commune 745.69
    primum 745.61
    secundum 745.5
  ovarian rests in fallopian tube 752.19
  pancreatic tissue in intestinal tract 751.5
  primary (deciduous)
    teeth 520.6
    vitreous hyperplasia 743.51
  pulmonary hypertension 747.83   ▲
  pupillary membrane 743.46
    iris 743.46
  Rhesus (Rh) titer 999.7
  right aortic arch 747.21
  sinus
    urogenitalis 752.8

Persistence, persistent — continued
  sinus — continued
    venosus with imperfect incorporation in
      right auricle 747.49
  thymus (gland) 254.8
    hyperplasia 254.0
  thyroglossal duct 759.2
  thyrolingual duct 759.2
  truncus arteriosus or communis 745.0
  tunica vasculosa lentis 743.39
  umbilical sinus 753.7
  urachus 753.7
  vegetative state 780.03
  vitelline duct 751.0
  wolffian duct 752.8
Person (with)
  admitted for clinical research, as participant or
    control subject V70.7
  awaiting admission to adequate facility
    elsewhere V63.2
    undergoing social agency investigation V63.8
  concern (normal) about sick person in family
    V61.49
  consulting on behalf of another V65.1
  feared
    complaint in whom no diagnosis was made
      V65.5
    condition not demonstrated V65.5
  feigning illness V65.2
  healthy, accompanying sick person V65.0
  living (in)
    alone V60.3
    boarding school V60.6
    residence remote from hospital or medical
      care facility V63.0
    residential institution V60.6
    without
      adequate
        financial resources V60.2
        housing (heating) (space) V60.1
      housing (permanent) (temporary) V60.0
      material resources V60.2
      person able to render necessary care
        V60.4
      shelter V60.0
  medical services in home not available V63.1
  on waiting list V63.2
    undergoing social agency investigation V63.8
  sick or handicapped in family V61.49
  "worried well" V65.5
Personality
  affective 301.10
  aggressive 301.3
  amoral 301.7
  anancastic, anankastic 301.4
  antisocial 301.7
  asocial 301.7
  asthenic 301.6
  avoidant 301.82
  borderline 301.83
  change 310.1
  compulsive 301.4
  cycloid 301.13
  cyclothymic 301.13
  dependent 301.6
  depressive (chronic) 301.12
  disorder, disturbance NEC 301.9
    with
      antisocial disturbance 301.7
      pattern disturbance NEC 301.9
      sociopathic disturbance 301.7
      trait disturbance 301.9
  dual 300.14
  dyssocial 301.7
  eccentric 301.89
    "haltlose" type 301.89
  emotionally unstable 301.59
  epileptoid 301.3
  explosive 301.3
  fanatic 301.0
  histrionic 301.50
  hyperthymic 301.11
  hypomanic 301.11
  hypothymic 301.12
  hysterical 301.50
  immature 301.89
  inadequate 301.6

Personality — *continued*
labile 301.59
masochistic 301.89
morally defective 301.7
multiple 300.14
narcissistic 301.81
obsessional 301.4
obsessive (-compulsive) 301.4
overconscientious 301.4
paranoid 301.0
passive (-dependent) 301.6
passive-aggressive 301.84
pathologic NEC 301.9
pattern defect or disturbance 301.9
pseudosocial 301.7
psychoinfantile 301.59
psychoneurotic NEC 301.89
psychopathic 301.9
  with
    amoral trend 301.7
    antisocial trend 301.7
    asocial trend 301.7
    pathologic sexuality (*see also* Deviation, sexual) 302.9
  mixed types 301.9
schizoid 301.20
  introverted 301.21
  schizotypal 301.22
  with sexual deviation (*see also* Deviation, sexual) 302.9
    antisocial 301.7
    dyssocial 301.7
type A 301.4
unstable (emotional) 301.59
Perthes' disease (capital femoral osteochondrosis) 732.1
Pertussis (*see also* Whooping cough) 033.9
vaccination, prophylactic (against) V03.6
Peruvian wart 088.0
Perversion, perverted
appetite 307.52
  hysterical 300.11
function
  pineal gland 259.8
  pituitary gland 253.9
    anterior lobe
      deficient 253.2
      excessive 253.1
    posterior lobe 253.6
  placenta — *see* Placenta, abnormal
sense of smell or taste 781.1
  psychogenic 306.7
sexual (*see also* Deviation, sexual) 302.9
Pervious, congenital — *see also* Imperfect, closure
ductus arteriosus 747.0
Pes (congenital) (*see also* Talipes) 754.70
abductus (congenital) 754.60
  acquired 736.79
acquired NEC 736.79
  planus 734
adductus (congenital) 754.79
  acquired 736.79
cavus 754.71
  acquired 736.73
planovalgus (congenital) 754.69
  acquired 736.79
planus (acquired) (any degree) 734
  congenital 754.61
  rachitic 268.1
valgus (congenital) 754.61
  acquired 736.79
varus (congenital) 754.50
  acquired 736.79
Pest (*see also* Plague) 020.9
Pestis (*see also* Plague) 020.9
bubonica 020.0
fulminans 020.0
minor 020.8
pneumonica — *see* Plague, pneumonic
Petechia, petechiae 782.7
fetus or newborn 772.6
Petechial
fever 036.0
typhus 081.9

Petges-Cléjat or Petges-Clégat syndrome (poikilodermatomyositis) 710.3
Petit's
disease (*see also* Hernia, lumbar) 553.8
Petit mal (idiopathic) (*see also* Epilepsy) 345.0 ☑5th
status 345.2
Petrellidosis 117.6
Petrositis 383.20
acute 383.21
chronic 383.22
Peutz-Jeghers disease or syndrome 759.6
Peyronie's disease 607.89
Pfeiffer's disease 075
Phacentocele 379.32
traumatic 921.3
Phacoanaphylaxis 360.19
Phacocele (old) 379.32
traumatic 921.3
Phaehyphomycosis 117.8
Phagedena (dry) (moist) (*see also* Gangrene) 785.4
arteriosclerotic 440.2 ☑5th [785.4]
geometric 686.09
penis 607.89
senile 440.2 ☑5th [785.4]
sloughing 785.4
tropical (*see also* Ulcer, skin) 707.9
vulva 616.50
Phagedenic — *see also* condition
abscess — *see also* Abscess
  chancroid 099.0
bubo NEC 099.8
chancre 099.0
ulcer (tropical) (*see also* Ulcer, skin) 707.9
Phagomania 307.52
Phakoma 362.89
Phantom limb (syndrome) 353.6
Pharyngeal — *see also* condition
arch remnant 744.41
pouch syndrome 279.11
Pharyngitis (acute) (catarrhal) (gangrenous) (infective) (malignant) (membranous) (phlegmonous) (pneumococcal) (pseudomembranous) (simple) (staphylococcal) (subacute) (suppurative) (ulcerative) (viral) 462
with influenza, flu, or grippe 487.1
aphthous 074.0
atrophic 472.1
chronic 472.1
chlamydial 099.51
coxsackie virus 074.0
diphtheritic (membranous) 032.0
follicular 472.1
fusospirochetal 101
gonococcal 098.6
granular (chronic) 472.1
herpetic 054.79
hypertrophic 472.1
infectional, chronic 472.1
influenzal 487.1
lymphonodular, acute 074.8
septic 034.0
streptococcal 034.0
tuberculous (*see also* Tuberculosis) 012.8 ☑5th
vesicular 074.0
Pharyngoconjunctival fever 077.2
Pharyngoconjunctivitis, viral 077.2
Pharyngolaryngitis (acute) 465.0
chronic 478.9
septic 034.0
Pharyngoplegia 478.29
Pharyngotonsillitis 465.8
tuberculous 012.8 ☑5th
Pharyngotracheitis (acute) 465.8
chronic 478.9
Pharynx, pharyngeal — *see* condition
Phase of life problem NEC V62.89
Phenomenon
Arthus' — *see* Arthus' phenomenon
flashback (drug) 292.89
jaw-winking 742.8
Jod-Basedow 242.8 ☑5th
L. E. cell 710.0
lupus erythematosus cell 710.0

Phenomenon — *continued*
Pelger-Huët (hereditary hyposegmentation) 288.2
Raynaud's (paroxysmal digital cyanosis) (secondary) 443.0
Reilly's (*see also* Neuropathy, peripheral, autonomic) 337.9
vasomotor 780.2
vasospastic 443.9
vasovagal 780.2
Wenckebach's, heart block (second degree) 426.13
Phenylketonuria (PKU) 270.1
Phenylpyruvicaciduria 270.1
Pheochromoblastoma (M8700/3)
specified site — *see* Neoplasm, by site, malignant
unspecified site 194.0
Pheochromocytoma (M8700/0)
malignant (M8700/3)
  specified site — *see* Neoplasm, by site, malignant
  unspecified site 194.0
specified site — *see* Neoplasm, by site, benign
unspecified site 227.0
Phimosis (congenital) 605
chancroidal 099.0
due to infection 605
Phlebectasia (*see also* Varicose, vein) 454.9
congenital 747.6 ☑5th
esophagus (*see also* Varix, esophagus) 456.1
  with hemorrhage (*see also* Varix, esophagus, bleeding) 456.0
Phlebitis (infective) (pyemic) (septic) (suppurative) 451.9
antecubital vein 451.82
arm NEC 451.84
  axillary vein 451.89
  basilic vey 451.82
  deep 451.83
  superficial 451.82
basilic vein 451.82
blue 451.19
brachial vein 451.83
breast, superficial 451.89
cavernous (venous) sinus — *see* Phlebitis, intracranial sinus
cephalic vein 451.82
cerebral (venous) sinus — *see* Phlebitis, intracranial sinus
chest wall, superficial 451.89
complicating pregnancy or puerperium 671.9 ☑5th
  affecting fetus or newborn 760.3
cranial (venous) sinus — *see* Phlebitis, intracranial sinus
deep (vessels) 451.19
  femoral vein 451.11
  specified vessel NEC 451.19
due to implanted device — *see* Complications, due to (presence of) any device, implant or graft classified to 996.0-996.5 NEC
during or resulting from a procedure 997.2
femoral vein (deep) 451.11
femoropopliteal 451.0
following infusion, perfusion, or transfusion 999.2
gouty 274.89 [451.9]
hepatic veins 451.89
iliac vein 451.81
iliofemoral 451.11
intracranial sinus (any) (venous) 325
  late effect — *see* category 326
  nonpyogenic 437.6
    in pregnancy or puerperium 671.5 ☑5th
jugular vein 451.89
lateral (venous) sinus — *see* Phlebitis, intracranial sinus
leg 451.2
  deep (vessels) 451.19
    femoral vein 451.11
    specified vessel NEC 451.19
  superficial (vessels) 451.0
    femoral vein 451.11
longitudinal sinus — *see* Phlebitis, intracranial sinus

Phlebitis — *continued*
  lower extremity 451.2
    deep (vessels) 451.19
      femoral vein 451.11
      specified vessel NEC 451.19
    superficial (vessels) 451.0
      femoral vein 451.11
    migrans, migrating (superficial) 453.1
  pelvic
    with
      abortion — *see* Abortion, by type, with
        sepsis
      ectopic pregnancy (*see also* categories
        633.0-633.9) 639.0
      molar pregnancy (*see also* categories 630-
        632) 639.0
    following
      abortion 639.0
      ectopic or molar pregnancy 639.0
    puerperal, postpartum 671.4 ✓5ᵗʰ
  popliteal vein 451.19
  portal (vein) 572.1
  postoperative 997.2
  pregnancy 671.9 ✓5ᵗʰ
    deep 671.3 ✓5ᵗʰ
    specified type NEC 671.5 ✓5ᵗʰ
    superficial 671.2 ✓5ᵗʰ
  puerperal, postpartum, childbirth 671.9 ✓5ᵗʰ
    deep 671.4 ✓5ᵗʰ
    lower extremities 671.2 ✓5ᵗʰ
    pelvis 671.4 ✓5ᵗʰ
    specified site NEC 671.5 ✓5ᵗʰ
    superficial 671.2 ✓5ᵗʰ
  radial vein 451.83
  retina 362.18
  saphenous (great) (long) 451.0
    accessory or small 451.0
  sinus (meninges) — *see* Phlebitis, intracranial
    sinus
  specified site NEC 451.89
  subclavian vein 451.89
  syphilitic 093.89
  tibial vein 451.19
  ulcer, ulcerative 451.9
    leg 451.2
      deep (vessels) 451.19
        femoral vein 451.11
        specified vessel NEC 451.19
      superficial (vessels) 451.0
        femoral vein 451.11
    lower extremity 451.2
      deep (vessels) 451.19
        femoral vein 451.11
        specified vessel NEC 451.19
      superficial (vessels) 451.0
  ulnar vein 451.83
  upper extremity — *see* Phlebitis, arm
  umbilicus 451.89
  uterus (septic) (*see also* Endometritis) 615.9
  varicose (leg) (lower extremity) (*see also*
    Varicose, vein) 454.1
Phlebofibrosis 459.89
Phleboliths 459.89
Phlebosclerosis 459.89
Phlebothrombosis — *see* Thrombosis
Phlebotomus fever 066.0
Phlegm, choked on 933.1
Phlegmasia
  alba dolens (deep vessels) 451.19
    complicating pregnancy 671.3 ✓5ᵗʰ
    nonpuerperal 451.19
    puerperal, postpartum, childbirth 671.4 ✓5ᵗʰ
  cerulea dolens 451.19
Phlegmon (*see also* Abscess) 682.9
  erysipelatous (*see also* Erysipelas) 035
  iliac 682.2
    fossa 540.1
  throat 478.29
Phlegmonous — *see* condition
Phlyctenulosis (allergic) (keratoconjuctivitis)
  (nontuberculous) 370.31
  cornea 370.31
    with ulcer (*see also* Ulcer, cornea) 370.00
  tuberculous (*see also* Tuberculosis) 017.3 ✓5ᵗʰ
    [370.31]

Phobia, phobic (reaction) 300.20
  animal 300.29
  isolated NEC 300.29
  obsessional 300.3
  simple NEC 300.29
  social 300.23
  specified NEC 300.29
  state 300.20
Phocas' disease 610.1
Phocomelia 755.4
  lower limb 755.32
    complete 755.33
    distal 755.35
    proximal 755.34
  upper limb 755.22
    complete 755.23
    distal 755.25
    proximal 755.24
Phoria (*see also* Heterophoria) 378.40
Phosphate-losing tubular disorder 588.0
Phosphatemia 275.3
Phosphaturia 275.3
Photoallergic response 692.72
Photocoproporphyria 277.1
Photodermatitis (sun) 692.72
  light other than sun 692.82
Photokeratitis 370.24
Photo-ophthalmia 370.24
Photophobia 368.13
Photopsia 368.15
Photoretinitis 363.31
Photoretinopathy 363.31
Photosensitiveness (sun) 692.72
  light other than sun 692.82
Photosensitization (sun) skin 692.72
  light other than sun 692.82
Phototoxic response 692.72
Phrenitis 323.9
Phrynoderma 264.8
Phthiriasis (pubis) (any site) 132.2
  with any infestation classifiable to 132.0, 132.1
    and 132.3
Phthirus infestation — *see* Phthiriasis
Phthisis (*see also* Tuberculosis) 011.9 ✓5ᵗʰ
  bulbi (infectional) 360.41
  colliers' 011.4 ✓5ᵗʰ
  cornea 371.05
  eyeball (due to infection) 360.41
  millstone makers' 011.4 ✓5ᵗʰ
  miners' 011.4 ✓5ᵗʰ
  potters' 011.4 ✓5ᵗʰ
  sandblasters' 011.4 ✓5ᵗʰ
  stonemasons' 011.4 ✓5ᵗʰ
Phycomycosis 117.7
Physalopteriasis 127.7
Physical therapy NEC V57.1
  breathing exercises V57.0
Physiological cup, optic papilla
  borderline, glaucoma suspect 365.00
  enlarged 377.14
  glaucomatous 377.14
Phytobezoar 938
  intestine 936
  stomach 935.2
Pian (*see also* Yaws) 102.9
Pianoma 102.1
Piarhemia, piarrhemia (*see also* Hyperlipemia)
  272.4
  bilharziasis 120.9
Pica 307.52
  hysterical 300.11
Pick's
  cerebral atrophy 331.1
    with dementia
      with behavioral disturbance 331.1
        [294.11]
      without behavioral disturbance 331.1
        [294.10]

Pick's — *continued*
  disease
    brain 331.1
      dementia in
        with behavioral disturbance 331.1
          [294.11]
        without behavioral disturbance 331.1
          [294.10]
    lipid histiocytosis 272.7
    liver (pericardial pseudocirrhosis of liver) 423.2
    pericardium (pericardial pseudocirrhosis of
      liver) 423.2
    polyserositis (pericardial pseudocirrhosis of
      liver) 423.2
    syndrome
      heart (pericardial pseudocirrhosis of liver)
        423.2
      liver (pericardial pseudocirrhosis of liver)
        423.2
    tubular adenoma (M8640/0)
      specified site — *see* Neoplasm, by site,
        benign
      unspecified site
        female 220
        male 222.0
Pick-Herxheimer syndrome (diffuse idiopathic
  cutaneous atrophy) 701.8
Pick-Niemann disease (lipid histiocytosis) 272.7
Pickwickian syndrome (cardiopulmonary obesity)
  278.8
Piebaldism, classic 709.09
Piedra 111.2
  beard 111.2
    black 111.3
    white 111.2
  black 111.3
  scalp 111.3
    black 111.3
    white 111.2
  white 111.2
Pierre Marie's syndrome (pulmonary
  hypertrophic osteoarthropathy) 731.2
Pierre Marie-Bamberger syndrome (hypertrophic
  pulmonary osteoarthropathy) 731.2
Pierre Mauriac's syndrome (diabetes-dwarfism-
  obesity) 258.1
Pierre Robin deformity or syndrome (congenital)
  756.0
Pierson's disease or osteochondrosis 732.1
Pigeon
  breast or chest (acquired) 738.3
    congenital 754.82
    rachitic (*see also* Rickets) 268.0
  breeders' disease or lung 495.2
  fanciers' disease or lung 495.2
  toe 735.8
Pigmentation (abnormal) 709.00
  anomaly 709.00
    congenital 757.33
    specified NEC 709.09
  conjunctiva 372.55
  cornea 371.10
    anterior 371.11
    posterior 371.13
    stromal 371.12
  lids (congenital) 757.33
    acquired 374.52
  limbus corneae 371.10
  metals 709.00
  optic papilla, congenital 743.57
  retina (congenital) (grouped) (nevoid) 743.53
    acquired 362.74
  scrotum, congenital 757.33
Piles — *see* Hemorrhoids
Pili
  annulati or torti (congenital) 757.4
  incarnati 704.8
Pill roller hand (intrinsic) 736.09
Pilomatrixoma (M8110/0) — *see* Neoplasm, skin,
  benign
Pilonidal — *see* condition
Pimple 709.8
PIN I (prostatic intraepithelial neoplasia
  I) 602.3

PIN II (prostatic intraepithelial neoplasia II) 602.3

PIN III (prostatic intraepithelial neoplasia III) 233.4

Pinched nerve — *see* Neuropathy, entrapment

Pineal body or gland — *see* condition

Pinealoblastoma (M9362/3) 194.4

Pinealoma (M9360/1) 237.1
    malignant (M9360/3) 194.4

Pineoblastoma (M9362/3) 194.4

Pineocytoma (M9361/1) 237.1

Pinguecula 372.51

Pinhole meatus (*see also* Stricture, urethra) 598.9

Pink
    disease 985.0
    eye 372.03
    puffer 492.8

Pinkus' disease (lichen nitidus) 697.1

Pinpoint
    meatus (*see also* Stricture, urethra) 598.9
    os uteri (*see also* Stricture, cervix) 622.4

Pinselhaare (congenital) 757.4

Pinta 103.9
    cardiovascular lesions 103.2
    chancre (primary) 103.0
    erythematous plaques 103.1
    hyperchromic lesions 103.1
    hyperkeratosis 103.1
    lesions 103.9
        cardiovascular 103.2
        hyperchromic 103.1
        intermediate 103.1
        late 103.2
        mixed 103.3
        primary 103.0
        skin (achromic) (cicatricial) (dyschromic) 103.2
            hyperchromic 103.1
            mixed (achromic and hyperchromic) 103.3
    papule (primary) 103.0
    skin lesions (achromic) (cicatricial) (dyschromic) 103.2
        hyperchromic 103.1
        mixed (achromic and hyperchromic) 103.3
    vitiligo 103.2

Pintid 103.0

Pinworms (disease) (infection) (infestation) 127.4

Piry fever 066.8

Pistol wound — *see* Gunshot wound

Pit, lip (mucus), congenital 750.25

Pitchers' elbow 718.82

Pithecoid pelvis 755.69
    with disproportion (fetopelvic) 653.2 ✓5ᵗʰ
        affecting fetus or newborn 763.1
        causing obstructed labor 660.1 ✓5ᵗʰ

Pithiatism 300.11

Pitted — *see also* Pitting
    teeth 520.4

Pitting (edema) (*see also* Edema) 782.3
    lip 782.3
    nail 703.8
        congenital 757.5

Pituitary gland — *see* condition

Pituitary snuff-takers' disease 495.8

Pityriasis 696.5
    alba 696.5
    capitis 690.11
    circinata (et maculata) 696.3
    Hebra's (exfoliative dermatitis) 695.89
    lichenoides et varioliformis 696.2
    maculata (et circinata) 696.3
    nigra 111.1
    pilaris 757.39
        acquired 701.1
        Hebra's 696.4
    rosea 696.3
    rotunda 696.3
    rubra (Hebra) 695.89
        pilaris 696.4
    sicca 690.18

Pityriasis — *continued*
    simplex 690.18
    specified type NEC 696.5
    streptogenes 696.5
    versicolor 111.0
        scrotal 111.0

Placenta, placental
    ablatio 641.2 ✓5ᵗʰ
        affecting fetus or newborn 762.1
    abnormal, abnormality 656.7 ✓5ᵗʰ
        with hemorrhage 641.8 ✓5ᵗʰ
            affecting fetus or newborn 762.1
        affecting fetus or newborn 762.2
    abruptio 641.2 ✓5ᵗʰ
        affecting fetus or newborn 762.1
    accessory lobe — *see* Placenta, abnormal
    accreta (without hemorrhage) 667.0 ✓5ᵗʰ
        with hemorrhage 666.0 ✓5ᵗʰ
    adherent (without hemorrhage) 667.0 ✓5ᵗʰ
        with hemorrhage 666.0 ✓5ᵗʰ
    apoplexy — *see* Placenta, separation
    battledore — *see* Placenta, abnormal
    bilobate — *see* Placenta, abnormal
    bipartita — *see* Placenta, abnormal
    carneous mole 631
    centralis — *see* Placenta, previa
    circumvallata — *see* Placenta, abnormal
    cyst (amniotic) — *see* Placenta, abnormal
    deficiency — *see* Placenta, insufficiency
    degeneration — *see* Placenta, insufficiency
    detachment (partial) (premature) (with hemorrhage) 641.2 ✓5ᵗʰ
        affecting fetus or newborn 762.1
    dimidiata — *see* Placenta, abnormal
    disease 656.7 ✓5ᵗʰ
        affecting fetus or newborn 762.2
    duplex — *see* Placenta, abnormal
    dysfunction — *see* Placenta, insufficiency
    fenestrata — *see* Placenta, abnormal
    fibrosis — *see* Placenta, abnormal
    fleshy mole 631
    hematoma — *see* Placenta, abnormal
    hemorrhage NEC — *see* Placenta, separation
    hormone disturbance or malfunction — *see* Placenta, abnormal
    hyperplasia — *see* Placenta, abnormal
    increta (without hemorrhage) 667.0 ✓5ᵗʰ
        with hemorrhage 666.0 ✓5ᵗʰ
    infarction 656.7 ✓5ᵗʰ
        affecting fetus or newborn 762.2
    insertion, vicious — *see* Placenta, previa
    insufficiency
        affecting
            fetus or newborn 762.2
            management of pregnancy 656.5 ✓5ᵗʰ
    lateral — *see* Placenta, previa
    low implantation or insertion — *see* Placenta, previa
    low-lying — *see* Placenta, previa
    malformation — *see* Placenta, abnormal
    malposition — *see* Placenta, previa
    marginalis, marginata — *see* Placenta, previa
    marginal sinus (hemorrhage) (rupture) 641.2 ✓5ᵗʰ
        affecting fetus or newborn 762.1
    membranacea — *see* Placenta, abnormal
    multilobed — *see* Placenta, abnormal
    multipartita — *see* Placenta, abnormal
    necrosis — *see* Placenta, abnormal
    percreta (without hemorrhage) 667.0 ✓5ᵗʰ
        with hemorrhage 666.0 ✓5ᵗʰ
    polyp 674.4 ✓5ᵗʰ
    previa (central) (centralis) (complete) (lateral) (marginal) (marginalis) (partial) (partialis) (total) (with hemorrhage) 641.1 ✓5ᵗʰ
        affecting fetus or newborn 762.0
        noted
            before labor, without hemorrhage (with cesarean delivery) 641.0 ✓5ᵗʰ
            during pregnancy (without hemorrhage) 641.0 ✓5ᵗʰ
            without hemorrhage (before labor and delivery) (during pregnancy) 641.0 ✓5ᵗʰ
    retention (with hemorrhage) 666.0 ✓5ᵗʰ
        fragments, complicating puerperium (delayed hemorrhage) 666.2 ✓5ᵗʰ

Placenta, placental — *continued*
    retention — *continued*
        fragments, complicating puerperium — *continued*
            without hemorrhage 667.1 ✓5ᵗʰ
        postpartum, puerperal 666.2 ✓5ᵗʰ
        without hemorrhage 667.0 ✓5ᵗʰ
    separation (normally implanted) (partial) (premature) (with hemorrhage) 641.2 ✓5ᵗʰ
        affecting fetus or newborn 762.1
    septuplex — *see* Placenta, abnormal
    small — *see* Placenta, insufficiency
    softening (premature) — *see* Placenta, abnormal
    spuria — *see* Placenta, abnormal
    succenturiata — *see* Placenta, abnormal
    syphilitic 095.8
    transfusion syndromes 762.3
    transmission of chemical substance — *see* Absorption, chemical, through placenta
    trapped (with hemorrhage) 666.0 ✓5ᵗʰ
        without hemorrhage 667.0 ✓5ᵗʰ
    trilobate — *see* Placenta, abnormal
    tripartita — *see* Placenta, abnormal
    triplex — *see* Placenta, abnormal
    varicose vessel — *see* Placenta, abnormal
    vicious insertion — *see* Placenta, previa

Placentitis
    affecting fetus or newborn 762.7
    complicating pregnancy 658.4 ✓5ᵗʰ

Plagiocephaly (skull) 754.0

Plague 020.9
    abortive 020.8
    ambulatory 020.8
    bubonic 020.0
    cellulocutaneous 020.1
    lymphatic gland 020.0
    pneumonic 020.5
        primary 020.3
        secondary 020.4
    pulmonary — *see* Plague, pneumonic
    pulmonic — *see* Plague, pneumonic
    septicemic 020.2
    tonsillar 020.9
        septicemic 020.2
    vaccination, prophylactic (against) V03.3

Planning, family V25.09
    contraception V25.9
    procreation V26.4

Plaque
    artery, arterial — *see* Arteriosclerosis
    calcareous — *see* Calcification
    Hollenhorst's (retinal) 362.33
    tongue 528.6

Plasma cell myeloma 203.0 ✓5ᵗʰ

Plasmacytoma, plasmocytoma (solitary) (M9731/1) 238.6
    benign (M9731/0) — *see* Neoplasm, by site, benign
    malignant (M9731/3) 203.8 ✓5ᵗʰ

Plasmacytosis 288.8

Plaster ulcer (*see also* Decubitus) 707.0

Platybasia 756.0

Platyonychia (congenital) 757.5
    acquired 703.8

Platypelloid pelvis 738.6
    with disproportion (fetopelvic) 653.2 ✓5ᵗʰ
        affecting fetus or newborn 763.1
        causing obstructed labor 660.1 ✓5ᵗʰ
            affecting fetus or newborn 763.1
    congenital 755.69

Platyspondylia 756.19

Plethora 782.62
    newborn 776.4

Pleura, pleural — *see* condition

Pleuralgia 786.52

Pleurisy (acute) (adhesive) (chronic) (costal) (diaphragmatic) (double) (dry) (fetid) (fibrinous) (fibrous) (interlobar) (latent) (lung) (old) (plastic) (primary) (residual) (sicca) (sterile) (subacute) (unresolved) (with adherent pleura) 511.0

Pleurisy — *continued*
with
effusion (without mention of cause) 511.9
bacterial, nontuberculous 511.1
nontuberculous NEC 511.9
bacterial 511.1
pneumococcal 511.1
specified type NEC 511.8
staphylococcal 511.1
streptococcal 511.1
tuberculous (*see also* Tuberculosis,
pleura) 012.0 ✓5ᵗʰ
primary, progressive 010.1 ✓5ᵗʰ
influenza, flu, or grippe 487.1
tuberculosis — *see* Pleurisy, tuberculous
encysted 511.8
exudative (*see also* Pleurisy, with effusion)
511.9
bacterial, nontuberculous 511.1
fibrinopurulent 510.9
with fistula 510.0
fibropurulent 510.9
with fistula 510.0
hemorrhagic 511.8
influenzal 487.1
pneumococcal 511.0
with effusion 511.1
purulent 510.9
with fistula 510.0
septic 510.9
with fistula 510.0
serofibrinous (*see also* Pleurisy, with effusion)
511.9
bacterial, nontuberculous 511.1
seropurulent 510.9
with fistula 510.0
serous (*see also* Pleurisy, with effusion) 511.9
bacterial, nontuberculous 511.1
staphylococcal 511.0
with effusion 511.1
streptococcal 511.0
with effusion 511.1
suppurative 510.9
with fistula 510.0
traumatic (post) (current) 862.29
with open wound into cavity 862.39
tuberculous (with effusion) (*see also*
Tuberculosis, pleura) 012.0 ✓5ᵗʰ
primary, progressive 010.1 ✓5ᵗʰ
Pleuritis sicca — *see* Pleurisy
Pleurobronchopneumonia (*see also* Pneumonia,
broncho-) 485
Pleurodynia 786.52
epidemic 074.1
viral 074.1
Pleurohepatitis 573.8
Pleuropericarditis (*see also* Pericarditis) 423.9
acute 420.90
Pleuropneumonia (acute) (bilateral) (double)
(septic) (*see also* Pneumonia) 486
chronic (*see also* Fibrosis, lung) 515
Pleurorrhea (*see also* Hydrothorax) 511.8
Plexitis, brachial 353.0
Plica
knee 727.83
polonica 132.0
tonsil 474.8
Plicae dysphonia ventricularis 784.49
Plicated tongue 529.5
congenital 750.13
Plug
bronchus NEC 519.1
meconium (newborn) NEC 777.1
mucus — *see* Mucus, plug
Plumbism 984.9
specified type of lead — *see* Table of Drugs and
Chemicals
Plummer's disease (toxic nodular goiter)
242.3 ✓5ᵗʰ
Plummer-Vinson syndrome (sideropenic
dysphagia) 280.8
Pluricarential syndrome of infancy 260
Plurideficiency syndrome of infancy 260

Plus (and minus) hand (intrinsic) 736.09
PMS 625.4
Pneumathemia — *see* Air, embolism, by type
Pneumatic drill or hammer disease 994.9
Pneumatocele (lung) 518.89
intracranial 348.8
tension 492.0
Pneumatosis
cystoides intestinalis 569.89
peritonei 568.89
pulmonum 492.8
Pneumaturia 599.84
Pneumoblastoma (M8981/3) — *see* Neoplasm,
lung, malignant
Pneumocephalus 348.8
Pneumococcemia 038.2
Pneumococcus, pneumococcal — *see* condition
Pneumoconiosis (due to) (inhalation of) 505
aluminum 503
asbestos 501
bagasse 495.1
bauxite 503
beryllium 503
carbon electrode makers' 503
coal
miners' (simple) 500
workers' (simple) 500
cotton dust 504
diatomite fibrosis 502
dust NEC 504
inorganic 503
lime 502
marble 502
organic NEC 504
fumes or vapors (from silo) 506.9
graphite 503
hard metal 503
mica 502
moldy hay 495.0
rheumatoid 714.81
silica NEC 502
and carbon 500
silicate NEC 502
talc 502
Pneumocystis carinii pneumonia 136.3
Pneumocystosis 136.3
with pneumonia 136.3
Pneumoenteritis 025
Pneumohemopericardium (*see also* Pericarditis)
423.9
Pneumohemothorax (*see also* Hemothorax) 511.8
traumatic 860.4
with open wound into thorax 860.5
Pneumohydropericardium (*see also* Pericarditis)
423.9
Pneumohydrothorax (*see also* Hydrothorax)
511.8
Pneumomediastinum 518.1
congenital 770.2
fetus or newborn 770.2
Pneumomycosis 117.9
Pneumonia (acute) (Alpenstich) (benign) (bilateral)
(brain) (cerebral) (circumscribed) (congestive
) (creeping) (delayed resolution) (double)
(epidemic) (fever) (flash) (fulminant) (fungoid)
(granulomatous) (hemorrhagic) (incipient)
(infantile) (infectious) (infiltration) (insular)
(intermittent) (latent) (lobe) (migratory)
(newborn) (organized) (overwhelming)
(primary) (progressive) (pseudolobar)
(purulent) (resolved) (secondary) (senile)
(septic) (suppurative) (terminal) (true)
(unresolved) (vesicular) 486
with influenza, flu, or grippe 487.0
adenoviral 480.0
adynamic 514
alba 090.0
allergic 518.3
alveolar — *see* Pneumonia, lobar
anaerobes 482.81
anthrax 022.1 [484.5]
apex, apical — *see* Pneumonia, lobar
ascaris 127.0 [484.8]

Pneumonia — *continued*
aspiration 507.0
due to
aspiration of microorganisms
bacterial 482.9
specified type NEC 482.89
specified organism NEC 483.8
bacterial NEC 482.89
viral 480.9
specified type NEC 480.8
food (regurgitated) 507.0
gastric secretions 507.0
milk 507.0
oils, essences 507.1
solids, liquids NEC 507.8
vomitus 507.0
newborn 770.1
asthenic 514
atypical (disseminated, focal) (primary) 486
with influenza 487.0
bacillus 482.9
specified type NEC 482.89
bacterial 482.9
specified type NEC 482.89
Bacteroides (fragilis) (oralis) (melaninogenicus)
482.81
basal, basic, basilar — *see* Pneumonia, lobar
broncho-, bronchial (confluent) (croupous)
(diffuse) (disseminated) (hemorrhagic)
(involving lobes) (lobar) (terminal) 485
with influenza 487.0
allergic 518.3
aspiration (*see also* Pneumonia, aspiration)
507.0
bacterial 482.9
specified type NEC 482.89
capillary 466.19
with bronchospasm or obstruction
466.19
chronic (*see also* Fibrosis, lung) 515
congenital (infective) 770.0
diplococcal 481
Eaton's agent 483.0
Escherichia coli (E. coli) 482.82
Friedländer's bacillus 482.0
Hemophilus influenzae 482.2
hiberno-vernal 083.0 [484.8]
hypostatic 514
influenzal 487.0
inhalation (*see also* Pneumonia, aspiration)
507.0
due to fumes or vapors (chemical) 506.0
Klebsiella 482.0
lipid 507.1
endogenous 516.8
Mycoplasma (pneumoniae) 483.0
ornithosis 073.0
pleuropneumonia-like organisms (PPLO)
483.0
pneumococcal 481
Proteus 482.83
pseudomonas 482.1
specified organism NEC 483.8
bacterial NEC 482.89
staphylococcal 482.40
aureus 482.41
specified type NEC 482.49
streptococcal — *see* Pneumonia,
streptococcal
typhoid 002.0 [484.8]
viral, virus (*see also* Pneumonia, viral) 480.9
butyrivibrio (fibriosolvens) 482.81
Candida 112.4
capillary 466.19
with bronchospasm or obstruction 466.19
caseous (*see also* Tuberculosis) 011.6 ✓5ᵗʰ
catarrhal — *see* Pneumonia, broncho-central —
see Pneumonia, lobar
Chlamydia, chlamydial 483.1
pneumoniae 483.1
psittaci 073.0
specified type NEC 483.1
trachomatis 483.1
cholesterol 516.8
chronic (*see also* Fibrosis, lung) 515
Clostridium (haemolyticum) (novyi) NEC 482.81
confluent — *see* Pneumonia, broncho-

Pneumonia — *continued*
congenital (infective) 770.0
  aspiration 770.1
croupous — *see* Pneumonia, lobar
cytomegalic inclusion 078.5 *[484.1]*
deglutition (*see also* Pneumonia, aspiration)
  507.0
desquamative interstitial 516.8
diffuse — *see* Pneumonia, broncho-
diplococcal, diplococcus (broncho-) (lobar) 481
disseminated (focal) — *see* Pneumonia,
  broncho-
due to
  adenovirus 480.0
  Bacterium anitratum 482.83
  Chlamydia, chlamydial 483.1
    pneumoniae 483.1
    psittaci 073.0
    specified type NEC 483.1
    trachomatis 483.1
  coccidioidomycosis 114.0
  Diplococcus (pneumoniae) 481
  Eaton's agent 483.0
  Escherichia coli (E. coli) 482.82
  Friedländer's bacillus 482.0
  fumes or vapors (chemical) (inhalation)
    506.0
  fungus NEC 117.9 *[484.7]*
    coccidioidomycosis 114.0
  Hemophilus influenzae (H. influenzae) 482.2
  Herellea 482.83
  influenza 487.0
  Klebsiella pneumoniae 482.0
  Mycoplasma (pneumoniae) 483.0
  parainfluenza virus 480.2
  pleuropneumonia-like organism (PPLO)
    483.0
  Pneumococcus 481
  Pneumocystis carinii 136.3
  Proteus 482.83
  pseudomonas 482.1
  respiratory syncytial virus 480.1
  rickettsia 083.9 *[484.8]*
  specified
    bacteria NEC 482.89
    organism NEC 483.8
    virus NEC 480.8
  Staphylococcus 482.40
    aureus 482.41
    specified type NEC 482.49
  Streptococcus — *see also* Pneumonia,
    streptococcal
    pneumoniae 481
  virus (*see also* Pneumonia, viral) 480.9
Eaton's agent 483.0
embolic, embolism (*see also* Embolism,
  pulmonary) 415.1 ✓5ᵗʰ
eosinophilic 518.3
Escherichia coli (E. coli) 482.82
Eubacterium 482.81
fibrinous — *see* Pneumonia, lobar
fibroid (chronic)(*see also* Fibrosis, lung) 515
fibrous (*see also* Fibrosis, lung) 515
Friedländer's bacillus 482.0
Fusobacterium (nucleatum) 482.81
gangrenous 513.0
giant cell (*see also* Pneumonia, viral) 480.9
gram-negative bacteria NEC 482.83
  anaerobic 482.81
grippal 487.0
Hemophilus influenzae (bronchial) (lobar) 482.2
hypostatic (broncho-) (lobar) 514
in
  actinomycosis 039.1
  anthrax 022.1 *[484.5]*
  aspergillosis 117.3 *[484.6]*
  candidiasis 112.4
  coccidioidomycosis 114.0
  cytomegalic inclusion disease 078.5 *[484.1]*
  histoplasmosis (*see also* Histoplasmosis)
    115.95
  infectious disease NEC 136.9 *[484.8]*
  measles 055.1
  mycosis, systemic NEC 117.9 *[484.7]*
  nocardiasis, nocardiosis 039.1
  ornithosis 073.0
  pneumocystosis 136.3

Pneumonia — *continued*
in — *continued*
  psittacosis 073.0
  Q fever 083.0 *[484.8]*
  salmonellosis 003.22
  toxoplasmosis 130.4
  tularemia 021.2
  typhoid (fever) 002.0 *[484.8]*
  varicella 052.1
  whooping cough (*see also* Whooping cough)
    033.9 *[484.3]*
infective, acquired prenatally 770.0
influenzal (broncho) (lobar) (virus) 487.0
inhalation (*see also* Pneumonia, aspiration)
  507.0
  fumes or vapors (chemical) 506.0
interstitial 516.8
  with influenzal 487.0
  acute 136.3
  chronic (*see also* Fibrosis, lung) 515
  desquamative 516.8
  hypostatic 514
  lipoid 507.1
  lymphoid 516.8
  plasma cell 136.3
  pseudomonas 482.1
intrauterine (infective) 770.0
  aspiration 770.1
Klebsiella pneumoniae 482.0
Legionnaires' 482.84
lipid, lipoid (exogenous) (interstitial) 507.1
  endogenous 516.8
lobar (diplococcal) (disseminated) (double)
  (interstitial) (pneumococcal, any type) 481
  with influenza 487.0
  bacterial 482.9
    specified type NEC 482.89
  chronic (*see also* Fibrosis, lung) 515
  Escherichia coli (E. coli) 482.82
  Friedländer's bacillus 482.0
  Hemophilus influenzae (H. influenzae) 482.2
  hypostatic 514
  influenzal 487.0
  Klebsiella 482.0
  ornithosis 073.0
  Proteus 482.83
  pseudomonas 482.1
  psittacosis 073.0
  specified organism NEC 483.8
    bacterial NEC 482.89
  staphylococcal 482.40
    aureus 482.41
    specified type NEC 482.49
  streptococcal — *see* Pneumonia,
    streptococcal
  viral, virus (*see also* Pneumonia, viral) 480.9
lobular (confluent) — *see* Pneumonia, broncho-
Löffler's 518.3
massive — *see* Pneumonia, lobar
meconium 770.1
metastatic NEC 038.8 *[484.8]*
Mycoplasma (pneumoniae) 483.0
necrotic 513.0
nitrogen dioxide 506.9
orthostatic 514
parainfluenza virus 480.2
parenchymatous (*see also* Fibrosis, lung) 515
passive 514
patchy — *see* Pneumonia, broncho-
Peptococcus 482.81
Peptostreptococcus 482.81
plasma cell 136.3
pleurolobar — see Pneumonia, lobar
pleuropneumonia-like organism (PPLO) 483.0
pneumococcal (broncho) (lobar) 481
Pneumocystis (carinii) 136.3
postinfectional NEC 136.9 *[484.8]*
postmeasles 055.1
postoperative 997.3
primary atypical 486
Proprionibacterium 482.81
Proteus 482.83
pseudomonas 482.1
psittacosis 073.0
radiation 508.0
respiratory syncytial virus 480.1
resulting from a procedure 997.3
rheumatic 390 *[517.1]*

Pneumonia — *continued*
Salmonella 003.22
segmented, segmental — *see* Pneumonia,
  broncho-
Serratia (marcescens) 482.83
specified
  bacteria NEC 482.89
  organism NEC 483.8
  virus NEC 480.8
spirochetal 104.8 *[484.8]*
staphylococcal (broncho) (lobar) 482.40
  aureus 482.41
  specified type NEC 482.49
static, stasis 514
streptococcal (broncho) (lobar) NEC 482.30
  Group
    A 482.31
    B 482.32
    specified NEC 482.39
  pneumoniae 481
  specified type NEC 482.39
Streptococcus pneumoniae 481
traumatic (complication) (early) (secondary)
  958.8
tuberculous (any) (*see also* Tuberculosis)
  011.6 ✓5ᵗʰ
tularemic 021.2
TWAR agent 483.1
varicella 052.1
Veillonella 482.81
viral, virus (broncho) (interstitial) (lobar) 480.9
  with influenza, flu, or grippe 487.0
  adenoviral 480.0
  parainfluenza 480.2
  respiratory syncytial 480.1
  specified type NEC 480.8
white (congenital) 090.0
Pneumonic — *see* condition
Pneumonitis (acute) (primary) (*see also*
  Pneumonia) 486
allergic 495.9
  specified type NEC 495.8
aspiration 507.0
  due to fumes or gases 506.0
  newborn 770.1
  obstetric 668.0 ✓5ᵗʰ
chemical 506.0
  due to fumes or gases 506.0
cholesterol 516.8
chronic (*see also* Fibrosis, lung) 515
congenital rubella 771.0
due to
  fumes or vapors 506.0
  inhalation
    food (regurgitated), milk, vomitus 507.0
    oils, essences 507.1
    saliva 507.0
    solids, liquids NEC 507.8
  toxoplasmosis (acquired) 130.4
    congenital (active) 771.2 *[484.8]*
eosinophilic 518.3
fetal aspiration 770.1
hypersensitivity 495.9
interstitial (chronic) (*see also* Fibrosis, lung)
  515
  lymphoid 516.8
lymphoid, interstitial 516.8
meconium 770.1
postanesthetic
  correct substance properly administered
    507.0
  obstetric 668.0 ✓5ᵗʰ
  overdose or wrong substance given 968.4
    specified anesthetic — *see* Table of Drugs
    and Chemicals
postoperative 997.3
  obstetric 668.0 ✓5ᵗʰ
radiation 508.0
rubella, congenital 771.0
"ventilation" 495.7
wood-dust 495.8
Pneumoconiosis — *see* Pneumoconiosis
Pneumoparotid 527.8
Pneumopathy NEC 518.89
alveolar 516.9
  specified NEC 516.8

Pneumopathy NEC — *continued*
  due to dust NEC 504
  parietoalveolar 516.9
    specified condition NEC 516.8
Pneumopericarditis (*see also* Pericarditis) 423.9
  acute 420.90
Pneumopericardium — *see also* Pericarditis
  congenital 770.2
  fetus or newborn 770.2
  traumatic (post) (*see also* Pneumothorax,
    traumatic) 860.0
    with open wound into thorax 860.1
Pneumoperitoneum 568.89
  fetus or newborn 770.2
Pneumophagia (psychogenic) 306.4
Pneumopleurisy, pneumopleuritis (*see also*
  Pneumonia) 486
Pneumopyopericardium 420.99
Pneumopyothorax (*see also* Pyopneumothorax)
  510.9
  with fistula 510.0
Pneumorrhagia 786.3
  newborn 770.3
  tuberculous (*see also* Tuberculosis, pulmonary)
    011.9 ✓5ᵗʰ
Pneumosiderosis (occupational) 503
Pneumothorax (acute) (chronic) 512.8
  congenital 770.2
  due to operative injury of chest wall or lung
    512.1
    accidental puncture or laceration 512.1
  fetus or newborn 770.2
  iatrogenic 512.1
  postoperative 512.1
  spontaneous 512.8
    fetus or newborn 770.2
    tension 512.0
  sucking 512.8
    iatrogenic 512.1
    postoperative 512.1
  tense valvular, infectional 512.0
  tension 512.0
    iatrogenic 512.1
    postoperative 512.1
    spontaneous 512.0
  traumatic 860.0
    with
      hemothorax 860.4
        with open wound into thorax 860.5
      open wound into thorax 860.1
  tuberculous (*see also* Tuberculosis) 011.7 ✓5ᵗʰ
Pocket(s)
  endocardial (*see also* Endocarditis) 424.90
  periodontal 523.8
Podagra 274.9
Podencephalus 759.89
Poikilocytosis 790.09
Poikiloderma 709.09
  Civatte's 709.09
  congenital 757.33
  vasculare atrophicans 696.2
Poikilodermatomyositis 710.3
Pointed ear 744.29
Poise imperfect 729.9
Poisoned — *see* Poisoning
Poisoning (acute) — *see also* Table of Drugs and
  Chemicals
  Bacillus, B.
    aertrycke (*see also* Infection, Salmonella)
      003.9
    botulinus 005.1
    cholerae (suis) (*see also* Infection,
      Salmonella) 003.9
    paratyphosus (*see also* Infection,
      Salmonella) 003.9
    suipestifer (*see also* Infection, Salmonella)
      003.9
  bacterial toxins NEC 005.9
  berries, noxious 988.2
  blood (general) — *see* Septicemia
  botulism 005.1
  bread, moldy, mouldy — *see* Poisoning, food
  damaged meat — *see* Poisoning, food

Poisoning (acute) — *see also* Table of Drugs and
  Chemicals — *continued*
  death-cap (Amanita phalloides) (Amanita verna)
    988.1
  decomposed food — *see* Poisoning, food
  diseased food — *see* Poisoning, food
  drug — *see* Table of Drugs and Chemicals
  epidemic, fish, meat, or other food — *see*
    Poisoning, food
  fava bean 282.2
  fish (bacterial) — *see also* Poisoning, food
    noxious 988.0
  food (acute) (bacterial) (diseased) (infected) NEC
    005.9
    due to
      bacillus
        aertrycke (*see also* Poisoning, food,
          due to Salmonella) 003.9
        botulinus 005.1
        cereus 005.89
        choleraesuis (*see also* Poisoning, food,
          due to Salmonella) 003.9
        paratyphosus (*see also* Poisoning,
          food, due to Salmonella) 003.9
        suipestifer (*see also* Poisoning, food,
          due to Salmonella) 003.9
      Clostridium 005.3
        botulinum 005.1
        perfringens 005.2
        welchii 005.2
      Salmonella (aertrycke) (callinarum)
        (choleraesuis) (enteritidis)
        (paratyphi) (suipestifer) 003.9
        with
          gastroenteritis 003.0
          localized infection(s) (*see also*
            Infection, Salmonella) 003.20
          septicemia 003.1
          specified manifestation NEC 003.8
      specified bacterium NEC 005.89
      Staphylococcus 005.0
      Streptococcus 005.8 ✓5ᵗʰ
      Vibrio parahaemolyticus 005.4
      Vibrio vulnificus 005.81
    noxious or naturally toxic 988.0
      berries 988.2
      fish 988.0
      mushroom 988.1
      plants NEC 988.2
  ice cream — *see* Poisoning, food
  ichthyotoxism (bacterial) 005.9
  kreotoxism, food 005.9
  malarial — *see* Malaria
  meat — *see* Poisoning, food
  mushroom (noxious) 988.1
  mussel — *see also* Poisoning, food
    noxious 988.0
  noxious foodstuffs (*see also* Poisoning, food,
    noxious) 988.9
    specified type NEC 988.8
  plants, noxious 988.2
  pork — *see also* Poisoning, food
    specified NEC 988.8
    Trichinosis 124
  ptomaine — *see* Poisoning, food
  putrefaction, food — *see* Poisoning, food
  radiation 508.0
  Salmonella (*see also* Infection, Salmonella)
    003.9
  sausage — *see also* Poisoning, food
    Trichinosis 124
  saxitoxin 988.0
  shellfish — *see also* Poisoning, food
    noxious 988.0
  Staphylococcus, food 005.0
  toxic, from disease NEC 799.8
  truffles — *see* Poisoning, food
  uremic — *see* Uremia
  uric acid 274.9
Poison ivy, oak, sumac or other plant
  dermatitis 692.6
Poker spine 720.0
Policeman's disease 729.2
Polioencephalitis (acute) (bulbar) (*see also*
  Poliomyelitis, bulbar) 045.0 ✓5ᵗʰ
  inferior 335.22

Polioencephalitis (*see also* Poliomyelitis, bulbar)
  — *continued*
  influenzal 487.8
  superior hemorrhagic (acute) (Wernicke's) 265.1
  Wernicke's (superior hemorrhagic) 265.1
Polioencephalomyelitis (acute) (anterior) (bulbar)
  (*see also* Polioencephalitis) 045.0 ✓5ᵗʰ
Polioencephalopathy, superior hemorrhagic
  265.1
  with
    beriberi 265.0
    pellagra 265.2
Poliomeningoencephalitis — *see*
  Meningoencephalitis
Poliomyelitis (acute) (anterior) (epidemic)
  045.9 ✓5ᵗʰ

> *Note* — Use the following fifth-digit
> subclassification with category 045:
>
>   0   poliovirus, unspecified type
>   1   poliovirus, type I
>   2   poliovirus, type II
>   3   poliovirus, type III

  with
    paralysis 045.1 ✓5ᵗʰ
      bulbar 045.0 ✓5ᵗʰ
  abortive 045.2 ✓5ᵗʰ
  ascending 045.9 ✓5ᵗʰ
    progressive 045.9 ✓5ᵗʰ
  bulbar 045.0 ✓5ᵗʰ
  cerebral 045.0 ✓5ᵗʰ
  chronic 335.21
  congenital 771.2
  contact V01.2
  deformities 138
  exposure to V01.2
  late effect 138
  nonepidemic 045.9 ✓5ᵗʰ
  nonparalytic 045.2 ✓5ᵗʰ
  old with deformity 138
  posterior, acute 053.19
  residual 138
  sequelae 138
  spinal, acute 045.9 ✓5ᵗʰ
  syphilitic (chronic) 094.89
  vaccination, prophylactic (against) V04.0
Poliosis (eyebrow) (eyelashes) 704.3
  circumscripta (congenital) 757.4
    acquired 704.3
  congenital 757.4
Pollakiuria 788.4 ✓5ᵗʰ
  psychogenic 306.53
Pollinosis 477.0
Pollitzer's disease (hidradenitis suppurativa)
  705.83
Polyadenitis (*see also* Adenitis) 289.3
  malignant 020.0
Polyalgia 729.9
Polyangiitis (essential) 446.0
Polyarteritis (nodosa) (renal) 446.0
Polyarthralgia 719.49
  psychogenic 306.0
Polyarthritis, polyarthropathy NEC 716.59
  due to or associated with other specified
    conditions — *see* Arthritis, due to or
    associated with
  endemic (*see also* Disease, Kaschin-Beck)
    716.0 ✓5ᵗʰ
  inflammatory 714.9
    specified type NEC 714.89
  juvenile (chronic) 714.30
    acute 714.31
  migratory — *see* Fever, rheumatic
  rheumatic 714.0
    fever (acute) — *see* Fever, rheumatic
Polycarential syndrome of infancy 260
Polychondritis (atrophic) (chronic) (relapsing)
  733.99
Polycoria 743.46
Polycystic (congenital) (disease) 759.89
  degeneration, kidney — *see* Polycystic, kidney

Polycystic — continued
  kidney (congenital) 753.12
    adult type (APKD) 753.13
    autosomal dominant 753.13
    autosomal recessive 753.14
    childhood type (CPKD) 753.14
    infantile type 753.14
  liver 751.62
  lung 518.89
    congenital 748.4
  ovary, ovaries 256.4
  spleen 759.0
Polycythemia (primary) (rubra) (vera) (M9950/1) 238.4
  acquired 289.0
  benign 289.0
    familial 289.6
  due to
    donor twin 776.4
    fall in plasma volume 289.0
    high altitude 289.0
    maternal-fetal transfusion 776.4
    stress 289.0
  emotional 289.0
  erythropoietin 289.0
  familial (benign) 289.6
  Gaisböck's (hypertonica) 289.0
  high altitude 289.0
  hypertonica 289.0
  hypoxemic 289.0
  neonatorum 776.4
  nephrogenous 289.0
  relative 289.0
  secondary 289.0
  spurious 289.0
  stress 289.0
Polycytosis cryptogenica 289.0
Polydactylism, polydactyly 755.00
  fingers 755.01
  toes 755.02
Polydipsia 783.5
Polydystrophic oligophrenia 277.5
Polyembryoma (M9072/3) — see Neoplasm, by site, malignant
Polygalactia 676.6 ✓5ᵗʰ
Polyglandular
  deficiency 258.9
  dyscrasia 258.9
  dysfunction 258.9
  syndrome 258.8
Polyhydramnios (see also Hydramnios) 657 ✓5ᵗʰ
Polymastia 757.6
Polymenorrhea 626.2
Polymicrogyria 742.2
Polymyalgia 725
  arteritica 446.5
  rheumatica 725
Polymyositis (acute) (chronic) (hemorrhagic) 710.4
  with involvement of
    lung 710.4 [517.8]
    skin 710.3
  ossificans (generalisata) (progressiva) 728.19
  Wagner's (dermatomyositis) 710.3
Polyneuritis, polyneuritic (see also Polyneuropathy) 356.9
  alcoholic 357.5
    with psychosis 291.1
  cranialis 352.6
  diabetic 250.6 ✓5ᵗʰ [357.2]
  demyelinating, chronic inflammatory 357.81▲
  due to lack of vitamin NEC 269.2 [357.4]
  endemic 265.0 [357.4]
  erythredema 985.0
  febrile 357.0
  hereditary ataxic 356.3
  idiopathic, acute 357.0
  infective (acute) 357.0
  nutritional 269.9 [357.4]
  postinfectious 357.0
Polyneuropathy (peripheral) 356.9
  alcoholic 357.5
  amyloid 277.3 [357.4]
  arsenical 357.7
  critical illness 357.82

Polyneuropathy — continued
  diabetic 250.6 ✓5ᵗʰ [357.2]
  due to
    antitetanus serum 357.6
    arsenic 357.7
    drug or medicinal substance 357.6
      correct substance properly administered 357.6
      overdose or wrong substance given or taken 977.9
        specified drug — see Table of Drugs and Chemicals
    lack of vitamin NEC 269.2 [357.4]
    lead 357.7
    organophosphate compounds 357.7
    pellagra 265.2 [357.4]
    porphyria 277.1 [357.4]
    serum 357.6
    toxic agent NEC 357.7
  hereditary 356.0
  idiopathic 356.9
    progressive 356.4
  in
    amyloidosis 277.3 [357.4]
    avitaminosis 269.2 [357.4]
      specified NEC 269.1 [357.4]
    beriberi 265.0 [357.4]
    collagen vascular disease NEC 710.9 [357.1]
    deficiency
      B-complex NEC 266.2 [357.4]
      vitamin B 266.9 [357.4]
      vitamin B 266.1 [357.4]
    diabetes 250.6 ✓5ᵗʰ [357.2]
    diphtheria (see also Diphtheria) 032.89 [357.4]
    disseminated lupus erythematosus 710.0 [357.1]
    herpes zoster 053.13
    hypoglycemia 251.2 [357.4]
    malignant neoplasm (M8000/3) NEC 199.1 [357.3]
    mumps 072.72
    pellagra 265.2 [357.4]
    polyarteritis nodosa 446.0 [357.1]
    porphyria 277.1 [357.4]
    rheumatoid arthritis 714.0 [357.1]
    sarcoidosis 135 [357.4]
    uremia 585 [357.4]
  lead 357.7
  nutritional 269.9 [357.4]
    specified NEC 269.8 [357.4]
  postherpetic 053.13
  progressive 356.4
  sensory (hereditary) 356.2
Polyonychia 757.5
Polyopia 368.2
  refractive 368.15
Polyorchism, polyorchidism (three testes) 752.8
Polyorrhymenitis (peritoneal) (see also Polyserositis) 568.82
  pericardial 423.2
Polyostotic fibrous dysplasia 756.54
Polyotia 744.1
Polyp, polypus

> Note — Polyps of organs or sites that do not appear in the list below should be coded to the residual category for diseases of the organ or site concerned.

  accessory sinus 471.8
  adenoid tissue 471.0
  adenomatous (M8210/0) — see also Neoplasm, by site, benign
    adenocarcinoma in (M8210/3) — see Neoplasm, by site, malignant
    carcinoma in (M8210/3) — see Neoplasm, by site, malignant
    multiple (M8221/0) — see Neoplasm, by site, benign
  antrum 471.8
  anus, anal (canal) (nonadenomatous) 569.0
    adenomatous 211.4
  Bartholin's gland 624.6
  bladder (M8120/1) 236.7
  broad ligament 620.8

Polyp, polypus — continued
  cervix (uteri) 622.7
    adenomatous 219.0
    in pregnancy or childbirth 654.6 ✓5ᵗʰ
      affecting fetus or newborn 763.89
      causing obstructed labor 660.2 ✓5ᵗʰ
    mucous 622.7
    nonneoplastic 622.7
  choanal 471.0
  cholesterol 575.6
  clitoris 624.6
  colon (M8210/0) (see also Polyp, adenomatous) 211.3
  corpus uteri 621.0
  dental 522.0
  ear (middle) 385.30
  endometrium 621.0
  ethmoidal (sinus) 471.8
  fallopian tube 620.8
  female genital organs NEC 624.8
  frontal (sinus) 471.8
  gallbladder 575.6
  gingiva 523.8
  gum 523.8
  labia 624.6
  larynx (mucous) 478.4
  malignant (M8000/3) — see Neoplasm, by site, malignant
  maxillary (sinus) 471.8
  middle ear 385.30
  myometrium 621.0
  nares
    anterior 471.9
    posterior 471.0
  nasal (mucous) 471.9
    cavity 471.0
    septum 471.9
  nasopharyngeal 471.0
  neoplastic (M8210/0) — see Neoplasm, by site, benign
  nose (mucous) 471.9
  oviduct 620.8
  paratubal 620.8
  pharynx 478.29
    congenital 750.29
  placenta, placental 674.4 ✓5ᵗʰ
  prostate 600.2
  pudenda 624.6
  pulp (dental) 522.0
  rectosigmoid 211.4
  rectum (nonadenomatous) 569.0
    adenomatous 211.4
  septum (nasal) 471.9
  sinus (accessory) (ethmoidal) (frontal) (maxillary) (sphenoidal) 471.8
  sphenoidal (sinus) 471.8
  stomach (M8210/0) 211.1
  tube, fallopian 620.8
  turbinate, mucous membrane 471.8
  ureter 593.89
  urethra 599.3
  uterine
    ligament 620.8
    tube 620.8
  uterus (body) (corpus) (mucous) 621.0
    in pregnancy or childbirth 654.1 ✓5ᵗʰ
      affecting fetus or newborn 763.89
      causing obstructed labor 660.2 ✓5ᵗʰ
  vagina 623.7
  vocal cord (mucous) 478.4
  vulva 624.6
Polyphagia 783.6
Polypoid — see condition
Polyposis — see also Polyp
  coli (adenomatous) (M8220/0) 211.3
    adenocarcinoma in (M8220/3) 153.9
    carcinoma in (M8220/3) 153.9
  familial (M8220/0) 211.3
  intestinal (adenomatous) (M8220/0) 211.3
  multiple (M8221/0) — see Neoplasm, by site, benign
Polyradiculitis (acute) 357.0
Polyradiculoneuropathy (acute) (segmentally demyelinating) 357.0
Polysarcia 278.00

Polyserositis — **Preauricular appendage**

Polyserositis (peritoneal) 568.82
  due to pericarditis 423.2
  paroxysmal (familial) 277.3
  pericardial 423.2
  periodic 277.3
  pleural — see Pleurisy
  recurrent 277.3
  tuberculous (see also Tuberculosis,
    polyserositis) 018.9 ✓5ᵗʰ
Polysialia 527.7
Polysplenia syndrome 759.0
Polythelia 757.6
Polytrichia (see also Hypertrichosis) 704.1
Polyunguia (congenital) 757.5
  acquired 703.8
Polyuria 788.42
Pompe's disease (glycogenosis II) 271.0
Pompholyx 705.81
Poncet's disease (tuberculous rheumatism) (see
  also Tuberculosis) 015.9 ✓5ᵗʰ
Pond fracture — see Fracture, skull, vault
Ponos 085.0
Pons, pontine — see condition
Poor
  contractions, labor 661.2 ✓5ᵗʰ
    affecting fetus or newborn 763.7
  fetal growth NEC 764.9 ✓5ᵗʰ
    affecting management of pregnancy
      656.5 ✓5ᵗʰ
  incorporation
    artificial skin graft 996.55
    decellularized allodermis graft 996.55
  obstetrical history V13.49 ●
    affecting management of current ●
      pregnancy V23.49 ●
      pre-term labor V23.41 ●
    pre-term labor V13.41 ●
  sucking reflex (newborn) 796.1
  vision NEC 369.9
Poradenitis, nostras 099.1
Porencephaly (congenital) (developmental) (true)
  742.4
  acquired 348.0
  nondevelopmental 348.0
  traumatic (post) 310.2
Porocephaliasis 134.1
Porokeratosis 757.39
  disseminated superficial actinic (DSAP) 692.75
Poroma, eccrine (M8402/0) — see Neoplasm,
  skin, benign
Porphyria (acute) (congenital) (constitutional)
  (erythropoietic) (familial) (hepatica)
  (idiopathic) (idiosyncratic) (intermittent)
  (latent) (mixed hepatic) (photosensitive)
  (South African genetic) (Swedish) 277.1
  acquired 277.1
  cutaneatarda
    hereditaria 277.1
    symptomatica 277.1
  due to drugs
    correct substance properly administered
      277.1
    overdose or wrong substance given or taken
      977.9
      specified drug — see Table of Drugs and
        Chemicals
  secondary 277.1
  toxic NEC 277.1
  variegata 277.1
Porphyrinuria (acquired) (congenital) (secondary)
  277.1
Porphyruria (acquired) (congenital) 277.1
Portal — see condition
Port wine nevus or mark 757.32
Posadas-Wernicke disease 114.9
Position
  fetus, abnormal (see also Presentation, fetal)
    652.9 ✓5ᵗʰ
  teeth, faulty 524.3
Positive
  culture (nonspecific) 795.39 ▲
    AIDS virus V08
    blood 790.7

Positive — continued
  culture — continued
    HIV V08
    human immunodeficiency virus V08
    nose 795.39 ▲
    skin lesion NEC 795.39 ▲
    spinal fluid 792.0
    sputum 795.39 ▲
    stool 792.1
    throat 795.39 ▲
    urine 791.9
    wound 795.39 ▲
  findings, anthrax 795.31 ●
  HIV V08
  human immunodeficiency virus (HIV) V08
  PPD 795.5
  serology
    AIDS virus V08
      inconclusive 795.71
    HIV V08
      inconclusive 795.71
    human immunodeficiency virus (HIV) V08
      inconclusive 795.71
    syphilis 097.1
      with signs or symptoms — see Syphilis,
        by site and stage
      false 795.6
    skin test 795.7
      tuberculin (without active tuberculosis)
        795.5
    VDRL 097.1
      with signs or symptoms — see Syphilis, by
        site and stage
      false 795.6
    Wassermann reaction 097.1
      false 795.6
Postcardiotomy syndrome 429.4
Postcaval ureter 753.4
Postcholecystectomy syndrome 576.0
Postclimacteric bleeding 627.1
Postcommissurotomy syndrome 429.4
Postconcussional syndrome 310.2
Postcontusional syndrome 310.2
Postcricoid region — see condition
Post-dates (pregnancy) — see Pregnancy
Postencephalitic — see also condition
  syndrome 310.8
Posterior — see condition
Posterolateral sclerosis (spinal cord) — see
  Degeneration, combined
Postexanthematous — see condition
Postfebrile — see condition
Postgastrectomy dumping syndrome 564.2
Posthemiplegic chorea 344.89
Posthemorrhagic anemia (chronic) 280.0
  acute 285.1
  newborn 776.5
Posthepatitis syndrome 780.79
Postherpetic neuralgia (intercostal) (syndrome)
  (zoster) 053.19
  geniculate ganglion 053.11
  ophthalmica 053.19
  trigeminal 053.12
Posthitis 607.1
Postimmunization complication or reaction —
  see Complications, vaccination
Postinfectious — see condition
Postinfluenzal syndrome 780.79
Postlaminectomy syndrome 722.80
  cervical, cervicothoracic 722.81
  kyphosis 737.12
  lumbar, lumbosacral 722.83
  thoracic, thoracolumbar 722.82
Postleukotomy syndrome 310.0
Postlobectomy syndrome 310.0
Postmastectomy lymphedema (syndrome) 457.0
Postmaturity, postmature (fetus or newborn)
  766.2
  affecting management of pregnancy
    post term pregnancy 645.1 ✓5ᵗʰ
    prolonged pregnancy 645.2 ✓5ᵗʰ
  syndrome 766.2

Postmeasles — see also condition
  complication 055.8
    specified NEC 055.79
Postmenopausal
  endometrium (atrophic) 627.8
    suppurative (see also Endometritis) 615.9
  hormone replacement V07.4
  status (age related) (natural) V49.81
Postnasal drip — see Sinusitis
Postnatal — see condition
Postoperative — see also condition
  confusion state 293.9
  psychosis 293.9
  status NEC (see also Status (post)) V45.89
Postpancreatectomy hyperglycemia 251.3
Postpartum — see also condition
  observation
    immediately after delivery V24.0
    routine follow-up V24.2
Postperfusion syndrome NEC 999.8
  bone marrow 996.85
Postpoliomyelitic — see condition
Postsurgery status NEC (see also Status (post))
  V45.89
Post-term (pregnancy) 645.1 ✓5ᵗʰ
  infant (294 days or more gestation) 766.2
Posttraumatic — see condition
Posttraumatic brain syndrome, nonpsychotic
  310.2
Post-typhoid abscess 002.0
Postures, hysterical 300.11
Postvaccinal reaction or complication — see
  Complications, vaccination
Postvagotomy syndrome 564.2
Postvalvulotomy syndrome 429.4
Postvasectomy sperm count V25.8
Potain's disease (pulmonary edema) 514
Potain's syndrome (gastrectasis with dyspepsia)
  536.1
Pott's
  curvature (spinal) (see also Tuberculosis)
    015.0 ✓5ᵗʰ [737.43]
  disease or paraplegia (see also Tuberculosis)
    015.0 ✓5ᵗʰ [730.88]
  fracture (closed) 824.4
    open 824.5
  gangrene 440.24
  osteomyelitis (see also Tuberculosis)
    015.0 ✓5ᵗʰ [730.88]
  spinal curvature (see also Tuberculosis)
    015.0 ✓5ᵗʰ [737.43]
  tumor, puffy (see also Osteomyelitis) 730.2 ✓5ᵗʰ
Potter's
  asthma 502
  disease 753.0
  facies 754.0
  lung 502
  syndrome (with renal agenesis) 753.0
Pouch
  bronchus 748.3
  Douglas' — see condition
  esophagus, esophageal (congenital) 750.4
    acquired 530.6
  gastric 537.1
  Hartmann's (abnormal sacculation of
    gallbladder neck) 575.8
    of intestine V44.3
      attention to V55.3
  pharynx, pharyngeal (congenital) 750.27
Poulet's disease 714.2
Poultrymen's itch 133.8
Poverty V60.2
Prader-Labhart-Willi-Fanconi syndrome
  (hypogenital dystrophy with diabetic
  tendency) 759.81
Prader-Willi syndrome (hypogenital dystrophy
  with diabetic tendency) 759.81
Preachers' voice 784.49
Pre-AIDS — see Human immunodeficiency virus
  (disease) (illness) (infection)
Preauricular appendage 744.1

✓4ᵗʰ Fourth-digit Required   ✓5ᵗʰ Fifth-digit Required   ▶◀ Revised Text   ● New Line   ▲ Revised Code

Prebetalipoproteinemia (acquired) (essential) (familial) (hereditary) (primary) (secondary) 272.1
  with chylomicronemia 272.3
Precipitate labor 661.3 ✓5ᵗʰ
  affecting fetus or newborn 763.6
Preclimacteric bleeding 627.0
  menorrhagia 627.0
Precocious
  adrenarche 259.1
  menarche 259.1
  menstruation 626.8
  pubarche 259.1
  puberty NEC 259.1
  sexual development NEC 259.1
  thelarche 259.1
Precocity, sexual (constitutional) (cryptogenic) (female) (idiopathic) (male) NEC 259.1
  with adrenal hyperplasia 255.2
Precordial pain 786.51
  psychogenic 307.89
Predeciduous teeth 520.2
Prediabetes, prediabetic 790.2
  complicating pregnancy, childbirth, or puerperium 648.8 ✓5ᵗʰ
  fetus or newborn 775.8
Predislocation status of hip, at birth (*See also* Subluxation, congenital, hip) 754.32
Preeclampsia (mild) 642.4 ✓5ᵗʰ
  with pre-existing hypertension 642.7 ✓5ᵗʰ
  affecting fetus or newborn 760.0
  severe 642.5 ✓5ᵗʰ
  superimposed on pre-existing hypertensive disease 642.7 ✓5ᵗʰ
Preeruptive color change, teeth, tooth 520.8
Preexcitation 426.7
  atrioventricular conduction 426.7
  ventricular 426.7
Preglaucoma 365.00
Pregnancy (single) (uterine) (without sickness) V22.2

  Note — Use the following fifth-digit subclassification with categories 640-648, 651-676:
  0   unspecified as to episode of care
  1   delivered, with or without mention of antepartum condition
  2   delivered, with mention of postpartum complication
  3   antepartum condition or complication
  4   postpartum condition or complication

  abdominal (ectopic) 633.00 ▲
    with intrauterine pregnancy 633.01 ●
    affecting fetus or newborn 761.4
  abnormal NEC 646.9 ✓5ᵗʰ
  ampullar — *see* Pregnancy, tubal
  broad ligament — *see* Pregnancy, cornual
  cervical — *see* Pregnancy, cornual
  combined (extrauterine and intrauterine) — *see* Pregnancy, cornual
  complicated (by)
    abnormal, abnormality NEC 646.9 ✓5ᵗʰ
      cervix 654.6 ✓5ᵗʰ
      cord (umbilical) 663.9 ✓5ᵗʰ
      glucose tolerance (conditions classifiable to 790.2) 648.8 ✓5ᵗʰ
      injury 648.9 ✓5ᵗʰ
        obstetrical NEC 665.9 ✓5ᵗʰ
      obstetrical trauma NEC 665.9 ✓5ᵗʰ
      pelvic organs or tissues NEC 654.9 ✓5ᵗʰ
      pelvis (bony) 653.0 ✓5ᵗʰ
      perineum or vulva 654.8 ✓5ᵗʰ
      placenta, placental (vessel) 656.7 ✓5ᵗʰ
      position
        cervix 654.4 ✓5ᵗʰ
        placenta 641.1 ✓5ᵗʰ
          without hemorrhage 641.0 ✓5ᵗʰ
        uterus 654.4 ✓5ᵗʰ

Pregnancy — *continued*
  complicated (by) — *continued*
    abnormal, abnormality NEC — *continued*
      size, fetus 653.5 ✓5ᵗʰ
      uterus (congenital) 654.0 ✓5ᵗʰ
    abscess or cellulitis
      bladder 646.6 ✓5ᵗʰ
      genitourinary tract (conditions classifiable to 590, 595, 597, 599.0, 614-616) 646.6 ✓5ᵗʰ
      kidney 646.6 ✓5ᵗʰ
      urinary tract NEC 646.6 ✓5ᵗʰ
    air embolism 673.0 ✓5ᵗʰ
    albuminuria 646.2 ✓5ᵗʰ
      with hypertension — *see* Toxemia, of pregnancy
    amnionitis 658.4 ✓5ᵗʰ
    amniotic fluid embolism 673.1 ✓5ᵗʰ
    anemia (conditions classifiable to 280-285) 648.2 ✓5ᵗʰ
    atrophy, yellow (acute) (liver) (subacute) 646.7 ✓5ᵗʰ
    bacilluria, asymptomatic 646.5 ✓5ᵗʰ
    bacteriuria, asymptomatic 646.5 ✓5ᵗʰ
    bicornis or bicornuate uterus 654.0 ✓5ᵗʰ
    bone and joint disorders (conditions classifiable to 720-724 or conditions affecting lower limbs classifiable to 711-719, 725-738) 648.7 ✓5ᵗʰ
    breech presentation 652.2 ✓5ᵗʰ
      with successful version 652.1 ✓5ᵗʰ
    cardiovascular disease (conditions classifiable to 390-398, 410-429) 648.6 ✓5ᵗʰ
      congenital (conditions classifiable to 745-747) 648.5 ✓5ᵗʰ
    cerebrovascular disorders (conditions classifiable to 430-434, 436-437) 674.0 ✓5ᵗʰ
    cervicitis (conditions classifiable to 616.0) 646.6 ✓5ᵗʰ
    chloasma (gravidarum) 646.8 ✓5ᵗʰ
    chorea (gravidarum) — *see* Eclampsia, pregnancy
    cholelithiasis 646.8 ✓5ᵗʰ ●
    contraction, pelvis (general) 653.1 ✓5ᵗʰ
      inlet 653.2 ✓5ᵗʰ
      outlet 653.3 ✓5ᵗʰ
    convulsions (eclamptic) (uremic) 642.6 ✓5ᵗʰ
      with pre-existing hypertension 642.7 ✓5ᵗʰ
    current disease or condition (nonobstetric)
      abnormal glucose tolerance 648.8 ✓5ᵗʰ
      anemia 648.2 ✓5ᵗʰ
      bone and joint (lower limb) 648.7 ✓5ᵗʰ
      cardiovascular 648.6 ✓5ᵗʰ
        congenital 648.5 ✓5ᵗʰ
      cerebrovascular 674.0 ✓5ᵗʰ
      diabetic 648.0 ✓5ᵗʰ
      drug dependence 648.3 ✓5ᵗʰ
      genital organ or tract 646.6 ✓5ᵗʰ
      gonorrheal 647.1 ✓5ᵗʰ
      hypertensive 642.2 ✓5ᵗʰ
        renal 642.1 ✓5ᵗʰ
      infectious 647.9 ✓5ᵗʰ
        specified type NEC 647.8 ✓5ᵗʰ
      liver 646.7 ✓5ᵗʰ
      malarial 647.4 ✓5ᵗʰ
      nutritional deficiency 648.9 ✓5ᵗʰ
      parasitic NEC 647.8 ✓5ᵗʰ
      renal 646.2 ✓5ᵗʰ
        hypertensive 642.1 ✓5ᵗʰ
      rubella 647.5 ✓5ᵗʰ
      specified condition NEC 648.9 ✓5ᵗʰ
      syphilitic 647.0 ✓5ᵗʰ
      thyroid 648.1 ✓5ᵗʰ
      tuberculous 647.3 ✓5ᵗʰ
      urinary 646.6 ✓5ᵗʰ
      venereal 647.2 ✓5ᵗʰ
      viral NEC 647.6 ✓5ᵗʰ
    cystitis 646.6 ✓5ᵗʰ
    cystocele 654.4 ✓5ᵗʰ
    death of fetus (near term) 656.4 ✓5ᵗʰ
      early pregnancy (before 22 completed weeks gestation) 632
    deciduitis 646.6 ✓5ᵗʰ
    decreased fetal movements 655.7

Pregnancy — *continued*
  complicated (by) — *continued*
    diabetes (mellitus) (conditions classifiable to 250) 648.0 ✓5ᵗʰ
    disorders of liver 646.7 ✓5ᵗʰ
    displacement, uterus NEC 654.4 ✓5ᵗʰ
    disproportion — *see* Disproportion
    double uterus 654.0 ✓5ᵗʰ
    drug dependence (conditions classifiable to 304) 648.3 ✓5ᵗʰ
    dysplasia, cervix 654.6 ✓5ᵗʰ
    early onset of delivery (spontaneous) 644.2 ✓5ᵗʰ
    eclampsia, eclamptic (coma) (convulsions) (delirium) (nephritis) (uremia) 642.6 ✓5ᵗʰ
      with pre-existing hypertension 642.7 ✓5ᵗʰ
    edema 646.1 ✓5ᵗʰ
      with hypertension — *see* Toxemia, of pregnancy
    effusion, amniotic fluid 658.1 ✓5ᵗʰ
      delayed delivery following 658.2 ✓5ᵗʰ
    embolism
      air 673.0 ✓5ᵗʰ
      amniotic fluid 673.1 ✓5ᵗʰ
      blood-clot 673.2 ✓5ᵗʰ
      cerebral 674.0 ✓5ᵗʰ
      pulmonary NEC 673.2 ✓5ᵗʰ
      pyemic 673.3 ✓5ᵗʰ
      septic 673.3 ✓5ᵗʰ
    emesis (gravidarum) — *see* Pregnancy, complicated, vomiting
    endometritis (conditions classifiable to 615.0-615.9) 646.6 ✓5ᵗʰ
      decidual 646.6 ✓5ᵗʰ
    excessive weight gain NEC 646.1 ✓5ᵗʰ
    face presentation 652.4 ✓5ᵗʰ
    failure, fetal head to enter pelvic brim 652.5 ✓5ᵗʰ
    false labor (pains) 644.1 ✓5ᵗʰ
    fatigue 646.8 ✓5ᵗʰ
    fatty metamorphosis of liver 646.7 ✓5ᵗʰ
    fetal
      death (near term) 656.4 ✓5ᵗʰ
        early (before 22 completed weeks gestation) 632
      deformity 653.7 ✓5ᵗʰ
      distress 656.8 ✓5ᵗʰ
    fibroid (tumor) (uterus) 654.1 ✓5ᵗʰ
    footling presentation 652.8 ✓5ᵗʰ
      with successful version 652.1 ✓5ᵗʰ
    gallbladder disease 646.8 ✓5ᵗʰ ●
    goiter 648.1 ✓5ᵗʰ
    gonococcal infection (conditions classifiable to 098) 647.1 ✓5ᵗʰ
    gonorrhea (conditions classifiable to 098) 647.1 ✓5ᵗʰ
    hemorrhage 641.9 ✓5ᵗʰ
      accidental 641.2 ✓5ᵗʰ
      before 22 completed weeks gestation NEC 640.9 ✓5ᵗʰ
      cerebrovascular 674.0 ✓5ᵗʰ
      due to
        afibrinogenemia or other coagulation defect (conditions classifiable to 286.0-286.9) 641.3 ✓5ᵗʰ
        leiomyoma, uterine 641.8 ✓5ᵗʰ
        marginal sinus (rupture) 641.2 ✓5ᵗʰ
        premature separation, placenta 641.2 ✓5ᵗʰ
        trauma 641.8 ✓5ᵗʰ
      early (before 22 completed weeks gestation) 640.9 ✓5ᵗʰ
      threatened abortion 640.0 ✓5ᵗʰ
      unavoidable 641.1 ✓5ᵗʰ
    hepatitis (acute) (malignant) (subacute) 646.7 ✓5ᵗʰ
      viral 647.6 ✓5ᵗʰ
    herniation of uterus 654.4 ✓5ᵗʰ
    high head at term 652.5 ✓5ᵗʰ
    hydatidiform mole (delivered) (undelivered) 630
    hydramnios 657 ✓5ᵗʰ
    hydrocephalic fetus 653.6 ✓5ᵗʰ
    hydrops amnii 657 ✓5ᵗʰ
    hydrorrhea 658.1 ✓5ᵗʰ
    hyperemesis (gravidarum) — *see* Hyperemesis, gravidarum

✓4ᵗʰ Fourth-digit Required   ✓5ᵗʰ Fifth-digit Required   ▶◀ Revised Text   ● New Line   ▲ Revised Code

Pregnancy — *continued*
  complicated (by) — *continued*
    hypertension — *see* Hypertension,
      complicating pregnancy
    hypertensive
      heart and renal disease 642.2 ✓5th
      heart disease 642.2 ✓5th
      renal disease 642.2 ✓5th
    hyperthyroidism 648.1 ✓5th
    hypothyroidism 648.1 ✓5th
    hysteralgia 646.8 ✓5th
    icterus gravis 646.7 ✓5th
    incarceration, uterus 654.3 ✓5th
    incompetent cervix (os) 654.5 ✓5th
    infection 647.9 ✓5th
      amniotic fluid 658.4 ✓5th
      bladder 646.6 ✓5th
      genital organ (conditions classifiable to
        614-616) 646.6 ✓5th
      kidney (conditions classifiable to 590.0-
        590.9) 646.6 ✓5th
      urinary (tract) 646.6 ✓5th
        asymptomatic 646.5 ✓5th
    infective and parasitic diseases NEC
      647.8 ✓5th
    inflammation
      bladder 646.6 ✓5th
      genital organ (conditions classifiable to
        614-616) 646.6 ✓5th
      urinary tract NEC 646.6 ✓5th
    insufficient weight gain 646.8 ✓5th
    intrauterine fetal death (near term) NEC
      656.4 ✓5th
      early (before 22 completed weeks'
        gestation) 632
    malaria (conditions classifiable to 084)
      647.4 ✓5th
    malformation, uterus (congenital) 654.0 ✓5th
    malnutrition (conditions classifiable to 260-
      269) 648.9 ✓5th
    malposition
      fetus — *see* Pregnancy, complicated,
        malpresentation
      uterus or cervix 654.4 ✓5th
    malpresentation 652.9 ✓5th
      with successful version 652.1 ✓5th
      in multiple gestation 652.6 ✓5th
      specified type NEC 652.8 ✓5th
    marginal sinus hemorrhage or rupture
      641.2 ✓5th
    maternal obesity syndrome 646.1 ✓5th
    menstruation 640.8 ✓5th
    mental disorders (conditions classifiable to
      290-303, 305-316, 317-319) 648.4 ✓5th
    mentum presentation 652.4 ✓5th
    missed
      abortion 632
      delivery (at or near term) 656.4 ✓5th
      labor (at or near term) 656.4 ✓5th
    necrosis
      genital organ or tract (conditions
        classifiable to 614-616) 646.6 ✓5th
      liver (conditions classifiable to 570)
        646.7 ✓5th
      renal, cortical 646.2 ✓5th
    nephritis or nephrosis (conditions
      classifiable to 580-589) 646.2 ✓5th
      with hypertension 642.1 ✓5th
    nephropathy NEC 646.2 ✓5th
    neuritis (peripheral) 646.4 ✓5th
    nutritional deficiency (conditions classifiable
      to 260-269) 648.9 ✓5th
    oblique lie or presentation 652.3 ✓5th
      with successful version 652.1 ✓5th
    obstetrical trauma NEC 665.9 ✓5th
    oligohydramnios NEC 658.0 ✓5th
    onset of contractions before 37 weeks
      644.0 ✓5th
    oversize fetus 653.5 ✓5th
    papyraceous fetus 646.0 ✓5th
    patent cervix 654.5 ✓5th
    pelvic inflammatory disease (conditions
      classifiable to 614-616) 646.6 ✓5th
    placenta, placental
      abnormality 656.7 ✓5th
      abruptio or ablatio 641.2 ✓5th
      detachment 641.2 ✓5th

Pregnancy — *continued*
  complicated (by) — *continued*
    placenta, placental — *continued*
      disease 656.7 ✓5th
      infarct 656.7 ✓5th
      low implantation 641.1 ✓5th
        without hemorrhage 641.0 ✓5th
      malformation 656.7 ✓5th
      malposition 641.1 ✓5th
        without hemorrhage 641.0 ✓5th
      marginal sinus hemorrhage 641.2 ✓5th
      previa 641.1 ✓5th
        without hemorrhage 641.0 ✓5th
      separation (premature) (undelivered)
        641.2 ✓5th
    placentitis 658.4 ✓5th
    polyhydramnios 657 ✓5th
    postmaturity
      post term 645.1 ✓5th
      prolonged 645.2 ✓5th
    prediabetes 648.8 ✓5th
    pre-eclampsia (mild) 642.4 ✓5th
      severe 642.5 ✓5th
      superimposed on pre-existing
        hypertensive disease 642.7 ✓5th
    premature rupture of membranes 658.1 ✓5th
      with delayed delivery 658.2 ✓5th
    previous
      infertility V23.0
      nonobstetric condition V23.8 ✓5th
      poor obstetrical history V23.49   ▲
      premature delivery V23.41   ▲
      trophoblastic disease (conditions
        classifiable to 630) V23.1
    prolapse, uterus 654.4 ✓5th
    proteinuria (gestational) 646.2 ✓5th
      with hypertension — *see* Toxemia, of
        pregnancy
    pruritus (neurogenic) 646.8 ✓5th
    psychosis or psychoneurosis 648.4 ✓5th
    ptyalism 646.8 ✓5th
    pyelitis (conditions classifiable to 590.0-
      590.9) 646.6 ✓5th
    renal disease or failure NEC 646.2 ✓5th
      with secondary hypertension 642.1 ✓5th
      hypertensive 642.2 ✓5th
    retention, retained dead ovum 631
    retroversion, uterus 654.3 ✓5th
    Rh immunization, incompatibility, or
      sensitization 656.1 ✓5th
    rubella (conditions classifiable to 056)
      647.5 ✓5th
    rupture
      amnion (premature) 658.1 ✓5th
        with delayed delivery 658.2 ✓5th
      marginal sinus (hemorrhage) 641.2 ✓5th
      membranes (premature) 658.1 ✓5th
        with delayed delivery 658.2 ✓5th
      uterus (before onset of labor) 665.0 ✓5th
    salivation (excessive) 646.8 ✓5th
    salpingo-oophoritis (conditions classifiable to
      614.0-614.2) 646.6 ✓5th
    septicemia (conditions classifiable to 038.0-
      038.9) 647.8 ✓5th
      postpartum 670 ✓4th
      puerperal 670 ✓4th
    spasms, uterus (abnormal) 646.8 ✓5th
    specified condition NEC 646.8 ✓5th
    spurious labor pains 644.1 ✓5th
    superfecundation 651.9 ✓5th
    superfetation 651.9 ✓5th
    syphilis (conditions classifiable to 090-097)
      647.0 ✓5th
    threatened
      abortion 640.0 ✓5th
      premature delivery 644.2 ✓5th
      premature labor 644.0 ✓5th
    thrombophlebitis (superficial) 671.2 ✓5th
      deep 671.3 ✓5th
    thrombosis 671.9 ✓5th
      venous (superficial) 671.2 ✓5th
      deep 671.3 ✓5th
    thyroid dysfunction (conditions classifiable
      to 240-246) 648.1 ✓5th
    thyroiditis 648.1 ✓5th
    thyrotoxicosis 648.1 ✓5th
    torsion of uterus 654.4 ✓5th

Pregnancy — *continued*
  complicated (by) — *continued*
    toxemia — *see* Toxemia, of pregnancy
    transverse lie or presentation 652.3 ✓5th
      with successful version 652.1 ✓5th
    tuberculosis (conditions classifiable to 010-
      018) 647.3 ✓5th
    tumor
      cervix 654.6 ✓5th
      ovary 654.4 ✓5th
      pelvic organs or tissue NEC 654.4 ✓5th
      uterus (body) 654.1 ✓5th
        cervix 654.6 ✓5th
      vagina 654.7 ✓5th
      vulva 654.8 ✓5th
    unstable lie 652.0 ✓5th
    uremia — *see* Pregnancy, complicated, renal
      disease
    urethritis 646.6 ✓5th
    vaginitis or vulvitis (conditions classifiable to
      616.1) 646.6 ✓5th
    varicose
      placental vessels 656.7 ✓5th
      veins (legs) 671.0 ✓5th
        perineum 671.1 ✓5th
        vulva 671.1 ✓5th
    varicosity, labia or vulva 671.1 ✓5th
    venereal disease NEC (conditions classifiable
      to 099) 647.2 ✓5th
    viral disease NEC (conditions classifiable to
      042, 050-055, 057-079) 647.6 ✓5th
    vomiting (incoercible) (pernicious)
      (persistent) (uncontrollable) (vicious)
      643.9 ✓5th
      due to organic disease or other cause
        643.8 ✓5th
      early — *see* Hyperemesis, gravidarum
      late (after 22 completed weeks gestation)
        643.2 ✓5th
    young maternal age 659.8 ✓5th
  complications NEC 646.9 ✓5th
  cornual 633.80   ▲
    with intrauterine pregnancy 633.81   ●
      affecting fetus or newborn 761.4
  death, maternal NEC 646.9 ✓5th
  delivered — *see* Delivery
  ectopic (ruptured) NEC 633.90   ▲
    with intrauterine pregnancy 633.91   ●
    abdominal — *see* Pregnancy, abdominal
    affecting fetus or newborn 761.4
    combined (extrauterine and intrauterine) —
      see Pregnancy, cornual
    ovarian — *see* Pregnancy, ovarian
    specified type NEC 633.80   ▲
      with intrauterine pregnancy 633.81   ●
      affecting fetus or newborn 761.4
    tubal — *see* Pregnancy, tubal
  examination, pregnancy not confirmed V72.4
  extrauterine — *see* Pregnancy, ectopic
  fallopian — *see* Pregnancy, tubal
  false 300.11
    labor (pains) 644.1 ✓5th
  fatigue 646.8 ✓5th
  illegitimate V61.6
  incidental finding V22.2
  in double uterus 654.0 ✓5th
  interstitial — *see* Pregnancy, cornual
  intraligamentous — *see* Pregnancy, cornual
  intramural — *see* Pregnancy, cornual
  intraperitoneal — *see* Pregnancy, abdominal
  isthmian — *see* Pregnancy, tubal
  management affected by
    abnormal, abnormality
      fetus (suspected) 655.9 ✓5th
        specified NEC 655.8 ✓5th
      placenta 656.7 ✓5th
    advanced maternal age NEC 659.6 ✓5th
      multigravida 659.6 ✓5th
      primigravida 659.5 ✓5th
    antibodies (maternal)
      anti-c 656.1 ✓5th
      anti-d 656.1 ✓5th
      anti-e 656.1 ✓5th
      blood group (ABO) 656.2 ✓5th
        Rh(esus) 656.1 ✓5th
    elderly multigravida 659.6 ✓5th
    elderly primigravida 659.5 ✓5th

✓4th Fourth-digit Required   ✓5th Fifth-digit Required   ►◄ Revised Text   ● New Line   ▲ Revised Code

Pregnancy — *continued*
  management affected by — *continued*
    fetal (suspected)
      abnormality 655.9 ✓5th
        acid-base balance 656.8 ✓5th
        heart rate or rhythm 659.7 ✓5th
        specified NEC 655.8 ✓5th
      acidemia 656.3 ✓5th
      anencephaly 655.0 ✓5th
      bradycardia 659.7 ✓5th
      central nervous system malformation 655.0 ✓5th
      chromosomal abnormalities (conditions classifiable to 758.0-758.9) 655.1 ✓5th
      damage from
        drugs 655.5 ✓5th
          obstetric, anesthetic, or sedative 655.5 ✓5th
        environmental toxins 655.8 ✓5th
        intrauterine contraceptive device 655.8 ✓5th
        maternal
          alcohol addiction 655.4 ✓5th
          disease NEC 655.4 ✓5th
          drug use 655.5 ✓5th
          listeriosis 655.4 ✓5th
          rubella 655.3 ✓5th
          toxoplasmosis 655.4 ✓5th
          viral infection 655.3 ✓5th
        radiation 655.6 ✓5th
      death (near term) 656.4 ✓5th
        early (before 22 completed weeks' gestation) 632
      distress 656.8 ✓5th
      excessive growth 656.6 ✓5th
      growth retardation 656.5 ✓5th
      hereditary disease 655.2 ✓5th
      hydrocephalus 655.0 ✓5th
      intrauterine death 656.4 ✓5th
      poor growth 656.5 ✓5th
      spina bifida (with myelomeningocele) 655.0 ✓5th
    fetal-maternal hemorrhage 656.0 ✓5th
    hereditary disease in family (possibly) affecting fetus 655.2 ✓5th
    incompatibility, blood groups (ABO) 656.2 ✓5th
      rh(esus) 656.1 ✓5th
    insufficient prenatal care V23.7
    intrauterine death 656.4 ✓5th
    isoimmunization (ABO) 656.2 ✓5th
      rh(esus) 656.1 ✓5th
    large-for-dates fetus 656.6 ✓5th
    light-for-dates fetus 656.5 ✓5th
    meconium in liquor 656.8 ✓5th
    mental disorder (conditions classifiable to 290-303, 305-316, 317-319) 648.4 ✓5th
    multiparity (grand) 659.4 ✓5th
    poor obstetric history V23.49 ▲
      pre-term labor V23.41 ●
    postmaturity
      post term 645.1 ✓5th
      prolonged 645.2 ✓5th
    post term pregnancy 645.1 ✓5th
    previous
      abortion V23.2
        habitual 646.3 ✓5th
      cesarean delivery 654.2 ✓5th
      difficult delivery V23.49 ▲
      forceps delivery V23.49 ▲
      habitual abortions 646.3 ✓5th
      hemorrhage, antepartum or postpartum V23.49 ▲
      hydatidiform mole V23.1
      infertility V23.0
      malignancy NEC V23.8 ✓5th
      nonobstetrical conditions V23.8 ✓5th
      premature delivery V23.41 ▲
      trophoblastic disease (conditions in 630) V23.1
      vesicular mole V23.1
    prolonged pregnancy 645.2 ✓5th
    small-for-dates fetus 656.5 ✓5th
    young maternal age 659.8 ✓5th
  maternal death NEC 646.9 ✓5th

Pregnancy — *continued*
  mesometric (mural) — *see* Pregnancy, cornual
  molar 631
    hydatidiform (*see also* Hydatidiform mole) 630
      previous, affecting management of pregnancy V23.1
    previous, affecting management of pregnancy V23.49 ▲
  multiple NEC 651.9 ✓5th
    with fetal loss and retention of one or more fetus(es) 651.6 ✓5th
    affecting fetus or newborn 761.5
    specified type NEC 651.8 ✓5th
      with fetal loss and retention of one or more fetus(es) 651.6 ✓5th
  mural — *see* Pregnancy, cornual
  observation NEC V22.1
    first pregnancy V22.0
    high-risk V23.9
      specified problem NEC V23.8 ✓5th
  ovarian 633.20 ▲
    with intrauterine pregnancy 633.21 ●
    affecting fetus or newborn 761.4
  postmature
    post term 645.1 ✓5th
    prolonged 645.2 ✓5th
  post term 645.1 ✓5th
  prenatal care only V22.1
    first pregnancy V22.0
    high-risk V23.9
      specified problem NEC V23.8 ✓5th
  prolonged 645.2 ✓5th
  quadruplet NEC 651.2 ✓5th
    with fetal loss and retention of one or more fetus(es) 651.5 ✓5th
    affecting fetus or newborn 761.5
  quintuplet NEC 651.8 ✓5th
    with fetal loss and retention of one or more fetus(es) 651.6 ✓5th
    affecting fetus or newborn 761.5
  sextuplet NEC 651.8 ✓5th
    with fetal loss and retention of one or more fetus(es) 651.6 ✓5th
    affecting fetus or newborn 761.5
  spurious 300.11
  superfecundation NEC 651.9 ✓5th
    with fetal loss and retention of one or more fetus(es) 651.6 ✓5th
  superfetation NEC 651.9 ✓5th
    with fetal loss and retention of one or more fetus(es) 651.6 ✓5th
  supervision (of) (for) — *see also* Pregnancy, management affected by
    elderly
      multigravida V23.82
      primigravida V23.81
    high-risk V23.9
      insufficient prenatal care V23.7
      specified problem NEC V23.8 ✓5th
    multiparity V23.3
    normal NEC V22.1
      first V22.0
    poor
      obstetric history V23.49 ▲
        pre-term labor V23.41 ●
      reproductive history V23.5
    previous
      abortion V23.2
      hydatidiform mole V23.1
      infertility V23.0
      neonatal death V23.5
      stillbirth V23.5
      trophoblastic disease V23.1
      vesicular mole V23.1
    specified problem NEC V23.8 ✓5th
    young
      multigravida V23.84
      primigravida V23.83
  triplet NEC 651.1 ✓5th
    with fetal loss and retention of one or more fetus(es) 651.4 ✓5th
    affecting fetus or newborn 761.5
  tubal (with rupture) 633.10 ▲
    with intrauterine pregnancy 633.11 ●
    affecting fetus or newborn 761.4

Pregnancy — *continued*
  twin NEC 651.0 ✓5th
    with fetal loss and retention of one fetus 651.3 ✓5th
    affecting fetus or newborn 761.5
  unconfirmed V72.4
  undelivered (no other diagnosis) V22.2
    with false labor 644.1 ✓5th
    high-risk V23.9
      specified problem NEC V23.8 ✓5th
  unwanted NEC V61.7

Pregnant uterus — *see* condition

Preiser's disease (osteoporosis) 733.09

Prekwashiorkor 260

Preleukemia 238.7

Preluxation of hip, congenital (*see also* Subluxation, congenital, hip) 754.32

Premature — *see also* condition
  beats (nodal) 427.60
    atrial 427.61
    auricular 427.61
    postoperative 997.1
    specified type NEC 427.69
    supraventricular 427.61
    ventricular 427.69
  birth NEC 765.1 ✓5th
  closure
    cranial suture 756.0
    fontanel 756.0
    foramen ovale 745.8
  contractions 427.60
    atrial 427.61
    auricular 427.61
    auriculoventricular 427.61
    heart (extrasystole) 427.60
    junctional 427.60
    nodal 427.60
    postoperative 997.1
    ventricular 427.69
  ejaculation 302.75
  infant NEC 765.1 ✓5th
    excessive 765.0 ✓5th
    light-for-dates — *see* Light-for-dates
  labor 644.2 ✓5th
    threatened 644.0 ✓5th
  lungs 770.4
  menopause 256.31
  puberty 259.1
  rupture of membranes or amnion 658.1 ✓5th
    affecting fetus or newborn 761.1
    delayed delivery following 658.2 ✓5th
  senility (syndrome) 259.8
  separation, placenta (partial) — *see* Placenta, separation
  ventricular systole 427.69

Prematurity NEC 765.1 ✓5th
  extreme 765.0 ✓5th

Premenstrual syndrome 625.4

Premenstrual tension 625.4

Premolarization, cuspids 520.2

Premyeloma 273.1

Prenatal
  care, normal pregnancy V22.1
    first V22.0
  death, cause unknown — *see* Death, fetus
  screening — *see* Antenatal, screening

Prepartum — *see* condition

Preponderance, left or right ventricular 429.3

Prepuce — *see* condition

Presbycardia 797
  hypertensive (*see also* Hypertension, heart) 402.90

Presbycusis 388.01

Presbyesophagus 530.89

Presbyophrenia 310.1

Presbyopia 367.4

Prescription of contraceptives NEC V25.02
  diaphragm V25.02
  oral (pill) V25.01
    repeat V25.41
  repeat V25.40
    oral (pill) V25.41

Pregnancy — Prescription

Presenile — see also condition
  aging 259.8
  dementia (see also Dementia, presenile) 290.10
Presenility 259.8
Presentation, fetal
  abnormal 652.9 ✓5ᵗʰ
    with successful version 652.1 ✓5ᵗʰ
      before labor, affecting fetus or newborn
        761.7
      causing obstructed labor 660.0 ✓5ᵗʰ
        affecting fetus or newborn, any, except
          breech 763.1
      in multiple gestation (one or more) 652.6 ✓5ᵗʰ
      specified NEC 652.8 ✓5ᵗʰ
    arm 652.7 ✓5ᵗʰ
      causing obstructed labor 660.0 ✓5ᵗʰ
    breech (buttocks) (complete) (frank) 652.2 ✓5ᵗʰ
      with successful version 652.1 ✓5ᵗʰ
        before labor, affecting fetus or newborn
          761.7
      before labor, affecting fetus or newborn
        761.7
    brow 652.4 ✓5ᵗʰ
      causing obstructed labor 660.0 ✓5ᵗʰ
    buttocks 652.2 ✓5ᵗʰ
    chin 652.4 ✓5ᵗʰ
    complete 652.2 ✓5ᵗʰ
    compound 652.8 ✓5ᵗʰ
    cord 663.0 ✓5ᵗʰ
    extended head 652.4 ✓5ᵗʰ
    face 652.4 ✓5ᵗʰ
      to pubes 652.8 ✓5ᵗʰ
    footling 652.8 ✓5ᵗʰ
    frank 652.2 ✓5ᵗʰ
    hand, leg, or foot NEC 652.8 ✓5ᵗʰ
    incomplete 652.8 ✓5ᵗʰ
    mentum 652.4 ✓5ᵗʰ
    multiple gestation (one fetus or more)
      652.6 ✓5ᵗʰ
    oblique 652.3 ✓5ᵗʰ
      with successful version 652.1 ✓5ᵗʰ
    shoulder 652.8 ✓5ᵗʰ
      affecting fetus or newborn 763.1
    transverse 652.3 ✓5ᵗʰ
      with successful version 652.1 ✓5ᵗʰ
    umbilical cord 663.0 ✓5ᵗʰ
    unstable 652.0 ✓5ᵗʰ
Prespondylolisthesis (congenital) (lumbosacral)
  756.11
Pressure
  area, skin ulcer (see also Decubitus) 707.0
  atrophy, spine 733.99
  birth, fetus or newborn NEC 767.9
  brachial plexus 353.0
  brain 348.4
    injury at birth 767.0
  cerebral — see Pressure, brain
  chest 786.59
  cone, tentorial 348.4
    injury at birth 767.0
  funis — see Compression, umbilical cord
  hyposystolic (see also Hypotension) 458.9
  increased
    intracranial 781.99
      due to
        benign intracranial hypertension 348.2
        hydrocephalus — see hydrocephalus
        injury at birth 767.8
    intraocular 365.00
  lumbosacral plexus 353.1
  mediastinum 519.3
  necrosis (chronic) (skin) (see also Decubitus)
    707.0
  nerve — see Compression, nerve
  paralysis (see also Neuropathy, entrapment)
    355.9
  sore (chronic) (see also Decubitus) 707.0
  spinal cord 336.9
  ulcer (chronic) (see also Decubitus) 707.0
  umbilical cord — see Compression, umbilical
    cord
  venous, increased 459.89
Pre-syncope 780.2
Preterm infant NEC 765.1 ✓5ᵗʰ
  extreme 765.0 ✓5ᵗʰ
Priapism (penis) 607.3

Prickling sensation (see also Disturbance,
  sensation) 782.0
Prickly heat 705.1
Primary — see condition
Primigravida, elderly
  affecting
    fetus or newborn 763.89
    management of pregnancy, labor, and
      delivery 659.5 ✓5ᵗʰ
Primipara, old
  affecting
    fetus or newborn 763.89
    management of pregnancy, labor, and
      delivery 659.5 ✓5ᵗʰ
Primula dermatitis 692.6
Primus varus (bilateral) (metatarsus) 754.52
P.R.I.N.D. 436
Pringle's disease (tuberous sclerosis) 759.5
Prinzmetal's angina 413.1
Prinzmetal-Massumi syndrome (anterior chest
  wall) 786.52
Prizefighter ear 738.7
Problem (with) V49.9
  academic V62.3
  acculturation V62.4
  adopted child V61.29
  aged
    in-law V61.3
    parent V61.3
    person NEC V61.8
  alcoholism in family V61.41
  anger reaction (see also Disturbance, conduct)
    312.0 ✓5ᵗʰ
  behavior, child 312.9
  behavioral V40.9
    specified NEC V40.3
  betting V69.3
  cardiorespiratory NEC V47.2
  care of sick or handicapped person in family or
    household V61.49
  career choice V62.2
  communication V40.1
  conscience regarding medical care V62.6
  delinquency (juvenile) 312.9
  diet, inappropriate V69.1
  digestive NEC V47.3
  ear NEC V41.3
  eating habits, inappropriate V69.1
  economic V60.2
    affecting care V60.9
      specified type NEC V60.8
  educational V62.3
  enuresis, child 307.6
  exercise, lack of V69.0
  eye NEC V41.1
  family V61.9
    specified circumstance NEC V61.8
  fear reaction, child 313.0
  feeding (elderly) (infant) 783.3
    newborn 779.3
    nonorganic 307.50
  fetal, affecting management of pregnancy
    656.9 ✓5ᵗʰ
    specified type NEC 656.8 ✓5ᵗʰ
  financial V60.2
  foster child V61.29
    specified NEC V41.8
  functional V41.9
    specified type NEC V41.8
  gambling V69.3
  genital NEC V47.5
  head V48.9
    deficiency V48.0
    disfigurement V48.6
    mechanical V48.2
    motor V48.2
    movement of V48.2
    sensory V48.4
    specified condition NEC V48.8
  hearing V41.2
  high-risk sexual behavior V69.2
  influencing health status NEC V49.89
  internal organ NEC V47.9
    deficiency V47.0

Problem (with) — continued
  internal organ NEC — continued
    mechanical or motor V47.1
  interpersonal NEC V62.81
  jealousy, child 313.3
  learning V40.0
  legal V62.5
  life circumstance NEC V62.89
  lifestyle V69.9
    specified NEC V69.8
  limb V49.9
    deficiency V49.0
    disfigurement V49.4
    mechanical V49.1
    motor V49.2
    movement, involving
      musculoskeletal system V49.1
      nervous system V49.2
    sensory V49.3
    specified condition NEC V49.5
  litigation V62.5
  living alone V60.3
  loneliness NEC V62.89
  marital V61.10
    involving
      divorce V61.0
      estrangement V61.0
      psychosexual disorder 302.9
      sexual function V41.7
  mastication V41.6
  medical care, within family V61.49
  mental V40.9
    specified NEC V40.2
  mental hygiene, adult V40.9
  multiparity V61.5
  nail biting, child 307.9
  neck V48.9
    deficiency V48.1
    disfigurement V48.7
    mechanical V48.3
    motor V48.3
    movement V48.3
    sensory V48.5
    specified condition NEC V48.8
  neurological NEC 781.99
  none (feared complaint unfounded) V65.5
  occupational V62.2
  parent-child V61.20
  partner V61.10
  personal NEC V62.89
    interpersonal conflict NEC V62.81
  personality (see also Disorder, personality)
    301.9
  phase of life V62.89
  placenta, affecting managment of pregnancy
    656.9 ✓5ᵗʰ
    specified type NEC 656.8 ✓5ᵗʰ
  poverty V60.2
  presence of sick or handicapped person in
    family or household V61.49
  psychiatric 300.9
  psychosocial V62.9
    specified type NEC V62.89
  relational NEC V62.81
  relationship, childhood 313.3
  religious or spiritual belief
    other than medical care V62.89
    regarding medical care V62.6
  self-damaging behavior V69.8
  sexual
    behavior, high-risk V69.2
    function NEC V41.7
  sibling relational V61.8
  sight V41.0
  sleep disorder, child 307.40
  smell V41.5
  speech V40.1
  spite reaction, child (see also Disturbance,
    conduct) 312.0 ✓5ᵗʰ
  spoiled child reaction (see also Disturbance,
    conduct) 312.1 ✓5ᵗʰ
  swallowing V41.6
  tantrum, child (see also Disturbance, conduct)
    312.1 ✓5ᵗʰ
  taste V41.5
  thumb sucking, child 307.9
  tic, child 307.21

Problem (with) — *continued*
  trunk V48.9
    deficiency V48.1
    disfigurement V48.7
    mechanical V48.3
    motor V48.3
    movement V48.3
    sensory V48.5
    specified condition NEC V48.8
  unemployment V62.0
  urinary NEC V47.4
  voice production V41.4
Procedure (surgical) not done NEC V64.3
  because of
    contraindication V64.1
    patient's decision V64.2
      for reasons of conscience or religion
        V62.6
    specified reason NEC V64.3
Procidentia
  anus (sphincter) 569.1
  rectum (sphincter) 569.1
  stomach 537.89
  uteri 618.1
Proctalgia 569.42
  fugax 564.6
  spasmodic 564.6
    psychogenic 307.89
Proctitis 569.49
  amebic 006.8
  chlamydial 099.52
  gonococcal 098.7
  granulomatous 555.1
  idiopathic 556.2
    with ulcerative sigmoiditis 556.3
  tuberculous (*see also* Tuberculosis) 014.8 ✔5ᵗʰ
  ulcerative (chronic) (nonspecific) 556.2
    with ulcerative sigmoiditis 556.3
Proctocele
  female (without uterine prolapse) 618.0
    with uterine prolapse 618.4
      complete 618.3
      incomplete 618.2
  male 569.49
Proctocolitis, idiopathic 556.2
  with ulcerative sigmoiditis 556.3
Proctoptosis 569.1
Proctosigmoiditis 569.89
  ulcerative (chronic) 556.3
Proctospasm 564.6
  psychogenic 306.4
Prodromal-AIDS — *see* Human immunodeficiency
  virus (disease) (illness) (infection)
Profichet's disease or syndrome 729.9
Progeria (adultorum) (syndrome) 259.8
Prognathism (mandibular) (maxillary) 524.00
Progonoma (melanotic) (M9363/0) — *see*
  Neoplasm, by site, benign
Progressive — *see* condition
Prolapse, prolapsed
  anus, anal (canal) (sphincter) 569.1
  arm or hand, complicating delivery 652.7 ✔5ᵗʰ
    causing obstructed labor 660.0 ✔5ᵗʰ
      affecting fetus or newborn 763.1
    fetus or newborn 763.1
  bladder (acquired) (mucosa) (sphincter)
    congenital (female) (male) 756.71
    female 618.0
    male 596.8
  breast implant (prosthetic) 996.54
  cecostomy 569.69
  cecum 569.89
  cervix, cervical (stump) (hypertrophied) 618.1
    anterior lip, obstructing labor 660.2 ✔5ᵗʰ
      affecting fetus or newborn 763.1
    congenital 752.49
    postpartal (old) 618.1
  ciliary body 871.1
  colon (pedunculated) 569.89
  colostomy 569.69
  conjunctiva 372.73
  cord — *see* Prolapse, umbilical cord
  disc (intervertebral) — *see* Displacement,
    intervertebral disc

Prolapse, prolapsed — *continued*
  duodenum 537.89
  eye implant (orbital) 996.59
    lens (ocular) 996.53
  fallopian tube 620.4
  fetal extremity, complicating delivery 652.8 ✔5ᵗʰ
    causing obstructed labor 660.0 ✔5ᵗʰ
    fetus or newborn 763.1
  funis — *see* Prolapse, umbilical cord
  gastric (mucosa) 537.89
  genital, female 618.9
    specified NEC 618.8
  globe 360.81
  ileostomy bud 569.69
  intervertebral disc — *see* Displacement,
    intervertebral disc
  intestine (small) 569.89
  iris 364.8
    traumatic 871.1
  kidney (*see also* Disease, renal) 593.0
    congenital 753.3
  laryngeal muscles or ventricle 478.79
  leg, complicating delivery 652.8 ✔5ᵗʰ
    causing obstructed labor 660.0 ✔5ᵗʰ
    fetus or newborn 763.1
  liver 573.8
  meatus urinarius 599.5
  mitral valve 424.0
  ocular lens implant 996.53
  organ or site, congenital NEC — *see*
    Malposition, congenital
  ovary 620.4
  pelvic (floor), female 618.8
  perineum, female 618.8
  pregnant uterus 654.4 ✔5ᵗʰ
  rectum (mucosa) (sphincter) 569.1
    due to Trichuris trichiuria 127.3
  spleen 289.59
  stomach 537.89
  umbilical cord
    affecting fetus or newborn 762.4
    complicating delivery 663.0 ✔5ᵗʰ
  ureter 593.89
    with obstruction 593.4
  ureterovesical orifice 593.89
  urethra (acquired) (infected) (mucosa) 599.5
    congenital 753.8
  uterovaginal 618.4
    complete 618.3
    incomplete 618.2
    specified NEC 618.8
  uterus (first degree) (second degree) (third
    degree) (complete) (without vaginal wall
    prolapse) 618.1
    with mention of vaginal wall prolapse — *see*
      Prolapse, uterovaginal
    congenital 752.3
    in pregnancy or childbirth 654.4 ✔5ᵗʰ
      affecting fetus or newborn 763.1
      causing obstructed labor 660.2 ✔5ᵗʰ
        affecting fetus or newborn 763.1
    postpartal (old) 618.1
  uveal 871.1
  vagina (anterior) (posterior) (vault) (wall)
    (without uterine prolapse) 618.0
    with uterine prolapse 618.4
      complete 618.3
      incomplete 618.2
    posthysterectomy 618.5
  vitreous (humor) 379.26
    traumatic 871.1
  womb — *see* Prolapse, uterus
Prolapsus, female 618.9
Proliferative — *see* condition
Prolinemia 270.8
Prolinuria 270.8
Prolonged, prolongation
  bleeding time (*see also* Defect, coagulation)
    790.92
    "idiopathic" (in von Willebrand's disease)
      286.4
  coagulation time (*see also* Defect, coagulation)
    790.92
  gestation syndrome 766.2
  labor 662.1 ✔5ᵗʰ
    affecting fetus or newborn 763.89
    first stage 662.0 ✔5ᵗʰ

Prolonged, prolongation — *continued*
  labor — *continued*
    second stage 662.2 ✔5ᵗʰ
  pregnancy 645.2 ✔5ᵗʰ
  PR interval 426.11
  prothrombin time (*see also* Defect, coagulation)
    790.92
  rupture of membranes (24 hours or more prior
    to onset of labor) 658.2 ✔5ᵗʰ
  uterine contractions in labor 661.4 ✔5ᵗʰ
    affecting fetus or newborn 763.7
Prominauris 744.29
Prominence
  auricle (ear) (congenital) 744.29
    acquired 380.32
  ischial spine or sacral promontory
    with disproportion (fetopelvic) 653.3 ✔5ᵗʰ
      affecting fetus or newborn 763.1
      causing obstructed labor 660.1 ✔5ᵗʰ
        affecting fetus or newborn 763.1
  nose (congenital) 748.1
    acquired 738.0
Pronation
  ankle 736.79
  foot 736.79
    congenital 755.67
Prophylactic
  administration of
    antibiotics V07.39
    antitoxin, any V07.2
    antivenin V07.2
    chemotherapeutic agent NEC V07.39
      fluoride V07.31
    diphtheria antitoxin V07.2
    gamma globulin V07.2
    immune sera (gamma globulin) V07.2
    RhoGAM V07.2
    tetanus antitoxin V07.2
  chemotherapy NEC V07.39
    fluoride V07.31
  immunotherapy V07.2
  measure V07.9
    specified type NEC V07.8
  postmenopausal hormone replacement V07.4
  sterilization V25.2
Proptosis (ocular) (*see also* Exophthalmos) 376.30
  thyroid 242.0 ✔5ᵗʰ
Propulsion
  eyeball 360.81
Prosecution, anxiety concerning V62.5
Prostate, prostatic — *see* condition
Prostatism 600.9
Prostatitis (congestive) (suppurative) 601.9
  acute 601.0
  cavitary 601.8
  chlamydial 099.54
  chronic 601.1
  diverticular 601.8
  due to Trichomonas (vaginalis) 131.03
  fibrous 600.9
  gonococcal (acute) 098.12
    chronic or duration of 2 months or over
      098.32
  granulomatous 601.8
  hypertrophic 600.0
  specified type NEC 601.8
  subacute 601.1
  trichomonal 131.03
  tuberculous (*see also* Tuberculosis)
    016.5 ✔5ᵗʰ *[601.4]*
Prostatocystitis 601.3
Prostatorrhea 602.8
Prostatoseminovesiculitis, trichomonal 131.03
Prostration 780.79
  heat 992.5
    anhydrotic 992.3
    due to
      salt (and water) depletion 992.4
      water depletion 992.3
  nervous 300.5
  newborn 779.89   ▲
  senile 797
Protanomaly 368.51

Protanopia (anomalous trichromat) (complete)
(incomplete) 368.51
Protein
deficiency 260
malnutrition 260
sickness (prophylactic) (therapeutic) 999.5
Proteinemia 790.99
Proteinosis
alveolar, lung or pulmonary 516.0
lipid 272.8
lipoid (of Urbach) 272.8
Proteinuria (*see also* Albuminuria) 791.0
Bence-Jones NEC 791.0
gestational 646.2 ☑5ᵗʰ
with hypertension — *see* Toxemia, of
pregnancy
orthostatic 593.6
postural 593.6
Proteolysis, pathologic 286.6
Protocoproporphyria 277.1
Protoporphyria (erythrohepatic) (erythropoietic)
277.1
Protrusio acetabuli 718.65
Protrusion
acetabulum (into pelvis) 718.65
device, implant, or graft — *see*
Complications, mechanical
ear, congenital 744.29
intervertebral disc — *see* Displacement,
intervertebral disc
nucleus pulposus — *see* Displacement,
intervertebral disc
Proud flesh 701.5
Prune belly (syndrome) 756.71
Prurigo (ferox) (gravis) (Hebra's) (hebrae) (mitis)
(simplex) 698.2
agria 698.3
asthma syndrome 691.8
Besnier's (atopic dermatitis) (infantile eczema)
691.8
eczematodes allergicum 691.8
estivalis (Hutchinson's) 692.72
Hutchinson's 692.72
nodularis 698.3
psychogenic 306.3
Pruritus, pruritic 698.9
ani 698.0
psychogenic 306.3
conditions NEC 698.9
psychogenic 306.3
due to Onchocerca volvulus 125.3
ear 698.9
essential 698.9
genital organ(s) 698.1
psychogenic 306.3
gravidarum 646.8 ☑5ᵗʰ
hiemalis 698.8
neurogenic (any site) 306.3
perianal 698.0
psychogenic (any site) 306.3
scrotum 698.1
psychogenic 306.3
senile, senilis 698.8
Trichomonas 131.9
vulva, vulvae 698.1
psychogenic 306.3
Psammocarcinoma (M8140/3) — *see* Neoplasm,
by site, malignant
Pseudarthrosis, pseudoarthrosis (bone) 733.82
joint following fusion V45.4
Pseudoacanthosis
nigricans 701.8
Pseudoaneurysm — *see* Aneurysm
Pseudoangina (pectoris) — *see* Angina
Pseudoangioma 452
Pseudo-Argyll-Robertson pupil 379.45
Pseudoarteriosus 747.89
Pseudoarthrosis — *see* Pseudarthrosis
Pseudoataxia 799.8
Pseudobursa 727.89
Pseudocholera 025
Pseudochromidrosis 705.89

Pseudocirrhosis, liver, pericardial 423.2
Pseudocoarctation 747.21
Pseudocowpox 051.1
Pseudocoxalgia 732.1
Pseudocroup 478.75
Pseudocyesis 300.11
Pseudocyst
lung 518.89
pancreas 577.2
retina 361.19
Pseudodementia 300.16
Pseudoelephantiasis neuroarthritica 757.0
Pseudoemphysema 518.89
Pseudoencephalitis
superior (acute) hemorrhagic 265.1
Pseudoerosion cervix, congenital 752.49
Pseudoexfoliation, lens capsule 366.11
Pseudofracture (idiopathic) (multiple)
(spontaneous) (symmetrical) 268.2
Pseudoglanders 025
Pseudoglioma 360.44
Pseudogout — *see* Chondrocalcinosis
Pseudohallucination 780.1
Pseudohemianesthesia 782.0
Pseudohemophilia (Bernuth's) (hereditary) (type
B) 286.4
type A 287.8
vascular 287.8
Pseudohermaphroditism 752.7
with chromosomal anomaly — *see* Anomaly,
chromosomal
adrenal 255.2
female (without adrenocortical disorder) 752.7
with adrenocortical disorder 255.2
adrenal 255.2
male (without gonadal disorder) 752.7
with
adrenocortical disorder 255.2
cleft scrotum 752.7
feminizing testis 257.8
gonadal disorder 257.9
adrenal 255.2
Pseudohole, macula 362.54
Pseudo-Hurler's disease (mucolipidosis III) 272.7
Pseudohydrocephalus 348.2
Pseudohypertrophic muscular dystrophy (Erb's)
359.1
Pseudohypertrophy, muscle 359.1
Pseudohypoparathyroidism 275.49
Pseudoinfluenza 487.1
Pseudoinsomnia 307.49
Pseudoleukemia 288.8
infantile 285.8
Pseudomembranous — *see* condition
Pseudomeningocele (cerebral) (infective) (surgical)
349.2
spinal 349.2
Pseudomenstruation 626.8
Pseudomucinous
cyst (ovary) (M8470/0) 220
peritoneum 568.89
Pseudomyeloma 273.1
Pseudomyxoma peritonei (M8480/6) 197.6
Pseudoneuritis optic (nerve) 377.24
papilla 377.24
congenital 743.57
Pseudoneuroma — *see* Injury, nerve, by site
Pseudo-obstruction
intestine 564.89
Pseudopapilledema 377.24.
Pseudoparalysis
arm or leg 781.4
atonic, congenital 358.8
Pseudopelade 704.09
Pseudophakia V43.1
Pseudopolycythemia 289.0
Pseudopolyposis, colon 556.4
Pseudoporencephaly 348.0

Pseudopseudohypoparathyroidism 275.49
Pseudopsychosis 300.16
Pseudopterygium 372.52
Pseudoptosis (eyelid) 374.34
Pseudorabies 078.89
Pseudoretinitis, pigmentosa 362.65
Pseudorickets 588.0
senile (Pozzi's) 731.0
Pseudorubella 057.8
Pseudoscarlatina 057.8
Pseudosclerema 778.1
Pseudosclerosis (brain)
Jakob's 046.1
of Westphal (-Strümpell) (hepatolenticular
degeneration) 275.1
spastic 046.1
with dementia
with behavioral disturbance 046.1
[294.11]
without behavioral disturbance 046.1
[294.10]
Pseudoseizure 780.39
non-psychiatric 780.39
psychiatric 300.11
Pseudotabes 799.8
diabetic 250.6 ☑5ᵗʰ [337.1]
Pseudotetanus (*see also* Convulsions) 780.39
Pseudotetany 781.7
hysterical 300.11
Pseudothalassemia 285.0
Pseudotrichinosis 710.3
Pseudotruncus arteriosus 747.29
Pseudotuberculosis, pasteurella (infection) 027.2
Pseudotumor
cerebri 348.2
orbit (inflammatory) 376.11
Pseudo-Turner's syndrome 759.89
Pseudoxanthoma elasticum 757.39
Psilosis (sprue) (tropical) 579.1
Monilia 112.89
nontropical 579.0
not sprue 704.00
Psittacosis 073.9
Psoitis 728.89
Psora NEC 696.1
Psoriasis 696.1
any type, except arthropathic 696.1
arthritic, arthropathic 696.0
buccal 528.6
flexural 696.1
follicularis 696.1
guttate 696.1
inverse 696.1
mouth 528.6
nummularis 696.1
psychogenic 316 [696.1]
punctata 696.1
pustular 696.1
rupioides 696.1
vulgaris 696.1
Psorospermiasis 136.4
Psorospermosis 136.4
follicularis (vegetans) 757.39
Psychalgia 307.80
Psychasthenia 300.89
compulsive 300.3
mixed compulsive states 300.3
obsession 300.3
Psychiatric disorder or problem NEC 300.9
Psychogenic — *see also* condition
factors associated with physical conditions 316
Psychoneurosis, psychoneurotic (*see also*
Neurosis) 300.9
anxiety (state) 300.00
climacteric 627.2
compensation 300.16
compulsion 300.3
conversion hysteria 300.11
depersonalization 300.6
depressive type 300.4
dissociative hysteria 300.15

Psychoneurosis, psychoneurotic (see also
　　Neurosis) — continued
　　hypochondriacal 300.7
　　hysteria 300.10
　　　conversion type 300.11
　　　dissociative type 300.15
　　mixed NEC 300.89
　　neurasthenic 300.5
　　obsessional 300.3
　　obsessive-compulsive 300.3
　　occupational 300.89
　　personality NEC 301.89
　　phobia 300.20
　　senile NEC 300.89

Psychopathic — see also condition
　　constitution, posttraumatic 310.2
　　　with psychosis 293.9
　　personality 301.9
　　　amoral trends 301.7
　　　antisocial trends 301.7
　　　asocial trends 301.7
　　　mixed types 301.7
　　state 301.9

Psychopathy, sexual (see also Deviation, sexual)
　　302.9

**Psychophysiologic, psychophysiological
　　condition** — see Reaction,
　　psychophysiologic

Psychose passionelle 297.8

Psychosexual identity disorder 302.6
　　adult-life 302.85
　　childhood 302.6

Psychosis 298.9
　　acute hysterical 298.1
　　affecting management of pregnancy, childbirth,
　　　or puerperium 648.4 ✓5ᵗʰ
　　affective NEC 296.90

> Note — Use the following fifth-digit
> subclassification with categories 296.0-
> 296.6:
>
> 　0　unspecified
> 　1　mild
> 　2　moderate
> 　3　severe, without mention of psychotic
> 　　behavior
> 　4　severe, specified as with psychotic
> 　　behavior
> 　5　in partial or unspecified remission
> 　6　in full remission

　　drug-induced 292.84
　　due to or associated with physical condition
　　　293.83
　　involutional 296.2 ✓5ᵗʰ
　　　recurrent episode 296.3 ✓5ᵗʰ
　　　single episode 296.2 ✓5ᵗʰ
　　manic-depressive 296.80
　　　circular (alternating) 296.7
　　　　currently depressed 296.5 ✓5ᵗʰ
　　　　currently manic 296.4 ✓5ᵗʰ
　　　depressed type 296.2 ✓5ᵗʰ
　　　　atypical 296.82
　　　　recurrent episode 296.3 ✓5ᵗʰ
　　　　single episode 296.2 ✓5ᵗʰ
　　　manic 296.0 ✓5ᵗʰ
　　　　atypical 296.81
　　　　recurrent episode 296.1 ✓5ᵗʰ
　　　　single episode 296.0 ✓5ᵗʰ
　　　mixed type NEC 296.89
　　　specified type NEC 296.89
　　senile 290.21
　　specified type NEC 296.99
　　alcoholic 291.9
　　　with
　　　　anxiety 291.89
　　　　delirium tremens 291.0
　　　　delusions 291.5
　　　　dementia 291.2
　　　　hallucinosis 291.3
　　　　mood disturbance 291.89
　　　　jealousy 291.5
　　　　paranoia 291.5
　　　　persisting amnesia 291.1

Psychosis — continued
　　alcoholic — continued
　　　with — continued
　　　　sexual dysfunction 291.89
　　　　sleep disturbance 291.89
　　　amnestic confabulatory 291.1
　　　delirium tremens 291.0
　　　hallucinosis 291.3
　　　Korsakoff's, Korsakov's, Korsakow's 291.1
　　　paranoid type 291.5
　　　pathological intoxication 291.4
　　　polyneuritic 291.1
　　　specified type NEC 291.89
　　alternating (see also Psychosis, manic-
　　　depressive, circular) 296.7
　　anergastic (see also Psychosis, organic) 294.9
　　arteriosclerotic 290.40
　　　with
　　　　acute confusional state 290.41
　　　　delirium 290.41
　　　　delusional features 290.42
　　　　depressive features 290.43
　　　depressed type 290.43
　　　paranoid type 290.42
　　　simple type 290.40
　　　uncomplicated 290.40
　　atypical 298.9
　　　depressive 296.82
　　　manic 296.81
　　borderline (schizophrenia) (see also
　　　Schizophrenia) 295.5 ✓5ᵗʰ
　　　of childhood (see also Psychosis, childhood)
　　　　299.8 ✓5ᵗʰ
　　　prepubertal 299.8 ✓5ᵗʰ
　　brief reactive 298.8
　　childhood, with origin specific to 299.9 ✓5ᵗʰ

> Note — Use the following fifth-digit
> subclassification with category 299:
>
> 　0　current or active state
> 　1　residual state

　　　atypical 299.8 ✓5ᵗʰ
　　　specified type NEC 299.8 ✓5ᵗʰ
　　circular (see also Psychosis, manic-depressive,
　　　circular) 296.7
　　climacteric (see also Psychosis, involutional)
　　　298.8
　　confusional 298.9
　　　acute 293.0
　　　reactive 298.2
　　　subacute 293.1
　　depressive (see also Psychosis, affective)
　　　296.2 ✓5ᵗʰ
　　　atypical 296.82
　　　involutional 296.2 ✓5ᵗʰ
　　　　recurrent episode 296.3 ✓5ᵗʰ
　　　　single episode 296.2 ✓5ᵗʰ
　　　psychogenic 298.0
　　　reactive (emotional stress) (psychological
　　　　trauma) 298.0
　　　recurrent episode 296.3 ✓5ᵗʰ
　　　　with hypomania (bipolar II) 296.89
　　　single episode 296.2 ✓5ᵗʰ
　　disintegrative (childhood) (see also Psychosis,
　　　childhood) 299.1 ✓5ᵗʰ
　　drug 292.9
　　　with
　　　　affective syndrome 292.84
　　　　amnestic syndrome 292.83
　　　　anxiety 292.89
　　　　delirium 292.81
　　　　　withdrawal 292.0
　　　　delusional syndrome 292.11
　　　　dementia 292.82
　　　　depressive state 292.84
　　　　hallucinosis 292.12
　　　　mood disturbance 292.84
　　　　organic personality syndrome NEC
　　　　　292.89
　　　　sexual dysfunction 292.89
　　　　sleep disturbance 292.89
　　　　withdrawal syndrome (and delirium)
　　　　　292.0
　　　affective syndrome 292.84
　　　delusional state 292.11
　　　hallucinatory state 292.12

Psychosis — continued
　　drug — continued
　　　hallucinosis 292.12
　　　paranoid state 292.11
　　　specified type NEC 292.89
　　　withdrawal syndrome (and delirium) 292.0
　　due to or associated with physical condition
　　　(see also Psychosis, organic) 293.9
　　epileptic NEC 294.8
　　excitation (psychogenic) (reactive) 298.1
　　exhaustive (see also Reaction, stress, acute)
　　　308.9
　　hypomanic (see also Psychosis, affective)
　　　296.0 ✓5ᵗʰ
　　　recurrent episode 296.1 ✓5ᵗʰ
　　　single episode 296.0 ✓5ᵗʰ
　　hysterical 298.8
　　　acute 298.1
　　incipient 298.8
　　　schizophrenic (see also Schizophrenia)
　　　　295.5 ✓5ᵗʰ
　　induced 297.3
　　infantile (see also Psychosis, childhood)
　　　299.0 ✓5ᵗʰ
　　infective 293.9
　　　acute 293.0
　　　subacute 293.1
　　in pregnancy, childbirth, or puerperium
　　　648.4 ✓5ᵗʰ
　　interactional (childhood) (see also Psychosis,
　　　childhood) 299.1 ✓5ᵗʰ
　　involutional 298.8
　　　depressive (see also Psychosis, affective)
　　　　296.2 ✓5ᵗʰ
　　　　recurrent episode 296.3 ✓5ᵗʰ
　　　　single episode 296.2 ✓5ᵗʰ
　　　melancholic 296.2 ✓5ᵗʰ
　　　　recurrent episode 296.3 ✓5ᵗʰ
　　　　single episode 296.2 ✓5ᵗʰ
　　　paranoid state 297.2
　　　paraphrenia 297.2
　　Korsakoff's, Korakov's, Korsakow's
　　　(nonalcoholic) 294.0
　　　alcoholic 291.1
　　mania (phase) (see also Psychosis, affective)
　　　296.0 ✓5ᵗʰ
　　　recurrent episode 296.1 ✓5ᵗʰ
　　　single episode 296.0 ✓5ᵗʰ
　　manic (see also Psychosis, affective) 296.0 ✓5ᵗʰ
　　　atypical 296.81
　　　recurrent episode 296.1 ✓5ᵗʰ
　　　single episode 296.0 ✓5ᵗʰ
　　manic-depressive 296.80
　　　circular 296.7
　　　　currently
　　　　　depressed 296.5 ✓5ᵗʰ
　　　　　manic 296.4 ✓5ᵗʰ
　　　　mixed 296.6 ✓5ᵗʰ
　　　depressive 296.2 ✓5ᵗʰ
　　　　recurrent episode 296.3 ✓5ᵗʰ
　　　　　with hypomania (bipolar II) 296.89
　　　　single episode 296.2 ✓5ᵗʰ
　　　hypomanic 296.0 ✓5ᵗʰ
　　　　recurrent episode 296.1 ✓5ᵗʰ
　　　　single episode 296.0 ✓5ᵗʰ
　　　manic 296.0 ✓5ᵗʰ
　　　　atypical 296.81
　　　　recurrent episode 296.1 ✓5ᵗʰ
　　　　single episode 296.0 ✓5ᵗʰ
　　　mixed NEC 296.89
　　　perplexed 296.89
　　　stuporous 296.89
　　menopausal (see also Psychosis, involutional)
　　　298.8
　　mixed schizophrenic and affective (see also
　　　Schizophrenia) 295.7 ✓5ᵗʰ
　　multi-infarct (cerebrovascular) (see also
　　　Psychosis, arteriosclerotic) 290.40
　　organic NEC 294.9
　　　due to or associated with
　　　　addiction
　　　　　alcohol (see also Psychosis, alcoholic)
　　　　　　291.9
　　　　　drug (see also Psychosis, drug) 292.9
　　　　alcohol intoxication, acute (see also
　　　　　Psychosis, alcoholic) 291.9

■✓4ᵗʰ Fourth-digit Required　　　■✓5ᵗʰ Fifth-digit Required　　　▶◀ Revised Text　　　● New Line　　　▲ Revised Code

Psychosis — *continued*
  organic NEC — *continued*
    due to or associated with — *continued*
      alcoholism (*see also* Psychosis, alcoholic)
        291.9
      arteriosclerosis (cerebral) (*see also*
        Psychosis, arteriosclerotic) 290.40
      cerebrovascular disease
        acute (psychosis) 293.0
        arteriosclerotic (*see also* Psychosis,
          arteriosclerotic) 290.40
      childbirth — *see* Psychosis, puerperal
      dependence
        alcohol (*see also* Psychosis, alcoholic)
          291.9
        drug 292.9
      disease
        alcoholic liver (*see also* Psychosis,
          alcoholic) 291.9
        brain
          arteriosclerotic (*see also* Psychosis,
            arteriosclerotic) 290.40
        cerebrovascular
          acute (psychosis) 293.0
          arteriosclerotic (*see also* Psychosis,
            arteriosclerotic) 290.40
        endocrine or metabolic 293.9
          acute (psychosis) 293.0
          subacute (psychosis) 293.1
        Jakob-Creutzfeldt
          with behavioral disturbance 046.1
            [294.11]
          without behavioral disturbance
            046.1 *[294.10]*
        liver, alcoholic (*see also* Psychosis,
          alcoholic) 291.9
      disorder
        cerebrovascular
          acute (psychosis) 293.0
        endocrine or metabolic 293.9
          acute (psychosis) 293.0
          subacute (psychosis) 293.1
      epilepsy
        with behavioral disturbance
          345.9 ✓5ᵗʰ *[294.11]*
        without behavioral disturbance
          345.9 ✓5ᵗʰ *[294.10]*
        transient (acute) 293.0
      Huntington's chorea
        with behavioral disturbance
          333.4 *[294.11]*
        without behavioral disturbance
          333.4 *[294.10]*
      infection
        brain 293.9
          acute (psychosis) 293.0
          chronic 294.8
          subacute (psychosis) 293.1
        intracranial NEC 293.9
          acute (psychosis) 293.0
          chronic 294.8
          subacute (psychosis) 293.1
      intoxication
        alcoholic (acute) (*see also* Psychosis,
          alcoholic) 291.9
        pathological 291.4
        drug (*see also* Psychosis, drug) 292.2
      ischemia
        cerebrovascular (generalized) (*see also*
          Psychosis, arteriosclerotic)
          290.40
      Jakob-Creutzfeldt disease or syndrome
        with behavioral disturbance
          046.1 *[294.11]*
        without behavioral disturbance
          046.1 *[294.10]*
      multiple sclerosis
        with behavioral disturbance
          340 *[294.11]*
        without behavioral disturbance
          340 *[294.10]*
      physical condition NEC 293.9
        with
          delusions 293.81
          hallucinations 293.82

Psychosis — *continued*
  organic NEC — *continued*
    due to or associated with — *continued*
      presenility 290.10
      puerperium — *see* Psychosis, puerperal
      sclerosis, multiple
        with behavioral disturbance
          340 *[294.11]*
        without behavioral disturbance
          340 *[294.10]*
      senility 290.20
      status epilepticus
        with behavioral disturbance
          345.3 ✓5ᵗʰ *[294.11]*
        without behavioral disturbance
          345.3 ✓5ᵗʰ *[294.10]*
      trauma
        brain (birth) (from electrical current)
          (surgical) 293.9
          acute (psychosis) 293.0
          chronic 294.8
          subacute (psychosis) 293.1
          unspecified physical condition
            294.9
      infective 293.9
        acute (psychosis) 293.0
        subacute 293.1
      posttraumatic 293.9
        acute 293.0
        subacute 293.1
      specified type NEC 294.8
      transient 293.9
        with
          anxiety 293.84
          delusions 293.81
          depression 293.83
          hallucinations 293.82
        depressive type 293.83
        hallucinatory type 293.82
        paranoid type 293.81
        specified type NEC 293.89
  paranoic 297.1
  paranoid (chronic) 297.9
    alcoholic 291.5
    chronic 297.1
    climacteric 297.2
    involutional 297.2
    menopausal 297.2
    protracted reactive 298.4
    psychogenic 298.4
      acute 298.3
    schizophrenic (*see also* Schizophrenia)
      295.3 ✓5ᵗʰ
    senile 290.20
  paroxysmal 298.9
    senile 290.20
  polyneuritic, alcoholic 291.1
  postoperative 293.9
  postpartum — *see* Psychosis, puerperal
  prepsychotic (*see also* Schizophrenia) 295.5 ✓5ᵗʰ
  presbyophrenic (type) 290.8
  presenile (*see also* Dementia, presenile) 290.10
  prison 300.16
  psychogenic 298.8
    depressive 298.0
    paranoid 298.4
      acute 298.3
  puerperal
    specified type — *see* categories 295-298 ✓5ᵗʰ
    unspecified type 293.89
      acute 293.0
      chronic 293.89
      subacute 293.1
  reactive (emotional stress) (psychological
    trauma) 298.8
    brief 298.8
    confusion 298.2
    depressive 298.0
    excitation 298.1
  schizo-affective (depressed) (excited) (*see also*
    Schizophrenia) 295.7 ✓5ᵗʰ
  schizophrenia, schizophrenic (*see also*
    Schizophrenia) 295.9 ✓5ᵗʰ
    borderline type 295.5 ✓5ᵗʰ
      of childhood (*see also* Psychosis,
        childhood) 299.8 ✓5ᵗʰ
    catatonic (excited) (withdrawn) 295.2 ✓5ᵗʰ

Psychosis — *continued*
  schizophrenia, schizophrenic (*see also*
    Schizophrenia) — *continued*
    childhood type (*see also* Psychosis,
      childhood) 299.9 ✓5ᵗʰ
      hebephrenic 295.1 ✓5ᵗʰ
      incipient 295.5 ✓5ᵗʰ
      latent 295.5 ✓5ᵗʰ
      paranoid 295.3 ✓5ᵗʰ
      prepsychotic 295.5 ✓5ᵗʰ
      prodromal 295.5 ✓5ᵗʰ
      pseudoneurotic 295.5 ✓5ᵗʰ
      pseudopsychopathic 295.5 ✓5ᵗʰ
      schizophreniform 295.4 ✓5ᵗʰ
      simple 295.0 ✓5ᵗʰ
    schizophreniform 295.4 ✓5ᵗʰ
    senile NEC 290.20
      with
        delusional features 290.20
        depressive features 290.21
      depressed type 290.21
      paranoid type 290.20
      simple deterioration 290.20
      specified type — *see* categories 295-298 ✓5ᵗʰ
    shared 297.3
    situational (reactive) 298.8
    symbiotic (childhood) (*see also* Psychosis,
      childhood) 299.1 ✓5ᵗʰ
    toxic (acute) 293.9
Psychotic (*see also* condition) 298.9
  episode 298.9
    due to or associated with physical
      conditions (*see also* Psychosis,
      organic) 293.9
Pterygium (eye) 372.40
  central 372.43
  colli 744.5
  double 372.44
  peripheral (stationary) 372.41
    progressive 372.42
  recurrent 372.45
Ptilosis 374.55
Ptomaine (poisoning) (*see also* Poisoning, food)
  005.9
Ptosis (adiposa) 374.30
  breast 611.8
  cecum 569.89
  colon 569.89
  congenital (eyelid) 743.61
    specified site NEC — *see* Anomaly, specified
      type NEC
  epicanthus syndrome 270.2
  eyelid 374.30
    congenital 743.61
    mechanical 374.33
    myogenic 374.32
    paralytic 374.31
  gastric 537.5
  intestine 569.89
  kidney (*see also* Disease, renal) 593.0
    congenital 753.3
  liver 573.8
  renal (*see also* Disease, renal) 593.0
    congenital 753.3
  splanchnic 569.89
  spleen 289.59
  stomach 537.5
  viscera 569.89
Ptyalism 527.7
  hysterical 300.11
  periodic 527.2
  pregnancy 646.8 ✓5ᵗʰ
  psychogenic 306.4
Ptyalolithiasis 527.5
Pubalgia 848.8
Pubarche, precocious 259.1
Pubertas praecox 259.1
Puberty V21.1
  abnormal 259.9
  bleeding 626.3
  delayed 259.0
  precocious (constitutional) (cryptogenic)
    (idiopathic) NEC 259.1

✓4ᵗʰ Fourth-digit Required   ✓5ᵗʰ Fifth-digit Required   ▶◀ Revised Text   ● New Line   ▲ Revised Code

Puberty — *continued*
  precocious — *continued*
    due to
      adrenal
        cortical hyperfunction 255.2
          hyperplasia 255.2
      cortical hyperfunction 255.2
      ovarian hyperfunction 256.1
        estrogen 256.0
      pineal tumor 259.8
      testicular hyperfunction 257.0
    premature 259.1
      due to
        adrenal cortical hyperfunction 255.2
        pineal tumor 259.8
        pituitary (anterior) hyperfunction 253.1
Puckering, macula 362.56
Pudenda, pudendum — *see* condition
Puente's disease (simple glandular cheilitis) 528.5
Puerperal
  abscess
    areola 675.1 ✓5ᵗʰ
    Bartholin's gland 646.6 ✓5ᵗʰ
    breast 675.1 ✓5ᵗʰ
    cervix (uteri) 670 ✓4ᵗʰ
    fallopian tube 670 ✓4ᵗʰ
    genital organ 670 ✓4ᵗʰ
    kidney 646.6 ✓5ᵗʰ
    mammary 675.1 ✓5ᵗʰ
    mesosalpinx 670 ✓4ᵗʰ
    nabothian 646.6 ✓5ᵗʰ
    nipple 675.0 ✓5ᵗʰ
    ovary, ovarian 670 ✓4ᵗʰ
    oviduct 670 ✓4ᵗʰ
    parametric 670 ✓4ᵗʰ
    para-uterine 670 ✓4ᵗʰ
    pelvic 670 ✓4ᵗʰ
    perimetric 670 ✓4ᵗʰ
    periuterine 670 ✓4ᵗʰ
    retro-uterine 670 ✓4ᵗʰ
    subareolar 675.1 ✓5ᵗʰ
    suprapelvic 670 ✓4ᵗʰ
    tubal (ruptured) 670 ✓4ᵗʰ
    tubo-ovarian 670 ✓4ᵗʰ
    urinary tract NEC 646.6 ✓5ᵗʰ
    uterine, uterus 670 ✓4ᵗʰ
    vagina (wall) 646.6 ✓5ᵗʰ
    vaginorectal 646.6 ✓5ᵗʰ
    vulvovaginal gland 646.6 ✓5ᵗʰ
  accident 674.9 ✓5ᵗʰ
  adnexitis 670 ✓4ᵗʰ
  afibrinogenemia, or other coagulation defect 666.3 ✓5ᵗʰ
  albuminuria (acute) (subacute) 646.2 ✓5ᵗʰ
    pre-eclamptic 642.4 ✓5ᵗʰ
  anemia (conditions classifiable to 280-285) 648.2 ✓5ᵗʰ
  anuria 669.3 ✓5ᵗʰ
  apoplexy 674.0 ✓5ᵗʰ
  asymptomatic bacteriuria 646.5 ✓5ᵗʰ
  atrophy, breast 676.3 ✓5ᵗʰ
  blood dyscrasia 666.3 ✓5ᵗʰ
  caked breast 676.2 ✓5ᵗʰ
  cardiomyopathy 674.8 ✓5ᵗʰ
  cellulitis — *see* Puerperal, abscess
  cerebrovascular disorder (conditions classifiable to 430-434, 436-437) 674.0 ✓5ᵗʰ
  cervicitis (conditions classifiable to 616.0) 646.6 ✓5ᵗʰ
  coagulopathy (any) 666.3 ✓5ᵗʰ
  complications 674.9 ✓5ᵗʰ
    specified type NEC 674.8 ✓5ᵗʰ
  convulsions (eclamptic) (uremic) 642.6 ✓5ᵗʰ
    with pre-existing hypertension 642.7 ✓5ᵗʰ
  cracked nipple 676.1 ✓5ᵗʰ
  cystitis 646.6 ✓5ᵗʰ
  cystopyelitis 646.6 ✓5ᵗʰ
  deciduitis (acute) 670 ✓4ᵗʰ
  delirium NEC 293.9
  diabetes (mellitus) (conditions classifiable to 250) 648.0 ✓5ᵗʰ
  disease 674.9 ✓5ᵗʰ
    breast NEC 676.3 ✓5ᵗʰ
    cerebrovascular (acute) 674.0 ✓5ᵗʰ

Puerperal — *continued*
  disease — *continued*
    nonobstetric NEC (*see also* Pregnancy, complicated, current disease or condition) 648.9 ✓5ᵗʰ
    pelvis inflammatory 670 ✓4ᵗʰ
    renal NEC 646.2 ✓5ᵗʰ
    tubo-ovarian 670 ✓4ᵗʰ
    Valsuani's (progressive pernicious anemia) 648.2 ✓5ᵗʰ
  disorder
    lactation 676.9 ✓5ᵗʰ
      specified type NEC 676.8 ✓5ᵗʰ
    nonobstetric NEC (*see also* Pregnancy, complicated, current disease or condition) 648.9 ✓5ᵗʰ
  disruption
    cesarean wound 674.1 ✓5ᵗʰ
    episiotomy wound 674.2 ✓5ᵗʰ
    perineal laceration wound 674.2 ✓5ᵗʰ
  drug dependence (conditions classifiable to 304) 648.3 ✓5ᵗʰ
  eclampsia 642.6 ✓5ᵗʰ
    with pre-existing hypertension 642.7 ✓5ᵗʰ
  embolism (pulmonary) 673.2 ✓5ᵗʰ
    air 673.0 ✓5ᵗʰ
    amniotic fluid 673.1 ✓5ᵗʰ
    blood-clot 673.2 ✓5ᵗʰ
    brain or cerebral 674.0 ✓5ᵗʰ
    cardiac 674.8 ✓5ᵗʰ
    fat 673.8 ✓5ᵗʰ
    intracranial sinus (venous) 671.5 ✓5ᵗʰ
    pyemic 673.3 ✓5ᵗʰ
    septic 673.3 ✓5ᵗʰ
    spinal cord 671.5 ✓5ᵗʰ
  endometritis (conditions classifiable to 615.0-615.9) 670 ✓4ᵗʰ
  endophlebitis — *see* Puerperal, phlebitis
  endotrachelitis 646.6 ✓5ᵗʰ
  engorgement, breasts 676.2 ✓5ᵗʰ
  erysipelas 670 ✓4ᵗʰ
  failure
    lactation 676.4 ✓5ᵗʰ
    renal, acute 669.3 ✓5ᵗʰ
  fever 670 ✓4ᵗʰ
    meaning pyrexia (of unknown origin) 672 ✓5ᵗʰ
    meaning sepsis 670 ✓4ᵗʰ
  fissure, nipple 676.1 ✓5ᵗʰ
  fistula
    breast 675.1 ✓5ᵗʰ
    mammary gland 675.1 ✓5ᵗʰ
    nipple 675.0 ✓5ᵗʰ
  galactophoritis 675.2 ✓5ᵗʰ
  galactorrhea 676.6 ✓5ᵗʰ
  gangrene
    gas 670 ✓4ᵗʰ
    uterus 670 ✓4ᵗʰ
  gonorrhea (conditions classifiable to 098) 647.1 ✓5ᵗʰ
  hematoma, subdural 674.0 ✓5ᵗʰ
  hematosalpinx, infectional 670 ✓4ᵗʰ
  hemiplegia, cerebral 674.0 ✓5ᵗʰ
  hemorrhage 666.1 ✓5ᵗʰ
    brain 674.0 ✓5ᵗʰ
    bulbar 674.0 ✓5ᵗʰ
    cerebellar 674.0 ✓5ᵗʰ
    cerebral 674.0 ✓5ᵗʰ
    cortical 674.0 ✓5ᵗʰ
    delayed (after 24 hours) (uterine) 666.2 ✓5ᵗʰ
    extradural 674.0 ✓5ᵗʰ
    internal capsule 674.0 ✓5ᵗʰ
    intracranial 674.0 ✓5ᵗʰ
    intrapontine 674.0 ✓5ᵗʰ
    meningeal 674.0 ✓5ᵗʰ
    pontine 674.0 ✓5ᵗʰ
    subarachnoid 674.0 ✓5ᵗʰ
    subcortical 674.0 ✓5ᵗʰ
    subdural 674.0 ✓5ᵗʰ
    uterine, delayed 666.2 ✓5ᵗʰ
    ventricular 674.0 ✓5ᵗʰ
  hemorrhoids 671.8 ✓5ᵗʰ
  hepatorenal syndrome 674.8 ✓5ᵗʰ
  hypertrophy
    breast 676.3 ✓5ᵗʰ
    mammary gland 676.3 ✓5ᵗʰ
  induration breast (fibrous) 676.3 ✓5ᵗʰ

Puerperal — *continued*
  infarction
    lung — *see* Puerperal, embolism
    pulmonary — *see* Puerperal, embolism
  infection
    Bartholin's gland 646.6 ✓5ᵗʰ
    breast 675.2 ✓5ᵗʰ
      with nipple 675.9 ✓5ᵗʰ
        specified type NEC 675.8 ✓5ᵗʰ
    cervix 646.6 ✓5ᵗʰ
    endocervix 646.6 ✓5ᵗʰ
    fallopian tube 670 ✓4ᵗʰ
    generalized 670 ✓4ᵗʰ
    genital tract (major) 670 ✓4ᵗʰ
      minor or localized 646.6 ✓5ᵗʰ
    kidney (bacillus coli) 646.6 ✓5ᵗʰ
    mammary gland 675.2 ✓5ᵗʰ
      with nipple 675.9 ✓5ᵗʰ
        specified type NEC 675.8 ✓5ᵗʰ
    nipple 675.0 ✓5ᵗʰ
      with breast 675.9 ✓5ᵗʰ
        specified type NEC 675.8 ✓5ᵗʰ
    ovary 670 ✓4ᵗʰ
    pelvic 670 ✓4ᵗʰ
    peritoneum 670 ✓4ᵗʰ
    renal 646.6 ✓5ᵗʰ
    tubo-ovarian 670 ✓4ᵗʰ
    urinary (tract) NEC 646.6 ✓5ᵗʰ
      asymptomatic 646.5 ✓5ᵗʰ
    uterus, uterine 670 ✓4ᵗʰ
    vagina 646.6 ✓5ᵗʰ
  inflammation — *see also* Puerperal, infection
    areola 675.1 ✓5ᵗʰ
    Bartholin's gland 646.6 ✓5ᵗʰ
    breast 675.2 ✓5ᵗʰ
    broad ligament 670 ✓4ᵗʰ
    cervix (uteri) 646.6 ✓5ᵗʰ
    fallopian tube 670 ✓4ᵗʰ
    genital organs 670 ✓4ᵗʰ
      localized 646.6 ✓5ᵗʰ
    mammary gland 675.2 ✓5ᵗʰ
    nipple 675.0 ✓5ᵗʰ
    ovary 670 ✓4ᵗʰ
    oviduct 670 ✓4ᵗʰ
    pelvis 670 ✓4ᵗʰ
    periuterine 670 ✓4ᵗʰ
    tubal 670 ✓4ᵗʰ
    vagina 646.6 ✓5ᵗʰ
    vein — *see* Puerperal, phlebitis
  inversion, nipple 676.3 ✓5ᵗʰ
  ischemia, cerebral 674.0 ✓5ᵗʰ
  lymphangitis 670 ✓4ᵗʰ
    breast 675.2 ✓5ᵗʰ
  malaria (conditions classifiable to 084) 647.4 ✓5ᵗʰ
  malnutrition 648.9 ✓5ᵗʰ
  mammillitis 675.0 ✓5ᵗʰ
  mammitis 675.2 ✓5ᵗʰ
  mania 296.0 ✓5ᵗʰ
    recurrent episode 296.1 ✓5ᵗʰ
    single episode 296.0 ✓5ᵗʰ
  mastitis 675.2 ✓5ᵗʰ
    purulent 675.1 ✓5ᵗʰ
    retromammary 675.1 ✓5ᵗʰ
    submammary 675.1 ✓5ᵗʰ
  melancholia 296.2 ✓5ᵗʰ
    recurrent episode 296.3 ✓5ᵗʰ
    single episode 296.2 ✓5ᵗʰ
  mental disorder (conditions classifiable to 290-303, 305-316, 317-319) 648.4 ✓5ᵗʰ
  metritis (septic) (suppurative) 670 ✓4ᵗʰ
  metroperitonitis 670 ✓4ᵗʰ
  metrorrhagia 666.2 ✓5ᵗʰ
  metrosalpingitis 670 ✓4ᵗʰ
  metrovaginitis 670 ✓4ᵗʰ
  milk leg 671.4 ✓5ᵗʰ
  monoplegia, cerebral 674.0 ✓5ᵗʰ
  necrosis
    kidney, tubular 669.3 ✓5ᵗʰ
    liver (acute) (subacute) (conditions classifiable to 570) 674.8 ✓5ᵗʰ
    ovary 670 ✓4ᵗʰ
    renal cortex 669.3 ✓5ᵗʰ
  nephritis or nephrosis (conditions classifiable to 580-589) 646.2 ✓5ᵗʰ
    with hypertension 642.1 ✓5ᵗʰ

Puerperal — *continued*
  nutritional deficiency (conditions classifiable to 260-269) 648.9 ✓5th
  occlusion, precerebral artery 674.0 ✓5th
  oliguria 669.3 ✓5th
  oophoritis 670 ✓4th
  ovaritis 670 ✓4th
  paralysis
    bladder (sphincter) 665.5 ✓5th
    cerebral 674.0 ✓5th
  paralytic stroke 674.0 ✓5th
  parametritis 670 ✓4th
  paravaginitis 646.6 ✓5th
  pelviperitonitis 670 ✓4th
  perimetritis 670 ✓4th
  perimetrosalpingitis 670 ✓4th
  perinephritis 646.6 ✓5th
  perioophoritis 670 ✓4th
  periphlebitis — *see* Puerperal, phlebitis
  perisalpingitis 670 ✓4th
  peritoneal infection 670 ✓4th
  peritonitis (pelvic) 670 ✓4th
  perivaginitis 646.6 ✓5th
  phlebitis 671.9 ✓5th
    deep 671.4 ✓5th
    intracranial sinus (venous) 671.5 ✓5th
    pelvic 671.4 ✓5th
    specified site NEC 671.5 ✓5th
    superficial 671.2 ✓5th
  phlegmasia alba dolens 671.4 ✓5th
  placental polyp 674.4 ✓5th
  pneumonia, embolic — *see* Puerperal, embolism
  prediabetes 648.8 ✓5th
  pre-eclampsia (mild) 642.4 ✓5th
    with pre-existing hypertension 642.7 ✓5th
    severe 642.5 ✓5th
  psychosis, unspecified (*see also* Psychosis, puerperal) 293.89
  pyelitis 646.6 ✓5th
  pyelocystitis 646.6 ✓5th
  pyelohydronephrosis 646.6 ✓5th
  pyelonephritis 646.6 ✓5th
  pyelonephrosis 646.6 ✓5th
  pyemia 670 ✓4th
  pyocystitis 646.6 ✓5th
  pyohemia 670 ✓4th
  pyometra 670 ✓4th
  pyonephritis 646.6 ✓5th
  pyonephrosis 646.6 ✓5th
  pyo-oophoritis 670 ✓4th
  pyosalpingitis 670 ✓4th
  pyosalpinx 670 ✓4th
  pyrexia (of unknown origin) 672 ✓5th
  renal
    disease NEC 646.2 ✓5th
    failure, acute 669.3 ✓5th
  retention
    decidua (fragments) (with delayed hemorrhage) 666.2 ✓5th
      without hemorrhage 667.1 ✓5th
    placenta (fragments) (with delayed hemorrhage) 666.2 ✓5th
      without hemorrhage 667.1 ✓5th
    secundines (fragments) (with delayed hemorrhage) 666.2 ✓5th
      without hemorrhage 667.1 ✓5th
  retracted nipple 676.0 ✓5th
  rubella (conditions classifiable to 056) 647.5 ✓5th
  salpingitis 670 ✓4th
  salpingo-oophoritis 670 ✓4th
  salpingo-ovaritis 670 ✓4th
  salpingoperitonitis 670 ✓4th
  sapremia 670 ✓4th
  secondary perineal tear 674.2 ✓5th
  sepsis (pelvic) 670 ✓4th
  septicemia 670 ✓4th
  subinvolution (uterus) 674.8 ✓5th
  sudden death (cause unknown) 674.9 ✓5th
  suppuration — *see* Puerperal, abscess
  syphilis (conditions classifiable to 090-097) 647.0 ✓5th
  tetanus 670 ✓4th
  thelitis 675.0 ✓5th
  thrombocytopenia 666.3 ✓5th
  thrombophlebitis (superficial) 671.2 ✓5th
    deep 671.4 ✓5th

Puerperal — *continued*
  thrombophlebitis — *continued*
    pelvic 671.4 ✓5th
    specified site NEC 671.5 ✓5th
  thrombosis (venous) — *see* Thrombosis, puerperal
  thyroid dysfunction (conditions classifiable to 240-246) 648.1 ✓5th
  toxemia (*see also* Toxemia, of pregnancy) 642.4 ✓5th
    eclamptic 642.6 ✓5th
      with pre-existing hypertension 642.7 ✓5th
    pre-eclamptic (mild) 642.4 ✓5th
      with
        convulsions 642.6 ✓5th
        pre-existing hypertension 642.7 ✓5th
      severe 642.5 ✓5th
  tuberculosis (conditions classifiable to 010-018) 647.3 ✓5th
  uremia 669.3 ✓5th
  vaginitis (conditions classifiable to 616.1) 646.6 ✓5th
  varicose veins (legs) 671.0 ✓5th
    vulva or perineum 671.1 ✓5th
  vulvitis (conditions classifiable to 616.1) 646.6 ✓5th
  vulvovaginitis (conditions classifiable to 616.1) 646.6 ✓5th
  white leg 671.4 ✓5th

Pulled muscle — *see* Sprain, by site

Pulmolithiasis 518.89

Pulmonary — *see* condition

Pulmonitis (unknown etiology) 486

Pulpitis (acute) (anachoretic) (chronic) (hyperplastic) (putrescent) (suppurative) (ulcerative) 522.0

Pulpless tooth 522.9

Pulse
  alternating 427.89
    psychogenic 306.2
  bigeminal 427.89
  fast 785.0
  feeble, rapid, due to shock following injury 958.4
  rapid 785.0
  slow 427.89
  strong 785.9
  trigeminal 427.89
  water-hammer (*see also* Insufficiency, aortic) 424.1
  weak 785.9

Pulseless disease 446.7

Pulsus
  alternans or trigeminy 427.89
    psychogenic 306.2

Punch drunk 310.2

Puncta lacrimalia occlusion 375.52

Punctiform hymen 752.49

Puncture (traumatic) — *see also* Wound, open, by site
  accidental, complicating surgery 998.2
  bladder, nontraumatic 596.6
  by
    device, implant, or graft — *see* Complications, mechanical
    foreign body
      internal organs — *see also* Injury, internal, by site
        by ingested object — *see* Foreign body
    left accidentally in operation wound 998.4
    instrument (any) during a procedure, accidental 998.2
  internal organs, abdomen, chest, or pelvis — *see* Injury, internal, by site
  kidney, nontraumatic 593.89

Pupil — *see* condition

Pupillary membrane 364.74
  persistent 743.46

Pupillotonia 379.46
  pseudotabetic 379.46

Purpura 287.2
  abdominal 287.0
  allergic 287.0

Purpura — *continued*
  anaphylactoid 287.0
  annularis telangiectodes 709.1
  arthritic 287.0
  autoerythrocyte sensitization 287.2
  autoimmune 287.0
  bacterial 287.0
  Bateman's (senile) 287.2
  capillary fragility (hereditary) (idiopathic) 287.8
  cryoglobulinemic 273.2
  devil's pinches 287.2
  fibrinolytic (*see also* Fibrinolysis) 286.6
  fulminans, fulminous 286.6
  gangrenous 287.0
  hemorrhagic (*see also* Purpura, thrombocytopenic) 287.3
    nodular 272.7
    nonthrombocytopenic 287.0
    thrombocytopenic 287.3
  Henoch's (purpura nervosa) 287.0
  Henoch-Schönlein (allergic) 287.0
  hypergammaglobulinemic (benign primary) (Waldenström's) 273.0
  idiopathic 287.3
    nonthrombocytopenic 287.0
    thrombocytopenic 287.3
  infectious 287.0
  malignant 287.0
  neonatorum 772.6
  nervosa 287.0
  newborn NEC 772.6
  nonthrombocytopenic 287.2
    hemorrhagic 287.0
    idiopathic 287.0
  nonthrombopenic 287.2
  peliosis rheumatica 287.0
  pigmentaria, progressiva 709.09
  posttransfusion 287.4
  primary 287.0
  primitive 287.0
  red cell membrane sensitivity 287.2
  rheumatica 287.0
  Schönlein (-Henoch) (allergic) 287.0
  scorbutic 267
  senile 287.2
  simplex 287.2
  symptomatica 287.0
  telangiectasia annularis 709.1
  thrombocytopenic (congenital) (essential) (hereditary) (idiopathic) (primary) (*see also* Thrombocytopenia) 287.3
    neonatal, transitory (*see also* Thrombocytopenia, neonatal transitory) 776.1
    puerperal, postpartum 666.3 ✓5th
    thrombotic 446.6
  thrombohemolytic (*see also* Fibrinolysis) 286.6
  thrombopenic (congenital) (essential) (*see also* Thrombocytopenia) 287.3
  thrombotic 446.6
    thrombocytic 446.6
    thrombocytopenic 446.6
  toxic 287.0
  variolosa 050.0
  vascular 287.0
  visceral symptoms 287.0
  Werlhof's (*see also* Purpura, thrombocytopenic) 287.3

Purpuric spots 782.7

Purulent — *see* condition

Pus
  absorption, general — *see* Septicemia
  in
    stool 792.1
    urine 791.9
  tube (rupture) (*see also* Salpingo-oophoritis) 614.2

Pustular rash 782.1

Pustule 686.9
  malignant 022.0
  nonmalignant 686.9

Putnam's disease (subacute combined sclerosis with pernicious anemia) 281.0 [336.2]

Putnam-Dana syndrome (subacute combined sclerosis with pernicious anemia) 281.0 [336.2]

Putrefaction, intestinal 569.89

✓4th Fourth-digit Required   ✓5th Fifth-digit Required   ▶◀ Revised Text   ● New Line   ▲ Revised Code

Putrescent pulp (dental) 522.1
Pyarthritis — *see* Pyarthrosis
Pyarthrosis (*see also* Arthritis, pyogenic)
711.0 ✓5ᵗʰ
   tuberculous — *see* Tuberculosis, joint
Pycnoepilepsy, pycnolepsy (idiopathic) (*see also*
   Epilepsy) 345.0 ✓5ᵗʰ
Pyelectasia 593.89
Pyelectasis 593.89
Pyelitis (congenital) (uremic) 590.80
   with
      abortion — *see* Abortion, by type, with
         specified complication NEC
      contracted kidney 590.00
      ectopic pregnancy (*see also* categories
         633.0-633.9) 639.8
      molar pregnancy (*see also* categories 630-
         632) 639.8
   acute 590.10
      with renal medullary necrosis 590.11
   chronic 590.00
      with
         renal medullary necrosis 590.01
   complicating pregnancy, childbirth, or
      puerperium 646.6 ✓5ᵗʰ
      affecting fetus or newborn 760.1
   cystica 590.3
      following
         abortion 639.8
         ectopic or molar pregnancy 639.8
   gonococcal 098.19
      chronic or duration of 2 months or over
         098.39
   tuberculous (*see also* Tuberculosis) 016.0 ✓5ᵗʰ
      [590.81]
Pyelocaliectasis 593.89
Pyelocystitis (*see also* Pyelitis) 590.80
Pyelohydronephrosis 591
Pyelonephritis (*see also* Pyelitis) 590.80
   acute 590.10
      with renal medullary necrosis 590.11
   chronic 590.00
   syphilitic (late) 095.4
   tuberculous (*see also* Tuberculosis) 016.0 ✓5ᵗʰ
      [590.81]
Pyelonephrosis (*see also* Pyelitis) 590.80
   chronic 590.00
Pyelophlebitis 451.89
Pyelo-ureteritis cystica 590.3
Pyemia, pyemic (purulent) (*see also* Septicemia)
   038.9
   abscess — *see* Abscess
   arthritis (*see also* Arthritis, pyogenic) 711.0 ✓5ᵗʰ
   Bacillus coli 038.42
   embolism — *see* Embolism, pyemic
   fever 038.9
   infection 038.9
   joint (*see also* Arthritis, pyogenic) 711.0 ✓5ᵗʰ
   liver 572.1
   meningococcal 036.2
   newborn 771.81 ▲
   phlebitis — *see* Phlebitis
   pneumococcal 038.2
   portal 572.1
   postvaccinal 999.3
   specified organism NEC 038.8
   staphylococcal 038.10
      aureus 038.11
      specified organism NEC 038.19
   streptococcal 038.0
   tuberculous — *see* Tuberculosis, miliary
Pygopagus 759.4
Pykno-epilepsy, pyknolepsy (idiopathic) (*see also*
   Epilepsy) 345.0 ✓5ᵗʰ
Pyle (-Cohn) disease (craniometaphyseal
   dysplasia) 756.89
Pylephlebitis (suppurative) 572.1
Pylethrombophlebitis 572.1
Pylethrombosis 572.1
Pyloritis (*see also* Gastritis) 535.5 ✓5ᵗʰ
Pylorospasm (reflex) 537.81
   congenital or infantile 750.5
   neurotic 306.4
   newborn 750.5
   psychogenic 306.4
Pylorus, pyloric — *see* condition
Pyoarthrosis — *see* Pyarthrosis

Pyocele
   mastoid 383.00
   sinus (accessory) (nasal) (*see also* Sinusitis)
      473.9
   turbinate (bone) 473.9
   urethra (*see also* Urethritis) 597.0
Pyococcal dermatitis 686.00
Pyococcide, skin 686.00
Pyocolpos (*see also* Vaginitis) 616.10
Pyocyaneus dermatitis 686.09
Pyocystitis (*see also* Cystitis) 595.9
Pyoderma, pyodermia 686.00
   gangrenosum 686.01
   specified type NEC 686.09
   vegetans 686.8
Pyodermatitis 686.00
   vegetans 686.8
Pyogenic — *see* condition
Pyohemia — *see* Septicemia
Pyohydronephrosis (*see also* Pyelitis) 590.80
Pyometra 615.9
Pyometritis (*see also* Endometritis) 615.9
Pyometrium (*see also* Endometritis) 615.9
Pyomyositis 728.0
   ossificans 728.19
   tropical (bungpagga) 040.81
Pyonephritis (*see also* Pyelitis) 590.80
   chronic 590.00
Pyonephrosis (congenital) (*see also* Pyelitis)
   590.80
   acute 590.10
Pyo-oophoritis (*see also* Salpingo-oophoritis)
   614.2
Pyo-ovarium (*see also* Salpingo-oophoritis) 614.2
Pyopericarditis 420.99
Pyopericardium 420.99
Pyophlebitis — *see* Phlebitis
Pyopneumopericardium 420.99
Pyopneumothorax (infectional) 510.9
   with fistula 510.0
   subdiaphragmatic (*see also* Peritonitis) 567.2
   subphrenic (*see also* Peritonitis) 567.2
   tuberculous (*see also* Tuberculosis, pleura)
      012.0 ✓5ᵗʰ
Pyorrhea (alveolar) (alveolaris) 523.4
   degenerative 523.5
Pyosalpingitis (*see also* Salpingo-oophoritis)
   614.2
Pyosalpinx (*see also* Salpingo-oophoritis) 614.2
Pyosepticemia — *see* Septicemia
Pyosis
   Corlett's (impetigo) 684
   Manson's (pemphigus contagiosus) 684
Pyothorax 510.9
   with fistula 510.0
   tuberculous (*see also* Tuberculosis, pleura)
      012.0 ✓5ᵗʰ
Pyoureter 593.89
   tuberculous (*see also* Tuberculosis) 016.2 ✓5ᵗʰ
Pyramidopallidonigral syndrome 332.0
Pyrexia (of unknown origin) (P.U.O.) 780.6
   atmospheric 992.0
   during labor 659.2 ✓5ᵗʰ
   environmentally-induced newborn 778.4
   heat 992.0
   newborn, environmentally-induced 778.4
   puerperal 672 ✓4ᵗʰ
Pyroglobulinemia 273.8
Pyromania 312.33
Pyrosis 787.1
Pyrroloporphyria 277.1
Pyuria (bacterial) 791.9

Q

Q fever 083.0
   with pneumonia 083.0 [484.8]
Quadricuspid aortic valve 746.89
Quadrilateral fever 083.0

Quadriparesis — *see* Quadriplegia
Quadriplegia 344.00
   with fracture, vertebra (process) — *see*
      Fracture, vertebra, cervical, with spinal
      cord injury
   brain (current episode) 437.8
   C1-C4
      complete 344.01
      incomplete 344.02
   C5-C7
      complete 344.03
      incomplete 344.04
   cerebral (current episode) 437.8
   congenital or infantile (cerebral) (spastic)
      (spinal) 343.2
   cortical 437.8
   embolic (current episode) (*see also* Embolism,
      brain) 434.1 ✓5ᵗʰ
   infantile (cerebral) (spastic) (spinal) 343.2
   newborn NEC 767.0
   specified NEC 344.09
   thrombotic (current episode) (*see also*
      Thrombosis, brain) 434.0 ✓5ᵗʰ
   traumatic — *see* Injury, spinal, cervical
Quadruplet
   affected by maternal complications of
      pregnancy 761.5
   healthy liveborn — *see* Newborn, multiple
   pregnancy (complicating delivery) NEC
      651.8 ✓5ᵗʰ
      with fetal loss and retention of one or more
         fetus(es) 651.5 ✓5ᵗʰ
Quarrelsomeness 301.3
Quartan
   fever 084.2
   malaria (fever) 084.2
Queensland fever 083.0
   coastal 083.0
   seven-day 100.89
Quervain's disease 727.04
   thyroid (subacute granulomatous thyroiditis)
      245.1
Queyrat's erythroplasia (M8080/2)
   specified site — *see* Neoplasm, skin, in situ
   unspecified site 233.5
Quincke's disease or edema — *see* Edema,
   angioneurotic
Quinquaud's disease (acne decalvans) 704.09
Quinsy (gangrenous) 475
Quintan fever 083.1
Quintuplet
   affected by maternal complications of
      pregnancy 761.5
   healthy liveborn — *see* Newborn, multiple
   pregnancy (complicating delivery) NEC
      651.2 ✓5ᵗʰ
      with fetal loss and retention of one or more
         fetus(es) 651.6 ✓5ᵗʰ
Quotidian
   fever 084.0
   malaria (fever) 084.0

R

Rabbia 071
Rabbit fever (*see also* Tularemia) 021.9
Rabies 071
   contact V01.5
   exposure to V01.5
   inoculation V04.5
      reaction — *see* Complications, vaccination
   vaccination, prophylactic (against) V04.5
Rachischisis (*see also* Spina bifida) 741.9 ✓5ᵗʰ
Rachitic — *see also* condition
   deformities of spine 268.1
   pelvis 268.1
      with disproportion (fetopelvic) 653.2 ✓5ᵗʰ
         affecting fetus or newborn 763.1
         causing obstructed labor 660.1 ✓5ᵗʰ
            affecting fetus or newborn 763.1
Rachitis, rachitism — *see also* Rickets
   acute 268.0
   fetalis 756.4

Rachitis, rachitism — *see also* Rickets —
   continued
   renalis 588.0
   tarda 268.0
Racket nail 757.5
Radial nerve — *see* condition
Radiation effects or sickness — *see also* Effect,
   adverse, radiation
   cataract 366.46
   dermatitis 692.82
    sunburn (*see also* Sunburn) 692.71
Radiculitis (pressure) (vertebrogenic) 729.2
   accessory nerve 723.4
   anterior crural 724.4
   arm 723.4
   brachial 723.4
   cervical NEC 723.4
   due to displacement of intervertebral disc —
    see Neuritis, due to, displacement
    intervertebral disc
   leg 724.4
   lumbar NEC 724.4
   lumbosacral 724.4
   rheumatic 729.2
   syphilitic 094.89
   thoracic (with visceral pain) 724.4
Radiculomyelitis 357.0
   toxic, due to
    Clostridium tetani 037
    Corynebacterium diphtheriae 032.89
Radiculopathy (*see also* Radiculitis) 729.2
Radioactive substances, adverse effect — *see*
   Effect, adverse, radioactive substance
Radiodermal burns (acute) (chronic)
   (occupational) — *see* Burn, by site
Radiodermatitis 692.82
Radionecrosis — *see* Effect, adverse, radiation
Radiotherapy session V58.0
Radium, adverse effect — *see* Effect, adverse,
   radioactive substance
Raeder-Harbitz syndrome (pulseless disease)
   446.7
Rage (*see also* Disturbance, conduct) 312.0 ✓5ᵗʰ
   meaning rabies 071
Rag sorters' disease 022.1
Raillietiniasis 123.8
Railroad neurosis 300.16
Railway spine 300.16
Raised — *see* Elevation
Raiva 071
Rake teeth, tooth 524.3
Rales 786.7
Ramifying renal pelvis 753.3
Ramsay Hunt syndrome (herpetic geniculate
   ganglionitis) 053.11
   meaning dyssynergia cerebellaris myoclonica
    334.2
Ranke's primary infiltration (*see also*
   Tuberculosis) 010.0 ✓5ᵗʰ
Ranula 527.6
   congenital 750.26
Rape — *see* Injury, by site
   alleged, observation or examination V71.5
Rapid
   feeble pulse, due to shock, following injury
    958.4
   heart (beat) 785.0
    psychogenic 306.2
   respiration 786.06
    psychogenic 306.1
   second stage (delivery) 661.3 ✓5ᵗʰ
    affecting fetus or newborn 763.6
   time-zone change syndrome 307.45
Rarefaction, bone 733.99
Rash 782.1
   canker 034.1
   diaper 691.0
   drug (internal use) 693.0
    contact 692.3
   ECHO 9 virus 078.89
   enema 692.89

Rash — *continued*
   food (*see also* Allergy, food) 693.1
   heat 705.1
   napkin 691.0
   nettle 708.8
   pustular 782.1
   rose 782.1
    epidemic 056.9
    of infants 057.8
   scarlet 034.1
   serum (prophylactic) (therapeutic) 999.5
   toxic 782.1
   wandering tongue 529.1
Rasmussen's aneurysm (*see also* Tuberculosis)
   011.2 ✓5ᵗʰ
Rat-bite fever 026.9
   due to Streptobacillus moniliformis 026.1 ✓5ᵗʰ
   spirochetal (morsus muris) 026.0 ✓5ᵗʰ
Rathke's pouch tumor (M9350/1) 237.0
Raymond (-Céstan) syndrome 433.8 ✓5ᵗʰ
Raynaud's
   disease or syndrome (paroxysmal digital
    cyanosis) 443.0
   gangrene (symmetric) 443.0 *[785.4]*
   phenomenon (paroxysmal digital cyanosis)
    (secondary) 443.0
RDS 769
Reaction
   acute situational maladjustment (*see also*
    Reaction, adjustment) 309.9
   adaptation (*see also* Reaction, adjustment)
    309.9
   adjustment 309.9
    with
     anxious mood 309.24
      with depressed mood 309.28
     conduct disturbance 309.3
      combined with disturbance of
       emotions 309.4
     depressed mood 309.0
      brief 309.0
       with anxious mood 309.28
      prolonged 309.1
     elective mutism 309.83
     mixed emotions and conduct 309.4
     mutism, elective 309.83
     physical symptoms 309.82
     predominant disturbance (of)
      conduct 309.3
      emotions NEC 309.29
       mixed 309.28
      mixed, emotions and conduct 309.4
      specified type NEC 309.89
     specific academic or work inhibition
      309.23
     withdrawal 309.83
    depressive 309.0
     with conduct disturbance 309.4
     brief 309.0
     prolonged 309.1
    specified type NEC 309.89
   adverse food NEC 995.7
   affective (*see also* Psychosis, affective) 296.90
    specified type NEC 296.99
   aggressive 301.3
    unsocialized (*see also* Disturbance, conduct)
     312.0 ✓5ᵗʰ
   allergic (*see also* Allergy) 995.3
    drug, medicinal substance, and biological —
     see Allergy, drug
    food — *see* Allergy, food
    serum 999.5
   anaphylactic — *see* Shock, anaphylactic
   anesthesia — *see* Anesthesia, complication
   anger 312.0 ✓5ᵗʰ
   antisocial 301.7
   antitoxin (prophylactic) (therapeutic) — *see*
    Complications, vaccination
   anxiety 300.00
   asthenic 300.5
   compulsive 300.3
   conversion (anesthetic) (autonomic)
    (hyperkinetic) (mixed paralytic)
    (paresthetic) 300.11
   deoxyribonuclease (DNA) (DNase)
    hypersensitivity NEC 287.2

Reaction — *continued*
   depressive 300.4
    acute 309.0
    affective (*see also* Psychosis, affective)
     296.2 ✓5ᵗʰ
     recurrent episode 296.3 ✓5ᵗʰ
     single episode 296.2 ✓5ᵗʰ
    brief 309.0
    manic (*see also* Psychosis, affective) 296.80
    neurotic 300.4
    psychoneurotic 300.4
    psychotic 298.0
   dissociative 300.15
   drug NEC (*see also* Table of Drugs and
    Chemicals) 995.2
    allergic — *see* Allergy, drug
    correct substance properly administered
     995.2
    obstetric anesthetic or analgesic NEC
     668.9 ✓5ᵗʰ
     affecting fetus or newborn 763.5
     specified drug — *see* Table of Drugs and
      Chemicals
    overdose or poisoning 977.9
     specified drug — *see* Table of Drugs and
      Chemicals
    specific to newborn 779.4
    transmitted via placenta or breast milk —
     see Absorption, drug, through
     placenta
    withdrawal NEC 292.0
     infant of dependent mother 779.5
    wrong substance given or taken in error
     977.9
     specified drug — *see* Table of Drugs and
      Chemicals
   dyssocial 301.7
   erysipeloid 027.1
   fear 300.20
    child 313.0
   fluid loss, cerebrospinal 349.0
   food — *see also* Allergy, food
    adverse NEC 995.7
    anaphylactic shock — *see* Anaphylactic
     shock, due to, food
   foreign
    body NEC 728.82
     in operative wound (inadvertently left)
      998.4
      due to surgical material intentionally
       left — *see* Complications, due to
       (presence of) any device, implant,
       or graft classified to 996.0-996.5
       NEC
    substance accidentally left during a
     procedure (chemical) (powder) (talc)
     998.7
     body or object (instrument) (sponge)
      (swab) 998.4
   graft-versus-host (GVH) 996.85
   grief (acute) (brief) 309.0
    prolonged 309.1
   gross stress (*see also* Reaction, stress, acute)
    308.9
   group delinquent (*see also* Disturbance,
    conduct) 312.2 ✓5ᵗʰ
   Herxheimer's 995.0
   hyperkinetic (*see also* Hyperkinesia) 314.9
   hypochondriacal 300.7
   hypoglycemic, due to insulin 251.0
    therapeutic misadventure 962.3
   hypomanic (*see also* Psychosis, affective)
    296.0 ✓5ᵗʰ
    recurrent episode 296.1 ✓5ᵗʰ
    single episode 296.0 ✓5ᵗʰ
   hysterical 300.10
    conversion type 300.11
    dissociative 300.15
   id (bacterial cause) 692.89
   immaturity NEC 301.89
    aggressive 301.3
    emotional instability 301.59
   immunization — *see* Complications,
    vaccination
   incompatibility
    blood group (ABO) (infusion) (transfusion)
     999.6

Reaction — *continued*
  incompatibility — *continued*
    Rh (factor) (infusion) (transfusion) 999.7
  inflammatory — *see* Infection
  infusion — *see* Complications, infusion
  inoculation (immune serum) — *see*
    Complications, vaccination
  insulin 995.2
  involutional
    paranoid 297.2
    psychotic (*see also* Psychosis, affective,
      depressive) 296.2 ✓5th
  leukemoid (lymphocytic) (monocytic)
    (myelocytic) 288.8
  LSD (*see also* Abuse, drugs, nondependent)
    305.3 ✓5th
  lumbar puncture 349.0
  manic-depressive (*see also* Psychosis, affective)
    296.80
    depressed 296.2 ✓5th
      recurrent episode 296.3 ✓5th
      single episode 296.2 ✓5th
    hypomanic 296.0 ✓5th
  neurasthenic 300.5
  neurogenic (*see also* Neurosis) 300.9
  neurotic NEC 300.9
  neurotic-depressive 300.4
  nitritoid — *see* Crisis, nitritoid
  obsessive (-compulsive) 300.3
  organic 293.9
    acute 293.0
    subacute 293.1
  overanxious, child or adolescent 313.0
  paranoid (chronic) 297.9
    acute 298.3
    climacteric 297.2
    involutional 297.2
    menopausal 297.2
    senile 290.20
    simple 297.0
  passive
    aggressive 301.84
    dependency 301.6
  personality (*see also* Disorder, personality)
    301.9
  phobic 300.20
  postradiation — *see* Effect, adverse, radiation
  psychogenic NEC 300.9
  psychoneurotic (*see also* Neurosis) 300.9
    anxiety 300.00
    compulsive 300.3
    conversion 300.11
    depersonalization 300.6
    depressive 300.4
    dissociative 300.15
    hypochondriacal 300.7
    hysterical 300.10
      conversion type 300.11
      dissociative type 300.15
    neurasthenic 300.5
    obsessive 300.3
    obsessive-compulsive 300.3
    phobic 300.20
    tension state 300.9
  psychophysiologic NEC (*see also* Disorder,
    psychosomatic) 306.9
    cardiovascular 306.2
    digestive 306.4
    endocrine 306.6
    gastrointestinal 306.4
    genitourinary 306.50
    heart 306.2
    hemic 306.8
    intestinal (large) (small) 306.4
    laryngeal 306.1
    lymphatic 306.8
    musculoskeletal 306.0
    pharyngeal 306.1
    respiratory 306.1
    skin 306.3
    special sense organs 306.7
  psychosomatic (*see also* Disorder,
    psychosomatic) 306.9
  psychotic (*see also* Psychosis) 298.9
    depressive 298.0
    due to or associated with physical condition
      (*see also* Psychosis, organic) 293.9

Reaction — *continued*
  psychotic (*see also* Psychosis) — *continued*
    involutional (*see also* Psychosis, affective)
      296.2 ✓5th
      recurrent episode 296.3 ✓5th
      single episode 296.2 ✓5th
  pupillary (myotonic) (tonic) 379.46
  radiation — *see* Effect, adverse, radiation
  runaway — *see also* Disturbance, conduct
    socialized 312.2 ✓5th
    undersocialized, unsocialized 312.1 ✓5th
  scarlet fever toxin — *see* Complications,
    vaccination
  schizophrenic (*see also* Schizophrenia)
    295.9 ✓5th
    latent 295.5 ✓5th
  serological for syphilis — *see* Serology for
    syphilis
  serum (prophylactic) (therapeutic) 999.5
    immediate 999.4
  situational (*see also* Reaction, adjustment)
    309.9
    acute, to stress 308.3
    adjustment (*see also* Reaction, adjustment)
      309.9
  somatization (*see also* Disorder, psychosomatic)
    306.9
  spinal puncture 349.0
  spite, child (*see also* Disturbance, conduct)
    312.0 ✓5th
  stress, acute 308.9
    with predominant disturbance (of)
      consciousness 308.1
      emotions 308.0
      mixed 308.4
      psychomotor 308.2
      specified type NEC 308.3
  bone or cartilage — *see* Fracture, stress
  surgical procedure — *see* Complications,
    surgical procedure
  tetanus antitoxin — *see* Complications,
    vaccination
  toxin-antitoxin — *see* Complications,
    vaccination
  transfusion (blood) (bone marrow)
    (lymphocytes) (allergic) — *see*
    Complications, transfusion
  tuberculin skin test, nonspecific (without active
    tuberculosis) 795.5
    positive (without active tuberculosis) 795.5
  ultraviolet — *see* Effect, adverse, ultraviolet
  undersocialized, unsocialized — *see also*
    Disturbance, conduct
    aggressive (type) 312.0 ✓5th
    unaggressive (type) 312.1 ✓5th
  vaccination (any) — *see* Complications,
    vaccination
  white graft (skin) 996.52
  withdrawing, child or adolescent 313.22
  x-ray — *see* Effect, adverse, x-rays

Reactive depression (*see also* Reaction,
  depressive) 300.4
  neurotic 300.4
  psychoneurotic 300.4
  psychotic 298.0

Rebound tenderness 789.6 ✓5th

Recalcitrant patient V15.81

Recanalization, thrombus — *see* Thrombosis

Recession, receding
  chamber angle (eye) 364.77
  chin 524.06
  gingival (generalized) (localized) (postinfective)
    (postoperative) 523.2

Recklinghausen's disease (M9540/1) 237.71
  bones (osteitis fibrosa cystica) 252.0

Recklinghausen-Applebaum disease
  (hemochromatosis) 275.0

Reclus' disease (cystic) 610.1

Recrudescent typhus (fever) 081.1

Recruitment, auditory 388.44

Rectalgia 569.42

Rectitis 569.49

Rectocele
  female (without uterine prolapse) 618.0
    with uterine prolapse 618.4
      complete 618.3
      incomplete 618.2
  in pregnancy or childbirth 654.4 ✓5th
    causing obstructed labor 660.2 ✓5th
      affecting fetus or newborn 763.1
  male 569.49
  vagina, vaginal (outlet) 618.0

Rectosigmoiditis 569.89
  ulcerative (chronic) 556.3

Rectosigmoid junction — *see* condition

Rectourethral — *see* condition

Rectovaginal — *see* condition

Rectovesical — *see* condition

Rectum, rectal — *see* condition

Recurrent — *see* condition

Red bugs 133.8

Red cedar asthma 495.8

Redness
  conjunctiva 379.93
  eye 379.93
  nose 478.1

Reduced ventilatory or vital capacity 794.2

Reduction
  function
    kidney (*see also* Disease, renal) 593.9
    liver 573.8
  ventilatory capacity 794.2
  vital capacity 794.2

Redundant, redundancy
  abdomen 701.9
  anus 751.5
  cardia 537.89
  clitoris 624.2
  colon (congenital) 751.5
  foreskin (congenital) 605
  intestine 751.5
  labia 624.3
  organ or site, congenital NEC — *see* Accessory
  panniculus (abdominal) 278.1
  prepuce (congenital) 605
  pylorus 537.89
  rectum 751.5
  scrotum 608.89
  sigmoid 751.5
  skin (of face) 701.9
    eyelids 374.30
  stomach 537.89
  uvula 528.9
  vagina 623.8

Reduplication — *see* Duplication

Referral
  adoption (agency) V68.89
  nursing care V63.8
  patient without examination or treatment
    V68.81
  social services V63.8

Reflex — *see also* condition
  blink, deficient 374.45
  hyperactive gag 478.29
  neurogenic bladder NEC 596.54
    atonic 596.54
      with cauda equina syndrome 344.61
  vasoconstriction 443.9
  vasovagal 780.2

Reflux
  esophageal 530.81
  esophagitis 530.11
  gastroesophageal 530.81
  mitral — *see* Insufficiency, mitral
  ureteral — *see* Reflux, vesicoureteral
  vesicoureteral 593.70
    with
      reflux nephropathy 593.73
        bilateral 593.72
        unilateral 593.71

Reformed gallbladder 576.0

Reforming, artificial openings (*see also*
  Attention to, artificial, opening) V55.9

Refractive error (*see also* Error, refractive) 367.9

✓4th Fourth-digit Required   ✓5th Fifth-digit Required   ►◄ Revised Text   ● New Line   ▲ Revised Code

Refsum's disease or syndrome (heredopathia
  atactica polyneuritiformis) 356.3
Refusal of
  food 307.59
    hysterical 300.11
  treatment because of, due to
    patient's decision NEC V64.2
    reason of conscience or religion V62.6
Regaud
  tumor (M8082/3) — see Neoplasm,
    nasopharynx, malignant
  type carcinoma (M8082/3) — see Neoplasm,
    nasopharynx, malignant
Regional — see condition
Regulation feeding (elderly) (infant) 783.3
  newborn 779.3
Regurgitated
  food, choked on 933.1
  stomach contents, choked on 933.1
Regurgitation
  aortic (valve) (see also Insufficiency, aortic)
    424.1
    congenital 746.4
    syphilitic 093.22
  food — see also Vomiting
    with reswallowing — see Rumination
    newborn 779.3
  gastric contents — see Vomiting
  heart — see Endocarditis
  mitral (valve) — see also Insufficiency, mitral
    congenital 746.6
  myocardial — see Endocarditis
  pulmonary (heart) (valve) (see also
    Endocarditis, pulmonary) 424.3
  stomach — see Vomiting
  tricuspid — see Endocarditis, tricuspid
  valve, valvular — see Endocarditis
  vesicoureteral — see Reflux, vesicoureteral
Rehabilitation V57.9
  multiple types V57.89
  occupational V57.21
  specified type NEC V57.89
  speech V57.3
  vocational V57.22
Reichmann's disease or syndrome
  (gastrosuccorrhea) 536.8
Reifenstein's syndrome (hereditary familial
  hypogonadism, male) 257.2
Reilly's syndrome or phenomenon (see also
  Neuropathy, peripheral, autonomic) 337.9
Reimann's periodic disease 277.3
Reinsertion, contraceptive device V25.42
Reiter's disease, syndrome, or urethritis
  099.3 [711.1] ✓5ᵗʰ
Rejection
  food, hysterical 300.11
  transplant 996.80
    bone marrow 996.85
    corneal 996.51
    organ (immune or nonimmune cause)
      996.80
      bone marrow 996.85
      heart 996.83
      intestines 996.87
      kidney 996.81
      liver 996.82
      lung 996.84
      pancreas 996.86
      specified NEC 996.89
    skin 996.52
      artificial 996.55
      decellularized allodermis 996.55
Relapsing fever 087.9
  Carter's (Asiatic) 087.0
  Dutton's (West African) 087.1
  Koch's 087.9
  louse-borne (epidemic) 087.0
  Novy's (American) 087.1
  Obermeyer's (European) 087.0
  Spirillum 087.9
  tick-borne (endemic) 087.1
Relaxation
  anus (sphincter) 569.49
    due to hysteria 300.11

Relaxation — continued
  arch (foot) 734
    congenital 754.61
  back ligaments 728.4
  bladder (sphincter) 596.59
  cardio-esophageal 530.89
  cervix (see also Incompetency, cervix) 622.5
  diaphragm 519.4
  inguinal rings — see Hernia, inguinal
  joint (capsule) (ligament) (paralytic) (see also
    Derangement, joint) 718.90
    congenital 755.8
  lumbosacral joint 724.6
  pelvic floor 618.8
  pelvis 618.8
  perineum 618.8
  posture 729.9
  rectum (sphincter) 569.49
  sacroiliac (joint) 724.6
  scrotum 608.89
  urethra (sphincter) 599.84
  uterus (outlet) 618.8
  vagina (outlet) 618.8
  vesical 596.59
Remains
  canal of Cloquet 743.51
  capsule (opaque) 743.51
Remittent fever (malarial) 084.6
Remnant
  canal of Cloquet 743.51
  capsule (opaque) 743.51
  cervix, cervical stump (acquired) (postoperative)
    622.8
  cystic duct, postcholecystectomy 576.0
  fingernail 703.8
    congenital 757.5
  meniscus, knee 717.5
  thyroglossal duct 759.2
  tonsil 474.8
    infected 474.00
  urachus 753.7
Remote effect of cancer — see condition
Removal (of)
  catheter (urinary) (indwelling) V53.6
    from artificial opening — see Attention to,
      artificial, opening
    non-vascular V58.82
    vascular V58.81
  cerebral ventricle (communicating) shunt
    V53.01
  device — see also Fitting (of)
    contraceptive V25.42
    fixation
      external V54.89   ▲
      internal V54.0
    traction V54.89   ▲
  dressing V58.3
  ileostomy V55.2
  Kirschner wire V54.89   ▲
  nonvascular catheter V58.82
  pin V54.0
  plaster cast V54.89   ▲
  plate (fracture) V54.0
  rod V54.0
  screw V54.0
  splint, external V54.89   ▲
  subdermal implantable contraceptive V25.43
  suture V58.3
  traction device, external V54.89   ▲
  vascular catheter V58.81
Ren
  arcuatus 753.3
  mobile, mobilis (see also Disease, renal) 593.0
    congenital 753.3
  unguliformis 753.3
Renal — see also condition
  glomerulohyalinosis-diabetic syndrome
    250.4 ✓5ᵗʰ [581.81]
Rendu-Osler-Weber disease or syndrome
  (familial hemorrhagic telangiectasia) 448.0
Reninoma (M8361/1) 236.91
Rénon-Delille syndrome 253.8

Repair
  pelvic floor, previous, in pregnancy or
    childbirth 654.4 ✓5ᵗʰ
    affecting fetus or newborn 763.89
  scarred tissue V51
**Replacement by artificial or mechanical device
  or prosthesis of** (see also Fitting (of))
  artificial skin V43.83
  bladder V43.5
  blood vessel V43.4
  breast V43.82
  eye globe V43.0
  heart V43.2
    valve V43.3
  intestine V43.89
  joint V43.60
    ankle V43.66
    elbow V43.62
    finger V43.69
    hip (partial) (total) V43.64
    knee V43.65
    shoulder V43.61
    specified NEC V43.69
    wrist V43.63
  kidney V43.89
  larynx V43.81
  lens V43.1
  limb(s) V43.7
  liver V43.89
  lung V43.89
  organ NEC V43.89
  pancreas V43.89
  skin (artificial) V43.83
  tissue NEC V43.89
Reprogramming
  cardiac pacemaker V53.31
Request for expert evidence V68.2
Reserve, decreased or low
  cardiac — see Disease, heart
  kidney (see also Disease, renal) 593.9
Residual — see also condition
  bladder 596.8
  foreign body — see Retention, foreign body
  state, schizophrenic (see also Schizophrenia)
    295.6 ✓5ᵗʰ
  urine 788.69
Resistance, resistant (to)

> Note — use the following subclassification for
> categories V09.5, V09.7, V09.8, V09.9:
>
> 0   without mention of resistance to
>   multiple drugs
> 1   with resistance to multiple drugs
>   V09.5   quinolones and
>   fluoroquinolones
>   V09.7   antimycobacterial agents
>   V09.8   specified drugs NEC
>   V09.9   unspecified drugs
> 9   multiple sites

  drugs by microorganisms V09.9 ✓5ᵗʰ
    Amikacin V09.4
    aminoglycosides V09.4
    Amodiaquine V09.5 ✓5ᵗʰ
    Amoxicillin V09.0
    Ampicillin V09.0
    antimycobacterial agents V09.7 ✓5ᵗʰ   ●
    Azithromycin V09.2
    Azlocillin V09.0
    Aztreonam V09.1
    B-lactam antibiotics V09.1
    bacampicillin V09.0
    Bacitracin V09.8 ✓5ᵗʰ
    Benznidazole V09.8 ✓5ᵗʰ
    Capreomycin V09.7 ✓5ᵗʰ
    Carbenicillin V09.0
    Cefaclor V09.1
    Cefadroxil V09.1
    Cefamandole V09.1
    Cefatetan V09.1
    Cefazolin V09.1
    Cefixime V09.1
    Cefonicid V09.1
    Cefoperazone V09.1
    Ceforanide V09.1

Resistance, resistant (to) — *continued*
  drugs by microorganisms — *continued*
    Cefotaxime V09.1
    Cefoxitin V09.1
    Ceftazidime V09.1
    Ceftizoxime V09.1
    Ceftriaxone V09.1
    Cefuroxime V09.1
    Cephalexin V09.1
    Cephaloglycin V09.1
    Cephaloridine V09.1
    Cephalosporins V09.1
    Cephalothin V09.1
    Cephapirin V09.1
    Cephradine V09.1
    Chloramphenicol V09.8 ✓5ᵗʰ
    Chloraquine V09.5 ✓5ᵗʰ
    Chlorguanide V09.8 ✓5ᵗʰ
    Chlorproguanil V09.8 ✓5ᵗʰ
    Chlortetracycline V09.3
    Cinoxacin V09.5 ✓5ᵗʰ
    Ciprofloxacin V09.5 ✓5ᵗʰ
    Clarithromycin V09.2
    Clindamycin V09.8 ✓5ᵗʰ
    Clioquinol V09.5 ✓5ᵗʰ
    Clofazimine V09.7 ✓5ᵗʰ
    Cloxacillin V09.0
    Cyclacillin V09.0
    Cycloserine V09.7 ✓5ᵗʰ
    Dapsone [DZ] V09.7 ✓5ᵗʰ
    Demeclocycline V09.3
    Dicloxacillin V09.0
    Doxycycline V09.3
    Enoxacin V09.5 ✓5ᵗʰ
    Erythromycin V09.2
    Ethambutol [EMB] V09.7 ✓5ᵗʰ
    Ethionamide [ETA] V09.7 ✓5ᵗʰ
    fluoroquinolones V09.5 ✓5ᵗʰ
    Gentamicin V09.4
    Halofantrine V09.8 ✓5ᵗʰ
    Imipenem V09.1
    Iodoquinol V09.5 ✓5ᵗʰ
    Isoniazid [INH] V09.7 ✓5ᵗʰ
    Kanamycin V09.4
    macrolides V09.2
    Mafenide V09.6
    Mefloquine V09.8 ✓5ᵗʰ
    Melasoprol V09.8 ✓5ᵗʰ
    Methacycline V09.3
    Methenamine V09.8 ✓5ᵗʰ
    Methicillin V09.0
    Metronidazole V09.8 ✓5ᵗʰ
    Mezlocillin V09.0
    Minocycline V09.3
    Nafcillin V09.0
    Nalidixic acid V09.5 ✓5ᵗʰ
    Natamycin V09.2
    Neomycin V09.4
    Netilmicin V09.4
    Nifurtimox V09.8 ✓5ᵗʰ
    Nimorazole V09.8 ✓5ᵗʰ
    Nitrofurantoin V09.8 ✓5ᵗʰ
    Norfloxacin V09.5 ✓5ᵗʰ
    Nystatin V09.2
    Ofloxacin V09.5 ✓5ᵗʰ
    Oleandomycin V09.2
    Oxacillin V09.0
    Oxytetracycline V09.3
    Para-amino salicylic acid [PAS] V09.7 ✓5ᵗʰ
    Paromomycin V09.4
    Penicillin (G) (V) (VK) V09.0
    penicillins V09.0
    Pentamidine V09.8 ✓5ᵗʰ
    Piperacillin V09.0
    Primaquine V09.5 ✓5ᵗʰ
    Proguanil V09.8 ✓5ᵗʰ
    Pyrazinamide [PZA] V09.7 ✓5ᵗʰ
    Pyrimethamine/sulfalene V09.8 ✓5ᵗʰ
    Pyrimethamine/sulfodoxine V09.8 ✓5ᵗʰ
    Quinacrine V09.5 ✓5ᵗʰ
    Quinidine V09.8 ✓5ᵗʰ
    Quinine V09.8 ✓5ᵗʰ
    quinolones V09.5 ✓5ᵗʰ
    Rifabutin V09.7 ✓5ᵗʰ
    Rifampin [RIF] V09.7 ✓5ᵗʰ
    Rifamycin V09.7 ✓5ᵗʰ
    Rolitetracycline V09.3

Resistance, resistant (to) — *continued*
  drugs by microorganisms — *continued*
    Specified drugs NEC V09.8 ✓5ᵗʰ
    Spectinomycin V09.8 ✓5ᵗʰ
    Spiramycin V09.2
    Streptomycin [SM] V09.4
    Sulfacetamide V09.6
    Sulfacytine V09.6
    Sulfadiazine V09.6
    Sulfadoxine V09.6
    Sulfamethoxazole V09.6
    Sulfapyridine V09.6
    Sulfasalizine V09.6
    Sulfasoxazone V09.6
    sulfonamides V09.6
    Sulfoxone V09.7 ✓5ᵗʰ
    tetracycline V09.3
    tetracyclines V09.3
    Thiamphenicol V09.8 ✓5ᵗʰ
    Ticarcillin V09.0
    Tinidazole V09.8 ✓5ᵗʰ
    Tobramycin V09.4
    Triamphenicol V09.8 ✓5ᵗʰ
    Trimethoprim V09.8 ✓5ᵗʰ
    Vancomycin V09.8 ✓5ᵗʰ
Resorption
  biliary 576.8
    purulent or putrid (*see also* Cholecystitis) 576.8
  dental (roots) 521.4
    alveoli 525.8
  septic — *see* Septicemia
  teeth (external) (internal) (pathological) (roots) 521.4
Respiration
  asymmetrical 786.09
  bronchial 786.09
  Cheyne-Stokes (periodic respiration) 786.04
  decreased, due to shock following injury 958.4
  disorder of 786.00
    psychogenic 306.1
    specified NEC 786.09
  failure 518.81
    acute 518.81
    acute and chronic 518.84
    chronic 518.83
    newborn 770.84 ▲
  insufficiency 786.09
    acute 518.82
    newborn NEC 770.89 ▲
  Kussmaul (air hunger) 786.09
  painful 786.52
  periodic 786.09
  poor 786.09
    newborn NEC 770.89 ▲
  sighing 786.7
    psychogenic 306.1
  wheezing 786.07
Respiratory — *see also* condition
  distress 786.09
    acute 518.82
    fetus or newborn NEC 770.89 ▲
    syndrome (newborn) 769
      adult (following shock, surgery, or trauma) 518.5
        specified NEC 518.82
  failure 518.81
    acute 518.81
    acute and chronic 518.8
    chronic 518.83
Respiratory syncytial virus (RSV) 079.6
  bronchiolitis 466.11
  pneumonia 480.1
Response
  photoallergic 692.72
  phototoxic 692.72
Rest, rests
  mesonephric duct 752.8
    fallopian tube 752.11
  ovarian, in fallopian tubes 752.19
  wolffian duct 752.8
Restless leg (syndrome) 333.99
Restlessness 799.2
Restoration of organ continuity from previous sterilization (tuboplasty) (vasoplasty) V26.0

Restriction of housing space V60.1
Restzustand, schizophrenic (*see also* Schizophrenia) 295.6 ✓5ᵗʰ
Retained — *see* Retention
Retardation
  development, developmental, specific (*see also* Disorder, development, specific) 315.9
    learning, specific 315.2
      arithmetical 315.1
      language (skills) 315.31
        expressive 315.31
        mixed receptive-expressive 315.32
      mathematics 315.1
      reading 315.00
        phonological 315.39
      written expression 315.2
    motor 315.4
  endochondral bone growth 733.91
  growth (physical) in childhood 783.43
    due to malnutrition 263.2
    fetal (intrauterine) 764.9 ✓5ᵗʰ
      affecting management of pregnancy 656.5 ✓5ᵗʰ
  intrauterine growth 764.9 ✓5ᵗʰ
    affecting management of pregnancy 656.5 ✓5ᵗʰ
  mental 319
    borderline V62.89
    mild, IQ 50-70 317
    moderate, IQ 35-49 318.0
    profound, IQ under 20 318.2
    severe, IQ 20-34 318.1
  motor, specific 315.4
  physical 783.43
    child 783.43
    due to malnutrition 263.2
    fetus (intrauterine) 764.9 ✓5ᵗʰ
      affecting management of pregnancy 656.5 ✓5ᵗʰ
  psychomotor NEC 307.9
  reading 315.00
Retching — *see* Vomiting
Retention, retained
  bladder NEC (*see also* Retention, urine) 788.20
    psychogenic 306.53
  carbon dioxide 276.2
  cyst — *see* Cyst
  dead
    fetus (after 22 completed weeks gestation) 656.4 ✓5ᵗʰ
      early fetal death (before 22 completed weeks gestation) 632
    ovum 631
  decidua (following delivery) (fragments) (with hemorrhage) 666.2 ✓5ᵗʰ
    without hemorrhage 667.1 ✓5ᵗʰ
  deciduous tooth 520.6
  dental root 525.3
  fecal (*see also* Constipation) 564.00
  fluid 276.6
  foreign body — *see also* Foreign body, retained
    bone 733.99
    current trauma — *see* Foreign body, by site or type
    middle ear 385.83
    muscle 729.6
    soft tissue NEC 729.6
  gastric 536.8
  membranes (following delivery) (with hemorrhage) 666.2 ✓5ᵗʰ
    with abortion — *see* Abortion, by type
    without hemorrhage 667.1 ✓5ᵗʰ
  menses 626.8
  milk (puerperal) 676.2 ✓5ᵗʰ
  nitrogen, extrarenal 788.9
  placenta (total) (with hemorrhage) 666.0 ✓5ᵗʰ
    with abortion — *see* Abortion, by type
    portions or fragments 666.2 ✓5ᵗʰ
      without hemorrhage 667.1 ✓5ᵗʰ
    without hemorrhage 667.0 ✓5ᵗʰ
  products of conception
    early pregnancy (fetal death before 22 completed weeks gestation) 632
    following
      abortion — *see* Abortion, by type

Retention — Rheumatism

Retention, retained — *continued*
products of conception — *continued*
following — *continued*
delivery 666.2 ✓5ᵗʰ
with hemorrhage 666.2 ✓5ᵗʰ
without hemorrhage 667.1 ✓5ᵗʰ
secundines (following delivery) (with hemorrhage) 666.2 ✓5ᵗʰ
with abortion — *see* Abortion, by type
complicating puerperium (delayed hemorrhage) 666.2 ✓5ᵗʰ
without hemorrhage 667.1 ✓5ᵗʰ
smegma, clitoris 624.8
urine NEC 788.20
bladder, incomplete emptying 788.21
psychogenic 306.53
specified NEC 788.29
water (in tissue) (*see also* Edema) 782.3
Reticulation, dust (occupational) 504
Reticulocytosis NEC 790.99
Reticuloendotheliosis
acute infantile (M9722/3) 202.5 ✓5ᵗʰ
leukemic (M9940/3) 202.4 ✓5ᵗʰ
malignant (M9720/3) 202.3 ✓5ᵗʰ
nonlipid (M9722/3) 202.5 ✓5ᵗʰ
Reticulohistiocytoma (giant cell) 277.8
Reticulohistiocytosis, multicentric 272.8
Reticulolymphosarcoma (diffuse) (M9613/3) 200.8 ✓5ᵗʰ
follicular (M9691/3) 202.0 ✓5ᵗʰ
nodular (M9691/3) 202.0 ✓5ᵗʰ
Reticulosarcoma (M9640/3) 200.0 ✓5ᵗʰ
nodular (M9642/3) 200.0 ✓5ᵗʰ
pleomorphic cell type (M9641/3) 200.0 ✓5ᵗʰ
Reticulosis (skin)
acute of infancy (M9722/3) 202.5 ✓5ᵗʰ
histiocytic medullary (M9721/3) 202.3 ✓5ᵗʰ
lipomelanotic 695.89
malignant (M9720/3) 202.3 ✓5ᵗʰ
Sézary's (M9701/3) 202.2 ✓5ᵗʰ
Retina, retinal — *see* condition
Retinitis (*see also* Chorioretinitis) 363.20
albuminurica 585 [363.10]
arteriosclerotic 440.8 [362.13]
central angiospastic 362.41
Coat's 362.12
diabetic 250.5 ✓5ᵗʰ [362.01]
disciformis 362.52
disseminated 363.10
metastatic 363.14
neurosyphilitic 094.83
pigment epitheliopathy 363.15
exudative 362.12
focal 363.00
in histoplasmosis 115.92
capsulatum 115.02
duboisii 115.12
juxtapapillary 363.05
macular 363.06
paramacular 363.06
peripheral 363.08
posterior pole NEC 363.07
gravidarum 646.8 ✓5ᵗʰ
hemorrhagica externa 362.12
juxtapapillary (Jensen's) 363.05
luetic — *see* Retinitis, syphilitic
metastatic 363.14
pigmentosa 362.74
proliferans 362.29
proliferating 362.29
punctata albescens 362.76
renal 585 [363.13]
syphilitic (secondary) 091.51
congenital 090.0 [363.13]
early 091.51
late 095.8 [363.13]
syphilitica, central, recurrent 095.8 [363.13]
tuberculous (*see also* Tuberculous) 017.3 ✓5ᵗʰ [363.13]
Retinoblastoma (M9510/3) 190.5
differentiated type (M9511/3) 190.5
undifferentiated type (M9512/3) 190.5

Retinochoroiditis (*see also* Chorioretinitis) 363.20
central angiospastic 362.41
disseminated 363.10
metastatic 363.14
neurosyphilitic 094.83
pigment epitheliopathy 363.15
syphilitic 094.83
due to toxoplasmosis (acquired) (focal) 130.2
focal 363.00
in histoplasmosis 115.92
capsulatum 115.02
duboisii 115.12
juxtapapillary (Jensen's) 363.05
macular 363.06
paramacular 363.06
peripheral 363.08
posterior pole NEC 363.07
juxtapapillaris 363.05
syphilitic (disseminated) 094.83
Retinopathy (background) 362.10
arteriosclerotic 440.8 [362.13]
atherosclerotic 440.8 [362.13]
central serous 362.41
circinate 362.10
Coat's 362.12
diabetic 250.5 ✓5ᵗʰ [362.01]
proliferative 250.5 ✓5ᵗʰ [362.02]
exudative 362.12
hypertensive 362.11
of prematurity 362.21
pigmentary, congenital 362.74
proliferative 362.29
diabetic 250.5 [362.02]
sickle-cell 282.60 [362.29]
solar 363.31
Retinoschisis 361.10
bullous 361.12
congenital 743.56
flat 361.11
juvenile 362.73
Retractile testis 752.52
Retraction
cervix (*see also* Retroversion, uterus) 621.6
drum (membrane) 384.82
eyelid 374.41
finger 736.29
head 781.0
lid 374.41
lung 518.89
mediastinum 519.3
nipple 611.79
congenital 757.6
puerperal, postpartum 676.0 ✓5ᵗʰ
palmar fascia 728.6
pleura (*see also* Pleurisy) 511.0
ring, uterus (Bandl's) (pathological) 661.4 ✓5ᵗʰ
affecting fetus or newborn 763.7
sternum (congenital) 756.3
acquired 738.3
during respiration 786.9
substernal 738.3
supraclavicular 738.8
syndrome (Duane's) 378.71
uterus (*see also* Retroversion, uterus) 621.6
valve (heart) — *see* Endocarditis
Retrobulbar — *see* condition
Retrocaval ureter 753.4
Retrocecal — *see also* condition
appendix (congenital) 751.5
Retrocession — *see* Retroversion
Retrodisplacement — *see* Retroversion
Retroflection, retroflexion — *see* Retroversion
Retrognathia, retrognathism (mandibular) (maxillary) 524.06
Retrograde
ejaculation 608.87
menstruation 626.8
Retroiliac ureter 753.4
Retroperineal — *see* condition
Retroperitoneal — *see* condition
Retroperitonitis (*see also* Peritonitis) 567.9
Retropharyngeal — *see* condition
Retroplacental — *see* condition

Retroposition — *see* Retroversion
Retrosternal thyroid (congenital) 759.2
Retroversion, retroverted
cervix (*see also* Retroversion, uterus) 621.6
female NEC (*see also* Retroversion, uterus) 621.6
iris 364.70
testis (congenital) 752.51
uterus, uterine (acquired) (acute) (adherent) (any degree) (asymptomatic) (cervix) (postinfectional) (postpartal, old) 621.6
congenital 752.3
in pregnancy or childbirth 654.3 ✓5ᵗʰ
affecting fetus or newborn 763.89
causing obstructed labor 660.2 ✓5ᵗʰ
affecting fetus or newborn 763.1
Retrusion, premaxilla (developmental) 524.04
Rett's syndrome 330.8
Reverse, reversed
peristalsis 787.4
Reye's syndrome 331.81
Reye-Sheehan syndrome (postpartum pituitary necrosis) 253.2
Rh (factor)
hemolytic disease 773.0
incompatibility, immunization, or sensitization
affecting management of pregnancy 656.1 ✓5ᵗʰ
fetus or newborn 773.0
transfusion reaction 999.7
negative mother, affecting fetus or newborn 773.0
titer elevated 999.7
transfusion reaction 999.7
Rhabdomyolysis (idiopathic) 728.89
Rhabdomyoma (M8900/0) — *see also* Neoplasm, connective tissue, benign
adult (M8904/0) — *see* Neoplasm, connective tissue, benign
fetal (M8903/0) — *see* Neoplasm, connective tissue, benign
glycogenic (M8904/0) — *see* Neoplasm, connective tissue, benign
Rhabdomyosarcoma (M8900/3) — *see also* Neoplasm, connective tissue, malignant
alveolar (M8920/3) — *see* Neoplasm, connective tissue, malignant
embryonal (M8910/3) — *see* Neoplasm, connective tissue, malignant
mixed type (M8902/3) — *see* Neoplasm, connective tissue, malignant
pleomorphic (M8901/3) — *see* Neoplasm, connective tissue, malignant
Rhabdosarcoma (M8900/3) — *see* Rhabdomyosarcoma
Rhesus (factor) (Rh) incompatibility — *see* Rh, incompatibility
Rheumaticosis — *see* Rheumatism
Rheumatism, rheumatic (acute NEC) 729.0
adherent pericardium 393
arthritis
acute or subacute — *see* Fever, rheumatic
chronic 714.0
spine 720.0
articular (chronic) NEC (*see also* Arthritis) 716.9 ✓5ᵗʰ
acute or subacute — *see* Fever, rheumatic
back 724.9
blennorrhagic 098.59
carditis — *see* Disease, heart, rheumatic
cerebral — *see* Fever, rheumatic
chorea (acute) — *see* Chorea, rheumatic
chronic NEC 729.0
coronary arteritis 391.9
chronic 398.99
degeneration, myocardium (*see also* Degeneration, myocardium, with rheumatic fever) 398.0
desert 114.0
febrile — *see* Fever, rheumatic
fever — *see* Fever, rheumatic
gonococcal 098.59
gout 274.0

Rheumatism, rheumatic — *continued*
heart
disease (*see also* Disease, heart, rheumatic)
398.90
failure (chronic) (congestive) (inactive)
398.91
hemopericardium — *see* Rheumatic,
pericarditis
hydropericardium — *see* Rheumatic,
pericarditis
inflammatory (acute) (chronic) (subacute) — *see*
Fever, rheumatic
intercostal 729.0
meaning Tietze's disease 733.6
joint (chronic) NEC (*see also* Arthritis)
716.9 ✓5ᵗʰ
acute — *see* Fever, rheumatic
mediastinopericarditis — *see* Rheumatic,
pericarditis
muscular 729.0
myocardial degeneration (*see also*
Degeneration, myocardium, with
rheumatic fever) 398.0
myocarditis (chronic) (inactive) (with chorea)
398.0
active or acute 391.2
with chorea (acute) (rheumatic)
(Sydenham's) 392.0
myositis 729.1
neck 724.9
neuralgic 729.0
neuritis (acute) (chronic) 729.2
neuromuscular 729.0
nodose — *see* Arthritis, nodosa
nonarticular 729.0
palindromic 719.30
ankle 719.37
elbow 719.32
foot 719.37
hand 719.34
hip 719.35
knee 719.36
multiple sites 719.39
pelvic region 719.35
shoulder (region) 719.31
specified site NEC 719.38
wrist 719.33
pancarditis, acute 391.8
with chorea (acute) (rheumatic)
(Sydenham's) 392.0
chronic or inactive 398.99
pericarditis (active) (acute) (with effusion) (with
pneumonia) 391.0
with chorea (acute) (rheumatic)
(Sydenham's) 392.0
chronic or inactive 393
pericardium — *see* Rheumatic, pericarditis
pleuropericarditis — *see* Rheumatic,
pericarditis
pneumonia 390 *[517.1]*
pneumonitis 390 *[517.1]*
pneumopericarditis — *see* Rheumatic,
pericarditis
polyarthritis
acute or subacute — *see* Fever, rheumatic
chronic 714.0
polyarticular NEC (*see also* Arthritis) 716.9 ✓5ᵗʰ
psychogenic 306.0
radiculitis 729.2
sciatic 724.3
septic — *see* Fever, rheumatic
spine 724.9
subacute NEC 729.0
torticollis 723.5
tuberculous NEC (*see also* Tuberculosis)
015.9 ✓5ᵗʰ
typhoid fever 002.0
Rheumatoid — *see also* condition
lungs 714.81
Rhinitis (atrophic) (catarrhal) (chronic) (croupous)
(fibrinous) (hyperplastic) (hypertrophic)
(membranous) (purulent) (suppurative)
(ulcerative) 472.0
with
hay fever (*see also* Fever, hay) 477.9
with asthma (bronchial) 493.0 ✓5ᵗʰ
sore throat — *see* Nasopharyngitis

Rhinitis — *continued*
acute 460
allergic (nonseasonal) (seasonal) (*see also* Fever,
hay) 477.9
with asthma (*see also* Asthma) 493.0 ✓5ᵗʰ
due to food 477.1
granulomatous 472.0
infective 460
obstructive 472.0
pneumococcal 460
syphilitic 095.8
congenital 090.0
tuberculous (*see also* Tuberculosis) 012.8 ✓5ᵗʰ
vasomotor (*see also* Fever, hay) 477.9
Rhinoantritis (chronic) 473.0
acute 461.0
Rhinodacryolith 375.57
Rhinolalia (aperta) (clausa) (open) 784.49
Rhinolith 478.1
nasal sinus (*see also* Sinusitis) 473.9
Rhinomegaly 478.1
Rhinopharyngitis (acute) (subacute) (*see also*
Nasopharyngitis) 460
chronic 472.2
destructive ulcerating 102.5
mutilans 102.5
Rhinophyma 695.3
Rhinorrhea 478.1
cerebrospinal (fluid) 349.81
paroxysmal (*see also* Fever, hay) 477.9
spasmodic (*see also* Fever, hay) 477.9
Rhinosalpingitis 381.50
acute 381.51
chronic 381.52
Rhinoscleroma 040.1
Rhinosporidiosis 117.0
Rhinovirus infection 079.3
Rhizomelique, pseudopolyarthritic 446.5
Rhoads and Bomford anemia (refractory) 284.9
Rhus
diversiloba dermatitis 692.6
radicans dermatitis 692.6
toxicodendron dermatitis 692.6
venenata dermatitis 692.6
verniciflua dermatitis 692.6
Rhythm
atrioventricular nodal 427.89
disorder 427.9
coronary sinus 427.89
ectopic 427.89
nodal 427.89
escape 427.89
heart, abnormal 427.9
fetus or newborn — *see* Abnormal, heart
rate
idioventricular 426.89
accelerated 427.89
nodal 427.89
sleep, inversion 780.55
nonorganic origin 307.45
Rhytidosis facialis 701.8
Rib — *see also* condition
cervical 756.2
Riboflavin deficiency 266.0
Rice bodies (*see also* Loose, body, joint) 718.1 ✓5ᵗʰ
knee 717.6
Richter's hernia — *see* Hernia, Richter's
Ricinism 988.2
Rickets (active) (acute) (adolescent) (adult) (chest
wall) (congenital) (current) (infantile)
(intestinal) 268.0
celiac 579.0
fetal 756.4
hemorrhagic 267
hypophosphatemic with nephroticglycosuric
dwarfism 270.0
kidney 588.0
late effect 268.1
renal 588.0
scurvy 267
vitamin D-resistant 275.3

Rickettsial disease 083.9
specified type NEC 083.8
Rickettsialpox 083.2
Rickettsiosis NEC 083.9
specified type NEC 083.8
tick-borne 082.9
specified type NEC 082.8
vesicular 083.2
Ricord's chancre 091.0
Riddoch's syndrome (visual disorientation)
368.16
Rider's
bone 733.99
chancre 091.0
Ridge, alveolus — *see also* condition
flabby 525.2
Ridged ear 744.29
Riedel's
disease (ligneous thyroiditis) 245.3
lobe, liver 751.69
struma (ligneous thyroiditis) 245.3
thyroiditis (ligneous) 245.3
Rieger's anomaly or syndrome (mesodermal
dysgenesis, anterior ocular segment) 743.44
Riehl's melanosis 709.09
Rietti-Greppi-Micheli anemia or syndrome
282.4
Rieux's hernia — *see* Hernia, Rieux's
Rift Valley fever 066.3
Riga's disease (cachectic aphthae) 529.0
Riga-Fede disease (cachectic aphthae) 529.0
Riggs' disease (compound periodontitis) 523.4
Right middle lobe syndrome 518.0
Rigid, rigidity — *see also* condition
abdominal 789.4 ✓5ᵗʰ
articular, multiple congenital 754.89
back 724.8
cervix uteri
in pregnancy or childbirth 654.6 ✓5ᵗʰ
affecting fetus or newborn 763.89
causing obstructed labor 660.2 ✓5ᵗʰ
affecting fetus or newborn 763.1
hymen (acquired) (congenital) 623.3
nuchal 781.6
pelvic floor
in pregnancy or childbirth 654.4 ✓5ᵗʰ
affecting fetus or newborn 763.89
causing obstructed labor 660.2 ✓5ᵗʰ
affecting fetus or newborn 763.1
perineum or vulva
in pregnancy or childbirth 654.8 ✓5ᵗʰ
affecting fetus or newborn 763.89
causing obstructed labor 660.2 ✓5ᵗʰ
affecting fetus or newborn 763.1
spine 724.8
vagina
in pregnancy or childbirth 654.7 ✓5ᵗʰ
affecting fetus or newborn 763.89
causing obstructed labor 660.2 ✓5ᵗʰ
affecting fetus or newborn 763.1
Rigors 780.99   ▲
Riley-Day syndrome (familial dysautonomia)
742.8
Ring(s)
aorta 747.21
Bandl's, complicating delivery 661.4 ✓5ᵗʰ
affecting fetus or newborn 763.7
contraction, complicating delivery 661.4 ✓5ᵗʰ
affecting fetus or newborn 763.7
esophageal (congenital) 750.3
Fleischer (-Kayser) (cornea) 275.1 *[371.14]*
hymenal, tight (acquired) (congenital) 623.3
Kayser-Fleischer (cornea) 275.1 *[371.14]*
retraction, uterus, pathological 661.4 ✓5ᵗʰ
affecting fetus or newborn 763.7
Schatzki's (esophagus) (congenital) (lower)
750.3
acquired 530.3
Soemmering's 366.51
trachea, abnormal 748.3
vascular (congenital) 747.21
Vossius' 921.3
late effect 366.21

✓4ᵗʰ Fourth-digit Required   ✓5ᵗʰ Fifth-digit Required   ▶◀ Revised Text   ● New Line   ▲ Revised Code

Ringed hair — Rupture

Ringed hair (congenital) 757.4
Ringing in the ear (see also Tinnitus) 388.30
Ringworm 110.9
  beard 110.0
  body 110.5
  Burmese 110.9
  corporeal 110.5
  foot 110.4
  groin 110.3
  hand 110.2
  honeycomb 110.0
  nails 110.1
  perianal (area) 110.3
  scalp 110.0
  specified site NEC 110.8
  Tokelau 110.5
Rise, venous pressure 459.89
Risk
  factor — see Problem
  suicidal 300.9
Ritter's disease (dermatitis exfoliativa neonatorum) 695.81
Rivalry, sibling 313.3
Rivalta's disease (cervicofacial actinomycosis) 039.3
River blindness 125.3 [360.13]
Robert's pelvis 755.69
  with disproportion (fetopelvic) 653.0 ✓5ᵗʰ
    affecting fetus or newborn 763.1
    causing obstructed labor 660.1 ✓5ᵗʰ
      affecting fetus or newborn 763.1
Robin's syndrome 756.0
Robinson's (hidrotic) ectodermal dysplasia 757.31
Robles' disease (onchocerciasis) 125.3 [360.13]
Rochalimea — see Rickettsial disease
Rocky Mountain fever (spotted) 082.0
Rodent ulcer (M8090/3) — see also Neoplasm, skin, malignant
  cornea 370.07
Roentgen ray, adverse effect — see Effect, adverse, x-ray
Roetheln 056.9
Roger's disease (congenital interventricular septal defect) 745.4
Rokitansky's
  disease (see also Necrosis, liver) 570
  tumor 620.2
Rokitansky-Aschoff sinuses (mucosal outpouching of gallbladder) (see also Disease, gallbladder) 575.8
Rokitansky-Kuster-Hauser syndrome (congenital absence vagina) 752.49
Rollet's chancre (syphilitic) 091.0
Rolling of head 781.0
Romano-Ward syndrome (prolonged Q-T interval) 794.31
Romanus lesion 720.1
Romberg's disease or syndrome 349.89
Roof, mouth — see condition
Rosacea 695.3
  acne 695.3
  keratitis 695.3 [370.49]
Rosary, rachitic 268.0
Rose
  cold 477.0
  fever 477.0
  rash 782.1
    epidemic 056.9
    of infants 057.8
Rosen-Castleman-Liebow syndrome (pulmonary proteinosis) 516.0
Rosenbach's erysipelatoid or erysipeloid 027.1
Rosenthal's disease (factor XI deficiency) 286.2
Roseola 057.8
  infantum, infantilis 057.8
Rossbach's disease (hyperchlorhydria) 536.8
  psychogenic 306.4
Rössle-Urbach-Wiethe lipoproteinosis 272.8
Ross river fever 066.3

Rostan's asthma (cardiac) (see also Failure, ventricular, left) 428.1
Rot
  Barcoo (see also Ulcer, skin) 707.9
  knife-grinders' (see also Tuberculosis) 011.4 ✓5ᵗʰ
Rot-Bernhardt disease 355.1
Rotation
  anomalous, incomplete or insufficient — see Malrotation
  cecum (congenital) 751.4
  colon (congenital) 751.4
  manual, affecting fetus or newborn 763.89
  spine, incomplete or insufficient 737.8
  tooth, teeth 524.3
  vertebra, incomplete or insufficient 737.8
Röteln 056.9
Roth's disease or meralgia 355.1
Roth-Bernhardt disease or syndrome 355.1
Rothmund (-Thomson) syndrome 757.33
Rotor's disease or syndrome (idiopathic hyperbilirubinemia) 277.4
Rotundum ulcus — see Ulcer, stomach
Round
  back (with wedging of vertebrae) 737.10
    late effect of rickets 268.1
  hole, retina 361.31
    with detachment 361.01
  ulcer (stomach) — see Ulcer, stomach
  worms (infestation) (large) NEC 127.0
Roussy-Lévy syndrome 334.3
Routine postpartum follow-up V24.2
Roy (-Jutras) syndrome (acropachyderma) 757.39
Rubella (German measles) 056.9
  complicating pregnancy, childbirth, or puerperium 647.5 ✓5ᵗʰ
  complication 056.8
    neurological 056.00
      encephalomyelitis 056.01
      specified type NEC 056.09
    specified type NEC 056.79
  congenital 771.0
  contact V01.4
  exposure to V01.4
  maternal
    with suspected fetal damage affecting management of pregnancy 655.3 ✓5ᵗʰ
    affecting fetus or newborn 760.2
      manifest rubella in infant 771.0
  specified complications NEC 056.79
  vaccination, prophylactic (against) V04.3
Rubeola (measles) (see also Measles) 055.9
  complicated 055.8
  meaning rubella (see also Rubella) 056.9
  scarlatinosis 057.8
Rubeosis iridis 364.42
  diabetica 250.5 ✓5ᵗʰ [364.42]
Rubinstein-Taybi's syndrome (brachydactylia, short stature, and mental retardation) 759.89
Rud's syndrome (mental deficiency, epilepsy, and infantilism) 759.89
Rudimentery (congenital) — see also Agenesis
  arm 755.22
  bone 756.9
  cervix uteri 752.49
  eye (see also Microphthalmos) 743.10
  fallopian tube 752.19
  leg 755.32
  lobule of ear 744.21
  patella 755.64
  respiratory organs in thoracopagus 759.4
  tracheal bronchus 748.3
  uterine horn 752.3
  uterus 752.3
    in male 752.7
    solid or with cavity 752.3
  vagina 752.49
Ruiter-Pompen (-Wyers) syndrome (angiokeratoma corporis diffusum) 272.7
Ruled out condition (see also Observation, suspected) V71.9

Rumination — see also Vomiting
  neurotic 300.3
  obsessional 300.3
  psychogenic 307.53
Runaway reaction — see also Disturbance, conduct
  socialized 312.2 ✓5ᵗʰ
  undersocialized, unsocialized 312.1 ✓5ᵗʰ
Runeberg's disease (progressive pernicious anemia) 281.0
Runge's syndrome (postmaturity) 766.2
Rupia 091.3
  congenital 090.0
  tertiary 095.9
Rupture, ruptured 553.9
  abdominal viscera NEC 799.8
    obstetrical trauma 665.5 ✓5ᵗʰ
  abscess (spontaneous) — see Abscess, by site
  amnion — see Rupture, membranes
  aneurysm — see Aneurysm
  anus (sphincter) — see Laceration, anus
  aorta, aortic 441.5
    abdominal 441.3
    arch 441.1
    ascending 441.1
    descending 441.5
      abdominal 441.3
      thoracic 441.1
    syphilitic 093.0
    thoracoabdominal 441.6
    thorax, thoracic 441.1
    transverse 441.1
    traumatic (thoracic) 901.0
      abdominal 902.0
    valve or cusp (see also Endocarditis, aortic) 424.1
  appendix (with peritonitis) 540.0
    with peritoneal abscess 540.1
    traumatic — see Injury, internal, gastrointestinal tract
  arteriovenous fistula, brain (congenital) 430
  artery 447.2
    brain (see also Hemorrhage, brain) 431
    coronary (see also Infarct, myocardium) 410.9 ✓5ᵗʰ
    heart (see also Infarct, myocardium) 410.9 ✓5ᵗʰ
    pulmonary 417.8
    traumatic (complication) (see also Injury, blood vessel, by site) 904.9
  bile duct, except cystic (see also Disease, biliary) 576.3
    cystic 575.4
    traumatic — see Injury, internal, intra-abdominal
  bladder (sphincter) 596.6
    with
      abortion — see Abortion, by type, with damage to pelvic organs
      ectopic pregnancy (see also categories 633.0-633.9) 639.2
      molar pregnancy (see also categories 630-632) 639.2
    following
      abortion 639.2
      ectopic or molar pregnancy 639.2
    nontraumatic 596.6
    obstetrical trauma 665.5 ✓5ᵗʰ
    spontaneous 596.6
    traumatic — see Injury, internal, bladder
  blood vessel (see also Hemorrhage) 459.0
    brain (see also Hemorrhage, brain) 431
    heart (see also Infarct, myocardium) 410.9 ✓5ᵗʰ
    traumatic (complication) (see also Injury, blood vessel, by site) 904.9
  bone — see Fracture, by site
  bowel 569.89
    traumatic — see Injury, internal, intestine
  Bowman's membrane 371.31
  brain
    aneurysm (congenital) (see also Hemorrhage, subarachnoid) 430
    late effect — see Late effect(s) (of) cerebrovascular disease
    syphilitic 094.87

✓4ᵗʰ Fourth-digit Required ✓5ᵗʰ Fifth-digit Required ►◄ Revised Text ● New Line ▲ Revised Code

Rupture, ruptured — *continued*
  brain — *continued*
    hemorrhagic (*see also* Hemorrhage, brain)
      431
    injury at birth 767.0
    syphilitic 094.89
  capillaries 448.9
  cardiac (*see also* Infarct, myocardium)
    410.9 ✓5ᵗʰ
  cartilage (articular) (current) — *see also* Sprain,
    by site
    knee — *see* Tear, meniscus
    semilunar — *see* Tear, meniscus
  cecum (with peritonitis) 540.0
    with peritoneal abscess 540.1
    traumatic 863.89
      with open wound into cavity 863.99
  cerebral aneurysm (congenital) (*see also*
    Hemorrhage, subarachnoid) 430
    late effect — *see* Late effect(s) (of)
      cerebrovascular disease
  cervix (uteri)
    with
      abortion — *see* Abortion, by type, with
        damage to pelvic organs
      ectopic pregnancy (*see also* categories
        633.0-633.9) 639.2
      molar pregnancy (*see also* categories 630-
        632) 639.2
    following
      abortion 639.2
      ectopic or molar pregnancy 639.2
    obstetrical trauma 665.3 ✓5ᵗʰ
    traumatic — *see* Injury, internal, cervix
  chordae tendineae 429.5
  choroid (direct) (indirect) (traumatic) 363.63
  circle of Willis (*see also* Hemorrhage,
    subarachnoid) 430
    late effect — *see* Late effect(s) (of)
      cerebrovascular disease
  colon 569.89
    traumatic — *see* Injury, internal, colon
  cornea (traumatic) — *see also* Rupture, eye
    due to ulcer 370.00
  coronary (artery) (thrombotic) (*see also* Infarct,
    myocardium) 410.9 ✓5ᵗʰ
  corpus luteum (infected) (ovary) 620.1
  cyst — *see* Cyst
  cystic duct (*see also* Disease, gallbladder) 575.4
  Descemet's membrane 371.33
    traumatic — *see* Rupture, eye
  diaphragm — *see also* Hernia, diaphragm
    traumatic — *see* Injury, internal, diaphragm
  diverticulum
    bladder 596.3
    intestine (large) (*see also* Diverticula) 562.10
      small 562.00
  duodenal stump 537.89
  duodenum (ulcer) — *see* Ulcer, duodenum, with
    perforation
  ear drum (*see also* Perforation, tympanum)
    384.20
    with otitis media — *see* Otitis media
    traumatic — *see* Wound, open, ear
  esophagus 530.4
    traumatic 862.22
      with open wound into cavity 862.32
      cervical region — *see* Wound, open,
        esophagus
  eye (without prolapse of intraocular tissue)
    871.0
    with
      exposure of intraocular tissue 871.1
      partial loss of intraocular tissue 871.2
      prolapse of intraocular tissue 871.1
    due to burn 940.5
  fallopian tube 620.8
    due to pregnancy — *see* Pregnancy, tubal
    traumatic — *see* Injury, internal, fallopian
      tube
  fontanel 767.3
  free wall (ventricle) (*see also* Infarct,
    myocardium) 410.9 ✓5ᵗʰ
  gallbladder or duct (*see also* Disease,
    gallbladder) 575.4
    traumatic — *see* Injury, internal, gallbladder

Rupture, ruptured — *continued*
  gastric (*see also* Rupture, stomach) 537.89
    vessel 459.0
  globe (eye) (traumatic) — *see* Rupture, eye
  graafian follicle (hematoma) 620.0
  heart (auricle) (ventricle) (*see also* Infarct,
    myocardium) 410.9 ✓5ᵗʰ
    infectional 422.90
    traumatic — *see* Rupture, myocardium,
      traumatic
  hymen 623.8
  internal
    organ, traumatic — *see also* Injury, internal,
      by site
      heart — *see* Rupture, myocardium,
        traumatic
      kidney — *see* Rupture, kidney
      liver — *see* Rupture, liver
      spleen — *see* Rupture, spleen, traumatic
    semilunar cartilage — *see* Tear, meniscus
  intervertebral disc — *see* Displacement,
    intervertebral disc
    traumatic (current) — *see* Dislocation,
      vertebra
  intestine 569.89
    traumatic — *see* Injury, internal, intestine
  intracranial, birth injury 767.0
  iris 364.76
    traumatic — *see* Rupture, eye
  joint capsule — *see* Sprain, by site
  kidney (traumatic) 866.03
    with open wound into cavity 866.13
    due to birth injury 767.8
    nontraumatic 593.89
  lacrimal apparatus (traumatic) 870.2
  lens (traumatic) 366.20
  ligament — *see also* Sprain, by site
    with open wound — *see* Wound, open, by
      site
    old (*see also* Disorder, cartilage, articular)
      718.0 ✓5ᵗʰ
  liver (traumatic) 864.04
    with open wound into cavity 864.14
    due to birth injury 767.8
    nontraumatic 573.8
  lymphatic (node) (vessel) 457.8
  marginal sinus (placental) (with hemorrhage)
    641.2 ✓5ᵗʰ
    affecting fetus or newborn 762.1
  meaning hernia — *see* Hernia
  membrana tympani (*see also* Perforation,
    tympanum) 384.20
    with otitis media — *see* Otitis media
    traumatic — *see* Wound, open, ear
  membranes (spontaneous)
    artificial
      delayed delivery following 658.3 ✓5ᵗʰ
        affecting fetus or newborn 761.1
      fetus or newborn 761.1
    delayed delivery following 658.2 ✓5ᵗʰ
      affecting fetus or newborn 761.1
    premature (less than 24 hours prior to onset
      of labor) 658.1 ✓5ᵗʰ
      affecting fetus or newborn 761.1
    delayed delivery following 658.2 ✓5ᵗʰ
      affecting fetus or newborn 761.1
  meningeal artery (*see also* Hemorrhage,
    subarachnoid) 430
    late effect — *see* Late effect(s) (of)
      cerebrovascular diseas
  meniscus (knee) — *see also* Tear, meniscus
    old (*see also* Derangement, meniscus) 717.5
      site other than knee — *see* Disorder,
        cartilage, articular
    site other than knee — *see* Sprain, by site
  mesentery 568.89
    traumatic — *see* Injury, internal, mesentery
  mitral — *see* Insufficiency, mitral
  muscle (traumatic) NEC — *see also* Sprain, by
    site
    with open wound — *see* Wound, open, by
      site
    nontraumatic 728.83
  musculotendinous cuff (nontraumatic)
    (shoulder) 840.4

Rupture, ruptured — *continued*
  mycotic aneurysm, causing cerebral
    hemorrhage (*see also* Hemorrhage,
    subarachnoid) 430
    late effect — *see* Late effect(s) (of)
      cerebrovascular disease
  myocardium, myocardial (*see also* Infarct,
    myocardium) 410.9 ✓5ᵗʰ
    traumatic 861.03
      with open wound into thorax 861.13
  nontraumatic (meaning hernia) (*see also*
    Hernia, by site) 553.9
    obstructed (*see also* Hernia, by site, with
      obstruction) 552.9
      gangrenous (*see also* Hernia, by site, with
        gangrene) 551.9
  operation wound 998.32 ▲
    internal 998.31 ●
  ovary, ovarian 620.8
    corpus luteum 620.1
    follicle (graafian) 620.0
  oviduct 620.8
    due to pregnancy — *see* Pregnancy, tubal
  pancreas 577.8
    traumatic — *see* Injury, internal, pancreas
  papillary muscle (ventricular) 429.6
  pelvic
    floor, complicating delivery 664.1 ✓5ᵗʰ
    organ NEC — *see* Injury, pelvic, organs
  penis (traumatic) — *see* Wound, open, penis
  perineum 624.8
    during delivery (*see also* Laceration,
      perineum, complicating delivery)
      664.4 ✓5ᵗʰ
  pharynx (nontraumatic) (spontaneous) 478.29
  pregnant uterus (before onset of labor)
    665.0 ✓5ᵗʰ
  prostate (traumatic) — *see* Injury, internal,
    prostate
  pulmonary
    artery 417.8
    valve (heart) (*see also* Endocarditis,
      pulmonary) 424.3
    vein 417.8
    vessel 417.8
  pupil, sphincter 364.75
  pus tube (*see also* Salpingo-oophoritis) 614.2
  pyosalpinx (*see also* Salpingo-oophoritis) 614.2
  rectum 569.49
    traumatic — *see* Injury, internal, rectum
  retina, retinal (traumatic) (without detachment)
    361.30
    with detachment (*see also* Detachment,
      retina, with retinal defect) 361.00
  rotator cuff (capsule) (traumatic) 840.4
    nontraumatic, complete 727.61
  sclera 871.0
  semilunar cartilage, knee (*see also* Tear,
    meniscus) 836.2
    old (*see also* Derangement, meniscus) 717.5
  septum (cardiac) 410.8 ✓5ᵗʰ
  sigmoid 569.89
    traumatic — *see* Injury, internal, colon,
      sigmoid
  sinus of Valsalva 747.29
  spinal cord — *see also* Injury, spinal, by site
    due to injury at birth 767.4
    fetus or newborn 767.4
    syphilitic 094.89
    traumatic — *see also* Injury, spinal, by site
      with fracture — *see* Fracture, vertebra,
        by site, with spinal cord injury
  spleen 289.59
    congenital 767.8
    due to injury at birth 767.8
    malarial 084.9
    nontraumatic 289.59
    spontaneous 289.59
    traumatic 865.04
      with open wound into cavity 865.14
  splenic vein 459.0
  stomach 537.89
    due to injury at birth 767.8
    traumatic — *see* Injury, internal, stomach
    ulcer — *see* Ulcer, stomach, with perforation
  synovium 727.50
    specified site NEC 727.59

Rupture, ruptured — *continued*
  tendon (traumatic) — *see also* Sprain, by site
    with open wound — *see* Wound, open, by
      site
    Achilles 845.09
      nontraumatic 727.67
    ankle 845.09
      nontraumatic 727.68
    biceps (long bead) 840.8
      nontraumatic 727.62
    foot 845.10
      interphalangeal (joint) 845.13
      metatarsophalangeal (joint) 845.12
      nontraumatic 727.68
      specified site NEC 845.19
      tarsometatarsal (joint) 845.11
    hand 842.10
      carpometacarpal (joint) 842.11
      interphalangeal (joint) 842.13
      metacarpophalangeal (joint) 842.12
      nontraumatic 727.63
        extensors 727.63
        flexors 727.64
      specified site NEC 842.19
      nontraumatic 727.60
      specified site NEC 727.69
    patellar 844.8
      nontraumatic 727.66
    quadriceps 844.8
      nontraumatic 727.65
    rotator cuff (capsule) 840.4
      nontraumatic, complete 727.61
    wrist 842.00
      carpal (joint) 842.01
      nontraumatic 727.63
        extensors 727.63
        flexors 727.64
      radiocarpal (joint) (ligament) 842.02
      radioulnar (joint), distal 842.09
      specified site NEC 842.09
  testis (traumatic) 878.2
    complicated 878.3
    due to syphilis 095.8
  thoracic duct 457.8
  tonsil 474.8
  traumatic
    with open wound — *see* Wound, open, by
      site
    aorta — *see* Rupture, aorta, traumatic
    ear drum — *see* Wound, open, ear, drum
    external site — *see* Wound, open, by site
    eye 871.2
    globe (eye) — *see* Wound, open, eyeball
    internal organ (abdomen, chest, or pelvis) —
      see also Injury, internal, by site
      heart — *see* Rupture, myocardium,
        traumatic
      kidney — *see* Rupture, kidney
      liver — *see* Rupture, liver
      spleen — *see* Rupture, spleen, traumatic
    ligament, muscle, or tendon — *see also*
      Sprain, by site
      with open wound — *see* Wound, open, by
        site
    meaning hernia — *see* Hernia
  tricuspid (heart) (valve) — *see* Endocarditis,
    tricuspid
  tube, tubal 620.8
    abscess (*see also* Salpingo-oophoritis) 614.2
    due to pregnancy — *see* Pregnancy, tubal
  tympanum, tympanic (membrane) (*see also*
    Perforation, tympanum) 384.20
    with otitis media — *see* Otitis media
    traumatic — *see* Wound, open, ear, drum
  umbilical cord 663.8 ☑5ᵗʰ
    fetus or newborn 772.0
  ureter (traumatic) (*see also* Injury, internal,
    ureter) 867.2
    nontraumatic 593.89
  urethra 599.84
    with
      abortion — *see* Abortion, by type, with
        damage to pelvic organs
      ectopic pregnancy (*see also* categories
        633.0-633.9) 639.2
      molar pregnancy (*see also* categories 630-
        632) 639.2

Rupture, ruptured — *continued*
  urethra — *continued*
    following
      abortion 639.2
      ectopic or molar pregnancy 639.2
    obstetrical trauma 665.5 ☑5ᵗʰ
    traumatic — *see* Injury, internal urethra
  uterosacral ligament 620.8
  uterus (traumatic) — *see also* Injury, internal
    uterus
    affecting fetus or newborn 763.89
    during labor 665.1 ☑5ᵗʰ
    nonpuerperal, nontraumatic 621.8
    nontraumatic 621.8
    pregnant (during labor) 665.1 ☑5ᵗʰ
      before labor 665.0 ☑5ᵗʰ
  vagina 878.6
    complicated 878.7
    complicating delivery — *see* Laceration,
      vagina, complicating delivery
  valve, valvular (heart) — *see* Endocarditis
  varicose vein — *see* Varicose, vein
  varix — *see* Varix
  vena cava 459.0
  ventricle (free wall) (left) (*see also* Infarct,
    myocardium) 410.9 ☑5ᵗʰ
  vesical (urinary) 596.6
    traumatic — *see* Injury, internal, bladder
  vessel (blood) 459.0
    pulmonary 417.8
  viscus 799.8
  vulva 878.4
    complicated 878.5
    complicating delivery 664.0 ☑5ᵗʰ

Russell's dwarf (uterine dwarfism and
  craniofacial dysostosis) 759.89

Russell's dysentery 004.8

Russell (-Silver) syndrome (congenital
  hemihypertrophy and short stature) 759.89

Russian spring-summer type encephalitis 063.0

Rust's disease (tuberculous spondylitis)
  015.0 ☑5ᵗʰ *[720.81]*

Rustitskii's disease (multiple myeloma)
  (M9730/3) 203.0 ☑5ᵗʰ

Ruysch's disease (Hirschsprung's disease) 751.3

Rytand-Lipsitch syndrome (complete
  atrioventricular bloc) 426.0

S

Saber
- shin 090.5
- tibia 090.5

Sac, lacrimal — *see* condition

Saccharomyces infection (*see also* Candidiasis) 112.9

Saccharopinuria 270.7

Saccular — *see* condition

Sacculation
- aorta (nonsyphilitic) (*see also* Aneurysm, aorta) 441.9
  - ruptured 441.5
  - syphilitic 093.0
- bladder 596.3
- colon 569.89
- intralaryngeal (congenital) (ventricular) 748.3
- larynx (congenital) (ventricular) 748.3
- organ or site, congenital — *see* Distortion
- pregnant uterus, complicating delivery 654.4 ✓5ᵗʰ
  - affecting fetus or newborn 763.1
    - causing obstructed labor 660.2 ✓5ᵗʰ
      - affecting fetus or newborn 763.1
- rectosigmoid 569.89
- sigmoid 569.89
- ureter 593.89
- urethra 599.2
- vesical 596.3

Sachs (-Tay) disease (amaurotic familial idiocy) 330.1

Sacks-Libman disease 710.0 [424.91]

Sacralgia 724.6

Sacralization
- fifth lumbar vertebra 756.15
- incomplete (vertebra) 756.15

Sacrodynia 724.6

Sacroiliac joint — *see* condition

Sacroiliitis NEC 720.2

Sacrum — *see* condition

Saddle
- back 737.8
- embolus, aorta 444.0
- nose 738.0
  - congenital 754.0
  - due to syphilis 090.5

Sadism (sexual) 302.84

Saemisch's ulcer 370.04

Saenger's syndrome 379.46

Sago spleen 277.3

Sailors' skin 692.74

Saint
- Anthony's fire (*see also* Erysipelas) 035
- Guy's dance — *see* Chorea
- Louis-type encephalitis 062.3
- triad (*see also* Hernia, diaphragm) 553.3
- Vitus' dance — *see* Chorea

Salicylism
- correct substance properly administered 535.4 ✓5ᵗʰ
- overdose or wrong substance given or taken 965.1

Salivary duct or gland — *see also* condition
- virus disease 078.5

Salivation (excessive) (*see also* Ptyalism) 527.7

Salmonella (aertrycke) (choleraesuis) (enteritidis) (gallinarum) (suipestifer) (typhimurium) (*see also* Infection, Salmonella) 003.9
- arthritis 003.23
- carrier (suspected) of V02.3
- meningitis 003.21
- osteomyelitis 003.24
- pneumonia 003.22
- septicemia 003.1
- typhosa 002.0
  - carrier (suspected) of V02.1

Salmonellosis 003.0
- with pneumonia 003.22

Salpingitis (catarrhal) (fallopian tube) (nodular) (pseudofollicular) (purulent) (septic) (*see also* Salpingo-oophoritis) 614.2
- ear 381.50
  - acute 381.51
  - chronic 381.52

Salpingitis
- Eustachian (tube) 381.50
  - acute 381.51
  - chronic 381.52
- follicularis 614.1
- gonococcal (chronic) 098.37
  - acute 098.17
- interstitial, chronic 614.1
- isthmica nodosa 614.1
- old — *see* Salpingo-oophoritis, chronic
- puerperal, postpartum, childbirth 670 ✓5ᵗʰ
- specific (chronic) 098.37
  - acute 098.17
- tuberculous (acute) (chronic) (*see also* Tuberculosis) 016.6 ✓5ᵗʰ
- venereal (chronic) 098.37
  - acute 098.17

Salpingocele 620.4

Salpingo-oophoritis (catarrhal) (purulent) (ruptured) (septic) (suppurative) 614.2
- acute 614.0
  - with
    - abortion — *see* Abortion, by type, with sepsis
    - ectopic pregnancy (*see also* categories 633.0-633.9) 639.0
    - molar pregnancy (*see also* categories 630-632) 639.0
  - following
    - abortion 639.0
    - ectopic or molar pregnancy 639.0
  - gonococcal 098.17
  - puerperal, postpartum, childbirth 670 ✓4ᵗʰ
  - tuberculous (*see also* Tuberculosis) 016.6 ✓5ᵗʰ
- chronic 614.1
  - gonococcal 098.37
  - tuberculous (see also Tuberculosis) 016.6 ✓5ᵗʰ
- complicating pregnancy 646.6 ✓5ᵗʰ
  - affecting fetus or newborn 760.8
- gonococcal (chronic) 098.37
  - acute 098.17
- old — *see* Salpingo-oophoritis, chronic
- puerperal 670 ✓4ᵗʰ
- specific — *see* Salpingo-oophoritis, gonococcal
- subacute (*see also* Salpingo-oophoritis, acute) 614.0
- tuberculous (acute) (chronic) (*see also* Tuberculosis) 016.6 ✓5ᵗʰ
- venereal — *see* Salpingo-oophoritis, gonococcal

Salpingo-ovaritis (*see also* Salpingooophoritis) 614.2

Salpingoperitonitis (*see also* Salpingo-oophoritis) 614.2

Salt-losing
- nephritis (*see also* Disease, renal) 593.9
- syndrome (*see also* Disease, renal) 593.9

Salt-rheum (*see also* Eczema) 692.9

Salzmann's nodular dystrophy 371.46

Sampson's cyst or tumor 617.1

Sandblasters'
- asthma 502
- lung 502

Sander's disease (paranoia) 297.1

Sandfly fever 066.0

Sandhoff's disease 330.1

Sanfilippo's syndrome (mucopolysaccharidosis III) 277.5

Sanger-Brown's ataxia 334.2

San Joaquin Valley fever 114.0

Sao Paulo fever or typhus 082.0

Saponification, mesenteric 567.8

Sapremia — *see* Septicemia

Sarcocele (benign)
- syphilitic 095.8
  - congenital 090.5

Sarcoepiplocele (*see also* Hernia) 553.9

Sarcoepiplomphalocele (*see also* Hernia, umbilicus) 553.1

Sarcoid (any site) 135
- with lung involvement 135 [517.8]
- Boeck's 135
- Darier-Roussy 135
- Spiegler-Fendt 686.8

Sarcoidosis 135
- cardiac 135 [425.8]
- lung 135 [517.8]

Sarcoma (M8800/3) — *see also* Neoplasm, connective tissue, malignant
- alveolar soft part (M9581/3) — *see* Neoplasm, connective tissue, malignant
- ameloblastic (M9330/3) 170.1
  - upper jaw (bone) 170.0
- botryoid (M8910/3) — *see* Neoplasm, connective tissue, malignant
- botryoides (M8910/3) — *see* Neoplasm, connective tissue, malignant
- cerebellar (M9480/3) 191.6
  - circumscribed (arachnoidal) (M9471/3) 191.6
- circumscribed (arachnoidal) cerebellar (M9471/3) 191.6
- clear cell, of tendons and aponeuroses (M9044/3) — *see* Neoplasm, connective tissue, malignant
- embryonal (M8991/3) — *see* Neoplasm, connective tissue, malignant
- endometrial (stromal) (M8930/3) 182.0
  - isthmus 182.1
- endothelial (M9130/3) — *see also* Neoplasm, connective tissue, malignant
  - bone (M9260/3) — *see* Neoplasm, bone, malignant
- epithelioid cell (M8804/3) — *see* Neoplasm, connective tissue, malignant
- Ewing's (M9260/3) — *see* Neoplasm, bone, malignant
- germinoblastic (diffuse) (M9632/3) 202.8 ✓5ᵗʰ
  - follicular (M9697/3) 202.0 ✓5ᵗʰ
- giant cell (M8802/3) — *see also* Neoplasm, connective tissue, malignant
  - bone (M9250/3) — *see* Neoplasm, bone, malignant
- glomoid (M8710/3) — *see* Neoplasm, connective tissue, malignant
- granulocytic (M9930/3) 205.3 ✓5ᵗʰ
- hemangioendothelial (M9130/3) — *see* Neoplasm, connective tissue, malignant
- hemorrhagic, multiple (M9140/3) — *see* Kaposi's, sarcoma
- Hodgkin's (M9662/3) 201.2 ✓5ᵗʰ
- immunoblastic (M9612/3) 200.8 ✓5ᵗʰ
- Kaposi's (M9140/3) — *see* Kaposi's, sarcoma
- Kupffer cell (M9124/3) 155.0
- leptomeningeal (M9530/3) — *see* Neoplasm, meninges, malignant
- lymphangioendothelial (M9170/3) — *see* Neoplasm, connective tissue, malignant
- lymphoblastic (M9630/3) 200.1 ✓5ᵗʰ
- lymphocytic (M9620/3) 200.1 ✓5ᵗʰ
- mast cell (M9740/3) 202.6 ✓5ᵗʰ
- melanotic (M8720/3) — *see* Melanoma
- meningeal (M9530/3) — *see* Neoplasm, meninges, malignant
- meningothelial (M9530/3) — *see* Neoplasm, meninges, malignant
- mesenchymal (M8800/3) — *see also* Neoplasm, connective tissue, malignant
  - mixed (M8990/3) — *see* Neoplasm, connective tissue, malignant
- mesothelial (M9050/3) — *see* Neoplasm, by site, malignant
- monstrocellular (M9481/3)
  - specified site — *see* Neoplasm, by site, malignant
  - unspecified site 191.9
- myeloid (M9930/3) 205.3 ✓5ᵗʰ
- neurogenic (M9540/3) — *see* Neoplasm, connective tissue, malignant
- odontogenic (M9270/3) 170.1
  - upper jaw (bone) 170.0
- osteoblastic (M9180/3) — *see* Neoplasm, bone, malignant

Saber — Sarcoma

Sarcoma — *see also* Neoplasm, connective tissue, malignant — *continued*
  osteogenic (M9180/3) — *see also* Neoplasm, bone, malignant
    juxtacortical (M9190/3) — *see* Neoplasm, bone, malignant
    periosteal (M9190/3) — *see* Neoplasm, bone, malignant
    periosteal (M8812/3) — *see also* Neoplasm, bone, malignant
    osteogenic (M9190/3) — *see* Neoplasm, bone, malignant
  plasma cell (M9731/3) 203.8 ✓5ᵗʰ
  pleomorphic cell (M8802/3) — *see* Neoplasm, connective tissue, malignant
  reticuloendothelial (M9720/3) 202.3 ✓5ᵗʰ
  reticulum cell (M9640/3) 200.0 ✓5ᵗʰ
    nodular (M9642/3) 200.0 ✓5ᵗʰ
    pleomorphic cell type (M9641/3) 200.0 ✓5ᵗʰ
  round cell (M8803/3) — *see* Neoplasm, connective tissue, malignant
  small cell (M8803/3) — *see* Neoplasm, connective tissue, malignant
  spindle cell (M8801/3) — *see* Neoplasm, connective tissue, malignant
  stromal (endometrial) (M8930/3) 182.0
    isthmus 182.1
  synovial (M9040/3) — *see also* Neoplasm, connective tissue, malignant
    biphasic type (M9043/3) — *see* Neoplasm, connective tissue, malignant
    epithelioid cell type (M9042/3) — *see* Neoplasm, connective tissue, malignant
    spindle cell type (M9041/3) — *see* Neoplasm, connective tissue, malignant

Sarcomatosis
  meningeal (M9539/3) — *see* Neoplasm, meninges, malignant
  specified site NEC (M8800/3) — *see* Neoplasm, connective tissue, malignant
  unspecified site (M8800/6) 171.9

Sarcosinemia 270.8

Sarcosporidiosis 136.5

Saturnine — *see* condition

Saturnism 984.9
  specified type of lead — *see* Table of Drugs and Chemicals

Satyriasis 302.89

Sauriasis — *see* Ichthyosis

Sauriderma 757.39

Sauriosis — *see* Ichthyosis

Savill's disease (epidemic exfoliative dermatitis) 695.89

SBE (subacute bacterial endocarditis) 421.0

Scabies (any site) 133.0

Scabs 782.8

Scaglietti-Dagnini syndrome (acromegalic macrospondylitis) 253.0

Scald, scalded — *see also* Burn, by site
  skin syndrome 695.1

Scalenus anticus (anterior) syndrome 353.0

Scales 782.8

Scalp — *see* condition

Scaphocephaly 756.0

Scaphoiditis, tarsal 732.5

Scapulalgia 733.90

Scapulohumeral myopathy 359.1

Scar, scarring (*see also* Cicatrix) 709.2
  adherent 709.2
  atrophic 709.2
  cervix
    in pregnancy or childbirth 654.6 ✓5ᵗʰ
      affecting fetus or newborn 763.89
      causing obstructed labor 660.2 ✓5ᵗʰ
        affecting fetus or newborn 763.1
  cheloid 701.4
  chorioretinal 363.30
    disseminated 363.35
    macular 363.32
    peripheral 363.34

Scar, scarring (*see also* Cicatrix) — *continued*
  chorioretinal — *continued*
    posterior pole NEC 363.33
  choroid (*see also* Scar, chorioretinal) 363.30
  compression, pericardial 423.9
  congenital 757.39
  conjunctiva 372.64
  cornea 371.00
    xerophthalmic 264.6
  due to previous cesarean delivery, complicating pregnancy or childbirth 654.2 ✓5ᵗʰ
    affecting fetus or newborn 763.89
  duodenal (bulb) (cap) 537.3
  hypertrophic 701.4
  keloid 701.4
  labia 624.4
  lung (base) 518.89
  macula 363.32
    disseminated 363.35
    peripheral 363.34
  muscle 728.89
  myocardium, myocardial 412
  painful 709.2
  papillary muscle 429.81
  posterior pole NEC 363.33
    macular — *see* Scar, macula
  postnecrotic (hepatic) (liver) 571.9
  psychic V15.49
  retina (*see also* Scar, chorioretinal) 363.30
  trachea 478.9
  uterus 621.8
    in pregnancy or childbirth NEC 654.9 ✓5ᵗʰ
      affecting fetus or newborn 763.89
      due to previous cesarean delivery 654.2 ✓5ᵗʰ
  vulva 624.4

Scarabiasis 134.1

Scarlatina 034.1
  anginosa 034.1
  maligna 034.1
  myocarditis, acute 034.1 *[422.0]*
    old (*see also* Myocarditis) 429.0
  otitis media 034.1 *[382.02]*
  ulcerosa 034.1

Scarlatinella 057.8

Scarlet fever (albuminuria) (angina) (convulsions) (lesions of lid) (rash) 034.1

Schamberg's disease, dermatitis, or dermatosis (progressive pigmentary dermatosis) 709.09

Schatzki's ring (esophagus) (lower) (congenital) 750.3
  acquired 530.3

Schaufenster krankheit 413.9

Schaumann's
  benign lymphogranulomatosis 135
  disease (sarcoidosis) 135
  syndrome (sarcoidosis) 135

Scheie's syndrome (mucopolysaccharidosis IS) 277.5

Schenck's disease (sporotrichosis) 117.1

Scheuermann's disease or osteochondrosis 732.0

Scheuthauer-Marie-Sainton syndrome (cleidocranialis dysostosis) 755.59

Schilder (-Flatau) disease 341.1

Schilling-type monocytic leukemia (M9890/3) 206.9 ✓5ᵗʰ

Schimmelbusch's disease, cystic mastitis, or hyperplasia 610.1

Schirmer's syndrome (encephalocutaneous angiomatosis) 759.6

Schistocelia 756.79

Schistoglossia 750.13

Schistosoma infestation — *see* Infestation, Schistosoma

Schistosomiasis 120.9
  Asiatic 120.2
  bladder 120.0
  chestermani 120.8
  colon 120.1
  cutaneous 120.3
  due to
    S. hematobium 120.0
    S. japonicum 120.2

Schistosomiasis — *continued*
  due to — *continued*
    S. mansoni 120.1
    S. mattheii 120.8
  eastern 120.2
  genitourinary tract 120.0
  intestinal 120.1
  lung 120.2
  Manson's (intestinal) 120.1
  Oriental 120.2
  pulmonary 120.2
  specified type NEC 120.8
  vesical 120.0

Schizencephaly 742.4

Schizo-affective psychosis (*see also* Schizophrenia) 295.7 ✓5ᵗʰ

Schizodontia 520.2

Schizoid personality 301.20
  introverted 301.21
  schizotypal 301.22

Schizophrenia, schizophrenic (reaction) 295.9 ✓5ᵗʰ

> *Note* — *Use the following fifth-digit subclassification with category 295:*
>
> 0   *unspecified*
> 1   *subchronic*
> 2   *chronic*
> 3   *subchronic with acute exacerbation*
> 4   *chronic with acute exacerbation*
> 5   *in remission*

  acute (attack) NEC 295.8 ✓5ᵗʰ
    episode 295.4 ✓5ᵗʰ
  atypical form 295.8 ✓5ᵗʰ
  borderline 295.5 ✓5ᵗʰ
  catalepsy 295.2 ✓5ᵗʰ
  catatonic (type) (acute) (excited) (withdrawn) 295.2 ✓5ᵗʰ
  childhood (type) (*see also* Psychosis, childhood) 299.9 ✓5ᵗʰ
  chronic NEC 295.6 ✓5ᵗʰ
  coenesthesiopathic 295.8 ✓5ᵗʰ
  cyclic (type) 295.7 ✓5ᵗʰ
  disorganized (type) 295.1 ✓5ᵗʰ
  flexibilitas cerea 295.2 ✓5ᵗʰ
  hebephrenic (type) (acute) 295.1 ✓5ᵗʰ
  incipient 295.5 ✓5ᵗʰ
  latent 295.5 ✓5ᵗʰ
  paranoid (type) (acute) 295.3 ✓5ᵗʰ
  paraphrenic (acute) 295.3 ✓5ᵗʰ
  prepsychotic 295.5 ✓5ᵗʰ
  primary (acute) 295.0 ✓5ᵗʰ
  prodromal 295.5 ✓5ᵗʰ
  pseudoneurotic 295.5 ✓5ᵗʰ
  pseudopsychopathic 295.5 ✓5ᵗʰ
  reaction 295.9 ✓5ᵗʰ
  residual (state) (type) 295.6 ✓5ᵗʰ
  restzustand 295.6 ✓5ᵗʰ
  schizo-affective (type) (depressed) (excited) 295.7 ✓5ᵗʰ
  schizophreniform type 295.4 ✓5ᵗʰ
  simple (type) (acute) 295.0 ✓5ᵗʰ
  simplex (acute) 295.0 ✓5ᵗʰ
  specified type NEC 295.8 ✓5ᵗʰ
  syndrome of childhood NEC (*see also* Psychosis, childhood) 299.9 ✓5ᵗʰ
  undifferentiated 295.9 ✓5ᵗʰ
    acute 295.8 ✓5ᵗʰ
    chronic 295.6 ✓5ᵗʰ

Schizothymia 301.20
  introverted 301.21
  schizotypal 301.22

Schlafkrankheit 086.5

Schlatter's tibia (osteochondrosis) 732.4

Schlatter-Osgood disease (osteochondrosis, tibial tubercle) 732.4

Schloffer's tumor (*see also* Peritonitis) 567.2

Schmidt's syndrome
  sphallo-pharyngo-laryngeal hemiplegia 352.6
  thyroid-adrenocortical insufficiency 258.1
  vagoaccessory 352.6

Schmincke
carcinoma (M8082/3) — *see* Neoplasm, nasopharynx, malignant
tumor (M8082/3) — *see* Neoplasm, nasopharynx, malignant
Schmitz (-Stutzer) dysentery 004.0
Schmorl's disease or nodes 722.30
lumbar, lumbosacral 722.32
specified region NEC 722.39
thoracic, thoracolumbar 722.31
Schneider's syndrome 047.9
Schneiderian
carcinoma (M8121/3)
specified site — *see* Neoplasm, by site, malignant
unspecified site 160.0
papilloma (M8121/0)
specified site — *see* Neoplasm, by site, benign
unspecified site 212.0
Schoffer's tumor (*see also* Peritonitis) 567.2
Scholte's syndrome (malignant carcinoid) 259.2
Scholz's disease 330.0
Scholz (-Bielschowsky-Henneberg) syndrome 330.0
Schönlein (-Henoch) disease (primary) (purpura) (rheumatic) 287.0
School examination V70.3
Schottmüller's disease (*see also* Fever, paratyphoid) 002.9
Schroeder's syndrome (endocrine-hypertensive) 255.3
Schüller-Christian disease or syndrome (chronic histiocytosis X) 277.8
Schultz's disease or syndrome (agranulocytosis) 288.0
Schultze's acroparesthesia, simple 443.89
Schwalbe-Ziehen-Oppenheimer disease 333.6
Schwannoma (M9560/0) — *see also* Neoplasm, connective tissue, benign
malignant (M9560/3) — *see* Neoplasm, connective tissue, malignant
Schwartz (-Jampel) syndrome 756.89
Schwartz-Bartter syndrome (inappropriate secretion of antidiuretic hormone) 253.6
Schweninger-Buzzi disease (macular atrophy) 701.3
Sciatic — *see* condition
Sciatica (infectional) 724.3
due to
displacement of intervertebral disc 722.10
herniation, nucleus pulposus 722.10
Scimitar syndrome (anomalous venous drainage, right lung to inferior vena cava) 747.49
Sclera — *see* condition
Sclerectasia 379.11
Scleredema
adultorum 710.1
Buschke's 710.1
newborn 778.1
Sclerema
adiposum (newborn) 778.1
adultorum 710.1
edematosum (newborn) 778.1
neonatorum 778.1
newborn 778.1
Scleriasis — *see* Scleroderma
Scleritis 379.00
with corneal involvement 379.05
anterior (annular) (localized) 379.03
brawny 379.06
granulomatous 379.09
posterior 379.07
specified NEC 379.09
suppurative 379.09
syphilitic 095.0
tuberculous (nodular) (*see also* Tuberculosis) 017.3 ☑5ᵗʰ [379.09]
Sclerochoroiditis (*see also* Scleritis) 379.00
Scleroconjunctivitis (*see also* Scleritis) 379.00
Sclerocystic ovary (syndrome) 256.4

Sclerodactylia 701.0
Scleroderma, sclerodermia (acrosclerotic) (diffuse) (generalized) (progressive) (pulmonary) 710.1
circumscribed 701.0
linear 701.0
localized (linear) 701.0
newborn 778.1
Sclerokeratitis 379.05
meaning sclerosing keratitis 370.54
tuberculous (*see also* Tuberculosis) 017.3 ☑5ᵗʰ [379.09]
Scleroma, trachea 040.1
Scleromalacia
multiple 731.0
perforans 379.04
Scleromyxedema 701.8
Scleroperikeratitis 379.05
Sclerose en plaques 340
Sclerosis, sclerotic
adrenal (gland) 255.8
Alzheimer's 331.0
with dementia — *see* Alzheimer's, dementia
amyotrophic (lateral) 335.20
annularis fibrosi
aortic 424.1
mitral 424.0
aorta, aortic 440.0
valve (*see also* Endocarditis, aortic) 424.1
artery, arterial, arteriolar, arteriovascular — *see* Arteriosclerosis
ascending multiple 340
Baló's (concentric) 341.1
basilar — *see* Sclerosis, brain
bone (localized) NEC 733.99
brain (general) (lobular) 341.9
Alzheimer's — *see* Alzheimer's, dementia
artery, arterial 437.0
atrophic lobar 331.0
with dementia
with behavioral disturbance 331.0 [294.11]
without behavioral disturbance 331.0 [294.10]
diffuse 341.1
familial (chronic) (infantile) 330.0
infantile (chronic) (familial) 330.0
Pelizaeus-Merzbacher type 330.0
disseminated 340
hereditary 334.2
infantile, (degenerative) (diffuse) 330.0
insular 340
Krabbe's 330.0
miliary 340
multiple 340
Pelizaeus-Merzbacher 330.0
progressive familial 330.0
senile 437.0
tuberous 759.5
bulbar, progressive 340
bundle of His 426.50
left 426.3
right 426.4
cardiac — *see* Arteriosclerosis, coronary
cardiorenal (*see also* Hypertension, cardiorenal) 404.90
cardiovascular (*see also* Disease, cardiovascular) 429.2
renal (*see also* Hypertension, cardiorenal) 404.90
centrolobar, familial 330.0
cerebellar — *see* Sclerosis, brain
cerebral — *see* Sclerosis, brain
cerebrospinal 340
disseminated 340
multiple 340
cerebrovascular 437.0
choroid 363.40
diffuse 363.56
combined (spinal cord) — *see also* Degeneration, combined
multiple 340
concentric, Baló's 341.1
cornea 370.54
coronary (artery) — *see* Arteriosclerosis, coronary

Sclerosis, sclerotic — *continued*
corpus cavernosum
female 624.8
male 607.89
Dewitzky's
aortic 424.1
mitral 424.0
diffuse NEC 341.1
disease, heart — *see* Arteriosclerosis, coronary
disseminated 340
dorsal 340
dorsolateral (spinal cord) — *see* Degeneration, combined
endometrium 621.8
extrapyramidal 333.90
eye, nuclear (senile) 366.16
Friedreich's (spinal cord) 334.0
funicular (spermatic cord) 608.89
gastritis 535.4 ☑5ᵗʰ
general (vascular) — *see* Arteriosclerosis
gland (lymphatic) 457.8
hepatic 571.9
hereditary
cerebellar 334.2
spinal 334.0
idiopathic cortical (Garré's) (*see also* Osteomyelitis) 730.1 ☑5ᵗʰ
ilium, piriform 733.5
insular 340
pancreas 251.8
Islands of Langerhans 251.8
kidney — *see* Sclerosis, renal
larynx 478.79
lateral 335.24
amyotrophic 335.20
descending 335.24
primary 335.24
spinal 335.24
liver 571.9
lobar, atrophic (of brain) 331.0
with dementia
with behavioral disturbance 331.0 [294.11]
without behavioral disturbance 331.0 [294.10]
lung (*see also* Fibrosis, lung) 515
mastoid 383.1
mitral — *see* Endocarditis, mitral
Mönckeberg's (medial) (*see also* Arteriosclerosis, extremities) 440.20
multiple (brain stem) (cerebral) (generalized) (spinal cord) 340
myocardium, myocardial — *see* Arteriosclerosis, coronary
nuclear (senile), eye 366.16
ovary 620.8
pancreas 577.8
penis 607.89
peripheral arteries NEC (*see also* Arteriosclerosis, extremities) 440.20
plaques 340
pluriglandular 258.8
polyglandular 258.8
posterior (spinal cord) (syphilitic) 094.0
posterolateral (spinal cord) — *see* Degeneration, combined
prepuce 607.89
primary lateral 335.24
progressive systemic 710.1
pulmonary (*see also* Fibrosis, lung) 515
artery 416.0
valve (heart) (*see also* Endocarditis, pulmonary) 424.3
renal 587
with
cystine storage disease 270.0
hypertension (*see also* Hypertension, kidney) 403.90
hypertensive heart disease (conditions classifiable to 402) (*see also* Hypertension, cardiorenal) 404.90
arteriolar (hyaline) (*see also* Hypertension, kidney) 403.90
hyperplastic (*see also* Hypertension, kidney) 403.90
retina (senile) (vascular) 362.17
rheumatic
aortic valve 395.9

Sclerosis, sclerotic — *continued*
  rheumatic — *continued*
    mitral valve 394.9
  Schilder's 341.1
  senile — *see* Arteriosclerosis
  spinal (cord) (general) (progressive) (transverse)
      336.8
    ascending 357.0
    combined — *see also* Degeneration,
        combined
      multiple 340
      syphilitic 094.89
    disseminated 340
    dorsolateral — *see* Degeneration, combined
    hereditary (Friedreich's) (mixed form) 334.0
    lateral (amyotrophic) 335.24
    multiple 340
    posterior (syphilitic) 094.0
  stomach 537.89
  subendocardial, congenital 425.3
  systemic (progressive) 710.1
    with lung involvement 710.1 *[517.2]*
  tricuspid (heart) (valve) — *see* Endocarditis,
      tricuspid
  tuberous (brain) 759.5
  tympanic membrane (*see also*
      Tympanosclerosis) 385.00
  valve, valvular (heart) — *see* Endocarditis
  vascular — *see* Arteriosclerosis
  vein 459.89
Sclerotenonitis 379.07
Sclerotitis (*see also* Scleritis) 379.00
  syphilitic 095.0
  tuberculous (*see also* Tuberculosis)
      017.3 ✓5ᵗʰ *[379.09]*
Scoliosis (acquired) (postural) 737.30
  congenital 754.2
  due to or associated with
    Charcôt-Marie-Tooth disease 356.1 *[737.43]*
    mucopolysaccharidosis 277.5 *[737.43]*
    neurofibromatosis 237.71 *[737.43]*
    osteitis
      deformans 731.0 *[737.43]*
      fibrosa cystica 252.0 *[737.43]*
    osteoporosis (*see also* Osteoporosis) 733.00
        [737.43]
    poliomyelitis 138 *[737.43]*
    radiation 737.33
    tuberculosis (*see also* Tuberculosis)
        015.0 ✓5ᵗʰ *[737.43]*
  idiopathic 737.30
    infantile
      progressive 737.32
      resolving 737.31
  paralytic 737.39
  rachitic 268.1
  sciatic 724.3
  specified NEC 737.39
  thoracogenic 737.34
  tuberculous (*see also* Tuberculosis)
      015.0 ✓5ᵗʰ *[737.43]*
Scoliotic pelvis 738.6
  with disproportion (fetopelvic) 653.0 ✓5ᵗʰ
    affecting fetus or newborn 763.1
    causing obstructed labor 660.1 ✓5ᵗʰ
      affecting fetus or newborn 763.1
Scorbutus, scorbutic 267
  anemia 281.8
Scotoma (ring) 368.44
  arcuate 368.43
  Bjerrum 368.43
  blind spot area 368.42
  central 368.41
  centrocecal 368.41
  paracecal 368.42
  paracentral 368.41
  scintillating 368.12
  Seidel 368.43
Scratch — *see* Injury, superficial, by site
Screening (for) V82.9
  alcoholism V79.1
  anemia, deficiency NEC V78.1
    iron V78.0
  anomaly, congenital V82.89
  antenatal V28.9
    alphafetoprotein levels, raised V28.1

Screening (for) — *continued*
  antenatal — *continued*
    based on amniocentesis V28.2
      chromosomal anomalies V28.0
      raised alphafetoprotein levels V28.1
    fetal growth retardation using
        ultrasonics V28.4
    isoimmunization V28.5
    malformations using ultrasonics V28.3
    raised alphafetoprotein levels V28.1
    specified condition NEC V28.8
    Streptococcus B V28.6
  arterial hypertension V81.1
  arthropod-borne viral disease NEC V73.5
  asymptomatic bacteriuria V81.5
  bacterial
    conjunctivitis V74.4
    disease V74.9
      specified condition NEC V74.8
  bacteriuria, asymptomatic V81.5
  blood disorder NEC V78.9
    specified type NEC V78.8
  bronchitis, chronic V81.3
  brucellosis V74.8
  cancer — *see* Screening, malignant neoplasm
  cardiovascular disease NEC V81.2
  cataract V80.2
  Chagas' disease V75.3
  chemical poisoning V82.5
  cholera V74.0
  cholesterol level V77.91
  chromosomal
    anomalies
      by amniocentesis, antenatal V28.0
      maternal postnatal V82.4
    athletes V70.3
  condition
    cardiovascular NEC V81.2
    eye NEC V80.2
    genitourinary NEC V81.6
    neurological V80.0
    respiratory NEC V81.4
    skin V82.0
    specified NEC V82.89
  congenital
    anomaly V82.89
      eye V80.2
    dislocation of hip V82.3
    eye condition or disease V80.2
  conjunctivitis, bacterial V74.4
  contamination NEC (*see also* Poisoning) V82.5
  coronary artery disease V81.0
  cystic fibrosis V77.6
  deficiency anemia NEC V78.1
    iron V78.0
  dengue fever V73.5
  depression V79.0
  developmental handicap V79.9
    in early childhood V79.3
    specified type NEC V79.8
  diabetes mellitus V77.1
  diphtheria V74.3
  disease or disorder V82.9
    bacterial V74.9
      specified NEC V74.8
    blood V78.9
      specified type NEC V78.8
    blood-forming organ V78.9
      specified type NEC V78.8
    cardiovascular NEC V81.2
      hypertensive V81.1
      ischemic V81.0
    Chagas' V75.3
    chlamydial V73.98
      specified NEC V73.88
    ear NEC V80.3
    endocrine NEC V77.99
    eye NEC V80.2
    genitourinary NEC V81.6
    heart NEC V81.2
      hypertensive V81.1
      ischemic V81.0
    immunity NEC V77.99
    infectious NEC V75.9
    lipoid NEC V77.91
    mental V79.9
      specified type NEC V79.8

Screening (for) — *continued*
  disease or disorder — *continued*
    metabolic NEC V77.99
      inborn NEC V77.7
    neurological V80.0
    nutritional NEC V77.99
    rheumatic NEC V82.2
    rickettsial V75.0
    sickle-cell V78.2
      trait V78.2
    specified type NEC V82.89
    thyroid V77.0
    vascular NEC V81.2
      ischemic V81.0
    venereal V74.5
    viral V73.99
      arthropod-borne NEC V73.5
      specified type NEC V73.89
  dislocation of hip, congenital V82.3
  drugs in athletes V70.3
  emphysema (chronic) V81.3
  encephalitis, viral (mosquito or tick borne)
      V73.5
  endocrine disorder NEC V77.99
  eye disorder NEC V80.2
    congenital V80.2
  fever
    dengue V73.5
    hemorrhagic V73.5
    yellow V73.4
  filariasis V75.6
  galactosemia V77.4
  genitourinary condition NEC V81.6
  glaucoma V80.1
  gonorrhea V74.5
  gout V77.5
  Hansen's disease V74.2
  heart disease NEC V81.2
    hypertensive V81.1
    ischemic V81.0
  heavy metal poisoning V82.5
  heiminthiasis, intestinal V75.7
  hematopoietic malignancy V76.89
  hemoglobinopathies NEC V78.3
  hemorrhagic fever V73.5
  Hodgkin's disease V76.89
  hormones in athletes V70.3
  hypercholesterolemia V77.91
  hyperlipdemia V77.91
  hypertension V81.1
  immunity disorder NEC V77.99
  inborn errors of metabolism NEC V77.7
  infection
    bacterial V74.9
      specified type NEC V74.8
    mycotic V75.4
    parasitic NEC V75.8
  infectious disease V75.9
    specified type NEC V75.8
  ingestion of radioactive substance V82.5
  intestinal helminthiasis V75.7
  iron deficiency anemia V78.0
  ischemic heart disease V81.0
  lead poisoning V82.5
  leishmaniasis V75.2
  leprosy V74.2
  leptospirosis V74.8
  leukemia V76.89
  lipoid disorder NEC V77.91
  lymphoma V76.89
  malaria V75.1
  malignant neoplasm (of) V76.9
    bladder V76.3
    blood V76.89
    breast V76.10
      mammogram NEC V76.12
        for high-risk patient V76.11
      specified type NEC V76.19
    cervix V76.2
    colon V76.51
    colorectal V76.51
    hematopoietic system V76.89
    intestine V76.50
      colon V76.51
      small V76.52
    lymph (glands) V76.89
    nervous system V76.81

Screening (for) — *continued*
  malignant neoplasm (of) — *continued*
    oral cavity V76.42
    other specified neoplasm NEC V76.89
    ovary V76.46
    prostate V76.44
    rectum V76.41
    respiratory organs V76.0
    skin V76.43
    specified sites NEC V76.49
    testis V76.45
    vagina V76.47
      following hysterectomy for malignant
        condition V67.01
  maternal postnatal chromosomal anomalies
    V82.4
  malnutrition V77.2
  mammogram NEC V76.12
    for high-risk patient V76.11
  measles V73.2
  mental
    disorder V79.9
      specified type NEC V79.8
    retardation V79.2
  metabolic disorder NEC V77.99
  metabolic errors, inborn V77.7
  mucoviscidosis V77.6
  multiphasic V82.6
  mycosis V75.4
  mycotic infection V75.4
  nephropathy V81.5
  neurological condition V80.0
  nutritional disorder V77.99
  obesity V77.8
  osteoporosis V82.81
  parasitic infection NEC V75.8
  phenylketonuria V77.3
  plague V74.8
  poisoning
    chemical NEC V82.5
      contaminated water supply V82.5
        heavy metal V82.5
  poliomyelitis V73.0
  postnatal chromosomal anomalies, maternal
    V82.4
  prenatal — *see* Screening, antenatal
  pulmonary tuberculosis V74.1
  radiation exposure V82.5
  renal disease V81.5
  respiratory condition NEC V81.4
  rheumatic disorder NEC V82.2
  rheumatoid arthritis V82.1
  rickettsial disease V75.0
  rubella V73.3
  schistosomiasis V75.5
  senile macular lesions of eye V80.2
  sickle-cell anemia, disease, or trait V78.2
  skin condition V82.0
  sleeping sickness V75.3
  smallpox V73.1
  special V82.9
    specified condition NEC V82.89
  specified type NEC V82.89
  spirochetal disease V74.9
    specified type NEC V74.8
  stimulants in athletes V70.3
  syphilis V74.5
  tetanus V74.8
  thyroid disorder V77.0
  trachoma V73.6
  trypanosomiasis V75.3
  tuberculosis, pulmonary V74.1
  venereal disease V74.5
  viral encephalitis
    mosquito-borne V73.5
    tick-borne V73.5
  whooping cough V74.8
  worms, intestinal V75.7
  yaws V74.6
  yellow fever V73.4
Scrofula (*see also* Tuberculosis) 017.2 ✓5ᵗʰ
Scrofulide (primary) (*see also* Tuberculosis)
  017.0 ✓5ᵗʰ
Scrofuloderma, scrofulodermia (any site)
  (primary) (*see also* Tuberculosis) 017.0 ✓5ᵗʰ
Scrofulosis (universal) (*see also* Tuberculosis)
  017.2 ✓5ᵗʰ

Scrofulosis lichen (primary) (*see also*
  Tuberculosis) 017.0 ✓5ᵗʰ
Scrofulous — *see* condition
Scrotal tongue 529.5
  congenital 750.13
Scrotum — *see* condition
Scurvy (gum) (infantile) (rickets) (scorbutic) 267
Sea-blue histiocyte syndrome 272.7
Seabright-Bantam syndrome
  (pseudohypoparathyroidism) 275.49
Seasickness 994.6
Seatworm 127.4
Sebaceous
  cyst (*see also* Cyst, sebaceous) 706.2
  gland disease NEC 706.9
Sebocystomatosis 706.2
Seborrhea, seborrheic 706.3
  adiposa 706.3
  capitis 690.11
  congestiva 695.4
  corporis 706.3
  dermatitis 690.10
    infantile 690.12
  diathesis in infants 695.89
  eczema 690.18
    infantile 691.12 ✓5ᵗʰ
  keratosis 702.19
    inflamed 702.11
  nigricans 705.89
  sicca 690.18
  wart 702.19
    inflamed 702.11
Seckel's syndrome 759.89
Seclusion pupil 364.74
Seclusiveness, child 313.22
Secondary — *see also* condition
  neoplasm — *see* Neoplasm, by site, malignant,
    secondary
Secretan's disease or syndrome (posttraumatic
  edema) 782.3
Secretion
  antidiuretic hormone, inappropriate (syndrome)
    253.6
  catecholamine, by pheochromocytoma 255.6
  hormone
    antidiuretic, inappropriate (syndrome) 253.6
    by
      carcinoid tumor 259.2
      pheochromocytoma 255.6
    ectopic NEC 259.3
  urinary
    excessive 788.42
    suppression 788.5
Section
  cesarean
    affecting fetus or newborn 763.4
    post mortem, affecting fetus or newborn
      761.6
    previous, in pregnancy or childbirth
      654.2 ✓5ᵗʰ
      affecting fetus or newborn 763.89
  nerve, traumatic — *see* Injury, nerve, by site
Seeligmann's syndrome (ichthyosis congenita)
  757.1
Segmentation, incomplete (congenital) — *see
  also* Fusion
  bone NEC 756.9
  lumbosacral (joint) 756.15
  vertebra 756.15
    lumbosacral 756.15
Seizure 780.39
  akinetic (idiopathic) (*see also* Epilepsy)
    345.0 ✓5ᵗʰ
    psychomotor 345.4 ✓5ᵗʰ
  apoplexy, apoplectic (*see also* Disease,
    cerebrovascular, acute) 436
  atonic (*see also* Epilepsy) 345.0 ✓5ᵗʰ
  autonomic 300.11
  brain or cerebral (*see also* Disease,
    cerebrovascular, acute) 436
  convulsive (*see also* Convulsions) 780.39
  cortical (focal) (motor) (*see also* Epilepsy)
    345.5 ✓5ᵗʰ

Seizure — *continued*
  epilepsy, epileptic (cryptogenic) (*see also*
    Epilepsy) 345.9 ✓5ᵗʰ
  epileptiform, epileptoid 780.39
    focal (*see also* Epilepsy) 345.5 ✓5ᵗʰ
  febrile 780.31
  heart — *see* Disease, heart
  hysterical 300.11
  Jacksonian (focal) (*see also* Epilepsy) 345.5 ✓5ᵗʰ
    motor type 345.5 ✓5ᵗʰ
    sensory type 345.5 ✓5ᵗʰ
  newborn 779.0
  paralysis (*see also* Disease, cerebrovascular,
    acute) 436
  recurrent 780.39
    epileptic — *see* Epilepsy
  repetitive 780.39
    epileptic — *see* Epilepsy
  salaam (*see also* Epilepsy) 345.6 ✓5ᵗʰ
  uncinate (*see also* Epilepsy) 345.4 ✓5ᵗʰ
Self-mutilation 300.9
Semicoma 780.09
Semiconsciousness 780.09
Seminal
  vesicle — *see* condition
  vesiculitis (*see also* Vesiculitis) 608.0
Seminoma (M9061/3)
  anaplastic type (M9062/3)
    specified site — *see* Neoplasm, by site,
      malignant
    unspecified site 186.9
  specified site — *see* Neoplasm, by site,
    malignant
  spermatocytic (M9063/3)
    specified site — *see* Neoplasm, by site,
      malignant
    unspecified site 186.9
  unspecified site 186.9
Semliki Forest encephalitis 062.8
Senear-Usher disease or syndrome (pemphigus
  erythematosus) 694.4
Senecio jacobae dermatitis 692.6
Senectus 797
Senescence 797
Senile (*see also* condition) 797
  cervix (atrophic) 622.8
  degenerative atrophy, skin 701.3
  endometrium (atrophic) 621.8
  fallopian tube (atrophic) 620.3
  heart (failure) 797
  lung 492.8
  ovary (atrophic) 620.3
  syndrome 259.8
  vagina, vaginitis (atrophic) 627.3
  wart 702.0
Senility 797
  with
    acute confusional state 290.3
    delirium 290.3
    mental changes 290.9
    psychosis NEC (*see also* Psychosis, senile)
      290.20
  premature (syndrome) 259.8
Sensation
  burning (*see also* Disturbance, sensation)
    782.0
    tongue 529.6
  choking 784.9
  loss of (*see also* Disturbance, sensation) 782.0
  prickling (*see also* Disturbance, sensation)
    782.0
  tingling (*see also* Disturbance, sensation) 782.0
Sense loss (touch) (*see also* Disturbance,
  sensation) 782.0
  smell 781.1
  taste 781.1
Sensibility disturbance NEC (cortical) (deep)
  (vibratory) (*see also* Disturbance, sensation)
  782.0
Sensitive dentine 521.8
Sensitiver Beziehungswahn 297.8
Sensitivity, sensitization — *see also* Allergy
  autoerythrocyte 287.2
  carotid sinus 337.0

Sensitivity, sensitization — *see also* Allergy —
 continued
  child (excessive) 313.21
  cold, autoimmune 283.0
  methemoglobin 289.7
  suxamethonium 289.8
  tuberculin, without clinical or radiological
   symptoms 795.5
Sensory
  extinction 781.8
  neglect 781.8
Separation
  acromioclavicular — *see* Dislocation,
   acromioclavicular
  anxiety, abnormal 309.21
  apophysis, traumatic — *see* Fracture, by site
  choroid 363.70
   hemorrhagic 363.72
   serous 363.71
  costochondral (simple) (traumatic) — *see*
   Dislocation, costochondral
  epiphysis, epiphyseal
   nontraumatic 732.9
    upper femoral 732.2
   traumatic — *see* Fracture, by site
  fracture — *see* Fracture, by site
  infundibulum cardiac from right ventricle by a
   partition 746.83
  joint (current) (traumatic) — *see* Dislocation, by
   site
  placenta (normally implanted) — *see* Placenta,
   separation
  pubic bone, obstetrical trauma 665.6 ☑5ᵗʰ
  retina, retinal (*see also* Detachment, retina)
   361.9
   layers 362.40
    sensory (*see also* Retinoschisis) 361.10
   pigment epithelium (exudative) 362.42
    hemorrhagic 362.43
  sternoclavicular (traumatic) — *see* Dislocation,
   sternoclavicular
  symphysis pubis, obstetrical trauma 665.6 ☑5ᵗʰ
  tracheal ring, incomplete (congenital) 748.3
Sepsis (generalized) (*see also* Septicemia) 038.9
  with
   abortion — *see* Abortion, by type, with
    sepsis
   ectopic pregnancy (*see also* categories
    633.0-633.9) 639.0
   molar pregnancy (*see also* categories 630-
    632) 639.0
  buccal 528.3
  complicating labor 659.3 ☑5ᵗʰ
  dental (pulpal origin) 522.4
  female genital organ NEC 614.9
  fetus (intrauterine) 771.81   ▲
  following
   abortion 639.0
   ectopic or molar pregnancy 639.0
   infusion, perfusion, or transfusion 999.3
  Friedländer's 038.49
  intraocular 360.00
  localized
   in operation wound 998.59
   skin (*see also* Abscess) 682.9
  malleus 024
  nadir 038.9
  newborn (organism unspecified) NEC 771.81▲
  oral 528.3
  puerperal, postpartum, childbirth (pelvic)
   670 ☑4ᵗʰ
  resulting from infusion, injection, transfusion,
   or vaccination 999.3
  severe 995.92   ●
  skin, localized (*see also* Abscess) 682.9
  umbilical (newborn) (organism unspecified)
   771.89   ▲
   tetanus 771.3
  urinary 599.0
Septate — *see also* Septum
Septic — *see also* condition
  adenoids 474.01
   and tonsils 474.02
  arm (with lymphangitis) 682.3
  embolus — *see* Embolism

Septic — *see also* condition — *continued*
  finger (with lymphangitis) 681.00
  foot (with lymphangitis) 682.7
  gallbladder (*see also* Cholecystitis) 575.8
  hand (with lymphangitis) 682.4
  joint (*see also* Arthritis, septic) 711.0 ☑5ᵗʰ
  kidney (*see also* Infection, kidney) 590.9
  leg (with lymphangitis) 682.6
  mouth 528.3
  nail 681.9
   finger 681.02
   toe 681.11
  shock (endotoxic) 785.59
  sore (*see also* Abscess) 682.9
   throat 034.0
    milk-borne 034.0
    streptococcal 034.0
  spleen (acute) 289.59
  teeth (pulpal origin) 522.4
  throat 034.0
  thrombus — *see* Thrombosis
  toe (with lymphangitis) 681.0 ☑5ᵗʰ
  tonsils 474.00
   and adenoids 474.02
  umbilical cord (newborn) (organism
   unspecified) 771.89   ▲
  uterus (*see also* Endometritis) 615.9
Septicemia, septicemic (generalized)
  (suppurative) 038.9
  with
   abortion — *see* Abortion, by type, with
    sepsis
   ectopic pregnancy (*see also* categories
    633.0-633.9) 639.0
   molar pregnancy (*see also* categories 630-
    632) 639.0
  Aerobacter aerogenes 038.49
  anaerobic 038.3
  anthrax 022.3
  Bacillus coli 038.42
  Bacteroides 038.3
  Clostridium 038.3
  complicating labor 659.3 ☑5ᵗʰ
  cryptogenic 038.9
  enteric gram-negative bacilli 038.40
  Enterobacter aerogenes 038.49
  Erysipelothrix (insidiosa) (rhusiopathiae) 027.1
  Escherichia coli 038.42
  following
   abortion 639.0
   ectopic or molar pregnancy 639.0
   infusion, injection, transfusion, or
    vaccination 999.3
  Friedländer's (bacillus) 038.49
  gangrenous 038.9
  gonococcal 098.89
  gram-negative (organism) 038.40
   anaerobic 038.3
  Hemophilus influenzae 038.41
  herpes (simplex) 054.5
  herpetic 054.5
  Listeria monocytogenes 027.0
  meningeal — *see* Meningitis
  meningococcal (chronic) (fulminating) 036.2
  navel, newborn (organism unspecified)
   771.89   ▲
  newborn (organism unspecified) 771.81   ▲
  plague 020.2
  pneumococcal 038.2
  postabortal 639.0
  postoperative 998.59
  Proteus vulgaris 038.49
  Pseudomonas (aeruginosa) 038.43
  puerperal, postpartum 670 ☑4ᵗʰ
  Salmonella (aertrycke) (callinarum)
   (choleraesuis) (enteritidis) (suipestifer)
   003.1
  Serratia 038.44
  Shigella (*see also* Dysentery, bacillary) 004.9
  specified organism NEC 038.8
  staphylococcal 038.10
   aureus 038.11
   specified organism NEC 038.19
  streptococcal (anaerobic) 038.0
  suipestifer 003.1

Septicemia, septicemic — *continued*
  umbilicus, newborn (organism unspecified)
   771.89   ▲
  viral 079.99
  Yersinia enterocolitica 038.49
Septum, septate (congenital) — *see also*
  Anomaly, specified type NEC
  anal 751.2
  aqueduct of Sylvius 742.3
   with spina bifida (*see also* Spina bifida)
    741.0 ☑5ᵗʰ
  hymen 752.49
  uterus (*see also* Double, uterus) 752.2
  vagina 752.49
   in pregnancy or childbirth 654.7 ☑5ᵗʰ
    affecting fetus or newborn 763.89
    causing obstructed labor 660.2 ☑5ᵗʰ
     affecting fetus or newborn 763.1
Sequestration
  lung (congenital) (extralobar) (intralobar) 748.5
  orbit 376.10
  pulmonary artery (congenital) 747.3
Sequestrum
  bone (*see also* Osteomyelitis) 730.1 ☑5ᵗʰ
   jaw 526.4
  dental 525.8
  jaw bone 526.4
  sinus (accessory) (nasal) (*see also* Sinusitis) 473.9
   maxillary 473.0
Sequoiosis asthma 495.8
Serology for syphilis
  doubtful
   with signs or symptoms — *see* Syphilis, by
    site and stage
   follow-up of latent syphilis — *see* Syphilis,
    latent
  false positive 795.6
  negative, with signs or symptoms — *see*
   Syphilis, by site and stage
  positive 097.1
   with signs or symptoms — *see* Syphilis, by
    site and stage
   false 795.6
   follow-up of latent syphilis — *see* Syphilis,
    latent
   only finding — *see* Syphilis, latent
  reactivated 097.1
Seroma (postoperative) (non-infected) 998.13
  infected 998.51
Seropurulent — *see* condition
Serositis, multiple 569.89
  pericardial 423.2
  peritoneal 568.82
  pleural — *see* Pleurisy
Serotonin syndrome 333.99
Serous — *see* condition
Sertoli cell
  adenoma (M8640/0)
   specified site — *see* Neoplasm, by site,
    benign
   unspecified site
    female 220
    male 222.0
  carcinoma (M8640/3)
   specified site — *see* Neoplasm, by site,
    malignant
   unspecified site 186.9
  syndrome (germinal aplasia) 606.0
  tumor (M8640/0)
   with lipid storage (M8641/0)
    specified site — *see* Neoplasm, by site,
     benign
    unspecified site
     female 220
     male 222.0
   specified site — *see* Neoplasm, by site,
    benign
   unspecified site
    female 220
    male 222.0
Sertoli-Leydig cell tumor (M8631/0)
  specified site — *see* Neoplasm, by site, benign
  unspecified site
   female 220
   male 222.0

Serum
   allergy, allergic reaction 999.5
      shock 999.4
   arthritis 999.5 *[713.6]*
   complication or reaction NEC 999.5
   disease NEC 999.5
   hepatitis 070.3 ✓5ᵗʰ
   intoxication 999.5
   jaundice (homologous) — *see* Hepatitis, viral
   neuritis 999.5
   poisoning NEC 999.5
   rash NEC 999.5
   reaction NEC 999.5
   sickness NEC 999.5
Sesamoiditis 733.99
Seven-day fever 061
   of
      Japan 100.89
      Queensland 100.89
Sever's disease or osteochondrosis (calcaneum)
   732.5
Sex chromosome mosaics 758.81
Sextuplet
   affected by maternal complications of
      pregnancy 761.5
   healthy liveborn — *see* Newborn, multiple
   pregnancy (complicating delivery) NEC
      651.8 ✓5ᵗʰ
      with fetal loss and retention of one or more
         fetus(es) 651.6 ✓5ᵗʰ
Sexual
   anesthesia 302.72
   deviation (*see also* Deviation, sexual) 302.9
   disorder (*see also* Deviation, sexual) 302.9
   frigidity (female) 302.72
   function, disorder of (psychogenic) 302.70
      specified type NEC 302.79
   immaturity (female) (male) 259.0
   impotence (psychogenic) 302.72
      organic origin NEC 607.84
   precocity (constitutional) (cryptogenic) (female)
      (idiopathic) (male) NEC 259.1
      with adrenal hyperplasia 255.2
   sadism 302.84
Sexuality, pathological (*see also* Deviation,
   sexual) 302.9
Sézary's disease, reticulosis, or syndrome
   (M9701/3) 202.2 ✓5ᵗʰ
Shadow, lung 793.1
Shaken infant syndrome 995.55
Shaking
   head (tremor) 781.0
   palsy or paralysis (*see also* Parkinsonism)
      332.0
Shallowness, acetabulum 736.39
Shaver's disease or syndrome (bauxite
   pneumoconiosis) 503
Shearing
   artificial skin graft 996.55
   decellularized allodermis graft 996.55
Sheath (tendon) — *see* condition
Shedding
   nail 703.8
   teeth, premature, primary (deciduous) 520.6
Sheehan's disease or syndrome (postpartum
   pituitary necrosis) 253.2
Shelf, rectal 569.49
Shell
   shock (current) (*see also* Reaction, stress,
      acute) 308.9
      lasting state 300.16
   teeth 520.5
Shield kidney 753.3
Shift, mediastinal 793.2
Shifting
   pacemaker 427.89
   sleep-work schedule (affecting sleep) 307.45
Shiga's
   bacillus 004.0
   dysentery 004.0
Shigella (dysentery) (*see also* Dysentery, bacillary)
   004.9
   carrier (suspected) of V02.3

Shigellosis (*see also* Dysentery, bacillary) 004.9
Shingles (*see also* Herpes, zoster) 053.9
   eye NEC 053.29
Shin splints 844.9
Shipyard eye or disease 077.1
Shirodkar suture, in pregnancy 654.5 ✓5ᵗʰ
Shock 785.50
   with
      abortion — *see* Abortion, by type, with
         shock
      ectopic pregnancy (*see also* categories
         633.0-633.9) 639.5
      molar pregnancy (*see also* categories 630-
         632) 639.5
   allergic — *see* Shock, anaphylactic
   anaclitic 309.21
   anaphylactic 995.0
      chemical — *see* Table of Drugs and
         Chemicals
      correct medicinal substance properly
         administered 995.0
      drug or medicinal substance
         correct substance properly administered
            995.0
         overdose or wrong substance given or
            taken 977.9
            specified drug — *see* Table of Drugs
               and Chemicals
      following sting(s) 989.5
      food — *see* Anaphylactic shock, due to, food
      immunization 999.4
      serum 999.4
   anaphylactoid — *see* Shock, anaphylactic
   anesthetic
      correct substance properly administered
         995.4
      overdose or wrong substance given 968.4
         specified anesthetic — *see* Table of Drugs
            and Chemicals
   birth, fetus or newborn NEC 779.89 ▲
   cardiogenic 785.51
   chemical substance — *see* Table of Drugs and
      Chemicals
   circulatory 785.59
   complicating
      abortion — *see* Abortion, by type, with
         shock
      ectopic pregnancy (*see also* categories
         633.0-633.9) 639.5
      labor and delivery 669.1 ✓5ᵗʰ
      molar pregnancy (*see also* categories 630-
         632) 639.5
   culture 309.29
   due to
      drug 995.0
         correct substance properly administered
            995.0
         overdose or wrong substance given or
            taken 977.9
            specified drug — *see* Table of Drugs
               and Chemicals
      food — *see* Anaphylactic shock, due to, food
   during labor and delivery 669.1 ✓5ᵗʰ
   electric 994.8
   endotoxic 785.59
      due to surgical procedure 998.0
   following
      abortion 639.5
      ectopic or molar pregnancy 639.5
      injury (immediate) (delayed) 958.4
      labor and delivery 669.1 ✓5ᵗʰ
   gram-negative 785.59
   hematogenic 785.59
   hemorrhagic
      due to
         disease 785.59
         surgery (intraoperative) (postoperative)
            998.0
         trauma 958.4
   hypovolemic NEC 785.59
      surgical 998.0
      traumatic 958.4
   insulin 251.0
      therapeutic misadventure 962.3
   kidney 584.5
   traumatic (following crushing) 958.5

Shock — *continued*
   lightning 994.0
   lung 518.5
   nervous (*see also* Reaction, stress, acute) 308.9
   obstetric 669.1 ✓5ᵗʰ
      with
         abortion — *see* Abortion, by type, with
            shock
         ectopic pregnancy (*see also* categories
            633.0-633.9) 639.5
         molar pregnancy (*see also* categories 630-
            632) 639.5
      following
         abortion 639.5
         ectopic or molar pregnancy 639.5
   paralysis, paralytic (*see also* Disease,
      cerebrovascular, acute) 436
      late effect — *see* Late effect(s) (of)
         cerebrovascular disease
   pleural (surgical) 998.0
      due to trauma 958.4
   postoperative 998.0
      with
         abortion — *see* Abortion, by type, with
            shock
         ectopic pregnancy (*see also* categories
            633.0-633.9) 639.5
         molar pregnancy (*see also* categories 630-
            632) 639.5
      following
         abortion 639.5
         ectopic or molar pregnancy 639.5
   psychic (*see also* Reaction, stress, acute) 308.9
      past history (of) V15.49
   psychogenic (*see also* Reaction, stress, acute)
      308.9
   septic 785.59
      with
         abortion — *see* Abortion, by type, with
            shock
         ectopic pregnancy (categories 633.0-
            633.9) 639.5
         molar pregnancy (*see also* categories 630-
            632) 639.5
      due to
         surgical procedure 998.0
         transfusion NEC 999.8
            bone marrow 996.85
      following
         abortion 639.5
         ectopic or molar pregnancy 639.5
         surgical procedure 998.0
         transfusion NEC 999.8
            bone marrow 996.85
   spinal — *see also* Injury, spinal, by site
      with spinal bone injury — *see* Fracture,
         vertebra, by site, with spinal cord
         injury
   surgical 998.0
   therapeutic misadventure NEC (*see also*
      Complications) 998.89
   thyroxin 962.7
   toxic 040.82 ▲
   transfusion — *see* Complications, transfusion
   traumatic (immediate) (delayed) 958.4
Shoemakers' chest 738.3
Short, shortening, shortness
   Achilles tendon (acquired) 727.81
   arm 736.89
      congenital 755.20
   back 737.9
   bowel syndrome 579.3
   breath 786.05
   common bile duct, congenital 751.69
   cord (umbilical) 663.4 ✓5ᵗʰ
      affecting fetus or newborn 762.6
   cystic duct, congenital 751.69
   esophagus (congenital) 750.4
   femur (acquired) 736.81
      congenital 755.34
   frenulum linguae 750.0
   frenum, lingual 750.0
   hamstrings 727.81
   hip (acquired) 736.39
      congenital 755.63
   leg (acquired) 736.81
      congenital 755.30

Short, shortening, shortness — *continued*
  metatarsus (congenital) 754.79
    acquired 736.79
  organ or site, congenital NEC — *see* Distortion
  palate (congenital) 750.26
  P-R interval syndrome 426.81
  radius (acquired) 736.09
    congenital 755.26
  round ligament 629.8
  sleeper 307.49
  stature, constitutional (hereditary) 783.43
  tendon 727.81
    Achilles (acquired) 727.81
      congenital 754.79
    congenital 756.89
  thigh (acquired) 736.81
    congenital 755.34
  tibialis anticus 727.81
  umbilical cord 663.4 ✓5ᵗʰ
    affecting fetus or newborn 762.6
  urethra 599.84
  uvula (congenital) 750.26
  vagina 623.8
Shortsightedness 367.1
Shoshin (acute fulminating beriberi) 265.0
Shoulder — *see* condition
Shovel-shaped incisors 520.2
Shower, thromboembolic — *see* Embolism
Shunt (status)
  aortocoronary bypass V45.81
  arterial-venous (dialysis) V45.1
  arteriovenous, pulmonary (acquired) 417.0
    congenital 747.3
    traumatic (complication) 901.40
  cerebral ventricle (communicating) in situ
    V45.2
  coronary artery bypass V45.81
  surgical, prosthetic, with complications — *see*
    Complications, shunt
  vascular NEC V45.89
Shutdown
  renal 586
    with
      abortion — *see* Abortion, by type, with
        renal failure
      ectopic pregnancy (*see also* categories
        633.0-633.9) 639.3
      molar pregnancy (*see also* categories 630-
        632) 639.3
    complicating
      abortion 639.3
      ectopic or molar pregnancy 639.3
    following labor and delivery 669.3 ✓5ᵗʰ
Shwachman's syndrome 288.0
Shy-Drager syndrome (orthostatic hypotension
  with multisystem degeneration) 333.0
Sialadenitis (any gland) (chronic) (suppurative)
  527.2
  epidemic — *see* Mumps
Sialadenosis, periodic 527.2
Sialaporia 527.7
Sialectasia 527.8
Sialitis 527.2
Sialoadenitis (*see also* Sialadenitis) 527.2
Sioloangitis 527.2
Sialodochitis (fibrinosa) 527.2
Sialodocholithiasis 527.5
Sialolithiasis 527.5
Sialorrhea (*see also* Ptyalism) 527.7
  periodic 527.2
Sialosis 527.8
  rheumatic 710.2
Siamese twin 759.4
Sicard's syndrome 352.6
Sicca syndrome (keratoconjunctivitis) 710.2
Sick 799.9
  cilia syndrome 759.89
  or handicapped person in family V61.49
Sickle-cell
  anemia (see also Disease, sickle-cell) 282.60
  disease (see also Disease, sickle-cell) 282.60

Sickle-cell — *continued*
  hemoglobin
    C disease 282.63
    D disease 282.69
    E disease 282.69
  thalassemia 282.4
  trait 282.5
Sicklemia (*see also* Disease, sickle-cell) 282.60
  trait 282.5
Sickness
  air (travel) 994.6
  airplane 994.6
  alpine 993.2
  altitude 993.2
  Andes 993.2
  aviators' 993.2
  balloon 993.2
  car 994.6
  compressed air 993.3
  decompression 993.3
  green 280.9
  harvest 100.89
  milk 988.8
  morning 643.0 ✓5ᵗʰ
  motion 994.6
  mountain 993.2
    acute 289.0
  protein (*see also* Complications, vaccination)
    999.5
  radiation NEC 990
  roundabout (motion) 994.6
  sea 994.6
  serum NEC 999.5
  sleeping (African) 086.5
    by Trypanosoma 086.5
      gambiense 086.3
      rhodesiense 086.4
    Gambian 086.3
    late effect 139.8
    Rhodesian 086.4
  sweating 078.2
  swing (motion) 994.6
  train (railway) (travel) 994.6
  travel (any vehicle) 994.6
Sick sinus syndrome 427.81
Sideropenia (*see also* Anemia, iron deficiency)
  280.9
Siderosis (lung) (occupational) 503
  cornea 371.15
  eye (bulbi) (vitreous) 360.23
  lens 360.23
Siegal-Cattan-Mamou disease (periodic) 277.3
Siemens' syndrome
  ectodermal dysplasia 757.31
  keratosis follicularis spinulosa (decalvans)
    757.39
Sighing respiration 786.7
Sigmoid
  flexure — *see* condition
  kidney 753.3
Sigmoiditis — *see* Enteritis
Silfverskiöld's syndrome 756.5 ✓5ᵗʰ
Silicosis, silicotic (complicated) (occupational)
  (simple) 502
  fibrosis, lung (confluent) (massive)
    (occupational) 502
  non-nodular 503
  pulmonum 502
Silicotuberculosis (*see also* Tuberculosis)
  011.4 ✓5ᵗʰ
Silo fillers' disease 506.9
Silver's syndrome (congenital hemihypertrophy
  and short stature) 759.89
Silver wire arteries, retina 362.13
Silvestroni-Bianco syndrome (thalassemia
  minima) 282.4
Simian crease 757.2
Simmonds' cachexia or disease (pituitary
  cachexia) 253.2
Simons' disease or syndrome (progressive
  lipodystrophy) 272.6
Simple, simplex — *see* condition

Sinding-Larsen disease (juvenile osteopathia
  patellae) 732.4
Singapore hemorrhagic fever 065.4
Singers' node or nodule 478.5
Single
  atrium 745.69
  coronary artery 746.85
  umbilical artery 747.5
  ventricle 745.3
Singultus 786.8
  epidemicus 078.89
Sinus — *see also* Fistula
  abdominal 569.81
  arrest 426.6
  arrhythmia 427.89
  bradycardia 427.89
    chronic 427.81
  branchial cleft (external) (internal) 744.41
  coccygeal (infected) 685.1
    with abscess 685.0
  dental 522.7
  dermal (congenital) 685.1
    with abscess 685.0
  draining — *see* Fistula
  infected, skin NEC 686.9
  marginal, ruptured or bleeding 641.2 ✓5ᵗʰ
    affecting fetus or newborn 762.1
  pause 426.6
  pericranii 742.0
  pilonidal (infected) (rectum) 685.1
    with abscess 685.0
  preauricular 744.46
  rectovaginal 619.1
  sacrococcygeal (dermoid) (infected) 685.1
    with abscess 685.0
  skin
    infected NEC 686.9
    noninfected — *see* Ulcer, skin
  tachycardia 427.89
  tarsi syndrome 726.79
  testis 608.89
  tract (postinfectional) — *see* Fistula
  urachus 753.7
Sinuses, Rokitansky-Aschoff (*see also* Disease,
  gallbladder) 575.8
Sinusitis (accessory) (nasal) (hyperplastic)
  (nonpurulent) (purulent) (chronic) 473.9
  with influenza, flu, or grippe 487.1
  acute 461.9
    ethmoidal 461.2
    frontal 461.1
    maxillary 461.0
    specified type NEC 461.8
    sphenoidal 461.3
  allergic (*see also* Fever, hay) 477.9
  antrum — *see* Sinusitis, maxillary
  due to
    fungus, any sinus 117.9
    high altitude 993.1
  ethmoidal 473.2
    acute 461.2
  frontal 473.1
    acute 461.1
  influenzal 478.1
  maxillary 473.0
    acute 461.0
  specified site NEC 473.8
  sphenoidal 473.3
    acute 461.3
  syphilitic, any sinus 095.8
  tuberculous, any sinus (*see also* Tuberculosis)
    012.8 ✓5ᵗʰ
Sinusitis-bronchiectasis-situs inversus
  (syndrome) (triad) 759.3
Sipple's syndrome (medullary thyroid carcinoma-
  pheochromocytoma) 193
Sirenomelia 759.89
Siriasis 992.0
Sirkari's disease 085.0
SIRS (systemic inflammatory response ●
  syndrome) 995.90 ●
  due to ●
    infectious process 995.91 ●
      with organ dysfunction 995.92 ●
    non-infectious process 995.93 ●
      with organ dysfunction 995.94 ●

Siti 104.0
Sitophobia 300.29
Situation, psychiatric 300.9
Situational
  disturbance (transient) (*see also* Reaction, adjustment) 309.9
    acute 308.3
  maladjustment, acute (*see also* Reaction, adjustment) 309.9
  reaction (*see also* Reaction, adjustment) 309.9
    acute 308.3
Situs inversus or transversus 759.3
  abdominalis 759.3
  thoracis 759.3
Sixth disease 057.8
Sjögren (-Gougerot) syndrome or disease (keratoconjunctivitis sicca) 710.2
  with lung involvement 710.2 *[517.8]*
Sjögren-Larsson syndrome (ichthyosis congenita) 757.1
Skeletal — *see* condition
Skene's gland — *see* condition
Skenitis (*see also* Urethritis) 597.89
  gonorrheal (acute) 098.0
    chronic or duration of 2 months or over 098.2
Skerljevo 104.0
Skevas-Zerfus disease 989.5
Skin — *see also* condition
  donor V59.1
  hidebound 710.9
SLAP lesion (superior glenoid labrum) 840.7
Slate-dressers' lung 502
Slate-miners' lung 502
Sleep
  disorder 780.50
    with apnea — *see* Apnea, sleep
    child 307.40
    nonorganic origin 307.40
      specified type NEC 307.49
  disturbance 780.50
    with apnea — *see* Apnea, sleep
    nonorganic origin 307.40
      specified type NEC 307.49
  drunkenness 307.47
  paroxysmal 347
  rhythm inversion 780.55
    nonorganic origin 307.45
  walking 307.46
    hysterical 300.13
Sleeping sickness 086.5
  late effect 139.8
Sleeplessness (*see also* Insomnia) 780.52
  menopausal 627.2
  nonorganic origin 307.41
Slipped, slipping
  epiphysis (postinfectional) 732.9
    traumatic (old) 732.9
      current — *see* Fracture, by site
    upper femoral (nontraumatic) 732.2
  intervertebral disc — *see* Displacement, intervertebral disc
  ligature, umbilical 772.3
  patella 717.89
  rib 733.99
  sacroiliac joint 724.6
  tendon 727.9
  ulnar nerve, nontraumatic 354.2
  vertebra NEC (*see also* Spondylolisthesis) 756.12
Slocumb's syndrome 255.3
Sloughing (multiple) (skin) 686.9
  abscess — *see* Abscess, by site
  appendix 543.9
  bladder 596.8
  fascia 728.9
  graft — *see* Complications, graft
  phagedena (*see also* Gangrene) 785.4
  reattached extremity (*see also* Complications, reattached extremity) 996.90
  rectum 569.49
  scrotum 608.89
  tendon 727.9

Sloughing — *continued*
  transplanted organ (*see also* Rejection, transplant, organ, by site) 996.80
  ulcer (*see also* Ulcer, skin) 707.9
Slow
  feeding newborn 779.3
  fetal, growth NEC 764.9 ✓5ᵗʰ
    affecting management of pregnancy 656.5 ✓5ᵗʰ
Slowing
  heart 427.89
  urinary stream 788.62
Sluder's neuralgia or syndrome 337.0
Slurred, slurring, speech 784.5
Small, smallness
  cardiac reserve — *see* Disease, heart
  for dates
    fetus or newborn 764.0 ✓5ᵗʰ
      with malnutrition 764.1 ✓5ᵗʰ
      affecting management of pregnancy 656.5 ✓5ᵗʰ
    infant, term 764.0 ✓5ᵗʰ
      with malnutrition 764.1 ✓5ᵗʰ
      affecting management of pregnancy 656.5 ✓5ᵗʰ
  introitus, vagina 623.3
  kidney, unknown cause 589.9
    bilateral 589.1
    unilateral 589.0
  ovary 620.8
  pelvis
    with disproportion (fetopelvic) 653.1 ✓5ᵗʰ
      affecting fetus or newborn 763.1
    causing obstructed labor 660.1 ✓5ᵗʰ
      affecting fetus or newborn 763.1
  placenta — *see* Placenta, insufficiency
  uterus 621.8
  white kidney 582.9
Small-for-dates (*see also* Light-for-dates) 764.0 ✓5ᵗʰ
  affecting management of pregnancy 656.5 ✓5ᵗʰ
Smallpox 050.9
  contact V01.3
  exposure to V01.3
  hemorrhagic (pustular) 050.0
  malignant 050.0
  modified 050.2
  vaccination
    complications — *see* Complications, vaccination
    prophylactic (against) V04.1
Smith's fracture (separation) (closed) 813.41
  open 813.51
Smith-Lemli Opitz syndrome (cerebrohepatorenal syndrome) 759.89
Smith-Strang disease (oasthouse urine) 270.2
Smokers'
  bronchitis 491.0
  cough 491.0
  syndrome (*see also* Abuse, drugs, nondependent) 305.1
  throat 472.1
  tongue 528.6
Smothering spells 786.09
Snaggle teeth, tooth 524.3
Snapping
  finger 727.05
  hip 719.65
  jaw 524.69
  knee 717.9
  thumb 727.05
Sneddon-Wilkinson disease or syndrome (subcorneal pustular dermatosis) 694.1
Sneezing 784.9
  intractable 478.1
Sniffing
  cocaine (*see also* Dependence) 304.2 ✓5ᵗʰ
  ether (*see also* Dependence) 304.6 ✓5ᵗʰ
  glue (airplane) (*see also* Dependence) 304.6 ✓5ᵗʰ
Snoring 786.09
Snow blindness 370.24
Snuffles (nonsyphilitic) 460
  syphilitic (infant) 090.0

Social migrant V60.0
Sodoku 026.0
Soemmering's ring 366.51
Soft — *see also* condition
  enlarged prostate 600.0
  nails 703.8
Softening
  bone 268.2
  brain (necrotic) (progressive) 434.9 ✓5ᵗʰ
    arteriosclerotic 437.0
    congenital 742.4
    embolic (*see also* Embolism, brain) 434.1 ✓5ᵗʰ
    hemorrhagic (*see also* Hemorrhage, brain) 431
    occlusive 434.9 ✓5ᵗʰ
    thrombotic (*see also* Thrombosis, brain) 434.0 ✓5ᵗʰ
  cartilage 733.92
  cerebellar — *see* Softening, brain
  cerebral — *see* Softening, brain
  cerebrospinal — *see* Softening, brain
  myocardial, heart (*see also* Degeneration, myocardial) 429.1
  nails 703.8
  spinal cord 336.8
  stomach 537.89
Solar fever 061
Soldier's
  heart 306.2
  patches 423.1
Solitary
  cyst
    bone 733.21
    kidney 593.2
  kidney (congenital) 753.0
  tubercle, brain (*see also* Tuberculosis, brain) 013.2 ✓5ᵗʰ
  ulcer, bladder 596.8
Somatization reaction, somatic reaction (*see also* Disorder, psychosomatic) 306.9
  disorder 300.81
Somatoform disorder 300.82
  atypical 300.82
  severe 300.81
  undifferentiated 300.82
Somnambulism 307.46
  hysterical 300.13
Somnolence 780.09
  nonorganic origin 307.43
  periodic 349.89
Sonne dysentery 004.3
Soor 112.0
Sore
  Delhi 085.1
  desert (*see also* Ulcer, skin) 707.9
  eye 379.99
  Lahore 085.1
  mouth 528.9
    canker 528.2
    due to dentures 528.9
  muscle 729.1
  Naga (*see also* Ulcer, skin) 707.9
  oriental 085.1
  pressure 707.0
    with gangrene 707.0 *[785.4]*
  skin NEC 709.9
  soft 099.0
  throat 462
    with influenza, flu, or grippe 487.1
    acute 462
    chronic 472.1
    clergyman's 784.49
    coxsackie (virus) 074.0
    diphtheritic 032.0
    epidemic 034.0
    gangrenous 462
    herpetic 054.79
    influenzal 487.1
    malignant 462
    purulent 462
    putrid 462
    septic 034.0
    streptococcal (ulcerative) 034.0
    ulcerated 462

✓4ᵗʰ Fourth-digit Required   ✓5ᵗʰ Fifth-digit Required   ►◄ Revised Text   ● New Line   ▲ Revised Code

Sore — _continued_
  throat — _continued_
    viral NEC 462
      Coxsackie 074.0
  tropical (_see also_ Ulcer, skin) 707.9
  veldt (_see also_ Ulcer, skin) 707.9
Sotos' syndrome (cerebral gigantism) 253.0
Sounds
  friction, pleural 786.7
  succussion, chest 786.7
South African cardiomyopathy syndrome 425.2
South American
  blastomycosis 116.1
  trypanosomiasis — _see_ Trypanosomiasis
Southeast Asian hemorrhagic fever 065.4
Spacing, teeth, abnormal 524.3
Spade-like hand (congenital) 754.89
Spading nail 703.8
  congenital 757.5
Spanemia 285.9
Spanish collar 605
Sparganosis 123.5
Spasm, spastic, spasticity (_see also_ condition)
  781.0
  accommodation 367.53
  ampulla of Vater (_see also_ Disease, gallbladder)
    576.8
  anus, ani (sphincter) (reflex) 564.6
    psychogenic 306.4
  artery NEC 443.9
    basilar 435.0
    carotid 435.8
    cerebral 435.9
      specified artery NEC 435.8
    retinal (_see also_ Occlusion, retinal, artery)
      362.30
    vertebral 435.1
    vertebrobasilar 435.3
  Bell's 351.0
  bladder (sphincter, external or internal) 596.8
  bowel 564.9
    psychogenic 306.4
  bronchus, bronchiole 519.1
  cardia 530.0
  cardiac — _see_ Angina
  carpopedal (_see also_ Tetany) 781.7
  cecum 564.9
    psychogenic 306.4
  cerebral (arteries) (vascular) 435.9
    specified artery NEC 435.8
  cerebrovascular 435.9
  cervix, complicating delivery 661.4 ✔5ᵗʰ
    affecting fetus or newborn 763.7
  ciliary body (of accommodation) 367.53
  colon 564.1
    psychogenic 306.4
  common duct (_see also_ Disease, biliary) 576.8
  compulsive 307.22
  conjugate 378.82
  convergence 378.84
  coronary (artery) — _see_ Angina
  diaphragm (reflex) 786.8
    psychogenic 306.1
  duodenum, duodenal (bulb) 564.89
  esophagus (diffuse) 530.5
    psychogenic 306.4
  facial 351.8
  fallopian tube 620.8
  gait 781.2
  gastrointestinal (tract) 536.8
    psychogenic 306.4
  glottis 478.75
    hysterical 300.11
    psychogenic 306.1
      specified as conversion reaction 300.11
    reflex through recurrent laryngeal nerve
      478.75
  habit 307.20
    chronic 307.22
    transient of childhood 307.21
  heart — _see_ Angina
  hourglass — _see_ Contraction, hourglass
  hysterical 300.11
  infantile (_see also_ Epilepsy) 345.6 ✔5ᵗʰ
  internal oblique, eye 378.51

Spasm, spastic, spasticity (_see also_ condition) —
  continued
  intestinal 564.9
    psychogenic 306.4
  larynx, laryngeal 478.75
    hysterical 300.11
    psychogenic 306.1
      specified as conversion reaction 300.11
  levator palpebrae superioris 333.81
  lightning (_see also_ Epilepsy) 345.6 ✔5ᵗʰ
  mobile 781.0
  muscle 728.85
    back 724.8
    psychogenic 306.0
  nerve, trigeminal 350.1
  nervous 306.0
  nodding 307.3
    infantile (_see also_ Epilepsy) 345.6 ✔5ᵗʰ
  occupational 300.89
  oculogyric 378.87
  ophthalmic artery 362.30
  orbicularis 781.0
  perineal 625.8
  peroneo-extensor (_see also_ Flat, foot) 734
  pharynx (reflex) 478.29
    hysterical 300.11
    psychogenic 306.1
      specified as conversion reaction 300.11
  pregnant uterus, complicating delivery
    661.4 ✔5ᵗʰ
  psychogenic 306.0
  pylorus 537.81
    adult hypertrophic 537.0
    congenital or infantile 750.5
    psychogenic 306.4
  rectum (sphincter) 564.6
    psychogenic 306.4
  retinal artery NEC (_see also_ Occlusion, retina,
    artery) 362.30
  sacroiliac 724.6
  salaam (infantile) (_see also_ Epilepsy) 345.6 ✔5ᵗʰ
  saltatory 781.0
  sigmoid 564.9
    psychogenic 306.4
  sphincter of Oddi (_see also_ Disease,
    gallbladder) 576.5
  stomach 536.8
    neurotic 306.4
  throat 478.29
    hysterical 300.11
    psychogenic 306.1
      specified as conversion reaction 300.11
  tic 307.20
    chronic 307.22
    transient of childhood 307.21
  tongue 529.8
  torsion 333.6
  trigeminal nerve 350.1
    postherpetic 053.12
  ureter 593.89
  urethra (sphincter) 599.84
  uterus 625.8
    complicating labor 661.4 ✔5ᵗʰ
      affecting fetus or newborn 763.7
  vagina 625.1
    psychogenic 306.51
  vascular NEC 443.9
  vasomotor NEC 443.9
  vein NEC 459.89
  vesical (sphincter, external or internal) 596.8
  viscera 789.0 ✔5ᵗʰ
Spasmodic — _see_ condition
Spasmophilia (_see also_ Tetany) 781.7
Spasmus nutans 307.3
Spastic — _see also_ Spasm
  child 343.9
Spasticity — _see also_ Spasm
  cerebral, child 343.9
Speakers' throat 784.49
Specific, specified — _see_ condition
Speech
  defect, disorder, disturbance, impediment NEC
    784.5
    psychogenic 307.9
  therapy V57.3

Spells 780.39
  breath-holding 786.9
Spencer's disease (epidemic vomiting) 078.82
Spens' syndrome (syncope with heart block)
  426.9
Spermatic cord — _see_ condition
Spermatocele 608.1
  congenital 752.8
Spermatocystitis 608.4
Spermatocytoma (M9063/3)
  specified site — _see_ Neoplasm, by site,
    malignant
  unspecified site 186.9
Spermatorrhea 608.89
Sperm counts
  fertility testing V26.21
  following sterilization reversal V26.22
  postvasectomy V25.8
Sphacelus (_see also_ Gangrene) 785.4
Sphenoidal — _see_ condition
Sphenoiditis (chronic) (_see also_ Sinusitis,
  sphenoidal) 473.3
Sphenopalatine ganglion neuralgia 337.0
Sphericity, increased, lens 743.36
Spherocytosis (congenital) (familial) (hereditary)
  282.0
  hemoglobin disease 282.7
  sickle-cell (disease) 282.60
Spherophakia 743.36
Sphincter — _see_ condition
Sphincteritis, sphincter of Oddi (_see also_
  Cholecystitis) 576.8
Sphingolipidosis 272.7
Sphingolipodystrophy 272.7
Sphingomyelinosis 272.7
Spicule tooth 520.2
Spider
  finger 755.59
  nevus 448.1
  vascular 448.1
Spiegler-Fendt sarcoid 686.8
Spielmeyer-Stock disease 330.1
Spielmeyer-Vogt disease 330.1
Spina bifida (aperta) 741.9 ✔5ᵗʰ

> Note — _Use the following fifth-digit_
> _subclassification with category 741:_
>
> 0   _unspecified region_
> 1   _cervical region_
> 2   _dorsal [thoracic] region_
> 3   _lumbar region_

  with hydrocephalus 741.0 ✔5ᵗʰ
    fetal (suspected), affecting management of
      pregnancy 655.0 ✔5ᵗʰ
  occulta 756.17
Spindle, Krukenberg's 371.13
Spine, spinal — _see_ condition
Spiradenoma (eccrine) (M8403/0) — _see_
  Neoplasm, skin, benign
Spirillosis NEC (_see also_ Fever, relapsing) 087.9
Spirillum minus 026.0
Spirillum obermeieri infection 087.0
Spirochetal — _see_ condition
Spirochetosis 104.9
  arthritic, arthritica 104.9 _[711.8]_ ✔5ᵗʰ
  bronchopulmonary 104.8
  icterohemorrhagica 100.0
  lung 104.8
Spitting blood (_see also_ Hemoptysis) 786.3
Splanchnomegaly 569.89
Splanchnoptosis 569.89
Spleen, splenic — _see also_ condition
  agenesis 759.0
  flexure syndrome 569.89
  neutropenia syndrome 288.0
  sequestration syndrome 282.60
Splenectasis (_see also_ Splenomegaly) 789.2

Sore — Splenectasis

Splenitis (interstitial) (malignant) (nonspecific) 289.59
  malarial (*see also* Malaria) 084.6
  tuberculous (*see also* Tuberculosis) 017.7 ✓5ᵗʰ
Splenocele 289.59
Splenomegalia — *see* Splenomegaly
Splenomegalic — *see* condition
Splenomegaly 789.2
  Bengal 789.2
  cirrhotic 289.51
  congenital 759.0
  congestive, chronic 289.51
  cryptogenic 789.2
  Egyptian 120.1
  Gaucher's (cerebroside lipidosis) 272.7
  idiopathic 789.2
  malarial (*see also* Malaria) 084.6
  neutropenic 288.0
  Niemann-Pick (lipid histiocytosis) 272.7
  siderotic 289.51
  syphilitic 095.8
    congenital 090.0
  tropical (Bengal) (idiopathic) 789.2
Splenopathy 289.50
Splenopneumonia — *see* Pneumonia
Splenoptosis 289.59
Splinter — *see* Injury, superficial, by site
Split, splitting
  heart sounds 427.89
  lip, congenital (*see also* Cleft, lip) 749.10
  nails 703.8
  urinary stream 788.61
Spoiled child reaction (*see also* Disturbance, conduct) 312.1 ✓5ᵗʰ
Spondylarthritis (*see also* Spondylosis) 721.90
Spondylarthrosis (*see also* Spondylosis) 721.90
Spondylitis 720.9
  ankylopoietica 720.0
  ankylosing (chronic) 720.0
  atrophic 720.9
    ligamentous 720.9
  chronic (traumatic) (*see also* Spondylosis) 721.90
  deformans (chronic) (*see also* Spondylosis) 721.90
  gonococcal 098.53
  gouty 274.0
  hypertrophic (*see also* Spondylosis) 721.90
  infectious NEC 720.9
  juvenile (adolescent) 720.0
  Kümmell's 721.7
  Marie-Strümpell (ankylosing) 720.0
  muscularis 720.9
  ossificans ligamentosa 721.6
  osteoarthritica (*see also* Spondylosis) 721.90
  posttraumatic 721.7
  proliferative 720.0
  rheumatoid 720.0
  rhizomelica 720.0
  sacroiliac NEC 720.2
  senescent (*see also* Spondylosis) 721.90
  senile (*see also* Spondylosis) 721.90
  static (*see also* Spondylosis) 721.90
  traumatic (chronic) (*see also* Spondylosis) 721.90
  tuberculous (*see also* Tuberculosis) 015.0 ✓5ᵗʰ [720.81]
  typhosa 002.0 [720.81]
Spondyloarthrosis (*see also* Spondylosis) 721.90
Spondylolisthesis (congenital) (lumbosacral) 756.12
  with disproportion (fetopelvic) 653.3 ✓5ᵗʰ
    affecting fetus or newborn 763.1
    causing obstructed labor 660.1 ✓5ᵗʰ
      affecting fetus or newborn 763.1
  acquired 738.4
  degenerative 738.4
  traumatic 738.4
    acute (lumbar) — *see* Fracture, vertebra, lumbar
    site other than lumbosacral — *see* Fracture, vertebra, by site
Spondylolysis (congenital) 756.11
  acquired 738.4
  cervical 756.19

Spondylolysis — *continued*
  lumbosacral region 756.11
    with disproportion (fetopelvic) 653.3 ✓5ᵗʰ
      affecting fetus or newborn 763.1
      causing obstructed labor 660.1 ✓5ᵗʰ
        affecting fetus or newborn 763.1
Spondylopathy
  inflammatory 720.9
    specified type NEC 720.89
  traumatic 721.7
Spondylose rhizomelique 720.0
Spondylosis 721.90
  with
    disproportion 653.3 ✓5ᵗʰ
      affecting fetus or newborn 763.1
      causing obstructed labor 660.1 ✓5ᵗʰ
        affecting fetus or newborn 763.1
    myelopathy NEC 721.91
  cervical, cervicodorsal 721.0
    with myelopathy 721.1
  inflammatory 720.9
  lumbar, lumbosacral 721.3
    with myelopathy 721.42
  sacral 721.3
    with myelopathy 721.42
  thoracic 721.2
    with myelopathy 721.41
  traumatic 721.7
Sponge
  divers' disease 989.5
  inadvertently left in operation wound 998.4
  kidney (medullary) 753.17
Spongioblastoma (M9422/3)
  multiforme (M9440/3)
    specified site — *see* Neoplasm, by site, malignant
    unspecified site 191.9
  polare (M9423/3)
    specified site — *see* Neoplasm, by site, malignant
    unspecified site 191.9
  primitive polar (M9443/3)
    specified site — *see* Neoplasm, by site, malignant
    unspecified site 191.9
  specified site — *see* Neoplasm, by site, malignant
  unspecified site 191.9
Spongiocytoma (M9400/3)
  specified site — *see* Neoplasm, by site, malignant
  unspecified site 191.9
Spongioneuroblastoma (M9504/3) — *see* Neoplasm, by site, malignant
Spontaneous — *see also* condition
  fracture — *see* Fracture, pathologic
Spoon nail 703.8
  congenital 757.5
Sporadic — *see* condition
Sporotrichosis (bones) (cutaneous) (disseminated) (epidermal) (lymphatic) (lymphocutaneous) (mucous membranes) (pulmonary) (skeletal) (visceral) 117.1
Sporotrichum schenckii infection 117.1
Spots, spotting
  atrophic (skin) 701.3
  Bitôt's (in the young child) 264.1
  café au lait 709.09
  cayenne pepper 448.1
  cotton wool (retina) 362.83
  de Morgan's (senile angiomas) 448.1
  Fuchs' black (myopic) 360.21
  intermenstrual
    irregular 626.6
    regular 626.5
  interpalpebral 372.53
  Koplik's 055.9
  liver 709.09
  Mongolian (pigmented) 757.33
  of pregnancy 641.9 ✓5ᵗʰ
  purpuric 782.7
  ruby 448.1
Spotted fever — *see* Fever, spotted

Sprain, strain (joint) (ligament) (muscle) (tendon) 848.9
  abdominal wall (muscle) 848.8
  Achilles tendon 845.09
  acromioclavicular 840.0
  ankle 845.00
    and foot 845.00
  anterior longitudinal, cervical 847.0
  arm 840.9
    upper 840.9
      and shoulder 840.9
  astragalus 845.00
  atlanto-axial 847.0
  atlanto-occipital 847.0
  atlas 847.0
  axis 847.0
  back (*see also* Sprain, spine) 847.9
  breast bone 848.40
  broad ligament — *see* Injury, internal, broad ligament
  calcaneofibular 845.02
  carpal 842.01
  carpometacarpal 842.11
  cartilage
    costal, without mention of injury to sternum 848.3
      involving sternum 848.42
    ear 848.8
    knee 844.9
      with current tear (*see also* Tear, meniscus) 836.2
    semilunar (knee) 844.8
      with current tear (*see also* Tear, meniscus) 836.2
    septal, nose 848.0
    thyroid region 848.2
    xiphoid 848.49
  cervical, cervicodorsal, cervicothoracic 847.0
  chondrocostal, without mention of injury to sternum 848.3
    involving sternum 848.42
  chondrosternal 848.42
  chronic (joint) — *see* Derangement, joint
  clavicle 840.9
  coccyx 847.4
  collar bone 840.9
  collateral, knee (medial) (tibial) 844.1
    lateral (fibular) 844.0
    recurrent or old 717.89
      lateral 717.81
      medial 717.82
  coracoacromial 840.8
  coracoclavicular 840.1
  coracohumeral 840.2
  coracoid (process) 840.9
  coronary, knee 844.8
  costal cartilage, without mention of injury to sternum 848.3
    involving sternum 848.42
  cricoarytenoid articulation 848.2
  cricothyroid articulation 848.2
  cruciate
    knee 844.2
    old 717.89
      anterior 717.83
      posterior 717.84
  deltoid
    ankle 845.01
    shoulder 840.8
  dorsal (spine) 847.1
  ear cartilage 848.8
  elbow 841.9
    and forearm 841.9
    specified site NEC 841.8
  femur (proximal end) 843.9
    distal end 844.9
  fibula (proximal end) 844.9
    distal end 845.00
  fibulocalcaneal 845.02
  finger(s) 842.10
  foot 845.10
    and ankle 845.00
  forearm 841.9
    and elbow 841.9
    specified site NEC 841.8
  glenoid (shoulder) (*see also* SLAP lesion) 840.8
  hand 842.10

Sprain, strain — *continued*
hip 843.9
and thigh 843.9
humerus (proximal end) 840.9
distal end 841.9
iliofemoral 843.0
infraspinatus 840.3
innominate
acetabulum 843.9
pubic junction 848.5
sacral junction 846.1
internal
collateral, ankle 845.01
semilunar cartilage 844.8
with current tear (*see also* Tear,
meniscus) 836.2
old 717.5
interphalangeal
finger 842.13
toe 845.13
ischiocapsular 843.1
jaw (cartilage) (meniscus) 848.1
old 524.69
knee 844.9
and leg 844.9
old 717.5
collateral
lateral 717.81
medial 717.82
cruciate
anterior 717.83
posterior 717.84
late effect — *see* Late, effects (of), sprain
lateral collateral, knee 844.0
old 717.81
leg 844.9
and knee 844.9
ligamentum teres femoris 843.8
low back 846.9
lumbar (spine) 847.2
lumbosacral 846.0
chronic or old 724.6
mandible 848.1
old 524.69
maxilla 848.1
medial collateral, knee 844.1
old 717.82
meniscus
jaw 848.1
old 524.69
knee 844.8
with current tear (*see also* Tear,
meniscus) 836.2
old 717.5
mandible 848.1
old 524.69
specified site NEC 848.8
metacarpal 842.10
distal 842.12
proximal 842.11
metacarpophalangeal 842.12
metatarsal 845.10
metatarsophalangeal 845.12
midcarpal 842.19
midtarsal 845.19
multiple sites, except fingers alone or toes
alone 848.8
neck 847.0
nose (septal cartilage) 848.0
occiput from atlas 847.0
old — *see* Derangement, joint
orbicular, hip 843.8
patella(r) 844.8
old 717.89
pelvis 848.5
phalanx
finger 842.10
toe 845.10
radiocarpal 842.02
radiohumeral 841.2
radioulnar 841.9
distal 842.09
radius, radial (proximal end) 841.9
and ulna 841.9
distal 842.09
collateral 841.0
distal end 842.00

Sprain, strain — *continued*
recurrent — *see* Sprain, by site
rib (cage), without mention of injury to sternum
848.3
involving sternum 848.42
rotator cuff (capsule) 840.4
round ligament — *see also* Injury, internal,
round ligament
femur 843.8
sacral (spine) 847.3
sacrococcygeal 847.3
sacroiliac (region) 846.9
chronic or old 724.6
ligament 846.1
specified site NEC 846.8
sacrospinatus 846.2
sacrospinous 846.2
sacrotuberous 846.3
scaphoid bone, ankle 845.00
scapula(r) 840.9
semilunar cartilage (knee) 844.8
with current tear (*see also* Tear, meniscus)
836.2
old 717.5
septal cartilage (nose) 848.0
shoulder 840.9
and arm, upper 840.9
blade 840.9
specified site NEC 848.8
spine 847.9
cervical 847.0
coccyx 847.4
dorsal 847.1
lumbar 847.2
lumbosacral 846.0
chronic or old 724.6
sacral 847.3
sacroiliac (*see also* Sprain, sacroiliac) 846.9
chronic or old 724.6
thoracic 847.1
sternoclavicular 848.41
sternum 848.40
subglenoid (*see also* SLAP lesion) 840.8
subscapularis 840.5
supraspinatus 840.6
symphysis
jaw 848.1
old 524.69
mandibular 848.1
old 524.69
pubis 848.5
talofibular 845.09
tarsal 845.10
tarsometatarsal 845.11
temporomandibular 848.1
old 524.69
teres
ligamentum femoris 843.8
major or minor 840.8
thigh (proximal end) 843.9
and hip 843.9
distal end 844.9
thoracic (spine) 847.1
thorax 848.8
thumb 842.10
thyroid cartilage or region 848.2
tibia (proximal end) 844.9
distal end 845.00
tibiofibular
distal 845.03
superior 844.3
toe(s) 845.10
trachea 848.8
trapezoid 840.8
ulna, ulnar (proximal end) 841.9
collateral 841.1
distal end 842.00
ulnohumeral 841.3
vertebrae (*see also* Sprain, spine) 847.9
cervical, cervicodorsal, cervicothoracic 847.0
wrist (cuneiform) (scaphoid) (semilunar) 842.00
xiphoid cartilage 848.49

Sprengel's deformity (congenital) 755.52

Spring fever 309.23

Sprue 579.1
celiac 579.0
idiopathic 579.0

Sprue — *continued*
meaning thrush 112.0
nontropical 579.0
tropical 579.1

Spur — *see also* Exostosis
bone 726.91
calcaneal 726.73
calcaneal 726.73
iliac crest 726.5
nose (septum) 478.1
bone 726.91
septal 478.1

Spuria placenta — *see* Placenta, abnormal

Spurway's syndrome (brittle bones and blue
sclera) 756.51

Sputum, abnormal (amount) (color) (excessive)
(odor) (purulent) 786.4
bloody 786.3

Squamous — *see also* condition
cell metaplasia
bladder 596.8
cervix — *see* condition
epithelium in
cervical canal (congenital) 752.49
uterine mucosa (congenital) 752.3
metaplasia
bladder 596.8
cervix — *see* condition

Squashed nose 738.0
congenital 754.0

Squeeze, divers' 993.3

Squint (*see also* Strabismus) 378.9
accommodative (*see also* Esotropia) 378.00
concomitant (*see also* Heterotropia) 378.30

Stab — *see also* Wound, open, by site
internal organs — *see* Injury, internal, by site,
with open wound

Staggering gait 781.2
hysterical 300.11

Staghorn calculus 592.0

Stälh's
ear 744.29
pigment line (cornea) 371.11

Stälhi's pigment lines (cornea) 371.11

Stain
port wine 757.32
tooth, teeth (hard tissues) 521.7
due to
accretions 523.6
deposits (betel) (black) (green) (materia
alba) (orange) (tobacco) 523.6
metals (copper) (silver) 521.7
nicotine 523.6
pulpal bleeding 521.7
tobacco 523.6

Stammering 307.0

Standstill
atrial 426.6
auricular 426.6
cardiac (*see also* Arrest, cardiac) 427.5
sinoatrial 429.6
sinus 426.6
ventricular (*see also* Arrest, cardiac) 427.5

Stannosis 503

Stanton's disease (melioidosis) 025

Staphylitis (acute) (catarrhal) (chronic)
(gangrenous) (membranous) (suppurative)
(ulcerative) 528.3

Staphylococcemia 038.10
aureus 038.11
specified organism NEC 038.19

Staphylococcus, staphylococcal — *see* condition

Staphyloderma (skin) 686.00

Staphyloma 379.11
anterior, localized 379.14
ciliary 379.11
cornea 371.73
equatorial 379.13
posterior 379.12
posticum 379.12
ring 379.15
sclera NEC 379.11

Starch eating 307.52

Stargardt's disease 362.75

Starvation (inanition) (due to lack of food) 994.2
  edema 262
  voluntary NEC 307.1

Stasis
  bile (duct) (*see also* Disease, biliary) 576.8
  bronchus (*see also* Bronchitis) 490
  cardiac (*see also* Failure, heart) 428.0
  cecum 564.89
  colon 564.89
  dermatitis (*see also* Varix, with stasis
    dermatitis) 454.1
  duodenal 536.8
  eczema (*see also* Varix, with stasis dermatitis)
    454.1
  edema (*see also* Hypertension, venous) ●
    459.30 ●
  foot 991.4
  gastric 536.3
  ileocecal coil 564.89
  ileum 564.89
  intestinal 564.89
  jejunum 564.89
  kidney 586
  liver 571.9
    cirrhotic — *see* Cirrhosis, liver
  lymphatic 457.8
  pneumonia 514
  portal 571.9
  pulmonary 514
  rectal 564.89
  renal 586
    tubular 584.5
  stomach 536.3
  ulcer
    with varicose veins 454.0
    without varicose veins 459.81
  urine NEC (*see also* Retention, urine) 788.20
  venous 459.81

State
  affective and paranoid, mixed, organic
    psychotic 294.8
  agitated 307.9
    acute reaction to stress 308.2
  anxiety (neurotic) (*see also* Anxiety) 300.00
    specified type NEC 300.09
  apprehension (*see also* Anxiety) 300.00
    specified type NEC 300.09
  climacteric, female 627.2
    following induced menopause 627.4
  clouded
    epileptic (*see also* Epilepsy) 345.9 ✓5ᵗʰ
    paroxysmal (idiopathic) (*see also* Epilepsy)
      345.9 ✓5ᵗʰ
  compulsive (mixed) (with obsession) 300.3
  confusional 298.9
    acute 293.0
      with
        arteriosclerotic dementia 290.41
        presenile brain disease 290.11
        senility 290.3
      alcoholic 291.0
      drug-induced 292.81
    epileptic 293.0
    postoperative 293.9
    reactive (emotional stress) (psychological
      trauma) 298.2
    subacute 293.1
  constitutional psychopathic 301.9
  convulsive (*see also* Convulsions) 780.39
  depressive NEC 311
    induced by drug 292.84
    neurotic 300.4
  dissociative 300.15
  hallucinatory 780.1
    induced by drug 292.12
  hyperdynamic beta-adrenergic circulatory
    429.82
  locked-in 344.81
  menopausal 627.2
    artificial 627.4
    following induced menopause 627.4
  neurotic NEC 300.9
    with depersonalization episode 300.6
  obsessional 300.3
  oneiroid (*see also* Schizophrenia) 295.4 ✓5ᵗʰ
  panic 300.01

State — *continued*
  paranoid 297.9
    alcohol-induced 291.5
    arteriosclerotic 290.42
    climacteric 297.2
    drug-induced 292.11
    in
      presenile brain disease 290.12
      senile brain disease 290.20
    involutional 297.2
    menopausal 297.2
    senile 290.20
    simple 297.0
  postleukotomy 310.0
  pregnant (*see also* Pregnancy) V22.2
  psychogenic, twilight 298.2
  psychotic, organic (*see also* Psychosis, organic)
    294.9
    mixed paranoid and affective 294.8
    senile or presenile NEC 290.9
    transient NEC 293.9
      with
        anxiety 293.84
        delusions 293.81
        depression 293.83
        hallucinations 293.82
  residual schizophrenic (*see also* Schizophrenia)
    295.6 ✓5ᵗʰ
  tension (*see also* Anxiety) 300.9
  transient organic psychotic 293.9
    anxiety type 293.84
    depressive type 293.83
    hallucinatory type 293.83
    paranoid type 293.81
    specified type NEC 293.89
  twilight
    epileptic 293.0
    psychogenic 298.2
  vegetative (persistent) 780.03

Status (post)
  absence
    epileptic (*see also* Epilepsy) 345.2
    of organ, acquired (postsurgical) — *see*
      Absence, by site, acquired
  anastomosis of intestine (for bypass) V45.3
  angioplasty, percutaneous transluminal
    coronary V45.82
  anginosus 413.9
  ankle prosthesis V43.66
  aortocoronary bypass or shunt V45.81
  arthrodesis V45.4
  artificially induced condition NEC V45.89
  artificial opening (of) V44.9
    gastrointestinal tract NEC V44.4
    specified site NEC V44.8
    urinary tract NEC V44.6
    vagina V44.7
  aspirator V46.0
  asthmaticus (*see also* Asthma) 493.9 ✓5ᵗʰ
  breast implant removal V45.83
  cardiac
    device (in situ) V45.00
      carotid sinus V45.09
        fitting or adjustment V53.39
      defibrillator, automatic implantable
        V45.02
      pacemaker V45.01
        fitting or adjustmanet V53.31
  carotid sinus stimulator V45.09
  cataract extraction V45.61
  chemotherapy V66.2
    current V58.69
  colostomy V44.3
  contraceptive device V45.59
    intrauterine V45.51
    subdermal V45.52
  convulsivus idiopathicus (*see also* Epilepsy)
    345.3
  coronary artery bypass or shunt V45.81
  cystostomy V44.50
    appendico-vesicostomy V44.52
    cutaneous-vesicostomy V44.51
    specified type NEC V44.59
  defibrillator, automatic implant-able cardiac
    V45.02
  dental crowns V45.84
  dental fillings V45.84

Status — *continued*
  dental restoration V45.84
  dental sealant V49.82
  dialysis V45.1
  donor V59.9
  drug therapy or regimen V67.59
    high-risk medication NEC V67.51
  elbow prosthesis V43.62
  enterostomy V44.4
  epileptic, epilepticus (absence) (grand mal) (*see*
    also Epilepsy) 345.3
    focal motor 345.7 ✓5ᵗʰ
    partial 345.7 ✓5ᵗʰ
    petit mal 345.2
    psychomotor 345.7 ✓5ᵗʰ
    temporal lobe 345.7 ✓5ᵗʰ
  eye (adnexa) surgery V45.69
  filtering bleb (eye) (postglaucoma) V45.69
    with rupture or complication 997.99
    pastcataract extraction (complication)
      997.99
  finger joint prosthesis V43.69
  gastrostomy V44.1
  grand mal 345.3
  heart valve prosthesis V43.3
  hip prosthesis (joint) (partial) (total) V43.64
  ileostomy V44.2
  intestinal bypass V45.3
  intrauterine contraceptive device V45.51
  jejunostomy V44.4
  knee joint prosthesis V43.65
  lacunaris 437.8
  lacunosis 437.8
  low birth weight V21.30
    less than 500 grams V21.31
    500-999 grams V21.32
    1000-1499 grams V21.33
    1500-1999 grams V21.34
    2000-2500 grams V21.35
  lymphaticus 254.8
  malignant neoplasm, ablated or excised — *see*
    History, malignant neoplasm
  marmoratus 333.7
  nephrostomy V44.6
  neuropacemaker NEC V45.89
    brain V45.89
    carotid sinus V45.09
    neurologic NEC V45.89
  organ replacement
    by artificial or mechanical device or
      prosthesis of
      artery V43.4
      artificial skin V43.83
      bladder V43.5
      blood vessel V43.4
      breast V43.82
      eye globe V43.0
      heart V43.2
        valve V43.3
      intestine V43.89
      joint V43.60
        ankle V43.66
        elbow V43.62
        finger V43.69
        hip (partial) (total) V43.64
        knee V43.65
        shoulder V43.61
        specified NEC V43.69
        wrist V43.63
      kidney V43.89
      larynx V43.81
      lens V43.1
      limb(s) V43.7
      liver V43.89
      lung V43.89
      organ NEC V43.89
      pancreas V43.89
      skin (artificial) V43.83
      tissue NEC V43.89
      vein V43.4
    by organ transplant (heterologous)
      (homologous) — *see* Status, transplant
  pacemaker
    brain V45.89
    cardiac V45.01
    carotid sinus V45.09
    neurologic NEC V45.89

Status — continued
  pacemaker — continued
    specified site NEC V45.89
  percutaneous transluminal coronary
    angioplasty V45.82
  petit mal 345.2
  postcommotio cerebri 310.2
  postmenopausal (age related) (natural) V49.81
  postoperative NEC V45.89
  postpartum NEC V24.2
    care immediately following delivery V24.0
    routine follow-up V24.2
  postsurgical NEC V45.89
  renal dialysis V45.1
  respirator V46.1
  reversed jejunal transposition (for bypass)
    V45.3
  shoulder prosthesis V43.61
  shunt
    aortocoronary bypass V45.81
    arteriovenous (for dialysis) V45.1
    cerebrospinal fluid V45.2
    vascular NEC V45.89
      aortocoronary (bypass) V45.81
    ventricular (communicating) (for drainage)
      V45.2
  sterilization
    tubal ligation V26.51
    vasectomy V26.52
  subdermal contraceptive device V45.52
  thymicolymphaticus 254.8
  thymicus 254.8
  thymolymphaticus 254.8
  tooth extraction 525.10
  tracheostomy V44.0
  transplant
    blood vessel V42.89
    bone V42.4
      marrow V42.81
    cornea V42.5
    heart V42.1
      valve V42.2
    intestine V42.84
    kidney V42.0
    liver V42.7
    lung V42.6
    organ V42.9
      specified site NEC V42.89
    pancreas V42.83
    peripheral stem cells V42.82
    skin V42.3
    stem cells, peripheral V42.82
    tissue V42.9
      specified type NEC V42.89
    vessel, blood V42.89
  tubal ligation V26.51
  ureterostomy V44.6
  urethrostomy V44.6
  vagina, artificial V44.7
  vascular shunt NEC V45.89
    aortocoronary (bypass) V45.81
  vasectomy V26.52
  ventilator V46.1
  wrist prosthesis V43.63
Stave fracture — see Fracture, metacarpus,
  metacarpal bone(s)
Steal
  subclavian artery 435.2
  vertebral artery 435.1
Stealing, solitary, child problem (see also
  Disturbance, conduct) 312.1 ☑5ᵗʰ
Steam burn — see Burn, by site
Steatocystoma multiplex 706.2
Steatoma (infected) 706.2
  eyelid (cystic) 374.84
    infected 373.13
Steatorrhea (chronic) 579.8
  with lacteal obstruction 579.2
  idiopathic 579.0
    adult 579.0
    infantile 579.0
  pancreatic 579.4
  primary 579.0
  secondary 579.8
  specified cause NEC 579.8
  tropical 579.1

Steatosis 272.8
  heart (see also Degeneration, myocardial) 429.1
  kidney 593.89
  liver 571.8
Steele-Richardson (-Olszewski) Syndrome 333.0
Stein's syndrome (polycystic ovary) 256.4
Stein-Leventhal syndrome (polycystic ovary)
  256.4
Steinbrocker's syndrome (see also Neuropathy,
  peripheral, autonomic) 337.9
Steinert's disease 359.2
Stenocardia (see also Angina) 413.9
Stenocephaly 756.0
Stenosis (cicatricial) — see also Stricture
  ampulla of Vater 576.2
    with calculus, cholelithiasis, or stones — see
      Choledocholithiasis
  anus, anal (canal) (sphincter) 569.2
    congenital 751.2
  aorta (ascending) 747.22
    arch 747.10
    arteriosclerotic 440.0
    calcified 440.0
  aortic (valve) 424.1
    with
      mitral (valve)
        insufficiency or incompetence 396.2
        stenosis or obstruction 396.0
    atypical 396.0
    congenital 746.3
    rheumatic 395.0
      with
        insufficiency, incompetency or
          regurgitation 395.2
          with mitral (valve) disease 396.8
        mitral (valve)
          disease (stenosis) 396.0
          insufficiency or incompetence 396.2
          stenosis or obstruction 396.0
    specified cause, except rheumatic 424.1
    syphilitic 093.22
  aqueduct of Sylvius (congenital) 742.3
    with spina bifida (see also Spina bifida)
      741.0 ☑5ᵗʰ
    acquired 331.4
  artery NEC 447.1
    basilar — see Narrowing, artery, basilar
    carotid (common) (internal) — see
      Narrowing, artery, carotid
    celiac 447.4
    cerebral 437.0
      due to
        embolism (see also Embolism, brain)
          434.1 ☑5ᵗʰ
        thrombus (see also Thrombosis, brain)
          434.0 ☑5ᵗʰ
    precerebral — see Narrowing, artery,
      precerebral
    pulmonary (congenital) 747.3
      acquired 417.8
    renal 440.1
    vertebral — see Narrowing, artery, vertebral
  bile duct or biliary passage (see also
    Obstruction, biliary) 576.2
    congenital 751.61
  bladder neck (acquired) 596.0
    congenital 753.6
  brain 348.8
  bronchus 519.1
    syphilitic 095.8
  cardia (stomach) 537.89
    congenital 750.7
  cardiovascular (see also Disease,
    cardiovascular) 429.2
  carotid artery — see Narrowing, artery, carotid
  cervix, cervical (canal) 622.4
    congenital 752.49
    in pregnancy or childbirth 654.6 ☑5ᵗʰ
      affecting fetus or newborn 763.89
      causing obstructed labor 660.2 ☑5ᵗʰ
        affecting fetus or newborn 763.1
  colon (see also Obstruction, intestine) 560.9
    congenital 751.2
  colostomy 569.62
  common bile duct (see also Obstruction,
    biliary) 576.2
    congenital 751.61

Stenosis — see also Stricture — continued
  coronary (artery) —see Arteriosclerosis,
    coronary
  cystic duct (see also Obstruction, gallbladder)
    575.2
    congenital 751.61
  due to (presence of) any device, implant, or
    graft classifiable to 996.0-996.5 — see
    Complications, due to (presence of) any
    device, implant, or graft classified to
    996.0-996.5 NEC
  duodenum 537.3
    congenital 751.1
  ejaculatory duct NEC 608.89
  endocervical os — see Stenosis, cervix
  enterostomy 569.62
  esophagus 530.3
    congenital 750.3
    syphilitic 095.8
      congenital 090.5
  external ear canal 380.50
    secondary to
      inflammation 380.53
      surgery 380.52
      trauma 380.51
  gallbladder (see also Obstruction, gallbladder)
    575.2
  glottis 478.74
  heart valve (acquired) — see also Endocarditis
    congenital NEC 746.89
      aortic 746.3
      mitral 746.5
      pulmonary 746.02
      tricuspid 746.1
  hepatic duct (see also Obstruction, biliary)
    576.2
  hymen 623.3
  hypertrophic subaortic (idiopathic) 425.1
  infundibulum cardiac 746.83
  intestine (see also Obstruction, intestine) 560.9
    congenital (small) 751.1
      large 751.2
  lacrimal
    canaliculi 375.53
    duct 375.56
      congenital 743.65
    punctum 375.52
      congenital 743.65
    sac 375.54
      congenital 743.65
  lacrimonasal duct 375.56
    congenital 743.65
    neonatal 375.55
  larynx 478.74
    congenital 748.3
    syphilitic 095.8
      congenital 090.5
  mitral (valve) (chronic) (inactive) 394.0
    with
      aortic (valve)
        disease (insufficiency) 396.1
        insufficiency or incompetence 396.1
        stenosis or obstruction 396.0
      incompetency, insufficiency or
        regurgitation 394.2
        with aortic valve disease 396.8
    active or acute 391.1
      with chorea (acute) (rheumatic)
        (Sydenham's) 392.0
    congenital 746.5
    specified cause, except rheumatic 424.0
    syphilitic 093.21
  myocardium, myocardial (see also
    Degeneration, myocardial) 429.1
    hypertrophic subaortic (idiopathic) 425.1
  nares (anterior) (posterior) 478.1
    congenital 748.0
  nasal duct 375.56
    congenital 743.65
  nasolacrimal duct 375.56
    congenital 743.65
    neonatal 375.55
  organ or site, congenital NEC — see Atresia
  papilla of Vater 576.2
    with calculus, cholelithiasis, or stones — see
      Choledocholithiasis

Stenosis — *see also* Stricture — *continued*
  pulmonary (artery) (congenital) 747.3
    with ventricular septal defect, dextraposition of aorta and hypertrophy of right ventricle 745.2
    acquired 417.8
    infundibular 746.83
    in tetralogy of Fallot 745.2
    subvalvular 746.83
    valve (*see also* Endocarditis, pulmonary) 424.3
      congenital 746.02
    vein 747.49
      acquired 417.8
    vessel NEC 417.8
  pulmonic (congenital) 746.02
    infundibular 746.83
    subvalvular 746.83
  pylorus (hypertrophic) 537.0
    adult 537.0
    congenital 750.5
    infantile 750.5
  rectum (sphincter) (*see also* Stricture, rectum) 569.2
  renal artery 440.1
  salivary duct (any) 527.8
  sphincter of Oddi (*see also* Obstruction, biliary) 576.2
  spinal 724.00
    cervical 723.0
    lumbar, lumbosacral 724.02
    nerve (root) NEC 724.9
    specified region NEC 724.09
    thoracic, thoracolumbar 724.01
  stomach, hourglass 537.6
  subaortic 746.81
    hypertrophic (idiopathic) 425.1
  supra (valvular)-aortic 747.22
  trachea 519.1
    congenital 748.3
    syphilitic 095.8
    tuberculous (*see also* Tuberculosis) 012.8 ✓5ᵗʰ
  tracheostomy 519.02
  tricuspid (valve) (*see also* Endocarditis, tricuspid) 397.0
    congenital 746.1
    nonrheumatic 424.2
  tubal 628.2
  ureter (*see also* Stricture, ureter) 593.3
    congenital 753.29
  urethra (*see also* Stricture, urethra) 598.9
  vagina 623.2
    congenital 752.49
    in pregnancy or childbirth 654.7 ✓5ᵗʰ
      affecting fetus or newborn 763.89
      causing obstructed labor 660.2 ✓5ᵗʰ
        affecting fetus or newborn 763.1
  valve (cardiac) (heart) (*see also* Endocarditis) 424.90
    congenital NEC 746.89
      aortic 746.3
      mitral 746.5
      pulmonary 746.02
      tricuspid 746.1
      urethra 753.6
  valvular (*see also* Endocarditis) 424.90
    congenital NEC 746.89
      urethra 753.6
  vascular graft or shunt 996.1
    atherosclerosis — *see* Arteriosclerosis, extremities
    embolism 996.74
    occlusion NEC 996.74
    thrombus 996.74
  vena cava (inferior) (superior) 459.2
    congenital 747.49
  ventricular shunt 996.2
  vulva 624.8
Stercolith (*see also* Fecalith) 560.39
  appendix 543.9
Stercoraceous, stercoral ulcer 569.82
  anus or rectum 569.41
Stereopsis, defective
  with fusion 368.33
  without fusion 368.32
Stereotypes NEC 307.3

Sterility
  female — *see* Infertility, female
  male (*see also* Infertility, male) 606.9
Sterilization, admission for V25.2
  status
    tubal ligation V26.51
    vasectomy V26.52
Sternalgia (*see also* Angina) 413.9
Sternopagus 759.4
Sternum bifidum 756.3
Sternutation 784.9
Steroid
  effects (adverse) (iatrogenic)
    cushingoid
      correct substance properly administered 255.0
      overdose or wrong substance given or taken 962.0
    diabetes
      correct substance properly administered 251.8
      overdose or wrong substance given or taken 962.0
    due to
      correct substance properly administered 255.8
      overdose or wrong substance given or taken 962.0
    fever
      correct substance properly administered 780.6
      overdose or wrong substance given or taken 962.0
    withdrawal
      correct substance properly administered 255.4
      overdose or wrong substance given or taken 962.0
  responder 365.03
Stevens-Johnson disease or syndrome (erythema multiforme exudativum) 695.1
Stewart-Morel syndrome (hyperostosis frontalis interna) 733.3
Sticker's disease (erythema infectiosum) 057.0
Sticky eye 372.03
Stieda's disease (calcification, knee joint) 726.62
Stiff
  back 724.8
  neck (*see also* Torticollis) 723.5
Stiff-man syndrome 333.91
Stiffness, joint NEC 719.50
  ankle 719.57
  back 724.8
  elbow 719.52
  finger 719.54
  hip 719.55
  knee 719.56
  multiple sites 719.59
  sacroiliac 724.6
  shoulder 719.51
  specified site NEC 719.58
  spine 724.9
  surgical fusion V45.4
  wrist 719.53
Stigmata, congenital syphilis 090.5
Still's disease or syndrome 714.30
Still-Felty syndrome (rheumatoid arthritis with splenomegaly and leukopenia) 714.1
Stillbirth, stillborn NEC 779.9
Stiller's disease (asthenia) 780.79
Stilling-Türk-Duane syndrome (ocular retraction syndrome) 378.71
Stimulation, ovary 256.1
Sting (animal) (bee) (fish) (insect) (jellyfish) (Portuguese man-o-war) (wasp) (venomous) 989.5
  anaphylactic shock or reaction 989.5
  plant 692.6
Stippled epiphyses 756.59

Stitch
  abscess 998.59
  burst (in ►external◄ operation wound) 998.32 ▲
    internal 998.31 ●
  in back 724.5
Stojano's (subcostal) syndrome 098.86
Stokes' disease (exophthalmic goiter) 242.0 ✓5ᵗʰ
Stokes-Adams syndrome (syncope with heart block) 426.9
Stokvis' (-Talma) disease (enterogenous cyanosis) 289.7
Stomach — *see* condition
Stoma malfunction
  colostomy 569.62
  cystostomy 997.5
  enterostomy 569.62
  gastrostomy 536.42
  ileostomy 569.62
  nephrostomy 997.5
  tracheostomy 519.02
  ureterostomy 997.5
Stomatitis 528.0
  angular 528.5
    due to dietary or vitamin deficiency 266.0
  aphthous 528.2
  candidal 112.0
  catarrhal 528.0
  denture 528.9
  diphtheritic (membranous) 032.0
  due to
    dietary deficiency 266.0
    thrush 112.0
    vitamin deficiency 266.0
  epidemic 078.4
  epizootic 078.4
  follicular 528.0
  gangrenous 528.1
  herpetic 054.2
  herpetiformis 528.2
  malignant 528.0
  membranous acute 528.0
  monilial 112.0
  mycotic 112.0
  necrotic 528.1
    ulcerative 101
  necrotizing ulcerative 101
  parasitic 112.0
  septic 528.0
  spirochetal 101
  suppurative (acute) 528.0
  ulcerative 528.0
    necrotizing 101
  ulceromembranous 101
  vesicular 528.0
    with exanthem 074.3
  Vincent's 101
Stomatocytosis 282.8
Stomatomycosis 112.0
Stomatorrhagia 528.9
Stone(s) — *see also* Calculus
  bladder 594.1
    diverticulum 594.0
  cystine 270.0
  heart syndrome (*see also* Failure, ventricular, left) 428.1
  kidney 592.0
  prostate 602.0
  pulp (dental) 522.2
  renal 592.0
  salivary duct or gland (any) 527.5
  ureter 592.1
  urethra (impacted) 594.2
  urinary (duct) (impacted) (passage) 592.9
    bladder 594.1
      diverticulum 594.0
    lower tract NEC 594.9
    specified site 594.8
  xanthine 277.2
Stonecutters' lung 502
  tuberculous (*see also* Tuberculosis) 011.4 ✓5ᵗʰ
Stonemasons'
  asthma, disease, or lung 502
  tuberculous (*see also* Tuberculosis) 011.4 ✓5ᵗʰ

✓4ᵗʰ Fourth-digit Required   ✓5ᵗʰ Fifth-digit Required   ►◄ Revised Text   ● New Line   ▲ Revised Code

Stonemasons' — *continued*
phthisis (*see also* Tuberculosis) 011.4 ✓5ᵗʰ

Stoppage
bowel (*see also* Obstruction, intestine) 560.9
heart (*see also* Arrest, cardiac) 427.5
intestine (*see also* Obstruction, intestine) 560.9
urine NEC (*see also* Retention, urine) 788.20

Storm, thyroid (apathetic) (*see also*
Thyrotoxicosis) 242.9 ✓5ᵗʰ

Strabismus (alternating) (congenital)
(nonparalytic) 378.9
concomitant (*see also* Heterotropia) 378.30
convergent (*see also* Esotropia) 378.00
divergent (*see also* Exotropia) 378.10
convergent (*see also* Esotropia) 378.00
divergent (*see also* Exotropia) 378.10
due to adhesions, scars — *see* Strabismus,
mechanical
in neuromuscular disorder NEC 378.73
intermittent 378.20
vertical 378.31
latent 378.40
convergent (esophoria) 378.41
divergent (exophoria) 378.42
vertical 378.43
mechanical 378.60
due to
Brown's tendon sheath syndrome 378.61
specified musculofascial disorder NEC
378.62
paralytic 378.50
third or oculomotor nerve (partial) 378.51
total 378.52
fourth or trochlear nerve 378.53
sixth or abducens nerve 378.54
specified type NEC 378.73
vertical (hypertropia) 378.31

Strain — *see also* Sprain, by site
eye NEC 368.13
heart — *see* Disease, heart
meaning gonorrhea — *see* Gonorrhea
physical NEC V62.89
postural 729.9
psychological NEC V62.89

Strands
conjunctiva 372.62
vitreous humor 379.25

Strangulation, strangulated 994.7
appendix 543.9
asphyxiation or suffocation by 994.7
bladder neck 596.0
bowel — *see* Strangulation, intestine
colon — *see* Strangulation, intestine
cord (umbilical) — *see* Compression, umbilical
cord
due to birth injury 767.8
food or foreign body (*see also* Asphyxia, food)
933.1
hemorrhoids 455.8
external 455.5
internal 455.2
hernia — *see also* Hernia, by site, with
obstruction
gangrenous — *see* Hernia, by site, with
gangrene
intestine (large) (small) 560.2
with hernia — *see also* Hernia, by site, with
obstruction
gangrenous — *see* Hernia, by site, with
gangrene
congenital (small) 751.1
large 751.2
mesentery 560.2
mucus (*see also* Asphyxia, mucus) 933.1
newborn 770.1
omentum 560.2
organ or site, congenital NEC — *see* Atresia
ovary 620.8
due to hernia 620.4
penis 607.89
foreign body 939.3
rupture (*see also* Hernia, by site, with
obstruction) 552.9
gangrenous (*see also* Hernia, by site, with
gangrene) 551.9

Strangulation, strangulated — *continued*
stomach, due to hernia (*see also* Hernia, by
site, with obstruction) 552.9
with gangrene (*see also* Hernia, by site, with
gangrene) 551.9
umbilical cord — *see* Compression, umbilical
cord
vesicourethral orifice 596.0

Strangury 788.1

Strawberry
gallbladder (*see also* Disease, gallbladder)
575.6
mark 757.32
tongue (red) (white) 529.3

Straw itch 133.8

Streak, ovarian 752.0

Strephosymbolia 315.01
secondary to organic lesion 784.69

Streptobacillary fever 026.1

Streptobacillus moniliformis 026.1

Streptococcemia 038.0

Streptococcicosis — *see* Infection, streptococcal

Streptococcus, streptococcal — *see* condition

Streptoderma 686.00

Streptomycosis — *see* Actinomycosis

Streptothricosis — *see* Actinomycosis

Streptothrix — *see* Actinomycosis

Streptotrichosis — *see* Actinomycosis

Stress
fracture — *see* Fracture, stress
polycythemia 289.0
reaction (gross) (*see also* Reaction, stress,
acute) 308.9

Stretching, nerve — *see* Injury, nerve, by site

Striae (albicantes) (atrophicae) (cutis distensae)
(distensae) 701.3

Striations of nails 703.8

Stricture (*see also* Stenosis) 799.8
ampulla of Vater 576.2
with calculus, cholelithiasis, or stones — *see*
Choledocholithiasis
anus (sphincter) 569.2
congenital 751.2
infantile 751.2
aorta (ascending) 747.22
arch 747.10
arteriosclerotic 440.0
calcified 440.0
aortic (valve) (*see also* Stenosis, aortic) 424.1
congenital 746.3
aqueduct of Sylvius (congenital) 742.3
with spina bifida (*see also* Spina bifida)
741.0 ✓5ᵗʰ
acquired 331.4
artery 447.1
basilar — *see* Narrowing, artery, basilar
carotid (common) (internal) — *see*
Narrowing, artery, carotid
celiac 447.4
cerebral 437.0
congenital 747.81
due to
embolism (*see also* Embolism, brain)
434.1 ✓5ᵗʰ
thrombus (*see also* Thrombosis, brain)
434.0 ✓5ᵗʰ
congenital (peripheral) 747.60
cerebral 747.81
coronary 746.85
gastrointestinal 747.61
lower limb 747.64
renal 747.62
retinal 743.58
specified NEC 747.69
spinal 747.82
umbilical 747.5
upper limb 747.63
coronary — *see* Arteriosclerosis, coronary
congenital 746.85
precerebral — *see* Narrowing, artery,
precerebral NEC
pulmonary (congenital) 747.3
acquired 417.8

Stricture (*see also* Stenosis) — *continued*
artery — *continued*
renal 440.1
vertebral — *see* Narrowing, artery, vertebral
auditory canal (congenital) (external) 744.02
acquired (*see also* Stricture, ear canal,
acquired) 380.50
bile duct or passage (any) (postoperative) (*see
also* Obstruction, biliary) 576.2
congenital 751.61
bladder 596.8
congenital 753.6
neck 596.0
congenital 753.6
bowel (*see also* Obstruction, intestine) 560.9
brain 348.8
bronchus 519.1
syphilitic 095.8
cardia (stomach) 537.89
congenital 750.7
cardiac — *see also* Disease, heart
orifice (stomach) 537.89
cardiovascular (*see also* Disease,
cardiovascular) 429.2
carotid artery — *see* Narrowing, artery, carotid
cecum (*see also* Obstruction, intestine) 560.9
cervix, cervical (canal) 622.4
congenital 752.49
in pregnancy or childbirth 654.6 ✓5ᵗʰ
affecting fetus or newborn 763.89
causing obstructed labor 660.2 ✓5ᵗʰ
affecting fetus or newborn 763.1
colon (*see also* Obstruction, intestine) 560.9
congenital 751.2
colostomy 569.62
common bile duct (*see also* Obstruction,
biliary) 576.2
congenital 751.61
coronary (artery) — *see* Arteriosclerosis,
coronary
congenital 746.85
cystic duct (*see also* Obstruction, gallbladder)
575.2
congenital 751.61
cystostomy 997.5
digestive organs NEC, congenital 751.8
duodenum 537.3
congenital 751.1
ear canal (external) (congenital) 744.02
acquired 380.50
secondary to
inflammation 380.53
surgery 380.52
trauma 380.51
ejaculatory duct 608.85
enterostomy 569.62
esophagus (corrosive) (peptic) 530.3
congenital 750.3
syphilitic 095.8
congenital 090.5
eustachian tube (*see also* Obstruction,
Eustachian tube) 381.60
congenital 744.24
fallopian tube 628.2
gonococcal (chronic) 098.37
acute 098.17
tuberculous (*see also* Tuberculosis)
016.6 ✓5ᵗʰ
gallbladder (*see also* Obstruction, gallbladder)
575.2
congenital 751.69
glottis 478.74
heart — *see also* Disease, heart
congenital NEC 746.89
valve — *see also* Endocarditis
congenital NEC 746.89
aortic 746.3
mitral 746.5
pulmonary 746.02
tricuspid 746.1
hepatic duct (*see also* Obstruction, biliary)
576.2
hourglass, of stomach 537.6
hymen 623.3
hypopharynx 478.29

Stricture (*see also* Stenosis) — *continued*
  intestine (*see also* Obstruction, intestine) 560.9
    congenital (small) 751.1
      large 751.2
    ischemic 557.1
  lacrimal
    canaliculi 375.53
      congenital 743.65
    punctum 375.52
      congenital 743.65
    sac 375.54
      congenital 743.65
  lacrimonasal duct 375.56
    congenital 743.65
    neonatal 375.55
  larynx 478.79
    congenital 748.3
    syphilitic 095.8
      congenital 090.5
  lung 518.89
  meatus
    ear (congenital) 744.02
      acquired (*see also* Stricture, ear canal, acquired) 380.50
    osseous (congenital) (ear) 744.03
      acquired (*see also* Stricture, ear canal, acquired) 380.50
    urinarius (*see also* Stricture, urethra) 598.9
      congenital 753.6
  mitral (valve) (*see also* Stenosis, mitral) 394.0
    congenital 746.5
    specified cause, except rheumatic 424.0
  myocardium, myocardial (*see also* Degeneration, myocardial) 429.1
    hypertrophic subaortic (idiopathic) 425.1
  nares (anterior) (posterior) 478.1
    congenital 748.0
  nasal duct 375.56
    congenital 743.65
    neonatal 375.55
  nasolacrimal duct 375.56
    congenital 743.65
    neonatal 375.55
  nasopharynx 478.29
    syphilitic 095.8
  nephrostomy 997.5
  nose 478.1
    congenital 748.0
  nostril (anterior) (posterior) 478.1
    congenital 748.0
  organ or site, congenital NEC — *see* Atresia
  osseous meatus (congenital) (ear) 744.03
    acquired (*see also* Stricture, ear canal, acquired) 380.50
  os uteri (*see also* Stricture, cervix) 622.4
  oviduct — *see* Stricture, fallopian tube
  pelviureteric junction 593.3
  pharynx (dilation) 478.29
  prostate 602.8
  pulmonary, pulmonic
    artery (congenital) 747.3
      acquired 417.8
      noncongenital 417.8
    infundibulum (congenital) 746.83
    valve (*see also* Endocarditis, pulmonary) 424.3
      congenital 746.02
    vein (congenital) 747.49
      acquired 417.8
    vessel NEC 417.8
  punctum lacrimale 375.52
    congenital 743.65
  pylorus (hypertrophic) 537.0
    adult 537.0
    congenital 750.5
    infantile 750.5
  rectosigmoid 569.89
  rectum (sphincter) 569.2
    congenital 751.2
    due to
      chemical burn 947.3
      irradiation 569.2
      lymphogranuloma venereum 099.1
    gonococcal 098.7
    inflammatory 099.1
    syphilitic 095.8

Stricture (*see also* Stenosis) — *continued*
  rectum — *continued*
    tuberculous (*see also* Tuberculosis) 014.8 ✓5ᵗʰ
  renal artery 440.1
  salivary duct or gland (any) 527.8
  sigmoid (flexure) (*see also* Obstruction, intestine) 560.9
  spermatic cord 608.85
  stoma (following) (of)
    colostomy 569.62
    cystostomy 997.5
    enterostomy 569.62
    gastrostomy 536.42
    ileostomy 569.62
    nephrostomy 997.5
    tracheostomy 519.02
    ureterostomy 997.5
  stomach 537.89
    congenital 750.7
    hourglass 537.6
  subaortic 746.81
    hypertrophic (acquired) (idiopathic) 425.1
  subglottic 478.74
  syphilitic NEC 095.8
  tendon (sheath) 727.81
  trachea 519.1
    congenital 748.3
    syphilitic 095.8
    tuberculous (*see also* Tuberculosis) 012.8 ✓5ᵗʰ
  tracheostomy 519.02
  tricuspid (valve) (*see also* Endocarditis, tricuspid) 397.0
    congenital 746.1
    nonrheumatic 424.2
  tunica vaginalis 608.85
  ureter (postoperative) 593.3
    congenital 753.29
    tuberculous (*see also* Tuberculosis) 016.2 ✓5ᵗʰ
  ureteropelvic junction 593.3
    congenital 753.21
  ureterovesical orifice 593.3
    congenital 753.22
  urethra (anterior) (meatal) (organic) (posterior) (spasmodic) 598.9
    associated with schistosomiasis (*see also* Schistosomiasis) 120.9 [598.01]
    congenital (valvular) 753.6
    due to
      infection 598.00
        syphilis 095.8 [598.01]
      trauma 598.1
    gonococcal 098.2 [598.01]
    gonorrheal 098.2 [598.01]
    infective 598.00
    late effect of injury 598.1
    postcatheterization 598.2
    postobstetric 598.1
    postoperative 598.2
    specified cause NEC 598.8
    syphilitic 095.8 [598.01]
    traumatic 598.1
    valvular, congenital 753.6
  urinary meatus (*see also* Stricture, urethra) 598.9
    congenital 753.6
  uterus, uterine 621.5
    os (external) (internal) — *see* Stricture, cervix
  vagina (outlet) 623.2
    congenital 752.49
  valve (cardiac) (heart) (*see also* Endocarditis) 424.90
    congenital (cardiac) (heart) NEC 746.89
      aortic 746.3
      mitral 746.5
      pulmonary 746.02
      tricuspid 746.1
      urethra 753.6
  valvular (*see also* Endocarditis) 424.90
  vascular graft or shunt 996.1
    atherosclerosis — *see* Arteriosclersis, extremities
    embolism 996.74
    occlusion NEC 996.74
    thrombus 996.74

Stricture (*see also* Stenosis) — *continued*
  vas deferens 608.85
    congenital 752.8
  vein 459.2
  vena cava (inferior) (superior) NEC 459.2
    congenital 747.49
  ventricular shunt 996.2
  vesicourethral orifice 596.0
    congenital 753.6
  vulva (acquired) 624.8
Stridor 786.1
  congenital (larynx) 748.3
Stridulous — *see* condition
Strippling of nails 703.8
Stroke (*see also* Disease, cerebrovascular, acute) 436
  apoplectic (*see also* Disease, cerebrovascular, acute) 436
  brain (*see also* Disease, cerebrovascular, acute) 436
  epileptic — *see* Epilepsy
  healed or old V12.59
  heart — *see* Disease, heart
  heat 992.0
  iatrogenic 997.02
  in evolution 435.9
  late effect — *see* Late effect(s) (of) cerebrovascular disease
  lightning 994.0
  paralytic (*see also* Disease, cerebrovascular, acute) 436
  postoperative 997.02
  progressive 435.9
Stromatosis, endometrial (M8931/1) 236.0
Strong pulse 785.9
Strongyloides stercoralis infestation 127.2
Strongyloidiasis 127.2
Strongyloidosis 127.2
Strongylus (gibsoni) infestation 127.7
Strophulus (newborn) 779.89 ▲
  pruriginosus 698.2
Struck by lightning 994.0
Struma (*see also* Goiter) 240.9
  fibrosa 245.3
  Hashimoto (struma lymphomatosa) 245.2
  lymphomatosa 245.2
  nodosa (simplex) 241.9
    endemic 241.9
    multinodular 241.1
    sporadic 241.9
    toxic or with hyperthyroidism 242.3 ✓5ᵗʰ
      multinodular 242.2 ✓5ᵗʰ
      uninodular 242.1 ✓5ᵗʰ
    toxicosa 242.3 ✓5ᵗʰ
      multinodular 242.2 ✓5ᵗʰ
      uninodular 242.1 ✓5ᵗʰ
    uninodular 241.0
  ovarii (M9090/0) 220
    and carcinoid (M9091/1) 236.2
    malignant (M9090/3) 183.0
  Riedel's (ligneous thyroiditis) 245.3
  scrofulous (*see also* Tuberculosis) 017.2 ✓5ᵗʰ
  tuberculous (*see also* Tuberculosis) 017.2 ✓5ᵗʰ
    abscess 017.2 ✓5ᵗʰ
    adenitis 017.2 ✓5ᵗʰ
    lymphangitis 017.2 ✓5ᵗʰ
    ulcer 017.2 ✓5ᵗʰ
Strumipriva cachexia (*see also* Hypothyroidism) 244.9
Strümpell-Marie disease or spine (ankylosing spondylitis) 720.0
Strümpell-Westphal pseudosclerosis (hepatolenticular degeneration) 275.1
Stuart's disease (congenital factor X deficiency) (*see also* Defect, coagulation) 286.3
Stuart-Power factor deficiency (congenital factor X deficiency) (*see also* Defect, coagulation) 286.3
Students' elbow 727.2
Stuffy nose 478.1
Stump — *see also* Amputation
  cervix, cervical (healed) 622.8

Stricture — Stump

Stupor 780.09
  catatonic (see also Schizophrenia) 295.2 ✓5ᵗʰ
  circular (see also Psychosis, manic-depressive,
      circular) 296.7
  manic 296.89
  manic-depressive (see also Psychosis, affective)
      296.89
  mental (anergic) (delusional) 298.9
  psychogenic 298.8
  reaction to exceptional stress (transient) 308.2
  traumatic NEC — see also Injury, intracranial
      with spinal (cord)
        lesion — see Injury, spinal, by site
        shock — see Injury, spinal, by site
Sturge (-Weber) (-Dimitri) disease or syndrome
    (encephalocutan-eous angiomatosis) 759.6
Sturge-Kalischer-Weber syndrome
    (encephalocutaneous angiomatosis) 759.6
Stuttering 307.0
Sty, stye 373.11
  external 373.11
  internal 373.12
  meibomian 373.12
Subacidity, gastric 536.8
  psychogenic 306.4
Subacute — see condition
Subarachnoid — see condition
Subclavian steal syndrome 435.2
Subcortical — see condition
Subcostal syndrome 098.86
  nerve compression 354.8
Subcutaneous, subcuticular — see condition
Subdelirium 293.1
Subdural — see condition
Subendocardium — see condition
Subependymoma (M9383/1) 237.5
Suberosis 495.3
Subglossitis — see Glossitis
Subhemophilia 286.0
Subinvolution (uterus) 621.1
  breast (postlactational) (postpartum) 611.8
  chronic 621.1
  puerperal, postpartum 674.8 ✓5ᵗʰ
Sublingual — see condition
Sublinguitis 527.2
Subluxation — see also Dislocation, by site
  congenital NEC — see also Malposition,
      congenital
    hip (unilateral) 754.32
      with dislocation of other hip 754.35
      bilateral 754.33
    joint
      lower limb 755.69
      shoulder 755.59
      upper limb 755.59
    lower limb (joint) 755.69
    shoulder (joint) 755.59
    upper limb (joint) 755.59
  lens 379.32
    anterior 379.33
    posterior 379.34
  rotary, cervical region of spine — see Fracture,
      vertebra, cervical
Submaxillary — see condition
Submersion (fatal) (nonfatal) 994.1
Submissiveness (undue), in child 313.0
Submucous — see condition
Subnormal, subnormality
  accommodation (see also Disorder,
      accommodation) 367.9
  mental (see also Retardation, mental) 319
    mild 317
    moderate 318.0
    profound 318.2
    severe 318.1
  temperature (accidental) 991.6
    not associated with low environmental
        temperature 780.99   ▲
Subphrenic — see condition
Subscapular nerve — see condition
Subseptus uterus 752.3
Subsiding appendicitis 542

Substernal thyroid (see also Goiter) 240.9
  congenital 759.2
Substitution disorder 300.11
Subtentorial — see condition
Subtertian
  fever 084.0
  malaria (fever) 084.0
Subthyroidism (acquired) (see also
    Hypothyroidism) 244.9
  congenital 243
Succenturiata placenta — see Placenta,
    abnormal
Succussion sounds, chest 786.7
Sucking thumb, child 307.9
Sudamen 705.1
Sudamina 705.1
Sudanese kala-azar 085.0
Sudden
  death, cause unknown (less than 24 hours)
      798.1
    during childbirth 669.9 ✓5ᵗʰ
    infant 798.0
    puerperal, postpartum 674.9 ✓5ᵗʰ
  hearing loss NEC 388.2
  heart failure (see also Failure, heart) 428.9
  infant death syndrome 798.0
Sudeck's atrophy, disease, or syndrome 733.7
SUDS (Sudden unexplained death) 798.2
Suffocation (see also Asphyxia) 799.0
  by
    bed clothes 994.7
    bunny bag 994.7
    cave-in 994.7
    constriction 994.7
    drowning 994.1
    inhalation
      food or foreign body (see also Asphyxia,
          food or foreign body) 933.1
      oil or gasoline (see also Asphyxia, food or
          foreign body) 933.1
    overlying 994.7
    plastic bag 994.7
    pressure 994.7
    strangulation 994.7
  during birth 768.1
  mechanical 994.7
Sugar
  blood
    high 790.2
    low 251.2
  in urine 791.5
Suicide, suicidal (attempted)
  by poisoning — see Table of Drugs and
      Chemicals
  risk 300.9
  tendencies 300.9
  trauma NEC (see also nature and site of injury)
      959.9
Suipestifer infection (see also Infection,
    Salmonella) 003.9
Sulfatidosis 330.0
Sulfhemoglobinemia, sulphemoglobinemia
    (acquired) (congenital) 289.7
Sumatran mite fever 081.2
Summer — see condition
Sunburn 692.71
  dermatitis 692.71
  due to
    other ultraviolet radiation 692.82
    tanning bed 692.82
  first degree 692.71
  second degree 692.76
  third degree 692.77
Sunken
  acetabulum 718.85
  fontanels 756.0
Sunstroke 992.0
Superfecundation 651.9 ✓5ᵗʰ
  with fetal loss and retention of one or more
      fetus(es) 651.6 ✓5ᵗʰ
Superfetation 651.9 ✓5ᵗʰ
  with fetal loss and retention of one or more
      fetus(es) 651.6 ✓5ᵗʰ

Superinvolution uterus 621.8
Supernumerary (congenital)
  aortic cusps 746.89
  auditory ossicles 744.04
  bone 756.9
  breast 757.6
  carpal bones 755.56
  cusps, heart valve NEC 746.89
    mitral 746.5
    pulmonary 746.09
  digit(s) 755.00
    finger 755.01
    toe 755.02
  ear (lobule) 744.1
  fallopian tube 752.19
  finger 755.01
  hymen 752.49
  kidney 753.3
  lacrimal glands 743.64
  lacrimonasal duct 743.65
  lobule (ear) 744.1
  mitral cusps 746.5
  muscle 756.82
  nipples 757.6
  organ or site NEC — see Accessory
  ossicles, auditory 744.04
  ovary 752.0
  oviduct 752.19
  pulmonic cusps 746.09
  rib 756.3
    cervical or first 756.2
        syndrome 756.2
  roots (of teeth) 520.2
  spinal vertebra 756.19
  spleen 759.0
  tarsal bones 755.67
  teeth 520.1
    causing crowding 524.3
  testis 752.8
  thumb 755.01
  toe 755.02
  uterus 752.2
  vagina 752.49
  vertebra 756.19
Supervision (of)
  contraceptive method previously prescribed
      V25.40
    intrauterine device V25.42
    oral contraceptive (pill) V25.41
    specified type NEC V25.49
    subdermal implantable contraceptive V25.43
  dietary (for) V65.3
    allergy (food) V65.3
    colitis V65.3
    diabetes mellitus V65.3
    food allergy intolerance V65.3
    gastritis V65.3
    hypercholesterolemia V65.3
    hypoglycemia V65.3
    intolerance (food) V65.3
    obesity V65.3
    specified NEC V65.3
  lactation V24.1
  pregnancy — see Pregnancy, supervision of
Supplemental teeth 520.1
  causing crowding 524.3
Suppression
  binocular vision 368.31
  lactation 676.5 ✓5ᵗʰ
  menstruation 626.8
  ovarian secretion 256.39
  renal 586
  urinary secretion 788.5
  urine 788.5
Suppuration, suppurative — see also condition
  accessory sinus (chronic) (see also Sinusitis)
      473.9
  adrenal gland 255.8
  antrum (chronic) (see also Sinusitis, maxillary)
      473.0
  bladder (see also Cystitis) 595.89
  bowel 569.89
  brain 324.0
    late effect 326
  breast 611.0
    puerperal, postpartum 675.1 ✓5ᵗʰ
  dental periosteum 526.5

Suppuration, suppurative — *see also* condition — *continued*
  diffuse (skin) 686.00
  ear (middle) (*see also* Otitis media) 382.4
    external (*see also* Otitis, externa) 380.10
    internal 386.33
  ethmoidal (sinus) (chronic) (*see also* Sinusitis, ethmoidal) 473.2
  fallopian tube (*see also* Salpingo-oophoritis) 614.2
  frontal (sinus) (chronic) (*see also* Sinusitis, frontal) 473.1
  gallbladder (*see also* Cholecystitis, acute) 575.0
  gum 523.3
  hernial sac — *see* Hernia, by site
  intestine 569.89
  joint (*see also* Arthritis, suppurative) 711.0 ✓5ᵗʰ
  labyrinthine 386.33
  lung 513.0
  mammary gland 611.0
    puerperal, postpartum 675.1 ✓5ᵗʰ
  maxilla, maxillary 526.4
    sinus (chronic) (*see also* Sinusitis, maxillary) 473.0
  muscle 728.0
  nasal sinus (chronic) (*see also* Sinusitis) 473.9
  pancreas 577.0
  parotid gland 527.2
  pelvis, pelvic
    female (*see also* Disease, pelvis, inflammatory) 614.4
      acute 614.3
    male (*see also* Peritonitis) 567.2
  pericranial (*see also* Osteomyelitis) 730.2 ✓5ᵗʰ
  salivary duct or gland (any) 527.2
  sinus (nasal) (*see also* Sinusitis) 473.9
  sphenoidal (sinus) (chronic) (*see also* Sinusitis, sphenoidal) 473.3
  thymus (gland) 254.1
  thyroid (gland) 245.0
  tonsil 474.8
  uterus (*see also* Endometritis) 615.9
  vagina 616.10
  wound — *see also* Wound, open, by site, complicated
    dislocation — *see* Dislocation, by site, compound
    fracture — *see* Fracture, by site, open
    scratch or other superficial injury — *see* Injury, superficial, by site
Supraglottitis 464.50
  with obstruction 464.51
Suprapubic drainage 596.8
Suprarenal (gland) — *see* condition
Suprascapular nerve — *see* condition
Suprasellar — *see* condition
Supraspinatus syndrome 726.10
Surfer knots 919.8
  infected 919.9
Surgery
  cosmetic NEC V50.1
    following healed injury or operation V51
    hair transplant V50.0
  elective V50.9
    breast augmentation or reduction V50.1
    circumcision, ritual or routine (in absence of medical indication) V50.2
    cosmetic NEC V50.1
    ear piercing V50.3
    face-lift V50.1
    following healed injury or operation V51
    hair transplant V50.0
  not done because of
    contraindication V64.1
    patient's decision V64.2
    specified reason NEC V64.3
  plastic
    breast augmentation or reduction V50.1
    cosmetic V50.1
    face-lift V50.1
    following healed injury or operation V51
    repair of scarred tissue (following healed injury or operation) V51
    specified type NEC V50.8

Surgery — *continued*
  previous, in pregnancy or childbirth
    cervix 654.6 ✓5ᵗʰ
      affecting fetus or newborn 763.89
      causing obstructed labor 660.2 ✓5ᵗʰ
        affecting fetus or newborn 763.1
    pelvic soft tissues NEC 654.9 ✓5ᵗʰ
      affecting fetus or newborn 763.89
      causing obstructed labor 660.2 ✓5ᵗʰ
        affecting fetus or newborn 763.1
    perineum or vulva 654.8 ✓5ᵗʰ
    uterus NEC 654.9 ✓5ᵗʰ
      affecting fetus or newborn 763.89
      causing obstructed labor 660.2 ✓5ᵗʰ
        affecting fetus or newborn 763.1
      due to previous cesarean delivery 654.2 ✓5ᵗʰ
    vagina 654.7 ✓5ᵗʰ
Surgical
  abortion — *see* Abortion, legal
  emphysema 998.81
  kidney (*see also* Pyelitis) 590.80
  operation NEC 799.9
  procedures, complication or misadventure — *see* Complications, surgical procedure
  shock 998.0
Suspected condition, ruled out (*see also* Observation, suspected) V71.9
  specified condition NEC V71.89
Suspended uterus, in pregnancy or childbirth 654.4 ✓5ᵗʰ
  affecting fetus or newborn 763.89
  causing obstructed labor 660.2 ✓5ᵗʰ
    affecting fetus or newborn 763.1
Sutton's disease 709.09
Sutton and Gull's disease (arteriolar nephrosclerosis) (*see also* Hypertension, kidney) 403.90
Suture
  burst (in ►external◄ operation wound) 998.32 ▲
    internal 998.31 ●
  inadvertently left in operation wound 998.4
  removal V58.3
  Shirodkar, in pregnancy (with or without cervical incompetence) 654.5 ✓5ᵗʰ
Swab inadvertently left in operation wound 998.4
Swallowed, swallowing
  difficulty (*see also* Dysphagia) 787.2
  foreign body NEC (*see also* Foreign body) 938
Swamp fever 100.89
Swan neck hand (intrinsic) 736.09
Sweat(s), sweating
  disease or sickness 078.2
  excessive 780.8
  fetid 705.89
  fever 078.2
  gland disease 705.9
    specified type NEC 705.89
  miliary 078.2
  night 780.8
Sweeley-Klionsky disease (angiokeratoma corporis diffusum) 272.7
Sweet's syndrome (acute febrile neutrophilic dermatosis) 695.89
Swelling
  abdominal (not referable to specific organ) 789.3 ✓5ᵗʰ
  adrenal gland, cloudy 255.8
  ankle 719.07
  anus 787.99
  arm 729.81
  breast 611.72
  Calabar 125.2
  cervical gland 785.6
  cheek 784.2
  chest 786.6
  ear 388.8
  epigastric 789.3 ✓5ᵗʰ
  extremity (lower) (upper) 729.81
  eye 379.92
  female genital organ 625.8
  finger 729.81
  foot 729.81

Swelling — *continued*
  glands 785.6
  gum 784.2
  hand 729.81
  head 784.2
  inflammatory — *see* Inflammation
  joint (*see also* Effusion, joint) 719.0 ✓5ᵗʰ
    tuberculous — *see* Tuberculosis, joint
  kidney, cloudy 593.89
  leg 729.81
  limb 729.81
  liver 573.8
  lung 786.6
  lymph nodes 785.6
  mediastinal 786.6
  mouth 784.2
  muscle (limb) 729.81
  neck 784.2
  nose or sinus 784.2
  palate 784.2
  pelvis 789.3 ✓5ᵗʰ
  penis 607.83
  perineum 625.8
  rectum 787.99
  scrotum 608.86
  skin 782.2
  splenic (*see also* Splenomegaly) 789.2
  substernal 786.6
  superficial, localized (skin) 782.2
  testicle 608.86
  throat 784.2
  toe 729.81
  tongue 784.2
  tubular (*see also* Disease, renal) 593.9
  umbilicus 789.3 ✓5ᵗʰ
  uterus 625.8
  vagina 625.8
  vulva 625.8
  wandering, due to Gnathostoma (spinigerum) 128.1
  white — *see* Tuberculosis, arthritis
Swift's disease 985.0
Swimmers'
  ear (acute) 380.12
  itch 120.3
Swimming in the head 780.4
Swollen — *see also* Swelling
  glands 785.6
Swyer-James syndrome (unilateral hyperlucent lung) 492.8
Swyer's syndrome (XY pure gonadal dysgenesis) 752.7
Sycosis 704.8
  barbae (not parasitic) 704.8
  contagiosa 110.0
  lupoid 704.8
  mycotic 110.0
  parasitic 110.0
  vulgaris 704.8
Sydenham's chorea — *see* Chorea, Sydenham's
Sylvatic yellow fever 060.0
Sylvest's disease (epidemic pleurodynia) 074.1
Symblepharon 372.63
  congenital 743.62
Symonds' syndrome 348.2
Sympathetic — *see* condition
Sympatheticotonia (*see also* Neuropathy, peripheral, autonomic) 337.9
Sympathicoblastoma (M9500/3)
  specified site — *see* Neoplasm, by site, malignant
  unspecified site 194.0
Sympathicogonioma (M9500/3) — *see* Sympathicoblastoma
Sympathoblastoma (M9500/3) — *see* Sympathicoblastoma
Sympathogonioma (M9500/3) — *see* Sympathicoblastoma
Symphalangy (*see also* Syndactylism) 755.10
Symptoms, specified (general) NEC 780.99 ▲
  abdomen NEC 789.9
  bone NEC 733.90
  breast NEC 611.79
  cardiac NEC 785.9

Suppuration — Symptoms, specified

Symptoms, specified — Syndrome

Symptoms, specified NEC — *continued*
  cardiovascular NEC 785.9
  chest NEC 786.9
  development NEC 783.9
  digestive system NEC 787.99
  eye NEC 379.99
  gastrointestinal tract NEC 787.99
  genital organs NEC
    female 625.9
    male 608.9
  head and neck NEC 784.9
  heart NEC 785.9
  joint NEC 719.60
    ankle 719.67
    elbow 719.62
    foot 719.67
    hand 719.64
    hip 719.65
    knee 719.66
    multiple sites 719.69
    pelvic region 719.65
    shoulder (region) 719.61
    specified site NEC 719.68
    wrist 719.63
  larynx NEC 784.9
  limbs NEC 729.89
  lymphatic system NEC 785.9
  menopausal 627.2
  metabolism NEC 783.9
  mouth NEC 528.9
  muscle NEC 728.9
  musculoskeletal NEC 781.99
    limbs NEC 729.89
  nervous system NEC 781.99
  neurotic NEC 300.9
  nutrition, metabolism, and development NEC
    783.9
  pelvis NEC 789.9
    female 625.9
  peritoneum NEC 789.9
  respiratory system NEC 786.9
  skin and integument NEC 782.9
  subcutaneous tissue NEC 782.9
  throat NEC 784.9
  tonsil NEC 784.9
  urinary system NEC 788.9
  vascular NEC 785.9
Sympus 759.89
Synarthrosis 719.80
  ankle 719.87
  elbow 719.82
  foot 719.87
  hand 719.84
  hip 719.85
  knee 719.86
  multiple sites 719.89
  pelvic region 719.85
  shoulder (region) 719.81
  specified site NEC 719.88
  wrist 719.83
Syncephalus 759.4
Synchondrosis 756.9
  abnormal (congenital) 756.9
  ischiopubic (van Neck's) 732.1
Synchysis (senile) (vitreous humor) 379.21
  scintillans 379.22
Syncope (near) (pre-) 780.2
  anginosa 413.9
  bradycardia 427.89
  cardiac 780.2
  carotid sinus 337.0
  complicating delivery 669.2 ✓5ᵗʰ
  due to lumbar puncture 349.0
  fatal 798.1
  heart 780.2
  heat 992.1
  laryngeal 786.2
  tussive 786.2
  vasoconstriction 780.2
  vasodepressor 780.2
  vasomotor 780.2
  vasovagal 780.2
Syncytial infarct — *see* Placenta, abnormal
Syndactylism, syndactyly (multiple sites) 755.10
  fingers (without fusion of bone) 755.11
    with fusion of bone 755.12

Syndactylism, syndactyly — *continued*
  toes (without fusion of bone) 755.13
    with fusion of bone 755.14
Syndrome — *see also* Disease
  abdominal
    acute 789.0 ✓5ᵗʰ
    migraine 346.2 ✓5ᵗʰ
    muscle deficiency 756.79
  Abercrombie's (amyloid degeneration) 277.3
  abnormal innervation 374.43
  abstinence
    alcohol 291.81
    drug 292.0
  Abt-Letterer-Siwe (acute histiocytosis X)
    (M9722/3) 202.5 ✓5ᵗʰ
  Achard-Thiers (adrenogenital) 255.2
  acid pulmonary aspiration 997.3
    obstetric (Mendelson's) 668.0 ✓5ᵗʰ
  acquired immune deficiency 042
  acquired immunodeficiency 042
  acrocephalosyndactylism 755.55
  acute abdominal 789.0 ✓5ᵗʰ
  acute chest 282.62 •
  acute coronary 411.1 •
  Adair-Dighton (brittle bones and blue sclera,
    deafness) 756.51
  Adams-Stokes (-Morgagni) (syncope with heart
    block) 426.9
  addisonian 255.4
  Adie (-Holmes) (pupil) 379.46
  adiposogenital 253.8
  adrenal
    hemorrhage 036.3
    meningococcic 036.3
  adrenocortical 255.3
  adrenogenital (acquired) (congenital) 255.2
    feminizing 255.2
    iatrogenic 760.79
    virilism (acquired) (congenital) 255.2
  affective organic NEC 293.89
    drug-induced 292.84
  afferent loop NEC 537.89
  African macroglobulinemia 273.3
  Ahumada-Del Castillo (nonpuerperal
    galactorrhea and amenorrhea) 253.1
  air blast concussion — *see* Injury, internal, by
    site
  Albright (-Martin) (pseudohypoparathyroidism)
    275.49
  Albright-McCune-Sternberg (osteitis fibrosa
    disseminata) 756.59
  alcohol withdrawal 291.81
  Alder's (leukocyte granulation anomaly) 288.2
  Aldrich (-Wiskott) (eczema-thrombocytopenia)
    279.12
  Alibert-Bazin (mycosis fungoides) (M9700/3)
    202.1 ✓5ᵗʰ
  Alice in Wonderland 293.89
  Allen-Masters 620.6
  Alligator baby (ichthyosis congenita) 757.1
  Alport's (hereditary hematuria-nephropathy-
    deafness) 759.89
  Alvarez (transient cerebral ischemia) 435.9
  alveolar capillary block 516.3
  Alzheimer's 331.0
    with dementia — *see* Alzheimer's, dementia
  amnestic (confabulatory) 294.0
    alcoholic 291.1
    drug-induced 292.83
    posttraumatic 294.0
  amotivational 292.89
  amyostatic 275.1
  amyotrophic lateral sclerosis 335.20
  angina (*see also* Angina) 413.9
  ankyloglossia superior 750.0
  anterior
    chest wall 786.52
    compartment (tibial) 958.8
    spinal artery 433.8 ✓5ᵗʰ
      compression 721.1
    tibial (compartment) 958.8
  antibody deficiency 279.00
    agammaglobulinemic 279.00
    congenital 279.04
    hypogammaglobulinemic 279.00
  anticardiolipin antibody 795.79
  antimongolism 758.3

Syndrome — *see also* Disease — *continued*
  antiphospholipid antibody 795.79
  Anton (-Babinski) (hemiasomatognosia) 307.9
  anxiety (*see also* Anxiety) 300.00
    organic 293.84
  aortic
    arch 446.7
    bifurcation (occlusion) 444.0
    ring 747.21
  Apert's (acrocephalosyndactyly) 755.55
  Apert-Gallais (adrenogenital) 255.2
  aphasia-apraxia-alexia 784.69
  "approximate answers" 300.16
  arcuate ligament (-celiac axis) 447.4
  arcus aortae 446.7
  arc-welders' 370.24
  argentaffin, argintaffinoma 259.2
  Argonz-Del Castillo (nonpuerperal galactorrhea
    and amenorrhea) 253.1
  Argyll Robertson's (syphilitic) 094.89
    nonsyphilitic 379.45
  arm-shoulder (*see also* Neuropathy, peripheral,
    autonomic) 337.9
  Arnold-Chiari (*see also* Spina bifida) 741.0 ✓5ᵗʰ
    type I 348.4
    type II 741.0 ✓5ᵗʰ
    type III 742.0
    type IV 742.2
  Arrillaga-Ayerza (pulmonary artery sclerosis
    with pulmonary hypertension) 416.0
  arteriomesenteric duodenum occlusion 537.89
  arteriovenous steal 996.73
  arteritis, young female (obliterative
    brachiocephalic) 446.7
  aseptic meningitis — *see* Meningitis, aseptic
  Asherman's 621.5
  asphyctic (*see also* Anxiety) 300.00
  aspiration, of newborn, massive or meconium
    770.1
  ataxia-telangiectasia 334.8
  Audry's (acropachyderma) 757.39
  auriculotemporal 350.8
  autosomal — *see also* Abnormal, autosomes
    NEC
    deletion 758.3
  Avellis' 344.89
  Axenfeld's 743.44
  Ayerza (-Arrillaga) (pulmonary artery sclerosis
    with pulmonary hypertension) 416.0
  Baader's (erythema multiforme exudativum)
    695.1
  Baastrup's 721.5
  Babinski (-Vaquez) (cardiovascular syphilis)
    093.89
  Babinski-Fröhlich (adiposogenital dystrophy)
    253.8
  Babinski-Nageotte 344.89
  Bagratuni's (temporal arteritis) 446.5
  Bakwin-Krida (craniometaphyseal dysplasia)
    756.89
  Balint's (psychic paralysis of visual
    disorientation) 368.16
  Ballantyne (-Runge) (postmaturity) 766.2
  ballooning posterior leaflet 424.0
  Banti's — *see* Cirrhosis, liver
  Bard-Pic's (carcinoma, head of pancreas) 157.0
  Bardet-Biedl (obesity, polydactyly, and mental
    retardation) 759.89
  Barlow's (mitral valve prolapse) 424.0
  Barlow (-Möller) (infantile scurvy) 267
  Baron Munchausen's 301.51
  Barré-Guillain 357.0
  Barré-Liéou (posterior cervical sympathetic)
    723.2
  Barrett's (chronic peptic ulcer of esophagus)
    530.2
  Bársony-Polgár (corkscrew esophagus) 530.5
  Bársony-Teschendorf (corkscrew esophagus)
    530.5
  Bartter's (secondary hyperaldosteronism with
    juxtaglomerular hyperplasia) 255.1
  Basedow's (exophthalmic goiter) 242.0 ✓5ᵗʰ
  basilar artery 435.0
  basofrontal 377.04
  Bassen-Kornzweig (abetalipoproteinemia) 272.5
  Batten-Steinert 359.2
  battered
    adult 995.81

Syndrome — *see also* Disease — *continued*
 battered — *continued*
  baby or child 995.54
  spouse 995.81
 Baumgarten-Cruveilhier (cirrhosis of liver)
   571.5
 Bearn-Kunkel (-Slater) (lupoid hepatitis) 571.49
 Beau's (*see also* Degeneration, myocardial)
   429.1
 Bechterew-Strümpell-Marie (ankylosing
   spondylitis) 720.0
 Beck's (anterior spinal artery occlusion)
   433.8 ✓5ᵗʰ
 Beckwith (-Wiedemann) 759.89
 Behçet's 136.1
 Bekhterev-Strümpell-Marie (ankylosing
   spondylitis) 720.0
 Benedikt's 344.89
 Béquez César (-Steinbrinck-Chédiak- Higashi)
   (congenital gigantism of peroxidase
   granules) 288.2
 Bernard-Horner (*see also* Neuropathy,
   peripheral, autonomic) 337.9
 Bernard-Sergent (acute adrenocortical
   insufficiency) 255.4
 Bernhardt-Roth 355.1
 Bernheim's (*see also* Failure, heart) 428.0
 Bertolotti's (sacralization of fifth lumbar
   vertebra) 756.15
 Besnier-Boeck-Schaumann (sarcoidosis) 135
 Bianchi's (aphasia-apraxia-alexia syndrome)
   784.69
 Biedl-Bardet (obesity, polydactyly, and mental
   retardation) 759.89
 Biemond's (obesity, polydactyly, and mental
   retardation) 759.89
 big spleen 289.4
 bilateral polycystic ovarian 256.4
 Bing-Horton's 346.2 ✓5ᵗʰ
 Biörck (-Thorson) (malignant carcinoid) 259.2
 Blackfan-Diamond (congenital hypoplastic
   anemia) 284.0
 black lung 500
 black widow spider bite 989.5
 bladder neck (*see also* Incontinence, urine)
   788.30
 blast (concussion) — *see* Blast, injury
 blind loop (postoperative) 579.2
 Bloch-Siemens (incontinentia pigmenti) 757.33
 Bloch-Sulzberger (incontinentia pigmenti)
   757.33
 Bloom (-Machacek) (-Torre) 757.39
 Blount-Barber (tibia vara) 732.4
 blue
  bloater 491.2 ✓5ᵗʰ
  diaper 270.0
  drum 381.02
  sclera 756.51
  toe — *see* Atherosclerosis
 Boder-Sedgwick (ataxia-telangiectasia) 334.8
 Boerhaave's (spontaneous esophageal rupture)
   530.4
 Bonnevie-Ullrich 758.6
 Bonnier's 386.19
 Bouillaud's (rheumatic heart disease) 391.9
 Bourneville (-Pringle) (tuberous sclerosis) 759.5
 Bouveret (-Hoffmann) (paroxysmal tachycardia)
   427.2
 brachial plexus 353.0
 Brachman-de Lange (Amsterdam dwarf, mental
   retardation, and brachycephaly) 759.89
 bradycardia-tachycardia 427.81
 Brailsford-Morquio (dystrophy)
   (mucopolysaccharidosis IV) 277.5
 brain (acute) (chronic) (nonpsychotic) (organic)
   (with behavioral reaction) (with neurotic
   reaction) 310.9
  with
   presenile brain disease (*see also*
    Dementia, presenile) 290.10
   psychosis, psychotic reaction (*see also*
    Psychosis, organic) 294.9
  chronic alcoholic 291.2
  congenital (*see also* Retardation, mental)
    319
  postcontusional 310.2
  posttraumatic
   nonpsychotic 310.2

Syndrome — *see also* Disease — *continued*
 brain — *continued*
  posttraumatic — *continued*
   psychotic 293.9
    acute 293.0
    chronic (*see also* Psychosis, organic)
      294.8
    subacute 293.1
  psycho-organic (*see also* Syndrome, psycho-
    organic) 310.9
   psychotic (*see also* Psychosis, organic) 294.9
   senile (*see also* Dementia, senile) 290.0
 branchial arch 744.41
 Brandt's (acrodermatitis enteropathica) 686.8
 Brennemann's 289.2
 Briquet's 300.81
 Brissaud-Meige (infantile myxedema) 244.9
 broad ligament laceration 620.6
 Brock's (atelectasis due to enlarged lymph
   nodes) 518.0
 Brown's tendon sheath 378.61
 Brown-Séquard 344.89
 brown spot 756.59
 Brugada 746.89
 Brugsch's (acropachyderma) 757.39
 bubbly lung 770.7
 Buchem's (hyperostosis corticalis) 733.3
 Budd-Chiari (hepatic vein thrombosis) 453.0
 Büdinger-Ludloff-Läwen 717.89
 bulbar 335.22
  lateral (*see also* Disease, cerebrovascular,
    acute) 436
 Bullis fever 082.8
 bundle of Kent (anomalous atrioventricular
   excitation) 426.7
 Bürger-Grütz (essential familial hyperlipemia)
   272.3
 Burke's (pancreatic insufficiency and chronic
   neutropenia) 577.8
 Burnett's (milk-alkali) 999.9
 Burnier's (hypophyseal dwarfism) 253.3
 burning feet 266.2
 Bywaters' 958.5
 Caffey's (infantile cortical hyperostosis) 756.59
 Calvé-Legg-Perthes (osteochrondrosis, femoral
   capital) 732.1
 Caplan (-Colinet) syndrome 714.81
 capsular thrombosis (*see also* Thrombosis,
   brain) 434.0 ✓5ᵗʰ
 carcinogenic thrombophlebitis 453.1
 carcinoid 259.2
 cardiac asthma (*see also* Failure, ventricular,
   left) 428.1
 cardiacos negros 416.0
 cardiopulmonary obesity 278.8
 cardiorenal (*see also* Hypertension, cardiorenal)
   404.90
 cardiorespiratory distress (idiopathic), newborn
   769
 cardiovascular renal (*see also* Hypertension,
   cardiorenal) 404.90
 cardiovasorenal 272.7
 Carini's (ichthyosis congenita) 757.1
 carotid
  artery (internal) 435.8
  body or sinus 337.0
 carpal tunnel 354.0
 Carpenter's 759.89
 Cassidy (-Scholte) (malignant carcinoid) 259.2
 cat-cry 758.3
 cauda equina 344.60
 causalgia 355.9
  lower limb 355.71
  upper limb 354.4
 cavernous sinus 437.6
 celiac 579.0
  artery compression 447.4
  axis 447.4
 cerebellomedullary malformation (*see also*
   Spina bifida) 741.0 ✓5ᵗʰ
 cerebral gigantism 253.0
 cerebrohepatorenal 759.89
 cervical (root) (spine) NEC 723.8
  disc 722.71
  posterior, sympathetic 723.2
  rib 353.0
  sympathetic paralysis 337.0
  traumatic (acute) NEC 847.0

Syndrome — *see also* Disease — *continued*
 cervicobrachial (diffuse) 723.3
 cervicocranial 723.2
 cervicodorsal outlet 353.2
 Céstan's 344.89
 Céstan (-Raymond) 433.8 ✓5ᵗʰ
 Céstan-Chenais 344.89
 chancriform 114.1
 Charcôt's (intermittent claudication) 443.9
  angina cruris 443.9
  due to atherosclerosis 440.21
 Charcôt-Marie-Tooth 356.1
 Charcôt-Weiss-Baker 337.0
 Cheadle (-Möller) (-Barlow) (infantile scurvy)
   267
 Chédiak-Higashi (-Steinbrinck) (congenital
   gigantism of peroxidase granules) 288.2
 chest wall 786.52
 Chiari's (hepatic vein thrombosis) 453.0
 Chiari-Frommel 676.6 ✓5ᵗʰ
 chiasmatic 368.41
 Chilaiditi's (subphrenic displacement, colon)
   751.4
 chondroectodermal dysplasia 756.55
 chorea-athetosis-agitans 275.1
 Christian's (chronic histiocytosis X) 277.8
 chromosome 4 short arm deletion 758.3
 Churg-Strauss 446.4
 Clarke-Hadfield (pancreatic infantilism) 577.8
 Claude's 352.6
 Claude Bernard-Horner (*see also* Neuropathy,
   peripheral, autonomic) 337.9
 Clérambault's
  automatism 348.8
  erotomania 297.8
 Clifford's (postmaturity) 766.2
 climacteric 627.2
 Clouston's (hidrotic ectodermal dysplasia)
   757.31
 clumsiness 315.4
 Cockayne's (microencephaly and dwarfism)
   759.89
 Cockayne-Weber (epidermolysis bullosa) 757.39
 Cogan's (nonsyphilitic interstitial keratitis)
   370.52
 cold injury (newborn) 778.2
 Collet (-Sicard) 352.6
 combined immunity deficiency 279.2
 compartment(al) (anterior) (deep) (posterior)
   (tibial) 958.8
  nontraumatic 729.9
 compression 958.5
  cauda equina 344.60
   with neurogenic bladder 344.61
 concussion 310.2
 congenital
  affecting more than one system 759.7
   specified type NEC 759.89
  facial diplegia 352.6
  muscular hypertrophy-cerebral 759.89
 congestion-fibrosis (pelvic) 625.5
 conjunctivourethrosynovial 099.3
 Conn (-Louis) (primary aldosteronism) 255.1
 Conradi (-Hünermann) (chondrodysplasia
   calcificans congenita) 756.59
 conus medullaris 336.8
 Cooke-Apert-Gallais (adrenogenital) 255.2
 Cornelia de Lange's (Amsterdam dwarf, mental
   retardation, and brachycephaly)
   759.8 ✓5ᵗʰ
 coronary insufficiency or intermediate 411.1
 cor pulmonale 416.9
 corticosexual 255.2
 Costen's (complex) 524.60
 costochondral junction 733.6
 costoclavicular 353.0
 costovertebral 253.0
 Cotard's (paranoia) 297.1
 craniovertebral 723.2
 Creutzfeldt-Jakob 046.1
  with dementia
   with behavioral disturbance 046.1
     [294.11]
   without behavioral disturbance 046.1
     [294.10]
 crib death 798.0
 cricopharyngeal 787.2
 cri-du-chat 758.3

Syndrome — Syndrome

Syndrome — *see also* Disease — *continued*
Crigler-Najjar (congenital hyperbilirubinemia)
277.4
crocodile tears 351.8
Cronkhite-Canada 211.3
croup 464.4
CRST (cutaneous systemic sclerosis) 710.1
crush 958.5
crushed lung (*see also* Injury, internal, lung)
861.20
Cruveilhier-Baumgarten (cirrhosis of liver)
571.5
cubital tunnel 354.2
Cuiffini-Pancoast (M8010/3) (carcinoma,
pulmonary apex) 162.3
Curschmann (-Batten) (-Steinert) 359.2
Cushing's (iatrogenic) (idiopathic) (pituitary
basophilism) (pituitary-dependent) 255.0
overdose or wrong substance given or taken
962.0
Cyriax's (slipping rib) 733.99
cystic duct stump 576.0
Da Costa's (neurocirculatory asthenia) 306.2
Dameshek's (erythroblastic anemia) 282.4
Dana-Putnam (subacute combined sclerosis
with pernicious anemia) 281.0 *[336.2]*
Danbolt (-Closs) (acrodermatitis enteropathica)
686.8
Dandy-Walker (atresia, foramen of Magendie)
742.3
with spina bifida (*see also* Spina bifida)
741.0 ✓5ᵗʰ
Danlos' 756.83
Davies-Colley (slipping rib) 733.99
dead fetus 641.3 ✓5ᵗʰ
defeminization 255.2
defibrination (*see also* Fibrinolysis) 286.6
Degos' 447.8
Deiters' nucleus 386.19
Déjérine-Roussy 348.8
Déjérine-Thomas 333.0
de Lange's (Amsterdam dwarf, mental
retardation, and brachycephaly)
(Cornelia) 759.89
Del Castillo's (germinal aplasia) 606.0
deletion chromosomes 758.3
delusional
induced by drug 292.11
dementia-aphonia, of childhood (*see also*
Psychosis, childhood) 299.1 ✓5ᵗʰ
demyelinating NEC 341.9
denial visual hallucination 307.9
depersonalization 300.6
Dercum's (adiposis dolorosa) 272.8
de Toni-Fanconi (-Debré) (cystinosis) 270.0
diabetes-dwarfism-obesity (juvenile) 258.1
diabetes mellitus-hypertension-nephrosis
250.4 ✓5ᵗʰ *[581.81]*
diabetes mellitus in newborn infant 775.1
diabetes-nephrosis 250.4 ✓5ᵗʰ *[581.81]*
diabetic amyotrophy 250.6 ✓5ᵗʰ *[358.1]*
Diamond-Blackfan (congenital hypoplastic
anemia) 284.0
Diamond-Gardener (autoerythrocyte
sensitization) 287.2
DIC (diffuse or disseminated intravascular
coagulopathy) (*see also* Fibrinolysis)
286.6
diencephalohypophyseal NEC 253.8
diffuse cervicobrachial 723.3
diffuse obstructive pulmonary 496
DiGeorge's (thymic hypoplasia) 279.11
Dighton's 756.51
Di Guglielmo's (erythremic myelosis) (M9841/3)
207.0 ✓5ᵗʰ
disc — *see* Displacement, intervertebral disc
discogenic — *see* Displacement, intervertebral
disc
disequilibrium 276.9
disseminated platelet thrombosis 446.6
Ditthomska 307.81
Doan-Wiseman (primary splenic neutropenia)
288.0
Döhle body-panmyelopathic 288.2
Donohue's (leprechaunism) 259.8
dorsolateral medullary (*see also* Disease,
cerebrovascular, acute) 436
double whammy 360.81

Syndrome — *see also* Disease — *continued*
Down's (mongolism) 758.0
Dresbach's (elliptocytosis) 282.1
Dressler's (postmyocardial infarction) 411.0
hemoglobinuria 283.2
drug withdrawal, infant, of dependent mother
779.5
dry skin 701.1
eye 375.15
DSAP (disseminated superficial actinic
porokeratosis) 692.75
Duane's (retraction) 378.71
Duane-Stilling-Türk (ocular retraction
syndrome) 378.71
Dubin-Johnson (constitutional
hyperbilirubinemia) 277.4
Dubin-Sprinz (constitutional
hyperbilirubinemia) 277.4
Duchenne's 335.22
due to abnormality
autosomal NEC (*see also* Abnormal,
autosomes NEC) 758.5
13 758.1
18 758.2
21 or 22 758.0
D 758.1
E 758.2
G 758.0
chromosomal 758.89
sex 758.81
dumping 564.2
nonsurgical 536.8
Duplay's 726.2
Dupré's (meningism) 781.6
Dyke-Young (acquired macrocytic hemolytic
anemia) 283.9
dyspraxia 315.4
dystocia, dystrophia 654.9 ✓5ᵗʰ
Eagle-Barret 756.71
Eales 362.18
Eaton-Lambert (*see also* Neoplasm, by site,
malignant) 199.1 *[358.1]*
Ebstein's (downward displacement, tricuspid
valve into right ventricle) 746.2
ectopic ACTH secretion 255.0
eczema-thrombocytopenia 279.12
Eddowes' (brittle bones and blue sclera) 756.51
Edwards' 758.2
efferent loop 537.89
effort (aviators') (psychogenic) 306.2
Ehlers-Danlos 756.83
Eisenmenger's (ventricular septal defect) 745.4
Ekbom's (restless legs) 333.99
Ekman's (brittle bones and blue sclera) 756.51
electric feet 266.2
Elephant man 237.71
Ellison-Zollinger (gastric hypersecretion with
pancreatic islet cell tumor) 251.5
Ellis-van Creveld (chondroectodermal
dysplasia) 756.55
embryonic fixation 270.2
empty sella (turcica) 253.8
endocrine-hypertensive 255.3
Engel-von Recklinghausen (osteitis fibrosa
cystica) 252.0
enteroarticular 099.3
entrapment — *see* Neuropathy, entrapment
eosinophilia myalgia 710.5
epidemic vomiting 078.82
Epstein's — *see* Nephrosis
Erb (-Oppenheim) — Goldflam 358.0
Erdheim's (acromegalic macrospondylitis) 253.0
Erlacher-Blount (tibia vara) 732.4
erythrocyte fragmentation 283.19
euthyroid sick 790.94
Evans' (thrombocytopenic purpura) 287.3
excess cortisol, iatrogenic 255.0
exhaustion 300.5
extrapyramidal 333.90
eyelid-malar-mandible 756.0
eye retraction 378.71
Faber's (achlorhydric anemia) 280.9
Fabry (-Anderson) (angiokeratoma corporis
diffusum) 272.7
facet 724.8
Fallot's 745.2
falx (*see also* Hemorrhage, brain) 431
familial eczema-thrombocytopenia 279.12

Syndrome — *see also* Disease — *continued*
Fanconi's (anemia) (congenital pancytopenia)
284.0
Fanconi (-de Toni) (-Debré) (cystinosis) 270.0
Farber (-Uzman) (disseminated
lipogranulomatosis) 272.8
fatigue NEC 300.5
chronic 780.71
faulty bowel habit (idiopathic megacolon) 564.7
FDH (focal dermal hypoplasia) 757.39
fecal reservoir 560.39
Feil-Klippel (brevicollis) 756.16
Felty's (rheumatoid arthritis with splenomegaly
and leukopenia) 714.1
fertile eunuch 257.2
fetal alcohol 760.71
late effect 760.71
fibrillation-flutter 427.32
fibrositis (periarticular) 729.0
Fiedler's (acute isolated myocarditis) 422.91
Fiessinger-Leroy (-Reiter) 099.3
Fiessinger-Rendu (erythema multiforme
exudativum) 695.1
first arch 756.0
Fisher's 357.0
Fitz's (acute hemorrhagic pancreatitis) 577.0
Fitz-Hugh and Curtis (gonococcal peritonitis)
098.86
Flajani (-Basedow) (exophthalmic goiter)
242.0 ✓5ᵗʰ
floppy
infant 781.99
valve (mitral) 424.0
flush 259.2
Foix-Alajouanine 336.1
Fong's (hereditary osteo-onychodysplasia)
756.89
foramen magnum 348.4
Forbes-Albright (nonpuerperal amenorrhea and
lactation associated with pituitary tumor)
253.1
Foster-Kennedy 377.04
Foville's (peduncular) 344.89
fragile X 759.83
Franceschetti's (mandibulofacial dysostosis)
756.0
Fraser's 759.89
Freeman-Sheldon 759.89
Frey's (auriculotemporal) 350.8
Friderichsen-Waterhouse 036.3
Friedrich-Erb-Arnold (acropachyderma) 757.39
Fröhlich's (adiposogenital dystrophy) 253.8
Froin's 336.8
Frommel-Chiari 676.6 ✓5ᵗʰ
frontal lobe 310.0
Fuller Albright's (osteitis fibrosa disseminata)
756.59
functional
bowel 564.9
prepubertal castrate 752.8
Gaisböck's (polycythemia hypertonica) 289.0
ganglion (basal, brain) 333.90
geniculi 351.1
Ganser's, hysterical 300.16
Gardner-Diamond (autoerythrocyte
sensitization) 287.2
gastroesophageal junction 530.0
gastroesophageal laceration-hemorrhage 530.7
gastrojejunal loop obstruction 537.89
Gayet-Wernicke's (superior hemorrhagic
polioencephalitis) 265.1
Gee-Herter-Heubner (nontropical sprue) 579.0
Gélineau's 347
genito-anorectal 099.1
Gerhardt's (vocal cord paralysis) 478.30
Gerstmann's (finger agnosia) 784.69
Gilbert's 277.4
Gilford (-Hutchinson) (progeria) 259.8
Gilles de la Tourette's 307.23
Gillespie's (dysplasia oculodentodigitalis)
759.89
Glénard's (enteroptosis) 569.89
Glinski-Simmonds (pituitary cachexia) 253.2
glucuronyl transferase 277.4
glue ear 381.20
Goldberg (-Maxwell) (-Morris) (testicular
feminization) 257.8

Syndrome — *see also* Disease — *continued*
  Goldenhar's (oculoauriculovertebral dysplasia) 756.0
  Goldflam-Erb 358.0
  Goltz-Gorlin (dermal hypoplasia) 757.39
  Goodpasture's (pneumorenal) 446.21
  Gopalan's (burning feet) 266.2
  Gorlin-Chaudhry-Moss 759.89
  Gougerot (-Houwer) — Sjögren (keratoconjunctivitis sicca) 710.2
  Gougerot-Blum (pigmented purpuric lichenoid dermatitis) 709.1
  Gougerot-Carteaud (confluent reticulate papillomatosis) 701.8
  Gouley's (constrictive pericarditis) 423.2
  Gowers' (vasovagal attack) 780.2
  Gowers-Paton-Kennedy 377.04
  Gradenigo's 383.02
  gray or grey (chloramphenicol) (newborn) 779.4
  Greig's (hypertelorism) 756.0
  Gubler-Millard 344.89
  Guérin-Stern (arthrogryposis multiplex congenita) 754.89
  Guillain-Barré (-Strohl) 357.0
  Gunn's (jaw-winking syndrome) 742.8
  Günther's (congenital erythropoietic porphyria) 277.1
  gustatory sweating 350.8
  H₃O 759.81
  Hadfield-Clarke (pancreatic infantilism) 577.8
  Haglund-Läwen-Fründ 717.89
  hairless women 257.8
  Hallermann-Streiff 756.0
  Hallervorden-Spatz 333.0
  Hamman's (spontaneous mediastinal emphysema) 518.1
  Hamman-Rich (diffuse interstitial pulmonary fibrosis) 516.3
  Hand-Schüller-Christian (chronic histiocytosis X) 277.8
  hand-foot 282.61
  Hanot-Chauffard (-Troisier) (bronze diabetes) 275.0
  Harada's 363.22
  Hare's (M8010/3) (carcinoma, pulmonary apex) 162.3
  Harkavy's 446.0
  harlequin color change 779.89 ▲
  Harris' (organic hyperinsulinism) 251.1
  Hart's (pellagra-cerebellar ataxia-renal aminoaciduria) 270.0
  Hayem-Faber (achlorhydric anemia) 280.9
  Hayem-Widal (acquired hemolytic jaundice) 283.9
  Heberden's (angina pectoris) 413.9
  Hedinger's (malignant carcinoid) 259.2
  Hegglin's 288.2
  Heller's (infantile psychosis) (*see also* Psychosis, childhood) 299.1 ✓5ᵗʰ
  H.E.L.L.P 642.5 ✓5ᵗʰ
  hemolytic-uremic (adult) (child) 283.11
  Hench-Rosenberg (palindromic arthritis) (*see also* Rheumatism, palindromic) 719.3 ✓5ᵗʰ
  Henoch-Schönlein (allergic purpura) 287.0
  hepatic flexure 569.89
  hepatorenal 572.4
    due to a procedure 997.4
    following delivery 674.8 ✓5ᵗʰ
  hepatourologic 572.4
  Herrick's (hemoglobin S disease) 282.61
  Herter (-Gee) (nontropical sprue) 579.0
  Heubner-Herter (nontropical sprue) 579.0
  Heyd's (hepatorenal) 572.4
  HHHO 759.81
  Hilger's 337.0
  Hoffa (-Kastert) (liposynovitis prepatellaris) 272.8
  Hoffmann's 244.9 [359.5]
  Hoffmann-Bouveret (paroxysmal tachycardia) 427.2
  Hoffmann-Werdnig 335.0
  Holländer-Simons (progressive lipodystrophy) 272.6
  Holmes' (visual disorientation) 368.16
  Holmes-Adie 379.46
  Hoppe-Goldflam 358.0

Syndrome — *see also* Disease — *continued*
  Horner's (*see also* Neuropathy, peripheral, autonomic) 337.9
    traumatic — *see* Injury, nerve, cervical sympathetic
  hospital addiction 301.51
  Hunt's (herpetic geniculate ganglionitis) 053.11
    dyssynergia cerebellaris myoclonica 334.2
  Hunter (-Hurler) (mucopolysaccharidosis II) 277.5
  hunterian glossitis 529.4
  Hurler (-Hunter) (mucopolysaccharidosis II) 277.5
  Hutchinson's incisors or teeth 090.5
  Hutchinson-Boeck (sarcoidosis) 135
  Hutchinson-Gilford (progeria) 259.8
  hydralazine
    correct substance properly administered 695.4
    overdose or wrong substance given or taken 972.6
  hydraulic concussion (abdomen) (*see also* Injury, internal, abdomen) 868.00
  hyperabduction 447.8
  hyperactive bowel 564.9
  hyperaldosteronism with hypokalemic alkalosis (Bartter's) 255.1
  hypercalcemic 275.42
  hypercoagulation NEC 289.8
  hypereosinophilic (idiopathic) 288.3
  hyperkalemic 276.7
  hyperkinetic — *see also* Hyperkinesia
    heart 429.82
  hyperlipemia-hemolytic anemia-icterus 571.1
  hypermobility 728.5
  hypernatremia 276.0
  hyperosmolarity 276.0
  hypersomnia-bulimia 349.89
  hypersplenic 289.4
  hypersympathetic (*see also* Neuropathy, peripheral, autonomic) 337.9
  hypertransfusion, newborn 776.4
  hyperventilation, psychogenic 306.1
  hyperviscosity (of serum) NEC 273.3
    polycythemic 289.0
    sclerothymic 282.8
  hypoglycemic (familial) (neonatal) 251.2
    functional 251.1
  hypokalemic 276.8
  hypophyseal 253.8
  hypophyseothalamic 253.8
  hypopituitarism 253.2
  hypoplastic left heart 746.7
  hypopotassemia 276.8
  hyposmolality 276.1
  hypotension, maternal 669.2 ✓5ᵗʰ
  hypotonia-hypomentia-hypogonadism-obesity 759.81
  ICF (intravascular coagulation-fibrinolysis) (*see also* Fibrinolysis) 286.6
  idiopathic cardiorespiratory distress, newborn 769
  idiopathic nephrotic (infantile) 581.9
  Imerslund (-Gräsbeck) (anemia due to familial selective vitamin B₁₂ malabsorption) 281.1
  immobility (paraplegic) 728.3
  immunity deficiency, combined 279.2
  impending coronary 411.1
  impingement
    shoulder 726.2
    vertebral bodies 724.4
  inappropriate secretion of antidiuretic hormone (ADH) 253.6
  incomplete
    mandibulofacial 756.0
  infant
    death, sudden (SIDS) 798.0
    Hercules 255.2
    of diabetic mother 775.0
    shaken 995.55
  infantilism 253.3
  inferior vena cava 459.2
  influenza-like 487.1
  inspissated bile, newborn 774.4
  intermediate coronary (artery) 411.1
  internal carotid artery (*see also* Occlusion, artery, carotid) 433.1 ✓5ᵗʰ

Syndrome — *see also* Disease — *continued*
  interspinous ligament 724.8
  intestinal
    carcinoid 259.2
    gas 787.3
    knot 560.2
  intravascular
    coagulation-fibrinolysis (ICF) (*see also* Fibrinolysis) 286.6
    coagulopathy (*see also* Fibrinolysis) 286.6
  inverted Marfan's 759.89
  IRDS (idiopathic respiratory distress, newborn) 769
  irritable
    bowel 564.1
    heart 306.2
    weakness 300.5
  ischemic bowel (transient) 557.9
    chronic 557.1
    due to mesenteric artery insufficiency 557.1
  Itsenko-Cushing (pituitary basophilism) 255.0
  IVC (intravascular coagulopathy) (*see also* Fibrinolysis) 286.6
  Ivemark's (asplenia with congenital heart disease) 759.0
  Jaccoud's 714.4
  Jackson's 344.89
  Jadassohn-Lewandowski (pachyonchia congenita) 757.5
  Jaffe-Lichtenstein (-Uehlinger) 252.0
  Jahnke's (encephalocutaneous angiomatosis) 759.6
  Jakob-Creutzfeldt 046.1
    with dementia
      with behavioral disturbance 046.1 [294.11]
      without behavioral disturbance 046.1 [294.10]
  Jaksch's (pseudoleukemia infantum) 285.8
  Jaksch-Hayem (-Luzet) (pseudoleukemia infantum) 285.8
  jaw-winking 742.8
  jejunal 564.2
  jet lag 307.45
  Jeune's (asphyxiating thoracic dystrophy of newborn) 756.4
  Job's (chronic granulomatous disease) 288.1
  Jordan's 288.2
  Joseph-Diamond-Blackfan (congenital hypoplastic anemia) 284.0
  Joubert 759.89
  jugular foramen 352.6
  Kahler's (multiple myeloma) (M9730/3) 203.0 ✓5ᵗʰ
  Kalischer's (encephalocutaneous angiomatosis) 759.6
  Kallmann's (hypogonadotropic hypogonadism with anosmia) 253.4
  Kanner's (autism) (*see also* Psychosis, childhood) 299.0 ✓5ᵗʰ
  Kartagener's (sinusitis, bronchiectasis, situs inversus) 759.3
  Kasabach-Merritt (capillary hemangioma associated with thrombocytopenic purpura) 287.3
  Kast's (dyschondroplasia with hemangiomas) 756.4
  Kaznelson's (congenital hypoplastic anemia) 284.0
  Kelly's (sideropenic dysphagia) 280.8
  Kimmelstiel-Wilson (intercapillary glomerulosclerosis) 250.4 ✓5ᵗʰ [581.81]
  Klauder's (erythema multiforme exudativum) 695.1
  Klein-Waardenburg (ptosis-epicanthus) 270.2
  Kleine-Levin 349.89
  Klinefelter's 758.7
  Klippel-Feil (brevicollis) 756.16
  Klippel-Trenaunay 759.89
  Klumpke (-Déjérine) (injury to brachial plexus at birth) 767.6
  Klüver-Bucy (-Terzian) 310.0
  Köhler-Pellegrini-Stieda (calcification, knee joint) 726.62
  König's 564.89
  Korsakoff's (nonalcoholic) 294.0
    alcoholic 291.1

Syndrome — Syndrome

Syndrome — *see also* Disease — *continued*
Korsakoff (-Wernicke) (nonalcoholic) 294.0
  alcoholic 291.1
Kostmann's (infantile genetic agranulocytosis) 288.0
Krabbe's
  congenital muscle hypoplasia 756.89
  cutaneocerebral angioma 759.6
Kunkel (lupoid hepatitis) 571.49
labyrinthine 386.50
laceration, broad ligament 620.6
Langdon Down (mongolism) 758.0
Larsen's (flattened facies and multiple congenital dislocations) 755.8
lateral
  cutaneous nerve of thigh 355.1
  medullary (*see also* Disease, cerebrovascular acute) 436
Launois' (pituitary gigantism) 253.0
Launois-Cléret (adiposogenital dystrophy) 253.8
Laurence-Moon (-Bardet) — Biedl (obesity, polydactyly, and mental retardation) 759.89
Lawford's (encephalocutaneous angiomatosis) 759.6
lazy
  leukocyte 288.0
  posture 728.3
Lederer-Brill (acquired infectious hemolytic anemia) 283.19
Legg-Calvé-Perthes (osteochondrosis capital femoral) 732.1
Lennox (*see also* Epilepsy) 345.0 ✓5ᵗʰ
lenticular 275.1
Léopold-Lévi's (paroxysmal thyroid instability) 242.9 ✓5ᵗʰ
Lepore hemoglobin 282.4
Léri-Weill 756.59
Leriche's (aortic bifurcation occlusion) 444.0
Lermoyez's (*see also* Disease, Ménière's) 386.00
Lesch-Nyhan (hypoxanthine-guanine-phosphoribosyltransferase deficiency) 277.2
Lev's (acquired complete heart block) 426.0
Levi's (pituitary dwarfism) 253.3
Lévy-Roussy 334.3
Lichtheim's (subacute combined sclerosis with pernicious anemia) 281.0 [336.2]
Li-Fraumeni 758.3
Lightwood's (renal tubular acidosis) 588.8
Lignac (-de Toni) (-Fanconi) (-Debré) (cystinosis) 270.0
Likoff's (angina in menopausal women) 413.9
liver-kidney 572.4
Lloyd's 258.1
lobotomy 310.0
Löffler's (eosinophilic pneumonitis) 518.3
Löfgren's (sarcoidosis) 135
long arm 18 or 21 deletion 758.3
Looser (-Debray) — Milkman (osteomalacia with pseudofractures) 268.2
Lorain-Levi (pituitary dwarfism) 253.3
Louis-Bar (ataxia-telangiectasia) 334.8
low
  atmospheric pressure 993.2
  back 724.2
    psychogenic 306.0
  output (cardiac) (*see also* Failure, heart) 428.9
Lowe's (oculocerebrorenal dystrophy) 270.8
Lowe-Terrey-MacLachlan (oculocerebrorenal dystrophy) 270.8
lower radicular, newborn 767.4
Lown (-Ganong)-Levine (short P-R interval, normal QRS complex, and supraventricular tachycardia) 426.81
Lucey-Driscoll (jaundice due to delayed conjugation) 774.30
Luetscher's (dehydration) 276.5
lumbar vertebral 724.4
Lutembacher's (atrial septal defect with mitral stenosis) 745.5
Lyell's (toxic epidermal necrolysis) 695.1
  due to drug
    correct substance properly administered 695.1
    overdose or wrong substance given or taken 977.9

Syndrome — *see also* Disease — *continued*
Lyell's — *continued*
  due to drug — *continued*
    overdose or wrong substance given or taken — *continued*
      specified drug — *see* Table of Drugs and Chemicals
MacLeod's 492.8
macrogenitosomia praecox 259.8
macroglobulinemia 273.3
Maffucci's (dyschondroplasia with hemangiomas) 756.4
Magenblase 306.4
magnesium-deficiency 781.7
malabsorption 579.9
  postsurgical 579.3
  spinal fluid 331.3
malignant carcinoid 259.2
Mallory-Weiss 530.7
mandibulofacial dysostosis 756.0
manic-depressive (*see also* Psychosis, affective) 296.80
Mankowsky's (familial dysplastic osteopathy) 731.2
maple syrup (urine) 270.3
Marable's (celiac artery compression) 447.4
Marchesani (-Weill) (brachymorphism and ectopia lentis) 759.89
Marchiafava-Bignami 341.8
Marchiafava-Micheli (paroxysmal nocturnal hemoglobinuria) 283.2
Marcus Gunn's (jaw-winking syndrome) 742.8
Marfan's (arachnodactyly) 759.82
  meaning congenital syphilis 090.49
  with luxation of lens 090.49 [379.32]
Marie's (acromegaly) 253.0
  primary or idiopathic (acropachyderma) 757.39
  secondary (hypertrophic pulmonary osteoarthropathy) 731.2
Markus-Adie 379.46
Maroteaux-Lamy (mucopolysaccharidosis VI) 277.5
Martin's 715.27
Martin-Albright (pseudohypoparathyroidism) 275.49
Martorell-Fabré (pulseless disease) 446.7
massive aspiration of newborn 770.1
Masters-Allen 620.6
mastocytosis 757.33
maternal hypotension 669.2 ✓5ᵗʰ
maternal obesity 646.1 ✓5ᵗʰ
May (-Hegglin) 288.2
McArdle (-Schmid) (-Pearson) (glycogenosis V) 271.0
McCune-Albright (osteitis fibrosa disseminata) 756.59
McQuarrie's (idiopathic familial hypoglycemia) 251.2
meconium
  aspiration 770.1
  plug (newborn) NEC 777.1
median arcuate ligament 447.4
mediastinal fibrosis 519.3
Meekeren-Ehlers-Danlos 756.83
Meige (blepharospasm-oromandibular dystonia) 333.82
  -Milroy (chronic hereditary edema) 757.0
MELAS 758.89
Melkersson (-Rosenthal) 351.8
Mende's (ptosis-epicanthus) 270.2
Mendelson's (resulting from a procedure) 997.3
  during labor 668.0 ✓5ᵗʰ
  obstetric 668.0 ✓5ᵗʰ
Ménétrier's (hypertrophic gastritis) 535.2 ✓5ᵗʰ
Ménière's (*see also* Disease, Ménière's) 386.00
meningo-eruptive 047.1
Menkes' 759.89
  glutamic acid 759.89
  maple syrup (urine) disease 270.3
menopause 627.2
  postartificial 627.4
menstruation 625.4
MERFF 758.89
mesenteric
  artery, superior 557.1
  vascular insufficiency (with gangrene) 557.1
metastatic carcinoid 259.2

Syndrome — *see also* Disease — *continued*
Meyenburg-Altherr-Uehlinger 733.99
Meyer-Schwickerath and Weyers (dysplasia oculodentodigitalis) 759.89
Micheli-Rietti (thalassemia minor) 282.4
Michotte's 721.5
micrognathia-glossoptosis 756.0
microphthalmos (congenital) 759.89
midbrain 348.8
middle
  lobe (lung) (right) 518.0
  radicular 353.0
Miescher's
  familial acanthosis nigricans 701.2
  granulomatosis disciformis 709.3
Mieten's 759.89
migraine 346.0 ✓5ᵗʰ
Mikity-Wilson (pulmonary dysmaturity) 770.7
Mikulicz's (dryness of mouth, absent or decreased lacrimation) 527.1
milk alkali (milk drinkers) 999.9
Milkman (-Looser) (osteomalacia with pseudofractures) 268.2
Millard-Gubler 344.89
Miller Fisher's 357.0
Milles' (encephalocutaneous angiomatosis) 759.6
Minkowski-Chauffard (*see also* Spherocytosis) 282.0
Mirizzi's (hepatic duct stenosis) 576.2
  with calculus, cholelithiasis, or stones — *see* Choledocholithiasis
mitral
  click (-murmur) 785.2
  valve prolapse 424.0
Möbius'
  congenital oculofacial paralysis 352.6
  ophthalmoplegic migraine 346.8 ✓5ᵗʰ
Mohr's (types I and II) 759.89
monofixation 378.34
Moore's (*see also* Epilepsy) 345.5 ✓5ᵗʰ
Morel-Moore (hyperostosis frontalis interna) 733.3
Morel-Morgagni (hyperostosis frontalis interna) 733.3
Morgagni (-Stewart-Morel) (hyperostosis frontalis interna) 733.3
Morgagni-Adams-Stokes (syncope with heart block) 426.9
Morquio (-Brailsford) (-Ullrich) (mucopolysaccharidosis IV) 277.5
Morris (testicular feminization) 257.8
Morton's (foot) (metatarsalgia) (metatarsal neuralgia) (neuralgia) (neuroma) (toe) 355.6
Moschcowitz (-Singer-Symmers) (thrombotic thrombocytopenic purpura) 446.6
Mounier-Kuhn 494.0
  with acute exacerbation 494.1
Mucha-Haberman (acute parapsoriasis varioliformis) 696.2
mucocutaneous lymph node (acute) (febrile) (infantile) (MCLS) 446.1
multiple
  deficiency 260
  operations 301.51
Munchausen's 301.51
Münchmeyer's (exostosis luxurians) 728.11
Murchison-Sanderson — *see* Disease, Hodgkin's
myasthenic — *see* Myasthenia, syndrome
myelodysplastic 238.7
myeloproliferative (chronic) (M9960/1) 238.7
myofascial pain NEC 729.1
Naffziger's 353.0
Nager-de Reynier (dysostosis mandibularis) 756.0
nail-patella (hereditary osteo-onychodysplasia) 756.89
Nebécourt's 253.3
Neill-Dingwall (microencephaly and dwarfism) 759.89
nephrotic (*see also* Nephrosis) 581.9
  diabetic 250.4 ✓5ᵗʰ [581.81]
Netherton's (ichthyosiform erythroderma) 757.1
neurocutaneous 759.6
neuroleptic mailgnant 333.92
Nezelof's (pure alymphocytosis) 279.13

Syndrome — *see also* Disease — *continued*
Niemann-Pick (lipid histiocytosis) 272.7
Nonne-Milroy-Meige (chronic hereditary edema) 757.0
nonsense 300.16
Noonan's 759.89
Nothnagel's
ophthalmoplegia-cerebellar ataxia 378.52
vasomotor acroparesthesia 443.89
nucleus ambiguous-hypoglossal 352.6
OAV (oculoauriculovertebral dysplasia) 756.0
obsessional 300.3
oculocutaneous 364.24
oculomotor 378.81
oculourethroarticular 099.3
Ogilvie's (sympathicotonic colon obstruction) 560.89
ophthalmoplegia-cerebellar ataxia 378.52
Oppenheim-Urbach (necrobiosis lipoidica diabeticorum) 250.8 ✓5ᵗʰ [709.3]
oral-facial-digital 759.89
organic
affective NEC 293.83
drug-induced 292.84
anxiety 293.84
delusional 293.81
alcohol-induced 291.5
drug-induced 292.11
due to or associated with
arteriosclerosis 290.42
presenile brain disease 290.12
senility 290.20
depressive 293.83
drug-induced 292.84
due to or associated with
arteriosclerosis 290.43
presenile brain disease 290.13
senile brain disease 290.21
hallucinosis 293.82
drug-induced 292.84
organic affective 293.83
induced by drug 292.84
organic personality 310.1
induced by drug 292.89
Ormond's 593.4
orodigitofacial 759.89
orthostatic hypotensive-dysautonomic dyskinetic 333.0
Osler-Weber-Rendu (familial hemorrhagic telangiectasia) 448.0
osteodermopathic hyperostosis 757.39
osteoporosis-osteomalacia 268.2
Österreicher-Turner (hereditary osteo-onychodysplasia) 756.89
Ostrum-Furst 756.59
otolith 386.19
otopalatodigital 759.89
outlet (thoracic) 353.0
ovarian remant 620.8
ovarian vein 593.4
Owren's (*see also* Defect, coagulation) 286.3
OX 758.6
pacemaker 429.4
Paget-Schroetter (intermittent venous claudication) 453.8
pain — *see* Pain
painful
apicocostal vertebral (M8010/3) 162.3
arc 726.19
bruising 287.2
feet 266.2
Pancoast's (carcinoma, pulmonary apex) (M8010/3) 162.3
panhypopituitary (postpartum) 253.2
papillary muscle 429.81
with myocardial infarction 410.8 ✓5ᵗʰ
Papillon-Léage and Psaume (orodigitofacial dysostosis) 759.89
parabiotic (transfusion)
donor (twin) 772.0
recipient (twin) 776.4
paralysis agitans 332.0
paralytic 344.9
specified type NEC 344.89
paraneoplastic — *see* condition
Parinaud's (paralysis of conjugate upward gaze) 378.81

Syndrome — *see also* Disease — *continued*
Parinaud's — *continued*
oculoglandular 372.02
Parkes Weber and Dimitri (encephalocutaneous angiomatosis) 759.6
Parkinson's (*see also* Parkinsonism) 332.0
parkinsonian (*see also* Parkinsonism) 332.0
Parry's (exophthalmic goiter) 242.0 ✓5ᵗʰ
Parry-Romberg 349.89
Parsonage-Aldren-Turner 353.5
Parsonage-Turner 353.5
Patau's (trisomy D) 758.1
patellofemoral 719.46
Paterson (-Brown) (-Kelly) (sideropenic dysphagia) 280.8
Payr's (splenic flexure syndrome) 569.89
pectoral girdle 447.8
pectoralis minor 447.8
Pelger-Huët (hereditary hyposegmentation) 288.2
pellagra-cerebellar ataxia-renal aminoaciduria 270.0
Pellegrini-Stieda 726.62
pellagroid 265.2
Pellizzi's (pineal) 259.8
pelvic congestion (-fibrosis) 625.5
Pendred's (familial goiter with deaf-mutism) 243
Penfield's (*see also* Epilepsy) 345.5 ✓5ᵗʰ
Penta X 758.81
peptic ulcer — *see* Ulcer, peptic 533.9 ✓5ᵗʰ
perabduction 447.8
periodic 277.3
periurethral fibrosis 593.4
persistent fetal circulation 747.83 ▲
Petges-Cléjat (poikilodermatomyositis) 710.3
Peutz-Jeghers 759.6
Pfeiffer (acrocephalosyndactyly) 755.55
phantom limb 353.6
pharyngeal pouch 279.11
Pick's (pericardial pseudocirrhosis of liver) 423.2
heart 423.2
liver 423.2
Pick-Herxheimer (diffuse idiopathic cutaneous atrophy) 701.8
Pickwickian (cardiopulmonary obesity) 278.8
PIE (pulmonary infiltration with eosinophilia) 518.3
Pierre Marie-Bamberger (hypertrophic pulmonary osteoarthropathy) 731.2
Pierre Mauriac's (diabetes-dwarfism-obesity) 258.1
Pierre Robin 756.0
pigment dispersion, iris 364.53
pineal 259.8
pink puffer 492.8
pituitary 253.0
placental
dysfunction 762.2
insufficiency 762.2
transfusion 762.3
plantar fascia 728.71
plica knee 727.83
Plummer-Vinson (sideropenic dysphagia) 280.8
pluricarential of infancy 260
plurideficiency of infancy 260
pluriglandular (compensatory) 258.8
polycarential of infancy 260
polyglandular 258.8
polysplenia 759.0
pontine 433.8 ✓5ᵗʰ
popliteal
artery entrapment 447.8
web 756.89
postartificial menopause 627.4
postcardiotomy 429.4
postcholecystectomy 576.0
postcommissurotomy 429.4
postconcussional 310.2
postcontusional 310.2
postencephalitic 310.8
posterior
cervical sympathetic 723.2
fossa compression 348.4
inferior cerebellar artery (*see also* Disease, cerebrovascular, acute) 436
postgastrectomy (dumping) 564.2

Syndrome — *see also* Disease — *continued*
post-gastric surgery 564.2
posthepatitis 780.79
postherpetic (neuralgia) (zoster) 053.19
geniculate ganglion 053.11
ophthalmica 053.19
postimmunization — *see* Complications, vaccination
postinfarction 411.0
postinfluenza (asthenia) 780.79
postirradiation 990
postlaminectomy 722.80
cervical, cervicothoracic 722.81
lumbar, lumbosacral 722.83
thoracic, thoracolumbar 722.82
postleukotomy 310.0
postlobotomy 310.0
postmastectomy lymphedema 457.0
postmature (of newborn) 766.2
postmyocardial infarction 411.0
postoperative NEC 998.9
blind loop 579.2
postperfusion NEC 999.8
bone marrow 996.85
postpericardiotomy 429.4
postphlebitic ▶(asymptomatic)◀ 459.10 ▲
with ●
complications NEC 459.19 ●
inflammation 459.12 ●
and ulcer 459.13 ●
stasis dermatitis 459.12 ●
with ulcer 459.13 ●
ulcer 459.11 ●
with inflammation 459.13 ●
postpolio (myelitis) 138
postvagotomy 564.2
postvalvulotomy 429.4
postviral (asthenia) NEC 780.79
Potain's (gastrectasis with dyspepsia) 536.1
potassium intoxication 276.7
Potter's 753.0
Prader (-Labhart) -Willi (-Fanconi) 759.81
preinfarction 411.1
preleukemic 238.7
premature senility 259.8
premenstrual 625.4
premenstrual tension 625.4
pre ulcer 536.9
Prinzmetal-Massumi (anterior chest wall syndrome) 786.52
Profichet's 729.9
progeria 259.8
progressive pallidal degeneration 333.0
prolonged gestation 766.2
Proteus (dermal hypoplasia) 757.39
prune belly 756.71
prurigo-asthma 691.8
pseudocarpal tunnel (sublimis) 354.0
pseudohermaphroditism-virilism-hirsutism 255.2
pseudoparalytica 358.0
pseudo-Turner's 759.89
psycho-organic 293.9
acute 293.0
anxiety type 293.84
depressive type 293.83
hallucinatory type 293.82
nonpsychotic severity 310.1
specified focal (partial) NEC 310.8
paranoid type 293.81
specified type NEC 293.89
subacute 293.1
pterygolymphangiectasia 758.6
ptosis-epicanthus 270.2
pulmonary 660.1 ✓5ᵗʰ
arteriosclerosis 416.0
hypoperfusion (idiopathic) 769
renal (hemorrhagic) 446.21
pulseless 446.7
Putnam-Dana (subacute combined sclerosis with pernicious anemia) 281.0 [336.2]
pyloroduodenal 537.89
pyramidopallidonigral 332.0
pyriformis 355.0
Q-T interval prolongation 794.31
radicular NEC 729.2
lower limbs 724.4

Syndrome — Syndrome

Syndrome — *see also* Disease — *continued*
  radicular NEC — *continued*
    upper limbs 723.4
      newborn 767.4
  Raeder-Harbitz (pulseless disease) 446.7
  Ramsay Hunt's
    dyssynergia cerebellaris myoclonica 334.2
    herpetic geniculate ganglionitis 053.11
  rapid time-zone change 307.45
  Raymond (-Céstan) 433.8 ✓5ᵗʰ
  Raynaud's (paroxysmal digital cyanosis) 443.0
  RDS (respiratory distress syndrome, newborn) 769
  Refsum's (heredopathia atactica polyneuritiformis) 356.3
  Reichmann's (gastrosuccorrhea) 536.8
  Reifenstein's (hereditary familial hypogonadism, male) 257.2
  Reilly's (*see also* Neuropathy, peripheral, autonomic) 337.9
  Reiter's 099.3
  renal glomerulohyalinosis-diabetic 250.4 ✓5ᵗʰ [581.81]
  Rendu-Osler-Weber (familial hemorrhagic telangiectasia) 448.0
  renofacial (congenital biliary fibroangiomatosis) 753.0
  Rénon-Delille 253.8
  respiratory distress (idiopathic) (newborn) 769
    adult (following shock, surgery, or trauma) 518.5
      specified NEC 518.82
  restless leg 333.99
  retraction (Duane's) 378.71
  retroperitoneal fibrosis 593.4
  Rett's 330.8
  Reye's 331.81
  Reye-Sheehan (postpartum pituitary necrosis) 253.2
  Riddoch's (visual disorientation) 368.16
  Ridley's (*see also* Failure, ventricular, left) 428.1
  Rieger's (mesodermal dysgenesis, anterior ocular segment) 743.44
  Rietti-Greppi-Micheli (thalassemia minor) 282.4
  right ventricular obstruction — *see* Failure, heart
  Riley-Day (familial dysautonomia) 742.8
  Robin's 756.0
  Rokitansky-Kuster-Hauser (congenital absence, vagina) 752.49
  Romano-Ward (prolonged Q-T interval) 794.31
  Romberg's 349.89
  Rosen-Castleman-Liebow (pulmonary proteinosis) 516.0
  rotator cuff, shoulder 726.10
  Roth's 355.1
  Rothmund's (congenital poikiloderma) 757.33
  Rotor's (idiopathic hyperbilirubinemia) 277.4
  Roussy-Lévy 334.3
  Roy (-Jutras) (acropachyderma) 757.39
  rubella (congenital) 771.0
  Rubinstein-Taybi's (brachydactylia, short stature, and mental retardation) 759.89
  Rud's (mental deficiency, epilepsy, and infantilism) 759.89
  Ruiter-Pompen (-Wyers) (angiokeratoma corporis diffusum) 272.7
  Runge's (postmaturity) 766.2
  Russell (-Silver) (congenital hemihypertrophy and short stature) 759.89
  Rytand-Lipsitch (complete atrioventricular block) 426.0
  sacralization-scoliosis-sciatica 756.15
  sacroiliac 724.6
  Saenger's 379.46
  salt
    depletion (*see also* Disease, renal) 593.9
      due to heat NEC 992.8
        causing heat exhaustion or prostration 992.4
    low (*see also* Disease, renal) 593.9
  salt-losing (*see also* Disease, renal) 593.9
  Sanfilippo's (mucopolysaccharidosis III) 277.5
  Scaglietti-Dagnini (acromegalic macrospondylitis) 253.0
  scalded skin 695.1
  scalenus anticus (anterior) 353.0

Syndrome — *see also* Disease — *continued*
  scapulocostal 354.8
  scapuloperoneal 359.1
  scapulovertebral 723.4
  Schaumann's (sarcoidosis) 135
  Scheie's (mucopolysaccharidosis IS) 277.5
  Scheuthauer-Marie-Sainton (cleidocranialis dysostosis) 755.59
  Schirmer's (encephalocutaneous angiomatosis) 759.6
  schizophrenic, of childhood NEC (*see also* Psychosis, childhood) 299.9 ✓5ᵗʰ
  Schmidt's
    sphallo-pharyngo-laryngeal hemiplegia 352.6
    thyroid-adrenocortical insufficiency 258.1
    vagoaccessory 352.6
  Schneider's 047.9
  Scholte's (malignant carcinoid) 259.2
  Scholz (-Bielschowsky-Henneberg) 330.0
  Schroeder's (endocrine-hypertensive) 255.3
  Schüller-Christian (chronic histiocytosis X) 277.8
  Schultz's (agranulocytosis) 288.0
  Schwartz (-Jampel) 756.89
  Schwartz-Bartter (inappropriate secretion of antidiuretic hormone) 253.6
  Scimitar (anomalous venous drainage, right lung to inferior vena cava) 747.49
  sclerocystic ovary 256.4
  sea-blue histiocyte 272.7
  Seabright-Bantam (pseudohypoparathyroidism) 275.49
  Seckel's 759.89
  Secretan's (posttraumatic edema) 782.3
  secretoinhibitor (keratoconjunctivitis sicca) 710.2
  Seeligmann's (ichthyosis congenita) 757.1
  Senear-Usher (pemphigus erythematosus) 694.4
  senilism 259.8
  serotonin 333.99
  serous meningitis 348.2
  Sertoli cell (germinal aplasia) 606.0
  sex chromosome mosaic 758.81
  Sézary's (reticulosis) (M9701/3) 202.2 ✓5ᵗʰ
  shaken infant 995.55
  Shaver's (bauxite pneumoconiosis) 503
  Sheehan's (postpartum pituitary necrosis) 253.2
  shock (traumatic) 958.4
    kidney 584.5
      following crush injury 958.5
    lung 518.5
    neurogenic 308.9
    psychic 308.9
  short
    bowel 579.3
    P-R interval 426.81
  shoulder-arm (*see also* Neuropathy, peripheral, autonomic) 337.9
  shoulder-girdle 723.4
  shoulder-hand (*see also* Neuropathy, peripheral, autonomic) 337.9
  Shwachman's 288.0
  Shy-Drager (orthostatic hypotension with multisystem degeneration) 333.0
  Sicard's 352.6
  sicca (keratoconjunctivitis) 710.2
  sick
    cell 276.1
    cilia 759.89
    sinus 427.81
  sideropenic 280.8
  Siemens'
    ectodermal dysplasia 757.31
    keratosis follicularis spinulosa (decalvans) 757.39
  Silfverskiöld's (osteochondrodystrophy, extremities) 756.50
  Silver's (congenital hemihypertrophy and short stature) 759.89
  Silvestroni-Bianco (thalassemia minima) 282.4
  Simons' (progressive lipodystrophy) 272.6
  sinus tarsi 726.79
  sinusitis-bronchiectasis-situs inversus 759.3
  Sipple's (medullary thyroid carcinoma-pheochromocytoma) 193

Syndrome — *see also* Disease — *continued*
  Sjögren (-Gougerot) (keratoconjunctivitis sicca) 710.2
    with lung involvement 710.2 [517.8]
  Sjögren-Larsson (ichthyosis congenita) 757.1
  Slocumb's 255.3
  Sluder's 337.0
  Smith-Lemli-Opitz (cerebrohepatorenal syndrome) 759.89
  smokers' 305.1
  Sneddon-Wilkinson (subcorneal pustular dermatosis) 694.1
  Sotos' (cerebral gigantism) 253.0
  South African cardiomyopathy 425.2
  spasmodic
    upward movement, eye(s) 378.82
    winking 307.20
  Spens' (syncope with heart block) 426.9
  spherophakia-brachymorphia 759.89
  spinal cord injury — *see also* Injury, spinal, by site
    with fracture, vertebra — *see* Fracture, vertebra, by site, with spinal cord injury
    cervical — *see* Injury, spinal, cervical
    fluid malabsorption (acquired) 331.3
  splenic
    agenesis 759.0
    flexure 569.89
    neutropenia 288.0
    sequestration 282.60
  Spurway's (brittle bones and blue sclera) 756.51
  staphylococcal scalded skin 695.1
  Stein's (polycystic ovary) 256.4
  Stein-Leventhal (polycystic ovary) 256.4
  Steinbrocker's (*see also* Neuropathy, peripheral, autonomic) 337.9
  Stevens-Johnson (erythema multiforme exudativum) 695.1
  Stewart-Morel (hyperostosis frontalis interna) 733.3
  stiff-man 333.91
  Still's (juvenile rheumatoid arthritis) 714.30
  Still-Felty (rheumatoid arthritis with splenomegaly and leukopenia) 714.1
  Stilling-Türk-Duane (ocular retraction syndrome) 378.71
  Stojano's (subcostal) 098.86
  Stokes (-Adams) (syncope with heart block) 426.9
  Stokvis-Talma (enterogenous cyanosis) 289.7
  stone heart (*see also* Failure, ventricular, left) 428.1
  straight-back 756.19
  stroke (*see also* Disease, cerebrovascular, acute) 436
    little 435.9
  Sturge-Kalischer-Weber (encephalotrigeminal angiomatosis) 759.6
  Sturge-Weber (-Dimitri) (encephalocutaneous angiomatosis) 759.6
  subclavian-carotid obstruction (chronic) 446.7
  subclavian steal 435.2
  subcoracoid-pectoralis minor 447.8
  subcostal 098.86
    nerve compression 354.8
  subperiosteal hematoma 267
  subphrenic interposition 751.4
  sudden infant death (SIDS) 798.0
  Sudeck's 733.7
  Sudeck-Leriche 733.7
  superior
    cerebellar artery (*see also* Disease, cerebrovascular, acute) 436
    mesenteric artery 557.1
    pulmonary sulcus (tumor) (M8010/3) 162.3
    vena cava 459.2
  suprarenal cortical 255.3
  supraspinatus 726.10
  swallowed blood 777.3
  sweat retention 705.1
  Sweet's (acute febrile neutrophilic dermatosis) 695.89
  Swyer-James (unilateral hyperlucent lung) 492.8
  Swyer's (XY pure gonadal dysgenesis) 752.7
  Symonds' 348.2

✓4ᵗʰ Fourth-digit Required   ✓5ᵗʰ Fifth-digit Required   ▶◀ Revised Text   ● New Line   ▲ Revised Code

Syndrome — *see also* Disease — *continued*
  sympathetic
    cervical paralysis 337.0
    pelvic 625.5
  syndactylic oxycephaly 755.55
  syphilitic-cardiovascular 093.89
  systemic
    fibrosclerosing 710.8
    inflammatory response (SIRS) 995.90 ●
      due to ●
        infectious process 995.91 ●
          with organ dysfunction 995.92 ●
        non-infectious process 995.93 ●
          with organ dysfunction 995.94 ●
  systolic click (-murmur) 785.2
  Tabagism 305.1
  tachycardia-bradycardia 427.81
  Takayasu (-Onishi) (pulseless disease) 446.7
  Tapia's 352.6
  tarsal tunnel 355.5
  Taussig-Bing (transposition, aorta and
    overriding pulmonary artery) 745.11
  Taybi's (otopalatodigital) 759.89
  Taylor's 625.5
  teething 520.7
  tegmental 344.89
  telangiectasis-pigmentation-cataract 757.33
  temporal 383.02
    lobectomy behavior 310.0
  temporomandibular joint-pain-dysfunction
    [TMJ] NEC 524.60
    specified NEC 524.69
  Terry's 362.21
  testicular feminization 257.8
  testis, nonvirilizing 257.8
  tethered (spinal) cord 742.59
  thalamic 348.8
  Thibierge-Weissenbach (cutaneous systemic
    sclerosis) 710.1
  Thiele 724.6
  thoracic outlet (compression) 353.0
  thoracogenous rheumatic (hypertrophic
    pulmonary osteoarthropathy) 731.2
  Thorn's (*see also* Disease, renal) 593.9
  Thorson-Biörck (malignant carcinoid) 259.2
  thrombopenia-hemangioma 287.3
  thyroid-adrenocortical insufficiency 258.1
  Tietze's 733.6
  time-zone (rapid) 307.45
  Tobias' (carcinoma, pulmonary apex)
    (M8010/3) 162.3
  toilet seat 926.0
  Tolosa-Hunt 378.55
  Toni-Fanconi (cystinosis) 270.0
  Touraine's (hereditary osteo-onychodysplasia)
    756.89
  Touraine-Solente-Golé (acropachyderma)
    757.39
  toxic
    oil 710.5
    shock 040.82 ▲
  transfusion
    fetal-maternal 772.0
    twin
      donor (infant) 772.0
      recipient (infant) 776.4
  Treacher Collins' (incomplete mandibulofacial
    dysostosis) 756.0
  trigeminal plate 259.8
  triple X female 758.81
  trisomy NEC 758.5
    13 or D₁ 758.1
    16-18 or E 758.2
    18 or E₃ 758.2
    20 758.5
    21 or G (mongolism) 758.0
    22 or G (mongolism) 758.0
    G 758.0
  Troisier-Hanot-Chauffard (bronze diabetes)
    275.0
  tropical wet feet 991.4
  Trousseau's (thrombophlebitis migrans visceral
    cancer) 453.1
  Türk's (ocular retraction syndrome) 378.71
  Turner's 758.6

Syndrome — *see also* Disease — *continued*
  Turner-Varny 758.6
  twin-to-twin transfusion 762.3
    recipient twin 776.4
  Uehlinger's (acropachyderma) 757.39
  Ullrich (-Bonnevie) (-Turner) 758.6
  Ullrich-Feichtiger 759.89
  underwater blast injury (abdominal) (*see also*
    Injury, internal, abdomen) 868.00
  universal joint, cervix 620.6
  Unverricht (-Lundborg) 333.2
  Unverricht-Wagner (dermatomyositis) 710.3
  upward gaze 378.81
  Urbach-Oppenheim (necrobiosis lipoidica
    diabeticorum) 250.8 ✓5ᵗʰ [709.3]
  Urbach-Wiethe (lipoid proteinosis) 272.8
  uremia, chronic 585
  urethral 597.81
  urethro-oculoarticular 099.3
  urethro-oculosynovial 099.3
  urohepatic 572.4
  uveocutaneous 364.24
  uveomeningeal, uveomeningitis 363.22
  vagohypoglossal 352.6
  vagovagal 780.2
  van Buchem's (hyperostosis corticalis) 733.3
  van der Hoeve's (brittle bones and blue sclera,
    deafness) 756.51
  van der Hoeve-Halbertsma-Waardenburg
    (ptosis-epicanthus) 270.2
  van der Hoeve-Waardenburg-Gualdi (ptosis-
    epicanthus) 270.2
  van Neck-Odelberg (juvenile osteochondrosis)
    732.1
  vanishing twin 651.33
  vascular splanchnic 557.0
  vasomotor 443.9
  vasovagal 780.2
  VATER 759.89
  Velo-cardio-facial 759.89 ●
    with chromosomal deletion 758.5 ●
  vena cava (inferior) (superior) (obstruction)
    459.2
  Verbiest's (claudicatio intermittens spinalis)
    435.1
  Vernet's 352.6
  vertebral
    artery 435.1
      compression 721.1
    lumbar 724.4
    steal 435.1
  vertebrogenic (pain) 724.5
  vertiginous NEC 386.9
  video display tube 723.8
  Villaret's 352.6
  Vinson-Plummer (sideropenic dysphagia) 280.8
  virilizing adrenocortical hyperplasia, congenital
    255.2
  virus, viral 079.99
  visceral larval migrans 128.0
  visual disorientation 368.16
  vitamin B₆ deficiency 266.1
  vitreous touch 997.99
  Vogt's (corpus striatum) 333.7
  Vogt-Koyanagi 364.24
  Volkmann's 958.6
  von Bechterew-Strümpell (ankylosing
    spondylitis) 720.0
  von Graefe's 378.72
  von Hippel-Lindau (angiomatosis
    retinocerebellosa) 759.6
  von Schroetter's (intermittent venous
    claudication) 453.8
  von Willebrand (-Jürgens) (angiohemophilia)
    286.4
  Waardenburg-Klein (ptosis epicanthus) 270.2
  Wagner (-Unverricht) (dermatomyositis) 710.3
  Waldenström's (macroglobulinemia) 273.3
  Waldenström-Kjellberg (sideropenic dysphagia)
    280.8
  Wallenberg's (posterior inferior cerebellar
    artery) (*see also* Disease, cerebrovascular,
    acute) 436
  Waterhouse (-Friderichsen) 036.3
  water retention 276.6
  Weber's 344.89
  Weber-Christian (nodular nonsuppurative
    panniculitis) 729.30

Syndrome — *see also* Disease — *continued*
  Weber-Cockayne (epidermolysis bullosa) 757.39
  Weber-Dimitri (encephalocutaneous
    angiomatosis) 759.6
  Weber-Gubler 344.89
  Weber-Leyden 344.89
  Weber-Osler (familial hemorrhagic
    telangiectasia) 448.0
  Wegener's (necrotizing respiratory
    granulomatosis) 446.4
  Weill-Marchesani (brachymorphism and ectopia
    lentis) 759.89
  Weingarten's (tropical eosinophilia) 518.3
  Weiss-Baker (carotid sinus syncope) 337.0
  Weissenbach-Thibierge (cutaneous systemic
    sclerosis) 710.1
  Werdnig-Hoffmann 335.0
  Werlhof-Wichmann (*see also* Purpura,
    thrombocytopenic) 287.3
  Wermer's (polyendocrine adenomatosis) 258.0
  Werner's (progeria adultorum) 259.8
  Wernicke's (nonalcoholic) (superior hemorrhagic
    polioencephalitis) 265.1
  Wernicke-Korsakoff (nonalcoholic) 294.0
    alcoholic 291.1
  Westphal-Strümpell (hepatolenticular
    degeneration) 275.1
  wet
    brain (alcoholic) 303.9 ✓5ᵗʰ
    feet (maceration) (tropical) 991.4
    lung
      adult 518.5
      newborn 770.6
  whiplash 847.0
  Whipple's (intestinal lipodystrophy) 040.2
  "whistling face" (craniocarpotarsal dystrophy)
    759.89
  Widal (-Abrami) (acquired hemolytic jaundice)
    283.9
  Wilkie's 557.1
  Wilkinson-Sneddon (subcorneal pustular
    dermatosis) 694.1
  Willan-Plumbe (psoriasis) 696.1
  Willebrand (-Jürgens) (angiohemophilia) 286.4
  Willi-Prader (hypogenital dystrophy with
    diabetic tendency) 759.81
  Wilson's (hepatolenticular degeneration) 275.1
  Wilson-Mikity 770.7
  Wiskott-Aldrich (eczema-thrombocytopenia)
    279.12
  withdrawal
    alcohol 291.81
    drug 292.0
    infant of dependent mother 779.5
  Woakes' (ethmoiditis) 471.1
  Wolff-Parkinson-White (anomalous
    atrioventricular excitation) 426.7
  Wright's (hyperabduction) 447.8
  X
    cardiac 413.9
    dysmetabolic 277.7
  xiphoidalgia 733.99
  XO 758.6
  XXX 758.81
  XXXXY 758.81
  XXY 758.7
  yellow vernix (placental dysfunction) 762.2
  Zahorsky's 074.0
  Zieve's (jaundice, hyperlipemia and hemolytic
    anemia) 571.1
  Zollinger-Ellison (gastric hypersecretion with
    pancreatic islet cell tumor) 251.5
  Zuelzer-Ogden (nutritional megaloblastic
    anemia) 281.2
Synechia (iris) (pupil) 364.70
  anterior 364.72
    peripheral 364.73
  intrauterine (traumatic) 621.5
  posterior 364.71
  vulvae, congenital 752.49
Synesthesia (*see also* Disturbance, sensation)
  782.0
Synodontia 520.2
Synophthalmus 759.89
Synorchidism 752.8
Synorchism 752.8

Syndrome — Synorchism

Synostosis (congenital) 756.59
  astragaloscaphoid 755.67
  radioulnar 755.53
  talonavicular (bar) 755.67
  tarsal 755.67
Synovial — *see* condition
Synovioma (M9040/3) — *see also* Neoplasm,
    connective tissue, malignant
  benign (M9040/0) — *see* Neoplasm, connective
    tissue, benign
Synoviosarcoma (M9040/3) — *see* Neoplasm,
    connective tissue, malignant
Synovitis 727.00
  chronic crepitant, wrist 727.2
  due to crystals — *see* Arthritis, due to crystals
  gonococcal 098.51
  gouty 274.0
  syphilitic 095.7
    congenital 090.0
  traumatic, current — *see* Sprain, by site
  tuberculous — *see* Tuberculosis, synovitis
  villonodular 719.20
    ankle 719.27
    elbow 719.22
    foot 719.27
    hand 719.24
    hip 719.25
    knee 719.26
    multiple sites 719.29
    pelvic region 719.25
    shoulder (region) 719.21
    specified site NEC 719.28
    wrist 719.23
Syphilide 091.3
  congenital 090.0
  newborn 090.0
  tubercular 095.8
    congenital 090.0
Syphilis, syphilitic (acquired) 097.9
  with lung involvement 095.1
  abdomen (late) 095.2
  acoustic nerve 094.86
  adenopathy (secondary) 091.4
  adrenal (gland) 095.8
    with cortical hypofunction 095.8
  age under 2 years NEC (*see also* Syphilis,
      congenital) 090.9 ✓5ᵗʰ
    acquired 097.9
  alopecia (secondary) 091.82
  anemia 095.8
  aneurysm (artery) (ruptured) 093.89
    aorta 093.0
    central nervous system 094.89
    congenital 090.5
  anus 095.8
    primary 091.1
    secondary 091.3
  aorta, aortic (arch) (abdominal) (insufficiency)
      (pulmonary) (regurgitation) (stenosis)
      (thoracic) 093.89
    aneurysm 093.0
  arachnoid (adhesive) 094.2
  artery 093.89
    cerebral 094.89
    spinal 094.89
  arthropathy (neurogenic) (tabetic) 094.0 [713.5]
  asymptomatic — *see* Syphilis, latent
  ataxia, locomotor (progressive) 094.0
  atrophoderma maculatum 091.3
  auricular fibrillation 093.89
  Bell's palsy 094.89
  bladder 095.8
  bone 095.5
    secondary 091.61
  brain 094.89
  breast 095.8
  bronchus 095.8
  bubo 091.0
  bulbar palsy 094.89
  bursa (late) 095.7
  cardiac decompensation 093.89
  cardiovascular (early) (late) (primary)
      (secondary) (tertiary) 093.9
    specified type and site NEC 093.89
  causing death under 2 years of age (*see also*
      Syphilis, congenital) 090.9 ✓5ᵗʰ
    stated to be acquired NEC 097.9

Syphilis, syphilitic — *continued*
  central nervous system (any site) (early) (late)
      (latent) (primary) (recurrent) (relapse)
      (secondary) (tertiary) 094.9
    with
      ataxia 094.0
      paralysis, general 094.1
        juvenile 090.40
      paresis (general) 094.1
        juvenile 090.40
      tabes (dorsalis) 094.0
        juvenile 090.40
      taboparesis 094.1
        juvenile 090.40
    aneurysm (ruptured) 094.87
    congenital 090.40
    juvenile 090.40
    remission in (sustained) 094.9
    serology doubtful, negative, or positive 094.9
    specified nature or site NEC 094.89
    vascular 094.89
  cerebral 094.89
    meningovascular 094.2
    nerves 094.89
    sclerosis 094.89
    thrombosis 094.89
  cerebrospinal 094.89
    tabetic 094.0
  cerebrovascular 094.89
  cervix 095.8
  chancre (multiple) 091.0
    extragenital 091.2
    Rollet's 091.0
  Charcôt's joint 094.0 [713.5]
  choked disc 094.89 [377.00]
  chorioretinitis 091.51
    congenital 090.0 [363.13]
    late 094.83
  choroiditis 091.51
    congenital 090.0 [363.13]
    late 094.83
    prenatal 090.0 [363.13]
  choroidoretinitis (secondary) 091.51
    congenital 090.0 [363.13]
    late 094.83
  ciliary body (secondary) 091.52
    late 095.8 [364.11]
  colon (late) 095.8
  combined sclerosis 094.89
  complicating pregnancy, childbirth or
      puerperium 647.0 ✓5ᵗʰ
    affecting fetus or newborn 760.2
  condyloma (latum) 091.3
  congenital 090.9 ✓5ᵗʰ
    with
      encephalitis 090.41
      paresis (general) 090.40
      tabes (dorsalis) 090.40
      taboparesis 090.40
    chorioretinitis, choroiditis 090.0 [363.13]
    early or less than 2 years after birth NEC
        090.2
      with manifestations 090.0
      latent (without manifestations) 090.1
        negative spinal fluid test 090.1
        serology, positive 090.1
      symptomatic 090.0
    interstitial keratitis 090.3
    juvenile neurosyphilis 090.40
    late or 2 years or more after birth NEC
        090.7 ✓5ᵗʰ
      chorioretinitis, choroiditis 090.5 [363.13]
      interstitial keratitis 090.3
      juvenile neurosyphilis NEC 090.40
      latent (without manifestations) 090.6 ✓5ᵗʰ
        negative spinal fluid test 090.6 ✓5ᵗʰ
        serology, positive 090.6 ✓5ᵗʰ
      symptomatic or with manifestations NEC
          090.5
        interstitial keratitis 090.3
  conjugal 097.9
    tabes 094.0
  conjunctiva 095.8 [372.10]
  contact V01.6
  cord, bladder 094.0
  cornea, late 095.8 [370.59]
  coronary (artery) 093.89
    sclerosis 093.89

Syphilis, syphilitic — *continued*
  coryza 095.8
    congenital 090.0
  cranial nerve 094.89
  cutaneous — *see* Syphilis, skin
  dacryocystitis 095.8
  degeneration, spinal cord 094.89
  d'emblée 095.8
  dementia 094.1
    paralytica 094.1
      juvenilis 090.40
  destruction of bone 095.5
  dilatation, aorta 093.0
  due to blood transfusion 097.9
  dura mater 094.89
  ear 095.8
    inner 095.8
      nerve (eighth) 094.86
      neurorecurrence 094.86
  early NEC 091.0
    cardiovascular 093.9
    central nervous system 094.9
      paresis 094.1
      tabes 094.0
    latent (without manifestations) (less than 2
        years after infection) 092.9
      negative spinal fluid test 092.9
      serological relapse following treatment
          092.0
      serology positive 092.9
    paresis 094.1
    relapse (treated, untreated) 091.7
    skin 091.3
    symptomatic NEC 091.89
      extragenital chancre 091.2
      primary, except extragenital chancre
          091.0
      secondary (*see also* Syphilis, secondary)
          091.3
        relapse (treated, untreated) 091.7
    tabes 094.0
    ulcer 091.3
  eighth nerve 094.86
  endemic, nonvenereal 104.0
  endocarditis 093.20
    aortic 093.22
    mitral 093.21
    pulmonary 093.24
    tricuspid 093.23
  epididymis (late) 095.8
  epiglottis 095.8
  epiphysitis (congenital) 090.0
  esophagus 095.8
  Eustachian tube 095.8
  exposure to V01.6
  eye 095.8 [363.13]
    neuromuscular mechanism 094.85
  eyelid 095.8 [373.5]
    with gumma 095.8 [373.5]
    ptosis 094.89
  fallopian tube 095.8
  fracture 095.5
  gallbladder (late) 095.8
  gastric 095.8
    crisis 094.0
    polyposis 095.8
  general 097.9
    paralysis 094.1
      juvenile 090.40
  genital (primary) 091.0
  glaucoma 095.8
  gumma (late) NEC 095.9
    cardiovascular system 093.9
    central nervous system 094.9
    congenital 090.5
    heart or artery 093.89
  heart 093.89
    block 093.89
    decompensation 093.89
    disease 093.89
    failure 093.89
    valve (*see also* Syphilis, endocarditis) 093.20
  hemianesthesia 094.89
  hemianopsia 095.8
  hemiparesis 094.89
  hemiplegia 094.89
  hepatic artery 093.89

Syphilis, syphilitic — *continued*
- hepatitis 095.3
- hepatomegaly 095.3
  - congenital 090.0
- hereditaria tarda (*see also* Syphilis, congenital, late) 090.7 ✓5ᵗʰ
- hereditary (*see also* Syphilis, congenital) 090.9 ✓5ᵗʰ
  - interstitial keratitis 090.3
- Hutchinson's teeth 090.5
- hyalitis 095.8
- inactive — *see* Syphilis, latent
- infantum NEC (*see also* Syphilis, congenital) 090.9 ✓5ᵗʰ
- inherited — *see* Syphilis, congenital
- internal ear 095.8
- intestine (late) 095.8
- iris, iritis (secondary) 091.52
  - late 095.8 [364.11]
- joint (late) 095.8
- keratitis (congenital) (early) (interstitial) (late) (parenchymatous) (punctata profunda) 090.3
- kidney 095.4
- lacrimal apparatus 095.8
- laryngeal paralysis 095.8
- larynx 095.8
- late 097.0
  - cardiovascular 093.9
  - central nervous system 094.9
  - latent or 2 years or more after infection (without manifestations) 096
    - negative spinal fluid test 096
    - serology positive 096
  - paresis 094.1
  - specified site NEC 095.8
  - symptomatic or with symptoms 095.9
  - tabes 094.0
- latent 097.1
  - central nervous system 094.9
  - date of infection unspecified 097.1
  - early or less than 2 years after infection 092.9
  - late or 2 years or more after infection 096
  - serology
    - doubtful
      - follow-up of latent syphilis 097.1
        - central nervous system 094 ✓4ᵗʰ
        - date of infection unspecified 097.1
        - early or less than 2 years after infection 092 ✓4ᵗʰ
        - late or 2 years or more after infection 096
    - positive, only finding 097.1
      - date of infection unspecified 097.1
      - early or less than 2 years after infection 097.1
      - late or 2 years or more after infection 097.1
- lens 095.8
- leukoderma 091.3
  - late 095.8
- lienis 095.8
- lip 091.3
  - chancre 091.2
  - late 095.8
  - primary 091.2
- Lissauer's paralysis 094.1
- liver 095.3
  - secondary 091.62
- locomotor ataxia 094.0
- lung 095.1
- lymphadenitis (secondary) 091.4
- lymph gland (early) (secondary) 091.4
  - late 095.8
- macular atrophy of skin 091.3
  - striated 095.8
- maternal, affecting fetus or newborn 760.2
  - manifest syphilis in newborn — *see* Syphilis, congenital
- mediastinum (late) 095.8
- meninges (adhesive) (basilar) (brain) (spinal cord) 094.2
- meningitis 094.2
  - acute 091.81
  - congenital 090.42
- meningoencephalitis 094.2

Syphilis, syphilitic — *continued*
- meningovascular 094.2
  - congenital 090.49
- mesarteritis 093.89
  - brain 094.89
  - spine 094.89
- middle ear 095.8
- mitral stenosis 093.21
- monoplegia 094.89
- mouth (secondary) 091.3
  - late 095.8
- mucocutaneous 091.3
  - late 095.8
- mucous
  - membrane 091.3
    - late 095.8
  - patches 091.3
    - congenital 090.0
- mulberry molars 090.5
- muscle 095.6
- myocardium 093.82
- myositis 095.6
- nasal sinus 095.8
- neonatorum NEC (*see also* Syphilis, congenital) 090.9 ✓5ᵗʰ
- nerve palsy (any cranial nerve) 094.89
- nervous system, central 094.9
- neuritis 095.8
  - acoustic nerve 094.86
- neurorecidive of retina 094.83
- neuroretinitis 094.85
- newborn (*see also* Syphilis, congenital) 090.9 ✓5ᵗʰ
- nodular superficial 095.8
- nonvenereal, endemic 104.0
- nose 095.8
  - saddle back deformity 090.5
  - septum 095.8
    - perforated 095.8
- occlusive arterial disease 093.89
- ophthalmic 095.8 [363.13]
- ophthalmoplegia 094.89
- optic nerve (atrophy) (neuritis) (papilla) 094.84
- orbit (late) 095.8
- orchitis 095.8
- organic 097.9
- osseous (late) 095.5
- osteochondritis (congenital) 090.0
- osteoporosis 095.5
- ovary 095.8
- oviduct 095.8
- palate 095.8
  - gumma 095.8
  - perforated 090.5
- pancreas (late) 095.8
- pancreatitis 095.8
- paralysis 094.89
  - general 094.1
  - juvenile 090.40
- paraplegia 094.89
- paresis (general) 094.1
  - juvenile 090.40
- paresthesia 094.89
- Parkinson's disease or syndrome 094.82
- paroxysmal tachycardia 093.89
- pemphigus (congenital) 090.0
- penis 091.0
  - chancre 091.0
  - late 095.8
- pericardium 093.81
- perichondritis, larynx 095.8
- periosteum 095.5
  - congenital 090.0
  - early 091.61
  - secondary 091.61
- peripheral nerve 095.8
- petrous bone (late) 095.5
- pharynx 095.8
  - secondary 091.3
- pituitary (gland) 095.8
- placenta 095.8
- pleura (late) 095.8
- pneumonia, white 090.0
- pontine (lesion) 094.89
- portal vein 093.89
- primary NEC 091.2
  - anal 091.1

Syphilis, syphilitic — *continued*
- primary NEC — *continued*
  - and secondary (*see also* Syphilis, secondary) 091.9
    - cardiovascular 093.9
    - central nervous system 094.9
    - extragenital chancre NEC 091.2
    - fingers 091.2
    - genital 091.0
    - lip 091.2
    - specified site NEC 091.2
    - tonsils 091.2
- prostate 095.8
- psychosis (intracranial gumma) 094.89
- ptosis (eyelid) 094.89
- pulmonary (late) 095.1
  - artery 093.89
- pulmonum 095.1
- pyelonephritis 095.4
- recently acquired, symptomatic NEC 091.89
- rectum 095.8
- respiratory tract 095.8
- retina
  - late 094.83
  - neurorecidive 094.83
- retrobulbar neuritis 094.85
- salpingitis 095.8
- sclera (late) 095.0
- sclerosis
  - cerebral 094.89
  - coronary 093.89
  - multiple 094.89
  - subacute 094.89
- scotoma (central) 095.8
- scrotum 095.8
- secondary (and primary) 091.9
  - adenopathy 091.4
  - anus 091.3
  - bone 091.61
  - cardiovascular 093.9
  - central nervous system 094.9
  - chorioretinitis, choroiditis 091.51
  - hepatitis 091.62
  - liver 091.62
  - lymphadenitis 091.4
  - meningitis, acute 091.81
  - mouth 091.3
  - mucous membranes 091.3
  - periosteum 091.61
  - periostitis 091.61
  - pharynx 091.3
  - relapse (treated) (untreated) 091.7
  - skin 091.3
  - specified form NEC 091.89
  - tonsil 091.3
  - ulcer 091.3
  - viscera 091.69
  - vulva 091.3
- seminal vesicle (late) 095.8
- seronegative
  - with signs or symptoms — *see* Syphilis, by site and stage
- seropositive
  - with signs or symptoms — *see* Syphilis, by site and stage
  - follow-up of latent syphilis — *see* Syphilis, latent
  - only finding — *see* Syphilis, latent
- seventh nerve (paralysis) 094.89
- sinus 095.8
- sinusitis 095.8
- skeletal system 095.5
- skin (early) (secondary) (with ulceration) 091.3
  - late or tertiary 095.8
- small intestine 095.8
- spastic spinal paralysis 094.0
- spermatic cord (late) 095.8
- spinal (cord) 094.89
  - with
    - paresis 094.1
    - tabes 094.0
- spleen 095.8
- splenomegaly 095.8
- spondylitis 095.5
- staphyloma 095.8
- stigmata (congenital) 090.5
- stomach 095.8
- synovium (late) 095.7

✓4ᵗʰ Fourth-digit Required　　　✓5ᵗʰ Fifth-digit Required　　　▶◀ Revised Text　　　● New Line　　　▲ Revised Code

Syphilis, syphilitic — *continued*
  tabes dorsalis (early) (late) 094.0
    juvenile 090.40
  tabetic type 094.0
    juvenile 090.40
  taboparesis 094.1
    juvenile 090.40
  tachycardia 093.89
  tendon (late) 095.7
  tertiary 097.0
    with symptoms 095.8
    cardiovascular 093.9
    central nervous system 094.9
    multiple NEC 095.8
    specified site NEC 095.8
  testis 095.8
  thorax 095.8
  throat 095.8
  thymus (gland) 095.8
  thyroid (late) 095.8
  tongue 095.8
  tonsil (lingual) 095.8
    primary 091.2
    secondary 091.3
  trachea 095.8
  tricuspid valve 093.23
  tumor, brain 094.89
  tunica vaginalis (late) 095.8
  ulcer (any site) (early) (secondary) 091.3
    late 095.9
      perforating 095.9
        foot 094.0
  urethra (stricture) 095.8
  urogenital 095.8
  uterus 095.8
  uveal tract (secondary) 091.50
    late 095.8 *[363.13]*
  uveitis (secondary) 091.50
    late 095.8 *[363.13]*
  uvula (late) 095.8
    perforated 095.8
  vagina 091.0
    late 095.8
  valvulitis NEC 093.20
  vascular 093.89
    brain or cerebral 094.89
  vein 093.89
    cerebral 094.89
  ventriculi 095.8
  vesicae urinariae 095.8
  viscera (abdominal) 095.2
    secondary 091.69
  vitreous (hemorrhage) (opacities) 095.8
  vulva 091.0
    late 095.8
    secondary 091.3
Syphiloma 095.9
  cardiovascular system 093.9
  central nervous system 094.9
  circulatory system 093.9
  congenital 090.5
Syphilophobia 300.29
Syringadenoma (M8400/0) — *see also* Neoplasm, skin, benign
  papillary (M8406/0) — *see* Neoplasm, skin, benign
Syringobulbia 336.0
Syringocarcinoma (M8400/3) — *see* Neoplasm, skin, malignant
Syringocystadenoma (M8400/0) — *see also* Neoplasm, skin, benign
  papillary (M8406/0) — *see* Neoplasm, skin, benign
Syringocystoma (M8407/0) — *see* Neoplasm, skin, benign
Syringoma (M8407/0) — *see also* Neoplasm, skin, benign
  chondroid (M8940/0) — *see* Neoplasm, by site, benign
Syringomyelia 336.0
Syringomyelitis 323.9
  late effect — *see* category 326
Syringomyelocele (*see also* Spina bifida) 741.9 ✓5ᵗʰ
Syringopontia 336.0

System, systemic — *see also* condition
  disease, combined — *see* Degeneration, combined
  fibrosclerosing syndrome 710.8
  inflammatory response syndrome (SIRS) ●
    995.90 ●
    due to ●
      infectious process 995.91 ●
        with organ dsfunction 995.92 ●
      non-infectious process 995.93 ●
        with organ dysfunction 995.94 ●
  lupus erythematosus 710.0
    inhibitor 286.5

T

Tab — *see* Tag
Tabacism 989.8 ✓5ᵗʰ
Tabacosis 989.8 ✓5ᵗʰ
Tabardillo 080
  flea-borne 081.0
  louse-borne 080
Tabes, tabetic
  with
    central nervous system syphilis 094.0
    Charcôt's joint 094.0 *[713.5]*
    cord bladder 094.0
    crisis, viscera (any) 094.0
    paralysis, general 094.1
    paresis (general) 094.1
    perforating ulcer 094.0
  arthropathy 094.0 *[713.5]*
  bladder 094.0
  bone 094.0
  cerebrospinal 094.0
  congenital 090.40
  conjugal 094.0
  dorsalis 094.0
    neurosyphilis 094.0
  early 094.0
  juvenile 090.40
  latent 094.0
  mesenterica (*see also* Tuberculosis) 014.8 ✓5ᵗʰ
  paralysis insane, general 094.1
  peripheral (nonsyphilitic) 799.8
  spasmodic 094.0
    not dorsal or dorsalis 343.9
  syphilis (cerebrospinal) 094.0
Taboparalysis 094.1
Taboparesis (remission) 094.1
  with
    Charcôt's joint 094.1 *[713.5]*
    cord bladder 094.1
    perforating ulcer 094.1
  juvenile 090.40
Tachyalimentation 579.3
Tachyarrhythmia, tachyrhythmia — *see also* Tachycardia
  paroxysmal with sinus bradycardia 427.81
Tachycardia 785.0
  atrial 427.89
  auricular 427.89
  newborn 779.82 ●
  nodal 427.89
  nonparoxysmal atrioventricular 426.89
  nonparoxysmal atrioventricular (nodal) 426.89
  paroxysmal 427.2
    with sinus bradycardia 427.81
    atrial (PAT) 427.0
      psychogenic 316 *[427.0]*
    atrioventricular (AV) 427.0
      psychogenic 316 *[427.0]*
    essential 427.2
    junctional 427.0
    nodal 427.0
    psychogenic 316 *[427.2]*
      atrial 316 *[427.0]*
      supraventricular 316 *[427.0]*
      ventricular 316 *[427.1]*
    supraventricular 427.0
      psychogenic 316 *[427.0]*
    ventricular 427.1
      psychogenic 316 *[427.1]*
  postoperative 997.1
  psychogenic 306.2
  sick sinus 427.81

Tachycardia — *continued*
  sinoauricular 427.89
  sinus 427.89
  supraventricular 427.89
  ventricular (paroxysmal) 427.1
    psychogenic 316 *[427.1]*
Tachypnea 786.06
  hysterical 300.11
  newborn (idiopathic) (transitory) 770.6
  psychogenic 306.1
  transitory, of newborn 770.6
Taenia (infection) (infestation) (*see also* Infestation, taenia) 123.3
  diminuta 123.6
  echinococcal infestation (*see also* Echinococcus) 122.9
  nana 123.6
  saginata infestation 123.2
  solium (intestinal form) 123.0
    larval form 123.1
Taeniasis (intestine) (*see also* Infestation, Taenia) 123.3
  saginata 123.2
  solium 123.0
Taenzer's disease 757.4
Tag (hypertrophied skin) (infected) 701.9
  adenoid 474.8
  anus 455.9
  endocardial (*see also* Endocarditis) 424.90
  hemorrhoidal 455.9
  hymen 623.8
  perineal 624.8
  preauricular 744.1
  rectum 455.9
  sentinel 455.9
  skin 701.9
    accessory 757.39
    anus 455.9
    congenital 757.39
    preauricular 744.1
    rectum 455.9
  tonsil 474.8
  urethra, urethral 599.84
  vulva 624.8
Tahyna fever 062.5
Takayasu (-Onishi) disease or syndrome (pulseless disease) 446.7
Talc granuloma 728.82
Talcosis 502
Talipes (congenital) 754.70
  acquired NEC 736.79
    planus 734
  asymmetric 754.79
    acquired 736.79
  calcaneovalgus 754.62
    acquired 736.76
  calcaneovarus 754.59
    acquired 736.76
  calcaneus 754.79
    acquired 736.76
  cavovarus 754.59
    acquired 736.75
  cavus 754.71
    acquired 736.73
  equinovalgus 754.69
    acquired 736.72
  equinovarus 754.51
    acquired 736.71
  equinus 754.79
    acquired, NEC 736.72
  percavus 754.71
    acquired 736.73
  planovalgus 754.69
    acquired 736.79
  planus (acquired) (any degree) 734
    congenital 754.61
    due to rickets 268.1
  valgus 754.60
    acquired 736.79
  varus 754.50
    acquired 736.79
Talma's disease 728.85
Tamponade heart (Rose's) (*see also* Pericarditis) 423.9
Tanapox 078.89

Tangier disease (familial high-density lipoprotein deficiency) 272.5

Tank ear 380.12

Tantrum (childhood) (see also Disturbance, conduct) 312.1 ✓5ᵗʰ

Tapeworm (infection) (infestation) (see also Infestation, tapeworm) 123.9

Tapia's syndrome 352.6

Tarantism 297.8

Target-oval cell anemia 282.4

Tarlov's cyst 355.9

Tarral-Besnier disease (pityriasis rubra pilaris) 696.4

Tarsalgia 729.2

Tarsal tunnel syndrome 355.5

Tarsitis (eyelid) 373.00
  syphilitic 095.8 [373.00]
  tuberculous (see also Tuberculosis) 017.0 ✓5ᵗʰ [373.4]

Tartar (teeth) 523.6

Tattoo (mark) 709.09

Taurodontism 520.2

Taussig-Bing defect, heart, or syndrome (transposition, aorta and overriding pulmonary artery) 745.11

Tay's choroiditis 363.41

Tay-Sachs
  amaurotic familial idiocy 330.1
  disease 330.1

Taybi's syndrome (otopalatodigital) 759.89

Taylor's
  disease (diffuse idiopathic cutaneous atrophy) 701.8
  syndrome 625.5

Tear, torn (traumatic) — see also Wound, open, by site
  anus, anal (sphincter) 863.89
    with open wound in cavity 863.99
    complicating delivery 664.2 ✓5ᵗʰ
      with mucosa 664.3 ✓5ᵗʰ
    nontraumatic, nonpuerperal 565.0
  articular cartilage, old (see also Disorder, cartilage, articular) 718.0 ✓5ᵗʰ
  bladder
    with
      abortion — see Abortion, by type, with damage to pelvic organs
      ectopic pregnancy (see also categories 633.0-633.9) 639.2
      molar pregnancy (see also categories 630-632) 639.2
    following
      abortion 639.2
      ectopic or molar pregnancy 639.2
    obstetrical trauma 665.5 ✓5ᵗʰ
  bowel
    with
      abortion — see Abortion, by type, with damage to pelvic organs
      ectopic pregnancy (see also categories 633.0-633.9) 639.2
      molar pregnancy (see also categories 630-632) 639.2
    following
      abortion 639.2
      ectopic or molar pregnancy 639.2
    obstetrical trauma 665.5 ✓5ᵗʰ
  broad ligament
    with
      abortion — see Abortion, by type, with damage to pelvic organs
      ectopic pregnancy (see also categories 633.0-633.9) 639.2
      molar pregnancy (see also categories 630-632) 639.2
    following
      abortion 639.2
      ectopic or molar pregnancy 639.2
    obstetrical trauma 665.6 ✓5ᵗʰ
  bucket handle (knee) (meniscus) — see Tear, meniscus

Tear, torn — see also Wound, open, by site — continued
  capsule
    joint — see Sprain, by site
    spleen — see Laceration, spleen, capsule
  cartilage — see also Sprain, by site
    articular, old (see also Disorder, cartilage, articular) 718.0 ✓5ᵗʰ
    knee — see Tear, meniscus
    semilunar (knee) (current injury) — see Tear, meniscus
  cervix
    with
      abortion — see Abortion, by type, with damage to pelvic organs
      ectopic pregnancy (see also categories 633.0-633.9) 639.2
      molar pregnancy (see also categories 630-632) 639.2
    following
      abortion 639.2
      ectopic or molar pregnancy 639.2
    obstetrical trauma (current) 665.3 ✓5ᵗʰ
    old 622.3
  internal organ (abdomen, chest, or pelvis) — see Injury, internal, by site
  ligament — see also Sprain, by site
    with open wound — see Wound, open by site
  meniscus (knee) (current injury) 836.2
    bucket handle 836.0
      old 717.0
    lateral 836.1
      anterior horn 836.1
        old 717.42
      bucket handle 836.1
        old 717.41
      old 717.40
      posterior horn 836.1
        old 717.43
      specified site NEC 836.1
        old 717.49
    medial 836.0
      anterior horn 836.0
        old 717.1
      bucket handle 836.0
        old 717.0
      old 717.3
      posterior horn 836.0
        old 717.2
    old NEC 717.5
    site other than knee — see Sprain, by site
  muscle — see also Sprain, by site
    with open wound — see Wound, open by site
  pelvic
    floor, complicating delivery 664.1 ✓5ᵗʰ
    organ NEC
      with
        abortion — see Abortion, by type, with damage to pelvic organs
        ectopic pregnancy (see also categories 633.0-633.9) 639.2
        molar pregnancy (see also categories 630-632) 639.2
      following
        abortion 639.2
        ectopic or molar pregnancy 639.2
      obstetrical trauma 665.5 ✓5ᵗʰ
  perineum — see also Laceration, perineum
    obstetrical trauma 665.5 ✓5ᵗʰ
  periurethral tissue
    with
      abortion — see Abortion, by type, with damage to pelvic organs
      ectopic pregnancy (see also categories 633.0-633.9) 639.2
      molar pregnancy (see also categories 630-632) 639.2
    following
      abortion 639.2
      ectopic or molar pregnancy 639.2
    obstetrical trauma 665.5 ✓5ᵗʰ
  rectovaginal septum — see Laceration, rectovaginal septum
  retina, retinal (recent) (with detachment) 361.00

Tear, torn — see also Wound, open, by site — continued
  retina, retinal — continued
    without detachment 361.30
    dialysis (juvenile) (with detachment) 361.04
    giant (with detachment) 361.03
    horseshoe (without detachment) 361.32
    multiple (with detachment) 361.02
      without detachment 361.33
    old
      delimited (partial) 361.06
      partial 361.06
      total or subtotal 361.07
    partial (without detachment)
      giant 361.03
      multiple defects 361.02
      old (delimited) 361.06
      single defect 361.01
    round hole (without detachment) 361.31
    single defect (with detachment) 361.01
    total or subtotal (recent) 361.05
      old 361.07
  rotator cuff (traumatic) 840.4
    current injury 840.4
    degenerative 726.10
    nontraumatic 727.61
  semilunar cartilage, knee (see also Tear, meniscus) 836.2
    old 717.5
  tendon — see also Sprain, by site
    with open wound — see Wound, open by site
  tentorial, at birth 767.0
  umbilical cord
    affecting fetus or newborn 772.0
    complicating delivery 663.8 ✓5ᵗʰ
  urethra
    with
      abortion — see Abortion, by type, with damage to pelvic organs
      ectopic pregnancy (see also categories 633.0-633.9) 639.2
      molar pregnancy (see also categories 630-632) 639.2
    following
      abortion 639.2
      ectopic or molar pregnancy 639.2
    obstetrical trauma 665.5 ✓5ᵗʰ
  uterus — see Injury, internal, uterus
  vagina — see Laceration, vagina
  vessel, from catheter 998.2
  vulva, complicating delivery 664.0 ✓5ᵗʰ

Tear stone 375.57

Teeth, tooth — see also condition
  grinding 306.8

Teething 520.7
  syndrome 520.7

Tegmental syndrome 344.89

Telangiectasia, telangiectasis (verrucous) 448.9
  ataxic (cerebellar) 334.8
  familial 448.0
  hemorrhagic, hereditary (congenital) (senile) 448.0
  hereditary hemorrhagic 448.0
  retina 362.15
  spider 448.1

Telecanthus (congenital) 743.63

Telescoped bowel or intestine (see also Intussusception) 560.0

Teletherapy, adverse effect NEC 990

Telogen effluvium 704.02

Temperature
  body, high (of unknown origin) (see also Pyrexia) 780.6
  cold, trauma from 991.9
    newborn 778.2
    specified effect NEC 991.8
  high
    body (of unknown origin) (see also Pyrexia) 780.6
    trauma from — see Heat

Temper tantrum (childhood) (see also Disturbance, conduct) 312.1 ✓5ᵗʰ

Temple — see condition

Temporal — *see also* condition
lobe syndrome 310.0
Temporomandibular joint-pain-dysfunction syndrome 524.60
Temporosphenoidal — *see* condition
Tendency
bleeding (*see also* Defect, coagulation) 286.9
homosexual, ego-dystonic 302.0
paranoid 301.0
suicide 300.9
Tenderness
abdominal (generalized) (localized) 789.6 ✓5ᵗʰ
rebound 789.6 ✓5ᵗʰ
skin 782.0
Tendinitis, tendonitis (*see also* Tenosynovitis) 726.90
Achilles 726.71
adhesive 726.90
shoulder 726.0
calcific 727.82
shoulder 726.11
gluteal 726.5
patellar 726.64
peroneal 726.79
pes anserinus 726.61
psoas 726.5
tibialis (anterior) (posterior) 726.72
trochanteric 726.5
Tendon — *see* condition
Tendosynovitis — *see* Tenosynovitis
Tendovaginitis — *see* Tenosynovitis
Tenesmus 787.99
rectal 787.99
vesical 788.9
Tenia — *see* Taenia
Teniasis — *see* Taeniasis
Tennis elbow 726.32
Tenonitis — *see also* Tenosynovitis
eye (capsule) 376.04
Tenontosynovitis — *see* Tenosynovitis
Tenontothecitis — *see* Tenosynovitis
Tenophyte 727.9
Tenosynovitis 727.00
adhesive 726.90
shoulder 726.0
ankle 727.06
bicipital (calcifying) 726.12
buttock 727.09
due to crystals — *see* Arthritis, due to crystals
elbow 727.09
finger 727.05
foot 727.06
gonococcal 098.51
hand 727.05
hip 727.09
knee 727.09
radial styloid 727.04
shoulder 726.10
adhesive 726.0
spine 720.1
supraspinatus 726.10
toe 727.06
tuberculous — *see* Tuberculosis, tenosynovitis
wrist 727.05
Tenovaginitis — *see* Tenosynovitis
Tension
arterial, high (*see also* Hypertension) 401.9
without diagnosis of hypertension 796.2
headache 307.81
intraocular (elevated) 365.00
nervous 799.2
ocular (elevated) 365.00
pneumothorax 512.0
iatrogenic 512.1
postoperative 512.1
spontaneous 512.0
premenstrual 625.4
state 300.9
Tentorium — *see* condition
Teratencephalus 759.89
Teratism 759.7
Teratoblastoma (malignant) (M9080/3) — *see* Neoplasm, by site, malignant

Teratocarcinoma (M9081/3) — *see also* Neoplasm, by site, malignant
liver 155.0
Teratoma (solid) (M9080/1) — *see also* Neoplasm, by site, uncertain behavior
adult (cystic) (M9080/0) — *see* Neoplasm, by site, benign
and embryonal carcinoma, mixed (M9081/3) — *see* Neoplasm, by site, malignant
benign (M9080/0) — *see* Neoplasm, by site, benign
combined with choriocarcinoma (M9101/3) — *see* Neoplasm, by site, malignant
cystic (adult) (M9080/0) — *see* Neoplasm, by site, benign
differentiated type (M9080/0) — *see* Neoplasm, by site, benign
embryonal (M9080/3) — *see also* Neoplasm, by site, malignant
liver 155.0
fetal
sacral, causing fetopelvic disproportion 653.7 ✓5ᵗʰ
immature (M9080/3) — *see* Neoplasm, by site, malignant
liver (M9080/3) 155.0
adult, benign, cystic, differentiated type or mature (M9080/0) 211.5
malignant (M9080/3) — *see also* Neoplasm, by site, malignant
anaplastic type (M9082/3) — *see* Neoplasm, by site, malignant
intermediate type (M9083/3) — *see* Neoplasm, by site, malignant
liver (M9080/3) 155.0
trophoblastic (M9102/3)
specified site — *see* Neoplasm, by site, malignant
unspecified site 186.9
undifferentiated type (M9082/3) — *see* Neoplasm, by site, malignant
mature (M9080/0) — *see* Neoplasm, by site, benign
ovary (M9080/0) 220
embryonal, immature, or malignant (M9080/3) 183.0
suprasellar (M9080/3) — *see* Neoplasm, by site, malignant
testis (M9080/3) 186.9
adult, benign, cystic, differentiated type or mature (M9080/0) 222.0
undescended 186.0
Terminal care V66.7
Termination
anomalous — *see also* Malposition, congenital
portal vein 747.49
right pulmonary vein 747.42
pregnancy (legal) (therapeutic) (*see* Abortion, legal) 635.9 ✓5ᵗʰ
fetus NEC 779.6
illegal (*see also* Abortion, illegal) 636.9 ✓5ᵗʰ
Ternidens diminutus infestation 127.7
Terrors, night (child) 307.46
Terry's syndrome 362.21
Tertiary — *see* condition
Tessellated fundus, retina (tigroid) 362.89
Test(s)
AIDS virus V72.6
adequacy
hemodialysis V56.31
peritoneal dialysis V56.32
allergen V72.7
bacterial disease NEC (*see also* Screening, by name of disease) V74.9
basal metabolic rate V72.6
blood-alcohol V70.4
blood-drug V70.4
for therapeutic drug monitoring V58.83
developmental, infant or child V20.2
Dick V74.8
fertility V26.21
genetic V26.3
hearing V72.1
HIV V72.6
human immunodeficiency virus V72.6
Kveim V82.89

Test(s) — *continued*
laboratory V72.6
for medicolegal reason V70.4
Mantoux (for tuberculosis) V74.1
mycotic organism V75.4
parasitic agent NEC V75.8
paternity V70.4
peritoneal equilibration V56.32
pregnancy
positive V22.1
first pregnancy V22.0
unconfirmed V72.4
preoperative V72.84
cardiovascular V72.81
respiratory V72.82
specified NEC V72.83
procreative management NEC V26.29
sarcoidosis V82.89
Schick V74.3
Schultz-Charlton V74.8
skin, diagnostic
allergy V72.7
bacterial agent NEC (*see also* Screening, by name of disease) V74.9
Dick V74.8
hypersensitivity V72.7
Kveim V82.89
Mantoux V74.1
mycotic organism V75.4
parasitic agent NEC V75.8
sarcoidosis V82.89
Schick V74.3
Schultz-Charlton V74.8
tuberculin V74.1
specified type NEC V72.8 ✓5ᵗʰ
tuberculin V74.1
vision V72.0
Wassermann
positive (*see also* Serology for syphilis, positive) 097.1
false 795.6
Testicle, testicular, testis — *see also* condition
feminization (syndrome) 257.8
Tetanus, tetanic (cephalic) (convulsions) 037
with
abortion — *see* Abortion, by type, with sepsis
ectopic pregnancy (*see also* categories 633.0-633.9) 639.0
molar pregnancy (*see* categories 630-632) 639.0
following
abortion 639.0
ectopic or molar pregnancy 639.0
inoculation V03.7
reaction (due to serum) — *see* Complications, vaccination
neonatorum 771.3
puerperal, postpartum, childbirth 670 ✓4ᵗʰ
Tetany, tetanic 781.7
alkalosis 276.3
associated with rickets 268.0
convulsions 781.7
hysterical 300.11
functional (hysterical) 300.11
hyperkinetic 781.7
hysterical 300.11
hyperpnea 786.01
hysterical 300.11
psychogenic 306.1
hyperventilation 786.01
hysterical 300.11
psychogenic 306.1
hypocalcemic, neonatal 775.4
hysterical 300.11
neonatal 775.4
parathyroid (gland) 252.1
parathyroprival 252.1
postoperative 252.1
postthyroidectomy 252.1
pseudotetany 781.7
hysterical 300.11
psychogenic 306.1
specified as conversion reaction 300.11
Tetralogy of Fallot 745.2
Tetraplegia — *see* Quadriplegia

Thailand hemorrhagic fever 065.4

Thalassanemia 282.4

Thalassemia (alpha) (beta) (disease) (Hb-C) (Hb-D) (Hb-E) (Hb-H) (Hb-I) (Hb-S) (high fetal gene) (high fetal hemoglobin) (intermedia) (major) (minima) (minor) (mixed) (sickle-cell) (trait) (with other hemoglobinopathy) 282.4

Thalassemic variants 282.4

Thaysen-Gee disease (nontropical sprue) 579.0

Thecoma (M8600/0) 220
malignant (M8600/3) 183.0

Thelarche, precocious 259.1

Thelitis 611.0
puerperal, postpartum 675.0 ☑5ᵗʰ

Therapeutic — *see* condition

Therapy V57.9
blood transfusion, without reported diagnosis V58.2
breathing V57.0
chemotherapy V58.1
fluoride V07.31
prophylactic NEC V07.39
dialysis (intermittent) (treatment)
extracorporeal V56.0
peritoneal V56.8
renal V56.0
specified type NEC V56.8
exercise NEC V57.1
breathing V57.0
extracorporeal dialysis (renal) V56.0
fluoride prophylaxis V07.31
hemodialysis V56.0
long term oxygen therapy V46.2 ●
occupational V57.21
orthoptic V57.4
orthotic V57.81
peritoneal dialysis V56.8
physical NEC V57.1
postmenopausal hormone replacement V07.4
radiation V58.0
speech V57.3
vocational V57.22

Thermalgesia 782.0

Thermalgia 782.0

Thermanalgesia 782.0

Thermanesthesia 782.0

Thermic — *see* condition

Thermography (abnormal) 793.9
breast 793.89

Thermoplegia 992.0

Thesaurismosis
amyloid 277.3
bilirubin 277.4
calcium 275.40
cystine 270.0
glycogen (*see also* Disease, glycogen storage) 271.0
kerasin 272.7
lipoid 272.7
melanin 255.4
phosphatide 272.7
urate 274.9

Thiaminic deficiency 265.1
with beriberi 265.0

Thibierge-Weissenbach syndrome (cutaneous systemic sclerosis) 710.1

Thickened endometrium 793.5

Thickening
bone 733.99
extremity 733.99
breast 611.79
hymen 623.3
larynx 478.79
nail 703.8
congenital 757.5
periosteal 733.99
pluera (*see also* Pleurisy) 511.0
skin 782.8
subepiglottic 478.79
tongue 529.8
valve, heart — *see* Endocarditis

Thiele syndrome 724.6

Thigh — *see* condition

Thinning vertebra (*see also* Osteoporosis) 733.00

Thirst, excessive 783.5
due to deprivation of water 994.3

Thomsen's disease 359.2

Thomson's disease (congenital poikiloderma) 757.33

Thoracic — *see also* condition
kidney 753.3
outlet syndrome 353.0
stomach — *see* Hernia, diaphragm

Thoracogastroschisis (congenital) 759.89

Thoracopagus 759.4

Thoracoschisis 756.3

Thorax — *see* condition

Thorn's syndrome (*see also* Disease, renal) 593.9

Thornwaldt's, Tornwaldt's
bursitis (pharyngeal) 478.29
cyst 478.26
disease (pharyngeal bursitis) 478.29

Thorson-Biörck syndrome (malignant carcinoid) 259.2

Threadworm (infection) (infestation) 127.4

Threatened
abortion or miscarriage 640.0 ☑5ᵗʰ
with subsequent abortion (*see also* Abortion, spontaneous) 634.9 ☑5ᵗʰ
affecting fetus 762.1
labor 644.1 ☑5ᵗʰ
affecting fetus or newborn 761.8
premature 644.0 ☑5ᵗʰ
miscarriage 640.0 ☑5ᵗʰ
affecting fetus 762.1
premature
delivery 644.2 ☑5ᵗʰ
affecting fetus or newborn 761.8
labor 644.0 ☑5ᵗʰ
before 22 completed weeks gestation 640.0 ☑5ᵗʰ

Three-day fever 066.0

Threshers' lung 495.0

Thrix annulata (congenital) 757.4

Throat — *see* condition

Thrombasthenia (Glanzmann's) (hemorrhagic) (hereditary) 287.1

Thromboangiitis 443.1
obliterans (general) 443.1
cerebral 437.1
vessels
brain 437.1
spinal cord 437.1

Thromboarteritis — *see* Arteritis

Thromboasthenia (Glanzmann's) (hemorrhagic) (hereditary) 287.1

Thrombocytasthenia (Glanzmann's) 287.1

Thrombocythemia (essential) (hemorrhagic) (primary) (M9962/1) 238.7
idiopathic (M9962/1) 238.7

Thrombocytopathy (dystrophic) (granulopenic) 287.1

Thrombocytopenia, thrombocytopenic 287.5
with giant hemangioma 287.3
amegakaryocytic, congenital 287.3
congenital 287.3
cyclic 287.3
dilutional 287.4
due to
drugs 287.4
extracorporeal circulation of blood 287.4
massive blood transfusion 287.4
platelet alloimmunization 287.4
essential 287.3
hereditary 287.3
Kasabach-Merritt 287.3
neonatal, transitory 776.1
due to
exchange transfusion 776.1
idiopathic maternal thrombocytopenia 776.1
isoimmunization 776.1
primary 287.3
puerperal, postpartum 666.3 ☑5ᵗʰ

Thrombocytopenia, thrombocytopenic — *continued*
purpura (*see also* Purpura, thrombocytopenic) 287.3
thrombotic 446.6
secondary 287.4
sex-linked 287.3

Thrombocytosis, essential 289.9

Thromboembolism — *see* Embolism

Thrombopathy (Bernard-Soulier) 287.1
constitutional 286.4
Willebrand-Jürgens (angiohemophilia) 286.4

Thrombopenia (*see also* Thrombocytopenia) 287.5

Thrombophlebitis 451.9
antecubital vein 451.82
antepartum (superficial) 671.2 ☑5ᵗʰ
affecting fetus or newborn 760.3
deep 671.3 ☑5ᵗʰ
arm 451.89
deep 451.83
superficial 451.82
breast, superficial 451.89
cavernous (venous) sinus — *see* Thrombophlebitis, intracranial venous sinus
cephalic vein 451.82
cerebral (sinus) (vein) 325
late effect — *see* category 326
nonpyogenic 437.6
in pregnancy or puerperium 671.5 ☑5ᵗʰ
late effect — *see* Late effect(s) (of) cerebrovascular disease
due to implanted device — *see* Complications, due to (presence of) any device, implant or graft classified to 996.0-996.5 NEC
during or resulting from a procedure NEC 997.2
femoral 451.11
femoropopliteal 451.19
following infusion, perfusion, or transfusion 999.2
hepatic (vein) 451.89
idiopathic, recurrent 453.1
iliac vein 451.81
iliofemoral 451.11
intracranial venous sinus (any) 325
late effect — *see* category 326
nonpyogenic 437.6
in pregnancy or puerperium 671.5 ☑5ᵗʰ
late effect — *see* Late effect(s) (of) cerebrovascular disease
jugular vein 451.89
lateral (venous) sinus — *see* Thrombophlebitis, intracranial venous sinus
leg 451.2
deep (vessels) 451.19
femoral vein 451.11
specified vessel NEC 451.19
superficial (vessels) 451.0
femoral vein 451.11
longitudinal (venous) sinus — *see* Thrombophlebitis, intracranial venous sinus
lower extremity 451.2
deep (vessels) 451.19
femoral vein 451.11
specified vessel NEC 451.19
superficial (vessels) 451.0
migrans, migrating 453.1
pelvic
with
abortion — *see* Abortion, by type, with sepsis
ectopic pregnancy — (*see also* categories 633.0-633.9) 639.0
molar pregnancy — (*see also* categories 630-632) 639.0
following
abortion 639.0
ectopic or molar pregnancy 639.0
puerperal 671.4 ☑5ᵗʰ
popliteal vein 451.19
portal (vein) 572.1
postoperative 997.2
pregnancy (superficial) 671.2 ☑5ᵗʰ
affecting fetus or newborn 760.3

Thrombophlebitis — *continued*
  pregnancy — *continued*
    deep 671.3 ☑5ᵗʰ
    puerperal, postpartum, childbirth (extremities)
      (superficial) 671.2 ☑5ᵗʰ
      deep 671.4 ☑5ᵗʰ
      pelvic 671.4 ☑5ᵗʰ
      specified site NEC 671.5 ☑5ᵗʰ
  radial vein 451.83
  saphenous (greater) (lesser) 451.0
  sinus (intracranial) — *see* Thrombophlebitis,
    intracranial venous sinus
    specified site NEC 451.89
  tibial vein 451.19

Thrombosis, thrombotic (marantic) (multiple)
  (progressive) (septic) (vein) (vessel) 453.9
  with childbirth or during the puerperium — *see*
    Thrombosis, puerperal, postpartum
  antepartum — *see* Thrombosis, pregnancy
  aorta, aortic 444.1
    abdominal 444.0
    bifurcation 444.0
    saddle 444.0
    terminal 444.0
    thoracic 444.1
    valve — *see* Endocarditis, aortic
  apoplexy (*see also* Thrombosis, brain)
    434.0 ☑5ᵗʰ
    late effect — *see* Late effect(s) (of)
      cerebrovascular disease
  appendix, septic — *see* Appendicitis, acute
  arteriolar-capillary platelet, disseminated 446.6
  artery, arteries (postinfectional) 444.9
    auditory, internal 433.8 ☑5ᵗʰ
    basilar (*see also* Occlusion, artery, basilar)
      433.0 ☑5ᵗʰ
    carotid (common) (internal) (*see also*
      Occlusion, artery, carotid) 433.1 ☑5ᵗʰ
      with other precerebral artery 433.3 ☑5ᵗʰ
    cerebellar (anterior inferior) (posterior
      inferior) (superior) 433.8 ☑5ᵗʰ
    cerebral (*see also* Thrombosis, brain)
      434.0 ☑5ᵗʰ
    choroidal (anterior) 433.8 ☑5ᵗʰ
    communicating posterior 433.8 ☑5ᵗʰ
    coronary (*see also* Infarct, myocardium)
      410.9 ☑5ᵗʰ
      without myocardial infarction 411.81
      due to syphilis 093.89
      healed or specified as old 412
    extremities 444.22
      lower 444.22
      upper 444.21
    femoral 444.22
    hepatic 444.89
    hypophyseal 433.8 ☑5ᵗʰ
    meningeal, anterior or posterior 433.8 ☑5ᵗʰ
    mesenteric (with gangrene) 557.0
    ophthalmic (*see also* Occlusion, retina)
      362.30
    pontine 433.8 ☑5ᵗʰ
    popliteal 444.22
    precerebral — *see* Occlusion, artery,
      precerebral NEC
    pulmonary 415.19
      iatrogenic 415.11
      postoperative 415.11
    renal 593.81
    retinal (*see also* Occlusion, retina) 362.30
    specified site NEC 444.89
    spinal, anterior or posterior 433.8 ☑5ᵗʰ
    traumatic (complication) (early) (*see also*
      Injury, blood vessel, by site) 904.9
    vertebral (*see also* Occlusion, artery,
      vertebral) 433.2 ☑5ᵗʰ
      with other precerebral artery 433.3 ☑5ᵗʰ
  atrial (endocardial) 424.90
    due to syphilis 093.89
  auricular (*see also* Infarct, myocardium)
    410.9 ☑5ᵗʰ
  axillary (vein) 453.8
  basilar (artery) (*see also* Occlusion, artery,
    basilar) 433.0 ☑5ᵗʰ
  bland NEC 453.9
  brain (artery) (stem) 434.0 ☑5ᵗʰ
    due to syphilis 094.89
    iatrogenic 997.02

Thrombosis, thrombotic — *continued*
  brain — *continued*
    late effect — *see* Late effect(s) (of)
      cerebrovascular disease
    postoperative 997.02
    puerperal, postpartum, childbirth 674.0 ☑5ᵗʰ
    sinus (*see also* Thrombosis, intracranial
      venous sinus) 325
  capillary 448.9
    arteriolar, generalized 446.6
  cardiac (*see also* Infarct, myocardium)
    410.9 ☑5ᵗʰ
    due to syphilis 093.89
    healed or specified as old 412
    valve — *see* Endocarditis
  carotid (artery) (common) (internal) (*see also*
    Occlusion, artery, carotid) 433.1 ☑5ᵗʰ
    with other precerebral artery 433.3 ☑5ᵗʰ
  cavernous sinus (venous) — *see* Thrombosis,
    intracranial venous sinus
  cerebellar artery (anterior inferior) (posterior
    inferior) (superior) 433.8 ☑5ᵗʰ
    late effect — *see* Late effect(s) (of)
      cerebrovascular disease
  cerebral (arteries) (*see also* Thrombosis, brain)
    434.0 ☑5ᵗʰ
    late effect — *see* Late effect(s) (of)
      cerebrovascular disese
  coronary (artery) (*see also* Infarct, myocardium)
    410.9 ☑5ᵗʰ
    without myocardial infarction 411.81
    due to syphilis 093.89
    healed or specified as old 412
  corpus cavernosum 607.82
  cortical (*see also* Thrombosis, brain) 434.0 ☑5ᵗʰ
  due to (presence of) any device, implant, or
    graft classifiable to 996.0-996.5— *see*
    Complications, due to (presence of) any
    device, implant, or graft classified to
    996.0-996.5 NEC
  effort 453.8
  endocardial — *see* Infarct, myocardium
  eye (*see also* Occlusion, retina) 362.30
  femoral (vein) (deep) 453.8
    with inflammation or phlebitis 451.11
    artery 444.22
  genital organ, male 608.83
  heart (chamber) (*see also* Infarct, myocardium)
    410.9 ☑5ᵗʰ
  hepatic (vein) 453.0
    artery 444.89
    infectional or septic 572.1
  iliac (vein) 453.8
    with inflammation or phlebitis 451.81
    artery (common) (external) (internal) 444.81
  inflammation, vein — *see* Thrombophlebitis
  internal carotid artery (*see also* Occlusion,
    artery, carotid) 433.1 ☑5ᵗʰ
    with other precerebral artery 433.3 ☑5ᵗʰ
  intestine (with gangrene) 557.0
  intracranial (*see also* Thrombosis, brain)
    434.0 ☑5ᵗʰ
    venous sinus (any) 325
      nonpyogenic origin 437.6
        in pregnancy or puerperium 671.5 ☑5ᵗʰ
  intramural (*see also* Infarct, myocardium)
    410.9 ☑5ᵗʰ
    without
      cardiac condition 429.89
      coronary artery disease 429.89
      myocardial infarction 429.89
    healed or specified as old 412
  jugular (bulb) 453.8
  kidney 593.81
    artery 593.81
  lateral sinus (venous) — *see* Thrombosis,
    intracranial venous sinus
  leg 453.8
    with inflammation or phlebitis — *see*
      Thrombophlebitis
    deep (vessels) 453.8
    superficial (vessels) 453.8
  liver (venous) 453.0
    artery 444.89
    infectional or septic 572.1
    portal vein 452
  longitudinal sinus (venous) — *see* Thrombosis,
    intracranial venous sinus

Thrombosis, thrombotic — *continued*
  lower extremity — *see* Thrombosis, leg
  lung 415.19
    iatrogenic 415.11
    postoperative 415.11
  marantic, dural sinus 437.6
  meninges (brain) (*see also* Thrombosis, brain)
    434.0 ☑5ᵗʰ
  mesenteric (artery) (with gangrene) 557.0
    vein (inferior) (superior) 557.0
  mitral — *see* Insufficiency, mitral
  mural (heart chamber) (*see also* Infarct,
    myocardium) 410.9 ☑5ᵗʰ
    without
      cardiac condition 429.89
      coronary artery disease 429.89
      myocardial infarction 429.89
    due to syphilis 093.89
    following myocardial infarction 429.79
    healed or specified as old 412
  omentum (with gangrene) 557.0
  ophthalmic (artery) (*see also* Occlusion, retina)
    362.30
  pampiniform plexus (male) 608.83
    female 620.8
  parietal (*see also* Infarct, myocardium)
    410.9 ☑5ᵗʰ
  penis, penile 607.82
  peripheral arteries 444.22
    lower 444.22
    upper 444.21
  platelet 446.6
  portal 452
    due to syphilis 093.89
    infectional or septic 572.1
  precerebral artery — *see also* Occlusion, artery,
    precerebral NEC
  pregnancy 671.9 ☑5ᵗʰ
    deep (vein) 671.3 ☑5ᵗʰ
    superficial (vein) 671.2 ☑5ᵗʰ
  puerperal, postpartum, childbirth 671.9 ☑5ᵗʰ
    brain (artery) 674.0 ☑5ᵗʰ
      venous 671.5 ☑5ᵗʰ
    cardiac 674.8 ☑5ᵗʰ
    cerebral (artery) 674.0 ☑5ᵗʰ
      venous 671.5 ☑5ᵗʰ
    deep (vein) 671.4 ☑5ᵗʰ
    intracranial sinus (nonpyogenic) (venous)
      671.5 ☑5ᵗʰ
    pelvic 671.4 ☑5ᵗʰ
    pulmonary (artery) 673.2 ☑5ᵗʰ
    specified site NEC 671.5 ☑5ᵗʰ
    superficial 671.2 ☑5ᵗʰ
  pulmonary (artery) (vein) 415.19
    iatrogenic 415.11
    postoperative 415.11
  renal (artery) 593.81
    vein 453.3
  resulting from presence of shunt or other
    internal prosthetic device — *see*
    Complications, due to (presence of) any
    device, implant, or graft classified to
    996.0-996.5 NEC
  retina, retinal (artery) 362.30
    arterial branch 362.32
    central 362.31
    partial 362.33
    vein
      central 362.35
      tributary (branch) 362.36
  scrotum 608.83
  seminal vesicle 608.83
  sigmoid (venous) sinus (*see* Thrombosis,
    intracranial venous sinus) 325
  silent NEC 453.9
  sinus, intracranial (venous) (any) (*see also*
    Thrombosis, intracranial venous sinus)
    325
  softening, brain (*see also* Thrombosis, brain)
    434.0 ☑5ᵗʰ
  specified site NEC 453.8
  spermatic cord 608.83
  spinal cord 336.1
    due to syphilis 094.89
    in pregnancy or puerperium 671.5 ☑5ᵗʰ
    pyogenic origin 324.1
      late effect — *see* category 326

Thrombosis, thrombotic — *continued*
   spleen, splenic 289.59
      artery 444.89
   testis 608.83
   traumatic (complication) (early) (*see also* Injury, blood vessel, by site) 904.9
   tricuspid — *see* Endocarditis, tricuspid
   tunica vaginalis 608.83
   umbilical cord (vessels) 663.6 ✓5ᵗʰ
      affecting fetus or newborn 762.6
   vas deferens 608.83
   vena cava (inferior) (superior) 453.2
Thrombus — *see* Thrombosis
Thrush 112.0
   newborn 771.7
Thumb — *see also* condition
   gamekeeper's 842.12
   sucking (child problem) 307.9
Thygeson's superficial punctate keratitis 370.21
Thymergasia (*see also* Psychosis, affective) 296.80
Thymitis 254.8
Thymoma (benign) (M8580/0) 212.6
   malignant (M8580/3) 164.0
Thymus, thymic (gland) — *see* condition
Thyrocele (*see also* Goiter) 240.9
Thyroglossal — *see also* condition
   cyst 759.2
   duct, persistent 759.2
Thyroid (body) (gland) — *see also* condition
   lingual 759.2
Thyroiditis 245.9
   acute (pyogenic) (suppurative) 245.0
      nonsuppurative 245.0
   autoimmune 245.2
   chronic (nonspecific) (sclerosing) 245.8
      fibrous 245.3
      lymphadenoid 245.2
      lymphocytic 245.2
      lymphoid 245.2
   complicating pregnancy, childbirth, or puerperium 648.1 ✓5ᵗʰ
   de Quervain's (subacute granulomatous) 245.1
   fibrous (chronic) 245.3
   giant (cell) (follicular) 245.1
   granulomatous (de Quervain's) (subacute) 245.1
   Hashimoto's (struma lymphomatosa) 245.2
   iatrogenic 245.4
   invasive (fibrous) 245.3
   ligneous 245.3
   lymphocytic (chronic) 245.2
   lymphoid 245.2
   lymphomatous 245.2
   pseudotuberculous 245.1
   pyogenic 245.0
   radiation 245.4
   Riedel's (ligneous) 245.3
   subacute 245.1
   suppurative 245.0
   tuberculous (*see also* Tuberculosis) 017.5 ✓5ᵗʰ
   viral 245.1
   woody 245.3
Thyrolingual duct, persistent 759.2
Thyromegaly 240.9
Thyrotoxic
   crisis or storm (*see also* Thyrotoxicosis) 242.9 ✓5ᵗʰ
   heart failure (*see also* Thyrotoxicosis) 242.9 ✓5ᵗʰ [425.7]
Thyrotoxicosis 242.9 ✓5ᵗʰ

> Note — Use the following fifth-digit subclassification with category 242:
>
> 0   without mention of thyrotoxic crisis or storm
>
> 1   with mention of thyrotoxic crisis or storm

   with
      goiter (diffuse) 242.0 ✓5ᵗʰ
         adenomatous 242.3 ✓5ᵗʰ
            multinodular 242.2 ✓5ᵗʰ

Thyrotoxicosis — *continued*
   with — *continued*
      goiter — *continued*
         adenomatous — *continued*
            uninodular 242.1 ✓5ᵗʰ
         nodular 242.3 ✓5ᵗʰ
            multinodular 242.2 ✓5ᵗʰ
            uninodular 242.1 ✓5ᵗʰ
      infiltrative
         dermopathy 242.0 ✓5ᵗʰ
         ophthalmopathy 242.0 ✓5ᵗʰ
      thyroid acropachy 242.0 ✓5ᵗʰ
   complicating pregnancy, childbirth, or puerperium 648.1 ✓5ᵗʰ
   due to
      ectopic thyroid nodule 242.4 ✓5ᵗʰ
      ingestion of (excessive) thyroid material 242.8 ✓5ᵗʰ
      specified cause NEC 242.8 ✓5ᵗʰ
   factitia 242.8 ✓5ᵗʰ
   heart 242.9 ✓5ᵗʰ [425.7]
   neonatal (transient) 775.3
TIA (transient ischemic attack) 435.9
   with transient neurologic deficit 435.9
   late effect — *see* Late effect(s) (of) cerebrovascular disease
Tibia vara 732.4
Tic 307.20
   breathing 307.20
   child problem 307.21
   compulsive 307.22
   convulsive 307.20
   degenerative (generalized) (localized) 333.3
      facial 351.8
   douloureux (*see also* Neuralgia, trigeminal) 350.1
      atypical 350.2
   habit 307.20
      chronic (motor or vocal) 307.22
      transient of childhood 307.21
   lid 307.20
      transient of childhood 307.21
   motor-verbal 307.23
   occupational 300.89
   orbicularis 307.20
      transient of childhood 307.21
   organic origin 333.3
   postchoreic — *see* Chorea
   psychogenic 307.20
      compulsive 307.22
   salaam 781.0
   spasm 307.20
      chronic (motor or vocal) 307.22
      transient of childhood 307.21
Tick (-borne) fever NEC 066.1
   American mountain 066.1
   Colorado 066.1
   hemorrhagic NEC 065.3
      Crimean 065.0
      Kyasanur Forest 065.2
      Omsk 065.1
   mountain 066.1
   nonxanthematous 066.1
Tick-bite fever NEC 066.1
   African 087.1
   Colorado (virus) 066.1
   Rocky Mountain 082.0
Tick paralysis 989.5
Tics and spasms, compulsive 307.22
Tietze's disease or syndrome 733.6
Tight, tightness
   anus 564.89
   chest 786.59
   fascia (lata) 728.9
   foreskin (congenital) 605
   hymen 623.3
   introitus (acquired) (congenital) 623.3
   rectal sphincter 564.89
   tendon 727.81
      Achilles (heel) 727.81
   urethral sphincter 598.9
Tilting vertebra 737.9
Timidity, child 313.21
Tinea (intersecta) (tarsi) 110.9
   amiantacea 110.0

Tinea — *continued*
   asbestina 110.0
   barbae 110.0
   beard 110.0
   black dot 110.0
   blanca 111.2
   capitis 110.0
   corporis 110.5
   cruris 110.3
   decalvans 704.09
   flava 111.0
   foot 110.4
   furfuracea 111.0
   imbricata (Tokelau) 110.5
   lepothrix 039.0
   manuum 110.2
   microsporic (*see also* Dermatophytosis) 110.9
   nigra 111.1
   nodosa 111.2
   pedis 110.4
   scalp 110.0
   specified site NEC 110.8
   sycosis 110.0
   tonsurans 110.0
   trichophytic (*see also* Dermatophytosis) 110.9
   unguium 110.1
   versicolor 111.0
Tingling sensation (*see also* Disturbance, sensation) 782.0
Tin-miners' lung 503
Tinnitus (aurium) 388.30
   audible 388.32
   objective 388.32
   subjective 388.31
Tipping pelvis 738.6
   with disproportion (fetopelvic) 653.0 ✓5ᵗʰ
      affecting fetus or newborn 763.1
      causing obstructed labor 660.1 ✓5ᵗʰ
         affecting fetus or newborn 763.1
Tiredness 780.79
Tissue — *see* condition
Tobacco
   abuse (affecting health) NEC (*see also* Abuse, drugs, nondependent) 305.1
   heart 989.8 ✓5ᵗʰ
Tobias' syndrome (carcinoma, pulmonary apex) (M8010/3) 162.3
Tocopherol deficiency 269.1
Todd's
   cirrhosis — *see* Cirrhosis, biliary
   paralysis (postepileptic transitory paralysis) 344.8 ✓5ᵗʰ
Toe — *see* condition
Toilet, artificial opening (*see also* Attention to, artificial, opening) V55.9
Tokelau ringworm 110.5
Tollwut 071
Tolosa-Hunt syndrome 378.55
Tommaselli's disease
   correct substance properly administered 599.7
   overdose or wrong substance given or taken 961.4
Tongue — *see also* condition
   worms 134.1
Tongue tie 750.0
Toni-Fanconi syndrome (cystinosis) 270.0
Tonic pupil 379.46
Tonsil — *see* condition
Tonsillitis (acute) (catarrhal) (croupous) (follicular) (gangrenous) (infective) (lacunar) (lingual) (malignant) (membranous) (phlegmonous) (pneumococcal) (pseudomembranous) (purulent) (septic) (staphylococcal) (subacute) (suppurative) (toxic) (ulcerative) (vesicular) (viral) 463
   with influenza, flu, or grippe 487.1
   chronic 474.00
   diphtheritic (membranous) 032.0
   hypertrophic 474.00
   influenzal 487.1
   parenchymatous 475
   streptococcal 034.0
   tuberculous (*see also* Tuberculosis) 012.8 ✓5ᵗʰ

Tonsillitis — *continued*
    Vincent's 101
Tonsillopharyngitis 465.8
Tooth, teeth — *see* condition
Toothache 525.9
Topagnosis 782.0
Tophi (gouty) 274.0
    ear 274.81
    heart 274.82
    specified site NEC 274.82
Torn — *see* Tear, torn
Tornwaldt's bursitis (disease) (pharyngeal
    bursitis) 478.29
    cyst 478.26
Torpid liver 573.9
Torsion
    accessory tube 620.5
    adnexa (female) 620.5
    aorta (congenital) 747.29
        acquired 447.1
    appendix epididymis 608.2
    bile duct 576.8
        with calculus, choledocholithiasis or stones
            — *see* Choledocholithiasis
        congenital 751.69
    bowel, colon, or intestine 560.2
    cervix (*see also* Malposition, uterus) 621.6
    duodenum 537.3
    dystonia — *see* Dystonia, torsion
    epididymis 608.2
        appendix 608.2
    fallopian tube 620.5
    gallbladder (*see also* Disease, gallbladder)
        575.8
        congenital 751.69
    gastric 537.89
    hydatid of Morgagni (female) 620.5
    kidney (pedicle) 593.89
    Meckel's diverticulum (congenital) 751.0
    mesentery 560.2
    omentum 560.2
    organ or site, congenital NEC — *see* Anomaly,
        specified type NEC
    ovary (pedicle) 620.5
        congenital 752.0
    oviduct 620.5
    penis 607.89
        congenital 752.69
    renal 593.89
    spasm — *see* Dystonia, torsion
    spermatic cord 608.2
    spleen 289.59
    testicle, testis 608.2
    tibia 736.89
    umbilical cord — *see* Compression, umbilical
        cord
    uterus (*see also* Malposition, uterus) 621.6
Torticollis (intermittent) (spastic) 723.5
    congenital 754.1
        sternomastoid 754.1
    due to birth injury 767.8
    hysterical 300.11
    ocular 781.93
    psychogenic 306.0
        specified as conversion reaction 300.11
    rheumatic 723.5
    rheumatoid 714.0
    spasmodic 333.83
    traumatic, current NEC 847.0
Tortuous
    artery 447.1
    fallopian tube 752.19
    organ or site, congenital NEC — *see* Distortion
    renal vessel, congenital 747.62
    retina vessel (congenital) 743.58
        acquired 362.17
    ureter 593.4
    urethra 599.84
    vein — *see* Varicose, vein
Torula, torular (infection) 117.5
    histolytica 117.5
    lung 117.5
Torulosis 117.5

Torus
    fracture   ●
        fibula 823.41   ●
            with tibia 823.42   ●
        radius 813.45   ●
        tibia 823.40   ●
            with fibula 823.42   ●
    mandibularis 526.81
    palatinus 526.81
Touch, vitreous 997.99
Touraine's syndrome (hereditary osteo-
    onychodysplasia) 756.89
Touraine-Solente-Golé syndrome
    (acropachyderma) 757.39
Tourette's disease (motor-verbal tic) 307.23
Tower skull 756.0
    with exophthalmos 756.0
Toxemia 799.8
    with
        abortion — *see* Abortion, by type, with
            toxemia
    bacterial — *see* Septicemia
    biliary (*see also* Disease, biliary) 576.8
    burn — *see* Burn, by site
    congenital NEC 779.89   ▲
    eclamptic 642.6 ✓5ᵗʰ
        with pre-existing hypertension 642.7 ✓5ᵗʰ
    erysipelatous (*see also* Erysipelas) 035
    fatigue 799.8
    fetus or newborn NEC 779.89   ▲
    food (*see also* Poisoning, food) 005.9
    gastric 537.89
    gastrointestinal 558.2
    intestinal 558.2
    kidney (*see also* Disease, renal) 593.9
    lung 518.89
    malarial NEC (*see also* Malaria) 084.6
    maternal (of pregnancy), affecting fetus or
        newborn 760.0
    myocardial — *see* Myocarditis, toxic
    of pregnancy (mild) (pre-eclamptic) 642.4 ✓5ᵗʰ
        with
            convulsions 642.6 ✓5ᵗʰ
            pre-existing hypertension 642.7 ✓5ᵗʰ
        affecting fetus or newborn 760.0
        severe 642.5 ✓5ᵗʰ
    pre-eclamptic — *see* Toxemia, of pregnancy
    puerperal, postpartum — *see* Toxemia, of
        pregnancy
    pulmonary 518.89
    renal (*see also* Disease, renal) 593.9
    septic (*see also* Septicemia) 038.9
    small intestine 558.2
    staphylococcal 038.10
        aureus 038.11
        due to food 005.0
        specified organism NEC 038.19
    stasis 799.8
    stomach 537.89
    uremic (*see also* Uremia) 586
    urinary 586
Toxemica cerebropathia psychica (nonalcoholic)
    294.0
    alcoholic 291.1
Toxic (poisoning) — *see also* condition
    from drug or poison — *see* Table of Drugs and
        Chemicals
    oil syndrome 710.5
    shock syndrome 040.82   ▲
    thyroid (gland) (*see also* Thyrotoxicosis)
        242.9 ✓5ᵗʰ
Toxicemia — *see* Toxemia
Toxicity
    dilantin
        asymptomatic 796.0
        symptomatic — *see* Table of Drugs and
            Chemicals
    drug
        asymptomatic 796.0
        symptomatic — *see* Table of Drugs and
            Chemicals
    fava bean 282.2
    from drug or poison
        asymptomatic 796.0
        symptomatic — *see* Table of Drugs and
            Chemicals

Toxicosis (*see also* Toxemia) 799.8
    capillary, hemorrhagic 287.0
Toxinfection 799.8
    gastrointestinal 558.2
Toxocariasis 128.0
Toxoplasma infection, generalized 130.9
Toxoplasmosis (acquired) 130.9
    with pneumonia 130.4
    congenital, active 771.2
    disseminated (multisystemic) 130.8
    maternal
        with suspected damage to fetus affecting
            management of pregnancy 655.4 ✓5ᵗʰ
        affecting fetus or newborn 760.2
            manifest toxoplasmosis in fetus or
                newborn 771.2
    multiple sites 130.8
    multisystemic disseminated 130.8
    specified site NEC 130.7
Trabeculation, bladder 596.8
Trachea — *see* condition
Tracheitis (acute) (catarrhal) (infantile)
    (membranous) (plastic) (pneumococcal)
    (septic) (suppurative) (viral) 464.10
    with
        bronchitis 490
            acute or subacute 466.0
            chronic 491.8
            tuberculosis — *see* Tuberculosis,
                pulmonary
        laryngitis (acute) 464.20
            with obstruction 464.21
            chronic 476.1
            tuberculous (*see also* Tuberculosis,
                larynx) 012.3 ✓5ᵗʰ
        obstruction 464.11
    chronic 491.8
        with
            bronchitis (chronic) 491.8
            laryngitis (chronic) 476.1
        due to external agent — *see* Condition,
            respiratory, chronic, due to
    diphtheritic (membranous) 032.3
    due to external agent — *see* Inflammation,
        respiratory, upper, due to
    edematous 464.11
    influenzal 487.1
    streptococcal 034.0
    syphilitic 095.8
    tuberculous (*see also* Tuberculosis) 012.8 ✓5ᵗʰ
Trachelitis (nonvenereal) (*see also* Cervicitis)
    616.0
    trichomonal 131.09
Tracheobronchial — *see* condition
Tracheobronchitis (*see also* Bronchitis) 490
    acute or subacute 466.0
        with bronchospasm or obstruction 466.0
    chronic 491.8
    influenzal 487.1
    senile 491.8
Tracheobronchomegaly (congenital) 748.3
Tracheobronchopneumonitis — *see* Pneumonia,
    broncho
Tracheocele (external) (internal) 519.1
    congenital 748.3
Tracheomalacia 519.1
    congenital 748.3
Tracheopharyngitis (acute) 465.8
    chronic 478.9
        due to external agent — *see* Condition,
            respiratory, chronic, due to
    due to external agent — *see* Inflammation,
        respiratory, upper, due to
Tracheostenosis 519.1
    congenital 748.3
Tracheostomy
    attention to V55.0
    complication 519.00
    hemorrhage 519.09
    infection 519.01
    malfunctioning 519.02
    obstruction 519.09
    sepsis 519.01
    status V44.0

Tonsillitis — Tracheostomy

Tracheostomy — *continued*
  stenosis 519.02
Trachoma, trachomatous 076.9
  active (stage) 076.1
  contraction of conjunctiva 076.1
  dubium 076.0
  healed or late effect 139.1
  initial (stage) 076.0
  Türck's (chronic catarrhal laryngitis) 476.0
Trachyphonia 784.49
Training
  orthoptic V57.4
  orthotic V57.81
Train sickness 994.6
Trait
  hemoglobin
    abnormal NEC 282.7
      with thalassemia 282.4
    C (*see also* Disease, hemoglobin, C) 282.7
      with elliptocytosis 282.7
    S (Hb-S) 282.5
  Lepore 282.4
    with other abnormal hemoglobin NEC 282.4
  paranoid 301.0
  sickle-cell 282.5
    with
      elliptocytosis 282.5
      spherocytosis 282.5
Traits, paranoid 301.0
Tramp V60.0
Trance 780.09
  hysterical 300.13
Transaminasemia 790.4
Transfusion, blood
  donor V59.01
    stem cells V59.02
  incompatible 999.6
  reaction or complication — *see* Complications, transfusion
  syndrome
    fetomaternal 772.0
    twin-to-twin
      blood loss (donor twin) 772.0
      recipient twin 776.4
  without reported diagnosis V58.2
Transient — *see also* condition
  alteration of awareness 780.02
  blindness 368.12
  deafness (ischemic) 388.02
  global amnesia 437.7
  person (homeless) NEC V60.0
Transitional, lumbosacral joint of vertebra 756.19
Translocation
  autosomes NEC 758.5
    13-15 758.1
    16-18 758.2
    21 or 22 758.0
    balanced in normal individual 758.4
    D₁ 758.1
    E₃ 758.2
    G 758.0
  balanced autosomal in normal individual 758.4
  chromosomes NEC 758.89
  Down's syndrome 758.0
Translucency, iris 364.53
Transmission of chemical substances through the placenta (affecting fetus or newborn) 760.70
  alcohol 760.71
  anti-infective agents 760.74
  cocaine 760.75
  "crack" 760.75
  diethylstilbestrol [DES] 760.76
  hallucinogenic agents 760.73
  medicinal agents NEC 760.79
  narcotics 760.72
  obstetric anesthetic or analgesic drug 763.5
  specified agent NEC 760.79
  suspected, affecting management of pregnancy 655.5 ☑5ᵗʰ
Transplant(ed)
  bone V42.4
    marrow V42.81

Transplant(ed) — *continued*
  complication — *see also* Complications, due to (presence of) any device, implant, or graft classified to 996.0-996.5 NEC
    bone marrow 996.85
    corneal graft NEC 996.79
      infection or inflammation 996.69
      reaction 996.51
      rejection 996.51
    organ (failure) (immune or nonimmune cause) (infection) (rejection) 996.87
      bone marrow 996.85
      heart 996.83
      intestines 996.87
      kidney 996.81
      liver 996.82
      lung 996.84
      pancreas 996.86
      specified NEC 996.89
    skin NEC 996.79
      infection or inflammation 996.69
      rejection 996.52
        artificial 996.55
        decellularized allodermis 996.55
  cornea V42.5
  hair V50.0
  heart V42.1
    valve V42.2
  intestine V42.84
  kidney V42.0
  liver V42.7
  lung V42.6
  organ V42.9
    specified NEC V42.89
  pancreas V42.83
  peripheral stem cells V42.82
  skin V42.3
  stem cells, peripheral V42.82
  tissue V42.9
    specified NEC V42.89
Transplants, ovarian, endometrial 617.1
Transposed — *see* Transposition
Transposition (congenital) — *see also* Malposition, congenital
  abdominal viscera 759.3
  aorta (dextra) 745.11
  appendix 751.5
  arterial trunk 745.10
  colon 751.5
  great vessels (complete) 745.10
    both originating from right ventricle 745.11
    corrected 745.12
    double outlet right ventricle 745.11
    incomplete 745.11
    partial 745.11
    specified type NEC 745.19
  heart 746.87
    with complete transposition of viscera 759.3
  intestine (large) (small) 751.5
  pulmonary veins 747.49
  reversed jejunal (for bypass) (status) V45.3
  stomach 750.7
    with general transposition of viscera 759.3
  teeth, tooth 524.3
  vessels (complete) 745.10
    partial 745.11
  viscera (abdominal) (thoracic) 759.3
Trans-sexualism 302.50
  with
    asexual history 302.51
    heterosexual history 302.53
    homosexual history 302.52
Transverse — *see also* condition
  arrest (deep), in labor 660.3 ☑5ᵗʰ
    affecting fetus or newborn 763.1
  lie 652.3 ☑5ᵗʰ
    before labor, affecting fetus or newborn 761.7
    causing obstructed labor 660.0 ☑5ᵗʰ
      affecting fetus or newborn 763.1
    during labor, affecting fetus or newborn 763.1
Transvestism, transvestitism (transvestic fetishism) 302.3
Trapped placenta (with hemorrhage) 666.0 ☑5ᵗʰ
  without hemorrhage 667.0 ☑5ᵗʰ

Trauma, traumatism (*see also* Injury, by site) 959.9
  birth — *see* Birth, injury NEC
  causing hemorrhage of pregnancy or delivery 641.8 ☑5ᵗʰ
  complicating
    abortion — *see* Abortion, by type, with damage to pelvic organs
    ectopic pregnancy (*see also* categories 633.0-633.9) 639.2
    molar pregnancy (*see also* categories 630-632) 639.2
  during delivery NEC 665.9 ☑5ᵗʰ
  following
    abortion 639.2
    ectopic or molar pregnancy 639.2
  maternal, during pregnancy, affecting fetus or newborn 760.5
  neuroma — *see* Injury, nerve, by site
  previous major, affecting management of pregnancy, childbirth, or puerperium V23.8 ☑5ᵗʰ
  psychic (current) — *see also* Reaction, adjustment
    previous (history) V15.49
  psychologic, previous (affecting health) V15.49
  transient paralysis — *see* Injury, nerve, by site
Traumatic — *see* condition
Treacher Collins' syndrome (incomplete facial dysostosis) 756.0
Treitz's hernia — *see* Hernia, Treitz's
Trematode infestation NEC 121.9
Trematodiasis NEC 121.9
Trembles 988.8
Trembling paralysis (*see also* Parkinsonism) 332.0
Tremor 781.0
  essential (benign) 333.1
  familial 333.1
  flapping (liver) 572.8
  hereditary 333.1
  hysterical 300.11
  intention 333.1
  mercurial 985.0
  muscle 728.85
  Parkinson's (*see also* Parkinsonism) 332.0
  psychogenic 306.0
    specified as conversion reaction 300.11
  senilis 797
  specified type NEC 333.1
Trench
  fever 083.1
  foot 991.4
  mouth 101
  nephritis — *see* Nephritis, acute
Treponema pallidum infection (*see also* Syphilis) 097.9
Treponematosis 102.9
  due to
    T. pallidum — *see* Syphilis
    T. pertenue (yaws) (*see also* Yaws) 102.9
Triad
  Kartagener's 759.3
  Reiter's (complete) (incomplete) 099.3
  Saint's (*see also* Hernia, diaphragm) 553.3
Trichiasis 704.2
  cicatricial 704.2
  eyelid 374.05
    with entropion (*see also* Entropion) 374.00
Trichinella spiralis (infection) (infestation) 124
Trichinelliasis 124
Trichinellosis 124
Trichiniasis 124
Trichinosis 124
Trichobezoar 938
  intestine 936
  stomach 935.2
Trichocephaliasis 127.3
Trichocephalosis 127.3
Trichocephalus infestation 127.3
Trichoclasis 704.2

Trichoepithelioma — Tuberculosis

Trichoepithelioma (M8100/0) — *see also* Neoplasm, skin, benign
  breast 217
  genital organ NEC — *see* Neoplasm, by site, benign
  malignant (M8100/3) — *see* Neoplasm, skin, malignant
Trichofolliculoma (M8101/0) — *see* Neoplasm, skin, benign
Tricholemmoma (M8102/0) — *see* Neoplasm, skin, benign
Trichomatosis 704.2
Trichomoniasis 131.9
  bladder 131.09
  cervix 131.09
  intestinal 007.3
  prostate 131.03
  seminal vesicle 131.09
  specified site NEC 131.8
  urethra 131.02
  urogenitalis 131.00
  vagina 131.01
  vulva 131.01
  vulvovaginal 131.01
Trichomycosis 039.0
  axillaris 039.0
  nodosa 111.2
  nodularis 111.2
  rubra 039.0
Trichonocardiosis (axillaris) (palmellina) 039.0
Trichonodosis 704.2
Trichophytid, trichophyton infection (*see also* Dermatophytosis) 110.9
Trichophytide — *see* Dermatophytosis
Trichophytobezoar 938
  intestine 936
  stomach 935.2
Trichophytosis — *see* Dermatophytosis
Trichoptilosis 704.2
Trichorrhexis (nodosa) 704.2
Trichosporosis nodosa 111.2
Trichostasis spinulosa (congenital) 757.4
Trichostrongyliasis (small intestine) 127.6
Trichostrongylosis 127.6
Trichostrongylus (instabilis) infection 127.6
Trichotillomania 312.39
Trichromat, anomalous (congenital) 368.59
Trichromatopsia, anomalous (congenital) 368.59
Trichuriasis 127.3
Trichuris trichiuria (any site) (infection) (infestation) 127.3
Tricuspid (valve) — *see* condition
Trifid — *see also* Accessory
  kidney (pelvis) 753.3
  tongue 750.13
Trigeminal neuralgia (*see also* Neuralgia, trigeminal) 350.1
Trigeminoencephaloangiomatosis 759.6
Trigeminy 427.89
  postoperative 997.1
Trigger finger (acquired) 727.03
  congenital 756.89
Trigonitis (bladder) (chronic) (pseudomembranous) 595.3
  tuberculous (*see also* Tuberculosis) 016.1 ✓5ᵗʰ
Trigonocephaly 756.0
Trihexosidosis 272.7
Trilobate placenta — *see* Placenta, abnormal
Trilocular heart 745.8
Tripartita placenta — *see* Placenta, abnormal
Triple — *see also* Accessory
  kidneys 753.3
  uteri 752.2
  X female 758.81
Triplegia 344.89
  congenital or infantile 343.8
Triplet
  affected by maternal complications of pregnancy 761.5
  healthy liveborn — *see* Newborn, multiple

Triplet — *continued*
  pregnancy (complicating delivery) NEC 651.1 ✓5ᵗʰ
    with fetal loss and retention of one or more fetus(es) 651.4 ✓5ᵗʰ
Triplex placenta — *see* Placenta, abnormal
Triplication — *see* Accessory
Trismus 781.0
  neonatorum 771.3
  newborn 771.3
Trisomy (syndrome) NEC 758.5
  13 (partial) 758.1
  16-18 758.2
  18 (partial) 758.2
  21 (partial) 758.0
  22 758.0
  autosomes NEC 758.5
  D₁ 758.1
  E₃ 758.2
  G (group) 758.0
  group D₁ 758.1
  group E 758.2
  group G 758.0
Tritanomaly 368.53
Tritanopia 368.53
Troisier-Hanot-Chauffard syndrome (bronze diabetes) 275.0
Trombidiosis 133.8
Trophedema (hereditary) 757.0
  congenital 757.0
Trophoblastic disease (*see also* Hydatidiform mole) 630
  previous, affecting management of pregnancy V23.1
Tropholymphedema 757.0
Trophoneurosis NEC 356.9
  arm NEC 354.9
  disseminated 710.1
  facial 349.89
  leg NEC 355.8
  lower extremity NEC 355.8
  upper extremity NEC 354.9
Tropical — *see also* condition
  maceration feet (syndrome) 991.4
  wet foot (syndrome) 991.4
Trouble — *see also* Disease
  bowel 569.9
  heart — *see* Disease, heart
  intestine 569.9
  kidney (*see also* Disease, renal) 593.9
  nervous 799.2
  sinus (*see also* Sinusitis) 473.9
Trousseau's syndrome (thrombophlebitis migrans) 453.1
Truancy, childhood — *see also* Disturbance, conduct
  socialized 312.2 ✓5ᵗʰ
  undersocialized, unsocialized 312.1 ✓5ᵗʰ
Truncus
  arteriosus (persistent) 745.0
  common 745.0
  communis 745.0
Trunk — *see* condition
Trychophytide — *see* Dermatophytosis
Trypanosoma infestation — *see* Trypanosomiasis
Trypanosomiasis 086.9
  with meningoencephalitis 086.9 [323.2]
  African 086.5
    due to Trypanosoma 086.5
      gambiense 086.3
      rhodesiense 086.4
  American 086.2
    with
      heart involvement 086.0
      other organ involvement 086.1
    without mention of organ involvement 086.2
  Brazilian — *see* Trypanosomiasis, American
  Chagas' — *see* Trypanosomiasis, American
  due to Trypanosoma
    cruzi — *see* Trypanosomiasis, American
    gambiense 086.3
    rhodesiense 086.4

Trypanosomiasis — *continued*
  gambiensis, Gambian 086.3
  North American — *see* Trypanosomiasis, American
  rhodesiensis, Rhodesian 086.4
  South American — *see* Trypanosomiasis, American
T-shaped incisors 520.2
Tsutsugamushi fever 081.2
Tube, tubal, tubular — *see also* condition
  ligation, admission for V25.2
Tubercle — *see also* Tuberculosis
  brain, solitary 013.2 ✓5ᵗʰ
  Darwin's 744.29
  epithelioid noncaseating 135
  Ghon, primary infection 010.0 ✓5ᵗʰ
Tuberculid, tuberculide (indurating) (lichenoid) (miliary) (papulonecrotic) (primary) (skin) (subcutaneous) (*see also* Tuberculosis) 017.0 ✓5ᵗʰ
Tuberculoma — *see also* Tuberculosis
  brain (any part) 013.2 ✓5ᵗʰ
  meninges (cerebral) (spinal) 013.1 ✓5ᵗʰ
  spinal cord 013.4 ✓5ᵗʰ
Tuberculosis, tubercular, tuberculous
  (calcification) (calcified) (caseous) (chromogenic acid-fast bacilli) (congenital) (degeneration) (disease) (fibrocaseous) (fistula) (gangrene) (interstitial) (isolated circumscribed lesions) (necrosis) (parenchymatous) (ulcerative) 011.9

> *Note* — *Use the following fifth-digit subclassification with categories 010-018:*
>
> *0   unspecified*
> *1   bacteriological or histological examination not done*
> *2   bacteriological or histological examination unknown (at present)*
> *3   tubercle bacilli found (in sputum) by microscopy*
> *4   tubercle bacilli not found (in sputum) by microscopy, but found by bacterial culture*
> *5   tubercle bacilli not found by bacteriological exam-ination, but tuberculosis confirmed histologically*
> *6   tubercle bacilli not found by bacteriological or histological examination, but tuberculosis confirmed by other methods [inoculation of animals]*
>
> *For tuberculous conditions specified as late effects or sequelae, see category 137.*

  abdomen 014.8 ✓5ᵗʰ
    lymph gland 014.8 ✓5ᵗʰ
  abscess 011.9 ✓5ᵗʰ
    arm 017.9 ✓5ᵗʰ
    bone (*see also* Osteomyelitis, due to, tuberculosis) 015.9 ✓5ᵗʰ *[730.8]* ✓5ᵗʰ
      hip 015.1 ✓5ᵗʰ *[730.85]*
      knee 015.2 ✓5ᵗʰ *[730.96]*
      sacrum 015.0 ✓5ᵗʰ *[730.88]*
      specified site NEC 015.7 ✓5ᵗʰ *[730.88]*
      spinal 015.0 ✓5ᵗʰ *[730.88]*
      vertebra 015.0 ✓5ᵗʰ *[730.88]*
    brain 013.3 ✓5ᵗʰ
    breast 017.9 ✓5ᵗʰ
    Cowper's gland 016.5 ✓5ᵗʰ
    dura (mater) 013.8 ✓5ᵗʰ
      brain 013.3 ✓5ᵗʰ
      spinal cord 013.5 ✓5ᵗʰ
    epidural 013.8 ✓5ᵗʰ
      brain 013.3 ✓5ᵗʰ
      spinal cord 013.5 ✓5ᵗʰ
    frontal sinus — *see* Tuberculosis, sinus
    genital organs NEC 016.9 ✓5ᵗʰ
      female 016.7 ✓5ᵗʰ
      male 016.5 ✓5ᵗʰ
    genitourinary NEC 016.9 ✓5ᵗʰ
    gland (lymphatic) — *see* Tuberculosis, lymph gland
    hip 015.1 ✓5ᵗʰ

Tuberculosis, tubercular, tuberculous —
continued
  abscess — continued
    iliopsoas 015.0 ✓5 [730.88]
    intestine 014.8 ✓5
    ischiorectal 014.8 ✓5
    joint 015.9 ✓5
      hip 015.1 ✓5
      knee 015.2 ✓5
      specified joint NEC 015.8 ✓5
      vertebral 015.0 ✓5 [730.88]
    kidney 016.0 ✓5 [590.81]
    knee 015.2 ✓5
    lumbar 015.0 ✓5 [730.88]
    lung 011.2 ✓5
      primary, progressive 010.8 ✓5
    meninges (cerebral) (spinal) 013.0 ✓5
    pelvic 016.9 ✓5
      female 016.7 ✓5
      male 016.5 ✓5
    perianal 014.8 ✓5
      fistula 014.8 ✓5
    perinephritic 016.0 ✓5 [590.81]
    perineum 017.9 ✓5
    perirectal 014.8 ✓5
    psoas 015.0 ✓5 [730.88]
    rectum 014.8 ✓5
    retropharyngeal 012.8 ✓5
    sacrum 015.0 ✓5 [730.88]
    scrofulous 017.2 ✓5
    scrotum 016.5 ✓5
    skin 017.0 ✓5
      primary 017.0 ✓5
    spinal cord 013.5 ✓5
    spine or vertebra (column)
        015.0 ✓5 [730.88]
    strumous 017.2 ✓5
    subdiaphragmatic 014.8 ✓5
    testis 016.5 ✓5
    thigh 017.9 ✓5
    urinary 016.3 ✓5
      kidney 016.0 ✓5 [590.81]
    uterus 016.7 ✓5
  accessory sinus — see Tuberculosis, sinus
  Addison's disease 017.6 ✓5
  adenitis (see also Tuberculosis, lymph gland)
      017.2 ✓5
  adenoids 012.8 ✓5
  adenopathy (see also Tuberculosis, lymph
      gland) 017.2 ✓5
    tracheobronchial 012.1 ✓5
      primary progressive 010.8 ✓5
  adherent pericardium 017.9 ✓5 [420.0]
  adnexa (uteri) 016.7 ✓5
  adrenal (capsule) (gland) 017.6 ✓5
  air passage NEC 012.8 ✓5
  alimentary canal 014.8 ✓5
  anemia 017.9 ✓5
  ankle (joint) 015.8 ✓5
    bone 015.5 ✓5 [730.87]
  anus 014.8 ✓5
  apex (see also Tuberculosis, pulmonary)
      011.9 ✓5
  apical (see also Tuberculosis, pulmonary)
      011.9 ✓5
  appendicitis 014.8 ✓5
  appendix 014.8 ✓5
  arachnoid 013.0 ✓5
  artery 017.9 ✓5
  arthritis (chronic) (synovial) 015.9 ✓5 [711.40]
    ankle 015.8 ✓5 [730.87]
    hip 015.1 ✓5 [711.45]
    knee 015.2 ✓5 [711.46]
    specified site NEC 015.8 ✓5 [711.48]
    spine or vertebra (column)
        015.0 ✓5 [720.81]
    wrist 015.8 ✓5 [730.83]
  articular — see Tuberculosis, joint
  ascites 014.0 ✓5
  asthma (see also Tuberculosis, pulmonary)
      011.9 ✓5
  axilla, axillary 017.2 ✓5
    gland 017.2 ✓5
  bilateral (see also Tuberculosis, pulmonary)
      011.9 ✓5
  bladder 016.1 ✓5

Tuberculosis, tubercular, tuberculous —
continued
  bone (see also Osteomyelitis, due to,
      tuberculosis) 015.9 ✓5 [730.8] ✓5
    hip 015.1 ✓5 [730.85]
    knee 015.2 ✓5 [730.86]
    limb NEC 015.5 ✓5 [730.88]
    sacrum 015.0 ✓5 [730.88]
    specified site NEC 015.7 ✓5 [730.88]
    spinal or vertebral column 015.0
        ✓5 [730.88]
  bowel 014.8 ✓5
    miliary 018.9 ✓5
  brain 013.2 ✓5
  breast 017.9 ✓5
  broad ligament 016.7 ✓5
  bronchi, bronchial, bronchus 011.3 ✓5
    ectasia, ectasis 011.5 ✓5
    fistula 011.3 ✓5
      primary, progressive 010.8 ✓5
    gland 012.1 ✓5
      primary, progressive 010.8 ✓5
    isolated 012.2 ✓5
    lymph gland or node 012.1 ✓5
      primary, progressive 010.8 ✓5
  bronchiectasis 011.5 ✓5
  bronchitis 011.3 ✓5
  bronchopleural 012.0 ✓5
  bronchopneumonia, bronchopneumonic
      011.6 ✓5
  bronchorrhagia 011.3 ✓5
  bronchotracheal 011.3 ✓5
    isolated 012.2 ✓5
  bronchus — see Tuberculosis, bronchi
  bronze disease (Addison's) 017.6 ✓5
  buccal cavity 017.9 ✓5
  bulbourethral gland 016.5 ✓5
  bursa (see also Tuberculosis, joint) 015.9 ✓5
  cachexia NEC (see also Tuberculosis,
      pulmonary) 011.9 ✓5
  cardiomyopathy 017.9 ✓5 [425.8]
  caries (see also Tuberculosis, bone)
      015.9 ✓5 [730.8] ✓5
  cartilage (see also Tuberculosis, bone)
      015.9 ✓5 [730.8] ✓5
    intervertebral 015.0 ✓5 [730.88]
  catarrhal (see also Tuberculosis, pulmonary)
      011.9 ✓5
  cecum 014.8 ✓5
  cellular tissue (primary) 017.0 ✓5
  cellulitis (primary) 017.0 ✓5
  central nervous system 013.9 ✓5
    specified site NEC 013.8 ✓5
  cerebellum (current) 013.2 ✓5
  cerebral (current) 013.2 ✓5
    meninges 013.0 ✓5
  cerebrospinal 013.6 ✓5
    meninges 013.0 ✓5
  cerebrum (current) 013.2 ✓5
  cervical 017.2 ✓5
    gland 017.2 ✓5
    lymph nodes 017.2 ✓5
  cervicitis (uteri) 016.7 ✓5
  cervix 016.7 ✓5
  chest (see also Tuberculosis, pulmonary)
      011.9 ✓5
  childhood type or first infection 010.0 ✓5
  choroid 017.3 ✓5 [363.13]
  choroiditis 017.3 ✓5 [363.13]
  ciliary body 017.3 ✓5 [364.11]
  colitis 014.8 ✓5
  colliers' 011.4 ✓5
  colliquativa (primary) 017.0 ✓5
  colon 014.8 ✓5
    ulceration 014.8 ✓5
  complex, primary 010.0 ✓5
  complicating pregnancy, childbirth, or
      puerperium 647.3 ✓5
    affecting fetus or newborn 760.2
  congenital 771.2
  conjunctiva 017.3 ✓5 [370.31]
  connective tissue 017.9 ✓5
    bone — see Tuberculosis, bone
  contact V01.1
  converter (tuberculin test) (without disease)
      795.5
  cornea (ulcer) 017.3 ✓5 [370.31]
  Cowper's gland 016.5 ✓5

Tuberculosis, tubercular, tuberculous —
continued
  coxae 015.1 ✓5 [730.85]
  coxalgia 015.1 ✓5 [730.85]
  cul-de-sac of Douglas 014.8 ✓5
  curvature, spine 015.0 ✓5 [737.40]
  cutis (colliquativa) (primary) 017.0 ✓5
  cyst, ovary 016.6 ✓5
  cystitis 016.1 ✓5
  dacryocystitis 017.3 ✓5 [375.32]
  dactylitis 015.5 ✓5
  diarrhea 014.8 ✓5
  diffuse (see also Tuberculosis, miliary)
      018.9 ✓5
    lung — see Tuberculosis, pulmonary
    meninges 013.0 ✓5
  digestive tract 014.8 ✓5
  disseminated (see also Tuberculosis, miliary)
      018.9 ✓5
    meninges 013.0 ✓5
  duodenum 014.8 ✓5
  dura (mater) 013.9 ✓5
    abscess 013.8 ✓5
      cerebral 013.3 ✓5
      spinal 013.5 ✓5
  dysentery 014.8 ✓5
  ear (inner) (middle) 017.4 ✓5
    bone 015.6 ✓5
    external (primary) 017.0 ✓5
    skin (primary) 017.0 ✓5
  elbow 015.8 ✓5
  emphysema — see Tuberculosis, pulmonary
  empyema 012.0 ✓5
  encephalitis 013.6 ✓5
  endarteritis 017.9 ✓5
  endocarditis (any valve) 017.9 ✓5 [424.91]
  endocardium (any valve) 017.9 ✓5 [424.91]
  endocrine glands NEC 017.9 ✓5
  endometrium 016.7 ✓5
  enteric, enterica 014.8 ✓5
  enteritis 014.8 ✓5
  enterocolitis 014.8 ✓5
  epididymis 016.4 ✓5
  epididymitis 016.4 ✓5
  epidural abscess 013.8 ✓5
    brain 013.3 ✓5
    spinal cord 013.5 ✓5
  epiglottis 012.3 ✓5
  episcleritis 017.3 ✓5 [379.00]
  erythema (induratum) (nodosum) (primary)
      017.1 ✓5
  esophagus 017.8 ✓5
  Eustachian tube 017.4 ✓5
  exposure to V01.1
  exudative 012.0 ✓5
    primary, progressive 010.1 ✓5
  eye 017.3 ✓5
    glaucoma 017.3 ✓5 [365.62]
  eyelid (primary) 017.0 ✓5
    lupus 017.0 ✓5 [373.4]
  fallopian tube 016.6 ✓5
  fascia 017.9 ✓5
  fauces 012.8 ✓5
  finger 017.9 ✓5
  first infection 010.0 ✓5
  fistula, perirectal 014.8 ✓5
  Florida 011.6 ✓5
  foot 017.9 ✓5
  funnel pelvis 137.3
  gallbladder 017.9 ✓5
  galloping (see also Tuberculosis, pulmonary)
      011.9 ✓5
  ganglionic 015.9 ✓5
  gastritis 017.9 ✓5
  gastrocolic fistula 014.8 ✓5
  gastroenteritis 014.8 ✓5
  gastrointestinal tract 014.8 ✓5
  general, generalized 018.9 ✓5
    acute 018.0 ✓5
    chronic 018.8 ✓5
  genital organs NEC 016.9 ✓5
    female 016.7 ✓5
    male 016.5 ✓5
  genitourinary NEC 016.9 ✓5
  genu 015.2 ✓5
  glandulae suprarenalis 017.6 ✓5
  glandular, general 017.2 ✓5
  glottis 012.3 ✓5

Tuberculosis — Tuberculosis

Tuberculosis, tubercular, tuberculous —
continued
grinders' 011.4 ✓5ᵗʰ
groin 017.2 ✓5ᵗʰ
gum 017.9 ✓5ᵗʰ
hand 017.9 ✓5ᵗʰ
heart 017.9 ✓5ᵗʰ [425.8]
hematogenous — *see* Tuberculosis, miliary
hemoptysis (*see also* Tuberculosis, pulmonary)
011.9 ✓5ᵗʰ
hemorrhage NEC (*see also* Tuberculosis,
pulmonary) 011.9 ✓5ᵗʰ
hemothorax 012.0 ✓5ᵗʰ
hepatitis 017.9 ✓5ᵗʰ
hilar lymph nodes 012.1 ✓5ᵗʰ
primary, progressive 010.8 ✓5ᵗʰ
hip (disease) (joint) 015.1 ✓5ᵗʰ
bone 015.1 ✓5ᵗʰ [730.85]
hydrocephalus 013.8 ✓5ᵗʰ
hydropneumothorax 012.0 ✓5ᵗʰ
hydrothorax 012.0 ✓5ᵗʰ
hypoadrenalism 017.6 ✓5ᵗʰ
hypopharynx 012.8 ✓5ᵗʰ
ileocecal (hyperplastic) 014.8 ✓5ᵗʰ
ileocolitis 014.8 ✓5ᵗʰ
ileum 014.8 ✓5ᵗʰ
iliac spine (superior) 015.0 ✓5ᵗʰ [730.88]
incipient NEC (*see also* Tuberculosis,
pulmonary) 011.9 ✓5ᵗʰ
indurativa (primary) 017.1 ✓5ᵗʰ
infantile 010.0 ✓5ᵗʰ
infection NEC 011.9 ✓5ᵗʰ
without clinical manifestation 010.0 ✓5ᵗʰ
infraclavicular gland 017.2 ✓5ᵗʰ
inguinal gland 017.2 ✓5ᵗʰ
inguinalis 017.2 ✓5ᵗʰ
intestine (any part) 014.8 ✓5ᵗʰ
iris 017.3 ✓5ᵗʰ [364.11]
iritis 017.3 ✓5ᵗʰ [364.11]
ischiorectal 014.8 ✓5ᵗʰ
jaw 015.7 ✓5ᵗʰ [730.88]
jejunum 014.8 ✓5ᵗʰ
joint 015.9 ✓5ᵗʰ
hip 015.1 ✓5ᵗʰ
knee 015.2 ✓5ᵗʰ
specified site NEC 015.8 ✓5ᵗʰ
vertebral 015.0 ✓5ᵗʰ [730.88]
keratitis 017.3 ✓5ᵗʰ [370.31]
interstitial 017.3 ✓5ᵗʰ [370.59]
keratoconjunctivitis 017.3 ✓5ᵗʰ [370.31]
kidney 016.0 ✓5ᵗʰ
knee (joint) 015.2 ✓5ᵗʰ
kyphoscoliosis 015.0 ✓5ᵗʰ [737.43]
kyphosis 015.0 ✓5ᵗʰ [737.41]
lacrimal apparatus, gland 017.3 ✓5ᵗʰ
laryngitis 012.3 ✓5ᵗʰ
larynx 012.3 ✓5ᵗʰ
leptomeninges, leptomeningitis (cerebral)
(spinal) 013.0 ✓5ᵗʰ
lichenoides (primary) 017.0 ✓5ᵗʰ
linguae 017.9 ✓5ᵗʰ
lip 017.9 ✓5ᵗʰ
liver 017.9 ✓5ᵗʰ
lordosis 015.0 ✓5ᵗʰ [737.42]
lung — *see* Tuberculosis, pulmonary
luposa 017.0 ✓5ᵗʰ
eyelid 017.0 ✓5ᵗʰ [373.4]
lymphadenitis — *see* Tuberculosis, lymph
gland
lymphangitis — *see* Tuberculosis, lymph gland
lymphatic (gland) (vessel) — *see* Tuberculosis,
lymph gland
lymph gland or node (peripheral) 017.2 ✓5ᵗʰ
abdomen 014.8 ✓5ᵗʰ
bronchial 012.1 ✓5ᵗʰ
primary, progressive 010.8 ✓5ᵗʰ
cervical 017.2 ✓5ᵗʰ
hilar 012.1 ✓5ᵗʰ
primary, progressive 010.8 ✓5ᵗʰ
intrathoracic 012.1 ✓5ᵗʰ
primary, progressive 010.8 ✓5ᵗʰ
mediastinal 012.1 ✓5ᵗʰ
primary, progressive 010.8 ✓5ᵗʰ
mesenteric 014.8 ✓5ᵗʰ
peripheral 017.2 ✓5ᵗʰ
retroperitoneal 014.8 ✓5ᵗʰ
tracheobronchial 012.1 ✓5ᵗʰ
primary, progressive 010.8 ✓5ᵗʰ

Tuberculosis, tubercular, tuberculous —
continued
malignant NEC (*see also* Tuberculosis,
pulmonary) 011.9 ✓5ᵗʰ
mammary gland 017.9 ✓5ᵗʰ
marasmus NEC (*see also* Tuberculosis,
pulmonary) 011.9 ✓5ᵗʰ
mastoiditis 015.6 ✓5ᵗʰ
maternal, affecting fetus or newborn 760.2
mediastinal (lymph) gland or node 012.1 ✓5ᵗʰ
primary, progressive 010.8 ✓5ᵗʰ
mediastinitis 012.8 ✓5ᵗʰ
primary, progressive 010.8 ✓5ᵗʰ
mediastinopericarditis 017.9 ✓5ᵗʰ [420.0]
mediastinum 012.8 ✓5ᵗʰ
primary, progressive 010.8 ✓5ᵗʰ
medulla 013.9 ✓5ᵗʰ
brain 013.2 ✓5ᵗʰ
spinal cord 013.4 ✓5ᵗʰ
melanosis, Addisonian 017.6 ✓5ᵗʰ
membrane, brain 013.0 ✓5ᵗʰ
meninges (cerebral) (spinal) 013.0 ✓5ᵗʰ
meningitis (basilar) (brain) (cerebral)
(cerebrospinal) (spinal) 013.0 ✓5ᵗʰ
meningoencephalitis 013.0 ✓5ᵗʰ
mesentery, mesenteric 014.8 ✓5ᵗʰ
lymph gland or node 014.8 ✓5ᵗʰ
miliary (any site) 018.9 ✓5ᵗʰ
acute 018.0 ✓5ᵗʰ
chronic 018.8 ✓5ᵗʰ
specified type NEC 018.8 ✓5ᵗʰ
millstone makers' 011.4 ✓5ᵗʰ
miners' 011.4 ✓5ᵗʰ
moulders' 011.4 ✓5ᵗʰ
mouth 017.9 ✓5ᵗʰ
multiple 018.9 ✓5ᵗʰ
acute 018.0 ✓5ᵗʰ
chronic 018.8 ✓5ᵗʰ
muscle 017.9 ✓5ᵗʰ
myelitis 013.6 ✓5ᵗʰ
myocarditis 017.9 ✓5ᵗʰ [422.0]
myocardium 017.9 ✓5ᵗʰ [422.0]
nasal (passage) (sinus) 012.8 ✓5ᵗʰ
nasopharynx 012.8 ✓5ᵗʰ
neck gland 017.2 ✓5ᵗʰ
nephritis 016.0 ✓5ᵗʰ [583.81] ✓5ᵗʰ
nerve 017.9 ✓5ᵗʰ
nose (septum) 012.8 ✓5ᵗʰ
ocular 017.3 ✓5ᵗʰ
old NEC 137.0
without residuals V12.01
omentum 014.8 ✓5ᵗʰ
oophoritis (acute) (chronic) 016.6 ✓5ᵗʰ
optic 017.3 ✓5ᵗʰ [377.39]
nerve trunk 017.3 ✓5ᵗʰ [377.39]
papilla, papillae 017.3 ✓5ᵗʰ [377.39]
orbit 017.3 ✓5ᵗʰ
orchitis 016.5 ✓5ᵗʰ [608.81]
organ, specified NEC 017.9 ✓5ᵗʰ
orificialis (primary) 017.0 ✓5ᵗʰ
osseous (*see also* Tuberculosis, bone)
015.9 ✓5ᵗʰ [730.8] ✓5ᵗʰ
osteitis (*see also* Tuberculosis, bone)
015.9 ✓5ᵗʰ [730.8] ✓5ᵗʰ
osteomyelitis (*see also* Tuberculosis, bone)
015.9 ✓5ᵗʰ [730.8] ✓5ᵗʰ
otitis (media) 017.4 ✓5ᵗʰ
ovaritis (acute) (chronic) 016.6 ✓5ᵗʰ
ovary (acute) (chronic) 016.6 ✓5ᵗʰ
oviducts (acute) (chronic) 016.6 ✓5ᵗʰ
pachymeningitis 013.0 ✓5ᵗʰ
palate (soft) 017.9 ✓5ᵗʰ
pancreas 017.9 ✓5ᵗʰ
papulonecrotic (primary) 017.0 ✓5ᵗʰ
parathyroid glands 017.9 ✓5ᵗʰ
paronychia (primary) 017.0 ✓5ᵗʰ
parotid gland or region 017.9 ✓5ᵗʰ
pelvic organ NEC 016.9 ✓5ᵗʰ
female 016.7 ✓5ᵗʰ
male 016.5 ✓5ᵗʰ
pelvis (bony) 015.7 ✓5ᵗʰ [730.85]
penis 016.5 ✓5ᵗʰ
peribronchitis 011.3 ✓5ᵗʰ
pericarditis 017.9 ✓5ᵗʰ [420.0]
pericardium 017.9 ✓5ᵗʰ [420.0]
perichondritis, larynx 012.3 ✓5ᵗʰ
perineum 017.9 ✓5ᵗʰ

Tuberculosis, tubercular, tuberculous —
continued
periostitis (*see also* Tuberculosis, bone)
015.9 ✓5ᵗʰ [730.8]
periphlebitis 017.9 ✓5ᵗʰ
eye vessel 017.3 ✓5ᵗʰ [362.18]
retina 017.3 ✓5ᵗʰ [362.18]
perirectal fistula 014.8 ✓5ᵗʰ
peritoneal gland 014.8 ✓5ᵗʰ
peritoneum 014.0 ✓5ᵗʰ
peritonitis 014.0 ✓5ᵗʰ
pernicious NEC (*see also* Tuberculosis,
pulmonary) 011.9 ✓5ᵗʰ
pharyngitis 012.8 ✓5ᵗʰ
pharynx 012.8 ✓5ᵗʰ
phlyctenulosis (conjunctiva) 017.3 ✓5ᵗʰ [370.31]
phthisis NEC (*see also* Tuberculosis,
pulmonary) 011.9 ✓5ᵗʰ
pituitary gland 017.9 ✓5ᵗʰ
placenta 016.7 ✓5ᵗʰ
pleura, pleural, pleurisy, pleuritis (fibrinous)
(obliterative) (purulent) (simple plastic)
(with effusion) 012.0 ✓5ᵗʰ
primary, progressive 010.1 ✓5ᵗʰ
pneumonia, pneumonic 011.6 ✓5ᵗʰ
pneumothorax 011.7 ✓5ᵗʰ
polyserositis 018.9 ✓5ᵗʰ
acute 018.0 ✓5ᵗʰ
chronic 018.8 ✓5ᵗʰ
potters' 011.4 ✓5ᵗʰ
prepuce 016.5 ✓5ᵗʰ
primary 010.9 ✓5ᵗʰ
complex 010.0 ✓5ᵗʰ
complicated 010.8 ✓5ᵗʰ
with pleurisy or effusion 010.1 ✓5ᵗʰ
progressive 010.8 ✓5ᵗʰ
with pleurisy or effusion 010.1 ✓5ᵗʰ
skin 017.0 ✓5ᵗʰ
proctitis 014.8 ✓5ᵗʰ
prostate 016.5 ✓5ᵗʰ [601.4]
prostatitis 016.5 ✓5ᵗʰ [601.4]
pulmonaris (*see also* Tuberculosis, pulmonary)
011.9 ✓5ᵗʰ
pulmonary (artery) (incipient) (malignant)
(multiple round foci) (pernicious)
(reinfection stage) 011.9 ✓5ᵗʰ
cavitated or with cavitation 011.2 ✓5ᵗʰ
primary, progressive 010.8 ✓5ᵗʰ
childhood type or first infection 010.0 ✓5ᵗʰ
chromogenic acid-fast bacilli 795.39 ▲
fibrosis or fibrotic 011.4 ✓5ᵗʰ
infiltrative 011.0 ✓5ᵗʰ
primary, progressive 010.9 ✓5ᵗʰ
nodular 011.1 ✓5ᵗʰ
specified NEC 011.8 ✓5ᵗʰ
sputum positive only 795.39 ▲
status following surgical collapse of lung
NEC 011.9 ✓5ᵗʰ
pyelitis 016.0 ✓5ᵗʰ [590.81]
pyelonephritis 016.0 ✓5ᵗʰ [590.81]
pyemia — *see* Tuberculosis, miliary
pyonephrosis 016.0 ✓5ᵗʰ
pyopneumothorax 012.0 ✓5ᵗʰ
pyothorax 012.0 ✓5ᵗʰ
rectum (with abscess) 014.8 ✓5ᵗʰ
fistula 014.8 ✓5ᵗʰ
reinfection stage (*see also* Tuberculosis,
pulmonary) 011.9 ✓5ᵗʰ
renal 016.0 ✓5ᵗʰ
renis 016.0 ✓5ᵗʰ
reproductive organ 016.7 ✓5ᵗʰ
respiratory NEC (*see also* Tuberculosis,
pulmonary) 011.9 ✓5ᵗʰ
specified site NEC 012.8 ✓5ᵗʰ
retina 017.3 ✓5ᵗʰ [363.13]
retroperitoneal (lymph gland or node) 014.8 ✓5ᵗʰ
gland 014.8 ✓5ᵗʰ
retropharyngeal abscess 012.8 ✓5ᵗʰ
rheumatism 015.9 ✓5ᵗʰ
rhinitis 012.8 ✓5ᵗʰ
sacroiliac (joint) 015.8 ✓5ᵗʰ
sacrum 015.0 ✓5ᵗʰ [730.88]
salivary gland 017.9 ✓5ᵗʰ
salpingitis (acute) (chronic) 016.6 ✓5ᵗʰ
sandblasters' 011.4 ✓5ᵗʰ
sclera 017.3 ✓5ᵗʰ [379.09]
scoliosis 015.0 ✓5ᵗʰ [737.43]
scrofulous 017.2 ✓5ᵗʰ

Tuberculosis, tubercular, tuberculous —
continued
  scrotum 016.5 ✓5th
  seminal tract or vesicle 016.5 ✓5th [608.81]
  senile NEC (*see also* Tuberculosis, pulmonary)
    011.9 ✓5th
  septic NEC (*see also* Tuberculosis, miliary)
    018.9 ✓5th
  shoulder 015.8 ✓5th
    blade 015.7 ✓5th [730.8] ✓5th
  sigmoid 014.8 ✓5th
  sinus (accessory) (nasal) 012.8 ✓5th
    bone 015.7 ✓5th [730.88]
    epididymis 016.4 ✓5th
  skeletal NEC (*see also* Osteomyelitis, due to
    tuberculosis) 015.9 ✓5th [730.8] ✓5th
  skin (any site) (primary) 017.0 ✓5th
  small intestine 014.8 ✓5th
  soft palate 017.9 ✓5th
  spermatic cord 016.5 ✓5th
  spinal
    column 015.0 ✓5th [730.88]
    cord 013.4 ✓5th
    disease 015.0 ✓5th [730.88]
    medulla 013.4 ✓5th
    membrane 013.0 ✓5th
    meninges 013.0 ✓5th
  spine 015.0 ✓5th [730.88]
  spleen 017.7 ✓5th
  splenitis 017.7 ✓5th
  spondylitis 015.0 ✓5th [720.81]
  spontaneous pneumothorax — *see*
    Tuberculosis, pulmonary
  sternoclavicular joint 015.8 ✓5th
  stomach 017.9 ✓5th
  stonemasons' 011.4 ✓5th
  struma 017.2 ✓5th
  subcutaneous tissue (cellular) (primary)
    017.0 ✓5th
  subcutis (primary) 017.0 ✓5th
  subdeltoid bursa 017.9 ✓5th
  submaxillary 017.9 ✓5th
    region 017.9 ✓5th
  supraclavicular gland 017.2 ✓5th
  suprarenal (capsule) (gland) 017.6 ✓5th
  swelling, joint (*see also* Tuberculosis, joint)
    015.9 ✓5th
  symphysis pubis 015.7 ✓5th [730.88]
  synovitis 015.9 ✓5th [727.01]
    hip 015.1 ✓5th [727.01]
    knee 015.2 ✓5th [727.01]
    specified site NEC 015.8 ✓5th [727.01]
    spine or vertebra 015.0 ✓5th [727.01]
  systemic — *see* Tuberculosis, miliary
  tarsitis (eyelid) 017.0 ✓5th [373.4]
    ankle (bone) 015.5 ✓5th [730.87]
  tendon (sheath) — *see* Tuberculosis,
    tenosynovitis
  tenosynovitis 015.9 ✓5th [727.01]
    hip 015.1 ✓5th [727.01]
    knee 015.2 ✓5th [727.01]
    specified site NEC 015.8 ✓5th [727.01]
    spine or vertebra 015.0 ✓5th [727.01]
  testis 016.5 ✓5th [608.81]
  throat 012.8 ✓5th
  thymus gland 017.9 ✓5th
  thyroid gland 017.5 ✓5th
  toe 017.9 ✓5th
  tongue 017.9 ✓5th
  tonsil (lingual) 012.8 ✓5th
  tonsillitis 012.8 ✓5th
  trachea, tracheal 012.8 ✓5th
    gland 012.1 ✓5th
      primary, progressive 010.8 ✓5th
      isolated 012.2 ✓5th
  tracheobronchial 011.3 ✓5th
    glandular 012.1 ✓5th
      primary, progressive 010.8 ✓5th
      isolated 012.2 ✓5th
    lymph gland or node 012.1 ✓5th
      primary, progressive 010.8 ✓5th
  tubal 016.6 ✓5th
  tunica vaginalis 016.5 ✓5th
  typhlitis 014.8 ✓5th
  ulcer (primary) (skin) 017.0 ✓5th
    bowel or intestine 014.8 ✓5th
    specified site NEC — *see* Tuberculosis, by
      site

Tuberculosis, tubercular, tuberculous —
continued
  unspecified site — *see* Tuberculosis, pulmonary
  ureter 016.2 ✓5th
  urethra, urethral 016.3 ✓5th
  urinary organ or tract 016.3 ✓5th
    kidney 016.0 ✓5th
  uterus 016.7 ✓5th
  uveal tract 017.3 ✓5th [363.13]
  uvula 017.9 ✓5th
  vaccination, prophylactic (against) V03.2
  vagina 016.7 ✓5th
  vas deferens 016.5 ✓5th
  vein 017.9 ✓5th
  verruca (primary) 017.0 ✓5th
  verrucosa (cutis) (primary) 017.0 ✓5th
  vertebra (column) 015.0 ✓5th [730.88]
  vesiculitis 016.5 ✓5th [608.81]
  viscera NEC 014.8 ✓5th
  vulva 016.7 ✓5th [616.51]
  wrist (joint) 015.8 ✓5th
    bone 015.5 ✓5th [730.83]
Tuberculum
  auriculae 744.29
  occlusal 520.2
  paramolare 520.2
Tuberous sclerosis (brain) 759.5
Tubo-ovarian — *see* condition
Tuboplasty, after previous sterilization V26.0
Tubotympanitis 381.10
Tularemia 021.9
  with
    conjunctivitis 021.3
    pneumonia 021.2
  bronchopneumonic 021.2
  conjunctivitis 021.3
  cryptogenic 021.1
  disseminated 021.8
  enteric 021.1
  generalized 021.8
  glandular 021.8
  intestinal 021.1
  oculoglandular 021.3
  ophthalmic 021.3
  pneumonia 021.2
  pulmonary 021.2
  specified NEC 021.8
  typhoidal 021.1
  ulceroglandular 021.0
  vaccination, prophylactic (against) V03.4
Tularensis conjunctivitis 021.3
Tumefaction — *see also* Swelling
  liver (*see also* Hypertrophy, liver) 789.1
Tumor (M8000/1) — *see also* Neoplasm, by site,
    unspecified nature
  Abrikossov's (M9580/0) — *see also* Neoplasm,
    connective tissue, benign
    malignant (M9580/3) — *see* Neoplasm,
      connective tissue, malignant
  acinar cell (M8550/1) — *see* Neoplasm, by site,
    uncertain behavior
  acinic cell (M8550/1) — *see* Neoplasm, by site,
    uncertain behavior
  adenomatoid (M9054/0) — *see also* Neoplasm,
    by site, benign
    odontogenic (M9300/0) 213.1
      upper jaw (bone) 213.0
  adnexal (skin) (M8390/0) — *see* Neoplasm,
    skin, benign
  adrenal
    cortical (benign) (M8370/0) 227.0
      malignant (M8370/3) 194.0
    rest (M8671/0) — *see* Neoplasm, by site,
      benign
  alpha cell (M8152/0)
    malignant (M8152/3)
      pancreas 157.4
      specified site NEC — *see* Neoplasm, by
        site, malignant
      unspecified site 157.4
    pancreas 211.7
    specified site NEC — *see* Neoplasm, by site,
      benign
    unspecified site 211.7
  aneurysmal (*see also* Aneurysm) 442.9

Tumor — *see also* Neoplasm, by site, unspecified
    nature — *continued*
  aortic body (M8691/1) 237.3
    malignant (M8691/3) 194.6
  argentaffin (M8241/1) — *see* Neoplasm, by site,
    uncertain behavior
  basal cell (M8090/1) — *see also* Neoplasm,
    skin, uncertain behavior
  benign (M8000/0) — *see* Neoplasm, by site,
    benign
  beta cell (M8151/0)
    malignant (M8151/3)
      pancreas 157.4
      specified site — *see* Neoplasm, by site,
        malignant
      unspecified site 157.4
    pancreas 211.7
    specified site NEC — *see* Neoplasm, by site,
      benign
    unspecified site 211.7
  blood — *see* Hematoma
  Brenner (M9000/0) 220
    borderline malignancy (M9000/1) 236.2
    malignant (M9000/3) 183.0
    proliferating (M9000/1) 236.2
  Brooke's (M8100/0) — *see* Neoplasm, skin,
    benign
  brown fat (M8880/0) — *see* Lipoma, by site
  Burkitt's (M9750/3) 200.2 ✓5th
  calcifying epithelial odontogenic (M9340/0)
    213.1
    upper jaw (bone) 213.0
  carcinoid (M8240/1) — *see* Carcinoid
  carotid body (M8692/1) 237.3
    malignant (M8692/3) 194.5
  Castleman's (mediastinal lymph node
    hyperplasia) 785.6
  cells (M8001/1) — *see also* Neoplasm, by site,
    unspecified nature
    benign (M8001/0) — *see* Neoplasm, by site,
      benign
    malignant (M8001/3) — *see* Neoplasm, by
      site, malignant
    uncertain whether benign or malignant
      (M8001/1) — *see* Neoplasm, by site,
      uncertain nature
  cervix
    in pregnancy or childbirth 654.6 ✓5th
      affecting fetus or newborn 763.89
      causing obstructed labor 660.2 ✓5th
        affecting fetus or newborn 763.1
  chondromatous giant cell (M9230/0) — *see*
    Neoplasm, bone, benign
  chromaffin (M8700/0) — *see also* Neoplasm, by
    site, benign
    malignant (M8700/3) — *see* Neoplasm, by
      site, malignant
  Cock's peculiar 706.2
  Codman's (benign chondroblastoma) (M9230/0)
    — *see* Neoplasm, bone, benign
  dentigerous, mixed (M9282/0) 213.1
    upper jaw (bone) 213.0
  dermoid (M9084/0) — *see* Neoplasm, by site,
    benign
    with malignant transformation (M9084/3)
      183.0
  desmoid (extra-abdominal) (M8821/1) — *see
    also* Neoplasm, connective tissue,
    uncertain behavior
    abdominal (M8822/1) — *see* Neoplasm,
      connective tissue, uncertain behavior
  embryonal (mixed) (M9080/1) — *see also*
    Neoplasm, by site, uncertain behavior
    liver (M9080/3) 155.0
  endodermal sinus (M9071/3)
    specified site — *see* Neoplasm, by site,
      malignant
    unspecified site
      female 183.0
      male 186.9
  epithelial
    benign (M8010/0) — *see* Neoplasm, by site,
      benign
    malignant (M8010/3) — *see* Neoplasm, by
      site, malignant
  Ewing's (M9260/3) — *see* Neoplasm, bone,
    malignant

Tumor *— see also* Neoplasm, by site, unspecified nature *— continued*
fatty *— see* Lipoma
fetal, causing disproportion 653.7 ☑5ᵗʰ
  causing obstructed labor 660.1 ☑5ᵗʰ
fibroid (M8890/0) *— see* Leiomyoma
G cell (M8153/1)
  malignant (M8153/3)
    pancreas 157.4
    specified site NEC *— see* Neoplasm, by site, malignant
    unspecified site 157.4
  specified site *— see* Neoplasm, by site, uncertain behavior
  unspecified site 235.5
giant cell (type) (M8003/1) *— see also* Neoplasm, by site, unspecified nature
  bone (M9250/1) 238.0
    malignant (M9250/3) *— see* Neoplasm, bone, malignant
  chondromatous (M9230/0) *— see* Neoplasm, bone, benign
  malignant (M8003/3) *— see* Neoplasm, by site, malignant
  peripheral (gingiva) 523.8
  soft parts (M9251/1) *— see also* Neoplasm, connective tissue, uncertain behavior
    malignant (M9251/3) *— see* Neoplasm, connective tissue, malignant
  tendon sheath 727.02
glomus (M8711/0) *— see also* Hemangioma, by site
jugulare (M8690/1) 237.3
  malignant (M8690/3) 194.6
gonadal stromal (M8590/1) *— see* Neoplasm, by site, uncertain behavior
granular cell (M9580/0) *— see also* Neoplasm, connective tissue, benign
  malignant (M9580/3) *— see* Neoplasm, connective tissue, malignant
granulosa cell (M8620/1) 236.2
  malignant (M8620/3) 183.0
granulosa cell-theca cell (M8621/1) 236.2
  malignant (M8621/3) 183.0
Grawitz's (hypernephroma) (M8312/3) 189.0
hazard-crile (M8350/3) 193
hemorrhoidal *— see* Hemorrhoids
hilar cell (M8660/0) 220
Hürthle cell (benign) (M8290/0) 226
  malignant (M8290/3) 193
hydatid (*see also* Echinococcus) 122.9
hypernephroid (M8311/1) *— see also* Neoplasm, by site, uncertain behavior
interstitial cell (M8650/1) *— see also* Neoplasm, by site, uncertain behavior
  benign (M8650/0) *— see* Neoplasm, by site, benign
  malignant (M8650/3) *— see* Neoplasm, by site, malignant
islet cell (M8150/0)
  malignant (M8150/3)
    pancreas 157.4
    specified site *— see* Neoplasm, by site, malignant
    unspecified site 157.4
  pancreas 211.7
  specified site NEC *— see* Neoplasm, by site, benign
  unspecified site 211.7
juxtaglomerular (M8361/1) 236.91
Krukenberg's (M8490/6) 198.6
Leydig cell (M8650/1)
  benign (M8650/0)
    specified site *— see* Neoplasm, by site, benign
    unspecified site
      female 220
      male 222.0
  malignant (M8650/3)
    specified site *— see* Neoplasm, by site, malignant
    unspecified site
      female 183.0
      male 186.9
  specified site *— see* Neoplasm, by site, uncertain behavior

Tumor *— see also* Neoplasm, by site, unspecified nature *— continued*
Leydig cell *— continued*
  unspecified site
    female 236.2
    male 236.4
lipid cell, ovary (M8670/0) 220
lipoid cell, ovary (M8670/0) 220
lymphomatous, benign (M9590/0) *— see also* Neoplasm, by site, benign
Malherbe's (M8110/0) *— see* Neoplasm, skin, benign
malignant (M8000/3) *— see also* Neoplasm, by site, malignant
  fusiform cell (type) (M8004/3) *— see* Neoplasm, by site, malignant
  giant cell (type) (M8003/3) *— see* Neoplasm, by site, malignant
  mixed NEC (M8940/3) *— see* Neoplasm, by site, malignant
  small cell (type) (M8002/3) *— see* Neoplasm, by site, malignant
  spindle cell (type) (M8004/3) *— see* Neoplasm, by site, malignant
mast cell (M9740/1) 238.5
  malignant (M9740/3) 202.6 ☑5ᵗʰ
melanotic, neuroectodermal (M9363/0) *— see* Neoplasm, by site, benign
Merkel cell *— see* Neoplasm, by site, malignant
mesenchymal
  malignant (M8800/3) *— see* Neoplasm, connective tissue, malignant
  mixed (M8990/1) *— see* Neoplasm, connective tissue, uncertain behavior
mesodermal, mixed (M8951/3) *— see also* Neoplasm, by site, malignant
  liver 155.0
mesonephric (M9110/1) *— see also* Neoplasm, by site, uncertain behavior
  malignant (M9110/3) *— see* Neoplasm, by site, malignant
metastatic
  from specified site (M8000/3) *— see* Neoplasm, by site, malignant
  to specified site (M8000/6) *— see* Neoplasm, by site, malignant, secondary
mixed NEC (M8940/0) *— see also* Neoplasm, by site, benign
  malignant (M8940/3) *— see* Neoplasm, by site, malignant
mucocarcinoid, malignant (M8243/3) *— see* Neoplasm, by site, malignant
mucoepidermoid (M8430/1) *— see* Neoplasm, by site, uncertain behavior
Mullerian, mixed (M8950/3) *— see* Neoplasm, by site, malignant
myoepithelial (M8982/0) *— see* Neoplasm, by site, benign
neurogenic olfactory (M9520/3) 160.0
nonencapsulated sclerosing (M8350/3) 193
odontogenic (M9270/1) 238.0
  adenomatoid (M9300/0) 213.1
    upper jaw (bone) 213.0
  benign (M9270/0) 213.1
    upper jaw (bone) 213.0
  calcifying epithelial (M9340/0) 213.1
    upper jaw (bone) 213.0
  malignant (M9270/3) 170.1
    upper jaw (bone) 170.0
  squamous (M9312/0) 213.1
    upper jaw (bone) 213.0
ovarian stromal (M8590/1) 236.2
ovary
  in pregnancy or childbirth 654.4 ☑5ᵗʰ
    affecting fetus or newborn 763.89
    causing obstructed labor 660.2 ☑5ᵗʰ
      affecting fetus or newborn 763.1
pacinian (M9507/0) *— see* Neoplasm, skin, benign
Pancoast's (M8010/3) 162.3
papillary *— see* Papilloma
pelvic, in pregnancy or childbirth 654.9 ☑5ᵗʰ
  affecting fetus or newborn 763.89
  causing obstructed labor 660.2 ☑5ᵗʰ
    affecting fetus or newborn 763.1
phantom 300.11

Tumor *— see also* Neoplasm, by site, unspecified nature *— continued*
plasma cell (M9731/1) 238.6
  benign (M9731/0) *— see* Neoplasm, by site, benign
  malignant (M9731/3) 203.8 ☑5ᵗʰ
polyvesicular vitelline (M9071/3)
  specified site *— see* Neoplasm, by site, malignant
  unspecified site
    female 183.0
    male 186.9
Pott's puffy (*see also* Osteomyelitis) 730.2 ☑5ᵗʰ
Rathke's pouch (M9350/1) 237.0
regaud's (M8082/3) *— see* Neoplasm, nasopharynx, malignant
rete cell (M8140/0) 222.0
retinal anlage (M9363/0) *— see* Neoplasm, by site, benign
Rokitansky's 620.2
salivary gland type, mixed (M8940/0) *— see also* Neoplasm, by site, benign
  malignant (M8940/3) *— see* Neoplasm, by site, malignant
Sampson's 617.1
Schloffer's (*see also* Peritonitis) 567.2
Schmincke (M8082/3) *— see* Neoplasm, nasopharynx, malignant
sebaceous (*see also* Cyst, sebaceous) 706.2
secondary (M8000/6) *— see* Neoplasm, by site, secondary
Sertoli cell (M8640/0)
  with lipid storage (M8641/0)
    specified site *— see* Neoplasm, by site, benign
    unspecified site
      female 220
      male 222.0
  specified site *— see* Neoplasm, by site, benign
  unspecified site
    female 220
    male 222.0
Sertoli-Leydig cell (M8631/0)
  specified site *— see* Neoplasm, by site, benign
  unspecified site
    female 220
    male 222.0
sex cord (-stromal) (M8590/1) *— see* Neoplasm, by site, uncertain behavior
skin appendage (M8390/0) *— see* Neoplasm, skin, benign
soft tissue
  benign (M8800/0) *— see* Neoplasm, connective tissue, benign
  malignant (M8800/3) *— see* Neoplasm, connective tissue, malignant
sternomastoid 754.1
superior sulcus (lung) (pulmonary) (syndrome) (M8010/3) 162.3
suprasulcus (M8010/3) 162.3
sweat gland (M8400/1) *— see also* Neoplasm, skin, uncertain behavior
  benign (M8400/0) *— see* Neoplasm, skin, benign
  malignant (M8400/3) *— see* Neoplasm, skin, malignant
syphilitic brain 094.89
  congenital 090.49
testicular stromal (M8590/1) 236.4
theca cell (M8600/0) 220
theca cell-granulosa cell (M8621/1) 236.2
theca-lutein (M8610/0) 220
turban (M8200/0) 216.4
uterus
  in pregnancy or childbirth 654.1 ☑5ᵗʰ
    affecting fetus or newborn 763.89
    causing obstructed labor 660.2 ☑5ᵗʰ
      affecting fetus or newborn 763.1
vagina
  in pregnancy or childbirth 654.7 ☑5ᵗʰ
    affecting fetus or newborn 763.89
    causing obstructed labor 660.2 ☑5ᵗʰ
      affecting fetus or newborn 763.1
varicose (*see also* Varicose, vein) 454.9
von Recklinghausen's (M9540/1) 237.71

Tumor — *see also* Neoplasm, by site, unspecified
  nature — *continued*
  vulva
    in pregnancy or childbirth 654.8 ✓5ᵗʰ
      affecting fetus or newborn 763.89
      causing obstructed labor 660.2 ✓5ᵗʰ
        affecting fetus or newborn 763.1
  Warthin's (salivary gland) (M8561/0) 210.2
  white — *see also* Tuberculosis, arthritis
  White-Darier 757.39
  Wilms' (nephroblastoma) (M8960/3) 189.0
  yolk sac (M9071/3)
    specified site — *see* Neoplasm, by site,
      malignant
    unspecified site
      female 183.0
      male 186.9
Tumorlet (M8040/1) — *see* Neoplasm, by site,
  uncertain behavior
Tungiasis 134.1
Tunica vasculosa lentis 743.39
Tunnel vision 368.45
Turban tumor (M8200/0) 216.4
Türck's trachoma (chronic catarrhal laryngitis)
  476.0
Türk's syndrome (ocular retraction syndrome)
  378.71
Turner's
  hypoplasia (tooth) 520.4
  syndrome 758.6
  tooth 520.4
Turner-Kieser syndrome (hereditary osteo-
  onychodysplasia) 756.89
Turner-Varny syndrome 758.6
Turricephaly 756.0
Tussis convulsiva (*see also* Whooping cough)
  033.9
Twin
  affected by maternal complications of
    pregnancy 761.5
  conjoined 759.4
  healthy liveborn — *see* Newborn, twin
  pregnancy (complicating delivery) NEC
    651.0 ✓5ᵗʰ
    with fetal loss and retention of one fetus
      651.3 ✓5ᵗʰ
Twinning, teeth 520.2
Twist, twisted
  bowel, colon, or intestine 560.2
  hair (congenital) 757.4
  mesentery 560.2
  omentum 560.2
  organ or site, congenital NEC — *see* Anomaly,
    specified type NEC
  ovarian pedicle 620.5
    congenital 752.0
  umbilical cord — *see* Compression, umbilical
    cord
Twitch 781.0
Tylosis 700
  buccalis 528.6
  gingiva 523.8
  linguae 528.6
  palmaris et plantaris 757.39
Tympanism 787.3
Tympanites (abdominal) (intestine) 787.3
Tympanitis — *see* Myringitis
Tympanosclerosis 385.00
  involving
    combined sites NEC 385.09
      with tympanic membrane 385.03
    tympanic membrane 385.01
      with ossicles 385.02
        and middle ear 385.03
Tympanum — *see* condition
Tympany
  abdomen 787.3
  chest 786.7
Typhlitis (*see also* Appendicitis) 541
Typhoenteritis 002.0
Typhogastric fever 002.0

Typhoid (abortive) (ambulant) (any site) (fever)
  (hemorrhagic) (infection) (intermittent)
  (malignant) (rheumatic) 002.0
  with pneumonia 002.0 *[484.8]*
  abdominal 002.0
  carrier (suspected) of V02.1
  cholecystitis (current) 002.0
  clinical (Widal and blood test negative) 002.0
  endocarditis 002.0 *[421.1]*
  inoculation reaction — *see* Complications,
    vaccination
  meningitis 002.0 *[320.7]*
  mesenteric lymph nodes 002.0
  myocarditis 002.0 *[422.0]*
  osteomyelitis (*see also* Osteomyelitis, due to,
    typhoid) 002.0 *[730.8]* ✓5ᵗʰ
  perichondritis, larynx 002.0 *[478.71]*
  pneumonia 002.0 *[484.8]*
  spine 002.0 *[720.81]*
  ulcer (perforating) 002.0
  vaccination, prophylactic (against) V03.1
  Widal negative 002.0
Typhomalaria (fever) (*see also* Malaria) 084.6
Typhomania 002.0
Typhoperitonitis 002.0
Typhus (fever) 081.9
  abdominal, abdominalis 002.0
  African tick 082.1
  amarillic (*see also* Fever, Yellow) 060.9
  brain 081.9
  cerebral 081.9
  classical 080
  endemic (flea-borne) 081.0
  epidemic (louse-borne) 080
  exanthematic NEC 080
  exanthematicus SAI 080
    brilli SAI 081.1
    Mexicanus SAI 081.0
    pediculo vestimenti causa 080
    typhus murinus 081.0
  flea-borne 081.0
  Indian tick 082.1
  Kenya tick 082.1
  louse-borne 080
  Mexican 081.0
    flea-borne 081.0
    louse-borne 080
    tabardillo 080
  mite-borne 081.2
  murine 081.0
  North Asian tick-borne 082.2
  petechial 081.9
  Queensland tick 082.3
  rat 081.0
  recrudescent 081.1
  recurrent (*see also* Fever, relapsing) 087.9
  São Paulo 082.0
  scrub (China) (India) (Malaya) (New Guinea)
    081.2
  shop (of Malaya) 081.0
  Siberian tick 082.2
  tick-borne NEC 082.9
  tropical 081.2
  vaccination, prophylactic (against) V05.8
Tyrosinemia 270.2
  neonatal 775.8
Tyrosinosis (Medes) (Sakai) 270.2
Tyrosinuria 270.2
Tyrosyluria 270.2

U

Uehlinger's syndrome (acropachyderma) 757.39
Uhl's anomaly or disease (hypoplasia of
  myocardium, right ventricle) 746.84
**Ulcer, ulcerated, ulcerating, ulceration,
  ulcerative** 707.9
  with gangrene 707.9 *[785.4]*
  abdomen (wall) (*see also* Ulcer, skin) 707.8
  ala, nose 478.1
  alveolar process 526.5
  amebic (intestine) 006.9
    skin 006.6
  anastomotic — *see* Ulcer, gastrojejunal
  anorectal 569.41

**Ulcer, ulcerated, ulcerating, ulceration,
  ulcerative** — *continued*
  antral — *see* Ulcer, stomach
  anus (sphincter) (solitary) 569.41
    varicose — *see* Varicose, ulcer, anus
  aphthous (oral) (recurrent) 528.2
    genital organ(s)
      female 616.8
      male 608.89
    mouth 528.2
  arm (*see also* Ulcer, skin) 707.8
  arteriosclerotic plaque — *see* Arteriosclerosis,
    by site
  artery NEC 447.2
    without rupture 447.8
  atrophic NEC — *see* Ulcer, skin
  Barrett's (chronic peptic ulcer of esophagus)
    530.2
  bile duct 576.8
  bladder (solitary) (sphincter) 596.8
    bilharzial (*see also* Schistosomiasis) 120.9
      [595.4]
    submucosal (*see also* Cystitis) 595.1
    tuberculous (*see also* Tuberculosis)
      016.1 ✓5ᵗʰ
  bleeding NEC — *see* Ulcer, peptic, with
    hemorrhage
  bone 730.9 ✓5ᵗʰ
  bowel (*see also* Ulcer, intestine) 569.82
  breast 611.0
  bronchitis 491.8
  bronchus 519.1
  buccal (cavity) (traumatic) 528.9
  burn (acute) — *see* Ulcer, duodenum
  Buruli 031.1
  buttock (*see also* Ulcer, skin) 707.8
    decubitus (*see also* Ulcer, decubitus) 707.0
  cancerous (M8000/3) — *see* Neoplasm, by site,
    malignant
  cardia — *see* Ulcer, stomach
  cardio-esophageal (peptic) 530.2
  cecum (*see also* Ulcer, intestine) 569.82
  cervix (uteri) (trophic) 622.0
    with mention of cervicitis 616.0
  chancroidal 099.0
  chest (wall) (*see also* Ulcer, skin) 707.8
  Chiclero 085.4
  chin (pyogenic) (*see also* Ulcer, skin) 707.8
  chronic (cause unknown) — *see also* Ulcer,
    skin
    penis 607.89
  Cochin-China 085.1
  colitis — *see* Colitis, ulcerative
  colon (*see also* Ulcer, intestine) 569.82
  conjunctiva (acute) (postinfectional) 372.00
  cornea (infectional) 370.00
    with perforation 370.06
    annular 370.02
    catarrhal 370.01
    central 370.03
    dendritic 054.42
    marginal 370.01
    mycotic 370.05
    phlyctenular, tuberculous (*see also*
      Tuberculosis) 017.3 ✓5ᵗʰ *[370.31]*
    ring 370.02
    rodent 370.07
    serpent, serpiginous 370.04
    superficial marginal 370.01
    tuberculous (*see also* Tuberculosis)
      017.3 ✓5ᵗʰ *[370.31]*
  corpus cavernosum (chronic) 607.89
  crural — *see* Ulcer, lower extremity
  Curling's — *see* Ulcer, duodenum
  Cushing's — *see* Ulcer, peptic
  cystitis (interstitial) 595.1
  decubitus (any site) 707.0
    with gangrene 707.0 *[785.4]*
  dendritic 054.42
  diabetes, diabetic (mellitus) 250.8 ✓5ᵗʰ *[707.9]*
    lower limb 250.8 ✓5ᵗʰ *[707.10]*
      ankle 250.8 ✓5ᵗʰ *[707.13]*
      calf 250.8 ✓5ᵗʰ *[707.12]*
      foot 250.8 ✓5ᵗʰ *[707.15]*
      heel 250.8 ✓5ᵗʰ *[707.14]*
      knee 250.8 ✓5ᵗʰ *[707.19]*
      specified site NEC 250.8 ✓5ᵗʰ *[707.19]*

Ulcer, ulcerated, ulcerating, ulceration, ulcerative — continued
diabetes, diabetic — continued
  lower limb — continued
    thigh 250.8 ✓5ᵗʰ [707.11]
    toes 250.8 ✓5ᵗʰ [707.15]
    specified site NEC 250.8 ✓5ᵗʰ [707.8]
Dieulafoy — see ►Lesion, Dieulafoy◄
due to
  infection NEC — see Ulcer, skin
  radiation, radium — see Ulcer, by site
  trophic disturbance (any region) — see
    Ulcer, skin
  x-ray — see Ulcer, by site
duodenum, duodenal (eroded) (peptic)
  532.9 ✓5ᵗʰ

Note — Use the following fifth-digit
subclassification with categories 531-534:

0   without mention of obstruction
1   with obstruction

  with
    hemorrhage (chronic) 532.4 ✓5ᵗʰ
      and perforation 532.6 ✓5ᵗʰ
    perforation (chronic) 532.5 ✓5ᵗʰ
      and hemorrhage 532.6 ✓5ᵗʰ
    acute 532.3 ✓5ᵗʰ
      with
        hemorrhage 532.0 ✓5ᵗʰ
          and perforation 532.2 ✓5ᵗʰ
        perforation 532.1 ✓5ᵗʰ
          and hemorrhage 532.2 ✓5ᵗʰ
    bleeding (recurrent) — see Ulcer, duodenum,
      with hemorrhage
    chronic 532.7 ✓5ᵗʰ
      with
        hemorrhage 532.4 ✓5ᵗʰ
          and perforation 532.6 ✓5ᵗʰ
        perforation 532.5 ✓5ᵗʰ
          and hemorrhage 532.6 ✓5ᵗʰ
    penetrating — see Ulcer, duodenum, with
      perforation
    perforating — see Ulcer, duodenum, with
      perforation
dysenteric NEC 009.0
elusive 595.1
endocarditis (any valve) (acute) (chronic)
  (subacute) 421.0
enteritis — see Colitis, ulcerative
enterocolitis 556.0
epiglottis 478.79
esophagus (peptic) 530.2
  due to ingestion
    aspirin 530.2
    chemicals 530.2
    medicinal agents 530.2
  fungal 530.2
  infectional 530.2
  varicose (see also Varix, esophagus) 456.1
    bleeding (see also Varix, esophagus,
      bleeding) 456.0
eye NEC 360.00
  dendritic 054.42
eyelid (region) 373.01
face (see also Ulcer, skin) 707.8
fauces 478.29
Fenwick (-Hunner) (solitary) (see also Cystitis)
  595.1
fistulous NEC — see Ulcer, skin
foot (indolent) (see also Ulcer, lower extremity)
  707.15
  perforating 707.15
    leprous 030.1
    syphilitic 094.0
  trophic 707.15
  varicose 454.0
    inflamed or infected 454.2
frambesial, initial or primary 102.0
gallbladder or duct 575.8
gall duct 576.8
gangrenous (see also Gangrene) 785.4
gastric — see Ulcer, stomach
gastrocolic — see Ulcer, gastrojejunal
gastroduodenal — see Ulcer, peptic
gastroesophageal — see Ulcer, stomach
gastrohepatic — see Ulcer, stomach

Ulcer, ulcerated, ulcerating, ulceration, ulcerative — continued
gastrointestinal — see Ulcer, gastrojejunal
gastrojejunal (eroded) (peptic) 534.9

Note — Use the following fifth-digit
subclassification with categories 531-534:

0   without mention of obstruction
1   with obstruction

  with
    hemorrhage (chronic) 534.4 ✓5ᵗʰ
      and perforation 534.6 ✓5ᵗʰ
    perforation 534.5 ✓5ᵗʰ
      and hemorrhage 534.6 ✓5ᵗʰ
    acute 534.3 ✓5ᵗʰ
      with
        hemorrhage 534.0 ✓5ᵗʰ
          and perforation 534.2 ✓5ᵗʰ
        perforation 534.1 ✓5ᵗʰ
          and hemorrhage 534.2 ✓5ᵗʰ
    bleeding (recurrent) — see Ulcer,
      gastrojejunal, with hemorrhage
    chronic 534.7 ✓5ᵗʰ
      with
        hemorrhage 534.4 ✓5ᵗʰ
          and perforation 534.6 ✓5ᵗʰ
        perforation 534.5 ✓5ᵗʰ
          and hemorrhage 534.6 ✓5ᵗʰ
    penetrating — see Ulcer, gastrojejunal, with
      perforation
    perforating — see Ulcer, gastrojejunal, with
      perforation
gastrojejunocolic — see Ulcer, gastrojejunal
genital organ
  female 629.8
  male 608.89
gingiva 523.8
gingivitis 523.1
glottis 478.79
granuloma of pudenda 099.2
groin (see also Ulcer, skin) 707.8
gum 523.8
gumma, due to yaws 102.4
hand (see also Ulcer, skin) 707.8
hard palate 528.9
heel (see also Ulcer, lower extremity) 707.14
  decubitus (see also Ulcer, decubitus) 707.0
hemorrhoids 455.8
  external 455.5
  internal 455.2
hip (see also Ulcer, skin) 707.8
  decubitus (see also Ulcer, decubitus) 707.0
Hunner's 595.1
hypopharynx 478.29
hypopyon (chronic) (subacute) 370.04
hypostaticum — see Ulcer, varicose
ileocolitis 556.1
ileum (see also Ulcer, intestine) 569.82
intestine, intestinal 569.82
  with perforation 569.83
  amebic 006.9
  duodenal — see Ulcer, duodenum
  granulocytopenic (with hemorrhage) 288.0
  marginal 569.82
  perforating 569.83
  small, primary 569.82
  stercoraceous 569.82
  stercoral 569.82
  tuberculous (see also Tuberculosis)
    014.8 ✓5ᵗʰ
  typhoid (fever) 002.0
  varicose 456.8
ischemic 707.9
  lower extremity (see also Ulcer, lower
    extremity) 707.10
    ankle 707.13
    calf 707.12
    foot 707.15
    heel 707.14
    knee 707.19
    specified site NEC 707.19
    thigh 707.11
    toes 707.15
jejunum, jejunal — see Ulcer, gastrojejunal
keratitis (see also Ulcer, cornea) 370.00
knee — see Ulcer, lower extremity

Ulcer, ulcerated, ulcerating, ulceration, ulcerative — continued
labium (majus) (minus) 616.50
laryngitis (see also Laryngitis) 464.00
  with obstruction 464.01
larynx (aphthous) (contact) 478.79
  diphtheritic 032.3
leg — see Ulcer, lower extremity
lip 528.5
Lipschütz's 616.50
lower extremity (atrophic) (chronic) (neurogenic)
  (perforating) (pyogenic) (trophic) (tropical)
  707.10
  with gangrene (see also Ulcer, lower
    extremity) 707.10 [785.4]
    arteriosclerotic 440.24
  ankle 707.13
  arteriosclerotic 440.23
    with gangrene 440.24
  calf 707.12
  decubitus 707.0
    with gangrene 707.0 [785.4]
  foot 707.15
  heel 707.14
  knee 707.19
  specified site NEC 707.19
  thigh 707.11
  toes 707.15
  varicose 454.0
    inflamed or infected 454.2
luetic — see Ulcer, syphilitic
lung 518.89
  tuberculous (see also Tuberculosis)
    011.2 ✓5ᵗʰ
malignant (M8000/3) — see Neoplasm, by site,
  malignant
marginal NEC — see Ulcer, gastrojejunal
meatus (urinarius) 597.89
Meckel's diverticulum 751.0
Meleney's (chronic undermining) 686.09
Mooren's (cornea) 370.07
mouth (traumatic) 528.9
mycobacterial (skin) 031.1
nasopharynx 478.29
navel cord (newborn) 771.4
neck (see also Ulcer, skin) 707.8
  uterus 622.0
neurogenic NEC — see Ulcer, skin
nose, nasal (infectional) (passage) 478.1
  septum 478.1
    varicose 456.8
  skin — see Ulcer, skin
  spirochetal NEC 104.8
oral mucosa (traumatic) 528.9
palate (soft) 528.9
penetrating NEC — see Ulcer, peptic, with
  perforation
penis (chronic) 607.89
peptic (site unspecified) 533.9

Note — Use the following fifth-digit
subclassification with categories 531-534:

0   without mention of obstruction
1   with obstruction

  with
    hemorrhage 533.4 ✓5ᵗʰ
      and perforation 533.6 ✓5ᵗʰ
    perforation (chronic) 533.5 ✓5ᵗʰ
      and hemorrhage 533.6 ✓5ᵗʰ
    acute 533.3 ✓5ᵗʰ
      with
        hemorrhage 533.0 ✓5ᵗʰ
          and perforation 533.2 ✓5ᵗʰ
        perforation 533.1 ✓5ᵗʰ
          and hemorrhage 533.2 ✓5ᵗʰ
    bleeding (recurrent) — see Ulcer, peptic,
      with hemorrhage
    chronic 533.7 ✓5ᵗʰ
      with
        hemorrhage 533.4 ✓5ᵗʰ
          and perforation 533.6 ✓5ᵗʰ
        perforation 533.5 ✓5ᵗʰ
          and hemorrhage 533.6 ✓5ᵗʰ
    penetrating — see Ulcer, peptic, with
      perforation

✓4ᵗʰ Fourth-digit Required   ✓5ᵗʰ Fifth-digit Required   ►◄ Revised Text   ● New Line   ▲ Revised Code

Ulcer, ulcerated, ulcerating, ulceration, ulcerative — *continued*

  perforating NEC (*see also* Ulcer, peptic, with perforation) 533.5 ✓5ᵗʰ
    skin 707.9
  perineum (*see also* Ulcer, skin) 707.8
  peritonsillar 474.8
  phagedenic (tropical) NEC — *see* Ulcer, skin
  pharynx 478.29
  phlebitis — *see* Phlebitis
  plaster (*see also* Ulcer, decubitus) 707.0
  popliteal space — *see* Ulcer, lower extremity
  postpyloric — *see* Ulcer, duodenum
  prepuce 607.89
  prepyloric — *see* Ulcer, stomach
  pressure (*see also* Ulcer, decubitus) 707.0
  primary of intestine 569.82
    with perforation 569.83
  proctitis 556.2
    with ulcerative sigmoiditis 556.3
  prostate 601.8
  pseudopeptic — *see* Ulcer, peptic
  pyloric — *see* Ulcer, stomach
  rectosigmoid 569.82
    with perforation 569.83
  rectum (sphincter) (solitary) 569.41
    stercoraceous, stercoral 569.41
    varicose — *see* Varicose, ulcer, anus
  retina (*see also* Chorioretinitis) 363.20
  rodent (M8090/3) — *see also* Neoplasm, skin, malignant
    cornea 370.07
  round — *see* Ulcer, stomach
  sacrum (region) (*see also* Ulcer, skin) 707.8
  Saemisch's 370.04
  scalp (*see also* Ulcer, skin) 707.8
  sclera 379.09
  scrofulous (*see also* Tuberculosis) 017.2 ✓5ᵗʰ
  scrotum 608.89
    tuberculous (*see also* Tuberculosis) 016.5 ✓5ᵗʰ
    varicose 456.4
  seminal vesicle 608.89
  sigmoid 569.82
    with perforation 569.83
  skin (atrophic) (chronic) (neurogenic) (non-healing) (perforating) (pyogenic) (trophic) 707.9
    with gangrene 707.9 *[785.4]*
    amebic 006.6
    decubitus 707.0
      with gangrene 707.0 *[785.4]*
    in granulocytopenia 288.0
    lower extremity (*see also* Ulcer, lower extremity) 707.10
      with gangrene 707.10 *[785.4]*
        arteriosclerotic 440.24
      ankle 707.13
      arteriosclerotic 440.23
        with gangrene 440.24
      calf 707.12
      foot 707.15
      heel 707.14
      knee 707.19
      specified site NEC 707.19
      thigh 707.11
      toes 707.15
    mycobacterial 031.1
    syphilitic (early) (secondary) 091.3
    tuberculous (primary) (*see also* Tuberculosis) 017.0 ✓5ᵗʰ
    varicose — *see* Ulcer, varicose
  sloughing NEC — *see* Ulcer, skin
  soft palate 528.9
  solitary, anus or rectum (sphincter) 569.41
  sore throat 462
    streptococcal 034.0
  spermatic cord 608.89
  spine (tuberculous) 015.0 ✓5ᵗʰ *[730.88]*
  stasis (leg) (venous) 454.0
    inflamed or infected 454.2
    without varicose veins 459.81 ●
  stercoral, stercoraceous 569.82
    with perforation 569.83
    anus or rectum 569.41
  stoma, stomal — *see* Ulcer, gastrojejunal

Ulcer, ulcerated, ulcerating, ulceration, ulcerative — *continued*

  stomach (eroded) (peptic) (round) 531.9

> *Note* — *Use the following fifth-digit subclassification with categories 531-534:*
>
>   0   *without mention of obstruction*
>   1   *with obstruction*

    with
      hemorrhage 531.4 ✓5ᵗʰ
        and perforation 531.6 ✓5ᵗʰ
      perforation (chronic) 531.5 ✓5ᵗʰ
        and hemorrhage 531.6 ✓5ᵗʰ
    acute 531.3 ✓5ᵗʰ
      with
        hemorrhage 531.0 ✓5ᵗʰ
          and perforation 531.2 ✓5ᵗʰ
        perforation 531.1 ✓5ᵗʰ
          and hemorrhage 531.2 ✓5ᵗʰ
    bleeding (recurrent) — *see* Ulcer, stomach, with hemorrhage
    chronic 531.7 ✓5ᵗʰ
      with
        hemorrhage 531.4 ✓5ᵗʰ
          and perforation 531.6 ✓5ᵗʰ
        perforation 531.5 ✓5ᵗʰ
          and hemorrhage 531.6 ✓5ᵗʰ
    penetrating — *see* Ulcer, stomach, with perforation
    perforating — *see* Ulcer, stomach, with perforation
  stomatitis 528.0
  stress — *see* Ulcer, peptic
  strumous (tuberculous) (*see also* Tuberculosis) 017.2 ✓5ᵗʰ
  submental (*see also* Ulcer, skin) 707.8
  submucosal, bladder 595.1
  syphilitic (any site) (early) (secondary) 091.3
    late 095.9
    perforating 095.9
      foot 094.0
  testis 608.89
  thigh — *see* Ulcer, lower extremity
  throat 478.29
    diphtheritic 032.0
  toe — *see* Ulcer, lower extremity
  tongue (traumatic) 529.0
  tonsil 474.8
    diphtheritic 032.0
  trachea 519.1
  trophic — *see* Ulcer, skin
  tropical NEC (*see also* Ulcer, skin) 707.9
  tuberculous — *see* Tuberculosis, ulcer
  tunica vaginalis 608.89
  turbinate 730.9 ✓5ᵗʰ
  typhoid (fever) 002.0
    perforating 002.0
  umbilicus (newborn) 771.4
  unspecified site NEC — *see* Ulcer, skin
  urethra (meatus) (*see also* Urethritis) 597.89
  uterus 621.8
    cervix 622.0
      with mention of cervicitis 616.0
    neck 622.0
      with mention of cervicitis 616.0
  vagina 616.8
  valve, heart 421.0
  varicose (lower extremity, any part) 454.0
    anus — *see* Varicose, ulcer, anus
    broad ligament 456.5
    esophagus (*see also* Varix, esophagus) 456.1
      bleeding (*see also* Varix, esophagus, bleeding) 456.0
    inflamed or infected 454.2
    nasal septum 456.8
    perineum 456.6
    rectum — *see* Varicose, ulcer, anus
    scrotum 456.4
    specified site NEC 456.8
    sublingual 456.3
    vulva 456.6
  vas deferens 608.89
  vesical (*see also* Ulcer, bladder) 596.8
  vulva (acute) (infectional) 616.50
    Behçet's syndrome 136.1 *[616.51]*

Ulcer, ulcerated, ulcerating, ulceration, ulcerative — *continued*

  vulva — *continued*
    herpetic 054.12
    tuberculous 016.7 ✓5ᵗʰ *[616.51]*
  vulvobuccal, recurring 616.50
  x-ray — *see* Ulcer, by site
  yaws 102.4

Ulcerosa scarlatina 034.1

Ulcus — *see also* Ulcer
  cutis tuberculosum (*see also* Tuberculosis) 017.0 ✓5ᵗʰ
  duodeni — *see* Ulcer, duodenum
  durum 091.0
    extragenital 091.2
  gastrojejunale — *see* Ulcer, gastrojejunal
  hypostaticum — *see* Ulcer, varicose
  molle (cutis) (skin) 099.0
  serpens corneae (pneumococcal) 370.04
  ventriculi — *see* Ulcer, stomach

Ulegyria 742.4

Ulerythema
  acneiforma 701.8
  centrifugum 695.4
  ophryogenes 757.4

Ullrich (-Bonnevie) (-Turner) syndrome 758.6

Ullrich-Feichtiger syndrome 759.89

Ulnar — *see* condition

Ulorrhagia 523.8

Ulorrhea 523.8

Umbilicus, umbilical — *see also* condition
  cord necrosis, affecting fetus or newborn 762.6

Unavailability of medical facilities (at) V63.9
  due to
    investigation by social service agency V63.8
    lack of services at home V63.1
    remoteness from facility V63.0
    waiting list V63.2
    home V63.1
    outpatient clinic V63.0
    specified reason NEC V63.8

Uncinaria americana infestion 126.1

Uncinariasis (*see also* Ancylostomiasis) 126.9

Unconscious, unconsciousness 780.09

Underdevelopment — *see also* Undeveloped
  sexual 259.0

Undernourishment 269.9

Undernutrition 269.9

Under observation — *see* Observation

Underweight 783.22
  for gestational age — *see* Light-for-dates

Underwood's disease (sclerema neonatorum) 778.1

Undescended — *see also* Malposition, congenital
  cecum 751.4
  colon 751.4
  testis 752.51

Undetermined diagnosis or cause 799.9

Undeveloped, undevelopment — *see also* Hypoplasia
  brain (congenital) 742.1
  cerebral (congenital) 742.1
  fetus or newborn 764.9 ✓5ᵗʰ
  heart 746.89
  lung 748.5
  testis 257.2
  uterus 259.0

Undiagnosed (disease) 799.9

Undulant fever (*see also* Brucellosis) 023.9

Unemployment, anxiety concerning V62.0

Unequal leg (acquired) (length) 736.81
  congenital 755.30

Unerupted teeth, tooth 520.6

Unextracted dental root 525.3

Unguis incarnatus 703.0

Unicornis uterus 752.3

Unicorporeus uterus 752.3

Uniformis uterus 752.3

Unilateral — *see also* condition
  development, breast 611.8
  organ or site, congenital NEC — *see* Agenesis

Ulcer — Unilateral

Unilateral — *see also* condition — *continued*
  vagina 752.49
Unilateralis uterus 752.3
Unilocular heart 745.8
Uninhibited bladder 596.54
  with cauda equina syndrome 344.61
  neurogenic — *see* Neurogenic, bladder 596.54
Union, abnormal — *see also* Fusion
  divided tendon 727.89
  larynx and trachea 748.3
Universal
  joint, cervix 620.6
  mesentery 751.4
Unknown
  cause of death 799.9
  diagnosis 799.9
Unna's disease (seborrheic dermatitis) 690.10
Unresponsiveness, adrenocorticotropin (ACTH) 255.4
Unsoundness of mind (*see also* Psychosis) 298.9
Unspecified cause of death 799.9
Unstable
  back NEC 724.9
  colon 569.89
  joint — *see* Instability, joint
  lie 652.0 ✓5ᵗʰ
    affecting fetus or newborn (before labor) 761.7
    causing obstructed labor 660.0 ✓5ᵗʰ
      affecting fetus or newborn 763.1
  lumbosacral joint (congenital) 756.19
    acquired 724.6
  sacroiliac 724.6
  spine NEC 724.9
Untruthfulness, child problem (*see also* Disturbance, conduct) 312.0 ✓5ᵗʰ
Unverricht (-Lundborg) disease, syndrome, or epilepsy 333.2
Unverricht-Wagner syndrome (dermatomyositis) 710.3
Upper respiratory — *see* condition
Upset
  gastric 536.8
    psychogenic 306.4
  gastrointestinal 536.8
    psychogenic 306.4
    virus (*see also* Enteritis, viral) 008.8
  intestinal (large) (small) 564.9
    psychogenic 306.4
  menstruation 626.9
  mental 300.9
  stomach 536.8
    psychogenic 306.4
Urachus — *see also* condition
  patent 753.7
  persistent 753.7
Uratic arthritis 274.0
Urbach's lipoid proteinosis 272.8
Urbach-Oppenheim disease or syndrome (necrobiosis lipoidica diabeticorum) 250.8 ✓5ᵗʰ [709.3]
Urbach-Wiethe disease or syndrome (lipoid proteinosis) 272.8
Urban yellow fever 060.1
Urea, blood, high — *see* Uremia
Uremia, uremic (absorption) (amaurosis) (amblyopia) (aphasia) (apoplexy) (coma) (delirium) (dementia) (dropsy) (dyspnea) (fever) (intoxication) (mania) (paralysis) (poisoning) (toxemia) (vomiting) 586
  with
    abortion — *see* Abortion, by type, with renal failure
    ectopic pregnancy (*see also* categories 633.0-633.9) 639.3
    hypertension (*see also* Hypertension, kidney) 403.91
    molar pregnancy (*see also* categories 630-632) 639.3
  chronic 585
  complicating
    abortion 639.3
    ectopic or molar pregnancy 639.3

Uremia, uremic — *continued*
  complicating — *continued*
    hypertension (*see also* Hypertension, kidney) 403.91
    labor and delivery 669.3 ✓5ᵗʰ
  congenital 779.89   ▲
  extrarenal 788.9
  hypertensive (chronic) (*see also* Hypertension, kidney) 403.91
  maternal NEC, affecting fetus or newborn 760.1
  neuropathy 585 [357.4]
  pericarditis 585 [420.0]
  prerenal 788.9
  pyelitic (*see also* Pyelitis) 590.80
Ureter, ureteral — *see* condition
Ureteralgia 788.0
Ureterectasis 593.89
Ureteritis 593.89
  cystica 590.3
  due to calculus 592.1
  gonococcal (acute) 098.19
    chronic or duration of 2 months or over 098.39
  nonspecific 593.89
Ureterocele (acquired) 593.89
  congenital 753.23
Ureterolith 592.1
Ureterolithiasis 592.1
Ureterostomy status V44.6
  with complication 997.5
Urethra, urethral — *see* condition
Urethralgia 788.9
Urethritis (abacterial) (acute) (allergic) (anterior) (chronic) (nonvenereal) (posterior) (recurrent) (simple) (subacute) (ulcerative) (undifferentiated) 597.80
  diplococcal (acute) 098.0
    chronic or duration of 2 months or over 098.2
  due to Trichomonas (vaginalis) 131.02
  gonococcal (acute) 098.0
    chronic or duration of 2 months or over 098.2
  nongonococcal (sexually transmitted) 099.40
    Chlamydia trachomatis 099.41
    Reiter's 099.3
    specified organism NEC 099.49
  nonspecific (sexually transmitted) (*see also* Urethritis, nongonococcal) 099.40
  not sexually transmitted 597.80
  Reiter's 099.3
  trichomonal or due to Trichomonas (vaginalis) 131.02
  tuberculous (*see also* Tuberculosis) 016.3 ✓5ᵗʰ
  venereal NEC (*see also* Urethritis, nongonococcal) 099.40
Urethrocele
  female 618.0
    with uterine prolapse 618.4
      complete 618.3
      incomplete 618.2
  male 599.5
Urethrolithiasis 594.2
Urethro-oculoarticular syndrome 099.3
Urethro-oculosynovial syndrome 099.3
Urethrorectal — *see* condition
Urethrorrhagia 599.84
Urethrorrhea 788.7
Urethrostomy status V44.6
  with complication 997.5
Urethrotrigonitis 595.3
Urethrovaginal — *see* condition
Urhidrosis, uridrosis 705.89
Uric acid
  diathesis 274.9
  in blood 790.6
Uricacidemia 790.6
Uricemia 790.6
Uricosuria 791.9

Urination
  frequent 788.41
  painful 788.1
Urine, urinary — *see also* condition
  abnormality NEC 788.69
  blood in (*see also* Hematuria) 599.7
  discharge, excessive 788.42
  enuresis 788.30
    nonorganic origin 307.6
  extravasation 788.8
  frequency 788.41
  incontinence 788.30
    active 788.30
    female 788.30
      stress 625.6
        and urge 788.33
    male 788.30
      stress 788.32
        and urge 788.33
    mixed (stress and urge) 788.33
    neurogenic 788.39
    nonorganic origin 307.6
    stress (female) 625.6
      male NEC 788.32
  intermittent stream 788.61
  pus in 791.9
  retention or stasis NEC 788.20
    bladder, incomplete emptying 788.21
    psychogenic 306.53
    specified NEC 788.29
  secretion
    deficient 788.5
    excessive 788.42
    frequency 788.41
  stream
    intermittent 788.61
    slowing 788.62
    splitting 788.61
    weak 788.62
Urinemia — *see* Uremia
Urinoma NEC 599.9
  bladder 596.8
  kidney 593.89
  renal 593.89
  ureter 593.89
  urethra 599.84
Uroarthritis, infectious 099.3
Urodialysis 788.5
Urolithiasis 592.9
Uronephrosis 593.89
Uropathy 599.9
  obstructive 599.6
Urosepsis 599.0
  meaning sepsis 038.9
  meaning urinary tract infection 599.0
Urticaria 708.9
  with angioneurotic edema 995.1
    hereditary 277.6
  allergic 708.0
  cholinergic 708.5
  chronic 708.8
  cold, familial 708.2
  dermatographic 708.3
  due to
    cold or heat 708.2
    drugs 708.0
    food 708.0
    inhalants 708.0
    plants 708.8
    serum 999.5
  factitial 708.3
  giant 995.1
    hereditary 277.6
  gigantea 995.1
    hereditary 277.6
  idiopathic 708.1
  larynx 995.1
    hereditary 277.6
  neonatorum 778.8
  nonallergic 708.1
  papulosa (Hebra) 698.2
  perstans hemorrhagica 757.39
  pigmentosa 757.33
  recurrent periodic 708.8
  serum 999.5
  solare 692.72

✓4ᵗʰ Fourth-digit Required   ✓5ᵗʰ Fifth-digit Required   ▶◀ Revised Text   ● New Line   ▲ Revised Code

Urticaria — *continued*
  specified type NEC 708.8
  thermal (cold) (heat) 708.2
  vibratory 708.4
Urticarioides acarodermatitis 133.9
Use of
  nonprescribed drugs (*see also* Abuse, drugs, nondependent) 305.9 ✓5ᵗʰ
  patent medicines (*see also* Abuse, drugs, nondependent) 305.9 ✓5ᵗʰ
Usher-Senear disease (pemphigus erythematosus) 694.4
Uta 085.5
Uterine size-date discrepancy 646.8 ✓5ᵗʰ
Uteromegaly 621.2
Uterovaginal — *see* condition
Uterovesical — *see* condition
Uterus — *see* condition
Utriculitis (utriculus prostaticus) 597.89
Uveal — *see* condition
Uveitis (anterior) (*see also* Iridocyclitis) 364.3
  acute or subacute 364.00
    due to or associated with
      gonococcal infection 098.41
      herpes (simplex) 054.44
        zoster 053.22
    primary 364.01
    recurrent 364.02
    secondary (noninfectious) 364.04
      infectious 364.03
  allergic 360.11
  chronic 364.10
    due to or associated with
      sarcoidosis 135 [364.11]
      tuberculosis (*see also* Tuberculosis) 017.3 ✓5ᵗʰ [364.11]
  due to
    operation 360.11
    toxoplasmosis (acquired) 130.2
      congenital (active) 771.2
  granulomatous 364.10
  heterochromic 364.21
  lens-induced 364.23
  nongranulomatous 364.00
  posterior 363.20
    disseminated — *see* Chorioretinitis, disseminated
    focal — *see* Chorioretinitis, focal
  recurrent 364.02
  sympathetic 360.11
  syphilitic (secondary) 091.50
    congenital 090.0 [363.13]
    late 095.8 [363.13]
  tuberculous (*see also* Tuberculosis) 017.3 ✓5ᵗʰ [364.11]
Uveoencephalitis 363.22
Uveokeratitis (*see also* Iridocyclitis) 364.3
Uveoparotid fever 135
Uveoparotitis 135
Uvula — *see* condition
Uvulitis (acute) (catarrhal) (chronic) (gangrenous) (membranous) (suppurative) (ulcerative) 528.3

V

Vaccination
complication or reaction — *see* Complications, vaccination
not done (contraindicated) V64.0
  because of patient's decision V64.2
prophylactic (against) V05.9
  arthropod-borne viral
    disease NEC V05.1
    encephalitis V05.0
  chickenpox V05.4
  cholera (alone) V03.0
    with typhoid-paratyphoid (cholera + TAB) V06.0
  common cold V04.7
  diphtheria (alone) V03.5
    with
      poliomyelitis (DTP+ polio) V06.3
      tetanus V06.5
        pertussis combined (DTP) V06.1
      typhoid-paratyphoid (DTP + TAB) V06.2
  disease (single) NEC V05.9
    bacterial NEC V03.9
      specified type NEC V03.89
    combinations NEC V06.9
      specified type NEC V06.8
    specified type NEC V05.8
  encephalitis, viral, arthropod-borne V05.0
  Hemophilus influenzae, type B [Hib] V03.81
  hepatitis, viral V05.3
  influenza V04.8
    with
      Streptococcus pneumoniae [pneumococcus] V06.6
  lileieshmaniasis V05.2
  measles (alone) V04.2
    with mumps-rubella (MMR) V06.4
  mumps (alone) V04.6
    with measles and rubella (MMR) V06.4
  pertussis alone V03.6
  plague V03.3
  poliomyelitis V04.0
    with diphtheria-tetanus-pertussis (DTP + polio) V06.3
  rabies V04.5
  rubella (alone) V04.3
    with measles and mumps (MMR) V06.4
  smallpox V04.1
  Streptococcus pneumoniae [pneumococcus] V03.82
    with
      influenza V06.6
  tetanus toxoid (alone) V03.7
    with diphtheria [Td] V06.5
      with
        pertussis (DTP) V06.1
          with poliomyelitis (DTP+polio) V06.3
  tuberculosis (BCG) V03.2
  tularemia V03.4
  typhoid-paratyphoid (TAB) (alone) V03.1
    with diphtheria-tetanus-pertussis (TAB + DTP) V06.2
  varicella V05.4
  viral
    encephalitis, arthropod-borne V05.0
    hepatitis V05.3
  yellow fever V04.4
Vaccinia (generalized) 999.0
congenital 771.2
conjunctiva 999.3
eyelids 999.0 [373.5]
localized 999.3
nose 999.3
not from vaccination 051.0
  eyelid 051.0 [373.5]
sine vaccinatione 051.0
without vaccination 051.0
Vacuum
extraction of fetus or newborn 763.3
in sinus (accessory) (nasal) (*see also* Sinusitis) 473.9
Vagabond V60.0
Vagabondage V60.0

Vagabonds' disease 132.1
Vagina, vaginal — *see* condition
Vaginalitis (tunica) 608.4
Vaginismus (reflex) 625.1
functional 306.51
hysterical 300.11
psychogenic 306.51
Vaginitis (acute) (chronic) (circumscribed) (diffuse) (emphysematous) (Hemophilus vaginalis) (nonspecific) (nonvenereal) (ulcerative) 616.10
with
  abortion — *see* Abortion, by type, with sepsis
  ectopic pregnancy (*see also* categories 633.0-633.9) 639.0
  molar pregnancy (*see also* categories 630-632) 639.0
adhesive, congenital 752.49
atrophic, postmenopausal 627.3
bacterial 616.10
blennorrhagic (acute) 098.0
  chronic or duration of 2 months or over 098.2
candidal 112.1
chlamydial 099.53
complicating pregnancy or puerperium 646.6 ✓5ᵗʰ
  affecting fetus or newborn 760.8
congenital (adhesive) 752.49
due to
  C. albicans 112.1
  Trichomonas (vaginalis) 131.01
following
  abortion 639.0
  ectopic or molar pregnancy 639.0
gonococcal (acute) 098.0
  chronic or duration of 2 months or over 098.2
granuloma 099.2
Monilia 112.1
mycotic 112.1
pinworm 127.4 [616.11]
postirradiation 616.10
postmenopausal atrophic 627.3
senile (atrophic) 627.3
syphilitic (early) 091.0
  late 095.8
trichomonal 131.01
tuberculous (*see also* Tuberculosis) 016.7 ✓5ᵗʰ
venereal NEC 099.8
Vaginosis — *see* Vaginitis
Vagotonia 352.3
Vagrancy V60.0
Vallecula — *see* condition
Valley fever 114.0
Valsuani's disease (progressive pernicious anemia, puerperal) 648.2 ✓5ᵗʰ
Valve, valvular (formation) — *see also* condition
cerebral ventricle (communicating) in situ V45.2
cervix, internal os 752.49
colon 751.5
congenital NEC — *see* Atresia
formation, congenital NEC — *see* Atresia
heart defect — *see* Anomaly, heart, valve
ureter 753.29
  pelvic junction 753.21
  vesical orifice 753.22
urethra 753.6
Valvulitis (chronic) (*see also* Endocarditis) 424.90
rheumatic (chronic) (inactive) (with chorea) 397.9
  active or acute (aortic) (mitral) (pulmonary) (tricuspid) 391.1
syphilitic NEC 093.20
  aortic 093.22
  mitral 093.21
  pulmonary 093.24
  tricuspid 093.23
Valvulopathy — *see* Endocarditis
van Bogaert's leukoencephalitis (sclerosing) (subacute) 046.2
van Bogaert-Nijssen (-Peiffer) disease 330.0

van Buchem's syndrome (hyperostosis corticalis) 733.3
van Creveld-von Gierke disease (glycogenosis I) 271.0
van den Bergh's disease (enterogenous cyanosis) 289.7
van der Hoeve's syndrome (brittle bones and blue sclera, deafness) 756.51
van der Hoeve-Halbertsma-Waardenburg syndrome (ptosis-epicanthus) 270.2
van der Hoeve-Waardenburg-Gualdi syndrome (ptosis epicanthus) 270.2
Vanillism 692.89
Vanishing lung 492.0
van Neck (-Odelberg) disease or syndrome (juvenile osteochondrosis) 732.1
Vanishing twin 651.33
Vapor asphyxia or suffocation NEC 987.9
specified agent — *see* Table of Drugs and Chemicals
Vaquez's disease (M9950/1) 238.4
Vaquez-Osler disease (polycythemia vera) (M9950/1) 238.4
Variance, lethal ball, prosthetic heart valve 996.02
Variants, thalassemic 282.4
Variations in hair color 704.3
Varicella 052.9
with
  complication 052.8
    specified NEC 052.7
  pneumonia 052.1
  vaccination and inoculation (prophylactic) V05.4
Varices — *see* Varix
Varicocele (scrotum) (thrombosed) 456.4
ovary 456.5
perineum 456.6
spermatic cord (ulcerated) 456.4
Varicose
aneurysm (ruptured) (*see also* Aneurysm) 442.9
dermatitis (lower extremity) — *see* Varicose, vein, inflamed or infected
eczema — *see* Varicose, vein
phlebitis — *see* Varicose, vein, inflamed or infected
placental vessel — *see* Placenta, abnormal
tumor — *see* Varicose, vein
ulcer (lower extremity, any part) 454.0
  anus 455.8
    external 455.5
    internal 455.2
  esophagus (*see also* Varix, esophagus) 456.1
    bleeding (*see also* Varix, esophagus, bleeding) 456.0
  inflamed or infected 454.2
  nasal septum 456.8
  perineum 456.6
  rectum — *see* Varicose, ulcer, anus
  scrotum 456.4
  specified site NEC 456.8
vein (lower extremity) (ruptured) (*see also* Varix) 454.9
  with
    complications NEC 454.8 ●
    edema 454.8 ●
    inflammation or infection 454.1
      ulcerated 454.2
    pain 454.8 ●
    stasis dermatitis 454.1
      with ulcer 454.2
    swelling 454.8 ●
    ulcer 454.0
      inflamed or infected 454.2
  anus — *see* Hemorrhoids
  broad ligament 456.5
  congenital (peripheral) NEC 747.60
    gastrointestinal 747.61
    lower limb 747.64
    renal 747.62
    specified NEC 747.69
    upper limb 747.63

Varicose — *continued*
  vein (*see also* Varix) — *continued*
    esophagus (ulcerated) (*see also* Varix, esophagus) 456.1
        bleeding (*see also* Varix, esophagus, bleeding) 456.0
      inflamed or infected 454.1
        with ulcer 454.2
      in pregnancy or puerperium 671.0 ✓5ᵗʰ
        vulva or perineum 671.1 ✓5ᵗʰ
      nasal septum (with ulcer) 456.8
      pelvis 456.5
      perineum 456.6
        in pregnancy, childbirth, or puerperium 671.1 ✓5ᵗʰ
      rectum — *see* Hemorrhoids
      scrotum (ulcerated) 456.4
      specified site NEC 456.8
      sublingual 456.3
      ulcerated 454.0
        inflamed or infected 454.2
      umbilical cord, affecting fetus or newborn 762.6
      urethra 456.8
      vulva 456.6
        in pregnancy, childbirth, or puerperium 671.1 ✓5ᵗʰ
    vessel — *see also* Varix
      placenta — *see* Placenta, abnormal

Varicosis, varicosities, varicosity (*see also* Varix) 454.9

Variola 050.9
  hemorrhagic (pustular) 050.0
  major 050.0
  minor 050.1
  modified 050.2

Varioloid 050.2

Variolosa, purpura 050.0

Varix (lower extremity) (ruptured) 454.9
  with
    complications NEC 454.8 ●
    edema 454.8 ●
    inflammation or infection 454.1
      with ulcer 454.2
    pain 454.8 ●
    stasis dermatitis 454.1
      with ulcer 454.2
    swelling 454.8 ●
    ulcer 454.0
      with inflammation or infection 454.2
  aneurysmal (*see also* Aneurysm) 442.9
  anus — *see* Hemorrhoids
  arteriovenous (congenital) (peripheral) NEC 747.60
    gastrointestinal 747.61
    lower limb 747.64
    renal 747.62
    specified NEC 747.69
    spinal 747.82
    upper limb 747.63
  bladder 456.5
  broad ligament 456.5
  congenital (peripheral) NEC 747.60
  esophagus (ulcerated) 456.1
    bleeding 456.0
      in
        cirrhosis of liver 571.5 [456.20]
        portal hypertension 572.3 [456.20]
    congenital 747.69
      in
        cirrhosis of liver 571.5 [456.21]
          with bleeding 571.5 [456.20]
        portal hypertension 572.3 [456.21]
          with bleeding 572.3 [456.20]
  gastric 456.8
  inflamed or infected 454.1
    ulcerated 454.2
  in pregnancy or puerperium 671.0 ✓5ᵗʰ
    perineum 671.1 ✓5ᵗʰ
    vulva 671.1 ✓5ᵗʰ
  labia (majora) 456.6
  orbit 456.8
    congenital 747.69
  ovary 456.5
  papillary 448.1
  pelvis 456.5

Varix — *continued*
  perineum 456.6
    in pregnancy or puerperium 671.1 ✓5ᵗʰ
  pharynx 456.8
  placenta — *see* Placenta, abnormal
  prostate 456.8
  rectum — *see* Hemorrhoids
  renal papilla 456.8
  retina 362.17
  scrotum (ulcerated) 456.4
  sigmoid colon 456.8
  specified site NEC 456.8
  spinal (cord) (vessels) 456.8
  spleen, splenic (vein) (with phlebolith) 456.8
  sublingual 456.3
  ulcerated 454.0
    inflamed or infected 454.2
  umbilical cord, affecting fetus or newborn 762.6
  uterine ligament 456.5
  vocal cord 456.8
  vulva 456.6
    in pregnancy, childbirth, or puerperium 671.1 ✓5ᵗʰ

Vasa previa 663.5 ✓5ᵗʰ
  affecting fetus or newborn 762.6
  hemorrhage from, affecting fetus or newborn 772.0

Vascular — *see also* condition
  loop on papilla (optic) 743.57
  sheathing, retina 362.13
  spasm 443.9
  spider 448.1

Vascularity, pulmonary, congenital 747.3

Vascularization
  choroid 362.16
  cornea 370.60
    deep 370.63
    localized 370.61
  retina 362.16
  subretinal 362.16

Vasculitis 447.6
  allergic 287.0
  cryoglobulinemic 273.2
  disseminated 447.6
  kidney 447.8
  leukocytoclastic 446.29
  nodular 695.2
  retinal 362.18
  rheumatic — *see* Fever, rheumatic

Vas deferens — *see* condition

Vas deferentitis 608.4

Vasectomy, admission for V25.2

Vasitis 608.4
  nodosa 608.4
  scrotum 608.4
  spermatic cord 608.4
  testis 608.4
  tuberculous (*see also* Tuberculosis) 016.5 ✓5ᵗʰ
  tunica vaginalis 608.4
  vas deferens 608.4

Vasodilation 443.9

Vasomotor — *see* condition

Vasoplasty, after previous sterilization V26.0

Vasoplegia, splanchnic (*see also* Neuropathy, peripheral, autonomic) 337.9

Vasospasm 443.9
  cerebral (artery) 435.9
    with transient neurologic deficit 435.9
  nerve
    arm NEC 354.9
    autonomic 337.9
    brachial plexus 353.0
    cervical plexus 353.2
    leg NEC 355.8
    lower extremity NEC 355.8
    peripheral NEC 355.9
    spinal NEC 355.9
    sympathetic 337.9
    upper extremity NEC 354.9
  peripheral NEC 443.9
  retina (artery) (*see also* Occlusion, retinal, artery) 362.30

Vasospastic — *see* condition

Vasovagal attack (paroxysmal) 780.2
  psychogenic 306.2

Vater's ampulla — *see* condition

VATER syndrome 759.89

Vegetation, vegetative
  adenoid (nasal fossa) 474.2
  consciousness (persistent) 780.03
  endocarditis (acute) (any valve) (chronic) (subacute) 421.0
  heart (mycotic) (valve) 421.0
  state (persistent) 780.03

Veil
  Jackson's 751.4
  over face (causing asphyxia) 768.9

Vein, venous — *see* condition

Veldt sore (*see also* Ulcer, skin) 707.9

Velpeau's hernia — *see* Hernia, femoral

Venereal
  balanitis NEC 099.8
  bubo 099.1
  disease 099.9
    specified nature or type NEC 099.8
  granuloma inguinale 099.2
  lymphogranuloma (Durand-Nicolas-Favre), any site 099.1
  salpingitis 098.37
  urethritis (*see also* Urethritis, nongonococcal) 099.40
  vaginitis NEC 099.8
  warts 078.19

Vengefulness, in child (*see also* Disturbance, conduct) 312.0 ✓5ᵗʰ

Venofibrosis 459.89

Venom, venomous
  bite or sting (animal or insect) 989.5
  poisoning 989.5

Venous — *see* condition

Ventouse delivery NEC 669.5 ✓5ᵗʰ
  affecting fetus or newborn 763.3

Ventral — *see* condition

Ventricle, ventricular — *see also* condition
  escape 427.69
  standstill (*see also* Arrest, cardiac) 427.5

Ventriculitis, cerebral (*see also* Meningitis) 322.9

Ventriculostomy status V45.2

Verbiest's syndrome (claudicatio intermittens spinalis) 435.1

Vernet's syndrome 352.6

Verneuil's disease (syphilitic bursitis) 095.7

Verruca (filiformis) 078.10
  acuminata (any site) 078.11
  necrogenica (primary) (*see also* Tuberculosis) 017.0 ✓5ᵗʰ
  plana (juvenilis) 078.19
  peruana 088.0
  peruviana 088.0
  plantaris 078.19
  seborrheica 702.19
    inflamed 702.11
  senilis 702.0
  tuberculosa (primary) (*see also* Tuberculosis) 017.0 ✓5ᵗʰ
  venereal 078.19
  viral NEC 078.10

Verrucosities (*see also* Verruca) 078.10

Verrucous endocarditis (acute) (any valve) (chronic) (subacute) 710.0 [424.91]
  nonbacterial 710.0 [424.91]

Verruga
  peruana 088.0
  peruviana 088.0

Verse's disease (calcinosis intervertebralis) 275.49 [722.90]

Version
  before labor, affecting fetus or newborn 761.7
  cephalic (correcting previous malposition) 652.1 ✓5ᵗʰ
    affecting fetus or newborn 763.1
  cervix (*see also* Malposition, uterus) 621.6
  uterus (postinfectional) (postpartal, old) (*see also* Malposition, uterus) 621.6
    forward — *see* Anteversion, uterus
    lateral — *see* Lateroversion, uterus

Vertebra, vertebral — *see* condition
Vertigo 780.4
  auditory 386.19
  aural 386.19
  benign paroxysmal positional 386.11
  central origin 386.2
  cerebral 386.2
  Dix and Hallpike (epidemic) 386.12
  endemic paralytic 078.81
  epidemic 078.81
    Dix and Hallpike 386.12
    Gerlier's 078.81
    Pedersen's 386.12
    vestibular neuronitis 386.12
  epileptic — *see* Epilepsy
  Gerlier's (epidemic) 078.81
  hysterical 300.11
  labyrinthine 386.10
  laryngeal 786.2
  malignant positional 386.2
  Ménière's (*see also* Disease, Ménière's) 386.00
  menopausal 627.2
  otogenic 386.19
  paralytic 078.81
  paroxysmal positional, benign 386.11
  Pedersen's (epidemic) 386.12
  peripheral 386.10
    specified type NEC 386.19
  positional
    benign paroxysmal 386.11
    malignant 386.2
Verumontanitis (chronic) (*see also* Urethritis) 597.89
Vesania (*see also* Psychosis) 298.9
Vesical — *see* condition
Vesicle
  cutaneous 709.8
  seminal — *see* condition
  skin 709.8
Vesicocolic — *see* condition
Vesicoperineal — *see* condition
Vesicorectal — *see* condition
Vesicourethrorectal — *see* condition
Vesicovaginal — *see* condition
Vesicular — *see* condition
Vesiculitis (seminal) 608.0
  amebic 006.8
  gonorrheal (acute) 098.14
    chronic or duration of 2 months or over 098.34
  trichomonal 131.09
  tuberculous (*see also* Tuberculosis) 016.5 ☑5ᵗʰ *[608.81]*
Vestibulitis (ear) (*see also* Labyrinthitis) 386.30
  nose (external) 478.1
  vulvar 616.10
Vestibulopathy, acute peripheral (recurrent) 386.12
Vestige, vestigial — *see also* Persistence
  branchial 744.41
  structures in vitreous 743.51
Vibriosis NEC 027.9
Vidal's disease (lichen simplex chronicus) 698.3
Video display tube syndrome 723.8
Vienna type encephalitis 049.8
Villaret's syndrome 352.6
Villous — *see* condition
VIN I (vulvar intraepithelial neoplasia I) 624.8
VIN II (vulvar intraepithelial neoplasia II) 624.8
VIN III (vulvar intraepithelial neoplasia III) 233.3
Vincent's
  angina 101
  bronchitis 101
  disease 101
  gingivitis 101
  infection (any site) 101
  laryngitis 101
  stomatitis 101
  tonsillitis 101
Vinson-Plummer syndrome (sideropenic dysphagia) 280.8

Viosterol deficiency (*see also* Deficiency, calciferol) 268.9
Virchow's disease 733.99
Viremia 790.8
Virilism (adrenal) (female) NEC 255.2
  with
    3-beta-hydroxysteroid dehydrogenase defect 255.2
    11-hydroxylase defect 255.2
    21-hydroxylase defect 255.2
    adrenal
      hyperplasia 255.2
      insufficiency (congenital) 255.2
    cortical hyperfunction 255.2
Virilization (female) (suprarenal) (*see also* Virilism) 255.2
  isosexual 256.4
Virulent bubo 099.0
Virus, viral — *see also* condition
  infection NEC (*see also* Infection, viral) 079.99
  septicemia 079.99
Viscera, visceral — *see* condition
Visceroptosis 569.89
Visible peristalsis 787.4
Vision, visual
  binocular, suppression 368.31
  blurred, blurring 368.8
    hysterical 300.11
  defect, defective (*see also* Impaired, vision) 369.9
  disorientation (syndrome) 368.16
  disturbance NEC (*see also* Disturbance, vision) 368.9
    hysterical 300.11
  examination V72.0
  field, limitation 368.40
  fusion, with defective steropsis 368.33
  hallucinations 368.16
  halos 368.16
  loss 369.9
    both eyes (*see also* Blindness, both eyes) 369.3
    complete (*see also* Blindness, both eyes) 369.00
    one eye 369.8
    sudden 368.16
  low (both eyes) 369.20
    one eye (other eye normal) (*see also* Impaired, vision) 369.70
      blindness, other eye 369.10
  perception, simultaneous without fusion 368.32
  tunnel 368.45
Vitality, lack or want of 780.79
  newborn 779.89 ▲
Vitamin deficiency NEC (*see also* Deficiency, vitamin) 269.2
Vitelline duct, persistent 751.0
Vitiligo 709.01
  due to pinta (carate) 103.2
  eyelid 374.53
  vulva 624.8
Vitium cordis — *see* Disease, heart
Vitreous — *see also* condition
  touch syndrome 997.99
Vocal cord — *see* condition
Vocational rehabilitation V57.22
Vogt's (Cecile) disease or syndrome 333.7
Vogt-Koyanagi syndrome 364.24
Vogt-Spielmeyer disease (amaurotic familial idiocy) 330.1
Voice
  change (*see also* Dysphonia) 784.49
  loss (*see also* Aphonia) 784.41
Volhard-Fahr disease (malignant nephrosclerosis) 403.0
Volhynian fever 083.1
Volkmann's ischemic contracture or paralysis (complicating trauma) 958.6
Voluntary starvation 307.1

Volvulus (bowel) (colon) (intestine) 560.2
  with
    hernia — *see also* Hernia, by site, with obstruction
    gangrenous — *see* Hernia, by site, with gangrene
    perforation 560.2
  congenital 751.5
  duodenum 537.3
  fallopian tube 620.5
  oviduct 620.5
  stomach (due to absence of gastrocolic ligament) 537.89
Vomiting 787.03
  with nausea 787.01
  allergic 535.4 ☑5ᵗʰ
  asphyxia 933.1
  bilious (cause unknown) 787.0
    following gastrointestinal surgery 564.3
  blood (*see also* Hematemesis) 578.0
  causing asphyxia, choking, or suffocation (*see also* Asphyxia, food) 933.1
  cyclical 536.2
    psychogenic 306.4
  epidemic 078.82
  fecal matter 569.89
  following gastrointestinal surgery 564.3
  functional 536.8
    psychogenic 306.4
  habit 536.2
  hysterical 300.11
  nervous 306.4
  neurotic 306.4
  newborn 779.3
  of or complicating pregnancy 643.9 ☑5ᵗʰ
    due to
      organic disease 643.8 ☑5ᵗʰ
      specific cause NEC 643.8 ☑5ᵗʰ
    early — *see* Hyperemesis, gravidarum
    late (after 22 completed weeks of gestation) 643.2 ☑5ᵗʰ
  pernicious or persistent 536.2
    complicating pregnancy — *see* Hyperemesis, gravidarum
    psychogenic 306.4
  physiological 787.0
  psychic 306.4
  psychogenic 307.54
  stercoral 569.89
  uncontrollable 536.2
    psychogenic 306.4
  uremic — *see* Uremia
  winter 078.82
von Bechterew (-Strumpell) disease or syndrome (ankylosing spondylitis) 720.0
von Bezold's abscess 383.01
von Economo's disease (encephalitis lethargica) 049.8
von Eulenburg's disease (congenital paramyotonia) 359.2
von Gierke's disease (glycogenosis I) 271.0
von Gies' joint 095.8
von Graefe's disease or syndrome 378.72
von Hippel (-Lindau) disease or syndrome (retinocerebral angiomatosis) 759.6
von Jaksch's anemia or disease (pseudoleukemia infantum) 285.8
von Recklinghausen's
  disease or syndrome (nerves) (skin) (M9540/1) 237.71
    bones (osteitis fibrosa cystica) 252.0
  tumor (M9540/1) 237.71
von Recklinghausen-Applebaum disease (hemochromatosis) 275.0
von Schroetter's syndrome (intermittent venous claudication) 453.8
von Willebrand (-Jürgens) (-Minot) disease or syndrome (angiohemophilia) 286.4
von Zambusch's disease (lichen sclerosus et atrophicus) 701.0
Voorhoeve's disease or dyschondroplasia 756.4
Vossius' ring 921.3
  late effect 366.21
Voyeurism 302.82

☑4ᵗʰ Fourth-digit Required   ☑5ᵗʰ Fifth-digit Required   ▶◀ Revised Text   ● New Line   ▲ Revised Code

Vrolik's disease — Wet

Vrolik's disease (osteogenesis imperfecta) 756.51

Vulva — *see* condition

Vulvismus 625.1

Vulvitis (acute) (allergic) (aphthous) (chronic) (gangrenous) (hypertrophic) (intertriginous) 616.10
  with
    abortion — *see* Abortion, by type, with sepsis
    ectopic pregnancy (*see also* categories 633.0-633.9) 639.0
    molar pregnancy (*see also* categories 630-632) 639.0
  adhesive, congenital 752.49
  blennorhagic (acute) 098.0
    chronic or duration of 2 months or over 098.2
  chlamydial 099.53
  complicating pregnancy or puerperium 646.6 ✔5ᵗʰ
  due to Ducrey's bacillus 099.0
  following
    abortion 639.0
    ectopic or molar pregnancy 639.0
  gonococcal (acute) 098.0
    chronic or duration of 2 months or over 098.2
  herpetic 054.11
  leukoplakic 624.0
  monilial 112.1
  puerperal, postpartum, childbirth 646.6 ✔5ᵗʰ
  syphilitic (early) 091.0
    late 095.8
  trichomonal 131.01

Vulvodynia 625.9

Vulvorectal — *see* condition

Vulvovaginitis (*see also* Vulvitis) 616.10
  amebic 006.8
  chlamydial 099.53
  gonococcal (acute) 098.0
    chronic or duration of 2 months or over 098.2
  herpetic 054.11
  monilial 112.1
  trichomonal (Trichomonas vaginalis) 131.01

W

Waardenburg's syndrome 756.89
  meaning ptosis-epicanthus 270.2

Waardenburg-Klein syndrome (ptosis-epicanthus) 270.2

Wagner's disease (colloid milium) 709.3

Wagner (-Unverricht) syndrome (dermatomyositis) 710.3

Waiting list, person on V63.2
  undergoing social agency investigation V63.8

Wakefulness disorder (*see also* Hypersomnia) 780.54
  nonorganic origin 307.43

Waldenström's
  disease (osteochondrosis, capital femoral) 732.1
  hepatitis (lupoid hepatitis) 571.49
  hypergammaglobulinemia 273.0
  macroglobulinemia 273.3
  purpura, hypergammaglobulinemic 273.0
  syndrome (macroglobulinemia) 273.3

Waldenström-Kjellberg syndrome (sideropenic dysphagia) 280.8

Walking
  difficulty 719.7 ✔5ᵗʰ
    psychogenic 307.9
  sleep 307.46
    hysterical 300.13

Wall, abdominal — *see* condition

Wallenberg's syndrome (posterior inferior cerebellar artery) (*see also* Disease, cerebrovascular, acute) 436

Wallgren's
  disease (obstruction of splenic vein with collateral circulation) 459.89
  meningitis (*see also* Meningitis, aseptic) 047.9

Wandering
  acetabulum 736.39
  gallbladder 751.69
  kidney, congenital 753.3
  organ or site, congenital NEC — *see* Malposition, congenital
  pacemaker (atrial) (heart) 427.89
  spleen 289.59

Wardrop's disease (with lymphangitis) 681.9
  finger 681.02
  toe 681.11

War neurosis 300.16

Wart (common) (digitate) (filiform) (infectious) (juvenile) (plantar) (viral) 078.10
  external genital organs (venereal) 078.19
  fig 078.19
  Hassall-Henle's (of cornea) 371.41
  Henle's (of cornea) 371.41
  juvenile 078.19
  moist 078.10
  Peruvian 088.0
  plantar 078.19
  prosector (*see also* Tuberculosis) 017.0 ✔5ᵗʰ
  seborrheic 702.19
    inflamed 702.11
  senile 702.0
  specified NEC 078.19
  syphilitic 091.3
  tuberculous (*see also* Tuberculosis) 017.0 ✔5ᵗʰ
  venereal (female) (male) 078.19

Warthin's tumor (salivary gland) (M8561/0) 210.2

Washerwoman's itch 692.4

Wassilieff's disease (leptospiral jaundice) 100.0

Wasting
  disease 799.4
    due to malnutrition 261
  extreme (due to malnutrition) 261
  muscular NEC 728.2
  palsy, paralysis 335.21

Water
  clefts 366.12
  deprivation of 994.3
  in joint (*see also* Effusion, joint) 719.0 ✔5ᵗʰ
  intoxication 276.6
  itch 120.3
  lack of 994.3
  loading 276.6
  on
    brain — *see* Hydrocephalus
    chest 511.8
  poisoning 276.6

Waterbrash 787.1

Water-hammer pulse (*see also* Insufficiency, aortic) 424.1

Waterhouse (-Friderichsen) disease or syndrome 036.3

Water-losing nephritis 588.8

Wax in ear 380.4

Waxy
  degeneration, any site 277.3
  disease 277.3
  kidney 277.3 [583.81]
  liver (large) 277.3
  spleen 277.3

Weak, weakness (generalized) 780.79
  arches (acquired) 734
    congenital 754.61
  bladder sphincter 596.59
  congenital 779.89 ▲
  eye muscle — *see* Strabismus
  foot (double) — *see* Weak, arches
  heart, cardiac (*see also* Failure, heart) 428.9
    congenital 746.9
  mind 317
  muscle 728.9
  myocardium (*see also* Failure, heart) 428.9
  newborn 779.89 ▲
  pelvic fundus 618.8
  pulse 785.9
  senile 797
  valvular — *see* Endocarditis

Wear, worn, tooth, teeth (approximal) (hard tissues) (interproximal) (occlusal) 521.1

Weather, weathered
  effects of
    cold NEC 991.9
      specified effect NEC 991.8
    hot (*see also* Heat) 992.9
  skin 692.74

Web, webbed (congenital) — *see also* Anomaly, specified type NEC
  canthus 743.63
  digits (*see also* Syndactylism) 755.10
  esophagus 750.3
  fingers (*see also* Syndactylism, fingers) 755.11
  larynx (glottic) (subglottic) 748.2
  neck (pterygium colli) 744.5
  Paterson-Kelly (sideropenic dysphagia) 280.8
  popliteal syndrome 756.89
  toes (*see also* Syndactylism, toes) 755.13

Weber's paralysis or syndrome 344.89

Weber-Christian disease or syndrome (nodular nonsuppurative panniculitis) 729.30

Weber-Cockayne syndrome (epidermolysis bullosa) 757.39

Weber-Dimitri syndrome 759.6

Weber-Gubler syndrome 344.89

Weber-Leyden syndrome 344.89

Weber-Osler syndrome (familial hemorrhagic telangiectasia) 448.0

Wedge-shaped or wedging vertebra (*see also* Osteoporosis) 733.00

Wegener's granulomatosis or syndrome 446.4

Wegner's disease (syphilitic osteochondritis) 090.0

Weight
  gain (abnormal) (excessive) 783.1
    during pregnancy 646.1 ✔5ᵗʰ
      insufficient 646.8 ✔5ᵗʰ
  less than 1000 grams at birth 765.0 ✔5ᵗʰ
  loss (cause unknown) 783.21

Weightlessness 994.9

Weil's disease (leptospiral jaundice) 100.0

Weill-Marchesani syndrome (brachymorphism and ectopia lentis) 759.89

Weingarten's syndrome (tropical eosinophilia) 518.3

Weir Mitchell's disease (erythromelalgia) 443.89

Weiss-Baker syndrome (carotid sinus syncope) 337.0

Weissenbach-Thibierge syndrome (cutaneous systemic sclerosis) 710.1

Wen (*see also* Cyst, sebaceous) 706.2

Wenckebach's phenomenon, heart block (second degree) 426.13

Werdnig-Hoffmann syndrome (muscular atrophy) 335.0

Werlhof's disease (*see also* Purpura, thrombocytopenic) 287.3

Werlhof-Wichmann syndrome (*see also* Purpura, thrombocytopenic) 287.3

Wermer's syndrome or disease (polyendocrine adenomatosis) 258.0

Werner's disease or syndrome (progeria adultorum) 259.8

Werner-His disease (trench fever) 083.1

Werner-Schultz disease (agranulocytosis) 288.0

Wernicke's encephalopathy, disease, or syndrome (superior hemorrhagic polioencephalitis) 265.1

Wernicke-Korsakoff syndrome or psychosis (nonalcoholic) 294.0
  alcoholic 291.1

Wernicke-Posadas disease (*see also* Coccidioidomycosis) 114.9

Wesselsbron fever 066.3

West African fever 084.8

West Nile fever 066.4 ▲

West Nile virus 066.4 ●

Westphal-Strümpell syndrome (hepatolenticular degeneration) 275.1

Wet
  brain (alcoholic) (*see also* Alcoholism) 303.9 ✔5ᵗʰ

Wet — *continued*
  feet, tropical (syndrome) (maceration) 991.4
  lung (syndrome)
    adult 518.5
    newborn 770.6
Wharton's duct — *see* condition
Wheal 709.8
Wheezing 786.07
Whiplash injury or syndrome 847.0
Whipple's disease or syndrome (intestinal lipodystrophy) 040.2
Whipworm 127.3
"Whistling face" syndrome (craniocarpotarsal dystrophy) 759.89
White — *see also* condition
  kidney
    large — *see* Nephrosis
    small 582.9
  leg, puerperal, postpartum, childbirth 671.4 ✓5ᵗʰ
    nonpuerperal 451.19
  mouth 112.0
  patches of mouth 528.6
  sponge nevus of oral mucosa 750.26
  spot lesions, teeth 521.01
White's disease (congenital) (keratosis follicularis) 757.39
Whitehead 706.2
Whitlow (with lymphangitis) 681.01
  herpetic 054.6
Whitmore's disease or fever (melioidosis) 025
Whooping cough 033.9
  with pneumonia 033.9 *[484.3]*
  due to
    Bordetella
      bronchoseptica 033.8
        with pneumonia 033.8 *[484.3]*
      parapertussis 033.1
        with pneumonia 033.1 *[484.3]*
      pertussis 033.0
        with pneumonia 033.0 *[484.3]*
    specified organism NEC 033.8
      with pneumonia 033.8 *[484.3]*
  vaccination, prophylactic (against) V03.6
Wichmann's asthma (laryngismus stridulus) 478.75
Widal (-Abrami) syndrome (acquired hemolytic jaundice) 283.9
Widening aorta (*see also* Aneurysm, aorta) 441.9
  ruptured 441.5
Wilkie's disease or syndrome 557.1
Wilkinson-Sneddon disease or syndrome (subcorneal pustular dermatosis) 694.1
Willan's lepra 696.1
Willan-Plumbe syndrome (psoriasis) 696.1
Willebrand (-Jürgens) syndrome or thrombopathy (angiohemophilia) 286.4
Willi-Prader syndrome (hypogenital dystrophy with diabetic tendency) 759.81
Willis' disease (diabetes mellitus) (*see also* Diabetes) 250.0 ✓5ᵗʰ
Wilms' tumor or neoplasm (nephroblastoma) (M8960/3) 189.0
Wilson's
  disease or syndrome (hepatolenticular degeneration) 275.1
  hepatolenticular degeneration 275.1
  lichen ruber 697.0
Wilson-Brocq disease (dermatitis exfoliativa) 695.89
Wilson-Mikity syndrome 770.7
Window — *see also* Imperfect, closure
  aorticopulmonary 745.0
Winged scapula 736.89
Winter — *see also* condition
  vomiting disease 078.82
Wise's disease 696.2
Wiskott-Aldrich syndrome (eczema-thrombocytopenia) 279.12

Withdrawal symptoms, syndrome
  alcohol 291.81
    delirium (acute) 291.0
      chronic 291.1
    newborn 760.71
  drug or narcotic 292.0
  newborn, infant of dependent mother 779.5
  steroid NEC
    correct substance properly administered 255.4
    overdose or wrong substance given or taken 962.0
Withdrawing reaction, child or adolescent 313.22
Witts' anemia (achlorhydric anemia) 280.9
Witzelsucht 301.9
Woakes' syndrome (ethmoiditis) 471.1
Wohlfart-Kugelberg-Welander disease 335.11
Woillez's disease (acute idiopathic pulmonary congestion) 518.5
Wolff-Parkinson-White syndrome (anomalous atrioventricular excitation) 426.7
Wolhynian fever 083.1
Wolman's disease (primary familial xanthomatosis) 272.7
Wood asthma 495.8
Woolly, wooly hair (congenital) (nevus) 757.4
Wool-sorters' disease 022.1
Word
  blindness (congenital) (developmental) 315.01
    secondary to organic lesion 784.61
  deafness (secondary to organic lesion) 784.69
    developmental 315.31
Worm(s) (colic) (fever) (infection) (infestation) (*see also* Infestation) 128.9
  guinea 125.7
  in intestine NEC 127.9
Worm-eaten soles 102.3
Worn out (*see also* Exhaustion) 780.79
"Worried well" V65.5
Wound, open (by cutting or piercing instrument) (by firearms) (cut) (dissection) (incised) (laceration) (penetration) (perforating) (puncture) (with initial hemorrhage, not internal) 879.8

Note — *For fracture with open wound, see Fracture.*

For laceration, traumatic rupture, tear or penetrating wound of internal organs, such as heart, lung, liver, kidney, pelvic organs, etc., whether or not accompanied by open wound or fracture in the same region, see Injury, internal.

For contused wound, see Contusion. For crush injury, see Crush. For abrasion, insect bite (nonvenomous), blister, or scratch, see Injury, superficial.

Complicated includes wounds with:
  delayed healing
  delayed treatment
  foreign body
  primary infection

For late effect of open wound, see Late, effect, wound, open, by site.

---

  abdomen, abdominal (external) (muscle) 879.2
    complicated 879.3
    wall (anterior) 879.2
      complicated 879.3
      lateral 879.4
        complicated 879.5
  alveolar (process) 873.62
    complicated 873.72
  ankle 891.0
    with tendon involvement 891.2
    complicated 891.1
  anterior chamber, eye (*see also* Wound, open, intraocular) 871.9
  anus 879.6
    complicated 879.7
  arm 884.0
    with tendon involvement 884.2

Wound, open — *continued*
  arm — *continued*
    complicated 884.1
    forearm 881.00
      with tendon involvement 881.20
      complicated 881.10
    multiple sites — *see* Wound, open, multiple, upper limb
    upper 880.03
      with tendon involvement 880.23
      complicated 880.13
      multiple sites (with axillary or shoulder regions) 880.09
        with tendon involvement 880.29
        complicated 880.19
  artery — *see* Injury, blood vessel, by site
  auditory
    canal (external) (meatus) 872.02
      complicated 872.12
    ossicles (incus) (malleus) (stapes) 872.62
      complicated 872.72
  auricle, ear 872.01
    complicated 872.11
  axilla 880.02
    with tendon involvement 880.22
    complicated 880.12
      with tendon involvement 880.29
    involving other sites of upper arm 880.09
      complicated 880.19
  back 876.0
    complicated 876.1
  bladder — *see* Injury, internal, bladder
  blood vessel — *see* Injury, blood vessel, by site
  brain — *see* Injury, intracranial, with open intracranial wound
  breast 879.0
    complicated 879.1
  brow 873.42
    complicated 873.52
  buccal mucosa 873.61
    complicated 873.71
  buttock 877.0
    complicated 877.1
  calf 891.0
    with tendon involvement 891.2
    complicated 891.1
  canaliculus lacrimalis 870.8
    with laceration of eyelid 870.2
  canthus, eye 870.8
    laceration — *see* Laceration, eyelid
  cavernous sinus — *see* Injury, intracranial
  cerebellum — *see* Injury, intracranial
  cervical esophagus 874.4
    complicated 874.5
  cervix — *see* Injury, internal, cervix
  cheek(s) (external) 873.41
    complicated 873.51
    internal 873.61
      complicated 873.71
  chest (wall) (external) 875.0
    complicated 875.1
  chin 873.44
    complicated 873.54
  choroid 363.63
  ciliary body (eye) (*see also* Wound, open, intraocular) 871.9
  clitoris 878.8
    complicated 878.9
  cochlea 872.64
    complicated 872.74
  complicated 879.9
  conjunctiva — *see* Wound, open, intraocular
  cornea (nonpenetrating) (*see also* Wound, open, intraocular) 871.9
  costal region 875.0
    complicated 875.1
  Descemet's membrane (*see also* Wound, open, intraocular) 871.9
  digit(s)
    foot 893.0
      with tendon involvement 893.2
      complicated 893.1
    hand 883.0
      with tendon involvement 883.2
      complicated 883.1
  drumhead, ear 872.61
    complicated 872.71

Wound, open — *continued*
ear 872.8
  canal 872.02
    complicated 872.12
  complicated 872.9
  drum 872.61
    complicated 872.71
  external 872.00
    complicated 872.10
  multiple sites 872.69
    complicated 872.79
  ossicles (incus) (malleus) (stapes) 872.62
    complicated 872.72
  specified part NEC 872.69
    complicated 872.79
elbow 881.01
  with tendon involvement 881.21
  complicated 881.11
epididymis 878.2
  complicated 878.3
epigastric region 879.2
  complicated 879.3
epiglottis 874.01
  complicated 874.11
esophagus (cervical) 874.4
  complicated 874.5
  thoracic — *see* Injury, internal, esophagus
Eustachian tube 872.63
  complicated 872.73
extremity
  lower (multiple) NEC 894.0
    with tendon involvement 894.2
    complicated 894.1
  upper (multiple) NEC 884.0
    with tendon involvement 884.2
    complicated 884.1
eye(s) (globe) — *see* Wound, open, intraocular
eyeball NEC 871.9
  laceration (*see also* Laceration, eyeball) 871.4
  penetrating (*see also* Penetrating wound, eyeball) 871.7
eyebrow 873.42
  complicated 873.52
eyelid NEC 870.8
  laceration — *see* Laceration, eyelid
face 873.40
  complicated 873.50
  multiple sites 873.49
    complicated 873.59
  specified part NEC 873.49
    complicated 873.59
fallopian tube — *see* Injury, internal, fallopian tube
finger(s) (nail) (subungual) 883.0
  with tendon involvement 883.2
  complicated 883.1
flank 879.4
  complicated 879.5
foot (any part except toe(s) alone) 892.0
  with tendon involvement 892.2
  complicated 892.1
forearm 881.00
  with tendon involvement 881.20
  complicated 881.10
forehead 873.42
  complicated 873.52
genital organs (external) NEC 878.8
  complicated 878.9
  internal — *see* Injury, internal, by site
globe (eye) (*see also* Wound, open, eyeball) 871.9
groin 879.4
  complicated 879.5
gum(s) 873.62
  complicated 873.72
hand (except finger(s) alone) 882.0
  with tendon involvement 882.2
  complicated 882.1
head NEC 873.8
  with intracranial injury — *see* Injury, intracranial
  due to or associated with skull fracture — *see* Fracture, skull
  complicated 873.9
  scalp — *see* Wound, open, scalp

Wound, open — *continued*
heel 892.0
  with tendon involvement 892.2
  complicated 892.1
high-velocity (grease gun) — *see* Wound, open, complicated, by site
hip 890.0
  with tendon involvement 890.2
  complicated 890.1
hymen 878.6
  complicated 878.7
hypochondrium 879.4
  complicated 879.5
hypogastric region 879.2
  complicated 879.3
iliac (region) 879.4
  complicated 879.5
incidental to
  dislocation — *see* Dislocation, open, by site
  fracture — *see* Fracture, open, by site
  intracranial injury — *see* Injury, intracranial, with open intracranial wound
  nerve injury — *see* Injury, nerve, by site
inguinal region 879.4
  complicated 879.5
instep 892.0
  with tendon involvement 892.2
  complicated 892.1
interscapular region 876.0
  complicated 876.1
intracranial — *see* Injury, intracranial, with open intracranial wound
intraocular 871.9
  with
    partial loss (of intraocular tissue) 871.2
    prolapse or exposure (of intraocular tissue) 871.1
  aceration (*see also* Laceration, eyeball) 871.4
  penetrating 871.7
    with foreign body (nonmagnetic) 871.6
      magnetic 871.5
  without prolapse (of intraocular tissue) 871.0
iris (*see also* Wound, open, eyeball) 871.9
jaw (fracture not involved) 873.44
  with fracture — *see* Fracture, jaw
  complicated 873.54
knee 891.0
  with tendon involvement 891.2
  complicated 891.1
labium (majus) (minus) 878.4
  complicated 878.5
lacrimal apparatus, gland, or sac 870.8
  with laceration of eyelid 870.2
larynx 874.01
  with trachea 874.00
    complicated 874.10
  complicated 874.11
leg (multiple) 891.0
  with tendon involvement 891.2
  complicated 891.1
  lower 891.0
    with tendon involvement 891.2
    complicated 891.1
  thigh 890.0
    with tendon involvement 890.2
    complicated 890.1
  upper 890.0
    with tendon involvement 890.2
    complicated 890.1
lens (eye) (alone) (*see also* Cataract, traumatic) 366.20
  with involvement of other eye structures — *see* Wound, open, eyeball
limb
  lower (multiple) NEC 894.0
    with tendon involvement 894.2
    complicated 894.1
  upper (multiple) NEC 884.0
    with tendon involvement 884.2
    complicated 884.1
lip 873.43
  complicated 873.53
loin 876.0
  complicated 876.1

Wound, open — *continued*
lumbar region 876.0
  complicated 876.1
malar region 873.41
  complicated 873.51
mastoid region 873.49
  complicated 873.59
mediastinum — *see* Injury, internal, mediastinum
midthoracic region 875.0
  complicated 875.1
mouth 873.60
  complicated 873.70
  floor 873.64
    complicated 873.74
  multiple sites 873.69
    complicated 873.79
  specified site NEC 873.69
    complicated 873.79
multiple, unspecified site(s) 879.8

> *Note* — *Multiple open wounds of sites classifiable to the same four-digit category should be classified to that category unless they are in different limbs.*
>
> *Multiple open wounds of sites classifiable to different four-digit categories, or to different limbs, should be coded separately.*

  complicated 879.9
  lower limb(s) (one or both) (sites classifiable to more than one three-digit category in 890 to 893) 894.0
    with tendon involvement 894.2
    complicated 894.1
  upper limb(s) (one or both) (sites classifiable to more than one three-digit category in 880 to 883) 884.0
    with tendon involvement 884.2
    complicated 884.1
muscle — *see* Sprain, by site
nail
  finger(s) 883.0
    complicated 883.1
  thumb 883.0
    complicated 883.1
  toe(s) 893.0
    complicated 893.1
nape (neck) 874.8
  complicated 874.9
  specified part NEC 874.8
    complicated 874.9
nasal — *see also* Wound, open, nose
  cavity 873.22
    complicated 873.32
  septum 873.21
    complicated 873.31
  sinuses 873.23
    complicated 873.33
nasopharynx 873.22
  complicated 873.32
neck 874.8
  complicated 874.9
  nape 874.8
    complicated 874.9
  specified part NEC 874.8
    complicated 874.9
nerve — *see* Injury, nerve, by site
non-healing surgical 998.83
nose 873.20
  complicated 873.30
  multiple sites 873.29
    complicated 873.39
  septum 873.21
    complicated 873.31
  sinuses 873.23
    complicated 873.33
occipital region — *see* Wound, open, scalp
ocular NEC 871.9
  adnexa 870.9
    specified region NEC 870.8
  laceration (*see also* Laceration, ocular) 871.4
  muscle (extraocular) 870.3
    with foreign body 870.4
    eyelid 870.1
    intraocular — *see* Wound, open, eyeball

Wound, open — *continued*
 ocular NEC — *continued*
  penetrating (*see also* Penetrating wound,
   ocular) 871.7
 orbit 870.8
  penetrating 870.3
   with foreign body 870.4
 orbital region 870.9
 ovary — *see* Injury, internal, pelvic organs
 palate 873.65
  complicated 873.75
 palm 882.0
  with tendon involvement 882.2
  complicated 882.1
 parathyroid (gland) 874.2
  complicated 874.3
 parietal region — *see* Wound, open, scalp
 pelvic floor or region 879.6
  complicated 879.7
 penis 878.0
  complicated 878.1
 perineum 879.6
  complicated 879.7
 periocular area 870.8
  laceration of skin 870.0
 pharynx 874.4
  complicated 874.5
 pinna 872.01
  complicated 872.11
 popliteal space 891.0
  with tendon involvement 891.2
  complicated 891.1
 prepuce 878.0
  complicated 878.1
 pubic region 879.2
  complicated 879.3
 pudenda 878.8
  complicated 878.9
 rectovaginal septum 878.8
  complicated 878.9
 sacral region 877.0
  complicated 877.1
 sacroiliac region 877.0
  complicated 877.1
 salivary (ducts) (glands) 873.69
  complicated 873.79
 scalp 873.0
  complicated 873.1
 scalpel, fetus or newborn 767.8
 scapular region 880.01
  with tendon involvement 880.21
  complicated 880.11
  involving other sites of upper arm 880.09
   with tendon involvement 880.29
   complicated 880.19
 sclera — (*see also* Wound, open, intraocular)
  871.9
 scrotum 878.2
  complicated 878.3
 seminal vesicle — *see* Injury, internal, pelvic
  organs
 shin 891.0
  with tendon involvement 891.2
  complicated 891.1
 shoulder 880.00
  with tendon involvement 880.20
  complicated 880.10
  involving other sites of upper arm 880.09
   with tendon involvement 880.29
   complicated 880.19
 skin NEC 879.8
  complicated 879.9
 skull — *see also* Injury, intracranial, with open
  intracranial wound
  with skull fracture — *see* Fracture, skull
 spermatic cord (scrotal) 878.2
  complicated 878.3
  pelvic region — *see* Injury, internal,
   spermatic cord
 spinal cord — *see* Injury, spinal
 sternal region 875.0
  complicated 875.1
 subconjunctival — *see* Wound, open,
  intraocular
 subcutaneous NEC 879.8
  complicated 879.9
 submaxillary region 873.44
  complicated 873.54

Wound, open — *continued*
 submental region 873.44
  complicated 873.54
 subungual
  finger(s) (thumb) — *see* Wound, open, finger
  toe(s) — *see* Wound, open, toe
 supraclavicular region 874.8
  complicated 874.9
 supraorbital 873.42
  complicated 873.52
 surgical, non-healing 998.83
 temple 873.49
  complicated 873.59
 temporal region 873.49
  complicated 873.59
 testis 878.2
  complicated 878.3
 thigh 890.0
  with tendon involvement 890.2
  complicated 890.1
 thorax, thoracic (external) 875.0
  complicated 875.1
 throat 874.8
  complicated 874.9
 thumb (nail) (subungual) 883.0
  with tendon involvement 883.2
  complicated 883.1
 thyroid (gland) 874.2
  complicated 874.3
 toe(s) (nail) (subungual) 893.0
  with tendon involvement 893.2
  complicated 893.1
 tongue 873.64
  complicated 873.74
 tonsil — *see* Wound, open, neck
 trachea (cervical region) 874.02
  with larynx 874.00
   complicated 874.10
  complicated 874.12
  intrathoracic — *see* Injury, internal, trachea
 trunk (multiple) NEC 879.6
  complicated 879.7
  specified site NEC 879.6
   complicated 879.7
 tunica vaginalis 878.2
  complicated 878.3
 tympanic membrane 872.61
  complicated 872.71
 tympanum 872.61
  complicated 872.71
 umbilical region 879.2
  complicated 879.3
 ureter — *see* Injury, internal, ureter
 urethra — *see* Injury, internal, urethra
 uterus — *see* Injury, internal, uterus
 uvula 873.69
  complicated 873.79
 vagina 878.6
  complicated 878.7
 vas deferens — *see* Injury, internal, vas
  deferens
 vitreous (humor) 871.2
 vulva 878.4
  complicated 878.5
 wrist 881.02
  with tendon involvement 881.22
  complicated 881.12

Wright's syndrome (hyperabduction) 447.8
 pneumonia 390 *[517.1]*

Wringer injury — *see* Crush injury, by site

Wrinkling of skin 701.8

Wrist — *see also* condition
 drop (acquired) 736.05

Wrong drug (given in error) NEC 977.9
 specified drug or substance — *see* Table of
  Drugs and Chemicals

Wry neck — *see also* Torticollis
 congenital 754.1

Wuchereria infestation 125.0
 bancrofti 125.0
 Brugia malayi 125.1
 malayi 125.1

Wuchereriasis 125.0

Wuchereriosis 125.0

Wuchernde struma langhans (M8332/3) 193

X

Xanthelasma 272.2
 eyelid 272.2 *[374.51]*
 palpebrarum 272.2 *[374.51]*

Xanthelasmatosis (essential) 272.2

Xanthelasmoidea 757.33

Xanthine stones 277.2

Xanthinuria 277.2

Xanthofibroma (M8831/0) — *see* Neoplasm,
 connective tissue, benign

Xanthoma(s), xanthomatosis 272.2
 with
  hyperlipoproteinemia
   type I 272.3
   type III 272.2
   type IV 272.1
   type V 272.3
 bone 272.7
 craniohypophyseal 277.8
 cutaneotendinous 272.7
 diabeticorum 250.8 ☑5ᵗʰ *[272.2]*
 disseminatum 272.7
 eruptive 272.2
 eyelid 272.2 *[374.51]*
 familial 272.7
 hereditary 272.7
 hypercholesterinemic 272.0
 hypercholesterolemic 272.0
 hyperlipemic 272.4
 hyperlipidemic 272.4
 infantile 272.7
 joint 272.7
 juvenile 272.7
 multiple 272.7
 multiplex 272.7
 primary familial 272.7
 tendon (sheath) 272.7
 tuberosum 272.2
 tuberous 272.2
 tubo-eruptive 272.2

Xanthosis 709.09
 surgical 998.81

Xenophobia 300.29

Xeroderma (congenital) 757.39
 acquired 701.1
 eyelid 373.33
 eyelid 373.33
 pigmentosum 757.33
 vitamin A deficiency 264.8

Xerophthalmia 372.53
 vitamin A deficiency 264.7

Xerosis
 conjunctiva 372.53
  with Bitôt's spot 372.53
   vitamin A deficiency 264.1
  vitamin A deficiency 264.0
 cornea 371.40
  with corneal ulceration 370.00
   vitamin A deficiency 264.3
  vitamin A deficiency 264.2
 cutis 706.8
 skin 706.8

Xerostomia 527.7

Xiphodynia 733.90

Xiphoidalgia 733.90

Xiphoiditis 733.99

Xiphopagus 759.4

XO syndrome 758.6

X-ray
 effects, adverse, NEC 990
 of chest
  for suspected tuberculosis V71.2
  routine V72.5

XXX syndrome 758.81

XXXXY syndrome 758.81

XXY syndrome 758.7

Xyloketosuria 271.8

Xylosuria 271.8

Xylulosuria 271.8

XYY syndrome 758.81

✔4ᵗʰ Fourth-digit Required   ✔5ᵗʰ Fifth-digit Required   ▶◀ Revised Text   ● New Line   ▲ Revised Code

Y

Yawning 786.09
  psychogenic 306.1
Yaws 102.9
  bone or joint lesions 102.6
  butter 102.1
  chancre 102.0
  cutaneous, less than five years after infection
      102.2
  early (cutaneous) (macular) (maculopapular)
      (micropapular) (papular) 102.2
    frambeside 102.2
    skin lesions NEC 102.2
  eyelid 102.9 [373.4]
  ganglion 102.6
  gangosis, gangosa 102.5
  gumma, gummata 102.4
    bone 102.6
  gummatous
    frambeside 102.4
    osteitis 102.6
    periostitis 102.6
  hydrarthrosis 102.6
  hyperkeratosis (early) (late) (palmar) (plantar)
      102.3
  initial lesions 102.0
  joint lesions 102.6
  juxta-articular nodules 102.7
  late nodular (ulcerated) 102.4
  latent (without clinical manifestations) (with
      positive serology) 102.8
  mother 102.0
  mucosal 102.7
  multiple papillomata 102.1
  nodular, late (ulcerated) 102.4
  osteitis 102.6
  papilloma, papillomata (palmar) (plantar) 102.1
  periostitis (hypertrophic) 102.6
  ulcers 102.4
  wet crab 102.1
Yeast infection (*see also* Candidiasis) 112.9
Yellow
  atrophy (liver) 570
    chronic 571.8
    resulting from administration of blood,
        plasma, serum, or other biological
        substance (within 8 months of
        administration) — *see* Hepatitis, viral
  fever — *see* Fever, yellow
  jack (*see also* Fever, yellow) 060.9
  jaundice (*see also* Jaundice) 782.4
Yersinia septica 027.8

Z

Zagari's disease (xerostomia) 527.7
Zahorsky's disease (exanthema subitum) 057.8
  syndrome (herpangina) 074.0
Zenker's diverticulum (esophagus) 530.6
Ziehen-Oppenheim disease 333.6
Zieve's syndrome (jaundice, hyperlipemia, and
      hemolytic anemia) 571.1
Zika fever 066.3
Zollinger-Ellison syndrome (gastric
      hypersecretion with pancreatic islet cell
      tumor) 251.5
Zona (*see also* Herpes, zoster) 053.9
Zoophilia (erotica) 302.1
Zoophobia 300.29
Zoster (herpes) (*see also* Herpes, zoster) 053.9
Zuelzer (-Ogden) anemia or syndrome
      (nutritional megaloblastic anemia) 281.2
Zygodactyly (*see also* Syndactylism) 755.10
Zygomycosis 117.7
Zymotic — *see* condition

SECTION 2

Alphabetic Index to Poisoning and External Causes of Adverse Effects of Drugs and Other Chemical Substances

TABLE OF DRUGS AND CHEMICALS

This table contains a classification of drugs and other chemical substances to identify poisoning states and external causes of adverse effects.

Each of the listed substances in the table is assigned a code according to the poisoning classification (960-989). These codes are used when there is a statement of poisoning, overdose, wrong substance given or taken, or intoxication.

The table also contains a listing of external causes of adverse effects. An adverse effect is a pathologic manifestation due to ingestion or exposure to drugs or other chemical substances (e.g., dermatitis, hypersensitivity reaction, aspirin gastritis). The adverse effect is to be identified by the appropriate code found in Section 1, Index to Diseases and Injuries. An external cause code can then be used to identify the circumstances involved. The table headings pertaining to external causes are defined below:

Accidental poisoning (E850-E869) — accidental overdose of drug, wrong substance given or taken, drug taken inadvertently, accidents in the usage of drugs and biologicals in medical and surgical procedures, and to show external causes of poisonings classifiable to 980-989.

Therapeutic use (E930-E949) — a correct substance properly administered in therapeutic or prophylactic dosage as the external cause of adverse effects.

Suicide attempt (E950-E952) — instances in which self-inflicted injuries or poisonings are involved.

Assault (E961-E962) — injury or poisoning inflicted by another person with the intent to injure or kill.

Undetermined (E980-E982) — to be used when the intent of the poisoning or injury cannot be determined whether it was intentional or accidental.

The American Hospital Formulary Service list numbers are included in the table to help classify new drugs not identified in the table by name. The AHFS list numbers are keyed to the continually revised American Hospital Formulary Service (AHFS).* These listings are found in the table under the main term **Drug.**

Excluded from the table are radium and other radioactive substances. The classification of adverse effects and complications pertaining to these substances will be found in Section 1, Index to Diseases and Injuries, and Section 3, Index to External Causes of Injuries.

Although certain substances are indexed with one or more subentries, the majority are listed according to one use or state. It is recognized that many substances may be used in various ways, in medicine and in industry, and may cause adverse effects whatever the state of the agent (solid, liquid, or fumes arising from a liquid). In cases in which the reported data indicates a use or state not in the table, or which is clearly different from the one listed, an attempt should be made to classify the substance in the form which most nearly expresses the reported facts.

*American Hospital Formulary Service, 2 vol. (Washington, D.C.: American Society of Hospital Pharmacists, 1959-)

		External Cause (E-Code)				
	Poisoning	Accident	Therapeutic Use	Suicide Attempt	Assault	Undetermined
1-propanol	980.3	E860.4	—	E950.9	E962.1	E980.9
2-propanol	980.2	E860.3	—	E950.9	E962.1	E980.9
2, 4-D (dichlorophenoxyacetic acid)	989.4	E863.5	—	E950.6	E962.1	E980.7
2, 4-toluene diisocyanate	983.0	E864.0	—	E950.7	E962.1	E980.6
2, 4, 5-T (trichlorophenoxyacetic acid)	989.2	E863.5	—	E950.6	E962.1	E980.7
14-hydroxydihydromorphinone	965.09	E850.2	E935.2	E950.0	E962.0	E980.0
ABOB	961.7	E857	E931.7	E950.4	E962.0	E980.4
Abrus (seed)	988.2	E865.3	—	E950.9	E962.1	E980.9
Absinthe	980.0	E860.1	—	E950.9	E962.1	E980.9
beverage	980.0	E860.0	—	E950.9	E962.1	E980.9
Acenocoumarin, acenocoumarol	964.2	E858.2	E934.2	E950.4	E962.0	E980.4
Acepromazine	969.1	E853.0	E939.1	E950.3	E962.0	E980.3
Acetal	982.8	E862.4	—	E950.9	E962.1	E980.9
Acetaldehyde (vapor)	987.8	E869.8	—	E952.8	E962.2	E982.8
liquid	989.89	E866.8	—	E950.9	E962.1	E980.9
Acetaminophen	965.4	E850.4	E935.4	E950.0	E962.0	E980.0
Acetaminosalol	965.1	E850.3	E935.3	E950.0	E962.0	E980.0
Acetanilid(e)	965.4	E850.4	E935.4	E950.0	E962.0	E980.0
Acetarsol, acetarsone	961.1	E857	E931.1	E950.4	E962.0	E980.4
Acetazolamide	974.2	E858.5	E944.2	E950.4	E962.0	E980.4
Acetic						
acid	983.1	E864.1	—	E950.7	E962.1	E980.6
with sodium acetate (ointment)	976.3	E858.7	E946.3	E950.4	E962.0	E980.4
irrigating solution	974.5	E858.5	E944.5	E950.4	E962.0	E980.4
lotion	976.2	E858.7	E946.2	E950.4	E962.0	E980.4
anhydride	983.1	E864.1	—	E950.7	E962.1	E980.6
ether (vapor)	982.8	E862.4	—	E950.9	E962.1	E980.9
Acetohexamide	962.3	E858.0	E932.3	E950.4	E962.0	E980.4
Acetomenaphthone	964.3	E858.2	E934.3	E950.4	E962.0	E980.4
Acetomorphine	965.01	E850.0	E935.0	E950.0	E962.0	E980.0
Acetone (oils) (vapor)	982.8	E862.4	—	E950.9	E962.1	E980.9
Acetophenazine (maleate)	969.1	E853.0	E939.1	E950.3	E962.0	E980.3
Acetophenetidin	965.4	E850.4	E935.4	E950.0	E962.0	E980.0
Acetophenone	982.0	E862.4	—	E950.9	E962.1	E980.9
Acetorphine	965.09	E850.2	E935.2	E950.0	E962.0	E980.0
Acetosulfone (sodium)	961.8	E857	E931.8	E950.4	E962.0	E980.4
Acetrizoate (sodium)	977.8	E858.8	E947.8	E950.4	E962.0	E980.4
Acetylcarbromal	967.3	E852.2	E937.3	E950.2	E962.0	E980.2
Acetylcholine (chloride)	971.0	E855.3	E941.0	E950.4	E962.0	E980.4
Acetylcysteine	975.5	E858.6	E945.5	E950.4	E962.0	E980.4
Acetyldigitoxin	972.1	E858.3	E942.1	E950.4	E962.0	E980.4
Acetyldihydrocodeine	965.09	E850.2	E935.2	E950.0	E962.0	E980.0
Acetyldihydrocodeinone	965.09	E850.2	E935.2	E950.0	E962.0	E980.0
Acetylene (gas) (industrial)	987.1	E868.1	—	E951.8	E962.2	E981.8
incomplete combustion of — *see* Carbon monoxide, fuel, utility						
tetrachloride (vapor)	982.3	E862.4	—	E950.9	E962.1	E980.9
Acetyliodosalicylic acid	965.1	E850.3	E935.3	E950.0	E962.0	E980.0
Acetylphenylhydrazine	965.8	E850.8	E935.8	E950.0	E962.0	E980.0
Acetylsalicylic acid	965.1	E850.3	E935.3	E950.0	E962.0	E980.0
Achromycin	960.4	E856	E930.4	E950.4	E962.0	E980.4
ophthalmic preparation	976.5	E858.7	E946.5	E950.4	E962.0	E980.4
topical NEC	976.0	E858.7	E946.0	E950.4	E962.0	E980.4
Acidifying agents	963.2	E858.1	E933.2	E950.4	E962.0	E980.4
Acids (corrosive) NEC	983.1	E864.1	—	E950.7	E962.1	E980.6
Aconite (wild)	988.2	E865.4	—	E950.9	E962.1	E980.9
Aconitine (liniment)	976.8	E858.7	E946.8	E950.4	E962.0	E980.4
Aconitum ferox	988.2	E865.4	—	E950.9	E962.1	E980.9
Acridine	983.0	E864.0	—	E950.7	E962.1	E980.6
vapor	987.8	E869.8	—	E952.8	E962.2	E982.8
Acriflavine	961.9	E857	E931.9	E950.4	E962.0	E980.4
Acrisorcin	976.0	E858.7	E946.0	E950.4	E962.0	E980.4
Acrolein (gas)	987.8	E869.8	—	E952.8	E962.2	E982.8
liquid	989.89	E866.8	—	E950.9	E962.1	E980.9
Actaea spicata	988.2	E865.4	—	E950.9	E962.1	E980.9
Acterol	961.5	E857	E931.5	E950.4	E962.0	E980.4
ACTH	962.4	E858.0	E932.4	E950.4	E962.0	E980.4
Acthar	962.4	E858.0	E932.4	E950.4	E962.0	E980.4
Actinomycin (C)(D)	960.7	E856	E930.7	E950.4	E962.0	E980.4
Adalin (acetyl)	967.3	E852.2	E937.3	E950.2	E962.0	E980.2
Adenosine (phosphate)	977.8	E858.8	E947.8	E950.4	E962.0	E980.4
Adhesives	989.89	E866.6	—	E950.9	E962.1	E980.9
ADH	962.5	E858.0	E932.5	E950.4	E962.0	E980.4
Adicillin	960.0	E856	E930.0	E950.4	E962.0	E980.4
Adiphenine	975.1	E855.6	E945.1	E950.4	E962.0	E980.4
Adjunct, pharmaceutical	977.4	E858.8	E947.4	E950.4	E962.0	E980.4
Adrenal (extract, cortex or medulla) (glucocorticoids) (hormones)						
(mineralocorticoids)	962.0	E858.0	E932.0	E950.4	E962.0	E980.4
ENT agent	976.6	E858.7	E946.6	E950.4	E962.0	E980.4
ophthalmic preparation	976.5	E858.7	E946.5	E950.4	E962.0	E980.4
topical NEC	976.0	E858.7	E946.0	E950.4	E962.0	E980.4
Adrenalin	971.2	E855.5	E941.2	E950.4	E962.0	E980.4

	Poisoning	External Cause (E-Code)				
		Accident	Therapeutic Use	Suicide Attempt	Assault	Undetermined
Adrenergic blocking agents	971.3	E855.6	E941.3	E950.4	E962.0	E980.4
Adrenergics	971.2	E855.5	E941.2	E950.4	E962.0	E980.4
Adrenochrome (derivatives)	972.8	E858.3	E942.8	E950.4	E962.0	E980.4
Adrenocorticotropic hormone	962.4	E858.0	E932.4	E950.4	E962.0	E980.4
Adrenocorticotropin	962.4	E858.0	E932.4	E950.4	E962.0	E980.4
Adriamycin	960.7	E856	E930.7	E950.4	E962.0	E980.4
Aerosol spray — *see* Sprays						
Aerosporin	960.8	E856	E930.8	E950.4	E962.0	E980.4
ENT agent	976.6	E858.7	E946.6	E950.4	E962.0	E980.4
ophthalmic preparation	976.5	E858.7	E946.5	E950.4	E962.0	E980.4
topical NEC	976.0	E858.7	E946.0	E950.4	E962.0	E980.4
Aethusa cynapium	988.2	E865.4	—	E950.9	E962.1	E980.9
Afghanistan black	969.6	E854.1	E939.6	E950.3	E962.0	E980.3
Aflatoxin	989.7	E865.9	—	E950.9	E962.1	E980.9
African boxwood	988.2	E865.4	—	E950.9	E962.1	E980.9
Agar (-agar)	973.3	E858.4	E943.3	E950.4	E962.0	E980.4
Agricultural agent NEC	989.89	E863.9	—	E950.6	E962.1	E980.7
Agrypnal	967.0	E851	E937.0	E950.1	E962.0	E980.1
Air contaminant(s), source or type not specified	987.9	E869.9	—	E952.9	E962.2	E982.9
specified type — *see* specific substance						
Akee	988.2	E865.4	—	E950.9	E962.1	E980.9
Akrinol	976.0	E858.7	E946.0	E950.4	E962.0	E980.4
Alantolactone	961.6	E857	E931.6	E950.4	E962.0	E980.4
Albamycin	960.8	E856	E930.8	E950.4	E962.0	E980.4
Albumin (normal human serum)	964.7	E858.2	E934.7	E950.4	E962.0	E980.4
Albuterol ●	975.7	E858.6	E945.7	E950.4	E962.0	E980.4
Alcohol	980.9	E860.9	—	E950.9	E962.1	E980.9
absolute	980.0	E860.1	—	E950.9	E962.1	E980.9
beverage	980.0	E860.0	E947.8	E950.9	E962.1	E980.9
amyl	980.3	E860.4	—	E950.9	E962.1	E980.9
antifreeze	980.1	E860.2	—	E950.9	E962.1	E980.9
butyl	980.3	E860.4	—	E950.9	E962.1	E980.9
dehydrated	980.0	E860.1	—	E950.9	E962.1	E980.9
beverage	980.0	E860.0	E947.8	E950.9	E862.1	E980.9
denatured	980.0	E860.1	—	E950.9	E962.1	E980.9
deterrents	977.3	E858.8	E947.3	E950.4	E962.0	E980.4
diagnostic (gastric function)	977.8	E858.8	E947.8	E950.4	E962.0	E980.4
ethyl	980.0	E860.1	—	E950.9	E962.1	E980.9
beverage	980.0	E860.0	E947.8	E950.9	E962.1	E980.9
grain	980.0	E860.1	—	E950.9	E962.1	E980.9
beverage	980.0	E860.0	E947.8	E950.9	E962.1	E980.9
industrial	980.9	E860.9	—	E950.9	E962.1	E980.9
isopropyl	980.2	E860.3	—	E950.9	E962.1	E980.9
methyl	980.1	E860.2	—	E950.9	E962.1	E980.9
preparation for consumption	980.0	E860.0	E947.8	E950.9	E962.1	E980.9
propyl	980.3	E860.4	—	E950.9	E962.1	E980.9
secondary	980.2	E860.3	—	E950.9	E962.1	E980.9
radiator	980.1	E860.2	—	E950.9	E962.1	E980.9
rubbing	980.2	E860.3	—	E950.9	E962.1	E980.9
specified type NEC	980.8	E860.8	—	E950.9	E962.1	E980.9
surgical	980.9	E860.9	—	E950.9	E962.1	E980.9
vapor (from any type of alcohol)	987.8	E869.8	—	E952.8	E962.2	E982.8
wood	980.1	E860.2	—	E950.9	E962.1	E980.9
Alcuronium chloride	975.2	E858.6	E945.2	E950.4	E962.0	E980.4
Aldactone	974.4	E858.5	E944.4	E950.4	E962.0	E980.4
Aldicarb	989.3	E863.2	—	E950.6	E962.1	E980.7
Aldomet	972.6	E858.3	E942.6	E950.4	E962.0	E980.4
Aldosterone	962.0	E858.0	E932.0	E950.4	E962.0	E980.4
Aldrin (dust)	989.2	E863.0	—	E950.6	E962.1	E980.7
Algeldrate	973.0	E858.4	E943.0	E950.4	E962.0	E980.4
Alidase	963.4	E858.1	E933.4	E950.4	E962.0	E980.4
Aliphatic thiocyanates	989.0	E866.8	—	E950.9	E962.1	E980.9
Alkaline antiseptic solution (aromatic)	976.6	E858.7	E946.6	E950.4	E962.0	E980.4
Alkalinizing agents (medicinal)	963.3	E858.1	E933.3	E950.4	E962.0	E980.4
Alkalis, caustic	983.2	E864.2	—	E950.7	E962.1	E980.6
Alkalizing agents (medicinal)	963.3	E858.1	E933.3	E950.4	E962.0	E980.4
Alka-seltzer	965.1	E850.3	E935.3	E950.0	E962.0	E980.0
Alkavervir	972.6	E858.3	E942.6	E950.4	E962.0	E980.4
Allegron	969.0	E854.0	E939.0	E950.3	E962.0	E980.3
Alleve — *see* Naproxen						
Allobarbital, allobarbitone	967.0	E851	E937.0	E950.1	E962.0	E980.1
Allopurinol	974.7	E858.5	E944.7	E950.4	E962.0	E980.4
Allylestrenol	962.2	E858.0	E932.2	E950.4	E962.0	E980.4
Allylisopropylacetylurea	967.8	E852.8	E937.8	E950.2	E962.0	E980.2
Allylisopropylmalonylurea	967.0	E851	E937.0	E950.1	E962.0	E980.1
Allyltribromide	967.3	E852.2	E937.3	E950.2	E962.0	E980.2
Aloe, aloes, aloin	973.1	E858.4	E943.1	E950.4	E962.0	E980.4
Alosetron	973.8	E858.4	E943.8	E950.4	E962.0	E980.4
Aloxidone	966.0	E855.0	E936.0	E950.4	E962.0	E980.4
Aloxiprin	965.1	E850.3	E935.3	E950.0	E962.0	E980.0
Alpha amylase	963.4	E858.1	E933.4	E950.4	E962.0	E980.4

		External Cause (E-Code)				
	Poisoning	Accident	Therapeutic Use	Suicide Attempt	Assault	Undetermined
Alphaprodine (hydrochloride)	965.09	E850.2	E935.2	E950.0	E962.0	E980.0
Alpha tocopherol	963.5	E858.1	E933.5	E950.4	E962.0	E980.4
Alseroxylon	972.6	E858.3	E942.6	E950.4	E962.0	E980.4
Alum (ammonium) (potassium)	983.2	E864.2	—	E950.7	E962.1	E980.6
medicinal (astringent) NEC	976.2	E858.7	E946.2	E950.4	E962.0	E980.4
Aluminium, aluminum (gel) (hydroxide)	973.0	E858.4	E943.0	E950.4	E962.0	E980.4
acetate solution	976.2	E858.7	E946.2	E950.4	E962.0	E980.4
aspirin	965.1	E850.3	E935.3	E950.0	E962.0	E980.0
carbonate	973.0	E858.4	E943.0	E950.4	E962.0	E980.4
glycinate	973.0	E858.4	E943.0	E950.4	E962.0	E980.4
nicotinate	972.2	E858.3	E942.2	E950.4	E962.0	E980.4
ointment (surgical) (topical)	976.3	E858.7	E946.3	E950.4	E962.0	E980.4
phosphate	973.0	E858.4	E943.0	E950.4	E962.0	E980.4
subacetate	976.2	E858.7	E946.2	E950.4	E962.0	E980.4
topical NEC	976.3	E858.7	E946.3	E950.4	E962.0	E980.4
Alurate	967.0	E851	E937.0	E950.1	E962.0	E980.1
Alverine (citrate)	975.1	E858.6	E945.1	E950.4	E962.0	E980.4
Alvodine	965.09	E850.2	E935.2	E950.0	E962.0	E980.0
Amanita phalloides	988.1	E865.5	—	E950.9	E962.1	E980.9
Amantadine (hydrochloride)	966.4	E855.0	E936.4	E950.4	E962.0	E980.4
Ambazone	961.9	E857	E931.9	E950.4	E962.0	E980.4
Ambenonium	971.0	E855.3	E941.0	E950.4	E962.0	E980.4
Ambutonium bromide	971.1	E855.4	E941.1	E950.4	E962.0	E980.4
Ametazole	977.8	E858.8	E947.8	E950.4	E962.0	E980.4
Amethocaine (infiltration) (topical)	968.5	E855.2	E938.5	E950.4	E962.0	E980.4
nerve block (peripheral) (plexus)	968.6	E855.2	E938.6	E950.4	E962.0	E980.4
spinal	968.7	E855.2	E938.7	E950.4	E962.0	E980.4
Amethopterin	963.1	E858.1	E933.1	E950.4	E962.0	E980.4
Amfepramone	977.0	E858.8	E947.0	E950.4	E962.0	E980.4
Amidon	965.02	E850.1	E935.1	E950.0	E962.0	E980.0
Amidopyrine	965.5	E850.5	E935.5	E950.0	E962.0	E980.0
Aminacrine	976.0	E858.7	E946.0	E950.4	E962.0	E980.4
Aminitrozole	961.5	E857	E931.5	E950.4	E962.0	E980.4
Aminoacetic acid	974.5	E858.5	E944.5	E950.4	E962.0	E980.4
Amino acids	974.5	E858.5	E944.5	E950.4	E962.0	E980.4
Aminocaproic acid	964.4	E858.2	E934.4	E950.4	E962.0	E980.4
Aminoethylisothiourium	963.8	E858.1	E933.8	E950.4	E962.0	E980.4
Aminoglutethimide	966.3	E855.0	E936.3	E950.4	E962.0	E980.4
Aminometradine	974.3	E858.5	E944.3	E950.4	E962.0	E980.4
Aminopentamide	971.1	E855.4	E941.1	E950.4	E962.0	E980.4
Aminophenazone	965.5	E850.5	E935.5	E950.0	E962.0	E980.0
Aminophenol	983.0	E864.0	—	E950.7	E962.1	E980.6
Aminophenylpyridone	969.5	E853.8	E939.5	E950.3	E962.0	E980.3
Aminophyllin	975.7	E858.6	E945.7	E950.4	E962.0	E980.4
Aminopterin	963.1	E858.1	E933.1	E950.4	E962.0	E980.4
Aminopyrine	965.5	E850.5	E935.5	E950.0	E962.0	E980.0
Aminosalicylic acid	961.8	E857	E931.8	E950.4	E962.0	E980.4
Amiphenazole	970.1	E854.3	E940.1	E950.4	E962.0	E980.4
Amiquinsin	972.6	E858.3	E942.6	E950.4	E962.0	E980.4
Amisometradine	974.3	E858.5	E944.3	E950.4	E962.0	E980.4
Amitriptyline	969.0	E854.0	E939.0	E950.3	E962.0	E980.3
Ammonia (fumes) (gas) (vapor)	987.8	E869.8	—	E952.8	E962.2	E982.8
liquid (household) NEC	983.2	E861.4	—	E950.7	E962.1	E980.6
spirit, aromatic	970.8	E854.3	E940.8	E950.4	E962.0	E980.4
Ammoniated mercury	976.0	E858.7	E946.0	E950.4	E962.0	E980.4
Ammonium						
carbonate	983.2	E864.2	—	E950.7	E962.1	E980.6
chloride (acidifying agent)	963.2	E858.1	E933.2	E950.4	E962.0	E980.4
expectorant	975.5	E858.6	E945.5	E950.4	E962.0	E980.4
compounds (household) NEC	983.2	E861.4	—	E950.7	E962.1	E980.6
fumes (any usage)	987.8	E869.8	—	E952.8	E962.2	E982.8
industrial	983.2	E864.2	—	E950.7	E962.1	E980.6
ichthyosulfonate	976.4	E858.7	E946.4	E950.4	E962.0	E980.4
mandelate	961.9	E857	E931.9	E950.4	E962.0	E980.4
Amobarbital	967.0	E851	E937.0	E950.1	E962.0	E980.1
Amodiaquin(e)	961.4	E857	E931.4	E950.4	E962.0	E980.4
Amopyroquin(e)	961.4	E857	E931.4	E950.4	E962.0	E980.4
Amphenidone	969.5	E853.8	E939.5	E950.3	E962.0	E980.3
Amphetamine	969.7	E854.2	E939.7	E950.3	E962.0	E980.3
Amphomycin	960.8	E856	E930.8	E950.4	E962.0	E980.4
Amphotericin B	960.1	E856	E930.1	E950.4	E962.0	E980.4
topical	976.0	E858.7	E946.0	E950.4	E962.0	E980.4
Ampicillin	960.0	E856	E930.0	E950.4	E962.0	E980.4
Amprotropine	971.1	E855.4	E941.1	E950.4	E962.0	E980.4
Amygdalin	977.8	E858.8	E947.8	E950.4	E962.0	E980.4
Amyl						
acetate (vapor)	982.8	E862.4	—	E950.9	E962.1	E980.9
alcohol	980.3	E860.4	—	E950.9	E962.1	E980.9
nitrite (medicinal)	972.4	E858.3	E942.4	E950.4	E962.0	E980.4
Amylase (alpha)	963.4	E858.1	E933.4	E950.4	E962.0	E980.4
Amylene hydrate	980.8	E860.8	—	E950.9	E962.1	E980.9

	Poisoning	External Cause (E-Code)				
		Accident	**Therapeutic Use**	**Suicide Attempt**	**Assault**	**Undetermined**
Amylobarbitone	967.0	E851	E937.0	E950.1	E962.0	E980.1
Amylocaine	968.9	E855.2	E938.9	E950.4	E962.0	E980.4
infiltration (subcutaneous)	968.5	E855.2	E938.5	E950.4	E962.0	E980.4
nerve block (peripheral) (plexus)	968.6	E855.2	E938.6	E950.4	E962.0	E980.4
spinal	968.7	E855.2	E938.7	E950.4	E962.0	E980.4
topical (surface)	968.5	E855.2	E938.5	E950.4	E962.0	E980.4
Amytal (sodium)	967.0	E851	E937.0	E950.1	E962.0	E980.1
Analeptics	970.0	E854.3	E940.0	E950.4	E962.0	E980.4
Analgesics	965.9	E850.9	E935.9	E950.0	E962.0	E980.0
aromatic NEC	965.4	E850.4	E935.4	E950.0	E962.0	E980.0
non-narcotic NEC	965.7	E850.7	E935.7	E950.0	E962.0	E980.0
specified NEC	965.8	E850.8	E935.8	E950.0	E962.0	E980.0
Anamirta cocculus	988.2	E865.3	—	E950.9	E962.1	E980.9
Ancillin	960.0	E856	E930.0	E950.4	E962.0	E980.4
Androgens (anabolic congeners)	962.1	E858.0	E932.1	E950.4	E962.0	E980.4
Androstalone	962.1	E858.0	E932.1	E950.4	E962.0	E980.4
Androsterone	962.1	E858.0	E932.1	E950.4	E962.0	E980.4
Anemone pulsatilla	988.2	E865.4	—	E950.9	E962.1	E980.9
Anesthesia, anesthetic (general) NEC	968.4	E855.1	E938.4	E950.4	E962.0	E980.4
block (nerve) (plexus)	968.6	E855.2	E938.6	E950.4	E962.0	E980.4
gaseous NEC	968.2	E855.1	E938.2	E950.4	E962.0	E980.4
halogenated hydrocarbon derivatives NEC	968.2	E855.1	E938.2	E950.4	E962.0	E980.4
infiltration (intradermal) (subcutaneous) (submucosal)	968.5	E855.2	E938.5	E950.4	E962.0	E980.4
intravenous	968.3	E855.1	E938.3	E950.4	E962.0	E980.4
local NEC	968.9	E855.2	E938.9	E950.4	E962.0	E980.4
nerve blocking (peripheral) (plexus)	968.6	E855.2	E938.6	E950.4	E962.0	E980.4
rectal NEC	968.3	E855.1	E938.3	E950.4	E962.0	E980.4
spinal	968.7	E855.2	E938.7	E950.4	E962.0	E980.4
surface	968.5	E855.2	E938.5	E950.4	E962.0	E980.4
topical	968.5	E855.2	E938.5	E950.4	E962.0	E980.4
Aneurine	963.5	E858.1	E933.5	E950.4	E962.0	E980.4
Angio-Conray	977.8	E858.8	E947.8	E950.4	E962.0	E980.4
Angiotensin	971.2	E855.5	E941.2	E950.4	E962.0	E980.4
Anhydrohydroxyprogesterone	962.2	E858.0	E932.2	E950.4	E962.0	E980.4
Anhydron	974.3	E858.5	E944.3	E950.4	E962.0	E980.4
Anileridine	965.09	E850.2	E935.2	E950.0	E962.0	E980.0
Aniline (dye) (liquid)	983.0	E864.0	—	E950.7	E962.1	E980.6
analgesic	965.4	E850.4	E935.4	E950.0	E962.0	E980.0
derivatives, therapeutic NEC	965.4	E850.4	E935.4	E950.0	E962.0	E980.0
vapor	987.8	E869.8	—	E952.8	E962.2	E982.8
Anisindione	964.2	E858.2	E934.2	E950.4	E962.0	E980.4
Aniscoropine	971.1	E855.4	E941.1	E950.4	E962.0	E980.4
Anorexic agents	977.0	E858.8	E947.0	E950.4	E962.0	E980.4
Ant (bite) (sting)	989.5	E905.5	—	E950.9	E962.1	E980.9
Antabuse	977.3	E858.8	E947.3	E950.4	E962.0	E980.4
Antacids	973.0	E858.4	E943.0	E950.4	E962.0	E980.4
Antazoline	963.0	E858.1	E933.0	E950.4	E962.0	E980.4
Anthelmintics	961.6	E857	E931.6	E950.4	E962.0	E980.4
Anthralin	976.4	E858.7	E946.4	E950.4	E962.0	E980.4
Anthramycin	960.7	E856	E930.7	E950.4	E962.0	E980.4
Antiadrenergics	971.3	E855.6	E941.3	E950.4	E962.0	E980.4
Antiallergic agents	963.0	E858.1	E933.0	E950.4	E962.0	E980.4
Antianemic agents NEC	964.1	E858.2	E934.1	E950.4	E962.0	E980.4
Antiaris toxicaria	988.2	E865.4	—	E950.9	E962.1	E980.9
Antiarteriosclerotic agents	972.2	E858.3	E942.2	E950.4	E962.0	E980.4
Antiasthmatics	975.7	E858.6	E945.7	E950.4	E962.0	E980.4
Antibiotics	960.9	E856	E930.9	E950.4	E962.0	E980.4
antifungal	960.1	E856	E930.1	E950.4	E962.0	E980.4
antimycobacterial	960.6	E856	E930.6	E950.4	E962.0	E980.4
antineoplastic	960.7	E856	E930.7	E950.4	E962.0	E980.4
cephalosporin (group)	960.5	E856	E930.5	E950.4	E962.0	E980.4
chloramphenicol (group)	960.2	E856	E930.2	E950.4	E962.0	E980.4
macrolides	960.3	E856	E930.3	E950.4	E962.0	E980.4
specified NEC	960.8	E856	E930.8	E950.4	E962.0	E980.4
tetracycline (group)	960.4	E856	E930.4	E950.4	E962.0	E980.4
Anticancer agents NEC	963.1	E858.1	E933.1	E950.4	E962.0	E980.4
antibiotics	960.7	E856	E930.7	E950.4	E962.0	E980.4
Anticholinergics	971.1	E855.4	E941.1	E950.4	E962.0	E980.4
Anticholinesterase (organophosphorus) (reversible)	971.0	E855.3	E941.0	E950.4	E962.0	E980.4
Anticoagulants	964.2	E858.2	E934.2	E950.4	E962.0	E980.4
antagonists	964.5	E858.2	E934.5	E950.4	E962.0	E980.4
Anti-common cold agents NEC	975.6	E858.6	E945.6	E950.4	E962.0	E980.4
Anticonvulsants NEC	966.3	E855.0	E936.3	E950.4	E962.0	E980.4
Antidepressants	969.0	E854.0	E939.0	E950.3	E962.0	E980.3
Antidiabetic agents	962.3	E858.0	E932.3	E950.4	E962.0	E980.4
Antidiarrheal agents	973.5	E858.4	E943.5	E950.4	E962.0	E980.4
Antidiuretic hormone	962.5	E858.0	E932.5	E950.4	E962.0	E980.4
Antidotes NEC	977.2	E858.8	E947.2	E950.4	E962.0	E980.4
Antiemetic agents	963.0	E858.1	E933.0	E950.4	E962.0	E980.4
Antiepilepsy agent NEC	966.3	E855.0	E936.3	E950.4	E962.0	E980.4
Antifertility pills	962.2	E858.0	E932.2	E950.4	E962.0	E980.4

✓4ᵗʰ Fourth-digit Required   ✓5ᵗʰ Fifth-digit Required   ►◄ Revised Text   ● New Line   ▲ Revised Code

	Poisoning	External Cause (E-Code)				
		Accident	**Therapeutic Use**	**Suicide Attempt**	**Assault**	**Undetermined**
Antiflatulents	973.8	E858.4	E943.8	E950.4	E962.0	E980.4
Antifreeze	989.89	E866.8	—	E950.9	E962.1	E980.9
alcohol	980.1	E860.2	—	E950.9	E962.1	E980.9
ethylene glycol	982.8	E862.4	—	E950.9	E962.1	E980.9
Antifungals (nonmedicinal) (sprays)	989.4	E863.6	—	E950.6	E962.1	E980.7
medicinal NEC	961.9	E857	E931.9	E950.4	E962.0	E980.4
antibiotic	960.1	E856	E930.1	E950.4	E962.0	E980.4
topical	976.0	E858.7	E946.0	E950.4	E962.0	E980.4
Antigastric secretion agents	973.0	E858.4	E943.0	E950.4	E962.0	E980.4
Anthelmintics	961.6	E857	E931.6	E950.4	E962.0	E980.4
Antihemophilic factor (human)	964.7	E858.2	E934.7	E950.4	E962.0	E980.4
Antihistamine	963.0	E858.1	E933.0	E950.4	E962.0	E980.4
Antihypertensive agents NEC	972.6	E858.3	E942.6	E950.4	E962.0	E980.4
Anti-infectives NEC	961.9	E857	E931.9	E950.4	E962.0	E980.4
antibiotics	960.9	E856	E930.9	E950.4	E962.0	E980.4
specified NEC	960.8	E856	E930.8	E950.4	E962.0	E980.4
anthelmintic	961.6	E857	E931.6	E950.4	E962.0	E980.4
antimalarial	961.4	E857	E931.4	E950.4	E962.0	E980.4
antimycobacterial NEC	961.8	E857	E931.8	E950.4	E962.0	E980.4
antibiotics	960.6	E856	E930.6	E950.4	E962.0	E980.4
antiprotozoal NEC	961.5	E857	E931.5	E950.4	E962.0	E980.4
blood	961.4	E857	E931.4	E950.4	E962.0	E980.4
antiviral	961.7	E857	E931.7	E950.4	E962.0	E980.4
arsenical	961.1	E857	E931.1	E950.4	E962.0	E980.4
ENT agents	976.6	E858.7	E946.6	E950.4	E962.0	E980.4
heavy metals NEC	961.2	E857	E931.2	E950.4	E962.0	E980.4
local	976.0	E858.7	E946.0	E950.4	E962.0	E980.4
ophthalmic preparation	976.5	E858.7	E946.5	E950.4	E962.0	E980.4
topical NEC	976.0	E858.7	E946.0	E950.4	E962.0	E980.4
Anti-inflammatory agents (topical)	976.0	E858.7	E946.0	E950.4	E962.0	E980.4
Antiknock (tetraethyl lead)	984.1	E862.1	—	E950.9	E962.1	E980.9
Antilipemics	972.2	E858.3	E942.2	E950.4	E962.0	E980.4
Antimalarials	961.4	E857	E931.4	E950.4	E962.0	E980.4
Antimony (compounds) (vapor) NEC	985.4	E866.2	—	E950.9	E962.1	E980.9
anti-infectives	961.2	E857	E931.2	E950.4	E962.0	E980.4
pesticides (vapor)	985.4	E863.4	—	E950.6	E962.2	E980.7
potassium tartrate	961.2	E857	E931.2	E950.4	E962.0	E980.4
tartrated	961.2	E857	E931.2	E950.4	E962.0	E980.4
Antimuscarinic agents	971.1	E855.4	E941.1	E950.4	E962.0	E980.4
Antimycobacterials NEC	961.8	E857	E931.8	E950.4	E962.0	E980.4
antibiotics	960.6	E856	E930.6	E950.4	E962.0	E980.4
Antineoplastic agents	963.1	E858.1	E933.1	E950.4	E962.0	E980.4
antibiotics	960.7	E856	E930.7	E950.4	E962.0	E980.4
Anti-Parkinsonism agents	966.4	E855.0	E936.4	E950.4	E962.0	E980.4
Antiphlogistics	965.69	E850.6	E935.6	E950.0	E962.0	E980.0
Antiprotozoals NEC	961.5	E857	E931.5	E950.4	E962.0	E980.4
blood	961.4	E857	E931.4	E950.4	E962.0	E980.4
Antipruritics (local)	976.1	E858.7	E946.1	E950.4	E962.0	E980.4
Antipsychotic agents NEC	969.3	E853.8	E939.3	E950.3	E962.0	E980.3
Antipyretics	965.9	E850.9	E935.9	E950.0	E962.0	E980.0
specified NEC	965.8	E850.8	E935.8	E950.0	E962.0	E980.0
Antipyrine	965.5	E850.5	E935.5	E950.0	E962.0	E980.0
Antirabies serum (equine)	979.9	E858.8	E949.9	E950.4	E962.0	E980.4
Antirheumatics	965.69	E850.6	E935.6	E950.0	E962.0	E980.0
Antiseborrheics	976.4	E858.7	E946.4	E950.4	E962.0	E980.4
Antiseptics (external) (medicinal)	976.0	E858.7	E946.0	E950.4	E962.0	E980.4
Antistine	963.0	E858.1	E933.0	E950.4	E962.0	E980.4
Antithyroid agents	962.8	E858.0	E932.8	E950.4	E962.0	E980.4
Antitoxin, any	979.9	E858.8	E949.9	E950.4	E962.0	E980.4
Antituberculars	961.8	E857	E931.8	E950.4	E962.0	E980.4
antibiotics	960.6	E856	E930.6	E950.4	E962.0	E980.4
Antitussives	975.4	E858.6	E945.4	E950.4	E962.0	E980.4
Antivaricose agents (sclerosing)	972.7	E858.3	E942.7	E950.4	E962.0	E980.4
Antivenin (crotaline) (spider-bite)	979.9	E858.8	E949.9	E950.4	E962.0	E980.4
Antivert	963.0	E858.1	E933.0	E950.4	E962.0	E980.4
Antivirals NEC	961.7	E857	E931.7	E950.4	E962.0	E980.4
Ant poisons — *see* Pesticides						
Antrol	989.4	E863.4	—	E950.6	E962.1	E980.7
fungicide	989.4	E863.6	—	E950.6	E962.1	E980.7
Apomorphine hydrochloride (emetic)	973.6	E858.4	E943.6	E950.4	E962.0	E980.4
Appetite depressants, central	977.0	E858.8	E947.0	E950.4	E962.0	E980.4
Apresoline	972.6	E858.3	E942.6	E950.4	E962.0	E980.4
Aprobarbital, aprobarbitone	967.0	E851	E937.0	E950.1	E962.0	E980.1
Apronalide	967.8	E852.8	E937.8	E950.2	E962.0	E980.2
Aqua fortis	983.1	E864.1	—	E950.7	E962.1	E980.6
Arachis oil (topical)	976.3	E858.7	E946.3	E950.4	E962.0	E980.4
cathartic	973.2	E858.4	E943.2	E950.4	E962.0	E980.4
Aralen	961.4	E857	E931.4	E950.4	E962.0	E980.4
Arginine salts	974.5	E858.5	E944.5	E950.4	E962.0	E980.4
Argyrol	976.0	E858.7	E946.0	E950.4	E962.0	E980.4
ENT agent	976.6	E858.7	E946.6	E950.4	E962.0	E980.4

	Poisoning	External Cause (E-Code)				
		Accident	Therapeutic Use	Suicide Attempt	Assault	Undetermined
Argyrol — *continued*						
ophthalmic preparation	976.5	E858.7	E946.5	E950.4	E962.0	E980.4
Aristocort	962.0	E858.0	E932.0	E950.4	E962.0	E980.4
ENT agent	976.6	E858.7	E946.6	E950.4	E962.0	E980.4
ophthalmic preparation	976.5	E858.7	E946.5	E950.4	E962.0	E980.4
topical NEC	976.0	E858.7	E946.0	E950.4	E962.0	E980.4
Aromatics, corrosive	983.0	E864.0	—	E950.7	E962.1	E980.6
disinfectants	983.0	E861.4	—	E950.7	E962.1	E980.6
Arsenate of lead (insecticide)	985.1	E863.4	—	E950.8	E962.1	E980.8
herbicide	985.1	E863.5	—	E950.8	E962.1	E980.8
Arsenic, arsenicals (compounds) (dust) (fumes) (vapor) NEC	985.1	E866.3	—	E950.8	E962.1	E980.8
anti-infectives	961.1	E857	E931.1	E950.4	E962.0	E980.4
pesticide (dust) (fumes)	985.1	E863.4	—	E950.8	E962.1	E980.8
Arsine (gas)	985.1	E866.3	—	E950.8	E962.1	E980.8
Arsphenamine (silver)	961.1	E857	E931.1	E950.4	E962.0	E980.4
Arsthinol	961.1	E857	E931.1	E950.4	E962.0	E980.4
Artane	971.1	E855.4	E941.1	E950.4	E962.0	E980.4
Arthropod (venomous) NEC	989.5	E905.5	—	E950.9	E962.1	E980.9
Asbestos	989.81	E866.8	—	E950.9	E962.1	E980.9
Ascaridole	961.6	E857	E931.6	E950.4	E962.0	E980.4
Ascorbic acid	963.5	E858.1	E933.5	E950.4	E962.0	E980.4
Asiaticoside	976.0	E858.7	E946.0	E950.4	E962.0	E980.4
Aspidium (oleoresin)	961.6	E857	E931.6	E950.4	E962.0	E980.4
Aspirin	965.1	E850.3	E935.3	E950.0	E962.0	E980.0
Astringents (local)	976.2	E858.7	E946.2	E950.4	E962.0	E980.4
Atabrine	961.3	E857	E931.3	E950.4	E962.0	E980.4
Ataractics	969.5	E853.8	E939.5	E950.3	E962.0	E980.3
Atonia drug, intestinal	973.3	E858.4	E943.3	E950.4	E962.0	E980.4
Atophan	974.7	E858.5	E944.7	E950.4	E962.0	E980.4
Atropine	971.1	E855.4	E941.1	E950.4	E962.0	E980.4
Attapulgite	973.5	E858.4	E943.5	E950.4	E962.0	E980.4
Attenuvax	979.4	E858.8	E949.4	E950.4	E962.0	E980.4
Aureomycin	960.4	E856	E930.4	E950.4	E962.0	E980.4
ophthalmic preparation	976.5	E858.7	E946.5	E950.4	E962.0	E980.4
topical NEC	976.0	E858.7	E946.0	E950.4	E962.0	E980.4
Aurothioglucose	965.69	E850.6	E935.6	E950.0	E962.0	E980.0
Aurothioglycanide	965.69	E850.6	E935.6	E950.0	E962.0	E980.0
Aurothiomalate	965.69	E850.6	E935.6	E950.0	E962.0	E980.0
Automobile fuel	981	E862.1	—	E950.9	E962.1	E980.9
Autonomic nervous system agents NEC	971.9	E855.9	E941.9	E950.4	E962.0	E980.4
Avlosulfon	961.8	E857	E931.8	E950.4	E962.0	E980.4
Avomine	967.8	E852.8	E937.8	E950.2	E962.0	E980.2
Azacyclonol	969.5	E853.8	E939.5	E950.3	E962.0	E980.3
Azapetine	971.3	E855.6	E941.3	E950.4	E962.0	E980.4
Azaribine	963.1	E858.1	E933.1	E950.4	E962.0	E980.4
Azaserine	960.7	E856	E930.7	E950.4	E962.0	E980.4
Azathioprine	963.1	E858.1	E933.1	E950.4	E962.0	E980.4
Azosulfamide	961.0	E857	E931.0	E950.4	E962.0	E980.4
Azulfidine	961.0	E857	E931.0	E950.4	E962.0	E980.4
Azuresin	977.8	E858.8	E947.8	E950.4	E962.0	E980.4
Bacimycin	976.0	E858.7	E946.0	E950.4	E962.0	E980.4
ophthalmic preparation	976.5	E858.7	E946.5	E950.4	E962.0	E980.4
Bacitracin	960.8	E856	E930.8	E950.4	E962.0	E980.4
ENT agent	976.6	E858.7	E946.6	E950.4	E962.0	E980.4
ophthalmic preparation	976.5	E858.7	E946.5	E950.4	E962.0	E980.4
topical NEC	976.0	E858.7	E946.0	E950.4	E962.0	E980.4
Baking soda	963.3	E858.1	E933.3	E950.4	E962.0	E980.4
BAL	963.8	E858.1	E933.8	E950.4	E962.0	E980.4
Bamethan (sulfate)	972.5	E858.3	E942.5	E950.4	E962.0	E980.4
Bamipine	963.0	E858.1	E933.0	E950.4	E962.0	E980.4
Baneberry	988.2	E865.4	—	E950.9	E962.1	E980.9
Banewort	988.2	E865.4	—	E950.9	E962.1	E980.9
Barbenyl	967.0	E851	E937.0	E950.1	E962.0	E980.1
Barbital, barbitone	967.0	E851	E937.0	E950.1	E962.0	E980.1
Barbiturates, barbituric acid	967.0	E851	E937.0	E950.1	E962.0	E980.1
anesthetic (intravenous)	968.3	E855.1	E938.3	E950.4	E962.0	E980.4
Barium (carbonate) (chloride) (sulfate)	985.8	E866.4	—	E950.9	E962.1	E980.9
diagnostic agent	977.8	E858.8	E947.8	E950.4	E962.0	E980.4
pesticide	985.8	E863.4	—	E950.6	E962.1	E980.7
rodenticide	985.8	E863.7	—	E950.6	E962.1	E980.7
Barrier cream	976.3	E858.7	E946.3	E950.4	E962.0	E980.4
Battery acid or fluid	983.1	E864.1	—	E950.7	E962.1	E980.6
Bay rum	980.8	E860.8	—	E950.9	E962.1	E980.9
BCG vaccine	978.0	E858.8	E948.0	E950.4	E962.0	E980.4
Bearsfoot	988.2	E865.4	—	E950.9	E962.1	E980.9
Beclamide	966.3	E855.0	E936.3	E950.4	E962.0	E980.4
Bee (sting) (venom)	989.5	E905.3	—	E950.9	E962.1	E980.9
Belladonna (alkaloids)	971.1	E855.4	E941.1	E950.4	E962.0	E980.4
Bemegride	970.0	E854.3	E940.0	E950.4	E962.0	E980.4
Benactyzine	969.8	E855.8	E939.8	E950.3	E962.0	E980.3
Benadryl	963.0	E858.1	E933.0	E950.4	E962.0	E980.4

✔4ᵗʰ Fourth-digit Required   ✔5ᵗʰ Fifth-digit Required   ▶◀ Revised Text   ● New Line   ▲ Revised Code

		External Cause (E-Code)				
	Poisoning	Accident	Therapeutic Use	Suicide Attempt	Assault	Undetermined
Bendrofluazide	974.3	E858.5	E944.3	E950.4	E962.0	E980.4
Bendroflumethiazide	974.3	E858.5	E944.3	E950.4	E962.0	E980.4
Benemid	974.7	E858.5	E944.7	E950.4	E962.0	E980.4
Benethamine penicillin G	960.0	E856	E930.0	E950.4	E962.0	E980.4
Benisone	976.0	E858.7	E946.0	E950.4	E962.0	E980.4
Benoquin	976.8	E858.7	E946.8	E950.4	E962.0	E980.4
Benoxinate	968.5	E855.2	E938.5	E950.4	E962.0	E980.4
Bentonite	976.3	E858.7	E946.3	E950.4	E962.0	E980.4
Benzalkonium (chloride)	976.0	E858.7	E946.0	E950.4	E962.0	E980.4
ophthalmic preparation	976.5	E858.7	E946.5	E950.4	E962.0	E980.4
Benzamidosalicylate (calcium)	961.8	E857	E931.8	E950.4	E962.0	E980.4
Benzathine penicillin	960.0	E856	E930.0	E950.4	E962.0	E980.4
Benzcarbimine	963.1	E858.1	E933.1	E950.4	E962.0	E980.4
Benzedrex	971.2	E855.5	E941.2	E950.4	E962.0	E980.4
Benzedrine (amphetamine)	969.7	E854.2	E939.7	E950.3	E962.0	E980.3
Benzene (acetyl) (dimethyl) (methyl) (solvent) (vapor)	982.0	E862.4	—	E950.9	E962.1	E980.9
hexachloride (gamma) (insecticide) (vapor)	989.2	E863.0	—	E950.6	E962.1	E980.7
Benzethonium	976.0	E858.7	E946.0	E950.4	E962.0	E980.4
Benzhexol (chloride)	966.4	E855.0	E936.4	E950.4	E962.0	E980.4
Benzilonium	971.1	E855.4	E941.1	E950.4	E962.0	E980.4
Benzin(e) — see Ligroin						
Benziodarone	972.4	E858.3	E942.4	E950.4	E962.0	E980.4
Benzocaine	968.5	E855.2	E938.5	E950.4	E962.0	E980.4
Benzodiapin	969.4	E853.2	E939.4	E950.3	E962.0	E980.3
Benzodiazepines (tranquilizers) NEC	969.4	E853.2	E939.4	E950.3	E962.0	E980.3
Benzoic acid (with salicylic acid) (anti-infective)	976.0	E858.7	E946.0	E950.4	E962.0	E980.4
Benzoin	976.3	E858.7	E946.3	E950.4	E962.0	E980.4
Benzol (vapor)	982.0	E862.4	—	E950.9	E962.1	E980.9
Benzomorphan	965.09	E850.2	E935.2	E950.0	E962.0	E980.0
Benzonatate	975.4	E858.6	E945.4	E950.4	E962.0	E980.4
Benzothiadiazides	974.3	E858.5	E944.3	E950.4	E962.0	E980.4
Benzoylpas	961.8	E857	E931.8	E950.4	E962.0	E980.4
Benzperidol	969.5	E853.8	E939.5	E950.3	E962.0	E980.3
Benzphetamine	977.0	E858.8	E947.0	E950.4	E962.0	E980.4
Benzpyrinium	971.1	E855.3	E941.0	E950.4	E962.0	E980.4
Benzquinamide	963.0	E858.1	E933.0	E950.4	E962.0	E980.4
Benzthiazide	974.3	E858.5	E944.3	E950.4	E962.0	E980.4
Benztropine	971.1	E855.4	E941.1	E950.4	E962.0	E980.4
Benzyl						
acetate	982.8	E862.4	—	E950.9	E962.1	E980.9
benzoate (anti-infective)	976.0	E858.7	E946.0	E950.4	E962.0	E980.4
morphine	965.09	E850.2	E935.2	E950.0	E962.0	E980.0
penicillin	960.0	E856	E930.0	E950.4	E962.0	E980.4
Bephenium hydroxynapthoate	961.6	E857	E931.6	E950.4	E962.0	E980.4
Bergamot oil	989.89	E866.8	—	E950.9	E962.1	E980.9
Berries, poisonous	988.2	E865.3	—	E950.9	E962.1	E980.9
Beryllium (compounds) (fumes)	985.3	E866.4	—	E950.9	E962.1	E980.9
Beta-carotene	976.3	E858.7	E946.3	E950.4	E962.0	E980.4
Beta-Chlor	967.1	E852.0	E937.1	E950.2	E962.0	E980.2
Betamethasone	962.0	E858.0	E932.0	E950.4	E962.0	E980.4
topical	976.0	E858.7	E946.0	E950.4	E962.0	E980.4
Betazole	977.8	E858.8	E947.8	E950.4	E962.0	E980.4
Bethanechol	971.0	E855.3	E941.0	E950.4	E962.0	E980.4
Bethanidine	972.6	E858.3	E942.6	E950.4	E962.0	E980.4
Betula oil	976.3	E858.7	E946.3	E950.4	E962.0	E980.4
Bhang	969.6	E854.1	E939.6	E950.3	E962.0	E980.3
Bialamicol	961.5	E857	E931.5	E950.4	E962.0	E980.4
Bichloride of mercury — see Mercury, chloride						
Bichromates (calcium) (crystals) (potassium) (sodium)	983.9	E864.3	—	E950.7	E962.1	E980.6
fumes	987.8	E869.8	—	E952.8	E962.2	E982.8
Biguanide derivatives, oral	962.3	E858.0	E932.3	E950.4	E962.0	E980.4
Biligrafin	977.8	E858.8	E947.8	E950.4	E962.0	E980.4
Bilopaque	977.8	E858.8	E947.8	E950.4	E962.0	E980.4
Bioflavonoids	972.8	E858.3	E942.8	E950.4	E962.0	E980.4
Biological substance NEC	979.9	E858.8	E949.9	E950.4	E962.0	E980.4
Biperiden	966.4	E855.0	E936.4	E950.4	E962.0	E980.4
Bisacodyl	973.1	E858.4	E943.1	E950.4	E962.0	E980.4
Bishydroxycoumarin	964.2	E858.2	E934.2	E950.4	E962.0	E980.4
Bismarsen	961.1	E857	E931.1	E950.4	E962.0	E980.4
Bismuth (compounds) NEC	985.8	E866.4	—	E950.9	E962.1	E980.9
anti-infectives	961.2	E857	E931.2	E950.4	E962.0	E980.4
subcarbonate	973.5	E858.4	E943.5	E950.4	E962.0	E980.4
sulfarsphenamine	961.1	E857	E931.1	E950.4	E962.0	E980.4
Bithionol	961.6	E857	E931.6	E950.4	E962.0	E980.4
Bitter almond oil	989.0	E866.8	—	E950.9	E962.1	E980.9
Bittersweet	988.2	E865.4	—	E950.9	E962.1	E930.9
Black						
flag	989.4	E863.4	—	E950.6	E962.1	E980.7
henbane	988.2	E865.4	—	E950.9	E962.1	E980.9
leaf (40)	989.4	E863.4	—	E950.6	E962.1	E980.7
widow spider (bite)	989.5	E905.1	—	E950.9	E962.1	E980.9

Fourth-digit Required   Fifth-digit Required   ►◄ Revised Text   ● New Line   ▲ Revised Code

	Poisoning	External Cause (E-Code)				
		Accident	Therapeutic Use	Suicide Attempt	Assault	Undetermined
Black — *continued*						
widow spider — *continued*						
antivenin	979.9	E858.8	E949.9	E950.4	E962.0	E980.4
Blast furnace gas (carbon monoxide from)	986	E868.8	—	E952.1	E962.2	E982.1
Bleach NEC	983.9	E864.3	—	E950.7	E962.1	E980.6
Bleaching solutions	983.9	E864.3	—	E950.7	E962.1	E980.6
Bleomycin (sulfate)	960.7	E856	E930.7	E950.4	E962.0	E980.4
Blockain	968.9	E855.2	E938.9	E950.4	E962.0	E980.4
infiltration (subcutaneous)	968.5	E855.2	E938.5	E950.4	E962.0	E980.4
nerve block (peripheral) (plexus)	968.6	E855.2	E938.6	E950.4	E962.0	E980.4
topical (surface)	968.5	E855.2	E938.5	E950.4	E962.0	E980.4
Blood (derivatives) (natural) (plasma) (whole)	964.7	E858.2	E934.7	E950.4	E962.0	E980.4
affecting agent	964.9	E858.2	E934.9	E950.4	E962.0	E980.4
specified NEC	964.8	E858.2	E934.8	E950.4	E962.0	E980.4
substitute (macromolecular)	964.8	E858.2	E934.8	E950.4	E962.0	E980.4
Blue velvet	965.09	E850.2	E935.2	E950.0	E962.0	E980.0
Bone meal	989.89	E866.5	—	E950.9	E962.1	E980.9
Bonine	963.0	E858.1	E933.0	E950.4	E962.0	E980.4
Boracic acid	976.0	E858.7	E946.0	E950.4	E962.0	E980.4
ENT agent	976.6	E858.7	E946.6	E950.4	E962.0	E980.4
ophthalmic preparation	976.5	E858.7	E946.5	E950.4	E962.0	E980.4
Borate (cleanser) (sodium)	989.6	E861.3	—	E950.9	E962.1	E980.9
Borax (cleanser)	989.6	E861.3	—	E950.9	E962.1	E980.9
Boric acid	976.0	E858.7	E946.0	E950.4	E962.0	E980.4
ENT agent	976.6	E858.7	E946.6	E950.4	E962.0	E980.4
ophthalmic preparation	976.5	E858.7	E946.5	E950.4	E962.0	E980.4
Boron hydride NEC	989.89	E866.8	—	E950.9	E962.1	E980.9
fumes or gas	987.8	E869.8	—	E952.8	E962.2	E982.8
Brake fluid vapor	987.8	E869.8	—	E952.8	E962.2	E982.8
Brass (compounds) (fumes)	985.8	E866.4	—	E950.9	E962.1	E980.9
Brasso	981	E861.3	—	E950.9	E962.1	E980.9
Bretylium (tosylate)	972.6	E858.3	E942.6	E950.4	E962.0	E980.4
Brevital (sodium)	968.3	E855.1	E938.3	E950.4	E962.0	E980.4
British antilewisite	963.8	E858.1	E933.8	E950.4	E962.0	E980.4
Bromal (hydrate)	967.3	E852.2	E937.3	E950.2	E962.0	E980.2
Bromelains	963.4	E858.1	E933.4	E950.4	E962.0	E980.4
Bromides NEC	967.3	E852.2	E937.3	E950.2	E962.0	E980.2
Bromine (vapor)	987.8	E869.8	—	E952.8	E962.2	E982.8
compounds (medicinal)	967.3	E852.2	E937.3	E950.2	E962.0	E980.2
Bromisovalum	967.3	E852.2	E937.3	E950.2	E962.0	E980.2
Bromobenzyl cyanide	987.5	E869.3	—	E952.8	E962.2	E982.8
Bromodiphenhydramine	963.0	E858.1	E933.0	E950.4	E962.0	E980.4
Bromoform	967.3	E852.2	E937.3	E950.2	E962.0	E980.2
Bromophenol blue reagent	977.8	E858.8	E947.8	E950.4	E962.0	E980.4
Bromosalicylhydroxamic acid	961.8	E857	E931.8	E950.4	E962.0	E980.4
Bromo-seltzer	965.4	E850.4	E935.4	E950.0	E962.0	E980.0
Brompheniramine	963.0	E858.1	E933.0	E950.4	E962.0	E980.4
Bromural	967.3	E852.2	E937.3	E950.2	E962.0	E980.2
Brown spider (bite) (venom)	989.5	E905.1	—	E950.9	E962.1	E980.9
Brucia	988.2	E865.3	—	E950.9	E962.1	E980.9
Brucine	989.1	E863.7	—	E950.6	E962.1	E980.7
Brunswick green — *see* Copper						
Bruten — *see* Ibuprofen						
Bryonia (alba) (dioica)	988.2	E865.4	—	E950.9	E962.1	E980.9
Buclizine	969.5	E853.8	E939.5	E950.3	E962.0	E980.3
Bufferin	965.1	E850.3	E935.3	E950.0	E962.0	E980.0
Bufotenine	969.6	E854.1	E939.6	E950.3	E962.0	E980.3
Buphenine	971.2	E855.5	E941.2	E950.4	E962.0	E980.4
Bupivacaine	968.9	E855.2	E938.9	E950.4	E962.0	E980.4
infiltration (subcutaneous)	968.5	E855.2	E938.5	E950.4	E962.0	E980.4
nerve block (peripheral) (plexus)	968.6	E855.2	E938.6	E950.4	E962.0	E980.4
Busulfan	963.1	E858.1	E933.1	E950.4	E962.0	E980.4
Butabarbital (sodium)	967.0	E851	E937.0	E950.1	E962.0	E980.1
Butabarbitone	967.0	E851	E937.0	E950.1	E962.0	E980.1
Butabarpal	967.0	E851	E937.0	E950.1	E962.0	E980.1
Butacaine	968.5	E855.2	E938.5	E950.4	E962.0	E980.4
Butallylonal	967.0	E851	E937.0	E950.1	E962.0	E980.1
Butane (distributed in mobile container)	987.0	E868.0	—	E951.1	E962.2	E981.1
distributed through pipes	987.0	E867	—	E951.0	E962.2	E981.0
incomplete combustion of — *see* Carbon monoxide, butane						
Butanol	980.3	E860.4	—	E950.9	E962.1	E980.9
Butanone	982.8	E862.4	—	E950.9	E962.1	E980.9
Butaperazine	969.1	E853.0	E939.1	E950.3	E962.0	E980.3
Butazolidin	965.5	E850.5	E935.5	E950.0	E962.0	E980.0
Butethal	967.0	E851	E937.0	E950.1	E962.0	E980.1
Butethamate	971.1	E855.4	E941.1	E950.4	E962.0	E980.4
Buthalitone (sodium)	968.3	E855.1	E938.3	E950.4	E962.0	E980.4
Butisol (sodium)	967.0	E851	E937.0	E950.1	E962.0	E980.1
Butobarbital, butobarbitone	967.0	E851	E937.0	E950.1	E962.0	E980.1
Butriptyline	969.0	E854.0	E939.0	E950.3	E962.0	E980.3
Buttercups	988.2	E865.4	—	E950.9	E962.1	E980.9

▣4ᵗʰ Fourth-digit Required   ▣5ᵗʰ Fifth-digit Required   ►◄ Revised Text   ● New Line   ▲ Revised Code

	Poisoning	Accident	Therapeutic Use	Suicide Attempt	Assault	Undetermined
Butter of antimony — *see* Antimony						
Butyl						
acetate (secondary)	982.8	E862.4	—	E950.9	E962.1	E980.9
alcohol	980.3	E860.4	—	E950.9	E962.1	E980.9
carbinol	980.8	E860.8	—	E950.9	E962.1	E980.9
carbitol	982.8	E862.4	—	E950.9	E962.1	E980.9
cellosolve	982.8	E862.4	—	E950.9	E962.1	E980.9
chloral (hydrate)	967.1	E852.0	E937.1	E950.2	E962.0	E980.2
formate	982.8	E862.4	—	E950.9	E962.1	E980.9
scopolammonium bromide	971.1	E855.4	E941.1	E950.4	E962.0	E980.4
Butyn	968.5	E855.2	E938.5	E950.4	E962.0	E980.4
Butyrophenone (-based tranquilizers)	969.2	E853.1	E939.2	E950.3	E962.0	E980.3
Cacodyl, cacodylic acid — *see* Arsenic						
Cactinomycin	960.7	E856	E930.7	E950.4	E962.0	E980.4
Cade oil	976.4	E858.7	E946.4	E950.4	E962.0	E980.4
Cadmium (chloride) (compounds) (dust) (fumes) (oxide)	985.5	E866.4	—	E950.9	E962.1	E980.9
sulfide (medicinal) NEC	976.4	E858.7	E946.4	E950.4	E962.0	E980.4
Caffeine	969.7	E854.2	E939.7	E950.3	E962.0	E980.3
Calabar bean	988.2	E865.4	—	E950.9	E962.1	E980.9
Caladium seguinium	988.2	E865.4	—	E950.9	E962.1	E980.9
Calamine (liniment) (lotion)	976.3	E858.7	E946.3	E950.4	E962.0	E980.4
Calciferol	963.5	E858.1	E933.5	E950.4	E962.0	E980.4
Calcium (salts) NEC	974.5	E858.5	E944.5	E950.4	E962.0	E980.4
acetylsalicylate	965.1	E850.3	E935.3	E950.0	E962.0	E980.0
benzamidosalicylate	961.8	E857	E931.8	E950.4	E962.0	E980.4
carbaspirin	965.1	E850.3	E935.3	E950.0	E962.0	E980.0
carbimide (citrated)	977.3	E858.8	E947.3	E950.4	E962.0	E980.4
carbonate (antacid)	973.0	E858.4	E943.0	E950.4	E962.0	E980.4
cyanide (citrated)	977.3	E858.8	E947.3	E950.4	E962.0	E980.4
dioctyl sulfosuccinate	973.2	E858.4	E943.2	E950.4	E962.0	E980.4
disodium edathamil	963.8	E858.1	E933.8	E950.4	E962.0	E980.4
disodium edetate	963.8	E858.1	E933.8	E950.4	E962.0	E980.4
EDTA	963.8	E858.1	E933.8	E950.4	E962.0	E980.4
hydrate, hydroxide	983.2	E864.2	—	E950.7	E962.1	E980.6
mandelate	961.9	E857	E931.9	E950.4	E962.0	E980.4
oxide	983.2	E864.2	—	E950.7	E962.1	E980.6
Calomel — *see* Mercury, chloride						
Caloric agents NEC	974.5	E858.5	E944.5	E950.4	E962.0	E980.4
Calusterone	963.1	E858.1	E933.1	E950.4	E962.0	E980.4
Camoquin	961.4	E857	E931.4	E950.4	E962.0	E980.4
Camphor (oil)	976.1	E858.7	E946.1	E950.4	E962.0	E980.4
Candeptin	976.0	E858.7	E946.0	E950.4	E962.0	E980.4
Candicidin	976.0	E858.7	E946.0	E950.4	E962.0	E980.4
Cannabinols	969.6	E854.1	E939.6	E950.3	E962.0	E980.3
Cannabis (derivatives) (indica) (sativa)	969.6	E854.1	E939.6	E950.3	E962.0	E980.3
Canned heat	980.1	E860.2	—	E950.9	E962.1	E980.9
Cantharides, cantharidin, cantharis	976.8	E858.7	E946.8	E950.4	E962.0	E980.4
Capillary agents	972.8	E858.3	E942.8	E950.4	E962.0	E980.4
Capreomycin	960.6	E856	E930.6	E950.4	E962.0	E980.4
Captodiame, captodiamine	969.5	E853.8	E939.5	E950.3	E962.0	E980.3
Caramiphen (hydrochloride)	971.1	E855.4	E941.1	E950.4	E962.0	E980.4
Carbachol	971.0	E855.3	E941.0	E950.4	E962.0	E980.4
Carbacrylamine resins	974.5	E858.5	E944.5	E950.4	E962.0	E980.4
Carbamate (sedative)	967.8	E852.8	E937.8	E950.2	E962.0	E980.2
herbicide	989.3	E863.5	—	E950.6	E962.1	E980.7
insecticide	989.3	E863.2	—	E950.6	E962.1	E980.7
Carbamazepine	966.3	E855.0	E936.3	E950.4	E962.0	E980.4
Carbamic esters	967.8	E852.8	E937.8	E950.2	E962.0	E980.2
Carbamide	974.4	E858.5	E944.4	E950.4	E962.0	E980.4
topical	976.8	E858.7	E946.8	E950.4	E962.0	E980.4
Carbamylcholine chloride	971.0	E855.3	E941.0	E950.4	E962.0	E980.4
Carbarsone	961.1	E857	E931.1	E950.4	E962.0	E980.4
Carbaryl	989.3	E863.2	—	E950.6	E962.1	E980.7
Carbaspirin	965.1	E850.3	E935.3	E950.0	E962.0	E980.0
Carbazochrome	972.8	E858.3	E942.8	E950.4	E962.0	E980.4
Carbenicillin	960.0	E856	E930.0	E950.4	E962.0	E980.4
Carbenoxolone	973.8	E858.4	E943.8	E950.4	E962.0	E980.4
Carbetapentane	975.4	E858.6	E945.4	E950.4	E962.0	E980.4
Carbimazole	962.8	E858.0	E932.8	E950.4	E962.0	E980.4
Carbinol	980.1	E860.2	—	E950.9	E962.1	E980.9
Carbinoxamine	963.0	E858.1	E933.0	E950.4	E962.0	E980.4
Carbitol	982.8	E862.4	—	E950.9	E962.1	E980.9
Carbocaine	968.9	E855.2	E938.9	E950.4	E962.0	E980.4
infiltration (subcutaneous)	968.5	E855.2	E938.5	E950.4	E962.0	E980.4
nerve block (peripheral) (plexus)	968.6	E855.2	E938.6	E950.4	E962.0	E980.4
topical (surface)	968.5	E855.2	E938.5	E950.4	E962.0	E980.4
Carbol-fuchsin solution	976.0	E858.7	E946.0	E950.4	E962.0	E980.4
Carbolic acid (*see also* Phenol)	983.0	E864.0	—	E950.7	E962.1	E980.6
Carbomycin	960.8	E856	E930.8	E950.4	E962.0	E980.4
Carbon						
bisulfide (liquid) (vapor)	982.2	E862.4	—	E950.9	E962.1	E980.9

	Poisoning	External Cause (E-Code)				
		Accident	Therapeutic Use	Suicide Attempt	Assault	Undetermined
Carbon — *continued*						
dioxide (gas)	987.8	E869.8	—	E952.8	E962.2	E982.8
disulfide (liquid) (vapor)	982.2	E862.4	—	E950.9	E962.1	E980.9
monoxide (from incomplete combustion of) (in) NEC	986	E868.9	—	E952.1	E962.2	E982.1
blast furnace gas	986	E868.8	—	E952.1	E962.2	E982.1
butane (distributed in mobile container)	986	E868.0	—	E951.1	E962.2	E981.1
distributed through pipes	986	E867	—	E951.0	E962.2	E981.0
charcoal fumes	986	E868.3	—	E952.1	E962.2	E982.1
coal						
gas (piped)	986	E867	—	E951.0	E962.2	E981.0
solid (in domestic stoves, fireplaces)	986	E868.3	—	E952.1	E962.2	E982.1
coke (in domestic stoves, fireplaces)	986	E868.3	—	E952.1	E962.2	E982.1
exhaust gas (motor) not in transit	986	E868.2	—	E952.0	E962.2	E982.0
combustion engine, any not in watercraft	986	E868.2	—	E952.0	E962.2	E982.0
farm tractor, not in transit	986	E868.2	—	E952.0	E962.2	E982.0
gas engine	986	E868.2	—	E952.0	E962.2	E982.0
motor pump	986	E868.2	—	E952.0	E962.2	E982.0
motor vehicle, not in transit	986	E868.2	—	E952.0	E962.2	E982.0
fuel (in domestic use)	986	E868.3	—	E952.1	E962.2	E982.1
gas (piped)	986	E867	—	E951.0	E962.2	E981.0
in mobile container	986	E868.0	—	E951.1	E962.2	E981.1
utility	986	E868.1	—	E951.8	E962.2	E981.1
in mobile container	986	E868.0	—	E951.1	E962.2	E981.1
piped (natural)	986	E867	—	E951.0	E962.2	E981.0
illuminating gas	986	E868.1	—	E951.8	E962.2	E981.8
industrial fuels or gases, any	986	E868.8	—	E952.1	E962.2	E982.1
kerosene (in domestic stoves, fireplaces)	986	E868.3	—	E952.1	E962.2	E982.1
kiln gas or vapor	986	E868.8	—	E952.1	E962.2	E982.1
motor exhaust gas, not in transit	986	E868.2	—	E952.0	E962.2	E982.0
piped gas (manufactured) (natural)	986	E867	—	E951.0	E962.2	E981.0
producer gas	986	E868.8	—	E952.1	E962.2	E982.1
propane (distributed in mobile container)	986	E868.0	—	E951.1	E962.2	E981.1
distributed through pipes	986	E867	—	E951.0	E962.2	E981.0
specified source NEC	986	E868.8	—	E952.1	E962.2	E982.1
stove gas	986	E868.1	—	E951.8	E962.2	E981.8
piped	986	E867	—	E951.0	E962.2	E981.0
utility gas	986	E868.1	—	E951.8	E962.2	E981.8
piped	986	E867	—	E951.0	E962.2	E981.0
water gas	986	E868.1	—	E951.8	E962.2	E981.8
wood (in domestic stoves, fireplaces)	986	E868.3	—	E952.1	E962.2	E982.1
tetrachloride (vapor) NEC	987.8	E869.8	—	E952.8	E962.2	E982.8
liquid (cleansing agent) NEC	982.1	E861.3	—	E950.9	E962.1	E980.9
solvent	982.1	E862.4	—	E950.9	E962.1	E980.9
Carbonic acid (gas)	987.8	E869.8	—	E952.8	E962.2	E982.8
anhydrase inhibitors	974.2	E858.5	E944.2	E950.4	E962.0	E980.4
Carbowax	976.3	E858.7	E946.3	E950.4	E962.0	E980.4
Carbrital	967.0	E851	E937.0	E950.1	E962.0	E980.1
Carbromal (derivatives)	967.3	E852.2	E937.3	E950.2	E962.0	E980.2
Cardiac						
depressants	972.0	E858.3	E942.0	E950.4	E962.0	E980.4
rhythm regulators	972.0	E858.3	E942.0	E950.4	E962.0	E980.4
Cardiografin	977.8	E858.8	E947.8	E950.4	E962.0	E980.4
Cardio-green	977.8	E858.8	E947.8	E950.4	E962.0	E980.4
Cardiotonic glycosides	972.1	E858.3	E942.1	E950.4	E962.0	E980.4
Cardiovascular agents NEC	972.9	E858.3	E942.9	E950.4	E962.0	E980.4
Cardrase	974.2	E858.5	E944.2	E950.4	E962.0	E980.4
Carfusin	976.0	E858.7	E946.0	E950.4	E962.0	E980.4
Carisoprodol	968.0	E855.1	E938.0	E950.4	E962.0	E980.4
Carmustine	963.1	E858.1	E933.1	E950.4	E962.0	E980.4
Carotene	963.5	E858.1	E933.5	E950.4	E962.0	E980.4
Carphenazine (maleate)	969.1	E853.0	E939.1	E950.3	E962.0	E980.3
Carter's Little Pills	973.1	E858.4	E943.1	E950.4	E962.0	E980.4
Cascara (sagrada)	973.1	E858.4	E943.1	E950.4	E962.0	E980.4
Cassava	988.2	E865.4	—	E950.9	E962.1	E980.9
Castellani's paint	976.0	E858.7	E946.0	E950.4	E962.0	E980.4
Castor						
bean	988.2	E865.3	—	E950.9	E962.1	E980.9
oil	973.1	E858.4	E943.1	E950.4	E962.0	E980.4
Caterpillar (sting)	989.5	E905.5	—	E950.9	E962.1	E980.9
Catha (edulis)	970.8	E854.3	E940.8	E950.4	E962.0	E980.4
Cathartics NEC	973.3	E858.4	E943.3	E950.4	E962.0	E980.4
contact	973.1	E858.4	E943.1	E950.4	E962.0	E980.4
emollient	973.2	E858.4	E943.2	E950.4	E962.0	E980.4
intestinal irritants	973.1	E858.4	E943.1	E950.4	E962.0	E980.4
saline	973.3	E858.4	E943.3	E950.4	E962.0	E980.4
Cathomycin	960.8	E856	E930.8	E950.4	E962.0	E980.4
Caustic(s)	983.9	E864.4	—	E950.7	E962.1	E980.6
alkali	983.2	E864.2	—	E950.7	E962.1	E980.6
hydroxide	983.2	E864.2	—	E950.7	E962.1	E980.6

	Poisoning	External Cause (E-Code)				
		Accident	Therapeutic Use	Suicide Attempt	Assault	Undetermined
Caustic(s) — continued						
potash	983.2	E864.2	—	E950.7	E962.1	E980.6
soda	983.2	E864.2	—	E950.7	E962.1	E980.6
specified NEC	983.9	E864.3	—	E950.7	E962.1	E980.6
Ceepryn	976.0	E858.7	E946.0	E950.4	E962.0	E980.4
ENT agent	976.6	E858.7	E946.6	E950.4	E962.0	E980.4
lozenges	976.6	E858.7	E946.6	E950.4	E962.0	E980.4
Celestone	962.0	E858.0	E932.0	E950.4	E962.0	E980.4
topical	976.0	E858.7	E946.0	E950.4	E962.0	E980.4
Cellosolve	982.8	E862.4	—	E950.9	E962.1	E980.9
Cell stimulants and proliferants	976.8	E858.7	E946.8	E950.4	E962.0	E980.4
Cellulose derivatives, cathartic	973.3	E858.4	E943.3	E950.4	E962.0	E980.4
nitrates (topical)	976.3	E858.7	E946.3	E950.4	E962.0	E980.4
Centipede (bite)	989.5	E905.4	—	E950.9	E962.1	E980.9
Central nervous system						
depressants	968.4	E855.1	E938.4	E950.4	E962.0	E980.4
anesthetic (general) NEC	968.4	E855.1	E938.4	E950.4	E962.0	E980.4
gases NEC	968.2	E855.1	E938.2	E950.4	E962.0	E980.4
intravenous	968.3	E855.1	E938.3	E950.4	E962.0	E980.4
barbiturates	967.0	E851	E937.0	E950.1	E962.0	E980.1
bromides	967.3	E852.2	E937.3	E950.2	E962.0	E980.2
cannabis sativa	969.6	E854.1	E939.6	E950.3	E962.0	E980.3
chloral hydrate	967.1	E852.0	E937.1	E950.2	E962.0	E980.2
hallucinogenics	969.6	E854.1	E939.6	E950.3	E962.0	E980.3
hypnotics	967.9	E852.9	E937.9	E950.2	E962.0	E980.2
specified NEC	967.8	E852.8	E937.8	E950.2	E962.0	E980.2
muscle relaxants	968.0	E855.1	E938.0	E950.4	E962.0	E980.4
paraldehyde	967.2	E852.1	E937.2	E950.2	E962.0	E980.2
sedatives	967.9	E852.9	E937.9	E950.2	E962.0	E980.2
mixed NEC	967.6	E852.5	E937.6	E950.2	E962.0	E980.2
specified NEC	967.8	E852.8	E937.8	E950.2	E962.0	E980.2
muscle-tone depressants	968.0	E855.1	E938.0	E950.4	E962.0	E980.4
stimulants	970.9	E854.3	E940.9	E950.4	E962.0	E980.4
amphetamines	969.7	E854.2	E939.7	E950.3	E962.0	E980.3
analeptics	970.0	E854.3	E940.0	E950.4	E962.0	E980.4
antidepressants	969.0	E854.0	E939.0	E950.3	E962.0	E980.3
opiate antagonists	970.1	E854.3	E940.1	E950.4	E962.0	E980.4
specified NEC	970.8	E854.3	E940.8	E950.4	E962.0	E980.4
Cephalexin	960.5	E856	E930.5	E950.4	E962.0	E980.4
Cephaloglycin	960.5	E856	E930.5	E950.4	E962.0	E980.4
Cephaloridine	960.5	E856	E930.5	E950.4	E962.0	E980.4
Cephalosporins NEC	960.5	E856	E930.5	E950.4	E962.0	E980.4
N (adicillin)	960.0	E856	E930.0	E950.4	E962.0	E980.4
Cephalothin (sodium)	960.5	E856	E930.5	E950.4	E962.0	E980.4
Cerbera (odallam)	988.2	E865.4	—	E950.9	E962.1	E980.9
Cerberin	972.1	E858.3	E942.1	E950.4	E962.0	E980.4
Cerebral stimulants	970.9	E854.3	E940.9	E950.4	E962.0	E980.4
psychotherapeutic	969.7	E854.2	E939.7	E950.3	E962.0	E980.3
specified NEC	970.8	E854.3	E940.8	E950.4	E962.0	E980.4
Cetalkonium (chloride)	976.0	E858.7	E946.0	E950.4	E962.0	E980.4
Cetoxime	963.0	E858.1	E933.0	E950.4	E962.0	E980.4
Cetrimide	976.2	E858.7	E946.2	E950.4	E962.0	E980.4
Cetylpyridinium	976.0	E858.7	E946.0	E950.4	E962.0	E980.4
ENT agent	976.6	E858.7	E946.6	E950.4	E962.0	E980.4
lozenges	976.6	E858.7	E946.6	E950.4	E962.0	E980.4
Cevadilla — *see* Sabadilla						
Cevitamic acid	963.5	E858.1	E933.5	E950.4	E962.0	E980.4
Chalk, precipitated	973.0	E858.4	E943.0	E950.4	E962.0	E980.4
Charcoal						
fumes (carbon monoxide)	986	E868.3	—	E952.1	E962.2	E982.1
industrial	986	E868.8	—	E952.1	E962.2	E982.1
medicinal (activated)	973.0	E858.4	E943.0	E950.4	E962.0	E980.4
Chelating agents NEC	977.2	E858.8	E947.2	E950.4	E962.0	E980.4
Chelidonium majus	988.2	E865.4	—	E950.9	E962.1	E980.9
Chemical substance	989.9	E866.9	—	E950.9	E962.1	E980.9
specified NEC	989.89	E866.8	—	E950.9	E962.1	E980.9
Chemotherapy, antineoplastic	963.1	E858.1	E933.1	E950.4	E962.0	E980.4
Chenopodium (oil)	961.6	E857	E931.6	E950.4	E962.0	E980.4
Cherry laurel	988.2	E865.4	—	E950.9	E962.1	E980.9
Chiniofon	961.3	E857	E931.3	E950.4	E962.0	E980.4
Chlophedianol	975.4	E858.6	E945.4	E950.4	E962.0	E980.4
Chloral (betaine) (formamide) (hydrate)	967.1	E852.0	E937.1	E950.2	E962.0	E980.2
Chloralamide	967.1	E852.0	E937.1	E950.2	E962.0	E980.2
Chlorambucil	963.1	E858.1	E933.1	E950.4	E962.0	E980.4
Chloramphenicol	960.2	E856	E930.2	E950.4	E962.0	E980.4
ENT agent	976.6	E858.7	E946.6	E950.4	E962.0	E980.4
ophthalmic preparation	976.5	E858.7	E946.5	E950.4	E962.0	E980.4
topical NEC	976.0	E858.7	E946.0	E950.4	E962.0	E980.4
Chlorate(s) (potassium) (sodium) NEC	983.9	E864.3	—	E950.7	E962.1	E980.6
herbicides	989.4	E863.5	—	E950.6	E962.1	E980.7

▨ Fourth-digit Required   ▨ Fifth-digit Required   ▶◀ Revised Text   ● New Line   ▲ Revised Code

	Poisoning	External Cause (E-Code)				
		Accident	Therapeutic Use	Suicide Attempt	Assault	Undetermined
Chlorcylizine	963.0	E858.1	E933.0	E950.4	E962.0	E980.4
Chlordan(e) (dust)	989.2	E863.0	—	E950.6	E962.1	E980.7
Chlordantoin	976.0	E858.7	E946.0	E950.4	E962.0	E980.4
Chlordiazepoxide	969.4	E853.2	E939.4	E950.3	E962.0	E980.3
Chloresium	976.8	E858.7	E946.8	E950.4	E962.0	E980.4
Chlorethiazol	967.1	E852.0	E937.1	E950.2	E962.0	E980.2
Chlorethyl — see Ethyl, chloride						
Chloretone	967.1	E852.0	E937.1	E950.2	E962.0	E980.2
Chlorex	982.3	E862.4	—	E950.9	E962.1	E980.9
Chlorhexadol	967.1	E852.0	E937.1	E950.2	E962.0	E980.2
Chlorhexidine (hydrochloride)	976.0	E858.7	E946.0	E950.4	E962.0	E980.4
Chlorhydroxyquinolin	976.0	E858.7	E946.0	E950.4	E962.0	E980.4
Chloride of lime (bleach)	983.9	E864.3	—	E950.7	E962.1	E980.6
Chlorinated						
camphene	989.2	E863.0	—	E950.6	E962.1	E980.7
diphenyl	989.89	E866.8	—	E950.9	E962.1	E980.9
hydrocarbons NEC	989.2	E863.0	—	E950.6	E962.1	E980.7
solvent	982.3	E862.4	—	E950.9	E962.1	E980.9
lime (bleach)	983.9	E864.3	—	E950.7	E962.1	E980.6
naphthalene — see Naphthalene						
pesticides NEC	989.2	E863.0	—	E950.6	E962.1	E980.7
soda — see Sodium, hypochlorite						
Chlorine (fumes) (gas)	987.6	E869.8	—	E952.8	E962.2	E982.8
bleach	983.9	E864.3	—	E950.7	E962.1	E980.6
compounds NEC	983.9	E864.3	—	E950.7	E962.1	E980.6
disinfectant	983.9	E861.4	—	E950.7	E962.1	E980.6
releasing agents NEC	983.9	E864.3	—	E950.7	E962.1	E980.6
Chlorisondamine	972.3	E858.3	E942.3	E950.4	E962.0	E980.4
Chlormadinone	962.2	E858.0	E932.2	E950.4	E962.0	E980.4
Chlormerodrin	974.0	E858.5	E944.0	E950.4	E962.0	E980.4
Chlormethiazole	967.1	E852.0	E937.1	E950.2	E962.0	E980.2
Chlormethylenecycline	960.4	E856	E930.4	E950.4	E962.0	E980.4
Chlormezanone	969.5	E853.8	E939.5	E950.3	E962.0	E980.3
Chloroacetophenone	987.5	E869.3	—	E952.8	E962.2	E982.8
Chloroaniline	983.0	E864.0	—	E950.7	E962.1	E980.6
Chlorobenzene, chlorobenzol	982.0	E862.4	—	E950.9	E962.1	E980.9
Chlorobutanol	967.1	E852.0	E937.1	E950.2	E962.0	E980.2
Chlorodinitrobenzene	983.0	E864.0	—	E950.7	E962.1	E980.6
dust or vapor	987.8	E869.8	—	E952.8	E962.2	E982.8
Chloroethane — see Ethyl, chloride						
Chloroform (fumes) (vapor)	987.8	E869.8	—	E952.8	E962.2	E982.8
anesthetic (gas)	968.2	E855.1	E938.2	E950.4	E962.0	E980.4
liquid NEC	968.4	E855.1	E938.4	E950.4	E962.0	E980.4
solvent	982.3	E862.4	—	E950.9	E962.1	E980.9
Chloroguanide	961.4	E857	E931.4	E950.4	E962.0	E980.4
Chloromycetin	960.2	E856	E930.2	E950.4	E962.0	E980.4
ENT agent	976.6	E858.7	E946.6	E950.4	E962.0	E980.4
ophthalmic preparation	976.5	E858.7	E946.5	E950.4	E962.0	E980.4
otic solution	976.6	E858.7	E946.6	E950.4	E962.0	E980.4
topical NEC	976.0	E858.7	E946.0	E950.4	E962.0	E980.4
Chloronitrobenzene	983.0	E864.0	—	E950.7	E962.1	E980.6
dust or vapor	987.8	E869.8	—	E952.8	E962.2	E982.8
Chlorophenol	983.0	E864.0	—	E950.7	E962.1	E980.6
Chlorophenothane	989.2	E863.0	—	E950.6	E962.1	E980.7
Chlorophyll (derivatives)	976.8	E858.7	E946.8	E950.4	E962.0	E980.4
Chloropicrin (fumes)	987.8	E869.8	—	E952.8	E962.2	E982.8
fumigant	989.4	E863.8	—	E950.6	E962.1	E980.7
fungicide	989.4	E863.6	—	E950.6	E962.1	E980.7
pesticide (fumes)	989.4	E863.4	—	E950.6	E962.1	E980.7
Chloroprocaine	968.9	E855.2	E938.9	E950.4	E962.0	E980.4
infiltration (subcutaneous)	968.5	E855.2	E938.5	E950.4	E962.0	E980.4
nerve block (peripheral) (plexus)	968.6	E855.2	E938.6	E950.4	E962.0	E980.4
Chloroptic	976.5	E858.7	E946.5	E950.4	E962.0	E980.4
Chloropurine	963.1	E858.1	E933.1	E950.4	E962.0	E980.4
Chloroquine (hydrochloride) (phosphate)	961.4	E857	E931.4	E950.4	E962.0	E980.4
Chlorothen	963.0	E858.1	E933.0	E950.4	E962.0	E980.4
Chlorothiazide	974.3	E858.5	E944.3	E950.4	E962.0	E980.4
Chlorotrianisene	962.2	E858.0	E932.2	E950.4	E962.0	E980.4
Chlorovinyldichloroarsine	985.1	E866.3	—	E950.8	E962.1	E980.8
Chloroxylenol	976.0	E858.7	E946.0	E950.4	E962.0	E980.4
Chlorphenesin (carbamate)	968.0	E855.1	E938.0	E950.4	E962.0	E980.4
topical (antifungal)	976.0	E858.7	E946.0	E950.4	E962.0	E980.4
Chlorpheniramine	963.0	E858.1	E933.0	E950.4	E962.0	E980.4
Chlorphenoxamine	966.4	E855.0	E936.4	E950.4	E962.0	E980.4
Chlorphentermine	977.0	E858.8	E947.0	E950.4	E962.0	E980.4
Chlorproguanil	961.4	E857	E931.4	E950.4	E962.0	E980.4
Chlorpromazine	969.1	E853.0	E939.1	E950.3	E962.0	E980.3
Chlorpropamide	962.3	E858.0	E932.3	E950.4	E962.0	E980.4
Chlorprothixene	969.3	E853.8	E939.3	E950.3	E962.0	E980.3
Chlorquinaldol	976.0	E858.7	E946.0	E950.4	E962.0	E980.4

✔4ᵗʰ Fourth-digit Required   ✔5ᵗʰ Fifth-digit Required   ▶◀ Revised Text   ● New Line   ▲ Revised Code

			External Cause (E-Code)			
	Poisoning	Accident	Therapeutic Use	Suicide Attempt	Assault	Undetermined
Chlortetracycline	960.4	E856	E930.4	E950.4	E962.0	E980.4
Chlorthalidone	974.4	E858.5	E944.4	E950.4	E962.0	E980.4
Chlortrianisene	962.2	E858.0	E932.2	E950.4	E962.0	E980.4
Chlor-Trimeton	963.0	E858.1	E933.0	E950.4	E962.0	E980.4
Chlorzoxazone	968.0	E855.1	E938.0	E950.4	E962.0	E980.4
Choke damp	987.8	E869.8	—	E952.8	E962.2	E982.8
Cholebrine	977.8	E858.8	E947.8	E950.4	E962.0	E980.4
Cholera vaccine	978.2	E858.8	E948.2	E950.4	E962.0	E980.4
Cholesterol-lowering agents	972.2	E858.3	E942.2	E950.4	E962.0	E980.4
Cholestyramine (resin)	972.2	E858.3	E942.2	E950.4	E962.0	E980.4
Cholic acid	973.4	E858.4	E943.4	E950.4	E962.0	E980.4
Choline	977.1	E858.8	E947.1	E950.4	E962.0	E980.4
dihydrogen citrate	965.1	E850.3	E935.3	E950.0	E962.0	E980.0
salicylate	974.1	E858.5	E944.1	E950.4	E962.0	E980.4
theophyllinate	971.0	E855.3	E941.0	E950.4	E962.0	E980.4
Cholinergics	977.8	E858.8	E947.8	E950.4	E962.0	E980.4
Cholografin	962.4	E858.0	E932.4	E950.4	E962.0	E980.4
Chorionic gonadotropin	983.9	E864.3	—	E950.7	E962.1	E980.6
Chromates	987.8	E869.8	—	E952.8	E962.2	E982.8
dust or mist	984.0	E866.0	—	E950.9	E962.1	E980.9
lead	984.0	E861.5	—	E950.9	E962.1	E980.9
paint	983.9	E864.3	—	E950.7	E962.1	E980.6
Chromic acid	987.8	E869.8	—	E952.8	E962.2	E982.8
dust or mist	985.6	E866.4	—	E950.9	E962.1	E980.9
Chromium						
compounds — see Chromates	972.4	E858.3	E942.4	E950.4	E962.0	E980.4
Chromonar	983.9	E864.3	—	E950.7	E962.1	E980.6
Chromyl chloride	976.4	E858.7	E946.4	E950.4	E962.0	E980.4
Chrysarobin (ointment)	973.1	E858.4	E943.1	E950.4	E962.0	E980.4
Chrysazin	963.4	E858.1	E933.4	E950.4	E962.0	E980.4
Chymar	976.5	E858.7	E946.5	E950.4	E962.0	E980.4
ophthalmic preparation	963.4	E858.1	E933.4	E950.4	E962.0	E980.4
Chymotrypsin	976.5	E858.7	E946.5	E950.4	E962.0	E980.4
ophthalmic preparation	988.2	E865.4	—	E950.9	E962.1	E980.9
Cicuta maculata or virosa	981	E862.1	—	E950.9	E962.1	E980.9
Cigarette lighter fluid	968.7	E855.2	E938.7	E950.4	E962.0	E980.4
Cinchocaine (spinal)	968.5	E855.2	E938.5	E950.4	E962.0	E980.4
topical (surface)	961.4	E857	E931.4	E950.4	E962.0	E980.4
Cinchona	961.4	E857	E931.4	E950.4	E962.0	E980.4
Cinchonine alkaloids	974.7	E858.5	E944.7	E950.4	E962.0	E980.4
Cinchophen	963.0	E858.1	E933.0	E950.4	E962.0	E980.4
Cinnarizine	968.9	E855.2	E938.9	E950.4	E962.0	E980.4
Citanest	968.5	E855.2	E938.5	E950.4	E962.0	E980.4
infiltration (subcutaneous)	968.6	E855.2	E938.6	E950.4	E962.0	E980.4
nerve block (peripheral) (plexus)	989.89	E866.8	—	E950.9	E962.1	E980.9
Citric acid	964.1	E858.2	E934.1	E950.4	E962.0	E980.4
Citrovorum factor	988.2	E865.4	—	E950.9	E962.1	E980.9
Claviceps purpurea	989.89	E861.3	—	E950.9	E962.1	E980.9
Cleaner, cleansing agent NEC	982.8	E862.9	—	E950.9	E962.1	E980.9
of paint or varnish	988.2	E865.4	—	E950.9	E962.1	E980.9
Clematis vitalba	963.0	E858.1	E933.0	E950.4	E962.0	E980.4
Clemizole	960.0	E856	E930.0	E950.4	E962.0	E980.4
penicillin	971.1	E855.4	E941.1	E950.4	E962.0	E980.4
Clidinium	960.8	E856	E930.8	E950.4	E962.0	E980.4
Clindamycin	965.09	E850.2	E935.2	E950.0	E962.0	E980.0
Cliradon	962.0	E858.0	E932.0	E950.4	E962.0	E980.4
Clocortolone	975.4	E858.6	E945.4	E950.4	E962.0	E980.4
Clofedanol	972.2	E858.3	E942.2	E950.4	E962.0	E980.4
Clofibrate	967.1	E852.0	E937.1	E950.2	E962.0	E980.2
Clomethiazole	977.8	E858.8	E947.8	E950.4	E962.0	E980.4
Clomiphene	969.4	E853.2	E939.4	E950.3	E962.0	E980.3
Clonazepam	972.6	E858.3	E942.6	E950.4	E962.0	E980.4
Clonidine	974.3	E858.5	E944.3	E950.4	E962.0	E980.4
Clopamide	969.4	E853.2	E939.4	E950.3	E962.0	E980.3
Clorazepate	974.4	E858.5	E944.4	E950.4	E962.0	E980.4
Clorexolone	983.9	E864.3	—	E950.7	E962.1	E980.6
Clorox (bleach)	977.0	E858.8	E947.0	E950.4	E962.0	E980.4
Clortermine	976.0	E858.7	E946.0	E950.4	E962.0	E980.4
Clotrimazole	960.0	E856	E930.0	E950.4	E962.0	E980.4
Cloxacillin	964.5	E858.2	E934.5	E950.4	E962.0	E980.4
Coagulants NEC						
Coal (carbon monoxide from) — see also Carbon, monoxide, coal						
oil — see Kerosene						
tar NEC	983.0	E864.0	—	E950.7	E962.1	E980.6
fumes	987.8	E869.8	—	E952.8	E962.2	E982.8
medicinal (ointment)	976.4	E858.7	E946.4	E950.4	E962.0	E980.4
analgesics NEC	965.5	E850.5	E935.5	E950.0	E962.0	E980.0
naphtha (solvent)	981	E862.0	—	E950.9	E962.1	E980.9
Cobalt (fumes) (industrial)	985.8	E866.4	—	E950.9	E962.1	E980.9
Cobra (venom)	989.5	E905.0	—	E950.9	E962.1	E980.9

	Poisoning	External Cause (E-Code)				
		Accident	Therapeutic Use	Suicide Attempt	Assault	Undetermined
Coca (leaf)	970.8	E854.3	E940.8	E950.4	E962.0	E980.4
Cocaine (hydrochloride) (salt)	970.8 ▲	E854.3 ▲	E940.8 ▲	E950.4	E962.0	E980.4
topical anesthetic ●	968.5	E855.2	E938.5	E950.4	E962.0	E980.4
Coccidioidin	977.8	E858.8	E947.8	E950.4	E962.0	E980.4
Cocculus indicus	988.2	E865.3	—	E950.9	E962.1	E980.9
Cochineal	989.89	E866.8	—	E950.9	E962.1	E980.9
medicinal products	977.4	E858.8	E947.4	E950.4	E962.0	E980.4
Codeine	965.09	E850.2	E935.2	E950.0	E962.0	E980.0
Coffee	989.89	E866.8	—	E950.9	E962.1	E980.9
Cogentin	971.1	E855.4	E941.1	E950.4	E962.0	E980.4
Coke fumes or gas (carbon monoxide)	986	E868.3	—	E952.1	E962.2	E982.1
industrial use	986	E868.8	—	E952.1	E962.2	E982.1
Colace	973.2	E858.4	E943.2	E950.4	E962.0	E980.4
Colchicine	974.7	E858.5	E944.7	E950.4	E962.0	E980.4
Colchicum	988.2	E865.3	—	E950.9	E962.1	E980.9
Cold cream	976.3	E858.7	E946.3	E950.4	E962.0	E980.4
Colestipol	972.2	E858.3	E942.2	E950.4	E962.0	E980.4
Colistimethate	960.8	E856	E930.8	E950.4	E962.0	E980.4
Colistin	960.8	E856	E930.8	E950.4	E962.0	E980.4
Collagenase	976.8	E858.7	E946.8	E950.4	E962.0	E980.4
Collagen	977.8	E866.8	E947.8	E950.9	E962.1	E980.9
Collodion (flexible)	976.3	E858.7	E946.3	E950.4	E962.0	E980.4
Colocynth	973.1	E858.4	E943.1	E950.4	E962.0	E980.4
Coloring matter — see Dye(s)						
Combustion gas — see Carbon, monoxide						
Compazine	969.1	E853.0	E939.1	E950.3	E962.0	E980.3
Compound						
42 (warfarin)	989.4	E863.7	—	E950.6	E962.1	E980.7
269 (endrin)	989.2	E863.0	—	E950.6	E962.1	E980.7
497 (dieldrin)	989.2	E863.0	—	E950.6	E962.1	E980.7
1080 (sodium fluoroacetate)	989.4	E863.7	—	E950.6	E962.1	E980.7
3422 (parathion)	989.3	E863.1	—	E950.6	E962.1	E980.7
3911 (phorate)	989.3	E863.1	—	E950.6	E962.1	E980.7
3956 (toxaphene)	989.2	E863.0	—	E950.6	E962.1	E980.7
4049 (malathion)	989.3	E863.1	—	E950.6	E962.1	E980.7
4124 (dicapthon)	989.4	E863.4	—	E950.6	E962.1	E980.7
E (cortisone)	962.0	E858.0	E932.0	E950.4	E962.0	E980.4
F (hydrocortisone)	962.0	E858.0	E932.0	E950.4	E962.0	E980.4
Congo red	977.8	E858.8	E947.8	E950.4	E962.0	E980.4
Coniine, conine	965.7	E850.7	E935.7	E950.0	E962.0	E980.0
Conium (maculatum)	988.2	E865.4	—	E950.9	E962.1	· E980.9
Conjugated estrogens (equine)	962.2	E858.0	E932.2	E950.4	E962.0	E980.4
Contac	975.6	E858.6	E945.6	E950.4	E962.0	E980.4
Contact lens solution	976.5	E858.7	E946.5	E950.4	E962.0	E980.4
Contraceptives (oral)	962.2	E858.0	E932.2	E950.4	E962.0	E980.4
vaginal	976.8	E858.7	E946.8	E950.4	E962.0	E980.4
Contrast media (roentgenographic)	977.8	E858.8	E947.8	E950.4	E962.0	E980.4
Convallaria majalis	988.2	E865.4	—	E950.9	E962.1	E980.9
Copper (dust) (fumes) (salts) NEC	985.8	E866.4	—	E950.9	E962.1	E980.9
arsenate, arsenite	985.1	E866.3	—	E950.8	E962.1	E980.8
insecticide	985.1	E863.4	—	E950.8	E962.1	E980.8
emetic	973.6	E858.4	E943.6	E950.4	E962.0	E980.4
fungicide	985.8	E863.6	—	E950.6	E962.1	E980.7
insecticide	985.8	E863.4	—	E950.6	E962.1	E980.7
oleate	976.0	E858.7	E946.0	E950.4	E962.0	E980.4
sulfate	983.9	E864.3	—	E950.7	E962.1	E980.6
fungicide	983.9	E863.6	—	E950.7	E962.1	E980.6
cupric	973.6	E858.4	E943.6	E950.4	E962.0	E980.4
cuprous	983.9	E864.3	—	E950.7	E962.1	E980.6
Copperhead snake (bite) (venom)	989.5	E905.0	—	E950.9	E962.1	E980.9
Coral (sting)	989.5	E905.6	—	E950.9	E962.1	E980.9
snake (bite) (venom)	989.5	E905.0	—	E950.9	E962.1	E980.9
Cordran	976.0	E858.7	E946.0	E950.4	E962.0	E980.4
Corn cures	976.4	E858.7	E946.4	E950.4	E962.0	E980.4
Cornhusker's lotion	976.3	E858.7	E946.3	E950.4	E962.0	E980.4
Corn starch	976.3	E858.7	E946.3	E950.4	E962.0	E980.4
Corrosive	983.9	E864.4	—	E950.7	E962.1	E980.6
acids NEC	983.1	E864.1	—	E950.7	E962.1	E980.6
aromatics	983.0	E864.0	—	E950.7	E962.1	E980.6
disinfectant	983.0	E861.4	—	E950.7	E962.1	E980.6
fumes NEC	987.9	E869.9	—	E952.9	E962.2	E982.9
specified NEC	983.9	E864.3	—	E950.7	E962.1	E980.6
sublimate — see Mercury, chloride						
Cortate	962.0	E858.0	E932.0	E950.4	E962.0	E980.4
Cort-Dome	962.0	E858.0	E932.0	E950.4	E962.0	E980.4
ENT agent	976.6	E858.7	E946.6	E950.4	E962.0	E980.4
ophthalmic preparation	976.5	E858.7	E946.5	E950.4	E962.0	E980.4
topical NEC	976.0	E858.7	E946.0	E950.4	E962.0	E980.4
Cortef	962.0	E858.0	E932.0	E950.4	E962.0	E980.4
ENT agent	976.6	E858.7	E946.6	E950.4	E962.0	E980.4
ophthalmic preparation	976.5	E858.7	E946.5	E950.4	E962.0	E980.4

		External Cause (E-Code)				
	Poisoning	Accident	Therapeutic Use	Suicide Attempt	Assault	Undetermined
Cortef — *continued*						
topical NEC	976.0	E858.7	E946.0	E950.4	E962.0	E980.4
Corticosteroids (fluorinated)	962.0	E858.0	E932.0	E950.4	E962.0	E980.4
ENT agent	976.6	E858.7	E946.6	E950.4	E962.0	E980.4
ophthalmic preparation	976.5	E858.7	E946.5	E950.4	E962.0	E980.4
topical NEC	976.0	E858.7	E946.0	E950.4	E962.0	E980.4
Corticotropin	962.4	E858.0	E932.4	E950.4	E962.0	E980.4
Cortisol	962.0	E858.0	E932.0	E950.4	E962.0	E980.4
ENT agent	976.6	E858.7	E946.6	E950.4	E962.0	E980.4
ophthalmic preparation	976.5	E858.7	E946.5	E950.4	E962.0	E980.4
topical NEC	976.0	E858.7	E946.0	E950.4	E962.0	E980.4
Cortisone derivatives (acetate)	962.0	E858.0	E932.0	E950.4	E962.0	E980.4
ENT agent	976.6	E858.7	E946.6	E950.4	E962.0	E980.4
ophthalmic preparation	976.5	E858.7	E946.5	E950.4	E962.0	E980.4
topical NEC	976.0	E858.7	E946.0	E950.4	E962.0	E980.4
Cortogen	962.0	E858.0	E932.0	E950.4	E962.0	E980.4
ENT agent	976.6	E858.7	E946.6	E950.4	E962.0	E980.4
ophthalmic preparation	976.5	E858.7	E946.5	E950.4	E962.0	E980.4
Cortone	962.0	E858.0	E932.0	E950.4	E962.0	E980.4
ENT agent	976.6	E858.7	E946.6	E950.4	E962.0	E980.4
ophthalmic preparation	976.5	E858.7	E946.5	E950.4	E962.0	E980.4
Cortril	962.0	E858.0	E932.0	E950.4	E962.0	E980.4
ENT agent	976.6	E858.7	E946.6	E950.4	E962.0	E980.4
ophthalmic preparation	976.5	E858.7	E946.5	E950.4	E962.0	E980.4
topical NEC	976.0	E858.7	E946.0	E950.4	E962.0	E980.4
Cosmetics	989.89	E866.7	—	E950.9	E962.1	E980.9
Cosyntropin	977.8	E858.8	E947.8	E950.4	E962.0	E980.4
Cotarnine	964.5	E858.2	E934.5	E950.4	E962.0	E980.4
Cottonseed oil	976.3	E858.7	E946.3	E950.4	E962.0	E980.4
Cough mixtures (antitussives)	975.4	E858.6	E945.4	E950.4	E962.0	E980.4
containing opiates	965.09	E850.2	E935.2	E950.0	E962.0	E980.0
expectorants	975.5	E858.6	E945.5	E950.4	E962.0	E980.4
Coumadin	964.2	E858.2	E934.2	E950.4	E962.0	E980.4
rodenticide	989.4	E863.7	—	E950.6	E962.1	E980.7
Coumarin	964.2	E858.2	E934.2	E950.4	E962.0	E980.4
Coumetarol	964.2	E858.2	E934.2	E950.4	E962.0	E980.4
Cowbane	988.2	E865.4	—	E950.9	E962.1	E980.9
Cozyme	963.5	E858.1	E933.5	E950.4	E962.0	E980.4
Crack ●	970.8	E854.3	E940.8	E950.4	E962.0	E980.4
Creolin	983.0	E864.0	—	E950.7	E962.1	E980.6
disinfectant	983.0	E861.4	—	E950.7	E962.1	E980.6
Creosol (compound)	983.0	E864.0	—	E950.7	E962.1	E980.6
Creosote (beechwood) (coal tar)	983.0	E864.0	—	E950.7	E962.1	E980.6
medicinal (expectorant)	975.5	E858.6	E945.5	E950.4	E962.0	E980.4
syrup	975.5	E858.6	E945.5	E950.4	E962.0	E980.4
Cresol	983.0	E864.0	—	E950.7	E962.1	E980.6
disinfectant	983.0	E861.4	—	E950.7	E962.1	E980.6
Cresylic acid	983.0	E864.0	—	E950.7	E962.1	E980.6
Cropropamide	965.7	E850.7	E935.7	E950.0	E962.0	E980.0
with crotethamide	970.0	E854.3	E940.0	E950.4	E962.0	E980.4
Crotamiton	976.0	E858.7	E946.0	E950.4	E962.0	E980.4
Crotethamide	965.7	E850.7	E935.7	E950.0	E962.0	E980.0
with cropropamide	970.0	E854.3	E940.0	E950.4	E962.0	E980.4
Croton (oil)	973.1	E858.4	E943.1	E950.4	E962.0	E980.4
chloral	967.1	E852.0	E937.1	E950.2	E962.0	E980.2
Crude oil	981	E862.1	—	E950.9	E962.1	E980.9
Cryogenine	965.8	E850.8	E935.8	E950.0	E962.0	E980.0
Cryolite (pesticide)	989.4	E863.4	—	E950.6	E962.1	E980.7
Cryptenamine	972.6	E858.3	E942.6	E950.4	E962.0	E980.4
Crystal violet	976.0	E858.7	E946.0	E950.4	E962.0	E980.4
Cuckoopint	988.2	E865.4	—	E950.9	E962.1	E980.9
Cumetharol	964.2	E858.2	E934.2	E950.4	E962.0	E980.4
Cupric sulfate	973.6	E858.4	E943.6	E950.4	E962.0	E980.4
Cuprous sulfate	983.9	E864.3	—	E950.7	E962.1	E980.6
Curare, curarine	975.2	E858.6	E945.2	E950.4	E962.0	E980.4
Cyanic acid — *see* Cyanide(s)						
Cyanide(s) (compounds) (hydrogen) (potassium) (sodium) NEC	989.0	E866.8	—	E950.9	E962.1	E980.9
dust or gas (inhalation) NEC	987.7	E869.8	—	E952.8	E962.2	E982.8
fumigant	989.0	E863.8	—	E950.6	E962.1	E980.7
mercuric — *see* Mercury						
pesticide (dust) (fumes)	989.0	E863.4	—	E950.6	E962.1	E980.7
Cyanocobalamin	964.1	E858.2	E934.1	E950.4	E962.0	E980.4
Cyanogen (chloride) (gas) NEC	987.8	E869.8	—	E952.8	E962.2	E982.8
Cyclaine	968.5	E855.2	E938.5	E950.4	E962.0	E980.4
Cyclamen europaeum	988.2	E865.4	—	E950.9	E962.1	E980.9
Cyclandelate	972.5	E858.3	E942.5	E950.4	E962.0	E980.4
Cyclazocine	965.09	E850.2	E935.2	E950.0	E962.0	E980.0
Cyclizine	963.0	E858.1	E933.0	E950.4	E962.0	E980.4
Cyclobarbital, cyclobarbitone	967.0	E851	E937.0	E950.1	E962.0	E980.1
Cycloguanil	961.4	E857	E931.4	E950.4	E962.0	E980.4
Cyclohexane	982.0	E862.4	—	E950.9	E962.1	E980.9

	Poisoning	External Cause (E-Code)				
		Accident	Therapeutic Use	Suicide Attempt	Assault	Undetermined
Cyclohexanol	980.8	E860.8	—	E950.9	E962.1	E980.9
Cyclohexanone	982.8	E862.4	—	E950.9	E962.1	E980.9
Cyclomethycaine	968.5	E855.2	E938.5	E950.4	E962.0	E980.4
Cyclopentamine	971.2	E855.5	E941.2	E950.4	E962.0	E980.4
Cyclopenthiazide	974.3	E858.5	E944.3	E950.4	E962.0	E980.4
Cyclopentolate	971.1	E855.4	E941.1	E950.4	E962.0	E980.4
Cyclophosphamide	963.1	E858.1	E933.1	E950.4	E962.0	E980.4
Cyclopropane	968.2	E855.1	E938.2	E950.4	E962.0	E980.4
Cycloserine	960.6	E856	E930.6	E950.4	E962.0	E980.4
Cyclothiazide	974.3	E858.5	E944.3	E950.4	E962.0	E980.4
Cycrimine	966.4	E855.0	E936.4	E950.4	E962.0	E980.4
Cymarin	972.1	E858.3	E942.1	E950.4	E962.0	E980.4
Cyproheptadine	963.0	E858.1	E933.0	E950.4	E962.0	E980.4
Cyprolidol	969.0	E854.0	E939.0	E950.3	E962.0	E980.3
Cytarabine	963.1	E858.1	E933.1	E950.4	E962.0	E980.4
Cytisus						
laburnum	988.2	E865.4	—	E950.9	E962.1	E980.9
scoparius	988.2	E865.4	—	E950.9	E962.1	E980.9
Cytomel	962.7	E858.0	E932.7	E950.4	E962.0	E980.4
Cytosine (antineoplastic)	963.1	E858.1	E933.1	E950.4	E962.0	E980.4
Cytoxan	963.1	E858.1	E933.1	E950.4	E962.0	E980.4
Dacarbazine	963.1	E858.1	E933.1	E950.4	E962.0	E980.4
Dactinomycin	960.7	E856	E930.7	E950.4	E962.0	E980.4
DADPS	961.8	E857	E931.8	E950.4	E962.0	E980.4
Dakin's solution (external)	976.0	E858.7	E946.0	E950.4	E962.0	E980.4
Dalmane	969.4	E853.2	E939.4	E950.3	E962.0	E980.3
DAM	977.2	E858.8	E947.2	E950.4	E962.0	E980.4
Danilone	964.2	E858.2	E934.2	E950.4	E962.0	E980.4
Danthron	973.1	E858.4	E943.1	E950.4	E962.0	E980.4
Dantrolene	975.2	E858.6	E945.2	E950.4	E962.0	E980.4
Daphne (gnidium) (mezereum)	988.2	E865.4	—	E950.9	E962.1	E980.9
berry	988.2	E865.3	—	E950.9	E962.1	E980.9
Dapsone	961.8	E857	E931.8	E950.4	E962.0	E980.4
Daraprim	961.4	E857	E931.4	E950.4	E962.0	E980.4
Darnel	988.2	E865.3	—	E950.9	E962.1	E980.9
Darvon	965.8	E850.8	E935.8	E950.0	E962.0	E980.0
Daunorubicin	960.7	E856	E930.7	E950.4	E962.0	E980.4
DBI	962.3	E858.0	E932.3	E950.4	E962.0	E980.4
D-Con (rodenticide)	989.4	E863.7	—	E950.6	E962.1	E980.7
DDS	961.8	E857	E931.8	E950.4	E962.0	E980.4
DDT	989.2	E863.0	—	E950.6	E962.1	E980.7
Deadly nightshade	988.2	E865.4	—	E950.9	E962.1	E980.9
berry	988.2	E865.3	—	E950.9	E962.1	E980.9
Deanol	969.7	E854.2	E939.7	E950.3	E962.0	E980.3
Debrisoquine	972.6	E858.3	E942.6	E950.4	E962.0	E980.4
Decaborane	989.89	E866.8	—	E950.9	E962.1	E980.9
fumes	987.8	E869.8	—	E952.8	E962.2	E982.8
Decadron	962.0	E858.0	E932.0	E950.4	E962.0	E980.4
ENT agent	976.6	E858.7	E946.6	E950.4	E962.0	E980.4
ophthalmic preparation	976.5	E858.7	E946.5	E950.4	E962.0	E980.4
topical NEC	976.0	E858.7	E946.0	E950.4	E962.0	E980.4
Decahydronaphthalene	982.0	E862.4	—	E950.9	E962.1	E980.9
Decalin	982.0	E862.4	—	E950.9	E962.1	E980.9
Decamethonium	975.2	E858.6	E945.2	E950.4	E962.0	E980.4
Decholin	973.4	E858.4	E943.4	E950.4	E962.0	E980.4
sodium (diagnostic)	977.8	E858.8	E947.8	E950.4	E962.0	E980.4
Declomycin	960.4	E856	E930.4	E950.4	E962.0	E980.4
Deferoxamine	963.8	E858.1	E933.8	E950.4	E962.0	E980.4
Dehydrocholic acid	973.4	E858.4	E943.4	E950.4	E962.0	E980.4
DeKalin	982.0	E862.4	—	E950.9	E962.1	E980.9
Delalutin	962.2	E858.0	E932.2	E950.4	E962.0	E980.4
Delphinium	988.2	E865.3	—	E950.9	E962.1	E980.9
Deltasone	962.0	E858.0	E932.0	E950.4	E962.0	E980.4
Deltra	962.0	E858.0	E932.0	E950.4	E962.0	E980.4
Delvinal	967.0	E851	E937.0	E950.1	E962.0	E980.1
Demecarium (bromide)	971.0	E855.3	E941.0	E950.4	E962.0	E980.4
Demeclocycline	960.4	E856	E930.4	E950.4	E962.0	E980.4
Demecolcine	963.1	E858.1	E933.1	E950.4	E962.0	E980.4
Demelanizing agents	976.8	E858.7	E946.8	E950.4	E962.0	E980.4
Demerol	965.09	E850.2	E935.2	E950.0	E962.0	E980.0
Demethylchlortetracycline	960.4	E856	E930.4	E950.4	E962.0	E980.4
Demethyltetracycline	960.4	E856	E930.4	E950.4	E962.0	E980.4
Demeton	989.3	E863.1	—	E950.6	E962.1	E980.7
Demulcents	976.3	E858.7	E946.3	E950.4	E962.0	E980.4
Demulen	962.2	E858.0	E932.2	E950.4	E962.0	E980.4
Denatured alcohol	980.0	E860.1	—	E950.9	E962.1	E980.9
Dendrid	976.5	E858.7	E946.5	E950.4	E962.0	E980.4
Dental agents, topical	976.7	E858.7	E946.7	E950.4	E962.0	E980.4
Deodorant spray (feminine hygiene)	976.8	E858.7	E946.8	E950.4	E962.0	E980.4
Deoxyribonuclease	963.4	E858.1	E933.4	E950.4	E962.0	E980.4

✔4ᵗʰ Fourth-digit Required	✔5ᵗʰ Fifth-digit Required	►◄ Revised Text	● New Line	▲ Revised Code

	Poisoning	External Cause (E-Code)				
		Accident	Therapeutic Use	Suicide Attempt	Assault	Undetermined
Depressants						
appetite, central	977.0	E858.8	E947.0	E950.4	E962.0	E980.4
cardiac	972.0	E858.3	E942.0	E950.4	E962.0	E980.4
central nervous system (anesthetic)	968.4	E855.1	E938.4	E950.4	E962.0	E980.4
psychotherapeutic	969.5	E853.9	E939.5	E950.3	E962.0	E980.3
Dequalinium	976.0	E858.7	E946.0	E950.4	E962.0	E980.4
Dermolate	976.2	E858.7	E946.2	E950.4	E962.0	E980.4
DES	962.2	E858.0	E932.2	E950.4	E962.0	E980.4
Desenex	976.0	E858.7	E946.0	E950.4	E962.0	E980.4
Deserpidine	972.6	E858.3	E942.6	E950.4	E962.0	E980.4
Desipramine	969.0	E854.0	E939.0	E950.3	E962.0	E980.3
Deslanoside	972.1	E858.3	E942.1	E950.4	E962.0	E980.4
Desocodeine	965.09	E850.2	E935.2	E950.0	E962.0	E980.0
Desomorphine	965.09	E850.2	E935.2	E950.0	E962.0	E980.0
Desonide	976.0	E858.7	E946.0	E950.4	E962.0	E980.4
Desoxycorticosterone derivatives	962.0	E858.0	E932.0	E950.4	E962.0	E980.4
Desoxyephedrine	969.7	E854.2	E939.7	E950.3	E962.0	E980.3
DET	969.6	E854.1	E939.6	E950.3	E962.0	E980.3
Detergents (ingested) (synthetic)	989.6	E861.0	—	E950.9	E962.1	E980.9
external medication	976.2	E858.7	E946.2	E950.4	E962.0	E980.4
Deterrent, alcohol	977.3	E858.8	E947.3	E950.4	E962.0	E980.4
Detrothyronine	962.7	E858.0	E932.7	E950.4	E962.0	E980.4
Dettol (external medication)	976.0	E858.7	E946.0	E950.4	E962.0	E980.4
Dexamethasone	962.0	E858.0	E932.0	E950.4	E962.0	E980.4
ENT agent	976.6	E858.7	E946.6	E950.4	E962.0	E980.4
ophthalmic preparation	976.5	E858.7	E946.5	E950.4	E962.0	E980.4
topical NEC	976.0	E858.7	E946.0	E950.4	E962.0	E980.4
Dexamphetamine	969.7	E854.2	E939.7	E950.3	E962.0	E980.3
Dexedrine	969.7	E854.2	E939.7	E950.3	E962.0	E980.3
Dexpanthenol	963.5	E858.1	E933.5	E950.4	E962.0	E980.4
Dextran	964.8	E858.2	E934.8	E950.4	E962.0	E980.4
Dextriferron	964.0	E858.2	E934.0	E950.4	E962.0	E980.4
Dextroamphetamine	969.7	E854.2	E939.7	E950.3	E962.0	E980.3
Dextro calcium pantothenate	963.5	E858.1	E933.5	E950.4	E962.0	E980.4
Dextromethorphan	975.4	E858.6	E945.4	E950.4	E962.0	E980.4
Dextromoramide	965.09	E850.2	E935.2	E950.0	E962.0	E980.0
Dextro pantothenyl alcohol	963.5	E858.1	E933.5	E950.4	E962.0	E980.4
topical	976.8	E858.7	E946.8	E950.4	E962.0	E980.4
Dextropropoxyphene (hydrochloride)	965.8	E850.8	E935.8	E950.0	E962.0	E980.0
Dextrorphan	965.09	E850.2	E935.2	E950.0	E962.0	E980.0
Dextrose NEC	974.5	E858.5	E944.5	E950.4	E962.0	E980.4
Dextrothyroxin	962.7	E858.0	E932.7	E950.4	E962.0	E980.4
DFP	971.0	E855.3	E941.0	E950.4	E962.0	E980.4
DHE-45	972.9	E858.3	E942.9	E950.4	E962.0	E980.4
Diabinese	962.3	E858.0	E932.3	E950.4	E962.0	E980.4
Diacetyl monoxime	977.2	E858.8	E947.2	E950.4	E962.0	E980.4
Diacetylmorphine	965.01	E850.0	E935.0	E950.0	E962.0	E980.0
Diagnostic agents	977.8	E858.8	E947.8	E950.4	E962.0	E980.4
Dial (soap)	976.2	E858.7	E946.2	E950.4	E962.0	E980.4
sedative	967.0	E851	E937.0	E950.1	E962.0	E980.1
Diallylbarbituric acid	967.0	E851	E937.0	E950.1	E962.0	E980.1
Diaminodiphenylsulfone	961.8	E857	E931.8	E950.4	E962.0	E980.4
Diamorphine	965.01	E850.0	E935.0	E950.0	E962.0	E980.0
Diamox	974.2	E858.5	E944.2	E950.4	E962.0	E980.4
Diamthazole	976.0	E858.7	E946.0	E950.4	E962.0	E980.4
Diaphenylsulfone	961.8	E857	E931.8	E950.4	E962.0	E980.4
Diasone (sodium)	961.8	E857	E931.8	E950.4	E962.0	E980.4
Diazepam	969.4	E853.2	E939.4	E950.3	E962.0	E980.3
Diazinon	989.3	E863.1	—	E950.6	E962.1	E980.7
Diazomethane (gas)	987.8	E869.8	—	E952.8	E962.2	E982.8
Diazoxide	972.5	E858.3	E942.5	E950.4	E962.0	E980.4
Dibenamine	971.3	E855.6	E941.3	E950.4	E962.0	E980.4
Dibenzheptropine	963.0	E858.1	E933.0	E950.4	E962.0	E980.4
Dibenzyline	971.3	E855.6	E941.3	E950.4	E962.0	E980.4
Diborane (gas)	987.8	E869.8	—	E952.8	E962.2	E982.8
Dibromomannitol	963.1	E858.1	E933.1	E950.4	E962.0	E980.4
Dibucaine (spinal)	968.7	E855.2	E938.7	E950.4	E962.0	E980.4
topical (surface)	968.5	E855.2	E938.5	E950.4	E962.0	E980.4
Dibunate sodium	975.4	E858.6	E945.4	E950.4	E962.0	E980.4
Dibutoline	971.1	E855.4	E941.1	E950.4	E962.0	E980.4
Dicapthon	989.4	E863.4	—	E950.6	E962.1	E980.7
Dichloralphenazone	967.1	E852.0	E937.1	E950.2	E962.0	E980.2
Dichlorodifluoromethane	987.4	E869.2	—	E952.8	E962.2	E982.8
Dichloroethane	982.3	E862.4	—	E950.9	E962.1	E980.9
Dichloroethylene	982.3	E862.4	—	E950.9	E962.1	E980.9
Dichloroethyl sulfide	987.8	E869.8	—	E952.8	E962.2	E982.8
Dichlorohydrin	982.3	E862.4	—	E950.9	E962.1	E980.9
Dichloromethane (solvent) (vapor)	982.3	E862.4	—	E950.9	E962.1	E980.9
Dichlorophen(e)	961.6	E857	E931.6	E950.4	E962.0	E980.4
Dichlorphenamide	974.2	E858.5	E944.2	E950.4	E962.0	E980.4
Dichlorvos	989.3	E863.1	—	E950.6	E962.1	E980.7

4ᵗʰ Fourth-digit Required   5ᵗʰ Fifth-digit Required   ▶◀ Revised Text   ● New Line   ▲ Revised Code

		External Cause (E-Code)				
	Poisoning	Accident	Therapeutic Use	Suicide Attempt	Assault	Undetermined
Diclofenac sodium	965.69	E850.6	E935.6	E950.0	E962.0	E980.0
Dicoumarin, dicumarol	964.2	E858.2	E934.2	E950.0	E962.0	E980.0
Dicyanogen (gas)	987.8	E869.8	—	E952.8	E962.2	E982.8
Dicyclomine	971.1	E855.4	E941.1	E950.4	E962.0	E980.4
Dieldrin (vapor)	989.2	E863.0	—	E950.6	E962.1	E980.7
Dienestrol	962.2	E858.0	E932.2	E950.4	E962.0	E980.4
Dietetics	977.0	E858.8	E947.0	E950.4	E962.0	E980.4
Diethazine	966.4	E855.0	E936.4	E950.4	E962.0	E980.4
Diethyl						
barbituric acid	967.0	E851	E937.0	E950.1	E962.0	E980.1
carbamazine	961.6	E857	E931.6	E950.4	E962.0	E980.4
carbinol	980.8	E860.8	—	E950.9	E962.1	E980.9
carbonate	982.8	E862.4	—	E950.9	E962.1	E980.9
ether (vapor) — see Ether(s)						
propion	977.0	E858.8	E947.0	E950.4	E962.0	E980.4
stilbestrol	962.2	E858.0	E932.2	E950.4	E962.0	E980.4
Diethylene						
dioxide	982.8	E862.4	—	E950.9	E962.1	E980.9
glycol (monoacetate) (monoethyl ether)	982.8	E862.4	—	E950.9	E962.1	E980.9
Diethylsulfone-diethylmethane	967.8	E852.8	E937.8	E950.2	E962.0	E980.2
Difencloxazine	965.09	E850.2	E935.2	E950.0	E962.0	E980.0
Diffusin	963.4	E858.1	E933.4	E950.4	E962.0	E980.4
Diflos	971.0	E855.3	E941.0	E950.4	E962.0	E980.4
Digestants	973.4	E858.4	E943.4	E950.4	E962.0	E980.4
Digitalin(e)	972.1	E858.3	E942.1	E950.4	E962.0	E980.4
Digitalis glycosides	972.1	E858.3	E942.1	E950.4	E962.0	E980.4
Digitoxin	972.1	E858.3	E942.1	E950.4	E962.0	E980.4
Digoxin	972.1	E858.3	E942.1	E950.4	E962.0	E980.4
Dihydrocodeine	965.09	E850.2	E935.2	E950.0	E962.0	E980.0
Dihydrocodeinone	965.09	E850.2	E935.2	E950.0	E962.0	E980.0
Dihydroergocristine	972.9	E858.3	E942.9	E950.4	E962.0	E980.4
Dihydroergotamine	972.9	E858.3	E942.9	E950.4	E962.0	E980.4
Dihydroergotoxine	972.9	E858.3	E942.9	E950.4	E962.0	E980.4
Dihydrohydroxycodeinone	965.09	E850.2	E935.2	E950.0	E962.0	E980.0
Dihydrohydroxymorphinone	965.09	E850.2	E935.2	E950.0	E962.0	E980.0
Dihydroisocodeine	965.09	E850.2	E935.2	E950.0	E962.0	E980.0
Dihydromorphine	965.09	E850.2	E935.2	E950.0	E962.0	E980.0
Dihydromorphinone	965.09	E850.2	E935.2	E950.0	E962.0	E980.0
Dihydrostreptomycin	960.6	E856	E930.6	E950.4	E962.0	E980.4
Dihydrotachysterol	962.6	E858.0	E932.6	E950.4	E962.0	E980.4
Dihydroxyanthraquinone	973.1	E858.4	E943.1	E950.4	E962.0	E980.4
Dihydroxycodeinone	965.09	E850.2	E935.2	E950.0	E962.0	E980.0
Diiodohydroxyquin	961.3	E857	E931.3	E950.4	E962.0	E980.4
topical	976.0	E858.7	E946.0	E950.4	E962.0	E980.4
Diiodohydroxyquinoline	961.3	E857	E931.3	E950.4	E962.0	E980.4
Dilantin	966.1	E855.0	E936.1	E950.4	E962.0	E980.4
Dilaudid	965.09	E850.2	E935.2	E950.0	E962.0	E980.0
Diloxanide	961.5	E857	E931.5	E950.4	E962.0	E980.4
Dimefline	970.0	E854.3	E940.0	E950.4	E962.0	E980.4
Dimenhydrinate	963.0	E858.1	E933.0	E950.4	E962.0	E980.4
Dimercaprol	963.8	E858.1	E933.8	E950.4	E962.0	E980.4
Dimercaptopropanol	963.8	E858.1	E933.8	E950.4	E962.0	E980.4
Dimetane	963.0	E858.1	E933.0	E950.4	E962.0	E980.4
Dimethicone	976.3	E858.7	E946.3	E950.4	E962.0	E980.4
Dimethindene	963.0	E858.1	E933.0	E950.4	E962.0	E980.4
Dimethisoquin	968.5	E855.2	E938.5	E950.4	E962.0	E980.4
Dimethisterone	962.2	E858.0	E932.2	E950.4	E962.0	E980.4
Dimethoxanate	975.4	E858.6	E945.4	E950.4	E962.0	E980.4
Dimethyl						
arsine, arsinic acid — see Arsenic						
carbinol	980.2	E860.3	—	E950.9	E962.1	E980.9
diguanide	962.3	E858.0	E932.3	E950.4	E962.0	E980.4
ketone	982.8	E862.4	—	E950.9	E962.1	E980.9
vapor	987.8	E869.8	—	E952.8	E962.2	E982.8
meperidine	965.09	E850.2	E935.2	E950.0	E962.0	E980.0
parathion	989.3	E863.1	—	E950.6	E962.1	E980.7
polysiloxane	973.8	E858.4	E943.8	E950.4	E962.0	E980.4
sulfate (fumes)	987.8	E869.8	—	E952.8	E962.2	E982.8
liquid	983.9	E864.3	—	E950.7	E962.1	E980.6
sulfoxide NEC	982.8	E862.4	—	E950.9	E962.1	E980.9
medicinal	976.4	E858.7	E946.4	E950.4	E962.0	E980.4
triptamine	969.6	E854.1	E939.6	E950.3	E962.0	E980.3
tubocurarine	975.2	E858.6	E945.2	E950.4	E962.0	E980.4
Dindevan	964.2	E858.2	E934.2	E950.4	E962.0	E980.4
Dinitro (-ortho-) cresol (herbicide) (spray)	989.4	E863.5	—	E950.6	E962.1	E980.7
insecticide	989.4	E863.4	—	E950.6	E962.1	E980.7
Dinitrobenzene	983.0	E864.0	—	E950.7	E962.1	E980.6
vapor	987.8	E869.8	—	E952.8	E962.2	E982.8
Dinitro-orthocresol (herbicide)	989.4	E863.5	—	E950.6	E962.1	E980.7
insecticide	989.4	E863.4	—	E950.6	E962.1	E980.7

	Poisoning	External Cause (E-Code)				
		Accident	Therapeutic Use	Suicide Attempt	Assault	Undetermined
Dinitrophenol (herbicide) (spray)	989.4	E863.5	—	E950.6	E962.1	E980.7
insecticide	989.4	E863.4	—	E950.6	E962.1	E980.7
Dinoprost	975.0	E858.6	E945.0	E950.4	E962.0	E980.4
Dioctyl sulfosuccinate (calcium) (sodium)	973.2	E858.4	E943.2	E950.4	E962.0	E980.4
Diodoquin	961.3	E857	E931.3	E950.4	E962.0	E980.4
Dione derivatives NEC	966.3	E855.0	E936.3	E950.4	E962.0	E980.4
Dionin	965.09	E850.2	E935.2	E950.0	E962.0	E980.0
Dioxane	982.8	E862.4	—	E950.9	E962.1	E980.9
Dioxin — *see* Herbicide						
Dioxyline	972.5	E858.3	E942.5	E950.4	E962.0	E980.4
Dipentene	982.8	E862.4	—	E950.9	E962.1	E980.9
Diphemanil	971.1	E855.4	E941.1	E950.4	E962.0	E980.4
Diphenadione	964.2	E858.2	E934.2	E950.4	E962.0	E980.4
Diphenhydramine	963.0	E858.1	E933.0	E950.4	E962.0	E980.4
Diphenidol	963.0	E858.1	E933.0	E950.4	E962.0	E980.4
Diphenoxylate	973.5	E858.4	E943.5	E950.4	E962.0	E980.4
Diphenylchloroarsine	985.1	E866.3	—	E950.8	E962.1	E980.8
Diphenylhydantoin (sodium)	966.1	E855.0	E936.1	E950.4	E962.0	E980.4
Diphenylpyraline	963.0	E858.1	E933.0	E950.4	E962.0	E980.4
Diphtheria						
antitoxin	979.9	E858.8	E949.9	E950.4	E962.0	E980.4
toxoid	978.5	E858.8	E948.5	E950.4	E962.0	E980.4
with tetanus toxoid	978.9	E858.8	E948.9	E950.4	E962.0	E980.4
with pertussis component	978.6	E858.8	E948.6	E950.4	E962.0	E980.4
vaccine	978.5	E858.8	E948.5	E950.4	E962.0	E980.4
Dipipanone	965.09	E850.2	E935.2	E950.0	E962.0	E980.0
Diplovax	979.5	E858.8	E949.5	E950.4	E962.0	E980.4
Diprophylline	975.1	E858.6	E945.1	E950.4	E962.0	E980.4
Dipyridamole	972.4	E858.3	E942.4	E950.4	E962.0	E980.4
Dipyrone	965.5	E850.5	E935.5	E950.0	E962.0	E980.0
Diquat	989.4	E863.5	—	E950.6	E962.1	E980.7
Disinfectant NEC	983.9	E861.4	—	E950.7	E962.1	E980.6
alkaline	983.2	E861.4	—	E950.7	E962.1	E980.6
aromatic	983.0	E861.4	—	E950.7	E962.1	E980.6
Disipal	966.4	E855.0	E936.4	E950.4	E962.0	E980.4
Disodium edetate	963.8	E858.1	E933.8	E950.4	E962.0	E980.4
Disulfamide	974.4	E858.5	E944.4	E950.4	E962.0	E980.4
Disulfanilamide	961.0	E857	E931.0	E950.4	E962.0	E980.4
Disulfiram	977.3	E858.8	E947.3	E950.4	E962.0	E980.4
Dithiazanine	961.6	E857	E931.6	E950.4	E962.0	E980.4
Dithioglycerol	963.8	E858.1	E933.8	E950.4	E962.0	E980.4
Dithranol	976.4	E858.7	E946.4	E950.4	E962.0	E980.4
Diucardin	974.3	E858.5	E944.3	E950.4	E962.0	E980.4
Diupres	974.3	E858.5	E944.3	E950.4	E962.0	E980.4
Diuretics NEC	974.4	E858.5	E944.4	E950.4	E962.0	E980.4
carbonic acid anhydrase inhibitors	974.2	E858.5	E944.2	E950.4	E962.0	E980.4
mercurial	974.0	E858.5	E944.0	E950.4	E962.0	E980.4
osmotic	974.4	E858.5	E944.4	E950.4	E962.0	E980.4
purine derivatives	974.1	E858.5	E944.1	E950.4	E962.0	E980.4
saluretic	974.3	E858.5	E944.3	E950.4	E962.0	E980.4
Diuril	974.3	E858.5	E944.3	E950.4	E962.0	E980.4
Divinyl ether	968.2	E855.1	E938.2	E950.4	E962.0	E980.4
D-lysergic acid diethylamide	969.6	E854.1	E939.6	E950.3	E962.0	E980.3
DMCT	960.4	E856	E930.4	E950.4	E962.0	E980.4
DMSO	982.8	E862.4	—	E950.9	E962.1	E980.9
DMT	969.6	E854.1	E939.6	E950.3	E962.0	E980.3
DNOC	989.4	E863.5	—	E950.6	E962.1	E980.7
DOCA	962.0	E858.0	E932.0	E950.4	E962.0	E980.4
Dolophine	965.02	E850.1	E935.1	E950.0	E962.0	E980.0
Doloxene	965.8	E850.8	E935.8	E950.0	E962.0	E980.0
DOM	969.6	E854.1	E939.6	E950.3	E962.0	E980.3
Domestic gas — *see* Gas, utility						
Domiphen (bromide) (lozenges)	976.6	E858.7	E946.6	E950.4	E962.0	E980.4
Dopa (levo)	966.4	E855.0	E936.4	E950.4	E962.0	E980.4
Dopamine	971.2	E855.5	E941.2	E950.4	E962.0	E980.4
Doriden	967.5	E852.4	E937.5	E950.2	E962.0	E980.2
Dormiral	967.0	E851	E937.0	E950.1	E962.0	E980.1
Dormison	967.8	E852.8	E937.8	E950.2	E962.0	E980.2
Dornase	963.4	E858.1	E933.4	E950.4	E962.0	E980.4
Dorsacaine	968.5	E855.2	E938.5	E950.4	E962.0	E980.4
Dothiepin hydrochloride	969.0	E854.0	E939.0	E950.3	E962.0	E980.3
Doxapram	970.0	E854.3	E940.0	E950.4	E962.0	E980.4
Doxepin	969.0	E854.0	E939.0	E950.3	E962.0	E980.3
Doxorubicin	960.7	E856	E930.7	E950.4	E962.0	E980.4
Doxycycline	960.4	E856	E930.4	E950.4	E962.0	E980.4
Doxylamine	963.0	E858.1	E933.0	E950.4	E962.0	E980.4
Dramamine	963.0	E858.1	E933.0	E950.4	E962.0	E980.4
Drano (drain cleaner)	983.2	E864.2	—	E950.7	E962.1	E980.6
Dromoran	965.09	E850.2	E935.2	E950.0	E962.0	E980.0
Dromostanolone	962.1	E858.0	E932.1	E950.4	E962.0	E980.4
Droperidol	969.2	E853.1	E939.2	E950.3	E962.0	E980.3

Drug	Poisoning	External Cause (E-Code)				
		Accident	Therapeutic Use	Suicide Attempt	Assault	Undetermined
Drug						
specified NEC	977.9	E858.9	E947.9	E950.5	E962.0	E980.5
AHFS List	977.8	E858.8	E947.8	E950.4	E962.0	E980.4
4:00 antihistamine drugs	963.0	E858.1	E933.0	E950.4	E962.0	E980.4
8:04 amebacides	961.5	E857	E931.5	E950.4	E962.0	E980.4
arsenical anti-infectives	961.1	E857	E931.1	E950.4	E962.0	E980.4
quinoline derivatives	961.3	E857	E931.3	E950.4	E962.0	E980.4
8:08 anthelmintics	961.6	E857	E931.6	E950.4	E962.0	E980.4
quinoline derivatives	961.3	E857	E931.3	E950.4	E962.0	E980.4
8:12.04 antifungal antibiotics	960.1	E856	E930.1	E950.4	E962.0	E980.4
8:12.06 cephalosporins	960.5	E856	E930.5	E950.4	E962.0	E980.4
8:12.08 chloramphenicol	960.2	E856	E930.2	E950.4	E962.0	E980.4
8:12.12 erythromycins	960.3	E856	E930.3	E950.4	E962.0	E980.4
8:12.16 penicillins	960.0	E856	E930.0	E950.4	E962.0	E980.4
8:12.20 streptomycins	960.6	E856	E930.6	E950.4	E962.0	E980.4
8:12.24 tetracyclines	960.4	E856	E930.4	E950.4	E962.0	E980.4
8:12.28 other antibiotics	960.8	E856	E930.8	E950.4	E962.0	E980.4
antimycobacterial	960.6	E856	E930.6	E950.4	E962.0	E980.4
macrolides	960.3	E856	E930.3	E950.4	E962.0	E980.4
8:16 antituberculars	961.8	E857	E931.8	E950.4	E962.0	E980.4
antibiotics	960.6	E856	E930.6	E950.4	E962.0	E980.4
8:18 antivirals	961.7	E857	E931.7	E950.4	E962.0	E980.4
8:20 plasmodicides (antimalarials)	961.4	E857	E931.4	E950.4	E962.0	E980.4
8:24 sulfonamides	961.0	E857	E931.0	E950.4	E962.0	E980.4
8:26 sulfones	961.8	E857	E931.8	E950.4	E962.0	E980.4
8:28 treponemicides	961.2	E857	E931.2	E950.4	E962.0	E980.4
8:32 trichomonacides	961.5	E857	E931.5	E950.4	E962.0	E980.4
quinoline derivatives	961.3	E857	E931.3	E950.4	E962.0	E980.4
nitrofuran derivatives	961.9	E857	E931.9	E950.4	E962.0	E980.4
8:36 urinary germicides	961.9	E857	E931.9	E950.4	E962.0	E980.4
quinoline derivatives	961.3	E857	E931.3	E950.4	E962.0	E980.4
8:40 other anti-infectives	961.9	E857	E931.9	E950.4	E962.0	E980.4
10:00 antineoplastic agents	963.1	E858.1	E933.1	E950.4	E962.0	E980.4
antibiotics	960.7	E856	E930.7	E950.4	E962.0	E980.4
progestogens	962.2	E858.0	E932.2	E950.4	E962.0	E980.4
12:04 parasympathomimetic (cholinergic) agents	971.0	E855.3	E941.0	E950.4	E962.0	E980.4
12:08 parasympatholytic (cholinergic-blocking) agents	971.1	E855.4	E941.1	E950.4	E962.0	E980.4
12:12 Sympathomimetic (adrenergic) agents	971.2	E855.5	E941.2	E950.4	E962.0	E980.4
12:16 sympatholytic (adrenergic-blocking) agents	971.3	E855.6	E941.3	E950.4	E962.0	E980.4
12:20 skeletal muscle relaxants						
central nervous system muscle-tone depressants	968.0	E855.1	E938.0	E950.4	E962.0	E980.4
myoneural blocking agents	975.2	E858.6	E945.2	E950.4	E962.0	E980.4
16:00 blood derivatives	964.7	E858.2	E934.7	E950.4	E962.0	E980.4
20:04 antianemia drugs	964.1	E858.2	E934.1	E950.4	E962.0	E980.4
20:04.04 iron preparations	964.0	E858.2	E934.0	E950.4	E962.0	E980.4
20:04.08 liver and stomach preparations	964.1	E858.2	E934.1	E950.4	E962.0	E980.4
20:12.04 anticoagulants	964.2	E858.2	E934.2	E950.4	E962.0	E980.4
20:12.08 antiheparin agents	964.5	E858.2	E934.5	E950.4	E962.0	E980.4
20:12.12 coagulants	964.5	E858.2	E934.5	E950.4	E962.0	E980.4
20:12.16 hemostatics NEC	964.5	E858.2	E934.5	E950.4	E962.0	E980.4
capillary active drugs	972.8	E858.3	E942.8	E950.4	E962.0	E980.4
24:04 cardiac drugs	972.9	E858.3	E942.9	E950.4	E962.0	E980.4
cardiotonic agents	972.1	E858.3	E942.1	E950.4	E962.0	E980.4
rhythm regulators	972.0	E858.3	E942.0	E950.4	E962.0	E980.4
24:06 antilipemic agents	972.2	E858.3	E942.2	E950.4	E962.0	E980.4
thyroid derivatives	962.7	E858.0	E932.7	E950.4	E962.0	E980.4
24:08 hypotensive agents	972.6	E858.3	E942.6	E950.4	E962.0	E980.4
adrenergic blocking agents	971.3	E855.6	E941.3	E950.4	E962.0	E980.4
ganglion blocking agents	972.3	E858.3	E942.3	E950.4	E962.0	E980.4
vasodilators	972.5	E858.3	E942.5	E950.4	E962.0	E980.4
24:12 vasodilating agents NEC	972.5	E858.3	E942.5	E950.4	E962.0	E980.4
coronary	972.4	E858.3	E942.4	E950.4	E962.0	E980.4
nicotinic acid derivatives	972.2	E858.3	E942.2	E950.4	E962.0	E980.4
24:16 sclerosing agents	972.7	E858.3	E942.7	E950.4	E962.0	E980.4
28:04 general anesthetics	968.4	E855.1	E938.4	E950.4	E962.0	E980.4
gaseous anesthetics	968.2	E855.1	E938.2	E950.4	E962.0	E980.4
halothane	968.1	E855.1	E938.1	E950.4	E962.0	E980.4
intravenous anesthetics	968.3	E855.1	E938.3	E950.4	E962.0	E980.4
28:08 analgesics and antipyretics	965.9	E850.9	E935.9	E950.0	E962.0	E980.0
antirheumatics	965.69	E850.6	E935.6	E950.0	E962.0	E980.0
aromatic analgesics	965.4	E850.4	E935.4	E950.0	E962.0	E980.0
non-narcotic NEC	965.7	E850.7	E935.7	E950.0	E962.0	E980.0
opium alkaloids	965.00	E850.2	E935.2	E950.0	E962.0	E980.0
heroin	965.01	E850.0	E935.0	E950.0	E962.0	E980.0
methadone	965.02	E850.1	E935.1	E950.0	E962.0	E980.0
specified type NEC	965.09	E850.2	E935.2	E950.0	E962.0	E980.0
pyrazole derivatives	965.5	E850.5	E935.5	E950.0	E962.0	E980.0
salicylates	965.1	E850.3	E935.3	E950.0	E962.0	E980.0
specified NEC	965.8	E850.8	E935.8	E950.0	E962.0	E980.0
28:10 narcotic antagonists	970.1	E854.3	E940.1	E950.4	E962.0	E980.4

		External Cause (E-Code)				
	Poisoning	Accident	Therapeutic Use	Suicide Attempt	Assault	Undetermined
Drug — *continued*	966.3	E855.0	E936.3	E950.4	E962.0	E980.4
28:12 anticonvulsants	967.0	E851	E937.0	E950.1	E962.0	E980.1
barbiturates	969.4	E853.2	E939.4	E950.3	E962.0	E980.3
benzodiazepine-based tranquilizers	967.3	E852.2	E937.3	E950.2	E962.0	E980.2
bromides	966.1	E855.0	E936.1	E950.4	E962.0	E980.4
hydantoin derivatives	966.0	E855.0	E936.0	E950.4	E962.0	E980.4
oxazolidine (derivatives)	966.2	E855.0	E936.2	E950.4	E962.0	E980.4
succinimides	969.0	E854.0	E939.0	E950.3	E962.0	E980.3
28:16.04 antidepressants	969.5	E853.9	E939.5	E950.3	E962.0	E980.3
28:16.08 tranquilizers	969.4	E853.2	E939.4	E950.3	E962.0	E980.3
benzodiazepine-based	969.2	E853.1	E939.2	E950.3	E962.0	E980.3
butyrophenone-based	969.3	E853.8	E939.3	E950.3	E962.0	E980.3
major NEC	969.1	E853.0	E939.1	E950.3	E962.0	E980.3
phenothiazine-based	969.8	E855.8	E939.8	E950.3	E962.0	E980.4
28:16.12 other psychotherapeutic agents	970.9	E854.3	E940.9	E950.4	E962.0	E980.4
28:20 respiratory and cerebral stimulants	970.0	E854.3	E940.0	E950.4	E962.0	E980.4
analeptics	977.0	E858.8	E947.0	E950.4	E962.0	E980.4
anorexigenic agents	969.7	E854.2	E939.7	E950.3	E962.0	E980.3
psychostimulants	970.8	E854.3	E940.8	E950.4	E962.0	E980.4
specified NEC	967.9	E852.9	E937.9	E950.2	E962.0	E980.2
28:24 sedatives and hypnotics	967.0	E851	E937.0	E950.1	E962.0	E980.1
barbiturates	969.4	E853.2	E939.4	E950.3	E962.0	E980.3
benzodiazepine-based tranquilizers	967.1	E852.0	E937.1	E950.2	E962.0	E980.2
chloral hydrate (group)	967.5	E852.4	E937.5	E950.2	E962.0	E980.2
glutethamide group	968.3	E855.1	E938.3	E950.4	E962.0	E980.4
intravenous anesthetics	967.4	E852.3	E937.4	E950.2	E962.0	E980.2
methaqualone (compounds)	967.2	E852.1	E937.2	E950.2	E962.0	E980.2
paraldehyde	969.1	E853.0	E939.1	E950.3	E962.0	E980.3
phenothiazine-based tranquilizers	967.8	E852.8	E937.8	E950.2	E962.0	E980.2
specified NEC	968.3	E855.1	E938.3	E950.4	E962.0	E980.4
thiobarbiturates	969.5	E853.9	E939.5	E950.3	E962.0	E980.3
tranquilizer NEC	977.8	E858.8	E947.8	E950.4	E962.0	E980.4
36:04 to 36:88 diagnostic agents	974.5	E858.5	E944.5	E950.4	E962.0	E980.4
40:00 electrolyte, caloric, and water balance agents NEC	963.2	E858.1	E933.2	E950.4	E962.0	E980.4
40:04 acidifying agents	963.3	E858.1	E933.3	E950.4	E962.0	E980.4
40:08 alkalinizing agents	974.5	E858.5	E944.5	E950.4	E962.0	E980.4
40:10 ammonia detoxicants	974.5	E858.5	E944.5	E950.4	E962.0	E980.4
40:12 replacement solutions	964.8	E858.2	E934.8	E950.4	E962.0	E980.4
plasma expanders	974.5	E858.5	E944.5	E950.4	E962.0	E980.4
40:16 sodium-removing resins	974.5	E858.5	E944.5	E950.4	E962.0	E980.4
40:18 potassium-removing resins	974.5	E858.5	E944.5	E950.4	E962.0	E980.4
40:20 caloric agents	974.5	E858.5	E944.5	E950.4	E962.0	E980.4
40:24 salt and sugar substitutes	974.4	E858.5	E944.4	E950.4	E962.0	E980.4
40:28 diuretics NEC	974.2	E858.5	E944.2	E950.4	E962.0	E980.4
carbonic acid anhydrase inhibitors	974.0	E858.5	E944.0	E950.4	E962.0	E980.4
mercurials	974.1	E858.5	E944.1	E950.4	E962.0	E980.4
purine derivatives	974.3	E858.5	E944.3	E950.4	E962.0	E980.4
saluretics	974.3	E858.5	E944.3	E950.4	E962.0	E980.4
thiazides	974.5	E858.5	E944.5	E950.4	E962.0	E980.4
40:36 irrigating solutions	974.7	E858.5	E944.7	E950.4	E962.0	E980.4
40:40 uricosuric agents	963.4	E858.1	E933.4	E950.4	E962.0	E980.4
44:00 enzymes	964.4	E858.2	E934.4	E950.4	E962.0	E980.4
fibrinolysis-affecting agents	973.4	E858.4	E943.4	E950.4	E962.0	E980.4
gastric agents	963.0	E858.1	E933.0	E950.4	E962.0	E980.4
48:00 expectorants and cough preparations	975.4	E858.6	E945.4	E950.4	E962.0	E980.4
antihistamine agents	965.09	E850.2	E935.2	E950.0	E962.0	E980.0
antitussives	975.5	E858.6	E945.5	E950.4	E962.0	E980.4
codeine derivatives	965.09	E850.2	E935.2	E950.0	E962.0	E980.0
expectorants						
narcotic agents NEC						
52:04 anti-infectives (EENT)	976.6	E858.7	E946.6	E950.4	E962.0	E980.4
ENT agent	976.5	E858.7	E946.5	E950.4	E962.0	E980.4
ophthalmic preparation						
52:04.04 antibiotics (EENT)	976.6	E858.7	E946.6	E950.4	E962.0	E980.4
ENT agent	976.5	E858.7	E946.5	E950.4	E962.0	E980.4
ophthalmic preparation						
52:04.06 antivirals (EENT)	976.6	E858.7	E946.6	E950.4	E962.0	E980.4
ENT agent	976.5	E858.7	E946.5	E950.4	E962.0	E980.4
ophthalmic preparation						
52:04.08 sulfonamides (EENT)	976.6	E858.7	E946.6	E950.4	E962.0	E980.4
ENT agent	976.5	E858.7	E946.5	E950.4	E962.0	E980.4
ophthalmic preparation						
52:04.12 miscellaneous anti-infectives (EENT)	976.6	E858.7	E946.6	E950.4	E962.0	E980.4
ENT agent	976.5	E858.7	E946.5	E950.4	E962.0	E980.4
ophthalmic preparation						
52:08 anti-inflammatory agents (EENT)	976.6	E858.7	E946.6	E950.4	E962.0	E980.4
ENT agent	976.5	E858.7	E946.5	E950.4	E962.0	E980.4
ophthalmic preparation	974.2	E858.5	E944.2	E950.4	E962.0	E980.4
52:10 carbonic anhydrase inhibitors	976.5	E858.7	E946.5	E950.4	E962.0	E980.4
52:12 contact lens solutions						

Drug — Drug

	Poisoning	External Cause (E-Code)				
		Accident	**Therapeutic Use**	**Suicide Attempt**	**Assault**	**Undetermined**
Drug — *continued*						
52:16 local anesthetics (EENT)	968.5	E855.2	E938.5	E950.4	E962.0	E980.4
52:20 miotics	971.0	E855.3	E941.0	E950.4	E962.0	E980.4
52:24 mydriatics						
adrenergics	971.2	E855.5	E941.2	E950.4	E962.0	E980.4
anticholinergics	971.1	E855.4	E941.1	E950.4	E962.0	E980.4
antimuscarinics	971.1	E855.4	E941.1	E950.4	E962.0	E980.4
parasympatholytics	971.1	E855.4	E941.1	E950.4	E962.0	E980.4
spasmolytics	971.1	E855.4	E941.1	E950.4	E962.0	E980.4
sympathomimetics	971.2	E855.5	E941.2	E950.4	E962.0	E980.4
52:28 mouth washes and gargles	976.6	E858.7	E946.6	E950.4	E962.0	E980.4
52:32 vasoconstrictors (EENT)	971.2	E855.5	E941.2	E950.4	E962.0	E980.4
52:36 unclassified agents (EENT)						
ENT agent	976.6	E858.7	E946.6	E950.4	E962.0	E980.4
ophthalmic preparation	976.5	E858.7	E946.5	E950.4	E962.0	E980.4
56:04 antacids and adsorbents	973.0	E858.4	E943.0	E950.4	E962.0	E980.4
56:08 antidiarrhea agents	973.5	E858.4	E943.5	E950.4	E962.0	E980.4
56:10 antiflatulents	973.8	E858.4	E943.8	E950.4	E962.0	E980.4
56:12 cathartics NEC	973.3	E858.4	E943.3	E950.4	E962.0	E980.4
emollients	973.2	E858.4	E943.2	E950.4	E962.0	E980.4
irritants	973.1	E858.4	E943.1	E950.4	E962.0	E980.4
56:16 digestants	973.4	E858.4	E943.4	E950.4	E962.0	E980.4
56:20 emetics and antiemetics						
antiemetics	963.0	E858.1	E933.0	E950.4	E962.0	E980.4
emetics	973.6	E858.4	E943.6	E950.4	E962.0	E980.4
56:24 lipotropic agents	977.1	E858.8	E947.1	E950.4	E962.0	E980.4
56:40 miscellaneous G.I. drugs	973.8	E858.4	E943.8	E950.4	E962.0	E980.4
60:00 gold compounds	965.69	E850.6	E935.6	E950.0	E962.0	E980.0
64:00 heavy metal antagonists	963.8	E858.1	E933.8	E950.4	E962.0	E980.4
68:04 adrenals	962.0	E858.0	E932.0	E950.4	E962.0	E980.4
68:08 androgens	962.1	E858.0	E932.1	E950.4	E962.0	E980.4
68:12 contraceptives, oral	962.2	E858.0	E932.2	E950.4	E962.0	E980.4
68:16 estrogens	962.2	E858.0	E932.2	E950.4	E962.0	E980.4
68:18 gonadotropins	962.4	E858.0	E932.4	E950.4	E962.0	E980.4
68:20 insulins and antidiabetic agents	962.3	E858.0	E932.3	E950.4	E962.0	E980.4
68:20.08 insulins	962.3	E858.0	E932.3	E950.4	E962.0	E980.4
68:24 parathyroid	962.6	E858.0	E932.6	E950.4	E962.0	E980.4
68:28 pituitary (posterior)	962.5	E858.0	E932.5	E950.4	E962.0	E980.4
anterior	962.4	E858.0	E932.4	E950.4	E962.0	E980.4
68:32 progestogens	962.2	E858.0	E932.2	E950.4	E962.0	E980.4
68:34 other corpus luteum						
hormones NEC	962.2	E858.0	E932.2	E950.4	E962.0	E980.4
68:36 thyroid and antithyroid						
antithyroid	962.8	E858.0	E932.8	E950.4	E962.0	E980.4
thyroid (derivatives)	962.7	E858.0	E932.7	E950.4	E962.0	E980.4
72:00 local anesthetics NEC	968.9	E855.2	E938.9	E950.4	E962.0	E980.4
topical (surface)	968.5	E855.2	E938.5	E950.4	E962.0	E980.4
infiltration (intradermal) (subcutaneous) (submucosal)	968.5	E855.2	E938.5	E950.4	E962.0	E980.4
nerve blocking (peripheral) (plexus) (regional)	968.6	E855.2	E938.6	E950.4	E962.0	E980.4
spinal	968.7	E855.2	E938.7	E950.4	E962.0	E980.4
76:00 oxytocics	975.0	E858.6	E945.0	E950.4	E962.0	E980.4
78:00 radioactive agents	990	—	—	—	—	—
80:04 serums NEC	979.9	E858.8	E949.9	E950.4	E962.0	E980.4
immune gamma globulin (human)	964.6	E858.2	E934.6	E950.4	E962.0	E980.4
80:08 toxoids NEC	978.8	E858.8	E948.8	E950.4	E962.0	E980.4
diphtheria	978.5	E858.8	E948.5	E950.4	E962.0	E980.4
and tetanus	978.9	E858.8	E948.9	E950.4	E962.0	E980.4
with pertussis component	978.6	E858.8	E948.6	E950.4	E962.0	E980.4
tetanus	978.4	E858.8	E948.4	E950.4	E962.0	E980.4
and diphtheria	978.9	E858.8	E948.9	E950.4	E962.0	E980.4
with pertussis component	978.6	E858.8	E948.6	E950.4	E962.0	E980.4
80:12 vaccines	979.9	E858.8	E949.9	E950.4	E962.0	E980.4
bacterial NEC	978.8	E858.8	E948.8	E950.4	E962.0	E980.4
with						
other bacterial components	978.9	E858.8	E948.9	E950.4	E962.0	E980.4
pertussis component	978.6	E858.8	E948.6	E950.4	E962.0	E980.4
viral and rickettsial components	979.7	E858.8	E949.7	E950.4	E962.0	E980.4
rickettsial NEC	979.6	E858.8	E949.6	E950.4	E962.0	E980.4
with						
bacterial component	979.7	E858.8	E949.7	E950.4	E962.0	E980.4
pertussis component	978.6	E858.8	E948.6	E950.4	E962.0	E980.4
viral component	979.7	E858.8	E949.7	E950.4	E962.0	E980.4
viral NEC	979.6	E858.8	E949.6	E950.4	E962.0	E980.4
with						
bacterial component	979.7	E858.8	E949.7	E950.4	E962.0	E980.4
pertussis component	978.6	E858.8	E948.6	E950.4	E962.0	E980.4
rickettsial component	979.7	E858.8	E949.7	E950.4	E962.0	E980.4
84:04.04 antibiotics (skin and mucous membrane)	976.0	E858.7	E946.0	E950.4	E962.0	E980.4
84:04.08 fungicides (skin and mucous membrane)	976.0	E858.7	E946.0	E950.4	E962.0	E980.4
84:04.12 scabicides and pediculicides (skin and mucous membrane)	976.0	E858.7	E946.0	E950.4	E962.0	E980.4

Drug — Drug

	Poisoning	Accident	Therapeutic Use	Suicide Attempt	Assault	Undetermined
Drug — *continued*						
84:04.16 miscellaneous local anti-infectives (skin and mucous membrane)	976.0	E858.7	E946.0	E950.4	E962.0	E980.4
84:06 anti-inflammatory agents (skin and mucous membrane)	976.0	E858.7	E946.0	E950.4	E962.0	E980.4
84:08 antipruritics and local anesthetics						
antipruritics	976.1	E858.7	E946.1	E950.4	E962.0	E980.4
local anesthetics	968.5	E855.2	E938.5	E950.4	E962.0	E980.4
84:12 astringents	976.2	E858.7	E946.2	E950.4	E962.0	E980.4
84:16 cell stimulants and proliferants	976.8	E858.7	E946.8	E950.4	E962.0	E980.4
84:20 detergents	976.2	E858.7	E946.2	E950.4	E962.0	E980.4
84:24 emollients, demulcents, and protectants	976.3	E858.7	E946.3	E950.4	E962.0	E980.4
84:28 keratolytic agents	976.4	E858.7	E946.4	E950.4	E962.0	E980.4
84:32 keratoplastic agents	976.4	E858.7	E946.4	E950.4	E962.0	E980.4
84:36 miscellaneous agents (skin and mucous membrane)	976.8	E858.7	E946.8	E950.4	E962.0	E980.4
86:00 spasmolytic agents	975.1	E858.6	E945.1	E950.4	E962.0	E980.4
antiasthmatics	975.7	E858.6	E945.7	E950.4	E962.0	E980.4
papaverine	972.5	E858.3	E942.5	E950.4	E962.0	E980.4
theophylline	974.1	E858.5	E944.1	E950.4	E962.0	E980.4
88:04 vitamin A	963.5	E858.1	E933.5	E950.4	E962.0	E980.4
88:08 vitamin B complex	963.5	E858.1	E933.5	E950.4	E962.0	E980.4
hematopoietic vitamin	964.1	E858.2	E934.1	E950.4	E962.0	E980.4
nicotinic acid derivatives	972.2	E858.3	E942.2	E950.4	E962.0	E980.4
88:12 vitamin C	963.5	E858.1	E933.5	E950.4	E962.0	E980.4
88:16 vitamin D	963.5	E858.1	E933.5	E950.4	E962.0	E980.4
88:20 vitamin E	963.5	E858.1	E933.5	E950.4	E962.0	E980.4
88:24 vitamin K activity	964.3	E858.2	E934.3	E950.4	E962.0	E980.4
88:28 multivitamin preparations	963.5	E858.1	E933.5	E950.4	E962.0	E980.4
92:00 unclassified therapeutic agents	977.8	E858.8	E947.8	E950.4	E962.0	E980.4
Duboisine	971.1	E855.4	E941.1	E950.4	E962.0	E980.4
Dulcolax	973.1	E858.4	E943.1	E950.4	E962.0	E980.4
Duponol (C) (EP)	976.2	E858.7	E946.2	E950.4	E962.0	E980.4
Durabolin	962.1	E858.0	E932.1	E950.4	E962.0	E980.4
Dyclone	968.5	E855.2	E938.5	E950.4	E962.0	E980.4
Dyclonine	968.5	E855.2	E938.5	E950.4	E962.0	E980.4
Dydrogesterone	962.2	E858.0	E932.2	E950.4	E962.0	E980.4
Dyes NEC	989.89	E866.8	—	E950.9	E962.1	E980.9
diagnostic agents	977.8	E858.8	E947.8	E950.4	E962.0	E980.4
pharmaceutical NEC	977.4	E858.8	E947.4	E950.4	E962.0	E980.4
Dyfols	971.0	E855.3	E941.0	E950.4	E962.0	E980.4
Dymelor	962.3	E858.0	E932.3	E950.4	E962.0	E980.4
Dynamite	989.89	E866.8	—	E950.9	E962.1	E980.9
fumes	987.8	E869.8		E952.8	E962.2	E982.8
Dyphylline	975.1	E858.6	E945.1	E950.4	E962.0	E980.4
Ear preparations	976.6	E858.7	E946.6	E950.4	E962.0	E980.4
Echothiopate, ecothiopate	971.0	E855.3	E941.0	E950.4	E962.0	E980.4
Ectylurea	967.8	E852.8	E937.8	E950.2	E962.0	E980.2
Edathamil disodium	963.8	E858.1	E933.8	E950.4	E962.0	E980.4
Edecrin	974.4	E858.5	E944.4	E950.4	E962.0	E980.4
Edetate, disodium (calcium)	963.8	E858.1	E933.8	E950.4	E962.0	E980.4
Edrophonium	971.0	E855.3	E941.0	E950.4	E962.0	E980.4
Elase	976.8	E858.7	E946.8	E950.4	E962.0	E980.4
Elaterium	973.1	E858.4	E943.1	E950.4	E962.0	E980.4
Elder	988.2	E865.4	—	E950.9	E962.1	E980.9
berry (unripe)	988.2	E865.3	—	E950.9	E962.1	E980.9
Electrolytes NEC	974.5	E858.5	E944.5	E950.4	E962.0	E980.4
Electrolytic agent NEC	974.5	E858.5	E944.5	E950.4	E962.0	E980.4
Embramine	963.0	E858.1	E933.0	E950.4	E962.0	E980.4
Emetics	973.6	E858.4	E943.6	E950.4	E962.0	E980.4
Emetine (hydrochloride)	961.5	E857	E931.5	E950.4	E962.0	E980.4
Emollients	976.3	E858.7	E946.3	E950.4	E962.0	E980.4
Emylcamate	969.5	E853.8	E939.5	E950.3	E962.0	E980.3
Encyprate	969.0	E854.0	E939.0	E950.3	E962.0	E980.3
Endocaine	968.5	E855.2	E938.5	E950.4	E962.0	E980.4
Endrin	989.2	E863.0	—	E950.6	E962.1	E980.7
Enflurane	968.2	E855.1	E938.2	E950.4	E962.0	E980.4
Enovid	962.2	E858.0	E932.2	E950.4	E962.0	E980.4
ENT preparations (anti-infectives)	976.6	E858.7	E946.6	E950.4	E962.0	E980.4
Enzodase	963.4	E858.1	E933.4	E950.4	E962.0	E980.4
Enzymes NEC	963.4	E858.1	E933.4	E950.4	E962.0	E980.4
Epanutin	966.1	E855.0	E936.1	E950.4	E962.0	E980.4
Ephedra (tincture)	971.2	E855.5	E941.2	E950.4	E962.0	E980.4
Ephedrine	971.2	E855.5	E941.2	E950.4	E962.0	E980.4
Epiestriol	962.2	E858.0	E932.2	E950.4	E962.0	E980.4
Epilim — *see* Sodium Valproate						
Epinephrine	971.2	E855.5	E941.2	E950.4	E962.0	E980.4
Epsom sait	973.3	E858.4	E943.3	E950.4	E962.0	E980.4
Equanil	969.5	E853.8	E939.5	E950.3	E962.0	E980.3
Equisetum (diuretic)	974.4	E858.5	E944.4	E950.4	E962.0	E980.4
Ergometrine	975.0	E858.6	E945.0	E950.4	E962.0	E980.4
Ergonovine	975.0	E858.6	E945.0	E950.4	E962.0	E980.4

✔4ᵈ Fourth-digit Required   ✔5ᵗʰ Fifth-digit Required   ▶◀ Revised Text   ● New Line   ▲ Revised Code

	Poisoning	External Cause (E-Code)				
		Accident	Therapeutic Use	Suicide Attempt	Assault	Undetermined
Ergot NEC	988.2	E865.4	—	E950.9	E962.1	E980.9
medicinal (alkaloids)	975.0	E858.6	E945.0	E950.4	E962.0	E980.4
Ergotamine (tartrate) (for migraine) NEC	972.9	E858.3	E942.9	E950.4	E962.0	E980.4
Ergotrate	975.0	E858.6	E945.0	E950.4	E962.0	E980.4
Erythrityl tetranitrate	972.4	E858.3	E942.4	E950.4	E962.0	E980.4
Erythrol tetranitrate	972.4	E858.3	E942.4	E950.4	E962.0	E980.4
Erythromycin	960.3	E856	E930.3	E950.4	E962.0	E980.4
ophthalmic preparation	976.5	E858.7	E946.5	E950.4	E962.0	E980.4
topical NEC	976.0	E858.7	E946.0	E950.4	E962.0	E980.4
Eserine	971.0	E855.3	E941.0	E950.4	E962.0	E980.4
Eskabarb	967.0	E851	E937.0	E950.1	E962.0	E980.1
Eskalith	969.8	E855.8	E939.8	E950.3	E962.0	E980.3
Estradiol (cypionate) (dipropionate) (valerate)	962.2	E858.0	E932.2	E950.4	E962.0	E980.4
Estriol	962.2	E858.0	E932.2	E950.4	E962.0	E980.4
Estrogens (with progestogens)	962.2	E858.0	E932.2	E950.4	E962.0	E980.4
Estrone	962.2	E858.0	E932.2	E950.4	E962.0	E980.4
Etafedrine	971.2	E855.5	E941.2	E950.4	E962.0	E980.4
Ethacrynate sodium	974.4	E858.5	E944.4	E950.4	E962.0	E980.4
Ethacrynic acid	974.4	E858.5	E944.4	E950.4	E962.0	E980.4
Ethambutol	961.8	E857	E931.8	E950.4	E962.0	E980.4
Ethamide	974.2	E858.5	E944.2	E950.4	E962.0	E980.4
Ethamivan	970.0	E854.3	E940.0	E950.4	E962.0	E980.4
Ethamsylate	964.5	E858.2	E934.5	E950.4	E962.0	E980.4
Ethanol	980.0	E860.1	—	E950.9	E962.1	E980.9
beverage	980.0	E860.0	—	E950.9	E962.1	E980.9
Ethchlorvynol	967.8	E852.8	E937.8	E950.2	E962.0	E980.2
Ethebenecid	974.7	E858.5	E944.7	E950.4	E962.0	E980.4
Ether(s) (diethyl) (ethyl) (vapor)	987.8	E869.8	—	E952.8	E962.2	E982.8
anesthetic	968.2	E855.1	E938.2	E950.4	E962.0	E980.4
petroleum — *see* Ligroin						
solvent	982.8	E862.4	—	E950.9	E962.1	E980.9
Ethidine chloride (vapor)	987.8	E869.8	—	E952.8	E962.2	E982.8
liquid (solvent)	982.3	E862.4	—	E950.9	E962.1	E980.9
Ethinamate	967.8	E852.8	E937.8	E950.2	E962.0	E980.2
Ethinylestradiol	962.2	E858.0	E932.2	E950.4	E962.0	E980.4
Ethionamide	961.8	E857	E931.8	E950.4	E962.0	E980.4
Ethisterone	962.2	E858.0	E932.2	E950.4	E962.0	E980.4
Ethobral	967.0	E851	E937.0	E950.1	E962.0	E980.1
Ethocaine (infiltration) (topical)	968.5	E855.2	E938.5	E950.4	E962.0	E980.4
nerve block (peripheral) (plexus)	968.6	E855.2	E938.6	E950.4	E962.0	E980.4
spinal	968.7	E855.2	E938.7	E950.4	E962.0	E980.4
Ethoheptazine (citrate)	965.7	E850.7	E935.7	E950.0	E962.0	E980.0
Ethopropazine	966.4	E855.0	E936.4	E950.4	E962.0	E980.4
Ethosuximide	966.2	E855.0	E936.2	E950.4	E962.0	E980.4
Ethotoin	966.1	E855.0	E936.1	E950.4	E962.0	E980.4
Ethoxazene	961.9	E857	E931.9	E950.4	E962.0	E980.4
Ethoxzolamide	974.2	E858.5	E944.2	E950.4	E962.0	E980.4
Ethyl						
acetate (vapor)	982.8	E862.4	—	E950.9	E962.1	E980.9
alcohol	980.0	E860.1	—	E950.9	E962.1	E980.9
beverage	980.0	E860.0	—	E950.9	E962.1	E980.9
aldehyde (vapor)	987.8	E869.8	—	E952.8	E962.2	E982.8
liquid	989.89	E866.8	—	E950.9	E962.1	E980.9
aminobenzoate	968.5	E855.2	E938.5	E950.4	E962.0	E980.4
biscoumacetate	964.2	E858.2	E934.2	E950.4	E962.0	E980.4
bromide (anesthetic)	968.2	E855.1	E938.2	E950.4	E962.0	E980.4
carbamate (antineoplastic)	963.1	E858.1	E933.1	E950.4	E962.0	E980.4
carbinol	980.3	E860.4	—	E950.9	E962.1	E980.9
chaulmoograte	961.8	E857	E931.8	E950.4	E962.0	E980.4
chloride (vapor)	987.8	E869.8	—	E952.8	E962.2	E982.8
anesthetic (local)	968.5	E855.2	E938.5	E950.4	E962.0	E980.4
inhaled	968.2	E855.1	E938.2	E950.4	E962.0	E980.4
solvent	982.3	E862.4	—	E950.9	E962.1	E980.9
estranol	962.1	E858.0	E932.1	E950.4	E962.0	E980.4
ether — *see* Ether(s)						
formate (solvent) NEC	982.8	E862.4	—	E950.9	E962.1	E980.9
iodoacetate	987.5	E869.3	—	E952.8	E962.2	E982.8
lactate (solvent) NEC	982.8	E862.4	—	E950.9	E962.1	E980.9
methylcarbinol	980.8	E860.8	—	E950.9	E962.1	E980.9
morphine	965.09	E850.2	E935.2	E950.0	E962.0	E980.0
Ethylene (gas)	987.1	E869.8	—	E952.8	E962.2	E982.8
anesthetic (general)	968.2	E855.1	E938.2	E950.4	E962.0	E980.4
chlorohydrin (vapor)	982.3	E862.4	—	E950.9	E962.1	E980.9
dichloride (vapor)	982.3	E862.4	—	E950.9	E962.1	E980.9
glycol(s) (any) (vapor)	982.8	E862.4	—	E950.9	E962.1	E980.9
Ethylidene						
chloride NEC	982.3	E862.4	—	E950.9	E962.1	E980.9
diethyl ether	982.8	E862.4	—	E950.9	E962.1	E980.9
Ethynodiol	962.2	E858.0	E932.2	E950.4	E962.0	E980.4
Etidocaine	968.9	E855.2	E938.9	E950.4	E962.0	E980.4
infiltration (subcutaneous)	968.5	E855.2	E938.5	E950.4	E962.0	E980.4

Ergot NEC — Etidocaine

	Poisoning	External Cause (E-Code)				
		Accident	Therapeutic Use	Suicide Attempt	Assault	Undetermined
Etidocaine — *continued*						
nerve (peripheral) (plexus)	968.6	E855.2	E938.6	E950.4	E962.0	E980.4
Etilfen	967.0	E851	E937.0	E950.1	E962.0	E980.1
Etomide	965.7	E850.7	E935.7	E950.0	E962.0	E980.0
Etorphine	965.09	E850.2	E935.2	E950.0	E962.0	E980.0
Etoval	967.0	E851	E937.0	E950.1	E962.0	E980.1
Etryptamine	969.0	E854.0	E939.0	E950.3	E962.0	E980.3
Eucaine	968.5	E855.2	E938.5	E950.4	E962.0	E980.4
Eucalyptus (oil) NEC	975.5	E858.6	E945.5	E950.4	E962.0	E980.4
Eucatropine	971.1	E855.4	E941.1	E950.4	E962.0	E980.4
Eucodal	965.09	E850.2	E935.2	E950.0	E962.0	E980.0
Euneryl	967.0	E851	E937.0	E950.1	E962.0	E980.1
Euphthalmine	971.1	E855.4	E941.1	E950.4	E962.0	E980.4
Eurax	976.0	E858.7	E946.0	E950.4	E962.0	E980.4
Euresol	976.4	E858.7	E946.4	E950.4	E962.0	E980.4
Euthroid	962.7	E858.0	E932.7	E950.4	E962.0	E980.4
Evans blue	977.8	E858.8	E947.8	E950.4	E962.0	E980.4
Evipal	967.0	E851	E937.0	E950.1	E962.0	E980.1
sodium	968.3	E855.1	E938.3	E950.4	E962.0	E980.4
Evipan	967.0	E851	E937.0	E950.1	E962.0	E980.1
sodium	968.3	E855.1	E938.3	E950.4	E962.0	E980.4
Exalgin	965.4	E850.4	E935.4	E950.0	E962.0	E980.0
Excipients, pharmaceutical	977.4	E858.8	E947.4	E950.4	E962.0	E980.4
Exhaust gas — *see* Carbon, monoxide						
Ex-Lax (phenolphthalein)	973.1	E858.4	E943.1	E950.4	E962.0	E980.4
Expectorants	975.5	E858.6	E945.5	E950.4	E962.0	E980.4
External medications (skin) (mucous membrane)	976.9	E858.7	E946.9	E950.4	E962.0	E980.4
dental agent	976.7	E858.7	E946.7	E950.4	E962.0	E980.4
ENT agent	976.6	E858.7	E946.6	E950.4	E962.0	E980.4
ophthalmic preparation	976.5	E858.7	E946.5	E950.4	E962.0	E980.4
specified NEC	976.8	E858.7	E946.8	E950.4	E962.0	E980.4
Eye agents (anti-infective)	976.5	E858.7	E946.5	E950.4	E962.0	E980.4
Factor IX complex (human)	964.5	E858.2	E934.5	E950.4	E962.0	E980.4
Fecal softeners	973.2	E858.4	E943.2	E950.4	E962.0	E980.4
Fenbutrazate	977.0	E858.8	E947.0	E950.4	E962.0	E980.4
Fencamfamin	970.8	E854.3	E940.8	E950.4	E962.0	E980.4
Fenfluramine	977.0	E858.8	E947.0	E950.4	E962.0	E980.4
Fenoprofen	965.61	E850.6	E935.6	E950.0	E962.0	E980.0
Fentanyl	965.09	E850.2	E935.2	E950.0	E962.0	E980.0
Fentazin	969.1	E853.0	E939.1	E950.3	E962.0	E980.3
Fenticlor, fentichlor	976.0	E858.7	E946.0	E950.4	E962.0	E980.4
Fer de lance (bite) (venom)	989.5	E905.0	—	E950.9	E962.1	E980.9
Ferric — *see* Iron						
Ferrocholinate	964.0	E858.2	E934.0	E950.4	E962.0	E980.4
Ferrous fumerate, gluconate, lactate, salt NEC, sulfate (medicinal)	964.0	E858.2	E934.0	E950.4	E962.0	E980.4
Ferrum — *see* Iron						
Fertilizers NEC	989.89	E866.5	—	E950.9	E962.1	E980.4
with herbicide mixture	989.4	E863.5	—	E950.6	E962.1	E980.7
Fibrinogen (human)	964.7	E858.2	E934.7	E950.4	E962.0	E980.4
Fibrinolysin	964.4	E858.2	E934.4	E950.4	E962.0	E980.4
Fibrinolysis-affecting agents	964.4	E858.2	E934.4	E950.4	E962.0	E980.4
Filix mas	961.6	E857	E931.6	E950.4	E962.0	E980.4
Fiorinal	965.1	E850.3	E935.3	E950.0	E962.0	E980.0
Fire damp	987.1	E869.8	—	E952.8	E962.2	E982.8
Fish, nonbacterial or noxious	988.0	E865.2	—	E950.9	E962.1	E980.9
shell	988.0	E865.1	—	E950.9	E962.1	E980.9
Flagyl	961.5	E857	E931.5	E950.4	E962.0	E980.4
Flavoxate	975.1	E858.6	E945.1	E950.4	E962.0	E980.4
Flaxedil	975.2	E858.6	E945.2	E950.4	E962.0	E980.4
Flaxseed (medicinal)	976.3	E858.7	E946.3	E950.4	E962.0	E980.4
Florantyrone	973.4	E858.4	E943.4	E950.4	E962.0	E980.4
Floraquin	961.3	E857	E931.3	E950.4	E962.0	E980.4
Florinef	962.0	E858.0	E932.0	E950.4	E962.0	E980.4
ENT agent	976.6	E858.7	E946.6	E950.4	E962.0	E980.4
ophthalmic preparation	976.5	E858.7	E946.5	E950.4	E962.0	E980.4
topical NEC	976.0	E858.7	E946.0	E950.4	E962.0	E980.4
Flowers of sulfur	976.4	E858.7	E946.4	E950.4	E962.0	E980.4
Floxuridine	963.1	E858.1	E933.1	E950.4	E962.0	E980.4
Flucytosine	961.9	E857	E931.9	E950.4	E962.0	E980.4
Fludrocortisone	962.0	E858.0	E932.0	E950.4	E962.0	E980.4
ENT agent	976.6	E858.7	E946.6	E950.4	E962.0	E980.4
ophthalmic preparation	976.5	E858.7	E946.5	E950.4	E962.0	E980.4
topical NEC	976.0	E858.7	E946.0	E950.4	E962.0	E980.4
Flumethasone	976.0	E858.7	E946.0	E950.4	E962.0	E980.4
Flumethiazide	974.3	E858.5	E944.3	E950.4	E962.0	E980.4
Flumidin	961.7	E857	E931.7	E950.4	E962.0	E980.4
Flunitrazepam	969.4	E853.2	E939.4	E950.3	E962.0	E980.3 ▲
Fluocinolone	976.0	E858.7	E946.0	E950.4	E962.0	E980.4
Fluocortolone	962.0	E858.0	E932.0	E950.4	E962.0	E980.4
Fluohydrocortisone	962.0	E858.0	E932.0	E950.4	E962.0	E980.4
ENT agent	976.6	E858.7	E946.6	E950.4	E962.0	E980.4

✓4ᵀᴴ Fourth-digit Required   ✓5ᵀᴴ Fifth-digit Required   ►◄ Revised Text   ● New Line   ▲ Revised Code

		External Cause (E-Code)				
	Poisoning	Accident	Therapeutic Use	Suicide Attempt	Assault	Undetermined
Fluohydrocortisone — *continued*						
ophthalmic preparation	976.5	E858.7	E946.5	E950.4	E962.0	E980.4
topical NEC	976.0	E858.7	E946.0	E950.4	E962.0	E980.4
Fluonid	976.0	E858.7	E946.0	E950.4	E962.0	E980.4
Fluopromazine	969.1	E853.0	E939.1	E950.3	E962.0	E980.3
Fluoracetate	989.4	E863.7	—	E950.6	E962.1	E980.7
Fluorescein (sodium)	977.8	E858.8	E947.8	E950.4	E962.0	E980.4
Fluoride(s) (pesticides) (sodium) NEC	989.4	E863.4	—	E950.6	E962.1	E980.7
hydrogen — *see* Hydrofluoric acid						
medicinal	976.7	E858.7	E946.7	E950.4	E962.0	E980.4
not pesticide NEC	983.9	E864.4	—	E950.7	E962.1	E980.6
stannous	976.7	E858.7	E946.7	E950.4	E962.0	E980.4
Fluorinated corticosteroids	962.0	E858.0	E932.0	E950.4	E962.0	E980.4
Fluorine (compounds) (gas)	987.8	E869.8	—	E952.8	E962.2	E982.8
salt — *see* Fluoride(s)						
Fluoristan	976.7	E858.7	E946.7	E950.4	E962.0	E980.4
Fluoroacetate	989.4	E863.7	—	E950.6	E962.1	E980.7
Fluorodeoxyuridine	963.1	E858.1	E933.1	E950.4	E962.0	E980.4
Fluorometholone (topical) NEC	976.0	E858.7	E946.0	E950.4	E962.0	E980.4
ophthalmic preparation	976.5	E858.7	E946.5	E950.4	E962.0	E980.4
Fluorouracil	963.1	E858.1	E933.1	E950.4	E962.0	E980.4
Fluothane	968.1	E855.1	E938.1	E950.4	E962.0	E980.4
Fluoxetine hydrochloride	969.0	E854.0	E939.0	E950.3	E962.0	E980.3
Fluoxymesterone	962.1	E858.0	E932.1	E950.4	E962.0	E980.4
Fluphenazine	969.1	E853.0	E939.1	E950.3	E962.0	E980.3
Fluprednisolone	962.0	E858.0	E932.0	E950.4	E962.0	E980.4
Flurandrenolide	976.0	E858.7	E946.0	E950.4	E962.0	E980.4
Flurazepam (hydrochloride)	969.4	E853.2	E939.4	E950.3	E962.0	E980.3
Flurbiprofen	965.61	E850.6	E935.6	E950.0	E962.0	E980.0
Flurobate	976.0	E858.7	E946.0	E950.4	E962.0	E980.4
Flurothyl	969.8	E855.8	E939.8	E950.3	E962.0	E980.3
Fluroxene	968.2	E855.1	E938.2	E950.4	E962.0	E980.4
Folacin	964.1	E858.2	E934.1	E950.4	E962.0	E980.4
Folic acid	964.1	E858.2	E934.1	E950.4	E962.0	E980.4
Follicle stimulating hormone	962.4	E858.0	E932.4	E950.4	E962.0	E980.4
Food, foodstuffs, nonbacterial or noxious	988.9	E865.9	—	E950.9	E962.1	E980.9
berries, seeds	988.2	E865.3	—	E950.9	E962.1	E980.9
fish	988.0	E865.2	—	E950.9	E962.1	E980.9
mushrooms	988.1	E865.5	—	E950.9	E962.1	E980.9
plants	988.2	E865.9	—	E950.9	E962.1	E980.9
specified type NEC	988.2	E865.4	—	E950.9	E962.1	E980.9
shellfish	988.0	E865.1	—	E950.9	E962.1	E980.9
specified NEC	988.8	E865.8	—	E950.9	E962.1	E980.9
Fool's parsley	988.2	E865.4	—	E950.9	E962.1	E980.9
Formaldehyde (solution)	989.89	E861.4	—	E950.9	E962.1	E980.9
fungicide	989.4	E863.6	—	E950.6	E962.1	E980.7
gas or vapor	987.8	E869.8	—	E952.8	E962.2	E982.8
Formalin	989.89	E861.4	—	E950.9	E962.1	E980.9
fungicide	989.4	E863.6	—	E950.6	E962.1	E980.7
vapor	987.8	E869.8	—	E952.8	E962.2	E982.8
Formic acid	983.1	E864.1	—	E950.7	E962.1	E980.6
vapor	987.8	E869.8	—	E952.8	E962.2	E982.8
Fowler's solution	985.1	E866.3	—	E950.8	E962.1	E980.8
Foxglove	988.2	E865.4	—	E950.9	E962.1	E980.9
Fox green	977.8	E858.8	E947.8	E950.4	E962.0	E980.4
Framycetin	960.8	E856	E930.8	E950.4	E962.0	E980.4
Frangula (extract)	973.1	E858.4	E943.1	E950.4	E962.0	E980.4
Frei antigen	977.8	E858.8	E947.8	E950.4	E962.0	E980.4
Freons	987.4	E869.2	—	E952.8	E962.2	E982.8
Fructose	974.5	E858.5	E944.5	E950.4	E962.0	E980.4
Frusemide	974.4	E858.5	E944.4	E950.4	E962.0	E980.4
FSH	962.4	E858.0	E932.4	E950.4	E962.0	E980.4
Fuel						
automobile	981	E862.1	—	E950.9	E962.1	E980.9
exhaust gas, not in transit	986	E868.2	—	E952.0	E962.2	E982.0
vapor NEC	987.1	E869.8	—	E952.8	E962.2	E982.8
gas (domestic use) — *see also* Carbon, monoxide, fuel						
utility	987.1	E868.1	—	E951.8	E962.2	E981.8
incomplete combustion of — *see* Carbon, monoxide, fuel, utility						
in mobile container	987.0	E868.0	—	E951.1	E962.2	E981.1
piped (natural)	987.1	E867	—	E951.0	E962.2	E981.0
industrial, incomplete combustion	986	E868.3	—	E952.1	E962.2	E982.1
Fugillin	960.8	E856	E930.8	E950.4	E962.0	E980.4
Fulminate of mercury	985.0	E866.1	—	E950.9	E962.1	E980.9
Fulvicin	960.1	E856	E930.1	E950.4	E962.0	E980.4
Fumadil	960.8	E856	E930.8	E950.4	E962.0	E980.4
Fumagillin	960.8	E856	E930.8	E950.4	E962.0	E980.4
Fumes (from)	987.9	E869.9	—	E952.9	E962.2	E982.9
carbon monoxide — *see* Carbon, monoxide						
charcoal (domestic use)	986	E868.3	—	E952.1	E962.2	E982.1

✓4ᵗʰ Fourth-digit Required   ✓5ᵗʰ Fifth-digit Required   ►◄ Revised Text   ● New Line   ▲ Revised Code

	Poisoning	External Cause (E-Code)				
		Accident	Therapeutic Use	Suicide Attempt	Assault	Undetermined
Fumes — *continued*						
chloroform — *see* Chloroform						
coke (in domestic stoves, fireplaces)	986	E868.3	—	E952.1	E962.2	E982.1
corrosive NEC	987.8	E869.8	—	E952.8	E962.2	E982.8
ether — *see* Ether(s)						
freons	987.4	E869.2	—	E952.8	E962.2	E982.8
hydrocarbons	987.1	E869.8	—	E952.8	E962.2	E982.8
petroleum (liquefied)	987.0	E868.0	—	E951.1	E962.2	E981.1
distributed through pipes (pure or mixed with air)	987.0	E867	—	E951.0	E962.2	E981.0
lead — *see* Lead						
metals — *see* specified metal						
nitrogen dioxide	987.2	E869.0	—	E952.8	E962.2	E982.8
pesticides — *see* Pesticides						
petroleum (liquefied)	987.0	E868.0	—	E951.1	E962.2	E981.1
distributed through pipes (pure or mixed with air)	987.0	E867	—	E951.0	E962.2	E981.0
polyester	987.8	E869.8	—	E952.8	E962.2	E982.8
specified source other (*see also* substance specified)	987.8	E869.8	—	E952.8	E962.2	E982.8
sulfur dioxide	987.3	E869.1	—	E952.8	E962.2	E982.8
Fumigants	989.4	E863.8	—	E950.6	E962.1	E980.7
Fungi, noxious, used as food	988.1	E865.5	—	E950.9	E962.1	E980.9
Fungicides (*see also* Antifungals)	989.4	E863.6	—	E950.6	E962.1	E980.7
Fungizone	960.1	E856	E930.1	E950.4	E962.0	E980.4
topical	976.0	E858.7	E946.0	E950.4	E962.0	E980.4
Furacin	976.0	E858.7	E946.0	E950.4	E962.0	E980.4
Furadantin	961.9	E857	E931.9	E950.4	E962.0	E980.4
Furazolidone	961.9	E857	E931.9	E950.4	E962.0	E980.4
Furnace (coal burning) (domestic), gas from	986	E868.3	—	E952.1	E962.2	E982.1
industrial	986	E868.8	—	E952.1	E962.2	E982.1
Furniture polish	989.89	E861.2	—	E950.9	E962.1	E980.9
Furosemide	974.4	E858.5	E944.4	E950.4	E962.0	E980.4
Furoxone	961.9	E857	E931.9	E950.4	E962.0	E980.4
Fusel oil (amyl) (butyl) (propyl)	980.3	E860.4	—	E950.9	E962.1	E980.9
Fusidic acid	960.8	E856	E930.8	E950.4	E962.0	E980.4
Gallamine	975.2	E858.6	E945.2	E950.4	E962.0	E980.4
Gallotannic acid	976.2	E858.7	E946.2	E950.4	E962.0	E980.4
Gamboge	973.1	E858.4	E943.1	E950.4	E962.0	E980.4
Gamimune	964.6	E858.2	E934.6	E950.4	E962.0	E980.4
Gamma-benzene hexachloride (vapor)	989.2	E863.0	—	E950.6	E962.1	E980.7
Gamma globulin	964.6	E858.2	E934.6	E950.4	E962.0	E980.4
Gamma Hydroxy Butyrate (GHB)	968.4	E855.1	E938.4	E950.4	E962.0	E980.4
Gamulin	964.6	E858.2	E934.6	E950.4	E962.0	E980.4
Ganglionic blocking agents	972.3	E858.3	E942.3	E950.4	E962.0	E980.4
Ganja	969.6	E854.1	E939.6	E950.3	E962.0	E980.3
Garamycin	960.8	E856	E930.8	E950.4	E962.0	E980.4
ophthalmic preparation	976.5	E858.7	E946.5	E950.4	E962.0	E980.4
topical NEC	976.0	E858.7	E946.0	E950.4	E962.0	E980.4
Gardenal	967.0	E851	E937.0	E950.1	E962.0	E980.1
Gardepanyl	967.0	E851	E937.0	E950.1	E962.0	E980.1
Gas	987.9	E869.9	—	E952.9	E962.2	E982.9
acetylene	987.1	E868.1	—	E951.8	E962.2	E981.8
incomplete combustion of — *see* Carbon, monoxide, fuel, utility						
air contaminants, source or type not specified	987.9	E869.9	—	E952.9	E962.2	E982.9
anesthetic (general) NEC	968.2	E855.1	E938.2	E950.4	E962.0	E980.4
blast furnace	986	E868.8	—	E952.1	E962.2	E982.1
butane — *see* Butane						
carbon monoxide — *see* Carbon, monoxide						
chlorine	987.6	E869.8	—	E952.8	E962.2	E982.8
coal — *see* Carbon, monoxide, coal						
cyanide	987.7	E869.8	—	E952.8	E962.2	E982.8
dicyanogen	987.8	E869.8	—	E952.8	E962.2	E982.8
domestic — *see* Gas, utility						
exhaust — *see* Carbon, monoxide, exhaust gas						
from wood- or coal-burning stove or fireplace	986	E868.3	—	E952.1	E962.2	E982.1
fuel (domestic use) — *see also* Carbon, monoxide, fuel						
industrial use	986	E868.8	—	E952.1	E962.2	E982.1
utility	987.1	E868.1	—	E951.8	E962.2	E981.8
incomplete combustion of — *see* Carbon, monoxide, fuel, utility						
in mobile container	987.0	E868.0	—	E951.1	E962.2	E981.1
piped (natural)	987.1	E867	—	E951.0	E962.2	E981.0
garage	986	E868.2	—	E952.0	E962.2	E982.0
hydrocarbon NEC	987.1	E869.8	—	E952.8	E962.2	E982.8
incomplete combustion of — *see* Carbon, monoxide, fuel, utility						
liquefied (mobile container)	987.0	E868.0	—	E951.1	E962.2	E981.1
piped	987.0	E867	—	E951.0	E962.2	E981.0
hydrocyanic acid	987.7	E869.8	—	E952.8	E962.2	E982.8
illuminating — *see* Gas, utility						
incomplete combustion, any — *see* Carbon, monoxide						
kiln	986	E868.8	—	E952.1	E962.2	E982.1
lacrimogenic	987.5	E869.3	—	E952.8	E962.2	E982.8
marsh	987.1	E869.8	—	E952.8	E962.2	E982.8

	Poisoning	Accident	Therapeutic Use	Suicide Attempt	Assault	Undetermined
				External Cause (E-Code)		
Gas — *continued*						
motor exhaust, not in transit	986	E868.8	—	E952.1	E962.2	E982.1
mustard — *see* Mustard, gas						
natural	987.1	E867	—	E951.0	E962.2	E981.0
nerve (war)	987.9	E869.9	—	E952.9	E962.2	E982.9
oils	981	E862.1	—	E950.9	E962.1	E980.9
petroleum (liquefied) (distributed in mobile containers)	987.0	E868.0	—	E951.1	E962.2	E981.1
piped (pure or mixed with air)	987.0	E867	—	E951.1	E962.2	E981.1
piped (manufactured) (natural) NEC	987.1	E867	—	E951.0	E962.2	E981.0
producer	986	E868.8	—	E952.1	E962.2	E982.1
propane — *see* Propane						
refrigerant (freon)	987.4	E869.2	—	E952.8	E962.2	E982.8
not freon	987.9	E869.9	—	E952.9	E962.2	E982.9
sewer	987.8	E869.8	—	E952.8	E962.2	E982.8
specified source NEC (*see also* substance specified)	987.8	E869.8	—	E952.8	E962.2	E982.8
stove — *see* Gas, utility						
tear	987.5	E869.3	—	E952.8	E962.2	E982.8
utility (for cooking, heating, or lighting) (piped) NEC	987.1	E868.1	—	E951.8	E962.2	E981.8
incomplete combustion of — *see* Carbon, monoxide, fuel, utility						
in mobile container	987.0	E868.0	—	E951.1	E962.2	E981.1
piped (natural)	987.1	E867	—	E951.0	E962.2	E981.0
water	987.1	E868.1	—	E951.8	E962.2	E981.8
incomplete combustion of — *see* Carbon, monoxide, fuel, utility						
Gaseous substance — *see* Gas						
Gasoline, gasolene	981	E862.1	—	E950.9	E962.1	E980.9
vapor	987.1	E869.8	—	E952.8	E962.2	E982.8
Gastric enzymes	973.4	E858.4	E943.4	E950.4	E962.0	E980.4
Gastrografin	977.8	E858.8	E947.8	E950.4	E962.0	E980.4
Gastrointestinal agents	973.9	E858.4	E943.9	E950.4	E962.0	E980.4
specified NEC	973.8	E858.4	E943.8	E950.4	E962.0	E980.4
Gaultheria procumbens	988.2	E865.4	—	E950.9	E962.1	E980.9
Gelatin (intravenous)	964.8	E858.2	E934.8	E950.4	E962.0	E980.4
absorbable (sponge)	964.5	E858.2	E934.5	E950.4	E962.0	E980.4
Gelfilm	976.8	E858.7	E946.8	E950.4	E962.0	E980.4
Gelfoam	964.5	E858.2	E934.5	E950.4	E962.0	E980.4
Gelsemine	970.8	E854.3	E940.8	E950.4	E962.0	E980.4
Gelsemium (sempervirens)	988.2	E865.4	—	E950.9	E962.1	E980.9
Gemonil	967.0	E851	E937.0	E950.1	E962.0	E980.1
Gentamicin	960.8	E856	E930.8	E950.4	E962.0	E980.4
ophthalmic preparation	976.5	E858.7	E946.5	E950.4	E962.0	E980.4
topical NEC	976.0	E858.7	E946.0	E950.4	E962.0	E980.4
Gentian violet	976.0	E858.7	E946.0	E950.4	E962.0	E980.4
Gexane	976.0	E858.7	E946.0	E950.4	E962.0	E980.4
Gila monster (venom)	989.5	E905.0	—	E950.9	E962.1	E980.9
Ginger, Jamaica	989.89	E866.8	—	E950.9	E962.1	E980.9
Gitalin	972.1	E858.3	E942.1	E950.4	E962.0	E980.4
Gitoxin	972.1	E858.3	E942.1	E950.4	E962.0	E980.4
Glandular extract (medicinal) NEC	977.9	E858.9	E947.9	E950.5	E962.0	E980.5
Glaucarubin	961.5	E857	E931.5	E950.4	E962.0	E980.4
Globin zinc insulin	962.3	E858.0	E932.3	E950.4	E962.0	E980.4
Glucagon	962.3	E858.0	E932.3	E950.4	E962.0	E980.4
Glucochloral	967.1	E852.0	E937.1	E950.2	E962.0	E980.2
Glucocorticoids	962.0	E858.0	E932.0	E950.4	E962.0	E980.4
Glucose	974.5	E858.5	E944.5	E950.4	E962.0	E980.4
oxidase reagent	977.8	E858.8	E947.8	E950.4	E962.0	E980.4
Glucosulfone sodium	961.8	E857	E931.8	E950.4	E962.0	E980.4
Glue(s)	989.89	E866.6	—	E950.9	E962.1	E980.9
Glutamic acid (hydrochloride)	973.4	E858.4	E943.4	E950.4	E962.0	E980.4
Glutathione	963.8	E858.1	E933.8	E950.4	E962.0	E980.4
Glutethimide (group)	967.5	E852.4	E937.5	E950.2	E962.0	E980.2
Glycerin (lotion)	976.3	E858.7	E946.3	E950.4	E962.0	E980.4
Glycerol (topical)	976.3	E858.7	E946.3	E950.4	E962.0	E980.4
Glyceryl						
guaiacolate	975.5	E858.6	E945.5	E950.4	E962.0	E980.4
triacetate (topical)	976.0	E858.7	E946.0	E950.4	E962.0	E980.4
trinitrate	972.4	E858.3	E942.4	E950.4	E962.0	E980.4
Glycine	974.5	E858.5	E944.5	E950.4	E962.0	E980.4
Glycobiarsol	961.1	E857	E931.1	E950.4	E962.0	E980.4
Glycols (ether)	982.8	E862.4	—	E950.9	E962.1	E980.9
Glycopyrrolate	971.1	E855.4	E941.1	E950.4	E962.0	E980.4
Glymidine	962.3	E858.0	E932.3	E950.4	E962.0	E980.4
Gold (compounds) (salts)	965.69	E850.6	E935.6	E950.0	E962.0	E980.0
Golden sulfide of antimony	985.4	E866.2	—	E950.9	E962.1	E980.9
Goldylocks	988.2	E865.4	—	E950.9	E962.1	E980.9
Gonadal tissue extract	962.9	E858.0	E932.9	E950.4	E962.0	E980.4
female	962.2	E858.0	E932.2	E950.4	E962.0	E980.4
male	962.1	E858.0	E932.1	E950.4	E962.0	E980.4
Gonadotropin	962.4	E858.0	E932.4	E950.4	E962.0	E980.4
Grain alcohol	980.0	E860.1	—	E950.9	E962.1	E980.9
beverage	980.0	E860.0	—	E950.9	E962.1	E980.9
Gramicidin	960.8	E856	E930.8	E950.4	E962.0	E980.4

Gas — Gramicidin

		External Cause (E-Code)				
	Poisoning	**Accident**	**Therapeutic Use**	**Suicide Attempt**	**Assault**	**Undetermined**
Gratiola officinalis	988.2	E865.4	—	E950.9	E962.1	E980.9
Grease	989.89	E866.8	—	E950.9	E962.1	E980.9
Green hellebore	988.2	E865.4	—	E950.9	E962.1	E980.9
Green soap	976.2	E858.7	E946.2	E950.4	E962.0	E980.4
Grifulvin	960.1	E856	E930.1	E950.4	E962.0	E980.4
Griseofulvin	960.1	E856	E930.1	E950.4	E962.0	E980.4
Growth hormone	962.4	E858.0	E932.4	E950.4	E962.0	E980.4
Guaiacol	975.5	E858.6	E945.5	E950.4	E962.0	E980.4
Guaiac reagent	977.8	E858.8	E947.8	E950.4	E962.0	E980.4
Guaifenesin	975.5	E858.6	E945.5	E950.4	E962.0	E980.4
Guaiphenesin	975.5	E858.6	E945.5	E950.4	E962.0	E980.4
Guanatol	961.4	E857	E931.4	E950.4	E962.0	E980.4
Guanethidine	972.6	E858.3	E942.6	E950.4	E962.0	E980.4
Guano	989.89	E866.5	—	E950.9	E962.1	E980.9
Guanochlor	972.6	E858.3	E942.6	E950.4	E962.0	E980.4
Guanoctine	972.6	E858.3	E942.6	E950.4	E962.0	E980.4
Guanoxan	972.6	E858.3	E942.6	E950.4	E962.0	E980.4
Hair treatment agent NEC	976.4	E858.7	E946.4	E950.4	E962.0	E980.4
Halcinonide	976.0	E858.7	E946.0	E950.4	E962.0	E980.4
Halethazole	976.0	E858.7	E946.0	E950.4	E962.0	E980.4
Hallucinogens	969.6	E854.1	E939.6	E950.3	E962.0	E980.3
Haloperidol	969.2	E853.1	E939.2	E950.3	E962.0	E980.3
Haloprogin	976.0	E858.7	E946.0	E950.4	E962.0	E980.4
Halotex	976.0	E858.7	E946.0	E950.4	E962.0	E980.4
Halothane	968.1	E855.1	E938.1	E950.4	E962.0	E980.4
Halquinols	976.0	E858.7	E946.0	E950.4	E962.0	E980.4
Harmonyl	972.6	E858.3	E942.6	E950.4	E962.0	E980.4
Hartmann's solution	974.5	E858.5	E944.5	E950.4	E962.0	E980.4
Hashish	969.6	E854.1	E939.6	E950.3	E962.0	E980.3
Hawaiian wood rose seeds	969.6	E854.1	E939.6	E950.3	E962.0	E980.3
Headache cures, drugs, powders NEC	977.9	E858.9	E947.9	E950.5	E962.0	E980.9
Heavenly Blue (morning glory)	969.6	E854.1	E939.6	E950.3	E962.0	E980.3
Heavy metal antagonists	963.8	E858.1	E933.8	E950.4	E962.0	E980.4
anti-infectives	961.2	E857	E931.2	E950.4	E962.0	E980.4
Hedaquinium	976.0	E858.7	E946.0	E950.4	E962.0	E980.4
Hedge hyssop	988.2	E865.4	—	E950.9	E962.1	E980.9
Heet	976.8	E858.7	E946.8	E950.4	E962.0	E980.4
Helenin	961.6	E857	E931.6	E950.4	E962.0	E980.4
Hellebore (black) (green) (white)	988.2	E865.4	—	E950.9	E962.1	E980.9
Hemlock	988.2	E865.4	—	E950.9	E962.1	E980.9
Hemostatics	964.5	E858.2	E934.5	E950.4	E962.0	E980.4
capillary active drugs	972.8	E858.3	E942.8	E950.4	E962.0	E980.4
Henbane	988.2	E865.4	—	E950.9	E962.1	E980.9
Heparin (sodium)	964.2	E858.2	E934.2	E950.4	E962.0	E980.4
Heptabarbital, heptabarbitone	967.0	E851	E937.0	E950.1	E962.0	E980.1
Heptachlor	989.2	E863.0	—	E950.6	E962.1	E980.7
Heptalgin	965.09	E850.2	E935.2	E950.0	E962.0	E980.0
Herbicides	989.4	E863.5	—	E950.6	E962.1	E980.7
Heroin	965.01	E850.0	E935.0	E950.0	E962.0	E980.0
Herplex	976.5	E858.7	E946.5	E950.4	E962.0	E980.4
HES	964.8	E858.2	E934.8	E950.4	E962.0	E980.4
Hetastarch	964.8	E858.2	E934.8	E950.4	E962.0	E980.4
Hexachlorocyclohexane	989.2	E863.0	—	E950.6	E962.1	E980.7
Hexachlorophene	976.2	E858.7	E946.2	E950.4	E962.0	E980.4
Hexadimethrine (bromide)	964.5	E858.2	E934.5	E950.4	E962.0	E980.4
Hexafluorenium	975.2	E858.6	E945.2	E950.4	E962.0	E980.4
Hexa-germ	976.2	E858.7	E946.2	E950.4	E962.0	E980.4
Hexahydrophenol	980.8	E860.8	—	E950.9	E962.1	E980.9
Hexalin	980.8	E860.8	—	E950.9	E962.1	E980.9
Hexamethonium	972.3	E858.3	E942.3	E950.4	E962.0	E980.4
Hexamethyleneamine	961.9	E857	E931.9	E950.4	E962.0	E980.4
Hexamine	961.9	E857	E931.9	E950.4	E962.0	E980.4
Hexanone	982.8	E862.4	—	E950.9	E962.1	E980.9
Hexapropymate	967.8	E852.8	E937.8	E950.2	E962.0	E980.2
Hexestrol	962.2	E858.0	E932.2	E950.4	E962.0	E980.4
Hexethal (sodium)	967.0	E851	E937.0	E950.1	E962.0	E980.1
Hexetidine	976.0	E858.7	E946.0	E950.4	E962.0	E980.4
Hexobarbital, hexobarbitone	967.0	E851	E937.0	E950.1	E962.0	E980.1
sodium (anesthetic)	968.3	E855.1	E938.3	E950.4	E962.0	E980.4
soluble	968.3	E855.1	E938.3	E950.4	E962.0	E980.4
Hexocyclium	971.1	E855.4	E941.1	E950.4	E962.0	E980.4
Hexoestrol	962.2	E858.0	E932.2	E950.4	E962.0	E980.4
Hexone	982.8	E862.4	—	E950.9	E962.1	E980.9
Hexylcaine	968.5	E855.2	E938.5	E950.4	E962.0	E980.4
Hexylresorcinol	961.6	E857	E931.6	E950.4	E962.0	E980.4
Hinkle's pills	973.1	E858.4	E943.1	E950.4	E962.0	E980.4
Histalog	977.8	E858.8	E947.8	E950.4	E962.0	E980.4
Histamine (phosphate)	972.5	E858.3	E942.5	E950.4	E962.0	E980.4
Histoplasmin	977.8	E858.8	E947.8	E950.4	E962.0	E980.4
Holly berries	988.2	E865.3	—	E950.9	E962.1	E980.9
Homatropine	971.1	E855.4	E941.1	E950.4	E962.0	E980.4

		External Cause (E-Code)				
	Poisoning	Accident	Therapeutic Use	Suicide Attempt	Assault	Undetermined
Homo-tet	964.6	E858.2	E934.6	E950.4	E962.0	E980.4
Hormones (synthetic substitute) NEC	962.9	E858.0	E932.9	E950.4	E962.0	E980.4
adrenal cortical steroids	962.0	E858.0	E932.0	E950.4	E962.0	E980.4
antidiabetic agents	962.3	E858.0	E932.3	E950.4	E962.0	E980.4
follicle stimulating	962.4	E858.0	E932.4	E950.4	E962.0	E980.4
gonadotropic	962.4	E858.0	E932.4	E950.4	E962.0	E980.4
growth	962.4	E858.0	E932.4	E950.4	E962.0	E980.4
ovarian (substitutes)	962.2	E858.0	E932.2	E950.4	E962.0	E980.4
parathyroid (derivatives)	962.6	E858.0	E932.6	E950.4	E962.0	E980.4
pituitary (posterior)	962.5	E858.0	E932.5	E950.4	E962.0	E980.4
anterior	962.4	E858.0	E932.4	E950.4	E962.0	E980.4
thyroid (derivative)	962.7	E858.0	E932.7	E950.4	E962.0	E980.4
Hornet (sting)	989.5	E905.3	—	E950.9	E962.1	E980.9
Horticulture agent NEC	989.4	E863.9	—	E950.6	E962.1	E980.7
Hyaluronidase	963.4	E858.1	E933.4	E950.4	E962.0	E980.4
Hyazyme	963.4	E858.1	E933.4	E950.4	E962.0	E980.4
Hycodan	965.09	E850.2	E935.2	E950.0	E962.0	E980.0
Hydantoin derivatives	966.1	E855.0	E936.1	E950.4	E962.0	E980.4
Hydeltra	962.0	E858.0	E932.0	E950.4	E962.0	E980.4
Hydergine	971.3	E855.6	E941.3	E950.4	E962.0	E980.4
Hydrabamine penicillin	960.0	E856	E930.0	E950.4	E962.0	E980.4
Hydralazine, hydrallazine	972.6	E858.3	E942.6	E950.4	E962.0	E980.4
Hydrargaphen	976.0	E858.7	E946.0	E950.4	E962.0	E980.4
Hydrazine	983.9	E864.3	—	E950.7	E962.1	E980.6
Hydriodic acid	975.5	E858.6	E945.5	E950.4	E962.0	E980.4
Hydrocarbon gas	987.1	E869.8	—	E952.8	E962.2	E982.8
incomplete combustion of — *see* Carbon, monoxide, fuel, utility						
liquefied (mobile container)	987.0	E868.0	—	E951.1	E962.2	E981.1
piped (natural)	987.0	E867	—	E951.0	E962.2	E981.0
Hydrochloric acid (liquid)	983.1	E864.1	—	E950.7	E962.1	E980.6
medicinal	973.4	E858.4	E943.4	E950.4	E962.0	E980.4
vapor	987.8	E869.8	—	E952.8	E962.2	E982.8
Hydrochlorothiazide	974.3	E858.5	E944.3	E950.4	E962.0	E980.4
Hydrocodone	965.09	E850.2	E935.2	E950.0	E962.0	E980.0
Hydrocortisone	962.0	E858.0	E932.0	E950.4	E962.0	E980.4
ENT agent	976.6	E858.7	E946.6	E950.4	E962.0	E980.4
ophthalmic preparation	976.5	E858.7	E946.5	E950.4	E962.0	E980.4
topical NEC	976.0	E858.7	E946.0	E950.4	E962.0	E980.4
Hydrocortone	962.0	E858.0	E932.0	E950.4	E962.0	E980.4
ENT agent	976.6	E858.7	E946.6	E950.4	E962.0	E980.4
ophthalmic preparation	976.5	E858.7	E946.5	E950.4	E962.0	E980.4
topical NEC	976.0	E858.7	E946.0	E950.4	E962.0	E980.4
Hydrocyanic acid — *see* Cyanide(s)						
Hydroflumethiazide	974.3	E858.5	E944.3	E950.4	E962.0	E980.4
Hydrofluoric acid (liquid)	983.1	E864.1	—	E950.7	E962.1	E980.6
vapor	987.8	E869.8	—	E952.8	E962.2	E982.8
Hydrogen	987.8	E869.8	—	E952.8	E962.2	E982.8
arsenide	985.1	E866.3	—	E950.8	E962.1	E980.8
arseniureted	985.1	E866.3	—	E950.8	E962.1	E980.8
cyanide (salts)	989.0	E866.8	—	E950.9	E962.1	E980.9
gas	987.7	E869.8	—	E952.8	E962.2	E982.8
fluoride (liquid)	983.1	E864.1	—	E950.7	E962.1	E980.6
vapor	987.8	E869.8	—	E952.8	E962.2	E982.8
peroxide (solution)	976.6	E858.7	E946.6	E950.4	E962.0	E980.4
phosphureted	987.8	E869.8	—	E952.8	E962.2	E982.8
sulfide (gas)	987.8	E869.8	—	E952.8	E962.2	E982.8
arseniureted	985.1	E866.3	—	E950.8	E962.1	E980.8
sulfureted	987.8	E869.8	—	E952.8	E962.2	E982.8
Hydromorphinol	965.09	E850.2	E935.2	E950.0	E962.0	E980.0
Hydromorphinone	965.09	E850.2	E935.2	E950.0	E962.0	E980.0
Hydromorphone	965.09	E850.2	E935.2	E950.0	E962.0	E980.0
Hydromox	974.3	E858.5	E944.3	E950.4	E962.0	E980.4
Hydrophilic lotion	976.3	E858.7	E946.3	E950.4	E962.0	E980.4
Hydroquinone	983.0	E864.0	—	E950.7	E962.1	E980.6
vapor	987.8	E869.8	—	E952.8	E962.2	E982.8
Hydrosulfuric acid (gas)	987.8	E869.8	—	E952.8	E962.2	E982.8
Hydrous wool fat (lotion)	976.3	E858.7	E946.3	E950.4	E962.0	E980.4
Hydroxide, caustic	983.2	E864.2	—	E950.7	E962.1	E980.6
Hydroxocobalamin	964.1	E858.2	E934.1	E950.4	E962.0	E980.4
Hydroxyamphetamine	971.2	E855.5	E941.2	E950.4	E962.0	E980.4
Hydroxychloroquine	961.4	E857	E931.4	E950.4	E962.0	E980.4
Hydroxydihydrocodeinone	965.09	E850.2	E935.2	E950.0	E962.0	E980.0
Hydroxyethyl starch	964.8	E858.2	E934.8	E950.4	E962.0	E980.4
Hydroxyphenamate	969.5	E853.8	E939.5	E950.3	E962.0	E980.3
Hydroxyphenylbutazone	965.5	E850.5	E935.5	E950.0	E962.0	E980.0
Hydroxyprogesterone	962.2	E858.0	E932.2	E950.4	E962.0	E980.4
Hydroxyquinoline derivatives	961.3	E857	E931.3	E950.4	E962.0	E980.4
Hydroxystilbamidine	961.5	E857	E931.5	E950.4	E962.0	E980.4
Hydroxyurea	963.1	E858.1	E933.1	E950.4	E962.0	E980.4
Hydroxyzine	969.5	E853.8	E939.5	E950.3	E962.0	E980.3
Hyoscine (hydrobromide)	971.1	E855.4	E941.1	E950.4	E962.0	E980.4

Homo-tet — Hyoscine

	Poisoning	External Cause (E-Code)				
		Accident	Therapeutic Use	Suicide Attempt	Assault	Undetermined
Hyoscyamine	971.1	E855.4	E941.1	E950.4	E962.0	E980.4
Hyoscyamus (albus) (niger)	988.2	E865.4	—	E950.9	E962.1	E980.9
Hypaque	977.8	E858.8	E947.8	E950.4	E962.0	E980.4
Hypertussis	964.6	E858.2	E934.6	E950.4	E962.0	E980.4
Hypnotics NEC	967.9	E852.9	E937.9	E950.2	E962.0	E980.2
Hypochlorites — *see* Sodium, hypochlorite						
Hypotensive agents NEC	972.6	E858.3	E942.6	E950.4	E962.0	E980.4
Ibufenac	965.69	E850.6	E935.6	E950.0	E962.0	E980.0
Ibuprofen	965.61	E850.6	E935.6	E950.0	E962.0	E980.0
ICG	977.8	E858.8	E947.8	E950.4	E962.0	E980.4
Ichthammol	976.4	E858.7	E946.4	E950.4	E962.0	E980.4
Ichthyol	976.4	E858.7	E946.4	E950.4	E962.0	E980.4
Idoxuridine	976.5	E858.7	E946.5	E950.4	E962.0	E980.4
IDU	976.5	E858.7	E946.5	E950.4	E962.0	E980.4
Iletin	962.3	E858.0	E932.3	E950.4	E962.0	E980.4
Ilex	988.2	E865.4	—	E950.9	E962.1	E980.9
Illuminating gas — *see* Gas, utility						
Ilopan	963.5	E858.1	E933.5	E950.4	E962.0	E980.4
Ilotycin	960.3	E856	E930.3	E950.4	E962.0	E980.4
ophthalmic preparation	976.5	E858.7	E946.5	E950.4	E962.0	E980.4
topical NEC	976.0	E858.7	E946.0	E950.4	E962.0	E980.4
Imipramine	969.0	E854.0	E939.0	E950.3	E962.0	E980.3
Immu-G	964.6	E858.2	E934.6	E950.4	E962.0	E980.4
Immuglobin	964.6	E858.2	E934.6	E950.4	E962.0	E980.4
Immune serum globulin	964.6	E858.2	E934.6	E950.4	E962.0	E980.4
Immunosuppressive agents	963.1	E858.1	E933.1	E950.4	E962.0	E980.4
Immu-tetanus	964.6	E858.2	E934.6	E950.4	E962.0	E980.4
Indandione (derivatives)	964.2	E858.2	E934.2	E950.4	E962.0	E980.4
Inderal	972.0	E858.3	E942.0	E950.4	E962.0	E980.4
Indian						
hemp	969.6	E854.1	E939.6	E950.3	E962.0	E980.3
tobacco	988.2	E865.4	—	E950.9	E962.1	E980.9
Indigo carmine	977.8	E858.8	E947.8	E950.4	E962.0	E980.4
Indocin	965.69	E850.6	E935.6	E950.0	E962.0	E980.0
Indocyanine green	977.8	E858.8	E947.8	E950.4	E962.0	E980.4
Indomethacin	965.69	E850.6	E935.6	E950.0	E962.0	E980.0
Industrial						
alcohol	980.9	E860.9	—	E950.9	E962.1	E980.9
fumes	987.8	E869.8	—	E952.8	E962.2	E982.8
solvents (fumes) (vapors)	982.8	E862.9	—	E950.9	E962.1	E980.9
Influenza vaccine	979.6	E858.8	E949.6	E950.4	E962.0	E982.8
Ingested substances NEC	989.9	E866.9	—	E950.9	E962.1	E980.9
INH (isoniazid)	961.8	E857	E931.8	E950.4	E962.0	E980.4
Inhalation, gas (noxious) — *see* Gas						
Ink	989.89	E866.8	—	E950.9	E962.1	E980.9
Innovar	967.6	E852.5	E937.6	E950.2	E962.0	E980.2
Inositol niacinate	972.2	E858.3	E942.2	E950.4	E962.0	E980.4
Inproquone	963.1	E858.1	E933.1	E950.4	E962.0	E980.4
Insect (sting), venomous	989.5	E905.5	—	E950.9	E962.1	E980.9
Insecticides (*see also* Pesticides)	989.4	E863.4	—	E950.6	E962.1	E980.7
chlorinated	989.2	E863.0	—	E950.6	E962.1	E980.7
mixtures	989.4	E863.3	—	E950.6	E962.1	E980.7
organochlorine (compounds)	989.2	E863.0	—	E950.6	E962.1	E980.7
organophosphorus (compounds)	989.3	E863.1	—	E950.6	E962.1	E980.7
Insular tissue extract	962.3	E858.0	E932.3	E950.4	E962.0	E980.4
Insulin (amorphous) (globin) (isophane) (Lente) (NPH) (protamine) (Semilente) (Ultralente) (zinc)	962.3	E858.0	E932.3	E950.4	E962.0	E980.4
Intranarcon	968.3	E855.1	E938.3	E950.4	E962.0	E980.4
Inulin	977.8	E858.8	E947.8	E950.4	E962.0	E980.4
Invert sugar	974.5	E858.5	E944.5	E950.4	E962.0	E980.4
Iodide NEC (*see also* Iodine)	976.0	E858.7	E946.0	E950.4	E962.0	E980.4
mercury (ointment)	976.0	E858.7	E946.0	E950.4	E962.0	E980.4
methylate	976.0	E858.7	E946.0	E950.4	E962.0	E980.4
potassium (expectorant) NEC	975.5	E858.6	E945.5	E950.4	E962.0	E980.4
Iodinated glycerol	975.5	E858.6	E945.5	E950.4	E962.0	E980.4
Iodine (antiseptic, external) (tincture) NEC	976.0	E858.7	E946.0	E950.4	E962.0	E980.4
diagnostic	977.8	E858.8	E947.8	E950.4	E962.0	E980.4
for thyroid conditions (antithyroid)	962.8	E858.0	E932.8	E950.4	E962.0	E980.4
vapor	987.8	E869.8	—	E952.8	E962.2	E982.8
Iodized oil	977.8	E858.8	E947.8	E950.4	E962.0	E980.4
Iodobismitol	961.2	E857	E931.2	E950.4	E962.0	E980.4
Iodochlorhydroxyquin	961.3	E857	E931.3	E950.4	E962.0	E980.4
topical	976.0	E858.7	E946.0	E950.4	E962.0	E980.4
Iodoform	976.0	E858.7	E946.0	E950.4	E962.0	E980.4
Iodopanoic acid	977.8	E858.8	E947.8	E950.4	E962.0	E980.4
Iodophthalein	977.8	E858.8	E947.8	E950.4	E962.0	E980.4
Ion exchange resins	974.5	E858.5	E944.5	E950.4	E962.0	E980.4
Iopanoic acid	977.8	E858.8	E947.8	E950.4	E962.0	E980.4
Iophendylate	977.8	E858.8	E947.8	E950.4	E962.0	E980.4
Iothiouracil	962.8	E858.0	E932.8	E950.4	E962.0	E980.4
Ipecac	973.6	E858.4	E943.6	E950.4	E962.0	E980.4

4ᵗʰ Fourth-digit Required   5ᵗʰ Fifth-digit Required   ►◄ Revised Text   ● New Line   ▲ Revised Code

	Poisoning	External Cause (E-Code)				
		Accident	Therapeutic Use	Suicide Attempt	Assault	Undetermined
Ipecacuanha	973.6	E858.4	E943.6	E950.4	E962.0	E980.4
Ipodate	977.8	E858.8	E947.8	E950.4	E962.0	E980.4
Ipral	967.0	E851	E937.0	E950.1	E962.0	E980.1
Ipratropium ●	975.1	E858.6	E945.1	E950.4	E962.0	E980.4
Iproniazid	969.0	E854.0	E939.0	E950.3	E962.0	E980.3
Iron (compounds) (medicinal) (preparations)	964.0	E858.2	E934.0	E950.4	E962.0	E980.4
dextran	964.0	E858.2	E934.0	E950.4	E962.0	E980.4
nonmedicinal (dust) (fumes) NEC	985.8	E866.4	—	E950.9	E962.1	E980.9
Irritant drug	977.9	E858.9	E947.9	E950.5	E962.0	E980.5
Ismelin	972.6	E858.3	E942.6	E950.4	E962.0	E980.4
Isoamyl nitrite	972.4	E858.3	E942.4	E950.4	E962.0	E980.4
Isobutyl acetate	982.8	E862.4	—	E950.9	E962.1	E980.9
Isocarboxazid	969.0	E854.0	E939.0	E950.3	E962.0	E980.3
Isoephedrine	971.2	E855.5	E941.2	E950.4	E962.0	E980.4
Isoetharine	971.2	E855.5	E941.2	E950.4	E962.0	E980.4
Isofluorophate	971.0	E855.3	E941.0	E950.4	E962.0	E980.4
Isoniazid (INH)	961.8	E857	E931.8	E950.4	E962.0	E980.4
Isopentaquine	961.4	E857	E931.4	E950.4	E962.0	E980.4
Isophane insulin	962.3	E858.0	E932.3	E950.4	E962.0	E980.4
Isopregnenone	962.2	E858.0	E932.2	E950.4	E962.0	E980.4
Isoprenaline	971.2	E855.5	E941.2	E950.4	E962.0	E980.4
Isopropamide	971.1	E855.4	E941.1	E950.4	E962.0	E980.4
Isopropanol	980.2	E860.3	—	E950.9	E962.1	E980.9
topical (germicide)	976.0	E858.7	E946.0	E950.4	E962.0	E980.4
Isopropyl						
acetate	982.8	E862.4	—	E950.9	E962.1	E980.9
alcohol	980.2	E860.3	—	E950.9	E962.1	E980.9
topical (germicide)	976.0	E858.7	E946.0	E950.4	E962.0	E980.4
ether	982.8	E862.4	—	E950.9	E962.1	E980.9
Isoproterenol	971.2	E855.5	E941.2	E950.4	E962.0	E980.4
Isosorbide dinitrate	972.4	E858.3	E942.4	E950.4	E962.0	E980.4
Isothipendyl	963.0	E858.1	E933.0	E950.4	E962.0	E980.4
Isoxazolyl penicillin	960.0	E856	E930.0	E950.4	E962.0	E980.4
Isoxsuprine hydrochloride	972.5	E858.3	E942.5	E950.4	E962.0	E980.4
l-thyroxine sodium	962.7	E858.0	E932.7	E950.4	E962.0	E980.4
Jaborandi (pilocarpus) (extract)	971.0	E855.3	E941.0	E950.4	E962.0	E980.4
Jalap	973.1	E858.4	E943.1	E950.4	E962.0	E980.4
Jamaica						
dogwood (bark)	965.7	E850.7	E935.7	E950.0	E962.0	E980.0
ginger	989.89	E866.8	—	E950.9	E962.1	E980.9
Jatropha	988.2	E865.4	—	E950.9	E962.1	E980.9
curcas	988.2	E865.3	—	E950.9	E962.1	E980.9
Jectofer	964.0	E858.2	E934.0	E950.4	E962.0	E980.4
Jellyfish (sting)	989.5	E905.6	—	E950.9	E962.1	E980.9
Jequirity (bean)	988.2	E865.3	—	E950.9	E962.1	E980.9
Jimson weed (seeds)	988.2	E865.4	—	E950.9	E962.1	E980.9
seeds	988.2	E865.3	—	E950.9	E962.1	E980.9
Juniper tar (oil) (ointment)	976.4	E858.7	E946.4	E950.4	E962.0	E980.4
Kallikrein	972.5	E858.3	E942.5	E950.4	E962.0	E980.4
Kanamycin	960.6	E856	E930.6	E950.4	E962.0	E980.4
Kantrex	960.6	E856	E930.6	E950.4	E962.0	E980.4
Kaolin	973.5	E858.4	E943.5	E950.4	E962.0	E980.4
Karaya (gum)	973.3	E858.4	E943.3	E950.4	E962.0	E980.4
Kemithal	968.3	E855.1	E938.3	E950.4	E962.0	E980.4
Kenacort	962.0	E858.0	E932.0	E950.4	E962.0	E980.4
Keratolytics	976.4	E858.7	E946.4	E950.4	E962.0	E980.4
Keratoplastics	976.4	E858.7	E946.4	E950.4	E962.0	E980.4
Kerosene, kerosine (fuel) (solvent) NEC	981	E862.1	—	E950.9	E962.1	E980.9
insecticide	981	E863.4	—	E950.6	E962.1	E980.7
vapor	987.1	E869.8	—	E952.8	E962.2	E982.8
Ketamine	968.3	E855.1	E938.3	E950.4	E962.0	E980.4
Ketobemidone	965.09	E850.2	E935.2	E950.0	E962.0	E980.0
Ketols	982.8	E862.4	—	E950.9	E962.1	E980.9
Ketone oils	982.8	E862.4	—	E950.9	E962.1	E980.9
Ketoprofen	965.61	E850.6	E935.6	E950.0	E962.0	E980.0
Kiln gas or vapor (carbon monoxide)	986	E868.8	—	E952.1	E962.2	E982.1
Konsyl	973.3	E858.4	E943.3	E950.4	E962.0	E980.4
Kosam seed	988.2	E865.3	—	E950.9	E962.1	E980.9
Krait (venom)	989.5	E905.0	—	E950.9	E962.1	E980.9
Kwell (insecticide)	989.2	E863.0	—	E950.6	E962.1	E980.7
anti-infective (topical)	976.0	E858.7	E946.0	E950.4	E962.0	E980.4
Laburnum (flowers) (seeds)	988.2	E865.3	—	E950.9	E962.1	E980.9
leaves	988.2	E865.4	—	E950.9	E962.1	E980.9
Lacquers	989.89	E861.6	—	E950.9	E962.1	E980.9
Lacrimogenic gas	987.5	E869.3	—	E952.8	E962.2	E982.8
Lactic acid	983.1	E864.1	—	E950.7	E962.1	E980.6
Lactobacillus acidophilus	973.5	E858.4	E943.5	E950.4	E962.0	E980.4
Lactoflavin	963.5	E858.1	E933.5	E950.4	E962.0	E980.4
Lactuca (virosa) (extract)	967.8	E852.8	E937.8	E950.2	E962.0	E980.2
Lactucarium	967.8	E852.8	E937.8	E950.2	E962.0	E980.2
Laevulose	974.5	E858.5	E944.5	E950.4	E962.0	E980.4

	Poisoning	External Cause (E-Code)				
		Accident	Therapeutic Use	Suicide Attempt	Assault	Undetermined
Lanatoside (C)	972.1	E858.3	E942.1	E950.4	E962.0	E980.4
Lanolin (lotion)	976.3	E858.7	E946.3	E950.4	E962.0	E980.4
Largactil	969.1	E853.0	E939.1	E950.3	E962.0	E980.3
Larkspur	988.2	E865.3	—	E950.9	E962.1	E980.9
Laroxyl	969.0	E854.0	E939.0	E950.3	E962.0	E980.3
Lasix	974.4	E858.5	E944.4	E950.4	E962.0	E980.4
Latex	989.82	E866.8	—	E950.9	E962.1	E980.9
Lathyrus (seed)	988.2	E865.3	—	E950.9	E962.1	E980.9
Laudanum	965.09	E850.2	E935.2	E950.0	E962.0	E980.0
Laudexium	975.2	E858.6	E945.2	E950.4	E962.0	E980.4
Laurel, black or cherry	988.2	E865.4	—	E950.9	E962.1	E980.9
Laurolinium	976.0	E858.7	E946.0	E950.4	E962.0	E980.4
Lauryl sulfoacetate	976.2	E858.7	E946.2	E950.4	E962.0	E980.4
Laxatives NEC	973.3	E858.4	E943.3	E950.4	E962.0	E980.4
emollient	973.2	E858.4	E943.2	E950.4	E962.0	E980.4
L-dopa	966.4	E855.0	E936.4	E950.4	E962.0	E980.4
Lead (dust) (fumes) (vapor) NEC	984.9	E866.0	—	E950.9	E962.1	E980.9
acetate (dust)	984.1	E866.0	—	E950.9	E962.1	E980.9
anti-infectives	961.2	E857	E931.2	E950.4	E962.0	E980.4
antiknock compound (tetraethyl)	984.1	E862.1	—	E950.9	E962.1	E980.9
arsenate, arsenite (dust) (insecticide) (vapor)	985.1	E863.4	—	E950.8	E962.1	E980.8
herbicide	985.1	E863.5	—	E950.8	E962.1	E980.8
carbonate	984.0	E866.0	—	E950.9	E962.1	E980.9
paint	984.0	E861.5	—	E950.9	E962.1	E980.9
chromate	984.0	E866.0	—	E950.9	E962.1	E980.9
paint	984.0	E861.5	—	E950.9	E962.1	E980.9
dioxide	984.0	E866.0	—	E950.9	E962.1	E980.9
inorganic (compound)	984.0	E866.0	—	E950.9	E962.1	E980.9
paint	984.0	E861.5	—	E950.9	E962.1	E980.9
iodide	984.0	E866.0	—	E950.9	E962.1	E980.9
pigment (paint)	984.0	E861.5	—	E950.9	E962.1	E980.9
monoxide (dust)	984.0	E866.0	—	E950.9	E962.1	E980.9
paint	984.0	E861.5	—	E950.9	E962.1	E980.9
organic	984.1	E866.0	—	E950.9	E962.1	E980.9
oxide	984.0	E866.0	—	E950.9	E962.1	E980.9
paint	984.0	E861.5	—	E950.9	E962.1	E980.9
paint	984.0	E861.5	—	E950.9	E962.1	E980.9
salts	984.0	E866.0	—	E950.9	E962.1	E980.9
specified compound NEC	984.8	E866.0	—	E950.9	E962.1	E980.9
tetra-ethyl	984.1	E862.1	—	E950.9	E962.1	E980.9
Lebanese red	969.6	E854.1	E939.6	E950.3	E962.0	E980.3
Lente Iletin (insulin)	962.3	E858.0	E932.3	E950.4	E962.0	E980.4
Leptazol	970.0	E854.3	E940.0	E950.4	E962.0	E980.4
Leritine	965.09	E850.2	E935.2	E950.0	E962.0	E980.0
Letter	962.7	E858.0	E932.7	E950.4	E962.0	E980.4
Lettuce opium	967.8	E852.8	E937.8	E950.2	E962.0	E980.2
Leucovorin (factor)	964.1	E858.2	E934.1	E950.4	E962.0	E980.4
Leukeran	963.1	E858.1	E933.1	E950.4	E962.0	E980.4
Levalbuterol ●	975.7	E858.6	E945.7	E950.4	E962.0	E980.4
Levallorphan	970.1	E854.3	E940.1	E950.4	E962.0	E980.4
Levanil	967.8	E852.8	E937.8	E950.2	E962.0	E980.2
Levarterenol	971.2	E855.5	E941.2	E950.4	E962.0	E980.4
Levodopa	966.4	E855.0	E936.4	E950.4	E962.0	E980.4
Levo-dromoran	965.09	E850.2	E935.2	E950.0	E962.0	E980.0
Levoid	962.7	E858.0	E932.7	E950.4	E962.0	E980.4
Levo-iso-methadone	965.02	E850.1	E935.1	E950.0	E962.0	E980.0
Levomepromazine	967.8	E852.8	E937.8	E950.2	E962.0	E980.2
Levoprome	967.8	E852.8	E937.8	E950.2	E962.0	E980.2
Levopropoxyphene	975.4	E858.6	E945.4	E950.4	E962.0	E980.4
Levorphan, levophanol	965.09	E850.2	E935.2	E950.0	E962.0	E980.0
Levothyroxine (sodium)	962.7	E858.0	E932.7	E950.4	E962.0	E980.4
Levsin	971.1	E855.4	E941.1	E950.4	E962.0	E980.4
Levulose	974.5	E858.5	E944.5	E950.4	E962.0	E980.4
Lewisite (gas)	985.1	E866.3	—	E950.8	E962.1	E980.8
Librium	969.4	E853.2	E939.4	E950.3	E962.0	E980.3
Lidex	976.0	E858.7	E946.0	E950.4	E962.0	E980.4
Lidocaine (infiltration) (topical)	968.5	E855.2	E938.5	E950.4	E962.0	E980.4
nerve block (peripheral) (plexus)	968.6	E855.2	E938.6	E950.4	E962.0	E980.4
spinal	968.7	E855.2	E938.7	E950.4	E962.0	E980.4
Lighter fluid	981	E862.1	—	E950.9	E962.1	E980.9
Lignocaine (infiltration) (topical)	968.5	E855.2	E938.5	E950.4	E962.0	E980.4
nerve block (peripheral) (plexus)	968.6	E855.2	E938.6	E950.4	E962.0	E980.4
spinal	968.7	E855.2	E938.7	E950.4	E962.0	E980.4
Ligroin(e) (solvent)	981	E862.0	—	E950.9	E962.1	E980.9
vapor	987.1	E869.8	—	E952.8	E962.2	E982.8
Ligustrum vulgare	988.2	E865.3	—	E950.9	E962.1	E980.9
Lily of the valley	988.2	E865.4	—	E950.9	E962.1	E980.9
Lime (chloride)	983.2	E864.2	—	E950.7	E962.1	E980.6
solution, sulferated	976.4	E858.7	E946.4	E950.4	E962.0	E980.4
Limonene	982.8	E862.4	—	E950.9	E962.1	E980.9
Lincomycin	960.8	E856	E930.8	E950.4	E962.0	E980.4

	Poisoning	External Cause (E-Code)				
		Accident	**Therapeutic Use**	**Suicide Attempt**	**Assault**	**Undetermined**
Lindane (insecticide) (vapor)	989.2	E863.0	—	E950.6	E962.1	E980.7
anti-infective (topical)	976.0	E858.7	E946.0	E950.4	E962.0	E980.4
Liniments NEC	976.9	E858.7	E946.9	E950.4	E962.0	E980.4
Linoleic acid	972.2	E858.3	E942.2	E950.4	E962.0	E980.4
Liothyronine	962.7	E858.0	E932.7	E950.4	E962.0	E980.4
Liotrix	962.7	E858.0	E932.7	E950.4	E962.0	E980.4
Lipancreatin	973.4	E858.4	E943.4	E950.4	E962.0	E980.4
Lipo-Lutin	962.2	E858.0	E932.2	E950.4	E962.0	E980.4
Lipotropic agents	977.1	E858.8	E947.1	E950.4	E962.0	E980.4
Liquefied petroleum gases	987.0	E868.0	—	E951.1	E962.2	E981.1
piped (pure or mixed with air)	987.0	E867	—	E951.0	E962.2	E981.0
Liquid petrolatum	973.2	E858.4	E943.2	E950.4	E962.0	E980.4
substance	989.9	E866.9	—	E950.9	E962.1	E980.9
specified NEC	989.89	E866.8	—	E950.9	E962.1	E980.9
Lirugen	979.4	E858.8	E949.4	E950.4	E962.0	E980.4
Lithane	969.8	E855.8	E939.8	E950.3	E962.0	E980.3
Lithium	985.8	E866.4	—	E950.9	E962.1	E980.9
carbonate	969.8	E855.8	E939.8	E950.3	E962.0	E980.3
Lithonate	969.8	E855.8	E939.8	E950.3	E962.0	E980.3
Liver (extract) (injection) (preparations)	964.1	E858.2	E934.1	E950.4	E962.0	E980.4
Lizard (bite) (venom)	989.5	E905.0	—	E950.9	E962.1	E980.9
LMD	964.8	E858.2	E934.8	E950.4	E962.0	E980.4
Lobelia	988.2	E865.4	—	E950.9	E962.1	E980.9
Lobeline	970.0	E854.3	E940.0	E950.4	E962.0	E980.4
Locorten	976.0	E858.7	E946.0	E950.4	E962.0	E980.4
Lolium temulentum	988.2	E865.3	—	E950.9	E962.1	E980.9
Lomotil	973.5	E858.4	E943.5	E950.4	E962.0	E980.4
Lomustine	963.1	E858.1	E933.1	E950.4	E962.0	E980.4
Lophophora williamsii	969.6	E854.1	E939.6	E950.3	E962.0	E980.3
Lorazepam	969.4	E853.2	E939.4	E950.3	E962.0	E980.3
Lotions NEC	976.9	E858.7	E946.9	E950.4	E962.0	E980.4
Lotronex	973.8	E858.4	E943.8	E950.4	E962.0	E980.4
Lotusate	967.0	E851	E937.0	E950.1	E962.0	E980.1
Lowila	976.2	E858.7	E946.2	E950.4	E962.0	E980.4
Loxapine	969.3	E853.8	E939.3	E950.3	E962.0	E980.3
Lozenges (throat)	976.6	E858.7	E946.6	E950.4	E962.0	E980.4
LSD (25)	969.6	E854.1	E939.6	E950.3	E962.0	E980.3
Lubricating oil NEC	981	E862.2	—	E950.9	E962.1	E980.9
Lucanthone	961.6	E857	E931.6	E950.4	E962.0	E980.4
Luminal	967.0	E851	E937.0	E950.1	E962.0	E980.1
Lung irritant (gas) NEC	987.9	E869.9	—	E952.9	E962.2	E982.9
Lutocylol	962.2	E858.0	E932.2	E950.4	E962.0	E980.4
Lutromone	962.2	E858.0	E932.2	E950.4	E962.0	E980.4
Lututrin	975.0	E858.6	E945.0	E950.4	E962.0	E980.4
Lye (concentrated)	983.2	E864.2	—	E950.7	E962.1	E980.6
Lygranum (skin test)	977.8	E858.8	E947.8	E950.4	E962.0	E980.4
Lymecycline	960.4	E856	E930.4	E950.4	E962.0	E980.4
Lymphogranuloma venereum antigen	977.8	E858.8	E947.8	E950.4	E962.0	E980.4
Lynestrenol	962.2	E858.0	E932.2	E950.4	E962.0	E980.4
Lyovac Sodium Edecrin	974.4	E858.5	E944.4	E950.4	E962.0	E980.4
Lypressin	962.5	E858.0	E932.5	E950.4	E962.0	E980.4
Lysergic acid (amide) (diethylamide)	969.6	E854.1	E939.6	E950.3	E962.0	E980.3
Lysergide	969.6	E854.1	E939.6	E950.3	E962.0	E980.3
Lysine vasopressin	962.5	E858.0	E932.5	E950.4	E962.0	E980.4
Lysol	983.0	E864.0	—	E950.7	E962.1	E980.6
Lytta (vitatta)	976.8	E858.7	E946.8	E950.4	E962.0	E980.4
Mace	987.5	E869.3	—	E952.8	E962.2	E982.8
Macrolides (antibiotics)	960.3	E856	E930.3	E950.4	E962.0	E980.4
Mafenide	976.0	E858.7	E946.0	E950.4	E962.0	E980.4
Magaldrate	973.0	E858.4	E943.0	E950.4	E962.0	E980.4
Magic mushroom	969.6	E854.1	E939.6	E950.3	E962.0	E980.3
Magnamycin	960.8	E856	E930.8	E950.4	E962.0	E980.4
Magnesia magma	973.0	E858.4	E943.0	E950.4	E962.0	E980.4
Magnesium (compounds) (fumes) NEC	985.8	E866.4	—	E950.9	E962.1	E980.9
antacid	973.0	E858.4	E943.0	E950.4	E962.0	E980.4
carbonate	973.0	E858.4	E943.0	E950.4	E962.0	E980.4
cathartic	973.3	E858.4	E943.3	E950.4	E962.0	E980.4
citrate	973.3	E858.4	E943.3	E950.4	E962.0	E980.4
hydroxide	973.0	E858.4	E943.0	E950.4	E962.0	E980.4
oxide	973.0	E858.4	E943.0	E950.4	E962.0	E980.4
sulfate (oral)	973.3	E858.4	E943.3	E950.4	E962.0	E980.4
intravenous	966.3	E855.0	E936.3	E950.4	E962.0	E980.4
trisilicate	973.0	E858.4	E943.0	E950.4	E962.0	E980.4
Malathion (insecticide)	989.3	E863.1	—	E950.6	E962.1	E980.7
Male fern (oleoresin)	961.6	E857	E931.6	E950.4	E962.0	E980.4
Mandelic acid	961.9	E857	E931.9	E950.4	E962.0	E980.4
Manganese compounds (fumes) NEC	985.2	E866.4	—	E950.9	E962.1	E980.9
Mannitol (diuretic) (medicinal) NEC	974.4	E858.5	E944.4	E950.4	E962.0	E980.4
hexanitrate	972.4	E858.3	E942.4	E950.4	E962.0	E980.4
mustard	963.1	E858.1	E933.1	E950.4	E962.0	E980.4

☑4ᵗʰ Fourth-digit Required   ☑5ᵗʰ Fifth-digit Required   ▶◀ Revised Text   ● New Line   ▲ Revised Code

	Poisoning	External Cause (E-Code)				
		Accident	Therapeutic Use	Suicide Attempt	Assault	Undetermined
Mannomustine	963.1	E858.1	E933.1	E950.4	E962.0	E980.4
MAO inhibitors	969.0	E854.0	E939.0	E950.3	E962.0	E980.3
Mapharsen	961.1	E857	E931.1	E950.4	E962.0	E980.4
Marcaine	968.9	E855.2	E938.9	E950.4	E962.0	E980.4
infiltration (subcutaneous)	968.5	E855.2	E938.5	E950.4	E962.0	E980.4
nerve block (peripheral) (plexus)	968.6	E855.2	E938.6	E950.4	E962.0	E980.4
Marezine	963.0	E858.1	E933.0	E950.4	E962.0	E980.4
Marihuana, marijuana (derivatives)	969.6	E854.1	E939.6	E950.3	E962.0	E980.3
Marine animals or plants (sting)	989.5	E905.6	—	E950.9	E962.1	E980.9
Marplan	969.0	E854.0	E939.0	E950.3	E962.0	E980.3
Marsh gas	987.1	E869.8	—	E952.8	E962.2	E982.8
Marsilid	969.0	E854.0	E939.0	E950.3	E962.0	E980.3
Matulane	963.1	E858.1	E933.1	E950.4	E962.0	E980.4
Mazindol	977.0	E858.8	E947.0	E950.4	E962.0	E980.4
Meadow saffron	988.2	E865.3	—	E950.9	E962.1	E980.9
Measles vaccine	979.4	E858.8	E949.4	E950.4	E962.0	E980.4
Meat, noxious or nonbacterial	988.8	E865.0	—	E950.9	E962.1	E980.9
Mebanazine	969.0	E854.0	E939.0	E950.3	E962.0	E980.3
Mebaral	967.0	E851	E937.0	E950.1	E962.0	E980.1
Mebendazole	961.6	E857	E931.6	E950.4	E962.0	E980.4
Mebeverine	975.1	E858.6	E945.1	E950.4	E962.0	E980.4
Mebhydroline	963.0	E858.1	E933.0	E950.4	E962.0	E980.4
Mebrophenhydramine	963.0	E858.1	E933.0	E950.4	E962.0	E980.4
Mebutamate	969.5	E853.8	E939.5	E950.3	E962.0	E980.3
Mecamylamine (chloride)	972.3	E858.3	E942.3	E950.4	E962.0	E980.4
Mechlorethamine hydrochloride	963.1	E858.1	E933.1	E950.4	E962.0	E980.4
Meclizene (hydrochloride)	963.0	E858.1	E933.0	E950.4	E962.0	E980.4
Meclofenoxate	970.0	E854.3	E940.0	E950.4	E962.0	E980.4
Meclozine (hydrochloride)	963.0	E858.1	E933.0	E950.4	E962.0	E980.4
Medazepam	969.4	E853.2	E939.4	E950.3	E962.0	E980.3
Medicine, medicinal substance	977.9	E858.9	E947.9	E950.5	E962.0	E980.5
specified NEC	977.8	E858.8	E947.8	E950.4	E962.0	E980.4
Medinal	967.0	E851	E937.0	E950.1	E962.0	E980.1
Medomin	967.0	E851	E937.0	E950.1	E962.0	E980.1
Medroxyprogesterone	962.2	E858.0	E932.2	E950.4	E962.0	E980.4
Medrysone	976.5	E858.7	E946.5	E950.4	E962.0	E980.4
Mefenamic acid	965.7	E850.7	E935.7	E950.0	E962.0	E980.0
Megahallucinogen	969.6	E854.1	E939.6	E950.3	E962.0	E980.3
Megestrol	962.2	E858.0	E932.2	E950.4	E962.0	E980.4
Meglumine	977.8	E858.8	E947.8	E950.4	E962.0	E980.4
Meladinin	976.3	E858.7	E946.3	E950.4	E962.0	E980.4
Melanizing agents	976.3	E858.7	E946.3	E950.4	E962.0	E980.4
Melarsoprol	961.1	E857	E931.1	E950.4	E962.0	E980.4
Melia azedarach	988.2	E865.3	—	E950.9	E962.1	E980.9
Mellaril	969.1	E853.0	E939.1	E950.3	E962.0	E980.3
Meloxine	976.3	E858.7	E946.3	E950.4	E962.0	E980.4
Melphalan	963.1	E858.1	E933.1	E950.4	E962.0	E980.4
Menadiol sodium diphosphate	964.3	E858.2	E934.3	E950.4	E962.0	E980.4
Menadione (sodium bisulfite)	964.3	E858.2	E934.3	E950.4	E962.0	E980.4
Menaphthone	964.3	E858.2	E934.3	E950.4	E962.0	E980.4
Meningococcal vaccine	978.8	E858.8	E948.8	E950.4	E962.0	E980.4
Menningovax-C	978.8	E858.8	E948.8	E950.4	E962.0	E980.4
Menotropins	962.4	E858.0	E932.4	E950.4	E962.0	E980.4
Menthol NEC	976.1	E858.7	E946.1	E950.4	E962.0	E980.4
Mepacrine	961.3	E857	E931.3	E950.4	E962.0	E980.4
Meparfynol	967.8	E852.8	E937.8	E950.2	E962.0	E980.2
Mepazine	969.1	E853.0	E939.1	E950.3	E962.0	E980.3
Mepenzolate	971.1	E855.4	E941.1	E950.4	E962.0	E980.4
Meperidine	965.09	E850.2	E935.2	E950.0	E962.0	E980.0
Mephenamin(e)	966.4	E855.0	E936.4	E950.4	E962.0	E980.4
Mephenesin (carbamate)	968.0	E855.1	E938.0	E950.4	E962.0	E980.4
Mephenoxalone	969.5	E853.8	E939.5	E950.3	E962.0	E980.3
Mephentermine	971.2	E855.5	E941.2	E950.4	E962.0	E980.4
Mephenytoin	966.1	E855.0	E936.1	E950.4	E962.0	E980.4
Mephobarbital	967.0	E851	E937.0	E950.1	E962.0	E980.1
Mepiperphenidol	971.1	E855.4	E941.1	E950.4	E962.0	E980.4
Mepivacaine	968.9	E855.2	E938.9	E950.4	E962.0	E980.4
infiltration (subcutaneous)	968.5	E855.2	E938.5	E950.4	E962.0	E980.4
nerve block (peripheral) (plexus)	968.6	E855.2	E938.6	E950.4	E962.0	E980.4
topical (surface)	968.5	E855.2	E938.5	E950.4	E962.0	E980.4
Meprednisone	962.0	E858.0	E932.0	E950.4	E962.0	E980.4
Meprobam	969.5	E853.8	E939.5	E950.3	E962.0	E980.3
Meprobamate	969.5	E853.8	E939.5	E950.3	E962.0	E980.3
Mepyramine (maleate)	963.0	E858.1	E933.0	E950.4	E962.0	E980.4
Meralluride	974.0	E858.5	E944.0	E950.4	E962.0	E980.4
Merbaphen	974.0	E858.5	E944.0	E950.4	E962.0	E980.4
Merbromin	976.0	E858.7	E946.0	E950.4	E962.0	E980.4
Mercaptomerin	974.0	E858.5	E944.0	E950.4	E962.0	E980.4
Mercaptopurine	963.1	E858.1	E933.1	E950.4	E962.0	E980.4
Mercumatilin	974.0	E858.5	E944.0	E950.4	E962.0	E980.4
Mercuramide	974.0	E858.5	E944.0	E950.4	E962.0	E980.4

▨4ᵗʰ Fourth-digit Required   ▨5ᵗʰ Fifth-digit Required   ▶◀ Revised Text   ● New Line   ▲ Revised Code

	Poisoning	External Cause (E-Code)				
		Accident	Therapeutic Use	Suicide Attempt	Assault	Undetermined
Mercuranin	976.0	E858.7	E946.0	E950.4	E962.0	E980.4
Mercurochrome	976.0	E858.7	E946.0	E950.4	E962.0	E980.4
Mercury, mercuric, mercurous (compounds) (cyanide) (fumes)						
(nonmedicinal) (vapor) NEC	985.0	E866.1	—	E950.9	E962.1	E980.9
ammoniated	976.0	E858.7	E946.0	E950.4	E962.0	E980.4
anti-infective	961.2	E857	E931.2	E950.4	E962.0	E980.4
topical	976.0	E858.7	E946.0	E950.4	E962.0	E980.4
chloride (antiseptic) NEC	976.0	E858.7	E946.0	E950.4	E962.0	E980.4
fungicide	985.0	E863.6	—	E950.6	E962.1	E980.7
diuretic compounds	974.0	E858.5	E944.0	E950.4	E962.0	E980.4
fungicide	985.0	E863.6	—	E950.6	E962.1	E980.7
organic (fungicide)	985.0	E863.6	—	E950.6	E962.1	E980.7
Merethoxylline	974.0	E858.5	E944.0	E950.4	E962.0	E980.4
Mersalyl	974.0	E858.5	E944.0	E950.4	E962.0	E980.4
Merthiolate (topical)	976.0	E858.7	E946.0	E950.4	E962.0	E980.4
ophthalmic preparation	976.5	E858.7	E946.5	E950.4	E962.0	E980.4
Meruvax	979.4	E858.8	E949.4	E950.4	E962.0	E980.4
Mescal buttons	969.6	E854.1	E939.6	E950.3	E962.0	E980.3
Mescaline (salts)	969.6	E854.1	E939.6	E950.3	E962.0	E980.3
Mesoridazine besylate	969.1	E853.0	E939.1	E950.3	E962.0	E980.3
Mestanolone	962.1	E858.0	E932.1	E950.4	E962.0	E980.4
Mestranol	962.2	E858.0	E932.2	E950.4	E962.0	E980.4
Metacresylacetate	976.0	E858.7	E946.0	E950.4	E962.0	E980.4
Metaldehyde (snail killer) NEC	989.4	E863.4	—	E950.6	E962.1	E980.7
Metals (heavy) (nonmedicinal) NEC	985.9	E866.4	—	E950.9	E962.1	E980.9
dust, fumes, or vapor NEC	985.9	E866.4	—	E950.9	E962.1	E980.9
light NEC	985.9	E866.4	—	E950.9	E962.1	E980.9
dust, fumes, or vapor NEC	985.9	E866.4	—	E950.9	E962.1	E980.9
pesticides (dust) (vapor)	985.9	E863.4	—	E950.6	E962.1	E980.7
Metamucil	973.3	E858.4	E943.3	E950.4	E962.0	E980.4
Metaphen	976.0	E858.7	E946.0	E950.4	E962.0	E980.4
Metaproterenol	975.1	E858.6	E945.1	E950.4	E962.0	E980.4
Metaraminol	972.8	E858.3	E942.8	E950.4	E962.0	E980.4
Metaxalone	968.0	E855.1	E938.0	E950.4	E962.0	E980.4
Metformin	962.3	E858.0	E932.3	E950.4	E962.0	E980.4
Methacycline	960.4	E856	E930.4	E950.4	E962.0	E980.4
Methadone	965.02	E850.1	E935.1	E950.0	E962.0	E980.0
Methallenestril	962.2	E858.0	E932.2	E950.4	E962.0	E980.4
Methamphetamine	969.7	E854.2	E939.7	E950.3	E962.0	E980.3
Methandienone	962.1	E858.0	E932.1	E950.4	E962.0	E980.4
Methandriol	962.1	E858.0	E932.1	E950.4	E962.0	E980.4
Methandrostenolone	962.1	E858.0	E932.1	E950.4	E962.0	E980.4
Methane gas	987.1	E869.8	—	E952.8	E962.2	E982.8
Methanol	980.1	E860.2	—	E950.9	E962.1	E980.9
vapor	987.8	E869.8	—	E952.8	E962.2	E982.8
Methantheline	971.1	E855.4	E941.1	E950.4	E962.0	E980.4
Methaphenilene	963.0	E858.1	E933.0	E950.4	E962.0	E980.4
Methapyrilene	963.0	E858.1	E933.0	E950.4	E962.0	E980.4
Methaqualone (compounds)	967.4	E852.3	E937.4	E950.2	E962.0	E980.2
Metharbital, metharbitone	967.0	E851	E937.0	E950.1	E962.0	E980.1
Methazolamide	974.2	E858.5	E944.2	E950.4	E962.0	E980.4
Methdilazine	963.0	E858.1	E933.0	E950.4	E962.0	E980.4
Methedrine	969.7	E854.2	E939.7	E950.3	E962.0	E980.3
Methenamine (mandelate)	961.9	E857	E931.9	E950.4	E962.0	E980.4
Methenolone	962.1	E858.0	E932.1	E950.4	E962.0	E980.4
Methergine	975.0	E858.6	E945.0	E950.4	E962.0	E980.4
Methiacil	962.8	E858.0	E932.8	E950.4	E962.0	E980.4
Methicillin (sodium)	960.0	E856	E930.0	E950.4	E962.0	E980.4
Methimazole	962.8	E858.0	E932.8	E950.4	E962.0	E980.4
Methionine	977.1	E858.8	E947.1	E950.4	E962.0	E980.4
Methisazone	961.7	E857	E931.7	E950.4	E962.0	E980.4
Methitural	967.0	E851	E937.0	E950.1	E962.0	E980.1
Methixene	971.1	E855.4	E941.1	E950.4	E962.0	E980.4
Methobarbital, methobarbitone	967.0	E851	E937.0	E950.1	E962.0	E980.1
Methocarbamol	968.0	E855.1	E938.0	E950.4	E962.0	E980.4
Methohexital, methohexitone (sodium)	968.3	E855.1	E938.3	E950.4	E962.0	E980.4
Methoin	966.1	E855.0	E936.1	E950.4	E962.0	E980.4
Methopholine	965.7	E850.7	E935.7	E950.0	E962.0	E980.0
Methorate	975.4	E858.6	E945.4	E950.4	E962.0	E980.4
Methoserpidine	972.6	E858.3	E942.6	E950.4	E962.0	E980.4
Methotrexate	963.1	E858.1	E933.1	E950.4	E962.0	E980.4
Methotrimeprazine	967.8	E852.8	E937.8	E950.2	E962.0	E980.2
Methoxa-Dome	976.3	E858.7	E946.3	E950.4	E962.0	E980.4
Methoxamine	971.2	E855.5	E941.2	E950.4	E962.0	E980.4
Methoxsalen	976.3	E858.7	E946.3	E950.4	E962.0	E980.4
Methoxybenzyl penicillin	960.0	E856	E930.0	E950.4	E962.0	E980.4
Methoxychlor	989.2	E863.0	—	E950.6	E962.1	E980.7
Methoxyflurane	968.2	E855.1	E938.2	E950.4	E962.0	E980.4
Methoxyphenamine	971.2	E855.5	E941.2	E950.4	E962.0	E980.4
Methoxypromazine	969.1	E853.0	E939.1	E950.3	E962.0	E980.3
Methoxypsoralen	976.3	E858.7	E946.3	E950.4	E962.0	E980.4

Mercuranin — Methoxypsoralen

Methscopolamine — Mitomycin

	Poisoning	External Cause (E-Code)				
		Accident	Therapeutic Use	Suicide Attempt	Assault	Undetermined
Methscopolamine (bromide)	971.1	E855.4	E941.1	E950.4	E962.0	E980.4
Methsuximide	966.2	E855.0	E936.2	E950.4	E962.0	E980.4
Methyclothiazide	974.3	E858.5	E944.3	E950.4	E962.0	E980.4
Methyl						
acetate	982.8	E862.4	—	E950.9	E962.1	E980.9
acetone	982.8	E862.4	—	E950.9	E962.1	E980.9
alcohol	980.1	E860.2	—	E950.9	E962.1	E980.9
amphetamine	969.7	E854.2	E939.7	E950.3	E962.0	E980.3
androstanolone	962.1	E858.0	E932.1	E950.4	E962.0	E980.4
atropine	971.1	E855.4	E941.1	E950.4	E962.0	E980.4
benzene	982.0	E862.4	—	E950.9	E962.1	E980.9
bromide (gas)	987.8	E869.8	—	E952.8	E962.2	E982.8
fumigant	987.8	E863.8	—	E950.6	E962.2	E980.7
butanol	980.8	E860.8	—	E950.9	E962.1	E980.9
carbinol	980.1	E860.2	—	E950.9	E962.1	E980.9
cellosolve	982.8	E862.4	—	E950.9	E962.1	E980.9
cellulose	973.3	E858.4	E943.3	E950.4	E962.0	E980.4
chloride (gas)	987.8	E869.8	—	E952.8	E962.2	E982.8
cyclohexane	982.8	E862.4	—	E950.9	E962.1	E980.9
cyclohexanone	982.8	E862.4	—	E950.9	E962.1	E980.9
dihydromorphinone	965.09	E850.2	E935.2	E950.0	E962.0	E980.0
ergometrine	975.0	E858.6	E945.0	E950.4	E962.0	E980.4
ergonovine	975.0	E858.6	E945.0	E950.4	E962.0	E980.4
ethyl ketone	982.8	E862.4	—	E950.9	E962.1	E980.9
hydrazine	983.9	E864.3	—	E950.7	E962.1	E980.6
isobutyl ketone	982.8	E862.4	—	E950.9	E962.1	E980.9
morphine NEC	965.09	E850.2	E935.2	E950.0	E962.0	E980.0
parafynol	967.8	E852.8	E937.8	E950.2	E962.0	E980.2
parathion	989.3	E863.1	—	E950.6	E962.1	E980.7
pentynol NEC	967.8	E852.8	E937.8	E950.2	E962.0	E980.2
peridol	969.2	E853.1	E939.2	E950.3	E962.0	E980.3
phenidate	969.7	E854.2	E939.7	E950.3	E962.0	E980.3
prednisolone	962.0	E858.0	E932.0	E950.4	E962.0	E980.4
ENT agent	976.6	E858.7	E946.6	E950.4	E962.0	E980.4
ophthalmic preparation	976.5	E858.7	E946.5	E950.4	E962.0	E980.4
topical NEC	976.0	E858.7	E946.0	E950.4	E962.0	E980.4
propylcarbinol	980.8	E860.8	—	E950.9	E962.1	E980.9
rosaniline NEC	976.0	E858.7	E946.0	E950.4	E962.0	E980.4
salicylate NEC	976.3	E858.7	E946.3	E950.4	E962.0	E980.4
sulfate (fumes)	987.8	E869.8	—	E952.8	E962.2	E982.8
liquid	983.9	E864.3	—	E950.7	E962.1	E980.6
sulfonal	967.8	E852.8	E937.8	E950.2	E962.0	E980.2
testosterone	962.1	E858.0	E932.1	E950.4	E962.0	E980.4
thiouracil	962.8	E858.0	E932.8	E950.4	E962.0	E980.4
Methylated spirit	980.0	E860.1	—	E950.9	E962.1	E980.9
Methyldopa	972.6	E858.3	E942.6	E950.4	E962.0	E980.4
Methylene						
blue	961.9	E857	E931.9	E950.4	E962.0	E980.4
chloride or dichloride (solvent) NEC	982.3	E862.4	—	E950.9	E962.1	E980.9
Methylhexabital	967.0	E851	E937.0	E950.1	E962.0	E980.1
Methylparaben (ophthalmic)	976.5	E858.7	E946.5	E950.4	E962.0	E980.4
Methyprylon	967.5	E852.4	E937.5	E950.2	E962.0	E980.2
Methysergide	971.3	E855.6	E941.3	E950.4	E962.0	E980.4
Metoclopramide	963.0	E858.1	E933.0	E950.4	E962.0	E980.4
Metofoline	965.7	E850.7	E935.7	E950.0	E962.0	E980.0
Metopon	965.09	E850.2	E935.2	E950.0	E962.0	E980.0
Metronidazole	961.5	E857	E931.5	E950.4	E962.0	E980.4
Metycaine	968.9	E855.2	E938.9	E950.4	E962.0	E980.4
infiltration (subcutaneous)	968.5	E855.2	E938.5	E950.4	E962.0	E980.4
nerve block (peripheral) (plexus)	968.6	E855.2	E938.6	E950.4	E962.0	E980.4
topical (surface)	968.5	E855.2	E938.5	E950.4	E962.0	E980.4
Metyrapone	977.8	E858.8	E947.8	E950.4	E962.0	E980.4
Mevinphos	989.3	E863.1	—	E950.6	E962.1	E980.7
Mezereon (berries)	988.2	E865.3	—	E950.9	E962.1	E980.9
Micatin	976.0	E858.7	E946.0	E950.4	E962.0	E980.4
Miconazole	976.0	E858.7	E946.0	E950.4	E962.0	E980.4
Midol	965.1	E850.3	E935.3	E950.0	E962.0	E980.0
Mifepristone	962.9	E858.0	E932.9	E950.4	E962.0	E980.4
Milk of magnesia	973.0	E858.4	E943.0	E950.4	E962.0	E980.4
Millipede (tropical) (venomous)	989.5	E905.4	—	E950.9	E962.1	E980.9
Miltown	969.5	E853.8	E939.5	E950.3	E962.0	E980.3
Mineral						
oil (medicinal)	973.2	E858.4	E943.2	E950.4	E962.0	E980.4
nonmedicinal	981	E862.1	—	E950.9	E962.1	E980.9
topical	976.3	E858.7	E946.3	E950.4	E962.0	E980.4
salts NEC	974.6	E858.5	E944.6	E950.4	E962.0	E980.4
spirits	981	E862.0	—	E950.9	E962.1	E980.9
Minocycline	960.4	E856	E930.4	E950.4	E962.0	E980.4
Mithramycin (antineoplastic)	960.7	E856	E930.7	E950.4	E962.0	E980.4
Mitobronitol	963.1	E858.1	E933.1	E950.4	E962.0	E980.4
Mitomycin (antineoplastic)	960.7	E856	E930.7	E950.4	E962.0	E980.4

✓4ᵗʰ Fourth-digit Required   ✓5ᵗʰ Fifth-digit Required   ▶◀ Revised Text   ● New Line   ▲ Revised Code

	Poisoning	External Cause (E-Code)				
		Accident	Therapeutic Use	Suicide Attempt	Assault	Undetermined
Mitotane	963.1	E858.1	E933.1	E950.4	E962.0	E980.4
Moderil	972.6	E858.3	E942.6	E950.4	E962.0	E980.4
Mogadon — *see* Nitrazepam						
Molindone	969.3	E853.8	E939.3	E950.3	E962.0	E980.3
Monistat	976.0	E858.7	E946.0	E950.4	E962.0	E980.4
Monkshood	988.2	E865.4	—	E950.9	E962.1	E980.9
Monoamine oxidase inhibitors	969.0	E854.0	E939.0	E950.3	E962.0	E980.3
Monochlorobenzene	982.0	E862.4	—	E950.9	E962.1	E980.9
Monosodium glutamate	989.89	E866.8	—	E950.9	E962.1	E980.9
Monoxide, carbon — *see* Carbon, monoxide						
Moperone	969.2	E853.1	E939.2	E950.3	E962.0	E980.3
Morning glory seeds	969.6	E854.1	E939.6	E950.3	E962.0	E980.3
Moroxydine (hydrochloride)	961.7	E857	E931.7	E950.4	E962.0	E980.4
Morphazinamide	961.8	E857	E931.8	E950.4	E962.0	E980.4
Morphinans	965.09	E850.2	E935.2	E950.0	E962.0	E980.0
Morphine NEC	965.09	E850.2	E935.2	E950.0	E962.0	E980.0
antagonists	970.1	E854.3	E940.1	E950.4	E962.0	E980.4
Morpholinylethylmorphine	965.09	E850.2	E935.2	E950.0	E962.0	E980.0
Morrhuate sodium	972.7	E858.3	E942.7	E950.4	E962.0	E980.4
Moth balls (*see also* Pesticides)	989.4	E863.4	—	E950.6	E962.1	E980.7
naphthalene	983.0	E863.4	—	E950.7	E962.1	E980.6
Motor exhaust gas — *see* Carbon, monoxide, exhaust gas						
Mouth wash	976.6	E858.7	E946.6	E950.4	E962.0	E980.4
Mucolytic agent	975.5	E858.6	E945.5	E950.4	E962.0	E980.4
Mucomyst	975.5	E858.6	E945.5	E950.4	E962.0	E980.4
Mucous membrane agents (external)	976.9	E858.7	E946.9	E950.4	E962.0	E980.4
specified NEC	976.8	E858.7	E946.8	E950.4	E962.0	E980.4
Mumps						
immune globulin (human)	964.6	E858.2	E934.6	E950.4	E962.0	E980.4
skin test antigen	977.8	E858.8	E947.8	E950.4	E962.0	E980.4
vaccine	979.6	E858.8	E949.6	E950.4	E962.0	E980.4
Mumpsvax	979.6	E858.8	E949.6	E950.4	E962.0	E980.4
Muriatic acid — *see* Hydrochloric acid						
Muscarine	971.0	E855.3	E941.0	E950.4	E962.0	E980.4
Muscle affecting agents NEC	975.3	E858.6	E945.3	E950.4	E962.0	E980.4
oxytocic	975.0	E858.6	E945.0	E950.4	E962.0	E980.4
relaxants	975.3	E858.6	E945.3	E950.4	E962.0	E980.4
central nervous system	968.0	E855.1	E938.0	E950.4	E962.0	E980.4
skeletal	975.2	E858.6	E945.2	E950.4	E962.0	E980.4
smooth	975.1	E858.6	E945.1	E950.4	E962.0	E980.4
Mushrooms, noxious	988.1	E865.5	—	E950.9	E962.1	E980.9
Mussel, noxious	988.0	E865.1	—	E950.9	E962.1	E980.9
Mustard (emetic)	973.6	E858.4	E943.6	E950.4	E962.0	E980.4
gas	987.8	E869.8	—	E952.8	E962.2	E982.8
nitrogen	963.1	E858.1	E933.1	E950.4	E962.0	E980.4
Mustine	963.1	E858.1	E933.1	E950.4	E962.0	E980.4
M-vac	979.4	E858.8	E949.4	E950.4	E962.0	E980.4
Mycifradin	960.8	E856	E930.8	E950.4	E962.0	E980.4
topical	976.0	E858.7	E946.0	E950.4	E962.0	E980.4
Mycitracin	960.8	E856	E930.8	E950.4	E962.0	E980.4
ophthalmic preparation	976.5	E858.7	E946.5	E950.4	E962.0	E980.4
Mycostatin	960.1	E856	E930.1	E950.4	E962.0	E980.4
topical	976.0	E858.7	E946.0	E950.4	E962.0	E980.4
Mydriacyl	971.1	E855.4	E941.1	E950.4	E962.0	E980.4
Myelobromal	963.1	E858.1	E933.1	E950.4	E962.0	E980.4
Myleran	963.1	E858.1	E933.1	E950.4	E962.0	E980.4
Myochrysin(e)	965.69	E850.6	E935.6	E950.0	E962.0	E980.0
Myoneural blocking agents	975.2	E858.6	E945.2	E950.4	E962.0	E980.4
Myristica fragrans	988.2	E865.3	—	E950.9	E962.1	E980.9
Myristicin	988.2	E865.3	—	E950.9	E962.1	E980.9
Mysoline	966.3	E855.0	E936.3	E950.4	E962.0	E980.4
Nafcillin (sodium)	960.0	E856	E930.0	E950.4	E962.0	E980.4
Nail polish remover	982.8	E862.4	—	E950.9	E962.1	E908.9
Nalidixic acid	961.9	E857	E931.9	E950.4	E962.0	E980.4
Nalorphine	970.1	E854.3	E940.1	E950.4	E962.0	E980.4
Naloxone	970.1	E854.3	E940.1	E950.4	E962.0	E980.4
Nandrolone (decanoate) (phenproprioate)	962.1	E858.0	E932.1	E950.4	E962.0	E980.4
Naphazoline	971.2	E855.5	E941.2	E950.4	E962.0	E980.4
Naphtha (painter's) (petroleum)	981	E862.0	—	E950.9	E962.1	E980.9
solvent	981	E862.0	—	E950.9	E962.1	E980.9
vapor	987.1	E869.8	—	E952.8	E962.2	E982.8
Naphthalene (chlorinated)	983.0	E864.0	—	E950.7	E962.1	E980.6
insecticide or moth repellent	983.0	E863.4	—	E950.7	E962.1	E980.6
vapor	987.8	E869.8	—	E952.8	E962.2	E982.8
Naphthol	983.0	E864.0	—	E950.7	E962.1	E980.6
Naphthylamine	983.0	E864.0	—	E950.7	E962.1	E980.6
Naprosyn — *see* Naproxen						
Naproxen	965.61	E850.6	E935.6	E950.0	E962.0	E980.0
Narcotic (drug)	967.9	E852.9	E937.9	E950.2	E962.0	E980.2
analgesic NEC	965.8	E850.8	E935.8	E950.0	E962.0	E980.0
antagonist	970.1	E854.3	E940.1	E950.4	E962.0	E980.4

Mitotane — Narcotic

		External Cause (E-Code)				
	Poisoning	Accident	Therapeutic Use	Suicide Attempt	Assault	Undetermined
Narcotic — *continued*						
specified NEC	967.8	E852.8	E937.8	E950.2	E962.0	E980.2
Narcotine	975.4	E858.6	E945.4	E950.4	E962.0	E980.4
Nardil	969.0	E854.0	E939.0	E950.3	E962.0	E980.3
Natrium cyanide — *see* Cyanide(s)						
Natural						
blood (product)	964.7	E858.2	E934.7	E950.4	E962.0	E980.4
gas (piped)	987.1	E867	—	E951.0	E962.2	E981.0
incomplete combustion	986	E867	—	E951.0	E962.2	E981.0
Nealbarbital, nealbarbitone	967.0	E851	E937.0	E950.1	E962.0	E980.1
Nectadon	975.4	E858.6	E945.4	E950.4	E962.0	E980.4
Nematocyst (sting)	989.5	E905.6	—	E950.9	E962.1	E980.9
Nembutal	967.0	E851	E937.0	E950.1	E962.0	E980.1
Neoarsphenamine	961.1	E857	E931.1	E950.4	E962.0	E980.4
Neocinchophen	974.7	E858.5	E944.7	E950.4	E962.0	E980.4
Neomycin	960.8	E856	E930.8	E950.4	E962.0	E980.4
ENT agent	976.6	E858.7	E946.6	E950.4	E962.0	E980.4
ophthalmic preparation	976.5	E858.7	E946.5	E950.4	E962.0	E980.4
topical NEC	976.0	E858.7	E946.0	E950.4	E962.0	E980.4
Neonal	967.0	E851	E937.0	E950.1	E962.0	E980.1
Neoprontosil	961.0	E857	E931.0	E950.4	E962.0	E980.4
Neosalvarsan	961.1	E857	E931.1	E950.4	E962.0	E980.4
Neosilversalvarsan	961.1	E857	E931.1	E950.4	E962.0	E980.4
Neosporin	960.8	E856	E930.8	E950.4	E962.0	E980.4
ENT agent	976.6	E858.7	E946.6	E950.4	E962.0	E980.4
opthalmic preparation	976.5	E858.7	E946.5	E950.4	E962.0	E980.4
topical NEC	976.0	E858.7	E946.0	E950.4	E962.0	E980.4
Neostigmine	971.0	E855.3	E941.0	E950.4	E962.0	E980.4
Neraval	967.0	E851	E937.0	E950.1	E962.0	E980.1
Neravan	967.0	E851	E937.0	E950.1	E962.0	E980.1
Nerium oleander	988.2	E865.4	—	E950.9	E962.1	E980.9
Nerve gases (war)	987.9	E869.9	—	E952.9	E962.2	E982.9
Nesacaine	968.9	E855.2	E938.9	E950.4	E962.0	E980.4
infiltration (subcutaneous)	968.5	E855.2	E938.5	E950.4	E962.0	E980.4
nerve block (peripheral) (plexus)	968.6	E855.2	E938.6	E950.4	E962.0	E980.4
Neurobarb	967.0	E851	E937.0	E950.1	E962.0	E980.1
Neuroleptics NEC	969.3	E853.8	E939.3	E950.3	E962.0	E980.3
Neuroprotective agent	977.8	E858.8	E947.8	E950.4	E962.0	E980.4
Neutral spirits	980.0	E860.1	—	E950.9	E962.1	E980.9
beverage	980.0	E860.0	—	E950.9	E962.1	E980.9
Niacin, niacinamide	972.2	E858.3	E942.2	E950.4	E962.0	E980.4
Nialamide	969.0	E854.0	E939.0	E950.3	E962.0	E980.3
Nickle (carbonyl) (compounds) (fumes) (tetracarbonyl) (vapor)	985.8	E866.4	—	E950.9	E962.1	E980.9
Niclosamide	961.6	E857	E931.6	E950.4	E962.0	E980.4
Nicomorphine	965.09	E850.2	E935.2	E950.0	E962.0	E980.0
Nicotinamide	972.2	E858.3	E942.2	E950.4	E962.0	E980.4
Nicotine (insecticide) (spray) (sulfate) NEC	989.4	E863.4	—	E950.6	E962.1	E980.7
not insecticide	989.89	E866.8	—	E950.9	E962.1	E980.9
Nicotinic acid (derivatives)	972.2	E858.3	E942.2	E950.4	E962.0	E980.4
Nicotinyl alcohol	972.2	E858.3	E942.2	E950.4	E962.0	E980.4
Nicoumalone	964.2	E858.2	E934.2	E950.4	E962.0	E980.4
Nifenazone	965.5	E850.5	E935.5	E950.0	E962.0	E980.0
Nifuraldezone	961.9	E857	E931.9	E950.4	E962.0	E980.4
Nightshade (deadly)	988.2	E865.4	—	E950.9	E962.1	E980.9
Nikethamide	970.0	E854.3	E940.0	E950.4	E962.0	E980.4
Nilstat	960.1	E856	E930.1	E950.4	E962.0	E980.4
topical	976.0	E858.7	E946.0	E950.4	E962.0	E980.4
Nimodipine	977.8	E858.8	E947.8	E950.4	E962.0	E980.4
Niridazole	961.6	E857	E931.6	E950.4	E962.0	E980.4
Nisentil	965.09	E850.2	E935.2	E950.0	E962.0	E980.0
Nitrates	972.4	E858.3	E942.4	E950.4	E962.0	E980.4
Nitrazepam	969.4	E853.2	E939.4	E950.3	E962.0	E980.3
Nitric						
acid (liquid)	983.1	E864.1	—	E950.7	E962.1	E980.6
vapor	987.8	E869.8	—	E952.8	E962.2	E982.8
oxide (gas)	987.2	E869.0	—	E952.8	E962.2	E982.8
Nitrite, amyl (medicinal) (vapor)	972.4	E858.3	E942.4	E950.4	E962.0	E980.4
Nitroaniline	983.0	E864.0	—	E950.7	E962.1	E980.6
vapor	987.8	E869.8	—	E952.8	E962.2	E982.8
Nitrobenzene, nitrobenzol	983.0	E864.0	—	E950.7	E962.1	E980.6
vapor	987.8	E869.8	—	E952.8	E962.2	E982.8
Nitrocellulose	976.3	E858.7	E946.3	E950.4	E962.0	E980.4
Nitrofuran derivatives	961.9	E857	E931.9	E950.4	E962.0	E980.4
Nitrofurantoin	961.9	E857	E931.9	E950.4	E962.0	E980.4
Nitrofurazone	976.0	E858.7	E946.0	E950.4	E962.0	E980.4
Nitrogen (dioxide) (gas) (oxide)	987.2	E869.0	—	E952.8	E962.2	E982.8
mustard (antineoplastic)	963.1	E858.1	E933.1	E950.4	E962.0	E980.4
Nitroglycerin, nitroglycerol (medicinal)	972.4	E858.3	E942.4	E950.4	E962.0	E980.4
nonmedicinal	989.89	E866.8	—	E950.9	E962.1	E980.9
fumes	987.8	E869.8	—	E952.8	E962.2	E982.8
Nitrohydrochloric acid	983.1	E864.1	—	E950.7	E962.1	E980.6

		External Cause (E-Code)				
	Poisoning	Accident	Therapeutic Use	Suicide Attempt	Assault	Undetermined
Nitromersol	976.0	E858.7	E946.0	E950.4	E962.0	E980.4
Nitronaphthalene	983.0	E864.0	—	E950.7	E962.2	E980.6
Nitrophenol	983.0	E864.0	—	E950.7	E962.2	E980.6
Nitrothiazol	961.6	E857	E931.6	E950.4	E962.0	E980.4
Nitrotoluene, nitrotoluol	983.0	E864.0	—	E950.7	E961.1	E980.6
vapor	987.8	E869.8	—	E952.8	E962.2	E982.8
Nitrous	968.2	E855.1	E938.2	E950.4	E962.0	E980.4
acid (liquid)	983.1	E864.1	—	E950.7	E962.1	E980.6
fumes	987.2	E869.0	—	E952.8	E962.2	E982.8
oxide (anesthetic) NEC	968.2	E855.1	E938.2	E950.4	E962.0	E980.4
Nitrozone	976.0	E858.7	E946.0	E950.4	E962.0	E980.4
Noctec	967.1	E852.0	E937.1	E950.2	E962.0	E980.2
Noludar	967.5	E852.4	E937.5	E950.2	E962.0	E980.2
Noptil	967.0	E851	E937.0	E950.1	E962.0	E980.1
Noradrenalin	971.2	E855.5	E941.2	E950.4	E962.0	E980.4
Noramidopyrine	965.5	E850.5	E935.5	E950.0	E962.0	E980.0
Norepinephrine	971.2	E855.5	E941.2	E950.4	E962.0	E980.4
Norethandrolone	962.1	E858.0	E932.1	E950.4	E962.0	E980.4
Norethindrone	962.2	E858.0	E932.2	E950.4	E962.0	E980.4
Norethisterone	962.2	E858.0	E932.2	E950.4	E962.0	E980.4
Norethynodrel	962.2	E858.0	E932.2	E950.4	E962.0	E980.4
Norlestrin	962.2	E858.0	E932.2	E950.4	E962.0	E980.4
Norlutin	962.2	E858.0	E932.2	E950.4	E962.0	E980.4
Normison — *see* Benzodiazepines						
Normorphine	965.09	E850.2	E935.2	E950.0	E962.0	E980.0
Nortriptyline	969.0	E854.0	E939.0	E950.3	E962.0	E980.3
Noscapine	975.4	E858.6	E945.4	E950.4	E962.0	E980.4
Nose preparations	976.6	E858.7	E946.6	E950.4	E962.0	E980.4
Novobiocin	960.8	E856	E930.8	E950.4	E962.0	E980.4
Novocain (infiltration) (topical)	968.5	E855.2	E938.5	E950.4	E962.0	E980.4
nerve block (peripheral) (plexus)	968.6	E855.2	E938.6	E950.4	E962.0	E980.4
spinal	968.7	E855.2	E938.7	E950.4	E962.0	E980.4
Noxythiolin	961.9	E857	E931.9	E950.4	E962.0	E980.4
NPH Iletin (insulin)	962.3	E858.0	E932.3	E950.4	E962.0	E980.4
Numorphan	965.09	E850.2	E935.2	E950.0	E962.0	E980.0
Nunol	967.0	E851	E937.0	E950.1	E962.0	E980.1
Nupercaine (spinal anesthetic)	968.7	E855.2	E938.7	E950.4	E962.0	E980.4
topical (surface)	968.5	E855.2	E938.5	E950.4	E962.0	E980.4
Nutmeg oil (liniment)	976.3	E858.7	E946.3	E950.4	E962.0	E980.4
Nux vomica	989.1	E863.7	—	E950.6	E962.1	E980.7
Nydrazid	961.8	E857	E931.8	E950.4	E962.0	E980.4
Nylidrin	971.2	E855.5	E941.2	E950.4	E962.0	E980.4
Nystatin	960.1	E856	E930.1	E950.4	E962.0	E980.4
topical	976.0	E858.7	E946.0	E950.4	E962.0	E980.4
Nytol	963.0	E858.2	E934.2	E950.4	E962.0	E980.4
Oblivion	967.8	E852.8	E937.8	E950.2	E962.0	E980.2
Octyl nitrite	972.4	E858.3	E942.4	E950.4	E962.0	E980.4
Oestradiol (cypionate) (dipropionate) (valerate)	962.2	E858.0	E932.2	E950.4	E962.0	E980.4
Oestriol	962.2	E858.0	E932.2	E950.4	E962.0	E980.4
Oestrone	962.2	E858.0	E932.2	E950.4	E962.0	E980.4
Oil (of) NEC	989.89	E866.8	—	E950.9	E962.1	E980.9
bitter almond	989.0	E866.8	—	E950.9	E962.1	E980.9
camphor	976.1	E858.7	E946.1	E950.4	E962.0	E980.4
colors	989.89	E861.6	—	E950.9	E962.1	E980.9
fumes	987.8	E869.8	—	E952.8	E962.2	E982.8
lubricating	981	E862.2	—	E950.9	E962.1	E980.9
specified source, other — *see* substance specified						
vitriol (liquid)	983.1	E864.1	—	E950.7	E962.1	E980.6
fumes	987.8	E869.8	—	E952.8	E962.2	E982.8
wintergreen (bitter) NEC	976.3	E858.7	E946.3	E950.4	E962.0	E980.4
Ointments NEC	976.9	E858.7	E946.9	E950.4	E962.0	E980.4
Oleander	988.2	E865.4	—	E950.9	E962.1	E980.9
Oleandomycin	960.3	E856	E930.3	E950.4	E962.0	E980.4
Oleovitamin A	963.5	E858.1	E933.5	E950.4	E962.0	E980.4
Oleum ricini	973.1	E858.4	E943.1	E950.4	E962.0	E980.4
Olive oil (medicinal) NEC	973.2	E858.4	E943.2	E950.4	E962.0	E980.4
OMPA	989.3	E863.1	—	E950.6	E962.1	E980.7
Oncovin	963.1	E858.1	E933.1	E950.4	E962.0	E980.4
Ophthaine	968.5	E855.2	E938.5	E950.4	E962.0	E980.4
Ophthetic	968.5	E855.2	E938.5	E950.4	E962.0	E980.4
Opiates, opioids, opium NEC	965.00	E850.2	E935.2	E950.0	E962.0	E980.0
antagonists	970.1	E854.3	E940.1	E950.4	E962.0	E980.4
Oracon	962.2	E858.0	E932.2	E950.4	E962.0	E980.4
Oragrafin	977.8	E858.8	E947.8	E950.4	E962.0	E980.4
Oral contraceptives	962.2	E858.0	E932.2	E950.4	E962.0	E980.4
Orciprenaline	975.1	E858.6	E945.1	E950.4	E962.0	E980.4
Organidin	975.5	E858.6	E945.5	E950.4	E962.0	E980.4
Organophosphates	989.3	E863.1	—	E950.6	E962.1	E980.7
Orimune	979.5	E858.8	E949.5	E950.4	E962.0	E980.4
Orinase	962.3	E858.0	E932.3	E950.4	E962.0	E980.4
Orphenadrine	966.4	E855.0	E936.4	E950.4	E962.0	E980.4

Nitromersol — Orphenadrine

	Poisoning	External Cause (E-Code)				
		Accident	Therapeutic Use	Suicide Attempt	Assault	Undetermined
Ortal (sodium)	967.0	E851	E937.0	E950.1	E962.0	E980.1
Orthoboric acid	976.0	E858.7	E946.0	E950.4	E962.0	E980.4
ENT agent	976.6	E858.7	E946.6	E950.4	E962.0	E980.4
ophthalmic preparation	976.5	E858.7	E946.5	E950.4	E962.0	E980.4
Orthocaine	968.5	E855.2	E938.5	E950.4	E962.0	E980.4
Ortho-Novum	962.2	E858.0	E932.2	E950.4	E962.0	E980.4
Orthotolidine (reagent)	977.8	E858.8	E947.8	E950.4	E962.0	E980.4
Osmic acid (liquid)	983.1	E864.1	—	E950.7	E962.1	E980.6
fumes	987.8	E869.8	—	E952.8	E962.2	E982.8
Osmotic diuretics	974.4	E858.5	E944.4	E950.4	E962.0	E980.4
Ouabain	972.1	E858.3	E942.1	E950.4	E962.0	E980.4
Ovarian hormones (synthetic substitutes)	962.2	E858.0	E932.2	E950.4	E962.0	E980.4
Ovral	962.2	E858.0	E932.2	E950.4	E962.0	E980.4
Ovulation suppressants	962.2	E858.0	E932.2	E950.4	E962.0	E980.4
Ovulen	962.2	E858.0	E932.2	E950.4	E962.0	E980.4
Oxacillin (sodium)	960.0	E856	E930.0	E950.4	E962.0	E980.4
Oxalic acid	983.1	E864.1	—	E950.7	E962.1	E980.6
Oxanamide	969.5	E853.8	E939.5	E950.3	E962.0	E980.3
Oxandrolone	962.1	E858.0	E932.1	E950.4	E962.0	E980.4
Oxaprozin	965.61	E850.6	E935.6	E950.0	E962.0	E980.
Oxazepam	969.4	E853.2	E939.4	E950.3	E962.0	E980.3
Oxazolidine derivatives	966.0	E855.0	E936.0	E950.4	E962.0	E980.4
Ox bile extract	973.4	E858.4	E943.4	E950.4	E962.0	E980.4
Oxedrine	971.2	E855.5	E941.2	E950.4	E962.0	E980.4
Oxeladin	975.4	E858.6	E945.4	E950.4	E962.0	E980.4
Oxethazaine NEC	968.5	E855.2	E938.5	E950.4	E962.0	E980.4
Oxidizing agents NEC	983.9	E864.3	—	E950.7	E962.1	E980.6
Oxolinic acid	961.3	E857	E931.3	E950.4	E962.0	E980.4
Oxophenarsine	961.1	E857	E931.1	E950.4	E962.0	E980.4
Oxsoralen	976.3	E858.7	E946.3	E950.4	E962.0	E980.4
Oxtriphylline	975.7	E858.6	E945.7	E950.4	E962.0	E980.4
Oxybuprocaine	968.5	E855.2	E938.5	E950.4	E962.0	E980.4
Oxybutynin	975.1	E858.6	E945.1	E950.4	E962.0	E980.0
Oxycodone	965.09	E850.2	E935.2	E950.0	E962.0	E980.0
Oxygen	987.8	E869.8	—	E952.8	E962.2	E982.8
Oxylone	976.0	E858.7	E946.0	E950.4	E962.0	E980.4
ophthalmic preparation	976.5	E858.7	E946.5	E950.4	E962.0	E980.4
Oxymesterone	962.1	E858.0	E932.1	E950.4	E962.0	E980.4
Oxymetazoline	971.2	E855.5	E941.2	E950.4	E962.0	E980.4
Oxymetholone	962.1	E858.0	E932.1	E950.4	E962.0	E980.4
Oxymorphone	965.09	E850.2	E935.2	E950.0	E962.0	E980.0
Oxypertine	969.0	E854.0	E939.0	E950.3	E962.0	E980.3
Oxyphenbutazone	965.5	E850.5	E935.5	E950.0	E962.0	E980.0
Oxyphencyclimine	971.1	E855.4	E941.1	E950.4	E962.0	E980.4
Oxyphenisatin	973.1	E858.4	E943.1	E950.4	E962.0	E980.4
Oxyphenonium	971.1	E855.4	E941.1	E950.4	E962.0	E980.4
Oxyquinoline	961.3	E857	E931.3	E950.4	E962.0	E980.4
Oxytetracycline	960.4	E856	E930.4	E950.4	E962.0	E980.4
Oxytocics	975.0	E858.6	E945.0	E950.4	E962.0	E980.4
Oxytocin	975.0	E858.6	E945.0	E950.4	E962.0	E980.4
Ozone	987.8	E869.8	—	E952.8	E962.2	E982.8
PABA	976.3	E858.7	E946.3	E950.4	E962.0	E980.4
Packed red cells	964.7	E858.2	E934.7	E950.4	E962.0	E980.4
Paint NEC	989.89	E861.6	—	E950.9	E962.1	E980.9
cleaner	982.8	E862.9	—	E950.9	E962.1	E980.9
fumes NEC	987.8	E869.8	—	E952.8	E962.1	E982.8
lead (fumes)	984.0	E861.5	—	E950.9	E962.1	E980.9
solvent NEC	982.8	E862.9	—	E950.9	E962.1	E980.9
stripper	982.8	E862.9	—	E950.9	E962.1	E980.9
Palfium	965.09	E850.2	E935.2	E950.0	E962.0	E980.0
Palivizumab	979.9	E858.8	E949.6	E950.4	E962.0	E980.4
Paludrine	961.4	E857	E931.4	E950.4	E962.0	E980.4
PAM	977.2	E855.8	E947.2	E950.4	E962.0	E980.4
Pamaquine (naphthoate)	961.4	E857	E931.4	E950.4	E962.0	E980.4
Pamprin	965.1	E850.3	E935.3	E950.0	E962.0	E980.0
Panadol	965.4	E850.4	E935.4	E950.0	E962.0	E980.0
Pancreatic dornase (mucolytic)	963.4	E858.1	E933.4	E950.4	E962.0	E980.4
Pancreatin	973.4	E858.4	E943.4	E950.4	E962.0	E980.4
Pancrelipase	973.4	E858.4	E943.4	E950.4	E962.0	E980.4
Pangamic acid	963.5	E858.1	E933.5	E950.4	E962.0	E980.4
Panthenol	963.5	E858.1	E933.5	E950.4	E962.0	E980.4
topical	976.8	E858.7	E946.8	E950.4	E962.0	E980.4
Pantopaque	977.8	E858.8	E947.8	E950.4	E962.0	E980.4
Pantopon	965.00	E850.2	E935.2	E950.0	E962.0	E980.0
Pantothenic acid	963.5	E858.1	E933.5	E950.4	E962.0	E980.4
Panwarfin	964.2	E858.2	E934.2	E950.4	E962.0	E980.4
Papain	973.4	E858.4	E943.4	E950.4	E962.0	E980.4
Papaverine	972.5	E858.3	E942.5	E950.4	E962.0	E980.4
Para-aminobenzoic acid	976.3	E858.7	E946.3	E950.4	E962.0	E980.4
Para-aminophenol derivatives	965.4	E850.4	E935.4	E950.0	E962.0	E980.0
Para-aminosalicylic acid (derivatives)	961.8	E857	E931.8	E950.4	E962.0	E980.4

	Poisoning	External Cause (E-Code)				
		Accident	Therapeutic Use	Suicide Attempt	Assault	Undetermined
Paracetaldehyde (medicinal)	967.2	E852.1	E937.2	E950.2	E962.0	E980.2
Paracetamol	965.4	E850.4	E935.4	E950.0	E962.0	E980.0
Paracodin	965.09	E850.2	E935.2	E950.0	E962.0	E980.0
Paradione	966.0	E855.0	E936.0	E950.4	E962.0	E980.4
Paraffin(s) (wax)	981	E862.3	—	E950.9	E962.1	E980.9
liquid (medicinal)	973.2	E858.4	E943.2	E950.4	E962.0	E980.4
nonmedicinal (oil)	981	E962.1	—	E950.9	E962.1	E980.9
Paraldehyde (medicinal)	967.2	E852.1	E937.2	E950.2	E962.0	E980.2
Paramethadione	966.0	E855.0	E936.0	E950.4	E962.0	E980.4
Paramethasone	962.0	E858.0	E932.0	E950.4	E962.0	E980.4
Paraquat	989.4	E863.5	—	E950.6	E962.1	E980.7
Parasympatholytics	971.1	E855.4	E941.1	E950.4	E962.0	E980.4
Parasympathomimetics	971.0	E855.3	E941.0	E950.4	E962.0	E980.4
Parathion	989.3	E863.1	—	E950.6	E962.1	E980.7
Parathormone	962.6	E858.0	E932.6	E950.4	E962.0	E980.4
Parathyroid (derivatives)	962.6	E858.0	E932.6	E950.4	E962.0	E980.4
Paratyphoid vaccine	978.1	E858.8	E948.1	E950.4	E962.0	E980.4
Paredrine	971.2	E855.5	E941.2	E950.4	E962.0	E980.4
Paregoric	965.00	E850.2	E935.2	E950.0	E962.0	E980.0
Pargyline	972.3	E858.3	E942.3	E950.4	E962.0	E980.4
Paris green	985.1	E866.3	—	E950.8	E962.1	E980.8
insecticide	985.1	E863.4	—	E950.8	E962.1	E980.8
Parnate	969.0	E854.0	E939.0	E950.3	E962.0	E980.3
Paromomycin	960.8	E856	E930.8	E950.4	E962.0	E980.4
Paroxypropione	963.1	E858.1	E933.1	E950.4	E962.0	E980.4
Parzone	965.09	E850.2	E935.2	E950.0	E962.0	E980.0
PAS	961.8	E857	E931.8	E950.4	E962.0	E980.4
PCBs	981	E862.3	—	E950.9	E962.1	E980.9
PCP (pentachlorophenol)	989.4	E863.6	—	E950.6	E962.1	E980.7
herbicide	989.4	E863.5	—	E950.6	E962.1	E980.7
insecticide	989.4	E863.4	—	E950.6	E962.1	E980.7
phencyclidine	968.3	E855.1	E938.3	E950.4	E962.0	E980.4
Peach kernel oil (emulsion)	973.2	E858.4	E943.2	E950.4	E962.0	E980.4
Peanut oil (emulsion) NEC	973.2	E858.4	E943.2	E950.4	E962.0	E980.4
topical	976.3	E858.7	E946.3	E950.4	E962.0	E980.4
Pearly Gates (morning glory seeds)	969.6	E854.1	E939.6	E950.3	E962.0	E980.3
Pecazine	969.1	E853.0	E939.1	E950.3	E962.0	E980.3
Pecilocin	960.1	E856	E930.1	E950.4	E962.0	E980.4
Pectin (with kaolin) NEC	973.5	E858.4	E943.5	E950.4	E962.0	E980.4
Pelletierine tannate	961.6	E857	E931.6	E950.4	E962.0	E980.4
Pemoline	969.7	E854.2	E939.7	E950.3	E962.0	E980.3
Pempidine	972.3	E858.3	E942.3	E950.4	E962.0	E980.4
Penamecillin	960.0	E856	E930.0	E950.4	E962.0	E980.4
Penethamate hydriodide	960.0	E856	E930.0	E950.4	E962.0	E980.4
Penicillamine	963.8	E858.1	E933.8	E950.4	E962.0	E980.4
Penicillin (any type)	960.0	E856	E930.0	E950.4	E962.0	E980.4
Penicillinase	963.4	E858.1	E933.4	E950.4	E962.0	E980.4
Pentachlorophenol (fungicide)	989.4	E863.6	—	E950.6	E962.1	E980.7
herbicide	989.4	E863.5	—	E950.6	E962.1	E980.7
insecticide	989.4	E863.4	—	E950.6	E962.1	E980.7
Pentaerythritol	972.4	E858.3	E942.4	E950.4	E962.0	E980.4
chloral	967.1	E852.0	E937.1	E950.2	E962.0	E980.2
tetranitrate NEC	972.4	E858.3	E942.4	E950.4	E962.0	E980.4
Pentagastrin	977.8	E858.8	E947.8	E950.4	E962.0	E980.4
Pentalin	982.3	E862.4	—	E950.9	E962.1	E980.9
Pentamethonium (bromide)	972.3	E858.3	E942.3	E950.4	E962.0	E980.4
Pentamidine	961.5	E857	E931.5	E950.4	E962.0	E980.4
Pentanol	980.8	E860.8	—	E950.9	E962.1	E980.9
Pentaquine	961.4	E857	E931.4	E950.4	E962.0	E980.4
Pentazocine	965.8	E850.8	E935.8	E950.0	E962.0	E980.0
Penthienate	971.1	E855.4	E941.1	E950.4	E962.0	E980.4
Pentobarbital, pentobarbitone (sodium)	967.0	E851	E937.0	E950.1	E962.0	E980.1
Pentolinium (tartrate)	972.3	E858.3	E942.3	E950.4	E962.0	E980.4
Pentothal	968.3	E855.1	E938.3	E950.4	E962.0	E980.4
Pentylenetetrazol	970.0	E854.3	E940.0	E950.4	E962.0	E980.4
Pentylsalicylamide	961.8	E857	E931.8	E950.4	E962.0	E980.4
Pepsin	973.4	E858.4	E943.4	E950.4	E962.0	E980.4
Peptavlon	977.8	E858.8	E947.8	E950.4	E962.0	E980.4
Percaine (spinal)	968.7	E855.2	E938.7	E950.4	E962.0	E980.4
topical (surface)	968.5	E855.2	E938.5	E950.4	E962.0	E980.4
Perchloroethylene (vapor)	982.3	E862.4	—	E950.9	E962.1	E980.9
medicinal	961.6	E857	E931.6	E950.4	E962.0	E980.4
Percodan	965.09	E850.2	E935.2	E950.0	E962.0	E980.0
Percogesic	965.09	E850.2	E935.2	E950.0	E962.0	E980.0
Percorten	962.0	E858.0	E932.0	E950.4	E962.0	E980.4
Pergonal	962.4	E858.0	E932.4	E950.4	E962.0	E980.4
Perhexiline	972.4	E858.3	E942.4	E950.4	E962.0	E980.4
Periactin	963.0	E858.1	E933.0	E950.4	E962.0	E980.4
Periclor	967.1	E852.0	E937.1	E950.2	E962.0	E980.2
Pericyazine	969.1	E853.0	E939.1	E950.3	E962.0	E980.3
Peritrate	972.4	E858.3	E942.4	E950.4	E962.0	E980.4

	Poisoning	External Cause (E-Code)				
		Accident	Therapeutic Use	Suicide Attempt	Assault	Undetermined
Permanganates NEC	983.9	E864.3	—	E950.7	E962.1	E980.6
potassium (topical)	976.0	E858.7	E946.0	E950.4	E962.0	E980.4
Pernocton	967.0	E851	E937.0	E950.1	E962.0	E980.1
Pernoston	967.0	E851	E937.0	E950.1	E962.0	E980.1
Peronin(e)	965.09	E850.2	E935.2	E950.0	E962.0	E980.0
Perphenazine	969.1	E853.0	E939.1	E950.3	E962.0	E980.3
Pertofrane	969.0	E854 ☑4ᵗʰ	E939.0	E950.3	E962.0	E980.3
Pertussis						
immune serum (human)	964.6	E858.2	E934.6	E950.4	E962.0	E980.4
vaccine (with diphtheria toxoid) (with tetanus toxoid)	978.6	E858.8	E948.6	E950.4	E962.0	E980.4
Peruvian balsam	976.8	E858.7	E946.8	E950.4	E962.0	E980.4
Pesticides (dust) (fumes) (vapor)	989.4	E863.4	—	E950.6	E962.1	E980.7
arsenic	985.1	E863.4	—	E950.8	E962.1	E980.8
chlorinated	989.2	E863.0	—	E950.6	E962.1	E980.7
cyanide	989.0	E863.4	—	E950.6	E962.1	E980.7
kerosene	981	E863.4	—	E950.6	E962.1	E980.7
mixture (of compounds)	989.4	E863.3	—	E950.6	E962.1	E980.7
naphthalene	983.0	E863.4	—	E950.7	E962.1	E980.6
organochlorine (compounds)	989.2	E863.0	—	E950.6	E962.1	E980.7
petroleum (distillate) (products) NEC	981	E863.4	—	E950.6	E962.1	E980.7
specified ingredient NEC	989.4	E863.4	—	E950.6	E962.1	E980.7
strychnine	989.1	E863.4	—	E950.6	E962.1	E980.7
thallium	985.8	E863.7	—	E950.6	E962.1	E980.7
Pethidine (hydrochloride)	965.09	E850.2	E935.2	E950.0	E962.0	E980.0
Petrichloral	967.1	E852.0	E937.1	E950.2	E962.0	E980.2
Petrol	981	E862.1	—	E950.9	E962.1	E980.9
vapor	987.1	E869.8	—	E952.8	E962.2	E982.8
Petrolatum (jelly) (ointment)	976.3	E858.7	E946.3	E950.4	E962.0	E980.4
hydrophilic	976.3	E858.7	E946.3	E950.4	E962.0	E980.4
liquid	973.2	E858.4	E943.2	E950.4	E962.0	E980.4
topical	976.3	E858.7	E946.3	E950.4	E962.0	E980.4
nonmedicinal	981	E862.1		E950.9	E962.1	E980.9
Petroleum (cleaners) (fuels) (products) NEC	981	E862.1		E950.9	E962.1	E980.9
benzin(e) — *see* Ligroin						
ether — *see* Ligroin						
jelly — *see* Petrolatum						
naphtha — *see* Ligroin						
pesticide	981	E863.4	—	E950.6	E962.1	E980.7
solids	981	E862.3	—	E950.9	E962.1	E980.9
solvents	981	E862.0	—	E950.9	E962.1	E980.9
vapor	987.1	E869.8	—	E952.8	E962.2	E982.8
Peyote	969.6	E854.1	E939.6	E950.3	E962.0	E980.3
Phanodorm, phanodorn	967.0	E851	E937.0	E950.1	E962.0	E980.1
Phanquinone, phanquone	961.5	E857	E931.5	E950.4	E962.0	E980.4
Pharmaceutical excipient or adjunct	977.4	E858.8	E947.4	E950.4	E962.0	E980.4
Phenacemide	966.3	E855.0	E936.3	E950.4	E962.0	E980.4
Phenacetin	965.4	E850.4	E935.4	E950.0	E962.0	E980.0
Phenadoxone	965.09	E850.2	E935.2	E950.0	E962.0	E980.0
Phenaglycodol	969.5	E853.8	E939.5	E950.3	E962.0	E980.3
Phenantoin	966.1	E855.0	E936.1	E950.4	E962.0	E980.4
Phenaphthazine reagent	977.8	E858.8	E947.8	E950.4	E962.0	E980.4
Phenazocine	965.09	E850.2	E935.2	E950.0	E962.0	E980.0
Phenazone	965.5	E850.5	E935.5	E950.0	E962.0	E980.0
Phenazopyridine	976.1	E858.7	E946.1	E950.4	E962.0	E980.4
Phenbenicillin	960.0	E856	E930.0	E950.4	E962.0	E980.4
Phenbutrazate	977.0	E858.8	E947.0	E950.4	E962.0	E980.4
Phencyclidine	968.3	E855.1	E938.3	E950.4	E962.0	E980.4
Phendimetrazine	977.0	E858.8	E947.0	E950.4	E962.0	E980.4
Phenelzine	969.0	E854.0	E939.0	E950.3	E962.0	E980.3
Phenergan	967.8	E852.8	E937.8	E950.2	E962.0	E980.2
Phenethicillin (potassium)	960.0	E856	E930.0	E950.4	E962.0	E980.4
Phenetsal	965.1	E850.3	E935.3	E950.0	E962.0	E980.0
Pheneturide	966.3	E855.0	E936.3	E950.4	E962.0	E980.4
Phenformin	962.3	E858.0	E932.3	E950.4	E962.0	E980.4
Phenglutarimide	971.1	E855.4	E941.1	E950.4	E962.0	E980.4
Phenicarbazide	965.8	E850.8	E935.8	E950.0	E962.0	E980.0
Phenindamine (tartrate)	963.0	E858.1	E933.0	E950.4	E962.0	E980.4
Phenindione	964.2	E858.2	E934.2	E950.4	E962.0	E980.4
Pheniprazine	969.0	E854.0	E939.0	E950.3	E962.0	E980.3
Pheniramine (maleate)	963.0	E858.1	E933.0	E950.4	E962.0	E980.4
Phenmetrazine	977.0	E858.8	E947.0	E950.4	E962.0	E980.4
Phenobal	967.0	E851	E937.0	E950.1	E962.0	E980.1
Phenobarbital	967.0	E851	E937.0	E950.1	E962.0	E980.1
Phenobarbitone	967.0	E851	E937.0	E950.1	E962.0	E980.1
Phenoctide	976	E858.7	E946.0	E950.4	E962.0	E980.4
Phenol (derivatives) NEC	983.0	E864.0	—	E950.7	E962.1	E980.6
disinfectant	983.0	E864.0	—	E950.7	E962.1	E980.6
pesticide	989.4	E863.4	—	E950.6	E962.1	E980.7
red	977.8	E858.8	E947.8	E950.4	E962.0	E980.4
Phenolphthalein	973.1	E858.4	E943.1	E950.4	E962.0	E980.4
Phenolsulfonphthalein	977.8	E858.8	E947.8	E950.4	E962.0	E980.4

	Poisoning	External Cause (E-Code)				
		Accident	Therapeutic Use	Suicide Attempt	Assault	Undetermined
Phenomorphan	965.09	E850.2	E935.2	E950.0	E962.0	E980.0
Phenonyl	967.0	E851	E937.0	E950.1	E962.0	E980.1
Phenoperidine	965.09	E850.2	E935.2	E950.0	E962.0	E980.0
Phenoquin	974.7	E858.5	E944.7	E950.4	E962.0	E980.4
Phenothiazines (tranquilizers) NEC	969.1	E853.0	E939.1	E950.3	E962.0	E980.3
insecticide	989.3	E863.4	—	E950.6	E962.1	E980.7
Phenoxybenzamine	971.3	E855.6	E941.3	E950.4	E962.0	E980.4
Phenoxymethyl penicillin	960.0	E856	E930.0	E950.4	E962.0	E980.4
Phenprocoumon	964.2	E858.2	E934.2	E950.4	E962.0	E980.4
Phensuximide	966.2	E855.0	E936.2	E950.4	E962.0	E980.4
Phentermine	977.0	E858.8	E947.0	E950.4	E962.0	E980.4
Phentolamine	971.3	E855.6	E941.3	E950.4	E962.0	E980.4
Phenyl						
butazone	965.5	E850.5	E935.5	E950.0	E962.0	E980.0
enediamine	983.0	E864.0	—	E950.7	E962.1	E980.6
hydrazine	983.0	E864.0	—	E950.7	E962.1	E980.6
antineoplastic	963.1	E858.1	E933.1	E950.4	E962.0	E980.4
mercuric compounds — see Mercury						
salicylate	976.3	E858.7	E946.3	E950.4	E962.0	E980.4
Phenylephrin	971.2	E855.5	E941.2	E950.4	E962.0	E980.4
Phenylethylbiguanide	962.3	E858.0	E932.3	E950.4	E962.0	E980.4
Phenylpropanolamine	971.2	E855.5	E941.2	E950.4	E962.0	E980.4
Phenylsulfthion	989.3	E863.1	—	E950.6	E962.1	E980.7
Phenyramidol, phenyramidon	965.7	E850.7	E935.7	E950.0	E962.0	E980.0
Phenytoin	966.1	E855.0	E936.1	E950.4	E962.0	E980.4
pHisoHex	976.2	E858.7	E946.2	E950.4	E962.0	E980.4
Pholcodine	965.09	E850.2	E935.2	E950.0	E962.0	E980.0
Phorate	989.3	E863.1	—	E950.6	E962.1	E980.7
Phosdrin	989.3	E863.1	—	E950.6	E962.1	E980.7
Phosgene (gas)	987.8	E869.8	—	E952.8	E962.2	E982.8
Phosphate (tricresyl)	989.89	E866.8	—	E950.9	E962.1	E980.9
organic	989.3	E863.1	—	E950.6	E962.1	E980.7
solvent	982.8	E862.4	—	E950.9	E926.1	E980.9
Phosphine	987.8	E869.8	—	E952.8	E962.2	E982.8
fumigant	987.8	E863.8	—	E950.6	E962.2	E980.7
Phospholine	971.0	E855.3	E941.0	E950.4	E962.0	E980.4
Phosphoric acid	983.1	E864.1	—	E950.7	E962.1	E980.6
Phosphorus (compounds) NEC	983.9	E864.3	—	E950.7	E962.1	E980.6
rodenticide	983.9	E863.7	—	E950.7	E962.1	E980.6
Phthalimidoglutarimide	967.8	E852.8	E937.8	E950.2	E962.0	E980.2
Phthalylsulfathiazole	961.0	E857	E931.0	E950.4	E962.0	E980.4
Phylloquinone	964.3	E858.2	E934.3	E950.4	E962.0	E980.4
Physeptone	965.02	E850.1	E935.1	E950.0	E962.0	E980.0
Physostigma venenosum	988.2	E865.4	—	E950.9	E962.1	E980.9
Physostigmine	971.0	E855.3	E941.0	E950.4	E962.0	E980.4
Phytolacca decandra	988.2	E865.4	—	E950.9	E962.1	E980.9
Phytomenadione	964.3	E858.2	E934.3	E950.4	E962.0	E980.4
Phytonadione	964.3	E858.2	E934.3	E950.4	E962.0	E980.4
Picric (acid)	983.0	E864.0	—	E950.7	E962.1	E980.6
Picrotoxin	970.0	E854.3	E940.0	E950.4	E962.0	E980.4
Pilocarpine	971.0	E855.3	E941.0	E950.4	E962.0	E980.4
Pilocarpus (jaborandi) extract	971.0	E855.3	E941.0	E950.4	E962.0	E980.4
Pimaricin	960.1	E856	E930.1	E950.4	E962.0	E980.4
Piminodine	965.09	E850.2	E935.2	E950.0	E962.0	E980.0
Pine oil, pinesol (disinfectant)	983.9	E861.4	—	E950.7	E962.1	E980.6
Pinkroot	961.6	E857	E931.6	E950.4	E962.0	E980.4
Pipadone	965.09	E850.2	E935.2	E950.0	E962.0	E980.0
Pipamazine	963.0	E858.1	E933.0	E950.4	E962.0	E980.4
Pipazethate	975.4	E858.6	E945.4	E950.4	E962.0	E980.4
Pipenzolate	971.1	E855.4	E941.1	E950.4	E962.0	E980.4
Piperacetazine	969.1	E853.0	E939.1	E950.3	E962.0	E980.3
Piperazine NEC	961.6	E857	E931.6	E950.4	E962.0	E980.4
estrone sulfate	962.2	E858.0	E932.2	E950.4	E962.0	E980.4
Piper cubeba	988.2	E865.4	—	E950.9	E962.1	E980.9
Piperidione	975.4	E858.6	E945.4	E950.4	E962.0	E980.4
Piperidolate	971.1	E855.4	E941.1	E950.4	E962.0	E980.4
Piperocaine	968.9	E855.2	E938.9	E950.4	E962.0	E980.4
infiltration (subcutaneous)	968.5	E855.2	E938.5	E950.4	E962.0	E980.4
nerve block (peripheral) (plexus)	968.6	E855.2	E938.6	E950.4	E962.0	E980.4
topical (surface)	968.5	E855.2	E938.5	E950.4	E962.0	E980.4
Pipobroman	963.1	E858.1	E933.1	E950.4	E962.0	E980.4
Pipradrol	970.8	E854.3	E940.8	E950.4	E962.0	E980.4
Piscidia (bark) (erythrina)	965.7	E850.7	E935.7	E950.0	E962.0	E980.0
Pitch	983.0	E864.0	—	E950.7	E962.1	E980.6
Pitkin's solution	968.7	E855.2	E938.7	E950.4	E962.0	E980.4
Pitocin	975.0	E858.6	E945.0	E950.4	E962.0	E980.4
Pitressin (tannate)	962.5	E858.0	E932.5	E950.4	E962.0	E980.4
Pituitary extracts (posterior)	962.5	E858.0	E932.5	E950.4	E962.0	E980.4
anterior	962.4	E858.0	E932.4	E950.4	E962.0	E980.4
Pituitrin	962.5	E858.0	E932.5	E950.4	E962.0	E980.4
Placental extract	962.9	E858.0	E932.9	E950.4	E962.0	E980.4

✓4ᵗʰ Fourth-digit Required   ✓5ᵗʰ Fifth-digit Required   ▶◀ Revised Text   ● New Line   ▲ Revised Code

	Poisoning	External Cause (E-Code)				
		Accident	Therapeutic Use	Suicide Attempt	Assault	Undetermined
Placidyl	967.8	E852.8	E937.8	E950.2	E962.0	E980.2
Plague vaccine	978.3	E858.8	E948.3	E950.4	E962.0	E980.4
Plant foods or fertilizers NEC	989.89	E866.5	—	E950.9	E962.1	E980.9
mixed with herbicides	989.4	E863.5	—	E950.6	E962.1	E980.7
Plants, noxious, used as food	988.2	E865.9	—	E950.9	E962.1	E980.9
berries and seeds	988.2	E865.3	—	E950.9	E962.1	E980.9
specified type NEC	988.2	E865.4	—	E950.9	E962.1	E980.9
Plasma (blood)	964.7	E858.2	E934.7	E950.4	E962.0	E980.4
expanders	964.8	E858.2	E934.8	E950.4	E962.0	E980.4
Plasmanate	964.7	E858.2	E934.7	E950.4	E962.0	E980.4
Plegicil	969.1	E853.0	E939.1	E950.3	E962.0	E980.3
Podophyllin	976.4	E858.7	E946.4	E950.4	E962.0	E980.4
Podophyllum resin	976.4	E858.7	E946.4	E950.4	E962.0	E980.4
Poison NEC	989.9	E866.9	—	E950.9	E962.1	E980.9
Poisonous berries	988.2	E865.3	—	E950.9	E962.1	E980.9
Pokeweed (any part)	988.2	E865.4	—	E950.9	E962.1	E980.9
Poldine	971.1	E855.4	E941.1	E950.4	E962.0	E980.4
Poliomyelitis vaccine	979.5	E858.8	E949.5	E950.4	E962.0	E980.4
Poliovirus vaccine	979.5	E858.8	E949.5	E950.4	E962.0	E980.4
Polish (car) (floor) (furniture) (metal) (silver)	989.89	E861.2	—	E950.9	E962.1	E980.9
abrasive	989.89	E861.3	—	E950.9	E962.1	E980.9
porcelain	989.89	E861.3	—	E950.9	E962.1	E980.9
Poloxalkol	973.2	E858.4	E943.2	E950.4	E962.0	E980.4
Polyaminostyrene resins	974.5	E858.5	E944.5	E950.4	E962.0	E980.4
Polychlorinated biphenyl — *see* PCBs						
Polycycline	960.4	E856	E930.4	E950.4	E962.0	E980.4
Polyester resin hardener	982.8	E862.4	—	E950.9	E962.1	E980.9
fumes	987.8	E869.8	—	E952.8	E962.2	E982.8
Polyestradiol (phosphate)	962.2	E858.0	E932.2	E950.4	E962.0	E980.4
Polyethanolamine alkyl sulfate	976.2	E858.7	E946.2	E950.4	E962.0	E980.4
Polyethylene glycol	976.3	E858.7	E946.3	E950.4	E962.0	E980.4
Polyferose	964.0	E858.2	E934.0	E950.4	E962.0	E980.4
Polymyxin B	960.8	E856	E930.8	E950.4	E962.0	E980.4
ENT agent	976.6	E858.7	E946.6	E950.4	E962.0	E980.4
ophthalmic preparation	976.5	E858.7	E946.5	E950.4	E962.0	E980.4
topical NEC	976.0	E858.7	E946.0	E950.4	E962.0	E980.4
Polynoxylin(e)	976.0	E858.7	E946.0	E950.4	E962.0	E980.4
Polyoxymethyleneurea	976.0	E858.7	E946.0	E950.4	E962.0	E980.4
Polytetrafluoroethylene (inhaled)	987.8	E869.8	—	E952.8	E962.2	E982.8
Polythiazide	974.3	E858.5	E944.3	E950.4	E962.0	E980.4
Polyvinylpyrrolidone	964.8	E858.2	E934.8	E950.4	E962.0	E980.4
Pontocaine (hydrochloride) (infiltration) (topical)	968.5	E855.2	E938.5	E950.4	E962.0	E980.4
nerve block (peripheral) (plexus)	968.6	E855.2	E938.6	E950.4	E962.0	E980.4
spinal	968.7	E855.2	E938.7	E950.4	E962.0	E980.4
Pot	969.6	E854.1	E939.6	E950.3	E962.0	E980.3
Potash (caustic)	983.2	E864.2	—	E950.7	E962.1	E980.6
Potassic saline injection (lactated)	974.5	E858.5	E944.5	E950.4	E962.0	E980.4
Potassium (salts) NEC	974.5	E858.5	E944.5	E950.4	E962.0	E980.4
aminosalicylate	961.8	E857	E931.8	E950.4	E962.0	E980.4
arsenite (solution)	985.1	E866.3	—	E950.8	E962.1	E980.8
bichromate	983.9	E864.3	—	E950.7	E962.1	E980.6
bisulfate	983.9	E864.3	—	E950.7	E962.1	E980.6
bromide (medicinal) NEC	967.3	E852.2	E937.3	E950.2	E962.0	E980.2
carbonate	983.2	E864.2	—	E950.7	E962.1	E980.6
chlorate NEC	983.9	E864.3	—	E950.7	E962.1	E980.6
cyanide — *see* Cyanide						
hydroxide	983.2	E864.2	—	E950.7	E962.1	E980.6
iodide (expectorant) NEC	975.5	E858.6	E945.5	E950.4	E962.0	E980.4
nitrate	989.89	E866.8	—	E950.9	E962.1	E980.9
oxalate	983.9	E864.3	—	E950.7	E962.1	E980.6
perchlorate NEC	977.8	E858.8	E947.8	E950.4	E962.0	E980.4
antithyroid	962.8	E858.0	E932.8	E950.4	E962.0	E980.4
permanganate	976.0	E858.7	E946.0	E950.4	E962.0	E980.4
nonmedicinal	983.9	E864.3	—	E950.7	E962.1	E980.6
Povidone-iodine (anti-infective) NEC	976.0	E858.7	E946.0	E950.4	E962.0	E980.4
Practolol	972.0	E858.3	E942.0	E950.4	E962.0	E980.4
Pralidoxime (chloride)	977.2	E858.8	E947.2	E950.4	E962.0	E980.4
Pramoxine	968.5	E855.2	E938.5	E950.4	E962.0	E980.4
Prazosin	972.6	E858.3	E942.6	E950.4	E962.0	E980.4
Prednisolone	962.0	E858.0	E932.0	E950.4	E962.0	E980.4
ENT agent	976.6	E858.7	E946.6	E950.4	E962.0	E980.4
ophthalmic preparation	976.5	E858.7	E946.5	E950.4	E962.0	E980.4
topical NEC	976.0	E858.7	E946.0	E950.4	E962.0	E980.4
Prednisone	962.0	E858.0	E932.0	E950.4	E962.0	E980.4
Pregnanediol	962.2	E858.0	E932.2	E950.4	E962.0	E980.4
Pregneninolone	962.2	E858.0	E932.2	E950.4	E962.0	E980.4
Preludin	977.0	E858.8	E947.0	E950.4	E962.0	E980.4
Premarin	962.2	E858.0	E932.2	E950.4	E962.0	E980.4
Prenylamine	972.4	E858.3	E942.4	E950.4	E962.0	E980.4
Preparation H	976.8	E858.7	E946.8	E950.4	E962.0	E980.4
Preservatives	989.89	E866.8	—	E950.9	E962.1	E980.9

Placidyl — Preservatives

	Poisoning	External Cause (E-Code)				
		Accident	Therapeutic Use	Suicide Attempt	Assault	Undetermined
Pride of China	988.2	E865.3	—	E950.9	E962.1	E980.9
Prilocaine	968.9	E855.2	E938.9	E950.4	E962.0	E980.4
infiltration (subcutaneous)	968.5	E855.2	E938.5	E950.4	E962.0	E980.4
nerve block (peripheral) (plexus)	968.6	E855.2	E938.6	E950.4	E962.0	E980.4
Primaquine	961.4	E857	E931.4	E950.4	E962.0	E980.4
Primidone	966.3	E855.0	E936.3	E950.4	E962.0	E980.4
Primula (veris)	988.2	E865.4	—	E950.9	E962.1	E980.9
Prinadol	965.09	E850.2	E935.2	E950.0	E962.0	E980.0
Priscol, Priscoline	971.3	E855.6	E941.3	E950.4	E962.0	E980.4
Privet	988.2	E865.4	—	E950.9	E962.1	E980.9
Privine	971.2	E855.5	E941.2	E950.4	E962.0	E980.4
Pro-Banthine	971.1	E855.4	E941.1	E950.4	E962.0	E980.4
Probarbital	967.0	E851	E937.0	E950.1	E962.0	E980.1
Probenecid	974.7	E858.5	E944.7	E950.4	E962.0	E980.4
Procainamide (hydrochloride)	972.0	E858.3	E942.0	E950.4	E962.0	E980.4
Procaine (hydrochloride) (infiltration) (topical)	968.5	E855.2	E938.5	E950.4	E962.0	E980.4
nerve block (peripheral) (plexus)	968.6	E855.2	E938.6	E950.4	E962.0	E980.4
penicillin G	960.0	E856	E930.0	E950.4	E962.0	E980.4
spinal	968.7	E855.2	E938.7	E950.4	E962.0	E980.4
Procalmidol	969.5	E853.8	E939.5	E950.3	E962.0	E980.3
Procarbazine	963.1	E858.1	E933.1	E950.4	E962.0	E980.4
Prochlorperazine	969.1	E853.0	E939.1	E950.3	E962.0	E980.3
Procyclidine	966.4	E855.0	E936.4	E950.4	E962.0	E980.4
Producer gas	986	E868.8	—	E952.1	E962.2	E982.1
Profenamine	966.4	E855.0	E936.4	E950.4	E962.0	E980.4
Profenil	975.1	E858.6	E945.1	E950.4	E962.0	E980.4
Progesterones	962.2	E858.0	E932.2	E950.4	E962.0	E980.4
Progestin	962.2	E858.0	E932.2	E950.4	E962.0	E980.4
Progestogens (with estrogens)	962.2	E858.0	E932.2	E950.4	E962.0	E980.4
Progestone	962.2	E858.0	E932.2	E950.4	E962.0	E980.4
Proguanil	961.4	E857	E931.4	E950.4	E962.0	E980.4
Prolactin	962.4	E858.0	E932.4	E950.4	E962.0	E980.4
Proloid	962.7	E858.0	E932.7	E950.4	E962.0	E980.4
Proluton	962.2	E858.0	E932.2	E950.4	E962.0	E980.4
Promacetin	961.8	E857	E931.8	E950.4	E962.0	E980.4
Promazine	969.1	E853.0	E939.1	E950.3	E962.0	E980.3
Promedol	965.09	E850.2	E935.2	E950.0	E962.0	E980.0
Promethazine	967.8	E852.8	E937.8	E950.2	E962.0	E980.2
Promin	961.8	E857	E931.8	E950.4	E962.0	E980.4
Pronestyl (hydrochloride)	972.0	E858.3	E942.0	E950.4	E962.0	E980.4
Pronetalol, pronethalol	972.0	E858.3	E942.0	E950.4	E962.0	E980.4
Prontosil	961.0	E857	E931.0	E950.4	E962.0	E980.4
Propamidine isethionate	961.5	E857	E931.5	E950.4	E962.0	E980.4
Propanal (medicinal)	967.8	E852.8	E937.8	E950.2	E962.0	E980.2
Propane (gas) (distributed in mobile container)	987.0	E868.0	—	E951.1	E962.2	E981.1
distributed through pipes	987.0	E867	—	E951.0	E962.2	E981.0
incomplete combustion of — see Carbon monoxide, Propane						
Propanidid	968.3	E855.1	E938.3	E950.4	E962.0	E980.4
Propanol	980.3	E860.4	—	E950.9	E962.1	E980.9
Propantheline	971.1	E855.4	E941.1	E950.4	E962.0	E980.4
Proparacaine	968.5	E855.2	E938.5	E950.4	E962.0	E980.4
Propatyl nitrate	972.4	E858.3	E942.4	E950.4	E962.0	E980.4
Propicillin	960.0	E856	E930.0	E950.4	E962.0	E980.4
Propiolactone (vapor)	987.8	E869.8	—	E952.8	E962.2	E982.8
Propiomazine	967.8	E852.8	E937.8	E950.2	E962.0	E980.2
Propionaldehyde (medicinal)	967.8	E852.8	E937.8	E950.2	E962.0	E980.2
Propionate compound	976.0	E858.7	E946.0	E950.4	E962.0	E980.4
Propion gel	976.0	E858.7	E946.0	E950.4	E962.0	E980.4
Propitocaine	968.9	E855.2	E938.9	E950.4	E962.0	E980.4
infiltration (subcutaneous)	968.5	E855.2	E938.5	E950.4	E962.0	E980.4
nerve block (peripheral) (plexus)	968.6	E855.2	E938.6	E950.4	E962.0	E980.4
Propoxur	989.3	E863.2	—	E950.6	E962.1	E980.7
Propoxycaine	968.9	E855.2	E938.9	E950.4	E962.0	E980.4
infiltration (subcutaneous)	968.5	E855.2	E938.5	E950.4	E962.0	E980.4
nerve block (peripheral) (plexus)	968.6	E855.2	E938.6	E950.4	E962.0	E980.4
topical (surface)	968.5	E855.2	E938.5	E950.4	E962.0	E980.4
Propoxyphene (hydrochloride)	965.8	E850.8	E935.8	E950.0	E962.0	E980.0
Propranolol	972.0	E858.3	E942.0	E950.4	E962.0	E980.4
Propyl						
alcohol	980.3	E860.4	—	E950.9	E962.1	E980.9
carbinol	980.3	E860.4	—	E950.9	E962.1	E980.9
hexadrine	971.2	E855.5	E941.2	E950.4	E962.0	E980.4
iodone	977.8	E858.8	E947.8	E950.4	E962.0	E980.4
thiouracil	962.8	E858.0	E932.8	E950.4	E962.0	E980.4
Propylene	987.1	E869.8	—	E952.8	E962.2	E982.8
Propylparaben (ophthalmic)	976.5	E858.7	E946.5	E950.4	E962.0	E980.4
Proscillaridin	972.1	E858.3	E942.1	E950.4	E962.0	E980.4
Prostaglandins	975.0	E858.6	E945.0	E950.4	E962.0	E980.4
Prostigmin	971.0	E855.3	E941.0	E950.4	E962.0	E980.4
Protamine (sulfate)	964.5	E858.2	E934.5	E950.4	E962.0	E980.4
zinc insulin	962.3	E858.0	E932.3	E950.4	E962.0	E980.4

	Poisoning	External Cause (E-Code)				
		Accident	Therapeutic Use	Suicide Attempt	Assault	Undetermined
Protectants (topical)	976.3	E858.7	E946.3	E950.4	E962.0	E980.4
Protein hydrolysate	974.5	E858.5	E944.5	E950.4	E962.0	E980.4
Prothiaden — see Dothiepin hydrochloride						
Prothionamide	961.8	E857	E931.8	E950.4	E962.0	E980.4
Prothipendyl	969.5	E853.8	E939.5	E950.3	E962.0	E980.3
Protokylol	971.2	E855.5	E941.2	E950.4	E962.0	E980.4
Protopam	977.2	E858.8	E947.2	E950.4	E962.0	E980.4
Protoveratrine(s) (A) (B)	972.6	E858.3	E942.6	E950.4	E962.0	E980.4
Protriptyline	969.0	E854.0	E939.0	E950.3	E962.0	E980.3
Provera	962.2	E858.0	E932.2	E950.4	E962.0	E980.4
Provitamin A	963.5	E858.1	E933.5	E950.4	E962.0	E980.4
Proxymetacaine	968.5	E855.2	E938.5	E950.4	E962.0	E980.4
Proxyphylline	975.1	E858.6	E945.1	E950.4	E962.0	E980.4
Prozac — see Fluoxetine hydrochloride						
Prunus	988.2	E865.4	—	E950.9	E962.1	E980.9
laurocerasus	988.2	E865.4	—	E950.9	E962.1	E980.9
virginiana	989.0	E866.8	—	E950.9	E962.1	E980.9
Prussic acid	987.7	E869.8	—	E952.8	E962.2	E982.8
vapor	971.2	E855.5	E941.2	E950.4	E962.0	E980.4
Pseudoephedrine	969.6	E854.1	E939.6	E950.3	E962.0	E980.3
Psilocin	969.6	E854.1	E939.6	E950.3	E962.0	E980.3
Psilocybin	977.8	E858.8	E947.8	E950.4	E962.0	E980.4
PSP	969.6	E854.1	E939.6	E950.3	E962.0	E980.3
Psychedelic agents	969.6	E854.1	E939.6	E950.3	E962.0	E980.3
Psychodysleptics	969.7	E854.2	E939.7	E950.3	E962.0	E980.3
Psychostimulants	969.9	E855.9	E939.9	E950.3	E962.0	E980.3
Psychotherapeutic agents	969.0	E854.0	E939.0	E950.3	E962.0	E980.3
antidepressants	969.8	E855.8	E939.8	E950.3	E962.0	E980.3
specified NEC	969.5	E853.9	E939.5	E950.3	E962.0	E980.3
tranquilizers NEC	969.6	E854.1	E939.6	E950.3	E962.0	E980.3
Psychotomimetic agents	969.9	E854.8	E939.9	E950.3	E962.0	E980.3
Psychotropic agents	969.8	E854.8	E939.8	E950.3	E962.0	E980.3
specified NEC	973.3	E858.4	E943.3	E950.4	E962.0	E980.4
Psyllium	964.1	E858.2	E934.1	E950.4	E962.0	E980.4
Pteroylglutamic acid	963.1	E858.1	E933.1	E950.4	E962.0	E980.4
Pteroyltriglutamate	987.8	E869.8	—	E952.8	E962.2	E982.8
PTFE	988.2	E865.4	—	E950.9	E962.1	E980.9
Pulsatilla	983.9	E864.3	—	E950.7	E962.1	E980.6
Purex (bleach)	974.1	E858.5	E944.1	E950.4	E962.0	E980.4
Purine diuretics	963.1	E858.1	E933.1	E950.4	E962.0	E980.4
Purinethol	964.8	E858.2	E934.8	E950.4	E962.0	E980.4
PVP	965.7	E850.7	E935.7	E950.0	E962.0	E980.0
Pyrabital	965.5	E850.5	E935.5	E950.0	E962.0	E980.0
Pyramidon	961.6	E857	E931.6	E950.4	E962.0	E980.4
Pyrantel (pamoate)	963.0	E858.1	E933.0	E950.4	E962.0	E980.4
Pyrathiazine	961.8	E857	E931.8	E950.4	E962.0	E980.4
Pyrazinamide	961.8	E857	E931.8	E950.4	E962.0	E980.4
Pyrazinoic acid (amide)	965.5	E850.5	E935.5	E950.0	E962.0	E980.0
Pyrazole (derivatives)	965.5	E850.5	E935.5	E950.0	E962.0	E980.0
Pyrazolone (analgesics)	989.4	E863.4	—	E950.6	E962.1	E980.7
Pyrethrins, pyrethrum	963.0	E858.1	E933.0	E950.4	E962.0	E980.4
Pyribenzamine	982.0	E862.4	—	E950.9	E962.1	E980.9
Pyridine (liquid) (vapor)	977.2	E858.8	E947.2	E950.4	E962.0	E980.4
aldoxime chloride	976.1	E858.7	E946.1	E950.4	E962.0	E980.4
Pyridium	971.0	E855.3	E941.0	E950.4	E962.0	E980.4
Pyridostigmine	963.5	E858.1	E933.5	E950.4	E962.0	E980.4
Pyridoxine	963.0	E858.1	E933.0	E950.4	E962.0	E980.4
Pyrilamine	961.4	E857	E931.4	E950.4	E962.0	E980.4
Pyrimethamine	983.0	E864.0	—	E950.7	E962.1	E980.6
Pyrogallic acid	976.3	E858.7	E946.3	E950.4	E962.0	E980.4
Pyroxylin	963.0	E858.1	E933.0	E950.4	E962.0	E980.4
Pyrrobutamine	968.5	E855.2	E938.5	E950.4	E962.0	E980.4
Pyrrocitine	961.6	E857	E931.6	E950.4	E962.0	E980.4
Pyrvinium (pamoate)	962.3	E858.0	E932.3	E950.4	E962.0	E980.4
PZI	967.4	E852.3	E937.4	E950.2	E962.0	E980.2
Quaalude	971.1	E855.4	E941.1	E950.4	E962.0	E980.4
Quaternary ammonium derivatives	983.2	E864.2	—	E950.7	E962.1	E980.6
Quicklime	961.3	E857	E931.3	E950.4	E962.0	E980.4
Quinacrine	972.0	E858.3	E942.0	E950.4	E962.0	E980.4
Quinaglute	967.0	E851	E937.0	E950.1	E962.0	E980.1
Quinalbarbitone	962.2	E858.0	E932.2	E950.4	E962.0	E980.4
Quinestradiol	974.3	E858.5	E944.3	E950.4	E962.0	E980.4
Quinethazone	972.0	E858.3	E942.0	E950.4	E962.0	E980.4
Quinidine (gluconate) (polygalacturonate) (salts) (sulfate)	961.4	E857	E931.4	E950.4	E962.0	E980.4
Quinine	961.3	E857	E931.3	E950.4	E962.0	E980.4
Quiniobine	961.3	E857	E931.3	E950.4	E962.0	E980.4
Quinolines	968.5	E855.2	E938.5	E950.4	E962.0	E980.4
Quotane						
Rabies						
immune globulin (human)	964.6	E858.2	E934.6	E950.4	E962.0	E980.4
vaccine	979.1	E858.8	E949.1	E950.4	E962.0	E980.4

✓4ᵗʰ Fourth-digit Required   ✓5ᵗʰ Fifth-digit Required   ►◄ Revised Text   ● New Line   ▲ Revised Code

	Poisoning	External Cause (E-Code)				
		Accident	Therapeutic Use	Suicide Attempt	Assault	Undetermined
Racemoramide	965.09	E850.2	E935.2	E950.0	E962.0	E980.0
Racemorphan	965.09	E850.2	E935.2	E950.0	E962.0	E980.0
Radiator alcohol	980.1	E860.2	—	E950.9	E962.1	E980.9
Radio-opaque (drugs) (materials)	977.8	E858.8	E947.8	E950.4	E962.0	E980.4
Ranunculus	988.2	E865.4	—	E950.9	E962.1	E980.9
Rat poison	989.4	E863.7	—	E950.6	E962.1	E980.7
Rattlesnake (venom)	989.5	E905.0	—	E950.9	E962.1	E980.9
Raudixin	972.6	E858.3	E942.6	E950.4	E962.0	E980.4
Rautensin	972.6	E858.3	E942.6	E950.4	E962.0	E980.4
Rautina	972.6	E858.3	E942.6	E950.4	E962.0	E980.4
Rautotal	972.6	E858.3	E942.6	E950.4	E962.0	E980.4
Rauwiloid	972.6	E858.3	E942.6	E950.4	E962.0	E980.4
Rauwoldin	972.6	E858.3	E942.6	E950.4	E962.0	E980.4
Rauwolfia (alkaloids)	972.6	E858.3	E942.6	E950.4	E962.0	E980.4
Realgar	985.1	E866.3	—	E950.8	E962.1	E980.8
Red cells, packed	964.7	E858.2	E934.7	E950.4	E962.0	E980.4
Reducing agents, industrial NEC	983.9	E864.3	—	E950.7	E962.1	E980.6
Refrigerant gas (freon)	987.4	E869.2	—	E952.8	E962.2	E982.8
not freon	987.9	E869.9	—	E952.9	E962.2	E982.9
Regroton	974.4	E858.5	E944.4	E950.4	E962.0	E980.4
Rela	968.0	E855.1	E938.0	E950.4	E962.0	E980.4
Relaxants, skeletal muscle (autonomic)	975.2	E858.6	E945.2	E950.4	E962.0	E980.4
central nervous system	968.0	E855.1	E938.0	E950.4	E962.0	E980.4
Renese	974.3	E858.5	E944.3	E950.4	E962.0	E980.4
Renografin	977.8	E858.8	E947.8	E950.4	E962.0	E980.4
Replacement solutions	974.5	E858.5	E944.5	E950.4	E962.0	E980.4
Rescinnamine	972.6	E858.3	E942.6	E950.4	E962.0	E980.4
Reserpine	972.6	E858.3	E942.6	E950.4	E962.0	E980.4
Resorcin, resorcinol	976.4	E858.7	E946.4	E950.4	E962.0	E980.4
Respaire	975.5	E858.6	E945.5	E950.4	E962.0	E980.4
Respiratory agents NEC	975.8	E858.6	E945.8	E950.4	E962.0	E980.4
Retinoic acid	976.8	E858.7	E946.8	E950.4	E962.0	E980.4
Retinol	963.5	E858.1	E933.5	E950.4	E962.0	E980.4
Rh (D) immune globulin (human)	964.6	E858.2	E934.6	E950.4	E962.0	E980.4
Rhodine	965.1	E850.3	E935.3	E950.0	E962.0	E980.0
RhoGAM	964.6	E858.2	E934.6	E950.4	E962.0	E980.4
Riboflavin	963.5	E858.1	E933.5	E950.4	E962.0	E980.4
Ricin	989.89	E866.8	—	E950.9	E962.1	E980.9
Ricinus communis	988.2	E865.3	—	E950.9	E962.1	E980.9
Rickettsial vaccine NEC	979.6	E858.8	E949.6	E950.4	E962.0	E980.4
with viral and bacterial vaccine	979.7	E858.8	E949.7	E950.4	E962.0	E980.4
Rifampin	960.6	E856	E930.6	E950.4	E962.0	E980.4
Rimifon	961.8	E857	E931.8	E950.4	E962.0	E980.4
Ringer's injection (lactated)	974.5	E858.5	E944.5	E950.4	E962.0	E980.4
Ristocetin	960.8	E856	E930.8	E950.4	E962.0	E980.4
Ritalin	969.7	E854.2	E939.7	E950.3	E962.0	E980.3
Roach killers — see Pesticides						
Rocky Mountain spotted fever vaccine	979.6	E858.8	E949.6	E950.4	E962.0	E980.4
Rodenticides	989.4	E863.7	—	E950.6	E962.1	E980.7
Rohypnol	969.4	E853.2	E939.4	E950.3	E962.0	E980.3 ▲
Rolaids	973.0	E858.4	E943.0	E950.4	E962.0	E980.4
Rolitetracycline	960.4	E856	E930.4	E950.4	E962.0	E980.4
Romilar	975.4	E858.6	E945.4	E950.4	E962.0	E980.4
Rose water ointment	976.3	E858.7	E946.3	E950.4	E962.0	E980.4
Rotenone	989.4	E863.7	—	E950.6	E962.1	E980.7
Rotoxamine	963.0	E858.1	E933.0	E950.4	E962.0	E980.4
Rough-on-rats	989.4	E863.7	—	E950.6	E962.1	E980.7
RU486	962.9	E858.0	E932.9	E950.4	E962.0	E980.4
Rubbing alcohol	980.2	E860.3	—	E950.9	E962.1	E980.9
Rubella virus vaccine	979.4	E858.8	E949.4	E950.4	E962.0	E980.4
Rubelogen	979.4	E858.8	E949.4	E950.4	E962.0	E980.4
Rubeovax	979.4	E858.8	E949.4	E950.4	E962.0	E980.4
Rubidomycin	960.7	E856	E930.7	E950.4	E962.0	E980.4
Rue	988.2	E865.4	—	E950.9	E962.1	E980.9
Ruta	988.2	E865.4	—	E950.9	E962.1	E980.9
Sabadilla (medicinal)	976.0	E858.7	E946.0	E950.4	E962.0	E980.4
pesticide	989.4	E863.4	—	E950.6	E962.1	E980.7
Sabin oral vaccine	979.5	E858.8	E949.5	E950.4	E962.0	E980.4
Saccharated iron oxide	964.0	E858.2	E934.0	E950.4	E962.0	E980.4
Saccharin	974.5	E858.5	E944.5	E950.4	E962.0	E980.4
Safflower oil	972.2	E858.3	E942.2	E950.4	E962.0	E980.4
Salbutamol sulfate	975.7	E858.6	E945.7	E950.4	E962.0	E980.4
Salicylamide	965.1	E850.3	E935.3	E950.0	E962.0	E980.0
Salicylate(s)	965.1	E850.3	E935.3	E950.0	E962.0	E980.0
methyl	976.3	E858.7	E946.3	E950.4	E962.0	E980.4
theobromine calcium	974.1	E858.5	E944.1	E950.4	E962.0	E980.4
Salicylazosulfapyridine	961.0	E857	E931.0	E950.4	E962.0	E980.4
Salicylhydroxamic acid	976.0	E858.7	E946.0	E950.4	E962.0	E980.4
Salicylic acid (keratolytic) NEC	976.4	E858.7	E946.4	E950.4	E962.0	E980.4
congeners	965.1	E850.3	E935.3	E950.0	E962.0	E980.0
salts	965.1	E850.3	E935.3	E950.0	E962.0	E980.0

Racemoramide — Salicylic acid

	Poisoning	External Cause (E-Code)				
		Accident	Therapeutic Use	Suicide Attempt	Assault	Undetermined
Saliniazid	961.8	E857	E931.8	E950.4	E962.0	E980.4
Salol	976.3	E858.7	E946.3	E950.4	E962.0	E980.4
Salt (substitute) NEC	974.5	E858.5	E944.5	E950.4	E962.0	E980.4
Saluretics	974.3	E858.5	E944.3	E950.4	E962.0	E980.4
Saluron	974.3	E858.5	E944.3	E950.4	E962.0	E980.4
Salvarsan 606 (neosilver) (silver)	961.1	E857	E931.1	E950.4	E962.0	E980.4
Sambucus canadensis	988.2	E865.4	—	E950.9	E962.1	E980.9
berry	988.2	E865.3	—	E950.9	E962.1	E980.9
Sandril	972.6	E858.3	E942.6	E950.4	E962.0	E980.4
Sanguinaria canadensis	988.2	E865.4	—	E950.9	E962.1	E980.9
Saniflush (cleaner)	983.9	E861.3	—	E950.7	E962.1	E980.6
Santonin	961.6	E857	E931.6	E950.4	E962.0	E980.4
Santyl	976.8	E858.7	E946.8	E950.4	E962.0	E980.4
Sarkomycin	960.7	E856	E930.7	E950.4	E962.0	E980.4
Saroten	969.0	E854.0	E939.0	E950.3	E962.0	E980.3
Saturnine — see Lead						
Savin (oil)	976.4	E858.7	E946.4	E950.4	E962.0	E980.4
Scammony	973.1	E858.4	E943.1	E950.4	E962.0	E980.4
Scarlet red	976.8	E858.7	E946.8	E950.4	E962.0	E980.4
Scheele's green	985.1	E866.3	—	E950.8	E962.1	E980.8
insecticide	985.1	E863.4	—	E950.8	E962.1	E980.8
Schradan	989.3	E863.1	—	E950.6	E962.1	E980.7
Schweinfurt(h) green	985.1	E866.3	—	E950.8	E962.1	E980.8
insecticide	985.1	E863.4	—	E950.8	E962.1	E980.8
Scilla — see Squill						
Sclerosing agents	972.7	E858.3	E942.7	E950.4	E962.0	E980.4
Scopolamine	971.1	E855.4	E941.1	E950.4	E962.0	E980.4
Scouring powder	989.89	E861.3	—	E950.9	E962.1	E980.9
Sea						
anemone (sting)	989.5	E905.6	—	E950.9	E962.1	E980.9
cucumber (sting)	989.5	E905.6	—	E950.9	E962.1	E980.9
snake (bite) (venom)	989.5	E905.0	—	E950.9	E962.1	E980.9
urchin spine (puncture)	989.5	E905.6	—	E950.9	E962.1	E980.9
Secbutabarbital	967.0	E851	E937.0	E950.1	E962.0	E980.1
Secbutabarbitone	967.0	E851	E937.0	E950.1	E962.0	E980.1
Secobarbital	967.0	E851	E937.0	E950.1	E962.0	E980.1
Seconal	967.0	E851	E937.0	E950.1	E962.0	E980.1
Secretin	977.8	E858.8	E947.8	E950.4	E962.0	E980.4
Sedatives, nonbarbiturate	967.9	E852.9	E937.9	E950.2	E962.0	E980.2
specified NEC	967.8	E852.8	E937.8	E950.2	E962.0	E980.2
Sedormid	967.8	E852.8	E937.8	E950.2	E962.0	E980.2
Seed (plant)	988.2	E865.3	—	E950.9	E962.1	E980.9
disinfectant or dressing	989.89	E866.5	—	E950.9	E962.1	E980.9
Selenium (fumes) NEC	985.8	E866.4	—	E950.9	E962.1	E980.9
disulfide or sulfide	976.4	E858.7	E946.4	E950.4	E962.0	E980.4
Selsun	976.4	E858.7	E946.4	E950.4	E962.0	E980.4
Senna	973.1	E858.4	E943.1	E950.4	E962.0	E980.4
Septisol	976.2	E858.7	E946.2	E950.4	E962.0	E980.4
Serax	969.4	E853.2	E939.4	E950.3	E962.0	E980.3
Serenesil	967.8	E852.8	E937.8	E950.2	E962.0	E980.2
Serenium (hydrochloride)	961.9	E857	E931.9	E950.4	E962.0	E980.4
Sernyl	968.3	E855.1	E938.3	E950.4	E962.0	E980.4
Serotonin	977.8	E858.8	E947.8	E950.4	E962.0	E980.4
Serpasil	972.6	E858.3	E942.6	E950.4	E962.0	E980.4
Sewer gas	987.8	E869.8	—	E952.8	E962.2	E982.8
Shampoo	989.6	E861.0	—	E950.9	E962.1	E980.9
Shellfish, nonbacterial or noxious	988.0	E865.1	—	E950.9	E962.1	E980.9
Silicones NEC	989.83	E866.8	E947.8	E950.9	E962.1	E980.9
Silvadene	976.0	E858.7	E946.0	E950.4	E962.0	E980.4
Silver (compound) (medicinal) NEC	976.0	E858.7	E946.0	E950.4	E962.0	E980.4
anti-infectives	976.0	E858.7	E946.0	E950.4	E962.0	E980.4
arsphenamine	961.1	E857	E931.1	E950.4	E962.0	E980.4
nitrate	976.0	E858.7	E946.0	E950.4	E962.0	E980.4
ophthalmic preparation	976.5	E858.7	E946.5	E950.4	E962.0	E980.4
toughened (keratolytic)	976.4	E858.7	E946.4	E950.4	E962.0	E980.4
nonmedicinal (dust)	985.8	E866.4	—	E950.9	E962.1	E980.9
protein (mild) (strong)	976.0	E858.7	E946.0	E950.4	E962.0	E980.4
salvarsan	961.1	E857	E931.1	E950.4	E962.0	E980.4
Simethicone	973.8	E858.4	E943.8	E950.4	E962.0	E980.4
Sinequan	969.0	E854.0	E939.0	E950.3	E962.0	E980.3
Singoserp	972.6	E858.3	E942.6	E950.4	E962.0	E980.4
Sintrom	964.2	E858.2	E934.2	E950.4	E962.0	E980.4
Sitosterols	972.2	E858.3	E942.2	E950.4	E962.0	E980.4
Skeletal muscle relaxants	975.2	E858.6	E945.2	E950.4	E962.0	E980.4
Skin						
agents (external)	976.9	E858.7	E946.9	E950.4	E962.0	E980.4
specified NEC	976.8	E858.7	E946.8	E950.4	E962.0	E980.4
test antigen	977.8	E858.8	E947.8	E950.4	E962.0	E980.4
Sleep-eze	963.0	E858.1	E933.0	E950.4	E962.0	E980.4
Sleeping draught (drug) (pill) (tablet)	967.9	E852.9	E937.9	E950.2	E962.0	E980.2
Smallpox vaccine	979.0	E858.8	E949.0	E950.4	E962.0	E980.4

	Poisoning	Accident	Therapeutic Use	Suicide Attempt	Assault	Undetermined
Smelter fumes NEC	985.9	E866.4	—	E950.9	E962.1	E980.9
Smog	987.3	E869.1	—	E952.8	E962.2	E982.8
Smoke NEC	987.9	E869.9	—	E952.9	E962.2	E982.9
Smooth muscle relaxant	975.1	E858.6	E945.1	E950.4	E962.0	E980.4
Snail killer	989.4	E863.4	—	E950.6	E962.1	E980.7
Snake (bite) (venom)	989.5	E905.0	—	E950.9	E962.1	E980.9
Snuff	989.89	E866.8	—	E950.9	E962.1	E980.9
Soap (powder) (product)	989.6	E861.1	—	E950.9	E962.1	E980.9
medicinal, soft	976.2	E858.7	E946.2	E950.4	E962.0	E980.4
Soda (caustic)	983.2	E864.2	—	E950.7	E962.1	E980.6
bicarb	963.3	E858.1	E933.3	E950.4	E962.0	E980.4
chlorinated — *see* Sodium, hypochlorite						
Sodium						
acetosulfone	961.8	E857	E931.8	E950.4	E962.0	E980.4
acetrizoate	977.8	E858.8	E947.8	E950.4	E962.0	E980.4
amytal	967.0	E851	E937.0	E950.1	E962.0	E980.1
arsenate — *see* Arsenic						
bicarbonate	963.3	E858.1	E933.3	E950.4	E962.0	E980.4
bichromate	983.9	E864.3	—	E950.7	E962.1	E980.6
biphosphate	963.2	E858.1	E933.2	E950.4	E962.0	E980.4
bisulfate	983.9	E864.3	—	E950.7	E962.1	E980.6
borate (cleanser)	989.6	E861.3	—	E950.9	E962.1	E980.9
bromide NEC	967.3	E852.2	E937.3	E950.2	E962.0	E980.2
cacodylate (nonmedicinal) NEC	978.8	E858.8	E948.8	E950.4	E962.0	E980.4
anti-infective	961.1	E857	E931.1	E950.4	E962.0	E980.4
herbicide	989.4	E863.5	—	E950.6	E962.1	E980.7
calcium edetate	963.8	E858.1	E933.8	E950.4	E962.0	E980.4
carbonate NEC	983.2	E864.2	—	E950.7	E962.1	E980.6
chlorate NEC	983.9	E864.3	—	E950.7	E962.1	E980.6
herbicide	983.9	E863.5	—	E950.7	E962.1	E980.6
chloride NEC	974.5	E858.5	E944.5	E950.4	E962.0	E980.4
chromate	983.9	E864.3	—	E950.7	E962.1	E980.6
citrate	963.3	E858.1	E933.3	E950.4	E962.0	E980.4
cyanide — *see* Cyanide(s)						
cyclamate	974.5	E858.5	E944.5	E950.4	E962.0	E980.4
diatrizoate	977.8	E858.8	E947.8	E950.4	E962.0	E980.4
dibunate	975.4	E858.6	E945.4	E950.4	E962.0	E980.4
dioctyl sulfosuccinate	973.2	E858.4	E943.2	E950.4	E962.0	E980.4
edetate	963.8	E858.1	E933.8	E950.4	E962.0	E980.4
ethacrynate	974.4	E858.5	E944.4	E950.4	E962.0	E980.4
fluoroacetate (dust) (rodenticide)	989.4	E863.7	—	E950.6	E962.1	E980.7
fluoride — *see* Fluoride(s)						
free salt	974.5	E858.5	E944.5	E950.4	E962.0	E980.4
glucosulfone	961.8	E857	E931.8	E950.4	E962.0	E980.4
hydroxide	983.2	E864.2	—	E950.7	E962.1	E980.6
hypochlorite (bleach) NEC	983.9	E864.3	—	E950.7	E962.1	E980.6
disinfectant	983.9	E861.4	—	E950.7	E962.1	E980.6
medicinal (anti-infective) (external)	976.0	E858.7	E946.0	E950.4	E962.0	E980.4
vapor	987.8	E869.8	—	E952.8	E962.2	E982.8
hyposulfite	976.0	E858.7	E946.0	E950.4	E962.0	E980.4
indigotindisulfonate	977.8	E858.8	E947.8	E950.4	E962.0	E980.4
iodide	977.8	E858.8	E947.8	E950.4	E962.0	E980.4
iothalamate	977.8	E858.8	E947.8	E950.4	E962.0	E980.4
iron edetate	964.0	E858.2	E934.0	E950.4	E962.0	E980.4
lactate	963.3	E858.1	E933.3	E950.4	E962.0	E980.4
lauryl sulfate	976.2	E858.7	E946.2	E950.4	E962.0	E980.4
L-triiodothyronine	962.7	E858.0	E932.7	E950.4	E962.0	E980.4
metrizoate	977.8	E858.8	E947.8	E950.4	E962.0	E980.4
monofluoroacetate (dust) (rodenticide)	989.4	E863.7	—	E950.6	E962.1	E980.7
morrhuate	972.7	E858.3	E942.7	E950.4	E962.0	E980.4
nafcillin	960.0	E856	E930.0	E950.4	E962.0	E980.4
nitrate (oxidizing agent)	983.9	E864.3	—	E950.7	E962.1	E980.6
nitrite (medicinal)	972.4	E858.3	E942.4	E950.4	E962.0	E980.4
nitroferricyanide	972.6	E858.3	E942.6	E950.4	E962.0	E980.4
nitroprusside	972.6	E858.3	E942.6	E950.4	E962.0	E980.4
para-aminohippurate	977.8	E858.8	E947.8	E950.4	E962.0	E980.4
perborate (nonmedicinal) NEC	989.89	E866.8	—	E950.9	E962.1	E980.9
medicinal	976.6	E858.7	E946.6	E950.4	E962.0	E980.4
soap	989.6	E861.1	—	E950.9	E962.1	E980.9
percarbonate — *see* Sodium, perborate						
phosphate	973.3	E858.4	E943.3	E950.4	E962.0	E980.4
polystyrene sulfonate	974.5	E858.5	E944.5	E950.4	E962.0	E980.4
propionate	976.0	E858.7	E946.0	E950.4	E962.0	E980.4
psylliate	972.7	E858.3	E942.7	E950.4	E962.0	E980.4
removing resins	974.5	E858.5	E944.5	E950.4	E962.0	E980.4
salicylate	965.1	E850.3	E935.3	E950.0	E962.0	E980.0
sulfate	973.3	E858.4	E943.3	E950.4	E962.0	E980.4
sulfoxone	961.8	E857	E931.8	E950.4	E962.0	E980.4
tetradecyl sulfate	972.7	E858.3	E942.7	E950.4	E962.0	E980.4
thiopental	968.3	E855.1	E938.3	E950.4	E962.0	E980.4
thiosalicylate	965.1	E850.3	E935.3	E950.0	E962.0	E980.0

External Cause (E-Code)

✓4ᵗʰ Fourth-digit Required   ✓5ᵗʰ Fifth-digit Required   ▶◀ Revised Text   ● New Line   ▲ Revised Code

	Poisoning	External Cause (E-Code)				
		Accident	Therapeutic Use	Suicide Attempt	Assault	Undetermined
Sodium — *continued*						
thiosulfate	976.0	E858.7	E946.0	E950.4	E962.0	E980.4
tolbutamide	977.8	E858.8	E947.8	E950.4	E962.0	E980.4
tyropanoate	977.8	E858.8	E947.8	E950.4	E962.0	E980.4
valproate	966.3	E855.0	E936.3	E950.4	E962.0	E980.4
Solanine	988.2	E865.4	—	E950.9	E962.1	E980.9
Solanum dulcamara	988.2	E865.4	—	E950.9	E962.1	E980.9
Solapsone	961.8	E857	E931.8	E950.4	E962.0	E980.4
Solasulfone	961.8	E857	E931.8	E950.4	E962.0	E980.4
Soldering fluid	983.1	E864.1	—	E950.7	E962.1	E980.6
Solid substance	989.9	E866.9	—	E950.9	E962.1	E980.9
specified NEC	989.9	E866.8	—	E950.9	E962.1	E980.9
Solvents, industrial	982.8	E862.9	—	E950.9	E962.1	E980.9
naphtha	981	E862.0	—	E950.9	E962.1	E980.9
petroleum	981	E862.0	—	E950.9	E962.1	E980.9
specified NEC	982.8	E862.4	—	E950.9	E962.1	E980.9
Soma	968.0	E855.1	E938.0	E950.4	E962.0	E980.4
Somatotropin	962.4	E858.0	E932.4	E950.4	E962.0	E980.4
Sominex	963.0	E858.1	E933.0	E950.4	E962.0	E980.4
Somnos	967.1	E852.0	E937.1	E950.2	E962.0	E980.2
Somonal	967.0	E851	E937.0	E950.1	E962.0	E980.1
Soneryl	967.0	E851	E937.0	E950.1	E962.0	E980.1
Soothing syrup	977.9	E858.9	E947.9	E950.5	E962.0	E980.5
Sopor	967.4	E852.3	E937.4	E950.2	E962.0	E980.2
Soporific drug	967.9	E852.9	E937.9	E950.2	E962.0	E980.2
specified type NEC	967.8	E852.8	E937.8	E950.2	E962.0	E980.2
Sorbitol NEC	977.4	E858.8	E947.4	E950.4	E962.0	E980.4
Sotradecol	972.7	E858.3	E942.7	E950.4	E962.0	E980.4
Spacoline	975.1	E858.6	E945.1	E950.4	E962.0	E980.4
Spanish fly	976.8	E858.7	E946.8	E950.4	E962.0	E980.4
Sparine	969.1	E853.0	E939.1	E950.3	E962.0	E980.3
Sparteine	975.0	E858.6	E945.0	E950.4	E962.0	E980.4
Spasmolytics	975.1	E858.6	E945.1	E950.4	E962.0	E980.4
anticholinergics	971.1	E855.4	E941.1	E950.4	E962.0	E980.4
Spectinomycin	960.8	E856	E930.8	E950.4	E962.0	E980.4
Speed	969.7	E854.2	E939.7	E950.3	E962.0	E980.3
Spermicides	976.8	E858.7	E946.8	E950.4	E962.0	E980.4
Spider (bite) (venom)	989.5	E905.1	—	E950.9	E962.1	E980.9
antivenin	979.9	E858.8	E949.9	E950.4	E962.0	E980.4
Spigelia (root)	961.6	E857	E931.6	E950.4	E962.0	E980.4
Spiperone	969.2	E853.1	E939.2	E950.3	E962.0	E980.3
Spiramycin	960.3	E856	E930.3	E950.4	E962.0	E980.4
Spirilene	969.5	E853.8	E939.5	E950.3	E962.0	E980.3
Spirit(s) (neutral) NEC	980.0	E860.1	—	E950.9	E962.1	E980.9
beverage	980.0	E860.0	—	E950.9	E962.1	E980.9
industrial	980.9	E860.9	—	E950.9	E962.1	E980.9
mineral	981	E862.0	—	E950.9	E962.1	E980.9
of salt — *see* Hydrochloric acid						
surgical	980.9	E860.9	—	E950.9	E962.1	E980.9
Spironolactone	974.4	E858.5	E944.4	E950.4	E962.0	E980.4
Sponge, absorbable (gelatin)	964.5	E858.2	E934.5	E950.4	E962.0	E980.4
Sporostacin	976.0	E858.7	E946.0	E950.4	E962.0	E980.4
Sprays (aerosol)	989.89	E866.8	—	E950.9	E962.1	E980.9
cosmetic	989.89	E866.7	—	E950.9	E962.1	E980.9
medicinal NEC	977.9	E858.9	E947.9	E950.5	E962.0	E980.5
pesticides — *see* Pesticides						
specified content — *see* substance specified						
Spurge flax	988.2	E865.4	—	E950.9	E962.1	E980.9
Spurges	988.2	E865.4	—	E950.9	E962.1	E980.9
Squill (expectorant) NEC	975.5	E858.6	E945.5	E950.4	E962.0	E980.4
rat poison	989.4	E863.7	—	E950.6	E962.1	E980.7
Squirting cucumber (cathartic)	973.1	E858.4	E943.1	E950.4	E962.0	E980.4
Stains	989.89	E866.8	—	E950.9	E962.1	E980.9
Stannous — *see also* Tin						
fluoride	976.7	E858.7	E946.7	E950.4	E962.0	E980.4
Stanolone	962.1	E858.0	E932.1	E950.4	E962.0	E980.4
Stanozolol	962.1	E858.0	E932.1	E950.4	E962.0	E980.4
Staphisagria or stavesacre (pediculicide)	976.0	E858.7	E946.0	E950.4	E962.0	E980.4
Stelazine	969.1	E853.0	E939.1	E950.3	E962.0	E980.3
Stemetil	969.1	E853.0	E939.1	E950.3	E962.0	E980.3
Sterculia (cathartic) (gum)	973.3	E858.4	E943.3	E950.4	E962.0	E980.4
Sternutator gas	987.8	E869.8	—	E952.8	E962.2	E982.8
Steroids NEC	962.0	E858.0	E932.0	E950.4	E962.0	E980.4
ENT agent	976.6	E858.7	E946.6	E950.4	E962.0	E980.4
ophthalmic preparation	976.5	E858.7	E946.5	E950.4	E962.0	E980.4
topical NEC	976.0	E858.7	E946.0	E950.4	E962.0	E980.4
Stibine	985.8	E866.4	—	E950.9	E962.1	E980.9
Stibophen	961.2	E857	E931.2	E950.4	E962.0	E980.4
Stilbamide, stilbamidine	961.5	E857	E931.5	E950.4	E962.0	E980.4
Stilbestrol	962.2	E858.0	E932.2	E950.4	E962.0	E980.4

Sodium — Stilbestrol

▪4ᵗʰ Fourth-digit Required ▪5ᵗʰ Fifth-digit Required ►◄ Revised Text ● New Line ▲ Revised Code

	Poisoning	External Cause (E-Code)				
		Accident	Therapeutic Use	Suicide Attempt	Assault	Undetermined
Stimulants (central nervous system)						
analeptics	970.9	E854.3	E940.9	E950.4	E962.0	E980.4
opiate antagonist	970.0	E854.3	E940.0	E950.4	E962.0	E980.4
psychotherapeutic NEC	970.1	E854.3	E940.1	E950.4	E962.0	E980.4
specified NEC	969.0	E854.0	E939.0	E950.3	E962.0	E980.3
	970.8	E854.3	E940.8	E950.4	E962.0	E980.4
Storage batteries (acid) (cells)	983.1	E864.1	—	E950.7	E962.1	E980.6
Stovaine	968.9	E855.2	E938.9	E950.4	E962.0	E980.4
infiltration (subcutaneous)	968.5	E855.2	E938.5	E950.4	E962.0	E980.4
nerve block (peripheral) (plexus)	968.6	E855.2	E938.6	E950.4	E962.0	E980.4
spinal	968.7	E855.2	E938.7	E950.4	E962.0	E980.4
topical (surface)	968.5	E855.2	E938.5	E950.4	E962.0	E980.4
Stovarsal	961.1	E857	E931.1	E950.4	E962.0	E980.4
Stove gas — *see* Gas, utility						
Stoxil	976.5	E858.7	E946.5	E950.4	E962.0	E980.4
STP	969.6	E854.1	E939.6	E950.3	E962.0	E980.3
Stramonium (medicinal) NEC	971.1	E855.4	E941.1	E950.4	E962.0	E980.4
natural state	988.2	E865.4		E950.9	E962.1	E980.9
Streptodornase	964.4	E858.2	E934.4	E950.4	E962.0	E980.4
Streptoduocin	960.6	E856	E930.6	E950.4	E962.0	E980.4
Streptokinase	964.4	E858.2	E934.4	E950.4	E962.0	E980.4
Streptomycin	960.6	E856	E930.6	E950.4	E962.0	E980.4
Streptozocin	960.7	E856	E930.7	E950.4	E962.0	E980.4
Stripper (paint) (solvent)	982.8	E862.9	—	E950.9	E962.1	E980.9
Strobane	989.2	E863.0	—	E950.6	E962.1	E980.7
Strophanthin	972.1	E858.3	E942.1	E950.4	E962.0	E980.4
Strophanthus hispidus or kombe	988.2	E865.4		E950.9	E962.1	E980.9
Strychnine (rodenticide) (salts)	989.1	E863.7	—	E950.6	E962.1	E980.7
medicinal NEC	970.8	E854.3	E940.8	E950.4	E962.0	E980.4
Strychnos (ignatii) — *see* Strychnine						
Styramate	968.0	E855.1	E938.0	E950.4	E962.0	E980.4
Styrene	983.0	E864.0	—	E950.7	E962.1	E980.6
Succinimide (anticonvulsant)	966.2	E855.0	E936.2	E950.4	E962.0	E980.4
mercuric — *see* Mercury						
Succinylcholine	975.2	E858.6	E945.2	E950.4	E962.0	E980.4
Succinylsulfathiazole	961.0	E857	E931.0	E950.4	E962.0	E980.4
Sucrose	974.5	E858.5	E944.5	E950.4	E962.0	E980.4
Sulfacetamide	961.0	E857	E931.0	E950.4	E962.0	E980.4
ophthalmic preparation	976.5	E858.7	E946.5	E950.4	E962.0	E980.4
Sulfachlorpyridazine	961.0	E857	E931.0	E950.4	E962.0	E980.4
Sulfacytine	961.0	E857	E931.0	E950.4	E962.0	E980.4
Sulfadiazine	961.0	E857	E931.0	E950.4	E962.0	E980.4
silver (topical)	976.0	E858.7	E946.0	E950.4	E962.0	E980.4
Sulfadimethoxine	961.0	E857	E931.0	E950.4	E962.0	E980.4
Sulfadimidine	961.0	E857	E931.0	E950.4	E962.0	E980.4
Sulfaethidole	961.0	E857	E931.0	E950.4	E962.0	E980.4
Sulfafurazole	961.0	E857	E931.0	E950.4	E962.0	E980.4
Sulfaguanidine	961.0	E857	E931.0	E950.4	E962.0	E980.4
Sulfamerazine	961.0	E857	E931.0	E950.4	E962.0	E980.4
Sulfameter	961.0	E857	E931.0	E950.4	E962.0	E980.4
Sulfamethizole	961.0	E857	E931.0	E950.4	E962.0	E980.4
Sulfamethoxazole	961.0	E857	E931.0	E950.4	E962.0	E980.4
Sulfamethoxydiazine	961.0	E857	E931.0	E950.4	E962.0	E980.4
Sulfamethoxypyridazine	961.0	E857	E931.0	E950.4	E962.0	E980.4
Sulfamethylthiazole	961.0	E857	E931.0	E950.4	E962.0	E980.4
Sulfamylon	976.0	E858.7	E946.0	E950.4	E962.0	E980.4
Sulfan blue (diagnostic dye)	977.8	E858.8	E947.8	E950.4	E962.0	E980.4
Sulfanilamide	961.0	E857	E931.0	E950.4	E962.0	E980.4
Sulfanilylguanidine	961.0	E857	E931.0	E950.4	E962.0	E980.4
Sulfaphenazole	961.0	E857	E931.0	E950.4	E962.0	E980.4
Sulfaphenylthiazole	961.0	E857	E931.0	E950.4	E962.0	E980.4
Sulfaproxyline	961.0	E857	E931.0	E950.4	E962.0	E980.4
Sulfapyridine	961.0	E857	E931.0	E950.4	E962.0	E980.4
Sulfapyrimidine	961.0	E857	E931.0	E950.4	E962.0	E980.4
Sulfarsphenamine	961.1	E857	E931.1	E950.4	E962.0	E980.4
Sulfasalazine	961.0	E857	E931.0	E950.4	E962.0	E980.4
Sulfasomizole	961.0	E857	E931.0	E950.4	E962.0	E980.4
Sulfasuxidine	961.0	E857	E931.0	E950.4	E962.0	E980.4
Sulfinpyrazone	974.7	E858.5	E944.7	E950.4	E962.0	E980.4
Sulfisoxazole	961.0	E857	E931.0	E950.4	E962.0	E980.4
ophthalmic preparation	976.5	E858.7	E946.5	E950.4	E962.0	E980.4
Sulfomyxin	960.8	E856	E930.8	E950.4	E962.0	E980.4
Sulfonal	967.8	E852.8	E937.8	E950.2	E962.0	E980.2
Sulfonamides (mixtures)	961.0	E857	E931.0	E950.4	E962.0	E980.4
Sulfones	961.8	E857	E931.8	E950.4	E962.0	E980.4
Sulfonethylmethane	967.8	E852.8	E937.8	E950.2	E962.0	E980.2
Sulfonmethane	967.8	E852.8	E937.8	E950.2	E962.0	E980.2
Sulfonphthal, sulfonphthol	977.8	E858.8	E947.8	E950.4	E962.0	E980.4
Sulfonylurea derivatives, oral	962.3	E858.0	E932.3	E950.4	E962.0	E980.4
Sulfoxone	961.8	E857	E931.8	E950.4	E962.0	E980.4
Sulfur, sulfureted, sulfuric, sulfurous, sulfuryl (compounds) NEC	989.89	E866.8	—	E950.9	E962.1	E980.9
acid	983.1	E864.1	—	E950.7	E962.1	E980.6

		External Cause (E-Code)				
	Poisoning	Accident	Therapeutic Use	Suicide Attempt	Assault	Undetermined
Sulfur, sulfureted, sulfuric, sulfurous, sulfuryl NEC — *continued*	987.3	E869.1	—	E952.8	E962.2	E982.8
dioxide						
ether — *see* Ether(s)	987.8	E869.8	—	E952.8	E962.2	E982.8
hydrogen	976.4	E858.7	E946.4	E950.4	E962.0	E980.4
medicinal (keratolytic) (ointment) NEC	989.4	E863.4	—	E950.6	E962.1	E980.7
pesticide (vapor)	987.8	E869.8	—	E952.8	E962.2	E982.8
vapor NEC	977.8	E858.8	E947.8	E950.4	E962.0	E980.4
Sulkowitch's reagent						
Sulph — *see also* Sulf-	961.8	E857	E931.8	E950.4	E962.0	E980.4
Sulphadione	966.3	E855.0	E936.3	E950.4	E962.0	E980.4
Sulthiame, sultiame	975.5	E858.6	E945.5	E950.4	E962.0	E980.4
Superinone	961.5	E857	E931.5	E950.4	E962.0	E980.4
Suramin	968.5	E855.2	E938.5	E950.4	E962.0	E980.4
Surfacaine	968.3	E855.1	E938.3	E950.4	E962.0	E980.4
Surital	976.8	E858.7	E946.8	E950.4	E962.0	E980.4
Sutilains	975.2	E858.6	E945.2	E950.4	E962.0	E980.4
Suxamethonium (bromide) (chloride) (iodide)	975.2	E858.6	E945.2	E950.4	E962.0	E980.4
Suxethonium (bromide)	976.3	E858.7	E946.3	E950.4	E962.0	E980.4
Sweet oil (birch)	982.3	E862.4	—	E950.9	E962.1	E980.9
Sym-dichloroethyl ether	971.3	E855.6	E941.3	E950.4	E962.0	E980.4
Sympatholytics	971.2	E855.5	E941.2	E950.4	E962.0	E980.4
Sympathomimetics	979.6 ▲	E858.8	E949.6	E950.4	E962.0	E980.4
Synagis	976.0	E858.7	E946.0	E950.4	E962.0	E980.4
Synalar	962.7	E858.0	E932.7	E950.4	E962.0	E980.4
Synthroid	975.0	E858.6	E945.0	E950.4	E962.0	E950.4
Syntocinon	972.6	E858.3	E942.6	E950.4	E962.0	E980.4
Syrosingopine	963.9	E858.1	E933.9	E950.4	E962.0	E980.4
Systemic agents (primarily)	963.8	E858.1	E933.8	E950.4	E962.0	E980.4
specified NEC	977.9	E858.9	E947.9	E950.5	E962.0	E980.5
Tablets (*see also* specified substance)	962.2	E858.0	E932.2	E950.4	E962.0	E980.4
Tace	971.0	E855.3	E941.0	E950.4	E962.0	E980.4
Tacrine	967.0	E851	E937.0	E950.1	E962.0	E980.1
Talbutal	976.3	E858.7	E946.3	E950.4	E962.0	E980.4
Talc	976.3	E858.7	E946.3	E950.4	E962.0	E980.4
Talcum	965.5	E850.5	E935.5	E950.0	E962.0	E980.0
Tandearil, tanderil	983.1	E864.1	—	E950.7	E962.1	E980.6
Tannic acid	976.2	E858.7	E946.2	E950.4	E962.0	E980.4
medicinal (astringent)						
Tannin — *see* Tannic acid	988.2	E865.4	—	E950.9	E962.1	E980.9
Tansy	960.3	E856	E930.3	E950.4	E962.0	E980.4
TAO	962.8	E858.0	E932.8	E950.4	E962.0	E980.4
Tapazole	983.0	E864.0	—	E950.7	E962.1	E980.6
Tar NEC						
camphor — *see* Naphthalene	987.8	E869.8	—	E952.8	E962.2	E982.8
fumes	969.3	E853.8	E939.3	E950.3	E962.0	E980.3
Taractan	989.5	E905.1	—	E950.9	E962.1	E980.9
Tarantula (venomous)	961.2	E857	E931.2	E950.4	E962.0	E980.4
Tartar emetic (anti-infective)	983.1	E864.1	—	E950.7	E962.1	E980.6
Tartaric acid	961.2	E857	E931.2	E950.4	E962.0	E980.4
Tartrated antimony (anti-infective)						
TCA — *see* Trichloroacetic acid	983.0	E864.0	—	E950.7	E962.1	E980.6
TDI	987.8	E869.8	—	E952.8	E962.2	E982.8
vapor	987.5	E869.3	—	E952.8	E962.2	E982.8
Tear gas	974.3	E858.5	E944.3	E950.4	E962.0	E980.4
Teclothiazide	966.3	E855.0	E936.3	E950.4	E962.0	E980.4
Tegretol	977.8	E858.8	E947.8	E950.4	E962.0	E980.4
Telepaque	985.8	E866.4	—	E950.9	E962.1	E980.9
Tellurium	985.8	E866.4	—	E950.9	E962.1	E980.9
fumes	963.1	E858.1	E933.1	E950.4	E962.0	E980.4
TEM						
Temazepan — *see* Benzodiazepines	963.1	E858.1	E933.1	E950.4	E962.0	E980.4
TEPA	989.3	E863.1	—	E950.6	E962.1	E980.7
TEPP	971.2	E855.5	E941.2	E950.4	E962.0	E980.4
Terbutaline	961.6	E857	E931.6	E950.4	E962.0	E980.4
Teroxalene	975.5	E858.6	E945.5	E950.4	E962.0	E980.4
Terpin hydrate	960.4	E856	E930.4	E950.4	E962.0	E980.4
Terramycin	975.4	E858.6	E945.4	E950.4	E962.0	E980.4
Tessalon	962.1	E858.0	E932.1	E950.4	E962.0	E980.4
Testosterone	978.4	E858.8	E948.4	E950.4	E962.0	E980.4
Tetanus (vaccine)	979.9	E858.8	E949.9	E950.4	E962.0	E980.4
antitoxin	964.6	E858.2	E934.6	E950.4	E962.0	E980.4
immune globulin (human)	978.4	E858.8	E948.4	E950.4	E962.0	E980.4
toxoid	978.9	E858.8	E948.9	E950.4	E962.0	E980.4
with diphtheria toxoid	978.6	E858.8	E948.6	E950.4	E962.0	E980.4
with pertussis	969.5	E853.8	E939.5	E950.3	E962.0	E980.3
Tetrabenazine	968.5	E855.2	E938.5	E950.4	E962.0	E980.4
Tetracaine (infiltration) (topical)	968.6	E855.2	E938.6	E950.4	E962.0	E980.4
nerve block (peripheral) (plexus)	968.7	E855.2	E938.7	E950.4	E962.0	E980.4
spinal						
Tetrachlorethylene — *see* Tetrachloroethylene						
Tetrachlormethiazide	974.3	E858.5	E944.3	E950.4	E962.0	E980.4

	Poisoning	External Cause (E-Code)				
		Accident	Therapeutic Use	Suicide Attempt	Assault	Undetermined
Tetrachloroethane (liquid) (vapor)	982.3	E862.4	—	E950.9	E962.1	E980.9
paint or varnish	982.3	E861.6	—	E950.9	E962.1	E980.9
Tetrachloroethylene (liquid) (vapor)	982.3	E862.4	—	E950.9	E962.1	E980.9
medicinal	961.6	E857	E931.6	E950.4	E962.0	E980.4
Tetrachloromethane — see Carbon, tetrachloride						
Tetracycline	960.4	E856	E930.4	E950.4	E962.0	E980.4
ophthalmic preparation	976.5	E858.7	E946.5	E950.4	E962.0	E980.4
topical NEC	976.0	E858.7	E946.0	E950.4	E962.0	E980.4
Tetraethylammonium chloride	972.3	E858.3	E942.3	E950.4	E962.0	E980.4
Tetraethyl lead (antiknock compound)	984.1	E862.1	—	E950.9	E962.1	E980.9
Tetraethyl pyrophosphate	989.3	E863.1	—	E950.6	E962.1	E980.7
Tetraethylthiuram disulfide	977.3	E858.8	E947.3	E950.4	E962.0	E980.4
Tetrahydroaminoacridine	971.0	E855.3	E941.0	E950.4	E962.0	E980.4
Tetrahydrocannabinol	969.6	E854.1	E939.6	E950.3	E962.0	E980.3
Tetrahydronaphthalene	982.0	E862.4	—	E950.9	E962.1	E980.9
Tetrahydrozoline	971.2	E855.5	E941.2	E950.4	E962.0	E980.4
Tetralin	982.0	E862.4	—	E950.9	E962.1	E980.9
Tetramethylthiuram (disulfide) NEC	989.4	E863.6	—	E950.6	E962.1	E980.7
medicinal	976.2	E858.7	E946.2	E950.4	E962.0	E980.4
Tetronal	967.8	E852.8	E937.8	E950.2	E962.0	E980.2
Tetryl	983.0	E864.0	—	E950.7	E962.1	E980.6
Thalidomide	967.8	E852.8	E937.8	E950.2	E962.0	E980.2
Thallium (compounds) (dust) NEC	985.8	E866.4	—	E950.9	E962.1	E980.9
pesticide (rodenticide)	985.8	E863.7	—	E950.6	E962.1	E980.7
THC	969.6	E854.1	E939.6	E950.3	E962.0	E980.3
Thebacon	965.09	E850.2	E935.2	E950.0	E962.0	E980.0
Thebaine	965.09	E850.2	E935.2	E950.0	E962.0	E980.0
Theobromine (calcium salicylate)	974.1	E858.5	E944.1	E950.4	E962.0	E980.4
Theophylline (diuretic)	974.1	E858.5	E944.1	E950.4	E962.0	E980.4
ethylenediamine	975.7	E858.6	E945.7	E950.4	E962.0	E980.4
Thiabendazole	961.6	E857	E931.6	E950.4	E962.0	E980.4
Thialbarbital, thialbarbitone	968.3	E855.1	E938.3	E950.4	E962.0	E980.4
Thiamine	963.5	E858.1	E933.5	E950.4	E962.0	E980.4
Thiamylal (sodium)	968.3	E855.1	E938.3	E950.4	E962.0	E980.4
Thiazesim	969.0	E854.0	E939.0	E950.3	E962.0	E980.3
Thiazides (diuretics)	974.3	E858.5	E944.3	E950.4	E962.0	E980.4
Thiethylperazine	963.0	E858.1	E933.0	E950.4	E962.0	E980.4
Thimerosal (topical)	976.0	E858.7	E946.0	E950.4	E962.0	E980.4
ophthalmic preparation	976.5	E858.7	E946.5	E950.4	E962.0	E980.4
Thioacetazone	961.8	E857	E931.8	E950.4	E962.0	E980.4
Thiobarbiturates	968.3	E855.1	E938.3	E950.4	E962.0	E980.4
Thiobismol	961.2	E857	E931.2	E950.4	E962.0	E980.4
Thiocarbamide	962.8	E858.0	E932.8	E950.4	E962.0	E980.4
Thiocarbarsone	961.1	E857	E931.1	E950.4	E962.0	E980.4
Thiocarlide	961.8	E857	E931.8	E950.4	E962.0	E980.4
Thioguanine	963.1	E858.1	E933.1	E950.4	E962.0	E980.4
Thiomercaptomerin	974.0	E858.5	E944.0	E950.4	E962.0	E980.4
Thiomerin	974.0	E858.5	E944.0	E950.4	E962.0	E980.4
Thiopental, thiopentone (sodium)	968.3	E855.1	E938.3	E950.4	E962.0	E980.4
Thiopropazate	969.1	E853.0	E939.1	E950.3	E962.0	E980.3
Thioproperazine	969.1	E853.0	E939.1	E950.3	E962.0	E980.3
Thioridazine	969.1	E853.0	E939.1	E950.3	E962.0	E980.3
Thio-TEPA, thiotepa	963.1	E858.1	E933.1	E950.4	E962.0	E980.4
Thiothixene	969.3	E853.8	E939.3	E950.3	E962.0	E980.3
Thiouracil	962.8	E858.0	E932.8	E950.4	E962.0	E980.4
Thiourea	962.8	E858.0	E932.8	E950.4	E962.0	E980.4
Thiphenamil	971.1	E855.4	E941.1	E950.4	E962.0	E980.4
Thiram NEC	989.4	E863.6	—	E950.6	E962.1	E980.7
medicinal	976.2	E858.7	E946.2	E950.4	E962.0	E980.4
Thonzylamine	963.0	E858.1	E933.0	E950.4	E962.0	E980.4
Thorazine	969.1	E853.0	E939.1	E950.3	E962.0	E980.3
Thornapple	988.2	E865.4	—	E950.9	E962.1	E980.9
Throat preparation (lozenges) NEC	976.6	E858.7	E946.6	E950.4	E962.0	E980.4
Thrombin	964.5	E858.2	E934.5	E950.4	E962.0	E980.4
Thrombolysin	964.4	E858.2	E934.4	E950.4	E962.0	E980.4
Thymol	983.0	E864.0	—	E950.7	E962.1	E980.6
Thymus extract	962.9	E858.0	E932.9	E950.4	E962.0	E980.4
Thyroglobulin	962.7	E858.0	E932.7	E950.4	E962.0	E980.4
Thyroid (derivatives) (extract)	962.7	E858.0	E932.7	E950.4	E962.0	E980.4
Thyrolar	962.7	E858.0	E932.7	E950.4	E962.0	E980.4
Thyrothrophin, thyrotropin	977.8	E858.8	E947.8	E950.4	E962.0	E980.4
Thyroxin(e)	962.7	E858.0	E932.7	E950.4	E962.0	E980.4
Tigan	963.0	E858.1	E933.0	E950.4	E962.0	E980.4
Tigloidine	968.0	E855.1	E938.0	E950.4	E962.0	E980.4
Tin (chloride) (dust) (oxide) NEC	985.8	E866.4	—	E950.9	E962.1	E980.9
anti-infectives	961.2	E857	E931.2	E950.4	E962.0	E980.4
Tinactin	976.0	E858.7	E946.0	E950.4	E962.0	E980.4
Tincture, iodine — see Iodine						
Tindal	969.1	E853.0	E939.1	E950.3	E962.0	E980.3
Titanium (compounds) (vapor)	985.8	E866.4	—	E950.9	E962.1	E980.9
ointment	976.3	E858.7	E946.3	E950.4	E962.0	E980.4

	Poisoning	External Cause (E-Code)				
		Accident	Therapeutic Use	Suicide Attempt	Assault	Undetermined
Titroid	962.7	E858.0	E932.7	E950.4	E962.0	E980.4
TMTD — *see* Tetramethylthiuram disulfide						
TNT	989.89	E866.8	—	E950.9	E962.1	E980.9
fumes	987.8	E869.8	—	E952.8	E962.2	E982.8
Toadstool	988.1	E865.5	—	E950.9	E962.1	E980.9
Tobacco NEC	989.84	E866.8	—	E950.9	E962.1	E980.9
Indian	988.2	E865.4	—	E950.9	E962.1	E980.9
smoke, second-hand	987.8	E869.4	—	—	—	—
Tocopherol	963.5	E858.1	E933.5	E950.4	E962.0	E980.4
Tocosamine	975.0	E858.6	E945.0	E950.4	E962.0	E980.4
Tofranil	969.0	E854.0	E939.0	E950.3	E962.0	E980.3
Toilet deodorizer	989.89	E866.8	—	E950.9	E962.1	E980.9
Tolazamide	962.3	E858.0	E932.3	E950.4	E962.0	E980.4
Tolazoline	971.3	E855.6	E941.3	E950.4	E962.0	E980.4
Tolbutamide	962.3	E858.0	E932.3	E950.4	E962.0	E980.4
sodium	977.8	E858.8	E947.8	E950.4	E962.0	E980.0
Tolmetin	965.69	E850.6	E935.6	E950.0	E962.0	E980.0
Tolnaftate	976.0	E858.7	E946.0	E950.4	E962.0	E980.4
Tolpropamine	976.1	E858.7	E946.1	E950.4	E962.0	E980.4
Tolserol	968.0	E855.1	E938.0	E950.4	E962.0	E980.4
Toluene (liquid) (vapor)	982.0	E862.4	—	E950.9	E962.1	E980.9
diisocyanate	983.0	E864.0	—	E950.7	E962.1	E980.6
Toluidine	983.0	E864.0	—	E950.7	E962.1	E980.6
vapor	987.8	E869.8	—	E952.8	E962.2	E982.8
Toluol (liquid) (vapor)	982.0	E862.4	—	E950.9	E962.1	E980.9
Tolylene-2, 4-diisocyanate	983.0	E864.0	—	E950.7	E962.1	E980.6
Tonics, cardiac	972.1	E858.3	E942.1	E950.4	E962.0	E980.4
Toxaphene (dust) (spray)	989.2	E863.0	—	E950.6	E962.1	E980.7
Toxoids NEC	978.8	E858.8	E948.8	E950.4	E962.0	E980.4
Tractor fuel NEC	981	E862.1	—	E950.9	E962.1	E980.9
Tragacanth	973.3	E858.4	E943.3	E950.4	E962.0	E980.4
Tramazoline	971.2	E855.5	E941.2	E950.4	E962.0	E980.4
Tranquilizers	969.5	E853.9	E939.5	E950.3	E962.0	E980.3
benzodiazepine-based	969.4	E853.2	E939.4	E950.3	E962.0	E980.3
butyrophenone-based	969.2	E853.1	E939.2	E950.3	E962.0	E980.3
major NEC	969.3	E853.8	E939.3	E950.3	E962.0	E980.3
phenothiazine-based	969.1	E853.0	E939.1	E950.3	E962.0	E980.3
specified NEC	969.5	E853.8	E939.5	E950.3	E962.0	E980.3
Trantoin	961.9	E857	E931.9	E950.4	E962.0	E980.4
Tranxene	969.4	E853.2	E939.4	E950.3	E962.0	E980.3
Tranylcypromine (sulfate)	969.0	E854.0	E939.0	E950.3	E962.0	E980.3
Trasentine	975.1	E858.6	E945.1	E950.4	E962.0	E980.4
Travert	974.5	E858.5	E944.5	E950.4	E962.0	E980.4
Trecator	961.8	E857	E931.8	E950.4	E962.0	E980.4
Tretinoin	976.8	E858.7	E946.8	E950.4	E962.0	E980.4
Triacetin	976.0	E858.7	E946.0	E950.4	E962.0	E980.4
Triacetyloleandomycin	960.3	E856	E930.3	E950.4	E962.0	E980.4
Triamcinolone	962.0	E858.0	E932.0	E950.4	E962.0	E980.4
ENT agent	976.6	E858.7	E946.6	E950.4	E962.0	E980.4
ophthalmic preparation	976.5	E858.7	E946.5	E950.4	E962.0	E980.4
topical NEC	976.0	E858.7	E946.0	E950.4	E962.0	E980.4
Triamterene	974.4	E858.5	E944.4	E950.4	E962.0	E980.4
Triaziquone	963.1	E858.1	E933.1	E950.4	E962.0	E980.4
Tribromacetaldehyde	967.3	E852.2	E937.3	E950.2	E962.0	E980.2
Tribromoethanol	968.2	E855.1	E938.2	E950.4	E962.0	E980.4
Tribromomethane	967.3	E852.2	E937.3	E950.2	E962.0	E980.2
Trichlorethane	982.3	E862.4	—	E950.9	E962.1	E980.9
Trichlormethiazide	974.3	E858.5	E944.3	E950.4	E962.0	E980.4
Trichloroacetic acid	983.1	E864.1	—	E950.7	E962.1	E980.6
medicinal (keratolytic)	976.4	E858.7	E946.4	E950.4	E962.0	E980.4
Trichloroethanol	967.1	E852.0	E937.1	E950.2	E962.0	E980.2
Trichloroethylene (liquid) (vapor)	982.3	E862.4	—	E950.9	E962.1	E980.9
anesthetic (gas)	968.2	E855.1	E938.2	E950.4	E962.0	E980.4
Trichloroethyl phosphate	967.1	E852.0	E937.1	E950.2	E962.0	E980.2
Trichlorofluoromethane NEC	987.4	E869.2	—	E952.8	E962.2	E982.8
Trichlorotriethylamine	963.1	E858.1	E933.1	E950.4	E962.0	E980.4
Trichomonacides NEC	961.5	E857	E931.5	E950.4	E962.0	E980.4
Trichomycin	960.1	E856	E930.1	E950.4	E962.0	E980.4
Triclofos	967.1	E852.0	E937.1	E950.2	E962.0	E980.2
Tricresyl phosphate	989.89	E866.8	—	E950.9	E962.1	E980.9
solvent	982.8	E862.4	—	E950.9	E962.1	E980.9
Tricyclamol	966.4	E855.0	E936.4	E950.4	E962.0	E980.4
Tridesilon	976.0	E858.7	E946.0	E950.4	E962.0	E980.4
Tridihexethyl	971.1	E855.4	E941.1	E950.4	E962.0	E980.4
Tridione	966.0	E855.0	E936.0	E950.4	E962.0	E980.4
Triethanolamine NEC	983.2	E864.2	—	E950.7	E962.1	E980.6
detergent	983.2	E861.0	—	E950.7	E962.1	E980.6
trinitrate	972.4	E858.3	E942.4	E950.4	E962.0	E980.4
Triethanomelamine	963.1	E858.1	E933.1	E950.4	E962.0	E980.4
Triethylene melamine	963.1	E858.1	E933.1	E950.4	E962.0	E980.4
Triethylenephosphoramide	963.1	E858.1	E933.1	E950.4	E962.0	E980.4

	Poisoning	External Cause (E-Code)				
		Accident	Therapeutic Use	Suicide Attempt	Assault	Undetermined
Triethylenethiophosphoramide	963.1	E858.1	E933.1	E950.4	E962.0	E980.4
Trifluoperazine	969.1	E853.0	E939.1	E950.3	E962.0	E980.3
Trifluperidol	969.2	E853.0	E939.2	E950.3	E962.0	E980.3
Triflupromazine	969.1	E853.0	E939.1	E950.3	E962.0	E980.3
Trihexyphenidyl	971.1	E855.4	E941.1	E950.4	E962.0	E980.4
Triiodothyronine	962.7	E858.0	E932.7	E950.4	E962.0	E980.4
Trilene	968.2	E855.1	E938.2	E950.4	E962.0	E980.4
Trimeprazine	963.0	E858.1	E933.0	E950.4	E962.0	E980.4
Trimetazidine	972.4	E858.3	E942.4	E950.4	E962.0	E980.4
Trimethadione	966.0	E855.0	E936.0	E950.4	E962.0	E980.4
Trimethaphan	972.3	E858.3	E942.3	E950.4	E962.0	E980.4
Trimethidinium	972.3	E858.3	E942.3	E950.4	E962.0	E980.4
Trimethobenzamide	963.0	E858.1	E933.0	E950.4	E962.0	E980.4
Trimethylcarbinol	980.8	E860.8	—	E950.9	E962.1	E980.9
Trimethylpsoralen	976.3	E858.7	E946.3	E950.4	E962.0	E980.4
Trimeton	963.0	E858.1	E933.0	E950.4	E962.0	E980.4
Trimipramine	969.0	E854.0	E939.0	E950.3	E962.0	E980.3
Trimustine	963.1	E858.1	E933.1	E950.4	E962.0	E980.4
Trinitrin	972.4	E858.3	E942.4	E950.4	E962.0	E980.4
Trinitrophenol	983.0	E864.0	—	E950.7	E962.1	E980.6
Trinitrotoluene	989.89	E866.8	—	E950.9	E962.1	E980.9
fumes	987.8	E869.8	—	E952.8	E962.2	E982.8
Trional	967.8	E852.8	E937.8	E950.2	E962.0	E980.2
Trioxide of arsenic — see Arsenic						
Trioxsalen	976.3	E858.7	E946.3	E950.4	E962.0	E980.4
Tripelennamine	963.0	E858.1	E933.0	E950.4	E962.0	E980.4
Triperidol	969.2	E853.1	E939.2	E950.3	E962.0	E980.3
Triprolidine	963.0	E858.1	E933.0	E950.4	E962.0	E980.4
Trisoralen	976.3	E858.7	E946.3	E950.4	E962.0	E980.4
Troleandomycin	960.3	E856	E930.3	E950.4	E962.0	E980.4
Trolnitrate (phosphate)	972.4	E858.3	E942.4	E950.4	E962.0	E980.4
Trometamol	963.3	E858.1	E933.3	E950.4	E962.0	E980.4
Tromethamine	963.3	E858.1	E933.3	E950.4	E962.0	E980.4
Tronothane	968.5	E855.2	E938.5	E950.4	E962.0	E980.4
Tropicamide	971.1	E855.4	E941.1	E950.4	E962.0	E980.4
Troxidone	966.0	E855.0	E936.0	E950.4	E962.0	E980.4
Tryparsamide	961.1	E857	E931.1	E950.4	E962.0	E980.4
Trypsin	963.4	E858.1	E933.4	E950.4	E962.0	E980.4
Tryptizol	969.0	E854.0	E939.0	E950.3	E962.0	E980.3
Tuaminoheptane	971.2	E855.5	E941.2	E950.4	E962.0	E980.4
Tuberculin (old)	977.8	E858.8	E947.8	E950.4	E962.0	E980.4
Tubocurare	975.2	E858.6	E945.2	E950.4	E962.0	E980.4
Tubocurarine	975.2	E858.6	E945.2	E950.4	E962.0	E980.4
Turkish green	969.6	E854.1	E939.6	E950.3	E962.0	E980.3
Turpentine (spirits of) (liquid) (vapor)	982.8	E862.4	—	E950.9	E962.1	E980.9
Tybamate	969.5	E853.8	E939.5	E950.3	E962.0	E980.3
Tyloxapol	975.5	E858.6	E945.5	E950.4	E962.0	E980.4
Tymazoline	971.2	E855.5	E941.2	E950.4	E962.0	E980.4
Typhoid vaccine	978.1	E858.8	E948.1	E950.4	E962.0	E980.4
Typhus vaccine	979.2	E858.8	E949.2	E950.4	E962.0	E980.4
Tyrothricin	976.0	E858.7	E946.0	E950.4	E962.0	E980.4
ENT agent	976.6	E858.7	E946.6	E950.4	E962.0	E980.4
ophthalmic preparation	976.5	E858.7	E946.5	E950.4	E962.0	E980.4
Undecenoic acid	976.0	E858.7	E946.0	E950.4	E962.0	E980.4
Undecylenic acid	976.0	E858.7	E946.0	E950.4	E962.0	E980.4
Unna's boot	976.3	E858.7	E946.3	E950.4	E962.0	E980.4
Uracil mustard	963.1	E858.1	E933.1	E950.4	E962.0	E980.4
Uramustine	963.1	E858.1	E933.1	E950.4	E962.0	E980.4
Urari	975.2	E858.6	E945.2	E950.4	E962.0	E980.4
Urea	974.4	E858.5	E944.4	E950.4	E962.0	E980.4
topical	976.8	E858.7	E946.8	E950.4	E962.0	E980.4
Urethan(e) (antineoplastic)	963.1	E858.1	E933.1	E950.4	E962.0	E980.4
Urginea (maritima) (scilla) — see Squill						
Uric acid metabolism agents NEC	974.7	E858.5	E944.7	E950.4	E962.0	E980.4
Urokinase	964.4	E858.2	E934.4	E950.4	E962.0	E980.4
Urokon	977.8	E858.8	E947.8	E950.4	E962.0	E980.4
Urotropin	961.9	E857	E931.9	E950.4	E962.0	E980.4
Urtica	988.2	E865.4	—	E950.9	E962.1	E980.9
Utility gas — see Gas, utility						
Vaccine NEC	979.9	E858.8	E949.9	E950.4	E962.0	E980.4
bacterial NEC	978.8	E858.8	E948.8	E950.4	E962.0	E980.4
with						
other bacterial component	978.9	E858.8	E948.9	E950.4	E962.0	E980.4
pertussis component	978.6	E858.8	E948.6	E950.4	E962.0	E980.4
viral-rickettsial component	979.7	E858.8	E949.7	E950.4	E962.0	E980.4
mixed NEC	978.9	E858.8	E948.9	E950.4	E962.0	E980.4
BCG	978.0	E858.8	E948.0	E950.4	E962.0	E980.4
cholera	978.2	E858.8	E948.2	E950.4	E962.0	E980.4
diphtheria	978.5	E858.8	E948.5	E950.4	E962.0	E980.4
influenza	979.6	E858.8	E949.6	E950.4	E962.0	E980.4
measles	979.4	E858.8	E949.4	E950.4	E962.0	E980.4

	Poisoning	External Cause (E-Code)				
		Accident	Therapeutic Use	Suicide Attempt	Assault	Undetermined
Vaccine NEC — *continued*						
meningococcal	978.8	E858.8	E948.8	E950.4	E962.0	E980.4
mumps	979.6	E858.8	E949.6	E950.4	E962.0	E980.4
paratyphoid	978.1	E858.8	E948.1	E950.4	E962.0	E980.4
pertussis (with diphtheria toxoid) (with tetanus toxoid)	978.6	E858.8	E948.6	E950.4	E962.0	E980.4
plague	978.3	E858.8	E948.3	E950.4	E962.0	E980.4
poliomyelitis	979.5	E858.8	E949.5	E950.4	E962.0	E980.4
poliovirus	979.5	E858.8	E949.5	E950.4	E962.0	E980.4
rabies	979.1	E858.8	E949.1	E950.4	E962.0	E980.4
respiratory syncytial virus	979.6 ▲	E858.8	E949.6	E950.4	E962.0	E980.4
rickettsial NEC	979.6	E858.8	E949.6	E950.4	E962.0	E980.4
with						
bacterial component	979.7	E858.8	E949.7	E950.4	E962.0	E980.4
pertussis component	978.6	E858.8	E948.6	E950.4	E962.0	E980.4
viral component	979.7	E858.8	E949.7	E950.4	E962.0	E980.4
Rocky mountain spotted fever	979.6	E858.8	E949.6	E950.4	E962.0	E980.4
rotavirus	979.6	E858.8	E949.6	E950.4	E962.0	E980.4
rubella virus	979.4	E858.8	E949.4	E950.4	E962.0	E980.4
sabin oral	979.5	E858.8	E949.5	E950.4	E962.0	E980.4
smallpox	979.0	E858.8	E949.0	E950.4	E962.0	E980.4
tetanus	978.4	E858.8	E948.4	E950.4	E962.0	E980.4
typhoid	978.1	E858.8	E948.1	E950.4	E962.0	E980.4
typhus	979.2	E858.8	E949.2	E950.4	E962.0	E980.4
viral NEC	979.6	E858.8	E949.6	E950.4	E962.0	E980.4
with						
bacterial component	979.7	E858.8	E949.7	E950.4	E962.0	E980.4
pertussis component	978.6	E858.8	E948.6	E950.4	E962.0	E980.4
rickettsial component	979.7	E858.8	E949.7	E950.4	E962.0	E980.4
yellow fever	979.3	E858.8	E949.3	E950.4	E962.0	E980.4
Vaccinia immune globulin (human)	964.6	E858.2	E934.6	E950.4	E962.0	E980.4
Vaginal contraceptives	976.8	E858.7	E946.8	E950.4	E962.0	E980.4
Valethamate	971.1	E855.4	E941.1	E950.4	E962.0	E980.4
Valisone	976.0	E858.7	E946.0	E950.4	E962.0	E980.4
Valium	969.4	E853.2	E939.4	E950.3	E962.0	E980.3
Valmid	967.8	E852.8	E937.8	E950.2	E962.0	E980.2
Vanadium	985.8	E866.4	—	E950.9	E962.1	E980.9
Vancomycin	960.8	E856	E930.8	E950.4	E962.0	E980.4
Vapor (*see also* Gas)	987.9	E869.9	—	E952.9	E962.2	E982.9
kiln (carbon monoxide)	986	E868.8	—	E952.1	E962.2	E982.1
lead — *see* Lead						
specified source NEC (*see also* specific substance)	987.8	E869.8	—	E952.8	E962.2	E982.8
Varidase	964.4	E858.2	E934.4	E950.4	E962.0	E980.4
Varnish	989.89	E861.6	—	E950.9	E962.1	E980.9
cleaner	982.8	E862.9	—	E950.9	E962.1	E980.9
Vaseline	976.3	E858.7	E946.3	E950.4	E962.0	E980.4
Vasodilan	972.5	E858.3	E942.5	E950.4	E962.0	E980.4
Vasodilators NEC	972.5	E858.3	E942.5	E950.4	E962.0	E980.4
coronary	972.4	E858.3	E942.4	E950.4	E962.0	E980.4
Vasopressin	962.5	E858.0	E932.5	E950.4	E962.0	E980.4
Vasopressor drugs	962.5	E858.0	E932.5	E950.4	E962.0	E980.4
Venom, venomous (bite) (sting)	989.5	E905.9	—	E950.9	E962.1	E980.9
arthropod NEC	989.5	E905.5	—	E950.9	E962.1	E980.9
bee	989.5	E905.3	—	E950.9	E962.1	E980.9
centipede	989.5	E905.4	—	E950.9	E962.1	E980.9
hornet	989.5	E905.3	—	E950.9	E962.1	E980.9
lizard	989.5	E905.0	—	E950.9	E962.1	E980.9
marine animals or plants	989.5	E905.6	—	E950.9	E962.1	E980.9
millipede (tropical)	989.5	E905.4	—	E950.9	E962.1	E980.9
plant NEC	989.5	E905.7	—	E950.9	E962.1	E980.9
marine	989.5	E905.6	—	E950.9	E962.1	E980.9
scorpion	989.5	E905.2	—	E950.9	E962.1	E980.9
snake	989.5	E905.0	—	E950.9	E962.1	E980.9
specified NEC	989.5	E905.8	—	E950.9	E962.1	E980.9
spider	989.5	E905.1	—	E950.9	E962.1	E980.9
wasp	989.5	E905.3	—	E950.9	E962.1	E980.9
Veramon	967.0	E851	E937.0	E950.1	E962.0	E980.1
Veratrum						
album	988.2	E865.4	—	E950.9	E962.1	E980.9
alkaloids	972.6	E858.3	E942.6	E950.4	E962.0	E980.4
viride	988.2	E865.4	—	E950.9	E962.1	E980.9
Verdigris (*see also* Copper)	985.8	E866.4	—	E950.9	E962.1	E980.9
Veronal	967.0	E851	E937.0	E950.1	E962.0	E980.1
Veroxil	961.6	E857	E931.6	E950.4	E962.0	E980.4
Versidyne	965.7	E850.7	E935.7	E950.0	E962.0	E980.0
Viagra	972.5	E858.3	E942.5	E950.4	E962.0	E980.4
Vienna						
green	985.1	E866.3	—	E950.8	E962.1	E980.8
insecticide	985.1	E863.4	—	E950.6	E962.1	E980.7
red	989.89	E866.8	—	E950.9	E962.1	E980.9
pharmaceutical dye	977.4	E858.8	E947.4	E950.4	E962.0	E980.4
Vinbarbital, vinbarbitone	967.0	E851	E937.0	E950.1	E962.0	E980.1

	Poisoning	External Cause (E-Code)				
		Accident	Therapeutic Use	Suicide Attempt	Assault	Undetermined
Vinblastine	963.1	E858.1	E933.1	E950.4	E962.0	E980.4
Vincristine	963.1	E858.1	E933.1	E950.4	E962.0	E980.4
Vinesthene, vinethene	968.2	E855.1	E938.2	E950.4	E962.0	E980.4
Vinyl						
bital	967.0	E851	E937.0	E950.1	E962.0	E980.1
ether	968.2	E855.1	E938.2	E950.4	E962.0	E980.4
Vioform	961.3	E857	E931.3	E950.4	E962.0	E980.4
topical	976.0	E858.7	E946.0	E930.4	E962.0	E980.4
Viomycin	960.6	E856	E930.6	E950.4	E962.0	E980.4
Viosterol	963.5	E858.1	E933.5	E950.4	E962.0	E980.4
Viper (venom)	989.5	E905.0	—	E950.9	E962.1	E980.9
Viprynium (embonate)	961.6	E857	E931.6	E950.4	E962.0	E980.4
Virugon	961.7	E857	E931.7	E950.4	E962.0	E980.4
Visine	976.5	E858.7	E946.5	E950.4	E962.0	E980.4
Vitamins NEC	963.5	E858.1	E933.5	E950.4	E962.0	E980.4
B12	964.1	E858.2	E934.1	E950.4	E962.0	E980.4
hematopoietic	964.1	E858.2	E934.1	E950.4	E962.0	E980.4
K	964.3	E858.2	E934.3	E950.4	E962.0	E980.4
Vleminckx's solution	976.4	E858.7	E946.4	E950.4	E962.0	E980.4
Voltaren — see Diclofenac sodium						
Ventolin — see Salbutamol sulfate						
Warfarin (potassium) (sodium)	964.2	E858.2	E934.2	E950.4	E962.0	E980.4
rodenticide	989.4	E863.7	—	E950.6	E962.1	E980.7
Wasp (sting)	989.5	E905.3	—	E950.9	E962.1	E980.9
Water						
balance agents NEC	974.5	E858.5	E944.5	E950.4	E962.0	E980.4
gas	987.1	E868.1	—	E951.8	E962.2	E981.8
incomplete combustion of — see Carbon, monoxide, fuel, utility						
hemlock	988.2	E865.4	—	E950.9	E962.1	E980.9
moccasin (venom)	989.5	E905.0	—	E950.9	E962.1	E980.9
Wax (paraffin) (petroleum)	981	E862.3	—	E950.9	E962.1	E980.9
automobile	989.89	E861.2	—	E950.9	E962.1	E980.9
floor	981	E862.0	—	E950.9	E962.1	E980.9
Weed killers NEC	989.4	E863.5	—	E950.6	E962.1	E980.7
Welldorm	967.1	E852.0	E937.1	E950.2	E962.0	E980.2
White						
arsenic — see Arsenic						
hellebore	988.2	E865.4	—	E950.9	E962.1	E980.9
lotion (keratolytic)	976.4	E858.7	E946.4	E950.4	E962.0	E980.4
spirit	981	E862.0	—	E950.9	E962.1	E980.9
Whitewashes	989.89	E861.6	—	E950.9	E962.1	E980.9
Whole blood	964.7	E858.2	E934.7	E950.4	E962.0	E980.4
Wild						
black cherry	988.2	E865.4	—	E950.9	E962.1	E980.9
poisonous plants NEC	988.2	E865.4	—	E950.9	E962.1	E980.9
Window cleaning fluid	989.89	E861.3	—	E950.9	E962.1	E980.9
Wintergreen (oil)	976.3	E858.7	E946.3	E950.4	E962.0	E980.4
Witch hazel	976.2	E858.7	E946.2	E950.4	E962.0	E980.4
Wood						
alcohol	980.1	E860.2	—	E950.9	E962.1	E980.9
spirit	980.1	E860.2	—	E950.9	E962.1	E980.9
Woorali	975.2	E858.6	E945.2	E950.4	E962.0	E980.4
Wormseed, American	961.6	E857	E931.6	E950.4	E962.0	E980.4
Xanthine diuretics	974.1	E858.5	E944.1	E950.4	E962.0	E980.4
Xanthocillin	960.0	E856	E930.0	E950.4	E962.0	E980.4
Xanthotoxin	976.3	E858.7	E946.3	E950.4	E962.0	E980.4
Xylene (liquid) (vapor)	982.0	E862.4	—	E950.9	E962.1	E980.9
Xylocaine (infiltration) (topical)	968.5	E855.2	E938.5	E950.4	E962.0	E980.4
nerve block (peripheral) (plexus)	968.6	E855.2	E938.6	E950.4	E962.0	E980.4
spinal	968.7	E855.2	E938.7	E950.4	E962.0	E980.4
Xylol (liquid) (vapor)	982.0	E862.4	—	E950.9	E962.1	E980.9
Xylometazoline	971.2	E855.5	E941.2	E950.4	E962.0	E980.4
Yellow						
fever vaccine	979.3	E858.8	E949.3	E950.4	E962.0	E980.4
jasmine	988.2	E865.4	—	E950.9	E962.1	E980.9
Yew	988.2	E865.4	—	E950.9	E962.1	E980.9
Zactane	965.7	E850.7	E935.7	E950.0	E962.0	E980.0
Zaroxolyn	974.3	E858.5	E944.3	E950.4	E962.0	E980.4
Zephiran (topical)	976.0	E858.7	E946.0	E950.4	E962.0	E980.4
ophthalmic preparation	976.5	E858.7	E946.5	E950.4	E962.0	E980.4
Zerone	980.1	E860.2	—	E950.9	E962.1	E980.9
Zinc (compounds) (fumes) (salts) (vapor) NEC	985.8	E866.4	—	E950.9	E962.1	E980.9
anti-infectives	976.0	E858.7	E946.0	E950.4	E962.0	E980.4
antivaricose	972.7	E858.3	E942.7	E950.4	E962.0	E980.4
bacitracin	976.0	E858.7	E946.0	E950.4	E962.0	E980.4
chloride	976.2	E858.7	E946.2	E950.4	E962.0	E980.4
gelatin	976.3	E858.7	E946.3	E950.4	E962.0	E980.4
oxide	976.3	E858.7	E946.3	E950.4	E962.0	E980.4
peroxide	976.0	E858.7	E946.0	E950.4	E962.0	E980.4
pesticides	985.8	E863.4	—	E950.6	E962.1	E980.7
phosphide (rodenticide)	985.8	E863.7	—	E950.6	E962.1	E980.7

		External Cause (E-Code)				
	Poisoning	Accident	Therapeutic Use	Suicide Attempt	Assault	Undetermined
Zinc NEC — *continued*						
stearate	976.3	E858.7	E946.3	E950.4	E962.0	E980.4
sulfate (antivaricose)	972.7	E858.3	E942.7	E950.4	E962.0	E980.4
ENT agent	976.6	E858.7	E946.6	E950.4	E962.0	E980.4
ophthalmic solution	976.5	E858.7	E946.5	E950.4	E962.0	E980.4
topical NEC	976.0	E858.7	E946.0	E950.4	E962.0	E980.4
undecylenate	976.0	E858.7	E946.0	E950.4	E962.0	E980.4
Zoxazolamine	968.0	E855.1	E938.0	E950.4	E962.0	E980.4
Zygadenus (venenosus)	988.2	E865.4	—	E950.9	E962.1	E980.9

SECTION 3
Alphabetic Index to External Causes of Injury and Poisoning (E Code)

This section contains the index to the codes which classify environmental events, circumstances, and other conditions as the cause of injury and other adverse effects. Where a code from the section Supplementary Classification of External Causes of Injury and Poisoning (E800-E998) is applicable, it is intended that the E code shall be used in addition to a code from the main body of the classification, Chapters 1 to 17.

The alphabetic index to the E codes is organized by main terms which describe the *accident, circumstance, event,* or *specific agent* which caused the injury or other adverse effect.

Note — Transport accidents (E800-E848) include accidents involving:
> *aircraft and spacecraft (E840-E845)*
> *watercraft (E830-E838)*
> *motor vehicle (E810-E825)*
> *railway (E800-E807)*
> *other road vehicles (E826-E829)*

For definitions and examples related to transport accidents — see Volume 1 code categories E800-E848.

The fourth-digit subdivisions for use with categories E800-E848 to identify the injured person are found at the end of this section.

For identifying the place in which an accident or poisoning occurred (circumstances classifiable to categories E850-E869 and E880-E928) — see the listing in this section under "Accident, occurring."

See the Table of Drugs and Chemicals (Section 2 of this volume) for identifying the specific agent involved in drug overdose or a wrong substance given or taken in error, and for intoxication or poisoning by a drug or other chemical substance.

The specific adverse effect, reaction, or localized toxic effect to a correct drug or substance properly administered in therapeutic or prophylactic dosage should be classified according to the nature of the adverse effect (e.g., allergy, dermatitis, tachycardia) listed in Section 1 of this volume.

Index to External Causes

A

Abandonment
  causing exposure to weather conditions — see
    Exposure
  child, with intent to injure or kill E968.4
  helpless person, infant, newborn E904.0
    with intent to injure or kill E968.4
Abortion, criminal, injury to child E968.8
Abuse (alleged) (suspected)
  adult
    by
      child E967.4
      ex-partner E967.3
      ex-spouse E967.3
      father E967.0
      grandchild E967.7
      grandparent E967.6
      mother E967.2
      non-related caregiver E967.8
      other relative E967.7
      other specified person E967.1
      partner E967.3
      sibling E967.5
      spouse E967.3
      stepfather E967.0
      stepmother E967.2
      unspecified person E967.9
  child
    by
      boyfriend of parent or guardian E967.0
      child E967.4
      father E967.0
      female partner of parent or guardian
        E967.2
      girlfriend of parent or guardian E967.2
      grandchild E967.7
      grandparent E967.6
      male partner of parent or guardian
        E967.2
      mother E967.2
      non-related caregiver E967.8
      other relative E967.7
      other specified person(s) E967.1
      sibling E967.5
      stepfather E967.0
      stepmother E967.2
      unspecified person E967.9
Accident (to) E928.9
  aircraft (in transit) (powered) E841 ✓4ᵗʰ
    at landing, take-off E840 ✓4ᵗʰ
    due to, caused by cataclysm — see
      categories E908 ✓4ᵗʰ, E909 ✓4ᵗʰ
    late effect of E929.1
    unpowered (see also Collision, aircraft,
      unpowered) E842 ✓4ᵗʰ
    while alighting, boarding E843 ✓4ᵗʰ
  amphibious vehicle
    on
      land — see Accident, motor vehicle
      water — see Accident, watercraft
  animal, ridden NEC E828 ✓4ᵗʰ
  animal-drawn vehicle NEC E827 ✓4ᵗʰ
  balloon (see also Collision, aircraft, unpowered)
    E842 ✓4ᵗʰ
  caused by, due to
    abrasive wheel (metalworking) E919.3
    animal NEC E906.9
      being ridden (in sport or transport)
        E828 ✓4ᵗʰ
    avalanche NEC E909.2
    band saw E919.4
    bench saw E919.4
    bore, earth-drilling or mining (land) (seabed)
      E919.1
    bulldozer E919.7
    cataclysmic
      earth surface movement or eruption
        E909.9
      storm E908.9
    chain
      hoist E919.2
        agricultural operations E919.0
        mining operations E919.1
      saw E920.1
    circular saw E919.4

Accident (to) — continued
  caused by, due to — continued
    cold (excessive) (see also Cold, exposure to)
      E901.9
    combine E919.0
    conflagration — see Conflagration
    corrosive liquid, substance NEC E924.1
    cotton gin E919.8
    crane E919.2
      agricultural operations E919.0
      mining operations E919.1
    cutting or piercing instrument (see also Cut)
      E920.9
    dairy equipment E919.8
    derrick E919.2
      agricultural operations E919.0
      mining operations E919.1
    drill E920.1
      earth (land) (seabed) E919.1
      hand (powered) E920.1
        not powered E920.4
      metalworking E919.3
      woodworking E919.4
    earth(-)
      drilling machine E919.1
      moving machine E919.7
      scraping machine E919.7
    electric
      current (see also Electric shock) E925.9
      motor — see also Accident, machine, by
        type of machine
        current (of) — see Electric shock
    elevator (building) (grain) E919.2
      agricultural operations E919.0
      mining operations E919.1
    environmental factors NEC E928.9
    excavating machine E919.7
    explosive material (see also Explosion)
      E923.9
    farm machine E919.0
    fire, flames — see also Fire
      conflagration — see Conflagration
    firearm missile — see Shooting
    forging (metalworking) machine E919.3
    forklift (truck) E919.2
      agricultural operations E919.0
      mining operations E919.1
    gas turbine E919.5
    harvester E919.0
    hay derrick, mower, or rake E919.0
    heat (excessive) (see also Heat) E900.9
    hoist (see also Accident, caused by, due to,
      lift) E919.2
      chain — see Accident, caused by, due to,
        chain
      shaft E919.1
    hot
      liquid E924.0
        caustic or corrosive E924.1
      object (not producing fire or flames)
        E924.8
      substance E924.9
        caustic or corrosive E924.1
        liquid (metal) NEC E924.0
        specified type NEC E924.8
    human bite E928.3
    ignition — see Ignition
    internal combustion engine E919.5
    landslide NEC E909.2
    lathe (metalworking) E919.3
      turnings E920.8
      woodworking E919.4
    lift, lifting (appliances) E919.2
      agricultural operations E919.0
      mining operations E919.1
      shaft E919.1
    lightning NEC E907
    machine, machinery — see also Accident,
      machine
      drilling, metal E919.3
      manufacturing, for manufacture of
        beverages E919.8
        clothing E919.8
        foodstuffs E919.8
        paper E919.8
        textiles E919.8

Accident (to) — continued
  caused by, due to — continued
    machine, machinery — see also Accident,
      machine — continued
      milling, metal E919.3
      moulding E919.4
      power press, metal E919.3
      printing E919.8
      rolling mill, metal E919.3
      sawing, metal E919.3
      specified type NEC E919.8
      spinning E919.8
      weaving E919.8
    natural factor NEC E928.9
    overhead plane E919.4
    plane E920.4
      overhead E919.4
    powered
      hand tool NEC E920.1
      saw E919.4
        hand E920.1
    printing machine E919.8
    pulley (block) E919.2
      agricultural operations E919.0
      mining operations E919.1
      transmission E919.6
    radial saw E919.4
    radiation — see Radiation
    reaper E919.0
    road scraper E919.7
      when in transport under its own power —
        see categories E810-E825 ✓4ᵗʰ
    roller coaster E919.8
    sander E919.4
    saw E920.4
      band E919.4
      bench E919.4
      chain E920.1
      circular E919.4
      hand E920.4
        powered E920.1
      powered, except hand E919.4
      radial E919.4
    sawing machine, metal E919.3
    shaft
      hoist E919.1
      lift E919.1
      transmission E919.6
    shears E920.4
      hand E920.4
        powered E920.1
      mechanical E919.3
    shovel E920.4
      steam E919.7
    spinning machine E919.8
    steam — see also Burning, steam
      engine E919.5
      shovel E919.7
    thresher E919.0
    thunderbolt NEC E907
    tractor E919.0
      when in transport under its own power —
        see categories E810-E825 ✓4ᵗʰ
    transmission belt, cable, chain, gear, pinion,
      pulley, shaft E919.6
    turbine (gas) (water driven) E919.5
    under-cutter E919.1
    weaving machine E919.8
    winch E919.2
      agricultural operations E919.0
      mining operations E919.1
  diving E883.0
    with insufficient air supply E913.2
  glider (hang) (see also Collision, aircraft,
    unpowered) E842 ✓4ᵗʰ
  hovercraft
    on
      land — see Accident, motor vehicle
      water — see Accident, watercraft
  ice yacht (see also Accident, vehicle NEC) E848
  in
    medical, surgical procedure
      as, or due to misadventure — see
        Misadventure

Accident (to) — *continued*
in — *continued*
medical, surgical procedure — *continued*
causing an abnormal reaction or later complication without mention of misadventure — *see* Reaction, abnormal
kite carrying a person (*see also* Collision, aircraft, unpowered) E842 ✓4ᵗʰ
land yacht (*see also* Accident, vehicle NEC) E848
late effect of — *see* Late effect
launching pad E845 ✓4ᵗʰ
machine, machinery (*see also* Accident, caused by, due to, by specific type of machine) E919.9
agricultural including animal-powered E919.0
earth-drilling E919.1
earth moving or scraping E919.7
excavating E919.7
involving transport under own power on highway or transport vehicle — *see* categories E810-E825 ✓4ᵗʰ, E840-E845 ✓4ᵗʰ
lifting (appliances) E919.2
metalworking E919.3
mining E919.1
prime movers, except electric motors E919.5
electric motors — *see* Accident, machine, by specific type of machine
recreational E919.8
specified type NEC E919.8
transmission E919.6
watercraft (deck) (engine room) (galley) (laundry) (loading) E836 ✓4ᵗʰ
woodworking or forming E919.4
motor vehicle (on public highway) (traffic) E819 ✓4ᵗʰ
due to cataclysm — *see* categories E908 ✓4ᵗʰ, E909 ✓4ᵗʰ
involving
collision (*see also* Collision, motor vehicle) E812 ✓4ᵗʰ
nontraffic, not on public highway — *see* categories E820-E825 ✓4ᵗʰ
not involving collision — *see* categories E816-E819 ✓4ᵗʰ
nonmotor vehicle NEC E829 ✓4ᵗʰ
nonroad — *see* Accident, vehicle NEC
road, except pedal cycle, animal-drawn vehicle, or animal being ridden E829 ✓4ᵗʰ
nonroad vehicle NEC — *see* Accident, vehicle NEC
not elsewhere classifiable involving
cable car (not on rails) E847
on rails E829 ✓4ᵗʰ
coal car in mine E846
hand truck — *see* Accident, vehicle NEC
logging car E846
sled(ge), meaning snow or ice vehicle E848
tram, mine or quarry E846
truck
mine or quarry E846
self-propelled, industrial E846
station baggage E846
tub, mine or quarry E846
vehicle NEC E848
snow and ice E848
used only on industrial premises E846
wheelbarrow E848
occurring (at) (in)
apartment E849.0
baseball field, diamond E849.4
construction site, any E849.3
dock E849.8
yard E849.3
dormitory E849.7
factory (building) (premises) E849.3
farm E849.1
buildings E849.1
house E849.0
football field E849.4
forest E849.8
garage (place of work) E849.3
private (home) E849.0

Accident (to) — *continued*
occurring (at) (in) — *continued*
gravel pit E849.2
gymnasium E849.4
highway E849.5
home (private) (residential) E849.0
institutional E849.7
hospital E849.7
hotel E849.6
house (private) (residential) E849.0
movie E849.6
public E849.6
institution, residential E849.7
jail E849.7
mine E849.2
motel E849.6
movie house E849.6
office (building) E849.6
orphanage E849.7
park (public) E849.4
mobile home E849.8
trailer E849.8
parking lot or place E849.8
place
industrial NEC E849.3
parking E849.8
public E849.8
specified place NEC E849.5
recreational NEC E849.4
sport NEC E849.4
playground (park) (school) E849.4
prison E849.6
public building NEC E849.6
quarry E849.2
railway
line NEC E849.8
yard E849.3
residence
home (private) E849.0
resort (beach) (lake) (mountain) (seashore) (vacation) E849.4
restaurant E849.6
sand pit E849.2
school (building) (private) (public) (state) E849.6
reform E849.7
riding E849.4
seashore E849.8
resort E849.4
shop (place of work) E849.3
commercial E849.6
skating rink E849.4
sports palace E849.4
stadium E849.4
store E849.6
street E849.5
swimming pool (public) E849.4
private home or garden E849.0
tennis court E849.4
theatre, theater E849.6
trailer court E849.8
tunnel E849.8
under construction E849.2
warehouse E849.3
yard
dock E849.3
industrial E849.3
private (home) E849.0
railway E849.3
off-road type motor vehicle (not on public highway) NEC E821 ✓4ᵗʰ
on public highway — *see* categories E810-E819 ✓4ᵗʰ
pedal cycle E826 ✓4ᵗʰ
railway E807 ✓4ᵗʰ
due to cataclysm — *see* categories E908 ✓4ᵗʰ, E909 ✓4ᵗʰ
involving
avalanche E909.2
burning by engine, locomotive, train (*see also* Explosion, railway engine) E803 ✓4ᵗʰ
collision (*see also* Collision, railway) E800 ✓4ᵗʰ
derailment (*see also* Derailment, railway) E802 ✓4ᵗʰ

Accident (to) — *continued*
railway — *continued*
involving — *continued*
explosion (*see also* Explosion, railway engine) E803 ✓4ᵗʰ
fall (*see also* Fall, from, railway rolling stock) E804 ✓4ᵗʰ
fire (*see also* Explosion, railway engine) E803 ✓4ᵗʰ
hitting by, being struck by
object falling in, on, from, rolling stock, train, vehicle E806 ✓4ᵗʰ
rolling stock, train, vehicle E805 ✓4ᵗʰ
overturning, railway rolling stock, train, vehicle (*see also* Derailment, railway) E802 ✓4ᵗʰ
running off rails, railway (*see also* Derailment, railway) E802 ✓4ᵗʰ
specified circumstances NEC E806 ✓4ᵗʰ
train or vehicle hit by
avalanche E909 ✓4ᵗʰ
falling object (earth, rock, tree) E806 ✓4ᵗʰ
due to cataclysm — *see* categories E908 ✓4ᵗʰ, E909 ✓4ᵗʰ
landslide E909 ✓4ᵗʰ
roller skate E885.1
scooter (nonmotorized) E885.0 ●
skateboard E885.2
ski(ing) E885.3
jump E884.9
lift or tow (with chair or gondola) E847
snow vehicle, motor driven (not on public highway) E820 ✓4ᵗʰ
on public highway — *see* catagories E810-E819 ✓4ᵗʰ
snowboard E885.4
spacecraft E845 ✓4ᵗʰ
specified cause NEC E928.8
street car E829 ✓4ᵗʰ
traffic NEC E819 ✓4ᵗʰ
vehicle NEC (with pedestrian) E848
battery powered
airport passenger vehicle E846
truck (baggage) (mail) E846
powered commercial or industrial (with other vehicle or object within commercial or industrial premises) E846
watercraft E838 ✓4ᵗʰ
with
drowning or submersion resulting from
accident other than to watercraft E832 ✓4ᵗʰ
accident to watercraft E830 ✓4ᵗʰ
injury, except drowning or submersion, resulting from
accident other than to watercraft — *see* categories E833-E838 ✓4ᵗʰ
accident to watercraft E831 ✓4ᵗʰ
due to, caused by cataclysm — *see* categories E908 ✓4ᵗʰ, E909 ✓4ᵗʰ
machinery E836 ✓4ᵗʰ

Acid throwing E961
Acosta syndrome E902.0
Aeroneurosis E902.1
Aero-otitis media — *see* Effects of, air pressure
Aerosinusitis — *see* Effects of, air pressure
After-effect, late — *see* Late effect
Air
blast
in
terrorism E979.2 ●
war operations E993
embolism (traumatic) NEC E928.9
in
infusion or transfusion E874.1
perfusion E874.2
sickness E903
Alpine sickness E902.0
Altitude sickness — *see* Effects of, air pressure
Anaphylactic shock, anaphylaxis (*see also* Table of Drugs and Chemicals) E947.9
due to bite or sting (venomous) — *see* Bite, venomous
Andes disease E902.0

✓4ᵗʰ Fourth-digit Required   ▶◀ Revised Text   ● New Line   ▲ Revised Code

Apoplexy
  heat — *see* Heat
Arachnidism E905.1
Arson E968.0
Asphyxia, asphyxiation
  by
    chemical
      in
        terrorism E979.7 ●
        war operations E997.2
    explosion — *see* Explosion
    food (bone) (regurgitated food) (seed) E911
    foreign object, except food E912
    fumes
      in
        terrorism (chemical weapons) ●
          E979.7
        war operations E997.2 ●
    gas — *see also* Table of Drugs and
      Chemicals
      in
        terrorism E979.7 ●
        war operations E997.2
      legal
        execution E978
        intervention (tear) E972
      tear E972
    mechanical means (*see also* Suffocation)
      E913.9
  from
    conflagration — *see* Conflagration
    fire — *see also* Fire E899 ▲
      in
        terrorism E979.3 ●
        war operations E990.9
    ignition — *see* Ignition
Aspiration
  foreign body — *see* Foreign body, aspiration
  mucus, not of newborn (with asphyxia,
    obstruction respiratory passage,
    suffocation) E912
  phlegm (with asphyxia, obstruction respiratory
    passage, suffocation) E912
  vomitus (with asphyxia, obstruction respiratory
    passage, suffocation) (*see also* Foreign
    body, aspiration, food) E911
Assassination (attempt) (*see also* Assault) E968.9
Assault (homicidal) (by) (in) E968.9
  acid E961
    swallowed E962.1
  air gun E968.6
  BB gun E968.6
  bite NEC E968.8
    of human being E968.7
  bomb ((placed in) car or house) E965.8
    antipersonnel E965.5
    letter E965.7
    petrol E965.7
  brawl (hand) (fists) (foot) E960.0
  burning, burns (by fire) E968.0
    acid E961
      swallowed E962.1
    caustic, corrosive substance E961
      swallowed E962.1
    chemical from swallowing caustic, corrosive
      substance NEC E962.1
    hot liquid E968.3
    scalding E968.3
    vitriol E961
      swallowed E962.1
  caustic, corrosive substance E961
    swallowed E962.1
  cut, any part of body E966
  dagger E966
  drowning E964
  explosive(s) E965.9
    bomb (*see also* Assault, bomb) E965.8
    dynamite E965.8
  fight (hand) (fists) (foot) E960.0
    with weapon E968.9
      blunt or thrown E968.2
      cutting or piercing E966
      firearm — *see* Shooting, homicide
  fire E968.0
  firearm(s) — *see* Shooting, homicide

Assault — *continued*
  garrotting E963
  gunshot (wound) — *see* Shooting, homicide
  hanging E963
  injury NEC E968.9
  knife E966
  late effect of E969
  ligature E963
  poisoning E962.9
    drugs or medicinals E962.0
    gas(es) or vapors, except drugs and
      medicinals E962.2
    solid or liquid substances, except drugs and
      medicinals E962.1
  puncture, any part of body E966
  pushing
    before moving object, train, vehicle E968.5
    from high place E968.1
  rape E960.1
  scalding E968.3
  shooting — *see* Shooting, homicide
  sodomy E960.1
  stab, any part of body E966
  strangulation E963
  submersion E964
  suffocation E963
  transport vehicle E968.5
  violence NEC E968.9
  vitriol E961
    swallowed E962.1
  weapon E968.9
    blunt or thrown E968.2
    cutting or piercing E966
    firearm — *see* Shooting, homicide
  wound E968.9
    cutting E966
    gunshot — *see* Shooting, homicide
    knife E966
    piercing E966
    puncture E966
    stab E966
Attack by animal NEC E906.9
Avalanche E909.2
  falling on or hitting
    motor vehicle (in motion) (on public
      highway) E909.2
    railway train E909.2
Aviators' disease E902.1

B

Barotitis, barodontalgia, barosinusitis,
  barotrauma (otitic) (sinus) — *see* Effects of,
  air pressure
Battered
  baby or child (syndrome) — *see* Abuse, child;
    category E967 ☑4ᵗʰ
  person other than baby or child — *see* Assault
Bayonet wound (*see also* Cut, by bayonet) E920.3
  in
    legal intervention E974
    terrorism E979.8 ●
    war operations E995
Bean in nose E912
Bed set on fire NEC E898.0
Beheading (by guillotine)
  homicide E966
  legal execution E978
Bending, injury in E927
Bends E902.0
Bite
  animal (nonvenomous) NEC E906.5
    other specified (except arthropod) E906.3
    venomous NEC E905.9
  arthropod (nonvenomous) NEC E906.4
    venomous — *see* Sting
  black widow spider E905.1
  cat E906.3
  centipede E905.4
  cobra E905.0
  copperhead snake E905.0
  coral snake E905.0
  dog E906.0
  fer de lance E905.0
  gila monster E905.0

Bite — *continued*
  human being
    accidental E928.3
    assault E968.7
  insect (nonvenomous) E906.4
    venomous — *see* Sting
  krait E905.0
  late effect of — *see* Late effect
  lizard E906.2
    venomous E905.0
  mamba E905.0
  marine animal
    nonvenomous E906.3
      snake E906.2
    venomous E905.6
      snake E905.0
  millipede E906.4
    venomous E905.4
  moray eel E906.3
  rat E906.1
  rattlesnake E905.0
  rodent, except rat E906.3
  serpent — *see* Bite, snake
  shark E906.3
  snake (venomous) E905.0
    nonvenomous E906.2
    sea E905.0
  spider E905.1
    nonvenomous E906.4
  tarantula (venomous) E905.1
  venomous NEC E905.9
    by specific animal — *see category* E905 ☑4ᵗʰ
  viper E905.0
  water moccasin E905.0
Blast (air)
  from nuclear explosion E996
  in
    terrorism E979.2 ●
      from nuclear explosion E979.5 ●
        underwater E979.0 ●
    war operations E993 ●
      from nuclear explosion E996 ●
        underwater E992 ●
  underwater E992
Blizzard E908.3
Blow E928.9
  by law-enforcing agent, police (on duty) E975
    with blunt object (baton) (nightstick) (stave)
      (truncheon) E973
Blowing up (*see also* Explosion) E923.9
Brawl (hand) (fists) (foot) E960.0
Breakage (accidental)
  cable of cable car not on rails E847
  ladder (causing fall) E881.0
  part (any) of
    animal-drawn vehicle E827 ☑4ᵗʰ
    ladder (causing fall) E881.0
    motor vehicle
      in motion (on public highway) E818 ☑4ᵗʰ
        not on public highway E825 ☑4ᵗʰ
    nonmotor road vehicle, except animal-drawn
      vehicle or pedal cycle E829 ☑4ᵗʰ
    off-road type motor vehicle (not on public
      highway) NEC E821 ☑4ᵗʰ
      on public highway E818 ☑4ᵗʰ
    pedal cycle E826 ☑4ᵗʰ
    scaffolding (causing fall) E881.1
    snow vehicle, motor-driven (not on public
      highway) E820 ☑4ᵗʰ
      on public highway E818 ☑4ᵗʰ
    vehicle NEC — *see* Accident, vehicle
Broken
  glass
    fall on E888.0
    injury by E920.8
  power line (causing electric shock) E925.1
Bumping against, into (accidentally)
  object (moving) E917.9
    caused by crowd E917.1
      with subsequent fall E917.6
    furniture E917.3
      with subsequent fall E917.7
    in
      running water E917.2
      sports E917.0
        with subsequent fall E917.5

Bumping against, into — *continued*
  object — *continued*
    stationary E917.4
      with subsequent fall E917.8
    person(s) E917.9
      with fall E886.9
        in sports E886.0
      as, or caused by, a crowd E917.1
        with subsequent fall E917.6
      in sports E917.0
        with fall E886.0

Burning, burns (accidental) (by) (from) (on) E899
  acid (any kind) E924.1
    swallowed — *see* Table of Drugs and Chemicals
  bedclothes (*see also* Fire, specified NEC) E898.0
  blowlamp (*see also* Fire, specified NEC) E898.1
  blowtorch (*see also* Fire, specified NEC) E898.1
  boat, ship, watercraft — *see* categories E830 ✓4ᵗʰ, E831 ✓4ᵗʰ, E837 ✓4ᵗʰ
  bonfire (controlled) E897
    uncontrolled E892
  candle (*see also* Fire, specified NEC) E898.1
  caustic liquid, substance E924.1
    swallowed — *see* Table of Drugs and Chemicals
  chemical E924.1
    from swallowing caustic, corrosive substance — *see* Table of Drugs and Chemicals
    in
      terrorism E979.7
      war operations E997.2
  cigar(s) or cigarette(s) (*see also* Fire, specified NEC) E898.1
  clothes, clothing, nightdress — *see* Ignition, clothes
    with conflagration — *see* Conflagration
  conflagration — *see* Conflagration
  corrosive liquid, substance E924.1
    swallowed — *see* Table of Drugs and Chemicals
  electric current (*see also* Electric shock) E925.9
  fire, flames (*see also* Fire) E899
  flare, Verey pistol E922.8
  heat
    from appliance (electrical) E924.8
    in local application, or packing during medical or surgical procedure E873.5
  homicide (attempt) (*see also* Assault, burning) E968.0
  hot
    liquid E924.0
      caustic or corrosive E924.1
    object (not producing fire or flames) E924.8
    substance E924.9
      caustic or corrosive E924.1
      liquid (metal) NEC E924.0
      specified type NEC E924.8
    tap water E924.2
  ignition — *see also* Ignition
    clothes, clothing, nightdress — *see also* Ignition, clothes
      with conflagration — *see* Conflagration
    highly inflammable material (benzine) (fat) (gasoline) (kerosene) (paraffin) (petrol) E894
  inflicted by other person
    stated as
      homicidal, intentional (*see also* Assault, burning) E968.0
      undetermined whether accidental or intentional (*see also* Burn, stated as undetermined whether accidental or intentional) E988.1
  internal, from swallowed caustic, corrosive liquid, substance — *see* Table of Drugs and Chemicals
  in
    terrorism E979.3 ●
      from nuclear explosion E979.5 ●
      petrol bomb E979.3 ●

Burning, burns — *continued*
  in — *continued*
    war operations (from fire-producing device or conventional weapon) E990.9 ● ● ●
      from nuclear explosion E996 ●
      petrol bomb E990.0 ●
  lamp (*see also* Fire, specified NEC) E898.1
  late effect of NEC E929.4
  lighter (cigar) (cigarette) (*see also* Fire, specified NEC) E898.1
  lightning E907
  liquid (boiling) (hot) (molten) E924.0
    caustic, corrosive (external) E924.1
      swallowed — *see* Table of Drugs and Chemicals
  local application of externally applied substance in medical or surgical care E873.5
  machinery — *see* Accident, machine
  matches (*see also* Fire, specified NEC) E898.1
  medicament, externally applied E873.5
  metal, molten E924.0
  object (hot) E924.8
    producing fire or flames — *see* Fire
  oven (electric) (gas) E924.8
  pipe (smoking) (*see also* Fire, specified NEC) E898.1
  radiation — *see* Radiation
  railway engine, locomotive, train (*see also* Explosion, railway engine) E803 ✓4ᵗʰ
  self-inflicted (unspecified whether accidental or intentional) E988.1
    caustic or corrosive substance NEC E988.7
    stated as intentional, purposeful E958.1
      caustic or corrosive substance NEC E958.7
  stated as undetermined whether accidental or intentional E988.1
    caustic or corrosive substance NEC E988.7
  steam E924.0
    pipe E924.8
  substance (hot) E924.9
    boiling or molten E924.0
    caustic, corrosive (external) E924.1
      swallowed — *see* Table of Drugs and Chemicals
  suicidal (attempt) NEC E958.1
    caustic substance E958.7
    late effect of E959
  tanning bed E926.2
  therapeutic misadventure
    overdose of radiation E873.2
  torch, welding (*see also* Fire, specified NEC) E898.1
  trash fire (*see also* Burning, bonfire) E897
  vapor E924.0
  vitriol E924.1
  x-rays E926.3
    in medical, surgical procedure — *see* Misadventure, failure, in dosage, radiation

Butted by animal E906.8

C

Cachexia, lead or saturnine E866.0
  from pesticide NEC (*see also* Table of Drugs and Chemicals) E863.4

Caisson disease E902.2

Capital punishment (any means) E978

Car sickness E903

Casualty (not due to war) NEC E928.9
  terrorism E979.8 ●
  war (*see also* War operations) E995

Cat
  bite E906.3
  scratch E906.8

Cataclysmic (any injury)
  earth surface movement or eruption E909.9
    specified type NEC E909.8
  storm or flood resulting from storm E908.9
    specified type NEC E909.8

Catching fire — *see* Ignition

Caught
  between
    objects (moving) (stationary and moving) E918
      and machinery — *see* Accident, machine
  by cable car, not on rails E847
  in
    machinery (moving parts of) — *see*, Accident, machine
    object E918

Cave-in (causing asphyxia, suffocation (by pressure)) (*see also* Suffocation, due to, cave-in) E913.3
  with injury other than asphyxia or suffocation E916
    with asphyxia or suffocation (*see also* Suffocation, due to, cave-in) E913.3
  struck or crushed by E916
    with asphyxia or suffocation (*see also* Suffocation, due to, cave-in) E913.3

Change(s) in air pressure — *see also* Effects of, air pressure
  sudden, in aircraft (ascent) (descent) (causing aeroneurosis or aviators' disease) E902.1

Chilblains E901.0
  due to manmade conditions E901.1

Choking (on) (any object except food or vomitus) E912
  apple E911
  bone E911
  food, any type (regurgitated) E911
  mucus or phlegm E912
  seed E911

Civil insurrection — *see* War operations

Cloudburst E908.8

Cold, exposure to (accidental) (excessive) (extreme) (place) E901.9
  causing chilblains or immersion foot E901.0
  due to
    manmade conditions E901.1
    specified cause NEC E901.8
    weather (conditions) E901.0
  late effect of NEC E929.5
  self-inflicted (undetermined whether accidental or intentional) E988.3
    suicidal E958.3
  suicide E958.3

Colic, lead, painter's, or saturnine — *see* category E866 ✓4ᵗʰ

Collapse
  building (moveable) E916
    burning ►(uncontrolled fire)◄ E891.8 ●
      in terrorism E979.3 ●
      private E890.8
  dam E909.3
  due to heat — *see* Heat
  machinery — *see* Accident, machine
  man-made structure E909.3
  postoperative NEC E878.9
  structure, burning NEC E891.8 ●
    burning (uncontrolled fire)
      in terrorism E979.3

✓4ᵗʰ Fourth-digit Required   ►◄ Revised Text   ● New Line   ▲ Revised Code

Collision (accidental)

> *Note* — *In the case of collisions between different types of vehicles, persons and objects, priority in classification is in the following order:*
>
> *Aircraft*
>
> *Watercraft*
>
> *Motor vehicle*
>
> *Railway vehicle*
>
> *Pedal cycle*
>
> *Animal-drawn vehicle*
>
> *Animal being ridden*
>
> *Streetcar or other nonmotor road vehicle*
>
> *Other vehicle*
>
> *Pedestrian or person using pedestrian conveyance*
>
> *Object (except where falling from or set in motion by vehicle etc. listed above)*
>
> *In the listing below, the combinations are listed only under the vehicle etc. having priority. For definitions, see Volume 1, page 247.*

aircraft (with object or vehicle) (fixed) (movable) (moving) E841 ✓4th
  with
    person (while landing, taking off) (without accident to aircraft) E844 ✓4th
  powered (in transit) (with unpowered aircraft) E841 ✓4th
    while landing, taking off E840 ✓4th
  unpowered E842 ✓4th
    while landing, taking off E840 ✓4th
animal being ridden (in sport or transport) E828 ✓4th
  and
    animal (being ridden) (herded) (unattended) E828 ✓4th
    nonmotor road vehicle, except pedal cycle or animal-drawn vehicle E828 ✓4th
    object (fallen) (fixed) (movable) (moving) not falling from or set in motion by vehicle of higher priority E828 ✓4th
    pedestrian (conveyance or vehicle) E828 ✓4th
animal-drawn vehicle E827 ✓4th
  and
    animal (being ridden) (herded) (unattended) E827 ✓4th
    nonmotor road vehicle, except pedal cycle E827 ✓4th
    object (fallen) (fixed) (movable) (moving) not falling from or set in motion by vehicle of higher priority E827 ✓4th
    pedestrian (conveyance or vehicle) E827 ✓4th
    streetcar E827 ✓4th
motor vehicle (on public highway) (traffic accident) E812 ✓4th
  after leaving, running off, public highway (without antecedent collision) (without re-entry) E816 ✓4th
  with antecedent collision on public highway — *see* categories E810-E815 ✓4th
  with re-entrance collision with another motor vehicle E811 ✓4th
  and
    abutment (bridge) (overpass) E815 ✓4th
    animal (herded) (unattended) E815 ✓4th
      carrying person, property E813 ✓4th
    animal-drawn vehicle E813 ✓4th
    another motor vehicle (abandoned) (disabled) (parked) (stalled) (stopped) E812 ✓4th

Collision — *continued*
  motor vehicle — *continued*
    and — *continued*
      another motor vehicle — *continued*
        with, involving re-entrance (on same roadway) (across median strip) E811 ✓4th
      any object, person, or vehicle off the public highway resulting from a noncollision motor vehicle nontraffic accident E816 ✓4th
      avalanche, fallen or not moving E815 ✓4th
        falling E909 ✓4th
      boundary fence E815 ✓4th
      culvert E815 ✓4th
      fallen
        stone E815 ✓4th
        tree E815 ✓4th
      falling E909.2
      guard post or guard rail E815 ✓4th
      inter-highway divider E815 ✓4th
      landslide, fallen or not moving E815 ✓4th
        moving E909 ✓4th
      machinery (road) E815 ✓4th
      moving E909.2
      nonmotor road vehicle NEC E813 ✓4th
      object (any object, person, or vehicle off the public highway resulting from a noncollision motor vehicle nontraffic accident) E815 ✓4th
        off, normally not on, public highway resulting from a noncollision motor vehicle traffic accident E816 ✓4th
      pedal cycle E813 ✓4th
      pedestrian (conveyance) E814 ✓4th
      person (using pedestrian conveyance) E814 ✓4th
      post or pole (lamp) (light) (signal) (telephone) (utility) E815 ✓4th
      railway rolling stock, train, vehicle E810 ✓4th
      safety island E815 ✓4th
      street car E813 ✓4th
      traffic signal, sign, or marker (temporary) E815 ✓4th
      tree E815 ✓4th
      tricycle E813 ✓4th
      wall of cut made for road E815 ✓4th
    due to cataclysm — *see* categories E908 ✓4th, E909 ✓4th
    not on public highway, nontraffic accident E822 ✓4th
    and
      animal (carrying person, property) (herded) (unattended) E822 ✓4th
      animal-drawn vehicle E822 ✓4th
      another motor vehicle (moving), except off-road motor vehicle E822 ✓4th
        stationary E823 ✓4th
      avalanche, fallen, not moving E823 ✓4th
        moving E909 ✓4th
      landslide, fallen, not moving E823 ✓4th
        moving E909 ✓4th
      nonmotor vehicle (moving) E822 ✓4th
        stationary E823 ✓4th
      object (fallen) (normally) (fixed) (movable but not in motion) (stationary) E823 ✓4th
        moving, except when falling from, set in motion by, aircraft or cataclysm E822 ✓4th
      pedal cycle (moving) E822 ✓4th
        stationary E823 ✓4th
      pedestrian (conveyance) E822 ✓4th
      person (using pedestrian conveyance) E822 ✓4th
      railway rolling stock, train, vehicle (moving) E822 ✓4th
        stationary E823 ✓4th
      road vehicle (any) (moving) E822 ✓4th
        stationary E823 ✓4th
      tricycle (moving) E822 ✓4th
        stationary E823 ✓4th
    moving E909.2

Collision — *continued*
  off-road type motor vehicle (not on public highway) E821 ✓4th
  and
    animal (being ridden) (-drawn vehicle) E821 ✓4th
    another off-road motor vehicle, except snow vehicle E821 ✓4th
    other motor vehicle, not on public highway E821 ✓4th
    other object or vehicle NEC, fixed or movable, not set in motion by aircraft, motor vehicle on highway, or snow vehicle, motor driven E821 ✓4th
    pedal cycle E821 ✓4th
    pedestrian (conveyance) E821 ✓4th
    railway train E821 ✓4th
  on public highway — *see* Collision, motor vehicle
  pedal cycle E826 ✓4th
  and
    animal (carrying person, property) (herded) (unherded) E826 ✓4th
    animal-drawn vehicle E826 ✓4th
    another pedal cycle E826 ✓4th
    nonmotor road vehicle E826 ✓4th
    object (fallen) (fixed) (movable) (moving) not falling from or set in motion by aircraft, motor vehicle, or railway train NEC E826 ✓4th
    pedestrian (conveyance) E826 ✓4th
    person (using pedestrian conveyance) E826 ✓4th
    street car E826 ✓4th
  pedestrian(s) (conveyance) E917.9
  with fall E886.9
    in sports E886.0
  and
    crowd, human stampede E917.1
      with subsequent fall E917.6
    furniture E917.3
      with subsequent fall E917.7
    machinery — *see* Accident, machine
    object (fallen) (moving) not falling from NEC, fixed or set in motion by any vehicle classifiable to E800-E848 E917.9
      with subsequent fall E917.6
      caused by a crowd E917.1
        with subsequent fall E917.6
      furniture E917.3
        with subsequent fall E917.7
      in
        running water E917.2
          with drowning or submersion — *see* Submersion
        sports E917.0
          with subsequent fall E917.5
        stationary E917.4
          with subsequent fall E917.8
    vehicle, nonmotor, nonroad E848
  in
    running water E917.2
      with drowning or submersion — *see* Submersion
    sports E917.0
      with fall E886.0
  person(s) (using pedestrian conveyance) (*see also* Collision, pedestrian) E917.9
  railway (rolling stock) (train) (vehicle) (with subsequent) derailment, explosion, fall or fire) E800 ✓4th
  with antecedent derailment E802 ✓4th
  and
    animal (carrying person) (herded) (unattended) E801 ✓4th
    another railway train or vehicle E800 ✓4th
    buffers E801 ✓4th
    fallen tree on railway E801 ✓4th
    farm machinery, nonmotor (in transport) (stationary) E801 ✓4th
    gates E801 ✓4th
    nonmotor vehicle E801 ✓4th

Collision — Collision

Collision — Cut

Collision — *continued*
  railway — *continued*
    and — *continued*
        object (fallen) (fixed) (movable) (moving)
          not falling from, set in motion by,
          aircraft or motor vehicle NEC
          E801 ✓4ᵗʰ
        pedal cycle E801 ✓4ᵗʰ
        pedestrian (conveyance) E805 ✓4ᵗʰ
        person (using pedestrian conveyance)
          E805 ✓4ᵗʰ
        platform E801 ✓4ᵗʰ
        rock on railway E801 ✓4ᵗʰ
        street car E801 ✓4ᵗʰ
    snow vehicle, motor-driven (not on public
      highway) E820 ✓4ᵗʰ
      and
        animal (being ridden) (-drawn vehicle)
          E820 ✓4ᵗʰ
        another off-road motor vehicle E820 ✓4ᵗʰ
        other motor vehicle, not on public
          highway E820 ✓4ᵗʰ
        other object or vehicle NEC, fixed or
          movable, not set in motion by
          aircraft or motor vehicle on highway
          E820 ✓4ᵗʰ
        pedal cycle E820 ✓4ᵗʰ
        pedestrian (conveyance) E820 ✓4ᵗʰ
        railway train E820 ✓4ᵗʰ
      on public highway — *see* Collision, motor
        vehicle
    street car(s) E829 ✓4ᵗʰ
      and
        animal, herded, not being ridden,
          unattended E829 ✓4ᵗʰ
        nonmotor road vehicle NEC E829 ✓4ᵗʰ
        object (fallen) (fixed) (movable) (moving)
          not falling from or set in motion by
          aircraft, animal-drawn vehicle,
          animal being ridden, motor vehicle,
          pedal cycle, or railway train
          E829 ✓4ᵗʰ
        pedestrian (conveyance) E829 ✓4ᵗʰ
        person (using pedestrian conveyance)
          E829 ✓4ᵗʰ
  vehicle
    animal-drawn — *see* Collision, animal-
      drawn vehicle
    motor — *see* Collision, motor vehicle
    nonmotor
      nonroad E848
        and
          another nonmotor, nonroad vehicle
            E848
          object (fallen) (fixed) (movable)
            (moving) not falling from or
            set in motion by aircraft,
            animal-drawn vehicle, animal
            being ridden, motor vehicle,
            nonmotor road vehicle, pedal
            cycle, railway train, or
            streetcar E848
      road, except animal being ridden, animal-
        drawn vehicle, or pedal cycle
        E829 ✓4ᵗʰ
        and
          animal, herded, not being ridden,
            unattended E829 ✓4ᵗʰ
          another nonmotor road vehicle,
            except animal being ridden,
            animal-drawn vehicle, or
            pedal cycle E829 ✓4ᵗʰ
          object (fallen) (fixed) (movable)
            (moving) not falling from or
            set in motion by, aircraft,
            animal-drawn vehicle, animal
            being ridden, motor vehicle,
            pedal cycle, or railway train
            E829 ✓4ᵗʰ
          pedestrian (conveyance) E829 ✓4ᵗʰ
          person (using pedestrian
            conveyance) E829 ✓4ᵗʰ
        vehicle, nonmotor, nonroad
          E829 ✓4ᵗʰ

Collision — *continued*
  watercraft E838 ✓4ᵗʰ
    and
      person swimming or water skiing
        E838 ✓4ᵗʰ
    causing
      drowning, submersion E830 ✓4ᵗʰ
      injury except drowning, submersion
        E831 ✓4ᵗʰ
Combustion, spontaneous — *see* Ignition
**Complication of medical or surgical procedure
  or treatment**
    as an abnormal reaction — *see* Reaction,
      abnormal
    delayed, without mention of misadventure —
      see Reaction, abnormal
    due to misadventure — *see* Misadventure
Compression
  divers' squeeze E902.2
  trachea by
    food E911
    foreign body, except food E912
Conflagration
  building or structure, except private dwelling
    (barn) (church) (convalescent or
    residential home) (factory) (farm
    outbuilding) (hospital) (hotel) (institution
    (educational) (domitory) (residential))
    (school) (shop) (store) (theatre) E891.9
    with or causing (injury due to)
      accident or injury NEC E891.9
        specified circumstance NEC E891.8
      burns, burning E891.3
      carbon monoxide E891.2
      fumes E891.2
        polyvinylchloride (PVC) or similar
          material E891.1
      smoke E891.2
    causing explosion E891.0
    in terrorism E979.3   ●
  not in building or structure E892
  private dwelling (apartment) (boarding house)
    (camping place) (caravan) (farmhouse)
    (home (private)) (house) (lodging house)
    (private garage) (rooming house)
    (tenement) E890.9
    with or causing (injury due to)
      accident or injury NEC E890.9
        specified circumstance NEC E890.8
      burns, burning E890.3
      carbon monoxide E890.2
      fumes E890.2
        polyvinylchloride (PVC) or similar
          material E890.1
      smoke E890.2
    causing explosion E890.0
Contact with
  dry ice E901.1
  liquid air, hydrogen, nitrogen E901.1
Cramp(s)
  Heat — *see* Heat
  swimmers (*see also* category E910 ✓4ᵗʰ) E910.2
    not in recreation or sport E910.3
Cranking (car) (truck) (bus) (engine), injury by
  E917.9
Crash
  aircraft (in transit) (powered) E841 ✓4ᵗʰ
    at landing, take-off E840 ✓4ᵗʰ
      in
        terrorism E979.1   ●
        war operations E994
    on runway NEC E840 ✓4ᵗʰ
    stated as
      homicidal E968.8
      suicidal E958.6
      undetermined whether accidental or
        intentional E988.6
    unpowered E842 ✓4ᵗʰ
  glider E842 ✓4ᵗʰ
  motor vehicle — *see also* Accident, motor
    vehicle
    homicidal E968.5
    suicidal E958.5
    undetermined whether accidental or
      intentional E988.5

Crushed (accidentally) E928.9
  between
    boat(s), ship(s), watercraft (and dock or pier)
      (without accident to watercraft)
      E838 ✓4ᵗʰ
      after accident to, or collision, watercraft
        E831 ✓4ᵗʰ
    objects (moving) (stationary and moving)
      E918
  by
    avalanche NEC E909.2
    boat, ship, watercraft after accident to,
      collision, watercraft E831 ✓4ᵗʰ
    cave-in E916
      with asphyxiation or suffocation (*see also*
        Suffocation, due to, cave-in) E913.3
    crowd, human stampede E917.1
    falling
      aircraft (*see also* Accident, aircraft)
        E841 ✓4ᵗʰ
        in
          terrorism E979.1   ●
          war operations E994
      earth, material E916
        with asphyxiation or suffocation (*see
          also* Suffocation, due to, cave-in)
          E913.3
      object E916
        on ship, watercraft E838 ✓4ᵗʰ
        while loading, unloading watercraft
          E838 ✓4ᵗʰ
    landslide NEC E909.2
    lifeboat after abandoning ship E831 ✓4ᵗʰ
    machinery — *see* Accident, machine
    railway rolling stock, train, vehicle (part of)
      E805 ✓4ᵗʰ
    street car E829 ✓4ᵗʰ
    vehicle NEC — *see* Accident, vehicle NEC
  in
    machinery — *see* Accident, machine
    object E918
    transport accident — *see* categories E800-
      E848
  late effect of NEC E929.9
Cut, cutting (any part of body) (accidental)
  E920.9
  by
    arrow E920.8
    axe E920.4
    bayonet (*see also* Bayonet wound) E920.3
    blender E920.2
    broken glass E920.8
      following fall E888.0
    can opener E920.4
      powered E920.2
    chisel E920.4
    circular saw E919.4
    cutting or piercing instrument — *see also*
      category E920 ✓4ᵗʰ
      following fall E888.0
      late effect of E929.8
    dagger E920.3
    dart E920.8
    drill — *see* Accident, caused by drill
    edge of stiff paper E920.8
    electric
      beater E920.2
      fan E920.2
      knife E920.2
      mixer E920.2
    fork E920.4
    garden fork E920.4
    hand saw or tool (not powered) E920.4
      powered E920.1
    hedge clipper E920.4
      powered E920.1
    hoe E920.4
    ice pick E920.4
    knife E920.3
      electric E920.2
    lathe turnings E920.8
    lawn mower E920.4
      powered E920.0
      riding E919.8
    machine — *see* Accident, machine
    meat
      grinder E919.8

Explosion — Fall (side tab)

Explosion — *continued*
- bomb — *continued*
  - in — *continued*
    - war operations — *continued*
      - injury by fragments from E991.9
        - antipersonnel bomb E991.3
- butane E923.2
- caused by
  - other person
    - stated as
      - intentional, homicidal — *see* Assault, explosive
      - undetermined whether accidental or homicidal E985.5
- coal gas E923.2
- detonator E923.1
- dyamite E923.1
- explosive (material) NEC E923.9
  - gas(es) E923.2
  - missile E923.8
    - in
      - terrorism E979.2 ●
      - war operations E993
        - injury by fragments from E991.9
          - antipersonnel bomb E991.3
  - used in blasting operations E923.1
- fire-damp E923.2
- fireworks E923.0
- gas E923.2
  - cylinder (in machinery) E921.1
  - pressure tank (in machinery) E921.1
- gasoline (fumes) (tank) not in moving motor vehicle E923.2
- grain store (military) (munitions) E923.8
- grenade E923.8
  - in
    - terrorism E979.2 ●
    - war operations E993
      - injury by fragments from E991.9
- homicide (attempt) — *see* Assault, explosive
- hot water heater, tank (in machinery) E921.0
- in mine (of explosive gases) NEC E923.2
- late effect of NEC E929.8
- machinery — *see also* Accident, machine
  - pressure vessel — *see* Explosion, pressure vessel
- methane E923.2
- missile E923.8
  - in
    - terrorism E979.2 ●
    - war operations E993
      - injury by fragments from E991.9
- motor vehicle (part of)
  - in motion (on public highway) E818 ☑4ᵗʰ
  - not on public highway E825 ☑4ᵗʰ
- munitions (dump) (factory) E923.8
  - in
    - terrorism E979.2 ●
    - war operations E993
- of mine E923.8
  - in
    - terrorism ●
      - at sea or in harbor E979.0 ●
      - land E979.2 ●
      - marine E979.0 ●
    - war operations
      - after cessation of hostilities E998
      - at sea or in harbor E992
      - land E993
        - after cessation of hostilities E998
        - injury by fragments from E991.9
      - marine E992
- own weapons
  - in
    - terrorism (*see also* Suicide) E979.2 ●
    - war operations E993
      - injury by fragments from E991.9
        - antipersonnel bomb E991.3
    - injury by fragments from E991.9
      - antipersonnel bomb E991.3
- pressure
  - cooker E921.8
  - gas tank (in machinery) E921.1
  - vessel (in machinery) E921.9
    - on transport vehicle — *see* categories E800-E848 ☑4ᵗʰ
  - specified type NEC E921.8

Explosion — *continued*
- propane E923.2
- railway engine, locomotive, train (boiler) (with subsequent collision, derailment, fall) E803 ☑4ᵗʰ
  - with
    - collision (antecedent) (*see also* Collision, railway) E800 ☑4ᵗʰ
    - derailment (antecedent) E802 ☑4ᵗʰ
    - fire (without antecedent collision or derailment) E803 ☑4ᵗʰ
- secondary fire resulting from — *see* Fire
- self-inflicted (unspecified whether accidental or intentional) E985.5
  - stated as intentional, purposeful E955.5
- shell (artillery) E923.8
  - in
    - terrorism E979.2 ●
    - war operations E993
      - injury by fragments from E991.9
- stated as undetermined whether caused accidentally or purposely inflicted E985.5
- steam or water lines (in machinery) E921.0
- suicide (attempted) E955.5
- terrorism — *see* Terrorism, explosion ●
- torpedo E923.8
  - in
    - terrorism E979.0 ●
    - war operations E992
- transport accident — *see* categories E800-E848 ☑4ᵗʰ
- war operations — *see* War operations, explosion
- watercraft (boiler) E837 ☑4ᵗʰ
  - causing drowning, submersion (after jumping from watercraft) E830 ☑4ᵗʰ

Exposure (weather) (conditions) (rain) (wind) E904.3
- with homicidal intent E968.4
- excessive E904.3
  - cold (*see also* Cold, exposure to) E901.9
    - self-inflicted — *see* Cold, exposure to, self-inflicted
  - heat (*see also* Heat) E900.9
- fire — *see* Fire ●
- helpless person, infant, newborn due to abandonment or neglect E904.0
- noise E928.1
- prolonged in deep-freeze unit or refrigerator E901.1
- radiation — *see* Radiation
- resulting from transport accident — *see* categories E800-E848 ☑4ᵗʰ
- smoke from, due to
  - fire — *see* Fire
  - tobacco, second-hand E869.4
- vibration E928.2

F

Fall, falling (accidental) E888.9
- building E916
  - burning E891.8
    - private E890.8
- down
  - escalator E880.0
  - ladder E881.0
    - in boat, ship, watercraft E833 ☑4ᵗʰ
  - staircase E880.9
  - stairs, steps — *see* Fall, from, stairs
- earth (with asphyxia or suffocation (by pressure)) (*see also* Earth, falling) E913.3
- from, off
  - aircraft (at landing, take-off) (in-transit) (while alighting, boarding) E843 ☑4ᵗʰ
    - resulting from accident to aircraft — *see* categories E840-E842 ☑4ᵗʰ
  - animal (in sport or transport) E828 ☑4ᵗʰ
  - animal-drawn vehicle E827 ☑4ᵗʰ
  - balcony E882
  - bed E884.4
  - bicycle E826 ☑4ᵗʰ
  - boat, ship, watercraft (into water) E832 ☑4ᵗʰ
    - after accident to, collision, fire on E830 ☑4ᵗʰ
      - and subsequently struck by (part of) boat E831 ☑4ᵗʰ

Fall, falling — *continued*
- from, off — *continued*
  - boat, ship, watercraft — *continued*
    - and subsequently struck by (part of) boat E831 ☑4ᵗʰ
    - burning, crushed, sinking E830 ☑4ᵗʰ
      - and subsequently struck by (part of) boat E831 ☑4ᵗʰ
  - bridge E882
  - building E882
    - burning ▶(uncontrolled fire)◀ E891.8
      - in terrorism E979.3 ●
    - private E890.8
  - bunk in boat, ship, watercraft E834 ☑4ᵗʰ
    - due to accident to watercraft E831 ☑4ᵗʰ
  - cable car (not on rails) E847
    - on rails E829 ☑4ᵗʰ
  - car — *see* Fall from motor vehicle
  - chair E884.2
  - cliff E884.1
  - commode E884.6
  - curb (sidewalk) E880.1
  - elevation aboard ship E834 ☑4ᵗʰ
    - due to accident to ship E831 ☑4ᵗʰ
  - embankment E884.9
  - escalator E880.0
  - fire escape E882
  - flagpole E882
  - furniture NEC E884.5
  - gangplank (into water) (*see also* Fall, from, boat) E832 ☑4ᵗʰ
    - to deck, dock E834 ☑4ᵗʰ
  - hammock on ship E834 ☑4ᵗʰ
    - due to accident to watercraft E831 ☑4ᵗʰ
  - haystack E884.9
  - high place NEC E884.9
    - stated as undetermined whether accidental or intentional — *see* Jumping, from, high place
  - horse (in sport or transport) E828 ☑4ᵗʰ
  - in-line skates E885.1
  - ladder E881.0
    - in boat, ship, watercraft E833 ☑4ᵗʰ
      - due to accident to watercraft E831 ☑4ᵗʰ
  - machinery — *see also* Accident, machine
    - not in operation E884.9
  - motor vehicle (in motion) (on public highway) E818 ☑4ᵗʰ
    - not on public highway E825 ☑4ᵗʰ
      - stationary, except while alighting, boarding, entering, leaving E884.9
    - while alighting, boarding, entering, leaving E824 ☑4ᵗʰ
    - stationary, except while alighting, boarding, entering, leaving E884.9
    - while alighting, boarding, entering, leaving, except off-road type motor vehicle E817 ☑4ᵗʰ
    - off-road type — *see* Fall, from, off-road type motor vehicle
  - nonmotor road vehicle (while alighting, boarding) NEC E829 ☑4ᵗʰ
    - stationary, except while alighting, boarding, entering, leaving E884.9
  - off road type motor vehicle (not on public highway) NEC E821 ☑4ᵗʰ
    - on public highway E818 ☑4ᵗʰ
      - while alighting, boarding, entering, leaving E817 ☑4ᵗʰ
  - snow vehicle — *see* Fall from snow vehicle, motor-driven
  - one
    - deck to another on ship E834 ☑4ᵗʰ
      - due to accident to ship E831 ☑4ᵗʰ
    - level to another NEC E884.9
      - boat, ship, or watercraft E834 ☑4ᵗʰ
        - due to accident to watercraft E831 ☑4ᵗʰ
  - pedal cycle E826 ☑4ᵗʰ
  - playground equipment E884.0
  - railway rolling stock, train, vehicle, (while alighting, boarding) E804 ☑4ᵗʰ
    - with
      - collision (*see also* Collision, railway) E800 ☑4ᵗʰ

Fall — Fire

Fire — *continued*
  specified — *continued*
    with — *continued*
      ignition (of)
        clothing — *see* Ignition, clothes
        highly inflammable material (benzine)
          (fat) (gasoline) (kerosene)
          (paraffin) (petrol) E894
  started by other person
    stated as
      with intent to injure or kill E968.0
      undetermined whether or not with intent
        to injure or kill E988.1
  suicide (attempted) E958.1
    late effect of E959
  tunnel (uncontrolled) E892
Fireball effects from nuclear explosion
  in
    terrorism E979.5 ●
    war operations E996
Fireworks (explosion) E923.0
Flash burns from explosion (*see also* Explosion)
  E923.9
Flood (any injury) (resulting from storm) E908.2
  caused by collapse of dam or manmade
    structure E909.3
Forced landing (aircraft) E840 ✓4ᵗʰ
Foreign body, object or material (entrance into
  (accidental))
  air passage (causing injury) E915
    with asphyxia, obstruction, suffocation E912
      food or vomitus E911
    nose (with asphyxia, obstruction,
      suffocation) E912
      causing injury without asphyxia,
        obstruction, suffocation E915
  alimentary canal (causing injury) (with
    obstruction) E915
    with asphyxia, obstruction respiratory
      passage, suffocation E912
      food E911
    mouth E915
      with asphyxia, obstruction, suffocation
        E912
        food E911
    pharynx E915
      with asphyxia, obstruction, suffocation
        E912
        food E911
    aspiration (with asphyxia, obstruction
      respiratory passage, suffocation) E912
    causing injury without asphyxia, obstruction
      respiratory passage, suffocation E915
    food (regurgitated) (vomited) E911
      causing injury without asphyxia,
        obstruction respiratory passage,
        suffocation E915
    mucus (not of newborn) E912
    phlegm E912
  bladder (causing injury or obstruction) E915
  bronchus, bronchi — *see* Foreign body, air
    passages
  conjunctival sac E914
  digestive system — *see* Foreign body,
    alimentary canal
  ear (causing injury or obstruction) E915
  esophagus (causing injury or obstruction) (*see
    also* Foreign body, alimentary canal)
    E915
  eye (any part) E914
  eyelid E914
  hairball (stomach) (with obstruction) E915
  ingestion — *see* Foreign body, alimentary canal
  inhalation — *see* Foreign body, aspiration
  intestine (causing injury or obstruction) E915
  iris E914
  lacrimal apparatus E914
  larynx — *see* Foreign body, air passage
  late effect of NEC E929.8
  lung — *see* Foreign body, air passage
  mouth — *see* Foreign body, alimentary canal,
    mouth
  nasal passage — *see* Foreign body, air passage,
    nose
  nose — *see* Foreign body, air passage, nose
  ocular muscle E914

Foreign body, object or material — *continued*
  operation wound (left in) — *see* Misadventure,
    foreign object
  orbit E914
  pharynx — *see* Foreign body, alimentary canal,
    pharynx
  rectum (causing injury or obstruction) E915
  stomach (hairball) (causing injury or
    obstruction) E915
  tear ducts or glands E914
  trachea — *see* Foreign body, air passage
  urethra (causing injury or obstruction) E915
  vagina (causing injury or obstruction) E915
Found dead, injured
  from exposure (to) — *see* Exposure
  on
    public highway E819 ✓4ᵗʰ
    railway right of way E807 ✓4ᵗʰ
Fracture (circumstances unknown or unspecified)
  E887
  due to specified external means — *see* manner
    of accident
  late effect of NEC E929.3
  occuring in water transport NEC E835 ✓4ᵗʰ
Freezing — *see* Cold, exposure to
Frostbite E901.0
  due to manmade conditions E901.1
Frozen — *see* Cold, exposure to

G

Garrotting, homicidal (attempted) E963
Gored E906.8
Gunshot wound (*see also* Shooting) E922.9

H

Hailstones, injury by E904.3
Hairball (stomach) (with obstruction) E915
Hanged himself (*see also* Hanging, self-inflicted)
  E983.0
Hang gliding E842 ✓4ᵗʰ
Hanging (accidental) E913.8
  caused by other person
    in accidental circumstances E913.8
    stated as
      intentional, homicidal E963
      undetermined whether accidental or
        intentional E983.0
  homicide (attempt) E963
  in bed or cradle E913.0
  legal execution E978
  self-inflicted (unspecified whether accidental or
    intentional) E983.0
    in accidental circumstances E913.8
    stated as intentional, purposeful E953.0
  stated as undetermined whether accidental or
    intentional E983.0
  suicidal (attempt) E953.0
Heat (apoplexy) (collapse) (cramps) (effects of)
  (excessive) (exhaustion) (fever) (prostration)
  (stroke) E900.9
  due to
    manmade conditions (as listed in E900.1,
      except boat, ship, watercraft) E900.1
    weather (conditions) E900.0
  from
    electric heating appartus causing burning
      E924.8
    nuclear explosion
      in
        terrorism E979.5 ●
        war operations E996
  generated in, boiler, engine, evaporator, fire
    room of boat, ship, watercraft E838 ✓4ᵗʰ
  inappropriate in local application or packing in
    medical or surgical procedure E873.5
  late effect of NEC E989
Hemorrhage
  delayed following medical or surgical treatment
    without mention of misadventure — *see*
    Reaction, abnormal
  during medical or surgical treatment as
    misadventure — *see* Misadventure, cut

High
  altitude, effects E902.9
  level of radioactivity, effects — *see* Radiation
  pressure effects — *see also* Effects of, air
    pressure
    from rapid descent in water (causing caisson
      or divers' disease, palsy, or paralysis)
      E902.2
  temperature, effects — *see* Heat
Hit, hitting (accidental) by
  aircraft (propeller) (without accident to aircraft)
    E844 ✓4ᵗʰ
    unpowered E842 ✓4ᵗʰ
  avalanche E909.2
  being thrown against object in or part of
    motor vehicle (in motion) (on public
      highway) E818 ✓4ᵗʰ
      not on public highway E825 ✓4ᵗʰ
    nonmotor road vehicle NEC E829 ✓4ᵗʰ
    street car E829 ✓4ᵗʰ
  boat, ship, watercraft
    after fall from watercraft E838 ✓4ᵗʰ
    damaged, involved in accident E831 ✓4ᵗʰ
    while swimming, water skiing E838 ✓4ᵗʰ
  bullet (*see also* Shooting) E922.9
    from air gun E922.4
    in
      terrorism E979.4 ●
      war operations E991.2
        rubber E991.0
  flare, Verey pistol (*see also* Shooting) E922.8
  hailstones E904.3
  landslide E909.2
  law-enforcing agent (on duty) E975
    with blunt object (baton) (night stick) (stave)
      (truncheon) E973
  machine — *see* Accident, machine
  missile
    firearm (*see also* Shooting) E922.9
    in
      terrorism — *see* Terrorism, mission ●
      war operations — *see* War operations,
        missile
  motor vehicle (on public highway) (traffic
    accident) E814 ✓4ᵗʰ
    not on public highway, nontraffic accident
      E822 ✓4ᵗʰ
  nonmotor road vehicle NEC E829 ✓4ᵗʰ
  object
    falling E916
      from, in, on
        aircraft E844 ✓4ᵗʰ
          due to accident to aircraft — *see*
            categories E840-E842 ✓4ᵗʰ
          unpowered E842 ✓4ᵗʰ
        boat, ship, watercraft E838 ✓4ᵗʰ
          due to accident to watercraft
          E831 ✓4ᵗʰ
        building E916
          burning (uncontrolled fire)
            E891.8
            in terrorism E979.3 ●
            private E890.8
        cataclysmic
          earth surface movement or eruption
            E909.9
          storm E908.9
        cave-in E916
          with asphyxiation or suffocation
            (*see also* Suffocation, due to,
            cave-in) E913.3
        earthquake E909.0
        motor vehicle (in motion) (on public
          highway) E818 ✓4ᵗʰ
          not on public highway E825 ✓4ᵗʰ
          stationary E916
        nonmotor road vehicle NEC E829 ✓4ᵗʰ
        pedal cycle E826 ✓4ᵗʰ
        railway rolling stock, train, vehicle
          E806 ✓4ᵗʰ
        street car E829 ✓4ᵗʰ
        structure, burning NEC E891.8
        vehicle, stationary E916
    moving NEC — *see* Striking against, object
    projected NEC — *see* Striking against, object

Fire — Hit

Hit, hitting — *continued*
  object — *continued*
    set in motion by
      compressed air or gas, spring, striking, throwing — *see* Striking against, object
      explosion — *see* Explosion
    thrown into, on, or towards
      motor vehicle (in motion) (on public highway) E818 ✓4ᵗʰ
        not on public highway E825 ✓4ᵗʰ
      nonmotor road vehicle NEC E829 ✓4ᵗʰ
      pedal cycle E826 ✓4ᵗʰ
      street car E829 ✓4ᵗʰ
    off-road type motor vehicle (not on public highway) E821 ✓4ᵗʰ
      on public highway E814 ✓4ᵗʰ
    other person(s) E917.9
      with blunt or thrown object E917.9
        in sports E917.0
          with subsequent fall E917.5
        intentionally, homicidal E968.2
      as, or caused by, a crowd E917.1
        with subsequent fall E917.6
        in sports E917.0
    pedal cycle E826 ✓4ᵗʰ
    police (on duty) E975
      with blunt object (baton) (nightstick) (stave) (truncheon) E973
    railway, rolling stock, train, vehicle (part of) E805 ✓4ᵗʰ
    shot — *see* Shooting
    snow vehicle, motor-driven (not on public highway) E820 ✓4ᵗʰ
      on public highway E814 ✓4ᵗʰ
    street car E829 ✓4ᵗʰ
    vehicle NEC — *see* Accident, vehicle NEC
Homicide, homicidal (attempt) (justifiable) (*also* Assault) E968.9
Hot
  liquid, object, substance, accident caused by — *see also* Accident, caused by, hot, by type of substance
    late effect of E929.8
  place, effects — *see* Heat
  weather, effects E900.0
Humidity, causing problem E904.3
Hunger E904.1
  resulting from
    abandonment or neglect E904.0
    transport accident — *see* categories E800-E848 ✓4ᵗʰ
Hurricane (any injury) E908.0
Hypobarism, hypobaropathy — *see* Effects of, air pressure
Hypothermia — *see* Cold, exposure to

I

Ictus
  caloris — *see* Heat
  solaris E900.0
Ignition (accidental)
  anesthetic gas in operating theatre E923.2
  bedclothes
    with
      conflagration — *see* Conflagration
      ignition (of)
        clothing — *see* Ignition, clothes
        highly inflammable material (benzine) (fat) (gasoline) (kerosene) (paraffin) (petrol) E894
  benzine E894
  clothes, clothing (from controlled fire) (in building) E893.9
    with conflagration — *see* Conflagration
    from
      bonfire E893.2
      highly inflammable material E894
      sources or material as listed in E893.8
      trash fire E893.2
      uncontrolled fire — *see* Conflagration

Ignition — *continued*
  clothes, clothing — *continued*
    in
      private dwelling E893.0
      specified building or structure, except private dwelling E893.1
    not in building or structure E893.2
  explosive material — *see* Explosion
  fat E894
  gasoline E894
  kerosene E894
  material
    explosive — *see* Explosion
    highly inflammable E894
      with conflagration — *see* Conflagration
      with explosion E923.2
  nightdress — *see* Ignition, clothes
  paraffin E894
  petrol E894
Immersion — *see* Submersion
Implantation of quills of porcupine E906.8
Inanition (from) E904.9
  hunger — *see* Lack of, food
  resulting from homicidal intent E968.4
  thirst — *see* Lack of, water
Inattention after, at birth E904.0
  homicidal, infanticidal intent E968.4
Infanticide (*see also* Assault)
Ingestion
  foreign body (causing injury) (with obstruction) — *see* Foreign body, alimentary canal
  poisonous substance NEC — *see* Table of Drugs and Chemicals
Inhalation
  excessively cold substance, manmade E901.1
  foreign body — *see* Foreign body, aspiration
  liquid air, hydrogen, nitrogen E901.1
  mucus, not of newborn (with asphyxia, obstruction respiratory passage, suffocation) E912
  phlegm (with asphyxia, obstruction respiratory passage, suffocation) E912
  poisonous gas — *see* Table of Drugs and Chemicals
  smoke from, due to
    fire — *see* Fire
    tobacco, second-hand E869.4
  vomitus (with asphyxia, obstruction respiratory passage, suffocation) E911
Injury, injured (accidental(ly)) NEC E928.9
  by, caused by, from
    air rifle (BB gun) E922.4
    animal (not being ridden) NEC E906.9
      being ridden (in sport or transport) E828 ✓4ᵗʰ
    assault (*see also* Assault) E968.9
    avalanche E909.2
    bayonet (*see also* Bayonet wound) E920.3
    being thrown against some part of, or object in
      motor vehicle (in motion) (on public highway) E818 ✓4ᵗʰ
        not on public highway E825 ✓4ᵗʰ
      nonmotor road vehicle NEC E829 ✓4ᵗʰ
      off-road motor vehicle NEC E821 ✓4ᵗʰ
      railway train E806 ✓4ᵗʰ
      snow vehicle, motor-driven E820 ✓4ᵗʰ
      street car E829 ✓4ᵗʰ
    bending E927
    broken glass E920.8
    bullet — *see* Shooting
    cave-in (*see also* Suffocation, due to, cave-in) E913.3
      earth surface movement or eruption E909.9
      earthquake E909.0
      flood E908.2
      hurricane E908.0
      landslide E909.2
      storm E908.9
      without asphyxiation or suffocation E916
    cloudburst E908.8
    cutting or piercing instrument (*see also* Cut) E920.9
    cyclone E908.1
    earth surface movement or eruption E909.9

Injury, injured — *continued*
  by, caused by, from — *continued*
    earthquake E909 ✓4ᵗʰ
    electric current (*see also* Electric shock) E925.9
    explosion (*see also* Explosion) E923.9
    fire — *see* Fire
    flare, Verey pistol E922.8
    flood E908
    foreign body — *see* Foreign body
    hailstones E904.3
    hurricane E908
    landslide E909 ✓4ᵗʰ
    law-enforcing agent, police, in course of legal intervention — *see* Legal intervention
    lightning E907
    live rail or live wire — *see* Electric shock
    machinery — *see also* Accident, machine
      aircraft, without accident to aircraft E844 ✓4ᵗʰ
      boat, ship, watercraft (deck) (engine room) (galley) (laundry) (loading) E836 ✓4ᵗʰ
    missile
      explosive E923.8
      firearm — *see* Shooting
      in
        terrorism — *see* Terrorism, missile ●
        war operations — *see* War operations, missile
    moving part of motor vehicle (in motion) (on public highway) E818 ✓4ᵗʰ
      not on public highway, nontraffic accident E825 ✓4ᵗʰ
      while alighting, boarding, entering, leaving — *see* Fall, from, motor vehicle, while alighting, boarding
    nail E920.8
    needle (sewing) E920.4
      hypodermic E920.5
    noise E928.1
    object
      fallen on
        motor vehicle (in motion) (on public highway) E818 ✓4ᵗʰ
          not on public highway E825 ✓4ᵗʰ
      falling — *see* Hit by, object, falling
    paintball gun E922.5 ●
    radiation — *see* Radiation
    railway rolling stock, train, vehicle (part of) E805 ✓4ᵗʰ
      door or window E806 ✓4ᵗʰ
    rotating propeller, aircraft E844 ✓4ᵗʰ
    rough landing of off-road type motor vehicle (after leaving ground or rough terrain) E821 ✓4ᵗʰ
    snow vehicle E820 ✓4ᵗʰ
    saber (*see also* Wound, saber) E920.3
    shot — *see* Shooting
    sound waves E928.1
    splinter or sliver, wood E920.8
    straining E927
    street car (door) E829 ✓4ᵗʰ
    suicide (attempt) E958.9
    sword E920.3
    terrorism — *see* Terrorism ●
    third rail — *see* Electric shock
    thunderbolt E907
    tidal wave E909.4
      caused by storm E908.0
    tornado E908.1
    torrential rain E908.2
    twisting E927
    vehicle NEC — *see* Accident, vehicle NEC
    vibration E928.2
    volcanic eruption E909.1
    weapon burst, in war operations E993
    weightlessness (in spacecraft, real or simulated) E928.0
    wood splinter or sliver E920.8
  due to
    civil insurrection — *see* War operations occurring after cessation of hostilities E998
    terrorism — *see* Terrorism ●

Hit — Injury (side tab)

Injury, injured — *continued*
due to — *continued*
war operations — *see* War operations
occurring after cessation of hostilities
E998
homicidal (*see also* Assault) E968.9
in, on
civil insurrection — *see* War operations
fight E960.0
parachute descent (voluntary) (without
accident to aircraft) E844 ✓4th
with accident to aircraft — *see* categories
E840-E842 ✓4th
public highway E819 ✓4th
railway right of way E807 ✓4th
terrorism — *see* Terrorism ●
war operations — *see* War operations
inflicted (by)
in course of arrest (attempted), suppression
of disturbance, maintenance of order,
by law enforcing agents — *see* Legal
intervention
law-enforcing agent (on duty) — *see* Legal
intervention
other person
stated as
accidental E928.9
homicidal, intentional — *see* Assault
undetermined whether accidental or
intentional — *see* Injury, stated
as undetermined
police (on duty) — *see* Legal intervention
late effect of E929.9
purposely (inflicted) by other person(s) — *see*
Assault
self-inflicted (unspecified whether accidental or
intentional) E988.9
stated as
accidental E928.9
intentionally, purposely E958.9
specified cause NEC E928.8
stated as
undetermined whether accidentally or
purposely inflicted (by) E988.9
cut (any part of body) E986
cutting or piercing instrument
(classifiable to E920) E986
drowning E984
explosive(s) (missile) E985.5
falling from high place E987.9
manmade structure, except residential
E987.1
natural site E987.2
residential premises E987.0
hanging E983.0
knife E986
late effect of E989
puncture (any part of body) E986
shooting — *see* Shooting, stated as
undetermined whether accidental or
intentional
specified means NEC E988.8
stab (any part of body) E986
strangulation — *see* Suffocation, stated as
undetermined whether accidental or
intentional
submersion E984
suffocation — *see* Suffocation, stated as
undetermined whether accidental or
intentional
to child due to criminal abortion E968.8
Insufficient nourishment — *see also* Lack of,
food
homicidal intent E968.4
Insulation, effects — *see* Heat
Interruption of respiration by
food lodged in esophagus E911
foreign body, except food, in esophagus E912
Intervention, legal — *see* Legal intervention
Intoxication, drug or poison — *see* Table of
Drugs and Chemicals
Irradiation — *see* Radiation

J

Jammed (accidentally)
between objects (moving) (stationary and
moving) E918
in object E918
Jumped or fell from high place, so stated —
see Jumping, from, high place, stated as
in undetermined circumstances
Jumping
before train, vehicle or other moving object
(unspecified whether accidental or
intentional) E988.0
stated as
intentional, purposeful E958.0
suicidal (attempt) E958.0
from
aircraft
by parachute (voluntarily) (without
accident to aircraft) E844 ✓4th
due to accident to aircraft — *see*
categories E840-E842 ✓4th
boat, ship, watercraft (into water)
after accident to, fire on, watercraft
E830 ✓4th
and subsequently struck by (part of)
boat E831 ✓4th
burning, crushed, sinking E830 ✓4th
and subsequently struck by (part of)
boat E831 ✓4th
voluntarily, without accident (to boat)
with injury other than drowning or
submersion E883.0
building ▶— *see also* Jumping, from, high
place◀
burning ▶(uncontrolled fire)◀ E891.8 ●
in terrorism E979.3
private E890.8
cable car (not on rails) E847
on rails E829 ✓4th
high place
in accidental circumstances or in sport —
see categories E880-E884 ✓4th
stated as
with intent to injure self E957.9
man-made structures NEC E957.1
natural sites E957.2
residential premises E957.0
in undetermined circumstances
E987.9
man-made structures NEC E987.1
natural sites E987.2
residential premises E987.0
suicidal (attempt) E957.9
man-made structures NEC E957.1
natural sites E957.1
residential premises E957.0
motor vehicle (in motion) (on public
highway) — *see* Fall, from, motor
vehicle
nonmotor road vehicle NEC E829 ✓4th
street car E829 ✓4th
structure ▶— *see also* Jumping, from, high
place◀
burning NEC (uncontrolled fire) ●
E891.8 ●
in terrorism E979.3 ●
into water
with injury other than drowning or
submersion E883.0
drowning or submersion — *see*
Submersion
from, off, watercraft — *see* Jumping, from,
boat
Justifiable homicide — *see* Assault

K

Kicked by
animal E906.8
person(s) (accidentally) E917.9
with intent to injure or kill E960.0
as, or caused by a crowd E917.1
with subsequent fall E917.6
in fight E960.0

Kicked by — *continued*
person(s) — *continued*
in sports E917.0
with subsequent fall E917.5
Kicking against
object (moving) E917.9
in sports E917.0
with subsequent fall E917.5
stationary E917.4
with subsequent fall E917.8
person — *see* Striking against, person
Killed, killing (accidentally) NEC (*see also* Injury)
E928.9
in
action — *see* War operations
brawl, fight (hand) (fists) (foot) E960.0
by weapon — *see also* Assault
cutting, piercing E966
firearm — *see* Shooting, homicide
self
stated as
accident E928.9
suicide — *see* Suicide
unspecified whether accidental or suicidal
E988.9
Knocked down (accidentally) (by) NEC E928.9
animal (not being ridden) E906.8
being ridden (in sport or transport) E828 ✓4th
blast from explosion (*see also* Explosion)
E923.9
crowd, human stampede E917.6
late effect of — *see* Late effect
person (accidentally) E917.9
in brawl, fight E960.0
in sports E917.5
transport vehicle — *see* vehicle involved under
Hit by
while boxing E917.5

L

Laceration NEC E928.9
Lack of
air (refrigerator or closed place), suffocation by
E913.2
care (helpless person) (infant) (newborn) E904.0
homicidal intent E968.4
food except as result of transport accident
E904.1
helpless person, infant, newborn due to
abandonment or neglect E904.0
water except as result of transport accident
E904.2
helpless person, infant, newborn due to
abandonment or neglect E904.0
Landslide E909.2
falling on, hitting
motor vehicle (any) (in motion) (on or off
public highway) E909.2
railway rolling stock, train, vehicle E909.2
Late effect of
accident NEC (accident classifiable to E928.9)
E929.9
specified NEC (accident classifiable to E910-
E928.8) E929.8
assault E969
fall, accidental (accident classifiable to E880-
E888) E929.3
fire, accident caused by (accident classifiable to
E890-E899) E929.4
homicide, attempt (any means) E969
injury due to terrorism E999.1 ●
injury undetermined whether accidentally or
purposely inflicted (injury classifiable to
E980-E988) E989
legal intervention (injury classifiable to E970-
E976) E977
medical or surgical procedure, test or therapy
as, or resulting in, or from
abnormal or delayed reaction or
complication — *see* Reaction,
abnormal
misadventure — *see* Misadventure
motor vehicle accident (accident classifiable to
E810-E825) E929.0

Late effect of — *continued*
  natural or environmental factor, accident due
    to (accident classifiable to E900-E909)
    E929.5
  poisoning, accidental (accident classifiable to
    E850-E858, E860-E869) E929.2
  suicide, attempt (any means) E959
  transport accident NEC (accident classifiable to
    E800-E807, E826-E838, E840-E848)
    E929.1
  war operations, injury due to (injury
    classifiable to E990-E998) E999.0 ▲
Launching pad accident E845 ☑4ᵗʰ
Legal
  execution, any method E978
  intervention (by) (injury from) E976
    baton E973
    bayonet E974
    blow E975
    blunt object (baton) (nightstick) (stave)
      (truncheon) E973
    cutting or piercing instrument E974
    dynamite E971
    execution, any method E973
    explosive(s) (shell) E971
    firearm(s) E970
    gas (asphyxiation) (poisoning) (tear) E972
    grenade E971
    late effect of E977
    machine gun E970
    manhandling E975
    mortar bomb E971
    nightstick E973
    revolver E970
    rifle E970
    specified means NEC E975
    stabbing E974
    stave E973
    truncheon E973
Lifting, injury in E927
Lightning (shock) (stroke) (struck by) E907
Liquid (noncorrosive) in eye E914
  corrosive E924.1
Loss of control
  motor vehicle (on public highway) (without
    antecedent collision) E816 ☑4ᵗʰ
    with
      antecedent collision on public highway —
        see Collision, motor vehicle
      involving any object, person or vehicle
        not on public highway E816 ☑4ᵗʰ
      on public highway — *see* Collision,
        motor vehicle
      not on public highway, nontraffic
        accident E825 ☑4ᵗʰ
        with antecedent collision — *see*
          Collision, motor vehicle, not
          on public highway
  off-road type motor vehicle (not on public
    highway) E821 ☑4ᵗʰ
    on public highway — *see* Loss of control,
      motor vehicle
  snow vehicle, motor-driven (not on public
    highway) E820 ☑4ᵗʰ
    on public highway — *see* Loss of control,
      motor vehicle
Lost at sea E832 ☑4ᵗʰ
  with accident to watercraft E830 ☑4ᵗʰ
  in war operations E995
Low
  pressure, effects — *see* Effects of, air pressure
  temperature, effects — *see* Cold, exposure to
**Lying before train, vehicle or other moving
  object** (unspecified whether accidental or
  intentional) E988.0
  stated as intentional, purposeful, suicidal
    (attempt) E958.0
Lynching (*see also* Assault) E968.9

M

**Malfunction, atomic power plant in water
  transport** E838 ☑4ᵗʰ
Mangled (accidentally) NEC E928.9

Manhandling (in brawl, fight) E960.0
  legal intervention E975
Manslaughter (nonaccidental) — *see* Assault
Marble in nose E912
Mauled by animal E906.8
Medical procedure, complication of
  delayed or as an abnormal reaction
    without mention of misadventure — *see*
      Reaction, abnormal
    due to or as a result of misadventure — *see*
      Misadventure
Melting of fittings and furniture in burning ●
  in terrorism E979.3 ●
Minamata disease E865.2
**Misadventure(s) to patient(s) during surgical or
  medical care** E876.9
  contaminated blood, fluid, drug or biological
    substance (presence of agents and toxins
    as listed in E875) E875.9
    administered (by) NEC E875.9
      infusion E875.0
      injection E875.1
      specified means NEC E875.2
      transfusion E875.0
      vaccination E875.1
  cut, cutting, puncture, perforation or
    hemorrhage (accidental) (inadvertent)
    (inappropriate) (during) E870.9
    aspiration of fluid or tissue (by puncture or
      catheterization, except heart) E870.5
    biopsy E870.8
      needle (aspirating) E870.5
    blood sampling E870.5
    catheterization E870.5
      heart E870.6
    dialysis (kidney) E870.2
    endoscopic examination E870.4
    enema E870.7
    infusion E870.1
    injection E870.3
    lumbar puncture E870.5
    needle biopsy E870.5
    paracentesis, abdominal E870.5
    perfusion E870.2
    specified procedure NEC E870.8
    surgical operation E870.0
    thoracentesis E870.5
    transfusion E870.1
    vaccination E870.3
  excessive amount of blood or other fluid during
    transfusion or infusion E873.0
  failure
    in dosage E873.9
      electroshock therapy E873.4
      inappropriate temperature (too hot or too
        cold) in local application and
        packing E873.5
      infusion
        excessive amount of fluid E873.0
        incorrect dilution of fluid E873.1
      insulin-shock therapy E873.4
      nonadministration of necessary drug or
        medicinal E873.6
      overdose — *see also* Overdose
        radiation, in therapy E873.2
      radiation
        inadvertent exposure of patient
          (receiving radiation for test or
          therapy) E873.3
        not receiving radiation for test or
          therapy — *see* Radiation
      overdose E873.2
      specified procedure NEC E873.8
      transfusion
        excessive amount of blood E873.0
    mechanical, of instrument or apparatus
      (during procedure) E874.9
      aspiration of fluid or tissue (by puncture
        or catheterization, except of heart)
        E874.4
      biopsy E874.8
        needle (aspirating) E874.4
      blood sampling E874.4
      catheterization E874.4
        heart E874.5

**Misadventure(s) to patient(s) during surgical or
  medical care** — *continued*
  failure — *continued*
    mechanical, of instrument or apparatus —
      continued
      dialysis (kidney) E874.2
      endoscopic examination E874.3
      enema E874.8
      infusion E874.1
      injection E874.8
      lumbar puncture E874.4
      needle biopsy E874.4
      paracentesis, abdominal E874.4
      perfusion E874.2
      specified procedure NEC E874.8
      surgical operation E874.0
      thoracentesis E874.4
      transfusion E874.1
      vaccination E874.8
    sterile precautions (during procedure)
      E872.9
      aspiration of fluid or tissue (by puncture
        or catheterization, except heart)
        E872.5
      biopsy E872.8
        needle (aspirating) E872.5
      blood sampling E872.5
      catheterization E872.5
        heart E872.6
      dialysis (kidney) E872.2
      endoscopic examination E872.4
      enema E872.8
      infusion E872.1
      injection E872.3
      lumbar puncture E872.5
      needle biopsy E872.5
      paracentesis, abdominal E872.5
      perfusion E872.2
      removal of catheter or packing E872.8
      specified procedure NEC E872.8
      surgical operation E872.0
      thoracentesis E872.5
      transfusion E872.1
      vaccination E872.3
    suture or ligature during surgical procedure
      E876.2
    to introduce or to remove tube or
      instrument E876.4
      foreign object left in body — *see*
        Misadventure, foreign object
  foreign object left in body (during procedure)
    E871.9
    aspiration of fluid or tissue (by puncture or
      catheterization, except heart) E871.5
    biopsy E871.8
      needle (aspirating) E871.5
    blood sampling E871.5
    catheterization E871.5
      heart E871.6
    dialysis (kidney) E871.2
    endoscopic examination E871.4
    enema E871.8
    infusion E871.1
    injection E871.3
    lumbar puncture E871.5
    needle biopsy E871.5
    paracentesis, abdominal E871.5
    perfusion E871.2
    removal of catheter or packing E871.7
    specified procedure NEC E871.8
    surgical operation E871.0
    thoracentesis E871.5
    transfusion E871.1
    vaccination E871.3
  hemorrhage — *see* Misadventure, cut
  inadvertent exposure of patient to radiation
    (being received for test or therapy) E873.3
  inappropriate
    operation performed E876.5
    temperature (too hot or too cold) in local
      application or packing E873.5
  infusion — *see also* Misadventure, by specific
    type, infusion
    excessive amount of fluid E873.0
    incorrect dilution of fluid E873.1
    wrong fluid E876.1
  mismatched blood in transfusion E876.0

Misadventure(s) — Puncture

Misadventure(s) to patient(s) during surgical or medical care — *continued*
  nonadministration of necessary drug or medicinal E873.6
  overdose — *see also* Overdose
    radiation, in therapy E873.2
  perforation — *see* Misadventure, cut
  performance of inappropriate operation E876.5
  puncture — *see* Misadventure, cut
  specified type NEC E876.8
    failure
      suture or ligature during surgical operation E876.2
      to introduce or to remove tube or instrument E876.4
      foreign object left in body E871.9
    infusion of wrong fluid E876.1
    performance of inappropriate operation E876.5
    transfusion of mismatched blood E876.0
    wrong
      fluid in infusion E876.1
      placement of endotracheal tube during anesthetic procedure E876.3
  transfusion — *see also* Misadventure, by specific type, transfusion
    excessive amount of blood E873.0
    mismatched blood E876.0
  wrong
    drug given in error — *see* Table of Drugs and Chemicals
    fluid in infusion E876.1
    placement of endotracheal tube during anesthetic procedure E876.3

Motion (effects) E903
  sickness E903

Mountain sickness E902.0

Mucus aspiration or inhalation, not of newborn (with asphyxia, obstruction respiratory passage, suffocation) E912

Mudslide of cataclysmic nature E909.2

Murder (attempt) (*see also* Assault) E968.9

N

Nail, injury by E920.8

Needlestick (sewing needle) E920.4
  hypodermic E920.5

Neglect — *see also* Privation
  criminal E968.4
  homicidal intent E968.4

Noise (causing injury) (pollution) E928.1

O

Object
  falling
    from, in, on, hitting
      aircraft E844 ☑4ᵗʰ
        due to accident to aircraft — *see* categories E840-E842 ☑4ᵗʰ
      machinery — *see* Accident, machine
        not in operation E916
      motor vehicle (in motion) (on public highway) E818 ☑4ᵗʰ
        not on public highway E825 ☑4ᵗʰ
        stationary E916
      nonmotor road vehicle NEC E829 ☑4ᵗʰ
      pedal cycle E826 ☑4ᵗʰ
      person E916
      railway rolling stock, train, vehicle E806 ☑4ᵗʰ
      street car E829 ☑4ᵗʰ
      watercraft E838 ☑4ᵗʰ
        due to accident to watercraft E831 ☑4ᵗʰ
  set in motion by
    accidental explosion of pressure vessel — *see* category E921 ☑4ᵗʰ
    firearm — *see* category E922 ☑4ᵗʰ
    machine(ry) — *see* Accident, machine
    transport vehicle — *see* categories E800-E848 ☑4ᵗʰ

Object — *continued*
  thrown from, in, on, towards
    aircraft E844 ☑4ᵗʰ
    cable car (not on rails) E847
      on rails E829 ☑4ᵗʰ
    motor vehicle (in motion) (on public highway) E818 ☑4ᵗʰ
      not on public highway E825 ☑4ᵗʰ
    nonmotor road vehicle NEC E829 ☑4ᵗʰ
    pedal cycle E826 ☑4ᵗʰ
    street car E829 ☑4ᵗʰ
    vehicle NEC — *see* Accident, vehicle NEC

Obstruction
  air passages, larynx, respiratory passages
    by
      external means NEC — *see* Suffocation
      food, any type (regurgitated) (vomited) E911
      material or object, except food E912
      mucus E912
      phlegm E912
      vomitus E911
  digestive tract, except mouth or pharynx
    by
      food, any type E915
      foreign body (any) E915
  esophagus
    food E911
    foreign body, except food E912
    without asphyxia or obstruction of respiratory passage E915
  mouth or pharynx
    by
      food, any type E911
      material or object, except food E912
  respiration — *see* Obstruction, air passages

Oil in eye E914

Overdose
  anesthetic (drug) — *see* Table of Drugs and Chemicals
  drug — *see* Table of Drugs and Chemicals

Overexertion (lifting) (pulling) (pushing) E927

Overexposure (accidental) (to)
  cold (*see also* Cold, exposure to) E901.9
    due to manmade conditions E901.1
  heat (*see also* Heat) E900.9
  radiation — *see* Radiation
  radioactivity — *see* Radiation
  sun, except sunburn E900.0
  weather — *see* Exposure
  wind — *see* Exposure

Overheated (*see also* Heat) E900.9

Overlaid E913.0

Overturning (accidental)
  animal-drawn vehicle E827 ☑4ᵗʰ
  boat, ship, watercraft
    causing
      drowning, submersion E830 ☑4ᵗʰ
      injury except drowning, submersion E831 ☑4ᵗʰ
  machinery — *see* Accident, machine
  motor vehicle (*see also* Loss of control, motor vehicle) E816 ☑4ᵗʰ
    with antecedent collision on public highway — *see* Collision, motor vehicle
    not on public highway, nontraffic accident E825 ☑4ᵗʰ
      with antecedent collision — *see* Collision, motor vehicle, not on public highway
  nonmotor road vehicle NEC E829 ☑4ᵗʰ
  off-road type motor vehicle — *see* Loss of control, off-road type motor vehicle
  pedal cycle E826 ☑4ᵗʰ
  railway rolling stock, train, vehicle (*see also* Derailment, railway) E802 ☑4ᵗʰ
  street car E829 ☑4ᵗʰ
  vehicle NEC — *see* Accident, vehicle NEC

P

Palsy, divers' E902.2

Parachuting (voluntary) (without accident to aircraft) E844 ☑4ᵗʰ

Parachuting — *continued*
  due to accident to aircraft — *see* categories E840-E842 ☑4ᵗʰ

Paralysis
  divers' E902.2
  lead or saturnine E866.0
    from pesticide NEC E863.4

Pecked by bird E906.8

Phlegm aspiration or inhalation (with asphyxia, obstruction respiratory passage, suffocation) E912

Piercing (*see also* Cut) E920.9

Pinched
  between objects (moving) (stationary and moving) E918
  in object E918

Pinned under
  machine(ry) — *see* Accident, machine

Place of occurrence of accident — *see* Accident (to), occurring (at) (in)

Plumbism E866.0
  from insecticide NEC E863.4

Poisoning (accidental) (by) — *see also* Table of Drugs and Chemicals
  carbon monoxide
    generated by
      aircraft in transit E844 ☑4ᵗʰ
      motor vehicle
        in motion (on public highway) E818 ☑4ᵗʰ
          not on public highway E825 ☑4ᵗʰ
      watercraft (in transit) (not in transit) E838 ☑4ᵗʰ
  caused by injection of poisons or toxins into or through skin by plant thorns, spines, or other mechanism E905.7
    marine or sea plants E905.6
  fumes or smoke due to
    conflagration — *see* Conflagration
    explosion or fire — *see* Fire
    ignition — *see* Ignition
  gas
    in legal intervention E972
    legal execution, by E978
    on watercraft E838 ☑4ᵗʰ
    used as anesthetic — *see* Table of Drugs and Chemicals
  in
    terrorism (chemical weapons) E979.7 ●
    war operations E997.2
  late effect of — *see* Late effect
  legal
    execution E978
    intervention
      by gas E972

Pressure, external, causing asphyxia, suffocation (*see also* Suffocation) E913.9

Privation E904.9
  food (*see also* Lack of, food) E904.1
  helpless person, infant, newborn due to abandonment or neglect E904.0
  late effect of NEC E929.5
  resulting from transport accident — *see* categories E800-E848 ☑4ᵗʰ
  water (*see also* Lack of, water) E904.2

Projected objects, striking against or struck by — *see* Striking against, object

Prolonged stay in
  high altitude (causing conditions as listed in E902.0) E902.0
  weightless environment E928.0

Prostration
  heat — *see* Heat

Pulling, injury in E927

Puncture, puncturing (*see also* Cut) E920.9
  by
    plant thorns or spines E920.8
      toxic reaction E905.7
        marine or sea plants E905.6
    sea-urchin spine E905.6

Scald — Sting

Scald, scalding — *continued*
  inflicted by other person
    stated as
      intentional or homicidal E968.3
      undetermined whether accidental or
        intentional E988.2
  late effect of NEC E929.8
  liquid (boiling) (hot) E924.0
  local application of externally applied
    substance in medical or surgical care
    E873.5
  molten metal E924.0
  self-inflicted (unspecified whether accidental or
    intentional) E988.2
    stated as intentional, purposeful E958.2
  stated as undetermined whether accidental or
    intentional E988.2
  steam E924.0
  tap water (boiling) E924.2
  transport accident — *see* catagories E800-E848
  vapor E924.0

Scratch, cat E906.8

Sea
  sickness E903

Self-mutilation — *see* Suicide

Sequelae (of)
  in
    terrorism E999.1
    war operations E999.0

Shock
  anaphylactic (*see also* Table of Drugs and
    Chemicals) E947.9
    due to
      bite (venomous) — *see* Bite, venomous
        NEC
      sting — *see* Sting
  electric (*see also* Electric shock) E925.9
  from electric appliance or current (*see also*
    Electric shock) E925.9

Shooting, shot (accidental(ly)) E922.9
  air gun E922.4
  BB gun E922.4
  hand gun (pistol) (revolver) E922.0
  himself (*see also* Shooting, self-inflicted)
    E985.4
    hand gun (pistol) (revolver) E985.0
    military firearm, except hand gun E985.3
      hand gun (pistol) (revolver) E985.0
    rifle (hunting) E985.2
      military E985.3
    shotgun (automatic) E985.1
    specified firearm NEC E985.4
    Verey pistol E985.4
  homicide (attempt) E965.4
    air gun E968.6
    BB gun E968.6
    hand gun (pistol) (revolver) E965.0
    military firearm, except hand gun E965.3
      hand gun (pistol) (revolver) E965.0
    paintball gun E965.4
    rifle (hunting) E965.2
      military E965.3
    shotgun (automatic) E965.1
    specified firearm NEC E965.4
    Verey pistol E965.4
  inflicted by other person
    in accidental circumstances E922.9
      hand gun (pistol) (revolver) E922.0
      military firearm, except hand gun E922.3
        hand gun (pistol) (revolver) E922.0
      rifle (hunting) E922.2
        military E922.3
      shotgun (automatic) E922.1
      specified firearm NEC E922.8
      Verey pistol E922.8
    stated as
      intentional, homicidal E965.4
        hand gun (pistol) (revolver) E965.0
        military firearm, except hand gun
          E965.3
          hand gun (pistol) (revolver) E965.0
        paintball gun E965.4
        rifle (hunting) E965.2
          military E965.3
        shotgun (automatic) E965.1
        specified firearm E965.4

Shooting, shot — *continued*
  inflicted by other person — *continued*
    stated as — *continued*
      intentional, homicidal — *continued*
        Verey pistol E965.4
      undetermined whether accidental or
        intentional E985.4
        air gun E985.6
        BB gun E985.6
        hand gun (pistol) (revolver) E985.0
        military firearm, except hand gun
          E985.3
          hand gun (pistol) (revolver) E985.0
        paintball gun E985.7
        rifle (hunting) E985.2
        shotgun (automatic) E985.1
        specified firearm NEC E985.4
        Verey pistol E985.4
  in
    terrorism — *see* Terrorism, shooting
    war operations — *see* War operations,
      shooting
  legal
    execution E978
    intervention E970
  military firearm, except hand gun E922.3
    hand gun (pistol) (revolver) E922.0
  paintball gun E922.5
  rifle (hunting) E922.2
    military E922.3
  self-inflicted (unspecified whether accidental or
    intentional) E985.4
    air gun E985.6
    BB gun E985.6
    hand gun (pistol) (revolver) E985.0
    military firearm, except hand gun E985.3
      hand gun (pistol) (revolver) E985.0
    paintball gun E985.7
    rifle (hunting) E985.2
      military E985.3
    shotgun (automatic) E985.1
    specified firearm NEC E985.4
    stated as
      accidental E922.9
        hand gun (pistol) (revolver) E922.0
        military firearm, except hand gun
          E922.3
          hand gun (pistol) (revolver) E922.0
        paintball gun E922.5
        rifle (hunting) E922.2
          military E922.3
        shotgun (automatic) E922.1
        specified firearm NEC E922.8
        Verey pistol E922.8
      intentional, purposeful E955.4
        hand gun (pistol) (revolver) E955.0
        military firearm, except hand gun
          E955.3
          hand gun (pistol) (revolver) E955.0
        paintball gun E955.7
        rifle (hunting) E955.2
          military E955.3
        shotgun (automatic) E955.1
        specified firearm NEC E955.4
        Verey pistol E955.4
    shotgun (automatic) E922.1
    specified firearm NEC E922.8
    stated as undetermined whether accidental or
      intentional E985.4
    hand gun (pistol) (revolver) E985.0
    military firearm, except hand gun E985.3
      hand gun (pistol) (revolver) E985.0
    paintball gun E985.7
    rifle (hunting) E985.2
      military E985.3
    shotgun (automatic) E985.1
    specified firearm NEC E985.4
    Verey pistol E985.4
  suicidal (attempt) E955.4
    air gun E955.6
    BB gun E955.6
    hand gun (pistol) (revolver) E955.0
    military firearm, except hand gun E955.3
      hand gun (pistol) (revolver) E955.0
    paintball gun E955.7
    rifle (hunting) E955.2
      military E955.3

Shooting, shot — *continued*
  suicidal — *continued*
    shotgun (automatic) E955.1
    specified firearm NEC E955.4
    Verey pistol E955.4
  Verey pistol E922.8

Shoving (accidentally) by other person (*see also*
  Pushing by other person) E917.9

Sickness
  air E903
  alpine E902.0
  car E903
  motion E903
  mountain E902.0
  sea E903
  travel E903

Sinking (accidental)
  boat, ship, watercraft (causing drowning,
    submersion) E830 ☑4ᵗʰ
    causing injury except drowning, submersion
      E831 ☑4ᵗʰ

Siriasis E900.0

Skydiving E844 ☑4ᵗʰ

Slashed wrists (*see also* Cut, self-inflicted) E986

Slipping (accidental)
  on
    deck (of boat, ship, watercraft) (icy) (oily)
      (wet) E835 ☑4ᵗʰ
    ice E885
    ladder of ship E833 ☑4ᵗʰ
      due to accident to watercraft E831 ☑4ᵗʰ
    mud E885
    oil E885
    snow E885
    stairs of ship E833 ☑4ᵗʰ
      due to accident to watercraft E831 ☑4ᵗʰ
    surface
      slippery E885
      wet E885

Sliver, wood, injury by E920.8

**Smouldering building or structure in
  terrorism** E979.3

Smothering, smothered (*see also* Suffocation)
  E913.9

Sodomy (assault) E960.1

Solid substance in eye (any part) or adnexa E914

Sound waves (causing injury) E928.1

Splinter, injury by E920.8

Stab, stabbing E966
  accidental — *see* Cut

Starvation E904.1
  helpless person, infant, newborn — *see* Lack of
    food
  homicidal intent E968.4
  late effect of NEC E929.5
  resulting from accident connected with
    transport — *see* catagories E800-E848

Stepped on
  by
    animal (not being ridden) E906.8
      being ridden (in sport or transport)
        E828 ☑4ᵗʰ
    crowd E917.1
    person E917.9
      in sports E917.0
    in sports E917.0

Stepping on
  object (moving) E917.9
    in sports E917.0
      with subsequent fall E917.5
    stationary E917.4
      with subsequent fall E917.8
  person E917.9
    as, or caused by a crowd E917.1
      with subsequent fall E917.6
    in sports E917.0

Sting E905.9
  ant E905.5
  bee E905.3
  caterpillar E905.5
  coral E905.6
  hornet E905.3
  insect NEC E905.5
  jellyfish E905.6

Sting — *continued*
  marine animal or plant E905.6
  nematocysts E905.6
  scorpion E905.2
  sea anemone E905.6
  sea cucumber E905.6
  wasp E905.3
  yellow jacket E905.3
Storm E908.9
  specified type NEC E908.8
Straining, injury in E927
Strangling — *see* Suffocation
Strangulation — *see* Suffocation
Strenuous movements (in recreational or other
  activities) E927
Striking against
  bottom (when jumping or diving into water)
    E883.0
  object (moving) E917.9
    caused by crowd E917.1
      with subsequent fall E917.6
    furniture E917.3
      with subsequent fall E917.7
    in
      running water E917.2
        with drowning or submersion — *see*
          Submersion
      sports E917.0
        with subsequent fall E917.5
    stationary E917.4
      with subsequent fall E917.8
  person(s) E917.9
    with fall E886.9
      in sports E886.0
    as, or caused by, a crowd E917.1
      with subsequent fall E917.6
        in sports E917.0
          with fall E886.0
Stroke
  heat — *see* Heat
  lightning E907
Struck by — *see also* Hit by
  bullet
    in
      terrorism E979.4
      war operations E991.2
        rubber E991.0
  lightning E907
  missile
    in terrorism — *see* Terrorism, missile
  object
    falling
      from, in, on
        building
          burning (uncontrolled fire)
            in terrorism E979.3
  thunderbolt E907
**Stumbling over animal, carpet, curb, rug or
  (small) object (with fall)** E885
  without fall — *see* Striking against, object
Submersion (accidental) E910.8
  boat, ship, watercraft (causing drowning,
    submersion) E830 ☑4ᵗʰ
    causing injury except drowning, submersion
      E831 ☑4ᵗʰ
  by other person
    in accidental circumstances — *see* category
      E910 ☑4ᵗʰ
    intentional, homicidal E964
    stated as undetermined whether due to
      accidental or intentional E984
  due to
    accident
      machinery — *see* Accident, machine
      to boat, ship, watercraft E830 ☑4ᵗʰ
      transport — *see* categories
        E800–E848 ☑4ᵗʰ
    avalanche E909.2
    cataclysmic
      earth surface movement or eruption E909.9
      storm E908.9
    cloudburst E908.8
    cyclone E908.1

Submersion — *continued*
  due to — *continued*
    fall
      from
        boat, ship, watercraft (not involved in
          accident) E832 ☑4ᵗʰ
          burning, crushed E830 ☑4ᵗʰ
          involved in accident, collision
            E830 ☑4ᵗʰ
        gangplank (into water) E832 ☑4ᵗʰ
        overboard NEC E832 ☑4ᵗʰ
    flood E908.2
    hurricane E908.0
    jumping into water E910.8
      from boat, ship, watercraft
        burning, crushed, sinking E830 ☑4ᵗʰ
        involved in accident, collision
          E830 ☑4ᵗʰ
        not involved in accident, for swim
          E910.2
      in recreational activity (without diving
        equipment) E910.2
        with or using diving equipment E910.1
      to rescue another person E910.3
  homicide (attempt) E964
  in
    bathtub E910.4
    specified activity, not sport, transport or
      recreational E910.3
    sport or recreational activity (without diving
      equipment) E910.2
      with or using diving equipment E910.1
    water skiing E910.0
    swimming pool NEC E910.8
  terrorism E979.8
  war operations E995
  water transport E832 ☑4ᵗʰ
    due to accident to boat, ship, watercraft
      E830 ☑4ᵗʰ
  landslide E909.2
    overturning boat, ship, watercraft E909.2
    sinking boat, ship, watercraft E909.2
    submersion boat, ship, watercraft E909.2
  tidal wave E909.4
    caused by storm E908.0
  torrential rain E908.2
  late effect of NEC E929.8
  quenching tank E910.8
  self-inflicted (unspecified whether accidental or
    intentional) E984
    in accidental circumstances — *see* category
      E910 ☑4ᵗʰ
    stated as intentional, purposeful E954
  stated as undetermined whether accidental or
    intentional E984
  suicidal (attempted) E954
  while
    attempting rescue of another person E910.3
    engaged in
      marine salvage E910.3
      underwater construction or repairs
        E910.3
    fishing, not from boat E910.2
    hunting, not from boat E910.2
    ice skating E910.2
    pearl diving E910.3
    placing fishing nets E910.3
    playing in water E910.2
    scuba diving E910.1
      nonrecreational E910.3
    skin diving E910.1
    snorkel diving E910.2
    spear fishing underwater E910.1
    surfboarding E910.2
    swimming (swimming pool) E910.2
    wading (in water) E910.2
    water skiing E910.0
Sucked
  into
    jet (aircraft) E844 ☑4ᵗʰ
Suffocation (accidental) (by external means) (by
  pressure) (mechanical) E913.9
  caused by other person
    in accidental circumstances — *see category*
      E913 ☑4ᵗʰ

Suffocation — *continued*
  caused by other person — *continued*
    stated as
      intentional, homicidal E963
      undetermined whether accidental or
        intentional E983.9
        by, in
          hanging E983.0
          plastic bag E983.1
          specified means NEC E983.8
  due to, by
    avalanche E909.2
    bedclothes E913.0
    bib E913.0
    blanket E913.0
    cave-in E913.3
      caused by cataclysmic earth surface
        movement or eruption E909.9
    conflagration — *see* Conflagration
    explosion — *see* Explosion
    falling earth, other substance E913.3
    fire — *see* Fire
    food, any type (ingestion) (inhalation)
      (regurgitated) (vomited) E911
    foreign body, except food (ingestion)
      (inhalation) E912
    ignition — *see* Ignition
    landslide E909.2
    machine(ry) — *see* Accident, machine
    material, object except food entering by nose
      or mouth, ingested, inhaled E912
    mucus (aspiration) (inhalation), not of
      newborn E912
    phlegm (aspiration) (inhalation) E912
    pillow E913.0
    plastic bag — *see* Suffocation, in, plastic bag
    sheet (plastic) E913.0
    specified means NEC E913.8
    vomitus (aspiration) (inhalation) E911
  homicidal (attempt) E963
  in
    airtight enclosed place E913.2
    baby carriage E913.0
    bed E913.0
    closed place E913.2
    cot, cradle E913.0
    perambulator E913.0
    plastic bag (in accidental circumstances)
      E913.1
      homicidal, purposely inflicted by other
        person E963
      self-inflicted (unspecified whether
        accidental or intentional) E983.1
        in accidental circumstances E913.1
        intentional, suicidal E953.1
      stated as undetermined whether
        accidentally or purposely inflicted
        E983.1
      suicidal, purposely self-inflicted E953.1
    refrigerator E913.2
  self-inflicted — *see also* Suffocation, stated as
    undetermined whether accidental or
    intentional E953.9
    in accidental circumstances — *see* category
      E913 ☑4ᵗʰ
    stated as intentional, purposeful — *see*
      Suicide, suffocation
  stated as undetermined whether accidental or
    intentional E983.9
    by, in
      hanging E983.0
      plastic bag E983.1
      specified means NEC E983.8
  suicidal — *see* Suicide, suffocation
Suicide, suicidal (attempted) (by) E958.9
  burning, burns E958.1
  caustic substance E958.7
    poisoning E950.7
    swallowed E950.7
  cold, extreme E958.3
  cut (any part of body) E956
  cutting or piercing instrument (classifiable to
    E920) E956
  drowning E954
  electrocution E958.4
  explosive(s) (classifiable to E923) E955.5
  fire E958.1

Suicide — Tripping

Suicide, suicidal — *continued*
firearm (classifiable to E922) — *see* Shooting, suicidal
hanging E953.0
jumping
before moving object, train, vehicle E958.0
from high place — *see* Jumping, from, high place, stated as, suicidal
knife E956
late effect of E959
motor vehicle, crashing of E958.5
poisoning — *see* Table of Drugs and Chemicals
puncture (any part of body) E956
scald E958.2
shooting — *see* Shooting, suicidal
specified means NEC E958.8
stab (any part of body) E956
strangulation — *see* Suicide, suffocation
submersion E954
suffocation E953.9
by, in
hanging E953.0
plastic bag E953.1
specified means NEC E953.8
wound NEC E958.9
Sunburn E926.2
Sunstroke E900.0
Supersonic waves (causing injury) E928.1
Surgical procedure, complication of
delayed or as an abnormal reaction without mention of misadventure — *see* Reaction, abnormal
due to or as a result of misadventure — *see* Misadventure
Swallowed, swallowing
foreign body — *see* Foreign body, alimentary canal
poison — *see* Table of Drugs and Chemicals
substance
caustic — *see* Table of Drugs and Chemicals
corrosive — *see* Table or drugs and chemicals
poisonous — *see* Table of Drugs and Chemicals
Swimmers cramp (*see also* category E910 ✓4ᵗʰ) E910.2
not in recreation or sport E910.3
Syndrome, battered
baby or child — *see* Abuse, child
wife — *see* Assault

T

Tackle in sport E886.0
Terrorism (injury) (by) (in) E979.8
air blast E979.2
aircraft burned, destroyed, exploded, shot down E979.1
used as a weapon E979.1
anthrax E979.6
asphyxia from
chemical (weapons) E979.7
fire, conflagration (caused by fire-producing device) E979.3
from nuclear explosion E979.5
gas or fumes E979.7
bayonet E979.8
biological agents E979.6
blast (air) (effects) E979.2
from nuclear explosion E979.5
underwater E979.0
bomb (antipersonnel) (mortar) (explosion) (fragments) E979.2
bullet(s) (from carbine, machine gun, pistol, rifle, shotgun) E979.4
burn from
chemical E979.7
fire, conflagration (caused by fire-producing device) E979.3
from nuclear explosion E979.5
gas E979.7
burning aircraft E979.1
chemical E9797.7
cholera E979.6
conflagration E9779.3
crushed by falling aircraft E979.1

Terrorism — *continued*
depth-charge E979.0
destruction of aircraft E979.1
disability, as sequelae one year or more after injury E999.1
drowning E979.8
effect
of nuclear weapon (direct) (secondary) E979.5
secondary NEC E979.9
sequelae E999.1
explosion (artillery shell) (breech-block) (cannon block) E979.2
aircraft E979.1
bomb (antipersonnel) (mortar) E979.2
nuclear (atom) (hydrogen) E979.5
depth-charge E979.0
grenade E979.2
injury by fragments from E979.2
land-mine E979.2
marine weapon E979.0
mine (land) E979.2
at sea or in harbor E979.0
marine E979.0
missile (explosive) NEC E979.2
munitions (dump) (factory) E979.2
nuclear (weapon) E979.5
other direct and secondary effects of E979.5
sea-based artillery shell E979.0
torpedo E979.0
exposure to ionizing radiation from nuclear explosion E979.5
falling aircraft E979.1
fire or fire-producing device E979.3
firearms E979.4
fireball effects from nuclear explosion E979.5
fragments from artillery shell, bomb NEC, grenade, guided missile, land-mine, rocket, shell, shrapnel E979.2
gas or fumes E979.7
grenade (explosion) (fragments) E979.2
guided missile (explosion) (fragments) E979.2
nuclear E979.5
heat from nuclear explosion E979.5
hot substances E979.3
hydrogen cyanide E979.7
land-mine (explosion) (fragments) E979.2
laser(s) E979.8
late effect of E999.1
lewisite E979.7
lung irritant (chemical) (fumes) (gas) E979.7
marine mine E979.0
mine E979.2
at sea E979.0
in harbor E979.0
land (explosion) (fragments) E979.2
marine E979.0
missile (explosion) (fragments) (guided) E979.2
marine E979.0
nuclear E979.5
mortar bomb (explosion) (fragments) E979.2
mustard gas E979.7
nerve gas E979.7
nuclear weapons E979.5
pellets (shotgun) E979.4
petrol bomb E979.3
piercing object E979.8
phosgene E979.7
poisoning (chemical) (fumes) (gas) E979.7
radiation, ionizing from nuclear explosion E979.5
rocket (explosion) (fragments) E979.2
saber, sabre E979.8
sarin E979.7
screening smoke E979.7
sequelae effect (of) E999.1
shell (aircraft) (artillery) (cannon) (land-based) (explosion) (fragments) E979.2
sea-based E979.0
shooting E979.4
bullet(s) E979.4
pellet(s) (rifle) (shotgun) E979.4
shrapnel E979.2

Terrorism — *continued*
smallpox E979.7
stabbing object(s) E979.8
submersion E979.8
torpedo E979.0
underwater blast E979.0
vesicant (chemical) (fumes) (gas) E979.7
weapon burst E979.2
Thermic fever E900.9
Thermoplegia E900.9
Thirst — *see also* Lack of water
resulting from accident connected with transport — *see* categories E800-E848 ✓4ᵗʰ
Thrown (accidently)
against object in or part of vehicle
by motion of vehicle
aircraft E844 ✓4ᵗʰ
boat, ship, watercraft E838 ✓4ᵗʰ
motor vehicle (on public highway) E818 ✓4ᵗʰ
not on public highway E825 ✓4ᵗʰ
off-road type (not on public highway) E821 ✓4ᵗʰ
on public highway E818 ✓4ᵗʰ
snow vehicle E820 ✓4ᵗʰ
on public high-way E818 ✓4ᵗʰ
nonmotor road vehicle NEC E829 ✓4ᵗʰ
railway rolling stock, train, vehicle E806 ✓4ᵗʰ
street car E829 ✓4ᵗʰ
from
animal (being ridden) (in sport or transport) E828 ✓4ᵗʰ
high place, homicide (attempt) E968.1
machinery — *see* Accident, machine
vehicle NEC — *see* Accident, vehicle NEC
off — *see* Thrown, from
overboard (by motion of boat, ship, watercraft) E832 ✓4ᵗʰ
by accident to boat, ship, watercraft E830 ✓4ᵗʰ
Thunderbolt NEC E907
Tidal wave (any injury) E909.4
caused by storm E908.0
Took
overdose of drug — *see* Table of Drugs and Chemicals
poison — *see* Table of Drugs and Chemicals
Tornado (any injury) E908.1
Torrential rain (any injury) E908.2
Traffic accident NEC E819 ✓4ᵗʰ
Trampled by animal E906.8
being ridden (in sport or transport) E828 ✓4ᵗʰ
Trapped (accidently)
between
objects (moving) (stationary and moving) E918
by
door of
elevator E918
motor vehicle (on public highway) (while alighting, boarding) — *see* Fall, from, motor vehicle, while alighting
railway train (underground) E806 ✓4ᵗʰ
street car E829 ✓4ᵗʰ
subway train E806 ✓4ᵗʰ
in object E918
Travel (effects) E903
sickness E903
Tree
falling on or hitting E916
motor vehicle (in motion) (on public highway) E818 ✓4ᵗʰ
not on public highway E825 ✓4ᵗʰ
nonmotor road vehicle NEC E829 ✓4ᵗʰ
pedal cycle E826 ✓4ᵗʰ
person E916
railway rolling stock, train, vehicle E806 ✓4ᵗʰ
street car E829 ✓4ᵗʰ
Trench foot E901.0
Tripping over animal, carpet, curb, rug, or small object (with fall) E885
without fall — *see* Striking against, object

Tsunami E909.4
Twisting, injury in E927

V

Violence, nonaccidental (*see also* Assault) E968.9
Volcanic eruption (any injury) E909.1
Vomitus in air passages (with asphyxia, obstruction or suffocation) E911

W

War operations (during hostilities) (injury) (by) (in) E995
  after cessation of hostilities, injury due to E998
  air blast E993
  aircraft burned, destroyed, exploded, shot down E994
  asphyxia from
    chemical E997.2
    fire, conflagration (caused by fire producing device or conventional weapon) E990.9
      from nuclear explosion E996
      petrol bomb E990.0
    fumes E997.2
    gas E997.2
  battle wound NEC E995
  bayonet E995
  biological warfare agents E997.1
  blast (air) (effects) E993
    from nuclear explosion E996
    underwater E992
  bomb (mortar) (explosion) E993
    after cessation of hostilities E998
    fragments, injury by E991.9
      antipersonnel E991.3
  bullet(s) (from carbine, machine gun, pistol, rifle, shotgun) E991.2
    rubber E991.0
  burn from
    chemical E997.2
    fire, conflagration (caused by fire-producing device or conventional weapon) E990.9
      from nuclear explosion E996
      petrol bomb E990.0
    gas E997.2
  burning aircraft E994
  chemical E997.2
  chlorine E997.2
  conventional warfare, specified from NEC E995
  crushing by falling aircraft E994
  depth charge E992
  destruction of aircraft E994
  disability as sequela one year or more after injury E999.0 ▲
  drowning E995
  effect (direct) (secondary) nuclear weapon E996
  explosion (artillery shell) (breech block) (cannon shell) E993
    after cessation of hostilities of bomb, mine placed in war E998
    aircraft E994
    bomb (mortar) E993
      atom E996
      hydrogen E996
      injury by fragments from E991.9
        antipersonnel E991.3
      nuclear E996
    depth charge E992
    injury by fragments from E991.9
      antipersonnel E991.3
    marine weapon E992
    mine
      at sea or in harbor E992
      land E993
        injury by fragments from E991.9
      marine E992
    munitions (accidental) (being used in war) (dump) (factory) E993
    nuclear (weapon) E996
    own weapons (accidental) E993
      injury by fragments from E991.9
        antipersonnel E991.3
    sea-based artillery shell E992
    torpedo E992

War operations — *continued*
  exposure to ionizing radiation from nuclear explosion E996
  falling aircraft E994
  fire or fire-producing device E990.9
    petrol bomb E990.0
  fireball effects from nuclear explosion E996
  fragments from
    antipersonnel bomb E991.3
    artillery shell, bomb NEC, grenade, guided missile, land mine, rocket, shell, shrapnel E991.9
  fumes E997.2
  gas E997.2
  grenade (explosion) E993
    fragments, injury by E991.9
  guided missile (explosion) E993
    fragments, injury by E991.9
    nuclear E996
  heat from nuclear explosion E996
  injury due to, but occurring after cessation of hostilities E998
  lacrimator (gas) (chemical) E997.2
  land mine (explosion) E993
    after cessation of hostilities E998
    fragments, injury by E991.9
  laser(s) E997.0
  late effect of E999.0 ▲
  lewisite E997.2
  lung irritant (chemical) (fumes) (gas) E997.2
  marine mine E992
  mine
    after cessation of hostilities E998
    at sea E992
    in harbor E992
    land (explosion) E993
      fragments, injury by E991.9
    marine E992
  missile (guided) (explosion) E993
    fragments, injury by E991.9
    marine E992
    nuclear E996
  mortar bomb (explosion) E993
    fragments, injury by E991.9
  mustard gas E997.2
  nerve gas E997.2
  phosgene E997.2
  poisoning (chemical) (fumes) (gas) E997.2
  radiation, ionizing from nuclear explosion E996
  rocket (explosion) E993
    fragments, injury by E991.9
  saber, sabre E995
  screening smoke E997.8
  shell (aircraft) (artillery) (cannon) (land based) (explosion) E993
    fragments, injury by E991.9
    sea-based E992
  shooting E991.2
    after cessation of hostilities E998
    bullet(s) E991.2
      rubber E991.0
    pellet(s) (rifle) E991.1
    shrapnel E991.9
    submersion E995
    torpedo E992
  unconventional warfare, except by nuclear weapon E997.9
    biological (warfare) E997.1
    gas, fumes, chemicals E997.2
    laser(s) E997.0
    specified type NEC E997.8
  underwater blast E992
  vesicant (chemical) (fumes) (gas) E997.2
  weapon burst E993

Washed
  away by flood — *see* Flood
  away by tidal wave — *see* Tidal wave
  off road by storm (transport vehicle) E908.9
  overboard E832

Weather exposure — *see also* Exposure
  cold E901.0
  hot E900.0

Weightlessness (causing injury) (effects of) (in spacecraft, real or simulated) E928.0

Wound (accidental) NEC (*see also* Injury) E928.9
  battle (*see also* War operations) E995
  bayonet E920.3
    in
      legal intervention E974
      war operations E995
  gunshot — *see* Shooting
  incised — *see* Cut
  saber, sabre E920.3
    in war operations E995

Tsunami — Wound

Railway Accidents (E800-E807)

The following fourth-digit subdivisions are for use with categories E800-E807 to identify the injured person:

.0 **Railway employee**
Any person who by virtue of his employment in connection with a railway, whether by the railway company or not, is at increased risk of involvement in a railway accident, such as:

> catering staff on train
> postal staff on train
> driver
> railway fireman
> guard
> shunter
> porter
>
> sleeping car attendant

.1 **Passenger on railway**
Any authorized person traveling on a train, except a railway employee
EXCLUDES intending passenger waiting at station (.8)
unauthorized rider on railway vehicle (.8)

.2 **Pedestrian**
See definition (r), Vol. 1, page 248

.3 **Pedal cyclist**
See definition (p), Vol. 1, page 248

.8 **Other specified person**
Intending passenger waiting at station
Unauthorized rider on railway vehicle

.9 **Unspecified person**

Motor Vehicle Traffic and Nontraffic Accidents (E810-E825)

The following fourth-digit subdivisions are for use with categories E810-E819 and E820-E825 to identify the injured person:

.0 **Driver of motor vehicle other than motorcycle**
See definition (1), Vol. 1, page 248

.1 **Passenger in motor vehicle other than motorcycle**
See definition (1), Vol. 1, page 248

.2 **Motorcyclist**
See definition (1), Vol. 1, page 248

.3 **Passenger on motorcycle**
See definition (1), Vol. 1, page 248

.4 **Occupant of streetcar**

.5 **Rider of animal; occupant of animal-drawn vehicle**

.6 **Pedal cyclist**
See definition (p), Vol. 1, page 248

.7 **Pedestrian**
See definition (r), Vol. 1, page 248

.8 **Other specified person**
Occupant of vehicle other than above
Person in railway train involved in accident
Unauthorized rider of motor vehicle

.9 **Unspecified person**

Other Road Vehicle Accidents (E826-E829)

(animal-drawn vehicle, streetcar, pedal cycle, and other nonmotor road vehicle accidents)

The following fourth-digit subdivisions are for use with categories E826-E829 to identify the injured person:

.0   **Pedestrian**
See definition (r), Vol. 1, page 248

.1   **Pedal cyclist** (does not apply to codes E827, E828, E829)
See definition (p), Vol. 1, page 248

.2   **Rider of animal** (does not apply to code E829)

.3   **Occupant of animal-drawn vehicle** (does not apply to codes E828, E829)

.4   **Occupant of streetcar**

.8   **Other specified person**

.9   **Unspecified person**

Water Transport Accidents (E830-E838)

The following fourth-digit subdivisions are for use with categories E830-E838 to identify the injured person:

.0   **Occupant of small boat, unpowered**

.1   **Occupant of small boat, powered**
See definition (t), Vol. 1, page 248

       EXCLUDES   water skier (.4)

.2   **Occupant of other watercraft — crew**
Persons:

        engaged in operation of watercraft

        providing passenger services [cabin attendants, ship's physician, catering personnel]

        working on ship during voyage in other capacity [musician in band, operators of shops and beauty parlors]

.3   **Occupant of other watercraft — other than crew**
Passenger
Occupant of lifeboat, other than crew, after abandoning ship

.4   **Water skier**

.5   **Swimmer**

.6   **Dockers, stevedores**
Longshoreman employed on the dock in loading and unloading ships

.8   **Other specified person**
Immigration and custom officials on board ship
Persons:

        accompanying passenger or member of crew visiting boat

Pilot (guiding ship into port)

.9   **Unspecified person**

Air and Space Transport Accidents (E840-E845)

The following fourth-digit subdivisions are for use with categories E840-E845 to identify the injured person:

.0   **Occupant of spacecraft**

.1   **Occupant of military aircraft, any**

Crew
Passenger (civilian) (military)
Troops
  } in military aircraft [air force] [army] [national guard] [navy]

> **EXCLUDES**   occupants of aircraft operated under jurisdiction of police departments (.5)
> parachutist (.7)

.2   **Crew of commercial aircraft (powered) in surface to surface transport**

.3   **Other occupant of commercial aircraft (powered) in surface to surface transport**

Flight personnel:
     not part of crew
     on familiarization flight

Passenger on aircraft

.4   **Occupant of commercial aircraft (powered) in surface to air transport**

Occupant [crew] [passenger] of aircraft (powered) engaged in activities, such as:

     air drops of emergency supplies
     air drops of parachutists, except from military craft
     crop dusting
     lowering of construction material [bridge or telephone pole]
     sky writing

.5   **Occupant of other powered aircraft**

Occupant [crew] [passenger] of aircraft (powered) engaged in activities, such as:

     aerial spraying (crops) (fire retardants)
     aerobatic flying
     aircraft racing
     rescue operation
     storm surveillance
     traffic suveillance

Occupant of private plane NOS

.6   **Occupant of unpowered aircraft, except parachutist**
Occupant of aircraft classifiable to E842

.7   **Parachutist (military) (other)**
Person making voluntary descent

> **EXCLUDES**   person making descent after accident to aircraft (.1-.6)

.8   **Ground crew, airline employee**
Persons employed at airfields (civil) (military) or launching pads, not occupants of aircraft

.9   **Other person**

---

1. INFECTIOUS AND PARASITIC DISEASES (001-139)

Note: Categories for "late effects" of infectious and parasitic diseases are to be found at 137-139.

> INCLUDES   diseases generally recognized as communicable or transmissible as well as a few diseases of unknown but possibly infectious origin

> EXCLUDES   acute respiratory infections (460-466)
> carrier or suspected carrier of infectious organism (V02.0-V02.9)
> certain localized infections
> influenza (487.0-487.8)

INTESTINAL INFECTIOUS DISEASES (001-009)

> EXCLUDES   helminthiases (120.0-129)

✓4th 001 Cholera

DEF: An acute infectious enteritis caused by a potent enterotoxin elaborated by *Vibrio cholerae*; the vibrio produces a toxin in the intestinal tract that changes the permeability of the mucosa leading to diarrhea and dehydration.

001.0   **Due to Vibrio cholerae**
001.1   **Due to Vibrio cholerae el tor**
001.9   **Cholera, unspecified**

✓4th 002 Typhoid and paratyphoid fevers

DEF: Typhoid fever: an acute generalized illness caused by *Salmonella typhi*; notable clinical features are fever, headache, abdominal pain, cough, toxemia, leukopenia, abnormal pulse, rose spots on the skin, bacteremia, hyperplasia of intestinal lymph nodes, mesenteric lymphadenopathy, and Peyer's patches in the intestines.

DEF: Paratyphoid fever: a prolonged febrile illness, much like typhoid but usually less severe; caused by salmonella serotypes other than *S. typhi*, especially *S. enteritidis* serotypes paratyphi A and B and *S. choleraesuis*.

002.0   **Typhoid fever**
     Typhoid (fever) (infection) [any site]
002.1   **Paratyphoid fever A**
002.2   **Paratyphoid fever B**
002.3   **Paratyphoid fever C**
002.9   **Paratyphoid fever, unspecified**

✓4th 003 Other salmonella infections

> INCLUDES   infection or food poisoning by Salmonella [any serotype]

DEF: Infections caused by a genus of gram-negative, anaerobic bacteria of the family *Enterobacteriaceae*; affecting warm-blooded animals, like humans; major symptoms are enteric fevers, acute gastroenteritis and septicemia.

003.0   **Salmonella gastroenteritis**
     Salmonellosis
003.1   **Salmonella septicemia**   `HIV`
✓5th 003.2   **Localized salmonella infections**
     003.20 Localized salmonella infection, unspecified   `HIV`
     003.21 Salmonella meningitis   `HIV`
     003.22 Salmonella pneumonia   `HIV`
     003.23 Salmonella arthritis   `HIV`
     003.24 Salmonella osteomyelitis   `HIV`
     003.29 Other   `HIV`
003.8   **Other specified salmonella infections**   `HIV`
003.9   **Salmonella infection, unspecified**   `HIV`

✓4th 004 Shigellosis

> INCLUDES   bacillary dysentery

DEF: Acute infectious dysentery caused by the genus *Shigella*, of the family *Enterobacteriaceae*; affecting the colon causing the release of blood-stained stools with accompanying tenesmus, abdominal cramps and fever.

004.0   **Shigella dysenteriae**
     Infection by group A Shigella (Schmitz) (Shiga)
004.1   **Shigella flexneri**
     Infection by group B Shigella
004.2   **Shigella boydii**
     Infection by group C Shigella

004.3   **Shigella sonnei**
     Infection by group D Shigella
004.8   **Other specified Shigella infections**
004.9   **Shigellosis, unspecified**

✓4th 005 Other food poisoning (bacterial)

> EXCLUDES   salmonella infections (003.0-003.9)
> toxic effect of:
>   food contaminants (989.7)
>   noxious foodstuffs (988.0-988.9)

DEF: Enteritis caused by ingesting contaminated foods and characterized by diarrhea, abdominal pain, vomiting; symptoms may be mild or life threatening.

005.0   **Staphylococcal food poisoning**
     Staphylococcal toxemia specified as due to food
005.1   **Botulism**
     Food poisoning due to Clostridium botulinum
005.2   **Food poisoning due to Clostridium perfringens [C. welchii]**
     Enteritis necroticans
005.3   **Food poisoning due to other Clostridia**
005.4   **Food poisoning due to Vibrio parahaemolyticus**
✓5th 005.8   **Other bacterial food poisoning**
> EXCLUDES   salmonella food poisoning (003.0-003.9)

     005.81 Food poisoning due to Vibrio vulnificus
     005.89 Other bacterial food poisoning
       Food poisoning due to Bacillus cereus
005.9   **Food poisoning, unspecified**

✓4th 006 Amebiasis

> INCLUDES   infection due to Entamoeba histolytica
> EXCLUDES   amebiasis due to organisms other than Entamoeba histolytica (007.8)

DEF: Infection of the large intestine caused by *Entamoeba histolytica*; usually asymptomatic but symptoms may range from mild diarrhea to profound life-threatening dysentery. Extraintestinal complications include hepatic abscess, which may rupture into the lung, pericardium or abdomen, causing life-threatening infections.

006.0   **Acute amebic dysentery without mention of abscess**
     Acute amebiasis

DEF: Sudden, severe *Entamoeba histolytica* infection causing bloody stools.

006.1   **Chronic intestinal amebiasis without mention of abscess**
     Chronic:
       amebiasis
       amebic dysentery
006.2   **Amebic nondysenteric colitis**

DEF: *Entamoeba histolytica* infection with inflamed colon but no dysentery.

006.3   **Amebic liver abscess**
     Hepatic amebiasis
006.4   **Amebic lung abscess**
     Amebic abscess of lung (and liver)
006.5   **Amebic brain abscess**
     Amebic abscess of brain (and liver) (and lung)
006.6   **Amebic skin ulceration**
     Cutaneous amebiasis
006.8   **Amebic infection of other sites**
     Amebic: Ameboma
       appendicitis
       balanitis
> EXCLUDES   specific infections by free-living amebae (136.2)

006.9   **Amebiasis, unspecified**
     Amebiasis NOS

✓4th ✓5th Additional Digit Required   Nonspecific PDx   Unacceptable PDx   Manifestation Code   `MSP` Medicare Secondary Payer   ►◄ Revised Text   ● New Code   ▲ Revised Code Title

2002 Ingenix, Inc.   Volume 1 — 1

Infectious and Parasitic Diseases 001–006.9

Infectious and Parasitc Diseases 007–008.8

✓4th **007 Other protozoal intestinal diseases**

INCLUDES   protozoal:
     colitis
     diarrhea
     dysentery

007.0 Balantidiasis
Infection by Balantidium coli

007.1 Giardiasis
Infection by Giardia lamblia   Lambliasis

007.2 Coccidiosis   HIV
Infection by Isospora belli and Isospora hominis
Isosporiasis

007.3 Intestinal trichomoniasis
DEF: Colitis, diarrhea, or dysentery caused by the protozoa *Trichomonas*.

007.4 Cryptosporidiosis
AHA: 4Q, '97, 30

DEF: An intestinal infection by protozoan parasites causing intractable diarrhea in patients with AIDS and other immunosuppressed individuals.

007.5 Cyclosporiasis
AHA: 4Q, '00, 38

DEF: An infection of the small intestine by the protozoal organism, *Cyclospora caytenanesis*, spread to humans though ingestion of contaminated water or food. Symptoms include watery diarrhea with frequent explosive bowel movements, loss of appetite, loss of weight, bloating, increased gas, stomach cramps, nausea, vomiting, muscle aches, low grade fever, and fatigue.

007.8 Other specified protozoal intestinal diseases
Amebiasis due to organisms other than Entamoeba histolytica

007.9 Unspecified protozoal intestinal disease
Flagellate diarrhea   Protozoal dysentery NOS

✓4th **008 Intestinal infections due to other organisms**

INCLUDES   any condition classifiable to 009.0-009.3 with mention of the responsible organisms

EXCLUDES   *food poisoning by these organisms (005.0-005.9)*

✓5th **008.0 Escherichia coli [E. coli]**
AHA: 4Q, '92, 17

008.00 E. coli, unspecified
E. coli enteritis NOS

008.01 Enteropathogenic E. coli
DEF: *E. coli* causing inflammation of intestines.

008.02 Enterotoxigenic E. coli
DEF: A toxic reaction to *E. coli* of the intestinal mucosa, causing voluminous watery secretions.

008.03 Enteroinvasive E. coli
DEF: *E. coli* infection penetrating intestinal mucosa.

008.04 Enterohemorrhagic E. coli
DEF: *E. coli* infection penetrating the intestinal mucosa, producing microscopic ulceration and bleeding.

008.09 Other intestinal E. coli infections

008.1 Arizona group of paracolon bacilli

008.2 Aerobacter aerogenes
Enterobacter aeogenes

008.3 Proteus (mirabilis) (morganii)

✓5th **008.4 Other specified bacteria**
AHA: 4Q, '92, 18

008.41 Staphylococcus   CC
Staphylococcal enterocolitis

CC Excl: 001.1, 002.0, 002.9, 003.0, 004.9, 005.0-005.2, 006.0-006.2, 006.9, 007.1-007.9, 008.00-008.49, 008.5, 008.61-008.69, 008.8, 009.0, 014.80-014.86, 112.85, 129, 487.8, 536.3, 536.8, 555.0-555.9, 556.0-556.9, 557.0-557.9, 558.2, 558.3, 558.9, 564.1, 775.0-775.9, 777.5, 777.8

008.42 Pseudomonas   CC
CC Excl: See code 008.41

AHA: 2Q, '89, 10

008.43 Campylobacter   CC
CC Excl: See code 008.41

008.44 Yersinia enterocolitica   CC
CC Excl: See code 008.41

008.45 Clostridium difficile   CC
Pseudomembranous colitis

CC Excl: See code 008.41

DEF: An overgrowth of a species of bacterium that is a part of the normal colon flora in human infants and sometimes in adults; produces a toxin that causes pseudomembranous enterocolitis.; typically is seen in patients undergoing antibiotic therapy.

008.46 Other anaerobes   CC
Anaerobic enteritis NOS
Bacteroides (fragilis)
Gram-negative anaerobes

CC Excl: See code 008.41

008.47 Other gram-negative bacteria   CC
Gram-negative enteritis NOS
EXCLUDES   *gram-negative anaerobes (008.46)*

CC Excl: See code 008.41

008.49 Other   CC
CC Excl: See code 008.41

AHA: 2Q, '89, 10; 1Q, '88, 6

008.5 Bacterial enteritis, unspecified

✓5th **008.6 Enteritis due to specified virus**
AHA: 4Q, '92, 18

008.61 Rotavirus

008.62 Adenovirus

008.63 Norwalk virus
Norwalk-like agent

008.64 Other small round viruses [SRVs]
Small round virus NOS

008.65 Calicivirus
DEF: Enteritis due to a subgroup of *Picornaviruses*.

008.66 Astrovirus

008.67 Enterovirus NEC
Coxsackie virus   Echovirus
EXCLUDES   *poliovirus (045.0-045.9)*

008.69 Other viral enteritis
Torovirus

008.8 Other organism, not elsewhere classified
Viral: Viral:
  enteritis NOS   gastroenteritis
EXCLUDES   *influenza with involvement of gastrointestinal tract (487.8)*

N Newborn Age: 0   P Pediatric Age: 0-17   M Maternity Age: 12-55   A Adult Age: 15-124   CC CC Condition   MC Major Complication   CD Complex Dx   HIV HIV Related Dx

2 — Volume 1   *2002 Ingenix, Inc.*

✓4ᵗʰ **009 Ill-defined intestinal infections**

> **EXCLUDES**   *diarrheal disease or intestinal infection due to specified organism (001.0-008.8)*
> *diarrhea following gastrointestinal surgery (564.4)*
> *intestinal malabsorption (579.0-579.9)*
> *ischemic enteritis (557.0-557.9)*
> *other noninfectious gastroenteritis and colitis (558.1-558.9)*
> *regional enteritis (555.0-555.9)*
> *ulcerative colitis (556)*

009.0   **Infectious colitis, enteritis, and gastroenteritis**

Colitis
Enteritis   } septic
Gastroenteritis

Dysentery: Dysentery:
   NOS   hemorrhagic
   catarrhal

AHA: 3Q, '99, 4

DEF: Colitis: An inflammation of mucous membranes of the colon
Enteritis: An inflammation of mucous membranes of the small intestine. Gastroenteritis: An inflammation of mucous membranes of stomach and intestines.

009.1   **Colitis, enteritis, and gastroenteritis of presumed infectious origin**

> **EXCLUDES**   *colitis NOS (558.9)*
> *enteritis NOS (558.9)*
> *gastroenteritis NOS (558.9)*

AHA: 3Q, '99, 6

009.2   **Infectious diarrhea**

Diarrhea:
   dysenteric
   epidemic
Infectious diarrheal disease NOS

009.3   **Diarrhea of presumed infectious origin**

> **EXCLUDES**   *diarrhea NOS (787.91)*

AHA: N-D, '87, 7

TUBERCULOSIS (010-018)

> **INCLUDES**   infection by Mycobacterium tuberculosis (human) (bovine)
> **EXCLUDES**   *congenital tuberculosis (771.2)*
> *late effects of tuberculosis (137.0-137.4)*

The following fifth-digit subclassification is for use with categories 010-018:

0   unspecified
1   bacteriological or histological examination not done
2   bacteriological or histological examination unknown (at present)
3   tubercle bacilli found (in sputum) by microscopy
4   tubercle bacilli not found (in sputum) by microscopy, but found by bacterial culture
5   tubercle bacilli not found by bacteriological examination, but tuberculosis confirmed histologically
6   tubercle bacilli not found by bacteriological or histological examination but tuberculosis confirmed by other methods [inoculation of animals]

DEF: An infection by *Mycobacterium tuberculosis* causing the formation of small, rounded nodules, called tubercles, that can disseminate throughout the body via lymph and blood vessels. Localized tuberculosis is most often seen in the lungs.

✓4ᵗʰ **010 Primary tuberculous infection**

DEF: Tuberculosis of the lungs occurring when the patient is first infected.

§ ✓5ᵗʰ **010.0**   **Primary tuberculous infection**   `HIV`

> **EXCLUDES**   *nonspecific reaction to tuberculin skin test without active tuberculosis (795.5)*
> *positive PPD (795.5)*
> *positive tuberculin skin test without active tuberculosis (795.5)*

DEF: Hilar or paratracheal lymph node enlargement in pulmonary tuberculosis.

§ ✓5ᵗʰ **010.1**   **Tuberculous pleurisy in primary progressive tuberculosis**   `HIV`

DEF: Inflammation and exudation in the lining of the tubercular lung.

§ ✓5ᵗʰ **010.8**   **Other primary progressive tuberculosis**   `HIV`

> **EXCLUDES**   *tuberculous erythema nodosum (017.1)*

§ ✓5ᵗʰ **010.9**   **Primary tuberculous infection, unspecified**   `HIV`

✓4ᵗʰ **011 Pulmonary tuberculosis**   `HIV`

Use additional code to identify any associated silicosis (502)

§ ✓5ᵗʰ **011.0**   **Tuberculosis of lung, infiltrative**   `CC` `HIV`

CC Excl: 011.00-011.96, 012.00-012.86, 017.90-017.96, 018.00-018.96, 031.0, 031.2, 031.8-031.9, 041.81-041.89, 041.9, 137.0, 139.8, 480.0-487.1, 494.0-494.1, 495.0-495.9, 496, 500-505, 506.0-506.9, 507.0-507.8, 508.0-508.9, 517.1, 518.89

§ ✓5ᵗʰ **011.1**   **Tuberculosis of lung, nodular**   `CC` `HIV`
CC Excl: See code 011.0

§ ✓5ᵗʰ **011.2**   **Tuberculosis of lung with cavitation**   `CC` `HIV`
CC Excl: See code 011.0

§ ✓5ᵗʰ **011.3**   **Tuberculosis of bronchus**   `CC` `HIV`

> **EXCLUDES**   *isolated bronchial tuberculosis (012.2)*

CC Excl: See code 011.0

§ ✓5ᵗʰ **011.4**   **Tuberculous fibrosis of lung**   `CC` `HIV`
CC Excl: See code 011.0

§ ✓5ᵗʰ **011.5**   **Tuberculous bronchiectasis**   `CC` `HIV`
CC Excl: See code 011.0

§ ✓5ᵗʰ **011.6**   **Tuberculous pneumonia [any form]**   `CC` `HIV`
CC Excl: For codes 011.60-011.65: See code 011.0

CC Excl: For code 011.66: 011.66, 139.8, 480.0-487.1, 494.0-494.1, 495.0-495.9, 496, 500-505, 506.0-506.9, 507.0-507.8, 508.0-508.9, 517.1, 518.89

DEF: Inflammatory pulmonary reaction to tuberculous cells.

§ ✓5ᵗʰ **011.7**   **Tuberculous pneumothorax**   `CC` `HIV`
CC Excl: See code 011.0

DEF: Spontaneous rupture of damaged tuberculous pulmonary tissue.

§ ✓5ᵗʰ **011.8**   **Other specified pulmonary tuberculosis**   `CC` `HIV`
CC Excl: See code 011.0

§ ✓5ᵗʰ **011.9**   **Pulmonary tuberculosis, unspecified**   `CC` `HIV`
Respiratory tuberculosis NOS
Tuberculosis of lung NOS
CC Excl: See code 011.0

---

§   Requires fifth-digit. See beginning of section 010-018 for codes and definitions.

✓4ᵗʰ Additional Digit Required   Nonspecific PDx   Unacceptable PDx   Manifestation Code   `MSP` Medicare Secondary Payer   ►◄ Revised Text   ● New Code   ▲ Revised Code Title
✓5ᵗʰ
2002 Ingenix, Inc.   **Volume 1 — 3**

Infectious and Parasitic Diseases 009-011.9

Infectious and Parasitic Diseases 012–016.3

✓4ᵗʰ **012 Other respiratory tuberculosis**
> **EXCLUDES**   respiratory tuberculosis, unspecified (011.9)

§ ✓5ᵗʰ **012.0 Tuberculous pleurisy**   CC HIV
> Tuberculosis of pleura
> Tuberculous empyema
> Tuberculous hydrothorax
>> **EXCLUDES**   pleurisy with effusion without mention of cause (511.9)
>> tuberculous pleurisy in primary progressive tuberculosis (010.1)
>
> CC Excl: See code 011.0
>
> DEF: Inflammation and exudation in the lining of the tubercular lung.

§ ✓5ᵗʰ **012.1 Tuberculosis of intrathoracic lymph nodes**   CC HIV
> Tuberculosis of lymph nodes:
>> hilar
>> mediastinal
>> tracheobronchial
> Tuberculous tracheobronchial adenopathy
>> **EXCLUDES**   that specified as primary (010.0-010.9)
>
> CC Excl: See code 011.0

§ ✓5ᵗʰ **012.2 Isolated tracheal or bronchial tuberculosis**   HIV

§ ✓5ᵗʰ **012.3 Tuberculous laryngitis**   HIV
> Tuberculosis of glottis

§ ✓5ᵗʰ **012.8 Other specified respiratory tuberculosis**   HIV
> Tuberculosis of: Tuberculosis of:
>> mediastinum   nose (septum)
>> nasopharynx   sinus [any nasal]

✓4ᵗʰ **013 Tuberculosis of meninges and central nervous system**

§ ✓5ᵗʰ **013.0 Tuberculous meningitis**   CC HIV
> Tuberculosis of meninges (cerebral) (spinal)
> Tuberculous:
>> leptomeningitis
>> meningoencephalitis
>> **EXCLUDES**   tuberculoma of meninges (013.1)
>
> CC Excl: 003.21, 013.00-013.16, 013.40-013.56, 013.80-013.96, 017.90-017.96, 031.2, 031.8-031.9, 036.0, 041.81-041.89, 041.9, 047.0-047.9, 049.0-049.1, 053.0, 054.72, 072.1, 090.42, 091.81, 094.2, 098.89, 100.81, 112.83, 114.2, 115.01, 115.11, 115.91, 130.0, 137.1, 139.8, 320.0-320.9, 321.0-321.8, 322.0-322.9, 349.89, 349.9, 357.0

§ ✓5ᵗʰ **013.1 Tuberculoma of meninges**   CC HIV
> CC Excl: See code 013.0

§ ✓5ᵗʰ **013.2 Tuberculoma of brain**   CC HIV
> Tuberculosis of brain (current disease)
> CC Excl: 013.20-013.36, 013.60-013.96, 017.90-017.96, 031.2, 031.8-031.9, 041.81-041.89, 041.9, 137.1, 139.8

§ ✓5ᵗʰ **013.3 Tuberculous abscess of brain**   CC HIV
> CC Excl: See code 013.2

§ ✓5ᵗʰ **013.4 Tuberculoma of spinal cord**   CC HIV
> CC Excl: 013.00-013.16, 013.40-013.56, 013.80-013.96, 017.90-017.96, 031.2, 031.8-031.9, 041.81-041.89, 041.9, 137.1, 139.8

§ ✓5ᵗʰ **013.5 Tuberculous abscess of spinal cord**   CC HIV
> CC Excl: See code 013.4

§ ✓5ᵗʰ **013.6 Tuberculous encephalitis or myelitis**   CC HIV
> CC Excl: 013.20-013.36, 013.60-013.96, 017.90-017.96, 031.2, 031.8-031.9, 041.81-041.89, 041.9, 137.1, 139.8

§ ✓5ᵗʰ **013.8 Other specified tuberculosis of central nervous system**   CC HIV
> CC Excl: 013.80-013.96, 017.90-017.96, 031.2, 031.8-031.9, 041.81-041.89, 041.9, 137.1, 139.8

§ ✓5ᵗʰ **013.9 Unspecified tuberculosis of central nervous system**   CC HIV
> Tuberculosis of central nervous system NOS
> CC Excl: See code 013.8

✓4ᵗʰ **014 Tuberculosis of intestines, peritoneum, and mesenteric glands**

§ ✓5ᵗʰ **014.0 Tuberculous peritonitis**   CC HIV
> Tuberculous ascites
> CC Excl: 014.00-014.86, 017.90-017.96, 031.2, 031.8-031.9, 041.81-041.89, 041.9, 139.8
>
> DEF: Tuberculous inflammation of the membrane lining the abdomen.

§ ✓5ᵗʰ **014.8 Other**   CC HIV
> Tuberculosis (of):
>> anus
>> intestine (large) (small)
>> mesenteric glands
>> rectum
>> retroperitoneal (lymph nodes)
> Tuberculous enteritis
> CC Excl: For code 014.80: See code 014.0
>
> CC Excl: For code 014.81: 014.81, 139.8
>
> CC Excl: For code 014.82: 014.00-014.86, 017.90-017.96, 031.2, 031.8-031.9, 041.81-041.89, 041.9, 139.8
>
> CC Excl: For code 014.83-014.86: See code 014.82

✓4ᵗʰ **015 Tuberculosis of bones and joints**
> Use additional code to identify manifestation, as:
>> tuberculous:
>>> arthropathy (711.4)
>>> necrosis of bone (730.8)
>>> osteitis (730.8)
>>> osteomyelitis (730.8)
>>> synovitis (727.01)
>>> tenosynovitis (727.01)

§ ✓5ᵗʰ **015.0 Vertebral column**   HIV
> Pott's disease
> Use additional code to identify manifestation, as:
>> curvature of spine [Pott's] (737.4)
>> kyphosis (737.4)
>> spondylitis (720.81)

§ ✓5ᵗʰ **015.1 Hip**   HIV

§ ✓5ᵗʰ **015.2 Knee**   HIV

§ ✓5ᵗʰ **015.5 Limb bones**   HIV
> Tuberculous dactylitis

§ ✓5ᵗʰ **015.6 Mastoid**   HIV
> Tuberculous mastoiditis

§ ✓5ᵗʰ **015.7 Other specified bone**   HIV

§ ✓5ᵗʰ **015.8 Other specified joint**   HIV

§ ✓5ᵗʰ **015.9 Tuberculosis of unspecified bones and joints**   HIV

✓4ᵗʰ **016 Tuberculosis of genitourinary system**

§ ✓5ᵗʰ **016.0 Kidney**   CC HIV
> Renal tuberculosis
> Use additional code to identify manifestation, as:
>> tuberculous:
>>> nephropathy (583.81)
>>> pyelitis (590.81)
>>> pyelonephritis (590.81)
> CC Excl: 016.00-016.36, 016.90-016.96, 017.90-017.96, 031.2, 031.8-031.9, 041.81-041.89, 041.9, 137.2, 139.8

§ ✓5ᵗʰ **016.1 Bladder**   CC HIV
> CC Excl: See code 016.0

§ ✓5ᵗʰ **016.2 Ureter**   CC HIV
> CC Excl: See code 016.0

§ ✓5ᵗʰ **016.3 Other urinary organs**   CC HIV
> CC Excl: See code 016.0

---

§   Requires fifth-digit. See beginning of section 010-018 for codes and definitions.

N Newborn Age: 0   **P** Pediatric Age: 0-17   **M** Maternity Age: 12-55   **A** Adult Age: 15-124   **CC** CC Condition   **MC** Major Complication   **CD** Complex Dx   **HIV** HIV Related Dx

§ ✓5ᵗʰ **016.4   Epididymis**   CC HIV ♂
   CC Excl: 016.40-016.56, 016.90-016.96, 017.90-017.96, 031.2,
   031.8-031.9, 041.81-041.89, 041.9, 137.2, 139.8

§ ✓5ᵗʰ **016.5   Other male genital organs**   CC HIV ♂
   Use additional code to identify manifestation, as:
      tuberculosis of:
         prostate (601.4)
         seminal vesicle (608.81)
         testis (608.81)
   CC Excl: See code 016.4

§ ✓5ᵗʰ **016.6   Tuberculous oophoritis and salpingitis**   CC HIV ♀
   CC Excl: 016.60-016.96, 017.90-017.96, 031.2, 031.8-031.9,
   041.81-041.89, 041.9, 137.2, 139.8

§ ✓5ᵗʰ **016.7   Other female genital organs**   CC HIV ♀
   Tuberculous:
      cervicitis
      endometritis
   CC Excl: See code 016.6

§ ✓5ᵗʰ **016.9   Genitourinary tuberculosis, unspecified**   CC HIV
   CC Excl: 016.90-016.96, 017.90-017.96, 031.2, 031.8-031.9,
   041.81-041.89, 041.9, 137.2, 139.8

✓4ᵗʰ **017 Tuberculosis of other organs**

§ ✓5ᵗʰ **017.0   Skin and subcutaneous cellular tissue**   HIV
   Lupus: Tuberculosis:
      exedens   cutis
      vulgaris   lichenoides
   Scrofuloderma   papulonecrotica
   Tuberculosis: verrucosa cutis
      colliquativa
      EXCLUDES   lupus erythematosus (695.4)
                        disseminated (710.0)
                     lupus NOS (710.0)
                     nonspecific reaction to tuberculin skin
                        test without active tuberculosis
                        (795.5)
                     positive PPD (795.5)
                     positive tuberculin skin test without
                        active tuberculosis (795.5)

§ ✓5ᵗʰ **017.1   Erythema nodosum with hypersensitivity**   HIV
           reaction in tuberculosis
   Bazin's disease   Erythema:
   Erythema: nodosum, tuberculous
      induratum   Tuberculosis indurativa
      EXCLUDES   erythema nodosum NOS (695.2)
   DEF: Tender, inflammatory, bilateral nodules appearing on the
   shins and thought to be an allergic reaction to tuberculotoxin.

§ ✓5ᵗʰ **017.2   Peripheral lymph nodes**   CC HIV
   Scrofula   Tuberculous adenitis
   Scrofulous abscess
      EXCLUDES   tuberculosis of lymph nodes:
                        bronchial and mediastinal (012.1)
                        mesenteric and retroperitoneal
                           (014.8)
                     tuberculous tracheobronchial
                        adenopathy (012.1)
   CC Excl: 017.20-017.26, 017.90-017.96, 031.2, 031.8-031.9,
   041.81-041.89, 041.9, 139.8
   DEF: Scrofula: Old name for tuberculous cervical lymphadenitis.

§ ✓5ᵗʰ **017.3   Eye**   CC HIV
   Use additional code to identify manifestation, as:
      tuberculous:
         chorioretinitis, disseminated (363.13)
         episcleritis (379.09)
         interstitial keratitis (370.59)
         iridocyclitis, chronic (364.11)
         keratoconjunctivitis (phlyctenular) (370.31)
   CC Excl: 017.30-017.36, 017.90-017.96, 031.2, 031.8-031.9,
   041.81-041.89, 041.9, 139.8

§ ✓5ᵗʰ **017.4   Ear**   CC HIV
   Tuberculosis of ear
   Tuberculous otitis media
      EXCLUDES   tuberculous mastoiditis (015.6)
   CC Excl: 017.40-017.46, 017.90-017.96, 031.2, 031.8-031.9,
   041.81-041.89, 041.9, 139.8

§ ✓5ᵗʰ **017.5   Thyroid gland**   CC HIV
   CC Excl: 017.50-017.56, 017.90-017.96, 031.2, 031.8-031.9,
   041.81-041.89, 041.9, 139.8

§ ✓5ᵗʰ **017.6   Adrenal glands**   CC HIV
   Addison's disease, tuberculous
   CC Excl: 017.60-017.66, 017.90-017.96, 031.2, 031.8-031.9,
   041.81-041.89, 041.9, 139.8

§ ✓5ᵗʰ **017.7   Spleen**   CC HIV
   CC Excl: 017.70-017.76, 017.90-017.96, 031.2, 031.8-031.9,
   041.81-041.89, 041.9, 139.8

§ ✓5ᵗʰ **017.8   Esophagus**   CC HIV
   CC Excl: 017.80-017.96, 031.2, 031.8-031.9, 041.81-041.89, 041.9, 139.8

§ ✓5ᵗʰ **017.9   Other specified organs**   CC HIV
   Use additional code to identify manifestation, as:
      tuberculosis of:
         endocardium [any valve] (424.91)
         myocardium (422.0)
         pericardium (420.0)
   CC Excl: 017.90-017.96, 031.2, 031.8-031.9, 041.81-041.89, 041.9, 139.8

✓4ᵗʰ **018 Miliary tuberculosis**
      INCLUDES   tuberculosis:
                        disseminated
                        generalized
                        miliary, whether of a single specified site,
                           multiple sites, or unspecified site
                        polyserositis
   DEF: A form of tuberculosis caused by caseous material carried through the
   bloodstream planting seedlike tubercles in various body organs.

§ ✓5ᵗʰ **018.0   Acute miliary tuberculosis**   CC HIV
   CC Excl: 017.90-017.96, 018.00-018.96, 031.2, 031.8-031.9,
   041.81-041.89, 041.9, 139.8

§ ✓5ᵗʰ **018.8   Other specified miliary tuberculosis**   CC HIV
   CC Excl: See code 018.0

§ ✓5ᵗʰ **018.9   Miliary tuberculosis, unspecified**   CC HIV
   CC Excl: See code 018.0

ZOONOTIC BACTERIAL DISEASES (020-027)

✓4ᵗʰ **020 Plague**
      INCLUDES   infection by Yersinia [Pasteurella] pestis

   020.0   Bubonic
   DEF: Most common acute and severe form of plague characterized
   by lymphadenopathy (buboes), chills, fever and headache.

   020.1   Cellulocutaneous
   DEF: Plague characterized by inflammation and necrosis of skin.

   020.2   Septicemic
   DEF: Plague characterized by massive infection in the
   bloodstream.

   020.3   Primary pneumonic
   DEF: Plague characterized by massive pulmonary infection.

   020.4   Secondary pneumonic
   DEF: Lung infection as a secondary complication of plague.

   020.5   Pneumonic, unspecified
   020.8   Other specified types of plague
      Abortive plague   Pestis minor
      Ambulatory plague
   020.9   Plague, unspecified

§ Requires fifth-digit. See beginning of section 010-018 for codes and definitions.

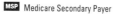

✓4ᵗʰ / ✓5ᵗʰ Additional Digit Required   Nonspecific PDx   Unacceptable PDx   Manifestation Code   **MSP** Medicare Secondary Payer   ▶◀ Revised Text   ● New Code   ▲ Revised Code Title

Infectious and Parasitic Diseases 016.4–020.9

✓4ᵗʰ **021 Tularemia**

> INCLUDES   deerfly fever
> infection by Francisella [Pasteurella] tularensis
> rabbit fever

DEF: A febrile disease transmitted by the bites of deer flies, fleas and ticks, by inhalations of aerosolized *F. tularensis* or by ingestion of contaminated food or water; patients quickly develop fever, chills, weakness, headache, backache and malaise.

021.0   Ulceroglandular tularemia

> **DEF:** Lesions occur at the site *Francisella tularensis* organism enters body, usually the fingers or hands.

021.1   Enteric tularemia

> Tularemia: Tularemia:
> cryptogenic   typhoidal
> intestinal

021.2   Pulmonary tularemia

> Bronchopneumonic tularemia

021.3   Oculoglandular tularemia

> **DEF:** Painful conjunctival infection by *Francisella tularensis* organism with possible corneal, preauricular lymph, or lacrimal involvement.

021.8   Other specified tularemia

> Tularemia: Tularemia:
> generalized or disseminated   glandular

021.9   Unspecified tularemia

✓4ᵗʰ **022 Anthrax**

DEF: An infectious bacterial disease usually transmitted by contact with infected animals or their discharges or products; it is classified by primary routes of inoculation as cutaneous, gastrointestinal and by inhalation.

022.0   Cutaneous anthrax

> Malignant pustule

022.1   Pulmonary anthrax

> Respiratory anthrax
> Wool-sorters' disease

022.2   Gastrointestinal anthrax

022.3   Anthrax septicemia

022.8   Other specified manifestations of anthrax

022.9   Anthrax, unspecified

✓4ᵗʰ **023 Brucellosis**

> INCLUDES   fever:
> Malta
> Mediterranean
> undulant

DEF: An infectious disease caused by gram-negative, aerobic coccobacilli organisms; it is transmitted to humans through contact with infected tissue or dairy products; fever, sweating, weakness and aching are symptoms.

023.0   Brucella melitensis

> **DEF:** Infection from direct or indirect contact with infected sheep or goats.

023.1   Brucella abortus

> **DEF:** Infection from direct or indirect contact with infected cattle.

023.2   Brucella suis

> **DEF:** Infection from direct or indirect contact with infected swine.

023.3   Brucella canis

> **DEF:** Infection from direct or indirect contact with infected dogs.

023.8   Other brucellosis

> Infection by more than one organism

023.9   Brucellosis, unspecified

024 Glanders

> Infection by:
> Actinobacillus mallei   Farcy
> Malleomyces mallei   Malleus
> Pseudomonas mallei

DEF: Equine infection causing mucosal inflammation and skin ulcers in humans.

025 Melioidosis

> Infection by: Infection by:
> Malleomyces pseudomallei   Pseudoglanders
> Pseudomonas pseudomallei   Whitmore's bacillus

DEF: Rare infection caused by *Pseudomonas pseudomallei*; clinical symptoms range from localized infection to fatal septicemia.

✓4ᵗʰ **026 Rat-bite fever**

026.0   Spirillary fever

> Rat-bite fever due to Spirillum minor [S. minus]
> Sodoku

026.1   Streptobacillary fever

> Epidemic arthritic erythema
> Haverhill fever
> Rat-bite fever due to Streptobacillus moniliformis

026.9   Unspecified rat-bite fever

✓4ᵗʰ **027 Other zoonotic bacterial diseases**

027.0   Listeriosis

> Infection   }
> Septicemia   } by Listeria monocytogenes

> Use additional code to identify manifestation, as meningitis (320.7)

> EXCLUDES   *congenital listeriosis (771.2)*

027.1   Erysipelothrix infection

> Erysipeloid (of Rosenbach)
> Infection   } by Erysipelothrix insidiosa
> Septicemia }   [E. rhusiopathiae]

> **DEF:** Usually associated with handling of fish, meat, or poultry; symptoms range from localized inflammation to septicemia.

027.2   Pasteurellosis

> Pasteurella pseudotuberculosis infection
> Mesenteric adenitis   }
> Septic infection (cat   } by Pasteurella multocida
> bite) (dog bite)   }   [P. septica]

> EXCLUDES   *infection by:*
> *Francisella [Pasteurella] tularensis*
> *(021.0-021.9)*
> *Yersinia [Pasteurella] pestis (020.0-*
> *020.9)*

> **DEF:** Swelling, abscesses, or septicemia from *Pasteurella multocida*, commonly transmitted to humans by a dog or cat scratch.

027.8   Other specified zoonotic bacterial diseases

027.9   Unspecified zoonotic bacterial disease

OTHER BACTERIAL DISEASES (030-041)

> EXCLUDES   *bacterial venereal diseases (098.0-099.9)*
> *bartonellosis (088.0)*

✓4ᵗʰ **030 Leprosy**

> INCLUDES   Hansen's disease
> infection by Mycobacterium leprae

030.0   Lepromatous [type L]

> Lepromatous leprosy (macular) (diffuse) (infiltrated) (nodular) (neuritic)

> **DEF:** Infectious, disseminated leprosy bacilli with lesions and deformities.

030.1   Tuberculoid [type T]

> Tuberculoid leprosy (macular) (maculoanesthetic) (major) (minor) (neuritic)

> **DEF:** Relatively benign, self-limiting leprosy with neuralgia and scales.

030.2   Indeterminate [group I]

> Indeterminate [uncharacteristic] leprosy (macular) (neuritic)

> **DEF:** Uncharacteristic leprosy, frequently an early manifestation.

030.3   Borderline [group B]

> Borderline or dimorphous leprosy (infiltrated) (neuritic)

> **DEF:** Transitional form of leprosy, neither lepromatous nor tuberculoid.

N Newborn Age: 0   P Pediatric Age: 0-17   M Maternity Age: 12-55   A Adult Age: 15-124   CC CC Condition   MC Major Complication   CD Complex Dx   HIV HIV Related Dx

6 — Volume 1   *2002 Ingenix, Inc.*

030.8 **Other specified leprosy**
030.9 **Leprosy, unspecified**

✓4ᵗʰ 031 **Diseases due to other mycobacteria**

031.0 **Pulmonary**   [CC]
Battey disease
Infection by Mycobacterium:
avium
intracellulare [Battey bacillus]
kansasii
CC Excl: 011.00-011.96, 012.00-012.86, 017.90-017.96, 031.0, 031.2, 031.8-031.9, 041.81-041.89, 041.9, 137.0, 139.8, 480.0-480.9, 481, 482.0-482.9, 483.0, 483.1, 483.8, 484.1-484.8, 485-486, 487.0-487.1, 494.0-494.1, 495.0-495.9, 496, 500-505, 506.0-506.9, 507.0-507.8, 508.0-508.9, 517.1, 518.89

031.1 **Cutaneous**
Buruli ulcer
Infection by Mycobacterium:
marinum [M. balnei]
ulcerans

031.2 **Disseminated**   [HIV]
Disseminated mycobacterium avium-intracellulare complex (DMAC)
Mycobacterium avium-intracellulare complex (MAC) bacteremia
AHA: 4Q, '97, 31

DEF: Disseminated mycobacterium avium-intracellulare complex (DMAC): A serious systemic form of MAC commonly observed in patients in the late course of AIDS.

DEF: Mycobacterium avium-intracellulare complex (MAC) bacterium: Human pulmonary disease, lymphadenitis in children and systemic disease in immunocompromised individuals caused by a slow growing, gram-positive, aerobic organism.

031.8 **Other specified mycobacterial diseases**   [HIV]
031.9 **Unspecified diseases due to mycobacteria**   [HIV]
Atypical mycobacterium infection NOS

✓4ᵗʰ 032 **Diphtheria**
INCLUDES   infection by Corynebacterium diphtheriae

032.0 **Faucial diphtheria**
Membranous angina, diphtheritic
DEF: Diphtheria of the throat.

032.1 **Nasopharyngeal diphtheria**
032.2 **Anterior nasal diphtheria**
032.3 **Laryngeal diphtheria**
Laryngotracheitis, diphtheritic

✓5ᵗʰ 032.8 **Other specified diphtheria**
032.81 **Conjunctival diphtheria**
Pseudomembranous diphtheritic conjunctivitis
032.82 **Diphtheritic myocarditis**
032.83 **Diphtheritic peritonitis**
032.84 **Diphtheritic cystitis**
032.85 **Cutaneous diphtheria**
032.89 **Other**
032.9 **Diphtheria, unspecified**

✓4ᵗʰ 033 **Whooping cough**
INCLUDES   pertussis
Use additional code to identify any associated pneumonia (484.3)
DEF: An acute, highly contagious respiratory tract infection caused by *Bordetella pertussis* and *B. bronchiseptica*; characteristic paroxysmal cough.

033.0 **Bordetella pertussis [B. pertussis]**
033.1 **Bordetella parapertussis [B. parapertussis]**
033.8 **Whooping cough due to other specified organism**
Bordetella bronchiseptica [B. bronchiseptica]
033.9 **Whooping cough, unspecified organism**

✓4ᵗʰ 034 **Streptococcal sore throat and scarlet fever**
034.0 **Streptococcal sore throat**

Septic:	Streptococcal:
angina	laryngitis
sore throat	pharyngitis
Streptococcal:	tonsillitis
angina	

034.1 **Scarlet fever**
Scarlatina
EXCLUDES   parascarlatina (057.8)
DEF: Streptococcal infection and fever with red rash spreading from trunk.

035 **Erysipelas**
EXCLUDES   postpartum or puerperal erysipelas (670)
DEF: An acute superficial cellulitis involving the dermal lymphatics; it is often caused by group A streptococci.

✓4ᵗʰ 036 **Meningococcal infection**
036.0 **Meningococcal meningitis**   [CC]
Cerebrospinal fever (meningococcal)
Meningitis:
cerebrospinal
epidemic
CC Excl: 003.21, 013.00-013.16, 036.0, 036.89, 036.9, 041.81-041.89, 041.9, 047.0-047.9, 049.0-049.1, 053.0, 054.72, 072.1, 090.42, 091.81, 094.2, 098.89, 100.81, 112.83, 114.2, 115.01, 115.11, 115.91, 130.0, 139.8, 320.0-320.9, 321.0-321.8, 322.0-322.9, 349.89, 349.9, 357.0

036.1 **Meningococcal encephalitis**   [CC]
CC Excl: 036.1, 036.89, 036.9, 041.81-041.89, 041.9, 139.8

036.2 **Meningococcemia**   [CC]
Meningococcal septicemia
CC Excl: 003.1, 020.2, 036.2, 036.89, 036.9, 038.0, 038.10-038.11, 038.19, 038.2-038.9, 041.81-041.89, 041.9, 054.5, 139.8, ▶995.90-995.94◀

036.3 **Waterhouse-Friderichsen syndrome, meningococcal**   [CC]
Meningococcal hemorrhagic adrenalitis
Meningococcic adrenal syndrome
Waterhouse-Friderichsen syndrome NOS
CC Excl: 036.3, 036.89, 036.9, 041.81-041.89, 041.9, 139.8

✓5ᵗʰ 036.4 **Meningococcal carditis**
036.40 **Meningococcal carditis, unspecified**   [CC]
CC Excl: 036.40, 036.89, 036.9, 041.81-041.89, 041.9, 139.8

036.41 **Meningococcal pericarditis**   [CC]
CC Excl: 036.41, 036.89, 036.9, 041.81-041.89, 041.9, 139.8
DEF: Meningococcal infection of the outer membrane of the heart.

036.42 **Meningococcal endocarditis**   [CC]
CC Excl: 036.42, 036.89, 036.9, 041.81-041.89, 041.9, 139.8
DEF: Meningococcal infection of the membranes lining the cavities of the heart.

036.43 **Meningococcal myocarditis**   [CC]
CC Excl: 036.43, 041.81-041.89, 041.9, 139.8
DEF: Meningococcal infection of the muscle of the heart.

✓5ᵗʰ 036.8 **Other specified meningococcal infections**
036.81 **Meningococcal optic neuritis**   [CC]
CC Excl: 036.81, 036.89, 036.9, 041.81-041.89, 041.9, 139.8

036.82 **Meningococcal arthropathy**   [CC]
CC Excl: 036.82, 036.89, 036.9, 041.81-041.89, 041.9, 139.8

036.89 **Other**   [CC]
CC Excl: 036.89, 036.9, 041.81-041.89, 041.9, 139.8

036.9 **Meningococcal infection, unspecified**   [CC]
Meningococcal infection NOS
CC Excl: See code 036.89

037 Tetanus   CC

> **EXCLUDES** tetanus:
>> complicating:
>>> abortion (634-638 with .0, 639.0)
>>> ectopic or molar pregnancy (639.0)
>> neonatorum (771.3)
>> puerperal (670)

CC Excl: 037, 139.8

DEF: An acute, often fatal, infectious disease caused by the anaerobic, spore-forming bacillus *Clostridium tetani*; the bacillus most often enters the body through a contaminated wound, burns, surgical wounds, or cutaneous ulcers. Symptoms include lockjaw, spasms, seizures, and paralysis.

√4th **038 Septicemia**

> **EXCLUDES** bacteremia (790.7)
> during labor (659.3)
> following ectopic or molar pregnancy (639.0)
> following infusion, injection, transfusion, or
>> vaccination (999.3)
> postpartum, puerperal (670)
> ▶septicemia (sepsis) of newborn (771.81)◄
> that complicating abortion (634-638
>> with .0, 639.0)

AHA: 4Q, '88, 10; 3Q, '88, 12

DEF: A systemic disease associated with the presence and persistence of pathogenic microorganisms or their toxins in the blood.

038.0   Streptococcal septicemia   CC HIV
  CC Excl: 003.1, 020.2, 036.2, 038.0-038.9, 040.82. 040.89, 041.00-041.05, 041.09-041.11, 041.19, 041.2-041.7, 041.81-041.86, 041.89, 041.9, 054.5, 139.8, V09.0-V09.91, ▶995.90-995.94◄

  AHA: 2Q, '96. 5

√5th **038.1   Staphylococcal septicemia**
  AHA: 4Q, '97, 32

   038.10 Staphylococcal septicemia,   CC HIV
   unspecified
     CC Excl: See code 038.0

   038.11 Staphylococcus aureus septicemia   CC HIV
     CC Excl: See code 038.0

     AHA: 2Q, '00, 5; 4Q, '98, 42

   038.19 Other staphylococcal septicemia   CC HIV
     CC Excl: See code 038.0

     AHA: 2Q, '00, 5

038.2   Pneumococcal septicemia [Streptococcus   CC HIV
pneumoniae septicemia]
  CC Excl: See code 038.0

  AHA: 2Q, '96, 5; 1Q, '91, 13

038.3   Septicemia due to anaerobes   CC HIV
  Septicemia due to bacteroides
  > **EXCLUDES** gas gangrene (040.0)
  > that due to anaerobic streptococci
  >> (038.0)

  CC Excl: See code 038.0

  DEF: Infection of blood by microorganisms that thrive without oxygen.

√5th **038.4   Septicemia due to other gram-negative organisms**
  DEF: Infection of blood by microorganisms categorized as gram-negative by Gram's method of staining for identification of bacteria.

   038.40 Gram-negative organism, unspecified CC HIV
     Gram-negative septicemia NOS
     CC Excl: See code 038.0

   038.41 Hemophilus influenzae   CC HIV
   [H. influenzae]
     CC Excl: See code 038.0

038.42 Escherichia coli [E. coli]   CC HIV
  CC Excl: See code 038.0

  ▽ **DRG** 416

038.43 Pseudomonas   CC HIV
  CC Excl: See code 038.0

038.44 Serratia   CC HIV
  CC Excl: See code 038.0

038.49 Other   CC HIV
  CC Excl: See code 038.0

  ▽ **DRG** 416

038.8   Other specified septicemias   CC HIV
  > **EXCLUDES** septicemia (due to):
  >> anthrax (022.3)
  >> gonococcal (098.89)
  >> herpetic (054.5)
  >> meningococcal (036.2)
  >> septicemic plague (020.2)

  CC Excl: See code 038.0

038.9   Unspecified septicemia   CC HIV
  Septicemia NOS
  > **EXCLUDES** bacteremia NOS (790.7)

  CC Excl: See code 038.0

  AHA: 2Q, '00, 3; 3Q, '99. 5. 9; 1Q, '98, 5; 3Q, '96, 16; 2Q, '96, 6

  ▽ **DRG** 416

√4th **039 Actinomycotic infections**
  > **INCLUDES** actinomycotic mycetoma
  > infection by Actinomycetales, such as species
  >> of Actinomyces, Actinomadura, Nocardia,
  >> Streptomyces
  > maduromycosis (actinomycotic)
  > schizomycetoma (actinomycotic)

  DEF: Inflammatory lesions and abscesses at site of infection by *Actinomyces israelii*.

039.0   Cutaneous   HIV
  Erythrasma   Trichomycosis axillaris

039.1   Pulmonary   HIV
  Thoracic actinomycosis

039.2   Abdominal   HIV

039.3   Cervicofacial

039.4   Madura foot   HIV
  > **EXCLUDES** madura foot due to mycotic infection
  >> (117.4)

039.8   Of other specified sites   HIV

039.9   Of unspecified site   HIV
  Actinomycosis NOS   Nocardiosis NOS
  Maduromycosis NOS

√4th **040 Other bacterial diseases**
  > **EXCLUDES** bacteremia NOS (790.7)
  > bacterial infection NOS (041.9)

040.0   Gas gangrene   CC
  Gas bacillus infection or gangrene
  Infection by Clostridium:
    histolyticum
    oedematiens
    perfringens [welchii]
    septicum
    sordellii
  Malignant edema
  Myonecrosis, clostridial
  Myositis, clostridial

  CC Excl: 040.0, 139.8

  AHA: 1Q, '95, 11

040.1   Rhinoscleroma
  DEF: Growths on the nose and nasopharynx caused by *Klebsiella rhinoscleromatis*.

040.2 Whipple's disease
Intestinal lipodystrophy

040.3 Necrobacillosis

DEF: Infection with *Fusobacterium necrophorum* causing abscess or necrosis.

✓5th **040.8 Other specified bacterial diseases**

040.81 Tropical pyomyositis

040.82 Toxic shock syndrome   CC
Use additional code to identify the organism
CC Excl: 040.82, 780.91-780.99, 785.50-785.59, 785.9, 799.8

040.89 Other
AHA: N-D, '86, 7

✓4th **041 Bacterial infection in conditions classified elsewhere and of unspecified site**

Note: This category is provided to be used as an additional code to identify the bacterial agent in diseases classified elsewhere. This category will also be used to classify bacterial infections of unspecified nature or site.

EXCLUDES   *bacteremia NOS (790.7)*
septicemia (038.0-038.9)

AHA: 2Q, '01, 12; J-A, '84, 19

✓5th **041.0 Streptococcus**

041.00 Streptococcus, unspecified

041.01 Group A
AHA: ▶1Q, '02, 3◀

041.02 Group B

041.03 Group C

041.04 Group D [Enterococcus]

041.05 Group G

041.09 Other Streptococcus

✓5th **041.1 Staphylococcus**

041.10 Staphylococcus, unspecified

041.11 Staphylococcus aureus
AHA: 2Q, '01, 11; 4Q, '98, 42, 54; 4Q, '97, 32

041.19 Other Staphylococcus

041.2 Pneumococcus

041.3 Friedländer's bacillus
Infection by Klebsiella pneumoniae

041.4 Escherichia coli [E. coli]

041.5 Hemophilus influenzae [H. influenzae]

041.6 Proteus (mirabilis) (morganii)

041.7 Pseudomonas

✓5th **041.8 Other specified bacterial infections**

041.81 Mycoplasma
Eaton's agent
Pleuropneumonia-like organisms [PPLO]

041.82 Bacillus fragilis

041.83 Clostridium perfringens

041.84 Other anaerobes
Bacteroides (fragilis)
Gram-negative anaerobes
EXCLUDES   *Helicobacter pylori (041.86)*

041.85 Other gram-negative organisms
Aerobacter aerogenes
Gram-negative bacteria NOS
Mima polymorpha
Serratia
EXCLUDES   *gram-negative anaerobes (041.84)*
AHA: 1Q, 95, 18

041.86 Helicobacter pylori (H. pylori)
AHA: 4Q, '95, 60

041.89 Other specified bacteria

041.9 Bacterial infection, unspecified
AHA: 2Q, '91, 9

HUMAN IMMUNODEFICIENCY VIRUS (HIV) INFECTION (042)

042 Human immunodeficiency virus [HIV] disease   CC
Acquired immune deficiency syndrome
Acquired immunodeficiency syndrome
AIDS
AIDS-like syndrome
AIDS-related complex
ARC
HIV infection, symptomatic
Use additional code(s) to identify all manifestations of HIV
Use additional code to identify HIV-2 infection (079.53)

EXCLUDES   *asymptomatic HIV infection status (V08)*
exposure to HIV virus (V01.7)
nonspecific serologic evidence of HIV (795.71)

CC Excl: 042, 139.8

AHA: 1Q, '99, 14, 4Q, '97, 30, 31; 1Q, '93, 21; 2Q, '92, 11; 3Q, '90, 17; J-A, '87, 8

POLIOMYELITIS AND OTHER NON-ARTHROPOD-BORNE VIRAL DISEASES OF CENTRAL NERVOUS SYSTEM (045-049)

✓4th **045 Acute poliomyelitis**

EXCLUDES   *late effects of acute poliomyelitis (138)*

The following fifth-digit subclassification is for use with category 045:

   0   **poliovirus, unspecified type**
   1   **poliovirus type I**
   2   **poliovirus type II**
   3   **poliovirus type III**

✓5th **045.0 Acute paralytic poliomyelitis specified as bulbar**
Infantile paralysis (acute)
Poliomyelitis (acute) (anterior)   } specified as bulbar

Polioencephalitis (acute) (bulbar)
Polioencephalomyelitis (acute) (anterior) (bulbar)

DEF: Acute paralytic infection occurring where the brain merges with the spinal cord; affecting breathing, swallowing, and heart rate.

✓5th **045.1 Acute poliomyelitis with other paralysis**
Paralysis: Paralysis:
   acute atrophic, spinal   infantile, paralytic
Poliomyelitis (acute)
anterior   } with paralysis except bulbar
epidemic

DEF: Paralytic infection affecting peripheral or spinal nerves.

✓5th **045.2 Acute nonparalytic poliomyelitis**
Poliomyelitis (acute)
anterior   } specified as nonparalytic
epidemic

DEF: Nonparalytic infection causing pain, stiffness, and paresthesias.

✓5th **045.9 Acute poliomyelitis, unspecified**
Infantile paralysis
Poliomyelitis (acute)
anterior   } unspecified whether paralytic or nonparalytic
epidemic

✓4th **046 Slow virus infection of central nervous system**

046.0 Kuru

DEF: A chronic, progressive, fatal nervous system disorder; clinical symptoms include cerebellar ataxia, trembling, spasticity and progressive dementia.

046.1 Jakob-Creutzfeldt disease
Subacute spongiform encephalopathy

DEF: Communicable, progressive spongiform encephalopathy thought to be caused by an infectious particle known as a "prion" (proteinaceous infection particle). This is a progressive, fatal disease manifested principally by mental deterioration.

✓4th ✓5th **Additional Digit Required**   Nonspecific PDx   Unacceptable PDx   Manifestation Code   MSP Medicare Secondary Payer   ▶◀ Revised Text   ● New Code   ▲ Revised Code Title

2002 Ingenix, Inc.   **October 2002 • Volume 1 — 9**

046.2 Subacute sclerosing panencephalitis `CC`
  Dawson's inclusion body encephalitis
  Van Bogaert's sclerosing leukoencephalitis
  CC Excl: 046.2, 139.8

  DEF: Progressive viral infection causing cerebral dysfunction, blindness, dementia, and death (SSPE).

046.3 Progressive multifocal leukoencephalopathy `HIV`
  Multifocal leukoencephalopathy NOS
  DEF: Infection affecting cerebral cortex in patients with weakened immune systems.

046.8 Other specified slow virus infection of central nervous system `HIV`

046.9 Unspecified slow virus infection of central nervous system `HIV`

✓4ᵗʰ 047 Meningitis due to enterovirus
  INCLUDES meningitis: meningitis:
            abacterial   viral
            aseptic
  EXCLUDES meningitis due to:
            adenovirus (049.1)
            arthropod-borne virus (060.0-066.9)
            leptospira (100.81)
            virus of:
              herpes simplex (054.72)
              herpes zoster (053.0)
              lymphocytic choriomeningitis (049.0)
              mumps (072.1)
              poliomyelitis (045.0-045.9)
            any other infection specifically classified elsewhere
  AHA: J-F, '87, 6

  047.0 Coxsackie virus
  047.1 ECHO virus
        Meningo-eruptive syndrome
  047.8 Other specified viral meningitis
  047.9 Unspecified viral meningitis
        Viral meningitis NOS

048 Other enterovirus diseases of central nervous system
  Boston exanthem

✓4ᵗʰ 049 Other non-arthropod-borne viral diseases of central nervous system
  EXCLUDES late effects of viral encephalitis (139.0)
  049.0 Lymphocytic choriomeningitis
        Lymphocytic:
          meningitis (serous) (benign)
          meningoencephalitis (serous) (benign)
  049.1 Meningitis due to adenovirus
        DEF: Inflammation of lining of brain caused by Arenaviruses and usually occurring in adults in fall and winter months.
  049.8 Other specified non-arthropod-borne viral diseases of central nervous system
        Encephalitis: Encephalitis:
        acute: lethargica
          inclusion body   Rio Bravo
          necrotizing   von Economo's disease
          epidemic
  049.9 Unspecified non-arthropod-borne viral diseases of central nervous system
        Viral encephalitis NOS

VIRAL DISEASES ACCOMPANIED BY EXANTHEM (050-057)
  EXCLUDES arthropod-borne viral diseases (060.0-066.9)
            Boston exanthem (048)

✓4ᵗʰ 050 Smallpox
  050.0 Variola major
        Hemorrhagic (pustular) smallpox
        Malignant smallpox
        Purpura variolosa
        DEF: Form of smallpox known for its high mortality; exists only in laboratories.

050.1 Alastrim
        Variola minor
        DEF: Mild form of smallpox known for its low mortality rate.

050.2 Modified smallpox
        Varioloid
        DEF: Mild form occurring in patients with history of infection or vaccination.

050.9 Smallpox, unspecified

✓4ᵗʰ 051 Cowpox and paravaccinia
  051.0 Cowpox
        Vaccinia not from vaccination
        EXCLUDES vaccinia (generalized) (from vaccination) (999.0)
        DEF: A disease contracted by milking infected cows; vesicles usually appear on the fingers, may spread to hands and adjacent areas and usually disappear without scarring; other associated features of the disease may include local edema, lymphangitis and regional lymphadenitis with or without fever.
  051.1 Pseudocowpox
        Milkers' node
        DEF: Hand lesions and mild fever in dairy workers caused by exposure to paravaccinia.
  051.2 Contagious pustular dermatitis
        Ecthyma contagiosum
        Orf
        DEF: Skin eruptions caused by exposure to poxvirus-infected sheep or goats.
  051.9 Paravaccinia, unspecified

✓4ᵗʰ 052 Chickenpox
  DEF: Contagious infection by *Varicella-zoster* virus causing rash with pustules and fever.
  052.0 Postvaricella encephalitis `CC`
        Postchickenpox encephalitis
        CC Excl: 051.9, 052.0, 052.7-052.9, 078.88-078.89, 079.81, 079.88-079.89, 079.98-079.99, 139.8
  052.1 Varicella (hemorrhagic) pneumonitis `CC`
        CC Excl: 051.9, 052.1, 052.7-052.9, 078.88-078.89, 079.81, 079.88-079.89, 079.98-079.99, 139.8
  052.7 With other specified complications `CC`
        CC Excl: 051.9, 052.7-052.9, 078.88-078.89, 079.81, 079.88-079.89, 079.98-079.99, 139.8
        AHA: ▶1Q, '02, 3◀
  052.8 With unspecified complication `CC`
        CC Excl: See code 052.7
  052.9 Varicella without mention of complication `CC`
        Chickenpox NOS   Varicella NOS
        CC Excl: See code 052.7

✓4ᵗʰ 053 Herpes zoster
  INCLUDES shingles
            zona
  DEF: Self-limiting infection by *varicella-zoster* virus causing unilateral eruptions and neuralgia along affected nerves.
  053.0 With meningitis `CC` `HIV`
        CC Excl: 003.21, 013.00-013.16, 036.0, 047.0-047.9, 049.0-049.1, 053.0-053.19, 053.79, 053.8-053.9, 054.72, 054.79, 054.8-054.9, 072.1, 078.88-078.89, 079.81, 079.88-079.89, 079.98-079.99, 090.42, 091.81, 094.2, 098.89, 100.81, 112.83, 114.2, 115.01, 115.11, 115.91, 130.0, 139.8, 320.0-320.9, 321.0-321.8, 322.0-322.9, 349.89, 349.9, 357.0
        DEF: *Varicella-zoster* virus infection causing inflammation of the lining of the brain and/or spinal cord.
  ✓5ᵗʰ 053.1 With other nervous system complications
        053.10 With unspecified nervous system complication `CC` `HIV`
              CC Excl: 053.0-053.19, 053.79, 053.8-053.9, 054.72, 054.79, 054.8-054.9, 078.88-078.89, 079.81, 079.88-079.89, 079.98-079.99, 139.8

N Newborn Age: 0   P Pediatric Age: 0-17   M Maternity Age: 12-55   A Adult Age: 15-124   CC CC Condition   MC Major Complication   CD Complex Dx   HIV HIV Related Dx

10 — Volume 1 • October 2002   2002 Ingenix, Inc.

053.11 Geniculate herpes zoster `CC` `HIV`
Herpetic geniculate ganglionitis
CC Excl: See code 053.10

DEF: Unilateral eruptions and neuralgia along the facial nerve geniculum affecting face and outer and middle ear.

053.12 Postherpetic trigeminal neuralgia `CC` `HIV`
CC Excl: See code 053.10

DEF: Severe oral or nasal pain following a herpes zoster infection.

053.13 Postherpetic polyneuropathy `CC` `HIV`
CC Excl: See code 053.10

DEF: Multiple areas of pain following a herpes zoster infection.

053.19 Other `CC` `HIV`
CC Excl: See code 053.10

√5th **053.2 With ophthalmic complications**
053.20 Herpes zoster dermatitis of eyelid `HIV`
Herpes zoster ophthalmicus
053.21 Herpes zoster keratoconjunctivitis `HIV`
053.22 Herpes zoster iridocyclitis `HIV`
053.29 Other `HIV`
√5th **053.7 With other specified complications**
053.71 Otitis externa due to herpes zoster `HIV`
053.79 Other `CC` `HIV`
CC Excl: 053.0-053.9, 054.0-054.71, 054.73, 054.79, 054.8-054.9, 078.88-078.89, 079.81, 079.88-079.89, 079.98-079.99, 139.8

053.8 With unspecified complication `CC` `HIV`
CC Excl: See code 053.79

053.9 Herpes zoster without mention of complication `HIV`
Herpes zoster NOS

√4th **054 Herpes simplex**
EXCLUDES congenital herpes simplex (771.2)
054.0 Eczema herpeticum `HIV`
Kaposi's varicelliform eruption
DEF: Herpes simplex virus invading site of preexisting skin inflammation.

√5th **054.1 Genital herpes**
AHA: J-F, '87, 15, 16

054.10 Genital herpes, unspecified `HIV`
Herpes progenitalis
054.11 Herpetic vulvovaginitis `HIV` ♀
054.12 Herpetic ulceration of vulva `HIV` ♀
054.13 Herpetic infection of penis `HIV` ♂
054.19 Other `HIV`
054.2 Herpetic gingivostomatitis `HIV`
054.3 Herpetic meningoencephalitis `CC` `HIV`
Herpes encephalitis   Simian B disease
CC Excl: 054.3, 054.79, 054.8-054.9, 139.8

DEF: Inflammation of the brain and its lining, caused by infection of herpes simplex 1 in adults and simplex 2 in newborns.

√5th **054.4 With ophthalmic complications**
054.40 With unspecified ophthalmic complication `HIV`
054.41 Herpes simplex dermatitis of eyelid `HIV`
054.42 Dendritic keratitis `HIV`
054.43 Herpes simplex disciform keratitis `HIV`
054.44 Herpes simplex iridocyclitis `HIV`
054.49 Other `HIV`
054.5 Herpetic septicemia `CC` `HIV`
CC Excl: 003.1, 020.2, 036.2, 038.0, 038.10-038.11, 038.19, 038.2-038.9, 054.5, 054.79, 054.8-054.9, 139.8, ▶995.90-995.94◀

AHA: 2Q, '00, 5

054.6 Herpetic whitlow `HIV`
Herpetic felon
DEF: A primary infection of the terminal segment of a finger by herpes simplex; intense itching and pain start the disease, vesicles form, and tissue ultimately is destroyed.

√5th **054.7 With other specified complications**
054.71 Visceral herpes simplex `CC` `HIV`
CC Excl: 054.71, 054.72, 054.79, 054.8-054.9, 139.8

054.72 Herpes simplex meningitis `CC` `HIV`
CC Excl: 003.21, 013.00-013.16, 036.0, 047.0-047.9, 049.0-049.1, 053.0, 054.72, 054.79, 054.8-054.9, 072.1, 090.42, 091.81, 094.2, 098.89, 100.81, 112.83, 114.2, 115.01, 115.11, 115.91, 130.0, 139.8, 320.0-320.9, 321.0-321.8, 322.0-322.9, 349.89, 349.9, 357.0

054.73 Herpes simplex otitis externa `HIV`
054.79 Other `CC` `HIV`
CC Excl: 054.79, 054.8-054.9, 078.88-078.89, 079.81, 079.88-079.89, 079.98-079.99, 139.8

054.8 With unspecified complication `CC` `HIV`
CC Excl: See code 054.79

054.9 Herpes simplex without mention of complication `HIV`

√4th **055 Measles**
INCLUDES morbilli   rubeola
055.0 Postmeasles encephalitis `CC`
CC Excl: 055.0, 055.79, 055.8-055.9, 078.88-078.89, 079.81, 079.88-079.89, 079.98-079.99, 139

055.1 Postmeasles pneumonia `CC`
CC Excl: 055.1, 055.79, 055.8-055.9, 078.88-078.89, 079.81, 079.88-079.89, 079.98-079.99, 139.8

055.2 Postmeasles otitis media `CC`
CC Excl: 055.2, 055.79, 055.8-055.9, 078.88-078.89, 079.81, 079.88-079.89, 079.98-079.99, 139.8

√5th **055.7 With other specified complications**
055.71 Measles keratoconjunctivitis `CC`
Measles keratitis
CC Excl: 055.71, 055.79, 055.8-055.9, 078.88-078.89, 079.81, 079.88-079.89, 079.98-079.99, 139.8

055.79 Other `CC`
CC Excl: 055.79, 055.8-055.9, 078.88-078.89, 079.81, 079.88-079.89, 079.98-079.99, 139.8

055.8 With unspecified complication `CC`
CC Excl: 055.79, 055.8-055.9, 056.09, 078.88-078.89, 079.81, 079.88-079.89, 079.98-079.99, 139.8

055.9 Measles without mention of complication
√4th **056 Rubella**
INCLUDES German measles
EXCLUDES congenital rubella (771.0)
DEF: Acute but usually benign togavirus infection causing fever, sore throat, and rash; associated with complications to fetus as a result of maternal infection.

√5th **056.0 With neurological complications**
056.00 With unspecified neurological complication `CC`
CC Excl: 056.00-056.09, 056.79, 056.8-056.9, 078.88-078.89, 079.81, 079.88-079.89, 079.98-079.99, 139.8

056.01 Encephalomyelitis due to rubella `CC`
Encephalitis
Meningoencephalitis } due to rubella
CC Excl: See code 056.00

056.09 Other `CC`
CC Excl: See code 056.00

√4th √5th Additional Digit Required   Nonspecific PDx   Unacceptable PDx   Manifestation Code   `MSP` Medicare Secondary Payer   ▶◀ Revised Text   ● New Code   ▲ Revised Code Title

2002 Ingenix, Inc.   **October 2002 • Volume 1 — 11**

Infectious and Parasitic Diseases 056.7–066.2

✓5ᵗʰ **056.7 With other specified complications**

056.71 Arthritis due to rubella `CC`

CC Excl: 056.71-056.9, 078.88-078.89, 079.81,
079.88-079.89, 079.98-079.99, 139.8

056.79 Other `CC`

CC Excl: See code 056.00

056.8 With unspecified complications `CC`

CC Excl: 056., 056.01, 056.79, 056.8-056.9, 078.88-078.89,
079.81, 079.88-079.89, 079.98-079.99, 139.8

056.9 Rubella without mention of complication

✓4ᵗʰ **057 Other viral exanthemata**

DEF: Skin eruptions or rashes and fever caused by viruses, including
poxviruses.

057.0 Erythema infectiosum [fifth disease]

DEF: A moderately contagious, benign, epidemic disease, usually
seen in children, and of probable viral etiology; a red macular rash
appears on the face and may spread to the limbs and trunk.

057.8 Other specified viral exanthemata

Dukes (-Filatow) disease
Exanthema subitum [sixth disease]
Fourth disease
Parascarlatina
Pseudoscarlatina
Roseola infantum

057.9 Viral exanthem, unspecified

ARTHROPOD-BORNE VIRAL DISEASES (060-066)

Use additional code to identify any associated meningitis
(321.2)

EXCLUDES   *late effects of viral encephalitis (139.0)*

✓4ᵗʰ **060 Yellow fever**

DEF: Fever and jaundice from infection by mosquito-borne virus of genus
Flavivirus.

060.0 Sylvatic

Yellow fever: Yellow fever:
jungle   sylvan

DEF: Yellow fever transmitted from animal to man, via mosquito.

060.1 Urban

DEF: Yellow fever transmitted from man to man, via mosquito.

060.9 Yellow fever, unspecified

061 Dengue

Breakbone fever

EXCLUDES   *hemorrhagic fever caused by dengue virus*
(065.4)

DEF: Acute, self-limiting infection by mosquito-borne virus characterized by
fever and generalized aches.

✓4ᵗʰ **062 Mosquito-borne viral encephalitis**

062.0 Japanese encephalitis

Japanese B encephalitis

DEF: Flavivirus causing inflammation of the brain, and Russia, with
a wide range of clinical manifestations.

062.1 Western equine encephalitis

DEF: Alphavirus WEE infection causing inflammation of the brain,
found in areas west of the Mississippi; transmitted horse to
mosquito to man.

062.2 Eastern equine encephalitis

EXCLUDES   *Venezuelan equine encephalitis (066.2)*

DEF: Alphavirus EEE causing inflammation of the brain and spinal
cord, found as far north as Canada and south into South America
and Mexico; transmitted horse to mosquito to man.

062.3 St. Louis encephalitis

DEF: Epidemic form caused by Flavivirus and transmitted by
mosquito, and characterized by fever, difficulty in speech, and
headache.

062.4 Australian encephalitis

Australian arboencephalitis   Murray Valley
Australian X disease   encephalitis

DEF: Flavivirus causing inflammation of the brain, occurring in
Australia and New Guinea.

062.5 California virus encephalitis

Encephalitis: Tahyna fever
California
La Crosse

DEF: Bunyamwere causing inflammation of the brain.

062.8 Other specified mosquito-borne viral encephalitis

Encephalitis by Ilheus virus

EXCLUDES   ▶*West Nile virus (066.4)*◄

062.9 Mosquito-borne viral encephalitis, unspecified

✓4ᵗʰ **063 Tick-borne viral encephalitis**

INCLUDES   diphasic meningoencephalitis

063.0 Russian spring-summer [taiga] encephalitis

063.1 Louping ill

DEF: Inflammation of brain caused by virus transmitted sheep to
tick to man; incidence usually limited to British Isles.

063.2 Central European encephalitis

DEF: Inflammation of brain caused by virus transmitted by tick;
limited to central Europe and presenting with two distinct phases.

063.8 Other specified tick-borne viral encephalitis

Langat encephalitis
Powassan encephalitis

063.9 Tick-borne viral encephalitis, unspecified

064 Viral encephalitis transmitted by other and unspecified arthropods

Arthropod-borne viral encephalitis, vector unknown
Negishi virus encephalitis

EXCLUDES   *viral encephalitis NOS (049.9)*

✓4ᵗʰ **065 Arthropod-borne hemorrhagic fever**

065.0 Crimean hemorrhagic fever [CHF Congo virus]

Central Asian hemorrhagic fever

065.1 Omsk hemorrhagic fever

065.2 Kyasanur Forest disease

065.3 Other tick-borne hemorrhagic fever

065.4 Mosquito-borne hemorrhagic fever

Chikungunya hemorrhagic fever
Dengue hemorrhagic fever

EXCLUDES   *Chikungunya fever (066.3)*
dengue (061)
yellow fever (060.0-060.9)

065.8 Other specified arthropod-borne hemorrhagic fever

Mite-borne hemorrhagic fever

065.9 Arthropod-borne hemorrhagic fever, unspecified

Arbovirus hemorrhagic fever NOS

✓4ᵗʰ **066 Other arthropod-borne viral diseases**

066.0 Phlebotomus fever

Changuinola fever
Sandfly fever

DEF: Sandfly-borne viral infection occurring in Asia, Mideast and
South America.

066.1 Tick-borne fever

Nairobi sheep disease
Tick fever:
American mountain
Colorado
Kemerovo
Quaranfil

066.2 Venezuelan equine fever

Venezuelan equine encephalitis

DEF: Alphavirus VEE infection causing inflammation of the brain,
usually limited to South America, Mexico, and Florida; transmitted
horse to mosquito to man

066.3 Other mosquito-borne fever

Fever (viral):	Fever (viral):
Bunyamwera	Oropouche
Bwamba	Pixuna
Chikungunya	Rift valley
Guama	Ross river
Mayaro	Wesselsbron
Mucambo	Zika
O'Nyong-Nyong	

> **EXCLUDES** dengue (061)
> yellow fever (060.0-060.9)

● **066.4 West Nile fever**
West Nile encephalitis
West Nile encephalomyelitis
West Nile virus

066.8 Other specified arthropod-borne viral diseases
Chandipura fever   Piry fever

066.9 Arthropod-borne viral disease, unspecified
Arbovirus infection NOS

OTHER DISEASES DUE TO VIRUSES AND CHLAMYDIAE (070-079)

✓4th **070 Viral hepatitis**

> **INCLUDES** viral hepatitis (acute) (chronic)
> **EXCLUDES** cytomegalic inclusion virus hepatitis (078.5)

DEF: Hepatitis A : HAV infection is self-limiting with flulike symptoms; transmission, fecal-oral.

DEF: Hepatitis B: HBV infection can be chronic and systemic; transmission, bodily fluids.

DEF: Hepatitis C: HCV infection can be chronic and systemic; transmission, blood transfusion and unidentified agents.

DEF: Hepatitis D (delta): HDV occurs only in the presence of hepatitis B virus.

DEF: Hepatitis E: HEV is epidemic form; transmission and nature under investigation.

070.0 Viral hepatitis A with hepatic coma

070.1 Viral hepatitis A without mention of hepatic coma
Infectious hepatitis

The following fifth-digit subclassification is for use with categories 070.2 and 070.3:

   0 acute or unspecified, without mention of hepatitis delta
   1 acute or unspecified, with hepatitis delta
   2 chronic, without mention of hepatitis delta
   3 chronic, with hepatitis delta

✓5th **070.2 Viral hepatitis B with hepatic coma** `CC`
CC Excl: 070.0-070.9, 078.88-078.89, 079.81, 079.88-079.89, 079.98-079.99, 139.8

AHA: 4Q, '91, 28

✓5th **070.3 Viral hepatitis B without mention of hepatic coma** `CC`
Serum hepatitis
CC Excl: See code 070.2

AHA: 1Q, '93, 28; 4Q, '91, 28

✓5th **070.4 Other specified viral hepatitis with hepatic coma**
AHA: 4Q, '91, 28

  070.41 Acute or unspecified hepatitis C with hepatic coma `CC`
  CC Excl: See code 070.2

  070.42 Hepatitis delta without mention of active hepatitis B disease with hepatic coma `CC`
    Hepatitis delta with hepatitis B carrier state
  CC Excl: See code 070.2

  070.43 Hepatitis E with hepatic coma `CC`
  CC Excl: See code 070.2

  070.44 Chronic hepatitis C with hepatic coma `CC`
  CC Excl: See code 070.2

  070.49 Other specified viral hepatitis with hepatic coma `CC`
  CC Excl: See code 070.2

✓5th **070.5 Other specified viral hepatitis without mention of hepatic coma**
AHA: 4Q, '91, 28

  070.51 Acute or unspecified hepatitis C without mention of hepatic coma `CC`
  CC Excl: See code 070.2

  070.52 Hepatitis delta without mention of active hepatititis B disease or hepatic coma `CC`
  CC Excl: See code 070.2

  070.53 Hepatitis E without mention of hepatic coma `CC`
  CC Excl: See code 070.2

  070.54 Chronic hepatitis C without mention of hepatic coma `CC`
  CC Excl: See code 070.2

  070.59 Other specified viral hepatitis without mention of hepatic coma `CC`
  CC Excl: See code 070.2

070.6 Unspecified viral hepatitis with hepatic coma `CC`
CC Excl: See code 070.2

070.9 Unspecified viral hepatitis without mention of hepatic coma `CC`
Viral hepatitis NOS
CC Excl: See code 070.2

071 Rabies
Hydrophobia
Lyssa

DEF: Acute infectious disease of the CNS caused by a rhabdovirus; usually spread by virus-laden saliva from bites by infected animals; it progresses from fever, restlessness, and extreme excitability, to hydrophobia, seizures, confusion and death.

✓4th **072 Mumps**

DEF: Acute infectious disease caused by paramyxovirus; usually seen in children less than 15 years of age; salivary glands are typically enlarged, and other organs, such as testes, pancreas and meninges, are often involved.

072.0 Mumps orchitis `CC` ♂
CC Excl: 072.0, 072.79, 072.8-072.9, 078.88-078.89, 079.81, 079.88-079.89, 079.98-079.99, 139.8

072.1 Mumps meningitis `CC`
CC Excl: 003.21, 013.00-013.16, 036.0, 047.0-047.9, 049.0-049.1, 053.0, 054.72, 072.1, 072.79, 072.8-072.9, 078.88-078.89, 079.81, 079.98-079.99, 090.42, 091.81, 094.2, 098.89, 100.81, 112.83, 114.2, 115.01, 115.11, 115.91, 130.0, 139.8, 320.0-320.9, 321.0-321.8, 322.0-322.9, 349.89, 349.9, 357.0

072.2 Mumps encephalitis `CC`
Mumps meningoencephalitis
CC Excl: 072.2, 072.79, 072.8-072.9, 078.88-078.89, 079.81, 079.88-079.89, 079.98-079.99, 139.8

072.3 Mumps pancreatitis `CC`
CC Excl: 072.3, 072.79, 072.8-072.9, 078.88-078.89, 079.81, 079.88-079.89, 079.98-079.99, 139.8

✓5th **072.7 Mumps with other specified complications**
  072.71 Mumps hepatitis `CC`
  CC Excl: 072.71, 072.79, 072.8-072.9, 078.88-078.89, 079.81, 079.88-079.89, 079.98-079.99, 139.8

  072.72 Mumps polyneuropathy `CC`
  CC Excl: 072.72, 072.79, 072.8-072.9, 078.88-078.89, 079.81, 079.88-079.89, 079.98-079.99, 139.8

  072.79 Other `CC`
  CC Excl: 072.79, 072.8-072.9, 078.88-078.89, 079.81, 079.88-079.89, 079.98-079.99, 139.8

✓4th ✓5th Additional Digit Required   Nonspecific PDx   Unacceptable PDx   Manifestation Code   **MSP** Medicare Secondary Payer   ►◄ Revised Text   ● New Code   ▲ Revised Code Title

2002 Ingenix, Inc.

October 2002 • Volume 1 — 13

Infectious and Parasitic Diseases 072.8–078.3

072.8   Mumps with unspecified complication   `CC`

CC Excl: 072.79, 072.8-072.9, 078.88-078.89, 079.81, 079.88-079.89, 079.98-079.99

072.9   Mumps without mention of complication
Epidemic parotitis   Infectious parotitis

✓4ᵗʰ **073   Ornithosis**

INCLUDES   parrot fever
            psittacosis

DEF: *Chlamydia psittaci* infection often transmitted from birds to humans.

073.0   With pneumonia
Lobular pneumonitis due to ornithosis

073.7   With other specified complications

073.8   With unspecified complication

073.9   Ornithosis, unspecified

✓4ᵗʰ **074   Specific diseases due to Coxsackie virus**

EXCLUDES   *Coxsackie virus:*
         infection NOS (079.2)
         meningitis (047.0)

074.0   Herpangina
Vesicular pharyngitis

DEF: Acute infectious coxsackie virus infection causing throat lesions, fever, and vomiting; generally affects children in summer.

074.1   Epidemic pleurodynia
Bornholm disease   Epidemic:
Devil's grip   myalgia
                     myositis

DEF: Paroxysmal pain in chest, accompanied by fever and usually limited to children and young adults; caused by coxsackie virus.

✓5ᵗʰ **074.2   Coxsackie carditis**

074.20   Coxsackie carditis, unspecified

074.21   Coxsackie pericarditis
DEF: Coxsackie infection of the outer lining of the heart.

074.22   Coxsackie endocarditis
DEF: Coxsackie infection within the heart's cavities.

074.23   Coxsackie myocarditis
Aseptic myocarditis of newborn
DEF: Coxsackie infection of the muscle of the heart.

074.3   Hand, foot, and mouth disease
Vesicular stomatitis and exanthem
DEF: Mild coxsackie infection causing lesions on hands, feet and oral mucosa, and most commonly seen in preschool children.

074.8   Other specified diseases due to Coxsackie virus
Acute lymphonodular pharyngitis

075   Infectious mononucleosis
Glandular fever   Pfeiffer's disease
Monocytic angina

AHA: ▶3Q, '01, 13;◄ M-A, '87, 8

DEF: Acute infection by Epstein-Barr virus causing fever, sore throat, enlarged lymph glands and spleen, and fatigue; usually seen in teens and young adults.

✓4ᵗʰ **076   Trachoma**

EXCLUDES   *late effect of trachoma (139.1)*

DEF: A chronic infectious disease of the cornea and conjunctiva caused by a strain of the bacteria *Chlamydia trachomatis*; the infection can cause photophobia, pain, excessive tearing and sometimes blindness.

076.0   Initial stage
Trachoma dubium

076.1   Active stage
Granular conjunctivitis (trachomatous)
Trachomatous:
    follicular conjunctivitis
    pannus

076.9   Trachoma, unspecified
Trachoma NOS

✓4ᵗʰ **077   Other diseases of conjunctiva due to viruses and Chlamydiae**

EXCLUDES   *ophthalmic complications of viral diseases*
                 classified elsewhere

077.0   Inclusion conjunctivitis
Paratrachoma   Swimming pool conjunctivitis

EXCLUDES   *inclusion blennorrhea (neonatal) (771.6)*

DEF: Pus in conjunctiva caused by *Chlamydiae trachomatis*.

077.1   Epidemic keratoconjunctivitis
Shipyard eye

DEF: Highly contagious corneal or conjunctival infection caused by adenovirus type 8; symptoms include inflammation and corneal infiltrates.

077.2   Pharyngoconjunctival fever
Viral pharyngoconjunctivitis

077.3   Other adenoviral conjunctivitis
Acute adenoviral follicular conjunctivitis

077.4   Epidemic hemorrhagic conjunctivitis
Apollo:
    conjunctivitis
    disease
Conjunctivitis due to enterovirus type 70
Hemorrhagic conjunctivitis (acute) (epidemic)

077.8   Other viral conjunctivitis
Newcastle conjunctivitis

✓5ᵗʰ **077.9   Unspecified diseases of conjunctiva due to viruses and Chlamydiae**

DEF: A genus of the family Chlamydiaceae; *C. psittaci* causes psittacosis in man and ornithosis in birds, and *C. trachomatis* causes trachoma, conjunctivitis, lymphogranuloma venereum, pneumonitis and pneumonia.

077.98   Due to Chlamydiae

077.99   Due to viruses
Viral conjunctivitis NOS

✓4ᵗʰ **078   Other diseases due to viruses and Chlamydiae**

EXCLUDES   *viral infection NOS (079.0-079.9)*
                 viremia NOS (790.8)

078.0   Molluscum contagiosum
DEF: Benign poxvirus infection causing small bumps on the skin or conjunctiva; transmitted by close contact.

✓5ᵗʰ **078.1   Viral warts**
Viral warts due to human papilloma virus

AHA: 2Q, '97, 9; 4Q, '93, 22

DEF: A keratotic papilloma of the epidermis caused by the human papilloma virus; the superficial vegetative lesions last for varying durations and eventually regress spontaneously.

078.10   Viral warts, unspecified
Condyloma NOS   Verruca:
Verruca: Vulgaris
    NOS   Warts (infectious)

078.11   Condyloma acuminatum
DEF: Clusters of mucosa or epidermal lesions on external genitalia; viral infection is sexually transmitted.

078.19   Other specified viral warts
Genital warts NOS   Verruca:
Verruca: plantaris
    plana

078.2   Sweating fever
Miliary fever   Sweating disease

DEF: A viral infection characterized by profuse sweating; various papular, vesicular and other eruptions cause the blockage of sweat glands.

078.3   Cat-scratch disease
Benign lymphoreticulosis (of inoculation)
Cat-scratch fever

`N` Newborn Age: 0   `P` Pediatric Age: 0-17   `M` Maternity Age: 12-55   `A` Adult Age: 15-124   `CC` CC Condition   `MC` Major Complication   `CD` Complex Dx   `HIV` HIV Related Dx

078.4 Foot and mouth disease
Aphthous fever   Epizootic:
Epizootic: stomatitis
    aphthae

DEF: Ulcers on oral mucosa, legs, and feet after exposure to infected animal.

078.5 Cytomegaloviral disease   **HIV**
Cytomegalic inclusion disease
Salivary gland virus disease
Use additional code to identify manifestation, as:
    cytomegalic inclusion virus:
       hepatitis (573.1)
       pneumonia (484.1)

EXCLUDES   *congenital cytomegalovirus infection (771.1)*

AHA: 3Q, '98, 4; 2Q, '93, 11; 1Q, '89, 9

DEF: A herpes virus inclusion associated with serious disease morbidity including fever, leukopenia, pneumonia, retinitis, hepatitis and organ transplant; often leads to syndromes such as hepatomegaly, splenomegaly and thrombocytopenia; a common post-transplant complication for organ transplant recipients.

078.6 Hemorrhagic nephrosonephritis
Hemorrhagic fever: Hemorrhagic fever:
    epidemic   Russian
    Korean   with renal syndrome

DEF: Viral infection causing kidney dysfunction and bleeding disorders.

078.7 Arenaviral hemorrhagic fever
Hemorrhagic fever: Hemorrhagic fever:
    Argentine   Junin virus
    Bolivian   Machupo virus

√5ᵗʰ 078.8 Other specified diseases due to viruses and Chlamydiae
EXCLUDES   *epidemic diarrhea (009.2)*
lymphogranuloma venereum (099.1)

078.81 Epidemic vertigo

078.82 Epidemic vomiting syndrome
Winter vomiting disease

078.88 Other specified diseases due to Chlamydiae
AHA: 4Q, '96, 22

078.89 Other specified diseases due to viruses
Epidemic cervical myalgia
Marburg disease
Tanapox

√4ᵗʰ 079 Viral and chlamydial infection in conditions classified elsewhere and of unspecified site
Note: This category is provided to be used as an additional code to identify the viral agent in diseases classifiable elsewhere. This category will also be used to classify virus infection of unspecified nature or site.

079.0 Adenovirus

079.1 ECHO virus
DEF: An "orphan" enteric RNA virus, certain serotypes of which are associated with human disease, especially aseptic meningitis.

079.2 Coxsackie virus
DEF: A heterogenous group of viruses associated with aseptic meningitis, myocarditis, pericarditis, and acute onset juvenile diabetes.

079.3 Rhinovirus
DEF: Rhinoviruses affect primarily the upper respiratory tract. Over 100 distinct types infect humans.

079.4 Human papillomavirus
AHA: 2Q, '97, 9; 4Q, '93, 22

DEF: Viral infection caused by the genus *Papillomavirus* causing cutaneous and genital warts, including verruca vulgaris and condyloma acuminatum; certain types are associated with cervical dysplasia, cancer and other genital malignancies.

√5ᵗʰ 079.5 Retrovirus
EXCLUDES   *human immunodeficiency virus, type 1 [HIV-1] (042)*
human T-cell lymphotrophic virus, type III [HTLV-III] (042)
lymphadenopathy-associated virus [LAV] (042)

AHA: 4Q, '93, 22, 23

DEF: A large group of RNA viruses that carry reverse transcriptase and include the leukoviruses and lentiviruses.

079.50 Retrovirus, unspecified

079.51 Human T-cell lymphotrophic virus, type I [HTLV-I]

079.52 Human T-cell lymphotrophic virus, type II [HTLV-II]

079.53 Human immunodeficiency virus, type 2 [HIV-2]

079.59 Other specified retrovirus

079.6 Respiratory syncytial virus (RSV)
AHA: 4Q, '96, 27, 28

DEF: The major respiratory pathogen of young children, causing severe bronchitis and bronchopneumonia, and minor infection in adults.

√5ᵗʰ 079.8 Other specified viral and chlamydial infections
AHA: 1Q, '88, 12

079.81 Hantavirus
AHA: 4Q, '95, 60

DEF: An infection caused by the Muerto Canyon virus whose primary rodent reservoir is the deer mouse *Peromyscus maniculatus*; commonly characterized by fever, myalgias, headache, cough and rapid decline.

079.88 Other specified chlamydial infection

079.89 Other specified viral infection

√5ᵗʰ 079.9 Unspecified viral and chlamydial infections
EXCLUDES   *viremia NOS (790.8)*

AHA: 2Q, '91, 8

079.98 Unspecified chlamydial infection
Chlamydial infections NOS

079.99 Unspecified viral infection
Viral infections NOS

RICKETTSIOSES AND OTHER ARTHROPOD-BORNE DISEASES (080-088)
EXCLUDES   *arthropod-borne viral diseases (060.0-066.9)*

080 Louse-borne [epidemic] typhus
Typhus (fever):   Typhus (fever):
    classical   exanthematic NOS
    epidemic   louse-borne

DEF: *Rickettsia prowazekii*; causes severe headache, rash, high fever.

√4ᵗʰ 081 Other typhus

081.0 Murine [endemic] typhus
Typhus (fever):   Typhus (fever):
    endemic   flea-borne

DEF: Milder typhus caused by *Rickettsia typhi (mooseri)*; transmitted by rat flea.

081.1 Brill's disease
Brill-Zinsser disease
Recrudescent typhus (fever)

081.2 Scrub typhus
Japanese river fever   Mite-borne typhus
Kedani fever   Tsutsugamushi

081.9 Typhus, unspecified
Typhus (fever) NOS

√4ᵗʰ 082 Tick-borne rickettsioses

082.0 Spotted fevers
Rocky mountain spotted fever
Sao Paulo fever

√4ᵗʰ Additional Digit Required   Nonspecific PDx   Unacceptable PDx   Manifestation Code   **MSP** Medicare Secondary Payer   ►◄ Revised Text   ● New Code   ▲ Revised Code Title
√5ᵗʰ

2002 Ingenix, Inc.   **Volume 1 — 15**

Infectious and Parasitic Diseases 082.1–086.0

082.1 **Boutonneuse fever**
     African tick typhus   Marseilles fever
     India tick typhus   Mediterranean tick fever
     Kenya tick typhus

082.2 **North Asian tick fever**
     Siberian tick typhus

082.3 **Queensland tick typhus**

✓5ᵗʰ 082.4 **Ehrlichiosis**
     AHA: 4Q, '00, 38

082.40 **Ehrlichiosis, unspecified**

082.41 **Ehrlichiosis chaffeensis [E. chaffeensis]**
     DEF: A febrile illness caused by bacterial infection, also
     called human monocytic ehrlichiosis (HME). Causal
     organism is *Ehrlichia chaffeensis*, transmitted by the
     Lone Star tick, *Amblyomma americanum.* Symptoms
     include fever, chills, myalgia, nausea, vomiting, diarrhea,
     confusion, and severe headache occurring one week
     after a tick bite. Clinical findings are lymphadenopathy,
     rash, thrombocytopenia, leukopenia, and abnormal liver
     function tests.

082.49 **Other ehrlichiosis**

082.8 **Other specified tick-borne rickettsioses**
     Lone star fever
     AHA: 4Q, '99, 19

082.9 **Tick-borne rickettsiosis, unspecified**
     Tick-borne typhus NOS

✓4ᵗʰ 083 **Other rickettsioses**

083.0 **Q fever**
     DEF: Infection of *Coxiella burnettii* usually acquired through
     airborne organisms.

083.1 **Trench fever**
     Quintan fever   Wolhynian fever

083.2 **Rickettsialpox**
     Vesicular rickettsiosis
     DEF: Infection of *Rickettsia akari* usually acquired through a mite
     bite.

083.8 **Other specified rickettsioses**

083.9 **Rickettsiosis, unspecified**

✓4ᵗʰ 084 **Malaria**
     Note: Subcategories 084.0-084.6 exclude the listed conditions
     with mention of pernicious complications (084.8-084.9).
     EXCLUDES *congenital malaria (771.2)*
     DEF: Mosquito-borne disease causing high fever and prostration and
     cataloged by species of *Plasmodium: P. falciparum, P. malariae, P. ovale, and*
     P. vivax.

084.0 **Falciparum malaria [malignant tertian]**
     Malaria (fever):
       by Plasmodium falciparum
       subtertian

084.1 **Vivax malaria [benign tertian]**
     Malaria (fever) by Plasmodium vivax

084.2 **Quartan malaria**
     Malaria (fever) by Plasmodium malariae
     Malariae malaria

084.3 **Ovale malaria**
     Malaria (fever) by Plasmodium ovale

084.4 **Other malaria**
     Monkey malaria

084.5 **Mixed malaria**
     Malaria (fever) by more than one parasite

084.6 **Malaria, unspecified**
     Malaria (fever) NOS

084.7 **Induced malaria**
     Therapeutically induced malaria
     EXCLUDES *accidental infection from syringe, blood*
       transfusion, etc. (084.0-084.6,
       above, according to parasite
       species)
       transmission from mother to child
       during delivery (771.2)

084.8 **Blackwater fever**
     Hemoglobinuric: Malarial hemoglobinuria
       fever (bilious)
       malaria
     DEF: Severe hemic and renal complication of *Plasmodium*
     falciparum infection.

084.9 **Other pernicious complications of malaria**
     Algid malaria
     Cerebral malaria
     Use additional code to identify complication, as:
       malarial:
         hepatitis (573.2)
         nephrosis (581.81)

✓4ᵗʰ 085 **Leishmaniasis**

085.0 **Visceral [kala-azar]**
     Dumdum fever   Leishmaniasis:
     Infection by Leishmania: dermal, post-kala-azar
       donovani   Mediterranean
       infantum   visceral (Indian)

085.1 **Cutaneous, urban**
     Aleppo boil   Leishmaniasis, cutaneous:
     Baghdad boil   dry form
     Delhi boil   late
     Infection by Leishmania   recurrent
       tropica (minor)   ulcerating
                     Oriental sore

085.2 **Cutaneous, Asian desert**
     Infection by Leishmania tropica major
     Leishmaniasis, cutaneous:
       acute necrotizing
       rural
       wet form
       zoonotic form

085.3 **Cutaneous, Ethiopian**
     Infection by Leishmania ethiopica
     Leishmaniasis, cutaneous:
       diffuse
       lepromatous

085.4 **Cutaneous, American**
     Chiclero ulcer
     Infection by Leishmania mexicana
     Leishmaniasis tegumentaria diffusa

085.5 **Mucocutaneous (American)**
     Espundia
     Infection by Leishmania braziliensis
     Uta

085.9 **Leishmaniasis, unspecified**

✓4ᵗʰ 086 **Trypanosomiasis**
     Use additional code to identify manifestations, as:
     trypanosomiasis:
     encephalitis (323.2)
     meningitis (321.3)

086.0 **Chagas' disease with heart involvement**   **CC**
     American trypanosomiasis   } with heart
     Infection by Trypanosoma   involvement
       cruzi
     Any condition classifiable to 086.2 with heart
       involvement
     CC Excl: 086.0, 139.8

N Newborn Age: 0   **P** Pediatric Age: 0-17   **M** Maternity Age: 12-55   **A** Adult Age: 15-124   **CC** CC Condition   **MC** Major Complication   **CD** Complex Dx   **HIV** HIV Related Dx

16 — Volume 1   *2002 Ingenix, Inc.*

086.1 **Chagas' disease with other organ involvement**

American trypanosomiasis
Infection by Trypanosoma cruzi } with heart involvement

Any condition classifiable to 086.2 with heart involvement

086.2 **Chagas' disease without mention of organ involvement**
American trypanosomiasis
Infection by Trypanosoma cruzi

086.3 **Gambian trypanosomiasis**
Gambian sleeping sickness
Infection by Trypanosoma gambiense

086.4 **Rhodesian trypanosomiasis**
Infection by Trypanosoma rhodesiense
Rhodesian sleeping sickness

086.5 **African trypanosomiasis, unspecified**
Sleeping sickness NOS

086.9 **Trypanosomiasis, unspecified**

√4ᵗʰ 087 **Relapsing fever**
　INCLUDES　recurrent fever

DEF: Infection of *Borrelia;* symptoms are episodic and include fever and arthralgia.

087.0 **Louse-borne**

087.1 **Tick-borne**

087.9 **Relapsing fever, unspecified**

√4ᵗʰ 088 **Other arthropod-borne diseases**

088.0 **Bartonellosis**
Carrión's disease　　　Verruga peruana
Oroya fever

√5ᵗʰ 088.8 **Other specified arthropod-borne diseases**

088.81 **Lyme disease**
Erythema chronicum migrans
AHA: 4Q, '91, 15; 3Q, '90, 14; 2Q, '89, 10

DEF: A recurrent multisystem disorder caused by the spirochete *Borrelia burgdorferi* with the carrier being the tick *Ixodes dammini;* the disease begins with lesions of erythema chronicum migrans; it is followed by arthritis of the large joints, myalgia, malaise, and neurological and cardiac manifestations.

088.82 **Babesiosis**
Babesiasis
AHA: 4Q, '93, 23

DEF: A tick-borne disease caused by infection of *Babesia,* characterized by fever, malaise, listlessness, severe anemia and hemoglobinuria.

088.89 **Other**

088.9 **Arthropod-borne disease, unspecified**

SYPHILIS AND OTHER VENEREAL DISEASES (090-099)
　EXCLUDES　nonvenereal endemic syphilis (104.0)
　　　　　　urogenital trichomoniasis (131.0)

√4ᵗʰ 090 **Congenital syphilis**

DEF: Infection by spirochete *Treponema pallidum* acquired in utero from the infected mother.

090.0 **Early congenital syphilis, symptomatic**
Congenital syphilitic:　Congenital syphilitic:
　choroiditis　　　　　　splenomegaly
　coryza (chronic)　　Syphilitic (congenital):
　hepatomegaly　　　　epiphysitis
　mucous patches　　　osteochondritis
　periostitis　　　　　　pemphigus
Any congenital syphilitic condition specified as early or manifest less than two years after birth

090.1 **Early congenital syphilis, latent**
Congenital syphilis without clinical manifestations, with positive serological reaction and negative spinal fluid test, less than two years after birth

090.2 **Early congenital syphilis, unspecified**
Congenital syphilis NOS, less than two years after birth

090.3 **Syphilitic interstitial keratitis**
Syphilitic keratitis:　Syphilitic keratitis:
　parenchymatous　　　punctata profunda
　EXCLUDES　*interstitial keratitis NOS (370.50)*

√5ᵗʰ 090.4 **Juvenile neurosyphilis**
Use additional code to identify any associated mental disorder

DEF: *Treponema pallidum* infection involving the nervous system.

090.40 **Juvenile neurosyphilis, unspecified**　CC
Congenital neurosyphilis
Dementia paralytica juvenilis
Juvenile:
　general paresis
　tabes
　taboparesis
CC Excl: 090.0-090.9, 091.0-091.9, 092.0, 092.9, 093.0-093.9, 094.0-094.9, 095.0-095.9, 096, 097.0-097.9, 099.40-099.59, 099.8, 099.9, 139.8

090.41 **Congenital syphilitic encephalitis**　CC
CC Excl: See code 090.40

DEF: Congenital *Treponema pallidum* infection involving the brain.

090.42 **Congenital syphilitic meningitis**　CC
CC Excl: 003.21, 013.00-013.16, 036.0, 047.0-047.9, 049.0-049.1, 053.0, 054.72, 072.1, 090.0-090.9, 091.0-091.9, 092.0, 092.9, 093.0-093.9, 094.0-094.9, 095.0-095.9, 096, 097.0-097.9, 098.89, 099.40-099.59, 099.8, 099.9, 100.81, 112.83, 114.2, 115.01, 115.11, 115.91, 130.0, 139.8, 320.0-320.9, 321.0-321.8, 322.0-322.9, 349.89, 349.9, 357.0

DEF: Congenital *Treponema pallidum* infection involving the lining of the brain and/or spinal cord.

090.49 **Other**　CC
CC Excl: See code 090.40

090.5 **Other late congenital syphilis, symptomatic**
Gumma due to congenital syphilis
Hutchinson's teeth
Syphilitic saddle nose
Any congenital syphilitic condition specified as late or manifest two years or more after birth

090.6 **Late congenital syphilis, latent**
Congenital syphilis without clinical manifestations, with positive serological reaction and negative spinal fluid test, two years or more after birth

090.7 **Late congenital syphilis, unspecified**
Congenital syphilis NOS, two years or more after birth

090.9 **Congenital syphilis, unspecified**

√4ᵗʰ 091 **Early syphilis, symptomatic**
　EXCLUDES　*early cardiovascular syphilis (093.0-093.9)*
　　　　　　early neurosyphilis (094.0-094.9)

091.0 **Genital syphilis (primary)**
Genital chancre

DEF: Genital lesion at the site of initial infection by *Treponema pallidum.*

091.1 **Primary anal syphilis**

DEF: Anal lesion at the site of initial infection by *Treponema pallidum.*

091.2 **Other primary syphilis**
Primary syphilis of:　Primary syphilis of:
　breast　　　　　　　　lip
　fingers　　　　　　　　tonsils

DEF: Lesion at the site of initial infection by *Treponema pallidum.*

√4ᵗʰ √5ᵗʰ Additional Digit Required　Nonspecific PDx　Unacceptable PDx　Manifestation Code　MSP Medicare Secondary Payer　▶◀ Revised Text　● New Code　▲ Revised Code Title

2002 Ingenix, Inc.　　　　　　　　　　　　　　　　　　　　　　　　　　　　　　　　　　　Volume 1 — 17

Infectious and Parasitc Diseases 091.3–094.84

091.3 Secondary syphilis of skin or mucous membranes
Condyloma latum   Secondary syphilis of:
Secondary syphilis of: skin
    anus   tonsils
    mouth   vulva
    pharynx
DEF: Transitory or chronic lesions following initial syphillis infection.

091.4 Adenopathy due to secondary syphilis
Syphilitic adenopathy (secondary)
Syphilitic lymphadenitis (secondary)

√5ᵗʰ 091.5 Uveitis due to secondary syphilis
091.50 Syphilitic uveitis, unspecified
091.51 Syphilitic chorioretinitis (secondary)
DEF: Inflammation of choroid and retina as a secondary infection.

091.52 Syphilitic iridocyclitis (secondary)
DEF: Inflammation of iris and ciliary body as a secondary infection.

√5ᵗʰ 091.6 Secondary syphilis of viscera and bone
091.61 Secondary syphilitic periostitis
DEF: Inflammation of outer layers of bone as a secondary infection.

091.62 Secondary syphilitic hepatitis
Secondary syphilis of liver
091.69 Other viscera

091.7 Secondary syphilis, relapse
Secondary syphilis, relapse (treated) (untreated)
DEF: Return of symptoms of syphillis following asymptomatic period.

√5ᵗʰ 091.8 Other forms of secondary syphilis
091.81 Acute syphilitic meningitis (secondary)
DEF: Sudden, severe inflammation of the lining of the brain and/or spinal cord as a secondary infection.

091.82 Syphilitic alopecia
DEF: Hair loss following initial syphillis infection.

091.89 Other
091.9 Unspecified secondary syphilis

√4ᵗʰ 092 Early syphilis, latent
    INCLUDES   syphilis (acquired) without clinical manifestations, with positive serological reaction and negative spinal fluid test, less than two years after infection

092.0 Early syphilis, latent, serological relapse after treatment
092.9 Early syphilis, latent, unspecified

√4ᵗʰ 093 Cardiovascular syphilis
093.0 Aneurysm of aorta, specified as syphilitic `CC`
Dilatation of aorta, specified as syphilitic
CC Excl: See code 090.40

093.1 Syphilitic aortitis `CC`
CC Excl: See code 090.40
DEF: Inflammation of the aorta – the main artery leading from the heart.

√5ᵗʰ 093.2 Syphilitic endocarditis
DEF: Inflammation of the tissues lining the cavities of the heart.

093.20 Valve, unspecified `CC`
Syphilitic ostial coronary disease
CC Excl: See code 090.40

093.21 Mitral valve `CC`
CC Excl: See code 090.40

093.22 Aortic valve `CC`
Syphilitic aortic incompetence or stenosis
CC Excl: See code 090.40

093.23 Tricuspid valve `CC`
CC Excl: See code 090.40

093.24 Pulmonary valve `CC`
CC Excl: See code 090.40

√5ᵗʰ 093.8 Other specified cardiovascular syphilis
093.81 Syphilitic pericarditis `CC`
CC Excl: See code 090.40
DEF: Inflammation of the outer lining of the heart.

093.82 Syphilitic myocarditis `CC`
CC Excl: See code 090.40
DEF: Inflammation of the muscle of the heart.

093.89 Other `CC`
CC Excl: See code 090.40

093.9 Cardiovascular syphilis, unspecified `CC`
CC Excl: See code 090.40

√4ᵗʰ 094 Neurosyphilis
Use additional code to identify any associated mental disorder

094.0 Tabes dorsalis `CC`
Locomotor ataxia (progressive)
Posterior spinal sclerosis (syphilitic)
Tabetic neurosyphilis
Use additional code to identify manifestation, as:
    neurogenic arthropathy [Charcot's joint disease] (713.5)
CC Excl: See code 090.40
DEF: Progressive degeneration of nerves associated with long-term syphillis; causing pain, wasting away, incontinence, and ataxia.

094.1 General paresis `CC`
Dementia paralytica
General paralysis (of the insane) (progressive)
Paretic neurosyphilis
Taboparesis
CC Excl: See code 090.40
DEF: Degeneration of brain associated with long-term syphillis, causing loss of brain function, progressive dementia, and paralysis.

094.2 Syphilitic meningitis `CC`
Meningovascular syphilis
   EXCLUDES   acute syphilitic meningitis (secondary) (091.81)
CC Excl: 003.21, 013.00-013.16, 036.0, 047.0-047.9, 049.0-049.1, 053.0, 054.72, 072.1, 090.0-090.9, 091.0-091.9, 092.0, 092.9, 093.0-093.9, 094.0-094.9, 095.0-095.9, 096, 097.0-097.9, 098.89, 099.40-099.59, 099.8, 099.9, 100.81, 112.83, 114.2, 115.01, 115.11, 115.91, 130.0, 139.8, 320.0-320.9, 321.0-321.8, 322.0-322.9, 349.89, 349.9, 357.0
DEF: Inflammation of the lining of the brain and/or spinal cord.

094.3 Asymptomatic neurosyphilis `CC`
CC Excl: See code 090.40

√5ᵗʰ 094.8 Other specified neurosyphilis
094.81 Syphilitic encephalitis `CC`
CC Excl: See code 090.40

094.82 Syphilitic Parkinsonism
DEF: Decreased motor function, tremors, and muscular rigidity.

094.83 Syphilitic disseminated retinochoroiditis
DEF: Inflammation of retina and choroid due to neurosyphillis.

094.84 Syphilitic optic atrophy
DEF: Degeneration of the eye and its nerves due to neurosyphillis.

`N` Newborn Age: 0   `P` Pediatric Age: 0-17   `M` Maternity Age: 12-55   `A` Adult Age: 15-124   `CC` CC Condition   `MC` Major Complication   `CD` Complex Dx   `HIV` HIV Related Dx

094.85 Syphilitic retrobulbar neuritis
DEF: Inflammation of the posterior optic nerve to neurosyphillis.

094.86 Syphilitic acoustic neuritis
DEF: Inflammation of acoustic nerve due to neurosyphillis.

094.87 Syphilitic ruptured cerebral aneurysm `CC`
CC Excl: See code 090.40

094.89 Other `CC`
CC Excl: See code 090.40

094.9 Neurosyphilis, unspecified `CC`
Gumma (syphilitic)
Syphilis (early) (late) } of central nervous system
Syphiloma   NOS

CC Excl: See code 090.40

✓4ᵗʰ **095 Other forms of late syphilis, with symptoms**
INCLUDES   gumma (syphilitic)
syphilis, late, tertiary, or unspecified stage

095.0 Syphilitic episcleritis

095.1 Syphilis of lung

095.2 Syphilitic peritonitis

095.3 Syphilis of liver

095.4 Syphilis of kidney

095.5 Syphilis of bone

095.6 Syphilis of muscle
Syphilitic myositis

095.7 Syphilis of synovium, tendon, and bursa
Syphilitic: Syphilitic:
bursitis   synovitis

095.8 Other specified forms of late symptomatic syphilis
EXCLUDES   *cardiovascular syphilis (093.0-093.9)*
neurosyphilis (094.0-094.9)

095.9 Late symptomatic syphilis, unspecified

096 Late syphilis, latent
Syphilis (acquired) without clinical manifestations, with positive serological reaction and negative spinal fluid test, two years or more after infection

✓4ᵗʰ **097 Other and unspecified syphilis**

097.0 Late syphilis, unspecified

097.1 Latent syphilis, unspecified
Positive serological reaction for syphilis

097.9 Syphilis, unspecified
Syphilis (acquired) NOS
EXCLUDES   *syphilis NOS causing death under two years of age (090.9)*

✓4ᵗʰ **098 Gonococcal infections**
DEF: *Neisseria gonorrhoeae* infection generally acquired in utero or in sexual congress.

098.0 Acute, of lower genitourinary tract `CC`
Gonococcal: Gonorrhea (acute):
Bartholinitis (acute)   NOS
urethritis (acute)   genitourinary (tract) NOS
vulvovaginitis (acute)
CC Excl: 098.0-098.39, 098.89, 099.40-099.59, 099.8, 099.9, 139.8

✓5ᵗʰ **098.1 Acute, of upper genitourinary tract**

098.10 Gonococcal infection (acute) of upper genitourinary tract, site unspecified `CC`
CC Excl: See code 098.0

098.11 Gonococcal cystitis (acute) `CC`
Gonorrhea (acute) of bladder
CC Excl: See code 098.0

098.12 Gonococcal prostatitis (acute) `CC`♂
CC Excl: See code 098.0

098.13 Gonococcal epididymo-orchitis (acute) `CC`♂
Gonococcal orchitis (acute)
CC Excl: See code 098.0
DEF: Acute inflammation of the testes.

098.14 Gonococcal seminal vesiculitis (acute) `CC`♂
Gonorrhea (acute) of seminal vesicle
CC Excl: See code 098.0

098.15 Gonococcal cervicitis (acute) `CC`♀
Gonorrhea (acute) of cervix
CC Excl: See code 098.0

098.16 Gonococcal endometritis (acute) `CC`♀
Gonorrhea (acute) of uterus
CC Excl: See code 098.0

098.17 Gonococcal salpingitis, specified as acute `CC`♀
CC Excl: See code 098.0
DEF: Acute inflammation of the fallopian tubes.

098.19 Other `CC`
CC Excl: See code 098.0

098.2 Chronic, of lower genitourinary tract
Gonococcal:
Bartholinitis   } specified as chronic
urethritis   or with
vulvovaginitis   duration of
Gonorrhea: two months
NOS   or more
genitourinary (tract)
Any condition classifiable to 098.0 specified as chronic or with duration of two months or more

✓5ᵗʰ **098.3 Chronic, of upper genitourinary tract**
INCLUDES   any condition classifiable to 098.1 stated as chronic or with a duration of two months or more

098.30 Chronic gonococcal infection of upper genitourinary tract, site unspecified

098.31 Gonococcal cystitis, chronic
Any condition classifiable to 098.11, specified as chronic
Gonorrhea of bladder, chronic

098.32 Gonococcal prostatitis, chronic ♂
Any condition classifiable to 098.12, specified as chronic

098.33 Gonococcal epididymo-orchitis, chronic ♂
Any condition classifiable to 098.13, specified as chronic
Chronic gonococcal orchitis
DEF: Chronic inflammation of the testes.

098.34 Gonococcal seminal vesiculitis, chronic ♂
Any condition classifiable to 098.14, specified as chronic
Gonorrhea of seminal vesicle, chronic

098.35 Gonococcal cervicitis, chronic ♀
Any condition classifiable to 098.15, specified as chronic
Gonorrhea of cervix, chronic

098.36 Gonococcal endometritis, chronic ♀
Any condition classifiable to 098.16, specified as chronic
DEF: Chronic inflammation of the uterus.

098.37 Gonococcal salpingitis (chronic) ♀
DEF: Chronic inflammation of the fallopian tubes.

098.39 Other

✓4ᵗʰ
✓5ᵗʰ Addiitional Digit Required   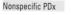 Nonspecific PDx   Unacceptable PDx   Manifestation Code   `MSP` Medicare Secondary Payer   ►◄ Revised Text   ● New Code   ▲ Revised Code Title

2002 Ingenix, Inc.   Volume 1 — 19

√5th **098.4 Gonococcal infection of eye**

098.40 Gonococcal conjunctivitis (neonatorum)
Gonococcal ophthalmia (neonatorum)
DEF: Infection of conjunctiva present at birth.

098.41 Gonococcal iridocyclitis
DEF: Inflammation and infection of iris and ciliary body.

098.42 Gonococcal endophthalmia
DEF: Inflammation and infection of contents of eyeball.

098.43 Gonococcal keratitis
DEF: Inflammation and infection of the cornea.

098.49 Other

√5th **098.5 Gonococcal infection of joint**

098.50 Gonococcal arthritis
Gonococcal infection of joint NOS

098.51 Gonococcal synovitis and tenosynovitis

098.52 Gonococcal bursitis
DEF: Inflammation of the sac-like cavities in a joint.

098.53 Gonococcal spondylitis

098.59 Other
Gonococcal rheumatism

098.6 Gonococcal infection of pharynx

098.7 Gonococcal infection of anus and rectum
Gonococcal proctitis

√5th **098.8 Gonococcal infection of other specified sites**

098.81 Gonococcal keratosis (blennorrhagica)
DEF: Pustular skin lesions caused by *Neisseria gonorrhoeae.*

098.82 Gonococcal meningitis
DEF: Inflammation of lining of brain and/or spinal cord.

098.83 Gonococcal pericarditis
DEF: Inflammation of the outer lining of the heart.

098.84 Gonococcal endocarditis
DEF: Inflammation of tissues lining the cavities of heart.

098.85 Other gonococcal heart disease

098.86 Gonococcal peritonitis
DEF: Inflammation of the membrane lining the abdomen.

098.89 Other
Gonococcemia

√4th **099 Other venereal diseases**

099.0 Chancroid

Bubo (inguinal): Chancre:
chancroidal Ducrey's
due to Hemophilus simple
ducreyi soft
 Ulcus molle (cutis) (skin)

DEF: A sexually transmitted disease caused by *Haemophilus ducreyi;* it is identified by a painful primary ulcer at the site of inoculation (usually external genitalia) with related lymphadenitis.

099.1 Lymphogranuloma venereum
Climatic or tropical bubo
(Durand-) Nicolas-Favre disease
Esthiomene
Lymphogranuloma inguinale
DEF: Sexually transmitted infection of *Chlamydia trachomatis* causing skin lesions.

099.2 Granuloma inguinale

Donovanosis Granuloma venereum
Granuloma pudendi Pudendal ulcer
(ulcerating)

DEF: Chronic, sexually transmitted infection of *Calymmatobacterium granulomatis* causing progressive, anogenital skin ulcers.

099.3 Reiter's disease
Reiter's syndrome
Use additional code for associated:
arthropathy (711.1)
conjunctivitis (372.33)
DEF: A symptom complex of unknown etiology consisting of urethritis, conjunctivitis, arthritis and myocutaneous lesions. It occurs most commonly in young men and patients with HIV and may precede or follow AIDS. Also a form of reactive arthritis.

√5th **099.4 Other nongonococcal urethritis [NGU]**

099.40 Unspecified
Nonspecific urethritis

099.41 Chlamydia trachomatis

099.49 Other specified organism

√5th **099.5 Other venereal diseases due to Chlamydia trachomatis**
EXCLUDES *Chlamydia trachomatis infection of conjunctiva (076.0-076.9, 077.0, 077.9)*
Lymphogranuloma venereum (099.1)
DEF: Venereal diseases caused by *Chlamydia trachomatis* at other sites besides the urethra (e.g., pharynx, anus and rectum, conjunctiva and peritoneum).

099.50 Unspecified site

099.51 Pharynx

099.52 Anus and rectum

099.53 Lower genitourinary sites
EXCLUDES *urethra (099.41)*
Use additional code to specify site of infection, such as:
bladder (595.4)
cervix (616.0)
vagina and vulva (616.11)

099.54 Other genitourinary sites
Use additional code to specify site of infection, such as:
pelvic inflammatory disease NOS (614.9)
testis and epididymis (604.91)

099.55 Unspecified genitourinary site

099.56 Peritoneum
Perihepatitis

099.59 Other specified site

099.8 Other specified venereal diseases

099.9 Venereal disease, unspecified

OTHER SPIROCHETAL DISEASES (100-104)

√4th **100 Leptospirosis**
DEF: An infection of any spirochete of the genus Leptospire in blood. This zoonosis is transmitted to humans most often by exposure with contaminated animal tissues or water and less often by contact with urine. Patients present with flulike symptoms, the most common being muscle aches involving the thighs and low back. Treatment is with hydration and antibiotics.

100.0 Leptospirosis icterohemorrhagica
Leptospiral or spirochetal jaundice (hemorrhagic)
Weil's disease

√5th **100.8 Other specified leptospiral infections**

100.81 Leptospiral meningitis (aseptic)

100.89 Other

Fever: Infection by Leptospira:
Fort Bragg australis
pretibial bataviae
swamp pyrogenes

100.9 Leptospirosis, unspecified

N Newborn Age: 0   P Pediatric Age: 0-17   M Maternity Age: 12-55   A Adult Age: 15-124   CC CC Condition   MC Major Complication   CD Complex Dx   HIV HIV Related Dx

20 — Volume 1   2002 Ingenix, Inc.

101 Vincent's angina

Acute necrotizing ulcerative: Trench mouth
    gingivitis   Vincent's:
    stomatitis   gingivitis
Fusospirochetal pharyngitis   infection [any site]
Spirochetal stomatitis

DEF: Painful ulceration with edema and hypermic patches of the oropharyngeal and throat membranes; it is caused by spreading of acute ulcerative gingivitis.

✓4th **102 Yaws**

INCLUDES   frambesia
                 pian

DEF: An infectious, endemic, tropical disease caused by *Treponema pertenue*; it usually affects persons 15 years old or younger; a primary cutaneous lesion develops, then a granulomatous skin eruption, and occasionally lesions that destroy skin and bone.

102.0 Initial lesions
Chancre of yaws
Frambesia, initial or primary
Initial frambesial ulcer
Mother yaw

102.1 Multiple papillomata and wet crab yaws
Butter yaws   Plantar or palmar
Frambesioma   papilloma of yaws
Pianoma

102.2 Other early skin lesions
Cutaneous yaws, less than five years after infection
Early yaws (cutaneous) (macular) (papular)
    (maculopapular) (micropapular)
Frambeside of early yaws

102.3 Hyperkeratosis
Ghoul hand
Hyperkeratosis, palmar or plantar (early) (late) due
    to yaws
Worm-eaten soles

DEF: Overgrowth of skin of palm of bottoms of feet, due to yaws.

102.4 Gummata and ulcers
Gummatous frambeside
Nodular late yaws (ulcerated)

DEF: Rubbery lesions and areas of dead skin caused by yaws.

102.5 Gangosa
Rhinopharyngitis mutilans

DEF: Massive, mutilating lesions of the nose and oral cavity caused by yaws.

102.6 Bone and joint lesions
Goundou
Gumma, bone
Gummatous osteitis or } of yaws (late)
    periostitis

Hydrarthrosis
Osteitis } of yaws (early) (late)
Periostitis (hypertrophic)

102.7 Other manifestations
Juxta-articular nodules of yaws
Mucosal yaws

102.8 Latent yaws
Yaws without clinical manifestations, with positive
    serology

102.9 Yaws, unspecified

✓4th ✓5th **103 Pinta**

DEF: A chronic form of treponema-tosis, endemic in areas of tropical America; it is identified by the presence of red, violet, blue, coffee-colored or white spots on the skin.

103.0 Primary lesions
Chancre (primary)
Papule (primary) } of pinta [carate]
Pintid

103.1 Intermediate lesions
Erythematous plaques
Hyperchromic lesions } of pinta [carate]
Hyperkeratosis

103.2 Late lesions
Cardiovascular lesions
Skin lesions:
    achromic
    cicatricial } of pinta [carate]
    dyschromic
Vitiligo

103.3 Mixed lesions
Achromic and hyperchromic skin lesions of pinta
    [carate]

103.9 Pinta, unspecified

✓4th **104 Other spirochetal infection**

104.0 Nonvenereal endemic syphilis
Bejel   Njovera

DEF: *Treponema pallidum, T. pertenue*, or *T. caroteum* infection transmitted non-sexually, causing lesions on mucosa and skin.

104.8 Other specified spirochetal infections
EXCLUDES   *relapsing fever (087.0-087.9)*
               syphilis (090.0-097.9)

104.9 Spirochetal infection, unspecified

MYCOSES (110-118)

Use additional code to identify manifestation as:
arthropathy (711.6)
meningitis (321.0-321.1)
otitis externa (380.15)
EXCLUDES   *infection by Actinomycetales, such as species of*
              Actinomyces, Actinomadura, Nocardia,
              Streptomyces (039.0-039.9)

✓4th **110 Dermatophytosis**

INCLUDES   infection by species of Epidermophyton,
              Microsporum, and Trichophyton
              tinea, any type except those in 111

DEF: Superficial infection of the skin caused by a parasitic fungus.

110.0 Of scalp and beard
Kerion   Trichophytic tinea
Sycosis, mycotic   [black dot tinea], scalp

110.1 Of nail
Dermatophytic onychia   Tinea unguium
Onychomycosis

110.2 Of hand
Tinea manuum

110.3 Of groin and perianal area
Dhobie itch   Tinea cruris
Eczema marginatum

110.4 Of foot
Athlete's foot   Tinea pedis

110.5 Of the body
Herpes circinatus   Tinea imbricata [Tokelau]

110.6 Deep seated dermatophytosis
Granuloma trichophyticum
Majocchi's granuloma

110.8 Of other specified sites

110.9 Of unspecified site
Favus NOS   Ringworm NOS
Microsporic tinea NOS

✓4th **111 Dermatomycosis, other and unspecified**

111.0 Pityriasis versicolor
Infection by Malassezia [Pityrosporum] furfur
Tinea flava
Tinea versicolor

✓4th ✓5th **Additional Digit Required**   Nonspecific PDx   Unacceptable PDx   Manifestation Code   **MSP** Medicare Secondary Payer   ►◄ Revised Text   ● New Code   ▲ Revised Code Title

2002 Ingenix, Inc.

Volume 1 — 21

Infectious and Parasitic Diseases 111.1–115.0

111.1   **Tinea nigra**
    Infection by Cladosporium species
    Keratomycosis nigricans
    Microsporosis nigra
    Pityriasis nigra
    Tinea palmaris nigra

111.2   **Tinea blanca**
    Infection by Trichosporon (beigelii) cutaneum
    White piedra

111.3   **Black piedra**
    Infection by Piedraia hortai

111.8   **Other specified dermatomycoses**

111.9   **Dermatomycosis, unspecified**

✓4th **112 Candidiasis**

    INCLUDES   infection by Candida species
                moniliasis
    EXCLUDES   *neonatal monilial infection (771.7)*

DEF: Fungal infection caused by Candida; usually seen in mucous membranes or skin.

112.0   **Of mouth**   **CC** **HIV**
    Thrush (oral)
    CC Excl: 112.0-112.9, 117.9, 139.8

112.1   **Of vulva and vagina**   ♀
    Candidal vulvovaginitis   Monilial vulvovaginitis

112.2   **Of other urogenital sites**
    Candidal balanitis
    AHA: 4Q, '96, 33

112.3   **Of skin and nails**   **HIV**
    Candidal intertrigo
    Candidal onychia
    Candidal perionyxis [paronychia]

112.4   **Of lung**   **CC** **HIV**
    Candidal pneumonia
    CC Excl: See code 112.0

    AHA: 2Q, '98, 7

112.5   **Disseminated**   **CC** **HIV**
    Systemic candidiasis
    CC Excl: See code 112.0

    AHA: 2Q, '00, 5; 2Q, '89, 10

✓5th **112.8**   **Of other specified sites**

    112.81 Candidal endocarditis   **CC** **HIV**
       CC Excl: See code 112.0

    112.82 Candidal otitis externa   **CC** **HIV**
       Otomycosis in moniliasis
       CC Excl: See code 112.0

    112.83 Candidal meningitis   **CC** **HIV**
       CC Excl: 003.21, 013.00-013.16, 036.0, 047.0-047.9,
       049.0-049.1, 053.0, 054.72, 072.1, 090.42, 091.81,
       094.2, 098.89, 100.81, 112.0-112.9, 114.2, 115.01,
       115.11, 115.91, 117.9, 130.0, 139.8, 320.0-320.9, 321.0-
       321.8, 322.0-322.9, 349.89, 349.9, 357.0

    112.84 Candidal esophagitis   **CC** **HIV**
       CC Excl: See code 112.0

       AHA: 4Q, '92, 19

    112.85 Candidal enteritis   **CC** **HIV**
       CC Excl: See code 112.0

       AHA: 4Q, '92, 19

    112.89 Other
       AHA: 1Q, '92, 17; 3Q, '91, 20

112.9   **Of unspecified site**   **HIV**

✓4th **114 Coccidioidomycosis**

    INCLUDES   infection by Coccidioides (immitis)
              Posada-Wernicke disease

    AHA: 4Q. '93, 23

DEF: A fungal disease caused by inhalation of dust particles containing arthrospores of *Coccidioides immitis*; a self-limited respiratory infection; the primary form is known as San Joaquin fever, desert fever or valley fever.

114.0   **Primary coccidioidomycosis (pulmonary)**   **CC** **HIV**
    Acute pulmonary coccidioidomycosis
    Coccidioidomycotic pneumonitis
    Desert rheumatism
    Pulmonary coccidioidomycosis
    San Joaquin Valley fever
    CC Excl: 114.0, 114.3, 114.4-114.5, 114.9, 117.9, 139.8

    DEF: Acute, self-limiting *Coccidioides immitis* infection of the lung.

114.1   **Primary extrapulmonary coccidioidomycosis**   **HIV**
    Chancriform syndrome
    Primary cutaneous coccidioidomycosis

    DEF: Acute, self-limiting *Coccidioides immitis* infection in nonpulmonary site.

114.2   **Coccidioidal meningitis**   **CC** **HIV**
    CC Excl: 003.21, 013.00-013.16, 036.0, 047.0-047.9, 049.0-049.1,
    053.0, 054.72, 072.1, 090.42, 091.81, 094.2, 098.89, 100.81, 112.83,
    114.2-114.9, 115.01, 115.11, 115.91, 117.9, 130.0, 139.8, 320.0-
    320.9, 321.0-321.8, 322.0-322.9, 349.89, 349.9, 357.0

    DEF: *Coccidioides immitis* infection of the lining of the brain and/or spinal cord.

114.3   **Other forms of progressive**   **CC** **HIV**
    coccidioidomycosis
    Coccidioidal granuloma
    Disseminated coccidioidomycosis
    CC Excl: 114.3, 114.9, 117.9, 139.8

114.4   **Chronic pulmonary coccidioidomycosis**   **HIV**
114.5   **Pulmonary coccidioidomycosis, unspecified**   **HIV**
114.9   **Coccidioidomycosis, unspecified**   **CC** **HIV**
    CC Excl: See code 114.3

✓4th **115 Histoplasmosis**

    The following fifth-digit subclassification is for use with category 115:
       0 without mention of manifestation
       1 meningitis
       2 retinitis
       3 pericarditis
       4 endocarditis
       5 pneumonia
       9 other

✓5th **115.0**   **Infection by Histoplasma capsulatum**   **CC 0-5** **HIV**
    American histoplasmosis
    Darling's disease
    Reticuloendothelial cytomycosis
    Small form histoplasmosis

    CC Excl: For code **115.00**: 115.00, 115.09, 115.90, 115.99, 117.9, 139.8;
    CC Excl: For code **115.01**: 003.21, 013.00-013.16, 036.0, 047.0-047.9,
    049.0-049.1, 053.0, 054.72, 072.1, 090.42, 091.81, 094.2, 098.89, 100.81,
    112.83, 114.2, 115.00-115.01, 115.09, 115.11, 115.90-115.91, 115.99,
    117.9, 130.0, 139.8, 320.0-320.9, 321.0-321.8, 322.0-322.9, 349.89, 349.9,
    357.0; CC Excl: For code **115.02**: 115.00, 115.02, 115.09, 115.90, 115.92,
    115.99, 117.9, 139.8; CC Excl: For code **115.03**: 115.00, 115.03, 115.09,
    115.90, 115.93, 115.99, 117.9, 139.8; CC Excl: For code **115.04**: 115.00,
    115.04, 115.09, 115.90, 115.94, 115.99, 117.9, 139.8; CC Excl: For code
    115.05: 115.00, 115.05, 115.09, 115.90, 115.95, 115.99, 117.9, 139.8, 480.0-
    480.9, 481, 482.0-482.7, 482.81-482.84, 482.89, 482.9, 483.0, 483.1, 483.8,
    484.1-484.8, 485-486, 487.0-487.1, 494.0-494.1, 495.0-495.9, 496, 500-
    505, 506.0-506.9, 507.0-507.8, 508.0-508.9, 517.1, 518.89

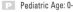 **N** Newborn Age: 0   **P** Pediatric Age: 0-17   **M** Maternity Age: 12-55   **A** Adult Age: 15-124   **CC** CC Condition   **MC** Major Complication   **CD** Complex Dx   **HIV** HIV Related Dx

22 — Volume 1   *2002 Ingenix, Inc.*

√5th **115.1 Infection by Histoplasma duboisii** `CC` `HIV`
African histoplasmosis
Large form histoplasmosis

CC Excl: For code 115.10: 115.10, 115.19, 115.90, 115.99, 117.9, 139.8; CC Excl: For code 115.11: 003.21, 013.00-013.16, 036.0, 047.0-047.9, 049.0-049.1, 053.0, 054.72, 072.1, 090.42, 091.81, 094.2, 098.89, 100.81, 112.83, 114.2, 115.01, 115.10-115.11, 115.19, 115.90-115.91, 115.99, 117.9, 130.0, 139.8, 320.0-320.9, 321.0-321.8, 322.0-322.9, 349.89, 349.9, 357.0; CC Excl: For code 115.12: 115.10, 115.12, 115.19, 115.90, 115.92, 115.99, 117.9, 139.8; CC Excl: For code 115.13: 115.10, 115.13, 115.19, 115.90, 115.93, 115.99, 117.9, 139.8; CC Excl: For code 115.14: 115.10, 115.14, 115.19, 115.90, 115.94, 115.99, 117.9, 139.8; CC Excl: For code 115.15: 115.05, 115.10, 115.15, 115.19, 115.90, 115.95, 115.99, 117.9, 139.8, 480.0-480.9, 481, 482.0-482.7, 482.81-482.83, 482.89, 482.9, 483.0, 483.1, 483.8, 484.1-484.8, 485-486,487.0-487.1, 494.0-494.1, 495.0-495.9, 496, 500-505, 506.0-506.9, 507.0-507.8, 508.0-508.9, 517.1, 518.89; CC Excl: For code 115.19: 115.10, 115.19, 115.90, 115.99, 117.9, 139.8

√5th **115.9 Histoplasmosis, unspecified** `CC` `HIV`
Histoplasmosis NOS

CC Excl: For code 115.90: 115.90, 115.99, 117.9, 139.8; CC Excl: For code 115.91: 003.21, 013.00-013.16, 036.0, 047.0-047.9, 049.0-049.1, 053.0, 054.72, 072.1, 090.42, 091.81, 094.2, 098.89, 100.81, 112.83, 114.2, 115.01, 115.11, 115.91, 115.99, 117.9, 130.0, 139.8, 320.0-320.9, 321.0-321.8, 322.0-322.9, 349.89, 349.9, 357.0; CC Excl: For code 115.92: 115.92, 115.99, 117.9, 139.8; CC Excl: For code 115.93: 115.93, 115.99, 117.9, 139.8; CC Excl: For code 115.94: 115.94, 115.99, 117.9, 139.8; CC Excl: For code 115.95: 115.05, 115.15, 115.95, 115.99, 117.9, 139.8; CC Excl: For code 115.99: 115.99, 117.9, 139.8

√4th **116 Blastomycotic infection**

116.0 Blastomycosis `CC`
Blastomycotic dermatitis
Chicago disease
Cutaneous blastomycosis
Disseminated blastomycosis
Gilchrist's disease
Infection by Blastomyces [Ajellomyces] dermatitidis
North American blastomycosis
Primary pulmonary blastomycosis

CC Excl: 116.0, 117.9, 139.8

116.1 Paracoccidioidomycosis `CC`
Brazilian blastomycosis
Infection by Paracoccidioides [Blastomyces] brasiliensis
Lutz-Splendore-Almeida disease
Mucocutaneous-lymphangitic paracoccidioidomycosis
Pulmonary paracoccidioidomycosis
South American blastomycosis
Visceral paracoccidioidomycosis

CC Excl: 116.1, 117.9, 139.8

116.2 Lobomycosis
Infections by Loboa [Blastomyces] loboi
Keloidal blastomycosis
Lobo's disease

√4th **117 Other mycoses**

117.0 Rhinosporidiosis
Infection by Rhinosporidium seeberi

117.1 Sporotrichosis
Cutaneous sporotrichosis
Disseminated sporotrichosis
Infection by Sporothrix [Sporotrichum] schenckii
Lymphocutaneous sporotrichosis
Pulmonary sporotrichosis
Sporotrichosis of the bones

117.2 Chromoblastomycosis
Chromomycosis
Infection by Cladosporidium carrionii, Fonsecaea compactum, Fonsecaea pedrosoi, Phialophora verrucosa

117.3 Aspergillosis `CC`
Infection by Aspergillus species, mainly A. fumigatus, A. flavus group, A. terreus group

CC Excl: 117.3, 117.9, 139.8

AHA: 4Q, '97, 40

117.4 Mycotic mycetomas `CC`
Infection by various genera and species of Ascomycetes and Deuteromycetes, such as Acremonium [Cephalosporium] falciforme, Neotestudina rosatii, Madurella grisea, Madurella mycetomii, Pyrenochaeta romeroi, Zopfia [Leptosphaeria] senegalensis
Madura foot, mycotic
Maduromycosis, mycotic
EXCLUDES actinomycotic mycetomas (039.0-039.9)

CC Excl: 117.4, 117.9, 139.8

117.5 Cryptococcosis `CC` `HIV`
Busse-Buschke's disease
European cryptococcosis
Infection by Cryptococcus neoformans
Pulmonary cryptococcosis
Systemic cryptococcosis
Torula

CC Excl: 117.5, 117.9, 139.8

117.6 Allescheriosis [Petriellidosis] `CC`
Infections by Allescheria [Petriellidium] boydii [Monosporium apiospermum]
EXCLUDES mycotic mycetoma (117.4)

CC Excl: 117.6, 117.9, 139.8

117.7 Zygomycosis [Phycomycosis or Mucormycosis] `CC`
Infection by species of Absidia, Basidiobolus, Conidiobolus, Cunninghamella, Entomophthora, Mucor, Rhizopus, Saksenaea

CC Excl: 117.7, 117.9, 139.8

117.8 Infection by dematiacious fungi, [Phaehyphomycosis]
Infection by dematiacious fungi, such as Cladosporium trichoides [bantianum], Dreschlera hawaiiensis, Phialophora gougerotii, Phialophora jeanselmi

117.9 Other and unspecified mycoses

118 Opportunistic mycoses `CC` `HIV`
Infection of skin, subcutaneous tissues, and/or organs by a wide variety of fungi generally considered to be pathogenic to compromised hosts only (e.g., infection by species of Alternaria, Dreschlera, Fusarium)

CC Excl: 117.9, 118, 139.8

HELMINTHIASES (120-129)

√4th **120 Schistosomiasis [bilharziasis]**

DEF: Infection caused by *Schistosoma*, a genus of flukes or trematode parasites.

120.0 Schistosoma haematobium
Vesical schistosomiasis NOS

120.1 Schistosoma mansoni
Intestinal schistosomiasis NOS

120.2 Schistosoma japonicum
Asiatic schistosomiasis NOS
Katayama disease or fever

120.3 Cutaneous
Cercarial dermatitis
Infection by cercariae of Schistosoma
Schistosome dermatitis
Swimmers' itch

√4th √5th **Additional Digit Required**   **Nonspecific PDx**   **Unacceptable PDx**   **Manifestation Code**   `MSP` Medicare Secondary Payer   ▶◀ Revised Text   ● New Code   ▲ Revised Code Title

120.8 Other specified schistosomiasis
Infection by Schistosoma:
bovis
intercalatum
mattheii
spindale
Schistosomiasis chestermani

120.9 Schistosomiasis, unspecified
Blood flukes NOS
Hemic distomiasis

✓4th **121 Other trematode infections**

121.0 Opisthorchiasis
Infection by:
cat liver fluke
Opisthorchis (felineus) (tenuicollis) (viverrini)

121.1 Clonorchiasis
Biliary cirrhosis due to clonorchiasis
Chinese liver fluke disease
Hepatic distomiasis due to Clonorchis sinensis
Oriental liver fluke disease

121.2 Paragonimiasis
Infection by Paragonimus
Lung fluke disease (oriental)
Pulmonary distomiasis

121.3 Fascioliasis
Infection by Fasciola:
gigantica
hepatica
Liver flukes NOS
Sheep liver fluke infection

121.4 Fasciolopsiasis
Infection by Fasciolopsis (buski)
Intestinal distomiasis

121.5 Metagonimiasis
Infection by Metagonimus yokogawai

121.6 Heterophyiasis
Infection by:
Heterophyes heterophyes
Stellantchasmus falcatus

121.8 Other specified trematode infections
Infection by:
Dicrocoelium dendriticum
Echinostoma ilocanum
Gastrodiscoides hominis

121.9 Trematode infection, unspecified
Distomiasis NOS
Fluke disease NOS

✓4th **122 Echinococcosis**
INCLUDES echinococciasis
hydatid disease
hydatidosis

DEF: Infection caused by larval forms of tapeworms of the genus *Echinococcus*.

122.0 Echinococcus granulosus infection of liver
122.1 Echinococcus granulosus infection of lung
122.2 Echinococcus granulosus infection of thyroid
122.3 Echinococcus granulosus infection, other
122.4 Echinococcus granulosus infection, unspecified
122.5 Echinococcus multilocularis infection of liver
122.6 Echinococcus multilocularis infection, other
122.7 Echinococcus multilocularis infection, unspecified
122.8 Echinococcosis, unspecified, of liver
122.9 Echinococcosis, other and unspecified

✓4th **123 Other cestode infection**

123.0 Taenia solium infection, intestinal form
Pork tapeworm (adult) (infection)

123.1 Cysticercosis
Cysticerciasis
Infection by Cysticercus cellulosae [larval form of Taenia solium]
AHA: 2Q, '97, 8

123.2 Taenia saginata infection
Beef tapeworm (infection)
Infection by Taeniarhynchus saginatus

123.3 Taeniasis, unspecified

123.4 Diphyllobothriasis, intestinal
Diphyllobothrium (adult) (latum) (pacificum) infection
Fish tapeworm (infection)

123.5 Sparganosis [larval diphyllobothriasis]
Infection by:
Diphyllobothrium larvae
Sparganum (mansoni) (proliferum)
Spirometra larvae

123.6 Hymenolepiasis
Dwarf tapeworm (infection)
Hymenolepis (diminuta) (nana) infection
Rat tapeworm (infection)

123.8 Other specified cestode infection
Diplogonoporus (grandis) } infection
Dipylidium (caninum)
Dog tapeworm (infection)

123.9 Cestode infection, unspecified
Tapeworm (infection) NOS

124 Trichinosis
Trichinella spiralis infection   Trichiniasis
Trichinellosis
DEF: Infection by *Trichinella spiralis*, the smallest of the parasitic nematodes.

✓4th **125 Filarial infection and dracontiasis**

125.0 Bancroftian filariasis
Chyluria
Elephantiasis
Infection } due to Wuchereria bancrofti
Lymphadenitis
Lymphangitis
Wuchereriasis

125.1 Malayan filariasis
Brugia filariasis
Chyluria
Elephantiasis } due to Brugia [Wuchereria] malayi
Infection
Lymphadenitis
Lymphangitis

125.2 Loiasis
Eyeworm disease of Africa   Loa loa infection

125.3 Onchocerciasis
Onchocerca volvulus infection
Onchocercosis

125.4 Dipetalonemiasis
Infection by:
Acanthocheilonema perstans
Dipetalonema perstans

125.5 Mansonella ozzardi infection
Filariasis ozzardi

125.6 Other specified filariasis
Dirofilaria infection
Infection by:
Acanthocheilonema streptocerca
Dipetalonema streptocerca

125.7 Dracontiasis
Guinea-worm infection
Infection by Dracunculus medinensis

125.9 Unspecified filariasis

✓4th **126 Ancylostomiasis and necatoriasis**
INCLUDES cutaneous larva migrans due to Ancylostoma
hookworm (disease) (infection)
uncinariasis

126.0 Ancylostoma duodenale
126.1 Necator americanus
126.2 Ancylostoma braziliense
126.3 Ancylostoma ceylanicum

N Newborn Age: 0   P Pediatric Age: 0-17   M Maternity Age: 12-55   A Adult Age: 15-124   CC CC Condition   MC Major Complication   CD Complex Dx   HIV HIV Related Dx

24 — Volume 1   *2002 Ingenix, Inc.*

126.8   **Other specified Ancylostoma**

126.9   **Ancylostomiasis and necatoriasis, unspecified**
     Creeping eruption NOS
     Cutaneous larva migrans NOS

√4ᵗʰ **127 Other intestinal helminthiases**

127.0   **Ascariasis**
     Ascaridiasis
     Infection by Ascaris lumbricoides
     Roundworm infection

127.1   **Anisakiasis**
     Infection by Anisakis larva

127.2   **Strongyloidiasis**   **HIV**
     Infection by Strongyloides stercoralis
     EXCLUDES   *trichostrongyliasis (127.6)*

127.3   **Trichuriasis**
     Infection by Trichuris trichiuria
     Trichocephaliasis
     Whipworm (disease) (infection)

127.4   **Enterobiasis**
     Infection by Enterobius vermicularis
     Oxyuriasis
     Oxyuris vermicularis infection
     Pinworm (disease) (infection)
     Threadworm infection

127.5   **Capillariasis**
     Infection by Capillaria philippinensis
     EXCLUDES   *infection by Capillaria hepatica (128.8)*

127.6   **Trichostrongyliasis**
     Infection by Trichostrongylus species

127.7   **Other specified intestinal helminthiasis**
     Infection by:
       Oesophagostomum apiostomum and related
         species
       Ternidens diminutus
       other specified intestinal helminth
     Physalopteriasis

127.8   **Mixed intestinal helminthiasis**
     Infection by intestinal helminths classified to more
       than one of the categories 120.0-127.7
     Mixed helminthiasis NOS

127.9   **Intestinal helminthiasis, unspecified**

√4ᵗʰ **128 Other and unspecified helminthiases**

128.0   **Toxocariasis**
     Larva migrans visceralis
     Toxocara (canis) (cati) infection
     Visceral larva migrans syndrome

128.1   **Gnathostomiasis**
     Infection by Gnathostoma spinigerum and related
       species

128.8   **Other specified helminthiasis**
     Infection by:
       Angiostrongylus cantonensis
       Capillaria hepatica
       other specified helminth

128.9   **Helminth infection, unspecified**
     Helminthiasis NOS   Worms NOS

129   **Intestinal parasitism, unspecified**

OTHER INFECTIOUS AND PARASITIC DISEASES (130–136)

√4ᵗʰ **130 Toxoplasmosis**
     INCLUDES   infection by toxoplasma gondii
       toxoplasmosis (acquired)
     EXCLUDES   *congenital toxoplasmosis (771.2)*

130.0   **Meningoencephalitis due to toxoplasmosis**   **CC** **HIV**
     Encephalitis due to acquired toxoplasmosis
     CC Excl: 130.0, 130.7-130.9, 139.8

130.1   **Conjunctivitis due to toxoplasmosis**   **CC** **HIV**
     CC Excl: 130.1, 130.7-130.9, 139.8

130.2   **Chorioretinitis due to toxoplasmosis**   **CC** **HIV**
     Focal retinochoroiditis due to acquired
       toxoplasmosis
     CC Excl: 130.2, 130.7-130.9, 139.8

130.3   **Myocarditis due to toxoplasmosis**   **CC** **HIV**
     CC Excl: 130.3, 130.7-130.9, 139.8

130.4   **Pneumonitis due to toxoplasmosis**   **CC** **HIV**
     CC Excl: 130.4, 130.7-130.9, 139.8, 480.0-480.9, 481, 482.0-482.7,
     |482.81-482.83, 482.89, 482.9, 483.0, 483.1, 483.8, 484.1-484.8,
     485-486, 487.0-487.1, 494.0-494.1, 495.0-495.9, 496, 500-505, 506.0-
     506.9, 507.0-507.8, 508.0-508.9, 517.1, 518.89

130.5   **Hepatitis due to toxoplasmosis**   **CC** **HIV**
     CC Excl: 130.5-130.9, 139.8

130.7   **Toxoplasmosis of other specified sites**   **CC** **HIV**
     CC Excl: 130.7-130.9, 139.8

130.8   **Multisystemic disseminated toxoplasmosis**   **CC** **HIV**
     Toxoplasmosis of multiple sites
     CC Excl: See code 130.7

130.9   **Toxoplasmosis, unspecified**   **HIV**

√4ᵗʰ **131 Trichomoniasis**
     INCLUDES   infection due to Trichomonas (vaginalis)

√5ᵗʰ 131.0   **Urogenital trichomoniasis**

131.00   **Urogenital trichomoniasis, unspecified**
     Fluor (vaginalis)   trichomonal or due to
     Leukorrhea   Trichomonas
     (vaginalis)   (vaginalis)
     DEF: *Trichomonas vaginalis* infection of reproductive
     and urinary organs, transmitted through coitus.

131.01   **Trichomonal vulvovaginitis**   ♀
     Vaginitis, trichomonal or due to
       Trichomonas (vaginalis)
     DEF: *Trichomonas vaginalis* infection of vulva and
     vagina; often asymptomatic, transmitted through coitus.

131.02   **Trichomonal urethritis**
     DEF: *Trichomonas vaginalis* infection of the urethra.

131.03   **Trichomonal prostatitis**   ♂
     DEF: *Trichomonas vaginalis* infection of the prostate.

131.09   **Other**

131.8   **Other specified sites**
     EXCLUDES   *intestinal (007.3)*

131.9   **Trichomoniasis, unspecified**

√4ᵗʰ **132 Pediculosis and phthirus infestation**

132.0   **Pediculus capitis [head louse]**

132.1   **Pediculus corporis [body louse]**

132.2   **Phthirus pubis [pubic louse]**
     Pediculus pubis

132.3   **Mixed infestation**
     Infestation classifiable to more than one of the
       categories 132.0-132.2

132.9   **Pediculosis, unspecified**

√4ᵗʰ **133 Acariasis**

133.0   **Scabies**
     Infestation by Sarcoptes scabiei   Sarcoptic itch
     Norwegian scabies

133.8   **Other acariasis**
     Chiggers   Infestation by:
     Infestation by: Trombicula
       Demodex folliculorum

133.9   **Acariasis, unspecified**
     Infestation by mites NOS

√4ᵗʰ / √5ᵗʰ Additional Digit Required   Nonspecific PDx   Unacceptable PDx   Manifestation Code   **MSP** Medicare Secondary Payer   ►◄ Revised Text   ● New Code   ▲ Revised Code Title

2002 Ingenix, Inc.   **Volume 1 — 25**

Infectious and Parasitic Diseases 134–139.8

✓4ᵗʰ **134 Other infestation**

134.0 Myiasis

Infestation by:
Dermatobia (hominis)
fly larvae
Gasterophilus (intestinalis)

Infestation by:
maggots
Oestrus ovis

134.1 Other arthropod infestation

Infestation by:
chigoe
sand flea
Tunga penetrans

Jigger disease
Scarabiasis
Tungiasis

134.2 Hirudiniasis

Hirudiniasis (external) (internal)
Leeches (aquatic) (land)

134.8 Other specified infestations

134.9 Infestation, unspecified

Infestation (skin) NOS   Skin parasites NOS

135 Sarcoidosis   CC

Besnier-Boeck-Schaumann disease
Lupoid (miliary) of Boeck
Lupus pernio (Besnier)
Lymphogranulomatosis, benign (Schaumann's)
Sarcoid (any site):
NOS
Boeck
Darier-Roussy
Uveoparotid fever

CC Excl: 135, 139.8

DEF: A chronic, granulomatous reticulosis (abnormal increase in cells), affecting any organ or tissue; acute form has high rate of remission; chronic form is progressive.

✓4ᵗʰ **136 Other and unspecified infectious and parasitic diseases**

136.0 Ainhum

Dactylolysis spontanea

DEF: A disease affecting the toes, especially the fifth digit, and sometimes the fingers, especially seen in black adult males; it is characterized by a linear constriction around the affected digit leading to spontaneous amputation of the distal part of the digit.

136.1 Behçet's syndrome

DEF: A chronic inflammatory disorder of unknown etiology involving the small blood vessels; it is characterized by recurrent aphthous ulceration of the oral and pharyngeal mucous membranes and the genitalia, skin lesions, severe uvetis, retinal vascularitis and optic atrophy.

136.2 Specific infections by free-living amebae

Meningoencephalitis due to Naegleria

136.3 Pneumocystosis   CC HIV

Pneumonia due to Pneumocystis carinii

CC Excl: 136.3, 139.8, 480.0-480.9, 481, 482.0-482.7, 482.81-482.83, 482.89, 482.9, 483.0, 483.1, 483.8, 484.1-484.8, 485-486, 487.0-487.1, 494.0-494.1, 495.0-495.9, 496, 500-505, 506.0-506.9, 507.0-507.8, 508.0-508.9, 517.1, 518.89

AHA: N-D, '87, 5, 6

DEF: Pneumocystis carinii fungus causing pneumonia in immunocompromised patients; a leading cause of death among AIDS patients.

136.4 Psorospermiasis

136.5 Sarcosporidiosis

Infection by Sarcocystis lindemanni

DEF: Sarcocystis infection causing muscle cysts of intestinal inflammation.

136.8 Other specified infectious and parasitic diseases HIV

Candiru infestation

136.9 Unspecified infectious and parasitic diseases

Infectious disease NOS   Parasitic disease NOS

AHA: 2Q, '91, 8

LATE EFFECTS OF INFECTIOUS AND PARASITIC DISEASES (137-139)

✓4ᵗʰ **137 Late effects of tuberculosis**

Note: This category is to be used to indicate conditions classifiable to 010-018 as the cause of late effects, which are themselves classified elsewhere. The "late effects" include those specified as such, as sequelae, or as due to old or inactive tuberculosis, without evidence of active disease.

137.0 Late effects of respiratory or unspecified tuberculosis   CC

CC Excl: 137.0, 139.8

137.1 Late effects of central nervous system tuberculosis   CC

CC Excl: 137.1, 139.8

137.2 Late effects of genitourinary tuberculosis   CC

CC Excl: 137.2, 139.8

137.3 Late effects of tuberculosis of bones and joints

137.4 Late effects of tuberculosis of other specified organs

138 Late effects of acute poliomyelitis   CC

Note: This category is to be used to indicate conditions classifiable to 045 as the cause of late effects, which are themselves classified elsewhere. The "late effects" include conditions specified as such, or as sequelae, or as due to old or inactive poliomyelitis, without evidence of active disease.

CC Excl: 138, 139.8

✓4ᵗʰ **139 Late effects of other infectious and parasitic diseases**

Note: This category is to be used to indicate conditions classifiable to categories 001-009, 020-041, 046-136 as the cause of late effects, which are themselves classified elsewhere. The "late effects" include conditions specified as such; they also include sequela of diseases classifiable to the above categories if there is evidence that the disease itself is no longer present.

139.0 Late effects of viral encephalitis

Late effects of conditions classifiable to 049.8-049.9, 062-064

139.1 Late effects of trachoma

Late effects of conditions classifiable to 076

139.8 Late effects of other and unspecified infectious and parasitic diseases

AHA: 4Q, '91, 15; 3Q, '90, 14; M-A, '87, 8

N Newborn Age: 0   P Pediatric Age: 0-17   M Maternity Age: 12-55   A Adult Age: 15-124   CC CC Condition   MC Major Complication   CD Complex Dx   HIV HIV Related Dx

2. NEOPLASMS (140-239)

Notes:

1. Content

This chapter contains the following broad groups:

140-195   Malignant neoplasms, stated or presumed to be primary, of specified sites, except of lymphatic and hematopoietic tissue

196-198   Malignant neoplasms, stated or presumed to be secondary, of specified sites

199   Malignant neoplasms, without specification of site

200-208   Malignant neoplasms, stated or presumed to be primary, of lymphatic and hematopoietic tissue

210-229   Benign neoplasms

230-234   Carcinoma in situ

235-238   Neoplasms of uncertain behavior [see Note, above category 235]

239   Neoplasms of unspecified nature

2. Functional activity

All neoplasms are classified in this chapter, whether or not functionally active. An additional code from Chapter 3 may be used to identify such functional activity associated with any neoplasm, e.g.:

    catecholamine-producing malignant pheochromocytoma of adrenal:

        code 194.0, additional code 255.6

    basophil adenoma of pituitary with Cushing's syndrome:

        code 227.3, additional code 255.0

3. Morphology [Histology]

For those wishing to identify the histological type of neoplasms, a comprehensive coded nomenclature, which comprises the morphology rubrics of the ICD-Oncology, is given in Appendix A.

4. Malignant neoplasms overlapping site boundaries

Categories 140-195 are for the classification of primary malignant neoplasms according to their point of origin. A malignant neoplasm that overlaps two or more subcategories within a three-digit rubric and whose point of origin cannot be determined should be classified to the subcategory .8 "Other."

For example, "carcinoma involving tip and ventral surface of tongue" should be assigned to 141.8. On the other hand, "carcinoma of tip of tongue, extending to involve the ventral surface" should be coded to 141.2, as the point of origin, the tip, is known. Three subcategories (149.8, 159.8, 165.8) have been provided for malignant neoplasms that overlap the boundaries of three-digit rubrics within certain systems.

Overlapping malignant neoplasms that cannot be classified as indicated above should be assigned to the appropriate subdivision of category 195 (Malignant neoplasm of other and ill-defined sites).

AHA: 2Q, '90, 7

DEF: An abnormal growth, such as a tumor. Morphology determines behavior, i.e., whether it will remain intact (benign) or spread to adjacent tissue (malignant). The term mass is not synonymous with neoplasm, as it is often used to describe cysts and thickenings such as those occurring with hematoma or infection.

MALIGNANT NEOPLASM OF LIP, ORAL CAVITY, AND PHARYNX (140-149)

> *EXCLUDES*   carcinoma in situ (230.0)

✓4ᵗʰ 140 Malignant neoplasm of lip

> *EXCLUDES*   skin of lip (173.0)

  140.0   Upper lip, vermilion border

Upper lip:	Upper lip:
NOS	lipstick area
external	

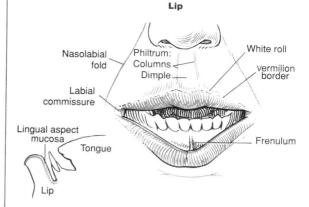

Lip

Nasolabial fold · Philtrum: Columns, Dimple · White roll · vermilion border · Labial commissure · Lingual aspect mucosa · Tongue · Frenulum · Lip

  140.1   Lower lip, vermilion border

Lower lip:	Lower lip:
NOS	lipstick area
external	

  140.3   Upper lip, inner aspect

Upper lip:	Upper lip:
buccal aspect	mucosa
frenulum	oral aspect

  140.4   Lower lip, inner aspect

Lower lip:	Lower lip:
buccal aspect	mucosa
frenulum	oral aspect

  140.5   Lip, unspecified, inner aspect

    Lip, not specified whether upper or lower:
      buccal aspect
      frenulum
      mucosa
      oral aspect

  140.6   Commissure of lip

    Labial commissure

  140.8   Other sites of lip

    Malignant neoplasm of contiguous or overlapping sites of lip whose point of origin cannot be determined

  140.9   Lip, unspecified, vermilion border

    Lip, not specified as upper or lower:
      NOS
      external
      lipstick area

✓4ᵗʰ 141 Malignant neoplasm of tongue

  141.0   Base of tongue

    Dorsal surface of base of tongue
    Fixed part of tongue NOS

  141.1   Dorsal surface of tongue

    Anterior two-thirds of tongue, dorsal surface
    Dorsal tongue NOS
    Midline of tongue

> *EXCLUDES*   dorsal surface of base of tongue (141.0)

  141.2   Tip and lateral border of tongue

  141.3   Ventral surface of tongue

    Anterior two-thirds of tongue, ventral surface
    Frenulum linguae

  141.4   Anterior two-thirds of tongue, part unspecified

    Mobile part of tongue NOS

  141.5   Junctional zone

    Border of tongue at junction of fixed and mobile parts at insertion of anterior tonsillar pillar

  141.6   Lingual tonsil

  141.8   Other sites of tongue

    Malignant neoplasm of contiguous or overlapping sites of tongue whose point of origin cannot be determined

  141.9   Tongue, unspecified

    Tongue NOS

✓4ᵗʰ Additional Digit Required   Nonspecific PDx   Unacceptable PDx   Manifestation Code   **MSP** Medicare Secondary Payer   ▶◀ Revised Text   ● New Code   ▲ Revised Code Title
✓5ᵗʰ
2002 Ingenix, Inc.

Volume 1 — 27

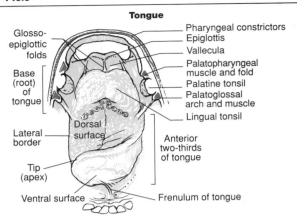

Tongue

Glosso-epiglottic folds
Pharyngeal constrictors
Epiglottis
Vallecula
Palatopharyngeal muscle and fold
Base (root) of tongue
Palatine tonsil
Palatoglossal arch and muscle
Lingual tonsil
Lateral border
Dorsal surface
Anterior two-thirds of tongue
Tip (apex)
Ventral surface
Frenulum of tongue

✓4th **142 Malignant neoplasm of major salivary glands**
INCLUDES   salivary ducts
EXCLUDES   malignant neoplasm of minor salivary glands:
NOS (145.9)
buccal mucosa (145.0)
soft palate (145.3)
tongue (141.0-141.9)
tonsil, palatine (146.0)

142.0   Parotid gland
142.1   Submandibular gland
Submaxillary gland
142.2   Sublingual gland
142.8   Other major salivary glands
Malignant neoplasm of contiguous or overlapping sites of salivary glands and ducts whose point of origin cannot be determined
142.9   Salivary gland, unspecified
Salivary gland (major) NOS

✓4th **143 Malignant neoplasm of gum**
INCLUDES   alveolar (ridge) mucosa
gingiva (alveolar) (marginal)
interdental papillae
EXCLUDES   malignant odontogenic neoplasms (170.0-170.1)

143.0   Upper gum
143.1   Lower gum
143.8   Other sites of gum
Malignant neoplasm of contiguous or overlapping sites of gum whose point of origin cannot be determined
143.9   Gum, unspecified

✓4th **144 Malignant neoplasm of floor of mouth**
144.0   Anterior portion
Anterior to the premolar-canine junction
144.1   Lateral portion
Other sites of floor of mouth
Malignant neoplasm of contiguous or overlapping sites of floor of mouth whose point of origin cannot be determined
144.9   Floor of mouth, part unspecified

✓4th **145 Malignant neoplasm of other and unspecified parts of mouth**
EXCLUDES   mucosa of lips (140.0-140.9)

145.0   Cheek mucosa
Buccal mucosa
Cheek, inner aspect
145.1   Vestibule of mouth
Buccal sulcus (upper) (lower)
Labial sulcus (upper) (lower)
145.2   Hard palate

145.3   Soft palate
EXCLUDES   nasopharyngeal [posterior] [superior] surface of soft palate (147.3)
145.4   Uvula
145.5   Palate, unspecified
Junction of hard and soft palate   Roof of mouth
145.6   Retromolar area
145.8   Other specified parts of mouth
Malignant neoplasm of contiguous or overlapping sites of mouth whose point of origin cannot be determined
145.9   Mouth, unspecified
Buccal cavity NOS
Minor salivary gland, unspecified site
Oral cavity NOS

✓4th **146 Malignant neoplasm of oropharynx**
146.0   Tonsil
Tonsil:
NOS
faucial
palatine
EXCLUDES   lingual tonsil (141.6)
pharyngeal tonsil (147.1)

AHA: S-O, '87, 8

146.1   Tonsillar fossa
146.2   Tonsillar pillars (anterior) (posterior)
Faucial pillar   Palatoglossal arch
Glossopalatine fold   Palatopharyngeal arch
146.3   Vallecula
Anterior and medial surface of the pharyngoepiglottic fold
146.4   Anterior aspect of epiglottis
Epiglottis, free border [margin]
Glossoepiglottic fold(s)
EXCLUDES   epiglottis:
NOS (161.1)
suprahyoid portion (161.1)
146.5   Junctional region
Junction of the free margin of the epiglottis, the aryepiglottic fold, and the pharyngoepiglottic fold
146.6   Lateral wall of oropharynx
146.7   Posterior wall of oropharynx
146.8   Other specified sites of oropharynx
Branchial cleft
Malignant neoplasm of contiguous or overlapping sites of oropharynx whose point of origin cannot be determined
146.9   Oropharynx, unspecified

Mouth

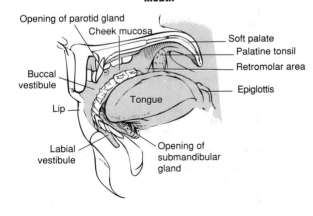

Opening of parotid gland
Cheek mucosa
Soft palate
Palatine tonsil
Retromolar area
Buccal vestibule
Epiglottis
Tongue
Lip
Labial vestibule
Opening of submandibular gland

N Newborn Age: 0   P Pediatric Age: 0-17   M Maternity Age: 12-55   A Adult Age: 15-124   CC CC Condition   MC Major Complication   CD Complex Dx   HIV HIV Related Dx

28 — Volume 1   2002 Ingenix, Inc.

Neoplasms 142-146.9 *(vertical sidebar text)*

Topical Sites in Oropharynx

Main Salivary Glands

Waldeyer's (Tonsillar) Ring

Nasopharynx

Hypopharynx

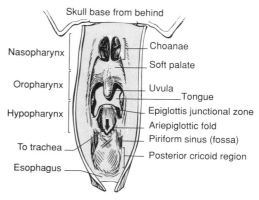

✓4th **147 Malignant neoplasm of nasopharynx**

    147.0   **Superior wall**
         Roof of nasopharynx

    147.1   **Posterior wall**
         Adenoid   Pharyngeal tonsil

    147.2   **Lateral wall**
         Fossa of Rosenmüller   Pharyngeal recess
         Opening of auditory tube

    147.3   **Anterior wall**
         Floor of nasopharynx
         Nasopharyngeal [posterior] [superior] surface of soft
           palate
         Posterior margin of nasal septum and choanae

    147.8   **Other specified sites of nasopharynx**
         Malignant neoplasm of contiguous or overlapping
           sites of nasopharynx whose point of origin
           cannot be determined

    147.9   **Nasopharynx, unspecified**
         Nasopharyngeal wall NOS

✓4th **148 Malignant neoplasm of hypopharynx**

    148.0   **Postcricoid region**

    148.1   **Pyriform sinus**
         Pyriform fossa

    148.2   **Aryepiglottic fold, hypopharyngeal aspect**
         Aryepiglottic fold or interarytenoid fold:
           NOS
           marginal zone
         EXCLUDES *aryepiglottic fold or interarytenoid fold,*
                   laryngeal aspect (161.1)

    148.3   **Posterior hypopharyngeal wall**

    148.8   **Other specified sites of hypopharynx**
         Malignant neoplasm of contiguous or overlapping
           sites of hypopharynx whose point of origin
           cannot be determined

    148.9   **Hypopharynx, unspecified**
         Hypopharyngeal wall NOS
         Hypopharynx NOS

✓4th **149 Malignant neoplasm of other and ill-defined sites within the lip, oral cavity, and pharynx**

    149.0   **Pharynx, unspecified**

    149.1   **Waldeyer's ring**

    149.8   **Other**
         Malignant neoplasms of lip, oral cavity, and pharynx
           whose point of origin cannot be assigned to
           any one of the categories 140-148
         EXCLUDES *"book leaf" neoplasm [ventral surface*
                   of tongue and floor of mouth]
                   (145.8)

    149.9   **Ill-defined**

MALIGNANT NEOPLASM OF DIGESTIVE ORGANS AND PERITONEUM (150-159)

       EXCLUDES *carcinoma in situ (230.1-230.9)*

✓4th **150 Malignant neoplasm of esophagus**

    150.0   **Cervical esophagus**   `CC`
         CC Excl: 150.0-150.9, 159.0, 159.8-159.9, 176.3, 195.8, 199.0-199.1,
         239.0, 239.8-239.9

    150.1   **Thoracic esophagus**   `CC`
         CC Excl: See code 150.0

    150.2   **Abdominal esophagus**   `CC`
         EXCLUDES *adenocarcinoma (151.0)*
                   cardio-esophageal junction (151.0)
         CC Excl: See code 150.0

    150.3   **Upper third of esophagus**   `CC`
         CC Excl: See code 150.0

         Proximal third of esophagus

    150.4   **Middle third of esophagus**   `CC`
         CC Excl: See code 150.0

✓4th Additional Digit Required   Nonspecific PDx   Unacceptable PDx   Manifestation Code   **MSP** Medicare Secondary Payer   ◄► Revised Text   ● New Code   ▲ Revised Code Title

2002 Ingenix, Inc.   Volume 1 — 29

150.5 Lower third of esophagus `CC`
   Distal third of esophagus
   EXCLUDES *adenocarcinoma (151.0)*
      cardio-esophageal junction (151.0)
   CC Excl: See code 150.0

150.8 Other specified part `CC`
   Malignant neoplasm of contiguous or overlapping sites of esophagus whose point of origin cannot be determined
   CC Excl: See code 150.0

150.9 Esophagus, unspecified `CC`
   CC Excl: See code 150.0

√4ᵗʰ 151 Malignant neoplasm of stomach

151.0 Cardia `CC`
   Cardiac orifice
   Cardio-esophageal junction
   EXCLUDES *squamous cell carcinoma (150.2, 150.5)*
   CC Excl: 151.0-151.9, 159.0, 159.8-159.9, 176.3, 195.8, 199.0-199.1, 239.0, 239.8-239.9

151.1 Pylorus `CC`
   Prepylorus   Pyloric canal
   CC Excl: See code 151.0

151.2 Pyloric antrum `CC`
   Antrum of stomach NOS
   CC Excl: See code 151.0

151.3 Fundus of stomach `CC`
   CC Excl: See code 151.0

151.4 Body of stomach `CC`
   CC Excl: See code 151.0

151.5 Lesser curvature, unspecified `CC`
   Lesser curvature, not classifiable to 151.1-151.4
   CC Excl: See code 151.0

151.6 Greater curvature, unspecified `CC`
   Greater curvature, not classifiable to 151.0-151.4
   CC Excl: See code 151.0

151.8 Other specified sites of stomach `CC`
   Anterior wall, not classifiable to 151.0-151.4
   Posterior wall, not classifiable to 151.0-151.4
   Malignant neoplasm of contiguous or overlapping sites of stomach whose point of origin cannot be determined
   CC Excl: See code 151.0

151.9 Stomach, unspecified `CC`
   Carcinoma ventriculi Gastric cancer
   CC Excl: See code 151.0
   AHA: 2Q, '01, 17

√4ᵗʰ 152 Malignant neoplasm of small intestine, including duodenum

152.0 Duodenum `CC`
   CC Excl: 152.0, 152.8-152.9, 159.0, 159.8-159.9, 176.3, 195.8, 199.0-199.1, 239.0, 239.8-239.9

152.1 Jejunum `CC`
   CC Excl: 152.1, 152.8-152.9, 159.0, 159.8-159.9, 176.3, 195.8, 199.0-199.1, 239.0, 239.8-239.9

152.2 Ileum `CC`
   EXCLUDES *ileocecal valve (153.4)*
   CC Excl: 152.2, 152.8-152.9, 159.0, 159.8-159.9, 176.3, 195.8, 199.0-199.1, 239.0, 239.8-239.9

152.3 Meckel's diverticulum `CC`
   CC Excl: 152.3-152.9, 159.0, 159.8-159.9, 176.3, 195.8, 199.0-199.1, 239.0, 239.8-239.9

152.8 Other specified sites of small intestine `CC`
   Duodenojejunal junction
   Malignant neoplasm of contiguous or overlapping sites of small intestine whose point of origin cannot be determined
   CC Excl: 152.8-152.9, 159.0, 159.8-159.9, 176.3, 195.8, 199.0-199.1, 239.0, 239.8-239.9

152.9 Small intestine, unspecified `CC`
   CC Excl: See code 152.8

√4ᵗʰ 153 Malignant neoplasm of colon

153.0 Hepatic flexure `CC`
   CC Excl: 153.0, 153.8-153.9, 159.0, 159.8-159.9, 176.3, 195.8, 199.0-199.1, 239.0, 239.8-239.9

153.1 Transverse colon `CC`
   CC Excl: 153.1, 153.8-153.9, 159.0, 159.8-159.9, 176.3, 195.8, 199.0-199.1, 239.0, 239.8-239.9

153.2 Descending colon `CC`
   Left colon
   CC Excl: 153.2, 153.8-153.9, 159.0, 159.8-159.9, 176.3, 195.8, 199.0-199.1, 239.0, 239.8-239.9

153.3 Sigmoid colon `CC`
   Sigmoid (flexure)
   EXCLUDES *rectosigmoid junction (154.0)*
   CC Excl: 153.3, 153.8-153.9, 159.0, 159.8-159.9, 176.3, 195.8, 199.0-199.1, 239.0, 239.8-239.9

153.4 Cecum `CC`
   Ileocecal valve
   CC Excl: 153.4, 153.8-153.9, 159.0, 159.8-159.9, 176.3, 195.8, 199.0-199.1, 239.0, 239.8-239.9

153.5 Appendix `CC`
   CC Excl: 153.5, 153.8-153.9, 159.0, 159.8-159.9, 176.3, 195.8, 199.0-199.1, 239.0, 239.8-239.9

153.6 Ascending colon `CC`
   Right colon
   CC Excl: 153.6, 153.8-153.9, 159.0, 159.8-159.9, 176.3, 195.8, 199.0-199.1, 239.0, 239.8-239.9

153.7 Splenic flexure `CC`
   CC Excl: 153.7-153.9, 159.0, 159.8-159.9, 176.3, 195.8, 199.0-199.1, 239.0, 239.8-239.9

153.8 Other specified sites of large intestine `CC`
   Malignant neoplasm of contiguous or overlapping sites of colon whose point of origin cannot be determined
   EXCLUDES *ileocecal valve (153.4)*
      rectosigmoid junction (154.0)
   CC Excl: 153.8-153.9, 159.0, 159.8-159.9, 176.3, 195.8, 199.0-199.1, 239.0, 239.8-239.9

153.9 Colon, unspecified `CC`
   Large intestine NOS
   CC Excl: See code 153.8

√4ᵗʰ 154 Malignant neoplasm of rectum, rectosigmoid junction, and anus

154.0 Rectosigmoid junction `CC`
   Colon with rectum
   Rectosigmoid (colon)
   CC Excl: 154.0, 154.8, 159.0, 159.8-159.9, 176.3, 195.8, 199.0-199.1, 239.0, 239.8-239.9

154.1 Rectum `CC`
   Rectal ampulla
   CC Excl: 154.1, 154.8, 159.0, 159.8-159.9, 176.3, 195.8, 199.0-199.1, 239.0, 239.8-239.9

N Newborn Age: 0 **P** Pediatric Age: 0-17 **M** Maternity Age: 12-55 **A** Adult Age: 15-124 `CC` CC Condition `MC` Major Complication `CD` Complex Dx `HIV` HIV Related Dx

30 — Volume 1   *2002 Ingenix, Inc.*

Colon

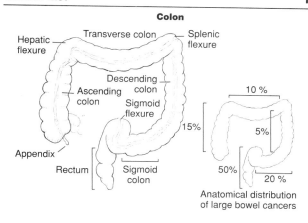

Anatomical distribution of large bowel cancers

154.2 **Anal canal** `CC`
Anal sphincter
> *EXCLUDES* skin of anus (172.5, 173.5)

CC Excl: 154.2-154.8, 159.0, 159.8-159.9, 176.3, 195.8, 199.0-199.1, 239.0, 239.8-239.9

AHA: 1Q, '01, 8

154.3 **Anus, unspecified** `CC`
> *EXCLUDES* anus:
> margin (172.5, 173.5)
> skin (172.5, 173.5)
> perianal skin (172.5, 173.5)

CC Excl: See code 154.2

154.8 **Other** `CC`
Anorectum
Cloacogenic zone
Malignant neoplasm of contiguous or overlapping sites of rectum, rectosigmoid junction, and anus whose point of origin cannot be determined

CC Excl: 154.8, 159.0, 159.8-159.9, 176.3, 195.8, 199.0-199.1, 239.0, 239.8-239.9

✓4ᵗʰ **155 Malignant neoplasm of liver and intrahepatic bile ducts**
155.0 **Liver, primary** `CC`
Carcinoma:
liver, specified as primary
hepatocellular
liver cell
Hepatoblastoma

CC Excl: 155.0-155.2, 159.0, 159.8-159.9, 176.3, 195.8, 199.0-199.1, 239.0, 239.8-239.9

155.1 **Intrahepatic bile ducts** `CC`
Canaliculi biliferi   Intrahepatic:
Interlobular: biliary passages
    bile ducts   canaliculi
    biliary canals   gall duct
> *EXCLUDES* hepatic duct (156.1)

CC Excl: See code 155.0

155.2 **Liver, not specified as primary or secondary** `CC`
CC Excl: See code 155.0

✓4ᵗʰ **156 Malignant neoplasm of gallbladder and extrahepatic bile ducts**
156.0 **Gallbladder** `CC`
CC Excl: 156.0, 156.8-156.9, 159.0, 159.8-159.9, 176.3, 195.8, 199.0-199.1, 239.0, 239.8-239.9

156.1 **Extrahepatic bile ducts** `CC`
Biliary duct or passage NOS
Common bile duct
Cystic duct
Hepatic duct
Sphincter of Oddi

CC Excl: 156.1, 156.8-156.9, 159.0, 159.8-159.9, 176.3, 195.8, 199.0-199.1, 239.0, 239.8-239.9

156.2 **Ampulla of Vater** `CC`
CC Excl: 156.2-156.9, 159.0, 159.8-159.9, 176.3, 195.8, 199.0-199.1, 239.0, 239.8-239.9

DEF: Malignant neoplasm in the area of dilation at the juncture of the common bile and pancreatic ducts near the opening into the lumen of the duodenum.

156.8 **Other specified sites of gallbladder and extrahepatic bile ducts** `CC`
Malignant neoplasm of contiguous or overlapping sites of gallbladder and extrahepatic bile ducts whose point of origin cannot be determined

CC Excl: 156.8-156.9, 159.0, 159.8-159.9, 176.3, 195.8, 199.0-199.1, 239.0, 239.8-239.9

156.9 **Biliary tract, part unspecified** `CC`
Malignant neoplasm involving both intrahepatic and extrahepatic bile ducts

CC Excl: See code 156.8

✓4ᵗʰ **157 Malignant neoplasm of pancreas**
157.0 **Head of pancreas** `CC`
CC Excl: 157.0-157.9, 159.0, 159.8-159.9, 176.3, 195.8, 199.0-199.1, 239.0, 239.8-239.9

AHA : 4Q, '00, 40

157.1 **Body of pancreas** `CC`
CC Excl: See code 157.0

157.2 **Tail of pancreas** `CC`
CC Excl: See code 157.0

157.3 **Pancreatic duct** `CC`
Duct of:
Santorini
Wirsung

CC Excl: See code 157.0

157.4 **Islets of Langerhans** `CC`
Islets of Langerhans, any part of pancreas
Use additional code to identify any functional activity

CC Excl: See code 157.0

DEF: Malignant neoplasm within the structures of the pancreas that produce insulin, somatostatin and glucagon.

157.8 **Other specified sites of pancreas** `CC`
Ectopic pancreatic tissue
Malignant neoplasm of contiguous or overlapping sites of pancreas whose point of origin cannot be determined

CC Excl: See code 157.0

157.9 **Pancreas, part unspecified** `CC`
CC Excl: See code 157.0

AHA: 4Q, '89, 11

✓4ᵗʰ **158 Malignant neoplasm of retroperitoneum and peritoneum**
158.0 **Retroperitoneum**
Periadrenal tissue   Perirenal tissue
Perinephric tissue   Retrocecal tissue

Retroperitoneum and Peritoneum

158.8 Specified parts of peritoneum
Cul-de-sac (of Douglas)
Mesentery
Mesocolon
Omentum
Peritoneum:
parietal
pelvic
Rectouterine pouch
Malignant neoplasm of contiguous or overlapping
sites of retroperitoneum and peritoneum whose
point of origin cannot be determined

158.9 Peritoneum, unspecified

✓4ᵗʰ 159 Malignant neoplasm of other and ill-defined sites within the digestive organs and peritoneum

159.0 Intestinal tract, part unspecified
Intestine NOS

159.1 Spleen, not elsewhere classified
Angiosarcoma
Fibrosarcoma } of spleen

> EXCLUDES *Hodgkin's disease (201.0-201.9)*
> *lymphosarcoma (200.1)*
> *reticulosarcoma (200.0)*

159.8 Other sites of digestive system and intra-abdominal organs
Malignant neoplasm of digestive organs and
peritoneum whose point of origin cannot be
assigned to any one of the categories 150-158

> EXCLUDES *anus and rectum (154.8)*
> *cardio-esophageal junction (151.0)*
> *colon and rectum (154.0)*

159.9 Ill-defined
Alimentary canal or tract NOS
Gastrointestinal tract NOS

> EXCLUDES *abdominal NOS (195.2)*
> *intra-abdominal NOS (195.2)*

MALIGNANT NEOPLASM OF RESPIRATORY AND INTRATHORACIC ORGANS (160-165)

> EXCLUDES *carcinoma in situ (231.0-231.9)*

✓4ᵗʰ 160 Malignant neoplasm of nasal cavities, middle ear, and accessory sinuses

160.0 Nasal cavities
Cartilage of nose   Septum of nose
Conchae, nasal   Vestibule of nose
Internal nose

> EXCLUDES *nasal bone (170.0)*
> *nose NOS (195.0)*
> *olfactory bulb (192.0)*
> *posterior margin of septum and*
> *choanae (147.3)*
> *skin of nose (172.3, 173.3)*
> *turbinates (170.0)*

160.1 Auditory tube, middle ear, and mastoid air cells
Antrum tympanicum   Tympanic cavity
Eustachian tube

> EXCLUDES *auditory canal (external) (172.2, 173.2)*
> *bone of ear (meatus) (170.0)*
> *cartilage of ear (171.0)*
> *ear (external) (skin) (172.2, 173.2)*

160.2 Maxillary sinus
Antrum (Highmore) (maxillary)

160.3 Ethmoidal sinus

160.4 Frontal sinus

160.5 Sphenoidal sinus

160.8 Other
Malignant neoplasm of contiguous or overlapping
sites of nasal cavities, middle ear, and
accessory sinuses whose point of origin cannot
be determined

160.9 Accessory sinus, unspecified

✓4ᵗʰ 161 Malignant neoplasm of larynx

161.0 Glottis
Intrinsic larynx
Laryngeal commissure (anterior) (posterior)
True vocal cord
Vocal cord NOS

161.1 Supraglottis
Aryepiglottic fold or interarytenoid fold, laryngeal
aspect
Epiglottis (suprahyoid portion) NOS
Extrinsic larynx
False vocal cords
Posterior (laryngeal) surface of epiglottis
Ventricular bands

> EXCLUDES *anterior aspect of epiglottis (146.4)*
> *aryepiglottic fold or interarytenoid fold:*
> *NOS (148.2)*
> *hypopharyngeal aspect (148.2)*
> *marginal zone (148.2)*

161.2 Subglottis

161.3 Laryngeal cartilages
Cartilage: Cartilage:
arytenoid   cuneiform
cricoid   thyroid

161.8 Other specified sites of larynx
Malignant neoplasm of contiguous or overlapping
sites of larynx whose point of origin cannot be
determined

161.9 Larynx, unspecified

✓4ᵗʰ 162 Malignant neoplasm of trachea, bronchus, and lung

162.0 Trachea
Cartilage
Mucosa } of trachea

162.2 Main bronchus `CC`
Carina
Hilus of lung
CC Excl: 162.2, 162.8-162.9, 165.8-165.9, 176.4, 195.8, 199.0-199.1,
239.1, 239.8-239.9

162.3 Upper lobe, bronchus or lung `CC`
CC Excl: 162.3, 162.8-162.9, 165.8-165.9, 176.4, 195.8, 199.0-199.1,
239.1, 239.8-239.9

162.4 Middle lobe, bronchus or lung `CC`
CC Excl: 162.4, 162.8-162.9, 165.8-165.9, 176.4, 195.8, 199.0-199.1,
239.1, 239.8-239.9

162.5 Lower lobe, bronchus or lung `CC`
CC Excl: 162.5-162.9, 165.8-165.9, 176.4, 195.8, 199.0-199.1, 239.1,
239.8-239.9

N Newborn Age: 0   P Pediatric Age: 0-17   M Maternity Age: 12-55   A Adult Age: 15-124   CC CC Condition   MC Major Complication   CD Complex Dx   HIV HIV Related Dx

32 — Volume 1   *2002 Ingenix, Inc.*

162.8 Other parts of bronchus or lung `CC`
Malignant neoplasm of contiguous or overlapping sites of bronchus or lung whose point of origin cannot be determined
CC Excl: 162.8-162.9, 165.8-165.9, 176.4, 195.8, 199.0-199.1, 239.1, 239.8-239.9

162.9 Bronchus and lung, unspecified `CC`
CC Excl: See code 162.8
AHA: 2Q, '97, 3; 4Q, '96, 48

✓4ᵗʰ **163 Malignant neoplasm of pleura**

163.0 Parietal pleura `CC`
CC Excl: 163.0-163.9, 165.8-165.9, 195.8, 199.0-199.1, 239.1, 239.8-239.9

163.1 Visceral pleura `CC`
CC Excl: See code 163.0

163.8 Other specified sites of pleura `CC`
Malignant neoplasm of contiguous or overlapping sites of pleura whose point of origin cannot be determined
CC Excl: See code 163.0

163.9 Pleura, unspecified `CC`
CC Excl: See code 163.0

✓4ᵗʰ **164 Malignant neoplasm of thymus, heart, and mediastinum**

164.0 Thymus `CC`
CC Excl: 164.0

164.1 Heart `CC`
Endocardium   Myocardium
Epicardium   Pericardium
EXCLUDES *great vessels (171.4)*
CC Excl: 164.1

164.2 Anterior mediastinum `CC`
CC Excl: 164.2-164.9, 165.8-165.9, 195.8, 199.0-199.1, 239.1, 239.8-239.9

164.3 Posterior mediastinum `CC`
CC Excl: See code 164.2

164.8 Other `CC`
Malignant neoplasm of contiguous or overlapping sites of thymus, heart, and mediastinum whose point of origin cannot be determined
CC Excl: See code 164.2

164.9 Mediastinum, part unspecified `CC`
CC Excl: See code 164.2

✓4ᵗʰ **165 Malignant neoplasm of other and ill-defined sites within the respiratory system and intrathoracic organs**

165.0 Upper respiratory tract, part unspecified

165.8 Other
Malignant neoplasm of respiratory and intrathoracic organs whose point of origin cannot be assigned to any one of the categories 160-164

165.9 Ill-defined sites within the respiratory system
Respiratory tract NOS
EXCLUDES *intrathoracic NOS (195.1)*
thoracic NOS (195.1)

MALIGNANT NEOPLASM OF BONE, CONNECTIVE TISSUE, SKIN, AND BREAST (170-176)
EXCLUDES *carcinoma in situ:*   *carcinoma in situ:*
breast (233.0)   *skin (232.0-232.9)*

✓4ᵗʰ **170 Malignant neoplasm of bone and articular cartilage**
INCLUDES cartilage (articular) (joint)
periosteum
EXCLUDES *bone marrow NOS (202.9)*
cartilage:
ear (171.0)
eyelid (171.0)
larynx (161.3)
nose (160.0)
synovia (171.0-171.9)

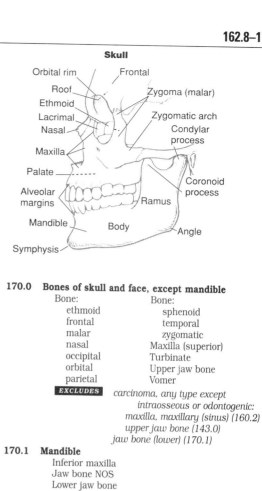

Skull

170.0 Bones of skull and face, except mandible
Bone: Bone:
ethmoid   sphenoid
frontal   temporal
malar   zygomatic
nasal   Maxilla (superior)
occipital   Turbinate
orbital   Upper jaw bone
parietal   Vomer
EXCLUDES *carcinoma, any type except intraosseous or odontogenic:*
maxilla, maxillary (sinus) (160.2)
upper jaw bone (143.0)
jaw bone (lower) (170.1)

170.1 Mandible
Inferior maxilla
Jaw bone NOS
Lower jaw bone
EXCLUDES *carcinoma, any type except intraosseous or odontogenic:*
jaw bone NOS (143.9)
lower (143.1)
upper jaw bone (170.0)

170.2 Vertebral column, excluding sacrum and coccyx
Spinal column   Vertebra
Spine
EXCLUDES *sacrum and coccyx (170.6)*

170.3 Ribs, sternum, and clavicle
Costal cartilage
Costovertebral joint
Xiphoid process

170.4 Scapula and long bones of upper limb
Acromion   Radius
Bones NOS of upper limb Ulna
Humerus
AHA: 2Q, '99, 9

170.5 Short bones of upper limb
Carpal   Scaphoid (of hand)
Cuneiform, wrist   Semilunar or lunate
Metacarpal   Trapezium
Navicular, of hand   Trapezoid
Phalanges of hand   Unciform
Pisiform

170.6 Pelvic bones, sacrum, and coccyx
Coccygeal vertebra   Pubic bone
Ilium   Sacral vertebra
Ischium

170.7 Long bones of lower limb
Bones NOS of lower limb
Femur
Fibula
Tibia

✓4ᵗʰ Additional Digit Required   Nonspecific PDx   Unacceptable PDx   Manifestation Code   `MSP` Medicare Secondary Payer   ►◄ Revised Text   ● New Code   ▲ Revised Code Title
✓5ᵗʰ
2002 Ingenix, Inc.

Volume 1 — 33

Neoplasms 170.8–173.5

170.8 Short bones of lower limb
 Astragalus [talus]   Navicular (of ankle)
 Calcaneus   Patella
 Cuboid   Phalanges of foot
 Cuneiform, ankle   Tarsal
 Metatarsal

170.9 Bone and articular cartilage, site unspecified

✓4ᵗʰ **171 Malignant neoplasm of connective and other soft tissue**

 INCLUDES
 blood vessel   muscle
 bursa   peripheral, sympathetic,
 fascia   and parasympathetic
 fat   nerves and ganglia
 ligament, except   synovia
    uterine   tendon (sheath)

 EXCLUDES
 cartilage (of):
   articular (170.0-170.9)
   larynx (161.3)
   nose (160.0)
 connective tissue:
   breast (174.0-175.9)
   internal organs—code to malignant neoplasm
     of the site [e.g., leiomyosarcoma of
     stomach, 151.9]
 heart (164.1)
 uterine ligament (183.4)

171.0 Head, face, and neck
 Cartilage of: Cartilage of:
   ear   eyelid
 AHA: 2Q, '99, 6

171.2 Upper limb, including shoulder
 Arm   Forearm
 Finger   Hand

171.3 Lower limb, including hip
 Foot   Thigh
 Leg   Toe
 Popliteal space

171.4 Thorax
 Axilla   Great vessels
 Diaphragm
   EXCLUDES *heart (164.1)*
             mediastinum (164.2-164.9)
             thymus (164.0)

171.5 Abdomen
 Abdominal wall   Hypochondrium
   EXCLUDES *peritoneum (158.8)*
             retroperitoneum (158.0)

171.6 Pelvis
 Buttock   Inguinal region
 Groin   Perineum
   EXCLUDES *pelvic peritoneum (158.8)*
             retroperitoneum (158.0)
             uterine ligament, any (183.3-183.5)

171.7 Trunk, unspecified
 Back NOS
 Flank NOS

171.8 Other specified sites of connective and other soft tissue
 Malignant neoplasm of contiguous or overlapping
   sites of connective tissue whose point of origin
   cannot be determined

171.9 Connective and other soft tissue, site unspecified

✓4ᵗʰ **172 Malignant melanoma of skin**
 INCLUDES
 melanocarcinoma
 melanoma (skin) NOS
 EXCLUDES
 skin of genital organs (184.0-184.9, 187.1-
   187.9)
 sites other than skin—code to malignant
   neoplasm of the site

 DEF: Malignant neoplasm of melanocytes; most common in skin, may involve oral cavity, esophagus, anal canal, vagina, leptomeninges, conjunctiva of the eye.

172.0 Lip
   EXCLUDES *vermilion border of lip (140.0-140.1,*
             140.9)

172.1 Eyelid, including canthus

172.2 Ear and external auditory canal
 Auricle (ear)
 Auricular canal, external
 External [acoustic] meatus
 Pinna

172.3 Other and unspecified parts of face
 Cheek (external)   Forehead
 Chin   Nose, external
 Eyebrow   Temple

172.4 Scalp and neck

172.5 Trunk, except scrotum
 Axilla   Perianal skin
 Breast   Perineum
 Buttock   Umbilicus
 Groin
   EXCLUDES *anal canal (154.2)*
             anus NOS (154.3)
             scrotum (187.7)

172.6 Upper limb, including shoulder
 Arm   Forearm
 Finger   Hand

172.7 Lower limb, including hip
 Ankle   Leg
 Foot   Popliteal area
 Heel   Thigh
 Knee   Toe

172.8 Other specified sites of skin
 Malignant melanoma of contiguous or overlapping
   sites of skin whose point of origin cannot be
   determined

172.9 Melanoma of skin, site unspecified

✓4ᵗʰ **173 Other malignant neoplasm of skin**
 INCLUDES
 malignant neoplasm of:
   sebaceous glands
   sudoriferous, sudoriparous glands
   sweat glands
 EXCLUDES
 Kaposi's sarcoma (176.0-176.9)
 malignant melanoma of skin (172.0-172.9)
 skin of genital organs (184.0-184.9, 187.1-
   187.9)

 AHA: 1Q, '00, 18; 2Q, '96, 12

173.0 Skin of lip
   EXCLUDES *vermilion border of lip (140.0-140.1,*
             140.9)

173.1 Eyelid, including canthus
   EXCLUDES *cartilage of eyelid (171.0)*

173.2 Skin of ear and external auditory canal
 Auricle (ear)   External meatus
 Auricular canal, external Pinna
   EXCLUDES *cartilage of ear (171.0)*

173.3 Skin of other and unspecified parts of face
 Cheek, external   Forehead
 Chin   Nose, external
 Eyebrow   Temple
 AHA: 1Q, '00, 3

173.4 Scalp and skin of neck

173.5 Skin of trunk, except scrotum
 Axillary fold   Skin of:
 Perianal skin   buttock
 Skin of: chest wall
   abdominal wall   groin
   anus   perineum
   back   Umbilicus
   breast
   EXCLUDES *anal canal (154.2)*
             anus NOS (154.3)
             skin of scrotum (187.7)

 AHA: 1Q, '01, 8

Ⓝ Newborn Age: 0   Ⓟ Pediatric Age: 0-17   Ⓜ Maternity Age: 12-55   Ⓐ Adult Age: 15-124   CC CC Condition   MC Major Complication   CD Complex Dx   HIV HIV Related Dx

Female Breast

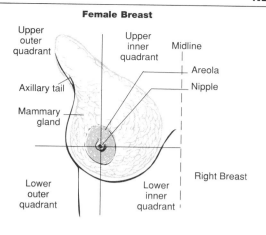

173.6   **Skin of upper limb, including shoulder**
    Arm   Forearm
    Finger   Hand

173.7   **Skin of lower limb, including hip**
    Ankle   Leg
    Foot   Popliteal area
    Heel   Thigh
    Knee   Toe

173.8   **Other specified sites of skin**
    Malignant neoplasm of contiguous or overlapping
        sites of skin whose point of origin cannot be
        determined

173.9   **Skin, site unspecified**

☑4ᵗʰ **174 Malignant neoplasm of female breast**
    INCLUDES   breast (female)   Paget's disease of:
        connective tissue   breast
        soft parts   nipple
    EXCLUDES   skin of breast (172.5, 173.5)
    AHA: 3Q, '97, 8; 4Q, '89, 11

174.0   **Nipple and areola**   ♀♂
174.1   **Central portion**   ♀♂
174.2   **Upper-inner quadrant**   ♀♂
174.3   **Lower-inner quadrant**   ♀♂
174.4   **Upper-outer quadrant**   ♀♂
174.5   **Lower-outer quadrant**   ♀♂
174.6   **Axillary tail**   ♀
174.8   **Other specified sites of female breast**   ♀
    Ectopic sites   Midline of breast
    Inner breast   Outer breast
    Lower breast   Upper breast
    Malignant neoplasm of contiguous or overlapping
        sites of breast whose point of origin cannot be
        determined

174.9   **Breast (female), unspecified**   ♀

☑4ᵗʰ **175 Malignant neoplasm of male breast**
    EXCLUDES   skin of breast (172.5,173.5)

175.0   **Nipple and areola**   ♂
175.9   **Other and unspecified sites of male breast**   ♂
    Ectopic breast tissue, male

☑4ᵗʰ **176 Kaposi's sarcoma**
    AHA: 4Q, '91, 24

176.0   **Skin**   HIV
176.1   **Soft tissue**   HIV
    INCLUDES   blood vessel
        connective tissue
        fascia
        ligament
        lymphatic(s) NEC
        muscle
    EXCLUDES   lymph glands and nodes (176.5)

176.2   **Palate**   HIV
176.3   **Gastrointestinal sites**   HIV
176.4   **Lung**   CC HIV
    CC Excl: 162.8-162.9, 165.8-165.9, 176.4, 195.8, 199.0-199.1,
    239.1, 239.8-239.9

176.5   **Lymph nodes**   CC HIV
    CC Excl: 176.5, 195.8, 196.0-196.9, 199.0-199.1, 239.8-239.9

176.8   **Other specified sites**   HIV
    INCLUDES   oral cavity NEC

176.9   **Unspecified**   HIV
    Viscera NOS

MALIGNANT NEOPLASM OF GENITOURINARY ORGANS (179-189)
    EXCLUDES   carcinoma in situ (233.1-233.9)

179 Malignant neoplasm of uterus, part unspecified   ♀

☑4ᵗʰ **180 Malignant neoplasm of cervix uteri**
    INCLUDES   invasive malignancy [carcinoma]
    EXCLUDES   carcinoma in situ (233.1)

180.0   **Endocervix**   ♀
    Cervical canal NOS   Endocervical gland
    Endocervical canal

180.1   **Exocervix**   ♀
180.8   **Other specified sites of cervix**   ♀
    Cervical stump
    Squamocolumnar junction of cervix
    Malignant neoplasm of contiguous or overlapping
        sites of cervix uteri whose point of origin
        cannot be determined

180.9   **Cervix uteri, unspecified**   ♀

181 Malignant neoplasm of placenta   ♀
    Choriocarcinoma NOS
    Chorioepithelioma NOS
    EXCLUDES   chorioadenoma (destruens) (236.1)
        hydatidiform mole (630)
            malignant (236.1)
        invasive mole (236.1)
        male choriocarcinoma NOS (186.0-186.9)

☑4ᵗʰ **182 Malignant neoplasm of body of uterus**
    EXCLUDES   carcinoma in situ (233.2)

182.0   **Corpus uteri, except isthmus**   ♀
    Cornu   Fundus
    Endometrium   Myometrium

182.1   **Isthmus**   ♀
    Lower uterine segment

182.8   **Other specified sites of body of uterus**   ♀
    Malignant neoplasm of contiguous or overlapping
        sites of body of uterus whose point of origin
        cannot be determined
    EXCLUDES   uterus NOS (179)

☑4ᵗʰ **183 Malignant neoplasm of ovary and other uterine adnexa**
    EXCLUDES   Douglas' cul-de-sac (158.8)

183.0   **Ovary**   ♀
    Use additional code to identify any functional
        activity

183.2   **Fallopian tube**   ♀
    Oviduct   Uterine tube

183.3   **Broad ligament**   ♀
    Mesovarium   Parovarian region

183.4   **Parametrium**   ♀
    Uterine ligament NOS Uterosacral ligament

183.5   **Round ligament**   ♀
    AHA: 3Q, '99, 5

183.8   **Other specified sites of uterine adnexa**   ♀
    Tubo-ovarian
    Utero-ovarian
    Malignant neoplasm of contiguous or overlapping
        sites of ovary and other uterine adnexa whose
        point of origin cannot be determined

183.9   **Uterine adnexa, unspecified**   ♀

☑4ᵗʰ Additional Digit Required   Nonspecific PDx   Unacceptable PDx   Manifestation Code   **MSP** Medicare Secondary Payer   ◄► Revised Text   ● New Code   ▲ Revised Code Title

2002 Ingenix, Inc.   **Volume 1 — 35**

Neoplasms 173.6–183.9

Neoplasms 184–191.3

✓4ᵗʰ **184 Malignant neoplasm of other and unspecified female genital organs**

> **EXCLUDES** *carcinoma in situ (233.3)*

184.0 Vagina ♀
Gartner's duct   Vaginal vault

184.1 Labia majora ♀
Greater vestibular [Bartholin's] gland

184.2 Labia minora ♀

184.3 Clitoris ♀

184.4 Vulva, unspecified ♀
External female genitalia NOS
Pudendum

184.8 Other specified sites of female genital organs ♀
Malignant neoplasm of contiguous or overlapping sites of female genital organs whose point of origin cannot be determined

184.9 Female genital organ, site unspecified ♀
Female genitourinary tract NOS

185 Malignant neoplasm of prostate ♂

> **EXCLUDES** *seminal vesicles (187.8)*

AHA: 3Q, '99, 5; 3Q, '92, 7

✓4ᵗʰ **186 Malignant neoplasm of testis**
Use additional code to identify any functional activity

186.0 Undescended testis ♂
Ectopic testis   Retained testis

186.9 Other and unspecified testis ♂
Testis: Testis:
NOS   scrotal
descended

✓4ᵗʰ **187 Malignant neoplasm of penis and other male genital organs**

187.1 Prepuce ♂
Foreskin

187.2 Glans penis ♂

187.3 Body of penis ♂
Corpus cavernosum

187.4 Penis, part unspecified ♂
Skin of penis NOS

187.5 Epididymis ♂

187.6 Spermatic cord ♂
Vas deferens

187.7 Scrotum ♂
Skin of scrotum

187.8 Other specified sites of male genital organs ♂
Seminal vesicle
Tunica vaginalis
Malignant neoplasm of contiguous or overlapping sites of penis and other male genital organs whose point of origin cannot be determined

187.9 Male genital organ, site unspecified ♂
Male genital organ or tract NOS

✓4ᵗʰ **188 Malignant neoplasm of bladder**

> **EXCLUDES** *carcinoma in situ (233.7)*

188.0 Trigone of urinary bladder

188.1 Dome of urinary bladder

188.2 Lateral wall of urinary bladder

188.3 Anterior wall of urinary bladder

188.4 Posterior wall of urinary bladder

188.5 Bladder neck
Internal urethral orifice

188.6 Ureteric orifice

188.7 Urachus

188.8 Other specified sites of bladder
Malignant neoplasm of contiguous or overlapping sites of bladder whose point of origin cannot be determined

188.9 Bladder, part unspecified
Bladder wall NOS

AHA: 1Q, '00, 5

✓4ᵗʰ **189 Malignant neoplasm of kidney and other and unspecified urinary organs**

189.0 Kidney, except pelvis `CC`
Kidney NOS   Kidney parenchyma
CC Excl: 189.0-189.1, 189.8-189.9, 195.8, 199.0-199.1, 239.5, 239.8-239.9

189.1 Renal pelvis `CC`
Renal calyces   Ureteropelvic junction
CC Excl: See code 189.0

189.2 Ureter `CC`
> **EXCLUDES** *ureteric orifice of bladder (188.6)*

CC Excl: 189.2, 189.8-189.9, 195.8, 199.0-199.1, 239.5, 239.8-239.9

189.3 Urethra
> **EXCLUDES** *urethral orifice of bladder (188.5)*

189.4 Paraurethral glands

189.8 Other specified sites of urinary organs
Malignant neoplasm of contiguous or overlapping sites of kidney and other urinary organs whose point of origin cannot be determined

189.9 Urinary organ, site unspecified
Urinary system NOS

MALIGNANT NEOPLASM OF OTHER AND UNSPECIFIED SITES (190-199)

> **EXCLUDES** *carcinoma in situ (234.0-234.9)*

✓4ᵗʰ **190 Malignant neoplasm of eye**

> **EXCLUDES** *carcinoma in situ (234.0)*
> *eyelid (skin) (172.1, 173.1)*
> *cartilage (171.0)*
> *optic nerve (192.0)*
> *orbital bone (170.0)*

190.0 Eyeball, except conjunctiva, cornea, retina, and choroid
Ciliary body   Sclera
Crystalline lens   Uveal tract
Iris

190.1 Orbit
Connective tissue of orbit
Extraocular muscle
Retrobulbar
> **EXCLUDES** *bone of orbit (170.0)*

190.2 Lacrimal gland

190.3 Conjunctiva

190.4 Cornea

190.5 Retina

190.6 Choroid

190.7 Lacrimal duct
Lacrimal sac   Nasolacrimal duct

190.8 Other specified sites of eye
Malignant neoplasm of contiguous or overlapping sites of eye whose point of origin cannot be determined

190.9 Eye, part unspecified

✓4ᵗʰ **191 Malignant neoplasm of brain**

> **EXCLUDES** *cranial nerves (192.0)*
> *retrobulbar area (190.1)*

191.0 Cerebrum, except lobes and ventricles `CC`
Basal ganglia   Globus pallidus
Cerebral cortex   Hypothalamus
Corpus striatum   Thalamus
CC Excl: 191.0-191.9, 192.0-192.1, 192.8-192.9, 195.8, 199.0-199.1, 239.6-239.9

191.1 Frontal lobe `CC`
CC Excl: See code 191.0

191.2 Temporal lobe `CC`
Hippocampus   Uncus
CC Excl: See code 191.0

191.3 Parietal lobe `CC`
CC Excl: See code 191.0

`N` Newborn Age: 0   `P` Pediatric Age: 0-17   `M` Maternity Age: 12-55   `A` Adult Age: 15-124   `CC` CC Condition   `MC` Major Complication   `CD` Complex Dx   `HIV` HIV Related Dx

36 — Volume 1   *2002 Ingenix, Inc.*

Brain and Meninges

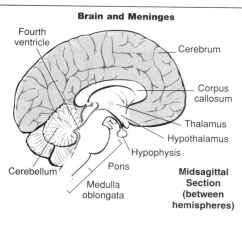

Fourth ventricle
Cerebrum
Corpus callosum
Thalamus
Hypothalamus
Hypophysis
Pons
Cerebellum
Medulla oblongata

Midsagittal Section (between hemispheres)

191.4   Occipital lobe   CC
CC Excl: See code 191.0

191.5   Ventricles   CC
Choroid plexus   Floor of ventricle
CC Excl: See code 191.0

191.6   Cerebellum NOS   CC
Cerebellopontine angle
CC Excl: See code 191.0

191.7   Brain stem   CC
Cerebral peduncle   Midbrain
Medulla oblongata   Pons
CC Excl: See code 191.0

191.8   Other parts of brain   CC
Corpus callosum
Tapetum
Malignant neoplasm of contiguous or overlapping sites of brain whose point of origin cannot be determined
CC Excl: See code 191.0

191.9   Brain, unspecified   CC
Cranial fossa NOS
CC Excl: See code 191.0

✓4ᵗʰ **192   Malignant neoplasm of other and unspecified parts of nervous system**
EXCLUDES   peripheral, sympathetic, and parasympathetic nerves and ganglia (171.0-171.9)

192.0   Cranial nerves   CC
Olfactory bulb
CC Excl: 192.0, 192.8-192.9, 195.8, 199.0-199.1, 239.6-239.9

192.1   Cerebral meninges   CC
Dura (mater)   Meninges NOS
Falx (cerebelli) (cerebri) Tentorium
CC Excl: 192.1, 192.8-192.9, 195.8, 199.0-199.1, 239.6-239.9

192.2   Spinal cord   CC
Cauda equina
CC Excl: 192.2, 192.8-192.9, 195.8, 199.0-199.1, 239.6-239.9

192.3   Spinal meninges   CC
CC Excl: 192.3-192.9, 195.8, 199.0-199.1, 239.6-239.9

192.8   Other specified sites of nervous system   CC
Malignant neoplasm of contiguous or overlapping sites of other parts of nervous system whose point of origin cannot be determined
CC Excl: 191.0-191.9, 192.0-192.9, 195.8, 199.0-199.1, 239.6-239.9

192.9   Nervous system, part unspecified
Nervous system (central) NOS
EXCLUDES   meninges NOS (192.1)

193   Malignant neoplasm of thyroid gland
Sipple's syndrome
Thyroglossal duct
Use additional code to identify any functional activity

✓4ᵗʰ **194   Malignant neoplasm of other endocrine glands and related structures**
Use additional code to identify any functional activity
EXCLUDES   islets of Langerhans (157.4)
ovary (183.0)
testis (186.0-186.9)
thymus (164.0)

194.0   Adrenal gland
Adrenal cortex   Suprarenal gland
Adrenal medulla

194.1   Parathyroid gland

194.3   Pituitary gland and craniopharyngeal duct
Craniobuccal pouch   Rathke's pouch
Hypophysis   Sella turcica
AHA: J-A, '85, 9

194.4   Pineal gland

194.5   Carotid body

194.6   Aortic body and other paraganglia
Coccygeal body   Para-aortic body
Glomus jugulare

194.8   Other
Pluriglandular involvement NOS
Note: If the sites of multiple involvements are known, they should be coded separately.

194.9   Endocrine gland, site unspecified

✓4ᵗʰ **195   Malignant neoplasm of other and ill-defined sites**
INCLUDES   malignant neoplasms of contiguous sites, not elsewhere classified, whose point of origin cannot be determined
EXCLUDES   malignant neoplasm:
lymphatic and hematopoietic tissue (200.0-208.9)
secondary sites (196.0-198.8)
unspecified site (199.0-199.1)

195.0   Head, face, and neck
Cheek NOS   Nose NOS
Jaw NOS   Supraclavicular region NOS

195.1   Thorax
Axilla   Intrathoracic NOS
Chest (wall) NOS

195.2   Abdomen
Intra-abdominal NOS
AHA: 2Q, '97, 3

195.3   Pelvis
Groin
Inguinal region NOS
Presacral region
Sacrococcygeal region
Sites overlapping systems within pelvis, as:
rectovaginal (septum)
rectovesical (septum)

195.4   Upper limb

195.5   Lower limb

195.8   Other specified sites
Back NOS   Trunk NOS
Flank NOS

✓4ᵗʰ **196   Secondary and unspecified malignant neoplasm of lymph nodes**
EXCLUDES   any malignant neoplasm of lymph nodes, specified as primary (200.0-202.9)
Hodgkin's disease (201.0-201.9)
lymphosarcoma (200.1)
other forms of lymphoma (202.0-202.9)
reticulosarcoma (200.0)
AHA: 2Q, '92, 3; M-J, '85, 3

Neoplasms 196.0–199.0

Lymph Nodes

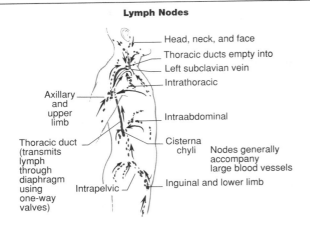

196.0 **Lymph nodes of head, face, and neck**   `CC`
    Cervical   Scalene
    Cervicofacial   Supraclavicular
    CC Excl: 176.5, 195.8, 196.0-196.9, 199.0-199.1, 239.8-239.9

196.1 **Intrathoracic lymph nodes**   `CC`
    Bronchopulmonary   Mediastinal
    Intercostal   Tracheobronchial
    CC Excl: See code 196.0

196.2 **Intra-abdominal lymph nodes**   `CC`
    Intestinal   Retroperitoneal
    Mesenteric
    CC Excl: See code 196.0

196.3 **Lymph nodes of axilla and upper limb**   `CC`
    Brachial   Infraclavicular
    Epitrochlear   Pectoral
    CC Excl: See code 196.0

196.5 **Lymph nodes of inguinal region and lower limb**   `CC`
    Femoral   Popliteal
    Groin   Tibial
    CC Excl: See code 196.0

196.6 **Intrapelvic lymph nodes**   `CC`
    Hypogastric   Obturator
    Iliac   Parametrial
    CC Excl: See code 196.0

196.8 **Lymph nodes of multiple sites**   `CC`
    CC Excl: See code 196.0

196.9 **Site unspecified**   `CC`
    Lymph nodes NOS
    CC Excl: See code 196.0

√4th **197 Secondary malignant neoplasm of respiratory and digestive systems**
    EXCLUDES   *lymph node metastasis (196.0-196.9)*
    AHA: M-J, '85, 3

197.0 **Lung**   `CC`
    Bronchus
    CC Excl: 195.8, 197.0, 197.3, 198.89, 199.0-199.1, 239.8-239.9
    AHA: 2Q, '99, 9

197.1 **Mediastinum**   `CC`
    CC Excl: 195.8, 197.1, 197.3, 198.89, 199.0-199.1, 239.8-239.9

197.2 **Pleura**   `CC`
    CC Excl: 195.8, 197.2-197.3, 198.89, 199.0-199.1, 239.8-239.9
    AHA: 4Q, '89, 11

197.3 **Other respiratory organs**   `CC`
    Trachea
    CC Excl: 195.8, 197.0-197.3, 198.89, 199.0-199.1, 239.8-239.9

197.4 **Small intestine, including duodenum**   `CC`
    CC Excl: 195.8, 197.4, 197.8, 198.89, 199.0-199.1, 239.8-239.9

197.5 **Large intestine and rectum**   `CC`
    CC Excl: 195.8, 197.5, 197.8, 198.89, 199.0-199.1, 239.8-239.9

197.6 **Retroperitoneum and peritoneum**   `CC`
    CC Excl: 195.8, 197.6, 197.8, 198.89, 199.0-199.1, 239.8-239.9
    AHA: 4Q, '89, 11

197.7 **Liver, specified as secondary**   `CC`
    CC Excl: 195.8, 197.7-197.8, 198.89, 199.0-199.1, 239.8-239.9

197.8 **Other digestive organs and spleen**   `CC`
    CC Excl: 195.8, 197.4-197.8, 198.89, 199.0-199.1, 239.8-239.9
    AHA: 2Q, '97, 3; 2Q, '92, 3

√4th **198 Secondary malignant neoplasm of other specified sites**
    EXCLUDES   *lymph node metastasis (196.0-196.9)*
    AHA: M-J, '85, 3

198.0 **Kidney**   `CC`
    CC Excl: 195.8, 198.0-198.1, 198.89, 199.0-199.1, 239.8-239.9

198.1 **Other urinary organs**   `CC`
    CC Excl: See code 198.0

198.2 **Skin**   `CC`
    Skin of breast
    CC Excl: 195.8, 198.2, 198.89, 199.0-199.1, 239.8-239.9

198.3 **Brain and spinal cord**   `CC`
    CC Excl: 195.8, 198.3, 198.89, 199.0-199.1, 239.8-239.9
    AHA: 3Q, '99, 7

198.4 **Other parts of nervous system**   `CC`
    Meninges (cerebral) (spinal)
    CC Excl: 195.8, 198.4, 198.89, 199.0-199.1, 239.8-239.9
    AHA: J-F, '87, 7

198.5 **Bone and bone marrow**   `CC`
    CC Excl: 195.8, 198.5, 198.89, 199.0-199.1, 239.8-239.9
    AHA: 3Q, '99, 5; 2Q, '92, 3; 1Q, '91, 16; 4Q, '89, 10
    DRG 239

198.6 **Ovary**   `CC` ♀
    CC Excl: 195.8, 198.6, 198.89, 199.0-199.1, 239.8-239.9

198.7 **Adrenal gland**   `CC`
    Suprarenal gland
    CC Excl: 195.8, 198.7, 198.89, 199.0-199.1, 239.8-239.9

√5th **198.8 Other specified sites**
    198.81 Breast   `CC`
        EXCLUDES   *skin of breast (198.2)*
        CC Excl: 195.8, 198.81, 198.89, 199.0-199.1, 239.8-239.9

    198.82 Genital organs   `CC`
        CC Excl: 195.8, 198.82, 198.89, 199.0-199.1, 239.8-239.9

    198.89 Other   `CC`
        EXCLUDES   *retroperitoneal lymph nodes (196.2)*
        CC Excl: 195.8, 198.89, 199.0-199.1, 239.8-239.9
        AHA: 2Q, '97, 4

√4th **199 Malignant neoplasm without specification of site**
    199.0 **Disseminated**   `CC`
        Carcinomatosis
        Generalized: unspecified site
          cancer   (primary)
          malignancy (secondary)
        Multiple cancer
        CC Excl: See code 198.89
        AHA: 4Q, '89, 10

| `N` Newborn Age: 0 | `P` Pediatric Age: 0-17 | `M` Maternity Age: 12-55 | `A` Adult Age: 15-124 | `CC` CC Condition | `MC` Major Complication | `CD` Complex Dx | `HIV` HIV Related Dx |

199.1 Other

Cancer   } unspecified site
Carcinoma   } (primary)
Malignancy   } (secondary)

MALIGNANT NEOPLASM OF LYMPHATIC AND HEMATOPOIETIC TISSUE (200-208)

EXCLUDES   secondary neoplasm of:
bone marrow (198.5)
spleen (197.8)
secondary and unspecified neoplasm of lymph nodes (196.0-196.9)

The following fifth-digit subclassification is for use with categories 200-202:

0 unspecified site, extranodal and solid organ sites
1 lymph nodes of head, face, and neck
2 intrathoracic lymph nodes
3 intra-abdominal lymph nodes
4 lymph nodes of axilla and upper limb
5 lymph nodes of inguinal region and lower limb
6 intrapelvic lymph nodes
7 spleen
8 lymph nodes of multiple sites

✓4th **200 Lymphosarcoma and reticulosarcoma**
     AHA: 2Q, '92, 3; N-D, '86, 5

§ ✓5th **200.0 Reticulosarcoma**   CC HIV
     Lymphoma (malignant):
       histiocytic (diffuse):
         nodular
         pleomorphic cell type
         reticulum cell type
       Reticulum cell sarcoma:
         NOS
         pleomorphic cell type

CC Excl: For code 200.00: 200.00-200.08, 239.8-239.9; **For code 200.01:** 200.00, 200.01, 200.08, 239.8-239.9; **For code 200.02:** 200.00, 200.02, 200.08, 239.8-239.9; **For code 200.03:** 200.00, 200.03, 200.08, 239.8-239.9; **For code 200.04:** 200.00, 200.04, 200.08, 239.8-239.9; **For code 200.05:** 200.00, 200.05, 200.08, 239.8-239.9; **For code 200.06:** 200.00, 200.06, 200.08, 239.8-239.9; **For code 200.07:** 200.00, 200.07-200.08, 239.8-239.9; **For code 200.08:** 200.00-200.08, 239.8-239.9

AHA: For Code 200.03: ▶3Q, '01, 12 ◀

DEF: Malignant lymphoma of primarily histolytic cells; commonly originates in reticuloendothelium of lymph nodes.

§ ✓5th **200.1 Lymphosarcoma**   CC
   Lymphoblastoma (diffuse)   Lymphosarcoma:
   Lymphoma (malignant):   NOS
     lymphoblastic (diffuse)   diffuse NOS
     lymphocytic (cell type)   lymphoblastic (diffuse)
       (diffuse)   lymphocytic (diffuse)
     lymphosarcoma type   prolymphocytic
EXCLUDES   lymphosarcoma:
     follicular or nodular (202.0)
     mixed cell type (200.8)
     lymphosarcoma cell leukemia (207.8)

CC Excl: For code 200.10: 200.10-200.18, 239.8-239.9; **For code 200.11:** 200.10, 200.11, 200.18, 239.8-239.9; **For code 200.12:** 200.10, 200.12, 200.18, 239.8-239.9; **For code 200.13:** 200.10, 200.13, 200.18, 239.8-239.9; **For code 200.14:** 200.10, 200.14, 200.18, 239.8-239.9; **For code 200.15:** 200.10, 200.15, 200.18, 239.8-239.9; **For code 200.16:** 200.10, 200.16, 200.18, 239.8-239.9; **For code 200.17:** 200.10, 200.17-200.18, 239.8-239.9; **For code 200.18:** 200.10-200.18, 239.8-239.9

DEF: Malignant lymphoma created from anaplastic lymphoid cells resembling lymphocytes or lymphoblasts.

§ ✓5th **200.2 Burkitt's tumor or lymphoma**   CC HIV
     Malignant lymphoma, Burkitt's type

CC Excl: For code 200.20: 200.20-200.28, 239.8-239.9; **For code 200.21:** 200.20, 200.21, 200.28, 239.8-239.9; **For code 200.22:** 200.20, 200.22, 200.28, 239.8-239.9; **For code 200.23:** 200.20, 200.23, 200.28, 239.8-239.9; **For code 200.24:** 200.20, 200.24, 200.28, 239.8-239.9; **For code 200.25:** 200.20, 200.25, 200.28, 239.8-239.9; **For code 200.26:** 200.20, 200.26, 200.28, 239.8-239.9; **For code 200.27:** 200.20, 200.27-200.28, 239.8-239.9; **For code 200.28:** 200.20-200.28, 239.8-239.9

DEF: Large osteolytic lesion most common in jaw or as abdominal mass; usually found in central Africa but reported elsewhere.

§ ✓5th **200.8 Other named variants**   CC HIV
     Lymphoma (malignant):
       lymphoplasmacytoid type
       mixed lymphocytic-histiocytic (diffuse)
     Lymphosarcoma, mixed cell type (diffuse)
     Reticulolymphosarcoma (diffuse)

CC Excl: For code 200.80: 200.80-200.88, 239.8-239.9; **For code 200.81:** 200.80, 200.81, 200.88, 239.8-239.9; **For code 200.82:** 200.80, 200.82, 200.88, 239.8-239.9; **For code 200.83:** 200.80, 200.83, 200.88, 239.8-239.9; **For code 200.84:** 200.80, 200.84, 200.88, 239.8-239.9; **For code 200.85:** 200.80, 200.85, 200.88, 239.8-239.9; **For code 200.86:** 200.80, 200.86, 200.88, 239.8-239.9; **For code 200.87:** 200.80, 200.87-200.88, 239.8-239.9; **For code 200.88:** 200.80-200.88, 239.8-239.9

✓4th **201 Hodgkin's disease**
     AHA: 2Q, '92, 3; N-D, '86, 5

DEF: Painless, progressive enlargement of lymph nodes, spleen and general lymph tissue; symptoms include anorexia, lassitude, weight loss, fever, pruritis, night sweats, anemia.

§ ✓5th **201.0 Hodgkin's paragranuloma**   CC
CC Excl: For code 201.00: 201.00-201.08, 201.90, 239.8-239.9; **For code 201.01:** 201.00, 201.01, 201.08, 201.90-201.91, 239.8-239.9; **For code 201.02:** 201.00, 201.02, 201.08, 201.90, 201.92, 239.8-239.9; **For code 201.03:** 201.00, 201.03, 201.08, 201.90, 201.93, 239.8-239.9; **For code 201.04:** 201.00, 201.04, 201.08, 201.90, 201.94, 239.8-239.9; **For code 201.05:** 201.00, 201.05, 201.08, 201.90, 201.95, 239.8-239.9; **For code 201.06:** 201.00, 201.06, 201.08, 201.90, 201.96, 239.8-239.9; **For code 201.07:** 201.00, 201.07-201.08, 201.90, 201.97, 239.8-239.9; **For code 201.08:** 201.00-201.08, 201.90, 201.98, 239.8-239.9

§ ✓5th **201.1 Hodgkin's granuloma**   CC
CC Excl: For code 201.10: 201.10-201.18, 201.90, 201.98, 239.8-239.9; **For code 201.11:** 201.10, 201.11, 201.18, 201.90-201.91, 201.98, 239.8-239.9; **For code 201.12:** 201.10, 201.12, 201.18, 201.90, 201.92, 201.98, 239.8-239.9; **For code 201.13:** 201.10, 201.13, 201.18, 201.90, 201.93, 201.98, 239.8-239.9; **For code 201.14:** 201.10, 201.14, 201.18, 201.90, 201.94, 201.98, 239.8-239.9; **For code 201.15:** 201.10, 201.15, 201.18, 201.90, 201.95, 201.98, 239.8-239.9; **For code 201.16:** 201.10, 201.16, 201.18, 201.90, 201.96, 201.98, 239.8-239.9; **For code 201.17:** 201.10, 201.17-201.18, 201.90, 201.97-201.98, 239.8-239.9; **For code 201.18:** 201.10-201.18, 201.90, 201.98, 239.8-239.9

AHA: 2Q, '99, 7

§ ✓5th **201.2 Hodgkin's sarcoma**   CC
CC Excl: For code 201.20: 201.20-201.28, 201.90, 201.98, 239.8-239.9; **For code 201.21:** 201.20, 201.21, 201.28, 201.90-201.91, 201.98, 239.8-239.9; **For code 201.22:** 201.20, 201.22, 201.28, 201.90, 201.92, 201.98, 239.8-239.9; **For code 201.23:** 201.20, 201.23, 201.28, 201.90, 201.93, 201.98, 239.8-239.9; **For code 201.24:** 201.20, 201.24, 201.28, 201.90, 201.94, 201.98, 239.8-239.9; **For code 201.25:** 201.20, 201.25, 201.28, 201.90, 201.95, 201.98, 239.8-239.9; **For code 201.26:** 201.20, 201.26, 201.28, 201.90, 201.96, 201.98, 239.8-239.9; **For code 201.27:** 201.20, 201.27-201.28, 201.90, 201.97-201.98, 239.8-239.9; **For code 201.28:** 201.20-201.28, 201.90, 201.98, 239.8-239.9

§   Requires fifth-digit. See beginning of section 200–208 for codes and definitions.

✓4th / ✓5th Additional Digit Required   Nonspecific PDx   Unacceptable PDx   Manifestation Code   MSP Medicare Secondary Payer   ▶◀ Revised Text   ● New Code   ▲ Revised Code Title

2002 Ingenix, Inc.   **January 2002 • Volume 1 — 39**

Neoplasms 199.1–201.2

Neoplasms 201.4–202.3

§ ✓5ᵗʰ **201.4**   **Lymphocytic-histiocytic predominance**   CC

CC Excl: For code **201.40:** 201.40-201.48, 201.90, 201.98, 239.8-239.9; For code **201.41:** 201.40, 201.41, 201.48, 201.90-201.91, 201.98, 239.8-239.9; For code **201.42:** 201.40, 201.42, 201.48, 201.90, 201.92, 201.98, 239.8-239.9; For code **201.43:** 201.40, 201.43, 201.48, 201.90, 201.93, 201.98, 239.8-239.9; For code **201.44:** 201.40, 201.44, 201.48, 201.90, 201.94, 201.98, 239.8-239.9; For code **201.45:** 201.40, 201.45, 201.48, 201.90, 201.95, 201.98, 239.8-239.9; For code **201.46:** 201.40, 201.46, 201.48, 201.90, 201.96, 201.98, 239.8-239.9; For code **201.47:** 201.40, 201.47-201.48, 201.90, 201.97-201.98, 239.8-239.9; For code **201.48:** 201.40-201.48, 201.90, 201.98, 239.8-239.9

§ ✓5ᵗʰ **201.5**   **Nodular sclerosis**   CC

Hodgkin's disease, nodular sclerosis:
    NOS
    cellular phase

CC Excl: For code **201.50:** 201.50-201.58, 201.90, 201.98, 239.8-239.9; For code **201.51:** 201.50, 201.51, 201.58, 201.90-201.91, 201.98, 239.8-239.9; For code **201.52:** 201.50, 201.52, 201.58, 201.90, 201.92, 201.98, 239.8-239.9; For code **201.53:** 201.50, 201.53, 201.58, 201.90, 201.93, 201.98, 239.8-239.9; For code **201.54:** 201.50, 201.54, 201.58, 201.90, 201.94, 201.98, 239.8-239.9; For code **201.55:** 201.50, 201.55, 201.58, 201.90, 201.95, 201.98, 239.8-239.9; For code **201.56:** 201.50, 201.56, 201.58, 201.90, 201.96, 201.98, 239.8-239.9; For code **201.57:** 201.50, 201.57-201.58, 201.90, 201.97-201.98, 239.8-239.9; For code **201.58:** 201.50-201.58, 201.90, 201.98, 239.8-239.9

§ ✓5ᵗʰ **201.6**   **Mixed cellularity**   CC

CC Excl: For code **201.60:** 201.60-201.68, 201.90, 201.98, 239.8-239.9; For code **201.61:** 201.60, 201.61, 201.68, 201.90-201.91, 201.98, 239.8-239.9; For code **201.62:** 201.60, 201.62, 201.68, 201.90, 201.92, 201.98, 239.8-239.9; For code **201.63:** 201.60, 201.63, 201.68, 201.90, 201.93, 201.98, 239.8-239.9; For code **201.64:** 201.60, 201.64, 201.68, 201.90, 201.94, 201.98, 239.8-239.9; For code **201.65:** 201.60, 201.65, 201.68, 201.90, 201.95, 201.98, 239.8-239.9; For code **201.66:** 201.60, 201.66, 201.68, 201.90, 201.96, 201.98, 239.8-239.9; For code **201.67:** 201.60, 201.67-201.68, 201.90, 201.97-201.98, 239.8-239.9; For code **201.68:** 201.60-201.68, 201.90, 201.98, 239.8-239.9

§ ✓5ᵗʰ **201.7**   **Lymphocytic depletion**   CC

Hodgkin's disease, lymphocytic depletion:
    NOS
    diffuse fibrosis
    reticular type

CC Excl: For code **201.70:** 201.70-201.78, 201.90, 201.98, 239.8-239.9; For code **201.71:** 201.70, 201.71, 201.78, 201.91, 201.98, 239.8-239.9; For code **201.72:** 201.70, 201.72, 201.78, 201.90, 201.92, 201.98, 239.8-239.9; For code **201.73:** 201.70, 201.73, 201.78, 201.90, 201.93, 201.98, 239.8-239.9; For code **201.74:** 201.70, 201.74, 201.78, 201.90, 201.94, 201.98, 239.8-239.9; For code **201.75:** 201.70, 201.75, 201.78, 201.90, 201.95, 201.98, 239.8-239.9; For code **201.76:** 201.70, 201.76, 201.78, 201.90, 201.96, 201.98, 239.8-239.9; For code **201.77:** 201.70, 201.77-201.78, 201.97-201.98, 239.8-239.9; For code **201.78:** 201.70-201.78, 201.90, 201.98, 239.8-239.9

§ ✓5ᵗʰ **201.9**   **Hodgkin's disease, unspecified**   CC

Hodgkin's: Malignant:
   disease NOS   lymphogranuloma
   lymphoma NOS   lymphogranulomatosis

CC Excl: For code **201.90:** 201.90-201.98, 239.8-239.9; For code **201.91:** 201.90, 201.91, 201.98, 239.8-239.9; For code **201.92:** 201.90, 201.92, 201.98, 239.8-239.9; For code **201.93:** 201.90, 201.93, 201.98, 239.8-239.9; For code **201.94:** 201.90, 201.94, 201.98, 239.8-239.9; For code **201.95:** 201.90, 201.95, 201.98, 239.8-239.9; For code **201.96:** 201.90, 201.96, 201.98, 239.8-239.9; For code **201.97:** 201.90, 201.97-201.98, 239.8-239.9; For code **201.98:** 201.90-201.98, 239.8-239.9

✓4ᵗʰ **202**   **Other malignant neoplasms of lymphoid and histiocytic tissue**

AHA: 2Q, '92, 3; N-D, '86, 5

§ ✓5ᵗʰ **202.0**   **Nodular lymphoma**   CC

Brill-Symmers disease   Lymphosarcoma:
Lymphoma: follicular (giant)
   follicular (giant)   nodular
   lymphocytic, nodular   Reticulosarcoma, follicular
                           or nodular

CC Excl: For code **202.00:** 202.00-202.08, 202.80, 202.90, 239.8-239.9; For code **202.01:** 202.00, 202.01, 202.08, 202.81, 202.91, 239.8-239.9; For code **202.02:** 202.00, 202.02, 202.08, 202.82, 202.92, 239.8-239.9; For code **202.03:** 202.00, 202.03, 202.08, 202.83, 202.93, 239.8-239.9; For code **202.04:** 202.00, 202.04, 202.08, 202.84, 202.94, 239.8-239.9; For code **202.05:** 202.00, 202.05, 202.08, 202.85, 202.95, 239.8-239.9; For code **202.06:** 202.00, 202.06, 202.08, 202.86, 202.96, 239.8-239.9; For code **202.07:** 202.00, 202.07-202.08, 202.87, 202.97, 239.8-239.9; For code **202.08:** 202.00-202.08, 202.88, 202.98, 239.8-239.9

DEF: Lymphomatous cells clustered into nodules within the lymph node; usually occurs in older adults and may involve all nodes and possibly extranodal sites.

§ ✓5ᵗʰ **202.1**   **Mycosis fungoides**   CC

CC Excl: For code **202.10:** 202.10-202.18, 202.80, 202.90, 239.8-239.9; For code **202.11:** 202.10, 202.11, 202.18, 202.81, 202.91, 239.8-239.9; For code **202.12:** 202.10, 202.12, 202.18, 202.82, 202.92, 239.8-239.9; For code **202.13:** 202.10, 202.13, 202.18, 202.83, 202.93, 239.8-239.9; For code **202.14:** 202.10, 202.14, 202.18, 202.84, 202.94, 239.8-239.9; For code **202.15:** 202.10, 202.15, 202.18, 202.85, 202.95, 239.8-239.9; For code **202.16:** 202.10, 202.16, 202.18, 202.86, 202.96, 239.8-239.9; For code **202.17:** 202.10, 202.17-202.18, 202.87, 202.97, 239.8-239.9; For code **202.18:** 202.10-202.18, 202.88, 202.98, 239.8-239.9

AHA: 2Q, '92, 4

DEF: Type of cutaneous T-cell lymphoma; may evolve into generalized lymphoma; formerly thought to be of fungoid origin.

§ ✓5ᵗʰ **202.2**   **Sézary's disease**   CC

CC Excl: For code **202.20:** 202.20-202.28, 202.80, 202.90, 239.8-239.9; For code **202.21:** 202.20, 202.21, 202.28, 202.81, 202.91, 239.8-239.9; For code **202.22:** 202.20, 202.22, 202.28, 202.82, 202.92, 239.8-239.9; For code **202.23:** 202.20, 202.23, 202.28, 202.83, 202.93, 239.8-239.9; For code **202.24:** 202.20, 202.24, 202.28, 202.84, 202.94, 239.8-239.9; For code **202.25:** 202.20, 202.25, 202.28, 202.85, 202.95, 239.8-239.9; For code **202.26:** 202.20, 202.26, 202.28, 202.86, 202.96, 239.8-239.9; For code **202.27:** 202.20, 202.27-202.28, 202.87, 202.97, 239.8-239.9; For code **202.28:** 202.20-202.28, 202.88, 202.98, 239.8-239.9

AHA: 2Q, '99, 7

DEF: Type of cutaneous T-cell lymphoma with erythroderma, intense pruritus, peripheral lymphadenopathy, abnormal hyperchromatic mononuclear cells in skin, lymph nodes and peripheral blood.

§ ✓5ᵗʰ **202.3**   **Malignant histiocytosis**   CC

Histiocytic medullary reticulosis
Malignant:
   reticuloendotheliosis
   reticulosis

CC Excl: For code **202.30:** 202.30-202.38, 202.80, 202.90, 239.8-239.9; For code **202.31:** 202.30, 202.31, 202.38, 202.81, 202.91, 239.8-239.9; For code **202.32:** 202.30, 202.32, 202.38, 202.82, 202.92, 239.8-239.9; For code **202.33:** 202.30, 202.33, 202.38, 202.83, 202.93, 239.8-239.9; For code **202.34:** 202.30, 202.34, 202.38, 202.84, 202.94, 239.8-239.9; For code **202.35:** 202.30, 202.35, 202.38, 202.85, 202.95, 239.8-239.9; For code **202.36:** 202.30, 202.36, 202.38, 202.86, 202.96, 239.8-239.9; For code **202.37:** 202.30, 202.37-202.38, 202.87, 202.97, 239.8-239.9; For code **202.38:** 202.30-202.38, 202.88, 202.98, 239.8-239.9

---

§   Requires fifth-digit. See beginning of section 200–208 for codes and definitions.

N Newborn Age: 0   P Pediatric Age: 0-17   M Maternity Age: 12-55   A Adult Age: 15-124   CC CC Condition   MC Major Complication   CD Complex Dx   HIV HIV Related Dx

§ ✓5ᵗʰ **202.4 Leukemic reticuloendotheliosis**   CC
    Hairy-cell leukemia

CC Excl: For code 202.40: 202.40-202.48, 202.80, 202.90, 239.8-239.9;
For code 202.41: 202.40, 202.41, 202.48, 202.81, 202.91, 239.8-239.9;
For code 202.42: 202.40, 202.42, 202.48, 202.82, 202.92, 239.8-239.9;
For code 202.43: 202.40, 202.43, 202.48, 202.83, 202.93, 239.8-239.9;
For code 202.44: 202.40, 202.44, 202.48, 202.84, 202.94, 239.8-239.9;
For code 202.45: 202.40, 202.45, 202.48, 202.85, 202.95, 239.8-239.9;
For code 202.46: 202.40, 202.46, 202.48, 202.86, 202.96, 239.8-239.9;
For code 202.47: 202.40, 202.47-202.48, 202.87, 202.97, 239.8-239.9;
For code 202.48: 202.40-202.48, 202.88, 202.98, 239.8-239.9

DEF: Chronic leukemia with large, mononuclear cells with "hairy" appearance in marrow, spleen, liver, blood.

§ ✓5ᵗʰ **202.5 Letterer-Siwe disease**   CC
    Acute:
        differentiated progressive histiocytosis
        histiocytosis X (progressive)
        infantile reticuloendotheliosis
        reticulosis of infancy

> **EXCLUDES**   *Hand-Schüller-Christian disease (277.8)*
> *histiocytosis (acute) (chronic) (277.8)*
> *histiocytosis X (chronic) (277.8)*

CC Excl: For code 202.50: 202.50-202.58, 202.80, 202.90, 239.8-239.9;
For code 202.51: 202.50, 202.51, 202.58, 202.81, 202.91, 239.8-239.9;
For code 202.52: 202.50, 202.52, 202.58, 202.82, 202.92, 239.8-239.9;
For code 202.53: 202.50, 202.53, 202.58, 202.83, 202.93, 239.8-239.9;
For code 202.54: 202.50, 202.54, 202.58, 202.84, 202.94, 239.8-239.9;
For code 202.55: 202.50, 202.55, 202.58, 202.85, 202.95, 239.8-239.9;
For code 202.56: 202.50, 202.56, 202.58, 202.86, 202.96, 239.8-239.9;
For code 202.57: 202.50, 202.57-202.58, 202.87, 202.97, 239.8-239.9;
For code 202.58: 202.50-202.58, 202.88, 202.98, 239.8-239.9

DEF: A recessive reticuloendotheliosis of early childhood, with a hemorrhagic tendency, eczema-like skin eruption, hepatosplenomegaly, including lymph node enlargement, and progressive anemia; it is often a fatal disease with no established cause.

§ ✓5ᵗʰ **202.6 Malignant mast cell tumors**   CC
    Malignant: Mast cell sarcoma
        mastocytoma   Systemic tissue mast
        mastocytosis   cell disease

> **EXCLUDES**   *mast cell leukemia (207.8)*

CC Excl: For code 202.60: 202.60-202.68, 202.80, 202.90, 239.8-239.9;
For code 202.61: 202.60, 202.61, 202.68, 202.81, 202.91, 239.8-239.9;
For code 202.62: 202.60, 202.62, 202.68, 202.82, 202.92, 239.8-239.9;
For code 202.63: 202.60, 202.63, 202.68, 202.83, 202.93, 239.8-239.9;
For code 202.64: 202.60, 202.64, 202.68, 202.84, 202.94, 239.8-239.9;
For code 202.65: 202.60, 202.65, 202.68, 202.85, 202.95, 239.8-239.9;
For code 202.66: 202.60, 202.66, 202.68, 202.86, 202.96, 239.8-239.9;
For code 202.67: 202.60, 202.67-202.68, 202.87, 202.97, 239.8-239.9;
For code 202.68: 202.60-202.68, 202.88, 202.98, 239.8-239.9

§ ✓5ᵗʰ **202.8 Other lymphomas**   CC HIV
    Lymphoma (malignant):
        NOS
        diffuse

> **EXCLUDES**   *benign lymphoma (229.0)*

CC Excl: For code 202.80: 202.80-202.88, 202.90, 239.8-239.9;
For code 202.81: 202.80, 202.81, 202.88, 202.91, 239.8-239.9; **For code 202.82:** 202.80, 202.82, 202.88, 202.92, 239.8-239.9; **For code 202.83:** 202.80, 202.83, 202.88, 202.93, 239.8-239.9; **For code 202.84:** 202.80, 202.84, 202.88, 202.94, 239.8-239.9; **For code 202.85:** 202.80, 202.85, 202.88, 202.95, 239.8-239.9; **For code 202.86:** 202.80, 202.86, 202.88, 202.96, 239.8-239.9; **For code 202.87:** 202.80, 202.87-202.88, 202.97, 239.8-239.9; **For code 202.88:** 202.80-202.88, 202.98, 239.8-239.9

AHA: 2Q, '92, 4

§ ✓5ᵗʰ **202.9 Other and unspecified malignant neoplasms of lymphoid and histiocytic tissue**   CC
    Malignant neoplasm of bone marrow NOS

CC Excl: For code 202.90: 202.90-202.98, 239.8-239.9; **For code 202.91:** 202.90, 202.91, 202.98, 239.8-239.9; **For code 202.92:** 202.90, 202.92, 202.98, 239.8-239.9; **For code 202.93:** 202.90, 202.93, 202.98, 239.8-239.9; **For code 202.94:** 202.90, 202.94, 202.98, 239.8-239.9; **For code 202.95:** 202.90, 202.95, 202.98, 239.8-239.9; **For code 202.96:** 202.90, 202.96, 202.98, 239.8-239.9; **For code 202.97:** 202.90, 202.97-202.98, 239.8-239.9; **For code 202.98:** 202.90-202.98, 239.8-239.9

✓4ᵗʰ **203 Multiple myeloma and immunoproliferative neoplasms**
AHA: 4Q, '91, 26

The following fifth-digit subclassification is for use with category 203:
    0 without mention of remission
    1 in remission

✓5ᵗʰ **203.0 Multiple myeloma**   CC
    Kahler's disease   Myelomatosis

> **EXCLUDES**   *solitary myeloma (238.6)*

CC Excl: 203.00-203.81, 204.00-204.91, 205.00-205.91, 206.00-206.91, 207.00-207.81, 208.00-208.91, 239.8-239.9

AHA: 1Q, '96, 16; 4Q, '89,10

✓5ᵗʰ **203.1 Plasma cell leukemia**   CC
    Plasmacytic leukemia
CC Excl: See code 203.0

AHA: 4Q, '90, 26; S-O, '86, 12

✓5ᵗʰ **203.8 Other immunoproliferative neoplasms**   CC
CC Excl: See code 203.0

AHA: 4Q, '90, 26; S-O, '86, 12

✓4ᵗʰ **204 Lymphoid leukemia**
> **INCLUDES**   leukemia:
>   lymphatic
>   lymphoblastic
>   lymphocytic
>   lymphogenous

AHA: 3Q, '93, 4

The following fifth-digit subclassification is for use with category 204:
    0 without mention of remission
    1 in remission

✓5ᵗʰ **204.0 Acute**   CC
> **EXCLUDES**   *acute exacerbation of chronic lymphoid leukemia (204.1)*

CC Excl: See code 203.0

AHA: 3Q, '99, 6

✓5ᵗʰ **204.1 Chronic**   CC
CC Excl: See code 203.0

✓5ᵗʰ **204.2 Subacute**   CC
CC Excl: See code 203.0

✓5ᵗʰ **204.8 Other lymphoid leukemia**   CC
    Aleukemic leukemia: Aleukemic leukemia:
        lymphatic   lymphoid
        lymphocytic
CC Excl: See code 203.0

✓5ᵗʰ **204.9 Unspecified lymphoid leukemia**   CC
CC Excl: See code 203.0

---

§ Requires fifth-digit. See beginning of section 200–208 for codes and definitions.

Neoplasms 205–210.1

✓4ᵗʰ **205 Myeloid leukemia**

INCLUDES   leukemia: leukemia:
granulocytic   myelomonocytic
myeloblastic   myelosclerotic
myelocytic   myelosis
myelogenous

AHA: 3Q, '93, 3; 4Q, '91, 26; 4Q, '90, 3; M-J, '85, 18

The following fifth-digit subclassification is for use with category 205:
0 **without mention of remission**
1 **in remission**

✓5ᵗʰ **205.0 Acute**   CC
Acute promyelocytic leukemia
EXCLUDES   *acute exacerbation of chronic myeloid leukemia (205.1)*
CC Excl: See code 203.0

✓5ᵗʰ **205.1 Chronic**   CC
Eosinophilic leukemia   Neutrophilic leukemia
CC Excl: See code 203.0
AHA: 1Q, 00, 6; J-A, '85, 13

✓5ᵗʰ **205.2 Subacute**   CC
CC Excl: See code 203.0

✓5ᵗʰ **205.3 Myeloid sarcoma**   CC
Chloroma   Granulocytic sarcoma
CC Excl: See code 203.0

✓5ᵗʰ **205.8 Other myeloid leukemia**   CC
Aleukemic leukemia: Aleukemic leukemia:
granulocytic   myeloid
myelogenous   Aleukemic myelosis
CC Excl: See code 203.0

✓5ᵗʰ **205.9 Unspecified myeloid leukemia**   CC
CC Excl: See code 203.0

✓4ᵗʰ **206 Monocytic leukemia**
INCLUDES   leukemia:
histiocytic
monoblastic
monocytoid

The following fifth-digit subclassification is for use with category 206:
0 **without mention of remission**
1 **in remission**

✓5ᵗʰ **206.0 Acute**   CC
EXCLUDES   *acute exacerbation of chronic monocytic leukemia (206.1)*
CC Excl: See code 203.0

✓5ᵗʰ **206.1 Chronic**   CC
CC Excl: See code 203.0

✓5ᵗʰ **206.2 Subacute**   CC
CC Excl: See code 203.0

✓5ᵗʰ **206.8 Other monocytic leukemia**   CC
Aleukemic:
monocytic leukemia
monocytoid leukemia
CC Excl: See code 203.0

✓5ᵗʰ **206.9 Unspecified monocytic leukemia**   CC
CC Excl: See code 203.0

✓4ᵗʰ **207 Other specified leukemia**
EXCLUDES   *leukemic reticuloendotheliosis (202.4)*
plasma cell leukemia (203.1)

The following fifth-digit subclassification is for use with category 207:
0 **without mention of remission**
1 **in remission**

✓5ᵗʰ **207.0 Acute erythremia and erythroleukemia**   CC
Acute erythremic myelosis
Di Guglielmo's disease
Erythremic myelosis
CC Excl: See code 203.0
DEF: Erythremia: polycythemia vera.
DEF: Erythroleukemia: a malignant blood dyscrasia (a myeloproliferative disorder).

✓5ᵗʰ **207.1 Chronic erythremia**   CC
Heilmeyer-Schöner disease
CC Excl: See code 203.0

✓5ᵗʰ **207.2 Megakaryocytic leukemia**   CC
Megakaryocytic myelosis   Thrombocytic leukemia
CC Excl: See code 203.0

✓5ᵗʰ **207.8 Other specified leukemia**   CC
Lymphosarcoma cell leukemia
CC Excl: See code 203.0

✓4ᵗʰ **208 Leukemia of unspecified cell type**
The following fifth-digit subclassification is for use with category 208:
0 **without mention of remission**
1 **in remission**

✓5ᵗʰ **208.0 Acute**   CC
Acute leukemia NOS   Stem cell leukemia
Blast cell leukemia
EXCLUDES   *acute exacerbation of chronic unspecified leukemia (208.1)*
CC Excl: See code 203.0

✓5ᵗʰ **208.1 Chronic**   CC
Chronic leukemia NOS
CC Excl: See code 203.0

✓5ᵗʰ **208.2 Subacute**   CC
Subacute leukemia NOS
CC Excl: See code 203.0

✓5ᵗʰ **208.8 Other leukemia of unspecified cell type**   CC
CC Excl: See code 203.0

✓5ᵗʰ **208.9 Unspecified leukemia**   CC
Leukemia NOS
CC Excl: See code 203.0

BENIGN NEOPLASMS (210-229)

✓4ᵗʰ **210 Benign neoplasm of lip, oral cavity, and pharynx**
EXCLUDES   *cyst (of):*
jaw (526.0-526.2,526.89)
oral soft tissue (528.4)
radicular (522.8)

210.0 Lip
Frenulum labii
Lip (inner aspect) (mucosa) (vermilion border)
EXCLUDES   *labial commissure (210.4)*
skin of lip (216.0)

210.1 Tongue
Lingual tonsil

 N Newborn Age: 0   P Pediatric Age: 0-17   M Maternity Age: 12-55   A Adult Age: 15-124   CC CC Condition   MC Major Complication   CD Complex Dx   HIV HIV Related Dx

42 — Volume 1   2002 Ingenix, Inc.

210.2 Major salivary glands

Gland: Gland:
   parotid   submandibular
   sublingual

EXCLUDES *benign neoplasms of minor salivary*
glands:
NOS (210.4)
buccal mucosa (210.4)
lips (210.0)
palate (hard) (soft) (210.4)
tongue (210.1)
tonsil, palatine (210.5)

210.3 Floor of mouth

210.4 Other and unspecified parts of mouth

Gingiva   Oral mucosa
Gum (upper) (lower)   Palate (hard) (soft)
Labial commissure   Uvula
Oral cavity NOS

EXCLUDES *benign odontogenic neoplasms of bone*
(213.0-213.1)
developmental odontogenic cysts
(526.0)
mucosa of lips (210.0)
nasopharyngeal [posterior] [superior]
surface of soft palate (210.7)

210.5 Tonsil

Tonsil (faucial) (palatine)

EXCLUDES *lingual tonsil (210.1)*
pharyngeal tonsil (210.7)
tonsillar:
fossa (210.6)
pillars (210.6)

210.6 Other parts of oropharynx

Branchial cleft or vestiges   Tonsillar:
Epiglottis, anterior aspect   fossa
Fauces NOS   pillars
Mesopharynx NOS   Vallecula

EXCLUDES *epiglottis:*
NOS (212.1)
suprahyoid portion (212.1)

210.7 Nasopharynx

Adenoid tissue   Pharyngeal tonsil
Lymphadenoid tissue   Posterior nasal septum

210.8 Hypopharynx

Arytenoid fold   Postcricoidregion
Laryngopharynx   Pyriform fossa

210.9 Pharynx, unspecified

Throat NOS

✓4ᵗʰ **211 Benign neoplasm of other parts of digestive system**

211.0 Esophagus

211.1 Stomach

Body
Cardia } of stomach
Fundus

Cardiac orifice
Pylorus

211.2 Duodenum, jejunum, and ileum

Small intestine NOS

EXCLUDES *ampulla of Vater (211.5)*
ileocecal valve (211.3)

211.3 Colon

Appendix   Ileocecal valve
Cecum   Large intestine NOS

EXCLUDES *rectosigmoid junction (211.4)*

AHA: ▶4Q, '01, 56◀

211.4 Rectum and anal canal

Anal canal or sphincter   Rectosigmoid junction
Anus NOS

EXCLUDES *anus:*
margin (216.5)
skin (216.5)
perianal skin (216.5)

211.5 Liver and biliary passages

Ampulla of Vater   Gallbladder
Common bile duct   Hepatic duct
Cystic duct   Sphincter of Oddi

211.6 Pancreas, except islets of Langerhans

211.7 Islets of Langerhans

Islet cell tumor
Use additional code to identify any functional
activity

211.8 Retroperitoneum and peritoneum

Mesentery   Omentum
Mesocolon   Retroperitoneal tissue

211.9 Other and unspecified site

Alimentary tract NOS
Digestive system NOS
Gastrointestinal tract NOS
Intestinal tract NOS
Intestine NOS
Spleen, not elsewhere classified

✓4ᵗʰ **212 Benign neoplasm of respiratory and intrathoracic organs**

212.0 Nasal cavities, middle ear, and accessory sinuses

Cartilage of nose   Sinus:
Eustachian tube   ethmoidal
Nares   frontal
Septum of nose   maxillary
                       sphenoidal

EXCLUDES *auditory canal (external) (216.2)*
bone of:
ear (213.0)
nose [turbinates] (213.0)
cartilage of ear (215.0)
ear (external) (skin) (216.2)
nose NOS (229.8)
skin (216.3)
olfactory bulb (225.1)
polyp of:
accessory sinus (471.8)
ear (385.30-385.35)
nasal cavity (471.0)
posterior margin of septum and
choanae (210.7)

212.1 Larynx

Cartilage: Epiglottis (suprahyoid portion) NOS
   arytenoid   Glottis
   cricoid   Vocal cords (false) (true)
   cuneiform
   thyroid

EXCLUDES *epiglottis, anterior aspect (210.6)*
polyp of vocal cord or larynx (478.4)

212.2 Trachea

212.3 Bronchus and lung

Carina   Hilus of lung

212.4 Pleura

212.5 Mediastinum

212.6 Thymus

212.7 Heart

EXCLUDES *great vessels (215.4)*

212.8 Other specified sites

212.9 Site unspecified

Respiratory organ NOS
Upper respiratory tract NOS

EXCLUDES *intrathoracic NOS (229.8)*
thoracic NOS (229.8)

✓4ᵗʰ **213 Benign neoplasm of bone and articular cartilage**

INCLUDES cartilage (articular) (joint)
periosteum

EXCLUDES *cartilage of:*   *cartilage of:*
ear (215.0)   *nose (212.0)*
eyelid (215.0)   *exostosis NOS (726.91)*
larynx (212.1)   *synovia (215.0-215.9)*

213.0 Bones of skull and face

EXCLUDES *lower jaw bone (213.1)*

✓4ᵗʰ Additional Digit Required   Nonspecific PDx   Unacceptable PDx   Manifestation Code   **MSP** Medicare Secondary Payer   ▶◀ Revised Text   ● New Code   ▲ Revised Code Title
✓5ᵗʰ

213.1   **Lower jaw bone**
213.2   **Vertebral column, excluding sacrum and coccyx**
213.3   **Ribs, sternum, and clavicle**
213.4   **Scapula and long bones of upper limb**
213.5   **Short bones of upper limb**
213.6   **Pelvic bones, sacrum, and coccyx**
213.7   **Long bones of lower limb**
213.8   **Short bones of lower limb**
213.9   **Bone and articular cartilage, site unspecified**

√4ᵗʰ **214 Lipoma**

INCLUDES   angiolipoma
fibrolipoma
hibernoma
lipoma (fetal) (infiltrating) (intramuscular)
myelolipoma
myxolipoma

DEF: Benign tumor frequently composed of mature fat cells; may occasionally be composed of fetal fat cells.

214.0   **Skin and subcutaneous tissue of face**
214.1   **Other skin and subcutaneous tissue**
214.2   **Intrathoracic organs**
214.3   **Intra-abdominal organs**
214.4   **Spermatic cord**   ♂
214.8   **Other specified sites**

AHA: 3Q, '94, 7

214.9   **Lipoma, unspecified site**

√4ᵗʰ **215 Other benign neoplasm of connective and other soft tissue**

INCLUDES   blood vessel
bursa
fascia
ligament
muscle
peripheral, sympathetic, and parasympathetic
    nerves and ganglia
synovia
tendon (sheath)

EXCLUDES   cartilage:
    articular (213.0-213.9)
    larynx (212.1)
    nose (212.0)
connective tissue of:
    breast (217)
    internal organ, except lipoma and
      hemangioma—code to benign neoplasm
      of the site
lipoma (214.0-214.9)

215.0   **Head, face, and neck**
215.2   **Upper limb, including shoulder**
215.3   **Lower limb, including hip**
215.4   **Thorax**

EXCLUDES   heart (212.7)
    mediastinum (212.5)
    thymus (212.6)

215.5   **Abdomen**
    Abdominal wall   Hypochondrium
215.6   **Pelvis**
    Buttock   Inguinal region
    Groin   Perineum

EXCLUDES   uterine:
    leiomyoma (218.0-218.9)
    ligament, any (221.0)

215.7   **Trunk, unspecified**
    Back NOS   Flank NOS
215.8   **Other specified sites**
215.9   **Site unspecified**

√4ᵗʰ **216 Benign neoplasm of skin**

INCLUDES   blue nevus   pigmented nevus
dermatofibroma   syringoadenoma
hydrocystoma   syringoma

EXCLUDES   skin of genital organs (221.0-222.9)

AHA: 1Q, '00, 21

216.0   **Skin of lip**

EXCLUDES   vermilion border of lip (210.0)

216.1   **Eyelid, including canthus**

EXCLUDES   cartilage of eyelid (215.0)

216.2   **Ear and external auditory canal**
    Auricle (ear)   External meatus
    Auricular canal, external   Pinna

EXCLUDES   cartilage of ear (215.0)

216.3   **Skin of other and unspecified parts of face**
    Cheek, external   Nose, external
    Eyebrow   Temple

216.4   **Scalp and skin of neck**

AHA: 3Q, '91, 12

216.5   **Skin of trunk, except scrotum**
    Axillary fold   Skin of:
    Perianal skin   buttock
    Skin of: chest wall
      abdominal wall   groin
      anus   perineum
      back   Umbilicus
      breast

EXCLUDES   anal canal (211.4)
    anus NOS (211.4)
    skin of scrotum (222.4)

216.6   **Skin of upper limb, including shoulder**
216.7   **Skin of lower limb, including hip**
216.8   **Other specified sites of skin**
216.9   **Skin, site unspecified**

217 Benign neoplasm of breast
    Breast (male) (female):   Breast (male) (female):
      connective tissue   soft parts
      glandular tissue

EXCLUDES   adenofibrosis (610.2)
    benign cyst of breast (610.0)
    fibrocystic disease (610.1)
    skin of breast (216.5)

AHA: 1Q, '00, 4

√4ᵗʰ **218 Uterine leiomyoma**

INCLUDES   fibroid (bleeding) (uterine)
uterine:
    fibromyoma
    myoma

DEF: Benign tumor primarily derived from uterine smooth muscle tissue; may contain fibrous, fatty, or epithelial tissue; also called uterine fibroid or myoma.

218.0   **Submucous leiomyoma of uterus**   ♀
218.1   **Intramural leiomyoma of uterus**   ♀
    Interstitial leiomyoma of uterus
218.2   **Subserous leiomyoma of uterus**   ♀

Types of Uterine Fibroids

Cornual — Pedunculated
Uterine cavity — Intramural
Subserosal — Submucosal
Cervical

N Newborn Age: 0   **P** Pediatric Age: 0-17   **M** Maternity Age: 12-55   **A** Adult Age: 15-124   **CC** CC Condition   **MC** Major Complication   **CD** Complex Dx   **HIV** HIV Related Dx

44 — Volume 1   *2002 Ingenix, Inc.*

218.9 Leiomyoma of uterus, unspecified   ♀

✓4ᵗʰ **219** Other benign neoplasm of uterus
    219.0 Cervix uteri   ♀
    219.1 Corpus uteri   ♀
        Endometrium   Myometrium
        Fundus
    219.8 Other specified parts of uterus   ♀
    219.9 Uterus, part unspecified   ♀
220 Benign neoplasm of ovary   ♀
    Use additional code to identify any functional activity
    (256.0-256.1)
    EXCLUDES   cyst:
        corpus albicans (620.2)
        corpus luteum (620.1)
        endometrial (617.1)
        follicular (atretic) (620.0)
        graafian follicle (620.0)
        ovarian NOS (620.2)
        retention (620.2)

✓4ᵗʰ **221** Benign neoplasm of other female genital organs
    INCLUDES   adenomatous polyp
        benign teratoma
    EXCLUDES   cyst:
        epoophoron (752.11)
        fimbrial (752.11)
        Gartner's duct (752.11)
        parovarian (752.11)

    221.0 Fallopian tube and uterine ligaments   ♀
        Oviduct
        Parametruim
        Uterine ligament (broad) (round) (uterosacral)
        Uterine tube
    221.1 Vagina   ♀
    221.2 Vulva   ♀
        Clitoris
        External female genitalia NOS
        Greater vestibular [Bartholin's] gland
        Labia (majora) (minora)
        Pudendum
        EXCLUDES   *Bartholin's (duct) (gland) cyst (616.2)*
    221.8 Other specified sites of female genital organs   ♀
    221.9 Female genital organ, site unspecified   ♀
        Female genitourinary tract NOS

✓4ᵗʰ **222** Benign neoplasm of male genital organs
    222.0 Testis   ♂
        Use additional code to identify any functional
        activity
    222.1 Penis   ♂
        Corpus cavernosum   Prepuce
        Glans penis
    222.2 Prostate   ♂
        EXCLUDES   *adenomatous hyperplasia of prostate*
            (600.2)
        prostatic:
            adenoma (600.2)
            enlargement (600.0)
            hypertrophy (600.0)
    222.3 Epididymis   ♂
    222.4 Scrotum   ♂
        Skin of scrotum
    222.8 Other specified sites of male genital organs   ♂
        Seminal vesicle
        Spermatic cord
    222.9 Male genital organ, site unspecified   ♂
        Male genitourinary tract NOS

✓4ᵗʰ **223** Benign neoplasm of kidney and other urinary organs
    223.0 Kidney, except pelvis
        Kidney NOS
        EXCLUDES   *renal:*
            calyces (223.1)
            pelvis (223.1)

Eyeball

    223.1 Renal pelvis
    223.2 Ureter
        EXCLUDES   *ureteric orifice of bladder (223.3)*
    223.3 Bladder
✓5ᵗʰ   **223.8** Other specified sites of urinary organs
        223.81 Urethra
            EXCLUDES   *urethral orifice of bladder*
                (223.3)
        223.89 Other
            Paraurethral glands
    223.9 Urinary organ, site unspecified
        Urinary system NOS

✓4ᵗʰ **224** Benign neoplasm of eye
    EXCLUDES   *cartilage of eyelid (215.0)*
        eyelid (skin) (216.1)
        optic nerve (225.1)
        orbital bone (213.0)
    224.0 Eyeball, except conjunctiva, cornea, retina, and choroid
        Ciliary body   Sclera
        Iris   Uveal tract
    224.1 Orbit
        EXCLUDES   *bone of orbit (213.0)*
    224.2 Lacrimal gland
    224.3 Conjunctiva
    224.4 Cornea
    224.5 Retina
        EXCLUDES   *hemangioma of retina (228.03)*
    224.6 Choroid
    224.7 Lacrimal duct
        Lacrimal sac   Nasolacrimal duct
    224.8 Other specified parts of eye
    224.9 Eye, part unspecified

✓4ᵗʰ **225** Benign neoplasm of brain and other parts of nervous system
    EXCLUDES   *hemangioma (228.02)*
        neurofibromatosis (237.7)
        peripheral, sympathetic, and parasympathetic
            nerves and ganglia (215.0-215.9)
        retrobulbar (224.1)
    225.0 Brain
    225.1 Cranial nerves
    225.2 Cerebral meninges
        Meninges NOS   Meningioma (cerebral)
    225.3 Spinal cord
        Cauda equina
    225.4 Spinal meninges
        Spinal meningioma
    225.8 Other specified sites of nervous system
    225.9 Nervous system, part unspecified
        Nervous system (central) NOS
        EXCLUDES   *meninges NOS (225.2)*
226 Benign neoplasm of thyroid glands
    Use additional code to identify any functional activity

Neoplasms 218.9–226

✓4ᵗʰ / ✓5ᵗʰ Additional Digit Required   Nonspecific PDx   Unacceptable PDx   Manifestation Code   **MSP** Medicare Secondary Payer   ►◄ Revised Text   ● New Code   ▲ Revised Code Title

2002 Ingenix, Inc.   **Volume 1 — 45**

Neoplasms 227–231.9

✓4ᵗʰ **227 Benign neoplasm of other endocrine glands and related structures**

Use additional code to identify any functional activity

EXCLUDES ovary (220) testis (222.0)
pancreas (211.6)

227.0 Adrenal gland
Suprarenal gland

227.1 Parathyroid gland

227.3 Pituitary gland and craniopharyngeal duct (pouch)
Craniobuccal pouch Rathke's pouch
Hypophysis Sella turcica

227.4 Pineal gland
Pineal body

227.5 Carotid body

227.6 Aortic body and other paraganglia
Coccygeal body Para-aortic body
Glomus jugulare

AHA: N-D, '84, 17

227.8 Other

227.9 Endocrine gland, site unspecified

✓4ᵗʰ **228 Hemangioma and lymphangioma, any site**

INCLUDES angioma (benign) (cavernous) (congenital) NOS
cavernous nevus
glomus tumor
hemangioma (benign) (congenital)

EXCLUDES benign neoplasm of spleen, except hemangioma
and lymphangioma (211.9)
glomus jugulare (227.6)
nevus:
NOS (216.0-216.9)
blue or pigmented (216.0-216.9)
vascular (757.32)

AHA: 1Q, '00, 21

✓5ᵗʰ **228.0 Hemangioma, any site**

AHA: J-F, '85, 19

DEF: A common benign tumor usually occurring in infancy; composed of newly formed blood vessels due to malformation of angioblastic tissue.

228.00 Of unspecified site

228.01 Of skin and subcutaneous tissue

228.02 Of intracranial structures

228.03 Of retina

228.04 Of intra-abdominal structures
Peritoneum Retroperitoneal tissue

228.09 Of other sites
Systemic angiomatosis

AHA: 3Q, '91, 20

228.1 Lymphangioma, any site
Congenital lymphangioma
Lymphatic nevus

✓4ᵗʰ **229 Benign neoplasm of other and unspecified sites**

229.0 Lymph nodes
EXCLUDES lymphangioma (228.1)

229.8 Other specified sites
Intrathoracic NOS Thoracic NOS

229.9 Site unspecified

CARCINOMA IN SITU (230-234)

INCLUDES Bowen's disease
erythroplasia
Queyrat's erythroplasia

EXCLUDES leukoplakia—see Alphabetic Index

DEF: A neoplastic type; with tumor cells confined to epithelium of origin; without further invasion.

✓4ᵗʰ **230 Carcinoma in situ of digestive organs**

230.0 Lip, oral cavity, and pharynx
Gingiva Oropharynx
Hypopharynx Salivary gland or duct
Mouth [any part] Tongue
Nasopharynx

EXCLUDES aryepiglottic fold or interarytenoid fold,
laryngeal aspect (231.0)
epiglottis:
NOS (231.0)
suprahyoid portion (231.0)
skin of lip (232.0)

230.1 Esophagus

230.2 Stomach
Body ⎫
Cardia ⎬ of stomach
Fundus ⎭
Cardiac orifice Pylorus

230.3 Colon
Appendix Ileocecal valve
Cecum Large intestine NOS
EXCLUDES rectosigmoid junction (230.4)

230.4 Rectum
Rectosigmoid junction

230.5 Anal canal
Anal sphincter

230.6 Anus, unspecified
EXCLUDES anus:
margin (232.5)
skin (232.5)
perianal skin (232.5)

230.7 Other and unspecified parts of intestine
Duodenum Jejunum
Ileum Small intestine NOS
EXCLUDES ampulla of Vater (230.8)

230.8 Liver and biliary system
Ampulla of Vater Gallbladder
Common bile duct Hepatic duct
Cystic duct Sphincter of Oddi

230.9 Other and unspecified digestive organs
Digestive organ NOS Pancreas
Gastrointestinal tract NOS Spleen

✓4ᵗʰ **231 Carcinoma in situ of respiratory system**

231.0 Larynx
Cartilage: Epiglottis:
arytenoid NOS
cricoid posterior surface
cuneiform suprahyoid portion
thyroid Vocal cords (false) (true)
EXCLUDES aryepiglottic fold or interarytenoid fold:
NOS (230.0)
hypopharyngeal aspect (230.0)
marginal zone (230.0)

231.1 Trachea

231.2 Bronchus and lung
Carina
Hilus of lung

231.8 Other specified parts of respiratory system
Accessory sinuses Nasal cavities
Middle ear Pleura
EXCLUDES ear (external) (skin) (232.2)
nose NOS (234.8)
skin (232.3)

231.9 Respiratory system, part unspecified
Respiratory organ NOS

N Newborn Age: 0 P Pediatric Age: 0-17 M Maternity Age: 12-55 A Adult Age: 15-124 CC CC Condition MC Major Complication CD Complex Dx HIV HIV Related Dx

✓4ᵗʰ **232 Carcinoma in situ of skin**

INCLUDES   pigment cells

232.0   Skin of lip

EXCLUDES   *vermilion border of lip (230.0)*

232.1   Eyelid, including canthus

232.2   Ear and external auditory canal

232.3   Skin of other and unspecified parts of face

232.4   Scalp and skin of neck

232.5   Skin of trunk, except scrotum

Anus, margin	Skin of:
Axillary fold	breast
Perianal skin	buttock
Skin of:	chest wall
abdominal wall	groin
anus	perineum
back	Umbilicus

EXCLUDES   *anal canal (230.5)*
anus NOS (230.6)
skin of genital organs (233.3, 233.5-233.6)

232.6   Skin of upper limb, including shoulder

232.7   Skin of lower limb, including hip

232.8   Other specified sites of skin

232.9   Skin, site unspecified

✓4ᵗʰ **233 Carcinoma in situ of breast and genitourinary system**

233.0   Breast

EXCLUDES   *Paget's disease (174.0-174.9)*
skin of breast (232.5)

233.1   Cervix uteri   ♀

AHA: 3Q, '92, 7; 3Q, '92, 8; 1Q, '91, 11

233.2   Other and unspecified parts of uterus   ♀

233.3   Other and unspecified female genital organs   ♀

233.4   Prostate   ♂

233.5   Penis   ♂

233.6   Other and unspecified male genital organs   ♂

233.7   Bladder

233.9   Other and unspecified urinary organs

✓4ᵗʰ **234 Carcinoma in situ of other and unspecified sites**

234.0   Eye

EXCLUDES   *cartilage of eyelid (234.8)*
eyelid (skin) (232.1)
optic nerve (234.8)
orbital bone (234.8)

234.8   Other specified sites

Endocrine gland [any]

234.9   Site unspecified

Carcinoma in situ NOS

NEOPLASMS OF UNCERTAIN BEHAVIOR (235-238)

Note: Categories 235–238 classify by site certain histomorphologically well-defined neoplasms, the subsequent behavior of which cannot be predicted from the present appearance.

✓4ᵗʰ **235 Neoplasm of uncertain behavior of digestive and respiratory systems**

235.0   Major salivary glands

Gland:	Gland:
parotid	submandibular
sublingual	

EXCLUDES   *minor salivary glands (235.1)*

235.1   Lip, oral cavity, and pharynx

Gingiva	Nasopharynx
Hypopharynx	Oropharynx
Minor salivary glands	Tongue
Mouth	

EXCLUDES   *aryepiglottic fold or interarytenoid fold, laryngeal aspect (235.6)*
epiglottis:
NOS (235.6)
suprahyoid portion (235.6)
skin of lip (238.2)

235.2   Stomach, intestines, and rectum

235.3   Liver and biliary passages

Ampulla of Vater	Gallbladder
Bile ducts [any]	Liver

235.4   Retroperitoneum and peritoneum

235.5   Other and unspecified digestive organs

Anal:	Esophagus
canal	Pancreas
sphincter	Spleen
Anus NOS	

EXCLUDES   *anus:*
margin (238.2)
skin (238.2)
perianal skin (238.2)

235.6   Larynx

EXCLUDES   *aryepiglottic fold or interarytenoid fold:*
NOS (235.1)
hypopharyngeal aspect (235.1)
marginal zone (235.1)

235.7   Trachea, bronchus, and lung

235.8   Pleura, thymus, and mediastinum

235.9   Other and unspecified respiratory organs

Accessory sinuses	Nasal cavities
Middle ear	Respiratory organ NOS

EXCLUDES   *ear (external) (skin) (238.2)*
nose (238.8)
skin (238.2)

✓4ᵗʰ **236 Neoplasm of uncertain behavior of genitourinary organs**

236.0   Uterus   ♀

236.1   Placenta   ♀

Chorioadenoma (destruens)
Invasive mole
Malignant hydatid(iform) mole

236.2   Ovary   ♀

Use additional code to identify any functional activity

236.3   Other and unspecified female genital organs   ♀

236.4   Testis   ♂

Use additional code to identify any functional activity

236.5   Prostate   ♂

236.6   Other and unspecified male genital organs   ♂

236.7   Bladder

✓5ᵗʰ **236.9   Other and unspecified urinary organs**

236.90   Urinary organ, unspecified

236.91   Kidney and ureter

236.99   Other

✓4ᵗʰ **237 Neoplasm of uncertain behavior of endocrine glands and nervous system**

237.0   Pituitary gland and craniopharyngeal duct

Use additional code to identify any functional activity

237.1   Pineal gland

237.2   Adrenal gland

Suprarenal gland
Use additional code to identify any functional activity

237.3   Paraganglia

Aortic body	Coccygeal body
Carotid body	Glomus jugulare

AHA: N-D, '84, 17

237.4   Other and unspecified endocrine glands

Parathyroid gland	Thyroid gland

237.5   Brain and spinal cord

237.6   Meninges

Meninges:	Meninges:
NOS	spinal
cerebral	

Neoplasms 237.7–239.9

√5ᵗʰ **237.7** **Neurofibromatosis**
von Recklinghausen's disease
DEF: An inherited condition with developmental changes in the nervous system, muscles, bones and skin; multiple soft tumors (neurofibromas) distributed over the entire body.

237.70 Neurofibromatosis, unspecified

237.71 Neurofibromatosis, type 1 [von Recklinghausen's disease]

237.72 Neurofibromatosis, type 2 [acoustic neurofibromatosis]
DEF: Inherited condition with cutaneous lesions, benign tumors of peripheral nerves and bilateral 8th nerve masses.

237.9 **Other and unspecified parts of nervous system**
Cranial nerves
EXCLUDES   peripheral, sympathetic, and parasympathetic nerves and ganglia (238.1)

√4ᵗʰ **238** **Neoplasm of uncertain behavior of other and unspecified sites and tissues**

238.0 **Bone and articular cartilage**
EXCLUDES   cartilage:
ear (238.1)
eyelid (238.1)
larynx (235.6)
nose (235.9)
synovia (238.1)

238.1 **Connective and other soft tissue**
Peripheral, sympathetic, and parasympathetic nerves and ganglia
EXCLUDES   cartilage (of):
articular (238.0)
larynx (235.6)
nose (235.9)
connective tissue of breast (238.3)

238.2 **Skin**
EXCLUDES   anus NOS (235.5)
skin of genital organs (236.3, 236.6)
vermilion border of lip (235.1)

238.3 **Breast**
EXCLUDES   skin of breast (238.2)

238.4 **Polycythemia vera**
DEF: Abnormal proliferation of all bone marrow elements, increased red cell mass and total blood volume; unknown etiology, frequently associated with splenomegaly, leukocytosis, and thrombocythemia.

238.5 **Histiocytic and mast cells**
Mast cell tumor NOS   Mastocytoma NOS

238.6 **Plasma cells**
Plasmacytoma NOS   Solitary myeloma

238.7 **Other lymphatic and hematopoietic tissues**
Disease:
lymphoproliferative (chronic) NOS
myeloproliferative (chronic) NOS
Idiopathic thrombocythemia
Megakaryocytic myelosclerosis
Myelodysplastic syndrome
Myelosclerosis with myeloid metaplasia
Panmyelosis (acute)
EXCLUDES   myelfibrosis (289.8)
myelosclerosis NOS (289.8)
myelosis:
NOS (205.9)
megakaryocytic (207.2)
AHA: ▶3Q, '01, 13;◀ 1Q, '97, 5; 2Q, '89, 8

238.8 **Other specified sites**
Eye   Heart
EXCLUDES   eyelid (skin) (238.2)
cartilage (238.1)

238.9 **Site unspecified**

NEOPLASMS OF UNSPECIFIED NATURE (239)

√4ᵗʰ **239** **Neoplasms of unspecified nature**
Note: Category 239 classifies by site neoplasms of unspecified morphology and behavior. The term "mass,"unless otherwise stated, is not to be regarded as a neoplastic growth.
INCLUDES   "growth" NOS   new growth NOS
neoplasm NOS   tumor NOS

239.0 **Digestive system**
EXCLUDES   anus:
margin (239.2)
skin (239.2)
perianal skin (239.2)

239.1 **Respiratory system**

239.2 **Bone, soft tissue, and skin**
EXCLUDES   anal canal (239.0)
anus NOS (239.0)
bone marrow (202.9)
cartilage:
larynx (239.1)
nose (239.1)
connective tissue of breast (239.3)
skin of genital organs (239.5)
vermilion border of lip (239.0)

239.3 **Breast**
EXCLUDES   skin of breast (239.2)

239.4 **Bladder**

239.5 **Other genitourinary organs**

239.6 **Brain**
EXCLUDES   cerebral meninges (239.7)
cranial nerves (239.7)

239.7 **Endocrine glands and other parts of nervous system**
EXCLUDES   peripheral, sympathetic, and parasympathetic nerves and ganglia (239.2)

239.8 **Other specified sites**
EXCLUDES   eyelid (skin) (239.2)
cartilage (239.2)
great vessels (239.2)
optic nerve (239.7)

239.9 **Site unspecified**

N Newborn Age: 0   P Pediatric Age: 0-17   M Maternity Age: 12-55   A Adult Age: 15-124   CC CC Condition   MC Major Complication   CD Complex Dx   HIV HIV Related Dx

48 — Volume 1 • January 2002   2002 Ingenix, Inc.

3. ENDOCRINE, NUTRITIONAL AND METABOLIC DISEASES, AND IMMUNITY DISORDERS (240-279)

EXCLUDES *endocrine and metabolic disturbances specific to the fetus and newborn (775.0-775.9)*

Note: All neoplasms, whether functionally active or not, are classified in Chapter 2. Codes in Chapter 3 (i.e., 242.8, 246.0, 251-253, 255-259) may be used to identify such functional activity associated with any neoplasm, or by ectopic endocrine tissue.

DISORDERS OF THYROID GLAND (240-246)

✓4th 240 Simple and unspecified goiter

DEF: An enlarged thyroid gland often caused by an inadequate dietary intake of iodine.

240.0 Goiter, specified as simple
Any condition classifiable to 240.9, specified as simple

240.9 Goiter, unspecified
Enlargement of thyroid
Goiter or struma:
  NOS
  diffuse colloid
  endemic
Goiter or struma:
  hyperplastic
  nontoxic (diffuse)
  parenchymatous
  sporadic

EXCLUDES *congenital (dyshormonogenic) goiter (246.1)*

✓4th 241 Nontoxic nodular goiter

EXCLUDES *adenoma of thyroid (226)*
cystadenoma of thyroid (226)

241.0 Nontoxic uninodular goiter
Thyroid nodule   Uninodular goiter (nontoxic)

DEF: Enlarged thyroid, commonly due to decreased thyroid production, with single nodule; no clinical hypothyroidism.

241.1 Nontoxic multinodular goiter
Multinodular goiter (nontoxic)

DEF: Enlarged thyroid, commonly due to decreased thyroid production with multiple nodules; no clinical hypothyroidism.

241.9 Unspecified nontoxic nodular goiter
Adenomatous goiter
Nodular goiter (nontoxic) NOS
Struma nodosa (simplex)

✓4th 242 Thyrotoxicosis with or without goiter

EXCLUDES *neonatal thyrotoxicosis (775.3)*

DEF: A condition caused by excess quantities of thyroid hormones being introduced into the tissues

The following fifth-digit subclassification is for use with category 242:

0 without mention of thyrotoxic crisis or storm
1 with mention of thyrotoxic crisis or storm

The Endocrine System

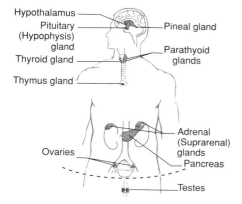

Hypothalamus
Pituitary (Hypophysis) gland
Thyroid gland
Thymus gland
Pineal gland
Parathyroid glands
Ovaries
Adrenal (Suprarenal) glands
Pancreas
Testes

✓5th 242.0 Toxic diffuse goiter   `CC`
Basedow's disease
Exophthalmic or toxic goiter NOS
Graves' disease
Primary thyroid hyperplasia

CC Excl: 017.50-017.56, 017.90-017.96, 240.0, 240.9, 241.0-241.9, 242.00-242.91,243, 244.0-244.9, 245.0-245.9, 246.0-246.9, 259.8-259.9

DEF: Diffuse thyroid enlargement accompanied by hyperthyroidism, bulging eyes, and dermopathy.

✓5th 242.1 Toxic uninodular goiter   `CC`
Thyroid nodule
Uninodular goiter } toxic or with hyperthyroidism

CC Excl: See code 242.0

DEF: Symptomatic hyperthyroidism with a single nodule on the enlarged thyroid gland. Abrupt onset of symptoms; including extreme nervousness, insomnia, weight loss, tremors, and psychosis or coma.

✓5th 242.2 Toxic multinodular goiter   `CC`
Secondary thyroid hyperplasia
CC Excl: See code 242.0

DEF: Symptomatic hyperthyroidism with multiple nodules on the enlarged thyroid gland. Abrupt onset of symptoms; including extreme nervousness, insomnia, weight loss, tremors, and psychosis or coma

✓5th 242.3 Toxic nodular goiter, unspecified   `CC`
Adenomatous goiter
Nodular goiter } toxic or with hyperthyroidism
Struma nodosa

Any condition classifiable to 241.9 specified as toxic or with hyperthyroidism
CC Excl: See code 242.0

✓5th 242.4 Thyrotoxicosis from ectopic thyroid nodule   `CC`
CC Excl: See code 242.0

✓5th 242.8 Thyrotoxicosis of other specified origin   `CC`
Overproduction of thyroid-stimulating hormone [TSH]
Thyrotoxicosis:
  factitia from ingestion of excessive thyroid material
Use additional E code to identify cause, if drug-induced
CC Excl: See code 242.0

✓5th 242.9 Thyrotoxicosis without mention of goiter or other cause   `CC`
Hyperthyroidism NOS
Thyrotoxicosis NOS
CC Excl: See code 242.0

243 Congenital hypothyroidism
Congenital thyroid insufficiency
Cretinism (athyrotic) (endemic)
Use additional code to identify associated mental retardation
EXCLUDES *congenital (dyshormonogenic) goiter (246.1)*

DEF: Underproduction of thyroid hormone present from birth.

✓4th 244 Acquired hypothyroidism
INCLUDES athyroidism (acquired)
hypothyroidism (acquired)
myxedema (adult) (juvenile)
thyroid (gland) insufficiency (acquired)

244.0 Postsurgical hypothyroidism
DEF: Underproduction of thyroid hormone due to surgical removal of all or part of the thyroid gland.

244.1 Other postablative hypothyroidism
Hypothyroidism following therapy, such as irradiation

✓4th ✓5th Additional Digit Required   Nonspecific PDx   Unacceptable PDx   Manifestation Code   **MSP** Medicare Secondary Payer   ◄► Revised Text   ● New Code   ▲ Revised Code Title

2002 Ingenix, Inc.

Volume 1 — 49

Endocrine, Nutritional, Metabolic, Immunity 244.2–250.2

244.2 Iodine hypothyroidism

Hypothyroidism resulting from administration or
ingestion of iodide

Use additional E code to identify drug

244.3 Other iatrogenic hypothyroidism

Hypothyroidism resulting from:

P-aminosalicylic acid [PAS]

Phenylbutazone

Resorcinol

Iatrogenic hypothyroidism NOS

Use additional E code to identify drug

244.8 Other specified acquired hypothyroidism

Secondary hypothyroidism NEC

AHA: J-A, '85, 9

244.9 Unspecified hypothyroidism

Hypothyroidism
Myxedema $\Big\}$ primary or NOS

AHA: 3Q, '99, 19; 4Q, '96, 29

✓4ᵗʰ **245 Thyroiditis**

245.0 Acute thyroiditis

Abscess of thyroid   Thyroiditis:
Thyroiditis: pyogenic
nonsuppurative, acute   suppurative

Use additional code to identify organism

DEF: Inflamed thyroid caused by infection, with abscess and liquid
puris.

245.1 Subacute thyroiditis

Thyroiditis: Thyroiditis:
de Quervain's   granulomatous
giant cell   viral

DEF: Inflammation of the thyroid, characterized by fever and painful
enlargement of the thyroid gland, with granulomas in the gland.

245.2 Chronic lymphocytic thyroiditis

Hashimoto's disease

Struma lymphomatosa

Thyroiditis:

autoimmune

lymphocytic (chronic)

DEF: Autoimmune disease of thyroid; lymphocytes infiltrate the
gland and thyroid antibodies are produced; women more often
affected.

245.3 Chronic fibrous thyroiditis

Struma fibrosa   Thyroiditis:
Thyroiditis: ligneous
invasive (fibrous)   Riedel's

DEF: Persistent fibrosing inflammation of thyroid with adhesions to
nearby structures; rare condition

245.4 Iatrogenic thyroiditis

Use additional code to identify cause

DEF: Thyroiditis resulting from treatment or intervention by
physician or in a patient intervention setting.

245.8 Other and unspecified chronic thyroiditis

Chronic thyroiditis:

NOS

nonspecific

245.9 Thyroiditis, unspecified

Thyroiditis NOS

✓4ᵗʰ **246 Other disorders of thyroid**

246.0 Disorders of thyrocalcitonin secretion

Hypersecretion of calcitonin or thyrocalcitonin

246.1 Dyshormonogenic goiter

Congenital (dyshormonogenic) goiter

Goiter due to enzyme defect in synthesis of thyroid
hormone

Goitrous cretinism (sporadic)

246.2 Cyst of thyroid

EXCLUDES   cystadenoma of thyroid (226)

246.3 Hemorrhage and infarction of thyroid

246.8 Other specified disorders of thyroid

Abnormality of thyroid-binding globulin

Atrophy of thyroid

Hyper-TBG-nemia

Hypo-TBG-nemia

246.9 Unspecified disorder of thyroid

DISEASES OF OTHER ENDOCRINE GLANDS (250-259)

✓4ᵗʰ **250 Diabetes mellitus**

EXCLUDES   gestational diabetes (648.8)
hyperglycemia NOS (790.6)
neonatal diabetes mellitus (775.1)
nonclinical diabetes (790.2)

The following fifth-digit subclassification is for use with
category 250:

**0 type II [non-insulin dependent type] [NIDDM
type] [adult-onset type] or unspecified
type, not stated as uncontrolled**

Fifth-digit 0 is for use for type II, adult-onset
diabetic patients, even if the patient requires
insulin

**1 type I [insulin dependent type] [IDDM] [juvenile
type], not stated as uncontrolled**

**2 type II [non-insulin dependent type] [NIDDM
type] [adult-onset type] or unspecified
type, uncontrolled**

Fifth-digit 2 is for use for type II, adult-onset
diabetic patients, even if the patient requires
insulin

**3 type I [insulin dependent type] [IDDM] [juvenile
type], uncontrolled**

AHA: 2Q,'01, 16; 2Q,'98, 15; 4Q, '97, 32; 2Q, '97, 14; 3Q, '96, 5; 4Q, '93,
19; 2Q, '92, 5; 3Q, '91, 3; 2Q, '90, 22; N-D, '85, 11

✓5ᵗʰ ⁸**250.0 Diabetes mellitus without mention**   CC 1-3
of complication

Diabetes mellitus without mention of complication or
manifestation classifiable to 250.1-250.9

Diabetes (mellitus) NOS

CC Excl: For code 250.01-250.03: 250.00-250.93, 251.0-251.3, 259.8-
259.9

AHA: 4Q, '97, 32; 3Q, '91, 3, 12; N-D, '85, 11; **For code 250.00:**
▶1Q, '02, 7, 11◄

✓5ᵗʰ **250.1 Diabetes with ketoacidosis**   CC 1-3

Diabetic:

acidosis
ketosis $\Big\}$ without mention of coma

CC Excl: For code 250.11-250.13: 250.00-250.93, 251.0-251.3,
259.8-259.9

AHA: 3Q, '91, 6

DEF: Diabetic hyperglycemic crisis causing ketone presence in
body fluids.

✓5ᵗʰ **250.2 Diabetes with hyperosmolarity**   CC 1-3

Hyperosmolar (nonketotic) coma

CC Excl: For code 250.21-250.23: 250.00-250.93, 251.0-251.3,
259.8-259.9

AHA: 4Q, '93, 19; 3Q, '91, 7

---

⁸   Questionable admission = 0

N Newborn Age: 0   P Pediatric Age: 0-17   M Maternity Age: 12-55   A Adult Age: 15-124   CC CC Condition   MC Major Complication   CD Complex Dx   HIV HIV Related Dx

50 — Volume 1 • October 2002   *2002 Ingenix, Inc.*

✓5th **250.3 Diabetes with other coma** CC 1-3
Diabetic coma (with ketoacidosis)
Diabetic hypoglycemic coma
Insulin coma NOS

> **EXCLUDES** *diabetes with hyperosmolar coma (250.2)*

CC Excl: For code 250.31-250.33: See code 250.01

AHA: 3Q, '91, 7,12

DEF: Coma (not hyperosmolar) caused by hyperglycemia or hypoglycemia as complication of diabetes.

✓5th **250.4 Diabetes with renal manifestations** CC 1-3
Use additional code to identify manifestation, as:
diabetic:
nephropathy NOS (583.81)
nephrosis (581.81)
intercapillary glomerulosclerosis (581.81)
Kimmelstiel-Wilson syndrome (581.81)

CC Excl: For code 250.41-250.43: See code 250.01

AHA: 3Q, '91, 8,12; S-O, '87, 9; S-O, '84, 3

✓5th **250.5 Diabetes with ophthalmic manifestations** CC 1-3
Use additional code to identify manifestation, as:
diabetic:
blindness (369.00-369.9)
cataract (366.41)
glaucoma (365.44)
retinal edema (362.83)
retinopathy (362.01-362.02)

CC Excl: For code 250.51-250.53: See code 250.01

AHA: 3Q, '91, 8; S-O, '85, 11

✓5th **250.6 Diabetes with neurological manifestations** CC 1-3
Use additional code to identify manifestation, as:
diabetic:
amyotrophy (358.1)
mononeuropathy (354.0-355.9)
neurogenic arthropathy (713.5)
peripheral autonomic neuropathy (337.1)
polyneuropathy (357.2)

CC Excl: For code 250.61-250.63: See code 250.01

AHA: 2Q, '93, 6; 2Q, '92, 15; 3Q, '91, 9; N-D, '84, 9

✓5th **250.7 Diabetes with peripheral circulatory disorders** CC 1-3
Use additional code to identify manifestation, as:
diabetic:
gangrene (785.4)
peripheral angiopathy (443.81)

CC Excl: For code 250.71-250.73: See code 250.01

AHA: 1Q, '96, 10; 3Q, '94, 5; 2Q, '94, 17; 3Q, '91, 10, 12; 3Q, '90, 15

DEF: Blood vessel damage or disease, usually in the feet, legs, or hands, as a complication of diabetes.

✓5th **250.8 Diabetes with other specified manifestations** CC 1-3
Diabetic hypoglycemia
Hypoglycemic shock
Use additional code to identify manifestation, as:
any associated ulceration (707.10-707.9)
diabetic bone changes (731.8)
Use additional E code to identify cause, if drug-induced

CC Excl: For code 250.81-250.83: See code 250.01

AHA: 4Q, '00, 44; 4Q, '97, 43; 2Q, '97, 16; 4Q, '93, 20; 3Q, '91, 10

✓5th **250.9 Diabetes with unspecified complication** CC 1-3
CC Excl: For code 250.91-250.93: See code 250.01

AHA: 2Q, '92, 15; 3Q, '91, 7, 12

✓4th **251 Other disorders of pancreatic internal secretion**

251.0 Hypoglycemic coma CC
Iatrogenic hyperinsulinism
Non-diabetic insulin coma
Use additional E code to identify cause, if drug-induced

> **EXCLUDES** *hypoglycemic coma in diabetes mellitus (250.3)*

CC Excl: 250.00-250.93, 251.0-251.3, 259.8-259.9

AHA: M-A, '85, 8

DEF: Coma induced by low blood sugar in non-diabetic patient.

251.1 Other specified hypoglycemia
Hyperinsulinism: Hyperplasia of pancreatic
NOS   islet beta cells NOS
ectopic
functional

> **EXCLUDES** *hypoglycemia:*
> *in diabetes mellitus (250.8)*
> *in infant of diabetic mother (775.0)*
> *hypoglycemic coma (251.0)*
> *neonatal hypoglycemia (775.6)*

Use additional E code to identify cause, if drug-induced.

DEF: Excessive production of insulin by the pancreas; associated with obesity and insulin-producing tumors.

251.2 Hypoglycemia, unspecified
Hypoglycemia: Hypoglycemia:
NOS   spontaneous
reactive

> **EXCLUDES** *hypoglycemia:*
> *with coma (251.0)*
> *in diabetes mellitus (250.8)*
> *leucine-induced (270.3)*

AHA: M-A, '85, 8

251.3 Postsurgical hypoinsulinemia CC
Hypoinsulinemia following complete or partial pancreatectomy
Postpancreatectomy hyperglycemia

CC Excl: See code 251.0

AHA: 3Q, '91, 6

251.4 Abnormality of secretion of glucagon
Hyperplasia of pancreatic islet alpha cells with glucagon excess

DEF: Production malfunction of a pancreatic hormone secreted by cells of the islets of Langerhans.

251.5 Abnormality of secretion of gastrin
Hyperplasia of pancreatic alpha cells with gastrin excess
Zollinger-Ellison syndrome

✓4th ✓5th Additional Digit Required   Nonspecific PDx   Unacceptable PDx   Manifestation Code   **MSP** Medicare Secondary Payer   ►◄ Revised Text   ● New Code   ▲ Revised Code Title

2002 Ingenix, Inc.   Volume 1 — 51

Endocrine, Nutritional, Metabolic, Immunity 250.3–251.5

Endocrine, Nutritional, Metabolic, Immunity 251.8–254.0

Dorsal View of Parathyroid Glands

251.8 Other specified disorders of pancreatic internal secretion
AHA: 2Q, '98, 15; 3Q, '91, 6

251.9 Unspecified disorder of pancreatic internal secretion
Islet cell hyperplasia NOS

✓4ᵗʰ **252 Disorders of parathyroid gland**

252.0 Hyperparathyroidism
Hyperplasia of parathyroid
Osteitis fibrosa cystica generalisata
von Recklinghausen's disease of bone
EXCLUDES *ectopic hyperparathyroidism (259.3)*
secondary hyperparathyroidism (of renal origin) (588.8)

DEF: Abnormally high secretion of parathyroid hormones causing bone deterioration, reduced renal function, kidney stones.

252.1 Hypoparathyroidism   CC
Parathyroiditis (autoimmune)
Tetany:
   parathyroid
   parathyroprival
EXCLUDES *pseudohypoparathyroidism (275.4)*
pseudopseudohypoparathyroidism (275.4)
tetany NOS (781.7)
transitory neonatal hypoparathyroidism (775.4)

CC Excl: 252.0-252.9, 259.8-259.9

DEF: Abnormally low secretion of parathyroid hormones which causes decreased calcium and increased phosphorus in the blood. Resulting in muscle cramps, tetany, urinary frequency and cataracts.

252.8 Other specified disorders of parathyroid gland
Cyst
Hemorrhage } of parathyroid gland

252.9 Unspecified disorder of parathyroid gland

✓4ᵗʰ **253 Disorders of the pituitary gland and its hypothalamic control**
INCLUDES the listed conditions whether the disorder is in the pituitary or the hypothalamus
EXCLUDES *Cushing's syndrome (255.0)*

253.0 Acromegaly and gigantism
Overproduction of growth hormone

DEF: Acromegaly: chronic, beginning in middle age; caused by hypersecretion of the pituitary growth hormone; produces enlarged parts of skeleton, especially the nose, ears, jaws, fingers and toes.

DEF: Gigantism: pituitary gigantism caused by excess growth of short flat bones; men may grow 78 to 80 inches tall.

253.1 Other and unspecified anterior pituitary hyperfunction
Forbes-Albright syndrome
EXCLUDES *overproduction of:*
ACTH (255.3)
thyroid-stimulating hormone [TSH] (242.8)

AHA: J-A, '85, 9

DEF: Spontaneous galactorrhea-amenorrhea syndrome unrelated to pregnancy; usually related to presence of pituitary tumor.

253.2 Panhypopituitarism   CC
Cachexia, pituitary
Necrosis of pituitary (postpartum)
Pituitary insufficiency NOS
Sheehan's syndrome
Simmonds' disease
EXCLUDES *iatrogenic hypopituitarism (253.7)*

CC Excl: 253.0-253.9, 259.8-259.9

DEF: Damage to or absence of pituitary gland leading to impaired sexual function, weight loss, fatigue, bradycardia, hypotension, pallor, depression, and impaired growth in children; called Simmonds' disease if cachexia is prominent.

253.3 Pituitary dwarfism
Isolated deficiency of (human) growth hormone [HGH]
Lorain-Levi dwarfism

DEF: Dwarfism with infantile physical characteristics due to abnormally low secretion of growth hormone and gonadotropin deficiency.

253.4 Other anterior pituitary disorders
Isolated or partial deficiency of an anterior pituitary hormone, other than growth hormone
Prolactin deficiency

AHA: J-A, '85, 9

253.5 Diabetes insipidus   CC
Vasopressin deficiency
EXCLUDES *nephrogenic diabetes insipidus (588.1)*

CC Excl: 253.1-253.2, 253.4-253.9, 259.8-259.9

DEF: Metabolic disorder causing insufficient antidiuretic hormone release; symptoms include frequent urination, thirst, ravenous hunger, loss of weight, fatigue.

253.6 Other disorders of neurohypophysis
Syndrome of inappropriate secretion of antidiuretic hormone [ADH]
EXCLUDES *ectopic antidiuretic hormone secretion (259.3)*

253.7 Iatrogenic pituitary disorders
Hypopituitarism: Hypopituitarism:
   hormone-induced   postablative
   hypophysectomy-induced   radiotherapy-induced
Use additional E code to identify cause

DEF: Pituitary dysfunction that results from drug therapy, radiation therapy, or surgery, causing mild to severe symptom.

253.8 Other disorders of the pituitary and other syndromes of diencephalohypophyseal origin
Abscess of pituitary   Cyst of Rathke's pouch
Adiposogenital dystrophy   Fröhlich's syndrome
EXCLUDES *craniopharyngioma (237.0)*

253.9 Unspecified
Dyspituitarism

✓4ᵗʰ **254 Diseases of thymus gland**
EXCLUDES *aplasia or dysplasia with immunodeficiency (279.2)*
hypoplasia with immunodeficiency (279.2)
myasthenia gravis (358.0)

254.0 Persistent hyperplasia of thymus
Hypertrophy of thymus

DEF: Continued abnormal growth of the twin lymphoid lobes that produce T lymphocytes.

N Newborn Age: 0   P Pediatric Age: 0-17   M Maternity Age: 12-55   A Adult Age: 15-124   CC CC Condition   MC Major Complication   CD Complex Dx   HIV HIV Related Dx

52 — Volume 1   *2002 Ingenix, Inc.*

254.1 Abscess of thymus `CC`
CC Excl: 254.0–254.1, 254.8–254.9, 259.8–259.9

254.8 Other specified diseases of thymus gland
Atrophy
Cyst } of thymus
EXCLUDES thymoma (212.6)

254.9 Unspecified disease of thymus gland

√4th **255 Disorders of adrenal glands**
INCLUDES the listed conditions whether the basic disorder is in the adrenals or is pituitary-induced

255.0 Cushing's syndrome `CC`
Adrenal hyperplasia due to excess ACTH
Cushing's syndrome:
NOS
iatrogenic
idiopathic
pituitary-dependent
Ectopic ACTH syndrome
Iatrogenic syndrome of excess cortisol
Overproduction of cortisol
Use additional E code to identify cause, if drug-induced
EXCLUDES congenital adrenal hyperplasia (255.2)
CC Excl: 255.0–255.2, 259.8–259.9

DEF: Due to adrenal cortisol oversecretion or glucocorticoid medications; may cause fatty tissue of the face, neck and body; osteoporosis and curvature of spine, hypertension, diabetes mellitus, female genitourinary problems, male impotence, degeneration of muscle tissues, weakness.

255.1 Hyperaldosteronism
Aldosteronism (primary) (secondary)
Bartter's syndrome
Conn's syndrome
DEF: Oversecretion of aldosterone causing fluid retention, hypertension.

255.2 Adrenogenital disorders
Achard-Thiers syndrome
Adrenogenital syndromes, virilizing or feminizing, whether acquired or associated with congenital adrenal hyperplasia consequent on inborn enzyme defects in hormone synthesis
Congenital adrenal hyperplasia
Female adrenal pseudohermaphroditism
Male:
macrogenitosomia praecox
sexual precocity with adrenal hyperplasia
Virilization (female) (suprarenal)
EXCLUDES adrenal hyperplasia due to excess ACTH (255.0)
isosexual virilization (256.4)

255.3 Other corticoadrenal overactivity `CC`
Acquired benign adrenal androgenic overactivity
Overproduction of ACTH
CC Excl: 017.60–017.66, 017.90–017.96, 255.3–255.9, 259.8–259.9

255.4 Corticoadrenal insufficiency `CC`
Addisonian crisis
Addison's disease NOS
Adrenal:
atrophy (autoimmune)
calcification
Adrenal:
crisis
hemorrhage
infarction
insufficiency NOS
EXCLUDES tuberculous Addison's disease (017.6)
CC Excl: See code 255.3

DEF: Underproduction of adrenal hormones causing low blood pressure.

255.5 Other adrenal hypofunction `CC`
Adrenal medullary insufficiency
EXCLUDES Waterhouse-Friderichsen syndrome (meningococcal) (036.3)
CC Excl: See code 255.3

255.6 Medulloadrenal hyperfunction `CC`
Catecholamine secretion by pheochromocytoma
CC Excl: See code 255.3

255.8 Other specified disorders of adrenal glands
Abnormality of cortisol-binding globulin

255.9 Unspecified disorder of adrenal glands

√4th **256 Ovarian dysfunction**
AHA: 4Q, '00, 51

256.0 Hyperestrogenism ♀
DEF: Excess secretion of estrogen by the ovaries; characterized by ovaries containing multiple follicular cysts filled with serous fluid.

256.1 Other ovarian hyperfunction ♀
Hypersecretion of ovarian androgens
AHA: 3Q, '95, 15

256.2 Postablative ovarian failure ♀
Ovarian failure:
iatrogenic
postirradiation
Ovarian failure:
postsurgical
▶Use additional code for states associated with artificial menopause (627.4)◀
EXCLUDES acquired absence of ovary (V45.77)
asymptomatic age-related (natural) postmenopausal status (V49.81)
DEF: Failed ovarian function after medical or surgical intervention.

√5th **256.3 Other ovarian failure**
Use additional code for states associated with ▶natural menopause (627.2)◀
EXCLUDES asymptomatic age-related (natural) postmenopausal status (V49.81)
AHA: 4Q, '01, 41

256.31 Premature menopause ♀
DEF: Permanent cessation of ovarian function before the age of 40 occuring naturally of unknown cause.

256.39 Other ovarian failure ♀
Delayed menarche
Ovarian hypofunction
Primary ovarian failure NOS

256.4 Polycystic ovaries ♀
Isosexual virilization   Stein-Leventhal syndrome
DEF: Multiple serous filled cysts of ovary; symptoms of infertility, hirsutism, oligomenorrhea or amenorrhea.

256.8 Other ovarian dysfunction ♀
256.9 Unspecified ovarian dysfunction ♀

√4th **257 Testicular dysfunction**
257.0 Testicular hyperfunction ♂
Hypersecretion of testicular hormones

257.1 Postablative testicular hypofunction ♂
Testicular hypofunction:
iatrogenic
postirradiation
Testicular hypofunction:
postsurgical

257.2 Other testicular hypofunction ♂
Defective biosynthesis of testicular androgen
Eunuchoidism:
NOS
hypogonadotropic
Failure:
Leydig's cell, adult
seminiferous tubule, adult
Testicular hypogonadism
EXCLUDES azoospermia (606.0)

257.8 Other testicular dysfunction ♂
Goldberg-Maxwell syndrome
Male pseudohermaphroditism with testicular feminization
Testicular feminization

257.9 Unspecified testicular dysfunction ♂

✓4th **258 Polyglandular dysfunction and related disorders**

258.0 Polyglandular activity in multiple endocrine adenomatosis `CC`
Wermer's syndrome

CC Excl: 240.0, 240.9, 241.0-241.9, 242.00-242.91, 243, 244.0-244.9, 245.0-245.9, 246.0-246.9, 250.00-250.93, 251.0-251.9, 252.0-252.9, 253.0-253.9, 254.0-254.9, 255.0-255.9, 256.0-256.2, 256.31-256.39, 256.4-256.9, 257.0-257.9, 258.0-258.9, 259.0-259.9

DEF: Wermer's syndrome: A rare hereditary condition characterized by the presence of adenomas or hyperplasia in more than one endocrine gland causing premature aging.

258.1 Other combinations of endocrine dysfunction `CC`
Lloyd's syndrome
Schmidt's syndrome
CC Excl: See code 258.0

258.8 Other specified polyglandular dysfunction `CC`
CC Excl: See code 258.0

258.9 Polyglandular dysfunction, unspecified `CC`
CC Excl: See code 258.0

✓4th **259 Other endocrine disorders**

259.0 Delay in sexual development and puberty, not elsewhere classified
Delayed puberty

259.1 Precocious sexual development and puberty, not elsewhere classified `P`
Sexual precocity: Sexual precocity:
    NOS   cryptogenic
    constitutional   idiopathic

259.2 Carcinoid syndrome `CC`
Hormone secretion by carcinoid tumors
CC Excl: 259.2-259.3, 259.8-259.9

DEF: Presence of carcinoid tumors that spread to liver; characterized by cyanotic flushing of skin, diarrhea, bronchospasm, acquired tricuspid and pulmonary stenosis, sudden drops in blood pressure, edema, ascites.

259.3 Ectopic hormone secretion, not elsewhere classified
Ectopic:
    antidiuretic hormone secretion [ADH]
    hyperparathyroidism
    EXCLUDES   ectopic ACTH syndrome (255.0)
AHA: N-D, '85, 4

259.4 Dwarfism, not elsewhere classified
Dwarfism:
    NOS
    constitutional
    EXCLUDES   dwarfism:
           achondroplastic (756.4)
           intrauterine (759.7)
           nutritional (263.2)
           pituitary (253.3)
           renal (588.0)
           progeria (259.8)

259.8 Other specified endocrine disorders
Pineal gland dysfunction   Werner's syndrome
Progeria

259.9 Unspecified endocrine disorder
Disturbance: Infantilism NOS
    endocrine NOS
    hormone NOS

NUTRITIONAL DEFICIENCIES (260-269)

> **EXCLUDES**   deficiency anemias (280.0-281.9)

260 Kwashiorkor `CC`
Nutritional edema with dyspigmentation of skin and hair
CC Excl: 260-262, 263.0-263.9

DEF: Syndrome, particularly children; excessive carbohydrate with inadequate protein intake, inhibited growth potential, anomalies in skin and hair pigmentation, edema and liver disease.

261 Nutritional marasmus `CC`
Nutritional atrophy
Severe calorie deficiency
Severe malnutrition NOS
CC Excl: See code 260

DEF: Protein-calorie malabsorption or malnutrition of children; characterized by tissue wasting, dehydration, and subcutaneous fat depletion; may occur with infectious disease; also called infantile atrophy.

262 Other severe, protein-calorie malnutrition `CC`
Nutritional edema without mention of dyspigmentation of skin and hair
CC Excl: See code 260

AHA: 4Q, '92, 24; J-A, '85, 12

✓4th **263 Other and unspecified protein-calorie malnutrition**
AHA: 4Q, '92, 24

263.0 Malnutrition of moderate degree `CC`
CC Excl: See code 260

AHA: J-A, '85, 1

DEF: Malnutrition characterized by biochemical changes in electrolytes, lipids, blood plasma.

263.1 Malnutrition of mild degree `CC`
CC Excl: See code 260

AHA: J-A, '85, 1

263.2 Arrested development following protein-calorie malnutrition `CC`
Nutritional dwarfism
Physical retardation due to malnutrition
CC Excl: See code 260

263.8 Other protein-calorie malnutrition `CC`
CC Excl: See code 260

263.9 Unspecified protein-calorie malnutrition `CC`
Dystrophy due to malnutrition
Malnutrition (calorie) NOS
    EXCLUDES   nutritional deficiency NOS (269.9)
CC Excl: See code 260

AHA: N-D, '84, 19

✓4th **264 Vitamin A deficiency**

264.0 With conjunctival xerosis
DEF: Vitamin A deficiency with conjunctival dryness.

264.1 With conjunctival xerosis and Bitot's spot
Bitot's spot in the young child
DEF: Vitamin A deficiency with conjunctival dryness, superficial spots of keratinized epithelium.

264.2 With corneal xerosis
DEF: Vitamin A deficiency with corneal dryness.

264.3 With corneal ulceration and xerosis
DEF: Vitamin A deficiency with corneal dryness, epithelial ulceration.

264.4 With keratomalacia
DEF: Vitamin A deficiency creating corneal dryness; progresses to corneal insensitivity, softness, necrosis; usually bilateral.

264.5 With night blindness
DEF: Vitamin A deficiency causing vision failure in dim light.

`N` Newborn Age: 0   `P` Pediatric Age: 0-17   `M` Maternity Age: 12-55   `A` Adult Age: 15-124   `CC` CC Condition   `MC` Major Complication   `CD` Complex Dx   `HIV` HIV Related Dx

264.6   With xerophthalmic scars of cornea

DEF: Vitamin A deficiency with corneal scars from dryness.

264.7   Other ocular manifestations of vitamin A deficiency

Xerophthalmia due to vitamin A deficiency

264.8   Other manifestations of vitamin A deficiency

Follicular keratosis ⎫ due to vitamin A
Xeroderma   ⎬ deficiency

264.9   Unspecified vitamin A deficiency

Hypovitaminosis A NOS

√4ᵗʰ **265   Thiamine and niacin deficiency states**

265.0   Beriberi

DEF: Inadequate vitamin B₁ (thiamine) intake, affects heart and peripheral nerves; individual may become edematous and develop cardiac disease due to the excess fluid; alcoholics and people with a diet of excessive polished rice prone to the disease.

265.1   Other and unspecified manifestations of thiamine deficiency

Other vitamin B₁ deficiency states

265.2   Pellagra

Deficiency: Deficiency:
  niacin (-tryptophan)   vitamin PP
  nicotinamide   Pellagra (alcoholic)
  nicotinic acid

DEF: Niacin deficiency causing dermatitis, inflammation of mucous membranes, diarrhea, and psychic disturbances.

√4ᵗʰ **266   Deficiency of B-complex components**

266.0   Ariboflavinosis

Riboflavin [vitamin B₂] deficiency

AHA: S-O, '86, 10

DEF: Vitamin B₂ (riboflavin) deficiency marked by swollen lips and tongue fissures, corneal vascularization, scaling lesions, and anemia.

266.1   Vitamin B₆ deficiency

Deficiency: Deficiency:
  pyridoxal   pyridoxine
  pyridoxamine   Vitamin B₆ deficiency
                                 syndrome

EXCLUDES *vitamin B₆-responsive sideroblastic anemia (285.0)*

DEF: Vitamin B₆ deficiency causing skin, lip, and tongue disturbances, peripheral neuropathy; and convulsions in infants.

266.2   Other B-complex deficiencies

Deficiency: Deficiency:
  cyanocobalamin   vitamin B₁₂
  folic acid

EXCLUDES *combined system disease with anemia (281.0-281.1)*
deficiency anemias (281.0-281.9)
subacute degeneration of spinal cord with anemia (281.0-281.1)

266.9   Unspecified vitamin B deficiency

267   Ascorbic acid deficiency

Deficiency of vitamin C
Scurvy

EXCLUDES *scorbutic anemia (281.8)*

DEF: Vitamin C deficiency causing swollen gums, myalgia, weight loss, and weakness.

√4ᵗʰ **268   Vitamin D deficiency**

EXCLUDES *vitamin D-resistant:*
osteomalacia (275.3)
rickets (275.3)

268.0   Rickets, active

EXCLUDES *celiac rickets (579.0)*
renal rickets (588.0)

DEF: Inadequate vitamin D intake, usually in pediatrics, that affects bones most involved with muscular action; may cause nodules on ends and sides of bones; delayed closure of fontanels in infants; symptoms may include muscle soreness, and profuse sweating.

268.1   Rickets, late effect

Any condition specified as due to rickets and stated to be a late effect or sequela of rickets
Use additional code to identify the nature of late effect

DEF: Distorted or demineralized bones as a result of vitamin D deficiency.

268.2   Osteomalacia, unspecified

DEF: Softening of bones due to decrease in calcium; marked by pain, tenderness, muscular weakness, anorexia, and weight loss.

268.9   Unspecified vitamin D deficiency

Avitaminosis D

√4ᵗʰ **269   Other nutritional deficiencies**

269.0   Deficiency of vitamin K   **CC**

EXCLUDES *deficiency of coagulation factor due to vitamin K deficiency (286.7)*
vitamin K deficiency of newborn (776.0)

CC Excl: 269.0

269.1   Deficiency of other vitamins

Deficiency: Deficiency:
  vitamin E   vitamin P

269.2   Unspecified vitamin deficiency

Multiple vitamin deficiency NOS

269.3   Mineral deficiency, not elsewhere classified

Deficiency: Deficiency:
  calcium, dietary   iodine

EXCLUDES *deficiency:*
calcium NOS (275.4)
potassium (276.8)
sodium (276.1)

269.8   Other nutritional deficiency

EXCLUDES *adult failure to thrive (783.7)*
failure to thrive in childhood (783.41)
feeding problems (783.3)
newborn (779.3)

269.9   Unspecified nutritional deficiency

OTHER METABOLIC AND IMMUNITY DISORDERS (270-279)

Use additional code to identify any associated mental retardation

√4ᵗʰ **270   Disorders of amino-acid transport and metabolism**

EXCLUDES *abnormal findings without manifest disease (790.0-796.9)*
disorders of purine and pyrimidine metabolism (277.1-277.2)
gout (274.0-274.9)

270.0   Disturbances of amino-acid transport

Cystinosis   Glycinuria (renal)
Cystinuria   Hartnup disease
Fanconi (-de Toni) (-Debré) syndrome

270.1   Phenylketonuria [PKU]

Hyperphenylalaninemia

DEF: Inherited metabolic condition causing excess phenylpyruvic and other acids in urine; results in mental retardation, neurological manifestations, including spasticity and tremors, light pigmentation, eczema, and mousy odor.

270.2   Other disturbances of aromatic amino-acid metabolism

Albinism   Hypertyrosinemia
Alkaptonuria   Indicanuria
Alkaptonuric ochronosis   Kynureninase defects
Disturbances of metabolism   Oasthouse urine disease
  of tyrosine and   Ochronosis
  tryptophan   Tyrosinosis
Homogentisic acid defects   Tyrosinuria
Hydroxykynureninuria   Waardenburg syndrome

EXCLUDES *vitamin B₆-deficiency syndrome (266.1)*

AHA: 3Q, '99, 20

√4ᵗʰ
√5ᵗʰ   Additional Digit Required   Nonspecific PDx   Unacceptable PDx   Manifestation Code   **MSP** Medicare Secondary Payer   ▶◀ Revised Text   ● New Code   ▲ Revised Code Title

2002 Ingenix, Inc.   **Volume 1 — 55**

270.3   Disturbances of branched-chain amino-acid metabolism
> Disturbances of metabolism of leucine, isoleucine, and valine
> Hypervalinemia
> Intermittent branched-chain ketonuria
> Leucine-induced hypoglycemia
> Leucinosis
> Maple syrup urine disease

AHA: 3Q, '00, 8

270.4   Disturbances of sulphur-bearing amino-acid metabolism
> Cystathioninemia
> Cystathioninuria
> Disturbances of metabolism of methionine, homocystine, and cystathionine
> Homocystinuria
> Hypermethioninemia
> Methioninemia

270.5   Disturbances of histidine metabolism
> Carnosinemia
> Histidinemia
> Hyperhistidinemia
> Imidazole aminoaciduria

270.6   Disorders of urea cycle metabolism
> Argininosuccinic aciduria
> Citrullinemia
> Disorders of metabolism of ornithine, citrulline, argininosuccinic acid, arginine, and ammonia
> Hyperammonemia
> Hyperomithinemia

270.7   Other disturbances of straight-chain amino-acid metabolism
> Glucoglycinuria
> Glycinemia (with methyl-malonic acidemia)
> Hyperglycinemia
> Hyperlysinemia
> Other disturbances of metabolism of glycine, threonine, serine, glutamine, and lysine
> Pipecolic acidemia
> Saccharopinuria

AHA: 3Q, '00, 8

270.8   Other specified disorders of amino-acid metabolism
> Alaninemia   Iminoacidopathy
> Ethanolaminuria   Prolinemia
> Glycoprolinuria   Prolinuria
> Hydroxyprolinemia   Sarcosinemia
> Hyperprolinemia

270.9   Unspecified disorder of amino-acid metabolism

√4th **271   Disorders of carbohydrate transport and metabolism**
> **EXCLUDES**   abnormality of secretion of glucagon (251.4)
>   diabetes mellitus (250.0-250.9)
>   hypoglycemia NOS (251.2)
>   mucopolysaccharidosis (277.5)

271.0   Glycogenosis
> Amylopectinosis
> Glucose-6-phosphatase deficiency
> Glycogen storage disease
> McArdle's disease
> Pompe's disease
> von Gierke's disease

AHA: 1Q, '98, 5

271.1   Galactosemia
> Galactose-1-phosphate uridyl transferase deficiency
> Galactosuria

DEF: Any of three genetic disorders due to defective galactose metabolism; symptoms include failure to thrive in infancy, jaundice, liver and spleen damage, cataracts, and mental retardation.

271.2   Hereditary fructose intolerance
> Essential benign fructosuria   Fructosemia

DEF: Chromosome recessive disorder of carbohydrate metabolism; in infants, occurs after dietary sugar introduced; characterized by enlarged spleen, yellowish cast to skin, and progressive inability to thrive.

Lipid Metabolism

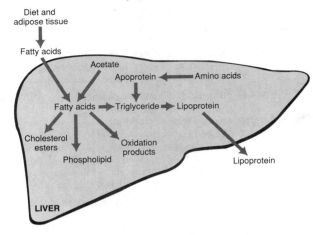

271.3   Intestinal disaccharidase deficiencies and disaccharide malabsorption
> Intolerance or malabsorption (congenital) (of):
>   glucose-galactose
>   lactose
>   sucrose-isomaltose

271.4   Renal glycosuria
> Renal diabetes

DEF: Persistent abnormal levels of glucose in urine, with normal blood glucose levels; caused by failure of the renal tubules to reabsorb glucose.

271.8   Other specified disorders of carbohydrate transport and metabolism
> Essential benign pentosuria   Mannosidosis
> Fucosidosis   Oxalosis
> Glycolic aciduria   Xylosuria
> Hyperoxaluria (primary)   Xylulosuria

271.9   Unspecified disorder of carbohydrate transport and metabolism

√4th **272   Disorders of lipoid metabolism**
> **EXCLUDES**   localized cerebral lipidoses (330.1)

272.0   Pure hypercholesterolemia
> Familial hypercholesterolemia
> Fredrickson Type IIa hyperlipoproteinemia
> Hyperbetalipoproteinemia
> Hyperlipidemia, Group A
> Low-density-lipoid-type [LDL] hyperlipoproteinemia

272.1   Pure hyperglyceridemia
> Endogenous hyperglyceridemia
> Fredrickson Type IV hyperlipoproteinemia
> Hyperlipidemia, Group B
> Hyperprebetalipoproteinemia
> Hypertriglyceridemia, essential
> Very-low-density-lipoid-type [VLDL] hyperlipoproteinemia

272.2   Mixed hyperlipidemia
> Broad- or floating-betalipoproteinemia
> Fredrickson Type IIb or III hyperlipoproteinemia
> Hypercholesterolemia with endogenous hyperglyceridemia
> Hyperbetalipoproteinemia with prebetalipoproteinemia
> Tubo-eruptive xanthoma
> Xanthoma tuberosum

DEF: Elevated levels of lipoprotein, a complex of fats and proteins, in blood due to inherited metabolic disorder.

272.3   Hyperchylomicronemia
> Bürger-Grütz syndrome
> Fredrickson type I or V hyperlipoproteinemia
> Hyperlipidemia, Group D
> Mixed hyperglyceridemia

N Newborn Age: 0   P Pediatric Age: 0-17   M Maternity Age: 12-55   A Adult Age: 15-124   CC CC Condition   MC Major Complication   CD Complex Dx   HIV HIV Related Dx

56 — Volume 1   *2002 Ingenix, Inc.*

272.4 Other and unspecified hyperlipidemia
Alpha-lipoproteinemia
Combined hyperlipidemia
Hyperlipidemia NOS
Hyperlipoproteinemia NOS
DEF: Hyperlipoproteinemia: elevated levels of transient chylomicrons in the blood which are a form of lipoproteins which transport dietary cholesterol and triglycerides from the small intestine to the blood.

272.5 Lipoprotein deficiencies
Abetalipoproteinemia
Bassen-Kornzweig syndrome
High-density lipoid deficiency
Hypoalphalipoproteinemia
Hypobetalipoproteinemia (familial)
DEF: Abnormally low levels of lipoprotein, a complex of fats and protein, in the blood.

272.6 Lipodystrophy
Barraquer-Simons disease
Progressive lipodystrophy
Use additional E code to identify cause, if iatrogenic
EXCLUDES   *intestinal lipodystrophy (040.2)*
DEF: Disturbance of fat metabolism resulting in loss of fatty tissue in some areas of the body.

272.7 Lipidoses
Chemically-induced lipidosis
Disease:
   Anderson's
   Fabry's
   Gaucher's
   I cell [mucolipidosis I]
   lipoid storage NOS
   Niemann-Pick
   pseudo-Hurler's or mucolipdosis III
   triglyceride storage, Type I or II
   Wolman's or triglyceride storage, Type III
Mucolipidosis II
Primary familial xanthomatosis
EXCLUDES   *cerebral lipidoses (330.1)*
                Tay-Sachs disease (330.1)
DEF: Lysosomal storage diseases marked by an abnormal amount of lipids in reticuloendothelial cells.

272.8 Other disorders of lipoid metabolism
Hoffa's disease or liposynovitis prepatellaris
Launois-Bensaude's lipomatosis
Lipoid dermatoarthritis

272.9 Unspecified disorder of lipoid metabolism

√4th **273 Disorders of plasma protein metabolism**
EXCLUDES   *agammaglobulinemia and*
                    hypogammaglobulinemia (279.0-279.2)
           coagulation defects (286.0-286.9)
           hereditary hemolytic anemias (282.0-282.9)

273.0 Polyclonal hypergammaglobulinemia
Hypergammaglobulinemic purpura:
   benign primary
   Waldenström's
DEF: Elevated blood levels of gamma globulins, frequently found in patients with chronic infectious diseases.

273.1 Monoclonal paraproteinemia
Benign monoclonal hypergammaglobulinemia [BMH]
Monoclonal gammopathy:
   NOS
   associated with lymphoplasmacytic dyscrasias
   benign
Paraproteinemia:
   benign (familial)
   secondary to malignant or inflammatory disease

273.2 Other paraproteinemias
Cryoglobulinemic: Mixed cryoglobulinemia
   purpura
   vasculitis

273.3 Macroglobulinemia   CC
Macroglobulinemia (idiopathic) (primary)
Waldenström's macroglobulinemia
CC Excl: 273.0-273.9
DEF: Elevated blood levels of macroglobulins (plasma globulins of high weight); characterized by malignant neoplasms of bone marrow, spleen, liver, or lymph nodes; symptoms include weakness, fatigue, bleeding disorders, and vision problems.

273.8 Other disorders of plasma protein metabolism
Abnormality of transport protein
Bisalbuminemia
AHA: 2Q, '98, 11

273.9 Unspecified disorder of plasma protein metabolism

√4th **274 Gout**
EXCLUDES   *lead gout (984.0-984.9)*
AHA: 2Q, '95, 4
DEF: Purine and pyrimidine metabolic disorders; manifested by hyperuricemia and recurrent acute inflammatory arthritis; monosodium urate or monohydrate crystals may be deposited in and around the joints, leading to joint destruction, and severe crippling.

274.0 Gouty arthropathy
√5th **274.1 Gouty nephropathy**
   274.10 Gouty nephropathy, unspecified
      AHA: N-D, '85, 15
   274.11 Uric acid nephrolithiasis
      DEF: Sodium urate stones in the kidney.
   274.19 Other
√5th **274.8 Gout with other specified manifestations**
   274.81 Gouty tophi of ear
      DEF: Chalky sodium urate deposit in the ear due to gout; produces chronic inflammation of external ear.
   274.82 Gouty tophi of other sites
      Gouty tophi of heart
   274.89 Other
      Use additional code to identify
         manifestations, as:
        gouty:
         iritis (364.11)   neuritis (357.4)

274.9 Gout, unspecified
√4th **275 Disorders of mineral metabolism**
EXCLUDES   *abnormal findings without manifest disease*
             (790.0-796.9)

275.0 Disorders of iron metabolism
Bronzed diabetes   Pigmentary cirrhosis (of liver)
Hemochromatosis
EXCLUDES   *anemia:*
        iron deficiency (280.0-280.9)
        sideroblastic (285.0)
AHA: 2Q, '97, 11

275.1 Disorders of copper metabolism
Hepatolenticular degeneration
Wilson's disease

275.2 Disorders of magnesium metabolism
Hypermagnesemia   Hypomagnesemia

275.3 Disorders of phosphorus metabolism
Familial hypophosphatemia   Vitamin D-resistant:
Hypophosphatasia   osteomalacia
                        rickets

√5th **275.4 Disorders of calcium metabolism**
EXCLUDES   *parathyroid disorders (252.0-252.9)*
           vitamin D deficiency (268.0-268.9)
AHA: 4Q, '97, 33

   275.40 Unspecified disorder of calcium metabolism
   275.41 Hypocalcemia
      DEF: Abnormally decreased blood calcium level; symptoms include hyperactive deep tendon reflexes, muscle, abdominal cramps, and carpedal spasm.

√4th √5th Additional Digit Required   Nonspecific PDx   Unacceptable PDx   Manifestation Code   MSP Medicare Secondary Payer   ►◄ Revised Text   ● New Code   ▲ Revised Code Title

2002 Ingenix, Inc.   **Volume 1 — 57**

Endocrine, Nutritional, Metabolic, Immunity 275.42–277.1

275.42 Hypercalcemia
DEF: Abnormally increased blood calcium level; symptoms include muscle weakness, fatigue, nausea, depression, and constipation.

275.49 Other disorders of calcium metabolism
Nephrocalcinosis
Pseudohypoparathyroidism
Pseudopseudohypoparathyroidism
DEF: Nephrocalcinosis: calcium phosphate deposits in the tubules of the kidney with resultant renal insufficiency.

DEF: Pseudohypoparathyroidism: inherited disorder with signs and symptoms of hypoparathyroidism; caused by inadequate response to parathyroid hormone, not hormonal deficiency. Symptoms include muscle cramps, tetany, urinary frequency, blurred vision due to cataracts, and dry scaly skin.

DEF: Pseudopseudohypoparathyroidism: clinical manifestations of hypoparathyroidism without affecting blood calcium levels.

275.8 Other specified disorders of mineral metabolism

275.9 Unspecified disorder of mineral metabolism

√4th **276 Disorders of fluid, electrolyte, and acid-base balance**
EXCLUDES diabetes insipidus (253.5)
familial periodic paralysis (359.3)

276.0 Hyperosmolality and/or hypernatremia CC
Sodium [Na] excess   Sodium [Na] overload
CC Excl: 276.0-276.9

276.1 Hyposmolality and/or hyponatremia CC
Sodium [Na] deficiency
CC Excl: See code 276.0
DRG 296

276.2 Acidosis CC
Acidosis: Acidosis:
    NOS   metabolic
    lactic   respiratory
EXCLUDES diabetic acidosis (250.1)
CC Excl: See code 276.0
AHA: J-F, '87, 15
DEF: Disorder involves decrease of pH (hydrogen ion) concentration in blood and cellular tissues; caused by increase in acid and decrease in bicarbonate.

276.3 Alkalosis CC
Alkalosis: Alkalosis:
    NOS   respiratory
    metabolic
CC Excl: See code 276.0
DEF: Accumulation of base (non-acid part of salt), or loss of acid without relative loss of base in body fluids; caused by increased arterial plasma bicarbonate concentration or loss of carbon dioxide due to hyperventilation.

276.4 Mixed acid-base balance disorder CC
Hypercapnia with mixed acid-base disorder
CC Excl: See code 276.0

276.5 Volume depletion CC
Dehydration
Depletion of volume of plasma or extracellular fluid
Hypovolemia
EXCLUDES hypovolemic shock:
    postoperative (998.0)
    traumatic (958.4)
CC Excl: See code 276.0
AHA: 4Q, '97, 30; 2Q, '88, 9
DRG 296

276.6 Fluid overload CC
Fluid retention
EXCLUDES ascites (789.5)
    localized edema (782.3)
CC Excl: See code 276.0

276.7 Hyperpotassemia CC
Hyperkalemia   Potassium [K]:
Potassium [K]:   intoxication
    excess   overload
CC Excl: See code 276.0
AHA: 2Q,'01, 12
DEF: Elevated blood levels of potassium; symptoms include abnormal EKG readings, weakness; related to defective renal excretion.

276.8 Hypopotassemia
Hypokalemia   Potassium [K] deficiency
DEF: Decreased blood levels of potassium; symptoms include neuromuscular disorders.

276.9 Electrolyte and fluid disorders not elsewhere classified CC
Electrolyte imbalance Hypochloremia
Hyperchloremia
EXCLUDES electrolyte imbalance:
    associated with hyperemesis
        gravidarum (643.1)
    complicating labor and delivery
        (669.0)
    following abortion and ectopic or
        molar pregnancy (634-638
        with .4, 639.4)
CC Excl: See code 276.0
AHA: J-F, '87, 15

√4th **277 Other and unspecified disorders of metabolism**
√5th **277.0 Cystic fibrosis**
Fibrocystic disease of the pancreas
Mucoviscidosis
AHA: 4Q, '90, 16; 3Q, '90, 18
DEF: Generalized, genetic disorder of infants, children, and young adults marked by exocrine gland dysfunction; characterized by chronic pulmonary disease with excess mucus production, pancreatic deficiency, high levels of electrolytes in the sweat.

277.00 Without mention of meconium ileus CC
▶Cystic fibrosis NOS◀
CC Excl: ▶277.00-277.09◀

277.01 With meconium ileus CC N
Meconium:
    ileus (of newborn)
    obstruction of intestine in mucoviscidosis
CC Excl: See code 277.00

277.02 With pulmonary manifestations CC
Cystic fibrosis with pulmonary exacerbation
Use additional code to identify any
    infectious organism present, such as:
    pseudomonas (041.7)
CC Excl: See code 277.00

277.03 With gastrointestinal manifestations CC
EXCLUDES with meconium ileus (277.01)
CC Excl: See code 277.00

277.09 With other manifestations CC
CC Excl: See code 277.00

277.1 Disorders of porphyrin metabolism
Hematoporphyria   Porphyrinuria
Hematoporphyrinuria   Protocoproporphyria
Hereditary coproporphyria Protoporphyria
Porphyria   Pyrroloporphyria

N Newborn Age: 0   P Pediatric Age: 0-17   M Maternity Age: 12-55   A Adult Age: 15-124   CC CC Condition   MC Major Complication   CD Complex Dx   HIV HIV Related Dx

58 — Volume 1 • October 2002   2002 Ingenix, Inc.

277.2 Other disorders of purine and pyrimidine metabolism
Hypoxanthine-guanine-phosphoribosyltransferase deficiency [HG-PRT deficiency]
Lesch-Nyhan syndrome
Xanthinuria
EXCLUDES gout (274.0-274.9)
orotic aciduric anemia (281.4)

277.3 Amyloidosis
Amyloidosis:
  NOS
  inherited systemic
  nephropathic
  neuropathic (Portuguese) (Swiss)
  secondary
Benign paroxysmal peritonitis
Familial Mediterranean fever
Hereditary cardiac amyloidosis

AHA: 1Q, '96, 16

DEF: Conditions of diverse etiologies characterized by the accumulation of insoluble fibrillar proteins (amyloid) in various organs and tissues of the body, compromising vital functions.

277.4 Disorders of bilirubin excretion
Hyperbilirubinemia:
  congenital
  constitutional
Syndrome:
  Crigler-Najjar
Syndrome:
  Dubin-Johnson
  Gilbert's
  Rotor's
EXCLUDES hyperbilirubinemias specific to the perinatal period (774.0-774.7)

277.5 Mucopolysaccharidosis
Gargoylism
Hunter's syndrome
Hurler's syndrome
Lipochondrodystrophy
Maroteaux-Lamy syndrome
Morquio-Brailsford disease
Osteochondrodystrophy
Sanfilippo's syndrome
Scheie's syndrome

DEF: Metabolism disorders evidenced by excretion of various mucopolysaccharides in urine and infiltration of these substances into connective tissue, with resulting various defects of bone, cartilage and connective tissue.

277.6 Other deficiencies of circulating enzymes
Alpha 1-antitrypsin deficiency
Hereditary angioedema

277.7 Dysmetabolic syndrome X [A]
Use additional code for associated manifestations, such as:
cardiovascular disease ▶(414.00-414.06)◀
obesity (278.00-278.01)
AHA: 4Q, '01, 42

DEF: A specific group of metabolic disorders that are related to the state of insulin resistance (decreased cellular response to insulin) without elevated blood sugars; often related to elevated cholesterol and triglycerides, obesity, cardiovascular disease, and high blood pressure.

277.8 Other specified disorders of metabolism
Hand-Schüller-Christian disease
Histiocytosis (acute) (chronic)
Histiocytosis X (chronic)
EXCLUDES histiocytosis:
acute differentiated progressive (202.5)
X, acute (progressive) (202.5)
AHA: 2Q,'01, 18; S-0, '87, 9

277.9 Unspecified disorder of metabolism
Enzymopathy NOS

√4ᵗʰ 278 Obesity and other hyperalimentation
EXCLUDES hyperalimentation NOS (783.6)
poisoning by vitamins NOS (963.5)
polyphagia (783.6)

√5ᵗʰ 278.0 Obesity
EXCLUDES adiposogenital dystrophy (253.8)
obesity of endocrine origin NOS (259.9)

278.00 Obesity, unspecified
Obesity NOS
AHA: 4Q, '01, 42;1Q, '99, 5, 6

278.01 Morbid obesity
DEF: Increased weight beyond limits of skeletal and physical requirements (125 percent or more over ideal body weight), as a result of excess fat in subcutaneous connective tissues.

278.1 Localized adiposity
Fat pad

278.2 Hypervitaminosis A
278.3 Hypercarotinemia
DEF: Elevated blood carotene level due to ingesting excess carotenoids or the inability to convert carotenoids to vitamin A.

278.4 Hypervitaminosis D
DEF: Weakness, fatigue, loss of weight, and other symptoms resulting from ingesting excessive amounts of vitamin D.

278.8 Other hyperalimentation

√4ᵗʰ 279 Disorders involving the immune mechanism
√5ᵗʰ 279.0 Deficiency of humoral immunity
DEF: Inadequate immune response to bacterial infections with potential reinfection by viruses due to lack of circulating immunoglobulins (acquired antibodies).

279.00 Hypogammaglobulinemia, unspecified
Agammaglobulinemia NOS
279.01 Selective IgA immunodeficiency
279.02 Selective IgM immunodeficiency [CC]
CC Excl: 279.02-279.9
279.03 Other selective immunoglobulin deficiencies [CC]
Selective deficiency of IgG
CC Excl: See code 279.02
279.04 Congenital hypogammaglobulinemia [CC]
Agammaglobulinemia:
Bruton's type
X-linked
CC Excl: See code 279.02
279.05 Immunodeficiency with increased IgM [CC]
Immunodeficiency with hyper-IgM:
autosomal recessive
X-linked
CC Excl: See code 279.02
279.06 Common variable immunodeficiency [CC]
Dysgammaglobulinemia (acquired) (congenital) (primary)
Hypogammaglobulinemia:
acquired primary
congenital non-sex-linked
sporadic
CC Excl: See code 279.02
279.09 Other [CC]
Transient hypogammaglobulinemia of infancy
CC Excl: See code 279.02

√5ᵗʰ 279.1 Deficiency of cell-mediated immunity
279.10 Immunodeficiency with predominant T-cell defect, unspecified [CC]
CC Excl: See code 279.02
AHA: S-0, '87, 10
279.11 DiGeorge's syndrome [CC]
Pharyngeal pouch syndrome
Thymic hypoplasia
CC Excl: See code 279.02

DEF: Congenital disorder due to defective development of the third and fourth pharyngeal pouches; results in hypoplasia or aplasia of the thymus, parathyroid glands; related to congenital heart defects, anomalies of the great vessels, esophageal atresia, and abnormalities of facial structures.

279.12 Wiskott-Aldrich syndrome `CC`
CC Excl: See code 279.02

DEF: A disease characterized by chronic conditions, such as eczema, suppurative otitis media and anemia; it results from an X-linked recessive gene and is classified as an immune deficiency syndrome.

279.13 Nezelof's syndrome `CC`
Cellular immunodeficiency with abnormal immunoglobulin deficiency
CC Excl: See code 279.02

DEF: Immune system disorder characterized by a pathological deficiency in cellular immunity and humoral antibodies resulting in inability to fight infectious diseases.

279.19 Other `CC`
EXCLUDES   ataxia-telangiectasia (334.8)
CC Excl: See code 279.02

279.2 Combined immunity deficiency `CC`
Agammaglobulinemia:
  autosomal recessive
  Swiss-type
  x-linked recessive
Severe combined immunodeficiency [SCID]
Thymic:
  alymphoplasia
  aplasia or dysplasia with immunodeficiency
  EXCLUDES   thymic hypoplasia (279.11)
CC Excl: See code 279.02

DEF: Agammaglobulinemia: No immunoglobulins in the blood.

DEF: Thymic alymphoplasia: Severe combined immunodeficiency; result of failed lymphoid tissue development.

279.3 Unspecified immunity deficiency `CC`
CC Excl: See code 279.02

279.4 Autoimmune disease, not elsewhere classified `CC`
Autoimmune disease NOS
EXCLUDES   transplant failure or rejection (996.80-996.89)
CC Excl: See code 279.02

279.8 Other specified disorders involving the immune `CC`
mechanism
Single complement [C$_1$-C$_9$] deficiency or dysfunction
CC Excl: See code 279.02

279.9 Unspecified disorder of immune mechanism `CC`
CC Excl: See code 279.02

AHA: 3Q, '92, 13

`N` Newborn Age: 0   `P` Pediatric Age: 0-17   `M` Maternity Age: 12-55   `A` Adult Age: 15-124   `CC` CC Condition   `MC` Major Complication   `CD` Complex Dx   `HIV` HIV Related Dx

60 — Volume 1   *2002 Ingenix, Inc.*

4. DISEASES OF THE BLOOD AND BLOOD-FORMING ORGANS (280-289)

EXCLUDES *anemia complicating pregnancy or the puerperium (648.2)*

√4th **280 Iron deficiency anemias**

INCLUDES anemia:
asiderotic
hypochromic-microcytic
sideropenic

EXCLUDES *familial microcytic anemia (282.4)*

280.0 **Secondary to blood loss (chronic)**   **cc**
Normocytic anemia due to blood loss
EXCLUDES *acute posthemorrhagic anemia (285.1)*

CC Excl: 280.0-280.9, 281.0-281.9, 282.0-282.9, 283.0-283.9, 284.0-284.9, 285.0-285.9, 289.8-289.9

AHA: 4Q, '93, 34

280.1 **Secondary to inadequate dietary iron intake**

280.8 **Other specified iron deficiency anemias**
Paterson-Kelly syndrome
Plummer-Vinson syndrome
Sideropenic dysphagia

280.9 **Iron deficiency anemia, unspecified**
Anemia:
achlorhydric
chlorotic
idiopathic hypochromic
iron [Fe] deficiency NOS

√4th **281 Other deficiency anemias**

281.0 **Pernicious anemia**
Anemia:
Addison's
Biermer's
congenital pernicious
Congenital intrinsic factor [Castle's] deficiency
EXCLUDES *combined system disease without mention of anemia (266.2)*
subacute degeneration of spinal cord without mention of anemia (266.2)

AHA: N-D, '84, 1; S-O, '84, 16

DEF: Chronic progressive anemia due to Vitamin B_{12} malabsorption; caused by lack of a secretion known as intrinsic factor, which is produced by the gastric mucosa of the stomach.

281.1 **Other vitamin B_{12} deficiency anemia**
Anemia:
vegan's
vitamin B_{12} deficiency (dietary)
due to selective vitamin B_{12} malabsorption with proteinuria
Syndrome:
Imerslund's
Imerslund-Gräsbeck
EXCLUDES *combined system disease without mention of anemia (266.2)*
subacute degeneration of spinal cord without mention of anemia (266.2)

281.2 **Folate-deficiency anemia**
Congenital folate malabsorption
Folate or folic acid deficiency anemia:
NOS
dietary
drug-induced
Goat's milk anemia
Nutritional megaloblastic anemia (of infancy)
Use additional E code to identify drug

DEF: Macrocytic anemia resembles pernicious anemia but without absence of hydrochloric acid secretions; responsive to folic acid therapy.

281.3 **Other specified megaloblastic anemias not elsewhere classified**
Combined B_{12} and folate-deficiency anemia
Refractory megaloblastic anemia
DEF: Megaloblasts predominant in bone marrow with few normoblasts; rare familial type associated with proteinuria and genitourinary tract anomalies.

281.4 **Protein-deficiency anemia**   **cc**
Amino-acid-deficiency anemia
CC Excl: See code 280.0

281.8 **Anemia associated with other specified nutritional deficiency**   **cc**
Scorbutic anemia
CC Excl: See code 280.0

281.9 **Unspecified deficiency anemia**
Anemia: Anemia:
dimorphic   nutritional NOS
macrocytic   simple chronic
megaloblastic NOS

√4th **282 Hereditary hemolytic anemias**
DEF: Escalated rate of erythrocyte destruction; similar to all anemias, occurs when imbalance exists between blood loss and blood production.

282.0 **Hereditary spherocytosis**
Acholuric (familial) jaundice
Congenital hemolytic anemia (spherocytic)
Congenital spherocytosis
Minkowski-Chauffard syndrome
Spherocytosis (familial)
EXCLUDES *hemolytic anemia of newborn (773.0-773.5)*
DEF: Hereditary, chronic illness marked by abnormal red blood cell membrane; symptoms include enlarged spleen, jaundice; and anemia in severe cases.

282.1 **Hereditary elliptocytosis**
Elliptocytosis (congenital)
Ovalocytosis (congenital) (hereditary)
DEF: Genetic hemolytic anemia characterized by malformed, elliptical erythrocytes; there is increased destruction of red cells with resulting anemia.

282.2 **Anemias due to disorders of glutathione metabolism**
Anemia:
6-phosphogluconic dehydrogenase deficiency
enzyme deficiency, drug-induced
erythrocytic glutathione deficiency
glucose-6-phosphate dehydrogenase [G-6-PD] deficiency
glutathione-reductase deficiency
hemolytic nonspherocytic (hereditary), type I
Disorder of pentose phosphate pathway
Favism

282.3 **Other hemolytic anemias due to enzyme deficiency**
Anemia:
hemolytic nonspherocytic (hereditary), type II
hexokinase deficiency
pyruvate kinase [PK] deficiency
triosephosphate isomerase deficiency

√4th √5th **Additional Digit Required** | **Nonspecific PDx** | **Unacceptable PDx** | **Manifestation Code** | **MSP** Medicare Secondary Payer | ►◄ Revised Text | ● New Code | ▲ Revised Code Title

2002 Ingenix, Inc.   **Volume 1 — 61**

Blood and Blood-Forming Organs 280–282.3

282.4   Thalassemias   `CC`
     Cooley's anemia
     Hereditary leptocytosis
     Mediterranean anemia (with other
        hemoglobinopathy)
     Microdrepanocytosis
     Sickle-cell thalassemia
     Thalassemia (alpha) (beta) (intermedia) (major)
        (minima) (minor) (mixed) (trait) (with other
        hemoglobinopathy)
     Thalassemia-Hb-S disease
     EXCLUDES   *sickle-cell:*
                  anemia (282.60-282.69)
                  trait (282.5)

     CC Excl: See code 280.0

282.5   Sickle-cell trait
     Hb-AS genotype   Heterozygous:
     Hemoglobin S [Hb-S] trait   hemoglobin S
                               Hb-S
     EXCLUDES   *that with other hemoglobinopathy*
                  (282.60-282.69)
                  that with thalassemia (282.4)

     DEF: Heterozygous genetic makeup characterized by one gene for
     normal hemoglobin and one for sickle-cell hemoglobin; clinical
     disease rarely present.

`√5ᵗʰ` **282.6   Sickle-cell anemia**
     EXCLUDES   *sickle-cell thalassemia (282.4)*
                  sickle-cell trait (282.5)

     DEF: Inherited blood disorder; sickle-shaped red blood cells are
     hard and pointed, clogging blood flow; anemia characterized by,
     periodic episodes of pain, acute abdominal discomfort, skin
     ulcerations of the legs, increased infections; occurs primarily in
     persons of African descent.

     282.60   Sickle-cell anemia, unspecified   `CC`
        CC Excl: See code 280.0

        AHA: 2Q, '97, 11

     282.61   Hb-S disease without mention of crisis   `CC`
        CC Excl: See code 280.0

     282.62   Hb-S disease with mention of crisis   `CC`
        Sickle-cell crisis NOS
        CC Excl: See code 280.0

        AHA: 2Q, '98, 8; 2Q, '91, 15

     282.63   Sickle-cell/Hb-C disease   `CC`
        Hb-S/Hb-C disease
        CC Excl: See code 280.0

     282.69   Other   `CC`
        Disease: Disease:
           Hb-S/Hb-D   sickle-cell/Hb-D
           Hb-S/Hb-E   sickle-cell/Hb-E
        CC Excl: See code 280.0

282.7   Other hemoglobinopathies
     Abnormal hemoglobin NOS
     Congenital Heinz-body anemia
     Disease:
       Hb-Bart's
       hemoglobin C [Hb-C]
       hemoglobin D [Hb-D]
       hemoglobin E [Hb-E]
       hemoglobin Zurich [Hb-Zurich]
     Hemoglobinopathy NOS
     Hereditary persistence of fetal hemoglobin[HPFH]
     Unstable hemoglobin hemolytic disease
     EXCLUDES   *familial polycythemia (289.6)*
                  hemoglobin M [Hb-M] disease (289.7)
                  high-oxygen-affinity hemoglobin (289.0)

     DEF: Any disorder of hemoglobin due to alteration of molecular
     structure; may include overt anemia.

282.8   Other specified hereditary hemolytic anemias
     Stomatocytosis

282.9   Hereditary hemolytic anemia, unspecified
     Hereditary hemolytic anemia NOS

`√4ᵗʰ` **283   Acquired hemolytic anemias**
     DEF: Non-heriditary anemia characterized by premature destruction of red
     blood cells; caused by infectious organisms, poisons, and physical agents

     AHA: N-D, '84, 1

     283.0   Autoimmune hemolytic anemias   `CC`
        Autoimmune hemolytic disease (cold type) (warm
          type)
        Chronic cold hemagglutinin disease
        Cold agglutinin disease or hemoglobinuria
        Hemolytic anemia:
          cold type (secondary) (symptomatic)
          drug-induced
          warm type (secondary) (symptomatic)
        Use additional E code to identify cause, if drug-
          induced
        EXCLUDES   *Evans' syndrome (287.3)*
                    hemolytic disease of newborn (773.0-
                       773.5)

        CC Excl: See code 280.0

`√5ᵗʰ`   **283.1   Non-autoimmune hemolytic anemias**
        Use additional E code to identify cause
        DEF: Hemolytic anemia and thrombocytopenia with acute renal
        failure; relatively rare condition; 50 percent of patients require
        renal dialysis.

        AHA: 4Q, '93, 25

     283.10   Non-autoimmune hemolytic   `CC`
           anemia, unspecified
        CC Excl: See code 280.0

     283.11   Hemolytic-uremic syndrome   `CC`
        CC Excl: See code 280.0

     283.19   Other non-autoimmune hemolytic   `CC`
           anemias
        Hemolytic anemia: Hemolytic anemia:
          mechanical   toxic
          microangiopathic
        CC Excl: See code 280.0

     283.2   Hemoglobinuria due to hemolysis from   `CC`
       external causes
        Acute intravascular hemolysis
        Hemoglobinuria:
          from exertion
          march
          paroxysmal (cold) (nocturnal)
          due to other hemolysis
        Marchiafava-Micheli syndrome
        Use additional E code to identify cause
        CC Excl: See code 280.0

     283.9   Acquired hemolytic anemia, unspecified   `CC`
        Acquired hemolytic anemia NOS
        Chronic idiopathic hemolytic anemia
        CC Excl: See code 280.0

`√4ᵗʰ` **284   Aplastic anemia**
     AHA: 1Q, '91, 14; N-D, '84, 1; S-O, '84, 16

     DEF: Bone marrow failure to produce the normal amount of blood
     components; generally non-responsive to usual therapy.

`N` Newborn Age: 0   `P` Pediatric Age: 0-17   `M` Maternity Age: 12-55   `A` Adult Age: 15-124   `CC` CC Condition   `MC` Major Complication   `CD` Complex Dx   `HIV` HIV Related Dx

62 — Volume 1   *2002 Ingenix, Inc.*

284.0 Constitutional aplastic anemia `CC`

Aplasia, (pure) red cell:
   congenital
   of infants
   primary
Blackfan-Diamond syndrome
Familial hypoplastic anemia
Fanconi's anemia
Pancytopenia with malformations

CC Excl: See code 280.0

AHA: 1Q, '91, 14

284.8 Other specified aplastic anemias `CC`

Aplastic anemia (due to):
   chronic systemic disease
   drugs
   infection
   radiation
   toxic (paralytic)
Pancytopenia (acquired)
Red cell aplasia (acquired) (adult) (pure) (with
   thymoma)
Use additional E code to identify cause

CC Excl: See code 280.0

AHA: 1Q, '97, 5; 1Q, '92, 15; 1Q, '91, 14

284.9 Aplastic anemia, unspecified `CC`

Anemia: Anemia:
   aplastic (idiopathic) NOS   nonregenerative
   aregenerative   refractory
   hypoplastic NOS   Medullary hypoplasia

CC Excl: See code 280.0

DEF: Group of hereditary anemias occurring in the Mediterranean and Southeast Asia; characterized by impaired hemoglobin synthesis; homozygous form may cause death in utero; mild red blood cell anomalies in heterozygous.

✓4ᵗʰ **285 Other and unspecified anemias**

AHA: 1Q, '91, 14; N-D, '84, 1

285.0 Sideroblastic anemia `CC`

Anemia:
   hypochromic with iron loading
   sideroachrestic
   sideroblastic
      acquired
      congenital
      hereditary
      primary
      refractory
      secondary (drug-induced) (due to disease)
      sex-linked hypochromic
      vitamin B_6-responsive
Pyridoxine-responsive (hypochromic) anemia
Use additional E code to identify cause, if drug
   induced

CC Excl: See code 280.0

DEF: Characterized by a disruption of final heme synthesis; results in iron overload of reticuloendothelial tissues.

285.1 Acute posthemorrhagic anemia `CC`

Anemia due to acute blood loss

    EXCLUDES   *anemia due to chronic blood loss
             (280.0)
           blood loss anemia NOS (280.0)*

CC Excl: 280.0-280.9, 281.0-281.9, 282.0-282.9, 283.0-283.9, 284.0, 284.8, 285.0-285.9, 289.8-289.9, 958.2

AHA: 2Q, '92, 15

✓5ᵗʰ **285.2 Anemia in chronic illness**

AHA: 4Q, '00, 39

285.21 Anemia in end-stage renal disease
285.22 Anemia in neoplastic disease
285.29 Anemia of other chronic illness

285.8 Other specified anemias

Anemia:
   dyserythropoietic (congenital)
   dyshematopoietic (congenital)
   leukoerythroblastic
   von Jaksch's
Infantile pseudoleukemia

AHA: 1Q, '91, 16

285.9 Anemia, unspecified

Anemia: Anemia:
   NOS   profound
   essential   progressive
   normocytic, not due secondary
     to blood loss Oligocythemia

    EXCLUDES   *anemia (due to):
       blood loss:
         acute (285.1)
         chronic or unspecified (280.0)
       iron deficiency (280.0-280.9)*

AHA: ▶1Q, '02, 14;◀ 2Q, '92, 16; M-A, '85, 13; N-D, '84, 1

✓4ᵗʰ **286 Coagulation defects**

286.0 Congenital factor VIII disorder `CC`

Antihemophilic globulin Hemophilia:
   [AHG] deficiency   A
Factor VIII (functional)   classical
   deficiency   familial
Hemophilia: hereditary
   NOS   Subhemophilia

    EXCLUDES   *factor VIII deficiency with vascular
          defect (286.4)*

CC Excl: 286.0-286.9, 287.0-287.9, 289.8-289.9

DEF: Hereditary, sex-linked, results in missing antihemophilic globulin (AHG) (factor VIII); causes abnormal coagulation characterized by increased tendency to bleeding, large bruises of skin, soft tissue; may also be bleeding in mouth, nose, gastrointestinal tract; after childhood, hemorrhages in joints, resulting in swelling and impaired function.

286.1 Congenital factor IX disorder `CC`

Christmas disease
Deficiency:
   factor IX (functional)
   plasma thromboplastin component [PTC]
Hemophilia B

CC Excl: See code 286.0

DEF: Deficiency of plasma thromboplastin component (PTC) (factor IX) and plasma thromboplastin antecedent (PTA); PTC deficiency clinically indistinguishable from classical hemophilia; PTA deficiency found in both sexes.

286.2 Congenital factor XI deficiency `CC`

Hemophilia C
Plasma thromboplastin antecedent [PTA] deficiency
Rosenthal's disease

CC Excl: See code 286.0

Blood and Blood-Forming Organs 284.0–286.2

✓4ᵗʰ Additional Digit Required   **Nonspecific PDx**   **Unacceptable PDx**   **Manifestation Code**   **MSP** Medicare Secondary Payer   ▶◀ Revised Text   ● New Code   ▲ Revised Code Title
✓5ᵗʰ

2002 Ingenix, Inc.   **October 2002 • Volume 1 — 63**

286.3   Congenital deficiency of other clotting factors `CC`
    Congenital afibrinogenemia
    Deficiency:
       AC globulin factor:
          I [fibrinogen]
          II [prothrombin]
          V [labile]
          VII [stable]
          X [Stuart-Prower]
          XII [Hageman]
          XIII [fibrin stabilizing]
       Laki-Lorand factor
       proaccelerin
    Disease
       Owren's
       Stuart-Prower
    Dysfibrinogenemia (congenital)
    Dysprothrombinemia (constitutional)
    Hypoproconvertinemia
    Hypoprothrmbinemia (hereditary)
    Parahemophilia
    CC Excl: See code 286.0

286.4   Von Willebrand's disease `CC`
    Angiohemophilia (A) (B)
    Constitutional thrombopathy
    Factor VIII deficiency with vascular defect
    Pseudohemophilia type B
    Vascular hemophilia
    von Willebrand's (-Jürgens') disease
       EXCLUDES   *factor VIII deficiency:*
          NOS (286.0)
          with functional defect (286.0)
       hereditary capillary fragility (287.8)
    CC Excl: See code 286.0

DEF: Abnormal blood coagulation caused by deficient blood Factor VII; congenital; symptoms include excess or prolonged bleeding, such as hemorrhage during menstruation, following birthing, or after surgical procedure.

286.5   Hemorrhagic disorder due to circulating anticoagulants `CC`
    Antithrombinemia
    Antithromboplastinemia
    Antithromboplastino-genemia
    Hyperheparinemia
    Increase in:
       anti-VIIIa
       anti-IXa
       anti-Xa
       anti-XIa
       antithrombin
    Systemic lupus erythematosus [SLE] inhibitor
    Use additional E code to identify cause, if drug
       induced
    CC Excl: See code 286.0

    AHA: 3Q, '92, 15; 3Q, '90, 14

286.6   Defibrination syndrome `CC`
    Afibrinogenemia, acquired
    Consumption coagulopathy
    Diffuse or disseminated intravascular coagulation
       [DIC syndrome]
    Fibrinolytic hemorrhage, acquired
    Hemorrhagic fibrinogenolysis
    Pathologic fibrinolysis
    Purpura:
       fibrinolytic
       fulminans
       EXCLUDES   *that complicating:*
          abortion (634-638 with .1, 639.1)
          pregnancy or the puerperium (641.3,
             666.3)
          disseminated intravascular coagulation
             in newborn (776.2)

    CC Excl: See code 286.0

    AHA: 4Q, '93, 29

DEF: Characterized by destruction of circulating fibrinogen; often precipitated by other conditions, such as injury, causing release of thromboplastic particles in blood stream.

286.7   Acquired coagulation factor deficiency `CC`
    Deficiency of coagulation factor due to:
       liver disease
       vitamin K deficiency
    Hypoprothrombinemia, acquired
    Use additional E code to identify cause, if drug
       induced
       EXCLUDES   *vitamin K deficiency of newborn*
          (776.0)

    CC Excl: See code 286.0

    AHA: 4Q, '93, 29

286.9   Other and unspecified coagulation defects `CC`
    Defective coagulation NOS
    Deficiency, coagulation factor NOS
    Delay, coagulation
    Disorder:
       coagulation
       hemostasis
       EXCLUDES   *abnormal coagulation profile (790.92)*
          hemorrhagic disease of newborn
             (776.0)
          that complicating:
          abortion (634-638 with .1, 639.1)
          pregnancy or the puerperium (641.3,
             666.3)

    CC Excl: See code 286.0

    AHA: 4Q, '99, 22; 4Q, '93, 29

☑4ᵗʰ **287 Purpura and other hemorrhagic conditions**
       EXCLUDES   *hemorrhagic thrombocythemia (238.7)*
          purpura fulminans (286.6)

    AHA: 1Q, '91, 14

287.0   Allergic purpura `CC`
    Peliosis rheumatica   Purpura:
    Purpura: rheumatica
       anaphylactoid   Schönlein-Henoch
       autoimmune   vascular
       Henoch's   Vasculitis, allergic
       nonthrombocytopenic:
          hemorrhagic
          idiopathic
       EXCLUDES   *hemorrhagic purpura (287.3)*
          purpura annularis telangiectodes
             (709.1)

    CC Excl: See code 286.0

DEF: Any hemorrhagic condition, thrombocytic or nonthrombocytopenic in origin, caused by a presumed allergic reaction.

`N` Newborn Age: 0   `P` Pediatric Age: 0-17   `M` Maternity Age: 12-55   `A` Adult Age: 15-124   `CC` CC Condition   `MC` Major Complication   `CD` Complex Dx   `HIV` HIV Related Dx

64 — Volume 1   *2002 Ingenix, Inc.*

287.1 **Qualitative platelet defects** `CC`
Thrombasthenia (hemorrhagic) (hereditary)
Thrombocytasthenia
Thrombocytopathy (dystrophic)
Thrombopathy (Bernard-Soulier)
EXCLUDES *von Willebrand's disease (286.4)*
CC Excl: See code 286.0

287.2 **Other nonthrombocytopenic purpuras** `CC`
Purpura: Purpura:
  NOS   simplex
  senile
CC Excl: See code 286.0

287.3 **Primary thrombocytopenia** `CC`
Evans' syndrome   Throbocytopenia:
Megakaryocytic hypoplasia   congenital
Purpura, thrombocytopenic   hereditary
  congenital   primary
  hereditary   Tidal platelet dysgenesis
  idiopathic
EXCLUDES *thrombotic thrombocytopenic purpura (446.6)*
transient thrombocytopenia of newborn (776.1)
CC Excl: See code 286.0

DEF: Decrease in number of blood platelets in circulating blood and purpural skin hemorrhages.

287.4 **Secondary thrombocytopenia** `CC`
Posttransfusion purpura
Thrombocytopenia (due to):
  dilutional
  drugs
  extracorporeal circulation of blood
  massive blood transfusion
  platelet alloimmunization
Use additional E code to identify cause
EXCLUDES *transient thrombocytopenia of newborn (776.1)*
CC Excl: See code 286.0

AHA: M-A, '85, 14

DEF: Reduced number of platelets in circulating blood as consequence of an underlying disease or condition.

287.5 **Thrombocytopenia, unspecified** `CC`
CC Excl: See code 286.0

287.8 **Other specified hemorrhagic conditions** `CC`
Capillary fragility (hereditary)
Vascular pseudohemophilia
CC Excl: See code 286.0

287.9 **Unspecified hemorrhagic conditions** `CC`
Hemorrhagic diathesis (familial)
CC Excl: See code 286.0

✓4ᵗʰ **288 Diseases of white blood cells**
EXCLUDES *leukemia (204.0-208.9)*
AHA: 1Q, '91, 14

288.0 **Agranulocytosis** `CC`
Infantile genetic agranulocytosis   Neutropenia:
Kostmann's syndrome   immune
Neutropenia: periodic
  NOS   toxic
  cyclic   Neutropenic
  drug-induced   splenomegaly
Use additional E code to identify drug or other cause
EXCLUDES *transitory neonatal neutropenia (776.7)*
CC Excl: 288.0-288.9, 289.8-289.9

AHA: 3Q, '99, 6; 2Q, '99, 9; 3Q, '96, 16; 2Q, '96, 6

DEF: Sudden, severe condition characterized by reduced number of white blood cells; results in sores in the throat, stomach or skin; symptoms include chills, fever; some drugs can bring on condition.

288.1 **Functional disorders of polymorphonuclear neutrophils** `CC`
Chronic (childhood) granulomatous disease
Congenital dysphagocytosis
Job's syndrome
Lipochrome histiocytosis (familial)
Progressive septic granulomatosis
CC Excl: See code 288.0

288.2 **Genetic anomalies of leukocytes**
Anomaly (granulation) (granulocyte) or syndrome:
  Alder's (-Reilly)
  Chédiak-Steinbrinck (-Higashi)
  Jordan's
  May-Hegglin
  Pelger-Huet
Hereditary:
  hypersegmentation
  hyposegmentation
  leukomelanopathy

288.3 **Eosinophilia**
Eosinophilia   Eosinophilia
  allergic   secondary
  hereditary   Eosinophilic leukocytosis
  idiopathic
EXCLUDES *Löffler's syndrome (518.3)*
pulmonary eosinophilia (518.3)
AHA: 3Q, '00, 11

DEF: Elevated number of eosinophils in the blood; characteristic of allergic states and various parasitic infections.

288.8 **Other specified disease of white blood cells**
Leukemoid reaction   Lymphocytopenia
  lymphocytic   Lymphocytosis (symptomatic)
  monocytic   Lymphopenia
  myelocytic   Monocytosis (symptomatic)
Leukocytosis   Plasmacytosis
EXCLUDES *immunity disorders (279.0-279.9)*
AHA: M-A, '87, 12

288.9 **Unspecified disease of white blood cells**

✓4ᵗʰ **289 Other diseases of blood and blood-forming organs**
289.0 **Polycythemia, secondary**
High-oxygen-affinity hemoglobin
Polycythemia:
  acquired
  benign
  due to:
    fall in plasma volume
    high altitude
  emotional
  erythropoietin
  hypoxemic
  nephrogenous
  relative
  spurious
  stress
EXCLUDES *polycythemia:*
neonatal (776.4)
primary (238.4)
vera (238.4)
DEF: Elevated number of red blood cells in circulating blood as result of reduced oxygen supply to the tissues.

289.1 **Chronic lymphadenitis**
Chronic:
  adenitis   } any lymph node, except
  lymphadenitis   mesenteric
EXCLUDES *acute lymphadenitis (683)*
mesenteric (289.2)
enlarged glands NOS (785.6)
DEF: Persistent inflammation of lymph node tissue; origin of infection is usually elsewhere.

✓4ᵗʰ
✓5ᵗʰ Additional Digit Required   Nonspecific PDx   Unacceptable PDx   Manifestation Code   `MSP` Medicare Secondary Payer   ▶◀ Revised Text   ● New Code   ▲ Revised Code Title
2002 Ingenix, Inc.   **Volume 1 — 65**

289.2 Nonspecific mesenteric lymphadenitis

Mesenteric lymphadenitis (acute) (chronic)

DEF: Inflammation of the lymph nodes in peritoneal fold that encases abdominal organs; disease resembles acute appendicitis; unknown etiology.

289.3 Lymphadenitis, unspecified, except mesenteric

AHA: 2Q, '92, 8

289.4 Hypersplenism

"Big spleen" syndrome   Hypersplenia
Dyssplenism

EXCLUDES   *primary splenic neutropenia (288.0)*

DEF: An overactive spleen; it causes a deficiency of the peripheral blood components, an increase in bone marrow cells and sometimes a notable increase in the size of the spleen.

√5ᵗʰ **289.5 Other diseases of spleen**

289.50 Disease of spleen, unspecified

289.51 Chronic congestive splenomegaly

289.59 Other

Lien migrans   Splenic:
Perisplenitis   fibrosis
Splenic: infarction
   abscess   rupture, nontraumatic
   atrophy   Splenitis
   cyst   Wandering spleen

EXCLUDES   *bilharzial splenic fibrosis*
               (120.0-120.9)
           hepatolienal fibrosis (571.5)
           splenomegaly NOS (789.2)

289.6 Familial polycythemia

Familial:
   benign polycythemia
   erythrocytosis

DEF: Elevated number of red blood cells.

289.7 Methemoglobinemia

Congenital NADH [DPNH]-methemoglobin-reductase deficiency
Hemoglobin M [Hb-M] disease
Methemoglobinemia:
   NOS
   acquired (with sulfhemoglobinemia)
   hereditary
   toxic
Stokvis' disease
Sulfhemoglobinemia
Use additional E code to identify cause

DEF: Presence in the blood of methemoglobin, a chemically altered form of hemoglobin; causes cyanosis, headache, dizziness, ataxia dyspnea, tachycardia, nausea, stupor, coma, and, rarely, death.

289.8 Other specified diseases of blood and blood-forming organs

Hypergammaglobulinemia
Myelofibrosis
Pseudocholinesterase deficiency

AHA: ▶1Q, '02, 16;◀ 2Q, '89, 8; M-A, '87, 12

289.9 Unspecified diseases of blood and blood-forming organs

Blood dyscrasia NOS
Erythroid hyperplasia

AHA: M-A, '85, 14

5. MENTAL DISORDERS (290-319)

In the International Classification of Diseases, 9th Revision (ICD-9), the corresponding Chapter V, "Mental Disorders," includes a glossary which defines the contents of each category. The introduction to Chapter V in ICD-9 indicates that the glossary is intended so that psychiatrists can make the diagnosis based on the descriptions provided rather than from the category titles. Lay coders are instructed to code whatever diagnosis the physician records.

Chapter 5, "Mental Disorders," in ICD-9-CM uses the standard classification format with inclusion and exclusion terms, omitting the glossary as part of the main text.

The mental disorders section of ICD-9-CM has been expanded to incorporate additional psychiatric disorders not listed in ICD-9. The glossary from ICD-9 does not contain all these terms. It now appears in Appendix B, which also contains descriptions and definitions for the terms added in ICD-9-CM. Some of these were provided by the American Psychiatric Association's Task Force on Nomenclature and Statistics who are preparing the Diagnostic and Statistical Manual, Third Edition (DSM-III), and others from A Psychiatric Glossary.

The American Psychiatric Association provided invaluable assistance in modifying Chapter 5 of ICD-9-CM to incorporate detail useful to American clinicians and gave permission to use material from the aforementioned sources.

1. Manual of the *International Statistical Classification of Diseases, Injuries, and Causes of Death*, 9th Revision, World Health Organization, Geneva, Switzerland, 1975.
2. American Psychiatric Association, Task Force on Nomenclature and Statistics, Robert L. Spitzer, M.D., Chairman.
3. *A Psychiatric Glossary*, Fourth Edition, American Psychiatric Association, Washington, D.C., 1975.

PSYCHOSES (290-299)
EXCLUDES   mental retardation (317-319)

ORGANIC PSYCHOTIC CONDITIONS (290-294)
INCLUDES   psychotic organic brain syndrome
EXCLUDES   nonpsychotic syndromes of organic etiology (310.0-310.9)
psychoses classifiable to 295-298 and without impairment of orientation, comprehension, calculation, learning capacity, and judgment, but associated with physical disease, injury, or condition affecting the brain [eg., following childbirth] (295.0-298.8)

AHA: 1Q, '88, 3

√4th 290 Senile and presenile organic psychotic conditions
Code first the associated neurological condition
EXCLUDES   dementia not classified as senile, presenile, or arteriosclerotic (294.10-294.11)
psychoses classifiable to 295-298 occurring in the senium without dementia or delirium (295.0-298.8)
senility with mental changes of nonpsychotic severity (310.1)
transient organic psychotic conditions (293.0-293.9)

290.0 Senile dementia, uncomplicated   A
Senile dementia:
NOS
simple type
EXCLUDES   mild memory disturbances, not amounting to dementia, associated with senile brain disease (310.1)
senile dementia with:
delirium or confusion (290.3)
delusional [paranoid] features (290.20)
depressive features (290.21)

AHA: 4Q, '99, 4

√5th 290.1 Presenile dementia
Brain syndrome with presenile brain disease
EXCLUDES   arteriosclerotic dementia (290.40-290.43)
dementia associated with other cerebral conditions (294.10-294.11)

AHA: N-D, '84, 20

290.10 Presenile dementia, uncomplicated   A HIV
Presenile dementia: Presenile dementia:
NOS   simple type

290.11 Presenile dementia with delirium   A HIV
Presenile dementia with acute confusional state

AHA: 1Q, '88, 3

290.12 Presenile dementia with delusional features   A HIV
Presenile dementia, paranoid type

290.13 Presenile dementia with depressive features   A HIV
Presenile dementia, depressed type

√5th 290.2 Senile dementia with delusional or depressive features
EXCLUDES   senile dementia:
NOS (290.0)
with delirium and/or confusion (290.3)

290.20 Senile dementia with delusional features   A
Senile dementia, paranoid type
Senile psychosis NOS

290.21 Senile dementia with depressive features   A

290.3 Senile dementia with delirium   A
Senile dementia with acute confusional state
EXCLUDES   senile:
dementia NOS (290.0)
psychosis NOS (290.20)

√5th 290.4 Arteriosclerotic dementia
Multi-infarct dementia or psychosis
Use additional code to identify cerebral atherosclerosis (437.0)
EXCLUDES   suspected cases with no clear evidence of arteriosclerosis (290.9)

290.40 Arteriosclerotic dementia, uncomplicated   A
Arteriosclerotic dementia:
NOS
simple type

290.41 Arteriosclerotic dementia with delirium   A
Arteriosclerotic dementia with acute confusional state

290.42 Arteriosclerotic dementia with delusional features   A
Arteriosclerotic dementia, paranoid type

290.43 Arteriosclerotic dementia with depressive features   A
Arteriosclerotic dementia, depressed type

290.8 Other specified senile psychotic conditions
Presbyophrenic psychosis

290.9 Unspecified senile psychotic condition   A

√4th 291 Alcoholic psychoses
EXCLUDES   alcoholism without psychosis (303.0-303.9)
AHA: S-O, '86, 3

291.0 Alcohol withdrawal delirium   CC
Alcoholic delirium   Delirium tremens
EXCLUDES   alcohol withdrawal (291.81)
CC Excl: 291.0-291.9, 292.0-292.9, 293.0-293.9, 294.0-294.9, 303.00-303.93, 304.00-304.91, 305.00-305.03, 305.20-305.93, 790.3

AHA: 2Q, '91, 11

 Additional Digit Required   Nonspecific PDx   Unacceptable PDx   Manifestation Code   Medicare Secondary Payer   ►◄ Revised Text   ● New Code   ▲ Revised Code Title

2002 Ingenix, Inc.

Volume 1 — 67

Mental Disorders 291.1–292.9

291.1 Alcohol amnestic syndrome `CC`
  Alcoholic polyneuritic psychosis
  Korsakoff's psychosis, alcoholic
  Wernicke-Korsakoff syndrome (alcoholic)
  CC Excl: See code 291.0

  AHA: 1Q, '88, 3

  DEF: Prominent and lasting reduced memory span, disordered time appreciation and confabulation, occurring in alcoholics, as sequel to acute alcoholic psychosis.

291.2 Other alcoholic dementia `CC`
  Alcoholic dementia NOS
  Alcoholism associated with dementia NOS
  Chronic alcoholic brain syndrome
  CC Excl: See code 291.0

291.3 Alcohol withdrawal hallucinosis `CC`
  Alcoholic: Alcoholic:
    hallucinosis (acute)   psychosis with hallucinosis
  EXCLUDES *alcohol withdrawal with delirium (291.0)*
                schizophrenia (295.0-295.9) and paranoid states (297.0-297.9) taking the form of chronic hallucinosis with clear consciousness in an alcoholic

  CC Excl: See code 291.0

  AHA: 2Q, '91, 11

  DEF: Psychosis lasting less than six months with slight or no clouding of consciousness in which auditory hallucinations predominate.

291.4 Idiosyncratic alcohol intoxication `CC`
  Pathologic: Pathologic:
    alcohol intoxication   drunkenness
  EXCLUDES *acute alcohol intoxication (305.0) in alcoholism (303.0) simple drunkenness (305.0)*

  CC Excl: See code 291.0

  DEF: Unique behavioral patterns, like belligerence, after intake of relatively small amounts of alcohol; behavior not due to excess consumption.

291.5 Alcoholic jealousy
  Alcoholic: Alcoholic:
    paranoia   psychosis, paranoid type
  EXCLUDES *nonalcoholic paranoid states (297.0-297.9)*
                schizophrenia, paranoid type (295.3)

√5th 291.8 Other specified alcoholic psychosis
  AHA: 3Q, '94, 13; J-A, '85, 10

  291.81 Alcohol withdrawal `CC`
    Alcohol:
      abstinence syndrome or symptoms
      withdrawal syndrome or symptoms
    EXCLUDES *alcohol withdrawal: delirium (291.0) hallucinosis (291.3) delirium tremens (291.0)*

    CC Excl: 291.0-291.9, 292.0-292.9, 293.0-293.9, 294.0-294.9, 303.00-303.93, 304.00-304.93, 305.00-305.03, 305.20-305.93, 790.3

    AHA: 4Q, '96, 28; 2Q, '91, 11

  291.89 Other `CC`
    CC Excl: See code 291.81

291.9 Unspecified alcoholic psychosis `CC`
  Alcoholic: Alcoholism (chronic) with
    mania NOS   psychosis
    psychosis NOS
  CC Excl: See code 291.0

√4th 292 Drug psychoses
  INCLUDES drug-induced mental disorders
              organic brain syndrome associated with consumption of drugs
  Use additional code for any associated drug dependence (304.0-304.9)
  Use additional E code to identify drug
  AHA: 2Q, '91, 11; S-O, '86, 3

  292.0 Drug withdrawal syndrome `CC`
    Drug:
      abstinence syndrome or symptoms
      withdrawal syndrome or symptoms
    CC Excl: See code 291.0

    AHA: 1Q, '97, 12

  √5th 292.1 Paranoid and/or hallucinatory states induced by drugs

    292.11 Drug-induced organic delusional syndrome `CC`
      Paranoid state induced by drugs
      CC Excl: See code 291.0

    292.12 Drug-induced hallucinosis `CC`
      Hallucinatory state induced by drugs
      EXCLUDES *states following LSD or other hallucinogens, lasting only a few days or less ["bad trips"] (305.3)*

      CC Excl: See code 291.0

  292.2 Pathological drug intoxication `CC`
    Drug reaction: ⎫
      NOS   ⎬ resulting in brief
      idiosyncratic   ⎪ psychotic
      pathologic   ⎭ states
    EXCLUDES *expected brief psychotic reactions to hallucinogens ["bad trips"] (305.3)*
                  physiological side-effects of drugs (e.g., dystonias)

    CC Excl: See code 291.0

  √5th 292.8 Other specified drug-induced mental disorders
    292.81 Drug-induced delirium `CC`
      CC Excl: See code 291.0

      AHA: 1Q, '88, 3

    292.82 Drug-induced dementia `CC`
      CC Excl: See code 291.0

    292.83 Drug-induced amnestic syndrome `CC`
      CC Excl: See code 291.0

    292.84 Drug-induced organic affective syndrome `CC`
      Depressive state induced by drugs
      CC Excl: See code 291.0

    292.89 Other `CC`
      Drug-induced organic personality syndrome
      CC Excl: See code 291.0

  292.9 Unspecified drug-induced mental disorder `CC`
    Organic psychosis NOS due to or associated with drugs
    CC Excl: See code 291.0

N Newborn Age: 0   **P** Pediatric Age: 0-17   **M** Maternity Age: 12-55   **A** Adult Age: 15-124   **CC** CC Condition   **MC** Major Complication   **CD** Complex Dx   **HIV** HIV Related Dx

2002 Ingenix, Inc.

√4th **293 Transient organic psychotic conditions**

     INCLUDES   transient organic mental disorders not associated with alcohol or drugs

Code first the associated physical or neurological condition

     EXCLUDES   *confusional state or delirium superimposed on senile dementia (290.3)*
dementia due to:
alcohol (291.0-291.9)
arteriosclerosis (290.40-290.43)
drugs (292.82)
senility (290.0)

293.0 Acute delirium
Acute:
confusional state
infective psychosis
organic reaction
posttraumatic organic psychosis
psycho-organic syndrome
Acute psychosis associated with endocrine, metabolic, or cerebrovascular disorder
Epileptic:
confusional state
twilight state

AHA: 1Q, '88, 3

293.1 Subacute delirium
Subacute:
confusional state
infective psychosis
organic reaction
posttraumatic organic psychosis
psycho-organic syndrome
psychosis associated with endocrine or metabolic disorder

AHA: 1Q, '88, 3

√5th **293.8 Other specified transient organic mental disorders**

    293.81 Organic delusional syndrome   CC
Transient organic psychotic condition, paranoid type

CC Excl: 291.0-291.7, 291.81, 291.89, 291.9, 292.0-292.9, 293.0, 293.9, 294.0-294.9, 303.00-303.93, 304.00-304.93, 305.00-305.03, 305.20-305.93, 790.3

    293.82 Organic hallucinosis syndrome   CC
Transient organic psychotic condition, hallucinatory type

CC Excl: See code 293.81

    293.83 Organic affective syndrome   CC
Transient organic psychotic condition, depressive type

CC Excl: See code 293.81

    293.84 Organic anxiety syndrome   CC
CC Excl: See code 293.81

      AHA: 4Q, '96, 29

    293.89 Other

293.9 Unspecified transient organic mental disorder
Organic psychosis: Organic psychosis:
infective NOS   transient NOS
posttraumatic NOS   Psycho-organic syndrome

√4th **294 Other organic psychotic conditions (chronic)**

     INCLUDES   organic psychotic brain syndromes (chronic), not elsewhere classified

AHA: M-A, '85, 12

294.0 Amnestic syndrome
Korsakoff's psychosis or syndrome (nonalcoholic)

     EXCLUDES   *alcoholic:*
amnestic syndrome (291.1)
Korsakoff's psychosis (291.1)

√5th **294.1 Dementia in conditions classified elsewhere**
Code first any underlying physical condition, as:
dementia in:
Alzheimer's disease (331.0)
cerebral lipidoses (330.1)
epilepsy (345.0-345.9)
general paresis [syphilis] (094.1)
hepatolenticular degeneration (275.1)
Huntington's chorea (333.4)
Jakob-Creutzfeldt disease (046.1)
multiple sclerosis (340)
Pick's disease of the brain (331.1)
polyarteritis nodosa (446.0)
syphilis (094.1)

     EXCLUDES   *dementia:*
arteriosclerotic (290.40-290.43)
presenile (290.10-290.13)
senile (290.0)
epileptic psychosis NOS (294.8)

AHA: 4Q, '00, 40; 1Q, '99, 14; N-D, '85, 5

    294.10 *Dementia in conditions classified elsewhere without behavioral disturbance*
Dementia in conditions classified elsewhere NOS

    294.11 *Dementia in conditions classified elsewhere with behavioral disturbance*
Aggressive behavior
Combative behavior
Violent behavior
Wandering off

AHA: 4Q, '00, 41

294.8 Other specified organic brain syndromes (chronic)
Epileptic psychosis NOS
Mixed paranoid and affective organic psychotic states
Use additional code for associated epilepsy (345.0-345.9)

     EXCLUDES   *mild memory disturbances, not amounting to dementia (310.1)*

AHA: 1Q, '88, 5

294.9 Unspecified organic brain syndrome (chronic)   HIV
Organic psychosis (chronic)

OTHER PSYCHOSES (295-299)

Use additional code to identify any associated physical disease, injury, or condition affecting the brain with psychoses classifiable to 295-298

√4th **295 Schizophrenic disorders**

     INCLUDES   schizophrenia of the types described in 295.0-295.9 occurring in children

     EXCLUDES   *childhood type schizophrenia (299.9)*
infantile autism (299.0)

The following fifth-digit subclassification is for use with category 295:

    0   unspecified
    1   subchronic
    2   chronic
    3   subchronic with acute exacerbation
    4   chronic with acute exacerbation
    5   in remission

DEF: Group of disorders with disturbances in thought (delusions, hallucinations), mood (blunted, flattened, inappropriate affect), sense of self, relationship to world; also bizarre, purposeless behavior, repetitious activity, or inactivity.

Mental Disorders 293-295

√4th √5th Additional Digit Required   Nonspecific PDx   Unacceptable PDx   Manifestation Code   **MSP** Medicare Secondary Payer   ◄► Revised Text   ● New Code   ▲ Revised Code Title

2002 Ingenix, Inc.   **Volume 1 — 69**

Mental Disorders 295.0–296.2

§ ✓5ᵗʰ **295.0 Simple type**   CC 0-4
Schizophrenia simplex
EXCLUDES   *latent schizophrenia (295.5)*
CC Excl: For codes 295.00-295.04: 295.00-295.95, 296.00-296.99, 297.0-297.9, 298.0-298.9, 299.00-299.91, 300.00-300.9, 301.0-301.9, 306.0-306.9, 307.0-307.9, 308.0-308.9, 309.0-309.9, 310.0-310.9, 311, 312.00-312.9, 313.0-313.9, 314.00-314.9, 315.00-315.9, 316-317, 318.0-318.2, 319

§ ✓5ᵗʰ **295.1 Disorganized type**   CC 0-4
Hebephrenia
Hebephrenic type schizophrenia
CC Excl: For codes 295.10-295.14: See code 295.0

DEF: Inappropriate behavior; results in extreme incoherence and disorganization of time, place and sense of social appropriateness; withdrawal from routine social interaction may occur.

§ ✓5ᵗʰ **295.2 Catatonic type**   CC 1-4
Catatonic (schizophrenia):   Schizophrenic:
  agitation   catalepsy
  excitation   catatonia
  excited type   flexibilitas cerea
  stupor
  withdrawn type
CC Excl: For codes 295.21-295.24: See code 295.0

DEF: Extreme changes in motor activity; one extreme is decreased response or reaction to the environment and the other is spontaneous activity.

§ ✓5ᵗʰ **295.3 Paranoid type**   CC 0-4
Paraphrenic schizophrenia
EXCLUDES   *involutional paranoid state (297.2)*
       paranoia (297.1)
       paraphrenia (297.2)
CC Excl: For codes 295.30–295.34: See code 295.0

DEF: Preoccupied with delusional suspicions and auditory hallucinations related to single theme; usually hostile, grandiose, overly religious, occasionally hypochondriacal.

§ ✓5ᵗʰ **295.4 Acute schizophrenic episode**   CC 0-4
Oneirophrenia   Schizophreniform:
Schizophreniform: disorder
  attack   psychosis, confusional type
EXCLUDES   *acute forms of schizophrenia of:*
     catatonic type (295.2)
     hebephrenic type (295.1)
     paranoid type (295.3)
     simple type (295.0)
     undifferentiated type (295.8)
CC Excl: For codes 295.40-295.44: See code 295.0

§ ✓5ᵗʰ **295.5 Latent schizophrenia**
Latent schizophrenic reaction
Schizophrenia:
  borderline
  incipient
  prepsychotic
  prodromal
  pseudoneurotic
  pseudopsychopathic
EXCLUDES   *schizoid personality (301.20-301.22)*

§ ✓5ᵗʰ **295.6 Residual schizophrenia**   CC 0-4
Chronic undifferentiated schizophrenia
Restzustand (schizophrenic)
Schizophrenic residual state
CC Excl: For codes 295.60-295.64: See code 295.0

§ ✓5ᵗʰ **295.7 Schizo-affective type**   CC 0-4
Cyclic schizophrenia
Mixed schizophrenic and affective psychosis
Schizo-affective psychosis
Schizophreniform psychosis, affective type
CC Excl: For codes 295.70-295.74: See code 295.0

§ ✓5ᵗʰ **295.8 Other specified types of schizophrenia**   CC 0-4
Acute (undifferentiated) schizophrenia
Atypical schizophrenia
Cenesthopathic schizophrenia
EXCLUDES   *infantile autism (299.0)*
CC Excl: For codes 295.80-295.84: See code 295.0

§ ✓5ᵗʰ **295.9 Unspecified schizophrenia**   CC 0-4
Schizophrenia:
  NOS
  mixed NOS
  undifferentiated NOS
Schizophrenic reaction NOS
Schizophreniform psychosis NOS
CC Excl: For codes 295.90-295.94: See code 295.0

AHA: 3Q, '95, 6

DRG 430 For code 295.90

✓4ᵗʰ **296 Affective psychoses**
INCLUDES   episodic affective disorders
EXCLUDES   *neurotic depression (300.4)*
     reactive depressive psychosis (298.0)
     reactive excitation (298.1)

The following fifth-digit subclassification is for use with categories 296.0-296.6:
  0 unspecified
  1 mild
  2 moderate
  3 severe, without mention of psychotic behavior
  4 severe, specified as with psychotic behavior
  5 in partial or unspecified remission
  6 in full remission

AHA: M-A, '85, 14

✓5ᵗʰ **296.0 Manic disorder, single episode**   CC 4
Hypomania (mild) NOS
Hypomanic psychosis
Mania (monopolar) NOS
Manic-depressive psychosis   } single episode or
  or reaction: unspecified
  hypomanic
  manic
EXCLUDES   *circular type, if there was a previous attack of depression (296.4)*
CC Excl: For code 296.04: See code 295.0

DEF: Mood disorder identified by hyperactivity; may show extreme agitation or exaggerated excitability; speech and thought processes may be accelerated.

✓5ᵗʰ **296.1 Manic disorder, recurrent episode**   CC 4
Any condition classifiable to 296.0, stated to be recurrent
EXCLUDES   *circular type, if there was a previous attack of depression (296.4)*
CC Excl: For code 296.14: See code 295.0

✓5ᵗʰ **296.2 Major depressive disorder, single episode**
Depressive psychosis
Endogenous depression
Involutional melancholia
Manic-depressive psychosis or } single episode or
  reaction, depressed type   unspecified
Monopolar depression
Psychotic depression
EXCLUDES   *circular type, if previous attack was of manic type (296.5)*
     depression NOS (311)
     reactive depression (neurotic) (300.4)
     psychotic (298.0)
DRG 430 For code 296.20

DEF: Mood disorder that produces depression; may exhibit as sadness, low self-esteem, or guilt feelings; other manifestations may be withdrawal from friends and family; interrupted sleep.

§   Requires fifth-digit. See category 295 for codes and definitions.

N Newborn Age: 0   P Pediatric Age: 0-17   M Maternity Age: 12-55   A Adult Age: 15-124   CC CC Condition   MC Major Complication   CD Complex Dx   HIV HIV Related Dx

§ ✓5th **296.3 Major depressive disorder, recurrent episode** CC 4
Any condition classifiable to 296.2, stated to be recurrent
    EXCLUDES   *circular type, if previous attack was of manic type (296.5)*
           depression NOS (311)
           reactive depression (neurotic) (300.4)
           psychotic (298.0)

CC Excl: For code 296.34: See code 295.0

▽ DRG 430 For code 296.30, 296.33 and 296.34

§ ✓5th **296.4 Bipolar affective disorder, manic** CC 4
Bipolar disorder, now manic
Manic-depressive psychosis, circular type but currently manic
    EXCLUDES   *brief compensatory or rebound mood swings (296.99)*

CC Excl: For code 296.44: See code 295.0

§ ✓5th **296.5 Bipolar affective disorder, depressed** CC 4
Bipolar disorder, now depressed
Manic-depressive psychosis, circular type but currently depressed
    EXCLUDES   *brief compensatory or rebound mood swings (296.99)*

CC Excl: For code 296.54: See code 295.0

§ ✓5th **296.6 Bipolar affective disorder, mixed** CC 4
Manic-depressive psychosis, circular type, mixed

CC Excl: For code 296.64: See code 295.0

296.7 Bipolar affective disorder, unspecified
Atypical bipolar affective disorder NOS
Manic-depressive psychosis, circular type, current condition not specified as either manic or depressive

DEF: Manic-depressive disorder referred to as bipolar because of the mood range from manic to depressive.

✓5th **296.8 Manic-depressive psychosis, other and unspecified**
    296.80 Manic-depressive psychosis, unspecified
         Manic-depressive:
           reaction NOS
           syndrome NOS
    296.81 Atypical manic disorder
    296.82 Atypical depressive disorder
    296.89 Other
         Manic-depressive psychosis, mixed type

✓5th **296.9 Other and unspecified affective psychoses**
    EXCLUDES   *psychogenic affective psychoses (298.0-298.8)*

    296.90 Unspecified affective psychosis
         Affective psychosis NOS
         Melancholia NOS

         AHA: M-A, '85, 14

    296.99 Other specified affective psychoses
         Mood swings: Mood swings:
           brief compensatory   rebound

✓4th **297 Paranoid states (Delusional disorders)**
    INCLUDES   paranoid disorders
    EXCLUDES   *acute paranoid reaction (298.3)*
           alcoholic jealousy or paranoid state (291.5)
           paranoid schizophrenia (295.3)

297.0 Paranoid state, simple
297.1 Paranoia
     Chronic paranoid psychosis
     Sander's disease
     Systematized delusions
    EXCLUDES   *paranoid personality disorder (301.0)*

297.2 Paraphrenia
     Involutional paranoid state
     Late paraphrenia
     Paraphrenia (involutional)

DEF: Paranoid schizophrenic disorder that persists over a prolonged period but does not distort personality despite persistent delusions.

297.3 Shared paranoid disorder
     Folie à deux
     Induced psychosis or paranoid disorder

DEF: Mental disorder two people share; first person with the delusional disorder convinces second person because of a close relationship and shared experiences to accept the delusions.

297.8 Other specified paranoid states
     Paranoia querulans
     Sensitiver Beziehungswahn
    EXCLUDES   *acute paranoid reaction or state (298.3)*
           senile paranoid state (290.20)

297.9 Unspecified paranoid state
     Paranoid: Paranoid:
       disorder NOS   reaction NOS
       psychosis NOS   state NOS

     AHA: J-A, '85, 9

✓4th **298 Other nonorganic psychoses**
    INCLUDES   psychotic conditions due to or provoked by:
           emotional stress
           environmental factors as major part of etiology

298.0 Depressive type psychosis CC
     Psychogenic depressive psychosis
     Psychotic reactive depression
     Reactive depressive psychosis
    EXCLUDES   *manic-depressive psychosis, depressed type (296.2-296.3)*
           neurotic depression (300.4)
           reactive depression NOS (300.4)

CC Excl: See code 295.0

298.1 Excitative type psychosis
     Acute hysterical psychosis   Reactive excitation
     Psychogenic excitation
    EXCLUDES   *manic-depressive psychosis, manic type (296.0-296.1)*

DEF: Affective disorder similar to manic-depressive psychosis, in the manic phase, seemingly brought on by stress.

298.2 Reactive confusion
     Psychogenic confusion   Psychogenic twilight state
    EXCLUDES   *acute confusional state (293.0)*

DEF: Confusion, disorientation, cloudiness in consciousness; brought on by severe emotional upheaval.

298.3 Acute paranoid reaction CC
     Acute psychogenic paranoid psychosis
     Bouffée délirante
    EXCLUDES   *paranoid states (297.0-297.9)*

CC Excl: See code 295.0

298.4 Psychogenic paranoid psychosis CC
     Protracted reactive paranoid psychosis

CC Excl: See code 295.0

298.8 Other and unspecified reactive psychosis
     Brief reactive psychosis NOS
     Hysterical psychosis
     Psychogenic psychosis NOS
     Psychogenic stupor
    EXCLUDES   *acute hysterical psychosis (298.1)*

298.9 Unspecified psychosis HIV
     Atypical psychosis
     Psychosis NOS
    ▽ DRG 430

---

§ Requires fifth-digit. See category 296 for codes and definitions.

Additional Digit Required   Nonspecific PDx   Unacceptable PDx   Manifestation Code   MSP Medicare Secondary Payer   ▶◀ Revised Text   ● New Code   ▲ Revised Code Title

Mental Disorders 299–300.20

√4th **299 Psychoses with origin specific to childhood**

INCLUDES   pervasive developmental disorders

EXCLUDES   *adult type psychoses occurring in childhood, as:*
affective disorders (296.0-296.9)
manic-depressive disorders (296.0-296.9)
schizophrenia (295.0-295.9)

The following fifth-digit subclassification is for use with category 299:

     0   current or active state
     1   residual state

√5th **299.0 Infantile autism**   CC 0
    Childhood autism   Kanner's syndrome
    Infantile psychosis

EXCLUDES   *disintegrative psychosis (299.1)*
Heller's syndrome (299.1)
schizophrenic syndrome of childhood (299.9)

CC Excl: For code **299.00**: See code 295.0

DEF: Severe mental disorder of children, results in impaired social behavior; abnormal development of communicative skills, appears to be unaware of the need for emotional support and offers little emotional response to family members.

√5th **299.1 Disintegrative psychosis**   CC 0
    Heller's syndrome
    Use additional code to identify any associated neurological disorder

EXCLUDES   *infantile autism (299.0)*
schizophrenic syndrome of childhood (299.9)

CC Excl: For code **299.10**: See code 295.0

DEF: Mental disease of children identified by impaired development of reciprocal social skills, verbal and nonverbal communication skills, imaginative play.

√5th **299.8 Other specified early childhood psychoses**   CC 0
    Atypical childhood psychosis
    Borderline psychosis of childhood

EXCLUDES   *simple stereotypes without psychotic disturbance (307.3)*

CC Excl: For code **299.80**: See code 295.0

√5th **299.9 Unspecified**   CC 0
    Child psychosis NOS
    Schizophrenia, childhood type NOS
    Schizophrenic syndrome of childhood NOS

EXCLUDES   *schizophrenia of adult type occurring in childhood (295.0-295.9)*

CC Excl: For code **299.90**: See code 295.0

NEUROTIC DISORDERS, PERSONALITY DISORDERS, AND OTHER NONPSYCHOTIC MENTAL DISORDERS (300-316)

√4th **300 Neurotic disorders**

√5th **300.0 Anxiety states**

EXCLUDES   *anxiety in:*
acute stress reaction (308.0)
transient adjustment reaction (309.24)
neurasthenia (300.5)
psychophysiological disorders (306.0-306.9)
separation anxiety (309.21)

DEF: Mental disorder characterized by anxiety and avoidance behavior not particularly related to any specific situation or stimulus; symptoms include emotional instability, apprehension, fatigue.

300.00 Anxiety state, unspecified
   Anxiety: Anxiety:
     neurosis   state (neurotic)
     reaction   Atypical anxiety disorder

AHA: ▶1Q, '02, 6◀

300.01 Panic disorder
   Panic: Panic:
     attack   state

DEF: Neurotic disorder characterized by recurrent panic or anxiety, apprehension, fear or terror; symptoms include shortness of breath, palpitations, dizziness, faintness or shakiness; fear of dying may persist or fear of other morbid consequences.

300.02 Generalized anxiety disorder

300.09 Other

√5th **300.1 Hysteria**

EXCLUDES   *adjustment reaction (309.0-309.9)*
anorexia nervosa (307.1)
gross stress reaction (308.0-308.9)
hysterical personality (301.50-301.59)
psychophysiologic disorders (306.0-306.9)

300.10 Hysteria, unspecified

300.11 Conversion disorder
   Astasia-abasia,   Hysterical
     hysterical   blindness
   Conversion hysteria   deafness
     or reaction   paralysis

AHA: N-D, '85, 15

DEF: Mental disorder that impairs physical functions with no physiological basis; sensory motor symptoms include seizures, paralysis, temporary blindness; increase in stress or avoidance of unpleasant responsibilities may precipitate.

300.12 Psychogenic amnesia
   Hysterical amnesia

300.13 Psychogenic fugue
   Hysterical fugue

DEF: Dissociative hysteria; identified by loss of memory, flight from familiar surroundings; conscious activity is not associated with perception of surroundings, no later memory of episode.

300.14 Multiple personality
   Dissociative identity disorder

300.15 Dissociative disorder or reaction, unspecified

DEF: Hysterical neurotic episode; sudden but temporary changes in perceived identity, memory, consciousness, segregated memory patterns exist separate from dominant personality.

300.16 Factitious illness with psychological symptoms
   Compensation neurosis
   Ganser's syndrome, hysterical

DEF: A disorder characterized by the purposeful assumption of mental illness symptoms; the symptoms are not real, possibly representing what the patient imagines mental illness to be like, and are acted out more often when another person is present.

300.19 Other and unspecified factitious illness
   Factitious illness (with physical symptoms) NOS

EXCLUDES   *multiple operations or hospital addiction syndrome (301.51)*

√5th **300.2 Phobic disorders**

EXCLUDES   *anxiety state not associated with a specific situation or object (300.00-300.09)*
obsessional phobias (300.3)

300.20 Phobia, unspecified
   Anxiety-hysteria NOS
   Phobia NOS

N Newborn Age: 0   P Pediatric Age: 0-17   M Maternity Age: 12-55   A Adult Age: 15-124   CC CC Condition   MC Major Complication   CD Complex Dx   HIV HIV Related Dx

72 — Volume 1 • October 2002   *2002 Ingenix, Inc.*

300.21 Agoraphobia with panic attacks
Fear of:
open spaces
streets } with panic attacks
travel

300.22 Agoraphobia without mention of panic attacks
Any condition classifiable to 300.21 without mention of panic attacks

300.23 Social phobia
Fear of: Fear of:
eating in public   washing in public
public speaking

300.29 Other isolated or simple phobias
Acrophobia   Claustrophobia
Animal phobias   Fear of crowds

300.3 Obsessive-compulsive disorders
Anancastic neurosis   Obsessional phobia [any]
Compulsive neurosis
EXCLUDES *obsessive-compulsive symptoms occurring in:*
endogenous depression (296.2-296.3)
organic states (eg., encephalitis)
schizophrenia (295.0-295.9)

300.4 Neurotic depression
Anxiety depression   Dysthymic disorder
Depression with anxiety Neurotic depressive state
Depressive reaction   Reactive depression
EXCLUDES *adjustment reaction with depressive symptoms (309.0-309.1)*
depression NOS (311)
manic-depressive psychosis, depressed type (296.2-296.3)
reactive depressive psychosis (298.0)

DEF: Depression without psychosis; less severe depression related to personal change or unexpected circumstances; also referred to as "reactional depression."

300.5 Neurasthenia
Fatigue neurosis   Psychogenic:
Nervous debility   general fatigue
Psychogenic:
asthenia
Use additional code to identify any associated physical disorder
EXCLUDES *anxiety state (300.00-300.09)*
neurotic depression (300.4)
psychophysiological disorders (306.0-306.9)
specific nonpsychotic mental disorders following organic brain damage (310.0-310.9)

DEF: Physical and mental symptoms caused primarily by what is known as mental exhaustion; symptoms include chronic weakness, fatigue.

300.6 Depersonalization syndrome
Depersonalization disorder
Derealization (neurotic)
Neurotic state with depersonalization episode
EXCLUDES *depersonalization associated with:*
anxiety (300.00-300.09)
depression (300.4)
manic-depressive disorder or psychosis (296.0-296.9)
schizophrenia (295.0-295.9)

DEF: Dissociative disorder characterized by feelings of strangeness about self or body image; symptoms include dizziness, anxiety, fear of insanity, loss of reality of surroundings.

300.7 Hypochondriasis
Body dysmorphic disorder
EXCLUDES *hypochondriasis in:*
hysteria (300.10-300.19)
manic-depressive psychosis, depressed type (296.2-296.3)
neurasthenia (300.5)
obsessional disorder (300.3)
schizophrenia (295.0-295.9)

√5th **300.8 Other neurotic disorders**
300.81 Somatization disorder
Briquet's disorder
Severe somatoform disorder

300.82 Undifferentiated somatoform disorder
Atypical somatoform disorder
Somatoform disorder NOS
AHA: 4Q, '96, 29
DEF: Disorders in which patients have symptoms that suggest an organic disease but no evidence of physical disorder after repeated testing.

300.89 Other
Occupational neurosis, including writers' cramp
Psychasthenia
Psychasthenic neurosis

300.9 Unspecified neurotic disorder
Neurosis NOS   Psychoneurosis NOS

√4th **301 Personality disorders**
INCLUDES character neurosis
Use additional code to identify any associated neurosis or psychosis, or physical condition
EXCLUDES *nonpsychotic personality disorder associated with organic brain syndromes (310.0-310.9)*

301.0 Paranoid personality disorder
Fanatic personality
Paranoid personality (disorder)
Paranoid traits
EXCLUDES *acute paranoid reaction (298.3)*
alcoholic paranoia (291.5)
paranoid schizophrenia (295.3)
paranoid states (297.0-297.9)
AHA: J-A, '85, 9

√5th **301.1 Affective personality disorder**
EXCLUDES *affective psychotic disorders (296.0-296.9)*
neurasthenia (300.5)
neurotic depression (300.4)
301.10 Affective personality disorder, unspecified
301.11 Chronic hypomanic personality disorder
Chronic hypomanic disorder
Hypomanic personality
301.12 Chronic depressive personality disorder
Chronic depressive disorder
Depressive character or personality
301.13 Cyclothymic disorder
Cycloid personality
Cyclothymia
Cyclothymic personality

√5th **301.2 Schizoid personality disorder**
EXCLUDES *schizophrenia (295.0-295.9)*
301.20 Schizoid personality disorder, unspecified
301.21 Introverted personality
301.22 Schizotypal personality

301.3 Explosive personality disorder
Aggressive: Emotional instability
personality   (excessive)
reaction   Pathological emotionality
Aggressiveness   Quarrelsomeness
EXCLUDES *dyssocial personality (301.7)*
hysterical neurosis (300.10-300.19)

√4th √5th Additional Digit Required   Nonspecific PDx   Unacceptable PDx   Manifestation Code   MSP Medicare Secondary Payer   ◄► Revised Text   ● New Code   ▲ Revised Code Title

2002 Ingenix, Inc.   Volume 1 — 73

301.4 Compulsive personality disorder
Anancastic personality
Obsessional personality
EXCLUDES *obsessive-compulsive disorder (300.3)*
phobic state (300.20-300.29)

√5th **301.5 Histrionic personality disorder**
EXCLUDES *hysterical neurosis (300.10-300.19)*
DEF: Extreme emotional behavior, often theatrical; often concerned about own appeal; may demand attention, exhibit seductive behavior.

301.50 Histrionic personality disorder, unspecified
Hysterical personality NOS

301.51 Chronic factitious illness with physical symptoms
Hospital addiction syndrome
Multiple operations syndrome
Munchausen syndrome

301.59 Other histrionic personality disorder
Personality: Personality:
emotionally unstable   psychoinfantile
labile

301.6 Dependent personality disorder
Asthenic personality
Inadequate personality
Passive personality
EXCLUDES *neurasthenia (300.5)*
passive-aggressive personality (301.84)
DEF: Overwhelming feeling of helplessness; fears of abandonment may persist; difficulty in making personal decisions without confirmation by others; low self-esteem due to irrational sensitivity to criticism.

301.7 Antisocial personality disorder
Amoral personality
Asocial personality
Dyssocial personality
Personality disorder with predominantly sociopathic or asocial manifestation
EXCLUDES *disturbance of conduct without specifiable personality disorder (312.0-312.9)*
explosive personality (301.3)
AHA: S-O, '84, 16
DEF: Continuous antisocial behavior that violates rights of others; social traits include extreme aggression, total disregard for traditional social rules.

√5th **301.8 Other personality disorders**
301.81 Narcissistic personality
DEF: Grandiose fantasy or behavior, lack of social empathy, hypersensitive to the lack of others' judgment, exploits others; also sense of entitlement to have expectations met, need for continual admiration.

301.82 Avoidant personality
DEF: Personality disorder marked by feelings of social inferiority; sensitivity to criticism, emotionally restrained due to fear of rejection.

301.83 Borderline personality
DEF: Personality disorder characterized by unstable moods, self-image, and interpersonal relationships; uncontrolled anger, impulsive and self-destructive acts, fears of abandonment, feelings of emptiness and boredom, recurrent suicide threats or self-mutilation.

301.84 Passive-aggressive personality
DEF: Pattern of procrastination and refusal to meet standards; introduce own obstacles to success and exploit failure.

301.89 Other
Personality: Personality:
eccentric   masochistic
"haltlose" type   psychoneurotic
immature
EXCLUDES *psychoinfantile personality (301.59)*

301.9 Unspecified personality disorder
Pathological personality NOS
Personality disorder NOS
Psychopathic:
constitutional state
personality (disorder)

√4th **302 Sexual deviations and disorders**
EXCLUDES *sexual disorder manifest in:*
organic brain syndrome (290.0-294.9, 310.0-310.9)
psychosis (295.0-298.9)

302.0 Ego-dystonic homosexuality
Ego-dystonic lesbianism
Homosexual conflict disorder
EXCLUDES *homosexual pedophilia (302.2)*

302.1 Zoophilia
Bestiality
DEF: A sociodeviant disorder marked by engaging in sexual intercourse with animals.

302.2 Pedophilia
DEF: A sociodeviant condition of adults characterized by sexual activity with children.

302.3 Transvestism
EXCLUDES *trans-sexualism (302.5)*
DEF: The desire to dress in clothing of opposite sex.

302.4 Exhibitionism
DEF: Sexual deviant behavior; exposure of genitals to strangers; behavior prompted by intense sexual urges and fantasies.

√5th **302.5 Trans-sexualism**
EXCLUDES *transvestism (302.3)*
DEF: Gender identity disturbance; overwhelming desire to change anatomic sex, due to belief that individual is a member of the opposite sex.

302.50 With unspecified sexual history
302.51 With asexual history
302.52 With homosexual history
302.53 With heterosexual history

302.6 Disorders of psychosexual identity
Feminism in boys
Gender identity disorder of childhood
EXCLUDES *gender identity disorder in adult (302.85)*
homosexuality (302.0)
trans-sexualism (302.50-302.53)
transvestism (302.3)

√5th **302.7 Psychosexual dysfunction**
EXCLUDES *impotence of organic origin (607.84)*
normal transient symptoms from ruptured hymen
transient or occasional failures of erection due to fatigue, anxiety, alcohol, or drugs

302.70 Psychosexual dysfunction, unspecified
302.71 With inhibited sexual desire
302.72 With inhibited sexual excitement
Frigidity   Impotence
302.73 With inhibited female orgasm ♀
302.74 With inhibited male orgasm ♂
302.75 With premature ejaculation ♂

N Newborn Age: 0   P Pediatric Age: 0-17   M Maternity Age: 12-55   A Adult Age: 15-124   CC CC Condition   MC Major Complication   CD Complex Dx   HIV HIV Related Dx

74 — Volume 1   2002 Ingenix, Inc.

302.76 With functional dyspareunia ♀

Dyspareunia, psychogenic

DEF: Difficult or painful sex due to psychosomatic state.

302.79 With other specified psychosexual dysfunctions

√5th **302.8 Other specified psychosexual disorders**

302.81 Fetishism

DEF: Psychosexual disorder noted for intense sexual urges and arousal precipitated by fantasies; use of inanimate objects, such as clothing, to stimulate sexual arousal, orgasm.

302.82 Voyeurism

DEF: Psychosexual disorder characterized by uncontrollable impulse to observe others, without their knowledge, who are nude or engaged in sexual activity.

302.83 Sexual masochism

DEF: Psychosexual disorder noted for need to achieve sexual gratification through humiliating or hurtful acts inflicted on self.

302.84 Sexual sadism

DEF: Psychosexual disorder noted for need to achieve sexual gratification through humiliating or hurtful acts inflicted on someone else.

302.85 Gender identity disorder of adolescent or adult life

302.89 Other

Nymphomania   Satyriasis

302.9 Unspecified psychosexual disorder

Pathologic sexuality NOS

Sexual deviation NOS

√4th **303 Alcohol dependence syndrome**

Use additional code to identify any associated condition, as:

alcoholic psychoses (291.0-291.9)

drug dependence (304.0-304.9)

physical complications of alcohol, such as:

cerebral degeneration (331.7)

cirrhosis of liver (571.2)

epilepsy (345.0-345.9)

gastritis (535.3)

hepatitis (571.1)

liver damage NOS (571.3)

EXCLUDES *drunkenness NOS (305.0)*

The following fifth-digit subclassification is for use with category 303:

0 unspecified

1 continuous

2 episodic

3 in remission

AHA: 3Q, '95, 6; 2Q, '91, 9; 4Q, '88, 8; S-O, '86, 3

√5th **303.0 Acute alcoholic intoxication** CC 0-2

Acute drunkenness in alcoholism

CC Excl: For codes 303.00-303.02: 291.0-291.9, 292.0-292.9, 303.00-303.93, 304.00-304.91, 305.00-305.03, 305.20-305.93, 790.3

√5th **303.9 Other and unspecified alcohol dependence** CC 0-2

Chronic alcoholism   Dipsomania

CC Excl: For codes 303.90-303.92: See code 303.0

AHA: 2Q, '89, 9

√4th **304 Drug dependence**

EXCLUDES *nondependent abuse of drugs (305.1-305.9)*

The following fifth-digit subclassification is for use with category 304:

0 unspecified

1 continuous

2 episodic

3 in remission

AHA: 2Q, '91, 10; 4Q, '88, 8; S-O, '86, 3

√5th **304.0 Opioid type dependence** CC 0-2

Heroin

Meperidine

Methadone

Morphine

Opium

Opium alkaloids and their derivatives

Synthetics with morphine-like effects

CC Excl: For codes 304.00-304.02: See code 303.0

√5th **304.1 Barbiturate and similarly acting sedative or hypnotic dependence** CC 0-2

Barbiturates

Nonbarbiturate sedatives and tranquilizers with a similar effect:

chlordiazepoxide

diazepam

glutethimide

meprobamate

methaqualone

CC Excl: For codes 304.10-304.12: See code 303.0

√5th **304.2 Cocaine dependence** CC 0-2

Coca leaves and derivatives

CC Excl: For codes 304.20-304.22: See code 303.0

√5th **304.3 Cannabis dependence**

Hashish   Marihuana

Hemp

√5th **304.4 Amphetamine and other psychostimulant dependence** CC 0-2

Methylphenidate   Phenmetrazine

CC Excl: For codes 304.40-304.42: See code 303.0

√5th **304.5 Hallucinogen dependence** CC 0-2

Dimethyltryptamine [DMT]

Lysergic acid diethylamide [LSD] and derivatives

Mescaline

Psilocybin

CC Excl: For codes 304.50-304.52: See code 303.0

√5th **304.6 Other specified drug dependence** CC 0-2

Absinthe addiction   Glue sniffing

EXCLUDES *tobacco dependence (305.1)*

CC Excl: For codes 304.60-304.62: See code 303.0

√5th **304.7 Combinations of opioid type drug with any other** CC 0-2

CC Excl: For codes 304.70-304.72: See code 303.0

AHA: M-A, '86, 12

√5th **304.8 Combinations of drug dependence excluding opioid type drug** CC 0-2

CC Excl: For codes 304.80-304.82: See code 303.0

AHA: M-A, '86, 12

√5th **304.9 Unspecified drug dependence** CC 0-2

Drug addiction NOS   Drug dependence NOS

CC Excl: For codes 304.90-304.92: See code 303.0

√4th **305 Nondependent abuse of drugs**

Note: Includes cases where a person, for whom no other diagnosis is possible, has come under medical care because of the maladaptive effect of a drug on which he is not dependent and that he has taken on his own initiative to the detriment of his health or social functioning.

EXCLUDES *alcohol dependence syndrome (303.0-303.9)*
drug dependence (304.0-304.9)
drug withdrawal syndrome (292.0)
poisoning by drugs or medicinal substances (960.0-979.9)

The following fifth-digit subclassification is for use with codes 305.0, 305.2-305.9:

0 unspecified

1 continuous

2 episodic

3 in remission

AHA: 2Q, '91, 10; 4Q, '88, 8; S-O, '86, 3

Mental Disorders 302.76–305

√4th √5th Additional Digit Required   Nonspecific PDx   Unacceptable PDx   Manifestation Code   MSP Medicare Secondary Payer   ◄► Revised Text   ● New Code   ▲ Revised Code Title

2002 Ingenix, Inc.

Volume 1 — 75

Mental Disorders 305.0–306.7

§ ✓5ᵗʰ **305.0 Alcohol abuse**   `CC 0-2`
  Drunkenness NOS
  Excessive drinking of alcohol NOS
  "Hangover" (alcohol)
  Inebriety NOS
    EXCLUDES *acute alcohol intoxication in alcoholism*
      (303.0)
      alcoholic psychoses (291.0-291.9)

  CC Excl: For codes 305.00-305.02: See code 303.0

  AHA: 3Q, '96, 16

305.1 Tobacco use disorder
  Tobacco dependence
    EXCLUDES *history of tobacco use (V15.82)*
  AHA: 2Q, '96, 10; N-D, '84, 12

§ ✓5ᵗʰ **305.2 Cannabis abuse**

§ ✓5ᵗʰ **305.3 Hallucinogen abuse**   `CC 0-2`
  Acute intoxication from hallucinogens ["bad trips"]
  LSD reaction

  CC Excl: For codes 305.30-305.32: See code 303.0

§ ✓5ᵗʰ **305.4 Barbiturate and similarly acting sedative**   `CC 0-2`
  or hypnotic abuse

  CC Excl: For codes 305.40-305.42: See code 303.0

§ ✓5ᵗʰ **305.5 Opioid abuse**   `CC 0-2`

  CC Excl: For codes 305.50-305.52: See code 303.0

§ ✓5ᵗʰ **305.6 Cocaine abuse**   `CC 0-2`

  CC Excl: For codes 305.60-305.62: See code 303.0

  AHA: 1Q, '93, 25

§ ✓5ᵗʰ **305.7 Amphetamine or related acting**   `CC 0-2`
  sympathomimetic abuse

  CC Excl: For codes 305.70-305.72: See code 303.0

§ ✓5ᵗʰ **305.8 Antidepressant type abuse**

§ ✓5ᵗʰ **305.9 Other, mixed, or unspecified drug abuse**   `CC 0-2`
  "Laxative habit"
  Misuse of drugs NOS
  Nonprescribed use of drugs or patent medicinals

  CC Excl: For codes 305.90-305.92: See code 303.0

  AHA: 3Q, '99, 20

✓4ᵗʰ **306 Physiological malfunction arising from mental factors**
    INCLUDES psychogenic:
      physical symptoms   } not involving
      physiological   tissue
        manifestations   damage

    EXCLUDES *hysteria (300.11-300.19)*
      physical symptoms secondary to a psychiatric
        disorder classified elsewhere
      psychic factors associated with physical
        conditions involving tissue damage
        classified elsewhere (316)
      specific nonpsychotic mental disorders following
        organic brain damage (310.0-310.9)

  DEF: Functional disturbances or interruptions due to mental or psychological
  causes; no tissue damage sustained in these conditions.

306.0 Musculoskeletal
  Psychogenic paralysis
  Psychogenic torticollis
    EXCLUDES *Gilles de la Tourette's syndrome*
      (307.23)
      paralysis as hysterical or conversion
        reaction (300.11)
      tics (307.20-307.22)

306.1 Respiratory
  Psychogenic: Psychogenic:
    air hunger   hyperventilation
    cough   yawning
    hiccough
    EXCLUDES *psychogenic asthma (316 and 493.9)*

306.2 Cardiovascular
  Cardiac neurosis
  Cardiovascular neurosis
  Neurocirculatory asthenia
  Psychogenic cardiovascular disorder
    EXCLUDES *psychogenic paroxysmal tachycardia*
      (316 and 427.2)

  AHA: J-A, '85, 14

  DEF: Neurocirculatory asthenia: functional nervous and circulatory
  irregularities with palpitations, dyspnea, fatigue, rapid pulse,
  precordial pain, fear of effort, discomfort during exercise, anxiety;
  also called DaCosta's syndrome, Effort syndrome, Irritable or
  Soldier's Heart.

306.3 Skin
  Psychogenic pruritus
    EXCLUDES *psychogenic:*
      alopecia (316 and 704.00)
      dermatitis (316 and 692.9)
      eczema (316 and 691.8 or 692.9)
      urticaria (316 and 708.0-708.9)

306.4 Gastrointestinal
  Aerophagy
  Cyclical vomiting, psychogenic
  Diarrhea, psychogenic
  Nervous gastritis
  Psychogenic dyspepsia
    EXCLUDES *cyclical vomiting NOS (536.2)*
      globus hystericus (300.11)
      mucous colitis (316 and 564.9)
      psychogenic:
        cardiospasm (316 and 530.0)
        duodenal ulcer (316 and 532.0-
          532.9)
        gastric ulcer (316 and 531.0-531.9)
        peptic ulcer NOS (316 and 533.0-
          533.9)
        vomiting NOS (307.54)

  AHA: 2Q, '89, 11

  DEF: Aerophagy: excess swallowing of air, usually unconscious;
  related to anxiety; results in distended abdomen or belching, often
  interpreted by the patient as a physical disorder.

✓5ᵗʰ **306.5 Genitourinary**
    EXCLUDES *enuresis, psychogenic (307.6)*
      frigidity (302.72)
      impotence (302.72)
      psychogenic dyspareunia (302.76)

306.50 Psychogenic genitourinary malfunction,
  unspecified

306.51 Psychogenic vaginismus   ♀
  Functional vaginismus

  DEF: Psychogenic response resulting in painful
  contractions of vaginal canal muscles; can be severe
  enough to prevent sexual intercourse.

306.52 Psychogenic dysmenorrhea   ♀
306.53 Psychogenic dysuria
306.59 Other
  AHA: M-A, '87, 11

306.6 Endocrine
306.7 Organs of special sense
    EXCLUDES *hysterical blindness or deafness*
      (300.11)
      psychophysical visual disturbances
        (368.16)

---

§   Requires fifth-digit. See category 305 for codes and definitions.

`N` Newborn Age: 0   `P` Pediatric Age: 0-17   `M` Maternity Age: 12-55   `A` Adult Age: 15-124   `CC` CC Condition   `MC` Major Complication   `CD` Complex Dx   `HIV` HIV Related Dx

306.8 Other specified psychophysiological malfunction

Bruxism   Teeth grinding

306.9 Unspecified psychophysiological malfunction

Psychophysiologic disorder NOS

Psychosomatic disorder NOS

√4th **307 Special symptoms or syndromes, not elsewhere classified**

Note: This category is intended for use if the psychopathology is manifested by a single specific symptom or group of symptoms which is not part of an organic illness or other mental disorder classifiable elsewhere.

     EXCLUDES *those due to mental disorders classified elsewhere*

those of organic origin

307.0 Stammering and stuttering

     EXCLUDES *dysphasia (784.5)*

lisping or lalling (307.9)

retarded development of speech (315.31-315.39)

307.1 Anorexia nervosa   CC

     EXCLUDES *eating disturbance NOS (307.50)*

feeding problem (783.3)

of nonorganic origin (307.59)

loss of appetite (783.0)

of nonorganic origin (307.59)

CC Excl: 306.4, 306.8-306.9, 307.1, 307.50-307.59, 309.22

AHA: 4Q, '89, 11

√5th **307.2 Tics**

     EXCLUDES *nail-biting or thumb-sucking (307.9)*

stereotypes occurring in isolation (307.3)

tics of organic origin (333.3)

DEF: Involuntary muscle response usually confined to the face, shoulders.

307.20 Tic disorder, unspecified

307.21 Transient tic disorder of childhood

307.22 Chronic motor tic disorder

307.23 Gilles de la Tourette's disorder

Motor-verbal tic disorder

DEF: Syndrome of facial and vocal tics in childhood; progresses to spontaneous or involuntary jerking, obscene utterances, other uncontrollable actions considered inappropriate.

307.3 Stereotyped repetitive movements

Body-rocking   Spasmus nutans

Head banging   Stereotypes NOS

     EXCLUDES *tics (307.20-307.23)*

of organic origin (333.3)

√5th **307.4 Specific disorders of sleep of nonorganic origin**

     EXCLUDES *narcolepsy (347)*

those of unspecified cause (780.50-780.59)

307.40 Nonorganic sleep disorder, unspecified

307.41 Transient disorder of initiating or maintaining sleep

Hyposomnia, Insomnia, Sleeplessness } associated with intermittent emotional reactions or conflicts

307.42 Persistent disorder of initiating or maintaining sleep

Hyposomnia, insomnia, or sleeplessness associated with:

anxiety

conditioned arousal

depression (major) (minor)

psychosis

307.43 Transient disorder of initiating or maintaining wakefulness

Hypersomnia associated with acute or intermittent emotional reactions or conflicts

307.44 Persistent disorder of initiating or maintaining wakefulness

Hypersomnia associated with depression (major) (minor)

307.45 Phase-shift disruption of 24-hour sleep-wake cycle

Irregular sleep-wake rhythm, nonorganic origin

Jet lag syndrome

Rapid time-zone change

Shifting sleep-work schedule

307.46 Somnambulism or night terrors

DEF: Sleepwalking marked by extreme terror, panic, screaming, confusion; no recall of event upon arousal; term may refer to simply the act of sleepwalking.

307.47 Other dysfunctions of sleep stages or arousal from sleep

Nightmares: Sleep drunkenness

NOS

REM-sleep type

307.48 Repetitive intrusions of sleep

Repetitive intrusion of sleep with:

atypical polysomnographic features

environmental disturbances

repeated REM-sleep interruptions

307.49 Other

"Short-sleeper"

Subjective insomnia complaint

√5th **307.5 Other and unspecified disorders of eating**

     EXCLUDES *anorexia:*

nervosa (307-1)

of unspecified cause (783.0)

overeating, of unspecified cause (783.6)

vomiting:

NOS (787.0)

cyclical (536.2)

psychogenic (306.4)

307.50 Eating disorder, unspecified

307.51 Bulimia

Overeating of nonorganic origin

DEF: Mental disorder commonly characterized by binge eating followed by self-induced vomiting; perceptions of being fat; and fear the inability to stop eating voluntarily.

307.52 Pica

Perverted appetite of nonorganic origin

DEF: Compulsive eating disorder characterized by craving for substances, other than food; such as paint chips or dirt.

307.53 Psychogenic rumination

Regurgitation, of nonorganic origin, of food with reswallowing

     EXCLUDES *obsessional rumination (300.3)*

307.54 Psychogenic vomiting

307.59 Other

Infantile feeding disturbances, Loss of appetite } of nonorganic origin

307.6 Enuresis

Enuresis (primary) (secondary) of nonorganic origin

     EXCLUDES *enuresis of unspecified cause (788.3)*

DEF: Involuntary urination past age of normal control; also called bedwetting; no trace to biological problem; focus on psychological issues.

307.7 Encopresis

Encopresis (continuous) (discontinuous) of nonorganic origin

     EXCLUDES *encopresis of unspecified cause (787.6)*

DEF: Inability to control bowel movements; cause traced to psychological, not biological, problems.

√4th √5th Additional Digit Required   Nonspecific PDx   Unacceptable PDx   Manifestation Code   **MSP** Medicare Secondary Payer   ►◄ Revised Text   ● New Code   ▲ Revised Code Title

Mental Disorders 307.8–310.0

✓5th **307.8 Psychalgia**

307.80 Psychogenic pain, site unspecified

307.81 Tension headache
> EXCLUDES *headache:*
> *NOS (784.0)*
> *migraine (346.0-346.9)*

AHA: N-D, '85, 16

307.89 Other
Psychogenic backache
> EXCLUDES *pains not specifically*
> *attributable to a*
> *psychological cause (in):*
> *back (724.5)*
> *joint (719.4)*
> *limb (729.5)*
> *lumbago (724.2)*
> *rheumatic (729.0)*

307.9 Other and unspecified special symptoms or syndromes, not elsewhere classified
Hair plucking   Masturbation
Lalling   Nail-biting
Lisping   Thumb-sucking

✓4th **308 Acute reaction to stress**
> INCLUDES   catastrophic stress
> combat fatigue
> gross stress reaction (acute)
> transient disorders in response to exceptional physical or mental stress which usually subside within hours or days
> EXCLUDES *adjustment reaction or disorder (309.0-309.9)*
> *chronic stress reaction (309.1-309.9)*

308.0 Predominant disturbance of emotions
Anxiety   } as acute reaction to
Emotional crisis   } exceptional
Panic state   } [gross] stress

308.1 Predominant disturbance of consciousness
Fugues as acute reaction to exceptional [gross] stress

308.2 Predominant psychomotor disturbance
Agitation states } as acute reaction to
Stupor   } exceptional [gross] stress

308.3 Other acute reactions to stress
Acute situational disturbance
Brief or acute posttraumatic stress disorder
> EXCLUDES *prolonged posttraumatic emotional disturbance (309.81)*

308.4 Mixed disorders as reaction to stress

308.9 Unspecified acute reaction to stress

✓4th **309 Adjustment reaction**
> INCLUDES   adjustment disorders
> reaction (adjustment) to chronic stress
> EXCLUDES *acute reaction to major stress (308.0-308.9)*
> *neurotic disorders (300.0-300.9)*

309.0 Brief depressive reaction
Adjustment disorder with depressed mood
Grief reaction
> EXCLUDES *affective psychoses (296.0-296.9)*
> *neurotic depression (300.4)*
> *prolonged depressive reaction (309.1)*
> *psychogenic depressive psychosis (298.0)*

309.1 Prolonged depressive reaction
> EXCLUDES *affective psychoses (296.0-296.9)*
> *brief depressive reaction (309.0)*
> *neurotic depression (300.4)*
> *psychogenic depressive psychosis (298.0)*

✓5th **309.2 With predominant disturbance of other emotions**

309.21 Separation anxiety disorder
> DEF: Abnormal apprehension by a child when physically separated from support environment; byproduct of abnormal symbiotic child-parent relationship.

309.22 Emancipation disorder of adolescence and early adult life
> DEF: Adjustment reaction of late adolescence; conflict over independence from parental supervision; symptoms include difficulty in making decisions, increased reliance on parental advice, deliberate adoption of values in opposition of parents.

309.23 Specific academic or work inhibition

309.24 Adjustment reaction with anxious mood

309.28 Adjustment reaction with mixed emotional features
Adjustment reaction with anxiety and depression

309.29 Other
Culture shock

309.3 With predominant disturbance of conduct
Conduct disturbance   } as adjustment reaction
Destructiveness   }
> EXCLUDES *destructiveness in child (312.9)*
> *disturbance of conduct NOS (312.9)*
> *dyssocial behavior without manifest psychiatric disorder (V71.01-V71.02)*
> *personality disorder with predominantly sociopathic or asocial manifestations (301.7)*

309.4 With mixed disturbance of emotions and conduct

✓5th **309.8 Other specified adjustment reactions**

309.81 Prolonged posttraumatic stress disorder
Chronic posttraumatic stress disorder
Concentration camp syndrome
> EXCLUDES *posttraumatic brain syndrome:*
> *nonpsychotic (310.2)*
> *psychotic (293.0-293.9)*

> DEF: Preoccupation with traumatic events beyond normal experience; events such as rape, personal assault, combat, natural disasters, accidents, torture precipitate disorder; also recurring flashbacks of trauma; symptoms include difficulty remembering, sleeping, or concentrating, and guilt feelings for surviving.

309.82 Adjustment reaction with physical symptoms

309.83 Adjustment reaction with withdrawal
Elective mutism as adjustment reaction
Hospitalism (in children) NOS

309.89 Other

309.9 Unspecified adjustment reaction
Adaptation reaction NOS
Adjustment reaction NOS

✓4th **310 Specific nonpsychotic mental disorders due to organic brain damage**
> EXCLUDES *neuroses, personality disorders, or other nonpsychotic conditions occurring in a form similar to that seen with functional disorders but in association with a physical condition (300.0-300.9, 301.0-301.9)*

310.0 Frontal lobe syndrome
Lobotomy syndrome
Postleucotomy syndrome [state]
> EXCLUDES *postcontusion syndrome (310.2)*

N Newborn Age: 0   P Pediatric Age: 0-17   M Maternity Age: 12-55   A Adult Age: 15-124   CC CC Condition   MC Major Complication   CD Complex Dx   HIV HIV Related Dx

2002 Ingenix, Inc.

310.1 Organic personality syndrome
Cognitive or personality change of other type, of nonpsychotic severity
Mild memory disturbance
Organic psychosyndrome of nonpsychotic severity
Presbyophrenia NOS
Senility with mental changes of nonpsychotic severity

DEF: Personality disorder caused by organic factors, such as brain lesions, head trauma, or cerebrovascular accident (CVA).

310.2 Postconcussion syndrome
Postcontusion syndrome or encephalopathy
Posttraumatic brain syndrome, nonpsychotic
Status postcommotio cerebri

EXCLUDES *frontal lobe syndrome (310.0)*
postencephalitic syndrome (310.8)
any organic psychotic conditions following head injury (293.0-294.0)

AHA: 4Q, '90, 24

DEF: Nonpsychotic disorder due to brain trauma, causes symptoms unrelated to any disease process; symptoms include amnesia, serial headaches, rapid heartbeat, fatigue, disrupted sleep patterns, inability to concentrate.

310.8 Other specified nonpsychotic mental disorders following organic brain damage
Postencephalitic syndrome
Other focal (partial) organic psychosyndromes

310.9 Unspecified nonpsychotic mental disorder **HIV** **following organic brain damage**

311 Depressive disorder, not elsewhere classified
Depressive disorder NOS   Depression NOS
Depressive state NOS

EXCLUDES *acute reaction to major stress with depressive symptoms (308.0)*
affective personality disorder (301.10-301.13)
affective psychoses (296.0-296.9)
brief depressive reaction (309.0)
depressive states associated with stressful events (309.0-309.1)
disturbance of emotions specific to childhood and adolescence, with misery and unhappiness (313.1)
mixed adjustment reaction with depressive symptoms (309.4)
neurotic depression (300.4)
prolonged depressive adjustment reaction (309.1)
psychogenic depressive psychosis (298.0)

✓4th 312 Disturbance of conduct, not elsewhere classified

EXCLUDES *adjustment reaction with disturbance of conduct (309.3)*
drug dependence (304.0-304.9)
dyssocial behavior without manifest psychiatric disorder (V71.01-V71.02)
personality disorder with predominantly sociopathic or asocial manifestations (301.7)
sexual deviations (302.0-302.9)

The following fifth-digit subclassification is for use with categories 312.0-312.2:
0 **unspecified**
1 **mild**
2 **moderate**
3 **severe**

✓5th 312.0 Undersocialized conduct disorder, aggressive type
Aggressive outburst   Unsocialized aggressive
Anger reaction   disorder

DEF: Mental condition identified by behaviors disrespectful of others' rights and of age-appropriate social norms or rules; symptoms include bullying, vandalism, verbal and physical abusiveness, lying, stealing, defiance.

✓5th 312.1 Undersocialized conduct disorder, unaggressive type
Childhood truancy, unsocialized
Solitary stealing
Tantrums

✓5th 312.2 Socialized conduct disorder
Childhood truancy, socialized   Group delinquency

EXCLUDES *gang activity without manifest psychiatric disorder (V71.01)*

✓5th 312.3 Disorders of impulse control, not elsewhere classified
312.30 Impulse control disorder, unspecified
312.31 Pathological gambling
312.32 Kleptomania
312.33 Pyromania
312.34 Intermittent explosive disorder
312.35 Isolated explosive disorder
312.39 Other

312.4 Mixed disturbance of conduct and emotions
Neurotic delinquency

EXCLUDES *compulsive conduct disorder (312.3)*

✓5th 312.8 Other specified disturbances of conduct, not elsewhere classified
312.81 Conduct disorder, childhood onset type
312.82 Conduct disorder, adolescent onset type
312.89 Other conduct disorder

312.9 Unspecified disturbance of conduct
Delinquency (juvenile)

✓4th 313 Disturbance of emotions specific to childhood and adolescence

EXCLUDES *adjustment reaction (309.0-309.9)*
emotional disorder of neurotic type (300.0-300.9)
masturbation, nail-biting, thumbsucking, and other isolated symptoms (307.0-307.9)

313.0 Overanxious disorder
Anxiety and fearfulness } of childhood and
Overanxious disorder   adolescence

EXCLUDES *abnormal separation anxiety (309.21)*
anxiety states (300.00-300.09)
hospitalism in children (309.83)
phobic state (300.20-300.29)

313.1 Misery and unhappiness disorder

EXCLUDES *depressive neurosis (300.4)*

✓5th 313.2 Sensitivity, shyness, and social withdrawal disorder

EXCLUDES *infantile autism (299.0)*
schizoid personality (301.20-301.22)
schizophrenia (295.0-295.9)

313.21 Shyness disorder of childhood
Sensitivity reaction of childhood or adolescence

313.22 Introverted disorder of childhood
Social withdrawal }
Withdrawal   } of childhood or
reaction   } adolescence

313.23 Elective mutism

EXCLUDES *elective mutism as adjustment reaction (309.83)*

✓4th ✓5th Additional Digit Required   Nonspecific PDx   Unacceptable PDx   Manifestation Code   **MSP** Medicare Secondary Payer   ►◄ Revised Text   ● New Code   ▲ Revised Code Title

2002 Ingenix, Inc.   **Volume 1 — 79**

Mental Disorders 313.3–319

313.3 Relationship problems
Sibling jealousy
> EXCLUDES *relationship problems associated with aggression, destruction, or other forms of conduct disturbance (312.0-312.9)*

√5th **313.8 Other or mixed emotional disturbances of childhood or adolescence**

313.81 Oppositional disorder
DEF: Mental disorder of children noted for pervasive opposition, defiance of authority.

313.82 Identity disorder
DEF: Distress of adolescents caused by inability to form acceptable self-identity; uncertainty about career choice, sexual orientation, moral values.

313.83 Academic underachievement disorder

313.89 Other P

313.9 Unspecified emotional disturbance of childhood or adolescence P

√4th **314 Hyperkinetic syndrome of childhood**
> EXCLUDES *hyperkinesis as symptom of underlying disorder—code the underlying disorder*

√5th **314.0 Attention deficit disorder**
Adult
Child
DEF: A behavioral disorder usually diagnosed at an early age; characterized by the inability to focus attention for a normal period of time.

314.00 Without mention of hyperactivity
Predominantly inattentive type
AHA: 1Q, '97, 8

314.01 With hyperactivity
Combined type
Overactivity NOS
Predominantly hyperactive/impulsive type
Simple disturbance of attention with overactivity
AHA: 1Q, '97, 8

314.1 Hyperkinesis with developmental delay
Developmental disorder of hyperkinesis
Use additional code to identify any associated neurological disorder

314.2 Hyperkinetic conduct disorder
Hyperkinetic conduct disorder without developmental delay
> EXCLUDES *hyperkinesis with significant delays in specific skills (314.1)*

314.8 Other specified manifestations of hyperkinetic syndrome

314.9 Unspecified hyperkinetic syndrome
Hyperkinetic reaction of childhood or adolescence NOS
Hyperkinetic syndrome NOS

√4th **315 Specific delays in development**
> EXCLUDES *that due to a neurological disorder (320.0-389.9)*

√5th **315.0 Specific reading disorder**

315.00 Reading disorder, unspecified

315.01 Alexia
DEF: Lack of ability to understand written language; manifestation of aphasia.

315.02 Developmental dyslexia
DEF: Serious impairment of reading skills unexplained in relation to general intelligence and teaching processes; it can be inherited or congenital.

315.09 Other
Specific spelling difficulty

315.1 Specific arithmetical disorder
Dyscalculia

315.2 Other specific learning difficulties
> EXCLUDES *specific arithmetical disorder (315.1)*
> *specific reading disorder (315.00-315.09)*

√5th **315.3 Developmental speech or language disorder**

315.31 Developmental language disorder
Developmental aphasia
Expressive language disorder
Word deafness
> EXCLUDES *acquired aphasia (784.3)*
> *elective mutism (309.83, 313.0, 313.23)*

315.32 Receptive language disorder (mixed)
Receptive expressive language disorder
AHA: 4Q, '96, 30

315.39 Other
Developmental articulation disorder
Dyslalia
> EXCLUDES *lisping and lalling (307.9)*
> *stammering and stuttering (307.0)*

315.4 Coordination disorder
Clumsiness syndrome   Specific motor development
Dyspraxia syndrome   disorder

315.5 Mixed development disorder

315.8 Other specified delays in development

315.9 Unspecified delay in development
Developmental disorder NOS

316 Psychic factors associated with diseases classified elsewhere
Psychologic factors in physical conditions classified elsewhere
Use additional code to identify the associated physical condition, as:
psychogenic:
asthma (493.9)
dermatitis (692.9)
duodenal ulcer (532.0-532.9)
eczema (691.8, 692.9)
gastric ulcer (531.0-531.9)
mucous colitis (564.9)
paroxysmal tachycardia (427.2)
ulcerative colitis (556)
urticaria (708.0-708.9)
psychosocial dwarfism (259.4)
> EXCLUDES *physical symptoms and physiological malfunctions, not involving tissue damage, of mental origin (306.0-306.9)*

MENTAL RETARDATION (317-319)
Use additional code(s) to identify any associated psychiatric or physical condition(s)

317 Mild mental retardation
High-grade defect
IQ 50-70
Mild mental subnormality

√4th **318 Other specified mental retardation**

318.0 Moderate mental retardation
IQ 35-49
Moderate mental subnormality

318.1 Severe mental retardation
IQ 20-34   Severe mental subnormality

318.2 Profound mental retardation
IQ under 20   Profound mental subnormality

319 Unspecified mental retardation
Mental deficiency NOS   Mental subnormality NOS

N Newborn Age: 0   P Pediatric Age: 0-17   M Maternity Age: 12-55   A Adult Age: 15-124   CC CC Condition   MC Major Complication   CD Complex Dx   HIV HIV Related Dx

80 — Volume 1   *2002 Ingenix, Inc.*

6. DISEASES OF THE NERVOUS SYSTEM AND SENSE ORGANS (320-389)

INFLAMMATORY DISEASES OF THE CENTRAL NERVOUS SYSTEM (320-326)

√4th **320 Bacterial meningitis**

INCLUDES
arachnoiditis
leptomeningitis
meningitis   } bacterial
meningoencephalitis
meningomyelitis
pachymeningitis

AHA: J-F, '87, 6

DEF: Bacterial infection causing inflammation of the lining of the brain and/or spinal cord.

320.0 **Hemophilus meningitis** CC
Meningitis due to Hemophilus influenzae [H. influenzae]
CC Excl: 003.21, 013.00-013.16, 036.0, 047.0-047.9, 049.0-049.1, 053.0, 054.72, 072.1, 090.42, 091.81, 094.2, 098.89, 100.81, 112.83, 114.2, 115.01, 115.11, 115.91, 130.0, 250.60-250.63, 250.80-250.93, 320.0-320.9, 321.0-321.8, 322.0-322.9, 349.89, 349.9, 357.0

320.1 **Pneumococcal meningitis** CC
CC Excl: See code 320.0

320.2 **Streptococcal meningitis** CC
CC Excl: See code 320.0

320.3 **Staphylococcal meningitis** CC
CC Excl: See code 320.0

320.7 *Meningitis in other bacterial diseases classified elsewhere* CC
Code first underlying disease, as:
actinomycosis (039.8)
listeriosis (027.0)
typhoid fever (002.0)
whooping cough (033.0-033.9)
EXCLUDES   *meningitis (in):*
epidemic (036.0)
gonococcal (098.82)
meningococcal (036.0)
salmonellosis (003.21)
syphilis:
NOS (094.2)
congenital (090.42)
meningovascular (094.2)
secondary (091.81)
tuberculous (013.0)
CC Excl: See code 320.0

√5th **320.8 Meningitis due to other specified bacteria**
320.81 Anaerobic meningitis CC
Bacteroides (fragilis)
Gram-negative anaerobes
CC Excl: See code 320.0

320.82 Meningitis due to gram-negative bacteria, not elsewhere classified CC
Aerobacter aerogenes   Klebsiella pneumoniae
Escherichia coli [E. coli] Proteus morganii
Friedländer bacillus   Pseudomonas
EXCLUDES   *gram-negative anaerobes (320.81)*
CC Excl: See code 320.0

320.89 Meningitis due to other specified bacteria CC
Bacillus pyocyaneus
CC Excl: See code 320.0

320.9 **Meningitis due to unspecified bacterium** CC
Meningitis: Meningitis:
bacterial NOS   pyogenic NOS
purulent NOS   suppurative NOS
CC Excl: See code 320.0

√4th **321 Meningitis due to other organisms**
AHA: J-F, '87, 6

DEF: Infection causing inflammation of the lining of the brain and/or spinal cord, due to organisms other than bacteria.

321.0 *Cryptococcal meningitis* CC
Code first underlying disease (117.5)
CC Excl: See code 320.0

321.1 *Meningitis in other fungal diseases* CC
Code first underlying disease (110.0-118)
EXCLUDES   *meningitis in:*
candidiasis (112.83)
coccidioidomycosis (114.2)
histoplasmosis (115.01, 115.11, 115.91)
CC Excl: See code 320.0

321.2 *Meningitis due to viruses not elsewhere classified* CC
Code first underlying disease, as:
meningitis due to arbovirus (060.0-066.9)
EXCLUDES   *meningitis (due to):*
abacterial (047.0-047.9)
adenovirus (049.1)
aseptic NOS (047.9)
Coxsackie (virus)(047.0)
ECHO virus (047.1)
enterovirus (047.0-047.9)
herpes simplex virus (054.72)
herpes zoster virus (053.0)
lymphocytic choriomeningitis virus (049.0)
mumps (072.1)
viral NOS (047.9)
meningo-eruptive syndrome (047.1)
CC Excl: 003.21, 013.00-013.16, 036.0, 047.0-047.9, 049.0-049.1, 053.0, 054.72, 072.1, 090.42, 091.81, 094.2, 098.89, 100.81, 112.83, 114.2, 115.01, 115.11, 115.91, 130.0, 320.0-320.9, 321.0-321.8, 322.0-322.9, 349.89, 349.9, 357.0

321.3 *Meningitis due to trypanosomiasis* CC
Code first underlying disease (086.0-086.9)
CC Excl: 003.21, 013.00-013.16, 036.0, 047.0-047.9, 049.0-049.1, 053.0, 054.72, 072.1, 090.42, 091.81, 094.2, 098.89, 100.81, 112.83, 114.2, 115.01, 115.11, 115.91, 130.0, 250.60-250.63, 250.80-250.93, 320.0-320.9, 321.0-321.8, 322.0-322.9, 349.89, 349.9, 357.0

321.4 *Meningitis in sarcoidosis* CC
Code first underlying disease (135)
CC Excl: See code 321.3

321.8 *Meningitis due to other nonbacterial organisms classified elsewhere* CC
Code first underlying disease
EXCLUDES   *leptospiral meningitis (100.81)*
CC Excl: See code 321.3

√4th **322 Meningitis of unspecified cause**
INCLUDES
arachnoiditis
leptomeningitis   } with no organism specified as cause
meningitis
pachymeningitis

AHA: J-F, '87, 6

DEF: Infection causing inflammation of the lining of the brain and/or spinal cord, due to unspecified cause.

322.0 **Nonpyogenic meningitis** CC
Meningitis with clear cerebrospinal fluid
CC Excl: See code 321.3

Nervous System and Sense Organs 320–322.0

√4th √5th Additional Digit Required   Nonspecific PDx   Unacceptable PDx   Manifestation Code   MSP Medicare Secondary Payer   ►◄ Revised Text   ● New Code   ▲ Revised Code Title
2002 Ingenix, Inc.

Volume 1 — 81

322.1   **Eosinophilic meningitis**   `CC`
CC Excl: See code 321.3

322.2   **Chronic meningitis**   `CC`
CC Excl: See code 321.3

322.9   **Meningitis, unspecified**   `CC`
CC Excl: See code 321.3

`✓4th` **323**   **Encephalitis, myelitis, and encephalomyelitis**

> `INCLUDES`   acute disseminated encephalomyelitis
> meningoencephalitis, except bacterial
> meningomyelitis, except bacterial
> myelitis (acute):
>   ascending
>   transverse

> `EXCLUDES`   bacterial:
>   meningoencephalitis (320.0-320.9)
>   meningomyelitis (320.0-320.9)

DEF: Encephalitis: inflammation of brain tissues.

DEF: Myelitis: inflammation of the spinal cord.

DEF: Encephalomyelitis: inflammation of brain and spinal cord.

323.0   **Encephalitis in viral diseases classified elsewhere**

> Code first underlying disease, as:
>   cat-scratch disease (078.3)
>   infectious mononucleosis (075)
>   ornithosis (073.7)

> `EXCLUDES`   encephalitis (in):
>   arthropod-borne viral (062.0-064)
>   herpes simplex (054.3)
>   mumps (072.2)
>   poliomyelitis (045.0-045.9)
>   rubella (056.01)
>   slow virus infections of central
>   nervous system (046.0-046.9)
>   other viral diseases of central
>   nervous system (049.8-049.9)
>   viral NOS (049.9)

323.1   **Encephalitis in rickettsial diseases classified elsewhere**

> Code first underlying disease (080-083.9)

DEF: Inflammation of the brain caused by rickettsial disease carried by louse, tick, or mite.

323.2   **Encephalitis in protozoal diseases classified elsewhere**

> Code first underlying disease, as:
>   malaria (084.0-084.9)
>   trypanosomiasis (086.0-086.9)

DEF: Inflammation of the brain caused by protozoal disease carried by mosquitoes and flies.

323.4   **Other encephalitis due to infection classified elsewhere**

> Code first underlying disease

> `EXCLUDES`   encephalitis (in):
>   meningococcal (036.1)
>   syphilis:
>   NOS (094.81)
>   congenital (090.41)
>   toxoplasmosis (130.0)
>   tuberculosis (013.6)
>   meningoencephalitis due to free-living
>   ameba [Naegleria] (136.2)

323.5   **Encephalitis following immunization procedures**

> Encephalitis   } postimmunization or
> Encephalomyelitis } postvaccinal

> Use additional E code to identify vaccine

323.6   **Postinfectious encephalitis**

> Code first underlying disease

> `EXCLUDES`   encephalitis:
>   postchickenpox (052.0)
>   postmeasles (055.0)

DEF: Infection, inflammation of brain several weeks following the outbreak of a systemic infection.

323.7   **Toxic encephalitis**

> Code first underlying cause, as:
>   carbon tetrachloride (982.1)
>   hydroxyquinoline derivatives (961.3)
>   lead (984.0-984.9)
>   mercury (985.0)
>   thallium (985.8)

AHA: 2Q, '97, 8

323.8   **Other causes of encephalitis**   `HIV`

323.9   **Unspecified cause of encephalitis**   `HIV`

`✓4th` **324**   **Intracranial and intraspinal abscess**

324.0   **Intracranial abscess**   `CC`

> Abscess (embolic):   Abscess (embolic) of brain
>   cerebellar   [any part]:
>   cerebral   epidural
>   extradural
>   otogenic
>   subdural

> `EXCLUDES`   tuberculous (013.3)

CC Excl: 006.5, 013.20-013.36, 250.60-250.63, 250.80-250.93, 324.0-324.9, 325, 348.8-348.9

324.1   **Intraspinal abscess**   `CC`

> Abscess (embolic) of spinal cord [any part]:
>   epidural
>   extradural
>   subdural

> `EXCLUDES`   tuberculous (013.5)

CC Excl: 006.5, 013.20-013.36, 250.60-250.63, 250.80-250.93, 324.1

324.9   **Of unspecified site**   `CC`

> Extradural or subdural abscess NOS

CC Excl: 006.5, 013.20-013.36, 250.60-250.63, 250.80-250.93, 324.0-324.9, 325

325   **Phlebitis and thrombophlebitis of intracranial venous sinuses**   `CC`

> Embolism   } of cavernous, lateral, or
> Endophlebitis   }   other intracranial
> Phlebitis, septic or suppurative } or unspecified
> Thrombophlebitis   }   intracranial
> Thrombosis   }   venous sinus

> `EXCLUDES`   that specified as:
>   complicating pregnancy, childbirth, or the
>   puerperium (671.5)
>   of nonpyogenic origin (437.6)

CC Excl: See code 324.9

DEF: Inflammation and formation of blood clot in a vein within the brain or its lining.

326   **Late effects of intracranial abscess or pyogenic infection**

> Note: This category is to be used to indicate conditions whose primary classification is to 320-325 [excluding 320.7, 321.0-321.8, 323.0-323.4, 323.6-323.7] as the cause of late effects, themselves classifiable elsewhere. The "late effects" include conditions specified as such, or as sequelae, which may occur at any time after the resolution of the causal condition.
> Use additional code to identify condition, as:
>   hydrocephalus (331.4)
>   paralysis (342.0-342.9, 344.0-344.9)

`N` Newborn Age: 0   `P` Pediatric Age: 0-17   `M` Maternity Age: 12-55   `A` Adult Age: 15-124   `CC` CC Condition   `MC` Major Complication   `CD` Complex Dx   `HIV` HIV Related Dx

HEREDITARY AND DEGENERATIVE DISEASES OF THE CENTRAL NERVOUS SYSTEM (330-337)

EXCLUDES　hepatolenticular degeneration (275.1)
multiple sclerosis (340)
other demyelinating diseases of central nervous system (341.0-341.9)

√4ᵗʰ **330 Cerebral degenerations usually manifest in childhood**
Use additional code to identify associated mental retardation

330.0 Leukodystrophy

Krabbe's disease
Leukodystrophy NOS
　globoid cell
　metachromatic
　sudanophilic

Pelizaeus-Merzbacher disease
Sulfatide lipidosis

DEF: Hereditary disease of arylsulfatase or cerebroside sulfatase; characterized by a diffuse loss of myelin in CNS; infantile form causes blindness, motor disturbances, rigidity, mental deterioration and, occasionally, convulsions.

330.1 Cerebral lipidoses

Amaurotic (familial) idiocy
Disease:
　Batten
　Jansky-Bielschowsky
　Kufs'

Disease:
　Spielmeyer-Vogt
　Tay-Sachs
Gangliosidosis

DEF: Genetic disorder causing abnormal lipid accumulation in the reticuloendothelial cells of the brain.

330.2 Cerebral degeneration in generalized lipidoses

Code first underlying disease, as:
　Fabry's disease (272.7)
　Gaucher's disease (272.7)
　Niemann-Pick disease (272.7)
　sphingolipidosis (272.7)

330.3 Cerebral degeneration of childhood in other diseases classified elsewhere

Code first underlying disease, as:
　Hunter's disease (277.5)
　mucopolysaccharidosis (277.5)

330.8 Other specified cerebral degenerations in childhood

Alpers' disease or gray-matter degeneration
Infantile necrotizing encephalomyelopathy
Leigh's disease
Subacute necrotizing encephalopathy or encephalomyelopathy

AHA: N-D, '85, 5

330.9 Unspecified cerebral degeneration in childhood

√4ᵗʰ **331 Other cerebral degenerations**

331.0 Alzheimer's disease

AHA: 4Q, '00, 41; 4Q, '99, 7; N-D, '84, 20

DEF: Diffuse atrophy of cerebral cortex; causing a progressive decline in intellectual and physical functions, including memory loss, personality changes and profound dementia.

331.1 Pick's disease

DEF: Rare, progressive degenerative brain disease, similar to Alzheimer's; cortical atrophy affects the frontal and temporal lobes.

331.2 Senile degeneration of brain
EXCLUDES　senility NOS (797)

331.3 Communicating hydrocephalus
EXCLUDES　congenital hydrocephalus (741.0, 742.3)

AHA: S-O, '85, 12

DEF: Subarachnoid hemorrhage and meningitis causing excess buildup of cerebrospinal fluid in cavities due to nonabsorption of fluid back through fluid pathways.

331.4 Obstructive hydrocephalus　　CC
Acquired hydrocephalus NOS
EXCLUDES　congenital hydrocephalus (741.0, 742.3)

CC Excl: 250.60-250.63, 250.80-250.93, 331.3-331.7, 331.89, 331.9, 348.8-348.9, 741.00-741.03, 742.3-742.4, 742.59, 742.8-742.9

AHA: 1Q, '99, 9

DEF: Obstruction of cerebrospinal fluid passage from brain into spinal canal.

331.7 Cerebral degeneration in diseases classified elsewhere

Code first underlying disease, as:
　alcoholism (303.0-303.9)
　beriberi (265.0)
　cerebrovascular disease (430-438)
　congenital hydrocephalus (741.0, 742.3)
　myxedema (244.0-244.9)
　neoplastic disease (140.0-239.9)
　vitamin B_{12} deficiency (266.2)
EXCLUDES　cerebral degeneration in:
　　Jakob-Creutzfeldt disease (046.1)
　　progressive multifocal leukoencephalopathy (046.3)
　　subacute spongiform encephalopathy (046.1)

√5ᵗʰ **331.8 Other cerebral degeneration**

331.81 Reye's syndrome　　A

DEF: Rare childhood illness, often developed after a bout of viral upper respiratory infection; characterized by vomiting, elevated serum transaminase, changes in liver and other viscera; symptoms may be followed by an encephalopathic phase with brain swelling, disturbances of consciousness and seizures; can be fatal.

331.89 Other
Cerebral ataxia

331.9 Cerebral degeneration, unspecified

√4ᵗʰ **332 Parkinson's disease**

332.0 Paralysis agitans

Parkinsonism or Parkinson's disease:
　NOS　　　　　primary
　idiopathic

AHA: M-A, '87, 7

DEF: Form of parkinsonism; progressive, occurs in senior years; characterized by masklike facial expression; condition affects ability to stand erect, walk smoothly; weakened muscles, also tremble and involuntarily movement.

332.1 Secondary Parkinsonism

Parkinsonism due to drugs
Use additional E code to identify drug, if drug-induced
EXCLUDES　Parkinsonism (in):
　　Huntington's disease (333.4)
　　progressive supranuclear palsy (333.0)
　　Shy-Drager syndrome (333.0)
　　syphilitic (094.82)

√4ᵗʰ **333 Other extrapyramidal disease and abnormal movement disorders**
INCLUDES　other forms of extrapyramidal, basal ganglia, or striatopallidal disease
EXCLUDES　abnormal movements of head NOS (781.0)

Nervous System and Sense Organs 330–333

√4ᵗʰ √5ᵗʰ Additional Digit Required　　Nonspecific PDx　　Unacceptable PDx　　Manifestation Code　　MSP Medicare Secondary Payer　　▶◀ Revised Text　　● New Code　　▲ Revised Code Title

2002 Ingenix, Inc.　　　　　　　　　　　　　　　　　　　　　　　　　　　　　**Volume 1 — 83**

Nervous System and Sense Organs 333.0–335.1

333.0 Other degenerative diseases of the basal ganglia
Atrophy or degeneration:
olivopontocerebellar [Déjérine-Thomas syndrome]
pigmentary pallidal [Hallervorden-Spatz disease]
striatonigral
Parkinsonian syndrome associated with:
idiopathic orthostatic hypotension
symptomatic orthostatic hypotension
Progressive supranuclear ophthalmoplegia
Shy-Drager syndrome

AHA: 3Q, '96, 8

333.1 Essential and other specified forms of tremor
Benign essential tremor
Familial tremor
Use additional E code to identify drug, if drug-induced
    EXCLUDES   tremor NOS (781.0)

333.2 Myoclonus
Familial essential myoclonus
Progressive myoclonic epilepsy
Unverricht-Lundborg disease
Use additional E code to identify drug, if drug-induced

AHA: 3Q, '97, 4; M-A, '87, 12

DEF: Spontaneous movements or contractions of muscles.

333.3 Tics of organic origin
Use additional E code to identify drug, if drug-induced
    EXCLUDES   Gilles de la Tourette's syndrome (307.23)
habit spasm (307.22)
tic NOS (307.20)

333.4 Huntington's chorea
DEF: Genetic disease characterized by chronic progressive mental deterioration; dementia and death within 15 years of onset.

333.5 Other choreas
Hemiballism(us)
Paroxysmal choreo-athetosis
Use additional E code to identify drug, if drug-induced
    EXCLUDES   Sydenham's or rheumatic chorea (392.0-392.9)

333.6 Idiopathic torsion dystonia
Dystonia:
deformans progressiva
musculorum deformans
(Schwalbe-) Ziehen-Oppenheim disease
DEF: Sustained muscular contractions, causing twisting and repetitive movements that result in abnormal postures of trunk and limbs; etiology unknown.

333.7 Symptomatic torsion dystonia
Athetoid cerebral palsy [Vogt's disease]
Double athetosis (syndrome)
Use additional E code to identify drug, if drug-induced

√5ᵗʰ 333.8 Fragments of torsion dystonia
Use additional E code to identify drug, if drug-induced

    333.81 Blepharospasm
       DEF: Uncontrolled winking or blinking due to orbicularis oculi muscle spasm.

    333.82 Orofacial dyskinesia
       DEF: Uncontrolled movement of mouth or facial muscles.

    333.83 Spasmodic torticollis
       EXCLUDES   torticollis:
         NOS (723.5)
         hysterical (300.11)
         psychogenic (306.0)
       DEF: Uncontrolled movement of head due to spasms of neck muscle.

    333.84 Organic writers' cramp
       EXCLUDES   pychogenic (300.89)
    333.89 Other

√5ᵗʰ 333.9 Other and unspecified extrapyramidal diseases and abnormal movement disorders

    333.90 Unspecified extrapyramidal disease and abnormal movement disorder

    333.91 Stiff-man syndrome

    333.92 Neuroleptic malignant syndrome
       Use additional E code to identify drug
       AHA: 4Q, '94, 37

    333.93 Benign shuddering attacks
       AHA: 4Q, '94, 37

    333.99 Other
       Restless legs
       AHA: 4Q, '94, 37

√4ᵗʰ 334 Spinocerebellar disease
    EXCLUDES   olivopontocerebellar degeneration (333.0)
          peroneal muscular atrophy (356.1)

334.0 Friedreich's ataxia
DEF: Genetic recessive disease of children; sclerosis of dorsal, lateral spinal cord columns; characterized by ataxia, speech impairment, swaying and irregular movements, with muscle paralysis, especially of lower limbs.

334.1 Hereditary spastic paraplegia

334.2 Primary cerebellar degeneration
Cerebellar ataxia:
Marie's
Sanger-Brown
Dyssynergia cerebellaris myoclonica
Primary cerebellar degeneration:
NOS
hereditary
sporadic
AHA: M-A, '87, 9

334.3 Other cerebellar ataxia
Cerebellar ataxia NOS
Use additional E code to identify drug, if drug-induced

334.4 Cerebellar ataxia in diseases classified elsewhere
Code first underlying disease, as:
alcoholism (303.0-303.9)
myxedema (244.0-244.9)
neoplastic disease (140.0-239.9)

334.8 Other spinocerebellar diseases
Ataxia-telangiectasia [Louis-Bar syndrome]
Corticostriatal-spinal degeneration

334.9 Spinocerebellar disease, unspecified

√4ᵗʰ 335 Anterior horn cell disease
335.0 Werdnig-Hoffmann disease   `CC`
Infantile spinal muscular atrophy
Progressive muscular atrophy of infancy
CC Excl: 250.60-250.63, 250.80-250.93, 334.8-334.9, 335.0, 335.10-335.9, 336.0-336.9, 337.0-337.9, 349.89, 349.9

DEF: Spinal muscle atrophy manifested in prenatal period or shortly after birth; symptoms include hypotonia, atrophy of skeletal muscle; death occurs in infancy.

√5ᵗʰ 335.1 Spinal muscular atrophy

    335.10 Spinal muscular atrophy, unspecified   `CC`
       CC Excl: See code 335.0

    335.11 Kugelberg-Welander disease   `CC`
       Spinal muscular atrophy:
         familial
         juvenile
       CC Excl: See code 335.0

       DEF: Hereditary; juvenile muscle atrophy; appears during first two decades of life; due to lesions of anterior horns of spinal cord; includes wasting, diminution of lower body muscles and twitching.

    335.19 Other   `CC`
       Adult spinal muscular atrophy
       CC Excl: See code 335.0

`N` Newborn Age: 0   `P` Pediatric Age: 0-17   `M` Maternity Age: 12-55   `A` Adult Age: 15-124   `CC` CC Condition   `MC` Major Complication   `CD` Complex Dx   `HIV` HIV Related Dx

✓5ᵗʰ **335.2 Motor neuron disease**

335.20 Amyotrophic lateral sclerosis `CC` `A`
Motor neuron disease (bulbar) (mixed type)
CC Excl: See code 335.0

AHA: 4Q, '95, 81

335.21 Progressive muscular atrophy `CC`
Duchenne-Aran muscular atrophy
Progressive muscular atrophy (pure)
CC Excl: See code 335.0

335.22 Progressive bulbar palsy `CC`
CC Excl: See code 335.0

335.23 Pseudobulbar palsy `CC`
CC Excl: See code 335.0

335.24 Primary lateral sclerosis `CC`
CC Excl: See code 335.0

335.29 Other `CC`
CC Excl: See code 335.0

335.8 Other anterior horn cell diseases `CC`
CC Excl: See code 335.0

335.9 Anterior horn cell disease, unspecified `CC`
CC Excl: See code 335.0

✓4ᵗʰ **336 Other diseases of spinal cord**

336.0 Syringomyelia and syringobulbia
AHA: 1Q, '89, 10

336.1 Vascular myelopathies
Acute infarction of spinal cord (embolic)
(nonembolic)
Arterial thrombosis of spinal cord
Edema of spinal cord
Hematomyelia
Subacute necrotic myelopathy

336.2 Subacute combined degeneration of spinalcord in diseases classified elsewhere
Code first underlying disease, as:
pernicious anemia (281.0)
other vitamin B_{12} deficiency anemia (281.1)
vitamin B_{12} deficiency (266.2)

336.3 Myelopathy in other diseases classified elsewhere
Code first underlying disease, as:
myelopathy in neoplastic disease (140.0-239.9)
EXCLUDES myelopathy in:
intervertebral disc disorder (722.70-722.73)
spondylosis (721.1, 721.41-721.42, 721.91)

AHA: 3Q, '99, 5

336.8 Other myelopathy
Myelopathy: Myelopathy:
drug-induced   radiation-induced
Use additonal E code to identify cause

336.9 Unspecified disease of spinal cord `HIV`
Cord compression NOS   Myelopathy NOS
EXCLUDES myelitis (323.0-323.9)
spinal (canal) stenosis (723.0, 724.00-724.09)

✓4ᵗʰ **337 Disorders of the autonomic nervous system**
INCLUDES disorders of peripheral autonomic, sympathetic, parasympathetic, or vegetative system
EXCLUDES familial dysautonomia [Riley-Day syndrome] (742.8)

337.0 Idiopathic peripheral autonomic neuropathy
Carotid sinus syncope or syndrome
Cervical sympathetic dystrophy or paralysis

337.1 Peripheral autonomic neuropathy in disorders classified elsewhere
Code first underlying disease, as:
amyloidosis (277.3)
diabetes (250.6)
AHA: 2Q, '93, 6; 3Q, '91, 9; N-D, '84, 9

✓5ᵗʰ **337.2 Reflex sympathetic dystrophy**
AHA: 4Q, '93, 24

DEF: Disturbance of the sympathetic nervous system evidenced by sweating, pain, pallor and edema following injury to nerves or blood vessels.

337.20 Reflex sympathetic dystrophy, unspecified
337.21 Reflex sympathetic dystrophy of the upper limb
337.22 Reflex sympathetic dystrophy of the lower limb
337.29 Reflex sympathetic dystrophy of other specified site

337.3 Autonomic dysreflexia
Use additional code to identify the cause, such as:
decubitus ulcer (707.0)
fecal impaction (560.39)
urinary tract infection (599.0)
AHA: 4Q, '98, 37

DEF: Noxious stimuli evokes paroxysmal hypertension, bradycardia, excess sweating, headache, pilomotor responses, facial flushing, and nasal congestion due to uncontrolled parasympathetic nerve response; usually occurs in patients with spinal cord injury above major sympathetic outflow tract (T_6).

337.9 Unspecified disorder of autonomic nervous system

OTHER DISORDERS OF THE CENTRAL NERVOUS SYSTEM (340-349)

340 Multiple sclerosis `CC` `A`
Disseminated or multiple sclerosis:
NOS   cord
brain stem   generalized
CC Excl: 250.60-250.63, 250.80-250.93, 340, 341.8-341.9

✓4ᵗʰ **341 Other demyelinating diseases of central nervous system**

341.0 Neuromyelitis optica

341.1 Schilder's disease
Baló's concentric sclerosis   Encephalitis periaxialis:
Encephalitis periaxialis: diffusa [Schilder's]
concentrica [Baló's]

DEF: Chronic leukoencephalopathy of children and adolescents; symptoms include blindness, deafness, bilateral spasticity and progressive mental deterioration.

341.8 Other demyelinating diseases of central nervous system
Central demyelination of corpus callosum
Central pontine myelinosis
Marchiafava (-Bignami) disease
AHA: N-D, '87, 6

341.9 Demyelinating disease of central nervous system, unspecified `HIV`

Nervous System and Sense Organs 335.2–341.9

✓4ᵗʰ ✓5ᵗʰ **Additional Digit Required**   Nonspecific PDx   Unacceptable PDx   **Manifestation Code**   `MSP` Medicare Secondary Payer   ▶◀ Revised Text   ● New Code   ▲ Revised Code Title

2002 Ingenix, Inc.   **Volume 1 — 85**

Nervous System and Sense Organs 342–344.9

√4th **342 Hemiplegia and hemiparesis**

Note: This category is to be used when hemiplegia (complete) (incomplete) is reported without further specification, or is stated to be old or long-standing but of unspecified cause. The category is also for use in multiple coding to identify these types of hemiplegia resulting from any cause.

EXCLUDES   *congenital (343.1)*
hemiplegia due to late effect of cerebrovascular accident (438.20-438.22)
infantile NOS (343.4)

The following fifth-digits are for use with codes 342.0-342.9:
   0 **affecting unspecified side**
   1 **affecting dominant side**
   2 **affecting nondominant side**

AHA: 4Q, '94, 38

√5th **342.0 Flaccid hemiplegia**
√5th **342.1 Spastic hemiplegia**
√5th **342.8 Other specified hemiplegia**
√5th **342.9 Hemiplegia, unspecified**
     AHA: 4Q, '98, 87

√4th **343 Infantile cerebral palsy**

INCLUDES   cerebral:
     palsy NOS
     spastic infantile paralysis
   congenital spastic paralysis (cerebral)
   Little's disease
   paralysis (spastic) due to birth injury:
     intracranial
     spinal

EXCLUDES   *hereditary cerebral paralysis, such as:*
hereditary spastic paraplegia (334.1)
Vogt's disease (333.7)
spastic paralysis specified as noncongenital or noninfantile (344.0-344.9)

343.0 Diplegic
   Congenital diplegia
   Congenital paraplegia
   DEF: Paralysis affecting both sides of the body simultaneously.

343.1 Hemiplegic
   Congenital hemiplegia
   EXCLUDES   *infantile hemiplegia NOS (343.4)*

343.2 Quadriplegic   CC
   Tetraplegic
   CC Excl: 250.60-250.63, 250.80-250.93, 342.00-342.92, 343.0-343.9, 344.00-344.61, 344.9, 348.8-348.9, 349.89, 349.9, 742.59, 742.8-742.9

343.3 Monoplegic
343.4 Infantile hemiplegia
   Infantile hemiplegia (postnatal) NOS

343.8 Other specified infantile cerebral palsy
343.9 Infantile cerebral palsy, unspecified
   Cerebral palsy NOS

√4th **344 Other paralytic syndromes**

Note: This category is to be used when the listed conditions are reported without further specification or are stated to be old or long-standing but of unspecified cause. The category is also for use in multiple coding to identify these conditions resulting from any cause.

INCLUDES   paralysis (complete) (incomplete), except as classifiable to 342 and 343

EXCLUDES   *congenital or infantile cerebral palsy (343.0-343.9)*
hemiplegia (342.0-342.9)
congenital or infantile (343.1, 343.4)

√5th **344.0 Quadriplegia and quadriparesis**
   344.00 Quadriplegia unspecified   CC
     CC Excl: See code 343.2
     AHA: 4Q, '98, 38

   344.01 C$_1$-C$_4$ complete   CC
     CC Excl: See code 343.2

   344.02 C$_1$-C$_4$ incomplete   CC
     CC Excl: See code 343.2

   344.03 C$_5$-C$_7$ complete   CC
     CC Excl: See code 343.2

   344.04 C$_5$-C$_7$ incomplete   CC
     CC Excl: See code 343.2

   344.09 Other   CC
     CC Excl: See code 343.2
     AHA: 1Q, '01, 12; 4Q, '98, 39

344.1 Paraplegia
   Paralysis of both lower limbs   Paraplegia (lower)
   AHA: M-A, '87, 10

344.2 Diplegia of upper limbs
   Diplegia (upper)   Paralysis of both upper limbs

√5th **344.3 Monoplegia of lower limb**
   Paralysis of lower limb
   EXCLUDES   *monoplegia of lower limb due to late effect of cerebrovascular accident (438.40-438.42)*

   344.30 Affecting unspecified side
   344.31 Affecting dominant side
   344.32 Affecting nondominant side

√5th **344.4 Monoplegia of upper limb**
   Paralysis of upper limb
   EXCLUDES   *monoplegia of upper limb due to late effect of cerebrovascular accident (438.30-438.32)*

   344.40 Affecting unspecified side
   344.41 Affecting dominant side
   344.42 Affecting nondominant side

344.5 Unspecified monoplegia

√5th **344.6 Cauda equina syndrome**
   DEF: Dull pain and paresthesias in sacrum, perineum and bladder due to compression of spinal nerve roots; pain radiates down buttocks, back of thigh, calf of leg and into foot with prickling, burning sensations.

   344.60 Without mention of neurogenic bladder
   344.61 With neurogenic bladder
     Acontractile bladder
     Autonomic hyperreflexia of bladder
     Cord bladder
     Detrusor hyperreflexia
     AHA: M-J, '87, 12; M-A, '87, 10

√5th **344.8 Other specified paralytic syndromes**
   344.81 Locked-in state
     AHA: 4Q, '93, 24

     DEF: State of consciousness where patients are paralyzed and unable to respond to environmental stimuli; patients have eye movements, and stimuli can enter the brain but patients cannot respond to stimuli.

   344.89 Other specified paralytic syndrome
     AHA: 2Q, '99, 4

344.9 Paralysis, unspecified

N Newborn Age: 0   P Pediatric Age: 0-17   M Maternity Age: 12-55   A Adult Age: 15-124   CC CC Condition   MC Major Complication   CD Complex Dx   HIV HIV Related Dx

86 — Volume 1   *2002 Ingenix, Inc.*

√4ᵗʰ **345 Epilepsy**

The following fifth-digit subclassification is for use with categories 345.0, .1, .4–.9:

    0 without mention of intractable epilepsy
    1 with intractable epilepsy

EXCLUDES   *progressive myoclonic epilepsy (333.2)*

AHA: 1Q, '93, 24; 2Q, '92, 8 4Q, '92, 23

DEF: Brain disorder characterized by electrical-like disturbances; may include occasional impairment or loss of consciousness, abnormal motor phenomena and psychic or sensory disturbances.

√5ᵗʰ **345.0 Generalized nonconvulsive epilepsy**   CC 1

Absences:	Seizures:
atonic	akinetic
typical	atonic
Minor epilepsy	
Petit mal	

CC Excl: For code 345.01: 250.60-250.63, 345.00-345.91, 348.8-348.9, 349.89, 349.9

√5ᵗʰ **345.1 Generalized convulsive epilepsy**   CC

Epileptic seizures:	Epileptic seizures:
clonic	tonic-clonic
myoclonic	Grand mal
tonic	Major epilepsy

EXCLUDES   *convulsions:*
        NOS (780.3)
        infantile (780.3)
        newborn (779.0)
    infantile spasms (345.6)

CC Excl: See code 345.01

AHA: 3Q, '97, 4

DEF: Convulsive seizures with tension of limbs (tonic) or rhythmic contractions (clonic).

345.2 Petit mal status   CC

Epileptic absence status

CC Excl: 250.60-250.63, 250.80-250.93, 345.00-345.91, 348.8-348.9, 349.89, 349.9

DEF: Minor myoclonic spasms and sudden momentary loss of consciousness in epilepsy.

345.3 Grand mal status   CC

Status epilepticus NOS

EXCLUDES   *epilepsia partialis continua (345.7)*
    status:
        psychomotor (345.7)
        temporal lobe (345.7)

CC Excl: See code 345.2

DEF: Sudden loss of consciousness followed by generalized convulsions in epilepsy.

√5ᵗʰ **345.4 Partial epilepsy, with impairment of consciousness**   CC 1

Epilepsy:
    limbic system
    partial:
        secondarily generalized
        with memory and ideational disturbances
    psychomotor
    psychosensory
    temporal lobe
Epileptic automatism

CC Excl: For code 345.41: 250.60-250.63, 345.00-345.91, 348.8-348.9, 349.89, 349.9

√5ᵗʰ **345.5 Partial epilepsy, without mention of impairment of consciousness**   CC 1

Epilepsy:	Epilepsy:
Bravais-Jacksonian NOS	sensory-induced
focal (motor) NOS	somatomotor
Jacksonian NOS	somatosensory
motor partial	visceral
partial NOS	visual

CC Excl: For code 345.51: See code 345.4

√5ᵗʰ **345.6 Infantile spasms**   CC 1

Hypsarrhythmia	Salaam attacks
Lightning spasms	

EXCLUDES   *salaam tic (781.0)*

CC Excl: For code 345.61: See code 345.4

AHA: N-D, '84, 12

√5ᵗʰ **345.7 Epilepsia partialis continua**   CC 1

Kojevnikov's epilepsy

CC Excl: For code 345.71: See code 345.4

DEF: Continuous muscle contractions and relaxation; result of abnormal neural discharge.

√5ᵗʰ **345.8 Other forms of epilepsy**   CC 1

Epilepsy:	Epilepsy:
cursive [running]	gelastic

CC Excl: For code 345.81: See code 345.4

√5ᵗʰ **345.9 Epilepsy, unspecified**   CC 1

Epileptic convulsions, fits, or seizures NOS

EXCLUDES   *convulsive seizure or fit NOS (780.3)*

CC Excl: For code 345.91: See code 345.4

AHA: N-D, '87, 12

√4ᵗʰ **346 Migraine**

DEF: Benign vascular headache of extreme pain; commonly associated with irritability, nausea, vomiting and often photophobia; premonitory visual hallucination of a crescent in the visual field (scotoma).

The following fifth-digit subclassification is for use with category 346:

    0 without mention of intractable migraine
    1 with intractable migraine, so stated

√5ᵗʰ **346.0 Classical migraine**

Migraine preceded or accompanied by transient focal neurological phenomena
Migraine with aura

√5ᵗʰ **346.1 Common migraine**

Atypical migraine	Sick headache

√5ᵗʰ **346.2 Variants of migraine**

Cluster headache	Migraine:
Histamine cephalgia	lower half
Horton's neuralgia	retinal
Migraine:	Neuralgia:
abdominal	ciliary
basilar	migrainous

√5ᵗʰ **346.8 Other forms of migraine**

Migraine:	Migraine:
hemiplegic	ophthalmoplegic

√5ᵗʰ **346.9 Migraine, unspecified**

AHA: N-D, '85, 16

347 Cataplexy and narcolepsy

DEF: Cataplexy: Sudden onset of muscle weakness with loss of tone and strength; caused by aggressive or spontaneous emotions.

DEF: Narcolepsy: Brief, recurrent, uncontrollable episodes of sound sleep.

√4ᵗʰ **348 Other conditions of brain**

348.0 Cerebral cysts

Arachnoid cyst	Porencephaly, acquired
Porencephalic cyst	Pseudoporencephaly

EXCLUDES   *porencephaly (congenital) (742.4)*

√4ᵗʰ
√5ᵗʰ   Additional Digit Required   Nonspecific PDx   Unacceptable PDx   Manifestation Code   **MSP** Medicare Secondary Payer   ◄ Revised Text   ● New Code   ▲ Revised Code Title

Nervous System and Sense Organs 348.1–349.9

348.1 Anoxic brain damage `CC`

> **EXCLUDES** *that occurring in:*
> *abortion (634-638 with .7, 639.8)*
> *ectopic or molar pregnancy (639.8)*
> *labor or delivery (668.2, 669.4)*
> *that of newborn (767.0, 768.0-768.9,*
> *772.1-772.2)*

Use additional E code to identify cause

CC Excl: 250.60-250.63, 250.80-250.93, 348.1-348.2, 349.89, 349.9

DEF: Brain injury due to lack of oxygen, other than birth trauma.

348.2 Benign intracranial hypertension

Pseudotumor cerebri

> **EXCLUDES** *hypertensive encephalopathy (437.2)*

DEF: Elevated pressure in brain due to fluid retention in brain cavities.

348.3 Encephalopathy, unspecified `HIV`

AHA: 3Q, '97, 4

348.4 Compression of brain

Compression ⎫
Herniation ⎬ brain (stem)

Posterior fossa compression syndrome

AHA: 4Q, '94, 37

DEF: Elevated pressure in brain due to blood clot, tumor, fracture, abscess, other condition.

348.5 Cerebral edema

DEF: Elevated pressure in the brain due to fluid retention in brain tissues.

348.8 Other conditions of brain

Cerebral: Cerebral:
   calcification   fungus

AHA: S-O, '87, 9

348.9 Unspecified condition of brain `HIV`

☑4ᵗʰ **349 Other and unspecified disorders of the nervous system**

349.0 Reaction to spinal or lumbar puncture

Headache following lumbar puncture

AHA: 2Q, '99, 9; 3Q, '90, 18

349.1 Nervous system complications from surgically implanted device `CC`

> **EXCLUDES** *immediate postoperative complications (997.00-997.09)*
> *mechanical complications of nervous system device (996.2)*

CC Excl: 250.60-250.63, 250.80-250.93, 349.1, 349.89, 349.9

Cranial Nerves

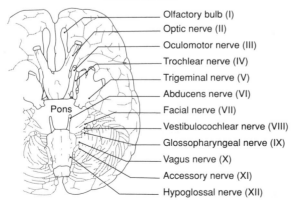

Olfactory bulb (I)
Optic nerve (II)
Oculomotor nerve (III)
Trochlear nerve (IV)
Trigeminal nerve (V)
Abducens nerve (VI)
Facial nerve (VII)
Vestibulocochlear nerve (VIII)
Glossopharyngeal nerve (IX)
Vagus nerve (X)
Accessory nerve (XI)
Hypoglossal nerve (XII)
Pons

349.2 Disorders of meninges, not elsewhere classified

Adhesions, meningeal (cerebral) (spinal)
Cyst, spinal meninges
Meningocele, acquired
Pseudomeningocele, acquired

AHA: 2Q, '98, 18; 3Q, '94, 4

☑5ᵗʰ **349.8 Other specified disorders of nervous system**

349.81 Cerebrospinal fluid rhinorrhea `CC`

> **EXCLUDES** *cerebrospinal fluid otorrhea (388.61)*

CC Excl: 250.60-250.63, 250.80-250.93, 349.81, 349.89, 349.9

DEF: Cerebrospinal fluid discharging from the nose; caused by fracture of frontal bone with tearing of dura mater and arachnoid.

349.82 Toxic encephalopathy `CC`

Use additional E code to identify cause

AHA: 4Q, '93, 29

CC Excl: 013.60-013.66, 017.90-017.96, 036.1, 049.8-049.9, 052.0, 054.3, 062.0-062.9, 063.0-063.9, 072.2, 090.41, 094.81, 130.0, 250.60-250.63, 250.80-250.93, 323.0-323.9, 348.3, 348.8-348.9, 349.82-349.89, 349.9

DEF: Brain tissue degeneration due to toxic substance.

349.89 Other

349.9 Unspecified disorders of nervous system `HIV`

Disorder of nervous system (central) NOS

Peripheral Nervous System

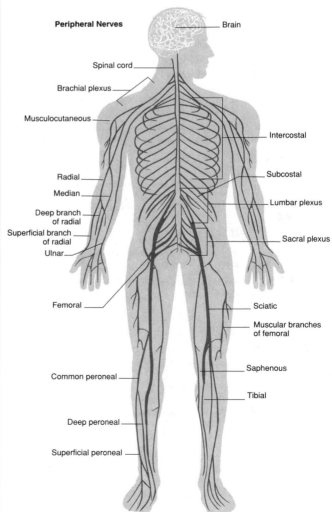

Peripheral Nerves
Brain
Spinal cord
Brachial plexus
Musculocutaneous
Intercostal
Radial
Subcostal
Median
Lumbar plexus
Deep branch of radial
Superficial branch of radial
Sacral plexus
Ulnar
Femoral
Sciatic
Muscular branches of femoral
Saphenous
Common peroneal
Tibial
Deep peroneal
Superficial peroneal

`N` Newborn Age: 0   `P` Pediatric Age: 0-17   `M` Maternity Age: 12-55   `A` Adult Age: 15-124   `CC` CC Condition   `MC` Major Complication   `CD` Complex Dx   `HIV` HIV Related Dx

DISORDERS OF THE PERIPHERAL NERVOUS SYSTEM (350-359)

EXCLUDES diseases of:
  acoustic [8th] nerve (388.5)
  oculomotor [3rd, 4th, 6th] nerves (378.0-378.9)
  optic [2nd] nerve (377.0-377.9)
  peripheral autonomic nerves (337.0-337.9)

neuralgia
neuritis   } NOS or "rheumatic"
radiculitis   (729.2)

peripheral neuritis in pregnancy (646.4)

✓4th **350 Trigeminal nerve disorders**
  INCLUDES   disorders of 5th cranial nerve

  350.1   Trigeminal neuralgia
      Tic douloureux   Trigeminal neuralgia NOS
      Trifacial neuralgia
      EXCLUDES   postherpetic (053.12)

  350.2   Atypical face pain
  350.8   Other specified trigeminal nerve disorders
  350.9   Trigeminal nerve disorder, unspecified

✓4th **351 Facial nerve disorders**
      INCLUDES   disorders of 7th cranial nerve
      EXCLUDES   that in newborn (767.5)

  351.0   Bell's palsy
      Facial palsy
      DEF: Unilateral paralysis of face due to lesion on facial nerve; produces facial distortion.

  351.1   Geniculate ganglionitis
      Geniculate ganglionitis NOS
      EXCLUDES   herpetic (053.11)
      DEF: Inflammation of tissue at bend in facial nerve.

  351.8   Other facial nerve disorders
      Facial myokymia   Melkersson's syndrome
  351.9   Facial nerve disorder, unspecified

✓4th **352 Disorders of other cranial nerves**
  352.0   Disorders of olfactory [lst] nerve
  352.1   Glossopharyngeal neuralgia
      DEF: Pain between throat and ear along petrosal and jugular ganglia.

  352.2   Other disorders of glossopharyngeal [9th] nerve
  352.3   Disorders of pneumogastric [10th] nerve
      Disorders of vagal nerve
      EXCLUDES   paralysis of vocal cords or larynx (478.30-478.34)
      DEF: Nerve disorder affecting ear, tongue, pharynx, larynx, esophagus, viscera and thorax.

  352.4   Disorders of accessory [11th] nerve
      DEF: Nerve disorder affecting palate, pharynx, larynx, thoracic viscera, sternocleidomastoid and trapezius muscles.

  352.5   Disorders of hypoglossal [12th] nerve
      DEF: Nerve disorder affecting tongue muscles.

  352.6   Multiple cranial nerve palsies
      Collet-Sicard syndrome
      Polyneuritis cranialis
  352.9   Unspecified disorder of cranial nerves

✓4th **353 Nerve root and plexus disorders**
      EXCLUDES   conditions due to:
          intervertebral disc disorders (722.0-722.9)
          spondylosis (720.0-721.9)
          vertebrogenic disorders (723.0-724.9)

  353.0   Brachial plexus lesions
      Cervical rib syndrome
      Costoclavicular syndrome
      Scalenus anticus syndrome
      Thoracic outlet syndrome
      EXCLUDES   brachial neuritis or radiculitis NOS (723.4)
          that in newborn (767.6)\
      DEF: Acquired disorder in tissue along nerves in shoulder; causes corresponding motor and sensory dysfunction.

▶ **Trigeminal and Facial Nerve Branches** ◀

  353.1   Lumbosacral plexus lesions
      DEF: Acquired disorder in tissue along nerves in lower back; causes corresponding motor and sensory dysfunction.

  353.2   Cervical root lesions, not elsewhere classified
  353.3   Thoracic root lesions, not elsewhere classified
  353.4   Lumbosacral root lesions, not elsewhere classified
  353.5   Neuralgic amyotrophy
      Parsonage-Aldren-Turner syndrome
  353.6   Phantom limb (syndrome)
      DEF: Abnormal tingling or a burning sensation, transient aches, and intermittent or continuous pain perceived as originating in the absent limb.

  353.8   Other nerve root and plexus disorders
  353.9   Unspecified nerve root and plexus disorder

✓4th **354 Mononeuritis of upper limb and mononeuritis multiplex**
      DEF: Inflammation of a single nerve; known as mononeuritis multiplex when several nerves in unrelated body areas are affected.

  354.0   Carpal tunnel syndrome
      Median nerve entrapment
      Partial thenar atrophy
      DEF: Compression of median nerve by tendons; causes pain, tingling, numbness and burning sensation in hand.

  354.1   Other lesion of median nerve
      Median nerve neuritis
  354.2   Lesion of ulnar nerve
      Cubital tunnel syndrome
      Tardy ulnar nerve palsy
  354.3   Lesion of radial nerve
      Acute radial nerve palsy
      AHA: N-D, '87, 6

  354.4   Causalgia of upper limb
      EXCLUDES   causalgia:
          NOS (355.9)
          lower limb (355.71)
      DEF: Peripheral nerve damage, upper limb; usually due to injury; causes burning sensation and trophic skin changes.

  354.5   Mononeuritis multiplex
      Combinations of single conditions classifiable to 354 or 355
  354.8   Other mononeuritis of upper limb
  354.9   Mononeuritis of upper limb, unspecified

✓4th **355 Mononeuritis of lower limb**
  355.0   Lesion of sciatic nerve
      EXCLUDES   sciatica NOS (724.3)
      AHA: 2Q, '89, 12
      DEF: Acquired disorder of sciatic nerve; causes motor and sensory dysfunction in back, buttock and leg.

  355.1   Meralgia paresthetica
      Lateral cutaneous femoral nerve of thigh compression or syndrome
      DEF: Inguinal ligament entraps lateral femoral cutaneous nerve; causes tingling, pain and numbness along outer thigh.

  355.2   Other lesion of femoral nerve

Nervous System and Sense Organs 350–355.2

✓4th ✓5th Additional Digit Required   Nonspecific PDx   Unacceptable PDx   Manifestation Code   MSP Medicare Secondary Payer   ▶◀ Revised Text   ● New Code   ▲ Revised Code Title

2002 Ingenix, Inc.   **January 2002 • Volume 1 — 89**

Nervous System and Sense Organs 355.3–359.0

355.3   **Lesion of lateral popliteal nerve**
Lesion of common peroneal nerve

355.4   **Lesion of medial popliteal nerve**

355.5   **Tarsal tunnel syndrome**
DEF: Compressed, entrapped posterior tibial nerve; causes tingling, pain and numbness in sole of foot.

355.6   **Lesion of plantar nerve**
Morton's metatarsalgia, neuralgia, or neuroma

✓5ᵗʰ **355.7**   **Other mononeuritis of lower limb**
    355.71 Causalgia of lower limb
      EXCLUDES   causalgia:
        NOS (355.9)
        upper limb (354.4)
      DEF: Dysfunction of lower limb peripheral nerve, usually due to injury; causes burning pain and trophic skin changes.

    355.79 Other mononeuritis of lower limb

355.8   **Mononeuritis of lower limb, unspecified**

355.9   **Mononeuritis of unspecified site**
Causalgia NOS
    EXCLUDES   causalgia:
      lower limb (355.71)
      upper limb (354.4)

✓4ᵗʰ **356 Hereditary and idiopathic peripheral neuropathy**

356.0   **Hereditary peripheral neuropathy**
Déjérine-Sottas disease

356.1   **Peroneal muscular atrophy**
Charcôt-Marie-Tooth disease
Neuropathic muscular atrophy
DEF: Genetic disorder, in muscles innervated by peroneal nerves; symptoms include muscle wasting in lower limbs and locomotor difficulties.

356.2   **Hereditary sensory neuropathy**
DEF: Inherited disorder in dorsal root ganglia, optic nerve, and cerebellum, causing sensory losses, shooting pains, and foot ulcers.

356.3   **Refsum's disease**
Heredopathia atactica polyneuritiformis
DEF: Genetic disorder of lipid metabolism; causes persistent, painful inflammation of nerves and retinitis pigmentosa.

356.4   **Idiopathic progressive polyneuropathy**

356.8   **Other specified idiopathic peripheral neuropathy**
Supranuclear paralysis

356.9   **Unspecified**

✓4ᵗʰ **357 Inflammatory and toxic neuropathy**

357.0   **Acute infective polyneuritis**   CC
Guillain-Barré syndrome Postinfectious polyneuritis
CC Excl: 003.21, 013.00-013.16, 036.0, 036.89, 036.9, 041.81-041.89, 041.9, 047.0-047.9, 049.0-049.1, 053.0, 054.72, 072.1, 090.42, 091.81, 094.2, 098.89, 100.81, 112.83, 114.2, 115.01, 115.11, 115.91, 130.0, 139.8, 320.0-320.9, 321.0-321.8, 322.0-322.9, 349.89, 349.9, 357.0

AHA: 2Q, '98, 12

DEF: Guillain-Barré syndrome: acute demyelinatry polyneuropathy preceded by viral illness (i.e., herpes, cytomegalovirus [CMV], Epstein-Barr virus [EBV]) or a bacterial illness; areflexic motor paralysis with mild sensory disturbance and acellular rise in spinal fluid protein.

357.1   *Polyneuropathy in collagen vasculardisease*
Code first underlying disease, as:
    disseminated lupus erythematosus (710.0)
    polyarteritis nodosa (446.0)
    rheumatoid arthritis (714.0)

357.2   *Polyneuropathy in diabetes*
Code first underlying disease (250.6)
AHA: 2Q, '92, 15; 3Q, '91, 9

357.3   *Polyneuropathy in malignant disease*
Code first underlying disease (140.0-208.9)

357.4   *Polyneuropathy in other diseases classified elsewhere*
Code first underlying disease, as:
    amyloidosis (277.3)
    beriberi (265.0)
    deficiency of B vitamins (266.0-266.9)
    diphtheria (032.0-032.9)
    hypoglycemia (251.2)
    pellagra (265.2)
    porphyria (277.1)
    sarcoidosis (135)
    uremia (585)
    EXCLUDES   polyneuropathy in:
      herpes zoster (053.13)
      mumps (072.72)

AHA: 2Q, '98, 15

357.5   **Alcoholic polyneuropathy**

357.6   **Polyneuropathy due to drugs**
Use additional E code to identify drug

357.7   **Polyneuropathy due to other toxic agents**
Use additional E code to identify toxic agent

✓5ᵗʰ **357.8**   **Other**
AHA: 2Q, '98, 12

DEF: Chronic inflammatory demyelinating polyneuritis: inflammation of peripheral nerves resulting in destruction of myelin sheath; associated with diabetes mellitus, dysproteinemias, renal failure and malnutrition; symptoms include tingling, numbness, burning pain, diminished tendon reflexes, weakness, and atrophy in lower extremities.

    357.81 Chronic inflammatory demyelinating polyneuritis

    357.82 Critical illness polyneuropathy
Acute motor neuropathy

    357.89 Other inflammatory and toxic neuropathy

357.9   **Unspecified**

✓4ᵗʰ **358 Myoneural disorders**

358.0   **Myasthenia gravis**   CC
CC Excl: 250.60-250.63, 250.80-250.93, 349.89, 349.9, 358.0-358.1

DEF: Autoimmune disorder of acetylcholine at neuromuscular junction; causing fatigue of voluntary muscles.

358.1   *Myasthenic syndromes in diseases classified elsewhere*   CC

Amyotrophy
Eaton-Lambert   }   from stated cause
syndrome   classified elsewhere

Code first underlying disease, as:
    botulism (005.1)
    diabetes mellitus (250.6)
    hypothyroidism (244.0-244.9)
    malignant neoplasm (140.0-208.9)
    pernicious anemia (281.0)
    thyrotoxicosis (242.0-242.9)

CC Excl: See code 358.0

358.2   **Toxic myoneural disorders**
Use additional E code to identify toxic agent

358.8   **Other specified myoneural disorders**

358.9   **Myoneural disorders, unspecified**

✓4ᵗʰ **359 Muscular dystrophies and other myopathies**
    EXCLUDES   idiopathic polymyositis (710.4)

359.0   **Congenital hereditary muscular dystrophy**   CC
Benign congenital myopathy   Myotubular myopathy
Central core disease   Nemaline body disease
Centronuclear myopathy
    EXCLUDES   arthrogryposis multiplex congenita (754.89)

CC Excl: 250.60-250.63, 250.80-250.93, 349.89, 349.9, 359.0-359.1

DEF: Genetic disorder; causing progressive or nonprogressive muscle weakness.

N Newborn Age: 0   P Pediatric Age: 0-17   M Maternity Age: 12-55   A Adult Age: 15-124   CC CC Condition   MC Major Complication   CD Complex Dx   HIV HIV Related Dx

359.1 Hereditary progressive muscular dystrophy `CC`

Muscular dystrophy:	Muscular dystrophy:
NOS	Gower's
distal	Landouzy-Déjérine
Duchenne	limb-girdle
Erb's	ocular
fascioscapulohumeral	oculopharyngeal

CC Excl: See code 359.0

DEF: Genetic degenerative, muscle disease; causes progressive weakness, wasting of muscle with no nerve involvement.

359.2 Myotonic disorders

Dystrophia myotonica	Paramyotonia congenita
Eulenburg's disease	Steinert's disease
Myotonia congenita	Thomsen's disease

DEF: Impaired movement due to spasmatic, rigid muscles.

359.3 Familial periodic paralysis

Hypokalemic familial periodic paralysis

DEF: Genetic disorder; characterized by rapidly progressive flaccid paralysis; attacks often occur after exercise or exposure to cold or dietary changes.

359.4 Toxic myopathy

Use additional E code to identify toxic agent

AHA: 1Q, '88, 5

DEF: Muscle disorder caused by toxic agent.

359.5 *Myopathy in endocrine diseases classified elsewhere*

Code first underlying disease, as:
Addison's disease (255.4)
Cushing's syndrome (255.0)
hypopituitarism (253.2)
myxedema (244.0-244.9)
thyrotoxicosis (242.0-242.9)

DEF: Muscle disorder secondary to dysfunction in hormone secretion.

359.6 *Symptomatic inflammatory myopathy in diseases classified elsewhere*

Code first underlying disease, as:
amyloidosis (277.3)
disseminated lupus erythematosus (710.0)
malignant neoplasm (140.0-208.9)
polyarteritis nodosa (446.0)
rheumatoid arthritis (714.0)
sarcoidosis (135)
scleroderma (710.1)
Sjögren's disease (710.2)

√5ᵗʰ 359.8 Other myopathies

AHA: 3Q, '90, 17

● **359.81 Critical illness myopathy**
Acute necrotizing myopathy
Acute quadriplegic myopathy
Intensive care (ICU) myopathy
Myopathy of critical illness

● **359.89 Other myopathies**

359.9 Myopathy, unspecified

DISORDERS OF THE EYE AND ADNEXA (360-379)

√4ᵗʰ 360 Disorders of the globe

`INCLUDES` disorders affecting multiple structures of eye

√5ᵗʰ 360.0 Purulent endophthalmitis

360.00 Purulent endophthalmitis, unspecified

360.01 Acute endophthalmitis

360.02 Panophthalmitis

360.03 Chronic endophthalmitis

360.04 Vitreous abscess

√5ᵗʰ 360.1 Other endophthalmitis

360.11 Sympathetic uveitis

DEF: Inflammation of vascular layer of uninjured eye; follows injury to other eye.

Eye

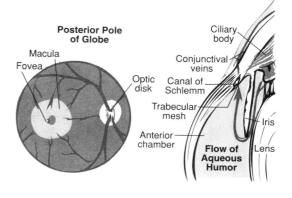

360.12 Panuveitis

DEF: Inflammation of entire vascular layer of eye, including choroid, iris and ciliary body.

360.13 Parasitic endophthalmitis NOS

DEF: Parasitic infection causing inflammation of the entire eye.

360.14 Ophthalmia nodosa

DEF: Conjunctival inflammation caused by embedded hairs.

360.19 Other

Phacoanaphylactic endophthalmitis

√5ᵗʰ 360.2 Degenerative disorders of globe

AHA: 3Q, '91, 3

360.20 Degenerative disorder of globe, unspecified

360.21 Progressive high (degenerative) myopia

Malignant myopia

DEF: Severe, progressive nearsightedness in adults, complicated by serious disease of the choroid; leads to retinal detachment and blindness.

360.23 Siderosis

DEF: Iron pigment deposits within tissue of eyeball; caused by high iron content of blood.

360.24 Other metallosis

Chalcosis

DEF: Metal deposits, other than iron, within eyeball tissues.

360.29 Other

`EXCLUDES` xerophthalmia (264.7)

√5ᵗʰ 360.3 Hypotony of eye

360.30 Hypotony, unspecified

DEF: Low osmotic pressure causing lack of tone, tension and strength.

360.31 Primary hypotony

√4ᵗʰ Additional Digit Required   Nonspecific PDx   Unacceptable PDx   Manifestation Code   **MSP** Medicare Secondary Payer   ►◄ Revised Text   ● New Code   ▲ Revised Code Title

2002 Ingenix, Inc.   **October 2002 • Volume 1 — 91**

Nervous System and Sense Organs 360.32–361.31

Adnexa

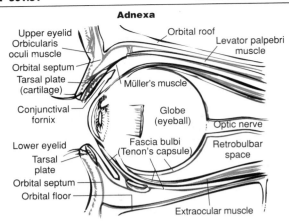

Upper eyelid
Orbicularis oculi muscle
Orbital septum
Tarsal plate (cartilage)
Conjunctival fornix
Lower eyelid
Tarsal plate
Orbital septum
Orbital floor

Orbital roof
Levator palpebri muscle
Müller's muscle
Globe (eyeball)
Optic nerve
Fascia bulbi (Tenon's capsule)
Retrobulbar space
Extraocular muscle

360.32 Ocular fistula causing hypotony

DEF: Low intraocular pressure due to leak through abnormal passage.

360.33 Hypotony associated with other ocular disorders

360.34 Flat anterior chamber

DEF: Low pressure behind cornea, causing compression.

√5th **360.4 Degenerated conditions of globe**

360.40 Degenerated globe or eye, unspecified

360.41 Blind hypotensive eye
Atrophy of globe
Phthisis bulbi

DEF: Vision loss due to extremely low intraocular pressure.

360.42 Blind hypertensive eye
Absolute glaucoma

DEF: Vision loss due to painful, high intraocular pressure.

360.43 Hemophthalmos, except current injury

EXCLUDES   traumatic (871.0-871.9, 921.0-921.9)

DEF: Pool of blood within eyeball, not from current injury.

360.44 Leucocoria

DEF: Whitish mass or reflex in the pupil behind lens; also called cat's eye reflex; often indicative of retinoblastoma.

√5th **360.5 Retained (old) intraocular foreign body, magnetic**

EXCLUDES   current penetrating injury with magnetic foreign body (871.5)
retained (old) foreign body of orbit (376.6)

360.50 Foreign body, magnetic, intraocular, unspecified

360.51 Foreign body, magnetic, in anterior chamber

360.52 Foreign body, magnetic, in iris or ciliary body

360.53 Foreign body, magnetic, in lens

360.54 Foreign body, magnetic, in vitreous

360.55 Foreign body, magnetic, in posterior wall

360.59 Foreign body, magnetic, in other or multiple sites

√5th **360.6 Retained (old) intraocular foreign body, nonmagnetic**
Retained (old) foreign body:
NOS
nonmagnetic

EXCLUDES   current penetrating injury with (nonmagnetic) foreign body (871.6)
retained (old) foreign body in orbit (376.6)

360.60 Foreign body, intraocular, unspecified

360.61 Foreign body in anterior chamber

360.62 Foreign body in iris or ciliary body

360.63 Foreign body in lens

360.64 Foreign body in vitreous

360.65 Foreign body in posterior wall

360.69 Foreign body in other or multiple sites

√5th **360.8 Other disorders of globe**

360.81 Luxation of globe

DEF: Displacement of eyeball.

360.89 Other

360.9 Unspecified disorder of globe

√4th **361 Retinal detachments and defects**

DEF: Light-sensitive layer at back of eye, separates from blood supply; disrupting vision.

√5th **361.0 Retinal detachment with retinal defect**
Rhegmatogenous retinal detachment

EXCLUDES   detachment of retinal pigment epithelium (362.42-362.43)
retinal detachment (serous) (without defect) (361.2)

361.00 Retinal detachment with retinal defect, unspecified

361.01 Recent detachment, partial, with single defect

361.02 Recent detachment, partial, with multiple defects

361.03 Recent detachment, partial, with giant tear

361.04 Recent detachment, partial, with retinal dialysis
Dialysis (juvenile) of retina (with detachment)

361.05 Recent detachment, total or subtotal

361.06 Old detachment, partial
Delimited old retinal detachment

361.07 Old detachment, total or subtotal

√5th **361.1 Retinoschisis and retinal cysts**

EXCLUDES   juvenile retinoschisis (362.73)
microcystoid degeneration of retina (362.62)
parasitic cyst of retina (360.13)

361.10 Retinoschisis, unspecified

DEF: Separation of retina due to degenerative process of aging; should not be confused with acute retinal detachment.

361.11 Flat retinoschisis

DEF: Slow, progressive split of retinal sensory layers

361.12 Bullous retinoschisis

DEF: Fluid retention between split retinal sensory layers.

361.13 Primary retinal cysts

361.14 Secondary retinal cysts

361.19 Other
Pseudocyst of retina

361.2 Serous retinal detachment
Retinal detachment without retinal defect

EXCLUDES   central serous retinopathy (362.41)
retinal pigment epithelium detachment (362.42-362.43)

√5th **361.3 Retinal defects without detachment**

EXCLUDES   chorioretinal scars after surgery for detachment (363.30-363.35)
peripheral retinal degeneration without defect (362.60-362.66)

361.30 Retinal defect, unspecified
Retinal break(s) NOS

361.31 Round hole of retina without detachment

N Newborn Age: 0   **P** Pediatric Age: 0-17   **M** Maternity Age: 12-55   **A** Adult Age: 15-124   **CC** CC Condition   **MC** Major Complication   **CD** Complex Dx   **HIV** HIV Related Dx

92 — Volume 1   *2002 Ingenix, Inc.*

361.32 Horseshoe tear of retina without detachment

Operculum of retina without mention of detachment

361.33 Multiple defects of retina without detachment

✓5th **361.8 Other forms of retinal detachment**

361.81 Traction detachment of retina

Traction detachment with vitreoretinal organization

361.89 Other

AHA: 3Q, '99, 12

361.9 Unspecified retinal detachment

AHA: N-D, '87, 10

✓4th **362 Other retinal disorders**

EXCLUDES chorioretinal scars (363.30-363.35)
chorioretinitis (363.0-363.2)

✓5th **362.0 Diabetic retinopathy**

Code first diabetes (250.5)

DEF: Retinal changes in diabetes of long duration; causes hemorrhages, microaneurysms, waxy deposits and proliferative noninflammatory degenerative disease of retina.

AHA: 3Q, '91, 8

362.01 Background diabetic retinopathy

Diabetic macular edema
Diabetic retinal edema
Diabetic retinal microaneurysms
Diabetic retinopathy NOS

362.02 Proliferative diabetic retinopathy

AHA: 3Q, '96, 5

✓5th **362.1 Other background retinopathy and retinal vascular changes**

362.10 Background retinopathy, unspecified

362.11 Hypertensive retinopathy

AHA: 3Q, '90, 3

DEF: Retinal irregularities caused by systemic hypertension.

362.12 Exudative retinopathy

Coats' syndrome

AHA: 3Q, '99, 12

362.13 Changes in vascular appearance

Vascular sheathing of retina
Use additional code for any associated atherosclerosis (440.8)

362.14 Retinal microaneurysms NOS

DEF: Microscopic dilation of retinal vessels in nondiabetic.

362.15 Retinal telangiectasia

DEF: Dilation of blood vessels of the retina.

362.16 Retinal neovascularization NOS

Neovascularization: Neovascularization:
choroidal   subretinal

DEF: New and abnormal vascular growth in the retina.

362.17 Other intraretinal microvascular abnormalities

Retinal varices

362.18 Retinal vasculitis

Eales' disease   Retinal:
Retinal: perivasculitis
arteritis   phlebitis
endarteritis

DEF: Inflammation of retinal blood vessels.

✓5th **362.2 Other proliferative retinopathy**

362.21 Retrolental fibroplasia

DEF: Fibrous tissue in vitreous, from retina to lens, causing blindness; associated with premature infants requiring high amounts of oxygen.

362.29 Other nondiabetic proliferative retinopathy

AHA: 3Q, '96, 5

✓5th **362.3 Retinal vascular occlusion**

DEF: Obstructed blood flow to and from retina.

362.30 Retinal vascular occlusion, unspecified

362.31 Central retinal artery occlusion

362.32 Arterial branch occlusion

362.33 Partial arterial occlusion

Hollenhorst plaque
Retinal microembolism

362.34 Transient arterial occlusion

Amaurosis fugax

AHA: 1Q, '00, 16

362.35 Central retinal vein occlusion

AHA: 2Q, '93, 6

362.36 Venous tributary (branch) occlusion

362.37 Venous engorgement

Occlusion:
incipient } of retinal vein
partial

✓5th **362.4 Separation of retinal layers**

EXCLUDES retinal detachment (serous) (361.2)
rhegmatogenous (361.00-361.07)

362.40 Retinal layer separation, unspecified

362.41 Central serous retinopathy

DEF: Serous-filled blister causing detachment of retina from pigment epithelium.

362.42 Serous detachment of retinal pigment epithelium

Exudative detachment of retinal pigment epithelium

DEF: Blister of fatty fluid causing detachment of retina from pigment epithelium.

362.43 Hemorrhagic detachment of retinal pigment epithelium

DEF: Blood-filled blister causing detachment of retina from pigment epithelium.

✓5th **362.5 Degeneration of macula and posterior pole**

EXCLUDES degeneration of optic disc (377.21-377.24)
hereditary retinal degeneration [dystrophy] (362.70-362.77)

362.50 Macular degeneration (senile), unspecified

362.51 Nonexudative senile macular degeneration

Senile macular degeneration:
atrophic
dry

362.52 Exudative senile macular degeneration

Kuhnt-Junius degeneration
Senile macular degeneration:
disciform
wet

DEF: Leakage in macular blood vessels with loss of visual acuity.

362.53 Cystoid macular degeneration

Cystoid macular edema

DEF: Retinal swelling and cyst formation in macula.

362.54 Macular cyst, hole, or pseudohole

362.55 Toxic maculopathy

Use additional E code to identify drug, if drug induced

362.56 Macular puckering

Preretinal fibrosis

362.57 Drusen (degenerative)

DEF: White, hyaline deposits on Bruch's membrane (lamina basalis choroideae).

Nervous System and Sense Organs 361.32–362.57

✓4th
✓5th
Additional Digit Required   Nonspecific PDx   Unacceptable PDx   Manifestation Code   MSP Medicare Secondary Payer   ►◄ Revised Text   ● New Code   ▲ Revised Code Title

2002 Ingenix, Inc.

Volume 1 — 93

√5th **362.6 Peripheral retinal degenerations**

EXCLUDES *hereditary retinal degeneration [dystrophy] (362.70-362.77)*
retinal degeneration with retinal defect (361.00-361.07)

362.60 Peripheral retinal degeneration, unspecified

362.61 Paving stone degeneration
DEF: Degeneration of peripheral retina; causes thinning through which choroid is visible.

362.62 Microcystoid degeneration
Blessig's cysts   Iwanoff's cysts

362.63 Lattice degeneration
Palisade degeneration of retina
DEF: Degeneration of retina; often bilateral, usually benign; characterized by lines intersecting at irregular intervals in peripheral retina; retinal thinning and retinal holes may occur.

362.64 Senile reticular degeneration
DEF: Net-like appearance of retina; sign of degeneration.

362.65 Secondary pigmentary degeneration
Pseudoretinitis pigmentosa

362.66 Secondary vitreoretinal degenerations

√5th **362.7 Hereditary retinal dystrophies**
DEF: Genetically induced progressive changes in retina.

362.70 Hereditary retinal dystrophy, unspecified

362.71 *Retinal dystrophy in systemic or cerebroretinal lipidoses*
Code first underlying disease, as:
cerebroretinal lipidoses (330.1)
systemic lipidoses (272.7)

362.72 *Retinal dystrophy in other systemic disorders and syndromes*
Code first underlying disease, as:
Bassen-Kornzweig syndrome (272.5)
Refsum's disease (356.3)

362.73 Vitreoretinal dystrophies
Juvenile retinoschisis

362.74 Pigmentary retinal dystrophy
Retinal dystrophy, albipunctate
Retinitis pigmentosa

362.75 Other dystrophies primarily involving the sensory retina
Progressive cone(-rod) dystrophy
Stargardt's disease

362.76 Dystrophies primarily involving the retinal pigment epithelium
Fundus flavimaculatus
Vitelliform dystrophy

362.77 Dystrophies primarily involving Bruch's membrane
Dystrophy:
hyaline
pseudoinflammatory foveal
Hereditary drusen

√5th **362.8 Other retinal disorders**
EXCLUDES *chorioretinal inflammations (363.0-363.2)*
chorioretinal scars (363.30-363.35)

362.81 Retinal hemorrhage
Hemorrhage:
preretinal
retinal (deep) (superficial)
subretinal
AHA: 4Q, '96, 43

362.82 Retinal exudates and deposits

362.83 Retinal edema
Retinal:
cotton wool spots
edema (localized) (macular) (peripheral)
DEF: Retinal swelling due to fluid accumulation.

362.84 Retinal ischemia
DEF: Reduced retinal blood supply.

362.85 Retinal nerve fiber bundle defects

362.89 Other retinal disorders

362.9 Unspecified retinal disorder

√4th **363 Chorioretinal inflammations, scars, and other disorders of choroid**

√5th **363.0 Focal chorioretinitis and focal retinochoroiditis**
EXCLUDES *focal chorioretinitis or retinochoroiditis in:*
histoplasmosis (115.02, 115.12, 115.92)
toxoplasmosis (130.2)
congenital infection (771.2)

363.00 Focal chorioretinitis, unspecified
Focal:
choroiditis or chorioretinitis NOS
retinitis or retinochoroiditis NOS

363.01 Focal choroiditis and chorioretinitis, juxtapapillary

363.03 Focal choroiditis and chorioretinitis of other posterior pole

363.04 Focal choroiditis and chorioretinitis, peripheral

363.05 Focal retinitis and retinochoroiditis, juxtapapillary
Neuroretinitis

363.06 Focal retinitis and retinochoroiditis, macular or paramacular

363.07 Focal retinitis and retinochoroiditis of other posterior pole

363.08 Focal retinitis and retinochoroiditis, peripheral

√5th **363.1 Disseminated chorioretinitis and disseminated retinochoroiditis**
EXCLUDES *disseminated choroiditis or chorioretinitis in secondary syphilis (091.51)*
neurosyphilitic disseminated retinitis or retinochoroiditis (094.83)
retinal (peri)vasculitis (362.18)

363.10 Disseminated chorioretinitis, unspecified
Disseminated:
choroiditis or chorioretinitis NOS
retinitis or retinochoroiditis NOS

363.11 Disseminated choroiditis and chorioretinitis, posterior pole

363.12 Disseminated choroiditis and chorioretinitis, peripheral

363.13 Disseminated choroiditis and chorioretinitis, generalized
Code first any underlying disease, as:
tuberculosis (017.3)

363.14 Disseminated retinitis and retinochoroiditis, metastatic

363.15 Disseminated retinitis and retinochoroiditis, pigment epitheliopathy
Acute posterior multifocal placoid pigment epitheliopathy
DEF: Widespread inflammation of retina and choroid; characterized by pigmented epithelium involvement.

√5th **363.2 Other and unspecified forms of chorioretinitis and retinochoroiditis**
EXCLUDES *panophthalmitis (360.02)*
sympathetic uveitis (360.11)
uveitis NOS (364.3)

363.20 Chorioretinitis, unspecified
Choroiditis NOS
Retinitis NOS
Uveitis, posterior NOS

N Newborn Age: 0   P Pediatric Age: 0-17   M Maternity Age: 12-55   A Adult Age: 15-124   CC CC Condition   MC Major Complication   CD Complex Dx   HIV HIV Related Dx

2002 Ingenix, Inc.

363.21 Pars planitis
Posterior cyclitis

DEF: Inflammation of peripheral retina and ciliary body; characterized by bands of white cells.

363.22 Harada's disease

DEF: Retinal detachment and bilateral widespread exudative choroiditis; symptoms include headache, vomiting, increased lymphocytes in cerebrospinal fluid; and temporary or permanent deafness may occur.

√5th **363.3 Chorioretinal scars**
Scar (postinflammatory) (postsurgical) (posttraumatic):
choroid
retina

363.30 Chorioretinal scar, unspecified

363.31 Solar retinopathy

DEF: Retinal scarring caused by solar radiation.

363.32 Other macular scars

363.33 Other scars of posterior pole

363.34 Peripheral scars

363.35 Disseminated scars

√5th **363.4 Choroidal degenerations**

363.40 Choroidal degeneration, unspecified
Choroidal sclerosis NOS

363.41 Senile atrophy of choroid

DEF: Wasting away of choroid; due to aging.

363.42 Diffuse secondary atrophy of choroid

DEF: Wasting away of choroid in systemic disease.

363.43 Angioid streaks of choroid

DEF: Degeneration of choroid; characterized by dark brown steaks radiating from optic disk; occurs with pseudoxanthoma, elasticum or Paget's disease.

√5th **363.5 Hereditary choroidal dystrophies**
Hereditary choroidal atrophy:
partial [choriocapillaris]
total [all vessels]

363.50 Hereditary choroidal dystrophy or atrophy, unspecified

363.51 Circumpapillary dystrophy of choroid, partial

363.52 Circumpapillary dystrophy of choroid, total
Helicoid dystrophy of choroid

363.53 Central dystrophy of choroid, partial
Dystrophy, choroidal:
central areolar
circinate

363.54 Central choroidal atrophy, total
Dystrophy, choroidal:
central gyrate
serpiginous

363.55 Choroideremia

DEF: Hereditary choroid degeneration, occurs in first decade; characterized by constricted visual field and ultimately blindness in males; less debilitating in females.

363.56 Other diffuse or generalized dystrophy, partial
Diffuse choroidal sclerosis

363.57 Other diffuse or generalized dystrophy, total
Generalized gyrate atrophy, choroid

√5th **363.6 Choroidal hemorrhage and rupture**

363.61 Choroidal hemorrhage, unspecified

363.62 Expulsive choroidal hemorrhage

363.63 Choroidal rupture

√5th **363.7 Choroidal detachment**

363.70 Choroidal detachment, unspecified

363.71 Serous choroidal detachment

DEF: Detachment of choroid from sclera; due to blister of serous fluid.

363.72 Hemorrhagic choroidal detachment

DEF: Detachment of choroid from sclera; due to blood-filled blister.

363.8 Other disorders of choroid

363.9 Unspecified disorder of choroid

√4th **364 Disorders of iris and ciliary body**

√5th **364.0 Acute and subacute iridocyclitis**
Anterior uveitis ⎫
Cyclitis ⎪ acute
Iridocyclitis ⎬ subacute
Iritis ⎭

EXCLUDES   gonococcal (098.41)
herpes simplex (054.44)
herpes zoster (053.22)

364.00 Acute and subacute iridocyclitis, unspecified

364.01 Primary iridocyclitis

364.02 Recurrent iridocyclitis

364.03 Secondary iridocyclitis, infectious

364.04 Secondary iridocyclitis, noninfectious
Aqueous: Aqueous:
cells   flare
fibrin

364.05 Hypopyon

DEF: Accumulation of white blood cells between cornea and lens.

√5th **364.1 Chronic iridocyclitis**
EXCLUDES   posterior cyclitis (363.21)

364.10 Chronic iridocyclitis, unspecified

364.11 Chronic iridocyclitis in diseases classified elsewhere
Code first underlying disease, as:
sarcoidosis (135)
tuberculosis (017.3)
EXCLUDES   *syphilitic iridocyclitis (091.52)*

DEF: Persistent inflammation of iris and ciliary body; due to underlying disease or condition.

√5th **364.2 Certain types of iridocyclitis**
EXCLUDES   posterior cyclitis (363.21)
sympathetic uveitis (360.11)

364.21 Fuchs' heterochromic cyclitis

DEF: Chronic cyclitis characterized by differences in the color of the two irises; the lighter iris appears in the inflamed eye.

364.22 Glaucomatocyclitic crises

DEF: One-sided form of secondary open angle glaucoma; recurrent, uncommon and of short duration; causes high intraocular pressure, rarely damage.

364.23 Lens-induced iridocyclitis

DEF: Inflammation of iris; due to immune reaction to proteins in lens following trauma or other lens abnormality.

364.24 Vogt-Koyanagi syndrome

DEF: Uveomeningitis with exudative iridocyclitis and choroiditis; causes depigmentation of hair and skin, detached retina; tinnitus and loss of hearing may occur.

364.3 Unspecified iridocyclitis
Uveitis NOS

√5th **364.4 Vascular disorders of iris and ciliary body**

364.41 Hyphema
Hemorrhage of iris or ciliary body

DEF: Hemorrhage in anterior chamber; also called hyphemia or "blood shot" eyes.

√4th Additional Digit Required   Nonspecific PDx   Unacceptable PDx   Manifestation Code   **MSP** Medicare Secondary Payer   ►◄ Revised Text   ● New Code   ▲ Revised Code Title

2002 Ingenix, Inc.   **Volume 1 — 95**

Nervous System and Sense Organs 364.42–365.42

364.42 Rubeosis iridis
Neovascularization of iris or ciliary body

DEF: Blood vessel and connective tissue formation on surface of iris; symptomatic of diabetic retinopathy, central retinal vein occlusion and retinal detachment.

√5th **364.5 Degenerations of iris and ciliary body**
364.51 Essential or progressive iris atrophy
364.52 Iridoschisis

DEF: Splitting of the iris into two layers.

364.53 Pigmentary iris degeneration
Acquired heterochromia
Pigment dispersion syndrome } of iris
Translucency

364.54 Degeneration of pupillary margin
Atrophy of sphincter }
Ectropion of pigment } of iris
epithelium

364.55 Miotic cysts of pupillary margin

DEF: Serous-filled sacs in pupillary margin of iris.

364.56 Degenerative changes of chamber angle
364.57 Degenerative changes of ciliary body
364.59 Other iris atrophy
Iris atrophy (generalized) (sector shaped)

√5th **364.6 Cysts of iris, ciliary body, and anterior chamber**
EXCLUDES   miotic pupillary cyst (364.55)
parasitic cyst (360.13)

364.60 Idiopathic cysts

DEF: Fluid-filled sacs in iris or ciliary body; unknown etiology.

364.61 Implantation cysts
Epithelial down-growth, anterior chamber
Implantation cysts (surgical) (traumatic)

364.62 Exudative cysts of iris or anterior chamber
364.63 Primary cyst of pars plana

DEF: Fluid-filled sacs of outermost ciliary ring.

364.64 Exudative cyst of pars plana

DEF: Protein, fatty-filled sacs of outermost ciliary ring; due to fluid lead from blood vessels.

√5th **364.7 Adhesions and disruptions of iris and ciliary body**
EXCLUDES   flat anterior chamber (360.34)

364.70 Adhesions of iris, unspecified
Synechiae (iris) NOS

364.71 Posterior synechiae

DEF: Adhesion binding iris to lens.

364.72 Anterior synechiae

DEF: Adhesion binding the iris to cornea.

364.73 Goniosynechiae
Peripheral anterior synechiae

DEF: Adhesion binding the iris to cornea at the angle of the anterior chamber.

364.74 Pupillary membranes
Iris bombé   Pupillary:
Pupillary: seclusion
occlusion

DEF: Membrane traversing the pupil and blocking vision.

364.75 Pupillary abnormalities
Deformed pupil   Rupture of sphincter, pupil
Ectopic pupil

364.76 Iridodialysis

DEF: Separation of the iris from the ciliary body base; due to trauma or surgical accident.

364.77 Recession of chamber angle

DEF: Receding of anterior chamber angle of the eye; restricts vision.

364.8 Other disorders of iris and ciliary body
Prolapse of iris NOS
EXCLUDES   prolapse of iris in recent wound (871.1)

364.9 Unspecified disorder of iris and ciliary body

√4th **365 Glaucoma**
EXCLUDES   blind hypertensive eye [absolute glaucoma] (360.42)
congenital glaucoma (743.20-743.22)

DEF: Rise in intraocular pressure which restricts blood flow; multiple causes.

√5th **365.0 Borderline glaucoma [glaucoma suspect]**
AHA: 1Q, '90, 8

365.00 Preglaucoma, unspecified
365.01 Open angle with borderline findings
Open angle with:
borderline intraocular pressure
cupping of optic discs

DEF: Minor block of aqueous outflow from eye.

365.02 Anatomical narrow angle
365.03 Steroid responders
365.04 Ocular hypertension

DEF: High fluid pressure within eye; no apparent cause.

√5th **365.1 Open-angle glaucoma**
365.10 Open-angle glaucoma, unspecified
Wide-angle glaucoma NOS

365.11 Primary open angle glaucoma
Chronic simple glaucoma

DEF: High intraocular pressure, despite free flow of aqueous.

365.12 Low tension glaucoma
365.13 Pigmentary glaucoma

DEF: High intraocular pressure; due to iris pigment granules blocking aqueous flow.

365.14 Glaucoma of childhood
Infantile or juvenile glaucoma

365.15 Residual stage of open angle glaucoma

√5th **365.2 Primary angle-closure glaucoma**
365.20 Primary angle-closure glaucoma, unspecified
365.21 Intermittent angle-closure glaucoma
Angle-closure glaucoma:
interval
subacute

DEF: Recurring attacks of high intraocular pressure; due to blocked aqueous flow.

365.22 Acute angle-closure glaucoma

DEF: Sudden, severe rise in intraocular pressure due to blockage in aqueous drainage.

365.23 Chronic angle-closure glaucoma
AHA: 2Q, '98, 16

365.24 Residual stage of angle-closure glaucoma

√5th **365.3 Corticosteroid-induced glaucoma**

DEF: Elevated intraocular pressure; due to long-term corticosteroid therapy.

365.31 Glaucomatous stage
365.32 Residual stage

√5th **365.4 Glaucoma associated with congenital anomalies, dystrophies, and systemic syndromes**

365.41 *Glaucoma associated with chamber angle anomalies*
Code first associated disorder, as:
Axenfeld's anomaly (743.44)
Rieger's anomaly or syndrome (743.44)

365.42 *Glaucoma associated with anomalies of iris*
Code first associated disorder, as:
aniridia (743.45)
essential iris atrophy (364.51)

N Newborn Age: 0   P Pediatric Age: 0-17   M Maternity Age: 12-55   A Adult Age: 15-124   CC CC Condition   MC Major Complication   CD Complex Dx   HIV HIV Related Dx

96 — Volume 1   2002 Ingenix, Inc.

365.43 *Glaucoma associated with other anterior segment anomalies*
> Code first associated disorder, as:
> microcornea (743.41)

365.44 *Glaucoma associated with systemic syndromes*
> Code first associated disease, as
> neurofibromatosis (237.7)
> Sturge-Weber (-Dimitri) syndrome (759.6)

√5ᵗʰ **365.5 Glaucoma associated with disorders of the lens**

365.51 Phacolytic glaucoma
> Use additional code for associated hypermature cataract (366.18)
> DEF: Elevated intraocular pressure; due to lens protein blocking aqueous flow.

365.52 Pseudoexfoliation glaucoma
> Use additional code for associated pseudoexfoliation of capsule (366.11)
> DEF: Glaucoma characterized by small grayish particles deposited on the lens.

365.59 Glaucoma associated with other lens disorders
> Use additional code for associated disorder, as:
> dislocation of lens (379.33-379.34)
> spherophakia (743.36)

√5ᵗʰ **365.6 Glaucoma associated with other ocular disorders**

365.60 Glaucoma associated with unspecified ocular disorder

365.61 Glaucoma associated with pupillary block
> Use additional code for associated disorder, as:
> seclusion of pupil [iris bombé] (364.74)
> DEF: Acute, open-angle glaucoma caused by mature cataract; aqueous flow is blocked by lens material and macrophages.

365.62 Glaucoma associated with ocular inflammations
> Use additional code for associated disorder, as:
> glaucomatocyclitic crises (364.22)
> iridocyclitis (364.0-364.3)

365.63 Glaucoma associated with vascular disorders
> Use additional code for associated disorder, as:
> central retinal vein occlusion (362.35)
> hyphema (364.41)

365.64 Glaucoma associated with tumors or cysts
> Use additional code for associated disorder, as:
> benign neoplasm (224.0-224.9)
> epithelial down-growth (364.61)
> malignant neoplasm (190.0-190.9)

365.65 Glaucoma associated with ocular trauma
> Use additional code for associated condition, as:
> contusion of globe (921.3)
> recession of chamber angle (364.77)

√5ᵗʰ **365.8 Other specified forms of glaucoma**

365.81 Hypersecretion glaucoma

365.82 Glaucoma with increased episcleral venous pressure

365.83 Aqueous misdirection
> Malignant glaucoma

365.89 Other specified glaucoma
> AHA: 2Q, '98, 16

365.9 Unspecified glaucoma
> AHA: 2Q, '01, 16

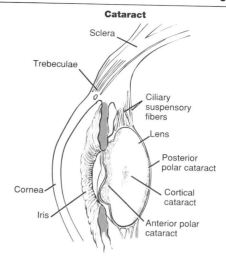

Cataract

√4ᵗʰ **366 Cataract**
> DEF: A variety of conditions that create a cloudy, or calcified lens that obstructs vision.
>
> **EXCLUDES**   congenital cataract (743.30-743.34)

√5ᵗʰ **366.0 Infantile, juvenile, and presenile cataract**

366.00 Nonsenile cataract, unspecified

366.01 Anterior subcapsular polar cataract
> DEF: Defect within the front, center lens surface.

366.02 Posterior subcapsular polar cataract
> DEF: Defect within the rear, center lens surface.

366.03 Cortical, lamellar, or zonular cataract
> DEF: Opacities radiating from center to edge of lens; appear as thin, concentric layers of lens.

366.04 Nuclear cataract

366.09 Other and combined forms of nonsenile cataract

√5ᵗʰ **366.1 Senile cataract**
> AHA: 3Q, '91, 9; S-O, '85, 10

366.10 Senile cataract, unspecified   🅰

366.11 Pseudoexfoliation of lens capsule   🅰

366.12 Incipient cataract   🅰
> Cataract: Cataract:
> coronary   punctate
> immature NOS   Water clefts
> DEF: Minor disorders of lens not affecting vision; due to aging.

366.13 Anterior subcapsular polar senile cataract   🅰

366.14 Posterior subcapsular polar senile cataract   🅰

366.15 Cortical senile cataract   🅰

366.16 Nuclear sclerosis   🅰
> Cataracta brunescens
> Nuclear cataract

366.17 Total or mature cataract   🅰

366.18 Hypermature cataract   🅰
> Morgagni cataract

366.19 Other and combined forms of senile cataract   🅰

√5ᵗʰ **366.2 Traumatic cataract**

366.20 Traumatic cataract, unspecified

366.21 Localized traumatic opacities
> Vossius' ring

366.22 Total traumatic cataract

366.23 Partially resolved traumatic cataract

√4ᵗʰ √5ᵗʰ Additional Digit Required   Nonspecific PDx   Unacceptable PDx   Manifestation Code   **MSP** Medicare Secondary Payer   ◄ Revised Text   ● New Code   ▲ Revised Code Title

2002 Ingenix, Inc.   **October 2002 • Volume 1 — 97**

Nervous System and Sense Organs 366.3–368.40

✓5ᵗʰ **366.3 Cataract secondary to ocular disorders**

366.30 Cataracta complicata, unspecified

366.31 Glaucomatous flecks (subcapsular)
*Code first underlying glaucoma
(365.0-365.9)*

366.32 Cataract in inflammatory disorders
Code first underlying condition, as:
chronic choroiditis (363.0-363.2)

366.33 Cataract with neovascularization
Code first underlying condition, as:
chronic iridocyclitis (364.10)

366.34 Cataract in degenerative disorders
Sunflower cataract
Code first underlying condition, as:
chalcosis (360.24)
degenerative myopia (360.21)
pigmentary retinal dystrophy (362.74)

✓5ᵗʰ **366.4 Cataract associated with other disorders**

366.41 *Diabetic cataract*
Code first diabetes (250.5)
AHA: 3Q, '91, 9; S-O, '85, 11

366.42 *Tetanic cataract*
Code first underlying disease, as:
calcinosis (275.4)
hypoparathyroidism (252.1)

366.43 *Myotonic cataract*
Code first underlying disorder (359.2)

366.44 *Cataract associated with other syndromes*
Code first underlying condition, as:
craniofacial dysostosis (756.0)
galactosemia (271.1)

366.45 Toxic cataract
Drug-induced cataract
Use additional E code to identify drug or
other toxic substance

**366.46 Cataract associated with radiation and
other physical influences**
Use additional E code to identify cause

✓5ᵗʰ **366.5 After-cataract**

366.50 After-cataract, unspecified
Secondary cataract NOS

366.51 Soemmering's ring
DEF: A donut-shaped lens remnant and a capsule behind
the pupil as a result of cataract surgery or trauma.

366.52 Other after-cataract, not obscuring vision

366.53 After-cataract, obscuring vision

366.8 Other cataract
Calcification of lens

366.9 Unspecified cataract

✓4ᵗʰ **367 Disorders of refraction and accommodation**

367.0 Hypermetropia
Far-sightedness   Hyperopia
DEF: Refraction error, called also hyperopia, focal point is posterior
to retina; abnormally short anteroposterior diameter or subnormal
refractive power; causes farsightedness.

367.1 Myopia
Near-sightedness
DEF: Refraction error, focal point is anterior to retina; causes near-
sightedness.

✓5ᵗʰ **367.2 Astigmatism**

367.20 Astigmatism, unspecified

367.21 Regular astigmatism

367.22 Irregular astigmatism

✓5ᵗʰ **367.3 Anisometropia and aniseikonia**

367.31 Anisometropia
DEF: Eyes with refractive powers that differ by at least
one diopter.

367.32 Aniseikonia
DEF: Eyes with unequal retinal imaging; usually due to
refractive error.

367.4 Presbyopia
DEF: Loss of crystalline lens elasticity; causes errors of
accommodation; due to aging.

✓5ᵗʰ **367.5 Disorders of accommodation**

367.51 Paresis of accommodation
Cycloplegia
DEF: Partial paralysis of ciliary muscle; causing focus
problems.

367.52 Total or complete internal ophthalmoplegia
DEF: Total paralysis of ciliary muscle; large pupil
incapable of focus.

367.53 Spasm of accommodation
DEF: Abnormal contraction of ciliary muscle; causes
focus problems.

✓5ᵗʰ **367.8 Other disorders of refraction and accommodation**

367.81 Transient refractive change

367.89 Other
Drug-induced ⎱ disorders of refraction
Toxic ⎰ and accommodation

**367.9 Unspecified disorder of refraction and
accommodation**

✓4ᵗʰ **368 Visual disturbances**
EXCLUDES *electrophysiological disturbances
(794.11-794.14)*

✓5ᵗʰ **368.0 Amblyopia ex anopsia**
DEF: Vision impaired due to disuse; esotropia often cause.

368.00 Amblyopia, unspecified

368.01 Strabismic amblyopia
Suppression amblyopia

368.02 Deprivation amblyopia
DEF: Decreased vision associated with suppressed
retinal image of one eye.

368.03 Refractive amblyopia

✓5ᵗʰ **368.1 Subjective visual disturbances**

368.10 Subjective visual disturbance, unspecified

368.11 Sudden visual loss

368.12 Transient visual loss
Concentric fading   Scintillating scotoma

368.13 Visual discomfort
Asthenopia   Photophobia
Eye strain

368.14 Visual distortions of shape and size
Macropsia   Micropsia
Metamorphopsia

**368.15 Other visual distortions and entoptic
phenomena**
Photopsia   Refractive:
Refractive: polyopia
diplopia   Visual halos

368.16 Psychophysical visual disturbances
Visual: Visual:
agnosia   hallucinations
disorientation syndrome

368.2 Diplopia
Double vision

✓5ᵗʰ **368.3 Other disorders of binocular vision**

368.30 Binocular vision disorder, unspecified

368.31 Suppression of binocular vision

**368.32 Simultaneous visual perception without
fusion**

368.33 Fusion with defective stereopsis
DEF: Faulty depth perception though normal ability to
focus.

368.34 Abnormal retinal correspondence

✓5ᵗʰ **368.4 Visual field defects**

368.40 Visual field defect, unspecified

N Newborn Age: 0   P Pediatric Age: 0-17   M Maternity Age: 12-55   A Adult Age: 15-124   CC CC Condition   MC Major Complication   CD Complex Dx   HIV HIV Related Dx

368.41 Scotoma involving central area

Scotoma:	Scotoma:
central	paracentral
centrocecal	

DEF: Vision loss (blind spot) in central five degrees of visual field.

368.42 Scotoma of blind spot area

Enlarged:	Paracecal scotoma
angioscotoma	
blind spot	

368.43 Sector or arcuate defects

Scotoma:	Scotoma:
arcuate	Seidel
Bjerrum	

DEF: Arc-shaped blind spot caused by retinal nerve damage.

368.44 Other localized visual field defect

Scotoma:	Visual field defect:
NOS	nasal step
ring	peripheral

368.45 Generalized contraction or constriction

368.46 Homonymous bilateral field defects
　　　Hemianopsia (altitudinal) (homonymous)
　　　Quadrant anopia

DEF: Disorders found in the corresponding vertical halves of the visual fields of both eyes.

368.47 Heteronymous bilateral field defects

Hemianopsia:	Hemianopsia:
binasal	bitemporal

DEF: Disorders in the opposite halves of the visual fields of both eyes.

√5ᵗʰ **368.5 Color vision deficiencies**
　　　Color blindness

368.51 Protan defect
　　　Protanomaly　　　Protanopia

DEF: Mild difficulty distinguishing green and red hues with shortened spectrum; sex-linked affecting one percent of males.

368.52 Deutan defect
　　　Deuteranomaly　　Deuteranopia

DEF: Male-only disorder; difficulty in distinguishing green and red, no shortened spectrum.

368.53 Tritan defect
　　　Tritanomaly　　　Tritanopia

DEF: Difficulty in distinguishing blue and yellow; occurs often due to drugs, retinal detachment and central nervous system diseases.

368.54 Achromatopsia
　　　Monochromatism (cone) (rod)

DEF: Complete color blindness; caused by disease, injury to retina, optic nerve or pathway.

368.55 Acquired color vision deficiencies

368.59 Other color vision deficiencies

√5ᵗʰ **368.6 Night blindness**
　　　Nyctalopia

DEF: Nyctalopia: disorder of vision in dim light or night blindness.

368.60 Night blindness, unspecified

368.61 Congenital night blindness
　　　Hereditary night blindness
　　　Oguchi's disease

368.62 Acquired night blindness
　　　EXCLUDES　　that due to vitamin A
　　　　　　　　　deficiency (264.5)

368.63 Abnormal dark adaptation curve

Abnormal threshold	} of cones or
Delayed adaptation	rods

368.69 Other night blindness

368.8 Other specified visual disturbances
　　　Blurred vision NOS

368.9 Unspecified visual disturbance

√4ᵗʰ **369 Blindness and low vision**

Note: Visual impairment refers to a functional limitation of the eye (e.g., limited visual acuity or visual field). It should be distinguished from visual disability, indicating a limitation of the abilities of the individual (e.g., limited reading skills, vocational skills), and from visual handicap, indicating a limitation of personal and socioeconomic independence (e.g., limited mobility, limited employability).

The levels of impairment defined in the table on the next page are based on the recommendations of the WHO Study Group on Prevention of Blindness (Geneva, November 6–10, 1972; WHO Technical Report Series 518), and of the International Council of Ophthalmology (1976).

Note that definitions of blindness vary in different settings.

For international reporting WHO defines blindness as profound impairment. This definition can be applied to blindness of one eye (369.1, 369.6) and to blindness of the individual (369.0).

For determination of benefits in the U.S.A., the definition of legal blindness as severe impairment is often used. This definition applies to blindness of the individual only.

　　EXCLUDES　　correctable impaired vision due to refractive
　　　　　　　　errors (367.0-367.9)

√5ᵗʰ **369.0 Profound impairment, both eyes**

369.00 Impairment level not further specified
　　　Blindness:
　　　　NOS according to WHO definition
　　　　both eyes

369.01 Better eye: total impairment; lesser eye: total impairment

369.02 Better eye: near-total impairment; lesser eye: not further specified

369.03 Better eye: near-total impairment; lesser eye: total impairment

369.04 Better eye: near-total impairment; lesser eye: near-total impairment

369.05 Better eye: profound impairment; lesser eye: not further specified

369.06 Better eye: profound impairment; lesser eye: total impairment

369.07 Better eye: profound impairment; lesser eye: near-total impairment

369.08 Better eye: profound impairment; lesser eye: profound impairment

√4ᵗʰ **369.1 Moderate or severe impairment, better eye, profound impairment lesser eye**

369.10 Impairment level not further specified
　　　Blindness, one eye, low vision other eye

369.11 Better eye: severe impairment; lesser eye: blind, not further specified

369.12 Better eye: severe impairment; lesser eye: total impairment

369.13 Better eye: severe impairment; lesser eye: near-total impairment

369.14 Better eye: severe impairment; lesser eye: profound impairment

369.15 Better eye: moderate impairment; lesser eye: blind, not further specified

369.16 Better eye: moderate impairment; lesser eye: total impairment

---

√4ᵗʰ √5ᵗʰ Additional Digit Required　　Nonspecific PDx　　Unacceptable PDx　　Manifestation Code　　**MSP** Medicare Secondary Payer　　►◄ Revised Text　　● New Code　　▲ Revised Code Title

2002 Ingenix, Inc.　　　　　　　　　　　　　　　　　　　　　　　　　　　　　　　　　　　　　**Volume 1 — 99**

369.17 Better eye: moderate impairment; lesser eye: near-total impairment

369.18 Better eye: moderate impairment; lesser eye: profound impairment

√5ᵗʰ **369.2** Moderate or severe impairment, both eyes

369.20 Impairment level not further specified
Low vision, both eyes NOS

369.21 Better eye: severe impairment; lesser eye: not further specified

369.22 Better eye: severe impairment; lesser eye: severe impairment

369.23 Better eye: moderate impairment; lesser eye: not further specified

369.24 Better eye: moderate impairment; lesser eye: severe impairment

369.25 Better eye: moderate impairment; lesser eye: moderate impairment

369.3 Unqualified visual loss, both eyes
EXCLUDES   blindness NOS:
legal [U.S.A. definition] (369.4)
WHO definition (369.00)

369.4 Legal blindness, as defined in U.S.A.
Blindness NOS according to U.S.A. definition
EXCLUDES   legal blindness with specification of
impairment level (369.01-369.08,
369.11-369.14, 369.21-369.22)

√5ᵗʰ **369.6** Profound impairment, one eye

369.60 Impairment level not further specified
Blindness, one eye

369.61 One eye: total impairment; other eye: not specified

369.62 One eye: total impairment; other eye: near-normal vision

369.63 One eye: total impairment; other eye: normal vision

369.64 One eye: near-total impairment; other eye: not specified

369.65 One eye: near-total impairment; other eye: near-normal vision

369.66 One eye: near-total impairment; other eye: normal vision

369.67 One eye: profound impairment; other eye: not specified

369.68 One eye: profound impairment; other eye: near-normal vision

369.69 One eye: profound impairment; other eye: normal vision

√5ᵗʰ **369.7** Moderate or severe impairment, one eye

369.70 Impairment level not further specified
Low vision, one eye

369.71 One eye: severe impairment; other eye: not specified

369.72 One eye: severe impairment; other eye: near-normal vision

369.73 One eye: severe impairment; other eye: normal vision

369.74 One eye: moderate impairment; other eye: not specified

369.75 One eye: moderate impairment; other eye: near-normal vision

369.76 One eye: moderate impairment; other eye: normal vision

369.8 Unqualified visual loss, one eye

369.9 Unspecified visual loss

Classification		LEVELS OF VISUAL IMPAIRMENT	Additional descriptors which may be encountered
"legal"	WHO	Visual acuity and/or visual field limitation (whichever is worse)	
(NEAR-) NORMAL VISION		RANGE OF NORMAL VISION 20/10 20/13 20/16 20/20 20/25 2.0 1.6 1.25 1.0 0.8	
		NEAR-NORMAL VISION 20/30 20/40 20/50 20/60 0.7 0.6 0.5 0.4 0.3	
LEGAL BLINDNESS (U.S.A.) both eyes	LOW VISION	MODERATE VISUAL IMPAIRMENT 20/70 20/80 20/100 20/125 20/160 0.25 0.20 0.16 0.12	Moderate low vision
		SEVERE VISUAL IMPAIRMENT 20/200 20/250 20/320 20/400 0.10 0.08 0.06 0.05 Visual field: 20 degrees or less	Severe low vision, "Legal" blindness
	BLINDNESS (WHO) one or both eyes	PROFOUND VISUAL IMPAIRMENT 20/500 20/630 20/800 20/1000 0.04 0.03 0.025 0.02 Count fingers at: less than 3m (10 ft.) Visual field: 10 degrees or less	Profound low vision, Moderate blindness
		NEAR-TOTAL VISUAL IMPAIRMENT Visual acuity: less than 0.02 (20/1000) Count fingers at: 1m (3 ft.) or less Hand movements: 5m (15 ft.) or less Light projection, light perception Visual field: 5 degrees or less	Severe blindness, Near-total blindness
		TOTAL VISUAL IMPAIRMENT No light perception (NLP)	Total blindness

Visual acuity refers to best achievable acuity with correction.
Non-listed Snellen fractions may be classified by converting to the nearest decimal equivalent, e.g. 10/200 = 0.05, 6/30 = 0.20.
CF (count fingers) without designation of distance, may be classified to profound impairment.
HM (hand motion) without designation of distance, may be classified to near-total impairment.
Visual field measurements refer to the largest field diameter for a 1/100 white test object.

√4ᵗʰ **370 Keratitis**

√5ᵗʰ **370.0 Corneal ulcer**
EXCLUDES   that due to vitamin A deficiency (264.3)

370.00 Corneal ulcer, unspecified

370.01 Marginal corneal ulcer

370.02 Ring corneal ulcer

370.03 Central corneal ulcer

370.04 Hypopyon ulcer
Serpiginous ulcer
DEF: Corneal ulcer with an accumulation of pus in the eye's anterior chamber..

370.05 Mycotic corneal ulcer
DEF: Fungal infection causing corneal tissue loss.

370.06 Perforated corneal ulcer
DEF: Tissue loss through all layers of cornea.

370.07 Mooren's ulcer
DEF: Tissue loss, with chronic inflammation, at junction of cornea and sclera; seen in elderly.

√5ᵗʰ **370.2 Superficial keratitis without conjunctivitis**
EXCLUDES   dendritic [herpes simplex] keratitis (054.42)

370.20 Superficial keratitis, unspecified

370.21 Punctate keratitis
Thygeson's superficial punctate keratitis

DEF: Formation of cellular and fibrinous deposits (keratic precipitates) on posterior surface; deposits develop after injury or iridocyclitis.

370.22 Macular keratitis
Keratitis: Keratitis:
   areolar   stellate
   nummular   striate

370.23 Filamentary keratitis
DEF: Keratitis characterized by twisted filaments of mucoid material on the cornea's surface.

370.24 Photokeratitis
Snow blindness
Welders' keratitis
AHA: 3Q, '96, 6

DEF: Painful, inflamed cornea; due to extended exposure to ultraviolet light.

√5th **370.3 Certain types of keratoconjunctivitis**

370.31 Phlyctenular keratoconjunctivitis
Phlyctenulosis
Use additional code for any associated tuberculosis (017.3)

DEF: Miniature blister on conjunctiva or cornea; associated with tuberculosis and malnutrition disorders.

370.32 Limbar and corneal involvement in vernal conjunctivitis
Use additional code for vernal conjunctivitis (372.13)

DEF: Corneal itching and inflammation in conjunctivitis; often limited to lining of eyelids.

370.33 Keratoconjunctivitis sicca, not specified as Sjögren's
EXCLUDES   Sjögren's syndrome (710.2)

DEF: Inflammation of conjunctiva and cornea; characterized by "horny" looking tissue and excess blood in these areas; decreased flow of lacrimal (tear) is a contributing factor.

370.34 Exposure keratoconjunctivitis
AHA: 3Q, '96, 6

DEF: Incomplete closure of eyelid causing dry, inflamed eye.

370.35 Neurotrophic keratoconjunctivitis

√5th **370.4 Other and unspecified keratoconjunctivitis**

370.40 Keratoconjunctivitis, unspecified
Superficial keratitis with conjunctivitis NOS

370.44 Keratitis or keratoconjunctivitis in exanthema
Code first underlying condition (050.0-052.9)
EXCLUDES   herpes simplex (054.43)
herpes zoster (053.21)
measles (055.71)

370.49 Other
EXCLUDES   epidemic keratoconjunctivitis (077.1)

√5th **370.5 Interstitial and deep keratitis**

370.50 Interstitial keratitis, unspecified

370.52 Diffuse interstitial keratitis
Cogan's syndrome

DEF: Inflammation of cornea; with deposits in middle corneal layers; may obscure vision.

370.54 Sclerosing keratitis
DEF: Chronic corneal inflammation leading to opaque scarring.

370.55 Corneal abscess
DEF: Pocket of pus and inflammation on the cornea.

370.59 Other
EXCLUDES   disciform herpes simplex keratitis (054.43)
syphilitic keratitis (090.3)

√5th **370.6 Corneal neovascularization**

370.60 Corneal neovascularization, unspecified

370.61 Localized vascularization of cornea
DEF: Limited infiltration of cornea by new blood vessels.

370.62 Pannus (corneal)
DEF: Buildup of superficial vascularization and granulated tissue under epithelium of cornea.

370.63 Deep vascularization of cornea
DEF: Deep infiltration of cornea by new blood vessels.

370.64 Ghost vessels (corneal)

370.8 Other forms of keratitis
AHA: 3Q, '94, 5

370.9 Unspecified keratitis

√4th **371 Corneal opacity and other disorders of cornea**

√5th **371.0 Corneal scars and opacities**
EXCLUDES   that due to vitamin A deficiency (264.6)

371.00 Corneal opacity, unspecified
Corneal scar NOS

371.01 Minor opacity of cornea
Corneal nebula

371.02 Peripheral opacity of cornea
Corneal macula not interfering with central vision

371.03 Central opacity of cornea
Corneal:
leucoma } interfering with central
macula } vision

371.04 Adherent leucoma
DEF: Dense, opaque corneal growth adhering to the iris; also spelled as leukoma.

371.05 Phthisical cornea
Code first underlying tuberculosis (017.3)

√5th **371.1 Corneal pigmentations and deposits**

371.10 Corneal deposit, unspecified

371.11 Anterior pigmentations
Stähli's lines

371.12 Stromal pigmentations
Hematocornea

371.13 Posterior pigmentations
Krukenberg spindle

371.14 Kayser-Fleischer ring
DEF: Copper deposits forming ring at outer edge of cornea; seen in Wilson's disease and other liver disorders.

371.15 Other deposits associated with metabolic disorders

371.16 Argentous deposits
DEF: Silver deposits in cornea.

√5th **371.2 Corneal edema**

371.20 Corneal edema, unspecified

371.21 Idiopathic corneal edema
DEF: Corneal swelling and fluid retention of unknown cause.

371.22 Secondary corneal edema
DEF: Corneal swelling and fluid retention caused by an underlying disease, injury, or condition.

371.23 Bullous keratopathy
DEF: Corneal degeneration; characterized by recurring, rupturing epithelial "blisters;" ruptured blebs expose corneal nerves, cause great pain; occurs in glaucoma, iridocyclitis and Fuchs' epithelial dystrophy.

Nervous System and Sense Organs 370.20–371.23

√4th √5th Additional Digit Required   Nonspecific PDx   Unacceptable PDx   Manifestation Code   MSP Medicare Secondary Payer   ►◄ Revised Text   ● New Code   ▲ Revised Code Title

2002 Ingenix, Inc.   **Volume 1 — 101**

371.24 Corneal edema due to wearing of contact lenses

√5th **371.3 Changes of corneal membranes**
371.30 Corneal membrane change, unspecified
371.31 Folds and rupture of Bowman's membrane
371.32 Folds in Descemet's membrane
371.33 Rupture in Descemet's membrane

√5th **371.4 Corneal degenerations**
371.40 Corneal degeneration, unspecified
371.41 Senile corneal changes
 Arcus senilis   Hassall-Henle bodies
371.42 Recurrent erosion of cornea
 EXCLUDES   *Mooren's ulcer (370.07)*
371.43 Band-shaped keratopathy
 DEF: Horizontal bands of superficial corneal calcium deposits.
371.44 Other calcerous degenerations of cornea
371.45 Keratomalacia NOS
 EXCLUDES   *that due to vitamin A deficiency (264.4)*
 DEF: Destruction of the cornea by keratinization of the epithelium with ulceration and perforation of the cornea; seen in cases of vitamin A deficiency.
371.46 Nodular degeneration of cornea
 Salzmann's nodular dystrophy
371.48 Peripheral degenerations of cornea
 Marginal degeneration of cornea [Terrien's]
371.49 Other
 Discrete colliquative keratopathy

√5th **371.5 Hereditary corneal dystrophies**
 DEF: Genetic disorder; leads to opacities, edema or lesions of cornea.
371.50 Corneal dystrophy, unspecified
371.51 Juvenile epithelial corneal dystrophy
371.52 Other anterior corneal dystrophies
 Corneal dystrophy: Corneal dystrophy:
 microscopic cystic   ring-like
371.53 Granular corneal dystrophy
371.54 Lattice corneal dystrophy
371.55 Macular corneal dystrophy
371.56 Other stromal corneal dystrophies
 Crystalline corneal dystrophy
371.57 Endothelial corneal dystrophy
 Combined corneal dystrophy
 Cornea guttata
 Fuchs' endothelial dystrophy
371.58 Other posterior corneal dystrophies
 Polymorphous corneal dystrophy

√5th **371.6 Keratoconus**
 DEF: Bilateral bulging protrusion of anterior cornea; often due to noninflammatory thinning.
371.60 Keratoconus, unspecified
371.61 Keratoconus, stable condition
371.62 Keratoconus, acute hydrops

√5th **371.7 Other corneal deformities**
371.70 Corneal deformity, unspecified
371.71 Corneal ectasia
 DEF: Bulging protrusion of thinned, scarred cornea.
371.72 Descemetocele
 DEF: Protrusion of Descemet's membrane into cornea.
371.73 Corneal staphyloma
 DEF: Protrusion of cornea into adjacent tissue.

√5th **371.8 Other corneal disorders**
371.81 Corneal anesthesia and hypoesthesia
 DEF: Decreased or absent sensitivity of cornea..

371.82 Corneal disorder due to contact lens
 EXCLUDES   *corneal edema due to contact lens (371.24)*
 DEF: Contact lens wear causing cornea disorder, excluding swelling.
371.89 Other
 AHA: 3Q, '99, 12

371.9 Unspecified corneal disorder

√4th **372 Disorders of conjunctiva**
 EXCLUDES   *keratoconjunctivitis (370.3-370.4)*

√5th **372.0 Acute conjunctivitis**
372.00 Acute conjunctivitis, unspecified
372.01 Serous conjunctivitis, except viral
 EXCLUDES   *viral conjunctivitis NOS (077.9)*
372.02 Acute follicular conjunctivitis
 Conjunctival folliculosis NOS
 EXCLUDES   *conjunctivitis:*
  adenoviral (acute follicular) (077.3)
  epidemic hemorrhagic (077.4)
  inclusion (077.0)
  Newcastle (077.8)
  epidemic keratoconjunctivitis (077.1)
  pharyngoconjunctival fever (077.2)
 DEF: Severe conjunctival inflammation with dense infiltrations of lymphoid tissues of inner eyelids; may be traced to a viral or chlamydial etiology.
372.03 Other mucopurulent conjunctivitis
 Catarrhal conjunctivitis
 EXCLUDES   *blennorrhea neonatorum (gonococcal) (098.40)*
  neonatal conjunctivitis(771.6)
  ophthalmia neonatorum NOS (771.6)
372.04 Pseudomembranous conjunctivitis
 Membranous conjunctivitis
 EXCLUDES   *diphtheritic conjunctivitis (032.81)*
 DEF: Severe inflammation of conjunctiva; false membrane develops on inner surface of eyelid; membrane can be removed without harming epithelium, due to bacterial infections, toxic and allergic factors, and viral infections.
372.05 Acute atopic conjunctivitis
 DEF: Sudden, severe conjunctivitis due to allergens.

√5th **372.1 Chronic conjunctivitis**
372.10 Chronic conjunctivitis, unspecified
372.11 Simple chronic conjunctivitis
372.12 Chronic follicular conjunctivitis
 DEF: Persistent conjunctival inflammation with dense, localized infiltrations of lymphoid tissues of inner eyelids.
372.13 Vernal conjunctivitis
 AHA: 3Q, '96, 8
372.14 Other chronic allergic conjunctivitis
 AHA: 3Q, '96, 8
372.15 Parasitic conjunctivitis
 Code first underlying disease, as:
 filariasis (125.0-125.9)
 mucocutaneous leishmaniasis (085.5)

√5th **372.2 Blepharoconjunctivitis**
372.20 Blepharoconjunctivitis, unspecified
372.21 Angular blepharoconjunctivitis
 DEF: Inflammation at junction of upper and lower eyelids; may block lacrimal secretions.

| N Newborn Age: 0 | P Pediatric Age: 0-17 | M Maternity Age: 12-55 | A Adult Age: 15-124 | CC CC Condition | MC Major Complication | CD Complex Dx | HIV HIV Related Dx |

2002 Ingenix, Inc.

372.22 Contact blepharoconjunctivitis

✓5th 372.3 **Other and unspecified conjunctivitis**
372.30 Conjunctivitis, unspecified
372.31 *Rosacea conjunctivitis*
　　Code first underlying rosacea dermatitis
　　(695.3)
372.33 *Conjunctivitis in mucocutaneous disease*
　　Code first underlying disease, as:
　　erythema multiforme (695.1)
　　Reiter's disease (099.3)
　　EXCLUDES　ocular pemphigoid (694.61)
372.39 Other

✓5th 372.4 **Pterygium**
　　EXCLUDES　pseudopterygium (372.52)
　　DEF: Wedge-shaped, conjunctival thickening that advances from
　　the inner corner of the eye toward the cornea.

372.40 Pterygium, unspecified
372.41 Peripheral pterygium, stationary
372.42 Peripheral pterygium, progressive
372.43 Central pterygium
372.44 Double pterygium
372.45 Recurrent pterygium

✓5th 372.5 **Conjunctival degenerations and deposits**
372.50 Conjunctival degeneration, unspecified
372.51 Pinguecula
　　DEF: Proliferative spot on the bulbar conjunctiva located
　　near the sclerocorneal junction, usually on the nasal
　　side; it is seen in elderly people.
372.52 Pseudopterygium
　　DEF: Conjunctival scar joined to the cornea; it looks like
　　a pterygium but is not attached to the tissue.
372.53 Conjunctival xerosis
　　EXCLUDES　conjunctival xerosis due to
　　vitamin A deficiency
　　(264.0, 264.1, 264.7)
　　DEF: Dry conjunctiva due to vitamin A deficiency; related
　　to Bitot's spots; may develop into xerophthalmia and
　　keratomalacia.
372.54 Conjunctival concretions
　　DEF: Calculus or deposit on conjunctiva.
372.55 Conjunctival pigmentations
　　Conjunctival argyrosis
　　DEF: Color deposits in conjunctiva.
372.56 Conjunctival deposits

✓5th 372.6 **Conjunctival scars**
372.61 Granuloma of conjunctiva
372.62 Localized adhesions and strands of
　　conjunctiva
　　DEF: Abnormal fibrous connections in conjunctiva.
372.63 Symblepharon
　　Extensive adhesions of conjunctiva
　　DEF: Adhesion of the eyelids to the eyeball.
372.64 Scarring of conjunctiva
　　Contraction of eye socket (after enucleation)

✓5th 372.7 **Conjunctival vascular disorders and cysts**
372.71 Hyperemia of conjunctiva
　　DEF: Conjunctival blood vessel congestion causing eye
　　redness.
372.72 Conjunctival hemorrhage
　　Hyposphagma Subconjunctival hemorrhage
372.73 Conjunctival edema
　　Chemosis of conjunctiva
　　Subconjunctival edema
　　DEF: Fluid retention and swelling in conjunctival
　　tissue.

372.74 Vascular abnormalities of conjunctiva
　　Aneurysm(ata) of conjunctiva
372.75 Conjunctival cysts
　　DEF: Abnormal sacs of fluid in conjunctiva.

✓5th 372.8 **Other disorders of conjunctiva**
372.81 Conjunctivochalasis
　　AHA: 4Q, '00, 41
　　DEF: Bilateral condition of redundant conjunctival tissue
　　between globe and lower eyelid margin; may cover
　　lower punctum, interferring with normal tearing.
372.89 Other disorders of conjunctiva
372.9 **Unspecified disorder of conjunctiva**

✓4th 373 **Inflammation of eyelids**
✓5th 373.0 **Blepharitis**
　　EXCLUDES　blepharoconjunctivitis (372.20-372.22)
373.00 Blepharitis, unspecified
373.01 Ulcerative blepharitis
373.02 Squamous blepharitis

✓5th 373.1 **Hordeolum and other deep inflammation of eyelid**
　　DEF: Purulent, localized, staphylococcal infection in sebaceous
　　glands of eyelids.
373.11 Hordeolum externum
　　Hordeolum NOS Stye
　　DEF: Infection of the oil glands in the eyelash follicles.
373.12 Hordeolum internum
　　Infection of meibomian gland
　　DEF: Infection of the oil gland of the eyelid margin.
373.13 Abscess of eyelid
　　Furuncle of eyelid
　　DEF: Inflamed pocket of pus on the eyelid.

373.2 **Chalazion**
　　Meibomian (gland) cyst
　　EXCLUDES　infected meibomian gland (373.12)
　　DEF: Chronic inflammation of the meibomian gland, causing an
　　eyelid mass.

✓5th 373.3 **Noninfectious dermatoses of eyelid**
373.31 Eczematous dermatitis of eyelid
373.32 Contact and allergic dermatitis of eyelid
373.33 Xeroderma of eyelid
373.34 Discoid lupus erythematosus of eyelid

373.4 *Infective dermatitis of eyelid of types resulting in deformity*
　　Code first underlying disease, as:
　　leprosy (030.0-030.9)
　　lupus vulgaris (tuberculous) (017.0)
　　yaws (102.0-102.9)

373.5 *Other infective dermatitis of eyelid*
　　Code first underlying disease, as:
　　actinomycosis (039.3)
　　impetigo (684)
　　mycotic dermatitis (110.0-111.9)
　　vaccinia (051.0)
　　postvaccination (999.0)
　　EXCLUDES　herpes:
　　simplex (054.41)
　　zoster (053.20)

373.6 *Parasitic infestation of eyelid*
　　Code first underlying disease, as:
　　leishmaniasis (085.0-085.9)
　　loiasis (125.2)
　　onchocerciasis (125.3)
　　pediculosis (132.0)
373.8 **Other inflammations of eyelids**
373.9 **Unspecified inflammation of eyelid**

Nervous System and Sense Organs 372.22–373.9

✓4th ✓5th Additional Digit Required　Nonspecific PDx　Unacceptable PDx　Manifestation Code　**MSP** Medicare Secondary Payer　►◄ Revised Text　● New Code　▲ Revised Code Title
2002 Ingenix, Inc.　　　　　　Volume 1 — 103

Nervous System and Sense Organs 374–375.13

Entropion and Ectropion

Normal eyelashes   Entropion   Ectropion

√4ᵗʰ **374 Other disorders of eyelids**

√5ᵗʰ **374.0 Entropion and trichiasis of eyelid**

DEF: Entropion: turning inward of eyelid edge toward eyeball.

DEF: Trichiasis: ingrowing eyelashes marked by irritation with possible distortion of sight.

374.00 Entropion, unspecified

374.01 Senile entropion   A

374.02 Mechanical entropion

374.03 Spastic entropion

374.04 Cicatricial entropion

374.05 Trichiasis without entropion

√5ᵗʰ **374.1 Ectropion**

DEF: Turning outward (eversion) of eyelid edge; exposes palpebral conjunctiva; dryness irritation result.

374.10 Ectropion, unspecified

374.11 Senile ectropion   A

374.12 Mechanical ectropion

374.13 Spastic ectropion

374.14 Cicatricial ectropion

√5ᵗʰ **374.2 Lagophthalmos**

DEF: Incomplete closure of eyes; causes dry eye and other complications.

374.20 Lagophthalmos, unspecified

374.21 Paralytic lagophthalmos

374.22 Mechanical lagophthalmos

374.23 Cicatricial lagophthalmos

√5ᵗʰ **374.3 Ptosis of eyelid**

374.30 Ptosis of eyelid, unspecified

AHA: 2Q, '96, 11

374.31 Paralytic ptosis

DEF: Drooping of upper eyelid due to nerve disorder.

374.32 Myogenic ptosis

DEF: Drooping of upper eyelid due to muscle disorder.

374.33 Mechanical ptosis

DEF: Outside force causes drooping of upper eyelid.

374.34 Blepharochalasis

Pseudoptosis

DEF: Loss of elasticity causing skin to hang over eyelid margin; due to intercellular tissue atrophy.

√5ᵗʰ **374.4 Other disorders affecting eyelid function**

EXCLUDES   blepharoclonus (333.81)
        blepharospasm (333.81)
        facial nerve palsy (351.0)
        third nerve palsy or paralysis (378.51-378.52)
        tic (psychogenic) (307.20-307.23)
        organic (333.3)

374.41 Lid retraction or lag

374.43 Abnormal innervation syndrome

Jaw-blinking

Paradoxical facial movements

374.44 Sensory disorders

374.45 Other sensorimotor disorders

Deficient blink reflex

374.46 Blepharophimosis

Ankyloblepharon

DEF: Narrowing of palpebral fissure horizontally; caused by laterally displaced inner canthi; either acquired or congenital.

√5ᵗʰ **374.5 Degenerative disorders of eyelid and periocular area**

374.50 Degenerative disorder of eyelid, unspecified

374.51 Xanthelasma

Xanthoma (planum) (tuberosum) of eyelid

Code first underlying condition (272.0-272.9)

DEF: Fatty tumors of the eyelid linked to high fat content of blood.

374.52 Hyperpigmentation of eyelid

Chloasma   Dyspigmentation

DEF: Excess pigment of eyelid.

374.53 Hypopigmentation of eyelid

Vitiligo of eyelid

DEF: Lack of color pigment of the eyelid.

374.54 Hypertrichosis of eyelid

DEF: Excessive eyelash growth.

374.55 Hypotrichosis of eyelid

Madarosis of eyelid

DEF: Less than normal, or absent, eyelashes.

374.56 Other degenerative disorders of skin affecting eyelid

√5ᵗʰ **374.8 Other disorders of eyelid**

374.81 Hemorrhage of eyelid

EXCLUDES   black eye (921.0)

374.82 Edema of eyelid

Hyperemia of eyelid

DEF: Swelling and fluid retention in eyelid.

374.83 Elephantiasis of eyelid

DEF: Filarial disease causing dermatitis and enlargement of eyelid.

374.84 Cysts of eyelids

Sebaceous cyst of eyelid

374.85 Vascular anomalies of eyelid

374.86 Retained foreign body of eyelid

374.87 Dermatochalasis

DEF: Loss of elasticity causing skin under eye to sag.

374.89 Other disorders of eyelid

374.9 Unspecified disorder of eyelid

√4ᵗʰ **375 Disorders of lacrimal system**

√5ᵗʰ **375.0 Dacryoadenitis**

375.00 Dacryoadenitis, unspecified

375.01 Acute dacryoadenitis

DEF: Severe, sudden inflammation of the lacrimal gland.

375.02 Chronic dacryoadenitis

DEF: Persistent inflammation of the lacrimal gland.

375.03 Chronic enlargement of lacrimal gland

√5ᵗʰ **375.1 Other disorders of lacrimal gland**

375.11 Dacryops

DEF: Overproduction and constant flow of tears; may cause distended lacrimal duct.

375.12 Other lacrimal cysts and cystic degeneration

375.13 Primary lacrimal atrophy

N Newborn Age: 0   P Pediatric Age: 0-17   M Maternity Age: 12-55   A Adult Age: 15-124   CC CC Condition   MC Major Complication   CD Complex Dx   HIV HIV Related Dx

104 — Volume 1   *2002 Ingenix, Inc.*

375.14 Secondary lacrimal atrophy
DEF: Wasting away of the lacrimal gland due to another disease.

375.15 Tear film insufficiency, unspecified
Dry eye syndrome
AHA: 3Q, '96, 6

DEF: Eye dryness and irritation from insufficient tear production.

375.16 Dislocation of lacrimal gland

√5th **375.2 Epiphora**
DEF: Abnormal development of tears due to stricture of lacrimal passages.

375.20 Epiphora, unspecified as to cause
375.21 Epiphora due to excess lacrimation
DEF: Tear overflow due to overproduction.

375.22 Epiphora due to insufficient drainage
DEF: Tear overflow due to blocked drainage.

√5th **375.3 Acute and unspecified inflammation of lacrimal passages**
EXCLUDES   *neonatal dacryocystitis (771.6)*
375.30 Dacryocystitis, unspecified
375.31 Acute canaliculitis, lacrimal
375.32 Acute dacryocystitis
Acute peridacryocystitis
375.33 Phlegmonous dacryocystitis
DEF: Infection of the tear sac with pockets of pus.

√5th **375.4 Chronic inflammation of lacrimal passages**
375.41 Chronic canaliculitis
375.42 Chronic dacryocystitis
375.43 Lacrimal mucocele
√5th **375.5 Stenosis and insufficiency of lacrimal passages**
375.51 Eversion of lacrimal punctum
DEF: Abnormal turning outward of the tear duct.

375.52 Stenosis of lacrimal punctum
DEF: Abnormal narrowing of the tear duct.

375.53 Stenosis of lacrimal canaliculi
375.54 Stenosis of lacrimal sac
DEF: Abnormal narrowing of the tear sac.

375.55 Obstruction of nasolacrimal duct, neonatal
EXCLUDES   *congenital anomaly of nasolacrimal duct (743.65)*
DEF: Acquired, abnormal obstruction of tear drainage system from the eye to the nose; in an infant.

375.56 Stenosis of nasolacrimal duct, acquired
375.57 Dacryolith
DEF: Concretion or stone anywhere in lacrimal system.

▶ **Lacrimal System** ◀

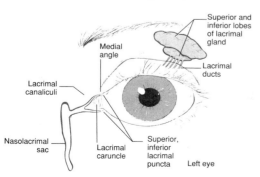

Superior and inferior lobes of lacrimal gland
Medial angle
Lacrimal ducts
Lacrimal canaliculi
Nasolacrimal sac
Lacrimal caruncle
Superior, inferior lacrimal puncta
Left eye

√5th **375.6 Other changes of lacrimal passages**
375.61 Lacrimal fistula
DEF: Abnormal communication from the lacrimal system.

375.69 Other
√5th **375.8 Other disorders of lacrimal system**
375.81 Granuloma of lacrimal passages
DEF: Abnormal nodules within lacrimal system.

375.89 Other
375.9 Unspecified disorder of lacrimal system
√4th **376 Disorders of the orbit**
√5th **376.0 Acute inflammation of orbit**
376.00 Acute inflammation of orbit, unspecified
376.01 Orbital cellulitis
Abscess of orbit
DEF: Infection of tissue between the orbital bone and eyeball.

376.02 Orbital periostitis
DEF: Inflammation of connective tissue covering the orbital bone.

376.03 Orbital osteomyelitis
DEF: Inflammation of the orbital bone.

376.04 Tenonitis
√5th **376.1 Chronic inflammatory disorders of orbit**
376.10 Chronic inflammation of orbit, unspecified
376.11 Orbital granuloma
Pseudotumor (inflammatory) of orbit
DEF: Abnormal nodule between orbital bone and eyeball.

376.12 Orbital myositis
DEF: Painful inflammation of the muscles of the eye.

376.13 *Parasitic infestation of orbit*
Code first underlying disease, as:
hydatid infestation of orbit (122.3, 122.6, 122.9)
myiasis of orbit (134.0)
√5th **376.2 Endocrine exophthalmos**
Code first underlying thyroid disorder (242.0-242.9)
376.21 *Thyrotoxic exophthalmos*
DEF: Painful inflammation of eye muscles.

376.22 *Exophthalmic ophthalmoplegia*
DEF: Inability to rotate eye as a result of bulging eyes.

√5th **376.3 Other exophthalmic conditions**
376.30 Exophthalmos, unspecified
DEF: Abnormal protrusion of eyeball.

376.31 Constant exophthalmos
DEF: Continuous, abnormal protrusion or bulging of eyeball.

376.32 Orbital hemorrhage
DEF: Bleeding behind the eyeball, causing it to bulge forward.

376.33 Orbital edema or congestion
DEF: Fluid retention behind eyeball, causing forward bulge.

376.34 Intermittent exophthalmos
376.35 Pulsating exophthalmos
DEF: Bulge or protrusion; associated with a carotid-cavernous fistula.

376.36 Lateral displacement of globe
DEF: Abnormal displacement of the eyeball away from nose, toward temple.

√5th **376.4 Deformity of orbit**
376.40 Deformity of orbit, unspecified

√4th √5th Additional Digit Required   Nonspecific PDx   Unacceptable PDx   Manifestation Code   **MSP** Medicare Secondary Payer   ▶◀ Revised Text   ● New Code   ▲ Revised Code Title

376.41 Hypertelorism of orbit
DEF: Abnormal increase in interorbital distance; associated with congenital facial deformities; may be accompanied by mental deficiency.

376.42 Exostosis of orbit
DEF: Abnormal bony growth of orbit.

376.43 Local deformities due to bone disease
DEF: Acquired abnormalities of orbit; due to bone disease.

376.44 Orbital deformities associated with craniofacial deformities

376.45 Atrophy of orbit
DEF: Wasting away of bone tissue of orbit.

376.46 Enlargement of orbit

376.47 Deformity due to trauma or surgery

√5th **376.5 Enophthalmos**
DEF: Recession of eyeball deep into eye socket.

376.50 Enophthalmos, unspecified as to cause

376.51 Enophthalmos due to atrophy of orbital tissue

376.52 Enophthalmos due to trauma or surgery

376.6 Retained (old) foreign body following penetrating wound of orbit
Retrobulbar foreign body

√5th **376.8 Other orbital disorders**
376.81 Orbital cysts
Encephalocele of orbit
AHA: 3Q, '99, 13

376.82 Myopathy of extraocular muscles
DEF: Disease in the muscles that control eyeball movement.

376.89 Other

376.9 Unspecified disorder of orbit

√4th **377 Disorders of optic nerve and visual pathways**

√5th **377.0 Papilledema**
377.00 Papilledema, unspecified `CC`
CC Excl: 017.30-017.36, 017.90-017.96, 036.81, 250.50-250.53, 250.80-250.93, 377.00-377.03, 377.14, 377.24, 379.8, 379.90, 379.99, 743.8-743.9

377.01 Papilledema associated with increased `CC` **intracranial pressure**
CC Excl: See code 377.00

377.02 Papilledema associated with decreased `CC` **ocular pressure**
CC Excl: See code 377.00

377.03 Papilledema associated with retinal disorder

377.04 Foster-Kennedy syndrome
DEF: Retrobulbar optic neuritis, central scotoma and optic atrophy; caused by tumors in frontal lobe of brain that press downward.

√5th **377.1 Optic atrophy**
377.10 Optic atrophy, unspecified
377.11 Primary optic atrophy
`EXCLUDES` *neurosyphilitic optic atrophy (094.84)*

377.12 Postinflammatory optic atrophy
DEF: : Adverse effect of inflammation causing wasting away of eye.

377.13 Optic atrophy associated with retinal dystrophies
DEF: Progressive changes in retinal tissue due to metabolic disorder causing wasting away of eye.

377.14 Glaucomatous atrophy [cupping] of optic disc

377.15 Partial optic atrophy
Temporal pallor of optic disc

377.16 Hereditary optic atrophy
Optic atrophy: Optic atrophy:
  dominant hereditary   Leber's

√5th **377.2 Other disorders of optic disc**
377.21 Drusen of optic disc
377.22 Crater-like holes of optic disc
377.23 Coloboma of optic disc
DEF: Ocular malformation caused by the failure of fetal fissure of optic stalk to close.

377.24 Pseudopapilledema

√5th **377.3 Optic neuritis**
`EXCLUDES` *meningococcal optic neuritis (036.81)*
377.30 Optic neuritis, unspecified
377.31 Optic papillitis
DEF: Swelling and inflammation of the optic disc.

377.32 Retrobulbar neuritis (acute)
`EXCLUDES` *syphilitic retrobulbar neuritis (094.85)*
DEF: Inflammation of optic nerve immediately behind the eyeball.

377.33 Nutritional optic neuropathy
DEF: Malnutrition causing optic nerve disorder.

377.34 Toxic optic neuropathy
Toxic amblyopia
DEF: Toxic substance causing optic nerve disorder.

377.39 Other
`EXCLUDES` *ischemic optic neuropathy (377.41)*

√5th **377.4 Other disorders of optic nerve**
377.41 Ischemic optic neuropathy
DEF: Decreased blood flow affecting optic nerve.

377.42 Hemorrhage in optic nerve sheaths
DEF: Bleeding in meningeal lining of optic nerve.

377.49 Other
Compression of optic nerve

√5th **377.5 Disorders of optic chiasm**
377.51 Associated with pituitary neoplasms and disorders
DEF: Abnormal pituitary growth causing disruption in nerve chain from retina to brain.

377.52 Associated with other neoplasms
DEF: Abnormal growth, other than pituitary, causing disruption in nerve chain from retina to brain.

377.53 Associated with vascular disorders
DEF: Vascular disorder causing disruption in nerve chain from retina to brain.

377.54 Associated with inflammatory disorders
DEF: Inflammatory disease causing disruption in nerve chain from retina to brain.

√5th **377.6 Disorders of other visual pathways**
377.61 Associated with neoplasms
377.62 Associated with vascular disorders
377.63 Associated with inflammatory disorders

√5th **377.7 Disorders of visual cortex**
`EXCLUDES` *visual:*
  agnosia (368.16)
  hallucinations (368.16)
  halos (368.15)
377.71 Associated with neoplasms
377.72 Associated with vascular disorders
377.73 Associated with inflammatory disorders

`N` Newborn Age: 0   `P` Pediatric Age: 0-17   `M` Maternity Age: 12-55   `A` Adult Age: 15-124   `CC` CC Condition   `MC` Major Complication   `CD` Complex Dx   `HIV` HIV Related Dx

377.75 Cortical blindness

DEF: Blindness due to brain disorder, rather than eye disorder.

377.9 Unspecified disorder of optic nerve and visual pathways

√4th **378 Strabismus and other disorders of binocular eye movements**

EXCLUDES *nystagmus and other irregular eye movements (379.50-379.59)*

DEF: Misalignment of the eyes due to imbalance in extraocular muscles.

√5th **378.0 Esotropia**

Convergent concomitant strabismus

EXCLUDES *intermittent esotropia (378.20-378.22)*

DEF: Visual axis deviation created by one eye fixing upon an image and the other eye deviating inward.

378.00 Esotropia, unspecified

378.01 Monocular esotropia

378.02 Monocular esotropia with A pattern

378.03 Monocular esotropia with V pattern

378.04 Monocular esotropia with other noncomitancies

Monocular esotropia with X or Y pattern

378.05 Alternating esotropia

378.06 Alternating esotropia with A pattern

378.07 Alternating esotropia with V pattern

378.08 Alternating esotropia with other noncomitancies

Alternating esotropia with X or Y pattern

√5th **378.1 Exotropia**

Divergent concomitant strabismus

EXCLUDES *intermittent exotropia (378.20, 378.23-378.24)*

DEF: Visual axis deviation created by one eye fixing upon an image and the other eye deviating outward.

378.10 Exotropia, unspecified

378.11 Monocular exotropia

378.12 Monocular exotropia with A pattern

378.13 Monocular exotropia with V pattern

378.14 Monocular exotropia with other noncomitancies

Monocular exotropia with X or Y pattern

378.15 Alternating exotropia

378.16 Alternating exotropia with A pattern

378.17 Alternating exotropia with V pattern

378.18 Alternating exotropia with other noncomitancies

Alternating exotropia with X or Y pattern

√5th **378.2 Intermittent heterotropia**

EXCLUDES *vertical heterotropia (intermittent) (378.31)*

DEF: Deviation of eyes seen only at intervals; it is also called strabismus.

Eye Musculature

Muscles and actions (right eye)

R.   L.
Monocular (one eye only) esotropia (inward)

Monocular exotropia (outward)

Monocular hypertropia (upward)

378.20 Intermittent heterotropia, unspecified

Intermittent: Intermittent:
esotropia NOS   exotropia NOS

378.21 Intermittent esotropia, monocular

378.22 Intermittent esotropia, alternating

378.23 Intermittent exotropia, monocular

378.24 Intermittent exotropia, alternating

√5th **378.3 Other and unspecified heterotropia**

378.30 Heterotropia, unspecified

378.31 Hypertropia

Vertical heterotropia (constant) (intermittent)

378.32 Hypotropia

378.33 Cyclotropia

378.34 Monofixation syndrome

Microtropia

378.35 Accommodative component in esotropia

√5th **378.4 Heterophoria**

DEF: Deviation occurring only when the other eye is covered..

378.40 Heterophoria, unspecified

378.41 Esophoria

378.42 Exophoria

378.43 Vertical heterophoria

378.44 Cyclophoria

378.45 Alternating hyperphoria

√5th **378.5 Paralytic strabismus**

DEF: Deviation of the eye due to nerve paralysis affecting muscle.

378.50 Paralytic strabismus, unspecified

378.51 Third or oculomotor nerve palsy, partial

AHA: 3Q, '91, 9

378.52 Third or oculomotor nerve palsy, total

AHA: 2Q, '89, 12

378.53 Fourth or trochlear nerve palsy

AHA: 2Q, '01, 21

378.54 Sixth or abducens nerve palsy

AHA: 2Q, '89, 12

378.55 External ophthalmoplegia

378.56 Total ophthalmoplegia

√5th **378.6 Mechanical strabismus**

DEF: Deviation of the eye due to an outside force upon the extraocular muscles.

378.60 Mechanical strabismus, unspecified

378.61 Brown's (tendon) sheath syndrome

DEF: Congenital or acquired shortening of the anterior sheath of the superior oblique muscle; the eye is unable to move upward and inward; it is usually unilateral.

378.62 Mechanical strabismus from other musculofascial disorders

378.63 Limited duction associated with other conditions

√5th **378.7 Other specified strabismus**

378.71 Duane's syndrome

DEF: Congenital, affects one eye; due to abnormal fibrous bands attached to rectus muscle; inability to abduct affected eye with retraction of globe.

378.72 Progressive external ophthalmoplegia

DEF: Paralysis progressing from one eye muscle to another.

378.73 Strabismus in other neuromuscular disorders

√5th **378.8 Other disorders of binocular eye movements**

EXCLUDES *nystagmus (379.50-379.56)*

378.81 Palsy of conjugate gaze

DEF: Paralysis progressing from one eye muscle to another.

√4th Additional Digit Required   Nonspecific PDx   Unacceptable PDx   Manifestation Code   MSP Medicare Secondary Payer   ◄► Revised Text   ● New Code   ▲ Revised Code Title
√5th

2002 Ingenix, Inc.   **Volume 1 — 107**

Nervous System and Sense Organs 378.82–379.50

378.82 Spasm of conjugate gaze
DEF: Muscle contractions impairing parallel movement of eye.

378.83 Convergence insufficiency or palsy

378.84 Convergence excess or spasm

378.85 Anomalies of divergence

378.86 Internuclear ophthalmoplegia
DEF: Eye movement anomaly due to brainstem lesion.

378.87 Other dissociated deviation of eye movements
Skew deviation

378.9 Unspecified disorder of eye movements
Ophthalmoplegia NOS   Strabismus NOS
AHA: 2Q, '01, 21

✓4th **379 Other disorders of eye**

✓5th **379.0 Scleritis and episcleritis**
EXCLUDES   syphilitic episcleritis (095.0)

379.00 Scleritis, unspecified
Episcleritis NOS

379.01 Episcleritis periodica fugax
DEF: Hyperemia (engorgement) of the sclera and overlying conjunctiva characterized by a sudden onset and short duration.

379.02 Nodular episcleritis
DEF: Inflammation of the outermost layer of the sclera, with formation of nodules.

379.03 Anterior scleritis

379.04 Scleromalacia perforans
DEF: Scleral thinning, softening and degeneration; seen with rheumatoid arthritis.

379.05 Scleritis with corneal involvement
Scleroperikeratitis

379.06 Brawny scleritis
DEF: Severe scleral inflammation with thickening corneal margins.

379.07 Posterior scleritis
Sclerotenonitis

379.09 Other
Scleral abscess

✓5th **379.1 Other disorders of sclera**
EXCLUDES   blue sclera (743.47)

379.11 Scleral ectasia
Scleral staphyloma NOS
DEF: Protrusion of the contents of the eyeball where the sclera has thinned.

379.12 Staphyloma posticum
DEF: Ring-shaped protrusion or bulging of sclera and uveal tissue at posterior pole of eye.

379.13 Equatorial staphyloma
DEF: Ring-shaped protrusion or bulging of sclera and uveal tissue midway between front and back of eye.

379.14 Anterior staphyloma, localized

379.15 Ring staphyloma

379.16 Other degenerative disorders of sclera

379.19 Other

✓5th **379.2 Disorders of vitreous body**
DEF: Disorder of clear gel that fills space between retina and lens.

379.21 Vitreous degeneration
Vitreous: Vitreous:
cavitation   liquefaction
detachment

379.22 Crystalline deposits in vitreous
Asteroid hyalitis   Synchysis scintillans

379.23 Vitreous hemorrhage
AHA: 3Q, '91, 15

379.24 Other vitreous opacities
Vitreous floaters

379.25 Vitreous membranes and strands

379.26 Vitreous prolapse
DEF: Slipping of vitreous from normal position.

379.29 Other disorders of vitreous
EXCLUDES   vitreous abscess (360.04)
AHA: 1Q, '99, 11

✓5th **379.3 Aphakia and other disorders of lens**
EXCLUDES   after-cataract (366.50-366.53)

379.31 Aphakia
EXCLUDES   cataract extraction status (V45.61)
DEF: Absence of eye's crystalline lens.

379.32 Subluxation of lens

379.33 Anterior dislocation of lens
DEF: Lens displaced toward iris.

379.34 Posterior dislocation of lens
DEF: Lens displaced backward toward vitreous.

379.39 Other disorders of lens

✓5th **379.4 Anomalies of pupillary function**

379.40 Abnormal pupillary function, unspecified

379.41 Anisocoria
DEF: Unequal pupil diameter.

379.42 Miosis (persistent), not due to miotics
DEF: Abnormal contraction of pupil less than 2 millimeters.

379.43 Mydriasis (persistent), not due to mydriatics
DEF: Morbid dilation of pupil.

379.45 Argyll Robertson pupil, atypical
Argyll Robertson phenomenon or pupil, nonsyphilitic
EXCLUDES   Argyll Robertson pupil (syphilitic) (094.89)
DEF: Failure of pupil to respond to light; affects both eyes; may be caused by diseases such as syphilis of the central nervous system or miosis.

379.46 Tonic pupillary reaction
Adie's pupil or syndrome

379.49 Other
Hippus   Pupillary paralysis

✓5th **379.5 Nystagmus and other irregular eye movements**

379.50 Nystagmus, unspecified
AHA: 2Q, '01, 21
DEF: Involuntary, rapid, rhythmic movement of eyeball; vertical, horizontal, rotatory or mixed; cause may be congenital, acquired, physiological, neurological, myopathic, or due to ocular diseases.

Ear and Mastoid Process

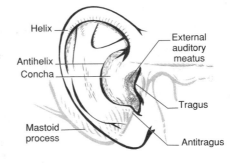

Helix   External auditory meatus   Antihelix   Concha   Tragus   Mastoid process   Antitragus

N Newborn Age: 0   P Pediatric Age: 0-17   M Maternity Age: 12-55   A Adult Age: 15-124   CC CC Condition   MC Major Complication   CD Complex Dx   HIV HIV Related Dx

108 — Volume 1   *2002 Ingenix, Inc.*

379.51 **Congenital nystagmus**

379.52 **Latent nystagmus**

379.53 **Visual deprivation nystagmus**

379.54 **Nystagmus associated with disorders of the vestibular system**

379.55 **Dissociated nystagmus**

379.56 **Other forms of nystagmus**

379.57 **Deficiencies of saccadic eye movements**
Abnormal optokinetic response
DEF: Saccadic eye movements; small, rapid, involuntary movements by both eyes simultaneously, due to changing point of fixation on visualized object.

379.58 **Deficiencies of smooth pursuit movements**

379.59 **Other irregularities of eye movements**
Opsoclonus

379.8 **Other specified disorders of eye and adnexa**

✓5ᵗʰ 379.9 **Unspecified disorder of eye and adnexa**

379.90 **Disorder of eye, unspecified**

379.91 **Pain in or around eye**

379.92 **Swelling or mass of eye**

379.93 **Redness or discharge of eye**

379.99 **Other ill-defined disorders of eye**
EXCLUDES   *blurred vision NOS (368.8)*

DISEASES OF THE EAR AND MASTOID PROCESS (380-389)

✓4ᵗʰ 380 **Disorders of external ear**

✓5ᵗʰ 380.0 **Perichondritis of pinna**
Perichondritis of auricle

380.00 **Perichondritis of pinna, unspecified**

380.01 **Acute perichondritis of pinna**

380.02 **Chronic perichondritis of pinna**

✓5ᵗʰ 380.1 **Infective otitis externa**

380.10 **Infective otitis externa, unspecified**
Otitis externa (acute):   Otitis externa (acute):
  NOS   hemorrhagica
  circumscribed   infective NOS
  diffuse

380.11 **Acute infection of pinna**
EXCLUDES   *furuncular otitis externa (680.0)*

380.12 **Acute swimmers' ear**
Beach ear   Tank ear
DEF: Otitis externa due to swimming.

380.13 *Other acute infections of external ear*
Code first underlying disease, as:
  erysipelas (035)
  impetigo (684)
  seborrheic dermatitis (690.10-690.18)
EXCLUDES   *herpes simplex (054.73)*
               herpes zoster (053.71)

380.14 **Malignant otitis externa**
DEF: Severe necrotic otitis externa; due to bacteria.

380.15 *Chronic mycotic otitis externa*
Code first underlying disease, as:
  aspergillosis (117.3)
  otomycosis NOS (111.9)
EXCLUDES   *candidal otitis externa (112.82)*

380.16 **Other chronic infective otitis externa**
Chronic infective otitis externa NOS

✓5ᵗʰ 380.2 **Other otitis externa**

380.21 **Cholesteatoma of external ear**
Keratosis obturans of external ear (canal)
EXCLUDES   *cholesteatoma NOS (385.30-385.35)*
               postmastoidectomy (383.32)
DEF: Cystlike mass filled with debris, including cholesterol; rare, congenital condition.

380.22 **Other acute otitis externa**
Acute otitis externa: Acute otitis externa:
  actinic   eczematoid
  chemical   reactive
  contact

380.23 **Other chronic otitis externa**
Chronic otitis externa NOS

✓5ᵗʰ 380.3 **Noninfectious disorders of pinna**

380.30 **Disorder of pinna, unspecified**

380.31 **Hematoma of auricle or pinna**

380.32 **Acquired deformities of auricle or pinna**
EXCLUDES   *cauliflower ear (738.7)*

380.39 **Other**
EXCLUDES   *gouty tophi of ear (274.81)*

380.4 **Impacted cerumen**
Wax in ear

✓5ᵗʰ 380.5 **Acquired stenosis of external ear canal**
Collapse of external ear canal

380.50 **Acquired stenosis of external ear canal, unspecified as to cause**

380.51 **Secondary to trauma**
DEF: Narrowing of the external ear canal; due to trauma.

380.52 **Secondary to surgery**
DEF: Postsurgical narrowing of the external ear canal.

380.53 **Secondary to inflammation**
DEF: Narrowing of the external ear canal; due to chronic inflammation.

✓5ᵗʰ 380.8 **Other disorders of external ear**

380.81 **Exostosis of external ear canal**

380.89 **Other**

380.9 **Unspecified disorder of external ear**

✓4ᵗʰ 381 **Nonsuppurative otitis media and Eustachian tube disorders**

✓5ᵗʰ 381.0 **Acute nonsuppurative otitis media**
Acute tubotympanic catarrh
Otitis media, acute or subacute:
  catarrhal
  exudative
  transudative
  with effusion
EXCLUDES   *otitic barotrauma (993.0)*

381.00 **Acute nonsuppurative otitis media, unspecified**

381.01 **Acute serous otitis media**
Acute or subacute secretory otitis media
DEF: Sudden, severe infection of the middle ear.

381.02 **Acute mucoid otitis media**
Acute or subacute seromucinous otitis media
Blue drum syndrome
DEF: Sudden, severe infection of the middle ear, with mucous.

381.03 **Acute sanguinous otitis media**
DEF: Sudden, severe infection of the middle ear, with blood.

381.04 **Acute allergic serous otitis media**

381.05 **Acute allergic mucoid otitis media**

381.06 **Acute allergic sanguinous otitis media**

✓5ᵗʰ 381.1 **Chronic serous otitis media**
Chronic tubotympanic catarrh

381.10 **Chronic serous otitis media, simple or unspecified**
DEF: Persistent infection of the middle ear, without pus.

381.19 **Other**
Serosanguinous chronic otitis media

Nervous System and Sense Organs 379.51–381.19

✓4ᵗʰ ✓5ᵗʰ Additional Digit Required   Nonspecific PDx   Unacceptable PDx   Manifestation Code   **MSP** Medicare Secondary Payer   ►◄ Revised Text   ● New Code   ▲ Revised Code Title

2002 Ingenix, Inc.   **Volume 1 — 109**

Nervous System and Sense Organs 381.2–383.1

√5ᵗʰ **381.2 Chronic mucoid otitis media**
Glue ear

> **EXCLUDES**   *adhesive middle ear disease (385.10-385.19)*

DEF: Chronic condition; characterized by viscous fluid in middle ear; due to obstructed Eustachian tube.

381.20 Chronic mucoid otitis media, simple or unspecified

381.29 Other
Mucosanguinous chronic otitis media

381.3 Other and unspecified chronic nonsuppurative otitis media

Otitis media, chronic: Otitis media, chronic:
allergic   seromucinous
exudative   transudative
secretory   with effusion

381.4 Nonsuppurative otitis media, not specified as acute or chronic

Otitis media: Otitis media:
allergic   seromucinous
catarrhal   serous
exudative   transudative
mucoid   with effusion
secretory

√5ᵗʰ **381.5 Eustachian salpingitis**

381.50 Eustachian salpingitis, unspecified

381.51 Acute Eustachian salpingitis
DEF: Sudden, severe inflammation of the Eustachian tube.

381.52 Chronic Eustachian salpingitis
DEF: Persistent inflammation of the Eustachian tube.

√5ᵗʰ **381.6 Obstruction of Eustachian tube**

Stenosis ⎫
Stricture ⎭ of Eustachian tube

381.60 Obstruction of Eustachian tube, unspecified

381.61 Osseous obstruction of Eustachian tube
Obstruction of Eustachian tube from cholesteatoma, polyp, or other osseous lesion

381.62 Intrinsic cartilagenous obstruction of Eustachian tube
DEF: Blockage of Eustachian tube; due to cartilage overgrowth.

381.63 Extrinsic cartilagenous obstruction of Eustachian tube
Compression of Eustachian tube

381.7 Patulous Eustachian tube
DEF: Distended, oversized Eustachian tube.

√5ᵗʰ **381.8 Other disorders of Eustachian tube**

381.81 Dysfunction of Eustachian tube

381.89 Other

381.9 Unspecified Eustachian tube disorder

√4ᵗʰ **382 Suppurative and unspecified otitis media**

√5ᵗʰ **382.0 Acute suppurative otitis media**

Otitis media, acute: Otitis media, acute:
necrotizing NOS   purulent

382.00 Acute suppurative otitis media without spontaneous rupture of ear drum
DEF: Sudden, severe inflammation of middle ear, with pus.

382.01 Acute suppurative otitis media with spontaneous rupture of ear drum
DEF: Sudden, severe inflammation of middle ear, with pressure tearing ear drum tissue.

382.02 *Acute suppurative otitis media in diseases classified elsewhere*

Code first underlying disease, as:
influenza (487.8)
scarlet fever (034.1)

> **EXCLUDES**   *postmeasles otitis (055.2)*

382.1 Chronic tubotympanic suppurative otitis media

Benign chronic
suppurative otitis ⎫ (with anterior
media ⎬ perforation of
Chronic tubotympanic ⎭ ear drum)
disease

DEF: Inflammation of tympanic cavity and auditory tube; with pus formation.

382.2 Chronic atticoantral suppurative otitis media

Chronic atticoantral ⎫ (with posterior or superior
disease ⎬ marginal perforation
Persistent mucosal ⎭ of ear drum)
disease

382.3 Unspecified chronic suppurative otitis media
Chronic purulent otitis media

> **EXCLUDES**   *tuberculous otitis media (017.4)*

DEF: Inflammation of upper tympanic membrane and mastoid antrum; with pus formation.

382.4 Unspecified suppurative otitis media
Purulent otitis media NOS

382.9 Unspecified otitis media

Otitis media: Otitis media:
NOS   chronic NOS
acute NOS

AHA: N-D, '84, 16

√4ᵗʰ **383 Mastoiditis and related conditions**

√5ᵗʰ **383.0 Acute mastoiditis**
Abscess of mastoid   Empyema of mastoid

383.00 Acute mastoiditis without complications
DEF: Sudden, severe inflammation of mastoid air cells.

383.01 Subperiosteal abscess of mastoid   **CC**
CC Excl: 015.60-015.66, 017.40-017.46, 017.90-017.96, 383.00-383.9, 388.71-388.72, 388.8-388.9, 744.00, 744.02, 744.09, 744.29, 744.3

DEF: Pocket of pus within the mastoid bone.

383.02 Acute mastoiditis with other complications
Gradenigo's syndrome

383.1 Chronic mastoiditis
Caries of mastoid
Fistula of mastoid

> **EXCLUDES**   *tuberculous mastoiditis (015.6)*

DEF: Persistent inflammation of the mastoid air cells.

Middle and Inner Ear

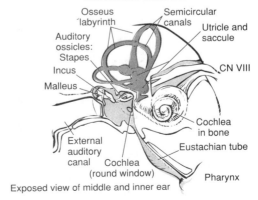

Exposed view of middle and inner ear

N Newborn Age: 0   **P** Pediatric Age: 0-17   **M** Maternity Age: 12-55   **A** Adult Age: 15-124   **CC** CC Condition   **MC** Major Complication   **CD** Complex Dx   **HIV** HIV Related Dx

110 — Volume 1   *2002 Ingenix, Inc.*

√5th **383.2 Petrositis**

Coalescing osteitis ⎫
Inflammation   ⎬ of petrous bone
Osteomyelitis   ⎭

383.20 Petrositis, unspecified

383.21 Acute petrositis

DEF: Sudden, severe inflammation of dense bone behind the ear.

383.22 Chronic petrositis

DEF: Persistent inflammation of dense bone behind the ear.

√5th **383.3 Complications following mastoidectomy**

383.30 Postmastoidectomy complication, unspecified   **CC**

CC Excl: See code 383.01

383.31 Mucosal cyst of postmastoidectomy cavity

DEF: Mucous-lined cyst cavity following removal of mastoid bone.

383.32 Recurrent cholesteatoma of postmastoidectomy cavity

DEF: Cystlike mass of cell debris in cavity following removal of mastoid bone.

383.33 Granulations of postmastoidectomy cavity

Chronic inflammation of postmastoidectomy cavity

DEF: Granular tissue in cavity following removal of mastoid bone.

√5th **383.8 Other disorders of mastoid**

383.81 Postauricular fistula   **CC**

CC Excl: See code 383.01

DEF: Abnormal passage behind mastoid cavity.

383.89 Other

383.9 Unspecified mastoiditis

√4th **384 Other disorders of tympanic membrane**

√5th **384.0 Acute myringitis without mention of otitis media**

384.00 Acute myringitis, unspecified

Acute tympanitis NOS

DEF: Sudden, severe inflammation of ear drum.

384.01 Bullous myringitis

Myringitis bullosa hemorrhagica

DEF: Type of viral otitis media characterized by the appearance of serous or hemorrhagic blebs on the tympanic membrane.

384.09 Other

384.1 Chronic myringitis without mention of otitis media

Chronic tympanitis

DEF: Persistent inflammation of ear drum; with no evidence of middle ear infection.

√5th **384.2 Perforation of tympanic membrane**

Perforation of ear drum: Perforation of ear drum:
  NOS   postinflammatory
  persistent posttraumatic

EXCLUDES   otitis media with perforation of tympanic membrane (382.00-382.9)
traumatic perforation [current injury] (872.61)

384.20 Perforation of tympanic membrane, unspecified

384.21 Central perforation of tympanic membrane

384.22 Attic perforation of tympanic membrane

Pars flaccida

384.23 Other marginal perforation of tympanic membrane

384.24 Multiple perforations of tympanic membrane

384.25 Total perforation of tympanic membrane

√5th **384.8 Other specified disorders of tympanic membrane**

384.81 Atrophic flaccid tympanic membrane

Healed perforation of ear drum

384.82 Atrophic nonflaccid tympanic membrane

384.9 Unspecified disorder of tympanic membrane

√4th **385 Other disorders of middle ear and mastoid**

EXCLUDES   mastoiditis (383.0-383.9)

√5th **385.0 Tympanosclerosis**

385.00 Tympanosclerosis, unspecified as to involvement

385.01 Tympanosclerosis involving tympanic membrane only

DEF: Tough, fibrous tissue impeding functions of ear drum.

385.02 Tympanosclerosis involving tympanic membrane and ear ossicles

DEF: Tough, fibrous tissue impeding functions of middle ear bones (stapes, malleus, incus).

385.03 Tympanosclerosis involving tympanic membrane, ear ossicles, and middle ear

DEF: Tough, fibrous tissue impeding functions of ear drum, middle ear bones and middle ear canal.

385.09 Tympanosclerosis involving other combination of structures

√5th **385.1 Adhesive middle ear disease**

Adhesive otitis   Otitis media:
Otitis media: fibrotic
  chronic adhesive

EXCLUDES   glue ear (381.20-381.29)

DEF: Adhesions of middle ear structures.

385.10 Adhesive middle ear disease, unspecified as to involvement

385.11 Adhesions of drum head to incus

385.12 Adhesions of drum head to stapes

385.13 Adhesions of drum head to promontorium

385.19 Other adhesions and combinations

√5th **385.2 Other acquired abnormality of ear ossicles**

385.21 Impaired mobility of malleus

Ankylosis of malleus

385.22 Impaired mobility of other ear ossicles

Ankylosis of ear ossicles, except malleus

385.23 Discontinuity or dislocation of ear ossicles

DEF: Disruption in auditory chain; created by malleus, incus and stapes.

385.24 Partial loss or necrosis of ear ossicles

DEF: Tissue loss in malleus, incus and stapes.

Cholesteatoma

Middle ear chamber

Cholesteatoma sac   Ear drum

√4th
√5th Additional Digit Required   Nonspecific PDx   Unacceptable PDx   Manifestation Code   **MSP** Medicare Secondary Payer   ◄► Revised Text   ● New Code   ▲ Revised Code Title

2002 Ingenix, Inc.   **Volume 1 — 111**

√5ᵗʰ **385.3 Cholesteatoma of middle ear and mastoid**

Cholesterosis
Epidermosis
Keratosis
Polyp } of (middle) ear

EXCLUDES cholesteatoma:
   external ear canal (380.21)
   recurrent of postmastoidectomy
      cavity (383.32)

DEF: Cystlike mass of middle ear and mastoid antrum filled with debris, including cholesterol.

   385.30 Cholesteatoma, unspecified
   385.31 Cholesteatoma of attic
   385.32 Cholesteatoma of middle ear
   385.33 Cholesteatoma of middle ear and mastoid
      AHA: 3Q, '00, 10

      DEF: Cystlike mass of cell debris in middle ear and mastoid air cells behind ear.

   385.35 Diffuse cholesteatosis

√5ᵗʰ **385.8 Other disorders of middle ear and mastoid**
   385.82 Cholesterin granuloma

      DEF: Granuloma formed of fibrotic tissue; contains cholesterol crystals surrounded by foreign-body cells; found in the middle ear and mastoid area.

   385.83 Retained foreign body of middle ear
      AHA: 3Q, '94, 7; N-D, '87, 9

   385.89 Other

   385.9 Unspecified disorder of middle ear and mastoid

√4ᵗʰ **386 Vertiginous syndromes and other disorders of vestibular system**
   EXCLUDES vertigo NOS (780.4)

   AHA: M-A, '85, 12

√5ᵗʰ **386.0 Ménière's disease**
   Endolymphatic hydrops
   Lermoyez's syndrome
   Ménière's syndrome or vertigo

   DEF: Distended membranous labyrinth of middle ear from endolymphatic hydrops; causes ischemia, failure of nerve function; hearing and balance dysfunction; symptoms include fluctuating deafness, ringing in ears and dizziness.

   386.00 Ménière's disease, unspecified
      Ménière's disease (active)
   386.01 Active Ménière's disease, cochleovestibular
   386.02 Active Ménière's disease, cochlear
   386.03 Active Ménière's disease, vestibular
   386.04 Inactive Ménière's disease
      Ménière's disease in remission

√5ᵗʰ **386.1 Other and unspecified peripheral vertigo**
   EXCLUDES epidemic vertigo (078.81)

   386.10 Peripheral vertigo, unspecified
   386.11 Benign paroxysmal positional vertigo
      Benign paroxysmal positional nystagmus
   386.12 Vestibular neuronitis
      Acute (and recurrent) peripheral vestibulopathy

      DEF: Transient benign vertigo, unknown cause; characterized by response to caloric stimulation on one side, nystagmus with rhythmic movement of eyes; normal auditory function present; occurs in young adults.

   386.19 Other
      Aural vertigo
      Otogenic vertigo

   386.2 Vertigo of central origin
      Central positional nystagmus
      Malignant positional vertigo

√5ᵗʰ **386.3 Labyrinthitis**
   386.30 Labyrinthitis, unspecified

   386.31 Serous labyrinthitis
      Diffuse labyrinthitis
      DEF: Inflammation of labyrinth; with fluid buildup.

   386.32 Circumscribed labyrinthitis
      Focal labyrinthitis
   386.33 Suppurative labyrinthitis
      Purulent labyrinthitis
      DEF: Inflammation of labyrinth; with pus.

   386.34 Toxic labyrinthitis
      DEF: Inflammation of labyrinth; due to toxic reaction.

   386.35 Viral labyrinthitis

√5ᵗʰ **386.4 Labyrinthine fistula**
   386.40 Labyrinthine fistula, unspecified
   386.41 Round window fistula
   386.42 Oval window fistula
   386.43 Semicircular canal fistula
   386.48 Labyrinthine fistula of combined sites

√5ᵗʰ **386.5 Labyrinthine dysfunction**
   386.50 Labyrinthine dysfunction, unspecified
   386.51 Hyperactive labyrinth, unilateral
      DEF: Oversensitivity of labyrinth to auditory signals; affecting one ear.

   386.52 Hyperactive labyrinth, bilateral
      DEF: Oversensitivity of labyrinth to auditory signals; affecting both ears.

   386.53 Hypoactive labyrinth, unilateral
      DEF: Reduced sensitivity of labyrinth to auditory signals; affecting one ear.

   386.54 Hypoactive labyrinth, bilateral
      DEF: Reduced sensitivity of labyrinth to auditory signals; affecting both ears.

   386.55 Loss of labyrinthine reactivity, unilateral
      DEF: Reduced reaction of labyrinth to auditory signals, affecting one ear.

   386.56 Loss of labyrinthine reactivity, bilateral
      DEF: Reduced reaction of labyrinth to auditory signals; affecting both ears.

   386.58 Other forms and combinations
   386.8 Other disorders of labyrinth
   386.9 Unspecified vertiginous syndromes and labyrinthine disorders

√4ᵗʰ **387 Otosclerosis**
   INCLUDES otospongiosis

   DEF: Synonym for otospongiosis, spongy bone formation in the labyrinth bones of the ear; it causes progressive hearing impairment.

   387.0 Otosclerosis involving oval window, nonobliterative
      DEF: Tough, fibrous tissue impeding functions of oval window.

   387.1 Otosclerosis involving oval window, obliterative
      DEF: Tough, fibrous tissue blocking oval window.

   387.2 Cochlear otosclerosis
      Otosclerosis involving: otic capsule   Otosclerosis involving: round window

      DEF: Tough, fibrous tissue impeding functions of cochlea.

   387.8 Other otosclerosis
   387.9 Otosclerosis, unspecified

√4ᵗʰ **388 Other disorders of ear**
√5ᵗʰ **388.0 Degenerative and vascular disorders of ear**
   388.00 Degenerative and vascular disorders, unspecified
   388.01 Presbyacusis

      DEF: Progressive, bilateral perceptive hearing loss caused by advancing age; it is also known as presbycusis.

N Newborn Age: 0   P Pediatric Age: 0-17   M Maternity Age: 12-55   A Adult Age: 15-124   CC CC Condition   MC Major Complication   CD Complex Dx   HIV HIV Related Dx

112 — Volume 1

2002 Ingenix, Inc.

388.02 Transient ischemic deafness
> DEF: Restricted blood flow to auditory organs causing temporary hearing loss.

√5ᵗʰ **388.1 Noise effects on inner ear**
    388.10 Noise effects on inner ear, unspecified
    388.11 Acoustic trauma (explosive) to ear
> Otitic blast injury

    388.12 Noise-induced hearing loss
388.2 Sudden hearing loss, unspecified
√5ᵗʰ **388.3 Tinnitus**
> DEF: Abnormal noises in ear; may be heard by others beside the affected individual; noises include ringing, clicking, roaring and buzzing.

    388.30 Tinnitus, unspecified
    388.31 Subjective tinnitus
    388.32 Objective tinnitus
√5ᵗʰ **388.4 Other abnormal auditory perception**
    388.40 Abnormal auditory perception, unspecified
    388.41 Diplacusis
> DEF: Perception of a single auditory sound as two sounds at two different levels of intensity.

    388.42 Hyperacusis
> DEF: Exceptionally acute sense of hearing caused by such conditions as Bell's palsy; this term may also refer to painful sensitivity to sounds.

    388.43 Impairment of auditory discrimination
> DEF: Impaired ability to distinguish tone of sound.

    388.44 Recruitment
> DEF: Perception of abnormally increased loudness caused by a slight increase in sound intensity; it is a term used in audiology.

388.5 Disorders of acoustic nerve
> Acoustic neuritis
> Degeneration ⎫
> Disorder   ⎬ of acoustic or eighth nerve

> EXCLUDES   *acoustic neuroma (225.1)*
> *syphilitic acoustic neuritis (094.86)*

AHA: M-A, '87, 8

√5ᵗʰ **388.6 Otorrhea**
    388.60 Otorrhea, unspecified
> Discharging ear NOS

    388.61 Cerebrospinal fluid otorrhea
> EXCLUDES   *cerebrospinal fluid rhinorrhea (349.81)*
> DEF: Spinal fluid leakage from ear.

    388.69 Other
> Otorrhagia

√5ᵗʰ **388.7 Otalgia**
    388.70 Otalgia, unspecified
> Earache NOS

    388.71 Otogenic pain
    388.72 Referred pain
388.8 Other disorders of ear
388.9 Unspecified disorder of ear
√4ᵗʰ **389 Hearing loss**
√5ᵗʰ **389.0 Conductive hearing loss**
> Conductive deafness

AHA: 4Q, '89, 5

> DEF: Dysfunction in sound-conducting structures of external or middle ear causing hearing loss.

    389.00 Conductive hearing loss, unspecified
    389.01 Conductive hearing loss, external ear
    389.02 Conductive hearing loss, tympanic membrane
    389.03 Conductive hearing loss, middle ear
    389.04 Conductive hearing loss, inner ear
    389.08 Conductive hearing loss of combined types
√5ᵗʰ **389.1 Sensorineural hearing loss**
> Perceptive hearing loss or deafness
> EXCLUDES   *abnormal auditory perception (388.40-388.44)*
> *psychogenic deafness (306.7)*

AHA: 4Q, '89, 5

> DEF: Nerve conduction causing hearing loss.

    389.10 Sensorineural hearing loss, unspecified
> **AHA:** 1Q, '93, 29

    389.11 Sensory hearing loss
    389.12 Neural hearing loss
    389.14 Central hearing loss
    389.18 Sensorineural hearing loss of combined types
389.2 Mixed conductive and sensorineural hearing loss
> Deafness or hearing loss of type classifiable to 389.0 with type classifiable to 389.1

389.7 Deaf mutism, not elsewhere classifiable
> Deaf, nonspeaking

389.8 Other specified forms of hearing loss
389.9 Unspecified hearing loss
> Deafness NOS

√4ᵗʰ / √5ᵗʰ Additional Digit Required   Nonspecific PDx   Unacceptable PDx   Manifestation Code   **MSP** Medicare Secondary Payer   ►◄ Revised Text   ● New Code   ▲ Revised Code Title

2002 Ingenix, Inc.   **Volume 1 — 113**

7. DISEASES OF THE CIRCULATORY SYSTEM (390-459)

ACUTE RHEUMATIC FEVER (390-392)

DEF: Febrile disease occurs mainly in children or young adults following throat infection by group A *streptococci*; symptoms include fever, joint pain, lesions of heart, blood vessels and joint connective tissue, abdominal pain, skin changes, and chorea.

390 Rheumatic fever without mention of heart involvement
Arthritis, rheumatic, acute or subacute
Rheumatic fever (active) (acute)
Rheumatism, articular, acute or subacute
> EXCLUDES   that with heart involvement (391.0-391.9)

✓4ᵗʰ **391 Rheumatic fever with heart involvement**
> EXCLUDES   chronic heart diseases of rheumatic origin
> (398.0-398.9) unless rheumatic fever is
> also present or there is evidence of
> recrudescence or activity of the rheumatic
> process

391.0   Acute rheumatic pericarditis
Rheumatic:
fever (active) (acute) with pericarditis
pericarditis (acute)
Any condition classifiable to 390 with pericarditis
> EXCLUDES   that not specified as rheumatic (420.0-
> 420.9)

DEF: Sudden, severe inflammation of heart lining due to rheumatic fever.

391.1   Acute rheumatic endocarditis
Rheumatic:
endocarditis, acute
fever (active) (acute) with endocarditis or valvulitis
valvulitis acute
Any condition classifiable to 390 with endocarditis
or valvulitis

DEF: Sudden, severe inflammation of heart cavities due to rheumatic fever.

391.2   Acute rheumatic myocarditis
Rheumatic fever (active) (acute) with myocarditis
Any condition classifiable to 390 with myocarditis

DEF: Sudden, severe inflammation of heart muscles due to rheumatic fever.

391.8   Other acute rheumatic heart disease
Rheumatic:
fever (active) (acute) with other or multiple types
of heart involvement
pancarditis, acute
Any condition classifiable to 390 with other or
multiple types of heart involvement

391.9   Acute rheumatic heart disease, unspecified
Rheumatic:
carditis, acute
fever (active) (acute) with unspecified type of heart
involvement
heart disease, active or acute
Any condition classifiable to 390 with unspecified
type of heart involvement

✓4ᵗʰ **392 Rheumatic chorea**
> INCLUDES   Sydenham's chorea
> EXCLUDES   chorea:
> NOS (333.5)
> Huntington's (333.4)

DEF: Childhood disease linked with rheumatic fever and streptococcal infections; symptoms include spasmodic, involuntary movements of limbs or facial muscles, psychic symptoms, and irritability.

392.0   With heart involvement
Rheumatic chorea with heart involvement of any
type classifiable to 391

392.9   Without mention of heart involvement

CHRONIC RHEUMATIC HEART DISEASE (393-398)

393 Chronic rheumatic pericarditis
Adherent pericardium, rheumatic
Chronic rheumatic:
mediastinopericarditis
myopericarditis
> EXCLUDES   pericarditis NOS or not specified as rheumatic
> (423.0-423.9)

DEF: Persistent inflammation of heart lining due to rheumatic heart disease.

✓4ᵗʰ **394 Diseases of mitral valve**
> EXCLUDES   that with aortic valve involvement (396.0-396.9)

394.0   Mitral stenosis   CC
Mitral (valve):   Mitral (valve):
obstruction (rheumatic)   stenosis NOS

CC Excl: 390, 391.8-391.9, 394.0-394.9, 396.0-396.9, 397.9, 398.90, 398.99, 424.0, 459.89, 459.9

DEF: Narrowing, of mitral valve between left atrium and left ventricle; due to rheumatic heart disease.

394.1   Rheumatic mitral insufficiency   CC
Rheumatic mitral: Rheumatic mitral:
incompetence   regurgitation
> EXCLUDES   that not specified as rheumatic (424.0)

CC Excl: See code 394.0

DEF: Malfunction of mitral valve between left atrium and left ventricle; due to rheumatic heart disease.

394.2   Mitral stenosis with insufficiency   CC
Mitral stenosis with incompetence or regurgitation

CC Excl: See code 394.0

DEF: A narrowing or stricture of the mitral valve situated between the left atrium and left ventricle. The stenosis interferes with blood flow from the atrium into the ventricle. If the valve does not completely close, it becomes insufficient (inadequate) and cannot prevent regurgitation (abnormal backward flow) into the atrium when the left ventricle contracts. This abnormal function is also called incompetence.

394.9   Other and unspecified mitral valve diseases   CC
Mitral (valve):   Mitral (valve):
disease (chronic)   failure

CC Excl: See code 394.0

✓4ᵗʰ **395 Diseases of aortic valve**
> EXCLUDES   that not specified as rheumatic (424.1)
> that with mitral valve involvement (396.0-396.9)

395.0   Rheumatic aortic stenosis   CC
Rheumatic aortic (valve) obstruction

CC Excl: 390, 391.8-391.9, 395.0-395.9, 396.0-396.9, 397.9, 398.90, 398.99, 424.1, 459.89, 459.9

AHA: 4Q, '88, 8

DEF: Narrowing of the aortic valve; results in backflow into ventricle; due to rheumatic heart disease.

395.1   Rheumatic aortic insufficiency   CC
Rheumatic aortic: Rheumatic aortic:
incompetence   regurgitation

CC Excl: See code 395.0

DEF: Malfunction of the aortic valve; results in backflow into left ventricle; due to rheumatic heart disease.

395.2   Rheumatic aortic stenosis with insufficiency   CC
Rheumatic aortic stenosis with incompetence or
regurgitation

CC Excl: See code 395.0

DEF: Malfunction and narrowing, of the aortic valve; results in backflow into left ventricle; due to rheumatic heart disease.

395.9   Other and unspecified rheumatic aortic diseases CC
Rheumatic aortic (valve) disease

CC Excl: See code 395.0

✓4ᵗʰ
✓5ᵗʰ Additional Digit Required   Nonspecific PDx   Unacceptable PDx   Manifestation Code   MSP Medicare Secondary Payer   ▶◀ Revised Text   ● New Code   ▲ Revised Code Title

2002 Ingenix, Inc.   Volume 1 — 115

Circulatory System 390–395.5

Circulatory System 396–402.00

√4ᵗʰ **396 Diseases of mitral and aortic valves**

> INCLUDES   involvement of both mitral and aortic valves, whether specified as rheumatic or not

AHA: N-D, '87, 8

396.0 Mitral valve stenosis and aortic valve stenosis CC
Atypical aortic (valve) stenosis
Mitral and aortic (valve) obstruction (rheumatic)
CC Excl: 390, 391.8-391.9, 394.0-394.9, 395.0-395.9, 396.0-396.9, 397.9, 398.90, 398.99, 424.0-424.1, 459.89, 459.9

396.1 Mitral valve stenosis and aortic valve insufficiency CC
CC Excl: See code 396.0

396.2 Mitral valve insufficiency and aortic valve stenosis CC
CC Excl: See code 396.0
AHA: 2Q, '00, 16

396.3 Mitral valve insufficiency and aortic valve insufficiency CC
Mitral and aortic (valve):   Mitral and aortic (valve):
incompetence   regurgitation
CC Excl: See code 396.0

396.8 Multiple involvement of mitral and aortic valves CC
Stenosis and insufficiency of mitral or aortic valve with stenosis or insufficiency, or both, of the other valve
CC Excl: See code 396.0

396.9 Mitral and aortic valve diseases, unspecified CC
CC Excl: See code 396.0

√4ᵗʰ **397 Diseases of other endocardial structures**
397.0 Diseases of tricuspid valve CC
Tricuspid (valve)   Tricuspid (valve)
(rheumatic):   (rheumatic):
disease   regurgitation
insufficiency   stenosis
obstruction
CC Excl: 397.0, 398.90, 398.99, 424.2, 459.89, 459.9
AHA: 2Q, '00, 16
DEF: Malfunction of the valve between right atrium and right ventricle; due to rheumatic heart disease.

397.1 Rheumatic diseases of pulmonary valve CC
> EXCLUDES   that not specified as rheumatic (424.3)
CC Excl: 397.1, 398.90, 398.99, 424.3, 459.89, 459.9

397.9 Rheumatic diseases of endocardium, valve unspecified CC
Rheumatic:
endocarditis (chronic)
valvulitis (chronic)
> EXCLUDES   that not specified as rheumatic (424.90-424.99)
CC Excl: 390, 391.1, 391.8-391.9, 394.0-394.9, 395.0-395.9, 397.1, 397.9, 398.90, 398.99, 421.0-421.9, 424.0-424.99, 459.89, 459.9

√4ᵗʰ **398 Other rheumatic heart disease**
398.0 Rheumatic myocarditis CC
Rheumatic degeneration of myocardium
> EXCLUDES   myocarditis not specified as rheumatic (429.0)
CC Excl: 390, 391.2-391.9, 398.0, 398.90, 398.99, 422.0, 422.90-422.99, 429.0, 429.71, 429.79, 459.89, 459.9
DEF: Chronic inflammation of heart muscle; due to rheumatic heart disease.

√5ᵗʰ **398.9 Other and unspecified rheumatic heart diseases**
398.90 Rheumatic heart disease, unspecified
Rheumatic:
carditis
heart disease NOS
> EXCLUDES   carditis not specified as rheumatic (429.89)
> heart disease NOS not specified as rheumatic (429.9)

398.91 Rheumatic heart failure (congestive) CC MC
Rheumatic left ventricular failure
CC Excl: 398.90-398.99, 402.01, 402.11, 402.91, 428.0-428.9, 459.89, 459.9
AHA: 1Q, '95, 6; 3Q, '88, 3
DEF: Decreased cardiac output, edema and hypertension; due to rheumatic heart disease.

398.99 Other

HYPERTENSIVE DISEASE (401-405)

> EXCLUDES   that complicating pregnancy, childbirth, or the puerperium (642.0-642.9)
> that involving coronary vessels (410.00-414.9)

AHA: 3Q, '90, 3; 2Q, '89, 12; S-O, '87, 9; J-A, '84, 11

√4ᵗʰ **401 Essential hypertension**
> INCLUDES   high blood pressure
> hyperpiesia
> hyperpiesis
> hypertension (arterial) (essential) (primary) (systemic)
> hypertensive vascular:
> degeneration
> disease
> EXCLUDES   elevated blood pressure without diagnosis of hypertension (796.2)
> pulmonary hypertension (416.0-416.9)
> that involving vessels of:
> brain (430-438)
> eye (362.11)

AHA: 2Q, '92, 5
DEF: Hypertension that occurs without apparent organic cause; idiopathic.

401.0 Malignant CC
CC Excl: 401.0-401.9, 402.00-402.91, 403.00-403.91, 404.00-404.93, 405.01-405.99, 459.89, 459.9
AHA: M-J, '85, 19
DEF: Severe high arterial blood pressure; results in necrosis in kidney, retina, etc.; hemorrhages occur and death commonly due to uremia or rupture of cerebral vessel.

401.1 Benign
DEF: Mildly elevated arterial blood pressure.

401.9 Unspecified
AHA: 4Q, '97, 37

√4ᵗʰ **402 Hypertensive heart disease**
> INCLUDES   hypertensive:
> cardiomegaly
> cardiopathy
> cardiovascular disease
> heart (disease) (failure)
> any condition classifiable to 428, 429.0-429.3, 429.8, 429.9 due to hypertension
▶Use additional code to specify type of heart failure (428.0, 428.20-428.23, 428.30-428.33, 428.40-428.43)◀
AHA: 2Q, '93, 9; N-D, '84, 18

√5ᵗʰ **402.0 Malignant**
402.00 Without heart failure CC
CC Excl: See code 401.0

N Newborn Age: 0   P Pediatric Age: 0-17   M Maternity Age: 12-55   A Adult Age :15-124   CC CC Condition   MC Major Complication   CD Complex Dx   HIV HIV Related Dx

116 — Volume 1 • October 2002   2002 Ingenix, Inc.

▲ 　　　　402.01　**With heart failure**　　`CC` `MC` `CD`
　　　　　　CC Excl: 398.91, 401.0-401.9, 402.00-402.91, 403.00-403.91, 404.00-404.93, 405.01-405.99, 428.0-428.9, 459.89, 459.9

✓5th　402.1　**Benign**
▲ 　　　　402.10　**Without heart failure**
▲ 　　　　402.11　**With heart failure**　　`CC` `MC` `CD`
　　　　　　CC Excl: See code 402.01

✓5th　402.9　**Unspecified**
▲ 　　　　402.90　**Without heart failure**
▲ 　　　　402.91　**With heart failure**　　`CC` `MC` `CD`
　　　　　　CC Excl: See code 402.01

　　　　　　AHA: 1Q, '93, 19; 2Q, '89, 12

　　　　　　▽ **DRG** 127

✓4th　**403　Hypertensive renal disease**
　　　INCLUDES　arteriolar nephritis
　　　　　　arteriosclerosis of:
　　　　　　　kidney
　　　　　　　renal arterioles
　　　　　　arteriosclerotic nephritis (chronic) (interstitial)
　　　　　　hypertensive:
　　　　　　　nephropathy
　　　　　　　renal failure
　　　　　　　uremia (chronic)
　　　　　　nephrosclerosis
　　　　　　renal sclerosis with hypertension
　　　　　　any condition classifiable to 585, 586, or 587
　　　　　　　　with any condition classifiable to 401
　　　EXCLUDES　*acute renal failure (584.5-584.9)*
　　　　　　renal disease stated as not due to hypertension
　　　　　　renovascular hypertension (405.0-405.9 with fifth-digit 1)

The following fifth-digit subclassification is for use with category 403:
　　　0　without mention of renal failure
　　　1　with renal failure

AHA: 4Q, '92, 22; 2Q, '92, 5

✓5th　**403.0　Malignant**　　`CC`
　　　CC Excl: 401.0-401.9, 402.00-402.91, 403.00-403.91, 404.00-404.93, 405.01-405.99, 459.89, 459.9

✓5th　**403.1　Benign**　　`CC 1`
　　　CC Excl: For code 403.11: See code 403.0

✓5th　**403.9　Unspecified**　　`CC 1`
　　　CC Excl: For code 403.91: See code 403.0

　　　AHA: For code 403.91: 2Q, '01, 11; 3Q, '91, 8

　　　▽ **DRG** 316 For code 403.91

✓4th　**404　Hypertensive heart and renal disease**
　　　INCLUDES　disease:
　　　　　　cardiorenal
　　　　　　cardiovascular renal
　　　　　　any condition classifiable to 402 with any condition classifiable to 403
　　　►Use additional code to specify type of heart failure (428.0, 428.20-428.23, 428.30-428.33, 428.40-428.43)◄

The following fifth-digit subclassification is for use with category 404:
▲　**0　without mention of heart failure or renal failure**
▲　**1　with heart failure**
　　2　with renal failure
▲　**3　with heart failure and renal failure**

AHA: 3Q, '90, 3; J-A, '84, 14

✓5th　**404.0　Malignant**　　`CC`
　　　CC Excl: See code 403.0

✓5th　**404.1　Benign**　　`CC 1-3`
　　　CC Excl: For codes 404.11-404.13: See code 403.0

✓5th　**404.9　Unspecified**　　`CC 1-3`
　　　CC Excl: For codes 404.91-404.93: See code 403.0

✓4th　**405　Secondary hypertension**
　　　AHA: 3Q, '90, 3; S-O, '87, 9, 11; J-A, '84, 14

　　　DEF: High arterial blood pressure due to or with a variety of primary diseases, such as renal disorders, CNS disorders, endocrine, and vascular diseases.

✓5th　**405.0　Malignant**
　　　　405.01　**Renovascular**　　`CC`
　　　　　CC Excl: 401.0-401.9, 402.00-402.91, 403.00-403.91, 404.00-404.93, 405.01-405.99, 459.89, 459.9
　　　　405.09　**Other**　　`CC`
　　　　　CC Excl: See code 405.01

✓5th　**405.1　Benign**
　　　　405.11　**Renovascular**
　　　　405.19　**Other**
✓5th　**405.9　Unspecified**
　　　　405.91　**Renovascular**
　　　　405.99　**Other**
　　　　　AHA: 3Q, '00, 4

ISCHEMIC HEART DISEASE (410-414)
　　　INCLUDES　that with mention of hypertension
　　　Use additional code to identify presence of hypertension (401.0-405.9)
　　　AHA: 3Q, '91, 10; J-A, '84, 5

✓4th　**410　Acute myocardial infarction**
　　　INCLUDES　cardiac infarction
　　　　　　coronary (artery):
　　　　　　　embolism
　　　　　　　occlusion
　　　　　　　rupture
　　　　　　　thrombosis
　　　　　　infarction of heart, myocardium, or ventricle
　　　　　　rupture of heart, myocardium, or ventricle
　　　　　　any condition classifiable to 414.1-414.9
　　　　　　　specified as acute or with a stated duration of 8 weeks or less

The following fifth-digit subclassification is for use with category 410:
　　　0　episode of care unspecified
　　　　Use when the source document does not contain sufficient information for the assignment of fifth digit 1 or 2.
　　　1　initial episode of care
　　　　Use fifth-digit 1 to designate the first episode of care (regardless of facility site) for a newly diagnosed myocardial infarction. The fifth-digit 1 is assigned regardless of the number of times a patient may be transferred during the initial episode of care.
　　　2　subsequent episode of care
　　　　Use fifth-digit 2 to designate an episode of care following the initial episode when the patient is admitted for further observation, evaluation or treatment for a myocardial infarction that has received initial treatment, but is still less than 8 weeks old.

AHA: 3Q, '01, 21; 3Q, '98, 15; 4Q, '97, 37; 3Q, '95, 9; 4Q, '92, 24; 1Q, '92,10; 3Q, '91, 18; 1Q, '91, 14; 3Q, '89, 3

DEF: A sudden insufficiency of blood supply to an area of the heart muscle; usually due to a coronary artery occlusion.

✓5th　**410.0　Of anterolateral wall**　　`CC 1` `A`
　　　CC Excl: For code 410.01: 410.00-410.92, 459.89, 459.9

✓4th ✓5th **Additional Digit Required**　　Nonspecific PDx　　Unacceptable PDx　　Manifestation Code　　`MSP` Medicare Secondary Payer　　►◄ Revised Text　　● New Code　　▲ Revised Code Title

2002 Ingenix, Inc.　　　　　　　　　　　　　　　　　　　　　　　**October 2002 • Volume 1 — 117**

Acute Myocardial Infarction

Anatomic Sites

Anterolateral 410.0   Other lateral 410.5

Posterobasal 410.6   Postero-lateral 410.5

Anteroseptal 410.1

Inferoposterior 410.3   Atrium only 410.8

Apical 410.1   Other and septum 410.4   Septum only / Papillary muscle

√5th **410.1 Of other anterior wall**   CC 1 A
Infarction:
anterior (wall) NOS
anteroapical } (with contiguous portion
anteroseptal } of intraventricular septum)

CC Excl: For code 410.11: See code 410.0

DRG 121 and 122 For code 410.11

√5th **410.2 Of inferolateral wall**   CC 1 A
CC Excl: For code 410.21: See code 410.0

√5th **410.3 Of inferoposterior wall**   CC 1 A
CC Excl: For code 410.31: See code 410.0

√5th **410.4 Of other inferior wall**   CC 1 A
Infarction:
diaphragmatic wall NOS } (with contiguous portion
inferior (wall) NOS } of intraventricular septum)

CC Excl: For code 410.41: See code 410.0

AHA: 1Q, '00, 7, 26; 4Q, '99, 9; 3Q, '97, 10

AHA: For code 410.41: 2Q, '01, 8, 9

DRG 121 and 122 For code 410.41

√5th **410.5 Of other lateral wall**   CC 1 A
Infarction: Infarction:
apical-lateral   high lateral
basal-lateral   posterolateral

CC Excl: For code 410.51: See code 410.0

√5th **410.6 True posterior wall infarction**   CC 1 A
Infarction: Infarction:
posterobasal   strictly posterior

CC Excl: For code 410.61: See code 410.0

√5th **410.7 Subendocardial infarction**   CC 1 A
Nontransmural infarction
CC Excl: For code 410.71: See code 410.0

AHA: 1Q, '00, 7

DRG 121 and 122 For code 410.71

√5th **410.8 Of other specified sites**   CC 1 A
Infarction of: Infarction of:
atrium   septum alone
papillary muscle

CC Excl: For code 410.81: See code 410.0

√5th **410.9 Unspecified site**   CC 1 A
Acute myocardial infarction NOS
Coronary occlusion NOS
CC Excl: For code 410.91: See code 410.0

AHA: 1Q, '96, 17; 1Q, '92, 9

DRG 121 and 122 For code 410.91

√4th **411 Other acute and subacute forms of ischemic heart disease**
AHA: 4Q, '94, 55; 3Q, '91, 24

411.0 Postmyocardial infarction syndrome CC MC CD A
Dressler's syndrome
CC Excl: 411.0, 411.81, 411.89, 459.89, 459.9

DEF: Complication developing several days/weeks after myocardial infarction; symptoms include fever, leukocytosis, chest pain, evidence of pericarditis, pleurisy, and pneumonitis; tendency to recur.

411.1 Intermediate coronary syndrome CC CD A
Impending infarction   Preinfarction syndrome
Preinfarction angina   Unstable angina
EXCLUDES   angina (pectoris) (413.9)
decubitus (413.0)

CC Excl: 410.00-410.92, 411.1-411.89, 413.0-413.9, 414.8-414.9, 459.89, 459.9

AHA: 3Q, '01, 15; 2Q, '01, 7, 9; 4Q, '98, 86; 2Q, '96, 10; 3Q, '91, 24; 1Q, '91, 14; 3Q, '90, 6; 4Q, '89, 10

DRG 140

DEF: A condition representing an intermediate stage between angina of effort and acute myocardial infarction. It is often documented by the physician as "unstable angina."

√5th **411.8 Other**
AHA: 3Q, '91, 18; 3Q, '89, 4

411.81 Acute coronary occlusion without myocardial infarction CC CD A
Acute coronary (artery):
embolism } without or not
obstruction } resulting in
occlusion } myocardial
thrombosis } infarction

EXCLUDES   obstruction without infarction due to atherosclerosis ▶(414.00-414.06)◄
occlusion without infarction due to atherosclerosis ▶(414.00-414.06)◄

CC Excl: 410.00-410.92, 411.0-411.89, 413.0-413.9, 414.8-414.9, 459.89, 459.9

AHA: 3Q, '91, 24; 1Q, '91, 14

DEF: Interrupted blood flow to a portion of the heart; without tissue death.

411.89 Other CC CD A
Coronary insufficiency (acute)
Subendocardial ischemia
CC Excl: See code 411.81

AHA: 3Q, '01, 14; 1Q, '92, 9

DRG 140

412 Old myocardial infarction A
Healed myocardial infarction
Past myocardial infarction diagnosed on ECG [EKG] or other special investigation, but currently presenting no symptoms
AHA: 2Q, '01, 9; 3Q, '98, 15; 2Q, '91, 22; 3Q, '90, 7

√4th **413 Angina pectoris**
DEF: Severe constricting pain in the chest, often radiating from the precordium to the left shoulder and down the arm, due to ischemia of the heart muscle; usually caused by coronary disease; pain is often precipitated by effort or excitement.

413.0 Angina decubitus CC A
Nocturnal angina
CC Excl: 410.00-410.92, 411.1-411.89, 413.0-413.9, 414.8-414.9, 459.89, 459.9
DEF: Angina occurring only in the recumbent position.

N Newborn Age: 0   P Pediatric Age: 0-17   M Maternity Age: 12-55   A Adult Age :15-124   CC CC Condition   MC Major Complication   CD Complex Dx   HIV HIV Related Dx

2002 Ingenix, Inc.

413.1　Prinzmetal angina　　CC　A
　　　Variant angina pectoris
　　CC Excl: See code 413.0

　　DEF Angina occurring when patient is recumbent; associated with ST-segment elevations.

413.9　Other and unspecified angina pectoris　　CC　A

Angina:	Anginal syndrome
NOS	Status anginosus
cardiac	Stenocardia
of effort	Syncope anginosa

　　EXCLUDES　*preinfarction angina (411.1)*

　　CC Excl: See code 413.0

　　AHA: 3Q, '91, 16; 3Q, '90, 6

　　▽ DRG 140

✓4ᵗʰ **414　Other forms of chronic ischemic heart disease**
　　EXCLUDES　*arteriosclerotic cardiovascular disease [ASCVD] (429.2)*
　　　　cardiovascular:
　　　　　arteriosclerosis or sclerosis (429.2)
　　　　　degeneration or disease (429.2)

✓5ᵗʰ **414.0　Coronary atherosclerosis**
　　　Arteriosclerotic heart disease [ASHD]
　　　Atherosclerotic heart disease
　　　Coronary (artery):
　　　　arteriosclerosis
　　　　arteritis or endarteritis
　　　　atheroma
　　　　sclerosis
　　　　stricture
　　EXCLUDES　*embolism of graft (996.72)*
　　　　occlusion NOS of graft (996.72)
　　　　thrombus of graft (996.72)

　　AHA: 2Q, '97, 13; 2Q, '95, 17; 4Q, '94, 49; 2Q, '94, 13; 1Q, '94, 6; 3Q, '90, 7

　　DEF: A chronic condition marked by thickening and loss of elasticity of the coronary artery; caused by deposits of plaque containing cholesterol, lipoid material and lipophages.

　　414.00　Of unspecified type of vessel, native or graft　　A
　　　　AHA: 3Q, '01, 15; 4Q, '99, 4; 3Q, '97, 15; 4Q, '96, 31
　　　　▽ DRG 132

　　414.01　Of native coronary artery　　A
　　　　AHA: 3Q, '01, 15; 2Q, '01, 8, 9; 3Q, '97, 15; 2Q, '96, 10; 4Q, '96, 31
　　　　▽ DRG 132
　　　　DEF: Plaque deposits in natural heart vessels.

　　414.02　Of autologous vein bypass graft　　A
　　　　DEF: Plaque deposit in grafted vein originating within patient.

　　414.03　Of nonautologous biological bypass graft　　A
　　　　DEF: Plaque deposits in grafted vessel originating outside patient.

　　414.04　Of artery bypass graft　　A
　　　　Internal mammary artery
　　　　AHA: 4Q, '96, 31
　　　　DEF: Plaque deposits in grafted artery originating within patient.

　　414.05　Of unspecified type of bypass graft　　A
　　　　Bypass graft NOS
　　　　AHA: 3Q, '97, 15; 4Q, '96, 31

● 　**414.06　Of coronary artery of transplanted heart**

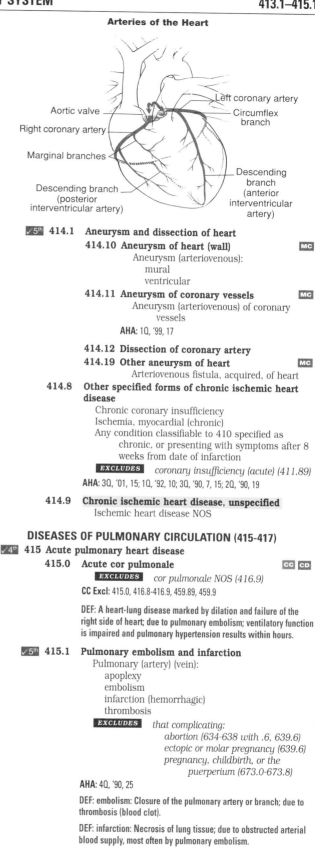

Arteries of the Heart

▲ ✓5ᵗʰ **414.1　Aneurysm and dissection of heart**
▲ 　　**414.10　Aneurysm of heart (wall)**　　MC
　　　　Aneurysm (arteriovenous):
　　　　　mural
　　　　　ventricular

▲ 　　**414.11　Aneurysm of coronary vessels**　　MC
　　　　Aneurysm (arteriovenous) of coronary vessels
　　　　AHA: 1Q, '99, 17

● 　　**414.12　Dissection of coronary artery**
▲ 　　**414.19　Other aneurysm of heart**　　MC
　　　　Arteriovenous fistula, acquired, of heart

　　414.8　Other specified forms of chronic ischemic heart disease
　　　Chronic coronary insufficiency
　　　Ischemia, myocardial (chronic)
　　　Any condition classifiable to 410 specified as chronic, or presenting with symptoms after 8 weeks from date of infarction
　　EXCLUDES　*coronary insufficiency (acute) (411.89)*
　　AHA: 3Q, '01, 15; 1Q, '92, 10; 3Q, '90, 7, 15; 2Q, '90, 19

　　414.9　Chronic ischemic heart disease, unspecified
　　　Ischemic heart disease NOS

DISEASES OF PULMONARY CIRCULATION (415-417)

✓4ᵗʰ **415　Acute pulmonary heart disease**
　　415.0　Acute cor pulmonale　　CC　CD
　　EXCLUDES　*cor pulmonale NOS (416.9)*
　　CC Excl: 415.0, 416.8-416.9, 459.89, 459.9

　　DEF: A heart-lung disease marked by dilation and failure of the right side of heart; due to pulmonary embolism; ventilatory function is impaired and pulmonary hypertension results within hours.

✓5ᵗʰ **415.1　Pulmonary embolism and infarction**
　　　Pulmonary (artery) (vein):
　　　　apoplexy
　　　　embolism
　　　　infarction (hemorrhagic)
　　　　thrombosis
　　EXCLUDES　*that complicating:*
　　　　abortion (634-638 with .6, 639.6)
　　　　ectopic or molar pregnancy (639.6)
　　　　pregnancy, childbirth, or the puerperium (673.0-673.8)

　　AHA: 4Q, '90, 25

　　DEF: embolism: Closure of the pulmonary artery or branch; due to thrombosis (blood clot).

　　DEF: infarction: Necrosis of lung tissue; due to obstructed arterial blood supply, most often by pulmonary embolism.

　　415.11　Iatrogenic pulmonary embolism　　CC　MC　CD
　　　　and infarction
　　　　CC Excl: 415.11, 415.19, 459.89, 459.9
　　　　AHA: 4Q, '95, 58

✓4ᵗʰ／✓5ᵗʰ Additional Digit Required　　Nonspecific PDx　　Unacceptable PDx　　Manifestation Code　　MSP Medicare Secondary Payer　　◀▶ Revised Text　　● New Code　　▲ Revised Code Title

2002 Ingenix, Inc.　　　　　　　　**October 2002 • Volume 1 — 119**

Circulatory System 415.19–421.0

415.19 Other   CC MC CD
     CC Excl: 415.11, 415.19, 459.89, 459.9

√4ᵗʰ **416 Chronic pulmonary heart disease**

416.0 Primary pulmonary hypertension   CC MC
     Idiopathic pulmonary arteriosclerosis
     Pulmonary hypertension (essential) (idiopathic)
     (primary)
     CC Excl: 416.0, 416.8-416.9, 417.8-417.9, 459.89, 459.9

     DEF: A rare increase in pulmonary circulation, often resulting in right ventricular failure or fatal syncope.

416.1 Kyphoscoliotic heart disease
     DEF: High blood pressure within the lungs as a result of curvature of the spine.

416.8 Other chronic pulmonary heart diseases
     Pulmonary hypertension, secondary

416.9 Chronic pulmonary heart disease, unspecified
     Chronic cardiopulmonary disease
     Cor pulmonale (chronic) NOS

√4ᵗʰ **417 Other diseases of pulmonary circulation**

417.0 Arteriovenous fistula of pulmonary vessels
     EXCLUDES   *congenital arteriovenous fistula (747.3)*
     DEF: Abnormal communication between blood vessels within lung.

417.1 Aneurysm of pulmonary artery
     EXCLUDES   *congenital aneurysm (747.3)*

417.8 Other specified diseases of pulmonary circulation
     Pulmonary: Pulmonary:
     arteritis   endarteritis
     Rupture
     Stricture } of pulmonary vessel

417.9 Unspecified disease of pulmonary circulation

OTHER FORMS OF HEART DISEASE (420-429)

√4ᵗʰ **420 Acute pericarditis**
     INCLUDES   acute:
         mediastinopericarditis
         myopericarditis
         pericardial effusion
         pleuropericarditis
         pneumopericarditis
     EXCLUDES   *acute rheumatic pericarditis (391.0)*
         postmyocardial infarction syndrome [Dressler's]
         (411.0)

     DEF: Inflammation of the pericardium (heart sac); pericardial friction rub results from this inflammation and is heard as a scratchy or leathery sound.

420.0 *Acute pericarditis in diseases classified elsewhere*   CC CD
     Code first underlying disease, as:
         actinomycosis (039.8)
         amebiasis (006.8)
         nocardiosis (039.8)
         tuberculosis (017.9)
         uremia (585)
     EXCLUDES   *pericarditis (acute) (in):*
         Coxsackie (virus) (074.21)
         gonococcal (098.83)
         histoplasmosis (115.0-115.9 with
           fifth-digit 3)
         meningococcal infection (036.41)
         syphilitic (093.81)
     CC Excl: 391.0, 393, 420.0-420.99, 423.8-423.9, 459.89, 459.9

Anatomy

Blood Flow

√5ᵗʰ **420.9 Other and unspecified acute pericarditis**

420.90 Acute pericarditis, unspecified   CC CD
     Pericarditis (acute):   Pericarditis (acute):
     NOS   sicca
     infective NOS
     CC Excl: See code 420.0
     AHA: 2Q, '89, 12

420.91 Acute idiopathic pericarditis   CC CD
     Pericarditis, acute: Pericarditis, acute:
     benign   viral
     nonspecific
     CC Excl: See code 420.0

420.99 Other   CC CD
     Pericarditis (acute):   Pericarditis (acute):
     pneumococcal   suppurative
     purulent   Pneumopyopericardium
     staphylococcal   Pyopericardium
     streptococcal
     EXCLUDES   *pericarditis in diseases*
         classified elsewhere
         (420.0)
     CC Excl: See code 420.0

√4ᵗʰ **421 Acute and subacute endocarditis**
     DEF: Bacterial inflammation of the endocardium (intracardiac area); major symptoms include fever, fatigue, heart murmurs, splenomegaly, embolic episodes and areas of infarction.

421.0 Acute and subacute bacterial endocarditis   CC CD HIV
     Endocarditis (acute)   Endocarditis (acute)
     (chronic) (subacute):   (chronic) (subacute):
     bacterial   ulcerative
     infective NOS   vegetative
     lenta   Infective aneurysm
     malignant   Subacute bacterial
     purulent   endocarditis [SBE]
     septic
     Use additional code to identify infectious organism
         [e.g., Streptococcus 041.0, Staphylococcus 041.1]
     CC Excl: 391.1, 397.9, 421.0-421.9, 424.90-424.99, 459.89, 459.9
     AHA: 1Q, '99, 12; 1Q, '91, 15

N Newborn Age: 0   P Pediatric Age: 0-17   M Maternity Age: 12-55   A Adult Age :15-124   CC CC Condition   MC Major Complication   CD Complex Dx   HIV HIV Related Dx

120 — Volume 1   *2002 Ingenix, Inc.*

421.1   *Acute and subacute infective endocarditis* `CC` `CD`
in diseases classified elsewhere
     Code first underlying disease, as:
       blastomycosis (116.0)
       Q fever (083.0)
       typhoid (fever) (002.0)
      EXCLUDES   *endocarditis (in):*
          Coxsackie (virus) (074.22)
          gonococcal (098.84)
          histoplasmosis (115.0-115.9 with
            fifth-digit 4)
          meningococcal infection (036.42)
          monilial (112.81)
    CC Excl: See code 421.0

421.9   **Acute endocarditis, unspecified** `CC` `CD` `HIV`
     Endocarditis
     Myoendocarditis } acute or subacute
     Periendocarditis
      EXCLUDES   *acute rheumatic endocarditis (391.1)*
    CC Excl: See code 421.0

`✓4ᵗʰ` **422 Acute myocarditis**
      EXCLUDES   *acute rheumatic myocarditis (391.2)*
    DEF: Acute inflammation of the muscular walls of the heart (myocardium).

422.0   *Acute myocarditis in diseases classified* `CC` `CD`
elsewhere
     Code first underlying disease, as:
       myocarditis (acute):
         influenzal (487.8)
         tuberculous (017.9)
      EXCLUDES   *myocarditis (acute) (due to):*
          aseptic, of newborn (074.23)
          Coxsackie (virus) (074.23)
          diphtheritic (032.82)
          meningococcal infection (036.43)
          syphilitic (093.82)
          toxoplasmosis (130.3)
    CC Excl: 391.2, 398.0, 422.0-422.99, 429.0, 429.71, 429.79, 459.89, 459.9

`✓5ᵗʰ` **422.9**   **Other and unspecified acute myocarditis**
    422.90 Acute myocarditis, unspecified `CC` `CD` `HIV`
       Acute or subacute (interstitial) myocarditis
      CC Excl: See code 422.0

    422.91 Idiopathic myocarditis `CC` `CD` `HIV`
       Myocarditis (acute or subacute):
         Fiedler's
         giant cell
         isolated (diffuse) (granulomatous)
         nonspecific granulomatous
      CC Excl: See code 422.0

    422.92 Septic myocarditis `CC` `CD` `HIV`
       Myocarditis, acute or subacute:
         pneumococcal
         staphylococcal
       Use additional code to identify infectious
         organism [e.g., Staphylococcus 041.1]
       EXCLUDES   *myocarditis, acute or*
          subacute:
          in bacterial diseases
            classified elsewhere
            (422.0)
          streptococcal (391.2)
      CC Excl: See code 422.0

    422.93 Toxic myocarditis `CC` `CD` `HIV`
      CC Excl: See code 422.0
      DEF: Inflammation of the heart muscle due to an adverse
      reaction to certain drugs or chemicals reaching the heart
      through the bloodstream.

    422.99 Other `CC` `CD` `HIV`
      CC Excl: See code 422.0

`✓4ᵗʰ` **423 Other diseases of pericardium**
      EXCLUDES   *that specified as rheumatic (393)*

423.0   **Hemopericardium** `CC` `CD`
    CC Excl: 423.0-423.9, 459.89, 459.9
    DEF: Blood in the pericardial sac (pericardium).

423.1   **Adhesive pericarditis** `CC`
     Adherent pericardium   Pericarditis:
     Fibrosis of pericardium   adhesive
     Milk spots   obliterative
                   Soldiers' patches
    CC Excl: See code 423.0
    DEF: Two layers of serous pericardium adhere to each other by
    fibrous adhesions.

423.2   **Constrictive pericarditis** `CC`
     Concato's disease   Pick's disease of heart (and liver)
    CC Excl: See code 423.0
    DEF: Inflammation identified by a rigid, thickened and sometimes
    calcified pericardium; ventricles of the heart cannot be adequately
    filled and congestive heart failure may result.

423.8   **Other specified diseases of pericardium**
     Calcification } of pericardium
     Fistula
    AHA: 2Q, '89, 12

423.9   **Unspecified disease of pericardium**

`✓4ᵗʰ` **424 Other diseases of endocardium**
      EXCLUDES   *bacterial endocarditis (421.0-421.9)*
          rheumatic endocarditis (391.1, 394.0-397.9)
          syphilitic endocarditis (093.20-093.24)

424.0   **Mitral valve disorders** `CC`
     Mitral (valve):
       incompetence } NOS of specified cause,
       insufficiency   except rheumatic
       regurgitation
      EXCLUDES   *mitral (valve):*
          disease (394.9)
          failure (394.9)
          stenosis (394.0)
          the listed conditions:
          specified as rheumatic (394.1)
          unspecified as to cause but with
            mention of:
            diseases of aortic valve (396.0-
             396.9)
            mitral stenosis or obstruction
             (394.2)
    CC Excl: 394.0-394.9, 396.0-396.9, 424.0, 459.89, 459.9
    AHA: 2Q, '00, 16; 3Q, '98, 11; N-D, '87, 8; N-D, '84, 8

424.1   **Aortic valve disorders** `CC`
     Aortic (valve):
       incompetence } NOS of specified
       insufficiency   cause, except
       regurgitation   rheumatic
       stenosis
      EXCLUDES   *hypertrophic subaortic stenosis (425.1)*
          that specified as rheumatic (395.0-
            395.9)
          that of unspecified cause but with
            mention of diseases of mitral
            valve (396.0-396.9)
    CC Excl: 395.0-395.9, 396.0-396.9, 424.1, 459.89, 459.9
    AHA: 4Q, '88, 8; N-D, '87, 8

`✓4ᵗʰ` `✓5ᵗʰ` Additional Digit Required   Nonspecific PDx   Unacceptable PDx   Manifestation Code   `MSP` Medicare Secondary Payer   ▶◀ Revised Text   ● New Code   ▲ Revised Code Title

2002 Ingenix, Inc.   **Volume 1 — 121**

Circulatory System 424.2–425.9

424.2 Tricuspid valve disorders, specified as nonrheumatic `CC`

Tricuspid valve:

incompetence
insufficiency ⎫ of specified cause,
regurgitation ⎬ except
stenosis ⎭ rheumatic

> **EXCLUDES** *rheumatic or of unspecified cause (397.0)*

CC Excl: 397.0, 424.2, 459.89, 459.9

424.3 Pulmonary valve disorders `CC`

Pulmonic: Pulmonic:
incompetence NOS   regurgitation NOS
insufficiency NOS   stenosis NOS

> **EXCLUDES** *that specified as rheumatic (397.1)*

CC Excl: 397.1, 424.3, 459.89, 459.9

√5th **424.9 Endocarditis, valve unspecified**

424.90 Endocarditis, valve unspecified, unspecified cause `CC` `CD`

Endocarditis (chronic):
    NOS
    nonbacterial thrombotic
Valvular:

incompetence ⎫ of unspecified
insufficiency ⎬ valve,
regurgitation ⎬ unspecified
stenosis ⎭ cause

Valvulitis (chronic)

CC Excl: 424.90-424.99, 459.89, 459.9

424.91 Endocarditis in diseases classified elsewhere `CC` `CD`

Code first underlying disease as:
atypical verrucous endocarditis [Libman-Sacks] (710.0)
disseminated lupus erythematosus (710.0)
tuberculosis (017.9)

> **EXCLUDES** *syphilitic (093.20-093.24)*

CC Excl: See code 424.90

424.99 Other `CC`

Any condition classifiable to 424.90 with specified cause, except rheumatic

> **EXCLUDES** *endocardial fibroelastosis (425.3)*
> *that specified as rheumatic (397.9)*

CC Excl: See code 424.90

√4th **425 Cardiomyopathy**

> **INCLUDES** myocardiopathy

AHA: J-A, '85, 15

425.0 Endomyocardial fibrosis `CC`

CC Excl: 425.0-425.9, 459.89, 459.9

Heart Valve Disorders

Valve stenosis (trouble opening)

Incompetent valve (trouble closing)

causes regurgitation (backflow of blood)

Insuficient valve (unable to close completely)

Shortened, fused chorda tendinae

Ventricular hypertrophy

Normal Heart Valve Function

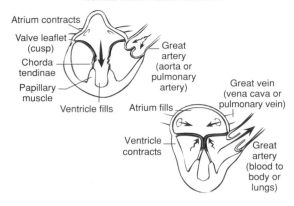

Atrium contracts
Valve leaflet (cusp)
Chorda tendinae
Papillary muscle
Ventricle fills
Great artery (aorta or pulmonary artery)
Atrium fills
Great vein (vena cava or pulmonary vein)
Ventricle contracts
Great artery (blood to body or lungs)

425.1 Hypertrophic obstructive cardiomyopathy `CC`

Hypertrophic subaortic stenosis (idiopathic)

CC Excl: See code 425.0

DEF: Cardiomyopathy marked by left ventricle hypertrophy, enlarged septum; results in obstructed blood flow.

425.2 Obscure cardiomyopathy of Africa `CC` `CD`

Becker's disease
Idiopathic mural endomyocardial disease

CC Excl: See code 425.0

425.3 Endocardial fibroelastosis `CC` `CD`

Elastomyofibrosis

CC Excl: See code 425.0

DEF: A condition marked by left ventricle hypertrophy and conversion of the endocardium into a thick fibroelastic coat; capacity of the ventricle may be reduced, but is often increased.

425.4 Other primary cardiomyopathies `CC` `CD`

Cardiomyopathy: Cardiomyopathy:
   NOS   idiopathic
   congestive   nonobstructive
   constrictive   obstructive
   familial   restrictive
   hypertrophic   Cardiovascular collagenosis

CC Excl: See code 425.0

AHA: 1Q, '00, 22; 4Q, '97, 55; 2Q, '90, 19

425.5 Alcoholic cardiomyopathy `CC` `CD`

CC Excl: See code 425.0

AHA: S-O, '85, 15

DEF: Heart disease as result of excess alcohol consumption.

425.7 Nutritional and metabolic cardiomyopathy `CC` `CD`

Code first underlying disease, as:
amyloidosis (277.3)
beriberi (265.0)
cardiac glycogenosis (271.0)
mucopolysaccharidosis (277.5)
thyrotoxicosis (242.0-242.9)

> **EXCLUDES** *gouty tophi of heart (274.82)*

CC Excl: See code 425.0

425.8 Cardiomyopathy in other diseases classified elsewhere `CC` `CD`

Code first underlying disease, as:
Friedreich's ataxia (334.0)
myotonia atrophica (359.2)
progressive muscular dystrophy (359.1)
sarcoidosis (135)

> **EXCLUDES** *cardiomyopathy in Chagas' disease (086.0)*

CC Excl: See code 425.0

AHA: 2Q, '93, 9

425.9 Secondary cardiomyopathy, unspecified `CC` `CD`

CC Excl: See code 425.0

N Newborn Age: 0   P Pediatric Age: 0-17   M Maternity Age: 12-55   A Adult Age :15-124   CC CC Condition   MC Major Complication   CD Complex Dx   HIV HIV Related Dx

Nerve Conduction of the Heart

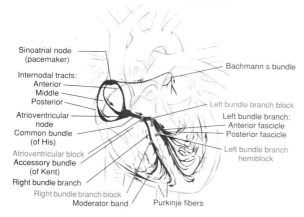

Sinoatrial node (pacemaker)
Bachmann s bundle
Internodal tracts:
  Anterior
  Middle
  Posterior
Atrioventricular node
Left bundle branch block
Left bundle branch:
  Anterior fascicle
  Posterior fascicle
Common bundle (of His)
Left bundle branch hemiblock
Atrioventricular block
Accessory bundle (of Kent)
Right bundle branch
Right bundle branch block
Moderator band
Purkinje fibers

✓4th **426 Conduction disorders**

DEF: Disruption or disturbance in the electrical impulses that regulate heartbeats.

426.0 Atrioventricular block, complete `CC` `MC`
    Third degree atrioventricular block
    CC Excl: 426.0-426.9, 427.0-427.5, 427.89, 459.89, 459.9

✓5th **426.1 Atrioventricular block, other and unspecified**
    426.10 Atrioventricular block, unspecified `MC`
        Atrioventricular [AV] block (incomplete) (partial)
    426.11 First degree atrioventricular block
        Incomplete atrioventricular block, first degree
        Prolonged P-R interval NOS
    426.12 Mobitz (type) II atrioventricular block `CC` `MC`
        Incomplete atrioventricular block:
            Mobitz (type) II
            second degree, Mobitz (type) II
        CC Excl: See code 426.0
        DEF: Impaired conduction of excitatory impulse from cardiac atrium to ventricle through AV node.
    426.13 Other second degree atrioventricular block `CC` `MC`
        Incomplete atrioventricular block:
            Mobitz (type) I [Wenckebach's]
            second degree:
                NOS
                Mobitz (type) I
                with 2:1 atrioventricular response [block]
            Wenckebach's phenomenon
        CC Excl: See code 426.0
        DEF: Wenckebach's phenomenon: impulses generated at constant rate to sinus node, P-R interval lengthens; results in cycle of ventricular inadequacy and shortened P-R interval; second-degree A-V block commonly called "Mobitz type 1."

    426.2 Left bundle branch hemiblock
        Block:
            left anterior fascicular
            left posterior fascicular
    426.3 Other left bundle branch block `MC`
        Left bundle branch block:
            NOS
            anterior fascicular with posterior fascicular
            complete
            main stem
    426.4 Right bundle branch block
        AHA: 3Q, '00, 3
✓5th **426.5 Bundle branch block, other and unspecified**
    426.50 Bundle branch block, unspecified
    426.51 Right bundle branch block and left posterior fascicular block `MC`

    426.52 Right bundle branch block and left anterior fascicular block `MC`
    426.53 Other bilateral bundle branch block `CC` `MC`
        Bifascicular block NOS
        Bilateral bundle branch block NOS
        Right bundle branch with left bundle branch block (incomplete) (main stem)
        CC Excl: See code 426.0
    426.54 Trifascicular block `CC` `MC`
        CC Excl: See code 426.0

    426.6 Other heart block `CC`
        Intraventricular block: Sinoatrial block
            NOS   Sinoauricular block
            diffuse
            myofibrillar
        CC Excl: See code 426.0
    426.7 Anomalous atrioventricular excitation `CC`
        Atrioventricular conduction:
            accelerated
            accessory
            pre-excitation
        Ventricular pre-excitation
        Wolff-Parkinson-White syndrome
        CC Excl: See code 426.0
        DEF: Wolff-Parkinson-White: normal conduction pathway is bypassed; results in short P-R interval on EKG; tendency to supraventricular tachycardia.
✓5th **426.8 Other specified conduction disorders**
    426.81 Lown-Ganong-Levine syndrome `CC`
        Syndrome of short P-R interval, normal QRS complexes, and supraventricular tachycardias
        CC Excl: See code 426.0
    426.89 Other `CC`
        Dissociation:
            atrioventricular [AV]
            interference
            isorhythmic
        Nonparoxysmal AV nodal tachycardia
        CC Excl: See code 426.0
    426.9 Conduction disorder, unspecified `CC`
        Heart block NOS   Stokes-Adams syndrome
        CC Excl: See code 426.0

✓4th **427 Cardiac dysrhythmias**
    EXCLUDES *that complicating:*
        abortion (634-638 with .7, 639.8)
        ectopic or molar pregnancy (639.8)
        labor or delivery (668.1, 669.4)
    AHA: J-A, '85, 15
    DEF: Disruption or disturbance in the rhythm of heartbeats.
    427.0 Paroxysmal supraventricular tachycardia `CC` `MC`
        Paroxysmal tachycardia: Paroxysmal tachycardia:
            atrial [PAT]   junctional
            atrioventricular [AV]   nodal
        CC Excl: See code 426.0
        `DRG` 138
        DEF: Rapid atrial rhythm.
    427.1 Paroxysmal ventricular tachycardia `CC` `MC` `CD`
        Ventricular tachycardia (paroxysmal)
        CC Excl: See code 426.0
        AHA: 3Q, '95, 9; M-A, '86, 11
        `DRG` 138
        DEF: Rapid ventricular rhythm.
    427.2 Paroxysmal tachycardia, unspecified `CC` `MC`
        Bouveret-Hoffmann syndrome
        Paroxysmal tachycardia:
            essential
            NOS
        CC Excl: See code 426.0

✓4th ✓5th Additional Digit Required   Nonspecific PDx   Unacceptable PDx   Manifestation Code   `MSP` Medicare Secondary Payer   ▶◀ Revised Text   ● New Code   ▲ Revised Code Title

2002 Ingenix, Inc.

Volume 1 — 123

Circulatory System 427.3–428.9

√5ᵗʰ 427.3 Atrial fibrillation and flutter

427.31 Atrial fibrillation `CC` `MC`

    CC Excl: See code 426.0

    AHA: 2Q, '99, 17; 3Q, '95, 8

    🔻 **DRG** 138

    DEF: Irregular, rapid atrial contractions.

427.32 Atrial flutter `CC` `MC`

    CC Excl: See code 426.0

    🔻 **DRG** 138

    DEF: Regular, rapid atrial contractions.

√5ᵗʰ 427.4 Ventricular fibrillation and flutter

427.41 Ventricular fibrillation `CC` `MC`

    CC Excl: See code 426.0

    DEF: Irregular, rapid ventricular contractions.

427.42 Ventricular flutter `CC` `MC`

    CC Excl: See code 426.0

    DEF: Regular, rapid, ventricular contractions.

427.5 Cardiac arrest `CC` `MC` `CD`

    Cardiorespiratory arrest

    CC Excl: 427.0-427.5, 459.89, 459.9

    AHA: 2Q, '00, 12; 3Q, '95, 8; 2Q, '88, 8

√5ᵗʰ 427.6 Premature beats

427.60 Premature beats, unspecified

    Ectopic beats   Premature contractions

    Extrasystoles   or systoles NOS

    Extrasystolic arrhythmia

427.61 Supraventricular premature beats

    Atrial premature beats, contractions, or

        systoles

427.69 Other

    Ventricular premature beats, contractions,

        or systoles

    AHA: 4Q, '93, 42

√5ᵗʰ 427.8 Other specified cardiac dysrhythmias

427.81 Sinoatrial node dysfunction

    Sinus bradycardia: Syndrome:

       persistent   sick sinus

       severe   tachycardia-

                         bradycardia

    EXCLUDES   *sinus bradycardia NOS*

                 (427.89)

    AHA: 3Q, '00, 8

    DEF: Complex cardiac arrhythmia; appears as severe sinus bradycardia, sinus bradycardia with tachycardia, or sinus bradycardia with atrioventricular block.

427.89 Other

    Rhythm disorder: Rhythm disorder:

       coronary sinus   nodal

       ectopic   Wandering (atrial)

                       pacemaker

    EXCLUDES   *carotid sinus syncope (337.0)*

                 ►*neonatal bradycardia*

                      (779.81)◄

                 ►*neonatal tachycardia*

                      (779.82)◄

                 reflex bradycardia (337.0)

                 tachycardia NOS (785.0)

    🔻 **DRG** 138

427.9 Cardiac dysrhythmia, unspecified

    Arrhythmia (cardiac) NOS

    AHA: 2Q, '89, 10

√4ᵗʰ 428 Heart failure

    EXCLUDES   *following cardiac surgery (429.4)*

                 rheumatic (398.91)

                 that complicating:

                    abortion (634-638 with .7, 639.8)

                    ectopic or molar pregnancy (639.8)

                    labor or delivery (668.1, 669.4)

    ►Code, if applicable, heart failure due to hypertension first (402.0-402.9, with fifth-digit 1 or 404.0-404.9 with fifth-digit 1 or 3)◄

    AHA: 3Q, '98, 5; 2Q, '90, 16; 2Q, '90, 19; 2Q, '89, 10; 3Q, '88, 3

428.0 Congestive heart failure, unspecified `CC` `MC` `CD`

    Congestive heart disease

    Right heart failure (secondary to left heart failure)

    EXCLUDES   ►*fluid overload NOS (276.6)*◄

    CC Excl: 398.91, 402.01, 402.11, 402.91, 428.0-428.9, 459.89, 459.9, 518.4

    AHA: 2Q, '01, 13; 4Q, '00, 48; 2Q, '00, 16; 1Q, '00, 22; 4Q, '99, 4; 1Q, '99, 11; 4Q, '97, 55; 3Q, '97, 10; 3Q, '96, 9; 3Q, '91, 18; 3Q, '91, 19; 2Q, '89, 12

    🔻 **DRG** 121 and127

    DEF: Mechanical inadequacy; caused by inability of heart to pump and circulate blood; results in fluid collection in lungs, hypertension, congestion and edema of tissue.

428.1 Left heart failure `CC` `MC` `CD`

    Acute edema of lung   ⎫   with heart disease

    Acute pulmonary   ⎬   NOS or heart

       edema   ⎭   failure

    Cardiac asthma   Left ventricular failure

    CC Excl: See code 428.0

    DEF: Mechanical inadequacy of left ventricle; causing fluid in lungs.

√5ᵗʰ 428.2 Systolic heart failure

    EXCLUDES   *combined systolic and diastolic heart*

                       failure (428.40-428.43)

428.20 Unspecified `CC`

    CC Excl: See code 428.0

428.21 Acute `CC`

    CC Excl: See code 428.0

428.22 Chronic `CC`

    CC Excl: See code 428.0

428.23 Acute on chronic `CC`

    CC Excl: See code 428.0

√5ᵗʰ 428.3 Diastolic heart failure `CC`

    EXCLUDES   *combined systolic and diastolic heart*

                       failure (428.40-428.43)

428.30 Unspecified `CC`

    CC Excl: See code 428.0

428.31 Acute `CC`

    CC Excl: See code 428.0

428.32 Chronic `CC`

    CC Excl: See code 428.0

428.33 Acute on chronic `CC`

    CC Excl: See code 428.0

√5ᵗʰ 428.4 Combined systolic and diastolic heart failure

428.40 Unspecified `CC`

    CC Excl: See code 428.0

428.41 Acute `CC`

    CC Excl: See code 428.0

428.42 Chronic `CC`

    CC Excl: See code 428.0

428.43 Acute on chronic `CC`

    CC Excl: See code 428.0

428.9 Heart failure, unspecified `CC` `MC` `CD`

    Cardiac failure NOS   Myocardial failure NOS

    Heart failure NOS   Weak heart

    CC Excl: See code 428.0

    AHA: 2Q, '89, 10; N-D, '85, 14

`N` Newborn Age: 0   `P` Pediatric Age: 0-17   `M` Maternity Age: 12-55   `A` Adult Age :15-124   `CC` CC Condition   `MC` Major Complication   `CD` Complex Dx   `HIV` HIV Related Dx

✓4th 429 Ill-defined descriptions and complications of heart disease

429.0 Myocarditis, unspecified

Myocarditis:
NOS
chronic (interstitial)
fibroid
senile
} (with mention of arteriosclerosis)

Use additional code to identify presence of arteriosclerosis

EXCLUDES   acute or subacute (422.0-422.9)
rheumatic (398.0)
acute (391.2)
that due to hypertension (402.0-402.9)

429.1 Myocardial degeneration

Degeneration of heart or myocardium:
fatty
mural
muscular
Myocardial:
degeneration
disease
} (with mention of arteriosclerosis)

Use additional code to identify presence of arteriosclerosis

EXCLUDES   that due to hypertension (402.0-402.9)

429.2 Cardiovascular disease, unspecified [A]

Arteriosclerotic cardiovascular disease [ASCVD]
Cardiovascular arteriosclerosis
Cardiovascular:
degeneration
disease
sclerosis
} (with mention of arteriosclerosis)

Use additional code to identify presence of arteriosclerosis

EXCLUDES   that due to hypertension (402.0-402.9)

429.3 Cardiomegaly

Cardiac: Ventricular dilatation
dilatation
hypertrophy
EXCLUDES   that due to hypertension (402.0-402.9)

429.4 Functional disturbances following cardiac surgery [CC] [CD]

Cardiac insufficiency
Heart failure
} following cardiac surgery or due to prosthesis

Postcardiotomy syndrome
Postvalvulotomy syndrome
EXCLUDES   cardiac failure in the immediate postoperative period (997.1)
CC Excl: 429.4, 429.71, 429.79, 459.89, 459.9
AHA: N-D, '85, 6

429.5 Rupture of chordae tendineae [CC] [MC] [CD]
CC Excl: 429.5, 429.71, 429.79, 459.89, 459.9
DEF: Torn tissue, between heart valves and papillary muscles.

429.6 Rupture of papillary muscle [CC] [MC] [CD]
CC Excl: 429.6, 429.71, 429.79, 429.81, 459.89, 459.9
DEF: Torn muscle, between chordae tendineae and heart wall.

✓5th 429.7 Certain sequelae of myocardial infarction, not elsewhere classified

Use additional code to identify the associated myocardial infarction:
with onset of 8 weeks or less (410.00-410.92)
with onset of more than 8 weeks (414.8)
EXCLUDES   congenital defects of heart (745, 746)
coronary aneurysm (414.11)
disorders of papillary muscle (429.6, 429.81)
postmyocardial infarction syndrome (411.0)
rupture of chordae tendineae (429.5)
AHA: 3Q, '89, 5

Berry Aneurysms

429.71 Acquired cardiac septal defect [CC] [CD] [A]
EXCLUDES   acute septal infarction (410.00-410.92)
CC Excl: 422.0-422.99, 429.0, 429.4-429.82, 459.89-459.9, 745.0-745.9, 746.89, 746.9, ▶747.83;◀ 747.89, 747.9, 759.7-759.89
DEF: Abnormal communication, between opposite heart chambers; due to defect of septum; not present at birth.

429.79 Other [CC] [CD] [A]
Mural thrombus (atrial) (ventricular), acquired, following myocardial infarction
CC Excl: See code 429.71
AHA: 1Q, '92, 10

✓5th 429.8 Other ill-defined heart diseases

429.81 Other disorders of papillary muscle [CC] [MC] [CD]
Papillary muscle: Papillary muscle:
atrophy   incompetence
degeneration   incoordination
dysfunction   scarring
CC Excl: 429.6, 429.71, 429.79, 429.81, 459.89, 459.9

429.82 Hyperkinetic heart disease [CC] [CD]
CC Excl: 429.71, 429.79, 429.82, 459.89, 459.9
DEF: Condition of unknown origin in young adults; marked by increased cardiac output at rest, increased rate of ventricular ejection; may lead to heart failure.

429.89 Other
Carditis
EXCLUDES   that due to hypertension (402.0-402.9)
AHA: 1Q, '92, 10

429.9 Heart disease, unspecified
Heart disease (organic) NOS   Morbus cordis NOS
EXCLUDES   that due to hypertension (402.0-402.9)
AHA: 1Q, '93, 19

✓4th ✓5th Additional Digit Required   Nonspecific PDx   Unacceptable PDx   Manifestation Code   MSP Medicare Secondary Payer   ▶◀ Revised Text   ● New Code   ▲ Revised Code Title

2002 Ingenix, Inc.   October 2002 • Volume 1 — 125

Circulatory System 430–435.8

CEREBROVASCULAR DISEASE (430-438)

| INCLUDES | with mention of hypertension (conditions classifiable to 401-405) |

Use additional code to identify presence of hypertension

| EXCLUDES | any condition classifiable to 430-434, 436, 437 occurring during pregnancy, childbirth, or the puerperium, or specified as puerperal (674.0) |
| | ▶iatrogenic cerebrovascular infarction or hemorrhage (997.02)◀ |

AHA: 1Q, '93, 27; 3Q, '91, 10; 3Q, '90, 3; 2Q, '89, 8; M-A, '85, 6

430 Subarachnoid hemorrhage   `CC` `MC`
Meningeal hemorrhage   Ruptured:
Ruptured: (congenital) cerebral
   berry aneurysm   aneurysm NOS

| EXCLUDES | syphilitic ruptured cerebral aneurysm (094.87) |

CC Excl: 430, 431, 432.0-432.9, 459.89, 459.9, 780.01-780.09, 800.00-800.99, 801.00-801.99, 803.00-803.99, 804.00-804.96, 850.0-850.9, 851.00-851.99, 852.00-852.19, 852.21-852.59, 853.00-853.19, 854.00-854.19

DEF: Bleeding in space between brain and lining.

431 Intracerebral hemorrhage   `CC` `MC`
Hemorrhage (of):   Hemorrhage (of):
   basilar   internal capsule
   bulbar   intrapontine
   cerebellar   pontine
   cerebral   subcortical
   cerebromeningeal   ventricular
   cortical   Rupture of blood vessel in
                       brain

CC Excl: See code 430

▽ **DRG** 014

DEF: Bleeding within the brain.

√4ʰ **432 Other and unspecified intracranial hemorrhage**

432.0 Nontraumatic extradural hemorrhage   `CC` `MC`
Nontraumatic epidural hemorrhage
CC Excl: See code 430

DEF: Bleeding, nontraumatic, between skull and brain lining.

432.1 Subdural hemorrhage   `CC` `MC`
Subdural hematoma, nontraumatic
CC Excl: See code 430

DEF: Bleeding, between outermost and other layers of brain lining.

432.9 Unspecified intracranial hemorrhage   `MC`
Intracranial hemorrhage NOS

√4ʰ **433 Occlusion and stenosis of precerebral arteries**

INCLUDES	embolism
	narrowing } of basilar, carotid, and
	obstruction vertebral arteries
	thrombosis

| EXCLUDES | insufficiency NOS of precerebral arteries (435.0-435.9) |

The following fifth-digit subclassification is for use with category 433:
   0 without mention of cerebral infarction
   1 with cerebral infarction

AHA: 2Q, '95, 14; 3Q, '90, 16

DEF: Blockage, stricture, arteries branching into brain.

√5ʰ **433.0 Basilar artery**   `CC 1`
CC Excl: For code 433.01: 250.70-250.93, 433.00-433.91, 435.0, 459.89, 459.9

√5ʰ **433.1 Carotid artery**   `CC 1`
CC Excl: For code 433.11: 250.70-250.93, 433.00-433.91, 459.89, 459.9
AHA: 1Q, '00, 16; **For code 433.10:** ▶1Q, '02, 7, 10◀

√5ʰ **433.2 Vertebral artery**   `CC 1`
CC Excl: For code 433.21: 250.70-250.93, 433.00-433.91, 435.1, 459.89, 459.9

¹ Nonspecific PDx = 0

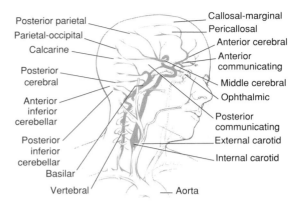

√5ʰ **433.3 Multiple and bilateral**   `CC 1`
CC Excl: For code 433.31: See code 433.11

√5ʰ **433.8 Other specified precerebral artery**   `CC 1`
CC Excl: For code 433.81: See code 433.01

√5ʰ ¹**433.9 Unspecified precerebral artery**   `CC 1`
Precerebral artery NOS
CC Excl: For code 433.91: See code 433.01

√4ʰ **434 Occlusion of cerebral arteries**

The following fifth-digit subclassification is for use with category 433:
   0 without mention of cerebral infarction
   1 with cerebral infarction

AHA: 2Q, '95, 14

√5ʰ **434.0 Cerebral thrombosis**   `CC 1` `MC`
Thrombosis of cerebral arteries
CC Excl: For code 434.01: 250.70-250.93, 434.00-434.91, 436, 459.89, 459.9

√5ʰ **434.1 Cerebral embolism**   `CC 1` `MC`
CC Excl: For code 434.11: See code 434.01
AHA: 3Q, '97, 11
▽ **DRG** 014 For code 434.11

√5ʰ ¹**434.9 Cerebral artery occlusion, unspecified**   `CC 1` `MC`
CC Excl: For code 434.91: See code 434.01
AHA: 4Q, '98, 87
▽ **DRG** 014 For code 434.91

√4ʰ **435 Transient cerebral ischemia**

INCLUDES	cerebrovascular insufficiency (acute) with transient focal neurological signs and symptoms
	insufficiency of basilar, carotid, and vertebral arteries
	spasm of cerebral arteries

| EXCLUDES | acute cerebrovascular insufficiency NOS (437.1) that due to any condition classifiable to 433 (433.0-433.9) |

DEF: Temporary restriction of blood flow, to arteries branching into brain.

435.0 Basilar artery syndrome
435.1 Vertebral artery syndrome
435.2 Subclavian steal syndrome
DEF: Cerebrovascular insufficiency, due to occluded subclavian artery; symptoms include pain in mastoid and posterior head regions, flaccid paralysis of arm and diminished or absent radical pulse on affected side.

435.3 Vertebrobasilar artery syndrome
AHA: 4Q, '95, 60

DEF: Transient ischemic attack; due to brainstem dysfunction; symptoms include confusion, vertigo, binocular blindness, diplopia, unilateral or bilateral weakness and paresthesis of extremities.

435.8 Other specified transient cerebral ischemias   `A`

`N` Newborn Age: 0   `P` Pediatric Age: 0-17   `M` Maternity Age: 12-55   `A` Adult Age :15-124   `CC` CC Condition   `MC` Major Complication   `CD` Complex Dx   `HIV` HIV Related Dx

435.9 Unspecified transient cerebral ischemia [A]
Impending cerebrovascular accident
Intermittent cerebral ischemia
Transient ischemic attack [TIA]
AHA: N-D, '85, 12

436 Acute, but ill-defined, cerebrovascular disease [CC] [MC]
Apoplexy, apoplectic: Cerebral seizure
  NOS   Cerebrovascular accident
  attack   [CVA] NOS
  cerebral   Stroke
  seizure
EXCLUDES   *any condition classifiable to categories 430-435*
           ▶*postoperative cerebrovascular accident*
           (997.02)◄
CC Excl: 250.70-250.93, 430-431, 432.0-432.9, 434.00-434.91, 436, 459.89, 459.9,
780.01-780.09, 800.00-800.99, 801.00-801.99, 803.00-803.99, 804.00-804.96, 850.0-
850.9, 851.00-851.99, 852.00-852.19, 852.21-852.59, 853.00-853.19, 854.00-854.19
AHA: 4Q, '99, 3
▽ **DRG** 014

✓4th **437 Other and ill-defined cerebrovascular disease**
437.0 Cerebral atherosclerosis [A]
Atheroma of cerebral arteries
Cerebral arteriosclerosis

437.1 Other generalized ischemic cerebrovascular disease
Acute cerebrovascular insufficiency NOS
Cerebral ischemia (chronic)

437.2 Hypertensive encephalopathy [CC]
CC Excl: 250.70-250.93, 437.2, 459.89, 459.9
AHA: J-A, '84, 14
DEF: Cerebral manifestations (such as visual disturbances and
headache) due to high blood pressure.

437.3 Cerebral aneurysm, nonruptured
Internal carotid artery, intracranial portion
Internal carotid artery NOS
EXCLUDES   *congenital cerebral aneurysm,*
           nonruptured (747.81)
           internal carotid artery, extracranial
           portion (442.81)

437.4 Cerebral arteritis [CC]
CC Excl: 250.70-250.93, 437.4, 459.89, 459.9
AHA: 4Q, '99, 21
DEF: Inflammation of a cerebral artery or arteries.

437.5 Moyamoya disease [CC]
CC Excl: 250.70-250.93, 437.5, 459.89, 459.9
DEF: Cerebrovascular ischemia; vessels occlude and rupture
causing tiny hemorrhages at base of brain; predominantly affects
Japanese.

437.6 Nonpyogenic thrombosis of intracranial [CC]
venous sinus
EXCLUDES   *pyogenic (325)*
CC Excl: 250.70-250.93, 437.6, 459.89, 459.9

437.7 Transient global amnesia
AHA: 4Q, '92, 20
DEF: Episode of short-term memory loss, not often recurrent;
pathogenesis unknown; with no signs or symptoms of neurological
disorder.
437.8 Other
437.9 Unspecified
Cerebrovascular disease or lesion NOS

✓4th **438 Late effects of cerebrovascular disease**
Note: This category is to be used to indicate conditions in
430-437 as the cause of late effects. The "late effects"
include conditions specified as such, as sequelae,
which may occur at any time after the onset of the
causal condition.
AHA: 4Q, '99, 4, 6, 7; 4Q, '98, 39, 88; 4Q, '97, 35, 37; 4Q, '92, 21; N-D, '86, 12;
M-A, '86, 7
438.0 Cognitive deficits

✓5th **438.1 Speech and language deficits**
438.10 Speech and language deficit, unspecified
438.11 Aphasia
AHA: 4Q, '97, 36
DEF: Impairment or absence of the ability to
communicate by speech, writing or signs or to
comprehend the spoken or written language due to
disease or injury to the brain. Total aphasia is the loss of
function of both sensory and motor areas of the brain.
438.12 Dysphasia
AHA: 4Q, '99, 3, 9
DEF: Impaired speech; marked by inability to sequence
language.
438.19 Other speech and language deficits
✓5th **438.2 Hemiplegia/hemiparesis**
DEF: Paralysis of one side of the body.
438.20 Hemiplegia affecting unspecified side
AHA: 4Q, '99, 3, 9
438.21 Hemiplegia affecting dominant side
438.22 Hemiplegia affecting nondominant side
AHA: ▶1Q, '02, 16◄
✓5th **438.3 Monoplegia of upper limb**
DEF: Paralysis of one limb or one muscle group.
438.30 Monoplegia of upper limb affecting
unspecified side
438.31 Monoplegia of upper limb affecting
dominant side
DEF: Inability to activate learned movements; no known
sensory or motor impairment.
438.32 Monoplegia of upper limb affecting
nondominant side
✓5th **438.4 Monoplegia of lower limb**
438.40 Monoplegia of lower limb affecting
unspecified side
438.41 Monoplegia of lower limb affecting
dominant side
438.42 Monoplegia of lower limb affecting
nondominant side
✓5th **438.5 Other paralytic syndrome**
Use additional code to identify type of paralytic
syndrome, such as:
  locked-in state (344.81)
  quadriplegia (344.00-344.09)
EXCLUDES   *late effects of cerebrovascular accident*
           with:
           hemiplegia/hemiparesis (438.20-
           438.22)
           monoplegia of lower limb (438.40-
           438.42)
           monoplegia of upper limb (438.30-
           438.32)
438.50 Other paralytic syndrome affecting
unspecified side
438.51 Other paralytic syndrome affecting
dominant side
438.52 Other paralytic syndrome affecting
nondominant side
438.53 Other paralytic syndrome, bilateral
AHA: 4Q, '98, 39
● **438.6 Alterations of sensations**
Use additional code to identify the altered sensation
● **438.7 Disturbances of vision**
Use additional code to identify the visual
disturbance
✓5th **438.8 Other late effects of cerebrovascular disease**
438.81 Apraxia
438.82 Dysphagia
DEF: Inability or difficulty in swallowing.
● **438.83 Facial weakness**
Facial droop

✓4th / ✓5th Additional Digit Required   Nonspecific PDx   Unacceptable PDx   Manifestation Code   [MSP] Medicare Secondary Payer   ▶◄ Revised Text   ● New Code   ▲ Revised Code Title

2002 Ingenix, Inc.   **October 2002 • Volume 1 — 127**

Map of Major Arteries

Major Arteries

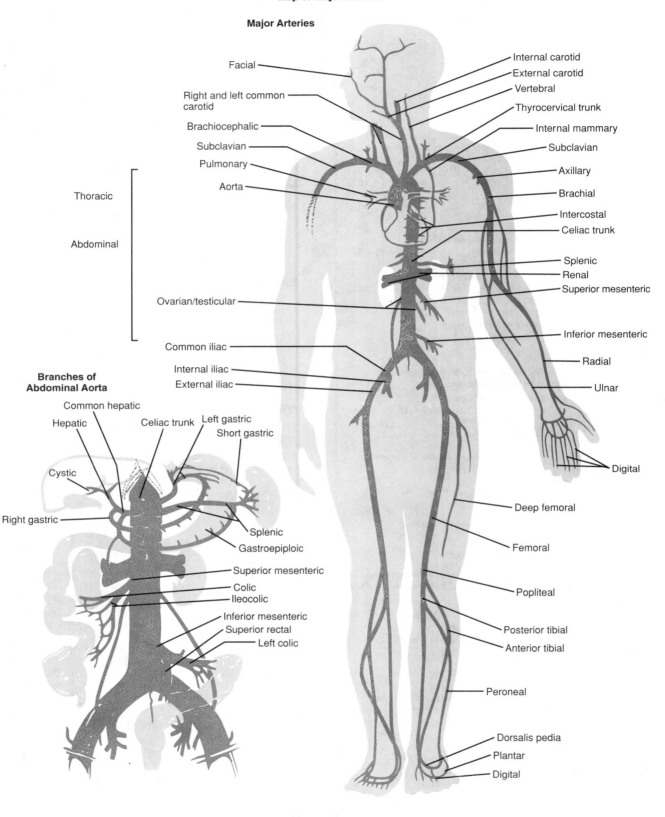

Thoracic

Abdominal

Facial

Right and left common carotid

Brachiocephalic

Subclavian

Pulmonary

Aorta

Ovarian/testicular

Common iliac

Internal iliac

External iliac

Internal carotid

External carotid

Vertebral

Thyrocervical trunk

Internal mammary

Subclavian

Axillary

Brachial

Intercostal

Celiac trunk

Splenic

Renal

Superior mesenteric

Inferior mesenteric

Radial

Ulnar

Digital

Deep femoral

Femoral

Popliteal

Posterior tibial

Anterior tibial

Peroneal

Dorsalis pedia

Plantar

Digital

Branches of Abdominal Aorta

Common hepatic

Hepatic

Celiac trunk

Left gastric

Short gastric

Cystic

Right gastric

Splenic

Gastroepiploic

Superior mesenteric

Colic

Ileocolic

Inferior mesenteric

Superior rectal

Left colic

N Newborn Age: 0   P Pediatric Age: 0-17   M Maternity Age: 12-55   A Adult Age :15-124   CC CC Condition   MC Major Complication   CD Complex Dx   HIV HIV Related Dx

2002 Ingenix, Inc.

Circulatory System

●   **438.84 Ataxia**

●   **438.85 Vertigo**

    438.89 Other late effects of cerebrovascular disease

       Use additional code to identify the late effect

       AHA: 4Q, '98, 39

438.9   Unspecified late effects of cerebrovascular disease

DISEASES OF ARTERIES, ARTERIOLES, AND CAPILLARIES (440-448)

√4th **440 Atherosclerosis**

    `INCLUDES`   arteriolosclerosis
               arteriosclerosis (obliterans) (senile)
               arteriosclerotic vascular disease
               atheroma
               degeneration:
                  arterial
                  arteriovascular
                  vascular
               endarteritis deformans or obliterans
               senile:
                  arteritis
                  endarteritis

    `EXCLUDES`   ▶*atheroembolism (445.01-445.89)*◀
             atherosclerosis of bypass graft of the extremities (403.30-403.32)

    DEF: Stricture and reduced elasticity of an artery; due to plaque deposits.

    440.0   Of aorta   `A`

       AHA: 2Q, '93, 7; 2Q, '93, 8; 4Q, '88, 8

    440.1   Of renal artery   `A`

       `EXCLUDES`   *atherosclerosis of renal arterioles (403.00-403.91)*

√5th **440.2   Of native arteries of the extremities**

       `EXCLUDES`   *atherosclerosis of bypass graft of the extremities (440.30-440.32)*

       AHA: 4Q, '94, 49; 4Q, '93, 27; 4Q, '92, 25; 3Q, '90, 15; M-A, '87, 6

       440.20 Atherosclerosis of the extremities, unspecified   `A`

       440.21 Atherosclerosis of the extremities with intermittent claudication   `A`

          DEF: Atherosclerosis; marked by pain, tension and weakness after walking; no symptoms while at rest.

       440.22 Atherosclerosis of the extremities with rest pain   `A`

          `INCLUDES`   any condition classifiable to 440.21

          DEF: Atherosclerosis, marked by pain, tension and weakness while at rest.

       440.23 Atherosclerosis of the extremities with ulceration

          Use additional code for any associated ulceration (707.10-707.9)

          `INCLUDES`   any condition classifiable to 440.21 and 440.22

          AHA: 4Q, '00, 44

       440.24 Atherosclerosis of the extremities with gangrene   `CC`

          `INCLUDES`   any condition classifiable to 440.21, 440.22, and 440.23 with ischemic gangrene 785.4

          `EXCLUDES`   *gas gangrene (040.0)*

          CC Excl: 440.24, ▶780.91-780.99,◀ 785.4, 799.8

          AHA: 4Q, '95, 54; 1Q, '95, 11

       440.29 Other   `A`

√5th **440.3   Of bypass graft of extremities**

       `EXCLUDES`   *atherosclerosis of native arteries of the extremities (440.21-440.24)*
             embolism [occlusion NOS] [thrombus] of graft (996.74)

       AHA: 4Q, '94, 49

    440.30 Of unspecified graft   `A`

    440.31 Of autologous vein bypass graft   `A`

    440.32 Of nonautologous biological bypass graft   `A`

    440.8   Of other specified arteries   `A`

       `EXCLUDES`   *basilar (433.0)*
             carotid (433.1)
             cerebral (437.0)
             coronary ▶(414.00-414.06)◀
             mesenteric (557.1)
             precerebral (433.0-433.9)
             pulmonary (416.0)
             vertebral (433.2)

    440.9   Generalized and unspecified atherosclerosis   `A`

       Arteriosclerotic vascular disease NOS

       `EXCLUDES`   *arteriosclerotic cardiovascular disease [ASCVD] (429.2)*

√4th **441 Aortic aneurysm and dissection**

    `EXCLUDES`   *syphilitic aortic aneurysm (093.0)*
            traumatic aortic aneurysm (901.0, 902.0)

√5th **441.0   Dissection of aorta**

       AHA: 4Q, '89, 10

       DEF: Dissection or splitting of wall of the aorta; due to blood entering through intimal tear or interstitial hemorrhage.

       441.00 Unspecified site   `CC` `MC` `A`

          CC Excl: 250.70-250.93, 441.00-441.9, 459.89, 459.9

       441.01 Thoracic   `CC` `MC` `A`

          CC Excl: See code 441.00

       441.02 Abdominal   `CC` `MC` `A`

          CC Excl: See code 441.00

       441.03 Thoracoabdominal   `CC` `MC` `A`

          CC Excl: See code 441.00

    441.1   Thoracic aneurysm, ruptured   `CC` `A`

       CC Excl: See code 441.00

    441.2   Thoracic aneurysm without mention of rupture   `A`

       AHA: 3Q, '92, 10

    441.3   Abdominal aneurysm, ruptured   `CC` `A`

       CC Excl: See code 441.00

    441.4   Abdominal aneurysm without mention of rupture   `CC` `A`

       AHA: 4Q, '00, 64; 1Q, '99, 15, 16, 17; 3Q, '92, 10

    441.5   Aortic aneurysm of unspecified site, ruptured   `CC` `A`

       Rupture of aorta NOS

       CC Excl: See code 441.00

    441.6   Thoracoabdominal aneurysm, ruptured   `CC` `A`

       CC Excl: See code 441.00

    441.7   Thoracoabdominal aneurysm, without mention of rupture   `A`

Thoracic and Abdominal Aortic Aneurysm

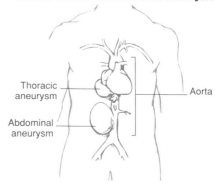

Thoracic aneurysm   Aorta

Abdominal aneurysm

√4th Additional Digit Required   `Nonspecific PDx`   `Unacceptable PDx`   `Manifestation Code`   `MSP` Medicare Secondary Payer   ▶◀ Revised Text   ● New Code   ▲ Revised Code Title
√5th

2002 Ingenix, Inc.   **October 2002 • Volume 1 — 129**

441.9   Aortic aneurysm of unspecified site without mention of rupture

Aneurysm
Dilatation   } of aorta
Hyaline necrosis

√4ᵗʰ **442 Other aneurysm**

INCLUDES   aneurysm (ruptured) (cirsoid) (false) (varicose)
aneurysmal varix

EXCLUDES   *arteriovenous aneurysm or fistula:*
acquired (447.0)
congenital (747.60-747.69)
traumatic (900.0-904.9)

DEF: Dissection or splitting of arterial wall; due to blood entering through intimal tear or interstitial hemorrhage.

442.0   Of artery of upper extremity A

442.1   Of renal artery A

442.2   Of iliac artery A

     AHA: 1Q, '99, 16, 17

442.3   Of artery of lower extremity A

Aneurysm:
femoral
popliteal   } artery

     AHA: 1Q, '99, 16

√5ᵗʰ **442.8   Of other specified artery**

442.81 Artery of neck A

Aneurysm of carotid artery (common) (external) (internal, extracranial portion)

EXCLUDES   *internal carotid artery, intra-cranial portion (437.3)*

442.82 Subclavian artery A

442.83 Splenic artery A

442.84 Other visceral artery A

Aneurysm:
celiac
gastroduodenal
gastroepiploic
hepatic   } artery
pancreaticoduodenal
superior mesenteric

442.89 Other A

Aneurysm:
mediastinal
spinal   } artery

EXCLUDES   *cerebral (nonruptured) (437.3)*
congenital (747.81)
ruptured (430)
coronary (414.11)
heart (414.10)
pulmonary (417.1)

442.9   Of unspecified site A

√4ᵗʰ **443 Other peripheral vascular disease**

443.0   Raynaud's syndrome

Raynaud's:
disease
phenomenon (secondary)
Use additional code to identify gangrene (785.4)

DEF: Constriction of the arteries, due to cold or stress; bilateral ischemic attacks of fingers, toes, nose or ears; symptoms include pallor, paresthesia and pain; more common in females.

443.1   Thromboangiitis obliterans [Buerger's disease]

Presenile gangrene

DEF: Inflammatory disease of extremity blood vessels, mainly the lower; occurs primarily in young men and leads to tissue ischemia and gangrene.

● √5ᵗʰ **443.2   Other arterial dissection**

EXCLUDES   *dissection of aorta (441.00-441.03)*
dissection of coronary arteries (414.12)

●   **443.21 Dissection of carotid artery**

Arterial Diseases and Disorders

Lipids
Calcium deposits

Atherosclerosis narrowing lumen

Thrombus (clot) forming in lumen

Organization of thrombus and recanalization

Intimal proliferation

Aneurysm bypasses lumen or...

Embolus (from elsewhere) occluding lumen

...bulges from arterial wall

Arteriovenous fistula

●   **443.22 Dissection of iliac artery**

●   **443.23 Dissection of renal artery**

●   **443.24 Dissection of vertebral artery**

●   **443.29 Dissection of other artery**

√5ᵗʰ **443.8   Other specified peripheral vascular diseases**

443.81 *Peripheral angiopathy in diseases classified elsewhere*

Code first underlying disease, as:
diabetes mellitus (250.7)

     AHA: 3Q, '91, 10

443.89 Other

Acrocyanosis   Erythrocyanosis
Acroparesthesia: Erythromelalgia
simple [Schultze's type]
vasomotor [Nothnagel's type]

EXCLUDES   *chilblains (991.5)*
frostbite (991.0-991.3)
immersion foot (991.4)

443.9   Peripheral vascular disease, unspecified

Intermittent claudication NOS
Peripheral:
angiopathy NOS
vascular disease NOS
Spasm of artery

EXCLUDES   *atherosclerosis of the arteries of the extremities (440.20-440.22)*
spasm of cerebral artery (435.0-435.9)

     AHA: 4Q, '92, 25; 3Q, '91, 10

√4ᵗʰ **444 Arterial embolism and thrombosis**

INCLUDES   infarction:
embolic
thrombotic
occlusion

EXCLUDES   *that complicating:*
abortion (634-638 with .6, 639.6)
▶*atheroembolism (445.01-445.89)*◀
ectopic or molar pregnancy (639.6)
pregnancy, childbirth, or the pueperium (673.0-673.8)

     AHA: 2Q, '92, 11; 4Q, '90, 27

444.0   Of abdominal aorta CC

Aortic bifurcation syndrome   Leriche's syndrome
Aortoiliac obstruction   Saddle embolus

     CC Excl: 250.70-250.93, 444.0, 444.89, 444.9, 459.89, 459.9

     AHA: 2Q, '93, 7; 4Q, '90, 27

444.1   Of thoracic aorta CC

Embolism or thrombosis of aorta (thoracic)

     CC Excl: 250.70-250.93, 444.1, 444.89, 444.9, 459.89, 459.9

√5ᵗʰ **444.2   Of arteries of the extremities**

     AHA: M-A, '87, 6

444.21 Upper extremity CC

     CC Excl: 250.70-250.93, 444.21, 444.89, 444.9, 459.89, 459.9

N Newborn Age: 0   P Pediatric Age: 0-17   M Maternity Age: 12-55   A Adult Age :15-124   CC CC Condition   MC Major Complication   CD Complex Dx   HIV HIV Related Dx

444.22 Lower extremity `CC`
Arterial embolism or thrombosis:
femoral
peripheral NOS
popliteal
EXCLUDES   *iliofemoral (444.81)*

CC Excl: 250.70-250.93, 444.22, 444.89, 444.9, 459.89, 459.9

AHA: 3Q, '90, 16

√5ᵗʰ **444.8 Of other specified artery**

444.81 Iliac artery `CC`

CC Excl: 250.70-250.93, 444.81-444.9, 459.89, 459.9

444.89 Other `CC`
EXCLUDES   *basilar (433.0)*
carotid (433.1)
cerebral (434.0-434.9)
coronary (410.00-410.92)
mesenteric (557.0)
ophthalmic (362.30-362.34)
precerebral (433.0-433.9)
pulmonary (415.19)
renal (593.81)
retinal (362.30-362.34)
vertebral (433.2)

CC Excl: 250.70-250.93, 444.89, 444.9, 459.89, 459.9

444.9 Of unspecified artery `CC`

CC Excl: See code 444.89

● √4ᵗʰ **445 Atheroembolism**
INCLUDES   atherothrombotic microembolism
cholesterol embolism

● √5ᵗʰ **445.0 Of extremities**

● **445.01 Upper extremity** `CC`

CC Excl: 250.70-250.73, 250.80-250.83, 250.90-250.93, 444.89, 444.9, 445.01, 459.89, 459.9

● **445.02 Lower extremity** `CC`

CC Excl: 250.70-250.73, 250.80-250.83, 250.90-250.93, 444.89, 444.9, 445.02, 459.89, 459.9

● √5ᵗʰ **445.8 Of other sites**

● **445.81 Kidney** `CC`
Use additional code for any associated kidney failure (584, 585)

CC Excl: 250.70-250.73, 250.80-250.83, 250.90-250.93, 444.89, 444.9, 445.81, 459.89, 459.9

● **445.89 Other site** `CC`

CC Excl: 250.70-250.73, 250.80-250.83, 250.90-250.93, 444.89, 444.9, 445.89, 459.9

√4ᵗʰ **446 Polyarteritis nodosa and allied conditions**

446.0 Polyarteritis nodosa `CC`
Disseminated necrotizing periarteritis
Necrotizing angiitis
Panarteritis (nodosa)
Periarteritis (nodosa)

CC Excl: 250.70-250.93, 446.0-446.7, 459.89, 459.9

DEF: Inflammation of small and mid-size arteries; symptoms related to involved arteries in kidneys, muscles, gastrointestinal tract and heart; results in tissue death.

446.1 Acute febrile mucocutaneous lymph node syndrome [MCLS]
Kawasaki disease

DEF: Acute febrile disease of children; marked by erythema of conjunctiva and mucous membranes of upper respiratory tract, skin eruptions and edema.

√5ᵗʰ **446.2 Hypersensitivity angiitis**
EXCLUDES   *antiglomerular basement membrane disease without pulmonary hemorrhage (583.89)*

446.20 Hypersensitivity angiitis, unspecified `CC`

CC Excl: See code 446.0

446.21 Goodpasture's syndrome `CC`
Antiglomerular basement membrane antibody-mediated nephritis with pulmonary hemorrhage
Use additional code to identify renal disease (583.81)

CC Excl: See code 446.0

DEF: Glomerulonephritis associated with hematuria, progresses rapidly; results in death from renal failure.

446.29 Other specified hypersensitivity angiitis `CC`

CC Excl: See code 446.0

AHA: 1Q, '95, 3

446.3 Lethal midline granuloma `CC`
Malignant granuloma of face

CC Excl: See code 446.0

DEF: Granulomatous lesion; in nose or paranasal sinuses; often fatal; occurs chiefly in males.

446.4 Wegener's granulomatosis `CC`
Necrotizing respiratory granulomatosis
Wegener's syndrome

CC Excl: See code 446.0

AHA: 3Q, '00, 11

DEF: A disease occurring mainly in men; marked by necrotizing granulomas and ulceration of the upper respiratory tract; underlying condition is a vasculitis affecting small vessels and is possibly due to an immune disorder.

446.5 Giant cell arteritis `CC`
Cranial arteritis   Temporal arteritis
Horton's disease

CC Excl: See code 446.0

DEF: Inflammation of arteries; due to giant cells affecting carotid artery branches, resulting in occlusion; symptoms include fever, headache and neurological problems; occurs in elderly.

446.6 Thrombotic microangiopathy `CC`
Moschcowitz's syndrome
Thrombotic thrombocytopenic purpura

CC Excl: See code 446.0

DEF: Blockage of small blood vessels; due to hyaline deposits; symptoms include purpura, CNS disorders; results in protracted disease or rapid death.

446.7 Takayasu's disease `CC`
Aortic arch arteritis
Pulseless disease

CC Excl: See code 446.0

DEF: Progressive obliterative arteritis of brachiocephalic trunk, left subclavian, and left common carotid arteries above aortic arch; results in ischemia in brain, heart and arm; pulses impalpable in head, neck and arms; more common in young adult females.

√4ᵗʰ **447 Other disorders of arteries and arterioles**

447.0 Arteriovenous fistula, acquired
Arteriovenous aneurysm, acquired
EXCLUDES   *cerebrovascular (437.3)*
coronary (414.19)
pulmonary (417.0)
surgically created arteriovenous shunt or fistula:
complication (996.1, 996.61-996.62)
status or presence (V45.1)
traumatic (900.0-904.9)

DEF: Communication between an artery and vein caused by error in healing.

447.1 Stricture of artery

AHA: 2Q, '93, 8; M-A, '87, 6

√4ᵗʰ √5ᵗʰ Additional Digit Required   Nonspecific PDx   Unacceptable PDx   Manifestation Code   `MSP` Medicare Secondary Payer   ►◄ Revised Text   ● New Code   ▲ Revised Code Title

Map of Major Veins

Circulatory System

External jugular

Internal jugular

Subclavian

Axillary

Brachial

Cephalic

Medial cubital

Cephalic

Basilic

Digital

Femoral

Great saphenous

Popliteal

Posterior tibial

Anterior tibial

Dorsal venous arch

Digital

Plantar

Brachiocephalic

Internal mammary

Superior vena cava

Azygos

Inferior vena cava

Hepatic

Renal

Ovarian/testicular

Portal

Common iliac

Internal iliac

External iliac

Hypogastric

Common femoral

Superficial femoral

Deep femoral

Femoral

Portal Venous Circulation

Inferior vena cava

Gastric

Portal

Splenic

Superior mesenteric

Right colic

Ileocolic

Inferior mesenteric

Left colic

| N | Newborn Age: 0 | P | Pediatric Age: 0-17 | M | Maternity Age: 12-55 | A | Adult Age :15-124 | CC | CC Condition | MC | Major Complication | CD | Complex Dx | HIV | HIV Related Dx |

132 — Volume 1   *2002 Ingenix, Inc.*

447.2   **Rupture of artery**

Erosion

Fistula, except arteriovenous } of artery

Ulcer

> EXCLUDES   *traumatic rupture of artery (900.0-904.9)*

447.3   **Hyperplasia of renal artery**

Fibromuscular hyperplasia of renal artery

DEF: Overgrowth of cells in muscular lining of renal artery.

447.4   **Celiac artery compression syndrome**

Celiac axis syndrome

Marable's syndrome

447.5   **Necrosis of artery**

447.6   **Arteritis, unspecified**

Aortitis NOS

Endarteritis NOS

> EXCLUDES   *arteritis, endarteritis:*
>   *aortic arch (446.7)*
>   *cerebral (437.4)*
>   *coronary ▶(414.00-414.06)◀*
>   *deformans (440.0-440.9)*
>   *obliterans (440.0-440.9)*
>   *pulmonary (417.8)*
>   *senile (440.0-440.9)*
>   *polyarteritis NOS (446.0)*
>   *syphilitic aortitis (093.1)*

AHA: 1Q, '95, 3

447.8   **Other specified disorders of arteries and arterioles**

Fibromuscular hyperplasia of arteries, except renal

447.9   **Unspecified disorders of arteries and arterioles**

√4th **448 Disease of capillaries**

448.0   **Hereditary hemorrhagic telangiectasia**

Rendu-Osler-Weber disease

DEF: Genetic disease with onset after puberty; results in multiple telangiectases, dilated venules on skin and mucous membranes; recurrent bleeding may occur.

448.1   **Nevus, non-neoplastic**

Nevus:

    araneus

    senile

    spider

    stellar

> EXCLUDES   *neoplastic (216.0-216.9)*
>   *port wine (757.32)*
>   *strawberry (757.32)*

DEF: Enlarged or malformed blood vessels of skin; results in reddish swelling, skin patch, or birthmark.

448.9   **Other and unspecified capillary diseases**

Capillary:

    hemorrhage

    hyperpermeability

    thrombosis

> EXCLUDES   *capillary fragility (hereditary) (287.8)*

DISEASES OF VEINS AND LYMPHATICS, AND OTHER DISEASES OF CIRCULATORY SYSTEM (451-459)

√4th **451 Phlebitis and thrombophlebitis**

> INCLUDES   endophlebitis   periphlebitis
>   inflammation, vein   suppurative phlebitis

Use additional E code to identify drug, if drug-induced

> EXCLUDES   *that complicating:*
>   *abortion (634-638 with .7, 639.8)*
>   *ectopic or molar pregnancy (639.8)*
>   *pregnancy, childbirth, or the puerperium (671.0-671.9)*
>   *that due to or following:*
>   *implant or catheter device (996.61-996.62)*
>   *infusion, perfusion, or transfusion (999.2)*

AHA: 1Q, '92, 16

DEF: Inflammation of a vein (phlebitis) with formation of a thrombus (thrombophlebitis).

451.0   **Of superficial vessels of lower extremities**   `CC`

Saphenous vein (greater) (lesser)

CC Excl: 250.70-250.93, 451.0-451.9, 459.89, 459.9

AHA: 3Q, '91, 16

√5th **451.1**   **Of deep vessels of lower extremities**

AHA: 3Q, '91, 16

   451.11 Femoral vein (deep) (superficial)   `CC`

     CC Excl: See code 451.0

   451.19 Other   `CC`

     Femoropopliteal vein   Tibial vein

     Popliteal vein

     CC Excl: See code 451.0

451.2   **Of lower extremities, unspecified**   `CC`

CC Excl: See code 451.0

√5th **451.8**   **Of other sites**

> EXCLUDES   *intracranial venous sinus (325)*
>   *nonpyogenic (437.6)*
>   *portal (vein) (572.1)*

   451.81 Iliac vein   `CC`

     CC Excl: See code 451.0

   451.82 Of superficial veins of upper extremities

     Antecubital vein   Cephalic vein

     Basilic vein

   451.83 Of deep veins of upper extremities

     Brachial vein   Ulnar vein

     Radial vein

   451.84 Of upper extremities, unspecified

   451.89 Other

     Axillary vein   Thrombophlebitis of

     Jugular vein   breast (Mondor's

     Subclavian vein   disease)

451.9   **Of unspecified site**

452 Portal vein thrombosis   `CC`

Portal (vein) obstruction

> EXCLUDES   *hepatic vein thrombosis (453.0)*
>   *phlebitis of portal vein (572.1)*

CC Excl: 250.70-250.93, 452, 453.8-453.9, 459.89, 459.9

DEF: Formation of a blood clot in main vein of liver.

√4th **453 Other venous embolism and thrombosis**

> EXCLUDES   *that complicating:*
>   *abortion (634-638 with .7, 639.8)*
>   *ectopic or molar pregnancy (639.8)*
>   *pregnancy, childbirth, or the puerperium (671.0-671.9)*
>   *that with inflammation, phlebitis, and thrombophlebitis (451.0-451.9)*

AHA: 1Q, '92, 16

453.0   **Budd-Chiari syndrome**   `CC`

Hepatic vein thrombosis

CC Excl: 250.70-250.93, 453.0, 453.8-453.9, 459.89, 459.9

DEF: Thrombosis or other obstruction of hepatic vein; symptoms include enlarged liver, extensive collateral vessels, intractable ascites and severe portal hypertension.

453.1   **Thrombophlebitis migrans**   `CC`

CC Excl: 250.70-250.93, 453.1, 453.8-453.9, 459.89, 459.9

DEF: Slow, advancing thrombophlebitis; appearing first in one vein then another.

453.2   **Of vena cava**   `CC`

CC Excl: 250.70-250.93, 453.2, 453.8-453.9, 459.89, 459.9

453.3   **Of renal vein**   `CC`

CC Excl: 250.70-250.93, 453.3, 453.8-453.9, 459.89, 459.9

√4th √5th Additional Digit Required   Nonspecific PDx   Unacceptable PDx   Manifestation Code   `MSP` Medicare Secondary Payer   ▶◀ Revised Text   ● New Code   ▲ Revised Code Title

2002 Ingenix, Inc.   **October 2002 • Volume 1 — 133**

453.8 Of other specified veins `CC`
EXCLUDES
    cerebral (434.0-434.9)
    coronary (410.00-410.92)
    intracranial venous sinus (325)
      nonpyogenic (437.6)
    mesenteric (557.0)
    portal (452)
    precerebral (433.0-433.9)
    pulmonary (415.19)

CC Excl: 250.70-250.93, 453.8-453.9, 459.89, 459.9

AHA: 3Q, '91, 16; M-A, '87, 6

DRG 130

453.9 Of unspecified site `CC`
Embolism of vein   Thrombosis (vein)
CC Excl: See code 453.8

454 Varicose veins of lower extremities
EXCLUDES *that complicating pregnancy, childbirth, or the puerperium (671.0)*
AHA: 2Q, '91, 20
DEF: Dilated leg veins; due to incompetent vein valves that allow reversed blood flow and cause tissue erosion or weakness of wall; may be painful.

454.0 With ulcer `A`
Varicose ulcer (lower extremity, any part)
Varicose veins with ulcer of lower extremity [any part] or of unspecified site
Any condition classifiable to 454.9 with ulcer or specified as ulcerated
AHA: 4Q, '99, 18

454.1 With inflammation `A`
Stasis dermatitis
Varicose veins with inflammation of lower extremity [any part] or of unspecified site
Any condition classifiable to 454.9 with inflammation or specified as inflamed

454.2 With ulcer and inflammation `A`
Varicose veins with ulcer and inflammation of lower extremity [any part] or of unspecified site
Any condition classifiable to 454.9 with ulcer and inflammation

454.8 With other complications
Edema
Pain
Swelling

454.9 Asymptomatic varicose veins `A`
Phlebectasia
Varicose veins } of lower extremity [any part] or of unspecified site
Varix
▶Varicose veins NOS◀

455 Hemorrhoids
INCLUDES hemorrhoids (anus) (rectum)
piles
varicose veins, anus or rectum
EXCLUDES *that complicating pregnancy, childbirth, or the puerperium (671.8)*
DEF: Varicose condition of external hemorrhoidal veins causing painful swellings at the anus.

455.0 Internal hemorrhoids without mention of complication
455.1 Internal thrombosed hemorrhoids
455.2 Internal hemorrhoids with other complication
Internal hemorrhoids: Internal hemorrhoids:
bleeding   strangulated
prolapsed   ulcerated
455.3 External hemorrhoids without mention of complication
455.4 External thrombosed hemorrhoids
455.5 External hemorrhoids with other complication
External hemorrhoids: External hemorrhoids:
bleeding   strangulated
prolapsed   ulcerated

455.6 Unspecified hemorrhoids without mention of complication
Hemorrhoids NOS
455.7 Unspecified thrombosed hemorrhoids
Thrombosed hemorrhoids, unspecified whether internal or external
455.8 Unspecified hemorrhoids with other complication
Hemorrhoids, unspecified whether internal or external:
bleeding   strangulated
prolapsed   ulcerated
455.9 Residual hemorrhoidal skin tags
Skin tags, anus or rectum

456 Varicose veins of other sites
456.0 Esophageal varices with bleeding `CC`
CC Excl: 251.5, 456.0, 456.20, 459.89, 459.9, 530.2, 530.7, 530.82, 531.00-531.91, 532.00-532.91, 533.00-533.91, 534.00-534.91, 535.01, 535.11, 535.21, 535.31, 535.41, 535.51, 535.61, 537.83, 562.02-562.03, 562.12-562.13, 569.3, 569.85, 578.0-578.9
DEF: Distended, tortuous, veins of lower esophagus, usually due to portal hypertension.
456.1 Esophageal varices without mention of bleeding
456.2 Esophageal varices in diseases classified elsewhere
Code first underlying cause, as:
cirrhosis of liver (571.0-571.9)
portal hypertension (572.3)
456.20 With bleeding `CC`
CC Excl: 456.0, 456.20, 459.89, 459.9, 530.82
AHA: N-D, '85, 14
456.21 Without mention of bleeding
456.3 Sublingual varices
DEF: Distended, tortuous veins beneath tongue.
456.4 Scrotal varices ♂
Varicocele
456.5 Pelvic varices
Varices of broad ligament
456.6 Vulval varices ♀
Varices of perineum
EXCLUDES *that complicating pregnancy, childbirth, or the puerperium (671.1)*
456.8 Varices of other sites
Varicose veins of nasal septum (with ulcer)
EXCLUDES *placental varices (656.7)*
retinal varices (362.17)
varicose ulcer of unspecified site (454.0)
varicose veins of unspecified site (454.9)

457 Noninfectious disorders of lymphatic channels
457.0 Postmastectomy lymphedema syndrome `A`
Elephantiasis
Obliteration of lymphatic vessel } due to mastectomy
DEF: Reduced lymphatic circulation following mastectomy; symptoms include swelling of the arm on the operative side.
457.1 Other lymphedema
Elephantiasis   Lymphedema:
(nonfilarial) NOS praecox
Lymphangiectasis   secondary
Lymphedema: Obliteration, lymphatic vessel
acquired (chronic)
EXCLUDES *elephantiasis (nonfilarial):*
congenital (757.0)
eyelid (374.83)
vulva (624.8)
DEF: Fluid retention due to reduced lymphatic circulation; due to other than mastectomy.

  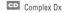

457.2 **Lymphangitis**

Lymphangitis: Lymphangitis:
    NOS   subacute
    chronic

> **EXCLUDES**   *acute lymphangitis (682.0-682.9)*

457.8 **Other noninfectious disorders of lymphatic channels**

Chylocele (nonfilarial)   Lymph node or vessel:
Chylous: fistula
    ascites   infarction
    cyst   rupture

> **EXCLUDES**   *chylocele:*
>   *filarial (125.0-125.9)*
>   *tunica vaginalis (nonfilarial) (608.84)*

457.9 **Unspecified noninfectious disorder of lymphatic channels**

✓4ᵗʰ 458 **Hypotension**

> **INCLUDES**   hypopiesis
> **EXCLUDES**   *cardiovascular collapse (785.50)*
>   *maternal hypotension syndrome (669.2)*
>   *shock (785.50-785.59)*
>   *Shy-Drager syndrome (333.0)*

458.0 **Orthostatic hypotension**

Hypotension: Hypotension:
    orthostatic (chronic)   postural

AHA: 3Q, '00, 8; 3Q, '91, 9

DEF: Low blood pressure; occurs when standing.

458.1 **Chronic hypotension**

Permanent idiopathic hypotension

DEF: Persistent low blood pressure.

458.2 **Iatrogenic hypotension**

Postoperative hypotension

AHA: 4Q, '95, 57

DEF: Abnormally low blood pressure; due to medical treatment.

458.8 **Other specified hypotension**   `MC`

AHA: 4Q, '97, 37

458.9 **Hypotension, unspecified**   `MC`

Hypotension (arterial) NOS

✓4ᵗʰ 459 **Other disorders of circulatory system**

459.0 **Hemorrhage, unspecified**   `CC`

Rupture of blood vessel NOS
Spontaneous hemorrhage NEC

> **EXCLUDES**   *hemorrhage:*
>   *gastrointestinal NOS (578.9)*
>   *in newborn NOS (772.9)*
>   *secondary or recurrent following trauma (958.2)*
>   *traumatic rupture of blood vessel (900.0-904.9)*

CC Excl: 459.0, 459.89, 459.9

AHA: 4Q, '90, 26

✓5ᵗʰ 459.1 **Postphlebitic syndrome**

▶Chronic venous hypertension due to deep vein thrombosis◀

> **EXCLUDES** ▶*chronic venous hypertension without deep vein thrombosis (459.30-459.39)*◀

AHA: 2Q, '91, 20

DEF: Various conditions following deep vein thrombosis; including edema, pain, stasis dermatitis, cellulitis, varicose veins and ulceration of the lower leg.

● **459.10** **Postphlebitic syndrome without complications**

Asymptomatic postphlebitic syndrome
Postphlebitic syndrome NOS

● **459.11** **Postphlebitic syndrome with ulcer**

● **459.12** **Postphlebitic syndrome with inflammation**

● **459.13** **Postphlebitic syndrome with ulcer and inflammation**

● **459.19** **Postphlebitic syndrome with other complication**

459.2 **Compression of vein**

Stricture of vein
Vena cava syndrome (inferior) (superior)

● **✓5ᵗʰ 459.3** **Chronic venous hypertension (idiopathic)**

Stasis edema

> **EXCLUDES**   *chronic venous hypertension due to deep vein thrombosis (459.10-459.9)*
>   *varicose veins (454.0-454.9)*

● **459.30** **Chronic venous hypertension without complications**

Asymptomatic chronic venous hypertension
Chronic venous hypertension NOS

● **459.31** **Chronic venous hypertension with ulcer**

● **459.32** **Chronic venous hypertension with inflammation**

● **459.33** **Chronic venous hypertension with ulcer and inflammation**

● **459.39** **Chronic venous hypertension with other complication**

✓5ᵗʰ 459.8 **Other specified disorders of circulatory system**

459.81 **Venous (peripheral) insufficiency, unspecified**

Chronic venous insufficiency NOS
Use additional code for any associated ulceration (707.10-707.9)

AHA: 2Q, '91, 20; M-A, '87, 6

DEF: Insufficient drainage, venous blood, any part of body, results in edema or dermatosis.

459.89 **Other**

Collateral circulation (venous), any site
Phlebosclerosis
Venofibrosis

459.9 **Unspecified circulatory system disorder**

✓4ᵗʰ
✓5ᵗʰ   Additional Digit Required   `Nonspecific PDx`   `Unacceptable PDx`   `Manifestation Code`   `MSP` Medicare Secondary Payer   ▶◀ Revised Text   ● New Code   ▲ Revised Code Title

2002 Ingenix, Inc.   October 2002 • Volume 1 — 135

8. DISEASES OF THE RESPIRATORY SYSTEM (460-519)

Use additional code to identify infectious organism

ACUTE RESPIRATORY INFECTIONS (460-466)

EXCLUDES *pneumonia and influenza (480.0-487.8)*

460 Acute nasopharyngitis [common cold]

Coryza (acute)
Nasal catarrh, acute
Nasopharyngitis:
  NOS
  acute
Nasopharyngitis:
  infective NOS
Rhinitis:
  acute
  infective

EXCLUDES *nasopharyngitis, chronic (472.2)*
pharyngitis:
  acute or unspecified (462)
  chronic (472.1)
rhinitis:
  allergic (477.0-477.9)
  chronic or unspecified (472.0)
sore throat:
  acute or unspecified (462)
  chronic (472.1)

AHA: 1Q, '88, 12

DEF: Acute inflammation of mucous membranes; extends from nares to pharynx.

✓4ᵗʰ 461 Acute sinusitis

INCLUDES abscess
empyema
infection
inflammation
suppuration
  acute, of sinus
  (accessory)
  (nasal)

EXCLUDES *chronic or unspecified sinusitis (473.0-473.9)*

461.0 Maxillary
Acute antritis

461.1 Frontal

461.2 Ethmoidal

461.3 Sphenoidal

461.8 Other acute sinusitis
Acute pansinusitis

461.9 Acute sinusitis, unspecified
Acute sinusitis NOS

462 Acute pharyngitis

Acute sore throat NOS
Pharyngitis (acute):
  NOS
  gangrenous
  infective
  phlegmonous
  pneumococcal
Pharyngitis (acute):
  staphylococcal
  suppurative
  ulcerative
Sore throat (viral) NOS
Viral pharyngitis

EXCLUDES *abscess:*
  peritonsillar [quinsy] (475)
  pharyngeal NOS (478.29)
  retropharyngeal (478.24)
chronic pharyngitis (472.1)
infectious mononucleosis (075)
that specified as (due to):
  Coxsackie (virus) (074.0)
  gonococcus (098.6)
  herpes simplex (054.79)
  influenza (487.1)
  septic (034.0)
  streptococcal (034.0)

AHA: 4Q, '99, 26; S-O, '85, 8

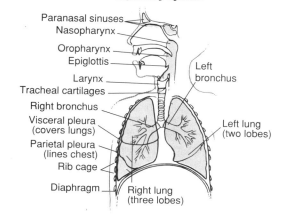

Respiratory System

Paranasal sinuses
Nasopharynx
Oropharynx
Epiglottis
Larynx
Tracheal cartilages
Right bronchus
Visceral pleura (covers lungs)
Parietal pleura (lines chest)
Rib cage
Diaphragm
Left bronchus
Left lung (two lobes)
Right lung (three lobes)

463 Acute tonsillitis

Tonsillitis (acute):
  NOS
  follicular
  gangrenous
  infective
  pneumococcal
Tonsillitis (acute):
  septic
  staphylococcal
  suppurative
  ulcerative
  viral

EXCLUDES *chronic tonsillitis (474.0)*
hypertrophy of tonsils (474.1)
peritonsillar abscess [quinsy] (475)
sore throat:
  acute or NOS (462)
  septic (034.0)
streptococcal tonsillitis (034.0)

AHA: N-D, '84, 16

✓4ᵗʰ 464 Acute laryngitis and tracheitis

EXCLUDES *that associated with influenza (487.1)*
that due to Streptococcus (034.0)

✓5ᵗʰ 464.0 Acute laryngitis
Laryngitis (acute):
  NOS
  edematous
  Hemophilus influenzae [H. influenzae]
  pneumococcal
  septic
  suppurative
  ulcerative

EXCLUDES *chronic laryngitis (476.0-476.1)*
influenzal laryngitis (487.1)

AHA: ▶4Q, '01, 42◀

DEF: ▶ A rapidly advancing generalized upper respiratory infection of the lingual tonsillar area, epiglottic folds, false vocal cords, and the epiglottis; seen most commonly in children, but can affect people of any age.◀

464.00 Without mention of obstruction

464.01 With obstruction

✓5ᵗʰ 464.1 Acute tracheitis
Tracheitis (acute):
  NOS
  catarrhal
Tracheitis (acute):
  viral

EXCLUDES *chronic tracheitis (491.8)*

464.10 Without mention of obstruction

464.11 With obstruction **CC**

CC Excl: 012.20-012.86, 017.90-017.96, 464.10-464.31, 519.8-519.9

✓5ᵗʰ 464.2 Acute laryngotracheitis
Laryngotracheitis (acute)
Tracheitis (acute) with laryngitis (acute)

EXCLUDES *chronic laryngotracheitis (476.1)*

464.20 Without mention of obstruction

464.21 With obstruction **CC**

CC Excl: See code 464.11

✓4ᵗʰ
✓5ᵗʰ Additional Digit Required   Nonspecific PDx   Unacceptable PDx   Manifestation Code   **MSP** Medicare Secondary Payer   ▶◀ Revised Text   ● New Code   ▲ Revised Code Title

Respiratory System 464.3–472.2

✓5ᵗʰ **464.3 Acute epiglottitis**
Viral epiglottitis
EXCLUDES *epiglottitis, chronic (476.1)*

464.30 Without mention of obstruction

464.31 With obstruction   CC
CC Excl: See code 464.11

464.4 Croup
Croup syndrome
DEF: Acute laryngeal obstruction due to allergy, foreign body or infection; symptoms include barking cough, hoarseness and harsh, persistent high-pitched respiratory sound.

✓5ᵗʰ **464.5 Supraglottitis, unspecified**
AHA: ▶4Q, '01, 42◀

DEF: A rapidly advancing generalized upper respiratory infection of the lingual tonsillar area, epiglottic folds, false vocal cords, and the epiglottis; seen most commonly in children, but can affect people of any age.

464.50 Without mention of obstruction
AHA: ▶4Q, '01, 43◀

464.51 With obstruction

✓4ᵗʰ **465 Acute upper respiratory infections of multiple or unspecified sites**
EXCLUDES *upper respiratory infection due to:*
influenza (487.1)
Streptococcus (034.0)

465.0 Acute laryngopharyngitis
DEF: Acute infection of the vocal cords and pharynx.

465.8 Other multiple sites
Multiple URI

465.9 Unspecified site
Acute URI NOS
Upper respiratory infection (acute)

✓4ᵗʰ **466 Acute bronchitis and bronchiolitis**
INCLUDES that with:
bronchospasm
obstruction

466.0 Acute bronchitis
Bronchitis, acute   Bronchitis, acute
or subacute: or subacute:
fibrinous   viral
membranous   with tracheitis
pneumococcal   Croupous bronchitis
purulent   Tracheobronchitis, acute
septic
EXCLUDES *acute bronchitis with:*
bronchiectasis (494.1)
chronic obstructive pulmonary
disease (491.21)

AHA: 4Q, '96, 28; 4Q, '91, 24; 1Q, '88, 12

DEF: Acute inflammation of main branches of bronchial tree due to infectious or irritant agents; symptoms include cough with a varied production of sputum, fever, substernal soreness, and lung rales.

✓5ᵗʰ **466.1 Acute bronchiolitis**
Bronchiolitis (acute)   Capillary pneumonia
DEF: Acute inflammation of finer subdivisions of bronchial tree due to infectious or irritant agents; symptoms include cough with a varied production of sputum, fever, substernal soreness, and lung rales.

466.11 Acute bronchiolitis due to respiratory syncytial virus (RSV)
AHA: 4Q, '96, 27

466.19 Acute bronchiolitis due to other infectious organisms
Use additional code to identify organism

OTHER DISEASES OF THE UPPER RESPIRATORY TRACT (470-478)

470 Deviated nasal septum
Deflected septum (nasal) (acquired)
EXCLUDES *congenital (754.0)*

✓4ᵗʰ **471 Nasal polyps**
EXCLUDES *adenomatous polyps (212.0)*

471.0 Polyp of nasal cavity
Polyp: Polyp:
choanal   nasopharyngeal

471.1 Polypoid sinus degeneration
Woakes' syndrome or ethmoiditis

471.8 Other polyp of sinus
Polyp of sinus:
accessory
ethmoidal
maxillary
sphenoidal

471.9 Unspecified nasal polyp
Nasal polyp NOS

✓4ᵗʰ **472 Chronic pharyngitis and nasopharyngitis**
472.0 Chronic rhinitis
Ozena   Rhinitis:
Rhinitis: hypertrophic
NOS   obstructive
atrophic   purulent
granulomatous   ulcerative
EXCLUDES *allergic rhinitis (477.0-477.9)*

DEF: Persistent inflammation of mucous membranes of nose.

472.1 Chronic pharyngitis
Chronic sore throat   Pharyngitis:
Pharyngitis: granular (chronic)
atrophic   hypertrophic

472.2 Chronic nasopharyngitis
EXCLUDES *acute or unspecified nasopharyngitis (460)*

DEF: Persistent inflammation of mucous membranes extending from nares to pharynx.

Upper Respiratory System

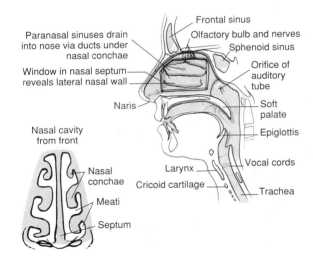

Paranasal sinuses drain into nose via ducts under nasal conchae
Window in nasal septum reveals lateral nasal wall
Naris
Nasal cavity from front
Nasal conchae
Meati
Septum
Frontal sinus
Olfactory bulb and nerves
Sphenoid sinus
Orifice of auditory tube
Soft palate
Epiglottis
Vocal cords
Larynx
Cricoid cartilage
Trachea

N Newborn Age: 0   P Pediatric Age: 0-17   M Maternity Age: 12-55   A Adult Age: 15-124   CC CC Condition   MC Major Complication   CD Complex Dx   HIV HIV Related Dx

138 — Volume 1 • January 2002   *2002 Ingenix, Inc.*

Paranasal Sinuses

Frontal
Ethmoid
Sphenoid
Maxillary
Frontal
Ethmoid
Sphenoid
Maxillary

✓4ᵗʰ **473 Chronic sinusitis**

INCLUDES
abscess
empyema   (chronic) of sinus
infection   (accessory) (nasal)
suppuration

EXCLUDES   *acute sinusitis (461.0-461.9)*

473.0   Maxillary
Antritis (chronic)

473.1   Frontal

473.2   Ethmoidal
EXCLUDES   *Woakes' ethmoiditis (471.1)*

473.3   Sphenoidal

473.8   Other chronic sinusitis
Pansinusitis (chronic)

473.9   Unspecified sinusitis (chronic)
Sinusitis (chronic) NOS

✓4ᵗʰ **474 Chronic disease of tonsils and adenoids**

✓5ᵗʰ **474.0   Chronic tonsillitis and adenoiditis**
EXCLUDES   *acute or unspecified tonsillitis (463)*
AHA: 4Q, '97, 38

474.00   Chronic tonsillitis

474.01   Chronic adenoiditis

474.02   Chronic tonsillitis and adenoiditis

✓5ᵗʰ **474.1   Hypertrophy of tonsils and adenoids**
Enlargement
Hyperplasia   of tonsils or adenoids
Hypertrophy

EXCLUDES   *that with:*
adenoiditis (474.01)
adenoiditis and tonsillitis (474.02)
tonsillitis (474.00)

474.10   Tonsils with adenoids

474.11   Tonsils alone

474.12   Adenoids alone

474.2   Adenoid vegetations
DEF: Fungus-like growth of lymph tissue between the nares and pharynx.

474.8   Other chronic disease of tonsils and adenoids
Amygdalolith   Tonsillar tag
Calculus, tonsil   Ulcer, tonsil
Cicatrix of tonsil (and adenoid)

474.9   Unspecified chronic disease of tonsils and adenoids
Disease (chronic) of tonsils (and adenoids)

475 Peritonsillar abscess   CC
Abscess of tonsil   Quinsy
Peritonsillar cellulitis
EXCLUDES   *tonsillitis:*
acute or NOS (463)
chronic (474.0)

CC Excl: 475, 519.8-519.9

✓4ᵗʰ **476 Chronic laryngitis and laryngotracheitis**

476.0   Chronic laryngitis
Laryngitis: Laryngitis:
catarrhal   sicca
hypertrophic

476.1   Chronic laryngotracheitis
Laryngitis, chronic, with tracheitis (chronic)
Tracheitis, chronic, with laryngitis
EXCLUDES   *chronic tracheitis (491.8)*
laryngitis and tracheitis, acute or
unspecified (464.00-464.51)

✓4ᵗʰ **477 Allergic rhinitis**
INCLUDES   allergic rhinitis (nonseasonal) (seasonal)
hay fever
spasmodic rhinorrhea
EXCLUDES   *allergic rhinitis with asthma (bronchial) (493.0)*

DEF: True immunoglobulin E (IgE)-mediated allergic reaction of nasal mucosa; seasonal (typical hay fever) or perennial (year-round allergens: dust, food, dander).

477.0   Due to pollen
Pollinosis

477.1   Due to food
AHA: 4Q, '00, 42

477.8   Due to other allergen

477.9   Cause unspecified
AHA: 2Q, '97, 9

✓4ᵗʰ **478 Other diseases of upper respiratory tract**

478.0   Hypertrophy of nasal turbinates
DEF: Overgrowth, enlargement of shell-shaped bones, in nasal cavity.

478.1   Other diseases of nasal cavity and sinuses
Abscess
Necrosis   of nose (septum)
Ulcer

Cyst or mucocele of sinus (nasal)
Rhinolith
EXCLUDES   *varicose ulcer of nasal septum (456.8)*

✓5ᵗʰ **478.2   Other diseases of pharynx, not elsewhere classified**

478.20   Unspecified disease of pharynx

478.21   Cellulitis of pharynx or nasopharynx   CC
CC Excl: 478.20-478.24, 519.8-519.9

478.22   Parapharyngeal abscess   CC
CC Excl: See code 478.21

478.24   Retropharyngeal abscess   CC
CC Excl: See code 478.21

DEF: Purulent infection, behind pharynx and front of precerebral fascia.

478.25   Edema of pharynx or nasopharynx

478.26   Cyst of pharynx or nasopharynx

478.29   Other
Abscess of pharynx or nasopharynx
EXCLUDES   *ulcerative pharyngitis (462)*

✓5ᵗʰ **478.3   Paralysis of vocal cords or larynx**
DEF: Loss of motor ability of vocal cords or larynx; due to nerve or muscle damage.

478.30   Paralysis, unspecified   CC
Laryngoplegia   Paralysis of glottis
CC Excl: 478.30-478.34, 478.5, 478.70, 519.8-519.9

✓4ᵗʰ
✓5ᵗʰ Additional Digit Required   Nonspecific PDx   Unacceptable PDx   Manifestation Code   MSP Medicare Secondary Payer   ▶◀ Revised Text   ● New Code   ▲ Revised Code Title

2002 Ingenix, Inc.   Volume 1 — 139

478.31 Unilateral, partial `CC`
    CC Excl: See code 478.30

478.32 Unilateral, complete `CC`
    CC Excl: See code 478.30

478.33 Bilateral, partial `CC`
    CC Excl: See code 478.30

478.34 Bilateral, complete `CC`
    CC Excl: See code 478.30

478.4 Polyp of vocal cord or larynx
    EXCLUDES *adenomatous polyps (212.1)*

478.5 Other diseases of vocal cords
    Abscess
    Cellulitis
    Granuloma } of vocal cords
    Leukoplakia

    Chorditis (fibrinous) (nodosa) (tuberosa)
    Singers' nodes

478.6 Edema of larynx
    Edema (of):   Edema (of):
      glottis   supraglottic
      subglottic

√5th **478.7 Other diseases of larynx, not elsewhere classified**
478.70 Unspecified disease of larynx
478.71 Cellulitis and perichondritis of larynx
    DEF: Inflammation of deep soft tissues or lining of bone of the larynx.

478.74 Stenosis of larynx
478.75 Laryngeal spasm
    Laryngismus (stridulus)
    DEF: Involuntary muscle contraction of the larynx.

478.79 Other
    Abscess
    Necrosis
    Obstruction } of larynx
    Pachyderma
    Ulcer
    EXCLUDES *ulcerative laryngitis (464.00-464.01)*
    AHA: 3Q, '91, 20

478.8 Upper respiratory tract hypersensitivity reaction, site unspecified
    EXCLUDES *hypersensitivity reaction of lower respiratory tract, as:*
        extrinsic allergic alveolitis (495.0-495.9)
        pneumoconiosis (500-505)

478.9 Other and unspecified diseases of upper respiratory tract
    Abscess } of trachea
    Cicatrix

Lungs

Right Lung (Three Lobes) — Trachea — **Left Lung (Two Lobes)**

Bronchopulmonary segments: S1   S3   Primary bronchus   Secondary bronchus

Upper lobe   S2   S1,2   S3 S4 S5   Upper lobe

Middle lobe   S5   S6

   S4   S7,8

Lower lobe   S8   S9 S10   S7 S10   Lower lobe   S9

Diaphragm

PNEUMONIA AND INFLUENZA (480-487)

    EXCLUDES *pneumonia:*
      allergic or eosinophilic (518.3)
      aspiration:
        NOS (507.0)
        newborn (770.1)
        solids and liquids (507.0-507.8)
      congenital (770.0)
      lipoid (507.1)
      passive (514)
      rheumatic (390)

√4th **480 Viral pneumonia**
480.0 Pneumonia due to adenovirus
480.1 Pneumonia due to respiratory syncytial virus
    AHA: 4Q, '96, 28; 1Q, '88, 12

480.2 Pneumonia due to parainfluenza virus
480.8 Pneumonia due to other virus not elsewhere classified `HIV`
    EXCLUDES *congenital rubella pneumonitis (771.0)*
      influenza with pneumonia, any form (487.0)
      pneumonia complicating viral diseases classified elsewhere (484.1-484.8)

480.9 Viral pneumonia, unspecified `HIV`
    AHA: 3Q, '98, 5

481 Pneumococcal pneumonia [Streptococcus pneumoniae pneumonia] `CC` `MC` `HIV`
    Lobar pneumonia, organism unspecified
    CC Excl: 011.00-011.06, 011.10-011.16, 011.20-011.26, 011.30-011.36, 011.40-011.46, 011.50-011.56, 011.60-011.66, 011.70-011.76, 011.80-011.86, 011.90-011.96, 012.00-012.06, 012.10-012.16, 012.80-012.86, 017.90-017.96, 021.2, 031.0, 039.1, 115.05, 115.15, 115.95, 122.1, 130.4, 136.3, 480.0-480.2, 480.8-480.9, 481, 482.0-482.2, 482.30-482.32, 482.39, 482.4, 482.81-482.84, 482.89, 482.9, 483.0-483.1, 483.8, 484.1, 484.3, 484.5-484.8, 485, 486, 487.0-487.1, 494.0-494.1, 495.0-495.9, 496, 500, 501, 502, 503, 504, 505, 506.0-506.4, 506.9, 507.0-507.1, 507.8, 508.0-508.1, 508.8, 508.9, 517.1-517.8, 18.89, 519.8, 519.9, 748.61

    AHA: 2Q, '98, 7; 4Q, '92, 19; 1Q, '92, 18; 1Q, '91, 13; 1Q, '88, 13; M-A, '85, 6

    DRG 089

√4th **482 Other bacterial pneumonia**
    AHA: 4Q, '93, 39

482.0 Pneumonia due to Klebsiella pneumoniae `CC` `MC` `HIV`
    CC Excl: See code 481

482.1 Pneumonia due to Pseudomonas `CC` `MC` `HIV`
    CC Excl: See code 481
    DRG 079

482.2 Pneumonia due to Hemophilus influenzae [H. influenzae] `CC` `MC` `HIV`
    CC Excl: See code 481

√5th **482.3 Pneumonia due to Streptococcus**
    EXCLUDES *Streptococcus pneumoniae (481)*
    AHA: 1Q, '88, 13

482.30 Streptococcus, unspecified `CC` `MC` `HIV`
    CC Excl: See code 481

482.31 Group A `CC` `MC` `HIV`
    CC Excl: See code 481

482.32 Group B `CC` `MC` `HIV`
    CC Excl: See code 481

482.39 Other Streptococcus `CC` `MC` `HIV`
    CC Excl: See code 481

`N` Newborn Age: 0   `P` Pediatric Age: 0-17   `M` Maternity Age: 12-55   `A` Adult Age: 15-124   `CC` CC Condition   `MC` Major Complication   `CD` Complex Dx   `HIV` HIV Related Dx

✓5ᵗʰ **482.4** **Pneumonia due to Staphylococcus**
AHA: 3Q, '91, 16

482.40 **Pneumonia due to** `CC` `MC` `HIV`
Staphylococcus unspecified
CC Excl: See code 481

▽ DRG 079

482.41 **Pneumonia due to** `CC` `MC` `HIV`
Staphylococcus aureus
CC Excl: See code 481

▽ DRG 079

482.49 **Other Staphylococcus** `CC` `MC` `HIV`
pneumonia
CC Excl: See code 481

▽ DRG 079

✓5ᵗʰ **482.8** **Pneumonia due to other specified bacteria**
EXCLUDES *pneumonia, complicating infectious*
disease classified elsewhere
(484.1-484.8)

AHA: 3Q, '88, 11

482.81 **Anaerobes** `CC` `MC` `HIV`
Bacteroides (melaninogenicus)
Gram-negative anaerobes
CC Excl: See code 481

482.82 **Escherichia coli [E. coli]** `CC` `MC` `HIV`
CC Excl: See code 481

482.83 **Other gram-negative bacteria** `CC` `MC` `HIV`
Gram-negative pneumonia NOS
Proteus
Serratia marcescens
EXCLUDES *gram-negative anaerobes*
(482.81)
Legionnaires' disease (482.84)
CC Excl: See code 481

AHA: 2Q, '98, 5; 3Q, '94, 9

▽ DRG 079

482.84 **Legionnaires' disease** `CC` `HIV`
CC Excl: See code 481

AHA: 4Q, '97, 38

DEF: Severe and often fatal infection by Legionella
pneumophilia; symptoms include high fever,
gastrointestinal pain, headache, myalgia, dry cough, and
pneumonia; transmitted airborne via air conditioning
systems, humidifiers, water faucets, shower heads; not
person-to-person contact.

482.89 **Other specified bacteria** `CC` `MC` `HIV`
CC Excl: See code 481

AHA: 2Q, '97, 6

482.9 **Bacterial pneumonia unspecified** `CC` `MC` `HIV`
CC Excl: See code 481

AHA: 2Q, '98, 6; 2Q, '97, 6; 1Q, '94, 17

✓4ᵗʰ **483** **Pneumonia due to other specified organism**
AHA: N-D, '87, 5

483.0 **Mycoplasma pneumoniae** `CC` `MC`
Eaton's agent
Pleuropneumonia-like organism [PPLO]
CC Excl: See code 481

483.1 **Chlamydia** `CC` `MC`
CC Excl: See code 481

AHA: 4Q, '96, 31

483.8 **Other specified organism** `CC` `MC`
CC Excl: See code 481

✓4ᵗʰ **484** **Pneumonia in infectious diseases classified elsewhere**
EXCLUDES *influenza with pneumonia, any form (487.0)*

484.1 **Pneumonia in cytomegalic inclusion disease** `CC` `MC`
Code first underlying disease (078.5)
CC Excl: See code 481

484.3 **Pneumonia in whooping cough** `CC` `MC`
Code first underlying disease (033.0-033.9)
CC Excl: See code 481

484.5 **Pneumonia in anthrax** `CC` `MC`
Code first underlying disease (022.1)
CC Excl: See code 481

484.6 **Pneumonia in aspergillosis** `CC` `MC`
Code first underlying disease (117.3)
CC Excl: See code 481

AHA: 4Q, '97, 40

484.7 **Pneumonia in other systemic mycoses** `CC` `MC`
Code first underlying disease
EXCLUDES *pneumonia in:*
candidiasis (112.4)
coccidioidomycosis (114.0)
histoplasmosis (115.0-115.9 with
fifth-digit 5)
CC Excl: See code 481

484.8 **Pneumonia in other infectious diseases** `CC` `MC`
classified elsewhere
Code first underlying disease, as:
Q fever (083.0)
typhoid fever (002.0)
EXCLUDES *pneumonia in:*
actinomycosis (039.1)
measles (055.1)
nocardiosis (039.1)
ornithosis (073.0)
Pneumocystis carinii (136.3)
salmonellosis (003.22)
toxoplasmosis (130.4)
tuberculosis (011.6)
tularemia (021.2)
varicella (052.1)
CC Excl: See code 481

485 **Bronchopneumonia, organism unspecified** `CC` `MC`
Bronchopneumonia: Pneumonia:
hemorrhagic   lobular
terminal   segmental
Pleurobronchopneumonia
EXCLUDES *bronchiolitis (acute) (466.11-466.19)*
chronic (491.8)
lipoid pneumonia (507.1)
CC Excl: See code 481

✓4ᵗʰ **Additional Digit Required**   **Nonspecific PDx**   **Unacceptable PDx**   **Manifestation Code**   `MSP` Medicare Secondary Payer   ▶◀ Revised Text   ● New Code   ▲ Revised Code Title
✓5ᵗʰ

2002 Ingenix, Inc.

Volume 1 — 141

486 Pneumonia, organism unspecified   `CC` `MC` `HIV`

> EXCLUDES   *hypostatic or passive pneumonia (514)*
> *influenza with pneumonia, any form (487.0)*
> *inhalation or aspiration pneumonia due to*
>   *foreign materials (507.0-507.8)*
> *pneumonitis due to fumes and vapors (506.0)*

CC Excl: See code 481

AHA: 4Q, '99, 6; 3Q, '99, 9; 3Q, '98, 7; 2Q, '98, 4, 5; 1Q, '98, 8; 3Q, '97, 9; 3Q, '94, 10; 3Q, '88, 11

▽ **DRG** 089 and 475

✓4ᵗʰ **487 Influenza**

> EXCLUDES   *Hemophilus influenzae [H. influenzae]:*
> *infection NOS (041.5)*
> *laryngitis (464.00-464.01)*
> *meningitis (320.0)*
> *pneumonia (482.2)*

487.0 With pneumonia   `CC` `MC`
> Influenza with pneumonia, any form
> Influenzal:
>   bronchopneumonia
>   pneumonia

CC Excl: See code 481

487.1 With other respiratory manifestations
> Influenza NOS
> Influenzal:
>   laryngitis
>   pharyngitis
>   respiratory infection (upper) (acute)

AHA: 4Q, '99, 26

487.8 With other manifestations
> Encephalopathy due to influenza
> Influenza with involvement of gastrointestinal tract
> EXCLUDES   *"intestinal flu" [viral gastroenteritis]*
>   *(008.8)*

CHRONIC OBSTRUCTIVE PULMONARY DISEASE AND ALLIED CONDITIONS (490-496)

AHA: 3Q, '88, 5

490 Bronchitis, not specified as acute or chronic
> Bronchitis NOS: Tracheobronchitis NOS
>   catarrhal
>   with tracheitis NOS
> EXCLUDES   *bronchitis:*
>   *allergic NOS (493.9)*
>   *asthmatic NOS (493.9)*
>   *due to fumes and vapors (506.0)*

✓4ᵗʰ **491 Chronic bronchitis**
> EXCLUDES   *chronic obstructive asthma (493.2)*

491.0 Simple chronic bronchitis
> Catarrhal bronchitis, chronic
> Smokers' cough

Bronchioli and Alveoli

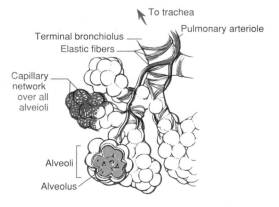

↖ To trachea

Pulmonary arteriole

Terminal bronchiolus

Elastic fibers

Capillary network over all alveioli

Alveoli

Alveolus

491.1 Mucopurulent chronic bronchitis   `CC`
> Bronchitis (chronic) (recurrent):
>   fetid
>   mucopurulent
>   purulent

CC Excl: 491.1-491.9, 493.20-493.21

AHA: 3Q, '88, 12

DEF: Chronic bronchial infection characterized by both mucus and pus secretions in the bronchial tree; recurs after asymptomatic periods; signs are coughing, expectoration and secondary changes in the lung.

✓5ᵗʰ **491.2 Obstructive chronic bronchitis**
> Bronchitis:
>   emphysematous
>   obstructive (chronic) (diffuse)
> Bronchitis with:
>   chronic airway obstruction
>   emphysema
> EXCLUDES   *asthmatic bronchitis (acute) NOS*
>   *(493.9)*
>   *chronic obstructive asthma (493.2)*

AHA: 3Q, '97, 9; 4Q, '91, 25; 2Q, '91, 21

491.20 Without mention of acute exacerbation   `CC`
> Emphysema with chronic bronchitis

CC Excl: See code 491.1

AHA: 3Q, '97, 9

491.21 With acute exacerbation   `CC`
> Acute and chronic obstructive bronchitis
> Acute bronchitis with chronic obstructive pulmonary disease [COPD]
> Acute exacerbation of chronic obstructive pulmonary disease [COPD]
> Emphysema with both acute and chronic bronchitis
> EXCLUDES   *chronic obstructive asthma*
>   *with acute exacerbation*
>   *(493.22)*

CC Excl: See code 491.1

AHA: ▶ 4Q, '01, 43; ◀ 2Q, '96, 10

▽ **DRG** 088 and 475

491.8 Other chronic bronchitis   `CC`
> Chronic:
>   tracheitis
>   tracheobronchitis

CC Excl: See code 491.1

491.9 Unspecified chronic bronchitis   `CC`
CC Excl: See code 491.1

✓4ᵗʰ **492 Emphysema**
AHA: 2Q, '91, 21

492.0 Emphysematous bleb
> Giant bullous emphysema
> Ruptured emphysematous bleb
> Tension pneumatocele
> Vanishing lung

AHA: 2Q, '93, 3

DEF: Formation of vesicle or bulla in emphysematous lung, more than one millimeter; contains serum or blood.

`N` Newborn Age: 0   `P` Pediatric Age: 0-17   `M` Maternity Age: 12-55   `A` Adult Age: 15-124   `CC` CC Condition   `MC` Major Complication   `CD` Complex Dx   `HIV` HIV Related Dx

492.8 Other emphysema `CC`

Emphysema (lung or pulmonary):
NOS
centriacinar
centrilobular
obstructive
panacinar
panlobular

Emphysema (lung or pulmonary):
unilateral
vesicular
MacLeod's syndrome
Swyer-James syndrome
Unilateral hyperlucent lung

EXCLUDES *emphysema:*
with both acute and chronic bronchitis (491.21)
with chronic bronchitis (491.2)
compensatory (518.2)
due to fumes and vapors (506.4)
interstitial (518.1)
newborn (770.2)
mediastinal (518.1)
surgical (subcutaneous) (998.81)
traumatic (958.7)

CC Excl: 492.0, 492.8, 493.20-493.21

AHA: 4Q, '93, 41; J-A, '84, 17

✓4th **493 Asthma**

EXCLUDES *wheezing NOS (786.07)*

The following fifth-digit subclassification is for use with category 493:

0 **without mention of status asthmaticus or acute exacerbation or unspecified**
1 **with status asthmaticus**
2 **with acute exacerbation**

AHA: 4Q, '01, 43; 4Q, '00, 42; 1Q, '91, 13; 3Q, '88, 9; J-A, '85, 8; N-D, '84, 17

DEF: Status asthmaticus: severe, intractable episode of asthma unresponsive to normal therapeutic measures.

✓5th **493.0 Extrinsic asthma** `CC 1-2`

Asthma:
allergic with
stated cause
atopic
childhood

Asthma:
hay
platinum
Hay fever with asthma

EXCLUDES *asthma:*
allergic NOS (493.9)
detergent (507.8)
miners' (500)
wood (495.8)

CC Excl: For code 493.01 and 493.02: 493.00-493.92, 517.8, 518.89, 519.8-519.9

DEF: Transient stricture of airway diameters of bronchi; due to environmental factor; also called allergic (bronchial) asthma.

✓5th **493.1 Intrinsic asthma** `CC 1-2`
Late-onset asthma
CC Excl: For code 493.11 and 493.12: See code 493.0

AHA: 3Q, '88, 9; M-A, '85, 7

DEF: Transient stricture, of airway diameters of bronchi; due to pathophysiological disturbances.

✓5th **493.2 Chronic obstructive asthma** `CC`
Asthma with chronic obstructive pulmonary disease [COPD]
▶Chronic asthmatic bronchitis◀

EXCLUDES *acute bronchitis (466.0)*

CC Excl: For code 493.20 and 493.21: 491.1-493.92, 517.8, 518.89, 519.8-519.9; For code 493.22: 493.00-493.92, 517.8, 518.89, 519.8-519.9

AHA: 2Q, '91, 21; 2Q, '90, 20

DRG 088 For code 493.20

DEF: Persistent narrowing of airway diameters in the bronchial tree, restricting airflow and causing constant labored breathing.

✓5th **493.9 Asthma, unspecified** `CC 1-2`
Asthma (bronchial) (allergic NOS)
Bronchitis:
allergic
asthmatic

CC Excl: For code 493.91 and 493.92: 493.00-493.92, 517.8, 518.89, 519.8-519.9

AHA: 4Q, '97, 40, For code 493.90: 4Q, '99, 25; 1Q, '97, 7

✓4th **494 Bronchiectasis**
Bronchiectasis (fusiform) (postinfectious) (recurrent)
Bronchiolectasis

EXCLUDES *congenital (748.61)*
tuberculous bronchiectasis (current disease) (011.5)

AHA: 4Q, '00, 42

DEF: Dilation of bronchi; due to infection or chronic conditions; causes decreased lung capacity and recurrent infections of lungs.

494.0 Bronchiectasis without acute exacerbation
494.1 Bronchiectasis with acute exacerbation `CC`
Acute bronchitis with bronchiectasis
CC Excl: 017.90-017.96, 487.1, 494.1, 496, 506.1, 506.4, 506.9, 748.61

✓4th **495 Extrinsic allergic alveolitis**

INCLUDES allergic alveolitis and pneumonitis due to inhaled organic dust particles of fungal, thermophilic actinomycete, or other origin

DEF: Pneumonitis due to particles inhaled into lung, often at workplace; symptoms include cough, chills, fever, increased heart and respiratory rates; develops within hours of exposure.

495.0 Farmers' lung `CC`
CC Excl: 011.00-011.96, 012.00-012.16, 012.80-012.86, 017.90-017.96, 021.2, 031.0, 039.1, 115.05, 115.15, 115.95, 122.1, 130.4, 136.3, 480.0-480.9, 481, 482.0-482.7, 482.81-482.84, 482.89, 482.9, 483.0, 483.1, 483.8, 484.1-484.8, 485-486, 487.0-487.1, 494.0-494.1, 495.0-495.9, 496, 500-505, 506.0-506.9, 507.0-507.8, 508.0-508.9, 517.1, 517.8, 518.89, 519.8-519.9, 748.61

495.1 Bagassosis `CC`
CC Excl: See code 495.0

495.2 Bird-fanciers' lung `CC`
Budgerigar-fanciers' disease or lung
Pigeon-fanciers' disease or lung
CC Excl: See code 495.0

495.3 Suberosis `CC`
Cork-handlers' disease or lung
CC Excl: See code 495.0

495.4 Malt workers' lung `CC`
Alveolitis due to Aspergillus clavatus
CC Excl: See code 495.0

495.5 Mushroom workers' lung `CC`
CC Excl: See code 495.0

495.6 Maple bark-strippers' lung `CC`
Alveolitis due to Cryptostroma corticale
CC Excl: See code 495.0

495.7 "Ventilation" pneumonitis `CC`
Allergic alveolitis due to fungal, thermophilic actinomycete, and other organisms growing in ventilation [air conditioning] systems
CC Excl: See code 495.0

Respiratory System 492.8–495.7

✓4th ✓5th Additional Digit Required   Nonspecific PDx   Unacceptable PDx   Manifestation Code   **MSP** Medicare Secondary Payer   ▶◀ Revised Text   ● New Code   ▲ Revised Code Title

495.8 Other specified allergic alveolitis and pneumonitis `CC`
  Cheese-washers' lung
  Coffee workers' lung
  Fish-meal workers' lung
  Furriers' lung
  Grain-handlers' disease or lung
  Pituitary snuff-takers' disease
  Sequoiosis or red-cedar asthma
  Wood asthma
  CC Excl: See code 495.0

495.9 Unspecified allergic alveolitis and pneumonitis `CC`
  Alveolitis, allergic (extrinsic)
  Hypersensitivity pneumonitis
  CC Excl: See code 495.0

496 Chronic airway obstruction, not elsewhere classified `CC` `A`
  Note: This code is not to be used with any code from categories 491-493
  Chronic:
    nonspecific lung disease
    obstructive lung disease
    obstructive pulmonary disease [COPD] NOS
    EXCLUDES chronic obstructive lung disease [COPD]
        specified (as) (with):
        allergic alveolitis (495.0-495.9)
        asthma (493.2)
        bronchiectasis (494.0-494.1)
        bronchitis (491.20-491.21)
          with emphysema (491.20-491.21)
        emphysema (492.0-492.8)
  CC Excl: 017.90-017.96, 487.1, 494.0-494.1, 496, 506.1, 506.4, 506.9, 748.61

  AHA: 2Q, '00, 15; 2Q, '92, 16; 2Q, '91, 21; 3Q, '88, 56

  `DRG` 088

PNEUMOCONIOSES AND OTHER LUNG DISEASES DUE TO EXTERNAL AGENTS (500-508)

  DEF: Permanent deposits of particulate matter, within lungs; due to occupational or environmental exposure; results in chronic induration and fibrosis. (See specific listings in 500-508 code range)

500 Coal workers' pneumoconiosis `A`
  Anthracosilicosis   Coal workers' lung
  Anthracosis   Miner's asthma
  Black lung disease

501 Asbestosis `A`

502 Pneumoconiosis due to other silica or silicates
  Pneumoconiosis due to talc
  Silicotic fibrosis (massive) of lung
  Silicosis (simple) (complicated)

503 Pneumoconiosis due to other inorganic dust
  Aluminosis (of lung)   Graphite fibrosis (of lung)
  Bauxite fibrosis (of lung) Siderosis
  Berylliosis   Stannosis

504 Pneumonopathy due to inhalation of other dust
  Byssinosis   Flax-dressers' disease
  Cannabinosis
    EXCLUDES allergic alveolitis (495.0-495.9)
        asbestosis (501)
        bagassosis (495.1)
        farmers' lung (495.0)

505 Pneumoconiosis, unspecified

√4th 506 Respiratory conditions due to chemical fumes and vapors
  Use additional E code to identify cause

506.0 Bronchitis and pneumonitis due to fumes and vapors `CC`
  Chemical bronchitis (acute)
  CC Excl: 011.00-011.96, 012.10-012.16, 012.80-012.86, 017.90-017.96, 021.2, 031.0, 039.1, 115.05, 115.15, 115.95, 122.1, 130.4, 136.3, 480.0-480.9, 481, 482.0-482.7, 482.81-482.84, 482.89, 482.9, 483.0, 483.1, 483.8, 484.1-484.8, 485-486, 487.0-487.1, 494.0-494.1, 495.0-495.9, 496, 500-505, 506.0-506.9, 507.0-507.8, 508.0-508.9, 517.1, 517.8, 518.89, 519.8-519.9, 748.61

506.1 Acute pulmonary edema due to fumes and vapors `CC`
  Chemical pulmonary edema (acute)
    EXCLUDES acute pulmonary edema NOS (518.4)
        chronic or unspecified pulmonary edema (514)
  CC Excl: See code 506.0

  AHA: 3Q, '88, 4

506.2 Upper respiratory inflammation due to fumes and vapors

506.3 Other acute and subacute respiratory conditions due to fumes and vapors

506.4 Chronic respiratory conditions due to fumes and vapors
  Emphysema (diffuse) (chronic)
  Obliterative bronchiolitis (chronic) (subacute)   due to inhalation of chemical fumes and vapors
  Pulmonary fibrosis (chronic)

506.9 Unspecified respiratory conditions due to fumes and vapors
  Silo-fillers' disease

√4th 507 Pneumonitis due to solids and liquids
  EXCLUDES fetal aspiration pneumonitis (770.1)
  AHA: 3Q, '91, 16

507.0 Due to inhalation of food or vomitus `CC` `MC`
  Aspiration pneumonia (due to):
    NOS
    food (regurgitated)
    gastric secretions
    milk
    saliva
    vomitus
  CC Excl: See code 506.0

  AHA: 1Q, '89, 10

  `DRG` 079 and 475

507.1 Due to inhalation of oils and essences `CC` `MC`
  Lipoid pneumonia (exogenous)
    EXCLUDES endogenous lipoid pneumonia (516.8)
  CC Excl: See code 506.0

507.8 Due to other solids and liquids `CC` `MC`
  Detergent asthma
  CC Excl: See code 506.0

√4th 508 Respiratory conditions due to other and unspecified external agents
  Use additional E code to identify cause

508.0 Acute pulmonary manifestations due to radiation `CC`
  Radiation pneumonitis
  CC Excl: See code 506.0

  AHA: 2Q, '88, 4

508.1 Chronic and other pulmonary manifestations due to radiation `CC`
  Fibrosis of lung following radiation
  CC Excl: See code 506.0

508.8 Respiratory conditions due to other specified external agents

---

508.9   Respiratory conditions due to unspecified external agent

OTHER DISEASES OF RESPIRATORY SYSTEM (510-519)

√4ᵗʰ **510 Empyema**

Use additional code to identify infectious organism (041.0-041.9)

EXCLUDES   *abscess of lung (513.0)*

DEF: Purulent infection, within pleural space.

510.0   With fistula   CC

Fistula:
bronchocutaneous
bronchopleural
hepatopleural
mediastinal
pleural
thoracic
Any condition classifiable to 510.9 with fistula

CC Excl: 510.0, 510.9, 517.8, 518.89, 519.8-519.9

DEF: Purulent infection of respiratory cavity; with communication from cavity to another structure.

510.9   Without mention of fistula   CC

Abscess: Pleurisy:
pleura   septic
thorax   seropurulent
Empyema (chest) (lung)   suppurative
(pleura)   Pyopneumothorax
Fibrinopurulent pleurisy Pyothorax
Pleurisy:
purulent

CC Excl: See code 510.0

AHA: 3Q, '94, 6

√4ᵗʰ **511 Pleurisy**

EXCLUDES   *malignant pleural effusion (197.2)*
pleurisy with mention of tuberculosis,
current disease (012.0)

DEF: Inflammation of serous membrane of lungs and lining of thoracic cavity; causes exudation in cavity or membrane surface.

511.0   Without mention of effusion or current tuberculosis

Adhesion, lung or pleura Pleurisy:
Calcification of pleura   NOS
Pleurisy (acute) (sterile): pneumococcal
diaphragmatic   staphylococcal
fibrinous   streptococcal
interlobar   Thickening of pleura

AHA: 3Q, '94, 5

511.1   With effusion, with mention of a bacterial cause other than tuberculosis   CC

Pleurisy with effusion (exudative) (serous):
pneumococcal
staphylococcal
streptococcal
other specified nontuberculous bacterial cause

CC Excl: 011.00-011.96, 012.00-012.16, 012.80-012.86, 017.90-017.96, 511.0-511.9, 517.8, 518.89, 519.8-519.9

511.8   Other specified forms of effusion, except tuberculous   CC

Encysted pleurisy
Hemopneumothorax
Hemothorax
Hydropneumothorax
Hydrothorax

EXCLUDES   *traumatic (860.2-860.5, 862.29, 862.39)*

CC Excl: See code 511.1

AHA: 1Q, '97, 10

511.9   Unspecified pleural effusion   CC

Pleural effusion NOS
Pleurisy:
exudative
serofibrinous
serous
with effusion NOS

CC Excl: See code 511.1

AHA: 3Q, '91, 19; 4Q, '89, 11

√4ᵗʰ **512 Pneumothorax**

DEF: Collapsed lung; due to gas or air in pleural space.

512.0   Spontaneous tension pneumothorax   CC

CC Excl: 512.0-512.1, 512.8, 517.8, 518.89, 519.8-519.9

AHA: 3Q, '94, 5

DEF: Leaking air from lung into lining causing collapse.

512.1   Iatrogenic pneumothorax   CC

Postoperative pneumothorax

CC Excl: See code 512.0

AHA: 4Q, '94, 40

DEF: Air trapped in the lining of the lung following surgery.

512.8   Other spontaneous pneumothorax   CC

Pneumothorax:
NOS
acute
chronic

EXCLUDES   *pneumothorax:*
congenital (770.2)
traumatic (860.0-860.1, 860.4-860.5)
tuberculous, current disease (011.7)

CC Excl: See code 512.0

AHA: 2Q, '93, 3

√4ᵗʰ **513 Abscess of lung and mediastinum**

513.0   Abscess of lung   CC

Abscess (multiple) of lung
Gangrenous or necrotic pneumonia
Pulmonary gangrene or necrosis

CC Excl: 006.4, 011.00-011.96, 012.00-012.16, 012.80-012.86, 017.90-017.96, 513.0, 519.8-519.9

AHA: 2Q, '98, 7

513.1   Abscess of mediastinum   CC

CC Excl: 513.1, 519.8-519.9

514 Pulmonary congestion and hypostasis

Hypostatic: Pulmonary edema:
bronchopneumonia   NOS
pneumonia   chronic
Passive pneumonia
Pulmonary congestion
(chronic) (passive)

EXCLUDES   *acute pulmonary edema:*
NOS (518.4)
with mention of heart disease or failure (428.1)

AHA: 2Q, '98, 6; 3Q, '88, 5

DEF: Excessive retention of interstitial fluid in the lungs and pulmonary vessels; due to poor circulation.

√4ᵗʰ √5ᵗʰ Additional Digit Required   Nonspecific PDx   Unacceptable PDx   Manifestation Code   MSP Medicare Secondary Payer   ►◄ Revised Text   ● New Code   ▲ Revised Code Title

2002 Ingenix, Inc.

Volume 1 — 145

Respiratory System 515–518.4

515 Postinflammatory pulmonary fibrosis `CC`

Cirrhosis of lung
Fibrosis of lung (atrophic)
  (confluent) (massive)   ⎫
  (perialveolar)   ⎬ chronic or unspecified
  (peribronchial)   ⎭
Induration of lung

CC Excl: 011.00-011.96, 012.00-012.16, 012.80-012.86, 017.90-017.96, 494.0-494.1, 495.0-495.9, 496, 500-505, 506.0-506.9, 507.0-507.8, 508.0-508.9, 515, 516.0-516.9, 517.2, 517.8, 518.89, 519.8-519.9, 748.61

DEF: Fibrosis and scarring of the lungs due to inflammatory reaction.

✓4ᵗʰ 516 Other alveolar and parietoalveolar pneumonopathy

516.0 Pulmonary alveolar proteinosis `CC`
CC Excl: See code 515

DEF: Reduced ventilation; due to proteinaceous deposits on alveoli; symptoms include dyspnea, cough, chest pain, weakness, weight loss, and hemoptysis.

516.1 *Idiopathic pulmonary hemosiderosis* `CC`
Code first underlying disease (275.0)
Essential brown induration of lung
CC Excl: See code 515

DEF: Fibrosis of alveolar walls; marked by abnormal amounts hemosiderin in lungs; primarily affects children; symptoms include anemia, fluid in lungs, and blood in sputum; etiology unknown.

516.2 Pulmonary alveolar microlithiasis `CC`
CC Excl: See code 515

DEF: Small calculi in pulmonary alveoli resembling sand-like particles on x-ray.

516.3 Idiopathic fibrosing alveolitis `CC`
Alveolar capillary block
Diffuse (idiopathic) (interstitial) pulmonary fibrosis
Hamman-Rich syndrome
CC Excl: See code 515

516.8 Other specified alveolar and parietoalveolar pneumonopathies `CC`
Endogenous lipoid pneumonia
Interstitial pneumonia (desquamative) (lymphoid)
> **EXCLUDES** *lipoid pneumonia, exogenous or unspecified (507.1)*

CC Excl: See code 515

AHA: 1Q, '92, 12

516.9 Unspecified alveolar and parietoalveolar pneumonopathy `CC`
CC Excl: See code 515

✓4ᵗʰ 517 Lung involvement in conditions classified elsewhere
> **EXCLUDES** *rheumatoid lung (714.81)*

517.1 *Rheumatic pneumonia* `CC`
Code first underlying disease (390)
CC Excl: 011.00-011.96, 012.00-012.16, 012.80-012.86, 017.90-017.96, 480.0-480.9, 481, 482.0-482.7, 482.81-482.84, 482.89, 482.9, 483.0, 483.1, 483.8, 484.1-484.8, 485-486, 487.0-487.1, 494.0-494.1, |495.0-495.9, 496, 500-505, 506.0-506.9, 507.0-507.8, 508.0-508.9, 515, 516.0-516.9, 517.1-517.8, 518.89, 519.8-519.9, 748.61

517.2 *Lung involvement in systemic sclerosis* `CC`
Code first underlying disease (710.1)
CC Excl: 011.00-011.96, 012.00-012.16, 012.80-012.86, 017.90-017.96, 494.0-494.1, 495.0-495.9, 496, 500-505, 506.0-506.9, 507.0-507.8, 508.0-508.9, 515, 516.0-516.9, 517.2, 517.8, 518.89, 519.8-519.9, 748.61

517.8 *Lung involvement in other diseases classified elsewhere* `CC`
Code first underlying disease, as:
  amyloidosis (277.3)
  polymyositis (710.4)
  sarcoidosis (135)
  Sjögren's disease (710.2)
  systemic lupus erythematosus (710.0)
> **EXCLUDES** *syphilis (095.1)*

CC Excl: See code 517.2

✓4ᵗʰ 518 Other diseases of lung

518.0 Pulmonary collapse `CC` `MC`
Atelectasis
Collapse of lung
Middle lobe syndrome
> **EXCLUDES** *atelectasis:*
> * congenital (partial) (770.5)*
> *   primary (770.4)*
> * tuberculous, current disease (011.8)*

CC Excl: 518.0, 519.8-519.9

AHA: 4Q, '90, 25

518.1 Interstitial emphysema `CC`
Mediastinal emphysema
> **EXCLUDES** *surgical (subcutaneous) emphysema (998.81)*
> *that in fetus or newborn (770.2)*
> *traumatic emphysema (958.7)*

CC Excl: 518.1, 519.8-519.9

DEF: Escaped air from the alveoli trapped in the interstices of the lung; trauma or cough may cause the disease.

518.2 Compensatory emphysema
DEF: Distention of all or part of the lung caused by disease processes or surgical intervention that decreased volume in another part of the lung; overcompensation reaction to the loss of capacity in another part of the lung.

518.3 Pulmonary eosinophilia
Eosinophilic asthma
Löffler's syndrome
Pneumonia:
  allergic
  eosinophilic
Tropical eosinophilia
DEF: Infiltration, into pulmonary parenchyma of eosinophilia; results in cough, fever, and dyspnea.

518.4 Acute edema of lung, unspecified `CC`
Acute pulmonary edema NOS
Pulmonary edema, postoperative
> **EXCLUDES** *pulmonary edema:*
> * acute, with mention of heart disease or failure (428.1)*
> * chronic or unspecified (514)*
> * due to external agents (506.0-508.9)*

CC Excl: 398.91, 428.0-428.9, 518.4, 519.8-519.9

▽ **DRG** 087

DEF: Severe, sudden fluid retention within lung tissues.

N Newborn Age: 0   **P** Pediatric Age: 0-17   **M** Maternity Age: 12-55   **A** Adult Age :15-124   **CC** CC Condition   **MC** Major Complication   **CD** Complex Dx   **HIV** HIV Related Dx

146 — Volume 1   *2002 Ingenix, Inc.*

518.5 Pulmonary insufficiency following trauma and surgery `CC` `MC`
Adult respiratory distress syndrome
Pulmonary insufficiency following:
shock
surgery
trauma
Shock lung
EXCLUDES adult respiratory distress syndrome
associated with other conditions
(518.82)
pneumonia:
aspiration (507.0)
hypostatic (514)
respiratory failure in other conditions
(518.81, 518.83-518.84)

CC Excl: 518.5, 519.8-519.9

AHA: 3Q, '88, 3; 3Q, '88, 7; S-O, '87, 1

518.6 Allergic bronchopulmonary aspergillosis `CC`
CC Excl: 518.6, 519.8-519.9

AHA: 4Q, '97, 39

DEF: Noninvasive hypersensitive reaction; due to allergic reaction to *Aspergillus fumigatus* (mold).

√5th 518.8 Acute respiratory failure
518.81 Acute respiratory failure `CC` `MC`
Respiratory failure NOS
EXCLUDES acute and chronic respiratory
failure (518.84)
acute respiratory distress
(518.82)
chronic respiratory failure
(518.83)
respiratory arrest (799.1)
respiratory failure, newborn
▶(770.84)◀

CC Excl: 518.81-518.89, 519.8-519.9, 799.1

AHA: 4Q, '98, 41; 3Q, '91, 14; 2Q, '91, 3; 4Q, '90, 25;
2Q, '90, 20; 3Q, '88, 7; 3Q, '88, 10; S-O, '87, 1

DRG 087 and 475

518.82 Other pulmonary insufficiency, not `CC`
elsewhere classified
Acute respiratory distress
Acute respiratory insufficiency
Adult respiratory distress syndrome NEC
EXCLUDES adult respiratory distress
syndrome associated
with trauma and surgery
(518.5)
pulmonary insufficiency
following trauma and
surgery (518.5)
respiratory distress:
NOS (786.09)
newborn ▶(770.89)◀
syndrome, newborn (769)
shock lung (518.5)

CC Excl: See code 518.81

AHA: 2Q, '91, 21; 3Q, '88, 7

518.83 Chronic respiratory failure `CC` `MC`
CC Excl: See code 518.81

518.84 Acute and chronic respiratory `CC` `MC`
failure
Acute on chronic respiratory failure
CC Excl: See code 518.81

518.89 Other diseases of lung, not elsewhere
classified
Broncholithiasis   Lung disease NOS
Calcification of lung   Pulmolithiasis
AHA: 3Q, '90, 18; 4Q, '88, 6

DEF: Broncholithiasis: calculi in lumen of transbronchial tree.

DEF: Pulmolithiasis: calculi in lung.

√4th 519 Other diseases of respiratory system
√5th 519.0 Tracheostomy complications
519.00 Tracheostomy complication, unspecified `CC`
CC Excl: 519.0-519.1, 519.8-519.9

519.01 Infection of tracheostomy `CC`
Use additional code to identify type of
infection, such as:
abscess or cellulitis of neck (682.1)
septicemia (038.0-038.9)
Use additional code to identify organism
(041.00-041.9)
CC Excl: See code 519.00

AHA: 4Q, '98, 41

519.02 Mechanical complication of `CC`
tracheostomy
Tracheal stenosis due to tracheostomy
CC Excl: See code 519.00

519.09 Other tracheostomy complications `CC`
Hemorrhage due to tracheostomy
Tracheoesophageal fistula due to
tracheostomy
CC Excl: See code 519.00

519.1 Other diseases of trachea and bronchus, not
elsewhere classified
Calcification ⎫
Stenosis   ⎬ of bronchus or trachea
Ulcer   ⎭

AHA: 3Q, '88, 6

519.2 Mediastinitis `CC`
CC Excl: 519.2-519.3, 519.8-519.9

DEF: Inflammation of tissue between organs behind sternum.

519.3 Other diseases of mediastinum, not elsewhere
classified
Fibrosis ⎫
Hernia   ⎬ of mediastinum
Retraction ⎭

519.4 Disorders of diaphragm
Diaphragmitis   Relaxation of diaphragm
Paralysis of diaphragm
EXCLUDES congenital defect of diaphragm (756.6)
diaphragmatic hernia (551-553 with .3)
congenital (756.6)

519.8 Other diseases of respiratory system, not elsewhere
classified
AHA: 4Q, '89, 12

519.9 Unspecified disease of respiratory system
Respiratory disease (chronic) NOS

9. DISEASES OF THE DIGESTIVE SYSTEM (520-579)

DISEASES OF ORAL CAVITY, SALIVARY GLANDS, AND JAWS (520-529)

✓4ᵗʰ **520 Disorders of tooth development and eruption**

520.0 Anodontia
Absence of teeth (complete) (congenital) (partial)
Hypodontia
Oligodontia
EXCLUDES *acquired absence of teeth (525.10-525.19)*

520.1 Supernumerary teeth
Distomolar
Fourth molar
Mesiodens
Paramolar
Supplemental teeth
EXCLUDES *supernumerary roots (520.2)*

520.2 Abnormalities of size and form
Concrescence
Fusion ⎫ of teeth
Gemination ⎭

Dens evaginatus   Microdontia
Dens in dente   Peg-shaped [conical] teeth
Dens invaginatus   Supernumerary roots
Enamel pearls   Taurodontism
Macrodontia   Tuberculum paramolare
EXCLUDES *that due to congenital syphilis (090.5) tuberculum Carabelli, which is regarded as a normal variation*

Digestive System

The Oral Cavity

Teeth

Maxillary view

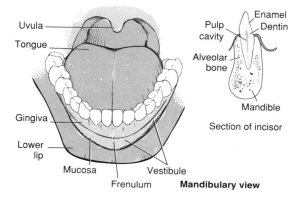

Mandibulary view

520.3 Mottled teeth
Mottling of enamel
Dental fluorosis   Nonfluoride enamel opacities

520.4 Disturbances of tooth formation
Aplasia and hypoplasia of cementum
Dilaceration of tooth
Enamel hypoplasia (neonatal) (postnatal) (prenatal)
Horner's teeth
Hypocalcification of teeth
Regional odontodysplasia
Turner's tooth
EXCLUDES *Hutchinson's teeth and mulberry molars in congenital syphilis (090.5)*
mottled teeth (520.3)

520.5 Hereditary disturbances in tooth structure, not elsewhere classified
Amelogenesis ⎫
Dentinogenesis ⎬ imperfecta
Odontogenesis ⎭

Dental dysplasia
Shell teeth

Digestive System 520–520.5

✓4ᵗʰ ✓5ᵗʰ Additional Digit Required   Nonspecific PDx   Unacceptable PDx   Manifestation Code   **MSP** Medicare Secondary Payer   ►◄ Revised Text   ● New Code   ▲ Revised Code Title

2002 Ingenix, Inc.

Volume 1 — 149

Digestive System 520.6–523.2

520.6 Disturbances in tooth eruption

Teeth:
  embedded
  impacted
  natal
  neonatal
  primary [deciduous]:
    persistent
    shedding, premature

Tooth eruption:
  late
  obstructed
  premature

EXCLUDES *exfoliation of teeth (attributable to disease of surrounding tissues) (525.0-525.19)*
impacted or embedded teeth with abnormal position of such teeth or adjacent teeth (524.3)

520.7 Teething syndrome

520.8 Other specified disorders of tooth development and eruption

Color changes during tooth formation
Pre-eruptive color changes

EXCLUDES *posteruptive color changes (521.7)*

520.9 Unspecified disorder of tooth development and eruption

✓4th **521 Diseases of hard tissues of teeth**

✓5th **521.0 Dental caries**

AHA: ▶4Q, '01, 44◀

521.00 Dental caries, unspecified

521.01 Dental caries limited to enamel
Initial caries
White spot lesion

521.02 Dental caries extending into dentine

521.03 Dental caries extending into pulp

521.04 Arrested dental caries

521.05 Odontoclasia
Infantile melanodontia
Melanodontoclasia

EXCLUDES *internal and external resorption of teeth (521.4)*

DEF: ▶ A pathological dental condition described as stained areas, loss of tooth substance, and hypoplasia linked to nutritional deficiencies during tooth development and to cariogenic oral conditions; synonyms are melanodontoclasia and infantile melanodontia.◀

521.09 Other dental caries

521.1 Excessive attrition
Approximal wear
Occlusal wear

521.2 Abrasion
Abrasion:
  dentifrice
  habitual
  occupational } of teeth
  ritual
  traditional
Wedge defect NOS

521.3 Erosion
Erosion of teeth:
  NOS
  due to:
    medicine
    persistent vomiting

Erosion of teeth:
  idiopathic
  occupational

521.4 Pathological resorption
Internal granuloma of pulp
Resorption of tooth or root (external) (internal)
DEF: Loss of dentin and cementum due to disease process.

521.5 Hypercementosis
Cementation hyperplasia
DEF: Excess deposits of cementum, on tooth root.

521.6 Ankylosis of teeth
DEF: Adhesion of tooth to surrounding bone.

521.7 Posteruptive color changes

Staining [discoloration] of teeth:
  NOS
  due to:
    drugs
    metals
    pulpal bleeding

EXCLUDES *accretions [deposits] on teeth (523.6)*
pre-eruptive color changes (520.8)

521.8 Other specified diseases of hard tissues of teeth
Irradiated enamel   Sensitive dentin

521.9 Unspecified disease of hard tissues of teeth

✓4th **522 Diseases of pulp and periapical tissues**

522.0 Pulpitis
Pulpal:
  abscess
  polyp
Pulpitis:
  acute
  chronic (hyperplastic) (ulcerative)
  suppurative

522.1 Necrosis of the pulp
Pulp gangrene
DEF: Death of pulp tissue.

522.2 Pulp degeneration
Denticles   Pulp stones
Pulp calcifications

522.3 Abnormal hard tissue formation in pulp
Secondary or irregular dentin

522.4 Acute apical periodontitis of pulpal origin
DEF: Severe inflammation of periodontal ligament due to pulpal inflammation or necrosis.

522.5 Periapical abscess without sinus
Abscess: Abscess:
  dental   dentoalveolar
EXCLUDES *periapical abscess with sinus (522.7)*

522.6 Chronic apical periodontitis
Apical or periapical granuloma
Apical periodontitis NOS

522.7 Periapical abscess with sinus
Fistula: Fistula:
  alveolar process   dental

522.8 Radicular cyst
Cyst: Cyst:
  apical (periodontal)   residual radicular
  periapical
  radiculodental
EXCLUDES *lateral developmental or lateral periodontal cyst (526.0)*
DEF: Cyst in tissue around tooth apex due to chronic infection of granuloma around root.

522.9 Other and unspecified diseases of pulp and periapical tissues

✓4th **523 Gingival and periodontal diseases**

523.0 Acute gingivitis
EXCLUDES *acute necrotizing ulcerative gingivitis (101)*
herpetic gingivostomatitis (054.2)

523.1 Chronic gingivitis
Gingivitis (chronic):   Gingivitis (chronic):
  NOS   simple marginal
  desquamative   ulcerative
  hyperplastic   Gingivostomatitis
EXCLUDES *herpetic gingivostomatitis (054.2)*

523.2 Gingival recession
Gingival recession (generalized) (localized) (postinfective) (postoperative)

N Newborn Age: 0   P Pediatric Age: 0-17   M Maternity Age: 12-55   A Adult Age: 15-124   CC CC Condition   MC Major Complication   CD Complex Dx   HIV HIV Related Dx

523.3 Acute periodontitis

Acute:
pericementitis
pericoronitis

Paradontal abscess
Periodontal abscess

EXCLUDES   *acute apical periodontitis (522.4)*
periapical abscess (522.5, 522.7)

DEF: Severe inflammation, of tissues supporting teeth.

523.4 Chronic periodontitis

Alveolar pyorrhea
Chronic pericoronitis
Pericementitis (chronic)
Periodontitis:
NOS

Periodontitis:
complex
simplex

EXCLUDES   *chronic apical periodontitis (522.6)*

523.5 Periodontosis

523.6 Accretions on teeth

Dental calculus:
subgingival
supragingival
Deposits on teeth:
betel

Deposits on teeth:
materia alba
soft
tartar
tobacco

DEF: Foreign material on tooth surface, usually plaque or calculus.

523.8 Other specified periodontal diseases

Giant cell:
epulis
peripheral granuloma
Gingival:
cysts
enlargement NOS
fibromatosis

Gingival polyp
Periodontal lesions due to
traumatic occlusion
Peripheral giant cell
granuloma

EXCLUDES   *leukoplakia of gingiva (528.6)*

523.9 Unspecified gingival and periodontal disease

✓4th **524 Dentofacial anomalies, including malocclusion**

✓5th **524.0 Major anomalies of jaw size**

EXCLUDES   *hemifacial atrophy or hypertrophy*
(754.0)
unilateral condylar hyperplasia or
hypoplasia of mandible (526.89)

524.00 Unspecified anomaly
DEF: Unspecified deformity of jaw size.

524.01 Maxillary hyperplasia
DEF: Overgrowth or over development of upper jaw bone.

524.02 Mandibular hyperplasia
DEF: Overgrowth or over development of lower jaw bone.

524.03 Maxillary hypoplasia
DEF: Incomplete or underdeveloped, upper jaw bone.

524.04 Mandibular hypoplasia
DEF: Incomplete or underdeveloped, lower jaw bone.

524.05 Macrogenia
DEF: Enlarged, jaw, especially chin; affects bone, soft tissue, or both.

524.06 Microgenia
DEF: Underdeveloped mandible, characterized by an extremely small chin.

524.09 Other specified anomaly

✓5th **524.1 Anomalies of relationship of jaw to cranial base**

524.10 Unspecified anomaly
Prognathism   Retrognathism
DEF: Prognathism: protrusion of lower jaw.

DEF: Retrognathism: jaw is located posteriorly to a normally positioned jaw; backward position of mandible.

524.11 Maxillary asymmetry
DEF: Absence of symmetry of maxilla.

524.12 Other jaw asymmetry
524.19 Other specified anomaly

524.2 Anomalies of dental arch relationship

Crossbite (anterior) (posterior)
Disto-occlusion
Mesio-occlusion
Midline deviation
Open bite (anterior) (posterior)
Overbite (excessive):
deep
horizontal
vertical
Overjet
Posterior lingual occlusion of mandibular teeth
Soft tissue impingement

EXCLUDES   *hemifacial atrophy or hypertrophy*
(754.0)
unilateral condylar hyperplasia or
hypoplasia of mandible (526.89)

524.3 Anomalies of tooth position

Crowding
Diastema
Displacement
Rotation
Spacing, abnormal
Transposition

} of tooth, teeth

Impacted or embedded teeth with abnormal position of such teeth or adjacent teeth

524.4 Malocclusion, unspecified
DEF: Malposition of top and bottom teeth; interferes with chewing.

524.5 Dentofacial functional abnormalities

Abnormal jaw closure
Malocclusion due to:
abnormal swallowing
mouth breathing
tongue, lip, or finger habits

✓5th **524.6 Temporomandibular joint disorders**

EXCLUDES   *current temporomandibular joint:*
dislocation (830.0-830.1)
strain (848.1)

524.60 Temporomandibular joint disorders, unspecified
Temporomandibular joint-pain-dysfunction syndrome [TMJ]

524.61 Adhesions and ankylosis (bony or fibrous)
DEF: Stiffening or union of temporomandibular joint due to bony or fibrous union across joint.

524.62 Arthralgia of temporomandibular joint
DEF: Pain in temporomandibular joint; not inflammatory in nature.

524.63 Articular disc disorder (reducing or non-reducing)

524.69 Other specified temporomandibular joint disorders

✓5th **524.7 Dental alveolar anomalies**

524.70 Unspecified alveolar anomaly

524.71 Alveolar maxillary hyperplasia
DEF: Excessive tissue formation in the dental alveoli of upper jaw.

524.72 Alveolar mandibular hyperplasia
DEF: Excessive tissue formation in the dental alveoli of lower jaw.

524.73 Alveolar maxillary hypoplasia
DEF: Incomplete or underdeveloped, alveolar tissue of upper jaw.

524.74 Alveolar mandibular hypoplasia
DEF: Incomplete or underdeveloped, alveolar tissue of lower jaw.

524.79 Other specified alveolar anomaly

524.8 Other specified dentofacial anomalies

524.9 Unspecified dentofacial anomalies

✓4th ✓5th   Additional Digit Required   Nonspecific PDx   Unacceptable PDx   Manifestation Code   **MSP** Medicare Secondary Payer   ►◄ Revised Text   ● New Code   ▲ Revised Code Title

Digestive System 525–528.2

√4ᵗʰ **525 Other diseases and conditions of the teeth and supporting structures**

525.0 Exfoliation of teeth due to systemic causes

DEF: Deterioration of teeth and surrounding structures due to systemic disease.

√5ᵗʰ **525.1 Loss of teeth due to trauma, extraction, or periodontal disease**

AHA: ▶4Q, '01, 44◄

525.10 Acquired absence of teeth, unspecified
Edentulism
Tooth extraction status, NOS

525.11 Loss of teeth due to trauma

525.12 Loss of teeth due to periodontal disease

525.13 Loss of teeth due to caries

525.19 Other loss of teeth

525.2 Atrophy of edentulous alveolar ridge

525.3 Retained dental root

525.8 Other specified disorders of the teeth and supporting structures
Enlargement of alveolar ridge NOS
Irregular alveolar process

525.9 Unspecified disorder of the teeth and supporting structures

√4ᵗʰ **526 Diseases of the jaws**

526.0 Developmental odontogenic cysts

Cyst:
dentigerous
eruption
follicular
lateral developmental

Cyst:
lateral periodontal
primordial
Keratocyst

EXCLUDES   radicular cyst (522.8)

526.1 Fissural cysts of jaw

Cyst:
globulomaxillary
incisor canal
median anterior maxillary

Cyst:
median palatal
nasopalatine
palatine of papilla

EXCLUDES   cysts of oral soft tissues (528.4)

526.2 Other cysts of jaws

Cyst of jaw:
NOS
aneurysmal

Cyst of jaw:
hemorrhagic
traumatic

526.3 Central giant cell (reparative) granuloma

EXCLUDES   peripheral giant cell granuloma (523.8)

526.4 Inflammatory conditions

Abscess
Osteitis
Osteomyelitis (neonatal)
Periostitis
} of jaw (acute) (chronic) (suppurative)

Sequestrum of jaw bone

EXCLUDES   alveolar osteitis (526.5)

526.5 Alveolitis of jaw

Alveolar osteitis   Dry socket

DEF: Inflammation, of alveoli or tooth socket.

√5ᵗʰ **526.8 Other specified diseases of the jaws**

526.81 Exostosis of jaw
Torus mandibularis   Torus palatinus

DEF: Spur or bony outgrowth on the jaw.

526.89 Other

Cherubism
Fibrous dysplasia
Latent bone cyst
Osteoradionecrosis
} of jaw(s)

Unilateral condylar hyperplasia or hypoplasia of mandible

526.9 Unspecified disease of the jaws

√4ᵗʰ **527 Diseases of the salivary glands**

527.0 Atrophy

DEF: Wasting away, necrosis of salivary gland tissue.

527.1 Hypertrophy

DEF: Overgrowth or overdeveloped salivary gland tissue.

527.2 Sialoadenitis

Parotitis:
NOS
allergic
toxic
Sialoangitis
Sialodochitis

EXCLUDES   epidemic or infectious parotitis (072.0-072.9)
uveoparotid fever (135)

DEF: Inflammation of salivary gland.

527.3 Abscess   **CC**

CC Excl: 527.0-527.9, 537.89, 537.9

527.4 Fistula   **CC**

EXCLUDES   congenital fistula of salivary gland (750.24)

CC Excl: See code 527.3

527.5 Sialolithiasis

Calculus
Stone
} of salivary gland or duct

Sialodocholithiasis

527.6 Mucocele

Mucous:
extravasation cyst of salivary gland
retention cyst of salivary gland
Ranula

DEF: Dilated salivary gland cavity filled with mucous.

527.7 Disturbance of salivary secretion

Hyposecretion
Ptyalism
Sialorrhea
Xerostomia

527.8 Other specified diseases of the salivary glands

Benign lymphoepithelial lesion of salivary gland
Sialectasia
Sialosis
Stenosis
Stricture
} of salivary duct

527.9 Unspecified disease of the salivary glands

√4ᵗʰ **528 Diseases of the oral soft tissues, excluding lesions specific for gingiva and tongue**

528.0 Stomatitis

Stomatitis:
NOS
ulcerative

Vesicular stomatitis

EXCLUDES   stomatitis:
acute necrotizing ulcerative (101)
aphthous (528.2)
gangrenous (528.1)
herpetic (054.2)
Vincent's (101)

AHA: 2Q, '99, 9

DEF: Inflammation of oral mucosa; labial and buccal mucosa, tongue, plate, floor of the mouth, and gingivae.

528.1 Cancrum oris

Gangrenous stomatitisNoma

DEF: A severely gangrenous lesion of mouth due to fusospirochetal infection; destroys buccal, labial and facial tissues; can be fatal; found primarily in debilitated and malnourished children.

528.2 Oral aphthae

Aphthous stomatitis
Canker sore
Periadenitis mucosa necrotica recurrens
Recurrent aphthous ulcer
Stomatitis herpetiformis

EXCLUDES   herpetic stomatitis (054.2)

DEF: Small oval or round ulcers of the mouth marked by a grayish exudate and a red halo effect.

| N Newborn Age: 0 | P Pediatric Age: 0-17 | M Maternity Age: 12-55 | A Adult Age: 15-124 | CC CC Condition | MC Major Complication | CD Complex Dx | HIV HIV Related Dx |

152 — Volume 1 • January 2002   *2002 Ingenix, Inc.*

528.3   Cellulitis and abscess   CC
   Cellulitis of mouth (floor)   Oral fistula
   Ludwig's angina
      EXCLUDES   abscess of tongue (529.0)
                 cellulitis or abscess of lip (528.5)
                 fistula (of):
                    dental (522.7)
                    lip (528.5)
                    gingivitis (523.0-523.1)
   CC Excl: 528.0, 528.3, 529.0, 529.2

528.4   Cysts
   Dermoid cyst   ⎫
   Epidermoid cyst   ⎪
   Epstein's pearl   ⎬ of mouth
   Lymphoepithelial cyst   ⎪
   Nasoalveolar cyst   ⎪
   Nasolabial cyst   ⎭
      EXCLUDES   cyst: cyst:
                 gingiva (523.8)   tongue (529.8)

528.5   Diseases of lips
   Abscess   ⎫
   Cellulitis   ⎬ of lip(s)
   Fistula   ⎪
   Hypertrophy   ⎭

   Cheilitis: Cheilodynia
      NOS   Cheilosis
      angular
      EXCLUDES   actinic cheilitis (692.79)
                 congenital fistula of lip (750.25)
                 leukoplakia of lips (528.6)
   AHA: S-O, '86, 10

528.6   Leukoplakia of oral mucosa, including tongue
   Leukokeratosis of oral   Leukoplakia of:
      mucosa   lips
   Leukoplakia of: tongue
      gingiva
      EXCLUDES   carcinoma in situ (230.0, 232.0)
                 leukokeratosis nicotina palati (528.7)
   DEF: Thickened white patches of epithelium on mucous membranes
   of mouth.

**528.7   Other disturbances of oral epithelium, including
          tongue**
   Erythroplakia   ⎫ of mouth or
   Focal epithelial hyperplasia ⎬ tongue
   Leukoedema   ⎭

   Leukokeratosis nicotina palati
      EXCLUDES   carcinoma in situ (230.0, 232.0)
                 leukokeratosis NOS (702)

528.8   Oral submucosal fibrosis, including of tongue
**528.9   Other and unspecified diseases of the oral soft
          tissues**
   Cheek and lip biting
   Denture sore mouth
   Denture stomatitis
   Melanoplakia
   Papillary hyperplasia of palate

   Eosinophilic granuloma ⎫
   Irritative hyperplasia ⎬ of oral mucosa
   Pyogenic granuloma   ⎪
   Ulcer (traumatic)   ⎭

☑4ᵗʰ **529   Diseases and other conditions of the tongue**
   529.0   Glossitis
      Abscess   ⎫ of tongue
      Ulceration (traumatic)⎭
         EXCLUDES   glossitis:
                    benign migratory (529.1)
                    Hunter's (529.4)
                    median rhomboid (529.2)
                    Moeller's (529.4)

529.1   Geographic tongue
   Benign migratory glossitis   Glossitis areata
      exfoliativa
   DEF: Chronic glossitis; marked by filiform papillae atrophy and
   inflammation; no known etiology.

529.2   Median rhomboid glossitis
   DEF: A noninflammatory, congenital disease characterized by
   rhomboid-like lesions at the middle third of the tongue's dorsal
   surface.

529.3   Hypertrophy of tongue papillae
   Black hairy tongue   Hypertrophy of foliate papillae
   Coated tongue   Lingua villosa nigra

529.4   Atrophy of tongue papillae
   Bald tongue   Glossitis:
   Glazed tongue   Moeller's
   Glossitis: Glossodynia exfoliativa
      Hunter's   Smooth atrophic tongue

529.5   Plicated tongue
   Fissured ⎫
   Furrowed ⎬ tongue
   Scrotal   ⎭
      EXCLUDES   fissure of tongue, congenital (750.13)
   DEF: Cracks, fissures or furrows, on dorsal surface of tongue.

529.6   Glossodynia
   Glossopyrosis   Painful tongue
      EXCLUDES   glossodynia exfoliativa (529.4)

529.8   Other specified conditions of the tongue
   Atrophy   ⎫
   Crenated   ⎬ (of) tongue
   Enlargement ⎪
   Hypertrophy ⎭

   Glossocele
   Glossoptosis
      EXCLUDES   erythroplasia of tongue (528.7)
                 leukoplakia of tongue (528.6)
                 macroglossia (congenital) (750.15)
                 microglossia (congenital) (750.16)
                 oral submucosal fibrosis (528.8)

529.9   Unspecified condition of the tongue

DISEASES OF ESOPHAGUS, STOMACH, AND DUODENUM (530-537)

☑4ᵗʰ **530   Diseases of esophagus**
      EXCLUDES   esophageal varices (456.0-456.2)

   530.0   Achalasia and cardiospasm
      Achalasia (of cardia)   Megaesophagus
      Aperistalsis of esophagus
         EXCLUDES   congenital cardiospasm (750.7)
      DEF: Failure of smooth muscle fibers to relax, at gastrointestinal
      junctures; such as esophagogastric sphincter when swallowing.

☑5ᵗʰ **530.1   Esophagitis**
      Abscess of esophagus   Esophagitis:
      Esophagitis: peptic
         NOS   postoperative
         chemical   regurgitant
      Use additional E code to identify cause, if induced
         by chemical
         EXCLUDES   tuberculous esophagitis (017.8)
      AHA: 4Q, '93, 27; 1Q, '92, 17; 3Q, '91, 20

   530.10   Esophagitis, unspecified
   530.11   Reflux esophagitis
      AHA: 4Q, '95, 82
      DEF: Inflammation of lower esophagus; due to
      regurgitated gastric acid.

   530.12   Acute esophagitis
      AHA: ▶4Q, '01, 45◀
      DEF: ▶ An acute inflammation of the mucous lining or
      submucosal coat of the esophagus. ◀

   530.19   Other esophagitis
      AHA: ▶3Q, '01, 10◀

☑4ᵗʰ / ☑5ᵗʰ Additional Digit Required | Nonspecific PDx | Unacceptable PDx | Manifestation Code | MSP Medicare Secondary Payer | ▶◀ Revised Text | ● New Code | ▲ Revised Code Title

Digestive System 530.2–531.4

530.2   **Ulcer of esophagus**
Ulcer of esophagus: Ulcer of esophagus:
   fungal   peptic
Ulcer of esophagus due to ingestion of:
   aspirin   chemicals
   medicines
Use additional E code to identify cause, if induced
   by chemical or drug

530.3   **Stricture and stenosis of esophagus**
Compression of esophagus
Obstruction of esophagus
> **EXCLUDES**   *congenital stricture of esophagus
> (750.3)*

AHA: 2Q, '01, 4; 2Q, '97, 3; 1Q, '88, 13

530.4   **Perforation of esophagus**   `CC`
Rupture of esophagus
> **EXCLUDES**   *traumatic perforation of esophagus
> (862.22, 862.32, 874.4-874.5)*

CC Excl: 530.4, 530.7-530.81, 530.83-530.9

530.5   **Dyskinesia of esophagus**
Corkscrew esophagus   Esophagospasm
Curling esophagus   Spasm of esophagus
> **EXCLUDES**   *cardiospasm (530.0)*

AHA: 1Q, '88, 13; N-D, '84, 19

DEF: Difficulty performing voluntary esophageal movements.

530.6   **Diverticulum of esophagus, acquired**
Diverticulum, acquired: Diverticulum, acquired:
   epiphrenic   traction
   pharyngoesophageal   Zenker's
   pulsion   (hypopharyngeal)
   subdiaphragmatic   Esophageal pouch, acquired
                   Esophagocele, acquired
> **EXCLUDES**   *congenital diverticulum of esophagus
> (750.4)*

AHA: J-F, '85, 3

530.7   **Gastroesophageal laceration-hemorrhage**   `CC`
syndrome
Mallory-Weiss syndrome
CC Excl: 251.5, 456.0, 530.2, 530.4, 530.7-530.9, 531.00-531.91, 532.00-
532.91, 533.00-533.91, 534.00-534.91, 535.01, 535.11, 535.21, 535.31,
535.41, 535.51, 535.61, 537.83, 562.02-562.03, 562.12-562.13, 569.3,
569.85, 578.0-578.9

DEF: Laceration of distal esophagus and proximal stomach due to
vomiting, hiccups or other sustained activity.

✓5th **530.8**   **Other specified disorders of esophagus**
     530.81   **Esophageal reflux**
         Gastroesophageal reflux
>   **EXCLUDES**   *reflux esophagitis (530.11)*

         AHA: 2Q, '01, 4; 1Q, '95, 7; 4Q, '92, 27

         DEF: Regurgitation of the gastric contents into esophagus
         and possibly pharynx; where aspiration may occur
         between the vocal cords and down into the trachea.

530.82   **Esophageal hemorrhage**   `CC`
> **EXCLUDES**   *hemorrhage due to esophageal
> varices (456.0-456.2)*

CC Excl: 251.5, 456.0, 456.20, 459.89-459.9, 530.2, 530.7,
530.82, 531.00-531.21, 531.30-531.31, 531.40-531.91, 532.00-
532.91, 533.00-533.91, 534.00-534.51, 534.61, 534.70-534.91,
535.01-535.11, 535.21, 535.31, 535.41, 535.51, 535.61, 537.83,
562.02-562.03, 562.12-562.13, 569.3, 569.85, 578.0-578.9

530.83   **Esophageal leukoplakia**
530.84   **Tracheoesophageal fistula**   `CC`
> **EXCLUDES**   *congenital tracheoesophageal
> fistula (750.3)*

CC Excl: 530.4, 530.7, 530.81, 530.83-530.9

530.89   **Other**
> **EXCLUDES**   *Paterson-Kelly syndrome
> (280.8)*

530.9   **Unspecified disorder of esophagus**

✓4th **531**   **Gastric ulcer**
> **INCLUDES**   ulcer (peptic):
>   prepyloric
>   pylorus
>   stomach
Use additional E code to identify drug, if drug-induced
> **EXCLUDES**   *peptic ulcer NOS (533.0-533.9)*

The following fifth-digit subclassification is for use with
category 531:
   0   **without mention of obstruction**
   1   **with obstruction**

AHA: 1Q, '91, 15; 4Q, '90, 27

DEF: Destruction of tissue in lumen of stomach due to action of gastric acid
and pepsin on gastric mucosa decreasing resistance to ulcers.

✓5th **531.0**   **Acute with hemorrhage**   `CC`
CC Excl: 251.5, 456.0, 530.2, 530.7, 530.82, 531.00-531.91, 532.00-532.91,
533.00-533.91, 534.00-534.91, 535.01, 535.11, 535.21, 535.31, 535.41,
535.51, 535.61, 537.83, 537.89, 537.9, 562.02-562.03, 562.12-562.13,
569.3, 569.85, 578.0-578.9

AHA: N-D, '84, 15

✓5th **531.1**   **Acute with perforation**   `CC`
CC Excl: See code 531.0

✓5th **531.2**   **Acute with hemorrhage and perforation**   `CC`
CC Excl: See code 531.0

✓5th **531.3**   **Acute without mention of hemorhage**   `CC 1`
orperforation
CC Excl: For code 531.31: see code 531.0

✓5th **531.4**   **Chronic or unspecified with hemorrhage**   `CC`
CC Excl: See code 531.0

AHA: 4Q, '90, 22

▽ **DRG** 174 For code 531.40

Esophagus

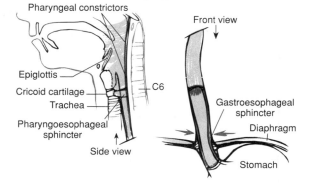

Pharyngeal constrictors
Front view
Epiglottis
Cricoid cartilage
Trachea
C6
Pharyngoesophageal
sphincter
Gastroesophageal
sphincter
Diaphragm
Side view
Stomach

Stomach

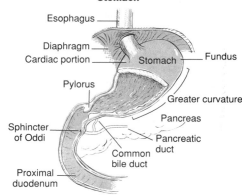

Esophagus
Diaphragm
Cardiac portion
Stomach
Fundus
Pylorus
Greater curvature
Pancreas
Sphincter
of Oddi
Pancreatic
duct
Common
bile duct
Proximal
duodenum

`N` Newborn Age: 0   `P` Pediatric Age: 0-17   `M` Maternity Age: 12-55   `A` Adult Age: 15-124   `CC` CC Condition   `MC` Major Complication   `CD` Complex Dx   `HIV` HIV Related Dx

154 — Volume 1   *2002 Ingenix, Inc.*

√5ᵗʰ **531.5 Chronic or unspecified with perforation** `CC`
CC Excl: See code 531.0

√5ᵗʰ **531.6 Chronic or unspecified with hemorrhage and perforation** `CC`
CC Excl: See code 531.0

√5ᵗʰ **531.7 Chronic without mention of hemorrhage or perforation** `CC 1`
CC Excl: For code 531.71: see code 531.0

√5ᵗʰ **531.9 Unspecified as acute or chronic, without mention of hemorrhage or perforation** `CC 1`
CC Excl: For code 531.91: see code 531.0

√4ᵗʰ **532 Duodenal ulcer**
> INCLUDES   erosion (acute) of duodenum
> ulcer (peptic):
>   duodenum
>   postpyloric
> Use additional E code to identify drug, if drug-induced
> EXCLUDES *peptic ulcer NOS (533.0-533.9)*

The following fifth-digit subclassification is for use with category 532:
0 without mention of obstruction
1 with obstruction

AHA: 4Q, '90, 27, 1Q, '91, 15

DEF: Ulcers in duodenum due to action of gastric acid and pepsin on mucosa decreasing resistance to ulcers.

√5ᵗʰ **532.0 Acute with hemorrhage** `CC`
CC Excl: 251.5, 456.0, 530.2, 530.7, 530.82, 531.00-531.91, 532.00-532.91, 533.00-533.91, 534.00-534.91, 535.01, 535.11, 535.21, 535.31, 535.41, 535.51, 535.61, 537.3, 537.83, 537.89, 537.9, 562.02-562.03, 562.12-562.13, 569.3, 569.85, 578.0-578.9

AHA: 4Q, '90, 22

√5ᵗʰ **532.1 Acute with perforation** `CC`
CC Excl: See code 532.0

√5ᵗʰ **532.2 Acute with hemorrhage and perforation** `CC`
CC Excl: See code 532.0

√5ᵗʰ **532.3 Acute without mention of hemorrhage or perforation** `CC 1`
CC Excl: For code 532.31: See code 532.0

√5ᵗʰ **532.4 Chronic or unspecified with hemorrhage** `CC`
CC Excl: See code 532.0

   ▽ DRG 174 For code 532.40

√5ᵗʰ **532.5 Chronic or unspecified with perforation** `CC`
CC Excl: See code 532.0

Duodenum

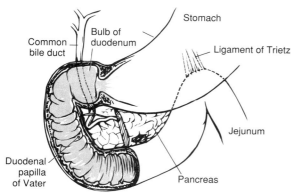

√5ᵗʰ **532.6 Chronic or unspecified with hemorrhage and perforation** `CC`
CC Excl: See code 532.0

√5ᵗʰ **532.7 Chronic without mention of hemorrhage or perforation** `CC 1`
CC Excl: For code 532.71: See code 532.0

√5ᵗʰ **532.9 Unspecified as acute or chronic, without mention of hemorrhage or perforation** `CC 1`
CC Excl: For code 532.91: See code 532.0

√4ᵗʰ **533 Peptic ulcer, site unspecified**
> INCLUDES   gastroduodenal ulcer NOS   stress ulcer NOS
> peptic ulcer NOS
> Use additional E code to identify drug, if drug-induced
> EXCLUDES *peptic ulcer:*
>   *duodenal (532.0-532.9)*
>   *gastric (531.0-531.9)*

The following fifth-digit subclassification is for use with category 533:
0 without mention of obstruction
1 with obstruction

AHA: 1Q, '91, 15; 4Q, '90, 27

DEF: Ulcer of mucous membrane of esophagus, stomach or duodenum due to gastric acid secretion.

√5ᵗʰ **533.0 Acute with hemorrhage** `CC`
CC Excl: See code 532.0

√5ᵗʰ **533.1 Acute with perforation** `CC`
CC Excl: See code 532.0

√5ᵗʰ **533.2 Acute with hemorrhage and perforation** `CC`
CC Excl: See code 532.0

√5ᵗʰ **533.3 Acute without mention of hemorrhage and perforation** `CC 1`
CC Excl: For code 533.31: See code 532.0

√5ᵗʰ **533.4 Chronic or unspecified with hemorrhage** `CC`
CC Excl: See code 532.0

√5ᵗʰ **533.5 Chronic or unspecified with perforation** `CC`
CC Excl: See code 532.0

√5ᵗʰ **533.6 Chronic or unspecified with hemorrhage and perforation** `CC`
CC Excl: See code 532.0

√5ᵗʰ **533.7 Chronic without mention of hemorrhage or perforation** `CC 1`
CC Excl: For code 533.71: See code 532.0

AHA: 2Q, '89, 16

√5ᵗʰ **533.9 Unspecified as acute or chronic, without mention of hemorrhage or perforation** `CC 1`
CC Excl: For code 533.91: See code 532.0

√4ᵗʰ **534 Gastrojejunal ulcer**
> INCLUDES   ulcer (peptic) or erosion: ulcer (peptic) or erosion:
>   anastomotic   jejunal
>   gastrocolic   marginal
>   gastrointestinal   stomal
>   gastrojejunal
> EXCLUDES *primary ulcer of small intestine (569.82)*

The following fifth-digit subclassification is for use with category 534:
0 without mention of obstruction
1 with obstruction

AHA: 1Q, '91, 15; 4Q, '90, 27

√4ᵗʰ Additional Digit Required   Nonspecific PDx   Unacceptable PDx   Manifestation Code   **MSP** Medicare Secondary Payer   ►◄ Revised Text   ● New Code   ▲ Revised Code Title
√5ᵗʰ
2002 Ingenix, Inc.

Digestive System 531.5–534

Volume 1 — 155

Digestive System 534.0–537.0

√5ᵗʰ **534.0 Acute with hemorrhage**   `CC`
  CC Excl: 251.5, 456.0, 530.2, 530.7, 530.82, 531.00-531.91,
  532.00-532.91, 533.00-533.91, 534.00-534.91, 535.01, 535.11,
  535.21, 535.31, 535.41, 535.51, 535.61, 537.83, 537.89, 537.9,
  562.02-562.03, 562.12-562.13, 569.3, 569.85, 578.0-578.9

√5ᵗʰ **534.1 Acute with perforation**   `CC`
  CC Excl: See code 534.0

√5ᵗʰ **534.2 Acute with hemorrhage and perforation**   `CC`
  CC Excl: See code 534.0

√5ᵗʰ **534.3 Acute without mention of hemorrhage or**   `CC`
      perforation
  CC Excl: For code 534.31: See code 534.0

√5ᵗʰ **534.4 Chronic or unspecified with hemorrhage**   `CC 1`
  CC Excl: See code 534.0

√5ᵗʰ **534.5 Chronic or unspecified with perforation**   `CC`
  CC Excl: See code 534.0

√5ᵗʰ **534.6 Chronic or unspecified with hemorrhage and**   `CC`
      perforation
  CC Excl: See code 534.0

√5ᵗʰ **534.7 Chronic without mention of hemorrhage or**   `CC 1`
      perforation
  CC Excl: For code 534.71: See code 534.0

√5ᵗʰ **534.9 Unspecified as acute or chronic, without**   `CC 1`
      mention of hemorrhage or perforation
  CC Excl: For code 534.91: See code 534.0

√4ᵗʰ **535 Gastritis and duodenitis**

  The following fifth-digit subclassification is for use with
  category 535:
    0 without mention of hemorrhage
    1 with hemorrhage

  AHA: 2Q, '92, 9; 4Q, '91, 25

√5ᵗʰ **535.0 Acute gastritis**   `CC 1`
  CC Excl: For code 535.01: 251.5, 456.0, 530.2, 530.7, 530.82,
  531.00-531.91, 532.00-532.91, 533.00-533.91, 534.00-534.91,
  535.01, 535.11, 535.21, 535.31, 535.41, 535.51, 535.61, 537.83,
  562.02-562.03, 562.12-562.13, 569.3, 569.85, 578.0-578.9

  AHA: 2Q, '92, 8; N-D, '86, 9

√5ᵗʰ **535.1 Atrophic gastritis**   `CC 1`
      Gastritis: Gastritis:
        atrophic-hyperplastic   chronic (atrophic)
  CC Excl: For code 535.11: See code 535.01

  AHA: 1Q, '94, 18

  DEF: Inflammation of stomach, with mucous membrane atrophy and
  peptic gland destruction.

√5ᵗʰ **535.2 Gastric mucosal hypertrophy**   `CC 1`
      Hypertrophic gastritis
  CC Excl: For code 535.21: See code 535.01

√5ᵗʰ **535.3 Alcoholic gastritis**   `CC 1`
  CC Excl: For code 535.31: See code 535.01

√5ᵗʰ **535.4 Other specified gastritis**   `CC 1`
      Gastritis:
        allergic
        bile induced
        irritant
        superficial
        toxic
  CC Excl: For code 535.41: See code 535.01

  AHA: 4Q, '90, 27

√5ᵗʰ **535.5 Unspecified gastritis and gastroduodenitis**   `CC 1`
  CC Excl: For code 535.51: See code 535.01

  AHA: For code 535.50: 4Q, '99, 25

√5ᵗʰ **535.6 Duodenitis**   `CC 1`
  CC Excl: For code 535.61: See code 535.01

  DEF: Inflammation of intestine, between pylorus and jejunum.

√4ᵗʰ **536 Disorders of function of stomach**
  EXCLUDES *functional disorders of stomach specified as*
                psychogenic (306.4)

  536.0 Achlorhydria
  DEF: Absence of gastric acid due to gastric mucosa atrophy;
  unresponsive to histamines; also known as gastric anacidity.

  536.1 Acute dilatation of stomach   `CC`
      Acute distention of stomach
  CC Excl: 536.1

  536.2 Persistent vomiting
      Habit vomiting   Uncontrollable vomiting
      Persistent vomiting [not of pregnancy]
      EXCLUDES *excessive vomiting in pregnancy*
                    (643.0-643.9)
                    vomiting NOS (787.0)

  536.3 Gastroparesis
  AHA: 2Q, '01, 4; 4Q, '94, 42

  DEF: Slight degree of paralysis within muscular coat of stomach.

√5ᵗʰ **536.4 Gastrostomy complications**
  AHA: 4Q, '98, 42

  536.40 Gastrostomy complication, unspecified `CC`
  CC Excl: 536.40-536.49, 997.4, 997.71, 997.91, 997.99,
  998.81, 998.83-998.9

  536.41 Infection of gastrostomy   `CC`
      Use additional code to specify type of
        infection, such as:
      abscess or cellulitis of abdomen (682.2)
      septicemia (038.0-038.9)
      Use additional code to identify organism
        (041.00-041.9)
  CC Excl: See code 536.40

  AHA: 4Q, '98, 42

  536.42 Mechanical complication of gastrostomy `CC`
  CC Excl: See code 536.40

  536.49 Other gastrostomy complications   `CC`
  CC Excl: See code 536.40

  AHA: 4Q, '98, 42

  536.8 Dyspepsia and other specified disorders of function
      of stomach
      Achylia gastrica   Hyperchlorhydria
      Hourglass contraction   Hypochlorhydria
        of stomach   Indigestion
      Hyperacidity
      EXCLUDES *achlorhydria (536.0)*
                    heartburn (787.1)

  AHA: 2Q, '93, 6; 2Q, '89, 16; N-D, '84, 9

  536.9 Unspecified functional disorder of stomach
      Functional gastrointestinal:
        disorder
        disturbance
        irritation

√4ᵗʰ **537 Other disorders of stomach and duodenum**

  537.0 Acquired hypertrophic pyloric stenosis   `CC`
      Constriction ⎫
      Obstruction ⎬ of pylorus, acquired or
      Stricture   ⎭   adult
      EXCLUDES *congenital or infantile pyloric stenosis*
                    (750.5)
  CC Excl: 536.3, 536.8-536.9, 537.0, 537.3, 750.5, 750.8-750.9, 751.1, 751.5

  AHA: 2Q, '01, 4; J-F, '85, 14

`N` Newborn Age: 0   `P` Pediatric Age: 0-17   `M` Maternity Age: 12-55   `A` Adult Age: 15-124   `CC` CC Condition   `MC` Major Complication   `CD` Complex Dx   `HIV` HIV Related Dx

537.1 Gastric diverticulum

> **EXCLUDES** *congenital diverticulum of stomach (750.7)*

AHA: J-F, '85, 4

DEF: Herniated sac or pouch, within stomach or duodenum.

537.2 Chronic duodenal ileus

DEF: Persistent obstruction between pylorus and jejunum.

537.3 Other obstruction of duodenum `CC`

Cicatrix
Stenosis
Stricture } of duodenum
Volvulus

> **EXCLUDES** *congenital obstruction of duodenum (751.1)*

CC Excl: 537.3, 750.8-750.9, 751.1, 751.5

537.4 Fistula of stomach or duodenum `CC`

Gastrocolic fistula   Gastrojejunocolic fistula

CC Excl: 537.4, 750.8-750.9, 751.5

537.5 Gastroptosis

DEF: Downward displacement of stomach.

537.6 Hourglass stricture or stenosis of stomach

Cascade stomach

> **EXCLUDES** *congenital hourglass stomach (750.7)*
> *hourglass contraction of stomach (536.8)*

√5ᵗʰ 537.8 Other specified disorders of stomach and duodenum

AHA: 4Q, '91, 25

> **537.81 Pylorospasm**
>
> > **EXCLUDES** *congenital pylorospasm (750.5)*
>
> DEF: Spasm of the pyloric sphincter.

> **537.82 Angiodysplasia of stomach and duodenum (without mention of hemorrhage)**
>
> **AHA:** 3Q, '96, 10; 4Q, '90, 4

> **537.83 Angiodysplasia of stomach and duodenum with hemorrhage** `CC`
>
> **CC Excl:** 251.5, 456.0, 530.2, 530.7, 530.82, 531.000-531.91, 532.00-532.91, 533.00-533.91, 534.00-534.91, 535.01, 535.11, 535.21, 535.31, 535.41, 535.51, 535.61, 537.83, 562.02-562.03, 562.12-562.13, 569.3, 569.85, 578.0-578.9
>
> DEF: Bleeding of stomach and duodenum due to vascular abnormalities.

> **537.84 Dieulafoy lesion (hemorrhagic) of stomach and duodenum** `CC`
>
> **CC Excl:** 251.5, 530.2, 530.7, 530.82, 531.00-531.91, 532.00-532.91, 533.00-533.91, 534.00-534.91, 535.01, 535.11, 535.21, 535.31, 535.41, 535.51, 535.61, 537.83-537.84, 562.02-562.03, 562.12-562.13, 569.3, 569.85-569.86, 578.0-578.1, 578.9

> **537.89 Other**
>
> Gastric or duodenal:
>   prolapse
>   rupture
> Intestinal metaplasia of gastric mucosa
> Passive congestion of stomach
>
> > **EXCLUDES** *diverticula of duodenum (562.00-562.01)*
> > *gastrointestinal hemorrhage (578.0-578.9)*
>
> **AHA:** N-D, '84, 7

537.9 Unspecified disorder of stomach and duodenum

APPENDICITIS (540-543)

√4ᵗʰ 540 Acute appendicitis

AHA: N-D, '84, 19

DEF: Inflammation of vermiform appendix due to fecal obstruction, neoplasm or foreign body of appendiceal lumen; causes infection, edema and infarction of appendiceal wall; may result in mural necrosis, and perforation.

540.0 With generalized peritonitis `CC`

Appendicitis (acute):
   fulminating
   gangrenous   with:
   obstructive   perforation
   Cecitis (acute)   peritonitis (generalized)
                          rupture

Rupture of appendix

> **EXCLUDES** *acute appendicitis with peritoneal abscess (540.1)*

CC Excl: 537.89, 537.9, 540.0-540.9, 541-542, 543.0, 543.9

540.1 With peritoneal abscess `CC`

With generalized peritonitis
Abscess of appendix

CC Excl: See code 540.0

AHA: N-D, '84, 19

540.9 Without mention of peritonitis `CC`

Acute:
   appendicitis:
      fulminating
      gangrenous   without mention of
      inflamed   perforation,
      obstructive   peritonitis, or rupture
      cecitis

CC Excl: See code 540.0

AHA: 1Q, '01, 15; 4Q, '97, 52

541 Appendicitis, unqualified

AHA: 2Q, '90, 26

542 Other appendicitis

Appendicitis: Appendicitis:
   chronic   relapsing
   recurrent   subacute

> **EXCLUDES** *hyperplasia (lymphoid) of appendix (543.0)*

AHA: 1Q, '01, 15

√4ᵗʰ 543 Other diseases of appendix

543.0 Hyperplasia of appendix (lymphoid)

DEF: Proliferation of cells in appendix tissue.

543.9 Other and unspecified diseases of appendix

Appendicular or appendiceal:
   colic
   concretion
   fistula
Diverticulum
Fecalith
Intussusception } of appendix
Mucocele
Stercolith

Appendix

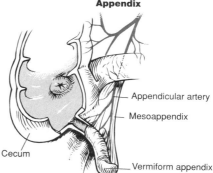

Appendicular artery

Mesoappendix

Cecum

Vermiform appendix

√4ᵗʰ √5ᵗʰ Additional Digit Required   Nonspecific PDx   Unacceptable PDx   Manifestation Code   **MSP** Medicare Secondary Payer   ▶◀ Revised Text   ● New Code   ▲ Revised Code Title

2002 Ingenix, Inc.

October 2002 • Volume 1 — 157

Digestive System 537.1–543.9

Digestive System 550–552.00

HERNIA OF ABDOMINAL CAVITY (550-553)

INCLUDES   hernia:
acquired
congenital, except diaphragmatic or hiatal

✓4th **550 Inguinal hernia**
INCLUDES   bubonocele
inguinal hernia (direct) (double) (indirect)
(oblique) (sliding)
scrotal hernia

The following fifth-digit subclassification is for use with
category 550:

  0 unilateral or unspecified (not specified as recurrent)
     Unilateral NOS
  1 unilateral or unspecified, recurrent
  2 bilateral (not specified as recurrent)
     Bilateral NOS
  3 bilateral, recurrent

AHA: N-D, '85, 12

DEF: Hernia protrusion of an abdominal organ or tissue through inguinal
canal.

DEF: Indirect inguinal hernia: (external or oblique) leaves abdomen through
deep inguinal ring, passes through inguinal canal lateral to the inferior
epigastric artery.

DEF: Direct inguinal hernia: (internal) emerges between inferior epigastric
artery and rectus muscle edge.

✓5th **550.0 Inguinal hernia, with gangrene**   CC
Inguinal hernia with gangrene (and obstruction)
CC Excl: 537.89, 537.9, 550.00-550.93, 552.8-552.9, 553.8-553.9

✓5th **550.1 Inguinal hernia, with obstruction, without**   CC
mention of gangrene
Inguinal hernia with mention of incarceration,
irreducibility, or strangulation
CC Excl: See code 550.0

Inguinal Hernias

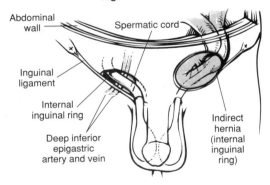

Abdominal wall
Spermatic cord
Inguinal ligament
Internal inguinal ring
Deep inferior epigastric artery and vein
Indirect hernia (internal inguinal ring)

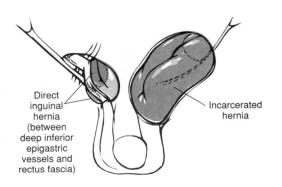

Direct inguinal hernia (between deep inferior epigastric vessels and rectus fascia)
Incarcerated hernia

✓5th **550.9 Inguinal hernia, without mention of obstruction or**
gangrene
Inguinal hernia NOS

✓4th **551 Other hernia of abdominal cavity, with gangrene**
INCLUDES   that with gangrene (and obstruction)

✓5th **551.0 Femoral hernia with gangrene**
551.00 Unilateral or unspecified (not specified   CC
as recurrent)
Femoral hernia NOS with gangrene
CC Excl: 537.89, 537.9, 551.00-551.03, 552.8-552.9,
553.00-553.03, 553.8-553.9

551.01 Unilateral or unspecified, recurrent   CC
CC Excl: See code 551.0

551.02 Bilateral (not specified as recurrent)   CC
CC Excl: See code 551.0

551.03 Bilateral, recurrent   CC
CC Excl: See code 551.0

551.1 Umbilical hernia with gangrene   CC
Parumbilical hernia specified as gangrenous
CC Excl: 537.89, 537.9, 551.1-551.29, 552.1-552.29, 552.8-552.9,
553.1-553.29, 553.8-553.9

✓5th **551.2 Ventral hernia with gangrene**
551.20 Ventral, unspecified, with gangrene   CC
CC Excl: See code 551.1

551.21 Incisional, with gangrene   CC
Hernia:
  postoperative   } specified as
  recurrent, ventral }   gangrenous
CC Excl: See code 551.1

551.29 Other   CC
Epigastric hernia specified as gangrenous
CC Excl: See code 551.1

551.3 Diaphragmatic hernia with gangrene   CC
Hernia:
  hiatal (esophageal) (sliding) } specified as
  paraesophageal   }   gangrenous
  Thoracic stomach
EXCLUDES   congenital diaphragmatic hernia
(756.6)
CC Excl: 551.3, 552.3, 552.8-552.9, 553.3, 553.8-553.9

551.8 Hernia of other specified sites, with gangrene CC
Any condition classifiable to 553.8 if specified as
gangrenous
CC Excl: 537.89, 537.9, 550.00-550.93, 551.00-551.9,
552.00-552.9, 553.00-553.9

551.9 Hernia of unspecified site, with gangrene   CC
Any condition classifiable to 553.9 if specified as
gangrenous
CC Excl: See code 551.8

✓4th **552 Other hernia of abdominal cavity, with obstruction, but**
without mention of gangrene
EXCLUDES   that with mention of gangrene (551.0-551.9)

✓5th **552.0 Femoral hernia with obstruction**
Femoral hernia specified as incarcerated,
irreducible, strangulated, or causing
obstruction
552.00 Unilateral or unspecified (not specified   CC
as recurrent)
CC Excl: 537.89, 537.9, 551.00-551.03, 552.00-552.03,
552.8-552.9, 553.00-553.03, 553.8-553.9

N Newborn Age: 0   P Pediatric Age: 0-17   M Maternity Age: 12-55   A Adult Age :15-124   CC CC Condition   MC Major Complication   CD Complex Dx   HIV HIV Related Dx

158 — Volume 1   2002 Ingenix, Inc.

552.01 Unilateral or unspecified, recurrent `CC`
CC Excl: See code 552.00

552.02 Bilateral (not specified as recurrent) `CC`
CC Excl: See code 552.00

552.03 Bilateral, recurrent `CC`
CC Excl: See code 552.00

552.1 Umbilical hernia with obstruction `CC`
Parumbilical hernia specified as incarcerated, irreducible, strangulated, or causing obstruction

CC Excl: 551.1-551.29, 552.1-552.29, 552.8-552.9, 553.8-553.9

√5ᵗʰ **552.2 Ventral hernia with obstruction**
Ventral hernia specified as incarcerated, irreducible, strangulated, or causing obstruction

552.20 Ventral, unspecified, with obstruction `CC`
CC Excl: See code 552.1

552.21 Incisional, with obstruction `CC`
Hernia:
postoperative
recurrent, ventral
} specified as incarcerated, irreducible, strangulated, or causing obstruction

CC Excl: See code 552.1

552.29 Other `CC`
Epigastric hernia specified as incarcerated, irreducible, strangulated, or causing obstruction

CC Excl: See code 552.1

552.3 Diaphragmatic hernia with obstruction `CC`
Hernia:
hiatal (esophageal)
(sliding)
paraesophageal
Thoracic stomach
} specified as incarcerated, irreducible, strangulated, or causing obstruction

EXCLUDES congenital diaphragmatic hernia (756.6)

CC Excl: 551.3, 552.3-552.9, 553.3-553.9

552.8 Hernia of other specified sites, with obstruction `CC`
Any condition classifiable to 553.8 if specified as incarcerated, irreducible, strangulated, or causing obstruction

CC Excl: 550.00-550.93, 551.00-551.9, 552.00-552.9, 553.00-553.9

552.9 Hernia of unspecified site, with obstruction `CC`
Any condition classifiable to 553.9 if specified as incarcerated, irreducible, strangulated, or causing obstruction

CC Excl: See code 552.8

√4ᵗʰ **553 Other hernia of abdominal cavity without mention of obstruction or gangrene**
EXCLUDES the listed conditions with mention of:
gangrene (and obstruction) (551.0-551.9)
obstruction (552.0-552.9)

√5ᵗʰ **553.0 Femoral hernia**
553.00 Unilateral or unspecified (not specified as recurrent)
Femoral hernia NOS

553.01 Unilateral or unspecified, recurrent
553.02 Bilateral (not specified as recurrent)
553.03 Bilateral, recurrent

553.1 Umbilical hernia
Parumbilical hernia

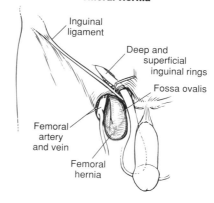

Femoral Hernia

Inguinal ligament
Deep and superficial inguinal rings
Fossa ovalis
Femoral artery and vein
Femoral hernia

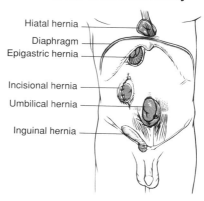

Hernias of Abdominal Cavity

Hiatal hernia
Diaphragm
Epigastric hernia
Incisional hernia
Umbilical hernia
Inguinal hernia

√5ᵗʰ **553.2 Ventral hernia**
553.20 Ventral, unspecified
553.21 Incisional
Hernia: Hernia:
postoperative   recurrent, ventral
553.29 Other
Hernia: Hernia:
epigastric   spigelian
553.3 Diaphragmatic hernia
Hernia: Thoracic stomach
hiatal (esophageal) (sliding)
paraesophageal
EXCLUDES congenital:
diaphragmatic hernia (756.6)
hiatal hernia (750.6)
esophagocele (530.6)

AHA: 2Q, '01, 6; 1Q, '00, 6

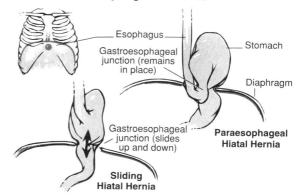

Diaphragmatic Hernias

Esophagus
Gastroesophageal junction (remains in place)
Stomach
Diaphragm
Gastroesophageal junction (slides up and down)
Paraesophageal Hiatal Hernia
Sliding Hiatal Hernia

√4ᵗʰ
√5ᵗʰ Additional Digit Required   Nonspecific PDx   Unacceptable PDx   Manifestation Code   `MSP` Medicare Secondary Payer   ◄ Revised Text   ● New Code   ▲ Revised Code Title

2002 Ingenix, Inc.

Volume 1 — 159

Digestive System 552.01–553.3

553.8　Hernia of other specified sites
　　Hernia:
　　　ischiatic
　　　ischiorectal
　　　lumbar
　　　obturator
　　　pudendal
　　　retroperitoneal
　　　sciatic
　　Other abdominal hernia of specified site
　　　　EXCLUDES　*vaginal enterocele (618.6)*

553.9　Hernia of unspecified site
　　Enterocele　　　　　　Hernia:
　　Epiplocele　　　　　　　intestinal
　　Hernia:　　　　　　　　intra-abdominal
　　　NOS　　　　　　　　Rupture (nontraumatic)
　　interstitial　　　　　Sarcoepiplocele

NONINFECTIOUS ENTERITIS AND COLITIS (555-558)

✓4ᵗʰ　555　Regional enteritis
　　　INCLUDES　Crohn's disease
　　　　　　　　Granulomatous enteritis
　　　EXCLUDES　*ulcerative colitis (556)*
　　DEF: Inflammation of intestine; classified to site.

555.0　Small intestine
　　Ileitis:　　　　　　　　Regional enteritis or
　　　regional　　　　　　　Crohn's disease of:
　　　segmental　　　　　　duodenum
　　　terminal　　　　　　　ileum
　　　　　　　　　　　　　　jejunum

555.1　Large intestine
　　Colitis:　　　　　　　　Regional enteritis or
　　　granulmatous　　　　　Crohn's disease of:
　　　regional　　　　　　　colon
　　　transmural　　　　　　large bowel
　　　　　　　　　　　　　　rectum
　　AHA: 3Q, '99, 8

555.2　Small intestine with large intestine
　　Regional ileocolitis

555.9　Unspecified site
　　Crohn's disease NOS
　　Regional enteritis NOS
　　AHA: 3Q, '99, 8; 4Q, '97, 42; 2Q, '97, 3

✓4ᵗʰ　556　Ulcerative colitis
　　AHA: 3Q, '99, 8

　　DEF: Chronic inflammation of mucosal lining of intestinal tract; may be single
　　area or entire colon.

556.0　Ulcerative (chronic) enterocolitis
556.1　Ulcerative (chronic) ileocolitis
556.2　Ulcerative (chronic) proctitis
556.3　Ulcerative (chronic) proctosigmoiditis

Large Intestine

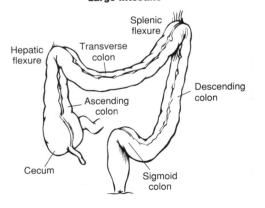

Splenic flexure
Transverse colon
Hepatic flexure
Descending colon
Ascending colon
Cecum
Sigmoid colon

556.4　Pseudopolyposis of colon
556.5　Left-sided ulcerative (chronic) colitis
556.6　Universal ulcerative (chronic) colitis
　　Pancolitis
556.8　Other ulcerative colitis
556.9　Ulcerative colitis, unspecified
　　Ulcerative enteritis NOS

✓4ᵗʰ　557　Vascular insufficiency of intestine
　　　EXCLUDES　*necrotizing enterocolitis of the newborn (777.5)*
　　DEF: Inadequacy of intestinal vessels.

557.0　Acute vascular insufficiency of intestine　　CC
　　Acute:
　　　hemorrhagic enterocolitis
　　　ischemic colitis, enteritis, or enterocolitis
　　　massive necrosis of intestine
　　Bowel infarction
　　Embolism of mesenteric artery
　　Fulminant enterocolitis
　　Hemorrhagic necrosis of intestine
　　Infarction of appendices epiploicae
　　Intestinal gangrene
　　Intestinal infarction (acute) (agnogenic)
　　　(hemorrhagic) (nonocclusive)
　　Mesenteric infarction (embolic) (thrombotic)
　　Necrosis of intestine
　　Terminal hemorrhagic enteropathy
　　Thrombosis of mesenteric artery
　　CC Excl: 557.0-557.1
　　　DRG 188
　　AHA: ▶4Q, '01, 53◀

557.1　Chronic vascular insufficiency of intestine
　　Angina, abdominal
　　Chronic ischemic colitis, enteritis, or enterocolitis
　　Ischemic stricture of intestine
　　Mesenteric:
　　　angina
　　　artery syndrome (superior)
　　　vascular insufficiency
　　AHA: 3Q, '96, 9; 4Q, '90, 4; N-D, '86, 11; N-D, '84, 7

557.9　Unspecified vascular insufficiency of intestine
　　Alimentary pain due to vascular insufficiency
　　Ischemic colitis, enteritis, or enterocolitis NOS
　　　DRG 188

✓4ᵗʰ　558　Other and unspecified noninfectious gastroenteritis and colitis
　　　EXCLUDES　*infectious:*
　　　　　　　colitis, enteritis, or gastroenteritis (009.0-
　　　　　　　009.1)
　　　　　　　diarrhea (009.2-009.3)

558.1　Gastroenteritis and colitis due to radiation　　CC
　　Radiation enterocolitis
　　CC Excl: 558.1

558.2　Toxic gastroenteritis and colitis　　CC
　　Use additional E code to identify cause
　　CC Excl: 558.2

558.3　Allergic gastroenteritis and colitis
　　AHA: 4Q, '00, 42

　　DEF: True immunoglobulin E (IgE)-mediated allergic reaction of the
　　lining of the stomach, intestines, or colon to food proteins; causes
　　nausea, vomiting, diarrhea, and abdominal cramping.

**558.9　Other and unspecified noninfectious gastroenteritis
and colitis**
　　Colitis
　　Enteritis
　　Gastroenteritis
　　Ileitis　　　　　　} NOS, dietetic, or
　　Jejunitis　　　　　　noninfectious
　　Sigmoiditis
　　AHA: 3Q, '99, 4, 6; N-D, '87, 7

N Newborn Age: 0　　P Pediatric Age: 0-17　　M Maternity Age: 12-55　　A Adult Age :15-124　　CC CC Condition　　MC Major Complication　　CD Complex Dx　　HIV HIV Related Dx

160 — Volume 1 • January 2002　　　　　　　　　　　　　　　　　　　　　　　　　　2002 Ingenix, Inc.

OTHER DISEASES OF INTESTINES AND PERITONEUM (560-569)

√4th **560 Intestinal obstruction without mention of hernia**

> EXCLUDES   duodenum (537.2-537.3)
> inguinal hernia with obstruction (550.1)
> intestinal obstruction complicating hernia
> (552.0-552.9)
> mesenteric:
>   embolism (557.0)
>   infarction (557.0)
>   thrombosis (557.0)
> neonatal intestinal obstruction (277.01, 777.1-
> 777.2, 777.4)

560.0 Intussusception cc

Intussusception (colon) (intestine) (rectum)
Invagination of intestine or colon

> EXCLUDES intussusception of appendix (543.9)

CC Excl: 560.0-560.9, 569.89, 569.9

AHA: 4Q, '98, 82

DEF: Prolapse of a bowel section into adjacent section; occurs primarily in children; symptoms include paroxysmal pain, vomiting, presence of lower abdominal tumor and blood, and mucous passage from rectum.

560.1 Paralytic ileus cc

Adynamic ileus
Ileus (of intestine) (of bowel) (of colon)
Paralysis of intestine or colon

> EXCLUDES gallstone ileus (560.31)

CC Excl: See code 560.0

AHA: J-F, '87, 13

DEF: Obstruction of ileus due to inhibited bowel motility.

560.2 Volvulus cc

Knotting
Strangulation } of intestine, bowel, or
Torsion   colon
Twist

CC Excl: See code 560.0

DEF: Entanglement of bowel; causes obstruction; may compromise bowel circulation.

√5th **560.3 Impaction of intestine**

560.30 Impaction of intestine, unspecified cc

Impaction of colon
CC Excl: See code 560.0

560.31 Gallstone ileus cc

Obstruction of intestine by gallstone
CC Excl: See code 560.0

Volvulus and Diverticulitis

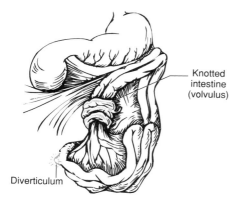

Knotted
intestine
(volvulus)

Diverticulum

560.39 Other cc

Concretion of intestine
Enterolith
Fecal impaction
CC Excl: See code 560.0

AHA: 4Q, '98, 38

√5th **560.8 Other specified intestinal obstruction**

560.81 Intestinal or peritoneal adhesions cc
with obstruction (postoperative)
(postinfection)

> EXCLUDES adhesions without obstruction
> (568.0)

CC Excl: See code 560.0

AHA: 4Q, '95, 55; 3Q, '95, 6; N-D, '87, 9

DEF: Obstruction of peritoneum or intestine due to abnormal union of tissues.

560.89 Other cc

Mural thickening causing obstruction

> EXCLUDES ischemic stricture of intestine
> (557.1)

CC Excl: See code 560.0

AHA: 2Q, '97, 3; 1Q, '88, 6

560.9 Unspecified intestinal obstruction cc

Enterostenosis
Obstruction
Occlusion } of intestine or colon
Stenosis
Stricture

> EXCLUDES congenital stricture or stenosis of
> intestine (751.1-751.2)

CC Excl: See code 560.0

√4th **562 Diverticula of intestine**

Use additional code to identify any associated:
peritonitis (567.0-567.9)

> EXCLUDES congenital diverticulum of colon (751.5)
> diverticulum of appendix (543.9)
> Meckel's diverticulum (751.0)

AHA: 4Q, '91, 25; J-F, '85, 1

√5th **562.0 Small intestine**

562.00 Diverticulosis of small intestine (without
mention of hemorrhage)

Diverticulosis:

duodenum }
ileum   } without mention of
jejunum } diverticulitis

DEF: Saclike herniations of mucous lining of small intestine.

562.01 Diverticulitis of small intestine (without
mention of hemorrhage)

Diverticulitis (with diverticulosis):
duodenum
ileum
jejunum
small intestine

DEF: Inflamed saclike herniations of mucous lining of small intestine.

562.02 Diverticulosis of small intestine with cc
hemorrhage

CC Excl: 251.5, 456.0, 530.2, 530.7, 530.82, 531.00-531.91, 532.00-532.91, 533.00-533.91, 534.00-534.91, 535.01, 535.11, 535.21, 535.31, 535.41, 535.51, 535.61, 537.83, 562.02-562.03, 562.12-562.13, 569.3, 569.85, 578.0-578.9

562.03 Diverticulitis of small intestine with cc
hemorrhage

CC Excl: See code 562.02

√4th √5th Additional Digit Required   Nonspecific PDx   Unacceptable PDx   Manifestation Code   MSP Medicare Secondary Payer   ►◄ Revised Text   ● New Code   ▲ Revised Code Title

2002 Ingenix, Inc.

Volume 1 — 161

Digestive System 562.1–566

√5ᵗʰ **562.1   Colon**

562.10   Diverticulosis of colon (without mention of hemorrhage)

Diverticulosis:
  NOS
  intestine (large)   } without mention
Diverticular disease   of diverticulitis
  (colon)

AHA: 4Q, '90, 21; J-F, '85, 5

DEF: Saclike herniations of mucous lining of large intestine

562.11   Diverticulitis of colon (without mention of hemorrhage)

Diverticulitis (with diverticulosis):
  NOS
  colon
  intestine (large)

AHA: 1Q, '96, 14; J-F, '85, 5

DEF: Inflamed saclike herniations of mucosal lining of large intestine.

562.12   Diverticulosis of colon with hemorrhage `CC`

CC Excl: See code 562.02

▽ **DRG** 174

562.13   Diverticulitis of colon with hemorrhage `CC`

CC Excl: See code 562.02

√4ᵗʰ **564   Functional digestive disorders, not elsewhere classified**

`EXCLUDES` *functional disorders of stomach (536.0-536.9)*
            those specified as psychogenic (306.4)

√5ᵗʰ **564.0   Constipation**

AHA: ▶4Q, '01, 45◀

564.00   Constipation, unspecified

564.01   Slow transit constipation

DEF:▶ Delay in the transit of fecal material through the colon secondary to smooth muscle dysfunction or decreased peristaltic contractions along the colon: also called colonic inertia or delayed transit. ◀

564.02   Outlet dysfunction constipation

DEF:▶ Failure to relax the paradoxical contractions of the striated pelvic floor muscles during the attempted defecation.◀

564.09   Other constipation

564.1   Irritable bowel syndrome

Irritable colon
Spastic colon

AHA: 1Q, '88, 6

DEF: Functional gastrointestinal disorder (FGID); symptoms following meals include diarrhea, constipation, abdominal pain; other symptoms include bloating, gas, distended abdomen, nausea, vomiting, appetite loss, emotional distress, and depression.

564.2   Postgastric surgery syndromes

Dumping syndrome   Postgastrectomy syndrome
Jejunal syndrome   Postvagotomy syndrome

`EXCLUDES` *malnutrition following gastrointestinal surgery (579.3)*
            postgastrojejunostomy ulcer (534.0-534.9)

AHA: 1Q, '95, 11

564.3   Vomiting following gastrointestinal surgery

Vomiting (bilious) following gastrointestinal surgery

564.4   Other postoperative functional disorders

Diarrhea following gastrointestinal surgery

`EXCLUDES` *colostomy and enterostomy complications (569.60-569.69)*

564.5   Functional diarrhea

`EXCLUDES` *diarrhea:*
            NOS (787.91)
            psychogenic (306.4)

DEF: Diarrhea with no detectable organic cause.

564.6   Anal spasm

Proctalgia fugax

564.7   Megacolon, other than Hirschsprung's

Dilatation of colon

`EXCLUDES` *megacolon:*
            congenital [Hirschsprung's] (751.3)
            toxic (556)

DEF: Enlarged colon; congenital or acquired; can occur acutely or become chronic.

√5ᵗʰ **564.8   Other specified functional disorders of intestine**

`EXCLUDES` *malabsorption (579.0-579.9)*

AHA: 1Q, '88, 6

564.81   Neurogenic bowel

AHA: 1Q, '01, 12; 4Q, '98, 45

DEF: Disorder of bowel due to spinal cord lesion above conus medullaris; symptoms include precipitous micturition, nocturia, catheter intolerance, headache, sweating, nasal obstruction and spastic contractions.

564.89   Other functional disorders of intestine

Atony of colon

564.9   Unspecified functional disorder of intestine

√4ᵗʰ **565   Anal fissure and fistula**

565.0   Anal fissure

Tear of anus, nontraumatic

`EXCLUDES` *traumatic (863.89, 863.99)*

DEF: Ulceration of cleft at anal mucosa; causes pain, itching, bleeding, infection, and sphincter spasm; may occur with hemorrhoids.

565.1   Anal fistula

Fistula:
  anorectal
  rectal
  rectum to skin

`EXCLUDES` *fistula of rectum to internal organs—*
            see Alphabetic Index
            ischiorectal fistula (566)
            rectovaginal fistula (619.1)

DEF: Abnormal opening on cutaneous surface near anus; may lack connection with rectum.

566   Abscess of anal and rectal regions   `CC`

Abscess:
  ischiorectal
  perianal
  perirectal
Cellulitis:
  anal
  perirectal
  rectal
Ischiorectal fistula

CC Excl: 566

Anal Fistula and Abscess

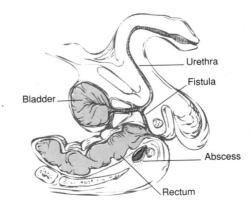

Urethra
Fistula
Bladder
Abscess
Rectum

`N` Newborn Age: 0   `P` Pediatric Age: 0-17   `M` Maternity Age: 12-55   `A` Adult Age: 15-124   `CC` CC Condition   `MC` Major Complication   `CD` Complex Dx   `HIV` HIV Related Dx

162 — Volume 1 • January 2002

2002 Ingenix, Inc.

✓4th **567 Peritonitis**

EXCLUDES peritonitis:
benign paroxysmal (277.3)
pelvic, female (614.5, 614.7)
periodic familial (277.3)
puerperal (670)
with or following:
abortion (634-638 with .0, 639.0)
appendicitis (540.0-540.1)
ectopic or molar pregnancy (639.0)

DEF: Inflammation of the peritoneal cavity.

567.0 **Peritonitis in infectious diseases classified elsewhere** CC
Code first underlying disease
EXCLUDES peritonitis:
gonococcal (098.86)
syphilitic (095.2)
tuberculous (014.0)
CC Excl: 567.0-567.9, 569.89, 569.9

567.1 **Pneumococcal peritonitis** CC
CC Excl: See code 567.0

567.2 **Other suppurative peritonitis** CC
Abscess (of):   Abscess (of):
  abdominopelvic   subhepatic
  mesenteric   subphrenic
  omentum   Peritonitis (acute):
  peritoneum   general
  retrocecal   pelvic, male
  retroperitoneal   subphrenic
  subdiaphragmatic   suppurative

CC Excl: See code 567.0

AHA: 2Q, '01, 11, 12; 3Q, '99, 9; 2Q, '98, 19

▽ DRG 188

567.8 **Other specified peritonitis** CC
Chronic proliferative   Peritonitis due to:
  peritonitis   bile
Fat necrosis of peritoneum   urine
Mesenteric saponification

CC Excl: See code 567.0

567.9 **Unspecified peritonitis** CC
Peritonitis: Peritonitis:
  NOS   of unspecified cause

CC Excl: See code 567.0

Rectum and Anus

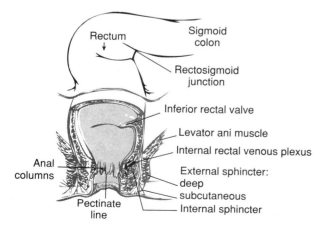

Rectum
Sigmoid colon
Rectosigmoid junction
Inferior rectal valve
Levator ani muscle
Internal rectal venous plexus
Anal columns
External sphincter:
  deep
  subcutaneous
Pectinate line
Internal sphincter

✓4th **568 Other disorders of peritoneum**

568.0 **Peritoneal adhesions (postoperative) (postinfection)**
Adhesions (of):   Adhesions (of):
  abdominal (wall)   mesenteric
  diaphragm   omentum
  intestine   stomach
  male pelvis   Adhesive bands

EXCLUDES adhesions:
pelvic, female (614.6)
with obstruction:
duodenum (537.3)
intestine (560.81)

AHA: 4Q, '95, 55; 3Q, '95, 7; S-O, '85, 11

DEF: Abnormal union of tissues in peritoneum.

✓5th **568.8** **Other specified disorders of peritoneum**
568.81 Hemoperitoneum (nontraumatic) CC
CC Excl: 568.81

568.82 Peritoneal effusion (chronic)
EXCLUDES *ascites NOS (789.5)*
DEF: Persistent leakage of fluid within peritoneal cavity.

568.89 Other
Peritoneal: Peritoneal:
  cyst   granuloma

568.9 **Unspecified disorder of peritoneum**

✓4th **569 Other disorders of intestine**

569.0 **Anal and rectal polyp**
Anal and rectal polyp NOS
EXCLUDES *adenomatous anal and rectal polyp (211.4)*

569.1 **Rectal prolapse**
Procidentia: Prolapse:
  anus (sphincter)   anal canal
  rectum (sphincter)   rectal mucosa
Proctoptosis
EXCLUDES *prolapsed hemorrhoids (455.2, 455.5)*

569.2 **Stenosis of rectum and anus**
Stricture of anus (sphincter)

569.3 **Hemorrhage of rectum and anus** CC
EXCLUDES *gastrointestinal bleeding NOS (578.9)*
melena (578.1)
CC Excl: 251.5, 456.0, 530.2, 530.7, 530.82, 531.00-531.91, 532.00-532.91, 533.00-533.91, 534.00-534.91, 535.01, 535.11, 535.21, 535.31, 535.41, 535.51, 535.61, 537.83, 562.02-562.03, 562.12-562.13, 569.3, 569.85, 578.0-578.9

✓5th **569.4** **Other specified disorders of rectum and anus**
569.41 Ulcer of anus and rectum
Solitary ulcer ⎫ of anus (sphincter) or
Stercoral ulcer ⎭   rectum (sphincter)

569.42 Anal or rectal pain
AHA: 1Q, '96, 13

569.49 Other
Granuloma ⎫ of rectum (sphincter)
Rupture ⎭

Hypertrophy of anal papillae
Proctitis NOS
EXCLUDES *fistula of rectum to:*
internal organs—see Alphabetic Index
skin (565.1)
hemorrhoids (455.0-455.9)
incontinence of sphincter ani (787.6)

Digestive System 567–569.49

✓4th ✓5th Additional Digit Required   Nonspecific PDx   Unacceptable PDx   Manifestation Code   MSP Medicare Secondary Payer   ►◄ Revised Text   ● New Code   ▲ Revised Code Title

2002 Ingenix, Inc.

Volume 1 — 163

Digestive System 569.5–571.4

569.5   Abscess of intestine `CC`
> **EXCLUDES**   appendiceal abscess (540.1)

CC Excl: 569.5

✓5ᵗʰ **569.6   Colostomy and enterostomy complications**

AHA: 4Q, '95, 58

DEF: Complication in a surgically created opening, from intestine to surface skin.

569.60   Colostomy and enterostomy complication, unspecified `CC`

CC Excl: 569.60-569.69

569.61   Infection of colostomy or enterostomy `CC`
> Use additional code to identify organism (041.00-041.9)
> Use additional code to specify type of infection, such as:
>> abscess or cellulitis of abdomen (682.2)
>> septicemia (038.0-038.9)

CC Excl: see code 596.60

569.62   Mechanical complication of colostomy and enterostomy `CC`
> Malfunction of colostomy and enterostomy

CC Excl: 536.40-536.49, 569.60-569.69, 997.4, 997.71, 997.91, 997.99, 998.81, 998.83-998.9

AHA: 4Q, '98, 44

569.69   Other complication `CC`
> Fistula   Prolapse
> Hernia

CC Excl: see code 596.60

AHA: 3Q, '98, 16

✓5ᵗʰ **569.8   Other specified disorders of intestine**

AHA: 4Q, '91, 25

569.81   Fistula of intestine, excluding rectum and anus
> Fistula: Fistula:
>> abdominal wall   enteroenteric
>> enterocolic   ileorectal
>
> **EXCLUDES**   fistula of intestine to internal organs—see Alphabetic Index
>> persistent postoperative fistula (998.6)

AHA: 3Q, '99, 8

569.82   Ulceration of intestine
> Primary ulcer of intestine
> Ulceration of colon
> **EXCLUDES**   that with perforation (569.83)

569.83   Perforation of intestine `CC`

CC Excl: 569.83

569.84   Angiodysplasia of intestine (without mention of hemorrhage)

AHA: 3Q, '96, 10; 4Q, '90, 4; 4Q, '90, 21

DEF: Small vascular abnormalities of the intestinal tract without bleeding problems.

569.85   Angiodysplasia of intestine with hemorrhage `CC`

CC Excl: 251.5, 456.0, 530.2, 530.7, 530.82, 531.00-531.91, 532.00-532.91, 533.00-533.91, 534.00-534.91, 535.01, 535.11, 535.21, 535.31, 535.41, 535.51, 535.61, 537.83, 562.02-562.03, 562.12-562.13, 569.3, 569.85, 578.0-578.9

AHA: 3Q, '96, 9

DEF: Small vascular abnormalities of the intestinal tract with bleeding problems.

569.86   Dieulafoy lesion (hemorrhagic) of intestine `CC`

CC Excl: 251.5, 530.2, 530.7, 530.82, 531.00-531.91, 532.00-532.91, 533.00-533.91, 534.00-534.91, 535.01, 535.11, 535.21, 535.31, 535.41, 535.51, 535.61, 537.83-537.84, 562.02-562.03, 562.12-562.13, 569.3, 569.85-569.86, 578.0-578.1, 578.9

569.89   Other
> Enteroptosis
> Granuloma   } of intestine
> Prolapse
>
> Pericolitis
> Perisigmoiditis
> Visceroptosis
> **EXCLUDES**   gangrene of intestine, mesentery, or omentum (557.0)
>> hemorrhage of intestine NOS (578.9)
>> obstruction of intestine (560.0-560.9)

AHA: 3Q, '96, 9

569.9   Unspecified disorder of intestine

OTHER DISEASES OF DIGESTIVE SYSTEM (570-579)

570   Acute and subacute necrosis of liver `CC`
> Acute hepatic failure
> Acute or subacute hepatitis, not specified as infective
> Necrosis of liver (acute) (diffuse) (massive) (subacute)
> Parenchymatous degeneration of liver
> Yellow atrophy (liver) (acute) (subacute)
> **EXCLUDES**   icterus gravis of newborn (773.0-773.2)
>> serum hepatitis (070.2-070.3)
>> that with:
>>> abortion (634-638 with .7, 639.8)
>>> ectopic or molar pregnancy (639.8)
>>> pregnancy, childbirth, or the puerperium (646.7)
>> viral hepatitis (070.0-070.9)

CC Excl: 570, 573.4-573.9

AHA: 1Q, '00, 22

✓4ᵗʰ **571   Chronic liver disease and cirrhosis**

571.0   Alcoholic fatty liver `A`

571.1   Acute alcoholic hepatitis `A`
> Acute alcoholic liver disease

571.2   Alcoholic cirrhosis of liver `CC` `A`
> Florid cirrhosis
> Laennec's cirrhosis (alcoholic)

CC Excl: 571.2, 573.8-573.9

AHA: ▶1Q, '02, 3;◀ N-D, '85, 14

DEF: Fibrosis and dysfunction, of liver; due to alcoholic liver disease.

571.3   Alcoholic liver damage, unspecified `A`

✓5ᵗʰ **571.4   Chronic hepatitis**
> **EXCLUDES**   viral hepatitis (acute) (chronic) (070.0-070.9)

Liver

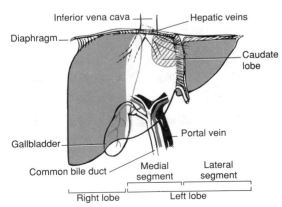

N Newborn Age: 0   **P** Pediatric Age: 0-17   **M** Maternity Age: 12-55   **A** Adult Age: 15-124   **CC** CC Condition   **MC** Major Complication   **CD** Complex Dx   **HIV** HIV Related Dx

164 — Volume 1 • October 2002   *2002 Ingenix, Inc.*

571.40 Chronic hepatitis, unspecified

571.41 Chronic persistent hepatitis

571.49 Other `CC`

Chronic hepatitis:
   active
   aggressive
Recurrent hepatitis

CC Excl: 571.49, 571.5-571.9, 573.8-573.9

AHA: 3Q, '99, 19; N-D, '85, 14

571.5 Cirrhosis of liver without mention of alcohol `CC`

Cirrhosis of liver: Cirrhosis of liver:
   NOS   postnecrotic
   cryptogenic   Healed yellow atrophy
   macronodular   (liver)
   micronodular   Portal cirrhosis
   posthepatitic

CC Excl: See code 571.49

DEF: Fibrosis and dysfunction of liver; not alcohol related.

571.6 Biliary cirrhosis `CC`

Chronic nonsuppurative destructive cholangitis
Cirrhosis:
   cholangitic
   cholestatic

CC Excl: See code 571.49

571.8 Other chronic nonalcoholic liver disease

Chronic yellow atrophy (liver)
Fatty liver, without mention of alcohol

AHA: 2Q, '96, 12

571.9 Unspecified chronic liver disease without mention of alcohol

√4ᵗʰ **572 Liver abscess and sequelae of chronic liver disease**

572.0 Abscess of liver `CC`

EXCLUDES   *amebic liver abscess (006.3)*

CC Excl: 006.3, 572.0-572.1, 573.8-573.9

572.1 Portal pyemia `CC`

Phlebitis of portal vein   Pylephlebitis
Portal thrombophlebitis   Pylethrombophlebitis

CC Excl: See code 572.0

DEF: Inflammation of portal vein or branches; may be due to intestinal disease; symptoms include fever, chills, jaundice, sweating, and abscess in various body parts.

572.2 Hepatic coma `CC`

Hepatic encephalopathy
Hepatocerebral intoxication
Portal-systemic encephalopathy

CC Excl: 572.2, 573.8-573.9

AHA: ▶1Q, '02, 3;◀ 3Q, '95, 14

572.3 Portal hypertension

DEF: Abnormally high blood pressure in the portal vein.

572.4 Hepatorenal syndrome `CC`

EXCLUDES   *that following delivery (674.8)*

CC Excl: 572.4, 573.8-573.9

AHA: 3Q, '93, 15

DEF: Hepatic and renal failure characterized by cirrhosis with ascites or obstructive jaundice, oliguria, and low sodium concentration.

572.8 Other sequelae of chronic liver disease

√4ᵗʰ **573 Other disorders of liver**

EXCLUDES   *amyloid or lardaceous degeneration of liver (277.3)*
congenital cystic disease of liver (751.62)
glycogen infiltration of liver (271.0)
hepatomegaly NOS (789.1)
portal vein obstruction (452)

573.0 Chronic passive congestion of liver

DEF: Blood accumulation in liver tissue.

573.1 Hepatitis in viral diseases classified elswhere `CC`

Code first underlying disease as:
   Coxsackie virus disease (074.8)
   cytomegalic inclusion virus disease (078.5)
   infectious mononucleosis (075)

EXCLUDES   *hepatitis (in):*
mumps (072.71)
viral (070.0-070.9)
yellow fever (060.0-060.9)

CC Excl: 573.1-573.3, 573.8-573.9

573.2 Hepatitis in other infectious diseases classified elsewhere `CC`

Code first underlying disease, as:
   malaria (084.9)

EXCLUDES   *hepatitis in:*
late syphilis (095.3)
secondary syphilis (091.62)
toxoplasmosis (130.5)

CC Excl: See code 573.1

573.3 Hepatitis, unspecified `CC`

Toxic (noninfectious) hepatitis
Use additional E code to identify cause

CC Excl: See code 573.1

AHA: 3Q, '98, 3, 4; 4Q, '90, 26

573.4 Hepatic infarction `CC`

CC Excl: 570, 573.4-573.9

573.8 Other specified disorders of liver

Hepatoptosis

573.9 Unspecified disorder of liver

√4ᵗʰ **574 Cholelithiasis**

The following fifth-digit subclassification is for use with category 574:

   0 without mention of obstruction
   1 with obstruction

√5ᵗʰ **574.0 Calculus of gallbladder with acute cholecystitis** `CC` `A`

Biliary calculus
Calculus of cystic duct   } with acute cholecystitis
Cholelithiasis

Any condition classifiable to 574.2 with acute cholecystitis

CC Excl: For code 574.00: 574.00-574.21, 574.40, 574.60-574.61, 574.80-574.81, 575.0, 575.10-575.12, 575.9, 576.8-576.9;
CC Excl: For code 574.01: 574.00-574.21, 574.60-574.61, 574.80-574.81, 575.0, 575.10-575.12, 575.9, 576.8-576.9

AHA: 4Q, '96, 32

√5ᵗʰ **574.1 Calculus of gallbladder with other cholecystitis** `CC` `A`

Biliary calculus
Calculus of cystic duct   } with cholecystitis
Cholelithiasis

Cholecystitis with cholelithiasis NOS
Any condition classifiable to 574.2 with cholecystitis (chronic)

CC Excl: See code 574.01

AHA: 3Q, '99, 9; 4Q, '96, 32, 69; 2Q, '96, 13

Digestive System 571.40–574.1

√4ᵗʰ
√5ᵗʰ
Additional Digit Required   Nonspecific PDx   Unacceptable PDx   Manifestation Code   `MSP` Medicare Secondary Payer   ▶◀ Revised Text   ● New Code   ▲ Revised Code Title

2002 Ingenix, Inc.   **October 2002 • Volume 1 — 165**

Gallbladder and Bile Ducts

Right hepatic artery
Cystic artery
Right and left bile ducts
Triangle of Calot
Common hepatic artery
Portal vein
Cystic duct
Gallstone in fundus
Hartmann s pouch (infundibulum)
Common bile duct empties into Duodenum

✓5th 574.2 Calculus of gallbladder without mention of cholecystitis CC 1 A

Biliary:
 calculus NOS
 colic NOS
Calculus of cystic duct

Cholelithiasis NOS
Colic (recurrent) of gallbladder
Gallstone (impacted)

CC Excl: For code 574.21: See code 574.01

AHA: For code 574.20: 1Q, '88, 14

✓5th 574.3 Calculus of bile duct with acute cholecystitis CC A

Calculus of bile duct [any]
Choledocholithiasis
} with acute cholecystitis

Any condition classifiable to 574.5 with acute cholecystitis

CC Excl: 574.30-574.51, 574.60-574.61, 574.70-574.71, 574.80-574.81, 574.90-574.91, 575.0, 575.10-575.12, 576.8-576.9

✓5th 574.4 Calculus of bile duct with other cholecystitis CC A

Calculus of bile duct [any]
Choledocholithiasis
} with cholecystitis (chronic)

Any condition classifiable to 574.5 with cholecystitis (chronic)

CC Excl: See code 574.3

✓5th 574.5 Calculus of bile duct without mention of cholecystitis CC A

Calculus of:
 bile duct [any]
 common duct
 hepatic duct

Choledocholithiasis
Hepatic:
 colic (recurrent)
 lithiasis

CC Excl: See code 574.3

AHA: 3Q, '94, 11

✓5th 574.6 Calculus of gallbladder and bile duct with acute cholecystitis CC A

Any condition classifiable to 574.0 and 574.3

CC Excl: 574.60-574.61, 575.0, 575.10-575.12, 575.9, 576.8-576.9

AHA: 4Q, '96, 32

✓5th 574.7 Calculus of gallbladder and bile duct with other cholecystitis CC A

Any condition classifiable to 574.1 and 574.4

CC Excl: 574.30-574.31, 574.40-574.41, 574.50-574.51, 574.60-574.61, 574.70-574.71, 574.80-574.81, 574.90-574.91, 575.0, 575.10-575.12, 576.8-576.9

AHA: 4Q, '96, 32

✓5th 574.8 Calculus of gallbladder and bile duct with acute and chronic cholecystitis CC A

Any condition classifiable to 574.6 and 574.7

CC Excl: 574.80-574.81, 575.0, 575.10-575.12, 575.9, 576.8-576.9

AHA: 4Q, '96, 32

✓5th 574.9 Calculus of gallbladder and bile duct without cholecystitis CC A

Any condition classifiable to 574.2 and 574.5

CC Excl: See code 574.7

AHA: 4Q, '96, 32

✓4th 575 Other disorders of gallbladder

575.0 Acute cholecystitis CC A

Abscess of gallbladder
Angiocholecystitis
Cholecystitis:
 emphysematous (acute)
 gangrenous
 suppurative
Empyema of gallbladder
Gangrene of gallbladder
} without mention of calculus

EXCLUDES that with:
 acute and chronic cholecystitis (575.12)
 choledocholithiasis (574.3)
 choledocholithiasis and cholelithiasis (574.6)
 cholelithiasis (574.0)

CC Excl: 574.60-574.61, 574.80-574.81, 575.0, 575.10-575.12, 575.9, 576.8-576.9

AHA: 3Q, '91, 17

✓5th 575.1 Other cholecystitis

Cholecystitis:
 NOS
 chronic
} without mention of calculus

EXCLUDES that with:
 choledocholithiasis (574.4)
 choledocholithiasis and cholelithiasis (574.8)
 cholelithiasis (574.1)

AHA: 4Q, '96, 32

575.10 Cholecystitis, unspecified A
Cholecystitis NOS

575.11 Chronic cholecystitis A

575.12 Acute and chronic cholecystitis CC A
CC Excl: 575.0, 575.10-575.12, 575.9, 576.8-576.9

AHA: 4Q, '97, 52; 4Q, '96, 32

575.2 Obstruction of gallbladder CC A

Occlusion
Stenosis
Stricture
} of cystic duct or gallbladder without mention of calculus

EXCLUDES that with calculus (574.0-574.2 with fifth-digit 1)

CC Excl: 575.2-575.9, 576.8-576.9

575.3 Hydrops of gallbladder CC A
Mucocele of gallbladder

CC Excl: See code 575.2

AHA: 2Q, '89, 13

DEF: Serous fluid accumulation in bladder.

575.4 Perforation of gallbladder CC
Rupture of cystic duct or gallbladder

CC Excl: See code 575.2

N Newborn Age: 0   P Pediatric Age: 0-17   M Maternity Age: 12-55   A Adult Age: 15-124   CC CC Condition   MC Major Complication   CD Complex Dx   HIV HIV Related Dx

2002 Ingenix, Inc.

575.5 **Fistula of gallbladder** `CC`
Fistula: Fistula:
cholecystoduodenal cholecystoenteric
CC Excl: See code 575.2

575.6 **Cholesterolosis of gallbladder**
Strawberry gallbladder
AHA: 4Q, '90, 17

DEF: Cholesterol deposits in gallbladder tissue.

575.8 **Other specified disorders of gallbladder**
Adhesions
Atrophy
Cyst
Hypertrophy } (of) cystic duct or
Nonfunctioning gallbladder
Ulcer

Biliary dyskinesia
EXCLUDES Hartmann's pouch of intestine (V44.3)
nonvisualization of gallbladder (793.3)

AHA: 4Q, '90, 26; 2Q, '89, 13

575.9 **Unspecified disorder of gallbladder**

√4ᵗʰ **576 Other disorders of biliary tract**
EXCLUDES that involving the:
cystic duct (575.0-575.9)
gallbladder (575.0-575.9)

576.0 **Postcholecystectomy syndrome** `A`
AHA: 1Q, '88, 10

DEF: Jaundice or abdominal pain following cholecystectomy.

576.1 **Cholangitis** `CC`
Cholangitis: Cholangitis:
NOS recurrent
acute sclerosing
ascending secondary
chronic stenosing
primary suppurative
CC Excl: 576.1, 576.8-576.9

AHA: 2Q, '99, 13

576.2 **Obstruction of bile duct**
Occlusion } of bile duct, except cystic
Stenosis } duct, without mention
Stricture } of calculus

EXCLUDES congenital (751.61)
that with calculus (574.3-574.5 with
fifth-digit 1)
AHA: 1Q, '01, 8; 2Q, '99, 13

576.3 **Perforation of bile duct** `CC`
Rupture of bile duct, except cystic duct
CC Excl: 576.3-576.4, 576.8-576.9

576.4 **Fistula of bile duct** `CC`
Choledochoduodenal fistula
CC Excl: See code 576.3

576.5 **Spasm of sphincter of Oddi**
576.8 **Other specified disorders of biliary tract**
Adhesions
Atrophy
Cyst
Hypertrophy } of bile duct [any]
Stasis
Ulcer

EXCLUDES congenital choledochal cyst (751.69)
AHA: 2Q, '99, 14

576.9 **Unspecified disorder of biliary tract**

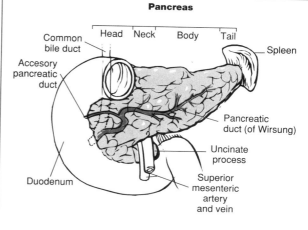

Pancreas

√4ᵗʰ **577 Diseases of pancreas**
577.0 **Acute pancreatitis** `CC`
Abscess of pancreas Pancreatitis:
Necrosis of pancreas: acute (recurrent)
acute apoplectic
infective hemorrhagic
Pancreatitis: subacute
NOS suppurative
EXCLUDES mumps pancreatitis (072.3)
CC Excl: 577.0-577.1, 577.8-577.9

AHA: 3Q, '99, 9; 2Q, '98, 19; 2Q, '96, 13; 2Q, '89, 9

577.1 **Chronic pancreatitis** `A`
Chronic pancreatitis: Pancreatitis:
NOS painless
infectious recurrent
interstitial relapsing
AHA: 1Q, '01, 8; 2Q, '96, 13; 3Q, '94, 11

577.2 **Cyst and pseudocyst of pancreas** `CC`
CC Excl: 577.2, 577.8-577.9

577.8 **Other specified diseases of pancreas**
Atrophy
Calculus
Cirrhosis } of pancreas
Fibrosis

Pancreatic: Pancreatic:
infantilism necrosis:
necrosis: fat
NOS Pancreatolithiasis
aseptic
EXCLUDES fibrocystic disease of pancreas
▶(277.00-277.09)◀
islet cell tumor of pancreas (211.7)
pancreatic steatorrhea (579.4)

AHA: 1Q, '01, 8

577.9 **Unspecified disease of pancreas**

√4ᵗʰ
√5ᵗʰ Additional Digit Required   Nonspecific PDx   Unacceptable PDx   Manifestation Code   **MSP** Medicare Secondary Payer   ▶◀ Revised Text   ● New Code   ▲ Revised Code Title

2002 Ingenix, Inc.

October 2002 • Volume 1 — 167

Digestive System 578–579.9

√4ᵗʰ **578 Gastrointestinal hemorrhage**

> EXCLUDES   *that with mention of:*
> *angiodysplasia of stomach and duodenum (537.83)*
> *angiodysplasia of intestine (569.85)*
> *diverticulitis, intestine:*
> *large (562.13)*
> *small (562.03)*
> *diverticulosis, intestine:*
> *large (562.12)*
> *small (562.02)*
> *gastritis and duodenitis (535.0-535.6)*
> *ulcer:*
> *duodenal, gastric, gastrojejuunal or peptic (531.00-534.91)*

AHA: 2Q, '92, 9; 4Q, '90, 20

578.0   Hematemesis   `CC`
> Vomiting of blood

CC Excl: 251.5, 456.0, 530.2, 530.7, 530.82, 531.00-531.91, 532.00-532.91, 533.00-533.91, 534.00-534.91, 535.01, 535.11, 535.21, 535.31, 535.41, 535.51, 535.61, 537.83, 562.02-562.03, 562.12-562.13, 569.3, 569.85, 578.0-578.9

578.1   Blood in stool   `CC`
> Melena
>
> > EXCLUDES   *melena of the newborn (772.4, 777.3)*
> > *occult blood (792.1)*

CC Excl: See code 578.0

AHA: 2Q, '92, 8

   `DRG` **174**

578.9   Hemorrhage of gastrointestinal tract, unspecified   `CC`
> Gastric hemorrhage
> Intestinal hemorrhage

CC Excl: See code 578.0

AHA: N-D, '86, 9

√4ᵗʰ **579 Intestinal malabsorption**

579.0   Celiac disease
> Celiac: Gee (-Herter) disease
>   crisis   Gluten enteropathy
>   infantilism   Idiopathic steatorrhea
>   rickets   Nontropical sprue

DEF: Malabsorption syndrome due to gluten consumption; symptoms include fetid, bulky, frothy, oily stools; distended abdomen, gas, weight loss, asthenia, electrolyte depletion and vitamin B, D and K deficiency.

579.1   Tropical sprue
> Sprue: Tropical steatorrhea
>   NOS
>   tropical

DEF: Diarrhea, occurs in tropics; may be due to enteric infection and malnutrition.

579.2   Blind loop syndrome
> Postoperative blind loop syndrome

DEF: Obstruction or impaired passage in small intestine due to alterations, from strictures or surgery; causes stasis, abnormal bacterial flora, diarrhea, weight loss, multiple vitamin deficiency, and megaloblastic anemia.

579.3   Other and unspecified postsurgical nonabsorption   `CC`
> Hypoglycemia   }   following gastrointestinal
> Malnutrition   surgery

CC Excl: 579.3-579.9

579.4   Pancreatic steatorrhea

DEF: Excess fat in feces due to absence of pancreatic juice in intestine.

579.8   Other specified intestinal malabsorption
> Enteropathy: Steatorrhea (chronic)
>   exudative
>   protein-losing

AHA: 1Q, '88, 6

579.9   Unspecified intestinal malabsorption
> Malabsorption syndrome NOS

| `N` Newborn Age: 0 | `P` Pediatric Age: 0-17 | `M` Maternity Age: 12-55 | `A` Adult Age: 15-124 | `CC` CC Condition | `MC` Major Complication | `CD` Complex Dx | `HIV` HIV Related Dx |

168 — Volume 1 • October 2002   *2002 Ingenix, Inc.*

10. DISEASES OF THE GENITOURINARY SYSTEM (580-629)

Kidney

Nephron

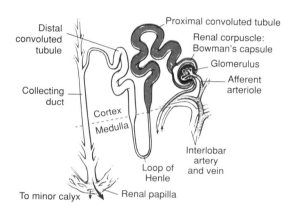

NEPHRITIS, NEPHROTIC SYNDROME, AND NEPHROSIS (580-589)

EXCLUDES　　hypertensive renal disease (403.00-403.91)

✓4ᵗʰ **580 Acute glomerulonephritis**

INCLUDES　acute nephritis

DEF: Acute, severe inflammation in tuft of capillaries that filter the kidneys.

580.0　With lesion of proliferative glomerulonephritis CC
Acute (diffuse) proliferative glomerulonephritis
Acute poststreptococcal glomerulonephritis

CC Excl: 016.00-016.06, 016.30-016.36, 016.90-016.96, 017.90-
017.96, 098.10, 098.19, 098.30-098.31, 098.89, 112.2, 131.00,
131.8-131.9, 250.40-250.43, 250.80-250.93, 274.10, 274.19,
580.0-580.9, 581.0-581.9, 582.0-582.9, 583.0-583.9, 584.5-584.9,
585-587, 588.0-588.9, 589.0-589.9, 590.00-590.9, 591, 593.0-593.2,
593.89, 593.9, 599.7-599.9

580.4　With lesion of rapidly progressive CC
glomerulonephritis
Acute nephritis with lesion of necrotizing
glomerulitis

CC Excl: See code 580.0

DEF: Acute glomerulonephritis; progresses to ESRD with diffuse
epithelial proliferation.

✓5ᵗʰ **580.8　With other specified pathological lesion in kidney**

580.81 *Acute glomerulonephritis in diseases* CC
classified elsewhere
Code first underlying disease, as:
infectious hepatitis (070.0-070.9)
mumps (072.79)
subacute bacterial endocarditis (421.0)
typhoid fever (002.0)

CC Excl: See code 580.0

580.89　Other CC
Glomerulonephritis, acute, with lesion of:
exudative nephritis
interstitial (diffuse) (focal) nephritis

CC Excl: 016.00-016.06, 016.30-016.36, 016.90-016.96,
017.90-017.96, 098.10, 098.19, 098.30-098.31, 098.89,
112.2, 131.00, 131.8-131.9, 274.10, 274.19, 580.0-580.9,
581.0-581.9, 582.0-582.9, 583.0-583.9, 584.5-584.9, 585-
587, 588.0-588.9, 589.0-589.9, 590.00-590.9, 591, 593.0-
593.2, 593.89, 593.9, 599.7-599.9

580.9　Acute glomerulonephritis with unspecified CC
pathological lesion in kidney
Glomerulonephritis:
NOS
hemorrhagic　} specified as acute
Nephritis
Nephropathy

CC Excl: 016.00-016.06, 016.30-016.36, 016.90-016.96, 017.90-
017.96, 098.10, 098.19, 098.30-098.31, 098.89, 112.2, 131.00,
131.8-131.9, 250.40-250.43, 250.80-250.93, 274.10, 274.19, 580.0-
580.9, 581.0-581.9, 582.0-582.9, 583.0-583.9, 584.5-584.9, 585-587,
588.0-588.9, 589.0-589.9, 590.00-590.09, 591, 593.0-593.2, 593.89,
593.9, 599.7-599.9

✓4ᵗʰ **581 Nephrotic syndrome**
DEF: Disease process marked by symptoms such as; extensive edema, notable
proteinuria, hypoalbuminemia, and susceptibility to intercurrent infections.

581.0　With lesion of proliferative glomerulonephritis CC
CC Excl: See code 580.9

581.1　With lesion of membranous glomerulonephritis CC
Epimembranous nephritis
Idiopathic membranous glomerular disease
Nephrotic syndrome with lesion of:
focal glomerulosclerosis
sclerosing membranous glomerulonephritis
segmental hyalinosis

CC Excl: See code 580.9

581.2　With lesion of membranoproliferative CC
glomerulonephritis
Nephrotic syndrome with lesion (of):
endothelial
hypocomplementemic
persistent
lobular　　　　　　} glomerulonephritis
mesangiocapillary
mixed membranous and
proliferative

CC Excl: See code 580.9

DEF: Glomerulonephritis combined with clinical features of
nephrotic syndrome; characterized by uneven thickening of
glomerular capillary walls and mesangial cell increase; slowly
progresses to ESRD.

581.3　With lesion of minimal change CC
glomerulonephritis
Foot process disease
Lipoid nephrosis
Minimal change:
glomerular disease
glomerulitis
nephrotic syndrome

CC Excl: See code 580.9

✓4ᵗʰ
✓5ᵗʰ Additional Digit Required　　Nonspecific PDx　　Unacceptable PDx　　Manifestation Code　　MSP Medicare Secondary Payer　　►◄ Revised Text　　● New Code　　▲ Revised Code Title

2002 Ingenix, Inc.　　　　　　　　　　　　　　　　　　　　　　　　　　　　　　　　　　　　Volume 1 — 169

Genitourinary System 580–581.3

Genitourinary System 581.8–583.81

✓4ᵗʰ **581.8** **With other specified pathological lesion in kidney**

     581.81 *Nephrotic syndrome in diseases* `CC`
         classified elsewhere

            Code first underlying disease, as:
               amyloidosis (277.3)
               diabetes mellitus (250.4)
               malaria (084.9)
               polyarteritis (446.0)
               systemic lupus erythematosus (710.0)

             EXCLUDES   *nephrosis in epidemic*
                          hemorrhagic fever
                          (078.6)

         CC Excl: See code 580.9

         AHA: 3Q, '91, 8,12; S-O, '85, 3

     581.89 **Other** `CC`
         Glomerulonephritis with edema and lesion
         of:
            exudative nephritis
            interstitial (diffuse) (focal) nephritis

         CC Excl: See code 580.9

     581.9 **Nephrotic syndrome with unspecified** `CC`
         pathological lesion in kidney
         Glomerulonephritis with edema NOS
         Nephritis:
            nephrotic NOS
            with edema NOS
         Nephrosis NOS
         Renal disease with edema NOS

         CC Excl: See code 580.9

✓4ᵗʰ **582** **Chronic glomerulonephritis**
         INCLUDES   chronic nephritis

   DEF: Slow progressive type of nephritis characterized by inflammation of the
   capillary loops in the glomeruli of the kidney, which leads to renal failure.

     582.0 **With lesion of proliferative glomerulonephritis**
         Chronic (diffuse) proliferative glomerulonephritis

     582.1 **With lesion of membranous glomerulonephritis**
         Chronic glomerulonephritis:
            membranous
            sclerosing
         Focal glomerulosclerosis
         Segmental hyalinosis

         AHA: S-O, '84, 16

     582.2 **With lesion of membranoproliferative**
         glomerulonephritis
         Chronic glomerulonephritis:
            endothelial
            hypocomplementemic persistent
            lobular
            membranoproliferative
            mesangiocapillary
            mixed membranous and proliferative

         DEF: Chronic glomerulonephritis with mesangial cell proliferation.

     582.4 **With lesion of rapidly progressive**
         glomerulonephritis
         Chronic nephritis with lesion of necrotizing
            glomerulitis

         DEF: Chronic glomerulonephritis rapidly progresses to ESRD;
         marked by diffuse epithelial proliferation.

✓5ᵗʰ **582.8** **With other specified pathological lesion in kidney**

     582.81 *Chronic glomerulonephritis in diseases*
         classified elsewhere

            Code first underlying disease, as:
               amyloidosis (277.3)
               systemic lupus erythematosus (710.0)

     582.89 **Other**
         Chronic glomerulonephritis with lesion of:
            exudative nephritis
            interstitial (diffuse) (focal) nephritis

     582.9 **Chronic glomerulonephritis with unspecified**
         pathological lesion in kidney
         Glomerulonephritis:
            NOS
            hemorrhagic   }   specified as chronic
         Nephritis
         Nephropathy

         AHA: 2Q, '01, 12

✓4ᵗʰ **583** **Nephritis and nephropathy, not specified as acute or chronic**
     INCLUDES   "renal disease" so stated, not specified as acute
                   or chronic but with stated pathology or
                   cause

     583.0 **With lesion of proliferative glomerulonephritis**
         Proliferative: Proliferative
            glomerulonephritis   nephritis NOS
            (diffuse) NOS   nephropathy NOS

     583.1 **With lesion of membranous glomerulonephritis**
         Membranous:
            glomerulonephritis NOS
            nephritis NOS
         Membranous nephropathy NOS

         DEF: Kidney inflammation or dysfunction with deposits on
         glomerular capillary basement membranes.

     583.2 **With lesion of membranoproliferative**
         glomerulonephritis
         Membranoproliferative:
            glomerulonephritis NOS
            nephritis NOS
            nephropathy NOS
         Nephritis NOS, with lesion of:
            hypocomplementemic
            persistent
            lobular   }
            mesangiocapillary   } glomerulonephritis
            mixed membranous   }
              and proliferative   }

         DEF: Kidney inflammation or dysfunction with mesangial cell
         proliferation.

     583.4 **With lesion of rapidly progressive** `CC`
         glomerulonephritis
         Necrotizing or rapidly progressive:
            glomerulitis NOS
            glomerulonephritis NOS
            nephritis NOS
            nephropathy NOS
         Nephritis, unspecified, with lesion of necrotizing
            glomerulitis

         CC Excl: See code 580.9

         DEF: Kidney inflammation or dysfunction; rapidly progresses to
         ESRD marked by diffuse epithelial proliferation.

     583.6 **With lesion of renal cortical necrosis**
         Nephritis NOS   } with (renal) cortical
         Nephropathy NOS   }   necrosis

         Renal cortical necrosis NOS

     583.7 **With lesion of renal medullary necrosis**
         Nephritis NOS   } with (renal) medullary
         Nephropathy NOS   }   [papillary] necrosis

✓5ᵗʰ **583.8** **With other specified pathological lesion in kidney**

     583.81 *Nephritis and nephropathy, not specified*
         as acute or chronic, in diseases classified
         elsewhere

            Code first underlying disease, as:
               amyloidosis (277.3)
               diabetes mellitus (250.4)
               gonococcal infection (098.19)
               Goodpasture's syndrome (446.21)
               systemic lupus erythematosus (710.0)
               tuberculosis (016.0)
             EXCLUDES   *gouty nephropathy (274.10)*
                          syphilitic nephritis (095.4)

         AHA: 3Q, '91, 8; S-O, '85, 3

N Newborn Age: 0   P Pediatric Age: 0-17   M Maternity Age: 12-55   A Adult Age: 15-124   CC CC Condition   MC Major Complication   CD Complex Dx   HIV HIV Related Dx

583.89 Other

Glomerulitis	with lesion of:
Glomerulonephritis	exudative
Nephritis	nephritis
Nephropathy	interstitial
Renal disease	nephritis

583.9 With unspecified pathological lesion in kidney

Glomerulitis	
Glomerulonephritis	NOS
Nephritis	
Nephropathy	

> EXCLUDES *nephropathy complicating pregnancy, labor, or the puerperium (642.0-642.9, 646.2)*
> *renal disease NOS with no stated cause (593.9)*

√4th **584 Acute renal failure**

> EXCLUDES *following labor and delivery (669.3)*
> *posttraumatic (958.5)*
> *that complicating:*
> *abortion (634-638 with .3, 639.3)*
> *ectopic or molar pregnancy (639.3)*

AHA: 1Q, '93, 18; 2Q, '92, 5; 4Q, '92, 22

DEF: State resulting from increasing urea and related substances from the blood (azotemia), often with urine output of less than 500 ml per day.

584.5 With lesion of tubular necrosis CC MC

Lower nephron nephrosis
Renal failure with (acute) tubular necrosis
Tubular necrosis:
  NOS
  acute

CC Excl: 250.40-250.43, 250.80-250.93, 274.10, 274.19, 580.0-580.9, 581.0-581.9, 582.0-582.9, 583.0-583.9, 584.5-584.9, 585-587, 588.0-588.9, 589.0-589.9, 590.00-590.9, 591, 593.0-593.2, 593.89, 593.9, 599.7-599.9, 753.0, 753.20-753.23, 753.29, 753.3, 753.9

DEF: Acute decline in kidney efficiency with destruction of tubules.

584.6 With lesion of renal cortical necrosis CC MC

CC Excl: See code 584.5

DEF: Acute decline in kidney efficiency with destruction of renal tissues that filter blood.

584.7 With lesion of renal medullary [papillary] necrosis CC MC

Necrotizing renal papillitis

CC Excl: See code 584.5

DEF: Acute decline in kidney efficiency with destruction of renal tissues that collect urine.

584.8 With other specified pathological lesion in kidney CC MC

CC Excl: 250.40-250.43, 250.80-250.93, 274.10, 274.19, 580.0-580.9, 581.0-581.9, 582.0-582.9, 583.0-583.9, 584.5-584.9, 585-587, 588.0-588.9, 589.0-589.9, 590.00-590.9, 591, 593.0-593.2, 593.89, 593.9, 599.7-599.9

AHA: N-D, '85, 1

584.9 Acute renal failure, unspecified CC MC

CC Excl: 250.40-250.43, 250.80-250.93, 274.10, 274.19, 580.0-580.9, 581.0-581.9, 582.0-582.9, 583.0-583.9, 584.5-584.9, 585-587, 588.0-588.9, 589.0-589.9, 590.00-590.9, 591, 593.0-593.2, 593.89, 593.9, 599.7-599.9, 753.0, 753.20-753.23, 753.29, 753.3, 753.9

AHA: 2Q, '01, 14; 1Q, '00, 22; 3Q, '96, 9; 4Q, '88, 1

▽ **DRG 316**

585 Chronic renal failure CC

Chronic uremia
Use additional code to identify manifestation as:
  uremic:
    neuropathy (357.4)
    pericarditis (420.0)

> EXCLUDES *that with any condition classifiable to 401 (403.0-403.9 with fifth-digit 1)*

CC Excl: See code 584.9

AHA: 2Q, '01, 12, 13; 1Q, '01, 3; 4Q, '98, 55; 3Q, '98, 6, 7; 2Q, '98, 20; 3Q, '96, 9; 1Q, '93, 18; 3Q, '91, 8; 4Q, '89, 1; N-D, '85, 15; S-O, '84, 3

▽ **DRG 316**

586 Renal failure, unspecified

Uremia NOS

> EXCLUDES *following labor and delivery (669.3)*
> *posttraumatic renal failure (958.5)*
> *that complicating:*
> *abortion (634-638 with .3, 639.3)*
> *ectopic or molar pregnancy (639.3)*
> *uremia:*
> *extrarenal (788.9)*
> *prerenal (788.9)*
> *with any condition classifiable to 401 (403.0-403.9 with fifth-digit 1)*

AHA: 3Q, '98, 6; 1Q, '93, 18

DEF: Renal failure: kidney functions cease; malfunction may be due to inability to excrete metabolized substances or retain level of electrolytes.

DEF: Uremia: excess urea, creatinine and other nitrogenous products of protein and amino acid metabolism in blood due to reduced excretory function in bilateral kidney disease; also called azotemia.

587 Renal sclerosis, unspecified

Atrophy of kidney	Renal:
Contracted kidney	cirrhosis
	fibrosis

> EXCLUDES *nephrosclerosis (arteriolar) (arteriosclerotic) (403.00-403.91)*
> *with hypertension (403.00-403.92)*

√4th **588 Disorders resulting from impaired renal function**

588.0 Renal osteodystrophy

Azotemic osteodystrophy
Phosphate-losing tubular disorders
Renal:
  dwarfism   infantilism
  rickets

DEF: Bone disorder that results in various bone diseases such as osteomalacia, osteoporosis or osteosclerosis; caused by impaired renal function, an abnormal level of phosphorus in the blood and impaired stimulation of the parathyroid.

588.1 Nephrogenic diabetes insipidus

> EXCLUDES *diabetes insipidus NOS (253.5)*

DEF: Type of diabetes due to renal tubules inability to reabsorb water; not responsive to vasopressin; may develop into chronic renal insufficiency.

588.8 Other specified disorders resulting from impaired renal function

Hypokalemic nephropathy
Secondary hyperparathyroidism (of renal origin)

> EXCLUDES *secondary hypertension (405.0-405.9)*

588.9 Unspecified disorder resulting from impaired renal function

√4th **589 Small kidney of unknown cause**

589.0 Unilateral small kidney

589.1 Bilateral small kidneys

589.9 Small kidney, unspecified

√4th √5th Additional Digit Required   Nonspecific PDx   Unacceptable PDx   Manifestation Code   MSP Medicare Secondary Payer   ▶◀ Revised Text   ● New Code   ▲ Revised Code Title

2002 Ingenix, Inc.   **Volume 1 — 171**

Genitourinary System 590–593.4 *(side tab)*

OTHER DISEASES OF URINARY SYSTEM (590-599)

✓4ᵗʰ 590 Infections of kidney
Use additional code to identify organism, such as Escherichia coli [E. coli] (041.4)

✓5ᵗʰ 590.0 Chronic pyelonephritis
Chronic pyelitis
Chronic pyonephrosis
►Code if applicable, any casual condition first◄

590.00 Without lesion of renal medullary necrosis
590.01 With lesion of renal medullary necrosis

✓5ᵗʰ 590.1 Acute pyelonephritis
Acute pyelitis   Acute pyonephrosis

590.10 Without lesion of renal medullary necrosis `CC`
CC Excl: 016.00-016.06, 016.30-016.36, 016.90-016.96, 017.90-017.96, 098.10, 098.19, 098.30-098.31, 098.89, 112.2, 131.00, 131.8-131.9, 250.40-250.43, 250.80-250.93, 274.10, 274.19, 580.0-580.9, 581.0-581.9, 582.0-582.9, 583.0-583.9, 584.5-584.9, 585-587, 588.0-588.9, 589.0-589.9, 590.00-590.9, 591, 593.0-593.2, 593.89, 593.9, 599.0, 599.7-599.9

▽ DRG 320

590.11 With lesion of renal medullary necrosis `CC`
CC Excl: See code 590.10

590.2 Renal and perinephric abscess `CC`
Abscess: Abscess:
kidney   perirenal
nephritic   Carbuncle of kidney
CC Excl: See code 590.10

590.3 Pyeloureteritis cystica `CC`
Infection of renal pelvis and ureter
Ureteritis cystica
CC Excl: 016.00-016.06, 016.30-016.36, 016.90-016.96, 017.90-017.96, 098.10, 098.19, 098.30-098.31, 098.89, 112.2, 131.00, 131.8-131.9, 274.10, 274.19, 580.0-580.9, 581.0-581.9, 582.0-582.9, 583.0-583.9, 584.5-584.9, 585-587, 588.0-588.9, 589.0-589.9, 590.00-590.9, 591, 593.0-593.2, 593.89, 593.9, 599.0, 599.7-599.9
DEF: Inflammation and formation of submucosal cysts in the kidney, pelvis, and ureter.

✓5ᵗʰ 590.8 Other pyelonephritis or pyonephrosis, not specified as acute or chronic

590.80 Pyelonephritis, unspecified `CC`
Pyelitis NOS
Pyelonephritis NOS
CC Excl: See code 590.3
AHA: 1Q, '98, 10; 4Q, '97, 40

590.81 Pyelitis or pyelonephritis in diseases classified elsewhere `CC`
Code first underlying disease, as:
tuberculosis (016.0)
CC Excl: See code 590.3
▽ DRG 320

590.9 Infection of kidney, unspecified `CC`
EXCLUDES urinary tract infection NOS (599.0)
CC Excl: See code 590.3

591 Hydronephrosis `CC`
Hydrocalycosis
Hydronephrosis
Hydroureteronephrosis
EXCLUDES congenital hydronephrosis (753.29)
hydroureter (593.5)
CC Excl: See code 590.3
AHA: 2Q, '98, 9
DEF: Distention of kidney and pelvis, with urine build-up due to ureteral obstruction; pyonephrosis may result.

Genitourinary System

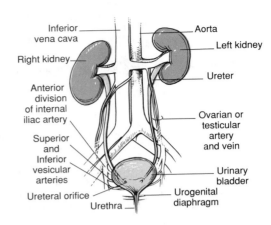

✓4ᵗʰ 592 Calculus of kidney and ureter
EXCLUDES nephrocalcinosis (275.4)

592.0 Calculus of kidney
Nephrolithiasis NOS
Renal calculus or stone
Staghorn calculus
Stone in kidney
EXCLUDES uric acid nephrolithiasis (274.11)
AHA: 1Q, '00, 4

592.1 Calculus of ureter `CC`
Ureteric stone
Ureterolithiasis
CC Excl: 592.0-592.9, 593.3-593.5, 593.89, 593.9, 594.0-594.9, 599.6-599.9
AHA: 2Q, '98, 9; 1Q, '98, 10; 1Q, '91, 11

592.9 Urinary calculus, unspecified
AHA: 1Q, '98, 10; 4Q, '97, 40

✓4ᵗʰ 593 Other disorders of kidney and ureter
593.0 Nephroptosis
Floating kidney
Mobile kidney

593.1 Hypertrophy of kidney

593.2 Cyst of kidney, acquired
Cyst (multiple) (solitary) of kidney, not congenital
Peripelvic (lymphatic) cyst
EXCLUDES calyceal or pyelogenic cyst of kidney (591)
congenital cyst of kidney (753.1)
polycystic (disease of) kidney (753.1)
AHA: 4Q, '90, 3
DEF: Abnormal, fluid-filled sac in the kidney, not present at birth.

593.3 Stricture or kinking of ureter
Angulation ⎫
Constriction ⎬ of ureter (post-operative)
Stricture of pelviureteric junction
AHA: 2Q, '98, 9
DEF: Stricture or knot in tube connecting kidney to bladder.

593.4 Other ureteric obstruction
Idiopathic retroperitoneal fibrosis
Occlusion NOS of ureter
EXCLUDES that due to calculus (592.1)
AHA: 2Q, '97, 4

N Newborn Age: 0   P Pediatric Age: 0-17   M Maternity Age: 12-55   A Adult Age: 15-124   CC CC Condition   MC Major Complication   CD Complex Dx   HIV HIV Related Dx

593.5 Hydroureter `cc`

> *EXCLUDES*   congenital hydroureter (753.22)
>   hydroureteronephrosis (591)

CC Excl: 593.3-593.5, 593.89, 593.9, 595.0-595.9, 596.8-596.9, 599.0, 599.6-599.9, 753.4-753.5, 753.9

593.6 Postural proteinuria

> Benign postural proteinuria   Orthostatic
> proteinuria
> *EXCLUDES*   proteinuria NOS (791.0)3

DEF: Excessive amounts of serum protein in the urine caused by the body position, e.g., orthostatic and lordotic.

✓5th **593.7 Vesicoureteral reflux**

AHA: 4Q, '94, 42

DEF: Backflow of urine, from bladder into ureter due to obstructed bladder neck.

> **593.70 Unspecified or without reflux nephropathy**
> **593.71 With reflux nephropathy, unilateral**
> **593.72 With reflux nephropathy, bilateral**
> **593.73 With reflux nephropathy NOS**

✓5th **593.8 Other specified disorders of kidney and ureter**

> **593.81 Vascular disorders of kidney**
> Renal (artery):   Renal (artery):
>   embolism   thrombosis
>   hemorrhage   Renal infarction
>
> **593.82 Ureteral fistula**
> Intestinoureteral fistula
> > *EXCLUDES*   fistula between ureter and
> >   female genital tract
> >   (619.0)
>
> **DEF:** Abnormal communication, between tube connecting kidney to bladder and another structure.
>
> **593.89 Other**
> Adhesions, kidney   Polyp of ureter
>   or ureter   Pyelectasia
> Periureteritis   Ureterocele
> > *EXCLUDES*   tuberculosis of ureter (016.2)
> >   ureteritis cystica (590.3)

593.9 Unspecified disorder of kidney and ureter

> Renal disease NOS
> Salt-losing nephritis or syndrome
> *EXCLUDES*   cystic kidney disease (753.1)
>   nephropathy, so stated (583.0-583.9)
>   renal disease:
>   acute (580.0-580.9)
>   arising in pregnancy or the
>   puerperium (642.1-642.2,
>   642.4-642.7, 646.2)
>   chronic (582.0-582.9)
>   not specified as acute or chronic, but
>   with stated pathology or cause
>   (583.0-583.9)

AHA: 1Q, '93, 17

✓4th **594 Calculus of lower urinary tract**

594.0 Calculus in diverticulum of bladder

DEF: Stone or mineral deposit in abnormal sac on the bladder wall.

594.1 Other calculus in bladder

> Urinary bladder stone
> *EXCLUDES*   staghorn calculus (592.0)

DEF: Stone or mineral deposit in bladder.

594.2 Calculus in urethra

DEF: Stone or mineral deposit in tube that empties urine from bladder.

594.8 Other lower urinary tract calculus

AHA: J-F, '85, 16

594.9 Calculus of lower urinary tract, unspecified

> *EXCLUDES*   calculus of urinary tract NOS (592.9)

✓4th **595 Cystitis**

> *EXCLUDES*   prostatocystitis (601.3)
> Use additional code to identify organism, such as Escherichia coli [E. coli] (041.4)

595.0 Acute cystitis `cc`

> *EXCLUDES*   trigonitis (595.3)

CC Excl: 016.10-016.16, 016.30-016.36, 016.90-016.96, 017.90-017.96, 098.0, 098.11, 098.2, 098.39, 098.89, 112.2, 131.00, 131.8-131.9, 593.3-593.5, 593.89, 593.9, 595.0-595.9, 596.8-596.9, 599.0, 599.6-599.9

AHA: 2Q, '99, 15

DEF: Acute inflammation of bladder.

595.1 Chronic interstitial cystitis `cc`

> Hunner's ulcer
> Panmural fibrosis of bladder
> Submucous cystitis

CC Excl: See code 595.0

DEF: Inflamed lesion affecting bladder wall; symptoms include urinary frequency, pain on bladder filling, nocturia, and distended bladder.

595.2 Other chronic cystitis `cc`

> Chronic cystitis NOS
> Subacute cystitis
> *EXCLUDES*   trigonitis (595.3)

CC Excl: See code 595.0

DEF: Persistent inflammation of bladder.

595.3 Trigonitis

> Follicular cystitis
> Trigonitis (acute) (chronic)
> Urethrotrigonitis

DEF: Inflammation of the triangular area of the bladder called the trigonum vesicae.

595.4 Cystitis in diseases classified elsewhere `cc`

> *Code first underlying disease, as:*
>   actinomycosis (039.8)
>   amebiasis (006.8)
>   bilharziasis (120.0-120.9)
>   Echinococcus infestation (122.3, 122.6)
> > *EXCLUDES*   cystitis:
> >   diphtheritic (032.84)
> >   gonococcal (098.11, 098.31)
> >   monilial (112.2)
> >   trichomonal (131.09)
> >   tuberculous (016.1)

CC Excl: See code 595.0

✓5th **595.8 Other specified types of cystitis**

> **595.81 Cystitis cystica** `cc`
> **CC Excl:** See code 595.0
>
> **DEF:** Inflammation of the bladder characterized by formation of multiple cysts.
>
> **595.82 Irradiation cystitis** `cc`
> Use additional E code to identify cause
> **CC Excl:** See code 595.0
>
> **DEF:** Inflammation of the bladder due to effects of radiation.
>
> **595.89 Other** `cc`
> Abscess of bladder   Cystitis:
> Cystitis: emphysematous
>   bullous   glandularis
> **CC Excl:** See code 595.0

595.9 Cystitis, unspecified `cc`

> **CC Excl:** See code 595.0

✓4th
✓5th **Additional Digit Required**   Nonspecific PDx   Unacceptable PDx   Manifestation Code   **MSP** Medicare Secondary Payer   ►◄ Revised Text   ● New Code   ▲ Revised Code Title

2002 Ingenix, Inc.

Volume 1 — 173

Bladder

Anterior View

Lateral View

√4ᵗʰ **596 Other disorders of bladder**

Use additional code to identify urinary incontinence (625.6, 788.30-788.39)

AHA: M-A, '87, 10

596.0 Bladder neck obstruction   **cc**

Contracture (acquired)   of bladder neck or
Obstruction (acquired) } vesicourethral
Stenosis (acquired)   orifice

EXCLUDES *congenital (753.6)*

CC Excl: 185, 188.0-188.9, 189.3-189.9, 596.0, 596.4, 596.51-596.59, 596.8-596.9, 600.0-600.9, 601.0-601.9, 602.0-602.9

AHA: 2Q, '01, 14; N-D, '86, 10

DEF: Bladder outlet and vesicourethral obstruction; occurs more often in males as a consequence of benign prostatic hypertrophy or prostatic cancer; may also occur in either sex due to strictures, following radiation, cystoscopy, catheterization, injury, infection, blood clots, bladder cancer, impaction or disease compressing bladder neck.

596.1 Intestinovesical fistula   **cc**

Fistula: Fistula:
   enterovesical   vesicoenteric
   vesicocolic   vesicorectal

CC Excl: 098.0, 098.2, 098.39, 098.89, 596.1-596.2, 596.8-596.9, 599.7-599.9, 788.1

DEF: Abnormal communication, between intestine and bladder.

596.2 Vesical fistula, not elsewhere classified   **cc**

Fistula: Fistula:
   bladder NOS   vesicocutaneous
   urethrovesical   vesicoperineal

EXCLUDES *fistula between bladder and female genital tract (619.0)*

CC Excl: See code 596.1

DEF: Abnormal communication between bladder and another structure.

596.3 Diverticulum of bladder

Diverticulitis   } of bladder
Diverticulum (acquired) (false) }

EXCLUDES *that with calculus in diverticulum of bladder (594.0)*

DEF: Abnormal pouch in bladder wall.

596.4 Atony of bladder   **cc**

High compliance bladder
Hypotonicity } of bladder
Inertia

EXCLUDES *neurogenic bladder (596.54)*

CC Excl: 596.4, 596.51-596.59, 596.8-596.9, 599.7-599.9, 788.1

DEF: Distended, bladder with loss of expulsive force; linked to CNS disease.

√5ᵗʰ **596.5 Other functional disorders of bladder**

EXCLUDES *cauda equina syndrome with neurogenic bladder (344.61)*

596.51 Hypertonicity of bladder

Hyperactivity
Overactive bladder

DEF: Abnormal tension of muscular wall of bladder; may appear after surgery of voluntary nerve.

596.52 Low bladder compliance

DEF: Low bladder capacity; causes increased pressure and frequent urination.

596.53 Paralysis of bladder

DEF: Impaired bladder motor function due to nerve or muscle damage.

596.54 Neurogenic bladder NOS

AHA: 1Q, '01, 12

DEF: Unspecified dysfunctional bladder due to lesion of central, peripheral nervous system; may result in incontinence, residual urine retention, urinary infection, stones and renal failure.

596.55 Detrusor sphincter dyssynergia

DEF: Instability of the urinary bladder sphincter muscle associated with urinary incontinence..

596.59 Other functional disorder of bladder

Detrusor instability

DEF: Detrusor instability: instability of bladder; marked by uninhibited contractions often leading to incontinence.

596.6 Rupture of bladder, nontraumatic   **cc**

CC Excl: 596.6-596.9, 599.7-599.9, 788.1

596.7 Hemorrhage into bladder wall   **cc**

Hyperemia of bladder

EXCLUDES *acute hemorrhagic cystitis (595.0)*

CC Excl: See code 596.6

596.8 Other specified disorders of bladder

Bladder: Bladder:
   calcified   hemorrhage
   contracted   hypertrophy

EXCLUDES *cystocele, female (618.0, 618.2-618.4) hernia or prolapse of bladder, female (618.0, 618.2-618.4)*

AHA: J-F, '85, 8

596.9 Unspecified disorder of bladder

AHA: J-F, '85, 8

√4ᵗʰ **597 Urethritis, not sexually transmitted, and urethral syndrome**

EXCLUDES *nonspecific urethritis, so stated (099.4)*

N Newborn Age: 0   **P** Pediatric Age: 0-17   **M** Maternity Age: 12-55   **A** Adult Age: 15-124   **CC** CC Condition   **MC** Major Complication   **CD** Complex Dx   **HIV** HIV Related Dx

597.0 Urethral abscess   `CC`
Abscess: Abscess of:
  periurethral   Cowper's gland
  urethral (gland)   Littré's gland
Abscess of: Periurethral cellulitis
  bulbourethral gland

   EXCLUDES *urethral caruncle (599.3)*

CC Excl: 098.0, 098.2, 098.39, 098.89, 099.40-099.49, 112.2, 131.00, 131.02, 131.8-131.9, 597.0-597.89, 598.00-598.01, 598.8-598.9, 599.0, 599.6-599.9, 607.1-607.83, 607.89, 607.9, 608.4, 608.81, 608.85, 608.87, 608.89, 752.61-752.65, 752.69, 752.8-752.9, 753.6-753.9, 788.1

DEF: Pocket of pus in tube that empties urine from the bladder.

√5ᵗʰ **597.8 Other urethritis**
  597.80 Urethritis, unspecified
  597.81 Urethral syndrome NOS
  597.89 Other
    Adenitis, Skene's glands
    Cowperitis
    Meatitis, urethral
    Ulcer, urethra (meatus)
    Verumontanitis
     EXCLUDES *trichomonal (131.02)*

√4ᵗʰ **598 Urethral stricture**
Use additional code to identify urinary incontinence (625.6, 788.30-788.39)
  INCLUDES pinhole meatus
        stricture of urinary meatus
  EXCLUDES *congenital stricture of urethra and urinary meatus (753.6)*

DEF: Narrowing of tube that empties urine from bladder.

√5ᵗʰ **598.0 Urethral stricture due to infection**
  598.00 Due to unspecified infection
  598.01 *Due to infective diseases classified elsewhere*
    Code first underlying disease, as:
      gonococcal infection (098.2)
      schistosomiasis (120.0-120.9)
      syphilis (095.8)

598.1 Traumatic urethral stricture   `CC`
Stricture of urethra: Stricture of urethra:
  late effect of injury   postobstetric
  EXCLUDES *postoperative following surgery on genitourinary tract (598.2)*

CC Excl: 098.0, 098.2, 098.39, 098.89, 131.02, 598.1-598.9, 599.6-599.9, 752.61-752.65, 752.69, 753.6-753.9, 788.1

598.2 Postoperative urethral stricture   `CC`
Postcatheterization stricture of urethra
CC Excl: See code 598.1

AHA: 3Q, '97, 6

598.8 Other specified causes of urethral stricture
AHA: N-D, '84, 9

598.9 Urethral stricture, unspecified

√4ᵗʰ **599 Other disorders of urethra and urinary tract**
599.0 Urinary tract infection, site not specified   `CC`
  EXCLUDES *candidiasis of urinary tract (112.2)*
        ▶*urinary tract infection of newborn (771.82)*◀
Use additional code to identify organism, such as Escherichia coli [E. coli] (041.4)

CC Excl: 098.2, 098.39, 098.89, 099.40-099.49, 112.2, 131.00, 131.8-131.9, 590.10-590.9, 591, 593.89, 593.9, 595.0-595.9, 599.0, 599.6-599.9, 788.1, 996.64

AHA: 4Q, '99, 6; 2Q, '99, 15;1Q, '98, 5; 2Q, '96, 7; 4Q, '96, 33; 2Q, '95, 7; 1Q, '92, 13

  ▽ **DRG** 320

599.1 Urethral fistula
Fistula:
  urethroperineal
  urethrorectal
Urinary fistula NOS
  EXCLUDES *fistula:*
      urethroscrotal (608.89)
      urethrovaginal (619.0)
      urethrovesicovaginal (619.0)

AHA: 3Q, '97, 6

599.2 Urethral diverticulum
DEF: Abnormal pouch in urethral wall.

599.3 Urethral caruncle
Polyp of urethra

599.4 Urethral false passage   `CC`
CC Excl: 597.0-597.89, 598.00-598.9, 599.1-599.9, 607.1-607.83, 607.89, 607.9, 608.4, 608.81, 608.85, 608.87, 608.89, 752.61-752.65, 752.69, 752.8-752.9, 753.9, 788.1

DEF: Abnormal opening in urethra due to surgery; trauma or disease.

599.5 Prolapsed urethral mucosa
Prolapse of urethra
Urethrocele
  EXCLUDES *urethrocele, female (618.0, 618.2-618.4)*

599.6 Urinary obstruction, unspecified   `CC`
Obstructive uropathy NOS
Urinary (tract) obstruction NOS
Use additional code to identify urinary incontinence (625.6, 788.30-788.39)
  EXCLUDES *obstructive nephropathy NOS (593.89)*

CC Excl: 185, 188.0-188.9, 189.2-189.9, 274.11, 344.61, 592.1, 592.9, 593.3-593.5, 593.89, 593.9, 594.0-594.9, 595.0-595.9, 596.0, 596.51-596.59, 596.8-596.9, 597.0-597.89, 598.00-598.9, 599.0-599.9, 600.0-600.9, 601.0-601.9, 602.0-602.9, 753.0-753.9, 788.1

599.7 Hematuria   `CC`
Hematuria (benign) (essential)
  EXCLUDES *hemoglobinuria (791.2)*

CC Excl: 592.0-592.9, 593.89, 593.9, 594.0-594.9, 596.6-596.7, 599.7-599.9

AHA: 1Q, '00, 5; 3Q, '95, 8

DEF: Blood in urine.

√5ᵗʰ **599.8 Other specified disorders of urethra and urinary tract**
Use additional code to identify urinary incontinence (625.6, 788.30-788.39), if present
  EXCLUDES *symptoms and other conditions classifiable to 788.0-788.2, 788.4-788.9, 791.0-791.9*

  599.81 Urethral hypermobility
    DEF: Hyperactive urethra.

  599.82 Intrinsic (urethral) spincter deficiency [ISD]
    AHA: 2Q, '96, 15
    DEF: Malfunctioning urethral sphincter.

  599.83 Urethral instability
    DEF: Inconsistent functioning of urethra.

  599.84 Other specified disorders of urethra
    Rupture of urethra (nontraumatic)
    Urethral:
      cyst
      granuloma
    DEF: Rupture of urethra due to herniation or breaking down of tissue; not due to trauma.
    DEF: Urethral cyst: abnormal sac in urethra; usually fluid filled.
    DEF: Granuloma: inflammatory cells forming small nodules in urethra.

  599.89 Other specified disorders of urinary tract

√4ᵗʰ √5ᵗʰ Additional Digit Required   Nonspecific PDx   Unacceptable PDx   Manifestation Code   **MSP** Medicare Secondary Payer   ▶◀ Revised Text   ● New Code   ▲ Revised Code Title

2002 Ingenix, Inc.   **October 2002 • Volume 1 — 175**

Genitourinary System 599.9–603.1

599.9   Unspecified disorder of urethra and urinary tract

DISEASES OF MALE GENITAL ORGANS (600-608)

✓4th **600 Hyperplasia of prostate**
> Use additional code to identify urinary incontinence (788.30-788.39)

AHA: 4Q, '00, 43; 3Q, '94, 12; 3Q, '92, 7; N-D, '86, 10

DEF: Fibrostromal proliferation in periurethral glands, causes blood in urine; etiology unknown.

600.0   **Hypertrophy (benign) of prostate**   A ♂
> Benign prostatic hypertrophy
> Enlargement of prostate
> Smooth enlarged prostate
> Soft enlarged prostate

         AHA: 2Q, '01, 14

600.1   **Nodular prostate**   A ♂
> Hard, firm prostate
> Multinodular prostate
> **EXCLUDES**   malignant neoplasm of prostate (185)

         DEF: Hard, firm nodule in prostate.

600.2   **Benign localized hyperplasia of prostate**   A ♂
> Adenofibromatous hypertrophy of prostate
> Adenoma of prostate
> Fibroadenoma of prostate
> Fibroma of prostate
> Myoma of prostate
> Polyp of prostate
> **EXCLUDES**   benign neoplasms of prostate (222.2)
>   hypertrophy of prostate (600.0)
>   malignant neoplasm of prostate (185)

         DEF: Benign localized hyperplasia is a clearly defined epithelial tumor. Other terms used for this condition are adenofibromatous hypertrophy of prostate, adenoma of prostate, fibroadenoma of prostate, fibroma of prostate, myoma of prostate, and polyp of prostate.

600.3   **Cyst of prostate**   ♂

         DEF: Sacs of fluid, which differentiate this from either nodular or adenomatous tumors.

600.9   **Hyperplasia of prostate, unspecified**   ♂
> Median bar
> Prostatic obstruction NOS

✓4th **601 Inflammatory diseases of prostate**
> Use additional code to identify organism, such as Staphylococcus (041.1), or Streptococcus (041.0)

601.0   **Acute prostatitis**   CC A ♂
> **CC Excl:** 098.12, 098.32, 098.89, 112.2, 131.00, 131.03, 131.8-131.9, 600.0-600.9, 601.0-601.9, 602.0-602.9

601.1   **Chronic prostatitis**   A ♂

601.2   **Abscess of prostate**   CC A ♂
> **CC Excl:** See code 601.0

601.3   **Prostatocystitis**   CC A ♂
> **CC Excl:** See code 601.0

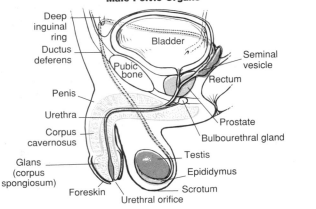
Male Pelvic Organs

Common Inguinal Canal Anomalies

601.4   *Prostatitis in diseases classified elsewhere*   A ♂
> *Code first underlying disease, as:*
> actinomycosis (039.8)
> blastomycosis (116.0)
> syphilis (095.8)
> tuberculosis (016.5)
> **EXCLUDES**   prostatitis:
>   gonococcal (098.12, 098.32)
>   monilial (112.2)
>   trichomonal (131.03)

601.8   **Other specified inflammatory diseases of prostate**   A ♂
> Prostatitis:
>   cavitary
>   diverticular
>   granulomatous

601.9   **Prostatitis, unspecified**   A ♂
> Prostatitis NOS

✓4th **602 Other disorders of prostate**

602.0   **Calculus of prostate**   A ♂
> Prostatic stone

         DEF: Stone or mineral deposit in prostate.

602.1   **Congestion or hemorrhage of prostate**   CC A ♂
> **CC Excl:** See code 601.0

         DEF: Bleeding or fluid collection in prostate.

602.2   **Atrophy of prostate**   A ♂

602.3   **Dysplasia of prostate**   ♂
> Prostatic intraepithelial ▶neoplasia◀ I (PIN I)
> Prostatic intraepithelial ▶neoplasia◀ II (PIN II)
> **EXCLUDES**   prostatic intraepithelial ▶neoplasia◀
>   III (PIN III) (233.4)

         AHA: 4Q, '01, 46

         DEF: Abnormality of shape and size of the intraepithelial tissues of the prostate; pre-malignant condition characterized by stalks and absence of a basilar cell layer; synonyms are intraductal dysplasia, large acinar atypical hyperplasia, atypical primary hyperplasia, hyperplasia with malignant changes, marked atypia, or duct-acinar dysplasia.

602.8   **Other specified disorders of prostate**   A ♂
> Fistula
> Infarction } of prostate
> Stricture
> Periprostatic adhesions

602.9   **Unspecified disorder of prostate**   A ♂

✓4th **603 Hydrocele**
> **INCLUDES**   hydrocele of spermatic cord, testis, or tunica vaginalis
> **EXCLUDES**   congenital (778.6)

         DEF: Circumscribed collection of fluid in tunica vaginalis, spermatic cord or testis.

603.0   **Encysted hydrocele**

603.1   **Infected hydrocele**   CC
> Use additional code to identify organism
> **CC Excl:** 112.2, 131.00, 131.8-131.9, 603.0-603.9

N Newborn Age: 0   P Pediatric Age: 0-17   M Maternity Age: 12-55   A Adult Age: 15-124   CC CC Condition   MC Major Complication   CD Complex Dx   HIV HIV Related Dx

603.8   **Other specified types of hydrocele**

603.9   **Hydrocele, unspecified**

✓4ᵗʰ **604 Orchitis and epididymitis**

Use additional code to identify organism, such as Escherichia coli [E. coli] (041.4), Staphylococcus (041.1), or Streptococcus (041.0)

604.0   **Orchitis, epididymitis, and epididymo-orchitis, with abscess**   CC A ♂

Abscess of epididymis or testis

CC Excl: 072.0, 098.13-098.14, 098.33-098.34, 098.89, 112.2, 131.00, 131.8-131.9, 604.0-604.99

✓5ᵗʰ **604.9 Other orchitis, epididymitis, and epididymo-orchitis, without mention of abscess**

604.90 Orchitis and epididymitis, unspecified   ♂

604.91 *Orchitis and epididymitis in diseases classified elsewhere*   ♂

Code first underlying disease, as:
diphtheria (032.89)
filariasis (125.0-125.9)
syphilis (095.8)

EXCLUDES   *orchitis:*
gonococcal (098.13, 098.33)
mumps (072.0)
tuberculous (016.5)
tuberculous epididymitis (016.4)

604.99 Other   ♂

605 Redundant prepuce and phimosis   ♂

Adherent prepuce   Phimosis (congenital)
Paraphimosis   Tight foreskin

DEF: Constriction of preputial orifice causing inability of the prepuce to be drawn back over the glans; it may be congenital or caused by infection.

✓4ᵗʰ **606 Infertility, male**

AHA: 2Q, '96, 9

606.0   **Azoospermia**   A ♂

Absolute infertility   Infertility due to:
Infertility due to: spermatogenic arrest
   germinal (cell) aplasia   (complete)

DEF: Absence of spermatozoa in the semen or inability to produce spermatozoa.

606.1   **Oligospermia**   A ♂

Infertility due to:
   germinal cell desquamation
   hypospermatogenesis
   incomplete spermatogenic arrest

DEF: Insufficient number of sperm in semen.

606.8   **Infertility due to extratesticular causes**   A ♂

Infertility due to: Infertility due to:
   drug therapy   radiation
   infection   systemic disease
   obstruction of efferent
     ducts

606.9   **Male infertility, unspecified**   A ♂

Torsion of Testes

Torsion of testis

Testes after correction showing bilateral fixation

✓4ᵗʰ **607 Disorders of penis**

EXCLUDES   *phimosis (605)*

607.0   **Leukoplakia of penis**   ♂

Kraurosis of penis

EXCLUDES   *carcinoma in situ of penis (233.5)*
erythroplasia of Queyrat (233.5)

DEF: White, thickened patches on glans penis.

607.1   **Balanoposthitis**   ♂

Balanitis

Use additional code to identify organism

DEF: Inflammation of glans penis and prepuce.

607.2   **Other inflammatory disorders of penis**   ♂

Abscess
Boil   } of corpus cavernosum
Carbuncle   or penis
Cellulitis

Cavernitis (penis)
Use additional code to identify organism

EXCLUDES   *herpetic infection (054.13)*

607.3   **Priapism**   ♂

Painful erection

DEF: Prolonged penile erection without sexual stimulation.

✓5ᵗʰ **607.8 Other specified disorders of penis**

607.81 Balanitis xerotica obliterans   ♂

Induratio penis plastica

DEF: Inflammation of the glans penis, caused by stricture of the opening of the prepuce.

607.82 Vascular disorders of penis   ♂

Embolism
Hematoma
   (nontraumatic)   } of corpus
Hemorrhage   cavernosum
Thrombosis   or penis

607.83 Edema of penis   ♂

DEF: Fluid retention within penile tissues.

607.84 Impotence of organic origin   A ♂

EXCLUDES   *nonorganic or unspecified (302.72)*

AHA: 3Q, '91, 11

DEF: Physiological cause interfering with erection.

607.89 Other   ♂

Atrophy
Fibrosis   } of corpus cavernosum
Hypertrophy   or penis
Ulcer (chronic)

607.9   **Unspecified disorder of penis**   ♂

✓4ᵗʰ **608 Other disorders of male genital organs**

608.0   **Seminal vesiculitis**   ♂

Abscess   } of seminal vesicle
Cellulitis

Vesiculitis (seminal)
Use additional code to identify organism

EXCLUDES   *gonococcal infection (098.14, 098.34)*

DEF: Inflammation of seminal vesicle.

608.1   **Spermatocele**   ♂

DEF: Cystic enlargement of the epididymis or the testis; the cysts contain spermatozoa.

608.2   **Torsion of testis**   ♂

Torsion of: Torsion of:
   epididymis   testicle
   spermatic cord

DEF: Twisted or rotated testis; may compromise blood flow.

608.3   **Atrophy of testis**   ♂

✓4ᵗʰ ✓5ᵗʰ **Additional Digit Required**   Nonspecific PDx   Unacceptable PDx   Manifestation Code   MSP Medicare Secondary Payer   ►◄ Revised Text   ● New Code   ▲ Revised Code Title

2002 Ingenix, Inc.   **Volume 1 — 177**

608.4 Other inflammatory disorders of male genital organs ♂

Abscess
Boil
Carbuncle
Cellulitis } of scrotum, spermatic cord, testis [except abscess], tunica vaginalis, or vas deferens

Vasitis
Use additional code to identify organism
EXCLUDES abscess of testis (604.0)

√5ᵗʰ **608.8 Other specified disorders of male genital organs**

608.81 Disorders of male genital organs in diseases classified elsewhere ♂
Code first underlying disease, as:
filariasis (125.0-125.9)
tuberculosis (016.5)

608.82 Hematospermia ♂
AHA: ▶4Q, '01, 46◀

DEF: ▶Presence of blood in the ejaculate; relatively common, affecting men of any age after puberty; cause is often difficult to determine since the semen originates in several organs, often the result of a viral bacterial infection and inflammation.◀

608.83 Vascular disorders ♂
Hematoma (nontraumatic)
Hemorrhage
Thrombosis } of seminal vesicle, spermatic cord, testis, scrotum, tunica vaginalis, or vas deferens

Hematocele NOS, male

608.84 Chylocele of tunica vaginalis ♂
DEF: Chylous effusion into tunica vaginalis; due to infusion of lymphatic fluids.

608.85 Stricture ♂
Stricture of:
spermatic cord
tunica vaginalis
Stricture of:
vas deferens

608.86 Edema ♂

608.87 Retrograde ejaculation ♂
AHA: ▶4Q, '01, 46◀

DEF: ▶Condition where the semen travels to the bladder rather than out through the urethra due to damaged nerves causing the bladder neck to remain open during ejaculation.◀

608.89 Other ♂
Atrophy
Fibrosis
Hypertrophy
Ulcer } of seminal vesicle, spermatic cord, testis, scrotum, tunica vaginalis, or vas deferens

EXCLUDES atrophy of testis (608.3)

608.9 Unspecified disorder of male genital organs ♂

DISORDERS OF BREAST (610-611)

√4ᵗʰ **610 Benign mammary dysplasias**

610.0 Solitary cyst of breast
Cyst (solitary) of breast

610.1 Diffuse cystic mastopathy Ⓐ
Chronic cystic mastitis
Cystic breast
Fibrocystic disease of breast

DEF: Extensive formation of nodular cysts in breast tissue; symptoms include tenderness, change in size and hyperplasia of ductal epithelium.

610.2 Fibroadenosis of breast
Fibroadenosis of breast:
NOS
chronic
cystic
Fibroadenosis of breast:
diffuse
periodic
segmental

DEF: Non-neoplastic nodular condition of breast.

610.3 Fibrosclerosis of breast
DEF: Fibrous tissue in breast.

610.4 Mammary duct ectasia
Comedomastitis
Duct ectasia
Mastitis:
periductal
plasma cell

DEF: Atrophy of duct epithelium; causes distended collecting ducts of mammary gland; drying up of breast secretion, intraductal inflammation and periductal and interstitial chronic inflammatory reaction.

610.8 Other specified benign mammary dysplasias
Mazoplasia
Sebaceous cyst of breast

610.9 Benign mammary dysplasia, unspecified

√4ᵗʰ **611 Other disorders of breast**
EXCLUDES that associated with lactation or the puerperium (675.0-676.9)

611.0 Inflammatory disease of breast
Abscess (acute) (chronic) (nonpuerperal) of:
areola
breast
Mammillary fistula
Mastitis (acute) (subacute) (nonpuerperal):
NOS
infective
retromammary
submammary

EXCLUDES carbuncle of breast (680.2)
chronic cystic mastitis (610.1)
neonatal infective mastitis (771.5)
thrombophlebitis of breast [Mondor's disease] (451.89)

611.1 Hypertrophy of breast
Gynecomastia
Hypertrophy of breast:
NOS
massive pubertal

611.2 Fissure of nipple

611.3 Fat necrosis of breast
Fat necrosis (segmental) of breast
DEF: Splitting of neutral fats in adipose tissue cells as a result of trauma; a firm circumscribed mass is then formed in the breast.

611.4 Atrophy of breast

611.5 Galactocele

611.6 Galactorrhea not associated with childbirth

√5ᵗʰ **611.7 Signs and symptoms in breast**
611.71 Mastodynia
Pain in breast

611.72 Lump or mass in breast CC
CC Excl: 610.0-610.9, 611.0-611.9

611.79 Other
Induration of breast
Inversion of nipple
Nipple discharge
Retraction of nipple

611.8 Other specified disorders of breast
Hematoma (nontraumatic)
Infarction } of breast

Occlusion of breast duct
Subinvolution of breast (postlactational) (postpartum)

611.9 Unspecified breast disorder

INFLAMMATORY DISEASE OF FEMALE PELVIC ORGANS (614-616)

Use additional code to identify organism, such as Staphylococcus (041.1), or Streptococcus (041.0)
EXCLUDES that associated with pregnancy, abortion, childbirth, or the puerperium (630-676.9)

√4ᵗʰ **614 Inflammatory disease of ovary, fallopian tube, pelvic cellular tissue, and peritoneum**
EXCLUDES endometritis (615.0-615.9)
major infection following delivery (670)
that complicating:
abortion (634-638 with .0, 639.0)
ectopic or molar pregnancy (639.0)
pregnancy or labor (646.6)

Ⓝ Newborn Age: 0   Ⓟ Pediatric Age: 0-17   Ⓜ Maternity Age: 12-55   Ⓐ Adult Age :15-124   **CC** CC Condition   **MC** Major Complication   **CD** Complex Dx   **HIV** HIV Related Dx

614.0 Acute salpingitis and oophoritis   CC ♀

Any condition classifiable to 614.2, specified as acute or subacute

CC Excl: 016.60-016.96, 017.90-017.96, 098.15-098.17, 098.35-098.37, 098.89, 112.2, 131.00, 131.8-131.9, 614.0-614.9, 615.0-615.9, 616.8-616.9, 625.8-625.9, 629.8-629.9, 752.8-752.9

DEF: Acute inflammation, of ovary and fallopian tube.

614.1 Chronic salpingitis and oophoritis   ♀

Hydrosalpinx
Salpingitis:
   follicularis
   isthmica nodosa
Any condition classifiable to 614.2, specified as chronic

DEF: Persistent inflammation of ovary and fallopian tube.

614.2 Salpingitis and oophoritis not specified as acute, subacute, or chronic   ♀

Abscess (of):   Pyosalpinx
  fallopian tube   Perisalpingitis
  ovary   Salpingitis
  tubo-ovarian   Salpingo-oophoritis
Oophoritis   Tubo-ovarian inflammatory
Perioophoritis   disease

EXCLUDES *gonococcal infection (chronic) (098.37)*
     acute (098.17)
   tuberculous (016.6)

AHA: 2Q, '91, 5

614.3 Acute parametritis and pelvic cellulitis   CC ♀

Acute inflammatory pelvic disease
Any condition classifiable to 614.4, specified as acute

CC Excl: See code 614.0

DEF: Parametritis: inflammation of the parametrium; pelvic cellulitis is a synonym for parametritis.

614.4 Chronic or unspecified parametritis and pelvic cellulitis   ♀

Abscess (of):
   broad ligament
   parametrium   } chronic or NOS
   pelvis, female
   pouch of Douglas

Chronic inflammatory pelvic disease
Pelvic cellulitis, female

EXCLUDES *tuberculous (016.7)*

614.5 Acute or unspecified pelvic peritonitis, female   CC ♀

CC Excl: See code 614.0

614.6 Pelvic peritoneal adhesions, female (postoperative) (postinfection)   ♀

Adhesions:
   peritubal
   tubo-ovarian
Use additional code to identify any associated infertility (628.2)

AHA: 3Q, '95, 7; 3Q, '94, 12

DEF: Fibrous scarring abnormally joining structures within abdomen.

614.7 Other chronic pelvic peritonitis, female   ♀
EXCLUDES *tuberculous(016.7)*

614.8 Other specified inflammatory disease of female pelvic organs and tissues   ♀

614.9 Unspecified inflammatory disease of female pelvic organs and tissues   ♀

Pelvic infection or inflammation, female NOS
Pelvic inflammatory disease [PID]

Female Genitourinary System

√4th **615 Inflammatory diseases of uterus, except cervix**

EXCLUDES *following delivery (670)*
hyperplastic endometritis (621.3)
that complicating:
  abortion (634-638 with .0, 639.0)
  ectopic or molar pregnancy (639.0)
  pregnancy or labor (646.6)

615.0 Acute   CC ♀

Any condition classifiable to 615.9, specified as acute or subacute

CC Excl: 016.60-016.96, 017.90-017.96, 098.15-098.17, 098.35-098.37, 098.89, 112.2, 131.00, 131.8-131.9, 614.0-614.9, 615.0-615.9, 616.0, 616.8-616.9, 621.8-621.9, 625.8-625.9, 629.8-629.9, 752.8-752.9

615.1 Chronic   ♀

Any condition classifiable to 615.9, specified as chronic

615.9 Unspecified inflammatory disease of uterus   ♀

Endometritis   Perimetritis
Endomyometritis   Pyometra
Metritis   Uterine abscess
Myometritis

√4th **616 Inflammatory disease of cervix, vagina, and vulva**

EXCLUDES *that complicating:*
  abortion (634-638 with .0, 639.0)
  ectopic or molar pregnancy (639.0)
  pregnancy, childbirth, or the puerperium (646.6)

616.0 Cervicitis and endocervicitis   ♀

Cervicitis   } with or without mention of
Endocervicitis }   erosion or ectropion

Nabothian (gland) cyst or follicle

EXCLUDES *erosion or ectropion without mention of cervicitis (622.0)*

√5th **616.1 Vaginitis and vulvovaginitis**

DEF: Inflammation or infection of vagina or external female genitalia.

616.10 Vaginitis and vulvovaginitis, unspecified   ♀

Vaginitis:
   NOS
   postirradiation
Vulvitis NOS
Vulvovaginitis NOS
Use additional code to identify organism, such as Escherichia coli [E. coli] (041.4), Staphylococcus (041.1), or Streptococcus (041.0)

EXCLUDES *noninfective leukorrhea (623.5)*
postmenopausal or senile vaginitis (627.3)

√4th √5th **Additional Digit Required**   **Nonspecific PDx**   **Unacceptable PDx**   **Manifestation Code**   MSP **Medicare Secondary Payer**   ►◄ Revised Text   ● New Code   ▲ Revised Code Title

2002 Ingenix, Inc.   **Volume 1 — 179**

Genitourinary System 614.0–616.10

616.11 Vaginitis and vulvovaginitis in diseases classified elsewhere ♀

Code first underlying disease, as:
pinworm vaginitis (127.4)

> EXCLUDES   herpetic vulvovaginitis (054.11)
> monilial vulvotaginitis (112.1)
> trichomonal vaginitis or vulvovaginitis (131.01)

616.2 Cyst of Bartholin's gland ♀

Bartholin's duct cyst

DEF: Fluid-filled sac within gland of vaginal orifice.

616.3 Abscess of Bartholin's gland CC ♀

Vulvovaginal gland abscess

CC Excl: 016.70-016.96, 017.90-017.96, 112.1-112.2, 131.00-131.01, 131.8-131.9, 616.10-616.9, 624.3-624.9, 625.8-625.9, 629.8-629.9, 752.8-752.9

616.4 Other abscess of vulva CC ♀

Abscess
Carbuncle } of vulva
Furuncle

CC Excl: See code 616.3

√5ᵗʰ 616.5 Ulceration of vulva

616.50 Ulceration of vulva, unspecified ♀
Ulcer NOS of vulva

616.51 Ulceration of vulva in diseases classified elsewhere ♀

Code first underlying disease, as:
Behçet's syndrome (136.1)
tuberculosis (016.7)

> EXCLUDES   vulvar ulcer (in):
> gonococcal (098.0)
> herpes simplex (054.12)
> syphilitic (091.0)

616.8 Other specified inflammatory diseases of cervix, vagina, and vulva ♀

Caruncle, vagina or labium
Ulcer, vagina

> EXCLUDES   noninflammatory disorders of:
> cervix (622.0-622.9)
> vagina (623.0-623.9)
> vulva (624.0-624.9)

616.9 Unspecified inflammatory disease of cervix, vagina, and vulva ♀

OTHER DISORDERS OF FEMALE GENITAL TRACT (617-629)

√4ᵗʰ 617 Endometriosis

DEF: What resembles uterine mucosa (endometrial tissue) is found in the pelvic cavity.

617.0 Endometriosis of uterus ♀
Adenomyosis
Endometriosis:
cervix

Endometriosis:
internal
myometrium

> EXCLUDES   stromal endometriosis (236.0)

AHA: 3Q, '92, 7

DEF: Aberrant uterine mucosal tissue; creating products of menses and inflamed uterine tissues.

617.1 Endometriosis of ovary ♀
Chocolate cyst of ovary
Endometrial cystoma of ovary
DEF: Aberrant uterine tissue; creating products of menses and inflamed ovarian tissues.

617.2 Endometriosis of fallopian tube ♀
DEF: Aberrant uterine tissue; creating products of menses and inflamed tissues of fallopian tubes.

Common Sites of Endometriosis

Common sites of endometriosis, in descending order of frequency:
(1) ovary
(2) cul de sac
(3) utersacral ligaments
(4) broad ligaments
(5) fallopian tube
(6) uterovesical fold
(7) round ligament
(8) vermiform appedix
(9) vagina
(10) rectovaginal septum

617.3 Endometriosis of pelvic peritoneum ♀
Endometriosis:
broad ligament
cul-de-sac (Douglas')

Endometriosis:
parametrium
round ligament

DEF: Aberrant uterine tissue; creating products of menses and inflamed peritoneum tissues.

617.4 Endometriosis of rectovaginal septum and vagina ♀
DEF: Aberrant uterine tissue; creating products of menses and inflamed tissues in and behind vagina.

617.5 Endometriosis of intestine ♀
Endometriosis:
appendix
colon

Endometriosis:
rectum

DEF: Aberrant uterine tissue; creating products of menses and inflamed intestinal tissues.

617.6 Endometriosis in scar of skin ♀
617.8 Endometriosis of other specified sites ♀
Endometriosis:
bladder
lung

Endometriosis:
umbilicus
vulva

617.9 Endometriosis, site unspecified ♀

√4ᵗʰ 618 Genital prolapse
Use additional code to identify urinary incontinence (625.6, 788.31, 788.33-788.39)

> EXCLUDES   that complicating pregnancy, labor, or delivery (654.4)

618.0 Prolapse of vaginal walls without mention of uterine prolapse ♀
Cystocele   Cystourethrocele

Proctocele, female
Rectocele
Urethrocele, female
Vaginal prolapse
} without mention of uterine prolapse

> EXCLUDES   that with uterine prolapse (618.2-618.4)
> enterocele (618.6)
> vaginal vault prolapse following hysterectomy (618.5)

618.1 Uterine prolapse without mention of vaginal wall prolapse ♀
Descensus uteri
Uterine prolapse:
NOS
complete

Uterine prolapse:
first degree
second degree
third degree

> EXCLUDES   that with mention of cystocele, urethrocele, or rectocele (618.2-618.4)

618.2 Uterovaginal prolapse, incomplete ♀
DEF: Downward displacement of uterus downward into vagina.

618.3 Uterovaginal prolapse, complete ♀
DEF: Downward displacement of uterus exposed within external genitalia.

N Newborn Age: 0   P Pediatric Age: 0-17   M Maternity Age: 12-55   A Adult Age: 15-124   CC CC Condition   MC Major Complication   CD Complex Dx   HIV HIV Related Dx

180 — Volume 1   2002 Ingenix, Inc.

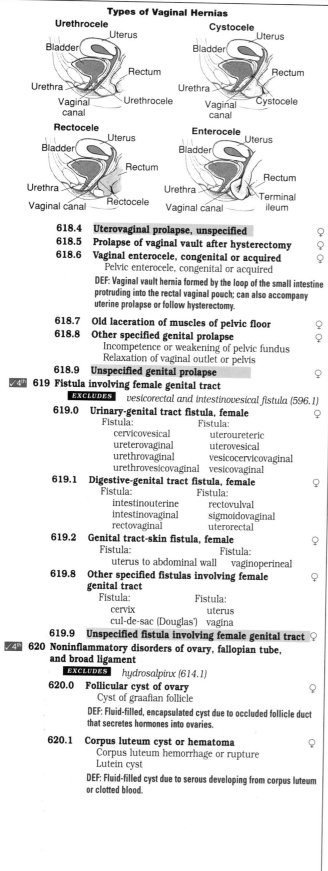

Types of Vaginal Hernias

Urethrocele

Cystocele

Rectocele

Enterocele

618.4 Uterovaginal prolapse, unspecified ♀

618.5 Prolapse of vaginal vault after hysterectomy ♀

618.6 Vaginal enterocele, congenital or acquired ♀
Pelvic enterocele, congenital or acquired

DEF: Vaginal vault hernia formed by the loop of the small intestine protruding into the rectal vaginal pouch; can also accompany uterine prolapse or follow hysterectomy.

618.7 Old laceration of muscles of pelvic floor ♀

618.8 Other specified genital prolapse ♀
Incompetence or weakening of pelvic fundus
Relaxation of vaginal outlet or pelvis

618.9 Unspecified genital prolapse ♀

✓4ᵗʰ **619 Fistula involving female genital tract**
EXCLUDES   vesicorectal and intestinovesical fistula (596.1)

619.0 Urinary-genital tract fistula, female ♀
Fistula: Fistula:
cervicovesical   uteroureteric
ureterovaginal   uterovesical
urethrovaginal   vesicocervicovaginal
urethrovesicovaginal vesicovaginal

619.1 Digestive-genital tract fistula, female ♀
Fistula: Fistula:
intestinouterine   rectovulval
intestinovaginal   sigmoidovaginal
rectovaginal   uterorectal

619.2 Genital tract-skin fistula, female ♀
Fistula: Fistula:
uterus to abdominal wall   vaginoperineal

619.8 Other specified fistulas involving female genital tract ♀
Fistula: Fistula:
cervix   uterus
cul-de-sac (Douglas') vagina

619.9 Unspecified fistula involving female genital tract ♀

✓4ᵗʰ **620 Noninflammatory disorders of ovary, fallopian tube, and broad ligament**
EXCLUDES   hydrosalpinx (614.1)

620.0 Follicular cyst of ovary ♀
Cyst of graafian follicle

DEF: Fluid-filled, encapsulated cyst due to occluded follicle duct that secretes hormones into ovaries.

620.1 Corpus luteum cyst or hematoma ♀
Corpus luteum hemorrhage or rupture
Lutein cyst

DEF: Fluid-filled cyst due to serous developing from corpus luteum or clotted blood.

620.2 Other and unspecified ovarian cyst ♀
Cyst:
NOS
corpus albicans
retention NOS   of ovary
serous
theca-lutein

Simple cystoma of ovary
EXCLUDES   cystadenoma (benign) (serous) (220)
developmental cysts (752.0)
neoplastic cysts (220)
polycystic ovaries (256.4)
Stein-Leventhal syndrome (256.4)

620.3 Acquired atrophy of ovary and fallopian tube ♀
Senile involution of ovary

620.4 Prolapse or hernia of ovary and fallopian tube ♀
Displacement of ovary and fallopian tube
Salpingocele

620.5 Torsion of ovary, ovarian pedicle, or fallopian tube ♀
Torsion: Torsion:
accessory tube   hydatid of Morgagni

620.6 Broad ligament laceration syndrome ♀
Masters-Allen syndrome

620.7 Hematoma of broad ligament CC ♀
Hematocele, broad ligament
CC Excl: 620.6-620.9, 625.8-625.9, 629.8-629.9, 752.8-752.9

DEF: Blood within peritoneal fold that supports uterus.

620.8 Other noninflammatory disorders of ovary, fallopian tube, and broad ligament ♀
Cyst
Polyp   of broad ligament or fallopian tube

Infarction
Rupture   of ovary or fallopian tube

Hematosalpinx
EXCLUDES   hematosalpinx in ectopic pregnancy (639.2)
peritubal adhesions (614.6)
torsion of ovary, ovarian pedicle, or fallopian tube (620.5)

620.9 Unspecified noninflammatory disorder of ovary, fallopian tube, and broad ligament ♀

✓4ᵗʰ **621 Disorders of uterus, not elsewhere classified**

621.0 Polyp of corpus uteri ♀
Polyp: Polyp:
endometrium   uterus NOS
EXCLUDES   cervical polyp NOS (622.7)

621.1 Chronic subinvolution of uterus ♀
EXCLUDES   puerperal (674.8)
AHA: 1Q, '91, 11

DEF: Abnormal size of uterus after delivery; the uterus does not return to its normal size after the birth of a child.

621.2 Hypertrophy of uterus ♀
Bulky or enlarged uterus
EXCLUDES   puerperal (674.8)

621.3 Endometrial cystic hyperplasia ♀
Hyperplasia (adenomatous) (cystic) (glandular) of endometrium

DEF: Abnormal cystic overgrowth of endometrial tissue.

621.4 Hematometra ♀
Hemometra
EXCLUDES   that in congenital anomaly (752.2-752.3)

DEF: Accumulated blood in uterus.

621.5 Intrauterine synechiae ♀
Adhesions of uterus   Band(s) of uterus

✓4ᵗʰ / ✓5ᵗʰ Additional Digit Required   Nonspecific PDx   Unacceptable PDx   Manifestation Code   MSP Medicare Secondary Payer   ▶◀ Revised Text   ● New Code   ▲ Revised Code Title

2002 Ingenix, Inc.   **Volume 1 — 181**

Genitourinary System 618.4–621.5

Uterus and Ovaries

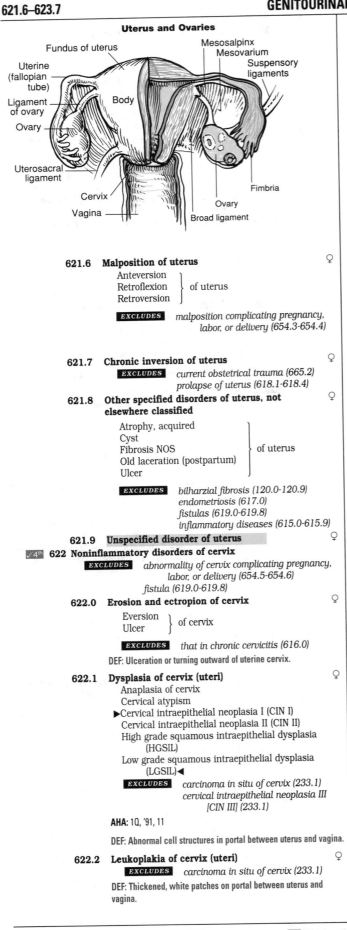

Fundus of uterus
Mesosalpinx
Mesovarium
Suspensory ligaments
Uterine (fallopian tube)
Ligament of ovary
Body
Ovary
Uterosacral ligament
Cervix
Vagina
Ovary
Fimbria
Broad ligament

621.6 Malposition of uterus ♀
Anteversion
Retroflexion } of uterus
Retroversion
EXCLUDES malposition complicating pregnancy, labor, or delivery (654.3-654.4)

621.7 Chronic inversion of uterus ♀
EXCLUDES current obstetrical trauma (665.2)
prolapse of uterus (618.1-618.4)

621.8 Other specified disorders of uterus, not elsewhere classified ♀
Atrophy, acquired
Cyst
Fibrosis NOS } of uterus
Old laceration (postpartum)
Ulcer
EXCLUDES bilharzial fibrosis (120.0-120.9)
endometriosis (617.0)
fistulas (619.0-619.8)
inflammatory diseases (615.0-615.9)

621.9 Unspecified disorder of uterus ♀

√4ᵗʰ **622 Noninflammatory disorders of cervix**
EXCLUDES abnormality of cervix complicating pregnancy, labor, or delivery (654.5-654.6)
fistula (619.0-619.8)

622.0 Erosion and ectropion of cervix ♀
Eversion } of cervix
Ulcer
EXCLUDES that in chronic cervicitis (616.0)
DEF: Ulceration or turning outward of uterine cervix.

622.1 Dysplasia of cervix (uteri) ♀
Anaplasia of cervix
Cervical atypism
▶Cervical intraepithelial neoplasia I (CIN I)
Cervical intraepithelial neoplasia II (CIN II)
High grade squamous intraepithelial dysplasia (HGSIL)
Low grade squamous intraepithelial dysplasia (LGSIL)◀
EXCLUDES carcinoma in situ of cervix (233.1)
cervical intraepithelial neoplasia III [CIN III] (233.1)
AHA: 1Q, '91, 11
DEF: Abnormal cell structures in portal between uterus and vagina.

622.2 Leukoplakia of cervix (uteri) ♀
EXCLUDES carcinoma in situ of cervix (233.1)
DEF: Thickened, white patches on portal between uterus and vagina.

622.3 Old laceration of cervix ♀
Adhesions
Band(s) } of cervix
Cicatrix (postpartum)
EXCLUDES current obstetrical trauma (665.3)
DEF: Scarring or other evidence of old wound on cervix.

622.4 Stricture and stenosis of cervix ♀
Atresia (acquired)
Contracture } of cervix
Occlusion
Pinpoint os uteri
EXCLUDES congenital (752.49)
that complicating labor (654.6)

622.5 Incompetence of cervix ♀
EXCLUDES complicating pregnancy (654.5)
that affecting fetus or newborn (761.0)
DEF: Inadequate functioning of cervix; marked by abnormal widening during pregnancy; causing miscarriage.

622.6 Hypertrophic elongation of cervix ♀
DEF: Overgrowth of cervix tissues extending down into vagina.

622.7 Mucous polyp of cervix ♀
Polyp NOS of cervix
EXCLUDES adenomatous polyp of cervix (219.0)

622.8 Other specified noninflammatory disorders of cervix ♀
Atrophy (senile)
Cyst } of cervix
Fibrosis
Hemorrhage
EXCLUDES endometriosis (617.0)
fistula (619.0-619.8)
inflammatory diseases (616.0)

622.9 Unspecified noninflammatory disorder of cervix ♀

√4ᵗʰ **623 Noninflammatory disorders of vagina**
EXCLUDES abnormality of vagina complicating pregnancy, labor, or delivery (654.7)
congenital absence of vagina (752.49)
congenital diaphragm or bands (752.49)
fistulas involving vagina (619.0-619.8)

623.0 Dysplasia of vagina ♀
EXCLUDES carcinoma in situ of vagina (233.3)

623.1 Leukoplakia of vagina ♀
DEF: Thickened white patches on vaginal canal.

623.2 Stricture or atresia of vagina ♀
Adhesions (postoperative) (postradiation) of vagina
Occlusion of vagina
Stenosis, vagina
Use additional E code to identify any external cause
EXCLUDES congenital atresia or stricture (752.49)

623.3 Tight hymenal ring ♀
Rigid hymen
Tight hymenal ring } acquired or congenital
Tight introitus
EXCLUDES imperforate hymen (752.42)

623.4 Old vaginal laceration ♀
EXCLUDES old laceration involving muscles of pelvic floor (618.7)
DEF: Scarring or other evidence of old wound on vagina.

623.5 Leukorrhea, not specified as infective ♀
Leukorrhea NOS of vagina
Vaginal discharge NOS
EXCLUDES trichomonal (131.00)
DEF: Viscid whitish discharge, from vagina.

623.6 Vaginal hematoma ♀
EXCLUDES current obstetrical trauma (665.7)

623.7 Polyp of vagina ♀

Ⓝ Newborn Age: 0 Ⓟ Pediatric Age: 0-17 Ⓜ Maternity Age: 12-55 Ⓐ Adult Age: 15-124 CC CC Condition MC Major Complication CD Complex Dx HIV HIV Related Dx

182 — Volume 1 • October 2002

2002 Ingenix, Inc.

623.8 Other specified noninflammatory disorders of vagina   ♀

Cyst
Hemorrhage } of vagina

623.9 Unspecified noninflammatory disorder of vagina   ♀

✓4ᵗʰ **624** Noninflammatory disorders of vulva and perineum

EXCLUDES abnormality of vulva and perineum complicating pregnancy, labor, or delivery (654.8)
condyloma acuminatum (078.1)
fistulas involving:
perineum — see Alphabetic Index
vulva (619.0-619.8)
vulval varices (456.6)
vulvar involvement in skin conditions (690-709.9)

624.0 Dystrophy of vulva   ♀

Kraurosis
Leukoplakia } of vulva

EXCLUDES carcinoma in situ of vulva (233.3)

624.1 Atrophy of vulva   ♀
624.2 Hypertrophy of clitoris   ♀

EXCLUDES that in endocrine disorders (255.2, 256.1)

624.3 Hypertrophy of labia   ♀

Hypertrophy of vulva NOS
DEF: Overgrowth of fleshy folds on either side of vagina.

624.4 Old laceration or scarring of vulva   ♀

DEF: Scarring or other evidence of old wound on external female genitalia.

624.5 Hematoma of vulva   ♀

EXCLUDES that complicating delivery (664.5)
DEF: Blood in tissue of external genitalia.

624.6 Polyp of labia and vulva   ♀
624.8 Other specified noninflammatory disorders of vulva and perineum   ♀

Cyst
Edema } of vulva
Stricture

AHA: 1Q, '95, 8

624.9 Unspecified noninflammatory disorder of vulva and perineum   ♀

✓4ᵗʰ **625** Pain and other symptoms associated with female genital organs

625.0 Dyspareunia   ♀

EXCLUDES psychogenic dyspareunia (302.76)
DEF: Difficult or painful sexual intercourse.

625.1 Vaginismus   ♀

Colpospasm
Vulvismus
EXCLUDES psychogenic vaginismus (306.51)
DEF: Vaginal spasms; due to involuntary contraction of musculature; prevents intercourse.

625.2 Mittelschmerz   ♀

Intermenstrual pain
Ovulation pain
DEF: Pain occurring between menstrual periods.

625.3 Dysmenorrhea   ♀

Painful menstruation
EXCLUDES psychogenic dysmenorrhea (306.52)
AHA: 2Q, '94, 12

625.4 Premenstrual tension syndromes   ♀

Menstrual:
migraine
molimen
Premenstual syndrome
Premenstrual tension NOS

625.5 Pelvic congestion syndrome   ♀

Congestion-fibrosis syndrome   Taylor's syndrome
DEF: Excessive accumulated of blood in vessels of pelvis; may occur after orgasm; causes abnormal menstruation, lower back pain and vaginal discharge.

625.6 Stress incontinence, female   ♀

EXCLUDES mixed incontinence (788.33)
stress incontinence, male (788.32)
DEF: Involuntary leakage of urine due to insufficient sphincter control; occurs upon sneezing, laughing, coughing, sudden movement or lifting.

625.8 Other specified symptoms associated with female genital organs   ♀

AHA: N-D, '85, 16

625.9 Unspecified symptom associated with female genital organs   ♀

✓4ᵗʰ **626** Disorders of menstruation and other abnormal bleeding from female genital tract

EXCLUDES menopausal and premenopausal bleeding (627.0)
pain and other symptoms associated with menstrual cycle (625.2-625.4)
postmenopausal bleeding (627.1)

626.0 Absence of menstruation   ♀

Amenorrhea (primary) (secondary)

626.1 Scanty or infrequent menstruation   ♀

Hypomenorrhea   Oligomenorrhea

626.2 Excessive or frequent menstruation   ♀

Heavy periods
Menometrorrhagia
Menorrhagia
Plymenorrhea
EXCLUDES premenopausal(627.0)
that in puberty (626.3)

626.3 Puberty bleeding   ♀

Excessive bleeding associated with onset of menstrual periods
Pubertal menorrhagia

626.4 Irregular menstrual cycle   ♀

Irregular:
bleeding NOS
menstruation
periods

626.5 Ovulation bleeding   ♀

Regular intermenstrual bleeding

626.6 Metrorrhagia   ♀

Bleeding unrelated to menstrual cycle
Irregular intermenstrual bleeding

626.7 Postcoital bleeding   ♀

DEF: Bleeding from vagina after sexual intercourse.

626.8 Other   ♀

Dysfunctional or functional uterine hemorrhage NOS
Menstruation:
retained
suppression of

626.9 Unspecified   ♀

✓4ᵗʰ **627** Menopausal and postmenopausal disorders

EXCLUDES asymptomatic age-related (natural) postmenopausal status (V49.81)

627.0 Premenopausal menorrhagia   ♀

Excessive bleeding associated with onset of menopause
Menorrhagia:
climacteric
menopausal
preclimacteric

627.1 Postmenopausal bleeding   ♀

▲ **627.2** **Symptomatic menopausal or female climacteric** ♀
states
Symptoms, such as flushing, sleeplessness,
headache, lack of concentration, associated
with the menopause

627.3 **Postmenopausal atrophic vaginitis** ♀
Senile (atrophic) vaginitis

▲ **627.4** **Symptomatic states associated with artificial** ♀
menopause
Postartificial menopause syndromes
Any condition classifiable to 627.1, 627.2, or 627.3
which follows induced menopause

DEF: Conditions arising after hysterectomy.

627.8 **Other specified menopausal and** ♀
postmenopausal disorders
EXCLUDES   *premature menopause NOS (256.31)*

627.9 **Unspecified menopausal and postmenopausal** ♀
disorder

√4ᵗʰ **628 Infertility, female**
INCLUDES   primary and secondary sterility

AHA: 2Q, '96, 9; 1Q, '95, 7

DEF: Infertility: inability to conceive for at least one year with regular
intercourse.

DEF: Primary infertility: occurring in patients who have never conceived.

DEF: Secondary infertility: occurring in patients who have previously
conceived.

628.0 **Associated with anovulation** ♀
Anovulatory cycle
Use additional code for any associated Stein-
Leventhal syndrome (256.4)

628.1 *Of pituitary-hypothalamic origin* ♀
Code first underlying cause, as:
adiposogenital dystrophy (253.8)
anterior pituitary disorder (253.0-253.4)

628.2 **Of tubal origin** ♀
Infertility associated with congenital anomaly of tube
Tubal:
block
occlusion
stenosis
Use additional code for any associated peritubal
adhesions (614.6)

628.3 **Of uterine origin** ♀
Infertility associated with congenital anomaly of
uterus
Nonimplantation
Use additional code for any associated tuberculous
endometritis (016.7)

628.4 **Of cervical or vaginal origin** ♀
Infertility associated with:
anomaly of cervical mucus
congenital structural anomaly
dysmucorrhea

628.8 **Of other specified origin** ♀

628.9 **Of unspecified origin** ♀

√4ᵗʰ **629 Other disorders of female genital organs**

629.0 **Hematocele, female, not elsewhere classified** ♀
EXCLUDES   *hematocele or hematoma:*
broad ligament (620.7)
fallopian tube (620.8)
that associated with ectopic
pregnancy ▶(633.00-633.91)◀
uterus (621.4)
vagina (623.6)
vulva (624.5)

629.1 **Hydrocele, canal of Nuck** ♀
Cyst of canal of Nuck (acquired)
EXCLUDES   *congenital (752.41)*

629.8 **Other specified disorders of female genital organs** ♀

629.9 **Unspecified disorder of female genital organs** ♀
Habitual aborter without current pregnancy

N Newborn Age: 0   P Pediatric Age: 0-17   M Maternity Age: 12-55   A Adult Age: 15-124   CC CC Condition   MC Major Complication   CD Complex Dx   HIV HIV Related Dx

184 — Volume 1 • October 2002
2002 Ingenix, Inc.

11. COMPLICATIONS OF PREGNANCY, CHILDBIRTH, AND THE PUERPERIUM (630-677)

ECTOPIC AND MOLAR PREGNANCY (630-633)

Use additional code from category 639 to identify any complications

630 Hydatidiform mole   M ♀

Trophoblastic disease NOS   Vesicularmole

EXCLUDES chorioadenoma (destruens) (236.1)
chorionepithelioma (181)
malignant hydatidiform mole (236.1)

DEF: Abnormal product of pregnancy; marked by mass of cysts resembling bunch of grapes due to chorionic villi proliferation, and dissolution; must be surgically removed.

631 Other abnormal product of conception   M ♀

Blighted ovum   Mole:
Mole: fleshy
  NOS   stone
  carneous

632 Missed abortion   M ♀

Early fetal death before completion of 22 weeks' gestation with retention of dead fetus

Retained products of conception, not following spontaneous or induced abortion or delivery

EXCLUDES failed induced abortion (638.0-638.9)
fetal death (intrauterine) (late) (656.4)
missed delivery (656.4)
that with abnormal product of conception (630, 631)

AHA: 1Q, '01, 5

√4ᵗʰ **633 Ectopic pregnancy**

INCLUDES ruptured ectopic pregnancy

DEF: Fertilized egg develops outside uterus.

√5ᵗʰ **633.0 Abdominal pregnancy**

Intraperitoneal pregnancy

- **633.00 Abdominal pregnancy without intrauterine pregnancy**   M ♀
- **633.01 Abdominal pregnancy with intrauterine pregnancy**   M ♀

√5ᵗʰ **633.1 Tubal pregnancy**

Fallopian pregnancy
Rupture of (fallopian) tube due to pregnancy
Tubal abortion

AHA: 2Q, '90, 27

- **633.10 Tubal pregnancy without intrauterine pregnancy**   M ♀
- **633.11 Tubal pregnancy with intrauterine pregnancy**   M ♀

√5ᵗʰ **633.2 Ovarian pregnancy**

- **633.20 Ovarian pregnancy without intrauterine pregnancy**   M ♀
- **633.21 Ovarian pregnancy with intrauterine pregnancy**   M ♀

√5ᵗʰ **633.8 Other ectopic pregnancy**

Pregnancy: Pregnancy:
  cervical   intraligamentous
  combined   mesometric
  cornual   mural

- **633.80 Other ectopic pregnancy without intrauterine pregnancy**   M ♀
- **633.81 Other ectopic pregnancy with intrauterine pregnancy**   ♀

√5ᵗʰ **633.9 Unspecified ectopic pregnancy**

- **633.90 Unspecified ectopic pregnancy without intrauterine pregnancy**   M ♀
- **633.91 Unspecified ectopic pregnancy with intrauterine pregnancy**   M ♀

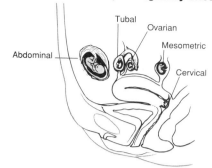

Ectopic Pregnancy Sites

Abdominal — Tubal — Ovarian — Mesometric — Cervical

OTHER PREGNANCY WITH ABORTIVE OUTCOME (634-639)

The following fourth-digit subdivisions are for use with categories 634-638:

.0 Complicated by genital tract and pelvic infection

Endometritis
Salpingo-oophoritis
Sepsis NOS
Septicemia NOS
Any condition classifiable to 639.0, with condition classifiable to 634-638

EXCLUDES urinary tract infection (634-638 with .7)

.1 Complicated by delayed or excessive hemorrhage

Afibrinogenemia
Defibrination syndrome
Intravascular hemolysis
Any condition classifiable to 639.1, with condition classifiable to 634-638
uterus

.2 Complicated by damage to pelvic organs and tissues

Laceration, perforation, or tear of:
  bladder
  uterus
Any condition classifiable to 639.2, with condition classifiable to 634-638

.3 Complicated by renal failure

Oliguria
Uremia
Any condition classifiable to 639.3, with condition classifiable to 634-638

.4 Complicated by metabolic disorder

Electrolyte imbalance with conditions classifiable to 634-638

.5 Complicated by shock

Circulatory collapse
Shock (postoperative) (septic)
Any condition classifiable to 639.5, with condition classifiable to 634-638

.6 Complicated by embolism

Embolism:
  NOS
  amniotic fluid
  pulmonary
Any condition classifiable to 639.6, with condition classifiable to 634-638

.7 With other specified complications

Cardiac arrest or failure
Urinary tract infection
Any condition classifiable to 639.8, with condition classifiable to 634-638

.8 With unspecified complication

.9 Without mention of complication

√4ᵗʰ √5ᵗʰ **Additional Digit Required**   Nonspecific PDx   Unacceptable PDx   Manifestation Code   MSP Medicare Secondary Payer   ►◄ Revised Text   ● New Code   ▲ Revised Code Title

Complications of Pregnancy, Childbirth, and the Puerperium 634–638.9

§ ✓4ᵗʰ **634 Spontaneous abortion**

Requires fifth-digit to identify stage:
  0 unspecified
  1 incomplete
  2 complete

INCLUDES   miscarriage
           spontaneous abortion

AHA: 2Q, '91, 16

DEF: Spontaneous premature expulsion of the products of conception from the uterus.

✓5ᵗʰ **634.0 Complicated by genital tract and pelvic infection**   CC M♀
     CC Excl: 634.00-634.92, 635.00-635.92, 636.00-636.92, 637.00-637.92, 638.0-638.9, 640.00-640.93, 641.00-641.23, 646.80-646.93, 648.90-648.94, 650, 669.40-669.44, 669.80-669.94

✓5ᵗʰ **634.1 Complicated by delayed or excessive hemorrhage**   CC M♀
     CC Excl: See code 634.0

✓5ᵗʰ **634.2 Complicated by damage to pelvic organs or tissues**   CC M♀
     CC Excl: See code 634.0

✓5ᵗʰ **634.3 Complicated by renal failure**   CC M♀
     CC Excl: See code 634.0

✓5ᵗʰ **634.4 Complicated by metabolic disorder**   CC M♀
     CC Excl: See code 634.0

✓5ᵗʰ **634.5 Complicated by shock**   CC M♀
     CC Excl: See code 634.0

✓5ᵗʰ **634.6 Complicated by embolism**   CC M♀
     CC Excl: See code 634.0

✓5ᵗʰ **634.7 With other specified complications**   CC M♀
     CC Excl: See code 634.0

✓5ᵗʰ **634.8 With unspecified complication**   CC M♀
     CC Excl: See code 634.0

✓5ᵗʰ **634.9 Without mention of complication**   CC M♀
     CC Excl: See code 634.0

§ ✓4ᵗʰ **635 Legally induced abortion**

Requires fifth-digit to identify stage:
  0 unspecified
  1 incomplete
  2 complete

INCLUDES   abortion or termination of pregnancy:
           elective
           legal
           therapeutic

EXCLUDES   *menstrual extraction or regulation (V25.3)*

AHA: 2Q, '94, 14

DEF: Intentional expulsion of products of conception from uterus performed by medical professionals inside boundaries of law.

✓5ᵗʰ **635.0 Complicated by genital tract and pelvic infection**   M♀

✓5ᵗʰ **635.1 Complicated by delayed or excessive hemorrhage**   M♀

✓5ᵗʰ **635.2 Complicated by damage to pelvic organs or tissues**   M♀

✓5ᵗʰ **635.3 Complicated by renal failure**   M♀

✓5ᵗʰ **635.4 Complicated by metabolic disorder**   M♀

✓5ᵗʰ **635.5 Complicated by shock**   M♀

✓5ᵗʰ **635.6 Complicated by embolism**   M♀

✓5ᵗʰ **635.7 With other specified complications**   M♀

✓5ᵗʰ **635.8 With unspecified complication**   M♀

✓5ᵗʰ **635.9 Without mention of complication**   M♀

§ ✓4ᵗʰ **636 Illegally induced abortion**

Requires fifth-digit to identify stage:
  0 unspecified
  1 incomplete
  2 complete

INCLUDES   abortion:
           criminal
           illegal
           self-induced

DEF: Intentional expulsion of products of conception from uterus; outside boundaries of law.

✓5ᵗʰ **636.0 Complicated by genital tract and pelvic infection**   M♀

✓5ᵗʰ **636.1 Complicated by delayed or excessive hemorrhage**   M♀

✓5ᵗʰ **636.2 Complicated by damage to pelvic organs or tissues**   M♀

✓5ᵗʰ **636.3 Complicated by renal failure**   M♀

✓5ᵗʰ **636.4 Complicated by metabolic disorder**   M♀

✓5ᵗʰ **636.5 Complicated by shock**   M♀

✓5ᵗʰ **636.6 Complicated by embolism**   M♀

✓5ᵗʰ **636.7 With other specified complications**   M♀

✓5ᵗʰ **636.8 With unspecified complication**   M♀

✓5ᵗʰ **636.9 Without mention of complication**   M♀

§ ✓4ᵗʰ **637 Unspecified abortion**

Requires fifth-digit to identify stage:
  0 unspecified
  1 incomplete
  2 complete

INCLUDES   abortion NOS
           retained products of conception following abortion, not classifiable elsewhere

✓5ᵗʰ **637.0 Complicated by genital tract and pelvic infection**   M♀

✓5ᵗʰ **637.1 Complicated by delayed or excessive hemorrhage**   M♀

✓5ᵗʰ **637.2 Complicated by damage to pelvic organs or tissues**   M♀

✓5ᵗʰ **637.3 Complicated by renal failure**   M♀

✓5ᵗʰ **637.4 Complicated by metabolic disorder**   M♀

✓5ᵗʰ **637.5 Complicated by shock**   M♀

✓5ᵗʰ **637.6 Complicated by embolism**   M♀

✓5ᵗʰ **637.7 With other specified complications**   M♀

✓5ᵗʰ **637.8 With unspecified complication**   M♀

✓5ᵗʰ **637.9 Without mention of complication**   M♀

§ ✓4ᵗʰ **638 Failed attempted abortion**

INCLUDES   failure of attempted induction of (legal) abortion

EXCLUDES   *incomplete abortion (634.0-637.9)*

DEF: Continued pregnancy despite an attempted legal abortion.

638.0 Complicated by genital tract and pelvic infection   M♀

638.1 Complicated by delayed or excessive hemorrhage   M♀

638.2 Complicated by damage to pelvic organs or tissues   M♀

638.3 Complicated by renal failure   M♀

638.4 Complicated by metabolic disorder   M♀

638.5 Complicated by shock   M♀

638.6 Complicated by embolism   M♀

638.7 With other specified complications   M♀

638.8 With unspecified complication   M♀

638.9 Without mention of complication   M♀

§   See beginning of section 634-639 for fourth-digit definitions.

N Newborn Age: 0   P Pediatric Age: 0-17   M Maternity Age: 12-55   A Adult Age: 15-124   CC CC Condition   MC Major Complication   CD Complex Dx   HIV HIV Related Dx

§ ☑4ᵗʰ **639 Complications following abortion and ectopic and molar pregnancies**

> Note: This category is provided for use when it is required to classify separately the complications classifiable to the fourth-digit level in categories 634-638; for example:
>
> a) when the complication itself was responsible for an episode of medical care, the abortion, ectopic or molar pregnancy itself having been dealt with at a previous episode
>
> b) when these conditions are immediate complications of ectopic or molar pregnancies classifiable to 630-633 where they cannot be identified at fourth-digit level.

639.0 Genital tract and pelvic infection   cc M ♀

Endometritis
Parametritis
Pelvic peritonitis
Salpingitis   } following conditions classifiable to 630-638
Salpingo-oophoritis
Sepsis NOS
Septicemia NOS

> **EXCLUDES** *urinary tract infection (639.8)*

CC Excl: 639.0, 639.2-639.9, 640.00-640.93, 641.00-641.23, 646.80-646.93, 648.90-648.94, 650, 669.40-669.44, 669.80-669.94

639.1 Delayed or excessive hemorrhage   cc M ♀

Afibrinogenemia   } following conditions classifiable to 630-638
Defibrination syndrome
Intravascular hemolysis

CC Excl: 639.1-639.9, 640.00-640.93, 641.00-641.23, 646.80-646.93, 648.90-648.94, 650, 669.40-669.44, 669.80-669.94

639.2 Damage to pelvic organs and tissues   cc M ♀

Laceration, perforation, or tear of:
bladder
bowel
broad ligament   } following conditions classifiable to 630-638
cervix
periurethral tissue
uterus
vagina

CC Excl: 639.2-639.9, 640.00-640.93, 641.00-641.23, 646.80-646.93, 648.90-648.94, 650, 669.40-669.44, 669.80-669.94

639.3 Renal failure   cc M ♀

Oliguria
Renal:
failure (acute) } following conditions classifiable to 630-638
shutdown
tubular necrosis
Uremia

CC Excl: See code 639.2

639.4 Metabolic disorders   cc M ♀

Electrolyte imbalance following conditions classifiable to 630-638

CC Excl: See code 639.2

639.5 Shock   cc M ♀

Circulatory collapse   } following conditions classifiable to 630-638
Shock (postoperative)
(septic)

CC Excl: See code 639.2

639.6 Embolism   cc M ♀

Embolism:
NOS
air
amniotic fluid
blood-clot
fat   } following conditions classifiable to 630-638
pulmonary
pyemic
septic
soap

CC Excl: See code 639.2

639.8 Other specified complications following abortionor ectopic and molar pregnancy   cc M ♀

Acute yellow atrophy or necrosis of liver
Cardiac arrest or failure   } following conditions classifiable to 630-638
Cerebral anoxia
Urinary tract infection

CC Excl: See code 639.2

639.9 Unspecified complication following abortion orectopic and molar pregnancy   cc M ♀

Complication(s) not further specified following conditions classifiable to 630-638

CC Excl: See code 639.2

COMPLICATIONS MAINLY RELATED TO PREGNANCY (640-648)

> **INCLUDES** the listed conditions even if they arose or were present during labor, delivery, or the puerperium

AHA: 2Q, '90, 11

The following fifth-digit subclassification is for use with categories 640-648 to denote the current episode of care. Valid fifth-digits are in [brackets] under each code.

   0 **unspecified as to episode of care or not applicable**
   1 **delivered, with or without mention of antepartum condition**

Antepartum condition with delivery
Delivery NOS (with mention of antepartum complication during current episode of care)
Intrapartum obstetric condition (with mention of antepartum complication during current episode of care)
Pregnancy, delivered (with mention of antepartum complication during current episode of care)

   2 **delivered, with mention of postpartum complication**

Delivery with mention of puerperal complication during current episode of care

   3 **antepartum condition or complication**

Antepartum obstetric condition, not delivered during the current episode of care

   4 **postpartum condition or complication**

Postpartum or puerperal obstetric condition or complication following delivery that occurred:
during previous episode of care
outside hospital, with subsequent admission for observation or care

☑4ᵗʰ **640 Hemorrhage in early pregnancy**

> **INCLUDES** hemorrhage before completion of 22 weeks' gestation

§ ☑5ᵗʰ **640.0 Threatened abortion**   cc M ♀
[0,1,3] **CC Excl:** 640.00-640.93, 641.00-641.13, 646.80-646.93, 648.90-648.94, 650, 669.40-669.44, 669.80-669.94

DEF: Bloody discharge during pregnancy; cervix may be dilated and pregnancy is threatened, but the pregnancy is not terminated.

§ ☑5ᵗʰ **640.8 Other specified hemorrhage in early**   cc M ♀
[0,1,3] **pregnancy**
CC Excl: See code 640.0

---

§ Requires fifth-digit. Valid digits are in [brackets] under each code. See beginning of section 640-648 for codes and definitions.

☑4ᵗʰ ☑5ᵗʰ **Additional Digit Required**   **Nonspecific PDx**   **Unacceptable PDx**   **Manifestation Code**   MSP Medicare Secondary Payer   ◄► Revised Text   ● New Code   ▲ Revised Code Title

2002 Ingenix, Inc.   **Volume 1 — 187**

Complications of Pregnancy, Childbirth, and the Puerperium 641.0–642.7

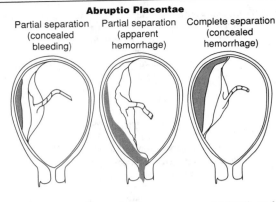

Placenta Previa
Low (marginal) implantation — Partial placenta previa — Total placenta previa

Abruptio Placentae
Partial separation (concealed bleeding) — Partial separation (apparent hemorrhage) — Complete separation (concealed hemorrhage)

§ √5th **640.9 Unspecified hemorrhage in early pregnancy** CC M ♀
[0,1,3]
CC Excl: See code 640.0

√4th **641 Antepartum hemorrhage, abruptio placentae, and placenta previa**

§ √5th **641.0 Placenta previa without hemorrhage** CC M ♀
[0,1,3]
Low impantation of placenta
Placenta previa noted:
   during pregnancy } without hemmorage
   before labor (and delivered
      by caesarean delivery.)

CC Excl: See code 640.0

DEF: Placenta implanted in lower segment of uterus; commonly causes hemorrhage in the last trimester of pregnancy.

§ √5th **641.1 Hemorrhage from placenta previa** CC M ♀
[0,1,3]
Low-lying placenta
Placenta previa
   incomplete } NOS or with
   marginal hemorrhage
   partial (intrapartum)
   total

EXCLUDES hemorrhage from vasa previa (663.5)

CC Excl: See code 640.0

§ √5th **641.2 Premature separation of placenta** M ♀
[0,1,3]
Ablatio placentae
Abruptio placentae
Accidental antepartum hemorrhage
Couvelaire uterus
Detachment of placenta (premature)
Premature separation of normally implanted placenta

DEF: Abruptio placentae: premature detachment of the placenta, characterized by shock, oliguria and decreased fibrinogen.

§ √5th **641.3 Antepartum hemorrhage associated with coagulation defects** CC M ♀
[0,1,3]
Antepartum or intrapartum hemorrhage associated with:
   afibrinogenemia
   hyperfibrinolysis
   hypofibrinogenemia

CC Excl: 641.30-641.93, 646.80-646.93, 648.90-648.94, 650, 669.40-669.44, 669.80-669.94

DEF: Uterine hemorrhage prior to delivery.

§ √5th **641.8 Other antepartum hemorrhage** CC M ♀
[0,1,3]
Antepartum or intrapartum hemorrhage associated with:
   trauma
   uterine leiomyoma

CC Excl: See code 641.3

§ √5th **641.9 Unspecified antepartum hemorrhage** CC M ♀
[0,1,3]
Hemorrhage: Hemorrhage:
   antepartum NOS   of pregnancy NOS
   intrapartum NOS

CC Excl: See code 641.3

√4th **642 Hypertension complicating pregnancy, childbirth, and the puerperium**

§ √5th **642.0 Benign essential hypertension complicating pregnancy, childbirth, and the puerperium** M ♀
[0-4]
Hypertension: specified as complicating,
   benign essential   or as a reason for
   chronic NOS   obstetric care during
   essential   pregnancy, childbirth,
   pre-existing NOS   or the puerperium

§ √5th **642.1 Hypertension secondary to renal disease, complicating pregnancy, childbirth, and the puerperium**
[0-4]
Hypertension secondary to renal disease, specified as complicating, or as a reason for obstetric care during pregnancy, childbirth, or the puerperium

§ √5th **642.2 Other pre-existing hypertension complicating pregnancy, childbirth, and the puerperium** M ♀
[0-4]
Hypertensive: specified as complicating,
   heart and renal   or as a reason for
      disease   obstetric care
   heart disease   during pregnancy,
   renal disease   childbirth, or the
Malignant   puerperium
   hypertension

§ √5th **642.3 Transient hypertension of pregnancy** M ♀
[0-4]
Gestational hypertension
Transient hypertension, so described, in pregnancy, childbirth, or the puerperium

AHA: 3Q, '90, 4

§ √5th **642.4 Mild or unspecified pre-eclampsia** CC M ♀
[0-4]
Hypertension in pregnancy, childbirth, or the puerperium, not specified as pre-existing, with either albuminuria or edema, or both; mild or unspecified
Pre-eclampsia: Toxemia (pre-eclamptic):
   NOS   NOS
   mild   mild

EXCLUDES albuminuria in pregnancy, without mention of hypertension (646.2)
edema in pregnancy, without mention of hypertension (646.1)

CC Excl: 642.00-642.94, 646.10-646.14, 646.80-646.93, 648.90-648.94, 650, 669.40-669.44, 669.80-669.94

§ √5th **642.5 Severe pre-eclampsia** CC M ♀
[0-4]
Hypertension in pregnancy, childbirth, or the puerperium, not specified as pre-existing, with either albuminuria or edema, or both; specified as severe
Pre-eclampsia, severe
Toxemia (pre-eclamptic), severe

CC Excl: See code 642.4

AHA: N-D, '85, 3

1 Nonspecific PDx=0
§ Requires fifth-digit. Valid digits are in [brackets] under each code. See beginning of section 640-648 for codes and definitions.

N Newborn Age: 0   P Pediatric Age: 0-17   M Maternity Age: 12-55   A Adult Age: 15-124   CC CC Condition   MC Major Complication   CD Complex Dx   HIV HIV Related Dx

§ ✓5th 1 **642.6**   **Eclampsia**   CC M ♀
[0-4]   Toxemia:
      eclamptic
      with convulsions
    CC Excl: See code 642.4

§ ✓5th 1 **642.7**   **Pre-eclampsia or eclampsia superimposed**   CC M ♀
[0-4]   **on pre-existing hypertension**
    Conditions classifiable to 642.4-642.6, with
      conditions classifiable to 642.0-642.2
    CC Excl: See code 642.4

§ ✓5th 1 **642.9**   **Unspecified hypertension complicating**   M ♀
[0-4]   **pregnancy, childbirth, or the puerperium**
    Hypertension NOS, without mention of albuminuria
      or edema, complicating pregnancy, childbirth,
      or the puerperium

✓4th **643**   **Excessive vomiting in pregnancy**
    INCLUDES   hyperemesis
       vomiting: arising during
         persistent   pregnancy
         vicious
      hyperemesis gravidarum

§ ✓5th 1 **643.0**   **Mild hyperemesis gravidarum**   M ♀
[0,1,3]   Hyperemesis gravidarum, mild or unspecified,
      starting before the end of the 22nd week of
      gestation
    DEF: Detrimental vomiting and nausea.

§ ✓5th 1 **643.1**   **Hyperemesis gravidarum with metabolic**   M ♀
[0,1,3]   disturbance
    Hyperemesis gravidarum, starting before the end of
      the 22nd week of gestation, with metabolic
      disturbance, such as:
       carbohydrate depletion
       dehydration
       electrolyte imbalance

§ ✓5th 1 **643.2**   **Late vomiting of pregnancy**   M ♀
[0,1,3]   Excessive vomiting starting after 22 completed
      weeks of gestation

§ ✓5th 1 **643.8**   **Other vomiting complicating pregnancy**   M ♀
[0,1,3]   Vomiting due to organic disease or other cause,
      specified as complicating pregnancy, or as a
      reason for obstetric care during pregnancy
    Use additional code to specify cause

§ ✓5th 1 **643.9**   **Unspecified vomiting of pregnancy**   M ♀
[0,1,3]   Vomiting as a reason for care during pregnancy,
      length of gestation unspecified

✓4th **644**   **Early or threatened labor**

§ ✓5th 1 **644.0**   **Threatened premature labor**   CC M ♀
[0,3]   Premature labor after 22 weeks, but before 37
      completed weeks of gestation without delivery
    EXCLUDES   *that occurring before 22 completed*
         weeks of gestation (640.0)
    CC Excl: 644.00-644.21, 646.80-646.93, 648.90-648.94,
    650, 669.40-669.44, 669.80-669.94

§ ✓5th 1 **644.1**   **Other threatened labor**   CC M ♀
[0,3]   False labor:
      NOS
      after 37 completed weeks of   without
        gestation   delivery
      Threatened labor NOS
    CC Excl: See code 644.0

§ ✓5th 1 **644.2**   **Early onset of delivery**   M ♀
[0,1]   Onset (spontaneous) of
      delivery   before 37 completed
    Premature labor with   weeks of gestation
      onset of delivery
    AHA: 2Q, '91, 16

✓4th **645**   **Late pregnancy**
    AHA: 4Q. '00, 43; 4Q, '91, 26

§ ✓5th 1 **645.1**   **Post term pregnancy**   M ♀
[0,1,3]   Pregnancy over 40 completed weeks to 42
      completed weeks gestation

§ ✓5th 1 **645.2**   **Prolonged pregnancy**   M ♀
[0,1,3]   Pregnancy which has advanced beyond 42
      completed weeks gestation

✓4th **646**   **Other complications of pregnancy, not elsewhere classified**
    Use additional code(s) to further specify complication
    AHA: 4Q, '95, 59

§ ✓5th 1 **646.0**   **Papyraceous fetus**   M ♀
[0,1,3]
    DEF: Fetus retained in the uterus beyond natural term, exhibits
    parchment-like skin.

§ ✓5th 1 **646.1**   **Edema or excessive weight gain in pregnancy,**   M ♀
[0-4]   **without mention of hypertension**
    Gestational edema
    Maternal obesity syndrome
    EXCLUDES   *that with mention of hypertension*
         (642.0-642.9)

§ ✓5th 1 **646.2**   **Unspecified renal disease in pregnancy,**   M ♀
[0-4]   **without mention of hypertension**
    Albuminuria   in pregnancy or the
    Nephropathy NOS   puerperium,
    Renal disease NOS   without mention
    Uremia   of hypertension
    Gestational proteinuria
    EXCLUDES   *that with mention of hypertension*
         (642.0-642.9)

§ ✓5th 1 **646.3**   **Habitual aborter**   M ♀
[0,1,3]   EXCLUDES   *with current abortion (634.0-634.9)*
         without current pregnancy (629.9)
    DEF: Three or more consecutive spontaneous abortions.

§ ✓5th 1 **646.4**   **Peripheral neuritis in pregnancy**   M ♀
[0-4]

§ ✓5th 1 **646.5**   **Asymptomatic bacteriuria in pregnancy**   M ♀
[0-4]

§ ✓5th 1 **646.6**   **Infections of genitourinary tract in**   CC M ♀
[0-4]   **pregnancy**
    Conditions classifiable to 590, 595, 597, 599.0, 616
      complicating pregnancy, childbirth, or the
      puerperium
    Conditions classifiable to ▶614.0-614.5, 614.7-
      614.9,◄ 615 complicating pregnancy or labor
    EXCLUDES   *major puerperal infection (670)*
    CC Excl: 646.60-646.64, 646.80-646.93, 648.90-648.94,
    650, 669.40-669.44, 669.80-669.94

§ ✓5th 1 **646.7**   **Liver disorders in pregnancy**   CC M ♀
[0,1,3]   Acute yellow atrophy of
      liver (obstetric) (true)
    Icterus gravis   of pregnancy
    Necrosis of liver
    EXCLUDES   *hepatorenal syndrome following*
         delivery (674.8)
         viral hepatitis (647.6)
    CC Excl: 646.70-646.93, 648.90-648.94, 650, 669.40-669.44,
    669.80-669.94

§ ✓5th 1 **646.8**   **Other specified complications of pregnancy**   M ♀
[0-4]   Fatigue during pregnancy
    Herpes gestationis
    Insufficient weight gain of pregnancy
    Uterine size-date discrepancy
    AHA: 3Q, '98, 16, J-F, '85, 15

§ ✓5th 1 **646.9**   **Unspecified complication of pregnancy**   M ♀
[0,1,3]

---

1   Nonspecific PDx=0

§   Requires fifth-digit. Valid digits are in [brackets] under each code. See beginning of section 640-648 for codes and definitions.

✓4th / ✓5th   Additional Digit Required   Nonspecific PDx   Unacceptable PDx   Manifestation Code   MSP Medicare Secondary Payer   ▶◀ Revised Text   ● New Code   ▲ Revised Code Title

2002 Ingenix, Inc.

October 2002 • Volume 1 — 189

Complications of Pregnancy, Childbirth, and the Puerperium 647–651.1

√4ᵗʰ **647 Infectious and parasitic conditions in the mother classifiable elsewhere, but complicating pregnancy, childbirth, or the puerperium**

> INCLUDES the listed conditions when complicating the pregnant state, aggravated by the pregnancy, or when a main reason for obstetric care
>
> EXCLUDES *those conditions in the mother known or suspected to have affected the fetus (655.0-655.9)*

Use additional code(s) to further specify complication Ⓜ♀

§ √5ᵗʰ¹ **647.0 Syphilis** Ⓜ♀
[0-4]   Conditions classifiable to 090-097

§ √5ᵗʰ¹ **647.1 Gonorrhea** Ⓜ♀
[0-4]   Conditions classifiable to 098

§ √5ᵗʰ¹ **647.2 Other venereal diseases** Ⓜ♀
[0-4]   Conditions classifiable to 099

§ √5ᵗʰ¹ **647.3 Tuberculosis** ⒸⒸ Ⓜ♀
[0-4]   Conditions classifiable to 010-018
CC Excl: 646.80-646.93, 647.30-647.34, 648.90-648.94, 650, 669.40-669.44, 669.80-669.94

§ √5ᵗʰ¹ **647.4 Malaria** ⒸⒸ Ⓜ♀
[0-4]   Conditions classifiable to 084
CC Excl: 646.80-646.93, 647.30-647.34, 648.90-648.94, 650, 669.40-669.44, 669.80-669.94

§ √5ᵗʰ¹ **647.5 Rubella** Ⓜ♀
[0-4]   Conditions classifiable to 056

§ √5ᵗʰ¹ **647.6 Other viral diseases** Ⓜ♀
[0-4]   Conditions classifiable to 042 and 050-079, except 056
AHA: J-F, '85, 15

§ √5ᵗʰ¹ **647.8 Other specified infectious and parasitic** Ⓜ♀
[0-4]   **diseases**

§ √5ᵗʰ **647.9 Unspecified infection or infestation** Ⓜ♀
[0-4]

√4ᵗʰ **648 Other current conditions in the mother classifiable elsewhere, but complicating pregnancy, childbirth, or the puerperium**

> INCLUDES the listed conditions when complicating the pregnant state, aggravated by the pregnancy, or when a main reason for obstetric care
>
> EXCLUDES *those conditions in the mother known or suspected to have affected the fetus (655.0-665.9)*

Use additional code(s) to identify the condition

§ √5ᵗʰ¹ **648.0 Diabetes mellitus** ⒸⒸ Ⓜ♀
[0-4]   Conditions classifiable to 250
> EXCLUDES *gestational diabetes (648.8)*

CC Excl: 646.80-646.93, 648.00-648.04, 648.90-648.94, 650, 669.40-669.44, 669.80-669.94
AHA: 3Q, '91, 5, 11

§ √5ᵗʰ¹ **648.1 Thyroid dysfunction** Ⓜ♀
[0-4]   Conditions classifiable to 240-246

§ √5ᵗʰ¹ **648.2 Anemia** ⒸⒸ Ⓜ♀
[0-4]   Conditions classifiable to 280-285
CC Excl: 646.80-646.93, 648.20-648.24, 648.90-648.94, 650, 669.40-669.44, 669.80-669.94
AHA: For Code 648.22: 1Q, '02, 14

§ √5ᵗʰ¹ **648.3 Drug dependence** ⒸⒸ Ⓜ♀
[0-4]   Conditions classifiable to 304
CC Excl: 646.80-646.93, 648.30-648.34, 648.90-648.94, 650, 669.40-669.44, 669.80-669.94
AHA: 2Q, '98, 13; 4Q, '88, 8

§ √5ᵗʰ¹ **648.4 Mental disorders** Ⓜ♀
[0-4]   Conditions classifiable to 290-303, 305-316, 317-319
AHA: 2Q, '98, 13; 4Q, '95, 63

§ √5ᵗʰ¹ **648.5 Congenital cardiovascular disorders** ⒸⒸ Ⓜ♀
[0-4]   Conditions classifiable to 745-747
CC Excl: 646.80-646.93, 648.50-648.64, 648.90-648.94, 650, 669.40-669.44, 669.80-669.94

§ √5ᵗʰ¹ **648.6 Other cardiovascular diseases** ⒸⒸ Ⓜ♀
[0-4]   Conditions classifiable to 390-398, 410-429
> EXCLUDES *cerebrovascular disorders in the puerperium (674.0)*
> *venous complications (671.0-671.9)*

CC Excl: See code 648.5
AHA: 3Q, '98, 11

§ √5ᵗʰ¹ **648.7 Bone and joint disorders of back, pelvis, and** Ⓜ♀
[0-4]   **lower limbs**
  Conditions classifiable to 720-724, and those classifiable to 711-719 or 725-738, specified as affecting the lower limbs

§ √5ᵗʰ¹ **648.8 Abnormal glucose tolerance** Ⓜ♀
[0-4]   Conditions classifiable to 790.2
  Gestational diabetes
AHA: 3Q, '91, 5

DEF: Glucose intolerance arising in pregnancy, resolving at end of pregnancy.

§ √5ᵗʰ¹ **648.9 Other current conditions classifiable elsewhere** Ⓜ♀
[0-4]   Conditions classifiable to 440-459
  Nutritional deficiencies [conditions classifiable to 260-269]
AHA: N-D, '87, 10; For code 648.91: 1Q, '02, 14

NORMAL DELIVERY, AND OTHER INDICATIONS FOR CARE IN PREGNANCY, LABOR, AND DELIVERY (650-659)

> The following fifth-digit subclassification is for use with categories 651-659 to denote the current episode of care. Valid fifth-digits are in [brackets] under each code.
>
> 0   **unspecified as to episode of care or not applicable**
> 1   **delivered, with or without mention of antepartum condition**
> 2   **delivered, with mention of postpartum complication**
> 3   **antepartum condition or complication**
> 4   **postpartum condition or complication**

650 Normal delivery Ⓜ♀
  Delivery requiring minimal or no assistance, with or without episiotomy, without fetal manipulation [e.g., rotation version] or instrumentation [forceps] of spontaneous, cephalic, vaginal, full-term, single, live-born infant. This code is for use as a single diagnosis code and is not to be used with any other code in the range 630-676.
> EXCLUDES *breech delivery (assisted) (spontaneous) NOS (652.2)*
> *delivery by vacuum extractor, forceps, cesarean section, or breech extraction, without specified complication (669.5-669.7)*

Use additional code to indicate outcome of delivery (V27.0)
AHA: ▶3Q, '01, 12;◀ 3Q, '00, 5; 4Q, '95, 28, 59

√4ᵗʰ **651 Multiple gestation**

§ √5ᵗʰ¹ **651.0 Twin pregnancy** Ⓜ♀
[0,1,3]

§ √5ᵗʰ¹ **651.1 Triplet pregnancy** Ⓜ♀
[0,1,3]

---

¹   Nonspecific PDx=0

§   Requires fifth-digit. Valid digits are in [brackets] under each code. See beginning of section 640-648 for codes and definitions.

Ⓝ Newborn Age: 0   Ⓟ Pediatric Age: 0-17   Ⓜ Maternity Age: 12-55   Ⓐ Adult Age :15-124   ⒸⒸ CC Condition   ⓂⒸ Major Complication   ⒸⒹ Complex Dx   ⒽⒾⓋ HIV Related Dx

190 — Volume 1 • January 2002   *2002 Ingenix, Inc.*

§ ✓5ᵗʰ ¹**651.2** **Quadruplet pregnancy** Ⓜ ♀
[0,1,3]

§ ✓5ᵗʰ ¹**651.3** **Twin pregnancy with fetal loss and retention** Ⓜ ♀
[0,1,3] **of one fetus**

§ ✓5ᵗʰ ¹**651.4** **Triplet pregnancy with fetal loss and** Ⓜ ♀

[0,1,3] **retention of one or more fetus(es)**

§ ✓5ᵗʰ ¹**651.5** **Quadruplet pregnancy with fetal loss and** Ⓜ ♀
[0,1,3] **retention of one or more fetus(es)**

§ ✓5ᵗʰ ¹**651.6** **Other multiple pregnancy with fetal loss and** Ⓜ ♀
[0,1,3] **retention of one or more fetus(es)**

§ ✓5ᵗʰ ¹**651.8** **Other specified multiple gestation** Ⓜ ♀
[0,1,3]

§ ✓5ᵗʰ **651.9** **Unspecified multiple gestation** Ⓜ ♀
[0,1,3]

✓4ᵗʰ **652 Malposition and malpresentation of fetus**
Code first any associated obstructed labor (660.0)

§ ✓5ᵗʰ ¹**652.0** **Unstable lie** Ⓜ ♀
[0,1,3]

DEF: Changing fetal position.

§ ✓5ᵗʰ ¹**652.1** **Breech or other malpresentation successfully** Ⓜ ♀
[0,1,3] **converted to cephalic presentation**
Cephalic version NOS

§ ✓5ᵗʰ ¹**652.2** **Breech presentation without mention of** Ⓜ ♀
[0,1,3] **version**
Breech delivery (assisted) (spontaneous) NOS
Buttocks presentation
Complete breech
Frank breech
EXCLUDES *footling presentation (652.8)*
incomplete breech (652.8)

DEF: Fetal presentation of buttocks or feet at birth canal.

§ ✓5ᵗʰ ¹**652.3** **Transverse or oblique presentation** Ⓜ ♀
[0,1,3] Oblique lie   Transverse lie
EXCLUDES *transverse arrest of fetal head (660.3)*

§ ✓5ᵗʰ ¹**652.4** **Face or brow presentation** Ⓜ ♀
[0,1,3] Mentum presentation

§ ✓5ᵗʰ ¹**652.5** **High head at term** Ⓜ ♀
[0,1,3] Failure of head to enter pelvic brim

§ ✓5ᵗʰ ¹**652.6** **Multiple gestation with malpresentation of** Ⓜ ♀
[0,1,3] **one fetus or more**

§ ✓5ᵗʰ ¹**652.7** **Prolapsed arm** Ⓜ ♀
[0,1,3]

§ ✓5ᵗʰ ¹**652.8** **Other specified malposition or** Ⓜ ♀
[0,1,3] **malpresentation**
Compound presentation

§ ✓5ᵗʰ **652.9** **Unspecified malposition or malpresentation** Ⓜ ♀
[0,1,3]

✓4ᵗʰ **653 Disproportion**
Code first any associated obstructed labor (660.1)

Malposition and Malpresentation

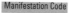

Breech

Shoulder
(arm
prolapse)

Mother's
pelvis

Face
(mentum)

Compound
(extremity
together
with head)

Oblique

Cephalopelvic Disproportion

Pubic symphysis

Ischial
tuberosity

Contraction of pelvic
outlet (from below)

Cephalopelvic disproportion
due to: Contraction of pelvic
inlet, or large fetus,
or hydrocephalus

Pubic symphysis

Pelvic inlet from above

§ ✓5ᵗʰ ¹**653.0** **Major abnormality of bony pelvis, not further** Ⓜ ♀
[0,1,3] **specified**
Pelvic deformity NOS

§ ✓5ᵗʰ ¹**653.1** **Generally contracted pelvis** Ⓜ ♀
[0,1,3] Contracted pelvis NOS

§ ✓5ᵗʰ ¹**653.2** **Inlet contraction of pelvis** Ⓜ ♀
[0,1,3] Inlet contraction (pelvis)

§ ✓5ᵗʰ ¹**653.3** **Outlet contraction of pelvis** Ⓜ ♀
[0,1,3] Outlet contraction (pelvis)

§ ✓5ᵗʰ ¹**653.4** **Fetopelvic disproportion** Ⓜ ♀
[0,1,3] Cephalopelvic disproportion NOS
Disproportion of mixed maternal and fetal origin,
with normally formed fetus

§ ✓5ᵗʰ ¹**653.5** **Unusually large fetus causing disproportion** Ⓜ ♀
[0,1,3] Disproportion of fetal origin with normally formed
fetus
Fetal disproportion NOS
EXCLUDES *that when the reason for medical care*
was concern for the fetus (656.6)

§ ✓5ᵗʰ ¹**653.6** **Hydrocephalic fetus causing disproportion** Ⓜ ♀
[0,1,3] **EXCLUDES** *that when the reason for medical care*
was concern for the fetus (655.0)

§ ✓5ᵗʰ ¹**653.7** **Other fetal abnormality causing disproportion** Ⓜ ♀
[0,1,3] Conjoined twins   Fetal:
Fetal: myelomeningocele
ascites   sacral teratoma
hydrops   tumor

§ ✓5ᵗʰ **653.8** **Disproportion of other origin** Ⓜ ♀
[0,1,3] **EXCLUDES** *shoulder (girdle) dystocia (660.4)*

§ ✓5ᵗʰ **653.9** **Unspecified disproportion** Ⓜ ♀
[0,1,3]

✓4ᵗʰ **654 Abnormality of organs and soft tissues of pelvis**
INCLUDES the listed conditions during pregnancy,
childbirth, or the puerperium
Code first any associated obstructed labor (660.2)

§ ✓5ᵗʰ ¹**654.0** **Congenital abnormalities of uterus** Ⓜ ♀
[0-4] Double uterus   Uterus bicornis

§ ✓5ᵗʰ ¹**654.1** **Tumors of body of uterus** Ⓜ ♀
[0-4] Uterine fibroids

§ ✓5ᵗʰ ¹**654.2** **Previous cesarean delivery** Ⓜ ♀
[0,1,3] Uterine scar from previous cesarean delivery
AHA: 1Q, '92, 8

§ ✓5ᵗʰ ¹**654.3** **Retroverted and incarcerated gravid uterus** Ⓜ ♀
[0-4]

DEF: Retroverted: tilted back uterus; no change in angle of
longitudinal axis.

DEF: Incarcerated: immobile, fixed uterus.

¹ Nonspecific PDx=0

§ Requires fifth-digit. Valid digits are in [brackets] under each code. See beginning of section 640-648 for codes and definitions.

✓4ᵗʰ / ✓5ᵗʰ Additional Digit Required   Nonspecific PDx   Unacceptable PDx   Manifestation Code   Ⓜ𝗦𝗣 Medicare Secondary Payer   ►◄ Revised Text   ● New Code   ▲ Revised Code Title

§ √5th **654.4** Other abnormalities in shape or position of gravid uterus and of neighboring structures Ⓜ♀
[0-4]
Cystocele Prolapse of gravid uterus
Pelvic floor repair Rectocele
Pendulous abdomen Rigid pelvic floor

§ √5th **654.5** Cervical incompetence Ⓜ♀
[0-4]
Presence of Shirodkar suture with or without mention of cervical incompetence

DEF: Abnormal cervix; tendency to dilate in second trimester; causes premature fetal expulsion.

DEF: Shirodkar suture: purse-string suture used to artificially close incompetent cervix.

§ √5th **654.6** Other congenital or acquired abnormality of cervix Ⓜ♀
[0-4]
Cicatricial cervix Rigid cervix (uteri)
Polyp of cervix Stenosis or stricture of cervix
Previous surgery to cervix Tumor of cervix

§ √5th **654.7** Congenital or acquired abnormality of vagina Ⓜ♀
[0-4]
Previous surgery to vagina Stricture of vagina
Septate vagina Tumor of vagina
Stenosis of vagina (acquired) (congenital)

§ √5th **654.8** Congenital or acquired abnormality of vulva Ⓜ♀
[0-4]
Fibrosis of perineum Rigid perineum
Persistent hymen Tumor of vulva
Previous surgery to perineum or vulva
EXCLUDES varicose veins of vulva (671.1)

§ √5th **654.9** Other and unspecified Ⓜ♀
[0-4]
Uterine scar NEC

√4th **655** Known or suspected fetal abnormality affecting management of mother
INCLUDES the listed conditions in the fetus as a reason for observation or obstetrical care of the mother, or for termination of pregnancy

AHA: 3Q, '90, 4

§ √5th **655.0** Central nervous system malformation in fetus Ⓜ♀
[0,1,3]
Fetal or suspected fetal:
anencephaly
hydrocephalus
spina bifida (with myelomeningocele)

§ √5th **655.1** Chromosomal abnormality in fetus Ⓜ♀
[0,1,3]

§ √5th **655.2** Hereditary disease in family possibly affecting fetus Ⓜ♀
[0,1,3]

§ √5th **655.3** Suspected damage to fetus from viral disease in the mother Ⓜ♀
[0,1,3]
Suspected damage to fetus from maternal rubella

§ √5th **655.4** Suspected damage to fetus from other disease in the mother Ⓜ♀
[0,1,3]
Suspected damage to fetus from maternal:
alcohol addiction
listeriosis
toxoplasmosis

§ √5th **655.5** Suspected damage to fetus from drugs Ⓜ♀
[0,1,3]

§ √5th **655.6** Suspected damage to fetus from radiation Ⓜ♀
[0,1,3]

§ √5th **655.7** Decreased fetal movements Ⓜ♀
[0,1,3]

AHA: 4Q, '97, 41

§ √5th **655.8** Other known or suspected fetal abnormality, not elsewhere classified Ⓜ♀
[0,1,3]
Suspected damage to fetus from:
environmental toxins
intrauterine contraceptive device

§ √5th **655.9** Unspecified Ⓜ♀
[0,1,3]

√4th **656** Other fetal and placental problems affecting management of mother

§ √5th **656.0** Fetal-maternal hemorrhage Ⓜ♀
[0,1,3]
Leakage (microscopic) of fetal blood into maternal circulation

§ √5th **656.1** Rhesus isoimmunization Ⓜ♀
[0,1,3]
Anti-D [Rh] antibodies
Rh incompatibility

DEF: Antibodies developing against Rh factor; mother with Rh negative develops antibodies against Rh positive fetus.

§ √5th **656.2** Isoimmunization from other and unspecified blood group incompatibility Ⓜ♀
[0,1,3]
ABO isoimmunization.

§ √5th **656.3** Fetal distress Ⓜ♀
[0,1,3]
Fetal metabolic acidemia
EXCLUDES abnormal fetal acid-base balance (656.8)
abnormality in fetal heart rate or rhythm (659.7)
fetal bradycardia (659.7)
fetal distress NOS (656.8)
fetal tachycardia (659.7)
meconium in liquor (656.8)

DEF: Life-threatening disorder; fetal anoxia, hemolytic disease and other miscellaneous diseases cause fetal distress.

AHA: N-D, '86, 4

§ √5th **656.4** Intrauterine death Ⓜ♀
[0,1,3]
Fetal death:
NOS
after completion of 22 weeks' gestation
late
Missed delivery
EXCLUDES missed abortion (632)

§ √5th **656.5** Poor fetal growth Ⓜ♀
[0,1,3]
"Light-for-dates"
"Placental insufficiency"
"Small-for-dates"

§ √5th **656.6** Excessive fetal growth Ⓜ♀
[0,1,3]
"Large-for-dates"

§ √5th **656.7** Other placental conditions Ⓜ♀
[0,1,3]
Abnormal placenta
Placental infarct
EXCLUDES placental polyp (674.4)
placentitis (658.4)

§ √5th **656.8** Other specified fetal and placental problems Ⓜ♀
[0,1,3]
Abnormal acid-base balance
Intrauterine acidosis
Lithopedian
Meconium in liquor

DEF: Lithopedion: Calcified fetus; not expelled by mother.

§ √5th **656.9** Unspecified fetal and placental problem Ⓜ♀
[0,1,3]

√4th **657** Polyhydramnios Ⓜ♀
[0,1,3] Hydramnios
§ √5th Use 0 as fourth-digit for this category
AHA: 4Q, '91, 26

DEF: Excess amniotic fluid.

√4th **658** Other problems associated with amniotic cavity and membranes
EXCLUDES amniotic fluid embolism (673.1)

§ √5th **658.0** Oligohydramnios Ⓜ♀
[0,1,3]
Oligohydramnios without mention of rupture of membranes

DEF: Deficient amount of amniotic fluid.

§ √5th **658.1** Premature rupture of membranes Ⓜ♀
[0,1,3]
Rupture of amniotic sac less than 24 hours prior to the onset of labor
AHA: For code 658.13: 1Q, '01, 5; 4Q, '98, 77

1 Nonspecific PDx=0
§ Requires fifth-digit. Valid digits are in [brackets] under each code. See beginning of section 640-648 for codes and definitions.

§ ✓5ᵗʰ¹ **658.2** **Delayed delivery after spontaneous or** M♀
[0,1,3]   **unspecified rupture of membranes**
     Prolonged rupture of membranes NOS
     Rupture of amniotic sac 24 hours or more prior to
       the onset of labor

§ ✓5ᵗʰ¹ **658.3** **Delayed delivery after artificial rupture of** M♀
[0,1,3]   **membranes**

§ ✓5ᵗʰ¹ **658.4** **Infection of amniotic cavity** M♀
[0,1,3]   Amnionitis   Membranitis
     Chorioamnionitis   Placentitis

§ ✓5ᵗʰ¹ **658.8** **Other** M♀
[0,1,3]   Amnion nodosum   Amniotic cyst

§ ✓5ᵗʰ¹ **658.9** **Unspecified** M♀
[0,1,3]

✓4ᵗʰ **659** **Other indications for care or intervention related to labor**
     and delivery, not elsewhere classified

§ ✓5ᵗʰ¹ **659.0** **Failed mechanical induction** M♀
[0,1,3]   Failure of induction of labor by surgical or other
       instrumental methods

§ ✓5ᵗʰ¹ **659.1** **Failed medical or unspecified induction** M♀
[0,1,3]   Failed induction NOS
     Failure of induction of labor by medical methods,
       such as oxytocic drugs

§ ✓5ᵗʰ¹ **659.2** **Maternal pyrexia during labor, unspecified** M♀
[0,1,3] **DEF:** Fever during labor.

§ ✓5ᵗʰ¹ **659.3** **Generalized infection during labor** CC M♀
[0,1,3]   Septicemia during labor
     CC Excl: 646.80-646.93, 648.90-648.94, 650, 659.30-659.33,
     669.40-669.44, 669.80-669.94

§ ✓5ᵗʰ¹ **659.4** **Grand multiparity** M♀
[0,1,3]   **EXCLUDES**   *supervision only, in pregnancy (V23.3)*
         without current pregnancy (V61.5)
     DEF: Having borne six or more children previously.

§ ✓5ᵗʰ¹ **659.5** **Elderly primigravida** M♀
[0,1,3]   First pregnancy in a woman who will be 35 years of
       age or older at expected date of delivery
     EXCLUDES   *supervision only, in pregnancy (V23.81)*
     AHA: ▶3Q, '01, 12◀

§ ✓5ᵗʰ¹ **659.6** **Elderly multigravida** M♀
[0,1,3]   Second or more pregnancy in a woman who will
       be 35 years of age or older at expected date
       of delivery
     EXCLUDES   *elderly primigravida 659.5*
         supervision only, in pregnancy (V23.82)
     AHA: ▶3Q, '01, 12◀

§ ✓5ᵗʰ¹ **659.7** **Abnormality in fetal heart rate or rhythm** M♀
[0,1,3]   Depressed fetal heart tones
     Fetal:
       bradycardia
       tachycardia
     Fetal heart rate decelerations
     Non-reassuring fetal heart rate or rhythm
     AHA: 4Q, '98, 48

§ ✓5ᵗʰ¹ **659.8** **Other specified indications for care or** M♀
[0,1,3]   **intervention related to labor and delivery**
     Pregnancy in a female less than 16 years old at
       expected date of delivery
     Very young maternal age
     AHA: ▶3Q, '01, 12◀

§ ✓5ᵗʰ¹ **659.9** **Unspecified indication for care or intervention** M♀

[0,1,3]   **related to labor and delivery**

COMPLICATIONS OCCURRING MAINLY IN THE COURSE OF LABOR AND DELIVERY (660-669)

The following fifth-digit subclassification is for use with
categories 660-669 to denote the current episode of care. Valid
fifth-digits are in [brackets] under each code.

   0   unspecified as to episode of care or not applicable
   1   delivered, with or without mention of antepartum
       condition
   2   delivered, with mention of postpartum
       complication
   3   antepartum condition or complication
   4   postpartum condition or complication

✓4ᵗʰ **660** **Obstructed labor**
     AHA: 3Q, '95, 10

§ ✓5ᵗʰ¹ **660.0** **Obstruction caused by malposition of fetus** M♀
[0,1,3]   **at onset of labor**
     Any condition classifiable to 652, causing
       obstruction during labor
     Use additional code from 652.0-652.9 to identify
       condition

§ ✓5ᵗʰ¹ **660.1** **Obstruction by bony pelvis** M♀
[0,1,3]   Any condition classifiable to 653, causing
       obstruction during labor
     Use additional code from 653.0-653.9 to identify
       condition

§ ✓5ᵗʰ¹ **660.2** **Obstruction by abnormal pelvic soft tissues** M♀
[0,1,3]   Prolapse of anterior lip of cervix
     Any condition classifiable to 654, causing
       obstruction during labor
     Use additional code from 654.0-654.9 to identify
       condition

§ ✓5ᵗʰ¹ **660.3** **Deep transverse arrest and persistent** M♀
[0,1,3]   **occipitoposterior position**

§ ✓5ᵗʰ¹ **660.4** **Shoulder (girdle) dystocia** M♀
[0,1,3]   Impacted shoulders
     DEF: Obstructed labor due to impacted fetal shoulders.

§ ✓5ᵗʰ¹ **660.5** **Locked twins** M♀
[0,1,3]

§ ✓5ᵗʰ¹ **660.6** **Failed trial of labor, unspecified** M♀
[0,1,3]   Failed trial of labor, without mention of condition or
       suspected condition

§ ✓5ᵗʰ¹ **660.7** **Failed forceps or vacuum extractor,** M♀
[0,1,3]   **unspecified**
     Application of ventouse or forceps, without mention
       of condition

§ ✓5ᵗʰ¹ **660.8** **Other causes of obstructed labor** M♀
[0,1,3]

§ ✓5ᵗʰ¹ **660.9** **Unspecified obstructed labor** M♀
[0,1,3]   Dystocia:
       NOS
       fetal NOS
       maternal NOS

✓4ᵗʰ **661** **Abnormality of forces of labor**

§ ✓5ᵗʰ¹ **661.0** **Primary uterine inertia** M♀
[0,1,3]   Failure of cervical dilation
     Hypotonic uterine dysfunction, primary
     Prolonged latent phase of labor
     DEF: Lack of efficient contractions during labor causing prolonged
     labor.

§ ✓5ᵗʰ¹ **661.1** **Secondary uterine inertia** M♀
[0,1,3]   Arrested active phase of labor
     Hypotonic uterine dysfunction, secondary

§ ✓5ᵗʰ¹ **661.2** **Other and unspecified uterine inertia** M♀
[0,1,3]   Desultory labor
     Irregular labor
     Poor contractions
     Slow slope active phase of labor

Complications of Pregnancy, Childbirth, and the Puerperium 658.2–661.2

---

¹   Nonspecific PDx=0

§   Requires fifth-digit. Valid digits are in [brackets] under each code. See beginning of section 640-648 for codes and definitions.

✓4ᵗʰ / ✓5ᵗʰ   Additional Digit Required   Nonspecific PDx   Unacceptable PDx   Manifestation Code   MSP Medicare Secondary Payer   ▶◀ Revised Text   ● New Code   ▲ Revised Code Title

2002 Ingenix, Inc.   **January 2002 • Volume 1 — 193**

§ √5ᵗʰ¹ **661.3 Precipitate labor** M ♀
[0,1,3] DEF: Rapid labor and delivery.

§ √5ᵗʰ¹ **661.4 Hypertonic, incoordinate, or prolonged** M ♀
[0,1,3] **uterine contractions**
Cervical spasm
Contraction ring (dystocia)
Dyscoordinate labor
Hourglass contraction of uterus
Hypertonic uterine dysfunction
Incoordinate uterine action
Retraction ring (Bandl's) (pathological)
Tetanic contractions
Uterine dystocia NOS
Uterine spasm

§ √5ᵗʰ¹ **661.9 Unspecified abnormality of labor** M ♀
[0,1,3]

√4ᵗʰ **662 Long labor**

§ √5ᵗʰ¹ **662.0 Prolonged first stage** M ♀
[0,1,3]

§ √5ᵗʰ¹ **662.1 Prolonged labor, unspecified** M ♀
[0,1,3]

§ √5ᵗʰ¹ **662.2 Prolonged second stage** M ♀
[0,1,3]

§ √5ᵗʰ¹ **662.3 Delayed delivery of second twin, triplet, etc.** M ♀
[0,1,3]

√4ᵗʰ **663 Umbilical cord complications**

§ √5ᵗʰ¹ **663.0 Prolapse of cord** M ♀
[0,1,3] Presentation of cord
DEF: Abnormal presentation of fetus; marked by protruding umbilical cord during labor; can cause fetal death.

§ √5ᵗʰ¹ **663.1 Cord around neck, with compression** M ♀
[0,1,3] Cord tightly around neck

§ √5ᵗʰ¹ **663.2 Other and unspecified cord entanglement,** M ♀
[0,1,3] **with compression**
Entanglement of cords of twins in mono-amniotic sac
Knot in cord (with compression)

§ √5ᵗʰ¹ **663.3 Other and unspecified cord entanglement,** M ♀
[0,1,3] **without mention of compression**

§ √5ᵗʰ¹ **663.4 Short cord** M ♀
[0,1,3]

§ √5ᵗʰ¹ **663.5 Vasa previa** M ♀
[0,1,3]
DEF: Abnormal presentation of fetus marked by blood vessels of umbilical cord in front of fetal head.

§ √5ᵗʰ¹ **663.6 Vascular lesions of cord** M ♀
[0,1,3] Bruising of cord
Hematoma of cord
Thrombosis of vessels of cord

§ √5ᵗʰ¹ **663.8 Other umbilical cord complications** M ♀
[0,1,3] Velamentous insertion of umbilical cord

§ √5ᵗʰ¹ **663.9 Unspecified umbilical cord complication** M ♀
[0,1,3]

√4ᵗʰ **664 Trauma to perineum and vulva during delivery**
INCLUDES damage from instruments
that from extension of episiotomy
AHA: 1Q, '92, 11; N-D, '84, 10

§ √5ᵗʰ¹ **664.0 First-degree perineal laceration** M ♀
[0,1,4] Perineal laceration, rupture, or tear involving:
fourchette
hymen
labia
skin
vagina
vulva

Perineal Lacerations

First degree
Anus
Second degree
Third degree
Fourth degree

§ √5ᵗʰ¹ **664.1 Second-degree perineal laceration** M ♀
[0,1,4] Perineal laceration, rupture, or tear (following episiotomy) involving:
pelvic floor
perineal muscles
vaginal muscles
EXCLUDES that involving anal sphincter (664.2)

§ √5ᵗʰ¹ **664.2 Third-degree perineal laceration** M ♀
[0,1,4] Perineal laceration, rupture, or tear (following episiotomy) involving:
anal sphincter
rectovaginal septum
sphincter NOS
EXCLUDES that with anal or rectal mucosal laceration (664.3)

§ √5ᵗʰ¹ **664.3 Fourth-degree perineal laceration** M ♀
[0,1,4] Perineal laceration, rupture, or tear as classifiable to 664.2 and involving also:
anal mucosa
rectal mucosa

§ √5ᵗʰ¹ **664.4 Unspecified perineal laceration** M ♀
[0,1,4] Central laceration
AHA: 1Q, '92, 8

§ √5ᵗʰ¹ **664.5 Vulval and perineal hematoma** M ♀
[0,1,4] AHA: N-D, '84, 10

§ √5ᵗʰ¹ **664.8 Other specified trauma to perineum and vulva** M ♀
[0,1,4]

§ √5ᵗʰ¹ **664.9 Unspecified trauma to perineum and vulva** M ♀
[0,1,4]

√4ᵗʰ **665 Other obstetrical trauma**
INCLUDES damage from instruments

§ √5ᵗʰ¹ **665.0 Rupture of uterus before onset of labor** CC M ♀
[0,1,3]
CC Excl: 646.80-646.93, 648.90-648.94, 650, 655.70-655.73, 665.00-665.11, 665.50-665.54, 665.80-665.94, 669.40-669.44, 669.80-669.94

§ √5ᵗʰ¹ **665.1 Rupture of uterus during labor** CC M ♀
[0,1] Rupture of uterus NOS
CC Excl: See code 665.0

§ √5ᵗʰ¹ **665.2 Inversion of uterus** M ♀
[0,2,4]

§ √5ᵗʰ¹ **665.3 Laceration of cervix** M ♀
[0,1,4]

§ √5ᵗʰ¹ **665.4 High vaginal laceration** M ♀
[0,1,4] Laceration of vaginal wall or sulcus without mention of perineal laceration

§ √5ᵗʰ¹ **665.5 Other injury to pelvic organs** M ♀
[0,1,4] Injury to: Injury to:
bladder   urethra
AHA: M-A, '87, 10

¹ Nonspecific PDx=0
§ Requires fifth-digit. Valid digits are in [brackets] under each code. See beginning of section 640-648 for codes and definitions.

N Newborn Age: 0   P Pediatric Age: 0-17   M Maternity Age: 12-55   A Adult Age :15-124   CC CC Condition   MC Major Complication   CD Complex Dx   HIV HIV Related Dx

2002 Ingenix, Inc.

§ ✓5th 1 **665.6 Damage to pelvic joints and ligaments** M ♀
[0,1,4]
    Avulsion of inner symphyseal cartilage
    Damage to coccyx
    Separation of symphysis (pubis)
    AHA: N-D, '84, 12

§ ✓5th 1 **665.7 Pelvic hematoma** M ♀
[0,1,2,4]
    Hematoma of vagina

§ ✓5th 1 **665.8 Other specified obstetrical trauma** M ♀
[0-4]

§ ✓5th 1 **665.9 Unspecified obstetrical trauma** M ♀
[0-4]

✓4th **666 Postpartum hemorrhage**
    AHA: 1Q, '88, 14

§ ✓5th 1 **666.0 Third-stage hemorrhage** M ♀
[0,2,4]
    Hemorrhage associated with retained, trapped, or
      adherent placenta
    Retained placenta NOS

§ ✓5th 1 **666.1 Other immediate postpartum hemorrhage** M ♀
[0,2,4]
    Atony of uterus
    Hemorrhage within the first 24 hours following
      delivery of placenta
    Postpartum hemorrhage (atonic) NOS

§ ✓5th 1 **666.2 Delayed and secondary postpartum** M ♀
[0,2,4] **hemorrhage**
    Hemorrhage:
      after the first 24 hours following delivery
      associated with retained portions of placenta or
        membranes
    Postpartum hemorrhage specified as delayed or
      secondary
    Retained products of conception NOS, following
      delivery

§ ✓5th 1 **666.3 Postpartum coagulation defects** CC 2,4 M ♀
[0,2,4]
    Postpartum: Postpartum:
      afibrinogenemia   fibrinolysis
    CC Excl: For codes 666.32-666.34: 646.80-646.93, 648.90-648.94,
    650, 666.00-666.34, 669.40-669.44, 669.80-669.94

✓4th **667 Retained placenta or membranes, without hemorrhage**
    AHA: 1Q, '88, 14

    DEF: Postpartum condition resulting from failure to expel placental membrane
    tissues due to failed contractions of uterine wall.

§ ✓5th 1 **667.0 Retained placenta without hemorrhage** M ♀
[0,2,4]
    Placenta accreta
    Retained placenta: } without
      NOS   } hemorrhage
      total

§ ✓5th 1 **667.1 Retained portions of placenta or membranes,** M ♀
[0,2,4] **Without hemorrhage**
    Retained products of conception following delivery,
      without hemorrhage

✓4th **668 Complications of the administration of anesthetic or other sedation in labor and delivery**
    INCLUDES complications arising from the administration
      of a general or local anesthetic, analgesic,
      or other sedation in labor and delivery
    EXCLUDES *reaction to spinal or lumbar puncture (349.0)*
    spinal headache (349.0)
    Use additional code(s) to further specify complication

§ ✓5th 1 **668.0 Pulmonary complications** CC M ♀
[0-4]
    Inhalation [aspiration] of   }
      stomach contents   } following anesthesia
      or secretions   } or other
    Mendelson's syndrome } sedation in labor
    Pressure collapse of lung } or delivery
    CC Excl: 646.80-646.93, 648.90-648.94, 650, 668.00-668.04,
    669.40-669.44, 669.80-669.94

§ ✓5th 1 **668.1 Cardiac complications** CC M ♀
[0-4]
    Cardiac arrest or failure following anesthesia or
      other sedation in labor and delivery
    CC Excl: 646.80-646.93, 648.90-648.94, 650, 668.10-668.14,
    669.40-669.44, 669.80-669.94

§ ✓5th 1 **668.2 Central nervous system complications** CC M ♀
[0-4]
    Cerebral anoxia following anesthesia or other
      sedation in labor and delivery
    CC Excl: 646.80-646.93, 648.90-648.94, 650, 668.20-668.24,
    669.40-669.44, 669.80-669.94

§ ✓5th 1 **668.8 Other complications of anesthesia or** CC M ♀
[0-4] **other sedation in labor and delivery**
    CC Excl: 646.80-646.93, 648.90-648.94, 650, 668.80-94, 668,
    669.40-669.44, 669.80-669.94
    AHA: 2Q, '99, 9

§ ✓5th 1 **668.9 Unspecified complication of anesthesia** CC M ♀
[0-4] **and other sedation**
    CC Excl: See code 668.8

✓4th **669 Other complications of labor and delivery, not elsewhere classified**

§ ✓5th 1 **669.0 Maternal distress** M ♀
[0-4]
    Metabolic disturbance in labor and delivery

§ ✓5th 1 **669.1 Shock during or following labor and** CC M ♀
[0-4] **delivery**
    Obstetric shock
    CC Excl: 646.80-646.93, 648.90-648.94, 650, 669.10-669.14,
    669.40-669.44, 669.80-669.94

§ ✓5th 1 **669.2 Maternal hypotension syndrome** M ♀
[0-4]
    DEF: Low arterial blood pressure, in mother, during labor and
    delivery.

§ ✓5th 1 **669.3 Acute renal failure following labor and** CC M ♀
[0,2,4] **delivery**
    CC Excl: 646.80-646.93, 648.90-648.94, 650, 669.30-669.44,
    669.80-669.94

§ ✓5th 1 **669.4 Other complications of obstetrical surgery** M ♀
[0-4] **and procedures**
    Cardiac: } following cesarean or other
      arrest   } obstetrical surgery or
      failure   } procedure, including
    Cerebral anoxia } delivery NOS
    EXCLUDES *complications of obstetrical surgical*
    wounds (674.1-674.3)

§ ✓5th 1 **669.5 Forceps or vacuum extractor delivery** M ♀
[0,1] **without mention of indication**
    Delivery by ventouse, without mention of indication

§ ✓5th 1 **669.6 Breech extraction, without mention of** M ♀
[0,1] **indication**
    EXCLUDES *breech delivery NOS (652.2)*

§ ✓5th 1 **669.7 Cesarean delivery, without mention of** M ♀
[0,1] **indication**
    AHA: For code 658.71: 1Q, '01, 11

§ ✓5th 1 **669.8 Other complications of labor and delivery** M ♀
[0-4]

§ ✓5th 1 **669.9 Unspecified complication of labor and delivery** M ♀
[0-4]

---

1 Nonspecific PDx=0
§ Requires fifth-digit. Valid digits are in [brackets] under each code. See beginning of section 640-648 for codes and definitions.

✓4th ✓5th Additional Digit Required   Nonspecific PDx   Unacceptable PDx   Manifestation Code   **MSP** Medicare Secondary Payer   ▶◀ Revised Text   ● New Code   ▲ Revised Code Title

2002 Ingenix, Inc.

Volume 1 — 195

COMPLICATIONS OF THE PUERPERIUM (670-677)

Note: Categories 671 and 673-676 include the listed conditions even if they occur during pregnancy or childbirth.

The following fifth-digit subclassification is for use with categories 670-676 to denote the current episode of care. Valid fifth-digits are in [brackets] under each code.

    0   **unspecified as to episode of care or not applicable**
    1   **delivered, with or without mention of antepartum condition**
    2   **delivered, with mention of postpartum complication**
    3   **antepartum condition or complication**
    4   **postpartum condition or complication**

✓4th 1 **670 Major puerperal infection**   cc M ♀
[0,2,4]

§ ✓5th Use 0 as fourth-digit for this category

Puerperal:
   endometritis
   fever (septic)
   pelvic:
     cellulitis
     sepsis

Puerperal:
   peritonitis
   pyemia
   salpingitis
   septicemia

EXCLUDES *infection following abortion (639.0)*
    minor genital tract infection following delivery (646.6)
    puerperal pyrexia NOS (672)
    puerperal fever NOS (672)
    puerperal pyrexia of unknown origin (672)
    urinary tract infection following delivery (646.6)

CC Excl: 646.80-646.93, 648.90-648.94, 650, 669.40-669.44, 669.80-669.94, 670.00-670.04

AHA: 4Q, '91, 26; 2Q, '91, 7

DEF: Infection and inflammation, following childbirth.

✓4th **671 Venous complications in pregnancy and the puerperium**

§ ✓5th 1 **671.0 Varicose veins of legs**   M ♀
[0-4]   Varicose veins NOS

DEF: Distended, tortuous veins on legs associated with pregnancy.

§ ✓5th 1 **671.1 Varicose veins of vulva and perineum**   M ♀
[0-4]

DEF: Distended, tortuous veins on external female genitalia associated with pregnancy.

§ ✓5th 1 **671.2 Superficial thrombophlebitis**   cc M ♀
[0-4]   Thrombophlebitis (superficial)

CC Excl: 646.80-646.93, 648.90-648.94, 650, 669.40-669.44, 669.80-669.94, 671.20-671.94

§ ✓5th 1 **671.3 Deep phlebothrombosis, antepartum**   cc M ♀
[0,1,3]   Deep-vein thrombosis, antepartum

CC Excl: See code 671.2

§ ✓5th 1 **671.4 Deep phlebothrombosis, postpartum**   cc M ♀
[0,2,4]   Deep-vein thrombosis, postpartum
   Pelvic thrombophlebitis, postpartum
   Phlegmasia alba dolens (puerperal)

CC Excl: See code 671.2

§ ✓5th 1 **671.5 Other phlebitis and thrombosis**   M ♀
[0-4]   Cerebral venous thrombosis
   Thrombosis of intracranial venous sinus

§ ✓5th 1 **671.8 Other venous complications**   M ♀
[0-4]   Hemorrhoids

§ ✓5th 1 **671.9 Unspecified venous complication**   M ♀
[0-4]   Phlebitis NOS
   Thrombosis NOS

✓4th 1 **672 Pyrexia of unknown origin during the puerperium**
[0,2,4]

§ ✓5th Use 0 as fourth-digit for this category

Postpartum fever NOS
Puerperal fever NOS
Puerperal pyrexia NOS

AHA: 4Q, '91, 26

DEF: Fever of unknown origin experienced by the mother after childbirth.

✓4th **673 Obstetrical pulmonary embolism**
   INCLUDES pulmonary emboli in pregnancy, childbirth, or the puerperium, or specified as puerperal
   EXCLUDES *embolism following abortion (639.6)*

§ ✓5th 1 **673.0 Obstetrical air embolism**   cc M ♀
[0-4]

CC Excl: 646.80-646.93, 648.90-648.94, 650, 669.40-669.44, 669.80-669.94, 673.00-673.84

DEF: Sudden blocking of pulmonary artery with air or nitrogen bubbles during puerperium.

§ ✓5th 1 **673.1 Amniotic fluid embolism**   cc M ♀
[0-4]

CC Excl: See code 673.0

DEF: Sudden onset of pulmonary artery blockage from amniotic fluid entering the mother's circulation near the end of pregnancy due to strong uterine contractions.

§ ✓5th 1 **673.2 Obstetrical blood-clot embolism**   cc M ♀
[0-4]   Puerperal pulmonary embolism NOS

CC Excl: See code 673.0

DEF: Blood clot blocking artery in the lung; associated with pregnancy.

§ ✓5th 1 **673.3 Obstetrical pyemic and septic embolism**   cc M ♀
[0-4]

CC Excl: See code 673.0

§ ✓5th 1 **673.8 Other pulmonary embolism**   cc M ♀
[0-4]   Fat embolism

CC Excl: See code 673.0

✓4th **674 Other and unspecified complications of the puerperium, not elsewhere classified**

§ ✓5th 1 **674.0 Cerebrovascular disorders in the puerperium**   cc M ♀
[0-4]   Any condition classifiable to 430-434, 436-437 occurring during pregnancy, childbirth, or the puerperium, or specified as puerperal
   EXCLUDES *intracranial venous sinus thrombosis (671.5)*

CC Excl: 646.80-646.93, 648.90-648.94, 650, 669.40-669.44, 669.80-669.94, 674.00-674.04

§ ✓5th 1 **674.1 Disruption of cesarean wound**   cc M ♀
[0,2,4]   Dehiscence or disruption of uterine wound
   EXCLUDES ▶ *uterine rupture before onset of labor (665.0)*
    uterine rupture during labor (665.1)◄

CC Excl: For Codes 674.10-674.12: 646.80-646.93, 648.90-648.94, 650, 669.40-669.44, 669.80-669.94, 674.10, 674.34

§ ✓5th 1 **674.2 Disruption of perineal wound**   cc M ♀
[0,2,4]   Breakdown of perineum   Disruption of wound of:
   Disruption of wound of: perineal laceration
    episiotomy   Secondary perineal tear

CC Excl: See code 674.1

AHA: For code 674.24: 1Q, '97, 9

---

1 Nonspecific PDx=0
§ Requires fifth-digit. Valid digits are in [brackets] under each code. See beginning of section 640-648 for codes and definitions.

N Newborn Age: 0   P Pediatric Age: 0-17   M Maternity Age: 12-55   A Adult Age :15-124   CC CC Condition   MC Major Complication   CD Complex Dx   HIV HIV Related Dx

§ ✓5th¹ **674.3**   **Other complications of obstetrical surgical**   M ♀
[0,2,4]   **wounds**

Hematoma
Hemorrhage   }   of cesarean section or perineal
Infection   wound

     EXCLUDES   damage from instruments in delivery
(664.0-665.9)

AHA: 2Q, '91, 7

§ ✓5th¹ **674.4**   **Placental polyp**   M ♀
[0,2,4]

§ ✓5th¹ **674.8**   **Other**   M ♀
[0,2,4]   Hepatorenal syndrome, following delivery
Postpartum:
   cardiomyopathy
   subinvolution of uterus
   uterine hypertrophy

AHA: 3Q, '98, 16

§ ✓5th¹ **674.9**   **Unspecified**   M ♀
[0,2,4]   Sudden death of unknown cause during the
     puerperium

✓4th **675**   **Infections of the breast and nipple associated with**
childbirth

    INCLUDES   the listed conditions during pregnancy,
                childbirth, or the puerperium

§ ✓5th¹ **675.0**   **Infections of nipple**   M ♀
[0-4]   Abscess of nipple

§ ✓5th¹ **675.1**   **Abscess of breast**   CC 0-2   M ♀
[0-4]   Abscess:
     mammary
     subareolar
     submammary
     purulent
     retromammary
     submammary

CC Excl: For codes 675.10-675.12: 646.80-646.93, 648.90-648.94, 650,
669.40-669.44, 669.80-669.94, 675.00-675.94

§ ✓5th¹ **675.2**   **Nonpurulent mastitis**   M ♀
[0-4]   Lymphangitis of breast
   Mastitis:
     NOS
     interstitial
     parenchymatous

§ ✓5th¹ **675.8**   **Other specified infections of the breast and**   M ♀
[0-4]   **nipple**

§ ✓5th¹ **675.9**   **Unspecified infection of the breast and nipple**   M ♀
[0-4]

✓4th **676**   **Other disorders of the breast associated with childbirth and**
disorders of lactation

    INCLUDES   the listed conditions during pregnancy, the
                puerperium, or lactation

§ ✓5th¹ **676.0**   **Retracted nipple**   M ♀
[0-4]

§ ✓5th¹ **676.1**   **Cracked nipple**   M ♀
[0-4]   Fissure of nipple

§ ✓5th¹ **676.2**   **Engorgement of breasts**   M ♀
[0-4]

DEF: Abnormal accumulation of milk in ducts of breast.

§ ✓5th¹ **676.3**   **Other and unspecified disorder of breast**   M ♀
[0-4]

§ ✓5th¹ **676.4**   **Failure of lactation**   M ♀
[0-4]   Agalactia

DEF: Abrupt ceasing of milk secretion by breast.

§ ✓5th¹ **676.5**   **Suppressed lactation**   M ♀
[0-4]

Lactation Process: Ejection Reflex Arc

Hypothalamus

Pituitary gland

Prolactin   Oxytocin
(stimulates milk   (stimulates
production)   contraction)

Myoepithelial   Uterus
cells of breast

Stimulation of
mechanoreceptors   Lacteal

§ ✓5th¹ **676.6**   **Galactorrhea**   M ♀
[0-4]   **EXCLUDES**   *galactorrhea not associated with*
                     childbirth (611.6)

DEF: Excessive or persistent milk secretion by breast; may be in
absence of nursing.

§ ✓5th¹ **676.8**   **Other disorders of lactation**   M ♀
[0-4]   Galactocele

DEF: Galactocele: Obstructed mammary gland, creating retention
cyst, results in milk-filled cysts enlarging mammary gland.

§ ✓5th¹ **676.9**   **Unspecified disorder of lactation**   M ♀
[0-4]

677   **Late effect of complication of pregnancy, childbirth,**   M ♀
and the puerperium

Note: This category is to be used to indicate conditions in
632-648.9 and 651-676.9 as the cause of the late
effect, themselves classifiable elsewhere. The "late
effects" include conditions specified as such, or as
sequelae, which may occur at any time after
puerperium.

Code first any sequelae

AHA: 1Q, '97, 9; 4Q, '94, 42

¹ Nonspecific PDx=0

§ Requires fifth-digit. Valid digits are in [brackets] under each code. See beginning of section 640-648 for codes and definitions.

✓4th ✓5th **Additional Digit Required**   **Nonspecific PDx**   **Unacceptable PDx**   **Manifestation Code**   **MSP** Medicare Secondary Payer   ►◄ Revised Text   ● New Code   ▲ Revised Code Title

2002 Ingenix, Inc.   **Volume 1 — 197**

Complications of Pregnancy, Childbirth, and the Puerperium 674.3–677

12. DISEASES OF THE SKIN AND SUBCUTANEOUS TISSUE
(680-709)

Skin and Subcutaneous Layer

Hair follicle

Epidermis

Dermis

Hypodermis (subcutaneous layer)

Bulb

Sebaceous gland

Arrector pili muscle

Thick-skin epidermis

Hair shaft

Pacinian corpuscle

Hair matrix

Sweat (eccrine gland)

Sensory nerve

Blood vessels

INFECTIONS OF SKIN AND SUBCUTANEOUS TISSUE (680-686)

EXCLUDES *certain infections of skin classified under "Infectious and Parasitic Diseases," such as:*
erysipelas (035)
erysipeloid of Rosenbach (027.1)
herpes:
   simplex (054.0-054.9)
   zoster (053.0-053.9)
molluscum contagiosum (078.0)
viral warts (078.1)

✓4th **680   Carbuncle and furuncle**
   INCLUDES   boil
             furunculosis

DEF: Carbuncle: necrotic boils in skin and subcutaneous tissue of neck or back mainly due to staphylococcal infection.

DEF: Furuncle: Circumscribed inflammation of corium and subcutaneous tissue due to staphylococcal infection.

680.0   Face   cc
   Ear [any part]
   Face [any part, except eye]
   Nose (septum)
   Temple (region)
     EXCLUDES   *eyelid (373.13)*
              lacrimal apparatus (375.31)
              orbit (376.01)
   CC Excl: 017.00-017.06, 017.90-017.96, ▶040.82,◀ 040.89, 041.00-041.89, 041.9, 680.0, 680.8-680.9, 686.00-686.01, 686.09, 686.1-686.9, 705.83, 709.8, V09.0-V09.91

680.1   Neck   cc
   CC Excl: 017.00-017.06, 017.90-017.96, ▶040.82,◀ 040.89, 041.00-041.89, 041.9, 680.1, 680.8-680.9, 686.00-686.01, 686.09, 686.1-686.9, 705.83, 709.8, V09.0-V09.91

680.2   Trunk   cc
   Abdominal wall
   Back [any part, except buttocks]
   Breast
   Chest wall
   Flank
   Groin
   Pectoral region
   Perineum
   Umbilicus
     EXCLUDES   *buttocks (680.5)*
              external genital organs:
                female (616.4)
                male (607.2, 608.4)
   CC Excl: 017.00-017.06, 017.90-017.96, ▶040.82,◀ 040.89, 041.00-041.89, 041.9, 680.2, 680.8-680.9, 686.00-686.01, 686.09, 686.1-686.9, 705.83, 709.8, V09.0-V09.91

680.3   Upper arm and forearm   cc
   Arm [any part, except hand]
   Axilla
   Shoulder
   CC Excl: 017.00-017.06, 017.90-017.96, ▶040.82,◀ 040.89, 041.00-041.89, 041.9, 680.0, 680.8-680.9, 686.00-686.01, 686.09, 686.1-686.9, 705.83, 709.8, V09.0-V09.91

680.4   Hand   cc
   Finger [any]
   Thumb
   Wrist
   CC Excl: 017.00-017.06, 017.90-017.96, ▶040.82,◀ 040.89, 041.00-041.89, 041.9, 680.0, 680.8-680.9, 686.00-686.01, 686.09, 686.1-686.9, 705.83, 709.8, V09.0-V09.91

680.5   Buttock   cc
   Anus
   Gluteal region
   CC Excl: 017.00-017.06, 017.90-017.96, ▶040.82,◀ 040.89, 041.00-041.89, 041.9, 680.0, 680.8-680.9, 686.00-686.01, 686.09, 686.1-686.9, 705.83, 709.8, V09.0-V09.91

680.6   Leg, except foot   cc
   Ankle   Knee
   Hip   Thigh
   CC Excl: 017.00-017.06, 017.90-017.96, ▶040.82,◀ 040.89, 041.00-041.89, 041.9, 680.0, 680.8-680.9, 686.00-686.01, 686.09, 686.1-686.9, 705.83, 709.8, V09.0-V09.91

680.7   Foot   cc
   Heel
   Toe
   CC Excl: 017.00-017.06, 017.90-017.96, ▶040.82,◀ 040.89, 041.00-041.89, 041.9, 680.0, 680.8-680.9, 686.00-686.01, 686.09, 686.1-686.9, 705.83, 709.8, V09.0-V09.91

680.8   Other specified sites   cc
   Head [any part, except face]
   Scalp
     EXCLUDES   *external genital organs:*
                female (616.4)
                male (607.2, 608.4)
   CC Excl: 017.00-017.06, 017.90-017.96, ▶040.82,◀ 040.89, 041.00-041.89, 041.9, 680.0, 680.8-680.9, 686.00-686.01, 686.09, 686.1-686.9, 705.83, 709.8, V09.0-V09.91

680.9   Unspecified site   cc
   Boil NOS   Furuncle NOS
   Carbuncle NOS
   CC Excl: See code 680.8

✓4th **681   Cellulitis and abscess of finger and toe**
   INCLUDES   that with lymphangitis
   Use additional code to identify organism, such as Staphylococcus (041.1)

AHA: 2Q, '91, 5; J-F, '87, 12

DEF: Acute suppurative inflammation and edema in subcutaneous tissue or muscle of finger or toe.

✓5th **681.0   Finger**
   681.00   Cellulitis and abscess, unspecified
   681.01   Felon
      Pulp abscess   Whitlow
      EXCLUDES   *herpetic whitlow (054.6)*
      DEF: Painful abscess of fingertips caused by infection in the closed space of terminal phalanx.

   681.02   Onychia and paronychia of finger
      Panaritium   } of finger
      Perionychia

      DEF: Onychia: inflammation of nail matrix; causes nail loss.

      DEF: Paronychia: inflammation of tissue folds around nail.

✓4th ✓5th **Additional Digit Required**   Nonspecific PDx   Unacceptable PDx   Manifestation Code   **MSP** Medicare Secondary Payer   ▶◀ Revised Text   ● New Code   ▲ Revised Code Title

2002 Ingenix, Inc.   **October 2002 • Volume 1 — 199**

☑5th **681.1　Toe**

　　　681.10　Cellulitis and abscess, unspecified

　　　681.11　Onychia and paronychia of toe

　　　　　Panaritium　} of toe
　　　　　Perionychia

681.9　Cellulitis and abscess of unspecified digit

　　　　Infection of nail NOS

☑4th **682　Other cellulitis and abscess**

　　INCLUDES　abscess (acute)　　} (with lymphangitis)
　　　　　　　cellulitis (diffuse)　} except of
　　　　　　　lymphangitis, acute　} finger or toe

　　Use additional code to identify organism, such as
　　　Staphylococcus (041.1)

　　EXCLUDES　lymphangitis (chronic) (subacute) (457.2)

　　AHA: 2Q, '91, 5; J-F, '87, 12; S-O, '85, 10

　　DEF: Cellulitis: Acute suppurative inflammation of deep subcutaneous tissue
　　and sometimes muscle due to infection of wound, burn or other lesion.

682.0　Face　　　　　　　　　　　　　　　CC

　　　Cheek, external　　Nose, external
　　　Chin　　　　　　　Submandibular
　　　Forehead　　　　　Temple (region)
　　　　EXCLUDES　ear [any part] (380.10-380.16)
　　　　　　　　　eyelid (373.13)
　　　　　　　　　lacrimal apparatus (375.31)
　　　　　　　　　lip (528.5)
　　　　　　　　　mouth (528.3)
　　　　　　　　　nose (internal) (478.1)
　　　　　　　　　orbit (376.01)
　　　CC Excl: 017.00-017.06, 017.90-017.96, 040.89, 041.00-041.89,
　　　041.9, 682.0, 682.8-682.9, 686.00-686.01, 686.09, 686.1-686.9,
　　　705.83, 709.8, V09.0-V09.91

682.1　Neck　　　　　　　　　　　　　　　CC

　　　CC Excl: 017.00-017.06, 017.90-017.96, 040.89, 041.00-041.89,
　　　041.9, 682.1, 682.8-682.9, 686.00-686.01, 686.09, 686.1-686.9,
　　　705.83, 709.8, V09.0-V09.91

682.2　Trunk　　　　　　　　　　　　　　　CC

　　　Abdominal wall　　Groin
　　　Back [any part, except　Pectoral region
　　　　buttock]　　　　Perineum
　　　Chest wall　　　　Umbilicus, except newborn
　　　Flank
　　　　EXCLUDES　anal and rectal regions (566)
　　　　　　　　　breast:
　　　　　　　　　　NOS (611.0)
　　　　　　　　　　puerperal (675.1)
　　　　　　　　　external genital organs:
　　　　　　　　　　female (616.3-616.4)
　　　　　　　　　　male (604.0, 607.2, 608.4)
　　　　　　　　　umbilicus, newborn (771.4)
　　　CC Excl: 017.00-017.06, 017.90-017.96, 040.89, 041.00-041.89,
　　　041.9, 682.2, 682.8-682.9, 686.00-686.01, 686.09, 686.1-686.9,
　　　705.83, 709.8, V09.0-V09.91

　　　AHA: 4Q, '98, 42

682.3　Upper arm and forearm　　　　　　CC

　　　Arm [any part, except hand]
　　　Axilla
　　　Shoulder
　　　　EXCLUDES　hand (682.4)
　　　CC Excl: 017.00-017.06, 017.90-017.96, 040.89, 041.00-041.89,
　　　041.9, 682.3, 682.8-682.9, 686.00-686.01, 686.09, 686.1-686.9,
　　　705.83, 709.8, V09.0-V09.91

682.4　Hand, except fingers and thumb
　　　Wrist
　　　　EXCLUDES　finger and thumb (681.00-681.02)

682.5　Buttock　　　　　　　　　　　　　CC
　　　Gluteal region
　　　　EXCLUDES　anal and rectal regions (566)
　　　CC Excl: 017.00-017.06, 017.90-017.96, 040.89, 041.00-041.89,
　　　041.9, 682.5, 682.8-682.9, 686.00-686.01, 686.09, 686.1-686.9,
　　　705.83, 709.8, V09.0-V09.91

682.6　Leg, except foot　　　　　　　　　CC
　　　Ankle　　　　　　Knee
　　　Hip　　　　　　　Thigh
　　　CC Excl: 017.00-017.06, 017.90-017.96, 040.89, 041.00-041.89,
　　　041.9, 682.6, 682.8-682.9, 686.00-686.01, 686.09, 686.1-686.9,
　　　705.83, 709.8, V09.0-V09.91

682.7　Foot, except toes　　　　　　　　CC
　　　Heel
　　　　EXCLUDES　toe (681.10-681.11)
　　　CC Excl: 017.00-017.06, 017.90-017.96, 040.89, 041.00-041.89,
　　　041.9, 682.7-682.9, 686.00-686.01, 686.09, 686.1-686.9, 705.83,
　　　709.8, V09.0-V09.91

682.8　Other specified sites　　　　　　CC
　　　Head [except face]
　　　Scalp
　　　　EXCLUDES　face (682.0)
　　　CC Excl: 017.00-017.06, 017.90-017.96, 040.89, 041.00-041.89,
　　　041.9, 682.8-682.9, 686.00-686.01, 686.09, 686.1-686.9, 705.83,
　　　709.8, V09.0-V09.91

682.9　Unspecified site　　　　　　　　　CC
　　　Abscess NOS　　　　Lymphangitis, acute NOS
　　　Cellulitis NOS
　　　　EXCLUDES　lymphangitis NOS (457.2)
　　　CC Excl: See code 682.8

683　Acute lymphadenitis

　　　Abscess (acute)　　　} lymph gland or node,
　　　Adenitis, acute　　　}   except mesenteric
　　　Lymphadenitis, acute　}

　　Use additional code to identify organism, such as
　　　Staphylococcus (041.1)
　　　EXCLUDES　enlarged glands NOS (785.6)
　　　　　　　　lymphadenitis:
　　　　　　　　　chronic or subacute, except mesenteric
　　　　　　　　　　(289.1)
　　　　　　　　　mesenteric (acute) (chronic) (subacute) (289.2)
　　　　　　　　　unspecified (289.3)

　　DEF: Acute inflammation of lymph nodes due to primary infection located
　　elsewhere in the body.

684　Impetigo　　　　　　　　　　　　　　CC
　　　Impetiginization of other dermatoses
　　　Impetigo (contagiosa) [any site] [any organism]:
　　　　bullous
　　　　circinate
　　　　neonatorum
　　　　simplex
　　　Pemphigus neonatorum
　　　　EXCLUDES　impetigo herpetiformis (694.3)

　　CC Excl: 684, 686.00-686.01, 686.09, 686.1-686.9, 709.8

　　DEF: Infectious skin disease commonly occurring in children; caused by
　　group A streptococci or *Staphylococcus aureus*; skin lesions usually appear
　　on the face and consist of subcorneal vesicles and bullae that burst and form
　　yellow crusts.

▶**Lymphatic System of Head and Neck**◀

Afferent
vessels (in)

Blood
vessels

Hilum

Efferent
vessel (out)

**Schematic
of lymph node**

Jugulodigastric
Submental
Submandibular
Jugulomyohyoid
Anterior cervical

Superficial
parotid

Occipital

**Lymphatic drainage of the
head, neck, and face**

N Newborn Age: 0　P Pediatric Age: 0-17　M Maternity Age: 12-55　A Adult Age: 15-124　CC CC Condition　MC Major Complication　CD Complex Dx　HIV HIV Related Dx

200 — Volume 1 • January 2002

2002 Ingenix, Inc.

Stages of Pilonidal Disease

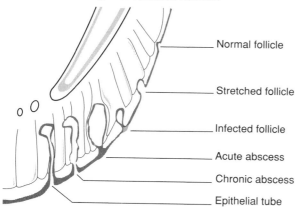

- Normal follicle
- Stretched follicle
- Infected follicle
- Acute abscess
- Chronic abscess
- Epithelial tube

✓4ᵗʰ **685 Pilonidal cyst**

INCLUDES   fistula } coccygeal or pilonidal
           sinus }

DEF: Hair-containing cyst or sinus in the tissues of the sacrococcygeal area; often drains through opening at the postanal dimple.

685.0   With abscess   CC

CC Excl: 685.0-685.1, 709.8

685.1   Without mention of abscess

✓4ᵗʰ **686 Other local infections of skin and subcutaneous tissue**

Use additional code to identify any infectious organism (041.0-041.8)

✓5ᵗʰ **686.0   Pyoderma**

Dermatitis: Dermatitis:
   purulent   suppurative
   septic

DEF: Nonspecific purulent skin disease related most to furuncles, pustules, or possibly carbuncles.

686.00   Pyoderma, unspecified

686.01   Pyoderma gangrenosum

AHA: 4Q, '97, 42

DEF: Persistent debilitating skin disease, characterized by irregular, boggy, blue-red ulcerations, with central healing and undermined edges.

686.09   Other pyoderma

686.1   Pyogenic granuloma

Granuloma:
   septic
   suppurative
   telangiectaticum

EXCLUDES   *pyogenic granuloma of oral mucosa (528.9)*

DEF: Solitary polypoid capillary hemangioma often associated with local irritation, trauma, and superimposed inflammation; located on the skin and gingival or oral mucosa.

686.8   Other specified local infections of skin and subcutaneous tissue

Bacterid (pustular)   Ecthyma
Dermatitis vegetans   Perlèche

EXCLUDES   *dermatitis infectiosa eczematoides (690.8)*
                 panniculitis (729.30-729.39)

686.9   Unspecified local infection of skin and subcutaneous tissue

Fistula of skin NOS
Skin infection NOS

EXCLUDES   *fistula to skin from internal organs — see Alphabetic Index*

OTHER INFLAMMATORY CONDITIONS OF SKIN AND SUBCUTANEOUS TISSUE (690-698)

EXCLUDES   *panniculitis (729.30-729.39)*

✓4ᵗʰ **690 Erythematosquamous dermatosis**

EXCLUDES   *eczematous dermatitis of eyelid (373.31)*
                 parakeratosis variegata (696.2)
                 psoriasis (696.0-696.1)
                 seborrheic keratosis (702.11-702.19)

✓5ᵗʰ **690.1   Seborrheic dermatitis**

AHA: 4Q, '95, 58

690.10   Seborrheic dermatitis, unspecified

Seborrheic dermatitis NOS

690.11   Seborrhea capitis   P

Cradle cap

690.12   Seborrheic infantile dermatitis   P

690.18   Other seborrheic dermatitis

690.8   Other erythematosquamous dermatosis

✓4ᵗʰ **691 Atopic dermatitis and related conditions**

DEF: Atopic dermatitis: chronic, pruritic, inflammatory skin disorder found on the face and antecubital and popliteal fossae; noted in persons with a hereditary predisposition to pruritus, and often accompanied by allergic rhinitis, hay fever, asthma, and extreme itching; also called allergic dermatitis, allergic or atopic eczema, or disseminated neurodermatitis.

691.0   Diaper or napkin rash

Ammonia dermatitis   Diaper or napkin:
Diaper or napkin: rash
   dermatitis   Psoriasiform napkin eruption
   erythema

691.8   Other atopic dermatitis and related conditions

Atopic dermatitis   Eczema:
Besnier's prurigo   intrinsic (allergic)
Eczema: Neurodermatitis:
   atopic   atopic
   flexural   diffuse (of Brocq)

✓4ᵗʰ **692 Contact dermatitis and other eczema**

INCLUDES   dermatitis: eczema (acute) (chronic):
            NOS   NOS
            contact   allergic
            occupational   erythematous
            venenata   occupational

EXCLUDES   *allergy NOS (995.3)*
                 contact dermatitis of eyelids (373.32)
                 dermatitis due to substances taken internally (693.0-693.9)
                 eczema of external ear (380.22)
                 perioral dermatitis (695.3)
                 urticarial reactions (708.0-708.9, 995.1)

DEF: Contact dermatitis: acute or chronic dermatitis caused by initial irritant effect of a substance, or by prior sensitization to a substance coming once again in contact with skin.

692.0   Due to detergents

692.1   Due to oils and greases

692.2   Due to solvents

Dermatitis due to solvents of:
   chlorocompound }
   cyclohexane   }
   ester   }
   glycol   } group
   hydrocarbon   }
   ketone   }

✓4ᵗʰ / ✓5ᵗʰ Additional Digit Required   Nonspecific PDx   Unacceptable PDx   Manifestation Code   MSP Medicare Secondary Payer   ►◄ Revised Text   ● New Code   ▲ Revised Code Title

2002 Ingenix, Inc.   **Volume 1 — 201**

Skin and Subcutaneous Tissue 692.3–692.83

692.3 Due to drugs and medicines in contact with skin

Dermatitis (allergic)   Dermatitis (allergic)
  (contact) due to: (contact) due to:
  arnica   neomycin
  fungicides   pediculocides
  iodine   phenols
  keratolytics   scabicides
  mercurials   any drug applied to skin
Dermatitis medicamentosa due to drug applied to
  skin
Use additional E code to identify drug

EXCLUDES   *allergy NOS due to drugs (995.2)*
          dermatitis due to ingested drugs
           (693.0)
          dermatitis medicamentosa NOS (693.0)

692.4 Due to other chemical products

Dermatitis due to:
  acids
  adhesive plaster
  alkalis
  caustics
  dichromate
  insecticide
  nylon
  plastic
  rubber

AHA: 2Q, '89, 16

692.5 Due to food in contact with skin

Dermatitis, contact,   Dermatitis, contact,
  due to: due to:
  cereals   fruit
  fish   meat
  flour   milk

EXCLUDES   *dermatitis due to:*
          dyes (692.89)
          ingested foods (693.1)
          preservatives (692.89)

692.6 Due to plants [except food]

Dermatitis due to:
  lacquer tree [Rhus verniciflua]
  poison:
    ivy [Rhus toxicodendron]
    oak [Rhus diversiloba]
    sumac [Rhus venenata]
    vine [Rhus radicans]
  primrose [Primula]
  ragweed [Senecio jacobae]
  other plants in contact with the skin

EXCLUDES   *allergy NOS due to pollen (477.0)*
          nettle rash (708.8)

√5th **692.7 Due to solar radiation**

EXCLUDES   *sunburn due to other ultraviolet*
          radiation exposure (692.82)

692.70 Unspecified dermatitis due to sun

692.71 Sunburn

First degree sunburn
Sunburn NOS

AHA: ▶4Q, '01, 47◀

692.72 Acute dermatitis due to solar radiation

Berlogue dermatitis
Photoallergic response
Phototoxic response
Polymorphus light eruption
Acute solar skin damage NOS

EXCLUDES   *sunburn (692.71, 692.76-*
          692.77)

Use additional E code to identify drug, if
  drug induced

DEF: Berloque dermatitis: Phytophotodermatitis due to
sun exposure after use of a product containing bergamot
oil; causes red patches, which may turn brown.

DEF: Photoallergic response: Dermatitis due to
hypersensitivity to the sun; causes papulovesicular,
eczematous or exudative eruptions.

DEF: Phototoxic response: Chemically induced sensitivity
to sun causes burn-like reaction, occasionally
vesiculation and subsequent hyperpigmentation.

DEF: Polymorphous light eruption: Inflammatory skin
eruptions due to sunlight exposure; eruptions differ in
size and shape.

DEF: Acute solar skin damage (NOS): Rapid, unspecified
injury to skin from sun.

692.73 Actinic reticuloid and actinic granuloma

DEF: Actinic reticuloid: Dermatosis aggravated by light,
causes chronic eczema-like eruption on exposed skin
which extends to other unexposed surfaces; occurs in
the eldery.

DEF: Actinic granuloma: Inflammatory response of skin to
sun causing small nodule of microphages.

**692.74 Other chronic dermatitis due to solar
radiation**

Chronic solar skin damage NOS
Solar elastosis

EXCLUDES   *actinic [solar] keratosis (702.0)*

DEF: Solar elastosis: Premature aging of skin of light-
skinned people; causes inelasticity, thinning or
thickening, wrinkling, dryness, scaling and
hyperpigmentation.

DEF: Chronic solar skin damage (NOS): Chronic skin
impairment due to exposure to the sun, not otherwise
specified.

**692.75 Disseminated superficial actinic
porokeratosis (DSAP)**

DEF: Autosomal dominant skin condition occurring in
skin that has been overexposed to the sun. Primarily
affects women over the age of 16; characterized by
numerous superficial annular, keratotic, brownish-red
spots or thickenings with depressed centers and sharp,
ridged borders. High risk that condition will evolve into
squamous cell carcinoma.

AHA: 4Q, '00, 43

692.76 Sunburn of second degree

AHA: ▶4Q, '01, 47◀

692.77 Sunburn of third degree

AHA: ▶4Q, '01, 47◀

692.79 Other dermatitis due to solar radiation

Hydroa aestivale
Photodermatitis   }
Photosensitiveness   } (due to sun)

Solar skin damage NOS

√5th **692.8 Due to other specified agents**

692.81 Dermatitis due to cosmetics

692.82 Dermatitis due to other radiation

Infrared rays   Tanning bed
Light, except   Ultraviolet rays, except
  from sun   from sun
Radiation NOS   X-rays

EXCLUDES   *solar radiation (692.70-692.79)*

AHA: ▶4Q, '01, 47;◀ 3Q, '00, 5

692.83 Dermatitis due to metals

Jewelry

N Newborn Age: 0   P Pediatric Age: 0-17   M Maternity Age: 12-55   A Adult Age: 15-124   CC CC Condition   MC Major Complication   CD Complex Dx   HIV HIV Related Dx

202 — Volume 1 • January 2002   *2002 Ingenix, Inc.*

692.89 Other

Dermatitis due to:	Dermatitis due to:
cold weather	hot weather
dyes	preservatives
furs	

> **EXCLUDES**   *allergy NOS due to animal hair, dander (animal), or dust (477.8)*
> *sunburn (692.71, 692.76-692.77)*

692.9 Unspecified cause
Dermatitis:
NOS
contact NOS
venenata NOS
Eczema NOS

√4th **693 Dermatitis due to substances taken internally**

> **EXCLUDES**   *adverse effect NOS of drugs and medicines (995.2)*
> *allergy NOS (995.3)*
> *contact dermatitis (692.0-692.9)*
> *urticarial reactions (708.0-708.9, 995.1)*

DEF: Inflammation of skin due to ingested substance.

693.0 Due to drugs and medicines
Dermatitis medicamentosa NOS
Use additional E code to identify drug

> **EXCLUDES**   *that due to drugs in contact with skin (692.3)*

693.1 Due to food

693.8 Due to other specified substances taken internally

693.9 Due to unspecified substance taken internally

> **EXCLUDES**   *dermatitis NOS (692.9)*

√4th **694 Bullous dermatoses**

694.0 Dermatitis herpetiformis
Dermatosis herpetiformis
Duhring's disease
Hydroa herpetiformis

> **EXCLUDES**   *herpes gestationis (646.8)*
> *dermatitis herpetiformis:*
> *juvenile (694.2)*
> *senile (694.5)*

DEF: Chronic, relapsing multisystem disease manifested most in the cutaneous system; seen as an extremely pruritic eruption of various combinations of lesions that frequently heal leaving hyperpigmentation or hypopigmentation and occasionally scarring; usually associated with an asymptomatic gluten-sensitive enteropathy, and immunogenic factors are believed to play a role in its origin.

694.1 Subcorneal pustular dermatosis
Sneddon-Wilkinson disease or syndrome

DEF: Chronic relapses of sterile pustular blebs beneath the horny skin layer of the trunk and skin folds; resembles dermatitis herpetiformis.

694.2 Juvenile dermatitis herpetiformis
Juvenile pemphigoid

694.3 Impetigo herpetiformis

DEF: Rare dermatosis associated with pregnancy; marked by itching pustules in third trimester, hypocalcemia, tetany, fever and lethargy; may result in maternal or fetal death.

694.4 Pemphigus   **CC**

Pemphigus:	Pemphigus:
NOS	malignant
erythematosus	vegetans
foliaceus	vulgaris

> **EXCLUDES**   *pemphigus neonatorum (684)*

CC Excl: 694.4-694.9, 709.8

DEF: Chronic, relapsing, sometimes fatal skin diseases; causes vesicles, bullae; autoantibodies against intracellular connections cause acantholysis.

694.5 Pemphigoid   **CC**
Benign pemphigus NOS
Bullous pemphigoid
Herpes circinatus bullosus
Senile dermatitis herpetiformis

CC Excl: See code 694.4

√5th **694.6 Benign mucous membrane pemphigoid**
Cicatricial pemphigoid
Mucosynechial atrophic bullous dermatitis

694.60 Without mention of ocular involvement

694.61 With ocular involvement
Ocular pemphigus

Mild self-limiting, subepidermal blistering of mucosa including the conjunctiva, seen predominantly in the elderly. It produces adhesions and scarring.

694.8 Other specified bullous dermatoses

> **EXCLUDES**   *herpes gestationis (646.8)*

694.9 Unspecified bullous dermatoses

√4th **695 Erythematous conditions**

695.0 Toxic erythema   **CC**
Erythema venenatum

CC Excl: 695.0-695.4, 709.8

695.1 Erythema multiforme
Erythema iris
Herpes iris
Lyell's syndrome
Scalded skin syndrome
Stevens-Johnson syndrome
Toxic epidermal necrolysis

DEF: Symptom complex with a varied skin eruption pattern of macular, bullous, papular, nodose, or vesicular lesions on the neck, face, and legs; gastritis and rheumatic pains are also noticeable, first-seen symptoms; complex is secondary to a number of factors, including infections, ingestants, physical agents, malignancy and pregnancy.

695.2 Erythema nodosum

> **EXCLUDES**   *tuberculous erythema nodosum (017.1)*

DEF: Panniculitis (an inflammatory reaction of the subcutaneous fat) of women, usually seen as a hypersensitivity reaction to various infections, drugs, sarcoidosis, and specific enteropathies; the acute stage is often associated with other symptoms, including fever, malaise, and arthralgia; the lesions are pink to blue in color, appear in crops as tender nodules and are found on the front of the legs below the knees.

695.3 Rosacea
Acne:
erythematosa
rosacea
Perioral dermatitis
Rhinophyma

DEF: Chronic skin disease, usually of the face, characterized by persistent erythema and sometimes by telangiectasis with acute episodes of edema, engorgement papules, and pustules.

695.4 Lupus erythematosus
Lupus:
erythematodes (discoid)
erythematosus (discoid), not disseminated

> **EXCLUDES**   *lupus (vulgaris) NOS (017.0)*
> *systemic [disseminated] lupus erythematosus (710.0)*

DEF: Group of connective tissue disorders occurring as various cutaneous diseases of unknown origin; it primarily affects women between the ages of 20 and 40.

√5th **695.8 Other specified erythematous conditions**

695.81 Ritter's disease
Dermatitis exfoliativa neonatorum

DEF: Infectious skin disease of infants and young children marked by eruptions ranging from a localized bullous type to widespread development of easily ruptured fine vesicles and bullae; results in exfoliation of large planes of skin and leaves raw areas; also called staphylococcal scalded skin syndrome.

√4th √5th **Additional Digit Required**   **Nonspecific PDx**   **Unacceptable PDx**   **Manifestation Code**   **MSP** Medicare Secondary Payer   ▶◀ Revised Text   ● New Code   ▲ Revised Code Title

2002 Ingenix, Inc.   **Volume 1 — 203**

695.89 Other
Erythema intertrigo
Intertrigo
Pityriasis rubra (Hebra)
EXCLUDES   *mycotic intertrigo (111.0-*
111.9)

AHA:: S-O, '86, 10

695.9 Unspecified erythematous condition
Erythema NOS   Erythroderma (secondary)

✓4ᵗʰ **696 Psoriasis and similar disorders**

696.0 Psoriatic arthropathy   CC
CC Excl: 015.80-015.96, 017.90-017.96, 036.82, 056.71, 098.50-
098.51, 098.59, 098.89, 696.0, 711.00-711.99, 712.10-712.99, 713.0-
713.8, 714.0, 715.00, 715.09-715.10, 715.18, 715.20-715.98, 716.00-
716.99, 718.00-718.08, 719.00-719.09, 719.10, 719.18-719.19, 719.20-
719.99

DEF: Psoriasis associated with inflammatory arthritis; often
involves interphalangeal joints.

696.1 Other psoriasis
Acrodermatitis continua   Psoriasis:
Dermatitis repens   any type, except
Psoriasis: arthropathic
   NOS
EXCLUDES   *psoriatic arthropathy (696.0)*

696.2 Parapsoriasis
Parakeratosis variegata
Parapsoriasis lichenoides chronica
Pityriasis lichenoides et varioliformis

DEF: Erythodermas similar to lichen, planus and psoriasis;
symptoms include redness and itching; resistant to treatment.

696.3 Pityriasis rosea
Pityriasis circinata (et maculata)

DEF: Common, self-limited rash of unknown etiology marked by a
solitary erythematous, salmon or fawn-colored herald plaque on
the trunk, arms or thighs; followed by development of papular or
macular lesions that tend to peel and form a scaly collarette.

696.4 Pityriasis rubra pilaris
Devergie's disease   Lichen ruber acuminatus
EXCLUDES   *pityriasis rubra (Hebra) (695.89)*

DEF: Inflammatory disease of hair follicles; marked by firm, red
lesions topped by horny plugs; may form patches; occurs on fingers
elbows, knees.

696.5 Other and unspecified pityriasis
Pityriasis: Pityriasis:
   NOS   streptogenes
   alba
EXCLUDES   *pityriasis:*
simplex (690.18)
versicolor (111.0)

696.8 Other

✓4ᵗʰ **697 Lichen**
EXCLUDES   *lichen:*
obtusus corneus (698.3)
pilaris (congenital) (757.39)
ruber acuminatus (696.4)
sclerosus et atrophicus (701.0)
scrofulosus (017.0)
simplex chronicus (698.3)
spinulosus (congenital) (757.39)
urticatus (698.2)

697.0 Lichen planus
Lichen: Lichen:
   planopilaris   ruber planus

DEF: Inflammatory, pruritic skin disease; marked by angular, flat-
top, violet-colored papules; may be acute and widespread or
chronic and localized.

697.1 Lichen nitidus
Pinkus' disease

DEF: Chronic, inflammatory, usually asymptomatic skin disorder,
characterized by numerous glistening, flat-topped, discrete,
smooth, skin-colored micropapules most often on penis, lower
abdomen, inner thighs, wrists, forearms, breasts and buttocks.

697.8 Other lichen, not elsewhere classified
Lichen: Lichen:
   ruber moniliforme   striata

697.9 Lichen, unspecified

✓4ᵗʰ **698 Pruritus and related conditions**
EXCLUDES   *pruritus specified as psychogenic (306.3)*

DEF: Pruritus: Intense, persistent itching due to irritation of sensory nerve
endings from organic or psychogenic causes.

698.0 Pruritus ani
Perianal itch

698.1 Pruritus of genital organs

698.2 Prurigo
Lichen urticatus   Prurigo:
Prurigo: mitis
   NOS   simplex
   Hebra's   Urticaria papulosa (Hebra)
EXCLUDES   *prurigo nodularis (698.3)*

698.3 Lichenification and lichen simplex chronicus
Hyde's disease
Neurodermatitis (circumscripta) (local)
Prurigo nodularis
EXCLUDES   *neurodermatitis, diffuse (of Brocq)*
(691.8)

DEF: Lichenification: thickening of skin due to prolonged rubbing or
scratching.

DEF: Lichen simplex chronicus: eczematous dermatitis, of face,
neck, extremities, scrotum, vulva, and perianal region due to
repeated itching, rubbing and scratching; spontaneous or evolves
with other dermatoses.

698.4 Dermatitis factitia [artefacta]
Dermatitis ficta
Neurotic excoriation
Use additional code to identify any associated
mental disorder

DEF: Various types of self-inflicted skin lesions characterized in
appearance as an erythema to a gangrene.

698.8 Other specified pruritic conditions
Pruritus: Winter itch
   hiemalis
   senilis

698.9 Unspecified pruritic disorder
Itch NOS   Pruritus NOS

OTHER DISEASES OF SKIN AND SUBCUTANEOUS TISSUE (700-709)
EXCLUDES   *conditions confined to eyelids (373.0-374.9)*
congenital conditions of skin, hair, and nails
(757.0-757.9)

700 Corns and callosities
Callus   Clavus

DEF: Corns: Conical or horny thickening of skin on toes, due to friction,
pressure from shoes and hosiery; pain and inflammation may develop.

DEF: Callosities: Localized overgrowth (hyperplasia) of the horny epidermal
layer due to pressure or friction.

✓4ᵗʰ **701 Other hypertrophic and atrophic conditions of skin**
EXCLUDES   *dermatomyositis (710.3)*
hereditary edema of legs (757.0)
scleroderma (generalized) (710.1)

701.0 Circumscribed scleroderma
Addison's keloid   Morphea
Dermatosclerosis, localized   Scleroderma, circum-
Lichen sclerosus   scribed or localized
   et atrophicus

DEF: Thickened, hardened, skin and subcutaneous tissue; may
involve musculoskeletal system.

701.1 Keratoderma, acquired
Acquired:
ichthyosis
keratoderma palmaris et plantaris
Elastosis perforans serpiginosa
Hyperkeratosis:
NOS
follicularis in cutem penetrans
palmoplantaris climacterica
Keratoderma:
climactericum
tylodes, progressive
Keratosis (blennorrhagica)

EXCLUDES *Darier's disease [keratosis follicularis]*
(congenital) (757.39)
keratosis:
arsenical (692.4)
gonococcal (098.81)

AHA: 4Q, '94, 48

701.2 Acquired acanthosis nigricans
Keratosis nigricans

DEF: Diffuse velvety hyperplasia of the spinous skin layer of the axilla and other body folds marked by gray, brown, or black pigmentation; in adult form it is often associated with an internal carcinoma (malignant acanthosis nigricans) in a benign, nevoid form it is relatively generalized; benign juvenile form with obesity is sometimes caused by an endocrine disturbance.

701.3 Striae atrophicae
Atrophic spots of skin
Atrophoderma maculatum
Atrophy blanche (of Milian)
Degenerative colloid atrophy
Senile degenerative atrophy
Striae distensae

DEF: Bands of atrophic, depressed, wrinkled skin associated with stretching of skin from pregnancy, obesity, or rapid growth during puberty.

701.4 Keloid scar
Cheloid
Hypertrophic scar
Keloid

DEF: Overgrowth of scar tissue due to excess amounts of collagen during connective tissue repair; occurs mainly on upper trunk, face.

701.5 Other abnormal granulation tissue
Excessive granulation

701.8 Other specified hypertrophic and atrophic conditions of skin
Acrodermatitis atrophicans chronica
Atrophia cutis senilis
Atrophoderma neuriticum
Confluent and reticulate papillomatosis
Cutis laxa senilis
Elastosis senilis
Folliculitis ulerythematosa reticulata
Gougerot-Carteaud syndrome or disease

701.9 Unspecified hypertrophic and atrophic conditions of skin
Atrophoderma

√4th **702 Other dermatoses**
EXCLUDES *carcinoma in situ (232.0-232.9)*

702.0 Actinic keratosis
AHA: 1Q, '92, 18

DEF: Wart-like growth, red or skin-colored; may form a cutaneous horn.

√5th **702.1 Seborrheic keratosis**
DEF: Common, benign, lightly pigmented, warty growth composed of basaloid cells.

702.11 Inflamed seborrheic keratosis
AHA: 4Q, '94, 48

702.19 Other seborrheic keratosis
Seborrheic keratosis NOS

702.8 Other specified dermatoses

√4th **703 Diseases of nail**
EXCLUDES *congenital anomalies (757.5)*
onychia and paronychia (681.02, 681.11)

703.0 Ingrowing nail
Ingrowing nail with infection   Unguis incarnatus
EXCLUDES *infection, nail NOS (681.9)*

703.8 Other specified diseases of nail
Dystrophia unguium   Onychauxis
Hypertrophy of nail   Onychogryposis
Koilonychia   Onycholysis
Leukonychia (punctata) (striata)

703.9 Unspecified disease of nail

√4th **704 Diseases of hair and hair follicles**
EXCLUDES *congenital anomalies (757.4)*

√5th **704.0 Alopecia**
EXCLUDES *madarosis (374.55)*
syphilitic alopecia (091.82)

DEF: Lack of hair, especially on scalp; often called baldness; may be partial or total; occurs at any age.

704.00 Alopecia, unspecified
Baldness
Loss of hair

704.01 Alopecia areata
Ophiasis

DEF: Alopecia areata: usually reversible, inflammatory, patchy hair loss found in beard or scalp.

DEF: Ophiasis: alopecia areata of children; marked by band around temporal and occipital scalp margins.

704.02 Telogen effluvium
DEF: Shedding of hair from premature telogen development in follicles due to stress, including shock, childbirth, surgery, drugs or weight loss.

704.09 Other
Folliculitis decalvans
Hypotrichosis:
NOS
postinfectional NOS
Pseudopelade

704.1 Hirsutism
Hypertrichosis: Polytrichia
NOS
lanuginosa, acquired
EXCLUDES *hypertrichosis of eyelid (374.54)*

DEF: Excess hair growth; often in unexpected places and amounts.

704.2 Abnormalities of the hair
Atrophic hair   Trichiasis:
Clastothrix   NOS
Fragilitas crinium   cicatrical
                     Trichorrhexis (nodosa)
EXCLUDES *trichiasis of eyelid (374.05)*

704.3 Variations in hair color
Canities (premature)   Poliosis:
Grayness, hair (premature) NOS
Heterochromia of hair   circumscripta, acquired

704.8 Other specified diseases of hair and hair follicles
Folliculitis: Sycosis:
NOS   NOS
abscedens et suffodiens   barbae [not parasitic]
pustular   lupoid
Perifolliculitis: vulgaris
NOS
capitis abscedens et suffodiens
scalp

704.9 Unspecified disease of hair and hair follicles

√4th **705 Disorders of sweat glands**
705.0 Anhidrosis
Hypohidrosis   Oligohidrosis
DEF: Lack or deficiency of ability to sweat.

√4th / √5th Additional Digit Required   Nonspecific PDx   Unacceptable PDx   Manifestation Code   **MSP** Medicare Secondary Payer   ►◄ Revised Text   ● New Code   ▲ Revised Code Title

2002 Ingenix, Inc.   **Volume 1 — 205**

Skin and Subcutaneous Tissue 705.1–707.19

705.1   **Prickly heat**
    Heat rash   Sudamina
    Miliaria rubra (tropicalis)

√5ᵗʰ **705.8**   **Other specified disorders of sweat glands**

    705.81 Dyshidrosis
       Cheiropompholyx   Pompholyx
       DEF: Vesicular eruption, on hands, feet causing itching and burning.

    705.82 Fox-Fordyce disease
       DEF: Chronic, usually pruritic disease chiefly of women evidenced by small follicular papular eruptions, especially in the axillary and pubic areas; develops from the closure and rupture of the affected apocrine glands' intraepidermal portion of the ducts.

    705.83 Hidradenitis
       Hidradenitis suppurativa
       DEF: Inflamed sweat glands.

    705.89 Other
       Bromhidrosis   Granulosis rubra nasi
       Chromhidrosis   Urhidrosis
       EXCLUDES   hidrocystoma (216.0-216.9)
               hyperhidrosis (780.8)

       DEF: Bromhidrosis: foul-smelling axillary sweat due to decomposed bacteria.

       DEF: Chromhidrosis: secretion of colored sweat.

       DEF: Granulosis rubra nasi: ideopathic condition of children; causes redness, sweating around nose, face and chin; tends to end by puberty.

       DEF: Urhidrosis: urinous substance, such as uric acid, in sweat; occurs in uremia.

705.9   **Unspecified disorder of sweat glands**
    Disorder of sweat glands NOS

√4ᵗʰ **706 Diseases of sebaceous glands**

    706.0   **Acne varioliformis**
       Acne: Acne:
         frontalis   necrotica
       DEF: Rare form of acne characterized by persistent brown papulopustules usually on the brow and temporoparietal part of the scalp.

    706.1   **Other acne**
       Acne: Acne:
         NOS   vulgaris
         conglobata   Blackhead
         cystic   Comedo
         pustular
       EXCLUDES   acne rosacea (695.3)

    706.2   **Sebaceous cyst**
       Atheroma, skin   Wen
       Keratin cyst
       DEF: Benign epidermal cyst, contains sebum and keratin; presents as firm, circumscribed nodule.

    706.3   **Seborrhea**
       EXCLUDES   seborrhea:
                capitis (690.11)
                sicca (690.18)
             seborrheic
                dermatitis (690.10)
                keratosis (702.11-702.19)
       DEF: Seborrheic dermatitis marked by excessive secretion of sebum; the sebum forms an oily coating, crusts, or scales on the skin; it is also called hypersteatosis.

    706.8   **Other specified diseases of sebaceous glands**
       Asteatosis (cutis)
       Xerosis cutis

    706.9   **Unspecified disease of sebaceous glands**

Six Stages of Decubitus Ulcers

First Stage — Skin is warm, firm, or stretched

Second Stage — Bacteria enter

Third Stage — Fat layer exposed

Fourth Stage — Muscle necrosis

Fifth Stage — Advanced muscle necrosis

Sixth Stage — Bone necrosis

√4ᵗʰ **707 Chronic ulcer of skin**
    INCLUDES   non-infected sinus of skin
               non-healing ulcer
    EXCLUDES   specific infections classified under "Infectious and Parasitic Diseases" (001.0-136.9)
               varicose ulcer (454.0, 454.2)

    707.0   **Decubitus ulcer**   CC MC
       Bed sore
       Decubitus ulcer [any site]
       Plaster ulcer
       Pressure ulcer
       CC Excl: 707.0, 707.8-707.9, 709.8

       AHA: 4Q, '99, 20; 1Q, '96, 15; 3Q, '90, 15; N-D, '87, 9

√5ᵗʰ **707.1**   **Ulcer of lower limbs, except decubitus**
       Ulcer, chronic:
         neurogenic } of lower limb
         trophic

       ▶Code, if applicable, any causal condition first:◀
         atherosclerosis of the extremities with ulceration (440.23)
       ▶chronic venous hypertension with ulcer (459.31)
         chronic venous hypertension with ulcer and inflammation (459.33)◀
         diabetes mellitus (250.80-250.83)
       ▶postphlebitic syndrome with ulcer (459.11)
         postphlebitic syndrome with ulcer and inflammation (459.13)◀

       AHA: 4Q, '00, 44; 4Q, '99, 15

    707.10 Ulcer of lower limb, unspecified   CC
       CC Excl: 440.23, 707.10-707.19, 707.8-707.9, 709.8

    707.11 Ulcer of thigh   CC
       CC Excl: See code 707.10

    707.12 Ulcer of calf   CC
       CC Excl: See code 707.10

    707.13 Ulcer of ankle   CC
       CC Excl: See code 707.10

    707.14 Ulcer of heel and midfoot   CC
       Plantar surface of midfoot
       CC Excl: See code 707.10

    707.15 Ulcer of other part of foot   CC
       Toes
       CC Excl: See code 707.10

    707.19 Ulcer of other part of lower limb   CC
       CC Excl: See code 707.10

N Newborn Age: 0   **P** Pediatric Age: 0-17   **M** Maternity Age: 12-55   **A** Adult Age: 15-124   **CC** CC Condition   **MC** Major Complication   **CD** Complex Dx   **HIV** HIV Related Dx

707.8 Chronic ulcer of other specified sites

Ulcer, chronic:
neurogenic ⎫
trophic ⎭ of other specified sites

707.9 Chronic ulcer of unspecified site

Chronic ulcer NOS
Trophic ulcer NOS
Tropical ulcer NOS
Ulcer of skin NOS

✓4ᵗʰ **708 Urticaria**

EXCLUDES   *edema:*
angioneurotic (995.1)
Quincke's (995.1)
hereditary angioedema (277.6)
urticaria:
giant (995.1)
papulosa (Hebra) (698.2)
pigmentosa (juvenile) (congenital) (757.33)

DEF: Skin disorder marked by raised edematous patches of skin or mucous membrane with intense itching; also called hives.

708.0 Allergic urticaria

708.1 Idiopathic urticaria

708.2 Urticaria due to cold and heat
Thermal urticaria

708.3 Dermatographic urticaria
Dermatographia   Factitial urticaria

708.4 Vibratory urticaria

708.5 Cholinergic urticaria

708.8 Other specified urticaria
Nettle rash   Urticaria:
Urticaria: recurrent periodic
chronic

708.9 Urticaria, unspecified
Hives NOS

✓4ᵗʰ **709 Other disorders of skin and subcutaneous tissue**

✓5ᵗʰ **709.0 Dyschromia**

EXCLUDES   *albinism (270.2)*
pigmented nevus (216.0-216.9)
that of eyelid (374.52-374.53)

DEF: Pigment disorder of skin or hair.

709.00 Dyschromia, unspecified

709.01 Vitiligo

DEF: Persistent, progressive development of nonpigmented white patches on otherwise normal skin.

709.09 Other

709.1 Vascular disorders of skin
Angioma serpiginosum
Purpura (primary)annularis telangiectodes

709.2 Scar conditions and fibrosis of skin
Adherent scar (skin)   Fibrosis, skin NOS
Cicatrix   Scar NOS
Disfigurement (due to scar)

EXCLUDES   *keloid scar (701.4)*

AHA: N-D, '84, 19

Cutaneous Lesions

Surface Lesions

Fissure   Polyp growth   Ulcer

Solid Lesions

Flat macule   Slightly elevated   Solid papule
                wheal

Sac Lesions

Cyst   Clear fluid vesicle   Pustule

709.3 Degenerative skin disorders
Calcinosis: Degeneration, skin
circumscripta   Deposits, skin
cutis   Senile dermatosis NOS
Colloid milium   Subcutaneous calcification

709.4 Foreign body granuloma of skin and subcutaneous tissue

EXCLUDES   *residual foreign body without granuloma of skin and subcutaneous tissue (729.6)*
that of muscle (728.82)

709.8 Other specified disorders of skin
Epithelial hyperplasia
Menstrual dermatosis
Vesicular eruption

AHA: N-D, '87, 6

DEF: Epithelial hyperplasia: increased number of epitheleal cells.

DEF: Vesicular eruption: liquid-filled structures appearing through skin.

709.9 Unspecified disorder of skin and subcutaneous tissue
Dermatosis NOS

✓4ᵗʰ ✓5ᵗʰ Additional Digit Required   Nonspecific PDx   Unacceptable PDx   Manifestation Code   MSP Medicare Secondary Payer   ►◄ Revised Text   ● New Code   ▲ Revised Code Title

2002 Ingenix, Inc.   **Volume 1 — 207**

13. DISEASES OF THE MUSCULOSKELETAL SYSTEM AND CONNECTIVE TISSUE (710-739)

Joint Structures

Muscle
Periosteum (covers bone)
Cortical bone
Medullary bone
Fascia over Muscle
Sesamoid bone
Bursa (with synovial fluid)
Tendon (muscle to bone)
Muscle insertion into bone (crosses one or more joints)

Retinaculum
Tendon sheath around
Tendon
Synovium lines
Joint capsule around
Synovial cavity (with fluid)
Articular cartilage
Ligament (bone to bone)
Bursa
Bone covered with periosteum

The following fifth-digit subclassification is for use with categories 711-712, 715-716, 718-719, and 730:

0 **site unspecified**
1 **shoulder region**
    Acromioclavicular joint(s)
    Clavicle
    Glenohumeral joint(s)
    Scapula
    Sternoclavicular joint(s)
2 **upper arm**
    Elbow joint
    Humerus
3 **forearm**
    Radius
    Ulna
    Wrist joint
4 **hand**
    Carpus
    Metacarpus
    Phalanges [fingers]
5 **pelvic region and thigh**
    Buttock
    Femur
    Hip (joint)
6 **lower leg**
    Fibula   Patella
    Knee joint   Tibia
7 **ankle and foot**
    Ankle joint   Phalanges, foot
    Digits [toes]   Tarsus
    Metatarsus   Other joints in foot
8 **other specified sites**
    Head   Skull
    Neck   Trunk
    Ribs   Vertebral column
9 **multiple sites**

ARTHROPATHIES AND RELATED DISORDERS (710-719)

> **EXCLUDES**   *disorders of spine (720.0-724.9)*

✓4th **710 Diffuse diseases of connective tissue**
> **INCLUDES**   all collagen diseases whose effects are not mainly confined to a single system
> **EXCLUDES**   *those affecting mainly the cardiovascular system, i.e., polyarteritis nodosa and allied conditions (446.0-446.7)*

710.0   **Systemic lupus erythematosus**   `CC`
    Disseminated lupus erythematosus
    Libman-Sacks disease
    Use additional code to identify manifestation, as:
      endocarditis (424.91)
      nephritis (583.81)
        chronic (582.81)
      nephrotic syndrome (581.81)
> **EXCLUDES**   *lupus erythematosus (discoid) NOS (695.4)*

CC Excl: 710.0

AHA: 2Q, '97, 8

DEF: A chronic multisystemic inflammatory disease affecting connective tissue; marked by anemia, leukopenia, muscle and joint pains, fever, rash of a butterfly pattern around cheeks and forehead area; of unknown etiology.

710.1   **Systemic sclerosis**   `CC`
    Acrosclerosis   Progressive systemic sclerosis
    CRST syndrome   Scleroderma
> **EXCLUDES**   *circumscribed scleroderma (701.0)*
▶Use additional code to identify manifestation, as:
    lung involvement (517.8)
    myopathy (359.6)◀
CC Excl: 710.1

AHA: 1Q, '88, 6

DEF: Systemic disease, involving excess fibrotic collagen build-up; symptoms include thickened skin; fibrotic degenerative changes in various organs; and vascular abnomalities; condition occurs more often in females.

710.2   **Sicca syndrome**
    Keratoconjunctivitis sicca   Sjögren's disease
DEF: Autoimmune disease; associated with keratoconjunctivitis, laryngopharyngitis, rhinitis, dry mouth, enlarged parotid gland, and chronic polyarthritis.

710.3   **Dermatomyositis**   `CC`
    Poikilodermatomyositis
    Polymyositis with skin involvement
CC Excl: 710.3

DEF: Polymyositis associated with flat-top purple papules on knuckles; marked by upper eyelid rash, edema of eyelids and orbit area, red rash on forehead, neck, shoulders, trunk and arms; symptoms include fever, weight loss aching muscles; visceral cancer (in individuals older than 40).

710.4   **Polymyositis**   `CC`
CC Excl: 710.4

DEF: Chronic, progressive, inflammatory skeletal muscle disease; causes weakness of limb girdles, neck, pharynx; may precede or follow scleroderma, Sjogren's disease, systemic lupus erythematosus, arthritis, or malignancy.

710.5   **Eosinophilia myalgia syndrome**   `CC`
    Toxic oil syndrome
    Use additional E code to identify drug, if drug induced
CC Excl: 292.0-292.9, 293.0-293.9, 710.5

AHA: 4Q, '92, 21

DEF: Eosinophilia myalgia syndrome (EMS): inflammatory, multisystem fibrosis; associated with ingesting elemetary L-tryptophan; symptoms include myalgia, weak limbs and bulbar muscles, distal sensory loss, areflexia, arthralgia, cough, fever, fatigue, skin rashes, myopathy, and eosinophil counts greater than 1000/microliter.

DEF: Toxic oil syndrome: syndrome silimar to EMS due to ingesting contaminated cooking oil.

✓4th ✓5th Additional Digit Required   Nonspecific PDx   Unacceptable PDx   Manifestation Code   `MSP` Medicare Secondary Payer   ▶◀ Revised Text   ● New Code   ▲ Revised Code Title

2002 Ingenix, Inc.

October 2002 • Volume 1 — 209

710.8 Other specified diffuse diseases of connective tissue `CC`
Multifocal fibrosclerosis (idiopathic) NEC
Systemic fibrosclerosing syndrome

CC Excl: 710.8

AHA: M-A, '87, 12

710.9 Unspecified diffuse connective tissue disease
Collagen disease NOS

✓4th **711 Arthropathy associated with infections**

INCLUDES	arthritis
	arthropathy
	polyarthritis
	polyarthropathy

associated with
conditions
classifiable below

EXCLUDES *rheumatic fever (390)*

The following fifth-digit subclassification is for use with category 711; valid digits are in [brackets] under each code.

0 site unspecified
1 shoulder region
2 upper arm
3 forearm
4 hand
5 pelvic region and thigh
6 lower leg
7 ankle and foot
8 other specified sites
9 multiple sites

AHA: 1Q, '92, 17

§ ✓5th **711.0 Pyogenic arthritis** `CC`
[0-9] Arthritis or polyarthritis (due to):
coliform [Escherichia coli]
Hemophilus influenzae [H. influenzae]
pneumococcal
Pseudomonas
staphylococcal
streptococcal
Pyarthrosis
Use additional code to identify infectious organism
(041.0-041.8)

CC Excl: For code 711.00: 015.80-015.96, 017.90-017.96, 036.82, 056.71, 098.50-098.51, 098.59, 098.89, 711.00-711.99, 712.10-712.99, 713.0-713.8, 714.0, 715.00, 715.09-715.10, 715.18-715.98, 716.00-716.99, 716.00-718.08, 719.00-719.10, 719.18-719.99 **For code 711.01:** 015.80-015.96, 017.90-017.96, 036.82, 056.71, 098.50-098.51, 098.59, 098.89, 711.00-711.01, 711.08-711.11, 711.18-711.21, 711.28-711.31, 711.38-711.41, 711.48-711.51, 711.58-711.61, 711.68-711.71, 711.78-711.81, 711.88-711.91, 711.98-711.99, 712.10-712.11, 712.18-712.21, 712.28-712.31, 712.38-712.81, 712.88-712.91, 712.98-712.99, 713.0-713.8, 714.0, 715.00, 715.09-715.11, 715.18-715.21, 715.28-715.31, 715.38-715.91, 715.98, 716.00-716.01, 716.08-716.11, 716.18-716.21, 716.28-716.31, 716.38-716.41, 716.48-716.51, 716.58-716.61, 716.68-716.81, 716.88-716.91, 716.98-716.99, 718.00-718.01, 718.08, 719.00-719.01, 719.08-719.11, 719.18-719.21, 719.28-719.31, 719.38-719.41, 719.48-719.51, 719.58-719.61, 719.68-719.70, 719.78-719.81, 719.88-719.91, 719.98-719.99 **For code 711.02:** 015.80-015.96, 017.90-017.96, 036.82, 056.71, 098.50-098.51, 098.59, 098.89, 711.00, 711.02, 711.08-711.10, 711.12, 711.18-711.20, 711.22, 711.28-711.30, 711.32, 711.38-711.40, 711.42, 711.48-711.50, 711.52, 711.58-711.60, 711.62, 711.68-711.70, 711.72, 711.78-711.80, 711.82, 711.88-711.90, 711.92, 711.98-711.99, 712.10, 712.12, 712.18-712.20, 712.22, 712.28-712.30, 712.32, 712.38-712.80, 712.82, 712.88-712.90, 712.92, 712.98-712.99, 713.0-713.8, 714.0, 715.00, 715.09-715.10, 715.12, 715.18, 715.20, 715.22, 715.28, 715.30, 715.32, 715.38-715.90, 715.92, 715.98, 716.00, 716.02, 716.08-716.10, 716.12, 716.18-716.20, 716.22, 716.28-716.30, 716.32, 716.38-716.40, 716.42, 716.48-716.50, 716.52, 716.58-716.60, 716.62, 716.68, 716.82, 716.88-716.90, 716.92, 716.98-716.99, 718.00, 718.02, 718.08, 719.00, 719.02, 719.08-719.10, 719.12, 719.18-719.20, 719.22, 719.28-719.30, 719.32, 719.38-719.40, 719.42, 719.48-719.50, 719.52, 719.58-719.60, 719.62, 719.68-719.70, 719.78-719.80, 719.82, 719.88-719.90, 719.92, 719.98-719.99 **For code 711.03:** 015.80-015.96, 017.90-017.96, 036.82, 056.71, 098.50-098.51, 098.59, 098.89, 711.00, 711.03, 711.08-711.10, 711.13, 711.18-711.20, 711.23, 711.28-711.30, 711.33, 711.38-711.40, 711.43, 711.48-711.50, 711.53, 711.58-711.60, 711.63, 711.68-711.70, 711.73,

711.78-711.80, 711.83, 711.88-711.90, 711.93, 711.98-711.99, 712.10, 712.13, 712.18-712.20, 712.23, 712.28-712.30, 712.33, 712.38-712.80, 712.83, 712.88-712.90, 712.93, 712.98-712.99, 713.0-713.8, 714.0, 715.00, 715.09-715.10, 715.13, 715.18, 715.20, 715.23, 715.28, 715.30, 715.33, 715.38-715.90, 715.93, 715.98, 716.00, 716.03, 716.08-716.10, 716.13, 716.18-716.20, 716.23, 716.28-716.30, 716.33, 716.38-716.40, 716.43, 716.48-716.50, 716.53, 716.58-716.60, 716.63, 716.68, 716.80, 716.83, 716.88-716.90, 716.93, 716.98-716.99, 718.00, 718.03, 718.08, 719.00, 719.03, 719.08-719.10, 719.13, 719.18-719.20, 719.23, 719.28-719.30, 719.33, 719.38-719.40, 719.43, 719.48-719.50, 719.53, 719.58-719.60, 719.63, 719.68-719.70, 719.78-719.80, 719.83, 719.88-719.90, 719.93, 719.98-719.99 **For code 711.04:** 015.80-015.96, 017.90-017.96, 036.82, 056.71, 098.50-098.51, 098.59, 098.89, 711.00, 711.04, 711.08-711.10, 711.14, 711.18-711.20, 711.24, 711.28-711.30, 711.34, 711.38-711.40, 711.44, 711.48-711.50, 711.54, 711.58-711.60, 711.64, 711.68-711.70, 711.74, 711.78-711.80, 711.84, 711.88-711.90, 711.94, 711.98-711.99, 712.10, 712.14, 712.18-712.20, 712.24, 712.28-712.30, 712.34, 712.38-712.80, 712.84, 712.88-712.90, 712.94, 712.98-712.99, 713.0-713.8, 714.0, 715.00-715.10, 715.14, 715.18, 715.20, 715.24, 715.28, 715.30, 715.34, 715.38-715.90, 715.94, 715.98, 716.00, 716.04, 716.08-716.10, 716.14, 716.18-716.20, 716.24, 716.28-716.30, 716.34, 716.38-716.40, 716.44, 716.48-716.50, 716.54, 716.58-716.60, 716.64, 716.68, 716.80, 716.84, 716.88-716.90, 716.94, 716.98-716.99, 718.00, 718.04, 718.08, 719.00, 719.04, 719.08-719.10, 719.14, 719.18-719.20, 719.24, 719.28-719.30, 719.34, 719.38-719.40, 719.44, 719.48-719.50, 719.54, 719.58-719.60, 719.64, 719.68-719.70, 719.78-719.80, 719.84, 719.88-719.90, 719.94, 719.98-719.99: **For code 711.05:** 015.80-015.96, 017.90-017.96, 036.82, 056.71, 098.50-098.51, 098.59, 098.89, 711.00, 711.05, 711.08-711.10, 711.15, 711.18-711.20, 711.25, 711.28-711.30, 711.35, 711.38-711.40, 711.45, 711.48-711.50, 711.55, 711.58-711.60, 711.65, 711.68-711.70, 711.75, 711.78-711.80, 711.85, 711.88-711.90, 711.95, 711.98-711.99, 712.10, 712.15, 712.18-712.20, 712.25, 712.28-712.30, 712.35, 712.38-712.80, 712.85, 712.88-712.90, 712.95, 712.98-712.99, 713.0-713.8, 714.0, 715.00, 715.09-715.10, 715.15, 715.18, 715.20, 715.25, 715.28, 715.30, 715.35, 715.38-715.90, 715.95, 715.98, 716.00, 716.05, 716.08-716.10, 716.15, 716.18-716.20, 716.25, 716.28-716.30, 716.35, 716.38-716.40, 716.45, 716.48-716.50, 716.55, 716.58-716.60, 716.65, 716.68, 716.80, 716.85, 716.88-716.90, 716.95, 716.98-716.99, 718.00, 718.05, 718.08, 719.00, 719.05, 719.08-719.10, 719.15, 719.18-719.20, 719.25, 719.28-719.30, 719.35, 719.38-719.40, 719.45, 719.48-719.50, 719.55, 719.58-719.60, 719.65, 719.68-719.70, 719.75, 719.78-719.80, 719.85, 719.88-719.90, 719.95, 719.98-719.99 **For code 711.06:** 015.80-015.96, 017.90-017.96, 036.82, 056.71, 098.50-098.51, 098.59, 098.89, 711.00, 711.06, 711.08-711.10, 711.16, 711.18-711.20, 711.26, 711.28-711.30, 711.36, 711.38-711.40, 711.46, 711.48-711.50, 711.56, 711.58-711.60, 711.66, 711.68-711.70, 711.76, 711.78-711.80, 711.86, 711.88-711.90, 711.96, 711.98-711.99, 712.10, 712.16, 712.18-712.20, 712.26, 712.28-712.30, 712.36, 712.38-712.80, 712.86, 712.88-712.90, 712.96, 712.98-712.99, 713.0-713.8, 714.0, 715.00, 715.09-715.10, 715.16, 715.18, 715.20, 715.26, 715.28, 715.30, 715.36, 715.38-715.90, 715.96, 715.98, 716.00, 716.06, 716.08-716.10, 716.16, 716.18-716.20, 716.26, 716.28-716.30, 716.36, 716.38-716.40, 716.46, 716.48-716.50, 716.56, 716.58-716.60, 716.66, 716.68, 716.80, 716.86, 716.88-716.90, 716.96, 716.98-716.99, 718.00, 718.08, 719.00, 719.06, 719.08-719.10, 719.16, 719.18-719.20, 719.26, 719.28-719.30, 719.36, 719.38-719.40, 719.46, 719.48-719.50, 719.56, 719.58-719.60, 719.66, 719.68-719.70, 719.76, 719.78-719.80, 719.86, 719.88-719.90, 719.96, 719.98-719.99 **For code 711.07:** 015.80-015.96, 017.90-017.96, 036.82, 056.71, 098.50-098.51, 098.59, 098.89, 711.00, 711.07-711.10, 711.17-711.20, 711.27-711.30, 711.37-711.40, 711.47-711.50, 711.57-711.60, 711.67-711.70, 711.77-711.80, 711.87-711.90, 711.97-711.99, 712.10, 712.17-712.20, 712.27-712.30, 712.37-712.80, 712.87-712.90, 712.97-712.99, 713.0-713.8, 714.0, 715.00, 715.09-715.10, 715.17-715.18, 715.20, 715.27-715.28, 715.30, 715.37-715.90, 715.97-715.98, 716.00, 716.07-716.10, 716.17-716.20, 716.27-716.30, 716.37-716.40, 716.47-716.50, 716.57-716.60, 716.67-716.68, 716.80, 716.87-716.90, 716.97-716.99, 718.00, 718.07-718.08, 719.00, 719.07-719.10, 719.17-719.20, 719.27-719.30, 719.37-719.40, 719.47-719.50, 719.57-719.60, 719.67-719.70, 719.77-719.80, 719.87-719.90, 719.97-719.99 **For code 711.08:** 015.80-015.96, 017.90-017.96, 036.82, 056.71, 098.50-098.51, 098.59, 098.89, 711.00-711.99, 712.10-712.99, 713.0-713.8, 714.0, 715.00, 715.09-715.10, 715.18-715.98, 716.00-716.99, 718.00-718.08, 719.00-719.10, 719.18-719.99 **For code 711.09:** See code 711.08

AHA: 1Q, '92, 16; 1Q, '91, 15

DEF: Infectious arthritis caused by various bacteria; marked by inflamed synovial membranes, and purulent effusion in joints.

---

§ Requires fifth-digit. Valid digits are in [brackets] under each code. See beginning of section 710-739 for codes and definitions.

`N` Newborn Age: 0   `P` Pediatric Age: 0-17   `M` Maternity Age: 12-55   `A` Adult Age: 15-124   `CC` CC Condition   `MC` Major Complication   `CD` Complex Dx   `HIV` HIV Related Dx

2002 Ingenix, Inc.

§ ✓5ᵗʰ **711.1**　**Arthropathy associated with Reiter's disease and**
[0-9]　　**nonspecific urethritis**
　　　　Code first underlying disease as:
　　　　　nonspecific urethritis (099.4)
　　　　　Reiter's disease (099.3)
　　DEF: Reiter's disease: joint disease marked by diarrhea, urethritis,
　　conjunctivitis, keratosis and arthritis; of unknown etiology; affects
　　young males.

　　DEF: Urethritis: inflamed urethra.

§ ✓5ᵗʰ **711.2**　**Arthropathy in Behçet's syndrome**
[0-9]　　　Code first underlying disease (136.1)
　　DEF: Behçet's syndrome: Chronic inflammatory disorder, of
　　unknown etiology; affects small blood vessels; causes ulcers of
　　oral and pharyngeal mucous membranes and genitalia, skin
　　lesions, retinal vasculitis, optic atrophy and severe uveitis.

§ ✓5ᵗʰ **711.3**　**Postdysenteric arthropathy**
[0-9]　　　Code first underlying disease as:
　　　　dysentery (009.0)
　　　　enteritis, infectious (008.0-009.3)
　　　　paratyphoid fever (002.1-002.9)
　　　　typhoid fever (002.0)
　　　EXCLUDES　salmonella arthritis (003.23)

§ ✓5ᵗʰ **711.4**　**Arthropathy associated with other bacterial**
[0-9]　　**diseases**
　　　　Code first underlying disease as:
　　　　diseases classifiable to 010-040, 090-099, except
　　　　　as in 711.1, 711.3, and 713.5
　　　　leprosy (030.0-030.9)
　　　　tuberculosis (015.0-015.9)
　　　EXCLUDES　gonococcal arthritis (098.50)
　　　　　　　meningococcal arthritis (036.82)

§ ✓5ᵗʰ **711.5**　**Arthropathy associated with other viral diseases**
[0-9]　　　Code first underlying disease as:
　　　　diseases classifiable to 045-049, 050-079, 480,
　　　　　487
　　　　O'nyong nyong (066.3)
　　　EXCLUDES　that due to rubella (056.71)

§ ✓5ᵗʰ **711.6**　**Arthropathy associated with mycoses**　　CC
[0-9]　　　Code first underlying disease (110.0-118)
　　CC Excl: For code 711.60: See code 711.08: **For code 711.61:** 015.80-
　　015.96, 017.90-017.96, 036.82, 056.71, 098.50-098.51, 098.59, 098.89,
　　711.00-711.01, 711.08-711.11, 711.18-711.21, 711.28-711.31, 711.38-
　　711.41, 711.48-711.51, 711.58-711.61, 711.68-711.71, 711.78-711.81,
　　711.88-711.91, 711.98-711.99, 712.10-712.11, 712.18-712.21, 712.28-
　　712.31, 712.38-712.81, 712.88-712.91, 712.98-712.99, 713.0-713.8, 714.0,
　　715.00, 715.09-715.11, 715.18-715.21, 715.28, 715.30-715.31, 715.38-
　　715.91, 715.98, 716.00-716.01, 716.08-716.11, 716.18-716.21, 716.28-
　　716.31, 716.38-716.41, 716.48-716.51, 716.58-716.61, 716.68, 716.80-
　　716.81, 716.88-716.91, 716.98-716.99, 718.00-718.01, 718.08, 719.00-
　　719.01, 719.08-719.11, 719.18-719.21, 719.28-719.31, 719.38-719.41,
　　719.48-719.51, 719.58-719.61, 719.68-719.70, 719.78-719.81, 719.88-
　　719.91, 719.98-719.99: **For code 711.62:** 015.80-015.96, 017.90-017.96,
　　036.82, 056.71, 098.50-098.51, 098.59, 098.89, 711.00, 711.02, 711.08-
　　711.10, 711.12, 711.18-711.20, 711.22, 711.28-711.30, 711.32, 711.38-
　　711.40, 711.42, 711.48-711.50, 711.52, 711.58-711.60, 711.62, 711.68-
　　711.70, 711.72, 711.78-711.80, 711.82, 711.88-711.90, 711.92,
　　711.98-711.99, 712.10, 712.12, 712.18-712.20, 712.22, 712.28-712.30,
　　712.32, 712.38-712.80, 712.82, 712.88-712.90, 712.92, 712.98-712.99,
　　713.0-713.8, 714.0, 715.00, 715.09-715.10, 715.12, 715.18, 715.22,
　　715.28, 715.30, 715.32, 715.38-715.90, 715.92, 715.98, 716.00, 716.02,
　　716.08-716.10, 716.12, 716.18-716.20, 716.22, 716.28-716.30, 716.32,
　　716.38-716.40, 716.42, 716.48-716.50, 716.52, 716.58-716.60, 716.62,
　　716.68, 716.80, 716.82, 716.88-716.90, 716.92, 716.98-716.99, 718.00,
　　718.02, 718.08, 719.00, 719.02, 719.08-719.10, 719.12, 719.18-719.20,
　　719.22, 719.28-719.30, 719.32, 719.38-719.40, 719.42, 719.48-719.50,
　　719.52, 719.58-719.60, 719.62, 719.68-719.70, 719.78-719.80, 719.82,
　　719.88-719.90, 719.92, 719.98-719.99: **For code 711.63:** 015.80-015.96,
　　017.90-017.96, 036.82, 056.71, 098.50-098.51, 098.59, 098.89, 711.00,
　　711.03, 711.08-711.10, 711.13, 711.18-711.20, 711.23, 711.28-711.30,

711.33, 711.38-711.40, 711.43, 711.48-711.50, 711.53, 711.58-711.60,
711.63, 711.68-711.70, 711.73, 711.78-711.80, 711.83, 711.88-711.90,
711.93, 711.98-711.99, 712.10, 712.13, 712.18-712.20, 712.23, 712.28-
712.30, 712.33, 712.38-712.80, 712.83, 712.88-712.90, 712.93, 712.98-
712.99, 713.0-713.8, 714.0, 715.00, 715.09-715.10, 715.13, 715.18, 715.20,
715.23, 715.28, 715.30, 715.33, 715.38-715.90, 715.93, 715.98, 716.00,
716.03, 716.08-716.10, 716.13, 716.18-716.20, 716.23, 716.28-716.30,
716.33, 716.38-716.40, 716.43, 716.48-716.50, 716.53, 716.58-716.60,
716.63, 716.68, 716.80, 716.83, 716.88-716.90, 716.93, 716.98-716.99,
718.00, 718.03, 718.08, 719.00, 719.03, 719.08-719.10, 719.13, 719.18-
719.20, 719.23, 719.28-719.30, 719.33, 719.38-719.40, 719.43, 719.48-
719.50, 719.53, 719.58-719.60, 719.63, 719.68-719.70, 719.78-719.80,
719.83, 719.88-719.90, 719.93, 719.98-719.99 **For code 711.64:** 015.80-
015.96, 017.90-017.96, 036.82, 056.71, 098.50-098.51, 098.59, 098.89,
711.00, 711.04, 711.08-711.10, 711.14, 711.18-711.20, 711.24, 711.28-
711.30, 711.34, 711.38-711.40, 711.44, 711.48-711.50, 711.5, 711.58-
711.60, 711.64, 711.68-711.70, 711.74, 711.78-711.80, 711.84, 711.88-
711.90, 711.94, 711.98-711.99, 712.10, 712.14, 712.18-712.20, 712.24,
712.28-712.30, 712.34, 712.38-712.80, 712.84, 712.88-712.90, 712.94,
712.98-712.99, 713.0-713.8, 714.0, 715.00-715.10, 715.14, 715.18, 715.20,
715.24, 715.28, 715.30, 715.34, 715.38-715.90, 715.94, 715.98, 716.00,
716.04, 716.08-716.10, 716.14, 716.18-716.20, 716.24, 716.28-716.30,
716.34, 716.38-716.40, 716.44, 716.48-716.50, 716.54, 716.58-716.60,
716.64, 716.68, 716.80, 716.84, 716.88-716.90, 716.94, 716.98-716.99,
718.00, 718.04, 718.08, 719.00, 719.04, 719.08-719.10, 719.14, 719.18-
719.20, 719.24, 719.28-719.30, 719.34, 719.38-719.40, 719.44, 719.48-
719.50, 719.54, 719.58-719.60, 719.64, 719.68-719.70, 719.78-719.80,
719.84, 719.88-719.90, 719.94, 719.98-719.99CC **For code 711.65:**
015.80-015.96, 017.90-017.96, 036.82, 056.71, 098.50-098.51, 098.59,
098.89, 711.00, 711.05, 711.08-711.10, 711.15, 711.18-711.20, 711.25,
711.28-711.30, 711.35, 711.38-711.40, 711.45, 711.48-711.50, 711.55,
711.58-711.60, 711.65, 711.68-711.70, 711.75, 711.78-711.80, 711.85,
711.88-711.90, 711.95, 711.98-711.99, 712.10, 712.15, 712.18-712.20,
712.25, 712.28-712.30, 712.35, 712.38-712.80, 712.85, 712.88-712.90,
712.95, 712.98-712.99, 713.0-713.8, 714.0, 715.00, 715.09-715.10, 715.15,
715.18, 715.20, 715.25, 715.28, 715.30, 715.35, 715.38-715.90, 715.95,
715.98, 716.00, 716.05, 716.08-716.10, 716.15, 716.18-716.20, 716.25,
716.28-716.30, 716.35, 716.38-716.40, 716.45, 716.48-716.50, 716.55,
716.58-716.60, 716.65, 716.68, 716.80, 716.85, 716.88-716.90, 716.95,
716.98-716.99, 718.00, 718.05, 718.08, 719.00, 719.05, 719.08-719.10,
719.15, 719.18-719.20, 719.25, 719.28-719.30, 719.35, 719.38-719.40,
719.45, 719.48-719.50, 719.55, 719.58-719.60, 719.65, 719.68-719.70,
719.75, 719.78-719.80, 719.85, 719.88-719.90, 719.95, 719.98-719.99
For code 711.66: 015.80-015.96, 017.90-017.96, 036.82, 056.71, 098.50-
098.51, 098.59, 098.89, 711.00, 711.06, 711.08-711.10, 711.16, 711.18-
711.20, 711.26, 711.28-711.30, 711.36, 711.38-711.40, 711.46, 711.48-
711.50, 711.56, 711.58-711.60, 711.66, 711.68-711.70, 711.76, 711.78-
711.80, 711.86, 711.88-711.90, 711.96, 711.98-711.99, 712.10, 712.16,
712.18-712.20, 712.26, 712.28-712.30, 712.36, 712.38-712.80, 712.86,
712.88-712.90, 712.96, 712.98-712.99, 713.0-713.8, 714.0, 715.00, 715.09-
715.10, 715.16, 715.18, 715.20, 715.26, 715.28, 715.30, 715.36, 715.38-
715.90, 715.96, 715.98, 716.00, 716.06, 716.08-716.10, 716.16, 716.18-
716.20, 716.26, 716.28-716.30, 716.36, 716.38-716.40, 716.46, 716.48-
716.50, 716.56, 716.58-716.60, 716.66, 716.68, 716.80, 716.86, 716.88-
716.90, 716.96, 716.98-716.99, 718.00, 718.08, 719.00, 719.06, 719.08-
719.10, 719.16, 719.18-719.20, 719.26, 719.28-719.30, 719.36, 719.38-
719.40, 719.46, 719.48-719.50, 719.56, 719.58-719.60, 719.66, 719.68-
719.70, 719.76, 719.78-719.80, 719.86, 719.88-719.90, 719.96, 719.98-
719.99 **For code 711.67:** 015.80-015.96, 017.90-017.96, 036.82, 056.71,
098.50-098.51, 098.59, 098.89, 711.00, 711.07-711.10, 711.17-711.20,
711.27-711.30, 711.37-711.40, 711.47-711.50, 711.57-711.60, 711.67-
711.70, 711.77-711.80, 711.87-711.90, 711.97-711.99, 712.10, 712.17-
712.20, 712.27-712.30, 712.37-712.80, 712.87-712.90, 712.97-712.99,
713.0-713.8, 714.0, 715.00, 715.09-715.10, 715.17-715.18, 715.20, 715.27-
715.28, 715.30, 715.37-715.90, 715.97-715.98, 716.00, 716.07-716.10,
716.17-716.20, 716.27-716.30, 716.37-716.40, 716.47-716.50, 716.57-
716.60, 716.67-716.80, 716.87-716.90, 716.97-716.99, 718.00, 718.07-
718.08, 719.00, 719.07-719.10, 719.17-719.20, 719.27-719.30, 719.37-
719.40, 719.47-719.50, 719.57-719.60, 719.67-719.70, 719.77-719.80,
719.87-719.90, 719.97-719.99 **For code 711.68:** 015.80-015.96, 017.90-
017.96, 036.82, 056.71, 098.50-098.51, 098.59, 098.89, 711.00-711.99,
712.10-712.99, 713.0-713.8, 714.0, 715.00, 715.09-715.10, 715.18-715.98,
716.00-716.99, 718.00-718.08, 719.00-719.10, 719.18-719.99 **For code
711.69:** See code 711.68

§ Requires fifth-digit. Valid digits are in [brackets] under each code. See beginning of section 710-739 for codes and definitions.

✓4ᵗʰ
✓5ᵗʰ Additional Digit Required　　Nonspecific PDx　　Unacceptable PDx　　Manifestation Code　　MSP Medicare Secondary Payer　　◄ Revised Text　　● New Code　　▲ Revised Code Title

2002 Ingenix, Inc.

Volume 1 — 211

§ ✓5ᵗʰ **711.7 Arthropathy associated with helminthiasis**
[0-9]
    Code first underlying disease as:
      filariasis (125.0-125.9)

§ ✓5ᵗʰ **711.8 Arthropathy associated with other infectious and parasitic diseases**
[0-9]
    Code first underlying disease as:
      diseases classifiable to 080-088, 100-104, 130-136

    EXCLUDES   *arthropathy associated with sarcoidosis (713.7)*

    AHA: 4Q, '91, 15; 3Q, '90, 14

§ ✓5ᵗʰ **711.9 Unspecified infective arthritis**
[0-9]
    Infective arthritis or polyarthritis (acute) (chronic) (subacute) NOS

✓4ᵗʰ **712 Crystal arthropathies**
    INCLUDES   crystal-induced arthritis and synovitis
    EXCLUDES   *gouty arthropathy (274.0)*
    DEF: Joint disease due to urate crystal deposit in joints or synovial membranes.

    The following fifth-digit subclassification is for use with category 712; valid digits are in [brackets] under each code. See above category 710 for definitions:

      0   **site unspecified**
      1   **shoulder region**
      2   **upper arm**
      3   **forearm**
      4   **hand**
      5   **pelvic region and thigh**
      6   **lower leg**
      7   **ankle and foot**
      8   **other specified sites**
      9   **multiple sites**

§ ✓5ᵗʰ **712.1 Chondrocalcinosis due to dicalcium phosphate crystals**
[0-9]
    Chondrocalcinosis due to dicalcium phosphate crystals (with other crystals)
    Code first underlying disease (275.4)

§ ✓5ᵗʰ **712.2 Chondrocalcinosis due to pyrophosphate crystals**
[0-9]
    Code first underlying disease (275.4)

§ ✓5ᵗʰ **712.3 Chondrocalcinosis, unspecified**
[0-9]
    Code first underlying disease (275.4)

§ ✓5ᵗʰ **712.8 Other specified crystal arthropathies**
[0-9]

§ ✓5ᵗʰ **712.9 Unspecified crystal arthropathy**
[0-9]

✓4ᵗʰ **713 Arthropathy associated with other disorders classified elsewhere**
    INCLUDES   arthritis
                 arthropathy   } associated with
                  polyarthritis   conditions classifiable
                  polyarthropathy   below

713.0 Arthropathy associated with other endocrine and metabolic disorders
    Code first underlying disease as:
      acromegaly (253.0)
      hemochromatosis (275.0)
      hyperparathyroidism (252.0)
      hypogammaglobulinemia (279.00-279.09)
      hypothyroidism (243-244.9)
      lipoid metabolism disorder (272.0-272.9)
      ochronosis (270.2)
    EXCLUDES   *arthropathy associated with:*
      amyloidosis (713.7)
      crystal deposition disorders, except gout (712.1-712.9)
      diabetic neuropathy (713.5)
      gouty arthropathy (274.0)

713.1 Arthropathy associated with gastrointestinal conditions other than infections
    Code first underlying disease as:
      regional enteritis (555.0-555.9)
      ulcerative colitis (556)

713.2 Arthropathy associated with hematological disorders
    Code first underlying disease as:
      hemoglobinopathy (282.4-282.7)
      hemophilia (286.0-286.2)
      leukemia (204.0-208.9)
      malignant reticulosis (202.3)
      multiple myelomatosis (203.0)
    EXCLUDES   *arthropathy associated with Henoch-Schönlein purpura (713.6)*

713.3 Arthropathy associated with dermatological disorders
    Code first underlying disease as:
      erythema multiforme (695.1)
      erythema nodosum (695.2)
    EXCLUDES   *psoriatic arthropathy (696.0)*

713.4 Arthropathy associated with respiratory disorders
    Code first underlying disease as:
      diseases classifiable to 490-519
    EXCLUDES   *arthropathy associated with respiratory infections (711.0, 711.4-711.8)*

713.5 Arthropathy associated with neurological disorders
    Charcôt's arthropathy } associated with diseases
    Neuropathic arthritis   classifiable elsewhere

    Code first underlying disease as:
      neuropathic joint disease [Charcôt's joints]:
        NOS (094.0)
        diabetic (250.6)
        syringomyelic (336.0)
        tabetic [syphilitic] (094.0)

713.6 Arthropathy associated with hypersensitivity reaction
    Code first underlying disease as:
      Henoch (-Schönlein) purpura (287.0)
      serum sickness (999.5)
    EXCLUDES   *allergic arthritis NOS (716.2)*

713.7 Other general diseases with articular involvement
    Code first underlying disease as:
      amyloidosis (277.3)
      familial Mediterranean fever (277.3)
      sarcoidosis (135)

    AHA: 2Q, '97, 12

713.8 Arthropathy associated with other condition classifiable elsewhere
    Code first underlying disease as:
      conditions classifiable elsewhere except as in 711.1-711.8, 712, and 713.0-713.7

✓4ᵗʰ **714 Rheumatoid arthritis and other inflammatory polyarthropathies**
    EXCLUDES   *rheumatic fever (390)*
               rheumatoid arthritis of spine NOS (720.0)

    AHA: 2Q, '95, 3

714.0 Rheumatoid arthritis
    Arthritis or polyarthritis:
      atrophic
      rheumatic (chronic)
    Use additional code to identify manifestation, as:
      myopathy (359.6)
      polyneuropathy (357.1)
    EXCLUDES   *juvenile rheumatoid arthritis NOS (714.30)*

    AHA: 1Q, '90, 5

    DEF: Chronic systemic disease principally of joints, manifested by inflammatory changes in articular structures and synovial membranes, atrophy, and loss in bone density.

---

§   Requires fifth-digit. Valid digits are in [brackets] under each code. See beginning of section 710-739 for codes and definitions.

N Newborn Age: 0   **P** Pediatric Age: 0-17   **M** Maternity Age: 12-55   **A** Adult Age: 15-124   **CC** CC Condition   **MC** Major Complication   **CD** Complex Dx   **HIV** HIV Related Dx

212 — Volume 1   *2002 Ingenix, Inc.*

714.1   **Felty's syndrome**   `CC`
Rheumatoid arthritis with splenoadenomegaly and
leukopenia
CC Excl: 036.82, 056.71, 711.00-711.99, 712.10-712.99, 713.0-713.8,
714.0-714.4, 715.00, 715.09-715.10, 715.18-715.98, 716.00-716.99,
718.00-718.08, 719.00-719.10, 719.18-719.70, 719.75-719.99

DEF: Syndrome marked by rheumatoid arthritis, splenomegaly,
leukopenia, pigmented spots on lower extremity skin, anemia, and
thrombocytopenia.

714.2   **Other rheumatoid arthritis with visceral or**   `CC`
systemic involvement
Rheumatoid carditis
CC Excl: See code 714.1

√5th **714.3**   **Juvenile chronic polyarthritis**
DEF: Rheumatoid arthritis of more than one joint; lasts longer than
six weeks in age 17 or younger; symptoms include fever,
erythematous rash, weight loss, lymphadenopathy,
hepatosplenomegaly and pericarditis.

    714.30   **Polyarticular juvenile rheumatoid**   `CC`
arthritis, chronic or unspecified
Juvenile rheumatoid arthritis NOS
Still's disease
CC Excl: See code 714.1

    714.31   **Polyarticular juvenile rheumatoid**   `CC`
arthritis, acute
CC Excl: See code 714.1

    714.32   **Pauciarticular juvenile rheumatoid**   `CC`
arthritis
CC Excl: See code 714.1

    714.33   **Monoarticular juvenile rheumatoid**   `CC`
arthritis
CC Excl: See code 714.1

714.4   **Chronic postrheumatic arthropathy**
Chronic rheumatoid nodular fibrositis
Jaccoud's syndrome
DEF: Persistent joint disorder; follows previous rheumatic infection.

√5th **714.8**   **Other specified inflammatory polyarthropathies**
    714.81   **Rheumatoid lung**
Caplan's syndrome
Diffuse interstitial rheumatoid disease of
lung
Fibrosing alveolitis, rheumatoid
DEF: Lung disorders associated with rheumatoid arthritis.

    714.89   **Other**
714.9   **Unspecified inflammatory polyarthropathy**
Inflammatory polyarthropathy or polyarthritis NOS
EXCLUDES   *polyarthropathy NOS (716.5)*

√4th **715**   **Osteoarthrosis and allied disorders**
Note: Localized, in the subcategories below, includes bilateral
involvement of the same site.
INCLUDES   arthritis or polyarthritis:
      degenerative
      hypertrophic
      degenerative joint disease
      osteoarthritis
EXCLUDES   *Marie-Strümpell spondylitis (720.0)*
osteoarthrosis [osteoarthritis] of spine (721.0-
721.9)

The following fifth-digit subclassification is for use with category
715; valid digits are in [brackets] under each code. See definitions
prior to category 710.
    0   **site unspecified**
    1   **shoulder region**
    2   **upper arm**
    3   **forearm**
    4   **hand**
    5   **pelvic region and thigh**
    6   **lower leg**
    7   **ankle and foot**
    8   **other specified sites**
    9   **multiple sites**

§ √5th **715.0**   **Osteoarthrosis, generalized**
[0,4,9]   Degenerative joint disease, involving multiple joints
Primary generalized hypertrophic osteoarthrosis
DEF: Chronic noninflammatory arthritis; marked by degenerated
articular cartilage and enlarged bone; symptoms include pain and
stiffness with activity; occurs among elderly.

§ √5th **715.1**   **Osteoarthrosis, localized, primary**
[0-8]   Localized osteoarthropathy, idiopathic
§ √5th **715.2**   **Osteoarthrosis, localized, secondary**
[0-8]   Coxae malum senilis
§ √5th **715.3**   **Osteoarthrosis, localized, not specified whether**
[0-8]   **primary or secondary**
Otto's pelvis
§ √5th **715.8**   **Osteoarthrosis involving, or with mention of more**
[0,9]   **than one site, but not specified as generalized**
§ √5th **715.9**   **Osteoarthrosis, unspecified whether generalized or**
[0-8]   **localized**
AHA: For code 715.90: 2Q, '97, 12

AHA: N-D, '87, 7

√4th **716**   **Other and unspecified arthropathies**
EXCLUDES   *cricoarytenoid arthropathy (478.79)*

The following fifth-digit subclassification is for use with
category 716; valid digits are in [brackets] under each code.
See above category 710 for definitions.
    0   **site unspecified**
    1   **shoulder region**
    2   **upper arm**
    3   **forearm**
    4   **hand**
    5   **pelvic region and thigh**
    6   **lower leg**
    7   **ankle and foot**
    8   **other specified sites**
    9   **multiple sites**

AHA: 2Q, '95, 3

§ √5th **716.0**   **Kaschin-Beck disease**
[0-9]   Endemic polyarthritis
DEF: Chronic degenerative disease of spine and peripheral joints;
occurs in eastern Siberian, northern Chinese, and Korean youth;
may be a mycotoxicosis caused by eating cereals infected with
fungus.

§ √5th **716.1**   **Traumatic arthropathy**
[0-9]   **AHA: For Code 716.11:** ▶ 1Q, '02, 9◀

¹   Nonspecific PDx=0
§   Requires fifth-digit. Valid digits are in [brackets] under each code. See beginning of section 710-739 for codes and definitions.

√4th / √5th Additional Digit Required   Nonspecific PDx   Unacceptable PDx   Manifestation Code   `MSP` Medicare Secondary Payer   ▶◀ Revised Text   ● New Code   ▲ Revised Code Title

§ √5ᵗʰ **716.2 Allergic arthritis**
[0-9]   EXCLUDES   *arthritis associated with Henoch-Schönlein purpura or serum sickness (713.6)*

§ √5ᵗʰ **716.3 Climacteric arthritis**   ♀
[0-9]   Menopausal arthritis

DEF: Ovarian hormone deficiency; causes pain in small joints, shoulders, elbows or knees; affects females at menopause; also called arthropathia ovaripriva.

§ √5ᵗʰ **716.4 Transient arthropathy**
[0-9]   EXCLUDES   *palindromic rheumatism (719.3)*

§ √5ᵗʰ **716.5 Unspecified polyarthropathy or polyarthritis**
[0-9]

§ √5ᵗʰ **716.6 Unspecified monoarthritis**
[0-8]   Coxitis

§ √5ᵗʰ **716.8 Other specified arthropathy**
[0-9]

§ √5ᵗʰ **716.9 Arthropathy, unspecified**
[0-9]   Arthritis ⎫
     Arthropathy ⎬ (acute) (chronic) (subacute)
     ⎭

    Articular rheumatism (chronic)
    Inflammation of joint NOS

√4ᵗʰ **717 Internal derangement of knee**

INCLUDES   degeneration ⎫
     rupture, old ⎬ of articular cartilage or
     tear, old ⎭ meniscus of knee

EXCLUDES   *acute derangement of knee (836.0-836.6)*
    ankylosis (718.5)
    contracture (718.4)
    current injury (836.0-836.6)
    deformity (736.4-736.6)
    recurrent dislocation (718.3)

717.0 Old bucket handle tear of medial meniscus
    Old bucket handle tear of unspecified cartilage

717.1 Derangement of anterior horn of medial meniscus

717.2 Derangement of posterior horn of medial meniscus

717.3 Other and unspecified derangement of medial meniscus
    Degeneration of internal semilunar cartilage

√5ᵗʰ **717.4 Derangement of lateral meniscus**
    717.40 Derangement of lateral meniscus, unspecified
    717.41 Bucket handle tear of lateral meniscus
    717.42 Derangement of anterior horn of lateral meniscus
    717.43 Derangement of posterior horn of lateral meniscus
    717.49 Other

717.5 Derangement of meniscus, not elsewhere classified
    Congenital discoid meniscus
    Cyst of semilunar cartilage
    Derangement of semilunar cartilage NOS

Disruption and Tears of Meniscus

Bucket-handle

Flap-type

Radial
Peripheral

Horizontal cleavage

Vertical

Congenital discoid meniscus

Internal Derangements of Knee

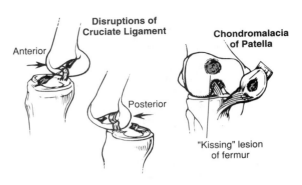

Disruptions of Cruciate Ligament

Anterior

Posterior

Chondromalacia of Patella

"Kissing" lesion of fermur

717.6 Loose body in knee
    Joint mice, knee
    Rice bodies, knee (joint)

DEF: The presence in the joint synovial area of a small, frequently calcified, loose body created from synovial membrane, organized fibrin fragments of articular cartilage or arthritis osteophytes.

717.7 Chondromalacia of patella
    Chondromalacia patellae
    Degeneration [softening] of articular cartilage of patella

AHA: M-A, '85, 14; N-D, '84, 9

DEF: Softened patella cartilage.

√5ᵗʰ **717.8 Other internal derangement of knee**
    717.81 Old disruption of lateral collateral ligament
    717.82 Old disruption of medial collateral ligament
    717.83 Old disruption of anterior cruciate ligament
    717.84 Old disruption of posterior cruciate ligament
    717.85 Old disruption of other ligaments of knee
       Capsular ligament of knee
    717.89 Other
       Old disruption of ligaments NOS

717.9 Unspecified internal derangement of knee
    Derangement NOS of knee

√4ᵗʰ **718 Other derangement of joint**
    EXCLUDES   *current injury (830.0-848.9)*
       jaw (524.6)

The following fifth-digit subclassification is for use with category 718; valid digits are in [brackets] under each code. See above category 710 for definitions.

    0 **site unspecified**
    1 **shoulder region**
    2 **upper arm**
    3 **forearm**
    4 **hand**
    5 **pelvic region and thigh**
    6 **lower leg**
    7 **ankle and foot**
    8 **other specified sites**
    9 **multiple sites**

§ √5ᵗʰ **718.0 Articular cartilage disorder**
[0-5,7-9]   Meniscus: Meniscus:
    disorder   tear, old
    rupture, old   Old rupture of ligament(s) of joint NOS

    EXCLUDES   *articular cartilage disorder:*
       in ochronosis (270.2)
       knee (717.0-717.9)
    chondrocalcinosis (275.4)
    metastatic calcification (275.4)

§ Requires fifth-digit. Valid digits are in [brackets] under each code. See beginning of section 710-739 for codes and definitions.

N Newborn Age: 0   P Pediatric Age: 0-17   M Maternity Age: 12-55   A Adult Age: 15-124   CC CC Condition   MC Major Complication   CD Complex Dx   HIV HIV Related Dx

§ ✓5ᵗʰ **718.1 Loose body in joint**
[0-5,7-9]   Joint mice

> EXCLUDES   knee (717.6)

AHA: For code 718.17: 2Q, '01, 15

DEF: Calcified loose bodies in synovial fluid; due to arthritic osteophytes.

§ ✓5ᵗʰ **718.2 Pathological dislocation**
[0-9]   Dislocation or displacement of joint, not recurrent
and not current injury
Spontaneous dislocation (joint)

§ ✓5ᵗʰ **718.3 Recurrent dislocation of joint**
[0-9]   **AHA:** N-D, '87, 7

§ ✓5ᵗʰ² **718.4 Contracture of joint**
[0-9]   **AHA:** 4Q, '98, 40

§ ✓5ᵗʰ¹ **718.5 Ankylosis of joint**
[0-9]   Ankylosis of joint (fibrous) (osseous)

> EXCLUDES   spine (724.9)
> stiffness of joint without mention of ankylosis (719.5)

DEF: Immobility and solidification, of joint; due to disease, injury or surgical procedure.

§ ✓5ᵗʰ **718.6 Unspecified intrapelvic protrusion of acetabulum**
[0,5]   Protrusio acetabuli, unspecified

DEF: Sinking of the floor of acetabulum; causing femoral head to protrude, limits hip movement; of unknown etiology.

§ ✓5ᵗʰ **718.7 Developmental dislocation of joint**
[0-9]
> EXCLUDES   ▶congenital dislocation of joint
> (754.0-755.8)
> traumatic dislocation of joint
> (830-839)◀

AHA: 4Q, '01, 48

§ ✓5ᵗʰ **718.8 Other joint derangement, not elsewhere classified**
[0-9]   Flail joint (paralytic)   Instability of joint

> EXCLUDES   deformities classifiable to 736 (736.0-736.9)

AHA: For code 718.81: 2Q, '00, 14

§ ✓5ᵗʰ **718.9 Unspecified derangement of joint**
[0-5,7-9]   EXCLUDES   knee (717.9)

✓4ᵗʰ **719 Other and unspecified disorders of joint**

> EXCLUDES   jaw (524.6)

The following fifth-digit subclassification is for use with category 719; valid digits are in [brackets] under each code. See above category 710 for definitions.

    0 site unspecified
    1 shoulder region
    2 upper arm
    3 forearm
    4 hand
    5 pelvic region and thigh
    6 lower leg /Knee
    7 ankle and foot
    8 other specified sites
    9 multiple sites

§ ✓5ᵗʰ **719.0 Effusion of joint**
[0-9]   Hydrarthrosis
Swelling of joint, with or without pain
> EXCLUDES   intermittent hydrarthrosis (719.3)

§ ✓5ᵗʰ **719.1 Hemarthrosis**
[0-9]   EXCLUDES   current injury (840.0-848.9)

§ ✓5ᵗʰ **719.2 Villonodular synovitis**
[0-9]

DEF: Overgrowth of synovial tissue, especially at knee joint; due to macrophage infiltration of giant cells in synovial villi and fibrous nodules.

Joint Derangements and Disorders

Loose body in joint — Dislocation of joint — Joint contracture — Ankylosis of joint — Synovial effusion (fluid) — Hemarthrosis (blood)

§ ✓5ᵗʰ **719.3 Palindromic rheumatism**
[0-9]   Hench-Rosenberg syndrome
Intermittent hydrarthrosis

DEF: Recurrent episodes of afebrile arthritis and periarthritis marked by their complete disappearance after a few days or hours; causes swelling, redness, and disability usually affecting only one joint; no known cause; affects adults of either sex.

§ ✓5ᵗʰ **719.4 Pain in joint**
[0-9]   Arthralgia
AHA: For code 719.46: 1Q, '01, 3

§ ✓5ᵗʰ **719.5 Stiffness of joint, not elsewhere classified**
[0-9]

§ ✓5ᵗʰ **719.6 Other symptoms referable to joint**
[0-9]   Joint crepitus   Snapping hip
AHA: 1Q, '94, 15

§ ✓5ᵗʰ **719.7 Difficulty in walking**
[0,5-9]   EXCLUDES   abnormality of gait (781.2)

§ ✓5ᵗʰ **719.8 Other specified disorders of joint**
[0-9]   Calcification of joint   Fistula of joint
> EXCLUDES   temporomandibular joint-pain-dysfunction syndrome [Costen's syndrome] (524.6)

(handwritten: 719.70 NOt PT justificat code)

§ ✓5ᵗʰ **719.9 Unspecified disorder of joint**
[0-9]

DORSOPATHIES (720-724)

> EXCLUDES   curvature of spine (737.0-737.9)
> osteochondrosis of spine (juvenile) (732.0)
> adult (732.8)

✓4ᵗʰ **720 Ankylosing spondylitis and other inflammatory spondylopathies**

720.0 Ankylosing spondylitis
Rheumatoid arthritis of spine NOS
Spondylitis:
    Marie-Strümpell
    rheumatoid

DEF: Rheumatoid arthritis of spine and sacroiliac joints; fusion and deformity in spine follows; affects mainly males; cause unknown.

720.1 Spinal enthesopathy
Disorder of peripheral ligamentous or muscular attachments of spine
Romanus lesion

DEF: Tendinous or muscular vertebral bone attachment abnormality.

720.2 Sacroiliitis, not elsewhere classified
Inflammation of sacroiliac joint NOS

DEF: Pain due to inflammation in joint, at juncture of sacrum and hip.

---

¹ Nonspecific PDx=0
² Nonspecific PDx=9
§ Requires fifth-digit. Valid digits are in [brackets] under each code. See beginning of section 710-739 for codes and definitions.

✓4ᵗʰ Additional Digit Required   Nonspecific PDx   Unacceptable PDx   Manifestation Code   **MSP** Medicare Secondary Payer   ▶◀ Revised Text   ● New Code   ▲ Revised Code Title

Musculoskeletal and Connective Tissue 720.8–722.52

√5th **720.8 Other inflammatory spondylopathies**

720.81 *Inflammatory spondylopathies in diseases classified elsewhere*

Code first underlying disease as:
tuberculosis (015.0)

720.89 Other

720.9 Unspecified inflammatory spondylopathy
Spondylitis NOS

√4th **721 Spondylosis and allied disorders**

AHA: 2Q, '89, 14

DEF: Degenerative changes in spinal joint.

721.0 Cervical spondylosis without myelopathy
Cervical or cervicodorsal: Cervical or cervicodorsal:
   arthritis   spondylarthritis
   osteoarthritis

721.1 Cervical spondylosis with myelopathy
Anterior spinal artery compression syndrome
Spondylogenic compression of cervical spinal cord
Vertebral artery compression syndrome

721.2 Thoracic spondylosis without myelopathy
Thoracic: Thoracic:
   arthritis   spondylarthritis
   osteoarthritis

721.3 Lumbosacral spondylosis without myelopathy
Lumbar or lumbosacral: Lumbar or lumbosacral:
   arthritis   spondylarthritis
   osteoarthritis

√5th **721.4 Thoracic or lumbar spondylosis with myelopathy**

721.41 Thoracic region
Spondylogenic compression of thoracic spinal cord

721.42 Lumbar region
Spondylogenic compression of lumbar spinal cord

721.5 Kissing spine
Baastrup's syndrome

DEF: Compression of spinous processes of adjacent vertebrae; due to mutual contact.

721.6 Ankylosing vertebral hyperostosis

721.7 Traumatic spondylopathy
Kümmell's disease or spondylitis

721.8 Other allied disorders of spine

√5th **721.9 Spondylosis of unspecified site**

721.90 Without mention of myelopathy
Spinal:
   arthritis (deformans) (degenerative)
     (hypertrophic)
   osteoarthritis NOS
Spondylarthrosis NOS

721.91 With myelopathy
Spondylogenic compression of spinal cord NOS

Normal Anatomy of Vertebral Disc

Normal Top View   Normal Side View

Derangement of Vertebral Disc

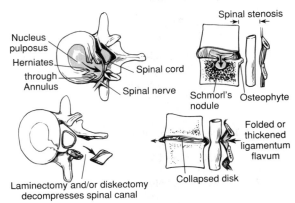

Laminectomy and/or diskectomy decompresses spinal canal

√4th **722 Intervertebral disc disorders**

AHA: 1Q, '88. 10

722.0 Displacement of cervical intervertebral disc without myelopathy   Ⓐ
Neuritis (brachial) or radiculitis due to displacement or rupture of cervical intervertebral disc
Any condition classifiable to 722.2 of the cervical or cervicothoracic intervertebral disc

√5th **722.1 Displacement of thoracic or lumbar intervertebral disc without myelopathy**

722.10 Lumbar intervertebral disc without myelopathy   Ⓐ
Lumbago or sciatica due to displacement of intervertebral disc
Neuritis or radiculitis due to displacement or rupture of lumbar intervertebral disc
Any condition classifiable to 722.2 of the lumbar or lumbosacral intervertebral disc

722.11 Thoracic intervertebral disc without myelopathy   Ⓐ
Any condition classifiable to 722.2 of thoracic intervertebral disc

722.2 Displacement of intervertebral disc, site unspecified, without myelopathy   Ⓐ
Discogenic syndrome NOS
Herniation of nucleus pulposus NOS
Intervertebral disc NOS:
   extrusion
   prolapse
   protrusion
   rupture
Neuritis or radiculitis due to displacement or rupture of intervertebral disc

√5th **722.3 Schmorl's nodes**

DEF: Irregular bone defect in the margin of the vertebral body; causes herniation into end plate of vertebral body.

722.30 Unspecified region   Ⓐ
722.31 Thoracic region   Ⓐ
722.32 Lumbar region   Ⓐ
722.39 Other   Ⓐ

722.4 Degeneration of cervical intervertebral disc   Ⓐ
Degeneration of cervicothoracic intervertebral disc

√5th **722.5 Degeneration of thoracic or lumbar intervertebral disc**

722.51 Thoracic or thoracolumbar intervertebral disc   Ⓐ

722.52 Lumbar or lumbosacral intervertebral disc   Ⓐ

Ⓝ Newborn Age: 0   Ⓟ Pediatric Age: 0-17   Ⓜ Maternity Age: 12-55   Ⓐ Adult Age: 15-124   **CC** CC Condition   **MC** Major Complication   **CD** Complex Dx   **HIV** HIV Related Dx

216 — Volume 1   *2002 Ingenix, Inc.*

722.6 Degeneration of intervertebral disc, site unspecified   A
  Degenerative disc disease NOS
  Narrowing of intervertebral disc or space NOS

✓5th **722.7 Intervertebral disc disorder with myelopathy**
  722.70 Unspecified region   A
  722.71 Cervical region   A
  722.72 Thoracic region   A
  722.73 Lumbar region   A

✓5th **722.8 Postlaminectomy syndrome**
  AHA: J-F, '87, 7

  DEF: Spinal disorder due to spinal laminectomy surgery.

  722.80 Unspecified region   CC A
    CC Excl: 722.51-722.93

  722.81 Cervical region   CC A
    CC Excl: See code 722.80

  722.82 Thoracic region   CC A
    CC Excl: See code 722.80

  722.83 Lumbar region   CC A
    CC Excl: See code 722.80

    AHA: 2Q, '97, 15

✓5th **722.9 Other and unspecified disc disorder**
  Calcification of intervertebral cartilage or disc
  Discitis
  722.90 Unspecified region   A
    AHA: N-D, '84, 19

  722.91 Cervical region   A
  722.92 Thoracic region   A
  722.93 Lumbar region   A

✓4th **723 Other disorders of cervical region**
  EXCLUDES   conditions due to:
    intervertebral disc disorders (722.0-722.9)
    spondylosis (721.0-721.9)

  AHA: 3Q, '94, 14; 2Q, '89, 14

  723.0 Spinal stenosis in cervical region
  723.1 Cervicalgia
    Pain in neck
    DEF: Pain in cervical spine or neck region.

  723.2 Cervicocranial syndrome
    Barré-Liéou syndrome
    Posterior cervical sympathetic syndrome
    DEF: Neurologic disorder of upper cervical spine and nerve roots.

Spinal Stenosis in Cervical Region

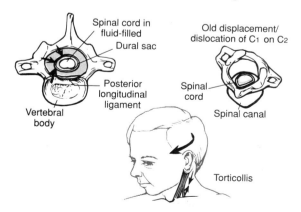

Spinal cord in fluid-filled Dural sac
Spinal cord
Posterior longitudinal ligament
Vertebral body
Old displacement/dislocation of C1 on C2
Spinal cord
Spinal canal
Torticollis

723.3 Cervicobrachial syndrome (diffuse)
  AHA: N-D, '85, 12

  DEF: Complex of symptoms due to scalenus anterior muscle compressing the brachial plexus; pain radiates from shoulder to arm or back of neck.

723.4 Brachial neuritis or radiculitis NOS   CC
  Cervical radiculitis
  Radicular syndrome of upper limbs
  CC Excl: 722.6-722.71, 722.80-722.81, 722.90-722.91, 723.0-723.9

723.5 Torticollis, unspecified   CC
  Contracture of neck
  EXCLUDES   congenital (754.1)
    due to birth injury (767.8)
    hysterical (300.11)
    ►ocular torticollis (781.93)◄
    psychogenic (306.0)
    spasmodic (333.83)
    traumatic, current (847.0)
  CC Excl: 053.71, 722.6-722.71, 722.80-722.81, 722.90-722.91, 723.0-723.9
  AHA: 2Q, '01, 21; 1Q, '95, 7

  DEF: Abnormally positioned neck relative to head; due to cervical muscle or fascia contractions; also called wryneck.

723.6 Panniculitis specified as affecting neck
  DEF: Inflammation of the panniculus adiposus (subcutaneous fat) in the neck.

723.7 Ossification of posterior longitudinal ligament in cervical region

723.8 Other syndromes affecting cervical region
  Cervical syndrome NEC
  Klippel's disease
  Occipital neuralgia
  AHA: 1Q, '00, 7

723.9 Unspecified musculoskeletal disorders and symptoms referable to neck
  Cervical (region) disorder NOS

✓4th **724 Other and unspecified disorders of back**
  EXCLUDES   collapsed vertebra (code to cause, e.g., osteoporosis, 733.00-733.09)
    conditions due to:
      intervertebral disc disorders (722.0-722.9)
      spondylosis (721.0-721.9)
  AHA: 2Q, '89, 14

✓5th **724.0 Spinal stenosis, other than cervical**
  724.00 Spinal stenosis, unspecified region   A
  724.01 Thoracic region   A
  724.02 Lumbar region   A
    AHA: 4Q, '99, 13

  724.09 Other   A

724.1 Pain in thoracic spine

724.2 Lumbago
  Low back pain   Lumbalgia
  Low back syndrome
  AHA: N-D, '85, 12

724.3 Sciatica
  Neuralgia or neuritis of sciatic nerve
  EXCLUDES   specified lesion of sciatic nerve (355.0)
  AHA: 2Q, '89, 12

724.4 Thoracic or lumbosacral neuritis or radiculitis, unspecified
  Radicular syndrome of lower limbs
  AHA: 2Q, '99, 3

724.5 Backache, unspecified
  Vertebrogenic (pain) syndrome NOS

724.6 Disorders of sacrum
  Ankylosis
  Instability } lumbosacral or sacroiliac (joint)

Musculoskeletal and Connective Tissue 722.6–724.6

Musculoskeletal and Connective Tissue 724.7–727.00

✓5ᵗʰ **724.7 Disorders of coccyx**
    724.70 Unspecified disorder of coccyx
    724.71 Hypermobility of coccyx
    724.79 Other
      Coccygodynia

724.8 Other symptoms referable to back
  Ossification of posterior longitudinal ligament NOS
  Panniculitis specified as sacral or affecting back

724.9 Other unspecified back disorders
  Ankylosis of spine NOS
  Compression of spinal nerve root NEC
  Spinal disorder NOS
  EXCLUDES sacroiliitis (720.2)

RHEUMATISM, EXCLUDING THE BACK (725-729)

INCLUDES disorders of muscles and tendons and their attachments, and of other soft tissues

725 Polymyalgia rheumatica
DEF: Joint and muscle pain, pelvis, and shoulder girdle stiffness, high sedimentation rate and temporal arteritis; occurs in elderly.

✓4ᵗʰ **726 Peripheral enthesopathies and allied syndromes**
Note: Enthesopathies are disorders of peripheral ligamentous or muscular attachments.
EXCLUDES spinal enthesopathy (720.1)

726.0 Adhesive capsulitis of shoulder

✓5ᵗʰ **726.1 Rotator cuff syndrome of shoulder and allied disorders**
  726.10 Disorders of bursae and tendons in shoulder region, unspecified
    Rotator cuff syndrome NOS
    Supraspinatus syndrome NOS
    AHA: 2Q, '01, 11

  726.11 Calcifying tendinitis of shoulder
  726.12 Bicipital tenosynovitis
  726.19 Other specified disorders
    EXCLUDES complete rupture of rotator cuff, nontraumatic (727.61)

726.2 Other affections of shoulder region, not elsewhere classified
  Periarthritis of shoulder
  Scapulohumeral fibrositis

✓5ᵗʰ **726.3 Enthesopathy of elbow region**
  726.30 Enthesopathy of elbow, unspecified
  726.31 Medial epicondylitis
  726.32 Lateral epicondylitis
    Epicondylitis NOS   Tennis elbow
    Golfers' elbow
  726.33 Olecranon bursitis
    Bursitis of elbow
  726.39 Other

726.4 Enthesopathy of wrist and carpus
  Bursitis of hand or wrist
  Periarthritis of wrist

726.5 Enthesopathy of hip region
  Bursitis of hip   Psoas tendinitis
  Gluteal tendinitis   Trochanteric tendinitis
  Iliac crest spur

✓5ᵗʰ **726.6 Enthesopathy of knee**
  726.60 Enthesopathy of knee, unspecified
    Bursitis of knee NOS
  726.61 Pes anserinus tendinitis or bursitis
    DEF: Inflamed tendons of sartorius, gracilis and semitendinosus muscles of medial aspect of knee.
  726.62 Tibial collateral ligament bursitis
    Pellegrini-Stieda syndrome
  726.63 Fibular collateral ligament bursitis
  726.64 Patellar tendinitis
  726.65 Prepatellar bursitis

726.69 Other
  Bursitis:
    infrapatellar
    subpatellar

✓5ᵗʰ **726.7 Enthesopathy of ankle and tarsus**
  726.70 Enthesopathy of ankle and tarsus, unspecified
    Metatarsalgia NOS
    EXCLUDES Morton's metatarsalgia (355.6)
  726.71 Achilles bursitis or tendinitis
  726.72 Tibialis tendinitis
    Tibialis (anterior) (posterior) tendinitis
  726.73 Calcaneal spur
    DEF: Overgrowth of calcaneous bone; causes pain on walking; due to chronic avulsion injury of plantar fascia from calcaneus.
  726.79 Other
    Peroneal tendinitis

726.8 Other peripheral enthesopathies

✓5ᵗʰ **726.9 Unspecified enthesopathy**
  726.90 Enthesopathy of unspecified site
    Capsulitis NOS
    Periarthritis NOS
    Tendinitis NOS
  726.91 Exostosis of unspecified site
    Bone spur NOS
    AHA: 2Q, '01, 15

✓4ᵗʰ **727 Other disorders of synovium, tendon, and bursa**

✓5ᵗʰ **727.0 Synovitis and tenosynovitis**
  727.00 Synovitis and tenosynovitis, unspecified
    Synovitis NOS
    Tenosynovitis NOS

Bunion

Ganglia

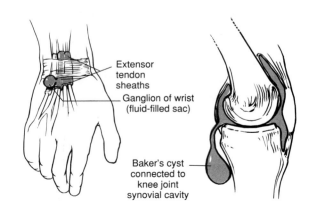

727.01 Synovitis and tenosynovitis in diseases classified elsewhere

Code first underlying disease as:
tuberculosis (015.0-015.9)

> **EXCLUDES**   crystal-induced (275.4)
> gonococcal (098.51)
> gouty (274.0)
> syphilitic (095.7)

727.02 Giant cell tumor of tendon sheath

727.03 Trigger finger (acquired)

> DEF: Stenosing tenosynovitis or nodule in flexor tendon; cessation of flexion or extension movement in finger, followed by snapping into place.

727.04 Radial styloid tenosynovitis
de Quervain's disease

727.05 Other tenosynovitis of hand and wrist

727.06 Tenosynovitis of foot and ankle

727.09 Other

727.1 Bunion

> DEF: Enlarged first metatarsal head due to inflamed bursa; results in laterally displaced great toe.

727.2 Specific bursitides often of occupational origin

Beat:
  elbow
  hand
  knee
Miners':
  elbow
  knee

Chronic crepitant synovitis of wrist

727.3 Other bursitis
Bursitis NOS

> **EXCLUDES**   bursitis:
> gonococcal (098.52)
> subacromial (726.19)
> subcoracoid (726.19)
> subdeltoid (726.19)
> syphilitic (095.7)
> "frozen shoulder" (726.0)

✓5ᵗʰ **727.4 Ganglion and cyst of synovium, tendon, and bursa**

727.40 Synovial cyst, unspecified

> **EXCLUDES**   that of popliteal space (727.51)

AHA: 2Q, '97, 6

727.41 Ganglion of joint

727.42 Ganglion of tendon sheath

727.43 Ganglion, unspecified

727.49 Other
Cyst of bursa

✓5ᵗʰ **727.5 Rupture of synovium**

727.50 Rupture of synovium, unspecified

727.51 Synovial cyst of popliteal space
Baker's cyst (knee)

727.59 Other

✓5ᵗʰ **727.6 Rupture of tendon, nontraumatic**

727.60 Nontraumatic rupture of unspecified tendon

727.61 Complete rupture of rotator cuff

727.62 Tendons of biceps (long head)

727.63 Extensor tendons of hand and wrist

727.64 Flexor tendons of hand and wrist

727.65 Quadriceps tendon

727.66 Patellar tendon

727.67 Achilles tendon

727.68 Other tendons of foot and ankle

727.69 Other

✓5ᵗʰ **727.8 Other disorders of synovium, tendon, and bursa**

727.81 Contracture of tendon (sheath)
Short Achilles tendon (acquired)

727.82 Calcium deposits in tendon and bursa
Calcification of tendon NOS
Calcific tendinitis NOS

> **EXCLUDES**   peripheral ligamentous or muscular attachments (726.0-726.9)

727.83 Plica syndrome
Plica knee

AHA: 4Q, '00, 44

> DEF: A fold in the synovial tissue that begins to form before birth, creating a septum between two pockets of synovial tissue; two most common plicae are the medial patellar plica and the suprapatellar plica. Plica syndrome, or plica knee, refers to symptomatic plica. Experienced by females more commonly than males.

727.89 Other
Abscess of bursa or tendon

> **EXCLUDES**   xanthomatosis localized to tendons (272.7)

AHA: 2Q, '89, 15

727.9 Unspecified disorder of synovium, tendon, and bursa

✓4ᵗʰ **728 Disorders of muscle, ligament, and fascia**

> **EXCLUDES**   enthesopathies (726.0-726.9)
> muscular dystrophies (359.0-359.1)
> myoneural disorders (358.0-358.9)
> myopathies (359.2-359.9)
> old disruption of ligaments of knee (717.81-717.89)

728.0 Infective myositis   **CC**
Myositis:
  purulent
  suppurative

> **EXCLUDES**   myositis:
> epidemic (074.1)
> interstitial (728.81)
> syphilitic (095.6)
> tropical (040.81)

CC Excl: 728.0, 728.11-728.3, 728.81, 728.86

> DEF: Inflamed connective septal tissue of muscle.

✓5ᵗʰ **728.1 Muscular calcification and ossification**

728.10 Calcification and ossification, unspecified
Massive calcification (paraplegic)

728.11 Progressive myositis ossificans

> DEF: Progressive myositic disease; marked by bony tissue formed by voluntary muscle; occurs among very young.

728.12 Traumatic myositis ossificans
Myositis ossificans (circumscripta)

728.13 Postoperative heterotopic calcification

> DEF: Abnormal formation of calcium deposits in muscular tissue after surgery, marked by a corresponding loss of muscle tone and tension.

728.19 Other
Polymyositis ossificans

728.2 Muscular wasting and disuse atrophy, not elsewhere classified
Amyotrophia NOS
Myofibrosis

> **EXCLUDES**   neuralgic amyotrophy (353.5)
> progressive muscular atrophy (335.0-335.9)

728.3 Other specific muscle disorders
Arthrogryposis
Immobility syndrome (paraplegic)

> **EXCLUDES**   arthrogryposis multiplex congenita (754.89)
> stiff-man syndrome (333.91)

728.4 Laxity of ligament

728.5 Hypermobility syndrome

✓4ᵗʰ ✓5ᵗʰ Additional Digit Required   Nonspecific PDx   Unacceptable PDx   Manifestation Code   **MSP** Medicare Secondary Payer   ▶◀ Revised Text   ● New Code   ▲ Revised Code Title

2002 Ingenix, Inc.   **Volume 1 — 219**

Musculoskeletal and Connective Tissue 728.6–729.9

728.6 Contracture of palmar fascia   A
Dupuytren's contracture

DEF: Dupuytren's contracture: flexion deformity of finger, due to shortened, thickened fibrosing of palmar fascia; cause unknown; associated with long-standing epilepsy; occurs more often in males.

√5ᵗʰ **728.7 Other fibromatoses**

728.71 Plantar fascial fibromatosis
Contracture of plantar fascia
Plantar fasciitis (traumatic)

DEF: Plantar fascia fibromatosis; causes nodular swelling and pain; not associated with contractures.

728.79 Other
Garrod's or knuckle pads
Nodular fasciitis
Pseudosarcomatous fibromatosis (proliferative) (subcutaneous)

DEF: Knuckle pads: Pea-size nodules on dorsal surface of interphalangeal joints; new growth of fibrous tissue with thickened dermis and epidermis.

√5ᵗʰ **728.8 Other disorders of muscle, ligament, and fascia**

728.81 Interstitial myositis
DEF: Inflammation of septal connective parts of muscle tissue.

728.82 Foreign body granuloma of muscle
Talc granuloma of muscle

728.83 Rupture of muscle, nontraumatic

728.84 Diastasis of muscle
Diastasis recti (abdomen)

EXCLUDES   *diastasis recti complicating pregnancy, labor, and delivery (665.8)*

DEF: Muscle separation, such as recti abdominis after repeated pregnancies.

728.85 Spasm of muscle

728.86 Necrotizing fasciitis   CC
Use additional code to identify:
infectious organism (041.00-041.89)
gangrene (785.4), if applicable

CC Excl: 728.0, 728.11-728.19, 728.2, 728.3, 728.82, 728.86

AHA: 4Q, '95, 54

DEF: Fulminating infection begins with extensive cellulitis, spreads to superficial and deep fascia; causes thrombosis of subcutaneous vessels, and gangrene of underlying tissue.

728.89 Other
Eosinophilic fasciitis
Use additional E code to identify drug, if drug induced

AHA: 2Q, '01, 14, 15

DEF: Eosinophilic fasciitis: inflammation of fascia of extremities associated with eosinophilia, edema, and swelling; occurs alone or as part of myalgia syndrome.

728.9 Unspecified disorder of muscle, ligament, and fascia
AHA: 4Q, '88, 11

√4ᵗʰ **729 Other disorders of soft tissues**
EXCLUDES   *acroparesthesia (443.89)*
carpal tunnel syndrome (354.0)
disorders of the back (720.0-724.9)
entrapment syndromes (354.0-355.9)
palindromic rheumatism (719.3)
periarthritis (726.0-726.9)
psychogenic rheumatism (306.0)

729.0 Rheumatism, unspecified and fibrositis
DEF: General term describes diseases of muscle, tendon, nerve, joint, or bone; symptoms include pain and stiffness.

729.1 Myalgia and myositis, unspecified
Fibromyositis NOS

DEF: Myalgia: muscle pain.

DEF: Myositis: inflamed voluntary muscle.

DEF: Fibromyositis: inflamed fibromuscular tissue.

729.2 Neuralgia, neuritis, and radiculitis, unspecified
EXCLUDES   *brachial radiculitis (723.4)*
cervical radiculitis (723.4)
lumbosacral radiculitis (724.4)
mononeuritis (354.0-355.9)
radiculitis due to intervertebral disc involvement (722.0-722.2, 722.7)
sciatica (724.3)

DEF: Neuralgia: paroxysmal pain along nerve symptoms include brief pain and tenderness at point nerve exits.

DEF: Neuritis: inflamed nerve, symptoms include paresthesia, paralysis and loss of reflexes at nerve site.

DEF: Radiculitis: inflamed nerve root.

√5ᵗʰ **729.3 Panniculitis, unspecified**
DEF: Inflammatory reaction of subcutaneous fat; causes nodules; often develops in abdominal region.

729.30 Panniculitis, unspecified site
Weber-Christian disease

DEF: Febrile, nodular, nonsuppurative, relapsing inflammation of subcutaneous fat.

729.31 Hypertrophy of fat pad, knee
Hypertrophy of infrapatellar fat pad

729.39 Other site
EXCLUDES   *panniculitis specified as (affecting):*
back (724.8)
neck (723.6)
sacral (724.8)

729.4 Fasciitis, unspecified
EXCLUDES   *necrotizing fasciitis (728.86)*
nodular fasciitis (728.79)

AHA: 2Q, '94, 13

729.5 Pain in limb

729.6 Residual foreign body in soft tissue
EXCLUDES   *foreign body granuloma:*
muscle (728.82)
skin and subcutaneous tissue (709.4)

√5ᵗʰ **729.8 Other musculoskeletal symptoms referable to limbs**

729.81 Swelling of limb
AHA: 4Q, '88, 6

729.82 Cramp

729.89 Other
EXCLUDES   *abnormality of gait (781.2)*
tetany (781.7)
transient paralysis of limb (781.4)

AHA: 4Q, '88, 12

729.9 Other and unspecified disorders of soft tissue
Polyalgia

N Newborn Age: 0   P Pediatric Age: 0-17   M Maternity Age: 12-55   A Adult Age :15-124   CC CC Condition   MC Major Complication   CD Complex Dx   HIV HIV Related Dx

2002 Ingenix, Inc.

220 — Volume 1

OSTEOPATHIES, CHONDROPATHIES, AND ACQUIRED MUSCULOSKELETAL DEFORMITIES (730-739)

√4th **730 Osteomyelitis, periostitis, and other infections involving bone**

> **EXCLUDES** jaw (526.4-526.5)
> petrous bone (383.2)

Use additional code to identify organism, such as Staphylococcus (041.1)

The following fifth-digit subclassification is for use with category 730; valid digits are in [brackets] under each code. See above category 710 for definitions.

    0   site unspecified
    1   shoulder region
    2   upper arm
    3   forearm
    4   hand
    5   pelvic region and thigh
    6   lower leg
    7   ankle and foot
    8   other specified sites
    9   multiple sites

AHA: 4Q, '97, 43

DEF: Osteomyelitis: bacterial inflammation of bone tissue and marrow.

DEF: Periostitis: inflammation of specialized connective tissue; causes swelling of bone and aching pain.

§ √5th ¹**730.0   Acute osteomyelitis**   CC
[0-9]
> Abscess of any bone except accessory sinus, jaw, or mastoid
> Acute or subacute osteomyelitis, with or without mention of periostitis

CC Excl: For code 730.00: 015.50-015.56, 015.70-015.76, 015.90-015.96, 017.90-017.96, 730.00-730.39, 730.80-730.99 **For code 730.01:** 015.50-015.56, 015.70-015.76, 015.90-015.96, 017.90-017.96, 730.00, 730.08-730.11, 730.18-730.21, 730.28-730.31, 730.38-730.39, 730.80-730.81, 730.88-730.91, 730.98-730.99 **For code 730.02:** 015.50-015.56, 015.70-015.76, 015.90-015.96, 017.90-017.96, 730.00, 730.08-730.10, 730.12, 730.18-730.20, 730.22, 730.28-730.30, 730.32, 730.38-730.39, 730.80, 730.82, 730.88-730.90, 730.92, 730.98-730.99 **For code 730.03:** 015.50-015.56, 015.70-015.76, 015.90-015.96, 017.90-017.96, 730.00, 730.08-730.10, 730.13, 730.18-730.20, 730.23, 730.28-730.30, 730.33, 730.38-730.39, 730.80, 730.83, 730.88-730.90, 730.93, 730.98-730.99 **For code 730.04:** 015.50-015.56, 015.70-015.76, 015.90-015.96, 017.90-017.96, 730.00, 730.08-730.10, 730.14, 730.18-730.20, 730.24, 730.28-730.30, 730.34, 730.38-730.39, 730.80, 730.84, 730.88-730.90, 730.94, 730.98-730.99 **For code 730.05:** 015.10-015.16, 015.50-015.56, 015.70-015.76, 015.90-015.96, 017.90-017.96, 730.00, 730.08-730.10, 730.15, 730.18-730.20, 730.25, 730.28-730.30, 730.35, 730.38-730.39, 730.80, 730.85, 730.88-730.90, 730.95, 730.98-730.99 **For code 730.06:** 015.20-015.56, 015.70-015.76, 015.90-015.96, 017.90-017.96, 730.00, 730.08-730.10, 730.16, 730.18-730.20, 730.26, 730.28-730.30, 730.36, 730.38-730.39, 730.80, 730.86, 730.88-730.90, 730.96, 730.98-730.99 **For code 730.07:** 015.50-015.56, 015.70-015.76, 015.90-015.96, 017.90-017.96, 730.00, 730.08-730.10, 730.17-730.20, 730.27-730.30, 730.37-730.39, 730.80, 730.87-730.90, 730.97-730.99 **For code 730.08:** 015.00-015.06, 015.50-015.56, 015.70-015.76, 015.90-015.96, 017.90-017.96, 730.00-730.39, 730.80-730.99 **For code 730.09:** 015.50-015.56, 015.70-015.76, 015.90-015.96, 017.90-017.96, 730.00-730.39, 730.80-730.99

AHA: For code 730.06: ▶1Q, '02, 4◀

§ √5th ¹**730.1   Chronic osteomyelitis**
[0-9]
> Brodie's abscess
> Chronic or old osteomyelitis, with or without mention of periostitis
> Sequestrum of bone
> Sclerosing osteomyelitis of Garré
> **EXCLUDES** aseptic necrosis of bone (733.40-733.49)

AHA: For code 730.17: 3Q, '00, 4

§ √5th ¹**730.2   Unspecified osteomyelitis**
[0-9]
> Osteitis or osteomyelitis NOS, with or without mention of periostitis

§ √5th ¹**730.3   Periostitis without mention of osteomyelitis**
[0-9]
> Abscess of periosteum } without mention of
> Periostosis   } osteomyelitis
>
> **EXCLUDES** that in secondary syphilis (091.61)

§ √5th **730.7   *Osteopathy resulting from poliomyelitis***
[0-9]
> *Code first underlying disease (045.0-045.9)*

§ √5th **730.8   *Other infections involving bone in diseases classified elsewhere***   CC
[0-9]
> *Code first underlying disease as:*
>   tuberculosis (015.0-015.9)
>   typhoid fever (002.0)
> **EXCLUDES** syphilis of bone NOS (095.5)

CC Excl: For code 730.80: See code 730.09 **CC Excl: For code 730.81:** 015.50-015.56, 015.70-015.76, 015.90-015.96, 017.90-017.96, 730.00-730.01, 730.08-730.11, 730.18-730.21, 730.28-730.31, 730.38-730.39, 730.80, 730.88-730.91, 730.98-730.99 **For code 730.82:** 015.50-015.56, 015.70-015.76, 015.90-015.96, 017.90-017.96, 730.00, 730.02, 730.08-730.10, 730.12, 730.18-730.20, 730.22, 730.28-730.30, 730.32, 730.38-730.39, 730.80, 730.88-730.90, 730.92, 730.98-730.99I: **For code 730.83:** 015.50-015.56, 015.70-015.76, 015.90-015.96, 017.90-017.96, 730.00, 730.03, 730.08-730.10, 730.13, 730.18-730.20, 730.23, 730.28-730.30, 730.33, 730.38-730.39, 730.80, 730.88-730.90, 730.93, 730.98-730.99: **For code 730.84:** 015.50-015.56, 015.70-015.76, 015.90-015.96, 017.90-017.96, 730.00, 730.08-730.10, 730.14, 730.18-730.20, 730.24, 730.28-730.30, 730.34, 730.38-730.39, 730.80, 730.88-730.90, 730.94, 730.98-730.99 **For code 730.85:** 015.10-015.16, 015.50-015.56, 015.70-015.76, 015.90-015.96, 017.90-017.96, 730.00, 730.05, 730.08-730.10, 730.15, 730.18-730.20, 730.25, 730.28-730.30, 730.35, 730.38-730.39, 730.80, 730.88-730.90, 730.95, 730.98-730.99 **For code 730.86:** 015.20-015.26, 015.50-015.56, 015.70-015.76, 015.90-015.96, 017.90-017.96, 730.00, 730.06, 730.08-730.10, 730.16, 730.18-730.20, 730.26, 730.28-730.30, 730.36, 730.38-730.39, 730.80, 730.88-730.90, 730.96, 730.98-730.99 **For code 730.87:** 015.50-015.56, 015.70-015.76, 015.90-015.96, 017.90-017.96, 730.00, 730.07-730.10, 730.17-730.20, 730.27-730.30, 730.37-730.39, 730.80, 730.88-730.90, 730.97-730.99 **For code 730.88:** 015.00-015.06, 015.50-015.56, 015.70-015.76, 015.90-015.96, 017.90-017.96, 730.00-730.39, 730.80-730.99: **For code 730.89:** 015.50-015.56, 015.70-015.76, 015.90-015.96, 017.90-017.96, 730.00-730.39, 730.80-730.99

AHA: 2Q, '97, 16; 3Q, '91, 10

§ √5th **730.9   Unspecified infection of bone**   CC
[0-9]
CC Excl: For code 730.90: See code 730.89 **For code 730.91:** 015.50-015.56, 015.70-015.76, 015.90-015.96, 017.90-017.96, 730.00-730.01, 730.08-730.11, 730.18-730.21, 730.28-730.31, 730.38-730.39, 730.80-730.81, 730.88-730.90, 730.98-730.99 **For code 730.92:** 015.50-015.56, 015.70-015.76, 015.90-015.96, 017.90-017.96, 730.00, 730.02, 730.08-730.10, 730.12, 730.18-730.20, 730.22, 730.28-730.30, 730.32, 730.38-730.39, 730.80, 730.82, 730.88-730.90, 730.98-730.99: **For code 730.93:** 015.50-015.56, 015.70-015.76, 015.90-015.96, 017.90-017.96, 730.00, 730.03, 730.08-730.10, 730.13, 730.18-730.20, 730.23, 730.28-730.30, 730.33, 730.38-730.39, 730.80, 730.83, 730.88-730.90, 730.98-730.99 **For code 730.94:** 015.50-015.56, 015.70-015.76, 015.90-015.96, 017.90-017.96, 730.00, 730.04, 730.08-730.10, 730.14, 730.18-730.20, 730.24, 730.28-730.30, 730.34, 730.38-730.39, 730.80, 730.84, 730.88-730.90, 730.98-730.99: **For code 730.95:** 015.10-015.16, 015.50-015.56, 015.70-015.76, 015.90-015.96, 017.90-017.96, 730.00, 730.05, 730.08-730.10, 730.15, 730.18-730.20, 730.25, 730.28-730.30, 730.35, 730.38-730.39, 730.80, 730.85, 730.88-730.90, 730.98-730.99 **For code 730.96:** 015.20-015.26, 015.50-015.56, 015.70-015.76, 015.90-015.96, 017.90-017.96, 730.00, 730.06, 730.08-730.10, 730.16, 730.18-730.20, 730.26, 730.28-730.30, 730.36, 730.38-730.39, 730.80, 730.86, 730.88-730.90, 730.98-730.99: **For code 730.97:** 015.50-015.56, 015.70-015.76, 015.90-015.96, 017.90-017.96, 730.00, 730.07-730.10, 730.17-730.20, 730.27-730.30, 730.37-730.39, 730.80, 730.87-730.90, 730.98-730.99: **For code 730.98:** 015.00-015.06, 015.50-015.56, 015.70-015.76, 015.90-015.96, 017.90-017.96, 730.00-730.39, 730.80-730.99 **For code 730.99:** 015.50-015.56, 015.70-015.76, 015.90-015.96, 017.90-017.96, 730.00-730.39, 730.80-730.99

¹ Nonspecific PDx=0

§ Requires fifth-digit. Valid digits are in [brackets] under each code. See beginning of section 710-739 for codes and definitions.

√4th √5th Additional Digit Required   Nonspecific PDx   Unacceptable PDx   Manifestation Code   **MSP** Medicare Secondary Payer   ▶◀ Revised Text   ● New Code   ▲ Revised Code Title

Musculoskeletal and Connective Tissue 731–733.09

Slipped Femoral Epiphysis

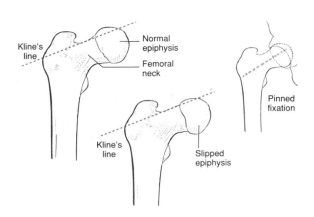

Kline's line — Normal epiphysis — Femoral neck — Pinned fixation — Kline's line — Slipped epiphysis

☑4ᵗʰ **731 Osteitis deformans and osteopathies associated with other disorders classified elsewhere**

DEF: Osteitis deformans: Bone disease marked by episodes of increased bone loss, excessive repair attempts follow; causes weakened, deformed bones with increased mass, bowed long bones, deformed flat bones, pain and pathological fractures; may be fatal if associated with congestive heart failure, giant cell tumors or bone sarcoma; also called Paget's disease.

731.0 Osteitis deformans without mention of bone tumor
Paget's disease of bone

731.1 Osteitis deformans in diseases classified elsewhere
Code first underlying disease as:
malignant neoplasm of bone (170.0-170.9)

731.2 Hypertrophic pulmonary osteoarthropathy
Bamberger-Marie disease
DEF: Clubbing, of fingers and toes; related to enlarged ends of long bones; due to chronic lung and heart disease.

731.8 Other bone involvement in diseases classified elsewhere
Code first underlying disease as:
diabetes mellitus (250.8)
Use additional code to specify bone condition, such as:
acute osteomyelitis (730.00-730.09)
AHA: 4Q, '97, 43; 2Q, '97, 16

☑4ᵗʰ **732 Osteochondropathies**
DEF: Conditions related to both bone and cartilage, or conditions in which cartilage is converted to bone (enchondral ossification).

732.0 Juvenile osteochondrosis of spine
Juvenile osteochondrosis (of):
marginal or vertebral epiphysis (of Scheuermann)
spine NOS
Vertebral epiphysitis
EXCLUDES   *adolescent postural kyphosis (737.0)*

732.1 Juvenile osteochondrosis of hip and pelvis
Coxa plana
Ischiopubic synchondrosis (of van Neck)
Osteochondrosis (juvenile) of:
acetabulum
head of femur (of Legg-Calvé-Perthes)
iliac crest (of Buchanan)
symphysis pubis (of Pierson)
Pseudocoxalgia

732.2 Nontraumatic slipped upper femoral epiphysis
Slipped upper femoral epiphysis NOS

732.3 Juvenile osteochondrosis of upper extremity
Osteochondrosis (juvenile) of:
capitulum of humerus (of Panner)
carpal lunate (of Kienbock)
hand NOS
head of humerus (of Haas)
heads of metacarpals (of Mauclaire)
lower ulna (of Burns)
radial head (of Brailsford)
upper extremity NOS

732.4 Juvenile osteochondrosis of lower extremity, excluding foot
Osteochondrosis (juvenile) of:
lower extremity NOS
primary patellar center (of Köhler)
proximal tibia (of Blount)
secondary patellar center (of Sinding-Larsen)
tibial tubercle (of Osgood-Schlatter)
Tibia vara

732.5 Juvenile osteochondrosis of foot
Calcaneal apophysitis
Epiphysitis, os calcis
Osteochondrosis (juvenile) of:
astragalus (of Diaz)
calcaneum (of Sever)
foot NOS
metatarsal
second (of Freiberg)
fifth (of Iselin)
os tibiale externum (of Haglund)
tarsal navicular (of Köhler)

732.6 Other juvenile osteochondrosis
Apophysitis ⎫
Epiphysitis ⎬ specified as juvenile,
Osteochondritis ⎪ of other site,
Osteochondrosis ⎭ or site NOS

732.7 Osteochondritis dissecans

732.8 Other specified forms of osteochondropathy
Adult osteochondrosis of spine

732.9 Unspecified osteochondropathy
Apophysitis ⎫ NOS
Epiphysitis ⎬ not specified as adult
Osteochondritis ⎪ or juvenile, of
Osteochondrosis ⎭ unspecified site

☑4ᵗʰ **733 Other disorders of bone and cartilage**
EXCLUDES   *bone spur (726.91)*
cartilage of, or loose body in, joint (717.0-717.9, 718.0-718.9)
giant cell granuloma of jaw (526.3)
osteitis fibrosa cystica generalisata (252.0)
osteomalacia (268.2)
polyostotic fibrous dysplasia of bone (756.54)
prognathism, retrognathism (524.1)
xanthomatosis localized to bone (272.7)

☑5ᵗʰ **733.0 Osteoporosis**
DEF: Bone mass reduction that ultimately results in fractures after minimal trauma; dorsal kyphosis or loss of height often occur.

733.00 Osteoporosis, unspecified
Wedging of vertebra NOS
AHA: ▶3Q, '01, 19;◀ 2Q, '98, 12

733.01 Senile osteoporosis
Postmenopausal osteoporosis

733.02 Idiopathic osteoporosis

733.03 Disuse osteoporosis

733.09 Other
Drug-induced osteoporosis
Use additional E code to identify drug

N Newborn Age: 0   P Pediatric Age: 0-17   M Maternity Age: 12-55   A Adult Age: 15-124   CC CC Condition   MC Major Complication   CD Complex Dx   HIV HIV Related Dx

√5ᵗʰ **733.1 Pathologic fracture**
Spontaneous fracture

EXCLUDES	stress fracture (733.93-733.95)
	traumatic fracture (800-829)

AHA: 4Q, '93, 25; N-D, '86, 10; N-D, '85, 16

DEF: Fracture due to bone structure weakening by pathological processes (e.g., osteoporosis, neoplasms and osteomalacia).

733.10 Pathologic fracture, unspecified site `CC`
CC Excl: 733.10-733.19, 733.93-733.95

733.11 Pathologic fracture of humerus `CC`
CC Excl: See code 733.10

733.12 Pathologic fracture of distal radius and ulna `CC`
Wrist NOS
CC Excl: See code 733.10

733.13 Pathologic fracture of vertebrae `CC`
Collapse of vertebra NOS
CC Excl: See code 733.10

AHA: 3Q, '99, 5

▽ **DRG** 239

733.14 Pathologic fracture of neck of femur `CC`
Femur NOS   Hip NOS
CC Excl: See code 733.10

AHA: 1Q, '01, 1; 1Q, '96, 16

733.15 Pathologic fracture of other specified part of femur `CC`
CC Excl: See code 733.10

AHA: 2Q, '98, 12

733.16 Pathologic fracture of tibia or fibula `CC`
Ankle NOS
CC Excl: See code 733.10

733.19 Pathologic fracture of other specified site `CC`
CC Excl: See code 733.10

√4ᵗʰ **733.2 Cyst of bone**
733.20 Cyst of bone (localized), unspecified
733.21 Solitary bone cyst
Unicameral bone cyst
733.22 Aneurysmal bone cyst
DEF: Solitary bone lesion, bulges into periosteum; marked by calcified rim.

733.29 Other
Fibrous dysplasia (monostotic)

EXCLUDES	cyst of jaw (526.0-526.2, 526.89)
	osteitis fibrosa cystica (252.0)
	polyostotic fibrousdyplasia of bone (756.54)

733.3 Hyperostosis of skull
Hyperostosis interna frontalis
Leontiasis ossium
DEF: Abnormal bone growth on inner aspect of cranial bones.

√5ᵗʰ **733.4 Aseptic necrosis of bone**

EXCLUDES	osteochondropathies (732.0-732.9)

DEF: Infraction of bone tissue due to a nonfectious etiology, such as a fracture, ischemic disorder or administration of immunosuppressive drugs; leads to degenerative joint disease or nonunion of fractures.

733.40 Aseptic necrosis of bone, site unspecified
733.41 Head of humerus
733.42 Head and neck of femur
Femur NOS

EXCLUDES	Legg-Calvé-Perthes disease (732.1)

733.43 Medial femoral condyle
733.44 Talus
733.49 Other
733.5 Osteitis condensans
Piriform sclerosis of ilium
DEF: Idiopathic condition marked by low back pain; associated with oval or triangular sclerotic, opaque bone next to sacroiliac joints in the ileum.

733.6 Tietze's disease
Costochondral junction syndrome
Costochondritis
DEF: Painful, idiopathic, nonsuppurative, swollen costal cartilage sometimes confused with cardiac symptoms because the anterior chest pain resembles that of coronary artery disease.

733.7 Algoneurodystrophy
Disuse atrophy of bone   Sudeck's atrophy
DEF: Painful, idiopathic.

√5ᵗʰ **733.8 Malunion and nonunion of fracture**
AHA: 2Q, '94, 5

733.81 Malunion of fracture `CC`
CC Excl: 733.81-733.82

733.82 Nonunion of fracture `CC`
Pseudoarthrosis (bone)
CC Excl: See code 733.81

√5ᵗʰ **733.9 Other and unspecified disorders of bone and cartilage**
733.90 Disorder of bone and cartilage, unspecified
733.91 Arrest of bone development or growth
Epiphyseal arrest
733.92 Chondromalacia
Chondromalacia:
NOS
localized, except patella
systemic
tibial plateau

EXCLUDES	chondromalacia of patella (717.7)

DEF: Articular cartilage softening.

733.93 Stress fracture of tibia or fibula `CC`
Stress reaction of tibia or fibula
CC Excl: 733.10-733.19, 733.93-733.95

AHA: ►4Q, '01, 48◄

733.94 Stress fracture of the metatarsals `CC`
Stress reaction of metatarsals
CC Excl: See code 733.93

AHA: ►4Q, '01, 48◄

733.95 Stress fracture of other bone `CC`
Stress reaction of other bone
CC Excl: See code 733.93

AHA: ►4Q, '01, 48◄

733.99 Other
Diaphysitis
Hypertrophy of bone
Relapsing polychondritis
AHA: J-F, '87, 14

734 Flat foot
Pes planus (acquired)
Talipes planus (acquired)

EXCLUDES	congenital (754.61)
	rigid flat foot (754.61)
	spastic (everted) flat foot (754.61)

√4ᵗʰ **735 Acquired deformities of toe**

EXCLUDES	congenital (754.60-754.69, 755.65-755.66)

735.0 Hallux valgus (acquired)
DEF: Angled displacement of the great toe, causing it to ride over or under other toes.

Acquired Deformities of Toe

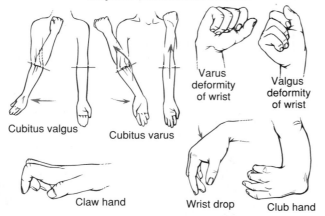

Hallux valgus

Hallux varus

Hallux malleus (hammer of big toe)

Hammertoe

735.1   Hallux varus (acquired)

DEF: Angled displacement of the great toe toward the body midline, away from the other toes.

735.2   Hallux rigidus

DEF: Limited flexion movement at metatarsophalangeal joint of great toe; due to degenerative joint disease.

735.3   Hallux malleus

DEF: Extended proximal phalanx, flexed distal phalanges, of great toe; foot resembles claw or hammer.

735.4   Other hammer toe (acquired)

735.5   Claw toe (acquired)

DEF: Hyperextended proximal phalanges, flexed middle and distal phalanges.

735.8   Other acquired deformities of toe

735.9   Unspecified acquired deformity of toe

√4ᵗʰ **736 Other acquired deformities of limbs**

> **EXCLUDES**   *congenital (754.3-755.9)*

√5ᵗʰ **736.0   Acquired deformities of forearm, excluding fingers**

736.00   Unspecified deformity

Deformity of elbow, forearm, hand, or wrist (acquired) NOS

736.01   Cubitus valgus (acquired)

DEF: Deviation of the elbow away from the body midline upon extension; it occurs when the palm is turning outward.

736.02   Cubitus varus (acquired)

DEF: Elbow joint displacement angled laterally; when the forearm is extended, it is deviated toward the midline of the body; also called "gun stock" deformity.

736.03   Valgus deformity of wrist (acquired)

DEF: Abnormal angulation away from the body midline.

Acquired Deformities of Forearm

Cubitus valgus

Cubitus varus

Varus deformity of wrist

Valgus deformity of wrist

Claw hand

Wrist drop

Club hand

736.04   Varus deformity of wrist (acquired)

DEF: Abnormal angulation toward the body midline.

736.05   Wrist drop (acquired)

DEF: Inability to extend the hand at the wrist due to extensor muscle paralysis

736.06   Claw hand (acquired)

DEF: Flexion and atrophy of the hand and fingers; found in ulnar nerve lesions, syringomyelia, and leprosy.

736.07   Club hand, acquired

DEF: Twisting of the hand out of shape or position; caused by the congenital absence of the ulna or radius.

736.09   Other

736.1   Mallet finger

DEF: Permanently flexed distal phalanx.

√5ᵗʰ **736.2   Other acquired deformities of finger**

736.20   Unspecified deformity

Deformity of finger (acquired) NOS

736.21   Boutonniere deformity

DEF: A complete or partial protrusion of a joint finger through a defect in the extensor aponeurosis; also called buttonhole deformity.

736.22   Swan-neck deformity

DEF: Flexed distal and hyperextended proximal interphalangeal joint.

736.29   Other

> **EXCLUDES**   *trigger finger (727.03)*

AHA: 2Q, '89, 13

√5ᵗʰ **736.3   Acquired deformities of hip**

736.30   Unspecified deformity

Deformity of hip (acquired) NOS

736.31   Coxa valga (acquired)

DEF: Increase of at least 140 degrees in the angle formed by the axis of the head and the neck of the femur, and the axis of its shaft.

736.32   Coxa vara (acquired)

DEF: The bending downward of the neck of the femur: causing difficulty in movement; a right angle or less may be formed by the axis of the head and neck of the femur, and the axis of its shaft.

736.39   Other

AHA: 2Q, '91, 18

√5ᵗʰ **736.4   Genu valgum or varum (acquired)**

736.41   Genu valgum (acquired)

DEF: Abnormally close together and an abnormally large space between the ankles; also called "knock-knees."

736.42   Genu varum (acquired)

DEF: Abnormally separated knees and the inward bowing of the legs; it is also called "bowlegs."

736.5   Genu recurvatum (acquired)

DEF: Hyperextended knees; also called "backknee."

736.6   Other acquired deformities of knee

Deformity of knee (acquired) NOS

Ⓝ Newborn Age: 0   Ⓟ Pediatric Age: 0-17   Ⓜ Maternity Age: 12-55   Ⓐ Adult Age: 15-124   **CC** CC Condition   **MC** Major Complication   **CD** Complex Dx   **HIV** HIV Related Dx

224 — Volume 1   *2002 Ingenix, Inc.*

Acquired Deformities of Hip

Genu valga (knock-knee)

Normal angle

Coxa valga

Coxa vara

Genu vara (bowleg)

Acquired Deformities of Lower Limb

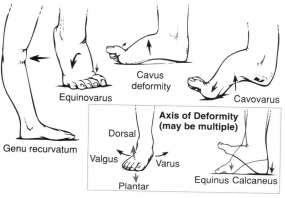

Equinovarus

Cavus deformity

Cavovarus

Genu recurvatum

Axis of Deformity (may be multiple)

Dorsal

Valgus | Varus

Plantar

Equinus Calcaneus

√5ᵗʰ **736.7** **Other acquired deformities of ankle and foot**

> **EXCLUDES** *deformities of toe (acquired) (735.0-735.9)*
> *pes planus (acquired) (734)*

736.70 Unspecified deformity of ankle and foot, acquired

736.71 Acquired equinovarus deformity
Clubfoot, acquired
> **EXCLUDES** *clubfoot not specified as acquired (754.5-754.7)*

736.72 Equinus deformity of foot, acquired
DEF: A plantar flexion deformity that forces people to walk on their toes.

736.73 Cavus deformity of foot
> **EXCLUDES** *that with claw foot (736.74)*
DEF: Abnormally high longitudinal arch of the foot.

Kyphosis and Lordosis

Kyphosis (hump)

Lordosis (concave)

736.74 **Claw foot, acquired**
DEF: High foot arch with hyperextended toes at metatarsophalangeal joint and flexed toes at distal joints; also called "main en griffe."

736.75 **Cavovarus deformity of foot, acquired**
DEF: Inward turning of the heel from the midline of the leg and an abnormally high longitudinal arch.

736.76 **Other calcaneus deformity**

736.79 **Other**
Acquired:
pes
talipes } not elsewhere classified

√5ᵗʰ **736.8** **Acquired deformities of other parts of limbs**

736.81 **Unequal leg length (acquired)**

736.89 **Other**
Deformity (acquired):
arm or leg, not elsewhere classified
shoulder

736.9 Acquired deformity of limb, site unspecified

√4ᵗʰ **737** **Curvature of spine**
> **EXCLUDES** *congenital (754.2)*

737.0 **Adolescent postural kyphosis**
> **EXCLUDES** *osteochondrosis of spine (juvenile) (732.0)*
> *adult (732.8)*

√5ᵗʰ **737.1** **Kyphosis (acquired)**

737.10 **Kyphosis (acquired) (postural)**

737.11 **Kyphosis due to radiation**

737.12 **Kyphosis, postlaminectomy**
AHA: J-F, '87, 7

737.19 **Other**
> **EXCLUDES** *that associated with conditions classifiable elsewhere (737.41)*

√5ᵗʰ **737.2** **Lordosis (acquired)**
DEF: Swayback appearance created by an abnormally increased spinal curvature; it is also referred to as "hollow back" or "saddle back."

737.20 **Lordosis (acquired) (postural)**

737.21 **Lordosis, postlaminectomy**

737.22 **Other postsurgical lordosis**

737.29 **Other**
> **EXCLUDES** *that associated with conditions classifiable elsewhere (737.42)*

√5ᵗʰ **737.3** **Kyphoscoliosis and scoliosis**
DEF: Kyphoscoliosis: backward and lateral curvature of the spinal column; it is found in vertebral osteochondrosis.

DEF: Scoliosis: an abnormal deviation of the spine to the left or right of the midline

737.30 **Scoliosis [and kyphoscoliosis], idiopathic**

737.31 **Resolving infantile idiopathic scoliosis**

737.32 **Progressive infantile idiopathic scoliosis**

737.33 **Scoliosis due to radiation**

737.34 **Thoracogenic scoliosis**

737.39 **Other**
> **EXCLUDES** *that associated with conditions classifiable elsewhere (737.43)*
> *that in kyphoscoliotic heart disease (416.1)*

√4ᵗʰ
√5ᵗʰ Additional Digit Required   Nonspecific PDx   Unacceptable PDx   Manifestation Code   **MSP** Medicare Secondary Payer   ▶◀ Revised Text   ● New Code   ▲ Revised Code Title

Musculoskeletal and Connective Tissue 737.4–739.9

Scoliosis and Kyphoscoliosis

Scoliosis

Kyphoscoliosis

✓5th **737.4 Curvature of spine associated with other conditions**
Code first associated condition as:
Charcôt-Marie-Tooth disease (356.1)
mucopolysaccharidosis (277.5)
neurofibromatosis (237.7)
osteitis deformans (731.0)
osteitis fibrosa cystica (252.0)
osteoporosis (733.00-733.09)
poliomyelitis (138)
tuberculosis [Pott's curvature] (015.0)

737.40 *Curvature of spine, unspecified*

737.41 *Kyphosis*

737.42 *Lordosis*

737.43 *Scoliosis*

737.8 **Other curvatures of spine**

737.9 **Unspecified curvature of spine**
Curvature of spine (acquired) (idiopathic) NOS
Hunchback, acquired
EXCLUDES   *deformity of spine NOS (738.5)*

✓4th **738 Other acquired deformity**
EXCLUDES   *congenital (754.0-756.9, 758.0-759.9)*
dentofacial anomalies (524.0-524.9)

738.0 **Acquired deformity of nose**
Deformity of nose (acquired)
Overdevelopment of nasal bones
EXCLUDES   *deflected or deviated nasal septum (470)*

✓5th **738.1 Other acquired deformity of head**

738.10 **Unspecified deformity**

738.11 **Zygomatic hyperplasia**
DEF: Abnormal enlargement of the zygoma (processus zygomaticus temporalis).

738.12 **Zygomatic hypoplasia**
DEF: Underdevelopment of the zygoma (processus zygomaticus temporalis).

738.19 **Other specified deformity**

738.2 **Acquired deformity of neck**

738.3 **Acquired deformity of chest and rib**
Deformity:	Pectus:
chest (acquired)	carinatum, acquired
rib (acquired)	excavatum, acquired

738.4 **Acquired spondylolisthesis**
Degenerative spondylolisthesis
Spondylolysis, acquired
EXCLUDES   *congenital (756.12)*

DEF: Vertebra displaced forward over another; due to bilateral defect in vertebral arch, eroded articular surface of posterior facts and elongated pedicle between fifth lumbar vertebra and sacrum.

738.5 **Other acquired deformity of back or spine**
Deformity of spine NOS
EXCLUDES   *curvature of spine (737.0-737.9)*

738.6 **Acquired deformity of pelvis**
Pelvic obliquity
EXCLUDES   *intrapelvic protrusion of acetabulum (718.6)*
that in relation to labor and delivery (653.0-653.4, 653.8-653.9)

DEF: Pelvic obliquity: slanting or inclination of the pelvis at an angle between 55 and 60 degrees between the plane of the pelvis and the horizontal plane.

738.7 **Cauliflower ear**
DEF: Abnormal external ear; due to injury, subsequent perichondritis.

738.8 **Acquired deformity of other specified site**
Deformity of clavicle
AHA: 2Q, '01, 15

738.9 **Acquired deformity of unspecified site**

✓4th **739 Nonallopathic lesions, not elsewhere classified**
INCLUDES   segmental dysfunction
somatic dysfunction

DEF: Disability, loss of function or abnormality of a body part that is neither classifiable to a particular system nor brought about therapeutically to counteract another disease.

739.0 **Head region**
Occipitocervical region

739.1 **Cervical region**
Cervicothoracic region

739.2 **Thoracic region**
Thoracolumbar region

739.3 **Lumbar region**
Lumbosacral region

739.4 **Sacral region**
Sacrococcygeal region   Sacroiliac region

739.5 **Pelvic region**
Hip region   Pubic region

739.6 **Lower extremities**

739.7 **Upper extremities**
Acromioclavicular region
Sternoclavicular region

739.8 **Rib cage**
Costochondral region   Sternochondral region
Costovertebral region

739.9 **Abdomen and other**
AHA: 2Q, '89, 14

N Newborn Age: 0	P Pediatric Age: 0-17	M Maternity Age: 12-55	A Adult Age: 15-124	CC CC Condition	MC Major Complication	CD Complex Dx	HIV HIV Related Dx

2002 Ingenix, Inc.

14. CONGENITAL ANOMALIES (740-759)

√4ᵗʰ **740 Anencephalus and similar anomalies**

740.0 Anencephalus

Acrania   Hemicephaly
Amyelencephalus   Hemianencephaly

DEF: Fetus without cerebrum, cerebellum and flat bones of skull.

740.1 Craniorachischisis

DEF: Congenital slit in cranium and vertebral column

740.2 Iniencephaly

DEF: Spinal cord passes through enlarged occipital bone (foramen magnum); absent vertebral bone layer and spinal processes; resulting in both reduction in number and proper fusion of the vertebrae.

√4ᵗʰ **741 Spina bifida**

EXCLUDES *spina bifida occulta (756.17)*

The following fifth-digit subclassification is for use with category 741:

0 unspecified region
1 cervical region
2 dorsal [thoracic] region
3 lumbar region

AHA: 3Q, '94, 7

DEF: Lack of closure of spinal cord's bony encasement; marked by cord protrusion into lumbosacral area; evident by elevated alpha-fetoprotein of amniotic fluid

√5ᵗʰ **741.0 With hydrocephalus**   **CC**
Arnold-Chiari syndrome, type II
Any condition classifiable to 741.9 with any condition classifiable to 742.3
Chiari malformation, type II

CC Excl: 741.00-741.93, 742.59, 742.8-742.9, 759.7-759.89

AHA: 4Q, '97, 51; 4Q, '94, 37; S-O, '87, 10

√5ᵗʰ **741.9 Without mention of hydrocephalus**   **CC**
Hydromeningocele (spinal)   Myelocystocele
Hydromyelocele   Rachischisis
Meningocele (spinal)   Spina bifida (aperta)
Meningomyelocele   Syringomyelocele
Myelocele

CC Excl: See code 741.0

√4ᵗʰ **742 Other congenital anomalies of nervous system**

742.0 Encephalocele
Encephalocystocele
Encephalomyelocele
Hydroencephalocele
Hydromeningocele, cranial
Meningocele, cerebral
Meningoencephalocele

AHA: 4Q, '94, 37

DEF: Brain tissue protrudes through skull defect.

Spina Bifida

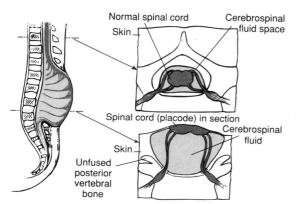

Normal spinal cord
Cerebrospinal fluid space
Skin
Normal spinal cord
Spinal cord (placode) in section
Cerebrospinal fluid
Skin
Unfused posterior vertebral bone

Normal Ventricles and Hydrocephalus

Cerebrospinal fluid in ventricles
Normal Ventricles
Third ventricle (III)
Choroid plexus produces Cerebrospinal fluid (CSF)
Lateral ventricles (I and II)
Fourth ventricle (IV)
Foramen of Monro
Foramen of Luschka
Cerebral aqueduct (Sylvius)
Foramen of Magendie

Hydrocephalus

Enlarged ventricles
Blockage of any CSF passage increases pressure in skull, which may push tissue through the Incisura tentorii or through the Foramen magnum

742.1 Microcephalus
Hydromicrocephaly
Micrencephaly

DEF: Extremely small head or brain.

742.2 Reduction deformities of brain
Absence
Agenesis   } of part of brain
Aplasia
Hypoplasia

Agyria   Holoprosencephaly
Arhinencephaly   Microgyria

AHA: 4Q, '94, 37

742.3 Congenital hydrocephalus
Aqueduct of Sylvius:
anomaly
obstruction, congenital
stenosis
Atresia of foramina of Magendie and Luschka
Hydrocephalus in newborn

EXCLUDES *hydrocephalus:*
acquired (331.3-331.4)
due to congenital toxoplasmosis (771.2)
with any condition classifiable to 741.9 (741.0)

DEF: Fluid accumulation within the skull; involves subarachnoid (external) or ventricular (internal) brain spaces.

742.4 Other specified anomalies of brain
Congenital cerebral cyst   Multiple anomalies of brain
Macroencephaly   NOS
Macrogyria   Porencephaly
Megalencephaly   Ulegyria

AHA: 1Q, '99, 9; 3Q, '92, 12

√5ᵗʰ **742.5 Other specified anomalies of spinal cord**
742.51 Diastematomyelia

DEF: Congenital anomaly often associated with spina bifida; the spinal cord is separated into halves by a bony tissue resembling a "spike" (a spicule), each half surrounded by a dural sac.

√4ᵗʰ √5ᵗʰ Additional Digit Required   **Nonspecific PDx**   **Unacceptable PDx**   **Manifestation Code**   **MSP** Medicare Secondary Payer   ▶◀ Revised Text   ● New Code   ▲ Revised Code Title

2002 Ingenix, Inc.   **Volume 1 — 227**

742.53 Hydromyelia
Hydrorhachis
DEF: Dilated central spinal cord canal; characterized by increased fluid accumulation.

742.59 Other
Amyelia
Atelomyelia
Congenital anomaly of spinal meninges
Defective development of cauda equina
Hypoplasia of spinal cord
Myelatelia
Myelodysplasia
AHA: 2Q, '91, 14; 1Q, '89, 10

742.8 Other specified anomalies of nervous system
Agenesis of nerve
Displacement of brachial plexus
Familial dysautonomia
Jaw-winking syndrome
Marcus-Gunn syndrome
Riley-Day syndrome
EXCLUDES *neurofibromatosis (237.7)*

742.9 Unspecified anomaly of brain, spinal cord, and nervous system
Anomaly
Congenital:
disease   } of: { brain
lesion   nervous system
Deformity   spinal cord

√4th **743 Congenital anomalies of eye**

√5th **743.0 Anophthalmos**
DEF: Complete absence of the eyes or the presence of vestigial eyes.

743.00 Clinical anophthalmos, unspecified
Agenesis   } of eye
Congenital absence
Anophthalmos NOS

743.03 Cystic eyeball, congenital

743.06 Cryptophthalmos
DEF: Eyelids continue over eyeball, results in apparent absence of eyelids.

√5th **743.1 Microphthalmos**
Dysplasia   } of eye
Hypoplasia
Rudimentary eye
DEF: Abnormally small eyeballs, may be opacities of cornea and lens, scarring of choroid and retina.

743.10 Microphthalmos, unspecified

743.11 Simple microphthalmos

743.12 Microphthalmos associated with other anomalies of eye and adnexa

√5th **743.2 Buphthalmos**
Glaucoma: Hydrophthalmos
congenital
newborn
EXCLUDES *glaucoma of childhood (365.14)*
traumatic glaucoma due to birth injury
(767.8)
DEF: Distended, enlarged fibrous coats of eye; due to intraocular pressure of congenital glaucoma.

743.20 Buphthalmos, unspecified

743.21 Simple buphthalmos

743.22 Buphthalmos associated with other ocular anomalies
Keratoglobus, congenital   } associated with
Megalocornea   buphthalmos

√5th **743.3 Congenital cataract and lens anomalies**
EXCLUDES *infantile cataract (366.00-366.09)*
DEF: Opaque eye lens.

743.30 Congenital cataract, unspecified

743.31 Capsular and subcapsular cataract

743.32 Cortical and zonular cataract

743.33 Nuclear cataract

743.34 Total and subtotal cataract, congenital

743.35 Congenital aphakia
Congenital absence of lens

743.36 Anomalies of lens shape
Microphakia   Spherophakia

743.37 Congenital ectopic lens

743.39 Other

√5th **743.4 Coloboma and other anomalies of anterior segment**
DEF: Coloboma: ocular tissue defect associated with defect of ocular fetal intraocular fissure; may cause small pit on optic disk, major defects of iris, ciliary body, choroid, and retina.

743.41 Anomalies of corneal size and shape
Microcornea
EXCLUDES *that associated with buphthalmos (743.22)*

743.42 Corneal opacities, interfering with vision, congenital

743.43 Other corneal opacities, congenital

743.44 Specified anomalies of anterior chamber, chamber angle, and related structures
Anomaly: Anomaly:
Axenfeld's   Rieger's
Peters'

743.45 Aniridia
DEF: Incompletely formed or absent iris; affects both eyes; dominant trait; also called congenital hyperplasia of iris.

743.46 Other specified anomalies of iris and ciliary body
Anisocoria, congenital   Coloboma of iris
Atresia of pupil   Corectopia

743.47 Specified anomalies of sclera

743.48 Multiple and combined anomalies of anterior segment

743.49 Other

√5th **743.5 Congenital anomalies of posterior segment**

743.51 Vitreous anomalies
Congenital vitreous opacity

743.52 Fundus coloboma
DEF: Absent retinal and choroidal tissue; occurs in lower fundus; a bright white ectatic zone of exposed sclera extends into and changes the optic disk.

743.53 Chorioretinal degeneration, congenital

743.54 Congenital folds and cysts of posterior segment

743.55 Congenital macular changes

743.56 Other retinal changes, congenital
AHA: 3Q, '99, 12

743.57 Specified anomalies of optic disc
Coloboma of optic disc (congenital)

743.58 Vascular anomalies
Congenital retinal aneurysm

743.59 Other

√5th **743.6 Congenital anomalies of eyelids, lacrimal system, and orbit**

743.61 Congenital ptosis
DEF: Drooping of eyelid.

743.62 Congenital deformities of eyelids
Ablepharon
Absence of eyelid
Accessory eyelid
Congenital:
ectropion
entropion
AHA: 1Q, '00, 22

| N Newborn Age: 0 | P Pediatric Age: 0-17 | M Maternity Age: 12-55 | A Adult Age: 15-124 | CC CC Condition | MC Major Complication | CD Complex Dx | HIV HIV Related Dx |

743.63 Other specified congenital anomalies of eyelid
Absence, agenesis, of cilia

743.64 Specified congenital anomalies of lacrimal gland

743.65 Specified congenital anomalies of lacrimal passages
Absence, agenesis of:
    lacrimal apparatus
    punctum lacrimale
    Accessory lacrimal canal

743.66 Specified congenital anomalies of orbit

743.69 Other
Accessory eye muscles

743.8 Other specified anomalies of eye
    EXCLUDES   congenital nystagmus (379.51)
                    ocular albinism (270.2)
                    retinitis pigmentosa (362.74)

743.9 Unspecified anomaly of eye
Congenital:
    anomaly NOS } of eye [any part]
    deformity NOS }

✓4th 744 Congenital anomalies of ear, face, and neck
    EXCLUDES   anomaly of:
                cervical spine (754.2, 756.10-756.19)
                larynx (748.2-748.3)
                nose (748.0-748.1)
                parathyroid gland (759.2)
                thyroid gland (759.2)
                cleft lip (749.10-749.25)

✓5th 744.0 Anomalies of ear causing impairment of hearing
    EXCLUDES   congenital deafness without mention of
                    cause (389.0-389.9)

744.00 Unspecified anomaly of ear with impairment of hearing

744.01 Absence of external ear
Absence of:
    auditory canal (external)
    auricle (ear) (with stenosis or atresia of auditory canal)

744.02 Other anomalies of external ear with impairment of hearing
Atresia or stricture of auditory canal (external)

744.03 Anomaly of middle ear, except ossicles
Atresia or stricture of osseous meatus (ear)

744.04 Anomalies of ear ossicles
Fusion of ear ossicles

744.05 Anomalies of inner ear
Congenital anomaly of:
    membranous labyrinth
    organ of Corti

744.09 Other
Absence of ear, congenital

744.1 Accessory auricle
Accessory tragus   Supernumerary:
Polyotia   ear
Preauricular appendage   lobule
DEF: Redundant tissue or structures of ear.

✓5th 744.2 Other specified anomalies of ear
    EXCLUDES   that with impairment of hearing
                    (744.00-744.09)

744.21 Absence of ear lobe, congenital

744.22 Macrotia
DEF: Abnormally large pinna of ear.

744.23 Microtia
DEF: Hypoplasia of pinna; associated with absent or closed auditory canal.

744.24 Specified anomalies of Eustachian tube
Absence of Eustachian tube

744.29 Other
Bat ear   Prominence of auricle
Darwin's tubercle   Ridge ear
Pointed ear
    EXCLUDES   preauricular sinus (744.46)

744.3 Unspecified anomaly of ear
Congenital:
    anomaly NOS } of ear, not elsewhere
    deformity NOS }   classified

✓5th 744.4 Branchial cleft cyst or fistula; preauricular sinus
DEF: Coloboma: malclosure of the intraoccular fissure in embryo resulting in defects to optic disk, iris, ciliary body, choroid, or retina.

744.41 Branchial cleft sinus or fistula
Branchial:
    sinus (external) (internal)
    vestige
DEF: Cyst due to failed closure of embryonic branchial cleft.

744.42 Branchial cleft cyst

744.43 Cervical auricle

744.46 Preauricular sinus or fistula

744.47 Preauricular cyst

744.49 Other
Fistula (of):   Fistula (of):
    auricle, congenital   cervicoaural

744.5 Webbing of neck
Pterygium colli
DEF: Thick, triangular skinfold, stretches from lateral side of neck across shoulder; associated with Turner's and Noonan's syndromes.

✓5th 744.8 Other specified anomalies of face and neck
744.81 Macrocheilia
Hypertrophy of lip, congenital
DEF: Abnormally large lips.

744.82 Microcheilia
DEF: Abnormally small lips.

744.83 Macrostomia
DEF: Bilateral or unilateral anomaly, of mouth due to malformed maxillary and mandibular processes; results in mouth extending toward ear.

744.84 Microstomia
DEF: Abnormally small mouth.

744.89 Other
    EXCLUDES   congenital fistula of lip
                    (750.25)
                    musculoskeletal anomalies
                    (754.0-754.1, 756.0)

744.9 Unspecified anomalies of face and neck
Congenital:
    anomaly NOS } of face [any part] or
    deformity NOS }   neck [any part]

✓4th 745 Bulbus cordis anomalies and anomalies of cardiac septal closure
745.0 Common truncus   CC
Absent septum   } between aorta and
Communication (abnormal) }   pulmonary artery

Aortic septal defect
Common aortopulmonary trunk
Persistent truncus arteriosus
CC Excl: 429.71, 429.79, 745.0-745.9, 746.89, 746.9, ▶ 747.83, ◀
747.89, 747.9, 759.7-759.89

✓5th 745.1 Transposition of great vessels
745.10 Complete transposition of great vessels CC
Transposition of great vessels:
    NOS
    classical
CC Excl: See code 745.0

✓4th / ✓5th Additional Digit Required   Nonspecific PDx   Unacceptable PDx   Manifestation Code   MSP Medicare Secondary Payer   ▶◀ Revised Text   ● New Code   ▲ Revised Code Title

2002 Ingenix, Inc.   October 2002 • Volume 1 — 229

Congenital Anomalies 745.11–746.4

Heart Defects

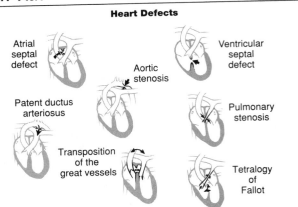

Atrial septal defect

Aortic stenosis

Ventricular septal defect

Patent ductus arteriosus

Pulmonary stenosis

Transposition of the great vessels

Tetralogy of Fallot

745.11 Double outlet right ventricle `CC`
Dextratransposition of aorta
Incomplete transposition of great vessels
Origin of both great vessels from right ventricle
Taussig-Bing syndrome or defect
CC Excl: See code 745.0

745.12 Corrected transposition of great vessels `CC`
CC Excl: See code 745.0

745.19 Other `CC`
CC Excl: See code 745.0

745.2 Tetralogy of Fallot `CC`
Fallot's pentalogy
Ventricular septal defect with pulmonary stenosis or atresia, dextraposition of aorta, and hypertrophy of right ventricle
EXCLUDES Fallot's triad (746.09)
CC Excl: See code 745.0
DEF: Obstructed cardiac outflow causes pulmonary stenosis, interventricular septal defect and right ventricular hypertrophy.

745.3 Common ventricle `CC`
Cor triloculare biatriatum
Single ventricle
CC Excl: See code 745.0

745.4 Ventricular septal defect `CC`
Eisenmenger's defect or complex
Gerbo dedefect
Interventricular septal defect
Left ventricular-right atrial communication
Roger's disease
EXCLUDES common atrioventricular canal type (745.69)
single ventricle (745.3)
CC Excl: See code 745.0

745.5 Ostium secundum type atrial septal defect
Defect: Patent or persistent:
atrium secundum   foramen ovale
fossa ovalis   ostium secundum
Lutembacher's syndrome
DEF: Opening in atrial septum due to failure of the septum secundum and the endocardial cushions to fuse; there is a rim of septum surrounding the defect.

√5th **745.6 Endocardial cushion defects**
DEF: Atrial and/or ventricular septa defects causing abnormal fusion of cushions in atrioventricular canal.

745.60 Endocardial cushion defect, unspecified type `CC`
CC Excl: See code 745.0
DEF: Septal defect due to imperfect fusion of endocardial cushions.

745.61 Ostium primum defect
Persistent ostium primum
DEF: Opening in low, posterior septum primum; causes cleft in basal portion of atrial septum; associated with cleft mitral valve.

745.69 Other `CC`
Absence of atrial septum
Atrioventricular canal type ventricular septal defect
Common atrioventricular canal
Common atrium
CC Excl: See code 745.0

745.7 Cor biloculare `CC`
Absence of atrial and ventricular septa
CC Excl: See code 745.0
DEF: Atrial and ventricular septal defect; marked by heart with two cardiac chambers (one atrium, one ventricle), and one atrioventricular valve.

745.8 Other

745.9 Unspecified defect of septal closure
Septal defect NOS

√4th **746 Other congenital anomalies of heart**
EXCLUDES endocardial fibroelastosis (425.3)

√5th **746.0 Anomalies of pulmonary valve**
EXCLUDES infundibular or subvalvular pulmonic stenosis (746.83)
tetralogy of Fallot (745.2)

746.00 Pulmonary valve anomaly, unspecified

746.01 Atresia, congenital `CC`
Congenital absence of pulmonary valve
CC Excl: 746.00-746.09, 746.89, 746.9, ▶ 747.83,◀
747.89, 747.9, 759.7-759.89

746.02 Stenosis, congenital `CC`
CC Excl: See code 746.01
DEF: Stenosis of opening between pulmonary artery and right ventricle; causes obstructed blood outflow from right ventricle.

746.09 Other
Congenital insufficiency of pulmonary valve
Fallot's triad or trilogy

746.1 Tricuspid atresia and stenosis, congenital `CC`
Absence of tricuspid valve
CC Excl: 746.1-746.7, 746.89, 746.9, ▶ 747.83,◀ 747.89, 747.9, 759.7-759.89

746.2 Ebstein's anomaly `CC`
CC Excl: See code 746.1
DEF: Malformation of the tricuspid valve characterized by septal and posterior leaflets attaching to the wall of the right ventricle; causing the right ventricle to fuse with the atrium producing a large right atrium and a small ventricle; causes a malfunction of the right ventricle with accompanying complications such as heart failure and abnormal cardiac rhythm.

746.3 Congenital stenosis of aortic valve `CC`
Congenital aortic stenosis
EXCLUDES congenital:
subaortic stenosis (746.81)
supravalvular aortic stenosis (747.22)
CC Excl: See code 746.1
AHA: 4Q, '88, 8
DEF: Stenosis of orifice of aortic valve; obstructs blood outflow from left ventricle.

746.4 Congenital insufficiency of aortic valve `CC`
Bicuspid aortic valve
Congenital aortic insufficiency
CC Excl: See code 746.1
DEF: Impaired functioning of aortic valve due to incomplete closure; causes backflow (regurgitation) of blood from aorta to left ventricle.

`N` Newborn Age: 0   `P` Pediatric Age: 0-17   `M` Maternity Age: 12-55   `A` Adult Age: 15-124   `CC` CC Condition   `MC` Major Complication   `CD` Complex Dx   `HIV` HIV Related Dx

230 — Volume 1 • October 2002

2002 Ingenix, Inc.

746.5   **Congenital mitral stenosis**   `CC`

Fused commissure
Parachute deformity   } of mitral valve
Supernumerary cusps

CC Excl: See code 746.1

DEF: Stenosis of left atrioventricular orifice.

746.6   **Congenital mitral insufficiency**   `CC`

CC Excl: See code 746.1

DEF: Impaired functioning of mitral valve due to incomplete closure; causes backflow of blood from left ventricle to left atrium.

746.7   **Hypoplastic left heart syndrome**   `CC`

Atresia, or marked hypoplasia, of aortic orifice or valve, with hypoplasia of ascending aorta and defective development of left ventricle (with mitral valve atresia)

CC Excl: See code 746.1

√5th **746.8**   **Other specified anomalies of heart**

746.81 Subaortic stenosis   `CC`

CC Excl: 746.81-746.84, 746.89, 746.9, ▶ 747.83,◄ 747.89, 747.9, 759.7-759.89

DEF: Stenosis, of left ventricular outflow tract due to fibrous tissue ring or septal hypertrophy below aortic valve.

746.82 Cor triatriatum   `CC`

CC Excl: See code 746.81

DEF: Transverse septum divides left atrium due to failed resorption of embryonic common pulmonary vein; results in three atrial chambers.

746.83 Infundibular pulmonic stenosis   `CC`

Subvalvular pulmonic stenosis

CC Excl: See code 746.81

DEF: Stenosis of right ventricle outflow tract within infundibulum due to fibrous diaphragm below valve or long, narrow fibromuscular channel.

746.84 Obstructive anomalies of heart, not elsewhere classified   `CC`

Uhl's disease

CC Excl: See code 746.81

746.85 Coronary artery anomaly

Anomalous origin or communication of coronary artery
Arteriovenous malformation of coronary artery
Coronary artery:
   absence
   arising from aorta or pulmonary trunk
   single

AHA: N-D, '85, 3

746.86 Congenital heart block   `CC`

Complete or incomplete atrioventricular [AV] block

CC Excl: 746.86, 746.89, 746.9, ▶ 747.83,◄ 747.89, 747.9, 759.7-759.89

DEF: Impaired conduction of electrical impulses; due to maldeveloped junctional tissue.

746.87 Malposition of heart and cardiac apex

Abdominal heart   Levocardia (isolated)
Dextrocardia   Mesocardia
Ectopia cordis

    EXCLUDES   *dextrocardia with complete transposition of viscera (759.3)*

746.89 Other

Atresia   } of cardiac vein
Hypoplasia

Congenital: Congenital:
  cardiomegaly   pericardial defect
  diverticulum, left ventricle

AHA: 3Q, '00, 3; 1Q, '99, 11; J-F, '85, 3

746.9   **Unspecified anomaly of heart**

Congenital:
  anomaly of heart NOS
  heart disease NOS

√4th **747 Other congenital anomalies of circulatory system**

747.0   **Patent ductus arteriosus**

Patent ductus Botalli
Persistent ductus arteriosus

DEF: Open lumen in ductus arteriosus causes arterial blood recirculation in lungs; inhibits blood supply to aorta; symptoms such as shortness of breath more noticeable upon activity.

√5th **747.1**   **Coarctation of aorta**

DEF: Localized deformity of aortic media seen as a severe constriction of the vessel lumen; major symptom is high blood pressure in the arms and low pressure in the legs; a CVA, rupture of the aorta, bacterial endocarditis or congestive heart failure can follow if left untreated.

747.10 Coarctation of aorta (preductal) (postductal)   `CC`

Hypoplasia of aortic arch

CC Excl: No Exclusions

AHA: 1Q, '99, 11; 4Q, '88, 8

747.11 Interruption of aortic arch   `CC`

CC Excl: 747.10-747.22, ▶ 747.83,◄ 747.89, 747.9, 759.7-759.89

√5th **747.2**   **Other anomalies of aorta**

747.20 Anomaly of aorta, unspecified

747.21 Anomalies of aortic arch

Anomalous origin, right subclavian artery
Dextraposition of aorta
Double aortic arch
Kommerell's diverticulum
Overriding aorta
Persistent:
  convolutions, aortic arch
  right aortic arch
Vascular ring

    EXCLUDES   *hypoplasia of aortic arch (747.10)*

747.22 Atresia and stenosis of aorta   `CC`

Absence   }
Aplasia   } of aorta
Hypoplasia   }
Stricture   }

Supra (valvular)-aortic stenosis

    EXCLUDES   *congenital aortic (valvular) stenosis or stricture, so stated (746.3)*
                  hypoplasia of aorta in hypoplastic left heart syndrome (746.7)

CC Excl: See code 747.11

747.29 Other

Aneurysm of sinus of Valsalva
Congenital:
  aneurysm   } of aorta
  dilation

747.3   **Anomalies of pulmonary artery**

Agenesis   }
Anomaly   }
Atresia   } of pulmonary artery
Coarctation   }
Hypoplasia   }
Stenosis   }

Pulmonary arteriovenous aneurysm

AHA: 1Q, '94, 15; 4Q, '88, 8

√5th **747.4**   **Anomalies of great veins**

747.40 Anomaly of great veins, unspecified

Anomaly NOS of: Anomaly NOS of:
  pulmonary veins   vena cava

√4th √5th Additional Digit Required   Nonspecific PDx   Unacceptable PDx   Manifestation Code   `MSP` Medicare Secondary Payer   ▶◄ Revised Text   ● New Code   ▲ Revised Code Title

747.41 Total anomalous pulmonary venous connection
Total anomalous pulmonary venous return [TAPVR]:
subdiaphragmatic
supradiaphragmatic

747.42 Partial anomalous pulmonary venous connection
Partial anomalous pulmonary venous return

747.49 Other anomalies of great veins
Absence | of vena cava
Congenital stenosis | (inferior)
| (superior)

Persistent:
left posterior cardinal vein
left superior vena cava
Scimitar syndrome
Transposition of pulmonary veins NOS

747.5 Absence or hypoplasia of umbilical artery
Single umbilical artery

✓5ᵗʰ **747.6 Other anomalies of peripheral vascular system**
Absence
Anomaly } of artery or vein, NEC
Atresia

Arteriovenous aneurysm (peripheral)
Arteriovenous malformation of the peripheral vascular system
Congenital:
  aneurysm (peripheral)   stricture, artery
  phlebectasia   varix
Multiple renal arteries

EXCLUDES   anomalies of:
cerebral vessels (747.81)
pulmonary artery (747.3)
congenital retinal aneurysm (743.58)
hemangioma (228.00-228.09)
lymphangioma (228.1)

747.60 Anomaly of the peripheral vascular system, unspecified site

747.61 Gastrointestinal vessel anomaly
AHA: 3Q '96, 10

747.62 Renal vessel anomaly

747.63 Upper limb vessel anomaly

747.64 Lower limb vessel anomaly

747.69 Anomalies of other specified sites of peripheral vascular system

✓5ᵗʰ **747.8 Other specified anomalies of circulatory system**

747.81 Anomalies of cerebrovascular system
Arteriovenous malformation of brain
Cerebral arteriovenous aneurysm, congenital
Congenital anomalies of cerebral vessels
EXCLUDES   ruptured cerebral (arteriovenous) aneurysm (430)

747.82 Spinal vessel anomaly
Arteriovenous malformation of spinal vessel
AHA: 3Q, '95, 5

● **747.83 Persistent fetal circulation**
Persistent pulmonary hypertension
Primary pulmonary hypertension of newborn

747.89 Other
Aneurysm, congenital, specified site not elsewhere classified
EXCLUDES   congenital aneurysm:
coronary (746.85)
peripheral (747.6)
pulmonary (747.3)
retinal (743.58)

747.9 Unspecified anomaly of circulatory system

✓4ᵗʰ **748 Congenital anomalies of respiratory system**
EXCLUDES   congenital defect of diaphragm (756.6)

748.0 Choanal atresia
Atresia } of nares (anterior)
Congenital stenosis } (posterior)

DEF: Occluded posterior nares (choana), bony or membranous due to failure of embryonic bucconasal membrane to rupture.

748.1 Other anomalies of nose
Absent nose   Congenital:
Accessory nose   notching of tip of nose
Cleft nose   perforation of wall of
Congenital: nasal sinus
  deformity of nose   Deformity of wall of nasal
       sinus
EXCLUDES   congenital deviation of nasal septum (754.0)

748.2 Web of larynx
Web of larynx: Web of larynx:
  NOS   subglottic
  glottic

DEF: Malformed larynx; marked by thin, translucent, or thick, fibrotic spread between vocal folds; affects speech.

748.3 Other anomalies of larynx, trachea, and bronchus
Absence or agenesis of: Congenital:
  bronchus   dilation, trachea
  larynx   stenosis:
  trachea   larynx
Anomaly(of):   trachea
  cricoid cartilage   tracheocele
  epiglottis   Diverticulum:
  thyroid cartilage   bronchus
  tracheal cartilage   trachea
Atresia (of):   Fissure of epiglottis
  epiglottis   Laryngocele
  glottis   Posterior cleft of cricoid
  larynx   cartilage (congenital)
  trachea   Rudimentary tracheal
Cleft thyroid, cartilage,   bronchus
  congenital   Stridor, laryngeal, congenital
AHA: 1Q, '99, 14

748.4 Congenital cystic lung   CC
Disease, lung: Honeycomb lung, congenital
  cystic, congenital
  polycystic, congenital
EXCLUDES   acquired or unspecified cystic lung (518.89)

CC Excl: 748.4-748.9

DEF: Enlarged air spaces of lung parenchyma.

748.5 Agenesis, hypoplasia, and dysplasia of lung   CC
Absence of lung (fissures) (lobe)
  (lobe)   Hypoplasia of lung
Aplasia of lung   Sequestration of lung
CC Excl: See code 748.4

✓5ᵗʰ **748.6 Other anomalies of lung**
748.60 Anomaly of lung, unspecified
748.61 Congenital bronchiectasis   CC
  CC Excl: 494.0-494.1, 496, 506.1, 506.4, 506.9, 748.61

748.69 Other
Accessory lung (lobe)
Azygos lobe (fissure), lung

748.8 Other specified anomalies of respiratory system
Abnormal communication between pericardial and pleural sacs
Anomaly, pleural folds
Atresia of nasopharynx
Congenital cyst of mediastinum

748.9 Unspecified anomaly of respiratory system
Anomaly of respiratory system NOS

✓4ᵗʰ **749 Cleft palate and cleft lip**

N Newborn Age: 0   P Pediatric Age: 0-17   M Maternity Age: 12-55   A Adult Age: 15-124   CC CC Condition   MC Major Complication   CD Complex Dx   HIV HIV Related Dx

Cleft Lip and Palate

Unilateral cleft lip — No cleft palate

Cleft lip with cleft alveolar ridge — No cleft palate

Unilateral cleft lip and cleft palate — Alveolar ridge — Cleft palate

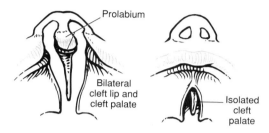

Prolabium

Bilateral cleft lip and cleft palate

Isolated cleft palate

✓5ᵗʰ **749.0 Cleft palate**

     749.00 Cleft palate, unspecified

     749.01 Unilateral, complete

     749.02 Unilateral, incomplete
         Cleft uvula

     749.03 Bilateral, complete

     749.04 Bilateral, incomplete

✓5ᵗʰ **749.1 Cleft lip**
         Cheiloschisis   Harelip
         Congenital fissure of lip   Labium leporinum

     749.10 Cleft lip, unspecified

     749.11 Unilateral, complete

     749.12 Unilateral, incomplete

     749.13 Bilateral, complete

     749.14 Bilateral, incomplete

✓5ᵗʰ **749.2 Cleft palate with cleft lip**
         Cheilopalatoschisis

     749.20 Cleft palate with cleft lip, unspecified

     749.21 Unilateral, complete

     749.22 Unilateral, incomplete

     749.23 Bilateral, complete
         AHA: 1Q, '96, 14

     749.24 Bilateral, incomplete

     749.25 Other combinations

✓4ᵗʰ **750 Other congenital anomalies of upper alimentary tract**
     EXCLUDES   dentofacial anomalies (524.0-524.9)

     750.0 Tongue tie
         Ankyloglossia

         DEF: Restricted tongue movement due to lingual frenum extending toward tip of tongue. Tongue may be fused to mouth floor affecting speech.

✓5ᵗʰ   **750.1 Other anomalies of tongue**

     750.10 Anomaly of tongue, unspecified

     750.11 Aglossia

         DEF: Absence of tongue.

     750.12 Congenital adhesions of tongue

     750.13 Fissure of tongue
         Bifid tongue   Double tongue

     750.15 Macroglossia
         Congenital hypertrophy of tongue

     750.16 Microglossia
         Hypoplasia of tongue

     750.19 Other

✓5ᵗʰ   **750.2 Other specified anomalies of mouth and pharynx**

     750.21 Absence of salivary gland

     750.22 Accessory salivary gland

     750.23 Atresia, salivary duct
         Imperforate salivary duct

     750.24 Congenital fistula of salivary gland

     750.25 Congenital fistula of lip
         Congenital (mucus) lip pits

     750.26 Other specified anomalies of mouth
         Absence of uvula

     750.27 Diverticulum of pharynx
         Pharyngeal pouch

     750.29 Other specified anomalies of pharynx
         Imperforate pharynx

     750.3 Tracheoesophageal fistula, esophageal atresia and stenosis

         Absent esophagus
         Atresia of esophagus
         Congenital:
           esophageal ring
           stenosis of esophagus
           stricture of esophagus

         Congenital fistula:
           esophagobronchial
           esophagotracheal
         Imperforate esophagus
         Webbed esophagus

     750.4 Other specified anomalies of esophagus

         Dilatation, congenital
         Displacement, congenital
         Diverticulum   } (of) esophagus
         Duplication
         Giant

         Esophageal pouch
         EXCLUDES   congenital hiatus hernia (750.6)

     AHA: J-F, '85, 3

     750.5 Congenital hypertrophic pyloric stenosis
         Congenital or infantile:
           constriction
           hypertrophy
           spasm   } of pylorus
           stenosis
           stricture

         DEF: Obstructed pylorus due to overgrowth of pyloric muscle.

     750.6 Congenital hiatus hernia
         Displacement of cardia through esophageal hiatus
         EXCLUDES   congenital diaphragmatic hernia (756.6)

     750.7 Other specified anomalies of stomach
         Congenital:
           cardiospasm
           hourglass stomach
         Displacement of stomach
         Diverticulum of stomach, congenital
         Duplication of stomach
         Megalogastria
         Microgastria
         Transposition of stomach

     750.8 Other specified anomalies of upper alimentary tract

     750.9 Unspecified anomaly of upper alimentary tract
         Congenital:
           anomaly NOS   } of upper alimentary tract
           deformity NOS   [any part, except tongue]

✓4ᵗʰ **751 Other congenital anomalies of digestive system**

     751.0 Meckel's diverticulum
         Meckel's diverticulum (displaced) (hypertrophic)
         Persistent:
           omphalomesenteric duct
           vitelline duct

         DEF: Malformed sacs or appendages of ileum of small intestine; can cause strangulation, volvulus and intussusception.

✓4ᵗʰ / ✓5ᵗʰ Additional Digit Required   Nonspecific PDx   Unacceptable PDx   Manifestation Code   **MSP** Medicare Secondary Payer   ►◄ Revised Text   ● New Code   ▲ Revised Code Title

2002 Ingenix, Inc.   **Volume 1 — 233**

751.1 Atresia and stenosis of small intestine [P]

Atresia of:
    duodenum
    ileum

Atresia of:
    intestine NOS

Congenital:
    absence
    obstruction } of small intestine or
    stenosis   intestine NOS
    stricture

Imperforate jejunum

751.2 Atresia and stenosis of large intestine, rectum, and anal canal [P]

Absence:
    anus (congenital)
    appendix, congenital
    large intestine, congenital
    rectum

Atresia of:
    anus
    colon
    rectum

Congenital or infantile:
    obstruction of large
        intestine
    occlusion of anus
    stricture of anus

Imperforate:
    anus
    rectum

Stricture of rectum, congenital

AHA: 2Q, '98, 16

751.3 Hirschsprung's disease and other congenital functional disorders of colon

Aganglionosis
Congenital dilation of colon

Congenital megacolon
Macrocolon

DEF: Hirschsprung's disease: enlarged or dilated colon (megacolon), with absence of ganglion cells in the narrowed wall distally; causes inability to defecate.

751.4 Anomalies of intestinal fixation

Congenital adhesions:
    omental, anomalous
    peritoneal
    Jackson's membrane
    Malrotation of colon

Rotation of cecum or colon:
    failure of
    incomplete
    insufficient
    Universal mesentery

751.5 Other anomalies of intestine

Congenital diverticulum, colon
Dolichocolon
Duplication of:
    anus
    appendix
    cecum
    intestine
Ectopic anus

Megaloappendix
Megaloduodenum
Microcolon
Persistent cloaca
Transposition of:
    appendix
    colon
    intestine

AHA: 3Q, '01, 8

√5th 751.6 Anomalies of gallbladder, bile ducts, and liver

751.60 Unspecified anomaly of gallbladder, bile ducts, and liver

751.61 Biliary atresia [P]

Congenital:
    absence
    hypoplasia } of bile duct (common)
    obstruction   or passage
    stricture

AHA: S-O, '87, 8

751.62 Congenital cystic disease of liver

Congenital polycystic disease of liver
Fibrocystic disease of liver

751.69 Other anomalies of gallbladder, bile ducts, and liver

Absence of:
    gallbladder, congenital
    liver (lobe)
Accessory:
    hepatic ducts
    liver
Congenital:
    choledochal cyst
    hepatomegaly

Duplication of:
    biliary duct
    cystic duct
    gallbladder
    liver
Floating:
    gallbladder
    liver
Intrahepatic
    gallbladder

AHA: S-O, '87, 8

751.7 Anomalies of pancreas

Absence
Accessory
Agenesis } (of) pancreas
Annular
Hypoplasia

Ectopic pancreatic tissue   Pancreatic heterotopia

EXCLUDES   *diabetes mellitus:*
        congenital (250.0-250.9)
        neonatal (775.1)
    fibrocystic disease of pancreas
    ▶*(277.00-277.09)◀*

751.8 Other specified anomalies of digestive system

Absence (complete) (partial) of alimentary tract NOS

Duplication } of digestive organs NOS
Malposition, congenital

EXCLUDES   *congenital diaphragmatic hernia (756.6)*
    congenital hiatus hernia (750.6)

751.9 Unspecified anomaly of digestive system

Congenital:
    anomaly NOS } of digestive system NOS
    deformity NOS

√4th 752 Congenital anomalies of genital organs

EXCLUDES   *syndromes associated with anomalies in the number and form of chromosomes (758.0-758.9)*
    testicular feminization syndrome (257.8)

752.0 Anomalies of ovaries ♀

Absence, congenital
Accessory } (of) ovary
Ectopic
Streak

√5th 752.1 Anomalies of fallopian tubes and broad ligaments

752.10 Unspecified anomaly of fallopian tubes and broad ligaments ♀

752.11 Embryonic cyst of fallopian tubes and broad ligaments ♀

Cyst:
    epoophoron
    fimbrial

Cyst:
    Gartner's duct
    parovarian

AHA: S-O, '85, 13

752.19 Other ♀

Absence
Accessory } (of) fallopian tube or
Atresia   broad ligament

752.2 Doubling of uterus ♀

Didelphic uterus
Doubling of uterus [any degree] (associated with doubling of cervix and vagina)

752.3 Other anomalies of uterus ♀

Absence, congenital
Agenesis } (of) uterus
Aplasia
Bicornuate

Uterus unicornis
Uterus with only one functioning horn

√5th 752.4 Anomalies of cervix, vagina, and external female genitalia

752.40 Unspecified anomaly of cervix, vagina, and external female genitalia ♀

752.41 Embryonic cyst of cervix, vagina, and external female genitalia ♀

Cyst of:
    canal of Nuck, congenital
    vagina, embryonal
    vulva, congenital

DEF: Embryonic fluid-filled cysts, of cervix, vagina or external female genitalia.

[N] Newborn Age: 0   [P] Pediatric Age: 0-17   [M] Maternity Age: 12-55   [A] Adult Age: 15-124   [CC] CC Condition   [MC] Major Complication   [CD] Complex Dx   [HIV] HIV Related Dx

234 — Volume 1 • October 2002   *2002 Ingenix, Inc.*

752.42 Imperforate hymen ♀

DEF: Complete closure of membranous fold around external opening of vagina.

752.49 Other anomalies of cervix, vagina, and external female genitalia ♀

Absence } of cervix, clitoris,
Agenesis } vagina, or vulva

Congenital stenosis or stricture of:
  cervical canal
  vagina

EXCLUDES *double vagina associated with total duplication (752.2)*

√5th **752.5 Undescended and retractile testicle**

AHA: 4Q, '96, 33

752.51 Undescended testis ♂
  Cryptorchism
  Ectopic testis

752.52 Retractile testis ♂

√5th **752.6 Hypospadias and epispadias and other penile anomalies**

AHA: 4Q, '96, 34, 35

752.61 Hypospadias ♂

AHA: 3Q, '97, 6

DEF: Hypospadias: abnormal opening of urethra on the ventral surface of the penis or perineum; also a rare defect of vagina.

752.62 Epispadias ♂
  Anaspadias

DEF: Epispadias: urethra opening on dorsal surface of penis; in females appears as a slit in the upper wall of urethra.

752.63 Congenital chordee ♂

DEF: Ventral bowing of penis due to fibrous band along corpus spongiosum; occurs with hypospadias.

752.64 Micropenis ♂

752.65 Hidden penis ♂

752.69 Other penile anomalies ♂

752.7 Indeterminate sex and pseudohermaphroditism

Gynandrism   Pseudohermaphroditism
Hermaphroditism   (male) (female)
Ovotestis   Pure gonadal dysgenesis

EXCLUDES *pseudohermaphroditism:*
  female, with adrenocortical disorder (255.2)
  male, with gonadal disorder (257.8)
  with specified chromosomal anomaly (758.0-758.9)
  testicular feminization syndrome (257.8)

DEF: Pseudohermaphroditism: presence of gonads of one sex and external genitalia of other sex.

752.8 Other specified anomalies of genital organs

Absence of: Atresia of:
  prostate   ejaculatory duct
  spermatic cord   vas deferens
  vas deferens   Fusion of testes
Anorchism   Hypoplasia of testis
Aplasia (congenital) of: Monorchism
  prostate   Polyorchism
  round ligament
  testicle

EXCLUDES *congenital hydrocele (778.6)*
  penile anomalies (752.61-752.69)
  phimosis or paraphimosis (605)

752.9 Unspecified anomaly of genital organs

Congenital:
  anomaly NOS } of genital organ,
  deformity NOS } not elsewhere classified

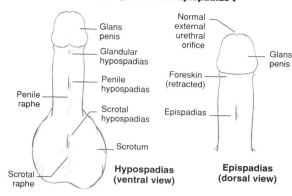

▶**Hypospadias and Epispadias**◀

Glans penis
Glandular hypospadias
Penile hypospadias
Scrotal hypospadias
Penile raphe
Scrotum
Scrotal raphe

Hypospadias (ventral view)

Normal external urethral orifice
Glans penis
Foreskin (retracted)
Epispadias

Epispadias (dorsal view)

√4th **753 Congenital anomalies of urinary system**

753.0 Renal agenesis and dysgenesis

Atrophy of kidney: Atrophy of kidney:
  congenital   infantile
Congenital absence of kidney(s)
Hypoplasia of kidney(s)

√5th **753.1 Cystic kidney disease**

EXCLUDES *acquired cyst of kidney (593.2)*

AHA: 4Q, '90. 3

753.10 Cystic kidney disease, unspecified

753.11 Congenital single renal cyst

753.12 Polycystic kidney, unspecified type

753.13 Polycystic kidney, autosomal dominant

DEF: Slow progressive disease characterized by bilateral cysts causing increased kidney size and impaired function.

753.14 Polycystic kidney, autosomal recessive

DEF: Rare disease characterized by multiple cysts involving kidneys and liver, producing renal and hepatic failure in childhood or adolescence.

753.15 Renal dysplasia

753.16 Medullary cystic kidney
  Nephronopthisis

DEF: Diffuse kidney disease results in uremia onset prior to age 20.

753.17 Medullary sponge kidney

DEF: Dilated collecting tubules; usually asymptomatic but calcinosis in tubules may cause renal insufficiency.

753.19 Other specified cystic kidney disease
  Multicystic kidney

√5th **753.2 Obstructive defects of renal pelvis and ureter**

AHA: 4Q, '96, 35

753.20 Unspecified obstructive defect of renal pelvis and ureter

753.21 Congenital obstruction of ureteropelvic junction

DEF: Stricture at junction of ureter and renal pelvis.

753.22 Congenital obstruction of ureterovesical junction
  Adynamic ureter
  Congenital hydroureter

DEF: Stricture at junction of ureter and bladder.

753.23 Congenital ureterocele

753.29 Other

753.3 Other specified anomalies of kidney

Accessory kidney   Fusion of kidneys
Congenital: Giant kidney
  calculus of kidney   Horseshoe kidney
  displaced kidney   Hyperplasia of kidney
Discoid kidney   Lobulation of kidney
Double kidney with   Malrotation of kidney
  double pelvis   Trifid kidney (pelvis)
Ectopic kidney

√4th √5th Additional Digit Required   Nonspecific PDx   Unacceptable PDx   **Manifestation Code**   MSP Medicare Secondary Payer   ►◄ Revised Text   ● New Code   ▲ Revised Code Title

2002 Ingenix, Inc.

January 2002 • Volume 1 — 235

Congenital Anomalies 753.4–755.01

753.4 Other specified anomalies of ureter
Absent ureter   Double ureter
Accessory ureter   Ectopic ureter
Deviation of ureter   Implantation, anomalous
Displaced ureteric   of ureter
   orifice

753.5 Exstrophy of urinary bladder
Ectopia vesicae
Extroversion of bladder
DEF: Absence of lower abdominal and anterior bladder walls with posterior bladder wall protrusion.

753.6 Atresia and stenosis of urethra and bladder neck
Congenital obstruction: Imperforate urinary
   bladder neck   meatus
   urethra   Impervious urethra
Congenital stricture of: Urethral valve formation
   urethra (valvular)
   urinary meatus
   vesicourethral orifice

753.7 Anomalies of urachus
Cyst
Fistula   } (of) urachussinus
Patent

Persistent umbilical sinus

753.8 Other specified anomalies of bladder and urethra
Absence, congenital of: Congenital urethrorectal
   bladder   fistula
   urethra   Congenital prolapse of:
Accessory: bladder (mucosa)
   bladder   urethra
   urethra   Double:
Congenital: urethra
   diverticulum of bladder   urinary meatus
   hernia of bladder

753.9 Unspecified anomaly of urinary system
Congenital:
   anomaly NOS   } of urinary system [any part,
   deformity NOS   except urachus]

✓4th **754 Certain congenital musculoskeletal deformities**
INCLUDES   nonteratogenic deformities which are considered to be due to intrauterine malposition and pressure

754.0 Of skull, face, and jaw
Asymmetry of face   Dolichocephaly
Compression facies   Plagiocephaly
Depressions in skull   Potter's facies
Deviation of nasal   Squashed or bent nose,
   septum, congenital   congenital
EXCLUDES   *dentofacial anomalies (524.0-524.9)*
     syphilitic saddle nose (090.5)

754.1 Of sternocleidomastoid muscle
Congenital sternomastoid torticollis
Congenital wryneck
Contracture of sternocleidomastoid (muscle)
Sternomastoid tumor

754.2 Of spine
Congenital postural:
   lordosis
   scoliosis

✓5th **754.3 Congenital dislocation of hip**
   754.30 Congenital dislocation of hip, unilateral
     Congenital dislocation of hip NOS
   754.31 Congenital dislocation of hip, bilateral
   754.32 Congenital subluxation of hip, unilateral
     Congenital flexion deformity, hip or thigh
     Predislocation status of hip at birth
     Preluxation of hip, congenital
   754.33 Congenital subluxation of hip, bilateral
   754.35 Congenital dislocation of one hip with subluxation of other hip

✓5th **754.4 Congenital genu recurvatum and bowing of long bones of leg**

754.40 Genu recurvatum
   DEF: Backward curving of knee joint.
754.41 Congenital dislocation of knee (with genu recurvatum)
754.42 Congenital bowing of femur
754.43 Congenital bowing of tibia and fibula
754.44 Congenital bowing of unspecified long bones of leg

✓5th **754.5 Varus deformities of feet**
   EXCLUDES   *acquired (736.71, 736.75, 736.79)*
   754.50 Talipes varus
     Congenital varus deformity of foot, unspecified
     Pes varus
     DEF: Inverted foot marked by outer sole resting on ground.
   754.51 Talipes equinovarus
     Equinovarus (congenital)
     DEF: Elevated, outward rotation of heel; also called clubfoot.
   754.52 Metatarsus primus varus
     DEF: Malformed first metatarsal bone, with bone angled toward body.
   754.53 Metatarsus varus
   754.59 Other
     Talipes calcaneovarus

✓5th **754.6 Valgus deformities of feet**
   EXCLUDES   *valgus deformity of foot (acquired) (736.79)*
   754.60 Talipes valgus
     Congenital valgus deformity of foot, unspecified
   754.61 Congenital pes planus
     Congenital rocker bottom flat foot
     Flat foot, congenital
     EXCLUDES   *pes planus (acquired) (734)*
   754.62 Talipes calcaneovalgus
   754.69 Other
     Talipes: Talipes:
     equinovalgus   planovalgus

✓5th **754.7 Other deformities of feet**
   EXCLUDES   *acquired (736.70-736.79)*
   754.70 Talipes, unspecified
     Congenital deformity of foot NOS
   754.71 Talipes cavus
     Cavus foot (congenital)
   754.79 Other
     Asymmetric talipes
     Talipes:
       calcaneus
       equinus

✓5th **754.8 Other specified nonteratogenic anomalies**
   754.81 Pectus excavatum
     Congenital funnel chest
   754.82 Pectus carinatum
     Congenital pigeon chest [breast]
   754.89 Other
     Club hand (congenital)
     Congenital:
       deformity of chest wall
       dislocation of elbow
     Generalized flexion contractures of lower limb joints, congenital
     Spade-like hand (congenital)

✓4th **755 Other congenital anomalies of limbs**
   EXCLUDES   *those deformities classifiable to 754.0-754.8*

✓5th **755.0 Polydactyly**
   755.00 Polydactyly, unspecified digits
     Supernumerary digits
   755.01 Of fingers
     Accessory fingers

N Newborn Age: 0   P Pediatric Age: 0-17   M Maternity Age: 12-55   A Adult Age: 15-124   CC CC Condition   MC Major Complication   CD Complex Dx   HIV HIV Related Dx

2002 Ingenix, Inc.

755.02 Of toes
Accessory toes

✓5th **755.1 Syndactyly**
Symphalangy   Webbing of digits

755.10 Of multiple and unspecified sites

755.11 Of fingers without fusion of bone

755.12 Of fingers with fusion of bone

755.13 Of toes without fusion of bone

755.14 Of toes with fusion of bone

✓5th **755.2 Reduction deformities of upper limb**

755.20 Unspecified reduction deformity of upper limb
Ectromelia NOS ⎫
Hemimelia NOS ⎬ of upper limb
Shortening of arm, congenital

755.21 Transverse deficiency of upper limb
Amelia of upper limb
Congenital absence of:
     fingers, all (complete or partial)
     forearm, including hand and fingers
     upper limb, complete
Congenital amputation of upper limb
Transverse hemimelia of upper limb

755.22 Longitudinal deficiency of upper limb, not elsewhere classified
Phocomelia NOS of upper limb
Rudimentary arm

755.23 Longitudinal deficiency, combined, involving humerus, radius, and ulna (complete or incomplete)
Congenital absence of arm and forearm (complete or incomplete) with or without metacarpal deficiency and/or phalangeal deficiency, incomplete
Phocomelia, complete, of upper limb

755.24 Longitudinal deficiency, humeral, complete or partial (with or without distal deficiencies, incomplete)
Congenital absence of humerus (with or without absence of some [but not all] distal elements)
Proximal phocomelia of upper limb

755.25 Longitudinal deficiency, radioulnar, complete or partial (with or without distal deficiencies, incomplete)
Congenital absence of radius and ulna (with or without absence of some [but not all] distal elements)
Distal phocomelia of upper limb

755.26 Longitudinal deficiency, radial, complete or partial (with or without distal deficiencies, incomplete)
Agenesis of radius
Congenital absence of radius (with or without absence of some [but not all] distal elements)

755.27 Longitudinal deficiency, ulnar, complete or partial (with or without distal deficiencies, incomplete)
Agenesis of ulna
Congenital absence of ulna (with or without absence of some [but not all] distal elements)

755.28 Longitudinal deficiency, carpals or metacarpals, complete or partial (with or without incomplete phalangeal deficiency)

755.29 Longitudinal deficiency, phalanges, complete or partial
Absence of finger, congenital
Aphalangia of upper limb, terminal, complete or partial
     EXCLUDES   *terminal deficiency of all five digits (755.21)*
                         transverse deficiency of phalanges (755.21)

✓5th **755.3 Reduction deformities of lower limb**

755.30 Unspecified reduction deformity of lower limb
Ectromelia NOS ⎫
Hemimelia NOS ⎬ of lower limb
Shortening of leg, congenital

755.31 Transverse deficiency of lower limb
Amelia of lower limb
Congenital absence of:
     foot
     leg, including foot and toes
     lower limb, complete
     toes, all, complete
Transverse hemimelia of lower limb

755.32 Longitudinal deficiency of lower limb, not elsewhere classified
Phocomelia NOS of lower limb

755.33 Longitudinal deficiency, combined, involving femur, tibia, and fibula (complete or incomplete)
Congenital absence of thigh and (lower) leg (complete or incomplete) with or without metacarpal deficiency and/or phalangeal deficiency, incomplete
Phocomelia, complete, of lower limb

755.34 Longitudinal deficiency, femoral, complete or partial (with or without distal deficiencies, incomplete)
Congenital absence of femur (with or without absence of some [but not all] distal elements)
Proximal phocomelia of lower limb

755.35 Longitudinal deficiency, tibiofibular, complete or partial (with or without distal deficiencies, incomplete)
Congenital absence of tibia and fibula (with or without absence of some [but not all] distal elements)
Distal phocomelia of lower limb

755.36 Longitudinal deficiency, tibia, complete or partial (with or without distal deficiencies, incomplete)
Agenesis of tibia
Congenital absence of tibia (with or without absence of some [but not all] distal elements)

755.37 Longitudinal deficiency, fibular, complete or partial (with or without distal deficiencies, incomplete)
Agenesis of fibula
Congenital absence of fibula (with or without absence of some [but not all] distal elements)

755.38 Longitudinal deficiency, tarsals or metatarsals, complete or partial (with or without incomplete phalangeal deficiency)

755.39 Longitudinal deficiency, phalanges, complete or partial
Absence of toe, congenital
Aphalangia of lower limb, terminal, complete or partial
     EXCLUDES   *terminal deficiency of all five digits (755.31)*
                         transverse deficiency of phalanges (755.31)

755.4 Reduction deformities, unspecified limb
Absence, congenital (complete or partial) of limb NOS
Amelia ⎫
Ectromelia ⎬ of unspecified limb
Hemimelia ⎪
Phocomelia ⎭

✓5th **755.5 Other anomalies of upper limb, including shoulder girdle**

755.50 Unspecified anomaly of upper limb

✓4th / ✓5th **Additional Digit Required**   Nonspecific PDx   Unacceptable PDx   Manifestation Code   **MSP** Medicare Secondary Payer   ▶◀ Revised Text   ● New Code   ▲ Revised Code Title

2002 Ingenix, Inc.   **Volume 1 — 237**

Congenital Anomalies 755.51–756.4

755.51 Congenital deformity of clavicle

755.52 Congenital elevation of scapula
Sprengel's deformity

755.53 Radioulnar synostosis
DEF: Osseous adhesion of radius and ulna.

755.54 Madelung's deformity
DEF: Distal ulnar overgrowth or radial shortening; also called carpus curvus.

755.55 Acrocephalosyndactyly
Apert's syndrome
DEF: Premature cranial suture fusion (craniostenosis); marked by cone-shaped or pointed (acrocephaly) head and webbing of the fingers (syndactyly); it is very similar to craniofacial dysostosis.

755.56 Accessory carpal bones

755.57 Macrodactylia (fingers)
DEF: Abnormally large fingers, toes.

755.58 Cleft hand, congenital
Lobster-claw hand
DEF: Extended separation between fingers into metacarpus; also may refer to large fingers and absent middle fingers of hand.

755.59 Other
Cleidocranial dysostosis
Cubitus:
    valgus, congenital
    varus, congenital
EXCLUDES *club hand (congenital) (754.89)*
congenital dislocation of elbow (754.89)

√5th **755.6 Other anomalies of lower limb, including pelvic girdle**

755.60 Unspecified anomaly of lower limb

755.61 Coxa valga, congenital
DEF: Abnormally wide angle between the neck and shaft of the femur.

755.62 Coxa vara, congenital
DEF: Diminished angle between neck and shaft of femur.

755.63 Other congenital deformity of hip (joint)
Congenital anteversion of femur (neck)
EXCLUDES *congenital dislocation of hip (754.30-754.35)*
AHA: 1Q, '94, 15; S-O, '84, 15

755.64 Congenital deformity of knee (joint)
Congenital:
    absence of patella
    genu valgum [knock-knee]
    genu varum [bowleg]
    Rudimentary patella

755.65 Macrodactylia of toes
DEF: Abnormally large toes.

755.66 Other anomalies of toes
Congenital: Congenital:
  hallux valgus   hammer toe
  hallux varus

755.67 Anomalies of foot, not elsewhere classified
Astragaloscaphoid synostosis
Calcaneonavicular bar
Coalition of calcaneus
Talonavicular synostosis
Tarsal coalitions

755.69 Other
Congenital:
    angulation of tibia
    deformity (of):
      ankle (joint)
      sacroiliac (joint)
    fusion of sacroiliac joint

755.8 Other specified anomalies of unspecified limb

755.9 Unspecified anomaly of unspecified limb
Congenital:
anomaly NOS
deformity NOS } of unspecified limb
EXCLUDES *reduction deformity of unspecified limb (755.4)*

√4th **756 Other congenital musculoskeletal anomalies**
EXCLUDES *those deformities classifiable to 754.0-754.8*

756.0 Anomalies of skull and face bones
Absence of skull bones   Imperfect fusion of skull
Acrocephaly   Oxycephaly
Congenital deformity   Platybasia
  of forehead   Premature closure of
Craniosynostosis   cranial sutures
Crouzon's disease   Tower skull
Hypertelorism   Trigonocephaly
EXCLUDES *acrocephalosyndactyly [Apert's syndrome] (755.55)*
dentofacial anomalies (524.0-524.9)
skull defects associated with brain anomalies, such as:
  anencephalus (740.0)
  encephalocele (742.0)
  hydrocephalus (742.3)
  microcephalus (742.1)
AHA: 3Q, '98, 9; 3Q, '96, 15

√5th **756.1 Anomalies of spine**

756.10 Anomaly of spine, unspecified

756.11 Spondylolysis, lumbosacral region
Prespondylolisthesis (lumbosacral)
DEF: Bilateral or unilateral defect through the pars interarticularis of a vertebra causes spondylolisthesis.

756.12 Spondylolisthesis
DEF: Downward slipping of lumbar vertebra over next vertebra; usually related to pelvic deformity.

756.13 Absence of vertebra, congenital

756.14 Hemivertebra
DEF: Incomplete development of one side of a vertebra.

756.15 Fusion of spine [vertebra], congenital

756.16 Klippel-Feil syndrome
DEF: Short, wide neck; limits range of motion due to abnormal number of cervical vertebra or fused hemivertebrae.

756.17 Spina bifida occulta
EXCLUDES *spina bifida (aperta) (741.0-741.9)*
DEF: Spina bifida marked by a bony spinal canal defect without a protrusion of the cord or meninges; it is diagnosed by radiography and has no symptoms.

756.19 Other
Platyspondylia   Supernumerary vertebra

756.2 Cervical rib
Supernumerary rib in the cervical region
DEF: Costa cervicalis: extra rib attached to cervical vertebra.

756.3 Other anomalies of ribs and sternum
Congenital absence of: Congenital:
  rib   fissure of sternum
  sternum   fusion of ribs
                      Sternum bifidum
EXCLUDES *nonteratogenic deformity of chest wall (754.81-754.89)*

756.4 Chondrodystrophy
Achondroplasia   Enchondromatosis
Chondrodystrophia (fetalis)   Ollier's disease
Dyschondroplasia
EXCLUDES *lipochondrodystrophy [Hurler's syndrome] (277.5)*
Morquio's disease (277.5)
AHA: S-O, '87, 10
DEF: Abnormal development of cartilage.

N Newborn Age: 0   P Pediatric Age: 0-17   M Maternity Age: 12-55   A Adult Age: 15-124   CC CC Condition   MC Major Complication   CD Complex Dx   HIV HIV Related Dx

√5th **756.5 Osteodystrophies**

756.50 Osteodystrophy, unspecified

756.51 Osteogenesis imperfecta
Fragilitas ossium
Osteopsathyrosis

DEF: A collagen disorder commonly characterized by brittle, osteoporotic, easily fractured bones, hypermobility of joints, blue sclerae, and a tendency to hemorrhage.

756.52 Osteopetrosis

DEF: Abnormally dense bone, optic atrophy, hepatosplenomegaly, deafness; sclerosing depletes bone marrow and nerve foramina of skull; often fatal.

756.53 Osteopoikilosis

DEF: Multiple sclerotic foci on ends of long bones, stippling in round, flat bones; identified by x-ray.

756.54 Polyostotic fibrous dysplasia of bone

DEF: Fibrous tissue displaces bone results in segmented ragged-edge café-au-lait spots; occurs in girls of early puberty.

756.55 Chondroectodermal dysplasia
Ellis-van Creveld syndrome

DEF: Inadequate enchondral bone formation; impaired development of hair and teeth, polydactyly, and cardiac septum defects.

756.56 Multiple epiphyseal dysplasia

756.59 Other
Albright (-McCune)-Sternberg syndrome

756.6 Anomalies of diaphragm
Absence of diaphragm
Congenital hernia:
diaphragmatic
foramen of Morgagni
Eventration of diaphragm
EXCLUDES   congenital hiatus hernia (750.6)

√5th **756.7 Anomalies of abdominal wall**

756.70 Anomaly of abdominal wall, unspecified

756.71 Prune belly syndrome
Eagle-Barrett syndrome
Prolapse of bladder mucosa

AHA: 4Q, '97, 44

DEF: Prune belly syndrome: absence of lower rectus abdominis muscle and lower and medial oblique muscles; results in dilated bladder and ureters, dysplastic kidneys and hydronephrosis; more common in male infants with undescended testicles.

756.79 Other congenital anomalies of abdominal wall
Exomphalos
Gastroschisis
Omphalocele
EXCLUDES   umbilical hernia (551-553 with .1)

DEF: Exomphalos: umbilical hernia prominent navel.

DEF: Gastroschisis: fissure of abdominal wall, results in protruding small or large intestine.

DEF: Omphalocele: hernia of umbilicus due to impaired abdominal wall; results in membrane-covered intestine protruding through peritoneum and amnion.

√5th **756.8 Other specified anomalies of muscle, tendon, fascia, and connective tissue**

756.81 Absence of muscle and tendon
Absence of muscle (pectoral)

756.82 Accessory muscle

756.83 Ehlers-Danlos syndrome

DEF: Danlos syndrome: connective tissue disorder causes hyperextended skin and joints; results in fragile blood vessels with bleeding, poor wound healing and subcutaneous pseudotumors.

756.89 Other
Amyotrophia congenita
Congenital shortening of tendon

AHA: 3Q, '99, 16

756.9 Other and unspecified anomalies of musculoskeletal system
Congenital:
anomaly NOS } of musculoskeletal system,
deformity NOS }   not elsewhere classified

√4th **757 Congenital anomalies of the integument**

INCLUDES   anomalies of skin, subcutaneous tissue, hair, nails, and breast

EXCLUDES   hemangioma (228.00-228.09)
pigmented nevus (216.0-216.9)

757.0 Hereditary edema of legs
Congenital lymphedema
Hereditary trophedema
Milroy's disease

757.1 Ichthyosis congenita
Congenital ichthyosis
Harlequin fetus
Ichthyosiform erythroderma

DEF: Overproduction of skin cells causes scaling of skin; may result in stillborn fetus or death soon after birth.

757.2 Dermatoglyphic anomalies
Abnormal palmar creases

DEF: Abnormal skin-line patterns of fingers, palms, toes and soles; initial finding of possible chromosomal abnormalities.

√5th **757.3 Other specified anomalies of skin**

757.31 Congenital ectodermal dysplasia

DEF: Tissues and structures originate in embryonic ectoderm; includes anhidrotic and hidrotic ectodermal dysplasia and EEC syndrome.

757.32 Vascular hamartomas
Birthmarks   Strawberry nevus
Port-wine stain

DEF: Benign tumor of blood vessels; due to malformed angioblastic tissues.

757.33 Congenital pigmentary anomalies of skin
Congenital poikiloderma
Urticaria pigmentosa
Xeroderma pigmentosum
EXCLUDES   albinism (270.2)

757.39 Other
Accessory skin tags, congenital
Congenital scar
Epidermolysis bullosa
Keratoderma (congenital)
EXCLUDES   pilonidal cyst (685.0-685.1)

757.4 Specified anomalies of hair
Congenital: Congenital:
alopecia   hypertrichosis
atrichosis   monilethrix
beaded hair   Persistent lanugo

757.5 Specified anomalies of nails
Anonychia   Congenital:
Congenital: leukonychia
clubnail   onychauxis
koilonychia   pachyonychia

757.6 Specified anomalies of breast
Absent   }
Accessory   } breast or nipple
Supernumerary }

Hypoplasia of breast
EXCLUDES   absence of pectoral muscle (756.81)

757.8 Other specified anomalies of the integument

757.9 Unspecified anomaly of the integument
Congenital:
anomaly NOS } of integument
deformity NOS }

√4th √5th Additional Digit Required   Nonspecific PDx   Unacceptable PDx   Manifestation Code   MSP Medicare Secondary Payer   ▶◀ Revised Text   ● New Code   ▲ Revised Code Title

Congenital Anomalies 758–759.9

✓4th 758 Chromosomal anomalies

INCLUDES   syndromes associated with anomalies in the number and form of chromosomes

758.0 Down's syndrome
Mongolism   Trisomy:
Translocation Down's   21 or 22
syndrome   G

758.1 Patau's syndrome
Trisomy: Trisomy:
13   D_1

DEF: Trisomy of 13th chromosome; characteristic failure to thrive, severe mental impairment, seizures, abnormal eyes, low-set ears and sloped forehead.

758.2 Edwards' syndrome
Trisomy:
18
E_3

DEF: Trisomy of 18th chromosome; characteristic mental and physical impairments; mainly affects females.

758.3 Autosomal deletion syndromes
Antimongolism syndrome
Cri-du-chat syndrome

DEF: Antimongolism syndrome: Deletions in 21st chromosome; characteristic oblique palpebral fissures, hypertonia, micrognathia, microcephaly, high-arched palate and impaired mental and physical growth.

DEF: Cri-du-chat syndrome: Abnormally large distance between two organs or parts, abnormally small brain and severe mental impairment; characteristic of abnormal 5th chromosome.

758.4 Balanced autosomal translocation in normal individual

758.5 Other conditions due to autosomal anomalies
Accessory autosomes NEC

758.6 Gonadal dysgenesis
Ovarian dysgenesis
Turner's syndrome
XO syndrome
EXCLUDES   pure gonadal dysgenesis (752.7)

758.7 Klinefelter's syndrome ♂
XXY syndrome

DEF: Impaired embryonic development of seminiferous tubes; results in small testes, azoospermia, infertility and enlarged mammary glands.

✓5th 758.8 Other conditions due to chromosome anomalies
758.81 Other conditions due to sex chromosome anomalies
758.89 Other

758.9 Conditions due to anomaly of unspecified chromosome

✓4th 759 Other and unspecified congenital anomalies

759.0 Anomalies of spleen
Aberrant ⎫
Absent ⎬ spleen
Accessory ⎭
Congenital splenomegaly
Ectopic spleen
Lobulation of spleen

759.1 Anomalies of adrenal gland
Aberrant ⎫
Absent ⎬ adrenal gland
Accessory ⎭
EXCLUDES   adrenogenital disorders (255.2)
congenital disorders of steroid metabolism (255.2)

759.2 Anomalies of other endocrine glands
Absent parathyroid gland
Accessory thyroid gland
Persistent thyroglossal or thyrolingual duct
Thyroglossal (duct) cyst
EXCLUDES   congenital:
goiter (246.1)
hypothyroidism (243)

759.3 Situs inversus
Situs inversus or transversus: Transposition of
abdominalis   viscera:
thoracis   abdominal
thoracic
EXCLUDES   dextrocardia without mention of complete transposition (746.87)

DEF: Laterally transposed thoracic and abdominal viscera.

759.4 Conjoined twins
Craniopagus   Thoracopagus
Dicephalus   Xiphopagus
Pygopagus

759.5 Tuberous sclerosis
Bourneville's disease   Epiloia

DEF: Hamartomas of brain, retina and viscera, impaired mental ability, seizures and adenoma sebaceum.

759.6 Other hamartoses, not elsewhere classified
Syndrome: Syndrome:
Peutz-Jeghers   von Hippel-Lindau
Sturge-Weber (-Dimitri)
EXCLUDES   neurofibromatosis (237.7)

AHA: 3Q, '92, 12

DEF: Peutz-Jeghers: hereditary syndrome characterized by hamartomas of small intestine

DEF: Sturge-Weber: congenital syndrome characterized by unilateral port-wine stain over trigeminal nerve, underlying meninges and cerebral cortex.

DEF: von Hipple-Lindau: hereditary syndrome of congenital angiomatosis of the retina and cerebellum.

759.7 Multiple congenital anomalies, so described
Congenital:
anomaly, multiple NOS
deformity, multiple NOS

✓5th 759.8 Other specified anomalies
AHA: S-O, '87, 9; S-O, '85, 11

759.81 Prader-Willi syndrome
759.82 Marfan syndrome
AHA: 3Q, '93, 11
759.83 Fragile X syndrome
AHA: 4Q, '94, 41
759.89 Other
Congenital malformation syndromes affecting multiple systems, not elsewhere classified
Laurence-Moon-Biedl syndrome
AHA: 1Q, '01, 3; 3Q, '99, 17, 18; 3Q, '98, 8

759.9 Congenital anomaly, unspecified

N Newborn Age: 0   P Pediatric Age: 0-17   M Maternity Age: 12-55   A Adult Age: 15-124   CC CC Condition   MC Major Complication   CD Complex Dx   HIV HIV Related Dx

240 — Volume 1   2002 Ingenix, Inc.

15. CERTAIN CONDITIONS ORIGINATING IN THE PERINATAL PERIOD (760-779)

> INCLUDES   conditions which have their origin in the perinatal period even though death or morbidity occurs later
> Use additional code(s) to further specify condition

MATERNAL CAUSES OF PERINATAL MORBIDITY AND MORTALITY (760-763)

AHA: 2Q, '89, 14; 3Q, '90, 5

√4th **760 Fetus or newborn affected by maternal conditions which may be unrelated to present pregnancy**

> INCLUDES   the listed maternal conditions only when specified as a cause of mortality or morbidity of the fetus or newborn
> EXCLUDES   *maternal endocrine and metabolic disorders affecting fetus or newborn (775.0-775.9)*

AHA: 1Q, '94, 8; 2Q, '92, 12; N-D, '84, 11

760.0 Maternal hypertensive disorders
Fetus or newborn affected by maternal conditions classifiable to 642

760.1 Maternal renal and urinary tract diseases
Fetus or newborn affected by maternal conditions classifiable to 580-599

760.2 Maternal infections
Fetus or newborn affected by maternal infectious disease classifiable to 001-136 and 487, but fetus or newborn not manifesting that disease
> EXCLUDES   *congenital infectious diseases (771.0-771.8)*
> *maternal genital tract and other localized infections (760.8)*

760.3 Other chronic maternal circulatory and respiratory diseases
Fetus or newborn affected by chronic maternal conditions classifiable to 390-459, 490-519, 745-748

760.4 Maternal nutritional disorders
Fetus or newborn affected by:
maternal disorders classifiable to 260-269
maternal malnutrition NOS
> EXCLUDES   *fetal malnutrition (764.10-764.29)*

760.5 Maternal injury
Fetus or newborn affected by maternal conditions classifiable to 800-995

760.6 Surgical operation on mother
> EXCLUDES   *cesarean section for present delivery (763.4)*
> *damage to placenta from amniocentesis, cesarean section, or surgical induction (762.1)*
> *previous surgery to uterus or pelvic organs (763.89)*

√5th **760.7 Noxious influences affecting fetus via placenta or breast milk**
Fetus or newborn affected by noxious substance transmitted via placenta or breast milk
> EXCLUDES   *anesthetic and analgesic drugs administered during labor and delivery (763.5)*
> *drug withdrawal syndrome in newborn (779.5)*

AHA: 3Q, '91, 21

760.70 Unspecified noxious substance
Fetus or newborn affected by:
Drug NEC

760.71 Alcohol
Fetal alcohol syndrome

760.72 Narcotics

760.73 Hallucinogenic agents

760.74 Anti-infectives
Antibiotics

760.75 Cocaine
AHA: 3Q, '94, 6; 2Q, '92, 12; 4Q, '91, 26

760.76 Diethylstilbestrol [DES]
AHA: 4Q, '94, 45

760.79 Other
Fetus or newborn affected by:
immune sera | transmitted via
medicinal agents NEC | placenta or
toxic substance NEC | breast milk

760.8 Other specified maternal conditions affecting fetus or newborn
Maternal genital tract and other localized infection affecting fetus or newborn, but fetus or newborn not manifesting that disease
> EXCLUDES   *maternal urinary tract infection affecting fetus or newborn (760.1)*

760.9 Unspecified maternal condition affecting fetus or newborn

√4th **761 Fetus or newborn affected by maternal complications of pregnancy**
> INCLUDES   the listed maternal conditions only when specified as a cause of mortality or morbidity of the fetus or newborn

761.0 Incompetent cervix
DEF: Inadequate functioning of uterine cervix.

761.1 Premature rupture of membranes
761.2 Oligohydramnios
> EXCLUDES   *that due to premature rupture of membranes (761.1)*
DEF: Deficient amniotic fluid.

761.3 Polyhydramnios
Hydramnios (acute) (chronic)
DEF: Excess amniotic fluid.

761.4 Ectopic pregnancy
Pregnancy: | Pregnancy:
abdominal | tubal
intraperitoneal

761.5 Multiple pregnancy
Triplet (pregnancy)   Twin (pregnancy)

761.6 Maternal death

761.7 Malpresentation before labor
Breech presentation
External version
Oblique lie
Transverse lie
Unstable lie
} before labor

761.8 Other specified maternal complications of pregnancy affecting fetus or newborn
Spontaneous abortion, fetus

761.9 Unspecified maternal complication of pregnancy affecting fetus or newborn

√4th **762 Fetus or newborn affected by complications of placenta, cord, and membranes**
> INCLUDES   the listed maternal conditions only when specified as a cause of mortality or morbidity in the fetus or newborn

AHA: 1Q, '94, 8

762.0 Placenta previa   N
DEF: Placenta developed in lower segment of uterus; causes hemorrhaging in last trimester.

√4th √5th Additional Digit Required   Nonspecific PDx   Unacceptable PDx   Manifestation Code   MSP Medicare Secondary Payer   ►◄ Revised Text   ● New Code   ▲ Revised Code Title

2002 Ingenix, Inc.

Volume 1 — 241

762.1 Other forms of placental separation and hemorrhage N
    Abruptio placentae
    Antepartum hemorrhage
    Damage to placenta from amniocentesis, cesarean section, or surgical induction
    Maternal blood loss
    Premature separation of placenta
    Rupture of marginal sinus

762.2 Other and unspecified morphological and functional abnormalities of placenta N
    Placental: Placental:
      dysfunction   insufficiency
      infarction

762.3 Placental transfusion syndromes N
    Placental and cord abnormality resulting in twin-to-twin or other transplacental transfusion
    Use additional code to indicate resultant condition in fetus or newborn:
      fetal blood loss (772.0)
      polycythemia neonatorum (776.4)

762.4 Prolapsed cord N
    Cord presentation

762.5 Other compression of umbilical cord N
    Cord around neck   Knot in cord
    Entanglement of cord Torsion of cord

762.6 Other and unspecified conditions of umbilical cord N
    Short cord
    Thrombosis
    Varices   } of umbilical cord
    Velamentous insertion
    Vasa previa

    EXCLUDES   infection of umbilical cord (771.4)
                 single umbilical artery (747.5)

762.7 Chorioamnionitis N
    Amnionitis
    Membranitis
    Placentitis
    DEF: Inflamed fetal membrane.

762.8 Other specified abnormalities of chorion and amnion N

762.9 Unspecified abnormality of chorion and amnion N

√4th **763 Fetus or newborn affected by other complications of labor and delivery**
    INCLUDES the listed conditions only when specified as a cause of mortality or morbidity in the fetus or newborn
    AHA: 1Q, '94, 8

763.0 Breech delivery and extraction N

763.1 Other malpresentation, malposition, and disproportion during labor and delivery N
    Fetus or newborn affected by:
      abnormality of bony pelvis
      contracted pelvis
      persistent occipitoposterior position
      shoulder presentation
      transverse lie
      conditions classifiable to 652, 653, and 660

763.2 Forceps delivery N
    Fetus or newborn affected by forceps extraction

763.3 Delivery by vacuum extractor N

763.4 Cesarean delivery N
    EXCLUDES placental separation or hemorrhage from cesarean section (762.1)

763.5 Maternal anesthesia and analgesia N
    Reactions and intoxications from maternal opiates and tranquilizers during labor and delivery
    EXCLUDES drug withdrawal syndrome in newborn (779.5)

763.6 Precipitate delivery N
    Rapid second stage

763.7 Abnormal uterine contractions N
    Fetus or newborn affected by:
      contraction ring
      hypertonic labor
      hypotonic uterine dysfunction
      uterine inertia or dysfunction
      conditions classifiable to 661, except 661.3

√5th **763.8 Other specified complications of labor and delivery affecting fetus or newborn**
    AHA: 4Q, '98, 46

    763.81 Abnormality in fetal heart rate or rhythm before the onset of labor N

    763.82 Abnormality in fetal heart rate or rhythm during labor N
      AHA: 4Q, '98, 46

    763.83 Abnormality in fetal heart rate or rhythm, unspecified as to time of onset N

    763.89 Other specified complications of labor and delivery affecting fetus or newborn N
      Fetus or newborn affected by:
        abnormality of maternal soft tissues
        destructive operation on live fetus to facilitate delivery
        induction of labor (medical)
        previous surgery to uterus or pelvic organs
        other conditions classifiable to 650-669
        other procedures used in labor and delivery

763.9 Unspecified complication of labor and delivery affecting fetus or newborn N

OTHER CONDITIONS ORIGINATING IN THE PERINATAL PERIOD (764-779)

The following fifth-digit subclassification is for use with ▶category 764 and codes 765.0-765.1◀ to denote birthweight:
  0 unspecified [weight]
  1 less than 500 grams
  2 500-749 grams
  3 750-999 grams
  4 1,000-1,249 grams
  5 1,250-1,499 grams
  6 1,500-1,749 grams
  7 1,750-1,999 grams
  8 2,000-2,499 grams
  9 2,500 grams and over

√4th **764 Slow fetal growth and fetal malnutrition**
    AHA: 1Q, '94, 8; 2Q, '91, 19; 2Q, '89, 15

√5th **764.0 "Light-for-dates" without mention of fetal malnutrition** N
    Infants underweight for gestational age
    "Small-for-dates"

√5th **764.1 "Light-for-dates" with signs of fetal malnutrition** N
    Infants "light-for-dates" classifiable to 764.0, who in addition show signs of fetal malnutrition, such as dry peeling skin and loss of subcutaneous tissue

√5th **764.2 Fetal malnutrition without mention of "light-for-dates"** N
    Infants, not underweight for gestational age, showing signs of fetal malnutrition, such as dry peeling skin and loss of subcutaneous tissue
    Intrauterine malnutrition

√5th **764.9 Fetal growth retardation, unspecified** N
    Intrauterine growth retardation
    AHA: For code 764.97: 1Q, '97, 6

N Newborn Age: 0   P Pediatric Age: 0-17   M Maternity Age: 12-55   A Adult Age: 15-124   CC CC Condition   MC Major Complication   CD Complex Dx   HIV HIV Related Dx

242 — Volume 1 • October 2002   2002 Ingenix, Inc.

✓4th **765 Disorders relating to short gestation and unspecified low birthweight**

INCLUDES   the listed conditions, without further specification, as causes of mortality, morbidity, or additional care, in fetus or newborn

AHA: 1Q, '97, 6; 1Q, '94, 8; 2Q, '91, 19; 2Q, '89, 15

§ ✓5th **765.0 Extreme immaturity**   CC 1-8 N

Note: Usually implies a birthweight of less than 1000 grams.

▶Use additional code for weeks of gestation (765.20-765.29)◀

CC Excl: For codes 765.01-765.08: 764.00-764.99, 765.00-765.19, ▶765.20-765.29,◀ 767.8-767.9, 779.8, ▶779.81-779.89◀

AHA: For code 756.03: 4Q, '01, 51

§ ✓5th **765.1 Other preterm infants**   N

Note: Usually implies a birthweight of 1000-2499 grams.
Prematurity NOS
Prematurity or small size, not classifiable to 765.0 or as "light-for-dates" in 764

▶Use additional code for weeks of gestation (765.20-765.29)◀

AHA: For code 765.10: 1Q, '94, 14

AHA: For code 765.17: 1Q, '97, 6

✓5th **765.2 Weeks of gestation**

765.20 Unspecified weeks of gestation   N
765.21 Less than 24 completed weeks of gestation   N
765.22 24 completed weeks of gestation   N
765.23 25-26 completed weeks of gestation   N
765.24 27-28 completed weeks of gestation   N
765.25 29-30 completed weeks of gestation   N
765.26 31-32 completed weeks of gestation   N
765.27 33-34 completed weeks of gestation   N
765.28 35-36 completed weeks of gestation   N
765.29 37 or more completed weeks of gestation   N

✓4th **766 Disorders relating to long gestation and high birthweight**

INCLUDES   the listed conditions, without further specification, as causes of mortality, morbidity, or additional care, in fetus or newborn

766.0 Exceptionally large baby   N

Note: Usually implies a birthweight of 4500 grams or more.

766.1 Other "heavy-for-dates" infants   N

Other fetus or infant "heavy-" or "large-for-dates" regardless of period of gestation

766.2 Post-term infant, not "heavy-for-dates"   N

Postmaturity NOS

✓4th **767 Birth trauma**

767.0 Subdural and cerebral hemorrhage   CC N

Subdural and cerebral hemorrhage, whether described as due to birth trauma or to intrapartum anoxia or hypoxia
Subdural hematoma (localized)
Tentorial tear
Use additional code to identify cause

EXCLUDES   intraventricular hemorrhage (772.10-772.14)
subarachnoid hemorrhage (772.2)

CC Excl: 767.0, 767.8-767.9, ▶779.81-779.89◀

767.1 Injuries to scalp   N

Caput succedaneum
Cephalhematoma
Chignon (from vacuum extraction)
Massive epicranial subaponeurotic hemorrhage

767.2 Fracture of clavicle   N

767.3 Other injuries to skeleton   N

Fracture of: Fracture of:
long bones   skull

EXCLUDES   congenital dislocation of hip (754.30-754.35)
fracture of spine, congenital (767.4)

767.4 Injury to spine and spinal cord   N

Dislocation
Fracture   of spine or spinal cord
Laceration   due to birth trauma
Rupture

767.5 Facial nerve injury   N

Facial palsy

767.6 Injury to brachial plexus   N

Palsy or paralysis: Palsy or paralysis:
brachial   Klumpke (-Déjérine)
Erb (-Duchenne)

767.7 Other cranial and peripheral nerve injuries   N

Phrenic nerve paralysis

767.8 Other specified birth trauma   N

Eye damage   Rupture of:
Hematoma of: liver
liver (subcapsular)   spleen
testes   Scalpel wound
vulva   Traumatic glaucoma

EXCLUDES   hemorrhage classifiable to 772.0-772.9

767.9 Birth trauma, unspecified   N

Birth injury NOS

✓4th **768 Intrauterine hypoxia and birth asphyxia**

Use only when associated with newborn morbidity classifiable elsewhere

AHA: 4Q, '92, 20

DEF: Oxygen intake insufficiency due to interrupted placental circulation or premature separation of placenta.

768.0 Fetal death from asphyxia or anoxia before onset of labor or at unspecified time   N

768.1 Fetal death from asphyxia or anoxia during labor   N

768.2 Fetal distress before onset of labor, in liveborn infant   N

Fetal metabolic acidemia before onset of labor, in liveborn infant

768.3 Fetal distress first noted during labor, in liveborn infant   N

Fetal metabolic acidemia first noted during labor, in liveborn infant

768.4 Fetal distress, unspecified as to time of onset, in liveborn infant   N

Fetal metabolic acidemia unspecified as to time of onset, in liveborn infant

AHA: N-D, '86, 10

768.5 Severe birth asphyxia   CC N

Birth asphyxia with neurologic involvement

CC Excl: 768.5-768.9, 769, 770.0-770.9, ▶779.81-779.89◀

AHA: N-D, '86, 3

768.6 Mild or moderate birth asphyxia   N

Birth asphyxia (without mention of neurologic nvolvement)

AHA: N-D, '86, 3

768.9 Unspecified birth asphyxia in liveborn infant   N

Anoxia
Asphyxia   NOS, in liveborn infant
Hypoxia

§ Requires fifth-digit. See beginning of section 764-779 for codes and definitions.

✓4th ✓5th Additional Digit Required   Nonspecific PDx   Unacceptable PDx   Manifestation Code   MSP Medicare Secondary Payer   ▶◀ Revised Text   ● New Code   ▲ Revised Code Title

2002 Ingenix, Inc.   October 2002 • Volume 1 — 243

Conditions in the Perinatal Period 765–768.9

Conditions in the Perinatal Period 769–771.7

769 Respiratory distress syndrome   `CC` `N`
Cardiorespiratory distress syndrome of newborn
Hyaline membrane disease (pulmonary)
Idiopathic respiratory distress syndrome [IRDS or RDS] of newborn
Pulmonary hypoperfusion syndrome
> EXCLUDES   *transient tachypnea of newborn (770.6)*

CC Excl: See code 768.5

AHA: 1Q, '89, 10; N-D, '86, 6

DEF: Severe chest contractions upon air intake and expiratory grunting; infant appears blue due to oxygen deficiency and has rapid respiratory rate; formerly called hyaline membrane disease.

✓4ᵗʰ 770 Other respiratory conditions of fetus and newborn

770.0 Congenital pneumonia   `CC` `N`
Infective pneumonia acquired prenatally
> EXCLUDES   *pneumonia from infection acquired after birth (480.0-486)*

CC Excl: See code 768.5

770.1 Meconium aspiration syndrome   `CC` `N`
Aspiration of contents of birth canal NOS
Meconium aspiration below vocal cords
Pneumonitis:
    fetal aspiration
    meconium

CC Excl: See code 768.5

DEF: Aspiration of meconium by the newborn infant prior to delivery. Presence of meconium in the trachea or chest x-ray indicating patchy infiltrates in conjunction with chest hyperextension establishes this diagnosis.

770.2 Interstitial emphysema and related conditions   `CC` `N`
Pneumomediastinum ⎫
Pneumopericardium ⎬ originating in the perinatal period
Pneumothorax ⎭

CC Excl: See code 768.5

770.3 Pulmonary hemorrhage   `CC` `N`
Hemorrhage:
    alveolar (lung) ⎫
    intra-alveolar (lung) ⎬ originating in the perinatal period
    massive pulmonary ⎭

CC Excl: See code 768.5

770.4 Primary atelectasis   `CC` `N`
Pulmonary immaturity NOS

CC Excl: See code 768.5

DEF: Alveoli fail to expand causing insufficient air intake by newborn.

770.5 Other and unspecified atelectasis   `CC` `N`
Atelectasis:
    NOS ⎫
    partial ⎬ originating in the perinatal period
    secondary ⎪
Pulmonary collapse ⎭

CC Excl: See code 768.5

770.6 Transitory tachypnea of newborn   `N`
Idiopathic tachypnea of newborn
Wet lung syndrome
> EXCLUDES   *respiratory distress syndrome (769)*

AHA: 4Q, '95, 4; 1Q, '94, 12; 3Q, '93, 7; 1Q, '89, 10; N-D, '86, 6

DEF: Quick, shallow breathing of newborn; short-term problem.

770.7 Chronic respiratory disease arising in the perinatal period   `CC`
Bronchopulmonary dysplasia
Interstitial pulmonary fibrosis of prematurity
Wilson-Mikity syndrome

CC Excl: See code 768.5

AHA: 2Q, '91, 19; N-D, '86, 11

✓5ᵗʰ 770.8 Other respiratory problems after birth
AHA: 2Q, '98, 10; 2Q, '96, 10

770.81 Primary apnea of newborn   `N`
Apneic spells of newborn NOS
Essential apnea of newborn
Sleep apnea of newborn

770.82 Other apnea of newborn   `N`
Obstructive apnea of newborn

770.83 Cyanotic attacks of newborn   `N`

770.84 Respiratory failure of newborn   `CC` `N`
> EXCLUDES   *respiratory distress syndrome (769)*

CC Excl: See code 768.5

770.89 Other respiratory problems after birth   `N`

770.9 Unspecified respiratory condition of fetus and newborn   `N`

✓4ᵗʰ 771 Infections specific to the perinatal period
> INCLUDES   infections acquired before or during birth or via the umbilicus
> EXCLUDES   *congenital pneumonia (770.0)*
> *congenital syphilis (090.0-090.9)*
> *maternal infectious disease as a cause of mortality or morbidity in fetus or newborn, but fetus or newborn not manifesting the disease (760.2)*
> *ophthalmia neonatorum due to gonococcus (098.40)*
> *other infections not specifically classified to this category*

AHA: N-D, '85, 4

771.0 Congenital rubella   `CC` `N`
Congenital rubella pneumonitis
CC Excl: 771.0-771.2, ▶779.81-779.89◀

771.1 Congenital cytomegalovirus infection   `CC` `N`
Congenital cytomegalic inclusion disease
CC Excl: See code 771.0

771.2 Other congenital infections   `N`
Congenital: Congenital:
  herpes simplex   toxoplasmosis
  listeriosis   tuberculosis
  malaria

771.3 Tetanus neonatorum   `CC` `N`
Tetanus omphalitis
> EXCLUDES   *hypocalcemic tetany (775.4)*

CC Excl: 771.3, ▶779.81-779.89◀

DEF: Severe infection of central nervous system; due to exotoxin of tetanus bacillus from navel infection prompted by nonsterile technique during umbilical ligation.

771.4 Omphalitis of the newborn   `N`
Infection:
  navel cord
  umbilical stump
> EXCLUDES   *tetanus omphalitis (771.3)*

DEF: Inflamed umbilicus.

771.5 Neonatal infective mastitis   `N`
> EXCLUDES   *noninfective neonatal mastitis (778.7)*

771.6 Neonatal conjunctivitis and dacryocystitis   `N`
Ophthalmia neonatorum NOS
> EXCLUDES   *ophthalmia neonatorum due to gonococcus (098.40)*

771.7 Neonatal Candida infection   `N`
Neonatal moniliasis
Thrush in newborn

`N` Newborn Age: 0   `P` Pediatric Age: 0-17   `M` Maternity Age: 12-55   `A` Adult Age: 15-124   `CC` CC Condition   `MC` Major Complication   `CD` Complex Dx   `HIV` HIV Related Dx

√5ᵗʰ 771.8 Other infection specific to the perinatal period
▶Use additional code to identify organism◀

● **771.81 Septicemia [sepsis] of newborn**   CC N
CC Excl: 771.4-771.89, 776.0-776.9, 779.81-779.89

● **771.82 Urinary tract infection of newborn**   N

● **771.83 Bacteremia of newborn**   CC N
CC Excl: See code 771.81

● **771.89 Other infections specific to the perinatal period**   N
Intra-amniotic infection of fetus NOS
Infection of newborn NOS

√4ᵗʰ 772 Fetal and neonatal hemorrhage
EXCLUDES hematological disorders of fetus and newborn (776.0-776.9)

772.0 Fetal blood loss   N
Fetal blood loss from: Fetal exsanguination
   cut end of co-twin's cord   Fetal hemorrhage
   placenta   into:
   ruptured cord   co-twin
   vasa previa   mother's circulation

√5ᵗʰ 772.1 Intraventricular hemorrhage
Intraventricular hemorrhage from any perinatal cause
AHA: 4Q, '01, 49; 3Q, '92, 8; 4Q, '88, 8

772.10 Unspecified grade   CC N
CC Excl: 772.0-772.2, 772.8-772.9, 776.0-776.9, ▶779.81-779.89◀

772.11 Grade I   CC N
Bleeding into germinal matrix
CC Excl: See code 772.10

772.12 Grade II   CC N
Bleeding into ventricle
CC Excl: See code 772.10

772.13 Grade III   CC N
Bleeding with enlargement of ventricle
CC Excl: See code 772.10
AHA: 4Q, '01, 51

772.14 Grade IV   CC N
Bleeding into cerebral cortex
CC Excl: See code 772.10

772.2 Subarachnoid hemorrhage   CC N
Subarachnoid hemorrhage from any perinatal cause
EXCLUDES subdural and cerebral hemorrhage (767.0)
CC Excl: 772.0-772.2, 772.8-772.9, 776.0-776.9, 779.7-779.89

772.3 Umbilical hemorrhage after birth   N
Slipped umbilical ligature

772.4 Gastrointestinal hemorrhage   CC N
EXCLUDES swallowed maternal blood (777.3)
CC Excl: 772.0, 772.4-772.5, 772.8-772.9, 776.0-776.9, ▶779.81-779.89◀

772.5 Adrenal hemorrhage   CC N
CC Excl: See code 772.4

772.6 Cutaneous hemorrhage   N
Bruising
Ecchymoses
Petechiae   ⎫ in fetus or newborn
Superficial hematoma

772.8 Other specified hemorrhage of fetus or newborn N
EXCLUDES hemorrhagic disease of newborn (776.0)
pulmonary hemorrhage (770.3)

772.9 Unspecified hemorrhage of newborn   N

√4ᵗʰ 773 Hemolytic disease of fetus or newborn, due to isoimmunization
DEF: Hemolytic anemia of fetus or newborn due to maternal antibody formation against fetal erythrocytes; infant blood contains nonmaternal antigen.

773.0 Hemolytic disease due to Rh isoimmunization   CC N
Anemia ⎫
Erythroblastosis (fetalis) ⎪ due to RH:
Hemolytic disease ⎬ antibodies
   (fetus) (newborn) ⎪ isoimmunization
Jaundice ⎭ maternal/fetal incompatibility
Rh hemolytic disease
Rh isoimmunization
CC Excl: 773.0-773.5, ▶779.81-779.89◀

773.1 Hemolytic disease due to ABO isoimmumization   CC N
ABO hemolytic disease   ABO isoimmunization
Anemia ⎫ due to ABO:
Erythroblastosis (fetalis) ⎪ antibodies
Hemolytic disease ⎬ isoimmunization
   (fetus) (newborn) ⎪ maternal/fetal
Jaundice ⎭ incompatibility
CC Excl: See code 773.0
AHA: 3Q, '92, 8
DEF: Incompatible Rh fetal-maternal blood grouping; prematurely destroys red blood cells; detected by Coombs test.

773.2 Hemolytic disease due to other and unspecified isoimmunization   CC N
Eythroblastosis (fetalis) (neonatorum) NOS
Hemolytic disease (fetus) (newborn) NOS
Jaundice or anemia due to other and unspecified blood-group incompatibility
CC Excl: See code 773.0
AHA: 1Q, '94, 13

773.3 Hydrops fetalis due to isoimmunization   CC N
Use additional code to identify type of isoimmunization (773.0-773.2)
CC Excl: See code 773.0
DEF: Massive edema of entire body and severe anemia; may result in fetal death or stillbirth.

773.4 Kernicterus due to isoimmunization   CC N
Use additional code to identify type of isoimmunization (773.0-773.2)
CC Excl: See code 773.0
DEF: Complication of erythroblastosis fetalis associated with severe neural symptoms, high blood bilirubin levels and nerve cell destruction; results in bilirubin-pigmented gray matter of central nervous system.

773.5 Late anemia due to isoimmunization   N

√4ᵗʰ 774 Other perinatal jaundice

774.0 *Perinatal jaundice from hereditary hemolyticanemias*   CC N
Code first underlying disease (282.0-282.9)
CC Excl: 774.0-774.7, ▶779.81-779.89◀

774.1 Perinatal jaundice from other excessive hemolysis   CC N
Fetal or neonatal jaundice from:
   bruising
   drugs or toxins transmitted from mother
   infection
   polycythemia
   swallowed maternal blood
Use additional code to identify cause
EXCLUDES jaundice due to isoimmunization (773.0-773.2)
CC Excl: See code 774.0

√4ᵗʰ √5ᵗʰ Additional Digit Required   Nonspecific PDx   Unacceptable PDx   Manifestation Code   **MSP** Medicare Secondary Payer   ▶◀ Revised Text   ● New Code   ▲ Revised Code Title

2002 Ingenix, Inc.   **October 2002 • Volume 1 — 245**

774.2 **Neonatal jaundice associated with preterm** `CC` `N`
delivery
Hyperbilirubinemia of prematurity
Jaundice due to delayed conjugation associated with
preterm delivery
CC Excl: See code 774.0

AHA: 3Q, '91, 21

✓5ᵗʰ **774.3** **Neonatal jaundice due to delayed conjugation from**
other causes
774.30 **Neonatal jaundice due to delayed** `CC` `N`
conjugation, cause unspecified
CC Excl: See code 774.0

DEF: Jaundice of newborn with abnormal bilirubin
metabolism; causes excess accumulated unconjugated
bilirubin in blood.

774.31 *Neonatal jaundice due to delayed* `CC` `N`
conjugation in diseases classified
elsewhere
Code first underlying diseases as:
congenital hypothyroidism (243)
Crigler-Najjar syndrome (277.4)
Gilbert's syndrome (277.4)
CC Excl: See code 774.0

774.39 **Other** `CC` `N`
Jaundice due to delayed conjugation from
causes, such as:
breast milk inhibitors
delayed development of conjugating
system
CC Excl: See code 774.0

774.4 **Perinatal jaundice due to hepatocellular** `CC` `N`
damage
Fetal or neonatal hepatitis
Giant cell hepatitis
Inspissated bile syndrome
CC Excl: See code 774.0

774.5 *Perinatal jaundice from other causes* `CC` `N`
Code first underlying cause as:
congenital obstruction of bile duct (751.61)
galactosemia (271.1)
mucoviscidosis ▶(277.00-277.09)◀
CC Excl: See code 774.0

774.6 **Unspecified fetal and neonatal jaundice** `N`
Icterus neonatorum
Neonatal hyperbilirubinemia (transient)
Physiologic jaundice NOS in newborn
EXCLUDES *that in preterm infants (774.2)*

AHA: 1Q, '94, 13; 2Q, '89, 15

774.7 **Kernicterus not due to isoimmunization** `CC` `N`
Bilirubin encephalopathy
Kernicterus of newborn NOS
EXCLUDES *kernicterus due to isoimmunization*
(773.4)
CC Excl: See code 774.0

✓4ᵗʰ **775** **Endocrine and metabolic disturbances specific to the fetus**
and newborn
INCLUDES transitory endocrine and metabolic
disturbances caused by the infant's
response to maternal endocrine and
metabolic factors, its removal from them,
or its adjustment to extrauterine
existence

775.0 **Syndrome of "infant of a diabetic mother"** `N`
Maternal diabetes mellitus affecting fetus or
newborn (with hypoglycemia)

AHA: 3Q, '91, 5

775.1 **Neonatal diabetes mellitus** `CC` `N`
Diabetes mellitus syndrome in newborn infant
CC Excl: 775.0-775.9, ▶779.81-779.89◀

AHA: 3Q, '91, 6

775.2 **Neonatal myasthenia gravis** `CC` `N`
CC Excl: See code 775.1

775.3 **Neonatal thyrotoxicosis** `CC` `N`
Neonatal hyperthyroidism (transient)
CC Excl: See code 775.1

775.4 **Hypocalcemia and hypomagnesemia of** `CC` `N`
newborn
Cow's milk hypocalcemia
Hypocalcemic tetany, neonatal
Neonatal hypoparathyroidism
Phosphate-loading hypocalcemia
CC Excl: See code 775.1

775.5 **Other transitory neonatal electrolyte** `CC` `N`
disturbances
Dehydration, neonatal
CC Excl: See code 775.1

775.6 **Neonatal hypoglycemia** `CC` `N`
EXCLUDES *infant of mother with diabetes mellitus*
(775.0)

CC Excl: See code 775.1

AHA: 1Q, '94, 8

775.7 **Late metabolic acidosis of newborn** `CC` `N`
CC Excl: See code 775.1

775.8 **Other transitory neonatal endocrine and** `N`
metabolic disturbances
Amino-acid metabolic disorders described as
transitory

775.9 **Unspecified endocrine and metabolic** `N`
disturbances specific to the fetus and newborn

✓4ᵗʰ **776** **Hematological disorders of fetus and newborn**
INCLUDES disorders specific to the fetus or newborn

776.0 **Hemorrhagic disease of newborn** `CC` `N`
Hemorrhagic diathesis of newborn
Vitamin K deficiency of newborn
EXCLUDES *fetal or neonatal hemorrhage (772.0-*
772.9)
CC Excl: 776.0-776.9, ▶771.81-771.82, 779.81-779.89◀

776.1 **Transient neonatal thrombocytopenia** `CC` `N`
Neonatal thrombocytopenia due to:
exchange transfusion
idiopathic maternal thrombocytopenia
isoimmunization
CC Excl: See code 776.0

DEF: Temporary decrease in blood platelets of newborn.

776.2 **Disseminated intravascular coagulation in** `CC` `N`
newborn
CC Excl: See code 776.0

DEF: Disseminated intravascular coagulation of newborn: clotting
disorder due to excess thromboplastic agents in blood as a result
of disease or trauma; causes blood clotting within vessels and
reduces available elements necessary for blood coagulation.

776.3 **Other transient neonatal disorders of** `CC` `N`
coagulation
Transient coagulation defect, newborn
CC Excl: See code 776.0

776.4 **Polycythemia neonatorum** `N`
Plethora of newborn   Polycythemia due to:
Polycythemia due to: maternal-fetal transfusion
donor twin transfusion

DEF: Abnormal increase of total red blood cells of newborn.

776.5 **Congenital anemia** `N`
Anemia following fetal blood loss
EXCLUDES *anemia due to isoimmunization (773.0-*
773.2, 773.5)
hereditary hemolytic anemias (282.0-
282.9)

`N` Newborn Age: 0   `P` Pediatric Age: 0-17   `M` Maternity Age: 12-55   `A` Adult Age: 15-124   `CC` CC Condition   `MC` Major Complication   `CD` Complex Dx   `HIV` HIV Related Dx

776.6   Anemia of prematurity   N

776.7   Transient neonatal neutropenia   N
Isoimmune neutropenia
Maternal transfer neutropenia

> EXCLUDES   *congenital neutropenia (nontransient)*
> *(288.0)*

DEF: Decreased neutrophilic leukocytes in blood of newborn.

776.8   Other specified transient hematological   N
disorders

776.9   Unspecified hematological disorder specific   N
to fetus or newborn

✓4th **777   Perinatal disorders of digestive system**

> INCLUDES   disorders specific to the fetus and newborn
> EXCLUDES   *intestinal obstruction classifiable to 560.0-560.9*

777.1   Meconium obstruction   CC N
Congenital fecaliths   Meconium ileus NOS
Delayed passage of meconium   Meconium plug
                              syndrome

> EXCLUDES   *meconium ileus in cystic fibrosis*
> *(277.01)*

CC Excl: 777.1-777.9, ▶779.81-779.89◀

DEF: Meconium blocked digestive tract of newborn.

777.2   Intestinal obstruction due to inspissated   CC N
milk

CC Excl: See code 777.1

777.3   Hematemesis and melena due to swallowed   N
maternal blood
Swallowed blood syndrome in newborn

> EXCLUDES   *that not due to swallowed maternal*
> *blood (772.4)*

777.4   Transitory ileus of newborn   N

> EXCLUDES   *Hirschsprung's disease (751.3)*

777.5   Necrotizing enterocolitis in fetus or   CC N
newborn
Pseudomembranous enterocolitis in newborn

CC Excl: See code 777.1

DEF: Acute inflammation of small intestine due to
pseudomembranous plaque over ulceration; may be due to
aggressive antibiotic therapy.

777.6   Perinatal intestinal perforation   CC N
Meconium peritonitis

CC Excl: See code 777.1

777.8   Other specified perinatal disorders of digestive
system

777.9   Unspecified perinatal disorder of digestive   N
system

✓4th **778   Conditions involving the integument and temperature**
regulation of fetus and newborn

778.0   Hydrops fetalis not due to isoimmunization   CC N
Idiopathic hydrops

> EXCLUDES   *hydrops fetalis due to isoimmunization*
> *(773.3)*

CC Excl: 778.0, ▶779.81-779.89◀

DEF: Edema of entire body, unrelated to immune response.

778.1   Sclerema neonatorum   N
Subcutaneous fat necrosis

DEF: Diffuse, rapidly progressing white, waxy, nonpitting hardening
of tissue, usually of legs and feet, life-threatening; found in preterm
or debilitated infants; unknown etiology.

778.2   Cold injury syndrome of newborn   N

778.3   Other hypothermia of newborn   N

778.4   Other disturbances of temperature regulation   N
of newborn
Dehydration fever in newborn
Environmentally-induced pyrexia
Hyperthermia in newborn
Transitory fever of newborn

778.5   Other and unspecified edema of newborn   N
Edema neonatorum

778.6   Congenital hydrocele   N
Congenital hydrocele of tunica vaginalis

778.7   Breast engorgement in newborn   N
Noninfective mastitis of newborn

> EXCLUDES   *infective mastitis of newborn (771.5)*

778.8   Other specified conditions involving the   N
integument of fetus and newborn
Urticaria neonatorum

> EXCLUDES   *impetigo neonatorum (684)*
> *pemphigus neonatorum (684)*

778.9   Unspecified condition involving the   N
integument and temperature regulation of
fetus and newborn

✓4th **779   Other and ill-defined conditions originating in the perinatal**
period

779.0   Convulsions in newborn   CC N
Fits   }
Seizures } in newborn

CC Excl: 779.0-779.1, ▶779.81-779.89◀

AHA: N-D, '94, 11

779.1   Other and unspecified cerebral irritability   CC N
in newborn

CC Excl: See code 779.0

779.2   Cerebral depression, coma, and other   N
abnormal cerebral signs
CNS dysfunction in newborn NOS

779.3   Feeding problems in newborn   CC N
Regurgitation of food }
Slow feeding   } in newborn
Vomiting   }

CC Excl: 779.3

AHA: 2Q, '89, 15

779.4   Drug reactions and intoxications specific   CC N
to newborn
Gray syndrome from chloramphenicol administration
in newborn

> EXCLUDES   *fetal alcohol syndrome (760.71)*
> *reactions and intoxications from*
> *maternal opiates and*
> *tranquilizers (763.5)*

CC Excl: 779.4-779.5

779.5   Drug withdrawal syndrome in newborn   N
Drug withdrawal syndrome in infant of dependent
mother

> EXCLUDES   *fetal alcohol syndrome (760.71)*

AHA: 3Q, '94, 6

779.6   Termination of pregnancy (fetus)   N
Fetal death due to: Fetal death due to:
induced abortion   termination of pregnancy

> EXCLUDES   *spontaneous abortion (fetus) (761.8)*

779.7   Periventricular leukomalacia   CC N

CC Excl: 772.0, 772.10-772.14, 772.2, 772.8, 772.9, 776.0-776.9, 779.7,
▶779.81-779.89◀

AHA: 4Q, '01, 50, 51

DEF: Necrosis of white matter adjacent to lateral ventricles with
the formation of cysts; cause of PVL has not been firmly
established, but thought to be related to inadequate blood flow in
certain areas of the brain.

✓5th **779.8   Other specified conditions originating in the**   N
perinatal period

AHA: 1Q, '94, 15

✓4th ✓5th Additional Digit Required   Nonspecific PDx   Unacceptable PDx   Manifestation Code   MSP Medicare Secondary Payer   ▶◀ Revised Text   ● New Code   ▲ Revised Code Title

2002 Ingenix, Inc.   October 2002 • Volume 1 — 247

Conditions in the Perinatal Period 776.6–779.8

●   **779.81 Neonatal bradycardia**   N

        EXCLUDES   *abnormality in fetal heart rate or rhythm complicating labor and delivery (763.81-763.83)*

                    bradycardia due to birth asphyxia (768.5-768.9)

●   **779.82 Neonatal tachycardia**   N

        EXCLUDES   *abnormality in fetal heart rate or rhythm complicating labor and delivery (763.81-763.83)*

779.89 Other specified conditions originating N
         in the perinatal period

779.9   Unspecified condition originating in the N
      perinatal period

       Congenital debility NOS
       Stillbirth NEC

N Newborn Age: 0   P Pediatric Age: 0-17   M Maternity Age: 12-55   A Adult Age: 15-124   CC CC Condition   MC Major Complication   CD Complex Dx   HIV HIV Related Dx

248 — Volume 1 • October 2002   *2002 Ingenix, Inc.*

16. SYMPTOMS, SIGNS, AND ILL-DEFINED CONDITIONS
(780-799)

This section includes symptoms, signs, abnormal results of laboratory or other investigative procedures, and ill-defined conditions regarding which no diagnosis classifiable elsewhere is recorded.

Signs and symptoms that point rather definitely to a given diagnosis are assigned to some category in the preceding part of the classification. In general, categories 780-796 include the more ill-defined conditions and symptoms that point with perhaps equal suspicion to two or more diseases or to two or more systems of the body, and without the necessary study of the case to make a final diagnosis. Practically all categories in this group could be designated as "not otherwise specified," or as "unknown etiology," or as "transient." The Alphabetic Index should be consulted to determine which symptoms and signs are to be allocated here and which to more specific sections of the classification; the residual subcategories numbered .9 are provided for other relevant symptoms which cannot be allocated elsewhere in the classification.

The conditions and signs or symptoms included in categories 780-796 consist of: (a) cases for which no more specific diagnosis can be made even after all facts bearing on the case have been investigated; (b) signs or symptoms existing at the time of initial encounter that proved to be transient and whose causes could not be determined; (c) provisional diagnoses in a patient who failed to return for further investigation or care; (d) cases referred elsewhere for investigation or treatment before the diagnosis was made; (e) cases in which a more precise diagnosis was not available for any other reason; (f) certain symptoms which represent important problems in medical care and which it might be desired to classify in addition to a known cause.

SYMPTOMS (780-789)

AHA: 1Q, '91, 12; 2Q, '90, 3; 2Q, '90, 5; 2Q, '90, 15; M-A, '85, 3

✓4ᵗʰ **780 General symptoms**

  ✓5ᵗʰ **780.0 Alteration of consciousness**

     EXCLUDES *coma:*
         diabetic (250.2-250.3)
         hepatic (572.2)
         originating in the perinatal period
             (779.2)

     AHA: 4Q, '92, 20

     780.01 Coma   CC

       CC Excl: 070.0-070.9, 250.00-250.93, 251.0-251.3, 348.8-348.9, 349.89, 349.9, 430-431, 432.0-432.9, 572.2, 780.01-780.09, 780.2, 780.4, ▶780.91-780.99,◀ 799.8, 800.00-800.99, 801.00-801.99, 803.00-803.99, 804.00-804.96, 850.0-850.9, 851.00-851.99, 852.00-852.19, 852.21-852.59, 853.00-853.19, 854.00-854.19

       AHA: 3Q, '96, 16

       DEF: State of unconsciousness from which the patient cannot be awakened.

     780.02 Transient alteration of awareness

       DEF: Temporary, recurring spells of reduced consciousness.

     780.03 Persistent vegetative state   CC
       CC Excl: See code 780.01

       DEF: Persistent wakefulness without consciousness due to nonfunctioning cerebral cortex.

     780.09 Other
       Drowsiness   Stupor
       Semicoma   Unconsciousness
       Somnolence

780.1 Hallucinations   CC
   Hallucinations: Hallucinations:
     NOS   olfactory
     auditory   tactile
     gustatory

     EXCLUDES *those associated with mental disorders, as functional psychoses (295.0-298.9) organic brain syndromes (290.0-294.9, 310.0-310.9) visual hallucinations (368.16)*

   CC Excl: 780.1, 780.4, ▶780.91-780.99,◀ 799.8

   DEF: Perception of external stimulus in absence of stimulus; inability to distinguish between real and imagined.

780.2 Syncope and collapse
   Blackout   (Near) (Pre) syncope
   Fainting   Vasovagal attack

     EXCLUDES *carotid sinus syncope (337.0) heat syncope (992.1) neurocirculatory asthenia (306.2) orthostatic hypotension (458.0) shock NOS (785.50)*

   AHA: ▶1Q, '02, 6;◀ 3Q, '00, 12; 3Q, '95, 14; N-D, '85, 12

   DEF: Sudden unconsciousness due to reduced blood flow to brain.

✓5ᵗʰ **780.3 Convulsions**

     EXCLUDES *convulsions: epileptic (345.10-345.91) in newborn (779.0)*

   AHA: 2Q, '97, 8; 1Q, '97, 12; 3Q, '94, 9; 1Q, '93, 24; 4Q, '92, 23; N-D, '87, 12

   DEF: Sudden, involuntary contractions of the muscles.

     780.31 Febrile convulsions   CC
       Febrile seizure

       CC Excl: 345.00-345.01, 345.10-345.11, 345.2-345.3, 345.40-345.41, 345.50-345.51, 345.60-345.61, 345.70-345.71, 345.80-345.81, 345.90-345.91, 348.8-348.9, 349.89, 349.9, 779.0-779.1, 780.31, 780.39, ▶780.91-780.99,◀ 799.8

       AHA: 4Q, '97, 45

     780.39 Other convulsions   CC
       Convulsive disorder NOS
       Fit NOS
       Seizure NOS
       CC Excl: See code 780.31

       AHA: 2Q, '99, 17; 4Q, '98, 39

780.4 Dizziness and giddiness
   Light-headedness   Vertigo NOS

     EXCLUDES *Ménière's disease and other specified vertiginous syndromes (386.0-386.9)*

   AHA: 3Q, '00, 12; 2Q, '97, 9; 2Q, '91, 17

   DEF: Whirling sensations in head with feeling of falling.

✓5ᵗʰ **780.5 Sleep disturbances**
     EXCLUDES *that of nonorganic origin (307.40-307.49)*

     780.50 Sleep disturbance, unspecified

     780.51 Insomnia with sleep apnea
       DEF: Transient cessation of breathing disturbing sleep.

     780.52 Other insomnia
       Insomnia NOS

       DEF: Inability to maintain adequate sleep cycle.

     780.53 Hypersomnia with sleep apnea
       AHA: 1Q, '93, 28; N-D, '85, 4

       DEF: Autonomic response inhibited during sleep; causes insufficient oxygen intake, acidosis and pulmonary hypertension.

✓4ᵗʰ ✓5ᵗʰ   Additional Digit Required   Nonspecific PDx   Unacceptable PDx   Manifestation Code   **MSP** Medicare Secondary Payer   ▶◀ Revised Text   ● New Code   ▲ Revised Code Title

2002 Ingenix, Inc.   **October 2002 • Volume 1 — 249**

780.54 Other hypersomnia
Hypersomnia NOS
DEF: Prolonged sleep cycle.

780.55 Disruptions of 24-hour sleep-wake cycle
Inversion of sleep rhythm
Irregular sleep-wake rhythm NOS
Non-24-hour sleep-wake rhythm

780.56 Dysfunctions associated with sleep stages or arousal from sleep

780.57 Other and unspecified sleep apnea
AHA: 1Q, '01, 6 ; 1Q, '97, 5; 1Q, '93, 28

780.59 Other

780.6 Fever
Chills with fever
Fever NOS
Fever of unknown origin (FUO)
Hyperpyrexia NOS
Pyrexia
Pyrexia of unknown origin
EXCLUDES pyrexia of unknown origin (during):
in newborn (778.4)
labor (659.2)
the puerperium (672)

AHA: 3Q, '00,13; 4Q, '99, 26; 2Q, '91, 8

DEF: Elevated body temperature; no known cause.

√5th 780.7 Malaise and fatigue
EXCLUDES debility, unspecified (799.3)
fatigue (during):
combat (308.0-308.9)
heat (992.6)
pregnancy (646.8)
neurasthenia (300.5)
senile asthenia (797)

AHA: 4Q, '88, 12; M-A, '87, 8

DEF: Indefinite feeling of debility or lack of good health.

780.71 Chronic fatigue syndrome
AHA: 4Q, '98, 48

DEF: Persistent fatigue, symptoms include weak muscles, sore throat, lymphadenitis, headache, depression and mild fever; no known cause; also called chronic mononucleosis, benign myalgic encephalomyelitis, Iceland disease and neurosthenia.

780.79 Other malaise and fatigue
Asthenia NOS   Postviral (asthenic) syndrome
Lethargy   Tiredness
AHA: 1Q, '00, 6; 4Q, '99, 26

DEF: Asthenia: Any weakness, lack of strength or loss of energy, especially neuromuscular.

DEF: Lethargy: Listlessness, drowsiness, stupor and apathy.

DEF: Postviral (asthenia) syndrome: Listlessness, drowsiness, stupor and apathy; follows acute viral infection.

DEF: Tiredness: General exhaustion or fatigue.

780.8 Hyperhidrosis
Diaphoresis
Excessive sweating
DEF: Excessive sweating, appears as droplets on skin; general or localized.

√5th 780.9 Other general symptoms
EXCLUDES hypothermia:
NOS (accidental) (991.6)
due to anesthesia (995.89)
of newborn (778.2-778.3)
memory disturbance as part of a
pattern of mental disorder

AHA: 4Q, '99, 10; 3Q, '93, 11; N-D, '85, 12

780.91 Fussy infant (baby)

780.92 Excessive crying of infant (baby)

780.99 Other general symptoms
Amnesia (retrograde)
Chill(s) NOS
Generalized pain
Hypothermia, not associated with low
environmental temperature

√4th 781 Symptoms involving nervous and musculoskeletal systems
EXCLUDES depression NOS (311)
disorders specifically relating to:
back (724.0-724.9)
hearing (388.0-389.9)
joint (718.0-719.9)
limb (729.0-729.9)
neck (723.0-723.9)
vision (368.0-369.9)
pain in limb (729.5)

781.0 Abnormal involuntary movements
Abnormal head movements   Spasms NOS
Fasciculation   Tremor NOS
EXCLUDES abnormal reflex (796.1)
chorea NOS (333.5)
infantile spasms (345.60-345.61)
spastic paralysis (342.1, 343.0-344.9)
specified movement disorders
classifiable to 333 (333.0-333.9)
that of nonorganic origin (307.2-307.3)

781.1 Disturbances of sensation of smell and taste
Anosmia   Parosmia
Parageusia

DEF: Anosmia: loss of sense of smell due to organic factors, including loss of olfactory nerve conductivity, cerebral disease, nasal fossae formation and peripheral olfactory nerve diseases; can also be psychological disorder.

DEF: Parageusia: distorted sense of taste, or bad taste in mouth.

DEF: Parosmia: distorted sense of smell.

781.2 Abnormality of gait
Gait: Gait:
ataxic   spastic
paralytic   staggering
EXCLUDES ataxia:
NOS (781.3)
locomotor (progressive) (094.0)
difficulty in walking (719.7)

DEF: Abnormal, asymmetric gait.

781.3 Lack of coordination
Ataxia NOS   Muscular incoordination
EXCLUDES ataxic gait (781.2)
cerebellar ataxia (334.0-334.9)
difficulty in walking (719.7)
vertigo NOS (780.4)

AHA: 3Q, '97, 12

781.4 Transient paralysis of limb
Monoplegia, transient NOS
EXCLUDES paralysis (342.0-344.9)

781.5 Clubbing of fingers
DEF: Enlarged soft tissue of distal fingers.

N Newborn Age: 0   P Pediatric Age: 0-17   M Maternity Age: 12-55   A Adult Age: 15-124   CC CC Condition   MC Major Complication   CD Complex Dx   HIV HIV Related Dx

781.6　Meningismus
Dupré's syndrome
Meningism
AHA: 3Q, '00,13; J-F, '87, 7

DEF: Condition with signs and symptoms that resemble meningeal irritation; it is associated with febrile illness and dehydration with no evidence of infection.

781.7　Tetany　　`cc`
Carpopedal spasm
　EXCLUDES　tetanus neonatorum (771.3)
　　　　tetany:
　　　　　hysterical (300.11)
　　　　　newborn (hypocalcemic) (775.4)
　　　　　parathyroid (252.1)
　　　　　psychogenic (306.0)
CC Excl: 037, 332.0-332.1, 333.0-333.99, 334.0-334.4, 342.10-342.12, 771.3, ▶780.91-780.99,◀ 781.7, 799.8

DEF: Nerve and muscle hyperexcitability; symptoms include muscle spasms, twitching, cramps, laryngospasm with inspiratory stridor, hyperreflexia and choreiform movements.

781.8　Neurologic neglect syndrome
Asomatognosia　　Left-sided neglect
Hemi-akinesia　　Sensory extinction
Hemi-inattention　　Sensory neglect
Hemispatial neglect　　Visuospatial neglect
AHA: 4Q, '94, 37

√5ᵗʰ **781.9　Other symptoms involving nervous and musculoskeletal systems**
AHA: 4Q, '00, 45

781.91　Loss of height
　EXCLUDES　osteoporosis (733.00-733.09)
781.92　Abnormal posture
781.93　Ocular torticollis
781.99　Other symptoms involving nervous and musculoskeletal systems

√4ᵗʰ **782　Symptoms involving skin and other integumentary tissue**
　EXCLUDES　symptoms relating to breast (611.71-611.79)

782.0　Disturbance of skin sensation
Anesthesia of skin　　Numbness
Burning or prickling sensation　　Paresthesia
Hyperesthesia　　Tingling
Hypoesthesia

782.1　Rash and other nonspecific skin eruption
Exanthem
　EXCLUDES　vesicular eruption (709.8)

782.2　Localized superficial swelling, mass, or lump
Subcutaneous nodules
　EXCLUDES　localized adiposity (278.1)

782.3　Edema
Anasarca
Dropsy
Localized edema NOS
　EXCLUDES　ascites (789.5)
　　　　edema of:
　　　　　newborn NOS (778.5)
　　　　　pregnancy (642.0-642.9, 646.1)
　　　　fluid retention (276.6)
　　　　hydrops fetalis (773.3, 778.0)
　　　　hydrothorax (511.8)
　　　　nutritional edema (260, 262)
AHA: 2Q, '00, 18

DEF: Edema: excess fluid in intercellular body tissue.

DEF: Anasarca: massive edema in all body tissues.

DEF: Dropsy: serous fluid accumulated in body cavity or cellular tissue.

DEF: Localized edema: edema in specific body areas.

782.4　Jaundice, unspecified, not of newborn
Cholemia NOS
Icterus NOS
　EXCLUDES　jaundice in newborn (774.0-774.7)
　　　　due to isoimmunization (773.0-773.2, 773.4)
DEF: Bilirubin deposits of skin, causing yellow cast.

782.5　Cyanosis
　EXCLUDES　newborn ▶(770.83)◀
DEF: Deficient oxygen of blood; causes blue cast to skin.

√5ᵗʰ **782.6　Pallor and flushing**
782.61　Pallor
782.62　Flushing
　　　　Excessive blushing

782.7　Spontaneous ecchymoses
Petechiae
　EXCLUDES　ecchymosis in fetus or newborn (772.6)
　　　　purpura (287.0-287.9)
DEF: Hemorrhagic spots of skin; resemble freckles.

782.8　Changes in skin texture
Induration ⎫
Thickening ⎬ of skin

782.9　Other symptoms involving skin and integumentary tissues

√4ᵗʰ **783　Symptoms concerning nutrition, metabolism, and development**
783.0　Anorexia
Loss of appetite
　EXCLUDES　anorexia nervosa (307.1)
　　　　loss of appetite of nonorganic origin (307.59)

783.1　Abnormal weight gain
　EXCLUDES　excessive weight gain in pregnancy (646.1)
　　　　obesity (278.00)
　　　　morbid (278.01)

√5ᵗʰ **783.2　Abnormal loss of weight and underweight**
AHA: 4Q, '00, 45

783.21　Loss of weight
783.22　Underweight

783.3　Feeding difficulties and mismanagement
Feeding problem (elderly) (infant)
　EXCLUDES　feeding disturbance or problems:
　　　　in newborn (779.3)
　　　　of nonorganic origin (307.50-307.59)
AHA: 3Q, '97, 12

√5ᵗʰ **783.4　Lack of expected normal physiological development in childhood**
　EXCLUDES　delay in sexual development and puberty (259.0)
　　　　gonadal dysgenesis (758.6)
　　　　pituitary dwarfism (253.3)
　　　　slow fetal growth and fetal malnutrition (764.00-764.99)
　　　　specific delays in mental development (315.0-315.9)
AHA: 4Q, '00, 45; 3Q, '97, 4

783.40　Lack of normal physiological development unspecified
Inadequate development
Lack of development

783.41　Failure to thrive　　`P`
Failure to gain weight

DEF: Organic failure to thrive: acute or chronic illness that interferes with nutritional intake, absorption, metabolism excretion and energy requirements. Nonorganic FTT is symptom of neglect or abuse.

783.42　Delayed milestones　　`P`
Late talker
Late walker

√4ᵗʰ / √5ᵗʰ Additional Digit Required　　Nonspecific PDx　　Unacceptable PDx　　Manifestation Code　　**MSP** Medicare Secondary Payer　　▶◀ Revised Text　　● New Code　　▲ Revised Code Title

Symptoms, Signs, and Ill-defined Conditions 783.43–785.51

783.43 Short stature
Growth failure
Growth retardation
Lack of growth
Physical retardation

DEF: Constitutional short stature: stature inconsistent with chronological age. Genetic short stature is when skeletal maturation matches chronological age.

783.5 Polydipsia
Excessive thirst

783.6 Polyphagia
Excessive eating   Hyperalimentation NOS
EXCLUDES   disorders of eating of nonorganic origin (307.50-307.59)

783.7 Adult failure to thrive   A

783.9 Other symptoms concerning nutrition, metabolism, and development
Hypometabolism
EXCLUDES   abnormal basal metabolic rate (794.7)
dehydration (276.5)
other disorders of fluid, electrolyte, and acid-base balance (276.0-276.9)

√4ᵗʰ **784 Symptoms involving head and neck**
EXCLUDES   encephalopathy NOS (348.3)
specific symptoms involving neck classifiable to 723 (723.0-723.9)

784.0 Headache
Facial pain   Pain in head NOS
EXCLUDES   atypical face pain (350.2)
migraine (346.0-346.9)
tension headache (307.81)

AHA: 3Q, '00, 13; 1Q, '90, 4; 3Q, '92, 14

784.1 Throat pain
EXCLUDES   dysphagia (787.2)
neck pain (723.1)
sore throat (462)
chronic (472.1)

784.2 Swelling, mass, or lump in head and neck
Space-occupying lesion, intracranial NOS

784.3 Aphasia
EXCLUDES   developmental aphasia (315.31)

AHA: 4Q, '98, 87; 3Q, '97, 12

DEF: Inability to communicate through speech, written word, or sign language.

√5ᵗʰ **784.4 Voice disturbance**
784.40 Voice disturbance, unspecified
784.41 Aphonia
Loss of voice
784.49 Other
Change in voice   Hypernasality
Dysphonia   Hyponasality
Hoarseness

784.5 Other speech disturbance
Dysarthria   Slurred speech
Dysphasia
EXCLUDES   stammering and stuttering (307.0)
that of nonorganic origin (307.0, 307.9)

√5ᵗʰ **784.6 Other symbolic dysfunction**
EXCLUDES   developmental learning delays (315.0-315.9)

784.60 Symbolic dysfunction, unspecified
784.61 Alexia and dyslexia
Alexia (with agraphia)

DEF: Alexia: Inability to understand written word due to central brain lesion.

DEF: Dyslexia: Ability to recognize letters but inability to read, spell, and write words; genetic.

784.69 Other
Acalculia   Agraphia NOS
Agnosia   Apraxia

784.7 Epistaxis
Hemorrhage from nose
Nosebleed

784.8 Hemorrhage from throat
EXCLUDES   hemoptysis (786.3)

784.9 Other symptoms involving head and neck
Choking sensation   Mouth breathing
Halitosis   Sneezing

√4ᵗʰ **785 Symptoms involving cardiovascular system**
EXCLUDES   heart failure NOS (428.9)

785.0 Tachycardia, unspecified
Rapid heart beat
EXCLUDES   ▶neonatal tachycardia (779.82)◄
paroxysmal tachycardia (427.0-427.2)

DEF: Excessively rapid heart rate.

785.1 Palpitations
Awareness of heart beat
EXCLUDES   specified dysrhythmias (427.0-427.9)

DEF: Shock syndrome: associated with myocardial infarction, cardiac tamponade and massive pulmonary embolism; symptoms include mental torpor, reduced blood pressure, tachycardia, pallor and cold, clammy skin.

785.2 Undiagnosed cardiac murmurs
Heart murmurs NOS
AHA: 4Q, '92, 16

785.3 Other abnormal heart sounds
Cardiac dullness, increased or decreased
Friction fremitus, cardiac
Precordial friction

785.4 Gangrene   CC
Gangrene:
NOS
spreading cutaneous
Gangrenous cellulitis
Phagedena
Code first any associated underlying condition:
diabetes (250.7)
Raynaud's syndrome (443.0)
EXCLUDES   gangrene of certain sites — see Alphabetic Index
gangrene with atherosclerosis of the extremities (440.24)
gas gangrene (040.0

CC Excl: 440.24, ▶780.91-780.99,◄ 785.4, 799.8

AHA: 3Q, '91, 12; 3Q, '90, 15; M-A, '86, 12

DEF: Gangrene: necrosis of skin tissue due to bacterial infection, diabetes, embolus and vascular supply loss.

DEF: Gangrenous cellulitis: group A streptococcal infection; begins with severe cellulitis, spreads to superficial and deep fascia; produces gangrene of underlying tissues.

√5ᵗʰ **785.5 Shock without mention of trauma**
785.50 Shock, unspecified   CC MC CD
Failure of peripheral circulation
CC Excl: ▶780.91-780.99,◄ 785.50-785.59, 785.9, 799.8

AHA: 2Q, '96, 10

785.51 Cardiogenic shock   CC MC CD
CC Excl: See code 785.50

DEF: Peripheral circulatory failure due to heart insufficiencies.

N Newborn Age: 0   P Pediatric Age: 0-17   M Maternity Age: 12-55   A Adult Age: 15-124   CC CC Condition   MC Major Complication   CD Complex Dx   HIV HIV Related Dx

252 — Volume 1 • October 2002

2002 Ingenix, Inc.

785.59 Other `CC`

Shock: Shock:
endotoxic   hypovolemic
gram-negative   septic

EXCLUDES   *shock (due to):*
anesthetic (995.4)
anaphylactic (995.0)
due to serum (999.4)
electric (994.8)
following abortion (639.5)
lightning (994.0)
obstetrical (669.1)
postoperative (998.0)
traumatic (958.4)

CC Excl: see code 785.50

AHA: 2Q, '00, 3

785.6 Enlargement of lymph nodes

Lymphadenopathy   "Swollen glands"

EXCLUDES   *lymphadenitis (chronic) (289.1-289.3)*
acute (683)

785.9 Other symptoms involving cardiovascular system

Bruit (arterial)   Weak pulse

√4th **786 Symptoms involving respiratory system and other chest symptoms**

√5th **786.0 Dyspnea and respiratory abnormalities**

786.00 Respiratory abnormality, unspecified

786.01 Hyperventilation

EXCLUDES   *hyperventilation, psychogenic (306.1)*

DEF: Rapid breathing causes carbon dioxide loss from blood.

786.02 Orthopnea

DEF: Difficulty breathing except in upright position.

786.03 Apnea `CC`

EXCLUDES   ▶ *apnea of newborn (770.81, 770.82)*◀
sleep apnea (780.51, 780.53, 780.57)

CC Excl: 518.81-518.84, 519.8, 519.9, 786.03, 786.04, 799.1

AHA: 4Q, '98, 50

DEF: Cessation of breathing.

786.04 Cheyne-Stokes respiration `CC`

CC Excl: 518.81-518.84, 519.8, 519.9, 786.03, 786.04, 799.1

AHA: 4Q, '98, 50

DEF: Rhythmic increase of depth and frequency of breathing with apnea; occurs in frontal lobe and diencephalic dysfunction.

786.05 Shortness of breath

AHA: 4Q, '99, 25; 1Q, '99, 6; 4Q, '98, 50

DEF: Inability to take in sufficient oxygen.

786.06 Tachypnea

EXCLUDES   *transitory tachypnea of newborn (770.6)*

AHA: 4Q, '98, 50

DEF: Abnormal rapid respiratory rate; called hyperventilation.

786.07 Wheezing

EXCLUDES   *asthma (493.00-493.92)*

AHA: 4Q, '98, 50

DEF: Stenosis of respiratory passageway; causes whistling sound; due to asthma, coryza, croup, emphysema, hay fever, edema, and pleural effusion.

786.09 Other

Respiratory:
distress
insufficiency

EXCLUDES   *respiratory distress:*
following trauma and surgery (518.5)
newborn ▶*(770.89)*◀
syndrome (newborn) (769)
adult (518.5)
respiratory failure (518.81, 518.83-518.84)
newborn ▶*(770.84)*◀

AHA: 2Q, '98, 10; 1Q, '97, 7; 1Q, '90, 9

786.1 Stridor

EXCLUDES   *congenital laryngeal stridor (748.3)*

DEF: Obstructed airway causes harsh sound.

786.2 Cough

EXCLUDES   *cough:*
psychogenic (306.1)
smokers' (491.0)
with hemorrhage (786.3)

AHA: 4Q, '99, 26

786.3 Hemoptysis `CC`

Cough with hemorrhage
Pulmonary hemorrhage NOS

EXCLUDES   *pulmonary hemorrhage of newborn (770.3)*

CC Excl: ▶780.91-780.99,◀ 786.3-786.4, 786.9, 799.8

AHA: 4Q, '90, 26

DEF: Coughing up blood or blood-stained sputum.

786.4 Abnormal sputum

Abnormal:
amount
color   } (of) sputum
odor
Excessive

√5th **786.5 Chest pain**

786.50 Chest pain, unspecified

AHA: ▶1Q, '02, 4;◀ 4Q, '99, 25

786.51 Precordial pain

DEF: Chest pain over heart and lower thorax.

786.52 Painful respiration

Pain: Pleurodynia
anterior chest wall
pleuritic

EXCLUDES   *epidemic pleurodynia (074.1)*

AHA: N-D, '84, 17

786.59 Other

Discomfort
Pressure   } in chest
Tightness

EXCLUDES   *pain in breast (611.71)*

AHA: ▶1Q, '02, 6◀

786.6 Swelling, mass, or lump in chest

EXCLUDES   *lump in breast (611.72)*

786.7 Abnormal chest sounds

Abnormal percussion, chest   Rales
Friction sounds, chest   Tympany, chest

EXCLUDES   *wheezing (786.07)*

786.8 Hiccough

EXCLUDES   *psychogenic hiccough (306.1)*

786.9 Other symptoms involving respiratory system and chest

Breath-holding spell

√4th
√5th Additional Digit Required   Nonspecific PDx   Unacceptable PDx   Manifestation Code   `MSP` Medicare Secondary Payer   ▶◀ Revised Text   ● New Code   ▲ Revised Code Title

Symptoms, Signs, and Ill-defined Conditions 785.59–786.9

Symptoms, Signs, and Ill-defined Conditions 787–788.41

√4th **787 Symptoms involving digestive system**

     EXCLUDES   constipation (564.00-564.09)
                pylorospasm (537.81)
                  congenital (750.5)

√5th **787.0 Nausea and vomiting**
     Emesis

     EXCLUDES   hematemesis NOS (578.0)
                vomiting:
                  bilious, following gastrointestinal
                     surgery (564.3)
                  cyclical (536.2)
                    psychogenic (306.4)
                  excessive, in pregnancy (643.0-
                    643.9)
                  habit (536.2)
                  of newborn (779.3)
                  psychogenic NOS (307.54)

     AHA: M-A, '85, 11

     787.01 Nausea with vomiting
     787.02 Nausea alone
         AHA: 3Q, '00, 12; 2Q, '97, 9

     787.03 Vomiting alone

787.1 Heartburn
     Pyrosis   Waterbrash
     EXCLUDES   dyspepsia or indigestion (536.8)

     AHA: 2Q, '01, 6

787.2 Dysphagia
     Difficulty in swallowing
     AHA: 2Q, '01, 4

787.3 Flatulence, eructation, and gas pain
     Abdominal distention (gaseous)
     Bloating
     Tympanites (abdominal) (intestinal)
     EXCLUDES   aerophagy (306.4)

     DEF: Flatulence: Excess air or gas in intestine or stomach.

     DEF: Eructation: Belching, expelling gas through mouth.

     DEF: Gas pain: Gaseous pressure affecting gastrointestinal system.

787.4 Visible peristalsis
     Hyperperistalsis
     DEF: Increase in involuntary movements of intestines.

787.5 Abnormal bowel sounds
     Absent bowel sounds
     Hyperactive bowel sounds

787.6 Incontinence of feces
     Encopresis NOS
     Incontinence of sphincter ani
     EXCLUDES   that of nonorganic origin (307.7)
     AHA: 1Q, '97, 9

787.7 Abnormal feces
     Bulky stools
     EXCLUDES   abnormal stool content (792.1)
                melena:
                  NOS (578.1)
                  newborn (772.4, 777.3)

√5th **787.9 Other symptoms involving digestive system**
     EXCLUDES   gastrointestinal hemorrhage (578.0-
                    578.9)
                intestinal obstruction (560.0-560.9)
                specific functional digestive disorders:
                  esophagus (530.0-530.9)
                  stomach and duodenum (536.0-
                    536.9)
                  those not elsewhere classified
                    (564.00-564.9)

     787.91 Diarrhea
         Diarrhea NOS
         AHA: 4Q, '95, 54

787.99 Other
     Change in bowel habits
     Tenesmus (rectal)
     DEF: Tenesmus: Painful, ineffective straining at the
     rectum with limited passage of fecal matter.

√4th **788 Symptoms involving urinary system**

     EXCLUDES   hematuria (599.7)
                nonspecific findings on examination of the urine
                  (791.0-791.9)
                small kidney of unknown cause (589.0-589.9)
                uremia NOS (586)

788.0 Renal colic
     Colic (recurrent) of: Colic (recurrent) of:
     kidney   ureter
     DEF: Kidney pain.

788.1 Dysuria
     Painful urination   Strangury

√5th **788.2 Retention of urine**
     DEF: Inability to void.

     788.20 Retention of urine, unspecified   `CC`
         CC Excl: 274.11, 344.61, 593.3-593.5, 596.0, 596.4-
         596.59, 596.8-596.9, 599.6, 600.1-600.9, 601.0-601.9,
         602.0-602.9, 753.0, 753.1, 753.20-753.23, 753.29,
         753.3-753.9, ▶780.91-780.99,◀ 788.20-788.29, 788.61-
         788.69, 788.9, 799.8

         AHA: 3Q, '96, 10

     788.21 Incomplete bladder emptying
     788.29 Other specified retention of urine   `CC`
         CC Excl: See code 788.20

√5th **788.3 Incontinence of urine**
     ▶Code, if applicable, any causal condition first,
         such as:◀
     congenital ureterocele (753.23)
     genital prolapse (618.0-618.9)
     EXCLUDES   that of nonorganic origin (307.6)

     AHA: 4Q, '92, 22

     788.30 Urinary incontinence, unspecified
         Enuresis NOS

     788.31 Urge incontinence
         AHA: 1Q, '00, 19

         DEF: Inability to control urination, upon urge to urinate.

     788.32 Stress incontinence, male   ♂
         EXCLUDES   stress incontinence, female
                    (625.6)

         DEF: Inability to control urination associated with weak
         sphincter in males.

     788.33 Mixed incontinence, (male) (female)
         Urge and stress
         DEF: Urge, stress incontinence: involuntary discharge of
         urine due to anatomic displacement.

     788.34 Incontinence without sensory awareness
         DEF: Involuntary discharge of urine without sensory
         warning.

     788.35 Post-void dribbling
         DEF: Involuntary discharge of residual urine after
         voiding.

     788.36 Nocturnal enuresis
         DEF: Involuntary discharge of urine during the night.

     788.37 Continuous leakage
         DEF: Continuous, involuntary urine seepage.

     788.39 Other urinary incontinence

√5th **788.4 Frequency of urination and polyuria**
     788.41 Urinary frequency
         Frequency of micturition

N Newborn Age: 0   P Pediatric Age: 0-17   M Maternity Age: 12-55   A Adult Age: 15-124   CC CC Condition   MC Major Complication   CD Complex Dx   HIV HIV Related Dx

788.42 Polyuria
DEF: Excessive urination.

788.43 Nocturia
DEF: Urination affecting sleep patterns.

788.5 Oliguria and anuria
Deficient secretion of urine
Suppression of urinary secretion
EXCLUDES that complicating:
abortion (634-638 with .3, 639.3)
ectopic or molar pregnancy (639.3)
pregnancy, childbirth, or the
puerperium (642.0-642.9,
646.2)
DEF: Oliguria: diminished urinary secretion related to fluid intake.
DEF: Anuria: lack of urinary secretion due to renal failure or obstructed urinary tract.

✓5th **788.6 Other abnormality of urination**
788.61 Splitting of urinary stream
Intermittent urinary stream
788.62 Slowing of urinary stream
Weak stream
788.69 Other
788.7 Urethral discharge
Penile discharge   Urethrorrhea
788.8 Extravasation of urine
DEF: Leaking or infiltration of urine into tissues.
788.9 Other symptoms involving urinary system
Extrarenal uremia   Vesical:
Vesical: tenesmus
pain
AHA: 4Q, '88, 1

✓4th **789 Other symptoms involving abdomen and pelvis**
EXCLUDES symptoms referable to genital organs:
female (625.0-625.9)
male (607.0-608.9)
psychogenic (302.70-302.79)

The following fifth-digit subclassification is to be used for codes 789.0, 789.3, 789.4, 789.6:
0 unspecified site
1 right upper quadrant
2 left upper quadrant
3 right lower quadrant
4 left lower quadrant
5 periumbilic
6 epigastric
7 generalized
9 other specified site
Multiple sites

✓5th **789.0 Abdominal pain**
Colic:
NOS   infantile
Cramps, abdominal
EXCLUDES renal colic (788.0)
AHA: 1Q, '95, 3; For code 789.06: ▶1Q, '02, 5◀

789.1 Hepatomegaly
Enlargement of liver
789.2 Splenomegaly
Enlargement of spleen
✓5th **789.3 Abdominal or pelvic swelling, mass, or lump**
Diffuse or generalized swelling or mass:
abdominal NOS
umbilical
EXCLUDES abdominal distention (gaseous) (787.3)
ascites (789.5)
✓5th **789.4 Abdominal rigidity**
789.5 Ascites   CC
Fluid in peritoneal cavity
CC Excl: ▶780.91-780.99,◀ 789.30-789.5, 789.9, 799.8
AHA: 4Q, '89, 11
DEF: Serous fluid effusion and accumulation in abdominal cavity.

✓5th **789.6 Abdominal tenderness**
Rebound tenderness
789.9 Other symptoms involving abdomen and pelvis
Umbilical: Umbilical:
bleeding   discharge

NONSPECIFIC ABNORMAL FINDINGS (790-796)
AHA: 2Q, '90, 16

✓4th **790 Nonspecific findings on examination of blood**
EXCLUDES abnormality of:
platelets (287.0-287.9)
thrombocytes (287.0-287.9)
white blood cells (288.0-288.9)
✓5th **790.0 Abnormality of red blood cells**
EXCLUDES anemia:
congenital (776.5)
newborn, due to isoimmunization
(773.0-773.2, 773.5)
of premature infant (776.6)
other specified types (280.0-285.9)
hemoglobin disorders (282.5-282.7)
polycythemia:
familial (289.6)
neonatorum (776.4)
secondary (289.0)
vera (238.4)
AHA: 4Q, '00, 46

790.01 Precipitous drop in hematocrit
Drop in hematocrit
790.09 Other abnormality of red blood cells
Abnormal red cell morphology NOS
Abnormal red cell volume NOS
Anisocytosis
Poikilocytosis
790.1 Elevated sedimentation rate
790.2 Abnormal glucose tolerance test
EXCLUDES that complicating pregnancy, childbirth,
or the puerperium (648.8)
AHA: 3Q, '91, 5
790.3 Excessive blood level of alcohol
Elevated blood-alcohol
AHA: S-O, '86, 3
790.4 Nonspecific elevation of levels of transaminase or lactic acid dehydrogenase [LDH]
790.5 Other nonspecific abnormal serum enzyme levels
Abnormal serum level of:
acid phosphatase
alkaline phosphatase
amylase
lipase
EXCLUDES deficiency of circulating enzymes (277.6)
790.6 Other abnormal blood chemistry
Abnormal blood level of: Abnormal blood level of:
cobalt   magnesium
copper   mineral
iron   zinc
lithium
EXCLUDES abnormality of electrolyte or acid-base
balance (276.0-276.9)
hypoglycemia NOS (251.2)
specific finding indicating abnormality
of:
amino-acid transport and
metabolism (270.0-270.9)
carbohydrate transport and
metabolism (271.0-271.9)
lipid metabolism (272.0-272.9)
uremia NOS (586)
AHA: 4Q, '88, 1

790.7 Bacteremia   `CC`
> EXCLUDES ▶ bacteremia of newborn (771.83)◀
> septicemia (038)

Use additional code to identify organism (041)

CC Excl: ▶780.91-780.99,◀ 790.7-790.99, 799.8

AHA: 4Q, '93, 29; 3Q, '88, 12

DEF: Bacterial infection of blood with no signs of infection.

790.8 Viremia, unspecified

AHA: 4Q, '88, 10

DEF: Presence of a virus in the blood stream.

√5ᵗʰ **790.9 Other nonspecific findings on examination of blood**

AHA: 4Q, '93, 29

790.91 Abnormal arterial blood gases

790.92 Abnormal coagulation profile
Abnormal or prolonged:
   bleeding time
   coagulation time
   partial thromboplastin time [PTT]
   prothrombintime [PT]
> EXCLUDES   coagulation (hemorrhagic)
> disorders (286.0-286.9)

790.93 Elevated prostate specific antigen, (PSA)   `A` ♂

790.94 Euthyroid sick syndrome

AHA: 4Q, '97, 45

DEF: Transient alteration of thyroid hormone metabolism due to nonthyroid illness or stress.

790.99 Other

√4ᵗʰ **791 Nonspecific findings on examination of urine**
> EXCLUDES   hematuria NOS (599.7)
> specific findings indicating abnormality of:
>   amino-acid transport and metabolism (270.0-270.9)
>   carbohydrate transport and metabolism (271.0-271.9)

791.0 Proteinuria
Albuminuria
Bence-Jones proteinuria
> EXCLUDES   postural proteinuria (593.6)
> that arising during pregnancy or the puerperium (642.0-642.9, 646.2)

AHA: 3Q, '91, 8

DEF: Excess protein in urine.

791.1 Chyluria   `CC`
> EXCLUDES   filarial (125.0-125.9)

CC Excl: ▶780.91-780.99,◀ 791.1, 791.9, 799.8

DEF: Excess chyle in urine.

791.2 Hemoglobinuria

DEF: Free hemoglobin in blood due to rapid hemolysis of red blood cells.

791.3 Myoglobinuria   `CC`

CC Excl: ▶780.91-780.99,◀ 791.2-791.3, 791.9, 799.8

DEF: Myoglobin (oxygen-transporting pigment) in urine.

791.4 Biliuria

DEF: Bile pigments in urine.

791.5 Glycosuria
> EXCLUDES   renal glycosuria (271.4)

DEF: Sugar in urine.

791.6 Acetonuria
Ketonuria

DEF: Excess acetone in urine.

791.7 Other cells and casts in urine

791.9 Other nonspecific findings on examination of urine
Crystalluria
Elevated urine levels of:
  17-ketosteroids
  catecholamines
Elevated urine levels of:
  indolacetic acid
  vanillylmandelic acid [VMA]
  Melanuria

√4ᵗʰ **792 Nonspecific abnormal findings in other body substances**
> EXCLUDES   that in chromosomal analysis (795.2)

792.0 Cerebrospinal fluid

792.1 Stool contents
Abnormal stool color
Fat in stool
Mucus in stool
Occult stool
Pus in stool
> EXCLUDES   blood in stool [melena] (578.1)
> newborn (772.4, 777.3)

AHA: 2Q, '92, 9

792.2 Semen   ♂
Abnormal spermatozoa
> EXCLUDES   azoospermia (606.0)
> oligospermia (606.1)

792.3 Amniotic fluid   `M`♀

AHA: N-D, '86, 4

DEF: Nonspecific abnormal findings in amniotic fluid.

792.4 Saliva
> EXCLUDES   that in chromosomal analysis (795.2)

792.5 Cloudy (hemodialysis) (peritoneal) dialysis effluent

792.9 Other nonspecific abnormal findings in body substances
Peritoneal fluid
Pleural fluid
Synovial fluid
Vaginal fluids

√4ᵗʰ **793 Nonspecific abnormal findings on radiological and other examination of body structure**
> INCLUDES   nonspecific abnormal findings of:
>   thermography
>   ultrasound examination [echogram]
>   x-ray examination
> EXCLUDES   abnormal results of function studies and radioisotope scans (794.0-794.9)

793.0 Skull and head
> EXCLUDES   nonspecific abnormal echoencephalogram (794.01)

793.1 Lung field
Coin lesion
Shadow } (of) lung

DEF: Coin lesion of lung: coin-shaped, solitary pulmonary nodule; diagnosis includes tuberculoma, histoplasmoma, blastomycoma, coccidioidomycoma, primary carcinoma of the lung, metastatic carcinoma and benign pulmonary tumor.

793.2 Other intrathoracic organ
Abnormal:
  echocardiogram
  heart shadow
Abnormal:
  ultrasound cardiogram
  Mediastinal shift

793.3 Biliary tract
Nonvisualization of gallbladder

793.4 Gastrointestinal tract

793.5 Genitourinary organs
Filling defect:
  bladder
  kidney
Filling defect:
  ureter

AHA: 4Q, '00, 46

793.6 Abdominal area, including retroperitoneum

793.7 Musculoskeletal system

√5ᵗʰ **793.8 Breast**

AHA: 4Q, '01, 51

793.80 Abnormal mammogram, unspecified

793.81 Mammographic microcalcification

DEF: Calcium and cellular debris deposits in the breast that cannot be felt but can be detected on a mammogram; can be a sign of cancer, benign conditions, or changes in the breast tissue as a result of inflammation, injury, or obstructed duct.

793.89 Other abnormal findings on radiological examination of breast

793.9 Other
Abnormal:
placental finding by x-ray or ultrasound method
radiological findings in skin and subcutaneous tissue
> EXCLUDES *abnormal finding by radioisotope localization of placenta (794.9)*

√4ᵗʰ **794 Nonspecific abnormal results of function studies**
INCLUDES radioisotope:
scans
uptake studies
scintiphotography

√5ᵗʰ **794.0 Brain and central nervous system**
794.00 Abnormal function study, unspecified
794.01 Abnormal echoencephalogram
794.02 Abnormal electroencephalogram [EEG]
794.09 Other
Abnormal brain scan

√5ᵗʰ **794.1 Peripheral nervous system and special senses**
794.10 Abnormal response to nerve stimulation, unspecified
794.11 Abnormal retinal function studies
Abnormal electroretinogram [ERG]
794.12 Abnormal electro-oculogram [EOG]
794.13 Abnormal visually evoked potential
794.14 Abnormal oculomotor studies
794.15 Abnormal auditory function studies
794.16 Abnormal vestibular function studies
794.17 Abnormal electromyogram [EMG]
> EXCLUDES *that of eye (794.14)*
794.19 Other

794.2 Pulmonary
Abnormal lung scan
Reduced:
ventilatory capacity
vital capacity

√5ᵗʰ **794.3 Cardiovascular**
794.30 Abnormal function study, unspecified
794.31 Abnormal electrocardiogram [ECG] [EKG]
794.39 Other
Abnormal:
ballistocardiogram
phonocardiogram
vectorcardiogram

794.4 Kidney
Abnormal renal function test

794.5 Thyroid
Abnormal thyroid:
scan
uptake

794.6 Other endocrine function study

794.7 Basal metabolism
Abnormal basal metabolic rate [BMR]

794.8 Liver
Abnormal liver scan

794.9 Other
Bladder
Pancreas
Placenta
Spleen

√4ᵗʰ **795 Nonspecific abnormal histological and immunological findings**
> EXCLUDES *nonspecific abnormalities of red blood cells (790.01-790.09)*

√5ᵗʰ **795.0 Nonspecific abnormal Papanicolaou smear of cervix** ♀
> EXCLUDES ▸carcinoma in-situ of cervix (233.1)
cervical intraepithelial neoplasia I (CIN I) (622.1)
cervical intraepithelial neoplasia II (CIN II) (622.1)
cervical intraepithelial neoplasia III (CIN III) (233.1)
dyplasia of cervix (uteri) (622.1)
high grade squamous intraepithelial dysplasia (HGSIL) (622.1)
low grade squamous intraepithelial dysplasia (LGSIL) (622.1)◂
795.00 Nonspecific abnormal Papanicolaou smear of cervix, unspecified
795.01 Atypical squamous cell changes of undetermined significance favor benign (ASCUS favor benign)
Atypical glandular cell changes of undetermined significance favor benign (AGCUS favor benign)
795.02 Atypical squamous cell changes of undetermined significance favor dysplasia (ASCUS favor dysplasia)
Atypical glandular cell changes of undetermined significance favor dysplasia (AGCUS favor dysplasia)
795.09 Other nonspecific abnormal Papanicolaou smear of cervix
Benign cellular chnages
Unsatisfactory smear

795.1 Nonspecific abnormal Papanicolaou smear of other site

795.2 Nonspecific abnormal findings on chromosomal analysis
Abnormal karyotype

√5ᵗʰ **795.3 Nonspecific positive culture findings**
Positive culture findings in:
nose
sputum
throat
wound
> EXCLUDES *that of:*
blood (790.7-790.8)
urine (791.9)
795.31 Nonspecific positive findings for anthrax
Positive findings by nasal swab
795.39 Other nonspecific positive culture findings

795.4 Other nonspecific abnormal histological findings

795.5 Nonspecific reaction to tuberculin skin test without active tuberculosis
Abnormal result of Mantoux test
PPD positive
Tuberculin (skin test):
positive
reactor

795.6 False positive serological test for syphilis
False positive Wassermann reaction

√5ᵗʰ **795.7 Other nonspecific immunological findings**
> EXCLUDES *isoimmunization, in pregnancy (656.1-656.2)*
affecting fetus or newborn (773.0-773.2)

AHA: 2Q, '93, 6

√4ᵗʰ √5ᵗʰ Additional Digit Required   Nonspecific PDx   Unacceptable PDx   Manifestation Code   MSP Medicare Secondary Payer   ▸◂ Revised Text   ● New Code   ▲ Revised Code Title

2002 Ingenix, Inc.

October 2002 • Volume 1 — 257

Symptoms, Signs, and Ill-defined Conditions 793.89–795.7

Symptoms, Signs, and Ill-defined Conditions 795.71–799.9

795.71 Nonspecific serologic evidence of human immunodeficiency virus [HIV]

Inclusive human immunodeficiency [HIV] test (adult) (infant)

Note: This code is **only** to be used when a test finding is reported as nonspecific. Asymptomatic positive findings are coded to V08. If any HIV infection symptom or condition is present, see code 042. Negative findings are not coded.

EXCLUDES   *acquired immunodeficiency syndrome [AIDS] (042)*
asymptomatic human immunodeficiency virus, [HIV] infection status (V08)
HIV infection, symptomatic (042)
human immunodeficiency virus [HIV] disease (042)
positive (status) NOS (V08)

AHA: 1Q, '93, 21; 1Q, '93, 22; 2Q, '92, 11; J-A, '87, 24

795.79 Other and unspecified nonspecific immunological findings

Raised antibody titer
Raised level of immunoglobulins

√4ᵗʰ **796 Other nonspecific abnormal findings**

796.0 Nonspecific abnormal toxicological findings

Abnormal levels of heavy metals or drugs in blood, urine, or other tissue

EXCLUDES   *excessive blood level of alcohol (790.3)*

AHA: 1Q, '97, 16

796.1 Abnormal reflex

796.2 Elevated blood pressure reading without diagnosis of hypertension

Note: This category is to be used to record an episode of elevated blood pressure in a patient in whom no formal diagnosis of hypertension has been made, or as an incidental finding.

AHA: 3Q, '90, 4; J-A, '84, 12

796.3 Nonspecific low blood pressure reading

796.4 Other abnormal clinical findings

AHA: 1Q, '97, 16

796.5 Abnormal finding on antenatal screening   M ♀

AHA: 4Q, '97, 46

796.9 Other

ILL-DEFINED AND UNKNOWN CAUSES OF MORBIDITY AND MORTALITY (797-799)

797 Senility without mention of psychosis

Old age
Senescence
Senile asthenia
Senile:
  debility
  exhaustion

EXCLUDES   *senile psychoses (290.0-290.9)*

√4ᵗʰ **798 Sudden death, cause unknown**

798.0 Sudden infant death syndrome   P

Cot death
Crib death
Sudden death of nonspecific cause in infancy

DEF: Death of infant under age one due to nonspecific cause.

798.1 Instantaneous death

798.2 Death occurring in less than 24 hours from onset of symptoms, not otherwise explained

Death known not to be violent or instantaneous, for which no cause could be discovered
Died without sign of disease

798.9 Unattended death

Death in circumstances where the body of the deceased was found and no cause could be discovered
Found dead

√4ᵗʰ **799 Other ill-defined and unknown causes of morbidity and mortality**

799.0 Asphyxia

EXCLUDES   *asphyxia (due to):*
    carbon monoxide (986)
    inhalation of food or foreign body (932-934.9)
    newborn (768.0-768.9)
    traumatic (994.7)

DEF: Lack of oxygen.

799.1 Respiratory arrest   CC

Cardiorespiratory failure

EXCLUDES   *cardiac arrest (427.5)*
failure of peripheral circulation (785.50)
respiratory distress:
  NOS (786.09)
  acute (518.82)
  following trauma and surgery (518.5)
  newborn ▶(770.89)◀
  syndrome (newborn) (769)
    adult (following trauma and surgery) (518.5)
  other (518.82)
respiratory failure (518.81, 518.83-518.84)
  newborn ▶(770.84)◀
respiratory insufficiency (786.09)
  acute (518.82)

CC Excl: 518.81-518.84, ▶780.91-780.99,◀ 798.0, 799.0-799.1, 799.8

799.2 Nervousness

"Nerves"

799.3 Debility, unspecified

EXCLUDES   *asthenia (780.79)*
nervous debility (300.5)
neurasthenia (300.5)
senile asthenia (797)

799.4 Cachexia   CC

Wasting disease

EXCLUDES   *nutritional marasmus (261)*

CC Excl: ▶780.91-780.99,◀ 799.3-799.4, 799.8

AHA: 3Q, '90, 17

DEF: General ill health and poor nutrition.

799.8 Other ill-defined conditions

799.9 Other unknown and unspecified cause

Undiagnosed disease, not specified as to site or system involved
Unknown cause of morbidity or mortality

AHA: 1Q, '98,.4; 1Q, '90, 20

N Newborn Age: 0   P Pediatric Age: 0-17   M Maternity Age: 12-55   A Adult Age: 15-124   CC CC Condition   MC Major Complication   CD Complex Dx   HIV HIV Related Dx

2002 Ingenix, Inc.

17. INJURY AND POISONING (800-999)

Use E code(s) to identify the cause and intent of the injury or poisoning (E800-E999)

Note:

1. The principle of multiple coding of injuries should be followed wherever possible. Combination categories for multiple injuries are provided for use when there is insufficient detail as to the nature of the individual conditions, or for primary tabulation purposes when it is more convenient to record a single code; otherwise, the component injuries should be coded separately.

   Where multiple sites of injury are specified in the titles, the word "with" indicates involvement of both sites, and the word "and" indicates involvement of either or both sites. The word "finger" includes thumb.

2. Categories for "late effect" of injuries are to be found at 905-909.

FRACTURES (800-829)

EXCLUDES malunion (733.81)
nonunion (733.82)
pathological or spontaneous fracture (733.10-733.19)
stress fractures (733.93-733.95)

The terms "condyle," "coronoid process," "ramus," and "symphysis" indicate the portion of the bone fractured, not the name of the bone involved.

The descriptions "closed" and "open" used in the fourth-digit subdivisions include the following terms:

closed (with or without delayed healing):
comminuted	impacted
depressed	linear
elevated	simple
fissured	slipped epiphysis
fracture NOS	spiral
greenstick	

open (with or without delayed healing):
compound	puncture
infected	with foreign body
missile	

A fracture not indicated as closed or open should be classified as closed.

AHA: 4Q, '90, 26; 3Q, '90, 5; 3Q, '90, 13; 2Q, '90, 7; 2Q, '89, 15, S-O, '85, 3

Fractures

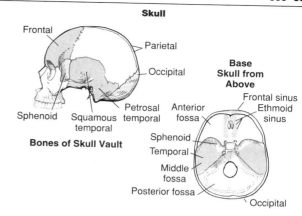

Skull

Bones of Skull Vault

Base Skull from Above

FRACTURE OF SKULL (800-804)

The following fifth-digit subclassification is for use with the appropriate codes in categories 800, 801, 803, and 804:

  0 unspecified state of consciousness
  1 with no loss of consciousness
  2 with brief [less than one hour] loss of consciousness
  3 with moderate [1-24 hours] loss of consciousness
  4 with prolonged [more than 24 hours] loss of consciousness and return to pre-existing conscious level
  5 with prolonged [more than 24 hours] loss of consciousness, without return to pre-existing conscious level

Use fifth-digit 5 to designate when a patient is unconscious and dies before regaining consciousness, regardless of the duration of the loss of consciousness

  6 with loss of consciousness of unspecified duration
  9 with concussion, unspecified

√4th **800 Fracture of vault of skull**

INCLUDES frontal bone
parietal bone

AHA: 4Q, '96, 36

DEF: Fracture of bone that forms skull dome and protects brain.

§ √5th **800.0 Closed without mention of intracranial injury** `CC` `MSP`
CC Excl: 800.00-801.99, 803.00-804.99, 829.0-829.1, 850.0-852.19, 852.21-854.19, 873.8-873.9, 879.8-879.9, 905.0, 925.1-925.2, 929.0-929.9, 958.8, 959.01, 959.09, 959.8-959.9

§ √5th **800.1 Closed with cerebral laceration and contusion** `CC` `MSP`
CC Excl: See code 800.0

§ √5th **800.2 Closed with subarachnoid, subdural, and extradural hemorrhage** `CC` `MSP`
CC Excl: See code 800.0

§ √5th **800.3 Closed with other and unspecified intracranial hemorrhage** `CC` `MSP`
CC Excl: See code 800.0

§ √5th **800.4 Closed with intracranial injury of other and unspecified nature** `CC` `MSP`
CC Excl: See code 800.0

§ √5th **800.5 Open without mention of intracranial injury** `CC` `MSP`
CC Excl: See code 800.0

§ √5th **800.6 Open with cerebral laceration and contusion** `CC` `MSP`
CC Excl: See code 800.0

§ Requires fifth-digit. See beginning of section 800-804 for codes and definitions.

√4th √5th Additional Digit Required   Nonspecific PDx   Unacceptable PDx   Manifestation Code   **MSP** Medicare Secondary Payer   ►◄ Revised Text   ● New Code   ▲ Revised Code Title

§ ✓5ᵗʰ **800.7 Open with subarachnoid, subdural, and extradural hemorrhage** `CC` `MSP`
CC Excl: See code 800.0

§ ✓5ᵗʰ **800.8 Open with other and unspecified intracranial hemorrhage** `CC` `MSP`
CC Excl: See code 800.0

§ ✓5ᵗʰ **800.9 Open with intracranial injury of other and unspecified nature** `CC` `MSP`
CC Excl: See code 800.0

✓4ᵗʰ **801 Fracture of base of skull**

INCLUDES
fossa:	sinus:
anterior	ethmoid
middle	frontal
posterior	sphenoid bone
occiput bone	temporal bone
orbital roof	

AHA: 4Q, '96, 36

DEF: Fracture of bone that forms skull floor.

§ ✓5ᵗʰ **801.0 Closed without mention of intracranial injury** `CC` `MSP`
CC Excl: See code 800.0

§ ✓5ᵗʰ **801.1 Closed with cerebral laceration and contusion** `CC` `MSP`
CC Excl: See code 800.0

AHA: 4Q, '96, 36

§ ✓5ᵗʰ **801.2 Closed with subarachnoid, subdural, and extradural hemorrhage** `CC` `MSP`
CC Excl: See code 800.0

§ ✓5ᵗʰ **801.3 Closed with other and unspecified intracranial hemorrhage** `CC` `MSP`
CC Excl: See code 800.0

§ ✓5ᵗʰ **801.4 Closed with intracranial injury of other and unspecified nature** `CC` `MSP`
CC Excl: See code 800.0

§ ✓5ᵗʰ **801.5 Open without mention of intracranial injury** `CC` `MSP`
CC Excl: See code 800.0

§ ✓5ᵗʰ **801.6 Open with cerebral laceration and contusion** `CC` `MSP`
CC Excl: See code 800.0

§ ✓5ᵗʰ **801.7 Open with subarachnoid, subdural, and extradural hemorrhage** `CC` `MSP`
CC Excl: See code 800.0

§ ✓5ᵗʰ **801.8 Open with other and unspecified intracranial hemorrhage** `CC` `MSP`
CC Excl: See code 800.0

§ ✓5ᵗʰ **801.9 Open with intracranial injury of other and unspecified nature** `CC` `MSP`
CC Excl: See code 800.0

✓4ᵗʰ **802 Fracture of face bones**
AHA: 4Q, '96, 36

802.0 Nasal bones, closed `MSP`
802.1 Nasal bones, open `CC` `MSP`
CC Excl: 800.00-800.99, 801.00-801.99, 802.0-802.1, 803.00-803.99, 804.00-804.99, 829.0-829.1, 850.0-850.9, 851.00-851.99, 852.00-852.19, 852.21-852.59, 853.00-853.19, 854.00-854.19, 873.8-873.9, 879.8-879.9, 905.0, 925.1-925.2, 929.0, 929.9, 958.8, 959.01, 959.09, 959.8-959.9

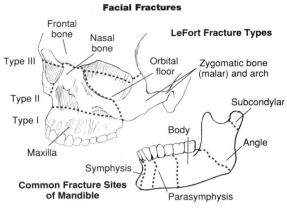

Facial Fractures

Frontal bone · Nasal bone · **LeFort Fracture Types** · Orbital floor · Zygomatic bone (malar) and arch · Type III · Type II · Type I · Maxilla · Subcondylar · Body · Angle · Symphysis · **Common Fracture Sites of Mandible** · Parasymphysis

✓5ᵗʰ **802.2 Mandible, closed**
Inferior maxilla   Lower jaw (bone)

802.20 Unspecified site `CC` `MSP`
CC Excl: 800.00-800.99, 801.00-801.99, 802.20-802.5, 803.00-803.99, 804.00-804.99, 829.0-829.1, 830.0-830.1, 850.0-850.9, 851.00-851.99, 852.00-852.19, 852.21-852.59, 853.00-853.19, 854.00-854.19, 873.8-873.9, 879.8-879.9, 905.0, 925.1, 925.2, 929.0, 929.9, 958.8, 959.01, 959.09, 959.8-959.9

802.21 Condylar process `CC` `MSP`
CC Excl: See code 802.20

802.22 Subcondylar `CC` `MSP`
CC Excl: See code 802.20

802.23 Coronoid process `CC` `MSP`
CC Excl: See code 802.20

802.24 Ramus, unspecified `CC` `MSP`
CC Excl: See code 802.20

802.25 Angle of jaw `CC` `MSP`
CC Excl: See code 802.20

802.26 Symphysis of body `CC` `MSP`
CC Excl: See code 802.20

802.27 Alveolar border of body `CC` `MSP`
CC Excl: See code 802.20

802.28 Body, other and unspecified `CC` `MSP`
CC Excl: See code 802.20

802.29 Multiple sites `CC` `MSP`
CC Excl: See code 802.20

✓5ᵗʰ **802.3 Mandible, open**
802.30 Unspecified site `CC` `MSP`
CC Excl: See code 802.20

802.31 Condylar process `CC` `MSP`
CC Excl: See code 802.20

802.32 Subcondylar `CC` `MSP`
CC Excl: See code 802.20

802.33 Coronoid process `CC` `MSP`
CC Excl: See code 802.20

802.34 Ramus, unspecified `CC` `MSP`
CC Excl: See code 802.20

802.35 Angle of jaw `CC` `MSP`
CC Excl: See code 802.20

802.36 Symphysis of body `CC` `MSP`
CC Excl: See code 802.20

802.37 Alveolar border of body `CC` `MSP`
CC Excl: See code 802.20

§   Requires fifth-digit. See beginning of section 800-804 for codes and definitions.

N Newborn Age: 0   P Pediatric Age: 0-17   M Maternity Age: 12-55   A Adult Age: 15-124   `CC` CC Condition   `MC` Major Complication   `CD` Complex Dx   `HIV` HIV Related Dx

802.38 **Body, other and unspecified** `CC` `MSP`
 CC Excl: See code 802.20

802.39 **Multiple sites** `CC` `MSP`
 CC Excl: See code 802.20

802.4 **Malar and maxillary bones, closed** `CC` `MSP`
 Superior maxilla Zygoma
 Upper jaw (bone) Zygomatic arch
 CC Excl: See code 802.20

802.5 **Malar and maxillary bones, open** `CC` `MSP`
 CC Excl: See code 802.20

802.6 **Orbital floor (blow-out), closed** `CC` `MSP`
 CC Excl: 800.00-800.99, 801.00-801.99, 802.6-802.9, 803.00-803.99,
 804.00-804.99, 829.0-829.1, 850.0-850.9, 851.00-851.99, 852.00-852.19,
 852.21-852.59, 853.00-853.19, 854.00-854.19, 873.8-873.9, 879.8-879.9,
 905.0, 925.1-925.2, 929.0, 929.9, 958.8, 959.01, 959.09, 959.8-959.9

802.7 **Orbital floor (blow-out), open** `CC` `MSP`
 CC Excl: See code 802.6

802.8 **Other facial bones, closed** `CC` `MSP`
 Alveolus   Palate
 Orbit:
  NOS
  part other than roof or floor
 EXCLUDES *orbital:*
   floor (802.6)
   roof (801.0-801.9)
 CC Excl: See code 802.6

802.9 **Other facial bones, open** `CC` `MSP`
 CC Excl: See code 802.6

✓4th **803 Other and unqualified skull fractures**
 INCLUDES skull NOS   skull multiple NOS
 AHA: 4Q, '96, 36

§ ✓5th 803.0 **Closed without mention of intracranial** `CC` `MSP`
 injury
 CC Excl: 800.00-800.99, 801.00-801.99, 803.00-803.99, 804.00-804.99,
 829.0-829.1, 850.0-850.9, 851.00-851.99, 852.00-852.19, 852.21-852.59,
 853.00-853.19, 854.00-854.19, 873.8-873.9, 879.8-879.9, 905.0, 925.1-
 925.2, 929.0, 929.9, 958.8, 959.01, 959.09, 959.8-959.9

§ ✓5th 803.1 **Closed with cerebral laceration and** `CC` `MSP`
 contusion
 CC Excl: See code 803.0

§ ✓5th 803.2 **Closed with subarachnoid, subdural, and** `CC` `MSP`
 extradural hemorrhage
 CC Excl: See code 803.0

§ ✓5th 803.3 **Closed with other and unspecified** `CC` `MSP`
 intracranial hemorrhage
 CC Excl: See code 803.0

§ ✓5th 803.4 **Closed with intracranial injury of other** `CC` `MSP`
 and unspecified nature
 CC Excl: See code 803.0

§ ✓5th 803.5 **Open without mention of intracranial injury** `CC` `MSP`
 CC Excl: See code 803.0

§ ✓5th 803.6 **Open with cerebral laceration and contusion** `CC` `MSP`
 CC Excl: See code 803.0

§ ✓5th 803.7 **Open with subarachnoid, subdural, and** `CC` `MSP`
 extradural hemorrhage
 CC Excl: See code 803.0

§ ✓5th 803.8 **Open with other and unspecified** `CC` `MSP`
 intracranial hemorrhage
 CC Excl: See code 803.0

§ ✓5th 803.9 **Open with intracranial injury of other and** `CC` `MSP`
 unspecified nature
 CC Excl: See code 803.0

✓4th **804 Multiple fractures involving skull or face with other bones**
 AHA: 4Q, '96, 36

§ ✓5th 804.0 **Closed without mention of intracranial** `CC` `MSP`
 injury
 CC Excl: See code 803.0

§ ✓5th 804.1 **Closed with cerebral laceration and** `CC` `MSP`
 contusion
 CC Excl: See code 803.0

§ ✓5th 804.2 **Closed with subarachnoid, subdural, and** `CC` `MSP`
 extradural hemorrhage
 CC Excl: See code 803.0

§ ✓5th 804.3 **Closed with other and unspecified** `CC` `MSP`
 intracranial hemorrhage
 CC Excl: See code 803.0

§ ✓5th 804.4 **Closed with intracranial injury of other** `CC` `MSP`
 and unspecified nature
 CC Excl: See code 803.0

§ ✓5th 804.5 **Open without mention of intracranial** `CC` `MSP`
 injury
 CC Excl: See code 803.0

§ ✓5th 804.6 **Open with cerebral laceration and** `CC` `MSP`
 contusion
 CC Excl: See code 803.0

§ ✓5th 804.7 **Open with subarachnoid, subdural, and** `CC` `MSP`
 extradural hemorrage
 CC Excl: See code 803.0

§ ✓5th 804.8 **Open with other and unspecified** `CC` `MSP`
 intracranial hemorrhage
 CC Excl: See code 803.0

§ ✓5th 804.9 **Open with intracranial injury of other and** `CC` `MSP`
 unspecified nature
 CC Excl: See code 803.0

FRACTURE OF NECK AND TRUNK (805-809)

✓4th **805 Fracture of vertebral column without mention of spinal cord**
 injury
 INCLUDES neural arch   transverse process
       spine   vertebra
       spinous process

 The following fifth-digit subclassification is for use with codes
 805.0-805.1:
   0 cervical vertebra, unspecified level
   1 first cervical vertebra
   2 second cervical vertebra
   3 third cervical vertebra
   4 fourth cervical vertebra
   5 fifth cervical vertebra
   6 sixth cervical vertebra
   7 seventh cervical vertebra
   8 multiple cervical vertebrae

✓5th 805.0 **Cervical, closed** `CC` `MSP`
 Atlas   Axis
 CC Excl: 805.00-805.18, 805.8-805.9, 806.00-806.19, 806.8-806.9, 829.0-
 829.1, 839.00-839.18, 839.40, 839.49-839.50, 839.59, 839.69, 839.79,
 839.8-839.9, 847.0, 847.9, 848.8-848.9, 879.8-879.9, 905.1, 926.11, 929.0,
 929.9, 952.00-952.09, 952.8-952.9, 958.8, 959.1, 959.8-959.9

✓5th 805.1 **Cervical, open** `CC` `MSP`
 CC Excl: See code 805.0

§ Requires fifth-digit. See beginning of section 800-804 for codes and definitions.

✓4th / ✓5th Additional Digit Required   Nonspecific PDx   Unacceptable PDx   Manifestation Code   `MSP` Medicare Secondary Payer   ►◄ Revised Text   ● New Code   ▲ Revised Code Title

2002 Ingenix, Inc.   **Volume 1 — 261**

Vertebral Column

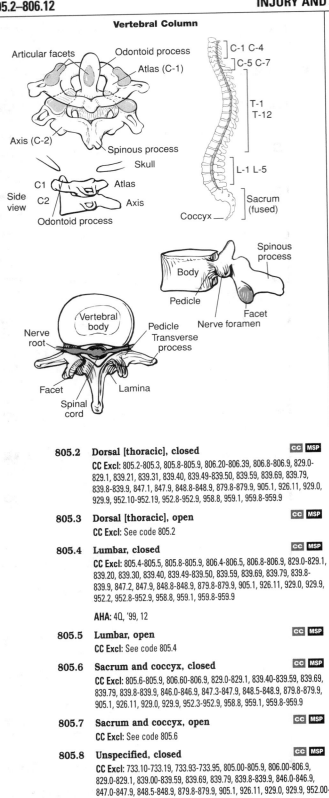

Articular facets

Odontoid process

Atlas (C-1)

Axis (C-2)

Spinous process

Skull

Side view

C1 — Atlas

C2 — Axis

Odontoid process

C-1 C-4
C-5 C-7
T-1 T-12
L-1 L-5
Sacrum (fused)
Coccyx

Body

Spinous process

Pedicle

Facet

Nerve foramen

Vertebral body

Pedicle

Transverse process

Nerve root

Facet

Lamina

Spinal cord

805.2   **Dorsal [thoracic], closed**   `CC` `MSP`
CC Excl: 805.2-805.3, 805.8-805.9, 806.20-806.39, 806.8-806.9, 829.0-829.1, 839.21, 839.31, 839.40, 839.49-839.50, 839.59, 839.69, 839.79, 839.8-839.9, 847.1, 847.9, 848.8-848.9, 879.8-879.9, 905.1, 926.11, 929.0, 929.9, 952.10-952.19, 952.8-952.9, 958.8, 959.1, 959.8-959.9

805.3   **Dorsal [thoracic], open**   `CC` `MSP`
CC Excl: See code 805.2

805.4   **Lumbar, closed**   `CC` `MSP`
CC Excl: 805.4-805.5, 805.8-805.9, 806.4-806.5, 806.8-806.9, 829.0-829.1, 839.20, 839.30, 839.40, 839.49-839.50, 839.59, 839.69, 839.79, 839.8-839.9, 847.2, 847.9, 848.8-848.9, 879.8-879.9, 905.1, 926.11, 929.0, 929.9, 952.2, 952.8-952.9, 958.8, 959.1, 959.8-959.9

AHA: 4Q, '99, 12

805.5   **Lumbar, open**   `CC` `MSP`
CC Excl: See code 805.4

805.6   **Sacrum and coccyx, closed**   `CC` `MSP`
CC Excl: 805.6-805.9, 806.60-806.9, 829.0-829.1, 839.40-839.59, 839.69, 839.79, 839.8-839.9, 846.0-846.9, 847.3-847.9, 848.5-848.9, 879.8-879.9, 905.1, 926.11, 929.0, 929.9, 952.3-952.9, 958.8, 959.1, 959.8-959.9

805.7   **Sacrum and coccyx, open**   `CC` `MSP`
CC Excl: See code 805.6

805.8   **Unspecified, closed**   `CC` `MSP`
CC Excl: 733.10-733.19, 733.93-733.95, 805.00-805.9, 806.00-806.9, 829.0-829.1, 839.00-839.59, 839.69, 839.79, 839.8-839.9, 846.0-846.9, 847.0-847.9, 848.5-848.9, 879.8-879.9, 905.1, 926.11, 929.0, 929.9, 952.00-952.9, 958.8, 959.1, 959.8-959.9

805.9   **Unspecified, open**   `CC` `MSP`
CC Excl: See code 805.8

√4th **806 Fracture of vertebral column with spinal cord injury**
   `INCLUDES`   any condition classifiable to 805 with:
       complete or incomplete transverse lesion (of cord)
       hematomyelia
       injury to:
          cauda equina
          nerve
       paralysis
       paraplegia
       quadriplegia
       spinal concussion

√5th **806.0**   **Cervical, closed**

806.00 C_1-C_4 **level with unspecified spinal cord injury**   `CC` `MSP`
Cervical region NOS with spinal cord injury NOS
CC Excl: 733.10-733.19, 733.93-733.95, 805.00-805.18, 805.8-805.9, 806.00-806.19, 806.8-806.9, 829.0-829.1, 839.00-839.18, 839.40, 839.49-839.50, 839.59, 839.69, 839.79, 839.8-839.9, 847.9, 848.8-848.9, 879.8-879.9, 905.1, 926.11, 929.0, 929.9, 952.00-952.09, 952.8-952.9, 958.8, 959.1, 959.8-959.9

806.01 C_1-C_4 **level with complete lesion of cord**   `CC` `MSP`
CC Excl: See code 806.00

806.02 C_1-C_4 **level with anterior cord syndrome**   `CC` `MSP`
CC Excl: See code 806.00

806.03 C_1-C_4 **level with central cord Syndrome**   `CC` `MSP`
CC Excl: See code 806.00

806.04 C_1-C_4 **level with other specified spinal cord injury**   `CC` `MSP`
C_1-C_4 level with:
    incomplete spinal cord lesion NOS
    posterior cord syndrome
CC Excl: See code 806.00

806.05 C_5-C_7 **level with unspecified spinal cord injury**   `CC` `MSP`
CC Excl: See code 806.00

806.06 C_5-C_7 **level with complete lesion of cord**   `CC` `MSP`
CC Excl: See code 806.00

806.07 C_5-C_7 **level with anterior cord syndrome**   `CC` `MSP`
CC Excl: See code 806.00

806.08 C_5-C_7 **level with central cord syndrome**   `CC` `MSP`
CC Excl: See code 806.00

806.09 C_5-C_7 **level with other specified spinal cord injury**   `CC` `MSP`
C_5-C_7 level with:
    incomplete spinal cord lesion NOS
    posterior cord syndrome
CC Excl: See code 806.00

√5th **806.1**   **Cervical, open**

806.10 C_1-C_4 **level with unspecified spinal cord injury**   `CC` `MSP`
CC Excl: See code 806.00

806.11 C_1-C_4 **level with complete lesion of cord**   `CC` `MSP`
CC Excl: See code 806.00

806.12 C_1-C_4 **level with anterior cord syndrome**   `CC` `MSP`
CC Excl: See code 806.00

`N` Newborn Age: 0   `P` Pediatric Age: 0-17   `M` Maternity Age: 12-55   `A` Adult Age: 15-124   `CC` CC Condition   `MC` Major Complication   `CD` Complex Dx   `HIV` HIV Related Dx

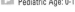

806.13 C₁-C₄ level with central cord syndrome `CC` `MSP`
CC Excl: See code 806.00

806.14 C₁-C₄ level with other specified spinal cord injury `CC` `MSP`
C₁-C₄ level with:
incomplete spinal cord lesion NOS
posterior cord syndrome
CC Excl: See code 806.00

806.15 C₅-C₇ level with unspecified spinal cord injury `CC` `MSP`
CC Excl: See code 806.00

806.16 C₅-C₇ level with complete lesion of cord `CC` `MSP`
CC Excl: See code 806.00

806.17 C₅-C₇ level with anterior cord syndrome `CC` `MSP`
CC Excl: See code 806.00

806.18 C₅-C₇ level with central cord syndrome `CC` `MSP`
CC Excl: See code 806.00

806.19 C₅-C₇ level with other specified spinal cord injury `CC` `MSP`
C₅-C₇ level with:
incomplete spinal cord lesion NOS
posterior cord syndrome
CC Excl: See code 806.00

√5th **806.2 Dorsal [thoracic], closed**

806.20 T₁-T₆ level with unspecified spinal cord injury `CC` `MSP`
Thoracic region NOS with spinal cord injury NOS
CC Excl: 733.10-733.19, 733.93-733.95, 805.2-805.3, 805.8-805.9, 806.20-806.39, 806.8-806.9, 829.0-829.1, 839.21, 839.31, 839.40, 839.49-839.50, 839.59, 839.69, 839.79, 839.8-839.9, 847.1, 847.9, 848.8-848.9, 879.8-879.9, 905.1, 926.11, 929.0, 929.9, 952.10-952.19, 952.8-952.9, 958.8, 959.1, 959.8-959.9

806.21 T₁-T₆ level with complete lesion of cord `CC` `MSP`
CC Excl: See code 806.20

806.22 T₁-T₆ level with anterior cord syndrome `CC` `MSP`
CC Excl: See code 806.20

806.23 T₁-T₆ level with central cord syndrome `CC` `MSP`
CC Excl: See code 806.20

806.24 T₁-T₆ level with other specified spinal cord injury `CC` `MSP`
T₁-T₆ level with:
incomplete spinal cord lesion NOS
posterior cord syndrome
CC Excl: See code 806.20

806.25 T₇-T₁₂ level with unspecified spinal cord injury `CC` `MSP`
CC Excl: See code 806.20

806.26 T₇-T₁₂ level with complete lesion of cord `CC` `MSP`
CC Excl: See code 806.20

806.27 T₇-T₁₂ level with anterior cord syndrome `CC` `MSP`
CC Excl: See code 806.20

806.28 T₇-T₁₂ level with central cord syndrome `CC` `MSP`
CC Excl: See code 806.20

806.29 T₇-T₁₂ level with other specified spinal cord injury `CC` `MSP`
T₇-T₁₂ level with:
incomplete spinal cord lesion NOS
posterior cord syndrome
CC Excl: See code 806.20

√5th **806.3 Dorsal [thoracic], open**

806.30 T₁-T₆ level with unspecified spinal cord injury `CC` `MSP`
CC Excl: See code 806.20

806.31 T₁-T₆ level with complete lesion of cord `CC` `MSP`
CC Excl: See code 806.20

806.32 T₁-T₆ level with anteriorr cord syndrome `CC` `MSP`
CC Excl: See code 806.20

806.33 T₁-T₆ level with centralr cord syndrome `CC` `MSP`
CC Excl: See code 806.20

806.34 T₁-T₆ level with other specified spinal cord injury `CC` `MSP`
T₁-T₆ level with:
incomplete spinal cord lesion NOS
posterior cord syndrome
CC Excl: See code 806.20

806.35 T₇-T₁₂ level with unspecified spinal cord injury `CC` `MSP`
CC Excl: See code 806.20

806.36 T₇-T₁₂ level with complete lesion of cord `CC` `MSP`
CC Excl: See code 806.20

806.37 T₇-T₁₂ level with anterior cord syndrome `CC` `MSP`
CC Excl: See code 806.20

806.38 T₇-T₁₂ level with central cord syndrome `CC` `MSP`
CC Excl: See code 806.20

806.39 T₇-T₁₂ level with other specified spinal cord injury `CC` `MSP`
T₇-T₁₂ level with:
incomplete spinal cord lesion NOS
posterior cord syndrome
CC Excl: See code 806.20

806.4 **Lumbar, closed** `CC` `MSP`
CC Excl: 733.10-733.19, 733.93-733.95, 805.4-805.5, 805.8-805.9, 806.4-806.5, 806.8-806.9, 829.0-829.1, 839.20, 839.30, 839.40, 839.49-839.50, 839.59, 839.69, 839.79, 839.8-839.9, 847.2, 847.9, 848.8-848.9, 879.8-879.9, 905.1, 926.11, 929.0, 929.9, 952.2, 952.8-952.9, 958.8, 959.1, 959.8-959.9
AHA: 4Q, '99, 11, 13

806.5 **Lumbar, open** `CC` `MSP`
CC Excl: See code 806.4

√5th **806.6 Sacrum and coccyx, closed**

806.60 With unspecified spinal spinal cord injury `CC` `MSP`
CC Excl: 733.10-733.19, 733.93-733.95, 805.6-805.9, 806.60-806.9, 829.0-829.1, 839.40-839.59, 839.69, 839.79, 839.8-839.9, 846.0-846.9, 847.0, 847.3-847.9, 848.5-848.9, 879.8-879.9, 905.1, 926.11, 929.0, 929.9, 952.3-952.9, 958.8, 959.1, 959.8-959.9

806.61 With complete cauda equina lesion `CC` `MSP`
CC Excl: See code 806.60

806.62 With other cauda equina injury `CC` `MSP`
CC Excl: See code 806.60

806.69 With other spinal cord injury `CC` `MSP`
CC Excl: See code 806.60

✓5th **806.7 Sacrum and coccyx, open**
806.70 With unspecified spinal cord injury `CC` `MSP`
CC Excl: See code 806.60

806.71 With complete cauda equina lesion `CC` `MSP`
CC Excl: See code 806.60

806.72 With other cauda equina injury `CC` `MSP`
CC Excl: See code 806.60

806.79 With other spinal cord injury `CC` `MSP`
CC Excl: See code 806.60

806.8 Unspecified, closed `CC` `MSP`
CC Excl: 733.10-733.19, 733.93-733.95, 805.00-805.09, 806.00-806.9, 829.0-829.1, 839.00-839.59, 839.69, 839.79, 839.8-839.9, 846.0-846.9, 847.0-847.9, 848.5-848.9, 879.8-879.9, 905.1, 926.11, 929.0, 929.9, 952.00-952.9, 958.8, 959.1, 959.8-959.9

806.9 Unspecified, open `CC` `MSP`
CC Excl: See code 806.8

✓4th **807 Fracture of rib(s), sternum, larynx, and trachea**

The following fifth-digit subclassification is for use with codes 807.0-807.1:

0 rib(s), unspecified
1 one rib
2 two ribs
3 three ribs
4 four ribs
5 five ribs
6 six ribs
7 seven ribs
8 eight or more ribs
9 multiple ribs, unspecified

✓5th **807.0 Rib(s), closed** `CC 4-9` `MSP`
CC Excl: For codes 807.04-807.09: 807.00-807.19, 807.4, 819.0-819.1, 828.0-828.1, 829.0-829.1, 848.8-848.9, 879.8-879.9, 929.0, 929.9, 958.8, 959.8-959.9

✓5th **807.1 Rib(s), open** `CC` `MSP`
CC Excl: See code 807.0

807.2 Sternum, closed `CC` `MSP`
CC Excl: 807.2-807.4, 829.0-829.1, 848.8-848.9, 879.8-879.9, 929.0, 929.9, 958.8, 959.8-959.9

DEF: Break in flat bone (breast bone) in anterior thorax.

807.3 Sternum, open `CC` `MSP`
CC Excl: See code 807.2

DEF: Break, with open wound, in flat bone in mid anterior thorax.

Ribs, Sternum, Larynx, and Trachea

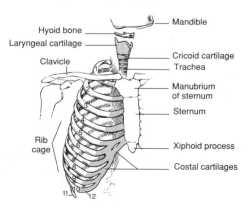

807.4 Flail chest `CC` `MSP`
CC Excl: 807.00-807.4, 829.0-829.1, 848.8-848.9, 879.8-879.9, 929.0, 929.9, 958.8, 959.8-959.9

807.5 Larynx and trachea, closed `CC` `MSP`
Hyoid bone   Trachea
Thyroid cartilage
CC Excl: 807.5-807.6, 829.0-829.1, 848.8-848.9, 879.8-879.9, 929.0, 929.9, 958.8, 959.8-959.9

807.6 Larynx and trachea, open `CC` `MSP`
CC Excl: See code 807.5

✓4th **808 Fracture of pelvis**
808.0 Acetabulum, closed `CC`
CC Excl: 733.10-733.19, 733.93-733.95, 808.0-808.1, 808.43, 808.49, 808.53, 808.59, 808.8-808.9, 809.0-809.1, 829.0-829.1, 835.00-835.13, 843.0-843.9, 846.0-846.9 848.5-848.9, 879.8-879.9, 929.0, 929.9, 958.8, 959.6, 959.8-959.9

808.1 Acetabulum, open `CC`
CC Excl: 808.0-808.1, 808.43, 808.49, 808.53, 808.59, 808.8-808.9, 809.0-809.1, 829.0-829.1, 835.00-835.13, 843.0-843.9, 846.0-846.9, 848.5-848.9, 879.8-879.9, 929.0, 929.9, 958.8, 959.6, 959.8-959.9

808.2 Pubis, closed `CC`
CC Excl: 733.10-733.19, 733.93-733.95, 808.2-808.3, 808.43, 808.49, 808.53, 808.59, 808.8-808.9, 809.0-809.1, 829.0-829.1, 835.00-835.13, 843.0-843.9, 846.0-846.9, 848.5-848.9, 879.8-879.9, 929.0, 929.9, 958.8, 959.6, 959.8-959.9

808.3 Pubis, open `CC`
CC Excl: See code 808.2

✓5th **808.4 Other specified part, closed**
808.41 Ilium
808.42 Ischium
808.43 Multiple pelvic fractures with `CC`
disruption of pelvic circle
CC Excl: 733.10-733.19, 733.93-733.95, 808.0-808.9, 809.0-809.1, 829.0-829.1, 835.00-835.13, 843.0-843.9, 846.0-846.9, 848.5-848.9, 879.8-879.9, 929.0, 929.9, 958.8, 959.6, 959.8-959.9

808.49 Other `CC`
Innominate bone
Pelvic rim
CC Excl: See code 808.43

✓5th **808.5 Other specified part, open**
808.51 Ilium `CC`
CC Excl: 733.10-733.19, 733.93-733.95, 808.41, 808.43, 808.49, 808.51, 808.53, 808.59, 808.8-808.9, 809.0-809.1, 829.0-829.1, 835.00-835.13, 843.0-843.9, 846.0-846.9, 848.5-848.9, 879.8-879.9, 929.0, 929.9, 958.8, 959.6, 959.8-959.9

Pelvis and Pelvic Fractures

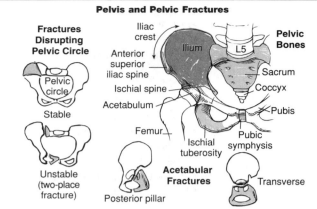

`N` Newborn Age: 0   `P` Pediatric Age: 0-17   `M` Maternity Age: 12-55   `A` Adult Age: 15-124   `CC` CC Condition   `MC` Major Complication   `CD` Complex Dx   `HIV` HIV Related Dx

808.52 **Ischium** `CC`
    CC Excl: 733.10-733.19, 733.93-733.95, 808.42-808.49, 808.52-808.59, 808.8-808.9, 809.0-809.1, 829.0-829.1, 835.00-835.13, 843.0-843.9, 846.0-846.9, 848.5-848.9, 879.8-879.9, 929.0, 929.9, 958.8, 959.6, 959.8-959.9

808.53 **Multiple pelvic fractures with disruption of pelvic circle** `CC`
    CC Excl: 733.10-733.19, 733.93-733.95, 808.0-808.9 809.0-809.1, 829.0-829.1, 835.00-835.13, 843.0-843.9, 846.0-846.9, 848.5-848.9, 879.8-879.9, 929.0, 929.9, 958.8, 959.6, 959.8-959.9

808.59 **Other** `CC`
    CC Excl: See code 808.53

808.8 **Unspecified, closed** `CC`
    CC Excl: See code 808.53

808.9 **Unspecified, open** `CC`
    CC Excl: See code 808.53

√4ᵗʰ **809 Ill-defined fractures of bones of trunk**
    `INCLUDES` bones of trunk with other bones except those of skull and face
    multiple bones of trunk
    `EXCLUDES` *multiple fractures of:*
        pelvic bones alone (808.0-808.9)
        ribs alone (807.0-807.1, 807.4)
        ribs or sternum with limb bones (819.0-819.1, 828.0-828.1)
        skull or face with other bones (804.0-804.9)

809.0 **Fracture of bones of trunk, closed**
809.1 **Fracture of bones of trunk, open**

FRACTURE OF UPPER LIMB (810-819)

√4ᵗʰ **810 Fracture of clavicle**
    `INCLUDES` collar bone
    interligamentous part of clavicle

The following fifth-digit subclassification is for use with category 810:
    0 unspecified part
        Clavicle NOS
    1 sternal end of clavicle
    2 shaft of clavicle
    3 acromial end of clavicle

√5ᵗʰ 810.0 **Closed** `MSP`

√5ᵗʰ 810.1 **Open** `MSP`

√4ᵗʰ **811 Fracture of scapula**
    `INCLUDES` shoulder blade

The following fifth-digit subclassification is for use with category 811:
    0 unspecified part
    1 acromial process
        Acromion (process)
    2 coracoid process
    3 glenoid cavity and neck of scapula
    9 other

√5ᵗʰ 811.0 **Closed** `MSP`

√5ᵗʰ 811.1 **Open** `MSP`

√4ᵗʰ **812 Fracture of humerus**

√5ᵗʰ 812.0 **Upper end, closed**
    812.00 **Upper end, unspecified part**
        Proximal end   Shoulder
    812.01 **Surgical neck**
        Neck of humerus NOS
    812.02 **Anatomical neck**
    812.03 **Greater tuberosity**
    812.09 **Other**
        Head   Upper epiphysis

Right Clavicle and Scapula, Anterior View

Right Humerus, Anterior View

√5ᵗʰ 812.1 **Upper end, open**
    812.10 **Upper end, unspecified part**
    812.11 **Surgical neck**
    812.12 **Anatomical neck**
    812.13 **Greater tuberosity**
    812.19 **Other**

√5ᵗʰ 812.2 **Shaft or unspecified part, closed**
    812.20 **Unspecified part of humerus**
        Humerus NOS   Upper arm NOS
    812.21 **Shaft of humerus**
        AHA: 3Q, '99, 14

√5ᵗʰ 812.3 **Shaft or unspecified part, open**
    812.30 **Unspecified part of humerus**
    812.31 **Shaft of humerus**

√5ᵗʰ 812.4 **Lower end, closed**
    Distal end of humerus   Elbow
    812.40 **Lower end, unspecified part**
    812.41 **Supracondylar fracture of humerus**
    812.42 **Lateral condyle**
        External condyle
    812.43 **Medial condyle**
        Internal epicondyle
    812.44 **Condyle(s), unspecified**
        Articular process NOS
        Lower epiphysis NOS
    812.49 **Other**
        Multiple fractures of lower end
        Trochlea

√5ᵗʰ 812.5 **Lower end, open**
    812.50 **Lower end, unspecified part**
    812.51 **Supracondylar fracture of humerus**
    812.52 **Lateral condyle**
    812.53 **Medial condyle**
    812.54 **Condyle(s), unspecified**
    812.59 **Other**

√4ᵗʰ √5ᵗʰ Additional Digit Required   Nonspecific PDx   Unacceptable PDx   Manifestation Code   `MSP` Medicare Secondary Payer   ▶◀ Revised Text   ● New Code   ▲ Revised Code Title

2002 Ingenix, Inc.   **Volume 1 — 265**

Injury and Poisoning 813–815.1

Right Radius and Ulna, Anterior View

- Olecranon process
- Coronoid process
- Radius
- Ulna
- Radius
- Shafts
- Colles fracture
- Humerus (lateral view)
- Radius dislocated
- Radial styloid process
- Ulnar styloid process
- Monteggia's fracture-dislocation

√4th **813 Fracture of radius and ulna**

√5th **813.0 Upper end, closed**
Proximal end

813.00 Upper end of forearm, unspecified

813.01 Olecranon process of ulna

813.02 Coronoid process of ulna

813.03 Monteggia's fracture
DEF: Fracture near the head of the ulnar shaft, causing dislocation of the radial head.

813.04 Other and unspecified fractures of proximal end of ulna (alone)
Multiple fractures of ulna, upper end

813.05 Head of radius

813.06 Neck of radius

813.07 Other and unspecified fractures of proximal end of radius (alone)
Multiple fractures of radius, upper end

813.08 Radius with ulna, upper end [any part]

√5th **813.1 Upper end, open**

813.10 Upper end of forearm, unspecified

813.11 Olecranon process of ulna

813.12 Coronoid process of ulna

813.13 Monteggia's fracture

813.14 Other and unspecified fractures of proximal end of ulna (alone)

813.15 Head of radius

813.16 Neck of radius

813.17 Other and unspecified fractures of proximal end of radius (alone)

813.18 Radius with ulna, upper end [any part]

√5th **813.2 Shaft, closed**

813.20 Shaft, unspecified

813.21 Radius (alone)

813.22 Ulna (alone)

813.23 Radius with ulna

√5th **813.3 Shaft, open**

813.30 Shaft, unspecified

813.31 Radius (alone)

813.32 Ulna (alone)

813.33 Radius with ulna

√5th **813.4 Lower end, closed**
Distal end

813.40 Lower end of forearm, unspecified

813.41 Colles' fracture
Smith's fracture
DEF: Break of lower end of radius; associated with backward movement of the radius lower section.

813.42 Other fractures of distal end of radius (alone)
Dupuytren's fracture, radius
Radius, lower end
DEF: Dupuytren's fracture: fracture and dislocation of the forearm; the fracture is of the radius above the wrist, and the dislocation is of the ulna at the lower end.

813.43 Distal end of ulna (alone)
Ulna:
head
lower end
lower epiphysis
styloid process

813.45 Torus fracture of radius

813.44 Radius with ulna, lower end

√5th **813.5 Lower end, open**

813.50 Lower end of forearm, unspecified

813.51 Colles' fracture

813.52 Other fractures of distal end of radius (alone)

813.53 Distal end of ulna (alone)

813.54 Radius with ulna, lower end

√5th **813.8 Unspecified part, closed**

813.80 Forearm, unspecified

813.81 Radius (alone)
AHA: 2Q, '98, 19

813.82 Ulna (alone)

813.83 Radius with ulna

√5th **813.9 Unspecified part, open**

813.90 Forearm, unspecified

813.91 Radius (alone)

813.92 Ulna (alone)

813.93 Radius with ulna

√4th **814 Fracture of carpal bone(s)**

The following fifth-digit subclassification is for use with category 814:
  0 carpal bone, unspecified
    Wrist NOS
  1 navicular [scaphoid] of wrist
  2 lunate [semilunar] bone of wrist
  3 triquetral [cuneiform] bone of wrist
  4 pisiform
  5 trapezium bone [larger multangular]
  6 trapezoid bone [smaller multangular]
  7 capitate bone [os magnum]
  8 hamate [unciform] bone
  9 other

√5th **814.0 Closed**

√5th **814.1 Open**

√4th **815 Fracture of metacarpal bone(s)**

INCLUDES   hand [except finger]
metacarpus

The following fifth-digit subclassification is for use with category 815:
  0 metacarpal bone(s), site unspecified
  1 base of thumb [first] metacarpal
    Bennett's fracture
  2 base of other metacarpal bone(s)
  3 shaft of metacarpal bone(s)
  4 neck of metacarpal bone(s)
  9 multiple sites of metacarpus

√5th **815.0 Closed**

√5th **815.1 Open**

N Newborn Age: 0   P Pediatric Age: 0-17   M Maternity Age: 12-55   A Adult Age: 15-124   CC CC Condition   MC Major Complication   CD Complex Dx   HIV HIV Related Dx

Hand Fractures

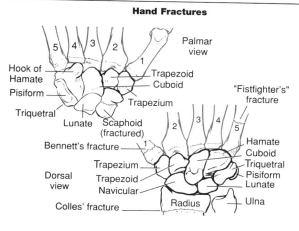

✓4th **816 Fracture of one or more phalanges of hand**

INCLUDES finger(s) thumb

The following fifth-digit subclassification is for use with category 816:

0 phalanx or phalanges, unspecified
1 middle or proximal phalanx or phalanges
2 distal phalanx or phalanges
3 multiple sites

✓5th **816.0 Closed**
✓5th **816.1 Open**

✓4th **817 Multiple fractures of hand bones**

INCLUDES metacarpal bone(s) with phalanx or phalanges of same hand

817.0 Closed
817.1 Open

✓4th **818 Ill-defined fractures of upper limb**

INCLUDES arm NOS
multiple bones of same upper limb

EXCLUDES multiple fractures of:
metacarpal bone(s) with phalanx or phalanges (817.0-817.1)
phalanges of hand alone (816.0-816.1)
radius with ulna (813.0-813.9)

818.0 Closed
818.1 Open

✓4th **819 Multiple fractures involving both upper limbs, and upper limb with rib(s) and sternum**

INCLUDES arm(s) with rib(s) or sternum
both arms [any bones]

819.0 Closed
819.1 Open

FRACTURE OF LOWER LIMB (820-829)

✓4th **820 Fracture of neck of femur**

✓5th **820.0 Transcervical fracture, closed**

820.00 Intracapsular section, unspecified CC

CC Excl: 733.10-733.19, 733.93-733.95, 820.00-820.9 821.00-821.39, 827.0-827.1, 828.0-828.1, 829.0-829.1, 843.0-843.9, 848.8-848.9, 879.8-879.9, 929.0, 929.9, 958.8, 959.6, 959.8-959.9

820.01 Epiphysis (separation) (upper) CC
Transepiphyseal
CC Excl: See code 820.00

820.02 Midcervical section CC
Transcervical NOS
CC Excl: See code 820.00

820.03 Base of neck CC
Cervicotrochanteric section
CC Excl: See code 820.00

820.09 Other CC
Head of femur
Subcapital
CC Excl: See code 820.00

✓5th **820.1 Transcervical fracture, open**

820.10 Intracapsular section, unspecified CC
CC Excl: See code 820.00

820.11 Epiphysis (separation) (upper) CC
CC Excl: See code 820.00

820.12 Midcervical section CC
CC Excl: See code 820.00

820.13 Base of neck CC
CC Excl: See code 820.00

820.19 Other CC
CC Excl: See code 820.00

✓5th **820.2 Pertrochanteric fracture, closed**

820.20 Trochanteric section, unspecified CC
Trochanter: Trochanter:
NOS   lesser
greater
CC Excl: See code 820.00

820.21 Intertrochanteric section CC
CC Excl: See code 820.00

820.22 Subtrochanteric section CC
CC Excl: See code 820.00

✓5th **820.3 Pertrochanteric fracture, open**

820.30 Trochanteric section, unspecified CC
CC Excl: See code 820.00

820.31 Intertrochanteric section CC
CC Excl: See code 820.00

820.32 Subtrochanteric section CC
CC Excl: See code 820.00

820.8 Unspecified part of neck of femur, closed CC
Hip NOS   Neck of femur NOS
CC Excl: See code 820.00

820.9 Unspecified part of neck of femur, open CC
CC Excl: See code 820.00

✓4th **821 Fracture of other and unspecified parts of femur**

✓5th **821.0 Shaft or unspecified part, closed**

821.00 Unspecified part of femur CC
Thigh   Upper leg
EXCLUDES hip NOS (820.8)
CC Excl: See code 820.00

821.01 Shaft CC
CC Excl: See code 820.00

AHA: 1Q, '99, 5

✓5th **821.1 Shaft or unspecified part, open**

821.10 Unspecified part of femur CC
CC Excl: See code 820.00

821.11 Shaft CC
CC Excl: See code 820.00

✓5th **821.2 Lower end, closed**
Distal end

821.20 Lower end, unspecified part
821.21 Condyle, femoral
821.22 Epiphysis, lower (separation)

✓4th
✓5th Additional Digit Required   Nonspecific PDx   Unacceptable PDx   Manifestation Code   MSP Medicare Secondary Payer   ◄► Revised Text   ● New Code   ▲ Revised Code Title

2002 Ingenix, Inc.

Volume 1 — 267

Right Femur, Anterior View

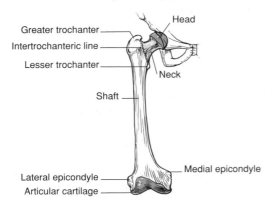

821.23 Supracondylar fracture of femur
821.29 Other
     Multiple fractures of lower end
√5th **821.3 Lower end, open**
     821.30 Lower end, unspecified part
     821.31 Condyle, femoral
     821.32 Epiphysis, lower (separation)
     821.33 Supracondylar fracture of femur
     821.39 Other
√4th **822 Fracture of patella**
     822.0 Closed
     822.1 Open
√4th **823 Fracture of tibia and fibula**

> **EXCLUDES** *Dupuytren's fracture (824.4-824.5)*
> *ankle (824.4-824.5)*
> *radius (813.42, 813.52)*
> *Pott's fracture (824.4-824.5)*
> *that involving ankle (824.0-824.9)*

The following fifth-digit subclassification is for use with category 823:
     0   tibia alone
     1   fibula alone
     2   fibula with tibia

√5th **823.0 Upper end, closed**
     Head   Tibia:
     Proximal end   condyles
                           tuberosity
√5th **823.1 Upper end, open**
√5th **823.2 Shaft, closed**
√5th **823.3 Shaft, open**
√5th **823.4 Torus fracture**
√5th **823.8 Unspecified part, closed**
     Lower leg NOS
     AHA: For code 823.82: 1Q, '97, 8

Right Tibula and Fibula, Anterior View

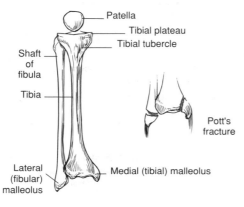

√5th **823.9 Unspecified part, open**
√4th **824 Fracture of ankle**
     824.0 Medial malleolus, closed
         Tibia involving: Tibia involving:
            ankle   malleolus
     824.1 Medial malleolus, open
     824.2 Lateral malleolus, closed
         Fibula involving:
            ankle
            malleolus
     824.3 Lateral malleolus, open
     824.4 Bimalleolar, closed
         Dupuytren's fracture, fibula   Pott's fracture
         DEF: Bimalleolar, closed: Breaking of both nodules (malleoli) on either side of ankle joint, without an open wound.

         DEF: Dupuytren's fracture (Pott's fracture): The breaking of the farthest end of the lower leg bone (fibula), with injury to the farthest end joint of the other lower leg bone (tibia).
     824.5 Bimalleolar, open
     824.6 Trimalleolar, closed
         Lateral and medial malleolus with anterior or posterior lip of tibia
     824.7 Trimalleolar, open
     824.8 Unspecified, closed
         Ankle NOS
         AHA: 3Q, '00, 12

     824.9 Unspecified, open
√4th **825 Fracture of one or more tarsal and metatarsal bones**
     825.0 Fracture of calcaneus, closed
         Heel bone   Os calcis
     825.1 Fracture of calcaneus, open
√5th **825.2 Fracture of other tarsal and metatarsal bones, closed**
     825.20 Unspecified bone(s) of foot [except toes]
         Instep
     825.21 Astragalus
         Talus
     825.22 Navicular [scaphoid], foot
     825.23 Cuboid
     825.24 Cuneiform, foot
     825.25 Metatarsal bone(s)
     825.29 Other
         Tarsal with metatarsal bone(s) only
         EXCLUDES *calcaneus (825.0)*
√5th **825.3 Fracture of other tarsal and metatarsal bones, open**
     825.30 Unspecified bone(s) of foot [except toes]
     825.31 Astragalus
     825.32 Navicular [scaphoid], foot
     825.33 Cuboid
     825.34 Cuneiform, foot
     825.35 Metatarsal bone(s)
     825.39 Other
√4th **826 Fracture of one or more phalanges of foot**
     INCLUDES   toe(s)
     826.0 Closed
     826.1 Open
√4th **827 Other, multiple, and ill-defined fractures of lower limb**
     INCLUDES   leg NOS
         multiple bones of same lower limb
     EXCLUDES   *multiple fractures of:*
         ankle bones alone (824.4-824.9)
         phalanges of foot alone (826.0-826.1)
         tarsal with metatarsal bones (825.29, 825.39)
         tibia with fibula (823.0-823.9 with fifth-digit 2)

N Newborn Age: 0   **P** Pediatric Age: 0-17   **M** Maternity Age: 12-55   **A** Adult Age: 15-124   **CC** CC Condition   **MC** Major Complication   **CD** Complex Dx   **HIV** HIV Related Dx

268 — Volume 1 • October 2002   **2002 Ingenix, Inc.**

Right Foot, Dorsal

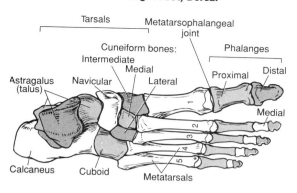

827.0   Closed

827.1   Open

✓4ᵗʰ 828   Multiple fractures involving both lower limbs, lower with upper limb, and lower limb(s) with rib(s) and sternum

INCLUDES   arm(s) with leg(s) [any bones]
both legs [any bones]
leg(s) with rib(s) or sternum

828.0   Closed   **MSP**

828.1   Open   **MSP**

✓4ᵗʰ 829   Fracture of unspecified bones

829.0   Unspecified bone, closed

829.1   Unspecified bone, open

DISLOCATION (830-839)

INCLUDES   displacement
subluxation

EXCLUDES   *congenital dislocation (754.0-755.8)*
pathological dislocation (718.2)
recurrent dislocation (718.3)

The descriptions "closed" and "open," used in the fourth-digit subdivisions, include the following terms:

closed:
  complete
  dislocation NOS
  partial
  simple
  uncomplicated

open:
  compound
  infected
  with foreign body

A dislocation not indicated as closed or open should be classified as closed.

AHA: 3Q, '90, 12

✓4ᵗʰ 830   Dislocation of jaw

INCLUDES   jaw (cartilage) (meniscus)
mandible
maxilla (inferior)
temporomandibular (joint)

830.0   Closed dislocation

830.1   Open dislocation

✓4ᵗʰ 831   Dislocation of shoulder

EXCLUDES   *sternoclavicular joint (839.61, 839.71)*
sternum (839.61, 839.71)

The following fifth-digit subclassification is for use with category 831:

0   shoulder, unspecified
Humerus NOS
1   anterior dislocation of humerus
2   posterior dislocation of humerus
3   inferior dislocation of humerus
4   acromioclavicular (joint)
Clavicle
9   other
Scapula

✓5ᵗʰ 831.0   Closed dislocation

✓5ᵗʰ 831.1   Open dislocation

✓4ᵗʰ 832   Dislocation of elbow

The following fifth-digit subclassification is for use with category 832:

0   elbow unspecified
1   anterior dislocation of elbow
2   posterior dislocation of elbow
3   medial dislocation of elbow
4   lateral dislocation of elbow
9   other

✓5ᵗʰ 832.0   Closed dislocation

✓5ᵗʰ 832.1   Open dislocation

✓4ᵗʰ 833   Dislocation of wrist

The following fifth-digit subclassification is for use with category 833:

0   wrist, unspecified part
Carpal (bone)
Radius, distal end
1   radioulnar (joint), distal
2   radiocarpal (joint)
3   midcarpal (joint)
4   carpometacarpal (joint)
5   metacarpal (bone), proximal end
9   other
Ulna, distal end

✓5ᵗʰ 833.0   Closed dislocation

✓5ᵗʰ 833.1   Open dislocation

✓4ᵗʰ 834   Dislocation of finger

INCLUDES   finger(s)   thumb
phalanx of hand

The following fifth-digit subclassification is for use with category 834:

0   finger, unspecified part
1   metacarpophalangeal (joint)
Metacarpal (bone), distal end
2   interphalangeal (joint), hand

✓5ᵗʰ 834.0   Closed dislocation

✓5ᵗʰ 834.1   Open dislocation

✓4ᵗʰ 835   Dislocation of hip

The following fifth-digit subclassification is for use with category 835:

0   dislocation of hip, unspecified
1   posterior dislocation
2   obturator dislocation
3   other anterior dislocation

✓5ᵗʰ 835.0   Closed dislocation

✓5ᵗʰ 835.1   Open dislocation

✓4ᵗʰ 836   Dislocation of knee

EXCLUDES   *dislocation of knee:*
old or pathological (718.2)
recurrent (718.3)
internal derangement of knee joint (717.0-717.5, 717.8-717.9)
old tear of cartilage or meniscus of knee (717.0-717.5, 717.8-717.9)

836.0   Tear of medial cartilage or meniscus of knee, current

Bucket handle tear:
NOS   } current injury
medial meniscus

836.1   Tear of lateral cartilage or meniscus of knee, current

836.2   Other tear of cartilage or meniscus of knee, current

Tear of:
cartilage
(semilunar)   } current injury, not specified
meniscus   as medial or lateral

✓4ᵗʰ ✓5ᵗʰ Additional Digit Required   Nonspecific PDx   Unacceptable PDx   Manifestation Code   **MSP** Medicare Secondary Payer   ►◄ Revised Text   ● New Code   ▲ Revised Code Title

2002 Ingenix, Inc.

Injury and Poisoning 827.0–836.2

Volume 1 — 269

Injury and Poisoning 836.3–839.9

	836.3	Dislocation of patella, closed
	836.4	Dislocation of patella, open
√5th	836.5	Other dislocation of knee, closed

836.50 Dislocation of knee, unspecified

836.51 Anterior dislocation of tibia, proximal end
Posterior dislocation of femur, distal end

836.52 Posterior dislocation of tibia, proximal end
Anterior dislocation of femur, distal end

836.53 Medial dislocation of tibia, proximal end

836.54 Lateral dislocation of tibia, proximal end

836.59 Other

√5th 836.6 Other dislocation of knee, open

836.60 Dislocation of knee, unspecified

836.61 Anterior dislocation of tibia, proximal end

836.62 Posterior dislocation of tibia, proximal end

836.63 Medial dislocation of tibia, proximal end

836.64 Lateral dislocation of tibia, proximal end

836.69 Other

√4th 837 Dislocation of ankle

> INCLUDES   astragalus
> fibula, distal end
> navicular, foot
> scaphoid, foot
> tibia, distal end

837.0 Closed dislocation

837.1 Open dislocation

√4th 838 Dislocation of foot

> The following fifth-digit subclassification is for use with category 838:
> 0 foot, unspecified
> 1 tarsal (bone), joint unspecified
> 2 midtarsal (joint)
> 3 tarsometatarsal (joint)
> 4 metatarsal (bone), joint unspecified
> 5 metatarsophalangeal (joint)
> 6 interphalangeal (joint), foot
> 9 other
> Phalanx of foot
> Toe(s)

√5th 838.0 Closed dislocation

√5th 838.1 Open dislocation   `CC 9`

√4th 839 Other, multiple, and ill-defined dislocations

√5th 839.0 Cervical vertebra, closed
Cervical spine   Neck

839.00 Cervical vertebra, unspecified   `CC` `MSP`
CC Excl: 805.00-805.18, 806.00-806.19, 806.8-806.9, 839.00-839.18, 847.0, 848.8-848.9, 879.8-879.9, 929.0, 929.9, 952.00-952.09, 958.8, 959.8-959.9

839.01 First cervical vertebra   `CC` `MSP`
CC Excl: See code 839.00

839.02 Second cervical vertebra   `CC` `MSP`
CC Excl: See code 839.00

839.03 Third cervical vertebra   `CC` `MSP`
CC Excl: See code 839.00

839.04 Fourth cervical vertebra   `CC` `MSP`
CC Excl: See code 839.00

839.05 Fifth cervical vertebra   `CC` `MSP`
CC Excl: See code 839.00

839.06 Sixth cervical vertebra   `CC` `MSP`
CC Excl: See code 839.00

839.07 Seventh cervical vertebra   `CC` `MSP`
CC Excl: See code 839.00

839.08 Multiple cervical vertebrae   `CC` `MSP`
CC Excl: See code 839.00

√5th 839.1 Cervical vertebra, open

839.10 Cervical vertebra, unspecified   `CC` `MSP`
CC Excl: See code 839.00

839.11 First cervical vertebra   `CC` `MSP`
CC Excl: See code 839.00

839.12 Second cervical vertebra   `CC` `MSP`
CC Excl: See code 839.00

839.13 Third cervical vertebra   `CC` `MSP`
CC Excl: See code 839.00

839.14 Fourth cervical vertebra   `CC` `MSP`
CC Excl: See code 839.00

839.15 Fifth cervical vertebra   `CC` `MSP`
CC Excl: See code 839.00

839.16 Sixth cervical vertebra   `CC` `MSP`
CC Excl: See code 839.00

839.17 Seventh cervical vertebra   `CC` `MSP`
CC Excl: See code 839.00

839.18 Multiple cervical vertebrae   `CC` `MSP`
CC Excl: See code 839.00

√5th 839.2 Thoracic and lumbar vertebra, closed

839.20 Lumbar vertebra   `MSP`

839.21 Thoracic vertebra   `MSP`
Dorsal [thoracic] vertebra

√5th 839.3 Thoracic and lumbar vertebra, open

839.30 Lumbar vertebra   `MSP`

839.31 Thoracic vertebra   `MSP`

√5th 839.4 Other vertebra, closed

839.40 Vertebra, unspecified site
Spine NOS

839.41 Coccyx

839.42 Sacrum
Sacroiliac (joint)

839.49 Other

√5th 839.5 Other vertebra, open

839.50 Vertebra, unspecified site

839.51 Coccyx

839.52 Sacrum

839.59 Other

√5th 839.6 Other location, closed

839.61 Sternum
Sternoclavicular joint

839.69 Other
Pelvis

√5th 839.7 Other location, open

839.71 Sternum   `MSP`

839.79 Other   `MSP`

839.8 Multiple and ill-defined, closed   `MSP`
Arm
Back
Hand
Multiple locations, except fingers or toes alone
Other ill-defined locations
Unspecified location

839.9 Multiple and ill-defined, open   `MSP`

`N` Newborn Age: 0   `P` Pediatric Age: 0-17   `M` Maternity Age: 12-55   `A` Adult Age: 15-124   `CC` CC Condition   `MC` Major Complication   `CD` Complex Dx   `HIV` HIV Related Dx

270 — Volume 1   *2002 Ingenix, Inc.*

SPRAINS AND STRAINS OF JOINTS AND ADJACENT MUSCLES
(840-848)

INCLUDES

avulsion
hemarthrosis
laceration   of:
rupture   joint capsule
sprain   ligament
strain   muscle
tear   tendon

EXCLUDES   *laceration of tendon in open wounds (880-884 and 890-894 with .2)*

✓4th **840 Sprains and strains of shoulder and upper arm**
- **840.0 Acromioclavicular (joint) (ligament)**
- **840.1 Coracoclavicular (ligament)**
- **840.2 Coracohumeral (ligament)**
- **840.3 Infraspinatus (muscle) (tendon)**
- **840.4 Rotator cuff (capsule)**

  EXCLUDES   *complete rupture of rotator cuff, nontraumatic (727.61)*

- **840.5 Subscapularis (muscle)**
- **840.6 Supraspinatus (muscle) (tendon)**
- **840.7 Superior glenoid labrum lesion**
  SLAP lesion

  AHA: ▶4Q,'01, 52 ◄

  DEF: ▶ Detachment injury of the superior aspect of the glenoid labrum which is the ring of fibrocartilage attached to the rim of the glenoid cavity of the scapula. ◄

- **840.8 Other specified sites of shoulder and upper arm**
- **840.9 Unspecified site of shoulder and upper arm**
  Arm NOS   Shoulder NOS

✓4th **841 Sprains and strains of elbow and forearm**
- **841.0 Radial collateral ligament**
- **841.1 Ulnar collateral ligament**
- **841.2 Radiohumeral (joint)**
- **841.3 Ulnohumeral (joint)**
- **841.8 Other specified sites of elbow and forearm**
- **841.9 Unspecified site of elbow and forearm**
  Elbow NOS

✓4th **842 Sprains and strains of wrist and hand**
- ✓5th **842.0 Wrist**
  - **842.00 Unspecified site**
  - **842.01 Carpal (joint)**
  - **842.02 Radiocarpal (joint) (ligament)**
  - **842.09 Other**
    Radioulnar joint, distal
- ✓5th **842.1 Hand**
  - **842.10 Unspecified site**
  - **842.11 Carpometacarpal (joint)**
  - **842.12 Metacarpophalangeal (joint)**
  - **842.13 Interphalangeal (joint)**
  - **842.19 Other**
    Midcarpal (joint)

✓4th **843 Sprains and strains of hip and thigh**
- **843.0 Iliofemoral (ligament)**
- **843.1 Ischiocapsular (ligament)**
- **843.8 Other specified sites of hip and thigh**
- **843.9 Unspecified site of hip and thigh**
  Hip NOS
  Thigh NOS

✓4th **844 Sprains and strains of knee and leg**
- **844.0 Lateral collateral ligament of knee**
- **844.1 Medial collateral ligament of knee**
- **844.2 Cruciate ligament of knee**
- **844.3 Tibiofibular (joint) (ligament), superior**
- **844.8 Other specified sites of knee and leg**
- **844.9 Unspecified site of knee and leg**
  Knee NOS   Leg NOS

✓4th **845 Sprains and strains of ankle and foot**
- ✓5th **845.0 Ankle**
  - **845.00 Unspecified site**
  - **845.01 Deltoid (ligament), ankle**
    Internal collateral (ligament), ankle
  - **845.02 Calcaneofibular (ligament)**
  - **845.03 Tibiofibular (ligament), distal**
  - **845.09 Other**
    Achilles tendon
- ✓5th **845.1 Foot**
  - **845.10 Unspecified site**
  - **845.11 Tarsometatarsal (joint) (ligament)**
  - **845.12 Metatarsophalangeal (joint)**
  - **845.13 Interphalangeal (joint), toe**
  - **845.19 Other**

✓4th **846 Sprains and strains of sacroiliac region**
- **846.0 Lumbosacral (joint) (ligament)**
- **846.1 Sacroiliac ligament**
- **846.2 Sacrospinatus (ligament)**
- **846.3 Sacrotuberous (ligament)**
- **846.8 Other specified sites of sacroiliac region**
- **846.9 Unspecified site of sacroiliac region**

✓4th **847 Sprains and strains of other and unspecified parts of back**

  EXCLUDES   *lumbosacral (846.0)*

- **847.0 Neck**   MSP
  Anterior longitudinal (ligament), cervical
  Atlanto-axial (joints)
  Atlanto-occipital (joints)
  Whiplash injury

  EXCLUDES   *neck injury NOS (959.0)*
  thyroid region (848.2)

- **847.1 Thoracic**
- **847.2 Lumbar**
- **847.3 Sacrum**
  Sacrococcygeal (ligament)
- **847.4 Coccyx**
- **847.9 Unspecified site of back**
  Back NOS

✓4th **848 Other and ill-defined sprains and strains**
- **848.0 Septal cartilage of nose**
- **848.1 Jaw**
  Temporomandibular (joint) (ligament)
- **848.2 Thyroid region**
  Cricoarytenoid (joint) (ligament)
  Cricothyroid (joint) (ligament)
  Thyroid cartilage
- **848.3 Ribs**

  Chondrocostal (joint) ⎫ without mention of
  Costal cartilage ⎭ injury to sternum

- ✓5th **848.4 Sternum**
  - **848.40 Unspecified site**
  - **848.41 Sternoclavicular (joint) (ligament)**
  - **848.42 Chondrosternal (joint)**
  - **848.49 Other**
    Xiphoid cartilage
- **848.5 Pelvis**
  Symphysis pubis

  EXCLUDES   *that in childbirth (665.6)*

- **848.8 Other specified sites of sprains and strains**
- **848.9 Unspecified site of sprain and strain**

Additional Digit Required   Nonspecific PDx   Unacceptable PDx   Manifestation Code   MSP Medicare Secondary Payer   ▶◄ Revised Text   ● New Code   ▲ Revised Code Title

INTRACRANIAL INJURY, EXCLUDING THOSE WITH SKULL FRACTURE (850-854)

> **EXCLUDES**   *intracranial injury with skull fracture (800-801 and 803-804, except .0 and .5)*
> *open wound of head without intracranial injury (870.0-873.9)*
> *skull fracture alone (800-801 and 803-804 with .0, .5)*

The description "with open intracranial wound," used in the fourth-digit subdivisions, includes those specified as open or with mention of infection or foreign body.

The following fifth-digit subclassification is for use with categories 851-854:

     0   unspecified state of consciousness
     1   with no loss of consciousness
     2   with brief [less than one hour] loss of consciousness
     3   with moderate [1-24 hours] loss of consciousness
     4   with prolonged [more than 24 hours] loss of consciousness and return to pre-existing conscious level
     5   with prolonged [more than 24 hours] loss of consciousness, without return to pre-existing conscious level

         Use fifth-digit 5 to designate when a patient is unconscious and dies before regaining consciousness, regardless of the duration of the loss of consciousness

     6   with loss of consciousness of unspecified duration
     9   with concussion, unspecified

AHA: 1Q, '93, 22

√4th **850 Concussion**

> **INCLUDES**   commotio cerebri
> **EXCLUDES**   *concussion with:*
> *cerebral laceration or contusion (851.0-851.9)*
> *cerebral hemorrhage (852-853)*
> *head injury NOS (959.01)*

AHA: 2Q, '96, 6; 4Q, '90, 24

850.0   With no loss of consciousness   `CC` `MSP`
     Concussion with mental confusion or disorientation, without loss of consciousness
     CC Excl: 800.00-800.99, 801.00-801.99, 803.00-803.99, 804.00-804.99, 850.0-850.9, 851.00-851.99, 852.00-852.19, 852.21-852.59, 853.00-853.19, 854.00-854.19, 873.8-873.9, 879.8-879.9, 905.0, 925.1-925.2, 929.0, 929.9, 958.8, 959.01, 959.09, 959.8-959.9

850.1   With brief loss of consciousness   `CC` `MSP`
     Loss of consciousness for less than one hour
     CC Excl: See code 850.0

     AHA: 1Q, '99, 10; 2Q, '92, 5

850.2   With moderate loss of consciousness   `CC` `MSP`
     Loss of consciousness for 1-24 hours
     CC Excl: See code 850.0

850.3   With prolonged loss of consciousness and return to pre-existing conscious level   `CC` `MSP`
     Loss of consciousness for more than 24 hours with complete recovery
     CC Excl: See code 850.0

850.4   With prolonged loss of consciousness, without return to pre-existing conscious level   `CC` `MSP`
     CC Excl: See code 850.0

850.5   With loss of consciousness of unspecified duration   `CC` `MSP`
     CC Excl: See code 850.0

850.9   Concussion, unspecified   `CC` `MSP`
     CC Excl: See code 850.0

Brain

√4th **851 Cerebral laceration and contusion**
     AHA: 4Q, '96, 36; 1Q, '93, 22; 4Q, '90, 24

§ √5th **851.0   Cortex (cerebral) contusion without mention of open intracranial wound**   `CC` `MSP`
     CC Excl: See code 850.0

§ √5th **851.1   Cortex (cerebral) contusion with open intracranial wound**   `CC` `MSP`
     CC Excl: See code 850.0

     AHA: 1Q, '92, 9

§ √5th **851.2   Cortex (cerebral) laceration without mention of open intracranial wound**   `CC` `MSP`
     CC Excl: See code 850.0

§ √5th **851.3   Cortex (cerebral) laceration with open intracranial wound**   `CC` `MSP`
     CC Excl: See code 850.0

§ √5th **851.4   Cerebellar or brain stem contusion without mention of open intracranial wound**   `CC` `MSP`
     CC Excl: See code 850.0

§ √5th **851.5   Cerebellar or brain stem contusion with open intracranial wound**   `CC` `MSP`
     CC Excl: See code 850.0

§ √5th **851.6   Cerebellar or brain stem laceration without mention of open intracranial wound**   `CC` `MSP`
     CC Excl: See code 850.0

§ √5th **851.7   Cerebellar or brain stem laceration with open intracranial wound**   `CC` `MSP`
     CC Excl: See code 850.0

§   Requires fifth-digit. See beginning of section 850-854 for codes and definitions.

`N` Newborn Age: 0   `P` Pediatric Age: 0-17   `M` Maternity Age: 12-55   `A` Adult Age: 15-124   `CC` CC Condition   `MC` Major Complication   `CD` Complex Dx   `HIV` HIV Related Dx

§ ✓5ᵗʰ **851.8** **Other and unspecified cerebral laceration** CC MSP
and contusion, without mention of open
intracranial wound
Brain (membrane) NOS
CC Excl: See code 850.0

AHA: 4Q, '96, 37

§ ✓5ᵗʰ **851.9** **Other and unspecified cerebral laceration** CC MSP
and contusion, with open intracranial wound
CC Excl: See code 850.0

✓4ᵗʰ **852** **Subarachnoid, subdural, and extradural hemorrhage,**
following injury
EXCLUDES Cerebral contusion or laceration (with
hemorrhage) (851.0-851.9)
DEF: Bleeding from lining of brain; due to injury.

§ ✓5ᵗʰ **852.0** **Subarachnoid hemorrhage following injury** CC MSP
without mention of open intracranial wound
Middle meningeal hemorrhage following injury
CC Excl: See code 850.0

§ ✓5ᵗʰ **852.1** **Subarachnoid hemorrhage following injury** CC MSP
with open intracranial wound
CC Excl: See code 850.0

§ ✓5ᵗʰ **852.2** **Subdural hemorrhage following injury** CC MSP
without mention of open intracranial wound
CC Excl: For code 852.20: 800.00-800.99, 801.00-801.99, 803.00-803.99,
804.00-804.99, 850.0-850.9, 851.00-851.99, 852.00-852.59, 853.00-853.19,
854.00-854.19, 873.8-873.9, 879.8-879.9, 905.0, 925.1-925.2, 929.0, 929.9,
958.8, 959.01, 959.09, 959.8-959.9 **For code 852.21:** 800.00-800.99,
801.00-801.99, 803.00-803.99, 804.00-804.99, 850.0-850.9, 851.00-851.99,
852.00-852.19, 852.21-852.59, 853.00-853.19, 854.00-854.19, 873.8-873.9,
879.8-879.9, 905.0, 925.1-925.2, 929.0, 929.9, 958.8, 959.01, 959.09, 959.8-
959.9 **For codes 852.22-852.29:** See code 852.21

AHA: 4Q, '96, 43

§ ✓5ᵗʰ **852.3** **Subdural hemorrhage following injury with** CC MSP
open intracranial wound
CC Excl: See code 852.21

§ ✓5ᵗʰ **852.4** **Extradural hemorrhage following injury** CC MSP
without mention of open intracranial wound
Epidural hematoma following injury
CC Excl: See code 852.21

§ ✓5ᵗʰ **852.5** **Extradural hemorrhage following injury** CC MSP
with open intracranial wound
CC Excl: See code 852.21

✓4ᵗʰ **853** **Other and unspecified intracranial hemorrhage following**
injury

§ ✓5ᵗʰ **853.0** **Without mention of open intracranial wound** CC MSP
Cerebral compression due to injury
Intracranial hematoma following injury
Traumatic cerebral hemorrhage
CC Excl: See code 852.21

AHA: 3Q, '90, 14

§ ✓5ᵗʰ **853.1** **With open intracranial wound** CC MSP
CC Excl: See code 852.21

✓4ᵗʰ **854** **Intracranial injury of other and unspecified nature**
INCLUDES brain injury NOS
cavernous sinus
intracranial injury
EXCLUDES any condition classifiable to 850-853
head injury NOS (959.01)
AHA: 1Q, '99, 10; 2Q, '92, 6

§ ✓5ᵗʰ **854.0** **Without mention of open intracranial wound** CC MSP
CC Excl: See code 852.21

§ ✓5ᵗʰ **854.1** **With open intracranial wound** CC MSP
CC Excl: See code 852.21

§ Requires fifth-digit. See beginning of section 850-854 for codes and definitions.

INTERNAL INJURY OF THORAX, ABDOMEN, AND PELVIS (860-869)

INCLUDES blast injuries
blunt trauma
bruise
concussion injuries
(except cerebral)
crushing } of internal organs
hematoma
laceration
puncture
tear
traumatic rupture

EXCLUDES concussion NOS (850.0-850.9)
flail chest (807.4)
foreign body entering through orifice (930.0-
939.9)
injury to blood vessels (901.0-902.9)
The description "with open wound," used in the fourth-digit
subdivisions, includes those with mention of infection
or foreign body.

✓4ᵗʰ **860** **Traumatic pneumothorax and hemothorax**
AHA: 2Q, '93, 4

DEF: Traumatic pneumothorax: air or gas leaking into pleural space of lung
due to trauma.

DEF: Traumatic hemothorax: blood buildup in pleural space of lung due to
trauma.

860.0 **Pneumothorax without mention of open** CC MSP
wound into thorax
CC Excl: 860.0-860.5, 861.20-861.32, 862.29, 862.39, 862.8-862.9, 875.0-
875.1, 879.8-879.9, 929.0, 929.9, 958.7-958.8, 959.8-959.9

860.1 **Pneumothorax with open wound into thorax** CC MSP
CC Excl: See code 860.0

860.2 **Hemothorax without mention of open wound** CC MSP
into thorax
CC Excl: See code 860.0

860.3 **Hemothorax with open wound into thorax** CC MSP
CC Excl: See code 860.0

860.4 **Pneumohemothorax without mention of** CC MSP
open wound into thorax
CC Excl: See code 860.0

860.5 **Pneumohemothorax with open wound into** CC MSP
thorax
CC Excl: See code 860.0

✓4ᵗʰ **861** **Injury to heart and lung**
EXCLUDES injury to blood vessels of thorax (901.0-901.9)

✓5ᵗʰ **861.0** **Heart, without mention of open wound into thorax**
AHA: 1Q, '92, 9

861.00 **Unspecified injury** MSP
861.01 **Contusion** CC MSP
Cardiac contusion   Myocardial contusion
CC Excl: 861.00-861.13, 862.29, 862.39, 862.8-862.9, 875.0-
875.1, 879.8-879.9, 929.0, 929.9, 958.7-958.8, 959.8-959.9

DEF: Bruising within the pericardium with no mention of
open wound.

861.02 **Laceration without penetration of** CC MSP
heart chambers
CC Excl: See code 861.01

DEF: Tearing injury of heart tissue, without penetration of
chambers; no open wound.

861.03 **Laceration with penetration of** CC MSP
heart chambers
CC Excl: See code 861.01

✓4ᵗʰ
✓5ᵗʰ **Additional Digit Required**   Nonspecific PDx   Unacceptable PDx   Manifestation Code   MSP Medicare Secondary Payer   ►◄ Revised Text   ● New Code   ▲ Revised Code Title

2002 Ingenix, Inc.

Injury and Poisoning 851.8-861.03

Volume 1 — 273

√5th 861.1 Heart, with open wound into thorax
861.10 Unspecified injury CC MSP
CC Excl: See code 861.01

861.11 Contusion CC MSP
CC Excl: See code 861.01

861.12 Laceration without penetration of CC MSP
heart chambers
CC Excl: See code 861.01

861.13 Laceration with penetration of heart CC MSP
chambers
CC Excl: See code 861.01

√5th 861.2 Lung, without mention of open wound into thorax
861.20 Unspecified injury MSP
861.21 Contusion MSP
DEF: Bruising of lung without mention of open wound.

861.22 Laceration CC MSP
CC Excl: 861.20-861.32, 862.29, 862.39, 862.8-862.9, 875.0-875.1, 879.8-879.9, 929.0, 929.9, 958.7-958.8, 959.8-959.9

√5th 861.3 Lung, with open wound into thorax
861.30 Unspecified injury CC MSP
CC Excl: See code 861.22

861.31 Contusion CC MSP
CC Excl: See code 861.22

861.32 Laceration CC MSP
CC Excl: See code 861.22

√4th 862 Injury to other and unspecified intrathoracic organs
EXCLUDES injury to blood vessels of thorax (901.0-901.9)

862.0 Diaphragm, without mention of open wound into cavity
862.1 Diaphragm, with open wound into cavity CC
CC Excl: 862.0-862.1, 862.29, 862.39, 862.8-862.9, 875.0-875.1, 879.8-879.9, 929.0, 929.9, 958.7-958.8, 959.8-959.9

√5th 862.2 Other specified intrathoracic organs, without mention of open wound into cavity
862.21 Bronchus CC
CC Excl: 862.21, 862.29, 862.31, 862.39, 862.8-862.9, 875.0-875.1, 879.8-879.9, 929.0, 929.9, 958.7-958.8, 959.8-959.9

862.22 Esophagus CC
CC Excl: 862.22, 862.29, 862.32, 862.39, 862.8-862.9, 875.0-875.1, 879.8-879.9, 929.0, 929.9, 958.7-958.8, 959.8-959.9

862.29 Other CC
Pleura
Thymus gland
CC Excl: 862.29, 862.39, 862.8-862.9, 875.0-875.1, 879.8-879.9, 929.0, 929.9, 958.7-958.8, 959.8-959.9

√5th 862.3 Other specified intrathoracic organs, with open wound into cavity
862.31 Bronchus CC
CC Excl: 862.21, 862.29, 862.31, 862.39, 862.8-862.9, 875.0-875.1, 879.8-879.9, 929.0, 929.9, 958.7-958.8, 959.8-959.9

862.32 Esophagus CC
CC Excl: 862.22, 862.29, 862.32, 862.39, 862.8-862.9, 875.0-875.1, 879.8-879.9, 929.0, 929.9, 958.7-958.8, 959.8-959.9

862.39 Other CC
CC Excl: 862.29, 862.39, 862.8-862.9, 875.0-875.1, 879.8-879.9, 929.0, 929.9, 958.7-958.8, 959.8-959.9

862.8 Multiple and unspecified intrathoracic organs, MSP
without mention of open wound into cavity
Crushed chest
Multiple intrathoracic organs

862.9 Multiple and unspecified intrathoracic organs, CC
with open wound into cavity
CC Excl: See code 862.39

√4th 863 Injury to gastrointestinal tract
EXCLUDES anal sphincter laceration during delivery (664.2)
bile duct (868.0-868.1 with fifth-digit 2)
gallbladder (868.0-868.1 with fifth-digit 2)

863.0 Stomach, without mention of open wound into MSP
cavity
863.1 Stomach, with open wound into cavity CC MSP
CC Excl: 863.0-863.1, 863.80, 863.89-863.90, 863.99, 868.00, 868.03-868.10, 868.13-868.19, 869.0-869.1, 879.2-879.9, 929.0, 929.9, 958.8, 959.8-959.9

√5th 863.2 Small intestine, without mention of open wound into cavity
863.20 Small intestine, unspecified site
863.21 Duodenum
863.29 Other

√5th 863.3 Small intestine, with open wound into cavity
863.30 Small intestine, unspecified site CC MSP
CC Excl: 863.20-863.39, 863.80, 863.89-863.90, 863.99, 868.00, 868.03-868.10, 868.13-868.19, 869.0-869.1, 879.2-879.9, 929.0, 929.9, 958.8, 959.8-959.9

863.31 Duodenum CC MSP
CC Excl: 863.21, 863.31, 863.39, 863.80, 863.89-863.90, 863.99, 868.00, 868.03-868.10, 868.13-868.19, 869.0-869.1, 879.2-879.9, 929.0, 929.9, 958.8, 959.8-959.9

863.39 Other CC MSP
CC Excl: 863.20-863.39, 863.80, 863.89-863.90, 863.99, 868.00, 868.03-868.10, 868.13-868.19, 869.0-869.1, 879.2-879.9, 929.0, 929.9, 958.8, 959.8-959.9

√5th 863.4 Colon or rectum, without mention of open wound into cavity
863.40 Colon, unspecified site
863.41 Ascending [right] colon
863.42 Transverse colon
863.43 Descending [left] colon
863.44 Sigmoid colon
863.45 Rectum
863.46 Multiple sites in colon and rectum
863.49 Other

√5th 863.5 Colon or rectum, with open wound into cavity
863.50 Colon, unspecified site CC MSP
CC Excl: 863.40-863.59, 863.80, 863.89-863.90, 863.99, 868.00, 868.03-868.10, 868.13-868.19, 869.0-869.1, 879.2-879.9, 929.0, 929.9, 958.8, 959.8-959.9

863.51 Ascending [right] colon CC MSP
CC Excl: See code 863.50

863.52 Transverse colon CC MSP
CC Excl: See code 863.50

863.53 Descending [left] colon CC MSP
CC Excl: See code 863.50

863.54 Sigmoid colon CC MSP
CC Excl: See code 863.50

863.55 Rectum CC MSP
CC Excl: See code 863.50

863.56 Multiple sites in colon and rectum CC MSP
CC Excl: See code 863.50

863.59 Other CC MSP
CC Excl: See code 863.50

N Newborn Age: 0 P Pediatric Age: 0-17 M Maternity Age: 12-55 A Adult Age: 15-124 CC CC Condition MC Major Complication CD Complex Dx HIV HIV Related Dx

274 — Volume 1 2002 Ingenix, Inc.

√5ᵗʰ **863.8** **Other and unspecified gastrointestinal sites, without mention of open wound into cavity**

863.80 Gastrointestinal tract, unspecified site `MSP`

863.81 Pancreas, head `MSP`

863.82 Pancreas, body `MSP`

863.83 Pancreas, tail `MSP`

863.84 Pancreas, multiple and unspecified sites `MSP`

863.85 Appendix `MSP`

863.89 Other `MSP`
> Intestine NOS

√5ᵗʰ **863.9** **Other and unspecified gastrointestinal sites, with open wound into cavity**

863.90 Gastrointestinal tract, unspecified site `CC` `MSP`
> **CC Excl:** 863.80-863.84, 863.89-863.94, 863.99, 868.00, 868.03-868.10, 868.13-868.19, 869.0-869.1, 879.2-879.9, 929.0, 929.9, 958.8, 959.8-959.9

863.91 Pancreas, head `CC` `MSP`
> **CC Excl:** 863.80-863.84, 863.91-863.94, 863.99, 868.00, 868.03-868.10, 868.13-868.19, 869.0-869.1, 879.2-879.9, 929.0, 929.9, 958.8, 959.8-959.9

863.92 Pancreas, body `CC` `MSP`
> **CC Excl:** See code 863.91

863.93 Pancreas, tail `CC` `MSP`
> **CC Excl:** See code 863.91

863.94 Pancreas, multiple and unspecified sites `CC` `MSP`
> **CC Excl:** See code 863.91

863.95 Appendix `CC` `MSP`
> **CC Excl:** 863.80, 863.85, 863.95, 863.99, 868.00, 868.03-868.10, 868.13-868.19, 869.0-869.1, 879.2-879.9, 929.0, 929.9, 958.8, 959.8-959.9

863.99 Other `CC` `MSP`
> **CC Excl:** 863.80, 863.99, 868.00, 868.03-868.10, 868.13-868.19, 869.0-869.1, 879.2-879.9, 929.0, 929.9, 958.8, 959.8-959.9

√4ᵗʰ **864 Injury to liver**

The following fifth-digit subclassification is for use with category 864:

0 unspecified injury

1 hematoma and contusion

2 laceration, minor
> Laceration involving capsule only, or without significant involvement of hepatic parenchyma [i.e., less than 1 cm deep]

3 laceration, moderate
> Laceration involving parenchyma but without major disruption of parenchyma [i.e., less than 10 cm long and less than 3 cm deep]

4 laceration, major
> Laceration with significant disruption of hepatic parenchyma [i.e., 10 cm long and 3 cm deep]
> Multiple moderate lacerations, with or without hematoma
> Stellate lacerations of liver

5 laceration, unspecified

9 other

√5ᵗʰ **864.0** **Without mention of open wound into cavity** `CC` `MSP`
> **CC Excl:** 863.80, 863.99, 864.00-864.19, 868.00, 868.03-868.10, 868.13-868.19, 869.0-869.1, 879.2-879.9, 929.0, 929.9, 958.8, 959.8-959.9

√5ᵗʰ **864.1** **With open wound into cavity** `CC` `MSP`
> **CC Excl:** See code 864.0

√4ᵗʰ **865 Injury to spleen**

The following fifth-digit subclassification is for use with category 865:

0 unspecified injury

1 hematoma without rupture of capsule

2 capsular tears, without major disruption of parenchyma

3 laceration extending into parenchyma

4 massive parenchymal disruption

9 other

√5ᵗʰ **865.0** **Without mention of open wound into cavity** `CC` `MSP`
> **CC Excl:** 865.00-865.19, 868.00, 868.03-868.10, 868.13-868.19, 869.0-869.1, 879.2-879.9, 929.0, 929.9, 958.8, 959.8-959.9

√5ᵗʰ **865.1** **With open wound into cavity** `CC` `MSP`
> **CC Excl:** See code 865.0

√4ᵗʰ **866 Injury to kidney**

The following fifth-digit subclassification is for use with category 866:

0 unspecified injury

1 hematoma without rupture of capsule

2 laceration

3 complete disruption of kidney parenchyma

√5ᵗʰ **866.0** **Without mention of open wound into cavity** `CC` `MSP`
> **CC Excl:** 866.00-866.13, 868.00, 868.03-868.10, 868.13-868.19, 869.0-869.1, 879.2-879.9, 929.0, 929.9, 958.8, 959.8-959.9

√5ᵗʰ **866.1** **With open wound into cavity** `CC` `MSP`
> **CC Excl:** See code 866.0

√4ᵗʰ **867 Injury to pelvic organs**
> `EXCLUDES` injury during delivery (664.0-665.9)

867.0 Bladder and urethra, without mention of open wound into cavity `CC` `MSP`
> **CC Excl:** 867.0-867.1, 867.6-867.9, 868.00, 868.03-868.10, 868.13-868.19, 869.0-869.1, 879.2-879.9, 929.0, 929.9, 958.8, 959.8-959.9
>
> **AHA:** N-D, '85, 15

867.1 Bladder and urethra, with open wound into cavity `CC` `MSP`
> **CC Excl:** See code 867.0

867.2 Ureter, without mention of open wound into cavity `CC` `MSP`
> **CC Excl:** 867.2-867.3, 867.6-867.9, 868.00, 868.03-868.10, 868.13-868.19, 869.0-869.1, 879.2-879.9, 929.0, 929.9, 958.8, 959.8-959.9

867.3 Ureter, with open wound into cavity `CC` `MSP`
> **CC Excl:** See code 867.2

867.4 Uterus, without mention of open wound intocavity `CC` `MSP` ♂
> **CC Excl:** 867.4-867.9, 868.00, 868.03-868.10, 868.13-868.19, 869.0-869.1, 879.2-879.9, 929.0, 929.9, 958.8, 959.8-959.9

867.5 Uterus, with open wound into cavity `CC` `MSP` ♂
> **CC Excl:** See code 867.4

867.6 Other specified pelvic organs, without mention of open wound into cavity `CC` `MSP`
> Fallopian tube   Seminal vesicle
> Ovary   Vas deferens
> Prostate
>
> **CC Excl:** 867.6-867.9, 868.00, 868.03-868.10, 868.13-868.19, 869.0-869.1, 879.2-879.9, 929.0, 929.9, 958.8, 959.8-959.9

867.7 Other specified pelvic organs, with open wound into cavity `CC` `MSP`
> **CC Excl:** See code 867.6

867.8 Unspecified pelvic organ, without mention of open wound into cavity `CC` `MSP`
> **CC Excl:** See code 867.6

√4ᵗʰ √5ᵗʰ Additional Digit Required   Nonspecific PDx   Unacceptable PDx   Manifestation Code   `MSP` Medicare Secondary Payer   ►◄ Revised Text   ● New Code   ▲ Revised Code Title

2002 Ingenix, Inc.

Injury and Poisoning 863.8–867.8

Volume 1 — 275

867.9   **Unspecified pelvic organ, with open wound into cavity** `CC` `MSP`

    CC Excl: See code 867.6

✓4th **868 Injury to other intra-abdominal organs**

    The following fifth-digit subclassification is for use with category 868:

      0   unspecified intra-abdominal organ
      1   adrenal gland
      2   bile duct and gallbladder
      3   peritoneum
      4   retroperitoneum
      9   other and multiple intra-abdominal organs

✓5th **868.0**   **Without mention of open wound into cavity** `CC` `MSP`

    CC Excl: For code **868.00**: 868.00, 868.03-868.10, 868.13-868.19, 869.0-869.1, 879.2-879.9, 929.0, 929.9, 958.8, 959.8-959.9 **For code 868.01**: 868.00, 868.01, 868.03-868.11, 868.13-868.19, 869.0-869.1, 879.2-879.9, 929.0, 929.9, 958.8, 959.8-959.9 **For code 868.02**: 868.00, 868.02-868.10, 868.13-868.19, 869.0-869.1, 879.2-879.9, 929.0, 929.9, 958.8, 959.8-959.9 **For codes 868.03-868.09**: 868.00, 868.03-868.10, 868.13-868.19, 869.0-869.1, 879.2-879.9, 929.0, 929.9, 958.8, 959.8-959.9

✓5th **868.1**   **With open wound into cavity** `CC` `MSP`

    CC Excl: For code **868.10**: See code 868.03 For code **868.11**: 868.00, 868.01, 868.03-868.11, 868.13-868.19, 869.0-869.1, 879.2-879.9, 929.0, 929.9, 958.8, 959.8-959.9 **For code 868.12**: 868.00, 868.03-868.10, 868.12-868.19, 869.0-869.1, 879.2-879.9, 929.0, 929.9, 958.8, 959.8-959.9 **For codes 868.13-868.19**: 868.00, 868.03-868.10, 868.13-868.19, 869.0-869.1, 879.2-879.9, 929.0, 929.9, 958.8, 959.8-959.9

✓4th **869 Internal injury to unspecified or ill-defined organs**

    INCLUDES   internal injury NOS
              multiple internal injury NOS

869.0   **Without mention of open wound into cavity** `CC` `MSP`

    CC Excl: See code 868.13

869.1   **With open wound into cavity** `CC` `MSP`

    CC Excl: See code 868.13

    AHA: 2Q, '89, 15

OPEN WOUND (870-897)

    INCLUDES   animal bite
              avulsion
              cut
              laceration
              puncture wound
              traumatic amputation

    EXCLUDES   *burn (940.0-949.5)*
              crushing (925-929.9)
              puncture of internal organs (860.0-869.1)
              superficial injury (910.0-919.9)
              that incidental to:
                 dislocation (830.0-839.9)
                 fracture (800.0-829.1)
                 internal injury (860.0-869.1)
                 intracranial injury (851.0-854.1)

    Note: The description "complicated" used in the fourth-digit subdivisions includes those with mention of delayed healing, delayed treatment, foreign body, or infection. Use additional code to identify infection

    AHA: ▶4Q, '01, 52 ◀

OPEN WOUND OF HEAD, NECK, AND TRUNK (870-879)

✓4th **870 Open wound of ocular adnexa**

    870.0   **Laceration of skin of eyelid and periocular area**

    870.1   **Laceration of eyelid, full-thickness, not involving lacrimal passages**

    870.2   **Laceration of eyelid involving lacrimal passages**

    870.3   **Penetrating wound of orbit, without mention of foreign body** `CC`

      CC Excl: 870.0-870.9, 871.0-871.9, 879.8-879.9, 929.0, 929.9, 958.8, 959.8-959.9

870.4   **Penetrating wound of orbit with foreign body** `CC`

    EXCLUDES   *retained (old) foreign body in orbit (376.6)*

    CC Excl: See code 870.3

870.8   **Other specified open wounds of ocular adnexa** `CC`

    CC Excl: See code 870.3

870.9   **Unspecified open wound of ocular adnexa** `CC`

    CC Excl: See code 870.3

✓4th **871 Open wound of eyeball**

    EXCLUDES   *2nd cranial nerve [optic] injury (950.0-950.9)*
              3rd cranial nerve [oculomotor] injury (951.0)

871.0   **Ocular laceration without prolapse of intraocular tissue** `CC`

    CC Excl: See code 870.3

    AHA: 3Q, '96, 7

    DEF: Tear in ocular tissue without displacing structures.

871.1   **Ocular laceration with prolapse or exposure of intraocular tissue** `CC`

    CC Excl: See code 870.3

871.2   **Rupture of eye with partial loss of intraocular tissue** `CC`

    DEF: Forcible tearing of eyeball, with tissue loss.

871.3   **Avulsion of eye** `CC`
      Traumatic enucleation

    CC Excl: See code 870.3

    DEF: Traumatic extraction of eyeball from socket.

871.4   **Unspecified laceration of eye** `CC`

    CC Excl: See code 870.3

871.5   **Penetration of eyeball with magnetic foreign body**

    EXCLUDES   *retained (old) magnetic foreign body in globe (360.50-360.59)*

871.6   **Penetration of eyeball with (nonmagnetic) foreign body**

    EXCLUDES   *retained (old) (nonmagnetic) foreign body in globe (360.60-360.69)*

871.7   **Unspecified ocular penetration**

871.9   **Unspecified open wound of eyeball** `CC`

    CC Excl: See code 870.3

✓4th **872 Open wound of ear**

✓5th **872.0**   **External ear, without mention of complication**
      872.00 External ear, unspecified site
      872.01 Auricle, ear
          Pinna
          DEF: Open wound of fleshy, outer ear.

      872.02 Auditory canal
          DEF: Open wound of passage from external ear to eardrum.

✓5th **872.1**   **External ear, complicated**
      872.10 External ear, unspecified site
      872.11 Auricle, ear
      872.12 Auditory canal

✓5th **872.6**   **Other specified parts of ear, without mention of complication**
      872.61 Ear drum
          Drumhead   Tympanic membrane

      872.62 Ossicles
      872.63 Eustachian tube
          DEF: Open wound of channel between nasopharynx and tympanic cavity.

872.64 Cochlea

DEF: Open wound of snail shell shaped tube of inner ear.

872.69 Other and multiple sites

✓5th **872.7 Other specified parts of ear, complicated**

872.71 Ear drum

872.72 Ossicles `CC`

CC Excl: 872.00-872.9, 879.8-879.9, 929.0, 929.9, 958.8, 959.8-959.9

872.73 Eustachian tube `CC`

CC Excl: See code 872.72

872.74 Cochlea `CC`

CC Excl: See code 872.72

872.79 Other and multiple sites

872.8 Ear, part unspecified, without mention of complication

Ear NOS

872.9 Ear, part unspecified, complicated

✓4th **873 Other open wound of head**

873.0 Scalp, without mention of complication

873.1 Scalp, complicated

✓5th **873.2 Nose, without mention of complication**

873.20 Nose, unspecified site

873.21 Nasal septum

DEF: Open wound between nasal passages.

873.22 Nasal cavity

DEF: Open wound of nostrils.

873.23 Nasal sinus

DEF: Open wound of mucous-lined respiratory cavities.

873.29 Multiple sites

✓5th **873.3 Nose, complicated**

873.30 Nose, unspecified site

873.31 Nasal septum

873.32 Nasal cavity

873.33 Nasal sinus `CC`

CC Excl: 873.20-873.39, 879.8-879.9, 929.0, 929.9, 958.8, 959.8-959.9

873.39 Multiple sites

✓5th **873.4 Face, without mention of complication**

873.40 Face, unspecified site

873.41 Cheek

873.42 Forehead

Eyebrow

AHA: 4Q, '96, 43

873.43 Lip

873.44 Jaw

873.49 Other and multiple sites

✓5th **873.5 Face, complicated**

873.50 Face, unspecified site

873.51 Cheek

873.52 Forehead

873.53 Lip

873.54 Jaw

873.59 Other and multiple sites

✓5th **873.6 Internal structures of mouth, without mention of complication**

873.60 Mouth, unspecified site

873.61 Buccal mucosa

DEF: Open wound of inside of cheek.

873.62 Gum (alveolar process)

873.63 Tooth (broken)

873.64 Tongue and floor of mouth

873.65 Palate

DEF: Open wound of roof of mouth.

873.69 Other and multiple sites

✓5th **873.7 Internal structures of mouth, complicated**

873.70 Mouth, unspecified site

873.71 Buccal mucosa

873.72 Gum (alveolar process)

873.73 Tooth (broken)

873.74 Tongue and floor of mouth

873.75 Palate

873.79 Other and multiple sites

873.8 Other and unspecified open wound of head without mention of complication

Head NOS

873.9 Other and unspecified open wound of head, complicated `CC`

CC Excl: 847.0, 873.40-873.79, 873.9, 874.8-874.9, 879.8-879.9, 929.0, 929.9, 958.8, 959.8-959.9

✓4th **874 Open wound of neck**

✓5th **874.0 Larynx and trachea, without mention of complication**

874.00 Larynx with trachea `CC`

CC Excl: 847.0, 874.00-874.12, 874.8-874.9, 879.8-879.9, 929.0, 929.9, 958.8, 959.8-959.9

874.01 Larynx `CC`

CC Excl: See code 874.00

874.02 Trachea `CC`

CC Excl: See code 874.00

✓5th **874.1 Larynx and trachea, complicated**

874.10 Larynx with trachea `CC`

CC Excl: See code 874.00

874.11 Larynx `CC`

CC Excl: See code 874.00

874.12 Trachea `CC`

CC Excl: See code 874.00

874.2 Thyroid gland, without mention of complication

874.3 Thyroid gland, complicated `CC`

CC Excl: 847.0, 874.2-874.3, 874.8-874.9, 879.8-879.9, 929.0, 929.9, 958.8, 959.8-959.9

874.4 Pharynx, without mention of complication

Cervical esophagus

874.5 Pharynx, complicated `CC`

CC Excl: 847.0, 874.4-874.9, 879.8-879.9, 929.0, 929.9, 958.8, 959.8-959.9

874.8 Other and unspecified parts, without mention of complication

Nape of neck   Throat NOS
Supraclavicular region

874.9 Other and unspecified parts, complicated

✓4th **875 Open wound of chest (wall)**

EXCLUDES   open wound into thoracic cavity (860.0-862.9)
traumatic pneumothorax and hemothorax
(860.1, 860.3, 860.5)

AHA: 3Q, '93, 17

875.0 Without mention of complication `CC`

CC Excl: 847.1, 862.29, 862.39, 862.8-862.9, 875.0-875.1, 879.8-879.9, 929.0, 929.9, 958.7-958.8, 959.8-959.9

875.1 Complicated `CC`

CC Excl: See code 875.0

✓4th **876 Open wound of back**

INCLUDES   loin
lumbar region

EXCLUDES   open wound into thoracic cavity (860.0-862.9)
traumatic pneumothorax and hemothorax
(860.1, 860.3, 860.5)

876.0 Without mention of complication

876.1 Complicated

✓4th ✓5th Additional Digit Required   Nonspecific PDx   Unacceptable PDx   Manifestation Code   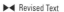 MSP Medicare Secondary Payer   ►◄ Revised Text   ● New Code   ▲ Revised Code Title

2002 Ingenix, Inc.

Volume 1 — 277

Injury and Poisoning 877–890.2

√4th **877 Open wound of buttock**
    INCLUDES   sacroiliac region

    877.0 **Without mention of complication**

    877.1 **Complicated**

√4th **878 Open wound of genital organs (external), including traumatic amputation**
    EXCLUDES *injury during delivery (664.0-665.9)*
            internal genital organs (867.0-867.9)

    878.0 **Penis, without mention of complication** ♂

    878.1 **Penis, complicated** ♂

    878.2 **Scrotum and testes, without mention of complication** ♂

    878.3 **Scrotum and testes, complicated** ♂

    878.4 **Vulva, without mention of complication** ♀
            Labium (majus) (minus)

    878.5 **Vulva, complicated** ♀

    878.6 **Vagina, without mention of complication** ♀

    878.7 **Vagina, complicated** ♀

    878.8 **Other and unspecified parts, without mention of complication**

    878.9 **Other and unspecified parts, complicated**

√4th **879 Open wound of other and unspecified sites, except limbs**

    879.0 **Breast, without mention of complication**

    879.1 **Breast, complicated**

    879.2 **Abdominal wall, anterior, without mention of complication**
        Abdominal wall NOS   Pubic region
        Epigastric region   Umbilical region
        Hypogastric region

        AHA: 2Q, '91, 22

    879.3 **Abdominal wall, anterior, complicated**

    879.4 **Abdominal wall, lateral, without mention of complication**
        Flank   Iliac (region)
        Groin   Inguinal region
        Hypochondrium

    879.5 **Abdominal wall, lateral, complicated**

    879.6 **Other and unspecified parts of trunk, without mention of complication**
        Pelvic region   Trunk NOS
        Perineum

    879.7 **Other and unspecified parts of trunk, complicated**

    879.8 **Open wound(s) (multiple) of unspecified site(s) without mention of complication**
        Multiple open wounds NOS   Open wound NOS

    879.9 **Open wound(s) (multiple) of unspecified site(s), complicated**

OPEN WOUND OF UPPER LIMB (880-887)

AHA: N-D, '85, 5

√4th **880 Open wound of shoulder and upper arm**

    The following fifth-digit subclassification is for use with category 880:
        0 shoulder region
        1 scapular region
        2 axillary region
        3 upper arm
        9 multiple sites

√5th 880.0 **Without mention of complication**

√5th 880.1 **Complicated**

√5th 880.2 **With tendon involvement**

√4th **881 Open wound of elbow, forearm, and wrist**

    The following fifth-digit subclassification is for use with category 881:
        0 forearm
        1 elbow
        2 wrist

√5th 881.0 **Without mention of complication**

√5th 881.1 **Complicated**

√5th 881.2 **With tendon involvement**

√4th **882 Open wound of hand except finger(s) alone**

    882.0 **Without mention of complication**

    882.1 **Complicated**

    882.2 **With tendon involvement**

√4th **883 Open wound of finger(s)**
    INCLUDES fingernail
            thumb (nail)

    883.0 **Without mention of complication**

    883.1 **Complicated**

    883.2 **With tendon involvement**

√4th **884 Multiple and unspecified open wound of upper limb**
    INCLUDES arm NOS
            multiple sites of one upper limb
            upper limb NOS

    884.0 **Without mention of complication**

    884.1 **Complicated**

    884.2 **With tendon involvement**

√4th **885 Traumatic amputation of thumb (complete) (partial)**
    INCLUDES thumb(s) (with finger(s) of either hand)

    885.0 **Without mention of complication**

    885.1 **Complicated**

√4th **886 Traumatic amputation of other finger(s) (complete) (partial)**
    INCLUDES finger(s) of one or both hands, without mention of thumb(s)

    886.0 **Without mention of complication**

    886.1 **Complicated**

√4th **887 Traumatic amputation of arm and hand (complete) (partial)**

    887.0 **Unilateral, below elbow, without mention of complication** CC MSP
        CC Excl: 880.00-880.29, 881.00-881.22, 882.0-882.2, 883.0-883.2, 884.0-884.2, 885.0-885.1, 886.0-886.1, 887.0-887.7, 929.0, 929.9, 958.8, 959.8-959.9

    887.1 **Unilateral, below elbow, complicated** CC MSP
        CC Excl: See code 887.0

    887.2 **Unilateral, at or above elbow, without mention of complication** CC MSP
        CC Excl: See code 887.0

    887.3 **Unilateral, at or above elbow, complicated** CC MSP
        CC Excl: See code 887.0

    887.4 **Unilateral, level not specified, without mention of complication** CC MSP
        CC Excl: See code 887.0

    887.5 **Unilateral, level not specified, complicated** CC MSP
        CC Excl: See code 887.0

    887.6 **Bilateral [any level], without mention of complication** CC MSP
        One hand and other arm
        CC Excl: See code 887.0

    887.7 **Bilateral [any level], complicated** CC MSP
        CC Excl: See code 887.0

OPEN WOUND OF LOWER LIMB (890-897)

AHA: N-D, '85, 5

√4th **890 Open wound of hip and thigh**

    890.0 **Without mention of complication**

    890.1 **Complicated**

    890.2 **With tendon involvement**

N Newborn Age: 0   P Pediatric Age: 0-17   M Maternity Age: 12-55   A Adult Age: 15-124   CC CC Condition   MC Major Complication   CD Complex Dx   HIV HIV Related Dx

278 — Volume 1   *2002 Ingenix, Inc.*

✓4th **891 Open wound of knee, leg [except thigh], and ankle**
> INCLUDES   leg NOS
> multiple sites of leg, except thigh
> EXCLUDES *that of thigh (890.0-890.2)*
> *with multiple sites of lower limb (894.0-894.2)*

891.0 Without mention of complication
891.1 Complicated
891.2 With tendon involvement

✓4th **892 Open wound of foot except toe(s) alone**
> INCLUDES   heel

892.0 Without mention of complication
892.1 Complicated
892.2 With tendon involvement

✓4th **893 Open wound of toe(s)**
> INCLUDES   toenail

893.0 Without mention of complication
893.1 Complicated
893.2 With tendon involvement

✓4th **894 Multiple and unspecified open wound of lower limb**
> INCLUDES   lower limb NOS
> multiple sites of one lower limb, with thigh

894.0 Without mention of complication
894.1 Complicated
894.2 With tendon involvement

✓4th **895 Traumatic amputation of toe(s) (complete) (partial)**
> INCLUDES   toe(s) of one or both feet

895.0 Without mention of complication
895.1 Complicated

✓4th **896 Traumatic amputation of foot (complete) (partial)**

896.0 Unilateral, without mention of complication CC MSP
> CC Excl: 890.0-890.2, 891.0-891.2, 892.0-892.2, 893.0-893.2, 894.0-894.2, 895.0-895.1, 896.0-896.3, 897.0-897.7, 929.0, 929.9, 958.8, 959.8-959.9

896.1 Unilateral, complicated CC MSP
> CC Excl: See code 896.0

896.2 Bilateral, without mention of complication CC MSP
> EXCLUDES *one foot and other leg (897.6-897.7)*
> CC Excl: See code 896.0

896.3 Bilateral, complicated CC MSP
> CC Excl: See code 896.0

✓4th **897 Traumatic amputation of leg(s) (complete) (partial)**

897.0 Unilateral, below knee, without mention of complication CC MSP
> CC Excl: See code 896.0

897.1 Unilateral, below knee, complicated CC MSP
> CC Excl: See code 896.0

897.2 Unilateral, at or above knee, without mention of complication CC MSP
> CC Excl: See code 896.0

897.3 Unilateral, at or above knee, complicated CC MSP
> CC Excl: See code 896.0

897.4 Unilateral, level not specified, without mention of complication CC MSP
> CC Excl: See code 896.0

897.5 Unilateral, level not specified, complicated CC MSP
> CC Excl: See code 896.0

897.6 Bilateral [any level], without mention of complication CC MSP
> One foot and other leg
> CC Excl: See code 896.0

897.7 Bilateral [any level], complicated CC MSP
> CC Excl: See code 896.0

> AHA: 3Q, '90, 5

INJURY TO BLOOD VESSELS (900-904)

> INCLUDES   arterial hematoma
> avulsion
> cut   of blood vessel,
> laceration   secondary to
> rupture   other injuries
> traumatic aneurysm   e.g., fracture
> or fistula (arteri-   or open
> ovenous)   wound

> EXCLUDES *accidental puncture or laceration during medical procedure (998.2)*
> *intracranial hemorrhage following injury (851.0-854.1)*

> AHA: 3Q, '90, 5

✓4th **900 Injury to blood vessels of head and neck**

✓5th **900.0 Carotid artery**

900.00 Carotid artery, unspecified CC MSP
> CC Excl: 900.00, 900.82, 900.89, 900.9, 904.9, 929.0, 929.9, 958.8, 959.8-959.9

900.01 Common carotid artery CC MSP
> CC Excl: See code 900.00

900.02 External carotid artery CC MSP
> CC Excl: See code 900.00

900.03 Internal carotid artery CC MSP
> CC Excl: See code 900.00

900.1 Internal jugular vein CC MSP
> CC Excl: 900.82, 900.89, 900.9, 904.9, 929.0, 929.9, 958.8, 959.8-959.9

✓5th **900.8 Other specified blood vessels of head and neck**

900.81 External jugular vein CC MSP
> Jugular vein NOS
> CC Excl: See code 900.1

900.82 Multiple blood vessels of head and neck CC MSP
> CC Excl: See code 900.1

900.89 Other CC MSP
> CC Excl: See code 900.1

900.9 Unspecified blood vessel of head and neck CC MSP
> CC Excl: See code 900.1

✓4th **901 Injury to blood vessels of thorax**
> EXCLUDES *traumatic hemothorax (860.2-860.5)*

901.0 Thoracic aorta CC
> CC Excl: 901.0, 904.9, 929.0, 929.9, 958.8, 959.8-959.9

901.1 Innominate and subclavian arteries CC
> CC Excl: 901.1, 904.9, 929.0, 929.9, 958.8, 959.8-959.9

901.2 Superior vena cava CC
> CC Excl: 901.2, 904.9, 929.0, 929.9, 958.8, 959.8-959.9

901.3 Innominate and subclavian veins CC
> CC Excl: 901.3, 904.9, 929.0, 929.9, 958.8, 959.8-959.9

✓5th **901.4 Pulmonary blood vessels**

901.40 Pulmonary vessel(s), unspecified

901.41 Pulmonary artery CC
> CC Excl: 901.40, 901.41, 904.9, 929.0, 929.9, 958.8, 959.8-959.9

901.42 Pulmonary vein CC
> CC Excl: 901.40, 901.42, 904.9, 929.0, 929.9, 958.8, 959.8-959.9

✓5th **901.8 Other specified blood vessels of thorax**

901.81 Intercostal artery or vein

901.82 Internal mammary artery or vein

901.83 Multiple blood vessels of thorax CC
> CC Excl: 904.9, 929.0, 929.9, 958.8, 959.8-959.9

901.89 Other
> Azygos vein
> Hemiazygos vein

✓4th ✓5th Additional Digit Required   Nonspecific PDx   Unacceptable PDx   Manifestation Code   MSP Medicare Secondary Payer   ►◄ Revised Text   ● New Code   ▲ Revised Code Title

2002 Ingenix, Inc.   **Volume 1 — 279**

Injury and Poisoning 901.9–904.1

901.9   Unspecified blood vessel of thorax

√4ᵗʰ **902 Injury to blood vessels of abdomen and pelvis**

902.0   Abdominal aorta   `CC`

CC Excl: 902.0, 902.87, 902.89, 902.9, 904.9, 929.0, 929.9, 958.8, 959.8-959.9

√5ᵗʰ **902.1   Inferior vena cava**

902.10   Inferior vena cava, unspecified   `CC`

CC Excl: 902.10, 902.87, 902.89, 902.9, 904.9, 929.0, 929.9, 958.8, 959.8-959.9

902.11   Hepatic veins   `CC`

CC Excl: 902.11, 902.87, 902.89, 902.9, 904.9, 929.0, 929.9, 958.8, 959.8-959.9

902.19   Other   `CC`

CC Excl: 902.19, 902.87, 902.89, 902.9, 904.9, 929.0, 929.9, 958.8, 959.8-959.9

√5ᵗʰ **902.2   Celiac and mesenteric arteries**

902.20   Celiac and mesenteric arteries, unspecified   `CC`

CC Excl: 902.20, 902.87, 902.89, 902.9, 904.9, 929.0, 929.9, 958.8, 959.8-959.9

902.21   Gastric artery

902.22   Hepatic artery   `CC`

CC Excl: 902.22, 902.87, 902.89, 902.9, 904.9, 929.0, 929.9, 958.8, 959.8-959.9

902.23   Splenic artery   `CC`

CC Excl: 902.23, 902.87, 902.89, 902.9, 904.9, 929.0, 929.9, 958.8, 959.8-959.9

902.24   Other specified branches of celiac axis   `CC`

CC Excl: 902.24, 902.87, 902.89, 902.9, 904.9, 929.0, 929.9, 958.8, 959.8-959.9

902.25   Superior mesenteric artery (trunk)   `CC`

CC Excl: 902.25, 902.87, 902.89, 902.9, 904.9, 929.0, 929.9, 958.8, 959.8-959.9

902.26   Primary branches of superior mesenteric artery   `CC`
          Ileocolic artery

CC Excl: 902.26, 902.87, 902.89, 902.9, 904.9, 929.0, 929.9, 958.8, 959.8-959.9

902.27   Inferior mesenteric artery   `CC`

CC Excl: 902.7, 902.87, 902.89, 902.9, 904.9, 929.0, 929.9, 958.8, 959.8-959.9

902.29   Other   `CC`

CC Excl: 902.29, 902.87, 902.89, 902.9, 904.9, 929.0, 929.9, 958.8, 959.8-959.9

√5ᵗʰ **902.3   Portal and splenic veins**

902.31   Superior mesenteric vein and primary subdivisions   `CC`
          Ileocolic vein

CC Excl: 902.31, 902.87, 902.89, 902.9, 904.9, 929.0, 929.9, 958.8, 959.8-959.9

902.32   Inferior mesenteric vein   `CC`

CC Excl: 902.32, 902.87, 902.89, 902.9, 904.9, 929.0, 929.9, 958.8, 959.8-959.9

902.33   Portal vein   `CC`

CC Excl: 902.33, 902.87, 902.89, 902.9, 904.9, 929.0, 929.9, 958.8, 959.8-959.9

902.34   Splenic vein   `CC`

CC Excl: 902.34, 902.87, 902.89, 902.9, 904.9, 929.0, 929.9, 958.8, 959.8-959.9

902.39   Other   `CC`
          Cystic vein   Gastric vein

CC Excl: 902.39, 902.87, 902.89, 902.9, 904.9, 929.0, 929.9, 958.8, 959.8-959.9

√5ᵗʰ **902.4   Renal blood vessels**

902.40   Renal vessel(s), unspecified   `CC`

CC Excl: 902.40, 902.87, 902.89, 902.9, 904.9, 929.0, 929.9, 958.8, 959.8-959.9

902.41   Renal artery   `CC`

CC Excl: 902.41, 902.87, 902.89, 902.9, 904.9, 929.0, 929.9, 958.8, 959.8-959.9

902.42   Renal vein   `CC`

CC Excl: 902.42, 902.87, 902.89, 902.9, 904.9, 929.0, 929.9, 958.8, 959.8-959.9

902.49   Other   `CC`
          Suprarenal arteries

CC Excl: 902.49, 902.87, 902.89, 902.9, 904.9, 929.0, 929.9, 958.8, 959.8-959.9

√5ᵗʰ **902.5   Iliac blood vessels**

902.50   Iliac vessel(s), unspecified   `CC`

CC Excl: 902.50, 902.53-902.54, 902.59, 902.87, 902.89, 902.9, 904.9, 929.0, 929.9, 958.8, 959.8-959.9

902.51   Hypogastric artery   `CC`

CC Excl: 902.51, 902.87, 902.89, 902.9, 904.9, 929.0, 929.9, 958.8, 959.8-959.9

902.52   Hypogastric vein   `CC`

CC Excl: 902.52, 902.87, 902.89, 902.9, 904.9, 929.0, 929.9, 958.8, 959.8-959.9

902.53   Iliac artery   `CC`

CC Excl: 902.50, 902.53, 902.59, 902.87, 902.89, 902.9, 904.9, 929.0, 929.9, 958.8, 959.8-959.9

902.54   Iliac vein   `CC`

CC Excl: 902.50, 902.54, 902.59, 902.87, 902.89, 902.9, 904.9, 929.0, 929.9, 958.8, 959.8-959.9

902.55   Uterine artery   ♀

902.56   Uterine vein   ♀

902.59   Other   `CC`

CC Excl: 902.50, 902.53-902.54, 902.59, 902.87, 902.89, 902.9, 904.9, 929.0, 929.9, 958.8, 959.8-959.9

√5ᵗʰ **902.8   Other specified blood vessels of abdomen and pelvis**

902.81   Ovarian artery   ♀

902.82   Ovarian vein   ♀

902.87   Multiple blood vessels of abdomen and pelvis   `CC`

CC Excl: 902.87, 902.89, 902.9, 904.9, 929.0, 929.9, 958.8, 959.8-959.9

902.89   Other

902.9   Unspecified blood vessel of abdomen and pelvis

√4ᵗʰ **903 Injury to blood vessels of upper extremity**

√5ᵗʰ **903.0   Axillary blood vessels**

903.00   Axillary vessel(s), unspecified

903.01   Axillary artery

903.02   Axillary vein

903.1   Brachial blood vessels

903.2   Radial blood vessels

903.3   Ulnar blood vessels

903.4   Palmar artery

903.5   Digital blood vessels

903.8   Other specified blood vessels of upper extremity
          Multiple blood vessels of upper extremity

903.9   Unspecified blood vessel of upper extremity

√4ᵗʰ **904 Injury to blood vessels of lower extremity and unspecified sites**

904.0   Common femoral artery   `CC`
          Femoral artery above profunda origin

CC Excl: No exclusions

904.1   Superficial femoral artery

N Newborn Age: 0   P Pediatric Age: 0-17   M Maternity Age: 12-55   A Adult Age: 15-124   `CC` CC Condition   `MC` Major Complication   `CD` Complex Dx   `HIV` HIV Related Dx

904.2 **Femoral veins**

904.3 **Saphenous veins**
Saphenous vein (greater) (lesser)

✓5th 904.4 **Popliteal blood vessels**
904.40 **Popliteal vessel(s), unspecified**
904.41 **Popliteal artery**
904.42 **Popliteal vein**

✓5th 904.5 **Tibial blood vessels**
904.50 **Tibial vessel(s), unspecified**
904.51 **Anterior tibial artery**
904.52 **Anterior tibial vein**
904.53 **Posterior tibial artery**
904.54 **Posterior tibial vein**

904.6 **Deep plantar blood vessels**

904.7 **Other specified blood vessels of lower extremity**
Multiple blood vessels of lower extremity

904.8 **Unspecified blood vessel of lower extremity**

904.9 **Unspecified site**
Injury to blood vessel NOS

LATE EFFECTS OF INJURIES, POISONINGS, TOXIC EFFECTS, AND OTHER EXTERNAL CAUSES (905-909)

Note: These categories are to be used to indicate conditions classifiable to 800-999 as the cause of late effects, which are themselves classified elsewhere. The "late effects" include those specified as such, or as sequelae, which may occur at any time after the acute injury.

✓4th **905 Late effects of musculoskeletal and connective tissue injuries**
AHA: 1Q, '95, 10; 2Q, '94, 3

905.0 **Late effect of fracture of skull and face bones**
Late effect of injury classifiable to 800-804
AHA: 3Q, '97, 12

905.1 **Late effect of fracture of spine and trunk without mention of spinal cord lesion**
Late effect of injury classifiable to 805, 807-809

905.2 **Late effect of fracture of upper extremities**
Late effect of injury classifiable to 810-819

905.3 **Late effect of fracture of neck of femur**
Late effect of injury classifiable to 820

905.4 **Late effect of fracture of lower extremities**
Late effect of injury classifiable to 821-827

905.5 **Late effect of fracture of multiple and unspecified bones**
Late effect of injury classifiable to 828-829

905.6 **Late effect of dislocation**
Late effect of injury classifiable to 830-839

905.7 **Late effect of sprain and strain without mention of tendon injury**
Late effect of injury classifiable to 840-848, except tendon injury

905.8 **Late effect of tendon injury**
Late effect of tendon injury due to:
open wound [injury classifiable to 880-884 with .2, 890-894 with .2]
sprain and strain [injury classifiable to 840-848]
AHA: 2Q, '89, 13; 2Q, '89, 15

905.9 **Late effect of traumatic amputation**
Late effect of injury classifiable to 885-887, 895-897
EXCLUDES late amputation stump complication (997.60-997.69)

✓4th **906 Late effects of injuries to skin and subcutaneous tissues**
906.0 **Late effect of open wound of head, neck, and trunk**
Late effect of injury classifiable to 870-879

906.1 **Late effect of open wound of extremities without mention of tendon injury**
Late effect of injury classifiable to 880-884, 890-894 except .2

906.2 **Late effect of superficial injury**
Late effect of injury classifiable to 910-919

906.3 **Late effect of contusion**
Late effect of injury classifiable to 920-924

906.4 **Late effect of crushing**
Late effect of injury classifiable to 925-929

906.5 **Late effect of burn of eye, face, head, and neck**
Late effect of injury classifiable to 940-941

906.6 **Late effect of burn of wrist and hand**
Late effect of injury classifiable to 944
AHA: 4Q, '94, 22

906.7 **Late effect of burn of other extremities**
Late effect of injury classifiable to 943 or 945
AHA: 4Q, '94, 22

906.8 **Late effect of burns of other specified sites**
Late effect of injury classifiable to 942, 946-947
AHA: 4Q, '94, 22

906.9 **Late effect of burn of unspecified site**
Late effect of injury classifiable to 948-949
AHA: 4Q, '94, 22

✓4th **907 Late effects of injuries to the nervous system**
907.0 **Late effect of intracranial injury without mention of skull fracture**
Late effect of injury classifiable to 850-854
AHA: 3Q, '90, 14

907.1 **Late effect of injury to cranial nerve**
Late effect of injury classifiable to 950-951

907.2 **Late effect of spinal cord injury**
Late effect of injury classifiable to 806, 952
AHA: 4Q, '98, 38

907.3 **Late effect of injury to nerve root(s), spinal plexus(es), and other nerves of trunk**
Late effect of injury classifiable to 953-954

907.4 **Late effect of injury to peripheral nerve of shoulder girdle and upper limb**
Late effect of injury classifiable to 955

907.5 **Late effect of injury to peripheral nerve of pelvic girdle and lower limb**
Late effect of injury classifiable to 956

907.9 **Late effect of injury to other and unspecified nerve**
Late effect of injury classifiable to 957

✓4th **908 Late effects of other and unspecified injuries**
908.0 **Late effect of internal injury to chest**
Late effect of injury classifiable to 860-862

908.1 **Late effect of internal injury to intra-abdominal organs**
Late effect of injury classifiable to 863-866, 868

908.2 **Late effect of internal injury to other internal organs**
Late effect of injury classifiable to 867 or 869

908.3 **Late effect of injury to blood vessel of head, neck, and extremities**
Late effect of injury classifiable to 900, 903-904

908.4 **Late effect of injury to blood vessel of thorax, abdomen, and pelvis**
Late effect of injury classifiable to 901-902

908.5 **Late effect of foreign body in orifice**
Late effect of injury classifiable to 930-939

908.6 **Late effect of certain complications of trauma**
Late effect of complications classifiable to 958

908.9 **Late effect of unspecified injury**
Late effect of injury classifiable to 959
AHA: 3Q, '00, 4

✓4th **909 Late effects of other and unspecified external causes**
909.0 **Late effect of poisoning due to drug, medicinal or biological substance**
Late effect of conditions classifiable to 960-979
EXCLUDES late effect of adverse effect of drug, medicinal or biological substance (909.5)

2002 Ingenix, Inc.

Additional Digit Required · Nonspecific PDx · Unacceptable PDx · Manifestation Code · **MSP** Medicare Secondary Payer · ▶◀ Revised Text · ● New Code · ▲ Revised Code Title

Injury and Poisoning 904.2–909.0

Volume 1 — 281

Injury and Poisoning 909.1–915.4

909.1 Late effect of toxic effects of nonmedical substances
    Late effect of conditions classifiable to 980-989

909.2 Late effect of radiation
    Late effect of conditions classifiable to 990

909.3 Late effect of complications of surgical and medical care
    Late effect of conditions classifiable to 996-999
    AHA: 1Q, '93, 29

909.4 Late effect of certain other external causes
    Late effect of conditions classifiable to 991-994

909.5 Late effect of adverse effect of drug, medical or biological substance
    EXCLUDES   *late effect of poisoning due to drug, medicinal or biological substance (909.0)*
    AHA: 4Q, '94, 48

909.9 Late effect of other and unspecified external causes

SUPERFICIAL INJURY (910-919)

EXCLUDES   *burn (blisters) (940.0-949.5)*
contusion (920-924.9)
foreign body:
    granuloma (728.82)
    inadvertently left in operative wound (998.4)
    residual in soft tissue (729.6)
insect bite, venomous (989.5)
open wound with incidental foreign body (870.0-897.7)

AHA: 2Q, '89, 15

√4th **910 Superficial injury of face, neck, and scalp except eye**
    INCLUDES   cheek   lip
                     ear   nose
                      gum   throat
    EXCLUDES   *eye and adnexa (918.0-918.9)*

910.0 Abrasion or friction burn without mention of infection

910.1 Abrasion or friction burn, infected

910.2 Blister without mention of infection

910.3 Blister, infected

910.4 Insect bite, nonvenomous, without mention of infection

910.5 Insect bite, nonvenomous, infected

910.6 Superficial foreign body (splinter) without major open wound and without mention of infection

910.7 Superficial foreign body (splinter) without major open wound, infected

910.8 Other and unspecified superficial injury of face, neck, and scalp without mention of infection

910.9 Other and unspecified superficial injury of face, neck, and scalp, infected

√4th **911 Superficial injury of trunk**
    INCLUDES   abdominal wall   interscapular region
                      anus   labium (majus) (minus)
                      back   penis
                      breast   perineum
                      buttock   scrotum
                      chest wall   testis
                      flank   vagina
                      groin   vulva
    EXCLUDES   *hip (916.0-916.9)*
                        scapular region (912.0-912.9)

911.0 Abrasion or friction burn without mention of infection
    AHA: ▶ 3Q, '01, 10 ◀

911.1 Abrasion or friction burn, infected

911.2 Blister without mention of infection

911.3 Blister, infected

911.4 Insect bite, nonvenomous, without mention of infection

911.5 Insect bite, nonvenomous, infected

911.6 Superficial foreign body (splinter) without major open wound and without mention of infection

911.7 Superficial foreign body (splinter) without major open wound, infected

911.8 Other and unspecified superficial injury of trunk without mention of infection

911.9 Other and unspecified superficial injury of trunk, infected

√4th **912 Superficial injury of shoulder and upper arm**
    INCLUDES   axilla   scapular region

912.0 Abrasion or friction burn without mention of infection

912.1 Abrasion or friction burn, infected

912.2 Blister without mention of infection

912.3 Blister, infected

912.4 Insect bite, nonvenomous, without mention of infection

912.5 Insect bite, nonvenomous, infected

912.6 Superficial foreign body (splinter) without major open wound and without mention of infection

912.7 Superficial foreign body (splinter) without major open wound, infected

912.8 Other and unspecified superficial injury of shoulder and upper arm without mention of infection

912.9 Other and unspecified superficial injury of shoulder and upper arm, infected

√4th **913 Superficial injury of elbow, forearm, and wrist**

913.0 Abrasion or friction burn without mention of infection

913.1 Abrasion or friction burn, infected

913.2 Blister without mention of infection

913.3 Blister, infected

913.4 Insect bite, nonvenomous, without mention of infection

913.5 Insect bite, nonvenomous, infected

913.6 Superficial foreign body (splinter) without major open wound and without mention of infection

913.7 Superficial foreign body (splinter) without major open wound, infected

913.8 Other and unspecified superficial injury of elbow, forearm, and wrist without mention of infection

913.9 Other and unspecified superficial injury of elbow, forearm, and wrist, infected

√4th **914 Superficial injury of hand(s) except finger(s) alone**

914.0 Abrasion or friction burn without mention of infection

914.1 Abrasion or friction burn, infected

914.2 Blister without mention of infection

914.3 Blister, infected

914.4 Insect bite, nonvenomous, without mention of infection

914.5 Insect bite, nonvenomous, infected

914.6 Superficial foreign body (splinter) without major open wound and without mention of infection

914.7 Superficial foreign body (splinter) without major open wound, infected

914.8 Other and unspecified superficial injury of hand without mention of infection

914.9 Other and unspecified superficial injury of hand, infected

√4th **915 Superficial injury of finger(s)**
    INCLUDES   fingernail   thumb (nail)

915.0 Abrasion or friction burn without mention of infection

915.1 Abrasion or friction burn, infected

915.2 Blister without mention of infection

915.3 Blister, infected

915.4 Insect bite, nonvenomous, without mention of infection

| N Newborn Age: 0 | P Pediatric Age: 0-17 | M Maternity Age: 12-55 | A Adult Age: 15-124 | CC CC Condition | MC Major Complication | CD Complex Dx | HIV HIV Related Dx |

282 — Volume 1 • January 2002   *2002 Ingenix, Inc.*

915.5   Insect bite, nonvenomous, infected

915.6   Superficial foreign body (splinter) without major open wound and without mention of infection

915.7   Superficial foreign body (splinter) without major open wound, infected

915.8   Other and unspecified superficial injury of fingers without mention of infection
> AHA: ▶3Q, '01, 10◀

915.9   Other and unspecified superficial injury of fingers, infected

✓4th **916 Superficial injury of hip, thigh, leg, and ankle**

916.0   Abrasion or friction burn without mention of infection

916.1   Abrasion or friction burn, infected

916.2   Blister without mention of infection

916.3   Blister, infected

916.4   Insect bite, nonvenomous, without mention of infection

916.5   Insect bite, nonvenomous, infected

916.6   Superficial foreign body (splinter) without major open wound and without mention of infection

916.7   Superficial foreign body (splinter) without major open wound, infected

916.8   Other and unspecified superficial injury of hip, thigh, leg, and ankle without mention of infection

916.9   Other and unspecified superficial injury of hip, thigh, leg, and ankle, infected

✓4th **917 Superficial injury of foot and toe(s)**
> INCLUDES   heel   toenail

917.0   Abrasion or friction burn without mention of infection

917.1   Abrasion or friction burn, infected

917.2   Blister without mention of infection

917.3   Blister, infected

917.4   Insect bite, nonvenomous, without mention of infection

917.5   Insect bite, nonvenomous, infected

917.6   Superficial foreign body (splinter) without major open wound and without mention of infection

917.7   Superficial foreign body (splinter) without major open wound, infected

917.8   Other and unspecified superficial injury of foot and toes without mention of infection

917.9   Other and unspecified superficial injury of foot and toes, infected

✓4th **918 Superficial injury of eye and adnexa**
> EXCLUDES   burn (940.0-940.9)
> foreign body on external eye (930.0-930.9)

918.0   Eyelids and periocular area
> Abrasion   Superficial foreign body
> Insect bite   (splinter)

918.1   Cornea
> Corneal abrasion   Superficial laceration
> EXCLUDES   corneal injury due to contact lens (371.82)

918.2   Conjunctiva

918.9   Other and unspecified superficial injuries of eye
> Eye (ball) NOS

✓4th **919 Superficial injury of other, multiple, and unspecified sites**
> EXCLUDES   multiple sites classifiable to the same three-digit category (910.0-918.9)

919.0   Abrasion or friction burn without mention of infection

919.1   Abrasion or friction burn, infected

919.2   Blister without mention of infection

919.3   Blister, infected

919.4   Insect bite, nonvenomous, without mention of infection

919.5   Insect bite, nonvenomous, infected

919.6   Superficial foreign body (splinter) without major open wound and without mention of infection

919.7   Superficial foreign body (splinter) without major open wound, infected

919.8   Other and unspecified superficial injury without mention of infection

919.9   Other and unspecified superficial injury, infected

CONTUSION WITH INTACT SKIN SURFACE (920-924)

> INCLUDES   bruise } without fracture or open
> hematoma }   wound

> EXCLUDES   concussion (850.0-850.9)
> hemarthrosis (840.0-848.9)
> internal organs (860.0-869.1)
> that incidental to:
>   crushing injury (925-929.9)
>   dislocation (830.0-839.9)
>   fracture (800.0-829.1)
>   internal injury (860.0-869.1)
>   intracranial injury (850.0-854.1)
>   nerve injury (950.0-957.9)
>   open wound (870.0-897.7)

920 Contusion of face, scalp, and neck except eye(s)
> Cheek   Mandibular joint area
> Ear (auricle)   Nose
> Gum   Throat
> Lip

✓4th **921 Contusion of eye and adnexa**

921.0   Black eye, not otherwise specified

921.1   Contusion of eyelids and periocular area

921.2   Contusion of orbital tissues

921.3   Contusion of eyeball
> AHA: J-A, '85, 16

921.9   Unspecified contusion of eye
> Injury of eye NOS

✓4th **922 Contusion of trunk**

922.0   Breast

922.1   Chest wall

922.2   Abdominal wall
> Flank   Groin

✓5th **922.3**   Back
> AHA: 4Q, '96, 39

     922.31 Back
> EXCLUDES   interscapular region (922.33)
> AHA: 3Q, '99, 14

     922.32 Buttock

     922.33 Interscapular region

922.4   Genital organs
> Labium (majus) (minus)   Vulva
> Penis   Vagina
> Perineum   Testis
> Scrotum

922.8   Multiple sites of trunk

922.9   Unspecified part
> Trunk NOS

✓4th **923 Contusion of upper limb**

✓5th **923.0**   Shoulder and upper arm

     923.00 Shoulder region

     923.01 Scapular region

     923.02 Axillary region

     923.03 Upper arm

     923.09 Multiple sites

✓5th **923.1**   Elbow and forearm

     923.10 Forearm

     923.11 Elbow

✓5th **923.2**   Wrist and hand(s), except finger(s) alone

     923.20 Hand(s)

     923.21 Wrist

Additional Digit Required   Nonspecific PDx   Unacceptable PDx   Manifestation Code   **MSP** Medicare Secondary Payer   ▶◀ Revised Text   ● New Code   ▲ Revised Code Title

2002 Ingenix, Inc.   **January 2002 • Volume 1 — 283**

923.3 **Finger**
Fingernail   Thumb (nail)
923.8 **Multiple sites of upper limb**
923.9 **Unspecified part of upper limb**
Arm NOS
√4ᵗʰ 924 **Contusion of lower limb and of other and unspecified sites**
√5ᵗʰ 924.0 **Hip and thigh**
924.00 **Thigh**
924.01 **Hip**
√5ᵗʰ 924.1 **Knee and lower leg**
924.10 **Lower leg**
924.11 **Knee**
√5ᵗʰ 924.2 **Ankle and foot, excluding toe(s)**
924.20 **Foot**
Heel
924.21 **Ankle**
924.3 **Toe**
Toenail
924.4 **Multiple sites of lower limb**
924.5 **Unspecified part of lower limb**
Leg NOS
924.8 **Multiple sites, not elsewhere classified**
924.9 **Unspecified site**

CRUSHING INJURY (925-929)

EXCLUDES concussion (850.0-850.9)
fractures (800-829)
internal organs (860.0-869.1)
that incidental to:
internal injury (860.0-869.1)
intracranial injury (850.0-854.1)

AHA: 2Q, '93, 7

√4ᵗʰ 925 **Crushing injury of face, scalp, and neck**
Cheek   Pharynx
Ear   Throat
Larynx
925.1 **Crushing injury of face and scalp**   CC MSP
Cheek   Ear
CC Excl: 873.8-873.9, 905.0, 925.1-925.2, 929.0, 929.9, 958.8, 959.01, 959.09, 959.8-959.9
925.2 **Crushing injury of neck**   CC MSP
Larynx   Throat
Pharynx
CC Excl: 873.8-873.9, 905.0, 925.1-925.2, 929.0, 929.9, 958.8, 959.01, 959.09, 959.8-959.9
√4ᵗʰ 926 **Crushing injury of trunk**
EXCLUDES crush injury of internal organs (860.0-869.1)
926.0 **External genitalia**
Labium (majus) (minus)   Testis
Penis   Vulva
Scrotum
√5ᵗʰ 926.1 **Other specified sites**
926.11 **Back**
926.12 **Buttock**
926.19 **Other**
Breast
EXCLUDES crushing of chest (860.0-862.9)
926.8 **Multiple sites of trunk**   MSP
926.9 **Unspecified site**
Trunk NOS
√4ᵗʰ 927 **Crushing injury of upper limb**
√5ᵗʰ 927.0 **Shoulder and upper arm**
927.00 **Shoulder region**
927.01 **Scapular region**
927.02 **Axillary region**
927.03 **Upper arm**
927.09 **Multiple sites**
√5ᵗʰ 927.1 **Elbow and forearm**

927.10 **Forearm**
927.11 **Elbow**
√5ᵗʰ 927.2 **Wrist and hand(s), except finger(s) alone**
927.20 **Hand(s)**
927.21 **Wrist**
927.3 **Finger(s)**
927.8 **Multiple sites of upper limb**
927.9 **Unspecified site**
Arm NOS
√4ᵗʰ 928 **Crushing injury of lower limb**
√5ᵗʰ 928.0 **Hip and thigh**
928.00 **Thigh**
928.01 **Hip**
√5ᵗʰ 928.1 **Knee and lower leg**
928.10 **Lower leg**
928.11 **Knee**
√5ᵗʰ 928.2 **Ankle and foot, excluding toe(s) alone**
928.20 **Foot**
Heel
928.21 **Ankle**
928.3 **Toe(s)**
928.8 **Multiple sites of lower limb**
928.9 **Unspecified site**
Leg NOS
√4ᵗʰ 929 **Crushing injury of multiple and unspecified sites**
EXCLUDES multiple internal injury NOS (869.0-869.1)
929.0 **Multiple sites, not elsewhere classified**   CC MSP
CC Excl: 929.0, 929.9, 958.8, 959.8-959.9
929.9 **Unspecified site**   MSP

EFFECTS OF FOREIGN BODY ENTERING THROUGH ORIFICE (930-939)

EXCLUDES foreign body:
granuloma (728.82)
inadvertently left in operative wound (998.4, 998.7)
in open wound (800-839, 851-897)
residual in soft tissues (729.6)
superficial without major open wound (910-919 with .6 or .7)

√4ᵗʰ 930 **Foreign body on external eye**
EXCLUDES foreign body in penetrating wound of:
eyeball (871.5-871.6)
retained (old) (360.5-360.6)
ocular adnexa (870.4)
retained (old) (376.6)
930.0 **Corneal foreign body**
930.1 **Foreign body in conjunctival sac**
930.2 **Foreign body in lacrimal punctum**
930.8 **Other and combined sites**
930.9 **Unspecified site**
External eye NOS
931 **Foreign body in ear**
Auditory canal   Auricle
932 **Foreign body in nose**
Nasal sinus   Nostril
√4ᵗʰ 933 **Foreign body in pharynx and larynx**
933.0 **Pharynx**
Nasopharynx   Throat NOS
933.1 **Larynx**
Asphyxia due to foreign body
Choking due to:
food (regurgitated)
phlegm
√4ᵗʰ 934 **Foreign body in trachea, bronchus, and lung**
934.0 **Trachea**
934.1 **Main bronchus**
934.8 **Other specified parts**
Bronchioles   Lung

N Newborn Age: 0   P Pediatric Age: 0-17   M Maternity Age: 12-55   A Adult Age: 15-124   CC CC Condition   MC Major Complication   CD Complex Dx   HIV HIV Related Dx

934.9   Respiratory tree, unspecified
Inhalation of liquid or vomitus, lower respiratory tract NOS

935 Foreign body in mouth, esophagus, and stomach
935.0   Mouth
935.1   Esophagus
AHA: 1Q, '88, 13

935.2   Stomach
936 Foreign body in intestine and colon
937 Foreign body in anus and rectum
Rectosigmoid (junction)
938 Foreign body in digestive system, unspecified
Alimentary tract NOS
Swallowed foreign body
939 Foreign body in genitourinary tract
939.0   Bladder and urethra
939.1   Uterus, any part ♀
EXCLUDES   intrauterine contraceptive device:
complications from (996.32, 996.65)
presence of (V45.51)

939.2   Vulva and vagina ♀
939.3   Penis ♂
939.9   Unspecified site

BURNS (940-949)

INCLUDES   burns from:
electrical heating appliance
electricity
flame
hot object
lightning
radiation
chemical burns (external) (internal)
scalds

EXCLUDES   friction burns (910-919 with .0, .1)
sunburn (692.71, 692.76-692.77)

AHA: 4Q, 94, 22; 2Q, '90, 7; 4Q, '88, 3; M-A, '86, 9

940 Burn confined to eye and adnexa
940.0   Chemical burn of eyelids and periocular area
940.1   Other burns of eyelids and periocular area
940.2   Alkaline chemical burn of cornea and conjunctival sac
940.3   Acid chemical burn of cornea and conjunctival sac
940.4   Other burn of cornea and conjunctival sac
940.5   Burn with resulting rupture and destruction of eyeball
940.9   Unspecified burn of eye and adnexa
941 Burn of face, head, and neck
EXCLUDES   mouth (947.0)
The following fifth-digit subclassification is for use with category 941:
0   face and head, unspecified site
1   ear [any part]
2   eye (with other parts of face, head, and neck)
3   lip(s)
4   chin
5   nose (septum)
6   scalp [any part]
    Temple (region)
7   forehead and cheek
8   neck
9   multiple sites [except with eye] of face, head, and neck

AHA: 4Q, '94, 22; M-A, '86, 9

941.0   Unspecified degree
941.1   Erythema [first degree]
941.2   Blisters, epidermal loss [second degree]
941.3   Full-thickness skin loss [third degree NOS]

941.4   Deep necrosis of underlying tissues [deep third degree] without mention of loss of a body part
941.5   Deep necrosis of underlying tissues [deep third degree] with loss of a body part
942 Burn of trunk
EXCLUDES   scapular region (943.0-943.5 with fifth-digit 6)
The following fifth-digit subclassification is for use with category 942:
0   trunk, unspecified site
1   breast
2   chest wall, excluding breast and nipple
3   abdominal wall
    Flank   Groin
4   back [any part]
    Buttock
    Interscapular region
5   genitalia
    Labium (majus) (minus)   Scrotum
    Penis   Testis
    Perineum   Vulva
9   other and multiple sites of trunk

AHA: 4Q, '94, 22; M-A, '86, 9

942.0   Unspecified degree
942.1   Erythema [first degree]
942.2   Blisters, epidermal loss [second degree]
942.3   Full-thickness skin loss [third degree NOS]
942.4   Deep necrosis of underlying tissues [deep third degree] without mention of loss of a body part
942.5   Deep necrosis of underlying tissues [deep third degree] with loss of a body part
943 Burn of upper limb, except wrist and hand
The following fifth-digit subclassification is for use with category 943:
0   upper limb, unspecified site
1   forearm
2   elbow
3   upper arm
4   axilla
5   shoulder
6   scapular region
9   multiple sites of upper limb, except wrist and hand

AHA: 4Q, '94, 22; M-A, '86, 9

943.0   Unspecified degree
943.1   Erythema [first degree]
943.2   Blisters, epidermal loss [second degree]
943.3   Full-thickness skin loss [third degree NOS]
943.4   Deep necrosis of underlying tissues [deep third degree] without mention of loss of a body part
943.5   Deep necrosis of underlying tissues [deep third degree] with loss of a body part
944 Burn of wrist(s) and hand(s)
The following fifth-digit subclassification is for use with category 944:
0   hand, unspecified site
1   single digit [finger (nail)] other than thumb
2   thumb (nail)
3   two or more digits, not including thumb
4   two or more digits including thumb
5   palm
6   back of hand
7   wrist
8   multiple sites of wrist(s) and hand(s)

944.0   Unspecified degree
944.1   Erythema [first degree]
944.2   Blisters, epidermal loss [second degree]
944.3   Full-thickness skin loss [third degree NOS]
944.4   Deep necrosis of underlying tissues [deep third degree] without mention of loss of a body part

✓5th **944.5** Deep necrosis of underlying tissues [deep third degree] with loss of a body part

✓4th **945** Burn of lower limb(s)

The following fifth-digit subclassification is for use with category 945:

  0 lower limb [leg], unspecified site
  1 toe(s) (nail)
  2 foot
  3 ankle
  4 lower leg
  5 knee
  6 thigh [any part]
  9 multiple sites of lower limb(s)

AHA: 4Q, '94, 22; M-A, '86, 9

✓5th **945.0** Unspecified degree
✓5th **945.1** Erythema [first degree]
✓5th **945.2** Blisters, epidermal loss [second degree]
✓5th **945.3** Full-thickness skin loss [third degree NOS]
✓5th **945.4** Deep necrosis of underlying tissues [deep third degree] without mention of loss of a body part
✓5th **945.5** Deep necrosis of underlying tissues [deep third degree] with loss of a body part

✓4th **946** Burns of multiple specified sites

INCLUDES burns of sites classifiable to more than one three-digit category in 940-945
EXCLUDES multiple burns NOS (949.0-949.5)

AHA: 4Q, '94, 22; M-A, '86, 9

946.0 Unspecified degree
946.1 Erythema [first degree]
946.2 Blisters, epidermal loss [second degree]
946.3 Full-thickness skin loss [third degree NOS]
946.4 Deep necrosis of underlying tissues [deep third degree] without mention of loss of a body part
946.5 Deep necrosis of underlying tissues [deep third degree] with loss of a body part

✓4th **947** Burn of internal organs

INCLUDES burns from chemical agents (ingested)
AHA: 4Q, '94, 22; M-A, '86, 9

947.0 Mouth and pharynx
  Gum　　　　Tongue
947.1 Larynx, trachea, and lung
947.2 Esophagus
947.3 Gastrointestinal tract
  Colon　　　　Small intestine
  Rectum　　　Stomach
947.4 Vagina and uterus　　　　♀
947.8 Other specified sites
947.9 Unspecified site

✓4th **948** Burns classified according to extent of body surface involved

Note: This category is to be used when the site of the burn is unspecified, or with categories 940-947 when the site is specified.
EXCLUDES sunburn (692.71, 692.76-692.77)

The following fifth-digit subclassification is for use with category 948 to indicate the percent of body surface with third degree burn; valid digits are in [brackets] under each code:

  0 less than 10 percent or unspecified
  1 10-19%
  2 20-29%
  3 30-39%
  4 40-49%
  5 50-59%
  6 60-69%
  7 70-79%
  8 80-89%
  9 90% or more of body surface

AHA: 4Q, '94, 22; 4Q, '88, 3; M-A, '86, 9; N-D, '84, 13

Burns
Degrees of Burns

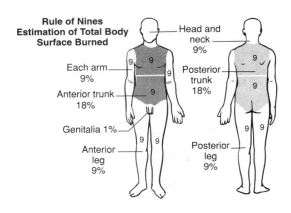

Rule of Nines
Estimation of Total Body Surface Burned

✓5th **948.0** [0] Burn [any degree] involving less than 10 percent of body surface
✓5th **948.1** [0-1] 10-19 percent of body surface
✓5th **948.2** [0-2] 20-29 percent of body surface
✓5th **948.3** [0-3] 30-39 percent of body surface
✓5th **948.4** [0-4] 40-49 percent of body surface
✓5th **948.5** [0-5] 50-59 percent of body surface
✓5th **948.6** [0-6] 60-69 percent of body surface
✓5th **948.7** [0-7] 70-79 percent of body surface
✓5th **948.8** [0-8] 80-89 percent of body surface
✓5th **948.9** [0-9] 90 percent or more of body surface

✓4th **949** Burn, unspecified

INCLUDES burn NOS multiple burns NOS
EXCLUDES burn of unspecified site but with statement of the extent of body surface involved (948.0-948.9)

AHA: 4Q, '94, 22; M-A, '86, 9

949.0 Unspecified degree
949.1 Erythema [first degree]
949.2 Blisters, epidermal loss [second degree]
949.3 Full-thickness skin loss [third degree NOS]
949.4 Deep necrosis of underlying tissues [deep third degree] without mention of loss of a body part
949.5 Deep necrosis of underlying tissues [deep third degree] with loss of a body part

INJURY TO NERVES AND SPINAL CORD (950-957)

INCLUDES division of nerve
lesion in continuity
traumatic neuroma
traumatic transient paralysis
(with open wound)

EXCLUDES accidental puncture or laceration during medical procedure (998.2)

√4ᵗʰ **950 Injury to optic nerve and pathways**

950.0 Optic nerve injury
Second cranial nerve

950.1 Injury to optic chiasm

950.2 Injury to optic pathways

950.3 Injury to visual cortex

950.9 Unspecified
Traumatic blindness NOS

√4ᵗʰ **951 Injury to other cranial nerve(s)**

951.0 Injury to oculomotor nerve
Third cranial nerve

951.1 Injury to trochlear nerve
Fourth cranial nerve

951.2 Injury to trigeminal nerve
Fifth cranial nerve

951.3 Injury to abducens nerve
Sixth cranial nerve

951.4 Injury to facial nerve
Seventh cranial nerve

951.5 Injury to acoustic nerve
Auditory nerve
Eighth cranial nerve
Traumatic deafness NOS

951.6 Injury to accessory nerve
Eleventh cranial nerve

951.7 Injury to hypoglossal nerve
Twelfth cranial nerve

951.8 Injury to other specified cranial nerves
Glossopharyngeal [9th cranial] nerve
Olfactory [1st cranial] nerve
Pneumogastric [10th cranial] nerve
Traumatic anosmia NOS
Vagus [10th cranial] nerve

951.9 Injury to unspecified cranial nerve

√4ᵗʰ **952 Spinal cord injury without evidence of spinal bone injury**

√5ᵗʰ **952.0 Cervical**

952.00 C_1-C_4 level with unspecified spinal cord cc
injury
Spinal cord injury, cervical region NOS
CC Excl: 805.00-805.18, 805.8-805.9, 806.00-806.19, 806.8-806.9, 839.00-839.18, 839.40, 839.49-839.50, 839.59, 839.69, 839.79, 839.8-839.9, 847.9, 905.1, 926.11, 952.00-952.09, 952.8-952.9, 958.8, 959.1, 959.8-959.9

Spinal Nerve Roots

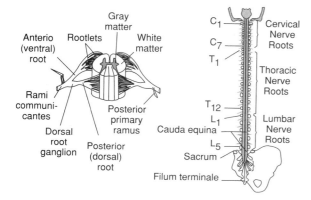

√5ᵗʰ **952.1 Dorsal [thoracic]**

952.10 T_1-T_6 level with unspecified spinal cord cc
injury
Spinal cord injury, thoracic region NOS
CC Excl: 805.8-805.9, 806.20-806.39, 839.40, 839.49-839.50, 839.59, 839.69, 839.79, 839.8-839.9, 847.9, 905.1, 926.11, 952.10-952.19, 952.8-952.9, 958.8, 959.1, 959.8-959.9

952.01 C_1-C_4 level with complete lesion of cc
spinal cord
CC Excl: See code 952.00

952.02 C_1-C_4 level with anterior cord syndrome cc
CC Excl: See code 952.00

952.03 C_1-C_4 level with central cord syndrome cc
CC Excl: See code 952.00

952.04 C_1-C_4 level with other specified spinal cc
cord injury
Incomplete spinal cord lesion at C_1-C_4 level:
NOS
with posterior cord syndrome
CC Excl: See code 952.00

952.05 C_5-C_7 level with unspecified spinal cord cc
injury
CC Excl: See code 952.00

952.06 C_5-C_7 level with complete lesion of cc
spinal cord
CC Excl: See code 952.00

952.07 C_5-C_7 level with anterior cord syndrome cc
CC Excl: See code 952.00

952.08 C_5-C_7 level with central cord syndrome cc
CC Excl: See code 952.00

952.09 C_5-C_7 level with other specified spinal cc
cord injury
Incomplete spinal cord lesion at C_5-C_7 level:
NOS
with posterior cord syndrome
CC Excl: See code 952.00

952.11 T_1-T_6 level with complete lesion of cc
spinal cord
CC Excl: See code 952.10

952.12 T_1-T_6 level with anterior cord syndrome cc
CC Excl: See code 952.10

952.13 T_1-T_6 level with central cord syndrome cc
CC Excl: See code 952.10

952.14 T_1-T_6 level with other specified spinal cc
cord injury
Incomplete spinal cord lesion at T_1-T_6 level:
NOS
with posterior cord syndrome
CC Excl: See code 952.10

952.15 T_7-T_{12} level with unspecified spinal cc
cord injury
CC Excl: See code 952.10

952.16 T_7-T_{12} level with complete lesion of cc
spinal cord
CC Excl: See code 952.10

952.17 T_7-T_{12} level with anterior cord syndrome cc
CC Excl: See code 952.10

952.18 T_7-T_{12} level with central cord syndrome cc
CC Excl: See code 952.10

√4ᵗʰ √5ᵗʰ Additional Digit Required   Nonspecific PDx   Unacceptable PDx   Manifestation Code   **MSP** Medicare Secondary Payer   ▶◀ Revised Text   ● New Code   ▲ Revised Code Title

2002 Ingenix, Inc.   **Volume 1 — 287**

Injury and Poisoning 950–952.18

Injury and Poisoning 952.19–958.4

952.19 **T$_7$-T$_{12}$ level with other specified spinal** `CC`
cord injury
> Incomplete spinal cord lesion at T$_7$-T$_{12}$ level: NOS
> with posterior cord syndrome

CC Excl: See code 952.10

952.2 **Lumbar** `CC`
CC Excl: 805.8-805.9, 806.4-806.5, 839.40, 839.49-839.50, 839.59, 839.69, 839.79, 839.8-839.9, 847.9, 905.1, 926.11, 952.2, 952.8-952.9, 958.8, 959.1, 959.8-959.9

952.3 **Sacral** `CC`
CC Excl: 805.8-805.9, 806.60-806.79, 839.40, 839.49-839.50, 839.59, 839.69, 839.79, 839.8-839.9, 847.9, 905.1, 926.11, 952.3-952.4, 952.8-952.9, 958.8, 959.1, 959.8-959.9

952.4 **Cauda equina** `CC`
CC Excl: See code 952.3

952.8 **Multiple sites of spinal cord** `CC`
CC Excl: 805.8-805.9, 839.40, 839.49-839.50, 839.59, 839.69, 839.79, 839.8-839.9, 847.9, 905.1, 926.11, 952.2-952.9, 958.8, 959.1, 959.8-959.9

952.9 **Unspecified site of spinal cord** `CC`
CC Excl: 805.8-805.9, 839.40, 839.49-839.50, 839.59, 839.69, 839.79, 839.8-839.9, 847.9, 905.1, 926.11, 952.2-952.9, 958.8, 959.1, 959.8-959.9

√4ᵗʰ 953 Injury to nerve roots and spinal plexus

953.0 **Cervical root** `CC`
CC Excl: 953.8-953.9, 958.8, 959.8-959.9

953.1 **Dorsal root** `CC`
CC Excl: See code 953.0

953.2 **Lumbar root** `CC`
CC Excl: See code 953.0

953.3 **Sacral root** `CC`
CC Excl: See code 953.0

953.4 **Brachial plexus** `CC`
CC Excl: See code 953.0

953.5 **Lumbosacral plexus** `CC`
CC Excl: See code 953.0

953.8 **Multiple sites** `CC`
CC Excl: See code 953.0

953.9 **Unspecified site** `CC`
CC Excl: See code 953.0

√4ᵗʰ 954 Injury to other nerve(s) of trunk, excluding shoulder and pelvic girdles

954.0 **Cervical sympathetic**
954.1 **Other sympathetic**
> Celiac ganglion or plexus   Splanchnic nerve(s)
> Inferior mesenteric plexus   Stellate ganglion

954.8 **Other specified nerve(s) of trunk**
954.9 **Unspecified nerve of trunk**

√4ᵗʰ 955 Injury to peripheral nerve(s) of shoulder girdle and upper limb

955.0 **Axillary nerve**
955.1 **Median nerve**
955.2 **Ulnar nerve**
955.3 **Radial nerve**
955.4 **Musculocutaneous nerve**
955.5 **Cutaneous sensory nerve, upper limb**
955.6 **Digital nerve**
955.7 **Other specified nerve(s) of shoulder girdle and upper limb**
955.8 **Multiple nerves of shoulder girdle and upper limb**
955.9 **Unspecified nerve of shoulder girdle and upper limb**

√4ᵗʰ 956 Injury to peripheral nerve(s) of pelvic girdle and lower limb
956.0 **Sciatic nerve**
956.1 **Femoral nerve**
956.2 **Posterior tibial nerve**
956.3 **Peroneal nerve**
956.4 **Cutaneous sensory nerve, lower limb**
956.5 **Other specified nerve(s) of pelvic girdle and lower limb**
956.8 **Multiple nerves of pelvic girdle and lower limb**
956.9 **Unspecified nerve of pelvic girdle and lower limb**

√4ᵗʰ 957 Injury to other and unspecified nerves
957.0 **Superficial nerves of head and neck**
957.1 **Other specified nerve(s)**
957.8 **Multiple nerves in several parts**
> Multiple nerve injury NOS

957.9 **Unspecified site**
> Nerve injury NOS

CERTAIN TRAUMATIC COMPLICATIONS AND UNSPECIFIED INJURIES (958-959)

√4ᵗʰ 958 Certain early complications of trauma
> *EXCLUDES* adult respiratory distress syndrome (518.5)
> flail chest (807.4)
> shock lung (518.5)
> that occurring during or following medical procedures (996.0-999.9)

958.0 **Air embolism** `CC`
> Pneumathemia
> *EXCLUDES* that complicating:
> abortion (634-638 with .6, 639.6)
> ectopic or molar pregnancy (639.6)
> pregnancy, childbirth, or the puerperium (673.0)

CC Excl: 958.0, 958.8, 959.8-959.9, 997.91, 997.99, 998.81, 998.83-998.9, 999.1

DEF: Arterial obstruction due to introduction of air bubbles into the veins following surgery or trauma.

958.1 **Fat embolism** `CC`
> *EXCLUDES* that complicating:
> abortion (634-638 with .6, 639.6)
> pregnancy, childbirth, or the puerperium (673.8)

CC Excl: 958.1, 958.8, 959.8-959.9, 997.91, 997.99, 998.81, 998.83-998.9

DEF: Arterial blockage due to the entrance of fat in circulatory system, after fracture of large bones or administration of corticosteroids.

958.2 **Secondary and recurrent hemorrhage** `CC`
CC Excl: 958.2, 958.8, 959.8-959.9, 997.91, 997.99, 998.81, 998.83-998.9

958.3 **Posttraumatic wound infection, not elsewhere classified** `CC`
> *EXCLUDES* infected open wounds–code to complicated open wound of site

CC Excl: 958.3, 958.8, 959.8-959.9, 997.91, 997.99, 998.81, 998.83-998.9

AHA: ▶4Q, '01, 53;◀ S-O, '85, 10

958.4 **Traumatic shock** `CC` `MSP`
> Shock (immediate) (delayed) following injury
> *EXCLUDES* shock:
> anaphylactic (995.0)
> due to serum (999.4)
> anesthetic (995.4)
> electric (994.8)
> following abortion (639.5)
> lightning (994.0)
> nontraumatic NOS (785.50)
> obstetric (669.1)
> postoperative (998.0)

CC Excl: 958.4, 958.8, 959.8-959.9, 997.91, 997.99, 998.81, 998.83-998.9

DEF: Shock, immediate or delayed following injury.

N Newborn Age: 0   P Pediatric Age: 0-17   M Maternity Age: 12-55   A Adult Age: 15-124   `CC` CC Condition   `MC` Major Complication   `CD` Complex Dx   `HIV` HIV Related Dx

288 — Volume 1 • January 2002   2002 Ingenix, Inc.

958.5   **Traumatic anuria**   `CC` `MSP`
        Crush syndrome
        Renal failure following crushing
        `EXCLUDES`   *that due to a medical procedure (997.5)*

        CC Excl: 958.5, 958.8, 959.8-959.9, 995.4, 997.91, 997.99, 998.0, 998.11-998.13, 998.81, 998.83-998.9

        DEF: Complete suppression of urinary secretion by kidneys due to trauma.

958.6   **Volkmann's ischemic contracture**
        Posttraumatic muscle contracture

        DEF: Muscle deterioration due to loss of blood supply from injury or tourniquet; causes muscle contraction and results in inability to extend the muscles fully.

958.7   **Traumatic subcutaneous emphysema**   `CC`
        `EXCLUDES`   *subcutaneous emphysema resulting from a procedure (998.81)*

        CC Excl: 860.0-860.5, 861.20-861.32, 862.0-862.1, 862.29, 862.31-862.9, 875.0-875.1, 958.7-958.8, 959.8-959.9, 997.91, 997.99, 998.81, 998.83-998.9

958.8   **Other early complications of trauma**
        AHA: 2Q, '92, 13

        DEF: Compartmental syndrome is abnormal pressure in confined anatomical space, as in swollen muscle restricted by fascia.

`✓4ᵗʰ` **959 Injury, other and unspecified**
        `INCLUDES`   injury NOS
        `EXCLUDES`   *injury NOS of:*
                blood vessels (900.0-904.9)
                eye (921.0-921.9)
                internal organs (860.0-869.1)
                intracranial sites (854.0-854.1)
                nerves (950.0-951.9, 953.0-957.9)
                spinal cord (952.0-952.9)

`✓5ᵗʰ` **959.0**   **Head, face, and neck**
        959.01   **Head injury, unspecified**   `MSP`
                `EXCLUDES`   *concussion (850.1-850.9)*
                         with head injury NOS (850.1-850.9)
                         ▶*head injury NOS with loss of consciousness (850.1-850.5)*◄
                         specified intracranial injuries (850.0-854.1)
                AHA: 4Q, '97, 46

        959.09   **Injury of face and neck**   `MSP`
                Cheek   Mouth
                Ear   Nose
                Eyebrow   Throat
                Lip
                AHA: 4Q, '97, 46

959.1   **Trunk**
        Abdominal wall   External genital organs
        Back   Flank
        Breast   Groin
        Buttock   Interscapular region
        Chest wall   Perineum
        `EXCLUDES`   *scapular region (959.2)*
        AHA: 1Q, '99, 10

959.2   **Shoulder and upper arm**
        Axilla   Scapular region

959.3   **Elbow, forearm, and wrist**
        AHA: 1Q, '97, 8

959.4   **Hand, except finger**

959.5   **Finger**
        Fingernail   Thumb (nail)

959.6   **Hip and thigh**
        Upper leg

959.7   **Knee, leg, ankle, and foot**

959.8   **Other specified sites, including multiple**
        `EXCLUDES`   *multiple sites classifiable to the same four-digit category (959.0-959.7)*

959.9   **Unspecified site**

POISONING BY DRUGS, MEDICINAL AND BIOLOGICAL SUBSTANCES (960-979)

   `INCLUDES`   overdose of these substances
                  wrong substance given or taken in error
   `EXCLUDES`   *adverse effects ["hypersensitivity," "reaction," etc.] of correct substance properly administered. Such cases are to be classified according to the nature of the adverse effect, such as:*
              adverse effect NOS (995.2)
              allergic lymphadenitis (289.3)
              aspirin gastritis (535.4)
              blood disorders (280.0-289.9)
              dermatitis:
                  contact (692.0-692.9)
                  due to ingestion (693.0-693.9)
              nephropathy (583.9)
              [The drug giving rise to the adverse effect may be identified by use of categories E930-E949.]
              drug dependence (304.0-304.9)
              drug reaction and poisoning affecting the newborn (760.0-779.9)
              nondependent abuse of drugs (305.0-305.9)
              pathological drug intoxication (292.2)
      Use additional code to specify the effects of the poisoning
   AHA: 2Q, '90, 11

`✓4ᵗʰ` **960 Poisoning by antibiotics**
        `EXCLUDES`   *antibiotics:*
                ear, nose, and throat (976.6)
                eye (976.5)
                local (976.0)

        960.0   **Penicillins**
                Ampicillin   Cloxacillin
                Carbenicillin   Penicillin G

        960.1   **Antifungal antibiotics**
                Amphotericin B   Nystatin
                Griseofulvin   Trichomycin
                `EXCLUDES`   *preparations intended for topical use (976.0-976.9)*

        960.2   **Chloramphenicol group**
                Chloramphenicol   Thiamphenicol

        960.3   **Erythromycin and other macrolides**
                Oleandomycin   Spiramycin

        960.4   **Tetracycline group**
                Doxycycline   Oxytetracycline
                Minocycline

        960.5   **Cephalosporin group**
                Cephalexin   Cephaloridine
                Cephaloglycin   Cephalothin

        960.6   **Antimycobacterial antibiotics**
                Cycloserine   Rifampin
                Kanamycin   Streptomycin

        960.7   **Antineoplastic antibiotics**
                Actinomycin such as:
                   Bleomycin   Daunorubicin
                   Cactinomycin   Mitomycin
                   Dactinomycin

        960.8   **Other specified antibiotics**
        960.9   **Unspecified antibiotic**

`✓4ᵗʰ` **961 Poisoning by other anti-infectives**
        `EXCLUDES`   *anti-infectives:*
                ear, nose, and throat (976.6)
                eye (976.5)
                local (976.0)

        961.0   **Sulfonamides**
                Sulfadiazine   Sulfamethoxazole
                Sulfafurazole

        961.1   **Arsenical anti-infectives**

        961.2   **Heavy metal anti-infectives**
                Compounds of: Compounds of:
                   antimony   lead
                   bismuth   mercury
                `EXCLUDES`   *mercurial diuretics (974.0)*

Injury and Poisoning 961.3–965.6

961.3 Quinoline and hydroxyquinoline derivatives
Chiniofon   Diiodohydroxyquin
EXCLUDES   *antimalarial drugs (961.4)*

961.4 Antimalarials and drugs acting on other blood protozoa
Chloroquine   Proguanil [chloroguanide]
Cycloguanil   Pyrimethamine
Primaquine   Quinine

961.5 Other antiprotozoal drugs
Emetine

961.6 Anthelmintics
Hexylresorcinol   Thiabendazole
Piperazine

961.7 Antiviral drugs
Methisazone
EXCLUDES   *amantadine (966.4)*
cytarabine (963.1)
idoxuridine (976.5)

961.8 Other antimycobacterial drugs
Ethambutol   Para-aminosalicylic acid
Ethionamide   derivatives
Isoniazid   Sulfones

961.9 Other and unspecified anti-infectives
Flucytosine
Nitrofuran derivatives

✓4ᵗʰ 962 Poisoning by hormones and synthetic substitutes
EXCLUDES   *oxytocic hormones (975.0)*

962.0 Adrenal cortical steroids
Cortisone derivatives   Fluorinated corticosteroids
Desoxycorticosterone derivatives

962.1 Androgens and anabolic congeners
Methandriol   Oxymetholone
Nandrolone   Testosterone

962.2 Ovarian hormones and synthetic substitutes
Contraceptives, oral
Estrogens
Estrogens and progestogens, combined
Progestogens

962.3 Insulins and antidiabetic agents
Acetohexamide   Insulin
Biguanide derivatives,   Phenformin
   oral   Sulfonylurea derivatives,
Chlorpropamide   oral
Glucagon   Tolbutamide
AHA: M-A, '85, 8

962.4 Anterior pituitary hormones
Corticotropin
Gonadotropin
Somatotropin [growth hormone]

962.5 Posterior pituitary hormones
Vasopressin
EXCLUDES   *oxytocic hormones (975.0)*

962.6 Parathyroid and parathyroid derivatives

962.7 Thyroid and thyroid derivatives
Dextrothyroxin
Levothyroxine sodium
Liothyronine
Thyroglobulin

962.8 Antithyroid agents
Iodides
Thiouracil
Thiourea

962.9 Other and unspecified hormones and synthetic substitutes

✓4ᵗʰ 963 Poisoning by primarily systemic agents

963.0 Antiallergic and antiemetic drugs
Antihistamines   Diphenylpyraline
Chlorpheniramine   Thonzylamine
Diphenhydramine   Tripelennamine
EXCLUDES   *phenothiazine-based tranquilizers (969.1)*

963.1 Antineoplastic and immunosuppressive drugs
Azathioprine   Cytarabine
Busulfan   Fluorouracil
Chlorambucil   Mercaptopurine
Cyclophosphamide   thio-TEPA
EXCLUDES   *antineoplastic antibiotics (960.7)*

963.2 Acidifying agents

963.3 Alkalizing agents

963.4 Enzymes, not elsewhere classified
Penicillinase

963.5 Vitamins, not elsewhere classified
Vitamin A   Vitamin D
EXCLUDES   *nicotinic acid (972.2)*
vitamin K (964.3)

963.8 Other specified systemic agents
Heavy metal antagonists

963.9 Unspecified systemic agent

✓4ᵗʰ 964 Poisoning by agents primarily affecting blood constituents

964.0 Iron and its compounds
Ferric salts
Ferrous sulfate and other ferrous salts

964.1 Liver preparations and other antianemic agents
Folic acid

964.2 Anticoagulants
Coumarin   Phenindione
Heparin   Warfarin sodium
AHA: 1Q, '94, 22

964.3 Vitamin K [phytonadione]

964.4 Fibrinolysis-affecting drugs
Aminocaproic acid   Streptokinase
Streptodornase   Urokinase

964.5 Anticoagulant antagonists and other coagulants
Hexadimethrine   Protamine sulfate

964.6 Gamma globulin

964.7 Natural blood and blood products
Blood plasma   Packed red cells
Human fibrinogen   Whole blood
EXCLUDES   *transfusion reactions (999.4-999.8)*

964.8 Other specified agents affecting blood constituents
Macromolecular blood substitutes
Plasma expanders

964.9 Unspecified agent affecting blood constituents

✓4ᵗʰ 965 Poisoning by analgesics, antipyretics, and antirheumatics
EXCLUDES   *drug dependence (304.0-304.9)*
nondependent abuse (305.0-305.9)

✓5ᵗʰ 965.0 Opiates and related narcotics
965.00 Opium (alkaloids), unspecified
965.01 Heroin
Diacetylmorphine
965.02 Methadone
965.09 Other
Codeine [methylmorphine]
Meperidine [pethidine]
Morphine

965.1 Salicylates
Acetylsalicylic acid [aspirin]
Salicylic acid salts
AHA: N-D, '94, 15

965.4 Aromatic analgesics, not elsewhere classified
Acetanilid   Phenacetin [acetophenetidin]
Paracetamol [acetaminophen]

965.5 Pyrazole derivatives
Aminophenazone [aminopyrine]
Phenylbutazone

✓5ᵗʰ 965.6 Antirheumatics [antiphlogistics]
EXCLUDES   *salicylates (965.1)*
steroids (962.0-962.9)
AHA: 4Q, '98, 50

N Newborn Age: 0   P Pediatric Age: 0-17   M Maternity Age: 12-55   A Adult Age: 15-124   CC CC Condition   MC Major Complication   CD Complex Dx   HIV HIV Related Dx

290 — Volume 1   *2002 Ingenix, Inc.*

965.61 Propionic acid derivatives
  Fenoprofen
  Flurbiprofen
  Ibuprofen
  Ketoprofen
  Naproxen
  Oxaprozin
  AHA: 4Q, '98, 50

965.69 Other antirheumatics
  Gold salts
  Indomethacin

965.7 Other non-narcotic analgesics
  Pyrabital

965.8 Other specified analgesics and antipyretics
  Pentazocine

965.9 Unspecified analgesic and antipyretic

✓4th **966 Poisoning by anticonvulsants and anti-Parkinsonism drugs**

966.0 Oxazolidine derivatives
  Paramethadione
  Trimethadione

966.1 Hydantoin derivatives
  Phenytoin

966.2 Succinimides
  Ethosuximide
  Phensuximide

966.3 Other and unspecified anticonvulsants
  Primidone
  EXCLUDES   *barbiturates (967.0)*
  sulfonamides (961.0)

966.4 Anti-Parkinsonism drugs
  Amantadine
  Ethopropazine [profenamine]
  Levodopa [L-dopa]

✓4th **967 Poisoning by sedatives and hypnotics**
  EXCLUDES   *drug dependence (304.0-304.9)*
  nondependent abuse (305.0-305.9)

967.0 Barbiturates
  Amobarbital [amylobarbitone]
  Barbital [barbitone]
  Butabarbital [butabarbitone]
  Pentobarbital [pentobarbitone]
  Phenobarbital [phenobarbitone]
  Secobarbital [quinalbarbitone]
  EXCLUDES   *thiobarbiturate anesthetics (968.3)*

967.1 Chloral hydrate group
967.2 Paraldehyde
967.3 Bromine compounds
  Bromide
  Carbromal (derivatives)

967.4 Methaqualone compounds
967.5 Glutethimide group
967.6 Mixed sedatives, not elsewhere classified
967.8 Other sedatives and hypnotics
967.9 Unspecified sedative or hypnotic
  Sleeping:
    drug
    pill } NOS
    tablet

✓4th **968 Poisoning by other central nervous system depressants and anesthetics**
  EXCLUDES   *drug dependence (304.0-304.9)*
  nondependent abuse (305.0-305.9)

968.0 Central nervous system muscle-tone depressants
  Chlorphenesin (carbamate)   Methocarbamol
  Mephenesin

968.1 Halothane
968.2 Other gaseous anesthetics
  Ether
  Halogenated hydrocarbon derivatives, except halothane
  Nitrous oxide

968.3 Intravenous anesthetics
  Ketamine
  Methohexital [methohexitone]
  Thiobarbiturates, such as thiopental sodium

968.4 Other and unspecified general anesthetics
968.5 Surface [topical] and infiltration anesthetics
  Cocaine   Procaine
  Lidocaine [lignocaine]   Tetracaine
  AHA: 1Q, '93, 25

968.6 Peripheral nerve- and plexus-blocking anesthetics
968.7 Spinal anesthetics
968.9 Other and unspecified local anesthetics

✓4th **969 Poisoning by psychotropic agents**
  EXCLUDES   *drug dependence (304.0-304.9)*
  nondependent abuse (305.0-305.9)

969.0 Antidepressants
  Amitriptyline
  Imipramine
  Monoamine oxidase [MAO] inhibitors

969.1 Phenothiazine-based tranquilizers
  Chlorpromazine   Prochlorperazine
  Fluphenazine   Promazine

969.2 Butyrophenone-based tranquilizers
  Haloperidol   Trifluperidol
  Spiperone

969.3 Other antipsychotics, neuroleptics, and major tranquilizers
969.4 Benzodiazepine-based tranquilizers
  Chlordiazepoxide   Lorazepam
  Diazepam   Medazepam
  Flurazepam   Nitrazepam

969.5 Other tranquilizers
  Hydroxyzine   Meprobamate

969.6 Psychodysleptics [hallucinogens]
  Cannabis (derivatives)   Mescaline
  Lysergide [LSD]   Psilocin
  Marihuana (derivatives)   Psilocybin

969.7 Psychostimulants
  Amphetamine
  Caffeine
  EXCLUDES   *central appetite depressants (977.0)*

969.8 Other specified psychotropic agents
969.9 Unspecified psychotropic agent

✓4th **970 Poisoning by central nervous system stimulants**

970.0 Analeptics
  Lobeline
  Nikethamide

970.1 Opiate antagonists
  Levallorphan
  Nalorphine
  Naloxone

970.8 Other specified central nervous system stimulants
970.9 Unspecified central nervous system stimulant

✓4th **971 Poisoning by drugs primarily affecting the autonomic nervous system**

971.0 Parasympathomimetics [cholinergics]
  Acetylcholine   Pilocarpine
  Anticholinesterase:
    organophosphorus
    reversible

971.1 Parasympatholytics [anticholinergics and antimuscarinics] and spasmolytics
  Atropine   Quaternary ammonium
  Homatropine   derivatives
  Hyoscine [scopolamine]
  EXCLUDES   *papaverine (972.5)*

971.2 Sympathomimetics [adrenergics]
  Epinephrine [adrenalin]   Levarterenol [noradrenalin]

971.3 Sympatholytics [antiadrenergics]
  Phenoxybenzamine   Tolazolinehydrochloride

971.9 Unspecified drug primarily affecting autonomic nervous system

---

✓4th ✓5th Additional Digit Required   Nonspecific PDx   Unacceptable PDx   Manifestation Code   **MSP** Medicare Secondary Payer   ►◄ Revised Text   ● New Code   ▲ Revised Code Title

2002 Ingenix, Inc.

✓4ᵗʰ 972 Poisoning by agents primarily affecting the cardiovascular system

972.0 Cardiac rhythm regulators
Practolol   Propranolol
Procainamide   Quinidine
EXCLUDES lidocaine (968.5)

972.1 Cardiotonic glycosides and drugs of similar action
Digitalis glycosides   Strophanthins
Digoxin

972.2 Antilipemic and antiarteriosclerotic drugs
Clofibrate   Nicotinic acid derivatives

972.3 Ganglion-blocking agents
Pentamethonium bromide

972.4 Coronary vasodilators
Dipyridamole   Nitrites
Nitrates [nitroglycerin]

972.5 Other vasodilators
Cyclandelate   Papaverine
Diazoxide
EXCLUDES nicotinic acid (972.2)

972.6 Other antihypertensive agents
Clonidine   Rauwolfia alkaloids
Guanethidine   Reserpine

972.7 Antivaricose drugs, including sclerosing agents
Sodium morrhuate   Zinc salts

972.8 Capillary-active drugs
Adrenochrome derivatives   Metaraminol

972.9 Other and unspecified agents primarily affecting the cardiovascular system

✓4ᵗʰ 973 Poisoning by agents primarily affecting the gastrointestinal system

973.0 Antacids and antigastric secretion drugs
Aluminum hydroxide   Magnesium trisilicate

973.1 Irritant cathartics
Bisacodyl   Phenolphthalein
Castor oil

973.2 Emollient cathartics
Dioctyl sulfosuccinates

973.3 Other cathartics, including intestinal atonia drugs
Magnesium sulfate

973.4 Digestants
Pancreatin   Pepsin
Papain

973.5 Antidiarrheal drugs
Kaolin   Pectin
EXCLUDES anti-infectives (960.0-961.9)

973.6 Emetics

973.8 Other specified agents primarily affecting the gastrointestinal system

973.9 Unspecified agent primarily affecting the gastrointestinal system

✓4ᵗʰ 974 Poisoning by water, mineral, and uric acid metabolism drugs

974.0 Mercurial diuretics
Chlormerodrin   Mersalyl
Mercaptomerin

974.1 Purine derivative diuretics
Theobromine   Theophylline
EXCLUDES aminophylline [theophylline ethylenediamine] (975.7)
caffeine (969.7)

974.2 Carbonic acid anhydrase inhibitors
Acetazolamide

974.3 Saluretics
Benzothiadiazides   Chlorothiazide group

974.4 Other diuretics
Ethacrynic acid   Furosemide

974.5 Electrolytic, caloric, and water-balance agents

974.6 Other mineral salts, not elsewhere classified

974.7 Uric acid metabolism drugs
Allopurinol   Probenecid
Colchicine

✓4ᵗʰ 975 Poisoning by agents primarily acting on the smooth and skeletal muscles and respiratory system

975.0 Oxytocic agents
Ergot alkaloids   Prostaglandins
Oxytocin

975.1 Smooth muscle relaxants
Adiphenine   Metaproterenol [orciprenaline]
EXCLUDES papaverine (972.5)

975.2 Skeletal muscle relaxants

975.3 Other and unspecified drugs acting on muscles

975.4 Antitussives
Dextromethorphan   Pipazethate

975.5 Expectorants
Acetylcysteine   Terpin hydrate
Guaifenesin

975.6 Anti-common cold drugs

975.7 Antiasthmatics
Aminophylline [theophylline ethylenediamine]

975.8 Other and unspecified respiratory drugs

✓4ᵗʰ 976 Poisoning by agents primarily affecting skin and mucous membrane, ophthalmological, otorhinolaryngological, and dental drugs

976.0 Local anti-infectives and anti-inflammatory drugs

976.1 Antipruritics

976.2 Local astringents and local detergents

976.3 Emollients, demulcents, and protectants

976.4 Keratolytics, keratoplastics, other hair treatment drugs and preparations

976.5 Eye anti-infectives and other eye drugs
Idoxuridine

976.6 Anti-infectives and other drugs and preparations for ear, nose, and throat

976.7 Dental drugs topically applied
EXCLUDES anti-infectives (976.0)
local anesthetics (968.5)

976.8 Other agents primarily affecting skin and mucous membrane
Spermicides [vaginal contraceptives]

976.9 Unspecified agent primarily affecting skin and mucous membrane

✓4ᵗʰ 977 Poisoning by other and unspecified drugs and medicinal substances

977.0 Dietetics
Central appetite depressants

977.1 Lipotropic drugs

977.2 Antidotes and chelating agents, not elsewhere classified

977.3 Alcohol deterrents

977.4 Pharmaceutical excipients
Pharmaceutical adjuncts

977.8 Other specified drugs and medicinal substances
Contrast media used for diagnostic x-ray procedures
Diagnostic agents and kits

977.9 Unspecified drug or medicinal substance

✓4ᵗʰ 978 Poisoning by bacterial vaccines

978.0 BCG

978.1 Typhoid and paratyphoid

978.2 Cholera

978.3 Plague

978.4 Tetanus

978.5 Diphtheria

978.6 Pertussis vaccine, including combinations with a pertussis component

978.8 Other and unspecified bacterial vaccines

978.9 Mixed bacterial vaccines, except combinations with a pertussis component

✓4ᵗʰ 979 Poisoning by other vaccines and biological substances
EXCLUDES gamma globulin (964.6)

979.0 Smallpox vaccine

979.1 Rabies vaccine

N Newborn Age: 0   **P** Pediatric Age: 0-17   **M** Maternity Age: 12-55   **A** Adult Age: 15-124   **CC** CC Condition   **MC** Major Complication   **CD** Complex Dx   **HIV** HIV Related Dx

292 — Volume 1   *2002 Ingenix, Inc.*

979.2 **Typhus vaccine**

979.3 **Yellow fever vaccine**

979.4 **Measles vaccine**

979.5 **Poliomyelitis vaccine**

979.6 **Other and unspecified viral and rickettsial vaccines**
Mumps vaccine

979.7 **Mixed viral-rickettsial and bacterial vaccines, except combinations with a pertussis component**
EXCLUDES   *combinations with a pertussis component (978.6)*

979.9 **Other and unspecified vaccines and biological substances**

TOXIC EFFECTS OF SUBSTANCES CHIEFLY NONMEDICINAL AS TO SOURCE (980-989)

EXCLUDES   *burns from chemical agents (ingested) (947.0-947.9)*
localized toxic effects indexed elsewhere (001.0-799.9)
respiratory conditions due to external agents (506.0-508.9)
Use additional code to specify the nature of the toxic effect

√4th 980 **Toxic effect of alcohol**

980.0 **Ethyl alcohol**
Denatured alcohol   Grain alcohol
Ethanol
Use additional code to identify any associated:
acute alcohol intoxication (305.0)
in alcoholism (303.0)
drunkenness (simple) (305.0)
pathological (291.4)

AHA: 3Q, '96, 16

980.1 **Methyl alcohol**
Methanol   Wood alcohol

980.2 **Isopropyl alcohol**
Dimethyl carbinol   Rubbing alcohol
Isopropanol

980.3 **Fusel oil**
Alcohol: Alcohol:
   amyl   propyl
   butyl

980.8 **Other specified alcohols**

980.9 Unspecified alcohol

981 **Toxic effect of petroleum products**
Benzine   Petroleum:
Gasoline   ether
Kerosene   naphtha
Paraffin wax   spirit

√4th 982 **Toxic effect of solvents other than petroleum-based**

982.0 **Benzene and homologues**

982.1 **Carbon tetrachloride**

982.2 **Carbon disulfide**
Carbon bisulfide

982.3 **Other chlorinated hydrocarbon solvents**
Tetrachloroethylene   Trichloroethylene
EXCLUDES   *chlorinated hydrocarbon preparations other than solvents (989.2)*

982.4 **Nitroglycol**

982.8 **Other nonpetroleum-based solvents**
Acetone

√4th 983 **Toxic effect of corrosive aromatics, acids, and caustic alkalis**

983.0 **Corrosive aromatics**
Carbolic acid or phenol
Cresol

983.1 **Acids**
Acid: Acid:
   hydrochloric   sulfuric
   nitric

983.2 **Caustic alkalis**
Lye   Sodium hydroxide
Potassium hydroxide

983.9 **Caustic, unspecified**

√4th 984 **Toxic effect of lead and its compounds (including fumes)**
INCLUDES   that from all sources except medicinal substances

984.0 **Inorganic lead compounds**
Lead dioxide   Lead salts

984.1 **Organic lead compounds**
Lead acetate
Tetraethyl lead

984.8 **Other lead compounds**

984.9 Unspecified lead compound

√4th 985 **Toxic effect of other metals**
INCLUDES   that from all sources except medicinal substances

985.0 **Mercury and its compounds**
Minamata disease

985.1 **Arsenic and its compounds**

985.2 **Manganese and its compounds**

985.3 **Beryllium and its compounds**

985.4 **Antimony and its compounds**

985.5 **Cadmium and its compounds**

985.6 **Chromium**

985.8 **Other specified metals**
Brass fumes   Iron compounds
Copper salts   Nickel compounds
AHA: 1Q, '88, 5

985.9 Unspecified metal

986 **Toxic effect of carbon monoxide**
Carbon monoxide from any source

√4th 987 **Toxic effect of other gases, fumes, or vapors**

987.0 **Liquefied petroleum gases**
Butane   Propane

987.1 **Other hydrocarbon gas**

987.2 **Nitrogen oxides**
Nitrogen dioxide   Nitrous fumes

987.3 **Sulfur dioxide**

987.4 **Freon**
Dichloromonofluoromethane

987.5 **Lacrimogenic gas**
Bromobenzyl cyanide   Ethyliodoacetate
Chloroacetophenone

987.6 **Chlorine gas**

987.7 **Hydrocyanic acid gas**

987.8 **Other specified gases, fumes, or vapors**
Phosgene   Polyester fumes

987.9 **Unspecified gas, fume, or vapor**

√4th 988 **Toxic effect of noxious substances eaten as food**
EXCLUDES   *allergic reaction to food, such as:*
gastroenteritis (558.3)
rash (692.5, 693.1)
food poisoning (bacterial) (005.0-005.9)
toxic effects of food contaminants, such as:
aflatoxin and other mycotoxin (989.7)
mercury (985.0)

988.0 **Fish and shellfish**

988.1 **Mushrooms**

988.2 **Berries and other plants**

988.8 **Other specified noxious substances eaten as food**

988.9 Unspecified noxious substance eaten as food

√4th 989 **Toxic effect of other substances, chiefly nonmedicinal as to source**

989.0 **Hydrocyanic acid and cyanides**
Potassium cyanide   Sodium cyanide
EXCLUDES   *gas and fumes (987.7)*

989.1 **Strychnine and salts**

989.2 **Chlorinated hydrocarbons**
Aldrin   DDT
Chlordane   Dieldrin
EXCLUDES   *chlorinated hydrocarbon solvents (982.0-982.3)*

√4th √5th Additional Digit Required   Nonspecific PDx   Unacceptable PDx   Manifestation Code   MSP Medicare Secondary Payer   ▶◀ Revised Text   ● New Code   ▲ Revised Code Title

2002 Ingenix, Inc.   **Volume 1 — 293**

Injury and Poisoning 979.2–989.2

Injury and Poisoning 989.3–994.3

989.3 **Organophosphate and carbamate**
Carbaryl   Parathion
Dichlorvos   Phorate
Malathion   Phosdrin

989.4 **Other pesticides, not elsewhere classified**
Mixtures of insecticides

989.5 **Venom**
Bites of venomous snakes, lizards, and spiders
Tick paralysis

989.6 **Soaps and detergents**

989.7 **Aflatoxin and other mycotoxin [food contaminants]**

✓5th **989.8** **Other substances, chiefly nonmedicinal as to source**
AHA: 4Q, '95, 60

     989.81 **Asbestos**
         EXCLUDES   *asbestosis (501)*
                    exposure to asbestos (V15.84)

     989.82 **Latex**

     989.83 **Silicone**
         EXCLUDES   *silicone used in medical*
                    devices, implants and
                    grafts (996.00-996.79)

     989.84 **Tobacco**
     989.89 **Other**

989.9 **Unspecified substance, chiefly nonmedicinal as to source**

OTHER AND UNSPECIFIED EFFECTS OF EXTERNAL CAUSES
(990-995)

990 **Effects of radiation, unspecified**
Complication of: Radiation sickness
phototherapy
radiation therapy
    EXCLUDES   *specified adverse effects of radiation. Such*
                conditions are to be classified according to
                the nature of the adverse effect, as:
                burns (940.0-949.5)
                dermatitis (692.7-692.8)
                leukemia (204.0-208.9)
                pneumonia (508.0)
                sunburn (692.71, 692.76-692.77)
                [The type of radiation giving rise to the adverse
                effect may be identified by use of the E
                codes.]

✓4th **991** **Effects of reduced temperature**

991.0 **Frostbite of face**

991.1 **Frostbite of hand**

991.2 **Frostbite of foot**

991.3 **Frostbite of other and unspecified sites**

991.4 **Immersion foot**
Trench foot
DEF: Paresthesia, edema, blotchy cyanosis of foot, the skin is soft (macerated), pale and wrinkled, and the sole is swollen with surface ridging and following sustained immersion in water.

991.5 **Chilblains**
Erythema pernio   Perniosis
DEF: Red, swollen, itchy skin; follows damp cold exposure; also associated with pruritus and a burning feeling, in hands, feet, ears, and face in children, legs and toes in women, and hands and fingers in men.

991.6 **Hypothermia**
Hypothermia (accidental)
    EXCLUDES   *hypothermia following anesthesia*
                (995.89)
                hypothermia not associated with low
                environmental temperature
                ▶*(780.99)*◀
DEF: Reduced body temperature due to low environmental temperatures.

991.8 **Other specified effects of reduced temperature**

991.9 **Unspecified effect of reduced temperature**
Effects of freezing or excessive cold NOS

✓4th **992** **Effects of heat and light**
    EXCLUDES   *burns (940.0-949.5)*
                diseases of sweat glands due to heat (705.0-
                705.9)
                malignant hyperpyrexia following anesthesia
                (995.86)
                sunburn (692.71, 692.76-692.77)

992.0 **Heat stroke and sunstroke**
Heat apoplexy   Siriasis
Heat pyrexia   Thermoplegia
Ictus solaris
DEF: Headache, vertigo, cramps and elevated body temperature due to high environmental temperatures.

992.1 **Heat syncope**
Heat collapse

992.2 **Heat cramps**

992.3 **Heat exhaustion, anhydrotic**
Heat prostration due to water depletion
    EXCLUDES   *that associated with salt depletion*
                (992.4)

992.4 **Heat exhaustion due to salt depletion**
Heat prostration due to salt (and water) depletion

992.5 **Heat exhaustion, unspecified**
Heat prostration NOS

992.6 **Heat fatigue, transient**

992.7 **Heat edema**
DEF: Fluid retention due to high environmental temperatures.

992.8 **Other specified heat effects**

992.9 **Unspecified**

✓4th **993** **Effects of air pressure**

993.0 **Barotrauma, otitic**
Aero-otitis media
Effects of high altitude on ears
DEF: Ringing ears, deafness, pain and vertigo due to air pressure changes.

993.1 **Barotrauma, sinus**
Aerosinusitis
Effects of high altitude on sinuses

993.2 **Other and unspecified effects of high altitude**
Alpine sickness   Hypobaropathy
Andes disease   Mountain sickness
Anoxia due to high altitude
AHA: 3Q, '88, 4

993.3 **Caisson disease**
Bends   Decompression sickness
Compressed-air disease   Divers' palsy or paralysis
DEF: Rapid reduction in air pressure while breathing compressed air; symptoms include skin lesions, joint pains, respiratory and neurological problems.

993.4 **Effects of air pressure caused by explosion**

993.8 **Other specified effects of air pressure**

993.9 **Unspecified effect of air pressure**

✓4th **994** **Effects of other external causes**
    EXCLUDES   *certain adverse effects not elsewhere classified*
                (995.0-995.8)

994.0 **Effects of lightning**
Shock from lightning   Struck by lightning NOS
    EXCLUDES   *burns (940.0-949.5)*

994.1 **Drowning and nonfatal submersion**
Bathing cramp
Immersion
AHA: 3Q, '88, 4

994.2 **Effects of hunger**
Deprivation of food
Starvation

994.3 **Effects of thirst**
Deprivation of water

N Newborn Age: 0   **P** Pediatric Age: 0-17   **M** Maternity Age: 12-55   **A** Adult Age: 15-124   **CC** CC Condition   **MC** Major Complication   **CD** Complex Dx   **HIV** HIV Related Dx

994.4   Exhaustion due to exposure

994.5   Exhaustion due to excessive exertion
　　Overexertion

994.6   Motion sickness
　　Air sickness
　　Seasickness
　　Travel sickness

994.7   Asphyxiation and strangulation
　　Suffocation (by):
　　　bedclothes
　　　cave-in
　　　constriction
　　　mechanical
　　　plastic bag
　　　pressure
　　　strangulation
　　EXCLUDES　*asphyxia from:*
　　　　　carbon monoxide (986)
　　　　　inhalation of food or foreign body
　　　　　(932-934.9)
　　　　　other gases, fumes, and vapors
　　　　　(987.0-987.9)

994.8   Electrocution and nonfatal effects of electric current
　　Shock from electric current
　　EXCLUDES　*electric burns (940.0-949.5)*

994.9   Other effects of external causes
　　Effects of:
　　　abnormal gravitational [G] forces or states
　　　weightlessness

✓4th **995   Certain adverse effects not elsewhere classified**
　　EXCLUDES　*complications of surgical and medical care (996.0-999.9)*

995.0   Other anaphylactic shock
　　Allergic shock
　　Anaphylactic　｝ NOS or due to adverse effect of
　　　reaction　　　correct medicinal substance
　　Anaphylaxis　　properly administered

　　Use additional E code to identify external cause,
　　　such as:
　　　adverse effects of correct medicinal substance
　　　properly administered [E930-E949]
　　EXCLUDES　*anaphylactic reaction to serum (999.4)*
　　　　anaphylactic shock due to adverse food
　　　　reaction (995.60-995.69)

　　AHA: 4Q, '93, 30

　　DEF: Immediate sensitivity response after exposure to specific
　　antigen; results in life-threatening respiratory distress; usually
　　followed by vascular collapse, shock , urticaria, angioedema and
　　pruritus.

995.1   Angioneurotic edema
　　Giant urticaria
　　EXCLUDES　*urticaria:*
　　　　due to serum (999.5)
　　　　other specified (698.2, 708.0-708.9,
　　　　757.33)
　　DEF: Circulatory response of deep dermis, subcutaneous or
　　submucosal tissues; causes localized edema and wheals.

995.2   Unspecified adverse effect of drug, medicinal and biological substance
　　Adverse effect　　｝
　　Allergic reaction　 (due) to correct medicinal
　　Hypersensitivity　　substance properly
　　Idiosyncrasy　　　 administered

　　Drug:　　　　　 Drug:
　　　hypersensitivity NOS　 reaction NOS
　　EXCLUDES　*pathological drug intoxication (292.2)*
　　AHA: 2Q, '97, 12; 3Q, '95, 13; 3Q, '92, 16

995.3   Allergy, unspecified
　　Allergic reaction NOS　　Idiosyncrasy NOS
　　Hypersensitivity NOS
　　EXCLUDES　*allergic reaction NOS to correct*
　　　　medicinal substance properly
　　　　administered (995.2)
　　　　specific types of allergic reaction, such
　　　　as:
　　　　　allergic diarrhea (558.3)
　　　　　dermatitis (691.0-693.9)
　　　　　hayfever (477.0-477.9)

995.4   Shock due to anesthesia　　　**CC**
　　Shock due to anesthesia in which the correct
　　　substance was properly administered
　　EXCLUDES　*complications of anesthesia in labor or*
　　　　delivery (668.0-668.9)
　　　　overdose or wrong substance given
　　　　(968.0-969.9)
　　　　postoperative shock NOS (998.0)
　　　　specified adverse effects of anesthesia
　　　　classified elsewhere, such as:
　　　　　anoxic brain damage (348.1)
　　　　　hepatitis (070.0-070.9), etc.
　　　　unspecified adverse effect of
　　　　anesthesia (995.2)

　　CC Excl: 958.4, 995.4, 997.91, 997.99, 998.0, 998.11-998.13,
　　998.81, 998.83-998.9

✓5th **995.5   Child maltreatment syndrome**
　　Use additional code(s), if applicable, to identify any
　　　associated injuries
　　Use additional E code to identify:
　　　nature of abuse (E960-E968)
　　　perpetrator (E967.0-E967.9)
　　AHA: 1Q, '98, 11

　　995.50   Child abuse, unspecified　　**P**
　　995.51   Child emotional/psychological abuse　**P**
　　　AHA: 4Q, '96, 38, 40

　　995.52   Child neglect (nutritional)　　**P**
　　　AHA: 4Q, '96, 38, 40

　　995.53   Child sexual abuse　　　**P**
　　　AHA: 4Q, '96, 39, 40

　　995.54   Child physical abuse　　　**P**
　　　Battered baby or child syndrome
　　　EXCLUDES　*shaken infant syndrome*
　　　　　(995.55)
　　　AHA: 3Q, '99, 14; 4Q, '96, 39, 40

　　995.55   Shaken infant syndrome　　**P**
　　　Use additional code(s) to identify any
　　　　associated injuries
　　　AHA: 4Q, '96, 40, 43

　　995.59   Other child abuse and neglect　**P**
　　　Multiple forms of abuse

✓5th **995.6   Anaphylactic shock due to adverse food reaction**
　　Anaphylactic shock due to nonpoisonous foods
　　AHA: 4Q, '93, 30

　　995.60   Due to unspecified food
　　995.61   Due to peanuts
　　995.62   Due to crustaceans
　　995.63   Due to fruits and vegetables
　　995.64   Due to tree nuts and seeds
　　995.65   Due to fish
　　995.66   Due to food additives
　　995.67   Due to milk products
　　995.68   Due to eggs
　　995.69   Due to other specified food

✓4th
✓5th Additional Digit Required　　Nonspecific PDx　　Unacceptable PDx　　Manifestation Code　　**MSP** Medicare Secondary Payer　　▶◀ Revised Text　　● New Code　　▲ Revised Code Title

2002 Ingenix, Inc.　　　　　　　　　　　　　　　　　　　　　　　　　　　　　　　　　**Volume 1 — 295**

995.7 Other adverse food reactions, not elsewhere classified
Use additional code to identify the type of reaction, such as:
hives (708.0)
wheezing (786.07)
EXCLUDES *anaphylactic shock due to adverse food reaction (995.60-995.69)*
asthma (493.0, 493.9)
dermatitis due to food (693.1)
in contact with skin (692.5)
gastroenteritis and colitis due to food (558.3)
rhinitis due to food (477.1)

√5th **995.8 Other specified adverse effects, not elsewhere classified**

995.80 Adult maltreatment, unspecified A
Abused person NOS
Use additional code to identify:
any associated injury
perpetrator (E967.0-E967.9)
AHA: 4Q, '96, 41, 43

995.81 Adult physical abuse A
Battered:
person syndrome NEC
man
spouse
woman
Use additional code to identify:
any association injury
nature of abuse (E960-E968)
perpetrator (E967.0-E967.9)
AHA: 4Q, '96, 42, 43

995.82 Adult emotional/psychological abuse A
Use additional E code to identify perpetrator (E967.0-E967.9)

995.83 Adult sexual abuse A
Use additional code(s) to identify:
any associated injury
perpetrator (E967.0-E967.9)

995.84 Adult neglect (nutritional) A
Use addition code(s) to identify:
intent of neglect (E904.0, E968.4)
perpetrator (E967.0-E967.9)

995.85 Other adult abuse and neglect A
Multiple forms of abuse and neglect
Use additional code(s) to identify
any associated injury
intent of neglect (E904.0, E968.4)
nature of abuse (E960-E968)
perpetrator (E967.0-E967.9)

995.86 Malignant hyperthermia CC
Malignant hyperpyrexia due to anesthesia
CC Excl: 958.4, 995.4, 995.86, 997.91, 997.99, 998.0, 998.11-998.13, 998.81, 998.83-998.9
AHA: 4Q, '98, 51

995.89 Other
Hypothermia due to anesthesia

● √5th **995.9 Systemic inflammatory response syndrome (SIRS)**

● **995.90 Systemic inflammatory response syndrome, unspecified** CC
SIRS NOS
CC Excl: 003.1, 020.2, 036.2, 038.0-038.9, 040.82, 040.89, 041.00-041.19, 041.2-041.7, 041.81-041.86, 041.89, 041.9, 054.5, 139.8, 995.90-995.94, V09.0-V09.91

● **995.91 Systemic inflammatory response syndrome due to infectious process without organ dysfunction** CC
CC Excl: See code 995.90

● **995.92 Systemic inflammatory response syndrome due to infectious process with organ dysfunction** CC
Severe sepsis
Use additional code to specify organ dysfunction, such as:
encephalopathy (348.3)
heart failure (428.0-428.9)
kidney failure (584.5-584.9, 585, 586)
CC Excl: See code 995.90

● **995.93 Systemic inflammatory response syndrome due to noninfectious process without organ dysfunction** CC
CC Excl: See code 995.90

● **995.94 Systemic inflammatory response syndrome due to noninfectious process with organ dysfunction** CC
Use additional code to specify organ dysfunction, such as:
encephalopathy (348.3)
heart failure (428.0-428.9)
kidney failure (584.5-584.9, 585, 586)
CC Excl: See code 995.90

COMPLICATIONS OF SURGICAL AND MEDICAL CARE, NOT ELSEWHERE CLASSIFIED (996-999)

EXCLUDES *adverse effects of medicinal agents (001.0-799.9, 995.0-995.8)*
burns from local applications and irradiation (940.0-949.5)
complications of:
conditions for which the procedure was performed
surgical procedures during abortion, labor, and delivery (630-676.9)
poisoning and toxic effects of drugs and chemicals (960.0-989.9)
postoperative conditions in which no complications are present, such as:
artificial opening status (V44.0-V44.9)
closure of external stoma (V55.0-V55.9)
fitting of prosthetic device (V52.0-V52.9)
specified complications classified elsewhere
anesthetic shock (995.4)
electrolyte imbalance (276.0-276.9)
postlaminectomy syndrome (722.80-722.83)
postmastectomy lymphedema syndrome (457.0)
postoperative psychosis (293.0-293.9)
any other condition classified elsewhere in the Alphabetic Index when described as due to a procedure

√4th **996 Complications peculiar to certain specified procedures**
INCLUDES complications, not elsewhere classified, in the use of artificial substitutes [e.g., Dacron, metal, Silastic, Teflon] or natural sources [e.g., bone] involving
anastomosis (internal)
graft (bypass) (patch)
implant
internal device:
catheter   fixation
electronic   prosthetic
reimplant
transplant
EXCLUDES *accidental puncture or laceration during procedure (998.2)*
complications of internal anastomosis of:
gastrointestinal tract (997.4)
urinary tract (997.5)
other specified complications classified elsewhere, such as:
hemolytic anemia (283.1)
functional cardiac disturbances (429.4)
serum hepatitis (070.2-070.3)
AHA: 1Q, '94, 3

N Newborn Age: 0   P Pediatric Age: 0-17   M Maternity Age: 12-55   A Adult Age: 15-124   CC CC Condition   MC Major Complication   CD Complex Dx   HIV HIV Related Dx

296 — Volume 1 • October 2002   2002 Ingenix, Inc.

✓5th **996.0 Mechanical complication of cardiac device, implant, and graft**

    Breakdown (mechanical)   Obstruction, mechanical
    Displacement   Perforation
    Leakage   Protrusion

    AHA: 2Q, '93, 9

996.00 Unspecified device, implant, and graft `CC` `MSP`

    CC Excl: 996.00, 996.04, 996.61-996.62, 996.70-996.74, 997.91, 997.99, 998.81, 998.83-998.9

996.01 Due to cardiac pacemaker (electrode) `CC` `MSP`

    CC Excl: 996.01, 997.91, 997.99, 998.81, 998.83-998.9

    AHA: 2Q, '99, 11

996.02 Due to heart valve prosthesis `CC` `MSP`

    CC Excl: 996.02, 997.91, 997.99, 998.81, 998.83-998.9

996.03 Due to coronary bypass graft `CC` `MSP`

    EXCLUDES atherosclerosis of graft (414.02, 414.03)
                 embolism [occlusion NOS] [thrombus] of graft (996.72)

    CC Excl: 996.03, 997.91, 997.99, 998.81, 998.83-998.9

    AHA: 2Q, '95, 17; N-D, '86, 5

996.04 Due to automatic implantable cardiac defibrillator `CC`

    CC Excl: 996.04, 997.91, 997.99, 998.81, 998.83-998.9

996.09 Other `CC` `MSP`

    CC Excl: 996.09, 997.91, 997.99, 998.81, 998.83-998.9

    AHA: 2Q, '93, 9

996.1 Mechanical complication of other vascular device, implant, and graft `CC` `MSP`

    Mechanical complications involving:
    aortic (bifurcation) graft (replacement)
    arteriovenous:
        dialysis catheter
        fistula   } surgically created
        shunt

    balloon (counterpulsation) device, intra-aortic
    carotid artery bypass graft
    femoral-popliteal bypass graft
    umbrella device, vena cava

    EXCLUDES atherosclerosis of biological graft (440.30-440.32)
              embolism [occulsion NOS] [thrombus] of (biological) (synthetic) graft (996.74)
              peritoneal dialysis catheter (996.56)

    CC Excl: 996.1, 997.91, 997.99, 998.81, 998.83-998.9

    AHA: ▶1Q, '02, 13;◀ 1Q, '95, 3

996.2 Mechanical complication of nervous system device, implant, and graft `CC`

    Mechanical complications involving:
    dorsal column stimulator
    electrodes implanted in brain [brain "pacemaker"]
    peripheral nerve graft
    ventricular (communicating) shunt

    CC Excl: 996.2, 996.63, 996.75, 997.91, 997.99, 998.81, 998.83-998.9

    AHA: 2Q, '99, 4; S-O, '87, 10

✓5th **996.3 Mechanical complication of genitourinary device, implant, and graft**

    AHA: 3Q, '01, 13; S-O, '85, 3

996.30 Unspecified device, implant, and graft `CC` `MSP`

    CC Excl: 996.30, 996.64-996.65, 996.76, 997.91, 997.99, 998.81, 998.83-998.9

996.31 Due to urethral [indwelling] catheter `MSP`

996.32 Due to intrauterine contraceptive device `MSP` ♂

996.39 Other `CC` `MSP`

    Cystostomy catheter
    Prosthetic reconstruction of vas deferens
    Repair (graft) of ureter without mention of resection

    EXCLUDES complications due to:
             external stoma of urinary tract (997.5)
             internal anastomosis of urinary tract (997.5)

    CC Excl: 996.39, 996.64-996.65, 996.76, 997.91, 997.99, 998.81, 998.83-998.9

996.4 Mechanical complication of internal orthopedic device, implant, and graft `CC` `MSP`

    Mechanical complications involving:
    external (fixation) device utilizing internal screw(s), pin(s) or other methods of fixation
    grafts of bone, cartilage, muscle, or tendon
    internal (fixation) device such as nail, plate, rod, etc.

    EXCLUDES complications of external orthopedic device, such as:
             pressure ulcer due to cast (707.0)

    CC Excl: 996.4, 996.66-996.67, 996.77-996.78, 997.91, 997.99, 998.81, 998.83-998.9

    AHA: 2Q, '99, 10; 2Q, '98, 19; 2Q, '96, 11; 3Q, '95, 16; N-D, '85, 11

✓5th **996.5 Mechanical complication of other specified prosthetic device, implant, and graft**

    Mechanical complications involving:
    prosthetic implant in:
        bile duct   chin
        breast   orbit of eye
    nonabsorbable surgical material NOS
    other graft, implant, and internal device, not elsewhere classified

    AHA: 1Q, '98, 11

996.51 Due to corneal graft `CC`

    CC Excl: 996.51, 997.91, 997.99

996.52 Due to graft of other tissue, not elsewhere classified `CC`

    Skin graft failure or rejection

    EXCLUDES failure of artificial skin graft (996.55)
             failure of decellularized allodermis (996.55)
             sloughing of temporary skin allografts or xenografts (pigskin)—omit code

    CC Excl: 996.52, 996.55, 997.91, 997.99

    AHA: 1Q, '96, 10

996.53 Due to ocular lens prosthesis `CC`

    EXCLUDES contact lenses—code to condition

    CC Excl: 996.53, 997.91, 997.99

    AHA: 1Q, '00, 9

996.54 Due to breast prosthesis `CC`

    Breast capsule (prosthesis)
    Mammary implant

    CC Excl: 996.54, 997.91, 997.99

    AHA: 2Q, '98, 14; 3Q, '92, 4

996.55 Due to artificial skin graft and decellularized allodermis `CC`

    Dislodgement   Non-adherence
    Displacement   Poor incorporation
    Failure   Shearing

    CC Excl: 996.52, 996.55-996.60, 996.68-996.69, 996.70, 996.79, 997.91, 997.99

    AHA: 4Q, '98, 52

996.56 Due to peritoneal dialysis catheter `CC`

> EXCLUDES   mechanical complication of arteriovenous dialysis catheter (996.1)

CC Excl: 996.56, 996.59, 996.60, 996.68-996.70, 996.79, 997.91, 997.99

AHA: 4Q, '98, 54

996.59 Due to other implant and internal device, not elsewhere classified `CC`

Nonabsorbable surgical material NOS
Prosthetic implant in:
  bile duct
  chin
  orbit of eye

CC Excl: 996.59, 996.60, 996.68-996.70, 996.79, 997.91, 997.99

AHA: 2Q, '99, 13; 3Q, '94, 7

√5th **996.6 Infection and inflammatory reaction due to internal prosthetic device, implant, and graft**

Infection (causing obstruction) ⎱ due to (presence of) any device,
Inflammation ⎰ implant, and graft classifiable to 996.0-996.5

Use additional code to identify specified infections

AHA: 2Q, '89, 16; J-F, '87, 14

996.60 Due to unspecified device, implant, and graft `CC`

CC Excl: 996.00-996.30, 996.39, 996.4-996.79, 997.91, 997.99, 998.81, 998.83-998.9

996.61 Due to cardiac device, implant, and graft `CC`

Cardiac pacemaker or defibrillator:
  electrode(s), lead(s)
  pulse generator
  subcutaneous pocket
Coronary artery bypass graft
Heart valve prosthesis

CC Excl: 996.00-996.1, 996.52, 996.55-996.62, 996.68-996.74, 996.79, 997.91, 997.99, 998.81, 998.83-998.9

996.62 Due to other vascular device, implant, and graft `CC` `MC`

Arterial graft
Arteriovenous fistula or shunt
Infusion pump
Vascular catheter (arterial) (dialysis) (venous)

CC Excl: See code 996.61

AHA: 2Q, '94, 13

996.63 Due to nervous system device, implant, and graft `CC`

Electrodes implanted in brain
Peripheral nerve graft
Spinal canal catheter
Ventricular (communicating) shunt (catheter)

CC Excl: 996.2, 996.52, 996.55-996.60, 996.63, 996.68-996.70, 996.75, 996.79, 997.91, 997.99, 998.81, 998.83-998.9

996.64 Due to indwelling urinary catheter `CC`

Use additional code to identify specified infections, such as:
  Cystitis (595.0-595.9)
  Sepsis (038.0-038.9)

CC Excl: 599.0, 996.30, 996.39, 996.56-996.60, 996.64-996.65, 996.68-996.70, 996.76, 996.79, 997.91, 997.99, 998.81, 998.83-998.9

996.65 Due to other genitourinary device, implant, and graft `CC`

Intrauterine contraceptive device

CC Excl: 996.30, 996.39, 996.52, 996.55-996.60, 996.64-996.65, 996.68-996.70, 996.76, 996.79, 997.91, 997.99, 998.81, 998.83-998.9

AHA: 1Q, '00, 15

996.66 Due to internal joint prosthesis `CC`

CC Excl: 996.4, 996.52, 996.55-996.60, 996.66-996.70, 996.77-996.79, 997.91, 997.99, 998.81, 998.83-998.9

AHA: 2Q, '91, 18

996.67 Due to other internal orthopedic device, implant, and graft `CC`

Bone growth stimulator (electrode)
Internal fixation device (pin) (rod) (screw)

CC Excl: See code 996.66

996.68 Due to peritoneal dialysis catheter `CC`

Exit-site infection or inflammation

CC Excl: 996.56, 996.59, 996.60, 996.68-996.70, 996.79, 997.91, 997.99

AHA: 4Q, '98, 54

996.69 Due to other internal prosthetic device, implant, and graft `CC`

Breast prosthesis
Ocular lens prosthesis
Prosthetic orbital implant

CC Excl: 996.00-996.30, 996.39, 996.4-996.79, 997.91, 997.99, 998.81, 998.83-998.9

AHA: 4Q, '98, 52

√5th **996.7 Other complications of internal (biological) (synthetic) prosthetic device, implant, and graft**

Complication NOS
  occlusion NOS
Embolism
Fibrosis   ⎱ due to (presence of) any
Hemorrhage   device, implant, and
Pain   graft classifiable to
Stenosis   996.0-996.5
Thrombus ⎰

> EXCLUDES   transplant rejection (996.8)

AHA: 1Q, '89, 9; N-D, '86, 5

996.70 Due to unspecified device, implant, and graft `CC`

CC Excl: See code 996.69

996.71 Due to heart valve prosthesis `CC`

CC Excl: 996.00, 996.02, 996.09, 996.1, 996.52, 996.55-996.62, 996.68-996.74, 996.79, 997.91-997.99, 998.81, 998.83-998.9

996.72 Due to other cardiac device, implant, and graft `CC` `MC`

Cardiac pacemaker or defibrillator:
  electrode(s), lead(s)
  subcutaneous pocket
Coronary artery bypass (graft)

> EXCLUDES   occlusion due to atherosclerosis ▶(414.02-414.06)◀

CC Excl: 996.00-996.02, 996.04, 996.09, 996.1, 996.52, 996.55-996.62, 996.68-996.74, 996.79, 997.91-997.99, 998.81, 998.83-998.9

AHA: ▶3Q, '01, 20 ◀

996.73 Due to renal dialysis device, implant, and graft `CC`

CC Excl: 996.1, 996.52, 996.55-996.60, 996.68-996.70, 996.73, 996.79, 997.91, 997.99, 998.81, 998.83-998.9

AHA: 2Q, '91, 18

996.74 Due to other vascular device, implant, and graft `CC`

> EXCLUDES   occlusion of biological graft due to atherosclerosis (440.30-440.32)

CC Excl: 996.00-996.1, 996.52, 996.55-996.62, 996.68-996.74, 996.79, 997.91, 997.99, 998.81, 998.83-998.9

`N` Newborn Age: 0   `P` Pediatric Age: 0-17   `M` Maternity Age: 12-55   `A` Adult Age: 15-124   `CC` CC Condition   `MC` Major Complication   `CD` Complex Dx   `HIV` HIV Related Dx

996.75 Due to nervous system device, implant, `CC`
and graft
CC Excl: 996.2, 996.52, 996.55-996.60, 996.63, 996.66-996.70, 996.75, 996.79, 997.91, 997.99, 998.81, 998.83-998.9

996.76 Due to genitourinary device, implant, `CC`
and graft
CC Excl: 996.30, 996.39, 996.52, 996.55-996.60, 996.64-996.65, 996.68-996.70, 996.76, 996.79, 997.91, 997.99, 998.81, 998.83-998.9

AHA: 1Q, '00, 15

996.77 Due to internal joint prosthesis `CC`
CC Excl: 996.4, 996.52, 996.55-996.60, 996.66-996.67, 996.69-996.70, 996.77-996.79, 997.91, 997.99, 998.81, 998.83-998.9

996.78 Due to other internal orthopedic `CC`
device, implant, and graft
CC Excl: See code 996.77

996.79 Due to other internal prosthetic `CC`
device, implant, and graft
CC Excl: 996.00-996.30, 996.39, 996.4-996.79, 997.91, 997.99, 998.81, 998.83-998.9

AHA: 1Q,'01, 8; 3Q, '95, 14; 3Q, '92, 4

√5ᵗʰ 996.8 Complications of transplanted organ
Transplant failure or rejection
Use additional code to identify nature of
complication, such as:
Cytomegalovirus (CMV) infection (078.5)
AHA: ▶3Q, '01, 12;◀ 3Q, '93, 3, 4; 2Q, '93, 11; 1Q, '93, 24

996.80 Transplanted organ, unspecified `CC`
CC Excl: 996.80, 996.87, 997.91, 997.99

996.81 Kidney `CC`
CC Excl: 996.81, 997.91, 997.99

AHA: 3Q, '98, 6, 7; 3Q, '94, 8; 2Q, '94, 9; 1Q, '93, 24

996.82 Liver `CC`
CC Excl: 996.82, 997.91, 997.99

AHA: 3Q, '98, 3, 4

996.83 Heart `CC`
CC Excl: 996.83, 997.91, 997.99

AHA: 3Q, '98, 5

996.84 Lung `CC`
CC Excl: 996.84, 997.91, 997.99

AHA: 3Q, '98, 5

996.85 Bone marrow `CC`
Graft-versus-host disease (acute) (chronic)
CC Excl: 996.85, 997.91, 997.99

AHA: 4Q, '90, 4

996.86 Pancreas `CC`
CC Excl: 996.86, 997.91, 997.99

996.87 Intestine `CC`
CC Excl: 996.80, 996.87, 997.91, 997.99

996.89 Other specified transplanted organ `CC`
CC Excl: 996.89, 997.91, 997.99

AHA: 3Q, '94, 5

√5ᵗʰ 996.9 Complications of reattached extremity or body part
996.90 Unspecified extremity `CC`
CC Excl: 996.90, 997.91, 997.99, 998.81, 998.83-998.9

996.91 Forearm `CC`
CC Excl: 996.91, 997.91, 997.99, 998.81, 998.83-998.9

996.92 Hand `CC`
CC Excl: 996.92, 997.91, 997.99, 998.81, 998.83-998.9

996.93 Finger(s) `CC`
CC Excl: 996.93, 997.91, 997.99, 998.81, 998.83-998.9

996.94 Upper extremity, other and unspecified `CC`
CC Excl: 996.94, 997.91, 997.99, 998.81, 998.83-998.9

996.95 Foot and toe(s) `CC`
CC Excl: 996.95, 997.91, 997.99, 998.81, 998.83-998.9

996.96 Lower extremity, other and unspecified `CC`
CC Excl: 996.96, 997.91, 997.99, 998.81, 998.83-998.9

996.99 Other specified body part `CC`
CC Excl: 996.99, 997.91, 997.99, 998.81, 998.83-998.9

√4ᵗʰ 997 Complications affecting specified body systems, not elsewhere classified
Use additional code to identify complications
EXCLUDES *the listed conditions when specified as:*
causing shock (998.0)
complications of:
anesthesia:
adverse effect (001.0-799.9, 995.0-995.8)
in labor or delivery (668.0-668.9)
poisoning (968.0-969.9)
implanted device or graft (996.0-996.9)
obstetrical procedures (669.0-669.4)
reattached extremity (996.90-996.96)
transplanted organ (996.80-996.89)
AHA: 1Q, '94, 4; 1Q, '93, 26

√5ᵗʰ 997.0 Nervous system complications
CC Excl: For codes 997.00-997.09: 997.00-997.09, 997.91, 997.99, 998.81, 998.83, 998.89, 998.9

997.00 Nervous system complication, unspecified `CC`

997.01 Central nervous system complication `CC`
Anoxic brain damage
Cerebral hypoxia
EXCLUDES *cerebrovascular hemorrhage or infarction (997.02)*

997.02 Iatrogenic cerbrovascular infarction or hemorrhage `CC`
Postoperative stroke
AHA: 4Q, '95, 57

997.09 Other nervous system complications `CC`

997.1 Cardiac complications `CC`
Cardiac:
arrest
insufficiency   } during or resulting from a procedure
Cardiorespiratory failure
Heart failure

EXCLUDES *the listed conditions as long-term effects of cardiac surgery or due to the presence of cardiac prosthetic device (429.4)*

CC Excl: 997.1, 997.91, 997.99, 998.81, 998.83-998.9

997.2 Peripheral vascular complications `CC`
Phlebitis or thrombophlebitis during or resulting from a procedure
EXCLUDES *the listed conditions due to:*
implant or catheter device (996.62)
infusion, perfusion, or transfusion (999.2)
complications affecting blood vessels (997.71-997.79)

CC Excl: 997.2, 997.79, 997.91, 997.99, 998.81, 998.83-998.9

▽ **DRG** 130

√4ᵗʰ √5ᵗʰ Additional Digit Required   Nonspecific PDx   Unacceptable PDx   Manifestation Code   **MSP** Medicare Secondary Payer   ►◄ Revised Text   ● New Code   ▲ Revised Code Title

997.3 Respiratory complications `CC`

Mendelson's syndrome ⎫ resulting from a proce-
Pooneumonia (aspiration) ⎭ dure

> **EXCLUDES** *iatrogenic [postoperative] pneumothorax*
> *(512.1)*
> *iatrogenic pulmonary embolism (415.11)*
> *Mendelson's syndrome in labor and*
> *delivery (668.0)*
> *specified complications classified*
> *elsewhere, such as:*
> *adult respiratory distress syndrome*
> *(518.5)*
> *pulmonary edema, postoperative*
> *(518.4)*
> *respiratory insufficiency, acute,*
> *postoperative (518.5)*
> *shock lung (518.5)*
> *tracheostomy complications*
> *(519.00-519.09)*

CC Excl: 997.3, 997.91, 997.99, 998.81, 998.83, 998.83-998.9

AHA: 1Q, '97, 10; 2Q, '93, 3; 2Q, '93, 9; 4Q, '90, 25

DEF: Mendelson's syndrome: acid pneumonitis due to aspiration of gastric acids, may occur after anesthesia or sedation.

997.4 Digestive system complications `CC`

Complications of:
intestinal (internal) anastomosis and bypass, not
elsewhere classified, except that involving
urinary tract

Hepatic failure ⎫
Hepatorenal syndrome ⎬ specified as due to
Intestinal obstruction NOS ⎭ a procedure

> **EXCLUDES** *gastrostomy complications*
> *(536.40-536.49)*
> *specified gastrointestinal complications*
> *classified elsewhere, such as:*
> *blind loop syndrome (579.2)*
> *colostomy and enterostomy*
> *complications (569.60-569.69)*
> *gastrojejunal ulcer (534.0-534.9)*
> *infection of external stoma (569.61)*
> *pelvic peritoneal adhesions, female*
> *(614.6)*
> *peritoneal adhesions (568.0)*
> *peritoneal adhesions with*
> *obstruction (560.81)*
> *postcholecystectomy syndrome*
> *(576.0)*
> *postgastric surgery syndromes*
> *(564.2)*

CC Excl: 536.40-536.49, 997.4, 997.71, 997.91, 997.99, 998.81, 998.83-998.9

AHA: 2Q, '01, 4-6; 3Q, '99, 4; 2Q, '99, 14; 3Q, '97, 7; 1Q, '97, 11; 2Q, '95, 7; 1Q, '93, 26; 3Q, '92, 15; 2Q, '89, 15; 1Q, '88, 14

▽ **DRG** 188

997.5 Urinary complications `CC`

Complications of:
external stoma of urinary tract
internal anastomosis and bypass of urinary tract,
including that involving intestinal tract

Oliguria or anuria ⎫
Renal: ⎪
failure (acute) ⎬ specified as due to
insufficiency (acute) ⎪ procedure
Tubular necrosis (acute) ⎭

> **EXCLUDES** *specified complications classified*
> *elsewhere, such as:*
> *postoperative stricture of:*
> *ureter (593.3)*
> *urethra (598.2)*

CC Excl: 997.5, 997.72, 997.91, 997.99, 998.81, 998.83-998.9

AHA: 3Q '96, 10, 15; 4Q, '95, 73; 1Q, '92, 13; 2Q, '89, 16; M-A, '87, 10; S-O, '85, 3

✓5th **997.6 Amputation stump complication**

> **EXCLUDES** *admission for treatment for a current*
> *traumatic amputation — code to*
> *complicated traumatic*
> *amputation*
> *phantom limb (syndrome) (353.6)*

AHA: 4Q, '95, 82

997.60 Unspecified complication

997.61 Neuroma of amputation stump

> **DEF:** Hyperplasia generated nerve cell mass following
> amputation.

997.62 Infection (chronic) `CC`

Use additional code to identify the organism

CC Excl: 997.60, 997.62, 997.69, 997.91, 997.99, 998.81, 998.83-998.9

AHA: 4Q, '96, 46

997.69 Other

✓5th **997.7 Vascular complications of other vessels**

> **EXCLUDES** *peripheral vascular complications*
> *(997.2)*

997.71 Vascular complications of mesenteric `CC`
artery

CC Excl: 997.2, 997.71-997.79, 997.91, 997.99, 998.81 998.83-998.9

AHA: ▶4Q, '01, 53 ◀

997.72 Vascular complications of renal artery `CC`

CC Excl: See code 997.71

997.79 Vascular complications of other vessels `CC`

CC Excl: See code 997.71

✓5th **997.9 Complications affecting other specified body**
systems, not elsewhere classified `CC`

> **EXCLUDES** *specified complications classified*
> *elsewhere, such as:*
> *broad ligament laceration syndrome*
> *(620.6)*
> *postartificial menopause syndrome*
> *(627.4)*
> *postoperative stricture of vagina*
> *(623.2)*

997.91 Hypertension

> **EXCLUDES** *essential hypertension (*
> *401.0-401.9)*

AHA: 4Q, '95, 57

997.99 Other `CC`

Vitreous touch syndrome

CC Excl: 997.91, 997.99, 998.81, 998.83-998.9

AHA: 2Q, '94, 12; 1Q, '94, 17

DEF: Vitreous touch syndrome: vitreous protruding
through pupil and attaches to corneal epithelium; causes
aqueous fluid in vitreous body; marked by corneal
edema, loss of lucidity; complication of cataract surgery.

✓4th **998 Other complications of procedures, not elsewhere classified**

AHA: 1Q, '94, 4

998.0 Postoperative shock `CC`

Collapse NOS ⎫ during or resulting
Shock (endotoxic) (hypo- ⎬ from a surgical
volemic) (septic) ⎭ procedure

> **EXCLUDES** *shock:*
> *anaphylactic due to serum (999.4)*
> *anesthetic (995.4)*
> *electric (994.8)*
> *following abortion (639.5)*
> *obstetric (669.1)*
> *traumatic (958.4)*

CC Excl: 958.4, 995.4, 997.91, 997.99, 998.0, 998.11-998.13, 998.81, 998.83-998.9

`N` Newborn Age: 0 `P` Pediatric Age: 0-17 `M` Maternity Age: 12-55 `A` Adult Age :15-124 `CC` CC Condition `MC` Major Complication `CD` Complex Dx `HIV` HIV Related Dx

√5ᵗʰ **998.1   Hemorrhage or hematoma or seroma complicating a procedure**

> **EXCLUDES**   *hemorrhage, hematoma, or seroma:*
> *complicating cesarean section or*
> *puerperal perineal wound*
> *(674.3)*

998.11 Hemorrhage complicating a procedure `CC`
CC Excl: 456.0, 456.20, 530.81-530.83, 530.89, 531.00-531.01, 531.20-531.21, 531.40-531.41, 531.60-531.61, 532.00-532.01, 532.20-532.21, 532.40-532.41, 532.60-532.61, 533.00-533.01, 533.20-533.21, 533.40-533.41, 533.60-533.61, 534.00-534.01, 534.20-534.21, 534.40-534.41, 534.60-534.61, 535.01, 535.11, 535.21, 535.31, 535.41, 535.51, 535.61, 537.83, 562.02-562.03, 562.12-562.13, 569.3, 569.85, 578.0-578.1, 578.9, 772.4, 997.91, 997.99, 998.0, 998.11-998.13, 998.81, 998.89, 998.9

AHA: 4Q, '97, 52; 1Q, '97, 10

998.12 Hematoma complicating a procedure `CC`
CC Excl: see code 998.11

998.13 Seroma complicating a procedure `CC`
CC Excl: See code 998.11

AHA: 4Q, '96, 46; 1Q, '93, 26; 2Q, '92, 15; S-O, '87, 8

998.2   Accidental puncture or laceration during a procedure `CC`
Accidental perforation by catheter or other instrument during a procedure on:
  blood vessel
  nerve
  organ

> **EXCLUDES**   *iatrogenic [postoperative] pneumothorax*
> *(512.1)*
> *puncture or laceration caused by*
> *implanted device intentionally left*
> *in operation wound (996.0-996.5)*
> *specified complications classified*
> *elsewhere, such as:*
> *broad ligament laceration syndrome*
> *(620.6)*
> *trauma from instruments during*
> *delivery (664.0-665.9)*

CC Excl: 997.91, 997.99, 998.2, 998.81, 998.83-998.9

AHA: 3Q, '94, 6; 3Q, '90, 17; 3Q, '90, 18

√5ᵗʰ **998.3   Disruption of operation wound** `CC`
Dehiscence } of operation wound
Rupture

> **EXCLUDES**   *disruption of:*
> *cesarean wound (674.1)*
> *perineal wound, puerperal (674.2)*

CC Excl: 997.91, 997.99, 998.3, 998.81, 998.83-998.9

AHA: 1Q, '93, 19

998.31 Disruption of internal operation wound `CC`
CC Excl: 997.91-997.99, 998.31, 998.32, 998.81-998.89, 998.9

998.32 Disruption of external operation wound `CC`
Disruption of operation wound NOS
CC Excl: See code 998.31

998.4   Foreign body accidentally left during a procedure `CC`
Adhesions   } due to foreign body accidentally left
Obstruction   in operative wound or body
Perforation   cavity during a procedure

> **EXCLUDES**   *obstruction or perforation caused by*
> *implanted device intentionally left*
> *in body (996.0-996.5)*

CC Excl: 997.91, 997.99, 998.4, 998.81, 998.83-998.9

AHA: 1Q, '89, 9

√5ᵗʰ **998.5   Postoperative infection**

> **EXCLUDES**   *infection due to:*
> *implanted device (996.60-996.69)*
> *infusion, perfusion, or transfusion*
> *(999.3)*
> *postoperative obstetrical wound*
> *infection (674.3)*

998.51 Infected postoperative seroma `CC`
Use additional code to identify organism
CC Excl: 997.91, 997.99, 998.51-998.59, 998.81, 998.83-998.9

AHA: 4Q, '96, 46

998.59 Other postoperative infection `CC`
Abscess:
  intra-abdominal   }
  stitch
  subphrenic   } postoperative
  wound
Septicemia   }

Use additional code to identify infection
CC Excl: See code 998.51

AHA: 3Q, '98, 3; 3Q, '95, 5; 2Q, '95, 7; 3Q, '94, 6; 1Q, '93, 19; J-F, '87, 14

998.6   Persistent postoperative fistula `CC`
CC Excl: 997.91, 997.99, 998.6, 998.81, 998.83-998.9

AHA: J-F, '87, 14

998.7   Acute reaction to foreign substance accidentally left during a procedure `CC`
Peritonitis: Peritonitis:
  aseptic   chemical
CC Excl: 997.91, 997.99, 998.7, 998.81, 998.83-998.9

√5ᵗʰ **998.8   Other specified complications of procedures, not elsewhere classified**
AHA: 4Q, '94, 46; 1Q, '89, 9

998.81 Emphysema (subcutaneous) (surgical) resulting from a procedure

998.82 Cataract fragments in eye following cataract surgery

998.83 Non-healing surgical wound `CC`
CC Excl: 997.91, 997.99, 998.81, 998.83, 998.89, 998.9

AHA: 4Q, '96, 47

998.89 Other specified complications `CC`
CC Excl: See code 998.83

AHA: 3Q, '99, 13; 2Q, '98, 16

998.9   Unspecified complication of procedure, not elsewhere classified `CC`
Postoperative complication NOS

> **EXCLUDES**   *complication NOS of obstetrical, surgery*
> *or procedure (669.4)*

CC Excl: See code 998.83

AHA: 4Q, '93, 37

√4ᵗʰ √5ᵗʰ Additional Digit Required   Nonspecific PDx   Unacceptable PDx   Manifestation Code   `MSP` Medicare Secondary Payer   ►◄ Revised Text   ● New Code   ▲ Revised Code Title

2002 Ingenix, Inc.   October 2002 • Volume 1 — 301

Injury and Poisoning 999–999.9

✓4th 999 Complications of medical care, not elsewhere classified

INCLUDES   complications, not elsewhere classified, of:
- dialysis (hemodialysis) (peritoneal) (renal)
- extracorporeal circulation
- hyperalimentation therapy
- immunization
- infusion
- inhalation therapy
- injection
- inoculation
- perfusion
- transfusion
- vaccination
- ventilation therapy

EXCLUDES   *specified complications classified elsewhere such as:*
- *complications of implanted device (996.0-996.9)*
- *contact dermatitis due to drugs (692.3)*
- *dementia dialysis (294.8)*
- *transient (293.9)*
- *dialysis disequilibrium syndrome (276.0-276.9)*
- *poisoning and toxic effects of drugs and chemicals (960.0-989.9)*
- *postvaccinal encephalitis (323.5)*
- *water and electrolyte imbalance (276.0-276.9)*

999.0 Generalized vaccinia

DEF: Skin eruption, self-limiting; follows vaccination; due to transient viremia with virus localized in skin.

999.1 Air embolism   `CC`

Air embolism to any site following infusion, perfusion, or transfusion

EXCLUDES   *embolism specified as:*
- *complicating:*
  - *abortion (634-638 with .6, 639.6)*
  - *ectopic or molar pregnancy (639.6)*
  - *pregnancy, childbirth, or the puerperium (673.0)*
- *due to implanted device (996.7)*
- *traumatic (958.0)*

CC Excl: 958.0, 999.1

999.2 Other vascular complications   `CC`

Phlebitis
Thromboembolism } following infusion, perfusion, or transfusion
Thrombophlebitis

EXCLUDES   *the listed conditions when specified as:*
- *due to implanted device (996.61-996.62, 996.72-996.74)*
- *postoperative NOS (997.2, 997.71-997.79)*

CC Excl: 999.2

AHA: 2Q, '97, 5

999.3 Other infection   `CC`

Infection
Sepsis } following infusion, injection, transfusion, or vaccination
Septicemia

EXCLUDES   *the listed conditions when specified as:*
- *due to implanted device (996.60-996.69)*
- *postoperative NOS (998.51-998.59)*

CC Excl: 999.3

AHA: 2Q, '01, 11, 12; 2Q, '97, 5; J-F, '87, 14

999.4 Anaphylactic shock due to serum   `CC`

EXCLUDES   *shock:*
- *allergic NOS (995.0)*
- *anaphylactic:*
  - *NOS (995.0)*
  - *due to drugs and chemicals (995.0)*

CC Excl: 999.4

DEF: Life-threatening hypersensitivity to foreign serum; causes respiratory distress, vascular collapse, and shock.

999.5 Other serum reaction   `CC`

Intoxication by serum   Serum sickness
Protein sickness   Urticaria due to serum
Serum rash

EXCLUDES   *serum hepatitis (070.2-070.3)*

CC Excl: 999.5

DEF: Serum sickness: Hypersensitivity to foreign serum; causes fever, hives, swelling, and lymphadenopathy.

999.6 ABO incompatibility reaction   `CC`

Incompatible blood transfusion
Reaction to blood group incompatibility in infusion or transfusion

CC Excl: 999.6

999.7 Rh incompatibility reaction   `CC`

Reactions due to Rh factor in infusion or transfusion

CC Excl: 999.7

999.8 Other transfusion reaction   `CC`

Septic shock due to transfusion
Transfusion reaction NOS

EXCLUDES   *postoperative shock (998.0)*

CC Excl: 999.8

AHA: 3Q, '00, 9

999.9 Other and unspecified complications of medical care, not elsewhere classified

Complications, not elsewhere classified, of:
- electroshock
- inhalation } therapy
- ultrasound
- ventilation

Unspecified misadventure of medical care

EXCLUDES   *unspecified complication of:*
- *phototherapy (990)*
- *radiation therapy (999)*

AHA: 2Q, '97, 5

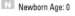
`N` Newborn Age: 0   `P` Pediatric Age: 0-17   `M` Maternity Age: 12-55   `A` Adult Age: 15-124   `CC` CC Condition   `MC` Major Complication   `CD` Complex Dx   `HIV` HIV Related Dx

302 — Volume 1   *2002 Ingenix, Inc.*

SUPPLEMENTARY CLASSIFICATION OF FACTORS INFLUENCING HEALTH STATUS AND CONTACT WITH HEALTH SERVICES (V01-V83)

This classification is provided to deal with occasions when circumstances other than a disease or injury classifiable to categories 001-999 (the main part of ICD) are recorded as "diagnoses" or "problems." This can arise mainly in three ways:

a) When a person who is not currently sick encounters the health services for some specific purpose, such as to act as a donor of an organ or tissue, to receive prophylactic vaccination, or to discuss a problem which is in itself not a disease or injury. This will be a fairly rare occurrence among hospital inpatients, but will be relatively more common among hospital outpatients and patients of family practitioners, health clinics, etc.

b) When a person with a known disease or injury, whether it is current or resolving, encounters the health care system for a specific treatment of that disease or injury (e.g., dialysis for renal disease; chemotherapy for malignancy; cast change).

c) When some circumstance or problem is present which influences the person's health status but is not in itself a current illness or injury. Such factors may be elicited during population surveys, when the person may or may not be currently sick, or be recorded as an additional factor to be borne in mind when the person is receiving care for some current illness or injury classifiable to categories 001-999.

In the latter circumstances the V code should be used only as a supplementary code and should not be the one selected for use in primary, single cause tabulations. Examples of these circumstances are a personal history of certain diseases, or a person with an artificial heart valve in situ.

AHA: J-F, '87, 8

PERSONS WITH POTENTIAL HEALTH HAZARDS RELATED TO COMMUNICABLE DISEASES (V01-V06)

EXCLUDES *family history of infectious and parasitic diseases (V18.8)*
personal history of infectious and parasitic diseases (V12.0)

√4th **V01 Contact with or exposure to communicable diseases**

V01.0 Cholera
Conditions classifiable to 001

V01.1 Tuberculosis
Conditions classifiable to 010-018

V01.2 Poliomyelitis
Conditions classifiable to 045

V01.3 Smallpox
Conditions classifiable to 050

V01.4 Rubella
Conditions classifiable to 056

V01.5 Rabies
Conditions classifiable to 071

V01.6 Venereal diseases
Conditions classifiable to 090-099

V01.7 Other viral diseases
Conditions classifiable to 042-078 and V08, except as above
AHA: 2Q, '92, 11

√5th **V01.8 Other communicable diseases**
Conditions classifiable to 001-136, except as above
AHA: J-A, '87, 24

● **V01.81 Anthrax**
● **V01.89 Other communicable diseases**

V01.9 Unspecified communicable disease

√4th **V02 Carrier or suspected carrier of infectious diseases**
AHA: 3Q, '95, 18; 3Q, '94, 4

V02.0 Cholera
V02.1 Typhoid
V02.2 Amebiasis
V02.3 Other gastrointestinal pathogens
V02.4 Diphtheria

√5th **V02.5 Other specified bacterial diseases**
V02.51 Group B streptococcus
AHA: ▶1Q, '02, 14;◀ 4Q, '98, 56

V02.52 Other streptococcus
V02.59 Other specified bacterial diseases
Meningococcal
Staphylococcal

√5th **V02.6 Viral hepatitis**
Hepatitis Australian-antigen [HAA] [SH] carrier
Serum hepatitis carrier
V02.60 Viral hepatitis carrier, unspecified
AHA: 4Q, '97, 47

V02.61 Hepatitis B carrier
AHA: 4Q, '97, 47

V02.62 Hepatitis C carrier
AHA: 4Q, '97, 47

V02.69 Other viral hepatitis carrier
AHA: 4Q, '97, 47

V02.7 Gonorrhea
V02.8 Other venereal diseases
V02.9 Other specified infectious organism
AHA: 3Q, '95, 18; 1Q, '93, 22; J-A, '87, 24

√4th **V03 Need for prophylactic vaccination and inoculation against bacterial diseases**
EXCLUDES *vaccination not carried out because of contraindication (V64.0)*
vaccines against combinations of diseases (V06.0-V06.9)

V03.0 Cholera alone
V03.1 Typhoid-paratyphoid alone [TAB]
V03.2 Tuberculosis [BCG]
V03.3 Plague
V03.4 Tularemia
V03.5 Diphtheria alone
V03.6 Pertussis alone
V03.7 Tetanus toxoid alone

√5th **V03.8 Other specified vaccinations against single bacterial diseases**
V03.81 Hemophilus influenza, type B [Hib]
V03.82 Streptococcus pneumoniae [pneumococcus]
V03.89 Other specified vaccination
AHA: 2Q, '00, 9

V03.9 Unspecified single bacterial disease

√4th **V04 Need for prophylactic vaccination and inoculation against certain viral diseases**
EXCLUDES *vaccines against combinations of diseases (V06.0-V06.9)*

V04.0 Poliomyelitis
V04.1 Smallpox
V04.2 Measles alone
V04.3 Rubella alone
V04.4 Yellow fever
V04.5 Rabies
V04.6 Mumps alone
V04.7 Common cold
V04.8 Influenza

√4th **V05 Need for other prophylactic vaccination and inoculation against single diseases**
EXCLUDES *vaccines against combinations of diseases (V06.0-V06.9)*

V05.0 Arthropod-borne viral encephalitis
V05.1 Other arthropod-borne viral diseases
V05.2 Leishmaniasis
V05.3 Viral hepatitis

V Codes V05.4–V10.09

V05.4   **Varicella**
     Chickenpox

V05.8   **Other specified disease**
     AHA: 1Q, '01, 4; 3Q, '91, 20

V05.9   **Unspecified single disease**

✓4ᵗʰ **V06**   **Need for prophylactic vaccination and inoculation against combinations of diseases**
     Note: Use additional single vaccination codes from categories V03-V05 to identify any vaccinations not included in a combination code.

V06.0   **Cholera with typhoid-paratyphoid [cholera+TAB]**

V06.1   **Diphtheria-tetanus-pertussis, combined [DTP]**
     AHA: 3Q, '98, 13

V06.2   **Diphtheria-tetanus-pertussis with typhoid-paratyphoid [DTP+TAB]**

V06.3   **Diphtheria-tetanus-pertussis with poliomyelitis [DTP+polio]**

V06.4   **Measles-mumps-rubella [MMR]**

V06.5   **Tetanus-diphtheria [Td]**

V06.6   **Streptococcus pneumoniae [pneumococcus] and influenza**

V06.8   **Other combinations**
     EXCLUDES   *multiple single vaccination codes (V03.0-V05.9)*
     AHA: 1Q, '94, 19

V06.9   **Unspecified combined vaccine**

PERSONS WITH NEED FOR ISOLATION, OTHER POTENTIAL HEALTH HAZARDS AND PROPHYLACTIC MEASURES (V07-V09)

✓4ᵗʰ **V07**   **Need for isolation and other prophylactic measures**
     EXCLUDES   *prophylactic organ removal (V50.41-V50.49)*

³ **V07.0**   **Isolation**
     Admission to protect the individual from his surroundings or for isolation of individual after contact with infectious diseases

V07.1   **Desensitization to allergens**

V07.2   **Prophylactic immunotherapy**
     Administration of:
       antivenin
       immune sera [gamma globulin]
       RhoGAM
       tetanus antitoxin

✓5ᵗʰ **V07.3**   **Other prophylactic chemotherapy**
     V07.31   **Prophylactic fluoride administration**
     ³ **V07.39**   **Other prophylactic chemotherapy**
       EXCLUDES   *maintenance chemotherapy following disease (V58.1)*

V07.4   **Postmenopausal hormone replacement therapy**   ♀

³ **V07.8**   **Other specified prophylactic measure**
     AHA: 1Q, '92, 11

V07.9   **Unspecified prophylactic measure**

³ **V08**   **Asymptomatic human immunodeficiency virus [HIV] infection status**
     HIV positive NOS
     Note: This code is *only* to be used when no HIV infection symptoms or conditions are present. If any HIV infection symptoms or conditions are present, see code 042.
     EXCLUDES   *AIDS (042)*
       human immunodeficiency virus [HIV] disease (042)
       exposure to HIV (V01.7)
       nonspecific serologic evidence of HIV (795.71)
       symptomatic human immunodeficiency virus [HIV] infection (042)
     AHA: 2Q, '99, 8; 3Q, '95, 18

³ These V codes may be used as principal diagnosis on Medicare patients.

✓4ᵗʰ **V09**   **Infection with drug-resistant microorganisms**
     Note: This category is intended for use as an additional code for infectious conditions classified elsewhere to indicate the presence of drug-resistance of the infectious organism.
     AHA: 3Q, '94, 4; 4Q, '93, 22

V09.0   **Infection with microorganisms resistant to penicillins**

V09.1   **Infection with microorganisms resistant to cephalosporins and other B-lactam antibiotics**

V09.2   **Infection with microorganisms resistant to macrolides**

V09.3   **Infection with microorganisms resistant to tetracyclines**

V09.4   **Infection with microorganisms resistant to aminoglycosides**

✓5ᵗʰ **V09.5**   **Infection with microorganisms resistant to quinolones and fluoroquinolones**
     V09.50   **Without mention of resistance to multiple quinolones and fluoroquinoles**
     V09.51   **With resistance to multiple quinolones and fluoroquinoles**

V09.6   **Infection with microorganisms resistant to sulfonamides**

✓5ᵗʰ **V09.7**   **Infection with microorganisms resistant to other specified antimycobacterial agents**
     EXCLUDES   *Amikacin (V09.4)*
       Kanamycin (V09.4)
       Streptomycin [SM] (V09.4)
     V09.70   **Without mention of resistance to multiple antimycobacterial agents**
     V09.71   **With resistance to multiple antimycobacterial agents**

✓5ᵗʰ **V09.8**   **Infection with microorganisms resistant to other specified drugs**
     V09.80   **Without mention of resistance to multiple drugs**
     V09.81   **With resistance to multiple drugs**

✓5ᵗʰ **V09.9**   **Infection with drug-resistant microorganisms, unspecified**
     Drug resistance, NOS
     V09.90   **Without mention of multiple drug resistance**
     V09.91   **With multiple drug resistance**
       Multiple drug resistance NOS

PERSONS WITH POTENTIAL HEALTH HAZARDS RELATED TO PERSONAL AND FAMILY HISTORY (V10-V19)

     EXCLUDES   *obstetric patients where the possibility that the fetus might be affected is the reason for observation or management during pregnancy (655.0-655.9)*
     AHA: J-F, '87, 1

✓4ᵗʰ **V10**   **Personal history of malignant neoplasm**
     AHA: 4Q, '98, 69; 1Q, '95, 4; 3Q, '92, 5; M-J, '85, 10; 2Q, '90, 9

✓5ᵗʰ **V10.0**   **Gastrointestinal tract**
     History of conditions classifiable to 140-159
     V10.00   **Gastrointestinal tract, unspecified**
     V10.01   **Tongue**
     V10.02   **Other and unspecified oral cavity and pharynx**
     V10.03   **Esophagus**
     V10.04   **Stomach**
     V10.05   **Large intestine**
       AHA: 3Q, '99, 7; 1Q, '95, 4
     V10.06   **Rectum, rectosigmoid junction, and anus**
     V10.07   **Liver**
     V10.09   **Other**

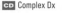

N Newborn Age: 0   P Pediatric Age: 0-17   M Maternity Age: 12-55   A Adult Age: 15-124   CC CC Condition   MC Major Complication   CD Complex Dx   HIV HIV Related Dx

✓5th **V10.1** **Trachea, bronchus, and lung**
     History of conditions classifiable to 162
     V10.11 **Bronchus and lung**
     V10.12 **Trachea**

✓5th **V10.2** **Other respiratory and intrathoracic organs**
     History of conditions classifiable to 160, 161, 163-165
     V10.20 **Respiratory organ, unspecified**
     V10.21 **Larynx**
     V10.22 **Nasal cavities, middle ear, and accessory sinuses**
     V10.29 **Other**

V10.3 **Breast**
     History of conditions classifiable to 174 and 175
     AHA: 4Q, '01, 66; 4Q, '98, 65; 4Q, '97, 50; 1Q, '91, 16; 1Q, '90, 21

✓5th **V10.4** **Genital organs**
     History of conditions classifiable to 179-187
     V10.40 **Female genital organ, unspecified** ♀
     V10.41 **Cervix uteri** ♀
     V10.42 **Other parts of uterus** ♀
     V10.43 **Ovary** ♀
     V10.44 **Other female genital organs** ♀
     V10.45 **Male genital organ, unspecified** ♂
     V10.46 **Prostate** ♂
     V10.47 **Testis** ♂
     V10.48 **Epididymis** ♂
     V10.49 **Other male genital organs** ♂

✓5th **V10.5** **Urinary organs**
     History of conditions classifiable to 188 and 189
     V10.50 **Urinary organ, unspecified**
     V10.51 **Bladder**
     V10.52 **Kidney**
       EXCLUDES *renal pelvis (V10.53)*
     V10.53 **Renal pelvis**
       AHA: 4Q, '01, 55
     V10.59 **Other**

✓5th **V10.6** **Leukemia**
     Conditions classifiable to 204-208
       EXCLUDES *leukemia in remission (204-208)*
     AHA: 2Q, '92, 13; 4Q, '91, 26; 4Q, '90, 3
     V10.60 **Leukemia, unspecified**
     V10.61 **Lymphoid leukemia**
     V10.62 **Myeloid leukemia**
     V10.63 **Monocytic leukemia**
     V10.69 **Other**

✓5th **V10.7** **Other lymphatic and hematopoietic neoplasms**
     Conditions classifiable to 200-203
       EXCLUDES *listed conditions in 200-203 in remission*
     AHA: M-J, '85, 18
     V10.71 **Lymphosarcoma and reticulosarcoma**
     V10.72 **Hodgkin's disease**
     V10.79 **Other**

✓5th **V10.8** **Personal history of malignant neoplasm of other sites**
     History of conditions classifiable to 170-173, 190-195
     V10.81 **Bone**
     V10.82 **Malignant melanoma of skin**
     V10.83 **Other malignant neoplasm of skin**
     V10.84 **Eye**
     V10.85 **Brain**
       AHA: 1Q, '01, 6
     V10.86 **Other parts of nervous system**
       EXCLUDES *peripheral sympathetic, and parasympa-thetic nerves (V10.89)*

     V10.87 **Thyroid**
     V10.88 **Other endocrine glands and related structures**
     V10.89 **Other**
V10.9 **Unspecified personal history of malignant neoplasm**

✓4th **V11** **Personal history of mental disorder**
     V11.0 **Schizophrenia**
       EXCLUDES *that in remission (295.0-295.9 with fifth-digit 5)*
     V11.1 **Affective disorders**
       Personal history of manic-depressive psychosis
       EXCLUDES *that in remission (296.0-296.6 with fifth-digit 5, 6)*
     V11.2 **Neurosis**
     V11.3 **Alcoholism**
     V11.8 **Other mental disorders**
     V11.9 **Unspecified mental disorder**

✓4th **V12** **Personal history of certain other diseases**
     AHA: 3Q, '92, 11

     ✓5th **V12.0** **Infectious and parasitic diseases**
     V12.00 **Unspecified infectious and parasitic disease**
     V12.01 **Tuberculosis**
     V12.02 **Poliomyelitis**
     V12.03 **Malaria**
     V12.09 **Other**
     V12.1 **Nutritional deficiency**
     V12.2 **Endocrine, metabolic, and immunity disorders**
       EXCLUDES *history of allergy (V14.0-V14.9, V15.01-V15.09)*
     V12.3 **Diseases of blood and blood-forming organs**

     ✓5th **V12.4** **Disorders of nervous system and sense organs**
     V12.40 **Unspecified disorder of nervous system and sense organs**
     V12.41 **Benign neoplasm of the brain**
       AHA: 4Q, '97, 48
     V12.49 **Other disorders of nervous system and sense organs**
       AHA: 4Q, '98, 59

     ✓5th **V12.5** **Diseases of circulatory system**
       AHA: 4Q, '95, 61
       EXCLUDES *old myocardial infarction (412) postmyocardial infarction syndrome (411.0)*
     V12.50 **Unspecified circulatory disease**
     V12.51 **Venous thrombosis and embolism**
       Pulmonary embolism
       AHA: ▶1Q, '02, 15◀
     V12.52 **Thrombophlebitis**
     V12.59 **Other**
       AHA: 4Q, '99, 4; 4Q, '98, 88; 4Q, '97, 37

     V12.6 **Diseases of respiratory system**
     ✓5th **V12.7** **Diseases of digestive system**
       AHA: 1Q, '95, 3; 2Q, '89, 16
     V12.70 **Unspecified digestive disease**
     V12.71 **Peptic ulcer disease**
     V12.72 **Colonic polyps**
     V12.79 **Other**

✓4th **V13** **Personal history of other diseases**
     ✓5th **V13.0** **Disorders of urinary system**
     V13.00 **Unspecified urinary disorder**
     V13.01 **Urinary calculi**
     V13.09 **Other**
     V13.1 **Trophoblastic disease** ♀
       EXCLUDES *supervision during a current pregnancy (V23.1)*

V Codes V10.1–V13.1

✓4th ✓5th Additional Digit Required   Nonspecific PDx   Unacceptable PDx   Manifestation Code   **MSP** Medicare Secondary Payer   ▶◀ Revised Text   ● New Code   ▲ Revised Code Title

V Codes V13.2–V16.6

√5ᵗʰ **V13.2 Other genital system and obstetric disorders**

> EXCLUDES   *supervision during a current pregnancy of a woman with poor obstetric history (V23.0-V23.9)*
> *habitual aborter (646.3)*
> *without current pregnancy (629.9)*

•   **V13.21 Personal history of pre-term labor**

> EXCLUDES   *current pregnancy with history of pre-term labor (V23.41)*

•   **V13.29 Other genital system and obstetric disorders**

V13.3 Diseases of skin and subcutaneous tissue

V13.4 Arthritis

V13.5 Other musculoskeletal disorders

√5ᵗʰ **V13.6 Congenital malformations**

> **AHA:** 4Q, '98, 63

V13.61 Hypospadias   ♂

V13.69 Other congenital malformations

V13.7 Perinatal problems

> EXCLUDES   *low birth weight status (V21.30-V21.35)*

V13.8 Other specified diseases

V13.9 Unspecified disease

√4ᵗʰ **V14 Personal history of allergy to medicinal agents**

V14.0 Penicillin

V14.1 Other antibiotic agent

V14.2 Sulfonamides

V14.3 Other anti-infective agent

V14.4 Anesthetic agent

V14.5 Narcotic agent

V14.6 Analgesic agent

V14.7 Serum or vaccine

V14.8 Other specified medicinal agents

V14.9 Unspecified medicinal agent

√4ᵗʰ **V15 Other personal history presenting hazards to health**

√5ᵗʰ **V15.0 Allergy, other than to medicinal agents**

> EXCLUDES   *allergy to food substance used as base for medicinal agent (V14.0-V14.9)*

> **AHA:** 4Q, '00, 42, 49

V15.01 Allergy to peanuts

V15.02 Allergy to milk products

> EXCLUDES   *lactose intolerance (271.3)*

V15.03 Allergy to eggs

V15.04 Allergy to seafood
> Seafood (octopus) (squid) ink
> Shellfish

V15.05 Allergy to other foods
> Food additives
> Nuts other than peanuts

V15.06 Allergy to insects
> Bugs
> Insect bites and stings
> Spiders

V15.07 Allergy to latex
> Latex sensitivity

V15.08 Allergy to radiographic dye
> Contrast media used for diagnostic x-ray procedures

V15.09 Other allergy, other than to medicinal agents

V15.1 Surgery to heart and great vessels

> EXCLUDES   *replacement by transplant or other means (V42.1-V42.2, V43.2-V43.4)*

V15.2 Surgery to other major organs

> EXCLUDES   *replacement by transplant or other means (V42.0-V43.8)*

V15.3 Irradiation
> Previous exposure to therapeutic or other ionizing radiation

√5ᵗʰ **V15.4 Psychological trauma**

> EXCLUDES   *history of condition classifiable to 290-316 (V11.0-V11.9)*

V15.41 History of physical abuse
> Rape
> **AHA:** 3Q, '99, 15

V15.42 History of emotional abuse
> Neglect
> **AHA:** 3Q, '99, 15

V15.49 Other
> **AHA:** 3Q, '99, 15

V15.5 Injury

V15.6 Poisoning

V15.7 Contraception

> EXCLUDES   *current contraceptive management (V25.0-V25.4)*
> *presence of intrauterine contraceptive device as incidental finding (V45.5)*

√5ᵗʰ **V15.8 Other specified personal history presenting hazards to health**

> **AHA:** 4Q, '95, 62

V15.81 Noncompliance with medical treatment
> **AHA:** 2Q, '01, 11; 12, 13; 2Q '99, 17; 2Q, '97, 11; 1Q, '97, 12; 3Q, '96, 9

V15.82 History of tobacco use
> EXCLUDES   *tobacco dependence (305.1)*

V15.84 Exposure to asbestos

V15.85 Exposure to potentially hazardous body fluids

V15.86 Exposure to lead

V15.89 Other
> **AHA:** 1Q, '90, 21; N-D, '84, 12

V15.9 Unspecified personal history presenting hazards to health

√4ᵗʰ **V16 Family history of malignant neoplasm**

V16.0 Gastrointestinal tract
> Family history of condition classifiable to 140-159
> **AHA:** 1Q, '99, 4

V16.1 Trachea, bronchus, and lung
> Family history of condition classifiable to 162

V16.2 Other respiratory and intrathoracic organs
> Family history of condition classifiable to 160-161, 163-165

V16.3 Breast
> Family history of condition classifiable to 174
> **AHA:** 2Q, '00, 8; 1Q, '92, 11

√5ᵗʰ **V16.4 Genital organs**
> Family history of condition classifiable to 179-187
> **AHA:** 4Q, '97, 48

V16.40 Genital organ, unspecified

V16.41 Ovary

V16.42 Prostate

V16.43 Testis

V16.49 Other

√5ᵗʰ **V16.5 Urinary organs**
> Family history of condition classifiable to 189

V16.51 Kidney

V16.59 Other

V16.6 Leukemia
> Family history of condition classifiable to 204-208

N Newborn Age: 0   P Pediatric Age: 0-17   M Maternity Age: 12-55   A Adult Age: 15-124   CC CC Condition   MC Major Complication   CD Complex Dx   HIV HIV Related Dx

V16.7 Other lymphatic and hematopoietic neoplasms
    Family history of condition classifiable to 200-203

V16.8 Other specified malignant neoplasm
    Family history of other condition classifiable to 140-199

V16.9 Unspecified malignant neoplasm

✓4th **V17 Family history of certain chronic disabling diseases**

V17.0 Psychiatric condition
> EXCLUDES   *family history of mental retardation (V18.4)*

V17.1 Stroke (cerebrovascular)

V17.2 Other neurological diseases
    Epilepsy
    Huntington's chorea

V17.3 Ischemic heart disease

V17.4 Other cardiovascular diseases

V17.5 Asthma

V17.6 Other chronic respiratory conditions

V17.7 Arthritis

V17.8 Other musculoskeletal diseases

✓4th **V18 Family history of certain other specific conditions**

V18.0 Diabetes mellitus

V18.1 Other endocrine and metabolic diseases

V18.2 Anemia

V18.3 Other blood disorders

V18.4 Mental retardation

V18.5 Digestive disorders

✓5th **V18.6 Kidney diseases**

    V18.61 Polycystic kidney

    V18.69 Other kidney diseases

V18.7 Other genitourinary diseases

V18.8 Infectious and parasitic diseases

✓4th **V19 Family history of other conditions**

V19.0 Blindness or visual loss

V19.1 Other eye disorders

V19.2 Deafness or hearing loss

V19.3 Other ear disorders

V19.4 Skin conditions

V19.5 Congenital anomalies

V19.6 Allergic disorders

V19.7 Consanguinity

V19.8 Other condition

PERSONS ENCOUNTERING HEALTH SERVICES IN CIRCUMSTANCES RELATED TO REPRODUCTION AND DEVELOPMENT (V20-V28)

✓4th **V20 Health supervision of infant or child**

³ **V20.0 Foundling**   P

V20.1 Other healthy infant or child receiving care   P
    Medical or nursing care supervision of healthy infant in cases of:
      maternal illness, physical or psychiatric
      socioeconomic adverse condition at home
      too many children at home preventing or interfering with normal care
    AHA: 1Q, '00, 25; 3Q, '89, 14

V20.2 Routine infant or child health check   P
    Developmental testing of infant or child
    Immunizations appropriate for age
    Routine vision and hearing testing
    Use additional code(s) to identify:
      special screening examination(s) performed (V73.0-V82.9)
> EXCLUDES   *special screening for developmental handicaps (V79.3)*

✓4th **V21 Constitutional states in development**

V21.0 Period of rapid growth in childhood

V21.1 Puberty

³ These V codes may be used as principal diagnosis on Medicare patients.

V21.2 Other adolescence

✓5th **V21.3 Low birth weight status**
> EXCLUDES   *history of perinatal problems*

    AHA: 4Q, '00, 51

    V21.30 Low birth weight status, unspecified

    V21.31 Low birth weight status, less than 500 grams

    V21.32 Low birth weight status, 500-999 grams

    V21.33 Low birth weight status, 1000-1499 grams

    V21.34 Low birth weight status, 1500-1999 grams

    V21.35 Low birth weight status, 2000-2500 grams

V21.8 Other specified constitutional states in development

V21.9 Unspecified constitutional state in development

✓4th **V22 Normal pregnancy**
> EXCLUDES   *pregnancy examination or test, pregnancy unconfirmed (V72.4)*

V22.0 Supervision of normal first pregnancy   ♀
    AHA: 3Q, '99, 16

V22.1 Supervision of other normal pregnancy   ♀
    AHA: 3Q, '99, 16

V22.2 Pregnant state, incidental   ♀
    Pregnant state NOS

✓4th **V23 Supervision of high-risk pregnancy**
    AHA: 1Q, 90, 10

V23.0 Pregnancy with history of infertility   M ♀

V23.1 Pregnancy with history of trophoblastic disease   M ♀
    Pregnancy with history of:
      hydatidiform mole
      vesicular mole
> EXCLUDES   *that without current pregnancy (V13.1)*

V23.2 Pregnancy with history of abortion   M ♀
    Pregnancy with history of conditions classifiable to 634-638
> EXCLUDES   *habitual aborter:*
>   *care during pregnancy (646.3)*
>   *that without current pregnancy (629.9)*

V23.3 Grand multiparity   M ♀
> EXCLUDES   *care in relation to labor and delivery (659.4)*
>   *that without current pregnancy (V61.5)*

✓5th **V23.4 Pregnancy with other poor obstetric history**
    Pregnancy with history of other conditions classifiable to 630-676

    V23.41 Pregnancy with history of pre-term labor   M ♀

    V23.49 Pregnancy with other poor obstetric history   M ♀

V23.5 Pregnancy with other poor reproductive history   M ♀
    Pregnancy with history of stillbirth or neonatal death

V23.7 Insufficient prenatal care   CC M ♀
    History of little or no prenatal care
    CC Excl: V22.0-V22.2, V23.0-V23.9

✓5th **V23.8 Other high-risk pregnancy**
    AHA: 4Q, '98, 56, 63

    V23.81 Elderly primigravida   CC M ♀
      First pregnancy in a woman who will be 35 years of age or older at expected date of delivery
> EXCLUDES   *elderly primigravida complicating pregnancy (659.5)*

      CC Excl: See code V23.7

✓4th ✓5th Additional Digit Required   Nonspecific PDx   Unacceptable PDx   Manifestation Code   MSP Medicare Secondary Payer   ►◄ Revised Text   ● New Code   ▲ Revised Code Title

2002 Ingenix, Inc.   October 2002 • Volume 1 — 307

V Codes V16.7–V23.81

V23.82 **Elderly multigravida**   CC M ♀
Second or more pregnancy in a woman who will be 35 years of age or older at expected date of delivery

> EXCLUDES   elderly multigravida complicating pregnancy (659.6)

CC Excl: See code V23.7

V23.83 **Young primigravida**   CC M ♀
First pregnancy in a female less than 16 years old at expected date of delivery

> EXCLUDES   young primigravida complicating pregnancy (659.8)

CC Excl: See code V23.7

V23.84 **Young multigravida**   CC M ♀
Second or more pregnancy in a female less than 16 years old at expected date of delivery

> EXCLUDES   young multigravida complicating pregnancy (659.8)

V23.89 **Other high-risk pregnancy**   CC M ♀
CC Excl: See code V23.7

V23.9 **Unspecified high-risk pregnancy**   CC M ♀
CC Excl: See code V23.7

✓4th **V24 Postpartum care and examination**
3   **V24.0** **Immediately after delivery**   M ♀
Care and observation in uncomplicated cases

V24.1 **Lactating mother**   ♀
Supervision of lactation

V24.2 **Routine postpartum follow-up**   ♀

✓4th **V25 Encounter for contraceptive management**
AHA: 4Q, '92, 24

✓5th **V25.0** **General counseling and advice**
V25.01 **Prescription of oral contraceptives**   ♀
V25.02 **Initiation of other contraceptive measures**
Fitting of diaphragm
Prescription of foams, creams, or other agents
AHA: 3Q, '97, 7

V25.09 **Other**
Family planning advice

V25.1 **Insertion of intrauterine contraceptive device**   ♀

3   **V25.2** **Sterilization**
Admission for interruption of fallopian tubes or vas deferens

3   **V25.3** **Menstrual extraction**   ♀
Menstrual regulation

✓5th **V25.4** **Surveillance of previously prescribed contraceptive methods**
Checking, reinsertion, or removal of contraceptive device
Repeat prescription for contraceptive method
Routine examination in connection with contraceptive maintenance

> EXCLUDES   presence of intrauterine contraceptive device as incidental finding (V45.5)

V25.40 **Contraceptive surveillance, unspecified**
V25.41 **Contraceptive pill**   ♀
V25.42 **Intrauterine contraceptive device**   ♀
Checking, reinsertion, or removal of intrauterine device
V25.43 **Implantable subdermal contraceptive**   ♀

V25.49 **Other contraceptive method**
AHA: 3Q, '97, 7

V25.5 **Insertion of implantable subdermal contraceptive**   ♀
AHA: 3Q, '92, 9

V25.8 **Other specified contraceptive management**
Postvasectomy sperm count

> EXCLUDES   sperm count following sterilization reversal (V26.22) sperm count for fertility testing (V26.21)

AHA: 3Q, '96, 9

V25.9 **Unspecified contraceptive management**

✓4th **V26 Procreative management**
3   **V26.0** **Tuboplasty or vasoplasty after previous sterilization**
AHA: 2Q, '95, 10

V26.1 **Artificial insemination**   ♀

✓5th **V26.2** **Investigation and testing**
> EXCLUDES   postvasectomy sperm count (V25.8)

AHA: 4Q, '00, 56

V26.21 **Fertility testing**
Fallopian insufflation
Sperm count for fertility testing
> EXCLUDES   genetic counseling and testing (V26.3)

V26.22 **Aftercare following sterilization reversal**
Fallopian insufflation following sterilization reversal
Sperm count following sterilization reversal

V26.29 **Other investigation and testing**
AHA: 2Q, '96, 9; N-D, '85, 15

V26.3 **Genetic counseling and testing**
> EXCLUDES   fertility testing (V26.21)

V26.4 **General counseling and advice**

✓5th **V26.5** **Sterilization status**
V26.51 **Tubal ligation status**   ♀
> EXCLUDES   infertility not due to previous tubal ligation (628.0-628.9)

V26.52 **Vasectomy status**   ♂
V26.8 **Other specified procreative management**
V26.9 **Unspecified procreative management**

✓4th **V27 Outcome of delivery**
Note: This category is intended for the coding of the outcome of delivery on the mother's record.

AHA: 2Q, '91, 16

V27.0 **Single liveborn**   M ♀
AHA: 1Q, '01, 10; 3Q, '00, 5; 4Q, '98, 77; 4Q, '95, 59; 1Q, '92, 9

V27.1 **Single stillborn**   M ♀
V27.2 **Twins, both liveborn**   M ♀
V27.3 **Twins, one liveborn and one stillborn**   M ♀
V27.4 **Twins, both stillborn**   M ♀
V27.5 **Other multiple birth, all liveborn**   M ♀
V27.6 **Other multiple birth, some liveborn**   M ♀
V27.7 **Other multiple birth, all stillborn**   M ♀
V27.9 **Unspecified outcome of delivery**   M ♀

Single birth } outcome to infant
Multiple birth } unspecified

---

3 These V codes may be used as principal diagnosis on Medicare patients.

| N Newborn Age: 0 | P Pediatric Age: 0-17 | M Maternity Age: 12-55 | A Adult Age: 15-124 | CC CC Condition | MC Major Complication | CD Complex Dx | HIV HIV Related Dx |

✓4ᵗʰ **V28 Antenatal screening**

    EXCLUDES   *abnormal findings on screening — code to findings*
            routine prenatal care (V22.0-V23.9)

    V28.0   Screening for chromosomal anomalies by amniocentesis   M ♀

    V28.1   Screening for raised alpha-fetoprotein levels in amniotic fluid   M ♀

    V28.2   Other screening based on amniocentesis   M ♀

    V28.3   Screening for malformation using ultrasonics   ♀

    V28.4   Screening for fetal growth retardation using ultrasonics   ♀

    V28.5   Screening for isoimmunization   ♀

    V28.6   Screening for Streptococcus B   M ♀
         AHA: 4Q, '97, 46

    V28.8   Other specified antenatal screening   ♀
         AHA: 3Q, '99, 16

    V28.9   Unspecified antenatal screening   ♀

✓4ᵗʰ **V29 Observation and evaluation of newborns and infants for suspected condition not found**

    Note: This category is to be used for newborns, within the neonatal period, (the first 28 days of life) who are suspected of having an abnormal condition resulting from exposure from the mother or the birth process, but without signs or symptoms, and, which after examination and observation, is found not to exist.

    AHA: 1Q, '00, 25; 4Q, '94, 47; 1Q, '94, 9; 4Q, '92, 21

  [3] **V29.0**   Observation for suspected infectious condition   N
         AHA: 1Q, '01, 10

  [3] **V29.1**   Observation for suspected neurological condition   N

  [3] **V29.2**   Observation for suspected respiratory condition   N

    V29.3   Observation for suspected genetic or metabolic condition   N
         AHA: 4Q, '98, 59, 68

  [3] **V29.8**   Observation for other specified suspected condition   N

    V29.9   Observation for unspecified suspected condition   N
         AHA: ▶1Q, '02, 6◀

LIVEBORN INFANTS ACCORDING TO TYPE OF BIRTH (V30-V39)

    Note: These categories are intended for the coding of liveborn infants who are consuming health care [e.g., crib or bassinet occupancy].

The following fourth-digit subdivisions are for use with categories V30-V39:   N

    ✓5ᵗʰ **0**   Born in hospital   N
        1   Born before admission to hospital
        2   Born outside hospital and not hospitalized

The following two fifth-digits are for use with the fourth-digit .0, Born in hospital:
        0   delivered without mention of cesarean delivery
        1   delivered by cesarean delivery

    AHA: 1Q, '01, 10

[4] ✓4ᵗʰ **V30 Single liveborn**
    AHA: 4Q, '98, 46, 59; 1Q, '94, 9

[4] ✓4ᵗʰ **V31 Twin, mate liveborn**
    AHA: 3Q, '92, 10

[4] ✓4ᵗʰ **V32 Twin, mate stillborn**

[4] ✓4ᵗʰ **V33 Twin, unspecified**

[4] ✓4ᵗʰ **V34 Other multiple, mates all liveborn**

[4] ✓4ᵗʰ **V35 Other multiple, mates all stillborn**

[4] ✓4ᵗʰ **V36 Other multiple, mates live- and stillborn**

[4] ✓4ᵗʰ **V37 Other multiple, unspecified**

[5] ✓4ᵗʰ **V39 Unspecified**

PERSONS WITH A CONDITION INFLUENCING THEIR HEALTH STATUS (V40-V49)

    Note: These categories are intended for use when these conditions are recorded as "diagnoses" or "problems."

✓4ᵗʰ **V40 Mental and behavioral problems**

    V40.0   Problems with learning
    V40.1   Problems with communication [including speech]
    V40.2   Other mental problems
    V40.3   Other behavioral problems
    V40.9   Unspecified mental or behavioral problem

✓4ᵗʰ **V41 Problems with special senses and other special functions**

    V41.0   Problems with sight
    V41.1   Other eye problems
    V41.2   Problems with hearing
    V41.3   Other ear problems
    V41.4   Problems with voice production
    V41.5   Problems with smell and taste
    V41.6   Problems with swallowing and mastication
    V41.7   Problems with sexual function

        EXCLUDES   *marital problems (V61.10)*
                 psychosexual disorders (302.0-302.9)

    V41.8   Other problems with special functions
    V41.9   Unspecified problem with special functions

✓4ᵗʰ **V42 Organ or tissue replaced by transplant**

    INCLUDES   homologous or heterologous (animal) (human) transplant organ status

    AHA: 3Q, '98, 3, 4

    V42.0   Kidney   CC
         CC Excl: 996.80-996.81, 996.87, V42.0, V42.89-V42.9
         AHA: 3Q, '01, 12

    V42.1   Heart   CC
         CC Excl: 996.80, 996.83, 996.87, V42.1, V42.89-V42.9
         AHA: 3Q, '01, 13

    V42.2   Heart valve   CC
         CC Excl: 996.71, V42.2, V42.89-V42.9

    V42.3   Skin
    V42.4   Bone
    V42.5   Cornea

    V42.6   Lung   CC
         CC Excl: 996.80, 996.84, 996.87, V42.6, V42.89-V42.9

    V42.7   Liver   CC
         CC Excl: 996.80, 996.82, 996.87, V42.7, V42.89-V42.9

    ✓5ᵗʰ **V42.8**   Other specified organ or tissue
         AHA: 4Q, '98, 64; 4Q, '97, 49

        V42.81   Bone marrow   CC
             CC Excl: 996.80, 996.85, 996.87, V42.9

        V42.82   Peripheral stem cells   CC
             CC Excl: 996.80, 996.87, V42.9

        V42.83   Pancreas   CC
             CC Excl: 996.80, 996.86-996.87, V42.83, V42.9
             AHA: 2Q, '01, 16

        V42.84   Intestines   CC
             CC Excl: 996.80, 996.89, V42.84-V42.9
             AHA: 4Q, '00, 48, 50

        V42.89   Other   CC
             CC Excl: 996.80, 996.87-996.89, V42.89-V42.9

---

[3] These V codes may be used as principal diagnosis on Medicare patients.
[4] These codes with the fourth digit of 0 or 1, may be used as a principal diagnosis for Medicare patients.
[5] These V codes are acceptable as principal diagnosis with the fourth digit of 0.

✓4ᵗʰ ✓5ᵗʰ **Additional Digit Required**   Nonspecific PDx   Unacceptable PDx   Manifestation Code   **MSP** Medicare Secondary Payer   ▶◀ Revised Text   ● New Code   ▲ Revised Code Title

2002 Ingenix, Inc.

October 2002 • Volume 1 — **309**

V Codes V42.9–V45.83

V42.9 Unspecified organ or tissue

√4th **V43 Organ or tissue replaced by other means**

    INCLUDES   replacement of organ by:
         artificial device
         mechanical device
         prosthesis

    EXCLUDES   *cardiac pacemaker in situ (V45.01)*
         fitting and adjustment of prosthetic device
         (V52.0-V52.9)
         renal dialysis status (V45.1)

V43.0 Eye globe

V43.1 Lens
     Pseudophakos
     AHA: 4Q, '98, 65

V43.2 Heart   CC
     CC Excl: 996.80, 996.83, 996.87, V42.1, V43.2

V43.3 Heart valve

V43.4 Blood vessel

V43.5 Bladder

√5th **V43.6 Joint**
     V43.60 Unspecified joint
     V43.61 Shoulder
     V43.62 Elbow
     V43.63 Wrist
     V43.64 Hip
     V43.65 Knee
     V43.66 Ankle
     V43.69 Other

V43.7 Limb

√5th **V43.8 Organ or tissue replaced by other means**
     V43.81 Larynx
         AHA: 4Q, '95, 55
     V43.82 Breast
         AHA: 4Q, '95, 55
     V43.83 Artificial skin
     V43.89 Other

√4th **V44 Artificial opening status**

    EXCLUDES   *artificial openings requiring attention or*
         management (V55.0-V55.9)

V44.0 Tracheostomy
     AHA: 1Q, '01, 6

V44.1 Gastrostomy
     AHA: 1Q, '01, 12; 3Q, '97, 12; 1Q, '93, 26

V44.2 Ileostomy

V44.3 Colostomy

V44.4 Other artificial opening of gastrointestinal tract

√5th **V44.5 Cystostomy**
     V44.50 Cystostomy, unspecified
     V44.51 Cutaneous-vesicostomy
     V44.52 Appendico-vesicostomy
     V44.59 Other cystostomy

V44.6 Other artificial opening of urinary tract
     Nephrostomy   Urethrostomy
     Ureterostomy

V44.7 Artificial vagina

V44.8 Other artificial opening status

V44.9 Unspecified artificial opening status

√4th **V45 Other postsurgical states**

    EXCLUDES   *aftercare management (V51-V58.9)*
         malfunction or other complication — code to
         condition

√5th **V45.0 Cardiac device in situ**
     V45.00 Unspecified cardiac device
     V45.01 Cardiac pacemaker
     V45.02 Automatic implantable cardiac defibrillator

     V45.09 Other specified cardiac device
         Carotid sinus pacemaker in situ

V45.1 Renal dialysis status   CC
     Patient requiring intermittent renal dialysis
     Presence of arterial-venous shunt (for dialysis)

    EXCLUDES   *admission for dialysis treatment or*
         session (V56.0)

     CC Excl: 996.73, V45.1

     AHA: 2Q, '01, 12, 13

V45.2 Presence of cerebrospinal fluid drainage device
     Cerebral ventricle (communicating) shunt, valve, or
     device in situ

    EXCLUDES   *malfunction (996.2)*

V45.3 Intestinal bypass or anastomosis status

V45.4 Arthrodesis status
     AHA: N-D, '84, 18

√5th **V45.5 Presence of contraceptive device**

    EXCLUDES   *checking, reinsertion, or removal of*
         device (V25.42)
         complication from device (996.32)
         insertion of device (V25.1)

     V45.51 Intrauterine contraceptive device   ♀
     V45.52 Subdermal contraceptive implant
     V45.59 Other

√5th **V45.6 States following surgery of eye and adnexa**
     Cataract extraction   ⎱
     Filtering bleb   ⎰ state following eye
     Surgical eyelid adhesion ⎰ surgery

    EXCLUDES   *aphakia (379.31)*
         artificial eye globe (V43.0)

     AHA: 4Q, '98, 65; 4Q, '97, 49

     V45.61 Cataract extraction status
         Use additional code for associated
         artificial lens status (V43.1)

     V45.69 Other states following surgery of eye and adnexa
         AHA: 2Q, '01, 16; 1Q, '98, 10; 4Q, '97, 19

√5th **V45.7 Acquired absence of organ**
     AHA: 4Q, '98, 65; 4Q, '97, 50

    ³ **V45.71 Acquired absence of breast**
         AHA: ▶4Q, '01, 66;◀ 4Q, '97, 50

     V45.72 Acquired absence of intestine (large) (small)
     V45.73 Acquired absence of kidney
     V45.74 Other parts of urinary tract
         Bladder
         AHA: 4Q, '00, 51

     V45.75 Stomach
         AHA: 4Q, '00, 51

     V45.76 Lung
         AHA: 4Q, '00, 51

     V45.77 Genital organs
         AHA: 4Q, '00, 51

     V45.78 Eye
         AHA: 4Q, '00, 51

     V45.79 Other acquired absence of organ
         AHA: 4Q, '00, 51

√5th **V45.8 Other postsurgical status**
     V45.81 Aortocoronary bypass status
         AHA: ▶3Q, '01, 15;◀ 3Q, '97, 16

     V45.82 Percutaneous transluminal coronary angioplasty status

     V45.83 Breast implant removal status
         AHA: 4Q, '95, 55

---

³ These V codes may be used as principal diagnosis on Medicare patients.

| N Newborn Age: 0 | P Pediatric Age: 0-17 | M Maternity Age: 12-55 | A Adult Age: 15-124 | CC CC Condition | MC Major Complication | CD Complex Dx | HIV HIV Related Dx |

V45.84 Dental restoration status
Dental crowns status
Dental fillings status
AHA: 4Q, '01, 54

V45.89 Other
Presence of neuropacemaker or other electronic device
EXCLUDES *artificial heart valve in situ (V43.3)*
vascular prosthesis in situ (V43.4)
AHA: 1Q, '95, 11

✓4ᵗʰ **V46 Other dependence on machines**

V46.0 Aspirator

V46.1 Respirator   CC
Iron lung
CC Excl: V46.0-V46.1, V46.8-V46.9
AHA: 1Q, '01, 12; J-F, '87, 7 3

● **V46.2 Supplemental oxygen**
Long-term oxygen therapy

V46.8 Other enabling machines
Hyperbaric chamber
Possum [Patient-Operated-Selector-Mechanism]
EXCLUDES *cardiac pacemaker (V45.0)*
kidney dialysis machine (V45.1)

V46.9 Unspecified machine dependence

✓4ᵗʰ **V47 Other problems with internal organs**

V47.0 Deficiencies of internal organs

V47.1 Mechanical and motor problems with internal organs

V47.2 Other cardiorespiratory problems
Cardiovascular exercise intolerance with pain (with):
at rest
less than ordinary activity
ordinary activity

V47.3 Other digestive problems

V47.4 Other urinary problems

V47.5 Other genital problems

V47.9 Unspecified

✓4ᵗʰ **V48 Problems with head, neck, and trunk**

V48.0 Deficiencies of head
EXCLUDES *deficiencies of ears, eyelids, and nose (V48.8)*

V48.1 Deficiencies of neck and trunk

V48.2 Mechanical and motor problems with head

V48.3 Mechanical and motor problems with neck and trunk

V48.4 Sensory problem with head

V48.5 Sensory problem with neck and trunk

V48.6 Disfigurements of head

V48.7 Disfigurements of neck and trunk

V48.8 Other problems with head, neck, and trunk

V48.9 Unspecified problem with head, neck, or trunk

✓4ᵗʰ **V49 Other conditions influencing health status**

V49.0 Deficiencies of limbs

V49.1 Mechanical problems with limbs

V49.2 Motor problems with limbs

V49.3 Sensory problems with limbs

V49.4 Disfigurements of limbs

V49.5 Other problems of limbs

✓5ᵗʰ **V49.6 Upper limb amputation status**
AHA: 4Q, '98, 42; 4Q, '94, 39

V49.60 Unspecified level

V49.61 Thumb

V49.62 Other finger(s)

V49.63 Hand

V49.64 Wrist
Disarticulation of wrist

V49.65 Below elbow

V49.66 Above elbow
Disarticulation of elbow

V49.67 Shoulder
Disarticulation of shoulder

✓5ᵗʰ **V49.7 Lower limb amputation status**
AHA: 4Q, '98, 42; 4Q, '94, 39

V49.70 Unspecified level

V49.71 Great toe

V49.72 Other toe(s)

V49.73 Foot

V49.74 Ankle
Disarticulation of ankle

V49.75 Below knee

V49.76 Above knee
Disarticulation of knee

V49.77 Hip
Disarticulation of hip

✓5ᵗʰ **V49.8 Other specified conditions influencing health status**
AHA: 4Q, '00, 51

V49.81 Postmenopausal status (age-related) (natural)   A ♀
EXCLUDES *menopausal and premenopausal disorder (627.0-627.9)*
postsurgical menopause (256.2)
premature menopause (256.31)
symptomatic menopause (627.0-627.9)
AHA: 4Q, '00, 54

▲ **V49.81 Asymptomatic postmenopausal status (age-related) (natural)**

V49.82 Dental sealant status
AHA: 4Q, '01, 54

V49.89 Other specified conditions influencing health status

V49.9 Unspecified

PERSONS ENCOUNTERING HEALTH SERVICES FOR SPECIFIC PROCEDURES AND AFTERCARE (V50-V59)

Note: Categories V51-V58 are intended for use to indicate a reason for care in patients who may have already been treated for some disease or injury not now present, or who are receiving care to consolidate the treatment, to deal with residual states, or to prevent recurrence.
EXCLUDES *follow-up examination for medical surveillance following treatment (V67.0-V67.9)*

✓4ᵗʰ **V50 Elective surgery for purposes other than remedying health states**

³ **V50.0 Hair transplant**

³ **V50.1 Other plastic surgery for unacceptable cosmetic appearance**
Breast augmentation or reduction
Face-lift
EXCLUDES *plastic surgery following healed injury or operation (V51)*

³ **V50.2 Routine or ritual circumcision**   ♂
Circumcision in the absence of significant medical indication

V50.3 Ear piercing

✓5ᵗʰ **V50.4 Prophylactic organ removal**
EXCLUDES *organ donations (V59.0-V59.9)*
therapeutic organ removal — code to condition
AHA: 4Q, '94, 44

³ **V50.41 Breast**

³ **V50.42 Ovary**   ♀

³ These V codes may be used as principal diagnosis on Medicare patients.

✓4ᵗʰ ✓5ᵗʰ Additional Digit Required | Nonspecific PDx | Unacceptable PDx | Manifestation Code | MSP Medicare Secondary Payer | ▶◀ Revised Text | ● New Code | ▲ Revised Code Title

2002 Ingenix, Inc.

October 2002 • Volume 1 — 311

V Codes V45.84–V50.42

[3] **V50.49 Other**

V50.8 Other

V50.9 Unspecified

[3] **V51 Aftercare involving the use of plastic surgery**

Plastic surgery following healed injury or operation

> EXCLUDES   cosmetic plastic surgery (V50.1)
> plastic surgery as treatment for current injury —
>   code to condition
> repair of scarred tissue — code to scar

√4th **V52 Fitting and adjustment of prosthetic device and implant**

> INCLUDES   removal of device
> EXCLUDES   malfunction or complication of prosthetic device
>   (996.0-996.7)
> status only, without need for care (V43.0-V43.8)

AHA: 4Q, '95, 55 ; 1Q, '90, 7

[3] **V52.0 Artificial arm (complete) (partial)**

[3] **V52.1 Artificial leg (complete) (partial)**

[3] **V52.2 Artificial eye**

[3] **V52.3 Dental prosthetic device**

[3] **V52.4 Breast prosthesis and implant**   ♀

> EXCLUDES   admission for implant insertion (V50.1)

AHA: 4Q, '95, 80, 81

[3] **V52.8 Other specified prosthetic device**

V52.9 Unspecified prosthetic device

√4th **V53 Fitting and adjustment of other device**

> INCLUDES   removal of device
>   replacement of device
> EXCLUDES   status only, without need for care (V45.0-V45.8)

√5th **V53.0 Devices related to nervous system and special senses**

AHA: 4Q, '98, 66; 4Q, '97, 51

V53.01 Fitting and adjustment of cerebral ventricular (communicating) shunt

AHA: 4Q, '97, 51

V53.02 Neuropacemaker (brain) (peripheral nerve) (spinal cord)

[3] **V53.09 Fitting and adjustment of other devices related to nervous system and special senses**

Auditory substitution device

Visual substitution device

AHA: 2Q '99, 4

V53.1 Spectacles and contact lenses

V53.2 Hearing aid

√5th **V53.3 Cardiac device**

Reprogramming

AHA: 3Q, '92, 3; 1Q, '90, 7; M-J, '87, 8 ; N-D, '84, 18

[3] **V53.31 Cardiac pacemaker**

> EXCLUDES   mechanical complication of
>   cardiac pacemaker
>   (996.01)

AHA: ▶1Q, '02, 3◀

[3] **V53.32 Automatic implantable cardiac defibrillator**

[3] **V53.39 Other cardiac device**

V53.4 Orthodontic devices

V53.5 Other intestinal appliance

> EXCLUDES   colostomy (V55.3)
> ileostomy (V55.2)
> other artificial opening of digestive tract
>   (V55.4)

V53.6 Urinary devices

Urinary catheter

> EXCLUDES   cystostomy (V55.5)
> nephrostomy (V55.6)
> ureterostomy (V55.6)
> urethrostomy (V55.6)

V53.7 Orthopedic devices

Orthopedic:	Orthopedic:
brace	corset
cast	shoes

> EXCLUDES   other orthopedic aftercare (V54)

V53.8 Wheelchair

V53.9 Other and unspecified device

√4th **V54 Other orthopedic aftercare**

> EXCLUDES   fitting and adjustment of orthopedic devices
>   (V53.7)
> malfunction of internal orthopedic device (996.4)
> other complication of nonmechanical nature
>   (996.60-996.79)

AHA: 3Q, '95, 3

[3] **V54.0 Aftercare involving removal of fracture plate or other internal fixation device**

Removal of:	Removal of:
pins	rods
plates	screws

> EXCLUDES   malfunction of internal orthopedic
>   device (996.4)
> other complication of nonmechanical
>   nature (996.60-996.79)
> removal of external fixation device
>   ▶(V54.89)◀

√5th **V54.1 Aftercare for healing traumatic fracture**

V54.10 Aftercare for healing traumatic fracture of arm, unspecified

V54.11 Aftercare for healing traumatic fracture of upper arm

V54.12 Aftercare for healing traumatic fracture of lower arm

V54.13 Aftercare for healing traumatic fracture of hip

V54.14 Aftercare for healing traumatic fracture of leg, unspecified

V54.15 Aftercare for healing traumatic fracture of upper leg

> EXCLUDES   aftercare for healing traumatic
>   fracture of hip (V54.13)

V54.16 Aftercare for healing traumatic fracture of lower leg

V54.17 Aftercare for healing traumatic fracture of vertebrae

V54.19 Aftercare for healing traumatic fracture of other bone

√5th **V54.2 Aftercare for healing pathologic fracture**

V54.20 Aftercare for healing pathologic fracture of arm, unspecified

V54.21 Aftercare for healing pathologic fracture of upper arm

V54.22 Aftercare for healing pathologic fracture of lower arm

V54.23 Aftercare for healing pathologic fracture of hip

V54.24 Aftercare for healing pathologic fracture of leg, unspecified

V54.25 Aftercare for healing pathologic fracture of upper leg

> EXCLUDES   aftercare for healing pathologic
>   fracture of hip (V54.23)

V54.26 Aftercare for healing pathologic fracture of lower leg

V54.27 Aftercare for healing pathologic fracture of vertebrae

V54.29 Aftercare for healing pathologic fracture of other bone

---

[3]   These V codes may be used as principal diagnosis on Medicare patients.

[6]   Rehabilitation codes acceptable as a principal diagnosis when accompanied by a secondary diagnosis reflection the condition treated.

N Newborn Age: 0   **P** Pediatric Age: 0-17   **M** Maternity Age: 12-55   **A** Adult Age: 15-124   **CC** CC Condition   **MC** Major Complication   **CD** Complex Dx   **HIV** HIV Related Dx

✓5th **V54.8 Other orthopedic aftercare**
AHA: 3Q, '01, 19; 4Q, '99, 5

● **V54.81 Aftercare following joint replacement**
Use additional code to identify joint
replacement site (V43.60-V43.69)

● **V54.89 Other orthopedic aftercare**
Aftercare for healing fracture NOS

V54.9 Unspecified orthopedic aftercare

✓4th **V55 Attention to artificial openings**
INCLUDES　adjustment or repositioning of catheter
closure
passage of sounds or bougies
reforming
removal or replacement of catheter
toilet or cleansing
EXCLUDES　complications of external stoma (519.00-
519.09, 569.60-569.69, 997.4,
997.5)
status only, without need for care (V44.0-V44.9)

3 **V55.0 Tracheostomy**

3 **V55.1 Gastrostomy**
AHA: 4Q, '99, 9; 3Q, '97, 7, 8; 1Q, '96, 14; 3Q, '95, 13

3 **V55.2 Ileostomy**

3 **V55.3 Colostomy**
AHA: 3Q, '97, 9

3 **V55.4 Other artificial opening of digestive tract**

3 **V55.5 Cystostomy**

3 **V55.6 Other artificial opening of urinary tract**
Nephrostomy　　　Urethrostomy
Ureterostomy

3 **V55.7 Artificial vagina**

3 **V55.8 Other specified artificial opening**

V55.9 Unspecified artificial opening

✓4th **V56 Encounter for dialysis and dialysis catheter care**
Use additional code to identify the associated condition
EXCLUDES　dialysis preparation — code to condition
AHA: 4Q, '98, 66; 1Q, '93, 29

3 **V56.0 Extracorporeal dialysis**
Dialysis (renal) NOS
EXCLUDES　dialysis status (V45.1)
AHA: 4Q, '00, 40; 3Q, '98, 6; 2Q, '98, 20

6 **V56.1 Fitting and adjustment of extracorporeal dialysis catheter**
Removal or replacement of catheter
Toilet or cleansing
Use additional code for any concurrent
extracorporeal dialysis (V56.0)
AHA: 2Q, '98, 20

V56.2 Fitting and adjustment of peritoneal dialysis catheter
Use additional code for any concurrent peritoneal
dialysis (V56.8)
AHA: 4Q, '98, 55

✓5th **V56.3 Encounter for adequacy testing for dialysis**
AHA: 4Q, '00, 55

V56.31 Encounter for adequacy testing for hemodialysis

V56.32 Encounter for adequacy testing for peritoneal dialysis
Peritoneal equilibration test

3 **V56.8 Other dialysis**
Peritoneal dialysis
AHA: 4Q, '98, 55

✓4th **V57 Care involving use of rehabilitation procedures**
Use additional code to identify underlying condition
AHA: ▶1Q, '02, 19;◀3Q, '97, 12; 1Q, '90, 6; S-O, '86, 3

V57.0 Breathing exercises

6 **V57.1 Other physical therapy**
Therapeutic and remedial exercises, except
breathing
AHA: 4Q, '99, 5

✓5th **V57.2 Occupational therapy and vocational rehabilitation**

6 **V57.21 Encounter for occupational therapy**
AHA: 4Q, '99, 7

6 **V57.22 Encounter for vocational therapy**

6 **V57.3 Speech therapy**
AHA: 4Q, '97, 36

V57.4 Orthoptic training

✓5th **V57.8 Other specified rehabilitation procedure**
V57.81 Orthotic training
Gait training in the use of artificial limbs

6 **V57.89 Other**
Multiple training or therapy
AHA:▶1Q, '02, 16;◀3Q, '01, 21; 3Q, '97, 11, 12; S-O, '86, 4

6 **V57.9 Unspecified rehabilitation procedure**

✓4th **V58 Encounter for other and unspecified procedures and aftercare**
EXCLUDES　convalescence and palliative care (V66)

3 **V58.0 Radiotherapy**
Encounter or admission for radiotherapy
EXCLUDES　encounter for radioactive implant —
code to condition
radioactive iodine therapy — code to
condition
AHA: 3Q, '92, 5; 2Q, '90, 7; J-F, '87, 13

3 **V58.1 Chemotherapy**
Encounter or admission for chemotherapy
EXCLUDES　prophylactic chemotherapy against
disease which has never been
present (V03.0-V07.9)
AHA: 3Q, '93, 4; 2Q, '92, 6; 2Q, '91, 17; 2Q, '90, 7; S-O, '84, 5

V58.2 Blood transfusion, without reported diagnosis
V58.3 Attention to surgical dressings and sutures
Change of dressings
Removal of sutures

✓5th **V58.4 Other aftercare following surgery**
▶Note: Codes from this subcategory should be used in
conjunction with other aftercare codes to fully
identify the reason for the aftercare encounter◀
EXCLUDES　aftercare following sterilization
reversal surgery (V26.22)
attention to artificial openings (V55.0-
V55.9)
orthopedic aftercare (V54.0-V54.9)
AHA: 4Q, '99, 9; N-D, '87, 9

3, 7 **V58.41 Encounter for planned postoperative wound closure**
EXCLUDES　disruption of operative wound (998.3)
AHA: 4Q, '99, 15

7 **V58.42 Aftercare following surgery for neoplasm**
Conditions classifiable to 140-239

3 These V codes may be used as principal diagnosis on Medicare patients.
6 Rehabilitation codes acceptable as a principal diagnosis when accompanied by a secondary diagnosis reflection the condition treated.
7 These V codes are acceptable as principal diagnosis when accompanied by a diagnosis of personal history of malignancy. These codes group to DRGs 465-466.

✓4th ✓5th Additional Digit Required　Nonspecific PDx　Unacceptable PDx　Manifestation Code　MSP Medicare Secondary Payer　▶◀ Revised Text　● New Code　▲ Revised Code Title

V Codes V54.8–V58.42

●   7 **V58.43 Aftercare following surgery for injury and trauma**
Conditions classifiable to 800-999
EXCLUDES *aftercare for healing traumatic fracture (V54.10-V54.19)*

3, 7 **V58.49 Other specified aftercare following surgery**
AHA: 1Q, '96, 8, 9

7 **V58.5 Orthodontics**
EXCLUDES *fitting and adjustment of orthodontic device (V53.4)*

✓5ᵗʰ **V58.6 Long-term (current) drug use**
EXCLUDES *drug abuse (305.00-305.93)*
drug dependence (304.00-304.93)

AHA: 4Q, '95, 61

3, 7 **V58.61 Long-term (current) use of anticoagulants**
AHA: ▶1Q, '02, 15, 16◀

7 **V58.62 Long-term (current) use of antibiotics**
AHA: 4Q, '98, 59

3, 7 **V58.69 Long-term (current) use of other medications**
High-risk medications
AHA: 2Q, '00, 8; 3Q, '99, 13; 2Q, '99, 17; 1Q, '97, 12; 2Q, '96, 7

● ✓5ᵗʰ **V58.7 Aftercare following surgery to specified body systems, not elsewhere classified**
Note: Codes from this subcategory should be used in conjunction with other aftercare codes to fully identify the reason for the aftercare encounter

● 7 **V58.71 Aftercare following surgery of the sense organs, NEC**
Conditions classifiable to 360-379, 380-389

● 7 **V58.72 Aftercare following surgery of the nervous system, NEC**
Conditions classifiable to 320-359
EXCLUDES *aftercare following surgery of the sense organs, NEC (V58.71)*

● 7 **V58.73 Aftercare following surgery of the circulatory system, NEC**
Conditions classifiable to 390-459

● 7 **V58.74 Aftercare following surgery of the respiratory system, NEC**
Conditions classifiable to 460-519

● 7 **V58.75 Aftercare following surgery of the teeth, oral cavity and digestive system, NEC**
Conditions classifiable to 520-579

● 7 **V58.76 Aftercare following surgery of the genitourinary system, NEC**
Conditions classifiable to 580-629
EXCLUDES *aftercare following sterilization reversal (V26.22)*

● 7 **V58.77 Aftercare following surgery of the skin and subcutaneous tissue, NEC**
Conditions classifiable to 680-709

● 7 **V58.78 Aftercare following surgery of the musculoskeletal system, NEC**
Conditions classifiable to 710-739

✓5ᵗʰ **V58.8 Other specified procedures and aftercare**
AHA: 4Q, '94, 45; 2Q, '94, 8

7 **V58.81 Fitting and adjustment of vascular catheter**
Removal or replacement of catheter
Toilet or cleansing
EXCLUDES *complication of renal dialysis (996.73)*
complication of vascular catheter (996.74)
dialysis preparation — code to condition
encounter for dialysis (V56.0-V56.8)
fitting and adjustment of dialysis catheter (V56.1)

7 **V58.82 Fitting and adjustment of nonvascular catheter, NEC**
Removal or replacement of catheter
Toilet or cleansing
EXCLUDES *fitting and adjustment of peritoneal dialysis catheter (V56.2)*
fitting and adjustment of urinary catheter (V53.6)

7 **V58.83 Encounter for therapeutic drug monitoring**
▶Use additional code for any associated long-term (current) drug use (V58.61-V58.69)◀
EXCLUDES *blood-drug testing for medicolegal reasons (V70.4)*

3, 7 **V58.89 Other specified aftercare**
AHA: 4Q, '98, 59

7 **V58.9 Unspecified aftercare**

✓4ᵗʰ **V59 Donors**
EXCLUDES *examination of potential donor (V70.8)*
self-donation of organ or tissue — code to condition
AHA: 4Q, '95, 62; 1Q, '90, 10; N-D, '84, 8

✓5ᵗʰ **V59.0 Blood**
V59.01 Whole blood
V59.02 Stem cells
V59.09 Other

3 **V59.1 Skin**
3 **V59.2 Bone**
3 **V59.3 Bone marrow**
3 **V59.4 Kidney**
3 **V59.5 Cornea**
3 **V59.6 Liver**
3 **V59.8 Other specified organ or tissue**
3 **V59.9 Unspecified organ or tissue**

PERSONS ENCOUNTERING HEALTH SERVICES IN OTHER CIRCUMSTANCES (V60-V68)

✓4ᵗʰ **V60 Housing, household, and economic circumstances**
V60.0 Lack of housing
Hobos   Transients
Social migrants   Vagabonds
Tramps

V60.1 Inadequate housing
Lack of heating   Technical defects in
Restriction of space   home preventing adequate care

V60.2 Inadequate material resources
Economic problem
Poverty NOS

V60.3 Person living alone

---

3   These V codes may be used as principal diagnosis on Medicare patients.
6   Rehabilitation codes acceptable as a principal diagnosis when accompanied by a secondary diagnosis reflection the condition treated.
7   These V codes are acceptable as principal diagnosis when accompanied by a diagnosis of personal history of malignancy. These codes group to DRGs 465-466.

N Newborn Age: 0   **P** Pediatric Age: 0-17   **M** Maternity Age: 12-55   **A** Adult Age: 15-124   **CC** CC Condition   **MC** Major Complication   **CD** Complex Dx   **HIV** HIV Related Dx

V60.4 No other household member able to render care
Person requiring care (has) (is):
  family member too handicapped, ill, or otherwise
    unsuited to render care
  partner temporarily away from home
  temporarily away from usual place of abode
  EXCLUDES   holiday relief care (V60.5)

V60.5 Holiday relief care
Provision of health care facilities to a person
  normally cared for at home, to enable relatives
  to take a vacation

V60.6 Person living in residential institution
Boarding school resident

V60.8 Other specified housing or economic circumstances

V60.9 Unspecified housing or economic circumstance

V61 Other family circumstances
INCLUDES   when these circumstances or fear of them,
  affecting the person directly involved or
  others, are mentioned as the reason,
  justified or not, for seeking or receiving
  medical advice or care

AHA: 1Q, '90, 9

V61.0 Family disruption
Divorce
Estrangement

V61.1 Counseling for marital and partner problems
EXCLUDES   problems related to:
  psychosexual disorders (302.0-
   302.9)
  sexual function (V41.7)

V61.10 Counseling for marital and partner problems, unspecified
Marital conflict
Partner conflict

V61.11 Counseling for victim of spousal and partner abuse
EXCLUDES   encounter for treatment of
  current injuries due to
  abuse (995.80-995.85)

V61.12 Counseling for perpetrator of spousal and partner abuse

V61.2 Parent-child problems

V61.20 Counseling for parent-child problem, unspecified
Concern about behavior of child
Parent-child conflict

³ **V61.21 Counseling for victim of child abuse**
Child battering   Child neglect
EXCLUDES   current injuries due to abuse
  (995.50-995.59)

V61.22 Counseling for perpetrator of parental child abuse
EXCLUDES   counseling for non-parental
  abuser (V62.83)

V61.29 Other
Problem concerning adopted or foster child
AHA: 3Q, '99, 16

V61.3 Problems with aged parents or in-laws

V61.4 Health problems within family
V61.41 Alcoholism in family
V61.49 Other
Care of   }   sick or handicapped
Presence of }   person in family
         or household

V61.5 Multiparity
V61.6 Illegitimacy or illegitimate pregnancy ♀
V61.7 Other unwanted pregnancy ♀
V61.8 Other specified family circumstances

Problems with family members NEC
V61.9 Unspecified family circumstance

V62 Other psychosocial circumstances
INCLUDES   those circumstances or fear of them, affecting
  the person directly involved or others,
  mentioned as the reason, justified or not,
  for seeking or receiving medical advice or
  care
EXCLUDES   previous psychological trauma (V15.41-V15.49)

V62.0 Unemployment
EXCLUDES   circumstances when main problem is
  economic inadequacy or poverty
  (V60.2)

V62.1 Adverse effects of work environment

V62.2 Other occupational circumstances or maladjustment
Career choice problem
Dissatisfaction with employment

V62.3 Educational circumstances
Dissatisfaction with school environment
Educational handicap

V62.4 Social maladjustment
Cultural deprivation
Political, religious, or sex discrimination
Social:
  isolation
  persecution

V62.5 Legal circumstances
Imprisonment   Litigation
Legal investigation   Prosecution

V62.6 Refusal of treatment for reasons of religion or conscience

V62.8 Other psychological or physical stress, not elsewhere classified
V62.81 Interpersonal problems, not elsewhere classified
V62.82 Bereavement, uncomplicated
EXCLUDES   bereavement as adjustment
  reaction (309.0)
V62.83 Counseling for perpetrator of physical/sexual abuse
EXCLUDES   counseling for perpetrator of
  parental child abuse
  (V61.22)
  counseling for perpetrator of
  spousal and partner
  abuse (V61.12)
V62.89 Other
Life circumstance problems
Phase of life problems

V62.9 Unspecified psychosocial circumstance

V63 Unavailability of other medical facilities for care
AHA: 1Q, '91, 21

V63.0 Residence remote from hospital or other health care facility

V63.1 Medical services in home not available
EXCLUDES   no other household member able to
  render care (V60.4)
AHA: ▶4Q, '01, 67;◀ 1Q, '01, 12

V63.2 Person awaiting admission to adequate facility elsewhere

V63.8 Other specified reasons for unavailability of medical facilities
Person on waiting list undergoing social agency
  investigation

V63.9 Unspecified reason for unavailability of medical facilities

V64 Persons encountering health services for specific procedures, not carried out

³ These V codes may be used as principal diagnosis on Medicare patients.

V64.0 Vaccination not carried out because of contraindication

V64.1 Surgical or other procedure not carried out because of contraindication

V64.2 Surgical or other procedure not carried out because of patient's decision
AHA: 2Q, '01, 8

V64.3 Procedure not carried out for other reasons

V64.4 Laparoscopic surgical procedure converted to open procedure
AHA: 4Q, '98, 68; 4Q, '97, 52

√4th **V65** Other persons seeking consultation without complaint or sickness

3　**V65.0** Healthy person accompanying sick person
　　　Boarder

V65.1 Person consulting on behalf of another person
　Advice or treatment for nonattending third party
　EXCLUDES　concern (normal) about sick person in family (V61.41-V61.49)

3　**V65.2** Person feigning illness
　　Malingerer　　　　　Peregrinating patient
　　AHA: 3Q, '99, 20

V65.3 Dietary surveillance and counseling
　Dietary surveillance and counseling (in):
　　　NOS　　　　　　gastritis
　　　colitis　　　　　hypercholesterolemia
　　　diabetes mellitus　hypoglycemia
　　　food allergies or　obesity
　　　　intolerance

√5th **V65.4** Other counseling, not elsewhere classified
　　Health:　　　　　　Health:
　　　advice　　　　　　instruction
　　　education
　　EXCLUDES　counseling (for):
　　　　　　　contraception (V25.40-V25.49)
　　　　　　　genetic (V26.3)
　　　　　　　on behalf of third party (V65.1)
　　　　　　　procreative management (V26.4)

　V65.40 Counseling NOS
　V65.41 Exercise counseling
　V65.42 Counseling on substance use and abuse
　V65.43 Counseling on injury prevention
　V65.44 Human immunodeficiency virus [HIV] counseling
　V65.45 Counseling on other sexually transmitted diseases
　V65.49 Other specified counseling
　　　AHA: 2Q, '00, 8

V65.5 Person with feared complaint in whom no diagnosis was made
　Feared condition not demonstrated
　Problem was normal state
　"Worried well"

V65.8 Other reasons for seeking consultation
　　EXCLUDES　specified symptoms
　AHA: 3Q, '92, 4

V65.9 Unspecified reason for consultation

√4th **V66** Convalescence and palliative care
3　**V66.0** Following surgery
3　**V66.1** Following radiotherapy
3　**V66.2** Following chemotherapy
3　**V66.3** Following psychotherapy and other treatment for mental disorder
3　**V66.4** Following treatment of fracture
　V66.5 Following other treatment
3　**V66.6** Following combined treatment

V66.7 Encounter for palliative care
　End of life care
　Hospice care
　Terminal care
　Code first underlying disease
　AHA: 1Q, '98, 11; 4Q, '96, 47, 48

V66.9 Unspecified convalescence
　AHA: 4Q, '99, 8

√4th **V67** Follow-up examination
　INCLUDES　surveillance only following completed treatment
　EXCLUDES　surveillance of contraception (V25.40-V25.49)
　AHA: 4Q, '94, 48

√5th **V67.0** Following surgery
　AHA: 4Q, '00, 56; 4Q, '98, 69; 4Q, '97, 50; 2Q, '95, 8;1Q, '95, 4; 3Q, '92, 11

3, 7　**V67.00** Following surgery, unspecified

3, 7　**V67.01** Follow-up vaginal pap smear　　　　♀
　Vaginal pap-smear, status-post hysterectomy for malignant condition
　Use additional code to identify:
　　acquired absence of uterus (V45.77)
　　personal history of malignant neoplasm (V10.40-V10.44)
　EXCLUDES　vaginal pap smear status-post hysterectomy for non-malignant condition (V76.47)

3, 7　**V67.09** Following other surgery
　EXCLUDES　sperm count following sterilization reversal (V26.22)
　　　　　　sperm count for fertility testing (V26.21)

3　**V67.1** Following radiotherapy
3　**V67.2** Following chemotherapy
　Cancer chemotherapy follow-up
3　**V67.3** Following psychotherapy and other treatment for mental disorder
3, 7　**V67.4** Following treatment of healed fracture
　EXCLUDES　current (healing) fracture aftercare (V54.0-V54.9)
　AHA: 1Q, '90, 7

√5th **V67.5** Following other treatment
3　**V67.51** Following completed treatment with high-risk medications, not elsewhere classified
　EXCLUDES　long-term (current) drug use (V58.61-V58.69)
　AHA: 1Q, '99, 5, 6;4Q, '95, 61 ; 1Q, '90, 18

3　**V67.59** Other

3　**V67.6** Following combined treatment
　V67.9 Unspecified follow-up examination

√4th **V68** Encounters for administrative purposes
　V68.0 Issue of medical certificates
　Issue of medical certificate of:
　　cause of death
　　fitness
　　incapacity
　EXCLUDES　encounter for general medical examination (V70.0-V70.9)

3　These V codes may be used as principal diagnosis on Medicare patients.
7　These V codes are acceptable as principal diagnosis when accompanied by a diagnosis of personal history of malignancy. These codes group to DRGs 465-466.

N Newborn Age: 0　P Pediatric Age: 0-17　M Maternity Age: 12-55　A Adult Age: 15-124　CC CC Condition　MC Major Complication　CD Complex Dx　HIV HIV Related Dx

V68.1 Issue of repeat prescriptions
Issue of repeat prescription for:
    appliance
    glasses
    medications
    EXCLUDES *repeat prescription for contraceptives (V25.41-V25.49)*

V68.2 Request for expert evidence

✓5ᵗʰ **V68.8 Other specified administrative purpose**

    V68.81 Referral of patient without examination or treatment

    V68.89 Other

V68.9 Unspecified administrative purpose

✓4ᵗʰ **V69 Problems related to lifestyle**
    AHA: 4Q, '94, 48

V69.0 Lack of physical exercise

V69.1 Inappropriate diet and eating habits
    EXCLUDES *anorexia nervosa (307.1)*
    bulimia (783.6)
    malnutrition and other nutritional deficiencies (260-269.9)
    other and unspecified eating disorders (307.50-307.59)

V69.2 High-risk sexual behavior

V69.3 Gambling and betting
    EXCLUDES *pathological gambling (312.31)*

V69.8 Other problems related to lifestyle
    Self-damaging behavior

V69.9 Problem related to lifestyle, unspecified

PERSONS WITHOUT REPORTED DIAGNOSIS ENCOUNTERED DURING EXAMINATION AND INVESTIGATION OF INDIVIDUALS AND POPULATIONS ▶(V70-V83)◀

Note: Nonspecific abnormal findings disclosed at the time of these examinations are classifiable to categories 790-796.

✓4ᵗʰ **V70 General medical examination**
Use additional code(s) to identify any special screening examination(s) performed (V73.0-V82.9)

V70.0 Routine general medical examination at a health care facility
    Health checkup
    EXCLUDES *health checkup of infant or child (V20.2)*

³ **V70.1 General psychiatric examination, requested by the authority**

V70.2 General psychiatric examination, other and unspecified

V70.3 Other medical examination for administrative purposes
    General medical examination for:
    admission to old age home
    adoption
    camp
    driving license
    immigration and naturalization
    insurance certification
    marriage
    prison
    school admission
    sports competition
    EXCLUDES *attendance for issue of medical certificates (V68.0)*
    pre-employment screening (V70.5)
    AHA: 1Q, '90, 6

³ **V70.4 Examination for medicolegal reasons**
    Blood-alcohol tests
    Blood-drug tests
    Paternity testing
    EXCLUDES *examination and observation following:*
    accidents (V71.3, V71.4)
    assault (V71.6)
    rape (V71.5)

³ **V70.5 Health examination of defined subpopulations**
    Armed forces personnel   Prisoners
    Inhabitants of institutions   Prostitutes
    Occupational health   Refugees
      examinations   School children
    Pre-employment screening   Students
    Preschool children

V70.6 Health examination in population surveys
    EXCLUDES *special screening (V73.0-V82.9)*

³ **V70.7 Examination of participant in clinical trial**
    Examination of participant or control in clinical research
    AHA: 4Q, '01, 55

V70.8 Other specified general medical examinations
    Examination of potential donor of organ or tissue

V70.9 Unspecified general medical examination

✓4ᵗʰ **V71 Observation and evaluation for suspected conditions not found**
    INCLUDES This category is to be used when persons without a diagnosis are suspected of having an abnormal condition, without signs or symptoms, which requires study, but after examination and observation, is found not to exist. This category is also for use for administrative and legal observation status.
    AHA: 4Q, '94, 47; 2Q, '90, 5; M-A, '87, 1

✓5ᵗʰ **V71.0 Observation for suspected mental condition**
    ³ **V71.01 Adult antisocial behavior**   Ⓐ
    Dyssocial behavior or gang activity in adult without manifest psychiatric disorder
    ³ **V71.02 Childhood or adolescent antisocial behavior**
    Dyssocial behavior or gang activity in child or adolescent without manifest psychiatric disorder
    ³ **V71.09 Other suspected mental condition**

³ **V71.1 Observation for suspected malignant neoplasm**

³ **V71.2 Observation for suspected tuberculosis**

³ **V71.3 Observation following accident at work**

³ **V71.4 Observation following other accident**
    Examination of individual involved in motor vehicle traffic accident

³ **V71.5 Observation following alleged rape or seduction**
    Examination of victim or culprit

³ **V71.6 Observation following other inflicted injury**
    Examination of victim or culprit

³ **V71.7 Observation for suspected cardiovascular disease**
    AHA: 3Q, '90, 10; S-O, '87, 10

▲ ✓5ᵗʰ **V71.8 Observation and evaluation for other specified suspected conditions**
    AHA: 4Q, '00, 54 ; 1Q, '90, 19

    ³ **V71.81 Abuse and neglect**
    EXCLUDES *adult abuse and neglect (995.80-995.85)*
    child abuse and neglect (995.50-995.59)
    AHA: 4Q, '00, 55

●   **V71.82 Observation and evaluation for suspected exposure to anthrax**

●   **V71.83 Observation and evaluation for suspected exposure to other biological agent**

³ These V codes may be used as principal diagnosis on Medicare patients.

Additional Digit Required   **Nonspecific PDx**   **Unacceptable PDx**   **Manifestation Code**   **MSP** Medicare Secondary Payer   ▶◀ Revised Text   ● New Code   ▲ Revised Code Title

2002 Ingenix, Inc.   **October 2002 • Volume 1 — 317**

³ **V71.89 Other specified suspected conditions**

V71.9 Observation for unspecified suspected condition

AHA: ▶1Q, '02, 6◀

✓4ᵗʰ **V72 Special investigations and examinations**

INCLUDES   routine examination of specific system

EXCLUDES   *general medical examination (V70.0-V70.4)*
general screening examination of defined population groups (V70.5, V70.6, V70.7)
routine examination of infant or child (V20.2)

Use additional code(s) to identify any special screening examination(s) performed (V73.0-V82.9)

³ **V72.0 Examination of eyes and vision**

V72.1 Examination of ears and hearing

V72.2 Dental examination

³ **V72.3 Gynecological examination**   ♀

Papanicolaou cervical smear as part of general gynecological examination
Pelvic examination (annual) (periodic)
Use additional code to identify routine vaginal Papanicolaou smear (V76.47)

EXCLUDES   *cervical Papanicolaou smear without general gynecological examination (V76.2)*
routine examination in contraceptive management (V25.40-V25.49)

V72.4 Pregnancy examination or test, pregnancy unconfirmed   ♀

Possible pregnancy, not (yet) confirmed

EXCLUDES   *pregnancy examination with immediate confirmation (V22.0-V22.1)*

V72.5 Radiological examination, not elsewhere classified

Routine chest x-ray

EXCLUDES   *examination for suspected tuberculosis (V71.2)*

AHA: 1Q, '90, 19

V72.6 Laboratory examination

EXCLUDES   *that for suspected disorder (V71.0-V71.9)*

AHA: 1Q, '90, 22

V72.7 Diagnostic skin and sensitization tests

Allergy tests   Skin tests for hypersensitivity

EXCLUDES   *diagnostic skin tests for bacterial diseases (V74.0-V74.9)*

✓5ᵗʰ **V72.8 Other specified examinations**

³ **V72.81 Pre-operative cardiovascular examination**

³ **V72.82 Pre-operative respiratory examination**

AHA: 3Q, '96, 14

³ **V72.83 Other specified pre-operative examination**

AHA: 3Q, '96, 14

V72.84 Pre-operative examination, unspecified

V72.85 Other specified examination

V72.9 Unspecified examination

✓4ᵗʰ **V73 Special screening examination for viral and chlamydial diseases**

V73.0 Poliomyelitis

V73.1 Smallpox

V73.2 Measles

V73.3 Rubella

V73.4 Yellow fever

V73.5 Other arthropod-borne viral diseases

Dengue fever   Viral encephalitis:
Hemorrhagic fever   mosquito-borne
    tick-borne

V73.6 Trachoma

✓5ᵗʰ **V73.8 Other specified viral and chlamydial diseases**

V73.88 Other specified chlamydial diseases

V73.89 Other specified viral diseases

✓5ᵗʰ **V73.9 Unspecified viral and chlamydial disease**

V73.98 Unspecified chlamydial disease

V73.99 Unspecified viral disease

✓4ᵗʰ **V74 Special screening examination for bacterial and spirochetal diseases**

INCLUDES   diagnostic skin tests for these diseases

V74.0 Cholera

V74.1 Pulmonary tuberculosis

V74.2 Leprosy [Hansen's disease]

V74.3 Diphtheria

V74.4 Bacterial conjunctivitis

V74.5 Venereal disease

V74.6 Yaws

V74.8 Other specified bacterial and spirochetal diseases

Brucellosis   Tetanus
Leptospirosis   Whooping cough
Plague

V74.9 Unspecified bacterial and spirochetal disease

✓4ᵗʰ **V75 Special screening examination for other infectious diseases**

V75.0 Rickettsial diseases

V75.1 Malaria

V75.2 Leishmaniasis

V75.3 Trypanosomiasis

Chagas' disease
Sleeping sickness

V75.4 Mycotic infections

V75.5 Schistosomiasis

V75.6 Filariasis

V75.7 Intestinal helminthiasis

V75.8 Other specified parasitic infections

V75.9 Unspecified infectious disease

✓4ᵗʰ **V76 Special screening for malignant neoplasms**

V76.0 Respiratory organs

✓5ᵗʰ **V76.1 Breast**

AHA: 4Q, '98, 67

V76.10 Breast screening, unspecified

V76.11 Screening mammogram for high-risk patient   ♀

V76.12 Other screening mammogram

V76.19 Other screening breast examination

V76.2 Cervix   ♀

Routine cervical Papanicolaou smear

EXCLUDES   *that as part of a general gynecological examination (V72.3)*

V76.3 Bladder

✓5ᵗʰ **V76.4 Other sites**

V76.41 Rectum

V76.42 Oral cavity

V76.43 Skin

V76.44 Prostate   ♀

V76.45 Testis   ♀

V76.46 Ovary

AHA: 4Q, '00, 52

V76.47 Vagina

Vaginal pap smear status-post hysterectomy for non-malignant condition
Use additional code to identify acquired absence of uterus (V45.77)

EXCLUDES   *vaginal pap smear status-post hysterectomy for malignant condition (V67.01)*

AHA: 4Q, '00, 52

V76.49 Other sites

AHA: 1Q, '99, 4

³ These V codes may be used as principal diagnosis on Medicare patients.

N Newborn Age: 0   **P** Pediatric Age: 0-17   **M** Maternity Age: 12-55   **A** Adult Age: 15-124   **CC** CC Condition   **MC** Major Complication   **CD** Complex Dx   **HIV** HIV Related Dx

√5ᵗʰ **V76.5 Intestine**
AHA: 4Q, '00, 52

V76.50 Intestine, unspecified
V76.51 Colon
    EXCLUDES   *rectum (V76.41)*
    AHA: 4Q, '01, 56

V76.52 Small intestine
√5ᵗʰ **V76.8 Other neoplasm**
AHA: 4Q, '00, 52

V76.81 Nervous system
V76.89 Other neoplasm
V76.9 Unspecified

√4ᵗʰ **V77 Special screening for endocrine, nutritional, metabolic, and immunity disorders**
V77.0 Thyroid disorders
V77.1 Diabetes mellitus
V77.2 Malnutrition
V77.3 Phenylketonuria [PKU]
V77.4 Galactosemia
V77.5 Gout
V77.6 Cystic fibrosis
     Screening for mucoviscidosis
V77.7 Other inborn errors of metabolism
V77.8 Obesity
√5ᵗʰ **V77.9 Other and unspecified endocrine, nutritional, metabolic, and immunity disorders**
AHA: 4Q, '00, 53

V77.91 Screening for lipid disorders
     Screening for cholesterol level
     Screening for hypercholesterolemia
     Screening for hyperlipidemia
V77.99 Other and unspecified endocrine, nutritional, metabolic, and immunity disorders

√4ᵗʰ **V78 Special screening for disorders of blood and blood-forming organs**
V78.0 Iron deficiency anemia
V78.1 Other and unspecified deficiency anemia
V78.2 Sickle cell disease or trait
V78.3 Other hemoglobinopathies
V78.8 Other disorders of blood and blood-forming organs
V78.9 Unspecified disorder of blood and blood-forming organs

√4ᵗʰ **V79 Special screening for mental disorders and developmental handicaps**
V79.0 Depression
V79.1 Alcoholism
V79.2 Mental retardation
V79.3 Developmental handicaps in early childhood
V79.8 Other specified mental disorders and developmental handicaps
V79.9 Unspecified mental disorder and developmental handicap

√4ᵗʰ **V80 Special screening for neurological, eye, and ear diseases**
V80.0 Neurological conditions
V80.1 Glaucoma

V80.2 Other eye conditions
   Screening for: Screening for:
     cataract   senile macular lesions
     congenital anomaly of eye
       EXCLUDES   *general vision examination (V72.0)*
V80.3 Ear diseases
       EXCLUDES   *general hearing examination (V72.1)*

√4ᵗʰ **V81 Special screening for cardiovascular, respiratory, and genitourinary diseases**
V81.0 Ischemic heart disease
V81.1 Hypertension
V81.2 Other and unspecified cardiovascular conditions
V81.3 Chronic bronchitis and emphysema
V81.4 Other and unspecified respiratory conditions
       EXCLUDES   *screening for:*
         lung neoplasm (V76.0)
         pulmonary tuberculosis (V74.1)
V81.5 Nephropathy
     Screening for asymptomatic bacteriuria
V81.6 Other and unspecified genitourinary conditions

√4ᵗʰ **V82 Special screening for other conditions**
V82.0 Skin conditions
V82.1 Rheumatoid arthritis
V82.2 Other rheumatic disorders
V82.3 Congenital dislocation of hip
V82.4 Maternal postnatal screening for chromosomal anomalies ♀
       EXCLUDES   *antenatal screening by amniocentesis (V28.0)*
V82.5 Chemical poisoning and other contamination
     Screening for:
       heavy metal poisoning
       ingestion of radioactive substance
       poisoning from contaminated water supply
       radiation exposure
V82.6 Multiphasic screening
√5ᵗʰ **V82.8 Other specified conditions**
AHA: 4Q, '00, 53

V82.81 Osteoporosis
     Use additional code to identify:
       postmenopausal hormone replacement therapy status (V07.4)
       postmenopausal (age-related) (natural) status (V49.81)
     AHA: 4Q, '00, 54

V82.89 Other specified conditions
V82.9 Unspecified condition

√4ᵗʰ **V83 Genetic carrier status**
AHA: 4Q, '01, 54

√5ᵗʰ **V83.0 Hemophilia A carrier**
   V83.01 Asymptomatic hemophilia A carrier
   V83.02 Symptomatic hemophilia A carrier
√5ᵗʰ **V83.8 Other genetic carrier status**
   V83.81 Cystic fibrosis gene carrier
   V83.89 Other genetic carrier status

V Codes V76.5–V83.89

√4ᵗʰ √5ᵗʰ Additional Digit Required   Nonspecific PDx   Unacceptable PDx   Manifestation Code   MSP Medicare Secondary Payer   ►◄ Revised Text   ● New Code   ▲ Revised Code Title

2002 Ingenix, Inc.   **October 2002 • Volume 1 — 319**

SUPPLEMENTARY CLASSIFICATION OF EXTERNAL CAUSES OF INJURY AND POISONING (E800-E999)

This section is provided to permit the classification of environmental events, circumstances, and conditions as the cause of injury, poisoning, and other adverse effects. Where a code from this section is applicable, it is intended that it shall be used in addition to a code from one of the main chapters of ICD-9-CM, indicating the nature of the condition. Certain other conditions which may be stated to be due to external causes are classified in Chapters 1 to 16 of ICD-9-CM. For these, the "E" code classification should be used as an additional code for more detailed analysis.

Machinery accidents [other than those connected with transport] are classifiable to category E919, in which the fourth-digit allows a broad classification of the type of machinery involved. If a more detailed classification of type of machinery is required, it is suggested that the "Classification of Industrial Accidents according to Agency," prepared by the International Labor Office, be used in addition. This is reproduced in Appendix D for optional use.

Categories for "late effects" of accidents and other external causes are to be found at E929, E959, E969, E977, E989, and E999.

DEFINITIONS AND EXAMPLES RELATED TO TRANSPORT ACCIDENTS

(a) A **transport accident** (E800-E848) is any accident involving a device designed primarily for, or being used at the time primarily for, conveying persons or goods from one place to another.

> **INCLUDES**   accidents involving:
> aircraft and spacecraft (E840-E845)
> watercraft (E830-E838)
> motor vehicle (E810-E825)
> railway (E800-E807)
> other road vehicles (E826-E829)

In classifying accidents which involve more than one kind of transport, the above order of precedence of transport accidents should be used.

Accidents involving agricultural and construction machines, such as tractors, cranes, and bulldozers, are regarded as transport accidents only when these vehicles are under their own power on a highway [otherwise the vehicles are regarded as machinery]. Vehicles which can travel on land or water, such as hovercraft and other amphibious vehicles, are regarded as watercraft when on the water, as motor vehicles when on the highway, and as off-road motor vehicles when on land, but off the highway.

> **EXCLUDES**   *accidents:*
> *in sports which involve the use of transport but where the transport vehicle itself was not involved in the accident*
> *involving vehicles which are part of industrial equipment used entirely on industrial premises*
> *occurring during transportation but unrelated to the hazards associated with the means of transportation [e.g., injuries received in a fight on board ship; transport vehicle involved in a cataclysm such as an earthquake]*
> *to persons engaged in the maintenance or repair of transport equipment or vehicle not in motion, unlesss injured by another vehicle in motion*

(b) A **railway accident** is a transport accident involving a railway train or other railway vehicle operated on rails, whether in motion or not.

> **EXCLUDES**   *accidents:*
> *in repair shops*
> *in roundhouse or on turntable*
> *on railway premises but not involving a train or other railway vehicle*

(c) A **railway train** or **railway vehicle** is any device with or without cars coupled to it, desiged for traffic on a railway.

> **INCLUDES**   interurban:
> electric car ⎫ (operated chiefly on its
> streetcar ⎬ own right-of-way,
>   ⎭ not open to other
>   traffic)
> railway train, any power [diesel] [electric] [steam]
> funicular
> monorail or two-rail
> subterranean or elevated
> other vehicle designed to run on a railway track

> **EXCLUDES**   *interurban electric cars [streetcars] specified to be operating on a right-of-way that forms part of the public street or highway [definition (n)]*

(d) A **railway** or **railroad** is a right-of-way designed for traffic on rails, which is used by carriages or wagons transporting passengers or freight, and by other rolling stock, and which is not open to other public vehicular traffic.

(e) A **motor vehicle accident** is a transport accident involving a motor vehicle. It is defined as a motor vehicle traffic accident or as a motor vehicle nontraffic accident according to whether the accident occurs on a public highway or elsewhere.

> **EXCLUDES**   *injury or damage due to cataclysm*
> *injury or damage while a motor vehicle, not under its own power, is being loaded on, or unloaded from, another conveyance*

(f) A **motor vehicle traffic accident** is any motor vehicle accident occurring on a public highway [i.e., originating, terminating, or involving a vehicle partially on the highway]. A motor vehicle accident is assumed to have occurred on the highway unless another place is specified, except in the case of accidents involving only off-road motor vehicles which are classified as nontraffic accidents unless the contrary is stated.

(g) A **motor vehicle nontraffic accident** is any motor vehicle accident which occurs entirely in any place other than a public highway.

(h) A **public highway [trafficway]** or **street** is the entire width between property lines [or other boundary lines] of every way or place, of which any part is open to the use of the public for purposes of vehicular traffic as a matter of right or custom. A **roadway** is that part of the public highway designed, improved, and ordinarily used, for vehicular travel.

> **INCLUDES**   approaches (public) to:
> docks
> public building
> station

> **EXCLUDES**   *driveway (private)*
> *parking lot*
> *ramp*
> *roads in:*
> *airfield*
> *farm*
> *industrial premises*
> *mine*
> *private grounds*
> *quarry*

(i) A **motor vehicle** is any mechanically or electrically powered device, not operated on rails, upon which any person or property may be transported or drawn upon a highway. Any object such as a trailer, coaster, sled, or wagon being towed by a motor vehicle is considerd a part of the motor vehicle.

INCLUDES   automobile [any type]
bus
construction machinery, farm and industrial machinery, steam roller, tractor, army tank, highway grader, or similar vehicle on wheels or treads, while in transport under own power
fire engine (motorized)
motorcycle
motorized bicycle [moped] or scooter
trolley bus not operating on rails
truck
van

EXCLUDES *devices used solely to move persons or materials within the confines of a building and its premises, such as:*
building elevator
coal car in mine
electric baggage or mail truck used solely within a railroad station
electric truck used solely within an industrial plant
moving overhead crane

(j) A **motorcycle** is a two-wheeled motor vehicle having one or two riding saddles and sometimes having a third wheel for the support of a sidecar. The sidecar is considered part of the motorcycle.

INCLUDES   motorized:
bicycle [moped]
scooter
tricycle

(k) An **off-road motor vehicle** is a motor vehicle of special design, to enable it to negotiate rough or soft terrain or snow. Examples of special design are high construction, special wheels and tires, driven by treads, or support on a cushion of air.

INCLUDES   all terrain vehicle [ATV]
army tank
hovercraft, on land or swamp
snowmobile

(l) A **driver** of a motor vehicle is the occupant of the motor vehicle operating it or intending to operate it. A **motorcyclist** is the driver of a motorcycle. Other authorized occupants of a motor vehicle are **passengers**.

(m) An **other road vehicle** is any device, except a motor vehicle, in, on, or by which any person or property may be transported on a highway.

INCLUDES   animal carrying a person or goods
animal-drawn vehicles
animal harnessed to conveyance
bicycle [pedal cycle]
streetcar
tricycle (pedal)

EXCLUDES *pedestrian conveyance [definition (q)]*

(n) A **streetcar** is a device designed and used primarily for transporting persons within a municipality, running on rails, usually subject to normal traffic control signals, and operated principally on a right-of-way that forms part of the traffic way. A trailer being towed by a streetcar is considered a part of the streetcar.

INCLUDES   interurban or intraurban electric or streetcar, when specified to be operating on a street or public highway
tram (car)
trolley (car)

(o) A **pedal cycle** is any road transport vehicle operated solely by pedals.

INCLUDES   bicycle
pedal cycle
tricycle

EXCLUDES *motorized bicycle [definition (i)]*

(p) A **pedal cyclist** is any person riding on a pedal cycle or in a sidecar attached to such a vehicle.

(q) A **pedestrian conveyance** is any human powered device by which a pedestrian may move other than by walking or by which a walking person may move another pedestrian.

INCLUDES   baby carriage
coaster wagon
ice skates
perambulator
pushcart
pushchair
roller skates
scooter
skateboard
skis
sled
wheelchair

(r) A **pedestrian** is any person involved in an accident who was not at the time of the accident riding in or on a motor vehicle, railroad train, streetcar, animal-drawn or other vehicle, or on a bicycle or animal.

INCLUDES   person:
changing tire of vehicle
in or operating a pedestrian conveyance
making adjustment to motor of vehicle
on foot

(s) A **watercraft** is any device for transporting passengers or goods on the water.

(t) A **small boat** is any watercraft propelled by paddle, oars, or small motor, with a passenger capacity of less than ten.

INCLUDES   boat NOS
canoe
coble
dinghy
punt
raft
rowboat
rowing shell
scull
skiff
small motorboat

EXCLUDES *barge*
lifeboat (used after abandoning ship)
raft (anchored) being used as a diving platform
yacht

(u) An **aircraft** is any device for transporting passengers or goods in the air.

INCLUDES   airplane [any type]
balloon
bomber
dirigible
glider (hang)
military aircraft
parachute

(v) A **commercial transport aircraft** is any device for collective passenger or freight transportation by air, whether run on commercial lines for profit or by government authorities, with the exception of military craft.

RAILWAY ACCIDENTS (E800-E807)

Note: For definitions of railway accident and related terms see definitions (a) to (d).

EXCLUDES *accidents involving railway train and:*
aircraft (E840.0-E845.9)
motor vehicle (E810.0-E825.9)
watercraft (E830.0-E838.9)

The following fourth-digit subdivisions are for use with categories E800-E807 to identify the injured person:

.0 Railway employee
Any person who by virtue of his employment in connection with a railway, whether by the railway company or not, is at increased risk of involvement in a railway accident, such as:
catering staff of train
driver
guard
porter
postal staff on train
railway fireman
shunter
sleeping car attendant

.1 Passenger on railway
Any authorized person traveling on a train, except a railway employee.

EXCLUDES *intending passenger waiting at station (.8)*
unauthorized rider on railway vehicle (.8)

.2 Pedestrian
See definition (r)

.3 Pedal cyclist
See definition (p)

.8 Other specified person
Intending passenger or bystander waiting at station
Unauthorized rider on railway vehicle

.9 Unspecified person

§ ✓4ᵗʰ **E800 Railway accident involving collision with rolling stock**

INCLUDES collision between railway trains or railway vehicles, any kind
collision NOS on railway
derailment with antecedent collision with rolling stock or NOS

§ ✓4ᵗʰ **E801 Railway accident involving collision with other object**

INCLUDES collision of railway train with:
buffers
fallen tree on railway
gates
platform
rock on railway
streetcar
other nonmotor vehicle
other object

EXCLUDES *collision with:*
aircraft (E840.0-E842.9)
motor vehicle (E810.0-E810.9, E820.0-E822.9)

§ ✓4ᵗʰ **E802 Railway accident involving derailment without antecedent collision**

§ ✓4ᵗʰ **E803 Railway accident involving explosion, fire, or burning**

EXCLUDES *explosion or fire, with antecedent derailment (E802.0-E802.9)*
explosion or fire, with mention of antecedent collision (E800.0-E801.9)

§ ✓4ᵗʰ **E804 Fall in, on, or from railway train**

INCLUDES fall while alighting from or boarding railway train

EXCLUDES *fall related to collision, derailment, or explosion of railway train (E800.0-E803.9)*

§ ✓4ᵗʰ **E805 Hit by rolling stock**

INCLUDES crushed
injured
killed   } by railway train or part
knocked down
run over

EXCLUDES *pedestrian hit by object set in motion by railway train (E806.0-E806.9)*

§ ✓4ᵗʰ **E806 Other specified railway accident**

INCLUDES hit by object falling in railway train
injured by door or window on railway train
nonmotor road vehicle or pedestrian hit by object set in motion by railway train
railway train hit by falling:
earth NOS
rock
tree
other object

EXCLUDES *railway accident due to cataclysm (E908-E909)*

§ ✓4ᵗʰ **E807 Railway accident of unspecified nature**

INCLUDES found dead   } on railway right-of-way
injured   } NOS

railway accident NOS

MOTOR VEHICLE TRAFFIC ACCIDENTS (E810-E819)

Note: For definitions of motor vehicle traffic accident, and related terms, see definitions (e) to (k).

EXCLUDES *accidents involving motor vehicle and aircraft (E840.0-E845.9)*

The following fourth-digit subdivisions are for use with categories E810-E819 to identify the injured person:

.0 Driver of motor vehicle other than motorcycle
See definition (1)

.1 Passenger in motor vehicle other than motorcycle
See definition (1)

.2 Motorcyclist
See definition (1)

.3 Passenger on motorcycle
See definition (1)

.4 Occupant of streetcar

.5 Rider of animal; occupant of animal-drawn vehicle

.6 Pedal cyclist
See definition (p)

.7 Pedestrian
See definition (r)

.8 Other specified person
Occupant of vehicle other than above
Person in railway train involved in accident
Unauthorized rider of motor vehicle

.9 Unspecified person

§§ ✓4ᵗʰ **E810 Motor vehicle traffic accident involving collision with train**

EXCLUDES *motor vehicle collision with object set in motion by railway train (E815.0-E815.9)*
railway train hit by object set in motion by motor vehicle (E818.0-E818.9)

§ Requires fourth-digit. See beginning of section E800-E807 for codes and definitions.
§§ Requires fourth-digit. See beginning of section E810-E819 for codes and definitions.

✓4ᵗʰ Fourth-digit Required   ►◄ Revised Text   ● New Code   ▲ Revised Code Title

§ ✓4ᵗʰ **E811 Motor vehicle traffic accident involving re-entrant collision with another motor vehicle**

INCLUDES   collision between motor vehicle which accidentally leaves the roadway then re-enters the same roadway, or the opposite roadway on a divided highway, and another motor vehicle

EXCLUDES   *collision on the same roadway when none of the motor vehicles involved have left and re-entered the highway (E812.0-E812.9)*

§ ✓4ᵗʰ **E812 Other motor vehicle traffic accident involving collision with motor vehicle**

INCLUDES   collision with another motor vehicle parked, stopped, stalled, disabled, or abandoned on the highway
motor vehicle collision NOS

EXCLUDES   *collision with object set in motion by another motor vehicle (E815.0-E815.9)*
re-entrant collision with another motor vehicle (E811.0-E811.9)

§ ✓4ᵗʰ **E813 Motor vehicle traffic accident involving collision with other vehicle**

INCLUDES   collision between motor vehicle, any kind, and:
other road (nonmotor transport) vehicle, such as:
    animal carrying a person
    animal-drawn vehicle
    pedal cycle
    streetcar

EXCLUDES   *collision with:*
object set in motion by nonmotor road vehicle (E815.0-E815.9)
pedestrian (E814.0-E814.9)
nonmotor road vehicle hit by object set in motion by motor vehicle (E818.0-E818.9)

§ ✓4ᵗʰ **E814 Motor vehicle traffic accident involving collision with pedestrian**

INCLUDES   collision between motor vehicle, any kind, and pedestrian
pedestrian dragged, hit, or run over by motor vehicle, any kind

EXCLUDES   *pedestrian hit by object set in motion by motor vehicle (E818.0-E818.9)*

§ ✓4ᵗʰ **E815 Other motor vehicle traffic accident involving collision on the highway**

INCLUDES   collision (due to loss of control) (on highway) between motor vehicle, any kind, and:
abutment (bridge) (overpass)
animal (herded) (unattended)
fallen stone, traffic sign, tree, utility pole
guard rail or boundary fence
interhighway divider
landslide (not moving)
object set in motion by railway train or road vehicle (motor) (nonmotor)
object thrown in front of motor vehicle
other object, fixed, movable, or moving
safety island
temporary traffic sign or marker
wall of cut made for road

EXCLUDES   *collision with:*
any object off the highway (resulting from loss of control) (E816.0-E816.9)
any object which normally would have been off the highway and is not stated to have been on it (E816.0-E816.9)
motor vehicle parked, stopped, stalled, disabled, or abandoned on highway (E812.0-E812.9)
moving landslide (E909)
motor vehicle hit by object:
set in motion by railway train or road vehicle (motor) (nonmotor) (E818.0-E818.9)
thrown into or on vehicle (E818.0-E818.9)

§ ✓4ᵗʰ **E816 Motor vehicle traffic accident due to loss of control, without collision on the highway**

INCLUDES   motor vehicle:
failing to make curve
going out of control (due to):
    blowout
    burst tire
    driver falling asleep
    driver inattention
    excessive speed
    failure of mechanical part
and:
    coliding with object off the highway
    overturning
    stopping abruptly off the highway

EXCLUDES   *collision on highway following loss of control (E810.0-E815.9)*
loss of control of motor vehicle following collision on the highway (E810.0-E815.9)

§ ✓4ᵗʰ **E817 Noncollision motor vehicle traffic accident while boarding or alighting**

INCLUDES   fall down stairs of motor bus
fall from car in street
injured by moving part of the vehicle
trapped by door of motor bus
while boarding or alighting

---

§   Requires fourth-digit. See beginning of section E810-E819 for codes and definitions.

§§ ☑4ᵗʰ **E818 Other noncollision motor vehicle traffic accident**

INCLUDES   accidental poisoning
                  from exhaust gas
                  generated by
               breakage of any part of
               explosion of any part of
               fall, jump, or being
                  accidentally pushed
                  from   } motor
               fire starting in   vehicle while
               hit by object thrown into   in motion
                  or on
               injured by being thrown
                  against some part
                  of, or object in
               injury from moving part
                  of
               object falling in or on
               object thrown on

            collision of railway train or road vehicle except
               motor vehicle, with object set in motion
               by motor vehicle
            motor vehicle hit by object set in motion by
               railway train or road vehicle (motor)
               (nonmotor)
            pedestrian, railway train, or road vehicle
               (motor) (nonmotor) hit by object set in
               motion by motor vehicle

EXCLUDES   *collision between motor vehicle and:*
               object set in motion by railway train or road
                  vehicle (motor) (nonmotor) (E815.0-
                  E815.9)
               object thrown towards the motor vehicle
                  (E815.0-E815.9)
            person overcome by carbon monoxide generated
               by stationary motor vehicle off the
               roadway with motor running (E868.2)

§§ ☑4ᵗʰ **E819 Motor vehicle traffic accident of unspecified nature**

INCLUDES   motor vehicle traffic accident NOS
            traffic accident NOS

MOTOR VEHICLE NONTRAFFIC ACCIDENTS (E820-E825)

Note: For definitions of motor vehicle nontraffic accident and
related terms see definition (a) to (k).

INCLUDES   accidents involving motor vehicles being used
               in recreational or sporting activities off
               the highway
            collision and noncollision motor vehicle
               accidents occurring entirely off the
               highway

EXCLUDES   *accidents involving motor vehicle and:*
               aircraft (E840.0-E845.9)
               watercraft (E830.0-E838.9)
            accidents, not on the public highway, involving
               agricultural and construction machinery
               but not involving another motor vehicle
               (E919.0, E919.2, E919.7)

The following fourth-digit subdivisions are for use with
categories E820-E825 to identify the injured person:

.0 Driver of motor vehicle other than motorcycle
   See definition (l)
.1 Passenger in motor vehicle other than
   motorcycle
   See definition (l)
.2 Motorcyclist
   See definition (l)
.3 Passenger on motorcycle
   See definition (l)
.4 Occupant of streetcar
.5 Rider of animal; occupant of animal-drawn
   vehicle
.6 Pedal cyclist
   See definition (p)
.7 Pedestrian
   See definition (r)
.8 Other specified person
   Occupant of vehicle other than above
   Person on railway train involved in accident
   Unauthorized rider of motor vehicle
.9 Unspecified person

§ ☑4ᵗʰ **E820 Nontraffic accident involving motor-driven snow vehicle**

INCLUDES   breakage of part of   } motor-driven
            fall from   snow
            hit by   vehicle (not
            overturning of   on public
            run over or dragged by   highway)

            collision of motor-driven snow vehicle with:
               animal (being ridden) (-drawn vehicle)
               another off-road motor vehicle
               other motor vehicle, not on public highway
               railway train
               other object, fixed or movable
            injury caused by rough landing of motor-
               driven snow vehicle (after leaving ground
               on rough terrain)

EXCLUDES   *accident on the public highway involving motor*
               driven snow vehicle (E810.0-E819.9)

§ ☑4ᵗʰ **E821 Nontraffic accident involving other off-road motor vehicle**

INCLUDES   breakage of part of   } off-road motor
            fall from   vehicle,
            hit by   except
            overturning of   snow
            run over or dragged by   vehicle (not
            thrown against some   on public
               part of or object in   highway)

            collision with:
               animal (being ridden) (-drawn vehicle)
               another off-road motor vehicle, except snow
                  vehicle
               other motor vehicle, not on public highway
               other object, fixed or movable

EXCLUDES   *accident on public highway involving off-road*
               motor vehicle (E810.0-E819.9)
            collision between motor driven snow vehicle and
               other off-road motor vehicle (E820.0-
               E820.9)
            hovercraft accident on water (E830.0-E838.9)

---

§ Requires fourth-digit. See beginning of section E820-E825 for codes and definitions.
§§ Requires fourth-digit. See beginning of section E810-E819 for codes and definitions

☑4ᵗʰ Fourth-digit Required   ►◄ Revised Text   ● New Code   ▲ Revised Code Title

§§ ☑4ᵗʰ **E822 Other motor vehicle nontraffic accident involving collision with moving object**

> INCLUDES   collision, not on public highway, between motor vehicle, except off-road motor vehicle and:
>   animal
>   nonmotor vehicle
>   other motor vehicle, except off-road motor vehicle
>   pedestrian
>   railway train
>   other moving object
>
> EXCLUDES   *collision with:*
>   *motor-driven snow vehicle (E820.0-E820.9)*
>   *other off-road motor vehicle (E821.0-E821.9)*

§§ ☑4ᵗʰ **E823 Other motor vehicle nontraffic accident involving collision with stationary object**

> INCLUDES   collision, not on public highway, between motor vehicle, except off-road motor vehicle, and any object, fixed or movable, but not in motion

§§ ☑4ᵗʰ **E824 Other motor vehicle nontraffic accident while boarding and alighting**

> INCLUDES   fall
> injury from moving part of motor vehicle
> trapped by door of motor vehicle
> } while boarding or alighting from motor vehicle, except off-road motor vehicle, not on public highway

§§ ☑4ᵗʰ **E825 Other motor vehicle nontraffic accident of other and unspecified nature**

> INCLUDES   accidental poisoning from carbon monoxide generated by
> breakage of any part of
> explosion of any part of
> fall, jump, or being accidentally pushed from
> fire starting in
> hit by object thrown into, towards, or on
> injured by being thrown against some part of, or object in
> injury from moving part of
> object falling in or on
> } motor vehicle while in motion, not on public highway
>
> motor vehicle nontraffic accident NOS
>
> EXCLUDES   *fall from or in stationary motor vehicle (E884.9, E885.9)*
> *overcome by carbon monoxide or exhaust gas generated by stationary motor vehicle off the roadway with motor running (E868.2)*
> *struck by falling object from or in stationary motor vehicle (E916)*

OTHER ROAD VEHICLE ACCIDENTS (E826-E829)

Note: Other road vehicle accidents are transport accidents involving road vehicles other than motor vehicles. For definitions of other road vehicle and related terms see definitions (m) to (o).

> INCLUDES   accidents involving other road vehicles being used in recreational or sporting activities
>
> EXCLUDES   *collision of other road vehicle [any] with:*
>   *aircraft (E840.0-E845.9)*
>   *motor vehicle (E813.0-E813.9, E820.0-E822.9)*
>   *railway train (E801.0-E801.9)*

The following fourth-digit subdivisions are for use with categories E826-E829 to identify the injured person.

.0 Pedestrian
     See definition (r)
.1 Pedal cyclist
     See definition (p)
.2 Rider of animal
.3 Occupant of animal-drawn vehicle
.4 Occupant of streetcar
.8 Other specified person
.9 Unspecified person

§ ☑4ᵗʰ **E826 Pedal cycle accident**
[0-9]

> INCLUDES   breakage of any part of pedal cycle
> collision between pedal cycle and:
>   animal (being ridden) (herded) (unattended)
>   another pedal cycle
>   any pedestrian
>   nonmotor road vehicle
>   other object, fixed, movable, or moving, not set in motion by motor vehicle, railway train, or aircraft
> entanglement in wheel of pedal cycle
> fall from pedal cycle
> hit by object falling or thrown on the pedal cycle
> pedal cycle accident NOS
> pedal cycle overturned

§ ☑4ᵗʰ **E827 Animal-drawn vehicle accident**
[0,2-4,8,9]

> INCLUDES   breakage of any part of vehicle
> collision between animal-drawn vehicle and:
>   animal (being ridden) (herded) (unattended)
>   nonmotor road vehicle, except pedal cycle
>   pedestrian, pedestrian conveyance, or pedestrian vehicle
>   other object, fixed, movable, or moving, not set in motion by motor vehicle, railway train, or aircraft
> fall from
> knocked down by
> overturning of
> run over by
> thrown from
> } animal-drawn vehicle
>
> EXCLUDES   *collision of animal-drawn vehicle with pedal cycle (E826.0-E826.9)*

---

§ Requires fourth-digit. Valid digits are in [brackets] under each code. See beginning of section E826-E829 for codes and definitions.
§§ Requires fourth-digit. See beginning of section E820-E825 for codes and definitions.

§§ ✓4ᵗʰ **E828 Accident involving animal being ridden**

[0,2,4,8,9] | INCLUDES | collision between animal being ridden and:
            another animal
            nonmotor road vehicle, except pedal cycle, and animal-drawn vehicle
            pedestrian, pedestrian conveyance, or pedestrian vehicle
            other object, fixed, movable, or moving, not set in motion by motor vehicle, railway train, or aircraft

fall from
knocked down by } animal being
thrown from   } ridden
trampled by

ridden animal stumbled and fell

| EXCLUDES | collision of animal being ridden with:
            animal-drawn vehicle (E827.0-E827.9)
            pedal cycle (E826.0-E826.9)

§§ ✓4ᵗʰ **E829 Other road vehicle accidents**

[0,4,8,9] | INCLUDES | accident while
            boarding or alighting from
            blow from object in   } streetcar
            breakage of any part of   } nonmotor road
            caught in door of-   } vehicle not
            derailment of   } classifiable
            fall in, on, or from   } to E826-
            fire in   } E828

collision between streetcar or nonmotor road vehicle, except as in E826-E828, and:
            animal (not being ridden)
            another nonmotor road vehicle not classifiable to E826-E828
            pedestrian
            other object, fixed, movable, or moving, not set in motion by motor vehicle, railway train, or aircraft
nonmotor road vehicle accident NOS
streetcar accident NOS

| EXCLUDES | collision with:
            animal being ridden (E828.0-E828.9)
            animal-drawn vehicle (E827.0-E827.9)
            pedal cycle (E826.0-E826.9)

WATER TRANSPORT ACCIDENTS (E830-E838)

Note: For definitions of water transport accident and related terms see definitions (a), (s), and (t).

| INCLUDES | watercraft accidents in the course of recreational activities

| EXCLUDES | accidents involving both aircraft, including objects set in motion by aircraft, and watercraft (E840.0-E845.9)

The following fourth-digit subdivisions are for use with categories E830-E838 to identify the injured person:

.0 Occupant of small boat, unpowered
.1 Occupant of small boat, powered
      See definition (t)
      | EXCLUDES | water skier (.4)
.2 Occupant of other watercraft — crew
      Persons:
            engaged in operation of watercraft
            providing passenger services [cabin attendants, ship's physician, catering personnel]
            working on ship during voyage in other capacity [musician in band, operators of shops and beauty parlors]
.3 Occupant of other watercraft — other than crew
      Passenger
      Occupant of lifeboat, other than crew, after abandoning ship
.4 Water skier
.5 Swimmer
.6 Dockers, stevedores
      Longshoreman employed on the dock in loading and unloading ships
.8 Other specified person
      Immigration and custom officials on board ship
      Person:
            accompanying passenger or member of crew visiting boat
      Pilot (guiding ship into port)
.9 Unspecified person

§ ✓4ᵗʰ **E830 Accident to watercraft causing submersion**

| INCLUDES | submersion and drowning due to:
            boat overturning
            boat submerging
            falling or jumping from burning ship
            falling or jumping from crushed watercraft
            ship sinking
            other accident to watercraft

§ ✓4ᵗʰ **E831 Accident to watercraft causing other injury**

| INCLUDES | any injury, except submersion and drowning, as a result of an accident to watercraft
            burned while ship on fire
            crushed between ships in collision
            crushed by lifeboat after abandoning ship
            fall due to collision or other accident to watercraft
            hit by falling object due to accident to watercraft
            injured in watercraft accident involving collision
            struck by boat or part thereof after fall or jump from damaged boat

| EXCLUDES | burns from localized fire or explosion on board ship (E837.0-E837.9)

§ ✓4ᵗʰ **E832 Other accidental submersion or drowning in water transport accident**

| INCLUDES | submersion or drowning as a result of an accident other than accident to the watercraft, such as:
            fall:
                from gangplank
                from ship
                overboard
            thrown overboard by motion of ship
            washed overboard

| EXCLUDES | submersion or drowning of swimmer or diver who voluntarily jumps from boat not involved in an accident (E910.0-E910.9)

§ Requires fourth-digit. See beginning of section E830-E838 for codes and definitions.
§§ Requires fourth-digit. Valid digits are in [brackets] under each code. See beginning of section E826-E829 for codes and definitions.

✓4ᵗʰ Fourth-digit Required   ▶◀ Revised Text   ● New Code   ▲ Revised Code Title

E Codes E828–E832

§§ ☑4ᵗʰ E833 Fall on stairs or ladders in water transport

> EXCLUDES   *fall due to accident to watercraft (E831.0-E831.9)*

§§ ☑4ᵗʰ E834 Other fall from one level to another in water transport

> EXCLUDES   *fall due to accident to watercraft (E831.0-E831.9)*

§§ ☑4ᵗʰ E835 Other and unspecified fall in water transport

> EXCLUDES   *fall due to accident to watercraft (E831.0-E831.9)*

§§ ☑4ᵗʰ E836 Machinery accident in water transport

> INCLUDES   injuries in water transport caused by:
>
> deck
> engine room
> galley } machinery
> laundry
> loading

§§ ☑4ᵗʰ E837 Explosion, fire, or burning in watercraft

> INCLUDES   explosion of boiler on steamship
> localized fire on ship
>
> EXCLUDES   *burning ship (due to collision or explosion) resulting in:*
> *submersion or drowning (E830.0-E830.9)*
> *other injury (E831.0-E831.9)*

§§ ☑4ᵗʰ E838 Other and unspecified water transport accident

> INCLUDES   accidental poisoning by gases or fumes on ship
> atomic power plant malfunction in watercraft
> crushed between ship and stationary object [wharf]
> crushed between ships without accident to watercraft
> crushed by falling object on ship or while loading or unloading
> hit by boat while water skiing
> struck by boat or part thereof (after fall from boat)
> watercraft accident NOS

AIR AND SPACE TRANSPORT ACCIDENTS (E840-E845)

Note: For definition of aircraft and related terms see definitions (u) and (v).

The following fourth-digit subdivisions are for use with categories E840-E845 to identify the injured person. Valid fourth digits are in [brackets] under codes E842-E845.

.0 Occupant of spacecraft
.1 Occupant of military aircraft, any
Crew in military aircraft [air force] [army] [national guard] [navy]
Passenger (civilian) (military) in military aircraft [air force] [army] [national guard] [navy]
Troops in military aircraft [air force] [army] [national guard] [navy]

> EXCLUDES   *occupants of aircraft operated under jurisdiction of police departments (.5)*
> *parachutist (.7)*

.2 Crew of commercial aircraft (powered) in surface to surface transport
.3 Other occupant of commercial aircraft (powered) in surface to surface transport
Flight personnel:
not part of crew
on familiarization flight
Passenger on aircraft (powered) NOS

.4 Occupant of commercial aircraft (powered) in surface to air transport
Occupant [crew] [passenger] of aircraft (powered) engaged in activities, such as:
aerial spraying (crops) (fire retardants)
air drops of emergency supplies
air drops of parachutists, except from military craft
crop dusting
lowering of construction material [bridge or telephone pole]
sky writing

.5 Occupant of other powered aircraft
Occupant [crew][passenger] of aircraft [powered] engaged in activities, such as:
aerobatic flying
aircraft racing
rescue operation
storm surveillance
traffic surveillance
Occupant of private plane NOS

.6 Occupant of unpowered aircraft, except parachutist
Occupant of aircraft classifiable to E842

.7 Parachutist (military) (other)
Person making voluntary descent

> EXCLUDES   *person making descent after accident to aircraft (.1-.6)*

.8 Ground crew, airline employee
Persons employed at airfields (civil) (military) or launching pads, not occupants of aircraft

.9 Other person

§ ☑4ᵗʰ E840 Accident to powered aircraft at takeoff or landing

> INCLUDES   collision of aircraft with any object, fixed, movable, or moving
> crash } while taking off or landing
> explosion on aircraft
> fire on aircraft
> forced landing

§ ☑4ᵗʰ E841 Accident to powered aircraft, other and unspecified

> INCLUDES   aircraft accident NOS
> aircraft crash or wreck NOS
> any accident to powered aircraft while in transit or when not specified whether in transit, taking off, or landing
> collision of aircraft with another aircraft, bird, or any object, while in transit
> explosion on aircraft while in transit
> fire on aircraft while in transit

§ ☑4ᵗʰ E842 Accident to unpowered aircraft

[6-9]
> INCLUDES   any accident, except collision with powered aircraft, to:
> balloon
> glider
> hang glider
> kite carrying a person
> hit by object falling from unpowered aircraft

§ ☑4ᵗʰ E843 Fall in, on, or from aircraft

[0-9]
> INCLUDES   accident in boarding or alighting from aircraft, any kind
> fall in, on, or from aircraft [any kind], while in transit, taking off, or landing, except when as a result of an accident to aircraft

---

§ Requires fourth-digit. See beginning of section E840-E845 for codes and definitions.
§§ Requires fourth-digit. See beginning of section E830-E838 for codes and definitions.

§ ☑4ᵗʰ **E844 Other specified air transport accidents**
[0-9]   INCLUDES hit by:

        aircraft
        object falling from
            aircraft
        injury by or from:
            machinery on
              aircraft   without
            rotating propeller   accident
            voluntary parachute   to aircraft
              descent
        poisoning by carbon
            monoxide from
            aircraft while in
            transit
        sucked into jet

        any accident involving other transport vehicle
           (motor) (nonmotor) due to being hit by
           object set in motion by aircraft (powered)

EXCLUDES *air sickness (E903)*
        effects of:
          high altitude (E902.0-E902.1)
          pressure change (E902.0-E902.1)
        injury in parachute descent due to accident to
          aircraft (E840.0-E842-9)

§ ☑4ᵗʰ **E845 Accident involving spacecraft**
[0,8,9]   INCLUDES launching pad accident
         EXCLUDES *effects of weightlessness in spacecraft (E928.0)*

VEHICLE ACCIDENTS NOT ELSEWHERE CLASSIFIABLE (E846-E848)

E846 Accidents involving powered vehicles used solely within the buildings and premises of industrial or commercial establishment
    Accident to, on, or involving:
        battery powered airport passenger vehicle
        battery powered trucks (baggage) (mail)
        coal car in mine
        logging car
        self propelled truck, industrial
        station baggage truck (powered)
        tram, truck, or tub (powered) in mine or quarry
    Collision with:
        pedestrian
        other vehicle or object within premises
    Explosion of
    Fall from   powered vehicle, industrial
    Overturning of   or commercial
    Struck by

        EXCLUDES *accidental poisoning by exhaust gas from*
            vehicle not elsewhere classifiable (E868.2)
           injury by crane, lift (fork), or elevator (E919.2)

E847 Accidents involving cable cars not running on rails
    Accident to, on, or involving:
        cable car, not on rails
        ski chair-lift
        ski-lift with gondola
        téléférique
    Breakage of cable
    Caught or dragged by
    Fall or jump from   cable car, not on rails
    Object thrown from or in

E848 Accidents involving other vehicles, not elsewhere classifiable
    Accident to, on, or involving:
        ice yacht
        land yacht
        nonmotor, nonroad vehicle NOS

☑4ᵗʰ **E849 Place of occurrence**
    The following category is for use to denote the place where
    the injury or poisoning occurred.

E849.0 Home
    Apartment   *Private:*
    Boarding house   *garage*
    Farm house   *garden*
    Home premises   *home*
    House (residential)   *walk*
    Noninstitutional   *Swimming pool in private*
      place of residence   *house or garden*
    Private: *Yard of home*
      driveway

    EXCLUDES *home under construction but not yet*
           occupied (E849.3)
        institutional place of residence (E849.7)

E849.1 Farm
    Farm:
      buildings
      land under cultivation

    EXCLUDES *farm house and home premises of farm*
           (E849.0)

E849.2 Mine and quarry
    Gravel pit   *Tunnel under*
    Sand pit   *construction*

E849.3 Industrial place and premises
    Building under   *Industrial yard*
      construction   *Loading platform (factory)*
    Dockyard   *(store)*
    Dry dock   *Plant, industrial*
    Factory   *Railway yard*
      building   *Shop (place of work)*
      premises   *Warehouse*
    Garage (place of work) *Workhouse*

E849.4 Place for recreation and sport
    Amusement park   *Public park*
    Baseball field   *Racecourse*
    Basketball court   *Resort NOS*
    Beach resort   *Riding school*
    Cricket ground   *Rifle range*
    Fives court   *Seashore resort*
    Football field   *Skating rink*
    Golf course   *Sports palace*
    Gymnasium   *Stadium*
    Hockey field   *Swimming pool, public*
    Holiday camp   *Tennis court*
    Ice palace   *Vacation resort*
    Lake resort
    Mountain resort
    Playground, including school playground
    EXCLUDES *that in private house or garden*
           (E849.0)

E849.5 Street and highway

E849.6 Public building
    Building (including adjacent grounds) used by the
      general public or by a particular group of the
      public, such as:
    airport   *music hall*
    bank   *nightclub*
    café   *office*
    casino   *office building*
    church   *opera house*
    cinema   *post office*
    clubhouse   *public hall*
    courthouse   *radio broadcasting station*
    dance hall   *restaurant*
    garage building (for   *school (state) (public)*
      car storage)   *(private)*
    hotel   *shop, commercial*
    market (grocery or   *station (bus) (railway)*
      other   *store*
      commodity)   *theater*
    movie house
    EXCLUDES *home garage (E849.0)*
        industrial building or workplace
          (E849.3)

---

§ Requires fourth-digit. See beginning of section E840-E845 for codes and definitions.

E Codes E844–E849.6

E849.7 Residential institution
Children's home   Old people's home
Dormitory   Orphanage
Hospital   Prison
Jail   Reform school

E849.8 Other specified places
Beach NOS   Pond or pool (natural)
Canal   Prairie
Caravan site NOS   Public place NOS
Derelict house   Railway line
Desert   Reservoir
Dock   River
Forest   Sea
Harbor   Seashore NOS
Hill   Stream
Lake NOS   Swamp
Mountain   Trailer court
Parking lot   Woods
Parking place

E849.9 Unspecified place

ACCIDENTAL POISONING BY DRUGS, MEDICINAL SUBSTANCES, AND BIOLOGICALS (E850-E858)

INCLUDES   accidental overdose of drug, wrong drug given
            or taken in error, and drug taken
            inadvertently
            accidents in the use of drugs and biologicals in
            medical and surgical procedures

EXCLUDES   *administration with suicidal or homicidal intent
            or intent to harm, or in circumstances
            classifiable to E980-E989 (E950.0-E950.5,
            E962.0, E980.0-E980.5)
            correct drug properly administered in
            therapeutic or prophylactic dosage, as the
            cause of adverse effect (E930.0-E949.9)*

See Alphabetic Index for more complete list of specific
drugs to be classified under the fourth-digit subdivisions.
The American Hospital Formulary numbers can be used to
classify new drugs listed by the American Hospital
Formulary Service (AHFS). See Appendix C.

☑4ᵗʰ **E850 Accidental poisoning by analgesics, antipyretics, and antirheumatics**

E850.0 Heroin
Diacetylmorphine

E850.1 Methadone

E850.2 Other opiates and related narcotics
Codeine [methylmorphine]   Morphine
Meperidine [pethidine]   Opium (alkaloids)

E850.3 Salicylates
Acetylsalicylic acid [aspirin]
Amino derivatives of salicylic acid
Salicylic acid salts

E850.4 Aromatic analgesics, not elsewhere classified
Acetanilid
Paracetamol [acetaminophen]
Phenacetin [acetophenetidin]

E850.5 Pyrazole derivatives
Aminophenazone [amidopyrine]
Phenylbutazone

E850.6 Antirheumatics [antiphlogistics]
Gold salts
Indomethacin
EXCLUDES   salicylates (E850.3)
            steroids (E858.0)

E850.7 Other non-narcotic analgesics
Pyrabital

E850.8 Other specified analgesics and antipyretics
Pentazocine

E850.9 Unspecified analgesic or antipyretic

E851 Accidental poisoning by barbiturates
Amobarbital [amylobarbitone]
Barbital [barbitone]
Butabarbital [butabarbitone]
Pentobarbital [pentobarbitone]
Phenobarbital [phenobarbitone]
Secobarbital [quinalbarbitone]
EXCLUDES   thiobarbiturates (E855.1)

☑4ᵗʰ **E852 Accidental poisoning by other sedatives and hypnotics**

E852.0 Chloral hydrate group

E852.1 Paraldehyde

E852.2 Bromine compounds
Bromides
Carbromal (derivatives)

E852.3 Methaqualone compounds

E852.4 Glutethimide group

E852.5 Mixed sedatives, not elsewhere classified

E852.8 Other specified sedatives and hypnotics

E852.9 Unspecified sedative or hypnotic
Sleeping:
drug
pill   } NOS
tablet

☑4ᵗʰ **E853 Accidental poisoning by tranquilizers**

E853.0 Phenothiazine-based tranquilizers
Chlorpromazine   Prochlorperazine
Fluphenazine   Promazine

E853.1 Butyrophenone-based tranquilizers
Haloperidol   Trifluperidol
Spiperone

E853.2 Benzodiazepine-based tranquilizers
Chlordiazepoxide   Lorazepam
Diazepam   Medazepam
Flurazepam   Nitrazepam

E853.8 Other specified tranquilizers
Hydroxyzine   Meprobamate

E853.9 Unspecified tranquilizer

☑4ᵗʰ **E854 Accidental poisoning by other psychotropic agents**

E854.0 Antidepressants
Amitriptyline
Imipramine
Monoamine oxidase [MAO] inhibitors

E854.1 Psychodysleptics [hallucinogens]
Cannabis derivatives   Mescaline
Lysergide [LSD]   Psilocin
Marihuana (derivatives)   Psilocybin

E854.2 Psychostimulants
Amphetamine   Caffeine
EXCLUDES   central appetite depressants (E858.8)

E854.3 Central nervous system stimulants
Analeptics   Opiate antagonists

E854.8 Other psychotropic agents

☑4ᵗʰ **E855 Accidental poisoning by other drugs acting on central and autonomic nervous system**

E855.0 Anticonvulsant and anti-Parkinsonism drugs
Amantadine
Hydantoin derivatives
Levodopa [L-dopa]
Oxazolidine derivatives [paramethadione]
    [trimethadione]
Succinimides

E855.1 Other central nervous system depressants
Ether
Gaseous anesthetics
Halogenated hydrocarbon derivatives
Intravenous anesthetics
Thiobarbiturates, such as thiopental sodium

E855.2 Local anesthetics
Cocaine   Procaine
Lidocaine [lignocaine]   Tetracaine

E Codes E849.7–E855.2

E855.3 Parasympathomimetics [cholinergics]
   Acetylcholine   Pilocarpine
   Anticholinesterase:
      organophosphorus
      reversible

E855.4 Parasympatholytics [anticholinergics and antimuscarinics] and spasmolytics
   Atropine
   Homatropine
   Hyoscine [scopolamine]
   Quaternary ammonium derivatives

E855.5 Sympathomimetics [adrenergics]
   Epinephrine [adrenalin]
   Levarterenol [noradrenalin]

E855.6 Sympatholytics [antiadrenergics]
   Phenoxybenzamine
   Tolazoline hydrochloride

E855.8 Other specified drugs acting on central and autonomic nervous systems

E855.9 Unspecified drug acting on central and autonomic nervous systems

E856 Accidental poisoning by antibiotics

E857 Accidental poisoning by other anti-infectives

☑4ᵗʰ **E858 Accidental poisoning by other drugs**

E858.0 Hormones and synthetic substitutes

E858.1 Primarily systemic agents

E858.2 Agents primarily affecting blood constituents

E858.3 Agents primarily affecting cardiovascular system

E858.4 Agents primarily affecting gastrointestinal system

E858.5 Water, mineral, and uric acid metabolism drugs

E858.6 Agents primarily acting on the smooth and skeletal muscles and respiratory system

E858.7 Agents primarily affecting skin and mucous membrane, ophthalmological, otorhinolaryngological, and dental drugs

E858.8 Other specified drugs
   Central appetite depressants

E858.9 Unspecified drug

ACCIDENTAL POISONING BY OTHER SOLID AND LIQUID SUBSTANCES, GASES, AND VAPORS (E860-E869)

Note: Categories in this section are intended primarily to indicate the external cause of poisoning states classifiable to 980-989. They may also be used to indicate external causes of localized effects classifiable to 001-799.

☑4ᵗʰ **E860 Accidental poisoning by alcohol, not elsewhere classified**

E860.0 Alcoholic beverages
   Alcohol in preparations intended for consumption

E860.1 Other and unspecified ethyl alcohol and its products
   Denatured alcohol   Grain alcohol NOS
   Ethanol NOS   Methylated spirit

E860.2 Methyl alcohol
   Methanol   Wood alcohol

E860.3 Isopropyl alcohol
   Dimethyl carbinol   Rubbing alcohol subsitute
   Isopropanol   Secondary propyl alcohol

E860.4 Fusel oil
   Alcohol: Alcohol:
      amyl   propyl
      butyl

E860.8 Other specified alcohols

E860.9 Unspecified alcohol

☑4ᵗʰ **E861 Accidental poisoning by cleansing and polishing agents, disinfectants, paints, and varnishes**

E861.0 Synthetic detergents and shampoos

E861.1 Soap products

E861.2 Polishes

E861.3 Other cleansing and polishing agents
   Scouring powders

E861.4 Disinfectants
   Household and other disinfectants not ordinarily used on the person
   EXCLUDES *carbolic acid or phenol (E864.0)*

E861.5 Lead paints

E861.6 Other paints and varnishes
   Lacquers   Paints, other than lead
   Oil colors   White washes

E861.9 Unspecified

☑4ᵗʰ **E862 Accidental poisoning by petroleum products, other solvents and their vapors, not elsewhere classified**

E862.0 Petroleum solvents
   Petroleum: Petroleum:
      ether   naphtha
      benzine

E862.1 Petroleum fuels and cleaners
   Antiknock additives to petroleum fuels
   Gas oils
   Gasoline or petrol
   Kerosene
   EXCLUDES *kerosene insecticides (E863.4)*

E862.2 Lubricating oils

E862.3 Petroleum solids
   Paraffin wax

E862.4 Other specified solvents
   Benzene

E862.9 Unspecified solvent

☑4ᵗʰ **E863 Accidental poisoning by agricultural and horticultural chemical and pharmaceutical preparations other than plant foods and fertilizers**
   EXCLUDES *plant foods and fertilizers (E866.5)*

E863.0 Insecticides of organochlorine compounds
   Benzene hexachloride   Dieldrin
   Chlordane   Endrine
   DDT   Toxaphene

E863.1 Insecticides of organophosphorus compounds
   Demeton   Parathion
   Diazinon   Phenylsulphthion
   Dichlorvos   Phorate
   Malathion   Phosdrin
   Methyl parathion

E863.2 Carbamates
   Aldicarb   Propoxur
   Carbaryl

E863.3 Mixtures of insecticides

E863.4 Other and unspecified insecticides
   Kerosene insecticides

E863.5 Herbicides
   2, 4-Dichlorophenoxyacetic acid [2, 4-D]
   2, 4, 5-Trichlorophenoxyacetic acid [2, 4, 5-T]
   Chlorates
   Diquat
   Mixtures of plant foods and fertilizers with herbicides
   Paraquat

E863.6 Fungicides
   Organic mercurials (used in seed dressing)
   Pentachlorophenols

E863.7 Rodenticides
   Fluoroacetates   Warfarin
   Squill and derivatives Zinc phosphide
   Thallium

E863.8 Fumigants
   Cyanides   Phosphine
   Methyl bromide

E863.9 Other and unspecified

E Codes E855.3–E863.9

✓4th **E864 Accidental poisoning by corrosives and caustics, not elsewhere classified**

> EXCLUDES　those as components of disinfectants (E861.4)

E864.0 Corrosive aromatics
> Carbolic acid or phenol

E864.1 Acids
> Acid:
>> hydrochloric
>> nitric
>> sulfuric

E864.2 Caustic alkalis
> Lye

E864.3 Other specified corrosives and caustics

E864.4 Unspecified corrosives and caustics

✓4th **E865 Accidental poisoning from poisonous foodstuffs and poisonous plants**

> INCLUDES　any meat, fish, or shellfish
> plants, berries, and fungi eaten as, or in mistake for, food, or by a child

> EXCLUDES　anaphylactic shock due to adverse food reaction (995.60-995.69)
> food poisoning (bacterial) (005.0-005.9)
> poisoning and toxic reactions to venomous plants (E905.6-E905.7)

E865.0 Meat

E865.1 Shellfish

E865.2 Other fish

E865.3 Berries and seeds

E865.4 Other specified plants

E865.5 Mushrooms and other fungi

E865.8 Other specified foods

E865.9 Unspecified foodstuff or poisonous plant

✓4th **E866 Accidental poisoning by other and unspecified solid and liquid substances**

> EXCLUDES　these substances as a component of:
>> medicines (E850.0-E858.9)
>> paints (E861.5-E861.6)
>> pesticides (E863.0-E863.9)
>> petroleum fuels (E862.1)

E866.0 Lead and its compounds and fumes

E866.1 Mercury and its compounds and fumes

E866.2 Antimony and its compounds and fumes

E866.3 Arsenic and its compounds and fumes

E866.4 Other metals and their compounds and fumes
> Beryllium (compounds)　　Iron (compounds)
> Brass fumes　　　　　　　Manganese (compounds)
> Cadmium (compounds)　　Nickel (compounds)
> Copper salts　　　　　　Thallium (compounds)

E866.5 Plant foods and fertilizers
> EXCLUDES　mixtures with herbicides (E863.5)

E866.6 Glues and adhesives

E866.7 Cosmetics

E866.8 Other specified solid or liquid substances

E866.9 Unspecified solid or liquid substance

E867 Accidental poisoning by gas distributed by pipeline
> Carbon monoxide from incomplete combustion of piped gas
> Coal gas NOS
> Liquefied petroleum gas distributed through pipes (pure or mixed with air)
> Piped gas (natural) (manufactured)

✓4th **E868 Accidental poisoning by other utility gas and other carbon monoxide**

E868.0 Liquefied petroleum gas distributed in mobile containers
> Butane
> Liquefied hydrocarbon gas NOS }　or carbon monoxide from incomplete conbustion of these gases
> Propane

E868.1 Other and unspecified utility gas
> Acetylene
> Gas NOS used for lighting, heating, or cooking }　or carbon monoxide from incomplete combustion of these gases
> Water gas

E868.2 Motor vehicle exhaust gas
> Exhaust gas from:
>> farm tractor, not in transit
>> gas engine
>> motor pump
>> motor vehicle, not in transit
>> any type of combustion engine not in watercraft
> EXCLUDES　poisoning by carbon monoxide from:
>> aircraft while in transit (E844.0-E844.9)
>> motor vehicle while in transit (E818.0-E818.9)
>> watercraft whether or not in transit (E838.0-E838.9)

E868.3 Carbon monoxide from incomplete combustion of other domestic fuels
> Carbon monoxide from incomplete combustion of:
>> coal
>> coke
>> kerosene }　in domestic stove or fireplace
>> wood
> EXCLUDES　carbon monoxide from smoke and fumes due to conflagration (E890.0-E893.9)

E868.8 Carbon monoxide from other sources
> Carbon monoxide from:
>> blast furnace gas
>> incomplete combustion of fuels in industrial use
>> kiln vapor

E868.9 Unspecified carbon monoxide

✓4th **E869 Accidental poisoning by other gases and vapors**
> EXCLUDES　effects of gases used as anesthetics (E855.1, E938.2)
> fumes from heavy metals (E866.0-E866.4)
> smoke and fumes due to conflagration or explosion (E890.0-E899)

E869.0 Nitrogen oxides

E869.1 Sulfur dioxide

E869.2 Freon

E869.3 Lacrimogenic gas [tear gas]
> Bromobenzyl cyanide　Ethyliodoacetate
> Chloroacetophenone

E869.4 Second-hand tobacco smoke

E869.8 Other specified gases and vapors
> Chlorine　　　　　　　　Hydrocyanic acid gas

E869.9 Unspecified gases and vapors

MISADVENTURES TO PATIENTS DURING SURGICAL AND MEDICAL CARE (E870-E876)

> EXCLUDES　accidental overdose of drug and wrong drug given in error (E850.0-E858.9)
> surgical and medical procedures as the cause of abnormal reaction by the patient, without mention of misadventure at the time of procedure (E878.0-E879.9)

✓4th **E870 Accidental cut, puncture, perforation, or hemorrhage during medical care**

E870.0 Surgical operation

E870.1 Infusion or transfusion

E870.2 Kidney dialysis or other perfusion

E870.3 Injection or vaccination

E870.4 Endoscopic examination

✓4th Fourth-digit Required　　►◄ Revised Text　　● New Code　　▲ Revised Code Title

E870.5 **Aspiration of fluid or tissue, puncture, and catheterization**

    Abdominal paracentesis   Lumbar puncture
    Aspirating needle biopsy   Thoracentesis
    Blood sampling

    EXCLUDES *heart catheterization (E870.6)*

E870.6 **Heart catheterization**

E870.7 **Administration of enema**

E870.8 **Other specified medical care**

E870.9 **Unspecified medical care**

✓4ᵗʰ **E871 Foreign object left in body during procedure**

E871.0 **Surgical operation**

E871.1 **Infusion or transfusion**

E871.2 **Kidney dialysis or other perfusion**

E871.3 **Injection or vaccination**

E871.4 **Endoscopic examination**

E871.5 **Aspiration of fluid or tissue, puncture, and catheterization**

    Abdominal paracentesis   Lumbar puncture
    Aspiration needle biopsy   Thoracentesis
    Blood sampling

    EXCLUDES *heart catheterization (E871.6)*

E871.6 **Heart catheterization**

E871.7 **Removal of catheter or packing**

E871.8 **Other specified procedures**

E871.9 **Unspecified procedure**

✓4ᵗʰ **E872 Failure of sterile precautions during procedure**

E872.0 **Surgical operation**

E872.1 **Infusion or transfusion**

E872.2 **Kidney dialysis and other perfusion**

E872.3 **Injection or vaccination**

E872.4 **Endoscopic examination**

E872.5 **Aspiration of fluid or tissue, puncture, and catheterization**

    Abdominal paracentesis   Lumbar puncture
    Aspiration needle biopsy   Thoracentesis
    Blood sampling

    EXCLUDES *heart catheterization (E872.6)*

E872.6 **Heart catheterization**

E872.8 **Other specified procedures**

E872.9 **Unspecified procedure**

✓4ᵗʰ **E873 Failure in dosage**

    EXCLUDES *accidental overdose of drug, medicinal or biological substance (E850.0-E858.9)*

E873.0 **Excessive amount of blood or other fluid during transfusion or infusion**

E873.1 **Incorrect dilution of fluid during infusion**

E873.2 **Overdose of radiation in therapy**

E873.3 **Inadvertent exposure of patient to radiation during medical care**

E873.4 **Failure in dosage in electroshock or insulin-shock therapy**

E873.5 **Inappropriate [too hot or too cold] temperature in local application and packing**

E873.6 **Nonadministration of necessary drug or medicinal substance**

E873.8 **Other specified failure in dosage**

E873.9 **Unspecified failure in dosage**

✓4ᵗʰ **E874 Mechanical failure of instrument or apparatus during procedure**

E874.0 **Surgical operation**

E874.1 **Infusion and transfusion**

    Air in system

E874.2 **Kidney dialysis and other perfusion**

E874.3 **Endoscopic examination**

E874.4 **Aspiration of fluid or tissue, puncture, and catheterization**

    Abdominal paracentesis   Lumbar puncture
    Aspiration needle biopsy   Thoracentesis
    Blood sampling

    EXCLUDES *heart catheterization (E874.5)*

E874.5 **Heart catheterization**

E874.8 **Other specified procedures**

E874.9 **Unspecified procedure**

✓4ᵗʰ **E875 Contaminated or infected blood, other fluid, drug, or biological substance**

    INCLUDES   presence of:
        bacterial pyrogens
        endotoxin-producing bacteria
        serum hepatitis-producing agent

E875.0 **Contaminated substance transfused or infused**

E875.1 **Contaminated substance injected or used for vaccination**

E875.2 **Contaminated drug or biological substance administered by other means**

E875.8 **Other**

E875.9 **Unspecified**

✓4ᵗʰ **E876 Other and unspecified misadventures during medical care**

E876.0 **Mismatched blood in transfusion**

E876.1 **Wrong fluid in infusion**

E876.2 **Failure in suture and ligature during surgical operation**

E876.3 **Endotracheal tube wrongly placed during anesthetic procedure**

E876.4 **Failure to introduce or to remove other tube or instrument**

    EXCLUDES *foreign object left in body during procedure (E871.0-E871.9)*

E876.5 **Performance of inappropriate operation**

E876.8 **Other specified misadventures during medical care**

    Performance of inappropriate treatment NEC

E876.9 **Unspecified misadventure during medical care**

SURGICAL AND MEDICAL PROCEDURES AS THE CAUSE OF ABNORMAL REACTION OF PATIENT OR LATER COMPLICATION, WITHOUT MENTION OF MISADVENTURE AT THE TIME OF PROCEDURE (E878-E879)

    INCLUDES   procedures as the cause of abnormal reaction, such as:
        displacement or malfunction of prosthetic device
        hepatorenal failure, postoperative
        malfunction of external stoma
        postoperative intestinal obstruction
        rejection of transplanted organ

    EXCLUDES *anesthetic management properly carried out as the cause of adverse effect (E937.0-E938.9)*

        infusion and transfusion, without mention of misadventure in the technique of procedure (E930.0-E949.9)

✓4ᵗʰ **E878 Surgical operation and other surgical procedures as the cause of abnormal reaction of patient, or of later complication, without mention of misadventure at the time of operation**

E878.0 **Surgical operation with transplant of whole organ**

    Transplantation of: Transplantation of:
      heart   liver
      kidney

E878.1 **Surgical operation with implant of artificial internal device**

    Cardiac pacemaker   Heart valve prosthesis
    Electrodes implanted in   Internal orthopedic
      brain   device

E878.2 Surgical operation with anastomosis, bypass, or graft, with natural or artificial tissues used as implant

Anastomosis: Graft of blood vessel,
    arteriovenous   tendon, or skin
    gastrojejunal

> EXCLUDES   *external stoma (E878.3)*

E878.3 Surgical operation with formation of external stoma

Colostomy   Gastrostomy
Cystostomy   Ureterostomy
Duodenostomy

E878.4 Other restorative surgery

E878.5 Amputation of limb(s)

E878.6 Removal of other organ (partial) (total)

E878.8 Other specified surgical operations and procedures

E878.9 Unspecified surgical operations and procedures

✓4ᵗʰ **E879 Other procedures, without mention of misadventure at the time of procedure, as the cause of abnormal reaction of patient, or of later complication**

E879.0 Cardiac catheterization

E879.1 Kidney dialysis

E879.2 Radiological procedure and radiotherapy

> EXCLUDES   *radio-opaque dyes for diagnostic x-ray procedures (E947.8)*

E879.3 Shock therapy

Electroshock therapy
Insulin-shock therapy

E879.4 Aspiration of fluid

Lumbar puncture
Thoracentesis

E879.5 Insertion of gastric or duodenal sound

E879.6 Urinary catheterization

E879.7 Blood sampling

E879.8 Other specified procedures

Blood transfusion

E879.9 Unspecified procedure

ACCIDENTAL FALLS (E880-E888)

> EXCLUDES   *falls (in or from):*
> *burning building (E890.8, E891.8)*
> *into fire (E890.0-E899)*
> *into water (with submersion or drowning) (E910.0-E910.9)*
> *machinery (in operation) (E919.0-E919.9)*
> *on edged, pointed, or sharp object (E920.0-E920.9)*
> *transport vehicle (E800.0-E845.9)*
> *vehicle not elsewhere classifiable (E846-E848)*

✓4ᵗʰ **E880 Fall on or from stairs or steps**

E880.0 Escalator

E880.1 Fall on or from sidewalk curb

> EXCLUDES   *fall from moving sidewalk (E885.9)*

E880.9 Other stairs or steps

✓4ᵗʰ **E881 Fall on or from ladders or scaffolding**

E881.0 Fall from ladder

E881.1 Fall from scaffolding

E882 Fall from or out of building or other structure

Fall from: Fall from:
    balcony   turret
    bridge   viaduct
    building   wall
    flagpole   window
    tower   Fall through roof

> EXCLUDES   *collapse of a building or structure (E916)*
> *fall or jump from burning building (E890.8, E891.8)*

✓4ᵗʰ **E883 Fall into hole or other opening in surface**

> INCLUDES   fall into: fall into:
>   cavity   shaft
>   dock   swimming pool
>   hole   tank
>   pit   well
>   quarry

> EXCLUDES   *fall into water NOS (E910.9)*
> *that resulting in drowning or submersion without mention of injury (E910.0-E910.9)*

E883.0 Accident from diving or jumping into water [swimming pool]

Strike or hit:
    against bottom when jumping or diving into water
    wall or board of swimming pool
    water surface

> EXCLUDES   *diving with insufficient air supply (E913.2)*
> *effects of air pressure from diving (E902.2)*

E883.1 Accidental fall into well

E883.2 Accidental fall into storm drain or manhole

E883.9 Fall into other hole or other opening in surface

✓4ᵗʰ **E884 Other fall from one level to another**

E884.0 Fall from playground equipment

> EXCLUDES   *recreational machinery (E919.8)*

E884.1 Fall from cliff

E884.2 Fall from chair

E884.3 Fall from wheelchair

E884.4 Fall from bed

E884.5 Fall from other furniture

E884.6 Fall from commode

Toilet

E884.9 Other fall from one level to another

Fall from:
    embankment
    haystack
    stationary vehicle
    tree

✓4ᵗʰ **E885 Fall on same level from slipping, tripping, or stumbling**

● **E885.0 Fall from (nonmotorized) scooter**

E885.1 Fall from roller skates

In-line skates

E885.2 Fall from skateboard

E885.3 Fall from skis

E885.4 Fall from snowboard

E885.9 Fall from other slipping, tripping, or stumbling

Fall on moving sidewalk

✓4ᵗʰ **E886 Fall on same level from collision, pushing, or shoving, by or with other person**

> EXCLUDES   *crushed or pushed by a crowd or human stampede (E917.1, E917.6)*

E886.0 In sports

Tackles in sports

> EXCLUDES   *kicked, stepped on, struck by object, in sports (E917.0, E917.5)*

E886.9 Other and unspecified

Fall from collision of pedestrian (conveyance) with another pedestrian (conveyance)

E887 Fracture, cause unspecified

✓4ᵗʰ **E888 Other and unspecified fall**

Accidental fall NOS
Fall on same level NOS

E888.0 Fall resulting in striking against sharp object

Use additional external cause code to identify object (E920)

E888.1 Fall resulting in striking against other object

E888.8 Other fall

E888.9 Unspecified fall

Fall NOS

ACCIDENTS CAUSED BY FIRE AND FLAMES (E890-E899)

INCLUDES   asphyxia or poisoning due to conflagration or ignition
burning by fire
secondary fires resulting from explosion

EXCLUDES   *arson (E968.0)*
fire in or on:
    machinery (in operation) (E919.0-E919.9)
    transport vehicle other than stationary vehicle (E800.0-E845.9)
    vehicle not elsewhere classifiable (E846-E848)

✓4ᵗʰ E890 Conflagration in private dwelling

INCLUDES   conflagration in: conflagration in:
   apartment   lodging house
   boarding house   mobile home
   camping place   private garage
   caravan   rooming house
   farmhouse   tenement
   house
conflagration originating from sources classifiable to E893-E898 in the above buildings

E890.0 Explosion caused by conflagration

E890.1 Fumes from combustion of polyvinylchloride [PVC] and similar material in conflagration

E890.2 Other smoke and fumes from conflagration
Carbon monoxide
Fumes NOS   } from conflagration in private building
Smoke NOS

E890.3 Burning caused by conflagration

E890.8 Other accident resulting from conflagration
Collapse of
Fall from   } burning private building
Hit by object falling from
Jump from

E890.9 Unspecified accident resulting from conflagration in private dwelling

✓4ᵗʰ E891 Conflagration in other and unspecified building or structure

Conflagration in: Conflagration in:
   barn   farm outbuildings
   church   hospital
   convalescent and other   hotel
      residential home   school
   dormitory of educational   store
      institution   theater
   factory
Conflagration originating from sources classifiable to E893-E898, in the above buildings

E891.0 Explosion caused by conflagration

E891.1 Fumes from combustion of polyvinylchloride [PVC] and similar material in conflagration

E891.2 Other smoke and fumes from conflagration
Carbon monoxide } from conflagration in
Fumes NOS   building or
Smoke NOS   structure

E891.3 Burning caused by conflagration

E891.8 Other accident resulting from conflagration
Collapse of
Fall from   } burning building or
Hit by object falling from   structure
Jump from

E891.9 Unspecified accident resulting from conflagration of other and unspecified building or structure

E892 Conflagration not in building or structure

Fire (uncontrolled) (in) (of):   Fire (uncontrolled) (in) (of):
   forest   prairie
   grass   transport vehicle [any],
   hay   except while in
   lumber   transit
   mine   tunnel

✓4ᵗʰ E893 Accident caused by ignition of clothing

EXCLUDES   *ignition of clothing:*
from highly inflammable material (E894)
with conflagration (E890.0-E892)

E893.0 From controlled fire in private dwelling
Ignition of clothing from:
   normal fire (charcoal)
     (coal) (electric)
     (gas) (wood) in:
   brazier   } in private dwelling
   fireplace   (as listed in
   furnace   E890)
   stove

E893.1 From controlled fire in other building or structure
Ignition of clothing from:
   normal fire (charcoal)
     (coal) (electric)
     (gas) (wood) in:
   brazier   } in other building or
   fireplace   structure (as
   furnace   listed in E81)
   stove

E893.2 From controlled fire not in building or structure
Ignition of clothing from:
   bonfire (controlled)
   brazier fire (controlled), not in building or structure
   trash fire (controlled)

EXCLUDES   *conflagration not in building (E892)*
trash fire out of control (E892)

E893.8 From other specified sources
Ignition of clothing from:
   blowlamp
   blowtorch
   burning bedspread
   candle
   cigar
   cigarette
   lighter
   matches
   pipe
   welding torch

E893.9 Unspecified source
Ignition of clothing (from controlled fire NOS) (in building NOS) NOS

E894 Ignition of highly inflammable material

Ignition of:
   benzine
   gasoline
   fat   } (with ignition of clothing)
   kerosene
   paraffin
   petrol

EXCLUDES   *ignition of highly inflammable material with:*
conflagration (E890.0-E892)
explosion (E923.0-E923.9)

E895 Accident caused by controlled fire in private dwelling

Burning by (flame of)
    normal fire (charcoal)
    (coal) (electric) (gas)
    (wood) in: } in private dwelling (as
    brazier   listed in E890)
    fireplace
    furnace
    stove

> **EXCLUDES** *burning by hot objects not producing fire or*
> *flames (E924.0-E924.9)*
> *ignition of clothing from these sources (E893.0)*
> *poisoning by carbon monoxide from incomplete*
> *combustion of fuel (E867-E868.9)*
> *that with conflagration (E890.0-E890.9)*

E896 Accident caused by controlled fire in other and unspecified building or structure

Burning by (flame of) normal fire (charcoal) (coal) (electric)
    (gas) (wood) in:
    brazier
    fireplace   } in other building or structure (as
    furnace   listed in E891)
    stove

> **EXCLUDES** *burning by hot objects not producing fire or*
> *flames (E924.0-E924.9)*
> *ignition of clothing from these sources (E893.1)*
> *poisoning by carbon monoxide from incomplete*
> *combustion of fuel (E867-E868.9)*
> *that with conflagration (E891.0-E891.9)*

E897 Accident caused by controlled fire not in building or structure

Burns from flame of:
    bonfire
    brazier fire, not in building   } controlled
        or structure
    trash fire

> **EXCLUDES** *ignition of clothing from these sources (E893.2)*
> *trash fire out of control (E892)*
> *that with conflagration (E892)*

✓4ᵗʰ E898 Accident caused by other specified fire and flames

> **EXCLUDES** *conflagration (E890.0-E892)*
> *that with ignition of:*
> *clothing (E893.0-E893.9)*
> *highly inflammable material (E894)*

E898.0 Burning bedclothes
Bed set on fire NOS

E898.1 Other
Burning by:	Burning by:
blowlamp	lamp
blowtorch	lighter
candle	matches
cigar	pipe
cigarette	welding torch
fire in room NOS	

E899 Accident caused by unspecified fire
Burning NOS

ACCIDENTS DUE TO NATURAL AND ENVIRONMENTAL FACTORS
(E900-E909)

✓4ᵗʰ E900 Excessive heat

E900.0 Due to weather conditions
Excessive heat as the external cause of:
    ictus solaris
    siriasis
    sunstroke

E900.1 Of man-made origin
Heat (in):	Heat (in):
boiler room	generated in transport
drying room	vehicle
factory	kitchen
furnace room	

E900.9 Of unspecified origin

✓4ᵗʰ E901 Excessive cold

E901.0 Due to weather conditions
Excessive cold as the cause of:
    chilblains NOS
    immersion foot

E901.1 Of man-made origin
Contact with or inhalation of:
    dry ice
    liquid air
    liquid hydrogen
    liquid nitrogen
Prolonged exposure in:
    deep freeze unit
    refrigerator

E901.8 Other specified origin

E901.9 Of unspecified origin

✓4ᵗʰ E902 High and low air pressure and changes in air pressure

E902.0 Residence or prolonged visit at high altitude
Residence or prolonged visit at high altitude as the
    cause of:
    Acosta syndrome
    Alpine sickness
    altitude sickness
    Andes disease
    anoxia, hypoxia
    barotitis, barodontalgia, barosinusitis, otitic
        barotrauma
    hypobarism, hypobaropathy
    mountain sickness
    range disease

E902.1 In aircraft
Sudden change in air pressure in aircraft during
    ascent or descent as the cause of:
    aeroneurosis
    aviators' disease

E902.2 Due to diving
High air pressure from
    rapid descent in water   } as the cause of:
Reduction in atmospheric   caisson disease
    pressure while   divers' disease
    surfacing from deep   divers' palsy or
    water diving   paralysis

E902.8 Due to other specified causes
Reduction in atmospheric pressure whilesurfacing
    from underground

E902.9 Unspecified cause

E903 Travel and motion

✓4ᵗʰ E904 Hunger, thirst, exposure, and neglect

> **EXCLUDES** *any condition resulting from homicidal intent*
> *(E968.0-E968.9)*
> *hunger, thirst, and exposure resulting from*
> *accidents connected with transport*
> *(E800.0-E848)*

E904.0 Abandonment or neglect of infants and helpless persons
Exposure to weather   } resulting from
    conditions   abandonment or
Hunger or thirst   neglect

Desertion of newborn
Inattention at or after birth
Lack of care (helpless person) (infant)

> **EXCLUDES** *criminal [purposeful] neglect (E968.4)*

E904.1 Lack of food
Lack of food as the cause of:
    inanition
    insufficient nourishment
    starvation

> **EXCLUDES** *hunger resulting from abandonment or*
> *neglect (E904.0)*

E904.2 Lack of water
Lack of water as the cause of:
　dehydration
　inanition
　EXCLUDES　*dehydration due to acute fluid loss (276.5)*

E904.3 Exposure (to weather conditions), not elsewhere classifiable
Exposure NOS
Humidity
Struck by hailstones
　EXCLUDES　*struck by lightning (E907)*

E904.9 Privation, unqualified
Destitution

✓4ᵗʰ E905 Venomous animals and plants as the cause of poisoning and toxic reactions
　INCLUDES　chemical released by animal
　　　　　insects
　　　　　release of venom through fangs, hairs, spines, tentacles, and other venom apparatus
　EXCLUDES　*eating of poisonous animals or plants (E865.0-E865.9)*

E905.0 Venomous snakes and lizards

Cobra	Mamba
Copperhead snake	Rattlesnake
Coral snake	Sea snake
Fer de lance	Snake (venomous)
Gila monster	Viper
Krait	Water moccasin

　EXCLUDES　*bites of snakes and lizards known to be nonvenomous (E906.2)*

E905.1 Venomous spiders

Black widow spider	Tarantula (venomous)
Brown spider	

E905.2 Scorpion

E905.3 Hornets, wasps, and bees
Yellow jacket

E905.4 Centipede and venomous millipede (tropical)

E905.5 Other venomous arthropods
Sting of:
　ant
　caterpillar

E905.6 Venomous marine animals and plants
Puncture by sea urchin spine
Sting of:
　coral
　jelly fish
　nematocysts
　sea anemone
　sea cucumber
　other marine animal or plant
　EXCLUDES　*bites and other injuries caused by nonvenomous marine animal (E906.2-E906.8)*
　　　　　bite of sea snake (venomous) (E905.0)

E905.7 Poisoning and toxic reactions caused by other plants
Injection of poisons or toxins into or through skin by plant thorns, spines, or other mechanisms
　EXCLUDES　*puncture wound NOS by plant thorns or spines (E920.8)*

E905.8 Other specified

E905.9 Unspecified
Sting NOS
Venomous bite NOS

✓4ᵗʰ E906 Other injury caused by animals
　EXCLUDES　*poisoning and toxic reactions caused by venomous animals and insects (E905.0-E905.9)*
　　　　　road vehicle accident involving animals (E827.0-E828.9)
　　　　　tripping or falling over an animal (E885.9)

E906.0 Dog bite

E906.1 Rat bite

E906.2 Bite of nonvenomous snakes and lizards

E906.3 Bite of other animal except arthropod

Cats	Rodents, except rats
Moray eel	Shark

E906.4 Bite of nonvenomous arthropod
Insect bite NOS

E906.5 Bite by unspecified animal
Animal bite NOS

E906.8 Other specified injury caused by animal
Butted by animal
Fallen on by horse or other animal, not being ridden
Gored by animal
Implantation of quills of porcupine
Pecked by bird
Run over by animal, not being ridden
Stepped on by animal, not being ridden
　EXCLUDES　*injury by animal being ridden (E828.0-E828.9)*

E906.9 Unspecified injury caused by animal

E907 Lightning
　EXCLUDES　*injury from:*
　　　　　fall of tree or other object caused by lightning (E916)
　　　　　fire caused by lightning (E890.0-E892)

✓4ᵗʰ E908 Cataclysmic storms, and floods resulting from storms
　EXCLUDES　*collapse of dam or man-made structure causing flood (E909.3)*

E908.0 Hurricane
Storm surge
"Tidal wave" caused by storm action
Typhoon

E908.1 Tornado
Cyclone
Twisters

E908.2 Floods
Torrential rainfall
Flash flood
　EXCLUDES　*collapse of dam or man-made structure causing flood (E909.3)*

E908.3 Blizzard (snow) (ice)

E908.4 Dust storm

E908.8 Other cataclysmic storms

E908.9 Unspecified cataclysmic storms, and floods resulting from storms
Storm NOS

✓4ᵗʰ E909 Cataclysmic earth surface movements and eruptions

E909.0 Earthquakes

E909.1 Volcanic eruptions
Burns from lava
Ash inhalation

E909.2 Avalanche, landslide, or mudslide

E909.3 Collapse of dam or man-made structure

E909.4 Tidalwave caused by earthquake
Tidalwave NOS
Tsunami
　EXCLUDES　*tidalwave caused by tropical storm (E908.0)*

E909.8 Other cataclysmic earth surface movements and eruptions

E909.9 Unspecified cataclysmic earth surface movements and eruptions

　　✓4ᵗʰ Fourth-digit Required　　▶◀ Revised Text　　● New Code　　▲ Revised Code Title

ACCIDENTS CAUSED BY SUBMERSION, SUFFOCATION, AND FOREIGN BODIES (E910-E915)

✓4ᵗʰ E910 Accidental drowning and submersion

INCLUDES
immersion
swimmers' cramp

EXCLUDES
diving accident (NOS) (resulting in injury except drowning) (E883.0)
diving with insufficient air supply (E913.2)
drowning and submersion due to:
cataclysm (E908-E909)
machinery accident (E919.0-E919.9)
transport accident (E800.0-E845.9)
effect of high and low air pressure (E902.2)
injury from striking against objects while in running water (E917.2)

E910.0 While water-skiing
Fall from water skis with submersion or drowning
EXCLUDES *accident to water-skier involving a watercraft and resulting in submersion or other injury (E830.4, E831.4)*

E910.1 While engaged in other sport or recreational activity with diving equipment
Scuba diving NOS   Underwater spear
Skin diving NOS   fishing NOS

E910.2 While engaged in other sport or recreational activity without diving equipment
Fishing or hunting, except from boat or with diving equipment
Ice skating
Playing in water
Surfboarding
Swimming NOS
Voluntarily jumping from boat, not involved in accident, for swim NOS
Wading in water
EXCLUDES *jumping into water to rescue another person (E910.3)*

E910.3 While swimming or diving for purposes other than recreation or sport
Marine salvage
Pearl diving
Placement of fishing nets
Rescue (attempt) of another person   (with diving equipment)
Underwater construction or repairs

E910.4 In bathtub

E910.8 Other accidental drowning or submersion
Drowning in: Drowning in:
quenching tank   swimming pool

E910.9 Unspecified accidental drowning or submersion
Accidental fall into water NOS
Drowning NOS

E911 Inhalation and ingestion of food causing obstruction of respiratory tract or suffocation
Aspiration and inhalation of food [any] (into respiratory tract) NOS
Asphyxia by
Choked on   food [including bone, seed in food, regurgitated food]
Suffocation by
Compression of trachea
Interruption of respiration   by food lodged in esophagus
Obstruction of respiration
Obstruction of pharynx by food (bolus)
EXCLUDES *injury, except asphyxia and obstruction of respiratory passage, caused by food (E915)*
obstruction of esophagus by food without mention of asphyxia or obstruction of respiratory passage (E915)

E912 Inhalation and ingestion of other object causing obstruction of respiratory tract or suffocation
Aspiration and inhalation of foreign body except food (into respiratory tract) NOS
Foreign object [bean] [marble] in nose
Obstruction of pharynx by foreign body
Compression
Interruption of respiration   by foreign body in esophagus
Obstruction of respiration
EXCLUDES *injury, except asphyxia and obstruction of respiratory passage, caused by foreign body (E915)*
obstruction of esophagus by foreign body without mention of asphyxia or obstruction in respiratory passage (E915)

✓4ᵗʰ E913 Accidental mechanical suffocation
EXCLUDES *mechanical suffocation from or by:*
accidental inhalation or ingestion of:
food (E911)
foreign object (E912)
cataclysm (E908-E909)
explosion (E921.0-E921.9, E923.0-E923.9)
machinery accident (E919.0-E919.9)

E913.0 In bed or cradle
EXCLUDES *suffocation by plastic bag (E913.1)*

E913.1 By plastic bag

E913.2 Due to lack of air (in closed place)
Accidentally closed up in refrigerator or other airtight enclosed space
Diving with insufficient air supply
EXCLUDES *suffocation by plastic bag (E913.1)*

E913.3 By falling earth or other substance
Cave-in NOS
EXCLUDES *cave-in caused by cataclysmic earth surface movements and eruptions (E909)*
struck by cave-in without asphyxiation or suffocation (E916)

E913.8 Other specified means
Accidental hanging, except in bed or cradle

E913.9 Unspecified means
Asphyxia, mechanical NOS   Suffocation NOS
Strangulation NOS

E914 Foreign body accidentally entering eye and adnexa
EXCLUDES *corrosive liquid (E924.1)*

E915 Foreign body accidentally entering other orifice
EXCLUDES *aspiration and inhalation of foreign body, any, (into respiratory tract) NOS (E911-E912)*

OTHER ACCIDENTS (E916-E928)

E916 Struck accidentally by falling object
Collapse of building, except on fire
Falling:
rock
snowslide NOS
stone
tree
Object falling from:
machine, not in operation
stationary vehicle
Code first:
collapse of building on fire (E890.0-E891.9)
falling object in:
cataclysm (E908-E909)
machinery accidents (E919.0-E919.9)
transport accidents (E800.0-E845.9)
vehicle accidents not elsewhere classifiable (E846-E848)
object set in motion by:
explosion (E921.0-E921.9, E923.0-E923.9)
firearm (E922.0-E922.9)
projected object (E917.0-E917.9)

☑4ᵗʰ **E917 Striking against or struck accidentally by objects or persons**

INCLUDES   bumping into or
against
colliding with   } object (moving)
kicking against   (projected)
stepping on   (stationary)
struck by   pedestrian conveyance
person

EXCLUDES   *fall from:*
collision with another person, except when
caused by a crowd (E886.0-E886.9)
stumbling over object (E885.9)
fall resulting in striking against object (E888.0,
E888.1)
injury caused by:
assault (E960.0-E960.1, E967.0-E967.9)
cutting or piercing instrument (E920.0-
E920.9)
explosion (E921.0-E921.9, E923.0-E923.9)
firearm (E922.0-E922.9)
machinery (E919.0-E919.9)
transport vehicle (E800.0-E845.9)
vehicle not elsewhere classifiable (E846-
E848)

E917.0 In sports without subsequent fall
Kicked or stepped on during game (football) (rugby)
Struck by hit or thrown ball
Struck by hockey stick or puck

E917.1 Caused by a crowd, by collective fear or panic
without subsequent fall
Crushed
Pushed   } by crowd or human stampede
Stepped on

E917.2 In running water without subsequent fall
EXCLUDES   *drowning or submersion (E910.0-*
E910.9)
that in sports (E917.0, E917.5)

E917.3 Furniture without subsequent fall
EXCLUDES   *fall from furniture (E884.2, E884.4-*
E884.5)

E917.4 Other stationary object without subsequent fall
Bath tub
Fence
Lamp-post

E917.5 Object in sports with subsequent fall
Knocked down while boxing

E917.6 Caused by a crowd, by collective fear or panic with
subsequent fall

E917.7 Furniture with subsequent fall
EXCLUDES   *fall from furniture (E884.2, E884.4-*
E884.5)

E917.8 Other stationary object with subsequent fall
Bath tub
Fence
Lamp-post

E917.9 Other striking against with or without subsequent
fall

E918 Caught accidentally in or between objects
Caught, crushed, jammed, or pinched in or between moving
or stationary objects, such as:
escalator
folding object
hand tools, appliances, or implements
sliding door and door frame
under packing crate
washing machine wringer
EXCLUDES   *injury caused by:*
cutting or piercing instrument (E920.0-
E920.9)
machinery (E919.0-E919.9)
transport vehicle (E800.0-E845.9)
vehicle not elsewhere classifiable (E846-
E848)
struck accidentally by:
falling object (E916)
object (moving) (projected) (E917.0-E917.9)

☑4ᵗʰ **E919 Accidents caused by machinery**

INCLUDES   burned by
caught in (moving
parts of)
collapse of
crushed by
cut or pierced by
drowning or
submersion
caused by
explosion of, on, in
fall from or into
moving part of   } machinery
fire starting in or on   (accident)
mechanical
suffocation
caused by
object falling from, on,
in motion by
overturning of
pinned under
run over by
struck by
thrown from

caught between machinery and other object
machinery accident NOS
EXCLUDES   *accidents involving machinery, not in operation*
(E884.9, E916-E918)
injury caused by:
electric current in connection with machinery
(E925.0-E925.9)
escalator (E880.0, E918)
explosion of pressure vessel in connection
with machinery (E921.0-E921.9)
moving sidewalk (E885.9)
powered hand tools, appliances, and
implements (E916-E918, E920.0-
E921.9, E923.0-E926.9)
transport vehicle accidents involving
machinery (E800.0-E848.9)
poisoning by carbon monoxide generated by
machine (E868.8)

☑4ᵗʰ Fourth-digit Required   ►◄ Revised Text   ● New Code   ▲ Revised Code Title

E919.0 Agricultural machines

Animal-powered agricultural machine
Combine
Derrick, hay
Farm machinery NOS
Farm tractor
Harvester
Hay mower or rake
Reaper
Thresher

> EXCLUDES   *that in transport under own power on the highway (E810.0-E819.9)*
> *that being towed by another vehicle on the highway (E810.0-E819.9, E827.0-E827.9, E829.0-E829.9)*
> *that involved in accident classifiable to E820-E829 (E820.0-E829.9)*

E919.1 Mining and earth-drilling machinery

Bore or drill (land) (seabed)   Shaft lift
Shaft hoist   Under-cutter

> EXCLUDES   *coal car, tram, truck, and tub in mine (E846)*

E919.2 Lifting machines and appliances

Chain hoist
Crane
Derrick
Elevator (building) (grain)   except in agricultural or mining operations
Forklift truck
Lift
Pulley block
Winch

> EXCLUDES   *that being towed by another vehicle on the highway (E810.0-E819.9, E827.0-E827.9, E829.0-829.9)*
> *that in transport under own power on the highway (E810.0-E819.9)*
> *that involved in accident classifiable to E820-E829 (E820.0-E829.9)*

E919.3 Metalworking machines

Abrasive wheel   Metal:
Forging machine   drilling machine
Lathe   milling machine
Mechanical shears   power press
                       rolling-mill
                       sawing machine

E919.4 Woodworking and forming machines

Band saw   Overhead plane
Bench saw   Powered saw
Circular saw   Radial saw
Molding machine   Sander

> EXCLUDES   *hand saw (E920.1)*

E919.5 Prime movers, except electrical motors

Gas turbine
Internal combustion engine
Steam engine
Water driven turbine

> EXCLUDES   *that being towed by other vehicle on the highway (E810.0-E819.9, E827.0-E827.9, E829.0-E829.9)*
> *that in transport under own power on the highway (E810.0-E819.9)*

E919.6 Transmission machinery

Transmission: Transmission:
   belt   pinion
   cable   pulley
   chain   shaft
   gear

E919.7 Earth moving, scraping, and other excavating machines

Bulldozer   Steam shovel
Road scraper

> EXCLUDES   *that being towed by other vehicle on the highway (E810.0-E819.9, E827.0-E827.9, E829.0-E829.9)*
> *that in transport under own power on the highway (E810.0-E819.9)*

E919.8 Other specified machinery

Machines for manufacture of:
   clothing
   foodstuffs and beverages
   paper
Printing machine
Recreational machinery
Spinning, weaving, and textile machines

E919.9 Unspecified machinery

√4ᵗʰ **E920 Accidents caused by cutting and piercing instruments or objects**

> INCLUDES   accidental injury (by) } object: edged pointed sharp

E920.0 Powered lawn mower

E920.1 Other powered hand tools

Any powered hand tool [compressed air] [electric] [explosive cartridge] [hydraulic power], such as:
   drill
   hand saw
   hedge clipper
   rivet gun
   snow blower
   staple gun

> EXCLUDES   *band saw (E919.4)*
> *bench saw (E919.4)*

E920.2 Powered household appliances and implements

Blender
Electric:
   beater or mixer
   can opener
   fan
   knife
   sewing machine
Garbage disposal appliance

E920.3 Knives, swords, and daggers

E920.4 Other hand tools and implements

Axe   Paper cutter
Can opener NOS   Pitchfork
Chisel   Rake
Fork   Scissors
Hand saw   Screwdriver
Hoe   Sewing machine, not powered
Ice pick   Shovel
Needle (sewing)

E920.5 Hypodermic needle

Contaminated needle
Needle stick

E920.8 Other specified cutting and piercing instruments or objects

Arrow   Nail
Broken glass   Plant thorn
Dart   Splinter
Edge of stiff paper   Tin can lid
Lathe turnings

> EXCLUDES   *animal spines or quills (E906.8)*
> *flying glass due to explosion (E921.0-E923.9)*

E920.9 Unspecified cutting and piercing instrument or object

✓4ᵗʰ **E921 Accident caused by explosion of pressure vessel**

    INCLUDES   accidental explosion of pressure vessels, whether or not part of machinery

    EXCLUDES   *explosion of pressure vessel on transport vehicle (E800.0-E845.9)*

E921.0 Boilers

E921.1 Gas cylinders
    Air tank
    Pressure gas tank

E921.8 Other specified pressure vessels
    Aerosol can   Pressure cooker
    Automobile tire

E921.9 Unspecified pressure vessel

✓4ᵗʰ **E922 Accident caused by firearm, and air gun missile**

E922.0 Handgun
    Pistol   Revolver

    EXCLUDES   *Verey pistol (E922.8)*

E922.1 Shotgun (automatic)

E922.2 Hunting rifle

E922.3 Military firearms
    Army rifle   Machine gun

E922.4 Air gun
    BB gun
    Pellet gun

● **E922.5 Paintball gun**

E922.8 Other specified firearm missile
    Verey pistol [flare]

E922.9 Unspecified firearm missile
    Gunshot wound NOS
    Shot NOS

✓4ᵗʰ **E923 Accident caused by explosive material**

    INCLUDES   flash burns and other injuries resulting from explosion of explosive material
    ignition of highly explosive material with explosion

    EXCLUDES   *explosion:*
       in or on machinery (E919.0-E919.9)
       on any transport vehicle, except stationary motor vehicle (E800.0-E848)
       with conflagration (E890.0, E891.0, E892)
       secondary fires resulting from explosion (E890.0-E899)

E923.0 Fireworks

E923.1 Blasting materials
    Blasting cap
    Detonator
    Dynamite
    Explosive [any] used in blasting operations

E923.2 Explosive gases
    Acetylene   Fire damp
    Butane   Gasoline fumes
    Coal gas   Methane
    Explosion in mine NOS   Propane

E923.8 Other explosive materials
    Bomb   Torpedo
    Explosive missile   Explosion in munitions:
    Grenade   dump
    Mine   factory
    Shell

E923.9 Unspecified explosive material
    Explosion NOS

✓4ᵗʰ **E924 Accident caused by hot substance or object, caustic or corrosive material, and steam**

    EXCLUDES   *burning NOS (E899)*
       chemical burn resulting from swallowing a corrosive substance (E860.0-E864.4)
       fire caused by these substances and objects (E890.0-E894)
       radiation burns (E926.0-E926.9)
       therapeutic misadventures (E870.0-E876.9)

E924.0 Hot liquids and vapors, including steam
    Burning or scalding by:
       boiling water
       hot or boiling liquids not primarily caustic or corrosive
       liquid metal
       steam
       other hot vapor

    EXCLUDES   *hot (boiling) tap water (E924.2)*

E924.1 Caustic and corrosive substances
    Burning by: Burning by:
       acid [any kind]   corrosive substance
       ammonia   lye
       caustic oven cleaner   vitriol
          or other substance

E924.2 Hot (boiling) tap water

E924.8 Other
    Burning by:
       heat from electric heating appliance
       hot object NOS
       light bulb
       steam pipe

E924.9 Unspecified

✓4ᵗʰ **E925 Accident caused by electric current**

    INCLUDES   electric current from exposed wire, faulty appliance, high voltage cable, live rail, or open electric socket as the cause of:
       burn
       cardiac fibrillation
       convulsion
       electric shock
       electrocution
       puncture wound
       respiratory paralysis

    EXCLUDES   *burn by heat from electrical appliance (E924.8)*
       lightning (E907)

E925.0 Domestic wiring and appliances

E925.1 Electric power generating plants, distribution stations, transmission lines
    Broken power line

E925.2 Industrial wiring, appliances, and electrical machinery
    Conductors
    Control apparatus
    Electrical equipment and machinery
    Transformers

E925.8 Other electric current
    Wiring and appliances in or on:
       farm [not farmhouse]
       outdoors
       public building
       residential institutions
       schools

E925.9 Unspecified electric current
    Burns or other injury from electric current NOS
    Electric shock NOS
    Electrocution NOS

✓4ᵗʰ **E926 Exposure to radiation**

    EXCLUDES   *abnormal reaction to or complication of treatment without mention of misadventure (E879.2)*
       atomic power plant malfunction in water transport (E838.0-E838.9)
       misadventure to patient in surgical and medical procedures (E873.2-E873.3)
       use of radiation in war operations (E996-E997.9)

E Codes E921–E926

E Codes E926.0–E930.3

E926.0 Radiofrequency radiation

Overexposure to:
microwave radiation
radar radiation
radiofrequency
radiofrequency radiation [any]

from:
high-powered radio and television transmitters
industrial radiofrequency induction heaters
radar installations

E926.1 Infrared heaters and lamps

Exposure to infrared radiation from heaters and lamps as the cause of:
blistering
burning
charring
inflammatory change

EXCLUDES *physical contact with heater or lamp (E924.8)*

E926.2 Visible and ultraviolet light sources

Arc lamps
Black light sources
Electrical welding arc

Oxygas welding torch
Sun rays
Tanning bed

EXCLUDES *excessive heat from these sources (E900.1-E900.9)*

E926.3 X-rays and other electromagnetic ionizing radiation

Gamma rays
X-rays (hard) (soft)

E926.4 Lasers

E926.5 Radioactive isotopes

Radiobiologicals
Radiopharmaceuticals

E926.8 Other specified radiation

Artificially accelerated beams of ionized particles generated by:
betatrons
synchrotrons

E926.9 Unspecified radiation

Radiation NOS

E927 Overexertion and strenuous movements

Excessive physical exercise
Overexertion (from):
lifting
pulling
pushing

Strenuous movements in:
recreational activities
other activities

✓4ᵗʰ **E928 Other and unspecified environmental and accidental causes**

E928.0 Prolonged stay in weightless environment

Weightlessness in spacecraft (simulator)

E928.1 Exposure to noise

Noise (pollution)
Sound waves

Supersonic waves

E928.2 Vibration

E928.3 Human bite

E928.8 Other

E928.9 Unspecified accident

Accident NOS
Blow NOS
Casualty (not due to war)
Decapitation

stated as accidentally inflicted

Knocked down
Killed
Injury [any part of body, or unspecified]
Mangled
Wound

stated as accidentally inflicted, but not otherwise specified

EXCLUDES *fracture, cause unspecified (E887)*
injuries undetermined whether accidentally or purposely inflicted (E980.0-E989)

LATE EFFECTS OF ACCIDENTAL INJURY (E929)

Note: This category is to beused to indicate accidental injury as the cause of death or disability from late effects, which are themselves classifiable elsewhere. The "late effects" include conditions reported as such, or as sequelae which may occur at any time after the attempted suicide or self-inflicted injury.

✓4ᵗʰ **E929 Late effects of accidental injury**

EXCLUDES *late effects of:*
surgical and medical procedures (E870.0-E879.9)
therapeutic use of drugs and medicines (E930.0-E949.9)

E929.0 Late effects of motor vehicle accident

Late effects of accidents classifiable to E810-E825

E929.1 Late effects of other transport accident

Late effects of accidents classifiable to E800-E807, E826-E838, E840-E848

E929.2 Late effects of accidental poisoning

Late effects of accidents classifiable to E850-E858, E860-E869

E929.3 Late effects of accidental fall

Late effects of accidents classifiable to E880-E888

E929.4 Late effects of accident caused by fire

Late effects of accidents classifiable to E890-E899

E929.5 Late effects of accident due to natural and environmental factors

Late effects of accidents classifiable to E900-E909

E929.8 Late effects of other accidents

Late effects of accidents classifiable to E910-E928.8

E929.9 Late effects of unspecified accident

Late effects of accidents classifiable to E928.9

DRUGS, MEDICINAL AND BIOLOGICAL SUBSTANCES CAUSING ADVERSE EFFECTS IN THERAPEUTIC USE (E930-E949)

INCLUDES correct drug properly administered in therapeutic or prophylactic dosage, as the cause of any adverse effect including allergic or hypersensitivity reactions

EXCLUDES *accidental overdose of drug and wrong drug given or taken in error (E850.0-E858.9)*
accidents in the technique of administration of drug or biological substance, such as accidental puncture during injection, or contamination of drug (E870.0-E876.9)
administration with suicidal or homicidal intent or intent to harm, or in circumstances classifiable to E980-E989 (E950.0-E950.5, E962.0, E980.0-E980.5)

See Alphabetic Index for more complete list of specific drugs to be classified under the fourth-digit subdivisions. The American Hospital Formulary numbers can be used to classify new drugs listed by the American Hospital Formulary Service (AHFS). See Appendix C.

✓4ᵗʰ **E930 Antibiotics**

EXCLUDES *that used as eye, ear, nose, and throat [ENT], and local anti-infectives (E946.0-E946.9)*

E930.0 Penicillins

Natural
Synthetic
Semisynthetic, such as:
ampicillin
cloxacillin

Semisynthetic, such as:
nafcillin
oxacillin

E930.1 Antifungal antibiotics

Amphotericin B
Griseofulvin

Hachimycin [trichomycin]
Nystatin

E930.2 Chloramphenicol group

Chloramphenicol

Thiamphenicol

E930.3 Erythromycin and other macrolides

Oleandomycin

Spiramycin

✓4ᵗʰ Fourth-digit Required   ▶◀ Revised Text   ● New Code   ▲ Revised Code Title

E930.4 **Tetracycline group**

Doxycycline   Oxytetracycline
Minocycline

E930.5 **Cephalosporin group**

Cephalexin   Cephaloridine
Cephaloglycin   Cephalothin

E930.6 **Antimycobacterial antibiotics**

Cycloserine   Rifampin
Kanamycin   Streptomycin

E930.7 **Antineoplastic antibiotics**

Actinomycins, such as: Actinomycins, such as:
   Bleomycin   Daunorubicin
   Cactinomycin   Mitomycin
   Dactinomycin

EXCLUDES   *other antineoplastic drugs (E933.1)*

E930.8 **Other specified antibiotics**

E930.9 **Unspecified antibiotic**

✓4ᵗʰ **E931 Other anti-infectives**

EXCLUDES   *ENT, and local anti-infectives (E946.0-E946.9)*

E931.0 **Sulfonamides**

Sulfadiazine   Sulfamethoxazole
Sulfafurazole

E931.1 **Arsenical anti-infectives**

E931.2 **Heavy metal anti-infectives**

Compounds of: Compounds of:
   antimony   lead
   bismuth   mercury

EXCLUDES   *mercurial diuretics (E944.0)*

E931.3 **Quinoline and hydroxyquinoline derivatives**

Chiniofon   Diiodohydroxyquin

EXCLUDES   *antimalarial drugs (E931.4)*

E931.4 **Antimalarials and drugs acting on other blood protozoa**

Chloroquine phosphate   Proguanil [chloroguanide]
Cycloguanil   Pyrimethamine
Primaquine   Quinine (sulphate)

E931.5 **Other antiprotozoal drugs**

Emetine

E931.6 **Anthelmintics**

Hexylresorcinol   Piperazine
Male fern oleoresin   Thiabendazole

E931.7 **Antiviral drugs**

Methisazone

EXCLUDES   *amantadine (E936.4)*
cytarabine (E933.1)
idoxuridine (E946.5)

E931.8 **Other antimycobacterial drugs**

Ethambutol   Para-aminosalicylic
Ethionamide   acid derivatives
Isoniazid   Sulfones

E931.9 **Other and unspecified anti-infectives**

Flucytosine   Nitrofuranderivatives

✓4ᵗʰ **E932 Hormones and synthetic substitutes**

E932.0 **Adrenal cortical steroids**

Cortisone derivatives
Desoxycorticosterone derivatives
Fluorinated corticosteroid

E932.1 **Androgens and anabolic congeners**

Nandrolone phenpropionate
Oxymetholone
Testosterone and preparations

E932.2 **Ovarian hormones and synthetic substitutes**

Contraceptives, oral
Estrogens
Estrogens and progestogens combined
Progestogens

E932.3 **Insulins and antidiabetic agents**

Acetohexamide   Phenformin
Biguanide derivatives, oral   Sulfonylurea
Chlorpropamide   derivatives,
Glucagon   oral
Insulin   Tolbutamide

EXCLUDES   *adverse effect of insulin administered for shock therapy (E879.3)*

E932.4 **Anterior pituitary hormones**

Corticotropin
Gonadotropin
Somatotropin [growth hormone]

E932.5 **Posterior pituitary hormones**

Vasopressin

EXCLUDES   *oxytocic agents (E945.0)*

E932.6 **Parathyroid and parathyroid derivatives**

E932.7 **Thyroid and thyroid derivatives**

Dextrothyroxine   Liothyronine
Levothyroxine sodium   Thyroglobulin

E932.8 **Antithyroid agents**

Iodides   Thiourea
Thiouracil

E932.9 **Other and unspecified hormones and synthetic substitutes**

✓4ᵗʰ **E933 Primarily systemic agents**

E933.0 **Antiallergic and antiemetic drugs**

Antihistamines   Diphenylpyraline
Chlorpheniramine   Thonzylamine
Diphenhydramine   Tripelennamine

EXCLUDES   *phenothiazine-based tranquilizers (E939.1)*

E933.1 **Antineoplastic and immunosuppressive drugs**

Azathioprine
Busulfan
Chlorambucil
Cyclophosphamide
Cytarabine
Fluorouracil
Mechlorethamine hydrochloride
Mercaptopurine
Triethylenethiophosphoramide [thio-TEPA]

EXCLUDES   *antineoplastic antibiotics (E930.7)*

E933.2 **Acidifying agents**

E933.3 **Alkalizing agents**

E933.4 **Enzymes, not elsewhere classified**

Penicillinase

E933.5 **Vitamins, not elsewhere classified**

Vitamin A   Vitamin D

EXCLUDES   *nicotinic acid (E942.2)*
vitamin K (E934.3)

E933.8 **Other systemic agents, not elsewhere classified**

Heavy metal antagonists

E933.9 **Unspecified systemic agent**

✓4ᵗʰ **E934 Agents primarily affecting blood constituents**

E934.0 **Iron and its compounds**

Ferric salts
Ferrous sulphate and other ferrous salts

E934.1 **Liver preparations and other antianemic agents**

Folic acid

E934.2 **Anticoagulants**

Coumarin
Heparin
Phenindione
Prothrombin synthesis inhibitor
Warfarin sodium

E934.3 **Vitamin K [phytonadione]**

E934.4 **Fibrinolysis-affecting drugs**

Aminocaproic acid   Streptokinase
Streptodornase   Urokinase

E Codes E930.4–E934.4

E934.5 **Anticoagulant antagonists and other coagulants**
    Hexadimethrine bromide
    Protamine sulfate

E934.6 **Gamma globulin**

E934.7 **Natural blood and blood products**
    Blood plasma   Packed red cells
    Human fibrinogen   Whole blood

E934.8 **Other agents affecting blood constituents**
    Macromolecular blood substitutes

E934.9 **Unspecified agent affecting blood constituents**

√4ᵗʰ **E935 Analgesics, antipyretics, and antirheumatics**

E935.0 **Heroin**
    Diacetylmorphine

E935.1 **Methadone**

E935.2 **Other opiates and related narcotics**
    Codeine [methylmorphine]   Morphine
    Meperidine [pethidine]   Opium (alkaloids)

E935.3 **Salicylates**
    Acetylsalicylic acid [aspirin]
    Amino derivatives of salicylic acid
    Salicylic acid salts

E935.4 **Aromatic analgesics, not elsewhere classified**
    Acetanilid
    Paracetamol [acetaminophen]
    Phenacetin [acetophenetidin]

E935.5 **Pyrazole derivatives**
    Aminophenazone [aminopyrine]
    Phenylbutazone

E935.6 **Antirheumatics [antiphlogistics]**
    Gold salts   Indomethacin
    EXCLUDES *salicylates (E935.3)*
                steroids (E932.0)

E935.7 **Other non-narcotic analgesics**
    Pyrabital

E935.8 **Other specified analgesics and antipyretics**
    Pentazocine

E935.9 **Unspecified analgesic and antipyretic**

√4ᵗʰ **E936 Anticonvulsants and anti-Parkinsonism drugs**

E936.0 **Oxazolidine derivatives**
    Paramethadione
    Trimethadione

E936.1 **Hydantoin derivatives**
    Phenytoin

E936.2 **Succinimides**
    Ethosuximide
    Phensuximide

E936.3 **Other and unspecified anticonvulsants**
    Beclamide
    Primidone

E936.4 **Anti-Parkinsonism drugs**
    Amantadine
    Ethopropazine [profenamine]
    Levodopa [L-dopa]

√4ᵗʰ **E937 Sedatives and hypnotics**

E937.0 **Barbiturates**
    Amobarbital [amylobarbitone]
    Barbital [barbitone]
    Butabarbital [butabarbitone]
    Pentobarbital [pentobarbitone]
    Phenobarbital [phenobarbitone]
    Secobarbital [quinalbarbitone]
    EXCLUDES *thiobarbiturates (E938.3)*

E937.1 **Chloral hydrate group**

E937.2 **Paraldehyde**

E937.3 **Bromine compounds**
    Bromide
    Carbromal (derivatives)

E937.4 **Methaqualone compounds**

E937.5 **Glutethimide group**

E937.6 **Mixed sedatives, not elsewhere classified**

E937.8 **Other sedatives and hypnotics**

E937.9 **Unspecified**
    Sleeping:
      drug
      pill } NOS
      tablet

√4ᵗʰ **E938 Other central nervous system depressants and anesthetics**

E938.0 **Central nervous system muscle-tone depressants**
    Chlorphenesin (carbamate)
    Mephenesin
    Methocarbamol

E938.1 **Halothane**

E938.2 **Other gaseous anesthetics**
    Ether
    Halogenated hydrocarbon derivatives, except
      halothane
    Nitrous oxide

E938.3 **Intravenous anesthetics**
    Ketamine
    Methohexital [methohexitone]
    Thiobarbiturates, such as thiopental sodium

E938.4 **Other and unspecified general anesthetics**

E938.5 **Surface and infiltration anesthetics**
    Cocaine   Procaine
    Lidocaine [lignocaine] Tetracaine

E938.6 **Peripheral nerve- and plexus-blocking anesthetics**

E938.7 **Spinal anesthetics**

E938.9 **Other and unspecified local anesthetics**

√4ᵗʰ **E939 Psychotropic agents**

E939.0 **Antidepressants**
    Amitriptyline
    Imipramine
    Monoamine oxidase [MAO] inhibitors

E939.1 **Phenothiazine-based tranquilizers**
    Chlorpromazine   Prochlorperazine
    Fluphenazine   Promazine
    Phenothiazine

E939.2 **Butyrophenone-based tranquilizers**
    Haloperidol   Trifluperidol
    Spiperone

E939.3 **Other antipsychotics, neuroleptics, and major tranquilizers**

E939.4 **Benzodiazepine-based tranquilizers**
    Chlordiazepoxide   Lorazepam
    Diazepam   Medazepam
    Flurazepam   Nitrazepam

E939.5 **Other tranquilizers**
    Hydroxyzine   Meprobamate

E939.6 **Psychodysleptics [hallucinogens]**
    Cannabis (derivatives)   Mescaline
    Lysergide [LSD]   Psilocin
    Marihuana (derivatives) Psilocybin

E939.7 **Psychostimulants**
    Amphetamine   Caffeine
    EXCLUDES *central appetite depressants (E947.0)*

E939.8 **Other psychotropic agents**

E939.9 **Unspecified psychotropic agent**

√4ᵗʰ **E940 Central nervous system stimulants**

E940.0 **Analeptics**
    Lobeline   Nikethamide

E940.1 **Opiate antagonists**
    Levallorphan   Naloxone
    Nalorphine

E940.8 **Other specified central nervous system stimulants**

E940.9 **Unspecified central nervous system stimulant**

√4ᵗʰ **E941 Drugs primarily affecting the autonomic nervous system**

E941.0 **Parasympathomimetics [cholinergics]**
    Acetylcholine
    Anticholinesterase:
      organophosphorus
      reversible
    Pilocarpine

√4ᵗʰ Fourth-digit Required   ►◄ Revised Text   ● New Code   ▲ Revised Code Title

E Codes E934.5–E941.0

E941.1 Parasympatholytics [anticholinergics and antimuscarinics] and spasmolytics

Atropine
Homatropine
Hyoscine [scopolamine]
Quaternary ammonium derivatives

EXCLUDES *papaverine (E942.5)*

E941.2 Sympathomimetics [adrenergics]

Epinephrine [adrenalin]   Levarterenol [noradrenalin]

E941.3 Sympatholytics [antiadrenergics]

Phenoxybenzamine
Tolazolinehydrochloride

E941.9 Unspecified drug primarily affecting the autonomic nervous system

✓4ᵗʰ **E942 Agents primarily affecting the cardiovascular system**

E942.0 Cardiac rhythm regulators

Practolol
Procainamide
Propranolol
Quinidine

E942.1 Cardiotonic glycosides and drugs of similar action

Digitalis glycosides   Strophanthins
Digoxin

E942.2 Antilipemic and antiarteriosclerotic drugs

Cholestyramine   Nicotinic acid derivatives
Clofibrate   Sitosterols

EXCLUDES *dextrothyroxine (E932.7)*

E942.3 Ganglion-blocking agents

Pentamethonium bromide

E942.4 Coronary vasodilators

Dipyridamole   Nitrites
Nitrates [nitroglycerin]   Prenylamine

E942.5 Other vasodilators

Cyclandelate   Hydralazine
Diazoxide   Papaverine

E942.6 Other antihypertensive agents

Clonidine   Rauwolfia alkaloids
Guanethidine   Reserpine

E942.7 Antivaricose drugs, including sclerosing agents

Monoethanolamine   Zinc salts

E942.8 Capillary-active drugs

Adrenochrome derivatives
Bioflavonoids
Metaraminol

E942.9 Other and unspecified agents primarily affecting the cardiovascular system

✓4ᵗʰ **E943 Agents primarily affecting gastrointestinal system**

E943.0 Antacids and antigastric secretion drugs

Aluminum hydroxide
Magnesium trisilicate

E943.1 Irritant cathartics

Bisacodyl   Phenolphthalein
Castor oil

E943.2 Emollient cathartics

Sodium dioctyl sulfosuccinate

E943.3 Other cathartics, including intestinal atonia drugs

Magnesium sulfate

E943.4 Digestants

Pancreatin   Pepsin
Papain

E943.5 Antidiarrheal drugs

Bismuth subcarbonatePectin
Kaolin

EXCLUDES *anti-infectives (E930.0-E931.9)*

E943.6 Emetics

E943.8 Other specified agents primarily affecting the gastrointestinal system

E943.9 Unspecified agent primarily affecting the gastrointestinal system

✓4ᵗʰ **E944 Water, mineral, and uric acid metabolism drugs**

E944.0 Mercurial diuretics

Chlormerodrin   Mercurophylline
Mercaptomerin   Mersalyl

E944.1 Purine derivative diuretics

Theobromine   Theophylline

EXCLUDES *aminophylline [theophylline ethylenediamine] (E945.7)*

E944.2 Carbonic acid anhydrase inhibitors

Acetazolamide

E944.3 Saluretics

Benzothiadiazides   Chlorothiazide group

E944.4 Other diuretics

Ethacrynic acid   Furosemide

E944.5 Electrolytic, caloric, and water-balance agents

E944.6 Other mineral salts, not elsewhere classified

E944.7 Uric acid metabolism drugs

Cinchophen and congeners   Phenoquin
Colchicine   Probenecid

✓4ᵗʰ **E945 Agents primarily acting on the smooth and skeletal muscles and respiratory system**

E945.0 Oxytocic agents

Ergot alkaloids
Prostaglandins

E945.1 Smooth muscle relaxants

Adiphenine
Metaproterenol [orciprenaline]

EXCLUDES *papaverine (E942.5)*

E945.2 Skeletal muscle relaxants

Alcuronium chloride
Suxamethonium chloride

E945.3 Other and unspecified drugs acting on muscles

E945.4 Antitussives

Dextromethorphan
Pipazethate hydrochloride

E945.5 Expectorants

Acetylcysteine   Ipecacuanha
Cocillana   Terpin hydrate
Guaifenesin [glyceryl guaiacolate]

E945.6 Anti-common cold drugs

E945.7 Antiasthmatics

Aminophylline [theophylline ethylenediamine]

E945.8 Other and unspecified respiratory drugs

✓4ᵗʰ **E946 Agents primarily affecting skin and mucous membrane, ophthalmological, otorhinolaryngological, and dental drugs**

E946.0 Local anti-infectives and anti-inflammatory drugs

E946.1 Antipruritics

E946.2 Local astringents and local detergents

E946.3 Emollients, demulcents, and protectants

E946.4 Keratolytics, kerstoplastics, other hair treatment drugs and preparations

E946.5 Eye anti-infectives and other eye drugs

Idoxuridine

E946.6 Anti-infectives and other drugs and preparations for ear, nose, and throat

E946.7 Dental drugs topically applied

E946.8 Other agents primarily affecting skin and mucous membrane

Spermicides

E946.9 Unspecified agent primarily affecting skin and mucous membrane

✓4ᵗʰ **E947 Other and unspecified drugs and medicinal substances**

E947.0 Dietetics

E947.1 Lipotropic drugs

E947.2 Antidotes and chelating agents, not elsewhere classified

E947.3 Alcohol deterrents

E947.4 Pharmaceutical excipients

E947.8 Other drugs and medicinal substances

Contrast media used for diagnostic x-ray procedures
Diagnostic agents and kits

E947.9 Unspecified drug or medicinal substance

✓4ᵗʰ **E948 Bacterial vaccines**

     E948.0 BCG vaccine

     E948.1 Typhoid and paratyphoid

     E948.2 Cholera

     E948.3 Plague

     E948.4 Tetanus

     E948.5 Diphtheria

     E948.6 Pertussis vaccine, including combinations with a pertussis component

     E948.8 Other and unspecified bacterial vaccines

     E948.9 Mixed bacterial vaccines, except combinations with a pertussis component

✓4ᵗʰ **E949 Other vaccines and biological substances**

     EXCLUDES *gamma globulin (E934.6)*

     E949.0 Smallpox vaccine

     E949.1 Rabies vaccine

     E949.2 Typhus vaccine

     E949.3 Yellow fever vaccine

     E949.4 Measles vaccine

     E949.5 Poliomyelitis vaccine

     E949.6 Other and unspecified viral and rickettsial vaccines
         Mumps vaccine

     E949.7 Mixed viral-rickettsial and bacterial vaccines, except combinations with a pertussis component

         EXCLUDES *combinations with a pertussis component (E948.6)*

     E949.9 Other and unspecified vaccines and biological substances

SUICIDE AND SELF-INFLICTED INJURY (E950-E959)

     INCLUDES injuries in suicide and attempted suicide
         self-inflicted injuries specified as intentional

✓4ᵗʰ **E950 Suicide and self-inflicted poisoning by solid or liquid substances**

     E950.0 Analgesics, antipyretics, and antirheumatics

     E950.1 Barbiturates

     E950.2 Other sedatives and hypnotics

     E950.3 Tranquilizers and other psychotropic agents

     E950.4 Other specified drugs and medicinal substances

     E950.5 Unspecified drug or medicinal substance

     E950.6 Agricultural and horticultural chemical and pharmaceutical preparations other than plant foods and fertilizers

     E950.7 Corrosive and caustic substances
         Suicide and self-inflicted poisoning by substances classifiable to E864

     E950.8 Arsenic and its compounds

     E950.9 Other and unspecified solid and liquid substances

✓4ᵗʰ **E951 Suicide and self-inflicted poisoning by gases in domestic use**

     E951.0 Gas distributed by pipeline

     E951.1 Liquefied petroleum gas distributed in mobile containers

     E951.8 Other utility gas

✓4ᵗʰ **E952 Suicide and self-inflicted poisoning by other gases and vapors**

     E952.0 Motor vehicle exhaust gas

     E952.1 Other carbon monoxide

     E952.8 Other specified gases and vapors

     E952.9 Unspecified gases and vapors

✓4ᵗʰ **E953 Suicide and self-inflicted injury by hanging, strangulation, and suffocation**

     E953.0 Hanging

     E953.1 Suffocation by plastic bag

     E953.8 Other specified means

     E953.9 Unspecified means

E954 Suicide and self-inflicted injury by submersion [drowning]

✓4ᵗʰ **E955 Suicide and self-inflicted injury by firearms, air guns and explosives**

     E955.0 Handgun

     E955.1 Shotgun

     E955.2 Hunting rifle

     E955.3 Military firearms

     E955.4 Other and unspecified firearm
         Gunshot NOS   Shot NOS

     E955.5 Explosives

     E955.6 Air gun
         BB gun
         Pellet gun

●   E955.7 Paintball gun

     E955.9 Unspecified

E956 Suicide and self-inflicted injury by cutting and piercing instrument

✓4ᵗʰ **E957 Suicide and self-inflicted injuries by jumping from high place**

     E957.0 Residential premises

     E957.1 Other man-made structures

     E957.2 Natural sites

     E957.9 Unspecified

✓4ᵗʰ **E958 Suicide and self-inflicted injury by other and unspecified means**

     E958.0 Jumping or lying before moving object

     E958.1 Burns, fire

     E958.2 Scald

     E958.3 Extremes of cold

     E958.4 Electrocution

     E958.5 Crashing of motor vehicle

     E958.6 Crashing of aircraft

     E958.7 Caustic substances, except poisoning
         EXCLUDES *poisoning by caustic substance (E950.7)*

     E958.8 Other specified means

     E958.9 Unspecified means

E959 Late effects of self-inflicted injury

     Note: This category is to be used to indicate circumstances classifiable to E950-E958 as the cause of death or disability from late effects, which are themselves classifiable elsewhere. The "late effects" include conditions reported as such, or as sequelae which may occur at any time after the attempted suicide or self-inflicted injury.

HOMICIDE AND INJURY PURPOSELY INFLICTED BY OTHER PERSONS (E960-E969)

     INCLUDES injuries inflicted by another person with intent to injure or kill, by any means

     EXCLUDES *injuries due to:*
         legal intervention (E970-E978)
         operations of war (E990-E999)
         ▶*terrorism (E979)*◀

✓4ᵗʰ **E960 Fight, brawl, rape**

     E960.0 Unarmed fight or brawl
         Beatings NOS
         Brawl or fight with hands, fists, feet
         Injured or killed in fight NOS
         EXCLUDES *homicidal:*
              injury by weapons (E965.0-E966, E969)
              strangulation (E963)
              submersion (E964)

     E960.1 Rape

E961 Assault by corrosive or caustic substance, except poisoning

Injury or death purposely caused by corrosive or caustic substance, such as:
acid [any]
corrosive substance
vitriol

> **EXCLUDES** *burns from hot liquid (E968.3)*
> *chemical burns from swallowing a corrosive substance (E962.0-E962.9)*

✓4ᵗʰ E962 Assault by poisoning

E962.0 Drugs and medicinal substances
Homicidal poisoning by any drug or medicinal substance

E962.1 Other solid and liquid substances

E962.2 Other gases and vapors

E962.9 Unspecified poisoning

E963 Assault by hanging and strangulation
Homicidal (attempt):
garrotting or ligature
hanging
Homicidal (attempt):
strangulation
suffocation

E964 Assault by submersion [drowning]

✓4ᵗʰ E965 Assault by firearms and explosives

E965.0 Handgun
Pistol   Revolver

E965.1 Shotgun

E965.2 Hunting rifle

E965.3 Military firearms

E965.4 Other and unspecified firearm

E965.5 Antipersonnel bomb

E965.6 Gasoline bomb

E965.7 Letter bomb

E965.8 Other specified explosive
Bomb NOS (placed in):   Dynamite
car
house

E965.9 Unspecified explosive

E966 Assault by cutting and piercing instrument
Assassination (attempt), homicide (attempt) by any instrument classifiable under E920
Homicidal:
cut
puncture
stab
Stabbed
} any part of body

✓4ᵗʰ E967 Perpetrator of child and adult abuse
Note: Selection of the correct perpetrator code is based on the relationship between the perpetrator and the victim

E967.0 By father, stepfather, or boyfriend
Male partner of child's parent or guardian

E967.1 By other specified person

E967.2 By mother, stepmother, or girlfriend
Female partner of child's parent or guardian

E967.3 By spouse or partner
Abuse of spouse or partner by ex-spouse or ex-partner

E967.4 By child

E967.5 By sibling

E967.6 By grandparent

E967.7 By other relative

E967.8 By non-related caregiver

E967.9 By unspecified person

✓4ᵗʰ E968 Assault by other and unspecified means

E968.0 Fire
Arson
Homicidal burns NOS
> **EXCLUDES** *burns from hot liquid (E968.3)*

E968.1 Pushing from a high place

E968.2 Striking by blunt or thrown object

E968.3 Hot liquid
Homicidal burns by scalding

E968.4 Criminal neglect
Abandonment of child, infant, or other helpless person with intent to injure or kill

E968.5 Transport vehicle
Being struck by other vehicle or run down with intent to injure
Pushed in front of, thrown from, or dragged by moving vehicle with intent to injure

E968.6 Air gun
BB gun
Pellet gun

E968.7 Human bite

E968.8 Other specified means

E968.9 Unspecified means
Assassination (attempt) NOS
Homicidal (attempt):
injury NOS
wound NOS
Manslaughter (nonaccidental)
Murder (attempt) NOS
Violence, non-accidental

E969 Late effects of injury purposely inflicted by other person
Note: This category is to be used to indicate circumstances classifiable to E960-E968 as the cause of death or disability from late effects, which are themselves classifiable elsewhere. The "late effects" include conditions reported as such, or as sequelae which may occur at any time after injury purposely inflicted by another person.

LEGAL INTERVENTION (E970-E978)

> **INCLUDES** injuries inflicted by the police or other law-enforcing agents, including military on duty, in the course of arresting or attempting to arrest lawbreakers, suppressing disturbances, maintaining order, and other legal action
> legal execution
> **EXCLUDES** *injuries caused by civil insurrections (E990.0-E999)*

E970 Injury due to legal intervention by firearms
Gunshot wound
Injury by:
machine gun
revolver
Injury by:
rifle pellet or rubber bullet
shot NOS

E971 Injury due to legal intervention by explosives
Injury by:
dynamite
explosive shell
Injury by:
grenade
mortar bomb

E972 Injury due to legal intervention by gas
Asphyxiation by gas
Injury by tear gas
Poisoning by gas

E973 Injury due to legal intervention by blunt object
Hit, struck by:
baton (nightstick)
blunt object
Hit, struck by:
stave

E974 Injury due to legal intervention by cutting and piercing instrument
Cut
Incised wound
Injured by bayonet
Stab wound

E975 Injury due to legal intervention by other specified means
Blow
Manhandling

E976 Injury due to legal intervention by unspecified means

E977 Late effects of injuries due to legal intervention
Note: This category is to be used to indicate circumstances classifiable to E970-E976 as the cause of death or disability from late effects, which are themselves classifiable elsewhere. The "late effects" include conditions reported as such, or as sequelae, which may occur at any time after the injury due to legal intervention.

E Codes E978–E993.9

E978 Legal execution
　　All executions performed at the behest of the judiciary or
　　　　ruling authority [whether permanent or temporary] as:
　　asphyxiation by gas
　　beheading, decapitation (by guillotine)
　　capital punishment
　　electrocution
　　hanging
　　poisoning
　　shooting
　　other specified means

TERRORISM (E979)

● ✓4ᵗʰ **E979 Terrorism**
　　Injuries resulting from the unlawful use of force or violence
　　　　against persons or property to intimidate or coerce a
　　　　Government, the civilian population, or any segment
　　　　thereof, in furtherance of political or social objective

● **E979.0 Terrorism involving explosion of marine weapons**
　　Depth-charge
　　Marine mine
　　Mine NOS, at sea or in harbour
　　Sea-based artillery shell
　　Torpedo
　　Underwater blast

● **E979.1 Terrorism involving destruction of aircraft**
　　Aircraft used as a weapon
　　Aircraft:
　　　burned
　　　exploded
　　　shot down
　　Crushed by falling aircraft

● **E979.2 Terrorism involving other explosions and fragments**
　　Antipersonnel bomb (fragments)
　　Blast NOS
　　Explosion (of):
　　　artillery shell
　　　breech-block
　　　cannon block
　　　mortar bomb
　　　munitions being used in terrorism
　　　NOS
　　Fragments from:
　　　artillery shell
　　　bomb
　　　grenade
　　　guided missile
　　　land-mine
　　　rocket
　　　shell
　　　shrapnel
　　Mine NOS

● **E979.3 Terrorism involving fires, conflagraton and hot substances**
　　Burning building or structure:
　　　collapse of
　　　fall from
　　　hit by falling object in
　　　jump from
　　Conflagraton NOS
　　Fire (causing):
　　　Asphyxia
　　　Burns
　　　NOS
　　　Other injury
　　Melting of fittings and furniture in burning
　　Petrol bomb
　　Smouldering building or structure

● **E979.4 Terrorism involving firearms**
　　Bullet:
　　　carbine
　　　machine gun
　　　pistol
　　　rifle
　　　rubber (rifle)
　　Pellets (shotgun)

● **E979.5 Terrorism involving nuclear weapons**
　　Blast effects
　　Exposure to ionizing radiation from nuclear weapon
　　Fireball effects
　　Heat from nuclear weapon
　　Other direct and secondary effects of nuclear
　　　weapons

● **E979.6 Terrorism involving biological weapons**
　　Anthrax
　　Cholera
　　Smallpox

● **E979.7 Terrorism involving chemical weapons**
　　Gases, fumes, chemicals
　　Hydrogen cyanide
　　Phosgene
　　Sarin

● **E979.8 Terrorism involving other means**
　　Drowning and submersion
　　Lasers
　　Piercing or stabbing instruments
　　Terrorism NOS

● **E979.9 Terrorism, secondary effects**
　　Note: This code is for use to identify conditions
　　　　occurring subsequent to a terrorist attack not
　　　　those that are due to the initial terrorist act
　　EXCLUDES *late effect of terrorist attack (E999.1)*

INJURY UNDETERMINED WHETHER ACCIDENTALLY OR PURPOSELY INFLICTED (E980–E989)

　　Note: Categories E980-E989 are for use when it is
　　　　unspecified or it cannot be determined whether the
　　　　injuries are accidental (unintentional), suicide
　　　　(attempted), or assault.

✓4ᵗʰ **E980 Poisoning by solid or liquid substances, undetermined whether accidentally or purposely inflicted**

E980.0 Analgesics, antipyretics, and antirheumatics

E980.1 Barbiturates

E980.2 Other sedatives and hypnotics

E980.3 Tranquilizers and other psychotropic agents

E980.4 Other specified drugs and medicinal substances

E980.5 Unspecified drug or medicinal substance

E980.6 Corrosive and caustic substances
　　Poisoning, undetermined whether accidental or
　　　　purposeful, by substances classifiable to E864

E980.7 Agricultural and horticultural chemical and pharmaceutical preparations other than plant foods and fertilizers

E980.8 Arsenic and its compounds

E980.9 Other and unspecified solid and liquid substances

✓4ᵗʰ **E981 Poisoning by gases in domestic use, undetermined whether accidentally or purposely inflicted**

E981.0 Gas distributed by pipeline

E981.1 Liquefied petroleum gas distributed in mobile containers

E981.8 Other utility gas

✓4ᵗʰ **E982 Poisoning by other gases, undetermined whether accidentally or purposely inflicted**

E982.0 Motor vehicle exhaust gas

E982.1 Other carbon monoxide

E982.8 Other specified gases and vapors

E982.9 Unspecified gases and vapors

✓4ᵗʰ **E983 Hanging, strangulation, or suffocation, undetermined whether accidentally or purposely inflicted**

E983.0 Hanging

E983.1 Suffocation by plastic bag

E983.8 Other specified means

E983.9 Unspecified means

✓4ᵗʰ Fourth-digit Required　　　▶◀ Revised Text　　　● New Code　　　▲ Revised Code Title

E984 Submersion [drowning], undetermined whether accidentally or purposely inflicted

✓4ᵗʰ E985 Injury by firearms, air guns and explosives, undetermined whether accidentally or purposely inflicted

E985.0 Handgun

E985.1 Shotgun

E985.2 Hunting rifle

E985.3 Military firearms

E985.4 Other and unspecified firearm

E985.5 Explosives

E985.6 Air gun

　　BB gun
　　Pellet gun

● E985.7 Paintball gun

E986 Injury by cutting and piercing instruments, undetermined whether accidentallyor purposely inflicted

✓4ᵗʰ E987 Falling from high place, undetermined whether accidentally or purposely inflicted

E987.0 Residential premises

E987.1 Other man-made structures

E987.2 Natural sites

E987.9 Unspecified site

✓4ᵗʰ E988 Injury by other and unspecified means, undetermined whether accidentally or purposely inflicted

E988.0 Jumping or lying before moving object

E988.1 Burns, fire

E988.2 Scald

E988.3 Extremes of cold

E988.4 Electrocution

E988.5 Crashing of motor vehicle

E988.6 Crashing of aircraft

E988.7 Caustic substances, except poisoning

E988.8 Other specified means

E988.9 Unspecified means

E989 Late effects of injury, undetermined whether accidentally or purposely inflicted

Note: This category is to be used to indicate circumstances classifiable to E980-E988 as the cause of death or disability from late effects, which are themselves classifiable elsewhere. The "late effects" include conditions reported as such, or as sequelae, which may occur at any time after injury, undetermined whether accidentally or purposely inflicted.

INJURY RESULTING FROM OPERATIONS OF WAR (E990-E999)

INCLUDES　injuries to military personnel and civilians caused by war and civil insurrections and occurring during the time of war and insurrection

EXCLUDES　*accidents during training of military personnel manufacture of war material and transport, unless attributable to enemy action*

✓4ᵗʰ E990 Injury due to war operations by fires and conflagrations

INCLUDES　asphyxia, burns, or other injury originating from fire caused by a fire-producing device or indirectly by any conventional weapon

E990.0 From gasoline bomb

E990.9 From other and unspecified source

✓4ᵗʰ E991 Injury due to war operations by bullets and fragments

E991.0 Rubber bullets (rifle)

E991.1 Pellets (rifle)

E991.2 Other bullets

　　Bullet [any, except rubber bullets and pellets]
　　　carbine
　　　machine gun
　　　pistol
　　　rifle
　　　shotgun

E991.3 Antipersonnel bomb (fragments)

E991.9 Other and unspecified fragments

Fragments from:	Fragments from:
artillery shell	land mine
bombs, except	rockets
anti-personnel	shell
grenade	Shrapnel
guided missile	

E992 Injury due to war operations by explosion of marine weapons

Depth charge	Sea-based artillery shell
Marine mines	Torpedo
Mine NOS, at sea or in harbor	Underwater blast

E993 Injury due to war operations by other explosion

Accidental explosion of munitions being used in war	Explosion of: artillery shell
	breech block
Accidental explosion of own weapons	cannon block
	mortar bomb
Air blast NOS	Injury by weapon burst
Blast NOS	
Explosion NOS	

E994 Injury due to war operations by destruction of aircraft

Airplane:	Airplane:
burned	shot down
exploded	Crushed by falling airplane

E995 Injury due to war operations by other and unspecified forms of conventional warfare

Battle wounds
Bayonet injury
Drowned in war operations

E996 Injury due to war operations by nuclear weapons

Blast effects
Exposure to ionizing radiation from nuclear weapons
Fireball effects
Heat
Other direct and secondary effects of nuclear weapons

✓4ᵗʰ E997 Injury due to war operations by other forms of unconventional warfare

E997.0 Lasers

E997.1 Biological warfare

E997.2 Gases, fumes, and chemicals

E997.8 Other specified forms of unconventional warfare

E997.9 Unspecified form of unconventional warfare

E998 Injury due to war operations but occurring after cessation of hostilities

Injuries due to operations of war but occurring after cessation of hostilities by any means classifiable under E990-E997

Injuries by explosion of bombs or mines placed in the course of operations of war, if the explosion occurred after cessation of hostilities

▲ ✓4ᵗʰ E999 Late effect of injury due to war operations and terrorism

Note: This category is to be used to indicate circumstances classifiable to ▶E979,◀ E990-E998 as the cause of death or disability from late effects, which are themselves classifiable elsewhere. The "late effects" include conditions reported as such, or as sequelae, which may occur at any time after the injury, resulting from operations of war ▶or terrorism◀.

● E999.0 Late effect of injury due to war operations

● E999.1 Late effect of injury due to terrorism

Official ICD•9•CM Government Appendixes

MORPHOLOGY OF NEOPLASMS

The World Health Organization has published an adaptation of the International Classification of Diseases for oncology (ICD-O). It contains a coded nomenclature for the morphology of neoplasms, which is reproduced here for those who wish to use it in conjunction with Chapter 2 of the International Classification of Diseases, 9th Revision, Clinical Modification.

The morphology code numbers consist of five digits; the first four identify the histological type of the neoplasm and the fifth indicates its behavior. The one-digit behavior code is as follows:

/0 Benign
/1 Uncertain whether benign or malignant
    Borderline malignancy
/2 Carcinoma in situ
    Intraepithelial
    Noninfiltrating
    Noninvasive
/3 Malignant, primary site
/6 Malignant, metastatic site
    Secondary site
/9 Malignant, uncertain whether primary or metastatic site

In the nomenclature below, the morphology code numbers include the behavior code appropriate to the histological type of neoplasm, but this behavior code should be changed if other reported information makes this necessary. For example, "chordoma (M9370/3)" is assumed to be malignant; the term "benign chordoma" should be coded M9370/0. Similarly, "superficial spreading adenocarcinoma (M8143/3)" described as "noninvasive" should be coded M8143/2 and "melanoma (M8720/3)" described as "secondary" should be coded M8720/6.

The following table shows the correspondence between the morphology code and the different sections of Chapter 2:

Morphology Code Histology/Behavior			ICD-9-CM Chapter 2
Any M8000-M8004	0	210-229	Benign neoplasms
	1	239	Neoplasms of unspecified nature
M8010+	1	235-238	Neoplasms of uncertain behavior
Any	2	230-234	Carcinoma in situ
Any	3	140-195	Malignant neoplasms, stated or presumed
		200-208	to be primary
Any	6	196-198	Malignant neoplasms, stated or presumed to be secondary

The ICD-O behavior digit /9 is inapplicable in an ICD context, since all malignant neoplasms are presumed to be primary (/3) or secondary (/6) according to other information on the medical record.

Only the first-listed term of the full ICD-O morphology nomenclature appears against each code number in the list below. The ICD-9-CM Alphabetical Index (Volume 2), however, includes all the ICD-O synonyms as well as a number of other morphological names still likely to be encountered on medical records but omitted from ICD-O as outdated or otherwise undesirable.

A coding difficulty sometimes arises where a morphological diagnosis contains two qualifying adjectives that have different code numbers. An example is "transitional cell epidermoid carcinoma." "Transitional cell carcinoma NOS" is M8120/3 and "epidermoid carcinoma NOS" is M8070/3. In such circumstances, the higher number (M8120/3 in this example) should be used, as it is usually more specific.

CODED NOMENCLATURE FOR MORPHOLOGY OF NEOPLASMS

M800	**Neoplasms NOS**
M8000/0	Neoplasm, benign
M8000/1	Neoplasm, uncertain whether benign or malignant
M8000/3	Neoplasm, malignant
M8000/6	Neoplasm, metastatic
M8000/9	Neoplasm, malignant, uncertain whether primary or metastatic
M8001/0	Tumor cells, benign
M8001/1	Tumor cells, uncertain whether benign or malignant
M8001/3	Tumor cells, malignant
M8002/3	Malignant tumor, small cell type
M8003/3	Malignant tumor, giant cell type
M8004/3	Malignant tumor, fusiform cell type
M801-M804	**Epithelial neoplasms NOS**
M8010/0	Epithelial tumor, benign
M8010/2	Carcinoma in situ NOS
M8010/3	Carcinoma NOS
M8010/6	Carcinoma, metastatic NOS
M8010/9	Carcinomatosis
M8011/0	Epithelioma, benign
M8011/3	Epithelioma, malignant
M8012/3	Large cell carcinoma NOS
M8020/3	Carcinoma, undifferentiated type NOS
M8021/3	Carcinoma, anaplastic type NOS
M8022/3	Pleomorphic carcinoma
M8030/3	Giant cell and spindle cell carcinoma
M8031/3	Giant cell carcinoma
M8032/3	Spindle cell carcinoma
M8033/3	Pseudosarcomatous carcinoma
M8034/3	Polygonal cell carcinoma
M8035/3	Spheroidal cell carcinoma
M8040/1	Tumorlet
M8041/3	Small cell carcinoma NOS
M8042/3	Oat cell carcinoma
M8043/3	Small cell carcinoma, fusiform cell type
M805-M808	**Papillary and squamous cell neoplasms**
M8050/0	Papilloma NOS (except Papilloma of urinary bladder M8120/1)
M8050/2	Papillary carcinoma in situ
M8050/3	Papillary carcinoma NOS
M8051/0	Verrucous papilloma
M8051/3	Verrucous carcinoma NOS
M8052/0	Squamous cell papilloma
M8052/3	Papillary squamous cell carcinoma
M8053/0	Inverted papilloma
M8060/0	Papillomatosis NOS
M8070/2	Squamous cell carcinoma in situ NOS
M8070/3	Squamous cell carcinoma NOS
M8070/6	Squamous cell carcinoma, metastatic NOS
M8071/3	Squamous cell carcinoma, keratinizing type NOS
M8072/3	Squamous cell carcinoma, large cell, nonkeratinizing type
M8073/3	Squamous cell carcinoma, small cell, nonkeratinizing type
M8074/3	Squamous cell carcinoma, spindle cell type
M8075/3	Adenoid squamous cell carcinoma
M8076/2	Squamous cell carcinoma in situ with questionable stromal invasion
M8076/3	Squamous cell carcinoma, microinvasive
M8080/2	Queyrat's erythroplasia
M8081/2	Bowen's disease
M8082/3	Lymphoepithelial carcinoma
M809-M811	**Basal cell neoplasms**
M8090/1	Basal cell tumor
M8090/3	Basal cell carcinoma NOS
M8091/3	Multicentric basal cell carcinoma
M8092/3	Basal cell carcinoma, morphea type
M8093/3	Basal cell carcinoma, fibroepithelial type
M8094/3	Basosquamous carcinoma
M8095/3	Metatypical carcinoma
M8096/0	Intraepidermal epithelioma of Jadassohn
M8100/0	Trichoepithelioma
M8101/0	Trichofolliculoma
M8102/0	Tricholemmoma
M8110/0	Pilomatrixoma
M812-M813	**Transitional cell papillomas and carcinomas**
M8120/0	Transitional cell papilloma NOS
M8120/1	Urothelial papilloma
M8120/2	Transitional cell carcinoma in situ
M8120/3	Transitional cell carcinoma NOS
M8121/0	Schneiderian papilloma
M8121/1	Transitional cell papilloma, inverted type
M8121/3	Schneiderian carcinoma
M8122/3	Transitional cell carcinoma, spindle cell type

M8123/3	Basaloid carcinoma
M8124/3	Cloacogenic carcinoma
M8130/3	Papillary transitional cell carcinoma

M814-M838 Adenomas and adenocarcinomas

M8140/0	Adenoma NOS
M8140/1	Bronchial adenoma NOS
M8140/2	Adenocarcinoma in situ
M8140/3	Adenocarcinoma NOS
M8140/6	Adenocarcinoma, metastatic NOS
M8141/3	Scirrhous adenocarcinoma
M8142/3	Linitis plastica
M8143/3	Superficial spreading adenocarcinoma
M8144/3	Adenocarcinoma, intestinal type
M8145/3	Carcinoma, diffuse type
M8146/0	Monomorphic adenoma
M8147/0	Basal cell adenoma
M8150/0	Islet cell adenoma
M8150/3	Islet cell carcinoma
M8151/0	Insulinoma NOS
M8151/3	Insulinoma, malignant
M8152/0	Glucagonoma NOS
M8152/3	Glucagonoma, malignant
M8153/1	Gastrinoma NOS
M8153/3	Gastrinoma, malignant
M8154/3	Mixed islet cell and exocrine adenocarcinoma
M8160/0	Bile duct adenoma
M8160/3	Cholangiocarcinoma
M8161/0	Bile duct cystadenoma
M8161/3	Bile duct cystadenocarcinoma
M8170/0	Liver cell adenoma
M8170/3	Hepatocellular carcinoma NOS
M8180/0	Hepatocholangioma, benign
M8180/3	Combined hepatocellular carcinoma and cholangiocarcinoma
M8190/0	Trabecular adenoma
M8190/3	Trabecular adenocarcinoma
M8191/0	Embryonal adenoma
M8200/0	Eccrine dermal cylindroma
M8200/3	Adenoid cystic carcinoma
M8201/3	Cribriform carcinoma
M8210/0	Adenomatous polyp NOS
M8210/3	Adenocarcinoma in adenomatous polyp
M8211/0	Tubular adenoma NOS
M8211/3	Tubular adenocarcinoma
M8220/0	Adenomatous polyposis coli
M8220/3	Adenocarcinoma in adenomatous polyposis coli
M8221/0	Multiple adenomatous polyps
M8230/3	Solid carcinoma NOS
M8231/3	Carcinoma simplex
M8240/1	Carcinoid tumor NOS
M8240/3	Carcinoid tumor, malignant
M8241/1	Carcinoid tumor, argentaffin NOS
M8241/3	Carcinoid tumor, argentaffin, malignant
M8242/1	Carcinoid tumor, nonargentaffin NOS
M8242/3	Carcinoid tumor, nonargentaffin, malignant
M8243/3	Mucocarcinoid tumor, malignant
M8244/3	Composite carcinoid
M8250/1	Pulmonary adenomatosis
M8250/3	Bronchiolo-alveolar adenocarcinoma
M8251/0	Alveolar adenoma
M8251/3	Alveolar adenocarcinoma
M8260/0	Papillary adenoma NOS
M8260/3	Papillary adenocarcinoma NOS
M8261/1	Villous adenoma NOS

M8261/3	Adenocarcinoma in villous adenoma
M8262/3	Villous adenocarcinoma
M8263/3	Tubulovillous adenoma
M8270/0	Chromophobe adenoma
M8270/3	Chromophobe carcinoma
M8280/0	Acidophil adenoma
M8280/3	Acidophil carcinoma
M8281/0	Mixed acidophil-basophil adenoma
M8281/3	Mixed acidophil-basophil carcinoma
M8290/0	Oxyphilic adenoma
M8290/3	Oxyphilic adenocarcinoma
M8300/0	Basophil adenoma
M8300/3	Basophil carcinoma
M8310/0	Clear cell adenoma
M8310/3	Clear cell adenocarcinoma NOS
M8311/1	Hypernephroid tumor
M8312/3	Renal cell carcinoma
M8313/0	Clear cell adenofibroma
M8320/3	Granular cell carcinoma
M8321/0	Chief cell adenoma
M8322/0	Water-clear cell adenoma
M8322/3	Water-clear cell adenocarcinoma
M8323/0	Mixed cell adenoma
M8323/3	Mixed cell adenocarcinoma
M8324/0	Lipoadenoma
M8330/0	Follicular adenoma
M8330/3	Follicular adenocarcinoma NOS
M8331/3	Follicular adenocarcinoma, well differentiated type
M8332/3	Follicular adenocarcinoma, trabecular type
M8333/0	Microfollicular adenoma
M8334/0	Macrofollicular adenoma
M8340/3	Papillary and follicular adenocarcinoma
M8350/3	Nonencapsulated sclerosing carcinoma
M8360/1	Multiple endocrine adenomas
M8361/1	Juxtaglomerular tumor
M8370/0	Adrenal cortical adenoma NOS
M8370/3	Adrenal cortical carcinoma
M8371/0	Adrenal cortical adenoma, compact cell type
M8372/0	Adrenal cortical adenoma, heavily pigmented variant
M8373/0	Adrenal cortical adenoma, clear cell type
M8374/0	Adrenal cortical adenoma, glomerulosa cell type
M8375/0	Adrenal cortical adenoma, mixed cell type
M8380/0	Endometrioid adenoma NOS
M8380/1	Endometrioid adenoma, borderline malignancy
M8380/3	Endometrioid carcinoma
M8381/0	Endometrioid adenofibroma NOS
M8381/1	Endometrioid adenofibroma, borderline malignancy
M8381/3	Endometrioid adenofibroma, malignant

M839-M842 Adnexal and skin appendage neoplasms

M8390/0	Skin appendage adenoma
M8390/3	Skin appendage carcinoma
M8400/0	Sweat gland adenoma
M8400/1	Sweat gland tumor NOS
M8400/3	Sweat gland adenocarcinoma
M8401/0	Apocrine adenoma
M8401/3	Apocrine adenocarcinoma
M8402/0	Eccrine acrospiroma
M8403/0	Eccrine spiradenoma
M8404/0	Hidrocystoma
M8405/0	Papillary hydradenoma

M8406/0	Papillary syringadenoma
M8407/0	Syringoma NOS
M8410/0	Sebaceous adenoma
M8410/3	Sebaceous adenocarcinoma
M8420/0	Ceruminous adenoma
M8420/3	Ceruminous adenocarcinoma

M843 Mucoepidermoid neoplasms

M8430/1	Mucoepidermoid tumor
M8430/3	Mucoepidermoid carcinoma

M844-M849 Cystic, mucinous, and serous neoplasms

M8440/0	Cystadenoma NOS
M8440/3	Cystadenocarcinoma NOS
M8441/0	Serous cystadenoma NOS
M8441/1	Serous cystadenoma, borderline malignancy
M8441/3	Serous cystadenocarcinoma NOS
M8450/0	Papillary cystadenoma NOS
M8450/1	Papillary cystadenoma, borderline malignancy
M8450/3	Papillary cystadenocarcinoma NOS
M8460/0	Papillary serous cystadenoma NOS
M8460/1	Papillary serous cystadenoma, borderline malignancy
M8460/3	Papillary serous cystadenocarcinoma
M8461/0	Serous surface papilloma NOS
M8461/1	Serous surface papilloma, borderline malignancy
M8461/3	Serous surface papillary carcinoma
M8470/0	Mucinous cystadenoma NOS
M8470/1	Mucinous cystadenoma, borderline malignancy
M8470/3	Mucinous cystadenocarcinoma NOS
M8471/0	Papillary mucinous cystadenoma NOS
M8471/1	Papillary mucinous cystadenoma, borderline malignancy
M8471/3	Papillary mucinous cystadenocarcinoma
M8480/0	Mucinous adenoma
M8480/3	Mucinous adenocarcinoma
M8480/6	Pseudomyxoma peritonei
M8481/3	Mucin-producing adenocarcinoma
M8490/3	Signet ring cell carcinoma
M8490/6	Metastatic signet ring cell carcinoma

M850-M854 Ductal, lobular, and medullary neoplasms

M8500/2	Intraductal carcinoma, noninfiltrating NOS
M8500/3	Infiltrating duct carcinoma
M8501/2	Comedocarcinoma, noninfiltrating
M8501/3	Comedocarcinoma NOS
M8502/3	Juvenile carcinoma of the breast
M8503/0	Intraductal papilloma
M8503/2	Noninfiltrating intraductal papillary adenocarcinoma
M8504/0	Intracystic papillary adenoma
M8504/2	Noninfiltrating intracystic carcinoma
M8505/0	Intraductal papillomatosis NOS
M8506/0	Subareolar duct papillomatosis
M8510/3	Medullary carcinoma NOS
M8511/3	Medullary carcinoma with amyloid stroma
M8512/3	Medullary carcinoma with lymphoid stroma
M8520/2	Lobular carcinoma in situ
M8520/3	Lobular carcinoma NOS

M8521/3	Infiltrating ductular carcinoma
M8530/3	Inflammatory carcinoma
M8540/3	Paget's disease, mammary
M8541/3	Paget's disease and infiltrating duct carcinoma of breast
M8542/3	Paget's disease, extramammary (except Paget's disease of bone)

M855   **Acinar cell neoplasms**

M8550/0	Acinar cell adenoma
M8550/1	Acinar cell tumor
M8550/3	Acinar cell carcinoma

M856-M858   **Complex epithelial neoplasms**

M8560/3	Adenosquamous carcinoma
M8561/0	Adenolymphoma
M8570/3	Adenocarcinoma with squamous metaplasia
M8571/3	Adenocarcinoma with cartilaginous and osseous metaplasia
M8572/3	Adenocarcinoma with spindle cell metaplasia
M8573/3	Adenocarcinoma with apocrine metaplasia
M8580/0	Thymoma, benign
M8580/3	Thymoma, malignant

M859-M867   **Specialized gonadal neoplasms**

M8590/1	Sex cord-stromal tumor
M8600/0	Thecoma NOS
M8600/3	Theca cell carcinoma
M8610/0	Luteoma NOS
M8620/1	Granulosa cell tumor NOS
M8620/3	Granulosa cell tumor, malignant
M8621/1	Granulosa cell-theca cell tumor
M8630/0	Androblastoma, benign
M8630/1	Androblastoma NOS
M8630/3	Androblastoma, malignant
M8631/0	Sertoli-Leydig cell tumor
M8632/1	Gynandroblastoma
M8640/0	Tubular androblastoma NOS
M8640/3	Sertoli cell carcinoma
M8641/0	Tubular androblastoma with lipid storage
M8650/0	Leydig cell tumor, benign
M8650/1	Leydig cell tumor NOS
M8650/3	Leydig cell tumor, malignant
M8660/0	Hilar cell tumor
M8670/0	Lipid cell tumor of ovary
M8671/0	Adrenal rest tumor

M868-M871   **Paragangliomas and glomus tumors**

M8680/1	Paraganglioma NOS
M8680/3	Paraganglioma, malignant
M8681/1	Sympathetic paraganglioma
M8682/1	Parasympathetic paraganglioma
M8690/1	Glomus jugulare tumor
M8691/1	Aortic body tumor
M8692/1	Carotid body tumor
M8693/1	Extra-adrenal paraganglioma NOS
M8693/3	Extra-adrenal paraganglioma, malignant
M8700/0	Pheochromocytoma NOS
M8700/3	Pheochromocytoma, malignant
M8710/3	Glomangiosarcoma
M8711/0	Glomus tumor
M8712/0	Glomangioma

M872-M879   **Nevi and melanomas**

M8720/0	Pigmented nevus NOS
M8720/3	Malignant melanoma NOS
M8721/3	Nodular melanoma
M8722/0	Balloon cell nevus
M8722/3	Balloon cell melanoma
M8723/0	Halo nevus
M8724/0	Fibrous papule of the nose
M8725/0	Neuronevus
M8726/0	Magnocellular nevus
M8730/0	Nonpigmented nevus
M8730/3	Amelanotic melanoma
M8740/0	Junctional nevus
M8740/3	Malignant melanoma in junctional nevus
M8741/2	Precancerous melanosis NOS
M8741/3	Malignant melanoma in precancerous melanosis
M8742/2	Hutchinson's melanotic freckle
M8742/3	Malignant melanoma in Hutchinson's melanotic freckle
M8743/3	Superficial spreading melanoma
M8750/0	Intradermal nevus
M8760/0	Compound nevus
M8761/1	Giant pigmented nevus
M8761/3	Malignant melanoma in giant pigmented nevus
M8770/0	Epithelioid and spindle cell nevus
M8771/3	Epithelioid cell melanoma
M8772/3	Spindle cell melanoma NOS
M8773/3	Spindle cell melanoma, type A
M8774/3	Spindle cell melanoma, type B
M8775/3	Mixed epithelioid and spindle cell melanoma
M8780/0	Blue nevus NOS
M8780/3	Blue nevus, malignant
M8790/0	Cellular blue nevus

M880   **Soft tissue tumors and sarcomas NOS**

M8800/0	Soft tissue tumor, benign
M8800/3	Sarcoma NOS
M8800/9	Sarcomatosis NOS
M8801/3	Spindle cell sarcoma
M8802/3	Giant cell sarcoma (except of bone M9250/3)
M8803/3	Small cell sarcoma
M8804/3	Epithelioid cell sarcoma

M881-M883   **Fibromatous neoplasms**

M8810/0	Fibroma NOS
M8810/3	Fibrosarcoma NOS
M8811/0	Fibromyxoma
M8811/3	Fibromyxosarcoma
M8812/0	Periosteal fibroma
M8812/3	Periosteal fibrosarcoma
M8813/0	Fascial fibroma
M8813/3	Fascial fibrosarcoma
M8814/3	Infantile fibrosarcoma
M8820/0	Elastofibroma
M8821/1	Aggressive fibromatosis
M8822/1	Abdominal fibromatosis
M8823/1	Desmoplastic fibroma
M8830/0	Fibrous histiocytoma NOS
M8830/1	Atypical fibrous histiocytoma
M8830/3	Fibrous histiocytoma, malignant
M8831/0	Fibroxanthoma NOS
M8831/1	Atypical fibroxanthoma
M8831/3	Fibroxanthoma, malignant
M8832/0	Dermatofibroma NOS
M8832/1	Dermatofibroma protuberans
M8832/3	Dermatofibrosarcoma NOS

M884   **Myxomatous neoplasms**

M8840/0	Myxoma NOS
M8840/3	Myxosarcoma

M885-M888   **Lipomatous neoplasms**

M8850/0	Lipoma NOS
M8850/3	Liposarcoma NOS
M8851/0	Fibrolipoma
M8851/3	Liposarcoma, well differentiated type
M8852/0	Fibromyxolipoma
M8852/3	Myxoid liposarcoma
M8853/3	Round cell liposarcoma
M8854/3	Pleomorphic liposarcoma
M8855/3	Mixed type liposarcoma
M8856/0	Intramuscular lipoma
M8857/0	Spindle cell lipoma

M8860/0	Angiomyolipoma
M8860/3	Angiomyoliposarcoma
M8861/0	Angiolipoma NOS
M8861/1	Angiolipoma, infiltrating
M8870/0	Myelolipoma
M8880/0	Hibernoma
M8881/0	Lipoblastomatosis

M889-M892   **Myomatous neoplasms**

M8890/0	Leiomyoma NOS
M8890/1	Intravascular leiomyomatosis
M8890/3	Leiomyosarcoma NOS
M8891/1	Epithelioid leiomyoma
M8891/3	Epithelioid leiomyosarcoma
M8892/1	Cellular leiomyoma
M8893/0	Bizarre leiomyoma
M8894/0	Angiomyoma
M8894/3	Angiomyosarcoma
M8895/0	Myoma
M8895/3	Myosarcoma
M8900/0	Rhabdomyoma NOS
M8900/3	Rhabdomyosarcoma NOS
M8901/3	Pleomorphic rhabdomyosarcoma
M8902/3	Mixed type rhabdomyosarcoma
M8903/0	Fetal rhabdomyoma
M8904/0	Adult rhabdomyoma
M8910/3	Embryonal rhabdomyosarcoma
M8920/3	Alveolar rhabdomyosarcoma

M893-M899   **Complex mixed and stromal neoplasms**

M8930/3	Endometrial stromal sarcoma
M8931/1	Endolymphatic stromal myosis
M8932/0	Adenomyoma
M8940/0	Pleomorphic adenoma
M8940/3	Mixed tumor, malignant NOS
M8950/3	Mullerian mixed tumor
M8951/3	Mesodermal mixed tumor
M8960/1	Mesoblastic nephroma
M8960/3	Nephroblastoma NOS
M8961/3	Epithelial nephroblastoma
M8962/3	Mesenchymal nephroblastoma
M8970/3	Hepatoblastoma
M8980/3	Carcinosarcoma NOS
M8981/3	Carcinosarcoma, embryonal type
M8982/0	Myoepithelioma
M8990/0	Mesenchymoma, benign
M8990/1	Mesenchymoma NOS
M8990/3	Mesenchymoma, malignant
M8991/3	Embryonal sarcoma

M900-M903   **Fibroepithelial neoplasms**

M9000/0	Brenner tumor NOS
M9000/1	Brenner tumor, borderline malignancy
M9000/3	Brenner tumor, malignant
M9010/0	Fibroadenoma NOS
M9011/0	Intracanalicular fibroadenoma NOS
M9012/0	Pericanalicular fibroadenoma
M9013/0	Adenofibroma NOS
M9014/0	Serous adenofibroma
M9015/0	Mucinous adenofibroma
M9020/0	Cellular intracanalicular fibroadenoma
M9020/1	Cystosarcoma phyllodes NOS
M9020/3	Cystosarcoma phyllodes, malignant
M9030/0	Juvenile fibroadenoma

M904   **Synovial neoplasms**

M9040/0	Synovioma, benign
M9040/3	Synovial sarcoma NOS
M9041/3	Synovial sarcoma, spindle cell type
M9042/3	Synovial sarcoma, epithelioid cell type
M9043/3	Synovial sarcoma, biphasic type
M9044/3	Clear cell sarcoma of tendons and aponeuroses

M905	**Mesothelial neoplasms**
M9050/0	Mesothelioma, benign
M9050/3	Mesothelioma, malignant
M9051/0	Fibrous mesothelioma, benign
M9051/3	Fibrous mesothelioma, malignant
M9052/0	Epithelioid mesothelioma, benign
M9052/3	Epithelioid mesothelioma, malignant
M9053/0	Mesothelioma, biphasic type, benign
M9053/3	Mesothelioma, biphasic type, malignant
M9054/0	Adenomatoid tumor NOS
M906-M909	**Germ cell neoplasms**
M9060/3	Dysgerminoma
M9061/3	Seminoma NOS
M9062/3	Seminoma, anaplastic type
M9063/3	Spermatocytic seminoma
M9064/3	Germinoma
M9070/3	Embryonal carcinoma NOS
M9071/3	Endodermal sinus tumor
M9072/3	Polyembryoma
M9073/1	Gonadoblastoma
M9080/0	Teratoma, benign
M9080/1	Teratoma NOS
M9080/3	Teratoma, malignant NOS
M9081/3	Teratocarcinoma
M9082/3	Malignant teratoma, undifferentiated type
M9083/3	Malignant teratoma, intermediate type
M9084/0	Dermoid cyst
M9084/3	Dermoid cyst with malignant transformation
M9090/0	Struma ovarii NOS
M9090/3	Struma ovarii, malignant
M9091/1	Strumal carcinoid
M910	**Trophoblastic neoplasms**
M9100/0	Hydatidiform mole NOS
M9100/1	Invasive hydatidiform mole
M9100/3	Choriocarcinoma
M9101/3	Choriocarcinoma combined with teratoma
M9102/3	Malignant teratoma, trophoblastic
M911	**Mesonephromas**
M9110/0	Mesonephroma, benign
M9110/1	Mesonephric tumor
M9110/3	Mesonephroma, malignant
M9111/1	Endosalpingioma
M912-M916	**Blood vessel tumors**
M9120/0	Hemangioma NOS
M9120/3	Hemangiosarcoma
M9121/0	Cavernous hemangioma
M9122/0	Venous hemangioma
M9123/0	Racemose hemangioma
M9124/3	Kupffer cell sarcoma
M9130/0	Hemangioendothelioma, benign
M9130/1	Hemangioendothelioma NOS
M9130/3	Hemangioendothelioma, malignant
M9131/0	Capillary hemangioma
M9132/0	Intramuscular hemangioma
M9140/3	Kaposi's sarcoma
M9141/0	Angiokeratoma
M9142/0	Verrucous keratotic hemangioma
M9150/0	Hemangiopericytoma, benign
M9150/1	Hemangiopericytoma NOS
M9150/3	Hemangiopericytoma, malignant
M9160/0	Angiofibroma NOS
M9161/1	Hemangioblastoma
M917	**Lymphatic vessel tumors**
M9170/0	Lymphangioma NOS
M9170/3	Lymphangiosarcoma
M9171/0	Capillary lymphangioma
M9172/0	Cavernous lymphangioma
M9173/0	Cystic lymphangioma
M9174/0	Lymphangiomyoma
M9174/1	Lymphangiomyomatosis
M9175/0	Hemolymphangioma
M918-M920	**Osteomas and osteosarcomas**
M9180/0	Osteoma NOS
M9180/3	Osteosarcoma NOS
M9181/3	Chondroblastic osteosarcoma
M9182/3	Fibroblastic osteosarcoma
M9183/3	Telangiectatic osteosarcoma
M9184/3	Osteosarcoma in Paget's disease of bone
M9190/3	Juxtacortical osteosarcoma
M9191/0	Osteoid osteoma NOS
M9200/0	Osteoblastoma
M921-M924	**Chondromatous neoplasms**
M9210/0	Osteochondroma
M9210/1	Osteochondromatosis NOS
M9220/0	Chondroma NOS
M9220/1	Chondromatosis NOS
M9220/3	Chondrosarcoma NOS
M9221/0	Juxtacortical chondroma
M9221/3	Juxtacortical chondrosarcoma
M9230/0	Chondroblastoma NOS
M9230/3	Chondroblastoma, malignant
M9240/3	Mesenchymal chondrosarcoma
M9241/0	Chondromyxoid fibroma
M925	**Giant cell tumors**
M9250/1	Giant cell tumor of bone NOS
M9250/3	Giant cell tumor of bone, malignant
M9251/1	Giant cell tumor of soft parts NOS
M9251/3	Malignant giant cell tumor of soft parts
M926	**Miscellaneous bone tumors**
M9260/3	Ewing's sarcoma
M9261/3	Adamantinoma of long bones
M9262/0	Ossifying fibroma
M927-M934	**Odontogenic tumors**
M9270/0	Odontogenic tumor, benign
M9270/1	Odontogenic tumor NOS
M9270/3	Odontogenic tumor, malignant
M9271/0	Dentinoma
M9272/0	Cementoma NOS
M9273/0	Cementoblastoma, benign
M9274/0	Cementifying fibroma
M9275/0	Gigantiform cementoma
M9280/0	Odontoma NOS
M9281/0	Compound odontoma
M9282/0	Complex odontoma
M9290/0	Ameloblastic fibro-odontoma
M9290/3	Ameloblastic odontosarcoma
M9300/0	Adenomatoid odontogenic tumor
M9301/0	Calcifying odontogenic cyst
M9310/0	Ameloblastoma NOS
M9310/3	Ameloblastoma, malignant
M9311/0	Odontoameloblastoma
M9312/0	Squamous odontogenic tumor
M9320/0	Odontogenic myxoma
M9321/0	Odontogenic fibroma NOS
M9330/0	Ameloblastic fibroma
M9330/3	Ameloblastic fibrosarcoma
M9340/0	Calcifying epithelial odontogenic tumor
M935-M937	**Miscellaneous tumors**
M9350/1	Craniopharyngioma
M9360/1	Pinealoma
M9361/1	Pineocytoma
M9362/3	Pineoblastoma
M9363/0	Melanotic neuroectodermal tumor
M9370/3	Chordoma
M938-M948	**Gliomas**
M9380/3	Glioma, malignant
M9381/3	Gliomatosis cerebri
M9382/3	Mixed glioma
M9383/1	Subependymal glioma
M9384/1	Subependymal giant cell astrocytoma
M9390/0	Choroid plexus papilloma NOS
M9390/3	Choroid plexus papilloma, malignant
M9391/3	Ependymoma NOS
M9392/3	Ependymoma, anaplastic type
M9393/1	Papillary ependymoma
M9394/1	Myxopapillary ependymoma
M9400/3	Astrocytoma NOS
M9401/3	Astrocytoma, anaplastic type
M9410/3	Protoplasmic astrocytoma
M9411/3	Gemistocytic astrocytoma
M9420/3	Fibrillary astrocytoma
M9421/3	Pilocytic astrocytoma
M9422/3	Spongioblastoma NOS
M9423/3	Spongioblastoma polare
M9430/3	Astroblastoma
M9440/3	Glioblastoma NOS
M9441/3	Giant cell glioblastoma
M9442/3	Glioblastoma with sarcomatous component
M9443/3	Primitive polar spongioblastoma
M9450/3	Oligodendroglioma NOS
M9451/3	Oligodendroglioma, anaplastic type
M9460/3	Oligodendroblastoma
M9470/3	Medulloblastoma NOS
M9471/3	Desmoplastic medulloblastoma
M9472/3	Medullomyoblastoma
M9480/3	Cerebellar sarcoma NOS
M9481/3	Monstrocellular sarcoma
M949-M952	**Neuroepitheliomatous neoplasms**
M9490/0	Ganglioneuroma
M9490/3	Ganglioneuroblastoma
M9491/0	Ganglioneuromatosis
M9500/3	Neuroblastoma NOS
M9501/3	Medulloepithelioma NOS
M9502/3	Teratoid medulloepithelioma
M9503/3	Neuroepithelioma NOS
M9504/3	Spongioneuroblastoma
M9505/1	Ganglioglioma
M9506/0	Neurocytoma
M9507/0	Pacinian tumor
M9510/3	Retinoblastoma NOS
M9511/3	Retinoblastoma, differentiated type
M9512/3	Retinoblastoma, undifferentiated type
M9520/3	Olfactory neurogenic tumor
M9521/3	Esthesioneurocytoma
M9522/3	Esthesioneuroblastoma
M9523/3	Esthesioneuroepithelioma
M953	**Meningiomas**
M9530/0	Meningioma NOS
M9530/1	Meningiomatosis NOS
M9530/3	Meningioma, malignant
M9531/0	Meningotheliomatous meningioma
M9532/0	Fibrous meningioma
M9533/0	Psammomatous meningioma
M9534/0	Angiomatous meningioma
M9535/0	Hemangioblastic meningioma
M9536/0	Hemangiopericytic meningioma
M9537/0	Transitional meningioma
M9538/1	Papillary meningioma
M9539/3	Meningeal sarcomatosis
M954-M957	**Nerve sheath tumor**
M9540/0	Neurofibroma NOS
M9540/1	Neurofibromatosis NOS
M9540/3	Neurofibrosarcoma
M9541/0	Melanotic neurofibroma
M9550/0	Plexiform neurofibroma
M9560/0	Neurilemmoma NOS

Appendix A: Morphology of Neoplasms

M9560/1	*Neurinomatosis*
M9560/3	*Neurilemmoma, malignant*
M9570/0	*Neuroma NOS*
M958	**Granular cell tumors and alveolar soft part sarcoma**
M9580/0	*Granular cell tumor NOS*
M9580/3	*Granular cell tumor, malignant*
M9581/3	*Alveolar soft part sarcoma*
M959-M963	**Lymphomas, NOS or diffuse**
M9590/0	*Lymphomatous tumor, benign*
M9590/3	*Malignant lymphoma NOS*
M9591/3	*Malignant lymphoma, non Hodgkin's type*
M9600/3	*Malignant lymphoma, undifferentiated cell type NOS*
M9601/3	*Malignant lymphoma, stem cell type*
M9602/3	*Malignant lymphoma, convoluted cell type NOS*
M9610/3	*Lymphosarcoma NOS*
M9611/3	*Malignant lymphoma, lymphoplasmacytoid type*
M9612/3	*Malignant lymphoma, immunoblastic type*
M9613/3	*Malignant lymphoma, mixed lymphocytic-histiocytic NOS*
M9614/3	*Malignant lymphoma, centroblastic-centrocytic, diffuse*
M9615/3	*Malignant lymphoma, follicular center cell NOS*
M9620/3	*Malignant lymphoma, lymphocytic, well differentiated NOS*
M9621/3	*Malignant lymphoma, lymphocytic, intermediate differentiation NOS*
M9622/3	*Malignant lymphoma, centrocytic*
M9623/3	*Malignant lymphoma, follicular center cell, cleaved NOS*
M9630/3	*Malignant lymphoma, lymphocytic, poorly differentiated NOS*
M9631/3	*Prolymphocytic lymphosarcoma*
M9632/3	*Malignant lymphoma, centroblastic type NOS*
M9633/3	*Malignant lymphoma, follicular center cell, noncleaved NOS*
M964	**Reticulosarcomas**
M9640/3	*Reticulosarcoma NOS*
M9641/3	*Reticulosarcoma, pleomorphic cell type*
M9642/3	*Reticulosarcoma, nodular*
M965-M966	**Hodgkin's disease**
M9650/3	*Hodgkin's disease NOS*
M9651/3	*Hodgkin's disease, lymphocytic predominance*
M9652/3	*Hodgkin's disease, mixed cellularity*
M9653/3	*Hodgkin's disease, lymphocytic depletion NOS*

M9654/3	*Hodgkin's disease, lymphocytic depletion, diffuse fibrosis*
M9655/3	*Hodgkin's disease, lymphocytic depletion, reticular type*
M9656/3	*Hodgkin's disease, nodular sclerosis NOS*
M9657/3	*Hodgkin's disease, nodular sclerosis, cellular phase*
M9660/3	*Hodgkin's paragranuloma*
M9661/3	*Hodgkin's granuloma*
M9662/3	*Hodgkin's sarcoma*
M969	**Lymphomas, nodular or follicular**
M9690/3	*Malignant lymphoma, nodular NOS*
M9691/3	*Malignant lymphoma, mixed lymphocytic-histiocytic, nodular*
M9692/3	*Malignant lymphoma, centroblastic-centrocytic, follicular*
M9693/3	*Malignant lymphoma, lymphocytic, well differentiated, nodular*
M9694/3	*Malignant lymphoma, lymphocytic, intermediate differentiation, nodular*
M9695/3	*Malignant lymphoma, follicular center cell, cleaved, follicular*
M9696/3	*Malignant lymphoma, lymphocytic, poorly differentiated, nodular*
M9697/3	*Malignant lymphoma, centroblastic type, follicular*
M9698/3	*Malignant lymphoma, follicular center cell, noncleaved, follicular*
M970	**Mycosis fungoides**
M9700/3	*Mycosis fungoides*
M9701/3	*Sezary's disease*
M971-M972	**Miscellaneous reticuloendothelial neoplasms**
M9710/3	*Microglioma*
M9720/3	*Malignant histiocytosis*
M9721/3	*Histiocytic medullary reticulosis*
M 722/3	*Letterer-Siwe's disease*
M973	**Plasma cell tumors**
M9730/3	*Plasma cell myeloma*
M9731/0	*Plasma cell tumor, benign*
M9731/1	*Plasmacytoma NOS*
M9731/3	*Plasma cell tumor, malignant*
M974	**Mast cell tumors**
M9740/1	*Mastocytoma NOS*
M9740/3	*Mast cell sarcoma*
M9741/3	*Malignant mastocytosis*
M975	**Burkitt's tumor**
M9750/3	*Burkitt's tumor*
M980-M994	**Leukemias**
M980	**Leukemias NOS**
M9800/3	*Leukemia NOS*
M9801/3	*Acute leukemia NOS*

M9802/3	*Subacute leukemia NOS*
M9803/3	*Chronic leukemia NOS*
M9804/3	*Aleukemic leukemia NOS*
M981	**Compound leukemias**
M9810/3	*Compound leukemia*
M982	**Lymphoid leukemias**
M9820/3	*Lymphoid leukemia NOS*
M9821/3	*Acute lymphoid leukemia*
M9822/3	*Subacute lymphoid leukemia*
M9823/3	*Chronic lymphoid leukemia*
M9824/3	*Aleukemic lymphoid leukemia*
M9825/3	*Prolymphocytic leukemia*
M983	**Plasma cell leukemias**
M9830/3	*Plasma cell leukemia*
M984	**Erythroleukemias**
M9840/3	*Erythroleukemia*
M9841/3	*Acute erythremia*
M9842/3	*Chronic erythremia*
M985	**Lymphosarcoma cell leukemias**
M9850/3	*Lymphosarcoma cell leukemia*
M986	**Myeloid leukemias**
M9860/3	*Myeloid leukemia NOS*
M9861/3	*Acute myeloid leukemia*
M9862/3	*Subacute myeloid leukemia*
M9863/3	*Chronic myeloid leukemia*
M9864/3	*Aleukemic myeloid leukemia*
M9865/3	*Neutrophilic leukemia*
M9866/3	*Acute promyelocytic leukemia*
M987	**Basophilic leukemias**
M9870/3	*Basophilic leukemia*
M988	**Eosinophilic leukemias**
M9880/3	*Eosinophilic leukemia*
M989	**Monocytic leukemias**
M9890/3	*Monocytic leukemia NOS*
M9891/3	*Acute monocytic leukemia*
M9892/3	*Subacute monocytic leukemia*
M9893/3	*Chronic monocytic leukemia*
M9894/3	*Aleukemic monocytic leukemia*
M990-M994	**Miscellaneous leukemias**
M9900/3	*Mast cell leukemia*
M9910/3	*Megakaryocytic leukemia*
M9920/3	*Megakaryocytic myelosis*
M9930/3	*Myeloid sarcoma*
M9940/3	*Hairy cell leukemia*
M995-M997	**Miscellaneous myeloproliferative and lymphoproliferative disorders**
M9950/1	*Polycythemia vera*
M9951/1	*Acute panmyelosis*
M9960/1	*Chronic myeloproliferative disease*
M9961/1	*Myelosclerosis with myeloid metaplasia*
M9962/1	*Idiopathic thrombocythemia*
M9970/1	*Chronic lymphoproliferative disease*

Glossary of Mental Disorders

The psychiatric terms which appear in Chapter 5, "Mental Disorders," are listed here in alphabetic sequence. Many of the glossary descriptions originally appeared in the section on Mental Disorders in the *International Classification of Diseases, 9th Revision,*[1] and others are included to define the psychiatric conditions added to *ICD-9-CM.* The additional definitions are based on material furnished by the *American Psychiatric Association's Task Force on Nomenclature and Statistics*[2] and from *A Psychiatric Glossary.*[3] In a few instances definitions were obtained from *Dorland's Illustrated Medical Dictionary*[4] and from *Stedman's Medical Dictionary, Illustrated.*[5]

1. *Manual of the International Classification of Diseases, Injuries, and Causes of Death,* 9th Revision. World Health Organization, Geneva, Switzerland, 1975.
2. American Psychiatric Association, Task Force on Nomenclature and Statistics, Robert L. Spitzer, Chairman.
3. *A Psychiatric Glossary,* Fourth Edition, American Psychiatric Association, Washington, D.C., 1975.
4. *Dorland's Illustrated Medical Dictionary,* Twenty-fifth Edition, W.B. Saunders Company, Philadelphia, 1974.
5. *Stedman's Medical Dictionary,* Illustrated, Twenty-third Edition, the Williams and Wilkins Company, Baltimore, 1976.

Academic underachievement disorder – Failure to achieve in most school tasks despite adequate intellectual capacity, a supportive and encouraging social environment, and apparent effort. The failure occurs in the absence of a demonstrable specific learning disability and is caused by emotional conflict not clearly associated with any other mental disorder.[2]

Adaptation reaction — *see* Adjustment reaction

Adjustment reaction or disorder – Mild or transient disorders lasting longer than acute stress reactions which occur in individuals of any age without any apparent pre-existing mental disorder. Such disorders are often relatively circumscribed or situation-specific, are generally reversible, and usually last only a few months. They are usually closely related in time and content to stresses such as bereavement, migration, or other experiences. Reactions to major stress that last longer than a few days are also included. In children such disorders are associated with no significant distortion of development.[1]

conduct disturbance – Mild or transient disorders in which the main disturbance predominantly involves a disturbance of conduct (e.g., an adolescent grief reaction resulting in aggressive or antisocial disorder).[1]

depressive reaction – States of depression, not specifiable as manic-depressive, psychotic, or neurotic.[1]

brief – Generally transient, in which the depressive symptoms are usually closely related in time and content to some stressful event.[1]

prolonged – Generally long-lasting, usually developing in association with prolonged exposure to a stressful situation.[1]

emotional disturbance – An adjustment disorder in which the main symptoms are emotional in type (e.g., anxiety, fear, worry) but not specifically depressive.[1]

mixed conduct and emotional disturbance – An adjustment reaction in which both emotional disturbance and disturbance of conduct are prominent features.[1]

Affective psychoses – Mental disorders, usually recurrent, in which there is a severe disturbance of mood (mostly compounded of depression and anxiety but also manifested as elation, and excitement) which is accompanied by one or more of the following – delusions, perplexity, disturbed attitude to self, disorder of perception and behavior; these are all in keeping with the individual's prevailing mood (as are hallucinations when they occur). There is a strong tendency to suicide. For practical reasons, mild disorders of mood may also be included here if the symptoms match closely the descriptions given; this applies particularly to mild hypomania.[1]

bipolar – A manic-depressive psychosis which has appeared in both the depressive and manic form, either alternating or separated by an interval of normality.[1]

atypical – An episode of affective psychosis with some, but not all, of the features of the one form of the disorder in individuals who have had a previous episode of the other form of the disorder.[2]

depressed – A manic-depressive psychosis, circular type, in which the depressive form is currently present.[1]

manic – A manic-depressive psychosis, circular type, in which the manic form is currently present.[1]

mixed – A manic-depressive psychosis, circular type, in which both manic and depressive symptoms are present at the same time.[1]

depressed type – A manic-depressive psychosis in which there is a widespread depressed mood of gloom and wretchedness with some degree of anxiety. There is often reduced activity but there may be restlessness and agitation. There is marked tendency to recurrence; in a few cases this may be at regular intervals.[1]

atypical – An affective depressive disorder that cannot be classified as a manic-depressive psychosis, depressed type, or chronic depressive personality disorder, or as an adjustment disorder.[2]

manic type – A manic-depressive psychosis characterized by states of elation or excitement out of keeping with the individual's circumstances and varying from enhanced liveliness (hypomania) to violent, almost uncontrollable, excitement. Aggression and anger, flight of ideas, distractibility,

impaired judgment, and grandiose ideas are common.[1]

mixed type – Manic-depressive psychosis syndromes corresponding to both the manic and depressed types, but which for other reasons cannot be classified more specifically.[1]

Aggressive personality — *see* Personality disorder, explosive type

Agoraphobia — *see* agoraphobia under Phobia

Alcohol dependence syndrome – A state, psychic and usually also physical, resulting from taking alcohol, characterized by behavioral and other responses that always include a compulsion to take alcohol on a continuous or periodic basis in order to experience its psychic effects, and sometimes to avoid the discomfort of its absence; tolerance may or may not be present. A person may be dependent on alcohol and other drugs; if so, also record the diagnosis of drug dependence to identify the agent. If alcohol dependence is associated with alcoholic psychosis or with physical complications, *both* diagnoses should be recorded.[1]

Alcohol intoxication

acute – A psychic and physical state resulting from alcohol ingestion characterized by slurred speech, unsteady gait, poor coordination, flushed facies, nystagmus, sluggish reflexes, fetor alcoholica, loud speech, emotional instability (e.g., jollity followed by lugubriousness), excessive conviviality, loquacity, and poorly inhibited sexual and aggressive behavior.[2]

idiosyncratic – Acute psychotic episodes induced by relatively small amounts of alcohol. These are regarded as individual idiosyncratic reactions to alcohol, not due to excessive consumption and without conspicuous neurological signs of intoxication.[1]

pathological – *see* Alcohol intoxication, idiosyncratic

Alcoholic psychoses – Organic psychotic states due mainly to excessive consumption of alcohol; defects of nutrition are thought to play an important role.[1]

alcohol abstinence syndrome — *see* alcohol withdrawal syndrome below

alcohol amnestic syndrome – A syndrome of prominent and lasting reduction of memory span, including striking loss of recent memory, disordered time appreciation and confabulation, occurring in alcoholics as the sequel to an acute alcoholic psychosis (especially delirium tremens) or, more rarely, in the course of chronic alcoholism. It is usually accompanied by peripheral neuritis and may be associated with Wernicke's encephalopathy.[1]

alcohol withdrawal delirium [delirium tremens] – Acute or subacute organic psychotic states in alcoholics, characterized by clouded consciousness, disorientation, fear, illusions, delusions, hallucinations of any kind, notably visual and tactile, and restlessness, tremor and sometimes fever.[1]

alcohol withdrawal hallucinosis – A psychosis usually of less than six months' duration, with slight or no clouding of consciousness and much anxious restlessness in which auditory hallucinations, mostly of voices uttering insults and threats, predominate.[1]

alcohol withdrawal syndrome – Tremor of hands, tongue, and eyelids following cessation of prolonged heavy drinking of alcohol. Nausea and vomiting, dry mouth, headache, heavy perspiration, fitful sleep, acute anxiety attacks, mood depression, feelings of guilt and remorse, and irritability are associated features.[2]

alcohol delirium — *see* alcohol withdrawal delirium above

alcoholic dementia – Nonhallucinatory dementias occurring in association with alcoholism, but not characterized by the features of either alcohol withdrawal delirium [delirium tremens] or alcohol amnestic syndrome [Korsakoff's alcoholic psychosis].[1]

alcoholic hallucinosis — *see* alcohol withdrawal hallucinosis above

alcoholic jealousy – Chronic paranoid psychosis characterized by delusional jealousy and associated with alcoholism.[1]

alcoholic paranoia — *see* Alcoholic jealousy

alcoholic polyneuritic psychosis — *see* alcohol amnestic syndrome above

Alcoholism

acute — *see* Alcohol intoxication, acute

chronic — *see* Alcohol dependence syndrome

Alexia – Loss of a previously possessed reading facility that cannot be explained by defective visual acuity.[3]

Amnesia, psychogenic – A form of dissociative hysteria in which there is a temporary disturbance in the ability to recall important personal information which has already been registered and stored in memory. The sudden onset of this disturbance in the absence of an underlying organic mental disorder, and the extent of the disturbance being too great to be explained by ordinary forgetfulness, are the essential features.[2]

Amnestic syndrome – A syndrome of prominent and lasting reduction of memory span, including striking loss of recent memory, disordered time appreciation, and confabulation. The commonest causes are chronic alcoholism [alcohol amnestic syndrome; Korsakoff's alcoholic psychosis], chronic barbiturate dependence, and malnutrition. An amnestic syndrome may be the predominating disturbance in the early states of presenile and senile dementia, arteriosclerotic dementia, and in encephalitis and other inflammatory and degenerative diseases in which there is particular bilateral involvement of the temporal lobes, and certain temporal lobe tumors.[2]

alcoholic — *see* alcohol amnestic syndrome under Alcoholic psychoses

Amoral personality — *see* Personality disorder, antisocial type

Anancastic [anankastic] neurosis — *see* Neurotic disorder, obsessive-compulsive

Anancastic [anankastic] personality — *see* Personality disorder, compulsive type

Anorexia nervosa – A disorder in which the main features are persistent active refusal to eat and marked loss of weight.

The level of activity and alertness is characteristically high in relation to the degree of emaciation. Typically the disorder begins in teenage girls but it may sometimes begin before puberty and rarely it occurs in males. Amenorrhea is usual and there may be a variety of other physiological changes including slow pulse and respiration, low body temperature, and dependent edema. Unusual eating habits and attitudes toward food are typical and sometimes starvation follows or alternates with periods of overeating. The accompanying psychiatric symptoms are diverse.[1]

Anxiety hysteria — *see* phobia under Neurotic disorders

Anxiety state (neurotic) – Apprehension, tension, or uneasiness that stems from the anticipation of danger, the source of which is largely unknown or unrecognized.[3]

atypical – An anxiety disorder that does not fulfill the criteria of generalized or panic attack anxiety. An example might be an individual with a single morbid fear.[2]

generalized – A disorder of at least six months' duration in which the predominant feature is limited to diffuse and persistent anxiety without the specific symptoms that characterize phobic disorders, panic disorder, or obsessive-compulsive disorder.[2]

panic attack – An episodic and often chronic, recurrent disorder in which the predominant features are anxiety attacks and nervousness. The anxiety attacks are manifested by discrete periods of sudden onset of intense apprehension, fearfulness, or terror often associated with feelings of impending doom.[2]

Aphasia, developmental – A delay in the production of spoken language. Rarely, there is also a developmental delay in the comprehension of speech sounds.[1]

Arteriosclerotic dementia – Dementia attributable, because of physical signs (on examination of the central nervous system), to degenerative arterial disease of the brain. Symptoms suggesting a focal lesion in the brain are common. There may be a fluctuating or patchy intellectual defect with insight, and an intermittent course is common. Clinical differentiation from senile or presenile dementia, which may coexist with it, may be very difficult or impossible. The diagnosis of cerebral atherosclerosis should also be recorded.[1]

Asocial personality — *see* Personality disorder, antisocial type

Astasia-abasia, hysterical – A form of conversion hysteria in which the individual is unable to stand or walk although the legs are otherwise under control.[4]

Asthenia, psychogenic — *see* neurasthenia under Neurotic disorders

Asthenic personality — *see* Personality disorder, dependent type

Attention deficit disorder — *see* Attention deficit disorder under Hyperkinetic syndrome of childhood.

Autism, infantile – A syndrome present from birth or beginning almost invariably in the first 30 months. Responses to

auditory and sometimes to visual stimuli are abnormal, and there are usually severe problems in the understanding of spoken language. Speech is delayed and, if it develops, is characterized by echolalia, the reversal of pronouns, immature grammatical structure, and inability to use abstract terms. There is generally an impairment in the social use of both verbal and gestural language. Problems in social relationships are most severe before the age of five years and include an impairment in the development of eye-to-eye gaze, social attachments, and cooperative play. Ritualistic behavior is usual and may include abnormal routines, resistance to change, attachment to odd objects, and stereotyped patterns of play. The capacity for abstract or symbolic thought and for imaginative play is diminished. Intelligence ranges from severely subnormal to normal or above. Performance is usually better on tasks involving rote memory or visuospatial skills than on those requiring symbolic or linguistic skills.[1]

Avoidant personality — *see* Personality disorder, avoidant type

"Bad trips" – Acute intoxication from hallucinogen abuse, manifested by hallucinatory states lasting only a few days or less.[1]

Barbiturate abuse – Cases where an individual has taken the drug to the detriment of his health or social functioning, in doses above or for periods beyond those normally regarded as therapeutic.[1]

Bestiality — *see* Zoophilia

Bipolar disorder — *see* Affective psychosis, bipolar

atypical — *see* Affective psychosis, bipolar, atypical

Body-rocking — *see* Stereotyped repetitive movements

Borderline personality — *see* Personality disorder, borderline type

Borderline psychosis of childhood — *see* Psychosis, atypical childhood

Borderline schizophrenia — *see* Schizophrenia, latent

Bouffée délirante — *see* Paranoid reaction, acute

Briquet's disorder — *see* Somatization disorder under Neurotic disorders

Bulimia – An episodic pattern of overeating [binge eating] accompanied by an awareness of the disordered eating pattern with a fear of not being able to stop eating voluntarily. Depressive moods and self-deprecating thoughts follow the episodes of binge eating.[2]

Catalepsy schizophrenia — *see* Schizophrenia, catatonic type

Catastrophic stress — *see* Gross stress reaction

Catatonia (schizophrenic) — *see* Schizophrenia, catatonic type

Character neurosis — *see* Personality disorders

Childhood autism — *see* Autism, infantile

Childhood type schizophrenia — *see* Psychosis, child

Chronic alcoholic brain syndrome — *see* Alcoholic dementia under Alcoholic psychoses

Clay-eating — *see* Pica

Clumsiness syndrome — *see* Coordination disorder under Developmental delay disorders, specific

Combat fatigue — *see* Posttraumatic disorder, acute

Compensation neurosis — *see* Compensation neurosis under Neurotic disorders

Compulsive conduct disorder — *see* Impulse control disorders under Conduct disorders

Compulsive neurosis — *see* Neurotic disorder, obsessive-compulsive

Compulsive personality — *see* Personality disorder, compulsive type

Concentration camp syndrome — *see* Posttraumatic stress disorder, prolonged

Conduct disorders – Disorders mainly involving aggressive and destructive behavior and disorders involving delinquency. It should be used for abnormal behavior, in individuals of any age, which gives rise to social disapproval but which is not part of any other psychiatric condition. Minor emotional disturbances may also be present. To be included, the behavior, as judged by its frequency, severity, and type of associations with other symptoms, must be abnormal in its context. Disturbances of conduct are distinguished from an adjustment reaction by a longer duration and by a lack of close relationship in time and content to some stress. They differ from a personality disorder by the absence of deeply ingrained maladaptive patterns of behavior present from adolescence or earlier.[1]

impulse control disorders – A failure to resist an impulse, drive, or temptation to perform some action which is harmful to the individual or to others. The impulse may or may not be consciously resisted, and the act may or may not be premeditated or planned. Prior to committing the act, there is an increasing sense of tension, and at the time of committing the act, there is an experience of either pleasure, gratification, or release. Immediately following the act, there may or may not be genuine regret, self-reproach, or guilt.[2] *See also* Intermittent explosive disorder, Isolated explosive disorder, Kleptomania, Pathological gambling, and Pyromania.

mixed disturbance of conduct and emotions – A disorder characterized by features of undersocialized and socialized disturbance of conduct, but in which there is also considerable emotional disturbance as shown, for example, by anxiety, misery, or obsessive manifestations.[1]

socialized conduct disorder – Conduct disorders in individuals who have acquired the values or behavior of a delinquent peer group to whom they are loyal and with whom they characteristically steal, play truant, and stay out late at night. There may also be sexual promiscuity.[1]

undersocialized conduct disturbance

aggressive type – A disorder characterized by a persistent pattern of disrespect for the feelings and well-being of others (bullying, physical aggression, cruel behavior, hostility, verbal abusiveness, impudence, defiance, negativism), aggressive antisocial behavior (destructiveness, stealing, persistent lying, frequent truancy, and vandalism), and failure to develop close and stable relationships with others.[2]

unaggressive type – A disorder in which there is a lack of concern for the rights and feelings of others to a degree which indicates a failure to establish a normal degree of affection, empathy, or bond with others. There are two patterns of behavior found. In one, the child is fearful and timid, lacking self-assertiveness, resorts to self-protective and manipulative lying, indulges in whining demandingness and temper tantrums, feels rejected and unfairly treated, and is mistrustful of others. In the other pattern of the disorder, the child approaches others strictly for his own gains and acts exclusively because of exploitative and extractive goals. The child lies brazenly and steals, appearing to feel no guilt, and forms no social bonds to other individuals.[2]

Confusion, psychogenic — *see* Psychosis, reactive confusion

Confusion, reactive — *see* Psychosis, reactive confusion

Confusional state

acute — *see* Delirium, acute

epileptic — *see* Delirium, acute

subacute — *see* Delirium, subacute

Conversion hysteria — *see* Hysteria, conversion type under Neurotic disorders

Coordination disorder — *see* Coordination disorder under Developmental delay disorders, specific

Culture shock – A form of stress reaction associated with an individual's assimilation into a new culture which is vastly different from that in which he was raised.[5]

Cyclic schizophrenia — *see* Schizophrenia, schizo-affective type

Cyclothymic personality or disorder — *see* Personality disorder, cyclothymic type

Delirium – Transient organic psychotic conditions with a short course in which there is a rapidly developing onset of disorganization of higher mental processes manifested by some degree of impairment of information processing, impaired or abnormal attention, perception, memory, and thinking. Clouded consciousness, confusion, disorientation, delusions, illusions, and often vivid hallucinations predominate in the clinical picture.[1, 2]

acute – short-lived states, lasting hours or days, of the above type.[1]

subacute – states of the above type in which the symptoms, usually less florid, last for several weeks or longer, during which they may show marked fluctuations in intensity.[1]

Delirium tremens — *see* Alcohol withdrawal delirium under Alcoholic psychoses

Delusions, systematized — *see* Paranoia

Dementia – A decrement in intellectual functioning of sufficient severity to interfere with occupational or social performance, or both. There is impairment of memory and abstract thinking, the ability to learn new skills, problem solving, and judgment. There is often also personality change or impairment in impulse control. Dementia in organic psychoses may be of a chronic or progressive nature, which if untreated are usually irreversible and terminal.[1, 2]

alcoholic — *see* Alcoholic dementia under Alcoholic psychoses

arteriosclerotic — *see* Arteriosclerotic dementia

multi-infarct — *see* Arteriosclerotic dementia

presenile — *see* Presenile dementia

repeated infarct — *see* Arteriosclerotic dementia

senile — *see* Senile dementia

Depersonalization syndrome — *see* Depersonalization syndrome under Neurotic disorders

Depression – States of depression, usually of moderate but occasionally of marked intensity, which have no specifically manic-depressive or other psychotic depressive features, and which do not appear to be associated with stressful events or other features specified under neurotic depression.[1]

anxiety — *see* Depression under Neurotic disorders

endogenous — *see* Affective psychosis, depressed type

monopolar — *see* Affective psychosis, depressed type

neurotic — *see* Depression under Neurotic disorders

psychotic — *see* Affective psychosis, depressed type

psychotic reactive — *see* Psychosis, depressive

reactive — *see* Depression under Neurotic disorders

reactive psychotic — *see* Psychosis, depressive

Depressive personality or character — *see* Personality disorder, chronic depressive type

Depressive reaction — *see* Depressive reaction under Adjustment reaction

Depressive psychosis — *see* Affective psychosis, depressed type

Derealization (neurotic) — *see* Depersonalization syndrome under Neurotic disorders

Developmental delay disorders, specific – A group of disorders in which a specific delay in development is the main feature. For many the delay is not explicable in terms of general intellectual retardation or of inadequate schooling. In each case development is related to biological maturation, but it is also influenced by nonbiological factors. A diagnosis of a specific developmental delay carries no etiological implications. A diagnosis of specific delay in development should not be made if it is due to a known neurological disorder.[1]

arithmetical disorder – Disorders in which the main feature is a serious impairment in the development of arithmetical skills.[1]

articulation disorder – A delay in the development of normal word-sound production resulting in defects of articulation. Omissions or substitutions of consonants are most frequent.[1]

Appendix B: Glossary of Mental Disorders

coordination disorder – Disorders in which the main feature is a serious impairment in the development of motor coordination which is not explicable in terms of general intellectual retardation. The clumsiness is commonly associated with perceptual difficulties.[1]

mixed development disorder – A delay in the development of one specific skill (e.g., reading, arithmetic, speech, or coordination) is frequently associated with lesser delays in other skills. When this occurs, the diagnosis should be made according to the skill most seriously impaired. The mixed category should be used only where the mixture of delayed skills is such that no one skill is preponderantly affected.[1]

motor retardation — see Coordination disorder above

reading disorder or retardation – Disorders in which the main feature is a serious impairment in the development of reading or spelling skills which is not explicable in terms of general intellectual retardation or of inadequate schooling. Speech or language difficulties, impaired right-left differentiation, perceptuo-motor problems, and coding difficulties are frequently associated. Similar problems are often present in other members of the family. Adverse psychosocial factors may be present.[1]

speech or language disorder – Disorders in which the main feature is a serious impairment in the development of speech or language (syntax or semantic) which is not explicable in terms of general intellectual retardation. Most commonly there is a delay in the development of normal word-sound production resulting in defects of articulation. Omissions or substitutions of consonants are most frequent. There may also be a delay in the production of spoken language. Rarely, there is also a developmental delay in the comprehension of sounds. Includes cases in which delay is largely due to environmental privation.[1]

Dipsomania — see Alcohol dependence syndrome

Disorganized schizophrenia — see Schizophrenia, disorganized type

Dissociative hysteria — see Hysteria, dissociative type under Neurotic disorders

Drug abuse – Includes cases where an individual, for whom no other diagnosis is possible, has come under medical care because of the maladaptive effect of a drug on which he is not dependent (see Drug dependence) and that he has taken on his own initiative to the detriment of his health or social functioning. When drug abuse is secondary to a psychiatric disorder, record the disorder as an additional diagnosis.[1]

Drug dependence – A state, psychic and sometimes also physical dependence, resulting from taking a drug, characterized by behavioral and other responses that always include a compulsion to take a drug on a continuous or periodic basis in order to experience its psychic effects, and sometimes to avoid the discomfort of its absence. Tolerance may or may not be present. A person may be dependent on more than one drug.[1]

Drug psychoses – Organic mental syndromes which are due to consumption of drugs (notably amphetamines, barbiturates, and opiate and LSD groups) and solvents. Some of the syndromes in this group are not as severe as most conditions labeled "psychotic," but they are included here for practical reasons. The drug should be identified, and also a diagnosis of drug dependence should be recorded, if present.[1]

drug-induced hallucinosis – Hallucinatory states of more than a few days, but not more than a few months' duration, associated with large or prolonged intake of drugs, notably of the amphetamine and LSD groups. Auditory hallucinations usually predominate and there may be anxiety or restlessness. States following LSD or other hallucinogens lasting only a few days or less ["bad trips"] are not included.[1]

drug-induced organic delusional syndrome – Paranoid states of more than a few days, but not more than a few months' duration, associated with large or prolonged intake of drugs, notably of the amphetamine and LSD groups.[1]

drug withdrawal syndrome – States associated with drug withdrawal ranging from severe, as specified for alcohol withdrawal delirium [delirium tremens], to less severe states characterized by one or more symptoms such as convulsions, tremor, anxiety, restlessness, gastrointestinal and muscular complaints, and mild disorientation and memory disturbance.[1]

Drunkenness

acute — see Alcohol intoxication, acute

pathologic — see Alcohol intoxication, idiosyncratic

simple – A state of inebriation due to alcohol consumption without conspicuous neurological signs of intoxication.[2]

sleep – An inability to fully arouse from the sleep state characterized by failure to attain full consciousness after arousal.[2]

Dyscalculia — see Arithmetical disorder under Developmental delay disorders, specific

Dyslalia — see Articulation disorder under Developmental delay disorders, specific

Dyslexia, developmental – A disorder in which the main feature is a serious impairment of reading skills which is not explicable in terms of general intellectual retardation or of inadequate schooling. Word-blindness and strephosymbolia (tendency to reverse letters and words in reading) are included.[1,3]

Dysmenorrhea, psychogenic – Painful menstruation due to disturbance of psychic control.[4]

Dyspareunia, functional — see Functional dyspareunia under Psychosexual dysfunctions

Dyspraxia syndrome — see Coordination disorder under Developmental delay disorders, specific

Dyssocial personality — see Personality disorder, antisocial type

Dysuria, psychogenic – Difficulty in passing urine due to psychic factors.[4]

Eating disorders – A group of disorders characterized by a conspicuous disturbance in eating behavior.[2] See also Bulimia, Pica, and Rumination, psychogenic.

Eccentric personality — see Personality disorder, eccentric type

Elective mutism – A pervasive and persistent refusal to speak in situations not attributable to a mental disorder. In some cases the behavior may manifest a form of withdrawal reaction to a specific stressful situation, or as a predominant feature in children exhibiting shyness or social withdrawal disorders.[2]

Emancipation disorder – An adjustment reaction in adolescents or young adults in which there is symptomatic expression (e.g., difficulty in making independent decisions, increased dependence on parental advice, adoption of values deliberately oppositional to parents) of a conflict over independence following the recent assumption of a status in which the individual is more independent of parental control or supervision.[2]

Emotional disturbances specific to childhood and adolescence – Less well-differentiated emotional disorders characteristic of the childhood period. When the emotional disorder takes the form of a neurosis, the appropriate diagnosis should be made. These disorders differ from adjustment reactions in terms of longer duration and by the lack of close relationship in time and content to some stress.[1] See also Academic underachievement disorder, Elective mutism, Identity disorder, Introverted disorder of childhood, Misery and unhappiness disorder, Oppositional disorder, Overanxious disorder, and Shyness disorder of childhood.

Encopresis – A disorder in which the main manifestation is the persistent voluntary or involuntary passage of formed stools of normal or near-normal consistency into places not intended for that purpose in the individual's own sociocultural setting. Sometimes the child has failed to gain bowel control, and sometimes he has gained control but then later again became encopretic. There may be a variety of associated psychiatric symptoms and there may be smearing of feces. The condition would not usually be diagnosed under the age of four years.[1]

Endogenous depression — see Affective psychosis, depressed type

Enuresis – A disorder in which the main manifestation is a persistent involuntary voiding of urine by day or night which is considered abnormal for the age of the individual. Sometimes the child will have failed to gain bladder control and in other cases he will have gained control and then lost it. Episodic or fluctuating enuresis should be included. The disorder would not usually be diagnosed under the age of four years.[1]

Epileptic confusional or twilight state — see Delirium, acute

Excitation

catatonic — *see* Schizophrenia, catatonic type

psychogenic — *see* Psychosis, excitative type

reactive — *see* Psychosis, excitative type

Exhaustion delirium — *see* Stress reaction, acute

Exhibitionism – Sexual deviation in which the main sexual pleasure and gratification is derived from exposure of the genitals to a person of the opposite sex.[1]

Explosive personality disorder — *see* Personality disorder, explosive type

Factitious illness – A form of hysterical neurosis in which there are physical or psychological symptoms that are not real, genuine, or natural, which are produced by the individual and are under his voluntary control.[2]

physical symptom type – The presentation of physical symptoms that may be total fabrication, self-inflicted, an exaggeration or exacerbation of a pre-existing physical condition, or any combination or variation of these.[2]

psychological symptom type – The voluntary production of symptoms suggestive of a mental disorder. Behavior may mimic psychosis or, rather, the individual's idea of psychosis.[2]

Fanatic personality — *see* Personality disorder, paranoid type

Fatigue neurosis — *see* Neurasthenia under Neurotic disorders

Feeble-minded — *see* Mental retardation, mild

Fetishism – A sexual deviation in which nonliving objects are utilized as a preferred or exclusive method of stimulating erotic arousal.[2]

Finger-flicking — *see* Stereotyped repetitive movements

Folie à deux — *see* Shared paranoid disorder

Frigidity – A psychosexual dysfunction in which there is partial or complete failure to attain or maintain the lubrication-swelling response of sexual excitement until completion of the sexual act.[2]

Frontal lobe syndrome – Changes in behavior following damage to the frontal areas of the brain or following interference with the connections of those areas. There is a general diminution of self-control, foresight, creativity, and spontaneity, which may be manifest as increased irritability, selfishness, restlessness, and lack of concern for others. Conscientiousness and powers of concentration are often diminished, but measurable deterioration of intellect or memory is not necessarily present. The overall picture is often one of emotional dullness, lack of drive, and slowness; but, particularly in persons previously with energetic, restless, or aggressive characteristics, there may be a change towards impulsiveness, boastfulness, temper outbursts, silly fatuous humor, and the development of unrealistic ambitions; the direction of change usually depends upon the previous personality. A considerable degree of recovery is possible and may continue over the course of several years.[1]

Fugue, psychogenic – A form of dissociative hysteria characterized by an episode of wandering with inability to recall one's prior identity. Both onset and recovery are rapid. Following recovery there is no recollection of events which took place during the fugue state.[2]

Ganser's syndrome (hysterical) – A form of factitious illness in which the patient voluntarily produces symptoms suggestive of a mental disorder.[2]

Gender identity disorder — *see* Gender identity disorder under Psychosexual identity disorders

Gilles de la Tourette's disorder or syndrome — *see* Gilles de la Tourette's disorder under Tics

Grief reaction — *see* Depressive reaction, brief under Adjustment reaction

Gross stress reaction — *see* Stress reaction, acute

Group delinquency — *see* Socialized conduct disorder under Conduct disorders

Habit spasm — *see* Chronic motor tic disorder under Tics

Hangover (alcohol) — *see* Drunkenness, simple

Head-banging — *see* Stereotyped repetitive movements

Hebephrenia — *see* Schizophrenia, disorganized type

Heller's syndrome — *see* Psychosis, disintegrative

High grade defect — *see* Mental retardation, mild

Homosexuality – Exclusive or predominant sexual attraction for persons of the same sex with or without physical relationship. Record homosexuality as a diagnosis whether or not it is considered as a mental disorder.[1]

Hospital addiction syndrome — *see* Munchausen syndrome

Hospital hoboes — *see* Munchausen syndrome

Hospitalism – A mild or transient adjustment reaction characterized by withdrawal seen in hospitalized patients. In young children this may be manifested by elective mutism.[1]

Hyperkinetic syndrome of childhood – Disorders in which the essential features are short attention span and distractibility. In early childhood the most striking symptom is disinhibited, poorly organized and poorly regulated extreme overactivity but in adolescence this may be replaced by underactivity. Impulsiveness, marked mood fluctuations, and aggression are also common symptoms. Delays in the development of specific skills are often present and disturbed, poor relationships are common. If the hyperkinesis is symptomatic of an underlying disorder, the diagnosis of the underlying disorder is recorded instead.[1]

attention deficit disorder – Cases of hyperkinetic syndrome in which short attention span, distractibility, and overactivity are the main manifestations without significant disturbance of conduct or delay in specific skills.[1]

hyperkinesis with developmental delay – Cases in which the hyperkinetic syndrome is associated with speech delay, clumsiness, reading difficulties, or other delays of specific skills.[1]

hyperkinetic conduct disorder – Cases in which the hyperkinetic syndrome is associated with marked conduct disturbance but not developmental delay.[1]

Hypersomnia – A disorder of initiating arousal from sleep or maintaining wakefulness.[2]

persistent – Chronic difficulty in initiating arousal from sleep or maintaining wakefulness associated with major or minor depressive mental disorders.[2]

transient – Episodes of difficulty in arousal from sleep or maintaining wakefulness associated with acute or intermittent emotional reactions or conflicts.[2]

Hypochondriasis — *see* Hypochondriasis under Neurotic disorders

Hypomania — *see* Affective psychosis, manic type

Hypomanic personality — *see* Personality disorder, chronic hypomanic type

Hyposomnia — *see* Insomnia

Hysteria — *see* Hysteria under Neurotic disorders

anxiety — *see* Phobia under Neurotic disorders

psychosis — *see* Psychosis, reactive
acute — *see* Psychosis, excitative type

Hysterical personality — *see* Personality disorder, histrionic type

Identity disorder – An emotional disorder caused by distress over the inability to reconcile aspects of the self into a relatively coherent and acceptable sense of self, not secondary to another mental disorder. The disturbance is manifested by intense subjective distress regarding uncertainty about a variety of issues relating to identity, including long-term goals, career choice, friendship patterns, values, and loyalties.[2]

Idiocy — *see* Mental retardation, profound

Imbecile — *see* Mental retardation, moderate

Impotence – A psychosexual dysfunction in which there is partial or complete failure to attain or maintain erection until completion of the sexual act.[2]

Impulse control disorder — *see* Impulse control disorders under Conduct disorders

Inadequate personality — *see* Personality disorder, dependent type

Induced paranoid disorder — *see* Shared paranoid disorder

Inebriety — *see* Drunkenness, simple

Infantile autism — *see* Autism, infantile

Insomnia – A disorder of initiating or maintaining sleep.[2]

persistent – A chronic state of sleeplessness associated with chronic anxiety, major or minor depressive disorders, or psychoses.[2]

transient – Episodes of sleeplessness associated with acute or intermittent emotional reactions or conflicts.[2]

Intermittent explosive disorder – Recurrent episodes of sudden and significant loss of control of aggressive impulses, not accounted for by any other mental disorder, which results in serious assault or destruction of property. The magnitude of the behavior during an episode is grossly out of proportion to any psychosocial stressors which may have played a role in eliciting the episode of lack of control. Following each episode there is genuine regret or self-reproach at the consequences of the action and the inability to control the aggressive impulse.[2]

Introverted disorder of childhood – An emotional disturbance in children chiefly manifested by a lack of interest in social relationships and indifference to social praise or criticism.[2]

Introverted personality — *see* Personality disorder, introverted type

Involutional melancholia — *see* Affective psychosis, depressed type

Involutional paranoid state — *see* Paraphrenia

Isolated explosive disorder – A disorder of impulse control in which there is a single discrete episode characterized by failure to resist an impulse which leads to a single, violent externally-directed act, which has a catastrophic impact on others, and for which the available information does not justify the diagnosis of another mental disorder.[2]

Isolated phobia — *see* Simple phobia under Phobia

Jet lag syndrome – A phase-shift disruption of the 24-hour sleep-wake cycle due to rapid time-zone changes experienced in long-distance travel.[2]

Kanner's syndrome — *see* Autism, infantile

Kleptomania – A disorder of impulse control characterized by a recurrent failure to resist impulses to steal objects not for immediate use or their monetary value. An increasing sense of tension is experienced prior to committing the act, with an intense experience of gratification at the time of committing the theft.[2]

Korsakoff's psychosis
  alcoholic — *see* Alcohol amnestic syndrome under Alcoholic psychoses
  nonalcoholic — *see* Amnestic syndrome

Latent schizophrenia — *see* Schizophrenia, latent

Lesbianism — *see* Homosexuality

Lobotomy syndrome — *see* Frontal lobe syndrome

LSD reaction – Acute intoxication from hallucinogen abuse, manifested by hallucinatory states lasting only a few days or less.[1]

Major depressive disorder — *see* Affective psychosis, depressed type

Malingering – A clinical picture in which the predominant feature is the presentation of fake or grossly exaggerated physical or psychiatric illness apparently under voluntary control. In contrast to factitious illness, the symptoms produced in malingering are in pursuit of a goal which, when known, is recognizable and obviously understandable in light of knowledge of the individual's circumstances. Examples of understandable goals include, but are not limited to, becoming a "patient" in order to avoid conscription or military duty, avoid work, obtain financial compensation, evade criminal prosecution, and obtain drugs.[2]

Mania (monopolar) — *see* Affective psychosis, manic type

Manic-depressive psychosis
  circular type — *see* Affective psychosis, bipolar

depressed type — *see* Affective psychosis, depressed type
  manic type — *see* Affective psychosis, manic type
  mixed type — *see* Affective psychosis, mixed type

Manic disorder — *see* Affective psychosis, manic type
  atypical — *see* Affective psychosis, manic type, atypical

Masochistic personality — *see* Personality disorder, masochistic type

Melancholia — *see* Affective psychoses
  involutional — *see* Affective psychosis, depressed type

Mental retardation – A condition of arrested or incomplete development of mind which is especially characterized by subnormality of intelligence. The coding should be made on the individual's *current* level of functioning *without regard to its nature* or causation, such as psychosis, cultural deprivation, Down's syndrome, etc. Where there is a specific cognitive handicap — such as in speech — the diagnosis of mental retardation should be based on assessments of cognition *outside the area of specific handicap*. The assessment of intellectual level should be based on whatever information is available, including clinical evidence, adaptive behavior, and psychometric findings. The IQ levels given are based on a test with a mean of 100 and a standard deviation of 15, such as the Wechsler scales. They are provided only as a guide and should not be applied rigidly. Mental retardation often involves psychiatric disturbances and may often develop as a result of some physical disease or injury. In these cases, an additional diagnosis should be recorded to identify any associated condition, psychiatric or physical.[1]

mild mental retardation – IQ criteria 50–70. Individuals with this level of retardation are usually educable. During the preschool period they can develop social and communication skills, have minimal retardation in sensorimotor areas, and often are not distinguished from normal children until a later age. During the school age period they can learn academic skills up to approximately the sixth-grade level. During the adult years, they can usually achieve social and vocational skills adequate for minimum self-support, but may need guidance and assistance when under social or economic stress.[1]

moderate mental retardation – IQ criteria 35–49. Individuals with this level of retardation are usually trainable. During the preschool period they can talk or learn to communicate. They have poor social awareness and fair motor development. During the school age period they can profit from training in social and occupational skills, but they are unlikely to progress beyond the second-grade level in academic subjects. During their adult years they may achieve self-maintenance in unskilled or semi-skilled work under sheltered conditions. They need supervision and guidance when under mild social or economic stress.[2]

severe mental retardation – IQ criteria 20–34. Individuals with this level of retardation evidence poor motor development, minimal speech, and are generally unable to profit from training and self-help during the preschool period. During the school age period they can talk or learn to communicate, can be trained in elementary health habits, and may profit from systematic habit training. During the adult years they may contribute partially to self-maintenance under complete supervision.[2]

profound mental retardation – IQ criteria under 20. Individuals with this level of retardation evidence minimal capacity for sensorimotor functioning and need nursing care during the preschool period. During the school age period some further motor development may occur, and they may respond to minimal or limited training in self-help. During the adult years some motor and speech development may occur, and they may achieve very limited self-care and need nursing care.[2]

Merycism — *see* Rumination, psychogenic

Minimal brain dysfunction [MBD] — *see* Hyperkinetic syndrome of childhood

Misery and unhappiness disorder – An emotional disorder characteristic of childhood in which the main symptoms involve misery and unhappiness. There may also be eating and sleep disturbances.

Mood swings (brief compensatory) (rebound) – Mild disorders of mood (depression and anxiety or elation and excitement, occurring alternatingly or episodically) seen in affective psychosis.[1]

Motor tic disorders — *see* Tics

Motor-verbal tic disorder — *see* Gilles de la Tourette's disorder under Tics

Multi-infarct dementia or psychosis — *see* Arteriosclerotic dementia

Multiple operations syndrome — *see* Munchausen syndrome

Multiple personality – A form of dissociative hysteria in which there is the domination of the individual at any one time by one of two or more distinct personalities. Each personality is a fully-integrated and complex unit with memories, behavior patterns, and social friendships which determine the nature of the individual's acts when uppermost in consciousness.[2]

Munchausen syndrome – A chronic form of factitious illness in which the individual demonstrates a plausible presentation of voluntarily produced physical symptomatology of such a degree that he is able to obtain and sustain multiple hospitalizations.[2]

Narcissistic personality — *see* Personality disorder, narcissistic type

Nervous debility — *see* Neurasthenia under Neurotic disorders

Neurasthenia — *see* Neurasthenia under Neurotic disorders

Neurotic delinquency — *see* Mixed disturbance of conduct and emotions under Conduct disorders

Neurotic disorders – Neurotic disorders are mental disorders without any demonstrable organic basis in which the individual may have considerable insight and has unimpaired reality testing, in that he usually does not confuse his morbid subjective experiences and fantasies with external reality. Behavior may be greatly affected although usually remaining within socially acceptable limits, but personality is not disorganized. The principal manifestations include excessive anxiety, hysterical symptoms, phobias, obsessional and compulsive symptoms, and depression.[1]

anxiety states – Various combinations of physical and mental manifestations of anxiety, not attributable to real danger and occurring either in attacks [see Anxiety state, panic attacks] or as a persisting state [see Anxiety state, generalized]. The anxiety is usually diffuse and may extend to panic. Other neurotic features such as obsessional or hysterical symptoms may be present but do not dominate the clinical picture.[1]

compensation neurosis – Certain unconscious neurotic reactions in which features of secondary gain, such as a situational or financial advantage, are prominent.[3]

depersonalization – A neurotic disorder with an unpleasant state of disturbed perception in which external objects or parts of one's own body are experienced as changed in their quality, unreal, remote, or automatized. The patient is aware of the subjective nature of the change he experiences. If depersonalization occurs as a feature of anxiety, schizophrenia, or other mental disorder, the condition is classified according to the major psychiatric disorder.[1]

depression – A neurotic disorder characterized by disproportionate depression which has usually recognizably ensued on a distressing experience; it does not include among its features delusions or hallucinations, and there is often preoccupation with the psychic trauma which preceded the illness, e.g., loss of a cherished person or possession. Anxiety is also frequently present and mixed states of anxiety and depression should be included here. The distinction between depressive neurosis and psychosis should be made not only upon the degree of depression but also on the presence or absence of other neurotic and psychotic characteristics, and upon the degree of disturbance of the individual's behavior.[1]

hypochondriasis – A neurotic disorder in which the conspicuous features are excessive concern with one's health in general or the integrity and functioning of some part of one's body, or less frequently, one's mind. It is usually associated with anxiety and depression. It may occur as a feature of some other severe mental disorder (e.g., manic-depressive psychosis, depressed type, schizophrenia, hysteria) and in that case should be classified according to the corresponding major disorder.[1]

hysteria – A neurotic mental disorder in which motives, of which the patient seems unaware, produce either a restriction of the field of consciousness or disturbances of motor or sensory function which may seem to have psychological advantage or symbolic value.[1] There are three subtypes –

conversion type – The chief or only symptoms of the hysterical neurosis consist of psychogenic disturbance of function in some part of the body, e.g., paralysis, tremor, blindness, deafness, seizures.[1]

dissociative type – The most prominent feature of the hysterical neurosis is a narrowing of the field of consciousness which seems to serve an unconscious purpose and is commonly accompanied or followed by a selective amnesia. There may be dramatic but essentially superficial changes of personality [multiple personality], or sometimes the patient enters into a wandering state [fugue].[1]

factitious illness – Physical or psychological symptoms that are not real, genuine, or natural, which are produced by the individual and are under his voluntary control.[2]

neurasthenia – A neurotic disorder characterized by fatigue, irritability, headache, depression, insomnia, difficulty in concentration, and lack of capacity for enjoyment [anhedonia]. It may follow or accompany an infection or exhaustion, or arise from continued emotional stress. If neurasthenia is associated with a physical disorder, the latter should also be recorded as a diagnosis.[1]

obsessive-compulsive – States in which the outstanding symptom is a feeling of subjective compulsion, which must be resisted, to carry out some action, to dwell on an idea, to recall an experience, or to ruminate on an abstract topic. Unwanted thoughts which intrude, the insistency of words or ideas, ruminations or trains of thought are perceived by the individual to be inappropriate or nonsensical. The obsessional urge or idea is recognized as alien to the personality but as coming from within the self. Obsessional actions may be quasi-ritual performances designed to relieve anxiety, e.g., washing the hands to cope with contamination. Attempts to dispel the unwelcome thoughts or urges may lead to a severe inner struggle, with intense anxiety.[1]

occupational – A neurosis characterized by a functional disorder of a group of muscles used chiefly in one's occupation, marked by the occurrence of spasm, paresis, or incoordination on attempt to repeat the habitual movements (e.g., writer's cramp).[5]

phobic disorders – Neurotic states with abnormally intense dread of certain objects or specific situations which would not normally have that effect. If the anxiety tends to spread from a specified situation or object to a wider range of circumstances, it becomes

akin to or identical with anxiety state and should be classified as such.[1] See also Phobia.

somatization disorder – A chronic, but fluctuating, neurotic disorder which begins early in life and is characterized by recurrent and multiple somatic complaints for which medical attention is sought but which are not apparently due to any physical illness. Complaints are presented in a dramatic, vague, or exaggerated way, or are part of a complicated medical history in which often many specific diagnoses have allegedly been made by other physicians. Complaints invariably refer to many organ systems (headache, fatigue, palpitations, fainting, nausea and vomiting, abdominal pains, bowel trouble, allergies, menstrual and sexual difficulties), and the individual frequently receives medical care from a number of physicians, sometimes simultaneously.[2]

Neurosis — see Neurotic disorders

Nightmares – Anxiety attacks occurring in dreams during REM sleep.[2]

Night terrors – A pathology of arousal from stage 4 sleep in which the individual experiences excessive terror and extreme panic (screaming, verbalizations), symptoms of autonomic activity, confusion, and poor recall for event.[2]

Nymphomania – Abnormal and excessive need or desire in the woman for sexual intercourse.[3]

Obsessional personality — see Personality disorder, compulsive type

Occupational neurosis — see Neurotic disorder, occupational

Oneirophrenia — see Schizophrenia, acute episode

Oppositional disorder of childhood or adolescence – A disorder characterized by pervasive opposition to all in authority regardless of self-interest, a continuous argumentativeness, and an unwillingness to respond to reasonable persuasion, not accounted for by a conduct disorder, adjustment disorder, or a psychosis of childhood. The oppositional behavior in this disorder is evoked by any demand, rule, suggestion, request, or admonishment placed on the individual.[2]

Organic affective syndrome – A clinical picture in which the predominating symptoms closely resemble those seen in either the depressive or manic affective disorders, occurring in the presence of evidence or history of a specific organic factor which is etiologically related to the disturbance, such as head trauma, endocranial tumors, and exocranial tumors secreting neurotoxic diatheses (e.g., pancreatic carcinoma). Excessive use of steroids, Cushing's syndrome, and other endocrine disorders may lead to an organic affective syndrome.[2]

Organic personality syndrome – Chronic, mild states of memory disturbance and intellectual deterioration, of nonpsychotic nature, often accompanied by increased irritability, querulousness, lassitude, and complaints of physical weakness. These states are often associated with old age, and may precede more severe states due to brain damage classifiable under senile

Appendix B: Glossary of Mental Disorders

or presenile dementia, dementia associated with other chronic organic psychotic brain syndromes, or delirium, delusions, hallucinosis, and depression in transient organic psychotic conditions.[1]

Organic psychosyndrome, focal (partial) – A nonpsychotic organic mental disorder resembling the postconcussion syndrome associated with localized diseases of the brain or surrounding tissues.[1]

Organic psychotic conditions – Syndromes in which there is impairment of orientation, memory, comprehension, calculation, learning capacity, and judgment. These are the essential features but there may also be shallowness or lability of affect, or a more persistent disturbance of mood, lowering of ethical standards and exaggeration or emergence of personality traits, and diminished capacity for independent decision.[1] *See also* Alcohol psychoses, Arteriosclerotic dementia, Drug psychoses, Presenile dementia, and Senile dementia.

mixed paranoid and affective – Organic psychosis in which depressive and paranoid symptoms are the main features.[1]

transient – States characterized by clouded consciousness, confusion, disorientation, illusions, and often vivid hallucinations. They are usually due to some intra- or extracerebral toxic, infectious, metabolic or other systemic disturbance and are generally reversible. Depressive and paranoid symptoms may also be present but are not the main feature. The diagnosis of the associated physical or neurological condition should also be recorded.[1]

acute delirium – Short-lived states, lasting hours or days, of the above type.[1]

subacute delirium – States of the above type in which the symptoms, usually less florid, last for several weeks or longer during which they may show marked fluctuations in intensity.[1]

Organic reaction — *see* Organic psychotic conditions, transient

Overanxious disorder – An ill-defined emotional disorder characteristic of childhood in which the main symptoms involve anxiety and fearfulness.[1]

Panic disorder — *see* Panic attack under Anxiety state

Paranoia – A rare chronic psychosis in which logically constructed systematized delusions have developed gradually without concomitant hallucinations or the schizophrenic type of disordered thinking. The delusions are mostly of grandeur (the paranoiac prophet or inventor), persecution, or somatic abnormality.[1]

alcoholic — *see* Alcoholic jealousy under Alcoholic psychoses

querulans – A paranoid state which, though in many ways akin to schizophrenic or affective states, differs from other paranoid states and psychogenic paranoid psychosis.[1]

senile — *see* Paraphrenia

Paranoid personality — *see* Personality disorder, paranoid type

Paranoid reaction, acute – Paranoid states apparently provoked by some emotional stress. The stress is often misconstrued as an attack or threat. Such states are particularly prone to occur in prisoners or as acute reactions to a strange and threatening environment, e.g., in immigrants.[1]

Paranoid schizophrenia — *see* Schizophrenia, paranoid type

Paranoid state

involutional — *see* Paraphrenia

senile — *see* Paraphrenia

simple – A psychosis, acute or chronic, not classifiable as schizophrenia or affective psychosis, in which delusions, especially of being influenced, persecuted, or treated in some special way, are the main symptoms. The delusions are of a fairly fixed, elaborate, and systematized kind.[1]

Paranoid traits — *see* Personality disorder, paranoid type

Paraphilia — *see* Sexual deviations

Paraphrenia – Paranoid psychosis in which there are conspicuous hallucinations, often in several modalities. Affective symptoms and disordered thinking, if present, do not dominate the clinical picture, and the personality is well preserved.[1]

Paraphrenic schizophrenia — *see* Schizophrenia, paranoid type

Passive-aggressive personality — *see* Personality disorder, passive-aggressive type

Passive personality — *see* Personality disorder, dependent type

Pathological

alcohol intoxication — *see* Alcohol intoxication, idiosyncratic

drug intoxication – Individual idiosyncratic reactions to comparatively small quantities of a drug, which take the form of acute, brief psychotic states of any type.[1]

drunkenness — *see* Alcohol intoxication, idiosyncratic

gambling – A disorder of impulse control characterized by a chronic and progressive preoccupation with gambling and urge to gamble, with subsequent gambling behavior that compromises, disrupts, or damages personal, family, and vocational pursuits.[2]

personality — *see* Personality disorder

Pedophilia – Sexual deviations in which an adult engages in sexual activity with a child of the same or opposite sex.[1]

Peregrinating patient — *see* Malingering

Personality disorders – Deeply ingrained maladaptive patterns of behavior generally recognizable by the time of adolescence or earlier and continuing throughout most of adult life, although often becoming less obvious in middle or old age. The personality is abnormal either in the balance of its components, their quality and expression, or in its total aspect. Because of this deviation or psychopathy the patient suffers or others have to suffer, and there is an adverse effect upon the individual or on society. It includes what is sometimes called psychopathic personality, but if this is determined primarily by malfunctioning of the brain, it should be classified as one of the nonpsychotic organic brain syndromes. When the patient exhibits an anomaly of personality directly related to his neurosis or psychosis, e.g., schizoid personality and schizophrenia or anancastic personality and obsessive compulsive neurosis, the relevant neurosis or psychosis which is in evidence should be diagnosed in addition.[1]

affective type – A chronic personality disorder characterized by lifelong predominance of a pronounced mood. The illness does not have a clear onset, and there may be intermittent periods of disturbed mood separated by periods of normal mood.[1]

anancastic [anankastic] type — *see* Personality disorder, compulsive type

antisocial type – A personality disorder characterized by disregard for social obligations, lack of feeling for others, and impetuous violence or callous unconcern. There is a gross disparity between behavior and the prevailing social norms. Behavior is not readily modifiable by experience, including punishment. People with this personality are often affectively cold, and may be abnormally aggressive or irresponsible. Their tolerance to frustration is low; they blame others or offer plausible rationalizations for the behavior which brings them into conflict with society.[1]

asthenic type — *see* Personality disorder, dependent type

avoidant type – Individuals with this disorder exhibit excessive social inhibitions and shyness, a tendency to withdraw from opportunities for developing close relationships, and a fearful expectation that they will be belittled and humiliated. Desires for affection and acceptance are strong, but they are unwilling to enter relationships unless given unusually strong guarantees that they will be uncritically accepted. Therefore, they have few close relationships and suffer from feelings of loneliness and isolation.[2]

borderline type – Individuals with this disorder are characterized by instability in a variety of areas, including interpersonal relationships, behavior, mood, and self image. Interpersonal relationships are often intense and unstable with marked shifts of attitude over time. Frequently there is impulsive and unpredictable behavior which is potentially physically self-damaging. There may be problems tolerating being alone, and chronic feelings of emptiness or boredom.[2]

chronic depressive type – An affective personality disorder characterized by lifelong predominance of a chronic nonpsychotic disturbance involving either intermittent or sustained periods of depressed mood (marked by worry, pessimism, low output of energy, and a sense of futility).[2]

chronic hypomanic type – An affective personality disorder characterized by lifelong predominance of a chronic nonpsychotic disturbance involving either intermittent or sustained periods of abnormally elevated mood (unshakable optimism and an enhanced zest for life and activity).[2]

compulsive type – A personality disorder characterized by feelings of personal insecurity, doubt, and incompleteness leading to excessive conscientiousness, checking, stubbornness, and caution. There may be insistent and unwelcome thoughts or impulses which do not attain the severity of an obsessional neurosis. There is perfectionism and meticulous accuracy and a need to check repeatedly in an attempt to ensure this. Rigidity and excessive doubt may be conspicuous.[1]

cyclothymic type – A chronic nonpsychotic disturbance involving depressed and elevated mood, lasting at least two years, separated by periods of normal mood.[2]

dependent type – A personality disorder characterized by passive compliance with the wishes of elders and others and a weak inadequate response to the demands of daily life. Lack of vigor may show itself in the intellectual or emotional spheres; there is little capacity for enjoyment.[1]

eccentric type – A personality disorder characterized by oddities of behavior which do not conform to the clinical syndromes of personality disorders described elsewhere.[2]

explosive type – A personality disorder characterized by instability of mood with liability to intemperate outbursts of anger, hate, violence, or affection. Aggression may be expressed in words or in physical violence. The outbursts cannot readily be controlled by the affected persons, who are not otherwise prone to antisocial behavior.[1]

histrionic type – A personality disorder characterized by shallow, labile affectivity, dependence on others, craving for appreciation and attention, suggestibility, and theatricality. There is often sexual immaturity, e.g., frigidity and over-responsiveness to stimuli. Under stress hysterical symptoms [neurosis] may develop.[1]

hysterical type — *see* Personality disorder, histrionic type

inadequate type — *see* Personality disorder, dependent type

introverted type – A form of schizoid personality in which the essential features are a profound defect in the ability to form social relationships and to respond to the usual forms of social reinforcements. Such patients are characteristically "loners" who do not appear distressed by their social distance and are not interested in greater social involvement.[2]

masochistic type – A personality disorder in which the individual appears to arrange life situations so as to be defeated and humiliated.[2]

narcissistic type – A personality disorder in which interpersonal difficulties are caused by an inflated sense of self-worth, and indifference to the welfare of others. Achievement deficits and social irresponsibilities are justified and sustained by a boastful arrogance, expansive fantasies, facile rationalization, and frank prevarication.[2]

paranoid type – A personality disorder in which there is excessive sensitiveness to setbacks or to what are taken to be humiliations and rebuffs, a tendency to distort experience by misconstruing the neutral or friendly actions of others as hostile or contemptuous, and a combative and tenacious sense of personal rights. There may be a proneness to jealousy or excessive self-importance. Such persons may feel helplessly humiliated and put upon; others, likewise excessively sensitive, are aggressive and insistent. In all cases there is excessive self-reference.[1]

passive-aggressive type – A personality disorder characterized by aggressive behavior manifested in passive ways, such as obstructionism, pouting, procrastination, intentional inefficiency, or stubbornness. The *aggression* often arises from resentment at failing to find gratification in a relationship with an individual or institution upon which the individual is overdependent.[3]

passive type — *see* Personality disorder, dependent type

schizoid type – A personality disorder in which there is withdrawal from affectional, social, and other contacts with autistic preference for fantasy and introspective reserve. Behavior may be slightly eccentric or indicate avoidance of competitive situations. Apparent coolness and detachment may mask an incapacity to express feeling.[1]

schizotypal type – A form of schizoid personality in which individuals with this disorder manifest various oddities of thinking, perception, communication, and behavior. The disturbance in thinking may be expressed as magical thinking, ideas of reference, or paranoid ideation. Perceptual disturbances may include recurrent illusions and derealization [depersonalization]. Frequently, but not invariably, the behavioral manifestations include social isolation and constricted or inappropriate affect which interferes with rapport in face-to-face interaction without any of the frank psychotic features which characterize schizophrenia.[2]

Phobia – Neurotic states with abnormally intense dread of certain objects or specific situations which would not normally have that effect. If the anxiety tends to spread from a specified situation or object to a wider range of circumstances, it becomes akin to or identical with anxiety state, and should be classified as such.[1]

acrophobia – Fear of heights[3]

agoraphobia – Fear of leaving the familiar setting of the home, and is almost always preceded by a phase during which there are recurrent panic attacks. Because of the anticipatory fear of helplessness when having a panic attack, the patient is reluctant or refuses to be alone, travel or walk alone, or to be in situations where there is no ready access to help, such as in crowds, closed or open spaces, or crowded stores.[2]

ailurophobia – Fear of cats[3]

algophobia – Fear of pain[3]

claustrophobia – Fear of closed spaces[3]

isolated phobia — *see* Simple phobia below

mysophobia – Fear of dirt or germs[3]

obsessional — *see* Neurotic disorder, obsessive-compulsive

panphobia – Fear of everything[3]

simple phobia – Fear of a discrete object or situation which is neither fear of leaving the familiar setting of the home [agoraphobia], or of being observed by others in certain situations [social phobia]. Examples of simple phobia are fear of animals, acrophobia, and claustrophobia.[2]

social phobia – Fear of situations in which the subject is exposed to possible scrutiny by others, and the possibility exists that he may act in a fashion that will be considered shameful. The most common social phobias are fears of public speaking, blushing, eating in public, writing in front of others, or using public lavatories.[2]

xenophobia – Fear of strangers[3]

Pica – Perverted appetite of nonorganic origin in which there is persistent eating of non-nutritional substances. Typically, infants ingest paint, plaster, string, hair, or cloth. Older children may have access to animal droppings, sand, bugs, leaves, or pebbles. In the adult, eating of starch or clay-earth has been observed.[2]

Postconcussion syndrome – States occurring after generalized contusion of the brain, in which the symptom picture may resemble that of the frontal lobe syndrome or that of any of the neurotic disorders, but in which in addition, headache, giddiness, fatigue, insomnia, and a subjective feeling of impaired intellectual ability are usually prominent. Mood may fluctuate, and quite ordinary stress may produce exaggerated fear and apprehension. There may be marked intolerance of mental and physical exertion, undue sensitivity to noise, and hypochondriacal preoccupation. The symptoms are more common in persons who have previously suffered from neurotic or personality disorders, or when there is a possibility of compensation. This syndrome is particularly associated with the closed type of head injury when signs of localized brain damage are slight or absent, but it may also occur in other conditions.[1]

Postcontusion syndrome or encephalopathy — *see* Postconcussion syndrome

Postencephalitic syndrome – A nonpsychotic organic mental disorder resembling the postconcussion syndrome associated with central nervous system infections.[1]

Postleucotomy syndrome — *see* Frontal lobe syndrome

Posttraumatic brain syndrome, nonpsychotic — *see* Postconcussion syndrome

Posttraumatic organic psychosis — *see* Organic psychotic conditions, transient

Posttraumatic stress disorder – The development of characteristic symptoms (re-experiencing the traumatic event, numbing of responsiveness to or involvement with the external world, and a variety of other autonomic, dysphoric, or cognitive symptoms) after experiencing a psychologically traumatic event or events outside the normal range of human experience (e.g., rape or assault, military combat, natural catastrophes such as flood or earthquake, or other disaster, such as airplane crash, fires, bombings).[2]

acute – Brief, episodic, or recurrent disorders lasting less than six months' duration after the onset of trauma.[2]

prolonged – Chronic disorders of the above type lasting six months or more following the trauma.[2]

Premature ejaculation — *see* Premature ejaculation under Psychosexual dysfunctions

Prepsychotic schizophrenia — *see* Schizophrenia, latent

Presbyophrenia — *see* Organic personality syndrome

Presenile dementia – Dementia occurring usually before the age of 65 in patients with the relatively rare forms of diffuse or lobar cerebral atrophy. The associated neurological condition (e.g., Alzheimer's disease, Pick's disease, Jakob-Creutzfeldt disease) should also be recorded as a diagnosis.[1]

Prodromal schizophrenia — *see* Schizophrenia, latent

Pseudoneurotic schizophrenia — *see* Schizophrenia, latent

Psychalgia – Pains of mental origin, e.g., headache or backache, for which a more precise medical or psychiatric diagnosis cannot be made.[1]

Psychasthenia – A functioning neurosis marked by stages of pathological fear or anxiety, obsessions, fixed ideas, tics, feelings of inadequacy, self-accusation, and pecular feelings of strangeness, unreality, and depersonalization.[4]

Psychic shock – A sudden disturbance of mental equilibrium produced by strong emotion in response to physical or mental stress.[4]

Psychic factors associated with physical diseases – Mental disturbances or psychic factors of any type thought to have played a major part in the etiology of physical conditions, usually involving tissue damage, classified elsewhere. The mental disturbance is usually mild and nonspecific, and the psychic factors (worry, fear, conflict, etc.) may be present without any overt psychiatric disorder. Examples of these conditions are asthma, dermatitis, eczema, duodenal ulcer, ulcerative colitis, and urticaria, specified as due to psychogenic factors. Use an additional diagnosis to identify the physical condition. In the rare instance that an overt psychiatric disorder is thought to have caused the physical condition, the psychiatric diagnosis should be recorded in addition.[1]

Psychoneurosis — *see* Neurotic disorders

Psycho-organic syndrome — *see* Organic psychotic conditions, transient

Psychopathic constitutional state — *see* Personality disorders

Psychopathic personality — *see* Personality disorders

Psychophysiological disorders – A variety of physical symptoms or types of physiological malfunctions of mental origin, not involving tissue damage, and usually mediated through the autonomic nervous system. The disorders are classified according to the body system involved. If the physical symptom is secondary to a psychiatric disorder classifiable elsewhere, the physical symptom is not classified as a psychophysiological disorder. If tissue damage is involved, then the diagnosis is classified as a *Psychic factor associated with diseases classified elsewhere*.[1]

Psychosexual dysfunctions – A group of disorders in which there is recurrent and persistent dysfunction encountered during sexual activity. The dysfunction may be lifelong or acquired, generalized or situational, and total or partial.[2]

functional dyspareunia – Recurrent and persistent genital pain associated with coitus.[2]

functional vaginismus – A history of recurrent and persistent involuntary spasm of the musculature of the outer one-third of the vagina that interferes with sexual activity.[2]

inhibited female orgasm – Recurrent and persistent inhibition of the female orgasm as manifested by a delay or absence of orgasm following a normal sexual excitement phase during sexual activity.[2]

inhibited male orgasm – Recurrent and persistent inhibition of the male orgasm as manifested by a delay or absence of either the emission or ejaculation phases, or more usually, both following an adequate phase of sexual excitement.[2]

inhibited sexual desire – Persistent inhibition of desire for engaging in a particular form of sexual activity.[2]

inhibited sexual excitement – Recurrent and persistent inhibition of sexual excitement during sexual activity, manifested either by partial or complete failure to attain or maintain erection until completion of the sexual act [impotence], or partial or complete failure to attain or maintain the lubrication-swelling response of sexual excitement until completion of the sexual act [frigidity].[2]

premature ejaculation – Ejaculation occurs before the individual wishes it, because of recurrent and persistent absence of reasonable voluntary control of ejaculation and orgasm during sexual activity.[2]

Psychosexual gender identity disorders – Behavior occurring in preadolescents of immature psychosexuality, or in adults, in which there is an incongruence between the individual's anatomic sex and gender identity.[2]

gender identity disorder – In children or in adults a condition in which the individual would prefer to be of the other sex, and strongly prefers the clothes, toys, activities, and companionship of the other sex. Cross-dressing is intermittent, although it may be frequent. In children the commonest form is feminism in boys.[2]

trans-sexualism – A psychosexual identity disorder centered around fixed beliefs that the overt bodily sex is wrong. The resulting behavior is directed towards either changing the sexual organs by operation, or completely concealing the bodily sex by adopting both the dress and behavior of the opposite sex.[1]

Psychosomatic disorders — *see* Psychophysiological disorders

Psychosis – Mental disorders in which impairment of mental function has developed to a degree that interferes grossly with insight, ability to meet some ordinary demands of life or to maintain adequate contact with reality. It is not an exact or well defined term. Mental retardation is excluded.[1]

affective — *see* Affective psychoses

alcoholic — *see* Alcoholic psychoses

atypical childhood – A variety of atypical infantile psychoses which may show some, but not all, of the features of infantile autism. Symptoms may include stereotyped repetitive movements, hyperkinesis, self-injury, retarded speech development, echolalia, and impaired social relationships. Such disorders may occur in children of any level of intelligence but are particularly common in those with mental retardation.[1]

borderline, of childhood — *see* Psychosis, atypical childhood

child – A group of disorders in children, characterized by distortions in the timing, rate, and sequence of many psychological functions involving language development and social relations in which the severe qualitative abnormalities are not normal for any stage of development.[2] *See also* Autism, infantile, Psychosis, disintegrative, Psychosis, atypical childhood.

depressive — *see* Affective psychosis, depressed type

depressive type – A depressive psychosis which can be similar in its symptoms to manic-depressive psychosis, depressed type but is apparently provoked by saddening stress such as a bereavement, or a severe disappointment or frustration. There may be less diurnal variation of symptoms than in manic-depressive psychosis, depressed type, and the delusions are more often understandable in the context of the life experiences. There is usually a serious disturbance of behavior, e.g., major suicidal attempt.[1]

disintegrative – A disorder in which normal or near-normal development for the first few years is followed by a loss of social skills and of speech, together with a severe disorder of emotions, behavior, and relationships. Usually this loss of speech and of social competence takes place over a period of a few months and is accompanied by the emergence of overactivity and of stereotypies. In most cases there is intellectual impairment, but this is not a necessary part of the disorder. The condition may follow overt brain disease, such as measles encephalitis, but it may also occur in the absence of any known organic brain disease or damage. Any associated neurological disorder should also be recorded.[1]

epileptic – An organic psychotic condition associated with epilepsy.[1]

excitative type – An affective psychosis similar in its symptoms to manic-depressive psychosis, manic type, but apparently provoked by emotional stress.[1]

hypomanic — see Affective psychosis, manic type

hysterical — see Psychosis, reactive
  acute — see Psychosis, excitative type

induced — see Shared paranoid disorder

infantile — see Autism, infantile

infective — see Organic psychotic conditions, transient

Korsakoff's
  alcoholic — see alcohol amnestic syndrome under Alcoholic psychoses
  nonalcoholic — see Amnestic syndrome

manic-depressive — see Affective psychoses

multi-infarct — see Arteriosclerotic dementia

paranoid
  chronic — see Paranoia
  protracted reactive — see Psychosis, paranoid, psychogenic
  psychogenic – Psychogenic or reactive paranoid psychosis of any type which is more protracted than the reactions described under Paranoid reaction, acute.[1]
    acute — see Paranoid reaction, acute

postpartum — see Psychosis, puerperal

psychogenic — see Psychosis, reactive
  depressive — see Psychosis, depressive type

puerperal – Any psychosis occurring within a fixed period (approximately 90 days) after childbirth.[3] The diagnosis should be classified according to the predominant symptoms or characteristics, such as schizophrenia, affective psychosis, paranoid states, or other specified psychosis.

reactive – A psychotic condition which is largely or entirely attributable to a recent life experience. This diagnosis is not used for the wider range of psychoses in which environmental factors play some, but not the *major*, part in etiology.[1]
  brief – A florid psychosis of at least a few hours' duration but lasting no more than two weeks, with sudden onset immediately following a severe environmental stress and eventually terminating in complete recovery to the pre-psychotic state.[2]
  confusion – Mental disorders with clouded consciousness, disorientation (though less marked than in organic confusion), and diminished accessibility often accompanied by excessive activity and apparently provoked by emotional stress.[1]
  depressive — see Psychosis, depressive type
  schizo-affective — see Schizophrenia, schizo-affective type

schizophrenic — see Schizophrenia

schizophreniform — see Schizophrenia
  affective type — see Schizophrenia, schizo-affective type
  confusional type — see Schizophrenia, acute episode
  senile — see Senile dementia, delusional type

Pyromania – A disorder of impulse control characterized by a recurrent failure to resist impulses to set fires without regard for the consequences, or with deliberate destructive intent. Invariably there is intense fascination with the setting of fires, seeing fires burn, and a satisfaction with the resultant destruction.[2]

Relationship problems of childhood – Emotional disorders characteristic of childhood in which the main symptoms involve relationship problems.[1]

Repeated infarct dementia — see Arteriosclerotic dementia

Residual schizophrenia — see Schizophrenia, residual type

Restzustand (schizophrenia) — see Schizophrenia, residual type

Rumination
  obsessional – The constant preoccupation with certain thoughts, with inability to dismiss them from the mind.[4] See Neurotic disorder, obsessive-compulsive.
  psychogenic – In children the regurgitation of food, with failure to thrive or weight loss developing after a period of normal functioning. Food is brought up without nausea, retching, or disgust. The food is then ejected from the mouth, or chewed and reswallowed.[2]

Sander's disease — see Paranoia

Satyriasis – Pathologic or exaggerated sexual desire or excitement in the man.[3]

Schizoid personality disorder — see Personality disorder, schizoid type

Schizophrenia – A group of psychoses in which there is a fundamental disturbance of personality, a characteristic distortion of thinking, often a sense of being controlled by alien forces, delusions which may be bizarre, disturbed perception, abnormal affect out of keeping with the real situation, and autism. Nevertheless, clear consciousness and intellectual capacity are usually maintained. The disturbance of personality involves its most basic functions which give the normal person his feeling of individuality, uniqueness, and self-direction. The most intimate thoughts, feelings, and acts are often felt to be known to or shared by others and explanatory delusions may develop, to the effect that natural or supernatural forces are at work to influence the schizophrenic person's thoughts and actions in ways that are often bizarre. He may see himself as the pivot of all that happens. Hallucinations, especially of hearing, are common and may comment on the patient or address him. Perception is frequently disturbed in other ways; there may be perplexity, irrelevant features may become all-important and accompanied by passivity feelings, may lead the patient to believe that everyday objects and situations possess a special, usually sinister, meaning intended for him. In the characteristic schizophrenic disturbance of thinking, peripheral and irrelevant features of a total concept, which are inhibited in normal directed mental activity, are brought to the forefront and utilized in place of the elements relevant and appropriate to the situation. Thus, thinking becomes vague, elliptical and obscure, and its expression in speech sometimes incomprehensible. Breaks and interpolations in the flow of consecutive thought are frequent, and the patient may be convinced that his thoughts are being withdrawn by some outside agency. Mood may be shallow, capricious, or incongruous. Ambivalence and disturbance of volition may appear as inertia, negativism, or stupor. Catatonia may be present. The diagnosis "schizophrenia" should not be made unless there is, or has been evident during the same illness, characteristic disturbance of thought, perception, mood, conduct, or personality — preferably in at least two of these areas. The diagnosis should not be restricted to conditions running a protracted, deteriorating, or chronic course. In addition to making the diagnosis on the criteria just given, effort should be made to specify one of the following subtypes of schizophrenia, according to the predominant symptoms.[1]
  acute (undifferentiated) – Schizophrenia of florid nature which cannot be classified as simple, catatonic, hebephrenic, paranoid, or any other types.[1]
  acute episode – Schizophrenic disorders, other than simple, hebephrenic, catatonic, and paranoid, in which there is a dream-like state with slight clouding of consciousness and perplexity. External things, people, and events may become charged with personal significance for the patient. There may be ideas of reference and emotional turmoil. In many such cases remission occurs within a few weeks or months, even without treatment.[1]
  atypical — see Schizophrenia, acute (undifferentiated)
  borderline — see Schizophrenia, latent
  catatonic type – Includes as an essential feature prominent psychomotor disturbances often alternating between extremes such as hyperkinesis and stupor, or automatic obedience and negativism. Constrained attitudes may be maintained for long periods – if the patient's limbs are put in some unnatural position, they may be held there for some time after the external force has been removed. Severe excitement may be a striking feature of the condition. Depressive or hypomanic concomitants may be present.[1]
  cenesthopathic — see Schizophrenia, acute (undifferentiated)
  childhood type — see Psychosis, child
  chronic undifferentiated — see Schizophrenia, residual
  cyclic — see Schizophrenia, schizo-affective type
  disorganized type – A form of schizophrenia in which affective changes are prominent, delusions and hallucinations fleeting and fragmentary, behav-

Appendix B: Glossary of Mental Disorders

ior irresponsible and unpredictable, and mannerisms common. The mood is shallow and inappropriate, accompanied by giggling or self-satisfied, self-absorbed smiling, or by a lofty manner, grimaces, mannerisms, pranks, hypochondriacal complaints, and reiterated phrases. Thought is disorganized. There is a tendency to remain solitary, and behavior seems empty of purpose and feeling. This form of schizophrenia usually starts between the ages of 15 and 25 years.[1]

hebephrenic type — see Schizophrenia, disorganized type

latent – It has not been possible to produce a generally acceptable description for this condition. It is not recommended for general use, but a description is provided for those who believe it to be useful – a condition of eccentric or inconsequent behavior and anomalies of affect which give the impression of schizophrenia though no definite and characteristic schizophrenic anomalies, present or past, have been manifest.[1]

paranoid type – The form of schizophrenia in which relatively stable delusions, which may be accompanied by hallucinations, dominate the clinical picture. The delusions are frequently of persecution, but may take other forms (for example, of jealousy, exalted birth, Messianic mission, or bodily change). Hallucinations and erratic behavior may occur; in some cases conduct is seriously disturbed from the outset, thought disorder may be gross, and affective flattening with fragmentary delusions and hallucinations may develop.[1]

prepsychotic — see Schizophrenia, latent

prodromal — see Schizophrenia, latent

pseudoneurotic — see Schizophrenia, latent

pseudopsychopathic — see Schizophrenia, latent

residual – A chronic form of schizophrenia in which the symptoms that persist from the acute phase have mostly lost their sharpness. Emotional response is blunted and thought disorder, even when gross, does not prevent the accomplishment of routine work.[1]

schizo-affective type – A psychosis in which pronounced manic or depressive features are intermingled with schizophrenic features and which tends towards remission without permanent defect, but which is prone to recur. The diagnosis should be made only when both the affective and schizophrenic symptoms are pronounced.[1]

simple type – A psychosis in which there is insidious development of oddities of conduct, inability to meet the demands of society, and decline in total performance. Delusions and hallucinations are not in evidence and the condition is less obviously psychotic than are the hebephrenic, catatonic, and paranoid types of schizophrenia. With increasing social impoverishment vagrancy may ensue and the patient becomes self-absorbed, idle, and aim-

less. Because the schizophrenic symptoms are not clear-cut, diagnosis of this form should be made sparingly, if at all.[1]

simplex — see Schizophrenia, simple type

Schizophrenic syndrome of childhood — see Psychosis, child

Schizophreniform

attack — see Schizophrenia, acute episode

disorder — see Schizophrenia, acute episode

psychosis — see Schizophrenia

affective type — see Schizophrenia, schizo-affective type

confusional type — see Schizophrenia, acute episode

Schizotypal personality — see Personality disorder, schizotypal type

Senile dementia – Dementia occurring usually after the age of 65 in which any cerebral pathology other than that of senile atrophic change can be reasonably excluded.[1]

delirium – Senile dementia with a superimposed reversible episode of acute confusional state.[1]

delusional type – A type of senile dementia characterized by development in advanced old age, progressive in nature, in which delusions, varying from simple poorly formed paranoid delusions to highly formed paranoid delusional states, and hallucinations are also present.[1, 2]

depressed type – A type of senile dementia characterized by development in advanced old age, progressive in nature, in which depressive features, ranging from mild to severe forms of manic-depressive affective psychosis, are also present. Disturbance of the sleep-waking cycle and preoccupation with dead people are often particularly prominent.[1, 2]

paranoid type — see Senile dementia, delusional type

simple type — see Senile dementia

Sensitiver Beziehungswahn – A paranoid state which, though in many ways akin to schizophrenic or affective states, differs from paranoia, simple paranoid state, shared paranoid disorder, or psychogenic psychosis.[1]

Sensitivity reaction of childhood or adolescence — see Shyness disorder of childhood

Separation anxiety disorder – A clinical disorder in children in which the predominant disturbance is exaggerated distress at separation from parents, home, or other familial surroundings. When separation is instituted, the child may experience anxiety to the point of panic. In adults a similar disorder is seen in agoraphobic reactions.[2]

Sexual deviations – Abnormal sexual inclinations or behavior which are part of a referral problem. The limits and features of normal sexual behavior have not been stated absolutely in different societies and cultures, but are broadly such as serve approved social and biological purposes. The sexual activity of affected persons is directed primarily either towards people not of the opposite sex, or

towards sexual acts not associated with coitus normally, or towards coitus performed under abnormal circumstances. If the anomalous behavior becomes manifest only during psychosis or other mental illness the condition should be classified under the major illness. It is common for more than one anomaly to occur together in the same individual; in that case the predominant deviation is classified. It is preferable not to diagnose sexual deviation in individuals who perform deviant sexual acts when normal sexual outlets are not available to them.[1] See also Exhibitionism, Fetishism, Homosexuality, Nymphomania, Pedophilia, Satyriasis, Sexual masochism, Sexual sadism, Transvestism, Voyeurism, and Zoophilia. Gender identity disorder and trans-sexualism are considered to be psychosexual gender identity disorders and are not included here.

Sexual masochism – A sexual deviation in which sexual arousal and pleasure is produced in an individual by his own physical or psychological suffering, and in which there are insistent and persistent fantasies wherein sexual excitement is produced as a result of suffering.[2]

Sexual sadism – A sexual deviation in which physical or psychological suffering inflicted on another person is utilized as a method of stimulating erotic excitement and orgasm, and in which there are insistent and persistent fantasies wherein sexual excitement is produced as a result of suffering inflicted on the partner.[2]

Shared paranoid disorder – Mainly delusional psychosis, usually chronic and often without florid features, which appears to have developed as a result of a close, if not dependent, relationship with another person who already has an established similar psychosis. The delusions are at least partly shared. The rare cases in which several persons are affected should also be included here.[1]

Shifting sleep-work schedule – A sleep disorder in which the phase-shift disruption of the 24-hour sleep-wake cycle occurs due to rapid changes in the individual's work schedule.[2]

Short sleeper – Individuals who typically need only 4–6 hours of sleep within the 24-hour cycle.[2]

Shyness disorder of childhood – A persistent and excessive shrinking from familiarity or contact with all strangers of sufficient severity as to interfere with peer functioning, yet there are warm and satisfying relationships with family members. A critical feature of this disorder is that the avoidant behavior with strangers persists even after prolonged exposure or contact.[2]

Sibling jealousy or rivalry – An emotional disorder related to competition between siblings for the love of a parent or for other recognition or gain.[3]

Simple phobia — see Simple phobia under Phobia

Situational disturbance, acute — see Stress reaction, acute

Social phobia — see Social phobia under Phobia

Social withdrawal of childhood — *see* Introverted disorder of childhood

Socialized conduct disorder — *see* Socialized conduct disorder under Conduct disorders

Somatization disorder — *see* Somatization disorder under Neurotic disorders

Somatoform disorder, atypical — *see* Hypochondriasis under Neurotic disorders

Spasmus nutans — *see* Stereotyped repetitive movements

Specific academic or work inhibition – An adjustment reaction in which a specific academic or work inhibition occurs in an individual whose intellectual capacity, skills, and previous academic or work performance have been at least adequate, and in which the inhibition occurs despite apparent effort and is not due to any other mental disorder.[2]

Stammering — *see* Stuttering

Starch-eating — *see* Pica

Status postcommotio cerebri — *see* Postconcussion syndrome

Stereotyped repetitive movements – Disorders in which voluntary repetitive stereotyped movements, which are not due to any psychiatric or neurological condition, constitute the main feature. Includes head-banging, spasmus nutans, rocking, twirling, finger-flicking mannerisms, and eye poking. Such movements are particularly common in cases of mental retardation with sensory impairment or with environmental monotony.[1]

Stereotypies — *see* Stereotyped repetitive movements

Stress reaction

  acute – Acute transient disorders of any severity and nature of emotions, consciousness, and psychomotor states (singly or in combination) which occur in individuals, without any apparent pre-existing mental disorder, in response to exceptional physical or mental stress, such as natural catastrophe or battle, and which usually subside within hours or days.[1]

  chronic — *see* Adjustment reaction

Stupor

  catatonic — *see* Schizophrenia, catatonic type

  psychogenic — *see* Psychosis, reactive

Stuttering – Disorders in the rhythm of speech, in which the individual knows precisely what he wishes to say, but at the time is unable to say it because of an involuntary, repetitive prolongation or cessation of a sound.[1]

Subjective insomnia complaint – A complaint of insomnia made by the individual, which has not been investigated or proven.[2]

Tension headache – Headache of mental origin for which a more precise medical or psychiatric diagnosis cannot be made.[1]

Systematized delusions — *see* Paranoia

Tics – Disorders of no known organic origin in which the outstanding feature consists of quick, involuntary, apparently purposeless, and frequently repeated movements which are not due to any neurological condition. Any part of the body may be involved but the face is most frequently affected. Only one form of tic may be present, or there may be a combination of tics which are carried out simultaneously, alternatively, or consecutively.[1]

  chronic motor tic disorder – A tic disorder starting in childhood and persisting into adult life. The tic is limited to no more than three motor areas, and rarely has a verbal component.[2]

  Gilles de la Tourette's disorder [motor-verbal tic disorder] – A rare disorder occurring in individuals of any level of intelligence in which facial tics and tic-like throat noises become more marked and more generalized, and in which later whole words or short sentences (often with obscene content) are ejaculated spasmodically and involuntarily. There is some overlap with other varieties of tic.[1]

  transient tic disorder of childhood – Facial or other tics beginning in childhood, but limited to one year in duration.[2]

Tobacco use disorder – Cases in which tobacco is used to the detriment of a person's health or social functioning or in which there is tobacco dependence. Dependence is included here rather than under drug dependence because tobacco differs from other drugs of dependence in its psychotoxic effects.[1]

Tranquilizer abuse – Cases where an individual has taken the drug to the detriment of his health or social functioning, in doses above or for periods beyond those normally regarded as therapeutic.[1]

Transient organic psychotic condition — *see* Organic psychotic conditions, transient

Trans-sexualism — *see* Trans-sexualism under Psychosexual identity disorders

Transvestism – Sexual deviation in which there is recurrent and persistent dressing in clothes of the opposite sex, and initially in the early stage of the illness, for the purpose of sexual arousal.[2]

Twilight state

  confusional — *see* Delirium, acute

  psychogenic — *see* Psychosis, reactive confusion

Undersocialized conduct disorder — *see* Undersocialized conduct disorder under Conduct disorders

Unsocialized aggressive disorder — *see* Undersocialized conduct disorder, aggressive type under Conduct disorders

Vaginismus, functional — *see* Functional vaginismus under Psychosexual dysfunctions

Vorbeireden – The symptom of the approximate answer or talking past the point, seen in the Ganser syndrome, a form of factitious illness.[2]

Voyeurism – A sexual deviation in which the individual repetitively seeks out situations in which he engages in looking at unsuspecting women who are either naked, in the act of disrobing, or engaging in sexual activity. The act of looking is accompanied by sexual excitement, frequently with orgasm. In its severe form, the act of peeping constitutes the preferred to exclusive sexual activity of the individual.[2]

Wernicke-Korsakoff syndrome — *see* Alcohol amnestic syndrome under Alcoholic psychoses

Withdrawal reaction of childhood or adolescence — *see* Introverted disorder of childhood

Word-deafness – A developmental delay in the comprehension of speech sounds.[1]

Zoophilia – Sexual or anal intercourse with animals.[1]

CLASSIFICATION OF DRUGS BY AMERICAN HOSPITAL FORMULARY SERVICE LIST NUMBER AND THEIR ICD-9-CM EQUIVALENTS

The coding of adverse effects of drugs is keyed to the continually revised Hospital Formulary of the American Hospital Formulary Service (AHFS) published under the direction of the American Society of Hospital Pharmacists.

The following section gives the ICD-9-CM diagnosis code for each AHFS list.

	AHFS* List	ICD-9-CM Diagnosis Code
4:00	ANTIHISTAMINE DRUGS	963.0
8:00	ANTI-INFECTIVE AGENTS	
8:04	Amebacides	961.5
	hydroxyquinoline derivatives	961.3
	arsenical anti-infectives	961.1
8:08	Anthelmintics	961.6
	quinoline derivatives	961.3
8:12.04	Antifungal Antibiotics	960.1
	nonantibiotics	961.9
8:12.06	Cephalosporins	960.5
8:12.08	Chloramphenicol	960.2
8:12.12	The Erythromycins	960.3
8:12.16	The Penicillins	960.0
8:12.20	The Streptomycins	960.6
8:12.24	The Tetracyclines	960.4
8:12.28	Other Antibiotics	960.8
	antimycobacterial antibiotics	960.6
	macrolides	960.3
8:16	Antituberculars	961.8
	antibiotics	960.6
8:18	Antivirals	961.7
8:20	Plasmodicides (antimalarials)	961.4
8:24	Sulfonamides	961.0
8:26	The Sulfones	961.8
8:28	Treponemicides	961.2
8:32	Trichomonacides	961.5
	hydroxyquinoline derivatives	961.3
	nitrofuran derivatives	961.9
8:36	Urinary Germicides	961.9
	quinoline derivatives	961.3
8:40	Other Anti-Infectives	961.9
10:00	ANTINEOPLASTIC AGENTS	963.1
	antibiotics	960.7
	progestogens	962.2
12:00	AUTONOMIC DRUGS	
12:04	Parasympathomimetic (Cholinergic) Agents	971.0
12:08	Parasympatholytic (Cholinergic Blocking) Agents	971.1
12:12	Sympathomimetic (Adrenergic) Agents	971.2
12:16	Sympatholytic (Adrenergic Blocking) Agents	971.3
12:20	Skeletal Muscle Relaxants	975.2
	central nervous system muscle-tone depressants	968.0
16:00	BLOOD DERIVATIVES	964.7
20:00	BLOOD FORMATION AND COAGULATION	
20:04	Antianemia Drugs	964.1
20:04.04	Iron Preparations	964.0
20:04.08	Liver and Stomach Preparations	964.1
20:12.04	Anticoagulants	964.2
20:12.08	Antiheparin Agents	964.5
20:12.12	Coagulants	964.5
20.12.16	Hemostatics	964.5
	capillary-active drugs	972.8
	fibrinolysis-affecting agents	964.4
	natural products	964.7
24:00	CARDIOVASCULAR DRUGS	
24:04	Cardiac Drugs	972.9
	cardiotonic agents	972.1
	rhythm regulators	972.0
24:06	Antilipemic Agents	972.2
	thyroid derivatives	962.7
24:08	Hypotensive Agents	972.6
	adrenergic blocking agents	971.3
	ganglion-blocking agents	972.3
	vasodilators	972.5

	AHFS* List	ICD-9-CM Diagnosis Code
24:12	Vasodilating Agents	972.5
	coronary	972.4
	nicotinic acid derivatives	972.2
24:16	Sclerosing Agents	972.7
28:00	CENTRAL NERVOUS SYSTEM DRUGS	
28:04	General Anesthetics	968.4
	gaseous anesthetics	968.2
	halothane	968.1
	intravenous anesthetics	968.3
28:08	Analgesics and Antipyretics	965.9
	antirheumatics	965.6
	aromatic analgesics	965.4
	non-narcotics NEC	965.7
	opium alkaloids	965.00
	heroin	965.01
	methadone	965.02
	specified type NEC	965.09
	pyrazole derivatives	965.5
	salicylates	965.1
	specified type NEC	965.8
28:10	Narcotic Antagonists	970.1
28:12	Anticonvulsants	966.3
	barbiturates	967.0
	benzodiazepine-based tranquilizers	969.4
	bromides	967.3
	hydantoin derivatives	966.1
	oxazolidine derivative	966.0
	succinimides	966.2
28:16.04	Antidepressants	969.0
28:16.08	Tranquilizers	969.5
	benzodiazepine-based	969.4
	butyrophenone-based	969.2
	major NEC	969.3
	phenothiazine-based	969.1
28:16.12	Other Psychotherapeutic Agents	969.8
28:20	Respiratory and Cerebral Stimulants	970.9
	analeptics	970.0
	anorexigenic agents	977.0
	psychostimulants	969.7
	specified type NEC	970.8
28:24	Sedatives and Hypnotics	967.9
	barbiturates	967.0
	benzodiazepine-based tranquilizers	969.4
	chloral hydrate group	967.1
	glutethamide group	967.5
	intravenous anesthetics	968.3
	methaqualone	967.4
	paraldehyde	967.2
	phenothiazine-based tranquilizers	969.1
	specified type NEC	967.8
	thiobarbiturates	968.3
	tranquilizer NEC	969.5
36:00	DIAGNOSTIC AGENTS	977.8
40:00	ELECTROLYTE, CALORIC, AND WATER BALANCE AGENTS NEC	974.5
40:04	Acidifying Agents	963.2
40:08	Alkalinizing Agents	963.3
40:10	Ammonia Detoxicants	974.5
40:12	Replacement Solutions NEC	974.5
	plasma volume expanders	964.8
40:16	Sodium-Removing Resins	974.5
40:18	Potassium-Removing Resins	974.5
40:20	Caloric Agents	974.5
40:24	Salt and Sugar Substitutes	974.5
40:28	Diuretics NEC	974.4
	carbonic acid anhydrase inhibitors	974.2
	mercurials	974.0
	purine derivatives	974.1
	saluretics	974.3
40:36	Irrigating Solutions	974.5
40:40	Uricosuric Agents	974.7
44:00	ENZYMES NEC	963.4
	fibrinolysis-affecting agents	964.4
	gastric agents	973.4

Appendix C: Classification of Drugs by AHFS List

AHFS* List	ICD-9-CM Diagnosis Code
48:00 EXPECTORANTS AND COUGH PREPARATIONS	
antihistamine agents	963.0
antitussives	975.4
codeine derivatives	965.09
expectorants	975.5
narcotic agents NEC	965.09
52:00 EYE, EAR, NOSE, AND THROAT PREPARATIONS	
52:04 Anti-Infectives	
ENT	976.6
ophthalmic	976.5
52:04.04 Antibiotics	
ENT	976.6
ophthalmic	976.5
52:04.06 Antivirals	
ENT	976.6
ophthalmic	976.5
52:04.08 Sulfonamides	
ENT	976.6
ophthalmic	976.5
52:04.12 Miscellaneous Anti-Infectives	
ENT	976.6
ophthalmic	976.5
52:08 Anti-Inflammatory Agents	
ENT	976.6
ophthalmic	976.5
52:10 Carbonic Anhydrase Inhibitors	974.2
52:12 Contact Lens Solutions	976.5
52:16 Local Anesthetics	968.5
52:20 Miotics	971.0
52:24 Mydriatics	
adrenergics	971.2
anticholinergics	971.1
antimuscarinics	971.1
parasympatholytics	971.1
spasmolytics	971.1
sympathomimetics	971.2
52:28 Mouth Washes and Gargles	976.6
52:32 Vasoconstrictors	971.2
52:36 Unclassified Agents	
ENT	976.6
ophthalmic	976.5
56:00 GASTROINTESTINAL DRUGS	
56:04 Antacids and Absorbents	973.0
56:08 Anti-Diarrhea Agents	973.5
56:10 Antiflatulents	973.8
56:12 Cathartics NEC	973.3
emollients	973.2
irritants	973.1
56:16 Digestants	973.4
56:20 Emetics and Antiemetics	
antiemetics	963.0
emetics	973.6
56:24 Lipotropic Agents	977.1
60:00 GOLD COMPOUNDS	965.6
64:00 HEAVY METAL ANTAGONISTS	963.8
68:00 HORMONES AND SYNTHETIC SUBSTITUTES	
68:04 Adrenals	962.0
68:08 Androgens	962.1
68:12 Contraceptives	962.2
68:16 Estrogens	962.2
68:18 Gonadotropins	962.4
68:20 Insulins and Antidiabetic Agents	962.3
68:20.08 Insulins	962.3
68:24 Parathyroid	962.6
68:28 Pituitary	
anterior	962.4
posterior	962.5
68:32 Progestogens	962.2
68:34 Other Corpus Luteum Hormones	962.2
68:36 Thyroid and Antithyroid	
antithyroid	962.8
thyroid	962.7

AHFS* List	ICD-9-CM Diagnosis Code
72:00 LOCAL ANESTHETICS NEC	968.9
topical (surface) agents	968.5
infiltrating agents (intradermal) (subcutaneous) (submucosal)	968.5
nerve blocking agents (peripheral) (plexus) (regional)	968.6
spinal	968.7
76:00 OXYTOCICS	975.0
78:00 RADIOACTIVE AGENTS	990
80:00 SERUMS, TOXOIDS, AND VACCINES	
80:04 Serums	979.9
immune globulin (gamma) (human)	964.6
80:08 Toxoids NEC	978.8
diphtheria	978.5
and tetanus	978.9
with pertussis component	978.6
tetanus	978.4
and diphtheria	978.9
with pertussis component	978.6
80:12 Vaccines NEC	979.9
bacterial NEC	978.8
with	
other bacterial component	978.9
pertussis component	978.6
viral and rickettsial component	979.7
rickettsial NEC	979.6
with	
bacterial component	979.7
pertussis component	978.6
viral component	979.7
viral NEC	979.6
with	
bacterial component	979.7
pertussis component	978.6
rickettsial component	979.7
84:00 SKIN AND MUCOUS MEMBRANE PREPARATIONS	
84:04 Anti-Infectives	976.0
84:04.04 Antibiotics	976.0
84:04.08 Fungicides	976.0
84:04.12 Scabicides and Pediculicides	976.0
84:04.16 Miscellaneous Local Anti-Infectives	976.0
84:06 Anti-Inflammatory Agents	976.0
84:08 Antipruritics and Local Anesthetics	
antipruritics	976.1
local anesthetics	968.5
84:12 Astringents	976.2
84:16 Cell Stimulants and Proliferants	976.8
84:20 Detergents	976.2
84:24 Emollients, Demulcents, and Protectants	976.3
84:28 Keratolytic Agents	976.4
84:32 Keratoplastic Agents	976.4
84:36 Miscellaneous Agents	976.8
86:00 SPASMOLYTIC AGENTS	975.1
antiasthmatics	975.7
papaverine	972.5
theophyllin	974.1
88:00 VITAMINS	
88:04 Vitamin A	963.5
88:08 Vitamin B Complex	963.5
hematopoietic vitamin	964.1
nicotinic acid derivatives	972.2
88:12 Vitamin C	963.5
88:16 Vitamin D	963.5
88:20 Vitamin E	963.5
88:24 Vitamin K Activity	964.3
88:28 Multivitamin Preparations	963.5
92:00 UNCLASSIFIED THERAPEUTIC AGENTS	977.8

* American Hospital Formulary Service

CLASSIFICATION OF INDUSTRIAL ACCIDENTS ACCORDING TO AGENCY

Annex B to the Resolution concerning Statistics of Employment Injuries adopted by the Tenth International Conference of Labor Statisticians on 12 October 1962

1 MACHINES

11 Prime-Movers, except Electrical Motors
111 *Steam engines*
112 *Internal combustion engines*
119 *Others*
12 Transmission Machinery
121 *Transmission shafts*
122 *Transmission belts, cables, pulleys, pinions, chains, gears*
129 *Others*
13 Metalworking Machines
131 *Power presses*
132 *Lathes*
133 *Milling machines*
134 *Abrasive wheels*
135 *Mechanical shears*
136 *Forging machines*
137 *Rolling-mills*
139 *Others*
14 Wood and Assimilated Machines
141 *Circular saws*
142 *Other saws*
143 *Molding machines*
144 *Overhand planes*
149 *Others*
15 Agricultural Machines
151 *Reapers (including combine reapers)*
152 *Threshers*
159 *Others*
16 Mining Machinery
161 *Under-cutters*
169 *Others*
19 Other Machines Not Elsewhere Classified
191 *Earth-moving machines, excavating and scraping machines, except means of transport*
192 *Spinning, weaving and other textile machines*
193 *Machines for the manufacture of foodstuffs and beverages*
194 *Machines for the manufacture of paper*
195 *Printing machines*
199 *Others*

2 MEANS OF TRANSPORT AND LIFTING EQUIPMENT

21 Lifting Machines and Appliances
211 *Cranes*
212 *Lifts and elevators*
213 *Winches*
214 *Pulley blocks*
219 *Others*
22 Means of Rail Transport
221 *Inter-urban railways*
222 *Rail transport in mines, tunnels, quarries, industrial establishments, docks, etc.*
229 *Others*
23 Other Wheeled Means of Transport, Excluding Rail Transport
231 *Tractors*
232 *Lorries*
233 *Trucks*
234 *Motor vehicles, not elsewhere classified*
235 *Animal-drawn vehicles*
236 *Hand-drawn vehicles*
239 *Others*
24 Means of Air Transport
25 Means of Water Transport
251 *Motorized means of water transport*
252 *Non-motorized means of water transport*
26 Other Means of Transport
261 *Cable-cars*
262 *Mechanical conveyors, except cable-cars*
269 *Others*

3 OTHER EQUIPMENT

31 Pressure Vessels
311 *Boilers*
312 *Pressurized containers*
313 *Pressurized piping and accessories*
314 *Gas cylinders*
315 *Caissons, diving equipment*
319 *Others*
32 Furnaces, Ovens, Kilns
321 *Blast furnaces*
322 *Refining furnaces*
323 *Other furnaces*
324 *Kilns*
325 *Ovens*
33 Refrigerating Plants
34 Electrical Installations, Including Electric Motors, but Excluding Electric Hand Tools
341 *Rotating machines*
342 *Conductors*
343 *Transformers*
344 *Control apparatus*
349 *Others*
35 Electric Hand Tools
36 Tools, Implements, and Appliances, Except Electric Hand Tools
361 *Power-driven hand tools, except electric hand tools*
362 *Hand tools, not power-driven*
369 *Others*
37 Ladders, Mobile Ramps
38 Scaffolding
39 Other Equipment, Not Elsewhere Classified

4 MATERIALS, SUBSTANCES AND RADIATIONS

41 Explosives
42 Dusts, Gases, Liquids and Chemicals, Excluding Explosives
421 *Dusts*
422 *Gases, vapors, fumes*
423 *Liquids, not elsewhere classified*
424 *Chemicals, not elsewhere classified*
43 Flying Fragments
44 Radiations
441 *Ionizing radiations*
449 *Others*
49 Other Materials and Substances Not Elsewhere Classified

5 WORKING ENVIRONMENT

51 Outdoor
511 *Weather*
512 *Traffic and working surfaces*
513 *Water*
519 *Others*
52 Indoor
521 *Floors*
522 *Confined quarters*
523 *Stairs*
524 *Other traffic and working surfaces*
525 *Floor openings and wall openings*
526 *Environmental factors (lighting, ventilation, temperature, noise, etc.)*
529 *Others*
53 Underground
531 *Roofs and faces of mine roads and tunnels, etc.*
532 *Floors of mine roads and tunnels, etc.*
533 *Working-faces of mines, tunnels, etc.*
534 *Mine shafts*
535 *Fire*
536 *Water*
539 *Others*

6 OTHER AGENCIES, NOT ELSEWHERE CLASSIFIED

61 Animals
611 *Live animals*
612 *Animal products*
69 Other Agencies, Not Elsewhere Classified

7 AGENCIES NOT CLASSIFIED FOR LACK OF SUFFICIENT DATA

LIST OF THREE-DIGIT CATEGORIES

1. INFECTIOUS AND PARASITIC DISEASES

Intestinal infectious diseases (001-009)
001 Cholera
002 Typhoid and paratyphoid fevers
003 Other salmonella infections
004 Shigellosis
005 Other food poisoning (bacterial)
006 Amebiasis
007 Other protozoal intestinal diseases
008 Intestinal infections due to other organisms
009 Ill-defined intestinal infections

Tuberculosis (010-018)
010 Primary tuberculous infection
011 Pulmonary tuberculosis
012 Other respiratory tuberculosis
013 Tuberculosis of meninges and central nervous system
014 Tuberculosis of intestines, peritoneum, and mesenteric glands
015 Tuberculosis of bones and joints
016 Tuberculosis of genitourinary system
017 Tuberculosis of other organs
018 Miliary tuberculosis

Zoonotic bacterial diseases (020-027)
020 Plague
021 Tularemia
022 Anthrax
023 Brucellosis
024 Glanders
025 Melioidosis
026 Rat-bite fever
027 Other zoonotic bacterial diseases

Other bacterial diseases (030-042)
030 Leprosy
031 Diseases due to other mycobacteria
032 Diphtheria
033 Whooping cough
034 Streptococcal sore throat and scarlatina
035 Erysipelas
036 Meningococcal infection
037 Tetanus
038 Septicemia
039 Actinomycotic infections
040 Other bacterial diseases
041 Bacterial infection in conditions classified elsewhere and of unspecified site

Human immunodeficiency virus (042)
042 Human immunodeficiency virus [HIV] disease

Poliomyelitis and other non-arthropod-borne viral diseases of central nervous system (045-049)
045 Acute poliomyelitis
046 Slow virus infection of central nervous system
047 Meningitis due to enterovirus
048 Other enterovirus diseases of central nervous system
049 Other non-arthropod-borne viral diseases of central nervous system

Viral diseases accompanied by exanthem (050-057)
050 Smallpox
051 Cowpox and paravaccinia
052 Chickenpox
053 Herpes zoster
054 Herpes simplex
055 Measles
056 Rubella
057 Other viral exanthemata

Arthropod-borne viral diseases (060-066)
060 Yellow fever
061 Dengue
062 Mosquito-borne viral encephalitis
063 Tick-borne viral encephalitis
064 Viral encephalitis transmitted by other and unspecified arthropods
065 Arthropod-borne hemorrhagic fever
066 Other arthropod-borne viral diseases

Other diseases due to viruses and Chlamydiae (070-079)
070 Viral hepatitis
071 Rabies
072 Mumps
073 Ornithosis
074 Specific diseases due to Coxsackievirus
075 Infectious mononucleosis
076 Trachoma
077 Other diseases of conjunctiva due to viruses and Chlamydiae
078 Other diseases due to viruses and Chlamydiae
079 Viral infection in conditions classified elsewhere and of unspecified site

Rickettsioses and other arthropod-borne diseases (080-088)
080 Louse-borne [epidemic] typhus
081 Other typhus
082 Tick-borne rickettsioses
083 Other rickettsioses
084 Malaria
085 Leishmaniasis
086 Trypanosomiasis
087 Relapsing fever
088 Other arthropod-borne diseases

Syphilis and other venereal diseases (090-099)
090 Congenital syphilis
091 Early syphilis, symptomatic
092 Early syphilis, latent
093 Cardiovascular syphilis
094 Neurosyphilis
095 Other forms of late syphilis, with symptoms
096 Late syphilis, latent
097 Other and unspecified syphilis
098 Gonococcal infections
099 Other venereal diseases

Other spirochetal diseases (100-104)
100 Leptospirosis
101 Vincent's angina
102 Yaws
103 Pinta
104 Other spirochetal infection

Mycoses (110-118)
110 Dermatophytosis
111 Dermatomycosis, other and unspecified
112 Candidiasis
114 Coccidioidomycosis
115 Histoplasmosis
116 Blastomycotic infection
117 Other mycoses
118 Opportunistic mycoses

Helminthiases (120-129)
120 Schistosomiasis [bilharziasis]
121 Other trematode infections
122 Echinococcosis
123 Other cestode infection
124 Trichinosis
125 Filarial infection and dracontiasis
126 Ancylostomiasis and necatoriasis
127 Other intestinal helminthiases
128 Other and unspecified helminthiases
129 Intestinal parasitism, unspecified

Other infectious and parasitic diseases (130-136)
130 Toxoplasmosis
131 Trichomoniasis
132 Pediculosis and phthirus infestation
133 Acariasis
134 Other infestation
135 Sarcoidosis
136 Other and unspecified infectious and parasitic diseases

Late effects of infectious and parasitic diseases (137-139)
137 Late effects of tuberculosis
138 Late effects of acute poliomyelitis
139 Late effects of other infectious and parasitic diseases

2. NEOPLASMS

Malignant neoplasm of lip, oral cavity, and pharynx (140-149)
140 Malignant neoplasm of lip
141 Malignant neoplasm of tongue
142 Malignant neoplasm of major salivary glands
143 Malignant neoplasm of gum
144 Malignant neoplasm of floor of mouth
145 Malignant neoplasm of other and unspecified parts of mouth
146 Malignant neoplasm of oropharynx
147 Malignant neoplasm of nasopharynx
148 Malignant neoplasm of hypopharynx
149 Malignant neoplasm of other and ill-defined sites within the lip, oral cavity, and pharynx

Malignant neoplasm of digestive organs and peritoneum (150-159)
150 Malignant neoplasm of esophagus
151 Malignant neoplasm of stomach
152 Malignant neoplasm of small intestine, including duodenum
153 Malignant neoplasm of colon
154 Malignant neoplasm of rectum, rectosigmoid junction, and anus
155 Malignant neoplasm of liver and intrahepatic bile ducts
156 Malignant neoplasm of gallbladder and extrahepatic bile ducts
157 Malignant neoplasm of pancreas
158 Malignant neoplasm of retroperitoneum and peritoneum
159 Malignant neoplasm of other and ill-defined sites within the digestive organs and peritoneum

Malignant neoplasm of respiratory and intrathoracic organs (160-165)
160 Malignant neoplasm of nasal cavities, middle ear, and accessory sinuses
161 Malignant neoplasm of larynx
162 Malignant neoplasm of trachea, bronchus, and lung
163 Malignant neoplasm of pleura
164 Malignant neoplasm of thymus, heart, and mediastinum
165 Malignant neoplasm of other and ill-defined sites within the respiratory system and intrathoracic organs

Malignant neoplasm of bone, connective tissue, skin, and breast (170-176)

170　Malignant neoplasm of bone and articular cartilage
171　Malignant neoplasm of connective and other soft tissue
172　Malignant melanoma of skin
173　Other malignant neoplasm of skin
174　Malignant neoplasm of female breast
175　Malignant neoplasm of male breast

Kaposi's sarcoma (176)

176　Kaposi's sarcoma

Malignant neoplasm of genitourinary organs (179-189)

179　Malignant neoplasm of uterus, part unspecified
180　Malignant neoplasm of cervix uteri
181　Malignant neoplasm of placenta
182　Malignant neoplasm of body of uterus
183　Malignant neoplasm of ovary and other uterine adnexa
184　Malignant neoplasm of other and unspecified female genital organs
185　Malignant neoplasm of prostate
186　Malignant neoplasm of testis
187　Malignant neoplasm of penis and other male genital organs
188　Malignant neoplasm of bladder
189　Malignant neoplasm of kidney and other unspecified urinary organs

Malignant neoplasm of other and unspecified sites (190-199)

190　Malignant neoplasm of eye
191　Malignant neoplasm of brain
192　Malignant neoplasm of other and unspecified parts of nervous system
193　Malignant neoplasm of thyroid gland
194　Malignant neoplasm of other endocrine glands and related structures
195　Malignant neoplasm of other and ill-defined sites
196　Secondary and unspecified malignant neoplasm of lymph nodes
197　Secondary malignant neoplasm of respiratory and digestive systems
198　Secondary malignant neoplasm of other specified sites
199　Malignant neoplasm without specification of site

Malignant neoplasm of lymphatic and hematopoietic tissue (200-208)

200　Lymphosarcoma and reticulosarcoma
201　Hodgkin's disease
202　Other malignant neoplasm of lymphoid and histiocytic tissue
203　Multiple myeloma and immunoproliferative neoplasms
204　Lymphoid leukemia
205　Myeloid leukemia
206　Monocytic leukemia
207　Other specified leukemia
208　Leukemia of unspecified cell type

Benign neoplasms (210-229)

210　Benign neoplasm of lip, oral cavity, and pharynx
211　Benign neoplasm of other parts of digestive system
212　Benign neoplasm of respiratory and intrathoracic organs
213　Benign neoplasm of bone and articular cartilage
214　Lipoma
215　Other benign neoplasm of connective and other soft tissue
216　Benign neoplasm of skin
217　Benign neoplasm of breast
218　Uterine leiomyoma
219　Other benign neoplasm of uterus
220　Benign neoplasm of ovary
221　Benign neoplasm of other female genital organs
222　Benign neoplasm of male genital organs
223　Benign neoplasm of kidney and other urinary organs
224　Benign neoplasm of eye
225　Benign neoplasm of brain and other parts of nervous system
226　Benign neoplasm of thyroid gland
227　Benign neoplasm of other endocrine glands and related structures
228　Hemangioma and lymphangioma, any site
229　Benign neoplasm of other and unspecified sites

Carcinoma in situ (230-234)

230　Carcinoma in situ of digestive organs
231　Carcinoma in situ of respiratory system
232　Carcinoma in situ of skin
233　Carcinoma in situ of breast and genitourinary system
234　Carcinoma in situ of other and unspecified sites

Neoplasms of uncertain behavior (235-238)

235　Neoplasm of uncertain behavior of digestive and respiratory systems
236　Neoplasm of uncertain behavior of genitourinary organs
237　Neoplasm of uncertain behavior of endocrine glands and nervous system
238　Neoplasm of uncertain behavior of other and unspecified sites and tissues

Neoplasms of unspecified nature (239)

239　Neoplasm of unspecified nature

3. ENDOCRINE, NUTRITIONAL AND METABOLIC DISEASES, AND IMMUNITY DISORDERS

Disorders of thyroid gland (240-246)

240　Simple and unspecified goiter
241　Nontoxic nodular goiter
242　Thyrotoxicosis with or without goiter
243　Congenital hypothyroidism
244　Acquired hypothyroidism
245　Thyroiditis
246　Other disorders of thyroid

Diseases of other endocrine glands (250-259)

250　Diabetes mellitus
251　Other disorders of pancreatic internal secretion
252　Disorders of parathyroid gland
253　Disorders of the pituitary gland and its hypothalamic control
254　Diseases of thymus gland
255　Disorders of adrenal glands
256　Ovarian dysfunction
257　Testicular dysfunction
258　Polyglandular dysfunction and related disorders
259　Other endocrine disorders

Nutritional deficiencies (260-269)

260　Kwashiorkor
261　Nutritional marasmus
262　Other severe protein-calorie malnutrition
263　Other and unspecified protein-calorie malnutrition
264　Vitamin A deficiency
265　Thiamine and niacin deficiency states
266　Deficiency of B-complex components
267　Ascorbic acid deficiency
268　Vitamin D deficiency
269　Other nutritional deficiencies

Other metabolic disorders and immunity disorders (270-279)

270　Disorders of amino-acid transport and metabolism
271　Disorders of carbohydrate transport and metabolism
272　Disorders of lipoid metabolism
273　Disorders of plasma protein metabolism
274　Gout
275　Disorders of mineral metabolism
276　Disorders of fluid, electrolyte, and acid-base balance
277　Other and unspecified disorders of metabolism
278　Obesity and other hyperalimentation
279　Disorders involving the immune mechanism

Diseases of blood and blood-forming organs (280-289)

280　Iron deficiency anemias
281　Other deficiency anemias
282　Hereditary hemolytic anemias
283　Acquired hemolytic anemias
284　Aplastic anemia
285　Other and unspecified anemias
286　Coagulation defects
287　Purpura and other hemorrhagic conditions
288　Diseases of white blood cells
289　Other diseases of blood and blood-forming organs

5.　MENTAL DISORDERS

Organic psychotic conditions (290-294)

290　Senile and presenile organic psychotic conditions
291　Alcoholic psychoses
292　Drug psychoses
293　Transient organic psychotic conditions
294　Other organic psychotic conditions (chronic)

Other psychoses (295-299)

295　Schizophrenic psychoses
296　Affective psychoses
297　Paranoid states
298　Other nonorganic psychoses
299　Psychoses with origin specific to childhood

Neurotic disorders, personality disorders, and other nonpsychotic mental disorders (300-316)

300　Neurotic disorders
301　Personality disorders
302　Sexual deviations and disorders
303　Alcohol dependence syndrome
304　Drug dependence
305　Nondependent abuse of drugs
306　Physiological malfunction arising from mental factors

307 Special symptoms or syndromes, not elsewhere classified
308 Acute reaction to stress
309 Adjustment reaction
310 Specific nonpsychotic mental disorders following organic brain damage
311 Depressive disorder, not elsewhere classified
312 Disturbance of conduct, not elsewhere classified
313 Disturbance of emotions specific to childhood and adolescence
314 Hyperkinetic syndrome of childhood
315 Specific delays in development
316 Psychic factors associated with diseases classified elsewhere

Mental retardation (317-319)
317 Mild mental retardation
318 Other specified mental retardation
319 Unspecified mental retardation

6. DISEASES OF THE NERVOUS SYSTEM AND SENSE ORGANS

Inflammatory diseases of the central nervous system (320-326)
320 Bacterial meningitis
321 Meningitis due to other organisms
322 Meningitis of unspecified cause
323 Encephalitis, myelitis, and encephalomyelitis
324 Intracranial and intraspinal abscess
325 Phlebitis and thrombophlebitis of intracranial venous sinuses
326 Late effects of intracranial abscess or pyogenic infection

Hereditary and degenerative diseases of the central nervous system (330-337)
330 Cerebral degenerations usually manifest in childhood
331 Other cerebral degenerations
332 Parkinson's disease
333 Other extrapyramidal diseases and abnormal movement disorders
334 Spinocerebellar disease
335 Anterior horn cell disease
336 Other diseases of spinal cord
337 Disorders of the autonomic nervous system

Other disorders of the central nervous system (340-349)
340 Multiple sclerosis
341 Other demyelinating diseases of central nervous system
342 Hemiplegia and hemiparesis
343 Infantile cerebral palsy
344 Other paralytic syndromes
345 Epilepsy
346 Migraine
347 Cataplexy and narcolepsy
348 Other conditions of brain
349 Other and unspecified disorders of the nervous system

Disorders of the peripheral nervous system (350-359)
350 Trigeminal nerve disorders
351 Facial nerve disorders
352 Disorders of other cranial nerves
353 Nerve root and plexus disorders
354 Mononeuritis of upper limb and mononeuritis multiplex
355 Mononeuritis of lower limb
356 Hereditary and idiopathic peripheral neuropathy
357 Inflammatory and toxic neuropathy
358 Myoneural disorders

359 Muscular dystrophies and other myopathies

Disorders of the eye and adnexa (360-379)
360 Disorders of the globe
361 Retinal detachments and defects
362 Other retinal disorders
363 Chorioretinal inflammations and scars and other disorders of choroid
364 Disorders of iris and ciliary body
365 Glaucoma
366 Cataract
367 Disorders of refraction and accommodation
368 Visual disturbances
369 Blindness and low vision
370 Keratitis
371 Corneal opacity and other disorders of cornea
372 Disorders of conjunctiva
373 Inflammation of eyelids
374 Other disorders of eyelids
375 Disorders of lacrimal system
376 Disorders of the orbit
377 Disorders of optic nerve and visual pathways
378 Strabismus and other disorders of binocular eye movements
379 Other disorders of eye

Diseases of the ear and mastoid process (380-389)
380 Disorders of external ear
381 Nonsuppurative otitis media and Eustachian tube disorders
382 Suppurative and unspecified otitis media
383 Mastoiditis and related conditions
384 Other disorders of tympanic membrane
385 Other disorders of middle ear and mastoid
386 Vertiginous syndromes and other disorders of vestibular system
387 Otosclerosis
388 Other disorders of ear
389 Hearing loss

7. DISEASES OF THE CIRCULATORY SYSTEM

Acute rheumatic fever (390-392)
390 Rheumatic fever without mention of heart involvement
391 Rheumatic fever with heart involvement
392 Rheumatic chorea

Chronic rheumatic heart disease (393-398)
393 Chronic rheumatic pericarditis
394 Diseases of mitral valve
395 Diseases of aortic valve
396 Diseases of mitral and aortic valves
397 Diseases of other endocardial structures
398 Other rheumatic heart disease

Hypertensive disease (401-405)
401 Essential hypertension
402 Hypertensive heart disease
403 Hypertensive renal disease
404 Hypertensive heart and renal disease
405 Secondary hypertension

Ischemic heart disease (410-414)
410 Acute myocardial infarction
411 Other acute and subacute form of ischemic heart disease

412 Old myocardial infarction
413 Angina pectoris
414 Other forms of chronic ischemic heart disease

Diseases of pulmonary circulation (415-417)
415 Acute pulmonary heart disease
416 Chronic pulmonary heart disease
417 Other diseases of pulmonary circulation

Other forms of heart disease (420-429)
420 Acute pericarditis
421 Acute and subacute endocarditis
422 Acute myocarditis
423 Other diseases of pericardium
424 Other diseases of endocardium
425 Cardiomyopathy
426 Conduction disorders
427 Cardiac dysrhythmias
428 Heart failure
429 Ill-defined descriptions and complications of heart disease

Cerebrovascular disease (430-438)
430 Subarachnoid hemorrhage
431 Intracerebral hemorrhage
432 Other and unspecified intracranial hemorrhage
433 Occlusion and stenosis of precerebral arteries
434 Occlusion of cerebral arteries
435 Transient cerebral ischemia
436 Acute but ill-defined cerebrovascular disease
437 Other and ill-defined cerebrovascular disease
438 Late effects of cerebrovascular disease

Diseases of arteries, arterioles, and capillaries (440-448)
440 Atherosclerosis
441 Aortic aneurysm and dissection
442 Other aneurysm
443 Other peripheral vascular disease
444 Arterial embolism and thrombosis
445 Atheroembolism
446 Polyarteritis nodosa and allied conditions
447 Other disorders of arteries and arterioles
448 Diseases of capillaries

Diseases of veins and lymphatics, and other diseases of circulatory system (451-459)
451 Phlebitis and thrombophlebitis
452 Portal vein thrombosis
453 Other venous embolism and thrombosis
454 Varicose veins of lower extremities
455 Hemorrhoids
456 Varicose veins of other sites
457 Noninfective disorders of lymphatic channels
458 Hypotension
459 Other disorders of circulatory system

8. DISEASES OF THE RESPIRATORY SYSTEM

Acute respiratory infections (460-466)
460 Acute nasopharyngitis [common cold]
461 Acute sinusitis
462 Acute pharyngitis
463 Acute tonsillitis
464 Acute laryngitis and tracheitis

465 Acute upper respiratory infections of multiple or unspecified sites
466 Acute bronchitis and bronchiolitis

Other diseases of upper respiratory tract (470-478)
470 Deviated nasal septum
471 Nasal polyps
472 Chronic pharyngitis and nasopharyngitis
473 Chronic sinusitis
474 Chronic disease of tonsils and adenoids
475 Peritonsillar abscess
476 Chronic laryngitis and laryngotracheitis
477 Allergic rhinitis
478 Other diseases of upper respiratory tract

Pneumonia and influenza (480-487)
480 Viral pneumonia
481 Pneumococcal pneumonia [Streptococcus pneumoniae pneumonia]
482 Other bacterial pneumonia
483 Pneumonia due to other specified organism
484 Pneumonia in infectious diseases classified elsewhere
485 Bronchopneumonia, organism unspecified
486 Pneumonia, organism unspecified
487 Influenza

Chronic obstructive pulmonary disease and allied conditions (490-496)
490 Bronchitis, not specified as acute or chronic
491 Chronic bronchitis
492 Emphysema
493 Asthma
494 Bronchiectasis
495 Extrinsic allergic alveolitis
496 Chronic airways obstruction, not elsewhere classified

Pneumoconioses and other lung diseases due to external agents (500-508)
500 Coal workers' pneumoconiosis
501 Asbestosis
502 Pneumoconiosis due to other silica or silicates
503 Pneumoconiosis due to other inorganic dust
504 Pneumopathy due to inhalation of other dust
505 Pneumoconiosis, unspecified
506 Respiratory conditions due to chemical fumes and vapors
507 Pneumonitis due to solids and liquids
508 Respiratory conditions due to other and unspecified external agents

Other diseases of respiratory system (510-519)
510 Empyema
511 Pleurisy
512 Pneumothorax
513 Abscess of lung and mediastinum
514 Pulmonary congestion and hypostasis
515 Postinflammatory pulmonary fibrosis
516 Other alveolar and parietoalveolar pneumopathy
517 Lung involvement in conditions classified elsewhere
518 Other diseases of lung

519 Other diseases of respiratory system

9. DISEASES OF THE DIGESTIVE SYSTEM

Diseases of oral cavity, salivary glands, and jaws (520-529)
520 Disorders of tooth development and eruption
521 Diseases of hard tissues of teeth
522 Diseases of pulp and periapical tissues
523 Gingival and periodontal diseases
524 Dentofacial anomalies, including malocclusion
525 Other diseases and conditions of the teeth and supporting structures
526 Diseases of the jaws
527 Diseases of the salivary glands
528 Diseases of the oral soft tissues, excluding lesions specific for gingiva and tongue
529 Diseases and other conditions of the tongue

Diseases of esophagus, stomach, and duodenum (530-537)
530 Diseases of esophagus
531 Gastric ulcer
532 Duodenal ulcer
533 Peptic ulcer, site unspecified
534 Gastrojejunal ulcer
535 Gastritis and duodenitis
536 Disorders of function of stomach
537 Other disorders of stomach and duodenum

Appendicitis (540-543)
540 Acute appendicitis
541 Appendicitis, unqualified
542 Other appendicitis
543 Other diseases of appendix

Hernia of abdominal cavity (550-553)
550 Inguinal hernia
551 Other hernia of abdominal cavity, with gangrene
552 Other hernia of abdominal cavity, with obstruction, but without mention of gangrene
553 Other hernia of abdominal cavity without mention of obstruction or gangrene

Noninfective enteritis and colitis (555-558)
555 Regional enteritis
556 Ulcerative colitis
557 Vascular insufficiency of intestine
558 Other noninfective gastroenteritis and colitis

Other diseases of intestines and peritoneum (560-569)
560 Intestinal obstruction without mention of hernia
562 Diverticula of intestine
564 Functional digestive disorders, not elsewhere classified
565 Anal fissure and fistula
566 Abscess of anal and rectal regions
567 Peritonitis
568 Other disorders of peritoneum
569 Other disorders of intestine

Other diseases of digestive system (570-579)
570 Acute and subacute necrosis of liver
571 Chronic liver disease and cirrhosis
572 Liver abscess and sequelae of chronic liver disease

573 Other disorders of liver
574 Cholelithiasis
575 Other disorders of gallbladder
576 Other disorders of biliary tract
577 Diseases of pancreas
578 Gastrointestinal hemorrhage
579 Intestinal malabsorption

10. DISEASES OF THE GENITOURINARY SYSTEM

Nephritis, nephrotic syndrome, and nephrosis (580-589)
580 Acute glomerulonephritis
581 Nephrotic syndrome
582 Chronic glomerulonephritis
583 Nephritis and nephropathy, not specified as acute or chronic
584 Acute renal failure
585 Chronic renal failure
586 Renal failure, unspecified
587 Renal sclerosis, unspecified
588 Disorders resulting from impaired renal function
589 Small kidney of unknown cause

Other diseases of urinary system (590-599)
590 Infections of kidney
591 Hydronephrosis
592 Calculus of kidney and ureter
593 Other disorders of kidney and ureter
594 Calculus of lower urinary tract
595 Cystitis
596 Other disorders of bladder
597 Urethritis, not sexually transmitted, and urethral syndrome
598 Urethral stricture
599 Other disorders of urethra and urinary tract

Diseases of male genital organs (600-608)
600 Hyperplasia of prostate
601 Inflammatory diseases of prostate
602 Other disorders of prostate
603 Hydrocele
604 Orchitis and epididymitis
605 Redundant prepuce and phimosis
606 Infertility, male
607 Disorders of penis
608 Other disorders of male genital organs

Disorders of breast (610-611)
610 Benign mammary dysplasias
611 Other disorders of breast

Inflammatory disease of female pelvic organs (614-616)
614 Inflammatory disease of ovary, fallopian tube, pelvic cellular tissue, and peritoneum
615 Inflammatory diseases of uterus, except cervix
616 Inflammatory disease of cervix, vagina, and vulva

Other disorders of female genital tract (617-629)
617 Endometriosis
618 Genital prolapse
619 Fistula involving female genital tract
620 Noninflammatory disorders of ovary, fallopian tube, and broad ligament
621 Disorders of uterus, not elsewhere classified
622 Noninflammatory disorders of cervix
623 Noninflammatory disorders of vagina
624 Noninflammatory disorders of vulva and perineum

625 Pain and other symptoms associated with female genital organs
626 Disorders of menstruation and other abnormal bleeding from female genital tract
627 Menopausal and postmenopausal disorders
628 Infertility, female
629 Other disorders of female genital organs

11. COMPLICATIONS OF PREGNANCY, CHILDBIRTH AND THE PUERPERIUM

Ectopic and molar pregnancy and other pregnancy with abortive outcome (630-639)
630 Hydatidiform mole
631 Other abnormal product of conception
632 Missed abortion
633 Ectopic pregnancy
634 Spontaneous abortion
635 Legally induced abortion
636 Illegally induced abortion
637 Unspecified abortion
638 Failed attempted abortion
639 Complications following abortion and ectopic and molar pregnancies

Complications mainly related to pregnancy (640-648)
640 Hemorrhage in early pregnancy
641 Antepartum hemorrhage, abruptio placentae, and placenta previa
642 Hypertension complicating pregnancy, childbirth, and the puerperium
643 Excessive vomiting in pregnancy
644 Early or threatened labor
645 Prolonged pregnancy
646 Other complications of pregnancy, not elsewhere classified
647 Infective and parasitic conditions in the mother classifiable elsewhere but complicating pregnancy, childbirth, and the puerperium
648 Other current conditions in the mother classifiable elsewhere but complicating pregnancy, childbirth, and the puerperium

Normal delivery, and other indications for care in pregnancy, labor, and delivery (650-659)
650 Normal delivery
651 Multiple gestation
652 Malposition and malpresentation of fetus
653 Disproportion
654 Abnormality of organs and soft tissues of pelvis
655 Known or suspected fetal abnormality affecting management of mother
656 Other fetal and placental problems affecting management of mother
657 Polyhydramnios
658 Other problems associated with amniotic cavity and membranes
659 Other indications for care or intervention related to labor and delivery and not elsewhere classified

Complications occurring mainly in the course of labor and delivery (660-669)
660 Obstructed labor
661 Abnormality of forces of labor
662 Long labor
663 Umbilical cord complications
664 Trauma to perineum and vulva during delivery

665 Other obstetrical trauma
666 Postpartum hemorrhage
667 Retained placenta or membranes, without hemorrhage
668 Complications of the administration of anesthetic or other sedation in labor and delivery
669 Other complications of labor and delivery, not elsewhere classified

Complications of the puerperium (670-677)
670 Major puerperal infection
671 Venous complications in pregnancy and the puerperium
672 Pyrexia of unknown origin during the puerperium
673 Obstetrical pulmonary embolism
674 Other and unspecified complications of the puerperium, not elsewhere classified
675 Infections of the breast and nipple associated with childbirth
676 Other disorders of the breast associated with childbirth, and disorders of lactation
677 Late effect of complication of pregnancy, childbirth, and the puerperium

12. DISEASES OF THE SKIN AND SUBCUTANEOUS TISSUE

Infections of skin and subcutaneous tissue (680-686)
680 Carbuncle and furuncle
681 Cellulitis and abscess of finger and toe
682 Other cellulitis and abscess
683 Acute lymphadenitis
684 Impetigo
685 Pilonidal cyst
686 Other local infections of skin and subcutaneous tissue

Other inflammatory conditions of skin and subcutaneous tissue (690-698)
690 Erythematosquamous dermatosis
691 Atopic dermatitis and related conditions
692 Contact dermatitis and other eczema
693 Dermatitis due to substances taken internally
694 Bullous dermatoses
695 Erythematous conditions
696 Psoriasis and similar disorders
697 Lichen
698 Pruritus and related conditions

Other diseases of skin and subcutaneous tissue (700-709)
700 Corns and callosities
701 Other hypertrophic and atrophic conditions of skin
702 Other dermatoses
703 Diseases of nail
704 Diseases of hair and hair follicles
705 Disorders of sweat glands
706 Diseases of sebaceous glands
707 Chronic ulcer of skin
708 Urticaria
709 Other disorders of skin and subcutaneous tissue

13. DISEASES OF THE MUSCULOSKELETAL SYSTEM AND CONNECTIVE TISSUE

Arthropathies and related disorders (710-719)
710 Diffuse diseases of connective tissue
711 Arthropathy associated with infections
712 Crystal arthropathies
713 Arthropathy associated with other disorders classified elsewhere
714 Rheumatoid arthritis and other inflammatory polyarthropathies
715 Osteoarthrosis and allied disorders
716 Other and unspecified arthropathies
717 Internal derangement of knee
718 Other derangement of joint
719 Other and unspecified disorder of joint

Dorsopathies (720-724)
720 Ankylosing spondylitis and other inflammatory spondylopathies
721 Spondylosis and allied disorders
722 Intervertebral disc disorders
723 Other disorders of cervical region
724 Other and unspecified disorders of back

Rheumatism, excluding the back (725-729)
725 Polymyalgia rheumatica
726 Peripheral enthesopathies and allied syndromes
727 Other disorders of synovium, tendon, and bursa
728 Disorders of muscle, ligament, and fascia
729 Other disorders of soft tissues

Osteopathies, chondropathies, and acquired musculoskeletal deformities (730-739)
730 Osteomyelitis, periostitis, and other infections involving bone
731 Osteitis deformans and osteopathies associated with other disorders classified elsewhere
732 Osteochondropathies
733 Other disorders of bone and cartilage
734 Flat foot
735 Acquired deformities of toe
736 Other acquired deformities of limbs
737 Curvature of spine
738 Other acquired deformity
739 Nonallopathic lesions, not elsewhere classified

14. CONGENITAL ANOMALIES
740 Anencephalus and similar anomalies
741 Spina bifida
742 Other congenital anomalies of nervous system
743 Congenital anomalies of eye
744 Congenital anomalies of ear, face, and neck
745 Bulbus cordis anomalies and anomalies of cardiac septal closure
746 Other congenital anomalies of heart
747 Other congenital anomalies of circulatory system
748 Congenital anomalies of respiratory system
749 Cleft palate and cleft lip
750 Other congenital anomalies of upper alimentary tract
751 Other congenital anomalies of digestive system

752 Congenital anomalies of genital organs
753 Congenital anomalies of urinary system
754 Certain congenital musculoskeletal deformities
755 Other congenital anomalies of limbs
756 Other congenital musculoskeletal anomalies
757 Congenital anomalies of the integument
758 Chromosomal anomalies
759 Other and unspecified congenital anomalies

15. CERTAIN CONDITIONS ORIGINATING IN THE PERINATAL PERIOD

Maternal causes of perinatal morbidity and mortality (760-763)
760 Fetus or newborn affected by maternal conditions which may be unrelated to present pregnancy
761 Fetus or newborn affected by maternal complications of pregnancy
762 Fetus or newborn affected by complications of placenta, cord, and membranes
763 Fetus or newborn affected by other complications of labor and delivery

Other conditions originating in the perinatal period (764-779)
764 Slow fetal growth and fetal malnutrition
765 Disorders relating to short gestation and unspecified low birthweight
766 Disorders relating to long gestation and high birthweight
767 Birth trauma
768 Intrauterine hypoxia and birth asphyxia
769 Respiratory distress syndrome
770 Other respiratory conditions of fetus and newborn
771 Infections specific to the perinatal period
772 Fetal and neonatal hemorrhage
773 Hemolytic disease of fetus or newborn, due to isoimmunization
774 Other perinatal jaundice
775 Endocrine and metabolic disturbances specific to the fetus and newborn
776 Hematological disorders of fetus and newborn
777 Perinatal disorders of digestive system
778 Conditions involving the integument and temperature regulation of fetus and newborn
779 Other and ill-defined conditions originating in the perinatal period

16. SYMPTOMS, SIGNS, AND ILL-DEFINED CONDITIONS

Symptoms (780-789)
780 General symptoms
781 Symptoms involving nervous and musculoskeletal systems
782 Symptoms involving skin and other integumentary tissue
783 Symptoms concerning nutrition, metabolism, and development
784 Symptoms involving head and neck
785 Symptoms involving cardiovascular system
786 Symptoms involving respiratory system and other chest symptoms
787 Symptoms involving digestive system
788 Symptoms involving urinary system
789 Other symptoms involving abdomen and pelvis

Nonspecific abnormal findings (790-796)
790 Nonspecific findings on examination of blood
791 Nonspecific findings on examination of urine
792 Nonspecific abnormal findings in other body substances
793 Nonspecific abnormal findings on radiological and other examination of body structure
794 Nonspecific abnormal results of function studies
795 Nonspecific abnormal histological and immunological findings
796 Other nonspecific abnormal findings

Ill-defined and unknown causes of morbidity and mortality (797-799)
797 Senility without mention of psychosis
798 Sudden death, cause unknown
799 Other ill-defined and unknown causes of morbidity and mortality

17. INJURY AND POISONING

Fracture of skull (800-804)
800 Fracture of vault of skull
801 Fracture of base of skull
802 Fracture of face bones
803 Other and unqualified skull fractures
804 Multiple fractures involving skull or face with other bones

Fracture of spine and trunk (805-809)
805 Fracture of vertebral column without mention of spinal cord lesion
806 Fracture of vertebral column with spinal cord lesion
807 Fracture of rib(s), sternum, larynx, and trachea
808 Fracture of pelvis
809 Ill-defined fractures of bones of trunk

Fracture of upper limb (810-819)
810 Fracture of clavicle
811 Fracture of scapula
812 Fracture of humerus
813 Fracture of radius and ulna
814 Fracture of carpal bone(s)
815 Fracture of metacarpal bone(s)
816 Fracture of one or more phalanges of hand
817 Multiple fractures of hand bones
818 Ill-defined fractures of upper limb
819 Multiple fractures involving both upper limbs, and upper limb with rib(s) and sternum

Fracture of lower limb (820-829)
820 Fracture of neck of femur
821 Fracture of other and unspecified parts of femur
822 Fracture of patella
823 Fracture of tibia and fibula
824 Fracture of ankle
825 Fracture of one or more tarsal and metatarsal bones
826 Fracture of one or more phalanges of foot
827 Other, multiple, and ill-defined fractures of lower limb
828 Multiple fractures involving both lower limbs, lower with upper limb, and lower limb(s) with rib(s) and sternum
829 Fracture of unspecified bones

Dislocation (830-839)
830 Dislocation of jaw
831 Dislocation of shoulder
832 Dislocation of elbow
833 Dislocation of wrist
834 Dislocation of finger
835 Dislocation of hip
836 Dislocation of knee
837 Dislocation of ankle
838 Dislocation of foot
839 Other, multiple, and ill-defined dislocations

Sprains and strains of joints and adjacent muscles (840-848)
840 Sprains and strains of shoulder and upper arm
841 Sprains and strains of elbow and forearm
842 Sprains and strains of wrist and hand
843 Sprains and strains of hip and thigh
844 Sprains and strains of knee and leg
845 Sprains and strains of ankle and foot
846 Sprains and strains of sacroiliac region
847 Sprains and strains of other and unspecified parts of back
848 Other and ill-defined sprains and strains

Intracranial injury, excluding those with skull fracture (850-854)
850 Concussion
851 Cerebral laceration and contusion
852 Subarachnoid, subdural, and extradural hemorrhage, following injury
853 Other and unspecified intracranial hemorrhage following injury
854 Intracranial injury of other and unspecified nature

Internal injury of chest, abdomen, and pelvis (860-869)
860 Traumatic pneumothorax and hemothorax
861 Injury to heart and lung
862 Injury to other and unspecified intrathoracic organs
863 Injury to gastrointestinal tract
864 Injury to liver
865 Injury to spleen
866 Injury to kidney
867 Injury to pelvic organs
868 Injury to other intra-abdominal organs
869 Internal injury to unspecified or ill-defined organs

Open wound of head, neck, and trunk (870-879)
870 Open wound of ocular adnexa
871 Open wound of eyeball
872 Open wound of ear
873 Other open wound of head
874 Open wound of neck
875 Open wound of chest (wall)
876 Open wound of back
877 Open wound of buttock

878 Open wound of genital organs (external), including traumatic amputation

879 Open wound of other and unspecified sites, except limbs

Open wound of upper limb (880-887)

880 Open wound of shoulder and upper arm

881 Open wound of elbow, forearm, and wrist

882 Open wound of hand except finger(s) alone

883 Open wound of finger(s)

884 Multiple and unspecified open wound of upper limb

885 Traumatic amputation of thumb (complete) (partial)

886 Traumatic amputation of other finger(s) (complete) (partial)

887 Traumatic amputation of arm and hand (complete) (partial)

Open wound of lower limb (890-897)

890 Open wound of hip and thigh

891 Open wound of knee, leg [except thigh], and ankle

892 Open wound of foot except toe(s) alone

893 Open wound of toe(s)

894 Multiple and unspecified open wound of lower limb

895 Traumatic amputation of toe(s) (complete) (partial)

896 Traumatic amputation of foot (complete) (partial)

897 Traumatic amputation of leg(s) (complete) (partial)

Injury to blood vessels (900-904)

900 Injury to blood vessels of head and neck

901 Injury to blood vessels of thorax

902 Injury to blood vessels of abdomen and pelvis

903 Injury to blood vessels of upper extremity

904 Injury to blood vessels of lower extremity and unspecified sites

Late effects of injuries, poisonings, toxic effects, and other external causes (905-909)

905 Late effects of musculoskeletal and connective tissue injuries

906 Late effects of injuries to skin and subcutaneous tissues

907 Late effects of injuries to the nervous system

908 Late effects of other and unspecified injuries

909 Late effects of other and unspecified external causes

Superficial injury (910-919)

910 Superficial injury of face, neck, and scalp except eye

911 Superficial injury of trunk

912 Superficial injury of shoulder and upper arm

913 Superficial injury of elbow, forearm, and wrist

914 Superficial injury of hand(s) except finger(s) alone

915 Superficial injury of finger(s)

916 Superficial injury of hip, thigh, leg, and ankle

917 Superficial injury of foot and toe(s)

918 Superficial injury of eye and adnexa

919 Superficial injury of other, multiple, and unspecified sites

Contusion with intact skin surface (920-924)

920 Contusion of face, scalp, and neck except eye(s)

921 Contusion of eye and adnexa

922 Contusion of trunk

923 Contusion of upper limb

924 Contusion of lower limb and of other and unspecified sites

Crushing injury (925-929)

925 Crushing injury of face, scalp, and neck

926 Crushing injury of trunk

927 Crushing injury of upper limb

928 Crushing injury of lower limb

929 Crushing injury of multiple and unspecified sites

Effects of foreign body entering through orifice (930-939)

930 Foreign body on external eye

931 Foreign body in ear

932 Foreign body in nose

933 Foreign body in pharynx and larynx

934 Foreign body in trachea, bronchus, and lung

935 Foreign body in mouth, esophagus, and stomach

936 Foreign body in intestine and colon

937 Foreign body in anus and rectum

938 Foreign body in digestive system, unspecified

939 Foreign body in genitourinary tract

Burns (940-949)

940 Burn confined to eye and adnexa

941 Burn of face, head, and neck

942 Burn of trunk

943 Burn of upper limb, except wrist and hand

944 Burn of wrist(s) and hand(s)

945 Burn of lower limb(s)

946 Burns of multiple specified sites

947 Burn of internal organs

948 Burns classified according to extent of body surface involved

949 Burn, unspecified

Injury to nerves and spinal cord (950-957)

950 Injury to optic nerve and pathways

951 Injury to other cranial nerve(s)

952 Spinal cord injury without evidence of spinal bone injury

953 Injury to nerve roots and spinal plexus

954 Injury to other nerve(s) of trunk excluding shoulder and pelvic girdles

955 Injury to peripheral nerve(s) of shoulder girdle and upper limb

956 Injury to peripheral nerve(s) of pelvic girdle and lower limb

957 Injury to other and unspecified nerves

Certain traumatic complications and unspecified injuries (958-959)

958 Certain early complications of trauma

959 Injury, other and unspecified

Poisoning by drugs, medicinals and biological substances (960-979)

960 Poisoning by antibiotics

961 Poisoning by other anti-infectives

962 Poisoning by hormones and synthetic substitutes

963 Poisoning by primarily systemic agents

964 Poisoning by agents primarily affecting blood constituents

965 Poisoning by analgesics, antipyretics, and antirheumatics

966 Poisoning by anticonvulsants and anti-Parkinsonism drugs

967 Poisoning by sedatives and hypnotics

968 Poisoning by other central nervous system depressants and anesthetics

969 Poisoning by psychotropic agents

970 Poisoning by central nervous system stimulants

971 Poisoning by drugs primarily affecting the autonomic nervous system

972 Poisoning by agents primarily affecting the cardiovascular system

973 Poisoning by agents primarily affecting the gastrointestinal system

974 Poisoning by water, mineral, and uric acid metabolism drugs

975 Poisoning by agents primarily acting on the smooth and skeletal muscles and respiratory system

976 Poisoning by agents primarily affecting skin and mucous membrane, ophthalmological, otorhinolaryngological, and dental drugs

977 Poisoning by other and unspecified drugs and medicinals

978 Poisoning by bacterial vaccines

979 Poisoning by other vaccines and biological substances

Toxic effects of substances chiefly non-medicinal as to source (980-989)

980 Toxic effect of alcohol

981 Toxic effect of petroleum products

982 Toxic effect of solvents other than petroleum-based

983 Toxic effect of corrosive aromatics, acids, and caustic alkalis

984 Toxic effect of lead and its compounds (including fumes)

985 Toxic effect of other metals

986 Toxic effect of carbon monoxide

987 Toxic effect of other gases, fumes, or vapors

988 Toxic effect of noxious substances eaten as food

989 Toxic effect of other substances, chiefly nonmedicinal as to source

Other and unspecified effects of external causes (990-995)

990 Effects of radiation, unspecified

991 Effects of reduced temperature

992 Effects of heat and light

993 Effects of air pressure

994 Effects of other external causes

995 Certain adverse effects, not elsewhere classified

Complications of surgical and medical care, not elsewhere classified (996-999)

996 Complications peculiar to certain specified procedures

997 Complications affecting specified body systems, not elsewhere classified

998 Other complications of procedures, not elsewhere classified

999 Complications of medical care, not elsewhere classified

SUPPLEMENTARY CLASSIFICATION OF FACTORS INFLUENCING HEALTH STATUS AND CONTACT WITH HEALTH SERVICES

Persons with potential health hazards related to communicable diseases (V01-V09)

V01 Contact with or exposure to communicable diseases
V02 Carrier or suspected carrier of infectious diseases
V03 Need for prophylactic vaccination and inoculation against bacterial diseases
V04 Need for prophylactic vaccination and inoculation against certain viral diseases
V05 Need for other prophylactic vaccination and inoculation against single diseases
V06 Need for prophylactic vaccination and inoculation against combinations of diseases
V07 Need for isolation and other prophylactic measures
V08 Asymptomatic human immunodeficiency virus [HIV] infection status
V09 Infection with drug-resistant microorganisms

Persons with potential health hazards related to personal and family history (V10-V19)

V10 Personal history of malignant neoplasm
V11 Personal history of mental disorder
V12 Personal history of certain other diseases
V13 Personal history of other diseases
V14 Personal history of allergy to medicinal agents
V15 Other personal history presenting hazards to health
V16 Family history of malignant neoplasm
V17 Family history of certain chronic disabling diseases
V18 Family history of certain other specific conditions
V19 Family history of other conditions

Persons encountering health services in circumstances related to reproduction and development (V20-V29)

V20 Health supervision of infant or child
V21 Constitutional states in development
V22 Normal pregnancy
V23 Supervision of high-risk pregnancy
V24 Postpartum care and examination
V25 Encounter for contraceptive management
V26 Procreative management
V27 Outcome of delivery
V28 Antenatal screening
V29 Observation and evaluation of newborns and infants for suspected condition not found

Liveborn infants according to type of birth (V30-V39)

V30 Single liveborn
V31 Twin, mate liveborn
V32 Twin, mate stillborn
V33 Twin, unspecified
V34 Other multiple, mates all liveborn
V35 Other multiple, mates all stillborn
V36 Other multiple, mates live- and stillborn
V37 Other multiple, unspecified
V39 Unspecified

Persons with a condition influencing their health status (V40-V49)

V40 Mental and behavioral problems
V41 Problems with special senses and other special functions
V42 Organ or tissue replaced by transplant
V43 Organ or tissue replaced by other means
V44 Artificial opening status
V45 Other postsurgical states
V46 Other dependence on machines
V47 Other problems with internal organs
V48 Problems with head, neck, and trunk
V49 Problems with limbs and other problems

Persons encountering health services for specific procedures and aftercare (V50-V59)

V50 Elective surgery for purposes other than remedying health states
V51 Aftercare involving the use of plastic surgery
V52 Fitting and adjustment of prosthetic device
V53 Fitting and adjustment of other device
V54 Other orthopedic aftercare
V55 Attention to artificial openings
V56 Encounter for dialysis and dialysis catheter care
V57 Care involving use of rehabilitation procedures
V58 Encounter for other and unspecified procedures and aftercare
V59 Donors

Persons encountering health services in other circumstances (V60-V69)

V60 Housing, household, and economic circumstances
V61 Other family circumstances
V62 Other psychosocial circumstances
V63 Unavailability of other medical facilities for care
V64 Persons encountering health services for specific procedures, not carried out
V65 Other persons seeking consultation without complaint or sickness
V66 Convalescence and palliative care
V67 Follow-up examination
V68 Encounters for administrative purposes
V69 Problems related to lifestyle

Persons without reported diagnosis encountered during examination and investigation of individuals and populations (V70-V83)

V70 General medical examination
V71 Observation and evaluation for suspected conditions not found
V72 Special investigations and examinations
V73 Special screening examination for viral and chlamydial diseases
V74 Special screening examination for bacterial and spirochetal diseases
V75 Special screening examination for other infectious diseases
V76 Special screening for malignant neoplasms
V77 Special screening for endocrine, nutritional, metabolic, and immunity disorders
V78 Special screening for disorders of blood and blood-forming organs
V79 Special screening for mental disorders and developmental handicaps
V80 Special screening for neurological, eye, and ear diseases
V81 Special screening for cardiovascular, respiratory, and genitourinary diseases
V82 Special screening for other conditions
V83 Genetic carrier status

SUPPLEMENTARY CLASSIFICATION OF EXTERNAL CAUSES OF INJURY AND POISONING

Railway accidents (E800-E807)

E800 Railway accident involving collision with rolling stock
E801 Railway accident involving collision with other object
E802 Railway accident involving derailment without antecedent collision
E803 Railway accident involving explosion, fire, or burning
E804 Fall in, on, or from railway train
E805 Hit by rolling stock
E806 Other specified railway accident
E807 Railway accident of unspecified nature

Motor vehicle traffic accidents (E810-E819)

E810 Motor vehicle traffic accident involving collision with train
E811 Motor vehicle traffic accident involving re-entrant collision with another motor vehicle
E812 Other motor vehicle traffic accident involving collision with another motor vehicle
E813 Motor vehicle traffic accident involving collision with other vehicle
E814 Motor vehicle traffic accident involving collision with pedestrian
E815 Other motor vehicle traffic accident involving collision on the highway
E816 Motor vehicle traffic accident due to loss of control, without collision on the highway
E817 Noncollision motor vehicle traffic accident while boarding or alighting
E818 Other noncollision motor vehicle traffic accident
E819 Motor vehicle traffic accident of unspecified nature

Motor vehicle nontraffic accidents (E820-E825)

E820 Nontraffic accident involving motor-driven snow vehicle
E821 Nontraffic accident involving other off-road motor vehicle
E822 Other motor vehicle nontraffic accident involving collision with moving object
E823 Other motor vehicle nontraffic accident involving collision with stationary object
E824 Other motor vehicle nontraffic accident while boarding and alighting
E825 Other motor vehicle nontraffic accident of other and unspecified nature

Other road vehicle accidents (E826-E829)

E826 Pedal cycle accident
E827 Animal-drawn vehicle accident

E828 Accident involving animal being ridden

E829 Other road vehicle accidents

Water transport accidents (E830-E838)

E830 Accident to watercraft causing submersion

E831 Accident to watercraft causing other injury

E832 Other accidental submersion or drowning in water transport accident

E833 Fall on stairs or ladders in water transport

E834 Other fall from one level to another in water transport

E835 Other and unspecified fall in water transport

E836 Machinery accident in water transport

E837 Explosion, fire, or burning in watercraft

E838 Other and unspecified water transport accident

Air and space transport accidents (E840-E845)

E840 Accident to powered aircraft at take-off or landing

E841 Accident to powered aircraft, other and unspecified

E842 Accident to unpowered aircraft

E843 Fall in, on, or from aircraft

E844 Other specified air transport accidents

E845 Accident involving spacecraft

Vehicle accidents, not elsewhere classifiable (E846-E849)

E846 Accidents involving powered vehicles used solely within the buildings and premises of an industrial or commercial establishment

E847 Accidents involving cable cars not running on rails

E848 Accidents involving other vehicles, not elsewhere classifiable

E849 Place of occurrence

Accidental poisoning by drugs, medicinal substances, and biologicals (E850-E858)

E850 Accidental poisoning by analgesics, antipyretics, and antirheumatics

E851 Accidental poisoning by barbiturates

E852 Accidental poisoning by other sedatives and hypnotics

E853 Accidental poisoning by tranquilizers

E854 Accidental poisoning by other psychotropic agents

E855 Accidental poisoning by other drugs acting on central and autonomic nervous systems

E856 Accidental poisoning by antibiotics

E857 Accidental poisoning by anti-infectives

E858 Accidental poisoning by other drugs

Accidental poisoning by other solid and liquid substances, gases, and vapors (E860-E869)

E860 Accidental poisoning by alcohol, not elsewhere classified

E861 Accidental poisoning by cleansing and polishing agents, disinfectants, paints, and varnishes

E862 Accidental poisoning by petroleum products, other solvents and their vapors, not elsewhere classified

E863 Accidental poisoning by agricultural and horticultural chemical and pharmaceutical preparations other than plant foods and fertilizers

E864 Accidental poisoning by corrosives and caustics, not elsewhere classified

E865 Accidental poisoning from poisonous foodstuffs and poisonous plants

E866 Accidental poisoning by other and unspecified solid and liquid substances

E867 Accidental poisoning by gas distributed by pipeline

E868 Accidental poisoning by other utility gas and other carbon monoxide

E869 Accidental poisoning by other gases and vapors

Misadventures to patients during surgical and medical care (E870-E876)

E870 Accidental cut, puncture, perforation, or hemorrhage during medical care

E871 Foreign object left in body during procedure

E872 Failure of sterile precautions during procedure

E873 Failure in dosage

E874 Mechanical failure of instrument or apparatus during procedure

E875 Contaminated or infected blood, other fluid, drug, or biological substance

E876 Other and unspecified misadventures during medical care

Surgical and medical procedures as the cause of abnormal reaction of patient or later complication, without mention of misadventure at the time of procedure (E878-E879)

E878 Surgical operation and other surgical procedures as the cause of abnormal reaction of patient, or of later complication, without mention of misadventure at the time of operation

E879 Other procedures, without mention of misadventure at the time of procedure, as the cause of abnormal reaction of patient, or of later complication

Accidental falls (E880-E888)

E880 Fall on or from stairs or steps

E881 Fall on or from ladders or scaffolding

E882 Fall from or out of building or other structure

E883 Fall into hole or other opening in surface

E884 Other fall from one level to another

E885 Fall on same level from slipping, tripping, or stumbling

E886 Fall on same level from collision, pushing or shoving, by or with other person

E887 Fracture, cause unspecified

E888 Other and unspecified fall

Accidents caused by fire and flames (E890-E899)

E890 Conflagration in private dwelling

E891 Conflagration in other and unspecified building or structure

E892 Conflagration not in building or structure

E893 Accident caused by ignition of clothing

E894 Ignition of highly inflammable material

E895 Accident caused by controlled fire in private dwelling

E896 Accident caused by controlled fire in other and unspecified building or structure

E897 Accident caused by controlled fire not in building or structure

E898 Accident caused by other specified fire and flames

E899 Accident caused by unspecified fire

Accidents due to natural and environmental factors (E900-E909)

E900 Excessive heat

E901 Excessive cold

E902 High and low air pressure and changes in air pressure

E903 Travel and motion

E904 Hunger, thirst, exposure, and neglect

E905 Venomous animals and plants as the cause of poisoning and toxic reactions

E906 Other injury caused by animals

E907 Lightning

E908 Cataclysmic storms, and floods resulting from storms

E909 Cataclysmic earth surface movements and eruptions

Accidents caused by submersion, suffocation, and foreign bodies (E910-E915)

E910 Accidental drowning and submersion

E911 Inhalation and ingestion of food causing obstruction of respiratory tract or suffocation

E912 Inhalation and ingestion of other object causing obstruction of respiratory tract or suffocation

E913 Accidental mechanical suffocation

E914 Foreign body accidentally entering eye and adnexa

E915 Foreign body accidentally entering other orifice

Other accidents (E916-E928)

E916 Struck accidentally by falling object

E917 Striking against or struck accidentally by objects or persons

E918 Caught accidentally in or between objects

E919 Accidents caused by machinery

E920 Accidents caused by cutting and piercing instruments or objects

E921 Accident caused by explosion of pressure vessel

E922 Accident caused by firearm missile

E923 Accident caused by explosive material

E924 Accident caused by hot substance or object, caustic or corrosive material, and steam

E925 Accident caused by electric current

E926 Exposure to radiation

E927 Overexertion and strenuous movements

E928   Other and unspecified environmental and accidental causes

Late effects of accidental injury (E929)
E929   Late effects of accidental injury

Drugs, medicinal and biological substances causing adverse effects in therapeutic use (E930-E949)
E930   Antibiotics
E931   Other anti-infectives
E932   Hormones and synthetic substitutes
E933   Primarily systemic agents
E934   Agents primarily affecting blood constituents
E935   Analgesics, antipyretics, and antirheumatics
E936   Anticonvulsants and anti-Parkinsonism drugs
E937   Sedatives and hypnotics
E938   Other central nervous system depressants and anesthetics
E939   Psychotropic agents
E940   Central nervous system stimulants
E941   Drugs primarily affecting the autonomic nervous system
E942   Agents primarily affecting the cardiovascular system
E943   Agents primarily affecting gastrointestinal system
E944   Water, mineral, and uric acid metabolism drugs
E945   Agents primarily acting on the smooth and skeletal muscles and respiratory system
E946   Agents primarily affecting skin and mucous membrane, ophthalmological, otorhinolaryngological, and dental drugs
E947   Other and unspecified drugs and medicinal substances
E948   Bacterial vaccines
E949   Other vaccines and biological substances

Suicide and self-inflicted injury (E950-E959)
E950   Suicide and self-inflicted poisoning by solid or liquid substances
E951   Suicide and self-inflicted poisoning by gases in domestic use
E952   Suicide and self-inflicted poisoning by other gases and vapors
E953   Suicide and self-inflicted injury by hanging, strangulation, and suffocation
E954   Suicide and self-inflicted injury by submersion [drowning]

E955   Suicide and self-inflicted injury by firearms and explosives
E956   Suicide and self-inflicted injury by cutting and piercing instruments
E957   Suicide and self-inflicted injuries by jumping from high place
E958   Suicide and self-inflicted injury by other and unspecified means
E959   Late effects of self-inflicted injury

Homicide and injury purposely inflicted by other persons (E960-E969)
E960   Fight, brawl, and rape
E961   Assault by corrosive or caustic substance, except poisoning
E962   Assault by poisoning
E963   Assault by hanging and strangulation
E964   Assault by submersion [drowning]
E965   Assault by firearms and explosives
E966   Assault by cutting and piercing instrument
E967   Child and adult battering and other maltreatment
E968   Assault by other and unspecified means
E969   Late effects of injury purposely inflicted by other person

Legal intervention (E970-E978)
E970   Injury due to legal intervention by firearms
E971   Injury due to legal intervention by explosives
E972   Injury due to legal intervention by gas
E973   Injury due to legal intervention by blunt object
E974   Injury due to legal intervention by cutting and piercing instruments
E975   Injury due to legal intervention by other specified means
E976   Injury due to legal intervention by unspecified means
E977   Late effects of injuries due to legal intervention
E978   Legal execution

Terrorism (E979)
E979   Terrorism

Injury undetermined whether accidentally or purposely inflicted (E980-E989)
E980   Poisoning by solid or liquid substances, undetermined whether accidentally or purposely inflicted
E981   Poisoning by gases in domestic use, undetermined whether accidentally or purposely inflicted

E982   Poisoning by other gases, undetermined whether accidentally or purposely inflicted
E983   Hanging, strangulation, or suffocation, undetermined whether accidentally or purposely inflicted
E984   Submersion [drowning], undetermined whether accidentally or purposely inflicted
E985   Injury by firearms and explosives, undetermined whether accidentally or purposely inflicted
E986   Injury by cutting and piercing instruments, undetermined whether accidentally or purposely inflicted
E987   Falling from high place, undetermined whether accidentally or purposely inflicted
E988   Injury by other and unspecified means, undetermined whether accidentally or purposely inflicted
E989   Late effects of injury, undetermined whether accidentally or purposely inflicted

Injury resulting from operations of war (E990-E999)
E990   Injury due to war operations by fires and conflagrations
E991   Injury due to war operations by bullets and fragments
E992   Injury due to war operations by explosion of marine weapons
E993   Injury due to war operations by other explosion
E994   Injury due to war operations by destruction of aircraft
E995   Injury due to war operations by other and unspecified forms of conventional warfare
E996   Injury due to war operations by nuclear weapons
E997   Injury due to war operations by other forms of unconventional warfare
E998   Injury due to war operations but occurring after cessation of hostilities
E999   Late effects of injury due to war operations

A

Abbe operation
construction of vagina 70.61
intestinal anastomosis — *see* Anastomosis, intestine

Abciximab, infusion 99.20

Abdominocentesis 54.91

Abdominohysterectomy 68.4

Abdominoplasty 86.83

Abdominoscopy 54.21

Abdominouterotomy 68.0
obstetrical 74.99

Abduction, arytenoid 31.69

Ablation
biliary tract (lesion) by ERCP 51.64
endometrial (hysteroscopic) 68.23
inner ear (cryosurgery) (ultrasound) 20.79
by injection 20.72
lesion
esophagus 42.39
endoscopic 42.33
heart (ventricular) 37.33
by cardiac catheter 37.34
intestine
large 45.49
endoscopic 45.43
large intestine 45.49
endoscopic 45.43
pituitary 07.69
by
cobalt 60 92.32
implantation (strontium-yttrium) (Y) NEC 07.68
transfrontal approach 07.64
transphenoidal approach 07.65
proton beam (Bragg peak) 92.33
prostate
by
cryoablation 60.62
laser, transurethral 60.21
radical cryosurgery ablation (RCSA) 60.62
radiofrequency thermotherapy 60.97
transurethral needle ablation (TUNA) 60.97

Abortion, therapeutic 69.51
by
aspiration curettage 69.51
dilation and curettage 69.01
hysterectomy — *see* Hysterectomy
hysterotomy 74.91
insertion
laminaria 69.93
prostaglandin suppository 96.49
intra-amniotic injection (saline) 75.0

Abrasion
corneal epithelium 11.41
for smear or culture 11.21
epicardial surface 36.39
pleural 34.6
skin 86.25

Abscission, cornea 11.49

Absorptiometry
photon (dual) (single) 88.98

Aburel operation (intra-amniotic injection for abortion) 75.0

Accouchement forcé 73.99

Acetabulectomy 77.85

Acetabuloplasty NEC 81.40
with prosthetic implant 81.52

Achillorrhaphy 83.64
delayed 83.62

Achillotenotomy 83.11
plastic 83.85

Achillotomy 83.11
plastic 83.85

Acid peel, skin 86.24

Acromionectomy 77.81

Acromioplasty 81.83
for recurrent dislocation of shoulder 81.82
partial replacement 81.81
total replacement 81.80

Actinotherapy 99.82

Activities of daily living (ADL)
therapy 93.83
training for the blind 93.78

Acupuncture 99.92
with smouldering moxa 93.35
for anesthesia 99.91

Adams operation
advancement of round ligament 69.22
crushing of nasal septum 21.88
excision of palmar fascia 82.35

Adenectomy — *see also* Excision, by site
prostate NEC 60.69
retropubic 60.4

Adenoidectomy (without tonsillectomy) 28.6
with tonsillectomy 28.3

Adhesiolysis — *see also* Lysis, adhesions
for collapse of lung 33.39
middle ear 20.23

Adipectomy 86.83

Adjustment
cardiac pacemaker program (reprogramming) — *omit code*
cochlear prosthetic device (external components) 95.49
dental 99.97
occlusal 24.8
spectacles 95.31

Administration (of) — *see also* Injection
adhesion barrier substance 99.77 ●
antitoxins NEC 99.58
botulism 99.57
diphtheria 99.58
gas gangrene 99.58
scarlet fever 99.58
tetanus 99.56
Bender Visual-Motor Gestalt test 94.02
Benton Visual Retention test 94.02
inhaled nitric oxide 00.12 ●
intelligence test or scale (Stanford-Binet) (Wechsler) (adult) (children) 94.01
Minnesota Multiphasic Personality Inventory (MMPI) 94.02
MMPI (Minnesota Multiphasic Personality Inventory) 94.02
neuroprotective agent 99.75
psychologic test 94.02
Stanford-Binet test 94.01
toxoid
diphtheria 99.36
with tetanus and pertussis, combined (DTP) 99.39
tetanus 99.38
with diphtheria and pertussis, combined (DTP) 99.39
vaccine — *see also* Vaccination
BCG 99.33
measles-mumps-rubella (MMR) 99.48
poliomyelitis 99.41
TAB 99.32
Wechsler
Intelligence Scale (adult) (children) 94.01
Memory Scale 94.02

Adrenalectomy (unilateral) 07.22
with partial removal of remaining gland 07.29
bilateral 07.3
partial 07.29
subtotal 07.29
complete 07.3
partial NEC 07.29
remaining gland 07.3
subtotal NEC 07.29
total 07.3

Adrenalorrhaphy 07.44

Adrenalotomy (with drainage) 07.41

Advancement
extraocular muscle 15.12
multiple (with resection or recession) 15.3
eyelid muscle 08.59
eye muscle 15.12
multiple (with resection or recession) 15.3
graft — *see* Graft
leaflet (heart) 35.10

Advancement — *continued*
pedicle (flap) 86.72
profundus tendon (Wagner) 82.51
round ligament 69.22
tendon 83.71
hand 82.51
profundus (Wagner) 82.51
Wagner (profundus tendon) 82.51

Albee operation
bone peg, femoral neck 78.05
graft for slipping patella 78.06
sliding inlay graft, tibia 78.07

Albert operation (arthrodesis of knee) 81.22

Aldridge (-Studdiford) operation (urethral sling) 59.5

Alexander operation
prostatectomy
perineal 60.62
suprapubic 60.3
shortening of round ligaments 69.22

Alexander-Adams operation (shortening of round ligaments) 69.22

Alimentation, parenteral 99.29

Allograft — *see* Graft

Almoor operation (extrapetrosal drainage) 20.22

Altemeier operation (perineal rectal pull-through) 48.49

Alveolectomy (interradicular) (intraseptal) (radical) (simple) (with graft) (with implant) 24.5

Alveoloplasty (with graft or implant) 24.5

Alveolotomy (apical) 24.0

Ambulatory cardiac monitoring (ACM) 89.50

Ammon operation (dacryocystotomy) 09.53

Amniocentesis (transuterine) (diagnostic) 75.1
with intra-amniotic injection of saline 75.0

Amniography 87.81

Amnioinfusion 75.37

Amnioscopy, internal 75.31

Amniotomy 73.09
to induce labor 73.01

Amputation (cineplastic) (closed flap) (guillotine) (kineplastic) (open) 84.91
abdominopelvic 84.19
above-elbow 84.07
above-knee (AK) 84.17
ankle (disarticulation) 84.13
through malleoli of tibia and fibula 84.14
arm NEC 84.00
through
carpals 84.03
elbow (disarticulation) 84.06
forearm 84.05
humerus 84.07
shoulder (disarticulation) 84.08
wrist (disarticulation) 84.04
upper 84.07
Batch-Spittler-McFaddin (knee disarticulation) 84.16
below-knee (BK) NEC 84.15
conversion into above-knee amputation 84.17
Boyd (hip disarticulation) 84.18
Callander's (knee disarticulation) 84.16
carpals 84.03
cervix 67.4
Chopart's (midtarsal) 84.12
clitoris 71.4
Dieffenbach (hip disarticulation) 84.18
Dupuytren's (shoulder disarticulation) 84.08
ear, external 18.39
elbow (disarticulation) 84.06
finger, except thumb 84.01
thumb 84.02
foot (middle) 84.12
forearm 84.05
forefoot 84.12
forequarter 84.09
Gordon-Taylor (hindquarter) 84.19
Gritti-Stokes (knee disarticulation) 84.16
Guyon (ankle) 84.13
hallux 84.11

✓4ᵗʰ Fourth-digit Required   ▶◀ Revised Text   ● New Line   ▲ Revised Code

Anastomosis — *continued*
  ureter (to) NEC — *continued*
    intestine 56.71
    skin 56.61
  ureterocalyceal 55.86
  ureterocolic 56.71
  ureterovesical 56.74
  urethra (end-to-end) 58.44
  vas deferens 63.82
  veins (suture of proximal to distal end) (with bypass graft) 39.29
    with excision or resection of vessel — *see* Phlebectomy, with anastomosis, by site
    mesenteric to vena cava 39.1
    portal to inferior vena cava 39.1
    revision 39.49
    splenic and renal 39.1
  ventricle, ventricular (intracerebral) (with valve) (*see also* Shunt, ventricular) 02.2
  ventriculoatrial (with valve) 02.32
  ventriculocaval (with valve) 02.32
  ventriculomastoid (with valve) 02.31
  ventriculopleural (with valve) 02.33
  vesicle — *see* Anastomosis, bladder

Anderson operation (tibial lengthening) 78.37

Anel operation (dilation of lacrimal duct) 09.42

Anesthesia
  acupuncture for 99.91
  cryoanalgesia, nerve (cranial) (peripheral) 04.2
  spinal — *omit code*

Aneurysmectomy 38.60
  with
    anastomosis 38.30
      abdominal
        artery 38.36
        vein 38.37
      aorta (arch) (ascending) (descending) 38.34
      head and neck NEC 38.32
      intracranial NEC 38.31
      lower limb
        artery 38.38
        vein 38.39
      thoracic NEC 38.35
      upper limb (artery) (vein) 38.33
    graft replacement (interposition) 38.40
      abdominal
        aorta 38.44
        artery 38.46
        vein 38.47
      aorta (arch) (ascending) (descending thoracic)
        abdominal 38.44
        thoracic 38.45
        thoracoabdominal 38.45 *[38.44]*
      head and neck NEC 38.42
      intracranial NEC 38.41
      lower limb
        artery 38.48
        vein 38.49
      thoracic NEC 38.45
      upper limb (artery) (vein) 38.43
  abdominal
    artery 38.66
    vein 38.67
  aorta (arch) (ascending) (descending) 38.64
  atrial, auricular 37.32
  head and neck NEC 38.62
  heart 37.32
  intracranial NEC 38.61
  lower limb
    artery 38.68
    vein 38.69
  sinus of Valsalva 35.39
  thoracic NEC 38.65
  upper limb (artery) (vein) 38.63
  ventricle (myocardium) 37.32

Aneurysmoplasty — *see* Aneurysmorrhaphy

Aneurysmorrhaphy NEC 39.52
  by or with
    anastomosis — *see* Aneurysmectomy, with anastomosis, by site
    clipping 39.51

Aneurysmorrhaphy NEC — *continued*
  by or with — *continued*
    coagulation 39.52
    electrocoagulation 39.52
    endovascular graft
      abdominal aorta 39.71
      lower extremity artery(s) 39.79
      thoracic aorta 39.79
      upper extremity artery(s) 39.79
    excision or resection — *see also* Aneurysmectomy, by site
      with
        anastomosis — *see* Aneurysmectomy, with anastomosis, by site
        graft replacement — *see* Aneurysmectomy, with graft replacement, by site
    filipuncture 39.52
    graft replacement — *see* Aneurysmectomy, with graft replacement, by site
    methyl methacrylate 39.52
    suture 39.52
    wiring 39.52
    wrapping 39.52
  Matas' 39.52

Aneurysmotomy — *see* Aneurysmectomy

Angiectomy
  with
    anastomosis 38.30
      abdominal
        artery 38.36
        vein 38.37
      aorta (arch) (ascending) (descending) 38.34
      head and neck NEC 38.32
      intracranial NEC 38.31
      lower limb
        artery 38.38
        vein 38.39
      thoracic vessel NEC 38.35
      upper limb (artery) (vein) 38.33
    graft replacement (interposition) 38.40
      abdominal
        aorta 38.44
        artery 38.46
        vein 38.47
      aorta (arch) (ascending) (descending thoracic)
        abdominal 38.44
        thoracic 38.45
        thoracoabdominal 38.45 *[38.44]*
      head and neck NEC 38.42
      intracranial NEC 38.41
      lower limb
        artery 38.48
        vein 38.49
      thoracic vessel NEC 38.45
      upper limb (artery) (vein) 38.43

Angiocardiography (selective) 88.50
  carbon dioxide (negative contrast) 88.58
  combined right and left heart 88.54
  left heart (aortic valve) (atrium) (ventricle) (ventricular outflow tract) 88.53
    combined with right heart 88.54
  right heart (atrium) (pulmonary valve) (ventricle) (ventricular outflow tract) 88.52
    combined with left heart 88.54
  vena cava (inferior) (superior) 88.51

Angiography (arterial) (*see also* Arteriography) 88.40
  by radioisotope — *see* Scan, radioisotope, by site
  by ultrasound — *see* Ultrasonography, by site
  basilar 88.41
  brachial 88.49
  carotid (internal) 88.41
  celiac 88.47
  cerebral (posterior circulation) 88.41
  coronary NEC 88.57
  eye (fluorescein) 95.12
  femoral 88.48
  heart 88.50
  intra-abdominal NEC 88.47
  intracranial 88.41

Angiography (*see also* Arteriography) — *continued*
  intrathoracic vessels NEC 88.44
  lower extremity NEC 88.48
  neck 88.41
  placenta 88.46
  pulmonary 88.43
  renal 88.45
  specified artery NEC 88.49
  transfemoral 88.48
  upper extremity NEC 88.49
  veins — *see* Phlebography
  vertebral 88.41

Angioplasty (laser) — *see also* Repair, blood vessel
  balloon (percutaneous transluminal) NEC 39.50
    coronary artery (single vessel) 36.01
      with thrombolytic agent infusion 36.02
      multiple vessels 36.05
    other sites (femoropopliteal) (iliac) (non-coronary) (renal) (vertebral) 39.50
  coronary 36.09
    open chest approach 36.03
    percutaneous transluminal (balloon) (single vessel) 36.01
      with thrombolytic agent infusion 36.02
      multiple vessels 36.05
  percutaneous transluminal (balloon) (single vessel) 39.50
    basilar 39.50
    carotid 39.50
    coronary (balloon) (single vessel) 36.01
      with thrombolytic agent infusion 36.02
      multiple vessels 36.05
    femoropopliteal 39.50
    head and neck 39.50
    iliac 39.50
    lower extremity NOS 39.50
    mesenteric 39.50
    renal 39.50
    upper extremity NOS 39.50
    vertebral 39.50
  specified site NEC 39.50

Angiorrhaphy 39.30
  artery 39.31
  vein 39.32

Angioscopy, percutaneous 38.22
  eye (fluorescein) 95.12

Angiotomy 38.00
  abdominal
    artery 38.06
    vein 38.07
  aorta (arch) (ascending) (descending) 38.04
  head and neck NEC 38.02
  intracranial NEC 38.01
  lower limb
    artery 38.08
    vein 38.09
  thoracic NEC 38.05
  upper limb (artery) (vein) 38.03

Angiotripsy 39.98

Ankylosis, production of — *see* Arthrodesis

Annuloplasty (heart) (posteromedial) 35.33

Anoplasty 49.79
  with hemorrhoidectomy 49.46

Anoscopy 49.21

Antibiogram — *see* Examination, microscopic

Antiembolic filter, vena cava 38.7

Antiphobic treatment 94.39

Antrectomy
  mastoid 20.49
  maxillary 22.39
    radical 22.31
  pyloric 43.6

Antrostomy — *see* Antrotomy

Antrotomy (exploratory) (nasal sinus) 22.2
  Caldwell-Luc (maxillary sinus) 22.39
    with removal of membrane lining 22.31
  intranasal 22.2
    with external approach (Caldwell-Luc) 22.39
      radical 22.31

Antrotomy — *continued*
  maxillary (simple) 22.2
    with Caldwell-Luc approach 22.39
      with removal of membrane lining 22.31
    external (Caldwell-Luc approach) 22.39
      with removal of membrane lining 22.31
    radical (with removal of membrane lining)
      22.31
Antrum window operation — *see* Antrotomy,
  maxillary
Aorticopulmonary window operation 39.59
Aortogram, aortography (abdominal) (retrograde)
  (selective) (translumbar) 88.42
Aortoplasty (aortic valve) (gusset type) 35.11
Aortotomy 38.04
Apexcardiogram (with ECG lead) 89.57
Apheresis, therapeutic — *see* category 99.7 ✓4ᵗʰ
Apicectomy
  lung 32.3
  petrous pyramid 20.59
  tooth (root) 23.73
    with root canal therapy 23.72
Apicoectomy 23.73
  with root canal therapy 23.72
Apicolysis (lung) 33.39
Apicostomy, alveolar 24.0
Aponeurectomy 83.42
  hand 82.33
Aponeurorrhaphy (*see also* Suture, tendon) 83.64
  hand (*see also* Suture, tendon, hand) 82.45
Aponeurotomy 83.13
  hand 82.11
Appendectomy (with drainage) 47.09
  incidental 47.19
    laparoscopic 47.11
  laparoscopic 47.01
Appendicectomy (with drainage) 47.09
  incidental 47.19
    laparoscopic 47.11
  laparoscopic 47.01
Appendicocecostomy 47.91
Appendicoenterostomy 47.91
Appendicolysis 54.59
  with appendectomy
    laparoscopic 47.01
    other 47.09
  laparoscopic 54.51
Appendicostomy 47.91
  closure 47.92
Appendicotomy 47.2
Application
  adhesion barrier ▶substance◀ 99.77   ▲
  anti-shock trousers 93.58
  arch bars (orthodontic) 24.7
    for immobilization (fracture) 93.55
  barrier substance, adhesion 99.77   ●
  Barton's tongs (skull) (with synchronous
    skeletal traction) 02.94
  bone growth stimulator (surface)
    (transcutaneous) 99.86
  bone morphogenetic protein (recombinant)   ●
    (rhBMP) 84.52   ●
  Bryant's traction 93.44
    with reduction of fracture or dislocation —
      see Reduction, fracture *and*
      Reduction, dislocation
  Buck's traction 93.46
  caliper tongs (skull) (with synchronous skeletal
    traction) 02.94
  cast (fiberglass) (plaster) (plastic) NEC 93.53
    with reduction of fracture or dislocation —
      see Reduction, fracture *and*
      Reduction, dislocation
    spica 93.51
  cervical collar 93.52
    with reduction of fracture or dislocation —
      see Reduction, fracture *and*
      Reduction, dislocation
  clamp, cerebral aneurysm (Crutchfield)
    (Silverstone) 39.51
  croupette, croup tent 93.94
  crown (artificial) 23.41

Application — *continued*
  Crutchfield tongs (skull) (with synchronous
    skeletal traction) 02.94
  Dunlop's traction 93.44
    with reduction of fracture or dislocation —
      see Reduction, fracture *and*
      Reduction, dislocation
  elastic stockings 93.59
  electronic gaiter 93.59
  external fixation device (bone) 78.10
    carpal, metacarpal 78.14
    clavicle 78.11
    femur 78.15
    fibula 78.17
    humerus 78.12
    patella 78.16
    pelvic 78.19
    phalanges (foot) (hand) 78.19
    radius 78.13
    scapula 78.11
    specified site NEC 78.19
    tarsal, metatarsal 78.18
    thorax (ribs) (sternum) 78.11
    tibia 78.17
    ulna 78.13
    vertebrae 78.19
  forceps, with delivery — *see* Delivery, forceps
  graft — *see* Graft
  gravity (G-) suit 93.59
  intermittent pressure device 93.59
  Jewett extension brace 93.59
  Jobst pumping unit (reduction of edema) 93.59
  Lyman Smith traction 93.44
    with reduction of fracture or dislocation —
      see Reduction, fracture *and*
      Reduction, dislocation
  MAST (military anti-shock trousers) 93.58
  Minerva jacket 93.52
  minifixator device (bone) — *see* category
    78.1 ✓4ᵗʰ
  neck support (molded) 93.52
  obturator (orthodontic) 24.7
  orthodontic appliance (obturator) (wiring) 24.7
  pelvic sling 93.44
    with reduction of fracture or dislocation —
      see Reduction, fracture *and*
      Reduction, dislocation
  peridontal splint (orthodontic) 24.7
  plaster jacket 93.51
    Minerva 93.52
  pressure
    dressing (bandage) (Gibney) (Robert Jones')
      (Shanz) 93.56
    trousers (anti-shock) (MAST) 93.58
  prosthesis for missing ear 18.71
  Russell's traction 93.44
    with reduction of fracture or dislocation —
      see Reduction, fracture *and*
      Reduction, dislocation
  splint, for immobilization (plaster) (pneumatic)
    (tray) 93.54
    with fracture reduction — *see* Reduction,
      fracture
  stereotactic head frame 93.59
  substance, adhesion barrier 99.77   ●
  Thomas collar 93.52
    with reduction of fracture or dislocation —
      see Reduction, fracture *and*
      Reduction, dislocation
  traction
    with reduction of fracture or dislocation —
      see Reduction, fracture *and*
      Reduction, dislocation
    adhesive tape (skin) 93.46
    boot 93.46
    Bryant's 93.44
    Buck's 93.46
    Cotrel's 93.42
    Dunlop's 93.44
    gallows 93.46
    Lyman Smith 93.44
    Russell's 93.44
    skeletal NEC 93.44
      intermittent 93.43
    skin, limbs NEC 93.46

Application — *continued*
  traction — *continued*
    spinal NEC 93.42
      with skull device (halo) (caliper)
        (Crutchfield) (Gardner-Wells) (Vinke)
        (tongs) 93.41
        with synchronous insertion 02.94
    Thomas' splint 93.45
  Unna's paste boot 93.53
  vasopneumatic device 93.58
  Velpeau dressing 93.59
  Vinke tongs (skull) (with synchronous skeletal
    traction) 02.94
  wound dressing NEC 93.57
Arc lamp — *see* Photocoagulation
Arrest
  bone growth (epiphyseal) 78.20
    by stapling — *see* Stapling, epiphyseal plate
    femur 78.25
    fibula 78.27
    humerus 78.22
    radius 78.23
    tibia 78.27
    ulna 78.23
  cardiac, induced (anoxic) (circulatory) 39.63
  circulatory, induced (anoxic) 39.63
  hemorrhage — *see* Control, hemorrhage
Arslan operation (fenestration of inner ear) 20.61
Arteriectomy 38.60
  with
    anastomosis 38.30
      abdominal 38.36
      aorta (arch) (ascending) (descending)
        38.34
      head and neck NEC 38.32
      intracranial NEC 38.31
      lower limb 38.38
      thoracic NEC 38.35
      upper limb 38.33
    graft replacement (interposition) 38.40
      abdominal
        aorta 38.44
      aorta (arch) (ascending) (descending
        thoracic)
        abdominal 38.44
        thoracic 38.45
        thoracoabdominal 38.45 *[38.44]*
      head and neck NEC 38.42
      intracranial NEC 38.41
      lower limb 38.48
      thoracic NEC 38.45
      upper limb 38.43
  abdominal 38.66
  aorta (arch) (ascending) (descending) 38.64
  head and neck NEC 38.62
  intracranial NEC 38.61
  lower limb 38.68
  thoracic NEC 38.65
  upper limb 38.63
Arteriography (contrast) (fluoroscopic)
  (retrograde) 88.40
  by
    radioisotope — *see* Scan, radioisotope
    ultrasound (Doppler) — *see*
      Ultrasonography, by site
  aorta (arch) (ascending) (descending) 88.42
  basilar 88.41
  brachial 88.49
  carotid (internal) 88.41
  cerebral (posterior circulation) 88.41
  coronary (direct) (selective) NEC 88.57
    double catheter technique (Judkins)
      (Ricketts and Abrams) 88.56
    single catheter technique (Sones) 88.55
  Doppler (ultrasonic) — *see* Ultrasonography, by
    site
  femoral 88.48
  head and neck 88.41
  intra-abdominal NEC 88.47
  intrathoracic NEC 88.44
  lower extremity 88.48
  placenta 88.46
  pulmonary 88.43
  radioisotope — *see* Scan, radioisotope
  renal 88.45

Arteriography — *continued*
    specified site NEC 88.49
    superior mesenteric artery 88.47
    transfemoral 88.48
    ultrasound — *see* Ultrasonography, by site
    upper extremity 88.49
Arterioplasty — *see* Repair, artery
Arteriorrhaphy 39.31
Arteriotomy 38.00
    abdominal 38.06
    aorta (arch) (ascending) (descending) 38.04
    head and neck NEC 38.02
    intracranial NEC 38.01
    lower limb 38.08
    thoracic NEC 38.05
    upper limb 38.03
Arteriovenostomy 39.29
    for renal dialysis 39.27
Arthrectomy 80.90
    ankle 80.97
    elbow 80.92
    foot and toe 80.98
    hand and finger 80.94
    hip 80.95
    intervertebral disc 80.5 ✓4ᵗʰ
    knee 80.96
        semilunar cartilage 80.6
    shoulder 80.91
    specified site NEC 80.99
    spine NEC 80.99
    wrist 80.93
Arthrocentesis 81.91
    for arthrography — *see* Arthrogram
Arthrodesis (compression) (extra-articular) (intra-
        articular) (with bone graft) (with fixation
        device) 81.20
    ankle 81.11
    carporadial 81.25
    cricoarytenoid 31.69
    elbow 81.24
    finger 81.28
    foot NEC 81.17
    hip 81.21
    interphalangeal
        finger 81.28
        toe NEC 77.58
            claw toe repair 77.57
            hammer toe repair 77.56
    ischiofemoral 81.21
    knee 81.22
    lumbosacral, lumbar NEC 81.08
        anterior (interbody), anterolateral technique
            81.06
        lateral transverse process technique 81.07
        posterior (interbody), posterolateral
            technique 81.08
    McKeever (metatarsophalangeal) 81.16
    metacarpocarpal 81.26
    metacarpophalangeal 81.27
    metatarsophalangeal 81.16
    midtarsal 81.14
    plantar 81.11
    sacroiliac 81.08
    shoulder 81.23
    specified joint NEC 81.29
    spinal (*see also* Fusion, spinal) 81.00
    subtalar 81.13
    tarsometatarsal 81.15
    tibiotalar 81.11
    toe NEC 77.58
        claw toe repair 77.57
        hammer toe repair 77.56
    triple 81.12
    wrist 81.26
Arthroendoscopy — *see* Arthroscopy
Arthrogram, arthrography 88.32
    temporomandibular 87.13
Arthrolysis 93.26
Arthroplasty (with fixation device) (with traction)
        81.96
    ankle 81.49
    carpals 81.75
        with prosthetic implant 81.74

Arthroplasty — *continued*
    carpocarpal, carpometacarpal 81.75
        with prosthetic implant 81.74
    Carroll and Taber (proximal interphalangeal
        joint) 81.72
    cup (partial hip) 81.52
    Curtis (interphalangeal joint) 81.72
    elbow 81.85
        with prosthetic replacement (total) 81.84
    femoral head NEC 81.40
        with prosthetic implant 81.52
    finger(s) 81.72
        with prosthetic implant 81.71
    foot (metatarsal) with joint replacement 81.57
    Fowler (metacarpophalangeal joint) 81.72
    hand (metacarpophalangeal) (interphalangeal)
        81.72
        with prosthetic implant 81.71
    hip (with bone graft) 81.40
        cup (partial hip) 81.52
        femoral head NEC 81.40
            with prosthetic implant 81.52
                with total replacement 81.51
        partial replacement 81.52
        total replacement 81.51
    interphalangeal joint 81.72
        with prosthetic implant 81.71
    Kessler (carpometacarpal joint) 81.74
    knee (*see also* Repair, knee) 81.47
        prosthetic replacement (bicompartmental)
            (hemijoint) (partial) (total)
            (tricompartmental) (unicompartmental)
            81.54
        revision 81.55
    metacarpophalangeal joint 81.72
        with prosthetic implant 81.71
    shoulder 81.83
        prosthetic replacement (partial) 81.81
            total 81.80
        for recurrent dislocation 81.82
    temporomandibular 76.5
    toe NEC 77.58
        with prosthetic replacement 81.57
        for hallux valgus repair 77.59
    wrist 81.75
        with prosthetic implant 81.74
            total replacement 81.73
Arthroscopy 80.20
    ankle 80.27
    elbow 80.22
    finger 80.24
    foot 80.28
    hand 80.24
    hip 80.25
    knee 80.26
    shoulder 80.21
    specified site NEC 80.29
    toe 80.28
    wrist 80.23
Arthrostomy (*see also* Arthrotomy) 80.10
Arthrotomy 80.10
    as operative approach — *omit code*
    with
        arthrography — *see* Arthrogram
        arthroscopy — *see* Arthroscopy
        injection of drug 81.92
        removal of prosthesis (*see also* Removal,
            prosthesis, joint structures) 80.00
    ankle 80.17
    elbow 80.12
    foot and toe 80.18
    hand and finger 80.14
    hip 80.15
    knee 80.16
    shoulder 80.11
    specified site NEC 80.19
    spine 80.19
    wrist 80.13
Artificial
    insemination 69.92
    kidney 39.95
    rupture of membranes 73.09
Arytenoidectomy 30.29
Arytenoidopexy 31.69

Asai operation (larynx) 31.75
Aspiration
    abscess — *see* Aspiration, by site
    anterior chamber, eye (therapeutic) 12.91
        diagnostic 12.21
    aqueous (eye) (humor) (therapeutic) 12.91
        diagnostic 12.21
    ascites 54.91
    Bartholin's gland (cyst) (percutaneous) 71.21
    biopsy — *see* Biopsy, by site
    bladder (catheter) 57.0
        percutaneous (needle) 57.11
    bone marrow (for biopsy) 41.31
        from donor for transplant 41.91
        stem cell 99.79
    branchial cleft cyst 29.0
    breast 85.91
    bronchus 96.05
        with lavage 96.56
    bursa (percutaneous) 83.94
        hand 82.92
    calculus, bladder 57.0
    cataract 13.3
        with
            phacoemulsification 13.41
            phacofragmentation 13.43
                posterior route 13.42
    chest 34.91
    cisternal 01.01
    cranial (puncture) 01.09
    craniobuccal pouch 07.72
    craniopharyngioma 07.72
    cul-de-sac (abscess) 70.0
    curettage, uterus 69.59
        after abortion or delivery 69.52
        diagnostic 69.59
        to terminate pregnancy 69.51
    cyst — *see* Aspiration, by site
    diverticulum, pharynx 29.0
    endotracheal 96.04
        with lavage 96.56
    extradural 01.09
    eye (anterior chamber) (therapeutic) 12.91
        diagnostic 12.21
    fallopian tube 66.91
    fascia 83.95
        hand 82.93
    gallbladder (percutaneous) 51.01
    hematoma — *see also* Aspiration, by site
        obstetrical 75.92
            incisional 75.91
    hydrocele, tunica vaginalis 61.91
    hygroma — *see* Aspiration, by site
    hyphema 12.91
    hypophysis 07.72
    intracranial space (epidural) (extradural)
        (subarachnoid) (subdural) (ventricular)
        01.09
        through previously implanted catheter or
            reservoir (Ommaya) (Rickham) 01.02
    joint 81.91
        for arthrography — *see* Arthrogram
    kidney (cyst) (pelvis) (percutaneous)
        (therapeutic) 55.92
        diagnostic 55.23
    liver (percutaneous) 50.91
    lung (percutaneous) (puncture) (needle) (trocar)
        33.93
    middle ear 20.09
        with intubation 20.01
    muscle 83.95
        hand 82.93
    nail 86.01
    nasal sinus 22.00
        by puncture 22.01
        through natural ostium 22.02
    nasotracheal 96.04
        with lavage 96.56
    orbit, diagnostic 16.22
    ovary 65.91
    percutaneous — *see* Aspiration, by site
    pericardium (wound) 37.0
    pituitary gland 07.72
    pleural cavity 34.91
    prostate (percutaneous) 60.91

Aspiration — Biopsy

Aspiration — continued
Rathke's pouch 07.72
seminal vesicles 60.71
seroma — see Aspiration, by site
skin 86.01
soft tissue NEC 83.95
    hand 82.93
spermatocele 63.91
spinal (puncture) 03.31
spleen (cyst) 41.1
stem cell 99.79
subarachnoid space (cerebral) 01.09
subcutaneous tissue 86.01
subdural space (cerebral) 01.09
tendon 83.95
    hand 82.93
testis 62.91
thymus 07.92
thyroid (field) (gland) 06.01
    postoperative 06.02
trachea 96.04
    with lavage 96.56
    percutaneous 31.99
tunica vaginalis (hydrocele) (percutaneous)
    61.91
vitreous (and replacement) 14.72
    diagnostic 14.11
Assessment
fitness to testify 94.11
mental status 94.11
nutritional status 89.39
personality 94.03
temperament 94.02
vocational 93.85
Assistance
cardiac (see also Resuscitation, cardiac)
    extracorporeal circulation 39.61
endotracheal respiratory — see category 96.7
hepatic, extracorporeal 50.92
respiratory (endotracheal) (mechanical) — see
    ventilation, mechanical
Astragalectomy 77.98
Asymmetrogammagram — see Scan,
    radioisotope
Atherectomy
coronary — see Angioplasty
peripheral 39.50
Atriocommissuropexy (mitral valve) 35.12
Atrioplasty NEC 37.99
combined with repair of valvular and
    ventricular septal defects — see Repair,
    endocardial cushion defect
septum (heart) NEC 35.71
Atrioseptopexy (see also Repair, atrial septal
    defect) 35.71
Atrioseptoplasty (see also Repair, atrial septal
    defect) 35.71
Atrioseptostomy (balloon) 35.41
Atriotomy 37.11
Atrioventriculostomy (cerebral-heart) 02.32
Attachment
eye muscle
    orbicularis oculi to eyebrow 08.36
    rectus to frontalis 15.9
pedicle (flap) graft 86.74
    hand 86.73
    lip 27.57
    mouth 27.57
pharyngeal flap (for cleft palate repair) 27.62
    secondary or subsequent 27.63
retina — see Reattachment, retina
Atticoantrostomy (ear) 20.49
Atticoantrotomy (ear) 20.49
Atticotomy (ear) 20.23
Audiometry (Békésy 5-tone) (impedance)
    (stapedial reflex response) (subjective) 95.41
Augmentation
bladder 57.87
breast — see Mammoplasty, augmentation
buttock ("fanny-lift") 86.89
chin 76.68
genioplasty 76.68

Augmentation — continued
mammaplasty — see Mammoplasty,
    augmentation
outflow tract (pulmonary valve) (gusset type)
    35.26
    in total repair of tetralogy of Fallot 35.81
vocal cord(s) 31.0
Auriculectomy 18.39
Autograft — see Graft
Autologous — see Blood, transfusion
Autopsy 89.8
Autotransfusion (whole blood) — see Blood,
    transfusion
Autotransplant, autotransplantation — see also
    Reimplantation
adrenal tissue (heterotopic) (orthotopic) 07.45
kidney 55.61
lung — see Transplant, transplantation, lung
    33.5 ☑4ᵗʰ
ovary 65.72
    laparoscopic 65.75
pancreatic tissue 52.81
parathyroid tissue (heterotopic) (orthotopic)
    06.95
thyroid tissue (heterotopic) (orthotopic) 06.94
tooth 23.5
Avulsion, nerve (cranial) (peripheral) NEC 04.07
acoustic 04.01
phrenic 33.31
sympathetic 05.29
Azygography 88.63

B

Bacterial smear — see Examination, microscopic
Baffes operation (interatrial transposition of
    venous return) 35.91
Baffle, atrial or interatrial 35.91
Balanoplasty 64.49
Baldy-Webster operation (uterine suspension)
    69.22
Ballistocardiography 89.59
Balloon
angioplasty — see Angioplasty, balloon
pump, intra-aortic 37.61
systostomy (atrial) 35.41
Ball operation
herniorrhaphy — see Repair, hernia, inguinal
undercutting 49.02
Bandage 93.57
elastic 93.56
Banding, pulmonary artery 38.85
Bankhart operation (capsular repair into glenoid,
    for shoulder dislocation) 81.82
Bardenheurer operation (ligation of innominate
    artery) 38.85
Barium swallow 87.61
Barkan operation (goniotomy) 12.52
    with goniopuncture 12.53
Barr operation (transfer of tibialis posterior
    tendon) 83.75
Barsky operation (closure of cleft hand) 82.82
Basal metabolic rate 89.39
Basiotripsy 73.8
Bassett operation (vulvectomy with inguinal
    lymph node dissection) 71.5 [40.3]
Bassini operation — see Repair, hernia, inguinal
Batch-Spittler-McFaddin operation (knee
    disarticulation) 84.16
Batista operation (partial ventriculectomy)
    (ventricular reduction) (ventricular
    remodeling) 37.35
Beck operation
aorta-coronary sinus shunt 36.39
epicardial poudrage 36.39
Beck-Jianu operation (permanent gastrostomy)
    43.19
Behavior modification 94.33

Bell-Beuttner operation (subtotal abdominal
    hysterectomy) 68.3
Belsey operation (esophagogastric sphincter)
    44.65
Benenenti operation (rotation of bulbous
    urethra) 58.49
Berke operation (levator resection of eyelid) 08.33
Bicuspidization of heart valve 35.10
aortic 35.11
mitral 35.12
Bicycle dynamometer 93.01
Biesenberger operation (size reduction of breast,
    bilateral) 85.32
unilateral 85.31
Bifurcation, bone (see also Osteotomy) 77.30
Bigelow operation (litholapaxy) 57.0
Bililite therapy (ultraviolet) 99.82
Billroth I operation (partial gastrectomy with
    gastroduodenostomy) 43.6
Billroth II operation (partial gastrectomy with
    gastrojejunostomy) 43.7
Binnie operation (hepatopexy) 50.69
Biofeedback, psychotherapy 94.39
Biopsy
abdominal wall 54.22
adenoid 28.11
adrenal gland NEC 07.11
    closed 07.11
    open 07.12
    percutaneous (aspiration) (needle) 07.11
alveolus 24.12
anus 49.23
appendix 45.26
artery (any site) 38.21
aspiration — see Biopsy, by site
bile ducts 51.14
    closed (endoscopic) 51.14
    open 51.13
    percutaneous (needle) 51.12
bladder 57.33
    closed 57.33
    open 57.34
    transurethral 57.33
blood vessel (any site) 38.21
bone 77.40
    carpal, metacarpal 77.44
    clavicle 77.41
    facial 76.11
    femur 77.45
    fibula 77.47
    humerus 77.42
    marrow 41.31
    patella 77.46
    pelvic 77.49
    phalanges (foot) (hand) 77.49
    radius 77.43
    scapula 77.41
    specified site NEC 77.49
    tarsal, metatarsal 77.48
    thorax (ribs) (sternum) 77.41
    tibia 77.47
    ulna 77.43
    vertebrae 77.49
bowel — see Biopsy, intestine
brain NEC 01.13
    closed 01.13
    open 01.14
    percutaneous (needle) 01.13
breast 85.11
    blind 85.11
    closed 85.11
    open 85.12
    percutaneous (needle) (Vimm-Silverman)
        85.11
bronchus NEC 33.24
    brush 33.24
    closed (endoscopic) 33.24
    open 33.25
    washings 33.24
bursa 83.21
cardioesophageal (junction) 44.14
    closed (endoscopic) 44.14
    open 44.15

Biopsy — *continued*
- cecum 45.25
  - brush 45.25
  - closed (endoscopic) 45.25
  - open 45.26
- cerebral meninges NEC 01.11
  - closed 01.11
  - open 01.12
  - percutaneous (needle) 01.11
- cervix (punch) 67.12
  - conization (sharp) 67.2
- chest wall 34.23
- clitoris 71.11
- colon 45.25
  - brush 45.25
  - closed (endoscopic) 45.25
  - open 45.26
- conjunctiva 10.21
- cornea 11.22
- cul-de-sac 70.23
- diaphragm 34.27
- duodenum 45.14
  - brush 45.14
  - closed (endoscopic) 45.14
  - open 45.15
- ear (external) 18.12
  - middle or inner 20.32
- endocervix 67.11
- endometrium NEC 68.16
  - by
    - aspiration curettage 69.59
    - dilation and curettage 69.09
  - closed (endoscopic) 68.16
  - open 68.13
- epididymis 63.01
- esophagus 42.24
  - closed (endoscopic) 42.24
  - open 42.25
- extraocular muscle or tendon 15.01
- eye 16.23
  - muscle (oblique) (rectus) 15.01
- eyelid 08.11
- fallopian tube 66.11
- fascia 83.21
- fetus 75.33
- gallbladder 51.12
  - closed (endoscopic) 51.14
  - open 51.13
  - percutaneous (needle) 51.12
- ganglion (cranial) (peripheral) NEC 04.11
  - closed 04.11
  - open 04.12
  - percutaneous (needle) 04.11
  - sympathetic nerve 05.11
- gum 24.11
- heart 37.25
- hypophysis (*see also* Biopsy, pituitary gland) 07.15
- ileum 45.14
  - brush 45.14
  - closed (endoscopic) 45.14
  - open 45.15
- intestine NEC 45.27
  - large 45.25
    - brush 45.25
    - closed (endoscopic) 45.25
    - open 45.26
  - small 45.14
    - brush 45.14
    - closed (endoscopic) 45.14
    - open 45.15
- intra-abdominal mass 54.24
  - closed 54.24
  - percutaneous (needle) 54.24
- iris 12.22
- jejunum 45.14
  - brush 45.14
  - closed (endoscopic) 45.14
  - open 45.15
- joint structure (aspiration) 80.30
  - ankle 80.37
  - elbow 80.32
  - foot and toe 80.38
  - hand and finger 80.34
  - hip 80.35
  - knee 80.36

Biopsy — *continued*
- joint structure — *continued*
  - shoulder 80.31
  - specified site NEC 80.39
  - spine 80.39
  - wrist 80.33
- kidney 55.23
  - closed 55.23
  - open 55.24
  - percutaneous (aspiration) (needle) 55.23
- labia 71.11
- lacrimal
  - gland 09.11
  - sac 09.12
- larynx 31.43
  - brush 31.43
  - closed (endoscopic) 31.43
  - open 31.45
- lip 27.23
- liver 50.11
  - closed 50.11
  - open 50.12
  - percutaneous (aspiration) (needle) 50.11
- lung NEC 33.27
  - brush 33.24
  - closed (percutaneous) (needle) 33.26
    - brush 33.24
    - endoscopic 33.27
      - brush 33.24
  - endoscopic 33.27
    - brush 33.24
  - open 33.28
  - transbronchial 33.27
- lymphatic structure (channel) (node) (vessel) 40.11
- mediastinum NEC 34.25
  - closed 34.25
  - open 34.26
  - percutaneous (needle) 34.25
- meninges (cerebral) NEC 01.11
  - closed 01.11
  - open 01.12
  - percutaneous (needle) 01.11
  - spinal 03.32
- mesentery 54.23
- mouth NEC 27.24
- muscle 83.21
  - extraocular 15.01
  - ocular 15.01
- nasopharynx 29.12
- nerve (cranial) (peripheral) NEC 04.11
  - closed 04.11
  - open 04.12
  - percutaneous (needle) 04.11
  - sympathetic 05.11
- nose, nasal 21.22
  - sinus 22.11
    - closed (endoscopic) (needle) 22.11
    - open 22.12
- ocular muscle or tendon 15.01
- omentum
  - closed 54.24
  - open 54.23
  - percutaneous (needle) 54.24
- orbit 16.23
  - by aspiration 16.22
- ovary 65.12
  - by aspiration 65.11
  - laparoscopic 65.13
- palate (bony) 27.21
  - soft 27.22
- pancreas 52.11
  - closed (endoscopic) 52.11
  - open 52.12
  - percutaneous (aspiration) (needle) 52.11
- pancreatic duct 52.14
  - closed (endoscopic) 52.14
- parathyroid gland 06.13
- penis 64.11
- perianal tissue 49.22
- pericardium 37.24
- periprostatic 60.15
- perirectal tissue 48.26
- perirenal tissue 59.21
- peritoneal implant
  - closed 54.24

Biopsy — *continued*
- peritoneal implant — *continued*
  - open 54.23
  - percutaneous (needle) 54.24
- peritoneum
  - closed 54.24
  - open 54.23
  - percutaneous (needle) 54.24
- periurethral tissue 58.24
- perivesical tissue 59.21
- pharynx, pharyngeal 29.12
- pineal gland 07.17
- pituitary gland 07.15
  - transfrontal approach 07.13
  - transsphenoidal approach 07.14
- pleura, pleural 34.24
- prostate NEC 60.11
  - closed (transurethral) 60.11
  - open 60.12
  - percutaneous (needle) 60.11
  - transrectal 60.11
- rectum 48.24
  - brush 48.24
  - closed (endoscopic) 48.24
  - open 48.25
- retroperitoneal tissue 54.24
- salivary gland or duct 26.11
  - closed (needle) 26.11
  - open 26.12
- scrotum 61.11
- seminal vesicle NEC 60.13
  - closed 60.13
  - open 60.14
  - percutaneous (needle) 60.13
- sigmoid colon 45.25
  - brush 45.25
  - closed (endoscopic) 45.25
  - open 45.26
- sinus, nasal 22.11
  - closed (endoscopic) (needle) 22.11
  - open 22.12
- skin (punch) 86.11
- skull 01.15
- soft palate 27.22
- soft tissue NEC 83.21
- spermatic cord 63.01
- sphincter of Oddi 51.14
  - closed (endoscopic) 51.14
  - open 51.13
- spinal cord (meninges) 03.32
- spleen 41.32
  - closed 41.32
  - open 41.33
  - percutaneous (aspiration) (needle) 41.32
- stomach 44.14
  - brush 44.14
  - closed (endoscopic) 44.14
  - open 44.15
- subcutaneous tissue (punch) 86.11
- supraglottic mass 29.12
- sympathetic nerve 05.11
- tendon 83.21
  - extraocular 15.01
  - ocular 15.01
- testis NEC 62.11
  - closed 62.11
  - open 62.12
  - percutaneous (needle) 62.11
- thymus 07.16
- thyroid gland NEC 06.11
  - closed 06.11
  - open 06.12
  - percutaneous (aspiration) (needle) 06.11
- tongue 25.01
  - closed (needle) 25.01
  - open 25.02
- tonsil 28.11
- trachea 31.44
  - brush 31.44
  - closed (endoscopic) 31.44
  - open 31.45
- tunica vaginalis 61.11
- umbilicus 54.22

✓4ᵗʰ Fourth-digit Required   ▶◀ Revised Text   ● New Line   ▲ Revised Code

Biopsy — Bypass

☑4ᵗʰ Fourth-digit Required ▶◀ Revised Text ● New Line ▲ Revised Code

Bypass — *continued*
  vascular NEC — *continued*
    aortofemoral-popliteal 39.25
    aortoiliac 39.25
      to popliteal 39.25
    aortoiliofemoral 39.25
    aortomesenteric 39.26
    aortopopliteal 39.25
    aortorenal 39.24
    aortosubclavian 39.22
    axillary-brachial 39.29
    axillary-femoral (superficial) 39.29
    axillofemoral (superficial) 39.29
    carotid-cerebral 39.28
    carotid-vertebral 39.28
    carotid to subclavian artery 39.22
    common hepatic-common iliac-renal 39.26
    coronary (*see also* Bypass, aortocoronary)
      36.10
    extracranial-intracranial [EC-IC] 39.28
    femoral-femoral 39.29
    femoroperoneal 39.29
    femoropopliteal (reversed saphenous vein)
      (saphenous) 39.29
    femorotibial (anterior) (posterior) 39.29
    iliofemoral 39.25
    ilioiliac 39.26
    internal mammary-coronary artery (single)
      36.15
      double vessel 36.16
    intra-abdominal (arterial) NEC 39.26
      venous NEC 39.1
    intrathoracic NEC 39.23
    peripheral artery NEC 39.29
    popliteal-tibial 39.29
    renal artery 39.24
    splenorenal (venous) 39.1
      arterial 39.26
    subclavian-axillary 39.29
    subclavian-carotid 39.22
    subclavian-subclavian 39.22
    Y graft to renal arteries 39.24

C

Caldwell operation (sulcus extension) 24.91
Caldwell-Luc operation (maxillary sinusotomy)
  22.39
  with removal of membrane lining 22.31
Calibration, urethra 89.29
Calicectomy (renal) 55.4
Callander operation (knee disarticulation) 84.16
Caloric test, vestibular function 95.44
Calycectomy (renal) 55.4
Calyco-ileoneocystostomy 55.86
Calycotomy (renal) 55.11
Campbell operation
  bone block, ankle 81.11
  fasciotomy (iliac crest) 83.14
  reconstruction of anterior cruciate ligament
    81.45
Campimetry 95.05
Canaliculodacryocystorhinostomy 09.81
Canaliculoplasty 09.73
Canaliculorhinostomy 09.81
Canaloplasty, external auditory meatus 18.6
Cannulation — *see also* Insertion, catheter
  ampulla of Vater 51.99
  antrum 22.01
  arteriovenous 39.93
  artery 38.91
  caval-mesenteric vein 39.1
  cisterna chyli 40.61
  Eustachian tube 20.8
  lacrimal apparatus 09.42
  lymphatic duct, left (thoracic) 40.61
  nasal sinus (by puncture) 22.01
    through natural ostium 22.02
  pancreatic duct 52.92
    by retrograde endoscopy (ERP) 52.93
  renoportal 39.1

Cannulation — *see also* Insertion, catheter —
    continued
  sinus (nasal) (by puncture) 22.01
    through natural ostium 22.02
  splenorenal (venous) 39.1
    arterial 39.26
  thoracic duct (cervical approach) (thoracic
    approach) 40.61
Cannulization — *see* Cannulation
Canthocystostomy 09.82
Canthoplasty 08.59
Canthorrhaphy 08.52
  division or severing 08.02
Canthotomy 08.51
Capsulectomy
  joint (*see also* Arthrectomy) 80.90
  kidney 55.91
  lens 13.65
    with extraction of lens 13.51
  ovary 65.29
    laparoscopic 65.25
Capsulo-iridectomy 13.65
Capsuloplasty — *see* Arthroplasty
Capsulorrhaphy 81.96
  with arthroplasty — *see* Arthroplasty
  ankle 81.94
  foot 81.94
  lower extremity NEC 81.95
  upper extremity 81.93
Capsulotomy
  joint (*see also* Division, joint capsule) 80.40
    for claw toe repair 77.57
  lens 13.64
    with
      discission of lens 13.2
      removal of foreign body 13.02
        by magnet extraction 13.01
Cardiac
  mapping 37.27
  massage (external) (closed chest) 99.63
    open chest 37.91
  retraining 93.36
Cardiectomy (stomach) 43.5
Cardiocentesis 37.0
Cardiography (*see also* Angiocardiography) 88.50
Cardiolysis 37.10
Cardiomyopexy 36.39
Cardiomyotomy 42.7
Cardio-omentopexy 36.39
Cardiopericardiopexy 36.39
Cardioplasty (stomach and esophagus) 44.65
  stomach alone 44.66
Cardioplegia 39.63
Cardiopneumopexy 36.39
Cardiorrhaphy 37.4
Cardioschisis 37.12
Cardiosplenopexy 36.39
Cardiotomy (exploratory) 37.11
Cardiovalvulotomy — *see* Valvulotomy, heart
Cardioversion (external) 99.62
  atrial 99.61
Carotid pulse tracing with ECG lead 89.56
Carpectomy (partial) 77.84
  total 77.94
Carroll and Taber arthroplasty (proximal
    interphalangeal joint) 81.72
Casting (for immobilization) NEC 93.53
  with fracture-reduction — *see* Reduction,
    fracture
Castration
  female (oophorectomy, bilateral) 65.51
    laparoscopic 65.53
  male 62.41
C.A.T. (computerized axial tomography) (*see also*
    Scan, C.A.T.) 88.38
Catheterization — *see also* Insertion, catheter
  arteriovenous 39.93
  artery 38.91

Catheterization — *see also* Insertion, catheter —
    continued
  bladder, indwelling 57.94
    percutaneous (cystostomy) 57.17
    suprapubic NEC 57.18
  bronchus 96.05
    with lavage 96.56
  cardiac (right) 37.21
    combined left and right 37.23
    left 37.22
      combined with right heart 37.23
    right 37.21
      combined with left heart 37.23
  central venous NEC 38.93
    peripherally inserted central catheter (PICC)
      38.93
  chest 34.04
    revision (with lysis of adhesions) 34.04
  Eustachian tube 20.8
  heart (right) 37.21
    combined left and right 37.23
    left 37.22
      combined with right heart 37.23
    right 37.21
      combined with left heart 37.23
  hepatic vein 38.93
  inferior vena cava 38.93
  intercostal space (with water seal), for drainage
    34.04
    revision (with lysis of adhesions) 34.04
  lacrimonasal duct 09.44
  laryngeal 96.05
  nasolacrimal duct 09.44
  pancreatic cyst 52.01
  renal vein 38.93
  Swan-Ganz (pulmonary) 89.64
  transtracheal for oxygenation 31.99
  umbilical vein 38.92
  ureter (to kidney) 59.8
    for retrograde pyelogram 87.74
  urethra, indwelling 57.94
  vein NEC 38.93
    for renal dialysis 38.95
Cattell operation (herniorrhaphy) 53.51
Cauterization — *see also* Destruction, lesion, by
    site
  anus NEC 49.39
    endoscopic 49.31
  Bartholin's gland 71.24
  broad ligament 69.19
  bronchus 32.09
    endoscopic 32.01
  canaliculi 09.73
  cervix 67.32
  chalazion 08.25
  choroid plexus 02.14
  conjunctiva 10.33
    lesion 10.32
  cornea (fistula) (ulcer) 11.42
  ear, external 18.29
  endometrial implant — *see* Excision, lesion, by
    site
  entropion 08.41
  esophagus 42.39
    endoscopic 42.33
  eyelid 08.25
    for entropion or ectropion 08.41
  fallopian tube 66.61
    by endoscopy (hysteroscopy) (laparoscopy)
      66.29
  hemorrhoids 49.43
  iris 12.41
  lacrimal
    gland 09.21
    punctum 09.72
      for eversion 09.71
    sac 09.6
  larynx 30.09
  liver 50.29
  lung 32.29
    endoscopic 32.28
  meibomian gland 08.25
  nose, for epistaxis (with packing) 21.03
  ovary 65.29
    laparoscopic 65.25

✔4ᵗʰ Fourth-digit Required   ▶◀ Revised Text   ● New Line   ▲ Revised Code

Closure — *see also* Repair — *continued*
  fistula — *continued*
    umbilicourinary 57.51
    ureter 56.84
    ureterocervical 56.84
    ureterorectal 56.84
    ureterosigmoidal 56.84
    ureterovaginal 56.84
    ureterovesical 56.84
    urethra 58.43
    urethroperineal 58.43
    urethroperineovesical 57.84
    urethrorectal 58.43
    urethroscrotal 58.43
    urethrovaginal 58.43
    uteroenteric 69.42
    uterointestinal 69.42
    uterorectal 69.42
    uteroureteric 56.84
    uterovaginal 69.42
    uterovesical 57.84
    vagina 70.8
    vaginocutaneous 70.75
    vaginoenteric 70.74
    vaginoperineal 70.75
    vaginovesical 57.84
    vesicocervicovaginal 57.84
    vesicocolic 57.83
    vesicocutaneous 57.84
    vesicoenteric 57.83
    vesicometrorectal 57.83
    vesicoperineal 57.84
    vesicorectal 57.83
    vesicosigmoidal 57.83
    vesicosigmoidovaginal 57.83
    vesicoureteral 56.84
    vesicoureterovaginal 56.84
    vesicourethral 57.84
    vesicourethrorectal 57.83
    vesicouterine 57.84
    vesicovaginal 57.84
    vulva 71.72
    vulvorectal 48.73
  foramen ovale (patent) 35.71
    with
      prosthesis (open heart technique) 35.51
        closed heart technique 35.52
      tissue graft 35.61
  gastroduodenostomy 44.5
  gastrojejunostomy 44.5
  gastrostomy 44.62
  ileostomy 46.51
  jejunostomy 46.51
  laceration — *see also* Suture, by site
    liver 50.61
  laparotomy, delayed 54.62
  meningocele (spinal) 03.51
    cerebral 02.12
  myelomeningocele 03.52
  nephrostomy 55.82
  palmar cleft 82.82
  patent ductus arteriosus 38.85
  pelviostomy 55.82
  peptic ulcer (bleeding) (perforated) 44.40
  perforation
    ear drum (*see also* Tympanoplasty) 19.4
    esophagus 42.82
    nasal septum 21.88
    tympanic membrane (*see also*
      Tympanoplasty) 19.4
  proctostomy 48.72
  punctum, lacrimal (papilla) 09.91
  pyelostomy 55.82
  rectostomy 48.72
  septum defect (heart) (*see also* Repair, heart, septum) 35.70
  sigmoidostomy 46.52
  skin (V-Y type) 86.59
  stoma
    bile duct 51.79
    bladder 57.82
    bronchus 33.42
    common duct 51.72
    esophagus 42.83
    gallbladder 51.92
    hepatic duct 51.79

Closure — *see also* Repair — *continued*
  stoma — *continued*
    intestine 46.50
      large 46.52
      small 46.51
    kidney 55.82
    larynx 31.62
    rectum 48.72
    stomach 44.62
    thorax 34.72
    trachea 31.72
    ureter 56.83
    urethra 58.42
  thoracostomy 34.72
  tracheostomy 31.72
  ulcer (bleeding) (peptic) (perforated) 44.40
    duodenum 44.42
    gastric 44.41
    intestine (perforated) 46.79
    skin 86.59
    stomach 44.41
  ureterostomy 56.83
  urethrostomy 58.42
  vagina 70.4
  vascular
    percutaneous puncture — *omit code*
  vesicostomy 57.22
  wound — *see also* Suture, by site
    with graft — *see* Graft
    with tissue adhesive 86.59

Coagulation, electrocoagulation — *see also* Destruction, lesion, by site
  aneurysm (cerebral) (peripheral vessel) 39.52
  arteriovenous fistula 39.53
  brain tissue (incremental) (radio-frequency) 01.59
  broad ligament 69.19
  cervix 67.32
  ear
    external 18.29
    inner 20.79
    middle 20.51
  fallopian tube 66.61
  gasserian ganglion 04.05
  nose for epistaxis (with packing) 21.03
  ovary 65.29
    laparoscopic 65.25
  pharynx (by diathermy) 29.39
  prostatic bed 60.94
  rectum (polyp) 48.32
    radical 48.31
  retina (for)
    destruction of lesion 14.21
    reattachment 14.51
    repair of tear 14.31
  round ligament 69.19
  semicircular canals 20.79
  spinal cord (lesion) 03.4
  urethrovesical junction, transurethral 57.49
  uterosacral ligament 69.19
  uterus 68.29
  vagina 70.33
  vulva 71.3

Coating, aneurysm of brain 39.52

Cobalt-60 therapy (treatment) 92.23

Coccygectomy (partial) 77.89
  total 77.99

Coccygotomy 77.39

"Cocked hat" procedure (metacarpal lengthening and transfer of local flap) 82.69

Cockett operation (varicose vein)
  lower limb 38.59
  upper limb 38.53

Cody tack (perforation of footplate) 19.0

Coffey operation (uterine suspension) (Meig's modification) 69.22

Cole operation (anterior tarsal wedge osteotomy) 77.28

Colectomy (partial) (segmental) (subtotal) 45.79
  cecum (with terminal ileum) 45.72
  left (Hartmann) (lower) (radical) 45.75
  multiple segmental 45.71
  right (radical) 45.73
  sigmoid 45.76

Colectomy — *continued*
  terminal ileum with cecum 45.72
  total 45.8
  transverse 45.74

Collapse, lung, surgical 33.39
  by
    destruction of phrenic nerve 33.31
    pneumoperitoneum 33.33
    pneumothorax, artificially-induced 33.32
    thoracoplasty 33.34

Collection, sperm for artificial insemination 99.96

Collis-Nissen operation (hiatal hernia repair with esophagogastroplasty) 53.80

Colocentesis 45.03

Colocolostomy 45.94
  proximal to distal segment 45.79

Colocystoplasty 57.87 *[45.52]*

Colofixation 46.64

Coloileotomy 45.00

Colonna operation
  adductor tenotomy (first stage) 83.12
  hip arthroplasty (second stage) 81.40
  reconstruction of hip (second stage) 81.40

Colonoscopy 45.23
  with biopsy 45.25
    rectum 48.24
  fiberoptic (flexible) 45.23
  intraoperative 45.21
  through stoma (artificial) 45.22
  transabdominal 45.21

Colopexy 46.63

Coloplication 46.64

Coloproctostomy 45.94

Colorectosigmoidostomy 45.94

Colorectostomy 45.94

Colorrhaphy 46.75

Coloscopy — *see* Colonoscopy

Colosigmoidostomy 45.94

Colostomy (ileo-ascending) (ileo-transverse) (perineal) (transverse) 46.10
  with anterior rectal resection 48.62
  delayed opening 46.14
  loop 46.03
  permanent (magnetic) 46.13
  temporary 46.11

Colotomy 45.03

Colpectomy 70.4

Colpoceliocentesis 70.0

Colpocentesis 70.0

Colpocleisis (complete) (partial) 70.8

Colpohysterectomy 68.59
  laparoscopically assisted (LAVH) 68.51

Colpoperineoplasty 70.79
  with repair of urethrocele 70.50

Colpoperineorrhaphy 70.71
  following delivery 75.69

Colpopexy 70.77

Colpoplasty 70.79

Colpopoiesis 70.61

Colporrhaphy 70.71
  anterior (cystocele repair) 70.51
  for repair of
    cystocele 70.51
      with rectocele 70.50
    enterocele 70.92
    rectocele 70.52
      with cystocele 70.50
    urethrocele 70.51
  posterior (rectocele repair) 70.52

Colposcopy 70.21

Colpotomy 70.14
  for pelvic peritoneal drainage 70.12

Commando operation (radical glossectomy) 25.4

Commissurotomy
  closed heart technique — *see* Valvulotomy, heart
  open heart technique — *see* Valvuloplasty, heart

Compression, trigeminal nerve 04.02
Conchectomy 21.69
Conchotomy 21.1
Conduction study, nerve 89.15
Conduitogram, ileum 87.78
Condylectomy — see category 77.8 ☑4ᵗʰ
  mandible 76.5
Condylotomy NEC (see also Division, joint
  capsule) 80.40
  mandible (open) 76.62
    closed 76.61
Conization
  cervix (knife) (sharp) (biopsy) 67.2
    by
      cryosurgery 67.33
      electroconization 67.32
Conjunctivocystorhinostomy 09.82
  with insertion of tube or stent 09.83
Conjunctivodacryocystorhinostomy (CDCR)
  09.82
  with insertion of tube or stent 09.83
Conjunctivodacryocystostomy 09.82
  with insertion of tube or stent 09.83
Conjunctivoplasty 10.49
Conjunctivorhinostomy 09.82
  with insertion of tube or stent 09.83
Constriction of globe, for scleral buckling (see
  also Buckling, scleral) 14.49
Construction
  auricle, ear (with graft) (with implant) 18.71
  ear
    auricle (with graft) (with implant) 18.71
    meatus (osseous) (side-lined) 18.6
  endorectal ileal pouch (J-pouch) (H-pouch) (S-
    pouch) (with anastomosis to anus) 45.95
  esophagus, artificial — see Anastomosis,
    esophagus
  ileal bladder (open) 56.51
    closed 57.87 [45.51]
  ileal conduit 56.51
  larynx, artificial 31.75
  patent meatus (ear) 18.6
  penis (rib graft) (skin graft) (myocutaneous flap)
    64.43
  pharyngeal valve, artificial 31.75
  urethra 58.46
  vagina, artificial 70.61
  venous valves (peripheral) 39.59
Consultation 89.09
  comprehensive 89.07
  limited (single organ system) 89.06
  specified type NEC 89.08
Continuous positive airway pressure (CPAP)
  93.90
Control
  atmospheric pressure and composition NEC
    93.98
    antigen-free air conditioning 93.98
    decompression chamber 93.97
    mountain sanatorium 93.98
  epistaxis 21.00
    by
      cauterization (and packing) 21.03
      coagulation (with packing) 21.03
      electrocoagulation (with packing) 21.03
      excision of nasal mucosa with grafting
        21.07
      ligation of artery 21.09
        ethmoidal 21.04
        external carotid 21.06
        maxillary (transantral) 21.05
      packing (nasal) (anterior) 21.01
        posterior (and anterior) 21.02
      specified means NEC 21.09
  hemorrhage 39.98
    abdominal cavity 54.19
    adenoids (postoperative) 28.7
    anus (postoperative) 49.95
    bladder (postoperative) 57.93
    chest 34.09
    colon 45.49
      endoscopic 45.43

Control — continued
  hemorrhage — continued
    duodenum (ulcer) 44.49
      by
        embolization (transcatheter) 44.44
        suture (ligation) 44.42
      endoscopic 44.43
    esophagus 42.39
      endoscopic 42.33
    gastric (ulcer) 44.49
      by
        embolization (transcatheter) 44.44
        suture (ligation) 44.41
      endoscopic 44.43
    intrapleural 34.09
      postoperative (recurrent) 34.03
    laparotomy site 54.12
    nose (see also Control, epistaxis) 21.00
    peptic (ulcer) 44.49
      by
        embolization (transcatheter) 44.44
        suture (ligation) 44.40
      endoscopic 44.43
    pleura, pleural cavity 34.09
      postoperative (recurrent) 34.03
    postoperative NEC 39.98
    postvascular surgery 39.41
    prostate 60.94
    specified site NEC 39.98
    stomach — see Control, hemorrhage, gastric
    thorax NEC 34.09
      postoperative (recurrent) 34.03
    thyroid (postoperative) 06.02
    tonsils (postoperative) 28.7
Conversion
  anastomosis — see Revision, anastomosis
  cardiac rhythm NEC 99.69
    to sinus rhythm 99.62
  gastrostomy to jejunostomy (endoscopic)
    44.32 ▲
  obstetrical position — see Version
Cooling, gastric 96.31
Cordectomy, vocal 30.22
Cordopexy, vocal 31.69
Cordotomy
  spinal (bilateral) NEC 03.29
    percutaneous 03.21
  vocal 31.3
Corectomy 12.12
Corelysis 12.35
Coreoplasty 12.35
Corneoconjunctivoplasty 11.53
Correction — see also Repair
  atresia
    esophageal 42.85
      by magnetic forces 42.99
    external meatus (ear) 18.6
    nasopharynx, nasopharyngeal 29.4
    rectum 48.0
    tricuspid 35.94
  atrial septal defect (see also Repair, atrial
    septal defect) 35.71
    combined with repair of valvular and
      ventricular septal defects — see
      Repair, endocardial cushion defect
  blepharoptosis (see also Repair, blepharoptosis)
    08.36
  bunionette (with osteotomy) 77.54
  chordee 64.42
  claw toe 77.57
  cleft
    lip 27.54
    palate 27.62
  clubfoot NEC 83.84
  coarctation of aorta
    with
      anastomosis 38.34
      graft replacement 38.44
  cornea NEC 11.59
    refractive NEC 11.79
      epikeratophakia 11.76
      keratomileusis 11.71
      keratophakia 11.72
      radial keratotomy 11.75

Correction — see also Repair — continued
  esophageal atresia 42.85
    by magnetic forces 42.99
  everted lacrimal punctum 09.71
  eyelid
    ptosis (see also Repair, blepharoptosis)
      08.36
    retraction 08.38
  fetal defect 75.36
  forcible, of musculoskeletal deformity NEC
    93.29
  hammer toe 77.56
  hydraulic pressure, open surgery for penile
    inflatable prosthesis 64.99
    urinary artificial sphincter 58.99
  intestinal malrotation 46.80
    large 46.82
    small 46.81
  inverted uterus — see Repair, inverted uterus
  lymphedema (of limb) 40.9
    excision with graft 40.9
    obliteration of lymphatics 40.9
    transplantation of autogenous lymphatics
      40.9
  nasopharyngeal atresia 29.4
  overlapping toes 77.58
  palate (cleft) 27.62
  prognathism NEC 76.64
  prominent ear 18.5
  punctum (everted) 09.71
  spinal pseudarthrosis — see Refusion, spinal
  syndactyly 86.85
  tetralogy of Fallot
    one-stage 35.81
    partial — see specific procedure
    total 35.81
  total anomalous pulmonary venous connection
    one-stage 35.82
    partial — see specific procedure
    total 35.82
  transposition, great arteries, total 35.84
  tricuspid atresia 35.94
  truncus arteriosus
    one-stage 35.83
    partial — see specific procedure
    total 35.83
  ureteropelvic junction 55.87
  ventricular septal defect (see also Repair,
    ventricular septal defect) 35.72
    combined with repair of valvular and atrial
      septal defects — see Repair,
      endocardial cushion defect
Costectomy 77.91
  with lung excision — see Excision, lung
  associated with thoracic operation — omit code
Costochondrectomy 77.91
  associated with thoracic operation — omit code
Costosternoplasty (pectus excavatum repair)
  34.74
Costotomy 77.31
Costotransversectomy 77.91
  associated with thoracic operation — omit code
Counseling (for) NEC 94.49
  alcoholism 94.46
  drug addiction 94.45
  employers 94.49
  family (medical) (social) 94.49
  marriage 94.49
  ophthalmologic (with instruction) 95.36
  pastoral 94.49
Countershock, cardiac NEC 99.62
Coventry operation (tibial wedge osteotomy)
  77.27
CPAP (continuous positive airway pressure) 93.90
Craniectomy 01.25
  linear (opening of cranial suture) 02.01
  reopening of site 01.23
  strip (opening of cranial suture) 02.01
Cranioclasis, fetal 73.8
Cranioplasty 02.06
  with synchronous repair of encephalocele 02.12
Craniotomy 01.24
  as operative approach — omit code

Craniotomy — *continued*
  fetal 73.8
  for decompression of fracture 02.02
  reopening of site 01.23
Craterization, bone (*see also* Excision, lesion, bone) 77.60
Crawford operation (tarso-frontalis sling of eyelid) 08.32
Creation — *see also* Formation
  cardiac pacemaker pocket
    with initial insertion of pacemaker — *omit code*
    new site (skin) (subcutaneous) 37.79
  conduit
    ileal (urinary) 56.51
    left ventricle and aorta 35.93
    right atrium and pulmonary artery 35.94
    right ventricle and pulmonary (distal) artery 35.92
      in repair of
        pulmonary artery atresia 35.92
        transposition of great vessels 35.92
        truncus arteriosus 35.83
  endorectal ileal pouch (J-pouch) (H-pouch) (S-pouch) (with anastomosis to anus) 45.95
  esophagogastric sphincteric competence NEC 44.66
  Hartmann pouch — *see* Colectomy, by site
  interatrial fistula 35.42
  pericardial window 37.12
  pleural window, for drainage 34.09
  pocket
    cardiac pacemaker
      with initial insertion of pacemaker — *omit code*
      new site (skin) (subcutaneous) 37.79
    loop recorder 86.09
    thalamic stimulator pulse generator
      with initial insertion of battery package — *omit code*
      new site (skin) (subcutaneous) 86.09
  shunt — *see also* Shunt
    arteriovenous fistula, for dialysis 39.93
    left-to-right (systemic to pulmonary circulation) 39.0
  subcutaneous tunnel for esophageal anastomosis 42.86
    with anastomosis — *see* Anastomosis, esophagus, antesternal
  syndactyly (finger) (toe) 86.89
  thalamic stimulator pulse generator pocket
    with initial insrtion of battery package — *omit code*
    new site (skin) (subcutaneous) 86.09
  tracheoesophageal fistula 31.95
  window
    pericardial 37.12
    pleura, for drainage 34.09
Credé maneuver 73.59
Cricoidectomy 30.29
Cricothyreotomy (for assistance in breathing) 31.1
Cricothyroidectomy 30.29
Cricothyrostomy 31.1
Cricothyrotomy (for assistance in breathing) 31.1
Cricotomy (for assistance in breathing) 31.1
Cricotracheotomy (for assistance in breathing) 31.1
Crisis intervention 94.35
Croupette, croup tent 93.94
Crown, dental (ceramic) (gold) 23.41
Crushing
  bone — *see* category 78.4 ☑4ᵗʰ
  calculus
    bile (hepatic) passage 51.49
      endoscopic 51.88
    bladder (urinary) 57.0
    pancreatic duct 52.09
      endoscopic 52.94
  fallopian tube (*see also* Ligation, fallopian tube) 66.39
  ganglion — *see* Crushing, nerve
  hemorrhoids 49.45

Crushing — *continued*
  nasal septum 21.88
  nerve (cranial) (peripheral) NEC 04.03
    acoustic 04.01
    auditory 04.01
    phrenic 04.03
      for collapse of lung 33.31
    sympathetic 05.0
    trigeminal 04.02
    vestibular 04.01
  vas deferens 63.71
Cryoablation — *see* Ablation
Cryoanalgesia
  nerve (cranial) (peripheral) 04.2
Cryoconization, cervix 67.33
Cryodestruction — *see* Destruction, lesion, by site
Cryoextraction, lens (*see also* Extraction, cataract, intracapsular) 13.19
Cryohypophysectomy (complete) (total) (*see also* Hypophysectomy) 07.69
Cryoleucotomy 01.32
Cryopexy, retinal — *see* Cryotherapy, retina
Cryoprostatectomy 60.62
Cryoretinopexy (for)
  reattachment 14.52
  repair of tear or defect 14.32
Cryosurgery — *see* Cryotherapy
Cryothalamectomy 01.41
Cryotherapy — *see also* Destruction, lesion, by site
  bladder 57.59
  brain 01.59
  cataract 13.19
  cervix 67.33
  choroid — *see* Cryotherapy, retina
  ciliary body 12.72
  corneal lesion (ulcer) 11.43
    to reshape cornea 11.79
  ear
    external 18.29
    inner 20.79
  esophagus 42.39
    endoscopic 42.33
  eyelid 08.25
  hemorrhoids 49.44
  iris 12.41
  nasal turbinates 21.61
  palate (bony) 27.31
  prostate 60.62
  retina (for)
    destruction of lesion 14.22
    reattachment 14.52
    repair of tear 14.32
  skin 86.3
  stomach 43.49
    endoscopic 43.41
  subcutaneous tissue 86.3
  turbinates (nasal) 21.61
  warts 86.3
    genital 71.3
Cryptectomy (anus) 49.39
  endoscopic 49.31
Cryptorchidectomy (unilateral) 62.3
  bilateral 62.41
Cryptotomy (anus) 49.39
  endoscopic 49.31
Cuirass 93.99
Culdocentesis 70.0
Culdoplasty 70.92
Culdoscopy (exploration) (removal of foreign body or lesion) 70.22
Culdotomy 70.12
Culp-Deweerd operation (spiral flap pyeloplasty) 55.87
Culp-Scardino operation (ureteral flap pyeloplasty) 55.87
Culture (and sensitivity) — *see* Examination, microscopic

Curettage (with packing) (with secondary closure) — *see also* Dilation and curettage
  adenoids 28.6
  anus 49.39
    endoscopic 49.31
  bladder 57.59
    transurethral 57.49
  bone (*see also* Excision, lesion, bone) 77.60
  brain 01.59
  bursa 83.39
    hand 82.29
  cartilage (*see also* Excision, lesion, joint) 80.80
  cerebral meninges 01.51
  chalazion 08.25
  conjunctiva (trachoma follicles) 10.33
  corneal epithelium 11.41
    for smear or culture 11.21
  ear, external 18.29
  eyelid 08.25
  joint (*see also* Excision, lesion, joint) 80.80
  meninges (cerebral) 01.51
    spinal 03.4
  muscle 83.32
    hand 82.22
  nerve (peripheral) 04.07
    sympathetic 05.29
  sclera 12.84
  skin 86.3
  spinal cord (meninges) 03.4
  subgingival 24.31
  tendon 83.39
    sheath 83.31
      hand 82.21
  uterus (with dilation) 69.09
    aspiration (diagnostic) NEC 69.59
      after abortion or delivery 69.52
      to terminate pregnancy 69.51
      following delivery or abortion 69.02
Curette evacuation, lens 13.2
Curtis operation (interphalangeal joint arthroplasty) 81.72
Cutaneolipectomy 86.83
Cutdown, venous 38.94
Cutting
  nerve (cranial) (peripheral) NEC 04.03
    acoustic 04.01
    auditory 04.01
    root, spinal 03.1
    sympathetic 05.0
    trigeminal 04.02
    vestibular 04.01
  pedicle (flap) graft 86.71
  pylorus (with wedge resection) 43.3
  spinal nerve root 03.1
  ureterovesical orifice 56.1
  urethral sphincter 58.5
CVP (central venous pressure monitoring) 89.62
Cyclectomy (ciliary body) 12.44
  eyelid margin 08.20
Cyclicotomy 12.55
Cycloanemization 12.74
Cyclocryotherapy 12.72
Cyclodialysis (initial) (subsequent) 12.55
Cyclodiathermy (penetrating) (surface) 12.71
Cycloelectrolysis 12.71
Cyclophotocoagulation 12.73
Cyclotomy 12.55
Cystectomy — *see also* Excision, lesion, by site
  gallbladder — *see* Cholecystectomy
  urinary (partial) (subtotal) 57.6
    complete (with urethrectomy) 57.79
    radical 57.71
      with pelvic exenteration (female) 68.8
    total (with urethrectomy) 57.79
Cystocolostomy 57.88
Cystogram, cystography NEC 87.77
Cystolitholapaxy 57.0
Cystolithotomy 57.19
Cystometrogram 89.22
Cystopexy NEC 57.89
Cystoplasty NEC 57.89

☑4ᵗʰ Fourth-digit Required   ▶◀ Revised Text   ● New Line   ▲ Revised Code

Cystoproctostomy 57.88
Cystoprostatectomy, radical 57.71
Cystopyelography 87.74
Cystorrhaphy 57.81
Cystoscopy (transurethral) 57.32
  with biopsy 57.33
  for
    control of hemorrhage
      bladder 57.93
      prostate 60.94
      retrograde pyelography 87.74
    ileal conduit 56.35
    through stoma (artificial) 57.31
Cystostomy
  closed (suprapubic) (percutaneous) 57.17
  open (suprapubic) 57.18
  percutaneous (closed) (suprapubic) 57.17
  suprapubic
    closed 57.17
    open 57.18
Cystotomy (open) (for removal of calculi) 57.19
Cystourethrogram (retrograde) (voiding) 87.76
Cystourethropexy (by) 59.79
  levator muscle sling 59.71
  retropubic suspension 59.5
  suprapubic suspension 59.4
Cystourethroplasty 57.85
Cystourethroscopy 57.32
  with biopsy
    bladder 57.33
    ureter 56.33
Cytology — see Examination, microscopic

D

Dacryoadenectomy 09.20
  partial 09.22
  total 09.23
Dacryoadenotomy 09.0
Dacryocystectomy (complete) (partial) 09.6
Dacryocystogram 87.05
Dacryocystorhinostomy (DCR) (by intubation) (external) (intranasal) 09.81
Dacryocystostomy 09.53
Dacryocystosyringotomy 09.53
Dacryocystotomy 09.53
Dahlman operation (excision of esophageal diverticulum) 42.31
Dana operation (posterior rhizotomy) 03.1
Danforth operation (fetal) 73.8
Darrach operation (ulnar resection) 77.83
Davis operation (intubated ureterotomy) 56.2
Deaf training 95.49
Debridement
  abdominal wall 54.3
  bone (see also Excision, lesion, bone) 77.60
    fracture — see Debridement, open fracture
  brain 01.59
  burn (skin) 86.28
    excisional 86.22
    nonexcisional 86.28
  cerebral meninges 01.51
  dental 96.54
  flap graft 86.75
  graft (flap) (pedicle) 86.75
  heart valve (calcified) — see Valvuloplasty, heart
  infection (skin) 86.28
    excisional 86.22
    nail bed or fold 86.27
    nonexcisional 86.28
  joint — see Excision, lesion, joint
  meninges (cerebral) 01.51
    spinal 03.4
  muscle 83.45
    hand 82.36
  nail 86.27
  nerve (peripheral) 04.07

Debridement — continued
  open fracture (compound) 79.60
    arm NEC 79.62
    carpal, metacarpal 79.63
    facial bone 76.2
    femur 79.65
    fibula 79.66
    foot NEC 79.67
    hand NEC 79.63
    humerus 79.61
    leg NEC 79.66
    phalanges
      foot 79.68
      hand 79.64
    radius 79.62
    specified site NEC 79.69
    tarsal, metatarsal 79.67
    tibia 79.66
    ulna 79.62
  patella 77.66
  pedicle graft 86.75
  skin or subcutaneous tissue (burn) (infection) (wound) 86.28
    cardioverter/defibrillator (automatic) pocket 37.99
    excisional 86.22
    graft 86.75
    nail, nail bed, or nail fold 86.27
    nonexcisional 86.28
    pacemaker pocket 37.79
    pocket
      cardiac pacemaker 37.79
      cardioverter/defibrillator (automatic) 37.99
  skull 01.25
    compound fracture 02.02
  spinal cord (meninges) 03.4
  wound (skin) 86.28
    excisional 86.22
    nonexcisional 86.28
Decapitation, fetal 73.8
Decapsulation, kidney 55.91
Declotting — see also Removal, thrombus
  arteriovenous cannula or shunt 39.49
Decompression
  anus (imperforate) 48.0
  biliary tract 51.49
    by intubation 51.43
      endoscopic 51.87
      percutaneous 51.98
  brain 01.24
  carpal tunnel 04.43
  cauda equina 03.09
  chamber 93.97
  colon 96.08
    by incision 45.03
    endoscopic (balloon) 46.85
  common bile duct 51.42
    by intubation 51.43
      endoscopic 51.87
      percutaneous 51.98
  cranial 01.24
    for skull fracture 02.02
  endolymphatic sac 20.79
  ganglion (peripheral) NEC 04.49
    cranial NEC 04.42
  gastric 96.07
  heart 37.0
  intestine 96.08
    by incision 45.00
    endoscopic (balloon) 46.85
  intracranial 01.24
  labyrinth 20.79
  laminectomy 03.09
  laminotomy 03.09
  median nerve 04.43
  muscle 83.02
    hand 82.02
  nerve (peripheral) NEC 04.49
    auditory 04.42
    cranial NEC 04.42
    median 04.43
    trigeminal (root) 04.41
  orbit (see also Orbitotomy) 16.09

Decompression — continued
  pancreatic duct 52.92
    endoscopic 52.93
  pericardium 37.0
  rectum 48.0
  skull fracture 02.02
  spinal cord (canal) 03.09
  tarsal tunnel 04.44
  tendon (sheath) 83.01
    hand 82.01
  thoracic outlet
    by
      myotomy (division of scalenus anticus muscle) 83.19
      tenotomy 83.13
  trigeminal (nerve root) 04.41
Decortication
  arterial 05.25
  brain 01.51
  cerebral meninges 01.51
  heart 37.31
  kidney 55.91
  lung (partial) (total) 34.51
  nasal turbinates — see Turbinectomy
  nose 21.89
  ovary 65.29
    laparoscopic 65.25
  periarterial 05.25
  pericardium 37.31
  ventricle. heart (complete) 37.31
Deepening
  alveolar ridge 24.5
  buccolabial sulcus 24.91
  lingual sulcus 24.91
Defatting, flap or pedicle graft 86.75
Defibrillation, electric (external) (internal) 99.62
  automatic cardioverter/defibrillator — see category 37.9 ☑4ᵗʰ
de Grandmont operation (tarsectomy) 08.35
Delaying of pedicle graft 86.71
Delivery (with)
  assisted spontaneous 73.59
  breech extraction (assisted) 72.52
    partial 72.52
      with forceps to aftercoming head 72.51
    total 72.54
      with forceps to aftercoming head 72.53
    unassisted (spontaneous delivery) — omit code
  cesarean section — see Cesarean section
  Credé maneuver 73.59
  De Lee maneuver 72.4
  forceps 72.9
    application to aftercoming head (Piper) 72.6
      with breech extraction
        partial 72.51
        total 72.53
    Barton's 72.4
    failed 73.3
    high 72.39
      with episiotomy 72.31
    low (outlet) 72.0
      with episiotomy 72.1
    mid 72.29
      with episiotomy 72.21
    outlet (low) 72.0
      with episiotomy 72.1
    rotation of fetal head 72.4
    trial 73.3
  instrumental NEC 72.9
    specified NEC 72.8
  key-in-lock rotation 72.4
  Kielland rotation 72.4
  Malström's extraction 72.79
    with episiotomy 72.71
  manually assisted (spontaneous) 73.59
  spontaneous (unassisted) 73.59
    assisted 73.59
  vacuum extraction 72.79
    with episiotomy 72.71
Delorme operation
  pericardiectomy 37.31
  proctopexy 48.76
  repair of prolapsed rectum 48.76

Delorme operation — *continued*
thoracoplasty 33.34

Denervation
aortic body 39.8
carotid body 39.8
facet, percutaneous (radiofrequency) 03.96
ovarian 65.94
paracervical uterine 69.3
uterosacral 69.3

Denker operation (radical maxillary antrotomy) 22.31

Dennis-Barco operation — *see* Repair, hernia, femoral

Denonvillier operation (limited rhinoplasty) 21.86

Densitometry, bone (serial) (radiographic) 88.98

Depilation, skin 86.92

Derlacki operation (tympanoplasty) 19.4

Dermabond 86.59

Dermabrasion (laser) 86.25
for wound debridement 86.28

Derotation — *see* Reduction, torsion

Desensitization
allergy 99.12
psychologic 94.33

Desmotomy (*see also* Division, ligament) 80.40

Destruction
breast 85.20
chorioretinopathy (*see also* Destruction, lesion, choroid) 14.29
ciliary body 12.74
epithelial downgrowth, anterior chamber 12.93
fallopian tube 66.39
with
crushing (and ligation) 66.31
by endoscopy (laparoscopy) 66.21
division (and ligation) 66.32
by endoscopy (culdoscopy)
(hysteroscopy) (laparoscopy)
(peritoneoscopy) 66.22
ligation 66.39
with
crushing 66.31
by endoscopy (laparoscopy) 66.21
division 66.32
by endoscopy (culdoscopy)
(hysteroscopy)
(laparoscopy)
(peritoneoscopy) 66.22
fetus 73.8
hemorrhoids 49.49
by
cryotherapy 49.44
sclerotherapy 49.42
inner ear (NEC) 20.79
by injection 20.72
intervertebral disc (NOS) 80.50
by injection 80.52
by other specified method 80.59
herniated (nucleus pulposus) 80.51
lacrimal sac 09.6
lesion (local)
anus 49.39
endoscopic 49.31
Bartholin's gland 71.24
by
aspiration 71.21
excision 71.24
incision 71.22
marsupialization 71.23
biliary ducts 51.69
endoscopic 51.64
bladder 57.59
transurethral 57.49
bone — *see* Excision, lesion, bone
bowel — *see* Destruction, lesion, intestine
brain (transtemporal approach) NEC 01.59
by stereotactic radiosurgery 92.30
cobalt 60 92.32
linear accelerator (LINAC) 92.31
multi-source 92.32
particle beam 92.33

Destruction — *continued*
lesion — *continued*
brain NEC — *continued*
by stereotactic radiosurgery — *continued*
particulate 92.33
radiosurgery NEC 92.39
single source photon 92.31
breast NEC 85.20
bronchus NEC 32.09
endoscopic 32.01
cerebral NEC 01.59
meninges 01.51
cervix 67.39
by
cauterization 67.32
cryosurgery, cryoconization 67.33
electroconization 67.32
choroid 14.29
by
cryotherapy 14.22
diathermy 14.21
implantation of radiation source 14.27
photocoagulation 14.25
laser 14.24
xenon arc 14.23
radiation therapy 14.26
ciliary body (nonexcisional) 12.43
by excision 12.44
conjunctiva 10.32
by excision 10.31
cornea NEC 11.49
by
cryotherapy 11.43
electrocauterization 11.42
thermocauterization 11.42
cul-de-sac 70.32
duodenum NEC 45.32
by excision 45.31
endoscopic 45.30
endoscopic 45.30
esophagus (chemosurgery) (cryosurgery)
(electroresection) (fulguration) NEC 42.39
by excision 42.32
endoscopic 42.33
endoscopic 42.33
eye NEC 16.93
eyebrow 08.25
eyelid 08.25
excisional — *see* Excision, lesion, eyelid
heart 37.33
by catheter ablation 37.34
intestine (large) 45.49
by excision 45.41
endoscopic 45.43
polypectomy 45.42
endoscopic 45.43
polypectomy 45.42
small 45.34
by excision 45.33
intranasal 21.31
iris (nonexcisional) NEC 12.41
by excision 12.42
kidney 55.39
by marsupialization 55.31
lacrimal sac 09.6
larynx 30.09
liver 50.29
lung 32.29
endoscopic 32.28
meninges (cerebral) 01.51
spinal 03.4
nerve (peripheral) 04.07
sympathetic 05.29
nose 21.30
intranasal 21.31
specified NEC 21.32
ovary
by
aspiration 65.91
excision 65.29
laparoscopic 65.25
cyst by rupture (manual) 65.93
palate (bony) (local) 27.31
wide 27.32

Destruction — *continued*
lesion — *continued*
pancreas 52.22
by marsupialization 52.3
endoscopic 52.21
pancreatic duct 52.22
endoscopic 52.21
penis 64.2
pharynx (excisional) NEC 29.39
pituitary gland
by stereotactic radiosurgery 92.30
cobalt 60 92.32
linear accelerator (LINAC) 92.31
multi-source 92.32
particle beam 92.33
particulate 92.33
radiosurgery NEC 92.39
single source photon 92.31
rectum (local) 48.32
by
cryosurgery 48.34
electrocoagulation 48.32
excision 48.35
fulguration 48.32
laser (Argon) 48.33
polyp 48.36
radical 48.31
retina 14.29
by
cryotherapy 14.22
diathermy 14.21
implantation of radiation source 14.27
photocoagulation 14.25
laser 14.24
xenon arc 14.23
radiation therapy 14.26
salivary gland NEC 26.29
by marsupialization 26.21
sclera 12.84
scrotum 61.3
skin NEC 86.3
sphincter of Oddi 51.69
endoscopic 51.64
spinal cord (meninges) 03.4
spleen 41.42
by marsupialization 41.41
stomach NEC 43.49
by excision 43.42
endoscopic 43.41
endoscopic 43.41
subcutaneous tissue NEC 86.3
testis 62.2
tongue 25.1
urethra (excisional) 58.39
endoscopic 58.31
uterus 68.29
nerve (cranial) (peripheral) (by cryoanalgesia) by radiofrequency) 04.2
sympathetic, by injection of neurolytic agent 05.32
neuroma
acoustic 04.01
by craniotomy 04.01
by stereotactic radiosurgery 92.30
cobalt 60 92.32
linear accelerator (LINAC) 92.31
multi-source 92.32
particle beam 92.33
particulate 92.33
radiosurgery NEC 92.39
single source photon 92.31
cranial 04.07
Morton's 04.07
peripheral
Morton's 04.07
prostate (prostatic tissue)
by
cryotherapy 60.62
microwave 60.96
radiofrequency 60.97
transurethral microwave thermotherapy (TUMT) 60.96
transurethral needle ablation (TUNA) 60.97
TULIP (transurethral (ultrasound) guided laser induced prostatectomy) 60.21

Destruction — *continued*
  prostate — *continued*
    TUMT (transurethral microwave thermotherapy) 60.96
    TUNA (transurethral needle ablation) 60.97
  semicircular canals, by injection 20.72
  vestibule, by injection 20.72

Detachment, uterosacral ligaments 69.3

Determination
  mental status (clinical) (medicolegal) (psychiatric) NEC 94.11
  psychologic NEC 94.09
  vital capacity (pulmonary) 89.37

Detorsion
  intestine (twisted) (volvulus) 46.80
    large 46.82
      endoscopic (balloon) 46.85
    small 46.81
  kidney 55.84
  ovary 65.95
  spermatic cord 63.52
    with orchiopexy 62.5
  testis 63.52
    with orchiopexy 62.5
  volvulus 46.80
    endoscopic (balloon) 46.85

Detoxification therapy 94.25
  alcohol 94.62
    with rehabilitation 94.63
    combined alcohol and drug 94.68
      with rehabilitation 94.69
  drug 94.65
    with rehabilitation 94.66
    combined alcohol and drug 94.68
      with rehabilitation 94.69

Devascularization, stomach 44.99

Dewebbing
  esophagus 42.01
  syndactyly (fingers) (toes) 86.85

Dextrorotation — *see* Reduction, torsion

Dialysis
  hemodiafiltration, hemofiltration (extracorporeal) 39.95
  kidney (extracorporeal) 39.95
  liver 50.92
  peritoneal 54.98
  renal (extracorporeal) 39.95

Diaphanoscopy
  nasal sinuses 89.35
  skull (newborn) 89.16

Diaphysectomy — *see* category 77.8 ☑4ᵗʰ

Diathermy 93.34
  choroid — *see* Diathermy, retina
  nasal turbinates 21.61
  retina
    for
      destruction of lesion 14.21
      reattachment 14.51
      repair of tear 14.31
  surgical — *see* Destruction, lesion, by site
  turbinates (nasal) 21.61

Dickson operation (fascial transplant) 83.82

Dickson-Diveley operation (tendon transfer and arthrodesis to correct claw toe) 77.57

Dieffenbach operation (hip disarticulation) 84.18

Dilation
  achalasia 42.92
  ampulla of Vater 51.81
    endoscopic 51.84
  anus, anal (sphincter) 96.23
  biliary duct
    endoscopic 51.84
    pancreatic duct 52.99
      endoscopic 52.98
    percutaneous (endoscopy) 51.98
    sphincter
      of Oddi 51.81
        endoscopic 51.84
        pancreatic 51.82
          endoscopic 51.85
  bladder 96.25
    neck 57.92
  bronchus 33.91

Dilation — *continued*
  cervix (canal) 67.0
    obstetrical 73.1
    to assist delivery 73.1
  choanae (nasopharynx) 29.91
  colon (endoscopic) (balloon) 46.85
  colostomy stoma 96.24
  duodenum (endoscopic) (balloon) 46.85
  endoscopic — *see* Dilation, by site
  enterostomy stoma 96.24
  esophagus (by bougie) (by sound) 42.92
  fallopian tube 66.96
  foreskin (newborn) 99.95
  frontonasal duct 96.21
  gastrojejunostomy site, endoscopic 44.22
  heart valve — *see* Valvulotomy, heart
  ileostomy stoma 96.24
  ileum (endoscopic) (balloon) 46.85
  intestinal stoma (artificial) 96.24
  intestine (endoscopic) (balloon) 46.85
  jejunum (endoscopic) (balloon) 46.85
  lacrimal
    duct 09.42
    punctum 09.41
  larynx 31.98
  lymphatic structure(s) (peripheral) 40.9
  nares 21.99
  nasolacrimal duct (retrograde) 09.43
    with insertion of tube or stent 09.44
  nasopharynx 29.91
  pancreatic duct 52.99
    endoscopic 52.98
  pharynx 29.91
  prostatic urethra (transurethral) (balloon) 60.95
  punctum, lacrimal papilla 09.41
  pylorus
    by incision 44.21
    endoscopic 44.22
  rectum 96.22
  salivary duct 26.91
  sphenoid ostia 22.52
  sphincter
    anal 96.23
    cardiac 42.92
    of Oddi 51.81
      endoscopic 51.84
    pancreatic 51.82
      endoscopic 51.85
    pylorus, endoscopic 44.22
      by incision 44.21
  Stenson's duct 26.91
  trachea 31.99
  ureter 59.8
    meatus 56.91
  ureterovesical orifice 59.8
  urethra 58.6
    prostatic (transurethral) (balloon) 60.95
  urethrovesical junction 58.6
  vagina (instrumental) (manual) NEC 96.16
  vesical neck 57.92
  Wharton's duct 26.91
  Wirsung's duct 52.99
    endoscopic 52.98

Dilation and curettage, uterus (diagnostic) 69.09
  after
    abortion 69.02
    delivery 69.02
  to terminate pregnancy 69.01

Diminution, ciliary body 12.74

Disarticulation 84.91
  ankle 84.13
  elbow 84.06
  finger, except thumb 84.01
    thumb 84.02
  hip 84.18
  knee 84.16
  shoulder 84.08
  thumb 84.02
  toe 84.11
  wrist 84.04

Discission
  capsular membrane 13.64
  cataract (Wheeler knife) (Ziegler knife) 13.2
    congenital 13.69
    secondary membrane 13.64

Discission — *continued*
  iris 12.12
  lens (capsule) (Wheeler knife) (Ziegler knife) (with capsulotomy) 13.2
  orbitomaxillary, radical 16.51
  pupillary 13.2
  secondary membrane (after cataract) 13.64
  vitreous strands (posterior approach) 14.74
    anterior approach 14.73

Discogram, diskogram 87.21

Discolysis (by injection) 80.52

Diskectomy, intervertebral 80.51
  herniated (nucleus pulposus) 80.51
  percutaneous 80.59

Dispensing (with fitting)
  contact lens 95.32
  low vision aids NEC 95.33
  spectacles 95.31

Dissection — *see also* Excision
  aneurysm 38.60
  artery-vein-nerve bundle 39.91
  branchial cleft fistula or sinus 29.52
  bronchus 32.1
  femoral hernia 53.29
  groin, radical 40.54
  larynx block (en bloc) 30.3
  mediastinum with pneumonectomy 32.5
  neck, radical 40.40
    with laryngectomy 30.4
    bilateral 40.42
    unilateral 40.41
  orbital fibrous bands 16.92
  pterygium (with reposition) 11.31
  radical neck — *see* Dissection, neck, radical
  retroperitoneal NEC 59.00
  thoracic structures (block) (en bloc) (radical) (brachial plexus, bronchus, lobe of lung, ribs, and sympathetic nerves) 32.6
  vascular bundle 39.91

Distention, bladder (therapeutic) (intermittent) 96.25

Diversion, urinary
  cutaneous 56.61
  ileal conduit 56.51
  internal NEC 56.71
  ureter to
    intestine 56.71
    skin 56.61
  uretero-ileostomy 56.51

Diversional therapy 93.81

Diverticulectomy
  bladder (suprapubic) 57.59
    transurethral approach 57.49
  duodenum 45.31
    endoscopic 45.30
  esophagus 42.31
    endoscopic 42.33
  esophagomyotomy 42.7
  hypopharyngeal (by cricopharyngeal myotomy) 29.32
  intestine
    large 45.41
      endoscopic 45.43
    small 45.33
  kidney 55.39
  Meckel's 45.33
  pharyngeal (by cricopharyngeal myotomy) 29.32
  pharyngoesophageal (by cricopharyngeal myotomy) 29.32
  stomach 43.42
    endoscopic 43.41
  urethra 58.39
    endoscopic 58.31

Division
  Achilles tendon 83.11
  adductor tendon (hip) 83.12
  adhesions — *see* Lysis, adhesions
  angle of mandible (open) 76.62
    closed 76.61
  anterior synechiae 12.32
  aponeurosis 83.13
  arcuate ligament (spine) — *omit code*
  arteriovenous fistula (with ligation) 39.53

☑4ᵗʰ Fourth-digit Required   ►◄ Revised Text   ● New Line   ▲ Revised Code

Division — Drainage

Division — *continued*
  artery (with ligation) 38.80
    abdominal 38.86
    aorta (arch) (ascending) (descending) 38.84
    head and neck NEC 38.82
    intracranial NEC 38.81
    lower limb 38.88
    thoracic NEC 38.85
    upper limb 38.83
  bladder neck 57.91
  blepharorrhaphy 08.02
  blood vessels, cornea 10.1
  bone (*see also* Osteotomy) 77.30
  brain tissue 01.32
    cortical adhesions 02.91
  canaliculus 09.52
  canthorrhaphy 08.02
  cartilage 80.40
    ankle 80.47
    elbow 80.42
    foot and toe 80.48
    hand and finger 80.44
    hip 80.45
    knee 80.46
    shoulder 80.41
    specified site NEC 80.49
    spine 80.49
    wrist 80.43
  cerebral tracts 01.32
  chordae tendineae 35.32
  common wall between posterior left atrium and coronary sinus (with roofing of resultant defect with patch graft) 35.82
  congenital web
    larynx 31.98
    pharynx 29.54
  endometrial synechiae 68.21
  fallopian tube — *see* Ligation, fallopian tube
  fascia 83.14
    hand 82.12
  frenulum, frenum
    labial 27.91
    lingual 25.91
    tongue 25.91
  ganglion, sympathetic 05.0
  glossopharyngeal nerve 29.92
  goniosynechiae 12.31
  hypophyseal stalk (*see also* Hypophysectomy, partial) 07.63
  iliotibial band 83.14
  isthmus
    horseshoe kidney 55.85
    thyroid 06.91
  joint capsule 80.40
    ankle 80.47
    elbow 80.42
    foot and toe 80.48
    hand and finger 80.44
    hip 80.45
    knee 80.46
    shoulder 80.41
    specified site NEC 80.49
    wrist 80.43
  labial frenum 27.91
  lacrimal ductules 09.0
  laryngeal nerve (external) (recurrent) (superior) 31.91
  ligament 80.40
    ankle 80.47
    arcuate (spine) — *omit code*
    canthal 08.36
    elbow 80.42
    foot and toe 80.48
    hand and finger 80.44
    hip 80.45
    knee 80.46
    palpebrae 08.36
    shoulder 80.41
    specified site NEC 80.49
    spine 80.49
      arcuate — *omit code*
      flavum — *omit code*
    uterosacral 69.3
    wrist 80.43
  ligamentum flavum (spine) — *omit code*
  meninges (cerebral) 01.31

Division — *continued*
  muscle 83.19
    hand 82.19
  nasolacrimal duct stricture (with drainage) 09.59
  nerve (cranial) (peripheral) NEC 04.03
    acoustic 04.01
    adrenal gland 07.42
    auditory 04.01
    glossopharyngeal 29.92
    lacrimal branch 05.0
    laryngeal (external) (recurrent) (superior) 31.91
    phrenic 04.03
      for collapse of lung 33.31
    root, spinal or intraspinal 03.1
    sympathetic 05.0
    tracts
      cerebral 01.32
      spinal cord 03.29
        percutaneous 03.21
    trigeminal 04.02
    vagus (*see also* Vagotomy) 44.00
    vestibular 04.01
  otosclerotic process or material, middle ear 19.0
  papillary muscle (heart) 35.31
  patent ductus arteriosus 38.85
  penile adhesions 64.93
  posterior synechiae 12.33
  pylorus (with wedge resection) 43.3
  rectum (stricture) 48.91
  scalenus anticus muscle 83.19
  Skene's gland 71.3
  soft tissue NEC 83.19
    hand 82.19
  sphincter
    anal (external) (internal) 49.59
      left lateral 49.51
      posterior 49.52
    cardiac 42.7
    of Oddi 51.82
      endoscopic 51.85
    pancreatic 51.82
      endoscopic 51.85
  spinal
    cord tracts 03.29
      percutaneous 03.21
    nerve root 03.1
  symblepharon (with insertion of conformer) 10.5
  synechiae
    endometrial 68.21
    iris (posterior) 12.33
      anterior 12.32
  tarsorrhaphy 08.02
  tendon 83.13
    Achilles 83.11
    adductor (hip) 83.12
    hand 82.11
  trabeculae carneae cordis (heart) 35.35
  tympanum 20.23
  uterosacral ligaments 69.3
  vaginal septum 70.14
  vas deferens 63.71
  vein (with ligation) 38.80
    abdominal 38.87
    head and neck NEC 38.82
    intracranial NEC 38.81
    lower limb 38.89
      varicose 38.59
    thoracic NEC 38.85
    upper limb 38.83
    varicose 38.50
      abdominal 38.57
      head and neck NEC 38.52
      intracranial NEC 38.51
      lower limb 38.59
      thoracic NEC 38.55
      upper limb 38.53
  vitreous, cicatricial bands (posterior approach) 14.74
    anterior approach 14.73
Doleris operation (shortening of round ligaments) 69.22

D'Ombrain operation (excision of pterygium with corneal graft) 11.32
Domestic tasks therapy 93.83
Dopplergram, Doppler flow mapping — *see also* Ultrasonography
  aortic arch 88.73
  head and neck 88.71
  heart 88.72
  thorax NEC 88.73
Dorrance operation (push-back operation for cleft palate) 27.62
Dotter operation (transluminal angioplasty) 39.59
Douche, vaginal 96.44
Douglas operation (suture of tongue to lip for micrognathia) 25.59
Doyle operation (paracervical uterine denervation) 69.3
Drainage
  by
    anastomosis — *see* Anastomosis
    aspiration — *see* Aspiration
    incision — *see* Incision
  abdomen 54.19
    percutaneous 54.91
  abscess — *see also* Drainage, by site *and* Incision, by site
    appendix 47.2
      with appendectomy 47.09
        laparoscopic 47.01
    parapharyngeal (oral) (transcervical) 28.0
    peritonsillar (oral) (transcervical) 28.0
    retropharyngeal (oral) (transcervical) 28.0
    thyroid (field) (gland) 06.09
      percutaneous (needle) 06.01
      postoperative 06.02
    tonsil, tonsillar (oral) (transcervical) 28.0
  antecubital fossa 86.04
  appendix 47.91
    with appendectomy 47.09
      laparoscopic 47.01
    abscess 47.2
      with appendectomy 47.09
        laparoscopic 47.01
  axilla 86.04
  bladder (without incision) 57.0
    by indwelling catheter 57.94
      percutaneous suprapubic (closed) 57.17
      suprapubic NEC 57.18
  buccal space 27.0
  bursa 83.03
    by aspiration 83.94
      hand 82.92
    hand 82.03
      by aspiration 82.92
    radial 82.03
    ulnar 82.03
  cerebrum, cerebral (meninges) (ventricle) (incision) (trephination) 01.39
    by
      anastomosis — *see* Shunt, ventricular
      aspiration 01.09
        through previously implanted catheter 01.02
  chest (closed) 34.04
    open (by incision) 34.09
  cranial sinus (incision) (trephination) 01.21
    by aspiration 01.09
  cul-de-sac 70.12
    by aspiration 70.0
  cyst — *see also* Drainage, by site *and* Incision, by site
    pancreas (by catheter) 52.01
      by marsupialization 52.3
      internal (anastomosis) 52.4
    pilonidal 86.03
    spleen, splenic (by marsupialization) 41.41
  duodenum (tube) 46.39
    by incision 45.01
  ear
    external 18.09
    inner 20.79
    middle (by myringotomy) 20.09
      with intubation 20.01

Drainage — *continued*
- epidural space cerebral (incision) (trephination) 01.24
  - by aspiration 01.09
- extradural space, cerebral (incision) (trephination) 01.24
  - by aspiration 01.09
- extraperitoneal 54.0
- facial region 27.0
- fascial compartments, head and neck 27.0
- fetal hydrocephalic head (needling) (trocar) 73.8
- gallbladder 51.04
  - by
    - anastomosis 51.35
    - aspiration 51.01
    - incision 51.04
- groin region (abdominal wall) (inguinal) 54.0
  - skin 86.04
  - subcutaneous tissue 86.04
- hematoma — *see* Drainage, by site *and* Incision, by site
- hydrocephalic head (needling) (trocar) 73.8
- hypochondrium 54.0
  - intra-abdominal 54.19
- iliac fossa 54.0
- infratemporal fossa 27.0
- intracranial space (epidural) (extradural) (incision) (trephination) 01.24
  - by aspiration 01.09
  - subarachnoid or subdural (incision) (trephination) 01.31
    - by aspiration 01.09
- intraperitoneal 54.19
  - percutaneous 54.91
- kidney (by incision) 55.01
  - by
    - anastomosis 55.86
    - catheter 59.8
  - pelvis (by incision) 55.11
- liver 50.0
  - by aspiration 50.91
- Ludwig's angina 27.0
- lung (by incision) 33.1
  - by punch (needle) (trocar) 33.93
- midpalmar space 82.04
- mouth floor 27.0
- mucocele, nasal sinus 22.00
  - by puncture 22.01
  - through natural ostium 22.02
- omentum 54.19
  - percutaneous 54.91
- ovary (aspiration) 65.91
  - by incision 65.09
  - laparoscopic 65.01
- palmar space (middle) 82.04
- pancreas (by catheter) 52.01
  - by anastomosis 52.96
- parapharyngeal 28.0
- paronychia 86.04
- parotid space 27.0
- pelvic peritoneum (female) 70.12
  - male 54.19
- pericardium 37.0
- perigastric 54.19
  - percutaneous 54.91
- perineum
  - female 71.09
  - male 86.04
- perisplenic tissue 54.19
  - percutaneous 54.91
- peritoneum 54.19
  - pelvic (female) 70.12
  - percutaneous 54.91
- peritonsillar 28.0
- pharyngeal space, lateral 27.0
- pilonidal cyst or sinus 86.03
- pleura (closed) 34.04
  - open (by incision) 34.09
- popliteal space 86.04
- postural 93.99
- postzygomatic space 27.0
- pseudocyst, pancreas 52.3
  - by anastomosis 52.4
- pterygopalatine fossa 27.0
- retropharyngeal 28.0
- scrotum 61.0

Drainage — *continued*
- skin 86.04
- spinal (canal) (cord) 03.09
  - by anastomosis — *see* Shunt, spinal
  - diagnostic 03.31
- spleen 41.2
  - cyst (by marsupialization) 41.41
- subarachnoid space, cerebral (incision) (trephination) 01.31
  - by aspiration 01.09
- subcutaneous tissue 86.04
- subdiaphragmatic 54.19
  - percutaneous 54.91
- subdural space, cerebral (incision) (trephination) 01.31
  - by aspiration 01.09
- subhepatic space 54.19
  - percutaneous 54.91
- sublingual space 27.0
- submental space 27.0
- subphrenic space 54.19
  - percutaneous 54.91
- supraclavicular fossa 86.04
- temporal pouches 27.0
- tendon (sheath) 83.01
  - hand 82.01
- thenar space 82.04
- thorax (closed) 34.04
  - open (by incision) 34.09
- thyroglossal tract (by incision) 06.09
  - by aspiration 06.01
- thyroid (field) (gland) (by incision) 06.09
  - by aspiration 06.01
  - postoperative 06.02
- tonsil 28.0
- tunica vaginalis 61.0
- ureter (by catheter) 59.8
  - by
    - anastomosis NEC (*see also* Anastomosis, ureter) 56.79
    - incision 56.2
- ventricle (cerebral) (incision) NEC 02.39
  - by
    - anastomosis — *see* Shunt, ventricular
    - aspiration 01.09
      - through previously implanted catheter 01.02
- vertebral column 03.09

Drawing test 94.08

Dressing
- burn 93.57
- ulcer 93.56
- wound 93.57

Drilling, bone (*see also* Incision, bone) 77.10

Ductogram, mammary 87.35

Duhamel operation (abdominoperineal pull-through) 48.65

Dührssen's
- incisions (cervix, to assist delivery) 73.93
- operation (vaginofixation of uterus) 69.22

Dunn operation (triple arthrodesis) 81.12

Duodenectomy 45.62
- with
  - gastrectomy — *see* Gastrectomy
  - pancreatectomy — *see* Pancreatectomy

Duodenocholedochotomy 51.51

Duodenoduodenostomy 45.91
- proximal to distal segment 45.62

Duodenoileostomy 45.91

Duodenojejunostomy 45.91

Duodenoplasty 46.79 ●

Duodenorrhaphy 46.71

Duodenoscopy 45.13
- through stoma (artificial) 45.12
- transabdominal (operative) 45.11

Duodenostomy 46.39

Duodenotomy 45.01

Dupuytren operation
- fasciectomy 82.35
- fasciotomy 82.12
  - with excision 82.35
- shoulder disarticulation 84.08

Durabond 86.59

Duraplasty 02.12

Durham (-Caldwell) operation (transfer of biceps femoris tendon) 83.75

DuToit and Roux operation (staple capsulorrhaphy of shoulder) 81.82

DuVries operation (tenoplasty) 83.88

Dwyer operation
- fasciotomy 83.14
- soft tissue release NEC 83.84
- wedge osteotomy, calcaneus 77.28

E

Eagleton operation (extrapetrosal drainage) 20.22

ECG — *see* Electrocardiogram

Echocardiography 88.72
- intracardiac (ICE) 37.28
- transesophageal 88.72
  - monitoring (Doppler) (ultrasound) 89.68

Echoencephalography 88.71

Echography — *see* Ultrasonography

Echogynography 88.79

Echoplacentogram 88.78

ECMO (extracorporeal membrane oxygenation) 39.65

Eden-Hybinette operation (glenoid bone block) 78.01

Educational therapy (bed-bound children) (handicapped) 93.82

EEG (electroencephalogram) 89.14
- monitoring (radiographic) (video) 89.19

Effler operation (heart) 36.2

Effleurage 93.39

EGD (esophagogastroduodenoscopy) 45.13
- with closed biopsy 45.16

Eggers operation
- tendon release (patellar retinacula) 83.13
- tendon transfer (biceps femoris tendon) (hamstring tendon) 83.75

EKG (*see also* Electrocardiogram) 89.52

Elastic hosiery 93.59

Electrocardiogram (with 12 or more leads) 89.52
- with vectorcardiogram 89.53
- fetal (scalp), intrauterine 75.32
- rhythm (with one to three leads) 89.51

Electrocautery — *see also* Cauterization
- cervix 67.32
- corneal lesion (ulcer) 11.42
- esophagus 42.39
  - endoscopic 42.33

Electrocoagulation — *see also* Destruction, lesion, by site
- aneurysm (cerebral) (peripheral vessels) 39.52
- cervix 67.32
- cystoscopic 57.49
- ear
  - external 18.29
  - inner 20.79
  - middle 20.51
- fallopian tube (lesion) 66.61
  - for tubal ligation — *see* Ligation, fallopian tube
- gasserian ganglion 04.02
- nasal turbinates 21.61
- nose, for epistaxis (with packing) 21.03
- ovary 65.29
  - laparoscopic 65.25
- prostatic bed 60.94
- rectum (polyp) 48.32
  - radical 48.31
- retina (for)
  - destruction of lesion 14.21
  - reattachment 14.51
  - repair of tear 14.31
- round ligament 69.19
- semicircular canals 20.79
- urethrovesical junction, transurethral 57.49

Drainage — Electrocoagulation

Enterocelectomy 53.9
  female 70.92
  vaginal 70.92
Enterocentesis 45.00
  duodenum 45.01
  large intestine 45.03
  small intestine NEC 45.02
Enterocholecystostomy 51.32
Enteroclysis (small bowel) 96.43
Enterocolectomy NEC 45.79
Enterocolostomy 45.93
Enteroentectropy 46.99
Enteroenterostomy 45.90
  small-to-large intestine 45.93
  small-to-small intestine 45.91
Enterogastrostomy 44.39
Enterolithotomy 45.00
Enterolysis 54.59
  laparoscopic 54.51
Enteropancreatostomy 52.96
Enterorrhaphy 46.79
  large intestine 46.75
  small intestine 46.73
Enterostomy NEC 46.39
  cecum (see also Colostomy) 46.10
  colon (transverse) (see also Colostomy) 46.10
    loop 46.03
  delayed opening 46.31
  duodenum 46.39
    loop 46.01
  feeding NEC 46.39
    percutaneous (endoscopic) 46.32
  ileum (Brooke) (Dragstedt) 46.20
    loop 46.01
  jejunum (feeding) 46.39
    loop 46.01
    percutaneous (endoscopic) 46.32
  sigmoid colon (see also Colostomy) 46.10
    loop 46.03
  transverse colon (see also Colostomy) 46.10
    loop 46.03
Enterotomy 45.00
  large intestine 45.03
  small intestine 45.02
Enucleation — see also Excision, lesion, by site
  cyst
    broad ligament 69.19
    dental 24.4
    liver 50.29
    ovarian 65.29
      laparoscopic 65.25
    parotid gland 26.29
    salivary gland 26.29
    skin 86.3
    subcutaneous tissue 86.3
  eyeball 16.49
    with implant (into Tenon's capsule) 16.42
      with attachment of muscles 16.41
EOG (electro-oculogram) 95.22
Epicardiectomy 36.39
Epididymectomy 63.4
  with orchidectomy (unilateral) 62.3
    bilateral 62.41
Epididymogram 87.93
Epididymoplasty 63.59
Epididymorrhaphy 63.81
Epididymotomy 63.92
Epididymovasostomy 63.83
Epiglottidectomy 30.21
Epikeratophakia 11.76
Epilation
  eyebrow (forceps) 08.93
    cryosurgical 08.92
    electrosurgical 08.91
  eyelid (forceps) NEC 08.93
    cryosurgical 08.92
    electrosurgical 08.91
  skin 86.92
Epiphysiodesis (see also Arrest, bone growth) — see category 78.2 ✓4th

Epiphysiolysis (see also Arrest, bone growth) — see category 78.2 ✓4th
Epiploectomy 54.4
Epiplopexy 54.74
Epiplorrhaphy 54.74
Episioperineoplasty 71.79
Episioperineorrhaphy 71.71
  obstetrical 75.69
Episioplasty 71.79
Episioproctotomy 73.6
Episiorrhaphy 71.71
  following routine episiotomy — see Episiotomy
  for obstetrical laceration 75.69
Episiotomy (with subsequent episiorrhaphy) 73.6
  high forceps 72.31
  low forceps 72.1
  mid forceps 72.21
  nonobstetrical 71.09
  outlet forceps 72.1
EPS (electrophysiologic stimulation) 37.26
Eptifibatide, infusion 99.20
Equalization, leg
  lengthening — see category 78.3 ✓4th
  shortening — see category 78.2 ✓4th
Equilibration (occlusal) 24.8
Equiloudness balance 95.43
ERC (endoscopic retrograde cholangiography) 51.11
ERCP (endoscopic retrograde cholangiopancreatography) 51.10
  cannulation of pancreatic duct 52.93
ERG (electroretinogram) 95.21
ERP (endoscopic retrograde pancreatography) 52.13
Eruption, tooth, surgical 24.6
Erythrocytapheresis, therapeutic 99.73
Escharectomy 86.22
Escharotomy 86.09
Esophageal voice training (post-laryngectomy) 93.73
Esophagectomy 42.40
  abdominothoracocervical (combined) (synchronous) 42.42
  partial or subtotal 42.41
  total 42.42
Esophagocologastrostomy (intrathoracic) 42.55
  antesternal or antethoracic 42.65
Esophagocolostomy (intrathoracic) NEC 42.56
  with interposition of colon 42.55
  antesternal or antethoracic NEC 42.66
    with interposition of colon 42.65
Esophagoduodenostomy (intrathoracic) NEC 42.54
  with
    complete gastrectomy 43.99
    interposition of small bowel 42.53
Esophagoenterostomy (intrathoracic) NEC (see also Anastomosis, esophagus, to intestinal segment) 42.54
  antesternal or antethoracic (see also Anastomosis, esophagus, antesternal, to intestinal segment) 42.64
Esophagoesophagostomy (intrathoracic) 42.51
  antesternal or antethoracic 42.61
Esophagogastrectomy 43.99
Esophagogastroduodenoscopy (EGD) 45.13
  with closed biopsy 45.16
  through stoma (artificial) 45.12
  transabdominal (operative) 45.11
Esophagogastromyotomy 42.7
Esophagogastropexy 44.65
Esophagogastroplasty 44.65
Esophagogastroscopy NEC 44.13
  through stoma (artificial) 44.12
  transabdominal (operative) 44.11
Esophagogastrostomy (intrathoracic) 42.52
  with partial gastrectomy 43.5
  antesternal or antethoracic 42.62

Esophagoileostomy (intrathoracic) NEC 42.54
  with interposition of small bowel 42.53
  antesternal or antethoracic NEC 42.64
    with interposition of small bowel 42.63
Esophagojejunostomy (intrathoracic) NEC 42.54
  with
    complete gastrectomy 43.99
    interposition of small bowel 42.53
  antesternal or antethoracic NEC 42.64
    with interposition of small bowel 42.63
Esophagomyotomy 42.7
Esophagoplasty NEC 42.89
Esophagorrhaphy 42.82
Esophagoscopy NEC 42.23
  by incision (operative) 42.21
  with closed biopsy 42.24
  through stoma (artificial) 42.22
  transabdominal (operative) 42.21
Esophagostomy 42.10
  cervical 42.11
  thoracic 42.19
Esophagotomy NEC 42.09
Estes operation (ovary) 65.72
  laparoscopic 65.75
Estlander operation (thoracoplasty) 33.34
ESWL (extracorporeal shockwave lithotripsy) NEC 98.59
  bile duct 98.52
  bladder 98.51
  gallbladder 98.52
  kidney 98.51
  Kock pouch (urinary diversion) 98.51
  renal pelvis 98.51
  specified site NEC 98.59
  ureter 98.51
Ethmoidectomy 22.63
Ethmoidotomy 22.51
Evacuation
  abscess — see Drainage, by site
  anterior chamber (eye) (aqueous) (hyphema) 12.91
  cyst — see also Excision, lesion, by site
    breast 85.91
    kidney 55.01
    liver 50.29
  hematoma — see also Incision, hematoma
    obstetrical 75.92
      incisional 75.91
  hemorrhoids (thrombosed) 49.47
  pelvic blood clot (by incision) 54.19
    by
      culdocentesis 70.0
      culdoscopy 70.22
  retained placenta
    with curettage 69.02
    manual 75.4
  streptothrix from lacrimal duct 09.42
Evaluation (of)
  audiological 95.43
  criminal responsibility, psychiatric 94.11
  functional (physical therapy) 93.01
  hearing NEC 95.49
  orthotic (for brace fitting) 93.02
  prosthetic (for artificial limb fitting) 93.03
  psychiatric NEC 94.19
    commitment 94.13
  psychologic NEC 94.08
  testimentary capacity, psychiatric 94.11
Evans operation (release of clubfoot) 83.84
Evisceration
  eyeball 16.39
    with implant (into scleral shell) 16.31
  ocular contents 16.39
    with implant (into scleral shell) 16.31
  orbit (see also Exenteration, orbit) 16.59
  pelvic (anterior) (posterior) (partial) (total) (female) 68.8
    male 57.71
Evulsion
  nail (bed) (fold) 86.23
  skin 86.3
  subcutaneous tissue 86.3

Enterocelectomy — Evulsion

Examination — Excision

Examination (for)
  breast
    manual 89.36
    radiographic NEC 87.37
    thermographic 88.85
    ultrasonic 88.73
  cervical rib (by x-ray) 87.43
  colostomy stoma (digital) 89.33
  dental (oral mucosa) (peridontal) 89.31
    radiographic NEC 87.12
  enterostomy stoma (digital) 89.33
  eye 95.09
    color vision 95.06
    comprehensive 95.02
    dark adaptation 95.07
    limited (with prescription of spectacles) 95.01
    under anesthesia 95.04
  fetus, intrauterine 75.35
  general physical 89.7
  glaucoma 95.03
  gynecological 89.26
  hearing 95.47
  microscopic (specimen) (of) 91.9 ✓4th

> *Note* — *Use the following fourth-digit*
> *subclassification with categories 90-91 to*
> *identify type of examination:*
>   *1 bacterial smear*
>   *2 culture*
>   *3 culture and sensitivity*
>   *4 parasitology*
>   *5 toxicology*
>   *6 cell block and Papanicolaou smear*
>   *9 other microscopic examination*

    adenoid 90.3 ✓4th
    adrenal gland 90.1 ✓4th
    amnion 91.4 ✓4th
    anus 90.9 ✓4th
    appendix 90.9 ✓4th
    bile ducts 91.0 ✓4th
    bladder 91.3 ✓4th
    blood 90.5 ✓4th
    bone 91.5 ✓4th
      marrow 90.6 ✓4th
    brain 90.0 ✓4th
    breast 91.6 ✓4th
    bronchus 90.4 ✓4th
    bursa 91.5 ✓4th
    cartilage 91.5 ✓4th
    cervix 91.4 ✓4th
    chest wall 90.4 ✓4th
    chorion 91.4 ✓4th
    colon 90.9 ✓4th
    cul-de-sac 91.1 ✓4th
    dental 90.8 ✓4th
    diaphragm 90.4 ✓4th
    duodenum 90.8 ✓4th
    ear 90.3 ✓4th
    endocrine gland NEC 90.1 ✓4th
    esophagus 90.8 ✓4th
    eye 90.2 ✓4th
    fallopian tube 91.4 ✓4th
    fascia 91.5 ✓4th
    female genital tract 91.4 ✓4th
    fetus 91.4 ✓4th
    gallbladder 91.0 ✓4th
    hair 91.6 ✓4th
    ileum 90.9 ✓4th
    jejunum 90.9 ✓4th
    joint fluid 91.5 ✓4th
    kidney 91.2 ✓4th
    large intestine 90.9 ✓4th
    larynx 90.3 ✓4th
    ligament 91.5 ✓4th
    liver 91.0 ✓4th
    lung 90.4 ✓4th
    lymph (node) 90.7 ✓4th
    meninges 90.0 ✓4th
    mesentery 91.1 ✓4th
    mouth 90.8 ✓4th
    muscle 91.5 ✓4th
    musculoskeletal system 91.5 ✓4th
    nails 91.6 ✓4th
    nerve 90.0 ✓4th

Examination (for) — *continued*
  microscopic — *continued*
    nervous system 90.0 ✓4th
    nose 90.3 ✓4th
    omentum 91.1 ✓4th
    operative wound 91.7 ✓4th
    ovary 91.4 ✓4th
    pancreas 91.0 ✓4th
    parathyroid gland 90.1 ✓4th
    penis 91.3 ✓4th
    perirenal tissue 91.2 ✓4th
    peritoneum (fluid) 91.1 ✓4th
    periureteral tissue 91.2 ✓4th
    perivesical (tissue) 91.3 ✓4th
    pharynx 90.3 ✓4th
    pineal gland 90.1 ✓4th
    pituitary gland 90.1 ✓4th
    placenta 91.4 ✓4th
    pleura (fluid) 90.4 ✓4th
    prostate 91.3 ✓4th
    rectum 90.9 ✓4th
    retroperitoneum 91.1 ✓4th
    semen 91.3 ✓4th
    seminal vesicle 91.3 ✓4th
    sigmoid 90.9 ✓4th
    skin 91.6 ✓4th
    small intestine 90.9 ✓4th
    specified site NEC 91.8 ✓4th
    spinal fluid 90.0 ✓4th
    spleen 90.6 ✓4th
    sputum 90.4 ✓4th
    stomach 90.8 ✓4th
    stool 90.9 ✓4th
    synovial membrane 91.5 ✓4th
    tendon 91.5 ✓4th
    thorax NEC 90.4 ✓4th
    throat 90.3 ✓4th
    thymus 90.1 ✓4th
    thyroid gland 90.1 ✓4th
    tonsil 90.3 ✓4th
    trachea 90.4 ✓4th
    ureter 91.2 ✓4th
    urethra 91.3 ✓4th
    urine 91.3 ✓4th
    uterus 91.4 ✓4th
    vagina 91.4 ✓4th
    vas deferens 91.3 ✓4th
    vomitus 90.8 ✓4th
    vulva 91.4 ✓4th
  neurologic 89.13
  neuro-ophthalmology 95.03
  opthalmoscopic 16.21
  panorex, mandible 87.12
  pelvic (manual) 89.26
    instrumental (by pelvimeter) 88.25
    pelvimetric 88.25
  physical, general 89.7
  postmortem 89.8
  rectum (digital) 89.34
    endoscopic 48.23
      through stoma (artificial) 48.22
      transabdominal 48.21
  retinal disease 95.03
  specified type (manual) NEC 89.39
  thyroid field, postoperative 06.02
  uterus (digital) 68.11
    endoscopic 68.12
  vagina 89.26
    endoscopic 70.21
  visual field 95.05
Exchange transfusion 99.01
  intrauterine 75.2
Excision
  aberrant tissue — *see* Excision, lesion, by site of tissue origin
  abscess — *see* Excision, lesion, by site
  accessory tissue — *see also* Excision, lesion, by site of tissue origin
    lung 32.29
      endoscopic 32.28
    spleen 41.93
  adenoids (tag) 28.6
    with tonsillectomy 28.3
  adenoma — *see* Excision, lesion, by site
  adrenal gland (*see also* Adrenalectomy) 07.22

Excision — *continued*
  ampulla of Vater (with reimplantation of common duct) 51.62
  anal papilla 49.39
    endoscopic 49.31
  aneurysm (arteriovenous) (*see also* Aneurysmectomy) 38.60
    coronary artery 36.91
    heart 37.32
    myocardium 37.32
    sinus of Valsalva 35.39
    ventricle (heart) 37.32
  anus (complete) (partial) 49.6
  aortic subvalvular ring 35.35
  apocrine gland 86.3
  aponeurosis 83.42
    hand 82.33
  appendiceal stump 47.01-47.09
  appendices epiploicae 54.4
  appendix (*see also* Appendectomy) 47.01, 47.09
    epididymis 63.3
    testis 62.2
  arcuate ligament (spine) — *omit code*
  arteriovenous fistula (*see also* Aneurysmectomy) 38.60
  artery (*see also* Arteriectomy) 38.60
  Baker's cyst, knee 83.39
  Bartholin's gland 71.24
  basal ganglion 01.59
  bile duct 51.69
    endoscopic 51.64
  bladder — *see also* Cystectomy
  bleb (emphysematous), lung 32.29
    endoscopic 32.28
  blood vessel (*see also* Angiectomy) 38.60
  bone (ends) (partial), except facial — *see* category 77.8 ✓4th
    facial NEC 76.39
      total 76.45
        with reconstruction 76.44
    for graft (autograft) (homograft) — *see* category 77.7 ✓4th
    fragments (chips) (*see also* Incision, bone) 77.10
      joint (*see also* Arthrotomy) 80.10
      necrotic (*see also* Sequestrectomy, bone) 77.00
    heterotopic, from
      muscle 83.32
        hand 82.22
      skin 86.3
      tendon 83.31
        hand 82.21
    mandible 76.31
      with arthrodesis — *see* Arthrodesis
      total 76.42
        with reconstruction 76.41
    spur — *see* Excision, lesion, bone
    total, except facial — *see* category 77.9 ✓4th
      facial NEC 76.45
        with reconstruction 76.44
      mandible 76.42
        with reconstruction 76.41
  brain 01.59
    hemisphere 01.52
    lobe 01.53
  branchial cleft cyst or vestige 29.2
  breast (*see also* Mastectomy) 85.41
    aberrant tissue 85.24
    accessory 85.24
    ectopic 85.24
    nipple 85.25
      accessory 85.24
    segmental 85.23
    supernumerary 85.24
    wedge 85.21
  broad ligament 69.19
  bronchogenic cyst 32.09
    endoscopic 32.01
  bronchus (wide sleeve) NEC 32.1
  buccal mucosa 27.49
  bulbourethral gland 58.92
  bulbous tuberosities (mandible) (maxilla) (fibrous) (osseous) 24.31
  bunion (*see also* Bunionectomy) 77.59
  bunionette (with osteotomy) 77.54

Excision — *continued*
  bursa 83.5
    hand 82.31
  canal of Nuck 69.19
  cardioma 37.33
  carotid body (lesion) (partial) (total) 39.8
  cartilage (*see also* Chondrectomy) 80.90
    intervertebral — *see* category 80.5 ☑4ᵗʰ
    knee (semilunar) 80.6
    larynx 30.29
    nasal (submucous) 21.5
  caruncle, urethra 58.39
    endoscopic 58.31
  cataract (*see also* Extraction, cataract) 13.19
    secondary membrane (after cataract) 13.65
  cervical
    rib 77.91
    stump 67.4
  cervix (stump) NEC 67.4
    cold (knife) 67.2
    conization 67.2
    cryoconization 67.33
    electroconizaton 67.32
  chalazion (multiple) (single) 08.21
  cholesteatoma — *see* Excision, lesion, by site
  choroid plexus 02.14
  cicatrix (skin) 86.3
  cilia base 08.20
  ciliary body, prolapsed 12.98
  clavicle (head) (partial) 77.81
    total (complete) 77.91
  clitoris 71.4
  coarctation of aorta (end-to-end anastomosis) 38.64
    with
      graft replacement (interposition)
        abdominal 38.44
        thoracic 38.45
        thoracoabdominal 38.45 *[38.44]*
  common
    duct 51.63
    wall between posterior and coronary sinus (with roofing of resultant defect with patch graft) 35.82
  condyle — *see* category 77.8 ☑4ᵗʰ
    mandible 76.5
  conjunctival ring 10.31
  cornea 11.49
    epithelium (with chemocauterization) 11.41
      for smear or culture 11.21
  costal cartilage 80.99
  cul-de-sac (Douglas) 70.92
  cusp, heart valve 35.10
    aortic 35.11
    mitral 35.12
    tricuspid 35.14
  cyst — *see also* Excision, lesion, by site
    apical (tooth) 23.73
      with root canal therapy 23.72
    Baker's (popliteal) 83.39
    breast 85.21
    broad ligament 69.19
    bronchogenic 32.09
      endoscopic 32.01
    cervix 67.39
    dental 24.4
    dentigerous 24.4
    epididymis 63.2
    fallopian tube 66.61
    Gartner's duct 70.33
    hand 82.29
    labia 71.3
    lung 32.29
      endoscopic 32.28
    mesonephric duct 69.19
    Morgagni
      female 66.61
      male 62.2
    müllerian duct 60.73
    nasolabial 27.49
    nasopalatine 27.31
      by wide excision 27.32
    ovary 65.29
      laparoscopic 65.25
    parovarian 69.19
    pericardium 37.31

Excision — *continued*
  cyst — *see also* Excision, lesion, by site — *continued*
    periodontal (apical) (lateral) 24.4
    popliteal (Baker's), knee 83.39
    radicular 24.4
    spleen 41.42
    synovial (membrane) 83.39
    thyroglossal (with resection of hyoid bone) 06.7
    urachal (bladder) 57.51
      abdominal wall 54.3
    vagina (Gartner's duct) 70.33
  cystic
    duct remnant 51.61
    hygroma 40.29
  dentinoma 24.4
  diaphragm 34.81
  disc, intervertebral (NOS) 80.50
    herniated (nucleus pulposus) 80.51
    other specified (diskectomy) 80.51
  diverticulum
    ampulla of Vater 51.62
    anus 49.39
      endoscopic 49.31
    bladder 57.59
      transurethral 57.49
    duodenum 45.31
      endoscopic 45.30
    esophagus (local) 42.31
      endoscopic 42.33
    hypopharyngeal (by cricopharyngeal myotomy) 29.32
    intestine
      large 45.41
        endoscopic 45.43
      small NEC 45.33
    Meckel's 45.33
    pharyngeal (by cricopharyngeal myotomy) 29.32
    pharyngoesophageal (by cricopharyngeal myotomy) 29.32
    stomach 43.42
      endoscopic 43.41
    urethra 58.39
      endoscopic 58.31
    ventricle, heart 37.33
  duct
    müllerian 69.19
    paramesonephric 69.19
    thyroglossal (with resection of hyoid bone) 06.7
  ear, external (complete) NEC 18.39
    partial 18.29
    radical 18.31
  ectopic
    abdominal fetus 74.3
    tissue — *see also* Excision, lesion, by site of tissue origin
      bone, from muscle 83.32
      breast 85.24
      lung 32.29
        endoscopic 32.28
      spleen 41.93
  empyema pocket, lung 34.09
  epididymis 63.4
  epiglottis 30.21
  epithelial downgrowth, anterior chamber (eye) 12.93
  epulis (gingiva) 24.31
  esophagus (*see also* Esophagectomy) 42.40
  exostosis (*see also* Excision, lesion, bone) 77.60
    auditory canal, external 18.29
    facial bone 76.2
    first metatarsal (hallux valgus repair) — *see* Bunionectomy
  eye 16.49
    with implant (into Tenon's capsule) 16.42
      with attachment of muscles 16.41
  eyelid 08.20
    redundant skin 08.86
  falciform ligament 54.4
  fallopian tube — *see* Salpingectomy
  fascia 83.44
    for graft 83.43
      hand 82.34

Excision — *continued*
  fascia — *continued*
    hand 82.35
      for graft 82.34
    fat pad NEC 86.3
      knee (infrapatellar) (prepatellar) 86.3
      scalene 40.21
  fibroadenoma, breast 85.21
  fissure, anus 49.39
    endoscopic 49.31
  fistula — *see also* Fistulectomy
    anal 49.12
    arteriovenous (*see also* Aneurysmectomy) 38.60
    ileorectal 46.74
    lacrimal
      gland 09.21
      sac 09.6
    rectal 48.73
    vesicovaginal 57.84
  frenulum, frenum
    labial (lip) 27.41
    lingual (tongue) 25.92
  ganglion (hand) (tendon sheath) (wrist) 82.21
    gasserian 04.05
    site other than hand or nerve 83.31
    sympathetic nerve 05.29
    trigeminal nerve 04.05
  gastrocolic ligament 54.4
  gingiva 24.31
  glomus jugulare tumor 20.51
  goiter — *see* Thyroidectomy
  gum 24.31
  hallux valgus — *see also* Bunionectomy
    with prosthetic implant 77.59
  hamartoma, mammary 85.21
  hematocele, tunica vaginalis 61.92
  hematoma — *see* Drainage, by site
  hemorrhoids (external) (internal) (tag) 49.46
  heterotopic bone, from
    muscle 83.32
      hand 82.22
    skin 86.3
    tendon 83.31
      hand 82.21
  hydatid of Morgagni
    female 66.61
    male 62.2
  hydatid cyst, liver 50.29
  hydrocele
    canal of Nuck (female) 69.19
    male 63.1
    round ligament 69.19
    spermatic cord 63.1
    tunica vaginalis 61.2
  hygroma, cystic 40.29
  hymen (tag) 70.31
  hymeno-urethral fusion 70.31
  intervertebral disc — *see* Excision, disc, intervertebral (NOS) 80.50
  intestine (*see also* Resection, intestine) 45.8
    for interposition 45.50
      large 45.52
      small 45.51
    large (total) 45.8
      for interposition 45.52
      local 45.41
        endoscopic 45.43
      segmental 45.79
        multiple 45.71
    small (total) 45.63
      for interposition 45.51
      local 45.33
      partial 45.62
      segmental 45.62
        multiple 45.61
  intraductal papilloma 85.21
  iris prolapse 12.13
  joint (*see also* Arthrectomy) 80.90
  keloid (scar), skin 86.3
  labia — *see* Vulvectomy
  lacrimal
    gland 09.20
      partial 09.22
      total 09.23
    passage 09.6

Excision — *continued*
  lacrimal — *continued*
    sac 09.6
  lesion (local)
    abdominal wall 54.3
    accessory sinus — *see* Excision, lesion,
        nasal sinus
    adenoids 28.92
    adrenal gland(s) 07.21
    alveolus 24.4
    ampulla of Vater 51.62
    anterior chamber (eye) NEC 12.40
    anus 49.39
      endoscopic 49.31
    apocrine gland 86.3
    artery 38.60
      abdominal 38.66
      aorta (arch) (ascending) (descending
          thoracic) 38.64
        with end-to-end anastomosis 38.45
          abdominal 38.44
          thoracic 38.45
          thoracoabdominal 38.45 [38.44]
        with graft interposition graft
            replacement 38.45
          abdominal 38.44
          thoracic 38.45
          thoracoabdominal 38.45 [38.44]
      head and neck NEC 38.62
      intracranial NEC 38.61
      lower limb 38.68
      thoracic NEC 38.65
      upper limb 38.63
    atrium 37.33
    auditory canal or meatus, external 18.29
      radical 18.31
    auricle, ear 18.29
      radical 18.31
    biliary ducts 51.69
      endoscopic 51.64
    bladder (transurethral) 57.49
      open 57.59
      suprapubic 57.59
    blood vessel 38.60
      abdominal
        artery 38.66
        vein 38.67
      aorta (arch) (ascending) (descending)
          38.64
      head and neck NEC 38.62
      intracranial NEC 38.61
      lower limb
        artery 38.68
        vein 38.69
      thoracic NEC 38.65
      upper limb (artery) (vein) 38.63
    bone 77.60
      carpal, metacarpal 77.64
      clavicle 77.61
      facial 76.2
      femur 77.65
      fibula 77.67
      humerus 77.62
      jaw 76.2
        dental 24.4
      patella 77.66
      pelvic 77.69
      phalanges (foot) (hand) 77.69
      radius 77.63
      scapula 77.61
      skull 01.6
      specified site NEC 77.69
      tarsal, metatarsal 77.68
      thorax (ribs) (sternum) 77.61
      tibia 77.67
      ulna 77.63
      vertebrae 77.69
    brain (transtemporal approach) NEC 01.59
      by stereotactic radiosurgery 92.30
        cobalt 60 92.32
        linear accelerator (LINAC) 92.31
        multi-source 92.32
        particle beam 92.33
        particulate 92.33
        radiosurgery NEC 92.39
        single source photon 92.31

Excision — *continued*
  lesion — *continued*
    breast (segmental) (wedge) 85.21
    broad ligament 69.19
    bronchus NEC 32.09
      endoscopic 32.01
    cerebral (cortex) NEC 01.59
      meninges 01.51
    cervix (myoma) 67.39
    chest wall 34.4
    choroid plexus 02.14
    ciliary body 12.44
    colon 45.41
      endoscopic NEC 45.43
        polypectomy 45.42
    conjunctiva 10.31
    cornea 11.49
    cranium 01.6
    cul-de-sac (Douglas') 70.32
    dental (jaw) 24.4
    diaphragm 34.81
    duodenum (local) 45.31
      endoscopic 45.30
    ear, external 18.29
      radical 18.31
    endometrium 68.29
    epicardium 37.31
    epididymis 63.3
    epiglottis 30.09
    esophagus NEC 42.32
      endoscopic 42.33
    eye, eyeball 16.93
      anterior segment NEC 12.40
    eyebrow (skin) 08.20
    eyelid 08.20
      by
        halving procedure 08.24
        wedge resection 08.24
      major
        full-thickness 08.24
        partial-thickness 08.23
      minor 08.22
    fallopian tube 66.61
    fascia 83.39
      hand 82.29
    groin region (abdominal wall) (inguinal) 54.3
      skin 86.3
      subcutaneous tissue 86.3
    gum 24.31
    heart 37.33
    hepatic duct 51.69
    inguinal canal 54.3
    intestine
      large 45.41
        endoscopic NEC 45.43
          polypectomy 45.42
      small NEC 45.33
    intracranial NEC 01.59
    intranasal 21.31
    intraspinal 03.4
    iris 12.42
    jaw 76.2
      dental 24.4
    joint 80.80
      ankle 80.87
      elbow 80.82
      foot and toe 80.88
      hand and finger 80.84
      hip 80.85
      knee 80.86
      shoulder 80.81
      specified site NEC 80.89
      spine 80.89
      wrist 80.83
    kidney 55.39
      with partial nephrectomy 55.4
    labia 71.3
    lacrimal
      gland (frontal approach) 09.21
      passage 09.6
      sac 09.6
    larynx 30.09
    ligament (joint) (*see also* Excision, lesion,
        joint) 80.80
      broad 69.19
      round 69.19

Excision — *continued*
  lesion — *continued*
    ligament (*see also* Excision, lesion, joint) —
        continued
      uterosacral 69.19
    lip 27.43
      by wide excision 27.42
    liver 50.29
    lung NEC 32.29
      by wide excision 32.3
      endoscopic 32.28
    lymph structure(s) (channel) (vessel) NEC
        40.29
      node — *see* Excision, lymph, node
    mammary duct 85.21
    mastoid (bone) 20.49
    mediastinum 34.3
    meninges (cerebral) 01.51
      spinal 03.4
    mesentery 54.4
    middle ear 20.51
    mouth NEC 27.49
    muscle 83.32
      hand 82.22
      ocular 15.13
    myocardium 37.33
    nail 86.23
    nasal sinus 22.60
      antrum 22.62
        with Caldwell-Luc approach 22.61
        specified approach NEC 22.62
      ethmoid 22.63
      frontal 22.42
      maxillary 22.62
        with Caldwell-Luc approach 22.61
        specified approach NEC 22.62
      sphenoid 22.64
    nasopharynx 29.3 ✔4ᵗʰ
    nerve (cranial) (peripheral) 04.07
      sympathetic 05.29
    nonodontogenic 24.31
    nose 21.30
      intranasal 21.31
      polyp 21.31
      skin 21.32
      specified site NEC 21.32
    odontogenic 24.4
    omentum 54.4
    orbit 16.92
    ovary 65.29
      by wedge resection 65.22
        laparoscopic 65.24
      that by laparoscope 65.25
    palate (bony) 27.31
      by wide excision 27.32
      soft 27.49
    pancreas (local) 52.22
      endoscopic 52.21
    parathyroid 06.89
    parotid gland or duct NEC 26.29
    pelvic wall 54.3
    pelvirectal tissue 48.82
    penis 64.2
    pericardium 37.31
    perineum (female) 71.3
      male 86.3
    periprostatic tissue 60.82
    perirectal tissue 48.82
    perirenal tissue 59.91
    peritoneum 54.4
    perivesical tissue 59.91
    pharynx 29.39
      diverticulum 29.32
    pineal gland 07.53
    pinna 18.29
      radical 18.31
    pituitary (gland) (*see also* Hypophysectomy,
        partial) 07.63
      by stereotactic radiosurgery 92.30
        cobalt 60 92.32
        linear accelerator (LINAC) 92.31
        multi-source 92.32
        particle beam 92.33
        particulate 92.33
        radiosurgery NEC 92.39
        single source photon 92.31

Excision — *continued*
  prolapsed iris (in wound) 12.13
  prostate — *see* Prostatectomy
  pterygium (simple) 11.39
    with corneal graft 11.32
  radius (head) (partial) 77.83
    total 77.93
  ranula, salivary gland NEC 26.29
  rectal mucosa 48.35
  rectum — *see* Resection, rectum
  redundant mucosa
    colostomy 45.41
      endoscopic 45.43
    duodenostomy 45.31
      endoscopic 45.30
    ileostomy 45.33
    jejunostomy 45.33
    perineum 71.3
    rectum 48.35
    vulva 71.3
  renal vessel, aberrant 38.66
  rib (cervical) 77.91
  ring of conjunctiva around cornea 10.31
  round ligament 69.19
  salivary gland 26.30
    complete 26.32
    partial 26.31
    radical 26.32
  scalene fat pad 40.21
  scar — *see also* Excision, lesion, by site
    epicardium 37.31
    mastoid 20.92
    pericardium 37.31
    pleura 34.59
    skin 86.3
    thorax 34.4
  secondary membrane, lens 13.65
  seminal vesicle 60.73
    with radical prostatectomy 60.5
  septum — *see also* Excision, by site
    uterus (congenital) 68.22
    vagina 70.33
  sinus — *see also* Excision, lesion, by site
    nasal — *see* Sinusectomy
    pilonidal 86.21
    preauricular (ear) (radical) 18.21
    tarsi 80.88
    thyroglossal (with resection of hyoid bone)
      06.7
    urachal (bladder) 57.51
      abdominal wall 54.3
  Skene's gland 71.3
  skin (local) 86.3
    for graft (with closure of donor site) 86.91
    radical (wide) (involving underlying or
      adjacent structure) (with flap closure)
      86.4
    tags
      perianal 49.03
      periauricular 18.29
  soft tissue NEC 83.49
    hand 82.39
  spermatocele 63.2
  spinous process 77.89
  spleen (total) 41.5
    accessory 41.93
    partial 41.43
  stomach — *see* Gastrectomy
  sublingual gland (salivary) (*see also* Excision,
    salivary gland) 26.30
  submaxillary gland (*see also* Excision, salivary
    gland) 26.30
  supernumerary
    breast 85.24
    digits 86.26
  sweat gland 86.3
  synechiae — *see also* Lysis, synechiae
    endometrial 68.21
  tarsal plate (eyelid) 08.20
    by wedge resection 08.24
  tattoo 86.3
    by dermabrasion 86.25
  tendon (sheath) 83.42
    for graft 83.41
      hand 82.32
    hand 82.33
      for graft 82.32

Excision — *continued*
  thymus (*see also* Thymectomy) 07.80
  thyroglossal duct or tract (with resection of
    hyoid bone) 06.7
  thyroid NEC (*see also* Thyroidectomy) 06.39
  tongue (complete) (total) 25.3
    partial or subtotal 25.2
    radical 25.4
  tonsil 28.2
    with adenoidectomy 28.3
    lingual 28.5
    tag 28.4
  tooth NEC (*see also* Removal, tooth, surgical)
    23.19
    from nasal sinus 22.60
  torus
    lingual 76.2
    mandible, mandibularis 76.2
    palate, palatinus 27.31
      by wide excision 27.32
  trabeculae carneae cordis (heart) 35.35
  trochanteric lipomatosis 86.83
  tumor — *see* Excision, lesion, by site
  ulcer — *see also* Excision, lesion, by site
    duodenum 45.31
      endoscopic 45.30
    stomach 43.42
      endoscopic 43.41
  umbilicus 54.3
  urachus, urachal (cyst) (bladder) 57.51
    abdominal wall 54.3
  ureter, ureteral 56.40
    with nephrectomy — *see* Nephrectomy
    partial 56.41
    stricture 56.41
    total 56.42
  ureterocele 56.41
  urethra, urethral 58.39
    with complete cystectomy 57.79
    endoscopic 58.31
    septum 58.0
    stricture 58.39
      endoscopic 58.31
    valve (congenital) 58.39
      endoscopic (transurethral) (transvesical)
        58.31
  urethrovaginal septum 70.33
  uterus (corpus) (*see also* Hysterectomy) 68.9
    cervix 67.4
      lesion 67.39
    lesion 68.29
    septum 68.22
  uvula 27.72
  vagina (total) 70.4
  varicocele, spermatic cord 63.1
  vein (*see also* Phlebectomy) 38.60
    varicose 38.50
      abdominal 38.57
      head and neck NEC 38.52
      intracranial NEC 38.51
      lower limb 38.59
      ovarian 38.67
      thoracic NEC 38.55
      upper limb 38.53
  verucca — *see also* Excision, lesion, by site
    eyelid 08.22
  vesicovaginal septum 70.33
  vitreous opacity 14.74
    anterior approach 14.73
  vocal cord(s) (submucous) 30.22
  vulva (bilateral) (simple) (*see also* Vulvectomy)
    71.62
  wart — *see also* Excision, lesion, by site
    eyelid 08.22
  wolffian duct 69.19
  xanthoma (tendon sheath, hand) 82.21
    site other than hand 83.31

Excisional biopsy — *see* Biopsy

Exclusion, pyloric 44.39

Exenteration
  ethmoid air cells 22.63
  orbit 16.59
    with
      removal of adjacent structures 16.51
      temporalis muscle transplant 16.59
      therapeutic removal of bone 16.52

Exenteration — *continued*
  pelvic (organs) (female) 68.8
    male 57.71
  petrous pyramid air cells 20.59

Exercise (physical therapy) NEC 93.19
  active musculoskeletal NEC 93.12
  assisting 93.11
    in pool 93.31
  breathing 93.18
  musculoskeletal
    active NEC 93.12
    passive NEC 93.17
  neurologic 89.13
  passive musculoskeletal NEC 93.17
  resistive 93.13

Exfoliation, skin, by chemical 86.24

Exostectomy (*see also* Excision, lesion, bone)
  77.60
  first metatarsal (hallux valgus repair) — *see*
    Bunionectomy
  hallux valgus repair (with wedge osteotomy) —
    see Bunionectomy

Expiratory flow rate 89.38

Exploration — *see also* Incision
  abdomen 54.11
  abdominal wall 54.0
  adrenal (gland) 07.41
    field 07.00
      bilateral 07.02
      unilateral 07.01
  artery 38.00
    abdominal 38.06
    aorta (arch) (ascending) (descending) 38.04
    head and neck NEC 38.02
    intracranial NEC 38.01
    lower limb 38.08
    thoracic NEC 38.05
    upper limb 38.03
  auditory canal, external 18.02
  axilla 86.09
  bile duct(s) 51.59
    common duct 51.51
      endoscopic 51.11
      for
        relief of obstruction 51.42
          endoscopic 51.84
        removal of calculus 51.41
          endoscopic 51.88
      laparoscopic 51.11
    for relief of obstruction 51.49
      endoscopic 51.84
  bladder (by incision) 57.19
    endoscopic 57.32
      through stoma (artificial) 57.31
  bone (*see also* Incision, bone) 77.10
  brain (tissue) 01.39
  breast 85.0
  bronchus 33.0
    endoscopic — *see* Bronchoscopy
  bursa 83.03
    hand 82.03
  carotid body 39.8
  carpal tunnel 04.43
  choroid 14.9
  ciliary body 12.44
  colon 45.03
  common bile duct 51.51
    endoscopic 51.11
    for
      relief of obstruction 51.42
        endoscopic 51.84
      removal of calculus 51.41
        endoscopic 51.88
  coronary artery 36.99
  cranium 01.24
  cul-de-sac 70.12
    endoscopic 70.22
  disc space 03.09
  duodenum 45.01
  endoscopic — *see* Endoscopy, by site
  epididymis 63.92
  esophagus (by incision) NEC 42.09
    endoscopic — *see* Esophagoscopy
  ethmoid sinus 22.51
  eyelid 08.09

Excision — Exploration

✔4ᵗʰ Fourth-digit Required   ▶◀ Revised Text   ● New Line   ▲ Revised Code

Exploration — *see also* Incision — *continued*
  fallopian tube 66.01
  fascia 83.09
    hand 82.09
  flank 54.0
  fossa (superficial) NEC 86.09
    pituitary 07.71
  frontal sinus 22.41
  frontonasal duct 96.21
  gallbladder 51.04
  groin (region) (abdominal wall) (inguinal) 54.0
    skin and subcutaneous tissue 86.09
  heart 37.11
  hepatic duct 51.59
  hypophysis 07.72
  ileum 45.02
  inguinal canal (groin) 54.0
  intestine (by incision) NEC 45.00
    large 45.03
    small 45.02
  intrathoracic 34.02
  jejunum 45.02
  joint structures (*see also* Arthrotomy) 80.10
  kidney 55.01
    pelvis 55.11
  labia 71.09
  lacrimal
    gland 09.0
    sac 09.53
  laparotomy site 54.12
  larynx (by incision) 31.3
    endoscopic 31.42
  liver 50.0
  lung (by incision) 33.1
  lymphatic structure(s) (channel) (node) (vessel) 40.0
  mastoid 20.21
  maxillary antrum or sinus (Caldwell-Luc approach) 22.39
  mediastinum 34.1
    endoscopic 34.22
  middle ear (transtympanic) 20.23
  muscle 83.02
    hand 82.02
  neck (*see also* Exploration, thyroid) 06.09
  nerve (cranial) (peripheral) NEC 04.04
    auditory 04.01
    root (spinal) 03.09
  nose 21.1
  orbit (*see also* Orbitotomy) 16.09
  pancreas 52.09
    endoscopic 52.13
  pancreatic duct 52.09
    endoscopic 52.13
  pelvis (by laparotomy) 54.11
    by colpotomy 70.12
  penis 64.92
  perinephric area 59.09
  perineum (female) 71.09
    male 86.09
  peripheral vessels
    lower limb
      artery 38.08
      vein 38.09
    upper limb (artery) (vein) 38.03
  periprostatic tissue 60.81
  perirenal tissue 59.09
  perivesical tissue 59.19
  petrous pyramid air cells 20.22
  pilonidal sinus 86.03
  pineal (gland) 07.52
    field 07.51
  pituitary (gland) 07.72
    fossa 07.71
  pleura 34.09
  popliteal space 86.09
  prostate 60.0
  rectum (*see also* Proctoscopy) 48.23
    by incision 48.0
  retroperitoneum 54.0
  retropubic 59.19
  salivary gland 26.0
  sclera (by incision) 12.89
  scrotum 61.0

Exploration — *see also* Incision — *continued*
  shunt
    ventriculoperitoneal at ●
      peritoneal site 54.95 ●
      ventricular site 02.41 ●
  sinus
    ethmoid 22.51
    frontal 22.41
    maxillary (Caldwell-Luc approach) 22.39
    sphenoid 22.52
    tract, skin and subcutaneous tissue 86.09
  skin 86.09
  soft tissue NEC 83.09
    hand 82.09
  spermatic cord 63.93
  sphenoidal sinus 22.52
  spinal (canal) (nerve root) 03.09
  spleen 41.2
  stomach (by incision) 43.0
    endoscopic — *see* Gastroscopy
  subcutaneous tissue 86.09
  subdiaphragmatic space 54.11
  superficial fossa 86.09
  tarsal tunnel 04.44
  tendon (sheath) 83.01
    hand 82.01
  testes 62.0
  thymus (gland) 07.92
    field 07.91
  thyroid (field) (gland) (by incision) 06.09
    postoperative 06.02
  trachea (by incision) 31.3
    endoscopic — *see* Tracheoscopy
  tunica vaginalis 61.0
  tympanum 20.09
    transtympanic route 20.23
  ureter (by incision) 56.2
    endoscopic 56.31
  urethra (by incision) 58.0
    endoscopic 58.22
  uterus (corpus) 68.0
    cervix 69.95
    digital 68.11
    postpartal, manual 75.7
  vagina (by incision) 70.14
    endoscopic 70.21
  vas deferens 63.6
  vein 38.00
    abdominal 38.07
    head and neck NEC 38.02
    intracranial NEC 38.01
    lower limb 38.09
    thoracic NEC 38.05
    upper limb 38.03
  vulva (by incision) 71.09

Exposure — *see also* Incision, by site
  tooth (for orthodontic treatment) 24.6

Expression, trachoma follicles 10.33

Exsanguination transfusion 99.01

Extension
  buccolabial sulcus 24.91
  limb, forced 93.25
  lingual sulcus 24.91
  mandibular ridge 76.43

Exteriorization
  esophageal pouch 42.12
  intestine 46.03
    large 46.03
    small 46.01
  maxillary sinus 22.9
  pilonidal cyst or sinus (open excision) (with partial closure) 86.21

Extirpation — *see also* Excision, by site
  aneurysm — *see* Aneurysmectomy
  arteriovenous fistula — *see* Aneurysmectomy
  lacrimal sac 09.6
  larynx 30.3
    with radical neck dissection (with synchronous thyroidectomy)(with synchronous tracheostomy) 30.4
  nerve, tooth (*see also* Therapy, root canal) 23.70
  varicose vein (peripheral) (lower limb) 38.59
    upper limb 38.53

Extracorporeal
  circulation (regional), except hepatic 39.61
    hepatic 50.92
    percutaneous 39.66
  hemodialysis 39.95
  membrane oxygenation (ECMO) 39.65
  photopheresis, therapeutic 99.88
  shockwave lithotripsy (ESWL) NEC 98.59
    bile duct 98.52
    bladder 98.51
    gallbladder 98.52
    kidney 98.51
    renal pelvis 98.51
    specified site NEC 98.59
    ureter 98.51

Extracranial-intracranial bypass [EC-IC] 39.28

Extraction
  breech (partial) 72.52
    with forceps to aftercoming head 72.51
    total 72.54
      with forceps to aftercoming head 72.53
  cataract 13.19
    after cataract (by)
      capsulectomy 13.65
      capsulotomy 13.64
      discission 13.64
      excision 13.65
      iridocapsulectomy 13.65
      mechanical fragmentation 13.66
      needling 13.64
      phacofragmentation (mechanical) 13.66
    aspiration (simple) (with irrigation) 13.3
    cryoextraction (intracapsular approach) 13.19
      temporal inferior route (in presence of fistulization bleb) 13.11
    curette evacuation (extracapsular approach) 13.2
    emulsification (and aspiration) 13.41
    erysiphake (intracapsular approach) 13.19
      temporal inferior route (in presence of fistulization bleb) 13.11
    extracapsular approach (with iridectomy) NEC 13.59
      by temporal inferior route (in presence of fistulization bleb) 13.51
      aspiration (simple) (with irrigation) 13.3
      curette evacuation 13.2
      emulsification (and aspiration) 13.41
      linear extraction 13.2
      mechanical fragmentation with aspiration by
        posterior route 13.42
        specified route NEC 13.43
      phacoemulsification (ultrasonic) (with aspiration) 13.41
      phacofragmentation (mechanical)
        with aspiration by
          posterior route 13.42
          specified route NEC 13.43
        ultrasonic (with aspiration) 13.41
      rotoextraction (mechanical) with aspiration by
        posterior route 13.42
        specified route NEC 13.43
    intracapsular (combined) (simple) (with iridectomy) (with suction) (with zonulolysis) 13.19
      by temporal inferior route (in presence of fistulization bleb) 13.11
    linear extraction (extracapsular approach) 13.2
    phacoemulsification (and aspiration) 13.41
    phacofragmentation (mechanical)
      with aspiration by
        posterior route 13.42
        specified route NEC 13.43
      ultrasonic 13.41
    rotoextraction (mechanical)
      with aspiration by
        posterior route 13.42
        specified route NEC 13.43
    secondary membranous (after cataract) (by)
      capsulectomy 13.65
      capsulotomy 13.64

Extraction — *continued*
  cataract — *continued*
    secondary membranous — *continued*
      discission 13.64
      excision 13.65
      iridocapsulectomy 13.65
      mechanical fragmentation 13.66
      needling 13.64
      phacofragmentation (mechanical) 13.66
  common duct stones (percutaneous) (through sinus tract) (with basket) 51.96
  foreign body — *see* Removal, foreign body
  kidney stone(s), percutaneous 55.03
    with fragmentation procedure 55.04
  lens (eye) (*see also* Extraction, cataract) 13.19
  Malström's 72.79
    with episiotomy 72.71
  menstrual, menses 69.6
  milk from lactating breast (manual) (pump) 99.98
  tooth (by forceps) (multiple) (single) NEC 23.09
    with mucoperiosteal flap elevation 23.19
    deciduous 23.01
    surgical NEC (*see also* Removal, tooth, surgical) 23.19
  vacuum, fetus 72.79
    with episiotomy 72.71
  vitreous (*see also* Removal, vitreous) 14.72

F

Face lift 86.82
Facetectomy 77.89
Facilitation, intraocular circulation NEC 12.59
Failed (trial) forceps 73.3
Family
  counselling (medical) (social) 94.49
  therapy 94.42
Farabeuf operation (ischiopubiotomy) 77.39
Fasanella-Servatt operation (blepharoptosis repair) 08.35
Fasciaplasty — *see* Fascioplasty
Fascia sling operation — *see* Operation, sling
Fasciectomy 83.44
  for graft 83.43
    hand 82.34
  hand 82.35
    for graft 82.34
  palmar (release of Dupuytren's contracture) 82.35
Fasciodesis 83.89
  hand 82.89
Fascioplasty (*see also* Repair, fascia) 83.89
  hand (*see also* Repair, fascia, hand) 82.89
Fasciorrhaphy — *see* Suture, fascia
Fasciotomy 83.14
  Dupuytren's 82.12
    with excision 82.35
  Dwyer 83.14
  hand 82.12
  Ober-Yount 83.14
  orbital (*see also* Orbitotomy) 16.09
  palmar (release of Dupuytren's contracture) 82.12
    with excision 82.35
Fenestration
  aneurysm (dissecting), thoracic aorta 39.54
  aortic aneurysm 39.54
  cardiac valve 35.10
  chest wall 34.01
  ear
    inner (with graft) 20.61
      revision 20.62
    tympanic 19.55
  labyrinth (with graft) 20.61
  Lempert's (endaural) 19.9
  operation (aorta) 39.54
  oval window, ear canal 19.55
  palate 27.1
  pericardium 37.12
  semicircular canals (with graft) 20.61

Fenestration — *continued*
  stapes foot plate (with vein graft) 19.19
    with incus replacement 19.11
  tympanic membrane 19.55
  vestibule (with graft) 20.61
Ferguson operation (hernia repair) 53.00
Fetography 87.81
Fetoscopy 75.31
Fiberoscopy — *see* Endoscopy, by site
Fibroidectomy, uterine 68.29
Fick operation (perforation of foot plate) 19.0
Filipuncture (aneurysm) (cerebral) 39.52
Filleting
  hammer toe 77.56
  pancreas 52.3
Filling, tooth (amalgam) (plastic) (silicate) 23.2
  root canal (*see also* therapy, root canal) 23.70
Fimbriectomy (*see also* Salpingectomy, partial) 66.69
  Uchida (with tubal ligation) 66.32
Finney operation (pyloroplasty) 44.29
Fissurectomy, anal 49.39
  endoscopic 49.31
  skin (subcutaneous tissue) 49.04
Fistulectomy — *see also* Closure, fistula, by site
  abdominothoracic 34.83
  abdominouterine 69.42
  anus 49.12
  appendix 47.92
  bile duct 51.79
  biliary tract NEC 51.79
  bladder (transurethral approach) 57.84
  bone (*see also* Excision, lesion, bone) 77.60
  branchial cleft 29.52
  bronchocutaneous 33.42
  bronchoesophageal 33.42
  bronchomediastinal 34.73
  bronchopleural 34.73
  bronchopleurocutaneous 34.73
  bronchopleuromediastinal 34.73
  bronchovisceral 33.42
  cervicosigmoidal 67.62
  cholecystogastroenteric 51.93
  cornea 11.49
  diaphragm 34.83
  enterouterine 69.42
  esophagopleurocutaneous 34.73
  esophagus NEC 42.84
  fallopian tube 66.73
  gallbladder 51.93
  gastric NEC 44.63
  hepatic duct 51.79
  hepatopleural 34.73
  hepatopulmonary 34.73
  intestine
    large 46.76
    small 46.74
  intestinouterine 69.42
  joint (*see also* Excision, lesion, joint) 80.80
  lacrimal
    gland 09.21
    sac 09.6
  laryngotracheal 31.62
  larynx 31.62
  mediastinocutaneous 34.73
  mouth NEC 27.53
  nasal 21.82
    sinus 22.71
  nasolabial 21.82
  nasopharyngeal 21.82
  oroantral 22.71
  oronasal 21.82
  pancreas 52.95
  perineorectal 71.72
  perineosigmoidal 71.72
  perirectal, not opening into rectum 48.93
  pharyngoesophageal 29.53
  pharynx NEC 29.53
  pleura 34.73
  rectolabial 71.72
  rectourethral 58.43
  rectouterine 69.42
  rectovaginal 70.73

Fistulectomy — *see also* Closure, fistula, by site — *continued*
  rectovesical 57.83
  rectovulvar 71.72
  rectum 48.73
  salivary (duct) (gland) 26.42
  scrotum 61.42
  skin 86.3
  stomach NEC 44.63
  subcutaneous tissue 86.3
  thoracoabdominal 34.83
  thoracogastric 34.83
  thoracointestinal 34.83
  thorax NEC 34.73
  trachea NEC 31.73
  tracheoesophageal 31.73
  ureter 56.84
  urethra 58.43
  uteroenteric 69.42
  uterointestinal 69.42
  uterorectal 69.42
  uterovaginal 69.42
  vagina 70.75
  vesicosigmoidovaginal 57.83
  vocal cords 31.62
  vulvorectal 71.72
Fistulization
  appendix 47.91
  arteriovenous 39.27
  cisterna chyli 40.62
  endolymphatic sac (for decompression) 20.79
  esophagus, external 42.10
    cervical 42.11
    specified technique NEC 42.19
  interatrial 35.41
  labyrinth (for decompression) 20.79
  lacrimal sac into nasal cavity 09.81
  larynx 31.29
  lymphatic duct, left (thoracic) 40.62
  orbit 16.09
  peritoneal 54.93
  salivary gland 26.49
  sclera 12.69
    by trephination 12.61
    with iridectomy 12.65
  sinus, nasal NEC 22.9
  subarachnoid space 02.2
  thoracic duct 40.62
  trachea 31.29
  tracheoesophageal 31.95
  urethrovaginal 58.0
  ventricle, cerebral (*see also* Shunt, ventricular) 02.2
Fistulogram
  abdominal wall 88.03
  chest wall 87.38
  retroperitoneum 88.14
Fistulotomy, anal 49.11
Fitting
  arch bars (orthodontic) 24.7
    for immobilization (fracture) 93.55
  artificial limb 84.40
  contact lens 95.32
  denture (total) 99.97
    bridge (fixed) 23.42
      removable 23.43
    partial (fixed) 23.42
      removable 23.43
  hearing aid 95.48
  obturator (orthodontic) 24.7
  ocular prosthetics 95.34
  orthodontic
    appliance 24.7
    obturator 24.7
    wiring 24.7
  orthotic device 93.23
  periodontal splint (orthodontic) 24.7
  prosthesis, prosthetic device
    above knee 84.45
    arm 84.43
      lower (and hand) 84.42
      upper (and shoulder) 84.41
    below knee 84.46
    hand (and lower arm) 84.42

Extraction — Fitting (side tab)

✓4ᵗʰ Fourth-digit Required   ▶◀ Revised Text   ● New Line   ▲ Revised Code

Fitting — *continued*
  prosthesis, prosthetic device — *continued*
    leg 84.47
      above knee 84.45
      below knee 84.46
    limb NEC 84.40
    ocular 95.34
    penis (external) 64.94
    shoulder (and upper arm) 84.41
  spectacles 95.31
Five-in-one repair, knee 81.42
Fixation
  bone
    external, without reduction 93.59
      with fracture reduction — *see* Reduction, fracture
      cast immobilization NEC 93.53
      splint 93.54
      traction (skeletal) NEC 93.44
        intermittent 93.43
    internal (without fracture reduction) 78.50
      with fracture-reduction — *see* Reduction, fracture
      carpal, metacarpal 78.54
      clavicle 78.51
      femur 78.55
      fibula 78.57
      humerus 78.52
      patella 78.56
      pelvic 78.59
      phalanges (foot) (hand) 78.59
      radius 78.53
      scapula 78.51
      specified site NEC 78.59
      tarsal, metatarsal 78.58
      thorax (ribs) (sternum) 78.51
      tibia 78.57
      ulna 78.53
      vertebrae 78.59
  breast (pendulous) 85.6
  cardinal ligaments 69.22
  duodenum 46.62
    to abdominal wall 46.61
  external (without manipulation for reduction) 93.59
    with fracture-reduction — *see* Reduction, fracture
    cast immobilization NEC 93.53
    pressure dressing 93.56
    splint 93.54
    traction (skeletal) NEC 93.44
      intermittent 93.43
  hip 81.40
  ileum 46.62
    to abdominal wall 46.61
  internal
    with fracture-reduction — *see* Reduction, fracture
    without fracture-reduction — *see* Fixation, bone, internal
  intestine 46.60
    large 46.64
      to abdominal wall 46.63
    small 46.62
      to abdominal wall 46.61
      to abdominal wall 46.60
  iris (bombé) 12.11
  jejunum 46.62
    to abdominal wall 46.61
  joint — *see* Arthroplasty
  kidney 55.7
  ligament
    cardinal 69.22
    palpebrae 08.36
  omentum 54.74
  parametrial 69.22
  rectum (sling) 48.76
  spine, with fusion (*see also* Fusion, spinal) 81.00
  spleen 41.95
  tendon 83.88
    hand 82.85
  testis in scrotum 62.5
  tongue 25.59
  urethrovaginal (to Cooper's ligament) 70.77

Fixation — *continued*
  uterus (abdominal) (vaginal) (ventrofixation) 69.22
  vagina 70.77
Flooding (psychologic desensitization) 94.33
Flowmetry, Doppler (ultrasonic) — *see also* Ultrasonography
  aortic arch 88.73
  head and neck 88.71
  heart 88.72
  thorax NEC 88.73
Fluoroscopy — *see* Radiography
Fog therapy (respiratory) 93.94
Folding, eye muscle 15.22
  multiple (two or more muscles) 15.4
Foley operation (pyeloplasty) 55.87
Fontan operation (creation of conduit between right atrium and pulmonary artery) 35.94
Foraminotomy 03.09
Forced extension, limb 93.25
Forceps delivery — *see* Delivery, forceps
Formation
  adhesions
    pericardium 36.39
    pleura 34.6
  anus, artificial (*see also* Colostomy) 46.13
    duodenostomy 46.39
    ileostomy (*see also* Ileostomy) 46.23
    jejunostomy 46.39
      percutaneous (endoscopic) (PEJ) 46.32
  arteriovenous fistula (for kidney dialysis) (peripheral) (shunt) 39.27
    external cannula 39.93
  bone flap, cranial 02.03
  cardiac pacemaker pocket
    with initial insertion of pacemaker — *omit code*
    new site (skin) (subcutaneous) 37.79
  colostomy (*see also* Colostomy) 46.13
  conduit
    ileal (urinary) 56.51
    left ventricle and aorta 35.93
    right atrium and pulmonary artery 35.94
    right ventricle and pulmonary (distal) artery 35.92
      in repair of
        pulmonary artery atresia 35.92
        transposition of great vessels 35.92
        truncus arteriosus 35.83
  endorectal ileal pouch (J-pouch) (H-pouch) (S-pouch) (with anastomosis to anus) 45.95
  fistula
    arteriovenous (for kidney dialysis) (peripheral shunt) 39.27
      external cannula 39.93
    bladder to skin NEC 57.18
      with bladder flap 57.21
      percutaneous 57.17
    cutaneoperitoneal 54.93
    gastric 43.19
      percutaneous (endoscopic) (transabdominal) 43.11
    mucous (*see also* Colostomy) 46.13
    rectovaginal 48.99
    tracheoesophageal 31.95
    tubulovalvular (Beck-Jianu) (Frank's) (Janeway) (Spivack's) (Ssabanejew-Frank) 43.19
    urethrovaginal 58.0
  ileal
    bladder
      closed 57.87 [45.51]
      open 56.51
    conduit 56.51
  interatrial fistula 35.42
  mucous fistula (*see also* Colostomy) 46.13
  pericardial
    baffle, interatrial 35.91
    window 37.12
  pleural window (for drainage) 34.09
  pocket
    cardiac pacemaker
      with initial insertion of pacemaker — *omit code*

Formation — *continued*
  pocket — *continued*
    cardiac pacemaker — *continued*
      new site (skin) (subcutaneous) 37.79
    thalamic stimulator pulse generator
      with initial insertion of battery package — *omit code*
      new site (skin) (subcutaneous) 86.09
  pupil 12.39
    by iridectomy 12.14
  rectovaginal fistula 48.99
  reversed gastric tube (intrathoracic) (retrosternal) 42.58
    antesternal or antethoracic 42.68
  septal defect, interatrial 35.42
  shunt
    abdominovenous 54.94
    arteriovenous 39.93
    peritoneojugular 54.94
    peritoneo-vascular 54.94
    pleuroperitoneal 34.05
    transjugular intrahepatic portosystemic [TIPS] 39.1
  subcutaneous tunnel
    esophageal 42.86
      with anastomosis — *see* Anastomosis, esophagus, antesternal
    pulse generator lead wire 86.99
      with initial procedure — *omit code*
    thalamic stimulator pulse generator pocket
      with initial insertion of battery package — *omit code*
      new site (skin) (subcutaneous) 86.09
  syndactyly (finger) (toe) 86.89
  tracheoesophageal 31.95
  tubulovalvular fistula (Beck-Jianu) (Frank's) (Janeway) (Spivack's) (Ssabanejew-Frank) 43.19
  uretero-ileostomy, cutaneous 56.51
  ureterostomy, cutaneous 56.61
    ileal 56.51
  urethrovaginal fistula 58.0
  window
    pericardial 37.12
    pleural (for drainage) 34.09
Fothergill (-Donald) operation (uterine suspension) 69.22
Fowler operation
  arthroplasty of metacarpophalangeal joint 81.72
  release (mallet finger repair) 82.84
  tenodesis (hand) 82.85
  thoracoplasty 33.34
Fox operation (entropion repair with wedge resection) 08.43
Fracture, surgical (*see also* Osteoclasis) 78.70
  turbinates (nasal) 21.62
Fragmentation
  lithotriptor — *see* Lithotripsy
  mechanical
    cataract (with aspiration) 13.43
      posterior route 13.42
      secondary membrane 13.66
    secondary membrane (after cataract) 13.66
  ultrasonic
    cataract (with aspiration) 13.41
    stones, urinary (Kock pouch) 59.95
    urinary stones 59.95
      percutaneous nephrostomy 55.04
Franco operation (suprapubic cystotomy) 57.18
Frank operation 43.19
Frazier (-Spiller) operation (subtemporal trigeminal rhizotomy) 04.02
Fredet-Ramstedt operation (pyloromyotomy) (with wedge resection) 43.3
Freeing
  adhesions — *see* Lysis, adhesions
  anterior synechiae (with injection of air or liquid) 12.32
  artery-vein-nerve bundle 39.91
  extraocular muscle, entrapped 15.7
  goniosynechiae (with injection of air or liquid) 12.31

G

Freeing — Gastroduodenoscopy

✓4ᵗʰ Fourth-digit Required　　▶◀ Revised Text　　● New Line　　▲ Revised Code

Gastroduodenostomy (bypass) (Jaboulay's) 44.39
  with partial gastrectomy 43.6
Gastroenterostomy (bypass) NEC 44.39
  with partial gastrectomy 43.7
Gastrogastrostomy (bypass) 44.39
  with partial gastrectomy 43.89
Gastrojejunostomy (bypass) 44.39
  with partial gastrectomy 43.7
  percutaneous (endoscopic) 44.32
Gastrolysis 54.59
  laparoscopic 54.51
Gastropexy 44.64
Gastroplasty NEC 44.69
Gastroplication 44.69
Gastropylorectomy 43.6
Gastrorrhaphy 44.61
Gastroscopy NEC 44.13
  through stoma (artificial) 44.12
  transabdominal (operative) 44.11
Gastrostomy (Brunschwig's) (decompression) (fine
  caliber tube) (Kader) (permanent) (Stamm)
  (Stamm-Kader) (temporary) (tube) (Witzel)
  43.19
  Beck-Jianu 43.19
  Frank's 43.19
  Janeway 43.19
  percutaneous (endoscopic) (PEG) 43.11
  Spivack's 43.19
  Ssabanejew-Frank 43.19
Gastrotomy 43.0
  for control of hemorrhage 44.49
Gavage, gastric 96.35
Gelman operation (release of clubfoot) 83.84
Genioplasty (augmentation) (with graft) (with
  implant) 76.68
  reduction 76.67
Ghormley operation (hip fusion) 81.21
Gifford operation
  destruction of lacrimal sac 09.6
  keratotomy (delimiting) 11.1
    radial (refractive) 11.75
Gill operation
  arthrodesis of shoulder 81.23
  laminectomy 03.09
Gill-Stein operation (carporadial arthrodesis)
  81.25
Gilliam operation (uterine suspension) 69.22
Gingivectomy 24.31
Gingivoplasty (with bone graft) (with soft tissue
  graft) 24.2
Girdlestone operation
  laminectomy with spinal fusion 81.00
  muscle transfer for claw toe repair 77.57
  resection of femoral head and neck 77.85
Girdlestone-Taylor operation (muscle transfer
  for claw toe repair) 77.57
Glenn operation (anastomosis of superior vena
  cava to right pulmonary artery) 39.21
Glenoplasty, shoulder 81.83
  with
    partial replacement 81.81
    total replacement 81.80
  for recurrent dislocation 81.82
Glomectomy
  carotid 39.8
  jugulare 20.51
Glossectomy (complete) (total) 25.3
  partial or subtotal 25.2
  radical 25.4
Glossopexy 25.59
Glossoplasty NEC 25.59
Glossorrhaphy 25.51
Glossotomy NEC 25.94
  for tongue tie 25.91
Glycoprotein IIB/IIIa inhibitor 99.20
Goebel-Frangenheim-Stoeckel operation
  (urethrovesical suspenion) 59.4
Goldner operation (clubfoot release) 80.48

Goldthwaite operation
  ankle stabilization 81.11
  patellar stabilization 81.44
  tendon transfer for stabilization of patella 81.44
Gonadectomy
  ovary
    bilateral 65.51
      laparoscopic 65.53
    unilateral 65.39
      laparoscopic 65.31
  testis 62.3
Goniopuncture 12.51
  with goniotomy 12.53
Gonioscopy 12.29
Goniospasis 12.59
Goniotomy (Barkan's) 12.52
  with goniopuncture 12.53
Goodal-Power operation (vagina) 70.8
Gordon-Taylor operation (hindquarter
  amputation) 84.19
GP IIb/IIIa inhibitor, infusion 99.20
Graber-Duvernay operation (drilling of femoral
  head) 77.15
Graft, grafting
  aneurysm 39.52
    endovascular
      abdominal aorta 39.71
      lower extremity artery(s) 39.79
      thoracic aorta 39.79
      upper extremity artery(s) 39.79
  artery, arterial (patch) 39.58
    with
      excision or resection of vessel — *see*
        Arteriectomy, with graft
        replacement
      synthetic patch (Dacron) (Teflon) 39.57
      tissue patch (vein) (autogenous)
        (homograft) 39.56
  blood vessel (patch) 39.58
    with
      excision or resection of vessel — *see*
        Angiectomy, with graft replacement
      synthetic patch (Dacron) (Teflon) 39.57
      tissue patch (vein) (autogenous)
        (homograft) 39.56
  bone (autogenous) (bone bank) (dual onlay)
    (heterogenous) (inlay) (massive onlay)
    (multiple) (osteoperiosteal) (peg)
    (subperiosteal) (with metallic fixation)
    78.00
    with
      arthrodesis — *see* Arthrodesis
      arthroplasty — *see* Arthroplasty
      gingivoplasty 24.2
      lengthening — *see* Lengthening, bone
    carpals, metacarpals 78.04
    clavicle 78.01
    facial NEC 76.91
      with total ostectomy 76.44
    femur 78.05
    fibula 78.07
    humerus 78.02
    joint — *see* Arthroplasty
    mandible 76.91
      with total mandibulectomy 76.41
    marrow — *see* Transplant, bone, marrow
    nose — *see* Graft, nose
    patella 78.06
    pelvic 78.09
    pericranial 02.04
    phalanges (foot) (hand) 78.09
    radius 78.03
    scapula 78.01
    skull 02.04
    specified site NEC 78.09
    spine 78.09
      with fusion — *see* Fusion, spinal
    tarsal, metatarsal 78.08
    thorax (ribs) (sternum) 78.01
    thumb (with transfer of skin flap) 82.69
    tibia 78.07
    ulna 78.03
    vertebrae 78.09
      with fusion — *see* Fusion, spinal

Graft, grafting — *continued*
  breast (*see also* Mammoplasty) 85.89
  buccal sulcus 27.99
  cartilage (joint) — *see also* Arthroplasty
    nose — *see* Graft, nose
  chest wall (mesh) (silastic) 34.79
  conjunctiva (free) (mucosa) 10.44
    for symblepharon repair 10.41
  cornea (*see also* Keratoplasty) 11.60
  dermal-fat 86.69
  dermal regenerative 86.67
  dura 02.12
  ear
    auricle 18.79
    external auditory meatus 18.6
      inner 20.61
      pedicle preparation 86.71
  esophagus NEC 42.87
    with interposition (intrathoracic) NEC 42.58
      antesternal or antethoracic NEC 42.68
      colon (intrathoracic) 42.55
        antesternal or antethoracic 42.65
      small bowel (intrathoracic) 42.53
        antesternal or antethoracic 42.63
  eyebrow (*see also* Reconstruction, eyelid, with
    graft) 08.69
  eyelid (*see also* Reconstruction, eyelid, with
    graft) 08.69
    free mucous membrane 08.62
  eye socket (skin) (cartilage) (bone) 16.63
  fallopian tube 66.79
  fascia 83.82
    with hernia repair — *see* Repair, hernia
    eyelid 08.32
    hand 82.72
    tarsal cartilage 08.69
  fat pad NEC 86.89
    with skin graft — *see* Graft, skin, full-
      thickness
  flap (advanced) (rotating) (sliding) — *see also*
    Graft, skin, pedicle
    tarsoconjunctival 08.64
  hair-bearing skin 86.64
  hand
    fascia 82.72
    free skin 86.62
    muscle 82.72
    pedicle (flap) 86.73
    tendon 82.79
  heart, for revascularization — *see* category
    36.3 ✔4ᵗʰ
  joint — *see* Arthroplasty
  larynx 31.69
  lip 27.56
    full-thickness 27.55
  lymphatic structure(s) (channel) (node) (vessel)
    40.9
  mediastinal fat to myocardium 36.39
  meninges (cerebral) 02.12
  mouth, except palate 27.56
    full-thickness 27.55
  muscle 83.82
    hand 82.72
  myocardium, for revascularization 36.39
  nasolabial flaps 21.86
  nerve (cranial) (peripheral) 04.5
  nipple 85.86
  nose 21.89
    with
      augmentation 21.85
      rhinoplasty — *see* Rhinoplasty
      total reconstruction 21.83
    septum 21.88
    tip 21.86
  omentum 54.74
    to myocardium 36.39
  orbit (bone) (cartilage) (skin) 16.63
  outflow tract (patch) (pulmonary valve) 35.26
    in total repair of tetralogy of Fallot 35.81
  ovary 65.92
  palate 27.69
    for cleft palate repair 27.62
  pedicle — *see* Graft, skin, pedicle
  penis (rib) (skin) 64.49
  pigskin 86.65
  pinch — *see* Graft, skin, free

Graft, grafting — *continued*
pocket — *see* Graft, skin, pedicle
porcine 86.65
postauricular (Wolff) 18.79
razor — *see* Graft, skin, free
rope — *see* Graft, skin, pedicle
saphenous vein in aortocoronary bypass — *see*
    Bypass, aortocoronary
scrotum 61.49
skin (partial-thickness) (split-thickness) 86.69
    amnionic membrane 86.66
    auditory meatus (ear) 18.6
    dermal-fat 86.69
        for breast augmentation 85.50
    dermal regenerative 86.67
    ear
        auditory meatus 18.6
        postauricular 18.79
    eyelid 08.61
    flap — *see* Graft, skin, pedicle
    free (autogenous) NEC 86.60
        lip 27.56
        thumb 86.62
            for
                pollicization 82.61
                reconstruction 82.69
    full-thickness 86.63
        breast 85.83
        hand 86.61
    hair-bearing 86.64
        eyelid or eyebrow 08.63
    hand 86.62
        full-thickness 86.61
    heterograft 86.65
    homograft 86.66
    island flap 86.70
    mucous membrane 86.69
        eyelid 08.62
    nose — *see* Graft, nose
    pedicle (flap) (tube) 86.70
        advancement 86.72
        attachment to site (advanced) (double)
            (rotating) (sliding) 86.74
            hand (cross finger) (pocket) 86.73
            lip 27.57
            mouth 27.57
            thumb 86.73
                for
                    pollicization 82.61
                    reconstruction NEC 82.69
        breast 85.84
            transverse rectus abdominis
                musculocutaneous (TRAM) 85.7
        defatting 86.75
        delayed 86.71
        design and raising 86.71
        elevation 86.71
        preparation of (cutting) 86.71
        revision 86.75
        sculpturing 86.71
        transection 86.71
        transfer 86.74
        trimming 86.71
    postauricular 18.79
    rotation flap 86.70
    specified site NEC 86.69
        full-thickness 86.63
    tarsal cartilage 08.69
    temporalis muscle to orbit 16.63
        with exenteration of orbit 16.59
    tendon 83.81
        for joint repair — *see* Arthroplasty
        hand 82.79
    testicle 62.69
    thumb (for reconstruction) NEC 82.69
    tongue (mucosal) (skin) 25.59
    trachea 31.79
    tubular (tube) — *see* Graft, skin, pedicle
    tunnel — *see* Graft, skin, pedicle
    tympanum (*see also* Tympanoplasty) 19.4
    ureter 56.89

Graft, grafting — *continued*
vein (patch) 39.58
    with
        excision or resection of vessel — *see*
            Phlebectomy, with graft
            replacement
        synthetic patch (Dacron) (Teflon) 39.57
        tissue patch (vein) (autogenous)
            (homograft) 39.56
    vermillion border (lip) 27.56
Grattage, conjunctiva 10.31
Green operation (scapulopexy) 78.41
Grice operation (subtalar arthrodesis) 81.13
Grip, strength 93.04
Gritti-Stokes operation (knee disarticulation)
    84.16
Gross operation (herniorrhaphy) 53.49
Group therapy 94.44
Guttering, bone (*see also* Excision, lesion, bone)
    77.60
Guyon operation (amputation of ankle) 84.13

H

Hagner operation (epididymotomy) 63.92
Halsted operation — *see* Repair, hernia, inguinal
Hampton operation (anastomosis small intestine
    to rectal stump) 45.92
Hanging hip operation (muscle release) 83.19
Harelip operation 27.54
Harrison-Richardson operation (vaginal
    suspension) 70.77
Hartmann resection (of intestine)(with pouch) —
    see Colectomy, by site
Harvesting
    bone marrow 41.91
    stem cells 99.79
Hauser operation
    achillotenotomy 83.11
    bunionectomy with adductor tendon transfer
        77.53
    stabilization of patella 81.44
Heaney operation (vaginal hysterectomy) 68.59
    laparoscopically assisted (LAVH) 68.51
Hearing aid (with battery replacement) 95.49
Hearing test 95.47
Hegar operation (perineorrhaphy) 71.79
Heine operation (cyclodialysis) 12.55
Heineke-Mikulicz operation (pyloroplasty) 44.29
Heller operation (esophagomyotomy) 42.7
Hellström operation (transplantation of aberrant
    renal vessel) 39.55
Hemicolectomy
    left 45.75
    right (extended) 45.73
Hemicystectomy 57.6
Hemigastrectomy — *see* Gastrectomy
Hemiglossectomy 25.2
Hemilaminectomy (decompression) (exploration)
    03.09
Hemilaryngectomy (anterior) (lateral) (vertical)
    30.1
Hemimandibulectomy 76.31
Hemimastectomy (radical) 85.23
Hemimaxillectomy (with bone graft) (with
    prosthesis) 76.39
Heminephrectomy 55.4
Hemipelvectomy 84.19
Hemispherectomy (cerebral) 01.52
Hemithyroidectomy (with removal of isthmus)
    (with removal of portion of remaining lobe)
    06.2
Hemodiafiltration (extracorporeal) 39.95
Hemodialysis (extracorporeal) 39.95
Hemodilution 99.03
Hemofiltration (extracorporeal) 39.95

Hemorrhage control — *see* Control, hemorrhage
Hemorrhoidectomy 49.46
    by
        cautery, cauterization 49.43
        crushing 49.45
        cryotherapy, cryosurgery 49.44
        excision 49.46
        injection 49.42
        ligation 49.45
Hemostasis — *see* Control, hemorrhage
Henley operation (jejunal transposition) 43.81
Hepatectomy (complete) (total) 50.4
    partial or subtotal 50.22
Hepatic assistance, extracorporeal 50.92
Hepatocholangiojejunostomy 51.37
Hepaticocystoduodenostomy 51.37
Hepaticodochotomy 51.59
Hepaticoduodenostomy 51.37
Hepaticojejunostomy 51.37
Hepaticolithectomy 51.49
    endoscopic 51.88
Hepaticolithotomy 51.49
    endoscopic 51.88
Hepaticostomy 51.59
Hepaticotomy 51.59
Hepatocholangiocystoduodenostomy 51.37
Hepatocholedochostomy 51.43
    endoscopic 51.87
Hepatoduodenostomy 50.69
Hepatogastrostomy 50.69
Hepatojejunostomy 50.69
Hepatolithotomy
    hepatic duct 51.49
    liver 50.0
Hepatopexy 50.69
Hepatorrhaphy 50.61
Hepatostomy (external) (internal) 50.69
Hepatotomy (with packing) 50.0
Hernioplasty — *see* Repair, hernia
Herniorrhaphy — *see* Repair, hernia
Herniotomy — *see* Repair, hernia
Heterograft — *see* Graft
Heterotransplant, heterotransplan-tation — *see*
    Transplant
Hey operation (amputation of foot) 84.12
Hey-Groves operation (reconstruction of anterior
    cruciate ligament) 81.45
Heymen operation (soft tissue release for
    clubfoot) 83.84
Heyman-Herndon (-Strong) **operation** (correction
    of metatarsus varus) 80.48
Hibbs operation (lumbar spinal fusion) — *see*
    Fusion, lumbar
Higgins operation — *see* Repair, hernia, femoral
High forceps delivery 72.39
    with episiotomy 72.31
Hill-Allison operation (hiatal hernia repair,
    transpleural approach) 53.80
Hinging, mitral valve 35.12
His bundle recording 37.29
Hitchcock operation (anchoring tendon of biceps)
    83.88
Hofmeister operation (gastrectomy) 43.7
Hoke operation
    midtarsal fusion 81.14
    triple arthrodesis 81.12
Holth operation
    iridencleisis 12.63
    sclerectomy 12.65
Homan operation (correction of lymphedema)
    40.9
Homograft — *see* Graft
Homotransplant, homotransplantation — *see*
    Transplant
Hosiery, elastic 93.59
Hutch operation (ureteroneo-cystostomy) 56.74

Hybinette-Eden operation (glenoid bone block) 78.01

Hydrocelectomy
canal of Nuck (female) 69.19
male 63.1
round ligament 69.19
spermatic cord 63.1
tunica vaginalis 61.2

Hydrotherapy 93.33
assisted exercise in pool 93.31
whirlpool 93.32

Hymenectomy 70.31

Hymenoplasty 70.76

Hymenorrhaphy 70.76

Hymenotomy 70.11

Hyperalimentation (parenteral) 99.15

Hyperbaric oxygenation 93.95
wound 93.59

Hyperextension, joint 93.25

Hyperthermia NEC 93.35
for cancer treatment (interstitial) (local)
(radiofrequency) (regional) (ultrasound)
(whole-body) 99.85

Hypnodrama, psychiatric 94.32

Hypnosis (psychotherapeutic) 94.32
for anesthesia — omit code

Hypnotherapy 94.32

Hypophysectomy (complete) (total) 07.69
partial or subtotal 07.63
transfrontal approach 07.61
transsphenoidal approach 07.62
specified approach NEC 07.68
transfrontal approach (complete) (total) 07.64
partial 07.61
transsphenoidal approach (complete) (total)
07.65
partial 07.62

Hypothermia (central) (local) 99.81
gastric (cooling) 96.31
freezing 96.32
systemic (in open heart surgery) 39.62

Hypotympanotomy 20.23

Hysterectomy 68.9
abdominal 68.4
partial or subtotal (supracervical)
(supravaginal) 68.3
radical (modified) (Wertheim's) 68.6
vaginal (complete) (partial) (subtotal) (total)
68.59
laparoscopically assisted (LAVH) 68.51
radical (Schauta) 68.7

Hysterocolpectomy (radical) (vaginal) 68.7
abdominal 68.6

Hysterogram NEC 87.85
percutaneous 87.84

Hysterolysis 54.59
laparoscopic 54.51

Hysteromyomectomy 68.29

Hysteropexy 69.22

Hysteroplasty 69.49

Hysterorrhaphy 69.41

Hysterosalpingography gas (contrast) 87.82
opaque dye (contrast) 87.83

Hysterosalpingostomy 66.74

Hysteroscopy 68.12
with
ablation
endometrial 68.23
biopsy 68.16

Hysterotomy (with removal of foreign body) (with
removal of hydatidiform mole) 68.0
for intrauterine transfusion 75.2
obstetrical 74.99
for termination of pregnancy 74.91

Hysterotrachelectomy 67.4

Hysterotracheloplasty 69.49

Hysterotrachelorrhaphy 69.41

Hysterotrachelotomy 69.95

I

ICCE (intracapsular cataract extraction) 13.19

Ileal
bladder
closed 57.87 [45.51]
open (ileoureterostomy) 56.51
conduit (ileoureterostomy) 56.51

Ileocecostomy 45.93

Ileocolectomy 45.73

Ileocolostomy 45.93

Ileocolotomy 45.00

Ileocystoplasty (isolated segment anastomosis)
(open loop) 57.87 [45.51]

Ileoduodenotomy 45.01

Ileoectomy (partial) 45.62
with cecectomy 45.72

Ileoentectropy 46.99

Ileoesophagostomy 42.54

Ileoileostomy 45.91
proximal to distal segment 45.62

Ileoloopogram 87.78

Ileopancreatostomy 52.96

Ileopexy 46.61

Ileoproctostomy 45.93

Ileorectostomy 45.93

Ileorrhaphy 46.73

Ileoscopy 45.13
through stoma (artificial) 45.12
transabdominal (operative) 45.11

Ileosigmoidostomy 45.93

Ileostomy 46.20
continent (permanent) 46.22
for urinary diversion 56.51
delayed opening 46.24
Hendon (temporary) 46.21
loop 46.01
Paul (temporary) 46.21
permanent 46.23
continent 46.22
repair 46.41
revision 46.41
tangential (temporary) 46.21
temporary 46.21
transplantation to new site 46.23
tube (temporary) 46.21
ureteral
external 56.51
internal 56.71

Ileotomy 45.02

Ileotransversostomy 45.93

Ileoureterostomy (Bricker's) (ileal bladder) 56.51

Imaging (diagnostic)
diagnostic, not elsewhere classified 88.90
intraoperative (iMRI) 88.96
magnetic resonance (nuclear) (proton) NEC
88.97
abdomen 88.97
bladder (urinary) 88.95
bone marrow blood supply 88.94
brain (brain stem) 88.91
intraoperative (iMRI) 88.96
real-time 88.96
chest (hilar) (mediastinal) 88.92
extremity (upper) (lower) 88.94
eye orbit 88.97
face 88.97
head NEC 88.97
musculoskeletal 88.94
myocardium 88.92
neck 88.97
orbit of eye 88.97
prostate 88.95
specified site NEC 88.97
spinal canal (cord) (spine) 88.93

Immobilization (by)
with fracture-reduction — see Reduction,
fracture
bandage 93.59
bone 93.53

Immobilization (by) — continued
cast NEC 93.53
with reduction of fracture or dislocation —
see Reduction, fracture, and
Reduction, dislocation
device NEC 93.59
pressure dressing 93.56
splint (plaster) (tray) 93.54
with reduction of fracture or dislocation —
see Reduction, fracture, and
Reduction, dislocation
stereotactic head frame 93.59

Immunization — see also Vaccination
allergy 99.12
autoimmune disease 99.13
BCG 99.33
brucellosis 99.55
cholera 99.31
diphtheria 99.36
DPT 99.39
epidemic parotitis 99.46
German measles 99.47
Hemophilus influenzae 99.52
influenza 99.52
measles 99.45
meningococcus 99.55
mumps 99.46
pertussis 99.37
plague 99.34
poliomyelitis 99.41
rabies 99.44
rubella 99.47
salmonella 99.55
smallpox 99.42
staphylococcus 99.55
TAB 99.32
tetanus 99.38
triple vaccine 99.48
tuberculosis 99.33
tularemia 99.35
typhoid-paratyphoid 99.32
typhus 99.55
viral NEC 99.55
whooping cough 99.37
yellow fever 99.43

Immunoadsorption
extracorporeal (ECI) 99.76

Immunotherapy, antineoplastic 99.28
C-Parvum 99.28
Interferon 99.28
Interleukin-2 99.28
Levamisole 99.28
Proleukin 99.28
Thymosin 99.28

Implant, implantation
abdominal artery to coronary artery 36.17
artery
aortic branches to heart muscle 36.2
mammary to ventricular wall (Vineberg) 36.2
baffle, atrial or interatrial 35.91
biliary fistulous tract into stomach or intestine
51.39
bipolar endoprosthesis (femoral head) 81.52
bladder sphincter, artificial (inflatable) 58.93
blood vessels to myocardium 36.2
bone growth stimulator (invasive)
(percutaneous) (semi-invasive) — see
category 78.9
bone morphogenetic protein (recombinant)
(rhBMP) 84.52
breast (for augmentation) (bilateral) 85.54
unilateral 85.53
cardiac resynchronization device
defibrillator (CRT-D) (total system) 00.51
left ventricular coronary venous lead
only 00.52
pulse generator only 00.54
pacemaker (CRT-P) (total system) 00.50
left ventricular coronary venous lead
only 00.52
pulse generator only 00.53
cardiomyostimulation system 37.67
cardioverter/defibrillator (automatic) 37.94
leads only (patch electrodes) (sensing)
(pacing) 37.95

✓4ᵗʰ Fourth-digit Required   ►◄ Revised Text   ● New Line   ▲ Revised Code

Implant — Implant

☑4ᵗʰ Fourth-digit Required　　▶◀ Revised Text　　● New Line　　▲ Revised Code

Incision (and drainage) — *continued*
- gallbladder 51.04
- gingiva 24.0
- gluteal 86.09
- groin region (abdominal wall) (inguinal) 54.0
  - skin 86.09
  - subcutaneous tissue 86.09
- gum 24.0
- hair follicles 86.09
- heart 37.10
  - valve — *see* Valvulotomy
- hematoma — *see also* Incision, by site
  - axilla 86.04
  - broad ligament 69.98
  - ear 18.09
  - episiotomy site 75.91
  - fossa (superficial) NEC 86.04
  - groin region (abdominal wall) (inguinal) 54.0
    - skin 86.04
    - subcutaneous tissue 86.04
  - laparotomy site 54.12
  - mediastinum 34.1
  - perineum (female) 71.09
    - male 86.04
  - popliteal space 86.04
  - scrotum 61.0
  - skin 86.04
  - space of Retzius 59.19
  - subcutaneous tissue 86.04
  - vagina (cuff) 70.14
    - episiotomy site 75.91
    - obstetrical NEC 75.92
- hepatic ducts 51.59
- hordeolum 08.09
- hygroma — *see also* Incision, by site
  - cystic 40.0
- hymen 70.11
- hypochondrium 54.0
  - intra-abdominal 54.19
- hypophysis 07.72
- iliac fossa 54.0
- infratemporal fossa 27.0
- ingrown nail 86.09
- intestine 45.00
  - large 45.03
  - small 45.02
- intracerebral 01.39
- intracranial (epidural space) (extradural space) 01.24
  - subarachnoid or subdural space 01.31
- intraperitoneal 54.19
- ischiorectal tissue 49.02
  - abscess 49.01
- joint structures (*see also* Arthrotomy) 80.10
- kidney 55.01
  - pelvis 55.11
- labia 71.09
- lacrimal
  - canaliculus 09.52
  - gland 09.0
  - passage NEC 09.59
  - punctum 09.51
  - sac 09.53
- larynx NEC 31.3
- ligamentum flavum (spine) — *omit code*
- liver 50.0
- lung 33.1
- lymphangioma 40.0
- lymphatic structure (channel) (node) (vessel) 40.0
- mastoid 20.21
- mediastinum 34.1
- meibomian gland 08.09
- meninges (cerebral) 01.31
  - spinal 03.09
- midpalmar space 82.04
- mouth NEC 27.92
  - floor 27.0
- muscle 83.02
  - with division 83.19
    - hand 82.19
  - hand 82.02
    - with division 82.19
- myocardium 37.11
- nailbed or nailfold 86.09
- nasolacrimal duct (stricture) 09.59

Incision (and drainage) — *continued*
- neck 86.09
- nerve (cranial) (peripheral) NEC 04.04
  - root (spinal) 03.1
- nose 21.1
- omentum 54.19
- orbit (*see also* Orbitotomy) 16.09
- ovary 65.09
  - laparoscopic 65.01
- palate 27.1
- palmar space (middle) 82.04
- pancreas 52.09
- pancreatic sphincter 51.82
  - endoscopic 51.85
- parapharyngeal (oral) (transcervical) 28.0
- paronychia 86.09
- parotid
  - gland or duct 26.0
  - space 27.0
- pelvirectal tissue 48.81
- penis 64.92
- perianal (skin) (tissue) 49.02
  - abscess 49.01
- perigastric 54.19
- perineum (female) 71.09
  - male 86.09
- peripheral vessels
  - lower limb
    - artery 38.08
    - vein 38.09
  - upper limb (artery) (vein) 38.03
- periprostatic tissue 60.81
- perirectal tissue 48.81
- perirenal tissue 59.09
- perisplenic 54.19
- peritoneum 54.95
  - by laparotomy 54.19
  - pelvic (female) 70.12
    - male 54.19
- periureteral tissue 59.09
- periurethral tissue 58.91
- perivesical tissue 59.19
- petrous pyramid (air cells) (apex) (mastoid) 20.22
- pharynx, pharyngeal (bursa) 29.0
  - space, lateral 27.0
- pilonidal sinus (cyst) 86.03
- pineal gland 07.52
- pituitary (gland) 07.72
- pleura NEC 34.09
- popliteal space 86.09
- postzygomatic space 27.0
- pouch of Douglas 70.12
- prostate (perineal approach) (transurethral approach) 60.0
- pterygopalatine fossa 27.0
- pulp canal (tooth) 24.0
- Rathke's pouch 07.72
- rectovaginal septum 48.81
- rectum 48.0
  - stricture 48.91
- renal pelvis 55.11
- retroperitoneum 54.0
- retropharyngeal (oral) (transcervical) 28.0
- salivary gland or duct 26.0
- sclera 12.89
- scrotum 61.0
- sebaceous cyst 86.04
- seminal vesicle 60.72
- sinus — *see* Sinusotomy
- Skene's duct or gland 71.09
- skin 86.09
  - with drainage 86.04
  - breast 85.0
  - cardiac pacemaker pocket, new site 37.79
  - ear 18.09
  - nose 21.1
  - subcutaneous tunnel for pulse generator lead wire 86.99
    - with initial procedure — *omit code*
  - thalamic stimulator pulse generator pocket, new site 86.09
    - with initial insertion of battery package — *omit code*
  - tunnel, subcutaneous for pulse generator lead wire 86.99
    - with initial procedure — *omit code*

Incision (and drainage) — *continued*
- skull (bone) 01.24
- soft tissue NEC 83.09
  - with division 83.19
    - hand 82.19
  - hand 82.09
    - with division 82.19
- space of Retzius 59.19
- spermatic cord 63.93
- sphincter of Oddi 51.82
  - endoscopic 51.85
- spinal
  - cord 03.09
  - nerve root 03.1
- spleen 41.2
- stomach 43.0
- stye 08.09
- subarachnoid space, cerebral 01.31
- subcutaneous tissue 86.09
  - with drainage 86.04
  - tunnel
    - esophageal 42.86
      - with anastomosis — *see* Anastomosis, esophagus, antesternal
    - pulse generator lead wire 86.99
      - with initial procedure — *omit code*
- subdiaphragmatic space 54.19
- subdural space, cerebral 01.31
- sublingual space 27.0
- submandibular space 27.0
- submaxillary 86.09
  - with drainage 86.04
- submental space 27.0
- subphrenic space 54.19
- supraclavicular fossa 86.09
  - with drainage 86.04
- sweat glands, skin 86.04
- temporal pouches 27.0
- tendon (sheath) 83.01
  - with division 83.13
    - hand 82.11
  - hand 82.01
    - with division 82.11
- testis 62.0
- thenar space 82.04
- thymus 07.92
- thyroid (field) (gland) NEC 06.09
  - postoperative 06.02
- tongue NEC 25.94
  - for tongue tie 25.91
- tonsil 28.0
- trachea NEC 31.3
- tunica vaginalis 61.0
- umbilicus 54.0
- urachal cyst 54.0
- ureter 56.2
- urethra 58.0
- uterus (corpus) 68.0
  - cervix 69.95
  - for termination of pregnancy 74.91
  - septum (congenital) 68.22
- uvula 27.71
- vagina (cuff) (septum) (stenosis) 70.14
  - for
    - incisional hematoma (episiotomy) 75.91
    - obstetrical hematoma NEC 75.92
    - pelvic abscess 70.12
- vas deferens 63.6 ✓4ᵗʰ
- vein 38.00
  - abdominal 38.07
  - head and neck NEC 38.02
  - intracranial NEC 38.01
  - lower limb 38.09
  - thoracic NEC 38.05
  - upper limb 38.03
- vertebral column 03.09
- vulva 71.09
  - obstetrical 75.92
- web, esophageal 42.01

Incudectomy NEC 19.3
- with
  - stapedectomy (*see also* Stapedectomy) 19.19
  - tympanoplasty — *see* Tympanoplasty

Incudopexy 19.19

✓4ᵗʰ Fourth-digit Required   ▶◀ Revised Text   ● New Line   ▲ Revised Code

Incudostapediopexy 19.19
 with incus replacement 19.11
Indentation, sclera, for buckling (*see also* Buckling, scleral) 14.49
Indicator dilution flow measurement 89.68
Induction
 abortion
  by
   D and C 69.01
    insertion of prostaglandin suppository 96.49
    intra-amniotic injection (prostaglandin) (saline) 75.0
  labor
   medical 73.4
   surgical 73.01
    intra- and extra-amniotic injection 73.1
    stripping of membranes 73.1
Inflation
 belt wrap 93.99
 Eustachian tube 20.8
 fallopian tube 66.8
  with injection of therapeutic agent 66.95
Infolding, sclera, for buckling (*see also* Buckling, scleral) 14.49
Infraction, turbinates (nasal) 21.62
Infundibulectomy
 hypophyseal (*see also* Hypophysectomy, partial) 07.63
 ventricle (heart) (right) 35.34
  in total repair of tetralogy of Fallot 35.81
Infusion (intra-arterial) (intravenous)
 Abciximab 99.20
 antibiotic
  oxazolidinone class 00.14 ●
 antineoplastic agent (chemotherapeutic) 99.25
  biological response modifier [BRM] 99.28
  high-dose interleukin-2 99.28 ●
 biological response modifier [BRM], antineoplastic agent 99.28
  high-dose interleukin-2 99.28 ●
 cancer chemotherapy agent NEC 99.25
 drotrecogin alfa (activated) 00.11 ●
 electrolytes 99.18
 enzymes, thrombolytic (streptokinase) (tissue plasminogen activator) (TPA) (urokinase)
  direct coronary artery 36.04
  intravenous 99.10
 Eptifibatide 99.20
 GB IIB/IIIa inhibitor 99.20
 hormone substance NEC 99.24
 human B-type natriuretic peptide (hBNP) 00.13 ●
 nesiritide 00.13 ●
 neuroprotective agent 99.75
 nimodipine 99.75
 nutritional substance — *see* Nutrition
 platelet inhibitor
  direct coronary artery 36.04
  intravenous 99.20
 prophylactic substance NEC 99.29
 recombinant protein 00.11 ●
 reteplase 99.10
 therapeutic substance NEC 99.29
 thrombolytic agent (enzyme) (streptokinase) 99.10
  with percutaneous transluminal angioplasty
   coronary (single vessel) 36.02
    multiple vessels 36.05
   non-coronary vessel(s) 39.50
    specified site NEC 39.50
   direct intracoronary artery 36.04
 tirofiban (HCl) 99.20
 vaccine
  tumor 99.28
Injection (into) (hypodermically) (intramuscularly) (intravenously) (acting locally or systemically)
 Actinomycin D, for cancer chemotherapy 99.25
 adhesion barrier ▶substance◀ 99.77 ▲
 alcohol
  nerve — *see* Injection, nerve
  spinal 03.8

Injection — *continued*
 anterior chamber, eye (air) (liquid) (medication) 12.92
 antibiotic 99.21
  oxazolidinone class 00.14 ●
 anticoagulant 99.19
 anti-D (Rhesus) globulin 99.11
 antidote NEC 99.16
 anti-infective NEC 99.22
 antineoplastic agent (chemotherapeutic) NEC 99.25
  biological response modifier [BRM] 99.28
  high-dose interleukin-2 99.28 ●
 antivenin 99.16
 barrier ▶substance,◀ adhesion 99.77 ▲
 BCG
  for chemotherapy 99.25
  vaccine 99.33
 biological response modifier [BRM], antineoplastic agent 99.28
  high-dose interleukin-2 99.28 ●
 bone marrow 41.92
  transplant — *see* Transplant, bone, marrow
 breast (therapeutic agent) 85.92
  inert material (silicone) (bilateral) 85.52
   unilateral 85.51
 bursa (therapeutic agent) 83.96
  hand 82.94
 cancer chemotherapeutic agent 99.25
 caudal — *see* Injection, spinal
 cortisone 99.23
 costochondral junction 81.92
 dinoprost-tromethine, intraamniotic 75.0
 ear, with alcohol 20.72
 electrolytes 99.18
 enzymes, thrombolytic (streptokinase) (tissue plasminogen activator) (TPA) (urokinase)
  direct coronary artery 36.04
  intravenous 99.10
 epidural, spinal — *see* Injection, spinal
 esophageal varices or blood vessel (endoscopic) (sclerosing agent) 42.33
 Eustachian tube (inert material) 20.8
 eye (orbit) (retrobulbar) 16.91
  anterior chamber 12.92
  subconjunctival 10.91
 fascia 83.98
  hand 82.96
 gamma globulin 99.14
 ganglion, sympathetic 05.39
  ciliary 12.79
  paravertebral stellate 05.39
 gel, adhesion barrier ▶— *see* Injection, adhesion barrier substance◀
 globulin
  anti-D (Rhesus) 99.11
  gamma 99.14
  Rh immune 99.11
 heart 37.92
 heavy metal antagonist 99.16
 hemorrhoids (sclerosing agent) 49.42
 hormone NEC 99.24
 human B-type natriuretic peptide (hBNP) 00.13 ●
 immune sera 99.14
 inert material — *see* Implant, inert material
 inner ear, for destruction 20.72
 insulin 99.17
 intervertebral space for herniated disc 80.52
 intra-amniotic
  for induction of
   abortion 75.0
   labor 73.1
 intrathecal — *see* Injection, spinal
 joint (therapeutic agent) 81.92
  temporomandibular 76.96
 kidney (cyst) (therapeutic substance) NEC 55.96
 larynx 31.0
 ligament (joint) (therapeutic substance) 81.92
 liver 50.94
 lung, for surgical collapse 33.32
 Methotrexate, for cancer chemotherapy 99.25
 nerve (cranial) (peripheral) 04.80
  agent NEC 04.89
   alcohol 04.2

Injection — *continued*
 nerve — *continued*
  agent NEC — *continued*
   anesthetic for analgesia 04.81
    for operative anesthesia — *omit code*
   neurolytic 04.2
   phenol 04.2
  laryngeal (external) (recurrent) (superior) 31.91
  optic 16.91
  sympathetic 05.39
   alcohol 05.32
   anesthetic for analgesia 05.31
   neurolytic agent 05.32
   phenol 05.32
 nesiritide 00.13 ●
 neuroprotective agent 99.75
 nimodipine 99.75
 orbit 16.91
 pericardium 37.93
 peritoneal cavity
  air 54.96
  locally-acting therapeutic substance 54.97
 platelet inhibitor
  direct coronary artery 36.04
  intravenous 99.20
 prophylactic substance NEC 99.29
 prostate 60.92
 radioisotopes (intracavitary) (intravenous) 92.28
 renal pelvis (cyst) 55.96
 retrobulbar (therapeutic substance) 16.91
  for anesthesia — *omit code*
 Rh immune globulin 99.11
 RhoGAM 99.11
 sclerosing agent NEC 99.29
  esophageal varices (endoscopic) 42.33
  hemorrhoids 49.42
  pleura 34.92
   treatment of malignancy (cytotoxic agent) 34.92 *[99.25]*
    with tetracycline 34.92 *[99.21]*
  varicose vein 39.92
  vein NEC 39.92
 semicircular canals, for destruction 20.72
 silicone — *see* Implant, inert material
 skin (sclerosing agent) (filling material) 86.02
 soft tissue 83.98
  hand 82.96
 spinal (canal) NEC 03.92
  alcohol 03.8
  anesthetic agent for analgesia 03.91
   for operative anesthesia — *omit code*
  contrast material (for myelogram) 87.21
  destructive agent NEC 03.8
  neurolytic agent NEC 03.8
  phenol 03.8
  proteolytic enzyme (chemopapain) (chemodiactin) 80.52
  saline (hypothermic) 03.92
  steroid 03.92
 spinal nerve root (intrathecal) — *see* Injection, spinal
 steroid NEC 99.23
 subarachnoid, spinal — *see* Injection, spinal
 subconjunctival 10.91
 tendon 83.97
  hand 82.95
 testis 62.92
 therapeutic agent NEC 99.29
 thoracic cavity 34.92
 thrombolytic agent (enzyme) (streptokinase) 99.10
  with percutaneous transluminal angioplasty
   coronary (single vessel) 36.02
    multiple vessels 36.05
   non-coronary vessel(s) 39.50
    specified site NEC 39.50
 trachea 31.94
 tranquilizer 99.26
 tunica vaginalis (with aspiration) 61.91
 tympanum 20.94
 urethra (inert material)
  for repair of urinary stress incontinence
   collagen implant 59.72
   endoscopic injection of implant 59.72
   fat implant 59.72

Injection — *continued*
  urethra — *continued*
    for repair of urinary stress incontinence — *continued*
      polytef implant 59.72
  vaccine
    tumor 99.28
  varices, esophagus (endoscopic) (sclerosing agent) 42.33
  varicose vein (sclerosing agent) 39.92
    esophagus (endoscopic) 42.33
  vestibule, for destruction 20.72
  vitreous substitute (silicone) 14.75
    for reattachment of retina 14.59
  vocal cords 31.0

Inlay, tooth 23.3

Inoculation
  antitoxins — *see* Administration, antitoxins
  toxoids — *see* Administration, toxoids
  vaccine — *see* Administration, vaccine

Insemination, artificial 69.92

Insertion
  airway
    esophageal obturator 96.03
    nasopharynx 96.01
    oropharynx 96.02
  Allen-Brown cannula 39.93
  arch bars (orthodontic) 24.7
    for immobilization (fracture) 93.55
  atrial septal umbrella 35.52
  Austin-Moore prosthesis 81.52
  baffle, heart (atrial) (interatrial) (intra-atrial) 35.91
  bag, cervix (nonobstetrical) 67.0
    after delivery or abortion 75.8
    to assist delivery or induce labor 73.1
  Baker's (tube) (for stenting) 46.85
  balloon
    gastric 44.93
    heart (pulsation-type) (Kantrowitz) 37.61
    intestine (for decompression) (for dilation) 46.85
  Barton's tongs (skull) (with synchronous skeletal traction) 02.94
  bipolar endoprosthesis (femoral head) 81.52
  Blakemore-Sengstaken tube 96.06
  bone growth stimulator (invasive) (percutaneous) (semi-invasive) — *see* category 78.9 ✓4ᵗʰ
  bone morphogenetic protein (recombinant) (rhBMP) 84.52 ●
  bougie, cervix, nonobstetrical 67.0
    to assist delivery or induce labor 73.1
  breast implant (for augmentation) (bilateral) 85.54
    unilateral 85.53
  bridge (dental) (fixed) 23.42
    removable 23.43
  bubble (balloon), stomach 44.93
  caliper tongs (skull) (with synchronous skeletal traction) 02.94
  cannula
    Allen-Brown 39.93
    for extracorporeal membrane oxygenation (ECMO) — *omit code*
    nasal sinus (by puncture) 22.01
      through natural ostium 22.02
    pancreatic duct 52.92
      endoscopic 52.93
    vessel to vessel 39.93
  cardiac resynchronization device ●
    defibrillator (CRT-D) (total system) 00.51 ●
      left ventricular coronary venous lead only 00.52 ●
      pulse generator only 00.54 ●
    pacemaker (CRT-P) (total system) 00.50 ●
      left ventricular coronary venous lead only 00.52 ●
      pulse generator only 00.53 ●
  catheter
    abdomen of fetus, for intrauterine transfusion 75.2
    anterior chamber (eye), for permanent drainage (glaucoma) 12.79

Insertion — *continued*
  catheter — *continued*
    artery 38.91
    bile duct(s) 51.59
      common 51.51
        endoscopic 51.87
      endoscopic 51.87
    bladder, indwelling 57.94
      suprapubic 57.18
        percutaneous (closed) 57.17
    bronchus 96.05
      with lavage 96.56
    central venous NEC 38.93
      for
        hemodialysis 38.95
        pressure monitoring 89.62
      peripherally inserted central catheter (PICC) 38.93
    chest 34.04
      revision (with lysis of adhesions) 34.04
    esophagus (nonoperative) 96.06
      permanent tube 42.81
    intercostal (with water seal), for drainage 34.04
      revision (with lysis of adhesions) 34.04
    spinal canal space (epidural) (subarachnoid) (subdural) for infusion of therapeutic or palliative substances 03.90
    Swan-Ganz (pulmonary) 89.64
    transtracheal for oxygenation 31.99
    vein NEC 38.93
      for renal dialysis 38.95
  chest tube 34.04
  choledochohepatic tube (for decompression) 51.43
    endoscopic 51.87
  cochlear prosthetic device — *see* Implant, cochlear prosthetic device
  contraceptive device (intrauterine) 69.7
  cordis cannula 54.98
  coronary (artery)
    stent (stent graft) 36.06
  Crosby-Cooney button 54.98
  CRT-D (cardiac resynchronization defibrillator) 00.51 ●
    left ventricular coronary venous lead only 00.52 ●
    pulse generator only 00.54 ●
  CRT-P (cardiac resynchronization pacemaker) 00.50 ●
    left ventricular coronary venous lead only 00.52 ●
    pulse generator only 00.53 ●
  Crutchfield tongs (skull) (with synchronous skeletal traction) 02.94
  Davidson button 54.98
  denture (total) 99.97
  device, vascular access 86.07
  diaphragm, vagina 96.17
  drainage tube
    kidney 55.02
      pelvis 55.12
    renal pelvis 55.12
  elbow prosthesis (total) 81.84
    revision 81.97
  electrode(s)
    bone growth stimulator (invasive) (percutaneous) (semi-invasive) — *see* category 78.9 ✓4ᵗʰ
    brain 02.93
      depth 02.93
      foramen ovale 02.93
      sphenoidal 02.96
    heart (initial) (transvenous) 37.70
      atrium (initial) 37.73
        replacement 37.76
      atrium and ventricle (initial) 37.72
        replacement 37.76
      epicardium (sternotomy or thoracotomy approach) 37.74
      left ventricular coronary venous system 00.52 ●
      temporary transvenous pacemaker system 37.78
        during and immediately following cardiac surgery 39.64

Insertion — *continued*
  electrode(s) — *continued*
    heart — *continued*
      ventricle (initial) 37.71
        replacement 37.76
    intracranial 02.93
    osteogenic (for bone growth stimulation) — *see* category 78.9 ✓4ᵗʰ
    peripheral nerve 04.92
    spine 03.93
  electroencephalographic receiver — *see* Implant, electroencephalographic receiver, by site
  electronic stimulator — *see* Implant, electronic stimulator, by site
  electrostimulator — *see* Implant, electronic stimulator, by site
  endograft(s), endovascular graft(s) ●
    endovascular, head and neck vessels 39.72 ●
    endovascular, other vessels (for aneurysm) 39.79 ●
  endoprosthesis
    bile duct 51.87
    femoral head (bipolar) 81.52
    pancreatic duct 52.93
  epidural pegs 02.93
  external fixation device (bone) — *see* category 78.1 ✓4ᵗʰ
  facial bone implant (alloplastic) (synthetic) 76.92
  filling material, skin (filling of defect) 86.02
  filter
    vena cava (inferior) (superior) (transvenous) 38.7
  fixator, mini device (bone) — *see* category 78.1 ✓4ᵗʰ
  frame (stereotactic)
    for radiosurgery 93.59
  Gardner Wells tongs (skull) (with synchronous skeletal traction) 02.94
  gastric bubble (balloon) 44.93
  globe, into eye socket 16.69
  Greenfield filter 38.7
  halo device (skull) (with synchronous skeletal traction) 02.94
  Harrington rod — *see also* Fusion, spinal, by level
    with dorsal, dorsolumbar fusion 81.05
  Harris pin 79.15
  heart
    pacemaker — *see* Insertion, pacemaker, cardiac
    pump (Kantrowitz) 37.62
    valve — *see* Replacement, heart valve
  hip prosthesis (partial) 81.52
    revision 81.53
    total 81.51
      revision 81.53
  Holter valve 02.2
  Hufnagel valve — *see* Replacement, heart valve
  implant — *see* Insertion, prosthesis
  infusion pump 86.06
  intercostal catheter (with water seal) for drainage 34.04
  intra-arterial blood gas monitoring system 89.60 ●
  intrauterine
    contraceptive device 69.7
    radium (intracavitary) 69.91
    tamponade (nonobstetric) 69.91
  Kantrowitz
    heart pump 37.62
    pulsation balloon (phase-shift) 37.61
  keratoprosthesis 11.73
  King-Mills umbrella device (heart) 35.52
  Kirschner wire 93.44
    with reduction of fracture or dislocation — *see* Reduction, fracture *and* Reduction, dislocation
  laminaria, cervix 69.93
  larynx, valved tube 31.75
  leads (cardiac) — *see* Insertion, electrode(s), heart
  lens, prosthetic (intraocular) 13.70
    with cataract extraction, one-stage 13.71

✓4ᵗʰ Fourth-digit Required   ▶◀ Revised Text   ● New Line   ▲ Revised Code

Insertion — Jejunocolostomy

Insertion — *continued*
  tube — *see also* Catheterization and
    Intubation — *continued*
    intercostal — *continued*
      revision (with lysis of adhesions) 34.04
    Miller-Abbott (for intestinal decompression)
      96.08
    nasobiliary (drainage) 51.86
    nasogastric (for intestinal decompression)
      NEC 96.07
    naso-intestinal 96.08   ●
    nasopancreatic drainage (endoscopic) 52.97
    pancreatic duct 52.92
      endoscopic 52.93
    rectum 96.09
    stomach (nasogastric) (for intestinal
      decompression) NEC 96.07
      for feeding 96.6
    tracheobronchial 96.05
  umbrella device
    atrial septum (King-Mills) 35.52
    vena cava (Mobitz-Uddin) 38.7
  ureteral stent (transurethral) 59.8
    with ureterotomy 59.8 *[56.2]*
  urinary sphincter, artificial (AUS) (inflatable)
    58.93
  vaginal mold 96.15
  valve
    Holter 02.2
    Hufnagel — *see* Replacement, heart valve
    pharyngeal (artificial) 31.75
    Spitz-Holter 02.2
    vas deferens 63.95
  vascular access device, totally implantable
    86.07
  vena cava sieve or umbrella 38.7
  Vinke tongs (skull) (with synchronous skeletal
    traction) 02.94
Instillation
  bladder 96.49
  digestive tract, except gastric gavage 96.43
  genitourinary NEC 96.49
  radioisotope (intracavitary) (intravenous) 92.28
Insufflation
  Eustachian tube 20.8
  fallopian tube (air) (dye) (gas) (saline) 66.8
    for radiography — *see*
      Hysterosalpingography
    therapeutic substance 66.95
  lumbar retroperitoneal, bilateral 88.15
Intercricothyroidotomy (for assistance in
  breathing) 31.1
Intermittent positive pressure breathing (IPPB)
  93.91
Interposition operation
  esophageal reconstruction (intrathoracic)
    (retrosternal) NEC (*see also* Anastomosis,
    esophagus, with, interposition) 42.58
  antesternal or antethoracic NEC (*see also*
    Anastomosis, esophagus, antesternal,
    with, interposition) 42.68
  uterine suspension 69.21
Interruption
  vena cava (inferior) (superior) 38.7
Interview (evaluation) (diagnostic)
  medical, except psychiatric 89.05
    brief (abbreviated history) 89.01
    comprehensive (history and evaluation of
      new problem) 89.03
    limited (interval history) 89.02
    specified type NEC 89.04
  psychiatric NEC 94.19
    follow-up 94.19
    initial 94.19
    pre-commitment 94.13
Intimectomy 38.10
  abdominal 38.16
  aorta (arch) (ascending) (descending) 38.14
  head and neck NEC 38.12
  intracranial NEC 38.11
  lower limb 38.18
  thoracic NEC 38.15
  upper limb 38.13

Introduction
  orthodontic appliance 24.7
  therapeutic substance (acting locally or
    systemically) NEC 99.29
    bursa 83.96
      hand 82.94
    fascia 83.98
      hand 82.96
    heart 37.92
    joint 81.92
      temporomandibular 76.96
    ligament (joint) 81.92
    pericardium 37.93
    soft tissue NEC 83.98
      hand 82.96
    tendon 83.97
      hand 82.95
    vein 39.92
Intubation — *see also* Catheterization and
  Insertion
  bile duct(s) 51.59
    common 51.51
      endoscopic 51.87
    endoscopic 51.87
  esophagus (nonoperative) (Sengstaken) 96.06
    permanent tube (silicone) (Souttar) 42.81
  Eustachian tube 20.8
  intestine (for decompression) 96.08
  lacrimal for
    dilation 09.42
    tear drainage, intranasal 09.81
  larynx 96.05
  nasobiliary (drainage) 51.86
  nasogastric
    for
      decompression, intestinal 96.07
      feeding 96.6
  nasolacrimal (duct) (with irrigation) 09.44
  nasopancreatic drainage (endoscopic) 52.97
  naso-intestinal 96.08   ●
  respiratory tract NEC 96.05
  small intestine (Miller-Abbott) 96.08
  stomach (nasogastric) (for intestinal
    decompression) NEC 96.07
    for feeding 96.6
  trachea 96.04
  ventriculocisternal 02.2
Invagination, diverticulum
  gastric 44.69
  pharynx 29.59
  stomach 44.69
Inversion
  appendix 47.99
  diverticulum
    gastric 44.69
    intestine
      large 45.49
        endoscopic 45.43
      small 45.34
    stomach 44.69
  tunica vaginalis 61.49
Ionization, medical 99.27
Iontherapy 99.27
Iontophoresis 99.27
Iridectomy (basal) (buttonhole) (optical)
  (peripheral) (total) 12.14
  with
    capsulectomy 13.65
    cataract extraction — *see* Extraction,
      cataract
    filtering operation (for glaucoma) NEC 12.65
    scleral
      fistulization 12.65
      thermocauterization 12.62
      trephination 12.61
Iridencleisis 12.63
Iridesis 12.63
Irido-capsulectomy 13.65
Iridocyclectomy 12.44
Iridocystectomy 12.42
Iridodesis 12.63
Iridoplasty NEC 12.39
Iridosclerectomy 12.65

Iridosclerotomy 12.69
Iridotasis 12.63
Iridotomy 12.12
  by photocoagulation 12.12
  with transfixion 12.11
  for iris bombé 12.11
  specified type NEC 12.12
Iron lung 93.99
Irradiation
  gamma, stereotactic 92.32
Irrigation
  anterior chamber (eye) 12.91
  bronchus NEC 96.56
  canaliculus 09.42
  catheter
    ureter 96.46
    urinary, indwelling NEC 96.48
    vascular 96.57
    ventricular 02.41
    wound 96.58
  cholecystostomy 96.41
  cornea 96.51
    with removal of foreign body 98.21
  corpus cavernosum 64.98
  cystostomy 96.47
  ear (removal of cerumen) 96.52
  enterostomy 96.36
  eye 96.51
    with removal of foreign body 98.21
  gastrostomy 96.36
  lacrimal
    canaliculi 09.42
    punctum 09.41
  muscle 83.02
    hand 82.02
  nasal
    passages 96.53
    sinus 22.00
  nasolacrimal duct 09.43
    with insertion of tube or stent 09.44
  nephrostomy 96.45
  peritoneal 54.25
  pyelostomy 96.45
  rectal 96.39
  stomach 96.33
  tendon (sheath) 83.01
    hand 82.01
  trachea NEC 96.56
  traumatic cataract 13.3
  tube
    biliary NEC 96.41
    nasogastric NEC 96.34
    pancreatic 96.42
  ureterostomy 96.46
  ventricular shunt 02.41
  wound (cleaning) NEC 96.59
Irving operation (tubal ligation) 66.32
Irwin operation (*see also* Osteotomy) 77.30
Ischiectomy (partial) 77.89
  total 77.99
Ischiopubiotomy 77.39
Isolation
  after contact with infectious disease 99.84
  ileal loop 45.51
  intestinal segment or pedicle flap
    large 45.52
    small 45.51
Isthmectomy, thyroid (*see also* Thyroidectomy,
  partial) 06.39

Jaboulay operation (gastroduodenostomy) 44.39
Janeway operation (permanent gastrostomy)
  43.19
Jatene operation (arterial switch) 35.84
Jejunectomy 45.62
Jejunocecostomy 45.93
Jejunocholecystostomy 51.32
Jejunocolostomy 45.93

Jejunoileostomy — Lengthening

Index to Procedures

Manipulation

Lower GI series (x-ray) 87.64
Lucas and Murray operation (knee arthrodesis with plate) 81.22
Lumpectomy
    breast 85.21
    specified site — *see* Excision, lesion, by site
Lymphadenectomy (simple) (*see also* Excision, lymph, node) 40.29
Lymphadenotomy 40.0
Lymphangiectomy (radical) (*see also* Excision, lymph, node, by site, radical) 40.50
Lymphangiogram
    abdominal 88.04
    cervical 87.08
    intrathoracic 87.34
    lower limb 88.36
    pelvic 88.04
    upper limb 88.34
Lymphangioplasty 40.9
Lymphangiorrhaphy 40.9
Lymphangiotomy 40.0
Lymphaticostomy 40.9
    thoracic duct 40.62
Lysis
    adhesions

> *Note:*
>
> blunt — omit code
> digital — omit code
> manual — omit code
> mechanical — omit code
> without instrumentation — omit code

    abdominal 54.59
        laparoscopic 54.51
    appendiceal 54.59
        laparoscopic 54.51
    artery-vein-nerve bundle 39.91
    biliary tract 54.59
        laparoscopic 54.51
    bladder (neck) (intraluminal) 57.12
        external 59.11
            laparoscopic 59.12
        transurethral 57.41
    blood vessels 39.91
    bone — *see* category 78.4 ☑4ᵗʰ
    bursa 83.91
        by stretching or manipulation 93.28
        hand 82.91
    cartilage of joint 93.26
    chest wall 33.99
    choanae (nasopharynx) 29.54
    conjunctiva 10.5
    corneovitreal 12.34
    cortical (brain) 02.91
    ear, middle 20.23
    Eustachean tube 20.8
    extraocular muscle 15.7
    extrauterine 54.59
        laparoscopic 54.51
    eyelid 08.09
        and conjunctiva 10.5
    eye muscle 15.7
    fallopian tube 65.89
        laparoscopic 65.81
    fascia 83.91
        hand 82.91
            by stretching or manipulation 93.26
    gallbladder 54.59
        laparoscopic 54.51
    ganglion (peripheral) NEC 04.49
        cranial NEC 04.42
    hand 82.91
        by stretching or manipulation 93.26
    heart 37.10
    intestines 54.59
        laparoscopic 54.51
    iris (posterior) 12.33
        anterior 12.32
    joint (capsule) (structure) (*see also* Division, joint capsule) 80.40
    kidney 59.02
        laparoscopic 59.03

Lysis — *continued*
    adhesions — *continued*
        labia (vulva) 71.01
        larynx 31.92
        liver 54.59
            laparoscopic 54.51
        lung (for collapse of lung) 33.39
        mediastinum 34.99
        meninges (spinal) 03.6
            cortical 02.91
        middle ear 20.23
        muscle 83.91
            by stretching or manipulation 93.27
            extraocular 15.7
            hand 82.91
                by stretching or manipulation 93.26
        nasopharynx 29.54
        nerve (peripheral) NEC 04.49
            cranial NEC 04.42
            roots, spinal 03.6
            trigeminal 04.41
        nose, nasal 21.91
        ocular muscle 15.7
        ovary 65.89
            laparoscopic 65.81
        pelvic 54.59
            laparoscopic 54.51
        penile 64.93
        pericardium 37.12
        perineal (female) 71.01
        peripheral vessels 39.91
        perirectal 48.81
        perirenal 59.02
            laparoscopic 59.03
        peritoneum (pelvic) 54.59
            laparoscopic 54.51
        periureteral 59.02
            laparoscopic 59.03
        perivesical 59.11
            laparoscopic 59.12
        pharynx 29.54
        pleura (for collapse of lung) 33.39
        spermatic cord 63.94
        spinal (cord) (meninges) (nerve roots) 03.6
        spleen 54.59
            laparoscopic 54.51
        tendon 83.91
            by stretching or manipulation 93.27
            hand 82.91
                by stretching or manipulation 93.26
        thorax 34.99
        tongue 25.93
        trachea 31.92
        tubo-ovarian 65.89
            laparoscopic 65.81
        ureter 59.02
            with freeing or repositioning of ureter 59.02
            intraluminal 56.81
            laparoscopic 59.03
        urethra (intraluminal) 58.5
        uterus 54.59
            intraluminal 68.21
            laparoscopic 54.51
            peritoneal 54.59
                laparoscopic 54.51
        vagina (intraluminal) 70.13
        vitreous (posterior approach) 14.74
            anterior approach 14.73
        vulva 71.01
    goniosynechiae (with injection of air or liquid) 12.31
    synechiae (posterior) 12.33
        anterior (with injection of air or liquid) 12.32

M

Madlener operation (tubal ligation) 66.31
Magnet extraction
    foreign body
        anterior chamber, eye 12.01
        choroid 14.01
        ciliary body 12.01

Magnet extraction — *continued*
    foreign body — *continued*
        conjunctiva 98.22
        cornea 11.0
        eye, eyeball NEC 98.21
            anterior segment 12.01
            posterior segment 14.01
        intraocular (anterior segment) 12.01
        iris 12.01
        lens 13.01
        orbit 98.21
        retina 14.01
        sclera 12.01
        vitreous 14.01
Magnetic resonance imaging (nuclear) — *see* Imaging, magnetic resonance
Magnuson (-Stack) operation (arthroplasty for recurrent shoulder dislocation) 81.82
Malleostapediopexy 19.19
    with incus replacement 19.11
Malström's vacuum extraction 72.79
    with episiotomy 72.71
Mammaplasty — *see* Mammoplasty
Mammectomy — *see also* Mastectomy
    subcutaneous (unilateral) 85.34
        bilateral 85.36
            with synchronous implant 85.35
Mammilliplasty 85.87
Mammography NEC 87.37
Mammoplasty 85.89
    with
        full-thickness graft 85.83
        muscle flap 85.85
        pedicle graft 85.84
        split-thickness graft 85.82
    amputative (reduction) (bilateral) 85.32
        unilateral 85.31
    augmentation 85.50
        with
            breast implant (bilateral) 85.54
                unilateral 85.53
            injection into breast (bilateral) 85.52
                unilateral 85.51
    reduction (bilateral) 85.32
        unilateral 85.31
    revision 85.89
    size reduction (gynecomastia) (bilateral) 85.32
        unilateral 85.31
Mammotomy 85.0
Manchester (-Donald) (-Fothergill) operation (uterine suspension) 69.22
Mandibulectomy (partial) 76.31
    total 76.42
        with reconstruction 76.41
Maneuver (method)
    Bracht 72.52
    Credé 73.59
    De Lee (key-in-lock) 72.4
    Kristeller 72.54
    Lovset's (extraction of arms in breech birth) 72.52
    Mauriceau (-Smellie-Veit) 72.52
    Pinard (total breech extraction) 72.54
    Prague 72.52
    Ritgen 73.59
    Scanzoni (rotation) 72.4
    Van Hoorn 72.52
    Wigand-Martin 72.52
Manipulation
    with reduction of fracture or dislocation — *see* Reduction, fracture *and* Reduction, dislocation
    enterostomy stoma (with dilation) 96.24
    intestine (intra-abdominal) 46.80
        large 46.82
        small 46.81
    joint
        adhesions 93.26
            temporomandibular 76.95
        dislocation — *see* Reduction, dislocation
    lacrimal passage (tract) NEC 09.49
    muscle structures 93.27
    musculoskeletal (physical therapy) NEC 93.29

Lower GI series — Manipulation

☑4ᵗʰ Fourth-digit Required   ▶◀ Revised Text   ● New Line   ▲ Revised Code

2002 Ingenix, Inc.

Volume 3 — 43

      ☑4ᵗʰ Fourth-digit Required   ►◄ Revised Text   ● New Line   ▲ Revised Code

Monitoring
cardiac output (by)
ambulatory (ACM) 89.50
electrographic 89.54
during surgery — *omit code*
Fick method 89.67
Holter-type device 89.50
indicator dilution technique 89.68
oxygen consumption technique 89.67
specified technique NEC 89.68
telemetry (cardiac) 89.54
thermodilution indicator 89.68
transesophageal (Doppler) (ultrasound) 89.68
central venous pressure 89.62
circulatory NEC 89.69
continuous intra-arterial bood gas 89.60 ●
coronary blood flow (coincidence counting technique) 89.69
electroencephalographic 89.19
radio-telemetered 89.19
video 89.19
fetus (fetal heart)
antepartum
nonstress (fetal activity acceleration determinations) 75.35
oxytocin challenge (contraction stress test) 75.35
ultrasonography (early pregnancy) (Doppler) 88.78
intrapartum (during labor) (extrauterine) (external) 75.34
ausculatory (stethoscopy) — *omit code*
internal (with contraction measurements) (ECG) 75.32
intrauterine (direct) (ECG) 75.32
phonocardiographic (extrauterine) 75.34
pulsed ultrasound (Doppler) 88.78
transcervical fetal oxygen saturation monitoring 75.38
transcervical fetal SpO$_2$ monitoring 75.38
Holter-type device (cardiac) 89.50
intracranial pressure 01.18
pulmonary artery
pressure 89.63
wedge 89.64
sleep (recording) — *see* categories 89.17-89.18
systemic arterial pressure 89.61
telemetry (cardiac) 89.54
transesophageal cardiac output (Doppler) 89.68
ventricular pressure (cardiac) 89.62
Moore operation (arthroplasty) 81.52
Moschowitz
enterocele repair 70.92
herniorrhaphy — *see* Repair, hernia, femoral
sigmoidopexy 46.63
Mountain resort sanitarium 93.98
Mouth-to-mouth resuscitation 93.93
Moxibustion 93.35
MRI — *see* Imaging, magnetic resonance
Muller operation (banding of pulmonary artery) 38.85
Multiple sleep latency test (MSLT) 89.18
Mumford operation (partial claviculectomy) 77.81
Musculoplasty (*see also* Repair, muscle) 83.87
hand (*see also* Repair, muscle, hand) 82.89
Music therapy 93.84
Mustard operation (interatrial transposition of venous return) 35.91
Myectomy 83.45
anorectal 48.92
eye muscle 15.13
multiple 15.3
for graft 83.43
hand 82.34
hand 82.36
for graft 82.34
levator palpebrae 08.33
rectal 48.92
Myelogram, myelography (air) (gas) 87.21
posterior fossa 87.02

Myelotomy
spine, spinal (cord) (tract) (one-stage) (two-stage) 03.29
percutaneous 03.21
Myocardiectomy (infarcted area) 37.33
Myocardiotomy 37.11
Myoclasis 83.99
hand 82.99
Myomectomy (uterine) 68.29
broad ligament 69.19
Myoplasty (*see also* Repair, muscle) 83.87
hand (*see also* Repair, muscle, hand) 82.89
mastoid 19.9
Myorrhaphy 83.65
hand 82.46
Myosuture 83.65
hand 82.46
Myotasis 93.27
Myotenontoplasty (*see also* Repair, tendon) 83.88
hand 82.86
Myotenoplasty (*see also* Repair, tendon) 83.88
hand 82.86
Myotenotomy 83.13
hand 82.11
Myotomy 83.02
with division 83.19
hand 82.19
colon NEC 46.92
sigmoid 46.91
cricopharyngeal 29.31
that for pharyngeal (pharyngoesophageal) diverticulectomy 29.32
esophagus 42.7
eye (oblique) (rectus) 15.21
multiple (two or more muscles) 15.4
hand 82.02
with division 82.19
levator palpebrae 08.38
sigmoid (colon) 46.91
Myringectomy 20.59
Myringodectomy 20.59
Myringomalleolabyrinthopexy 19.52
Myringoplasty (epitympanic, type I) (by cauterization) (by graft) 19.4
revision 19.6
Myringostapediopexy 19.53
Myringostomy 20.01
Myringotomy (with aspiration) (with drainage) 20.09
with insertion of tube or drainage device (button) (grommet) 20.01

N

Nailing, intramedullary — *see* Reduction, fracture with internal fixation
Narcoanalysis 94.21
Narcosynthesis 94.21
Narrowing, palpebral fissure 08.51
Nasopharyngogram 87.09
contrast 87.06
Necropsy 89.8
Needleoscopy (fetus) 75.31
Needling
Bartholin's gland (cyst) 71.21
cataract (secondary) 13.64
fallopian tube 66.91
hydrocephalic head 73.8
lens (capsule) 13.2
pupillary membrane (iris) 12.35
Nephrectomy (complete) (total) (unilateral) 55.51
bilateral 55.54
partial (wedge) 55.4
remaining or solitary kidney 55.52
removal transplanted kidney 55.53
Nephrocolopexy 55.7
Nephrocystanastomosis NEC 56.73
Nephrolithotomy 55.01

Nephrolysis 59.02
laparoscopic 59.03
Nephropexy 55.7
Nephroplasty 55.89
Nephropyeloplasty 55.87
Nephropyeloureterostomy 55.86
Nephrorrhaphy 55.81
Nephroscopy 55.21
Nephrostolithotomy, percutaneous 55.03
Nephrostomy (with drainage tube) 55.02
closure 55.82
percutaneous 55.03
with fragmentation (ultrasound) 55.04
Nephrotomogram, nephrotomography NEC 87.72
Nephrotomy 55.01
Nephroureterectomy (with bladder cuff) 55.51
Nephroureterocystectomy 55.51 *[57.79]*
Nerve block (cranial) (peripheral) NEC (*see also* Block, by site) 04.81
Neurectasis (cranial) (peripheral) 04.91
Neurectomy (cranial) (infraorbital) (occipital) (peripheral) (spinal) NEC 04.07
gastric (vagus) (*see also* Vagotomy) 44.00
opticociliary 12.79
paracervical 05.22
presacral 05.24
retrogasserian 04.07
sympathetic — *see* Sympathectomy
trigeminal 04.07
tympanic 20.91
Neurexeresis NEC 04.07
Neuroablation ●
radiofrequency 04.2 ●
Neuroanastomosis (cranial) (peripheral) NEC 04.74
accessory-facial 04.72
accessory-hypoglossal 04.73
hypoglossal-facial 04.71
Neurolysis (peripheral nerve) NEC 04.49
carpal tunnel 04.43
cranial nerve NEC 04.42
spinal (cord) (nerve roots) 03.6
tarsal tunnel 04.44
trigeminal nerve 04.41
Neuroplasty (cranial) (peripheral) NEC 04.79
of old injury (delayed repair) 04.76
revision 04.75
Neurorrhaphy (cranial) (peripheral) 04.3
Neurotomy (cranial) (peripheral) (spinal) NEC 04.04
acoustic 04.01
glossopharyngeal 29.92
lacrimal branch 05.0
retrogasserian 04.02
sympathetic 05.0
vestibular 04.01
Neurotripsy (peripheral) NEC 04.03
trigeminal 04.02
Nicola operation (tenodesis for recurrent dislocation of shoulder) 81.82
Nimodipine, infusion 99.75
NIPS (non-invasive programmed electrical stimulation) 37.26 ●
Nissen operation (fundoplication of stomach) 44.66
Noble operation (plication of small intestine) 46.62
Norman Miller operation (vaginopexy) 70.77
Norton operation (extraperitoneal cesarean section) 74.2
Nuclear magnetic resonance imaging — *see* Imaging, magnetic resonance
Nutrition, concentrated substances
enteral infusion (of) 96.6
parenteral, total 99.15
peripheral parenteral 99.15

✓4ᵀᴴ Fourth-digit Required　　▶◀ Revised Text　　● New Line　　▲ Revised Code

O

Ober (-Yount) operation (glutealiliotibial fasciotomy) 83.14

Obliteration
bone cavity (*see also* Osteoplasty) 78.40
calyceal diverticulum 55.39
canaliculi 09.6
cerebrospinal fistula 02.12
cul-de-sac 70.92
frontal sinus (with fat) 22.42
lacrimal punctum 09.91
lumbar pseudomeningocele 03.51
lymphatic structure(s) (peripheral) 40.9
maxillary sinus 22.31
meningocele (sacral) 03.51
pelvic 68.8
pleural cavity 34.6
sacral meningocele 03.51
Skene's gland 71.3
tympanomastoid cavity 19.9
vagina, vaginal (partial) (total) 70.4
vault 70.8

Occlusal molds (dental) 89.31

Occlusion
artery
by embolization — *see* Embolization, artery
by endovascular approach — *see* ●
Embolization, artery ●
by ligation — *see* Ligation, artery
fallopian tube — *see* Ligation, fallopian tube
patent ductus arteriosus (PDA) 38.85
vein
by embolization — *see* Embolization, vein
by endovascular approach — *see* ●
Embolization, vein ●
by ligation — *see* Ligation, vein
vena cava (surgical) 38.7

Occupational therapy 93.83

O'Donoghue operation (triad knee repair) 81.43

Odontectomy NEC (*see also* Removal, tooth, surgical) 23.19

Oleothorax 33.39

Olshausen operation (uterine suspension) 69.22

Omentectomy 54.4

Omentofixation 54.74

Omentopexy 54.74

Omentoplasty 54.74

Omentorrhaphy 54.74

Omentotomy 54.19

Omphalectomy 54.3

Onychectomy 86.23

Onychoplasty 86.86

Onychotomy 86.09
with drainage 86.04

Oophorectomy (unilateral) 65.39
with salpingectomy 65.49
laparoscopic 65.41
bilateral (same operative episode) 65.51
laparoscopic 65.53
with salpingectomy 65.61
laparoscopic 65.63
laparoscopic 65.31
partial 65.29
laparoscopic 65.25
wedge 65.22
that by laparoscope 65.24
remaining ovary 65.52
laparoscopic 65.54
with tube 65.62
laparoscopic 65.64

Oophorocystectomy 65.29
laparoscopic 65.25

Oophoropexy 65.79

Oophoroplasty 65.79

Oophororrhaphy 65.71
laparoscopic 65.74

Oophorostomy 65.09
laparoscopic 65.01

Oophorotomy 65.09
laparoscopic 65.01

Opening
bony labyrinth (ear) 20.79
cranial suture 02.01
heart valve
closed heart technique — *see* Valvulotomy, by site
open heart technique — *see* Valvuloplasty, by site
spinal dura 03.09

Operation
Abbe
construction of vagina 70.61
intestinal anastomosis — *see* Anastomosis, intestine
abdominal (region) NEC 54.99
abdominoperineal NEC 48.5
Aburel (intra-amniotic injection for abortion) 75.0
Adams
advancement of round ligament 69.22
crushing of nasal septum 21.88
excision of palmar fascia 82.35
adenoids NEC 28.99
adrenal (gland) (nerve) (vessel) NEC 07.49
Albee
bone peg, femoral neck 78.05
graft for slipping patella 78.06
sliding inlay graft, tibia 78.07
Albert (arthrodesis, knee) 81.22
Aldridge (-Studdiford) (urethral sling) 59.5
Alexander
prostatectomy
perineal 60.62
suprapubic 60.3
shortening of round ligaments of uterus 69.22
Alexander-Adams (shortening of round ligaments of uterus) 69.22
Almoor (extrapetrosal drainage) 20.22
Altemeier (perineal rectal pull-through) 48.49
Ammon (dacryocystotomy) 09.53
Anderson (tibial lengthening) 78.37
Anel (dilation of lacrimal duct) 09.42
anterior chamber (eye) NEC 12.99
anti-incontinence NEC 59.79
antrum window (nasal sinus) 22.2
with Caldwell-Luc approach 22.39
anus NEC 49.99
aortic body NEC 39.8
aorticopulmonary window 39.59
appendix NEC 47.99
Arslan (fenestration of inner ear) 20.61
artery NEC 39.99
Asai (larynx) 31.75
Baffes (interatrial transposition of venous return) 35.91
Baldy-Webster (uterine suspension) 69.22
Ball
herniorrhaphy — *see* Repair, hernia, inguinal
undercutting 49.02
Bankhart (capsular repair into glenoid, for shoulder dislocation) 81.82
Bardenheurer (ligation of innominate artery) 38.85
Barkan (goniotomy) 12.52
with goniopuncture 12.53
Barr (transfer of tibialis posterior tendon) 83.75
Barsky (closure of cleft hand) 82.82
Bassett (vulvectomy with inguinal lymph node dissection) 71.5 *[40.3]*
Bassini (herniorrhaphy) — *see* Repair, hernia, inguinal
Batch-Spittler-McFaddin (knee disarticulation) 84.16
Batista (partial ventriculectomy) (ventricular reduction) (ventricular remodeling) 37.35
Beck I (epicardial poudrage) 36.39
Beck II (aorta-coronary sinus shunt) 36.39
Beck-Jianu (permanent gastrostomy) 43.19
Bell-Beuttner (subtotal abdominal hysterectomy) 68.3
Belsey (esophagogastric sphincter) 44.65
Benenenti (rotation of bulbous urethra) 58.49
Berke (levator resection eyelid) 08.33

Operation — *continued*
Biesenberger (size reduction of breast, bilateral) 85.32
unilateral 85.31
Bigelow (litholapaxy) 57.0
biliary (duct) (tract) NEC 51.99
Billroth I (partial gastrectomy with gastroduodenostomy) 43.6
Billroth II (partial gastrectomy with gastrojejunostomy) 43.7
Binnie (hepatopexy) 50.69
Bischoff (ureteroneocystostomy) 56.74
bisection hysterectomy 68.3
Bishoff (spinal myelotomy) 03.29
bladder NEC 57.99
flap 56.74
Blalock (systemic-pulmonary anastomosis) 39.0
Blalock-Hanlon (creation of atrial septal defect) 35.42
Blalock-Taussig (subclavian-pulmonary anastomosis) 39.0
Blascovic (resection and advancement of levator palpebrae superioris) 08.33
blood vessel NEC 39.99
Blount
femoral shortening (with blade plate) 78.25
by epiphyseal stapling 78.25
Boari (bladder flap) 56.74
Bobb (cholelithotomy) 51.04
bone NEC — *see* category 78.4 ✓4ᵗʰ
facial 76.99
injury NEC — *see* category 79.9 ✓4ᵗʰ
marrow NEC 41.98
skull NEC 02.99
Bonney (abdominal hysterectomy) 68.4
Borthen (iridotasis) 12.63
Bost
plantar dissection 80.48
radiocarpal fusion 81.26
Bosworth
arthroplasty for acromioclavicular separation 81.83
fusion of posterior lumbar spine 81.08
for pseudarthrosis 81.38
resection of radial head ligaments (for tennis elbow) 80.92
shelf procedure, hip 81.40
Bottle (repair of hydrocele of tunica vaginalis) 61.2
Boyd (hip disarticulation) 84.18
brain NEC 02.99
Brauer (cardiolysis) 37.10
breast NEC 85.99
Bricker (ileoureterostomy) 56.51
Bristow (repair of shoulder dislocation) 81.82
Brock (pulmonary valvulotomy) 35.03
Brockman (soft tissue release for clubfoot) 83.84
bronchus NEC 33.98
Browne (-Denis) (hypospadias repair) 58.45
Brunschwig (temporary gastrostomy) 43.19
buccal cavity NEC 27.99
Bunnell (tendon transfer) 82.56
Burch procedure (retropubic urethral suspension for urinary stress incontinence) 59.5
Burgess (amputation of ankle) 84.14
bursa NEC 83.99
hand 82.99
bypass — *see* Bypass
Caldwell (sulcus extension) 24.91
Caldwell-Luc (maxillary sinusotomy) 22.39
with removal of membrane lining 22.31
Callander (knee disarticulation) 84.16
Campbell
bone block, ankle 81.11
fasciotomy (iliac crest) 83.14
reconstruction of anterior cruciate ligaments 81.45
canthus NEC 08.99
cardiac NEC 37.99
septum NEC 35.98
valve NEC 35.99
carotid body or gland NEC 39.8
Carroll and Taber (arthroplasty proximal interphalangeal joint) 81.72

Ober (-Yount) operation — Operation

Index to Procedures

Operation — *continued*

Cattell (herniorrhaphy) 53.51
Cecil (urethral reconstruction) 58.46
cecum NEC 46.99
cerebral (meninges) NEC 02.99
cervix NEC 69.99
Chandler (hip fusion) 81.21
Charles (correction of lymphedema) 40.9
Charnley (compression arthrodesis)
  ankle 81.11
  hip 81.21
  knee 81.22
Cheatle-Henry — *see* Repair, hernia, femoral
chest cavity NEC 34.99
Chevalier-Jackson (partial laryngectomy) 30.29
Child (radical subtotal pancreatectomy) 52.53
Chopart (midtarsal amputation) 84.12
chordae tendineae NEC 35.32
choroid NEC 14.9
ciliary body NEC 12.98
cisterna chyli NEC 40.69
Clagett (closure of chest wall following open flap drainage) 34.72
Clayton (resection of metatarsal heads and bases of phalanges) 77.88
clitoris NEC 71.4
cocked hat (metacarpal lengthening and transfer of local flap) 82.69
Cockett (varicose vein)
  lower limb 38.59
  upper limb 38.53
Cody tack (perforation of footplate) 19.0
Coffey (uterine suspension) (Meigs' modification) 69.22
Cole (anterior tarsal wedge osteotomy) 77.28
Collis-Nissen (hiatal hernia repair) 53.80
colon NEC 46.99
Colonna
  adductor tenotomy (first stage) 83.12
  hip arthroplasty (second stage) 81.40
  reconstruction of hip (second stage) 81.40
commando (radical glossectomy) 25.4
conjunctiva NEC 10.99
  destructive NEC 10.33
cornea NEC 11.99
Coventry (tibial wedge osteotomy) 77.27
Crawford (tarso-frontalis sling of eyelid) 08.32
cul-de-sac NEC 70.92
Culp-Deweerd (spiral flap pyeloplasty) 55.87
Culp-Scardino (ureteral flap pyeloplasty) 55.87
Curtis (interphalangeal joint arthroplasty) 81.72
cystocele NEC 70.51
Dahlman (excision of esophageal diverticulum) 42.31
Dana (posterior rhizotomy) 03.1
Danforth (fetal) 73.8
Darrach (ulnar resection) 77.83
Davis (intubated ureterotomy) 56.2
de Grandmont (tarsectomy) 08.35
Delorme
  pericardiectomy 37.31
  proctopexy 48.76
  repair of prolapsed rectum 48.76
  thoracoplasty 33.34
Denker (radical maxillary antrotomy) 22.31
Dennis-Varco (herniorrhaphy) — *see* Repair, hernia, femoral
Denonvillier (limited rhinoplasty) 21.86
dental NEC 24.99
  orthodontic NEC 24.8
Derlacki (tympanoplasty) 19.4
diaphragm NEC 34.89
Dickson (fascial transplant) 83.82
Dickson-Diveley (tendon transfer and arthrodesis to correct claw toe) 77.57
Dieffenbach (hip disarticulation) 84.18
digestive tract NEC 46.99
Doléris (shortening of round ligaments) 69.22
D'Ombrain (excision of pterygium with corneal graft) 11.32
Dorrance (push-back operation for cleft palate) 27.62
Dotter (transluminal angioplasty) 39.59
Douglas (suture of tongue to lip for micrognathia) 25.59

Operation — *continued*

Doyle (paracervical uterine denervation) 69.3
Duhamel (abdominoperineal pull-through) 48.65
Dührssen (vaginofixation of uterus) 69.22
Dunn (triple arthrodesis) 81.12
duodenum NEC 46.99
Dupuytren
  fasciectomy 82.35
  fasciotomy 82.12
    with excision 82.35
  shoulder disarticulation 84.08
Durham (-Caldwell) (transfer of biceps femoris tendon) 83.75
DuToit and Roux (staple capsulorrhaphy of shoulder) 81.82
DuVries (tenoplasty) 83.88
Dwyer
  fasciotomy 83.14
  soft tissue release NEC 83.84
  wedge osteotomy, calcaneus 77.28
Eagleton (extrapetrosal drainage) 20.22
ear (external) NEC 18.9
  middle or inner NEC 20.99
Eden-Hybinette (glenoid bone block) 78.01
Effler (heart) 36.2
Eggers
  tendon release (patellar retinacula) 83.13
  tendon transfer (biceps femoris tendon) (hamstring tendon) 83.75
Elliot (scleral trephination with iridectomy) 12.61
Ellis Jones (repair of peroneal tendon) 83.88
Ellison (reinforcement of collateral ligament) 81.44
Elmslie-Cholmeley (tarsal wedge osteotomy) 77.28
Eloesser
  thoracoplasty 33.34
  thoracostomy 34.09
Emmet (cervix) 67.61
endorectal pull-through 48.41
epididymis NEC 63.99
esophagus NEC 42.99
Estes (ovary) 65.72
  laparoscopic 65.75
Estlander (thoracoplasty) 33.34
Evans (release of clubfoot) 83.84
extraocular muscle NEC 15.9
  multiple (two or more muscles) 15.4
    with temporary detachment from globe 15.3
  revision 15.6
  single 15.29
    with temporary detachment from globe 15.19
eyeball NEC 16.99
eyelid(s) NEC 08.99
face NEC 27.99
facial bone or joint NEC 76.99
fallopian tube NEC 66.99
Farabeuf (ischiopubiotomy) 77.39
Fasanella-Servatt (blepharoptosis repair) 08.35
fascia NEC 83.99
  hand 82.99
female (genital organs) NEC 71.9
  hysterectomy NEC 68.9
fenestration (aorta) 39.54
Ferguson (hernia repair) 53.00
Fick (perforation of footplate) 19.0
filtering (for glaucoma) 12.79
  with iridectomy 12.65
Finney (pyloroplasty) 44.2 ✓4ᵗʰ
fistulizing, sclera NEC 12.69
Foley (pyeloplasty) 55.87
Fontan (creation of conduit between right atrium and pulmonary artery) 35.94
Fothergill (-Donald) (uterine suspension) 69.22
Fowler
  arthroplasty of metacarpophalangeal joint 81.72
  release (mallet finger repair) 82.84
  tenodesis (hand) 82.85
  thoracoplasty 33.34
Fox (entropion repair with wedge resection) 08.43

Operation — *continued*

Franco (suprapubic cystotomy) 57.19
Frank (permanent gastrostomy) 43.19
Frazier (-Spiller) (subtemporal trigeminal rhizotomy) 04.02
Fredet-Ramstedt (pyloromyotomy) (with wedge resection) 43.3
Frenckner (intrapetrosal drainage) 20.22
Frickman (abdominal proctopexy) 48.75
Frommel (shortening of uterosacral ligaments) 69.22
Gabriel (abdominoperineal resection of rectum) 48.5
gallbladder NEC 51.99
ganglia NEC 04.99
  sympathetic 05.89
Gant (wedge osteotomy of trochanter) 77.25
Garceau (tibial tendon transfer) 83.75
Gardner (spinal meningocele repair) 03.51
gastric NEC 44.99
Gelman (release of clubfoot) 83.84
genital organ NEC
  female 71.9
  male 64.99
Ghormley (hip fusion) 81.21
Gifford
  destruction of lacrimal sac 09.6
  keratotomy (delimiting) 11.1
Gill
  arthrodesis of shoulder 81.23
  laminectomy 03.09
Gill-Stein (carporadial arthrodesis) 81.25
Gilliam (uterine suspension) 69.22
Girdlestone
  laminectomy with spinal fusion 81.00
  muscle transfer for claw toe 77.57
  resection of femoral head and neck 77.85
Girdlestone-Taylor (muscle transfer for claw toe repair) 77.57
glaucoma NEC 12.79
Glenn (anastomosis of superior vena cava to right pulmonary artery) 39.21
globus pallidus NEC 01.42
Goebel-Frangenheim-Stoeckel (urethrovesical suspension) 59.4
Goldner (clubfoot release) 80.48
Goldthwait
  ankle stabilization 81.11
  patella stabilization 81.44
  tendon transfer for patella dislocation 81.44
Goodall-Power (vagina) 70.4
Gordon-Taylor (hindquarter amputation) 84.19
Graber-Duvernay (drilling femoral head) 77.15
Green (scapulopexy) 78.41
Grice (subtalar arthrodesis) 81.13
Gritti-Stokes (knee disarticulation) 84.16
Gross (herniorrhaphy) 53.49
gum NEC 24.39
Guyon (amputation of ankle) 84.13
Hagner (epididymotomy) 63.92
Halsted — *see* Repair, hernia, inguinal
Hampton (anastomosis small intestine to rectal stump) 45.92
hanging hip (muscle release) 83.19
harelip 27.54
Harrison-Richardson (vaginal suspension) 70.77
Hartmann — *see* Colectomy, by site
Hauser
  achillotenotomy 83.11
  bunionectomy with adductor tendon transfer 77.53
  stabilization of patella 81.44
Heaney (vaginal hysterectomy) 68.59
  laparoscopically assisted (LAVH) 68.51
heart NEC 37.99
  valve NEC 35.99
    adjacent structure NEC 35.39
Hegar (perineorrhaphy) 71.79
Heine (cyclodialysis) 12.55
Heineke-Mikulicz (pyloroplasty) 44.2 ✓4ᵗʰ
Heller (esophagomyotomy) 42.7
Hellström (transplantation of aberrant renal vessel) 39.55
hemorrhoids NEC 49.49
Henley (jejunal transposition) 43.81

Operation — *continued*
hepatic NEC 50.99
hernia — *see* Repair, hernia
Hey (amputation of foot) 84.12
Hey-Groves (reconstruction of anterior cruciate
 ligament) 81.45
Heyman (soft tissue release for clubfoot) 83.84
Heyman-Herndon (-Strong) (correction of
 metatarsus varus) 80.48
Hibbs (lumbar spinal fusion) — *see* Fusion,
 lumbar
Higgins — *see* Repair, hernia, femoral
Hill-Allison (hiatal hernia repair, transpleural
 approach) 53.80
Hitchcock (anchoring tendon of biceps) 83.88
Hofmeister (gastrectomy) 43.7
Hoke
 midtarsal fusion 81.14
 triple arthrodesis 81.12
Holth
 iridencleisis 12.63
 sclerectomy 12.65
Homan (correction of lymphedema) 40.9
Hutch (ureteroneocystostomy) 56.74
Hybinette-eden (glenoid bone block) 78.01
hymen NEC 70.91
hypopharynx NEC 29.99
hypophysis NEC 07.79
ileal loop 56.51
ileum NEC 46.99
intestine NEC 46.99
iris NEC 12.97
 inclusion 12.63
Irving (tubal ligation) 66.32
Irwin (*see also* Osteotomy) 77.30
Jaboulay (gastroduodenostomy) 44.39
Janeway (permanent gastrostomy) 43.19
Jatene (arterial switch) 35.84
jejunum NEC 46.99
Johanson (urethral reconstruction) 58.46
joint (capsule) (ligament) (structure) NEC 81.99
 facial NEC 76.99
Jones
 claw toe (transfer of extensor hallucis longus
  tendon) 77.57
  modified (with arthrodesis) 77.57
 dacryocystorhinostomy 09.81
 hammer toe (interphalangeal fusion) 77.56
 modified (tendon transfer with arthrodesis)
  77.57
 repair of peroneal tendon 83.88
Joplin (exostectomy with tendon transfer) 77.53
Kader (temporary gastrostomy) 43.19
Kaufman (for urinary stress incontinence)
 59.79
Kazanjiian (buccal vestibular sulcus extension)
 24.91
Kehr (hepatopexy) 50.69
Keller (bunionectomy) 77.59
Kelly (-Kennedy) (urethrovesical plication) 59.3
Kelly-Stoeckel (urethrovesical plication) 59.3
Kerr (cesarean section) 74.1
Kessler (arthroplasty, carpometacarpal joint)
 81.74
Kidner (excision of accessory navicular bone)
 (with tendon transfer) 77.98
kidney NEC 55.99
Killian (frontal sinusotomy) 22.41
King-Steelquist (hindquarter amputation) 84.19
Kirk (amputation through thigh) 84.17
Kock pouch
 bowel anastomosis — *omit code*
 continent ileostomy 46.22
 cutaneous uretero-ileostomy 56.51
 ESWL (electrocorporeal shockwave
  lithotripsy) 98.51
 removal, calculus 57.19
 revision, cutaneous uretero-ileostomy 56.52
 urinary diversion procedure 56.51
Kondoleon (correction of lymphedema) 40.9
Krause (sympathetic denervation) 05.29
Kroener (partial salpingectomy) 66.69
Kroenlein (lateral orbitotomy) 16.01
Krönig (low cervical cesarean section) 74.1
Krukenberg (reconstruction of below-elbow
 amputation) 82.89

Operation — *continued*
Kuhnt-Szymanowski (ectropion repair with lid
 reconstruction) 08.44
Labbe (gastrotomy) 43.0
labia NEC 71.8
lacrimal
 gland 09.3
 system NEC 09.99
Ladd (mobilization of intestine) 54.95
Lagrange (iridosclerectomy) 12.65
Lambrinudi (triple arthrodesis) 81.12
Langenbeck (cleft palate repair) 27.62
Lapidus (bunionectomy with metatarsal
 osteotomy) 77.51
Larry (shoulder disarticulation) 84.08
larynx NEC 31.98
Lash operation (internal cervical os repair)
 67.59
Latzko
 cesarean section, extraperitoneal 74.2
 colpocleisis 70.8
Leadbetter (urethral reconstruction) 58.46
Leadbetter-Politano (ureteroneocystostomy)
 56.74
Le Fort (colpocleisis) 70.8
LeMesurier (cleft lip repair) 27.54
lens NEC 13.9
Leriche (periarterial sympathectomy) 05.25
levator muscle sling
 eyelid ptosis repair 08.33
 urethrovesical suspension 59.71
 urinary stress incontinence 59.71
lid suture (blepharoptosis) 08.31
ligament NEC 81.99
 broad NEC 69.98
 round NEC 69.98
 uterine NEC 69.98
Lindholm (repair of ruptured tendon) 83.88
Linton (varicose vein) 38.59
lip NEC 27.99
Lisfranc
 foot amputation 84.12
 shoulder disarticulation 84.08
Littlewood (forequarter amputation) 84.09
 liver NEC 50.99
 Lloyd-Davies (abdominoperineal resection)
  48.5
Longmire (bile duct anastomosis) 51.39
Lord
 dilation of anal canal for hemorrhoids 49.49
 hemorrhoidectomy 49.49
 orchidopexy 62.5
Lucas and Murray (knee arthrodesis with plate)
 81.22
lung NEC 33.99
lung volume reduction 32.22
lymphatic structure(s) NEC 40.9
 duct, left (thoracic) NEC 40.69
Madlener (tubal ligation) 66.31
Magnuson (-Stack) (arthroplasty for recurrent
 shoulder dislocation) 81.82
male genital organs NEC 64.99
Manchester (-Donald) (-Fothergill), (uterine
 suspension) 69.22
mandible NEC 76.99
 orthognathic 76.64
Marckwald operation (cervical os repair) 67.59
Marshall-Marchetti (-Krantz) (retropubic
 urethral suspension) 59.5
Matas (aneurysmorrhaphy) 39.52
Mayo
 bunionectomy 77.59
 herniorrhaphy 53.49
 vaginal hysterectomy 68.59
  laparoscopically assisted (LAVH) 68.51
Mazet (knee disarticulation) 84.16
McBride (bunionectomy with soft tissue
 correction) 77.53
McBurney — *see* Repair, hernia, inguinal
McCall (enterocele repair) 70.92
McCauley (release of clubfoot) 83.84
McDonald (encirclement suture, cervix)
 67.59
McIndoe (vaginal construction) 70.61
McKeever (fusion of first metatarsophalangeal
 joint for hallux valgus repair) 77.52

Operation — *continued*
McKissock (breast reduction) 85.33
McReynolds (transposition of pterygium) 11.31
McVay
 femoral hernia — *see* Repair hernia, femoral
 inguinal hernia — *see* Repair hernia,
  inguinal
meninges (spinal) NEC 03.99
 cerebral NEC 02.99
mesentery NEC 54.99
Mikulicz (exteriorization of intestine) (first
 stage) 46.03
 second stage 46.04
Miles (complete proctectomy) 48.5
Millard (cheiloplasty) 27.54
Miller
 midtarsal arthrodesis 81.14
 urethrovesical suspension 59.4
Millin-Read (urethrovesical suspension) 59.4
Mitchell (hallux valgus repair) 77.51
Mohs (chemosurgical excision of skin) 86.24
Moore (arthroplasty) 81.52
Moschowitz
 enterocele repair 70.92
 herniorrhaphy — *see* Repair, hernia, femoral
 sigmoidopexy 46.63
mouth NEC 27.99
Muller (banding of pulmonary artery) 38.85
Mumford (partial claviculectomy) 77.81
muscle NEC 83.99
 extraocular — *see* Operation, extraocular
 hand NEC 82.99
 papillary heart NEC 35.31
musculoskeletal system NEC 84.99
Mustard (interatrial transposition of venous
 return) 35.91
nail (finger) (toe) NEC 86.99
nasal sinus NEC 22.9
nasopharynx NEC 29.99
nerve (cranial) (peripheral) NEC 04.99
 adrenal NEC 07.49
 sympathetic NEC 05.89
nervous system NEC 05.9
Nicola (tenodesis for recurrent dislocation of
 shoulder) 81.82
nipple NEC 85.99
Nissen (fundoplication of stomach) 44.66
Noble (plication of small intestine) 46.62
node (lymph) NEC 40.9
Norman Miller (vaginopexy) 70.77
Norton (extraperitoneal cesarean operation)
 74.2
nose, nasal NEC 21.99
 sinus NEC 22.9
Ober (-Yount) (gluteal-iliotibial fasciotomy)
 83.14
obstetric NEC 75.99
ocular NEC 16.99
 muscle — *see* Operation, extraocular muscle
O'Donoghue (triad knee repair) 81.43
Olshausen (uterine suspension) 69.22
omentum NEC 54.99
ophthalmologic NEC 16.99
oral cavity NEC 27.99
orbicularis muscle sling 08.36
orbit NEC 16.98
oropharynx NEC 29.99
orthodontic NEC 24.8
orthognathic NEC 76.69
Oscar Miller (midtarsal arthrodesis) 81.14
Osmond-Clark (soft tissue release with
 peroneus brevis tendon transfer) 83.75
ovary NEC 65.99
Oxford (for urinary incontinence) 59.4
palate NEC 27.99
palpebral ligament sling 08.36
Panas (linear proctotomy) 48.0
Pancoast (division of trigeminal nerve at
 foramen ovale) 04.02
pancreas NEC 52.99
pantaloon (revision of gastic anastomosis) 44.5
papillary muscle (heart) NEC 35.31
Paquin (ureteroneocystostomy) 56.74
parathyroid gland(s) NEC 06.99
parotid gland or duct NEC 26.99
Partsch (marsupialization of dental cyst) 24.4

☑4ᵗʰ Fourth-digit Required   ▶◀ Revised Text   ● New Line   ▲ Revised Code

✓4ᵗʰ Fourth-digit Required　　▶◀ Revised Text　　● New Line　　▲ Revised Code

Operation — Osteotomy

Operation — *continued*
tongue NEC 25.99
flap, palate 27.62
tie 25.91
tonsil NEC 28.99
Torek (-Bevan) (orchidopexy) (first stage) (second stage) 62.5
Torkildsen (ventriculocisternal shunt) 02.2
Torpin (cul-de-sac resection) 70.92
Toti (dacryocystorhinostomy) 09.81
Touchas 86.83
Touroff (ligation of subclavian artery) 38.85
trabeculae corneae cordis (heart) NEC 35.35
trachea NEC 31.99
Trauner (lingual sulcus extension) 24.91
truncus arteriosus NEC 35.83
Tsuge (macrodactyly repair) 82.83
Tudor "rabbit ear" (anterior urethropexy) 59.79
Tuffier
apicolysis of lung 33.39
vaginal hysterectomy 68.59
laparoscopically assisted (LAVH) 68.51
tunica vaginalis NEC 61.99
Turco (release of joint capsules in clubfoot) 80.48
Uchida (tubal ligation with or without fimbriectomy) 66.32
umbilicus NEC 54.99
urachus NEC 57.51
Urban (mastectomy) (unilateral) 85.47
bilateral 85.48
ureter NEC 56.99
urethra NEC 58.99
urinary system NEC 59.99
uterus NEC 69.99
supporting structures NEC 69.98
uvula NEC 27.79
vagina NEC 70.91
vascular NEC 39.99
vas deferens NFC 63.99
ligation NEC 63.71
vein NEC 39.99
vena cava sieve 38.7
vertebra NEC 78.49
vesical (bladder) NEC 57.99
vessel NEC 39.99
cardiac NEC 36.99
Vicq d'Azyr (larynx) 31.1
Vidal (varicocele ligation) 63.1
Vineberg (implantation of mammary artery into ventricle) 36.2
vitreous NEC 14.79
vocal cord NEC 31.98
von Kraske (proctectomy) 48.64
Voss (hanging hip operation) 83.19
Vulpius (-Compere) (lengthening of gastrocnemius muscle) 83.85
vulva NEC 71.8
Ward-Mayo (vaginal hysterectomy) 68.59
laparoscopically assisted (LAVH) 68.51
Wardill (cleft palate) 27.62
Waters (extraperitoneal cesarean section) 74.2
Waterston (aorta-right pulmonary artery anastomosis) 39.0
Watkins (-Wertheim) (uterus interposition) 69.21
Watson-Jones
hip arthrodesis 81.21
reconstruction of lateral ligaments, ankle 81.49
shoulder arthrodesis (extra-articular) 81.23
tenoplasty 83.88
Weir
appendicostomy 47.91
correction of nostrils 21.86
Wertheim (radical hysterectomy) 68.6
West (dacryocystorhinostomy) 09.81
Wheeler
entropion repair 08.44
halving procedure (eyelid) 08.24
Whipple (radical pancreaticoduodenectomy) 52.7
Child modification (radical subtotal pancreatectomy) 52.53
Rodney Smith modification (radical subtotal pancreatectomy) 52.53

Operation — *continued*
White (lengthening of tendo calcaneus by incomplete tenotomy) 83.11
Whitehead
glossectomy, radical 25.4
hemorrhoidectomy 49.46
Whitman
foot stabilization (talectomy) 77.98
hip reconstruction 81.40
repair of serratus anterior muscle 83.87
talectomy 77.98
trochanter wedge osteotomy 77.25
Wier (entropion repair) 08.44
Williams-Richardson (vaginal construction) 70.61
Wilms (thoracoplasty) 33.34
Wilson (angulation osteotomy for hallux valgus) 77.51
window
antrum (nasal sinus) — *see* Antrotomy, maxillary
aorticopulmonary 39.59
bone cortex (*see also* Incision, bone) 77.10
facial 76.09
nasoantral — *see* Antrotomy, maxillary
pericardium 37.12
pleural 34.09
Winiwarter (cholecystoenterostomy) 51.32
Witzel (temporary gastrostomy) 43.19
Woodward (release of high riding scapula) 81.83
Young
epispadias repair 58.45
tendon transfer (anterior tibialis) (repair of flat foot) 83.75
Yount (division of iliotibial band) 83.14
Zancolli
capsuloplasty 81.72
tendon transfer (biceps) 82.56
Ziegler (iridectomy) 12.14
Operculectomy 24.6
Ophthalmectomy 16.49
with implant (into Tenon's capsule) 16.42
with attachment of muscles 16.41
Ophthalmoscopy 16.21
Opponensplasty (hand) 82.56
Orbitomaxillectomy, radical 16.51
Orbitotomy (anterior) (frontal) (temporofrontal) (transfrontal) NEC 16.09
with
bone flap 16.01
insertion of implant 16.02
Kroenlein (lateral) 16.01
lateral 16.01
Orchidectomy (with epididymectomy) (unilateral) 62.3
bilateral (radical) 62.41
remaining or solitary testis 62.42
Orchidopexy 62.5
Orchidoplasty 62.69
Orchidorrhaphy 62.61
Orchidotomy 62.0
Orchiectomy (with epididymectomy) (unilateral) 62.3
bilateral (radical) 62.41
remaining or solitary testis 62.42
Orchiopexy 62.5
Orchioplasty 62.69
Orthoroentgenography — *see* Radiography
Oscar Miller operation (midtarsal arthrodesis) 81.14
Osmond-Clark operation (soft tissue release with peroneus brevis tendon transfer) 83.75
Ossiculectomy NEC 19.3
with
stapedectomy (*see also* Stapedectomy) 19.19
stapes mobilization 19.0
tympanoplasty 19.53
revision 19.6
Ossiculotomy NEC 19.3

Ostectomy (partial), except facial — *see also* category 77.8 ✓4ᵗʰ
facial NEC 76.39
total 76.45
with reconstruction 76.44
first metatarsal head — *see* Bunionectomy
for graft (autograft) (homograft) — *see also* category 77.7 ✓4ᵗʰ
mandible 76.31
total 76.42
with reconstruction 76.41
total, except facial — *see also* category 77.9 ✓4ᵗʰ
facial NEC 76.45
with reconstruction 76.44
mandible 76.42
with reconstruction 76.41
Osteoarthrotomy (*see also* Osteotomy) 77.30
Osteoclasis 78.70
carpal, metacarpal 78.74
clavicle 78.71
ear 20.79
femur 78.75
fibula 78.77
humerus 78.72
patella 78.76
pelvic 78.79
phalanges (foot) (hand) 78.79
radius 78.73
scapula 78.71
specified site NEC 78.79
tarsal, metatarsal 78.78
thorax (ribs) (sternum) 78.71
tibia 78.77
ulna 78.73
vertebrae 78.79
Osteolysis — *see* category 78.4 ✓4ᵗʰ
Osteopathic manipulation (*see also* Manipulation, osteopathic) 93.67
Osteoplasty NEC — *see* category 78.4 ✓4ᵗʰ
with bone graft — *see* Graft, bone
for
bone lengthening — *see* Lengthening, bone
bone shortening — *see* Shortening, bone
repair of malunion or nonunion of fracture — *see* Repair, fracture, malunion or nonunion
carpal, metacarpal 78.44
clavicle 78.41
cranium NEC 02.06
with
flap (bone) 02.03
graft (bone) 02.04
facial bone NEC 76.69
femur 78.45
fibula 78.47
humerus 78.42
mandible, mandibular NEC 76.64
body 76.63
ramus (open) 76.62
closed 76.61
maxilla (segmental) 76.65
total 76.66
nasal bones 21.89
patella 78.46
pelvic 78.49
phalanges (foot) (hand) 78.49
radius 78.43
scapula 78.41
skull NEC 02.06
with
flap (bone) 02.03
graft (bone) 02.04
specified site NEC 78.49
tarsal, metatarsal 78.48
thorax (ribs) (sternum) 78.41
tibia 78.47
ulna 78.43
vertebrae 78.49
Osteorrhaphy (*see also* Osteoplasty) 78.40
Osteosynthesis (fracture) — *see* Reduction, fracture
Osteotomy (adduction) (angulation) (block) (derotational) (displacement) (partial) (rotational) 77.30

✓4ᵗʰ Fourth-digit Required　▶◀ Revised Text　● New Line　▲ Revised Code

Osteotomy — *continued*
carpals, metacarpals 77.34
wedge 77.24
clavicle 77.31
wedge 77.21
facial bone NEC 76.69
femur 77.35
wedge 77.25
fibula 77.37
wedge 77.27
humerus 77.32
wedge 77.22
mandible (segmental) (subapical) 76.64
angle (open) 76.62
closed 76.61
body 76.63
Gigli saw 76.61
ramus (open) 76.62
closed 76.61
maxilla (segmental) 76.65
total 76.66
metatarsal 77.38
wedge 77.28
for hallux valgus repair 77.51
patella 77.36
wedge 77.26
pelvic 77.39
wedge 77.29
phalanges (foot) (hand) 77.39
for repair of
bunion — *see* Bunionectomy
bunionette 77.54
hallux valgus — *see* Bunionectomy
wedge 77.29
for repair of
bunion — *see* Bunionectomy
bunionette 77.54
hallux valgus — *see* Bunionectomy
radius 77.33
wedge 77.23
scapula 77.31
wedge 77.21
specified site NEC 77.39
wedge 77.29
tarsal 77.38
wedge 77.28
thorax (ribs) (sternum) 77.31
wedge 77.21
tibia 77.37
wedge 77.27
toe 77.39
for repair of
bunion — *see* Bunionectomy
bunionette 77.54
hallux valgus — *see* Bunionectomy
wedge 77.29
for repair of
bunion — *see* Bunionectomy
bunionette 77.54
hallux valgus — *see* Bunionectomy
ulna 77.33
wedge 77.23
vertebrae 77.39
wedge 77.29
Otonecrectomy (inner ear) 20.79
Otoplasty (external) 18.79
auditory canal or meatus 18.6
auricle 18.79
cartilage 18.79
reconstruction 18.71
prominent or protruding 18.5
Otoscopy 18.11
Outfolding, sclera, for buckling (*see also* Buckling, scleral) 14.49
Outfracture, turbinates (nasal) 21.62
Output and clearance, circulatory 92.05
Overdistension, bladder (therapeutic) 96.25
Overlapping, sclera, for buckling (*see also* Buckling, scleral) 14.49
Oversewing
pleural bleb 32.21
ulcer crater (peptic) 44.40
duodenum 44.42
stomach 44.41

Oxford operation (for urinary incontinence) 59.4
Oximetry
fetal pulse 75.38
Oxygenation 93.96
extracorporeal membrane (ECMO) 39.65
hyperbaric 93.95
wound 93.59
Oxygen therapy (catalytic) (pump) 93.96
hyperbaric 93.95

P

Pacemaker
cardiac — *see also* Insertion, pacemaker, cardiac
intraoperative (temporary) 39.64
temporary (during and immediately following cardiac surgery) 39.64
Packing — *see also* Insertion, pack
auditory canal 96.11
nose, for epistaxis (anterior) 21.01
posterior (and anterior) 21.02
rectal 96.19
sella turcica 07.79
vaginal 96.14
Palatoplasty 27.69
for cleft palate 27.62
secondary or subsequent 27.63
Palatorrhaphy 27.61
for cleft palate 27.62
Pallidectomy 01.42
Pallidoansotomy 01.42
Pallidotomy 01.42
by stereotactic radiosurgery 92.32
cobalt 60 92.32
linear accelerator (LINAC) 92.31
multi-source 92.32
particle beam 92.33
particulate 92.33
radiosurgery NEC 92.39
single source photon 92.31
Panas operation (linear proctotomy) 48.0
Pancoast operation (division of trigeminal nerve at foramen ovale) 04.02
Pancreatectomy (total) (with synchronous duodenectomy) 52.6
partial NEC 52.59
distal (tail) (with part of body) 52.52
proximal (head) (with part of body) (with synchronous duodenectomy) 52.51
radical 52.53
subtotal 52.53
radical 52.7
subtotal 52.53
Pancreaticocystoduodenostomy 52.4
Pancreaticocystoenterostomy 52.4
Pancreaticocystogastrostomy 52.4
Pancreaticocystojejunostomy 52.4
Pancreaticoduodenectomy (total) 52.6
partial NEC 52.59
proximal 52.51
radical subtotal 52.53
radical (one-stage) (two-stage) 52.7
subtotal 52.53
Pancreaticoduodenostomy 52.96
Pancreaticoenterostomy 52.96
Pancreaticogastrostomy 52.96
Pancreaticoileostomy 52.96
Pancreaticojejunostomy 52.96
Pancreatoduodenectomy (total) 52.6
partial NEC 52.59
radical (one-stage) (two-stage) 52.7
subtotal 52.53
Pancreatogram 87.66
endoscopic retrograde (ERP) 52.13
Pancreatolithotomy 52.09
endoscopic 52.94
Pancreatotomy 52.09

Pancreolithotomy 52.09
endoscopic 52.94
Panendoscopy 57.32
specified site, other than bladder — *see* Endoscopy, by site
through artificial stoma 57.31
Panhysterectomy (abdominal) 68.4
vaginal 68.59
laparoscopically assisted (LAVH) 68.51
Panniculectomy 86.83
Panniculotomy 86.83
Pantaloon operation (revision of gastric anastomosis) 44.5
Papillectomy, anal 49.39
endoscopic 49.31
Papillotomy (pancreas) 51.82
endoscopic 51.85
Paquin operation (ureteroneocystostomy) 56.74
Paracentesis
abdominal (percutaneous) 54.91
anterior chamber, eye 12.91
bladder 57.11
cornea 12.91
eye (anterior chamber) 12.91
thoracic, thoracis 34.91
tympanum 20.09
with intubation 20.01
Parasitology — *see* Examination, microscopic
Parathyroidectomy (partial) (subtotal) NEC 06.89
complete 06.81
ectopic 06.89
global removal 06.81
mediastinal 06.89
total 06.81
Parenteral nutrition, total 99.15
peripheral 99.15
Parotidectomy 26.30
complete 26.32
partial 26.31
radical 26.32
Partsch operation (marsupialization of dental cyst) 24.4
Passage — *see* Insertion and Intubation
Passage of sounds, urethra 58.6
Patch
blood, spinal (epidural) 03.95
graft — *see* Graft
spinal, blood (epidural) 03.95
subdural, brain 02.12
Patellapexy 78.46
Patellaplasty NEC 78.46
Patellectomy 77.96
partial 77.86
Pattee operation (auditory canal) 18.6
Pectenotomy (*see also* Sphincterotomy, anal) 49.59
Pedicle flap — *see* Graft, skin, pedicle
Peet operation (splanchnic resection) 05.29
PEG (percutaneous endoscopic gastrostomy) 43.11
PEJ (percutaneous endoscopic jejunostomy) 46.32
Pelvectomy, kidney (partial) 55.4
Pelvimetry 88.25
gynecological 89.26
Pelviolithotomy 55.11
Pelvioplasty, kidney 55.87
Pelviostomy 55.12
closure 55.82
Pelviotomy 77.39
to assist delivery 73.94
Pelvi-ureteroplasty 55.87
Pemberton operation
osteotomy of ilium 77.39
rectum (mobilization and fixation for prolapse repair) 48.76
Penectomy 64.3
Pereyra operation (paraurethral suspension) 59.6
Perforation
stapes footplate 19.0

Perfusion — Plexectomy

✔4ᵗʰ Fourth-digit Required   ▶◀ Revised Text   ● New Line   ▲ Revised Code

Index to Procedures

Procedure — Quotient, respiratory (side tab)

Procedure — *see also* specific procedure — *continued*
  diagnostic NEC — *continued*
    pituitary gland 07.19
    pleura 34.28
    posterior chamber, eye 14.19
    prostate 60.18
    pulmonary 33.29
    rectosigmoid 48.29
    rectum 48.29
    renal 55.29
    respiratory 33.29
    retina 14.19
    retroperitoneum 59.29
    salivary gland or duct 26.19
    sclera 12.29
    scrotum 61.19
    seminal vesicle 60.19
    sigmoid 45.28
    sinus, nasal 22.19
    skin 86.19
    skull 01.19
    soft tissue 83.29
    spermatic cord 63.09
    sphincter of Oddi 51.19
    spine, spinal (canal) (cord) (meninges) (structure) 03.39
    spleen 41.39
    stomach 44.19
    subcutaneous tissue 86.19
    sympathetic nerve 05.19
    tarsus 09.19
    tendon NEC 83.29
      extraocular 15.09
    testicle 62.19
    thalamus 01.18
    thoracic duct 40.19
    thorax 34.28
    thymus 07.19
    thyroid gland 06.19
    tongue 25.09
    tonsils 28.19
    tooth 24.19
    trachea 31.49
    tunica vaginalis 61.19
    ureter 56.39
    urethra 58.29
    uterus and supporting structures 68.19
    uvula 27.29
    vagina 70.29
    vas deferens 63.09
    vesical 57.39
    vessel (blood) (any site) 38.2
    vitreous 14.19
    vulva 71.19
  fistulizing, sclera NEC 12.69
  miscellaneous (nonoperative) NEC 99.99
  respiratory (nonoperative) NEC 93.99
  surgical — *see* Operation
Proctectasis 96.22
Proctectomy (partial) (*see also* Resection, rectum) 48.69
  abdominoperineal 48.5
  complete (Miles) (Rankin) 48.5
  pull-through 48.49
Proctoclysis 96.37
Proctolysis 48.99
Proctopexy (Delorme) 48.76
  abdominal (Ripstein) 48.75
Proctoplasty 48.79
Proctorrhaphy 48.71
Proctoscopy 48.23
  with biopsy 48.24
  through stoma (artificial) 48.22
  transabdominal approach 48.21
Proctosigmoidectomy (*see also* Resection, rectum) 48.69
Proctosigmoidopexy 48.76
Proctosigmoidoscopy (rigid) 48.23
  with biopsy 48.24
  flexible 45.24
  through stoma (artificial) 48.22
  transabdominal approach 48.21

Proctostomy 48.1
Proctotomy (decompression) (linear) 48.0
Production — *see also* Formation and Creation
  atrial septal defect 35.42
  subcutaneous tunnel for esophageal anastomosis 42.86
    with anastomosis — *see* Anastomosis, esophagus, antesternal
Prognathic recession 76.64
Prophylaxis, dental (scaling) (polishing) 96.54
Prostatectomy (complete) (partial) NEC 60.69
  loop 60.29
  perineal 60.62
  radical (any approach) 60.5
  retropubic (punch) (transcapsular) 60.4
  suprapubic (punch) (transvesical) 60.3
  transcapsular NEC 60.69
    retropubic 60.4
  transperineal 60.62
  transurethral 60.29
    ablation (contact) (noncontact) by laser 60.21
    electrovaporization 60.29
    enucleative 60.29
    resection of prostate (TURP) 60.29
    ultrasound guided laser induced (TULIP) 60.21
  transvesical punch (suprapubic) 60.3
Prostatocystotomy 60.0
Prostatolithotomy 60.0
Prostatotomy (perineal) 60.0
Prostatovesiculectomy 60.5
Protection (of)
  individual from his surroundings 99.84
  surroundings from individual 99.84
Psychoanalysis 94.31
Psychodrama 94.43
Psychotherapy NEC 94.39
  biofeedback 94.39
  exploratory verbal 94.37
  group 94.44
    for psychosexual dysfunctions 94.41
  play 94.36
  psychosexual dysfunctions 94.34
  supportive verbal 94.38
PTCA (percutaneous transluminal coronary angioplasty) — *see* Angioplasty, balloon, coronary
Ptyalectasis 26.91
Ptyalithotomy 26.0
Ptyalolithotomy 26.0
Pubiotomy 77.39
  assisting delivery 73.94
Pubococcygeoplasty 59.71
Puestow operation (pancreaticojejunostomy) 52.96
Pull-through
  abdomino-anal 48.49
  abdominoperineal 48.49
    Duhamel type 48.65
  endorectal 48.41
Pulmowrap 93.99
Pulpectomy (*see also* Therapy, root canal) 23.70
Pulpotomy (*see also* Therapy, root canal) 23.70
Pump-oxygenator, for extracorporeal circulation 39.61
  percutaneous 39.66
Punch
  operation
    bladder neck, transurethral 57.49
    prostate — *see* Prostatectomy
  resection, vocal cords 30.22
Puncture
  antrum (nasal) (bilateral) (unilateral) 22.01
  artery NEC 38.98
    for
      arteriography (*see also* Arteriography) 88.40
      coronary arteriography (*see also* Arteriography, coronary) 88.57
      percutanous vascular closure — *omit code*

Puncture — *continued*
  bladder, suprapubic (for drainage) NEC 57.18
    needle 57.11
    percutaneous (suprapubic) 57.17
  bursa 83.94
    hand 82.92
  cisternal 01.01
    with contrast media 87.02
  cranial 01.09
    with contrast media 87.02
  craniobuccal pouch 07.72
  craniopharyngioma 07.72
  fallopian tube 66.91
  fontanel, anterior 01.09
  heart 37.0
    for intracardiac injection 37.92
  hypophysis 07.72
  iris 12.12
  joint 81.91
  kidney (percutaneous) 55.92
  larynx 31.98
  lumbar (diagnostic) (removal of dye) 03.31
  lung (for aspiration) 33.93
  nasal sinus 22.01
  pericardium 37.0
  pituitary gland 07.72
  pleural cavity 34.91
  Rathke's pouch 07.72
  spinal 03.31
  spleen 41.1
    for biopsy 41.32
  sternal (for bone marrow biopsy) 41.31
    donor for bone marrow transplant 41.91
  vein NEC 38.99
    for
      phlebography (*see also* Phlebography) 88.60
      transfusion — *see* Transfusion
  ventricular shunt tubing 01.02
Pupillotomy 12.35
Push-back operation (cleft palate repair) 27.62
Putti-Platt operation (capsulorrhaphy of shoulder for recurrent dislocation) 81.82
Pyelogram (intravenous) 87.73
  infusion (continuous) (diuretic) 87.73
  percutaneous 87.75
  retrograde 87.74
Pyeloileostomy 56.71
Pyelolithotomy 55.11
Pyeloplasty 55.87
Pyelorrhaphy 55.81
Pyeloscopy 55.22
Pyelostolithotomy, percutaneous 55.03
Pyelostomy 55.12
  closure 55.82
Pyelotomy 55.11
Pyeloureteroplasty 55.87
Pylorectomy 43.6
Pyloroduodenotomy — *see category* 44.2 ✔4ᵗʰ
Pyloromyotomy (Ramstedt) (with wedge resection) 43.3
Pyloroplasty (Finney) (Heineke-Mikulicz) 44.29
  dilation, endoscopic 44.22
    by incision 44.21
  not elsewhere classified 44.29
  revision 44.29
Pylorostomy — *see* Gastrostomy

Q

Quadrant resection of breast 85.22
Quadricepsplasty (Thompson) 83.86
Quarantine 99.84
Quenuthoracoplasty 77.31
Quotient, respiratory 89.38

R

Rachicentesis 03.31

Rachitomy 03.09

Radiation therapy — *see also* Therapy, radiation
  teleradiotheraphy — *see* Teleradiotheraphy

Radical neck dissection — *see* Dissection, neck

Radicotomy 03.1

Radiculectomy 03.1

Radiculotomy 03.1

Radiography (diagnostic) NEC 88.39
  abdomen, abdominal (flat plate) NEC 88.19
    wall (soft tissue) NEC 88.09
  adenoid 87.09
  ankle (skeletal) 88.28
    soft tissue 88.37
  bone survey 88.31
  bronchus 87.49
  chest (routine) 87.44
    wall NEC 87.39
  clavicle 87.43
  contrast (air) (gas) (radio-opaque substance)
      NEC
    abdominal wall 88.03
    arteries (by fluoroscopy) — *see* Arteriography
    bile ducts NEC 87.54
    bladder NEC 87.77
    brain 87.02
    breast 87.35
    bronchus NEC (transcricoid) 87.32
      endotracheal 87.31
    epididymis 87.93
    esophagus 87.61
    fallopian tubes
      gas 87.82
      opaque dye 87.83
    fistula (sinus tract) — *see also* Radiography,
        contrast, by site
      abdominal wall 88.03
      chest wall 87.38
    gallbladder NEC 87.59
    intervertebral disc(s) 87.21
    joints 88.32
    larynx 87.07
    lymph — *see* Lymphangiogram
    mammary ducts 87.35
    mediastinum 87.33
    nasal sinuses 87.15
    nasolacrimal ducts 87.05
    nasopharynx 87.06
    orbit 87.14
    pancreas 87.66
    pelvis
      gas 88.12
      opaque dye 88.11
    peritoneum NEC 88.13
    retroperitoneum NEC 88.15
    seminal vesicles 87.91
    sinus tract — *see also* Radiography,
        contrast, by site
      abdominal wall 88.03
      chest wall 87.38
      nose 87.15
    skull 87.02
    spinal disc(s) 87.21
    trachea 87.32
    uterus
      gas 87.82
      opaque dye 87.83
    vas deferens 87.94
    veins (by fluoroscopy) — *see* Phlebography
    vena cava (inferior) (superior) 88.51
  dental NEC 87.12
  diaphragm 87.49
  digestive tract NEC 87.69
    barium swallow 87.61
    lower GI series 87.64
    small bowel series 87.63
    upper GI series 87.62
  elbow (skeletal) 88.22
    soft tissue 88.35
  epididymis NEC 87.95
  esophagus 87.69
    barium-swallow 87.61
  eye 95.14

Radiography NEC — *continued*
  face, head, and neck 87.09
  facial bones 87.16
  fallopian tubes 87.85
  foot 88.28
  forearm (skeletal) 88.22
    soft tissue 88.35
  frontal area, facial 87.16
  genital organs
    female NEC 87.89
    male NEC 87.99
  hand (skeletal) 88.23
    soft tissue 88.35
  head NEC 87.09
  heart 87.49
  hip (skeletal) 88.26
    soft tissue 88.37
  intestine NEC 87.65
  kidney-ureter-bladder (KUB) 87.79
  knee (skeletal) 88.27
    soft tissue 88.37
  KUB (kidney-ureter-bladder) 87.79
  larynx 87.09
  lower leg (skeletal) 88.27
    soft tissue 88.37
  lower limb (skeletal) NEC 88.29
    soft tissue NEC 88.37
  lung 87.49
  mandible 87.16
  maxilla 87.16
  mediastinum 87.49
  nasal sinuses 87.16
  nasolacrimal duct 87.09
  nasopharynx 87.09
  neck NEC 87.09
  nose 87.16
  orbit 87.16
  pelvis (skeletal) 88.26
    pelvimetry 88.25
    soft tissue 88.19
  prostate NEC 87.92
  retroperitoneum NEC 88.16
  ribs 87.43
  root canal 87.12
  salivary gland 87.09
  seminal vesicles NEC 87.92
  shoulder (skeletal) 88.21
    soft tissue 88.35
  skeletal NEC 88.33
    series (whole or complete) 88.31
  skull (lateral, sagittal or tangential projection)
      NEC 87.17
  spine NEC 87.29
    cervical 87.22
    lumbosacral 87.24
    sacrococcygeal 87.24
    thoracic 87.23
  sternum 87.43
  supraorbital area 87.16
  symphysis menti 87.16
  teeth NEC 87.12
    full-mouth 87.11
  thigh (skeletal) 88.27
    soft tissue 88.37
  thyroid region 87.09
  tonsils and adenoids 87.09
  trachea 87.49
  ultrasonic — *see* Ultrasonography
  upper arm (skeletal) 88.21
    soft tissue 88.35
  upper limb (skeletal) NEC 88.24
    soft tissue NEC 88.35
  urinary system NEC 87.79
  uterus NEC 87.85
    gravid 87.81
  uvula 87.09
  vas deferens NEC 87.95
  wrist 88.23
  zygomaticomaxillary complex 87.16

Radioisotope
  scanning — *see* Scan, radioisotope
  therapy — *see* Therapy, radioisotope

Radiology
  diagnostic — *see* Radiography
  therapeutic — *see* Therapy, radiation

Radiosurgery, stereotactic 92.30
  cobalt 60 92.32
  linear accelerator (LINAC) 92.31
  multi-source 92.32
  particle beam 92.33
  particulate 92.33
  radiosurgery NEC 92.39
  single source photon 92.31

Raising, pedicle graft 86.71

Ramadier operation (intrapetrosal drainage)
    20.22

Ramisection (sympathetic) 05.0

Ramstedt operation (pyeloromyotomy) (with
    wedge resection) 43.3

Range of motion testing 93.05

Rankin operation
  exteriorization of intestine 46.03
  proctectomy (complete) 48.5

Rashkind operation (balloon septostomy) 35.41

Rastelli operation (creation of conduit between
    right ventricle and pulmonary artery) 35.92
  in repair of
    pulmonary artery atresia 35.92
    transposition of great vessels 35.92
    truncus arteriosus 35.83

Raz-Pereyra procedure (Bladder neck
    suspension) 59.79

RCSA (radical cryosurgical ablation) of prostate
    60.62

Readjustment — *see* Adjustment

Reamputation, stump 84.3

Reanastomosis — *see* Anastomosis

Reattachment
  amputated ear 18.72
  ankle 84.27
  arm (upper) NEC 84.24
  choroid and retina NEC 14.59
    by
      cryotherapy 14.52
      diathermy 14.51
      electrocoagulation 14.51
      photocoagulation 14.55
        laser 14.54
        xenon arc 14.53
  ear (amputated) 18.72
  extremity 84.29
    ankle 84.27
    arm (upper) NEC 84.24
    fingers, except thumb 84.22
      thumb 84.21
    foot 84.26
    forearm 84.23
    hand 84.23
    leg (lower) NEC 84.27
    thigh 84.28
    thumb 84.21
    toe 84.25
    wrist 84.23
  finger 84.22
    thumb 84.21
  foot 84.26
  forearm 84.23
  hand 84.23
  joint capsule (*see also* Arthroplasty) 81.96
  leg (lower) NEC 84.27
  ligament — *see also* Arthroplasty
    uterosacral 69.22
  muscle 83.74
    hand 82.54
    papillary (heart) 35.31
  nerve (peripheral) 04.79
  nose (amputated) 21.89
  papillary muscle (heart) 35.31
  penis (amputated) 64.45
  retina (and choroid) NEC 14.59
    by
      cryotherapy 14.52
      diathermy 14.51
      electrocoagulation 14.51
      photocoagulation 14.55
        laser 14.54
        xenon arc 14.53

Reattachment — *continued*
tendon (to tendon) 83.73
hand 82.53
to skeletal attachment 83.88
hand 82.85
thigh 84.28
thumb 84.21
toe 84.25
tooth 23.5
uterosacral ligament(s) 69.22
vessels (peripheral) 39.59
renal, aberrant 39.55
wrist 84.23
Recession
extraocular muscle 15.11
multiple (two or more muscles) (with advancement or resection) 15.3
gastrocnemius tendon (Strayer operation) 83.72
levator palpebrae (superioris) muscle 08.38
prognathic jaw 76.64
tendon 83.72
hand 82.52
Reclosure — *see also* Closure
disrupted abdominal wall (postoperative) 54.61
Reconstruction (plastic) — *see also* Construction *and* Repair, by site
alveolus, alveolar (process) (ridge) (with graft or implant) 24.5
artery (graft) — *see* Graft, artery
artificial stoma, intestine 46.40
auditory canal (external) 18.6
auricle (ear) 18.71
bladder 57.87
with
ileum 57.87 [45.51]
sigmoid 57.87 [45.52]
bone, except facial (*see also* Osteoplasty) 78.40
facial NEC 76.46
with total ostectomy 76.44
mandible 76.43
with total mandibulectomy 76.41
breast, total 85.7
bronchus 33.48
canthus (lateral) 08.59
cardiac annulus 35.33
chest wall (mesh) (silastic) 34.79
cleft lip 27.54
conjunctival cul-de-sac 10.43
with graft (buccal mucous membrane) (free) 10.42
cornea NEC 11.79
diaphragm 34.84
ear (external) (auricle) 18.71
external auditory canal 18.6
meatus (new) (osseous skin-lined) 18.6
ossicles 19.3
prominent or protruding 18.5
eyebrow 08.70
eyelid 08.70
with graft or flap 08.69
hair follicle 08.63
mucous membrane 08.62
skin 08.61
tarsoconjunctival (one-stage) (two-stage) 08.64
full-thickness 08.74
involving lid margin 08.73
partial-thickness 08.72
involving lid margin 08.71
eye socket 16.64
with graft 16.63
fallopian tube 66.79
foot and toes (with fixation device) 81.57
with prosthetic implant 81.57
frontonasal duct 22.79
hip (total) (with prosthesis) 81.51
intraoral 27.59
joint — *see* Arthroplasty
lymphatic (by transplantation) 40.9
mandible 76.43
with total mandibulectomy 76.41
mastoid cavity 19.9
mouth 27.59
nipple NEC 85.87

Reconstruction (plastic) — *see also* Construction *and* Repair, by site — *continued*
nose (total) (with arm flap) (with forehead flap) 21.83
ossicles (graft) (prosthesis) NEC 19.3
with
stapedectomy 19.19
tympanoplasty 19.53
pelvic floor 71.79
penis (rib graft) (skin graft) (myocutaneous flap) 64.44
pharynx 29.4
scrotum (with pedicle flap) (with rotational flap) 61.49
skin (plastic) (without graft) NEC 86.89
with graft — *see* Graft, skin
subcutaneous tissue (plastic) (without skin graft) NEC 86.89
with graft — *see* Graft, skin
tendon pulley —(with graft) (with local tissue) 83.83
for opponensplasty 82.71
hand 82.71
thumb (osteoplastic) (with bone graft) (with skin graft) 82.69
trachea (with graft) 31.75
umbilicus 53.49
ureteropelvic junction 55.87
urethra 58.46
vagina 70.62
vas deferens, surgically divided 63.82
Recontour, gingiva 24.2
Recreational therapy 93.81
Rectectomy (*see also* Resection, rectum) 48.69
Rectopexy (Delorme) 48.76
abdominal (Ripstein) 48.75
Rectoplasty 48.79
Rectorectostomy 48.74
Rectorrhaphy 48.71
Rectosigmoidectomy (*see also* Resection, rectum) 48.69
transsacral 48.61
Rectosigmoidostomy 45.94
Rectostomy 48.1
closure 48.72
Red cell survival studies 92.05
Reduction
adipose tissue 86.83
batwing arms 86.83
breast (bilateral) 85.32
unilateral 85.31
bulbous tuberosities (mandible) (maxilla) (fibrous) (osseous) 24.31
buttocks 86.83
diastasis, ankle mortise (closed) 79.77
open 79.87
dislocation (of joint) (manipulation) (with cast) (with splint) (with traction device) (closed) 79.70
with fracture — *see* Reduction, fracture, by site
ankle (closed) 79.77
open 79.87
elbow (closed) 79.72
open 79.82
finger (closed) 79.74
open 79.84
foot (closed) 79.78
open 79.88
hand (closed) 79.74
open 79.84
hip (closed) 79.75
open 79.85
knee (closed) 79.76
open 79.86
open (with external fixation) (with internal fixation) 79.80
specified site NEC 79.89
shoulder (closed) 79.71
open 79.81
specified site (closed) NEC 79.79
open 79.89

Reduction — *continued*
dislocation — *continued*
temporomandibular (closed) 76.93
open 76.94
toe (closed) 79.78
open 79.88
wrist (closed) 79.73
open 79.83
elephantiasis, scrotum 61.3
epistaxis (*see also* Control, epistaxis) 21.00
fracture (bone) (with cast) (with splint) (with traction device) 79.00
with internal fixation 79.10
alveolar process (with stabilization of teeth)
mandible (closed) 76.75
open 76.77
maxilla (closed) 76.73
open 76.77
ankle — *see* Reduction, fracture, leg
arm (closed) NEC 79.02
with internal fixation 79.12
open 79.22
with internal fixation 79.32
blow-out — *see* Reduction, fracture, orbit
carpal, metacarpal (closed) 79.03
with internal fixation 79.13
open 79.23
with internal fixation 79.33
epiphysis — *see* Reduction, separation
facial (bone) NEC 76.70
closed 76.78
open 76.79
femur (closed) 79.05
with internal fixation 79.15
open 79.25
with internal fixation 79.35
fibula (closed) 79.06
with internal fixation 79.16
open 79.26
with internal fixation 79.36
foot (closed) NEC 79.07
with internal fixation 79.17
open 79.27
with internal fixation 79.37
hand (closed) NEC 79.03
with internal fixation 79.13
open 79.23
with internal fixation 79.33
humerus (closed) 79.01
with internal fixation 79.11
open 79.21
with internal fixation 79.31
jaw (lower) — *see also* Reduction, fracture, mandible
upper — *see* Reduction, fracture, maxilla
larynx 31.64
leg (closed) NEC 79.06
with internal fixation 79.16
open 79.26
with internal fixation 79.36
malar (closed) 76.71
open 76.72
mandible (with dental wiring) (closed) 76.75
open 76.76
maxilla (with dental wiring) (closed) 76.73
open 76.74
nasal (closed) 21.71
open 21.72
open 79.20
with internal fixation 79.30
specified site NEC 79.29
with internal fixation 79.39
orbit (rim) (wall) (closed) 76.78
open 76.79
patella (open) (with internal fixation) 79.36
phalanges
foot (closed) 79.08
with internal fixation 79.18
open 79.28
with internal fixation 79.38
hand (closed) 79.04
with internal fixation 79.14
open 79.24
with internal fixation 79.34

✔4ᵗ Fourth-digit Required   ▶◀ Revised Text   ● New Line   ▲ Revised Code

Release — Removal

Release — *continued*
tenosynovitis — *continued*
de Quervain's 82.01
external pollicis brevis 82.01
hand 82.01
torsion
intestine 46.80
large 46.82
endoscopic (balloon) 46.85
small 46.81
kidney pedicle 55.84
ovary 65.95
testes 63.52
transverse carpal ligament (for nerve
decompression) 04.43
trigger finger or thumb 82.01
urethral stricture 58.5
Volkmann's contracture
excision of scar, muscle 83.32
fasciotomy 83.14
muscle transplantation 83.77
web contracture (skin) 86.84

Relief — *see* Release

Relocation — *see also* Revision
cardiac pacemaker pocket, new site (skin)
(subcutaneous) 37.79
CRT-D pocket 37.99   ●
CRT-P pocket 37.79   ●

Remobilization
joint 93.16
stapes 19.0

Remodel
ventricle 37.35

Removal — *see also* Excision
Abrams bar (chest wall) 34.01
abscess — *see* Incision, by site
adenoid tag(s) 28.6
anal sphincter   ●
with revision 49.75   ●
without revision 49.76   ●
arch bars (orthodontic) 24.8
immobilization device 97.33
arterial graft or prosthesis 39.49
arteriovenous shunt (device) 39.43
with creation of new shunt 39.42
Barton's tongs (skull) 02.95
with synchronous replacement 02.94
bladder sphincter, artificial 58.99
with replacement 58.93
blood clot — *see also* Incision, by site
bladder (by incision) 57.19
without incision 57.0
kidney (without incision) 56.0
by incision 55.01
ureter
by incision 56.2
bone fragment (chip) (*see also* Incision, bone)
77.10
joint (*see also* Arthrotomy) 80.10
necrotic (*see also* Sequestrectomy, bone)
77.00
joint (*see also* Arthrotomy) 80.10
skull 01.25
with debridement compound fracture
02.02
bone growth stimulator — *see* category
78.6 ✓4ᵗʰ
bony spicules, spinal canal 03.53
brace 97.88
breast implant 85.94
tissue expander 85.96
calcareous deposit
bursa 83.03
hand 82.03
tendon, intratendinous 83.39
hand 82.29
calcification, heart valve leaflets —*see*
Valvuloplasty, heart
calculus
bile duct (by incision) 51.49
endoscopic 51.88
laparoscopic 51.88
percutaneous 51.98
bladder (by incision) 57.19
without incision 57.0

Removal — *see also* Excision — *continued*
calculus — *continued*
common duct (by incision) 51.41
endoscopic 51.88
laparoscopic 51.88
percutaneous 51.96
gallbladder 51.04
endoscopic 51.88
laparoscopic 51.88
kidney (by incision) 55.01
without incision 56.0
percutaneous 55.03
with fragmentation (ultrasound) 55.04
renal pelvis (by incision) 55.11
percutaneous nephrostomy 55.03
with fragmentation 55.04
transurethral 56.0
lacrimal
canaliculi 09.42
by incision 09.52
gland 09.3
by incision 09.0
passage(s) 09.49
by incision 09.59
punctum 09.41
by incision 09.51
sac 09.49
by incision 09.53
pancreatic duct (by incision) 52.09
endoscopic 52.94
perirenal tissue 59.09
pharynx 29.39
prostate 60.0
salivary gland (by incision) 26.0
by probe 26.91
ureter (by incision) 56.2
without incision 56.0
urethra (by incision) 58.0
without incision 58.6
caliper tongs (skull) 02.95
cannula
for extracorporeal membrane
oxygenation (ECMO) — *omit code*
cardiac pacemaker (device) (initial) (permanent)
▶(cardiac resynchronization device,
CRT-P)◀ 37.89
with replacement
cardiac resynchronization pacemaker ●
(CRT-P)
device only 00.53   ●
total system 00.50   ●
dual-chamber 37.87
single-chamber device 37.85
rate responsive 37.86
cardioverter/defibrillator pulse generator
without replacement ▶(cardiac
resynchronization defibrillator device
(CRT-D)◀ 37.99
cast 97.88
with reapplication 97.13
lower limb 97.12
upper limb 97.11
catheter (indwelling) — *see also* Removal, tube
bladder 97.64
middle ear (tympanum) 20.1
ureter 97.62
urinary 97.64
ventricular (cerebral) 02.43
with synchronous replacement 02.42
cerclage material, cervix 69.96
cerumen, ear 96.52
corneal epithelium 11.41
for smear or culture 11.21
coronary artery obstruction (thrombus) 36.09
direct intracoronary artery infusion 36.04
open chest approach 36.03
percutaneous transluminal (balloon) (single
vessel) 36.01
with thrombolytic agent infusion 36.02
multiple vessels 36.05
Crutchfield tongs (skull) 02.95
with synchronous replacement 02.94
cyst — *see also* Excision, lesion, by site
dental 24.4
lung 32.29
endoscopic 32.28

Removal — *see also* Excision — *continued*
cystic duct remnant 51.61
decidua (by)
aspiration curettage 69.52
curettage (D and C) 69.02
manual 75.4
dental wiring (immobilization device) 97.33
orthodontic 24.8
device (therapeutic) NEC 97.89
abdomen NEC 97.86
digestive system NEC 97.59
drainage — *see* Removal, tube
external fixation device 97.88
mandibular NEC 97.36
minifixator (bone) — *see* category
78.6 ✓4ᵗʰ
for musculoskeletal immobilization NEC
97.88
genital tract NEC 97.79
head and neck NEC 97.39
intrauterine contraceptive 97.71
thorax NEC 97.49
trunk NEC 97.87
urinary system NEC 97.69
diaphragm, vagina 97.73
drainage device — *see* Removal, tube
dye, spinal canal 03.31
ectopic fetus (from) 66.02
abdominal cavity 74.3
extraperitoneal (intraligamentous) 74.3
fallopian tube (by salpingostomy) 66.02
by salpingotomy 66.01
with salpingectomy 66.62
intraligamentous 74.3
ovarian 74.3
peritoneal (following uterine or tubal
rupture) 74.3
site NEC 74.3
tubal (by salpingostomy) 66.02
by salpingotomy 66.01
with salpingectomy 66.62
electrodes
bone growth stimulator — *see* category
78.6 ✓4ᵗʰ
brain 01.22
depth 01.22
with synchronous replacement 02.93
foramen ovale 01.22
with synchronous replacement 02.93
sphenoidal — *omit code*
with synchronous replacement 02.96
cardiac pacemaker (atrial) (transvenous)
(ventricular) 37.77
with replacement 37.76
depth 01.22
with synchronous replacement 02.93
epicardial (myocardial) 37.77
with replacement (by)
atrial and/or ventricular lead(s)
(electrode) 37.76
epicardial lead 37.74
epidural pegs 01.22
with synchronous replacement 02.93
foramen ovale 01.22
with synchronous replacement 02.93
intracranial 01.22
with synchronous replacement 02.93
peripheral nerve 04.93
with synchronous replacement 04.92
sphenoidal — *omit code*
with synchronous replacement 02.96
spinal 03.94
with synchronous replacement 03.93
temporary transvenous pacemaker system
— *omit code*
electroencephalographic receiver (brain)
(intracranial) 01.22
with synchronous replacement 02.93
electronic
stimulator
bladder 57.98
bone 78.6 ✓4ᵗʰ
brain 01.22
with synchronous replacement 02.93
intracranial 01.22
with synchronous replacement 02.93

Removal — Removal

✔4ᵗʰ Fourth-digit Required   ▶◀ Revised Text   ● New Line   ▲ Revised Code

Removal — *see also* Excision — *continued*
  foreign body NEC (*see also* Incision, by site) —
     continued
    sinus — *continued*
     sphenoid 22.52
    skin NEC 98.20
     by incision 86.05
    skull 01.24
     with incision into brain 01.39
    small intestine (intraluminal) 98.03
     by incision 45.02
    soft tissue NEC 83.09
     hand 82.09
    spermatic cord 63.93
    spinal (canal) (cord) (meninges) 03.01
    stomach (intraluminal) 98.03
     bubble (balloon) 44.94
     by incision 43.0
    subconjunctival (by magnet) 98.22
     by incision 10.0
    subcutaneous tissue NEC 98.20
     by incision 86.05
    supraclavicular fossa 98.27
     by incision 86.05
    tendon (sheath) 83.01
     hand 82.01
    testis 62.0
    thorax (by incision) 34.09
    thyroid (field) (gland) (by incision) 06.09
    tonsil 98.13
     by incision 28.91
    trachea (intraluminal) 98.15
     by incision 31.3
    trunk NEC 98.25
    tunica vaginalis 98.24
    upper limb, except hand 98.27
     hand 98.26
    ureter (transurethral) 56.0
     by incision 56.2
    urethra (intraluminal) 98.19
     by incision 58.0
    uterus (intraluminal) 98.16
    vagina (intraluminal) 98.17
     by incision 70.14
    vas deferens 63.6
    vitreous (by incision) 14.00
     with use of magnet 14.01
     without use of magnet 14.02
    vulva 98.23
     by incision 71.09
  gallstones
    bile duct (by incision) NEC 51.49
     endoscopic 51.88
    common duct (by incision) 51.41
     endoscopic 51.88
     percutaneous 51.96
    duodenum 45.01
    gallbladder 51.04
     endoscopic 51.88
     laparoscopic 51.88
    hepatic ducts 51.49
     endoscopic 51.88
    intestine 45.00
     large 45.03
     small NEC 45.02
    liver 50.0
  Gardner Wells tongs (skull) 02.95
    with synchronous replacement 02.94
  gastric bubble (balloon) 44.94
  granulation tissue — *see also* Excision, lesion,
    by site
    with repair — *see* Repair, by site
    cranial 01.6
    skull 01.6
  halo traction device (skull) 02.95
    with synchronous replacement 02.94
  heart assist system 37.64
    with replacement 37.63
    intra-aortic balloon pump (IABP) 97.44
    nonoperative 97.44
  hematoma — *see* Drainage, by site
  Hoffman minifixator device (bone) — *see*
    category 78.6 ✔4ᵗʰ
  hydatidiform mole 68.0
  impacted
    feces (rectum) (by flushing) (manual) 96.38

Removal — *see also* Excision — *continued*
  impacted — *continued*
    tooth 23.19
     from nasal sinus (maxillary) 22.61
  implant
    breast 85.94
    cochlear prosthetic device 20.99
    cornea 11.92
    lens (prosthetic) 13.8
    middle ear NEC 20.99
    ocular 16.71
     posterior segment 14.6
    orbit 16.72
    retina 14.6
    tympanum 20.1
  internal fixation device — *see* Removal, fixation
    device, internal
  intra-aortic balloon pump (IABP) 97.44
  intrauterine contraceptive device (IUD) 97.71
  joint (structure) NOS 80.90
    ankle 80.97
    elbow 80.92
    foot and toe 80.98
    hand and finger 80.94
    hip 80.95
    knee 80.96
    other specified sites 80.99
    shoulder 80.91
    spine 80.99
    toe 80.98
    wrist 80.93
  Kantrowitz heart pump 37.64
    nonoperative 97.44
  keel (tantalum plate), larynx 31.98
  kidney — *see also* Nephrectomy
    mechanical 55.98
    transplanted or rejected 55.53
  laminaria (tent), uterus 97.79
  leads (cardiac) — *see* Removal, electrodes,
    cardiac pacemaker
  lesion — *see* Excision, lesion, by site
  ligamentum flavum (spine) — *omit code*
  ligature
    fallopian tube 66.79
    ureter 56.86
    vas deferens 63.84
  loop recorder 86.05
  loose body
    bone — *see* Sequestrectomy, bone
    joint 80.10
    mesh (surgical) — *see* Removal, foreign
     body, by site
  lymph node — *see* Excision, lymph, node
  minifixator device (bone) — *see* category
    78.6 ✔4ᵗʰ
    external fixation device 97.88
  Mulligan hood, fallopian tube 66.94
    with synchronous replacement 66.93
  muscle stimulator (skeletal) 83.93
    with replacement 83.92
  myringotomy device or tube 20.1
  nail (bed) (fold) 86.23
    internal fixation device — *see* Removal,
     fixation device, internal
  necrosis
    skin 86.28
     excisional 86.22
  neuropacemaker
    brain 01.22
     with synchronous replacement 02.93
    intracranial 01.22
     with synchronous replacement 02.93
    peripheral nerve 04.93
     with synchronous replacement 04.92
    spinal 03.94
     with synchronous replacement 03.93
  neurostimulator
    brain 01.22
     with synchronous replacement 02.93
    intracranial 01.22
     with synchronous replacement 02.93
    peripheral nerve 04.93
     with synchronous replacement 04.92
    spinal 03.94
     with synchronous replacement 03.93

Removal — *see also* Excision — *continued*
  nonabsorbable surgical material NEC — *see*
    Removal, foreign body, by site
  odontoma (tooth) 24.4
  orbital implant 16.72
  osteocartilagenous loose body, joint structures
    (*see also* Arthrotomy) 80.10
  outer attic wall (middle ear) 20.59
  ovo-testis (unilateral) 62.3
    bilateral 62.41
  pacemaker
    brain (intracranial) 01.22
     with synchronous replacement 02.93
    cardiac (device) (initial) (permanent) 37.89
     with replacement
      dual-chamber device 37.87
      single-chamber device 37.85
       rate responsive 37.86
     electrodes (atrial) (transvenous)
      (ventricular) 37.77
      with replacement 37.76
     epicardium (myocardium) 37.77
      with replacement (by)
       atrial and/or ventricular lead(s)
        (electrode) 37.76
       epicardial lead 37.74
     temporary transvenous pacemaker
      system — *omit code*
    intracranial 01.22
     with synchronous replacement 02.93
    neural
     brain 01.22
      with synchronous replacement 02.93
     peripheral nerve 04.93
      with synchronous replacement 04.92
     spine 03.94
      with synchronous replacement 03.93
    spinal 03.94
     with synchronous replacement 03.93
  pack, packing
    dental 97.34
    intrauterine 97.72
    nasal 97.32
    rectum 97.59
    trunk NEC 97.85
    vagina 97.75
    vulva 97.75
  pantopaque dye, spinal canal 03.31
  patella (complete) 77.96
    partial 77.86
  pectus deformity implant device 34.01
  pelvic viscera, en masse (female) 68.8
    male 57.71
  pessary, vagina NEC 97.74
  pharynx (partial) 29.33
  phlebolith — *see* Removal, embolus
  placenta (by)
    aspiration curettage 69.52
    D and C 69.02
    manual 75.4
  plaque, dental 96.54
  plate, skull 02.07
    with synchronous replacement 02.05
  polyp — *see also* Excision, lesion, by site
    esophageal 42.32
     endoscopic 42.33
    gastric (endoscopic) 43.41
    intestine 45.41
     endoscopic 45.42
    nasal 21.31
  prosthesis
    bile duct 51.95
     nonoperative 97.55
    cochlear prosthetic device 20.99
    dental 97.35
    eye 97.31
    facial bone 76.99
    fallopian tube 66.94
     with synchronous replacement 66.93
    joint structures 80.00
     ankle 80.07
     elbow 80.02
     foot and toe 80.08
     hand and finger 80.04
     hip 80.05
     knee 80.06

Removal — *see also* Excision — *continued*
  prosthesis — *continued*
    joint structures — *continued*
      shoulder 80.01
      specified site NEC 80.09
      spine 80.09
      wrist 80.03
    lens 13.8
    penis (internal) without replacement 64.96
    Rosen (urethra) 59.99
    testicular, by incision 62.0
    urinary sphincter, artificial 58.99
      with replacement 58.93
  pseudophakos 13.8
  pterygium 11.39
    with corneal graft 11.32
  pulse generator
    cardiac pacemaker 37.86
    cardioverter/defibrillator 37.99
  pump assist device, heart 37.64
    with replacement 37.63
    nonoperative 97.44
  radioactive material — *see* Removal, foreign
    body, by site
  redundant skin, eyelid 08.86
  rejected organ
    kidney 55.53
    testis 62.42
  reservoir, ventricular (Ommaya) (Rickham)
    02.43
    with synchronous replacement 02.42
  retained placenta (by)
    aspiration curettage 69.52
    D and C 69.02
    manual 75.4
  retinal implant 14.6
  rhinolith 21.31
  rice bodies, tendon sheaths 83.01
    hand 82.01
  Roger-Anderson minifixator device (bone) — *see*
    category 78.6 ✓4ᵗʰ
  root, residual (tooth) (buried) (retained) 23.11
  Rosen prosthesis (urethra) 59.99
  Scribner shunt 39.43
  scleral buckle or implant 14.6
  secondary membranous cataract (with
    iridectomy) 13.65
  secundines (by)
    aspiration curettage 69.52
    D and C 69.02
    manual 75.4
  sequestrum — *see* Sequestrectomy
  seton, anus 49.93
  Shepard's tube (ear) 20.1
  Shirodkar suture, cervix 69.96
  shunt
    arteriovenous 39.43
      with creation of new shunt 39.42
    lumbar-subarachnoid NEC 03.98
    pleurothecal 03.98
    salpingothecal 03.98
    spinal (thecal) NEC 03.98
    subarachnoid-peritoneal 03.98
    subarachnoid-ureteral 03.98
  silastic tubes
    ear 20.1
    fallopian tubes 66.94
      with synchronous replacement 66.93
  skin
    necrosis or slough 86.28
      excisional 86.22
      superficial layer (by dermabrasion) 86.25
  skull tongs 02.95
    with synchronous replacement 02.94
  splint 97.88
  stent
    bile duct 97.55
    larynx 31.98
    ureteral 97.62
    urethral 97.65
  stimoceiver (brain) (intracranial) 01.22
    with synchronous replacement 02.93
  subdural
    grids 01.22
    strips 01.22
  supernumerary digit(s) 86.26

Removal — *see also* Excision — *continued*
  suture(s) NEC 97.89
    abdominal wall 97.83
    by incision — *see* Incision, by site
    genital tract 97.79
    head and neck 97.38
    thorax 97.43
    trunk NEC 97.84
  symblepharon — *see* Repair, symblepharon
  temporary transvenous pacemaker system —
    omit code
  testis (unilateral) 62.3
    bilateral 62.41
    remaining or solitary 62.42
  thrombus 38.00
    with endarterectomy — *see* Endarterectomy
    abdominal
      artery 38.06
      vein 38.07
    aorta (arch) (ascending) (descending) 38.04
    arteriovenous shunt or cannula 39.49
    bovine graft 39.49
    coronary artery 36.09
    head and neck vessel NEC 38.02
    intracranial vessel NEC 38.01
    lower limb
      artery 38.08
      vein 38.09
    pulmonary (artery) (vein) 38.05
    thoracic vessel NEC 38.05
    upper limb (artery) (vein) 38.03
  tissue expander (skin) NEC 86.05
    breast 85.96
  toes, supernumerary 86.26
  tongs, skull 02.95
    with synchronous replacement 02.94
  tonsil tag 28.4
  tooth (by forceps) (multiple) (single) NEC 23.09
    deciduous 23.01
    surgical NEC 23.19
      impacted 23.19
      residual root 23.11
      root apex 23.73
        with root canal therapy 23.72
  trachoma follicles 10.33
  T-tube (bile duct) 97.55
  tube
    appendix 97.53
    bile duct (T-tube) NEC 97.55
    cholecystostomy 97.54
    cystostomy 97.63
    ear (button) 20.1
    gastrostomy 97.51
    large intestine 97.53
    liver 97.55
    mediastinum 97.42
    nephrostomy 97.61
    pancreas 97.56
    peritoneum 97.82
    pleural cavity 97.41
    pyelostomy 97.61
    retroperitoneum 97.81
    small intestine 97.52
    thoracotomy 97.41
    tracheostomy 97.37
    tympanostomy 20.1
    tympanum 20.1
    ureterostomy 97.62
  ureteral splint (stent) 97.62
  urethral sphincter, artificial 58.99
    with replacement 58.93
  urinary sphincter, artificial 58.99
    with replacement 58.93
  utricle 20.79
  valve
    vas deferens 63.85
    ventricular (cerebral) 02.43
  vascular graft or prosthesis 39.49
  ventricular shunt or reservoir 02.43
    with synchronous replacement 02.42
  Vinke tongs (skull) 02.95
    with synchronous replacement 02.94
  vitreous (with replacement) 14.72
    anterior approach (partial) 14.71
    open sky technique 14.71

Removal — *see also* Excision — *continued*
  Wagner-Brooker minifixator device (bone) —
    see category 78.6 ✓4ᵗʰ
  wiring, dental (immobilization device) 97.33
    orthodontic 24.8
Renipuncture (percutaneous) 55.92
Renogram 92.03
Renotransplantation NEC 55.69
Reopening — *see also* Incision, by site
  blepharorrhaphy 08.02
  canthorrhaphy 08.02
  cilia base 08.71
  craniotomy or craniectomy site 01.23
  fallopian tube (divided) 66.79
  iris in anterior chambers 12.97
  laminectomy or laminotomy site 03.02
  laparotomy site 54.12
  osteotomy site (*see also* Incision, bone) 77.10
    facial bone 76.09
  tarsorrhaphy 08.02
  thoracotomy site (for control of hemorrhage)
    (for examination) (for exploration) 34.03
  thyroid field wound (for control of hemorrhage)
    (for examination) (for exploration) (for
    removal of hematoma) 06.02
Repacking — *see* Replacement, pack, by site
Repair
  abdominal wall 54.72
  adrenal gland 07.44
  alveolus, alveolar (process) (ridge) (with graft)
    (with implant) 24.5
  anal sphincter 49.79
    artificial sphincter
      implantation 49.75 ●
      revision 49.75 ●
    laceration (by suture) 49.71
      obstetric (current) 75.62
      old 49.79
  aneurysm (false) (true) 39.52
    by or with
      clipping 39.51
      coagulation 39.52
      coil (endovascular approach) 39.79 ●
        head and neck 39.72 ●
      electrocoagulation 39.52
        excision or resection of vessel — *see*
          also Aneurysmectomy, by site
      with
        anastomosis — *see* Aneurysmectomy,
          with anastomosis, by site
        graft replacement — *see*
          Aneurysmectomy, with graft
          replacement, by site
      endovascular graft 39.79
        abdominal aorta 39.71
        head and neck 39.72 ●
        lower extremity artery(s) 39.79
        thoracic aorta 39.79
        upper extremity artery(s) 39.79
      filipuncture 39.52
      graft replacement — *see*
        Aneurysmectomy, with graft
        replacement, by site
      ligation 39.52
      liquid tissue adhesive (glue) 39.79 ●
        endovascular approach 39.79 ●
          head and neck 39.72 ●
      methyl methacrylate 39.52
        endovascular approach 39.79 ●
          head and neck 39.72 ●
      occlusion 39.52
        endovascular approach 39.79 ●
          head and neck 39.72 ●
      suture 39.52
      trapping 39.52
      wiring 39.52
      wrapping (gauze) (methyl methacrylate)
        (plastic) 39.52
  coronary artery 36.91
  heart 37.32
  sinus of Valsalva 35.39
  thoracic aorta (dissecting), by fenestration
    39.54

✓4ᵗʰ Fourth-digit Required   ▶◀ Revised Text   ● New Line   ▲ Revised Code

Repair — Repair

◢4ᵗʰ Fourth-digit Required   ►◄ Revised Text   ● New Line   ▲ Revised Code

Replacement — *continued*

Replacement — *continued*
cast NEC 97.13
  lower limb 97.12
  upper limb 97.11
catheter
  bladder (indwelling) 57.95
  cystostomy 59.94
  ventricular shunt (cerebral) 02.42
  wound 97.15
CRT-D (cardiac resynchronization   ●
    defibrillator) 00.51   ●
  left ventricular coronary venous lead ●
    only 00.52   ●
  pulse generator only 00.54   ●
CRT-P (cardiac resynchronization   ●
    pacemaker) 00.50   ●
  left ventricular coronary venous lead ●
    only 00.52   ●
  pulse generator only 00.53   ●
Crutchfield tongs (skull) 02.94
cystostomy tube (catheter) 59.94
diaphragm, vagina 97.24
drain — *see also* Replacement, tube
  vagina 97.26
  vulva 97.26
  wound musculoskeletal or skin 97.16
ear (prosthetic) 18.71
elbow (joint), total 81.84
electrode(s) — *see* Implant, electrode or lead by
    site or name of device
  brain
    depth 02.93
    foramen ovale 02.93
    sphenoidal 02.96
  depth 02.93
  foramen ovale 02.93
  sphenoidal 02.96
electroencephalographic receiver (brain)
    (intracranial) 02.93
electronic
  cardioverter/defibrillator — *see*
    Replacement, cardioverter/defibrillator
  leads (electrode)(s) — *see* Replacement,
    pacemaker, electrode(s), cardiac
  stimulator — *see also* Implant, electronic
    stimulator, by site
    bladder 57.97
    muscle (skeletal) 83.92
    ureter 56.93
electrostimulator — *see* Implant, electronic
    stimulator by site
enterostomy device (tube)
  large intestine 97.04
  small intestine 97.03
epidural pegs 02.93
femoral head, by prosthesis 81.52
  revision 81.53
Gardner Wells tongs (skull) 02.94
graft — *see* Graft
halo traction device (skull) 02.94
Harrington rod (with refusion of spine) — *see*
    Refusion, spinal
heart
  artificial 37.63
  valve (with prosthesis) (with tissue graft)
    35.20
    aortic (with prosthesis) 35.22
      with tissue graft 35.21
    mitral (with prosthesis) 35.24
      with tissue graft 35.23
    poppet (prosthetic) 35.95
    pulmonary (with prosthesis) 35.26
      with tissue graft 35.25
      in total repair of tetralogy of Fallot
        35.81
    tricuspid (with prosthesis) 35.28
      with tissue graft 35.27
hip (partial) (with fixation device) (with
    prosthesis) (with traction) 81.52
  acetabulum 81.52
    revision 81.53
  femoral head 81.52
    revision 81.53
  total 81.51
    revision 81.53
inverted uterus — *see* Repair, inverted uterus

Replacement — *continued*
iris NEC 12.39
kidney, mechanical 55.97
knee (bicompartmental) (hemijoint) (partial)
    (total) (tricompartmental)
    (unicompartmental) 81.54
  revision 81.55
laryngeal stent 31.93
leads (electrode)(s) — *see* Replacement,
    pacemaker, electrode(s), cardiac
mechanical kidney 55.97
mitral valve (with prosthesis) 35.24
  with tissue graft 35.23
Mulligan hood, fallopian tube 66.93
muscle stimulator (skeletal) 83.92
nephrostomy tube 55.93
neuropacemaker — *see* Implant,
    neuropacemaker, by site
neurostimulator — *see also* implant,
    neurostimulator, by site
  peripheral nerve 04.92
  skeletal muscle 83.92
pacemaker
  brain 02.93
  cardiac device (initial) (permanent)
    dual-chamber device 37.87
    resynchronization — *see* Replacement, ●
      CRT-P   ●
    single-chamber device 37.85
      rate responsive 37.86
  electrode(s), cardiac (atrial) (transvenous)
    (ventricular) 37.76
    epicardium (myocardium) 37.74
    left ventricular coronary venous   ●
      system 00.52   ●
  intracranial 02.93
  neural
    brain 02.93
    intracranial 02.93
    peripheral nerve 04.92
    spine 03.93
  spine 03.93
  temporary transvenous pacemaker system
    37.78
pack or bag
  nose 97.21
  teeth, tooth 97.22
  vagina 97.26
  vulva 97.26
  wound 97.16
pessary, vagina NEC 97.25
prosthesis
  acetabulum 81.53
  arm (bioelectric) (cineplastic) (kineplastic)
    84.44
  biliary tract 51.99
  cochlear 20.96
  channel (single) 20.97
    multiple 20.98
  elbow 81.97
  extremity (bioelectric) (cineplastic)
    (kineplastic) 84.40
    lower 84.48
    upper 84.44
  fallopian tube (Mulligan hood) (stent) 66.93
  femur 81.53
  knee 81.55
  leg (bioelectric) (cineplastic) (kineplastic)
    84.48
  penis (internal) (non-inflatable) 64.95
    inflatable (internal) 64.97
  pulmonary valve (with prosthesis) 35.26
    with tissue graft 35.25
    in total repair of tetralogy of Fallot 35.81
  pyelostomy tube 55.94
  rectal tube 96.09
  shoulder NEC 81.83
    partial 81.81
    total 81.80
  skull
    plate 02.05
    tongs 02.94
  specified appliance or device NEC 97.29
stent
  bile duct 97.05
  fallopian tube 66.93

Replacement — *continued*
stent — *continued*
  larynx 31.93
  pancreatic duct 97.05
  trachea 31.93
stimoceiver — *see* Implant, stimoceiver, by site
subdural
  grids 02.93
  strips 02.93
testis in scrotum 62.5
tongs, skull 02.94
tracheal stent 31.93
tricuspid valve (with prosthesis) 35.28
  with tissue graft 35.27
tube
  bile duct 97.05
  bladder 57.95
  cystostomy 59.94
  esophagostomy 97.01
  gastrostomy 97.02
  large intestine 97.04
  nasogastric 97.01
  nephrostomy 55.93
  pancreatic duct 97.05
  pyelostomy 55.94
  rectal 96.09
  small intestine 97.03
  tracheostomy 97.23
  ureterostomy 59.93
  ventricular (cerebral) 02.42
umbilical cord, prolapsed 73.92
ureter
  bladder flap 56.74
  ileal segment implanted into bladder 56.89
    [45.51]
ureterostomy tube 59.93
urethral sphincter, artificial 58.93
urinary sphincter, artificial 58.93
valve
  heart — *see also* Replacement, heart valve
    poppet (prosthetic) 35.95
  ventricular (cerebral) 02.42
ventricular shunt (catheter) (valve) 02.42
Vinke tongs (skull) 02.94
vitreous (silicone) 14.75
  for retinal reattachment 14.59

Replant, replantation — *see also* Reattachment
extremity — *see* Reattachment, extremity
penis 64.45
scalp 86.51
tooth 23.5

Reposition
cardiac pacemaker
  electrode(s) (atrial) (transvenous)
    (ventricular) 37.75
  pocket 37.79
cardioverter/defibrillator
  lead(s) (sensing) (pacing) (epicardial patch)
    37.99
  pocket 37.99
  pulse generator 37.99
cilia base 08.71
iris 12.39
renal vessel, aberrant 39.55
thyroid tissue 06.94
tricuspid valve (with plication) 35.14

Resection — *see also* Excision, by site
abdominoendorectal (combined) 48.5
abdominoperineal (rectum) 48.5
  pull-through (Altmeier) (Swenson) NEC
    48.49
    Duhamel type 48.65
alveolar process and palate (en bloc) 27.32
aneurysm — *see* Aneurysmectomy
aortic valve (for subvalvular stenosis) 35.11
artery — *see* Arteriectomy
bile duct NEC 51.69
  common duct NEC 51.63
bladder (partial) (segmental) (transvesical)
    (wedge) 57.6
  complete or total 57.79
  lesionNEC 57.59
    transurethral approach 57.49
  neck 57.59
    transurethral approach 57.49

Resection — *see also* Excision, by site — *continued*

blood vessel — *see* Angiectomy
brain 01.59
  by
    stereotactic radiosurgery 92.30
      cobalt 80 92.32
      linear accelerator (LINAC) 92.31
      multi-source 92.32
      particle beam 92.33
      particulate 92.33
      radiosurgery NEC 92.39
      single source photon 92.31
  hemisphere 01.52
  lobe 01.53
breast — *see also* Mastectomy
  quadrant 85.22
  segmental 85.23
broad ligament 69.19
bronchus (sleeve) (wide sleeve) 32.1
  block (en bloc) (with radical dissection of brachial plexus, bronchus, lobe of lung, ribs, and sympathetic nerves) 32.6
bursa 83.5
  hand 82.31
cecum (and terminal ileum) 45.72
cerebral meninges 01.51
chest wall 34.4
clavicle 77.81
clitoris 71.4
colon (partial) (segmental) 45.79
  ascending (cecum and terminal ileum) 45.72
  cecum (and terminal ileum) 45.72
  complete 45.8
  descending (sigmoid) 45.76
  for interposition 45.52
  Hartmann 45.75
  hepatic flexure 45.73
  left radical (hemicolon) 45.75
  multiple segmental 45.71
  right radical (hemicolon) (ileocolectomy) 45.73
  segmental NEC 45.79
    multiple 45.71
  sigmoid 45.76
  splenic flexure 45.75
  total 45.8
  transverse 45.74
conjunctiva, for pterygium 11.39
  corneal graft 11.32
cornual (fallopian tube) (unilateral) 66.69
  bilateral 66.63
diaphragm 34.81
endaural 20.79
endorectal (pull-through) (Soave) 48.41
  combined abdominal 48.5
esophagus (partial) (subtotal) (*see also* Esophagectomy) 42.41
  total 42.42
exteriorized intestine — *see* Resection, intestine, exteriorized
fascia 83.44
  for graft 83.43
    hand 82.34
  hand 82.35
    for graft 82.34
gallbladder (total) 51.22
gastric (partial) (sleeve) (subtotal) NEC (*see also* Gastrectomy) 43.89
  with anastomosis NEC 43.89
    esophagogastric 43.5
    gastroduodenal 43.6
    gastrogastric 43.89
    gastrojejunal 43.7
  complete or total NEC 43.99
    with intestinal interposition 43.91
  radical NEC 43.99
    with intestinal interposition 43.91
  wedge 43.42
    endoscopic 43.41
hallux valgus (joint) — *see also* Bunionectomy
  with prosthetic implant 77.59
hepatic
  duct 51.69
  flexure (colon) 45.73

Resection — *see also* Excision, by site — *continued*

infundibula, heart (right) 35.34
intestine (partial) NEC 45.79
  cecum (with terminal ileum) 45.72
  exteriorized (large intestine) 46.04
    small intestine 46.02
  for interposition 45.50
    large intestine 45.52
    small intestine 45.51
  hepatic flexure 45.73
  ileum 45.62
    with cecum 45.72
  large (partial) (segmental) NEC 45.79
    for interposition 45.52
    multiple segmental 45.71
    total 45.8
  left hemicolon 45.75
  multiple segmental (large intestine) 45.71
    small intestine 45.61
  right hemicolon 45.73
  segmental (large intestine) 45.79
    multiple 45.71
    small intestine 45.62
      multiple 45.61
  sigmoid 45.76
  small (partial) (segmental) NEC 45.62
    for interposition 45.51
    multiple segmental 45.61
    total 45.63
  total
    large intestine 45.8
    small intestine 45.63
joint structure NEC (*see also* Arthrectomy) 80.90
kidney (segmental) (wedge) 55.4
larynx — *see also* Laryngectomy
  submucous 30.29
lesion — *see* Excision, lesion, by site
levator palpebrae muscle 08.33
ligament (*see also* Arthrectomy) 80.90
  broad 69.19
  round 69.19
  uterine 69.19
lip (wedge) 27.43
liver (partial) (wedge) 50.22
  lobe (total) 50.3
  total 50.4
lung (wedge) NEC 32.29
  endoscopic 32.28
  segmental (any part) 32.3
  volume reduction 32.22
meninges (cerebral) 01.51
  spinal 03.4
mesentery 54.4
muscle 83.45
  extraocular 15.13
    with
      advancement or recession of other eye muscle 15.3
      suture of original insertion 15.13
    levator palpebrae 08.33
    Müller's, for blepharoptosis 08.35
    orbicularis oculi 08.20
    tarsal, for blepharoptosis 08.35
  for graft 83.43
    hand 82.34
  hand 82.36
    for graft 82.34
  ocular — *see* Resection, muscle, extraocular
myocardium 37.33
nasal septum (submucous) 21.5
nerve (cranial) (peripheral) NEC 04.07
  phrenic 04.03
    for collapse of lung 33.31
  sympathetic 05.29
  vagus — *see* Vagotomy
nose (complete) (extended) (partial) (radical) 21.4
omentum 54.4
orbitomaxillary, radical 16.51
ovary (*see also* Oophorectomy wedge) 65.22
  laparoscopic 65.24
palate (bony) (local) 27.31
  by wide excision 27.32
  soft 27.49

Resection — *see also* Excision, by site — *continued*

pancreas (total) (with synchronous duodenectomy) 52.6
  partial NEC 52.59
    distal (tail) (with part of body) 52.52
    proximal (head) (with part of body) (with synchronous duodenectomy) 52.51
    radical subtotal 52.53
  radical (one-stage) (two-stage) 52.7
  subtotal 52.53
pancreaticoduodenal (*see also* Pancreatectomy) 52.6
pelvic viscera (en masse) (female) 68.8
  male 57.71
penis 64.3
pericardium (partial) (for)
  chronic constrictive pericarditis 37.31
  drainage 37.12
  removal of adhesions 37.31
peritoneum 54.4
pharynx (partial) 29.33
phrenic nerve 04.03
  for collapse of lung 33.31
prostate — *see also* Prostatectomy
  transurethral (punch) 60.29
pterygium 11.39
radial head 77.83
rectosigmoid (*see also* Resection, rectum) 48.69
rectum (partial) NEC 48.69
  with
    pelvic exenteration 68.8
    transsacral sigmoidectomy 48.61
  abdominoendorectal (combined) 48.5
  abdominoperineal 48.5
    pull-through NEC 48.49
      Duhamel type 48.65
  anterior 48.63
    with colostomy (synchronous) 48.62
  Duhamel 48.65
  endorectal 48.41
    combined abdominal 48.5
  posterior 48.64
  pull-through NEC 48.49
    endorectal 48.41
  submucosal (Soave) 48.41
    combined abdominal 48.5
rib (transaxillary) 77.91
  as operative approach — *omit code*
  incidental to thoracic operation — *omit code*
right ventricle (heart), for infundibular stenosis 35.34
root (tooth) (apex) 23.73
  with root canal therapy 23.72
  residual or retained 23.11
round ligament 69.19
sclera 12.65
  with scleral buckling (*see also* Buckling, scleral) 14.49
  lamellar (for retinal reattachment) 14.49
    with implant 14.41
scrotum 61.3
soft tissue NEC 83.49
  hand 82.39
sphincter of Oddi 51.89
spinal cord (meninges) 03.4
splanchnic 05.29
splenic flexure (colon) 45.75
sternum 77.81
stomach (partial) (sleeve) (subtotal) NEC (*see also* Gastrectomy) 43.89
  with anastomosis NEC 43.89
    esophagogastric 43.5
    gastroduodenal 43.6
    gastrogastric 43.89
    gastrojejunal 43.7
  complete or total NEC 43.99
    with intestinal interposition 43.91
  fundus 43.89
  radical NEC 43.99
    with intestinal interposition 43.91
  wedge 43.42
    endoscopic 43.41
submucous
  larynx 30.29
  nasal septum 21.5

■✓4■ Fourth-digit Required   ▶◀ Revised Text   ● New Line   ▲ Revised Code

Resection — *see also* Excision, by site —
   continued
  submucous — *continued*
    vocal cords 30.22
  synovial membrane (complete) (partial) (*see also*
    Synovectomy) 80.70
  tarsolevator 08.33
  tendon 83.42
    hand 82.33
  thoracic structures (block) (en bloc) (radical)
    (brachial plexus, bronchus, lobes of lung,
    ribs, and sympathetic nerves) 32.6
  thorax 34.4
  tongue 25.2
    wedge 25.1
  tooth root 23.73
    with root canal therapy 23.72
    apex (abscess) 23.73
      with root canal therapy 23.72
    residual or retained 23.11
  trachea 31.5
  transurethral
    bladder NEC 57.49
    prostate 60.29
  transverse colon 45.74
  turbinates — *see* Turbinectomy
  ureter (partial) 56.41
    total 56.42
  uterus — *see* Hysterectomy
  vein — *see* Phlebectomy
  ventricle (heart) 37.35
    infundibula 35.34
  vesical neck 57.59
    transurethral 57.49
  vocal cords (punch) 30.22

Respirator, volume-controlled (Bennett) (Byrd) —
  see Ventilation

Restoration
  cardioesophageal angle 44.66
  dental NEC 23.49
    by
      application of crown (artificial) 23.41
      insertion of bridge (fixed) 23.42
        removable 23.43
  extremity — *see* Reattachment, extremity
  eyebrow 08.70
    with graft 08.63
  eye socket 16.64
    with graft 16.63
  tooth NEC 23.2
    by
      crown (artificial) 23.41
      filling (amalgam) (plastic) (silicate) 23.2
      inlay 23.3

Resuscitation
  artificial respiration 93.93
  cardiac 99.60
    cardioversion 99.62
      atrial 99.61
    defibrillation 99.62
    external massage 99.63
      open chest 37.91
    intracardiac injection 37.92
  cardiopulmonary 99.60
  endotracheal intubation 96.04
  manual 93.93
  mouth-to-mouth 93.93
  pulmonary 93.93

Resuture
  abdominal wall 54.61
  cardiac septum prosthesis 35.95
  chest wall 34.71
  heart valve prosthesis (poppet) 35.95
  wound (skin and subcutaneous tissue) (without
    graft) NEC 86.59

Retavase, infusion 99.10
Reteplase, infusion 99.10
Retinaculotomy NEC (*see also* Division, ligament)
  80.40
  carpal tunnel (flexor) 04.43

Retraining
  cardiac 93.36
  vocational 93.85

Retrogasserian neurotomy 04.02

Revascularization
  cardiac (heart muscle) (myocardium) (direct)
    36.10
    with
      bypass anastomosis
        abdominal artery to coronary artery
          36.17
        aortocoronary (catheter stent)
          (homograft) (prosthesis)
          (saphenous vein graft) 36.10
        one coronary vessel 36.11
        two coronary vessels 36.12
        three coronary vessels 36.13
        four coronary vessels 36.14
        gastroepiploic artery to coronary artery
          36.17
        internal mammary-coronary artery
          (single vessel) 36.15
          double vessel 36.16
        specified type NEC 36.19
        thoracic artery-coronary artery (single
          vessel) 36.15
          double vessel 36.16
      implantation of artery into heart (muscle)
        (myocardium) (ventricle) 36.2
    indirect 36.2
    specified type NEC 36.39
    transmyocardial open chest 36.31
      percutaneous 36.32
      specified type NEC 36.32
      thoracoscopic 36.32

Reversal, intestinal segment 45.50
  large 45.52
  small 45.51

Revision
  amputation stump 84.3
    current traumatic — *see* Amputation
  anastomosis
    biliary tract 51.94
    blood vessel 39.49
    gastric, gastrointestinal (with jejunal
      interposition) 44.5
    intestine (large) 46.94
      small 46.93
    pleurothecal 03.97
    pyelointestinal 56.72
    salpingothecal 03.97
    subarachnoid-peritoneal 03.97
    subarachnoid-ureteral 03.97
    ureterointestinal 56.72
  ankle replacement (prosthesis) 81.59
  anterior segment (eye) wound (operative) NEC
    12.83
  arteriovenous shunt (cannula) (for dialysis)
    39.42
  arthroplasty — *see* Arthroplasty
  bone flap, skull 02.06
  breast implant 85.93
  bronchostomy 33.42
  bypass graft (vascular) 39.49
    abdominal-coronary artery 36.17
    aortocoronary (catheter stent) (with
      prosthesis) (with saphenous vein graft)
      (with vein graft) 36.10
    one coronary vessel 36.11
    two coronary vessels 36.12
    three coronary vessels 36.13
    four coronary vessels 36.14
    CABG — *see* Revision, aortocoronary bypass
      graft
    chest tube — *see* intercostal catheter
    coronary artery bypass graft (CABG) — *see*
      Revision, aortocoronary bypass graft,
      abdominal-coronary artery bypass,
      and internal mammary-coronary
      artery bypass
    intercostal catheter (with lysis of adhesions)
      34.04
    internal mammary-coronary artery (single)
      36.15
      double vessel 36.16
  cannula, vessel-to-vessel (arteriovenous) 39.94
  canthus, lateral 08.59
  cardiac pacemaker
    device (permanent) 37.89

Revision — *continued*
  cardiac pacemaker — *continued*
    electrode(s) (atrial) (transvenous)
      (ventricular) 37.75
    pocket 37.79
  cardioverter/defibrillator (automatic) pocket
    37.99
  cholecystostomy 51.99
  cleft palate repair 27.63
  colostomy 46.43
  conduit, urinary 56.52
  cystostomy (stoma) 57.22
  elbow replacement (prosthesis) 81.97
  enterostomy (stoma) 46.40
    large intestine 46.43
    small intestine 46.41
  enucleation socket 16.64
    with graft 16.63
  esophagostomy 42.83
  exenteration cavity 16.66
    with secondary graft 16.65
  extraocular muscle surgery 15.6
  fenestration, inner ear 20.62
  filtering bleb 12.66
  fixation device (broken) (displaced) (*see also*
    Fixation, bone, internal) 78.50
  flap or pedicle graft (skin) 86.75
  foot replacement (prosthesis) 81.59
  gastric anastomosis (with jejunal interposition)
    44.5
  gastroduodenostomy (with jejunal interposition)
    44.5
  gastrointestinal anastomosis (with jejunal
    interposition) 44.5
  gastrojejunostomy 44.5
  gastrostomy 44.69
  hand replacement (prosthesis) 81.97
  heart procedure NEC 35.95
  hip replacement (acetabulum) (femoral head)
    (partial) (total) 81.53
  Holter (-Spitz) valve 02.42
  ileal conduit 56.52
  ileostomy 46.41
  jejunoileal bypass 46.93
  jejunostomy 46.41
  joint replacement
    acetabulum 81.53
    ankle 81.59
    elbow 81.97
    femoral head 81.53
    foot 81.59
    hand 81.97
    hip (partial) (total) 81.53
    knee 81.55
    lower extremity NEC 81.59
    toe 81.59
    upper extremity 81.97
    wrist 81.97
  knee replacement (prosthesis) 81.55
  laryngostomy 31.63
  lateral canthus 08.59
  mallet finger 82.84
  mastoid antrum 19.9
  mastoidectomy 20.92
  nephrostomy 55.89
  neuroplasty 04.75
  ocular implant 16.62
  orbital implant 16.62
  pocket
    cardiac pacemaker
      with initial insertion of pacemaker — *omit*
        code
      new site (skin) (subcutaneous) 37.79
    thalamic stimulator pulse generator
      with initial insertion of battery package —
        omit code
      new site (skin) (subcutaneous) 86.09
  previous mastectomy site — *see* category
    85.0-85.99
  proctostomy 48.79
  prosthesis
    acetabulum
      hip 81.53
    ankle 81.59
    breast 85.93
    elbow 81.97

Index to Procedures

Revision — *continued*
  prosthesis — *continued*
    femoral head 81.53
    foot 81.59
    hand 81.97
    heart valve (poppet) 35.95
    hip (partial) (total) 81.53
    knee 81.55
    lower extremity NEC 81.59
    shoulder 81.97
    toe 81.59
    upper extremity NEC 81.97
    wrist 81.97
  ptosis overcorrection 08.37
  pyelostomy 55.12
  pyloroplasty 44.29
  rhinoplasty 21.84
    scar
      skin 86.84
        with excision 86.3
  scleral fistulization 12.66
  shoulder replacement (prosthesis) 81.97
  shunt
    arteriovenous (cannula) (for dialysis) 39.42
    lumbar-subarachnoid NEC 03.97
    peritoneojugular 54.99
    peritoneovascular 54.99
    pleurothecal 03.97
    salpingothecal 03.97
    spinal (thecal) NEC 03.97
    subarachnoid-peritoneal 03.97
    subarachnoid-ureteral 03.97
    ventricular (cerebral) 02.42
    ventriculoperitoneal
      at peritoneal site 54.95
      at ventricular site 02.42
  stapedectomy NEC 19.29
    with incus replacement (homograft)
      (prosthesis) 19.21
  stoma
    bile duct 51.79
    bladder (vesicostomy) 57.22
    bronchus 33.42
    common duct 51.72
    esophagus 42.89
    gallbladder 51.99
    hepatic duct 51.79
    intestine 46.40
      large 46.43
      small 46.41
    kidney 55.89
    larynx 31.63
    rectum 48.79
    stomach 44.69
    thorax 34.79
    trachea 31.74
    ureter 56.62
    urethra 58.49
  tack operation 20.79
  toe replacement (prosthesis) 81.59
  tracheostomy 31.74
  tunnel
    pulse generator lead wire 86.99
      with initial procedure — *omit code*
  tympanoplasty 19.6
  uretero-ileostomy, cutaneous 56.52
  ureterostomy (cutaneous) (stoma) NEC 56.62
    ileal 56.52
  urethrostomy 58.49
  urinary conduit 56.52
  vascular procedure (previous) NEC 39.49
  ventricular shunt (cerebral) 02.42
  vesicostomy stoma 57.22
  wrist replacement (prosthesis) 81.97
Rhinectomy 21.4
Rhinocheiloplasty 27.59
  cleft lip 27.54
Rhinomanometry 89.12
Rhinoplasty (external) (internal) NEC 21.87
  augmentation (with graft) (with synthetic
    implant) 21.85
  limited 21.86
  revision 21.84
  tip 21.86
  twisted nose 21.84

Rhinorrhaphy (external) (internal) 21.81
  for epistaxis 21.09
Rhinoscopy 21.21
Rhinoseptoplasty 21.84
Rhinotomy 21.1
Rhizotomy (radiofrequency) (spinal) 03.1
  acoustic 04.01
  trigeminal 04.02
Rhytidectomy (facial) 86.82
  eyelid
    lower 08.86
    upper 08.87
Rhytidoplasty (facial) 86.82
Ripstein operation (repair of prolapsed rectum)
  48.75
Rodney Smith operation (radical subtotal
  pancreatectomy) 52.53
Roentgenography — *see also* Radiography
  cardiac, negative contrast 88.58
Rolling of conjunctiva 10.33
Root
  canal (tooth) (therapy) 23.70
    with
      apicoectomy 23.72
      irrigation 23.71
    resection (tooth) (apex) 23.73
      with root canal therapy 23.72
      residual or retained 23.11
Rotation of fetal head
  forceps (instrumental) (Kielland) (Scanzoni)
    (key-in-lock) 72.4
  manual 73.51
Routine
  chest x-ray 87.44
  psychiatric visit 94.12
Roux-en-Y operation
  bile duct 51.36
  cholecystojejunostomy 51.32
  esophagus (intrathoracic) 42.54
  pancreaticojejunostomy 52.96
Roux-Goldthwait operation (repair of recurrent
  patellar dislocation) 81.44
Roux-Herzen-Judine operation (jejunal loop
  interposition) 42.63
Rubin test (insufflation of fallopian tube) 66.8
Ruiz-Mora operation (proximal phalangectomy
  for hammer toe) 77.99
Rupture
  esophageal web 42.01
  joint adhesions, manual 93.26
  membranes, artificial 73.09
    for surgical induction of labor 73.01
  ovarian cyst, manual 65.93
Russe operation (bone graft of scaphoid) 78.04

S

Sacculotomy (tack) 20.79
Sacrectomy (partial) 77.89
  total 77.99
Saemisch operation (corneal section) 11.1
Salpingectomy (bilateral) (total) (transvaginal)
  66.51
  with oophorectomy 65.61
    laparoscopic 65.63
  partial (unilateral) 66.69
    with removal of tubal pregnancy 66.62
    bilateral 66.63
      for sterilization 66.39
        by endoscopy 66.29
  remaining or solitary tube 66.52
    with ovary 65.62
      laparoscopic 65.64
  unilateral (total) 66.4
    with
      oophorectomy 65.49
        laparoscopic 65.41
      removal of tubal pregnancy 66.62
    partial 66.69

Salpingography 87.85
Salpingohysterostomy 66.74
Salpingo-oophorectomy (unilateral) 65.49
  that by laparoscope 65.41
  bilateral (same operative episode) 65.61
    laparoscopic 65.63
  remaining or solitary tube and ovary 65.62
    laparoscopic 65.64
Salpingo-oophoroplasty 65.73
  laparoscopic 65.76
Salpingo-oophororrhaphy 65.79
Salpingo-oophorostomy 66.72
Salpingo-oophorotomy 65.09
  laparoscopic 65.01
Salpingoplasty 66.79
Salpingorrhaphy 66.71
Salpingosalpingostomy 66.73
Salpingostomy (for removal of non-ruptured
  ectopic pregnancy) 66.02
Salpingotomy 66.01
Salpingo-uterostomy 66.74
Salter operation (innominate osteotomy) 77.39
Salvage (autologous blood) (intraoperative)
  (perioperative) (postoperative) 99.00
**Sampling, blood for genetic determination of
  fetus** 75.33
Sandpapering (skin) 86.25
Saucerization
  bone (*see also* Excision, lesion, bone) 77.60
  rectum 48.99
Sauer-Bacon operation (abdominoperineal
  resection) 48.5
Scalenectomy 83.45
Scalenotomy 83.19
Scaling and polishing, dental 96.54
Scan, scanning
  C.A.T. (computerized axial tomography) 88.38
    abdomen 88.01
    bone 88.38
      mineral density 88.98
    brain 87.03
    head 87.03
    kidney 87.71
    skeletal 88.38
      mineral density 88.98
    thorax 87.41
  computerized axial tomography (C.A.T.) (*see
    also* Scan, C.A.T.) 88.38
  C.T. — *see* Scan, C.A.T.
  gallium — *see* Scan, radioisotope
  liver 92.02
  positron emission tomography (PET) — *see*
    Scan, radioisotope
  radioisotope
    adrenal 92.09
    bone 92.14
      marrow 92.05
    bowel 92.04
    cardiac output 92.05
    cardiovascular 92.05
    cerebral 92.11
    circulation time 92.05
    eye 95.16
    gastrointestinal 92.04
    head NEC 92.12
    hematopoietic 92.05
    intestine 92.04
    iodine-131 92.01
    kidney 92.03
    liver 92.02
    lung 92.15
    lymphatic system 92.16
    myocardial infarction 92.05
    pancreatic 92.04
    parathyroid 92.13
    pituitary 92.11
    placenta 92.17
    protein-bound iodine 92.01
    pulmonary 92.15
    radio-iodine uptake 92.01
    renal 92.03
    specified site NEC 92.19

Scan, scanning — *continued*
  radioisotope — *continued*
    spleen 92.05
    thyroid 92.01
    total body 92.18
    uterus 92.19
  renal 92.03
  thermal — *see* Thermography
Scapulectomy (partial) 77.81
  total 77.91
Scapulopexy 78.41
Scarification
  conjunctiva 10.33
  nasal veins (with packing) 21.03
  pericardium 36.39
  pleura 34.6
    chemical 34.92
      with cancer chemotherapy substance
        34.92 [99.25]
        tetracycline 34.92 [99.21]
Schanz operation (femoral osteotomy) 77.35
Schauta (-Amreich) operation (radical vaginal
  hysterectomy) 68.7
Schede operation (thoracoplasty) 33.34
Scheie operation
  cautery of sclera 12.62
  sclerostomy 12.62
Schlatter operation (total gastrectomy) 43.99
Schroeder operation (endocervical excision)
  67.39
Schuchardt operation (nonobstetrical episiotomy)
  71.09
Schwartze operation (simple mastoidectomy)
  20.41
Scintiphotography — *see* Scan, radioisotope
Scintiscan — *see* Scan, radioisotope
Sclerectomy (punch) (scissors) 12.65
  for retinal reattachment 14.49
  Holth's 12.65
  trephine 12.61
    with implant 14.41
Scleroplasty 12.89
Sclerosis — *see* Sclerotherapy
Sclerostomy (Scheie's) 12.62
Sclerotherapy
  esophageal varices (endoscopic) 42.33
  hemorrhoids 49.42
  pleura 34.92
    treatment of malignancy (cytotoxic agent)
      34.92 [99.25]
      with tetracycline 34.92 [99.21]
  varicose vein 39.92
  vein NEC 39.92
Sclerotomy (exploratory) 12.89
  anterior 12.89
    with
      iridectomy 12.65
      removal of vitreous 14.71
  posterior 12.89
    with
      iridectomy 12.65
      removal of vitreous 14.72
Scott operation
  intestinal bypass for obesity 45.93
  jejunocolostomy (bypass) 45.93
Scraping
  corneal epithelium 11.41
    for smear or culture 11.21
  trachoma follicles 10.33
Scrotectomy (partial) 61.3
Scrotoplasty 61.49
Scrotorrhaphy 61.41
Scrototomy 61.0
Scrub, posterior nasal (adhesions) 21.91
Sculpturing, heart valve — *see* Valvuloplasty,
  heart
Section — *see also* Division *and* Incision
  cesarean — *see* Cesarean section
  ganglion, sympathetic 05.0

Section — *see also* Division *and* Incision —
  continued
  hypophyseal stalk (*see also* Hypophysectomy,
    partial) 07.63
  ligamentum flavum (spine) — *omit code*
  nerve (cranial) (peripheral) NEC 04.03
    acoustic 04.01
    spinal root (posterior) 03.1
    sympathetic 05.0
    trigeminal tract 04.02
  Saemisch (corneal) 11.1
  spinal ligament 80.49
    arcuate — *omit code*
    flavum — *omit code*
  tooth (impacted) 23.19
Sedden-Brooks operation (transfer of pectoralis
  major tendon) 83.75
Semb operation (apicolysis of lung) 33.39
Senning operation (correction of transposition of
  great vessels) 35.91
Separation
  twins (attached) (conjoined) (Siamese) 84.93
    asymmetrical (unequal) 84.93
    symmetrical (equal) 84.92
Septectomy
  atrial (closed) 35.41
    open 35.42
    transvenous method (balloon) 35.41
  submucous (nasal) 21.5
Septoplasty NEC 21.88
  with submucous resection of septum 21.5
Septorhinoplasty 21.84
Septostomy (atrial) (balloon) 35.41
Septotomy, nasal 21.1
Sequestrectomy
  bone 77.00
    carpals, metacarpals 77.04
    clavicle 77.01
    facial 76.01
    femur 77.05
    fibula 77.07
    humerus 77.02
    nose 21.32
    patella 77.06
    pelvic 77.09
    phalanges (foot) (hand) 77.09
    radius 77.03
    scapula 77.01
    skull 01.25
    specified site NEC 77.09
    tarsals, metatarsals 77.08
    thorax (ribs) (sternum) 77.01
    tibia 77.07
    ulna 77.03
    vertebrae 77.09
  nose 21.32
  skull 01.25
Sesamoidectomy 77.98
Setback, ear 18.5
Sever operation (division of soft tissue of arm)
  83.19
Severing of blepharorrhaphy 08.02
Sewell operation (heart) 36.2
Sharrard operation (iliopsoas muscle transfer)
  83.77
Shaving
  bone (*see also* Excision, lesion, bone) 77.60
  cornea (epithelium) 11.41
    for smear or culture 11.21
  patella 77.66
Shelf operation (hip arthroplasty) 81.40
Shirodkar operation (encirclement suture, cervix)
  67.59
Shock therapy
  chemical 94.24
  electroconvulsive 94.27
  electrotonic 94.27
  insulin 94.24
  subconvulsive 94.26
Shortening
  bone (fusion) 78.20
    femur 78.25

Shortening — *continued*
  bone — *continued*
    specified site NEC (*see* category 78.2 ✔4ᵗʰ)
    tibia 78.27
    ulna 78.23
  endopelvic fascia 69.22
  extraocular muscle NEC 15.22
    multiple (two of more muscles) 15.4
  eyelid margin 08.71
  eye muscle NEC 15.22
    multiple (two or more muscles) (with
      lengthening) 15.4
  finger (macrodactyly repair) 82.83
  heel cord 83.85
  levator palpebrae muscle 08.33
  ligament — *see also* Arthroplasty
    round 69.22
    uterosacral 69.22
  muscle 83.85
    extraocular 15.22
      multiple (two or more muscles) 15.4
    hand 82.55
  sclera (for repair of retinal detachment) 14.59
    by scleral buckling (*see also* Buckling,
      scleral) 14.49
  tendon 83.85
    hand 82.55
  ureter (with reimplantation) 56.41
Shunt — *see also* Anastomosis and Bypass,
  vascular
  abdominovenous 54.94
  aorta-coronary sinus 36.39
  aorta (descending)-pulmonary (artery) 39.0
  aortocarotid 39.22
  aortoceliac 39.26
  aortofemoral 39.25
  aortoiliac 39.25
  aortoiliofemoral 39.25
  aortomesenteric 39.26
  aorto-myocardial (graft) 36.2
  aortorenal 39.24
  aortosubclavian 39.22
  apicoaortic 35.93
  arteriovenous NEC 39.29
    for renal dialysis (by)
      anastomosis 39.27
      external cannula 39.93
  ascending aorta to pulmonary artery
    (Waterston) 39.0
  axillary-femoral 39.29
  carotid-carotid 39.22
  carotid-subclavian 39.22
  caval-mesenteric 39.1
  corpora cavernosa-corpus spongiosum 64.98
  corpora-saphenous 64.98
  descending aorta to pulmonary artery (Potts-
    Smith) 39.0
  endolymphatic (-subarachnoid) 20.71
  endolymph-perilymph 20.71
  extracranial-intracranial (EC-IC) 39.28
  femoroperoneal 39.29
  femoropopliteal 39.29
  iliofemoral 39.25
  ilioiliac 39.25
  intestinal
    large-to-large 45.94
    small-to-large 45.93
    small-to-small 45.91
  left subclavian to descending aorta (Blalock-
    Park) 39.0
  left-to-right (systemic-pulmonary artery) 39.0
  left ventricle (heart) (apex) and aorta 35.93
  lienorenal 39.1
  lumbar-subarachnoid (with valve) NEC 03.79
  mesocaval 39.1
  peritoneal-jugular 54.94
  peritoneo-vascular 54.94
  peritoneovenous 54.94
  pleuroperitoneal 34.05
  pleurothecal (with valve) 03.79
  portacaval (double) 39.1
  portal-systemic 39.1
  portal vein to vena cava 39.1
  pulmonary-innominate 39.0
  pulmonary vein to atrium 35.82

✔4ᵗʰ Fourth-digit Required   ▶◀ Revised Text   ● New Line   ▲ Revised Code

4ᵗʰ Fourth-digit Required ▶◀ Revised Text ● New Line ▲ Revised Code

Stapling — Suture (side tab)

Stapling
- artery 39.31
- blebs, lung (emphysematous) 32.21
- diaphysis (*see also* Stapling, epiphyseal plate) 78.20
- epiphyseal plate 78.20
  - femur 78.25
  - fibula 78.27
  - humerus 78.22
  - radius 78.23
  - specified site NEC 78.29
  - tibia 78.27
  - ulna 78.23
- gastric varices 44.91
- graft — *see* Graft
- vein 39.32

Steinberg operation 44.5

Steindler operation
- fascia stripping (for cavus deformity) 83.14
- flexorplasty (elbow) 83.77
- muscle transfer 83.77

Stereotactic head frame application 93.59

Stereotactic radiosurgery 92.30
- cobalt 60 92.32
- linear accelerator (LINAC) 92.31
- multi-source 92.32
- particle beam 92.33
- particulate 92.33
- radiosurgery NEC 92.39
- single source photon 92.31

Sterilization
- female (*see also* specific operation) 66.39
- male NEC (*see also* Ligation, vas deferens) 63.70

Sternotomy 77.31
- as operative approach — *omit code*
- for bone marrow biopsy 41.31

Stewart operation (renal plication with pyeloplasty) 55.87

Stimulation (electronic) — *see also* Implant, electronic stimulator
- bone growth (percutaneous) — *see category* 78.9 ✓4ᵗʰ
  - transcutaneous (surface) 99.86
- cardiac (external) 99.62
  - internal 37.91
- carotid sinus 99.64
- defibrillator ●
  - non-invasive programmed electrical stimulation (NIPS) 37.26 ●
- electrophysiologic, cardiac 37.26
- nerve, peripheral or spinal cord, transcutaneous 93.39

Stitch, Kelly-Stoeckel (urethra) 59.3
Stomatoplasty 27.59
Stomatorrhaphy 27.52
Stone operation (anoplasty) 49.79
Strassman operation (metroplasty) 69.49
Strayer operation (gastrocnemius recession) 83.72

Stretching
- eyelid (with elongation) 08.71
- fascia 93.28
- foreskin 99.95
- iris 12.63
- muscle 93.27
- nerve (cranial) (peripheral) 04.91
- tendon 93.27

Stripping
- bone (*see also* Incision, bone) 77.10
- carotid sinus 39.8
- cranial suture 02.01
- fascia 83.14
  - hand 82.12
- membranes for surgical induction of labor 73.1
- meninges (cerebral) 01.51
  - spinal 03.4
- saphenous vein, varicose 38.59
- subdural membrane (cerebral) 01.51
  - spinal 03.4
- varicose veins (lower limb) 38.59
  - upper limb 38.53
- vocal cords 30.09

Stromeyer-Little operation (hepatotomy) 50.0
Strong operation (unbridling of celiac artery axis) 39.91
Stryker frame 93.59

Study
- bone mineral density 88.98
- bundle of His 37.29
- color vision 95.06
- conduction, nerve (median) 89.15
- dark adaptation, eye 95.07
- electrophysiologic stimulation and recording, cardiac 37.26
- function — *see also* Function, study
  - radioisotope — *see* Scan, radioisotope
- lacrimal flow (radiographic) 87.05
- ocular motility 95.15
- pulmonary function — *see categories* 89.37-89.38
- radiographic — *see* Radiography
- radio-iodinated triolein 92.04
- renal clearance 92.03
- spirometer 89.37
- tracer — *see also* Scan, radioisotope eye (P³²) 95.16
- ultrasonic — *see* Ultrasonography
- visual field 95.05
- xenon flow NEC 92.19
  - cardiovascular 92.05
  - pulmonary 92.15

Sturmdorf operation (conization of cervix) 67.2

Submucous resection
- larynx 30.29
- nasal septum 21.5

Summerskill operation (dacryocystorhinostomy by intubation) 09.81

Surmay operation (jejunostomy) 46.39

Suspension
- balanced, for traction 93.45
- bladder NEC 57.89
- diverticulum, pharynx 29.59
- kidney 55.7
- Olshausen (uterus) 69.22
- ovary 65.79
- paraurethral (Pereyra) 59.6
- periurethral 59.6
- urethra (retropubic) (sling) 59.5
- urethrovesical
  - Goebel-Frangenheim-Stoeckel 59.4
  - gracilis muscle transplant 59.71
  - levator muscle sling 59.71
  - Marshall-Marchetti (-Krantz) 59.5
  - Millin-Read 59.4
  - suprapubic 59.4
- uterus (abdominal or vaginal approach) 69.22
- vagina 70.77

Suture (laceration)
- abdominal wall 54.63
  - secondary 54.61
- adenoid fossa 28.7
- adrenal (gland) 07.44
- aneurysm (cerebral) (peripheral) 39.52
- anus 49.71
  - obstetric laceration (current) 75.62
  - old 49.79
- aorta 39.31
- aponeurosis (*see also* Suture, tendon) 83.64
- arteriovenous fistula 39.53
- artery 39.31
  - percutaneous puncture closure — *omit code*
- bile duct 51.79
- bladder 57.81
  - obstetric laceration (current) 75.61
- blood vessel NEC 39.30
  - artery 39.31
  - percutaneous puncture closure — *omit code*
  - vein 39.32
- breast (skin) 85.81
- bronchus 33.41
- bursa 83.99
  - hand 82.99
- canaliculus 09.73
- cecum 46.75
- cerebral meninges 02.11

Suture — *continued*
- cervix (traumatic laceration) 67.61
  - internal os, encirclement 67.59
  - obstetric laceration (current) 75.51
  - old 67.69
- chest wall 34.71
- cleft palate 27.62
- clitoris 71.4
- colon 46.75
- common duct 51.71
- conjunctiva 10.6
- cornea 11.51
  - with conjunctival flap 11.53
- corneoscleral 11.51
  - with conjunctival flap 11.53
- diaphragm 34.82
- duodenum 46.71
  - ulcer (bleeding) (perforated) 44.42
    - endoscopic 44.43
- dura mater (cerebral) 02.11
  - spinal 03.59
- ear, external 18.4
- enterocele 70.92
- entropion 08.42
- epididymis (and)
  - spermatic cord 63.51
  - vas deferens 63.81
- episiotomy — *see* Episiotomy
- esophagus 42.82
- eyeball 16.89
- eyebrow 08.81
- eyelid 08.81
  - with entropion or ectropion repair 08.42
- fallopian tube 66.71
- fascia 83.65
  - hand 82.46
  - to skeletal attachment 83.89
    - hand 82.89
- gallbladder 51.91
- ganglion, sympathetic 05.81
- gingiva 24.32
- great vessel 39.30
  - artery 39.31
  - vein 39.32
- gum 24.32
- heart 37.4
- hepatic duct 51.79
- hymen 70.76
- ileum 46.73
- intestine 46.79
  - large 46.75
  - small 46.73
- jejunum 46.73
- joint capsule 81.96
  - with arthroplasty — *see* Arthroplasty
    - ankle 81.94
    - foot 81.94
    - lower extremity NEC 81.95
    - upper extremity 81.93
- kidney 55.81
- labia 71.71
- laceration — *see* Suture, by site
- larynx 31.61
- ligament 81.96
  - with arthroplasty — *see* Arthroplasty
    - ankle 81.94
    - broad 69.29
    - Cooper's 54.64
    - foot and toes 81.94
    - gastrocolic 54.73
    - knee 81.95
    - lower extremity NEC 81.95
    - sacrouterine 69.29
    - upper extremity 81.93
    - uterine 69.29
- ligation — *see* Ligation
- lip 27.51
- liver 50.61
- lung 33.43
- meninges (cerebral) 02.11
  - spinal 03.59
- mesentery 54.75
- mouth 27.52
- muscle 83.65
  - hand 82.46
  - ocular (oblique) (rectus) 15.7

Suture — *continued*
  nerve (cranial) (peripheral) 04.3
    sympathetic 05.81
  nose (external) (internal) 21.81
    for epistaxis 21.09
  obstetric laceration NEC 75.69
    bladder 75.61
    cervix 75.51
    corpus uteri 75.52
    pelvic floor 75.69
    perineum 75.69
    rectum 75.62
    sphincter ani 75.62
    urethra 75.61
    uterus 75.50
    vagina 75.69
    vulva 75.69
  omentum 54.64
  ovary 65.71
    laparoscopic 65.74
  palate 27.61
    cleft 27.62
  palpebral fissure 08.59
  pancreas 52.95
  pelvic floor 71.71
    obstetric laceration (current) 75.69
  penis 64.41
  peptic ulcer (bleeding) (perforated) 44.40
  pericardium 37.4
  perineum (female) 71.71
    after delivery 75.69
      episiotomy repair — *see* Episiotomy
    male 86.59
  periosteum 78.20
    carpal, metacarpal 78.24
    femur 78.25
    fibula 78.27
    humerus 78.22
    pelvic 78.29
    phalanges (foot) (hand) 78.29
    radius 78.23
    specified site NEC 78.29
    tarsal, metatarsal 78.28
    tibia 78.27
    ulna 78.23
    vertebrae 78.24
  peritoneum 54.64
  periurethral tissue to symphysis pubis 59.5
  pharynx 29.51
  pleura 34.93
  rectum 48.71
    obstetric laceration (current) 75.62
  retina (for reattachment) 14.59
  sacrouterine ligament 69.29
  salivary gland 26.41
  scalp 86.59
    replantation 86.51
  sclera (with repair of conjunctiva) 12.81
  scrotum (skin) 61.41
  secondary
    abdomninal wall 54.61
    episiotomy 75.69
    peritoneum 54.64
  sigmoid 46.75
  skin (mucous membrane) (without graft) 86.59
    with graft — *see* Graft, skin
    breast 85.81
    ear 18.4
    eyebrow 08.81
    eyelid 08.81
    nose 21.81
    penis 64.41
    scalp 86.59
      replantation 86.51
    scrotum 61.41
    vulva 71.71
  specified site NEC — *see* Repair, by site
  spermatic cord 63.51
  sphincter ani 49.71
    obstetric laceration (current) 75.62
    old 49.79
  spinal meninges 03.59
  spleen 41.95
  stomach 44.61
    ulcer (bleeding) (perforated) 44.41
      endoscopic 44.43

Suture — *continued*
  subcutaneous tissue (without skin graft) 86.59
    with graft — *see* Graft, skin
  tendon (direct) (immediate) (primary) 83.64
    delayed (secondary) 83.62
      hand NEC 82.43
        flexors 82.42
    hand NEC 82.45
      delayed (secondary) 82.43
      flexors 82.44
        delayed (secondary) 82.42
    ocular 15.7
    rotator cuff 83.63
    sheath 83.61
      hand 82.41
    supraspinatus (rotator cuff repair) 83.63
    to skeletal attachment 83.88
      hand 82.85
  Tenon's capsule 15.7
  testis 62.61
  thymus 07.93
  thyroid gland 06.93
  tongue 25.51
  tonsillar fossa 28.7
  trachea 31.71
  tunica vaginalis 61.41
  ulcer (bleeding) (perforated) (peptic) 44.40
    duodenum 44.42
      endoscopic 44.43
    gastric 44.41
      endoscopic 44.43
    intestine 46.79
    skin 86.59
    stomach 44.41
      endoscopic 44.43
  ureter 56.82
  urethra 58.41
    obstetric laceration (current) 75.61
  uterosacral ligament 69.29
  uterus 69.41
    obstetric laceration (current) 75.50
    old 69.49
  uvula 27.73
  vagina 70.71
    obstetric laceration (current) 75.69
    old 70.79
  vas deferens 63.81
  vein 39.32
  vulva 71.71
    obstetric laceration (current) 75.69
    old 71.79

Suture-ligation — *see also* Ligation
  blood vessel — *see* Ligation, blood vessel
Sweep, anterior iris 12.97
Swenson operation
  bladder reconstruction 57.87
  proctectomy 48.49
Swinney operation (urethral reconstruction) 58.46
Switch, switching
  coronary arteries 35.84
  great arteries, total 35.84
Syme operation
  ankle amputation through malleoli of tibia and fibula 84.14
  urethrotomy, external 58.0
Sympathectomy NEC 05.29
  cervical 05.22
  cervicothoracic 05.22
  lumbar 05.23
  periarterial 05.25
  presacral 05.24
  renal 05.29
  thoracolumbar 05.23
  tympanum 20.91
Sympatheticotripsy 05.0
Symphysiotomy 77.39
  assisting delivery (obstetrical) 73.94
  kidney (horseshoe) 55.85
Symphysis, pleural 34.6
Synchondrotomy (*see also* Division, cartilage) 80.40
Syndactylization 86.89

Syndesmotomy (*see also* Division, ligament) 80.40
Synechiotomy
  endometrium 68.21
  iris (posterior) 12.33
    anterior 12.32
Synovectomy (joint) (complete) (partial) 80.70
  ankle 80.77
  elbow 80.72
  foot and toe 80.78
  hand and finger 80.74
  hip 80.75
  knee 80.76
  shoulder 80.71
  specified site NEC 80.79
  spine 80.79
  tendon sheath 83.42
    hand 82.33
  wrist 80.73
Syringing
  lacrimal duct or sac 09.43
  nasolacrimal duct 09.43
    with
      dilation 09.43
      insertion of tube or stent 09.44

T

Taarnhoj operation (trigeminal nerve root decompression) 04.41
Tack operation (sacculotomy) 20.79
Take-down
  anastomosis
    arterial 39.49
    blood vessel 39.49
    gastric, gastrointestinal 44.5
    intestine 46.93
    stomach 44.5
    vascular 39.49
    ventricular 02.43
  arterial bypass 39.49
  arteriovenous shunt 39.43
    with creation of new shunt 39.42
  cecostomy 46.52
  colostomy 46.52
  duodenostomy 46.51
  enterostomy 46.50
  esophagostomy 42.83
  gastroduodenostomy 44.5
  gastrojejunostomy 44.5
  ileostomy 46.51
  intestinal stoma 46.50
    large 46.52
    small 46.51
  jejunoileal bypass 46.93
  jejunostomy 46.51
  laryngostomy 31.62
  sigmoidostomy 46.52
  stoma
    bile duct 51.79
    bladder 57.82
    bronchus 33.42
    common duct 51.72
    esophagus 42.83
    gall bladder 51.92
    hepatic duct 51.79
    intestine 46.50
      large 46.52
      small 46.51
    kidney 55.82
    larynx 31.62
    rectum 48.72
    stomach 44.62
    thorax 34.72
    trachea 31.72
    ureter 56.83
    urethra 58.42
  systemic-pulmonary artery anastomosis 39.49
    in total repair of tetralogy of Fallot 35.81
  tracheostomy 31.72
  vascular anastomosis or bypass 39.49
  ventricular shunt (cerebral) 02.43
Talectomy 77.98

✔4ᵗʰ Fourth-digit Required   ▶◀ Revised Text   ● New Line   ▲ Revised Code

Therapy — Tracheloplasty

✓4ᵀᴴ Fourth-digit Required   ►◄ Revised Text   ● New Line   ▲ Revised Code

Transplant, transplantation — *continued*
- hair follicles
  - eyebrow 08.63
  - eyelid 08.63
  - scalp 86.64
- heart (orthotopic) 37.5
  - combined with lung 33.6
- ileal stoma to new site 46.23
- intestine 46.97
- islets of Langerhans (cells) 52.86
  - allotransplantation of cells 52.85
  - autotransplantation of cells 52.84
  - heterotransplantation of cells 52.85
  - homotransplantation of cells 52.84
- kidney NEC 55.69
- liver 50.59
  - auxiliary (permanent) (temporary) (recipient's liver in situ) 50.51
  - cells into spleen via percutaneous catheterization 38.91
- lung 33.50
  - bilateral 33.52
  - combined with heart 33.6
  - double 33.52
  - single 33.51
  - unilateral 33.51
- lymphatic structure(s) (peripheral) 40.9
- mammary artery to myocardium or ventricular wall 36.2
- muscle 83.77
  - gracilis (for) 83.77
    - anal incontinence 49.74
    - urethrovesical suspension 59.71
  - hand 82.58
  - temporalis 83.77
    - with orbital exenteration 16.59
- nerve (cranial) (peripheral) 04.6
- ovary 65.92
- pancreas 52.80
  - heterotransplant 52.83
  - homotransplant 52.82
  - islets of Langerhans (cells) 52.86
    - allotransplantation of cells 52.85
    - autotransplanation of cells 52.84
  - islets of Langerhans — *continued*
    - heterotransplantation of cells 52.85
    - homotransplantation of cells 52.84
  - reimplantation 52.81
- pes anserinus (tendon) (repair of knee) 81.47
- renal NEC 55.69
  - vessel, aberrant 39.55
- salivary duct opening 26.49
- skin — *see* Graft skin
- spermatic cord 63.53
- spleen 41.94
- stem cell
  - allogeneic (hematopoietic) 41.05
    - with purging 41.08
  - autologous (hematopoietic) 41.04
    - with purging 41.07
  - cord blood 41.06
- tendon 83.75
  - hand 82.56
  - pes anserinus (repair of knee) 81.47
  - superior rectus (blepharoptosis) 08.36
- testis to scrotum 62.5
- thymus 07.94
- thyroid tissue 06.94
- toe (replacing absent thumb) (with amputation) 82.69 [84.11]
  - to finger, except thumb 82.81 [84.11]
- tooth 23.5
- ureter to
  - bladder 56.74
  - ileum (external diversion) 56.51
    - internal diversion only 56.71
  - intestine 56.71
  - skin 56.61
- vein (peripheral) 39.59
  - renal, aberrant 39.55
- vitreous 14.72
  - anterior approach 14.71

Transposition
- extraocular muscles 15.5

Transposition — *continued*
- eyelash flaps 08.63
  - eye muscle (oblique) (rectus) 15.5
- finger (replacing absent thumb) (same hand) 82.61
  - to
    - finger, except thumb 82.81
    - opposite hand (with amputation) 82.69 [84.01]
- interatrial venous return 35.91
- jejunal (Henley) 43.81
- joint capsule (*see also* Arthroplasty) 81.96
- muscle NEC 83.79
  - extraocular 15.5
  - hand 82.59
- nerve (cranial) (peripheral) (radial anterior) (ulnar) 04.6
- nipple 85.86
- pterygium 11.31
- tendon NEC 83.76
  - hand 82.57
- vocal cords 31.69

Transureteroureterostomy 56.75

Transversostomy (*see also* Colostomy) 46.10

Trapping, aneurysm (cerebral) 39.52

Trauner operation (lingual sulcus extension) 24.91

Trephination, trephining
- accessory sinus — *see* Sinusotomy
- corneoscleral 12.89
- cranium 01.24
- nasal sinus — *see* Sinusotomy
- sclera (with iridectomy) 12.61

Trial (failed) forceps 73.3

Trigonectomy 57.6

Trimming, amputation stump 84.3

Triple arthrodesis 81.12

Trochanterplasty 81.40

Tsuge operation (macrodactyly repair) 82.83

Tuck, tucking — *see also* Plication
- eye muscle 15.22
  - multiple (two or more muscles) 15.4
- levator palpebrac, for blepharoptosis 08.34

Tudor "rabbit ear" operation (anterior urethropexy) 59.79

Tuffier operation
- apicolysis of lung 33.39
- vaginal hysterectomy 68.59
  - laparoscopically assisted (LAVH) 68.51

TULIP (transurethral ultrasound guided laser induced prostatectomy) 60.21

TUMT (transurethral microwave thermotherapy) of prostate 60.96

TUNA (transurethral needle ablation) of prostate 60.97

Tunnel, subcutaneous (antethoracic) 42.86
- esophageal 42.86
  - with anastomosis — *see* Anastomosis, esophagus, antesternal
- pulse generator lead wire 86.99
  - with initial procedure — *omit code*
- with esophageal anastomosis 42.68

Turbinectomy (complete) (partial) NEC 21.69
- by
  - cryosurgery 21.61
  - diathermy 21.61
- with sinusectomy — *see* Sinusectomy

Turco operation (release of joint capsules in clubfoot) 80.48

TURP (transurethral resection of prostate) 60.29

Tylectomy (breast)(partial) 85.21

Tympanectomy 20.59
- with tympanoplasty — *see* Tympanoplasty

Tympanogram 95 .41

Tympanomastoidectomy 20.42

Tympanoplasty (type I) (with graft) 19.4
- with
  - air pocket over round window 19.54
  - fenestra in semicircular canal 19.55
  - graft against
    - incus or malleus 19.52

Tympanoplasty — *continued*
- with — *continued*
  - mobile and intact stapes 19.53
  - incudostapediopexy 19.52
- epitympanic, type I 19.4
- revision 19.6
- type
  - II (graft against incus or malleus) 19.52
  - III (graft against mobile and intact stapes) 19.53
  - IV (air pocket over round window) 19.54
  - V (fenestra in semicircular canal) 19.55

Tympanosympathectomy 20.91

Tympanotomy 20.09
- with intubation 20.01

U

Uchida operation (tubal ligation with or without fimbriectomy) 66.32

UFR (uroflowmetry) 89.24

Ultrasonography
- abdomen 88.76
- aortic arch 88.73
- biliary tract 88.74
- breast 88.73
- deep vein thrombosis 88.77
- digestive system 88.74
- eye 95.13
- head and neck 88.71
- heart (intravascular) 88.72
- intestine 88.74
- lung 88.73
- midline shift, brain 88.71
- multiple sites 88.79
- peripheral vascular system 88.77
- retroperitoneum 88.76
- therapeutic — *see* Ultrasound
- thorax NEC 88.73
- total body 88.79
- urinary system 88.75
- uterus 88.79
  - gravid 88.78

Ultrasound
- diagnostic — *see* Ultrasonography
- fragmentation (of)
  - cataract (with aspiration) 13.41
  - urinary calculus, stones (Kock pouch) 59.95
- heart (intravascular) 88.72
- inner ear 20.79
- therapeutic
  - head 00.01
  - heart 00.02
  - neck 00.01
  - other therapeutic ultrasound 00.09
  - peripheral vascular vessels 00.03
  - vessels of head and neck 00.01
- therapy 93.35

Umbilectomy 54.3

Unbridling
- blood vessel, peripheral 39.91
- celiac artery axis 39.91

Uncovering — *see* Incision, by site

Undercutting
- hair follicle 86.09
- perianal tissue 49.02

Unroofing — *see also* Incision, by site
- external
  - auditory canal 18.02
  - ear NEC 18.09
- kidney cyst 55.39

UPP (urethral pressure profile) 89.25

Upper GI series (x-ray) 87.62

UPPP (uvulopalatopharyngoplasty) 27.69 [29.4]

Uranoplasty (for cleft palate repair) 27.62

Uranorrhaphy (for cleft palate repair) 27.62

Uranostaphylorrhaphy 27.62

Urban operation (mastectomy) (unilateral) 85.47
- bilateral 85.48

✓4ᵗʰ Fourth-digit Required   ►◄ Revised Text   ● New Line   ▲ Revised Code

Transplant — Urban operation

Ureterectomy 56.40
  with nephrectomy 55.51
    partial 56.41
    total 56.42
Ureterocecostomy 56.71
Ureterocelectomy 56.41
Ureterocolostomy 56.71
Ureterocystostomy 56.74
Ureteroenterostomy 56.71
Ureteroileostomy (internal diversion) 56.71
  external diversion 56.51
Ureterolithotomy 56.2
Ureterolysis 59.02
  with freeing or repositioning of ureter 59.02
  laparoscopic 59.03
Ureteroneocystostomy 56.74
Ureteropexy 56.85
Ureteroplasty 56.89
Ureteroplication 56.89
Ureteroproctostomy 56.71
Ureteropyelography (intravenous) (diuretic
    infusion) 87.73
  percutaneous 87.75
  retrograde 87.74
Ureteropyeloplasty 55.87
Ureteropyelostomy 55.86
Ureterorrhaphy 56.82
Ureteroscopy 56.31
  with biopsy 56.33
Ureterosigmoidostomy 56.71
Ureterostomy (cutaneous) (external) (tube) 56.61
  closure 56.83
  ileal 56.51
Ureterotomy 56.2
Ureteroureterostomy (crossed) 56.75
  lumbar 56.41
  resection with end-to-end anastomosis 56.41
  spatulated 56.41
Urethral catheterization, indwelling 57.94
Urethral pressure profile (UPP) 89.25
Urethrectomy (complete) (partial) (radical) 58.39
  with
    complete cystectomy 57.79
    pelvic exenteration 68.8
    radical cystectomy 57.71
Urethrocystography (retrograde) (voiding) 87.76
Urethrocystopexy (by) 59.79
  levator muscle sling 59.71
  retropubic suspension 59.5
  suprapubic suspension 59.4
Urethrolithotomy 58.0
Urethrolysis 58.5
Urethropexy 58.49
  anterior 59.79
Urethroplasty 58.49
  augmentation 59.79
  collagen implant 59.72
  fat implant 59.72
  injection (endoscopic) of implant into urethra
    59.72
  polytef implant 59.72
Urethrorrhaphy 58.41
Urethroscopy 58.22
  for control of hemorrhage of prostate 60.94
  perineal 58.21
Urethrostomy (perineal) 58.0
Urethrotomy (external) 58.0
  internal (endoscopic) 58.5
Uroflowmetry (UFR) 89.24
Urography (antegrade) (excretory) (intravenous)
    87.73
  retrograde 87.74
Uteropexy (abdominal approach) (vaginal
    approach) 69.22
UVP (uvulopalatopharyngoplasty) 27.69 *[29.4]*
Uvulectomy 27.72
Uvulopalatopharyngoplasty (UPPP) 27.69 *[29.4]*
Uvulotomy 27.71

V

Vaccination (prophylactic) (against) 99.59
  anthrax 99.55
  brucellosis 99.55
  cholera 99.31
  common cold 99.51
  disease NEC 99.55
    arthropod-borne viral NEC 99.54
  encephalitis, arthropod-borne viral 99.53
  German measles 99.47
  hydrophobia 99.44
  infectious parotitis 99.46
  influenza 99.52
  measles 99.45
  mumps 99.46
  paratyphoid fever 99.32
  pertussis 99.37
  plague 99.34
  poliomyelitis 99.41
  rabies 99.44
  Rocky Mountain spotted fever 99.55
  rubella 99.47
  rubeola 99.45
  smallpox 99.42
  Staphylococcus 99.55
  Streptococcus 99.55
  tuberculosis 99.33
  tularemia 99.35
  tumor 99.28
  typhoid 99.32
  typhus 99.55
  undulant fever 99.55
  yellow fever 99.43
Vacuum extraction, fetal head 72.79
  with episiotomy 72.71
Vagectomy (subdiaphragmatic) (*see also*
    Vagotomy) 44.00
Vaginal douche 96.44
Vaginectomy 70.4
Vaginofixation 70.77
Vaginoperineotomy 70.14
Vaginoplasty 70.79
Vaginorrhaphy 70.71
  obstetrical 75.69
Vaginoscopy 70.21
Vaginotomy 70.14
  for
    culdocentesis 70.0
    pelvic abscess 70.12
Vagotomy (gastric) 44.00
  parietal cell 44.02
  selective NEC 44.03
    highly 44.02
    Holle's 44.02
    proximal 44.02
  truncal 44.01
Valvotomy — *see* Valvulotomy
Valvulectomy, heart — *see* Valvuloplasty, heart
Valvuloplasty
  heart (open heart technique) (without valve
      replacement) 35.10
    with prosthesis or tissue graft — *see*
        Replacement, heart, valve, by site
    aortic valve 35.11
      percutaneous (balloon) 35.96
    combined with repair of atrial and
        ventricular septal defects — *see*
        Repair, endocardial cushion defect
    mitral valve 35.12
      percutaneous (balloon) 35.96
    pulmonary valve 35.13
      in total repair of tetralogy of Fallot 35.81
      percutaneous (balloon) 35.96
    tricuspid valve 35.14
Valvulotomy
  heart (closed heart technique) (transatrial)
      (transventricular) 35.00
    aortic valve 35.01
    mitral valve 35.02
    open heart technique — *see* Valvuloplasty,
        heart

Valvulotomy — *continued*
  heart — *continued*
    pulmonary valve 35.03
      in total repair of tetralogy of Fallot 35.81
    tricuspid valve 35.04
Varicocelectomy, spermatic cord 63.1
Varicotomy, peripheral vessels (lower limb)
    38.59
  upper limb 38.53
Vascular closure, percutaneous puncture —
    omit code
Vascularization — *see* Revascularization
Vasectomy (complete) (partial) 63.73
Vasogram 87.94
Vasoligation 63.71
  gastric 38.86
Vasorrhaphy 63.81
Vasostomy 63.6
Vasotomy 63.6
Vasotripsy 63.71
Vasovasostomy 63.82
Vectorcardiogram (VCG) (with ECG) 89.53
Venectomy — *see* Phlebectomy
Venipuncture NEC 38.99
  for injection of contrast material — *see*
      Phlebography
Venography — *see* Phlebography
Venorrhaphy 39.32
Venotomy 38.00
  abdominal 38.07
  head and neck NEC 38.02
  intracranial NEC 38.01
  lower limb 38.09
  thoracic NEC 38.05
  upper limb 38.03
Venotripsy 39.98
Venovenostomy 39.29
Ventilation
  bi-level airway pressure 93.90
  continuous positive airway pressure [CPAP]
      93.90
  endotracheal respiratory assistance — *see*
      category 96.7 ✓4ᵗʰ
  intermittent mandatory ventilation [IMV] — *see*
      category 96.7 ✓4ᵗʰ
  intermittent positive pressure breathing [IPPB]
      93.91
  mechanical
    endotracheal respiratory assistance — *see*
        category 96.7 ✓4ᵗʰ
    intermittent mandatory ventilation [IMV] —
        see category 96.7 ✓4ᵗʰ
    other continuous (unspecified duration)
        96.70
      for less than 96 consecutive hours 96.71
      for 96 consecutive hours or more 96.72
    positive and expiratory pressure [PEEP] —
        see category 96.7
    pressure support ventilation [PSV] —*see*
        category 96.7
  negative pressure (continuous) [CNP] 93.99
Ventriculectomy, heart
  partial 37.35
Ventriculocholecystostomy 02.34
Ventriculocisternostomy 02.2
Ventriculocordectomy 30.29
Ventriculogram, Ventriculography (cerebral)
    87.02
  cardiac
    left ventricle (outflow tract) 88.53
      combined with right heart 88.54
    right ventricle (outflow tract) 88.52
      combined with left heart 88.54
    radionuclide cardiac 92.05
Ventriculomyocardiotomy 37.11
Ventriculoperitoneostomy 02.34
Ventriculopuncture 01.09
  through previously implanted catheter or
      reservoir (Ommaya) (Rickham) 01.02

Index to Procedures

Ventriculoseptopexy (*see also* Repair, ventricular septal defect) 35.72

Ventriculoseptoplasty (*see also* Repair, ventricular septal defect) 35.72

Ventriculostomy 02.2

Ventriculotomy
cerebral 02.2
heart 37.11

Ventriculoureterostomy 02.35

Ventriculovenostomy 02.32

Ventrofixation, uterus 69.22

Ventrohysteropexy 69.22

Ventrosuspension, uterus 69.22

VEP (visual evoked potential) 95.23

Version, obstetrical (bimanual) (cephalic) (combined) (internal) (podalic) 73.21
with extraction 73.22
Braxton Hicks 73.21
with extraction 73.22
external (bipolar) 73.91
Potter's (podalic) 73.21
with extraction 73.22
Wigand's (external) 73.91
Wright's (cephalic) 73.21
with extraction 73.22

Vesicolithotomy (suprapubic) 57.19

Vesicostomy 57.21

Vesicourethroplasty 57.85

Vesiculectomy 60.73
with radical prostatectomy 60.5

Vesiculogram, seminal 87.92
contrast 87.91

Vesiculotomy 60.72

Vestibuloplasty (buccolabial) (lingual) 24.91

Vestibulotomy 20.79

Vicq D'azyr operation (larynx) 31.1

Vidal operation (variocele ligation) 63.1

Vidianectomy 05.21

Villusectomy (*see also* Synovectomy) 80.70

Vision check 95.09

Visual evoked potential (VEP) 95.23

Vitrectomy (mechanical) (posterior approach) 14.74
with scleral buckling 14.49
anterior approach 14.73

Vocational
assessment 93.85
retraining 93.85
schooling 93.82

Voice training (postlaryngectomy) 93.73

von Kraske operation (proctectomy) 48.64

Voss operation (hanging hip operation) 83.19

Vulpius (-Compere) operation (lengthening of gastrocnemius muscle) 83.85

Vulvectomy (bilateral) (simple) 71.62
partial (unilateral) 71.61
radical (complete) 71.5
unilateral 71.61

V-Y operation (repair)
bladder 57.89
neck 57.85
ectropion 08.44
lip 27.59
skin (without graft) 86.89
subcutaneous tissue (without skin graft) 86.89
tongue 25.59

W

Wada test (hemispheric function) 89.10

Ward-Mayo operation (vaginal hysterectomy) 68.59
laparoscopically assisted (LAVH) 68.51

Washing — *see* Lavage *and* Irrigation

Waterston operation (aorta-right pulmonary artery anastomosis) 39.0

Watkins (-Wertheim) operation (uterus interposition) 69.21

Watson-Jones operation
hip arthrodesis 81.21
reconstruction of lateral ligaments, ankle 81.49
shoulder arthrodesis (extra-articular) 81.23
tenoplasty 83.88

Webbing (syndactylization) 86.89

Weir operation
appendicostomy 47.91
correction of nostrils 21.86

Wertheim operation (radical hysterectomy) 68.6

West operation (dacryocystorhinostomy) 09.81

Wheeler operation
entropion repair 08.44
halving procedure (eyelid) 08.24

Whipple operation (radical pancreaticoduodenectomy) 52.7
Child modification (radical subtotal pancreatectomy) 52.53
Rodney Smith modification (radical subtotal pancreatectomy) 52.53

White operation (lengthening of tendo calcaneus by incomplete tenotomy) 83.11

Whitehead operation
glossectomy, radical 25.4
hemorrhoidectomy 49.46

Whitman operation
foot stabilization (talectomy) 77.98
hip reconstruction 81.40
repair of serratus anterior muscle 83.87
talectomy 77.98
trochanter wedge osteotomy 77.25

Wier operation (entropion repair) 08.44

Williams-Richardson operation (vaginal construction) 70.61

Wilms operation (thoracoplasty) 33.34

Wilson operation (angulation osteotomy for hallux valgus) 77.51

Window operation
antrum (nasal sinus) — *see* Antrotomy, maxillary
aorticopulmonary 39.59
bone cortex (*see also* Incision, bone) 77.10
facial 76.09
nasoantral — *see* Antrotomy, maxillary
pericardium 37.12
pleura 34.09

Winiwarter operation (cholecystoenterostomy) 51.32

Wiring
aneurysm 39.52
dental (for immobilization) 93.55
with fracture-reduction — *see* Reduction, fracture
orthodontic 24.7

Wirsungojejunostomy 52.96

Witzel operation (temporary gastrostomy) 43.19

Woodward operation (release of high riding scapula) 81.83

Wrapping, aneurysm (gauze) (methyl methacrylate) (plastic) 39.52

X

Xenograft 86.65

Xerography, breast 87.36

Xeromammography 87.36

Xiphoidectomy 77.81

X-ray
chest (routine) 87.44
wall NEC 87.39
contrast — *see* Radiography, contrast
diagnostic — *see* Radiography
injection of radio-opaque substance — *see* Radiography, contrast
skeletal series, whole or complete 88.31
therapeutic — *see* Therapy, radiation

Y

Young operation
epispadias repair 58.45
tendon transfer (anterior tibialis) (repair of flat foot) 83.75

Yount operation (division of iliotibial band) 83.14

Z

Zancolli operation
capsuloplasty 81.72
tendon transfer (biceps) 82.56

Ziegler operation (iridectomy) 12.14

Zonulolysis (with lens extraction) (*see also* Extraction, cataract, intracapsular) 13.19

Z-plasty
epicanthus 08.59
eyelid (*see also* Reconstruction, eyelid) 08.70
hypopharynx 29.4
skin (scar) (web contracture) 86.84
with excision of lesion 86.3

00. PROCEDURES AND INTERVENTIONS, NOT ELSEWHERE CLASSIFIED (00)

● ✓3rd **00 Procedures and interventions, not elsewhere classified**

● ✓4th **00.0 Therapeutic ultrasound**

● **00.01 Therapeutic ultrasound of vessels of head and neck**
Anti-restenotic ultrasound
Intravascular non-ablative ultrasound
EXCLUDES   *diagnostic ultrasound of:*
eye (95.13)
head and neck (88.71)
that of inner ear (20.79)
ultrasonic:
angioplasty of non-coronary vessel (39.50)
embolectomy (38.01, 38.02)
endarterectomy (38.11, 38.12)
thrombectomy (38.01, 38.02)

● **00.02 Therapeutic ultrasound of heart**
Anti-restenotic ultrasound
Intravascular non-ablative ultrasound
EXCLUDES   *diagnostic ultrasound of heart (88.72)*
ultrasonic ablation of heart lesion (37.34)
ultrasonic angioplasty of coronary vessels (36.01, 36.02, 36.05, 36.09)

● **00.03 Therapeutic ultrasound of peripheral vascular vessels**
Anti-restenotic ultrasound
Intravascular non-ablative ultrasound
EXCLUDES   *diagnostic ultrasound of peripheral vascular system (88.77)*
ultrasonic angioplasty of: non-coronary vessel (39.50)

● **00.09 Other therapeutic ultrasound**
EXCLUDES   *ultrasonic:*
fragmentation of urinary stones (59.95)
percutaneous nephrostomy with fragmentation (55.04)
physical therapy (93.35)
transurethral guided laser induced prostatectomy (TULIP) (60.21)

● ✓4th **00.1 Pharmaceuticals**

● **00.10 Implantation of chemotherapeutic agent**
Brain wafer chemotherapy
Interstitial/intracavitary
EXCLUDES   *injection or infusion of cancer chemotherapeutic substance (99.25)*

● **00.11 Infusion of drotrecogin alfa (activated)**
Infusion of recombinant protein

● **00.12 Administration of inhaled nitric oxide**
Nitric oxide therapy

● **00.13 Injection or infusion of nesiritide**
Human B-type natriuretic peptide (hBNP)

● **00.14 Injection or infusion of oxazolidinone class of antibiotics**
Linezolid injection

● ✓4th **00.5 Other cardiovascular procedures**

● **00.50 Implantation of cardiac resynchronization pacemaker without mention of defibrillation, total system [CRT-P]**
Biventricular pacing without internal cardiac defibrillator
Implantation of cardiac resynchronization (biventricular) pulse generator pacing device, formation of pocket, transvenous leads including placement of lead into left ventricular coronary venous system, and intraoperative procedures for evaluation of lead signals
EXCLUDES   *implantation of cardiac resynchronization defibrillator, total system [CRT-D] (00.51)*
insertion or replacement of any type pacemaker device (37.80-37.87)
replacement of cardiac resynchronization: defibrillator, pulse generator only [CRT-D] (00.54)
pacemaker, pulse generator only [CRT-P] (00.53)

● **00.51 Implantation of cardiac resynchronization defibrillator, total system [CRT-D]**
Biventricular pacing with internal cardiac defibrillator
Implantation of cardiac resynchronization (biventricular) pulse generator with defibrillator [AICD], formation of pocket, transvenous leads, including placement of lead into left ventricular coronary venous system, intraoperative procedures for evaluation of lead signals, and obtaining defibrillator threshold measurements
EXCLUDES   *implantation of cardiac resynchronization pacemaker, total system [CRT-P] (00.50)*
implantation or replacement of automatic cardioverter/defibrillator, total system [AICD] (37.94)
replacement of cardiac resynchronization defibrillator, pulse generator only [CRT-D] (00.54)

● **00.52 Implantation or replacement of transvenous lead [electrode] into left ventricular coronary venous system**
EXCLUDES   *implantation of cardiac resynchronization: defibrillator, total system [CRT-D] (00.51)*
pacemaker, total system [CRT-P] (00.50)
initial insertion of transvenous lead [electrode] (37.70-37.72)
replacement of transvenous atrial and/or ventricular lead(s) [electrodes] (37.76)

Procedures and Interventions, NEC 00.53–00.55

00.53   **Implantation or replacement of cardiac resynchronization pacemaker, pulse generator only [CRT-P]**

Implantation of CRT-P device with removal of any existing CRT-P or other pacemaker device

EXCLUDES   *implantation of cardiac resynchronization pacemaker, total system [CRT-P] (00.50)*

implantation or replacement of cardiac resynchronization defibrillator, pulse generator only [CRT-D] (00.54)

insertion or replacement of any type pacemaker device (37.80-37.87)

00.54   **Implantation or replacement of cardiac resynchronization defibrillator, pulse generator device only [CRT-D]**

Implantation of CRT-D device with removal of any existing CRT-D, CRT-P, pacemaker, or defibrillator device

EXCLUDES   *implantation of automatic cardioverter/defibrillator pulse generator only (37.96)*

implantation of cardiac resynchronization defibrillator, total system [CRT-D] (00.51)

implantation or replacement of cardiac resynchronization pacemaker, pulse generator only [CRT-P] (00.53)

00.55   **Insertion of drug-eluting non-coronary artery stent(s)**

Endograft(s)

Endovascular graft(s)

Stent graft(s)

Code also any non-coronary angioplasty or atherectomy (39.50)

EXCLUDES   *drug-coated stents, e.g., heparin coated (39.90)*

insertion of drug-eluting coronary artery stent (36.07)

insertion of non-drug-eluting stent(s):

coronary artery (36.06)

non-coronary artery (39.90)

that for aneurysm repair (39.71-39.79)

1. OPERATIONS ON THE NERVOUS SYSTEM (01-05)

√3rd **01 Incision and excision of skull, brain, and cerebral meninges**

√4th **01.0 Cranial puncture**

01.01 Cisternal puncture
Cisternal tap
EXCLUDES pneumocisternogram (87.02)

DEF: Needle insertion through subarachnoid space to withdraw cerebrospinal fluid.

01.02 Ventriculopuncture through previously implanted catheter
Puncture of ventricular shunt tubing

DEF: Piercing of artificial, fluid-diverting tubing in the brain for withdrawal of cerebrospinal fluid.

01.09 Other cranial puncture
Aspiration of:
subarachnoid space
subdural space
Cranial aspiration NOS
Puncture of anterior fontanel
Subdural tap (through fontanel)

√4th **01.1 Diagnostic procedures on skull, brain, and cerebral meninges**

01.11 Closed [percutaneous] [needle] biopsy of cerebral meninges
Burr hole approach

DEF: Needle excision of tissue sample through skin into cerebral membranes; no other procedure performed.

01.12 Open biopsy of cerebral meninges

DEF: Open surgical excision of tissue sample from cerebral membrane.

01.13 Closed [percutaneous] [needle] biopsy of brain
Burr hole approach
Stereotactic method
AHA: M-A, '87, 9

DEF: Removal by needle of brain tissue sample through skin.

01.14 Open biopsy of brain

DEF: Open surgical excision of brain tissue sample.

01.15 Biopsy of skull

01.18 Other diagnostic procedures on brain and cerebral meninges
EXCLUDES cerebral:
arteriography (88.41)
thermography (88.81)
contrast radiogram of brain (87.01-87.02)
echoencephalogram (88.71)
electroencephalogram (89.14)
microscopic examination of specimen from nervous system and of spinal fluid (90.01-90.09)
neurologic examination (89.13)
phlebography of head and neck (88.61)
pneumoencephalogram (87.01)
radioisotope scan:
cerebral (92.11)
head NEC (92.12)
tomography of head:
C.A.T. scan (87.03)
other (87.04)

AHA: 3Q, '98, 12

01.19 Other diagnostic procedures on skull
EXCLUDES transillumination of skull (89.16)
x-ray of skull (87.17)

√4th **01.2 Craniotomy and craniectomy**
EXCLUDES decompression of skull fracture (02.02)
exploration of orbit (16.01-16.09)
that as operative approach — omit code

AHA: 1Q, '91, 1

DEF: Craniotomy: Incision into skull.

DEF: Craniectomy: Excision of part of skull.

01.21 Incision and drainage of cranial sinus

DEF: Incision for drainage, including drainage of air cavities in skull bones.

01.22 Removal of intracranial neurostimulator
EXCLUDES removal with synchronous replacement (02.93)

01.23 Reopening of craniotomy site

DEF: Reopening of skull incision.

01.24 Other craniotomy
Cranial:
decompression
exploration
trephination
Craniotomy NOS
Craniotomy with removal of:
epidural abscess
extradural hematoma
foreign body of skull
EXCLUDES removal of foreign body with incision into brain (01.39)

AHA: 2Q, '91, 14

01.25 Other craniectomy
Debridement of skull NOS
Sequestrectomy of skull
EXCLUDES debridement of compound fracture of skull (02.02)
strip craniectomy (02.01)

√4th **01.3 Incision of brain and cerebral meninges**

01.31 Incision of cerebral meninges
Drainage of:
intracranial hygroma
subarachnoid abscess (cerebral)
subdural empyema

01.32 Lobotomy and tractotomy
Division of:
brain tissue
cerebral tracts
Percutaneous (radiofrequency)
cingulotomy

DEF: Lobotomy: Incision of nerve fibers of brain lobe, usually frontal.

DEF: Tractotomy: Severing of a nerve fiber group to relieve pain.

01.39 Other incision of brain
Amygdalohippocampotomy
Drainage of intracerebral hematoma
Incision of brain NOS
EXCLUDES division of cortical adhesions (02.91)

√4th **01.4 Operations on thalamus and globus pallidus**

01.41 Operations on thalamus
Chemothalamectomy Thalamotomy
EXCLUDES that by stereotactic radiosurgery (92.30-92.39)

01.42 Operations on globus pallidus
Pallidoansectomy Pallidotomy
EXCLUDES that by stereotactic radiosurgery (92.30-92.39)

Operations on the Nervous System 01–01.42

√3rd
√4th **Additional Digit Required**

2002 Ingenix, Inc.

Nonspecific OR Procedure   Valid OR Procedure   Non-OR Procedure

Volume 3 —83

Operations on the Nervous System 01.5–02.43

✓4th **01.5 Other excision or destruction of brain and meninges**
AHA: 4Q, '93, 33

01.51 Excision of lesion or tissue of cerebral meninges

Decortication
Resection   } of (cerebral)
Stripping of subdural   meninges
    membrane

EXCLUDES   biopsy of cerebral meninges
(01.11-01.12)

01.52 Hemispherectomy
DEF: Removal of one half of the brain. Most often performed for malignant brain tumors or intractable epilepsy.

01.53 Lobectomy of brain
DEF: Excision of a brain lobe.

01.59 Other excision or destruction of lesion or tissue of brain
Curettage of brain
Debridement of brain
Marsupialization of brain cyst
Transtemporal (mastoid) excision of brain
    tumor

EXCLUDES   biopsy of brain (01.13-01.14)
that by stereotactic radiosurgery (92.30-92.39)

AHA: 3Q, '99, 7; 1Q, '99, 9; 3Q, '98, 12; 1Q, '98, 6

01.6 Excision of lesion of skull
Removal of granulation tissue of cranium

EXCLUDES   biopsy of skull (01.15)
sequestrectomy (01.25)

✓3rd **02 Other operations on skull, brain, and cerebral meninges**

✓4th **02.0 Cranioplasty**

EXCLUDES   that with synchronous repair of
encephalocele (02.12)

02.01 Opening of cranial suture
Linear craniectomy
Strip craniectomy
DEF: Opening of the lines of junction between the bones of the skull for removal of strips of skull bone.

02.02 Elevation of skull fracture fragments
Debridement of compound fracture of skull
Decompression of skull fracture
Reduction of skull fracture
Code also any synchronous debridement of
    brain (01.59)

EXCLUDES   debridement of skull NOS
(01.25)
removal of granulation tissue
of cranium (01.6)

02.03 Formation of cranial bone flap
Repair of skull with flap

02.04 Bone graft to skull
Pericranial graft (autogenous)
(heterogenous)

02.05 Insertion of skull plate
Replacement of skull plate

02.06 Other cranial osteoplasty
Repair of skull NOS
Revision of bone flap of skull
AHA: 3Q, '98, 9

DEF: Plastic surgery repair of skull bones.

02.07 Removal of skull plate

EXCLUDES   removal with synchronous
replacement (02.05)

✓4th **02.1 Repair of cerebral meninges**

EXCLUDES   marsupialization of cerebral lesion
(01.59)

02.11 Simple suture of dura mater of brain

02.12 Other repair of cerebral meninges
Closure of fistula of cerebrospinal fluid
Dural graft
Repair of encephalocele including
    synchronous cranioplasty
Repair of meninges NOS
Subdural patch

02.13 Ligation of meningeal vessel
Ligation of:
    longitudinal sinus
    middle meningeal artery

02.14 Choroid plexectomy
Cauterization of choroid plexus
DEF: Excision or destruction of the ependymal cells that form the membrane lining in the third, fourth, and lateral ventricles of the brain and secrete cerebrospinal fluid.

02.2 Ventriculostomy
Anastomosis of ventricle to:
    cervical subarachnoid space
    cisterna magna
Insertion of Holter valve
Ventriculocisternal intubation
DEF: Surgical creation of an opening of ventricle; often performed to drain cerebrospinal fluid in treating hydrocephalus.

✓4th **02.3 Extracranial ventricular shunt**

INCLUDES   that with insertion of valve
DEF: Placement of shunt or creation of artificial passage leading from skull cavities to site outside skull to relieve excess cerebrospinal fluid created in the chorioid plexuses of the third and fourth ventricles of the brain.

02.31 Ventricular shunt to structure in head and neck
Ventricle to nasopharynx shunt
Ventriculomastoid anastomosis

02.32 Ventricular shunt to circulatory system
Ventriculoatrial anastomosis
Ventriculocaval shunt

02.33 Ventricular shunt to thoracic cavity
Ventriculopleural anastomosis

02.34 Ventricular shunt to abdominal cavity and organs
Ventriculocholecystostomy
Ventriculoperitoneostomy

02.35 Ventricular shunt to urinary system
Ventricle to ureter shunt

02.39 Other operations to establish drainage of ventricle
Ventricle to bone marrow shunt
Ventricular shunt to extracranial site NEC

✓4th **02.4 Revision, removal, and irrigation of ventricular shunt**

EXCLUDES   revision of distal catheter of ventricular
shunt (54.95)

▲   **02.41 Irrigation and exploration of ventricular shunt**
▶Exploration and ventriculoperitoneal shunt
    at ventricular site◀

02.42 Replacement of ventricular shunt
Reinsertion of Holter valve
Replacement of ventricular catheter
Revision of ventriculoperitoneal shunt at
    ventricular site
AHA: N-D, '86, 8

02.43 Removal of ventricular shunt
AHA: N-D, '86, 8

BI Bilateral Procedure   **NC** Non-covered Procedure   ▶◀ Revised Text   ● New Code   ▲ Revised Code Title

✓4ᵗʰ **02.9**   **Other operations on skull, brain, and cerebral meninges**

> **EXCLUDES**   operations on:
> pineal gland (07.17, 07.51-07.59)
> pituitary gland [hypophysis] (07.13-07.15, 07.61-07.79)

02.91   **Lysis of cortical adhesions**

DEF: Breaking up of fibrous structures in brain outer layer.

02.92   **Repair of brain**

02.93   **Implantation of intracranial neurostimulator**

Implantation, insertion, placement, or replacement of intracranial:
brain pacemaker [neuropacemaker]
depth electrodes
epidural pegs
electroencephalographic receiver
foramen ovale electrodes
intracranial electrostimulator
subdural grids
subdural strips

AHA: 4Q, '97, 57; 4Q, '92, 28

02.94   **Insertion or replacement of skull tongs or halo traction device**

AHA: 3Q, '01, 8; 3Q, '96, 14

DEF: Halo traction device: Metal or plastic band encircles the head or neck secured to the skull with four pins and attached to a metal chest plate by rods; provides support and stability for the head and neck.

DEF: Skull tongs: Device inserted into each side of the skull used to apply parallel traction to the long axis of the cervical spine.

02.95   **Removal of skull tongs or halo traction device**

02.96   **Insertion of sphenoidal electrodes**

AHA: 4Q, '92, 28

02.99   **Other**

> **EXCLUDES**   chemical shock therapy (94.24)
> electroshock therapy:
> subconvulsive (94.26)
> other (94.27)

✓3ʳᵈ **03**   **Operations on spinal cord and spinal canal structures**

▶Code also any application or administration of an adhesion barrier substance (99.77)◀

✓4ᵗʰ **03.0**   **Exploration and decompression of spinal canal structures**

03.01   **Removal of foreign body from spinal canal**

03.02   **Reopening of laminectomy site**

03.09   **Other exploration and decompression of spinal canal**

Decompression:
laminectomy   laminotomy
▶Expansile laminoplasty◀
Exploration of spinal nerve root
Foraminotomy

> **EXCLUDES**   drainage of spinal fluid by anastomosis (03.71-03.79)
> laminectomy with excision of intervertebral disc (80.51)
> spinal tap (03.31)
> that as operative approach — omit code

AHA: 4Q, '99, 14; 2Q, '97, 6; 2Q, '95, 9; 2Q, '95, 10; 2Q, '90, 22, S-Q, '86, 12

DEF: Decompression of spinal canal: Excision of bone pieces, hematoma or other lesion to relieve spinal cord pressure.

DEF: Foraminotomy: Removal of root opening between vertebrae to relieve nerve root pressure.

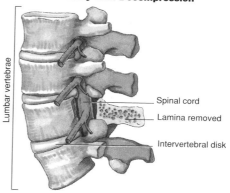

Laminotomy with Decompression

Lumbar vertebrae
Spinal cord
Lamina removed
Intervertebral disk

03.1   **Division of intraspinal nerve root**

Rhizotomy

DEF: Rhizotomy: Surgical severing of spinal nerve roots within spinal canal for pain relief.

✓4ᵗʰ **03.2**   **Chordotomy**

DEF: Chordotomy: Surgical cutting of lateral spinothalamic tract of spinal cord to relieve pain.

03.21   **Percutaneous chordotomy**

Stereotactic chordotomy

DEF: Percutaneous chordotomy: Insertion of hollow needle through skin to interrupt spinal nerve root.

DEF: Stereotactic chordotomy: Use of three-dimensional imaging to locate spinal nerve root for surgical interruption.

03.29   **Other chordotomy**

Chordotomy NOS
Tractotomy (one-stage) (two-stage) of spinal cord
Transection of spinal cord tracts

DEF: Tractotomy (one stage) (two stages) of the spinal cord: Surgical incision or severing of a nerve tract of spinal cord.

DEF: Transection of spinal cord tracts: Use of transverse incision to divide spinal nerve root.

✓4ᵗʰ **03.3**   **Diagnostic procedures on spinal cord and spinal canal structures**

03.31   **Spinal tap**

Lumbar puncture for removal of dye

> **EXCLUDES**   lumbar puncture for injection of dye [myelogram] (87.21)

AHA: 2Q, '90, 22

DEF: Puncture into lumbar subarachnoid space to tap cerebrospinal fluid.

03.32   **Biopsy of spinal cord or spinal meninges**

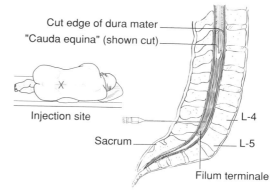

Lumbar Spinal Puncture

Cut edge of dura mater
"Cauda equina" (shown cut)
Injection site
Sacrum
Filum terminale
L-4
L-5

Operations on the Nervous System 02.9–03.32

Operations on the Nervous System 03.39–04.06

03.39 Other diagnostic procedures on spinal cord and spinal canal structures
> EXCLUDES microscopic examination of specimen from nervous system or of spinal fluid (90.01-90.09)
> x-ray of spine (87.21-87.29)

03.4 Excision or destruction of lesion of spinal cord or spinal meninges
Curettage
Debridement
Marsupialization of cyst
Resection
} of spinal cord or spinal meninges
> EXCLUDES biopsy of spinal cord or meninges (03.32)
AHA: 3Q, '95, 5

✓4th **03.5 Plastic operations on spinal cord structures**
03.51 Repair of spinal meningocele
Repair of meningocele NOS
DEF: Restoration of hernial protrusion of spinal meninges through defect in vertebral column.

03.52 Repair of spinal myelomeningocele
DEF: Restoration of hernial protrusion of spinal cord and meninges through defect in vertebral column.

03.53 Repair of vertebral fracture
Elevation of spinal bone fragments
Reduction of fracture of vertebrae
Removal of bony spicules from spinal canal
AHA: 4Q, '99, 11, 12, 13; 3Q, '96, 14

03.59 Other repair and plastic operations on spinal cord structures
Repair of:
diastematomyelia
spina bifida NOS
spinal cord NOS
spinal meninges NOS
vertebral arch defect

03.6 Lysis of adhesions of spinal cord and nerve roots
AHA: 2Q, '98, 18

✓4th **03.7 Shunt of spinal theca**
> INCLUDES that with valve
DEF: Surgical passage created from spinal cord dura mater to another channel.
03.71 Spinal subarachnoid-peritoneal shunt
03.72 Spinal subarachnoid-ureteral shunt
03.79 Other shunt of spinal theca
Lumbar-subarachnoid shunt NOS
Pleurothecal anastomosis
Salpingothecal anastomosis
AHA: 1Q, '97, 7

03.8 Injection of destructive agent into spinal canal
✓4th **03.9 Other operations on spinal cord and spinal canal structures**
03.90 Insertion of catheter into spinal canal for infusion of therapeutic or palliative substances
Insertion of catheter into epidural, subarachnoid, or subdural space of spine with intermittent or continuous infusion of drug (with creation of any reservoir)
Code also any implantation of infusion pump (86.06)
03.91 Injection of anesthetic into spinal canal for analgesia
> EXCLUDES that for operative anesthesia — omit code
AHA: 3Q, '00, 15; 1Q, '99, 8; 2Q, '98, 18

03.92 Injection of other agent into spinal canal
Intrathecal injection of steroid
Subarachnoid perfusion of refrigerated saline
> EXCLUDES injection of:
> contrast material for myelogram (87.21)
> destructive agent into spinal canal (03.8)
AHA: 3Q, '00, 15; 2Q, '98, 18

03.93 Insertion or replacement of spinal neurostimulator
AHA: 1Q, '00, 19
03.94 Removal of spinal neurostimulator
03.95 Spinal blood patch
DEF: Injection of blood into epidural space to patch hole in outer spinal membrane when blood clots.
03.96 Percutaneous denervation of facet
03.97 Revision of spinal thecal shunt
AHA: 2Q, '99, 4
03.98 Removal of spinal thecal shunt
03.99 Other

✓3rd **04 Operations on cranial and peripheral nerves**
✓4th **04.0 Incision, division, and excision of cranial and peripheral nerves**
> EXCLUDES opticociliary neurectomy (12.79)
> sympathetic ganglionectomy (05.21-05.29)
04.01 Excision of acoustic neuroma
That by craniotomy
> EXCLUDES that by stereotactic radiosurgery (92.3)
AHA: 2Q, '98, 20; 2Q, '95, 8; 4Q, '92, 26
04.02 Division of trigeminal nerve
Retrogasserian neurotomy
DEF: Transection of sensory root fibers of trigeminal nerve for relief of trigeminal neuralgia.
04.03 Division or crushing of other cranial and peripheral nerves
> EXCLUDES that of:
> glossopharyngeal nerve (29.92)
> laryngeal nerve (31.91)
> nerves to adrenal glands (07.42)
> phrenic nerve for collapse of lung (33.31)
> vagus nerve (44.00-44.03)
AHA: 2Q, '98, 20
04.04 Other incision of cranial and peripheral nerves
04.05 Gasserian ganglionectomy
04.06 Other cranial or peripheral ganglionectomy
> EXCLUDES sympathetic ganglionectomy (05.21-05.29)

Release of Carpal Tunnel
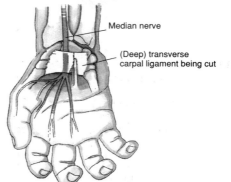
Median nerve
(Deep) transverse carpal ligament being cut

04.07 **Other excision or avulsion of cranial and peripheral nerves**

Curettage
Debridement ⎫ of peripheral nerve
Resection ⎭

Excision of peripheral neuroma [Morton's]

EXCLUDES *biopsy of cranial or peripheral nerve (04.11-04.12)*

AHA: 2Q, '95, 8; 4Q, '92, 26

✓4th **04.1** **Diagnostic procedures on peripheral nervous system**

04.11 **Closed [percutaneous] [needle] biopsy of cranial or peripheral nerve or ganglion**

04.12 **Open biopsy of cranial or peripheral nerve or ganglion**

04.19 **Other diagnostic procedures on cranial and peripheral nerves and ganglia**

EXCLUDES *microscopic examination of specimen from nervous system (90.01-90.09)*
neurologic examination (89.13)

04.2 **Destruction of cranial and peripheral nerves**

Destruction of cranial or peripheral nerves by:
cryoanalgesia
injection of neurolytic agent
radiofrequency
▶Radiofrequency ablation◀

AHA: 4Q, '95, 74

04.3 **Suture of cranial and peripheral nerves**

✓4th **04.4** **Lysis of adhesions and decompression of cranial and peripheral nerves**

04.41 **Decompression of trigeminal nerve root**
04.42 **Other cranial nerve decompression**
04.43 **Release of carpal tunnel**
04.44 **Release of tarsal tunnel**
04.49 **Other peripheral nerve or ganglion decompression or lysis of adhesions**
Peripheral nerve neurolysis NOS

04.5 **Cranial or peripheral nerve graft**

04.6 **Transposition of cranial and peripheral nerves**
Nerve transplantation
DEF: Relocation of cranial or peripheral nerves without detaching or severing them.

✓4th **04.7** **Other cranial or peripheral neuroplasty**

04.71 **Hypoglossal-facial anastomosis**
DEF: Surgical connection of hypoglossal nerve to facial nerve.

04.72 **Accessory-facial anastomosis**
DEF: Surgical connection of accessory nerve to facial nerve.

04.73 **Accessory-hypoglossal anastomosis**
DEF: Surgical connection of accessory nerve to hypoglossal nerve.

04.74 **Other anastomosis of cranial or peripheral nerve**

04.75 **Revision of previous repair of cranial and peripheral nerves**

04.76 **Repair of old traumatic injury of cranial and peripheral nerves**

04.79 **Other neuroplasty**

✓4th **04.8** **Injection into peripheral nerve**

EXCLUDES *destruction of nerve (by injection of neurolytic agent) (04.2)*

04.80 **Peripheral nerve injection, not otherwise specified**

04.81 **Injection of anesthetic into peripheral nerve for analgesia**

EXCLUDES *that for operative anesthesia — omit code*

AHA: 1Q, '00, 7

04.89 **Injection of other agent, except neurolytic**

EXCLUDES *injection of neurolytic agent (04.2)*

✓4th **04.9** **Other operations on cranial and peripheral nerves**

04.91 **Neurectasis**
DEF: Surgical stretching of peripheral or cranial nerve.

04.92 **Implantation or replacement of peripheral neurostimulator**
AHA: 3Q, '01, 16; 2Q, '00, 22; 3Q, '96, 12

DEF: Placement of or removal and replacement of test neurostimulator or permanent neurostimulator during the same episode.

04.93 **Removal of peripheral neurostimulator**
AHA: 3Q, '01, 16

DEF: Removal of test neurostimulator or permanent neurostimulator when a permanent device is not placed during the same episode.

04.99 **Other**

✓3rd **05** **Operations on sympathetic nerves or ganglia**

EXCLUDES *paracervical uterine denervation (69.3)*

05.0 **Division of sympathetic nerve or ganglion**

EXCLUDES *that of nerves to adrenal glands (07.42)*

✓4th **05.1** **Diagnostic procedures on sympathetic nerves or ganglia**

05.11 **Biopsy of sympathetic nerve or ganglion**
05.19 **Other diagnostic procedures on sympathetic nerves or ganglia**

✓4th **05.2** **Sympathectomy**

DEF: Sympathectomy: Division of nerve pathway at a specific site of a sympathetic nerve.

05.21 **Sphenopalatine ganglionectomy**
05.22 **Cervical sympathectomy**
05.23 **Lumbar sympathectomy**
DEF: Excision, resection of lumber chain nerve group to relieve causalgia, Raynaud's disease, or lower extremity thromboangiitis.

05.24 **Presacral sympathectomy**
DEF: Excision or resection of hypogastric nerve network.

05.25 **Periarterial sympathectomy**
DEF: Removal of arterial sheath containing sympathetic nerve fibers.

05.29 **Other sympathectomy and ganglionectomy**
Excision or avulsion of sympathetic nerve NOS
Sympathetic ganglionectomy NOS

EXCLUDES *biopsy of sympathetic nerve or ganglion (05.11)*
opticociliary neurectomy (12.79)
periarterial sympathectomy (05.25)
tympanosympathectomy (20.91)

✓4th **05.3** **Injection into sympathetic nerve or ganglion**

EXCLUDES *injection of ciliary sympathetic ganglion (12.79)*

05.31 **Injection of anesthetic into sympathetic nerve for analgesia**

05.32 **Injection of neurolytic agent into sympathetic nerve**

05.39 **Other injection into sympathetic nerve or ganglion**

✓4th **05.8** **Other operations on sympathetic nerves or ganglia**

05.81 **Repair of sympathetic nerve or ganglion**
05.89 **Other**

05.9 **Other operations on nervous system**

✓3rd
✓4th **Additional Digit Required**

Nonspecific OR Procedure

Valid OR Procedure

Non-OR Procedure

Operations on the Endocrine System 06–06.99

2. OPERATIONS ON THE ENDOCRINE SYSTEM (06-07)

√3rd **06 Operations on thyroid and parathyroid glands**
     INCLUDES   incidental resection of hyoid bone

√4th **06.0 Incision of thyroid field**
     EXCLUDES   *division of isthmus (06.91)*

06.01 Aspiration of thyroid field
Percutaneous or needle drainage of thyroid field
   EXCLUDES   *aspiration biopsy of thyroid (06.11)*
drainage by incision (06.09)
postoperative aspiration of field (06.02)

06.02 Reopening of wound of thyroid field
Reopening of wound of thyroid field for:
control of (postoperative) hemorrhage
examination
exploration
removal of hematoma

06.09 Other incision of thyroid field
Drainage of hematoma
Drainage of thyroglossal tract
Exploration:
neck
thyroid (field)
Removal of foreign body
Thyroidotomy NOS
   } by incision
   EXCLUDES   *postoperative exploration (06.02)*
removal of hematoma by aspiration (06.01)

√4th **06.1 Diagnostic procedures on thyroid and parathyroid glands**
DEF: Insertion of needle to draw or drain fluid from around thyroid.

06.11 Closed [percutaneous] [needle] biopsy of thyroid gland
Aspiration biopsy of thyroid
DEF: Insertion of needle-type device for removal of thyroid tissue sample.

06.12 Open biopsy of thyroid gland
06.13 Biopsy of parathyroid gland
06.19 Other diagnostic procedures on thyroid and parathyroid glands
   EXCLUDES   *radioisotope scan of:*
parathyroid (92.13)
thyroid (92.01)
soft tissue x-ray of thyroid field (87.09)

Thyroidectomy

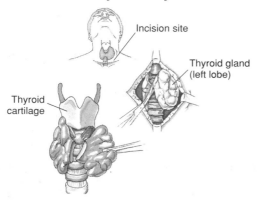
Incision site
Thyroid gland (left lobe)
Thyroid cartilage

06.2 Unilateral thyroid lobectomy
Complete removal of one lobe of thyroid (with removal of isthmus or portion of other lobe)
Hemithyroidectomy
   EXCLUDES   *partial substernal thyroidectomy (06.51)*
DEF: Excision of thyroid lobe.

√4th **06.3 Other partial thyroidectomy**
06.31 Excision of lesion of thyroid
   EXCLUDES   *biopsy of thyroid (06.11-06.12)*
DEF: Removal of growth on thyroid.

06.39 Other
Isthmectomy   Partial thyroidectomy NOS
   EXCLUDES   *partial substernal thyroidectomy (06.51)*

06.4 Complete thyroidectomy
   EXCLUDES   *complete substernal thyroidectomy (06.52)*
that with laryngectomy (30.3-30.4)

√4th **06.5 Substernal thyroidectomy**
DEF: Removal of thyroid tissue below breastbone.

06.50 Substernal thyroidectomy, not otherwise specified
06.51 Partial substernal thyroidectomy
06.52 Complete substernal thyroidectomy

06.6 Excision of lingual thyroid
Excision of thyroid by:
submental route
transoral route
DEF: Excision of thyroid tissue at base of tongue.

06.7 Excision of thyroglossal duct or tract
√4th **06.8 Parathyroidectomy**
DEF: Removal of parathyroid glands.

06.81 Complete parathyroidectomy
06.89 Other parathyroidectomy
Parathyroidectomy NOS
Partial parathyroidectomy
   EXCLUDES   *biopsy of parathyroid (06.13)*

√4th **06.9 Other operations on thyroid (region) and parathyroid**
06.91 Division of thyroid isthmus
Transection of thyroid isthmus
DEF: Cutting or division of tissue at narrowest point of thyroid.

06.92 Ligation of thyroid vessels
06.93 Suture of thyroid gland
06.94 Thyroid tissue reimplantation
Autotransplantation of thyroid tissue
DEF: Placement of thyroid tissue graft into functional site.
DEF: Autotransplantation of thyroid tissue: Tissue graft from patient thyroid tissue to another site on thyroid.

06.95 Parathyroid tissue reimplantation
Autotransplantation of parathyroid tissue
DEF: Placement of parathyroid tissue graft into functional site.
DEF: Autotransplantation of parathyroid tissue: Use of patient parathyroid tissue for graft.

06.98 Other operations on thyroid glands
06.99 Other operations on parathyroid glands

BI Bilateral Procedure   NC Non-covered Procedure   ►◄ Revised Text   ● New Code   ▲ Revised Code Title

√3rd **07 Operations on other endocrine glands**

INCLUDES operations on:
adrenal glands   pituitary gland
pineal gland   thymus

EXCLUDES operations on:
aortic and carotid bodies (39.8)
ovaries (65.0-65.99)
pancreas (52.01-52.99)
testes (62.0-62.99)

√4th **07.0 Exploration of adrenal field**
EXCLUDES incision of adrenal (gland) (07.41)

07.00 **Exploration of adrenal field, not otherwise specified**

07.01 **Unilateral exploration of adrenal field**
DEF: Investigation of one adrenal gland for diagnostic reasons.

07.02 **Bilateral exploration of adrenal field**
DEF: Investigation of both adrenal glands for diagnostic reasons.

√4th **07.1 Diagnostic procedures on adrenal glands, pituitary gland, pineal gland, and thymus**

07.11 **Closed [percutaneous] [needle] biopsy of adrenal gland**

07.12 **Open biopsy of adrenal gland**

07.13 **Biopsy of pituitary gland, transfrontal approach**
DEF: Excision of pituitary gland tissue for exam through frontal bone.

07.14 **Biopsy of pituitary gland, transsphenoidal approach**
DEF: Excision of pituitary gland tissue for exam through sphenoid bone.

07.15 **Biopsy of pituitary gland, unspecified approach**

07.16 **Biopsy of thymus**

07.17 **Biopsy of pineal gland**

07.19 **Other diagnostic procedures on adrenal glands, pituitary gland, pineal gland, and thymus**
EXCLUDES microscopic examination of specimen from endocrine gland (90.11-90.19)
radioisotope scan of pituitary gland (92.11)

√4th **07.2 Partial adrenalectomy**

07.21 **Excision of lesion of adrenal gland**
EXCLUDES biopsy of adrenal gland (07.11-07.12)

07.22 **Unilateral adrenalectomy**
Adrenalectomy NOS
EXCLUDES excision of remaining adrenal gland (07.3)
DEF: Excision of one adrenal gland.

07.29 **Other partial adrenalectomy**
Partial adrenalectomy NOS

07.3 **Bilateral adrenalectomy**
Excision of remaining adrenal gland
EXCLUDES bilateral partial adrenalectomy (07.29)

√4th **07.4 Other operations on adrenal glands, nerves, and vessels**

07.41 **Incision of adrenal gland**
Adrenalotomy (with drainage)

07.42 **Division of nerves to adrenal glands**

07.43 **Ligation of adrenal vessels**

07.44 **Repair of adrenal gland**

07.45 **Reimplantation of adrenal tissue**
Autotransplantation of adrenal tissue
DEF: Placement of adrenal tissue graft into functional site.
DEF: Autotransplantation of adrenal tissue: Use of tissue graft from the patient's own body.

07.49 **Other**

√4th **07.5 Operations on pineal gland**

07.51 **Exploration of pineal field**
EXCLUDES that with incision of pineal gland (07.52)

07.52 **Incision of pineal gland**

07.53 **Partial excision of pineal gland**
EXCLUDES biopsy of pineal gland (07.17)

07.54 **Total excision of pineal gland**
Pinealectomy (complete) (total)

07.59 **Other operations on pineal gland**

√4th **07.6 Hypophysectomy**
DEF: Excision, destruction of pituitary gland.

07.61 **Partial excision of pituitary gland, transfrontal approach**
Cryohypophysectomy, partial
Division of hypophyseal stalk
Excision of lesion of pituitary [hypophysis] } transfrontal approach
Hypophysectomy, subtotal
Infundibulectomy, hypophyseal
EXCLUDES biopsy of pituitary gland, transfrontal approach (07.13)
DEF: Removal of pituitary gland, partial, through frontal bone.

07.62 **Partial excision of pituitary gland, transsphenoidal approach**
EXCLUDES biopsy of pituitary gland, transsphenoidal approach (07.14)
DEF: Removal of pituitary gland, partial, through sphenoid bone.

07.63 **Partial excision of pituitary gland, unspecified approach**
EXCLUDES biopsy of pituitary gland NOS (07.15)

07.64 **Total excision of pituitary gland, transfrontal approach**
Ablation of pituitary by implantation (strontium-yttrium) } transfrontal approach
Cryohypophysectomy, complete
DEF: Removal of pituitary gland, total, through frontal bone.

07.65 **Total excision of pituitary gland, transsphenoidal approach**
DEF: Removal of pituitary gland, total, through sphenoid bone.

07.68 **Total excision of pituitary gland, other specified approach**
DEF: Destroy or remove pituitary gland by a specified approach, other than those listed.

07.69 **Total excision of pituitary gland, unspecified approach**

Hypophysectomy NOS
Pituitectomy NOS

☑4th **07.7** **Other operations on hypophysis**

07.71 **Exploration of pituitary fossa**

EXCLUDES   *exploration with incision of pituitary gland (07.72)*

DEF: Exploration of region of pituitary gland.

07.72 **Incision of pituitary gland**

Aspiration of: Aspiration of:
   craniobuccal pouch   pituitary gland
   craniopharyngioma   Rathke's pouch
   hypophysis

07.79 **Other**

Insertion of pack into sella turcica

☑4th **07.8** **Thymectomy**

07.80 **Thymectomy, not otherwise specified**

07.81 **Partial excision of thymus**

EXCLUDES   *biopsy of thymus (07.16)*

07.82 **Total excision of thymus**

☑4th **07.9** **Other operations on thymus**

07.91 **Exploration of thymus field**

EXCLUDES   *exploration with incision of thymus (07.92)*

07.92 **Incision of thymus**

07.93 **Repair of thymus**

07.94 **Transplantation of thymus**

DEF: Placement of thymus tissue grafts into functional area of gland.

07.99 **Other**

Thymopexy

---

3. OPERATIONS ON THE EYE (08-16)

√3rd **08 Operations on eyelids**

INCLUDES   operations on the eyebrow

√4th **08.0 Incision of eyelid**

08.01 Incision of lid margin
DEF: Cutting into eyelid edge.

08.02 Severing of blepharorrhaphy
DEF: Freeing of eyelids previously sutured shut.

08.09 Other incision of eyelid

√4th **08.1 Diagnostic procedures on eyelid**

08.11 Biopsy of eyelid

08.19 Other diagnostic procedures on eyelid

√4th **08.2 Excision or destruction of lesion or tissue of eyelid**
Code also any synchronous reconstruction (08.61-08.74)

EXCLUDES   biopsy of eyelid (08.11)

08.20 Removal of lesion of eyelid, not otherwise specified
Removal of meibomian gland NOS

08.21 Excision of chalazion

08.22 Excision of other minor lesion of eyelid
Excision of: Excision of:
verruca   wart

08.23 Excision of major lesion of eyelid, partial-thickness
Excision involving one-fourth or more of lid margin, partial-thickness
DEF: Excision of lesion not in all eyelid layers.

08.24 Excision of major lesion of eyelid, full-thickness
Excision involving one-fourth or more of lid margin, full-thickness
Wedge resection of eyelid
DEF: Excision of growth in all eyelid layers, full thickness.

08.25 Destruction of lesion of eyelid

√4th **08.3 Repair of blepharoptosis and lid retraction**

08.31 Repair of blepharoptosis by frontalis muscle technique with suture
DEF: Correction of drooping upper eyelid with suture of frontalis muscle.

08.32 Repair of blepharoptosis by frontalis muscle technique with fascial sling
DEF: Correction of drooping upper eyelid with fascial tissue sling of frontalis muscle.

08.33 Repair of blepharoptosis by resection or advancement of levator muscle or aponeurosis
DEF: Correction of drooping upper eyelid with levator muscle, extended, cut, or by expanded tendon.

08.34 Repair of blepharoptosis by other levator muscle techniques

08.35 Repair of blepharoptosis by tarsal technique
DEF: Correction of drooping upper eyelid with tarsal muscle.

08.36 Repair of blepharoptosis by other techniques
Correction of eyelid ptosis NOS
Orbicularis oculi muscle sling for correction of blepharoptosis

08.37 Reduction of overcorrection of ptosis
DEF: Correction, release of previous plastic repair of drooping eyelid.

08.38 Correction of lid retraction
DEF: Fixing of withdrawn eyelid into normal position.

√4th **08.4 Repair of entropion or ectropion**

08.41 Repair of entropion or ectropion by thermocauterization
DEF: Restoration of eyelid margin to normal position with heat cautery.

08.42 Repair of entropion or ectropion by suture technique
DEF: Restoration of eyelid margin to normal position by suture.

08.43 Repair of entropion or ectropion with wedge resection
DEF: Restoration of eyelid margin to normal position by removing tissue.

08.44 Repair of entropion or ectropion with lid reconstruction
DEF: Reconstruction of eyelid margin.

08.49 Other repair of entropion or ectropion

√4th **08.5 Other adjustment of lid position**

08.51 Canthotomy
DEF: Incision into outer canthus of eye.

08.52 Blepharorrhaphy
Canthorrhaphy Tarsorrhaphy
DEF: Suture together of eyelids, partial or repair; done to shorten palpebral fissure or protect cornea.

08.59 Other
Canthoplasty NOS
Repair of epicanthal fold

√4th **08.6 Reconstruction of eyelid with flaps or grafts**
EXCLUDES   that associated with repair of entropion and ectropion (08.44)

08.61 Reconstruction of eyelid with skin flap or graft
DEF: Rebuild of eyelid by graft or flap method.

08.62 Reconstruction of eyelid with mucous membrane flap or graft
DEF: Rebuild of eyelid with mucous membrane by graft or flap method.

08.63 Reconstruction of eyelid with hair follicle graft
DEF: Rebuild of eyelid with hair follicle graft.

08.64 Reconstruction of eyelid with tarsoconjunctival flap
Transfer of tarsoconjunctival flap from opposing lid
DEF: Recreation of eyelid with tarsoconjunctival tissue.

08.69 Other reconstruction of eyelid with flaps or grafts

√4th **08.7 Other reconstruction of eyelid**
EXCLUDES   that associated with repair of entropion and ectropion (08.44)

08.70 Reconstruction of eyelid, not otherwise specified
AHA: 2Q, '96, 11

08.71 Reconstruction of eyelid involving lid margin, partial-thickness
DEF: Repair of eyelid margin not using all lid layers.

08.72 Other reconstruction of eyelid, partial-thickness
DEF: Reshape of eyelid not using all lid layers.

Operations on the Eye 08.73–10.1

08.73 Reconstruction of eyelid involving lid margin, full-thickness
DEF: Repair of eyelid and margin using all tissue layers.

08.74 Other reconstruction of eyelid, full-thickness
DEF: Other repair of eyelid using all tissue layers.

√4th **08.8 Other repair of eyelid**

08.81 Linear repair of laceration of eyelid or eyebrow

08.82 Repair of laceration involving lid margin, partial-thickness
DEF: Repair of laceration not involving all layers of eyelid margin.

08.83 Other repair of laceration of eyelid, partial thickness
DEF: Repair of eyelid tear not involving all eyelid layers.

08.84 Repair of laceration involving lid margin, full-thickness
DEF: Repair of eyelid margin tear involving all margin layers.

08.85 Other repair of laceration of eyelid, full-thickness
DEF: Repair of eyelid tear involving all layers.

08.86 Lower eyelid rhytidectomy
DEF: Removal of wrinkles from lower eyelid.

08.87 Upper eyelid rhytidectomy
AHA: 2Q, '96, 11
DEF: Removal of wrinkles from upper eyelid.

08.89 Other eyelid repair
AHA: 1Q, '00, 22

√4th **08.9 Other operations on eyelids**

08.91 Electrosurgical epilation of eyelid
DEF: Electrical removal of eyelid hair roots.

08.92 Cryosurgical epilation of eyelid
DEF: Removal of eyelid hair roots by freezing.

08.93 Other epilation of eyelid

08.99 Other

√3rd **09 Operations on lacrimal system**

√4th **09.0 Incision of lacrimal gland**
Incision of lacrimal cyst (with drainage)

√4th **09.1 Diagnostic procedures on lacrimal system**

09.11 Biopsy of lacrimal gland

09.12 Biopsy of lacrimal sac

09.19 Other diagnostic procedures on lacrimal system
EXCLUDES   contrast dacryocystogram (87.05)
soft tissue x-ray of nasolacrimal duct (87.09)

√4th **09.2 Excision of lesion or tissue of lacrimal gland**

09.20 Excision of lacrimal gland, not otherwise specified

09.21 Excision of lesion of lacrimal gland
EXCLUDES   biopsy of lacrimal gland (09.11)

09.22 Other partial dacryoadenectomy
EXCLUDES   biopsy of lacrimal gland (09.11)
DEF: Excision, partial, of tear gland.

09.23 Total dacryoadenectomy
DEF: Excision, total, of tear gland.

09.3 Other operations on lacrimal gland

√4th **09.4 Manipulation of lacrimal passage**
INCLUDES   removal of calculus
that with dilation
EXCLUDES   contrast dacryocystogram (87.05)

09.41 Probing of lacrimal punctum
DEF: Exploration of tear duct entrance with flexible rod.

09.42 Probing of lacrimal canaliculi
DEF: Exploration of tear duct with flexible rod.

09.43 Probing of nasolacrimal duct
EXCLUDES   that with insertion of tube or stent (09.44)
DEF: Exploration of passage between tear sac and nose with flexible rod.

09.44 Intubation of nasolacrimal duct
Insertion of stent into nasolacrimal duct
AHA: 2Q, '94, 11

09.49 Other manipulation of lacrimal passage

√4th **09.5 Incision of lacrimal sac and passages**

09.51 Incision of lacrimal punctum

09.52 Incision of lacrimal canaliculi

09.53 Incision of lacrimal sac
DEF: Cutting into lacrimal pouch of tear gland.

09.59 Other incision of lacrimal passages
Incision (and drainage) of nasolacrimal duct NOS

09.6 Excision of lacrimal sac and passage
EXCLUDES   biopsy of lacrimal sac (09.12)
DEF: Removal of pouch and passage of tear gland.

09.7 Repair of canaliculus and punctum
EXCLUDES   repair of eyelid (08.81-08.89)

09.71 Correction of everted punctum
DEF: Repair of an outwardly turned tear duct entrance.

09.72 Other repair of punctum

09.73 Repair of canaliculus

√4th **09.8 Fistulization of lacrimal tract to nasal cavity**

09.81 Dacryocystorhinostomy [DCR]
DEF: Creation of entrance between tear gland and nasal passage for tear flow.

09.82 Conjunctivocystorhinostomy
Conjunctivodacryocystorhinostomy [CDCR]
EXCLUDES   that with insertion of tube or stent (09.83)
DEF: Creation of tear drainage path from lacrimal sac to nasal cavity through conjunctiva.

09.83 Conjunctivorhinostomy with insertion of tube or stent
DEF: Creation of passage between eye sac membrane and nasal cavity with tube or stent.

√4th **09.9 Other operations on lacrimal system**

09.91 Obliteration of lacrimal punctum
DEF: Destruction, total of tear gland opening in eyelid.

09.99 Other
AHA: 2Q, '94, 11

√3rd **10 Operations on conjunctiva**

10.0 Removal of embedded foreign body from conjunctiva by incision
EXCLUDES   removal of:
embedded foreign body without incision (98.22)
superficial foreign body (98.21)

10.1 Other incision of conjunctiva

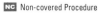

√4th **10.2** Diagnostic procedures on conjunctiva

10.21 Biopsy of conjunctiva

10.29 Other diagnostic procedures on conjunctiva

√4th **10.3** Excision or destruction of lesion or tissue of conjunctiva

10.31 Excision of lesion or tissue of conjunctiva

Excision of ring of conjunctiva around cornea

EXCLUDES biopsy of conjunctiva (10.21)

AHA: 4Q, '00, 41; 3Q, '96, 7

DEF: Removal of growth or tissue from eye membrane.

10.32 Destruction of lesion of conjunctiva

EXCLUDES excision of lesion (10.31)
thermocauterization for entropion (08.41)

DEF: Destruction of eye membrane growth; not done by excision.

10.33 Other destructive procedures on conjunctiva

Removal of trachoma follicles

√4th **10.4** Conjunctivoplasty

DEF: Correction of conjunctiva by plastic surgery.

10.41 Repair of symblepharon with free graft

AHA: 3Q, '96, 7

10.42 Reconstruction of conjunctival cul-de-sac with free graft

EXCLUDES revision of enucleation socket with graft (16.63)

DEF: Rebuilding of eye membrane fold with graft of unattached tissue.

10.43 Other reconstruction of conjunctival cul-de-sac

EXCLUDES revision of enucleation socket (16.64)

10.44 Other free graft to conjunctiva

10.49 Other conjunctivoplasty

EXCLUDES repair of cornea with conjunctival flap (11.53)

10.5 Lysis of adhesions of conjunctiva and eyelid

Division of symblepharon (with insertion of conformer)

10.6 Repair of laceration of conjunctiva

EXCLUDES that with repair of sclera (12.81)

√4th **10.9** Other operations on conjunctiva

10.91 Subconjunctival injection

AHA: 3Q, '96, 7

10.99 Other

√3rd **11** Operations on cornea

11.0 Magnetic removal of embedded foreign body from cornea

EXCLUDES that with incision (11.1)

11.1 Incision of cornea

Incision of cornea for removal of foreign body

√4th **11.2** Diagnostic procedures on cornea

11.21 Scraping of cornea for smear or culture

11.22 Biopsy of cornea

11.29 Other diagnostic procedures on cornea

√4th **11.3** Excision of pterygium

11.31 Transposition of pterygium

DEF: Cutting into membranous structure extending from eye membrane to cornea and suturing it in a downward position.

11.32 Excision of pterygium with corneal graft

DEF: Surgical removal and repair of membranous structure extending from eye membrane to cornea using corneal tissue transplant.

11.39 Other excision of pterygium

√4th **11.4** Excision or destruction of tissue or other lesion of cornea

11.41 Mechanical removal of corneal epithelium

That by chemocauterization

EXCLUDES that for smear or culture (11.21)

DEF: Removal of outer layer of cornea by mechanical means.

11.42 Thermocauterization of corneal lesion

DEF: Destruction of corneal lesion by electrical cautery.

11.43 Cryotherapy of corneal lesion

DEF: Destruction of corneal lesion with cold therapy.

11.49 Other removal or destruction of corneal lesion

Excision of cornea NOS

EXCLUDES biopsy of cornea (11.22)

√4th **11.5** Repair of cornea

11.51 Suture of corneal laceration

AHA: 3Q, '96, 7

11.52 Repair of postoperative wound dehiscence of cornea

DEF: Repair of ruptured postoperative corneal wound.

11.53 Repair of corneal laceration or wound with conjunctival flap

DEF: Correction corneal wound or tear with conjunctival tissue.

11.59 Other repair of cornea

√4th **11.6** Corneal transplant

EXCLUDES excision of pterygium with corneal graft (11.32)

11.60 Corneal transplant, not otherwise specified

Keratoplasty NOS

11.61 Lamellar keratoplasty with autograft

DEF: Restoration of sight using patient's own corneal tissue, partial thickness.

11.62 Other lamellar keratoplasty

AHA: S-O, '85, 6

DEF: Restoration of sight using donor corneal tissue, partial thickness.

11.63 Penetrating keratoplasty with autograft

Perforating keratoplasty with autograft

11.64 Other penetrating keratoplasty

Perforating keratoplasty (with homograft)

11.69 Other corneal transplant

√4th **11.7** Other reconstructive and refractive surgery on cornea

11.71 Keratomileusis [NC]

DEF: Restoration of corneal shape by removing portion of cornea, freezing, reshaping curve and reattaching it.

11.72 Keratophakia [NC]

DEF: Correction of eye lens loss by by dissecting the central zone of the cornea and replacing it with a thickened graft of the cornea.

11.73 Keratoprosthesis

DEF: Placement of corneal artificial implant.

11.74 Thermokeratoplasty

DEF: Reshaping and reforming cornea by heat application.

√3rd
√4th Additional Digit Required

2002 Ingenix, Inc.

Nonspecific OR Procedure   Valid OR Procedure   Non-OR Procedure

Operations on the Eye 10.2–11.74

Volume 3 —93

Operations on the Eye 11.75–12.64

11.75 Radial keratotomy   NC
DEF: Incisions around cornea radius to correct nearsightedness.

11.76 Epikeratophakia   NC
DEF: Repair lens loss by cornea graft sutured to central corneal zone.

11.79 Other

√4th **11.9 Other operations on cornea**
11.91 Tattooing of cornea
11.92 Removal of artificial implant from cornea
11.99 Other

√3rd **12 Operations on iris, ciliary body, sclera, and anterior chamber**

    EXCLUDES   *operations on cornea (11.0-11.99)*

√4th **12.0 Removal of intraocular foreign body from anterior segment of eye**

12.00 Removal of intraocular foreign body from anterior segment of eye, not otherwise specified

12.01 Removal of intraocular foreign body from anterior segment of eye with use of magnet

12.02 Removal of intraocular foreign body from anterior segment of eye without use of magnet

√4th **12.1 Iridotomy and simple iridectomy**

    EXCLUDES   *iridectomy associated with:*
       cataract extraction (13.11-13.69)
       removal of lesion (12.41-12.42)
       scleral fistulization (12.61-12.69)

12.11 Iridotomy with transfixion
12.12 Other iridotomy
    Corectomy
    Discission of iris
    Iridotomy NOS

DEF: Corectomy: Incision into iris (also called iridectomy).

12.13 Excision of prolapsed iris
DEF: Removal of downwardly placed portion of iris.

12.14 Other iridectomy
    Iridectomy (basal) (peripheral) (total)
DEF: Removal, partial or total of iris.

√4th **12.2 Diagnostic procedures on iris, ciliary body, sclera, and anterior chamber**

12.21 Diagnostic aspiration of anterior chamber of eye
DEF: Suction withdrawal of fluid from anterior eye chamber for diagnostic reasons.

12.22 Biopsy of iris
12.29 Other diagnostic procedures on iris, ciliary body, sclera, and anterior chamber

√4th **12.3 Iridoplasty and coreoplasty**
DEF: Correction or abnormal iris or pupil by plastic surgery.

12.31 Lysis of goniosynechiae
    Lysis of goniosynechiae by injection of air or liquid
DEF: Freeing of fibrous structures between cornea and iris by injecting air or liquid.

12.32 Lysis of other anterior synechiae
    Lysis of anterior synechiae:
      NOS
      by injection of air or liquid

12.33 Lysis of posterior synechiae
    Lysis of iris adhesions NOS

12.34 Lysis of corneovitreal adhesions
DEF: Release of adhesions of cornea and vitreous body.

12.35 Coreoplasty
    Needling of pupillary membrane
DEF: Correction of an iris defect.

12.39 Other iridoplasty

√4th **12.4 Excision or destruction of lesion of iris and ciliary body**

12.40 Removal of lesion of anterior segment of eye, not otherwise specified

12.41 Destruction of lesion of iris, nonexcisional
    Destruction of lesion of iris by:
      cauterization
      cryotherapy
      photocoagulation

12.42 Excision of lesion of iris
    EXCLUDES   *biopsy of iris (12.22)*

12.43 Destruction of lesion of ciliary body, nonexcisional

12.44 Excision of lesion of ciliary body

√4th **12.5 Facilitation of intraocular circulation**

12.51 Goniopuncture without goniotomy
DEF: Stab incision into anterior chamber of eye to relieve optic pressure.

12.52 Goniotomy without goniopuncture
DEF: Incision into Schlemm's canal to drain aqueous and relieve pressure.

12.53 Goniotomy with goniopuncture
12.54 Trabeculotomy ab externo
DEF: Incision into supporting connective tissue strands of eye capsule, via exterior approach.

12.55 Cyclodialysis
DEF: Creation of passage between anterior chamber and suprachoroidal space.

12.59 Other facilitation of intraocular circulation

√4th **12.6 Scleral fistulization**
    EXCLUDES   *exploratory sclerotomy (12.89)*

12.61 Trephination of sclera with iridectomy
DEF: Cut around sclerocornea to remove part of the iris.

12.62 Thermocauterization of sclera with iridectomy
DEF: Destruction of outer eyeball layer with partial excision of iris using heat.

12.63 Iridencleisis and iridotasis
DEF: Creation of permanent drain in iris by transposing or stretching iris tissue.

12.64 Trabeculectomy ab externo
DEF: Excision of supporting connective tissue strands of eye capsule, via exterior approach.

Trabeculectomy Ab Externo

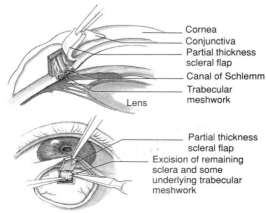

Cornea
Conjunctiva
Partial thickness scleral flap
Canal of Schlemm
Trabecular meshwork
Lens

Partial thickness scleral flap
Excision of remaining sclera and some underlying trabecular meshwork

---

12.65 Other scleral fistulization with iridectomy

DEF: Creation of outer eyeball layer passage with partial excision of iris.

12.66 Postoperative revision of scleral fistulization procedure

Revision of filtering bleb

EXCLUDES   *repair of fistula (12.82)*

AHA: 2Q, '01, 16

12.69 Other fistulizing procedure

√4th 12.7 Other procedures for relief of elevated intraocular pressure

12.71 Cyclodiathermy

DEF: Destruction of ciliary body tissue with heat.

12.72 Cyclocryotherapy

DEF: Destruction of ciliary body tissue by freezing.

12.73 Cyclophotocoagulation

DEF: Destruction of ciliary body tissue by high energy light source.

12.74 Diminution of ciliary body, not otherwise specified

12.79 Other glaucoma procedures

AHA: 2Q, '98, 16

√4th 12.8 Operations on sclera

EXCLUDES   *those associated with:*
retinal reattachment (14.41-14.59)
scleral fistulization (12.61-12.69)

12.81 Suture of laceration of sclera

Suture of sclera with synchronous repair of conjunctiva

12.82 Repair of scleral fistula

EXCLUDES   *postoperative revision of scleral fistulization procedure (12.66)*

12.83 Revision of operative wound of anterior segment, not elsewhere classified

EXCLUDES   *postoperative revision of scleral fistulization procedure (12.66)*

12.84 Excision or destruction of lesion of sclera

12.85 Repair of scleral staphyloma with graft

DEF: Repair of protruding outer eyeball layer with a graft.

12.86 Other repair of scleral staphyloma

12.87 Scleral reinforcement with graft

DEF: Restoration of outer eyeball shape with tissue graft.

12.88 Other scleral reinforcement

12.89 Other operations on sclera

Exploratory sclerotomy

√4th 12.9 Other operations on iris, ciliary body, and anterior chamber

12.91 Therapeutic evacuation of anterior chamber

Paracentesis of anterior chamber

EXCLUDES   *diagnostic aspiration (12.21)*

12.92 Injection into anterior chamber

Injection of:
air
liquid   } into anterior chamber
medication

AHA: J-A, '84, 1

12.93 Removal or destruction of epithelial downgrowth from anterior chamber

EXCLUDES   *that with iridectomy (12.41-12.42)*

DEF: Excision or destruction of epithelial overgrowth in anterior eye chamber.

12.97 Other operations on iris

12.98 Other operations on ciliary body

12.99 Other operations on anterior chamber

√3rd 13 Operations on lens

√4th 13.0 Removal of foreign body from lens

EXCLUDES   *removal of pseudophakos (13.8)*

13.00 Removal of foreign body from lens, not otherwise specified

13.01 Removal of foreign body from lens with use of magnet

13.02 Removal of foreign body from lens without use of magnet

√4th 13.1 Intracapsular extraction of lens

Code also any synchronous insertion of pseudophakos (13.71)

AHA: S-O, '85, 6

13.11 Intracapsular extraction of lens by temporal inferior route

DEF: Extraction of lens and capsule via anterior approach through outer side of eyeball.

13.19 Other intracapsular extraction of lens

Cataract extraction NOS
Cryoextraction of lens
Erysiphake extraction of cataract
Extraction of lens NOS

13.2 Extracapsular extraction of lens by linear extraction technique

AHA: S-O, '85, 6

DEF: Excision of lens without the posterior capsule at junction between the cornea and outer eyeball layer by means of a linear incision.

13.3 Extracapsular extraction of lens by simple aspiration (and irrigation) technique

Irrigation of traumatic cataract

AHA: S-O, '85, 6

DEF: Removal of lens without the posterior capsule by suctioning and flushing out the area.

√4th 13.4 Extracapsular extraction of lens by fragmentation and aspiration technique

AHA: S-O, '85, 6

DEF: Removal of lens after division into smaller pieces with posterior capsule left intact.

13.41 Phacoemulsification and aspiration of cataract

AHA: 3Q, '96, 4; 1Q, '94, 16

13.42 Mechanical phacofragmentation and aspiration of cataract by posterior route

Code also any synchronous vitrectomy (14.74)

Extraction of Lens
(with insertion of intraocular lens prosthesis)

Iris
Lens cataract removed
Iris
Lens
Intraocular lens insertion

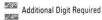
Operations on the Eye 12.65–13.42

Operations on the Eye 13.43–14.49

Laser Surgery (YAG)

13.43   **Mechanical phacofragmentation and other aspiration of cataract**

✓4th **13.5**   **Other extracapsular extraction of lens**
Code also any synchronous insertion of pseudophakos (13.71)

AHA: S-O, '85, 6

13.51   **Extracapsular extraction of lens by temporal inferior route**
DEF: Removal of lens through outer eyeball with posterior capsule left intact.

13.59   **Other extracapsular extraction of lens**

✓4th **13.6**   **Other cataract extraction**
Code also any synchronous insertion of pseudophakos (13.71)

AHA: S-O, '85, 6

13.64   **Discision of secondary membrane [after cataract]**
DEF: Breaking up of fibrotic lens capsule developed after previous lens extraction.

13.65   **Excision of secondary membrane [after cataract]**
Capsulectomy
DEF: Capsulectomy: Excision of lens capsule membrane after previous lens extraction.

13.66   **Mechanical fragmentation of secondary membrane [after cataract]**
DEF: Breaking up and removal of fibrotic lens capsule developed after previous lens extraction.

13.69   **Other cataract extraction**

✓4th **13.7**   **Insertion of prosthetic lens [pseudophakos]**

AHA: J-A, '84, 1

DEF: Insertion of ocular implant, following lens extraction.

13.70   **Insertion of pseudophakos, not otherwise specified**

13.71   **Insertion of intraocular lens prosthesis at time of cataract extraction, one-stage**
Code also synchronous extraction of cataract (13.11-13.69)

AHA: 3Q, '96, 4

13.72   **Secondary insertion of intraocular lens prosthesis**

13.8   **Removal of implanted lens**
Removal of pseudophakos

13.9   **Other operations on lens**

AHA: 1Q, '00, 9

✓3rd **14**   **Operations on retina, choroid, vitreous, and posterior chamber**

✓4th **14.0**   **Removal of foreign body from posterior segment of eye**
EXCLUDES   removal of surgically implanted material (14.6)

14.00   **Removal of foreign body from posterior segment of eye, not otherwise specified**

14.01   **Removal of foreign body from posterior segment of eye with use of magnet**

14.02   **Removal of foreign body from posterior segment of eye without use of magnet**

✓4th **14.1**   **Diagnostic procedures on retina, choroid, vitreous, and posterior chamber**

14.11   **Diagnostic aspiration of vitreous**

14.19   **Other diagnostic procedures on retina, choroid, vitreous, and posterior chamber**

✓4th **14.2**   **Destruction of lesion of retina and choroid**
INCLUDES   destruction of chorioretinopathy or isolated chorioretinal lesion
EXCLUDES   that for repair of retina (14.31-14.59)
DEF: Destruction of damaged retina and choroid tissue.

14.21   **Destruction of chorioretinal lesion by diathermy**

14.22   **Destruction of chorioretinal lesion by cryotherapy**

14.23   **Destruction of chorioretinal lesion by xenon arc photocoagulation**

14.24   **Destruction of chorioretinal lesion by laser photocoagulation**

14.25   **Destruction of chorioretinal lesion by photocoagulation of unspecified type**

14.26   **Destruction of chorioretinal lesion by radiation therapy**

14.27   **Destruction of chorioretinal lesion by implantation of radiation source**

14.29   **Other destruction of chorioretinal lesion**
Destruction of lesion of retina and choroid NOS

✓4th **14.3**   **Repair of retinal tear**
INCLUDES   repair of retinal defect
EXCLUDES   repair of retinal detachment (14.41-14.59)

14.31   **Repair of retinal tear by diathermy**

14.32   **Repair of retinal tear by cryotherapy**

14.33   **Repair of retinal tear by xenon arc photocoagulation**

14.34   **Repair of retinal tear by laser photocoagulation**

AHA: 1Q, '94, 17

14.35   **Repair of retinal tear by photocoagulation of unspecified type**

14.39   **Other repair of retinal tear**

✓4th **14.4**   **Repair of retinal detachment with scleral buckling and implant**
DEF: Placement of material around eye to indent sclera and close a hole or tear or to reduce vitreous traction.

14.41   **Scleral buckling with implant**

AHA: 3Q, '96, 6

14.49   **Other scleral buckling**
Scleral buckling with:
air tamponade
resection of sclera
vitrectomy

AHA: 1Q, '94, 16

BI Bilateral Edit   NC Non-covered Procedure   ▶◀ Revised Text   ● New Code   ▲ Revised Code Title

✓4th **14.5** **Other repair of retinal detachment**
INCLUDES that with drainage

14.51 **Repair of retinal detachment with diathermy**

14.52 **Repair of retinal detachment with cryotherapy**

14.53 **Repair of retinal detachment with xenon arc photocoagulation**

14.54 **Repair of retinal detachment with laser photocoagulation**
AHA: N-D, '87, 10

14.55 **Repair of retinal detachment with photocoagulation of unspecified type**

14.59 **Other**

14.6 **Removal of surgically implanted material from posterior segment of eye**

✓4th **14.7** **Operations on vitreous**

14.71 **Removal of vitreous, anterior approach**
Open sky technique
Removal of vitreous, anterior approach (with replacement)
DEF: Removal of all or part of the eyeball fluid via the anterior segment of the eyeball.

14.72 **Other removal of vitreous**
Aspiration of vitreous by posterior sclerotomy

14.73 **Mechanical vitrectomy by anterior approach**
AHA: 3Q, '96, 4, 5
DEF: Removal of abnormal tissue in eyeball fluid to control fibrotic overgrowth in severe intraocular injury.

14.74 **Other mechanical vitrectomy**
AHA: 3Q, '96, 4, 5

14.75 **Injection of vitreous substitute**
EXCLUDES that associated with removal (14.71-14.72)
AHA: 1Q, '98, 6; 3Q, '96, 4, 5; 1Q, '94, 17

14.79 **Other operations on vitreous**
AHA: 3Q, '99, 12; 1Q, '99, 11; 1Q, '98, 6

14.9 **Other operations on retina, choroid, and posterior chamber**
AHA: 3Q, '96, 5

✓3rd **15** **Operations on extraocular muscles**

✓4th **15.0** **Diagnostic procedures on extraocular muscles or tendons**

15.01 **Biopsy of extraocular muscle or tendon**

15.09 **Other diagnostic procedures on extraocular muscles and tendons**

✓4th **15.1** **Operations on one extraocular muscle involving temporary detachment from globe**

15.11 **Recession of one extraocular muscle**
AHA: 3Q, '96, 3
DEF: Detachment of exterior eye muscle with posterior reattachment to correct strabismus.

15.12 **Advancement of one extraocular muscle**
DEF: Detachment of exterior eye muscle with forward reattachment to correct strabismus.

15.13 **Resection of one extraocular muscle**

15.19 **Other operations on one extraocular muscle involving temporary detachment from globe**
EXCLUDES transposition of muscle (15.5)

✓4th **15.2** **Other operations on one extraocular muscle**

15.21 **Lengthening procedure on one extraocular muscle**
DEF: Extension of exterior eye muscle length.

Lengthening Procedure on One Extraocular Muscle

Proposed second cut
Extraocular muscle
Lengthened muscle

Shortening Procedure on One Extraocular Muscle

To be resected
Muscle advanced and reattached
Iris

15.22 **Shortening procedure on one extraocular muscle**
DEF: Shortening of exterior eye muscle.

15.29 **Other**

15.3 **Operations on two or more extraocular muscles involving temporary detachment from globe, one or both eyes**
AHA: 3Q, '96, 3

15.4 **Other operations on two or more extraocular muscles, one or both eyes**

15.5 **Transposition of extraocular muscles**
EXCLUDES that for correction of ptosis (08.31-08.36)
DEF: Relocation of exterior eye muscle to a more functional site.

15.6 **Revision of extraocular muscle surgery**
DEF: Repair of previous exterior eye muscle surgery.

15.7 **Repair of injury of extraocular muscle**
Freeing of entrapped extraocular muscle
Lysis of adhesions of extraocular muscle
Repair of laceration of extraocular muscle, tendon, or Tenon's capsule

15.9 **Other operations on extraocular muscles and tendons**

✓3rd **16** **Operations on orbit and eyeball**
EXCLUDES reduction of fracture of orbit (76.78-76.79)

✓4th **16.0** **Orbitotomy**

16.01 **Orbitotomy with bone flap**
Orbitotomy with lateral approach
DEF: Incision into orbital bone with insertion of small bone piece.

16.02 **Orbitotomy with insertion of orbital implant**
EXCLUDES that with bone flap (16.01)

16.09 **Other orbitotomy**

✓3rd
✓4th Additional Digit Required

2002 Ingenix, Inc.

Nonspecific OR Procedure   Valid OR Procedure   Non-OR Procedure

Operations on the Eye 16.1–16.99

16.1   Removal of penetrating foreign body from eye, not otherwise specified

EXCLUDES   removal of nonpenetrating foreign body (98.21)

DEF: Removal of foreign body from an unspecified site in eye.

✓4th **16.2   Diagnostic procedures on orbit and eyeball**

16.21   Ophthalmoscopy

16.22   Diagnostic aspiration of orbit

16.23   Biopsy of eyeball and orbit

16.29   Other diagnostic procedures on orbit and eyeball

EXCLUDES   examination of form and structure of eye (95.11-95.16)
general and subjective eye examination (95.01-95.09)
microscopic examination of specimen from eye (90.21-90.29)
objective functional tests of eye (95.21-95.26)
ocular thermography (88.82)
tonometry (89.11)
x-ray of orbit (87.14, 87.16)

✓4th **16.3   Evisceration of eyeball**

DEF: Removal of eyeball, leaving sclera and occasionally cornea.

16.31   Removal of ocular contents with synchronous implant into scleral shell

DEF: Removal of eyeball leaving outer eyeball layer with ocular implant into shell.

16.39   Other evisceration of eyeball

✓4th **16.4   Enucleation of eyeball**

DEF: Removal of entire eyeball after severing eye muscles and optic nerves.

16.41   Enucleation of eyeball with synchronous implant into Tenon's capsule with attachment of muscles

Integrated implant of eyeball

DEF: Removal of eyeball with insertion of ocular implant and muscle attachment.

16.42   Enucleation of eyeball with other synchronous implant

16.49   Other enucleation of eyeball

Removal of eyeball NOS

✓4th **16.5   Exenteration of orbital contents**

16.51   Exenteration of orbit with removal of adjacent structures

Radical orbitomaxillectomy

DEF: Removal of contents of bony cavity of eye as well as related tissues and structures.

DEF: Radical orbitomaxillectomy: Removal of contents of bony cavity of eye, related tissues and structures, and a portion of maxillary bone.

16.52   Exenteration of orbit with therapeutic removal of orbital bone

16.59   Other exenteration of orbit

Evisceration of orbit NOS
Exenteration of orbit with temporalis muscle transplant

✓4th **16.6   Secondary procedures after removal of eyeball**

EXCLUDES   that with synchronous:
enucleation of eyeball (16.41-16.42)
evisceration of eyeball (16.31)

16.61   Secondary insertion of ocular implant

DEF: Insertion of ocular implant after previous eye removal.

16.62   Revision and reinsertion of ocular implant

DEF: Reimplant or correction of ocular implant.

16.63   Revision of enucleation socket with graft

DEF: Implant of tissue to correct socket after eye removal.

16.64   Other revision of enucleation socket

16.65   Secondary graft to exenteration cavity

DEF: Implant of tissue in place of eye after removal.

16.66   Other revision of exenteration cavity

16.69   Other secondary procedures after removal of eyeball

✓4th **16.7   Removal of ocular or orbital implant**

16.71   Removal of ocular implant

16.72   Removal of orbital implant

✓4th **16.8   Repair of injury of eyeball and orbit**

16.81   Repair of wound of orbit

EXCLUDES   reduction of orbital fracture (76.78-76.79)
repair of extraocular muscles (15.7)

16.82   Repair of rupture of eyeball

Repair of multiple structures of eye

EXCLUDES   repair of laceration of:
cornea (11.51-11.59)
sclera (12.81)

16.89   Other repair of injury of eyeball or orbit

✓4th **16.9   Other operations on orbit and eyeball**

EXCLUDES   irrigation of eye (96.51)
prescription and fitting of low vision aids (95.31-95.33)
removal of:
eye prosthesis NEC (97.31)
nonpenetrating foreign body from eye without incision (98.21)

16.91   Retrobulbar injection of therapeutic agent

EXCLUDES   injection of radiographic contrast material (87.14)
opticociliary injection (12.79)

16.92   Excision of lesion of orbit

EXCLUDES   biopsy of orbit (16.23)

16.93   Excision of lesion of eye, unspecified structure

EXCLUDES   biopsy of eye NOS (16.23)

16.98   Other operations on orbit

16.99   Other operations on eyeball

---

4. OPERATIONS ON THE EAR (18-20)

✓3rd **18** **Operations on external ear**

INCLUDES   operations on:
  external auditory canal
  skin and cartilage of:
    auricle
    meatus

✓4th **18.0** **Incision of external ear**

EXCLUDES   *removal of intraluminal foreign body (98.11)*

18.01 **Piercing of ear lobe**
  Piercing of pinna

18.02 **Incision of external auditory canal**

18.09 **Other incision of external ear**

✓4th **18.1** **Diagnostic procedures on external ear**

18.11 **Otoscopy**
  DEF: Exam of the ear with instrument designed for visualization.

18.12 **Biopsy of external ear**

18.19 **Other diagnostic procedures on external ear**
  EXCLUDES   *microscopic examination of specimen from ear (90.31-90.39)*

✓4th **18.2** **Excision or destruction of lesion of external ear**

18.21 **Excision of preauricular sinus**
  Radical excision of preauricular sinus or cyst
  EXCLUDES   *excision of preauricular remnant [appendage] (18.29)*
  DEF: Excision of preauricular sinus or cyst with adjacent tissues.

18.29 **Excision or destruction of other lesion of external ear**
  Cauterization
  Coagulation
  Cryosurgery   } of external ear
  Curettage
  Electrocoagulation
  Enucleation

  Excision of:
    exostosis of external auditory canal
    preauricular remnant [appendage]
  Partial excision of ear
  EXCLUDES   *biopsy of external ear (18.12)*
             radical excision of lesion (18.31)
             removal of cerumen (96.52)

✓4th **18.3** **Other excision of external ear**
  EXCLUDES   *biopsy of external ear (18.12)*

18.31 **Radical excision of lesion of external ear**
  EXCLUDES   *radical excision of preauricular sinus (18.21)*
  DEF: Removal of damaged, diseased ear and adjacent tissue.

18.39 **Other**
  Amputation of external ear
  EXCLUDES   *excision of lesion (18.21-18.29, 18.31)*

18.4 **Suture of laceration of external ear**

18.5 **Surgical correction of prominent ear**
  Ear:
    pinning
    setback
  DEF: Reformation of protruding outer ear.

18.6 **Reconstruction of external auditory canal**
  Canaloplasty of external auditory meatus
  Construction [reconstruction] of external meatus of ear:
    osseous portion
    skin-lined portion (with skin graft)
  DEF: Repair of outer ear canal.

✓4th **18.7** **Other plastic repair of external ear**

18.71 **Construction of auricle of ear**
  Prosthetic appliance for absent ear
  Reconstruction:
    auricle
    ear
  DEF: Reformation or repair of external ear flap.

18.72 **Reattachment of amputated ear**

18.79 **Other plastic repair of external ear**
  Otoplasty NOS   Repair of lop ear
  Postauricular skin graft
  DEF: Postauricular skin graft: Graft repair behind ear.

  DEF: Repair of lop ear: Reconstruction of ear that is at right angle to head.

18.9 **Other operations on external ear**
  EXCLUDES   *irrigation of ear (96.52)*
             packing of external auditory canal (96.11)
             removal of:
               cerumen (96.52)
               foreign body (without incision) (98.11)

✓3rd **19** **Reconstructive operations on middle ear**

19.0 **Stapes mobilization**
  Division, otosclerotic:
    material
    process
  Remobilization of stapes
  Stapediolysis
  Transcrural stapes mobilization
  EXCLUDES   *that with synchronous stapedectomy (19.11-19.19)*
  DEF: Repair of innermost bone of middle ear to enable movement and response to sound.

✓4th **19.1** **Stapedectomy**
  EXCLUDES   *revision of previous stapedectomy (19.21-19.29)*
             stapes mobilization only (19.0)
  DEF: Removal of innermost bone of middle ear.

19.11 **Stapedectomy with incus replacement**
  Stapedectomy with incus:
    homograft
    prosthesis
  DEF: Removal of innermost bone of middle ear with autograft or prosthesis replacement.

19.19 **Other stapedectomy**

✓4th **19.2** **Revision of stapedectomy**

19.21 **Revision of stapedectomy with incus replacement**

19.29 **Other revision of stapedectomy**

19.3 **Other operations on ossicular chain**
  Incudectomy NOS
  Ossiculectomy NOS
  Reconstruction of ossicles, second stage
  DEF: Incudectomy: Excision of middle bone of middle ear, not otherwise specified.

  DEF: Ossiculectomy: Excision of middle ear bones, not otherwise specified.

  DEF: Reconstruction of ossicles, second stage: Repair of middle ear bones following previous surgery.

Operations on the Ear 18–19.3

Operations on the Ear 19.4–20.72

Stapedectomy with Incus Replacement

Incus
Malleus
Stapes with footplate in oval window
Handle of malleus
Wire piston
Tympanic membrane
Cochlea
Tissue seal on oval window

■ Area excised

19.4 Myringoplasty

Epitympanic, type I	Myringoplasty by:
Myringoplasty by:	graft
cauterization	Tympanoplasty (type I)

DEF: Epitympanic, type I: Repair over or upon eardrum.

DEF: Myringoplasty by cauterization: Plastic repair of tympanic membrane of eardrum by heat.

DEF: Graft: Plastic repair using implanted tissue.

DEF: Tympanoplasty (type I): Reconstruction of eardrum to restore hearing.

✓4th 19.5 Other tympanoplasty

19.52 **Type II tympanoplasty**
Closure of perforation with graft against incus or malleus

19.53 **Type III tympanoplasty**
Graft placed in contact with mobile and intact stapes

AHA: M-A, '85, 15

19.54 **Type IV tympanoplasty**
Mobile footplate left exposed with air pocket between round window and graft

19.55 **Type V tympanoplasty**
Fenestra in horizontal semicircular canal covered by graft

19.6 Revision of tympanoplasty

DEF: Repair or correction of previous plastic surgery on eardrum.

19.9 Other repair of middle ear
Closure of mastoid fistula
Mastoid myoplasty
Obliteration of tympanomastoid cavity

DEF: Closure of mastoid fistula: Closing of abnormal channel in mastoid.

DEF: Mastoid myoplasty: Restoration or repair of mastoid muscle.

DEF: Obliteration of tympanomastoid cavity: Removal, total, of functional elements of middle ear.

✓3rd 20 Other operations on middle and inner ear

✓4th 20.0 Myringotomy

DEF: Myringotomy: Puncture of tympanic membrane or eardrum, also called tympanocentesis.

20.01 **Myringotomy with insertion of tube**
Myringostomy

20.09 **Other myringotomy**
Aspiration of middle ear NOS

20.1 Removal of tympanostomy tube

✓4th 20.2 Incision of mastoid and middle ear
20.21 **Incision of mastoid**
20.22 **Incision of petrous pyramid air cells**

20.23 **Incision of middle ear**
Atticotomy
Division of tympanum
Lysis of adhesions of middle ear
EXCLUDES division of otosclerotic process (19.0)
stapediolysis (19.0)
that with stapedectomy (19.11-19.19)

✓4th 20.3 Diagnostic procedures on middle and inner ear
20.31 **Electrocochleography**
DEF: Measure of electric potential of eighth cranial nerve by electrode applied sound.

20.32 **Biopsy of middle and inner ear**
20.39 **Other diagnostic procedures on middle and inner ear**
EXCLUDES auditory and vestibular function tests (89.13, 95.41-95.49)
microscopic examination of specimen from ear (90.31-90.39)

✓4th 20.4 Mastoidectomy
Code also any:
skin graft (18.79)
tympanoplasty (19.4-19.55)
EXCLUDES that with implantation of cochlear prosthetic device (20.96-20.98)
DEF: Mastoidectomy: Excision of bony protrusion behind ear.

20.41 **Simple mastoidectomy**
20.42 **Radical mastoidectomy**
20.49 **Other mastoidectomy**
Atticoantrostomy
Mastoidectomy:
NOS
modified radical
DEF: Atticoantrotomy: Opening of cavity of mastoid bone and middle ear.

✓4th 20.5 Other excision of middle ear
EXCLUDES that with synchronous mastoidectomy (20.41-20.49)
20.51 **Excision of lesion of middle ear**
EXCLUDES biopsy of middle ear (20.32)
20.59 **Other**
Apicectomy of petrous pyramid
Tympanectomy

✓4th 20.6 Fenestration of inner ear
20.61 **Fenestration of inner ear (initial)**
Fenestration of:
labyrinth
semicircular canals
vestibule
} with graft (skin) (vein)
EXCLUDES that with tympanoplasty, type V (19.55)
DEF: Creation of inner ear opening.

20.62 **Revision of fenestration of inner ear**

✓4th 20.7 Incision, excision, and destruction of inner ear
20.71 **Endolymphatic shunt**
DEF: Insertion of tube to drain fluid in inner ear cavities.

20.72 **Injection into inner ear**
Destruction by injection (alcohol):
inner ear
semicircular canals
vestibule

B1 Bilateral Edit   NC Non-covered Procedure   ▶◀ Revised Text   ● New Code   ▲ Revised Code Title

20.79 **Other incision, excision, and destruction of inner ear**

Decompression of labyrinth
Drainage of inner ear
Fistulization:
    endolymphatic sac
    labyrinth
Incision of endolymphatic sac
Labyrinthectomy (transtympanic)
Opening of bony labyrinth
Perilymphatic tap

EXCLUDES *biopsy of inner ear (20.32)*

DEF: Decompression of labyrinth: Controlled relief of pressure in cavities of inner ear.

DEF: Drainage of inner ear: Removal of fluid from inner ear.

DEF: Fistulization of endolymphatic sac: Creation of passage to fluid sac in inner ear cavities.

DEF: Fistulization of labyrinth: Creation of passage to inner ear cavities.

DEF: Incision of endolymphatic sac: Cutting into fluid sac in inner ear cavities.

DEF: Labyrinthectomy (transtympanic): Excision of cavities across eardrum.

DEF: Opening of bony labyrinth: Cutting into inner ear bony cavities.

DEF: Perilymphatic tap: Puncture or incision into fluid sac of inner ear cavities.

20.8 **Operations on Eustachian tube**

Catheterization
Inflation
Injection (Teflon paste)
Insufflation (boric acid-salicylic acid)
Intubation
Politzerization
    of Eustachian tube

DEF: Catheterization: Passing catheter into passage between pharynx and middle ear.

DEF: Inflation: Blowing air, gas or liquid into passage between pharynx and middle ear to inflate.

DEF: Injection (Teflon paste): Forcing fluid (Teflon paste) into passage between pharynx and middle ear.

DEF: Insufflation (boric acid-salicylic acid): Blowing gas or liquid into passage between pharynx and middle ear.

DEF: Intubation: Placing tube into passage between pharynx and middle ear.

DEF: Politzerization: Inflating passage between pharynx and middle ear with Politzer bag.

√4ᵗʰ 20.9 **Other operations on inner and middle ear**

20.91 **Tympanosympathectomy**

DEF: Excision or chemical suppression of impulses of middle ear nerves.

20.92 **Revision of mastoidectomy**

AHA: 2Q, '98, 20

DEF: Correction of previous removal of mastoid cells from temporal or mastoid bone.

20.93 **Repair of oval and round windows**

Closure of fistula: Closure of fistula:
  oval window   round window
  perilymph

DEF: Restoration of middle ear openings.

20.94 **Injection of tympanum**

20.95 **Implantation of electromagnetic hearing device**

Bone conduction hearing device

EXCLUDES *cochlear prosthetic device (20.96-20.98)*

AHA: 4Q, '89, 5

20.96 **Implantation or replacement of cochlear prosthetic device, not otherwise specified**

Implantation of receiver (within skull) and insertion of electrode(s) in the cochlea

INCLUDES mastoidectomy

EXCLUDES *electromagnetic hearing device (20.95)*

AHA: 4Q, '89, 5

20.97 **Implantation or replacement of cochlear prosthetic device, single channel**

Implantation of receiver (within skull) and insertion of electrode in the cochlea

INCLUDES mastoidectomy

EXCLUDES *electromagnetic hearing device (20.95)*

AHA: 4Q, '89, 5

20.98 **Implantation or replacement of cochlear prosthetic device, multiple channel**

Implantation of receiver (within skull) and insertion of electrodes in the cochlea

INCLUDES mastoidectomy

EXCLUDES *electromagnetic hearing device (20.95)*

AHA: 4Q, '89, 5

20.99 **Other operations on middle and inner ear**

Repair or removal of cochlear prosthetic device (receiver) (electrode)

EXCLUDES *adjustment (external components) of cochlear prosthetic device (95.49)*
fitting of hearing aid (95.48)

AHA: 4Q, '89, 7

Operations on the Ear 20.79–20.99

Operations on Nose, Mouth, and Pharynx 21–21.87

5. OPERATIONS ON THE NOSE, MOUTH, AND PHARYNX (21-29)

√3rd **21   Operations on nose**

INCLUDES   operations on:
bone
skin } of nose

AHA: 1Q, '94, 5

√4th **21.0   Control of epistaxis**
21.00   Control of epistaxis, not otherwise specified
21.01   Control of epistaxis by anterior nasal packing
21.02   Control of epistaxis by posterior (and anterior) packing
21.03   Control of epistaxis by cauterization (and packing)
21.04   Control of epistaxis by ligation of ethmoidal arteries
21.05   Control of epistaxis by (transantral) ligation of the maxillary artery
21.06   Control of epistaxis by ligation of the external carotid artery
21.07   Control of epistaxis by excision of nasal mucosa and skin grafting of septum and lateral nasal wall
21.09   Control of epistaxis by other means

21.1   Incision of nose
Chondrotomy   Nasal septotomy
Incision of skin of nose

DEF: Chondrotomy: Incision or division of nasal cartilage.

DEF: Nasal septotomy: Incision into bone dividing nose into two chambers.

√4th **21.2   Diagnostic procedures on nose**
21.21   Rhinoscopy
DEF: Visualization of nasal passage with nasal speculum.

21.22   Biopsy of nose
21.29   Other diagnostic procedures on nose
EXCLUDES   microscopic examination of specimen from nose (90.31-90.39)
nasal:
function study (89.12)
x-ray (87.16)
rhinomanometry (89.12)

√4th **21.3   Local excision or destruction of lesion of nose**
EXCLUDES   biopsy of nose (21.22)
nasal fistulectomy (21.82)

21.30   Excision or destruction of lesion of nose, not otherwise specified
21.31   Local excision or destruction of intranasal lesion
Nasal polypectomy
21.32   Local excision or destruction of other lesion of nose
AHA: 2Q, '89, 16

21.4   Resection of nose
Amputation of nose
21.5   Submucous resection of nasal septum
DEF: Resection, partial, of nasal septum with mucosa reimplanted after excision.

√4th **21.6   Turbinectomy**
DEF: Removal, partial, or total of turbinate bones; inferior turbinate is most often excised.

21.61   Turbinectomy by diathermy or cryosurgery
DEF: Destruction of turbinate bone by heat or freezing.

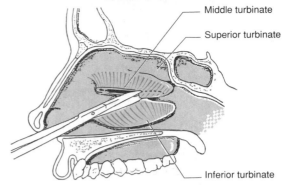

Excision of Turbinate

Middle turbinate
Superior turbinate
Inferior turbinate

21.62   Fracture of the turbinates
DEF: Surgical breaking of turbinate bones.

21.69   Other turbinectomy
EXCLUDES   turbinectomy associated with sinusectomy (22.31-22.39, 22.42, 22.60-22.64)

√4th **21.7   Reduction of nasal fracture**
21.71   Closed reduction of nasal fracture
21.72   Open reduction of nasal fracture

√4th **21.8   Repair and plastic operations on the nose**
21.81   Suture of laceration of nose
21.82   Closure of nasal fistula
Nasolabial
Nasopharyngeal } fistulectomy
Oronasal

DEF: Sealing off crack or hole between nose and lip, nose and pharynx, or nose and mouth.

21.83   Total nasal reconstruction
Reconstruction of nose with:
arm flap
forehead flap

DEF: Reformation, plastic, of nasal structure with tissue flap from arm or forehead.

21.84   Revision rhinoplasty
Rhinoseptoplasty
Twisted nose rhinoplasty

DEF: Rhinoseptoplasty: Repair of nose and the bone dividing the nose into two chambers.

DEF: Twisted nose rhinoplasty: Repair of nose alignment following reconstructive surgery.

21.85   Augmentation rhinoplasty
Augmentation rhinoplasty with:
graft
synthetic implant

DEF: Implant of tissue or synthetic graft to enlarge nose.

21.86   Limited rhinoplasty
Plastic repair of nasolabial flaps
Tip rhinoplasty

DEF: Plastic repair of nasolabial flaps: Reconstruction of nasal area above lips.

DEF: Tip rhinoplasty: Reconstruction or restoration of nasal tip.

21.87   Other rhinoplasty
Rhinoplasty NOS

21.88 Other septoplasty
Crushing of nasal septum
Repair of septal perforation

EXCLUDES   *septoplasty associated with submucous resection of septum (21.5)*

DEF: Crushing of nasal septum: Division and reconstruction of defects in bone dividing nasal chambers.

DEF: Repair of septal perforation: Repair of hole in bone dividing nasal chambers with adjacent tissue.

21.89 Other repair and plastic operations on nose
Reattachment of amputated nose

✓4th **21.9 Other operations on nose**

21.91 Lysis of adhesions of nose
Posterior nasal scrub

DEF: Posterior nasal scrub: Clearing out of abnormal adhesions in posterior nasal area.

21.99 Other

EXCLUDES   *dilation of frontonasal duct (96.21)*
irrigation of nasal passages (96.53)
removal of:
intraluminal foreign body without incision (98.12)
nasal packing (97.32)
replacement of nasal packing (97.21)

✓3rd **22 Operations on nasal sinuses**

✓4th **22.0 Aspiration and lavage of nasal sinus**

22.00 Aspiration and lavage of nasal sinus, not otherwise specified

22.01 Puncture of nasal sinus for aspiration or lavage

22.02 Aspiration or lavage of nasal sinus through natural ostium

DEF: Withdrawal of fluid and washing of nasal cavity through natural opening.

✓4th **22.1 Diagnostic procedures on nasal sinus**

22.11 Closed [endoscopic] [needle] biopsy of nasal sinus

22.12 Open biopsy of nasal sinus

22.19 Other diagnostic procedures on nasal sinuses
Endoscopy without biopsy

EXCLUDES   *transillumination of sinus (89.35)*
x-ray of sinus (87.15-87.16)

22.2 Intranasal antrotomy

EXCLUDES   *antrotomy with external approach (22.31-22.39)*

DEF: Incision of intranasal sinus.

✓4th **22.3 External maxillary antrotomy**

22.31 Radical maxillary antrotomy
Removal of lining membrane of maxillary sinus using Caldwell-Luc approach

DEF: Caldwell-Luc approach: Removal of membrane lining the maxillary cavity through incision above canine teeth.

22.39 Other external maxillary antrotomy
Exploration of maxillary antrum with Caldwell-Luc approach

✓4th **22.4 Frontal sinusotomy and sinusectomy**

22.41 Frontal sinusotomy

22.42 Frontal sinusectomy
Excision of lesion of frontal sinus
Obliteration of frontal sinus (with fat)

EXCLUDES   *biopsy of nasal sinus (22.11-22.12)*

✓4th **22.5 Other nasal sinusotomy**

22.50 Sinusotomy, not otherwise specified

22.51 Ethmoidotomy

22.52 Sphenoidotomy

22.53 Incision of multiple nasal sinuses

✓4th **22.6 Other nasal sinusectomy**

INCLUDES   that with incidental turbinectomy
EXCLUDES   *biopsy of nasal sinus (22.11-22.12)*

22.60 Sinusectomy, not otherwise specified

22.61 Excision of lesion of maxillary sinus with Caldwell-Luc approach

22.62 Excision of lesion of maxillary sinus with other approach

22.63 Ethmoidectomy

DEF: Removal of ethmoid cells and bone, partial or total includes excising mucosal lining, partial or total.

22.64 Sphenoidectomy

DEF: Removal of wedge shaped sphenoid bone at base of brain.

✓4th **22.7 Repair of nasal sinus**

22.71 Closure of nasal sinus fistula
Repair of oro-antral fistula

22.79 Other repair of nasal sinus
Reconstruction of frontonasal duct
Repair of bone of accessory sinus

22.9 Other operations on nasal sinuses
Exteriorization of maxillary sinus
Fistulization of sinus

EXCLUDES   *dilation of frontonasal duct (96.21)*

DEF: Exteriorization of maxillary sinus: Creation of external maxillary cavity opening.

DEF: Fistulization of sinus: Creation of fistula canal in nasal cavity.

✓3rd **23 Removal and restoration of teeth**

✓4th **23.0 Forceps extraction of tooth**

23.01 Extraction of deciduous tooth

23.09 Extraction of other tooth
Extraction of tooth NOS

✓4th **23.1 Surgical removal of tooth**

23.11 Removal of residual root

23.19 Other surgical extraction of tooth
Odontectomy NOS
Removal of impacted tooth
Tooth extraction with elevation of mucoperiosteal flap

23.2 Restoration of tooth by filling

23.3 Restoration of tooth by inlay

DEF: Restoration of tooth by cementing in a molded filling.

✓4th **23.4 Other dental restoration**

23.41 Application of crown

23.42 Insertion of fixed bridge

23.43 Insertion of removable bridge

23.49 Other

23.5 Implantation of tooth

DEF: Insertion of a sound tooth to replace extracted tooth.

23.6 Prosthetic dental implant
Endosseous dental implant

DEF: Implant of artificial denture within bone covering tooth socket.

✓4th **23.7 Apicoectomy and root canal therapy**

23.70 Root canal, not otherwise specified

23.71 Root canal therapy with irrigation

Operations on Nose, Mouth, and Pharynx 21.88–23.71

Operations on Nose, Mouth, and Pharynx 23.72–26.0

23.72   Root canal therapy with apicoectomy
DEF: Removal of tooth root to treat damaged root canal tissue.

23.73   Apicoectomy

√3rd **24**   **Other operations on teeth, gums, and alveoli**

24.0   **Incision of gum or alveolar bone**
Apical alveolotomy

√4th **24.1**   **Diagnostic procedures on teeth, gums, and alveoli**

24.11   **Biopsy of gum**

24.12   **Biopsy of alveolus**

24.19   **Other diagnostic procedures on teeth, gums, and alveoli**
EXCLUDES   *dental:*
examination (89.31)
x-ray:
full-mouth (87.11)
other (87.12)
microscopic examination of dental specimen (90.81-90.89)

24.2   **Gingivoplasty**
Gingivoplasty with bone or soft tissue graft
DEF: Repair of gum tissue.

√4th **24.3**   **Other operations on gum**

24.31   **Excision of lesion or tissue of gum**
EXCLUDES   *biopsy of gum (24.11)*
excision of odontogenic lesion (24.4)

24.32   **Suture of laceration of gum**

24.39   **Other**

24.4   **Excision of dental lesion of jaw**
Excision of odontogenic lesion

24.5   **Alveoloplasty**
Alveolectomy (interradicular) (intraseptal) (radical) (simple) (with graft or implant)
EXCLUDES   *biopsy of alveolus (24.12)*
en bloc resection of alveolar process and palate (27.32)
DEF: Repair or correction of bony tooth socket.

24.6   **Exposure of tooth**

24.7   **Application of orthodontic appliance**
Application, insertion, or fitting of:
arch bars   orthodontic wiring
orthodontic obturator   periodontal splint
EXCLUDES   *nonorthodontic dental wiring (93.55)*

24.8   **Other orthodontic operation**
Closure of diastema   Removal of arch bars
(alveolar) (dental)   Repair of dental arch
Occlusal adjustment
EXCLUDES   *removal of nonorthodontic wiring (97.33)*

√4th **24.9**   **Other dental operations**

24.91   **Extension or deepening of buccolabial or lingual sulcus**

24.99   **Other**
EXCLUDES   *dental:*
debridement (96.54)
examination (89.31)
prophylaxis (96.54)
scaling and polishing (96.54)
wiring (93.55)
fitting of dental appliance [denture] (99.97)
microscopic examination of dental specimen (90.81-90.89)
removal of dental:
packing (97.34)
prosthesis (97.35)
wiring (97.33)
replacement of dental packing (97.22)

√3rd **25**   **Operations on tongue**

√4th **25.0**   **Diagnostic procedures on tongue**

25.01   **Closed [needle] biopsy of tongue**

25.02   **Open biopsy of tongue**
Wedge biopsy

25.09   **Other diagnostic procedures on tongue**

25.1   **Excision or destruction of lesion or tissue of tongue**
EXCLUDES   *biopsy of tongue (25.01-25.02)*
frenumectomy:
labial (27.41)
lingual (25.92)

25.2   **Partial glossectomy**

25.3   **Complete glossectomy**
Glossectomy NOS
Code also any neck dissection (40.40-40.42)

25.4   **Radical glossectomy**
Code also any:
neck dissection (40.40-40.42)
tracheostomy (31.1-31.29)

√4th **25.5**   **Repair of tongue and glossoplasty**

25.51   **Suture of laceration of tongue**

25.59   **Other repair and plastic operations on tongue**
Fascial sling of tongue
Fusion of tongue (to lip)
Graft of mucosa or skin to tongue
EXCLUDES   *lysis of adhesions of tongue (25.93)*

AHA: 1Q, '97, 5

√4th **25.9**   **Other operations on tongue**

25.91   **Lingual frenotomy**
EXCLUDES   *labial frenotomy (27.91)*
DEF: Extension of groove between cheek and lips or cheek and tongue.

25.92   **Lingual frenectomy**
EXCLUDES   *labial frenectomy (27.41)*
DEF: Frenectomy: Removal of vertical membrane attaching tongue to floor mouth.

25.93   **Lysis of adhesions of tongue**

25.94   **Other glossotomy**

25.99   **Other**

√3rd **26**   **Operations on salivary glands and ducts**
INCLUDES   operations on:
lesser salivary
parotid
sublingual } gland and duct
submaxillary
Code also any neck dissection (40.40-40.42)

26.0   **Incision of salivary gland or duct**

BI Bilateral Edit   NC Non-covered Procedure   ►◄ Revised Text   ● New Code   ▲ Revised Code Title

✓4th **26.1** Diagnostic procedures on salivary glands and ducts

26.11 Closed [needle] biopsy of salivary gland or duct

26.12 Open biopsy of salivary gland or duct

26.19 Other diagnostic procedures on salivary glands and ducts

EXCLUDES *x-ray of salivary gland (87.09)*

✓4th **26.2** Excision of lesion of salivary gland

26.21 Marsupialization of salivary gland cyst

DEF: Creation of pouch of salivary gland cyst to drain and promote healing.

26.29 Other excision of salivary gland lesion

EXCLUDES *biopsy of salivary gland (26.11-26.12)*
salivary fistulectomy (26.42)

✓4th **26.3** Sialoadenectomy

DEF: Removal of salivary gland.

26.30 Sialoadenectomy, not otherwise specified

26.31 Partial sialoadenectomy

26.32 Complete sialoadenectomy

En bloc excision of salivary gland lesion
Radical sialoadenectomy

✓4th **26.4** Repair of salivary gland or duct

26.41 Suture of laceration of salivary gland

26.42 Closure of salivary fistula

DEF: Closing of abnormal opening in salivary gland.

26.49 Other repair and plastic operations on salivary gland or duct

Fistulization of salivary gland
Plastic repair of salivary gland or duct NOS
Transplantation of salivary duct opening

✓4th **26.9** Other operations on salivary gland or duct

26.91 Probing of salivary duct

26.99 Other

✓3rd **27** Other operations on mouth and face

INCLUDES operations on:
lips
palate
soft tissue of face and mouth, except tongue and gingiva

EXCLUDES operations on:
gingiva (24.0-24.99)
tongue (25.01-25.99)

27.0 Drainage of face and floor of mouth

Drainage of: Drainage of:
facial region (abscess)   Ludwig's angina
fascial compartment of face

EXCLUDES *drainage of thyroglossal tract (06.09)*

27.1 Incision of palate

✓4th **27.2** Diagnostic procedures on oral cavity

27.21 Biopsy of bony palate

27.22 Biopsy of uvula and soft palate

27.23 Biopsy of lip

27.24 Biopsy of mouth, unspecified structure

27.29 Other diagnostic procedures on oral cavity

EXCLUDES *soft tissue x-ray (87.09)*

✓4th **27.3** Excision of lesion or tissue of bony palate

27.31 Local excision or destruction of lesion or tissue of bony palate

Local excision or destruction of palate by:
cautery   cryotherapy
chemotherapy

EXCLUDES *biopsy of bony palate (27.21)*

27.32 Wide excision or destruction of lesion or tissue of bony palate

En bloc resection of alveolar process and palate

✓4th **27.4** Excision of other parts of mouth

27.41 Labial frenectomy

EXCLUDES *division of labial frenum (27.91)*

DEF: Removal of mucous membrane fold of lip.

27.42 Wide excision of lesion of lip

27.43 Other excision of lesion or tissue of lip

27.49 Other excision of mouth

EXCLUDES *biopsy of mouth NOS (27.24)*
excision of lesion of:
palate (27.31-27.32)
tongue (25.1)
uvula (27.72)
fistulectomy of mouth (27.53)
frenectomy of:
lip (27.41)
tongue (25.92)

✓4th **27.5** Plastic repair of mouth

EXCLUDES *palatoplasty (27.61-27.69)*

27.51 Suture of laceration of lip

27.52 Suture of laceration of other part of mouth

27.53 Closure of fistula of mouth

EXCLUDES *fistulectomy:*
nasolabial (21.82)
oro-antral (22.71)
oronasal (21.82)

27.54 Repair of cleft lip

27.55 Full-thickness skin graft to lip and mouth

27.56 Other skin graft to lip and mouth

27.57 Attachment of pedicle or flap graft to lip and mouth

AHA: 1Q, '96, 14

DEF: Repair of lip or mouth with tissue pedicle or flap still connected to original vascular base.

27.59 Other plastic repair of mouth

✓4th **27.6** Palatoplasty

27.61 Suture of laceration of palate

27.62 Correction of cleft palate

Correction of cleft palate by push-back operation

EXCLUDES *revision of cleft palate repair (27.63)*

27.63 Revision of cleft palate repair

Secondary:
attachment of pharyngeal flap
lengthening of palate

AHA: 1Q, '96, 14

27.69 Other plastic repair of palate

EXCLUDES *fistulectomy of mouth (27.53)*

AHA: 3Q, '99, 22; 1Q, '97, 14; 3Q, '92, 18

✓4th **27.7** Operations on uvula

27.71 Incision of uvula

27.72 Excision of uvula

EXCLUDES *biopsy of uvula (27.22)*

27.73 Repair of uvula

EXCLUDES *that with synchronous cleft palate repair (27.62)*
uranostaphylorrhaphy (27.62)

27.79 Other operations on uvula

AHA: 3Q, '92, 18

✓4th **27.9** Other operations on mouth and face

27.91 Labial frenotomy

Division of labial frenum

EXCLUDES *lingual frenotomy (25.91)*

DEF: Division of labial frenum: Cutting and separating mucous membrane fold of lip.

Operations on Nose, Mouth, and Pharynx 26.1–27.91

✓3rd
✓4th
Additional Digit Required

Nonspecific OR Procedure

Valid OR Procedure

Non-OR Procedure

2002 Ingenix, Inc.

Volume 3 —105

Operations on Nose, Mouth, and Pharynx 27.92–29.99

27.92   **Incision of mouth, unspecified structure**

   EXCLUDES   incision of:
     gum (24.0)
     palate (27.1)
     salivary gland or duct
      (26.0)
     tongue (25.94)
     uvula (27.71)

27.99   **Other operations on oral cavity**

   Graft of buccal sulcus

   EXCLUDES   removal of:
     intraluminal foreign body
      (98.01)
     penetrating foreign body
      from mouth without
      incision (98.22)

   DEF: Graft of buccal sulcus: Implant of tissue into groove of interior cheek lining.

√3rd 28   **Operations on tonsils and adenoids**

28.0   **Incision and drainage of tonsil and peritonsillar structures**

   Drainage (oral) (transcervical) of:
     parapharyngeal
     peritonsillar
     retropharyngeal   } abscess
     tonsillar

√4th 28.1   **Diagnostic procedures on tonsils and adenoids**

28.11   **Biopsy of tonsils and adenoids**

28.19   **Other diagnostic procedures on tonsils and adenoids**

   EXCLUDES   soft tissue x-ray (87.09)

28.2   **Tonsillectomy without adenoidectomy**

   AHA: 1Q, '97, 5; 2Q, '90, 23

28.3   **Tonsillectomy with adenoidectomy**

28.4   **Excision of tonsil tag**

28.5   **Excision of lingual tonsil**

28.6   **Adenoidectomy without tonsillectomy**

   Excision of adenoid tag

28.7   **Control of hemorrhage after tonsillectomy and adenoidectomy**

√4th 28.9   **Other operations on tonsils and adenoids**

28.91   **Removal of foreign body from tonsil and adenoid by incision**

   EXCLUDES   that without incision (98.13)

28.92   **Excision of lesion of tonsil and adenoid**

   EXCLUDES   biopsy of tonsil and adenoid
     (28.11)

28.99   **Other**

√3rd 29   **Operations on pharynx**

   INCLUDES   operations on: operations on:
     hypopharynx   pharyngeal pouch
     nasopharynx   pyriform sinus
     oropharynx

29.0   **Pharyngotomy**

   Drainage of pharyngeal bursa

   EXCLUDES   incision and drainage of
     retropharyngeal abscess (28.0)
     removal of foreign body (without
     incision) (98.13)

√4th 29.1   **Diagnostic procedures on pharynx**

29.11   **Pharyngoscopy**

29.12   **Pharyngeal biopsy**

   Biopsy of supraglottic mass

29.19   **Other diagnostic procedures on pharynx**

   EXCLUDES   x-ray of nasopharynx:
     contrast (87.06)
     other (87.09)

29.2   **Excision of branchial cleft cyst or vestige**

   EXCLUDES   branchial cleft fistulectomy (29.52)

√4th 29.3   **Excision or destruction of lesion or tissue of pharynx**

   AHA: 2Q, '89, 18

29.31   **Cricopharyngeal myotomy**

   EXCLUDES   that with pharyngeal
     diverticulectomy (29.32)

   DEF: Removal of outward pouching of throat.

29.32   **Pharyngeal diverticulectomy**

29.33   **Pharyngectomy (partial)**

   EXCLUDES   laryngopharyngectomy (30.3)

29.39   **Other excision or destruction of lesion or tissue of pharynx**

29.4   **Plastic operation on pharynx**

   Correction of nasopharyngeal atresia

   EXCLUDES   pharyngoplasty associated with cleft
     palate repair (27.62-27.63)

   AHA: 3Q, '99, 22; 1Q, '97, 5; 3Q, '92, 18

   DEF: Correction of nasopharyngeal atresia: Construction of normal opening for throat stricture behind nose.

√4th 29.5   **Other repair of pharynx**

29.51   **Suture of laceration of pharynx**

29.52   **Closure of branchial cleft fistula**

   DEF: Sealing off an abnormal opening of the branchial fissure in throat.

29.53   **Closure of other fistula of pharynx**

   Pharyngoesophageal fistulectomy

29.54   **Lysis of pharyngeal adhesions**

29.59   **Other**

   AHA: 2Q, '89, 18

√4th 29.9   **Other operations on pharynx**

29.91   **Dilation of pharynx**

   Dilation of nasopharynx

29.92   **Division of glossopharyngeal nerve**

29.99   **Other**

   EXCLUDES   insertion of radium into
     pharynx and
     nasopharynx (92.27)
     removal of intraluminal foreign
     body (98.13)

BI Bilateral Edit   **NC** Non-covered Procedure   ▶◀ Revised Text   ● New Code   ▲ Revised Code Title

6. OPERATIONS ON THE RESPIRATORY SYSTEM (30-34)

√3rd **30 Excision of larynx**

√4th **30.0 Excision or destruction of lesion or tissue of larynx**

30.01 Marsupialization of laryngeal cyst

DEF: Incision of cyst of larynx with the edges sutured open to create pouch.

30.09 Other excision or destruction of lesion or tissue of larynx

Stripping of vocal cords

EXCLUDES   *biopsy of larynx (31.43)*
laryngeal fistulectomy (31.62)
laryngotracheal fistulectomy (31.62)

30.1 Hemilaryngectomy

DEF: Excision of one side (half) of larynx.

√4th **30.2 Other partial laryngectomy**

30.21 Epiglottidectomy

DEF: Placement of artificial breathing tube in windpipe through mediastinum, for long-term use.

30.22 Vocal cordectomy

Excision of vocal cords

30.29 Other partial laryngectomy

Excision of laryngeal cartilage

30.3 Complete laryngectomy

Block dissection of larynx (with thyroidectomy) (with synchronous tracheostomy)
Laryngopharyngectomy

EXCLUDES   *that with radical neck dissection (30.4)*

30.4 Radical laryngectomy

Complete [total] laryngectomy with radical neck dissection (with thyroidectomy) (with synchronous tracheostomy)

√3rd **31 Other operations on larynx and trachea**

31.0 Injection of larynx

Injection of inert material into larynx or vocal cords

31.1 Temporary tracheostomy

Tracheotomy for assistance in breathing

AHA: 1Q, '97, 6

√4th **31.2 Permanent tracheostomy**

31.21 Mediastinal tracheostomy

31.29 Other permanent tracheostomy

EXCLUDES   *that with laryngectomy (30.3-30.4)*

31.3 Other incision of larynx or trachea

EXCLUDES   *that for assistance in breathing (31.1-31.29)*

√4th **31.4 Diagnostic procedures on larynx and trachea**

31.41 Tracheoscopy through artificial stoma

EXCLUDES   *that with biopsy (31.43-31.44)*

DEF: Exam by scope of trachea through an artificial opening.

Temporary Tracheostomy

Trachea
Tracheostomy tube
In place

Closed Endoscopic Biopsy of Larynx

Laryngoscope
Trachea
Palate

Growth on vocal cord

31.42 Laryngoscopy and other tracheoscopy

EXCLUDES   *that with biopsy (31.43-31.44)*

31.43 Closed [endoscopic] biopsy of larynx

31.44 Closed [endoscopic] biopsy of trachea

31.45 Open biopsy of larynx or trachea

31.48 Other diagnostic procedures on larynx

EXCLUDES   *contrast laryngogram (87.07)*
microscopic examination of specimen from larynx (90.31-90.39)
soft tissue x-ray of larynx NEC (87.09)

31.49 Other diagnostic procedures on trachea

EXCLUDES   *microscopic examination of specimen from trachea (90.41-90.49)*
x-ray of trachea (87.49)

31.5 Local excision or destruction of lesion or tissue of trachea

EXCLUDES   *biopsy of trachea (31.44-31.45)*
laryngotracheal fistulectomy (31.62)
tracheoesophageal fistulectomy (31.73)

√4th **31.6 Repair of larynx**

31.61 Suture of laceration of larynx

31.62 Closure of fistula of larynx

Laryngotracheal fistulectomy
Take-down of laryngostomy

DEF: Laryngotracheal fistulectomy: Excision and closing of passage between voice box and trachea.

DEF: Take-down of laryngostomy: Removal of laryngostomy tube and restoration of voice box.

31.63 Revision of laryngostomy

31.64 Repair of laryngeal fracture

DEF: Alignment and positioning of harder structures of larynx such as hyoid bone; following fracture.

31.69 Other repair of larynx

Arytenoidopexy
Graft of larynx
Transposition of vocal cords

EXCLUDES   *construction of artificial larynx (31.75)*

DEF: Arytenoidopexy: Fixation of pitcher-shaped cartilage in voice box.

DEF: Graft of larynx: Implant of graft tissue into voice box.

DEF: Transposition of the vocal cords: Placement of vocal cords into more functional positions.

√4th **31.7 Repair and plastic operations on trachea**

31.71 Suture of laceration of trachea

Operations on the Respiratory System 30–31.71

Operations on the Respiratory System 31.72–32.6

31.72   **Closure of external fistula of trachea**
Closure of tracheotomy

31.73   **Closure of other fistula of trachea**
Tracheoesophageal fistulectomy

> **EXCLUDES**   *laryngotracheal fistulectomy (31.62)*

DEF: Tracheoesophageal fistulectomy: Excision and closure of abnormal opening between windpipe and esophagus.

31.74   **Revision of tracheostomy**

31.75   **Reconstruction of trachea and construction of artificial larynx**
Tracheoplasty with artificial larynx

31.79   **Other repair and plastic operations on trachea**

√4ᵗʰ **31.9**   **Other operations on larynx and trachea**

31.91   **Division of laryngeal nerve**

31.92   **Lysis of adhesions of trachea or larynx**

31.93   **Replacement of laryngeal or tracheal stent**

DEF: Removal and substitution of tubed molding into larynx or trachea.

31.94   **Injection of locally-acting therapeutic substance into trachea**

31.95   **Tracheoesophageal fistulization**

DEF: Creation of passage between trachea and esophagus.

31.98   **Other operations on larynx**

Dilation
Division of congenital web } of larynx
Removal of keel or stent

> **EXCLUDES**   *removal of intraluminal foreign body from larynx without incision (98.14)*

DEF: Dilation: Increasing larynx size by stretching.

DEF: Division of congenital web: Cutting and separating congenital membranes around larynx.

DEF: Removal of keel or stent: Removal of prosthetic device from larynx.

31.99   **Other operations on trachea**

> **EXCLUDES**   *removal of:*
> *intraluminal foreign body from trachea without incision (98.15)*
> *tracheostomy tube (97.37)*
> *replacement of tracheostomy tube (97.23)*
> *tracheostomy toilette (96.55)*

AHA: 1Q, '97, 14

√3ʳᵈ **32**   **Excision of lung and bronchus**

> **INCLUDES**   rib resection
> sternotomy
> sternum-splitting } as operative
> incision   approach
> thoracotomy

Code also any synchronous bronchoplasty (33.48)

DEF: Rib resection: Cutting of ribs to access operative field.

DEF: Sternotomy: Cut through breastbone as an operative approach.

DEF: Sternum-splitting incision: Breaking through breastbone to access operative field.

√4ᵗʰ **32.0**   **Local excision or destruction of lesion or tissue of bronchus**

> **EXCLUDES**   *biopsy of bronchus (33.24-33.25)*
> *bronchial fistulectomy (33.42)*

AHA: 4Q, '88, 11

Lung Volume Reduction

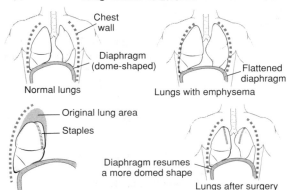

32.01   **Endoscopic excision or destruction of lesion or tissue of bronchus**

32.09   **Other local excision or destruction of lesion or tissue of bronchus**

> **EXCLUDES**   *that by endoscopic approach (32.01)*

32.1   **Other excision of bronchus**
Resection (wide sleeve) of bronchus

> **EXCLUDES**   *radical dissection [excision] of bronchus (32.6)*

DEF: Resection (wide sleeve) of bronchus: Excision and partial, lengthwise removal of a lung branch.

√4ᵗʰ **32.2**   **Local excision or destruction of lesion or tissue of lung**

32.21   **Plication of emphysematous bleb**

DEF: Stitching of a swollen vesicle into folds or tuck.

32.22   **Lung volume reduction surgery**   **NC**

AHA: 1Q, '97, 6; 3Q, '96, 20; 4Q, '95, 64

DEF: Excision of portion of lung(s) to reduce respiratory effort in moderate to severe emphysema.

32.28   **Endoscopic excision or destruction of lesion or tissue of lung**

> **EXCLUDES**   *biopsy of lung (33.26-33.27)*

32.29   **Other local excision or destruction of lesion or tissue of lung**
Resection of lung:
NOS
wedge

> **EXCLUDES**   *biopsy of lung (33.26-33.27)*
> *that by endoscopic approach (32.28)*
> *wide excision of lesion of lung (32.3)*

AHA: 3Q, '99, 3

32.3   **Segmental resection of lung**
Partial lobectomy

32.4   **Lobectomy of lung**
Lobectomy with segmental resection of adjacent lobes of lung

> **EXCLUDES**   *that with radical dissection [excision] of thoracic structures (32.6)*

32.5   **Complete pneumonectomy**
Excision of lung NOS
Pneumonectomy (with mediastinal dissection)

AHA: 1Q, '99, 6

32.6   **Radical dissection of thoracic structures**
Block [en bloc] dissection of bronchus, lobe of lung, brachial plexus, intercostal structure, ribs (transverse process), and sympathetic nerves

---

32.9   **Other excision of lung**

> EXCLUDES   *biopsy of lung and bronchus (33.24-33.27)*
> *pulmonary decortication (34.51)*

√3rd **33**   **Other operations on lung and bronchus**

> INCLUDES   rib resection
> sternotomy   } as operative
> sternum-splitting incision   approach
> thoracotomy

33.0   **Incision of bronchus**

33.1   **Incision of lung**

> EXCLUDES   *puncture of lung (33.93)*

√4th **33.2**   **Diagnostic procedures on lung and bronchus**

33.21   **Bronchoscopy through artificial stoma**

> EXCLUDES   *that with biopsy (33.24, 33.27)*

DEF: Visual exam of lung and its branches via tube through artificial opening.

33.22   **Fiber-optic bronchoscopy**

> EXCLUDES   *that with biopsy (33.24, 33.27)*

DEF: Exam of lung and bronchus via flexible optical instrument for visualization.

33.23   **Other bronchoscopy**

> EXCLUDES   *that for:*
> *aspiration (96.05)*
> *biopsy (33.24, 33.27)*

AHA: 1Q, '99, 6

33.24   **Closed [endoscopic] biopsy of bronchus**

Bronchoscopy (fiberoptic) (rigid) with:
brush biopsy of "lung"
brushing or washing for specimen collection
excision (bite) biopsy
►Diagnostic bronchoalveolar lavage (BAL)◄

> EXCLUDES   *closed biopsy of lung, other than brush biopsy of "lung" (33.26, 33.27)*
> ►*whole lung lavage (33.99)*◄

AHA: 4Q, '92, 27; 3Q, '91, 15

DEF: Brush biopsy: Obtaining cell or tissue samples via bristled instrument without incision.

33.25   **Open biopsy of bronchus**

> EXCLUDES   *open biopsy of lung (33.28)*

33.26   **Closed [percutaneous] [needle] biopsy of lung**

> EXCLUDES   *endoscopic biopsy of lung (33.27)*

AHA: 3Q, '92, 12

33.27   **Closed endoscopic biopsy of lung**

Fiber-optic (flexible) bronchoscopy with fluoroscopic guidance with biopsy
Transbronchial lung biopsy

> EXCLUDES   *brush biopsy of "lung" (33.24)*
> *percutaneous biopsy of lung (33.26)*

AHA: 4Q, '92, 27; 3Q, '91, 15; S-O, '86, 11

Bronchoscopy with Bite Biopsy

33.28   **Open biopsy of lung**

AHA: 3Q, '99, 3; 3Q, '92, 12

33.29   **Other diagnostic procedures on lung and bronchus**

> EXCLUDES   *contrast bronchogram:*
> *endotracheal (87.31)*
> *other (87.32)*
> *lung scan (92.15)*
> *magnetic resonance imaging (88.92)*
> *microscopic examination of specimen from bronchus or lung (90.41-90.49)*
> *routine chest x-ray (87.44)*
> *ultrasonography of lung (88.73)*
> *vital capacity determination (89.37)*
> *x-ray of bronchus or lung NOS (87.49)*

√4th **33.3**   **Surgical collapse of lung**

33.31   **Destruction of phrenic nerve for collapse of lung**

DEF: Therapeutic deadening or destruction of diaphragmatic nerve to collapse the lung.

33.32   **Artificial pneumothorax for collapse of lung**

Thoracotomy for collapse of lung

DEF: Forcing air or gas into diaphragmatic space to achieve therapeutic collapse of lung.

DEF: Thoracotomy for collapse of lung: Incision into chest for therapeutic collapse of lung.

33.33   **Pneumoperitoneum for collapse of lung**

DEF: Forcing air or gas into abdominal serous membrane to achieve therapeutic collapse of lung.

33.34   **Thoracoplasty**

DEF: Removal of ribs for therapeutic collapse of lungs.

33.39   **Other surgical collapse of lung**

Collapse of lung NOS

√4th **33.4**   **Repair and plastic operation on lung and bronchus**

33.41   **Suture of laceration of bronchus**

33.42   **Closure of bronchial fistula**

Closure of bronchostomy
Fistulectomy:
bronchocutaneous
bronchoesophageal
bronchovisceral

> EXCLUDES   *closure of fistula:*
> *bronchomediastinal (34.73)*
> *bronchopleural (34.73)*
> *bronchopleuromediastinal (34.73)*

DEF: Closure of bronchostomy: Removal of bronchostomy tube and repair of surgical wound.

DEF: Fistulectomy: Closure of abnormal passage.
Bronchocutaneous: Between skin and lung branch.
Bronchoesophagus: Between esophagus and lung branch.
Bronchovisceral: Between an internal organ and lung branch.

33.43   **Closure of laceration of lung**

33.48   **Other repair and plastic operations on bronchus**

33.49   **Other repair and plastic operations on lung**

> EXCLUDES   *closure of pleural fistula (34.73)*

✓4th **33.5 Lung transplant**
> EXCLUDES *combined heart-lung transplantation (33.6)*
> Code also cardiopulmonary bypass [extracorporeal circulation] [heart-lung machine] 39.61
> AHA: 4Q, '95, 75

33.50 Lung transplantation, not otherwise specified NC
33.51 Unilateral lung transplantation NC
33.52 Bilateral lung transplantation NC
> Double-lung transplantation
> En bloc transplantation
> DEF: Sequential excision and implant of both lungs.

33.6 Combined heart-lung transplantation NC
> Code also cardiopulmonary bypass [extracorporeal circulation] [heart-lung machine] (39.61)

✓4th **33.9 Other operations on lung and bronchus**
33.91 Bronchial dilation
> AHA: 1Q, '97, 14

33.92 Ligation of bronchus
> DEF: Tying off of a lung branch.

33.93 Puncture of lung
> EXCLUDES *needle biopsy (33.26)*
> DEF: Piercing of lung with surgical instrument.

33.98 Other operations on bronchus
> EXCLUDES *bronchial lavage (96.56)*
> *removal of intraluminal foreign body from bronchus without incision (98.15)*

33.99 Other operations on lung
> ▶Whole lung lavage◀
> EXCLUDES *other continuous mechanical ventilation (96.70-96.72)*
> *respiratory therapy (93.90-93.99)*

✓3rd **34 Operations on chest wall, pleura, mediastinum, and diaphragm**
> EXCLUDES *operations on breast (85.0-85.99)*

✓4th **34.0 Incision of chest wall and pleura**
> EXCLUDES *that as operative approach — omit code*
34.01 Incision of chest wall
> Extrapleural drainage
> EXCLUDES *incision of pleura (34.09)*
> AHA: 3Q, '00, 12; 1Q, '92, 13
> DEF: Extrapleural drainage: Incision to drain fluid from external pleura.

34.02 Exploratory thoracotomy
34.03 Reopening of recent thoracotomy site
34.04 Insertion of intercostal catheter for drainage
> Chest tube
> Closed chest drainage
> Revision of intercostal catheter (chest tube) (with lysis of adhesions)
> AHA: 1Q, '99, 10; 2Q, '99, 12; 1Q, '95, 5; 1Q, '92, 12
> DEF: Insertion of catheter between ribs for drainage.

34.05 Creation of pleuroperitoneal shunt
> AHA: 4Q, '94, 50

34.09 Other incision of pleura
> Creation of pleural window for drainage
> Intercostal stab
> Open chest drainage
> EXCLUDES *thoracoscopy (34.21)*
> *thoracotomy for collapse of lung (33.32)*
> AHA: 1Q, '94, 7; 4Q, '94, 50
> DEF: Creation of pleural window: Creation of circumscribed drainage hole in serous membrane of chest.
> DEF: Intercostal stab: Creation of penetrating stab wound between ribs.
> DEF: Open chest drainage: Insertion of tube through ribs and serous membrane of chest for drainage.

34.1 Incision of mediastinum
> EXCLUDES *mediastinoscopy (34.22)*
> *mediastinotomy associated with pneumonectomy (32.5)*

✓4th **34.2 Diagnostic procedures on chest wall, pleura, mediastinum, and diaphragm**
34.21 Transpleural thoracoscopy
> DEF: Exam of chest through serous membrane using scope.
34.22 Mediastinoscopy
> Code also any lymph node biopsy (40.11)
> DEF: Exam of lung cavity and heart using scope.
34.23 Biopsy of chest wall
34.24 Pleural biopsy
> AHA: 1Q, '92, 14
34.25 Closed [percutaneous] [needle] biopsy of mediastinum
34.26 Open biopsy of mediastinum
34.27 Biopsy of diaphragm
34.28 Other diagnostic procedures on chest wall, pleura, and diaphragm
> EXCLUDES *angiocardiography (88.50-88.58)*
> *aortography (88.42)*
> *arteriography of:*
> *intrathoracic vessels NEC (88.44)*
> *pulmonary arteries (88.43)*
> *microscopic examination of specimen from chest wall, pleura, and diaphragm (90.41-90.49)*
> *phlebography of:*
> *intrathoracic vessels NEC (88.63)*
> *pulmonary veins (88.62)*
> *radiological examinations of thorax:*
> *C.A.T. scan (87.41)*
> *diaphragmatic x-ray (87.49)*
> *intrathoracic lymphangiogram (87.34)*
> *routine chest x-ray (87.44)*
> *sinogram of chest wall (87.38)*
> *soft tissue x-ray of chest wall NEC (87.39)*
> *tomogram of thorax NEC (87.42)*
> *ultrasonography of thorax (88.73)*

34.29   Other diagnostic procedures on mediastinum

> EXCLUDES   mediastinal:
> pneumogram (87.33)
> x-ray NEC (87.49)

34.3   Excision or destruction of lesion or tissue of mediastinum

> EXCLUDES   biopsy of mediastinum (34.25-34.26)
> mediastinal fistulectomy (34.73)

34.4   Excision or destruction of lesion of chest wall

Excision of lesion of chest wall NOS (with excision of ribs)

> EXCLUDES   biopsy of chest wall (34.23)
> costectomy not incidental to thoracic procedure (77.91)
> excision of lesion of:
> breast (85.20-85.25)
> cartilage (80.89)
> skin (86.2-86.3)
> fistulectomy (34.73)

√4th   34.5   Pleurectomy

34.51   Decortication of lung

DEF: Removal of thickened serous membrane for lung expansion.

34.59   Other excision of pleura

Excision of pleural lesion

> EXCLUDES   biopsy of pleura (34.24)
> pleural fistulectomy (34.73)

34.6   Scarification of pleura

Pleurosclerosis

> EXCLUDES   injection of sclerosing agent (34.92)

AHA: 1Q, '92, 12

√4th   34.7   Repair of chest wall

DEF: Destruction of fluid-secreting serous membrane cells of chest.

34.71   Suture of laceration of chest wall

> EXCLUDES   suture of skin and subcutaneous tissue alone (86.59)

34.72   Closure of thoracostomy

34.73   Closure of other fistula of thorax

Closure of:
bronchopleural
bronchopleurocutaneous } fistula
bronchopleuromediastinal

34.74   Repair of pectus deformity

Repair of:
pectus carinatum
pectus excavatum } (with implant)

DEF: Pectus carinatum repair: Restoration of prominent chest bone defect with implant.

DEF: Pectus excavatum: Restoration of depressed chest bone defect with implant.

34.79   Other repair of chest wall

Repair of chest wall NOS

AHA: J-F, '87, 13

√4th   34.8   Operations on diaphragm

34.81   Excision of lesion or tissue of diaphragm

> EXCLUDES   biopsy of diaphragm (34.27)

34.82   Suture of laceration of diaphragm

34.83   Closure of fistula of diaphragm

Thoracicoabdominal
Thoracicogastric } fistulectomy
Thoracicointestinal

DEF: Fistulectomy: Closure of abnormal passage.

34.84   Other repair of diaphragm

> EXCLUDES   repair of diaphragmatic hernia (53.7-53.82)

34.85   Implantation of diaphragmatic pacemaker

34.89   Other operations on diaphragm

√4th   34.9   Other operations on thorax

34.91   Thoracentesis

AHA: S-O, '85, 6

DEF: Puncture of pleural cavity for fluid aspiration, also called pleurocentesis.

34.92   Injection into thoracic cavity

Chemical pleurodesis
Injection of cytotoxic agent or tetracycline
Requires additional code for any cancer chemotherapeutic substance (99.25)

> EXCLUDES   that for collapse of lung (33.32)

AHA: 1Q, '92, 12; 2Q, '89, 17

DEF: Chemical pleurodesis: Tetracycline hydrochloride injections to create adhesions between parietal and visceral pleura for treatment of pleural effusion.

34.93   Repair of pleura

34.99   Other

> EXCLUDES   removal of:
> mediastinal drain (97.42)
> sutures (97.43)
> thoracotomy tube (97.41)

AHA: 1Q, '00, 17; 1Q, '88, 9

DEF: Pleural tent: Extrapleural mobilization of parietal pleura that allows draping of membrane over visceral pleura to eliminate intrapleural dead space and seal visceral pleura.

Operations on the Respiratory System 34.29–34.99

Operations on the Cardiovascular System 35–35.41

7. OPERATIONS ON THE CARDIOVASCULAR SYSTEM (35-39)

√3rd **35   Operations on valves and septa of heart**

     INCLUDES   sternotomy (median)
                   (transverse) } as operative
                   thoractotomy   approach

     Code also cardiopulmonary bypass [extracorporeal circulation] [heart-lung machine] (39.61)

√4th **35.0   Closed heart valvotomy**

     EXCLUDES   *percutaneous (balloon) valvuloplasty (35.96)*

     DEF: Incision into valve to restore function.

     35.00   Closed heart valvotomy, unspecified valve
     35.01   Closed heart valvotomy, aortic valve
     35.02   Closed heart valvotomy, mitral valve
     35.03   Closed heart valvotomy, pulmonary valve
     35.04   Closed heart valvotomy, tricuspid valve

√4th **35.1   Open heart valvuloplasty without replacement**

     INCLUDES   open heart valvotomy

     EXCLUDES   *that associated with repair of:*
         endocardial cushion defect (35.54,35.63,35.73)
         percutaneous (balloon) valvuloplasty (35.96)
         valvular defect associated with atrial and ventricular septal defects (35.54, 35.63, 35.73)

     Code also cardiopulmonary bypass, if performed [extracorporeal circulation] [heart-lung machine] (39.61)

     DEF: Incision into heart for plastic repair of valve without replacing valve.

     35.10   Open heart valvuloplasty without replacement, unspecified valve
     35.11   Open heart valvuloplasty of aortic valve without replacement
     35.12   Open heart valvuloplasty of mitral valve without replacement
         AHA: 1Q, '97, 13
     35.13   Open heart valvuloplasty of pulmonary valve without replacement
     35.14   Open heart valvuloplasty of tricuspid valve without replacement

√4th **35.2   Replacement of heart valve**

     INCLUDES   excision of heart valve with replacement

     Code also cardiopulmonary bypass [extracorporeal circulation] [heart-lung machine] (39.61)

     EXCLUDES   *that associated with repair of:*
         endocardial cushion defect (35.54,35.63, 35.73)
         valvular defect associated with atrial and ventricular septal defects (35.54, 35.63, 35.73)

     DEF: Removal and replacement of valve with tissue from patient, animal, other human, or prosthetic (synthetic) valve.

     35.20   Replacement of unspecified heart valve
         Repair of unspecified heart valve with tissue graft or prosthetic implant
     35.21   Replacement of aortic valve with tissue graft
         Repair of aortic valve with tissue graft (autograft) (heterograft) (homograft)
         AHA: 2Q, '97, 8
     35.22   Other replacement of aortic valve
         Repair of aortic valve with replacement:
           NOS
           prosthetic (partial) (synthetic) (total)
         AHA: 1Q, '96, 11

     35.23   Replacement of mitral valve with tissue graft
         Repair of mitral valve with tissue graft (autograft) (heterograft) (homograft)
     35.24   Other replacement of mitral valve
         Repair of mitral valve with replacement:
           NOS
           prosthetic (partial) (synthetic) (total)
         AHA: 4Q, '97, 55
     35.25   Replacement of pulmonary valve with tissue graft
         Repair of pulmonary valve with tissue graft (autograft) (heterograft) (homograft)
         AHA: 2Q, '97, 8
     35.26   Other replacement of pulmonary valve
         Repair of pulmonary valve with replacement:
           NOS
           prosthetic (partial) (synthetic) (total)
     35.27   Replacement of tricuspid valve with tissue graft
         Repair of tricuspid valve with tissue graft (autograft) (heterograft) (homograft)
     35.28   Other replacement of tricuspid valve
         Repair of tricuspid valve with replacement:
           NOS
           prosthetic (partial) (synthetic) (total)

√4th **35.3   Operations on structures adjacent to heart valves**

     Code also cardiopulmonary bypass [extracorporeal circulation] [heart-lung machine] (39.61)

     35.31   Operations on papillary muscle
         Division
         Reattachment } of papillary
         Repair   muscle

     35.32   Operations on chordae tendineae
         Division } chordae tendineae
         Repair

     35.33   Annuloplasty
         Plication of annulus
         AHA: 1Q, '97, 13; 1Q, '88, 10

         DEF: Plication of annulus: Tuck stitched in valvular ring for tightening.

     35.34   Infundibulectomy
         Right ventricular infundibulectomy

         DEF: Infundibulectomy: Excision of funnel-shaped heart passage.

         DEF: Right ventricular infundibulectomy: Excision of funnel-shaped passage in right upper heart chamber.

     35.35   Operations on trabeculae carneae cordis
         Division } of trabeculae carneae
         Excision   cordis
         Excision of aortic subvalvular ring

     35.39   Operations on other structures adjacent to valves of heart
         Repair of sinus of Valsalva (aneurysm)

√4th **35.4   Production of septal defect in heart**

     35.41   Enlargement of existing atrial septal defect
         Rashkind procedure
         Septostomy (atrial) (balloon)

         DEF: Enlargement of partition wall defect in lower heart chamber to improve function.

         DEF: Rashkind procedure: Enlargement of partition wall defect between the two lower heart chambers by balloon catheter.

BI Bilateral Edit   NC Non-covered Procedure   ◀▶ Revised Text   ● New Code   ▲ Revised Code Title

35.42 Creation of septal defect in heart
Blalock-Hanlon operation

DEF: Blalock-Hanlon operation: Removal of partition wall defect in lower heart chamber.

√4ᵗʰ 35.5 Repair of atrial and ventricular septa with prosthesis

INCLUDES repair of septa with synthetic implant or patch

Code also cardiopulmonary bypass [extracorporeal circulation] [heart-lung machine] (39.61)

35.50 Repair of unspecified septal defect of heart with prosthesis

EXCLUDES that associated with repair of:
endocardial cushion defect (35.54)
septal defect associated with valvular defect (35.54)

35.51 Repair of atrial septal defect with prosthesis, open technique

Atrioseptoplasty
Correction of atrial septal defect
Repair:
foramen ovale (patent)
ostium secundum defect
} with prosthesis

EXCLUDES that associated with repair of:
atrial septal defect associated with valvular and ventricular septal defects (35.54)
endocardial cushion defect (35.54)

DEF: Repair of opening or weakening in septum separating the atria; prosthesis implanted through heart incision.

35.52 Repair of atrial septal defect with prosthesis, closed technique

Insertion of atrial septal umbrella [King-Mills]

AHA: 3Q, '98, 11

DEF: Correction of partition wall defect in lower heart chamber with artificial material; without incision into heart.

DEF: Insertion of atrial septal umbrella (King-Mills): Correction of partition wall defect in lower heart chamber with atrial septal umbrella.

35.53 Repair of ventricular septal defect with prosthesis

Correction of ventricular septal defect
Repair of supracristal defect
} with prosthesis

EXCLUDES that associated with repair of:
endocardial cushion defect (35.54)
ventricular defect associated with valvular and atrial septal defects (35.54)

35.54 Repair of endocardial cushion defect with prosthesis

Repair:
atrioventricular canal
ostium primum defect
valvular defect associated with atrial and ventricular septal defects
} with prosthesis (grafted to septa)

EXCLUDES repair of isolated:
atrial septal defect (35.51-35.52)
valvular defect (35.20, 35.22, 35.24, 35.26, 35.28)
ventricular septal defect (35.53)

√4ᵗʰ 35.6 Repair of atrial and ventricular septa with tissue graft

Code also cardiopulmonary bypass [extracorporeal circulation] [heart-lung machine] (39.61)

35.60 Repair of unspecified septal defect of heart with tissue graft

EXCLUDES that associated with repair of:
endocardial cushion defect (35.63)
septal defect associated with valvular defect (35.63)

35.61 Repair of atrial septal defect with tissue graft

Atrioseptoplasty
Correction of atrial septal defect
Repair:
foramen ovale (patent)
ostium secundum defect
} with tissue graft

EXCLUDES that associated with repair of:
atrial septal defect associated with valvular and ventricular septal defects (35.63)
endocardial cushion defect (35.63)

35.62 Repair of ventricular septal defect with tissue graft

Correction of ventricular septal defect
Repair of supracristal defect
} with tissue graft

EXCLUDES that associated with repair of:
endocardial cushion defect (35.63)
ventricular defect associated with valvular and atrial septal defects (35.63)

Operations on the Cardiovascular System 35.63–35.9

35.63 Repair of endocardial cushion defect with tissue graft

Repair of:
atrioventricular canal ⎫
ostium primum defect ⎪ with tissue
valvular defect ⎬ graft
  associated with ⎪
  atrial and ⎪
  ventricular septal ⎪
  defects ⎭

EXCLUDES repair of isolated:
  atrial septal defect (35.61)
  valvular defect (35.20-
    35.21, 35.23, 35.25,
    35.27)
  ventricular septal defect
    (35.62)

✓4th 35.7 Other and unspecified repair of atrial and ventricular septa

Code also cardiopulmonary bypass [extracorporeal circulation] [heart-lung machine] (39.61)

35.70 Other and unspecified repair of unspecified septal defect of heart

Repair of septal defect NOS
EXCLUDES that associated with repair of:
  endocardial cushion defect
    (35.73)
  septal defect associated
    with valvular defect
    (35.73)

35.71 Other and unspecified repair of atrial septal defect

Repair NOS:
atrial septum
foramen ovale (patent)
ostium secundum defect
EXCLUDES that associated with repair of:
  atrial septal defect
    associated with
    valvular and
    ventricular septal
    defects (35.73)
  endocardial cushion defect
    (35.73)

35.72 Other and unspecified repair of ventricular septal defect

Repair NOS:
supracristal defect
ventricular septum
EXCLUDES that associated with repair of:
  endocardial cushion defect
    (35.73)
  ventricular septal defect
    associated with valvular
    and atrial septal defects
    (35.73)

35.73 Other and unspecified repair of endocardial cushion defect

Repair NOS:
atrioventricular canal
ostium primum defect
valvular defect associated with atrial and
  ventricular septal defects
EXCLUDES repair of isolated:
  atrial septal defect (35.71)
  valvular defect (35.20,
    35.22, 35.24, 35.26,
    35.28)
  ventricular septal defect
    (35.72)

✓4th 35.8 Total repair of certain congenital cardiac anomalies

Note: For partial repair of defect [e.g. repair of atrial septal defect in tetralogy of Fallot] — code to specific procedure

35.81 Total repair of tetralogy of Fallot

One-stage total correction of tetralogy of
  Fallot with or without:
commissurotomy of pulmonary valve
infundibulectomy
outflow tract prosthesis
patch graft of outflow tract
prosthetic tube for pulmonary artery
repair of ventricular septal defect (with
  prosthesis)
take-down of previous systemic-
  pulmonary artery anastomosis

35.82 Total repair of total anomalous pulmonary venous connection

One-stage total correction of total
  anomalous pulmonary venous
  connection with or without:
anastomosis between (horizontal)
  common pulmonary trunk and
  posterior wall of left atrium (side-
  to-side)
enlargement of foramen ovale
incision [excision] of common wall
  between posterior left atrium and
  coronary sinus and roofing of
  resultant defect with patch graft
  (synthetic)
ligation of venous connection (descending
  anomalous vein) (to left innominate
  vein) (to superior vena cava)
repair of atrial septal defect (with
  prosthesis)

35.83 Total repair of truncus arteriosus

One-stage total correction of truncus
  arteriosus with or without:
construction (with aortic homograft) (with
  prosthesis) of a pulmonary artery
  placed from right ventricle to
  arteries supplying the lung
ligation of connections between aorta and
  pulmonary artery
repair of ventricular septal defect (with
  prosthesis)

35.84 Total correction of transposition of great vessels, not elsewhere classified

Arterial switch operation [Jatene]
Total correction of transposition of great
  arteries at the arterial level by
  switching the great arteries, including
  the left or both coronary arteries,
  implanted in the wall of the
  pulmonary artery
EXCLUDES baffle operation [Mustard]
  [Senning] (35.91)
  creation of shunt between
    right ventricle and
    pulmonary artery
    [Rastelli] (35.92)

✓4th 35.9 Other operations on valves and septa of heart

Code also cardiopulmonary bypass, if performed
[extracorporeal circulation] [heart-lung
machine] (39.61)

35.91 **Interatrial transposition of venous return**

Baffle:
 atrial
 interatrial
Mustard's operation
Resection of atrial septum and insertion of patch to direct systemic venous return to tricuspid valve and pulmonary venous return to mitral valve

DEF: Atrial baffle: Correction of venous flow of abnormal or deviated lower heart chamber.

DEF: Interatrial baffle: Correction of venous flow between abnormal lower heart chambers.

DEF: Mustard's operation: Creates intra-atrial baffle using pericardial tissue to correct transposition of the great vessels.

35.92 **Creation of conduit between right ventricle and pulmonary artery**

Creation of shunt between right ventricle and (distal) pulmonary artery
EXCLUDES *that associated with total repair of truncus arteriosus (35.83)*

35.93 **Creation of conduit between left ventricle and aorta**

Creation of apicoaortic shunt
Shunt between apex of left ventricle and aorta

35.94 **Creation of conduit between atrium and pulmonary artery**

Fontan procedure

35.95 **Revision of corrective procedure on heart**

Replacement of prosthetic heart valve poppet
Resuture of prosthesis of:
 septum
 valve
EXCLUDES *complete revision — code to specific procedure*
replacement of prosthesis or graft of:
septum (35.50-35.63)
valve (35.20-35.28)

DEF: Replacement of prosthetic heart valve poppet: Removal and replacement of valve-supporting prosthesis.

DEF: Resuture of prosthesis of septum: Restitching of prosthesis in partition wall.

DEF: Resuture of prosthesis of valve: Restitching of prosthetic valve.

35.96 **Percutaneous valvuloplasty**

Percutaneous balloon valvuloplasty
AHA: M-J, '86, 6; N-D, '85, 10

DEF: Repair of valve with catheter.

DEF: Percutaneous balloon valvuloplasty: Repair of valve with inflatable catheter.

35.98 **Other operations on septa of heart**

35.99 **Other operations on valves of heart**

√3rd **36** **Operations on vessels of heart**

INCLUDES sternotomy (median)
 (transverse) } as operative
 thoracotomy approach

Code also any injection or infusion of platelet inhibitor (99.20)
Code also cardiopulmonary bypass, if performed [extracorporeal circulation] [heart-lung machine] (39.61)

√4th **36.0** **Removal of coronary artery obstruction and insertion of stent(s)**

AHA: 4Q, '95, 66; 2Q, '94, 13; 1Q, '94, 3; 2Q, '90, 23; N-D, '86, 8

36.01 **Single vessel percutaneous transluminal coronary angioplasty [PTCA] or coronary atherectomy without mention of thrombolytic agent**

Balloon angioplasty of coronary artery
Coronary atherectomy
Percutaneous coronary angioplasty NOS
PTCA NOS
EXCLUDES *multiple vessel percutaneous transluminal coronary angioplasty [PTCA] or coronary atherectomy performed during the same operation (36.05)*
Code also any insertion of coronary stent(s) (36.06)

AHA: 1Q, '01, 9; 2Q, '01, 24; 1Q, '00, 11; 1Q, '99, 17; 4Q, '98, 74, 85; 3Q, '91, 24

DEF: Balloon angioplasty: Insertion of catheter with inflation of balloon to flatten plaque and widen vessels.

36.02 **Single vessel percutaneous transluminal coronary angioplasty [PTCA] or coronary atherectomy with mention of thrombolytic agent**

Balloon angioplasty of coronary artery with infusion of thrombolytic agent [streptokinase]
Coronary atherectomy
EXCLUDES *multiple vessel percutaneous transluminal coronary angioplasty [PTCA] or coronary atherectomy performed during the same operation (36.05)*
single vessel PTCA or coronary atherectomy without mention of thrombolytic agent (36.01)
Code also any insertion of coronary stent(s) (36.06)

AHA: 2Q, '01, 24; 1Q, '97, 3

36.03 **Open chest coronary artery angioplasty**

Coronary (artery):
 endarterectomy (with patch graft)
 thromboendarterectomy (with patch graft)
Open surgery for direct relief of coronary artery obstruction
EXCLUDES *that with coronary artery bypass graft (36.10-36.19)*
Code also any insertion of coronary stent(s) (36.06)

AHA: 2Q, '01, 24; 3Q, '93, 7

DEF: Endarterectomy (with patch graft): Excision of thickened material within coronary artery; repair with patch graft.

DEF: Thromboendarterectomy (with patch graft): Excision of blood clot and thickened material within artery; repair with patch graft.

DEF: Open surgery for direct relief of coronary artery obstruction: Removal of coronary artery obstruction through opening in chest.

Operations on the Cardiovascular System 35.91–36.03

Operations on the Cardiovascular System 36.04–36.14

PTCA (Balloon Angioplasty)

Coronary Bypass

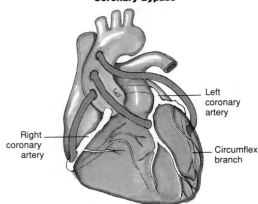

36.04   **Intracoronary artery thrombolytic infusion**
That by direct coronary artery injection, infusion, or catheterization
enzyme infusion
platelet inhibitor

> **EXCLUDES**   *infusion of platelet inhibitor(99.20)*
> *infusion of thrombolytic agent (99.10)*
> *that associated with any procedure in 36.02, 36.03*

AHA: 2Q, '01, 24; 4Q, '98, 85; 1Q, '97, 3; 4Q, '95, 67

DEF: Infusion of clot breaking solution into intracoronary artery.

36.05   **Multiple vessel percutaneous transluminal coronary angioplasty [PTCA] or coronary atherectomy performed during the same operation, with or without mention of thrombolytic agent**
Balloon angioplasty of multiple coronary arteries
Coronary atherectomy
Code also any:
   insertion of coronary artery stent(s) (36.06)
   intracoronary artery thrombolytic infusion (36.04)

> **EXCLUDES**   *single vessel [PTCA] or coronary atherectomy without mention of thrombolytic agent (36.01)*
> *with mention of thrombolytic agent (36.02)*

AHA: 2Q, '01, 24; 1Q, '94, 3

36.06   **Insertion of non-drug-eluting coronary artery stent(s)**
▶Bare stent(s)
Bonded stent(s)
Drug-coated stent(s), e.g., heparin coated
Endograft(s)
Endovascular graft(s)
Stent graft(s)◀
Code also any:
   open chest coronary artery angioplasty (36.03)
   percutaneous transluminal coronary angioplasty [PTCA] or coronary atherectomy (36.01, 36.02, 36.05)

> **EXCLUDES**   ▶ *insertion of drug-eluting coronary artery stent(s) (36.07)*◀

AHA: 1Q,'01, 9; 2Q, '01, 24; 1Q, '00, 11; 1Q, '99, 17

DEF: Percutaneous implant via catheter of metal stent, to enlarge, maintain lumen size of coronary artery.

● **36.07**   **Insertion of drug-eluting coronary artery stent(s)**
Endograft(s)
Endovascular graft(s)
Stent graft(s)
Code also any:
   open chest coronary artery angioplasty (36.03)
   percutaneous transluminal coronary angioplasty [PTCA] or coronary atherectomy (36.01, 36.02, 36.05)

> **EXCLUDES**   *drug-coated stents, e.g., heparin coated (36.06)*
> *insertion of non-drug-eluting coronary artery stent(s) (36.06)*

36.09   **Other removal of coronary artery obstruction**
Coronary angioplasty NOS

> **EXCLUDES**   *that by open angioplasty (36.03)*
> *that by percutaneous transluminal coronary angioplasty [PTCA] or coronary atherectomy (36.01-36.02, 36.05)*

√4ᵗʰ **36.1**   **Bypass anastomosis for heart revascularization**
Code also cardiopulmonary bypass [extracorporeal circulation] [heart-lung machine] (39.61)

AHA: 2Q, '96, 7; 3Q, '95, 7; 3Q, '93, 8; 1Q, '91, 7; 2Q, '90, 24; 4Q, '89, 3

DEF: Insertion of tube to bypass blocked coronary artery, correct coronary blood flow.

36.10   **Aortocoronary bypass for heart revascularization, not otherwise specified**
Direct revascularization:
   cardiac
   coronary   } with catheter stent,
   heart muscle   prosthesis, or
   myocardial   vein graft

Heart revascularization NOS
AHA: 2Q, '96, 7

36.11   **Aortocoronary bypass of one coronary artery**
AHA: 4Q, '89, 3

36.12   **Aortocoronary bypass of two coronary arteries**
AHA: 4Q, '99, 15; 2Q, '96, 7; 3Q, '97, 14; 4Q, '89, 3

36.13   **Aortocoronary bypass of three coronary arteries**
AHA: 2Q, '96, 7; 4Q, '89, 3

36.14   **Aortocoronary bypass of four or more coronary arteries**
AHA: 2Q, '96, 7; 4Q, '89, 3

BI Bilateral Edit   **NC** Non-covered Procedure   ▶◀ Revised Text   ● New Code   ▲ Revised Code Title

36.15 Single internal mammary-coronary artery bypass

Anastomosis (single):
mammary artery to coronary artery
thoracic artery to coronary artery

AHA: 4Q, '99, 15; 3Q, '97, 14; 2Q, '96, 7

36.16 Double internal mammary-coronary artery bypass

Anastomosis, double:
mammary artery to coronary artery
thoracic artery to coronary artery

AHA: 2Q, '96, 7

36.17 Abdominal-coronary artery bypass

Anastomosis:
gastroepiploic artery to coronary artery

AHA: 3Q, '97, 14; 4Q, '96, 64

36.19 Other bypass anastomosis for heart revascularization

AHA: 2Q, '96, 7

36.2 Heart revascularization by arterial implant

Implantation of:
aortic branches [ascending aortic branches] into
heart muscle
blood vessels into myocardium
internal mammary artery [internal thoracic
artery] into:
heart muscle
myocardium
ventricle
ventricular wall
Indirect heart revascularization NOS

√4ᵗʰ 36.3 Other heart revascularization

36.31 Open chest transmyocardial revascularization

DEF: Transmyocardial revascularization (TMR): Laser
creation of channels through myocardium allows
oxygenated blood flow from sinusoids to myocardial
tissue.

36.32 Other transmyocardial revascularization `NC`

Percutaneous transmyocardial
revascularization
Thoracoscopic transmyocardial
revascularization

AHA: 4Q, '98, 74

36.39 Other heart revascularization

Abrasion of epicardium
Cardio-omentopexy
Intrapericardial poudrage
Myocardial graft:
mediastinal fat
omentum
pectoral muscles

DEF: Cardio-omentopexy: Suture of omentum segment to heart after
drawing segment through incision in diaphragm.

DEF: Intrapericardial poudrage: Application of powder to heart
lining to promote fusion.

DEF: Myocardial graft:

Mediastinal fat: Implantation in heart muscle of fat from cavity
containing heart and structures.

Omentopexy: Suture of omentum to heart.

√4ᵗʰ 36.9 Other operations on vessels of heart

Code also cardiopulmonary bypass [extracorporeal
circulation] [heart-lung machine] (39.61)

36.91 Repair of aneurysm of coronary vessel

36.99 Other operations on vessels of heart

Exploration
Incision   of coronary
Ligation   artery

Repair of arteriovenous fistula

AHA: 1Q, '94, 3

Transmyocardial Revascularization

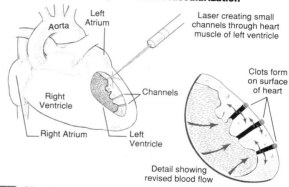

√3ʳᵈ 37 Other operations on heart and pericardium

Code also any injection or infusion of platelet inhibitor
(99.20)

37.0 Pericardiocentesis

DEF: Puncture of the heart lining to withdraw fluid.

√4ᵗʰ 37.1 Cardiotomy and pericardiotomy

Code also cardiopulmonary bypass [extracorporeal
circulation] [heart-lung machine] (39.61)

37.10 Incision of heart, not otherwise specified

Cardiolysis NOS

37.11 Cardiotomy

Incision of: Incision of:
atrium   myocardium
endocardium   ventricle

37.12 Pericardiotomy

Pericardial window   Pericardiolysis
operation   Pericardiotomy

DEF: Pericardial window operation: Incision into heart
lining for drainage.

DEF: Pericardiolysis: Destruction of heart tissue lining.

√4ᵗʰ 37.2 Diagnostic procedures on heart and pericardium

37.21 Right heart cardiac catheterization

Cardiac catheterization NOS

EXCLUDES *that with catheterization of left
heart (37.23)*

AHA: 2Q, '90, 23; M-J, '87, 11

37.22 Left heart cardiac catheterization

EXCLUDES *that with catheterization of
right heart (37.23)*

AHA: 1Q, '00, 21; 2Q, '90, 23; 4Q, '88, 4; M-J, '87, 11

37.23 Combined right and left heart cardiac catheterization

AHA: 2Q, '01, 8; 1Q, '00, 20; 3Q, '98, 11; 2Q, '90, 23;
M-J, '87, 11

37.24 Biopsy of pericardium

37.25 Biopsy of heart

AHA: 3Q, '94, 8

37.26 Cardiac electrophysiologic stimulation and recording studies

Electrophysiologic studies [EPS]
▶Non-invasive programmed electrical
stimulation (NIPS)◀
Programmed electrical stimulation
Code also any concomitant procedure

EXCLUDES *His bundle recording (37.29)*

AHA: ▶ 1Q, '02, 8, 9◀ 1Q, '99, 3; 2Q, '97, 10; 3Q, '90, 11

DEF: Diagnostic mapping and measurement of
intracardiac electrical activity; requires inserting three
to six catheters into heart blood vessels and positioning
catheters under fluoroscopic guidance to determine site
of the tachycardia or abnormal impulse pathway; may
also be used to terminate arrhythmias.

Operations on the Cardiovascular System 36.15–37.26

Intracardiac Echocardiography

Superior vena cava · Aorta · Inferior vena cava · Left atrium · Right atrium · Left ventricle · Femoral vein access · Right ventricle · Inferior vena cava · Miniaturized ultrasound transducer

37.27 Cardiac mapping
Code also any concomitant procedure
EXCLUDES   electrocardiogram (89.52)
His bundle recording (37.29)

37.28 Intracardiac echocardiography
ICE
Code also any synchronous Doppler flow mapping (88.72)

DEF: Creation of a two-dimensional graphic of heart using endoscopic echocardiographic equipment.

AHA: 4Q, '01, 62

37.29 Other diagnostic procedures on heart and pericardium
EXCLUDES   angiocardiography (88.50-88.58)
cardiac function tests (89.41-89.69)
cardiovascular radioisotopic scan and function study (92.05)
coronary arteriography (88.55-88.57)
diagnostic pericardiocentesis (37.0)
diagnostic ultrasound of heart (88.72)
x-ray of heart (87.49)

AHA: S-O, '87, 3

✓4ᵗʰ 37.3 Pericardiectomy and excision of lesion of heart
Code also cardiopulmonary bypass [extracorporeal circulation] [heart-lung machine] (39.61)

37.31 Pericardiectomy
Excision of:
adhesions of pericardium
constricting scar of:
epicardium
pericardium

DEF: Excision of a portion of heart lining.

37.32 Excision of aneurysm of heart
Repair of aneurysm of heart

37.33 Excision or destruction of other lesion or tissue of heart
EXCLUDES   catheter ablation of lesion or tissues of heart (37.34)

AHA: 2Q, '94, 12

37.34 Catheter ablation of lesion or tissues of heart
Cryoablation } of lesion or
Electrocurrent } tissues of
Resection } heart

AHA: 1Q, '00, 20

DEF: Destruction of heart tissue or lesion by freezing, electric current or resection.

37.35 Partial ventriculectomy   [NC]
Ventricular reduction surgery
Ventricular remodeling
Code also any synchronous:
mitral valve repair (35.02, 35.12)
mitral valve replacement (35.23-35.24)

AHA: 4Q, '97, 54, 55

DEF: Removal of elliptical slice of ventricle between anterior and posterior papillary muscle; also called Batiste operation.

37.4 Repair of heart and pericardium
AHA: 2Q, '90, 24

37.5 Heart transplantation   [NC]
EXCLUDES   combined heart-lung transplantation (33.6)

✓4ᵗʰ 37.6 Implantation of heart assist system
AHA: 4Q, '95, 68

DEF: Implant of device for assisting heart in circulating blood.

37.61 Implant of pulsation balloon
37.62 Implant of other heart assist system
Insertion of centrifugal pump
Insertion of heart assist system, not specified as pulsatile
Insertion of heart assist system, NOS
Insertion of heart pump

AHA: 2Q, '90, 25

37.63 Replacement and repair of heart assist system
37.64 Removal of heart assist system
EXCLUDES   that with replacement of implant (37.63)
nonoperative removal of heart assist system (97.44)

37.65 Implant of an external, pulsatile heart assist system
Note: Device not implantable (outside the body but connected to heart) with external circulation and pump
EXCLUDES   implant of pulsation balloon (37.61)

DEF: Insertion of short-term circulatory support device with pump outside body.

37.66 Implant of an implantable, pulsatile heart assist system   [NC]
Note: Device directly connected to the heart and implanted in the upper left quadrant of peritoneal cavity
Transportable, implantable heart assist system
EXCLUDES   implant of pulsation balloon (37.61)

AHA: 1Q, '98, 8

DEF: Insertion of long-term circulatory support device with pump in body.

Ventricular Reduction Surgery

Superior vena cava · Aorta · Pulmonary artery · Left atrium · Left ventricle · Shape of heart after reduction · Anterior interventricular branch of left coronary artery · Right atrium · Right coronary artery · Right ventricle · New apex · Apex · Superior vena cava · Aorta · Posterior interventricular branch of right coronary artery · Circumflex branch

Enlarged Heart

37.67 Implantation of cardiomyostimulation system

Note: Two-step open procedure consisting of tranfer of one end of the latissimus dorsi muscle; wrapping it around the heart; rib resection; implantation of epicardial cardiac pacing leads into the right ventricle; tunneling and pocket creation for the cardiomyostimulator.

AHA: 4Q, '98, 75; 1Q, '98, 8

✓4th **37.7 Insertion, revision, replacement, and removal of pacemaker leads; insertion of temporary pacemaker system; or revision of pocket**

Code also any insertion and replacement of pacemaker device (37.80-37.87)

EXCLUDES ▶ *implantation or replacement of transvenous lead [electrode] into left ventricular cardiac venous system (00.52)* ◀

AHA: 1Q, '94, 16; 3Q, '92, 3; M-J, '87, 1

10 **37.70 Initial insertion of lead [electrode], not otherwise specified**

EXCLUDES *insertion of temporary transvenous pacemaker system (37.78)*
replacement of atrial and/or ventricular lead(s) (37.76)

10 **37.71 Initial insertion of transvenous lead [electrode] into ventricle**

EXCLUDES *insertion of temporary transvenous pacemaker system (37.78)*
replacement of atrial and/or ventricular lead(s) (37.76)

11 **37.72 Initial insertion of transvenous leads [electrodes] into atrium and ventricle**

EXCLUDES *insertion of temporary transvenous pacemaker system (37.78)*
replacement of atrial and/or ventricular lead(s) (37.76)

AHA: 2Q, '97, 4

10 **37.73 Initial insertion of transvenous lead [electrode] into atrium**

EXCLUDES *insertion of temporary transvenous pacemaker system (37.78)*
replacement of atrial and/or ventricular lead(s) (37.76)

13 **37.74 Insertion or replacement of epicardial lead [electrode] into epicardium**

Insertion or replacement of epicardial lead by:
sternotomy
thoracotomy

EXCLUDES *replacement of atrial and/or ventricular lead(s) (37.76)*

Insertion of Pacemaker

Lead
Subclavian vein
Pulse generator (pacemaker)
Electrode

37.75 Revision of lead [electrode]

Repair of electrode [removal with re-insertion]
Repositioning of lead [electrode]
Revision of lead NOS

EXCLUDES *repositioning of temporary transvenous pacemaker system — omit code*

AHA: 2Q, '99, 12

12 **37.76 Replacement of transvenous atrial and/or ventricular lead(s) [electrode]**

Removal or abandonment of existing transvenous or epicardial lead(s) with transvenous lead(s) replacement

EXCLUDES *replacement of epicardial lead [electrode] (37.74)*

37.77 Removal of lead(s) [electrode] without replacement

Removal:
epicardial lead (transthoracic approach)
transvenous lead(s)

EXCLUDES *removal of temporary transvenous pacemaker system — omit code*
that with replacement of:
atrial and/or ventricular lead(s) [electrode] (37.76)
epicardial lead [electrode] (37.74)

37.78 Insertion of temporary transvenous pacemaker system

EXCLUDES *intraoperative cardiac pacemaker (39.64)*

AHA: 3Q, '93, 12; 1Q, '89, 2

37.79 Revision or relocation of pacemaker pocket

Debridement and reforming pocket (skin and subcutaneous tissue)
Relocation of pocket [creation of new pocket] ▶pacemaker or CRT-P◀

✓4th **37.8 Insertion, replacement, removal, and revision of pacemaker device**

Code also any lead insertion, lead replacement, lead removal and/or lead revision (37.70-37.77)

EXCLUDES ▶ *implantation of cardiac resynchronization pacemaker, total system [CRT-P] (00.50)*
implantation or replacement of cardiac resynchronization pacemaker pulse generator only [CRT-P] (00.53) ◀

AHA: M-J, '87, 1

37.80 Insertion of permanent pacemaker, initial or replacement, type of device not specified

10 Valid OR procedure code if accompanied by one of the following codes: 37.80, 37.81, 37.82, 37.85, 37.86, 37.87
11 Valid OR procedure code if accompanied by one of the following codes: 37.80, 37.83
12 Valid OR procedure code if accompanied by one of the following codes: 37.80, 37.85, 37.86, 37.87
13 Valid OR procedure code if accompanied by one of the following codes: 37.80, 37.81, 37.82, 37.83, 37.85, 37.86, 37.87

✓3rd
✓4th Additional Digit Required

Nonspecific OR Procedure | Valid OR Procedure | Non-OR Procedure

[14] **37.81** **Initial insertion of single-chamber device, not specified as rate responsive**

> **EXCLUDES** *replacement of existing pacemaker device (37.85-37.87)*

[14] **37.82** **Initial insertion of a single-chamber device, rate responsive**

Rate responsive to physiologic stimuli other than atrial rate

> **EXCLUDES** *replacement of existing pacemaker device (37.85-37.87)*

[15] **37.83** **Initial insertion of dual-chamber device**

Atrial ventricular sequential device

> **EXCLUDES** *replacement of existing pacemaker device (37.85-37.87)*

AHA: 2Q, '97, 4

37.85 **Replacement of any type pacemaker device with single-chamber device, not specified as rate responsive**

37.86 **Replacement of any type pacemaker device with single-chamber device, rate responsive**

Rate responsive to physiologic stimuli other than atrial rate

37.87 **Replacement of any type pacemaker device with dual-chamber device**

Atrial ventricular sequential device

37.89 **Revision or removal of pacemaker device**

►Removal without replacement of cardiac resynchronization pacemaker device [CRT-P]◄

Repair of pacemaker device

> **EXCLUDES** *removal of temporary transvenous pacemaker system — omit code*
> *replacement of existing pacemaker device (37.85-37.87)*
> ►*replacement of existing pacemaker device with CRT-P pacemaker device (00.53)*◄

AHA: N-D, '86, 1

✓4ᵗʰ **37.9** **Other operations on heart and pericardium**
AHA: 3Q, '90, 11

37.91 **Open chest cardiac massage**

> **EXCLUDES** *closed chest cardiac massage (99.63)*

AHA: 4Q, '88, 12

DEF: Massage of heart through opening in chest wall to reinstate or maintain circulation.

37.92 **Injection of therapeutic substance into heart**

Automatic Implantable Cardioverter/Defibrillator

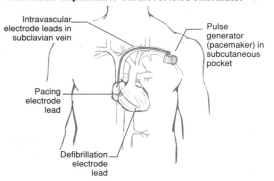

Intravascular electrode leads in subclavian vein

Pulse generator (pacemaker) in subcutaneous pocket

Pacing electrode lead

Defibrillation electrode lead

Endarterectomy of Aortic Bifurcation

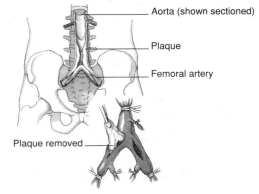

Aorta (shown sectioned)

Plaque

Femoral artery

Plaque removed

37.93 **Injection of therapeutic substance into pericardium**

37.94 **Implantation or replacement of automatic cardioverter/defibrillator, total system [AICD]**

Implantation of defibrillator with leads (epicardial patches), formation of pocket (abdominal fascia) (subcutaneous), any transvenous leads, intraoperative procedures for evaluation of lead signals, and obtaining defibrillator threshold measurements

Techniques: lateral thoracotomy
medial sternotomy
subxiphoid procedure

Code also extracorporeal circulation, if performed (39.61)

Code also any concomitant procedure [e.g., coronary bypass] (36.01-36.19)

> **EXCLUDES** ►*implantation of cardiac resynchronization defibrillator, total system [CRT-D] (00.51)* ◄

AHA: 3Q, '01, 5-7; 3Q, '99, 12; 1Q, '99, 3; 3Q, '90, 11; S-O, '87, 5

DEF: Direct insertion, of defibrillator/cardioverter system to deliver shock and restore heart rhythm.

37.95 **Implantation of automatic cardioverter/defibrillator lead(s) only**

AHA: 3Q, '90, 11

37.96 **Implantation of automatic cardioverter/defibrillator pulse generator only**

> **EXCLUDES** ►*implantation or replacement of cardiac resynchronization defibrillator, pulse generator device only [CRT-D] (00.54)*◄

AHA: 3Q, '90, 11

37.97 **Replacement of automatic cardioverter/defibrillator lead(s) only**

AHA: 3Q, '90, 11

37.98 **Replacement of automatic cardioverter/defibrillator pulse generator only**

AHA: 1Q, '99, 3; 3Q, '90, 11

> **EXCLUDES** ►*replacement of cardiac resynchronization defibrillator, pulse generator device only [CRT-D] (00.54)*◄

[14] Valid OR procedure code if accompanied by one of the following codes: 37.72, 37.76
[15] Valid OR procedure code if accompanied by one of the following codes: 37.70, 37.71, 37.73, 37.76

BI Bilateral Edit | **NC** Non-covered Procedure | ►◄ Revised Text | ● New Code | ▲ Revised Code Title

37.99 **Other**

Removal of cardioverter/defibrillator pulse generator only without replacement

►Removal without replacement of cardiac resynchronization defibrillator device [CRT-D]◄

Repositioning of lead(s) (sensing) (pacing) [electrode]

Repositioning of pulse generator

Revision of cardioverter/defibrillator (automatic) pocket

►Revision or relocation of CRT-D pocket◄

EXCLUDES *cardiac retraining (93.36)*
conversion of cardiac rhythm (99.60-99.69)

AHA: 1Q, '97, 12; 1Q, '94, 19; 3Q, '90, 11; 1Q, '89, 11

√3rd **38** **Incision, excision, and occlusion of vessels**

►Code also any application or administration of an adhesion barrier substance (99.77)◄

Code also cardiopulmonary bypass [extracorporeal circulation] [heart-lung machine] (39.61)

EXCLUDES *that of coronary vessels (36.01-36.99)*

The following fourth-digit subclassification is for use with appropriate categories in section 38.0, 38.1, 38.3, 38.5, 38.6, and 38.8 according to site. Valid fourth-digits are in [brackets] under each code.

0 **unspecified**

1 **intracranial vessels**
Cerebral (anterior) (middle)
Circle of Willis
Posterior communicating artery

2 **other vessels of head and neck**
Carotid artery (common) (external) (internal)
Jugular vein (external) (internal)

3 **upper limb vessels**
Axillary   Radial
Brachial   Ulnar

4 **aorta**

5 **other thoracic vessels**
Innominate   Vena cava, superior
Pulmonary (artery) (vein)
Subclavian

6 **abdominal arteries**
Celiac   Mesenteric
Gastric   Renal
Hepatic   Splenic
Iliac   Umbilical
EXCLUDES *abdominal aorta (4)*

7 **abdominal veins**
Iliac   Splenic
Portal   Vena cava (inferior)
Renal

8 **lower limb arteries**
Femoral (common) (superficial)
Popliteal
Tibial

9 **lower limb veins**
Femoral   Saphenous
Popliteal   Tibial

§ √4th 16**38.0** **Incision of vessel**
[0-9]   Embolectomy
Thrombectomy
EXCLUDES *puncture or catheterization of any:*
artery (38.91, 38.98)
vein (38.92-38.95, 38.99)

AHA: 2Q, '98, 23

DEF: Incision into vessel to remove mobile or stationary blood clot.

§ √4th 16**38.1** **Endarterectomy**
[0-6,8]   Endarterectomy with:
embolectomy
patch graft
temporary bypass during procedure
thrombectomy

AHA: 1Q, '00, 16; 2Q, '99, 5; 2Q, '95, 16; ►For code 38.12: 1Q, '02, 10◄

DEF: Excision of tunica intima of artery to relieve arterial walls thickened by plaque or chronic inflammation.

√4th **38.2** **Diagnostic procedures on blood vessels**

38.21 **Biopsy of blood vessel**

38.22 **Percutaneous angioscopy**
EXCLUDES *angioscopy of eye (95.12)*

38.29 **Other diagnostic procedures on blood vessels**
EXCLUDES *blood vessel thermography (88.86)*
circulatory monitoring (89.61-89.69)
contrast:
angiocardiography (88.50-88.58)
arteriography (88.40-88.49)
phlebography (88.60-88.67)
impedance phlebography (88.68)
peripheral vascular ultrasonography (88.77)
plethysmogram (89.58)

AHA: 3Q, '00, 16; 1Q, '99, 7

DEF: Exam, with fiberoptic catheter inserted through peripheral artery to visualize inner lining of blood vessels.

§ √4th 16**38.3** **Resection of vessel with anastomosis**
[0-9]   Angiectomy
Excision of:
aneurysm
(arteriovenous)   } with anastomosis
blood vessel (lesion)

DEF: Reconstruction and reconnection of vessel after partial excision.

Methods of Vessel Anastomoses

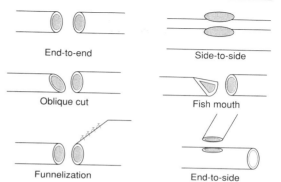

End-to-end   Side-to-side

Oblique cut   Fish mouth

Funnelization   End-to-side

§ Requires fourth-digit. Valid digits are in [brackets] under each code. See category 38 for definitions.
16 Nonspecific OR procedure = 0

√3rd
√4th
Additional Digit Required

Nonspecific OR Procedure

Valid OR Procedure

Non-OR Procedure

Operations on the Cardiovascular System 37.99–38.3

Operations on the Cardiovascuolar System 38.4–38.94

§§ ☑4th16 **38.4**   **Resection of vessel with replacement**
[0-9]

Angiectomy
Excision of:
  aneurysm
    (arteriovenous) or   ⎫
    blood vessel   ⎬ with replacement
    (lesion)   ⎭

> **EXCLUDES**   *endovascular repair of aneurysm (39.71-39.79)*

Requires the use of one of the following fourth-digit subclassifications to identify site:

0   unspecified site
1   intracranial vessels
  Cerebral (anterior) (middle)
  Circle of Willis
  Posterior communicating artery
2   other vessels of head and neck
  Carotid artery (common) (external) (internal)
  Jugular vein (external) (internal)
3   upper limb vessels
  Axillary   Radial
  Brachial   Ulnar
4   aorta, abdominal
  Code also any thoracic vessel involvement
    (thoracoabdominal procedure) (38.45)
5   thoracic vessel
  Aorta (thoracic)
  Innominate   Subclavian
  Pulmonary (artery) (vein)   Vena cava, superior
  Code also any abdominal aorta involvement
    (thoracoabdominal procedure) (38.44)
6   abdominal arteries
  Celiac   Mesenteric
  Gastric   Renal
  Hepatic   Splenic
  Iliac   Umbilical
> **EXCLUDES**   *abdominal aorta (4)*
7   abdominal veins
  Iliac   Splenic
  Portal   Vena cava (inferior)
  Renal
8   lower limb arteries
  Femoral (common) (superficial)
  Tibial
9   lower limb veins
  Femoral   Saphenous
  Popliteal   Tibial

AHA: 2Q, '99, 5, 6

DEF: Excision of aneurysm (arteriovenous): Excision and replacement of segment of stretched or bulging blood vessel.

DEF: Excision of blood vessel (lesion): Excision and replacement of segment of vessel containing lesion.

§ ☑4th16 **38.5**   **Ligation and stripping of varicose veins**
[0-3,5,7,9]   **EXCLUDES**   *ligation of varices:*
                esophageal (42.91)
                gastric (44.91)

AHA: For code 38.59: 2Q, '97, 7

DEF: Ligation of varicose veins: Typing off vein with thread or wire to eliminate blood flow; stripping involves excising length of vein.

§ ☑4th16 **38.6**   **Other excision of vessels**
[0-9]

Excision of blood vessel (lesion) NOS
> **EXCLUDES**   *excision of vessel for aortocoronary bypass (36.10-36.14)*
> *excision with:*
>   *anastomosis (38.30-38.39)*
>   *graft replacement (38.40-38.49)*
>   *implant (38.40-38.49)*

AHA: 3Q, '90, 17

38.7   **Interruption of the vena cava**

Insertion of implant or sieve in vena cava
Ligation of vena cava (inferior) (superior)
Plication of vena cava

AHA: 2Q, '94, 9; S-O, '85, 5

DEF: Interruption of the blood flow through the venous heart vessels to prevent clots from reaching the chambers of the heart by means of implanting a sieve or implant, separating off a portion or by narrowing the venous blood vessels.

§ ☑4th16 **38.8**   **Other surgical occlusion of vessels**
[0-9]

Clamping   ⎫
Division   ⎬ of blood vessel
Ligation   ⎪
Occlusion ⎭

> **EXCLUDES**   *adrenal vessels (07.43)*
> *esophageal varices (42.91)*
> *gastric or duodenal vessel for ulcer (44.40-44.49)*
> *gastric varices (44.91)*
> *meningeal vessel (02.13)*
> *percutaneous transcatheter infusion embolization (99.29)*
> *spermatic vein for varicocele (63.1)*
> *surgical occlusion of vena cava (38.7)*
> *that for chemoembolization (99.25)*
> *that for control of (postoperative) hemorrhage:*
>   *anus (49.95)*
>   *bladder (57.93)*
>   *following vascular procedure (39.41)*
>   *nose (21.00-21.09)*
>   *prostate (60.94)*
>   *tonsil (28.7)*
>   *thyroid vessel (06.92)*

AHA: 2Q, '90, 23; M-A, '87, 9; For code 38.86: N-D, '87, 4

☑4th **38.9**   **Puncture of vessel**
> **EXCLUDES**   *that for circulatory monitoring ▶(89.60-89.69)◀*

38.91   **Arterial catheterization**
  AHA: 1Q, '97, 3; 1Q, '95, 3; 2Q, '91, 15; 2Q, '90, 23

38.92   **Umbilical vein catheterization**

38.93   **Venous catheterization, not elsewhere classified**
> **EXCLUDES**   *that for cardiac catheterization (37.21-37.23)*
> *that for renal dialysis (38.95)*

  AHA: 3Q, '00, 9; 2Q, '98, 24; 1Q, '96, 3; 2Q, '96, 15; 3Q, '91, 13; 4Q, '90, 14; 2Q, '90, 24; 3Q, '88, 13

38.94   **Venous cutdown**
  DEF: Incision of vein to place needle or cathete.

Typical Venous Cutdown

Vein mobilized, opened by oblique cut, catheter inserted

Distal vein tied

Saphenous vein (typical site) accessed by transverse incision

---

§   Requires fourth-digit. Valid digits are in [brackets] under each code. See category 38 for definitions.
§§ Requires fourth-digit. Valid digits are in [brackets] under each code. See subcategory 38.4 for definitions.
16   Nonspecific OR procedure = 0

38.95   **Venous catheterization for renal dialysis**
> EXCLUDES   *insertion of totally implantable vascular access device [VAD] (86.07)*

AHA: 3Q, '98, 13; 2Q, '94, 11

38.98   **Other puncture of artery**
> EXCLUDES   *that for:*
> *arteriography (88.40-88.49)*
> *coronary arteriography (88.55-88.57)*

38.99   **Other puncture of vein**
Phlebotomy
> EXCLUDES   *that for:*
> *angiography (88.60-88.68)*
> *extracorporeal circulation (39.61, 50.92)*
> *injection or infusion of:*
> *sclerosing solution (39.92)*
> *therapeutic or prophylactic substance (99.11-99.29)*
> *perfusion (39.96, 39.97)*
> *phlebography (88.60-88.68)*
> *transfusion (99.01-99.09)*

AHA: 4Q, '94, 50; 1Q, '88, 11

√3rd **39**   **Other operations on vessels**
> EXCLUDES   *those on coronary vessels (36.0-36.99)*

39.0   **Systemic to pulmonary artery shunt**

Descending aorta-pulmonary artery
Left to right   }   anastomosis (graft)
Subclavian-pulmonary

Code also cardiopulmonary bypass [extracorporeal circulation] [heart-lung machine] (39.61)

DEF: Descending aorta-pulmonary artery anastomosis (graft): Connection of descending main heart artery to pulmonary artery.

DEF: Left to right anastomosis (graft): Connection of systemic arterial blood vessel to venous pulmonary system.

DEF: Subclavian-pulmonary anastomosis (graft): Connection of subclavian artery to pulmonary artery

39.1   **Intra-abdominal venous shunt**
Anastomosis:
mesocaval
portacaval
portal vein to inferior vena cava
splenic and renal veins
transjugular intrahepatic portosystemic shunt [TIPS]
> EXCLUDES   *peritoneovenous shunt (54.94)*

AHA: 4Q, '94, 50; 4Q, '93, 31; 2Q, '93, 8

DEF: Connection of two venous blood vessels within abdominal cavity.

√4th **39.2**   **Other shunt or vascular bypass**
DEF: Creation of supplemental blood flow to area with inadequate blood supply due to disease or injury of vessels.

39.21   **Caval-pulmonary artery anastomosis**
Code also cardiopulmonary bypass (39.61)

39.22   **Aorta-subclavian-carotid bypass**
Bypass (arterial):
aorta to carotid and brachial
aorta to subclavian and carotid
carotid to subclavian

39.23   **Other intrathoracic vascular shunt or bypass**
Intrathoracic (arterial) bypass graft NOS
> EXCLUDES   *coronary artery bypass (36.10-36.19)*

39.24   **Aorta-renal bypass**

39.25   **Aorta-iliac-femoral bypass**
Bypass:
aortofemoral
aortoiliac
aortoiliac to popliteal
aortopopliteal
iliofemoral [iliac-femoral]

AHA: 4Q, '90, 27; 1Q, '88, 10

39.26   **Other intra-abdominal vascular shunt or bypass**
Bypass:
aortoceliac
aortic-superior mesenteric
common hepatic-common iliac-renal
Intra-abdominal arterial bypass graft NOS
> EXCLUDES   *peritoneovenous shunt (54.94)*

39.27   **Arteriovenostomy for renal dialysis**
Anastomosis for renal dialysis
Formation of (peripheral) arteriovenous fistula for renal [kidney] dialysis
Code also any renal dialysis (39.95)

39.28   **Extracranial-intracranial (EC-IC) vascular bypass**   NC

AHA: 2Q, '92, 7; 4Q, '91, 22

39.29   **Other (peripheral) vascular shunt or bypass**
Bypass (graft):
axillary-brachial
axillary-femoral [axillofemoral] (superficial)
brachial
femoral-femoral
femoroperoneal
femoropopliteal (arteries)
femorotibial (anterior) (posterior)
popliteal
vascular NOS
> EXCLUDES   *peritoneovenous shunt (54.94)*

AHA: ▶1Q, '02, 13;◀ S-O, '85, 13

√4th **39.3**   **Suture of vessel**
Repair of laceration of blood vessel
> EXCLUDES   *any other vascular puncture closure device — omit code*
> *suture of aneurysm (39.52)*
> *that for control of hemorrhage (postoperative):*
> *anus (49.95)*
> *bladder (57.93)*
> *following vascular procedure (39.41)*
> *nose (21.00-21.09)*
> *prostate (60.94)*
> *tonsil (28.7)*

39.30   **Suture of unspecified blood vessel**
39.31   **Suture of artery**
39.32   **Suture of vein**

√4th **39.4**   **Revision of vascular procedure**

39.41   **Control of hemorrhage following vascular surgery**
> EXCLUDES   *that for control of hemorrhage (postoperative):*
> *anus (49.95)*
> *bladder (57.93)*
> *nose (21.00-21.09)*
> *prostate (60.94)*
> *tonsil (28.7)*

Operations on the Cardiovascuolar System 38.95–39.41

39.42 Revision of arteriovenous shunt for renal dialysis

Conversion of renal dialysis:
  end-to-end anastomosis to end-to-side
  end-to-side anastomosis to end-to-end
  vessel-to-vessel cannula to arteriovenous shunt
Removal of old arteriovenous shunt and creation of new shunt

EXCLUDES *replacement of vessel-to-vessel cannula (39.94)*

AHA: 2Q, '94, 15; 4Q, '93, 33

39.43 Removal of arteriovenous shunt for renal dialysis

EXCLUDES *that with replacement [revision] of shunt (39.42)*

39.49 Other revision of vascular procedure

Declotting (graft)
Revision of:
  anastomosis of blood vessel
  vascular procedure (previous)

AHA: 2Q, '98, 17; 1Q, '97, 3; 2Q, '94, 15

DEF: Declotting (graft): Removal of clot from graft.

✓4ᵗʰ 39.5 Other repair of vessels

39.50 Angioplasty or atherectomy of non-coronary vessel

Code also any:
  Insertion of non-coronary stent(s) or stent graft(s) (39.90)
  Injection or infusion of thrombolytic agent (99.10)
Percutaneous transluminal angioplasty (PTA) of non-coronary vessels:
  head and neck arteries:
    basilar
    carotid
    vertebral
  lower extremity vessels
  mesenteric artery
  renal artery
  upper extremity vessels

AHA: 1Q, '02, 13; 2Q, '01, 23; 2Q, '00, 10; 1Q, '00, 12; 2Q, '98, 17; 1Q, '97, 3; 4Q, '96, 63; 4Q, '95, 66

39.51 Clipping of aneurysm

EXCLUDES *clipping of arteriovenous fistula (39.53)*

39.52 Other repair of aneurysm

Repair of aneurysm by:
  coagulation
  electrocoagulation
  filipuncture
  methyl methacrylate
  suture
  wiring
  wrapping

EXCLUDES *endovascular repair of aneurysm (39.71-39.79)*
re-entry operation (aorta) (39.54)
that with:
  graft replacement (38.40-38.49)
  resection (38.30-38.49, 38.60-38.69)

AHA: 1Q, '99, 15, 16, 17; 1Q, '88, 10

DEF: Application of device in abnormally stretched blood vessel to prevent movement of material collected in vessel.

DEF: Repair of aneurysm by: Coagulation: Clotting or solidifying. Electrocoagulation: Electrically produced clotting. Filipuncture: Insertion of wire or thread. Methyl methacrylate: Injection or insertion of plastic material. Suture: Stitching. Wiring: Insertion of wire. Wrapping: Compression.

39.53 Repair of arteriovenous fistula

Embolization of carotid cavernous fistula
Repair of arteriovenous fistula by:
  clipping
  coagulation
  ligation and division

EXCLUDES *repair of:*
  arteriovenous shunt for renal dialysis (39.42)
  ▶*head and neck vessels, endovascular approach (39.72)*◀
  that with:
    graft replacement (38.40-38.49)
    resection (38.30-38.49, 38.60-38.69)

AHA: 1Q, '00, 8

DEF: Correction of arteriovenous fistula by application of clamps, causing coagulation or by tying off and dividing the connection.

39.54 Re-entry operation (aorta)

Fenestration of dissecting aneurysm of thoracic aorta
Code also cardiopulmonary bypass [extracorporeal circulation] [heart-lung machine] (39.61)

DEF: Re-entry operation: Creation of passage between stretched wall of the vessel and major arterial channel to heart.

DEF: Fenestration of dissecting aneurysm of thoracic aorta: Creation of passage between stretched arterial heart vessel and functional part of vessel.

39.55 Reimplantation of aberrant renal vessel

DEF: Reimplant of renal vessel into normal position.

39.56 Repair of blood vessel with tissue patch graft

EXCLUDES *that with resection (38.40-38.49)*

39.57 Repair of blood vessel with synthetic patch graft

EXCLUDES *that with resection (38.40-38.49)*

39.58 Repair of blood vessel with unspecified type of patch graft

EXCLUDES *that with resection (38.40-38.49)*

39.59 Other repair of vessel

Aorticopulmonary window operation
Arterioplasty NOS
Construction of venous valves (peripheral)
Plication of vein (peripheral)
Reimplantation of artery
Code also cardiopulmonary bypass [extracorporeal circulation] [heart-lung machine] (39.61)

EXCLUDES *interruption of the vena cava (38.7)*
reimplantation of renal artery (39.55)
that with:
  graft (39.56-39.58)
  resection (38.30-38.49, 38.60-38.69)

AHA: 4Q, '93, 31; 2Q, '89, 17; N-D, '86, 8; S-O, '85, 5; M-A, '85, 15

DEF: Aorticopulmonary window operation: Repair of abnormal opening between major heart arterial vessel above valves and pulmonary artery.

DEF: Construction of venous valves (peripheral): Reconstruction of valves within peripheral veins.

DEF: Plication of vein (peripheral): Shortening of peripheral vein.

DEF: Reimplantation of artery: Reinsertion of artery into its normal position.

BI Bilateral Edit   NC Non-covered Procedure   ▶◀ Revised Text   ● New Code   ▲ Revised Code Title

√4ᵗʰ **39.6** **Extracorporeal circulation and procedures auxiliary to heart surgery**

AHA: 1Q, '95, 5

39.61 **Extracorporeal circulation auxiliary to open heart surgery**
Artificial heart and lung
Cardiopulmonary bypass
Pump oxygenator

EXCLUDES *extracorporeal hepatic assistance (50.92)*
extracorporeal membrane oxygenation [ECMO] (39.65)
hemodialysis (39.95)
percutaneous cardiopulmonary bypass (39.66)

AHA: 4Q, '97, 55; 3Q, '97, 14; 2Q, '97, 8; 2Q, '90, 24

39.62 **Hypothermia (systemic) incidental to open heart surgery**

39.63 **Cardioplegia**
Arrest:
anoxic
circulatory

DEF: Purposely inducing electromechanical cardiac arrest.

39.64 **Intraoperative cardiac pacemaker**
Temporary pacemaker used during and immediately following cardiac surgery

AHA: 1Q, '89, 2; M-J, '87, 3

39.65 **Extracorporeal membrane oxygenation [ECMO]**

EXCLUDES *extracorporeal circulation auxiliary to open heart surgery (39.61)*
percutaneous cardiopulmonary bypass (39.66)

AHA: 2Q, '90, 23; 2Q, '89, 17; 4Q, '88, 5

DEF: Creation of closed-chest, heart-lung bypass or Bard cardiopulmonary assist system with tube insertion.

39.66 **Percutaneous cardiopulmonary bypass**
Closed chest

EXCLUDES *extracorporeal circulation auxiliary to open heart surgery (39.61)*
extracorporeal hepatic assistance (50.92)
extracorporeal membrane oxygenation [ECMO] (39.65)
hemodialysis (39.95)

AHA: 3Q, '96, 11

DEF: Use of mechanical pump system to oxygenate and pump blood throughout the body via catheter in the femoral artery and vein.

√4ᵗʰ **39.7** **Endovascular repair of vessel**
Endoluminal repair

EXCLUDES *angioplasty or atherectomy of non-coronary vessel (39.50)*
insertion of non-coronary stent or stents (39.90)
other repair of aneurysm (39.52)
resection of abdominal aorta with replacement (38.44)
resection of lower limb arteries with replacement (38.48)
resection of thoracic aorta with replacement (38.45)
resection of upper limb vessels with replacement (38.43)

39.71 **Endovascular implantation of graft in abdominal aorta**
Endovascular repair of abdominal aortic aneurysm with graft
Stent graft(s)

AHA: ▶1Q, '02, 13;◀ 4Q, '00, 63, 64

DEF: Replacement of a section of abdominal aorta with mesh graft; via catheters inserted through femoral arteries.

39.72 **Endovascular repair or occlusion of head and neck vessels**
Coil embolization or occlusion
Endograft(s)
Endovascular graft(s)
Liquid tissue adhesive (glue) embolization or occlusion
Other implant or substance for repair, embolization or occlusion
That for repair of aneurysm, arteriovenous malformation [AVM] or fistula

39.79 **Other endovascular repair of aneurysm of other vessels**
▶Coil embolization or occlusion
Endograft(s)
Endovascular graft(s)
Liquid tissue adhesive (glue) embolization or occlusion
Other implant or substance for repair, embolization or occlusion◀

EXCLUDES ▶ *endovascular repair or occlusion of head and neck vessels (39.72)*
insertion of drug-eluting non-coronary artery stent(s) (00.55)
insertion of non-coronary artery stent(s) (for other than aneurysm repair) (39.90)
non-endovascular repair of arteriovenous fistula (39.53)
other surgical occlusion of vessels–see category 38.8
percutaneous transcatheter infusion (99.29)
transcatheter embolization for gastric or duodenal bleeding (44.44) ◀

AHA: 3Q, '01, 17,18; 4Q, '00, 64

39.8 **Operations on carotid body and other vascular bodies**

Chemodectomy	Glomectomy, carotid
Denervation of:	Implantation into carotid body:
aortic body	electronic stimulator
carotid body	pacemaker

EXCLUDES *excision of glomus jugulare (20.51)*

DEF: Chemodectomy: Removal of a chemoreceptor vascular body.

DEF: Denervation of aortic body: Destruction of nerves attending the major heart blood vessels.

DEF: Destruction of carotid body: Destruction of nerves of carotid artery.

DEF: Glomectomy, carotid: Removal of the carotid artery framework.

Operations on the Cardiovascular System 39.6–39.8

Endovascular Repair of Abdominal Aortic Aneurysm

External Arteriovenous Shunt

√4ᵗʰ 39.9 Other operations on vessels

▲ **39.90 Insertion of non-drug-eluting, non-coronary artery stent(s)**

▶Bare stent(s)
Bonded stent(s)
Drug-coated stent(s), i.e., heparin coated
Endograft(s)
Endovascular graft(s)◀
Endovascular recanalization techniques
Stent graft(s)
Code also any:
    non-coronary angioplasty or atherectomy (39.50)

> **EXCLUDES** ▶ insertion of drug-eluting, non-coronary artery stent(s) (00.55)◀
> that for aneurysm repair (39.71-39.79)

AHA: 1Q, '00, 12; 4Q, '96, 63

39.91 Freeing of vessel

Dissection and freeing of adherent tissue:
    artery-vein-nerve bundle
    vascular bundle

39.92 Injection of sclerosing agent into vein

> **EXCLUDES** injection:
> esophageal varices (42.33)
> hemorrhoids (49.42)

AHA: 2Q, '92, 17

39.93 Insertion of vessel-to-vessel cannula

Formation of:
    arteriovenous:
        fistula   } by external
        shunt   } cannula

Code also any renal dialysis (39.95)

AHA: 3Q, '88, 13; S-O, '85, 5 & 12

39.94 Replacement of vessel-to-vessel cannula

Revision of vessel-to-vessel cannula

39.95 Hemodialysis

Artificial kidney   Hemodiafiltration
Hemofiltration   Renal dialysis

> **EXCLUDES** peritoneal dialysis (54.98)

AHA: 2Q, '01, 2-14; 4Q, '00, 40; 2Q, '98, 20; S-O, '86, 11

DEF: Filtration process to treats acute and chronic renal failure by eliminating toxic end products of nitrogen metabolism from blood.

39.96 Total body perfusion

Code also substance perfused (99.21-99.29)

39.97 Other perfusion

Perfusion NOS   Perfusion, local
Perfusion, local   [regional] of:
    [regional] of: lower limb
    carotid artery   neck
    coronary artery   upper limb
    head
Code also substance perfused (99.21-99.29)

> **EXCLUDES** perfusion of:
> kidney (55.95)
> large intestine (46.96)
> liver (50.93)
> small intestine (46.95)

AHA: 3Q, '96, 11

39.98 Control of hemorrhage, not otherwise specified

Angiotripsy
Control of postoperative hemorrhage NOS
Venotripsy

> **EXCLUDES** control of hemorrhage (postoperative):
> anus (49.95)
> bladder (57.93)
> following vascular procedure (39.41)
> nose (21.00-21.09)
> prostate (60.94)
> tonsil (28.7)
> that by:
> ligation (38.80-38.89)
> suture (39.30-39.32)

DEF: Angiotripsy: Clamping of tissue to stop arterial blood flow.

DEF: Venotripsy: Clamping of tissue to stop venous blood flow.

39.99 Other operations on vessels

> **EXCLUDES** injection or infusion of therapeutic or prophylactic substance (99.11-99.29)
> transfusion of blood and blood components (99.01-99.09)

AHA: 1Q, '89, 11

8. OPERATIONS ON THE HEMIC AND LYMPHATIC SYSTEM
(40-41)

√3rd **40 Operations on lymphatic system**

40.0 Incision of lymphatic structures

√4th **40.1 Diagnostic procedures on lymphatic structures**

40.11 Biopsy of lymphatic structure

40.19 Other diagnostic procedures on lymphatic structures

EXCLUDES   *lymphangiogram:*
abdominal (88.04)
cervical (87.08)
intrathoracic (87.34)
lower limb (88.36)
upper limb (88.34)
microscopic examination of
specimen (90.71-90.79)
radioisotope scan (92.16)
thermography (88.89)

√4th **40.2 Simple excision of lymphatic structure**

EXCLUDES   *biopsy of lymphatic structure (40.11)*

DEF: Removal of lymphatic structure only.

40.21 Excision of deep cervical lymph node

AHA: 4Q, '99, 16

40.22 Excision of internal mammary lymph node

40.23 Excision of axillary lymph node

40.24 Excision of inguinal lymph node

40.29 Simple excision of other lymphatic structure

Excision of:
cystic hygroma
lymphangioma
Simple lymphadenectomy

AHA: 1Q, '99, 6

DEF: Lymphangioma: Removal of benign congenital lymphatic malformation.

DEF: Simple lymphadenectomy: Removal of lymph node.

40.3 Regional lymph node excision

Extended regional lymph node excision
Regional lymph node excision with excision of
lymphatic drainage area including skin,
subcutaneous tissue, and fat

AHA: 2Q, '92, 7

DEF: Extended regional lymph node excision: Removal of lymph node group, including area around nodes.

√4th **40.4 Radical excision of cervical lymph nodes**

Resection of cervical lymph nodes down to muscle
and deep fascia

EXCLUDES   *that associated with radical*
laryngectomy (30.4)

40.40 Radical neck dissection, not otherwise specified

40.41 Radical neck dissection, unilateral

AHA: 2Q, '99, 6

DEF: Dissection, total, of cervical lymph nodes on one side of neck.

40.42 Radical neck dissection, bilateral

DEF: Dissection, total, of cervical lymph nodes on both sides of neck.

√4th **40.5 Radical excision of other lymph nodes**

EXCLUDES   *that associated with radical*
mastectomy (85.45-85.48)

40.50 Radical excision of lymph nodes, not otherwise specified

Radical (lymph) node dissection NOS

40.51 Radical excision of axillary lymph nodes

40.52 Radical excision of periaortic lymph nodes

40.53 Radical excision of iliac lymph nodes

40.54 Radical groin dissection

40.59 Radical excision of other lymph nodes

EXCLUDES   *radical neck dissection (40.40-40.42)*

√4th **40.6 Operations on thoracic duct**

40.61 Cannulation of thoracic duct

DEF: Placement of cannula in main lymphatic duct of chest.

40.62 Fistulization of thoracic duct

DEF: Creation of passage in main lymphatic duct of chest.

40.63 Closure of fistula of thoracic duct

DEF: Closure of fistula in main lymphatic duct of chest.

40.64 Ligation of thoracic duct

DEF: Tying off main lymphatic duct of chest.

40.69 Other operations on thoracic duct

40.9 Other operations on lymphatic structures

Anastomosis
Dilation
Ligation
Obliteration   } of peripheral lymphatics
Reconstruction
Repair
Transplantation

Correction of lymphedema of limb, NOS

EXCLUDES   *reduction of elephantiasis of scrotum*
(61.3)

√3rd **41 Operations on bone marrow and spleen**

√4th **41.0 Bone marrow or hematopoietic stem cell transplant**

EXCLUDES   *aspiration of bone marrow from donor*
(41.91)

AHA: 4Q, '00, 64; 1Q, '91, 3; 4Q, '91, 26

[17] **41.00 Bone marrow transplant, not otherwise specified**   NC

[17] **41.01 Autologous bone marrow transplant without purging**   NC

EXCLUDES   *that with purging (41.09)*

DEF: Transplant of patient's own bone marrow.

[18] **41.02 Allogeneic bone marrow transplant with purging**   NC

Allograft of bone marrow with in vitro
removal (purging) of T-cells

DEF: Transplant of bone marrow from donor to patient after donor marrow purged of undesirable cells.

[18] **41.03 Allogeneic bone marrow transplant without purging**   NC

Allograft of bone marrow NOS

[17] **41.04 Autologous hematopoietic stem cell transplant without purging**   NC

EXCLUDES   *that with purging (41.07)*

AHA: 4Q, '94, 52

[18] **41.05 Allogeneic hematopoietic stem cell transplant without purging**   NC

EXCLUDES   *that with purging (41.08)*

AHA: 4Q, '97, 55

[17] Covered procedure only when any of the following codes are present as either principal or secondary diagnosis: 200.00-202.8, 202.80-202.98, 204.01, 205.01, 206.01, 207.01, 208.01

[18] Covered procedure only when any of the following codes are present as either principal or secondary diagnosis: 204.00-208.91, 279.12, 279.2, 284.0-284.9

√3rd √4th Additional Digit Required   Nonspecific OR Procedure   Valid OR Procedure   Non-OR Procedure

Operations on Hemic and Lymphatic Systems 40-41.05

Partial Splenectomy

Total Splenectomy

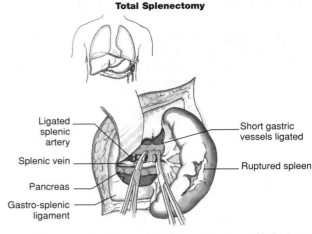

¹⁸ **41.06** **Cord blood stem cell transplant** `NC`
AHA: 4Q, '97, 56

¹⁷ **41.07** **Autologous hematopoietic stem cell transplant with purging** `NC`
Cell depletion

¹⁸ **41.08** **Allogeneic hematopoietic stem cell transplant with purging** `NC`
Cell depletion

¹⁷ **41.09** **Autologous bone marrow transplant with purging** `NC`
With extracorporeal purging of malignant cells from marrow
Cell depletion

41.1 **Puncture of spleen**
> EXCLUDES   aspiration biopsy of spleen (41.32)

41.2 **Splenotomy**

√4ᵗʰ **41.3** **Diagnostic procedures on bone marrow and spleen**

41.31 **Biopsy of bone marrow**

41.32 **Closed [aspiration] [percutaneous] biopsy of spleen**
Needle biopsy of spleen

41.33 **Open biopsy of spleen**

41.38 **Other diagnostic procedures on bone marrow**
> EXCLUDES   microscopic examination of specimen from bone marrow (90.61-90.69)
> radioisotope scan (92.05)

41.39 **Other diagnostic procedures on spleen**
> EXCLUDES   microscopic examination of specimen from spleen (90.61-90.69)
> radioisotope scan (92.05)

√4ᵗʰ **41.4** **Excision or destruction of lesion or tissue of spleen**
▶Code also any application or administration of an adhesion barrier substance (99.77)◀
> EXCLUDES   excision of accessory spleen (41.93)

41.41 **Marsupialization of splenic cyst**
DEF: Incision of cyst of spleen with edges sutured open to create pouch.

41.42 **Excision of lesion or tissue of spleen**
> EXCLUDES   biopsy of spleen (41.32-41.33)

41.43 **Partial splenectomy**
DEF: Removal of spleen, partial.

41.5 **Total splenectomy**
Splenectomy NOS
▶Code also any application or administration of an adhesion barrier substance (99.77)◀

√4ᵗʰ **41.9** **Other operations on spleen and bone marrow**
▶Code also any application or administration of an adhesion barrier substance (99.77)◀

41.91 **Aspiration of bone marrow from donor for transplant**
> EXCLUDES   biopsy of bone marrow (41.31)

AHA: 1Q, '91, 3

41.92 **Injection into bone marrow**
> EXCLUDES   bone marrow transplant (41.00-41.03)

AHA: 3Q, '96, 17

41.93 **Excision of accessory spleen**
41.94 **Transplantation of spleen**
41.95 **Repair and plastic operations on spleen**
41.98 **Other operations on bone marrow**
41.99 **Other operations on spleen**

---

¹⁷ Covered procedure only when any of the following codes are present as either principal or secondary diagnosis: 200.00-202.8, 202.80-202.98, 204.01, 205.01, 206.01, 207.01, 208.01

¹⁸ Covered procedure only when any of the following codes are present as either principal or secondary diagnosis: 204.00-208.91, 279.12, 279.2, 284.0-284.9

`BI` Bilateral Edit   `NC` Non-covered Procedure   ▶◀ Revised Text   ● New Code   ▲ Revised Code Title

9. OPERATIONS ON THE DIGESTIVE SYSTEM (42-54)

√3rd **42   Operations on esophagus**

√4th **42.0   Esophagotomy**

42.01   Incision of esophageal web

DEF: Cutting into congenital esophageal membrane.

42.09   Other incision of esophagus

Esophagotomy NOS

EXCLUDES   *esophagomyotomy (42.7)*
esophagostomy (42.10-42.19)

√4th **42.1   Esophagostomy**

42.10   Esophagostomy, not otherwise specified

42.11   Cervical esophagostomy

DEF: Creation of opening into upper region of esophagus.

42.12   Exteriorization of esophageal pouch

DEF: Transfer of section of esophageal pouch to exterior of the body.

42.19   Other external fistulization of esophagus

Thoracic esophagostomy
Code also any resection (42.40-42.42)

√4th **42.2   Diagnostic procedures on esophagus**

42.21   Operative esophagoscopy by incision

DEF: Esophageal examination with an endoscope through incision.

42.22   Esophagoscopy through artificial stoma

EXCLUDES   *that with biopsy (42.24)*

42.23   Other esophagoscopy

EXCLUDES   *that with biopsy (42.24)*

AHA: 1Q, '00, 20; 3Q, '98, 11

42.24   Closed [endoscopic] biopsy of esophagus

Brushing or washing for specimen collection
Esophagoscopy with biopsy
Suction biopsy of the esophagus

EXCLUDES   *esophagogastroduodenoscopy [EGD] with closed biopsy (45.16)*

DEF: Scope passed through mouth and throat to obtain biopsy specimen, usually by brushing and swabbing.

42.25   Open biopsy of esophagus

42.29   Other diagnostic procedures on esophagus

EXCLUDES   *barium swallow (87.61)*
esophageal manometry (89.32)
microscopic examination of specimen from esophagus (90.81-90.89)

AHA: 3Q, '96, 12

√4th **42.3   Local excision or destruction of lesion or tissue of esophagus**

42.31   Local excision of esophageal diverticulum

42.32   Local excision of other lesion or tissue of esophagus

EXCLUDES   *biopsy of esophagus (42.24-42.25)*
esophageal fistulectomy (42.84)

42.33   Endoscopic excision or destruction of lesion or tissue of esophagus

Ablation of esophageal neoplasm
Control of esophageal bleeding
Esophageal polypectomy
Esophageal varices
Injection of esophageal varices

} by endoscopic approach

EXCLUDES   *biopsy of esophagus (42.24-42.25)*
fistulectomy (42.84)
open ligation of esophageal varices (42.91)

42.39   Other destruction of lesion or tissue of esophagus

EXCLUDES   *that by endoscopic approach (42.33)*

√4th **42.4   Excision of esophagus**

EXCLUDES   *esophagogastrectomy NOS (43.99)*

42.40   Esophagectomy, not otherwise specified

42.41   Partial esophagectomy

Code also any synchronous:
anastomosis other than end-to-end (42.51-42.69)
esophagostomy (42.10-42.19)
gastrostomy (43.11-43.19)

DEF: Surgical removal of any part of esophagus.

42.42   Total esophagectomy

Code also any synchronous:
gastrostomy (43.11-43.19)
interposition or anastomosis other than end-to-end (42.51-42.69)

EXCLUDES   *esophagogastrectomy (43.99)*

AHA: 4Q, '88, 11

DEF: Surgical removal of entire esophagus.

√4th **42.5   Intrathoracic anastomosis of esophagus**

Code also any synchronous:
esophagectomy (42.40-42.42)
gastrostomy (43.1)

DEF: Connection of esophagus to conduit within chest.

42.51   Intrathoracic esophagoesophagostomy

DEF: Connection of both ends of esophagus within chest cavity.

42.52   Intrathoracic esophagogastrostomy

DEF: Connection of esophagus to stomach within chest; follows esophagogastrectomy.

42.53   Intrathoracic esophageal anastomosis with interposition of small bowel

42.54   Other intrathoracic esophagoenterostomy

Anastomosis of esophagus to intestinal segment NOS

42.55   Intrathoracic esophageal anastomosis with interposition of colon

42.56   Other intrathoracic esophagocolostomy

Esophagocolostomy NOS

42.58   Intrathoracic esophageal anastomosis with other interposition

Construction of artificial esophagus
Retrosternal formation of reversed gastric tube

DEF: Construction of artificial esophagus: Creation of artificial esophagus.

DEF: Retrosternal anastomosis of reversed gastric tube: Formation of gastric tube behind breastbone.

Operations on the Digestive System 42–42.58

Operations on the Digestive System 42.59–43.5

42.59   Other intrathoracic anastomosis of esophagus
AHA: 4Q, '88, 11

✓4th **42.6   Antesternal anastomosis of esophagus**
Code also any synchronous:
esophagectomy (42.40-42.42)
gastrostomy (43.1)

42.61   Antesternal esophagoesophagostomy

42.62   Antesternal esophagogastrostomy

42.63   Antesternal esophageal anastomosis with interposition of small bowel

42.64   Other antesternal esophagoenterostomy
Antethoracic:
esophagoenterostomy
esophagoileostomy
esophagojejunostomy

42.65   Antesternal esophageal anastomosis with interposition of colon
DEF: Connection of esophagus with colon segment.

42.66   Other antesternal esophagocolostomy
Antethoracic esophagocolostomy

42.68   Other antesternal esophageal anastomosis with interposition

42.69   Other antesternal anastomosis of esophagus

42.7   Esophagomyotomy
DEF: Division of esophageal muscle, usually distal.

✓4th **42.8   Other repair of esophagus**

42.81   Insertion of permanent tube into esophagus
AHA: 1Q, '97, 15

42.82   Suture of laceration of esophagus

42.83   Closure of esophagostomy

42.84   Repair of esophageal fistula, not elsewhere classified
EXCLUDES   repair of fistula:
bronchoesophageal (33.42)
esophagopleurocutaneous (34.73)
pharyngoesophageal (29.53)
tracheoesophageal (31.73)

42.85   Repair of esophageal stricture

42.86   Production of subcutaneous tunnel without esophageal anastomosis
DEF: Surgical formation of esophageal passage, without cutting, and reconnection.

42.87   Other graft of esophagus
EXCLUDES   antesternal esophageal anastomosis with interposition of:
colon (42.65)
small bowel (42.63)
antesternal esophageal anastomosis with other interposition (42.68)
intrathoracic esophageal anastomosis with interposition of:
colon (42.55)
small bowel (42.53)
intrathoracic esophageal anastomosis with other interposition (42.58)

42.89   Other repair of esophagus

✓4th **42.9   Other operations on esophagus**

42.91   Ligation of esophageal varices
EXCLUDES   that by endoscopic approach (42.33)
DEF: Destruction of dilated veins by suture strangulation.

42.92   Dilation of esophagus
Dilation of cardiac sphincter
EXCLUDES   intubation of esophagus (96.03, 96.06-96.08)
DEF: Passing of balloon or hydrostatic dilators through esophagus to enlarge esophagus and relieve obstruction.

42.99   Other
EXCLUDES   insertion of Sengstaken tube (96.06)
intubation of esophagus (96.03, 96.06-96.08)
removal of intraluminal foreign body from esophagus without incision (98.02)
tamponade of esophagus (96.06)

✓3rd **43   Incision and excision of stomach**
►Code also any application or administration of an adhesion barrier substance (99.77)◄

43.0   Gastrotomy
EXCLUDES   gastrostomy (43.11-43.19)
that for control of hemorrhage (44.49)
AHA: 3Q, '89, 14

✓4th **43.1   Gastrostomy**
AHA: S-O, '85, 5

43.11   Percutaneous [endoscopic] gastrostomy [PEG]
Percutaneous transabdominal gastrostomy
DEF: Endoscopic positioning of tube through abdominal wall into stomach.

43.19   Other gastrostomy
EXCLUDES   percutaneous [endoscopic] gastrostomy [PEG] (43.11)
AHA: 1Q, '92, 14; 3Q, '89, 14

43.3   Pyloromyotomy
DEF: Cutting into longitudinal and circular muscular membrane between stomach and small intestine.

✓4th **43.4   Local excision or destruction of lesion or tissue of stomach**

43.41   Endoscopic excision or destruction of lesion or tissue of stomach
Gastric polypectomy by endoscopic approach
Gastric varices by endoscopic approach
EXCLUDES   biopsy of stomach (44.14-44.15)
control of hemorrhage (44.43)
open ligation of gastric varices (44.91)
AHA: 3Q, '96, 10

43.42   Local excision of other lesion or tissue of stomach
EXCLUDES   biopsy of stomach (44.14-44.15)
gastric fistulectomy (44.62-44.63)
partial gastrectomy (43.5-43.89)

43.49   Other destruction of lesion or tissue of stomach
EXCLUDES   that by endoscopic approach (43.41)
AHA: N-D, '87, 5; S-O, '85, 6

43.5   Partial gastrectomy with anastomosis to esophagus
Proximal gastrectomy

B1 Bilateral Edit   NC Non-covered Procedure   ►◄ Revised Text   ● New Code   ▲ Revised Code Title

Billroth II Operation

Types of Vagotomy Procedures

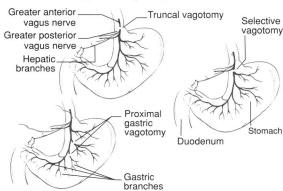

43.6   **Partial gastrectomy with anastomosis to duodenum**
Billroth I operation   Gastropylorectomy
Distal gastrectomy

43.7   **Partial gastrectomy with anastomosis to jejunum**
Billroth II operation

√4th **43.8**   **Other partial gastrectomy**

    43.81   **Partial gastrectomy with jejunal transposition**
Henley jejunal transposition operation
Code also any synchronous intestinal resection (45.51)

    43.89   **Other**
Partial gastrectomy with bypass gastrogastrostomy
Sleeve resection of stomach

√4th **43.9**   **Total gastrectomy**

    43.91   **Total gastrectomy with intestinal interposition**

    43.99   **Other total gastrectomy**
Complete gastroduodenectomy
Esophagoduodenostomy with complete gastrectomy
Esophagogastrectomy NOS
Esophagojejunostomy with complete gastrectomy
Radical gastrectom

√3rd **44**   **Other operations on stomach**
▶Code also any application or administration of an adhesion barrier substance (99.77)◀

√4th **44.0**   **Vagotomy**

    44.00   **Vagotomy, not otherwise specified**
Division of vagus nerve NOS
DEF: Cutting of vagus nerve to reduce acid production.

    44.01   **Truncal vagotomy**
DEF: Surgical removal of vagus nerve segment near stomach branches.

Partial Gastrectomy with Anastomosis to Duodenum

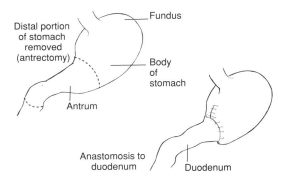

44.02   **Highly selective vagotomy**
Parietal cell vagotomy
Selective proximal vagotomy
DEF: Cutting select gastric branches of vagus nerve to reduce acid production and preserve other nerve functions.

44.03   **Other selective vagotomy**

√4th **44.1**   **Diagnostic procedures on stomach**

    44.11   **Transabdominal gastroscopy**
Intraoperative gastroscopy
EXCLUDES   that with biopsy (44.14)

    44.12   **Gastroscopy through artificial stoma**
EXCLUDES   that with biopsy (44.14)

    44.13   **Other gastroscopy**
EXCLUDES   that with biopsy (44.14)
AHA: 1Q, '88, 15; N-D, '87, 5

    44.14   **Closed [endoscopic] biopsy of stomach**
Brushing or washing for specimen collection
EXCLUDES   esophagogastroduodenoscopy [EGD] with closed biopsy (45.16)
AHA: 1Q, '88, 15; N-D, '87, 5

    44.15   **Open biopsy of stomach**

    44.19   **Other diagnostic procedures on stomach**
EXCLUDES   gastric lavage (96.33)
microscopic examination of specimen from stomach (90.81-90.89)
upper GI series (87.62)

√4th **44.2**   **Pyloroplasty**

    44.21   **Dilation of pylorus by incision**
DEF: Cutting and suturing pylorus to relieve obstruction.

    44.22   **Endoscopic dilation of pylorus**
Dilation with balloon endoscope
Endoscopic dilation of gastrojejunostomy site
AHA: 2Q, '01, 17

    44.29   **Other pyloroplasty**
Pyloroplasty NOS
Revision of pylorus
AHA: 3Q, '99, 3

√4th **44.3**   **Gastroenterostomy without gastrectomy**

    44.31   **High gastric bypass**
Printen and Mason gastric bypass
AHA: M-J, '85, 17
DEF: Connection of middle part of small intestine to upper stomach to divert food passage from upper intestine.

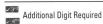 Additional Digit Required   Nonspecific OR Procedure   Valid OR Procedure   Non-OR Procedure

Operations on the Digestive System 44.32–45.12

44.32　Percutaneous [endoscopic] gastrojejunostomy
　　▶Endoscopic conversion of gastrostomy to jejunostomy◀

DEF: Percutaneous placement of a thin feeding tube through a gastrostomy tube and then pulling the tube into the proximal end of the jejunum.

44.39　Other gastroenterostomy
　　Bypass:
　　　gastroduodenostomy
　　　gastroenterostomy
　　　gastrogastrostomy
　　Gastrojejunostomy without gastrectomy NOS

AHA: 1Q, '01, 16, 17

✓4th **44.4　Control of hemorrhage and suture of ulcer of stomach or duodenum**

44.40　Suture of peptic ulcer, not otherwise specified

44.41　Suture of gastric ulcer site
　　EXCLUDES　ligation of gastric varices (44.91)

44.42　Suture of duodenal ulcer site
　　AHA: J-F, '87, 11

44.43　Endoscopic control of gastric or duodenal bleeding
　　AHA: 2Q, '92, 17; N-D, '87, 4

44.44　Transcatheter embolization for gastric or duodenal bleeding
　　EXCLUDES　surgical occlusion of abdominal vessels (38.86-38.87)

AHA: 1Q, '88, 15; N-D, '87, 4

DEF: Therapeutic blocking of stomach or upper small intestine blood vessel to stop hemorrhaging; accomplished by introducing various substances using a catheter.

44.49　Other control of hemorrhage of stomach or duodenum
　　That with gastrotomy

44.5　Revision of gastric anastomosis
　　Closure of:　　　　　　Closure of:
　　　gastric anastomosis　　gastrojejunostomy
　　　gastroduodenostomy　　Pantaloon operation

✓4th **44.6　Other repair of stomach**

44.61　Suture of laceration of stomach
　　EXCLUDES　that of ulcer site (44.41)

44.62　Closure of gastrostomy

44.63　Closure of other gastric fistula
　　Closure of:
　　　gastrocolic fistula
　　　gastrojejunocolic fistula

44.64　Gastropexy
　　AHA: M-J, '85, 17

DEF: Suturing of stomach into position.

44.65　Esophagogastroplasty
　　Belsey operation
　　Esophagus and stomach cardioplasty
　　AHA: M-J, '85, 17

44.66　Other procedures for creation of esophagogastric sphincteric competence
　　Fundoplication
　　Gastric cardioplasty
　　Nissen's fundoplication
　　Restoration of cardio-esophageal angle
　　AHA: 2Q, '01, 3, 5, 6; 3Q, '98, 10; M-J, '85, 17

44.69　Other
　　Inversion of gastric diverticulum
　　Repair of stomach NOS
　　AHA: 2Q, '01, 3; 3Q, '99, 3; M-J, '85, 17; N-D, '84, 13

DEF: Inversion of gastric diverticulum: Turning stomach inward to repair outpouch of wall.

✓4th **44.9　Other operations on stomach**

44.91　Ligation of gastric varices
　　EXCLUDES　that by endoscopic approach (43.41)

DEF: Destruction of dilated veins by suture or strangulation.

44.92　Intraoperative manipulation of stomach
　　Reduction of gastric volvulus

44.93　Insertion of gastric bubble (balloon)　NC

44.94　Removal of gastric bubble (balloon)

44.99　Other
　　EXCLUDES　change of gastrostomy tube (97.02)
　　　　　　　dilation of cardiac sphincter (42.92)
　　　　　　　gastric:
　　　　　　　　cooling (96.31)
　　　　　　　　freezing (96.32)
　　　　　　　　gavage (96.35)
　　　　　　　　hypothermia (96.31)
　　　　　　　　lavage (96.33)
　　　　　　　insertion of nasogastric tube (96.07)
　　　　　　　irrigation of gastrostomy (96.36)
　　　　　　　irrigation of nasogastric tube (96.34)
　　　　　　　removal of:
　　　　　　　　gastrostomy tube (97.51)
　　　　　　　　intraluminal foreign body from stomach without incision (98.03)
　　　　　　　replacement of:
　　　　　　　　gastrostomy tube (97.02)
　　　　　　　　(naso-)gastric tube (97.01)

✓3rd **45　Incision, excision, and anastomosis of intestine**
　　▶Code also any application or administration of an adhesion barrier substance (99.77)◀

✓4th **45.0　Enterotomy**
　　EXCLUDES　duodenocholedochotomy (51.41-51.42, 51.51)
　　　　　　　that for destruction of lesion (45.30-45.34)
　　　　　　　that of exteriorized intestine (46.14, 46.24, 46.31)

45.00　Incision of intestine not otherwise specified

45.01　Incision of duodenum

45.02　Other incision of small intestine

45.03　Incision of large intestine
　　EXCLUDES　proctotomy (48.0)

✓4th **45.1　Diagnostic procedures on small intestine**
　　Code also any laparotomy (54.11-54.19)

45.11　Transabdominal endoscopy of small intestine
　　Intraoperative endoscopy of small intestine
　　EXCLUDES　that with biopsy (45.14)

DEF: Endoscopic exam of small intestine through abdominal wall.

DEF: Intraoperative endoscope of small intestine: Endoscopic exam of small intestine during surgery.

45.12　Endoscopy of small intestine through artificial stoma
　　EXCLUDES　that with biopsy (45.14)

AHA: M-J, '85, 17

BI　Bilateral Edit　　　NC　Non-covered Procedure　　　▶◀ Revised Text　　　● New Code　　　▲ Revised Code Title

45.13 Other endoscopy of small intestine
Esophagogastroduodenoscopy [EGD]
> **EXCLUDES** that with biopsy (45.14, 45.16)

AHA: N-D, '87, 5

45.14 Closed [endoscopic] biopsy of small intestine
Brushing or washing for specimen collection
> **EXCLUDES** esophagogastroduodenoscopy [EGD] with closed biopsy (45.16)

45.15 Open biopsy of small intestine

45.16 Esophagogastroduodenoscopy [EGD] with closed biopsy
Biopsy of one or more sites involving esophagus, stomach, and/or duodenum

AHA: 2Q, '01, 9

45.19 Other diagnostic procedures on small intestine
> **EXCLUDES** microscopic examination of specimen from small intestine (90.91-90.99)
> radioisotope scan (92.04)
> ultrasonography (88.74)
> x-ray (87.61-87.69)

✓4ᵗʰ 45.2 Diagnostic procedures on large intestine
Code also any laparotomy (54.11-54.19)

45.21 Transabdominal endoscopy of large intestine
Intraoperative endoscopy of large intestine
> **EXCLUDES** that with biopsy (45.25)

DEF: Endoscopic exam of large intestine through abdominal wall.

DEF: Intraoperative endoscopy of large intestine: Endoscopic exam of large intestine during surgery.

45.22 Endoscopy of large intestine through artificial stoma
> **EXCLUDES** that with biopsy (45.25)

DEF: Endoscopic exam of large intestine lining from rectum to cecum via colostomy stoma.

45.23 Colonoscopy
Flexible fiberoptic colonoscopy
> **EXCLUDES** endoscopy of large intestine through artificial stoma (45.22)
> flexible sigmoidoscopy (45.24)
> rigid proctosigmoidoscopy (48.23)
> transabdominal endoscopy of large intestine (45.21)

AHA: S-O, '85, 5

DEF: Endoscopic exam of descending colon, splenic flexure, transverse colon, hepatic flexure and cecum.

Esophagogastroduodenoscopy

45.24 Flexible sigmoidoscopy
Endoscopy of descending colon
> **EXCLUDES** rigid proctosigmoidoscopy (48.23)

DEF: Endoscopic exam of anus, rectum and sigmoid colon.

45.25 Closed [endoscopic] biopsy of large intestine
Biopsy, closed, of unspecified intestinal site
Brushing or washing for specimen collection
Colonoscopy with biopsy
> **EXCLUDES** proctosigmoidoscopy with biopsy (48.24)

45.26 Open biopsy of large intestine

45.27 Intestinal biopsy, site unspecified

45.28 Other diagnostic procedures on large intestine

45.29 Other diagnostic procedures on intestine, site unspecified
> **EXCLUDES** microscopic examination of specimen (90.91-90.99)
> scan and radioisotope function study (92.04)
> ultrasonography (88.74)
> x-ray (87.61-87.69)

✓4ᵗʰ 45.3 Local excision or destruction of lesion or tissue of small intestine

45.30 Endoscopic excision or destruction of lesion of duodenum
> **EXCLUDES** biopsy of duodenum (45.14-45.15)
> control of hemorrhage (44.43)
> fistulectomy (46.72)

45.31 Other local excision of lesion of duodenum
> **EXCLUDES** biopsy of duodenum (45.14-45.15)
> fistulectomy (46.72)
> multiple segmental resection (45.61)
> that by endoscopic approach (45.30)

45.32 Other destruction of lesion of duodenum
> **EXCLUDES** that by endoscopic approach (45.30)

AHA: N-D, '87, 5; S-O, '85, 6

45.33 Local excision of lesion or tissue of small intestine, except duodenum
Excision of redundant mucosa of ileostomy
> **EXCLUDES** biopsy of small intestine (45.14-45.15)
> fistulectomy (46.74)
> multiple segmental resection (45.61)

45.34 Other destruction of lesion of small intestine, except duodenum

✓4ᵗʰ 45.4 Local excision or destruction of lesion or tissue of large intestine
AHA: N-D, '87, 11

45.41 Excision of lesion or tissue of large intestine
Excision of redundant mucosa of colostomy
> **EXCLUDES** biopsy of large intestine (45.25-45.27)
> endoscopic polypectomy of large intestine (45.42)
> fistulectomy (46.76)
> multiple segmental resection (45.71)
> that by endoscopic approach (45.42-45.43)

45.42 Endoscopic polypectomy of large intestine
> **EXCLUDES** that by open approach (45.41)

AHA: 2Q, '90, 25

DEF: Endoscopic removal of polyp from large intestine.

Operations on the Digestive System 45.43–45.95

45.43 Endoscopic destruction of other lesion or tissue of large intestine
Endoscopic ablation of tumor of large intestine
Endoscopic control of colonic bleeding
> **EXCLUDES** *endoscopic polypectomy of large intestine (45.42)*

45.49 Other destruction of lesion of large intestine
> **EXCLUDES** *that by endoscopic approach (45.43)*

√4th 45.5 Isolation of intestinal segment
Code also any synchronous:
anastomosis other than end-to-end (45.90-45.94)
enterostomy (46.10-46.39)

45.50 Isolation of intestinal segment, not otherwise specified
Isolation of intestinal pedicle flap
Reversal of intestinal segment
DEF: Isolation of small intestinal pedicle flap: Separation of intestinal pedicle flap.
DEF: Reversal of intestinal segment: Separation of intestinal segment.

45.51 Isolation of segment of small intestine
Isolation of ileal loop
Resection of small intestine for interposition
AHA: 3Q, '00, 7

45.52 Isolation of segment of large intestine
Resection of colon for interposition

√4th 45.6 Other excision of small intestine
Code also any synchronous:
anastomosis other than end-to-end (45.90-45.93, 45.95)
colostomy (46.10-46.13)
enterostomy (46.10-46.39)
> **EXCLUDES** *cecectomy (45.72)*
> *enterocolectomy (45.79)*
> *gastroduodenectomy (43.6-43.99)*
> *ileocolectomy (45.73)*
> *pancreatoduodenectomy (52.51-52.7)*

45.61 Multiple segmental resection of small intestine
Segmental resection for multiple traumatic lesions of small intestine

45.62 Other partial resection of small intestine
Duodenectomy   Jejunectomy
Ileectomy
> **EXCLUDES** *duodenectomy with synchronous pancreatectomy (52.51-52.7)*
> *resection of cecum and terminal ileum (45.72)*

45.63 Total removal of small intestine

Colectomy

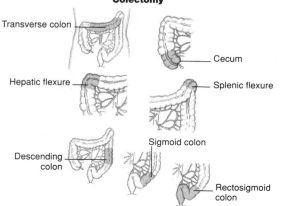

Transverse colon
Hepatic flexure
Descending colon
Cecum
Splenic flexure
Sigmoid colon
Rectosigmoid colon

Intestinal Anastomosis

Area to be excised

End-to-end anastomosis

√4th 45.7 Partial excision of large intestine
Code also any synchronous:
anastomosis other than end-to-end (45.92-45.94)
enterostomy (46.10-46.39)
AHA: 4Q, '92, 27

45.71 Multiple segmental resection of large intestine
Segmental resection for multiple traumatic lesions of large intestine

45.72 Cecectomy
Resection of cecum and terminal ileum

45.73 Right hemicolectomy
Ileocolectomy
Right radical colectomy
AHA: 3Q, '99, 10

45.74 Resection of transverse colon

45.75 Left hemicolectomy
> **EXCLUDES** *proctosigmoidectomy (48.41-48.69)*
> *second stage Mikulicz operation (46.04)*

DEF: Excision of left descending large intestine.

45.76 Sigmoidectomy
AHA: 1Q, '96, 9; 3Q, '89, 15

45.79 Other partial excision of large intestine
Enterocolectomy NEC
AHA: 3Q, '97, 9; 2Q, '91, 16

45.8 Total intra-abdominal colectomy
Excision of cecum, colon, and sigmoid
> **EXCLUDES** *coloproctectomy (48.41-48.69)*

√4th 45.9 Intestinal anastomosis
Code also any synchronous resection (45.31-45.8, 48.41-48.69)
> **EXCLUDES** *end-to-end anastomosis — omit code*

45.90 Intestinal anastomosis, not otherwise specified

45.91 Small-to-small intestinal anastomosis
AHA: M-J, '85, 17

45.92 Anastomosis of small intestine to rectal stump
Hampton procedure

45.93 Other small-to-large intestinal anastomosis
AHA: N-D, '86, 11

45.94 Large-to-large intestinal anastomosis
> **EXCLUDES** *rectorectostomy (48.74)*

AHA: 3Q, '89, 15

45.95 Anastomosis to anus
Formation of endorectal ileal pouch (J-pouch) (H-pouch) (S-pouch) with anastomosis of small intestine to anus

√3rd **46　Other operations on intestine**
▶Code also any application or administration of an adhesion barrier substance (99.77)◀

√4th **46.0　Exteriorization of intestine**
INCLUDES　loop enterostomy
multiple stage resection of intestine
DEF: Bringing intestinal segment to body surface.

46.01　Exteriorization of small intestine
Loop ileostomy

46.02　Resection of exteriorized segment of small intestine

46.03　Exteriorization of large intestine
Exteriorization of intestine NOS
First stage Mikulicz exteriorization of intestine
Loop colostomy

46.04　Resection of exteriorized segment of large intestine
Resection of exteriorized segment of intestine NOS
Second stage Mikulicz operation

√4th **46.1　Colostomy**
Code also any synchronous resection (45.49, 45.71-45.79, 45.8)
EXCLUDES　loop colostomy (46.03)
that with abdominoperineal resection of rectum (48.5)
that with synchronous anterior rectal resection (48.62)
DEF: Creation of opening from large intestine through abdominal wall to body surface.

46.10　Colostomy, not otherwise specified
46.11　Temporary colostomy
46.13　Permanent colostomy
46.14　Delayed opening of colostomy

√4th **46.2　Ileostomy**
Code also any synchronous resection (45.34, 45.61-45.63)
EXCLUDES　loop ileostomy (46.01)
DEF: Creation of artificial anus by bringing ileum through abdominal wall to body surface.

46.20　Ileostomy, not otherwise specified
46.21　Temporary ileostomy
46.22　Continent ileostomy
AHA: M-J, '85, 17

DEF: Creation of opening from third part of small intestine through abdominal wall, with pouch outside abdomen.

46.23　Other permanent ileostomy
46.24　Delayed opening of ileostomy

√4th **46.3　Other enterostomy**
Code also any synchronous resection (45.61-45.8)

46.31　Delayed opening of other enterostomy
46.32　Percutaneous (endoscopic) jejunostomy [PEJ]
DEF: Endoscopic placement of tube in midsection of small intestine through abdominal wall.

46.39　Other
Duodenostomy　Feeding enterostomy
AHA: 3Q, '89, 15

√4th **46.4　Revision of intestinal stoma**
DEF: Revision of opening surgically created from intestine through abdominal wall, to skin surface.

46.40　Revision of intestinal stoma, not otherwise specified
Plastic enlargement of intestinal stoma
Reconstruction of stoma of intestine
Release of scar tissue of intestinal stoma
EXCLUDES　excision of redundant mucosa (45.41)

46.41　Revision of stoma of small intestine
EXCLUDES　excision of redundant mucosa (45.33)
46.42　Repair of pericolostomy hernia
46.43　Other revision of stoma of large intestine
EXCLUDES　excision of redundant mucosa (45.41)

√4th **46.5　Closure of intestinal stoma**
Code also any synchronous resection (45.34, 45.49, 45.61-45.8)

46.50　Closure of intestinal stoma, not otherwise specified
46.51　Closure of stoma of small intestine
46.52　Closure of stoma of large intestine
Closure or take-down of cecostomy
Closure or take-down of colostomy
Closure or take-down of sigmoidostomy
AHA: 3Q, '97, 9; 2Q, '91, 16; N-D, '87, 8

√4th **46.6　Fixation of intestine**
46.60　Fixation of intestine not otherwise specified
Fixation of intestine to abdominal wall

46.61　Fixation of small intestine to abdominal wall
Ileopexy

46.62　Other fixation of small intestine
Noble plication of small intestine
Plication of jejunum
DEF: Noble plication of small intestine: Fixing small intestine into place with tuck in small intestine.

DEF: Plication of jejunum: Fixing small intestine into place with tuck in midsection.

46.63　Fixation of large intestine to abdominal wall
Cecocoloplicopexy
Sigmoidopexy　(Moschowitz)

46.64　Other fixation of large intestine
Cecofixation　Colofixation

√4th **46.7　Other repair of intestine**
EXCLUDES　closure of:
ulcer of duodenum (44.42)
vesicoenteric fistula (57.83)

46.71　Suture of laceration of duodenum
46.72　Closure of fistula of duodenum
46.73　Suture of laceration of small intestine, except duodenum
46.74　Closure of fistula of small intestine, except duodenum
EXCLUDES　closure of:
artificial stoma (46.51)
vaginal fistula (70.74)
repair of gastrojejunocolic fistula (44.63)

46.75　Suture of laceration of large intestine
46.76　Closure of fistula of large intestine
EXCLUDES　closure of:
gastrocolic fistula (44.63)
rectal fistula (48.73)
sigmoidovesical fistula (57.83)
stoma (46.52)
vaginal fistula (70.72-70.73)
vesicocolic fistula (57.83)
vesicosigmoidovaginal fistula (57.83)
AHA: 3Q, '99, 8

46.79　Other repair of intestine
▶Duodenoplasty◀

√3rd
√4th Additional Digit Required　　　Nonspecific OR Procedure　　　Valid OR Procedure　　　Non-OR Procedure

√4th **46.8   Dilation and manipulation of intestine**

46.80   Intra-abdominal manipulation of intestine, not otherwise specifie

Correction of intestinal malrotation
Reduction of:
    intestinal torsion
    intestinal volvulus
    intussusception

EXCLUDES   *reduction of intussusception with:*
    fluoroscopy (96.29)
    ionizing radiation enema (96.29)
    ultrasonography guidance (96.29)

AHA: 4Q, '98, 82

DEF: Correction of intestinal malrotation: Repair of abnormal rotation.

DEF: Reduction of:
    Intestinal torsion: Repair of twisted segment.
    Intestinal volvulus: Repair of a knotted segment.
    Intussusception: Repair of prolapsed segment.

46.81   Intra-abdominal manipulation of small intestine

46.82   Intra-abdominal manipulation of large intestine

46.85   Dilation of intestine

Dilation (balloon) of duodenum
Dilation (balloon) of jejunum
Endoscopic dilation (balloon) of large intestine
That through rectum or colostomy

AHA: 3Q, '89, 15

√4th **46.9   Other operations on intestines**

46.91   Myotomy of sigmoid colon

46.92   Myotomy of other parts of colon

46.93   Revision of anastomosis of small intestine

46.94   Revision of anastomosis of large intestine

46.95   Local perfusion of small intestine

Code also substance perfused (99.21-99.29)

46.96   Local perfusion of large intestine

Code also substance perfused (99.21-99.29)

46.97   Transplant of intestine   NC

AHA: 4Q, '00, 66

46.99   Other

Ileoentectropy

EXCLUDES   *diagnostic procedures on intestine (45.11-45.29)*
dilation of enterostomy stoma (96.24)
intestinal intubation (96.08)
removal of:
    intraluminal foreign body from large intestine without incision (98.04)
    intraluminal foreign body from small intestine without incision (98.03)
    tube from large intestine (97.53)
    tube from small intestine (97.52)
replacement of:
    large intestine tube or enterostomy device (97.04)
    small intestine tube or enterostomy device (97.03)

AHA: 3Q, '99, 11; 1Q, '89, 11

√3rd **47   Operations on appendix**

►Code also any application or administration of an adhesion barrier substance (99.77)◄

INCLUDES   appendiceal stump

√4th **47.0   Appendectomy**

EXCLUDES   *incidental appendectomy, so described (47.11, 47.19)*

AHA: 4Q, '96, 64; 3Q, '92, 12

47.01   Laparoscopic appendectomy

AHA: 1Q, '01, 15; 4Q, '96, 64

47.09   Other appendectomy

AHA: 4Q, '97, 52

√4th **47.1   Incidental appendectomy**

DEF: Removal of appendix during abdominal surgery as prophylactic measure, without significant appendiceal pathology.

47.11   Laparoscopic incidental appendectomy

47.19   Other incidental appendectomy

AHA: 4Q, '96, 65

47.2   Drainage of appendiceal abscess

EXCLUDES   *that with appendectomy (47.0)*

√4th **47.9   Other operations on appendix**

47.91   Appendicostomy

47.92   Closure of appendiceal fistula

47.99   Other

Anastomosis of appendix

EXCLUDES   *diagnostic procedures on appendix (45.21-45.29)*

AHA: 3Q, '01, 16

√3rd **48   Operations on rectum, rectosigmoid, and perirectal tissue**

►Code also any application or administration of an adhesion barrier substance (99.77)◄

48.0   Proctotomy

Decompression of imperforate anus
Panas' operation [linear proctotomy]

EXCLUDES   *incision of perirectal tissue (48.81)*

AHA: 3Q, '99, 8

DEF: Incision into rectal portion of large intestine.

DEF: Decompression of imperforate anus: opening a closed anus by means of an incision.

DEF: Panas' operation (linear proctotomy): Linear incision into rectal portion of large intestine

48.1   Proctostomy

√4th **48.2   Diagnostic procedures on rectum, rectosigmoid, and perirectal tissue**

48.21   Transabdominal proctosigmoidoscopy

Intraoperative proctosigmoidoscopy

EXCLUDES   *that with biopsy (48.24)*

48.22   Proctosigmoidoscopy through artificial stoma

EXCLUDES   *that with biopsy (48.24)*

48.23   Rigid proctosigmoidoscopy

EXCLUDES   *flexible sigmoidoscopy (45.24)*

AHA: 1Q, '01, 8

DEF: Endoscopic exam of anus, rectum and lower sigmoid colon.

48.24   Closed [endoscopic] biopsy of rectum

Brushing or washing for specimen collection
Proctosigmoidoscopy with biopsy

48.25   Open biopsy of rectum

48.26   Biopsy of perirectal tissue

48.29 **Other diagnostic procedures on rectum, rectosigmoid, and perirectal tissue**

> EXCLUDES   digital examination of rectum (89.34)
> lower GI series (87.64)
> microscopic examination of specimen from rectum (90.91-90.99)

✓4ᵗʰ **48.3** **Local excision or destruction of lesion or tissue of rectum**

48.31 **Radical electrocoagulation of rectal lesion or tissue**

> DEF: Destruction of lesion or tissue of large intestine, rectal part.

48.32 **Other electrocoagulation of rectal lesion or tissue**

> AHA: 2Q, '98, 18

48.33 **Destruction of rectal lesion or tissue by laser**

48.34 **Destruction of rectal lesion or tissue by cryosurgery**

48.35 **Local excision of rectal lesion or tissue**

> EXCLUDES   biopsy of rectum (48.24-48.25)
> [endoscopic] polypectomy of rectum (48.36)
> excision of perirectal tissue (48.82)
> hemorrhoidectomy (49.46)
> rectal fistulectomy (48.73)

48.36 **[Endoscopic] polypectomy of rectum**

> AHA: 4Q, '95, 65

✓4ᵗʰ **48.4** **Pull-through resection of rectum**

> Code also any synchronous anastomosis other than end-to-end (45.90, 45.92-45.95)

48.41 **Soave submucosal resection of rectum**

> Endorectal pull-through operation
>
> DEF: Soave submucosal resection: Resection of submucosal rectal part of large intestine by pull-through technique.
>
> DEF: Endorectal pull-through operation: Resection of interior large intestine by pull through technique.

48.49 **Other pull-through resection of rectum**

> Abdominoperineal pull-through
> Altemeier operation
> Swenson proctectomy
> EXCLUDES   Duhamel abdominoperineal pull-through (48.65)
>
> AHA: ▶3Q, '01, 8;◀ 2Q, '99, 13
>
> DEF: Abdominoperineal pull-through: Resection of large intestine, latter part, by pull-through of abdomen, scrotum or vulva and anus.
>
> DEF: Swenson proctectomy: Excision of large intestine, rectal by pull-through and preserving muscles that close the anus.

48.5 **Abdominoperineal resection of rectum**

> Combined abdominoendorectal resection
> Complete proctectomy
> Code also any synchronous anastomosis other than end-to-end (45.90, 45.92-45.95)
> INCLUDES   with synchronous colostomy
> EXCLUDES   Duhamel abdominoperineal pull-through (48.65)
> that as part of pelvic exenteration (68.8)
>
> AHA: 2Q, '97, 5
>
> DEF: Rectal excision through cavities formed by abdomen, anus, vulva or scrotum.

✓4ᵗʰ **48.6** **Other resection of rectum**

> Code also any synchronous anastomosis other than end-to-end (45.90, 45.92-45.95)

48.61 **Transsacral rectosigmoidectomy**

> DEF: Excision through sacral bone area of sigmoid and last parts of large intestine.

48.62 **Anterior resection of rectum with synchronous colostomy**

> DEF: Resection of front terminal end of large intestine and creation of colostomy.

48.63 **Other anterior resection of rectum**

> EXCLUDES   that with synchronous colostomy (48.62)
>
> AHA: 1Q, '96, 9

48.64 **Posterior resection of rectum**

48.65 **Duhamel resection of rectum**

> Duhamel abdominoperineal pull-through

48.69 **Other**

> Partial proctectomy
> Rectal resection NOS
>
> AHA: J-F, '87, 11; N-D, '86, 11

✓4ᵗʰ **48.7** **Repair of rectum**

> EXCLUDES   repair of:
> current obstetric laceration (75.62)
> vaginal rectocele (70.50, 70.52)

48.71 **Suture of laceration of rectum**

48.72 **Closure of proctostomy**

48.73 **Closure of other rectal fistula**

> EXCLUDES   fistulectomy:
> perirectal (48.93)
> rectourethral (58.43)
> rectovaginal (70.73)
> rectovesical (57.83)
> rectovesicovaginal (57.83)

48.74 **Rectorectostomy**

> Rectal anastomosis NOS
>
> DEF: Connection of two cut portions of large intestine, rectal end.

48.75 **Abdominal proctopexy**

> Frickman procedure
> Ripstein repair of rectal prolapse
>
> DEF: Fixation of rectum to adjacent abdominal structures.

48.76 **Other proctopexy**

> Delorme repair of prolapsed rectum
> Proctosigmoidopexy
> Puborectalis sling operation
> EXCLUDES   manual reduction of rectal prolapse (96.26)
>
> DEF: Delorme repair of prolapsed rectum: Fixation of collapsed large intestine, rectal part.
>
> DEF: Proctosigmoidopexy: Suturing of twisted large intestine, rectal part.
>
> DEF: Puborectalis sling operation: Fixation of large intestine, rectal part by forming puborectalis muscle into sling.

48.79 **Other repair of rectum**

> Repair of old obstetric laceration of rectum
> EXCLUDES   anastomosis to:
> large intestine (45.94)
> small intestine (45.92-45.93)
> repair of:
> current obstetrical laceration (75.62)
> vaginal rectocele (70.50, 70.52)

✓4ᵗʰ **48.8** **Incision or excision of perirectal tissue or lesion**

> INCLUDES   pelvirectal tissue
> rectovaginal septum

48.81 **Incision of perirectal tissue**

> Incision of rectovaginal septum

Operations on the Digestive System 48.82–49.93

48.82 Excision of perirectal tissue
> EXCLUDES   perirectal biopsy (48.26)
> perirectofistulectomy (48.93)
> rectal fistulectomy (48.73)

✓4th **48.9 Other operations on rectum and perirectal tissue**

48.91 Incision of rectal stricture

48.92 Anorectal myectomy
DEF: Excision of anorectal muscle.

48.93 Repair of perirectal fistula
> EXCLUDES   that opening into rectum
> (48.73)

DEF: Closure of abdominal passage in tissue around large intestine, rectal part.

48.99 Other
> EXCLUDES   digital examination of rectum
> (89.34)
> dilation of rectum (96.22)
> insertion of rectal tube (96.09)
> irrigation of rectum (96.38-
> 96.39)
> manual reduction of rectal
> prolapse (96.26)
> proctoclysis (96.37)
> rectal massage (99.93)
> rectal packing (96.19)
> removal of:
> impacted feces (96.38)
> intraluminal foreign body
> from rectum without
> incision (98.05)
> rectal packing (97.59)
> transanal enema (96.39)

✓3rd **49 Operations on anus**
► Code also any application or administration of an adhesion barrier substance (99.77) ◄

✓4th **49.0 Incision or excision of perianal tissue**

49.01 Incision of perianal abscess

49.02 Other incision of perianal tissue
Undercutting of perianal tissue
> EXCLUDES   anal fistulotomy (49.11)

49.03 Excision of perianal skin tags

49.04 Other excision of perianal tissue
> EXCLUDES   anal fistulectomy (49.12)
> biopsy of perianal tissue
> (49.22)

AHA: 1Q, '01, 8

✓4th **49.1 Incision or excision of anal fistula**
> EXCLUDES   closure of anal fistula (49.73)

49.11 Anal fistulotomy

49.12 Anal fistulectomy

✓4th **49.2 Diagnostic procedures on anus and perianal tissue**

49.21 Anoscopy

49.22 Biopsy of perianal tissue

49.23 Biopsy of anus

49.29 Other diagnostic procedures on anus and perianal tissue
> EXCLUDES   microscopic examination of
> specimen from anus
> (90.91-90.99)

✓4th **49.3 Local excision or destruction of other lesion or tissue of anus**
Anal cryptotomy
Cauterization of lesion of anus
> EXCLUDES   biopsy of anus (49.23)
> control of (postoperative) hemorrhage of
> anus (49.95)
> hemorrhoidectomy (49.46)

49.31 Endoscopic excision or destruction of lesion or tissue of anus

49.39 Other local excision or destruction of lesion or tissue of anus
> EXCLUDES   that by endoscopic approach
> (49.31)

AHA: 1Q, '01, 8

✓4th **49.4 Procedures on hemorrhoids**

49.41 Reduction of hemorrhoids
DEF: Manual manipulation to reduce hemorrhoids.

49.42 Injection of hemorrhoids

49.43 Cauterization of hemorrhoids
Clamp and cautery of hemorrhoids

49.44 Destruction of hemorrhoids by cryotherapy

49.45 Ligation of hemorrhoids

49.46 Excision of hemorrhoids
Hemorrhoidectomy NOS

49.47 Evacuation of thrombosed hemorrhoids
DEF: Removal of clotted material from hemorrhoid.

49.49 Other procedures on hemorrhoids
Lord procedure

✓4th **49.5 Division of anal sphincter**

49.51 Left lateral anal sphincterotomy

49.52 Posterior anal sphincterotomy

49.59 Other anal sphincterotomy
Division of sphincter NOS

49.6 Excision of anus

✓4th **49.7 Repair of anus**
> EXCLUDES   repair of current obstetric laceration
> (75.62)

49.71 Suture of laceration of anus

49.72 Anal cerclage
DEF: Encircling anus with ring or sutures.

49.73 Closure of anal fistula
> EXCLUDES   excision of anal fistula (49.12)

49.74 Gracilis muscle transplant for anal incontinence
DEF: Moving pubic attachment of gracilis muscle to restores anal control.

● **49.75 Implantation or revision of artificial anal sphincter**
Removal with subsequent replacement
Replacement during same or subsequent operative episode

● **49.76 Removal of artificial anal sphincter**
Explantation or removal without replacement
> EXCLUDES   revision with implantation
> during same operative
> episode (49.75)

49.79 Other repair of anal sphincter
Repair of old obstetric laceration of anus
> EXCLUDES   anoplasty with synchronous
> hemorrhoidectomy
> (49.46)
> repair of current obstetric
> laceration (75.62)

AHA: 2Q, '98, 16; 1Q, '97, 9

✓4th **49.9 Other operations on anus**
> EXCLUDES   dilation of anus (sphincter) (96.23)

49.91 Incision of anal septum

49.92 Insertion of subcutaneous electrical anal stimulator

49.93 Other incision of anus
Removal of:
foreign body from anus with incision
seton from anus
> EXCLUDES   anal fistulotomy (49.11)
> removal of intraluminal foreign
> body without incision
> (98.05)

49.94 **Reduction of anal prolapse**

> **EXCLUDES** *manual reduction of rectal prolapse (96.26)*

DEF: Manipulation of displaced anal tissue to normal position.

49.95 **Control of (postoperative) hemorrhage of anus**

49.99 **Other**

√3rd **50 Operations on liver**

▶Code also any application or administration of an adhesion barrier substance (99.77)◀

50.0 **Hepatotomy**

Incision of abscess of liver
Removal of gallstones from liver
Stromeyer-Little operation

√4th **50.1** **Diagnostic procedures on liver**

50.11 **Closed (percutaneous) [needle] biopsy of liver**

Diagnostic aspiration of liver

AHA: 4Q, '88, 12

50.12 **Open biopsy of liver**

Wedge biopsy

50.19 **Other diagnostic procedures on liver**

> **EXCLUDES** *liver scan and radioisotope function study (92.02)*
> *microscopic examination of specimen from liver (91.01-91.09)*

√4th **50.2** **Local excision or destruction of liver tissue or lesion**

50.21 **Marsupialization of lesion of liver**

DEF: Exteriorizing lesion by incision and suturing cut edges to skin to create opening.

Closed Liver Biopsy

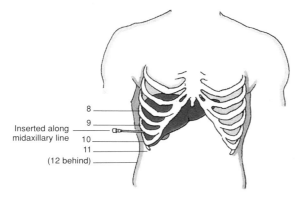

Inserted along midaxillary line
8
9
10
11
(12 behind)

Liver Biopsy (Open, Wedge)

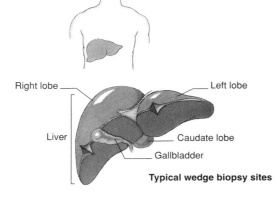

Right lobe
Left lobe
Liver
Caudate lobe
Gallbladder

Typical wedge biopsy sites

50.22 **Partial hepatectomy**

Wedge resection of liver

> **EXCLUDES** *biopsy of liver (50.11-50.12)*
> *hepatic lobectomy (50.3)*

50.29 **Other destruction of lesion of liver**

Cauterization
Enucleation } of hepatic lesion
Evacuation

> **EXCLUDES** *percutaneous aspiration of lesion (50.91)*

50.3 **Lobectomy of liver**

Total hepatic lobectomy with partial excision of other lobe

50.4 **Total hepatectomy**

√4th **50.5** **Liver transplant**

50.51 **Auxiliary liver transplant** NC

Auxiliary hepatic transplantation leaving patient's own liver in situ

50.59 **Other transplant of liver** NC

√4th **50.6** **Repair of liver**

50.61 **Closure of laceration of liver**

50.69 **Other repair of liver**

Hepatopexy

√4th **50.9** **Other operations on liver**

> **EXCLUDES** *lysis of adhesions (54.5)*

50.91 **Percutaneous aspiration of liver**

> **EXCLUDES** *percutaneous biopsy (50.11)*

DEF: Incision into liver through body wall to withdraw fluid.

50.92 **Extracorporeal hepatic assistance**

Liver dialysis

AHA: 2Q, '01, 21

DEF: Devices used outside body to assist liver function.

50.93 **Localized perfusion of liver**

50.94 **Other injection of therapeutic substance into liver**

50.99 **Other**

√3rd **51 Operations on gallbladder and biliary tract**

▶Code also any application or administration of an adhesion barrier substance (99.77)◀

> **INCLUDES** operations on:
> ampulla of Vater
> common bile duct
> cystic duct
> hepatic duct
> intrahepatic bile duct
> sphincter of Oddi

√4th **51.0** **Cholecystotomy and cholecystostomy**

51.01 **Percutaneous aspiration of gallbladder**

▶Percutaneous cholecystotomy for drainage
That by: needle or catheter◀

> **EXCLUDES** *needle biopsy (51.12)*

51.02 **Trocar cholecystostomy**

AHA: 3Q, '89, 18

DEF: Creating opening in gallbladder with catheter.

51.03 **Other cholecystostomy**

51.04 **Other cholecystotomy**

Cholelithotomy NOS

√4th **51.1** **Diagnostic procedures on biliary tract**

> **EXCLUDES** *that for endoscopic procedures classifiable to 51.64, 51.84-51.88, 52.14, 52.21, 52.93-52.94, 52.97-52.98*

AHA: 2Q, '97, 7

Operations on the Digestive System 51.10–51.62

51.10　Endoscopic retrograde cholangiopancreatography [ERCP]
> EXCLUDES　*endoscopic retrograde:*
> *cholangiography [ERC]*
> *(51.11)*
> *pancreatography [ERP]*
> *(52.13)*

AHA: 1Q, '01, 8; 2Q, '99, 13

DEF: Endoscopic and radioscopic exam of pancreatic and common bile ducts with contrast material injected in opposite direction of normal flow through catheter.

51.11　Endoscopic retrograde cholangiography [ERC]
Laparoscopic exploration of common bile duct
> EXCLUDES　*endoscopic retrograde:*
> *cholangiopancreatography*
> *[ERCP] (51.10)*
> *pancreatography [ERP]*
> *(52.13)*

AHA: 1Q, '96, 12; 3Q, '89, 18; 4Q, '88, 7

DEF: Endoscopic and radioscopic exam of common bile ducts with contrast material injected in opposite direction of normal flow through catheter.

51.12　Percutaneous biopsy of gallbladder or bile ducts
Needle biopsy of gallbladder

51.13　Open biopsy of gallbladder or bile ducts

51.14　Other closed [endoscopic] biopsy of biliary duct or sphincter of Oddi
Brushing or washing for specimen collection
Closed biopsy of biliary duct or sphincter of Oddi by procedures classifiable to 51.10-51.11, 52.13

DEF: Endoscopic biopsy of muscle tissue around pancreatic and common bile ducts.

51.15　Pressure measurement of sphincter of Oddi
Pressure measurement of sphincter by procedures classifiable to 51.10-51.11, 52.13

DEF: Pressure measurement tests of muscle tissue surrounding pancreatic and common bile ducts.

51.19　Other diagnostic procedures on biliary tract
> EXCLUDES　*biliary tract x-ray (87.51-*
> *87.59)*
> *microscopic examination of*
> *specimen from biliary*
> *tract (91.01-91.09)*

✓4ᵗʰ　**51.2　Cholecystectomy**
AHA: 1Q, '93, 17; 4Q, '91, 26; 3Q, '89, 18

51.21　Other partial cholecystectomy
Revision of prior cholecystectomy
> EXCLUDES　*that by laparoscope (51.24)*

AHA: 4Q, '96, 69

51.22　Cholecystectomy
> EXCLUDES　*laparoscopic cholecystectomy*
> *(51.23)*

AHA: 4Q, '97, 52; 2Q, '91, 16

51.23　Laparoscopic cholecystectomy
That by laser
AHA: 3Q, '98, 10; 4Q, '97, 52; 1Q, '96, 12; 2Q, '95, 11; 4Q, '91, 26

DEF: Endoscopic removal of gallbladder.

51.24　Laparoscopic partial cholecystectomy
AHA: 4Q, '96, 69

✓4ᵗʰ　**51.3　Anastomosis of gallbladder or bile duct**
> EXCLUDES　*resection with end-to-end anastomosis*
> *(51.61-51.69)*

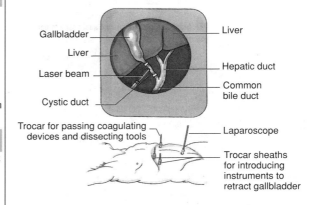

Laparoscopic Cholecystectomy by Laser

Gallbladder — Liver
Liver — Hepatic duct
Laser beam — Common bile duct
Cystic duct

Trocar for passing coagulating devices and dissecting tools — Laparoscope
Trocar sheaths for introducing instruments to retract gallbladder

51.31　Anastomosis of gallbladder to hepatic ducts
51.32　Anastomosis of gallbladder to intestine
51.33　Anastomosis of gallbladder to pancreas
51.34　Anastomosis of gallbladder to stomach
51.35　Other gallbladder anastomosis
Gallbladder anastomosis NOS

51.36　Choledochoenterostomy
DEF: Connection of common bile duct to intestine.

51.37　Anastomosis of hepatic duct to gastrointestinal tract
►Kasai portoenterostomy◄

51.39　Other bile duct anastomosis
Anastomosis of bile duct NOS
Anastomosis of unspecified bile duct to:
intestine　　　pancreas
liver　　　　　stomach

✓4ᵗʰ　**51.4　Incision of bile duct for relief of obstruction**

51.41　Common duct exploration for removal of calculus
> EXCLUDES　*percutaneous extraction*
> *(51.96)*

AHA: 1Q, '96, 12; 3Q, '89, 18; 4Q, '88, 7

51.42　Common duct exploration for relief of other obstruction
AHA: 3Q, '89, 18

51.43　Insertion of choledochohepatic tube for decompression
Hepatocholedochostomy
AHA: 3Q, '89, 18; 4Q, '88, 7

51.49　Incision of other bile ducts for relief of obstruction
AHA: 3Q, '89, 18

✓4ᵗʰ　**51.5　Other incision of bile duct**
> EXCLUDES　*that for relief of obstruction (51.41-*
> *51.49)*

51.51　Exploration of common duct
Incision of common bile duct
AHA: 2Q, '97, 16; 1Q, '96, 12

51.59　Incision of other bile duct
AHA: 2Q, '97, 16; 3Q, '89, 18

✓4ᵗʰ　**51.6　Local excision or destruction of lesion or tissue of biliary ducts and sphincter of Oddi**
Code also anastomosis other than end-to-end (51.31, 51.36-51.39)
> EXCLUDES　*biopsy of bile duct (51.12-51.13)*

51.61　Excision of cystic duct remnant
AHA: 3Q, '89, 18

51.62　Excision of ampulla of Vater (with reimplantation of common duct)

BI　Bilateral Edit　　　NC　Non-covered Procedure　　　►◄ Revised Text　　　● New Code　　　▲ Revised Code Title

51.63 **Other excision of common duct**
Choledochectomy
EXCLUDES *fistulectomy (51.72)*

51.64 **Endoscopic excision or destruction of lesion of biliary ducts or sphincter of Oddi**
Excision or destruction of lesion of biliary duct by procedures classifiable to 51.10-51.11, 52.13

51.69 **Excision of other bile duct**
Excision of lesion of bile duct NOS
EXCLUDES *fistulectomy (51.79)*

✓4ᵗʰ **51.7** **Repair of bile ducts**

51.71 **Simple suture of common bile duct**

51.72 **Choledochoplasty**
Repair of fistula of common bile duct

51.79 **Repair of other bile ducts**
Closure of artificial opening of bile duct NOS
Suture of bile duct NOS
EXCLUDES *operative removal of prosthetic device (51.95)*

✓4ᵗʰ **51.8** **Other operations on biliary ducts and sphincter of Oddi**

51.81 **Dilation of sphincter of Oddi**
Dilation of ampulla of Vater
EXCLUDES *that by endoscopic approach (51.84)*

DEF: Dilation of muscle around common bile and pancreatic ducts; to mitigate constriction obstructing bile flow.

51.82 **Pancreatic sphincterotomy**
Incision of pancreatic sphincter
Transduodenal ampullary sphincterotomy
EXCLUDES *that by endoscopic approach (51.85)*

DEF: Pancreatic sphincterotomy: Division of muscle around common bile and pancreatic ducts.

DEF: Transduodenal ampullary sphincterotomy: Incision into muscle around common bile and pancreatic ducts; closing approach through first section of small intestine.

51.83 **Pancreatic sphincteroplasty**

51.84 **Endoscopic dilation of ampulla and biliary duct**
Dilation of ampulla and biliary duct by procedures classifiable to 51.10-51.11, 52.13

51.85 **Endoscopic sphincterotomy and papillotomy**
Sphincterotomy and papillotomy by procedures classifiable to 51.10-51.11, 52.13

AHA: 2Q, '97, 7

DEF: Incision of muscle around common bile and pancreatic ducts and closing the duodenal papilla.

51.86 **Endoscopic insertion of nasobiliary drainage tube**
Insertion of nasobiliary tube by procedures classifiable to 51.10-51.11, 52.13

51.87 **Endoscopic insertion of stent (tube) into bile duct**
Endoprosthesis of bile duct
Insertion of stent into bile duct by procedures classifiable to 51.10-51.11, 52.13
EXCLUDES *nasobiliary drainage tube (51.86)*
replacement of stent (tube) (97.05)

51.88 **Endoscopic removal of stone(s) from biliary tract**
Laparoscopic removal of stone(s) from biliary tract
Removal of biliary tract stone(s) by procedures classifiable to 51.10-51.11, 52.13
EXCLUDES *percutaneous extraction of common duct stones (51.96)*

AHA: 2Q, '00, 11; 2Q, '97, 7

51.89 **Other operations on sphincter of Oddi**

✓4ᵗʰ **51.9** **Other operations on biliary tract**

51.91 **Repair of laceration of gallbladder**

51.92 **Closure of cholecystostomy**

51.93 **Closure of other biliary fistula**
Cholecystogastroenteric fistulectomy

51.94 **Revision of anastomosis of biliary tract**

51.95 **Removal of prosthetic device from bile duct**
EXCLUDES *nonoperative removal (97.55)*

51.96 **Percutaneous extraction of common duct stones**
AHA: 4Q, '88, 7

51.98 **Other percutaneous procedures on biliary tract**
Percutaneous biliary endoscopy via existing T-tube or other tract for:
dilation of biliary duct stricture
removal of stone(s) except common duct stone
exploration (postoperative)
Percutaneous transhepatic biliary drainage
EXCLUDES *percutaneous aspiration of gallbladder (51.01)*
percutaneous biopsy and/or collection of specimen by brushing or washing (51.12)
percutaneous removal of common duct stone(s) (51.96)

AHA: 1Q, '97, 14; 3Q, '89, 18; N-D, '87, 1

51.99 **Other**
Insertion or replacement of biliary tract prosthesis
EXCLUDES *biopsy of gallbladder (51.12-51.13)*
irrigation of cholecystostomy and other biliary tube (96.41)
lysis of peritoneal adhesions (54.5)
nonoperative removal of:
cholecystostomy tube (97.54)
tube from biliary tract or liver (97.55)

✓3ʳᵈ **52** **Operations on pancreas**
▶Code also any application or administration of an adhesion barrier substance (99.77)◄
INCLUDES operations on pancreatic duct

✓4ᵗʰ **52.0** **Pancreatotomy**

52.01 **Drainage of pancreatic cyst by catheter**

52.09 **Other pancreatotomy**
Pancreatolithotomy
EXCLUDES *drainage by anastomosis (52.4, 52.96)*
incision of pancreatic sphincter (51.82)
marsupialization of cyst (52.3)

DEF: Pancreatolithotomy: Incision into pancreas to remove stones.

Operations on the Digestive System 52.1–52.95

✓4th **52.1**   **Diagnostic procedures on pancreas**

52.11   **Closed [aspiration] [needle] [percutaneous] biopsy of pancreas**

52.12   **Open biopsy of pancreas**

52.13   **Endoscopic retrograde pancreatography [ERP]**

EXCLUDES   *endoscopic retrograde:*
cholangiography [ERC]
(51.11)
cholangiopancreatography
[ERCP] (51.10)
that for procedures classifiable
to 51.14-51.15, 51.64,
51.84-51.88, 52.14,
52.21, 52.92-52.94,
52.97-52.98

52.14   **Closed [endoscopic] biopsy of pancreatic duct**

Closed biopsy of pancreatic duct by procedures classifiable to 51.10-51.11, 52.13

52.19   **Other diagnostic procedures on pancreas**

EXCLUDES   *contrast pancreatogram*
(87.66)
endoscopic retrograde
pancreatography [ERP]
(52.13)
microscopic examination of
specimen from pancreas
(91.01-91.09)

✓4th **52.2**   **Local excision or destruction of pancreas and pancreatic duct**

EXCLUDES   *biopsy of pancreas (52.11-52.12,*
52.14)
pancreatic fistulectomy (52.95)

52.21   **Endoscopic excision or destruction of lesion or tissue of pancreatic duct**

Excision or destruction of lesion or tissue of pancreatic duct by procedures classifiable to 51.10-51.11, 52.13

52.22   **Other excision or destruction of lesion or tissue of pancreas or pancreatic duct**

52.3   **Marsupialization of pancreatic cyst**

EXCLUDES   *drainage of cyst by catheter (52.01)*

DEF: Incision into pancreas and suturing edges to form pocket; promotes drainage and healing.

52.4   **Internal drainage of pancreatic cyst**

Pancreaticocystoduodenostomy
Pancreaticocystogastrostomy
Pancreaticocystojejunostomy

DEF: Withdrawing fluid from pancreatic cyst by draining it through a created passage to another organ.

DEF: Pancreaticocystoduodenostomy: Creation of passage from pancreatic cyst to first portion of small intestine.

DEF: Pancreaticocystogastrostomy: Creation of passage from pancreatic cyst to stomach.

DEF: Pancreaticocystojejunostomy: Creation of passage from pancreatic cyst to midsection of small intestine.

✓4th **52.5**   **Partial pancreatectomy**

EXCLUDES   *pancreatic fistulectomy (52.95)*

52.51   **Proximal pancreatectomy**

Excision of head of pancreas (with part of body)
Proximal pancreatectomy with synchronous duodenectomy

52.52   **Distal pancreatectomy**

Excision of tail of pancreas (with part of body)

52.53   **Radical subtotal pancreatectomy**

52.59   **Other partial pancreatectomy**

52.6   **Total pancreatectomy**

Pancreatectomy with synchronous duodenectomy

AHA: 4Q, '96, 71

52.7   **Radical pancreaticoduodenectomy**

One-stage pancreaticoduodenal resection with choledochojejunal anastomosis, pancreaticojejunal anastomosis, and gastrojejunostomy
Two-stage pancreaticoduodenal resection (first stage) (second stage)
Radical resection of the pancreas
Whipple procedure

EXCLUDES   *radical subtotal pancreatectomy (52.53)*

AHA: 1Q, '01, 13

DEF: ▶Whipple procedure: pancreaticoduodenectomy involving the removal of the head of the pancreas and part of the small intestines; pancreaticojejeunostomy, choledochojejunal anastomosis, and gastrojejunostomy included in the procedure.◀

✓4th **52.8**   **Transplant of pancreas**

[19] **52.80**   **Pancreatic transplant, not otherwise specified**   NC

52.81   **Reimplantation of pancreatic tissue**

[19] **52.82**   **Homotransplant of pancreas**   NC

52.83   **Heterotransplant of pancreas**   NC

52.84   **Autotransplantation of cells of islets of Langerhans**

Homotransplantation of islet cells of pancreas

AHA: 4Q, '96, 70, 71

DEF: Transplantation of Islet cells from pancreas to another location of same patient.

52.85   **Allotransplantation of cells of islets of Langerhans**

Heterotransplantation of islet cells of pancreas

AHA: 4Q, '96, 70, 71

DEF: Transplantation of Islet cells from one individual to another.

52.86   **Transplantation of cells of islets of Langerhans, not otherwise specified**

AHA: 4Q, '96, 70

✓4th **52.9**   **Other operations on pancreas**

DEF: Placement of tube into pancreatic duct, without an endoscope.

52.92   **Cannulation of pancreatic duct**

EXCLUDES   *that by endoscopic approach*
(52.93)

52.93   **Endoscopic insertion of stent (tube) into pancreatic duct**

Insertion of cannula or stent into pancreatic duct by procedures classifiable to 51.10-51.11, 52.13

EXCLUDES   *endoscopic insertion of*
nasopancreatic drainage
tube (52.97)
replacement of stent (tube)
(97.05)

AHA: 2Q, '97, 7

52.94   **Endoscopic removal of stone(s) from pancreatic duct**

Removal of stone(s) from pancreatic duct by procedures classifiable to 51.10-51.11, 52.13

52.95   **Other repair of pancreas**

Fistulectomy⎫
Simple suture⎭ of pancreas

[19]   Covered procedure when a diagnosis code is present from 250.00-250.93 and 585, V42.0, or V42.89

BI Bilateral Edit   NC Non-covered Procedure   ▶◀ Revised Text   ● New Code   ▲ Revised Code Title

Indirect Repair of Hernia

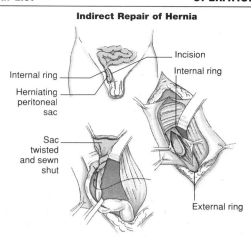

Internal ring
Herniating peritoneal sac
Incision
Internal ring
Sac twisted and sewn shut
External ring

52.96 Anastomosis of pancreas

Anastomosis of pancreas (duct) to:
intestine   stomach
jejunum

EXCLUDES   *anastomosis to:*
bile duct (51.39)
gallbladder (51.33)

52.97 Endoscopic insertion of nasopancreatic drainage tube

Insertion of nasopancreatic drainage tube by procedures classifiable to 51.10-51.11, 52.13

EXCLUDES   *drainage of pancreatic cyst by catheter (52.01)*
replacement of stent (tube) (97.05)

52.98 Endoscopic dilation of pancreatic duct

Dilation of Wirsung's duct by procedures classifiable to 51.10-51.11, 52.13

52.99 Other

Dilation of pancreatic [Wirsung's] duct   } by open
Repair of pancreatic [Wirsung's] duct   } approach

EXCLUDES   *irrigation of pancreatic tube (96.42)*
removal of pancreatic tube (97.56)

✓3rd **53   Repair of hernia**

▶Code also any application or administration of an adhesion barrier substance (99.77)◀

INCLUDES   hernioplasty   herniotomy
herniorrhaphy

EXCLUDES   *manual reduction of hernia (96.27)*

AHA: 3Q, '94, 8

DEF: Repair of hernia: Restoration of abnormally protruding organ or tissue.

DEF: Herniorrhaphy: Repair of hernia.

DEF: Herniotomy: Division of constricted, strangulated, irreducible hernia.

✓4th **53.0   Unilateral repair of inguinal hernia**

53.00   Unilateral repair of inguinal hernia, not otherwise specified

Inguinal herniorrhaphy NOS

53.01   Repair of direct inguinal hernia

AHA: 4Q, '96, 66

53.02   Repair of indirect inguinal hernia

53.03   Repair of direct inguinal hernia with graft or prosthesis

53.04   Repair of indirect inguinal hernia with graft or prosthesis

53.05   Repair of inguinal hernia with graft or prosthesis, not otherwise specified

✓4th **53.1   Bilateral repair of inguinal hernia**

53.10   Bilateral repair of inguinal hernia, not otherwise specified

53.11   Bilateral repair of direct inguinal hernia

53.12   Bilateral repair of indirect inguinal hernia

53.13   Bilateral repair of inguinal hernia, one direct and one indirect

53.14   Bilateral repair of direct inguinal hernia with graft or prosthesis

53.15   Bilateral repair of indirect inguinal hernia with graft or prosthesis

53.16   Bilateral repair of inguinal hernia, one direct and one indirect, with graft or prosthesis

53.17   Bilateral inguinal hernia repair with graft or prosthesis, not otherwise specified

✓4th **53.2   Unilateral repair of femoral hernia**

53.21   Unilateral repair of femoral hernia with graft or prosthesis

53.29   Other unilateral femoral herniorrhaphy

✓4th **53.3   Bilateral repair of femoral hernia**

53.31   Bilateral repair of femoral hernia with graft or prosthesis

53.39   Other bilateral femoral herniorrhaphy

✓4th **53.4   Repair of umbilical hernia**

EXCLUDES   *repair of gastroschisis (54.71)*

53.41   Repair of umbilical hernia with prosthesis

53.49   Other umbilical herniorrhaphy

✓4th **53.5   Repair of other hernia of anterior abdominal wall (without graft or prosthesis)**

53.51   Incisional hernia repair

53.59   Repair of other hernia of anterior abdominal wall

Repair of hernia: Repair of hernia:
epigastric   spigelian
hypogastric   ventral

AHA: 3Q, '96, 15

✓4th **53.6   Repair of other hernia of anterior abdominal wall with graft or prosthesis**

53.61   Incisional hernia repair with prosthesis

53.69   Repair of other hernia of anterior abdominal wall with prosthesis

53.7   Repair of diaphragmatic hernia, abdominal approach

✓4th **53.8   Repair of diaphragmatic hernia, thoracic approach**

DEF: Repair of diaphragmatic hernia though abdomen and thorax.

53.80   Repair of diaphragmatic hernia with thoracic approach, not otherwise specified

Thoracoabdominal repair of diaphragmatic hernia

53.81   Plication of the diaphragm

DEF: Tuck repair of diaphragmatic hernia.

53.82   Repair of parasternal hernia

DEF: Repair of hernia protruding into breastbone area.

53.9   Other hernia repair

Repair of hernia: Repair of hernia:
ischiatic   omental
ischiorectal   retroperitoneal
lumbar   sciatic
obturator

EXCLUDES   *relief of strangulated hernia with exteriorization of intestine (46.01, 46.03)*
repair of pericolostomy hernia (46.42)
repair of vaginal enterocele (70.92)

✓3rd **54**   **Other operations on abdominal region**
     ►Code also any application or administration of an adhesion barrier substance (99.77)◄

INCLUDES   operations on: operations on:
       epigastric region   male pelvic cavity
       flank   mesentery
       groin region   omentum
       hypochondrium   peritoneum
       inguinal region   retroperitoneal
       loin region   tissue space

EXCLUDES   *female pelvic cavity (69.01-70.92)*
               hernia repair (53.00-53.9)
               obliteration of cul-de-sac (70.92)
               retroperitoneal tissue dissection (59.00-59.09)
               skin and subcutaneous tissue of abdominal wall (86.01-86.99)

54.0   **Incision of abdominal wall**
     Drainage of:
       abdominal wall
       extraperitoneal abscess
       retroperitoneal abscess
     EXCLUDES   *incision of peritoneum (54.95)*
               laparotomy (54.11-54.19)

AHA: 1Q, '97, 11; N-D, '87, 12

✓4th **54.1**   **Laparotomy**

AHA: 1Q, '92, 13

DEF: Incision into abdomen.

54.11   **Exploratory laparotomy**
     EXCLUDES   *exploration incidental to intra-abdominal surgery — omit code*

AHA: 3Q, '89, 14; 4Q, '88, 12

DEF: Exam of peritoneal cavity through incision into abdomen.

54.12   **Reopening of recent laparotomy site**
     Reopening of recent laparotomy site for:
       control of hemorrhage
       exploration
       incision of hematoma

54.19   **Other laparotomy**
     Drainage of intraperitoneal abscess or hematoma
     EXCLUDES   *culdocentesis (70.0)*
               drainage of appendiceal abscess (47.2)
               exploration incidental to intra-abdominal surgery — omit code
               Ladd operation (54.95)
               percutaneous drainage of abdomen (54.91)
               removal of foreign body (54.92)

✓4th **54.2**   **Diagnostic procedures of abdominal region**

54.21   **Laparoscopy**
     Peritoneoscopy
     EXCLUDES   *laparoscopic cholecystectomy (51.23)*
               that incidental to destruction of fallopian tubes (66.21-66.29)

DEF: Endoscopic exam of peritoneal cavity through abdominal incision.

54.22   **Biopsy of abdominal wall or umbilicus**

54.23   **Biopsy of peritoneum**
     Biopsy of:
       mesentery
       omentum
       peritoneal implant
     EXCLUDES   *closed biopsy of:*
               omentum (54.24)
               peritoneum (54.24)

54.24   **Closed [percutaneous] [needle] biopsy of intra-abdominal mass**
     Closed biopsy of:
       omentum
       peritoneal implant
       peritoneum
     EXCLUDES   *that of:*
               fallopian tube (66.11)
               ovary (65.11)
               uterine ligaments (68.15)
               uterus (68.16)

AHA: 4Q, '97, 57

54.25   **Peritoneal lavage**
     Diagnostic peritoneal lavage
     EXCLUDES   *peritoneal dialysis (54.98)*

AHA: 2Q, '98, 19; 4Q, '93, 28

DEF: Irrigation of peritoneal cavity with siphoning of liquid contents for analysis.

54.29   **Other diagnostic procedures on abdominal region**
     EXCLUDES   *abdominal lymphangiogram (88.04)*
               abdominal x-ray NEC (88.19)
               angiocardiography of venae cavae (88.51)
               C.A.T. scan of abdomen (88.01)
               contrast x-ray of abdominal cavity (88.11-88.15)
               intra-abdominal arteriography NEC (88.47)
               microscopic examination of peritoneal and retroperitoneal specimen (91.11-91.19)
               phlebography of:
               intra-abdominal vessels NEC (88.65)
               portal venous system (88.64)
               sinogram of abdominal wall (88.03)
               soft tissue x-ray of abdominal wall NEC (88.09)
               tomography of abdomen NEC (88.02)
               ultrasonography of abdomen and retroperitoneum (88.76)

54.3   **Excision or destruction of lesion or tissue of abdominal wall or umbilicus**
     Debridement of abdominal wall
     Omphalectomy
     EXCLUDES   *biopsy of abdominal wall or umbilicus (54.22)*
               size reduction operation (86.83)
               that of skin of abdominal wall (86.22, 86.26, 86.3)

AHA: 1Q, '89, 11

54.4   **Excision or destruction of peritoneal tissue**
     Excision of:
       appendices epiploicae
       falciform ligament
       gastrocolic ligament
       lesion of:
         mesentery
         omentum
         peritoneum
       presacral lesion NOS
       retroperitoneal lesion NOS
     EXCLUDES   *biopsy of peritoneum (54.23)*
               endometrectomy of cul-de-sac (70.32)

✓4th **54.5** **Lysis of peritoneal adhesions**
Freeing of adhesions of:
   biliary tract
   intestines
   liver
   pelvic peritoneum
   peritoneum
   spleen
   uterus
   EXCLUDES   *lysis of adhesions of:*
      bladder (59.11)
      fallopian tube and ovary (65.81, 65.89)
      kidney (59.02)
      ureter (59.02-59.03)

AHA: 3Q, '94, 8; 4Q, '90, 18

   54.51 **Laparoscopic lysis of peritoneal adhesions**
      AHA: 4Q, '96, 65

   54.59 **Other lysis of peritoneal adhesions**
      AHA: 4Q, '96, 66

✓4th **54.6** **Suture of abdominal wall and peritoneum**
   54.61 **Reclosure of postoperative disruption of abdominal wall**
   54.62 **Delayed closure of granulating abdominal wound**
      Tertiary subcutaneous wound closure
      DEF: Closure of outer layers of abdominal wound; follows procedure to close initial layers of wound.
   54.63 **Other suture of abdominal wall**
      Suture of laceration of abdominal wall
      EXCLUDES   *closure of operative wound — omit code*
   54.64 **Suture of peritoneum**
      Secondary suture of peritoneum
      EXCLUDES   *closure of operative wound — omit code*

✓4th **54.7** **Other repair of abdominal wall and peritoneum**
   54.71 **Repair of gastroschisis**
      DEF: Repair of congenital fistula of abdominal wall.
   54.72 **Other repair of abdominal wall**
   54.73 **Other repair of peritoneum**
      Suture of gastrocolic ligament
   54.74 **Other repair of omentum**
      Epiplorrhaphy
      Graft of omentum
      Omentopexy
      Reduction of torsion of omentum
      EXCLUDES   *cardio-omentopexy (36.39)*

      AHA: J-F, '87, 11

      DEF: Epiplorrhaphy: Suture of abdominal serous membrane.

      DEF: Graft of omentum: Implantation of tissue into abdominal serous membrane.

      DEF: Omentopexy: Anchoring of abdominal serous membrane.

      DEF: Reduction of torsion of omentum: Reduction of twisted abdominal serous membrane.

   54.75 **Other repair of mesentery**
      Mesenteric plication
      Mesenteropexy
      DEF: Creation of folds in mesentery for shortening.

      DEF: Mesenteriopexy: Fixation of torn, incised mesentery.

✓4th **54.9** **Other operations of abdominal region**
   EXCLUDES   *removal of ectopic pregnancy (74.3)*

54.91 **Percutaneous abdominal drainage**
   Paracentesis
   EXCLUDES   *creation of cutaneoperitoneal fistula (54.93)*

AHA: 3Q, '99, 9; 2Q, '99, 14; 3Q, '98, 12; 1Q, '92, 14; 2Q, '90, 25

DEF: Puncture for removal of fluid.

54.92 **Removal of foreign body from peritoneal cavity**
   AHA: 1Q, '89, 11

54.93 **Creation of cutaneoperitoneal fistula**
   AHA: 2Q, '95, 10; N-D, '84, 6

   DEF: Creation of opening between skin and peritoneal cavity.

54.94 **Creation of peritoneovascular shunt**
   Peritoneovenous shunt
   AHA: 1Q, '94, 7; 1Q, '88, 9; S-O, '85, 6

   DEF: Construction of shunt to connect peritoneal cavity with vascular system.

   DEF: Peritoneovenous shunt: Construction of shunt to connect peritoneal cavity with vein.

54.95 **Incision of peritoneum**
   ►Exploration of ventriculoperitoneal shunt at peritoneal site◄
   Ladd operation
   Revision of distal catheter of ventricular shunt
   Revision of ventriculoperitoneal shunt at peritoneal site
   EXCLUDES   *that incidental to laparotomy (54.11-54.19)*

AHA: 4Q, '95, 65

DEF: Ladd operation: Peritoneal attachment of incompletely rotated cecum, obstructing duodenum.

54.96 **Injection of air into peritoneal cavity**
   Pneumoperitoneum
   EXCLUDES   *that for:*
      collapse of lung (33.33)
      radiography (88.12-88.13, 88.15)

54.97 **Injection of locally-acting therapeutic substance into peritoneal cavity**
   EXCLUDES   *peritoneal dialysis (54.98)*

54.98 **Peritoneal dialysis**
   EXCLUDES   *peritoneal lavage (diagnostic) (54.25)*

AHA: 4Q, '93, 28; N-D, '84, 6

DEF: Separation of blood elements by diffusion through membrane.

54.99 **Other**
   EXCLUDES   *removal of:*
      abdominal wall sutures (97.83)
      peritoneal drainage device (97.82)
      retroperitoneal drainage device (97.81)

AHA: 1Q, '99, 4

Operations on the Urinary System 55–55.53

10. OPERATIONS ON THE URINARY SYSTEM (55-59)

✓3rd 55   Operations on kidney
> ►Code also any application or administration of an adhesion barrier substance (99.77)◄

    INCLUDES   operations on renal pelvis

    EXCLUDES   *perirenal tissue (59.00-59.09, 59.21-59.29, 59.91-59.92)*

✓4th 55.0   Nephrotomy and nephrostomy

    EXCLUDES   *drainage by:*
          anastomosis (55.86)
          aspiration (55.92)

55.01   Nephrotomy
Evacuation of renal cyst
Exploration of kidney
Nephrolithotomy

DEF: Nephrotomy: Incision into kidney.

DEF: Evacuation of renal cyst: Draining contents of cyst.

DEF: Exploration of kidney: Exploration through incision.

DEF: Nephrolithotomy: Removal of kidney stone through incision.

55.02   Nephrostomy
AHA: 2Q, '97, 4

55.03   Percutaneous nephrostomy without fragmentation
Nephrostolithotomy, percutaneous (nephroscopic)
Percutaneous removal of kidney stone(s) by:
    forceps extraction (nephroscopic)
    basket extraction
Pyelostolithotomy, percutaneous (nephroscopic)
With placement of catheter down ureter

    EXCLUDES   *percutaneous removal by fragmentation (55.04)*
repeat nephroscopic removal during current episode (55.92)

AHA: 2Q, '96, 5

DEF: Insertion of tube through abdominal wall without breaking up stones.

DEF: Nephrostolithotomy: Insertion of tube through the abdominal wall to remove stones.

DEF: Basket extraction: Removal, percutaneous of stone with grasping forceps.

DEF: Pyelostolithotomy: Removal, percutaneous of stones from funnel-shaped portion of kidney.

55.04   Percutaneous nephrostomy with fragmentation
Percutaneous nephrostomy with disruption of kidney stone by ultrasonic energy and extraction (suction) through endoscope
With placement of catheter down ureter
With fluoroscopic guidance

    EXCLUDES   *repeat fragmentation during current episode (59.95)*

AHA: 1Q, '89, 1; S-O, '86, 11

DEF: Insertion of tube through abdominal wall into kidney to break up stones.

✓4th 55.1   Pyelotomy and pyelostomy

    EXCLUDES   *drainage by anastomosis (55.86)*
percutaneous pyelostolithotomy (55.03)
removal of calculus without incision (56.0)

55.11   Pyelotomy
Exploration of renal pelvis
Pyelolithotomy

55.12   Pyelostomy
Insertion of drainage tube into renal pelvis

✓4th 55.2   Diagnostic procedures on kidney

55.21   Nephroscopy
DEF: Endoscopic exam of renal pelvis; retrograde through ureter, percutaneous or open exposure.

55.22   Pyeloscopy
DEF: Fluoroscopic exam of kidney pelvis, calyces and ureters; follows IV or retrograde injection of contrast.

55.23   Closed [percutaneous] [needle] biopsy of kidney
Endoscopic biopsy via existing nephrostomy, nephrotomy, pyelostomy, or pyelotomy

55.24   Open biopsy of kidney

55.29   Other diagnostic procedures on kidney

    EXCLUDES   *microscopic examination of specimen from kidney (91.21-91.29)*
pyelogram:
    intravenous (87.73)
    percutaneous (87.75)
    retrograde (87.74)
radioisotope scan (92.03)
renal arteriography (88.45)
tomography:
    C.A.T scan (87.71)
    other (87.72)

✓4th 55.3   Local excision or destruction of lesion or tissue of kidney

55.31   Marsupialization of kidney lesion
DEF: Exteriorization of lesion by incising anterior wall and suturing cut edges to create open pouch.

55.39   Other local destruction or excision of renal lesion or tissue
Obliteration of calyceal diverticulum

    EXCLUDES   *biopsy of kidney (55.23-55.24)*
partial nephrectomy (55.4)
percutaneous aspiration of kidney (55.92)
wedge resection of kidney (55.4)

55.4   Partial nephrectomy
Calycectomy
Wedge resection of kidney
Code also any synchronous resection of ureter (56.40-56.42)

DEF: Surgical removal of a part of the kidney.

DEF: Calycectomy: Removal of indentations in kidney.

✓4th 55.5   Complete nephrectomy
Code also any synchronous excision of:
    bladder segment (57.6)
    lymph nodes (40.3, 40.52-40.59)

55.51   Nephroureterectomy
Nephroureterectomy with bladder cuff
Total nephrectomy (unilateral)

    EXCLUDES   *removal of transplanted kidney (55.53)*

DEF: Complete removal of the kidney and all or portion of the ureter.

DEF: Nephroureterectomy with bladder cuff: Removal of kidney, ureter, and portion of bladder attached to ureter.

DEF: Total nephrectomy (unilateral): Complete excision of one kidney.

55.52   Nephrectomy of remaining kidney
Removal of solitary kidney

    EXCLUDES   *removal of transplanted kidney (55.53)*

55.53   Removal of transplanted or rejected kidney

| BI Bilateral Edit | NC Non-covered Procedure | ►◄ Revised Text | ● New Code | ▲ Revised Code Title |

55.54 Bilateral nephrectomy
    EXCLUDES   *complete nephrectomy NOS (55.51)*
    DEF: Removal of both kidneys same operative session.

✓4ᵗʰ **55.6 Transplant of kidney**
    55.61 Renal autotransplantation
    55.69 Other kidney transplantation
    AHA: 4Q, '96, 71

55.7 Nephropexy
    Fixation or suspension of movable [floating] kidney

✓4ᵗʰ **55.8 Other repair of kidney**
    55.81 Suture of laceration of kidney
    55.82 Closure of nephrostomy and pyelostomy
    DEF: Removal of tube from kidney and closure of site of tube insertion.

    55.83 Closure of other fistula of kidney
    55.84 Reduction of torsion of renal pedicle
    DEF: Restoration of twisted renal pedicle into normal position.

    55.85 Symphysiotomy for horseshoe kidney
    DEF: Division of congenitally malformed kidney into two parts.

    55.86 Anastomosis of kidney
       Nephropyeloureterostomy
       Pyeloureterovesical anastomosis
       Ureterocalyceal anastomosis
       EXCLUDES   *nephrocystanastomosis NOS (56.73)*
    DEF: Nephropyeloureterostomy: Creation of passage between kidney and ureter.
    DEF: Pyeloureterovesical anastomosis: Creation of passage between kidney and bladder.
    DEF: Ureterocalyceal anastomosis: Creation of passage between ureter and kidney indentations.

    55.87 Correction of ureteropelvic junction
    55.89 Other

✓4ᵗʰ **55.9 Other operations on kidney**
    EXCLUDES   *lysis of perirenal adhesions (59.02)*
    55.91 Decapsulation of kidney
       Capsulectomy
       Decortication   } of kidney

    55.92 Percutaneous aspiration of kidney (pelvis)
       Aspiration of renal cyst   Renipuncture
       EXCLUDES   *percutaneous biopsy of kidney (55.23)*
    AHA: N-D, '84, 20
    DEF: Insertion of needle into kidney to withdraw fluid.

Symphysiostomy for Horseshoe Kidney

Inferior Vena Cava
Aorta
Ureter
Sutures
Horseshoe kidney joined at inferior poles

55.93 Replacement of nephrostomy tube
55.94 Replacement of pyelostomy tube
55.95 Local perfusion of kidney
    DEF: Fluid passage through kidney.

55.96 Other injection of therapeutic substance into kidney
    Injection into renal cyst

55.97 Implantation or replacement of mechanical kidney
55.98 Removal of mechanical kidney
55.99 Other
    EXCLUDES   *removal of pyelostomy or nephrostomy tube (97.61)*

✓3ʳᵈ **56 Operations on ureter**
    ►Code also any application or administration of an adhesion barrier substance (99.77)◄

    56.0 Transurethral removal of obstruction from ureter and renal pelvis
       Removal of:
         blood clot
         calculus   } from ureter or renal pelvis
         foreign body   } without incision
       EXCLUDES   *manipulation without removal of obstruction (59.8)*
           that by incision (55.11, 56.2)
           transurethral insertion of ureteral stent for passage of calculus (59.8)
    AHA: 1Q, '89, 1; S-O, '86, 12
    DEF: Removal of obstruction by tube inserted through urethra to ureter.

    56.1 Ureteral meatotomy
    DEF: Incision into ureteral meatus to enlarge passage.

    56.2 Ureterotomy
       Incision of ureter for: Incision of ureter for:
         drainage   removal of calculus
         exploration
       EXCLUDES   *cutting of ureterovesical orifice (56.1)*
           removal of calculus without incision (56.0)
           transurethral insertion of ureteral stent for passage of calculus (59.8)
           urinary diversion (56.51-56.79)
    AHA: S-O, '86, 10

✓4ᵗʰ **56.3 Diagnostic procedures on ureter**
    56.31 Ureteroscopy
    56.32 Closed percutaneous biopsy of ureter
       EXCLUDES   *endoscopic biopsy of ureter (56.33)*
    56.33 Closed endoscopic biopsy of ureter
       Cystourethroscopy with ureteral biopsy
       Transurethral biopsy of ureter
       Ureteral endoscopy with biopsy through ureterotomy
       Ureteroscopy with biopsy
       EXCLUDES   *percutaneous biopsy of ureter (56.32)*
    56.34 Open biopsy of ureter
    56.35 Endoscopy (cystoscopy) (looposcopy) of ileal conduit
    DEF: Endoscopic exam of created opening between ureters and one end of small intestine; other end used to form artificial opening.

    56.39 Other diagnostic procedures on ureter
       EXCLUDES   *microscopic examination of specimen from ureter (91.21-91.29)*

Operations on the Urinary System 56.4–57.12

✓4ᵗʰ **56.4 Ureterectomy**
Code also anastomosis other than end-to-end
(56.51-56.79)
EXCLUDES   *fistulectomy (56.84)*
             nephroureterectomy (55.51-55.54)

     56.40 Ureterectomy, not otherwise specified
     56.41 Partial ureterotomy
         Excision of lesion of ureter
         Shortening of ureter with reimplantation
         EXCLUDES   *biopsy of ureter (56.32-56.34)*

     56.42 Total ureterectomy

✓4ᵗʰ **56.5 Cutaneous uretero-ileostomy**
     56.51 Formation of cutaneous uretero-ileostomy
         Construction of ileal conduit
         External ureteral ileostomy
         Formation of open ileal bladder
         Ileal loop operation
         Ileoureterostomy (Bricker's) (ileal bladder)
         Transplantation of ureter into ileum with
             external diversion
         EXCLUDES   *closed ileal bladder (57.87)*
             replacement of ureteral defect by ileal
               segment (56.89)

         DEF: Creation of urinary passage by connecting the
         terminal end of small intestine to ureter then connected
         to opening through abdominal wall.

         DEF: Construction of ileal conduit: Formation of conduit
         from terminal end of small intestine.

     56.52 Revision of cutaneous uretero-ileostomy
         AHA: 3Q, '96, 15; 4Q, '88, 7

✓4ᵗʰ **56.6 Other external urinary diversion**
     56.61 Formation of other cutaneous ureterostomy
         Anastomosis of ureter to skin
         Ureterostomy NOS
     56.62 Revision of other cutaneous ureterostomy
         Revision of ureterostomy stoma
         EXCLUDES   *nonoperative removal of*
             ureterostomy tube
             (97.62)

✓4ᵗʰ **56.7 Other anastomosis or bypass of ureter**
         EXCLUDES   *ureteropyelostomy (55.86)*
     56.71 Urinary diversion to intestine
         Anastomosis of ureter to intestine
         Internal urinary diversion NOS
         Code also any synchronous colostomy
         (46.10-46.13)
         EXCLUDES   *external ureteral ileostomy*
             (56.51)
     56.72 Revision of ureterointestinal anastomosis
         EXCLUDES   *revision of external ureteral*
             ileostomy (56.52)
     56.73 Nephrocystanastomosis, not otherwise
         specified
         DEF: Connection of kidney to bladder.
     56.74 Ureteroneocystostomy
         Replacement of ureter with bladder flap
         Ureterovesical anastomosis
         DEF: Transfer of ureter to another site in bladder.

         DEF: Ureterovesical anastomosis: Implantation of ureter
         into bladder.
     56.75 Transureteroureterostomy
         EXCLUDES   *ureteroureterostomy*
             associated with partial
             resection (56.41)
         DEF: Separating one ureter and joining the ends to the
         opposite ureter.

     56.79 Other

✓4ᵗʰ **56.8 Repair of ureter**
     56.81 Lysis of intraluminal adhesions of ureter
         EXCLUDES   *lysis of periureteral adhesions*
             (59.01-59.02)
             ureterolysis (59.02-59.03)
         DEF: Destruction of adhesions within urethral cavity.

     56.82 Suture of laceration of ureter
     56.83 Closure of ureterostomy
     56.84 Closure of other fistula of ureter
     56.85 Ureteropexy
     56.86 Removal of ligature from ureter
     56.89 Other repair of ureter
         Graft of ureter
         Replacement of ureter with ileal segment
             implanted into bladder
         Ureteroplication
         DEF: Graft of ureter: Tissue from another site for graft
         replacement or repair of ureter.

         DEF: Replacement of ureter with ileal segment implanted
         into bladder and ureter replacement with terminal end of
         small intestine.

         DEF: Ureteroplication: Creation of tucks in ureter.

✓4ᵗʰ **56.9 Other operations on ureter**
     56.91 Dilation of ureteral meatus
     56.92 Implantation of electronic ureteral
         stimulator
     56.93 Replacement of electronic ureteral
         stimulator
     56.94 Removal of electronic ureteral stimulator
         EXCLUDES   *that with synchronous*
             replacement (56.93)
     56.95 Ligation of ureter
     56.99 Other
         EXCLUDES   *removal of ureterostomy tube*
             and ureteral catheter
             (97.62)
             ureteral catheterization (59.8)

✓3ʳᵈ **57 Operations on urinary bladder**
▶Code also any application or administration of an adhesion
barrier substance (99.77)◀
EXCLUDES   *perivesical tissue (59.11-59.29, 59.91-59.92)*
             ureterovesical orifice (56.0-56.99)

     57.0 Transurethral clearance of bladder
         Drainage of bladder without incision
         Removal of:
             blood clot ⎫ from bladder
             calculus ⎬ without
             foreign body ⎭ incision
         EXCLUDES   *that by incision (57.19)*
         AHA: S-O, '86, 11

         DEF: Insertion of device through urethra to cleanse bladder.

✓4ᵗʰ **57.1 Cystotomy and cystostomy**
         EXCLUDES   *cystotomy and cystostomy as operative*
             approach — omit code
         DEF: Cystotomy: Incision of bladder.

         DEF: Cystostomy: Creation of opening into bladder.

     57.11 Percutaneous aspiration of bladder
     57.12 Lysis of intraluminal adhesions with
         incision into bladder
         EXCLUDES   *transurethral lysis of*
             intraluminal adhesions
             (57.41)
         DEF: Incision into bladder to destroy lesions.

BI Bilateral Edit   NC Non-covered Procedure   ▶◀ Revised Text   ● New Code   ▲ Revised Code Title

57.17　**Percutaneous cystostomy**
Closed cystostomy
Percutaneous suprapubic cystostomy
> **EXCLUDES**　removal of cystostomy tube
> (97.63)
> replacement of cystostomy
> tube (59.94)

DEF: Incision through body wall into bladder to insert tube.

DEF: Percutaneous (closed) suprapubic cystostomy: Incision above pubic arch, through body wall, into the bladder to insert tube.

57.18　**Other suprapubic cystostomy**
> **EXCLUDES**　percutaneous cystostomy
> (57.17)
> removal of cystostomy tube
> (97.63)
> replacement of cystostomy
> tube (59.94)

57.19　**Other cystotomy**
Cystolithotomy
> **EXCLUDES**　percutaneous cystostomy
> (57.17)
> suprapubic cystostomy (57.18)

AHA: 4Q, '95, 73; S-O, '86, 11

✓4th　**57.2**　**Vesicostomy**
> **EXCLUDES**　percutaneous cystostomy (57.17)
> suprapubic cystostomy (57.18)

57.21　**Vesicostomy**
Creation of permanent opening from
bladder to skin using a bladder flap

DEF: Creation of opening from the bladder to the skin.

DEF: Creation of permanent opening from the bladder to the skin using a bladder flap to create conduit from bladder to skin using bladder tissue.

57.22　**Revision or closure of vesicostomy**
> **EXCLUDES**　closure of cystostomy (57.82)

✓4th　**57.3**　**Diagnostic procedures on bladder**
57.31　**Cystoscopy through artificial stoma**
57.32　**Other cystoscopy**
Transurethral cystoscopy
> **EXCLUDES**　cystourethroscopy with
> ureteral biopsy (56.33)
> retrograde pyelogram (87.74)
> that for control of hemorrhage
> (postoperative):
> bladder (57.93)
> prostate (60.94)

AHA: 1Q, '01, 14

57.33　**Closed [transurethral] biopsy of bladder**
57.34　**Open biopsy of bladder**
Transurethral Cystourethroscopy

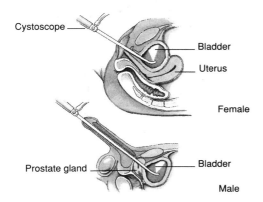

Cystoscope — Bladder
Uterus

Female

Prostate gland — Bladder

Male

57.39　**Other diagnostic procedures on bladder**
> **EXCLUDES**　cystogram NEC (87.77)
> microscopic examination of
> specimen from bladder
> (91.31-91.39)
> retrograde cystourethrogram
> (87.76)
> therapeutic distention of
> bladder
> (96.25)

✓4th　**57.4**　**Transurethral excision or destruction of bladder tissue**
DEF: Destruction of bladder tissue with instrument inserted into urethra.

57.41　**Transurethral lysis of intraluminal adhesions**
57.49　**Other transurethral excision or destruction of lesion or tissue of bladder**
Endoscopic resection of bladder lesion
> **EXCLUDES**　transurethral biopsy of
> bladder (57.33)
> transurethral fistulectomy
> (57.83-57.84)

✓4th　**57.5**　**Other excision or destruction of bladder tissue**
> **EXCLUDES**　that with transurethral approach
> (57.41-57.49)

57.51　**Excision of urachus**
Excision of urachal sinus of bladder
> **EXCLUDES**　excision of urachal cyst of
> abdominal wall (54.3)

57.59　**Open excision or destruction of other lesion or tissue of bladder**
Endometrectomy of bladder
Suprapubic excision of bladder lesion
> **EXCLUDES**　biopsy of bladder (57.33-
> 57.34)
> fistulectomy of bladder (57.83-
> 57.84)

DEF: Endometrectomy of bladder: Removal of inner lining.

DEF: Suprapubic excision of bladder lesion: Removal of lesion by excision above suprapubic bone arch.

57.6　**Partial cystectomy**
Excision of bladder dome　　Wedge resection of
　　　　　　　　　　　　　　　　bladder
Trigonectomy

✓4th　**57.7**　**Total cystectomy**
> **INCLUDES**　total cystectomy with urethrectomy

57.71　**Radical cystectomy**
Pelvic exenteration in male
Removal of bladder, prostate, seminal
vesicles and fat
Removal of bladder, urethra, and fat in a
female
Code also any:
lymph node dissection (40.3, 40.5)
urinary diversion (56.51-56.79)
> **EXCLUDES**　that as part of pelvic
> exenteration in female
> (68.8)

DEF: Radical cystectomy: Removal of bladder and surrounding tissue.

DEF: Pelvic exenteration in male: Excision of bladder, prostate, seminal vessels and fat.

57.79　**Other total cystectomy**
✓4th　**57.8**　**Other repair of urinary bladder**
> **EXCLUDES**　repair of:
> current obstetric laceration (75.61)
> cystocele (70.50-70.51)
> that for stress incontinence (59.3-59.79)

57.81　**Suture of laceration of bladder**

Operations on the Urinary System 57.82–58.39

57.82 **Closure of cystostomy**

57.83 **Repair of fistula involving bladder and intestine**

Rectovesicovaginal
Vesicosigmoidovaginal } fistulectomy

57.84 **Repair of other fistula of bladder**

Cervicovesical
Urethroperineovesical
Uterovesical
Vaginovesical } fistulectomy

EXCLUDES *vesicoureterovaginal fistulectomy (56.84)*

57.85 **Cystourethroplasty and plastic repair of bladder neck**

Plication of sphincter of urinary bladder
V-Y plasty of bladder neck

DEF: Cystourethroplasty: Reconstruction of narrowed portion of bladder.

DEF: Plication of sphincter or urinary bladder: Creation of tuck in bladder sphincter.

DEF: V-Y plasty of bladder neck: Surgical reconstruction of the narrowed portion of bladder by V-Y technique.

57.86 **Repair of bladder exstrophy**

DEF: Surgical connection of a congenital bladder wall defect.

57.87 **Reconstruction of urinary bladder**

Anastomosis of bladder with isolated segment of ileum
Augmentation of bladder
Replacement of bladder with ileum or sigmoid [closed ileal bladder]
Code also resection of intestine (45.50-45.52)

AHA: 3Q, '00, 7

DEF: Anastomosis of bladder with isolated segment of ileum: Creation of connection between bladder and separated terminal end of small intestine.

57.88 **Other anastomosis of bladder**

Anastomosis of bladder to intestine NOS
Cystocolic anastomosis

EXCLUDES *formation of closed ileal bladder (57.87)*

57.89 **Other repair of bladder**

Bladder suspension, not elsewhere classified
Cystopexy NOS
Repair of old obstetric laceration of bladder

EXCLUDES *repair of current obstetric laceration (75.61)*

√4ᵗʰ 57.9 **Other operations on bladder**

57.91 **Sphincterotomy of bladder**

Division of bladder neck

AHA: 2Q, '90, 26

57.92 **Dilation of bladder neck**

57.93 **Control of (postoperative) hemorrhage of bladder**

57.94 **Insertion of indwelling urinary catheter**

57.95 **Replacement of indwelling urinary catheter**

57.96 **Implantation of electronic bladder stimulator** NC

57.97 **Replacement of electronic bladder stimulator** NC

57.98 **Removal of electronic bladder stimulator**

EXCLUDES *that with synchronous replacement (57.97)*

57.99 **Other**

EXCLUDES *irrigation of:*
cystostomy (96.47)
other indwelling urinary catheter (96.48)
lysis of external adhesions (59.11)
removal of:
cystostomy tube (97.63)
other urinary drainagedevice (97.64)
therapeutic distention of bladder (96.25)

√3ʳᵈ 58 **Operations on urethra**

▶Code also any application or administration of an adhesion barrier substance (99.77)◀

INCLUDES operations on:
bulbourethral gland [Cowper's gland]
periurethral tissue

58.0 **Urethrotomy**

Excision of urethral septum
Formation of urethrovaginal fistula
Perineal urethrostomy
Removal of calculus from urethra by incision

EXCLUDES *drainage of bulbourethral gland or periurethral tissue (58.91)*
internal urethral meatotomy (58.5)
removal of urethral calculus without incision (58.6)

58.1 **Urethral meatotomy**

EXCLUDES *internal urethral meatotomy (58.5)*

DEF: Incision of urethra to enlarge passage.

√4ᵗʰ 58.2 **Diagnostic procedures on urethra**

58.21 **Perineal urethroscopy**

58.22 **Other urethroscopy**

58.23 **Biopsy of urethra**

58.24 **Biopsy of periurethral tissue**

DEF: Removal for biopsy of tissue around urethra.

58.29 **Other diagnostic procedures on urethra and periurethral tissue**

EXCLUDES *microscopic examination of specimen from urethra (91.31-91.39)*
retrograde cystourethrogram (87.76)
urethral pressure profile (89.25)
urethral sphincter electromyogram (89.23)

√4ᵗʰ 58.3 **Excision or destruction of lesion or tissue of urethra**

EXCLUDES *biopsy of urethra (58.23)*
excision of bulbourethral gland (58.92)
fistulectomy (58.43)
urethrectomy as part of:
complete cystectomy (57.79)
pelvic evisceration (68.8)
radical cystectomy (57.71)

58.31 **Endoscopic excision or destruction of lesion or tissue of urethra**

Fulguration of urethral lesion

58.39 **Other local excision or destruction of lesion or tissue of urethra**

Excision of:
congenital valve
lesion
stricture } of urethra

Urethrectomy

EXCLUDES *that by endoscopic appoach (58.31)*

✓4th **58.4**   **Repair of urethra**

EXCLUDES   *repair of current obstetric laceration (75.61)*

58.41   Suture of laceration of urethra

58.42   Closure of urethrostomy

58.43   Closure of other fistula of urethra

EXCLUDES   *repair of urethroperineovesical fistula (57.84)*

58.44   Reanastomosis of urethra

Anastomosis of urethra

DEF: Repair of severed urethra.

58.45   Repair of hypospadias or epispadias

AHA: 3Q, '97, 6; 4Q, '96, 35

DEF: Repair of abnormal urethral opening.

58.46   Other reconstruction of urethra

Urethral construction

58.47   Urethral meatoplasty

DEF: Reconstruction of urethral opening.

58.49   Other repair of urethra

Benenenti rotation of bulbous urethra
Repair of old obstetric laceration of urethra
Urethral plication

EXCLUDES   *repair of:*
   current obstetric laceration (75.61)
   urethrocele (70.50-70.51)

58.5   **Release of urethral stricture**

Cutting of urethral sphincter
Internal urethral meatotomy
Urethrolysis

AHA: 1Q, '97, 13

58.6   **Dilation of urethra**

Dilation of urethrovesical junction
Passage of sounds through urethra
Removal of calculus from urethra without incision

EXCLUDES   *urethral calibration (89.29)*

AHA: 1Q, '01, 14; 1Q, '97, 13

✓4th **58.9**   **Other operations on urethra and periurethral tissue**

58.91   Incision of periurethral tissue

Drainage of bulbourethral gland

DEF: Incision of tissue around urethra.

58.92   Excision of periurethral tissue

EXCLUDES   *biopsy of periurethral tissue (58.24)*
   lysis of periurethral adhesions (59.11-59.12)

58.93   Implantation of artificial urinary sphincter [AUS]

Placement of inflatable:
   urethral sphincter
   bladder sphincter
Removal with replacement of sphincter device [AUS]
With pump and/or reservoir

58.99   Other

Repair of inflatable sphincter pump and/or reservoir
Surgical correction of hydraulic pressure of inflatable sphincter device
Removal of inflatable urinary sphincter without replacement

EXCLUDES   *removal of:*
   intraluminal foreign body from urethra without incision (98.19)
   urethral stent (97.65)

✓3rd **59**   **Other operations on urinary tract**

►Code also any application or administration of an adhesion barrier substance (99.77)◄

✓4th **59.0**   **Dissection of retroperitoneal tissue**

59.00   Retroperitoneal dissection, not otherwise specified

59.02   Other lysis of perirenal or periureteral adhesions

EXCLUDES   *that by laparoscope (59.03)*

59.03   Laparoscopic lysis of perirenal or periureteral adhesions

59.09   Other incision of perirenal or periureteral tissue

Exploration of perinephric area
Incision of perirenal abscess

DEF: Exploration of the perinephric area: Exam of tissue around the kidney by incision.

DEF: Incision of perirenal abscess: Incising abscess in tissue around kidney.

✓4th **59.1**   **Incision of perivesical tissue**

DEF: Incising tissue around bladder.

59.11   Other lysis of perivesical adhesions

59.12   Laparoscopic lysis of perivesical adhesions

59.19   Other incision of perivesical tissue

Exploration of perivesical tissue
Incision of hematoma of space of Retzius
Retropubic exploration

✓4th **59.2**   **Diagnostic procedures on perirenal and perivesical tissue**

59.21   Biopsy of perirenal or perivesical tissue

59.29   Other diagnostic procedures on perirenal tissue, perivesical tissue, and retroperitoneum

EXCLUDES   *microscopic examination of specimen from:*
   perirenal tissue (91.21-91.29)
   perivesical tissue (91.31-91.39)
   retroperitoneum NEC (91.11-91.19)
   retroperitoneal x-ray (88.14-88.16)

59.3   **Plication of urethrovesical junction**

Kelly-Kennedy operation on urethra
Kelly-Stoeckel urethral plication

DEF: Suturing a tuck in tissues around urethra at junction with bladder; changes angle of junction and provides support.

59.4   **Suprapubic sling operation**

Goebel-Frangenheim-Stoeckel urethrovesical suspension
Millin-Read urethrovesical suspension
Oxford operation for urinary incontinence
Urethrocystopexy by suprapubic suspension

DEF: Suspension of urethra from suprapubic periosteum to restore support to bladder and urethra.

59.5   **Retropubic urethral suspension**

Burch procedure
Marshall-Marchetti-Krantz operation
Suture of periurethral tissue to symphysis pubis
Urethral suspension NOS

AHA: 1Q, '97, 11

DEF: Suspension of urethra from pubic bone with suture placed from symphysis pubis to paraurethral tissues; elevates urethrovesical angle, restores urinary continence.

59.6   **Paraurethral suspension**

Pereyra paraurethral suspension
Periurethral suspension

DEF: Suspension of bladder neck from fibrous membranes of anterior abdominal wall; upward traction applied; changes angle of urethra, improves urinary control.

Operations on the Urinary System 59.7–59.99

✓4ᵗʰ **59.7**   **Other repair of urinary stress incontinence**

59.71   **Levator muscle operation for urethrovesical suspension**
    Cystourethropexy with levator muscle sling
    Gracilis muscle transplant for
        urethrovesical suspension
    Pubococcygeal sling

59.72   **Injection of implant into urethra and/or bladder neck**
    Collagen implant
    Endoscopic injection of implant
    Fat implant
    Polytef implant
    AHA: 4Q, '95, 72, 73

    DEF: Injection of collagen into submucosal tissues to increase tissue bulk and improve urinary control.

59.79   **Other**
    Anterior urethropexy
    Repair of stress incontinence NOS
    Tudor "rabbit ear" urethropexy
    AHA: 2Q, '01, 20; 1Q, '00, 14, 15, 19

    DEF: Pubovaginal sling for treatment of stress incontinence: A strip of fascia is harvested and the vaginal epithelium is mobilized and then sutured to the midline at the urethral level to the rectus muscle to create a sling supporting the bladder.

    DEF: Vaginal wall sling with bone anchors for treatment of stress incontinence: A sling for the bladder is formed by a suture attachment of vaginal wall to the abdominal wall. In addition, a suture is run from the vagina to a bone anchor placed in the pubic bone.

    DEF: Transvaginal endoscopic bladder neck suspension for treatment of stress incontinence: Endoscopic surgical suturing of the vaginal epithelium and the pubocervical fascia at the bladder neck level on both sides of the urethra. Two supporting sutures are run from the vagina toan anchor placed in the pubic bone on each side.

59.8   **Ureteral catheterization**
    Drainage of kidney by catheter
    Insertion of ureteral stent
    Ureterovesical orifice dilation
    Code also any ureterotomy (56.2)
    EXCLUDES   *that for:*
            transurethral removal of calculus or clot from ureter and renal pelvis (56.0)
            retrograde pyelogram (87.74)
    AHA: 3Q, '00, 7; 1Q, '89, 1; S-O, '86, 10

✓4ᵗʰ **59.9**   **Other operations on urinary system**
    EXCLUDES   *nonoperative removal of therapeutic device (97.61-97.69)*

59.91   **Excision of perirenal or perivesical tissue**
    EXCLUDES   *biopsy of perirenal or perivesical tissue (59.21)*

59.92   **Other operations on perirenal or perivesical tissue**

59.93   **Replacement of ureterostomy tube**
    Change of ureterostomy tube
    Reinsertion of ureterostomy tube
    EXCLUDES   *nonoperative removal of ureterostomy tube (97.62)*

59.94   **Replacement of cystostomy tube**
    EXCLUDES   *nonoperative removal of cystostomy tube (97.63)*

59.95   **Ultrasonic fragmentation of urinary stones**
    Shattered urinary stones
    EXCLUDES   *percutaneous nephrostomy with fragmentation (55.04)*
            shockwave disintegration (98.51)
    AHA: 1Q, '89, 1; S-O, '86, 11

59.99   **Other**
    EXCLUDES   *instillation of medication into urinary tract (96.49)*
            irrigation of urinary tract (96.45-96.48)

11. OPERATIONS ON THE MALE GENITAL ORGANS (60-64)

√3rd **60** **Operations on prostate and seminal vesicles**
▶Code also any application or administration of an adhesion barrier substance (99.77)◀
|INCLUDES| operations on periprostatic tissue
|EXCLUDES| *that associated with radical cystectomy (57.71)*

60.0 **Incision of prostate**   ♂
Drainage of prostatic abscess
Prostatolithotomy
|EXCLUDES| *drainage of periprostatic tissue only (60.81)*

√4th **60.1** **Diagnostic procedures on prostate and seminal vesicles**

60.11 **Closed [percutaneous] [needle] biopsy of** ♂
prostate
Approach:
  transrectal   Punch biopsy
  transurethral

DEF: Excision of prostate tissue by closed technique for biopsy.

60.12 **Open biopsy of prostate**   ♂
60.13 **Closed [percutaneous] biopsy of seminal** ♂
vesicles
Needle biopsy of seminal vesicles

60.14 **Open biopsy of seminal vesicles**   ♂
60.15 **Biopsy of periprostatic tissue**   ♂
60.18 **Other diagnostic procedures on prostate** ♂
and periprostatic tissue
|EXCLUDES| *microscopic examination of specimen from prostate (91.31-91.39)*
x-ray of prostate (87.92)

60.19 **Other diagnostic procedures on seminal** ♂
vesicles
|EXCLUDES| *microscopic examination of specimen from seminal vesicles (91.31-91.39)*
x-ray:
contrast seminal vesiculogram (87.91)
other (87.92)

√4th **60.2** **Transurethral prostatectomy**
|EXCLUDES| *local excision of lesion of prostate (60.61)*

AHA: 2Q, '94, 9; 3Q, '92, 13

60.21 **Transurethral (ultrasound) guided laser** ♂
induced prostatectomy (TULIP)
Ablation (contact) (noncontact) by laser

AHA: 4Q, '95, 7

60.29 **Other transurethral prostatectomy**   ♂
Excision of median bar by transurethral approach
Transurethral electrovaporization of prostate (TEVAP)
Transurethral enucleative procedure
Transurethral prostatectomy NOS
Transurethral resection of prostate (TURP)

DEF: Excision of median bar by transurethral approach: Removal of fibrous structure of prostate.

DEF: Transurethral enucleate procedure: Transurethral prostatectomy.

AHA: 3Q, '97, 3

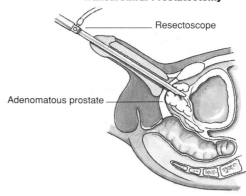

Transurethral Prostatectomy

Resectoscope

Adenomatous prostate

60.3 **Suprapubic prostatectomy**   ♂
Transvesical prostatectomy
|EXCLUDES| *local excision of lesion of prostate (60.61)*
radical prostatectomy (60.5)

DEF: Resection of prostate through incision in abdomen above pubic arch.

60.4 **Retropubic prostatectomy**   ♂
|EXCLUDES| *local excision of lesion of prostate (60.61)*
radical prostatectomy (60.5)

DEF: Removal of the prostate using an abdominal approach with direct cutting into prostatic capsule.

60.5 **Radical prostatectomy**   ♂
Prostatovesiculectomy
Radical prostatectomy by any approach
|EXCLUDES| *cystoprostatectomy (57.71)*

AHA: 3Q, '93, 12

DEF: Removal of prostate, epididymis and vas ampullae.

DEF: Prostatovesiculectomy: Removal of prostate and epididymis.

√4th **60.6** **Other prostatectomy**

60.61 **Local excision of lesion of prostate**   ♂
Excision of prostatic lesion by any approach
|EXCLUDES| *biopsy of prostate (60.11-60.12)*

60.62 **Perineal prostatectomy**   ♂
Cryoablation of prostate
Cryoprostatectomy
Cryosurgery of prostate
Radical cryosurcial ablation of prostate (RCSA)
|EXCLUDES| *local excision of lesion of prostate (60.61)*

AHA: 4Q, '95, 71

DEF: Excision of prostate tissue through incision between scrotum and anus.

60.69 **Other**   ♂
√4th **60.7** **Operations on seminal vesicles**

60.71 **Percutaneous aspiration of seminal**   ♂
vesicle
|EXCLUDES| *needle biopsy of seminal vesicle (60.13)*

60.72 **Incision of seminal vesicle**   ♂
60.73 **Excision of seminal vesicle**   ♂
Excision of Müllerian duct cyst
Spermatocystectomy
|EXCLUDES| *biopsy of seminal vesicle (60.13-60.14)*
prostatovesiculectomy (60.5)

60.79 **Other operations on seminal vesicles** ♂

Operations on Male Genital Organs 60–60.79

Operations on Male Genital Organs 60.8–62.41

✓4th **60.8** **Incision or excision of periprostatic tissue**

     60.81 **Incision of periprostatic tissue** ♂

         Drainage of periprostatic abscess

     60.82 **Excision of periprostatic tissue** ♂

         Excision of lesion of periprostatic tissue

         EXCLUDES *biopsy of periprostatic tissue (60.15)*

✓4th **60.9** **Other operations on prostate**

     60.91 **Percutaneous aspiration of prostate** ♂

         EXCLUDES *needle biopsy of prostate (60.11)*

     60.92 **Injection into prostate** ♂

     60.93 **Repair of prostate** ♂

     60.94 **Control of (postoperative) hemorrhage of prostate** ♂

         Coagulation of prostatic bed

         Cystoscopy for control of prostatic hemorrhage

     60.95 **Transurethral balloon dilation of the prostatic urethra** ♂

         AHA: 4Q, '91, 23

         DEF: Insertion and inflation of balloon to stretch prostate passage.

     60.96 **Transurethral destruction of prostate tissue by microwave thermotherapy** ♂

         Transurethral microwave thermotherapy (TUMT) of prostate

         EXCLUDES *Prostatectomy:*
             other (60.61-60.69)
             radical (60.5)
             retropubic (60.4)
             suprapubic (60.3)
             transurethral (60.21-60.29)

         AHA: 4Q, '00, 67

     60.97 **Other transurethral destruction of prostate tissue by other thermotherapy** ♂

         Radiofrequency thermotherapy

         Transurethral needle ablation (TUNA) of prostate

         EXCLUDES *Prostatectomy:*
             other (60.61-60.69)
             radical (60.5)
             retropubic (60.4)
             suprapubic (60.3)
             transurethral (60.21-60.29)

         AHA: 4Q, '00, 67

     60.99 **Other** ♂

         EXCLUDES *prostatic massage (99.94)*

         AHA: 3Q, '90, 12

✓3rd **61** **Operations on scrotum and tunica vaginalis**

     61.0 **Incision and drainage of scrotum and tunica vaginalis** ♂

         EXCLUDES *percutaneous aspiration of hydrocele (61.91)*

✓4th **61.1** **Diagnostic procedures on scrotum and tunica vaginalis**

     61.11 **Biopsy of scrotum or tunica vaginalis** ♂

     61.19 **Other diagnostic procedures on scrotum and tunica vaginalis** ♂

     61.2 **Excision of hydrocele (of tunica vaginalis)** ♂

         Bottle repair of hydrocele of tunica vaginalis

         EXCLUDES *percutaneous aspiration of hydrocele (61.91)*

         DEF: Removal of fluid collected in serous membrane of testes.

Hydrocelectomy

Scrotal skin incised
Sac opened
Fluid-filled sac mobilized
Excess tissue trimmed
Testis
Remaining sacular tissue folded back and sewn to itself to preclude recurrence ("bottle" procedure)

     61.3 **Excision or destruction of lesion or tissue of scrotum** ♂

         Fulguration of lesion
         Reduction of elephantiasis } of scrotum
         Partial scrotectomy

         EXCLUDES *biopsy of scrotum (61.11)*
                scrotal fistulectomy (61.42)

✓4th **61.4** **Repair of scrotum and tunica vaginalis**

     61.41 **Suture of laceration of scrotum and tunica vaginalis** ♂

     61.42 **Repair of scrotal fistula** ♂

     61.49 **Other repair of scrotum and tunica vaginalis** ♂

         Reconstruction with rotational or pedicle flaps

✓4th **61.9** **Other operations on scrotum and tunica vaginalis**

     61.91 **Percutaneous aspiration of tunica vaginalis** ♂

         Aspiration of hydrocele of tunica vaginalis

     61.92 **Excision of lesion of tunica vaginalis other than hydrocele** ♂

         Excision of hematocele of tunica vaginalis

         DEF: Removal of blood collected in tunica vaginalis.

     61.99 **Other** ♂

         EXCLUDES *removal of foreign body from scrotum without incision (98.24)*

✓3rd **62** **Operations on testes**

     62.0 **Incision of testis** ♂

✓4th **62.1** **Diagnostic procedures on testes**

     62.11 **Closed [percutaneous] [needle] biopsy of testis** ♂

     62.12 **Open biopsy of testis** ♂

     62.19 **Other diagnostic procedures on testes** ♂

     62.2 **Excision or destruction of testicular lesion** ♂

         Excision of appendix testis

         Excision of cyst of Morgagni in the male

         EXCLUDES *biopsy of testis (62.11-62.12)*

     62.3 **Unilateral orchiectomy** ♂

         Orchidectomy (with epididymectomy) NOS

✓4th **62.4** **Bilateral orchiectomy**

         Male castration

         Radical bilateral orchiectomy (with epididymectomy)

         Code also any synchronous lymph node dissection (40.3, 40.5)

         DEF: Removal of both testes.

         DEF: Radical bilateral orchiectomy (with epididymectomy): Excision of both testes and structures that store sperm.

     62.41 **Removal of both testes at same operative episode** ♂

         Bilateral orchiectomy NOS

BI Bilateral Edit   **NC** Non-covered Procedure   ▶◀ Revised Text   ● New Code   ▲ Revised Code Title

62.42   **Removal of remaining testis**   ♂
Removal of solitary testis

62.5   **Orchiopexy**   ♂
Mobilization and replacement of testis in scrotum
Orchiopexy with detorsion of testis
Torek (-Bevan) operation (orchidopexy) (first stage)
(second stage)
Transplantation to and fixation of testis in scrotum

DEF: Fixation of testis in scrotum.

DEF: Orchiopexy with detorsion of testis: Fixation and placement of testis in scrotum after correcting angle.

DEF: Torek operation (first stage) (second stage): Transfer of congenitally undescended testis from inguinal canal to scrotum.

DEF: Transplantation to and fixation of testis in scrotum: Transfer of displaced testis to scrotum.

√4th **62.6**   **Repair of testes**
EXCLUDES   reduction of torsion (63.52)
62.61   **Suture of laceration of testis**   ♂
62.69   **Other repair of testis**   ♂
Testicular graft

62.7   **Insertion of testicular prosthesis**   ♂

√4th **62.9**   **Other operations on testes**
62.91   **Aspiration of testis**   ♂
EXCLUDES   percutaneous biopsy of testis (62.11)
62.92   **Injection of therapeutic substance into**   ♂
testis
62.99   **Other**   ♂

√3rd **63**   **Operations on spermatic cord, epididymis, and vas deferens**

√4th **63.0**   **Diagnostic procedures on spermatic cord, epididymis, and vas deferens**
63.01   **Biopsy of spermatic cord, epididymis,**   ♂
or vas deferens
63.09   **Other diagnostic procedures on**   ♂
spermatic cord, epididymis, and vas
deferens
EXCLUDES   contrast epididymogram (87.93)
contrast vasogram (87.94)
other x-ray of epididymis and vas deferens (87.95)

63.1   **Excision of varicocele and hydrocele of**   ♂
spermatic cord
High ligation of spermatic vein
Hydrocelectomy of canal of Nuck

DEF: Removal of a swollen vein and collected fluid from spermatic cord.

DEF: High ligation of spermatic vein: Tying off of spermatic vein.

DEF: Hydrocelectomy of canal of Nuck: Removal of fluid collected from serous membrane of inguinal canal.

Varicocelectomy

Ligated veins
Pampiniform plexus
Ligated veins
Vas deferens
Artery

63.2   **Excision of cyst of epididymis**   ♂
Spermatocelectomy

63.3   **Excision of other lesion or tissue of spermatic**   ♂
cord and epididymis
Excision of appendix epididymis
EXCLUDES   biopsy of spermatic cord or epididymis (63.01)

63.4   **Epididymectomy**   ♂
EXCLUDES   that synchronous with orchiectomy (62.3-62.42)

√4th **63.5**   **Repair of spermatic cord and epididymis**
63.51   **Suture of laceration of spermatic cord**   ♂
and epididymis
63.52   **Reduction of torsion of testis or**   ♂
spermatic cord
EXCLUDES   that associated with orchiopexy (62.5)

DEF: Correction of twisted testicle or spermatic cord.

63.53   **Transplantation of spermatic cord**   ♂
63.59   **Other repair of spermatic cord and**   ♂
epididymis

63.6   **Vasotomy**   ♂
Vasostomy

DEF: Vasotomy: Incision of ducts carrying sperm from testicles.

DEF: Vasostomy: Creation of an opening into duct.

√4th **63.7**   **Vasectomy and ligation of vas deferens**
63.70   **Male sterilization procedure, not**   NC ♂
otherwise specified
63.71   **Ligation of vas deferens**   NC ♂
Crushing of vas deferens
Division of vas deferens
63.72   **Ligation of spermatic cord**   NC ♂
63.73   **Vasectomy**   NC ♂
AHA: 2Q, '98, 13

√4th **63.8**   **Repair of vas deferens and epididymis**
63.81   **Suture of laceration of vas deferens**   ♂
and epididymis
63.82   **Reconstruction of surgically divided vas**   ♂
deferens
63.83   **Epididymovasostomy**   ♂

DEF: Creation of new connection between vas deferens and epididymis.

63.84   **Removal of ligature from vas deferens**   ♂
63.85   **Removal of valve from vas deferens**   ♂
63.89   **Other repair of vas deferens and**   ♂
epididymis

√4th **63.9**   **Other operations on spermatic cord, epididymis, and vas deferens**
63.91   **Aspiration of spermatocele**   ♂

DEF: Puncture of cystic distention of epididymis.

63.92   **Epididymotomy**   ♂

DEF: Incision of epididymis.

63.93   **Incision of spermatic cord**   ♂

DEF: Incision into sperm storage structure.

63.94   **Lysis of adhesions of spermatic cord**   ♂
63.95   **Insertion of valve in vas deferens**   ♂
63.99   **Other**   ♂

√3rd **64**   **Operations on penis**
INCLUDES   operations on:
corpora cavernosa
glans penis
prepuce

64.0   **Circumcision**   ♂

DEF: Removal of penis foreskin.

√3rd√4th Additional Digit Required   Nonspecific OR Procedure   Valid OR Procedure   Non-OR Procedure

√4ᵗʰ 64.1　Diagnostic procedures on the penis
64.11　**Biopsy of penis**　♂
64.19　Other diagnostic procedures on penis　♂

64.2　Local excision or destruction of lesion of penis　♂
　　　　EXCLUDES　biopsy of penis (64.11)

64.3　Amputation of penis　♂

√4ᵗʰ 64.4　Repair and plastic operation on penis
64.41　**Suture of laceration of penis**　♂
64.42　**Release of chordee**　♂
　　　　AHA: 4Q, '96, 34

　　　　DEF: Correction of downward displacement of penis.

64.43　**Construction of penis**　♂
64.44　**Reconstruction of penis**　♂
64.45　**Replantation of penis**　♂
　　　　Reattachment of amputated penis
64.49　**Other repair of penis**　♂
　　　　EXCLUDES　repair of epispadias and
　　　　　　　　　　hypospadias (58.45)

64.5　Operations for sex transformation, not　NC ♂
elsewhere classified

√4ᵗʰ 64.9　Other operations on male genital organs
64.91　**Dorsal or lateral slit of prepuce**　♂
64.92　**Incision of penis**　♂
64.93　**Division of penile adhesions**　♂
64.94　**Fitting of external prosthesis of penis**　♂
　　　　Penile prosthesis NOS
64.95　**Insertion or replacement of non-inflatable** ♂
penile prosthesis
　　　　Insertion of semi-rigid rod prosthesis into
　　　　　shaft of penis
　　　　EXCLUDES　external penile prosthesis
　　　　　　　　　　(64.94)
　　　　　　　　　inflatable penile prosthesis
　　　　　　　　　　(64.97)
　　　　　　　　　plastic repair, penis (64.43-
　　　　　　　　　　64.49)
　　　　　　　　　that associated with:
　　　　　　　　　　construction (64.43)
　　　　　　　　　　reconstruction (64.44)

64.96　**Removal of internal prosthesis of penis**　♂
　　　　Removal without replacement of non-
　　　　　inflatable or inflatable penile
　　　　　prosthesis

64.97　Insertion or replacement of inflatable　♂
penile prosthesis
　　　Insertion of cylinders into shaft of penis and
　　　　placement of pump and reservoir
　　　EXCLUDES　external penile prosthesis
　　　　　　　　　(64.94)
　　　　　　　　non-inflatable penile
　　　　　　　　　prosthesis (64.95)
　　　　　　　　plastic repair, penis (64.43-
　　　　　　　　　64.49)

64.98　Other operations on penis　♂
　　　Corpora cavernosa-corpus spongiosum
　　　　shunt
　　　Corpora-saphenous shunt
　　　Irrigation of corpus cavernosum
　　　EXCLUDES　removal of foreign body:
　　　　　　　　　intraluminal (98.19)
　　　　　　　　　without incision (98.24)
　　　　　　　　stretching of foreskin (99.95)

　　　AHA: 3Q, '92, 9

　　　DEF: Corpora cavernosa-corpus spongiosum shunt:
　　　Insertion of shunt between erectile tissues of penis.

　　　DEF: Corpora-saphenous shunt: Insertion of shunt
　　　between erectile tissue and vein of penis.

　　　DEF: Irrigation of corpus cavernosum: Washing of
　　　erectile tissue forming dorsum and side of penis.

64.99　Other　♂
　　　EXCLUDES　collection of sperm for artificial
　　　　　　　　　insemination (99.96)

BI　Bilateral Edit　　　NC　Non-covered Procedure　　　►◄ Revised Text　　　● New Code　　　▲ Revised Code Title

12. OPERATIONS ON THE FEMALE GENITAL ORGANS (65–71)

✓3rd 65 Operations on ovary
▶Code also any application or administration of an adhesion barrier substance (99.77)◀

✓4th 65.0 Oophorotomy
Salpingo-oophorotomy

DEF: Incision into ovary.

DEF: Salpingo-oophorotomy: Incision into ovary and the fallopian tube.

65.01 **Laparoscopic oophorotomy** ♀
65.09 **Other oophorotomy** ♀

✓4th 65.1 Diagnostic procedures on ovaries
65.11 **Aspiration biopsy of ovary** ♀
65.12 **Other biopsy of ovary** ♀
65.13 **Laparoscopic biopsy of ovary** ♀
AHA: 4Q, '96, 67

65.14 **Other laparoscopic diagnostic procedures on ovaries** ♀
65.19 **Other diagnostic procedures on ovaries** ♀
EXCLUDES microscopic examination of specimen from ovary (91.41-91.49)

✓4th 65.2 Local excision or destruction of ovarian lesion or tissue
65.21 **Marsupialization of ovarian cyst** ♀
EXCLUDES that by laparoscope (65.23)
DEF: Exteriorized cyst to outside by incising anterior wall and suturing cut edges to create open pouch.

65.22 **Wedge resection of ovary** ♀
EXCLUDES that by laparoscope (65.24)
65.23 **Laparoscopic marsupialization of ovarian cyst** ♀
65.24 **Laparoscopic wedge resection of ovary** ♀
65.25 **Other laparoscopic local excision or destruction of ovary** ♀
65.29 **Other local excision or destruction of ovary** ♀

Bisection ⎫
Cauterization ⎬ of ovary
Partial excision ⎭

EXCLUDES biopsy of ovary (65.11-65.13) that by laparoscope (65.25)

✓4th 65.3 Unilateral oophorectomy
65.31 **Laparoscopic unilateral oophorectomy** ♀
65.39 **Other unilateral oophorectomy** ♀
EXCLUDES that by laparoscope (65.31)
AHA: 4Q, '96, 66

✓4th 65.4 Unilateral salpingo-oophorectomy
65.41 **Laparoscopic unilateral salpingo-oophorectomy** ♀
AHA: 4Q, '96, 67

65.49 **Other unilateral salpingo-oophorectomy** ♀

Oophorectomy

Fallopian tube
Fimbria
Ovary
Ovarian cyst

✓4th 65.5 Bilateral oophorectomy
65.51 **Other removal of both ovaries at same operative episode** ♀
Female castration
EXCLUDES that by laparoscope (65.53)
65.52 **Other removal of remaining ovary** ♀
Removal of solitary ovary
EXCLUDES that by laparoscope (65.54)
65.53 **Laparoscopic removal of both ovaries at same operative eisode** ♀
65.54 **Laparoscopic removal of remaining ovary** ♀

✓4th 65.6 Bilateral salpingo-oophorectomy
65.61 **Other removal of both ovaries and tubes at same operative episode** ♀
EXCLUDES that by laparoscope (65.53)
AHA: 4Q, '96, 65

65.62 **Other removal of remaining ovary and tube** ♀
Removal of solitary ovary and tube
EXCLUDES that by laparoscope (65.54)
65.63 **Laparoscopic removal of both ovaries and tubes at the same operative episode** ♀
AHA: 4Q, '96, 68

65.64 **Laparoscopic removal of remaining ovary and tube** ♀

✓4th 65.7 Repair of ovary
EXCLUDES salpingo-oophorostomy (66.72)
65.71 **Other simple suture of ovary** ♀
EXCLUDES that by laparoscope (65.74)
65.72 **Other reimplantation of ovary** ♀
EXCLUDES that by laparoscope (65.75)
DEF: Grafting and repositioning of ovary at same site.

65.73 **Other salpingo-oophoroplasty** ♀
EXCLUDES that by laparoscope (65.76)
65.74 **Laparoscopic simple suture of ovary** ♀
65.75 **Laparoscopic reimplantation of ovary** ♀
65.76 **Laparoscopic salpingo-oophoroplasty** ♀
65.79 **Other repair of ovary** ♀
Oophoropexy

✓4th 65.8 Lysis of adhesions of ovary and fallopian tube
65.81 **Laparoscopic lysis of adhesions of ovary and fallopian tube** ♀
AHA: 4Q, '96, 67

65.89 **Other lysis of adhesions of ovary and fallopian tube** ♀
EXCLUDES that by laparoscope (65.81)

✓4th 65.9 Other operations on ovary
65.91 **Aspiration of ovary** ♀
EXCLUDES aspiration biopsy of ovary (65.11)
65.92 **Transplantation of ovary** ♀
EXCLUDES reimplantation of ovary (65.72, 65.75)
65.93 **Manual rupture of ovarian cyst** ♀
DEF: Breaking up an ovarian cyst using manual technique or blunt instruments.

65.94 **Ovarian denervation** ♀
DEF: Destruction of nerve tracts to ovary.

65.95 **Release of torsion of ovary** ♀

Operations on the Female Genital System 65.99–66.9

Endoscopic Ligation of Fallopian Tubes

Ligated fallopian tube

Uterus
Ovary

Monitor view

Laparoscopic
procedure

65.99   **Other**   ♀
AHA: N-D, '86, 9

√3rd **66**   **Operations on fallopian tubes**
▶Code also any application or administration of an adhesion barrier substance (99.77)◀

√4th **66.0**   **Salpingotomy and salpingostomy**
   66.01   **Salpingotomy**   ♀
   66.02   **Salpingostomy**   ♀

√4th **66.1**   **Diagnostic procedures on fallopian tubes**
   66.11   **Biopsy of fallopian tube**   ♀
   66.19   **Other diagnostic procedures on fallopian tubes**   ♀
     EXCLUDES   *microscopic examination of specimen from fallopian tubes (91.41-91.49)*
       radiography of fallopian tubes (87.82-87.83, 87.85)
       Rubin's test (66.8)

√4th **66.2**   **Bilateral endoscopic destruction or occlusion of fallopian tubes**
     INCLUDES   bilateral endoscopic destruction or occlusion of fallopian tubes by:
     culdoscopy   laparoscopy
     endoscopy   peritoneoscopy
     hysteroscopy
     endoscopic destruction of solitary fallopian tube

DEF: Endoscopic blockage or destruction of both fallopian tubes.

DEF: Bilateral endoscopic destruction or occlusion of fallopian tubes by:

Culdoscopy: Endoscopic insertion through posterior structure of vagina.

Hysteroscopy: Endoscopic insertion through uterus.

Laparoscopy: Endoscopic insertion through abdomen.

Peritoneoscopy: Endoscopic insertion through abdominal serous membrane cavity.

Endoscopic destruction of solitary fallopian tube: Endoscopic destruction of one fallopian tube.

   66.21   **Bilateral endoscopic ligation and crushing of fallopian tubes**   NC ♀
   66.22   **Bilateral endoscopic ligation and division of fallopian tubes**   NC ♀
   66.29   **Other bilateral endoscopic destruction or occlusion of fallopian tubes**   NC ♀

√4th **66.3**   **Other bilateral destruction or occlusion of fallopian tubes**
     INCLUDES   destruction of solitary fallopian tube

     EXCLUDES   *endoscopic destruction or occlusion of fallopian tubes (66.21-66.29)*
   66.31   **Other bilateral ligation and crushing of fallopian tubes**   NC ♀
   66.32   **Other bilateral ligation and division of fallopian tubes**   NC ♀
     Pomeroy operation
   66.39   **Other bilateral destruction or occlusion of fallopian tubes**   NC ♀
     Female sterilization operation NOS

  66.4   **Total unilateral salpingectomy**   ♀

√4th **66.5**   **Total bilateral salpingectomy**
     EXCLUDES   *bilateral partial salpingectomy for sterilization (66.39)*
       that with oophorectomy (65.61-65.64)
   66.51   **Removal of both fallopian tubes at same operative episode**   ♀
   66.52   **Removal of remaining fallopian tube**   ♀
     Removal of solitary fallopian tube

√4th **66.6**   **Other salpingectomy**
     INCLUDES   salpingectomy by:
       cauterization
       coagulation
       electrocoagulation
       excision
     EXCLUDES   *fistulectomy (66.73)*
   66.61   **Excision or destruction of lesion of fallopian tube**   ♀
     EXCLUDES   *biopsy of fallopian tube (66.11)*
   66.62   **Salpingectomy with removal of tubal pregnancy**   ♀
     Code also any synchronous oophorectomy (65.31, 65.39)
     AHA: 3Q, '95, 15; S-O, '85, 14
   66.63   **Bilateral partial salpingectomy, not otherwise specified**   ♀
   66.69   **Other partial salpingectomy**   ♀

√4th **66.7**   **Repair of fallopian tube**
   66.71   **Simple suture of fallopian tube**   ♀
   66.72   **Salpingo-oophorostomy**   ♀
   66.73   **Salpingo-salpingostomy**   ♀
   66.74   **Salpingo-uterostomy**   ♀
   66.79   **Other repair of fallopian tube**   ♀
     Graft of fallopian tube
     Reopening of divided fallopian tube
     Salpingoplasty
     AHA: 2Q, '95, 10

DEF: Graft of fallopian: Repair of fallopian tube with implanted graft.

DEF: Reopening of divided fallopian tube: Reconnection of severed fallopian tube to restore patency.

DEF: Salpingoplasty: Plastic reconstruction of fallopian tube defect.

  66.8   **Insufflation of fallopian tube**
     Insufflation of fallopian tube with:
       air
       dye
       gas
       saline
     Rubin's test
     EXCLUDES   *insufflation of therapeutic agent (66.95)*
       that for hysterosalpingography (87.82-87.83)

DEF: Forceful blowing of gas or liquid into fallopian tubes.

DEF: Rubin's test: Introduction of carbon dioxide gas into fallopian tubes.

√4th **66.9**   **Other operations on fallopian tubes**

BI Bilateral Edit   NC Non-covered Procedure   ▶◀ Revised Text   ● New Code   ▲ Revised Code Title

66.91   Aspiration of fallopian tube

66.92   Unilateral destruction or occlusion of fallopian tube   ♀
   EXCLUDES   that of solitary tube (66.21-66.39)

66.93   Implantation or replacement of prosthesis of fallopian tube   ♀

66.94   Removal of prosthesis of fallopian tube   ♀

66.95   Insufflation of therapeutic agent into fallopian tubes   ♀

66.96   Dilation of fallopian tube   ♀

66.97   Burying of fimbriae in uterine wall   ♀
   DEF: Implantation of fallopian tube, fringed edges into uterine wall.

66.99   Other   ♀
   EXCLUDES   lysis of adhesions of ovary and tube (65.81, 65.89)

   AHA: 2Q, '94, 11

√3rd **67   Operations on cervix**
   ▶Code also any application or administration of an adhesion barrier substance (99.77)◄

67.0   Dilation of cervical canal   ♀
   EXCLUDES   dilation and curettage (69.01-69.09)
   that for induction of labor (73.1)

√4th **67.1**   Diagnostic procedures on cervix

67.11   Endocervical biopsy   ♀
   EXCLUDES   conization of cervix (67.2)

67.12   Other cervical biopsy   ♀
   Punch biopsy of cervix NOS
   EXCLUDES   conization of cervix (67.2)

67.19   Other diagnostic procedures on cervix   ♀
   EXCLUDES   microscopic examination of specimen from cervix (91.41-91.49)

67.2   Conization of cervix   ♀
   EXCLUDES   that by:
   cryosurgery (67.33)
   electrosurgery (67.32)
   DEF: Removal of cone-shaped section from distal cervix; cervical function preserved.

√4th **67.3**   Other excision or destruction of lesion or tissue of cervix

67.31   Marsupialization of cervical cyst   ♀
   DEF: Incision and then suturing open of a cyst in the neck of the uterus.

67.32   Destruction of lesion of cervix by cauterization   ♀
   Electroconization of cervix
   LEEP (loop electrosurgical excision procedure)
   LLETZ (large loop excision of the transformation zone)
   AHA: 1Q, '98, 3
   DEF: Destruction of lesion of uterine neck by applying intense heat.
   DEF: Electroconization of cervix: Electrocautery excision of multilayer cone-shaped section from uterine neck.

67.33   Destruction of lesion of cervix by cryosurgery   ♀
   Cryoconization of cervix
   DEF: Destruction of lesion of uterine neck by freezing.
   DEF: Cryoconization of cervix: Excision by freezing of multilayer cone-shaped section of abnormal tissue in uterine neck.

67.39   Other excision or destruction of lesion or tissue of cervix   ♀
   EXCLUDES   biopsy of cervix (67.11-67.12)
   cervical fistulectomy (67.62)
   conization of cervix (67.2)

Cerclage of Cervix

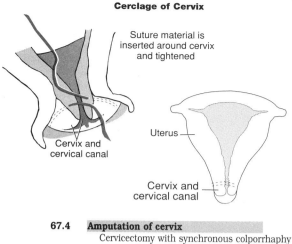

Suture material is inserted around cervix and tightened

Uterus

Cervix and cervical canal

Cervix and cervical canal

67.4   Amputation of cervix   ♀
   Cervicectomy with synchronous colporrhaphy
   DEF: Excision of lower uterine neck.
   DEF: Cervicectomy with synchronous colporrhaphy: Excision of lower uterine neck with suture of vaginal stump.

√4th **67.5**   Repair of internal cervical os
   AHA: 4Q, '01, 63; 3Q, '00; 11
   DEF: Repair of cervical opening defect.

67.51   Transabdominal cerclage of cervix

67.59   Other repair of internal cervical os
   Cerclage of isthmus uteri
   McDonald operation
   Shirodkar operation
   Transvaginal cerclage
   EXCLUDES   transabdominal cerclage of cervix (67.51)
   DEF: Cerclage of isthmus uteri: Placement of encircling suture in the constricted part of the between neck and body of uterus.
   DEF: Shirodkar operation: Placement of purse-string suture in internal cervical opening.

√4th **67.6**   Other repair of cervix
   EXCLUDES   repair of current obstetric laceration (75.51)

67.61   Suture of laceration of cervix   ♀

67.62   Repair of fistula of cervix   ♀
   Cervicosigmoidal fistulectomy
   EXCLUDES   fistulectomy:
   cervicovesical (57.84)
   ureterocervical (56.84)
   vesicocervicovaginal (57.84)
   DEF: Closure of fistula in lower uterus.
   DEF: Cervicosigmoidal fistulectomy: Excision of abnormal passage between uterine neck and torsion of large intestine.

67.69   Other repair of cervix   ♀
   Repair of old obstetric laceration of cervix

√3rd **68   Other incision and excision of uterus**
   ▶Code also any application or administration of an adhesion barrier substance (99.77)◄

68.0   Hysterotomy   ♀
   Hysterotomy with removal of hydatidiform mole
   EXCLUDES   hysterotomy for termination of pregnancy (74.91)
   DEF: Incision into the uterus

√4th **68.1**   Diagnostic procedures on uterus and supporting structures

Operations on the Female Genital System 68.11–68.9

68.11   **Digital examination of uterus**   ♀
> EXCLUDES   pelvic examination, so described (89.26)
> postpartal manual exploration of uterine cavity (75.7)

68.12   **Hysteroscopy**   ♀
> EXCLUDES   that with biopsy (68.16)

68.13   **Open biopsy of uterus**   ♀
> EXCLUDES   closed biopsy of uterus (68.16)

68.14   **Open biopsy of uterine ligaments**   ♀
> EXCLUDES   closed biopsy of uterine ligaments (68.15)

68.15   **Closed biopsy of uterine ligaments**   ♀
> Endoscopic (laparoscopy) biopsy of uterine adnexa, except ovary and fallopian tube

68.16   **Closed biopsy of uterus**   ♀
> Endoscopic (laparoscopy) (hysteroscopy) biopsy of uterus
> EXCLUDES   open biopsy of uterus (68.13)

68.19   **Other diagnostic procedures on uterus and supporting structures**   ♀
> EXCLUDES   diagnostic:
> aspiration curettage (69.59)
> dilation and curettage (69.09)
> microscopic examination of specimen from uterus (91.41-91.49)
> pelvic examination (89.26)
> radioisotope scan of:
> placenta (92.17)
> uterus (92.19)
> ultrasonography of uterus (88.78-88.79)
> x-ray of uterus (87.81-87.89)

✓4th **68.2**   **Excision or destruction of lesion or tissue of uterus**

68.21   **Division of endometrial synechiae**   ♀
> Lysis of intraluminal uterine adhesions

DEF: Separation of uterine adhesions.

DEF: Lysis of intraluminal uterine adhesion: Surgical destruction of adhesive, fibrous structures inside uterine cavity.

68.22   **Incision or excision of congenital septum of uterus**   ♀

68.23   **Endometrial ablation**   ♀
> Dilation and curettage
> Hysteroscopic endometrial ablation

AHA: 4Q, '96, 68

DEF: Removal or destruction of uterine lining; usually by electrocautery or loop electrosurgical excision procedure (LEEP).

68.29   **Other excision or destruction of lesion of uterus**   ♀
> Uterine myomectomy
> EXCLUDES   biopsy of uterus (68.13)
> uterine fistulectomy (69.42)

AHA: 1Q, '96, 14

68.3   **Subtotal abdominal hysterectomy**   ♀
> Supracervical hysterectomy

DEF: Excision of uterus, except lowest part, through abdominal incision.

Vaginal Hysterectomy

Total hysterectomy (uterus only removed)

Total hysterectomy with bilateral salpingectomy (uterus and tubes removed)

Total hysterectomy with bilateral salpingo-oophorectomy (uterus, tubes, and ovaries removed)

68.4   **Total abdominal hysterectomy**   ♀
> Hysterectomy:
> extended
> Code also any synchronous removal of tubes and ovaries (65.3-65.6)

AHA: 4Q, '96, 65

DEF: Complete excision of uterus and uterine neck through abdominal incision.

✓4th **68.5**   **Vaginal hysterectomy**
> Code also any synchronous:
> removal of tubes and ovaries (65.31-65.64)
> repair of cystocele or rectocele (70.50-70.52)
> repair of pelvic floor (70.79)

DEF: Complete excision of the uterus by a vaginal approach.

68.51   **Laparoscopically assisted vaginal hysterectomy (LAVH)**   ♀

AHA: 4Q, '96, 68

68.59   **Other vaginal hysterectomy**   ♀
> EXCLUDES   laparoscopically assisted vaginal hysterectomy (68.51)
> radical vaginal hysterectomy (68.7)

68.6   **Radical abdominal hysterectomy**   ♀
> Modified radical hysterectomy
> Wertheim's operation
> Code also any synchronous:
> lymph gland dissection (40.3, 40.5)
> removal of tubes and ovaries (65.61-65.64)
> EXCLUDES   pelvic evisceration (68.8)

DEF: Excision of uterus, loose connective tissue and smooth muscle around uterus and vagina via abdominal approach.

68.7   **Radical vaginal hysterectomy**   ♀
> Schauta operation
> Code also any synchronous:
> lymph gland dissection (40.3, 40.5)
> removal of tubes and ovaries (65.61-65.64)

DEF: Excision of uterus, loose connective tissue and smooth muscle around uterus and vagina via vaginal approach.

68.8   **Pelvic evisceration**   ♀
> Removal of ovaries, tubes, uterus, vagina, bladder, and urethra (with removal of sigmoid colon and rectum)
> Code also any synchronous:
> colostomy (46.10-46.13)
> lymph gland dissection (40.3, 40.5)
> urinary diversion (56.51-56.79)

68.9   **Other and unspecified hysterectomy**   ♀
> Hysterectomy NOS
> EXCLUDES   abdominal hysterectomy, any approach (68.3, 68.4, 68.6)
> vaginal hysterectomy, any approach (68.51, 68.59, 68.7)

BI Bilateral Edit   NC Non-covered Procedure   ►◄ Revised Text   ● New Code   ▲ Revised Code Title

Dilation and Curettage

Cervix (being dilated)

Fallopian tube

Ovary

Curetting endometrium

Cervix

Vagina

✓3rd **69 Other operations on uterus and supporting structures**
▶Code also any application or administration of an adhesion barrier substance (99.77)◀

✓4th **69.0 Dilation and curettage of uterus**
  EXCLUDES aspiration curettage of uterus (69.51-69.59)
  DEF: Stretching of uterine neck to scrape tissue from walls.

  69.01 Dilation and curettage for termination of pregnancy ♀
    AHA: 1Q, '98, 4

  69.02 Dilation and curettage following delivery or abortion ♀
    AHA: 3Q, '93, 6

  69.09 Other dilation and curettage ♀
    Diagnostic D and C
    AHA: 1Q, '98, 4

✓4th **69.1 Excision or destruction of lesion or tissue of uterus and supporting structures**

  69.19 Other excision or destruction of uterus and supporting structures ♀
    EXCLUDES biopsy of uterine ligament (68.14)

✓4th **69.2 Repair of uterine supporting structures**

  69.21 Interposition operation ♀
    Watkins procedure
    DEF: Repositioning or realignment of bladder and uterus.

  69.22 Other uterine suspension ♀
    Hysteropexy
    Manchester operation
    Plication of uterine ligament
    DEF: Hysteropexy: Fixation or anchoring of uterus.

    DEF: Manchester operation: Fixation or anchoring of uterus with suppurative banding tissue of uterine neck and vagina.

    DEF: Plication of uterine ligament: Creation of tucks in suppurative uterine banding tissue.

  69.23 Vaginal repair of chronic inversion of uterus ♀
    DEF: Repositioning of inverted uterus via vaginal approach.

  69.29 Other repair of uterus and supporting structures ♀

  69.3 Paracervical uterine denervation ♀

✓4th **69.4 Uterine repair**
    EXCLUDES repair of current obstetric laceration (75.50-75.52)

  69.41 Suture of laceration of uterus ♀

  69.42 Closure of fistula of uterus ♀
    EXCLUDES uterovesical fistulectomy (57.84)

  69.49 Other repair of uterus ♀
    Repair of old obstetric laceration of uterus

✓4th **69.5 Aspiration curettage of uterus**
    EXCLUDES menstrual extraction (69.6)

  69.51 Aspiration curettage of uterus for termination of pregnancy ♀
    Therapeutic abortion NOS

  69.52 Aspiration curettage following delivery or abortion ♀

  69.59 Other aspiration curettage of uterus ♀
    AHA: 1Q, '98, 7

  69.6 Menstrual extraction or regulation ♀
    DEF: Induction of menstruation by low pressure suction.

  69.7 Insertion of intrauterine contraceptive device ♀

✓4th **69.9 Other operations on uterus, cervix, and supporting structures** ♀
    EXCLUDES obstetric dilation or incision of cervix (73.1, 73.93)

  69.91 Insertion of therapeutic device into uterus ♀
    EXCLUDES insertion of:
      intrauterine contraceptive device (69.7)
      laminaria (69.93)
      obstetric insertion of bag, bougie, or pack (73.1)

  69.92 Artificial insemination ♀

  69.93 Insertion of laminaria ♀
    DEF: Placement of laminaria, a sea kelp, in cervical os to induce labor; applied for six to 12 hours.

  69.94 Manual replacement of inverted uterus ♀
    EXCLUDES that in immediate postpartal period (75.94)

  69.95 Incision of cervix ♀
    EXCLUDES that to assist delivery (73.93)

  69.96 Removal of cerclage material from cervix
    DEF: Removal of ring inserted to restore uterine neck competency.

  69.97 Removal of other penetrating foreign body from cervix ♀
    EXCLUDES removal of intraluminal foreign body from cervix (98.16)

  69.98 Other operations on supporting structures of uterus ♀
    EXCLUDES biopsy of uterine ligament (68.14)

  69.99 Other operations on cervix and uterus ♀
    EXCLUDES removal of:
      foreign body (98.16)
      intrauterine contraceptive device (97.71)
      obstetric bag, bougie, or pack (97.72)
      packing (97.72)

✓3rd **70 Operations on vagina and cul-de-sac**
    ▶Code also any application or administration of an adhesion barrier substance (99.77)◀

  70.0 Culdocentesis ♀
    AHA: 2Q, '90, 26
    DEF: Insertion of needle into upper vaginal vault encircling cervix to withdraw fluid.

✓4th **70.1 Incision of vagina and cul-de-sac**

  70.11 Hymenotomy ♀

  70.12 Culdotomy ♀
    DEF: Incision into pocket between terminal end of large intestine and posterior uterus.

✓3rd ✓4th Additional Digit Required

2002 Ingenix, Inc.

Nonspecific OR Procedure

Valid OR Procedure

Non-OR Procedure

October 2002 • Volume 3 —161

Operations on the Female Genital System 69–70.12

Operations on the Female Genital System 70.13–71.22

70.13   **Lysis of intraluminal adhesions of vagina** ♀

70.14   **Other vaginotomy** ♀
Division of vaginal septum
Drainage of hematoma of vaginal cuff

DEF: Division of vaginal septum: Incision into partition of vaginal walls.

DEF: Drainage of hematoma of vaginal cuff: Incision into vaginal tissue to drain collected blood.

✓4th **70.2**   **Diagnostic procedures on vagina and cul-de-sac**

70.21   **Vaginoscopy** ♀
70.22   **Culdoscopy** ♀

DEF: Endoscopic exam of pelvic viscera through incision in posterior vaginal wall.

70.23   **Biopsy of cul-de-sac** ♀
70.24   **Vaginal biopsy** ♀
70.29   **Other diagnostic procedures on vagina and cul-de-sac** ♀

✓4th **70.3**   **Local excision or destruction of vagina and cul-de-sac**

70.31   **Hymenectomy** ♀
70.32   **Excision or destruction of lesion of cul-de-sac** ♀
Endometrectomy of cul-de-sac
EXCLUDES   biopsy of cul-de-sac (70.23)

70.33   **Excision or destruction of lesion of vagina** ♀
EXCLUDES   biopsy of vagina (70.24)
vaginal fistulectomy (70.72-70.75)

70.4   **Obliteration and total excision of vagina** ♀
Vaginectomy
EXCLUDES   obliteration of vaginal vault (70.8)

DEF: Vaginectomy: Removal of vagina.

✓4th **70.5**   **Repair of cystocele and rectocele**

70.50   **Repair of cystocele and rectocele** ♀
DEF: Repair of anterior and posterior vaginal wall bulges.

70.51   **Repair of cystocele** ♀
Anterior colporrhaphy (with urethrocele repair)
AHA: N-D, '84, 20

70.52   **Repair of rectocele** ♀
Posterior colporrhaphy

✓4th **70.6**   **Vaginal construction and reconstruction**

70.61   **Vaginal construction** ♀
70.62   **Vaginal reconstruction** ♀
AHA: N-D, '84, 20

✓4th **70.7**   **Other repair of vagina**
EXCLUDES   lysis of intraluminal adhesions (70.13)
repair of current obstetric laceration (75.69)
that associated with cervical amputation (67.4)

70.71   **Suture of laceration of vagina** ♀
AHA: N-D, '84, 20

70.72   **Repair of colovaginal fistula** ♀
DEF: Correction of abnormal opening between midsection of large intestine and vagina.

70.73   **Repair of rectovaginal fistula** ♀
DEF: Correction of abnormal opening between last section of large intestine and vagina.

70.74   **Repair of other vaginoenteric fistula** ♀
DEF: Correction of abnormal opening between vagina and intestine; other than mid or last sections.

70.75   **Repair of other fistula of vagina** ♀
EXCLUDES   repair of fistula:
rectovesicovaginal (57.83)
ureterovaginal (56.84)
urethrovaginal (58.43)
uterovaginal (69.42)
vesicocervicovaginal (57.84)
vesicosigmoidovaginal (57.83)
vesicoureterovaginal (56.84)
vesicovaginal (57.84)

70.76   **Hymenorrhaphy** ♀
DEF: Closure of vagina with suture of hymenal ring or hymenal remnant flaps.

70.77   **Vaginal suspension and fixation** ♀
DEF: Repair of vaginal protrusion, sinking or laxity by suturing vagina into position.

70.79   **Other repair of vagina** ♀
Colpoperineoplasty
Repair of old obstetric laceration of vagina

70.8   **Obliteration of vaginal vault** ♀
LeFort operation

DEF: LeFort operation: Uniting or sewing together vaginal walls.

✓4th **70.9**   **Other operations on vagina and cul-de-sac**

70.91   **Other operations on vagina** ♀
EXCLUDES   insertion of:
diaphragm (96.17)
mold (96.15)
pack (96.14)
pessary (96.18)
suppository (96.49)
removal of:
diaphragm (97.73)
foreign body (98.17)
pack (97.75)
pessary (97.74)
replacement of:
diaphragm (97.24)
pack (97.26)
pessary (97.25)
vaginal dilation (96.16)
vaginal douche (96.44)

70.92   **Other operations on cul-de-sac** ♀
Obliteration of cul-de-sac
Repair of vaginal enterocele
AHA: 4Q, '94, 54

DEF: Repair of vaginal enterocele: Elimination of herniated cavity within pouch between last part of large intestine and posterior uterus.

✓3rd **71**   **Operations on vulva and perineum**
►Code also any application or administration of an adhesion barrier substance (99.77)◄

✓4th **71.0**   **Incision of vulva and perineum**

71.01   **Lysis of vulvar adhesions** ♀
71.09   **Other incision of vulva and perineum** ♀
Enlargement of introitus NOS
EXCLUDES   removal of foreign body without incision (98.23)

✓4th **71.1**   **Diagnostic procedures on vulva**

71.11   **Biopsy of vulva** ♀
71.19   **Other diagnostic procedures on vulva** ♀

✓4th **71.2**   **Operations on Bartholin's gland**

71.21   **Percutaneous aspiration of Bartholin's gland (cyst)**
71.22   **Incision of Bartholin's gland (cyst)** ♀

BI Bilateral Edit   NC Non-covered Procedure   ►◄ Revised Text   ● New Code   ▲ Revised Code Title

Marsupialization

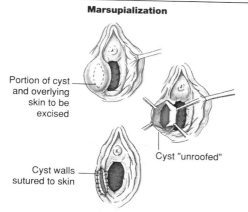

Portion of cyst and overlying skin to be excised

Cyst "unroofed"

Cyst walls sutured to skin

71.23 **Marsupialization of Bartholin's gland (cyst)** ♀

DEF: Incision and suturing opening of a cyst in Bartholin's gland.

71.24 **Excision or other destruction of Bartholin's gland (cyst)** ♀

71.29 **Other operations on Bartholin's gland** ♀

71.3 **Other local excision or destruction of vulva and perineum** ♀

Division of Skene's gland

EXCLUDES biopsy of vulva (71.11)
vulvar fistulectomy (71.72)

71.4 **Operations on clitoris** ♀

Amputation of clitoris
Clitoridotomy
Female circumcision

DEF: Amputation of clitoris: Removal of clitoris.

DEF: Clitoridotomy: Incision into clitoris.

DEF: Female circumcision: Incision of skin fold over clitoris.

71.5 **Radical vulvectomy** ♀

Code also any synchronous lymph gland dissection (40.3, 40.5)

DEF: Removal of over 80 percent of deep tissue from vulva, including tissue of abdomen, groin, labia minora, labia majora, clitoris, mons veneris, and terminal portions of urethra, vagina and other vulvar organs.

✓4th **71.6** **Other vulvectomy**

71.61 **Unilateral vulvectomy** ♀

71.62 **Bilateral vulvectomy** ♀
Vulvectomy NOS

✓4th **71.7** **Repair of vulva and perineum**

EXCLUDES repair of current obstetric laceration (75.69)

71.71 **Suture of laceration of vulva or perineum** ♀

71.72 **Repair of fistula of vulva or perineum** ♀

EXCLUDES repair of fistula:
urethroperineal (58.43)
urethroperineovesical (57.84)
vaginoperineal (70.75)

71.79 **Other repair of vulva and perineum** ♀
Repair of old obstetric laceration of vulva or perineum

AHA: 1Q, '97, 9

71.8 **Other operations on vulva** ♀

EXCLUDES removal of:
foreign body without incision (98.23)
packing (97.75)
replacement of packing (97.26)

71.9 **Other operations on female genital organs** ♀

Operations on the Female Genital System 71.23–71.9

✓3rd
✓4th Additional Digit Required

2002 Ingenix, Inc.

Nonspecific OR Procedure

Valid OR Procedure

Non-OR Procedure

Volume 3 —163

Obstetrical Procedures 72–74.2

13. OBSTETRICAL PROCEDURES (72-75)

√3rd **72 Forceps, vacuum, and breech delivery**

72.0 Low forceps operation ♀
Outlet forceps operation

72.1 Low forceps operation with episiotomy ♀
Outlet forceps operation with episiotomy

√4th **72.2 Mid forceps operation**

72.21 Mid forceps operation with episiotomy ♀

72.29 Other mid forceps operation ♀

√4th **72.3 High forceps operation**

72.31 High forceps operation with episiotomy ♀

72.39 Other high forceps operation ♀

72.4 Forceps rotation of fetal head ♀
DeLee maneuver
Key-in-lock rotation
Kielland rotation
Scanzoni's maneuver
Code also any associated forceps extraction (72.0-72.39)

√4th **72.5 Breech extraction**

72.51 Partial breech extraction with forceps to aftercoming head ♀

72.52 Other partial breech extraction ♀

72.53 Total breech extraction with forceps to aftercoming head ♀

72.54 Other total breech extraction ♀

72.6 Forceps application to aftercoming head ♀
Piper forceps operation
EXCLUDES partial breech extraction with forceps to aftercoming head (72.51)
total breech extraction with forceps to aftercoming head (72.53)

√4th **72.7 Vacuum extraction**
INCLUDES Malstöm's extraction

72.71 Vacuum extraction with episiotomy ♀

72.79 Other vacuum extraction ♀

72.8 Other specified instrumental delivery ♀

72.9 Unspecified instrumental delivery ♀

√3rd **73 Other procedures inducing or assisting delivery**

√4th **73.0 Artificial rupture of membranes**

73.01 Induction of labor by artificial rupture of membranes ♀
Surgical induction NOS
EXCLUDES artificial rupture of membranes after onset of labor (73.09)

AHA: 3Q, '00, 5

73.09 Other artificial rupture of membranes ♀
Artificial rupture of membranes at time of delivery

Breech Extraction

Breech presentation
Delivery of legs
Baby rotated for delivery of arms
Umbilicus

73.1 Other surgical induction of labor ♀
Induction by cervical dilation
EXCLUDES injection for abortion (75.0)
insertion of suppository for abortion (96.49)

√4th **73.2 Internal and combined version and extraction**

73.21 Internal and combined version without extraction ♀
Version NOS

73.22 Internal and combined version with extraction ♀

73.3 Failed forceps ♀
Application of forceps without delivery
Trial forceps

73.4 Medical induction of labor ♀
EXCLUDES medication to augment active labor — omit code

√4th **73.5 Manually assisted delivery** ♀

73.51 Manual rotation of fetal head ♀

73.59 Other manually assisted delivery ♀
Assisted spontaneous delivery
Credé maneuver
AHA: 4Q, '98, 76

73.6 Episiotomy ♀
Episioproctotomy
Episiotomy with subsequent episiorrhaphy
EXCLUDES that with:
high forceps (72.31)
low forceps (72.1)
mid forceps (72.21)
outlet forceps (72.1)
vacuum extraction (72.71)

AHA: 1Q, '92, 10

73.8 Operations on fetus to facilitate delivery ♀
Clavicotomy on fetus
Destruction of fetus
Needling of hydrocephalic head

√4th **73.9 Other operations assisting delivery**

73.91 External version ♀

73.92 Replacement of prolapsed umbilical cord ♀

73.93 Incision of cervix to assist delivery ♀
Dührssen's incisions

73.94 Pubiotomy to assist delivery ♀
Obstetrical symphysiotomy

73.99 Other ♀
EXCLUDES dilation of cervix, obstetrical, to induce labor (73.1)
insertion of bag or bougie to induce labor (73.1)
removal of cerclage material (69.96)

√3rd **74 Cesarean section and removal of fetus**
Code also any synchronous:
hysterectomy (68.3-68.4, 68.6, 68.8)
myomectomy (68.29)
sterilization (66.31-66.39, 66.63)

74.0 Classical cesarean section ♀
Transperitoneal classical cesarean section

74.1 Low cervical cesarean section ♀
Lower uterine segment cesarean section
AHA: 1Q, '01, 11

74.2 Extraperitoneal cesarean section ♀
Supravesical cesarean section

BI Bilateral Edit   NC Non-covered Procedure   ▶◀ Revised Text   ● New Code   ▲ Revised Code List

74.3 **Removal of extratubal ectopic pregnancy** ♀

Removal of:
 ectopic abdominal pregnancy
 fetus from peritoneal or extraperitoneal cavity
  following uterine or tubal rupture

> **EXCLUDES** *that by salpingostomy (66.02)*
> *that by salpingotomy (66.01)*
> *that with synchronous salpingectomy*
> *(66.62)*

AHA: 4Q, '92, 25; 2Q, '90, 25; 2Q, '90, 27; 1Q, '89, 11

74.4 **Cesarean section of other specified type** ♀

Peritoneal exclusion cesareansection
Transperitoneal cesarean section NOS
Vaginal cesarean section

✓4ᵗʰ **74.9** **Cesarean section of unspecified type**

74.91 **Hysterotomy to terminate pregnancy** ♀
 Therapeutic abortion by hysterotomy

74.99 **Other cesarean section of unspecified** ♀
type

 Cesarean section NOS
 Obstetrical abdominouterotomy
 Obstetrical hysterotomy

✓3ʳᵈ **75** **Other obstetric operations**

75.0 **Intra-amniotic injection for abortion** ♀

Injection of:
 prostaglandin ⎫ for induction of
 saline ⎭ abortion

Termination of pregnancy by intrauterine injection

> **EXCLUDES** *insertion of prostaglandin suppository*
> *for abortion (96.49)*

75.1 **Diagnostic amniocentesis** ♀

75.2 **Intrauterine transfusion** ♀

Exchange transfusion in utero
Insertion of catheter into abdomen of fetus for
 transfusion
Code also any hysterotomy approach (68.0)

✓4ᵗʰ **75.3** **Other intrauterine operations on fetus and amnion**

Code also any hysterotomy approach (68.0)

75.31 **Amnioscopy** ♀
 Fetoscopy
 Laparoamnioscopy

75.32 **Fetal EKG (scalp)** ♀

75.33 **Fetal blood sampling and biopsy** ♀

75.34 **Other fetal monitoring** ♀
 Fetal monitoring, not otherwise specified
 > **EXCLUDES** *fetal pulse oximetry (75.38)*

Amniocentesis

Aspiration of amniotic fluid

75.35 **Other diagnostic procedures on fetus** ♀
and amnion

Intrauterine pressure determination

> **EXCLUDES** *amniocentesis (75.1)*
> *diagnostic procedures on*
> *gravid uterus and*
> *placenta (87.81, 88.46,*
> *88.78, 92.17)*

75.36 **Correction of fetal defect** ♀

75.37 **Amnioinfusion**

Code also injection of antibiotic (99.21)

AHA: 4Q, '98, 76

75.38 **Fetal pulse oximetry**

Transcervical fetal oxygen saturation
 monitoring
Transcervical fetal SpO₂ monitoring

DEF: ▶Single-use sensor inserted through the birth
canal and positioned to rest against the fetal cheek,
forehead, or temple; infrared beam of light aimed at the
fetal skin is reflected back through the sensor for
analysis.◀

AHA: ▶4Q, '01, 64◀

75.4 **Manual removal of retained placenta**

> **EXCLUDES** *aspiration curettage (69.52)*
> *dilation and curettage (69.02)*

✓4ᵗʰ **75.5** **Repair of current obstetric laceration of uterus**

75.50 **Repair of current obstetric laceration of**
uterus, not otherwise specified

75.51 **Repair of current obstetric laceration of**
cervix

75.52 **Repair of current obstetric laceration of**
corpus uteri

✓4ᵗʰ **75.6** **Repair of other current obstetric laceration**

AHA: 1Q, '92, 11

75.61 **Repair of current obstetric laceration of**
bladder and urethra

75.62 **Repair of current obstetric laceration of**
rectum and sphincter ani

75.69 **Repair of other current obstetric laceration**
 Episioperineorrhaphy Repair of:
 Repair of: vagina
  pelvic floor vulva
  perineum
 Secondary repair of episiotomy
 > **EXCLUDES** *repair of routine episiotomy*
 > *(73.6)*

75.7 **Manual exploration of uterine cavity, postpartum**

75.8 **Obstetric tamponade of uterus or vagina**

> **EXCLUDES** *antepartum tamponade (73.1)*

✓4ᵗʰ **75.9** **Other obstetric operations**

75.91 **Evacuation of obstetrical incisional**
hematoma of perineum
 Evacuation of hematoma of:
  episiotomy
  perineorrhaphy

75.92 **Evacuation of other hematoma of vulva or**
vagina

75.93 **Surgical correction of inverted uterus**
 Spintelli operation
 > **EXCLUDES** *vaginal repair of chronic*
 > *inversion of uterus*
 > *(69.23)*

75.94 **Manual replacement of inverted uterus**

75.99 **Other**

Obstetrical Procedures 74.3–75.99

✓3ʳᵈ
✓4ᵗʰ Additional Digit Required

Nonspecific OR Procedure

Valid OR Procedure

Non-OR Procedure

2002 Ingenix, Inc.

Volume 3 —165

Operations on the Musculoskeletal System 76–76.92

14. OPERATIONS ON THE MUSCULOSKELETAL SYSTEM
(76-84)

√3ʳᵈ **76**   **Operations on facial bones and joints**

> EXCLUDES   *accessory sinuses (22.00-22.9)*
> *nasal bones (21.00-21.99)*
> *skull (01.01-02.99)*

√4ᵗʰ **76.0**   **Incision of facial bone without division**

76.01   **Sequestrectomy of facial bone**
Removal of necrotic bone chip from facial bone

76.09   **Other incision of facial bone**
Reopening of osteotomy site of facial bone

> EXCLUDES   *osteotomy associated with orthognathic surgery (76.61-76.69)*
> *removal of internal fixation device (76.97)*

√4ᵗʰ **76.1**   **Diagnostic procedures on facial bones and joints**

76.11   **Biopsy of facial bone**

76.19   **Other diagnostic procedures on facial bones and joints**

> EXCLUDES   *contrast arthrogram of temporomandibular joint (87.13)*
> *other x-ray (87.11-87.12, 87.14-87.16)*

AHA: N-D, '87, 12

76.2   **Local excision or destruction of lesion of facial bone**

> EXCLUDES   *biopsy of facial bone (76.11)*
> *excision of odontogenic lesion (24.4)*

√4ᵗʰ **76.3**   **Partial ostectomy of facial bone**

76.31   **Partial mandibulectomy**
Hemimandibulectomy

> EXCLUDES   *that associated with temporomandibular arthroplasty (76.5)*

DEF: Excision, partial of lower jawbone.

DEF: Hemimandibulectomy: Excision of one-half of lower jawbone.

76.39   **Partial ostectomy of other facial bone**
Hemimaxillectomy (with bonegraft or prosthesis)

AHA: J-F, '87, 14

DEF: Excision, partial of facial bone; other than lower jawbone.

DEF: Hemimaxillectomy (with bone graft or prosthesis): Excision of one side of upper jawbone and restoration with bone graft or prosthesis.

√4ᵗʰ **76.4**   **Excision and reconstruction of facial bones**

76.41   **Total mandibulectomy with synchronous reconstruction**

76.42   **Other total mandibulectomy**

76.43   **Other reconstruction of mandible**

> EXCLUDES   *genioplasty (76.67-76.68)*
> *that with synchronous total mandibulectomy (76.41)*

76.44   **Total ostectomy of other facial bone with synchronous reconstruction**

AHA: 3Q, '93, 6

DEF: Excision, facial bone, total with reconstruction during same operative session.

76.45   **Other total ostectomy of other facial bone**

76.46   **Other reconstruction of other facial bone**

> EXCLUDES   *that with synchronous total ostectomy (76.44)*

76.5   **Temporomandibular arthroplasty**

AHA: 4Q, '99, 20

√4ᵗʰ **76.6**   **Other facial bone repair and orthognathic surgery**
Code also any synchronous:
bone graft (76.91)
synthetic implant (76.92)

> EXCLUDES   *reconstruction of facial bones (76.41-76.46)*

76.61   **Closed osteoplasty [osteotomy] of mandibular ramus**
Gigli saw osteotomy

DEF: Reshaping and restoration of lower jawbone projection; closed surgical field.

DEF: Gigli saw osteotomy: Plastic repair using a flexible wire with saw teeth.

76.62   **Open osteoplasty [osteotomy] of mandibular ramus**

76.63   **Osteoplasty [osteotomy] of body of mandible**

76.64   **Other orthognathic surgery on mandible**
Mandibular osteoplasty NOS
Segmental or subapical osteotomy

76.65   **Segmental osteoplasty [osteotomy] of maxilla**
Maxillary osteoplasty NOS

76.66   **Total osteoplasty [osteotomy] of maxilla**

76.67   **Reduction genioplasty**
Reduction mentoplasty

DEF: Reduction of protruding chin or lower jawbone.

76.68   **Augmentation genioplasty**
Mentoplasty:
NOS
with graft or implant

DEF: Extension of the lower jawbone to a functional position by means of plastic surgery.

76.69   **Other facial bone repair**
Osteoplasty of facial bone NOS

√4ᵗʰ **76.7**   **Reduction of facial fracture**

> INCLUDES   internal fixation

Code also any synchronous:
bone graft (76.91)
synthetic implant (76.92)

> EXCLUDES   *that of nasal bones (21.71-21.72)*

76.70   **Reduction of facial fracture, not otherwise specified**

76.71   **Closed reduction of malar and zygomatic fracture**

76.72   **Open reduction of malar and zygomatic fracture**

76.73   **Closed reduction of maxillary fracture**

76.74   **Open reduction of maxillary fracture**

76.75   **Closed reduction of mandibular fracture**

76.76   **Open reduction of mandibular fracture**

76.77   **Open reduction of alveolar fracture**
Reduction of alveolar fracture with stabilization of teeth

76.78   **Other closed reduction of facial fracture**
Closed reduction of orbital fracture

> EXCLUDES   *nasal bone (21.71)*

76.79   **Other open reduction of facial fracture**
Open reduction of orbit rim or wall

> EXCLUDES   *nasal bone (21.72)*

√4ᵗʰ **76.9**   **Other operations on facial bones and joints**

76.91   **Bone graft to facial bone**

Autogenous
Bone bank   } graft to facial bone
Heterogenous

76.92   **Insertion of synthetic implant in facial bone**
Alloplastic implant to facial bone

| BI | Bilateral Edit | NC | Non-covered Procedure | ►◄ Revised Text | ● New Code | ▲ Revised Code Title |

76.93 Closed reduction of temporomandibular dislocation

76.94 Open reduction of temporomandibular dislocation

76.95 Other manipulation of temporomandibular joint

76.96 Injection of therapeutic substance into temporomandibular joint

76.97 Removal of internal fixation device from facial bone
> EXCLUDES   removal of:
> dental wiring (97.33)
> external mandibular fixation device NEC (97.36)

76.99 Other

77 Incision, excision, and division of other bones
> EXCLUDES   laminectomy for decompression (03.09)
> operations on:
> accessory sinuses (22.00-22.9)
> ear ossicles (19.0-19.55)
> facial bones (76.01-76.99)
> joint structures (80.00-81.99)
> mastoid (19.9-20.99)
> nasal bones (21.00-21.99)
> skull (01.01-02.99)

The following fourth-digit subclassification is for use with appropriate categories in section 77 to identify the site. Valid fourth-digit categories are in [brackets] under each code.

- 0 unspecified site
- 1 scapula, clavicle, and thorax [ribs and sternum]
- 2 humerus
- 3 radius and ulna
- 4 carpals and metacarpals
- 5 femur
- 6 patella
- 7 tibia and fibula
- 8 tarsals and metatarsals
- 9 other
  Pelvic bones
  Phalanges (of foot) (of hand)
  Vertebrae

§ 77.0 Sequestrectomy [0-9]
DEF: Excision and removal of dead bone.

§ 77.1 Other incision of bone without division [0-9]
Reopening of osteotomy site
> EXCLUDES   aspiration of bone marrow, (41.31, 41.91)
> removal of internal fixation device (78.60-78.69)
AHA: For code 77.17: ▶1Q, '02, 3◀
DEF: Incision into bone without division of site.

§ 77.2 Wedge osteotomy [0-9]
> EXCLUDES   that for hallux valgus (77.51)
DEF: Removal of wedge-shaped piece of bone.

§ 77.3 Other division of bone [0-9]
Osteoarthrotomy
> EXCLUDES   clavicotomy of fetus (73.8)
> laminotomy or incision of vertebra (03.01-03.09)
> pubiotomy to assist delivery (73.94)
> sternotomy incidental to thoracic operation — omit code

§ 77.4 Biopsy of bone [0-9]
AHA: 2Q, '98, 12

77.5 Excision and repair of bunion and other toe deformities

Repair of Hammertoes

77.51 Bunionectomy with soft tissue correction and osteotomy of the first metatarsal
DEF: Incision and removal of big toe bony prominence and reconstruction with soft tissue.

77.52 Bunionectomy with soft tissue correction and arthrodesis
DEF: Removal of big toe bony prominence and reconstruction with soft tissue and joint fixation.

77.53 Other bunionectomy with soft tissue correction

77.54 Excision or correction of bunionette
That with osteotomy
DEF: Resection of fifth metatarsal head via exposure of joint; includes imbrication of capsule.

77.56 Repair of hammer toe
Fusion
Phalangectomy (partial) } of hammer toe
Filleting
DEF: Repair of clawlike toe defect by joint fusion, partial removal of toe or via traction technique.

77.57 Repair of claw toe
Fusion
Phalangectomy (partial)
Capsulotomy } of claw toe
Tendon lengthening
DEF: Repair of clawlike toe defect by joint fusion, partial removal of toe, joint capsule incision or lengthening of fibrous muscle attachment.

77.58 Other excision, fusion, and repair of toes
Cockup toe repair
Overlapping toe repair
That with use of prosthetic materials

77.59 Other bunionectomy
Resection of hallux valgus joint with insertion of prosthesis
DEF: Resection of hallux valgus joint with insertion of prosthesis: Cutting away part of big toe with prosthesis insertion to correct bony prominence.

§ 77.6 Local excision of lesion or tissue of bone [0-9]
> EXCLUDES   biopsy of bone (77.40-77.49)
> debridement of compound fracture (79.60-79.69)
AHA: For code 77.61: 3Q, '01, 9; For code 77.65: S-O, '85, 4; For code 77.67: ▶1Q, '02, 3; ◀1Q, '99, 8; For code 77.69: 2Q, '00, 18

§ 77.7 Excision of bone for graft [0-9]
AHA: 4Q, '99, 11, 13; For code 77.79: 2Q, '00 12, 13; 4Q, '99, 11, 13

§ Requires fourth-digit. Valid digits are in [brackets] under each code. See code 77 for definitions.
16 Nonspecific OR procedure=0

Operations on the Musculoskeletal System 77.8–78.9

§ ✓4ᵗʰ ¹⁶ **77.8** **Other partial ostectomy**
[0-9]   Condylectomy

> **EXCLUDES**   *amputation (84.00-84.19, 84.91)*
> *arthrectomy (80.90-80.99)*
> *excision of bone ends associated with:*
>   *arthrodesis (81.00-81.29)*
>   *arthroplasty (81.51-81.59, 81.71-*
>   *81.81, 81.84)*
> *excision of cartilage (80.5-80.6, 80.80-*
>   *80.99)*
> *excision of head of femur with*
>   *synchronous replacement (81.51-*
>   *81.53)*
> *hemilaminectomy (03.01-03.09)*
> *laminectomy (03.01-03.09)*
> *ostectomy for hallux valgus (77.51-*
>   *77.59)*
> *partial amputation:*
>   *finger (84.01)*
>   *thumb (84.02)*
>   *toe (84.11)*
> *resection of ribs incidental to thoracic*
>   *operation — omit code*
> *that incidental to other operation —*
>   *omit code*

§ ✓4ᵗʰ ¹⁶ **77.9** **Total ostectomy**
[0-9]
> **EXCLUDES**   *amputation of limb (84.00-84.19,*
>   *84.91)*
> *that incidental to other operation —*
>   *omit code*

✓3ʳᵈ **78** **Other operations on bones, except facial bones**
> **EXCLUDES**   *operations on:*
>   *accessory sinuses (22.00-22.9)*
>   *facial bones (76.01-76.99)*
>   *joint structures (80.00-81.99)*
>   *nasal bones (21.00-21.99)*
>   *skull (01.01-02.99)*

The following fourth-digit subclassification is for use with categories in section 78 to identify the site. Valid fourth-digit categories are in [brackets] under each code.

0   **unspecified site**
1   **scapula, clavicle, and thorax [ribs and sternum]**
2   **humerus**
3   **radius and ulna**
4   **carpals and metacarpals**
5   **femur**
6   **patella**
7   **tibia and fibula**
8   **tarsals and metatarsals**
9   **other**
     Pelvic bones   Vertebrae
     Phalanges (of foot) (of hand)

§§ ✓4ᵗʰ ¹⁶ **78.0** **Bone graft**
[0-9]   Bone:
         bank graft
         graft (autogenous) (heterogenous)
     That with debridement of bone graft site (removal of
         sclerosed, fibrous, or necrotic bone or tissue)
     Transplantation of bone
     Code also any excision of bone for graft (77.70-
         77.79)
> **EXCLUDES**   *that for bone lengthening (78.30-78.39)*

AHA: 2Q, '98, 12' 3Q, '94, 10; 1Q, '91, 3

§§ ✓4ᵗʰ ¹⁶ **78.1** **Application of external fixation device**
[0-9]   Minifixator with insertion of pins/wires/screws into
     bone
> **EXCLUDES**   *other immobilization, pressure, and*
>   *attention to wound (93.51-93.59)*

AHA: 2Q, '94, 4

§§ ✓4ᵗʰ ¹⁶ **78.2** **Limb shortening procedures**
[0,2-5,7-9]   Epiphyseal stapling
     Open epiphysiodesis
     Percutaneous epiphysiodesis
     Resection/osteotomy

§§ ✓4ᵗʰ ¹⁶ **78.3** **Limb lengthening procedures**
[0,2-5,7-9]   Bone graft with or without internal fixation devices
     or osteotomy
     Distraction technique with or without
         corticotomy/osteotomy
     Code also any application of an external fixation
         device (78.10-78.19)

§§ ✓4ᵗʰ ¹⁶ **78.4** **Other repair or plastic operations on bone**
[0-9]   Other operation on bone NEC
     Repair of malunion or nonunion fracture NEC
> **EXCLUDES**   *application of external fixation device (78.10-*
>   *78.19)*
> *limb lengthening procedures (78.30-78.39)*
> *limb shortening procedures (78.20-78.29)*
> *osteotomy (77.3)*
> *reconstruction of thumb (82.61-82.69)*
> *repair of pectus deformity (34.74)*
> *repair with bone graft (78.00-78.09)*

AHA: 3Q, '92, 20; 4Q, '88, 11; **For code 78.47:** 3Q, '91, 20; **For code 78.49:** 4Q, '99, 22; 1Q, '97, 5

§§ ✓4ᵗʰ ¹⁶ **78.5** **Internal fixation of bone without fracture reduction**
[0-9]   Internal fixation of bone (prophylactic)
     Reinsertion of internal fixation device
     Revision of displaced or broken fixation device
> **EXCLUDES**   *arthroplasty and arthrodesis*
>   *(81.00-81.85)*
> *bone graft (78.00-78.09)*
> *limb shortening procedures (78.20-*
>   *78.29)*
> *that for fracture reduction (79.10-79.19,*
>   *79.30-79.59)*

AHA: 2Q, '99, 11; 2Q, '94, 4; **For Code 78.59:** 4Q, '99, 13

§§ ✓4ᵗʰ **78.6** **Removal of implanted devices from bone**
[0-9]   External fixator device (invasive)
     Internal fixation device
     Removal of bone growth stimulator (invasive)
> **EXCLUDES**   *removal of cast, splint, and traction*
>   *device (Kirschner wire)*
>   *(Steinmann pin) (97.88)*
> *removal of skull tongs or halo traction*
>   *device (02.95)*

AHA: 1Q, '00, 15; For Code 78.69: 2Q, '00, 18

§§ ✓4ᵗʰ ¹⁶ **78.7** **Osteoclasis**
[0-9]   **DEF: Surgical breaking or rebreaking of bone.**

§§ ✓4ᵗʰ ¹⁶ **78.8** **Diagnostic procedures on bone, not elsewhere classified**
[0-9]
> **EXCLUDES**   *biopsy of bone (77.40-77.49)*
> *magnetic resonance imaging (88.94)*
> *microscopic examination of specimen*
>   *from bone (91.51-91.59)*
> *radioisotope scan (92.14)*
> *skeletal x-ray (87.21-87.29, 87.43,*
>   *88.21-88.33)*
> *thermography (88.83)*

§§ ✓4ᵗʰ ¹⁶ **78.9** **Insertion of bone growth stimulator**
[0-9]   Insertion of:
         bone stimulator (electrical) to aid bone healing
         osteogenic electrodes for bone growth stimulation
         totally implanted device (invasive)
> **EXCLUDES**   *non-invasive (transcutaneous) (surface)*
>   *stimulator (99.86)*

---

§   Requires fourth-digit. Valid digits are in [brackets] under each code. See code 77 for definitions.
§§ Requires fourth-digit. Valid digits are in [brackets] under each code. See code 78 for definitions.
¹⁶ Nonspecific OR procedure=0

BI Bilateral Edit   **NC** Non-covered Procedure   ▶◀ Revised Text   ● New Code   ▲ Revised Code Title

✓3rd **79 Reduction of fracture and dislocation**

INCLUDES   application of cast or splint
reduction with insertion of traction device
(Kirschner wire) (Steinmann pin)

Code also any application of external fixation device (78.10-78.19)

EXCLUDES   external fixation alone for immobilization of fracture (93.51-93.56, 93.59)
internal fixation without reduction of fracture (78.50-78.59)
operations on:
facial bones(76.70-76.79)
nasal bones (21.71-21.72)
orbit (76.78-76.79)
skull (02.02)
vertebrae (03.53)
removal of cast or splint (97.88)
replacement of cast or splint (97.11-97.14)
traction alone for reduction of fracture (93.41-93.46)

The following fourth-digit subclassification is for use with appropriate categories in section 79 to identify the site. Valid fourth-digit categories are in [brackets] under each code.

0 **unspecified site**
1 **humerus**
2 **radius and ulna**
    Arm NOS
3 **carpals and metacarpals**
    Hand NOS
4 **phalanges of hand**
5 **femur**
6 **tibia and fibula**
    Leg NOS
7 **tarsals and metatarsals**
    Foot NOS
8 **phalanges of foot**
9 **other specified bone**

✓4th **79.0 Closed reduction of fracture without internal fixation**
[0-9]
EXCLUDES   that for separation of epiphysis (79.40-79.49)

AHA: 2Q, '94, 3; 3Q, '89, 17; 4Q, '88, 11; **For code 79.05:** 3Q, '89, 16

DEF: Manipulative realignment of fracture; without incision or internal fixation.

✓4th 16 **79.1 Closed reduction of fracture with internal fixation**
[0-9]
EXCLUDES   that for separation of epiphysis (79.40-79.49)

AHA: 2Q, '94, 4; 4Q, '93, 35; 1Q, '93, 27

DEF: Manipulative realignment of fracture; with internal fixation but without incision.

✓4th 16 **79.2 Open reduction of fracture without internal fixation**
[0-9]
EXCLUDES   that for separation of epiphysis (79.50-79.59)

AHA: 2Q, '94, 3

✓4th 16 **79.3 Open reduction of fracture with internal fixation**
[0-9]
EXCLUDES   that for separation of epiphysis (79.50-79.59)

AHA: 2Q, '98, 12; 3Q, '94, 10; 2Q, '94, 3; 4Q, '93, 35

DEF: Realignment of fracture with incision and internal fixation.

✓4th 16 **79.4 Closed reduction of separated epiphysis**
[0-2,5,6,9] Reduction with or without internal fixation

DEF: Manipulative reduction of expanded joint end of long bone to normal position without incision.

✓4th 16 **79.5 Open reduction of separated epiphysis**
[0-2,5,6,9] Reduction with or without internal fixation

DEF: Reduction of expanded joint end of long bone with incision.

✓4th 16 **79.6 Debridement of open fracture site**
[0-9] Debridement of compound fracture

AHA: 3Q, '95, 12; 3Q, '89, 16

DEF: Removal of damaged tissue at fracture site.

✓4th **79.7 Closed reduction of dislocation**
INCLUDES   closed reduction (with external traction device)
EXCLUDES   closed reduction of dislocation of temporomandibular joint (76.93)

DEF: Manipulative reduction of displaced joint without incision; with or without external traction.

79.70 **Closed reduction of dislocation of unspecified site**
79.71 **Closed reduction of dislocation of shoulder**
79.72 **Closed reduction of dislocation of elbow**
79.73 **Closed reduction of dislocation of wrist**
79.74 **Closed reduction of dislocation of hand and finger**
79.75 **Closed reduction of dislocation of hip**
79.76 **Closed reduction of dislocation of knee**
    AHA: N-D, '86, 7
79.77 **Closed reduction of dislocation of ankle**
79.78 **Closed reduction of dislocation of foot and toe**
79.79 **Closed reduction of dislocation of other specified sites**

✓4th 16 **79.8 Open reduction of dislocation**
INCLUDES   open reduction (with internal and external fixation devices)
EXCLUDES   open reduction of dislocation of temporomandibular joint (76.94)

DEF: Reduction of displaced joint via incision; with or without internal and external fixation.

79.80 **Open reduction of dislocation of unspecified site**
79.81 **Open reduction of dislocation of shoulder**
79.82 **Open reduction of dislocation of elbow**
79.83 **Open reduction of dislocation of wrist**
79.84 **Open reduction of dislocation of hand and finger**
79.85 **Open reduction of dislocation of hip**
79.86 **Open reduction of dislocation of knee**
79.87 **Open reduction of dislocation of ankle**
79.88 **Open reduction of dislocation of foot and toe**
79.89 **Open reduction of dislocation of other specified sites**

✓4th 16 **79.9 Unspecified operation on bone injury**
[0-9]

16 Nonspecific OR procedure=0

✓3rd ✓4th Additional Digit Required   Nonspecific OR Procedure   Valid OR Procedure   Non-OR Procedure

√3ʳᵈ **80**   **Incision and excision of joint structures**

INCLUDES   operations on:
- capsule of joint
- cartilage
- condyle
- ligament
- meniscus
- synovial membrane

EXCLUDES   *cartilage of:*
- *ear (18.01-18.9)*
- *nose (21.00-21.99)*
- *temporomandibular joint (76.01-76.99)*

The following fourth-digit subclassification is for use with appropriate categories in section 80 to identify the site:

- **0**   **unspecified site**
- **1**   **shoulder**
- **2**   **elbow**
- **3**   **wrist**
- **4**   **hand and finger**
- **5**   **hip**
- **6**   **knee**
- **7**   **ankle**
- **8**   **foot and toe**
- **9**   **other specified sites**
  - Spine

√4ᵗʰ¹⁶ **80.0**   **Arthrotomy for removal of prosthesis**

INCLUDES   cement spacer

AHA: For code 80.06: 2Q, '97, 10

DEF: Incision into joint to remove prosthesis.

√4ᵗʰ¹⁶ **80.1**   **Other arthrotomy**

Arthrostomy

EXCLUDES   *that for:*
- *arthrography (88.32)*
- *arthroscopy (80.20-80.29)*
- *injection of drug (81.92)*
- *operative approach — omit code*

DEF: Incision into joint; other than to remove prosthesis.

DEF: Arthrostomy: Creation of opening into joint.

√4ᵗʰ¹⁶ **80.2**   **Arthroscopy**

AHA: 3Q, '93, 5

√4ᵗʰ **80.3**   **Biopsy of joint structure**

Aspiration biopsy

√4ᵗʰ¹⁶ **80.4**   **Division of joint capsule, ligament, or cartilage**

Goldner clubfoot release
Heyman-Herndon(-Strong) correction of metatarsus varus
Release of:
- adherent or constrictive joint capsule
- joint
- ligament

EXCLUDES   *symphysiotomy to assist delivery (73.94)*
that for:
- *carpal tunnel syndrome (04.43)*
- *tarsal tunnel syndrome (04.44)*

DEF: Incision and separation of joint tissues, including capsule, fibrous bone attachment or cartilage.

√4ᵗʰ **80.5**   **Excision or destruction of intervertebral disc**

80.50   **Excision or destruction of intervertebral disc, unspecified**

Unspecified asto excision or destruction

80.51   **Excision of intervertebral disc**

Code also any concurrent spinal fusion (81.00-81.09)
Diskectomy
Level:
- cervical
- thoracic
- lumbar (lumbosacral)

Removal of herniated nucleus pulposus
That by laminotomy or hemilaminectomy
That with decompression of spinal nerve root at same level
Requires additional code for any concomitant decompression of spinal nerve root at different level from excision site

EXCLUDES   *intervertebral chemonucleolysis (80.52)*
laminectomy for exploration of intraspinal canal (03.09)
laminotomy for decompression of spinal nerve root only (03.09)

AHA: 1Q, '96, 7; 2Q, '95, 9; 2Q, '90, 27; S-O, '86, 12

DEF: Removal of intervertebral disc.

DEF: Removal of a herniated nucleus pulposus: Removal of displaced intervertebral disc, central part.

80.52   **Intervertebral chemonucleolysis**

With aspiration of disc fragments
With diskography
Injection of proteolytic enzyme into intervertebral space (chymopapain)

EXCLUDES   *injection of anesthestic substance (03.91)*
injection of other substances (03.92)

DEF: Destruction of intervertebral disc via injection of enzyme.

80.59   **Other destruction of intervertebral disc**

Destruction NEC
That by laser

80.6   **Excision of semilunar cartilage of knee**

Excision of meniscus of knee

AHA: 3Q, '00, 4; 2Q, '96, 3; 1Q, '93, 23

√4ᵗʰ¹⁶ **80.7**   **Synovectomy**

Complete or partial resection of synovial membrane

EXCLUDES   *excision of Baker's cyst (83.39)*

DEF: Excision of inner membrane of joint capsule.

√4ᵗʰ¹⁶ **80.8**   **Other local excision or destruction of lesion of joint**

√4ᵗʰ¹⁶ **80.9**   **Other excision of joint**

EXCLUDES   *cheilectomy of joint (77.80-77.89)*
excision of bone ends (77.80-77.89)

---

¹⁶ Nonspecific OR procedure=0

BI Bilateral Edit   NC Non-covered Procedure   ►◄ Revised Text   ● New Code   ▲ Revised Code Title

√3ʳᵈ **81 Repair and plastic operations on joint structures**

√4ᵗʰ **81.0 Spinal fusion**

▶Code also any 360 degree spinal fusion by a single incision (81.61)
Code also any insertion of interbody spinal fusion device (84.51)
Code also any insertion of recombinant bone morphogenetic protein (84.52)◀

INCLUDES   arthrodesis of spine with:
bone graft
internal fixation

EXCLUDES   *corrections of pseudarthrosis of spine (81.30-81.39)*
refusion of spine (81.30-81.39)

DEF: Immobilization of spinal column.

DEF: Anterior interbody fusion: Arthrodesis by excising disc and cartilage end plates with bone graft insertion between two vertebrae.

DEF: Lateral fusion: Arthrodesis by decorticating and bone grafting lateral surface of zygapophysial joint, pars interarticularis and transverse process.

DEF: Posterior fusion: Arthrodesis by decorticating and bone grafting of neural arches between right and left zygapophysial joints.

DEF: Posterolateral fusion: Arthrodesis by decorticating and bone grafting zygapophysial joint, pars interarticularis and transverse processes

81.00 Spinal fusion, not otherwise specified

81.01 Atlas-axis spinal fusion

Craniocervical fusion ⎫ by anterior
C₁-C₂ fusion   ⎬ transoral
Occiput C₂ fusion   ⎭ or posterior technique

81.02 Other cervical fusion, anterior technique
Arthrodesis of C₂ level or below:
anterior (interbody) technique
anterolateral technique
AHA: 1Q, '01, 6; 1Q, '96, 7

81.03 Other cervical fusion, posterior technique
Arthrodesis of C₂ level or below:
posterior (interbody) technique
posterolateral technique

81.04 Dorsal and dorsolumbar fusion, anterior technique
Arthrodesis of thoracic or thoracolumbar region:
anterior (interbody) technique
anterolateral technique

81.05 Dorsal and dorsolumbar fusion, posterior technique
Arthrodesis of thoracic or thoracolumbar region:
posterior (interbody) technique
posterolateral technique
AHA: 4Q, '99, 11

81.06 Lumbar and lumbosacral fusion, anterior technique
Arthrodesis of lumbar or lumbosacral region:
anterior (interbody) technique
anterolateral technique
AHA: 4Q, '99, 11

81.07 Lumbar and lumbosacral fusion, lateral transverse process technique

Types of Grafts for Anterior Arthrodesis

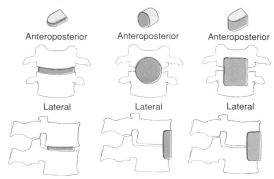

81.08 Lumbar and lumbosacral fusion, posterior technique
Arthrodesis of lumbar or lumbosacral region:
posterior (interbody) technique
posterolateral technique
AHA: 2Q, '00, 12, 13; 4Q, '99, 13; 2Q, '95, 9

√4ᵗʰ **81.1 Arthrodesis of foot and ankle**
INCLUDES   arthrodesis of foot and ankle with:
bone graft
external fixation device
DEF: Fixation of foot or ankle joints.

81.11 Ankle fusion
Tibiotalar fusion

81.12 Triple arthrodesis
Talus to calcaneus and calcaneus to cuboid and navicular

81.13 Subtalar fusion
81.14 Midtarsal fusion
81.15 Tarsometatarsal fusion
81.16 Metatarsophalangeal fusion
81.17 Other fusion of foot

√4ᵗʰ **81.2 Arthrodesis of other joint**
INCLUDES   arthrodesis with:
bone graft
external fixation device
excision of bone ends and compression

81.20 Arthrodesis of unspecified joint
81.21 Arthrodesis of hip
81.22 Arthrodesis of knee
81.23 Arthrodesis of shoulder
81.24 Arthrodesis of elbow
81.25 Carporadial fusion
81.26 Metacarpocarpal fusion
81.27 Metacarpophalangeal fusion
81.28 Interphalangeal fusion
81.29 Arthrodesis of other specified joints

√4ᵗʰ **81.3 Refusion of spine**
INCLUDES ▶ arthrodesis of spine with:
bone graft
internal fixation◀
correction of pseudarthrosis of spine
▶Code also any 360 degree spinal fusion by a single incision (81.61)
Code also any insertion of interbody spinal fusion device (84.51)
Code also any insertion of recombinant bone morphogenetic protein (84.52)◀
AHA: 4Q, '01, 64

81.30 Refusion of spine, not otherwise specified

81.31   Refusion of atlas-axis spine

Craniocervical fusion ⎫ by anterior
C₁-C₂ fusion   ⎬ transoral
Occiput C₂ fusion ⎭ or
                              posterior
                              technique

81.32   Refusion of other cervical spine, anterior technique

Arthrodesis of C₂ level or below:
    anterior (interbody) technique
    anterolateral technique

81.33   Refusion of other cervical spine, posterior technique

Arthrodesis of C₂ level or below:
    posterior (interbody) technique
    posterolateral technique

81.34   Refusion of dorsal and dorsolumbar spine, anterior technique

Arthrodesis of thoracic or thoracolumbar
    region:
    anterior (interbody) technique
    anterolateral technique

81.35   Refusion of dorsal and dorsolumbar spine, posterior technique

Arthrodesis of thoracic or thoracolumbar
    region:
    posterior (interbody) technique
    posterolateral technique

81.36   Refusion of lumbar and lumbosacral spine, anterior technique

Arthrodesis of lumbar or lumbosacral region
    anterior (interbody) technique
    anterolateral technique

81.37   Refusion of lumbar and lumbosacral spine, lateral transverse process technique

81.38   Refusion of lumbar and lumbosacral spine, posterior technique

Arthrodesis of lumbar or lumbosacral
    region:
    posterior (interbody) technique
    posterolateral technique

81.39   Refusion of spine, not elsewhere classified

√4ᵗʰ **81.4   Other repair of joint of lower extremity**

INCLUDES   arthroplasty of lower extremity with:
        external traction or fixation
        graft of bone (chips) or cartilage
        internal fixation device

AHA: S-O, '85, 4

81.40   Repair of hip, not elsewhere classified

81.42   Five-in-one repair of knee

Medial meniscectomy, medial collateral
    ligament repair, vastus medialis
    advancement, semitendinosus
    advancement, and pes anserinus
    transfer

81.43   Triad knee repair

Medial meniscectomy with repair of the
    anterior cruciate ligament and the
    medial collateral ligament
O'Donoghue procedure

81.44   Patellar stabilization

Roux-Goldthwait operation for recurrent
    dislocation of patella

DEF: Roux-Goldthwait operation: Stabilization of patella
via lateral ligament transposed at insertion beneath
undisturbed medial insertion; excision of capsule ellipse
and medial patella retinaculum; capsule reefed for
lateral patella hold.

81.45   Other repair of the cruciate ligaments

AHA: M-A, '87, 12

Partial Hip Replacement

Acetabulum remains intact

Prosthesis

Total Hip Replacement

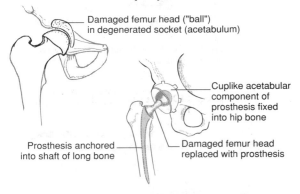

Damaged femur head ("ball") in degenerated socket (acetabulum)

Cuplike acetabular component of prosthesis fixed into hip bone

Prosthesis anchored into shaft of long bone

Damaged femur head replaced with prosthesis

81.46   Other repair of the collateral ligaments

81.47   Other repair of knee

AHA: 1Q, '00, 12, 13; 1Q, '96, 3; 3Q, '93, 5

81.49   Other repair of ankle

AHA: 2Q, '01, 15; 3Q, '00, 4

√4ᵗʰ **81.5   Joint replacement of lower extremity**

INCLUDES   arthroplasty of lower extremity with:
        external traction or fixation
        graft of bone (chips) or cartilage
        internal fixation device or
            prosthesis
        removal of cement spacer

AHA: S-O, '85, 4

81.51   Total hip replacement   BI

Replacement of both femoral head and
    acetabulum by prosthesis
Total reconstruction of hip

AHA: 2Q, '91, 18

DEF: Repair of both surfaces of hip joint with prosthesis.

81.52   Partial hip replacement   BI

Bipolar endoprosthesis

AHA: 2Q, '91, 18

DEF: Repair of single surface of hip joint with prosthesis.

81.53   Revision of hip replacement   BI

Partial
Total

AHA: 3Q, '97, 12

81.54   Total knee replacement   BI

Bicompartmental
Tricompartmental
Unicompartmental (hemijoint)

DEF: Repair of a knee joint with prosthetic implant in
one, two, or three compartments.

Total Knee Replacement

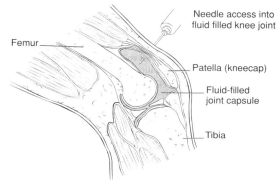

81.55   **Revision of knee replacement**   BI
           EXCLUDES   arthrodesis of knee (81.22)
           AHA: 2Q, '97, 10

81.56   **Total ankle replacement**   BI
81.57   **Replacement of joint of foot and toe**
81.59   **Revision of joint replacement of lower
           extremity, not elsewhere classified**

● ✓4ᵗʰ 81.6   **Other procedures on spine**
●   81.61   **360 degree spinal fusion, single incision
                   approach**
                   That by single incision but fusing or
                       refusing both anterior and posterior
                       spine
                   Code also refusion of spine (81.30-81.39)
                   Code also spinal fusion (81.00-81.08)

✓4ᵗʰ 81.7   **Arthroplasty and repair of hand, fingers, and wrist**
           INCLUDES   arthroplasty of hand and finger with:
                           external traction or fixation
                           graft of bone (chips) or cartilage
                           internal fixation device or
                               prosthesis
           EXCLUDES   operations on muscle, tendon, and
                           fascia of hand (82.01-82.99)
           DEF: Plastic surgery of hand, fingers and wrist joints.

81.71   **Arthroplasty of metacarpophalangeal and
           interphalangeal joint with implant**
81.72   **Arthroplasty of metacarpophalangeal and
           interphalangeal joint without implant**
           AHA: 1Q, '93, 28

81.73   **Total wrist replacement**
81.74   **Arthroplasty of carpocarpal or
           carpometacarpal joint with implant**
81.75   **Arthroplasty of carpocarpal or
           carpometacarpal joint without implant**
           AHA: 3Q, '93, 8

81.79   **Other repair of hand, fingers, and wrist**
✓4ᵗʰ 81.8   **Arthroplasty and repair of shoulder and elbow**
           INCLUDES   arthroplasty of upper limb NEC with:
                           external traction or fixation
                           graft of bone (chips) or cartilage
                           internal fixation device or
                               prosthesis
81.80   **Total shoulder replacement**
81.81   **Partial shoulder replacement**
81.82   **Repair of recurrent dislocation of shoulder**
           AHA: 3Q, '95, 15

81.83   **Other repair of shoulder**
           Revision of arthroplasty of shoulder
           AHA: ▶1Q, '02, 9;◀ 4Q, '01, 51; 2Q, '00, 14; 3Q, '93, 5

81.84   **Total elbow replacement**
81.85   **Other repair of elbow**

✓4ᵗʰ 81.9   **Other operations on joint structures**
       81.91   **Arthrocentesis**
                   Joint aspiration
                   EXCLUDES   that for:
                                   arthrography (88.32)
                                   biopsy of joint structure
                                       (80.30-80.39)
                                   injection of drug (81.92)
                   DEF: Insertion of needle to withdraw fluid from joint.

       81.92   **Injection of therapeutic substance into joint
                   or ligament**
                   AHA: 2Q, '00, 14; 3Q, '89, 16

       81.93   **Suture of capsule or ligament of upper
                   extremity**
                   EXCLUDES   that associated with
                                   arthroplasty (81.71-
                                   81.75, 81.80-81.81,
                                   81.84)

       81.94   **Suture of capsule or ligament of ankle and
                   foot**
                   EXCLUDES   that associated with
                                   arthroplasty (81.56-
                                   81.59)

       81.95   **Suture of capsule or ligament of other lower
                   extremity**
                   EXCLUDES   that associated with
                                   arthroplasty (81.51-
                                   81.55, 81.59)

       81.96   **Other repair of joint**
       81.97   **Revision of joint replacement of upper
                   extremity**
                   Partial
                   Removal of cement spacer
                   Total

       81.98   **Other diagnostic procedures on joint
                   structures**
                   EXCLUDES   arthroscopy (80.20-80.29)
                                   biopsy of joint structure
                                       (80.30-80.39)
                                   microscopic examination of
                                       specimen from joint
                                       (91.51-91.59)
                                   thermography (88.83)
                                   x-ray (87.21-87.29, 88.21-
                                       88.33)

       81.99   **Other**
✓3ʳᵈ 82   **Operations on muscle, tendon, and fascia of hand**
           INCLUDES   operations on:
                           aponeurosis
                           synovial membrane (tendon sheath)
                           tendon sheath

Arthrocentesis

Operations on the Musculoskeletal System 82.0–82.79

√4ᵗʰ **82.0 Incision of muscle, tendon, fascia, and bursa of hand**

82.01 Exploration of tendon sheath of hand

Incision of / Removal of rice bodies in } tendon sheath of hand

EXCLUDES   *division of tendon (82.11)*

DEF: Incision into and exploring the hand's muscle and its accompanying supportive, connective tissue, bands, and sacs.

82.02 Myotomy of hand

EXCLUDES   *myotomy for division (82.19)*

DEF: Incision into hand muscle.

82.03 Bursotomy of hand

82.04 Incision and drainage of palmar or thenar space

82.09 Other incision of soft tissue of hand

EXCLUDES   *incision of skin and subcutaneous tissue alone (86.01-86.09)*

AHA: N-D, '87, 10

√4ᵗʰ **82.1 Division of muscle, tendon, and fascia of hand**

82.11 Tenotomy of hand
Division of tendon of hand

82.12 Fasciotomy of hand
Division of fascia of hand

82.19 Other division of soft tissue of hand
Division of muscle of hand

√4ᵗʰ **82.2 Excision of lesion of muscle, tendon, and fascia of hand**

82.21 Excision or lesion of tendon sheath of hand
Ganglionectomy of tendon sheath (wrist)

82.22 Excision of lesion of muscle of hand

82.29 Excision of other lesion of soft tissue of hand

EXCLUDES   *excision of lesion of skin and subcutaneous tissue (86.21-86.3)*

√4ᵗʰ **82.3 Other excision of soft tissue of hand**
Code also any skin graft (86.61-86.62, 86.73)

EXCLUDES   *excision of skin and subcutaneous tissue (86.21-86.3)*

82.31 Bursectomy of hand

82.32 Excision of tendon of hand for graft

DEF: Resection and excision of fibrous tissue connecting bone to hand muscle for grafting.

82.33 Other tenonectomy of hand
Tenosynovectomy of hand

EXCLUDES   *excision of lesion of: tendon (82.29) sheath (82.21)*

DEF: Removal of fibrous bands connecting muscle to bone of hand.

DEF: Tenosynovectomy of hand: Excision of fibrous band connecting muscle and bone of hand and removal of coverings.

82.34 Excision of muscle or fascia of hand for graft

82.35 Other fasciectomy of hand
Release of Dupuytren's contracture

EXCLUDES   *excision of lesion of fascia (82.29)*

DEF: Excision of fibrous connective tissue; other than for grafting or removing lesion.

DEF: Release of Dupuytren's contracture: Excision of fibrous connective tissue to correct flexion of fingers.

82.36 Other myectomy of hand

EXCLUDES   *excision of lesion of muscle (82.22)*

82.39 Other excision of soft tissue of hand

EXCLUDES   *excision of skin (86.21-86.3) excision of soft tissue lesion (82.29)*

√4ᵗʰ **82.4 Suture of muscle, tendon, and fascia of hand**

82.41 Suture of tendon sheath of hand

82.42 Delayed suture of flexor tendon of hand

DEF: Suture of fibrous band between flexor muscle and bone; following initial repair.

82.43 Delayed suture of other tendon of hand

82.44 Other suture of flexor tendon of hand

EXCLUDES   *delayed suture of flexor tendon of hand (82.42)*

82.45 Other suture of other tendon of hand

EXCLUDES   *delayed suture of other tendon of hand (82.43)*

82.46 Suture of muscle or fascia of hand

√4ᵗʰ **82.5 Transplantation of muscle and tendon of hand**
AHA: 1Q, '93, 28

82.51 Advancement of tendon of hand

DEF: Detachment of fibrous connective muscle band and bone with reattachment at advanced point of hand.

82.52 Recession of tendon of hand

DEF: Detachment of fibrous band of muscle and bone with reattachment at drawn-back point of hand.

82.53 Reattachment of tendon of hand

82.54 Reattachment of muscle of hand

82.55 Other change in hand muscle or tendon length

82.56 Other hand tendon transfer or transplantation

EXCLUDES   *pollicization of thumb (82.61) transfer of finger, except thumb (82.81)*

AHA: 2Q, '99, 10; 4Q, '98, 40

82.57 Other hand tendon transposition
AHA: 1Q, '93, 28; 3Q, '93, 8

82.58 Other hand muscle transfer or transplantation

82.59 Other hand muscle transposition

√4ᵗʰ **82.6 Reconstruction of thumb**

INCLUDES   digital transfer to act as thumb
Code also any amputation for digital transfer (84.01, 84.11)

82.61 Pollicization operation carrying over nerves and blood supply

DEF: Creation or reconstruction of a thumb with another digit, commonly the index finger.

82.69 Other reconstruction of thumb
"Cocked-hat" procedure [skin flap and bone]
Grafts: bone / skin (pedicle) } to thumb

√4ᵗʰ **82.7 Plastic operation on hand with graft or implant**

82.71 Tendon pulley reconstruction
Reconstruction for opponensplasty

DEF: Reconstruction of fibrous band between muscle and bone of hand.

82.72 Plastic operation on hand with graft of muscle or fascia

82.79 Plastic operation on hand with other graft or implant
Tendon graft to hand
AHA: J-F, '87, 6

√4th **82.8　Other plastic operations on hand**

82.81　Transfer of finger, except thumb

EXCLUDES　*pollicization of thumb (82.61)*

82.82　Repair of cleft hand

DEF: Correction of fissure defect of hand.

82.83　Repair of macrodactyly

DEF: Reduction in size of abnormally large fingers.

82.84　Repair of mallet finger

DEF: Repair of flexed little finger.

82.85　Other tenodesis of hand

Tendon fixation of hand NOS

DEF: Fixation of fibrous connective band between muscle and bone of hand.

82.86　Other tenoplasty of hand

Myotenoplasty of hand

DEF: Myotenoplasty of hand: Plastic repair of muscle and fibrous band connecting muscle to bone.

82.89　Other plastic operations on hand

Plication of fascia
Repair of fascial hernia

EXCLUDES　*that with graft or implant (82.71-82.79)*

√4th **82.9　Other operations on muscle, tendon, and fascia of hand**

EXCLUDES　*diagnostic procedures on soft tissue of hand (83.21-83.29)*

82.91　Lysis of adhesions of hand

Freeing of adhesions of fascia, muscle, and tendon of hand

EXCLUDES　*decompression of carpal tunnel (04.43)*
that by stretching or manipulation only (93.26)

82.92　Aspiration of bursa of hand

82.93　Aspiration of other soft tissue of hand

EXCLUDES　*skin and subcutaneous tissue (86.01)*

82.94　Injection of therapeutic substance into bursa of hand

82.95　Injection of therapeutic substance into tendon of hand

82.96　Other injection of locally-acting therapeutic substance into soft tissue of hand

EXCLUDES　*subcutaneous or intramuscular injection (99.11-99.29)*

82.99　Other operations on muscle, tendon, and fascia of hand

√3rd **83　Operations on muscle, tendon, fascia, and bursa, except hand**

INCLUDES　operations on:
　　aponeurosis
　　synovial membrane of bursa and tendon sheaths
　　tendon sheaths

EXCLUDES　*diaphragm (34.81-34.89)*
hand (82.01-82.99)
muscles of eye (15.01-15.9)

√4th **83.0　Incision of muscle, tendon, fascia, and bursa**

83.01　Exploration of tendon sheath

Incision of tendon sheath
Removal of rice bodies from tendon sheath

DEF: Incision of external covering of fibrous cord for exam.

DEF: Removal of rice bodies from tendon sheath: Incision and removal of small bodies resembling grains of rice.

83.02　Myotomy

EXCLUDES　*cricopharyngeal myotomy (29.31)*

AHA: 2Q, '89, 18

83.03　Bursotomy

Removal of calcareous deposit of bursa

EXCLUDES　*aspiration of bursa (percutaneous) (83.94)*

83.09　Other incision of soft tissue

Incision of fascia

EXCLUDES　*incision of skin and subcutaneous tissue alone (86.01-86.09)*

√4th **83.1　Division of muscle, tendon, and fascia**

83.11　Achillotenotomy

DEF: Incision into fibrous connective cord between adductor muscle and hip bone.

83.12　Adductor tenotomy of hip

DEF: Incision into fibrous attachment between adductor muscle and hip bone.

83.13　Other tenotomy

Aponeurotomy
Division of tendon
Tendon release
Tendon transection
Tenotomy for thoracic outlet decompression

DEF: Aponeurotomy: Incision and separation of fibrous cords attaching a muscle to bone to aid movement.

DEF: Division of tendon: Separation of fibrous band connecting muscle to bone.

DEF: Tendon release: Surgical detachment of fibrous band from muscle and/or bone.

DEF: Tendon transection: Incision across width of fibrous bands between muscle and bone.

DEF: Tenotomy for thoracic outlet decompression: Incision of fibrous muscle with separation from bone to relieve compressed thoracic outlet..

83.14　Fasciotomy

Division of fascia
Division of iliotibial band
Fascia stripping
Release of Volkmann's contracture by fasciotomy

AHA: 3Q, '98, 8

DEF: Division of fascia: Incision to separate fibrous connective tissue.

DEF: Division of iliotibial band: Incision to separate fibrous band connecting tibial bone to muscle in flank.

DEF: Fascia stripping: Incision and lengthwise separation of fibrous connective tissue.

DEF: Release of Volkmann's contracture by fasciotomy: Divisional incision of connective tissue to correct defect in flexion of finger(s).

83.19　Other division of soft tissue

Division of muscle
Muscle release
Myotomy for thoracic outlet decompression
Myotomy with division
Scalenotomy
Transection of muscle

√4th **83.2　Diagnostic procedures on muscle, tendon, fascia, and bursa, including that of hand**

83.21　Biopsy of soft tissue

EXCLUDES　*biopsy of chest wall (34.23)*
biopsy of skin and subcutaneous tissue (86.11)

83.29   **Other diagnostic procedures on muscle, tendon, fascia, and bursa, including that of hand**

EXCLUDES   *microscopic examination of specimen (91.51-91.-59)*
soft tissue x-ray (87.09, 87.38-87.39, 88.09, 88.35, 88.37)
thermography of muscle (88.84)

√4th **83.3**   **Excision of lesion of muscle, tendon, fascia, and bursa**

EXCLUDES   *biopsy of soft tissue (83.21)*

83.31   **Excision of lesion of tendon sheath**
Excision of ganglion of tendon sheath, except of hand

83.32   **Excision of lesion of muscle**
Excision of:
   heterotopic bone
   muscle scar for release of Volkmann's contracture
   myositis ossificans

DEF: Heterotopic bone: Bone lesion in muscle.

DEF: Muscle scar for release of Volkmann's contracture: Scarred muscle tissue interfering with finger flexion.

DEF: Myositis ossificans: Bony deposits in muscle.

83.39   **Excision of lesion of other soft tissue**
Excision of Baker's cyst

EXCLUDES   *bursectomy (83.5)*
excision of lesion of skin and subcutaneous tissue (86.3)
synovectomy (80.70-80.79)

AHA: 2Q, '97, 6

√4th **83.4**   **Other excision of muscle, tendon, and fascia**

83.41   **Excision of tendon for graft**

83.42   **Other tenonectomy**
Excision of:
   aponeurosis
   tendon sheath
Tenosynovectomy

83.43   **Excision of muscle or fascia for graft**

83.44   **Other fasciectomy**

DEF: Excision of fascia; other than for graft.

83.45   **Other myectomy**
Debridement of muscle NOS
Scalenectomy

AHA: 1Q, '99, 8

DEF: Scalenectomy: Removal of thoracic scaleni muscle tissue.

83.49   **Other excision of soft tissue**

83.5   **Bursectomy**

AHA: 2Q, '99, 11

√4th **83.6**   **Suture of muscle, tendon, and fascia**

83.61   **Suture of tendon sheath**

83.62   **Delayed suture of tendon**

83.63   **Rotator cuff repair**

AHA: 2Q, '93, 8

DEF: Repair of musculomembranous structure around shoulder joint capsule.

83.64   **Other suture of tendon**
Achillorrhaphy
Aponeurorrhaphy

EXCLUDES   *delayed suture of tendon (83.62)*

DEF: Achillorrhaphy: Suture of fibrous band connecting Achilles tendon to heel bone.

DEF: Aponeurorraphy: Suture of fibrous cords connecting muscle to bone.

83.65   **Other suture of muscle or fascia**
Repair of diastasis recti

√4th **83.7**   **Reconstruction of muscle and tendon**

EXCLUDES   *reconstruction of muscle and tendon associated with arthroplasty*

83.71   **Advancement of tendon**

DEF: Detaching fibrous cord between muscle and bone with reattachment at advanced point.

83.72   **Recession of tendon**

DEF: Detaching fibrous cord between muscle and bone with reattachment at drawn-back point.

83.73   **Reattachment of tendon**

83.74   **Reattachment of muscle**

83.75   **Tendon transfer or transplantation**

83.76   **Other tendon transposition**

83.77   **Muscle transfer or transplantation**
Release of Volkmann's contracture by muscle transplantation

83.79   **Other muscle transposition**

√4th **83.8**   **Other plastic operations on muscle, tendon, and fascia**

EXCLUDES   *plastic operations on muscle, tendon, and fascia associated with arthroplasty*

83.81   **Tendon graft**

83.82   **Graft of muscle or fascia**

AHA: ▶3Q, '01, 9◀

83.83   **Tendon pulley reconstruction**

DEF: Reconstruction of fibrous cord between muscle and bone; at any site other than hand.

83.84   **Release of clubfoot, not elsewhere classified**
Evans operation on clubfoot

83.85   **Other change in muscle or tendon length**
Hamstring lengthening
Heel cord shortening
Plastic achillotenotomy
Tendon plication

DEF: Plastic achillotenotomy: Increase in heel cord length.

DEF: Tendon plication: Surgical tuck of tendon.

83.86   **Quadricepsplasty**

DEF: Correction of quadriceps femoris muscle.

83.87   **Other plastic operations on muscle**
Musculoplasty   Myoplasty

AHA: 1Q, '97, 9

83.88   **Other plastic operations on tendon**
Myotenoplasty
Tendon fixation
Tenodesis
Tenoplasty

83.89   **Other plastic operations on fascia**
Fascia lengthening
Fascioplasty
Plication of fascia

√4th **83.9**   **Other operations on muscle, tendon, fascia, and bursa**

EXCLUDES   *nonoperative:*
manipulation (93.25-93.29)
stretching (93.27-93.29)

83.91   **Lysis of adhesions of muscle, tendon, fascia, and bursa**

EXCLUDES   *that for tarsal tunnel syndrome (04.44)*

DEF: Separation of created fibrous structures from muscle, connective tissues, bands and sacs.

83.92   **Insertion or replacement of skeletal muscle stimulator**

Implantation, insertion, placement, or replacement of skeletal muscle:
electrodes
stimulator

AHA: 2Q, '99, 10

83.93   **Removal of skeletal muscle stimulator**

83.94   **Aspiration of bursa**

83.95   **Aspiration of other soft tissue**

EXCLUDES   *that of skin and subcutaneous tissue (86.01)*

83.96   **Injection of therapeutic substance into bursa**

83.97   **Injection of therapeutic substance into tendon**

83.98   **Injection of locally-acting therapeutic substance into other soft tissue**

EXCLUDES   *subcutaneous or intramuscular injection (99.11-99.29)*

83.99   **Other operations on muscle, tendon, fascia, and bursa**

Suture of bursa

√3ʳᵈ **84**   **Other procedures on musculoskeletal system**

√4ᵗʰ **84.0**   **Amputation of upper limb**

EXCLUDES   *revision of amputation stump (84.3)*

84.00   **Upper limb amputation, not otherwise specified**

Closed flap amputation
Kineplastic amputation
Open or guillotine amputation
Revision of current traumatic amputation
} of upper limb NOS

DEF: Closed flap amputation: Sewing a created skin flap over stump end of upper limb.

DEF: Kineplastic amputation: Amputation and preparation of stump of upper limb to permit movement.

DEF: Open or guillotine amputation: Straight incision across upper limb; used when primary closure is contraindicated.

DEF: Revision of current traumatic amputation: Reconstruction of traumatic amputation of upper limb to enable closure.

84.01   **Amputation and disarticulation of finger**

EXCLUDES   *ligation of supernumerary finger (86.26)*

84.02   **Amputation and disarticulation of thumb**

84.03   **Amputation through hand**

Amputation through carpals

84.04   **Disarticulation of wrist**

84.05   **Amputation through forearm**

Forearm amputation

84.06   **Disarticulation of elbow**

DEF: Amputation of forearm through elbow joint.

84.07   **Amputation through humerus**

Upper arm amputation

84.08   **Disarticulation of shoulder**

DEF: Amputation of arm through shoulder joint.

84.09   **Interthoracoscapular amputation**

Forequarter amputation

DEF: Removal of upper arm, shoulder bone and collarbone.

√4ᵗʰ **84.1**   **Amputation of lower limb**

EXCLUDES   *revision of amputation stump (84.3)*

84.10   **Lower limb amputation, not otherwise specified**

Closed flap amputation
Kineplastic amputation
Open or guillotine amputation
Revision of current traumatic amputation
} of lower limb NOS

DEF: Closed flap amputation: Sewing a created skin flap over stump of lower limb.

DEF: Kineplastic amputation: Amputation and preparation of stump of lower limb to permit movement.

DEF: Open or guillotine amputation: Straight incision across lower limb; used when primary closure is contraindicated.

DEF: Revision of current traumatic amputation: Reconstruction of traumatic amputation of lower limb to enable closure.

84.11   **Amputation of toe**

Amputation through metatarsophalangeal joint
Disarticulation of toe
Metatarsal head amputation
Ray amputation of foot (disarticulation of the metatarsal head of the toe extending across the forefoot, just proximal to the metatarsophalangeal crease)

EXCLUDES   *ligation of supernumerary toe (86.26)*

AHA: 4Q, '99, 19

84.12   **Amputation through foot**

Amputation of forefoot
Amputation through middle of foot
Chopart's amputation
Midtarsal amputation
Transmetatarsal amputation (amputation of the forefoot, including the toes)

EXCLUDES   *Ray amputation of foot (84.11)*

AHA: 4Q, '99, 19

DEF: Amputation of forefoot: Removal of foot in front of joint between toes and body of foot.

DEF: Chopart's amputation: Removal of foot with retention of heel, ankle and other associated ankle bones.

DEF: Midtarsal amputation: Amputation of foot through tarsals.

DEF: Transmetatarsal amputation: Amputation of foot through metatarsals.

84.13   **Disarticulation of ankle**

DEF: Removal of foot through ankle bone.

84.14   **Amputation of ankle through malleoli of tibia and fibula**

84.15   **Other amputation below knee**

Amputation of leg through tibia and fibula NOS

84.16   **Disarticulation of knee**

Batch, Spitler, and McFaddin amputation
Mazet amputation
S.P. Roger's amputation

DEF: Removal of lower leg through knee joint.

84.17 Amputation above knee
Amputation of leg through femur
Amputation of thigh
Conversion of below-knee amputation into
    above-knee amputation
Supracondylar above-knee amputation

84.18 Disarticulation of hip
DEF: Removal of leg through hip joint.

84.19 Abdominopelvic amputation
Hemipelvectomy
Hindquarter amputation
DEF: Removal of leg and portion of pelvic bone.

DEF: Hemipelvectomy: Removal of leg and lateral pelvis.

✓4ᵗʰ **84.2 Reattachment of extremity**
AHA: 1Q, '95, 8

84.21 Thumb reattachment
84.22 Finger reattachment
84.23 Forearm, wrist, or hand reattachment
84.24 Upper arm reattachment
Reattachment of arm NOS
84.25 Toe reattachment
84.26 Foot reattachment
84.27 Lower leg or ankle reattachment
Reattachment of leg NOS
84.28 Thigh reattachment
84.29 Other reattachment

84.3 Revision of amputation stump

Reamputation
Secondary closure } of stump
Trimming

EXCLUDES *revision of current traumatic
amputation [revision by further
amputation of current injury]
(84.00-84.19, 84.91)*

AHA: 4Q, '99; 15; 2Q, '98, 15; 4Q, '88, 12

✓4ᵗʰ **84.4 Implantation or fitting of prosthetic limb device**
**84.40 Implantation or fitting of prosthetic
limb device, not otherwise specified**
**84.41 Fitting of prosthesis of upper arm and
shoulder**
84.42 Fitting of prosthesis of lower arm and hand
**84.43 Fitting of prosthesis of arm, not otherwise
specified**
84.44 Implantation of prosthetic device of arm
84.45 Fitting of prosthesis above knee
84.46 Fitting of prosthesis below knee
**84.47 Fitting of prosthesis of leg, not otherwise
specified**
84.48 Implantation of prosthetic device of leg

✓4ᵗʰ **84.5 Implantation of other musculoskeletal devices and
substances**
84.51 Insertion of interbody spinal fusion device
Insertion of:
    cages (carbon, ceramic, metal, plastic or
        titanium)
    interbody fusion cage
    synthetic cages or spacers
    threaded bone dowels
Code also refusion of spine (81.30-81.39)
Code also spinal fusion (81.00-81.08)

**84.52 Insertion of recombinant bone
morphogenetic protein rhBMP**
That via collagen sponge, coral, ceramic and
    other carriers
Code also primary procedure performed:
    fracture repair (79.00-79.99)
    spinal fusion (81.00-81.08)
    spinal refusion (81.30-81.39)

✓4ᵗʰ **84.9 Other operations on musculoskeletal system**
EXCLUDES *nonoperative manipulation (93.25-
93.29)*
84.91 Amputation, not otherwise specified
84.92 Separation of equal conjoined twins
84.93 Separation of unequal conjoined twins
Separation of conjoined twins NOS
84.99 Other

15. OPERATIONS ON THE INTEGUMENTARY SYSTEM (85-86)

√3rd **85 Operations on the breast**

INCLUDES   operations on the skin and subcutaneous tissue of:

breast   } female or
previous mastectomy site   } male

revision of previous mastectomy site

85.0 Mastotomys
Incision of breast (skin)
Mammotomy

EXCLUDES   *aspiration of breast (85.91)*
removal of implant (85.94)AHA: 2Q, '90, 27

AHA: 2Q, '90, 27

√4th **85.1 Diagnostic procedures on breast**

85.11 Closed [percutaneous] [needle] biopsy of breast
AHA: 2Q, '00, 10; 3Q, '89, 17

DEF: Mammatome biopsy: Excision of breast tissue using a needle inserted through a small incision; followed by a full cut circle of tissue surrounding the core biopsy to obtain; multiple contiguous directional sampling for definitive diagnosis and staging of cancer

85.12 Open biopsy of breast
AHA: 3Q, '89, 17; M-A, '86, 11

DEF: Excision of breast tissue for examination.

85.19 Other diagnostic procedures on breast

EXCLUDES   *mammary ductogram (87.35)*
mammography NEC (87.37)
manual examination (89.36)
microscopic examination of specimen (91.61-91.69)
thermography (88.85)
ultrasonography (88.73)
xerography (87.36)

√4th **85.2 Excision or destruction of breast tissue**

EXCLUDES   *mastectomy (85.41-85.48)*
reduction mammoplasty (85.31-85.32)

85.20 Excision or destruction of breast tissue, not otherwise specified

85.21 Local excision of lesion of breast
Lumpectomy
Removal of area of fibrosis from breast

EXCLUDES   *biopsy of breast (85.11-85.12)*

AHA: 2Q, '90, 27; 3Q, '89, 17; M-A, '86, 11

85.22 Resection of quadrant of breast
85.23 Subtotal mastectomy

EXCLUDES   *quadrant resection (85.22)*

AHA: 2Q, '92, 7

DEF: Excision of a large portion of breast tissue.

85.24 Excision of ectopic breast tissue
Excision of accessory nipple

DEF: Excision of breast tissue outside normal breast region.

85.25 Excision of nipple

EXCLUDES   *excision of accessory nipple (85.24)*

√4th **85.3 Reduction mammoplasty and subcutaneous mammectomy**
AHA: 4Q, '95, 79, 80

85.31 Unilateral reduction mammoplasty
Unilateral:
amputative mammoplasty
size reduction mammoplasty

85.32 Bilateral reduction mammoplasty
Amputative mammoplasty
Reduction mammoplasty (for gynecomastia)

85.33 Unilateral subcutaneous mammectomy with synchronous implant

EXCLUDES   *that without synchronous implant (85.34)*

DEF: Removal of mammary tissue, leaving skin and nipple intact with implant of prosthesis.

85.34 Other unilateral subcutaneous mammectomy
Removal of breast tissue with preservation of skin and nipple
Subcutaneous mammectomy NOS

DEF: Excision of mammary tissue, leaving skin and nipple intact.

85.35 Bilateral subcutaneous mammectomy with synchronous implant

EXCLUDES   *that without synchronous implant (85.36)*

DEF: Excision of mammary tissue, both breasts, leaving skin and nipples intact; with prosthesis.

85.36 Other bilateral subcutaneous mammectomy

√4th **85.4 Mastectomy**

85.41 Unilateral simple mastectomy
Mastectomy: Mastectomy:
NOS   complete
DEF: Removal of one breast.

85.42 Bilateral simple mastectomy
Bilateral complete mastectomy
DEF: Removal of both breasts.

85.43 Unilateral extended simple mastectomy
Extended simple mastectomy NOS
Modified radical mastectomy
Simple mastectomy with excision of regional lymph nodes
AHA: 2Q, '92, 7; 3Q, '91, 24; 2Q, '91, 21

DEF: Removal of one breast and lymph nodes under arm.

85.44 Bilateral extended simple mastectomy
AHA: 2Q, '92, 7; 3Q, '91, 24; 2Q, '91, 21

85.45 Unilateral radical mastectomy
Excision of breast, pectoral muscles, and regional lymph nodes [axillary, clavicular, supraclavicular]
Radical mastectomy NOS
AHA: 2Q, '91, 21

DEF: Removal of one breast and regional lymph nodes, pectoral muscle and adjacent tissue.

Mastectomy

Partial mastectomy (lumpectomy): skin left intact

Simple mastectomy

Lymph nodes

Radical mastectomy

√3rd
√4th Additional Digit Required   Nonspecific OR Procedure   Valid OR Procedure   Non-OR Procedure

85.46   Bilateral radical mastectomy

     AHA: 2Q, '91, 21

85.47   Unilateral extended radical mastectomy

     Excision of breast, muscles, and lymph nodes [axillary, clavicular, supraclavicular, internal mammary, and mediastinal]

     Extended radical mastectomy NOS

     DEF: Removal of one breast, regional and middle chest lymph nodes, chest muscle and adjacent tissue.

85.48   Bilateral extended radical mastectomy

     DEF: Removal of both breasts, regional and middle chest lymph nodes, chest muscle and adjacent tissue.

√4ᵗʰ 85.5   Augmentation mammoplasty

     EXCLUDES   *that associated with subcutaneous mammectomy (85.33, 85.35)*

     AHA: 3Q, '97, 12; 4Q, '95, 76, 80

     DEF: Plastic surgery to increase breast size.

85.50   Augmentation mammoplasty, not otherwise specified

85.51   Unilateral injection into breast for augmentation

85.52   Bilateral injection into breast for augmentation

     Injection into breast for augmentation NOS

85.53   Unilateral breast implant

     AHA: 2Q, '00 18; 2Q, '98, 14

85.54   Bilateral breast implant

     Breast implant NOS

85.6   Mastopexy

     DEF: Anchoring of pendulous breast.

85.7   Total reconstruction of breast

     AHA: 4Q, '95, 77; 1Q, '93, 27

√4ᵗʰ 85.8   Other repair and plastic operations on breast

     EXCLUDES   *that for:*

         augmentation (85.50-85.54)

         reconstruction (85.7)

         reduction (85.31-85.32)

     AHA: 4Q, '95, 77

85.81   Suture of laceration of breast

85.82   Split-thickness graft to breast

85.83   Full-thickness graft to breast

     AHA: 4Q, '95, 77

85.84   Pedicle graft to breast

     AHA: 4Q, '95, 77

     DEF: Implantation of transferred muscle tissue still connected to vascular source.

85.85   Muscle flap graft to breast

     AHA: 4Q, '95, 77

     DEF: Relocation of nipple.

85.86   Transposition of nipple

     AHA: 4Q, '95, 78

85.87   Other repair or reconstruction of nipple

     AHA: 4Q, '95, 78

85.89   Other mammoplasty

√4ᵗʰ 85.9   Other operations on the breast

85.91   Aspiration of breast

     EXCLUDES   *percutaneous biopsy of breast (85.11)*

85.92   Injection of therapeutic agent into breast

     EXCLUDES   *that for augmentation of breast (85.51-85.52)*

85.93   Revision of implant of breast

     AHA: 2Q, '98, 14; 4Q, '95, 76

85.94   Removal of implant of breast

     AHA: 2Q, '98, 14; 3Q, '92, 4

85.95   Insertion of breast tissue expander

     Insertion (soft tissue) of tissue expander (one or more) under muscle or platysma to develop skin flaps for donor use

85.96   Removal of breast tissue expander(s)

     AHA: 2Q, '00, 18; 4Q, '95, 77

85.99   Other

√3ʳᵈ 86   Operations on skin and subcutaneous tissue

     INCLUDES   operations on: operations on:

         hair follicles   subcutaneous fat pads

         male perineum   sudoriferous glands

         nails   superficial fossae

         sebaceous glands

     EXCLUDES   *those on skin of:*

         anus (49.01-49.99)

         breast (mastectomy site) (85.0-85.99)

         ear (18.01-18.9)

         eyebrow (08.01-08.99)

         eyelid (08.01-08.99)

         female perineum (71.01-71.9)

         lips (27.0-27.99)

         nose (21.00-21.99)

         penis (64.0-64.99)

         scrotum (61.0-61.99)

         vulva (71.01-71.9)

√4ᵗʰ 86.0   Incision of skin and subcutaneous tissue

86.01   Aspiration of skin and subcutaneous tissue

     Aspiration of:

         abscess   } of nail, skin, or

         hematoma   subcutaneous

         seroma   tissue

     AHA: 3Q, '89, 16

86.02   Injection or tattooing of skin lesion or defect

     Insertion   } of filling material

     Injection

     Pigmenting of skin

     DEF: Pigmenting of skin: Adding color to skin.

86.03   Incision of pilonidal sinus or cyst

     EXCLUDES   *marsupialization (86.21)*

86.04   Other incision with drainage of skin and subcutaneous tissue

     EXCLUDES   *drainage of:*

         fascial compartments of face and mouth (27.0)

         palmar or thenar space (82.04)

         pilonidal sinus or cyst (86.03)

86.05   Incision with removal of foreign body from skin and subcutaneous tissue

     Removal of loop recorder

     Removal of tissue expander(s) from skin or soft tissue other than breast tissue

     EXCLUDES   *removal of foreign body without incision (98.20-98.29)*

     AHA: 2Q, '96, 15; N-D, '87, 10; N-D, '86, 9

86.06 **Insertion of totally implantable infusion pump**

Code also any associated catheterization

EXCLUDES *insertion of totally implantable vascular access device (86.07)*

AHA: 2Q, '99, 4; 4Q, '90, 14

86.07 **Insertion of totally implantable vascular access device [VAD]**

Totally implanted port

EXCLUDES *insertion of totally implantable infusion pump (86.06)*

AHA: 1Q, '01, 13; 1Q, '96, 3; 2Q, '94, 11; 3Q, '91, 13; 4Q, '90, 15

DEF: Placement of vascular access infusion catheter system under skin to allow for frequent manual infusions into blood vessel.

86.09 **Other incision of skin and subcutaneous tissue**

Creation of loop recorder pocket, new site, and insertion/relocation of device
Creation of pocket for implantable, patient-activated cardiac event recorder and insertion/relocation of device
Creation of thalamic stimulator pulse generator pocket, new site
Escharotomy
Exploration:
  sinus tract, skin
  superficial fossa
Undercutting of hair follicle

EXCLUDES *that of:*
  cardiac pacemaker pocket, new site (37.79)
  fascial compartments of face and mouth (27.0)

AHA: 4Q, '00, 68; 4Q, '99, 21; 4Q, '97, 57; 3Q, '89, 17; N-D, '86, 1; N-D, '84, 6

√4ᵗʰ **86.1** **Diagnostic procedures on skin and subcutaneous tissue**

86.11 **Biopsy of skin and subcutaneous tissue**

86.19 **Other diagnostic procedures on skin and subcutaneous tissue**

EXCLUDES *microscopic examination of specimen from skin and subcutaneous tissue (91.61-91.79)*

√4ᵗʰ **86.2** **Excision or destruction of lesion or tissue of skin and subcutaneous tissue**

86.21 **Excision of pilonidal cyst or sinus**

Marsupialization of cyst

EXCLUDES *incision of pilonidal cyst or sinus (86.03)*

DEF: Marsupialization of cyst: Incision of cyst and suturing edges to skin to open site.

86.22 **Excisional debridement of wound, infection, or burn**

Removal by excision of:
  devitalized tissue
  necrosis
  slough

EXCLUDES *debridement of:*
  abdominal wall (wound) (54.3)
  bone (77.60-77.69)
  muscle (83.45)
  of hand (82.36)
  nail (bed) (fold) (86.27)
  nonexcisional debridement of wound, infection, or burn (86.28)
  open fracture site (79.60-79.69)
  pedicle or flap graft (86.75)

AHA: 2Q, '00, 9; 1Q, '99, 8; 2Q, '92, 17; 3Q, '91, 18; 3Q, '89, 16; 4Q, '88, 5; N-D, '86, 1

86.23 **Removal of nail, nailbed, or nail fold**

86.24 **Chemosurgery of skin**

Chemical peel of skin

DEF: Chemicals applied to destroy skin tissue.

DEF: Chemical peel of skin: Chemicals used to peel skin layers.

86.25 **Dermabrasion**

That with laser

EXCLUDES *dermabrasion of wound to remove embedded debris (86.28)*

DEF: Removal of wrinkled or scarred skin; with fine sandpaper, wire, brushes or laser.

86.26 **Ligation of dermal appendage**

EXCLUDES *excision of preauricular appendage (18.29)*

DEF: Tying off extra skin.

86.27 **Debridement of nail, nail bed, or nail fold**

Removal of:
  necrosis
  slough

EXCLUDES *removal of nail, nail bed, or nail fold (86.23)*

86.28 **Nonexcisional debridement of wound, infection, or burn**

Debridement NOS
▶Maggot therapy◀
Removal of devitalized tissue, necrosis, and slough by such methods as:
  brushing
  irrigation (under pressure)
  scrubbing
  washing

AHA: 2Q, '01, 18; 3Q, '91, 18; 4Q, '88, 5

DEF: Removal of damaged skin; by methods other than excision.

86.3 **Other local excision or destruction of lesion or tissue of skin and subcutaneous tissue**

Destruction of skin by: Destruction of skin by:
  cauterization   fulguration
  cryosurgery   laser beam
That with Z-plasty

EXCLUDES *adipectomy (86.83)*
  biopsy of skin (86.11)
  wide or radical excision of skin (86.4)
  Z-plasty without excision (86.84)

AHA: 1Q, '96, 15; 2Q, '90, 27; 1Q, '89, 12; 3Q, '89, 18; 4Q, '88, 7

Operations on the Integumentary System 86.06–86.3

86.4   Radical excision of skin lesion
Wide excision of skin lesion involving underlying or adjacent structure
Code also any lymph node dissection (40.3-40.5)

√4ᵗʰ 86.5   Suture or other closure of skin and subcutaneous tissue

86.51   Replantation of scalp

86.59   Closure of skin and subcutaneous tissue of other sites
Adhesives (surgical) (tissue)
Staples
Sutures

> **EXCLUDES**   application of adhesive strips (butterfly) — omit code

AHA: 4Q, '99, 23

√4ᵗʰ 86.6   Free skin graft

> **INCLUDES**   excision of skin for autogenous graft
> **EXCLUDES**   construction or reconstruction of:
>   penis (64.43-64.44)
>   trachea (31.75)
>   vagina (70.61-70.62)

DEF: Transplantation of skin to another site.

86.60   Free skin graft, not otherwise specified

86.61   Full-thickness skin graft to hand

> **EXCLUDES**   heterograft (86.65)
>   homograft (86.66)

86.62   Other skin graft to hand

> **EXCLUDES**   heterograft (86.65)
>   homograft (86.66)

86.63   Full-thickness skin graft to other sites

> **EXCLUDES**   heterograft (86.65)
>   homograft (86.66)

86.64   Hair transplant

> **EXCLUDES**   hair follicle transplant to eyebrow or eyelash (08.63)

86.65   Heterograft to skin
Pigskin graft   Porcine graft

> **EXCLUDES** ► application of dressing only (93.57)◄

DEF: Implantation of nonhuman tissue.

86.66   Homograft to skin
Graft to skin of:
     amnionic membrane   } from donor
     skin

DEF: Implantation of tissue from human donor.

86.67   Dermal regenerative graft
Artificial skin, NOS
Creation of "neodermis"
Decellularized allodermis
Integumentary matrix implants
Prosthetic implant of dermal layer of skin
Regenerate dermal layer of skin

> **EXCLUDES**   heterograft to skin (86.65)
>   homograft to skin (86.66)

AHA: 4Q, '98, 76, 79

DEF: Replacement of dermis and epidermal layer of skin by cultured or regenerated autologous tissue; used to treat full-thickness or deep partial-thickness burns; also called cultured epidermal autograft (CEA).

86.69   Other skin graft to other sites

> **EXCLUDES**   heterograft (86.65)
>   homograft (86.66)

AHA: 4Q, '99, 15

√4ᵗʰ 86.7   Pedicle grafts or flaps

> **EXCLUDES**   construction or reconstruction of:
>   penis (64.43-64.44)
>   trachea (31.75)
>   vagina (70.61-70.62)

DEF: Full thickness skin and subcutaneous tissue partially attached to the body by a narrow strip of tissue so that it retains its blood supply. The unattached portion is sutured to the defect.

86.70   Pedicle or flap graft, not otherwise specified

86.71   Cutting and preparation of pedicle grafts or flaps
Elevation of pedicle from its bed
Flap design and raising
Partial cutting of pedicle or tube
Pedicle delay

> **EXCLUDES**   pollicization or digital transfer (82.61, 82.81)
>   revision of pedicle (86.75)

AHA: ►4Q, '01, 66◄

DEF: Elevation and preparation of tissue still attached to vascular bed; delayed implant.

DEF: Elevation of pedicle from its bed: Separation of tissue implanted from its bed.

DEF: Flap design and raising: Planing and elevation of tissue to be implanted.

86.72   Advancement of pedicle graft
AHA: 3Q, '99, 9, 10

86.73   Attachment of pedicle or flap graft to hand

> **EXCLUDES**   pollicization or digital transfer (82.61, 82.81)

86.74   Attachment of pedicle or flap graft to other sites
Attachment by   Attachment by
   advanced flap   rotating flap
   double pedicled flap   sliding flap
   pedicle graft   tube graft
AHA: 3Q, '99, 9; 1Q, '96, 15

DEF: Fixation of tissue implant still connected to original site, other than hand.

DEF: Attachment by:

Advanced flap: Sliding tissue implant into new position.

Double pedicle flap: Implant connected to two vascular beds.

Pedicle graft: Implant connected to vascular bed.

Rotating flap: Implant rotated along curved incision.

Sliding flap: Sliding implant to site.

Tube graft: Double tissue implant to form tube with base connected to original site.

86.75   Revision of pedicle or flap graft
Debridement   } of pedicle or flap
Defatting   }   graft

DEF: Connection of implant still attached to its vascular tissue.

√4ᵗʰ 86.8   Other repair and reconstruction of skin and subcutaneous tissue
DEF: Revision and tightening of excess, wrinkled facial skin.

86.81   Repair for facial weakness

86.82   Facial rhytidectomy
Face lift

> **EXCLUDES**   rhytidectomy of eyelid (08.86-08.87)

86.83   **Size reduction plastic operation**
Liposuction
Reduction of adipose tissue of:
   abdominal wall (pendulous)
   arms (batwing)
   buttock
   thighs (trochanteric lipomatosis)
EXCLUDES   breast (85.31-85.32)
DEF: Excision and plastic repair of excess skin and underlying tissue.

86.84   **Relaxation of scar or web contracture of skin**
Z-plasty of skin
EXCLUDES   Z-plasty with excision of lesion (86.3)

86.85   **Correction of syndactyly**
DEF: Plastic repair of webbed fingers or toes.

86.86   **Onychoplasty**
DEF: Plastic repair of nail or nail bed.

86.89   **Other repair and reconstruction of skin and subcutaneous tissue**
EXCLUDES   mentoplasty (76.67-76.68)
AHA: 1Q, '00, 26; 2Q, '98, 20; 2Q, '93, 11; 2Q, '92, 17

✓4ᵗʰ **86.9**   **Other operations on skin and subcutaneous tissue**
86.91   **Excision of skin for graft**
Excision of skin with closure of donor site
EXCLUDES   that with graft at same operative episode (86.60-86.69)

86.92   **Electrolysis and other epilation of skin**
EXCLUDES   epilation of eyelid (08.91-08.93)

86.93   **Insertion of tissue expander**
Insertion (subcutaneous) (soft tissue) of expander (one or more) in scalp (subgaleal space), face, neck, trunk except breast, and upper and lower extremities for development of skin flaps for donor use
EXCLUDES   flap graft preparation (86.71)
tissue expander, breast (85.95)

86.99   **Other**
EXCLUDES   removal of sutures from:
   abdomen (97.83)
   head and neck (97.38)
   thorax (97.43)
   trunk NEC (97.84)
wound catheter:
   irrigation (96.58)
   replacement (97.15)
AHA: 4Q, '97, 57; N-D, '86, 1

Diagnostic and Therapeutic Procedures 87–87.41

16. MISCELLANEOUS DIAGNOSTIC AND THERAPEUTIC PROCEDURES (87-99)

√3rd **87 Diagnostic radiology**

√4th **87.0 Soft tissue x-ray of face, head, and neck**
EXCLUDES *angiography (88.40-88.68)*

87.01 Pneumoencephalogram
DEF: Radiographic exam of cerebral ventricles and subarachnoid spaces; with injection of air or gas for contrast.

87.02 Other contrast radiogram of brain and skull
Pneumocisternogram
Pneumoventriculogram
Posterior fossa myelogram
DEF: Pneumocisternogram: Radiographic exam of subarachnoid spaces after injection of gas for contrast.

DEF: Pneumoventriculography: Radiographic exam of cerebral ventricles after injection of gas for contrast.

DEF: Posterior fossa myelogram: Radiographic exam of posterior channel of spinal cord after injection of gas or contrast.

87.03 Computerized axial tomography of head
C.A.T. scan of head
AHA: 3Q, '99, 7

87.04 Other tomography of head

87.05 Contrast dacryocystogram
DEF: Radiographic exam of tear sac after injection of contrast.

87.06 Contrast radiogram of nasopharynx

87.07 Contrast laryngogram

87.08 Cervical lymphangiogram
DEF: Radiographic exam of lymph vessels of neck; with or without contrast.

87.09 Other soft tissue x-ray of face, head, and neck
Noncontrast x-ray of: Noncontrast x-ray of:
adenoid   salivary gland
larynx   thyroid region
nasolacrimal duct   uvula
nasopharynx
EXCLUDES *x-ray study of eye (95.14)*

√4th **87.1 Other x-ray of face, head, and neck**
EXCLUDES *angiography (88.40-88.68)*

87.11 Full-mouth x-ray of teeth

87.12 Other dental x-ray
Orthodontic cephalogram or cephalometrics
Panorex examination of mandible
Root canal x-ray

87.13 Temporomandibular contrast arthrogram

87.14 Contrast radiogram of orbit

87.15 Contrast radiogram of sinus

87.16 Other x-ray of facial bones
X-ray of: X-ray of:
frontal area   orbit
mandible   supraorbital area
maxilla   symphysis menti
nasal sinuses   zygomaticomaxillary
nose   complex

87.17 Other x-ray of skull
Lateral projection
Sagittal projection } of skull
Tangential projection
DEF: Lateral projection: Side to side view of head.

DEF: Sagittal projection: View of body in plane running midline from front to back.

DEF: Tangential projection: Views from adjacent skull surfaces.

√4th **87.2 X-ray of spine**

87.21 Contrast myelogram
DEF: Radiographic exam of space between middle and outer spinal cord coverings after injection of contrast.

87.22 Other x-ray of cervical spine

87.23 Other x-ray of thoracic spine

87.24 Other x-ray of lumbosacral spine
Sacrococcygeal x-ray

87.29 Other x-ray of spine
Spinal x-ray NOS

√4th **87.3 Soft tissue x-ray of thorax**
EXCLUDES *angiocardiography (88.50-88.58)*
angiography (88.40-88.68)

87.31 Endotracheal bronchogram
DEF: Radiographic exam of lung, main branch, with contrast introduced through windpipe.

87.32 Other contrast bronchogram
Transcricoid bronchogram
DEF: Triscrichoid bronchogram: Radiographic exam of lung, main branch, with contrast introduced through cartilage of neck.

87.33 Mediastinal pneumogram
DEF: Radiographic exam of cavity containing heart, esophagus and adjacent structures.

87.34 Intrathoracic lymphangiogram
DEF: Radiographic exam of lymphatic vessels within chest; with or without contrast.

87.35 Contrast radiogram of mammary ducts
DEF: Radiographic exam of mammary ducts; with contrast.

87.36 Xerography of breast
DEF: Radiographic exam of breast via selenium-coated plates.

87.37 Other mammography
AHA: 3Q, '89, 17; 2Q, '90, 28; N-D, '87, 1

87.38 Sinogram of chest wall
Fistulogram of chest wall
DEF: Radiographic exam of chest cavity.

DEF: Fistulogram of chest wall: Radiographic exam of abnormal opening in chest.

87.39 Other soft tissue x-ray of chest wall

√4th **87.4 Other x-ray of thorax**
EXCLUDES *angiocardiography (88.50-88.58)*
angiography (88.40-88.68)

87.41 Computerized axial tomography of thorax
C.A.T. scan
Crystal linea scan of x-ray beam
Electronic subtraction } of thorax
Photoelectric response
Tomography with use of computer, x-rays, and camera

87.42   Other tomography of thorax
Cardiac tomogram
DEF: Radiographic exam of chest plane.

87.43   X-ray of ribs, sternum, and clavicle
Examination for:
    cervical rib
    fracture

87.44   Routine chest x-ray, so described
X-ray of chest NOS

87.49   Other chest x-ray
X-ray of: X-ray of:
    bronchus NOS   lung NOS
    diaphragm NOS   mediastinum NOS
    heart NOS   trachea NOS

✓4th **87.5   Biliary tract x-ray**

87.51   Percutaneous hepatic cholangiogram
AHA: 2Q, '90, 28; N-D, '87, 1

DEF: Radiographic exam of bile tract of gallbladder; with
needle injection of contrast into bile duct of liver.

87.52   Intravenous cholangiogram
DEF: Radiographic exam of bile ducts; with intravenous
contrast injection.

87.53   Intraoperative cholangiogram
AHA: 1Q, '96, 12; 2Q, '90, 28; 3Q, '89, 18; 4Q, '88, 7

DEF: Radiographic exam of bile ducts; with contrast;
following gallbladder removal.

87.54   Other cholangiogram

87.59   Other biliary tract x-ray
Cholecystogram

✓4th **87.6   Other x-ray of digestive system**

87.61   Barium swallow

87.62   Upper GI series

87.63   Small bowel series

87.64   Lower GI series

87.65   Other x-ray of intestine

87.66   Contrast pancreatogram

87.69   Other digestive tract x-ray

✓4th **87.7   X-ray of urinary system**
        EXCLUDES   *angiography of renal vessels (88.45,
                        88.65)*

87.71   Computerized axial tomography of kidney
C.A.T. scan of kidney

87.72   Other nephrotomogram
DEF: Radiographic exam of kidney plane.

Ureteropyelography

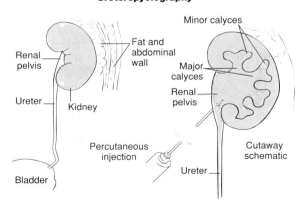

Minor calyces
Fat and abdominal wall
Major calyces
Renal pelvis
Renal pelvis
Ureter
Kidney
Percutaneous injection
Cutaway schematic
Ureter
Bladder

87.73   Intravenous pyelogram
Diuretic infusion pyelogram
DEF: Radiographic exam of lower kidney, with
intravenous contrast injection.

DEF: Diuretic infusion pyelogram: Radiographic exam of
lower kidney with diuretic contrast.

87.74   Retrograde pyelogram

87.75   Percutaneous pyelogram

87.76   Retrograde cystourethrogram
DEF: Radiographic exam of bladder and urethra with
contrast injected through catheter into bladder.

87.77   Other cystogram

87.78   Ileal conduitogram
AHA: M-J, '87, 11

DEF: Radiographic exam of passage created between
ureter and artificial opening into abdomen.

87.79   Other x-ray of the urinary system
KUB x-ray

✓4th **87.8   X-ray of female genital organs**

87.81   X-ray of gravid uterus   ♀
Intrauterine cephalometry by x-ray

87.82   Gas contrast hysterosalpingogram   ♀
DEF: Radiographic exam of uterus and fallopian tubes;
with gas contrast.

87.83   Opaque dye contrast hysterosal-   ♀
pingogram

87.84   Percutaneous hysterogram   ♀
DEF: Radiographic exam of uterus with contrast injected
through body wall.

87.85   Other x-ray of fallopian tubes and uterus ♀

87.89   Other x-ray of female genital organs   ♀

✓4th **87.9   X-ray of male genital organs**

87.91   Contrast seminal vesiculogram   ♂

87.92   Other x-ray of prostate and seminal   ♂
vesicles

87.93   Contrast epididymogram   ♂

87.94   Contrast vasogram   ♂

87.95   Other x-ray of epididymis and vas   ♂
deferens

87.99   Other x-ray of male genital organs   ♂

✓3rd **88   Other diagnostic radiology and related techniques**

✓4th **88.0   Soft tissue x-ray of abdomen**
        EXCLUDES   *angiography (88.40-88.68)*

88.01   Computerized axial tomography of abdomen
C.A.T. scan of abdomen
        EXCLUDES   *C.A.T. scan of kidney (87.71)*
AHA: 2Q, '98, 13

88.02   Other abdomen tomography
        EXCLUDES   *nephrotomogram (87.72)*

88.03   Sinogram of abdominal wall
Fistulogram of abdominal wall
DEF: Radiographic exam of abnormal abdominal
passage.

88.04   Abdominal lymphangiogram
DEF: Radiographic exam of abdominal lymphatic vessels;
with contrast.

88.09   Other soft tissue x-ray of abdominal wall

✓4th **88.1   Other x-ray of abdomen**

88.11   Pelvic opaque dye contrast radiography

88.12   Pelvic gas contrast radiography
Pelvic pneumoperitoneum

88.13   Other peritoneal pneumogram

88.14   Retroperitoneal fistulogram

88.15   Retroperitoneal pneumogram

88.16 Other retroperitoneal x-ray

88.19 Other x-ray of abdomen
Flat plate of abdomen
AHA: 3Q, '99, 9

√4ᵗʰ **88.2** Skeletal x-ray of extremities and pelvis
> **EXCLUDES** *contrast radiogram of joint (88.32)*

88.21 Skeletal x-ray of shoulder and upper arm

88.22 Skeletal x-ray of elbow and forearm

88.23 Skeletal x-ray of wrist and hand

88.24 Skeletal x-ray of upper limb, not otherwise specified

88.25 Pelvimetry
DEF: Imaging of pelvic bones to measure pelvic capacity.

88.26 Other skeletal x-ray of pelvis and hip

88.27 Skeletal x-ray of thigh, knee, and lower leg

88.28 Skeletal x-ray of ankle and foot

88.29 Skeletal x-ray of lower limb, not otherwise specified

√4ᵗʰ **88.3** Other x-ray

88.31 Skeletal series
X-ray of whole skeleton

88.32 Contrast arthrogram
> **EXCLUDES** *that of temporomandibular joint (87.13)*

88.33 Other skeletal x-ray
> **EXCLUDES** *skeletal x-ray of:*
> *extremities and pelvis (88.21-88.29)*
> *face, head, and neck (87.11-87.17)*
> *spine (87.21-87.29)*
> *thorax (87.43)*

88.34 Lymphangiogram of upper limb

88.35 Other soft tissue x-ray of upper limb

88.36 Lymphangiogram of lower limb

88.37 Other soft tissue x-ray of lower limb
> **EXCLUDES** *femoral angiography (88.48, 88.66)*

88.38 Other computerized axial tomography
C.A.T. scan NOS
> **EXCLUDES** *C.A.T. scan of:*
> *abdomen (88.01)*
> *head (87.03)*
> *kidney (87.71)*
> *thorax (87.41)*

88.39 X-ray, other and unspecified

√4ᵗʰ **88.4** Arteriography using contrast material
> **INCLUDES** angiography of arteries
> arterial puncture for injection of contrast material
> radiography of arteries (by fluoroscopy)
> retrograde arteriography

Note: The fourth-digit subclassification identifies the site to be viewed, not the site of injection.
> **EXCLUDES** *arteriography using:*
> *radioisotopes or radionuclides (92.01-92.19)*
> *ultrasound (88.71-88.79)*
> *fluorescein angiography of eye (95.12)*

AHA: N-D, '85, 14

DEF: Electromagnetic wave photography of arteries; with contrast.

88.40 Arteriography using contrast material, unspecified site

88.41 Arteriography of cerebral arteries
Angiography of:
basilar artery
carotid (internal)
posterior cerebral circulation
vertebral artery
AHA: 1Q, '00, 16; 1Q, '99, 7; 1Q, '97, 3

88.42 Aortography
Arteriography of aorta and aortic arch
AHA: 1Q, '99, 17

88.43 Arteriography of pulmonary arteries

88.44 Arteriography of other intrathoracic vessels
> **EXCLUDES** *angiocardiography (88.50-88.58)*
> *arteriography of coronary arteries (88.55-88.57)*

88.45 Arteriography of renal arteries

88.46 Arteriography of placenta
Placentogram using contrast material

88.47 Arteriography of other intra-abdominal arteries
AHA: 1Q, '00, 18; N-D, '87, 4

88.48 Arteriography of femoral and other lower extremity arteries
AHA: 2Q, '96, 6; 2Q, '89, 17

88.49 Arteriography of other specified sites

√4ᵗʰ **88.5** Angiocardiography using contrast material
> **INCLUDES** arterial puncture and insertion of arterial catheter for injection of contrast material
> cineangiocardiography
> selective angiocardiography
Code also synchronous cardiac catheterization (37.21-37.23)
> **EXCLUDES** *angiography of pulmonary vessels (88.43, 88.62)*

AHA: 3Q, '92, 10; M-J, '87, 11

DEF: Electromagnetic wave photography of heart and great vessels; with contrast.

88.50 Angiocardiography, not otherwise specified

88.51 Angiocardiography of venae cavae
Inferior vena cavography
Phlebography of vena cava (inferior) (superior)

88.52 Angiocardiography of right heart structures
Angiocardiography of:
pulmonary valve
right atrium
right ventricle (outflow tract)
> **EXCLUDES** *that combined with left heart angiocardiography (88.54)*

88.53 Angiocardiography of left heart structures
Angiocardiography of:
aortic valve
left atrium
left ventricle (outflow tract)
> **EXCLUDES** *that combined with right heart angiocardiography (88.54)*

AHA: 1Q, '00, 20; 4Q, '88, 4

88.54 Combined right and left heart angiocardiography

88.55 Coronary arteriography using a single catheter
 Coronary arteriography by Sones technique
 Direct selective coronary arteriography using a single catheter

88.56 Coronary arteriography using two catheters
 Coronary arteriography by:
  Judkins technique
  Ricketts and Abrams technique
 Direct selective coronary arteriography using two catheters
 AHA: 1Q, '00, 20; 4Q, '88, 4

88.57 Other and unspecified coronary arteriography
 Coronary arteriography NOS
 AHA: 1Q, '00, 21

88.58 Negative-contrast cardiac roentgenography
 Cardiac roentgenography with injection of carbon dioxide

√3rd **88.6** Phlebography

> INCLUDES angiography of veins
>   radiography of veins (by fluoroscopy)
>   retrograde phlebography
>   venipuncture for injection of contrast material
>   venography using contrast material

Note: The fourth-digit subclassification (88.60-88.67) identifies the site to be viewed, not the site of injection.

> EXCLUDES *angiography using:*
>   *radioisotopes or radionuclides (92.01-92.19)*
>   *ultrasound (88.71-88.79)*
>   *fluorescein angiography of eye (95.12)*

DEF: Electromagnetic wave photography of veins; with contrast.

88.60 Phlebography using contrast material, unspecified site

88.61 Phlebography of veins of head and neck using contrast material

88.62 Phlebography of pulmonary veins using contrast material

88.63 Phlebography of other intrathoracic veins using contrast material

88.64 Phlebography of the portal venous system using contrast material
 Splenoportogram (by splenic arteriography)

88.65 Phlebography of other intra-abdominal veins using contrast material

88.66 Phlebography of femoral and other lower extremity veins using contrast material

88.67 Phlebography of other specified sites using contrast material

88.68 Impedance phlebography

√4th **88.7** Diagnostic ultrasound

> INCLUDES echography
>   ultrasonic angiography
>   ultrasonography

> EXCLUDES ▶*therapeutic ultrasound (00.01-00.09)*◀

DEF: Graphic recording of anatomical structures via high frequency, sound-wave imaging and computer graphics.

88.71 Diagnostic ultrasound of head and neck
 Determination of midline shift of brain
 Echoencephalography

> EXCLUDES *eye (95.13)*

 AHA: ▶1Q, '02, 10;◀ 1Q, '92, 11

88.72 Diagnostic ultrasound of heart
 Echocardiography
 Intravascular ultrasound of heart
 AHA: 1Q, '00, 20, 21; 1Q, '99, 6; 3Q, '98, 11

88.73 Diagnostic ultrasound of other sites of thorax
 Aortic arch
 Breast } ultrasonography
 Lung

88.74 Diagnostic ultrasound of digestive system

88.75 Diagnostic ultrasound of urinary system

88.76 Diagnostic ultrasound of abdomen and retroperitoneum
 AHA: 2Q, '99, 14

88.77 Diagnostic ultrasound of peripheral vascular system
 Deep vein thrombosis ultrasonic scanning
 AHA: 4Q, '99, 17; 1Q, '99, 12; 1Q, '92, 11

88.78 Diagnostic ultrasound of gravid uterus ♀
 Intrauterine cephalometry:
  echo
  ultrasonic
 Placental localization by ultrasound

88.79 Other diagnostic ultrasound
 Ultrasonography of:
  multiple sites
  nongravid uterus
  total body

√4th **88.8** Thermography

DEF: Infrared photography to determine various body temperatures.

88.81 Cerebral thermography

88.82 Ocular thermography

88.83 Bone thermography
 Osteoarticular thermography

88.84 Muscle thermography

88.85 Breast thermography

88.86 Blood vessel thermography
 Deep vein thermography

88.89 Thermographay of other sites
 Lymph gland thermography
 Thermography NOS

√4th **88.9** Other diagnostic imaging

88.90 Diagnostic imaging, not elsewhere classified

88.91 Magnetic resonance imaging of brain and brain stem

> EXCLUDES ▶*intraoperative magnetic resonance imaging (88.96)*
>   *real-time magnetic resonance imaging (88.96)*◀

88.92 Magnetic resonance imaging of chest and myocardium
 For evaluation of hilar and mediastinal lymphadenopathy

88.93 Magnetic resonance imaging of spinal canal
 Spinal cord levels:
  cervical
  thoracic
  lumbar (lumbosacral)
 Spinal cord
 Spine

88.94 Magnetic resonance imaging of musculoskeletal
 Bone marrow blood supply
 Extremities (upper) (lower)

88.95 Magnetic resonance imaging of pelvis, prostate, and bladder

88.96 Other intraoperative magnetic resonance imaging
 iMRI
 Real-time magnetic resonance imaging

88.97 Magnetic resonance imaging of other and unspecified sites
 Abdomen   Face
 Eye orbit   Neck

√3rd
√4th Additional Digit Required

Nonspecific OR Procedure Valid OR Procedure Non-OR Procedure

88.98 **Bone mineral density studies**
Dual photon absorptiometry
Quantitative computed tomography (CT) studies
Radiographic densitometry
Single photon absorptiometry

DEF: Dual photon absorptiometry: Measurement of bone mineral density by comparing dissipation of emission from two separate photoelectric energy peaks.

DEF: Quantitative computed tomography (CT) studies: Computer assisted analysis of x-ray absorption through bone to determine density.

DEF: Radiographic densiometry: Measurement of bone mineral density by degree of bone radiopacity.

DEF: Single photon absorptiometry: Measurement of bone mineral density by degree of dissipation of emission from one photoelectric energy peaks emitted by gadolinium 153.

√3rd **89** **Interview, evaluation, consultation, and examination**

√4th **89.0** **Diagnostic interview, consultation, and evaluation**
EXCLUDES *psychiatric diagnostic interview (94.11-94.19)*

89.01 **Interview and evaluation, described as brief**
Abbreviated history and evaluation

89.02 **Interview and evaluation, described as limited**
Interval history and evaluation

89.03 **Interview and evaluation, described as comprehensive**
History and evaluation of new problem

89.04 **Other interview and evaluation**

89.05 **Diagnostic interview and evaluation, not otherwise specified**

89.06 **Consultation, described as limited**
Consultation on a single organ system

89.07 **Consultation, described as comprehensive**

89.08 **Other consultation**

89.09 **Consulation, not otherwise specified**

√4th **89.1** **Anatomic and physiologic measurements and manual examinations — nervous system and sense organs**
EXCLUDES *ear examination (95.41-95.49)*
eye examination (95.01-95.26)
the listed procedures when done as part of a general physical examination (89.7)

89.10 **Intracarotid amobarbital test**
Wada test

DEF: Amobarbital injections into internal carotid artery to induce hemiparalysis to determine the hemisphere that controls speech and language.

89.11 **Tonometry**
DEF: Pressure measurements inside eye.

89.12 **Nasal function study**
Rhinomanometry
DEF: Rhinomanometry: Measure of degree of nasal cavity obstruction.

89.13 **Neurologic examination**

89.14 **Electroencephalogram**
EXCLUDES *that with polysomnogram (89.17)*
DEF: Recording of electrical currents in brain via electrodes to detect epilepsy, lesions and other encephalopathies.

89.15 **Other nonoperative neurologic function tests**
AHA: 3Q, '95, 5; 2Q, '91, 14; J-F, '87, 16; N-D, '84, 6

89.16 **Transillumination of newborn skull**
DEF: Light passed through newborn skull for diagnostic purposes.

89.17 **Polysomnogram**
Sleep recording
DEF: Graphic studies of sleep patterns.

89.18 **Other sleep disorder function tests**
Multiple sleep latency test [MSLT]

89.19 **Video and radio-telemetered electroencephalographic monitoring**
Radiographic
Video } EEG Monitoring

AHA: 1Q, '92, 17; 2Q, '90, 27

√4th **89.2** **Anatomic and physiologic measurements and manual examinations — genitourinary system**
EXCLUDES *the listed procedures when done as part of a general physical examination (89.7)*

AHA: 1Q, '90, 27

89.21 **Urinary manometry**
Manometry through:
indwelling ureteral catheter
nephrostomy
pyelostomy
ureterostomy
DEF: Measurement of urinary pressure.

DEF: Manometry through:

Indwelling urinary catheter: Semipermanent urinary catheter.

Nephrostomy: Opening into pelvis of kidney.

Pyelostomy: Opening in lower kidney.

Ureterostomy: Opening into ureter.

89.22 **Cystometrogram**
DEF: Pressure recordings at various stages of bladder filling.

89.23 **Urethral sphincter electromyogram**

89.24 **Uroflowmetry [UFR]**
DEF: Continuous recording of urine flow.

89.25 **Urethral pressure profile [UPP]**

89.26 **Gynecological examination** ♀
Pelvic examination

89.29 **Other nonoperative genitourinary system measurements**
Bioassay of urine   Urine chemistry
Renal clearance
AHA: N-D, '84, 6

√4th **89.3** **Other anatomic and physiologic measurements and manual examinations**
EXCLUDES *the listed procedures when done as part of a general physical examination (89.7)*

89.31 **Dental examination**
Oral mucosal survey
Periodontal survey

89.32 **Esophageal manometry**
AHA: 3Q, '96, 13

DEF: Measurement of esophageal fluid and gas pressures.

89.33 **Digital examination of enterostomy stoma**
Digital examination of colostomy stoma

89.34 **Digital examination of rectum**

89.35 **Transillumination of nasal sinuses**

89.36 **Manual examination of breast**

BI Bilateral Edit   NC Non-covered Procedure   ◄► Revised Text   ● New Code   ▲ Revised Code Title

89.37   **Vital capacity determination**

DEF: Measurement of expelled gas volume after full inhalation.

89.38   **Other nonoperative respiratory measurements**

Plethysmography for measurement of respiratory function
Thoracic impedance plethysmography

AHA: S-O, '87, 6

DEF: Plethysmography for measurement of respiratory function: Registering changes in respiratory function as noted in blood circulation.

89.39   **Other nonoperative measurements and examinations**

14 C-Urea breath test
Basal metabolic rate [BMR]
Gastric:
    analysis
    function NEC

> **EXCLUDES**   body measurement (93.07)
> cardiac tests (89.41-89.69)
> fundus photography (95.11)
> limb length measurement (93.06)

AHA: 2Q, '01, 9; 3Q, '00, 9; 3Q, '96, 12; 1Q, '94, 18; N-D, '84, 6

✓4th **89.4**   **Cardiac stress tests and pacemaker checks**

89.41   **Cardiovascular stress test using treadmill**

AHA: 1Q, '88, 11

89.42   **Masters' two-step stress test**

AHA: 1Q, '88, 11

89.43   **Cardiovascular stress test using bicycle ergometer**

AHA: 1Q, '88, 11

DEF: Electrocardiogram during exercise on bicycle with device capable of measuring muscular, metabolic and respiratory effects of exercise.

89.44   **Other cardiovascular stress test**

Thallium stress test with or without transesophageal pacing

89.45   **Artificial pacemaker rate check**

Artificial pacemaker function check NOS

AHA: ▶1Q, '02, 3◀

89.46   **Artificial pacemaker artifact wave form check**

89.47   **Artificial pacemaker electrode impedance check**

89.48   **Artificial pacemaker voltage or amperage threshold check**

✓4th **89.5**   **Other nonoperative cardiac and vascular diagnostic procedures**

> **EXCLUDES**   fetal EKG (75.32)

89.50   **Ambulatory cardiac monitoring**

Analog devices [Holter-type]

AHA: 4Q, '99, 21; 4Q, '91, 23

89.51   **Rhythm electrocardiogram**

Rhythm EKG (with one to three leads)

89.52   **Electrocardiogram**

ECG NOS
EKG (with 12 or more leads)

AHA: 1Q, '88, 11; S-O, '87, 6

89.53   **Vectorcardiogram (with ECG)**

89.54   **Electrographic monitoring**

Telemetry

> **EXCLUDES**   ambulatory cardiac monitoring (89.50)
> electrographic monitoring during surgery — omit code

AHA: 4Q, '91, 23; 1Q, '88, 11

DEF: Evaluation of heart electrical activity by continuous screen monitoring.

DEF: Telemetry: Evaluation of heart electrical activity; with radio signals at distance from patient.

89.55   **Phonocardiogram with ECG lead**

89.56   **Carotid pulse tracing with ECG lead**

> **EXCLUDES**   oculoplethysmography (89.58)

89.57   **Apexcardiogram (with ECG lead)**

AHA: J-F, '87, 16

89.58   **Plethysmogram**

Penile plethysmography with nerve stimulation

> **EXCLUDES**   plethysmography (for):
> measurement of respiratory function (89.38)
> thoracic impedance (89.38)

AHA: S-O, '87, 7

DEF: Determination and recording of blood variations present or passing through an organ.

89.59   **Other nonoperative cardiac and vascular measurements**

AHA: 2Q, '92, 12

DEF: Monitoring pulmonary artery pressure via catheter inserted through right lower and upper heart chambers into pulmonary artery and advancing the balloon-tip to wedge it in the distal pulmonary artery branch.

✓4th **89.6**   **Circulatory monitoring**

> **EXCLUDES**   electrocardiographic monitoring during surgery — omit code

AHA: M-J, '87, 11

89.60   **Continuous intra-arterial blood gas monitoring**

Insertion of blood gas monitoring system and continuous monitoring of blood gases through an intra-arterial sensor

89.61   **Systemic arterial pressure monitoring**

89.62   **Central venous pressure monitoring**

89.63   **Pulmonary artery pressure monitoring**

> **EXCLUDES**   pulmonary artery wedge monitoring (89.64)

89.64   **Pulmonary artery wedge monitoring**

Pulmonary capillary wedge [PCW] monitoring
Swan-Ganz catheterization

89.65   **Measurement of systemic arterial blood gases**

> **EXCLUDES** ▶ continuous intra-arterial blood gas monitoring (89.60)◀

89.66   **Measurement of mixed venous blood gases**

89.67   **Monitoring of cardiac output by oxygen consumption technique**

Fick method

DEF: Fick method: Indirect measure of cardiac output through blood volume flow over pulmonary capillaries; determines oxygen absorption by measure of arterial oxygen content versus venous blood content.

Diagnostic and Therapeutic Procedures 89.37–89.67

Diagnostic and Therapeutic Procedures 89.68–92.1

Central Venous Pressure Monitoring

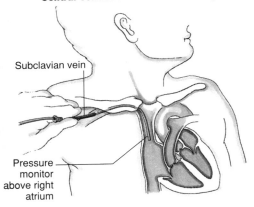

Subclavian vein

Pressure monitor above right atrium

89.68   **Monitoring of cardiac output by other technique**

Cardiac output monitor by thermodilution indicator

DEF: Cardiac output monitor by thermodilution indicator: Injection of ice cold dextrose solution into right lower heart chamber; temperature sensitive catheter monitors disappearance from beat to beat to measure expelled blood volume.

89.69   **Monitoring of coronary blood flow**

Coronary blood flow monitoring by coincidence counting technique

89.7   **General physical examination**

89.8   **Autopsy**

√3ʳᵈ   **90**   **Microscopic examination - I**

The following fourth-digit subclassification is for use with categories in section 90 to identify type of examination:

1   **bacterial smear**
2   **culture**
3   **culture and sensitivity**
4   **parasitology**
5   **toxicology**
6   **cell block and Papanicolaou smear**
9   **other microscopic examination**

√4ᵗʰ   **90.0**   **Microscopic examination of specimen from nervous system and of spinal fluid**

√4ᵗʰ   **90.1**   **Microscopic examination of specimen from endocrine gland, not elsewhere classified**

√4ᵗʰ   **90.2**   **Microscopic examination of specimen from eye**

√4ᵗʰ   **90.3**   **Microscopic examination of specimen from ear, nose, throat, and larynx**

√4ᵗʰ   **90.4**   **Microscopic examination of specimen from trachea, bronchus, pleura, lung, and other thoracic specimen, and of sputum**

√4ᵗʰ   **90.5**   **Microscopic examination of blood**

√4ᵗʰ   **90.6**   **Microscopic examination of specimen from spleen and of bone marrow**

√4ᵗʰ   **90.7**   **Microscopic examination of specimen from lymph node and of lymph**

√4ᵗʰ   **90.8**   **Microscopic examination of specimen from upper gastrointestinal tract and of vomitus**

√4ᵗʰ   **90.9**   **Microscopic examination of specimen from lower gastrointestinal tract and of stool**

√3ʳᵈ   **91**   **Microscopic examination - II**

The following fourth-digit subclassification is for use with categories in section 91 to identify type of examination:

1   **bacterial smear**
2   **culture**
3   **culture and sensitivity**
4   **parasitology**
5   **toxicology**
6   **cell block and Papanicolaou smear**
9   **other microscopic examination**

√4ᵗʰ   **91.0**   **Microscopic examination of specimen from liver, biliary tract, and pancreas**

√4ᵗʰ   **91.1**   **Microscopic examination of peritoneal and retroperitoneal specimen**

√4ᵗʰ   **91.2**   **Microscopic examination of specimen from kidney, ureter, perirenal and periureteral tissue**

√4ᵗʰ   **91.3**   **Microscopic examination of specimen from bladder, urethra, prostate, seminal vesicle, perivesical tissue, and of urine and semen**

√4ᵗʰ   **91.4**   **Microscopic examination of specimen from female genital tract**

Amnionic sac
Fetus

√4ᵗʰ   **91.5**   **Microscopic examination of specimen from musculoskeletal system and of joint fluid**

Microscopic examination of:

bone	ligament
bursa	muscle
cartilage	synovial membrane
fascia	tendon

√4ᵗʰ   **91.6**   **Microscopic examination of specimen from skin and other integument**

Microscopic examination of:
hair
nails
skin

EXCLUDES   *mucous membrane — code to organ site that of operative wound (91.71-91.79)*

√4ᵗʰ   **91.7**   **Microscopic examination of specimen from operative wound**

√4ᵗʰ   **91.8**   **Microscopic examination of specimen from other site**

√4ᵗʰ   **91.9**   **Microscopic examination of specimen from unspecified site**

√3ʳᵈ   **92**   **Nuclear medicine**

√4ᵗʰ   **92.0**   **Radioisotope scan and function study**

92.01   **Thyroid scan and radioisotope function studies**

Iodine-131 uptake
Protein-bound iodine
Radio-iodine uptake

92.02   **Liver scan and radioisotope function study**

92.03   **Renal scan and radioisotope function study**

Renal clearance study

92.04   **Gastrointestinal scan and radioisotope function study**

Radio-cobalt B_{12} Schilling test
Radio-iodinated triolein study

92.05   **Cardiovascular and hematopoietic scan and radioisotope function study**

Bone marrow
Cardiac output
Circulation time   } scan or function study
Radionuclide cardiac ventriculogram
Spleen

AHA: 2Q, '92, 7; 1Q, '88, 11

92.09   **Other radioisotope function studies**

√4ᵗʰ   **92.1**   **Other radioisotope scan**

92.11 **Cerebral scan**
Pituitary
92.12 **Scan of other sites of head**
EXCLUDES *eye (95.16)*
92.13 **Parathyroid scan**
92.14 **Bone scan**
92.15 **Pulmonary scan**
92.16 **Scan of lymphatic system**
92.17 **Placental scan**
92.18 **Total body scan**
92.19 **Scan of other sites**

√4th 92.2 **Therapeutic radiology and nuclear medicine**
EXCLUDES *that for:*
ablation of pituitary gland (07.64-07.69)
destruction of chorioretinal lesion (14.26-14.27)

AHA: 3Q, '92, 5

DEF: Radiation and nuclear isotope treatment of diseased tissue.

92.21 **Superficial radiation**
Contact radiation [up to 150 KVP]
92.22 **Orthovoltage radiation**
Deep radiation [200-300 KVP]
92.23 **Radioisotopic teleradiotherapy**
Teleradiotherapy using:
cobalt-60
iodine-125
radioactive cesium
92.24 **Teleradiotherapy using photons**
Megavoltage NOS
Supervoltage NOS
Use of:
Betatron
linear accelerator
92.25 **Teleradiotherapy using electrons**
Beta particles
92.26 **Teleradiotherapy of other particulate radiation**
Neutrons
Protons NOS
92.27 **Implantation or insertion of radioactive elements**
Intravascular brachytherapy
Code also incision of site
AHA: 1Q, '00, 11, 12; 3Q, '94, 11; 1Q, '88, 4

92.28 **Injection or instillation of radioisotopes**
Intracavitary } injection or
Intravenous } instillation
92.29 **Other radiotherapeutic procedure**

√4th 92.3 **Stereotactic radiosurgery**
Code also stereotactic head frame application (93.59)
EXCLUDES *stereotactic biopsy*
AHA: 4Q, '98, 79; 4Q, '95, 70

DEF: Ablation of deep intracranial lesions; single procedure; placement of head frame for 3-D analysis of lesion, followed by radiation treatment from helmet attached to frame.

92.30 **Stereotactic radiosurgery, not otherwise specified**
92.31 **Single source photon radiosurgery**
High energy x-rays
Linear accelerator (LINAC)
92.32 **Multi-source photon radiosurgery**
Cobalt 60 radiation
Gamma irradiation
92.33 **Particulate radiosurgery**
Particle beam radiation (cyclotron)
Proton accelerator
92.39 **Stereotactic radiosurgery, not elsewhere classified**

√3rd 93 **Physical therapy, respiratory therapy, rehabilitation, and related procedures**

√4th 93.0 **Diagnostic physical therapy**
AHA: N-D, '86, 7

93.01 **Functional evaluation**
93.02 **Orthotic evaluation**
93.03 **Prosthetic evaluation**
93.04 **Manual testing of muscle function**
AHA: J-F, '87, 16
93.05 **Range of motion testing**
AHA: J-F, '87, 16
93.06 **Measurement of limb length**
93.07 **Body measurement**
Girth measurement
Measurement of skull circumference
93.08 **Electromyography**
EXCLUDES *eye EMG (95.25)*
that with polysomnogram (89.17)
urethral sphincter EMG (89.23)

AHA: J-F, '87, 16

DEF: Graphic recording of electrical activity of muscle.

93.09 **Other diagnostic physical therapy procedure**
√4th 93.1 **Physical therapy exercises**
AHA: J-F, '87, 16; N-D, '86, 7

93.11 **Assisting exercise**
EXCLUDES *assisted exercise in pool (93.31)*
93.12 **Other active musculoskeletal exercise**
93.13 **Resistive exercise**
93.14 **Training in joint movements**
93.15 **Mobilization of spine**
93.16 **Mobilization of other joints**
EXCLUDES *manipulation of temporomandibular joint (76.95)*
93.17 **Other passive musculoskeletal exercise**
93.18 **Breathing exercise**
93.19 **Exercise, not elsewhere classified**
√4th 93.2 **Other physical therapy musculoskeletal manipulation**
AHA: N-D, '86, 7

93.21 **Manual and mechanical traction**
EXCLUDES *skeletal traction (93.43-93.44)*
skin traction (93.45-93.46)
spinal traction (93.41-93.42)
93.22 **Ambulation and gait training**
93.23 **Fitting of orthotic device**
93.24 **Training in use of prosthetic or orthotic device**
Training in crutch walking
93.25 **Forced extension of limb**
93.26 **Manual rupture of joint adhesions**
DEF: Therapeutic application of force to rupture adhesions restricting movement.
93.27 **Stretching of muscle or tendon**
93.28 **Stretching of fascia**
93.29 **Other forcible correction of deformity**
AHA: N-D, 85, 11
√4th 93.3 **Other physical therapy therapeutic procedures**
93.31 **Assisted exercise in pool**
93.32 **Whirlpool treatment**
93.33 **Other hydrotherapy**
93.34 **Diathermy**

√3rd
√4th Additional Digit Required

Nonspecific OR Procedure   Valid OR Procedure   Non-OR Procedure

Diagnostic and Therapeutic Procedures 93.35–93.82

93.35 Other heat therapy
Acupuncture with smouldering moxa
Hot packs
Hyperthermia NEC
Infrared irradiation
Moxibustion
Paraffin bath

> **EXCLUDES** hyperthermia for treatment of cancer (99.85)

DEF: Moxibustion: Igniting moxa, a Chinese plant, for counterirritation of skin.

DEF: Paraffin bath: Hot wax treatment.

93.36 Cardiac retraining
DEF: Cardiac rehabilitation regimen following myocardial infarction or coronary bypass graft procedure.

93.37 Prenatal training
Training for natural childbirth

93.38 Combined physical therapy without mention of the components

93.39 Other physical therapy
AHA: 3Q, '97, 12; 3Q, '91, 15

✓4ᵗʰ 93.4 Skeletal traction and other traction

93.41 Spinal traction using skull device
Traction using: Traction using:
   caliper tongs   halo device
   Crutchfield tongs   Vinke tongs

> **EXCLUDES** insertion of tongs or halo traction device (02.94)

AHA: ▶ 3Q, '01, 8;◀ 3Q, '96, 14; 2Q, '94, 3

DEF: Applying device to head to exert pulling force on spine.

93.42 Other spinal traction
Cotrel's traction

> **EXCLUDES** cervical collar (93.52)

DEF: Pulling force exerted on spine without skull device.

93.43 Intermittent skeletal traction

93.44 Other skeletal traction
Bryant's
Dunlop's   } traction
Lyman Smith
Russell's

93.45 Thomas' splint traction
DEF: Thomas splint: Placement of ring around thigh, attached to rods running length of leg for therapeutic purposes.

93.46 Other skin traction of limbs
Adhesive tape traction   Buck's traction
Boot traction   Gallows traction

✓4ᵗʰ 93.5 Other immobilization, pressure, and attention to wound

> **EXCLUDES** wound cleansing (96.58-96.59)

93.51 Application of plaster jacket

> **EXCLUDES** Minerva jacket (93.52)

93.52 Application of neck support
Application of:
   cervical collar
   Minerva jacket
   molded neck support

93.53 Application of other cast

93.54 Application of splint
Plaster splint
Tray splint

> **EXCLUDES** periodontal splint (24.7)

93.55 Dental wiring

> **EXCLUDES** that for orthodontia (24.7)

93.56 Application of pressure dressing
Application of:
   Gibney bandage
   Robert Jones' bandage
   Shanz dressing

93.57 Application of other wound dressing
▶Porcine wound dressing◀

93.58 Application of pressure trousers
Application of:
   anti-shock trousers
   MAST trousers
   vasopneumatic device

AHA: 3Q, '96, 13

93.59 Other immobilization, pressure, and attention to wound
Elastic stockings
Electronic gaiter
Intermittent pressure device
Oxygenation of wound (hyperbaric)
Stereotactic head frame application
Velpeau dressing

AHA: 3Q, '99, 7; 1Q, '99, 12, 13; 1Q, '91, 11; 1Q, '89, 12

✓4ᵗʰ 93.6 Osteopathic manipulative treatment

93.61 Osteopathic manipulative treatment for general mobilization
General articulatory treatment

93.62 Osteopathic manipulative treatment using high-velocity, low-amplitude forces
Thrusting forces

93.63 Osteopathic manipulative treatment using low-velocity, high-amplitude forces
Springing forces

93.64 Osteopathic manipulative treatment using isotonic, isometric forces

93.65 Osteopathic manipulative treatment using indirect forces

93.66 Osteopathic manipulative treatment to move tissue fluids
Lymphatic pump

93.67 Other specified osteopathic manipulative treatment

✓4ᵗʰ 93.7 Speech and reading rehabilitation and rehabilitation of the blind

93.71 Dyslexia training

93.72 Dysphasia training
DEF: Speech training to coordinate and arrange words in proper sequence.

93.73 Esophageal speech training
DEF: Speech training after voice box removal; sound is produced by vibration of air column in esophagus against the cricopharangeal sphincter.

93.74 Speech defect training

93.75 Other speech training and therapy
AHA: 4Q, '97, 36; 3Q, '97, 12

93.76 Training in use of lead dog for the blind

93.77 Training in braille or Moon

93.78 Other rehabilitation for the blind

✓4ᵗʰ 93.8 Other rehabilitation therapy

93.81 Recreational therapy
Diversional therapy
Play therapy

> **EXCLUDES** play psychotherapy (94.36)

93.82 Educational therapy
Education of bed-bound children
Special schooling for the handicapped

93.83   Occupational therapy
Daily living activities therapy
EXCLUDES   *training in activities of daily*
living for the blind
(93.78)

AHA: 3Q, '97, 12

93.84   Music therapy
93.85   Vocational rehabilitation
Sheltered employment
Vocational:
assessment
retraining
training

93.89   Rehabilitation, not elsewhere classified
✓4ᵗʰ **93.9   Respiratory therapy**
EXCLUDES   *insertion of airway (96.01-96.05)*
other continuous mechanical
ventilation (96.70-96.72)

93.90   Continuous positive airway pressure [CPAP]
AHA: ▶1Q, '02, 12, 13;◄ 3Q, '98, 14; 4Q, '91, 21

DEF: Noninvasive ventilation support system that
augments the ability to breathe spontaneously without
the insertion of an endotracheal tube or tracheostomy.

93.91   Intermittent positive pressure breathing [IPPB]
AHA: 4Q, '91, 21

93.93   Nonmechanical methods of resuscitation
Artificial respiration
Manual resuscitation
Mouth-to-mouth resuscititión

93.94   Respiratory medication administered by nebulizer
Mist therapy

93.95   Hyperbaric oxygenation
EXCLUDES   *oxygenation of wound (93.59)*

93.96   Other oxygen enrichment
Catalytic oxygen therapy
Cytoreductive effect
Oxygenators
Oxygen therapy
EXCLUDES   *oxygenation of wound (93.59)*

93.97   Decompression chamber
93.98   Other control of atmospheric pressure and composition
Antigen-free air conditioning
Helium therapy
EXCLUDES ▶ *inhaled nitric oxide therapy*
(INO) (00.12)◄

AHA: ▶1Q, '02, 14◄

93.99   Other respiratory procedures
Continuous negative pressure ventilation [CNP]
Postural drainage
AHA: 3Q, '99, 11; 4Q, '91, 22

✓3ʳᵈ **94   Procedures related to the psyche**
✓4ᵗʰ **94.0   Psychologic evaluation and testing**
94.01   Administration of intelligence test
Administration of:
Stanford-Binet
Wechsler Adult Intelligence Scale
Wechsler Intelligence Scale for Children

94.02   Administration of psychologic test
Administration of:
Bender Visual-Motor Gestalt Test
Benton Visual Retention Test
Minnesota Multiphasic Personality
Inventory
Wechsler Memory Scale

94.03   Character analysis
94.08   Other psychologic evaluation and testing
94.09   Psychologic mental status determination, not otherwise specified
✓4ᵗʰ **94.1   Psychiatric interviews, consultations, and evaluations**
94.11   Psychiatric mental status determination
Clinical psychiatric mental status
determination
Evaluation for criminal responsibility
Evaluation for testimentary capacity
Medicolegal mental status determination
Mental status determination NOS

94.12   Routine psychiatric visit, not otherwise specified
94.13   Psychiatric commitment evaluation
Pre-commitment interview
94.19   Other psychiatric interview and evaluation
Follow-up psychiatric interview NOS

✓4ᵗʰ **94.2   Psychiatric somatotherapy**
DEF: Biological treatment of mental disorders.

94.21   Narcoanalysis
Narcosynthesis
94.22   Lithium therapy
94.23   Neuroleptic therapy
94.24   Chemical shock therapy
94.25   Other psychiatric drug therapy
AHA: S-O, '86, 4

94.26   Subconvulsive electroshock therapy
94.27   Other electroshock therapy
Electroconvulsive therapy (ECT)
EST
94.29   Other psychiatric somatotherapy
✓4ᵗʰ **94.3   Individual psychotherapy**
94.31   Psychoanalysis
94.32   Hypnotherapy
Hypnodrome
Hypnosis
94.33   Behavior therapy
Aversion therapy
Behavior modification
Desensitization therapy
Extinction therapy
Relaxation training
Token economy
94.34   Individual therapy for psychosexual dysfunction
EXCLUDES   *that performed in group*
setting (94.41)

94.35   Crisis intervention
94.36   Play psychotherapy
94.37   Exploratory verbal psychotherapy
94.38   Supportive verbal psychotherapy
94.39   Other individual psychotherapy
Biofeedback
✓4ᵗʰ **94.4   Other psychotherapy and counselling**
94.41   Group therapy for psychosexual dysfunction
94.42   Family therapy
94.43   Psychodrama
94.44   Other group therapy
94.45   Drug addiction counselling
94.46   Alcoholism counselling
94.49   Other counselling
✓4ᵗʰ **94.5   Referral for psychologic rehabilitation**
94.51   Referral for psychotherapy
94.52   Referral for psychiatric aftercare
That in:
halfway house
outpatient (clinic) facility

Diagnostic and Therapeutic Procedures 93.83–94.52

94.53 Referral for alcoholism rehabilitation
94.54 Referral for drug addiction rehabilitation
94.55 Referral for vocational rehabilitation
94.59 Referral for other psychologic rehabilitation

✓4th **94.6 Alcohol and drug rehabilitation and detoxification**
AHA: 2Q, '91, 12

94.61 Alcohol rehabilitation
DEF: Program designed to restore social and physical functioning, free of the dependence of alcohol.

94.62 Alcohol detoxification
DEF: Treatment of physical symptoms during withdrawal from alcohol dependence.

94.63 Alcohol rehabilitation and detoxification

94.64 Drug rehabilitation
DEF: Program designed to restore social and physical functioning, free of the dependence of drugs.

94.65 Drug detoxification
DEF: Treatment of physical symptoms during withdrawal from drug dependence.

94.66 Drug rehabilitation and detoxification

94.67 Combined alcohol and drug rehabilitation

94.68 Combined alcohol and drug detoxification

94.69 Combined alcohol and drug rehabilitation and detoxification

✓3rd **95 Ophthalmologic and otologic diagnosis and treatment**

✓4th **95.0 General and subjective eye examination**

95.01 Limited eye examination
Eye examination with prescription of spectacles

95.02 Comprehensive eye examination
Eye examination covering all aspects of the visual system

95.03 Extended ophthalmologic work-up
Examination (for):
glaucoma
neuro-ophthalmology
retinal disease

95.04 Eye examination under anesthesia
Code also type of examination

95.05 Visual field study

95.06 Color vision study

95.07 Dark adaptation study
DEF: Exam of eye's adaption to dark.

95.09 Eye examination, not otherwise specified
Vision check NOS

✓4th **95.1 Examinations of form and structure of eye**

95.11 Fundus photography

95.12 Fluorescein angiography or angioscopy of eye

95.13 Ultrasound study of eye

95.14 X-ray study of eye

95.15 Ocular motility study

95.16 P$_{32}$ and other tracer studies of eye

✓4th **95.2 Objective functional tests of eye**
EXCLUDES that with polysomnogram (89.17)

95.21 Electroretinogram [ERG]

95.22 Electro-oculogram [EOG]

95.23 Visual evoked potential [VEP]
DEF: Measuring and recording evoked visual responses of body and senses.

95.24 Electronystagmogram [ENG]
DEF: Monitoring of brain waves to record induced and spontaneous eye movements.

95.25 Electromyogram of eye [EMG]

95.26 Tonography, provocative tests, and other glaucoma testing

✓4th **95.3 Special vision services**

95.31 Fitting and dispensing of spectacles

95.32 Prescription, fitting, and dispensing of contact lens

95.33 Dispensing of other low vision aids

95.34 Ocular prosthetics

95.35 Orthoptic training

95.36 Ophthalmologic counselling and instruction
Counselling in:
adaptation to visual loss
use of low vision aids

✓4th **95.4 Nonoperative procedures related to hearing**

95.41 Audiometry
Békésy 5-tone audiometry
Impedance audiometry
Stapedial reflex response
Subjective audiometry
Tympanogram

95.42 Clinical test of hearing
Tuning fork test
Whispered speech test

95.43 Audiological evaluation
Audiological evaluation by:
Bárány noise machine
blindfold test
delayed feedback
masking
Weber lateralization

95.44 Clinical vestibular function tests
Thermal test of vestibular function

95.45 Rotation tests
Bárány chair
DEF: Irrigation of ear canal with warm or cold water to evaluate vestibular function.

95.46 Other auditory and vestibular function tests

95.47 Hearing examination, not otherwise specified

95.48 Fitting of hearing aid
EXCLUDES implantation of electromagnetic hearing device (20.95)
AHA: 4Q, '89, 5

95.49 Other nonoperative procedures related to hearing
Adjustment (external components) of cochlear prosthetic device

✓3rd **96 Nonoperative intubation and irrigation**

✓4th **96.0 Nonoperative intubation of gastrointestinal and respiratory tracts**

96.01 Insertion of nasopharyngeal airway

96.02 Insertion of oropharyngeal airway

96.03 Insertion of esophageal obturator airway

96.04 Insertion of endotracheal tube

Endotracheal Intubation

Laryngoscope
Larynx
Trachea
Balloon inflated above carina

96.05 **Other intubation of respiratory tract**
AHA: 1Q, '97, 14

96.06 **Insertion of Sengstaken tube**
Esophageal tamponade

DEF: Insertion of Sengstaken tube: Nonsurgical emergency measure to stop esophageal bleeding using compression exerted by inflated balloons; additional tube ports to aspirate blood and clots.

96.07 **Insertion of other (naso-) gastric tube**
Intubation for decompression

EXCLUDES that for enteral infusion of nutritional substance (96.6)

96.08 **Insertion of (naso-) intestinal tube**
Miller-Abbott tube (for decompression)

96.09 **Insertion of rectal tube**
Replacement of rectal tube

✓4th **96.1** **Other nonoperative insertion**

EXCLUDES nasolacrimal intubation (09.44)

96.11 **Packing of external auditory canal**
96.14 **Vaginal packing** ♀
96.15 **Insertion of vaginal mold** ♀
96.16 **Other vaginal dilation** ♀
96.17 **Insertion of vaginal diaphragm** ♀
96.18 **Insertion of other vaginal pessary** ♀
96.19 **Rectal packing**

✓4th **96.2** **Nonoperative dilation and manipulation**

96.21 **Dilation of frontonasal duct**
96.22 **Dilation of rectum**
96.23 **Dilation of anal sphincter**
96.24 **Dilation and manipulation of enterostomy stoma**
96.25 **Therapeutic distention of bladder**
Intermittent distention of bladder
96.26 **Manual reduction of rectal prolapse**
96.27 **Manual reduction of hernia**
96.28 **Manual reduction of enterostomy prolapse**
AHA: N-D, '87, 11

96.29 **Reduction of intussusception of alimentary tract**
With:
    fluoroscopy
    ionizing radiation enema
    ultrasonography guidance
Hydrostatic reduction
Pneumatic reduction

EXCLUDES intra-abdominal manipulation of intestine, not otherwise specified (46.80)

AHA: 4Q, '98, 82

✓4th **96.3** **Nonoperative alimentary tract irrigation, cleaning, and local instillation**

96.31 **Gastric cooling**
Gastric hypothermia

DEF: Reduction of internal stomach temperature.

96.32 **Gastric freezing**
96.33 **Gastric lavage**
96.34 **Other irrigation of (naso-)gastric tube**
96.35 **Gastric gavage**

DEF: Food forced into stomach.

96.36 **Irrigation of gastrostomy or enterostomy**
96.37 **Proctoclysis**

DEF: Slow introduction of large amounts of fluids into lower large intestine.

96.38 **Removal of impacted feces**
Removal of impaction:
    by flushing manually
96.39 **Other transanal enema**
Rectal irrigation

EXCLUDES reduction of intussusception of alimentary tract by ionizing radiation enema (96.29)

✓4th **96.4** **Nonoperative irrigation, cleaning, and local instillation of other digestive and genitourinary organs**

96.41 **Irrigation of cholecystostomy and other biliary tube**
96.42 **Irrigation of pancreatic tube**
96.43 **Digestive tract instillation, except gastric gavage**
96.44 **Vaginal douche** ♀
96.45 **Irrigation of nephrostomy and pyelostomy**
96.46 **Irrigation of ureterostomy and ureteral catheter**
96.47 **Irrigation of cystostomy**
96.48 **Irrigation of other indwelling urinary catheter**
96.49 **Other genitourinary instillation**
Insertion of prostaglandin suppository
AHA: 1Q, '01, 5

✓4th **96.5** **Other nonoperative irrigation and cleaning**

96.51 **Irrigation of eye**
Irrigation of cornea

EXCLUDES irrigation with removal of foreign body (98.21)

96.52 **Irrigation of ear**
Irrigation with removal of cerumen
96.53 **Irrigation of nasal passages**
96.54 **Dental scaling, polishing, and debridement**
Dental prophylaxis   Plaque removal
96.55 **Tracheostomy toilette**
96.56 **Other lavage of bronchus and trachea**

EXCLUDES ▶ diagnostic bronchoalveolar lavage (BAL) (33.24) whole lung lavage (33.99)◀

96.57 **Irrigation of vascular catheter**
AHA: 3Q, '93, 5

96.58 **Irrigation of wound catheter**
96.59 **Other irrigation of wound**
Wound cleaning NOS

EXCLUDES debridement (86.22, 86.27-86.28)

AHA: S-O, '85, 7

96.6 **Enteral infusion of concentrated-nutritional substances**

✓3rd
✓4th Additional Digit Required

2002 Ingenix, Inc.

Nonspecific OR Procedure

Valid OR Procedure

Non-OR Procedure

October 2002 • Volume 3 —195

Diagnostic and Therapeutic Procedures 96.7–97.43

√4th **96.7**   **Other continuous mechanical ventilation**
    INCLUDES   Endotracheal respiratory assistance
                Intermittent mandatory ventilation
                [IMV]
                Positive end expiratory pressure
                [PEEP]
                Pressure support ventilation [PSV]
                That by tracheostomy
                Weaning of an intubated (endotracheal
                tube) patient
    EXCLUDES   *bi-level airway pressure (93.90)*
                *continuous negative pressure
                ventilation [CNP] (iron lung)
                (cuirass) (93.99)*
                *continuous positive airway pressure
                [CPAP] (93.90)*
                *intermittent positive pressure breathing
                [IPPB] (93.91)*
                that by face mask (93.90-93.99)
                that by nasal cannula (93.90-93.99)
                that by nasal catheter (93.90-93.99)
        Code also any associated:
            endotracheal tube insertion (96.04)
            tracheostomy (31.1-31.29)

Note: **Endotracheal intubation**
    To calculate the number of hours (duration) of continuous
    mechanical ventilation during a hospitalization, begin the
    count from the start of the (endotracheal) intubation. The
    duration ends with (endotracheal) extubation.

    If a patient is intubated prior to admission, begin counting
    the duration from the time of the admission. If a patient is
    transferred (discharged) while intubated, the duration would
    end at the time of transfer (discharge).

    For patients who begin on (endotracheal) intubation and
    subsequently have a tracheostomy performed for mechanical
    ventilation, the duration begins with the (endotracheal)
    intubation and ends when the mechanical ventilation is
    turned off (after the weaning period).

        Tracheostomy
    To calculate the number of hours of continuous mechanical
    ventilation during a hospitalization, begin counting the
    duration when mechanical ventilation is started. The
    duration ends when the mechanical ventilator is turned off
    (after the weaning period).

    If a patient has received a tracheostomy prior to admission
    and is on mechanical ventilation at the time of admission,
    begin counting the duration from the time of admission. If a
    patient is transferred (discharged) while still on mechanical
    ventilation via tracheostomy, the duration would end at the
    time of the transfer (discharge).

    AHA: 2Q, '92, 13; 4Q, '91, 16; 4Q, '91, 18; 4Q, '91, 21

    96.70   **Continuous mechanical ventilation of
                unspecified duration**
                Mechanical ventilation NOS

    96.71   **Continuous mechanical ventilation for less
                than 96 consecutive hours**
                AHA: ▶1Q, '02, 12;◀ 1Q, '01, 6

    96.72   **Continuous mechanical ventilation for 96
                consecutive hours or more**

√3rd **97**   **Replacement and removal of therapeutic appliances**
    √4th **97.0**   **Nonoperative replacement of gastrointestinal
                appliance**
        97.01   **Replacement of (naso-)gastric or
                    esophagostomy tube**
        97.02   **Replacement of gastrostomy tube**
                    AHA: 1Q, '97, 11
        97.03   **Replacement of tube or enterostomy device
                    of small intestine**
        97.04   **Replacement of tube or enterostomy device
                    of large intestine**

        97.05   Replacement of stent (tube) in biliary or
                pancreatic duct
                AHA: 2Q, '99, 13

√4th **97.1**   **Nonoperative replacement of musculoskeletal and
            integumentary system appliance**
        97.11   Replacement of cast on upper limb
        97.12   Replacement of cast on lower limb
        97.13   Replacement of other cast
        97.14   Replacement of other device for
                musculoskeletal immobilization
        97.15   Replacement of wound catheter
        97.16   Replacement of wound packing or drain
            EXCLUDES   *repacking of:*
                        dental wound (97.22)
                        vulvar wound (97.26)

√4th **97.2**   **Other nonoperative replacement**
        97.21   Replacement of nasal packing
        97.22   Replacement of dental packing
        97.23   Replacement of tracheostomy tube
                AHA: N-D, '87, 11

        97.24   Replacement and refitting of vaginal
                diaphragm
        97.25   Replacement of other vaginal pessary
        97.26   Replacement of vaginal or vulvar packing or
                drain
        97.29   Other nonoperative replacements
                AHA: 3Q, '99, 9; 3Q, '98, 12

√4th **97.3**   **Nonoperative removal of therapeutic device from
            head and neck**
        97.31   Removal of eye prosthesis
            EXCLUDES   *removal of ocular implant
                        (16.71)*
                        *removal of orbital implant
                        (16.72)*
        97.32   Removal of nasal packing
        97.33   Removal of dental wiring
        97.34   Removal of dental packing
        97.35   Removal of dental prosthesis
        97.36   Removal of other external mandibular
                fixation device
        97.37   Removal of tracheostomy tube
        97.38   Removal of sutures from head and neck
        97.39   Removal of other therapeutic device from
                head and neck
            EXCLUDES   *removal of skull tongs (02.94)*

√4th **97.4**   **Nonoperative removal of therapeutic device from
            thorax**
        97.41   Removal of thoracotomy tube or pleural
                cavity drain
                AHA: 1Q, '99, 10

        97.42   Removal of mediastinal drain
        97.43   Removal of sutures from thorax

            Intraaortic Balloon Pump

97.44   Nonoperative removal of heart assist system
Intra-aortic balloon pump (IABP)
AHA: ▶4Q, '01, 65◀

DEF: Non-invasive removal of ventricular assist systems, or intraaortic balloon pump, which is a balloon catheter placed into the descending thoracic aorta and timed to inflate and deflate with the patient's own heart rhythm to aid in blood circulation.

97.49   Removal of other device from thorax
AHA: N-D, '86, 9

√4th 97.5   Nonoperative removal of therapeutic device from digestive system
97.51   Removal of gastrostomy tube
97.52   Removal of tube from small intestine
97.53   Removal of tube from large intestine or appendix
97.54   Removal of cholecystostomy tube
97.55   Removal of T-tube, other bile duct tube, or liver tube
Removal of bile duct stent
AHA: 1Q, '01, 8

97.56   Removal of pancreatic tube or drain
97.59   Removal of other device from digestive system
Removal of rectal packing

√4th 97.6   Nonoperative removal of therapeutic device from urinary system
97.61   Removal of pyelostomy and nephrostomy tube
DEF: Nonsurgical removal of tubes from lower part of kidney.

97.62   Removal of ureterostomy tube and ureteral catheter
97.63   Removal of cystostomy tube
97.64   Removal of other urinary drainage device
Removal of indwelling urinary catheter
97.65   Removal of urethral stent
97.69   Removal of other device from urinary system

√4th 97.7   Nonoperative removal of therapeutic device from genital system
97.71   Removal of intrauterine contraceptive device   ♀
97.72   Removal of intrauterine pack   ♀
97.73   Removal of vaginal diaphragm   ♀
97.74   Removal of other vaginal pessary   ♀
97.75   Removal of vaginal or vulvar packing   ♀
97.79   Removal of other device from genital tract
Removal of sutures

√4th 97.8   Other nonoperative removal of therapeutic device
97.81   Removal of retroperitoneal drainage device
97.82   Removal of peritoneal drainage device
AHA: 2Q, '90, 28; S-O, '86, 12

97.83   Removal of abdominal wall sutures
97.84   Removal of sutures from trunk, not elsewhere classified
97.85   Removal of packing from trunk, not elsewhere classified
97.86   Removal of other device from abdomen
97.87   Removal of other device from trunk
97.88   Removal of external immobilization device
Removal of:
brace
cast
splint
97.89   Removal of other therapeutic device

√3rd 98   Nonoperative removal of foreign body or calculus
√4th 98.0   Removal of intraluminal foreign body from digestive system without incision
EXCLUDES   removal of therapeutic device (97.51-97.59)
DEF: Retrieval of foreign body from digestive system lining without incision.

98.01   Removal of intraluminal foreign body from mouth without incision
98.02   Removal of intraluminal foreign body from esophagus without incision
98.03   Removal of intraluminal foreign body from stomach and small intestine without incision
98.04   Removal of intraluminal foreign body from large intestine without incision
98.05   Removal of intraluminal foreign body from rectum and anus without incision

√4th 98.1   Removal of intraluminal foreign body from other sites without incision
EXCLUDES   removal of therapeutic device (97.31-97.49, 97.61-97.89)
98.11   Removal of intraluminal foreign body from ear without incision
98.12   Removal of intraluminal foreign body from nose without incision
98.13   Removal of intraluminal foreign body from pharynx without incision
98.14   Removal of intraluminal foreign body from larynx without incision
98.15   Removal of intraluminal foreign body from trachea and bronchus without incision
98.16   Removal of intraluminal foreign body from uterus without incision   ♀
EXCLUDES   removal of intrauterine contraceptive device (97.71)
98.17   Removal of intraluminal foreign body from vagina without incision   ♀
98.18   Removal of intraluminal foreign body from artificial stoma without incision
98.19   Removal of intraluminal foreign body from urethra without incision

√4th 98.2   Removal of other foreign body without incision
EXCLUDES   removal of intraluminal foreign body (98.01-98.19)
98.20   Removal of foreign body, not otherwise specified
98.21   Removal of superficial foreign body from eye without incision
98.22   Removal of other foreign body without incision from head and neck
Removal of embedded foreign body from eyelid or conjunctiva without incision
98.23   Removal of foreign body from vulva without incision   ♀
98.24   Removal of foreign body from scrotum or penis without incision   ♂
98.25   Removal of other foreign body without incision from trunk except scrotum, penis, or vulva
98.26   Removal of foreign body from hand without incision
AHA: N-D, '87, 10

98.27   Removal of foreign body without incision from upper limb, except hand
98.28   Removal of foreign body from foot without incision
98.29   Removal of foreign body without incision from lower limb, except foot

Extracorporeal Shock Wave Lithotripsy

✓4ᵗʰ 98.5   Extracorporeal shockwave lithotripsy [ESWL]
Lithotriptor tank procedure
Disintegration of stones by extracorporeal
   induced shockwaves
That with insertion of stent

DEF: Breaking of stones with high voltage condenser device synchronized with patient R waves.

98.51   Extracorporeal shockwave lithotripsy [ESWL] of the kidney, ureter and/or bladder
AHA: 4Q, '95, 73; 1Q, '89, 2

98.52   Extracorporeal shockwave lithotripsy `NC`
[ESWL] of the gallbladder and/or bile duct

98.59   Extracorporeal shockwave lithotripsy `NC`
of other sites

✓3ʳᵈ 99   Other nonoperative procedures

✓4ᵗʰ 99.0   Transfusion of blood and blood components
Use additional code for that done via catheter or
   cutdown (38.92-38.94)

DEF: Salvaging patient blood and reinfusing it during perioperative period.

99.00   Perioperative autologous transfusion of whole blood or blood components
Intraoperative blood collection
Postoperative blood collection
Salvage
AHA: 4Q, '95, 69

99.01   Exchange transfusion
Transfusion:
   exsanguination
   replacement
AHA: 2Q, '89, 15

DEF: Repetitive withdrawal of blood, replaced by donor blood.

99.02   Transfusion of previously collected autologous blood
Blood component
AHA: 4Q, '95, 69; 1Q, '90, 10; J-A, '85, 16

DEF: Transfusion with patient's own previously withdrawn and stored blood.

99.03   Other transfusion of whole blood
Transfusion:
   blood NOS
   hemodilution
   NOS

99.04   Transfusion of packed cells

99.05   Transfusion of platelets
Transfusion of thrombocytes

99.06   Transfusion of coagulation factors
Transfusion of antihemophilic factor

99.07   Transfusion of other serum
Transfusion of plasma
`EXCLUDES`   injection [transfusion] of:
   antivenin (99.16)
   gamma globulin (99.14)

99.08   Transfusion of blood expander
Transfusion of Dextran

99.09   Transfusion of other substance
Transfusion of:
   blood surrogate
   granulocytes
`EXCLUDES`   transplantation [transfusion] of
   bone marrow (41.0)

✓4ᵗʰ 99.1   Injection or infusion of therapeutic or prophylactic substance
`INCLUDES`   injection or infusion given:
   hypodermically
   intramuscularly } acting locally or
   intravenously   systemically

99.10   Injection or infusion of thrombolytic agent
Streptokinase
Tissue plasminogen activator (TPA)
Urokinase
`EXCLUDES`   aspirin — omit code
   GP IIB/IIIa platelet inhibitors
      (99.20)
   heparin (99.19)
   single vessel percutaneous
      transluminal coronary
      angioplasty [PTCA] or
      coronary atherectomy
      with mention of
      thrombolytic agent (36.02)
   warfarin — omit code
AHA: 2Q, '01, 7-9, 23; 4Q, '98, 83

99.11   Injection of Rh immune globulin
Injection of:
   Anti-D (Rhesus) globulin
   RhoGAM

99.12   Immunization for allergy
Desensitization

99.13   Immunization for autoimmune disease

99.14   Injection of gamma globulin
Injection of immune sera

99.15   Parenteral infusion of concentrated nutritional substances
Hyperalimentation
Total parenteral nutrition [TPN]
Peripheral parenteral nutrition [PPN]

DEF: Administration of greater than necessary amount of nutrients via other than the alimentary canal (e.g., infusion).

99.16   Injection of antidote
Injection of:
   antivenin
   heavy metal antagonist

99.17   Injection of insulin

99.18   Injection or infusion of electrolytes

99.19   Injection of anticoagulant
`EXCLUDES` ▶ infusion of drotrecogin alfa
   (activated) (00.11)◀

✓4ᵗʰ 99.2   Injection or infusion of other therapeutic or prophylactic substance
`INCLUDES`   injection or infusion given:
   hypodermically
   intramuscularly } acting locally or
   intravenously   systemically

Use additional code for:
injection (into):   injection (into):
   breast (85.92)   kidney (55.96)
   bursa (82.94, 83.96)   liver (50.94)
   intraperitoneal   orbit (16.91)
      (cavity) (54.97)   other sites — see
   intrathecal (03.92)   Alphabetic Index
   joint (76.96, 81.92)
perfusion: perfusion:
   NOS (39.97)   liver (50.93)
   intestine (46.95, 46.96)   total body (39.96)
   kidney (55.95)

99.20 Injection or infusion of platelet inhibitor
Glycoprotein IIB/IIIa inhibitor
GP IIB-IIIa inhibitor
GP IIB/IIIa inhibitor
EXCLUDES infusion of heparin (99.19)
injection or infusion of thrombolytic agent (99.10)
AHA: 4Q, '98, 85

99.21 Injection of antibiotic
EXCLUDES ▶ injection or infusion of oxazolidinone class of antibiotics (00.14)◄
AHA: 4Q, '98, 76; 2Q, '90, 24; M-A, '87, 9

99.22 Injection of other anti-infective
EXCLUDES ▶ injection or infusion of oxazolidinone class of antibiotics (00.14)◄

99.23 Injection of steroid
Injection of cortisone
Subdermal implantation of progesterone
AHA: 3Q, '00, 15; 1Q, '99, 8; 3Q, 96, 7; 3Q, '92, 9; S-O, '85, 7

99.24 Injection of other hormone

99.25 Injection or infusion of cancer chemotherapeutic substance
Chemoembolization
Injection or infusion of antineoplastic agent
EXCLUDES immunotherapy, antineoplastic (99.28)
▶implantation of chemotherapeutic agent (00.10)◄
injection of radioisotope (92.28)
injection or infusion of biological response modifier [BRM] as an antineoplastic agent (99.28)
AHA: 1Q, '99, 4; 1Q, '98, 6; 3Q, '96, 11; 4Q, '95, 67; 2Q, '92, 7; 1Q, '92, 12; 1Q, '88, 8; N-D, '86, 11

99.26 Injection of tranquilizer

99.27 Iontophoresis
DEF: Iontophoresis: Introduction of soluble salts into tissues via electric current.

99.28 Injection or infusion of biological response modifier [BRM] as an antineoplastic agent
▶High-dose interleukin-2 (IL-2) therapy◄
Immunotherapy, antineoplastic
▶Interleukin therapy◄
Tumor vaccine
AHA: 2Q, '99, 8; 2Q, '98, 10; 4Q, '94, 51

99.29 Injection or infusion of other therapeutic or prophylactic substance
EXCLUDES administration of neuroprotective agent (99.75)
immunization (99.31-99.59)
injection of sclerosing agent into:
esophageal varices (42.33)
hemorrhoids (49.42)
veins (39.92)
injection or infusion of:
▶human B-type natriuretic peptide (hBNP) (00.13)
nesiritide (00.13)◄
platelet inhibitor (99.20)
thrombolytic agent (99.10)
AHA: 1Q, '01, 15; 2Q, '00, 14; 1Q, '00, 8, 18, 23; 4Q, '99, 17; 3Q, '99, 21; 4Q, '98, 83; 2Q, '98, 17, 18, 23, 24; 1Q, '98, 6; 2Q, '97, 11; 1Q, '97, 3; 4Q, '95, 67; 2Q, '95, 12; 4Q, '90, 14; 2Q, '90, 23; 2Q, '89, 17; 1Q, '88, 9; N-D, '87, 4; S-O, '87, 11

✓4th **99.3 Prophylactic vaccination and inoculation against certain bacterial diseases**
DEF: Administration of a killed bacteria suspension to produce immunity.
99.31 Vaccination against cholera
99.32 Vaccination against typhoid and paratyphoid fever
Administration of TAB vaccine
99.33 Vaccination against tuberculosis
Administration of BCG vaccine
99.34 Vaccination against plague
99.35 Vaccination against tularemia
99.36 Administration of diphtheria toxoid
EXCLUDES administration of:
diphtheria antitoxin (99.58)
diphtheria-tetanus-pertussis, combined (99.39)
99.37 Vaccination against pertussis
EXCLUDES administration of diphtheria-tetanus-pertussis, combined (99.39)
99.38 Administration of tetanus toxoid
EXCLUDES administration of:
diphtheria-tetanus-pertussis, combined (99.39)
tetanus antitoxin (99.56)
99.39 Administration of diphtheria-tetanus-pertussis, combined

✓4th **99.4 Prophylactic vaccination and inoculation against certain viral diseases**
DEF: Administration of a killed virus suspension to produce immunity.
99.41 Administration of poliomyelitis vaccine
99.42 Vaccination against smallpox
99.43 Vaccination against yellow fever
99.44 Vaccination against rabies
99.45 Vaccination against measles
EXCLUDES administration of measles-mumps-rubella vaccine (99.48)
99.46 Vaccination against mumps
EXCLUDES administration of measles-mumps-rubella vaccine (99.48)
99.47 Vaccination against rubella
EXCLUDES administration of measles-mumps-rubella vaccine (99.48)
99.48 Administration of measles-mumps-rubella vaccine

✓4th **99.5 Other vaccination and inoculation**
99.51 Prophylactic vaccination against the common cold
99.52 Prophylactic vaccination against influenza
99.53 Prophylactic vaccination against arthropod-borne viral encephalitis
99.54 Prophylactic vaccination against other arthropod-borne viral diseases
99.55 Prophylactic administration of vaccine against other diseases
Vaccination against: anthrax, brucellosis, Rocky Mountain spotted fever
Vaccination against: Staphylococcus, Streptococcus, typhus
AHA: 2Q, '00, 9; 1Q, '94, 10
99.56 Administration of tetanus antitoxin
99.57 Administration of botulism antitoxin

99.58 Administration of other antitoxins
Administration of:
   diphtheria antitoxin
   gas gangrene antitoxin
   scarlet fever antitoxin

99.59 Other vaccination and inoculation
Vaccination NOS
> EXCLUDES   *injection of:*
>   *gamma globulin (99.14)*
>   *Rh immune globulin (99.11)*
>   *immunization for:*
>   *allergy (99.12)*
>   *autoimmune disease*
>   *(99.13)*

√4th 99.6 Conversion of cardiac rhythm
> EXCLUDES   *open chest cardiac:*
>   *electric stimulation (37.91)*
>   *massage (37.91)*

DEF: Correction of cardiac rhythm.

99.60 Cardiopulmonary resuscitation, not otherwise specified
AHA: 1Q, '94, 16

99.61 Atrial cardioversion
DEF: Application of electric shock to upper heart chamber to restore normal heart rhythm.

99.62 Other electric countershock of heart
Cardioversion:
   NOS
   external
Conversion to sinus rhythm
Defibrillation
External electrode stimulation

99.63 Closed chest cardiac massage
Cardiac massage NOS
Manual external cardiac massage
DEF: Application of alternating manual pressure over breastbone to restore normal heart rhythm.

99.64 Carotid sinus stimulation

99.69 Other conversion of cardiac rhythm
AHA: 4Q, '88, 11

√4th 99.7 Therapeutic apheresis or other injection, administration, or infusion of other therapeutic or prophylactic substance
DEF: Blood withdrawal from donor with desired portion removed (e.g., plasma, leukocytes, platelets, etc.) and retained; remainder transfused back into donor.

99.71 Therapeutic plasmapheresis
> EXCLUDES ► *extracorporeal*
>   *immunoadsorption [ECI]*
>   *(99.76)*◄

99.72 Therapeutic leukopheresis
Therapeutic leukocytapheresis

99.73 Therapeutic erythrocytapheresis
Therapeutic erythropheresis
AHA: 1Q, '94, 20

99.74 Therapeutic plateletpheresis

99.75 Administration of neuroprotective agent
AHA: 4Q, '00, 68

DEF: Direct application of neuroprotective agent (e.g., nimodipine) to miinimize ischemic injury by inhibiting toxic neurotransmitters, blocking free ions, removing free radicals, and causing vasodilation.

● **99.76 Extracorporeal immunoadsorption**
Removal of antibodies from plasma with protein A columns

● **99.77 Application or administration of adhesion barrier substance**

99.79 Other
Apheresis (harvest) of stem cells
AHA: 4Q, '97, 55

√4th 99.8 Miscellaneous physical procedures

99.81 Hypothermia (central) (local)
> EXCLUDES   *gastric cooling (96.31)*
>   *gastric freezing (96.32)*
>   *that incidental to open heart*
>   *surgery (39.62)*

99.82 Ultraviolet light therapy
Actinotherapy

99.83 Other phototherapy
Phototherapy of the newborn
> EXCLUDES   *extracorporeal*
>   *photochemotherapy*
>   *(99.88)*
>   *photocoagulation of retinal*
>   *lesion (14.23-14.25,*
>   *14.33-14.35, 14.53-*
>   *14.55)*

AHA: 2Q, '89, 15

DEF: Treating disease with light rays of various concentrations.

99.84 Isolation
Isolation after contact with infectious disease
Protection of individual from his surroundings
Protection of surroundings from individual

99.85 Hyperthermia for treatment of cancer
Hyperthermia (adjunct therapy) induced by microwave, ultrasound, low energy radio frequency, probes (interstitial), or other means in the treatment of cancer
Code also any concurrent chemotherapy or radiation therapy
AHA: 3Q, '96, 11; 3Q, '89, 17

99.86 Non-invasive placement of bone growth stimulator
Transcutaneous (surface) placement of pads or patches for stimulation to aid bone healing
> EXCLUDES   *insertion of invasive or semi-invasive bone growth stimulators (device) (percutaneous electrodes) (78.90-78.99)*

99.88 Therapeutic photopheresis
Extracorporeal photochemotherapy
Extracorporeal photopheresis
> EXCLUDES   *other phototherapy (99.83)*
>   *ultraviolet light therapy (99.82)*

AHA: 2Q, '99, 7

DEF: Extracorporeal photochemotherapy: Treating disease with drugs that react to ultraviolet radiation or sunlight.

√4th 99.9 Other miscellaneous procedures

99.91 Acupuncture for anesthesia

99.92 Other acupuncture
> EXCLUDES   *that with smouldering r (93.35)*

99.93 Rectal massage (for levator spasm)

99.94 Prostatic massage

99.95 Stretching of foreskin

99.96 Collection of sperm for artificia insemination

99.97 Fitting of denture

99.98 Extraction of milk from lact

99.99 Other
►Leech therapy◄
